Contents in Brief

Maternal & Child Health Nursing:

Care of the Childbearing & Childrearing Family

Adele Pillitteri, PhD, RN, PNP
Former Associate Professor
University of Southern California
Los Angeles, California

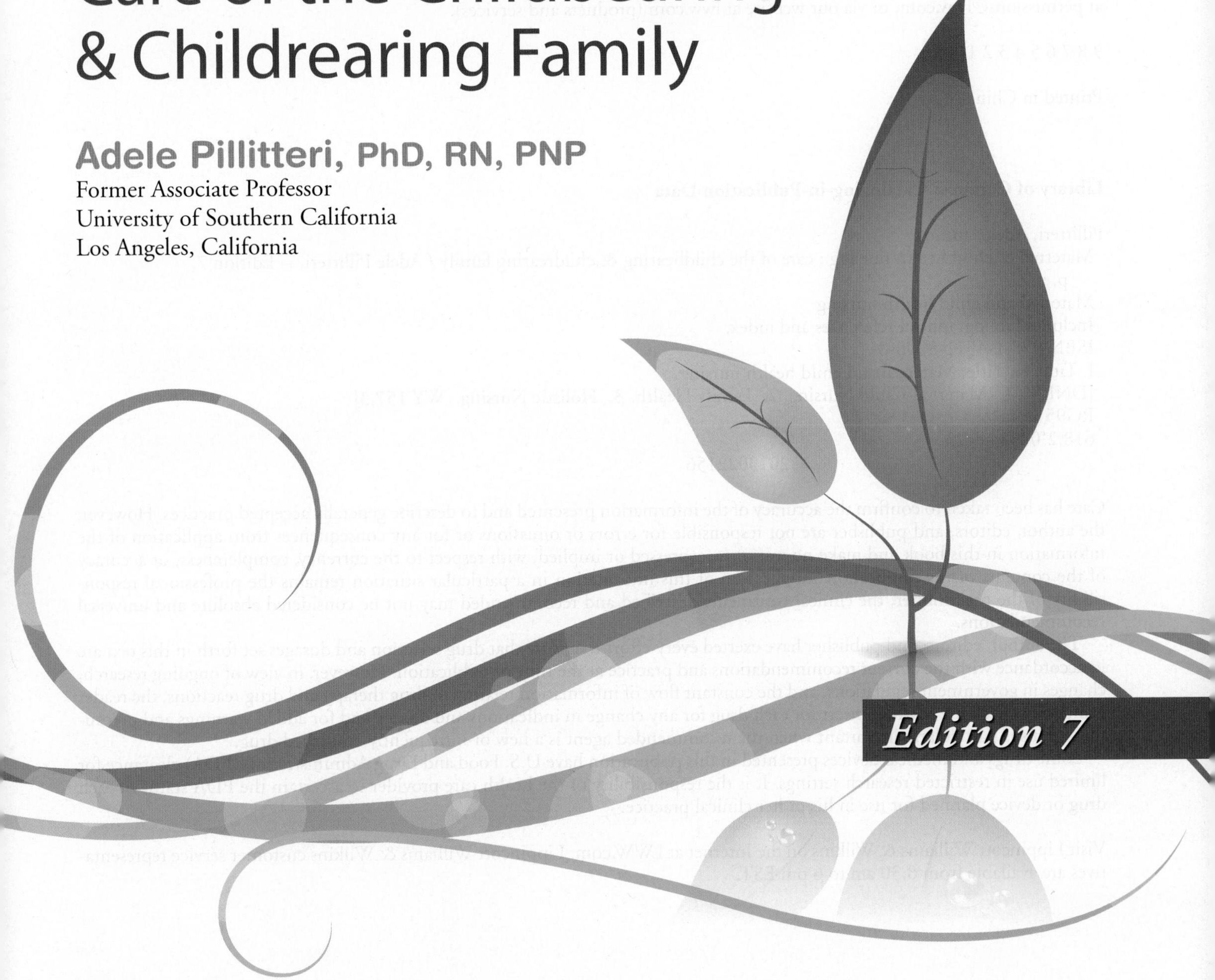

Edition 7

Wolters Kluwer | Lippincott Williams & Wilkins
Health
Philadelphia • Baltimore • New York • London
Buenos Aires • Hong Kong • Sydney • Tokyo

Acquisitions Editor: Patrick Barbera
Product Manager: Dawn Lagrosa
Production Project Manager: Marian Bellus
Marketing Manager: Nicole Dunlap
Manufacturing Manager: Karin Duffield
Design Coordinator: Joan Wendt
Production Services: Absolute Service, Inc.

7th edition

9 8 7 6 5 4 3 2 1

Printed in China

Library of Congress Cataloging-in-Publication Data

Pillitteri, Adele, author.
Maternal & child health nursing : care of the childbearing & childrearing family / Adele Pillitteri. -- Edition 7.
p. ; cm.
Maternal and child health nursing
Includes bibliographical references and index.
ISBN 978-1-4511-8790-8
I. Title. II. Title: Maternal and child health nursing.
[DNLM: 1. Maternal-Child Nursing. 2. Family Health. 3. Holistic Nursing. WY 157.3]
RG951
618.2′0231--dc23

2013022156

My son was born with cerebral palsy plus a severe cognitive challenge. I wrote the first edition of this book to help students learn the compassionate level of nursing care I wanted for him. Since then, I have been rewarded many times over by the excellent care he has received. In memory, this 7th edition is dedicated to him.

To Rusty, with love:

> *When we first learned of Rusty's diagnosis,*
> *we said to the doctor,*
> *"One of our families would like him to become a teacher.*
> *The other would like him to excel at a sport.*
> *He's not going to do either of those things, is he?"*
>
> *"Keep it in perspective,"*
> *was the doctor's reply.*
> *"Learning to speak will be so difficult for him, accomplishing that will be harder than the average person lecturing to an auditorium of students.*
> *Learning to walk will be so difficult, it will be harder than learning to swing a bat.*
> *If he's able to hold down a simple job, it will be a greater triumph than running into an end zone."*
>
> *In perspective:*
> *Rusty has lectured to thousands of students, has hit many home runs, and has scored many, many touchdowns.*

A son much to be admired, he will be greatly missed.

Contributors

Sharon Armstrong, NP, RNC, MSN
Nursing Professor
St. Clair County Community College
Port Huron, Michigan

Susan J. Brillhart, PhD, RN, PNP-BC
Assistant Professor
Borough of Manhattan Community College/CUNY
New York, New York

Laura Candelaria RN, MS, FNP
Professor of Nursing and Nutrition
Molloy College
Rockville Centre, New York

Darlene Nebel Cantu, RNC-NIC, C-EFM, MSN
Faculty
San Antonio College
San Antonio, Texas
University of Phoenix—Bachelor's and Master's online programs
Chamberlain College of Nursing—RN to BSN online program

Malinda Forsythe Carmouche, RN, MSN
Assistant Professor
Southern University
School of Nursing
Baton Rouge, Louisiana

Claudette Gordon, EdD, MS, RN
Assistant Professor
Nursing & Allied Health Sciences
Bronx Community College/CUNY
Bronx, New York

Marcia Jones, MA, PhD
Associate Professor
Nursing & Allied Health Sciences
Bronx Community College/CUNY
Bronx, New York

Debbie McGregor, EdD, RNC
Assistant Professor
Barry University
College of Health Sciences
Division of Nursing
Miami Shores, Florida

Nancy M. Peifer-Neil, BSN, MSN, PhD
Professor II
Palm Beach State College
Lake Worth, Florida

Kathleen Sebrey (Kit) Schafer, DNP, MSN, RNC, NP
Clinical Associate Professor
Purdue University
School of Nursing
West Lafayette, Indiana

Lynn M. Stover, RN, BC, DSN, SANE
Associate Professor of Nursing
Clayton State University
School of Nursing
Morrow, Georgia

Shawn Little, RN, BSN, MSN
Chamberlain College of Nursing
Atlanta, Georgia

Reviewers

Sharon Armstrong, NP, RNC, MSN
Nursing Professor
St. Clair County Community College
Port Huron, Michigan

Sandra L. Baker, DNP, RN, CNE
Dean
Riverside Community College
Associate Professor
California State University—Fullerton
Riverside, California

Colleen Battista, MSN
Nursing Faculty
North Island College
Vancouver Island, British Columbia

Ferrona Beason, PhD, ARNP
Instructor of Nursing
Barry University Division of Nursing
Miami Shores, Florida

Angela M. Berger, ADN, BSN, MSN
Manager of Staff Development
Soin Medical Center (Kettering Health Network)
Beavercreek, Ohio

Elizabeth W. Black, MSN, RN
Assistant Professor
Gwynedd-Mercy College
Gwynedd Valley, Pennsylvania

Landyn Blais
Instructor
Algonquin College of Applied Arts and Technology
Ottawa, Ontario

Kathleen Cahill, MSN, RN
Instructor
Saint Anselm College Department of Nursing
Manchester, New Hampshire

Darlene Nebel Cantu, RNC-NIC, C-EFM, MSN
Faculty
San Antonio College
San Antonio, Texas
University of Phoenix—Bachelor's and Master's online programs
Chamberlain College of Nursing—RN to BSN online program

Deborah Campagna, MS, BS, RN
Professor
Hudson Valley Community College
Troy, New York

Bonnie Carmack, MN, ARNP
Adjunct Faculty
Seminole State College
Oviedo, Florida

Malinda Forsythe Carmouche, RN, MSN
Assistant Professor
Southern University
School of Nursing
Baton Rouge, Louisiana

Lori Clay, MSN, RN, CPN
Arkansas State University
College of Nursing and Health Professions
Jonesboro, Arkansas

Diane Frances Colizza, RNC, MN
Assistant Professor, Clinical Track
Duquesne University School of Nursing
Pittsburgh, Pennsylvania

Carla Crider, MSN
Instructor
Weatherford College
Weatherford, Texas

Kelly L. Davis, BSN, MSN
Instructor, Nursing
Delaware Technical and Community College
Dover, Delaware

Margot R. De Sevo, PhD, LCCE, IBCLC, RNC
Associate Professor
Adelphi University
Garden City, New York

Elizabeth Allen DiFabio, MSN, RN
Nursing Faculty
Anoka-Ramsey Community College
Coon Rapids, Minnesota

Victoria Evans, BSN, MSN, MPH
Assistant Professor of Nursing
University of Maine at Augusta
Augusta, Maine

Dawn Garrett-Wright, PhD, RN, CNE
Assistant Professor and Program Coordinator
Western Kentucky University
Bowling Green, Kentucky

Linda Nicholson Grinstead, PhD, RN
Professor (retired)
Grand Valley State University
Grand Rapids, Michigan

Anna Gryczman, DNP, RN, PHN, AHN-BC, CNE
Nurse Educator
Century College
White Bear Lake, Minnesota

Michelle Gulbransen, RN, MN
Sessional Professor
St. Clair College
Windsor, Ontario

Margaret Harrison, MSN, RN
Baptist Health System School of Health Professions
Department of Professional Nursing
San Antonio, Texas

Sandra Kellogg, MSN
Nursing Department Director
Treasure Valley Community College
Ontario, Oregon

Katherine Kniest, BSN, MSN
Professor of Nursing
Harper College
Palatine, Illinois

Denise Callahan Long, MSN, NP
Faculty
Our Lady of Lourdes School of Nursing
Camden, New Jersey

Maria A. Marconi, RN, MS
Assistant Professor of Clinical Nursing
University of Rochester School of Nursing
Rochester, New York

Judy McAulay, RN, BN, MEd
Associate Professor
University of British Columbia—Okanagan School of Nursing
Kelowna, British Columbia

Paulette Melanson
Adjunct Faculty
Massachusetts College of Pharmacy and Health Sciences School of Nursing
Boston, Massachusetts

Debra Miller, BSN, MSN
Instructor
Southern Union State Community College
Opelika, Alabama

Karen Miller, MSN
Faculty II
Carolinas College of Health Sciences School of Nursing
Charlotte, North Carolina

Patricia A. Morgan, PhD, RN, CNE
Associate Professor, Director, Department of Nursing
University of New England
Portland, Maine

Lucille Morrison, BSN, MEd, MSN, CNRP, DNP
Assistant Professor of Nursing
Mercyhurst University
North East, Pennsylvania

Joan Murphy, RN, MSN, MACM
Adjunct Faculty, Associate Degree Nursing
Santa Rosa Junior College
Santa Rosa, California

Jan Marie Nick, PhD, RNC
Associate Professor, School of Nursing
Loma Linda University
Loma Linda, California

Sharon McCleave, BSc(Hons) Ost, MEd, PhD(c)
Professor, Human Biology
Seneca College
King City, Ontario

Rita Nutt, DNP, RN
Assistant Professor
Salisbury University
Salisbury, Maryland

Susan A. Orshan, PhD, RN, FACCE
Faculty
University of Phoenix School of Advanced Studies
Phoenix, Arizona

Nancy M. Peifer-Neil, BSN, MSN, PhD
Professor II
Palm Beach State College
Lake Worth, Florida

Patricia Perry, RN, MSN
Instructor, Associate Degree Nursing
Galveston College
Galveston, Texas

Sharon Puchalski, AAS, BS, MSN
Assistant Professor
Bergen Community College Division of Health Professions
Paramus, New Jersey

Justina Reinckens, RN, MA
Assistant Professor
Coppin State University
College of Health Professions
Helene Fuld School of Nursing
Baltimore, Maryland

Karen Rousseau, MSN
Director and Associate Professor of Nursing
American International College
Springfield, Massachusetts

Elizabeth B. Rudolf, MS, RN, CPN
Clinical Assistant Professor
Towson University
Towson, Maryland

Carolyn Santiago, NP
Director
Santa Barbara Business College
Vocational Nursing Program
Bakersfield, California

Ann D. H. Schide, MS
Associate Professor, Nursing—Nursing/Allied Health
Chattanooga State Community College
Chattanooga, Tennessee

Suzan Sherman, MS
Minnesota State University, Mankato
Mankato, Minnesota

Joy Shewchuk, RN, BSc, BSN, MSN
Professor
Humber College School of Health Sciences
Toronto, Ontario

Lynn M. Stover, RN, BC, DSN, SANE
Associate Professor of Nursing
Clayton State University
School of Nursing
Morrow, Georgia

Kelly Tobar, RN, MS, EdD
Faculty
California State University, Sacramento
Sacramento, California

Maureen Waller, MSN, RNC
Professor
College of DuPage
Glen Ellyn, Illinois

Carol M. Wiggs, PhD, RN, CNM
Associate Professor
The University of Texas Medical Branch
School of Nursing
Galveston, Texas

Barbara Wilford, MSN, MBA, RN
Assistant Professor of Nursing
Lorain County Community College
Elyria, Ohio

Michele Wolff, RN, MSN
Professor of Nursing
Saddleback College
Mission Viejo, California

Hollace Yowler, MSN, RN
Ivy Tech Community College
Madison, Indiana

Kathy Zimmerman, MSN, APN, FNP-BC, AHN-BC
Assistant Professor
Austin Peay State University
Clarksville, Tennessee

Rebecca Zuzik
Assistant Professor, Nursing
Westmoreland County Community College
Youngwood, Pennsylvania

Preface

Both maternal and child health nursing are expanding areas as a result of the broadening scope of practice within the nursing profession and the recognized need for better preventive and restorative care in these areas. The importance of this need is reflected in the fact that many of the health goals for the nation focus on these areas of nursing.

At the same time that the information in these areas of nursing is increasing, less time is available in nursing programs for teaching it. It's difficult for students to read all of the material contained in overlapping textbooks.

Maternal & Child Health Nursing: Care of the Childbearing and Childrearing Family, Seventh Edition, is written with this challenge in mind. It views maternal–child health care not as two separate disciplines but as a continuum of knowledge. It is designed to present the content of the two disciplines comprehensively but not redundantly. It is based on a philosophy of nursing care that respects clients as individuals, yet views them as part of families and society.

The book is designed for undergraduate student use in either a combined course in maternal–child health or for a curriculum in which these courses are taught separately. It provides a comprehensive, in-depth discussion of the many facets of maternal and child health nursing, while promoting a sensitive, holistic outlook on nursing practice. As such, the book will also be useful for practicing nurses or graduate students who are interested in reviewing or expanding their knowledge in these areas.

Basic themes that are integrated into this text include the experience of wellness and illness as family-centered events, the perception of pregnancy and childbirth as periods of wellness, and the importance of knowing normal child development in the planning of nursing care. Also included are themes reflective of changes in health care delivery and the importance of meeting the needs of a culturally diverse population.

The Changing Health Care Scene

The Patient Protection and Affordable Care Act has drastically changed the health care insurance and delivery system, increasing the availability of health care services to many more Americans. With 22 newly covered preventive health services for women, including pregnant women, and 27 newly covered preventive health services for children, the need for maternal–child health nurses has never been greater.

The move of the nurse from a minor to a major player in health care has made understanding interprofessional approaches to care more important than ever before. An increasingly multicultural population is reflected among both nurses and the clients they care for, necessitating care that respects cultural diversity. In order that nurses can be prepared for this new level of responsibility, educational changes have to keep pace with health care reform by emphasizing interprofessional care planning, a greater focus on communication, evidence-based therapeutic interventions, and critical thinking.

Nursing issues that grow out of the current climate of change include:

- The accentuation of Interprofessional Care Planning and the Nursing Process: The care planning process provides the structuring framework for coordinating communication that will result in safe and effective care. By structuring the text to reflect this process, students can begin to conceptualize how they will use textbook knowledge in nursing practice to diagnose, plan, care for, and monitor patients to maximize optimal outcomes. In addition, Nursing Process Overview boxes included at the beginning of each chapter provide a strong theoretical underpinning for nursing process and ways to use the nursing process in clinical practice.
- An emphasis on 2020 National Health Goals: As a way to focus care and research, National Health Goals have gained wider attention at a time when there is a greater need than ever to be wise in the choice of how dollars are spent. Students can familiarize themselves with how these goals can be applied directly to maternal and child health care by referring to the Nursing Care Planning Based on 2020 National Health Goals displays that appear in each chapter.
- The necessity for nurses to be active participants in redefining quality in health care. A major way nurses can do this is by joining with the Institute of Medicine to help define required competencies for practice. Included in each chapter are multiple choice questions based on the QSEN (Quality and Safety Education for Nurses) competencies so students can better envision how these competencies can be applied to practice.
- The importance of basing nursing care on evidence-based practice: The variety of new care settings, as well as the diversity of roles in which nurses practice, is reflected both in the proliferation of community-based nursing facilities and also in the increase in the numbers of nurse-midwives and women's health, pediatric and neonatal nurse practitioners. This new edition places emphasis on the need for nurses to read and apply research to practice by demonstrating how recent research applies directly to a patient scenario woven throughout each chapter. In addition, boxes on Nursing Care Planning Using Assessment, Nursing Care Planning Based on Responsibility for Pharmacology, and Nursing Care Planning Using Procedures illustrate how medical science is applied to care.
- The need to coordinate care: With a growing ambulatory population, nurses assume the increasingly important role as coordinators for health care teams. Interprofessional Care Maps in each chapter demonstrate how the nursing process works for a specific patient throughout the care cycle.
- The responsibility of health teaching with families as a cornerstone of nursing: The teaching role of the nurse has greater significance in the new health care milieu as the emphasis on preventive care and short stays in acute care settings create the need for families to be better educated in their own care. Nursing Care Planning Based on Family Teaching displays present detailed health information for the family, emphasizing the importance of a partnership between nurses and clients in the management of health and illness. Nursing Care Planning to Empower a Family boxes provide students with the type of information families need to learn how to participate in and improve both family and individual health.

- The obligation to individualize care according to sociocultural uniqueness: This is a reflection of both greater cultural sensitivity and an increasingly diverse population of caregivers and care recipients. Greater emphasis is being placed on the implications of multiple sociocultural factors in how they affect responses to health and illness. Nursing Care Planning Based on Effective Communication boxes give examples of ways to improve nurse–client communication. Nursing Care Planning to Respect Cultural Diversity displays demonstrate solutions in areas of caregiving that differ among patients of various cultures.

Organization of the Text

Maternal & Child Health Nursing follows the family from prepregnancy through pregnancy, labor, birth, and the postpartal period; it then follows the child and the family from birth through adolescence. Coverage includes ambulatory and inpatient care and focuses on primary as well as secondary and tertiary care.

The book is organized in eight units:

Unit 1 provides an introduction to maternal and child health nursing. A framework for practice is presented, as well as current trends and the importance of considering childbearing and childrearing within a diverse socioeconomic and family/community context.

Unit 2 examines the nursing role in preparing families for childbearing and childrearing, and discusses reproductive and sexual health, the role of the nurse in genetic counseling, reproductive life planning, and the concerns of the family having difficulty conceiving a child.

Unit 3 presents the nursing role in caring for a pregnant family during pregnancy, birth and the postpartal period and serving as a fetal advocate. A separate chapter details the role of the nurse in providing comfort during labor and birth.

Unit 4 addresses the nursing role when a woman develops a complication of pregnancy, labor or birth, or has a complication during the postpartal period. Separate chapters address the role of the nurse when a woman has a preexisting illness, develops a complication during pregnancy or the postpartal period, has a unique concern, or chooses or needs a cesarean birth. A final chapter details care of the high-risk newborn or a child born with a physical or a developmental challenge.

Unit 5 discusses the nursing role in health promotion during childhood. The chapters in this unit cover principles of growth and development and care of the child from infancy through adolescence, including child health assessment and communication and health teaching with children and families.

Unit 6 presents the nursing role in supporting the health of children and their families. The effects of illness on children and their families, diagnostic and therapeutic procedures, medication administration, and pain management are addressed, with respect to care of the child and family in hospital, home, and ambulatory settings.

Unit 7 examines the nursing role in restoring and maintaining the health of children and families when illness occurs. Disorders are presented according to body systems so that students have a ready orientation for locating content.

Unit 8 discusses the nursing role in restoring and maintaining the mental health of children and families. Separate chapters discuss the role of the nurse when intimate partner violence; child maltreatment; or mental, long-term, or fatal illness is present.

Pedagogic Features

Each chapter in the text is organized to provide a complete learning experience for the student. Numerous pedagogic features are included to help a student understand and increase retention. Important elements include:

- **Chapter Objectives:** Learning objectives are included at the beginning of each chapter to identify outcomes expected after the material in the chapter has been mastered.
- **Key Terms:** Terms that would be new to a student are listed at the beginning of each chapter in a ready reference list. When the terms first appear in the text, they are shown in boldface type and then defined. Definitions also appear online in the Glossary at http://www.thePoint.lww.com/Pillitteri7e.
- **Chapter-Opening Scenarios:** Short scenarios appear at the beginning of each chapter. These vignettes are designed to help students appreciate that nursing care is always individualized and provide a taste of what is to come in the chapter. Throughout the chapter, open-ended and multiple choice questions related to the scenario connect learning with patient care.
- **Nursing Process Overview:** Each chapter begins with a review of nursing process in which specific suggestions, such as examples of nursing diagnoses and outcome criteria helpful to modifying care in the area under discussion, are presented. These reviews are designed to improve students' preparation in clinical areas so they can focus their care planning and apply principles to practice.
- **Nursing Diagnoses and Related Interventions:** A consistent format highlights the nursing diagnoses and related interventions throughout the text. A special heading draws the students' attention to these sections where individual nursing diagnoses and outcome evaluation are detailed for the major conditions and disorders discussed.
- **NEW! QSEN Checkpoint Questions:** Throughout the text, multiple-choice QSEN Checkpoint Questions appear to help students check their progress and reward them for their comprehension. They relate the chapter-opening scenario to the six QSEN competencies: safety, quality improvement, evidence-based practice, teamwork and collaboration, informatics, and patient-centered care. Students can check their work by reading the answers provided in the Appendix A.
- **What If. . . Questions:** These critical-thinking questions also appear throughout each chapter in the text. They ask readers to apply the information just acquired in the patient scenario presented in the chapter opening, thus maximizing learning and emphasizing critical thinking. Suggested solutions are supplied at http://www.thePoint.lww.com/Pillitteri7e.
- **Tables and Displays:** Numerous tables and displays summarize important information or provide extra detail on topics so that a student has ready references to this information.
  - **Nursing Care Planning Based on 2020 National Health Goals:** To emphasize the nursing role in accomplishing the health care goals of our nation, these displays state specific ways in which maternal and child health nurses can provide better outcomes for families. They help the student to appreciate the importance of national health care planning and the influence that nurses can have in creating a healthier nation.

- **Nursing Care Planning Based on Effective Communication:** This feature presents case examples of less effective communication and more effective communication, illustrating for the student how an awareness of communication can improve the patient's understanding and positively impact outcomes.
- **Nursing Care Planning Based on Family Teaching:** These boxes present detailed health teaching information for the family, emphasizing the importance of a partnership between nurses and clients in the management of health and illness.
- **Nursing Care Planning Based on Responsibility for Pharmacology:** These boxes provide quick reference for medications that are commonly used for the health problems described in the text. They give the drug name (brand and generic, if applicable), dosage, pregnancy category, side effects, and nursing implications.
- **Nursing Care Planning Using Procedures:** Techniques of procedures specific to maternal and child health care are boxed in an easy-to-follow two-column format, often enhanced with color figures.
- **Nursing Care Planning Using Assessment:** These visual guides provide head-to-toe assessment information for overall health status or specific disorders or conditions.
- **Nursing Care Planning: Interprofessional Care Maps:** Because nurses rarely work in isolation, but rather as a member of a health care team or unit, interprofessional care maps written for specific clients are included in each chapter to demonstrate the use of the nursing process, provide examples of critical thinking, and clarify nursing care for specific client needs. These Interprofessional Care Maps not only demonstrate nursing process but also accentuate the increasingly important role of the nurse as a coordinator of client care.
  - NEW! **Nursing Care Planning to Respect Cultural Diversity:** These boxes help students appreciate how care delivery should alter to meet the needs of each patient in a country that continually attracts immigrants from throughout the world.
  - NEW! **Nursing Care Planning to Empower a Family:** Because patient education is an important nursing responsibility, these boxes provide students with the type of information families need to learn how to participate in improving their health.
- **Key Points:** A review of important points is highlighted at the end of each chapter to help students monitor their own comprehension.
- NEW! **Critical Thinking Care Studies:** To involve a student in the decision-making realities of the clinical setting, each chapter ends with an additional case scenario, followed by several thought-provoking questions. These could also serve as a basis for conference or class discussion. Suggested answers are supplied on thePoint.
- **Patient Scenarios.** Students are directed in each chapter to read a Patient Scenario related to the content of the chapter (found at http://thePoint.lww.com/Pillitteri7e). Following a full health history, physical examination, and pertinent laboratory work, the student is presented with 25 questions to test knowledge of the chapter's content. The scenarios are not only a good review of the chapter content but also instructive in how to word health histories related to a specific health concern.

Teaching and Learning Package

Resources for Instructors

Tools to assist you with teaching your course are available upon adoption of this text at http://thePoint.lww.com/Pillitteri7e/Pillitteri7e.

NEW! to This Edition

- **Pre-Lecture Quizzes:** These exercises ask students to recall information. Based on the main points of the chapter, each of the five true/false statements and five fill-in-the-blank questions will help you determine whether students have read the chapters. Answers are provided.
- **Assignments:** Grouped into Written Assignments, Group Assignments, Clinical Assignments, and Web Assignments, the Assignments package will give you a means to gauge students' understanding of the textbook material. The Assignments give students many chances to test their own knowledge of the chapter concepts as well as their developing critical thinking skills. Suggested answers are provided.
- **Discussion Topics:** With these topics, you can initiate and foster classroom discussion or assign them for use outside the classroom. Each Discussion Topic is designed to help students make a connection between the textbook and application. Suggested answers are provided.

Updated for This Edition

- **E-Book:** Online access to the book's full text and images gives you an easy-to-transport format.
- **PowerPoint Presentations With Guided Lecture Notes:** The PowerPoint presentations provide you with visual aids to support your lectures or classroom lessons. The accompanying Guided Lecture Notes offer brief talking points you can use along with the presentations.
- **Test Generator:** The Test Generator lets you put together exclusive new tests from a bank containing hundreds of questions to help you in assessing your students' understanding of the material. Test questions link to chapter learning objectives. This test generator comes with a bank of more than 1,100 questions.
- **Image Bank:** Access to downloadable photographs and illustrations from this textbook offer you the ability to use them in your PowerPoint slides or as you see fit throughout your course.

Resources for Students

Students can access all these learning tools using the code printed in the front of their textbooks by visiting http://thePoint.lww.com/Pillitteri7e.

NEW! to This Edition

- **NCLEX-Style Review Questions:** These *application-level* questions provide students the opportunity to test themselves on their ability to apply specific nursing actions based on what a nurse should know and what a nurse should do in a specific situation related to the chapter content. They also give students experience in answering questions of the type that will appear on the NCLEX.
- **Suggested Readings:** This list of journal articles provides students with the information needed to do more in-depth reading relevant to the topics included in the chapter.

- **Answers and Rationales:** Suggested Answers to teach chapter's What If. . . and Critical Thinking Care Study questions allow students to gauge whether they are on the right track by providing the main points that they are expected to address in answering these questions.

Updated for This Edition

- **E-Book:** Online access to the book's full text and images gives you an easy-to-transport format.
- **Patient Scenarios:** A patient care scenario details a full health history and examination findings pertinent to each chapter's content. Each scenario includes 25 related NCLEX-style questions to help students sharpen their skills and grow more familiar with NCLEX-type questions. Completing these exercises serve as an excellent review of the chapter content.
- **Journal Articles:** Updated for the new edition, online articles offer students the opportunity to read current research related to each chapter's material, as available in Lippincott Williams & Wilkins journals.
- **Watch & Learn Video Clips:** These audiovisual aides cover both maternal and child care topics:
  - Developmental Tasks of Pregnancy: 1st Trimester, Accepting the Pregnancy
  - Developmental Tasks of Pregnancy: 2nd Trimester, Accepting the Baby
  - Developmental Tasks of Pregnancy: 3rd Trimester, Preparing for Parenthood
  - Vaginal Birth
  - Scheduled Cesarean Birth
  - Assisting the Client With Breastfeeding
  - Developmental Considerations in Caring for Children: Infants
  - Developmental Considerations in Caring for Children: Toddlers
  - Developmental Considerations in Caring for Children: Preschoolers
  - Developmental Considerations in Caring for Children: School Agers
  - Developmental Considerations in Caring for Children: Adolescents
  - Care of the Hospitalized Child: Introduction
  - Care of the Hospitalized Child: Medication Administration
  - Care of the Hospitalized Child: Play
  - Care of the Hospitalized Child: Pain Management
  - Care of the Hospitalized Child: Parent and Family Participation
- **Spanish–English Audio Glossary:** This auditory aide provides helpful terms and phrases for communicating with patients who speak Spanish.

Companion Products for Instructors and Students

From traditional texts to interactive products, companion materials to *Maternal & Child Health Nursing* are tailored to fit every learning style. These integrated products offer students a seamless learning experience they won't find anywhere else.

- **PrepU:** *Practice makes perfect. And this is the perfect practice.* This adaptive, personalized learning tool determines what students know *as* they are learning and focuses them on what they are struggling with so they don't spend time on what they already know. Feedback is immediate and remediates students back to this specific text so they know where to go back to the text, read, and help understand a concept. No student has the same experience—PrepU recognizes when a student has reached mastery of a concept before moving them on to higher levels of learning. This will be a different experience for each student based on the number of questions he or she answers and whether he or she answers them correctly. Students get individual feedback about their performance, and instructors can track class statistics to gauge the level of understanding. Both students and instructors get a window into performance to help identify areas for remediation. Instructors can access the average mastery level of the class, students' strengths and weaknesses, and how often students use PrepU. The system is Mobile optimized, which means both students and instructors can access PrepU anytime, anywhere. For more information, visit http://thePoint.lww.com/Pillitteri7e/PrepU.
- **Study Guide:** This guide reinforces the text by offering exercises and study review tools to enhance the learning process. It also includes hundreds of NCLEX-style questions in both multiple choice and the alternate format.

Adele Pillitteri, PhD, RN, PNP

Acknowledgments

I would like to express my sincere appreciation to the contributors and reviewers who, by their hard work, made this edition of the book possible. I am also deeply grateful for the assistance and guidance throughout the project of Patrick Barbera, Acquisitions Editor; Nicky Dunlap, Marketing Manager; Dawn Lagrosa, Product Manager; Marian Bellus, Production Product Manager; and Joan Wendt, Design Director.

A.P.

Contents

Unit 1

Maternal and Child Health Nursing Practice

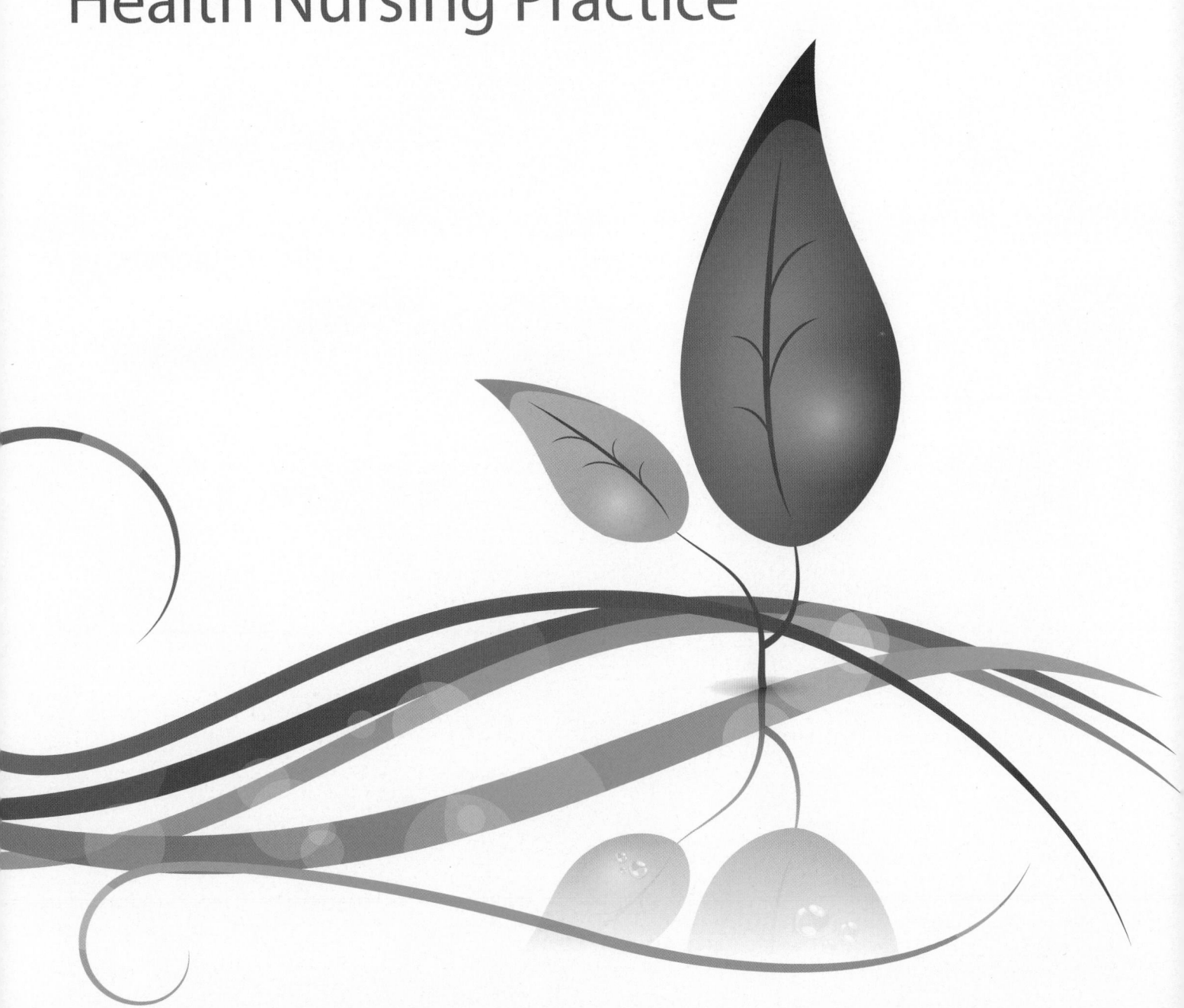

Chapter 1

A Framework for Maternal and Child Health Nursing

KEY TERMS

- client advocacy
- evidence-based practice
- fertility rate
- maternal and child health nursing
- mortality rate
- neonate
- nursing research
- Quality & Safety Education for Nurses (QSEN)
- scope of practice

OBJECTIVES

After mastering the contents of this chapter, you should be able to:

1. View the areas of maternal and child health as a continuum with a seamless flow between the two areas.
2. Identify the specific goals and philosophies of maternal and child health nursing and apply these to nursing practice.
3. Identify 2020 National Health Goals as an important guide to understanding the health of the nation and goals that nurses can help the nation achieve.
4. Describe the evolution, scope, competencies, and professional roles of nurses in maternal and child health nursing.
5. Describe family-centered care and ways maternal and child health nursing could be made both more family centered and respectful of diversity.
6. Using the nursing process, plan nursing care that includes the six competencies of Quality & Safety Education for Nurses (QSEN): Patient-Centered Care, Teamwork & Collaboration, Evidence-Based Practice (EBP), Quality Improvement (QI), Safety, and Informatics.
7. Define and use common statistical terms used in the field, such as infant and maternal mortality.
8. Use critical thinking to identify areas of nursing care that could benefit from additional research or application of evidence-based practice.
9. Integrate knowledge of maternal and child health nursing with the interplay of nursing process, the six competencies of QSEN, and Family Nursing to achieve quality maternal and child health nursing care.

Anna Chung is an early premature **neonate** who will be transported to a regional center for care about 30 miles from the community where she was born. Her parents, Melissa and Robert, tell you they are worried about their tiny daughter being cared for by strangers so many miles away. They're also concerned how they will be able to pay for or give informed consent for this special level of care. Melissa, 42 years old, feels too exhausted to leave the hospital only 2 days after having a cesarean birth. She wonders how she and her husband will be able to visit the new baby because of her exhaustion and because their first child, Miecko, 6 years old, is on home care for pneumonia. Robert wonders how Miecko will react to having an ill rather than a healthy sister.

This chapter discusses competencies, philosophies, challenges, and new roles for nurses in maternal–child health care and how these challenges and changes mold and affect care.

What are some health care issues evident in the previous scenario? What would be your nursing role with Mrs. Chung? With her two children?

GOALS AND PHILOSOPHIES OF MATERNAL AND CHILD HEALTH NURSING

The medical term "obstetrics," or care of women during childbirth, is derived from the Greek word *obstare*, which means "to keep watch." "Pediatrics" is a word derived from the Greek word *pais*, meaning "child." In nursing, these terms are seldom used in preference to "maternity" and "child health" to stress the importance of the nurse as a partner in care (not just keeping watch) and to stress the child's family is also included.

The area of childbearing and childrearing families is a major focus of nursing practice today because to have healthy adults, you must promote healthy lifestyles of childbearing women and their families from the time before children are born until they reach adulthood. This makes preconceptual and prenatal care and helping a family achieve emotional preparation for childbearing and childrearing essential to the health of a woman and her family.

As children grow, families need continued health supervision and support to ensure children remain well. As teenagers or young adults reach maturity and begin to plan for their own families, the cycle repeats and a new generation of support becomes necessary.

Although nursing has, in the past, typically divided its concerns for families during childbearing and childrearing into two separate entities, maternity care and child health care are not two separate entities, but a continuum (Fig. 1.1) (Burkhard, 2013).

The primary goal of both maternal and child health nursing can be stated simply as the promotion and maintenance of optimal family health to ensure cycles of optimal childbearing and childrearing. Major philosophical assumptions about combined maternal and child health nursing are listed in Box 1.1. Because the ages covered in this area are so large, concerns and goals of maternal and child health nursing care are also broad. Examples of the scope of practice include:

- Preconceptual health care
- Care of women during three trimesters of pregnancy and the puerperium (the 6 weeks after childbirth, sometimes termed the fourth trimester of pregnancy)

BOX 1.1 A Philosophy of Maternal and Child Health Nursing

Maternal and child health nursing is:

- Family centered; assessment should always include the family as well as an individual.
- Community centered; the health of families is both affected by and influences the health of communities.
- Evidence based; this is the means whereby critical knowledge increases.
- A challenging role for nurses and a major factor in keeping families well and optimally functioning.

A maternal and child health nurse:

- Considers the family as a whole and as a partner in care when planning or implementing or evaluating the effectiveness of care.
- Serves as an advocate to protect the rights of all family members, including the fetus.
- Demonstrates a high degree of independent nursing functions, because teaching and counseling are major interventions.
- Promotes health and disease prevention because these protect the health of the next generation.
- Serves as an important resource for families during childbearing and childrearing as these can be extremely stressful times in a life cycle.
- Respects personal, cultural, and religious attitudes and beliefs as these so strongly influence the meaning and impact of childbearing and childrearing.
- Encourages developmental stimulation during both health and illness so children can reach their ultimate capacity in adult life.
- Assesses families for strengths as well as specific needs or challenges.
- Encourages family bonding through rooming-in and family visiting in maternal and child health care settings.
- Encourages early hospital discharge options to reunite families as soon as possible in order to create a seamless, helpful transition process.
- Encourages families to reach out to their community so the family can develop a wealth of support people they can call on in a time of family crisis.

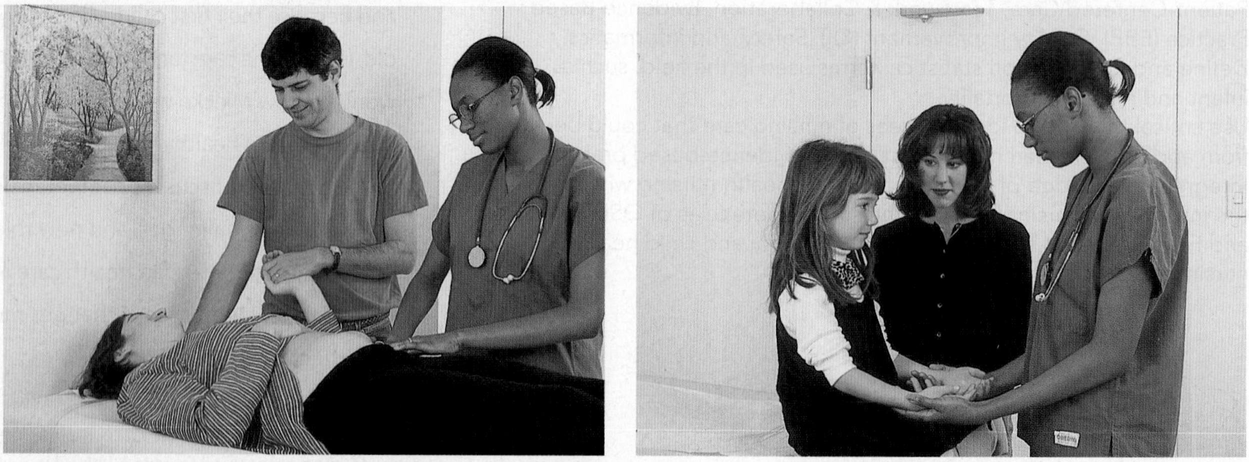

A B

FIGURE 1.1 Maternal and child health nursing includes care of the pregnant woman, child, and family. **(A)** During a prenatal visit, a nurse assesses that a pregnant woman's uterus is expanding normally. **(B)** During a health maintenance visit, a nurse assesses a child's growth and development. (© Barbara Proud.)

- Care of infants during the perinatal period (the time span beginning at 20 weeks of pregnancy to 4 weeks [28 days] after birth)
- Care of children from birth through young adulthood
- Care in settings as diverse as a birthing room, a pediatric intensive care unit, or the home

In all settings and types of care, keeping the family at the center of care or considering the family as the primary unit of care is important because the level of a family's functioning is so important to the health status of its members (Papp, 2012).

A healthy family establishes an environment conducive to growth and health-promoting behaviors to sustain family members during crises. Conversely, if a family's level of functioning is found to be low, the emotional, physical, and social health and potential of individuals in that family may also fall below a healthy level. Similarly, the health of an individual and his or her ability to function as a member of a family can strongly influence and improve overall family functioning. Some men, for example, relate so closely during their wife's or partner's pregnancy, they experience morning sickness at the same level as she does (Paulson & Bazemore, 2010).

For all these reasons, a family-centered or relationship approach enables nurses to better understand individuals and their effect on others and, in turn, to provide more holistic care (Hedges, Nichols, & Filoteo, 2012).

Family-centered care includes when children must be admitted to a hospital, respecting open visiting hours so parents can visit as much as possible, as well as a parent's bed placed next to the child's so a parent can sleep over. An important nursing role is to encourage parents to do as much for their child as they wish, such as feeding and bathing or administering oral medicine. Most of a parent's time, however, should be spent simply being close by to provide a comfortable, secure influence on their child (Fig. 1.2). For the same reasons, the most important role of parents on a family-centered maternity unit is to room-in and give total care to their newborn.

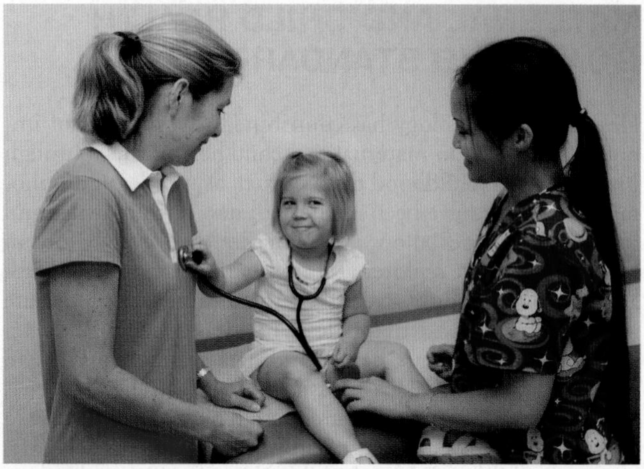

FIGURE 1.2 A nurse involves the mother in a physical exam to promote family-centered care.

Family-centered nursing care increases the number of clients a nurse cares for—that is, not four children, for example, but four children plus four sets of parents; not just a single newborn, but his or her parents as well. Caring for families this way, rather than just an individual newborn or child, has an immeasurable effect on the health of children and parents as well as client satisfaction (H. A. Adams, 2011).

Box 1.2 provides tips on how to help a family chose a health care setting that is family centered. Family Teaching boxes of this kind are found in all chapters as examples of the type of health teaching important in maternal and child health care.

BOX 1.2 Nursing Care Planning Based on Family Teaching

TIPS FOR SELECTING A FAMILY-CENTERED HEALTH CARE SETTING

Q. Melissa Chung asks you, "With so many health care settings available, how do we know which one to choose?"

A. When selecting a setting, asking the following questions can help you decide what is best for your family:

- If the setting is for child care, are personnel interested in you as well as your child? If the setting is a maternal care site, do they ask about family concerns as well as individual ones?
- Can the setting be reached easily? (Going for preventive care when well or for continuing care when ill should not be a chore.)
- Will the staff provide continuity of care so you'll always see the same primary care provider if possible?
- Does the physical setup of the facility provide for a sense of privacy, yet a sense that health care providers share pertinent information so you do not have to repeat your history at each visit?
- Is the cost of care and the number of referrals to specialists explained clearly?
- Are preventive care and health education stressed? (Keeping well is as important as recovering from illness.)
- Is health education done at your learning level?
- Do health care providers respect your opinion and ask for your input on health care decisions?
- Will the facility still be accessible if a family member becomes disabled?

MATERNAL AND CHILD HEALTH GOALS AND STANDARDS

Health care technology has contributed to a number of important advances in maternal and child health care. Through immunization, childhood diseases such as measles and poliomyelitis almost have been eradicated; new fertility drugs and fertility techniques allow more couples than ever before to conceive and have children; the ability to delay preterm birth and improve life for both early-premature and late-premature infants has increased dramatically; and as specific genes responsible for children's health disorders are identified, stem cell therapy may make it possible to replace diseased cells with new growth cells and cure these illnesses. In addition, a growing trend toward health care consumerism, or self-care, has made childbearing and childrearing families active participants in their own health monitoring.

Even in light of these changes, much more needs to be done. Health care may be more advanced, but it is still not accessible to everyone. These and other social changes and trends have expanded the roles of nurses in maternal and child health and, at the same time, made the delivery of quality maternal and child health nursing care a continuing challenge.

2020 National Health Goals

The importance a society assigns to human life can best be measured by the concern a nation places on its most vulnerable members—its elderly, its disadvantaged, and its youngest citizens. In light of this, in 1979, the U.S. Public Health Service first formulated health care objectives for the nation. Health care goals are reviewed every 10 years. In 2010, new goals to be achieved by 2020 were set (U.S. Department of Health and Human Services [DHHS], 2010). Many of these objectives directly involve maternal and child health care, because improving the health of these age groups will have long-term effects. The two main overarching national health goals are:

- Increase quality and years of healthy life.
- Eliminate health disparities.

A new objective added in 2010 recommends that 100% of prelicensure programs in nursing include core content on counseling for health promotion and disease prevention, cultural diversity, evaluation of health sciences literature, environmental health, public health systems, and global health, all important areas for maternal and child health and discussed throughout this text (DHHS, 2010).

The 2020 National Health Goals are intended to help citizens more easily understand the importance of health promotion and disease prevention and to encourage wide participation in improving health in the next decade. It's important for maternal and child health nurses to be familiar with these goals because nurses play such a vital role in helping the nation achieve these objectives through both practice and research (see www.healthypeople.gov). The goals also serve as the basis for grant funding and financing of evidence-based practice. Each of the following sections highlights goals as they relate to that specific area of care.

Global Health Goals

The United Nations (UN) and the World Health Organization (WHO) established millennium health goals in 2000 in an effort to improve health worldwide. As with 2020 National Health Goals, these concentrate on improving the health of women and children because increasing the health in these two populations can have such long-ranging effects on general health. These Global Health Goals are:

- End poverty and hunger.
- Achieve universal primary education.
- Promote gender equality and empower women.
- Reduce child mortality.
- Improve maternal health.
- Combat HIV/AIDS, malaria, and other diseases.
- Ensure environmental sustainability.
- Develop a global partnership for development.

The establishment of global health goals is a major step forward in improving the health of all people, as contagious diseases, poverty, and gender inequality do not respect national boundaries but follow people across the world and into all nations (UN, 2000).

Health Setting Magnet Status

Magnet status is a credential furnished by the American Nurses Credentialing Center (ANCC), an affiliate of the American Nurses Association, to hospitals that meet a rigorous set of criteria designed to improve the strength and quality of nursing care. Hospitals who achieve Magnet status meet criteria in five major categories:

- Transformational leadership. This is the ability of nurses in the designated organization to convert their organization's values, beliefs, and behaviors in order to create a high professional level of nursing care.
- Structural empowerment. This refers to the ability to provide an innovative environment where strong professional practice can flourish with regard to the hospital's mission, vision, and values.
- Exemplary professional practice. The setting demonstrates a comprehensive understanding of the role of nursing; the application of that role with patients, families, communities, and the interdisciplinary team is clear, so new knowledge and evidence can be applied to nursing care.
- New knowledge, innovation, and improvements. The organization demonstrates strong nursing leadership, empowered professionals, and exemplary practice while contributing to patient care.
- Empirical quality results. The hospital demonstrates solid structure and processes where strong professional practice can flourish and where the mission, vision, and values come to life as the organization achieves the outcomes believed to be important for the organization (ANCC, 2012).

Magnet hospitals typically demonstrate a high level of nursing job satisfaction and a low staff nurse turnover rate, and have policies in place that include nurses in data collection and decision making about patient care. These hospitals demonstrate they value staff nurses, involve them in research-based practice, and encourage and reward them for obtaining additional degrees in nursing. By 2013, all nurse managers and nurse leaders in Magnet designated hospitals must have either a Baccalaureate or Master's degree in nursing.

Not all hospitals can qualify for Magnet status; the desirability of being named a Magnet Hospital, however, has encouraged all hospitals to examine their nursing environment and bring about changes that improve working conditions, stress evidence-based practice, and improve the education level of their nurses (Hess, Desroches, Donelan, et al., 2011).

A FRAMEWORK FOR MATERNAL AND CHILD HEALTH NURSING CARE

Maternal and child health nursing can be visualized within a framework in which nurses use nursing process, nursing theory, and Quality & Safety Education for Nurses (QSEN) competencies to care for families during childbearing and childrearing years and through the four phases of health care:

- Health promotion
- Health maintenance
- Health restoration
- Health rehabilitation

Examples of these phases of health care as they relate to maternal and child health are shown in Table 1.1.

Nursing Process

Nursing care, at its best, is designed and implemented in a thorough manner, using an organized series of steps, to ensure quality and consistency of care (Carpenito, 2012). The nursing process, a scientific form of problem solving, serves as the basis for assessing, making a nursing diagnosis, planning, implementing, and evaluating care. It is a process broad enough to serve as the basis for modern nursing care because it is applicable to all health care settings, from the home to ambulatory clinics to intensive care units.

Because nurses rarely work in isolation, but rather as a member of an interprofessional team, interprofessional care maps and checkpoint questions on teamwork and collaboration are included throughout the text to demonstrate the use of the nursing process as well as to provide examples of critical thinking, clarify nursing care for specific client needs, and accentuate the increasingly important role of nurses as coordinators of care for a collaborative team.

Nursing Theory

One of the requirements of a profession (together with other critical determinants, such as members set their own standards, self-monitor their practice quality, and participate in research) is that a discipline's knowledge flows from a base of established theory.

Nursing theories are designed to offer helpful ways to view clients so nursing activities can be created to best meet client needs—for example, Calistra Roy's theory stresses that an important role of the nurse is to help patients adapt to change caused by illness or other stressors (Roy, 2011); Dorothea Orem's theory concentrates on examining patients' ability to perform self-care (Orem & Taylor, 2011); Patricia Benner's theory describes the way nurses move from novice to expert as they become more experienced and prepared to give interprofessional care (Benner, 2011). Using a theoretical basis such as these can help you appreciate the significant effect of a child's illness or the introduction of a new member on the total family.

Other issues most nursing theorists address include how nurses should be viewed or what should be the goals of nursing care. Extensive changes in the scope of maternal and child health nursing have occurred as health promotion (teaching, counseling, supporting, and advocacy, or keeping parents and children well) has become a greater priority in care (Salsman, Grunberg, Beaumont, et al., 2012). As promoting healthy pregnancies and keeping children well protects not only clients at present but the health of the next generation, maternal–child health nurses fill these expanded roles to a unique and special degree.

QSEN: Quality & Safety Education for Nurses

In 2007, the Robert Wood Johnson Foundation challenged nursing leaders to improve the quality of nursing care by describing what constitutes good nursing care, as well as to build into prelicensure and graduate programs in nursing the knowledge, skills, and attitudes necessary to help achieve that level of care (Disch, 2012).

TABLE 1.1 Definitions and Examples of Phases of Health Care

Term	Definition	Examples
Health promotion	Educating parents and children to follow sound health practices through teaching and role modeling	Teaching women the importance of rubella immunization before pregnancy; teaching adolescents the importance of safer sex practices
Health maintenance	Intervening to maintain health when risk of illness is present	Encouraging women to be partners in prenatal care; teaching parents the importance of safeguarding their home by childproofing against poisoning
Health restoration	Using conscientious assessment to be certain that symptoms of illness are identified and interventions are begun to return client to wellness most rapidly	Caring for a woman during a complication of pregnancy such as gestational diabetes or a child during an acute illness such as pneumonia
Health rehabilitation	Helping prevent complications from illness; helping a client with residual effects achieve an optimal state of wellness and independence; helping a client to accept inevitable death	Encouraging a woman with gestational trophoblastic disease (abnormal placenta growth) to continue therapy or a child with a renal transplant to continue to take necessary medications

Because of this challenge, the QSEN Learning Collaborative originated six competencies deemed necessary for quality care (Cronenwett, Sherwood, & Gelmon, 2009). These competencies incorporated five that were included in a study by the Institute of Medicine (IOM): patient-centered care, teamwork and collaboration, quality improvement, informatics, and evidence-based practice, plus an added sixth competency: safety.

The overall goal through all phases of QSEN is to address the challenge of preparing future nurses with the abilities necessary to continuously improve the quality and safety of the health care systems in which they work. Definitions of the six competencies and examples of the knowledge, skills, and attitudes necessary to achieve quality maternal and child health care are shown in Box 1.3.

Evidence-Based Practice

Evidence-based practice is the conscientious, explicit, and judicious use of current best evidence in making decisions about the care of patients (Falk, Wongsa, Dang, et al., 2012). Evidence can be a combination of research, clinical expertise, and patient preferences or values.

Use of evidence such as that obtained from randomized controlled trials helps to move health care actions from "just tradition" to a more solid, and therefore safer, scientific basis. The Cochrane Database (listed in PubMed, Ovid, and Medline) is a good source for discovering evidence-based practices as the organization consistently reviews, evaluates, and reports the strength of health-related research (Dong, Chen, & Yu, 2012).

QSEN Checkpoint Questions: Evidence-Based Practice are included in chapters throughout the text and contain summaries of current maternal and child health research followed by questions to assist you in developing a questioning attitude regarding current nursing practice or in thinking of ways to incorporate research findings into care.

Nursing Research

Nursing research (the systematic investigation of problems that have implications for nursing practice and usually carried out by nurses) plays an important role in evidence-based practice as bodies of professional knowledge only grow and expand to the extent people in that profession are able to carry out research (Christian, 2012). Examining nursing care in this way results in improved and cost-effective patient care as it provides evidence for action and justification for implementing activities.

A classic example of how the results of nursing research can influence nursing practice is the application of research carried out by Rubin (1963) concerning mothers' initial approaches to their newborns. Before the publication of this study, nurses assumed a woman who did not immediately hold and cuddle her infant at birth was a "cold" or unfeeling mother. After observing a multitude of new mothers, Rubin concluded attachment is not a spontaneous procedure; rather, it more commonly begins with only fingertip touching, then over the next few days, moves to "motherly" actions such as hugging and kissing. Armed with Rubin's findings, nurses today are better able to differentiate healthy from unhealthy bonding behavior in new mothers. Additional nursing research in this area (discussed in Chapter 17) has provided further substantiation regarding the importance of this original investigation.

Some examples of current questions that warrant nursing investigation in the area of maternal and child health nursing include:

- What is the most effective stimulus to encourage women to come for prenatal care or parents to bring children for health maintenance visits?
- How can nurses be instrumental in fostering diversity in care?
- How much self-care should young children be expected (or encouraged) to provide during an illness?
- What is the effect of market-driven health care on the quality of maternal–child nursing care?
- What active measures can nurses take to reduce the incidence of child or intimate partner violence?
- How can nurses best help families cope with the stress of a complication of pregnancy or a child's long-term illness?
- How can nurses help prevent violence such as homicide in communities and modify the effects of violence on families?
- What information do maternal and child health nurses need to know about alternative therapies, such as herbal remedies, so their practices remain current?

✔ *QSEN Checkpoint Question 1.1*

Teamwork & Collaboration

A nursing assistant has told you that Mr. Chung asked why the hospital where his baby is being cared for is termed a "Magnet hospital." You would want your team members to know which rationale?

a. Magnet hospitals are those who care for the most acutely ill patients.
b. The designation is one assigned by the American Medical Association.
c. The hospital has met high standards for nursing competency.
d. The term refers to hospitals that only admit a limited number of patients.

Look in Appendix A for the best answer and rationale.

A CHANGING DISCIPLINE

Maternal and child health is an ever-changing area of nursing. This happens because childhood infections, such as pertussis (whooping cough) and measles (Rubeola), can now be prevented so children no longer need care for these conditions. At the same time, illnesses that could not be treated before, such as cystic fibrosis or hypertension of pregnancy, can now be treated, so the number of settings and critical aspects of care increases.

Trends in the Maternal and Child Health Nursing Population

Not only patterns of illness but also variations in social structure, family lifestyle, and responsibilities continue to constantly change. Table 1.2 summarizes some of these changes that have directly altered assessment and planning care for maternal and child health nurses.

BOX 1.3 QSEN Competencies in Relation to the Chung Family

Competency	Knowledge	Skills	Attitudes
Patient-Centered Care			
The patient or designee is thought of as the source of control and full partner in the provision of compassionate and coordinated care based on respect for the patient's preferences, values, and needs.	Take an admission history detailing the Chung family's composition. Document the roles of family members and who will be the chief childcare provider.	Encourage Anna's family to spend as much time as possible with her while she is hospitalized; assess that she will have family support on transition to home.	Don't think of admitting Anna to the neonatal care nursery as a single patient, but rather, as admitting her family to the setting.
Teamwork and Collaboration			
Nurses function effectively within nursing and interprofessional teams, fostering open communication, mutual respect, and shared decision making as they achieve quality patient care.	Familiarize yourself with how many other health care providers will be interacting with Anna (e.g., neonatologist, nurse practitioner, nutritionist) to help appreciate how frightening having to meet so many people could be to a family.	Discuss with Anna's parents what problems, if any, they will have visiting so other team members can help reassure and support them when they visit.	Consider and respect Anna's parents as integrative members of her health care team.
Evidence-Based Practice			
Nurses integrate the best current evidence with clinical expertise and patient/family preferences and values for delivery of optimal health care.	Read journal articles related to new evidence about healthy families or neonatal care to be better prepared to help Anna seamlessly transition from one setting to the next.	Implement evidence-based practice so Anna's family are confident that care is based on credible research.	Value the need for change based on new evidence so you can explain to Anna's family with confidence any need for change in care.
Quality Improvement (QI)			
Nurses use data to monitor the outcomes of care and use improvement methods to design and test changes to continuously improve the quality and safety of health care systems.	View QI as an important role for all health care professionals beginning with prelicensure students.	Use whatever aids, such as checklists, flow sheets, or patient information forms, necessary in order to provide seamless nursing care from nursery admission to home.	Appreciate that continuous QI is an essential part of successful working with and respecting families.
Safety			
Nurses minimize the risk of harm to patients and providers through both system effectiveness and individual performance.	Learn the requirements for a safe health care setting for a vulnerable preterm infant.	Be certain Anna receives developmental stimuli as well as is cared for in an environment that promotes a sense of security and is as free from pain as possible.	Recognize families under stress do not "hear" instructions well and so may need these repeated or provided in a written form as well as orally.
Informatics			
Nurses use information and technology to communicate, manage knowledge, mitigate error, and support decision making.	Keep records and documentation current so various health care providers can keep informed in order to provide seamless care shifts and setting shifts in care.	Document care in an electronic health record so it can be available to various health care providers.	Recognize that documentation must be complete to be valuable (in audit reviews, what wasn't documented as being done is considered as not done).

TABLE 1.2 Trends in Maternal and Child Health Care and Implications for Nursing

Trend	Implications for Nursing
Families are not as extended as in previous generations, so contain fewer members.	Fewer family members are available as support people in a time of crisis. Nurses are called on to fulfill this role more than ever before.
The number of single-parent families is increasing so rapidly it now equals the number of nuclear families in the United States.	A single parent may have fewer financial resources than dual-employed parents. Nurses need to be aware of alternative care options and available to provide a backup opinion as needed.
Ninety percent of women in the United States work outside their home at least part time; many women are the main wage earner for their family.	Health care must be scheduled at times a working parent can come for care for herself or can bring a child for care. Problems of latchkey (self-care) children and the number and safety of child care centers need to be addressed.
Families are more mobile than previously; there is an increase in the number of homeless women and children.	Good interviewing and health monitoring are necessary with mobile families so a health database can be established and there can be continuity of care.
Both child and intimate partner violence is increasing in incidence.	Screening for child or intimate partner violence should be included in all family assessments. Nurses must be aware of the legal responsibilities for reporting violence.
Families are more health conscious than ever before; the use of Internet sites to monitor their health or ask health questions is rapidly increasing.	Families are ripe for health education; providing evidence-based information can be a major nursing role.
Health care must respect cost containment by creating "health care homes" or "medical homes."	Comprehensive care is necessary in primary care settings because referral to specialists may not be an option depending on a family's type or lack of health insurance.
Client advocacy is necessary as it is easy for families to feel lost in the health care system.	**Advocacy** is safeguarding and advancing the interests of clients and their families. Familiarity with the health care services available in a community, establishing and maintaining a relationship with families, as well as helping them make informed choices about what course of action to take or what services would be best to use are important nursing roles.

Measuring Maternal and Child Health

Measuring what constitutes the area of maternal and child health is not as simple as defining whether clients are ill or well because individual clients and health care practitioners can maintain different perspectives on illness and wellness. For example, some children with chronic but controllable asthma think of themselves as well; others with the same degree of involvement consider themselves ill. Although pregnancy is generally considered a well state, some women think of themselves as ill and needing special considerations during this time.

A more objective view of health can be provided by using national or regional health statistics to describe degrees of illness (Box 1.4). Such statistics are useful for comparisons among states and nations and for anticipating future health care needs of a community. Statistics require accurate recording, collection, and analysis and, because nurses play such a major role in the accurate collection and recording of health-related data, nurses play a major role in allowing the nation's present and future health to be described in these ways.

Birth Rate

The birth rate in the United States has decreased gradually over the past 10 years from a high of 30.2 per 1,000 population in 1909 to 13.5 per 1,000 population at present (Fig. 1.3). Currently, the average family in the United States has 1.2 children. Boys are born more often than girls at a rate of 1,050 boys to every 1,000 girls. Early in the century, births to teenage girls were steadily increasing; however, due to additional counseling and publicity of the risks of teenage birth, this rate is now steadily declining (presently at 34.3/1,000 from a high of 618/1,000 in 1961) (Alio, Mbah, Grunsten, et al., 2011).

The birth rate for women 20 to 24 years of age (90.0/1,000) is gradually declining as well, as women choose to postpone having children until past college age. In contrast, the number of children born to women older than 40 years of age is steadily increasing (presently at 10.2/1,000 from a low of almost no births in this age group in 1901 (Hamilton, Martin, & Ventura, 2011).

Fertility Rate

The fertility rate tends to be low in countries where there is famine because poor nutrition makes conceiving difficult, as well as in countries where the proportion of young adult men is low because of war or disease. This rate tends to be high in countries where the average woman has access to good nutrition and feels safe to begin a family. The U.S. fertility rate is currently at 66.7%, a rate typical of a healthy postindustrial country (Hamilton et al., 2011)

Fetal Death Rate

Fetal deaths occur because of maternal factors (such as premature cervical dilation and maternal hypertension) and also because of

BOX 1.4 Common Statistical Terms Used to Report Maternal and Child Health

Birth rate:	The number of births per 1,000 population.
Fertility rate:	The number of pregnancies per 1,000 women of childbearing age.
Fetal death rate:	The number of fetal deaths (over 500 g) per 1,000 live births.
Neonatal death rate:	The number of deaths per 1,000 live births occurring at birth or in the first 28 days of life.
Perinatal death rate:	The number of deaths during the perinatal time period (beginning when a fetus reaches 500 g, about week 20 of pregnancy, and ending about 4 to 6 weeks after birth); it is the sum of the fetal and neonatal rates.
Maternal mortality rate:	The number of maternal deaths per 100,000 live births that occur as a direct result of the reproductive process.
Infant mortality rate:	The number of deaths per 1,000 live births occurring at birth or in the first 12 months of life.
Childhood mortality rate:	The number of deaths per 1,000 population in children aged 1 to 14 years.

fetal factors (perhaps chromosomal abnormalities or poor placental attachment). The cause of many fetal deaths cannot be documented or occur for unknown reasons. Fetal death rate is important in evaluating the health of a nation because it reflects the overall quality of maternal health and whether common services such as prenatal care are available. A renewed emphasis on both preconceptual and prenatal care has helped to reduce the U.S. rate from a number as high as 18% in 1950 to 6.2% at present (National Center for Health Statistics [NCHS], 2012).

Neonatal Death Rate

This rate reflects not only the quality of care available to women during pregnancy and childbirth but also the quality of care available to infants during the first month of life. The leading causes of death during this time are prematurity with associated low birth weight or congenital malformations (NCHS, 2012).

The proportion of infants born with low birth weight is about 12.5% of all births (about 80% of infants who die within 48 hours after birth weigh less than 2,500 g [5.5 lb]). The number of low–birth-weight infants rises slightly each year due to an increase in multiple births in which children tend to be born prematurely and also because of better prenatal care that allows infants who would have died in utero (fetal death) to be born and survive. Even with this increase in low–birth-weight infants being born, the neonatal death rate has decreased 85%, from 28.8 in 1940 to as few as 4.5 deaths per 1,000 live births today (NCHS, 2012).

Infant Mortality Rate

The infant mortality rate of a country is a good index of its general health because it measures the quality of pregnancy

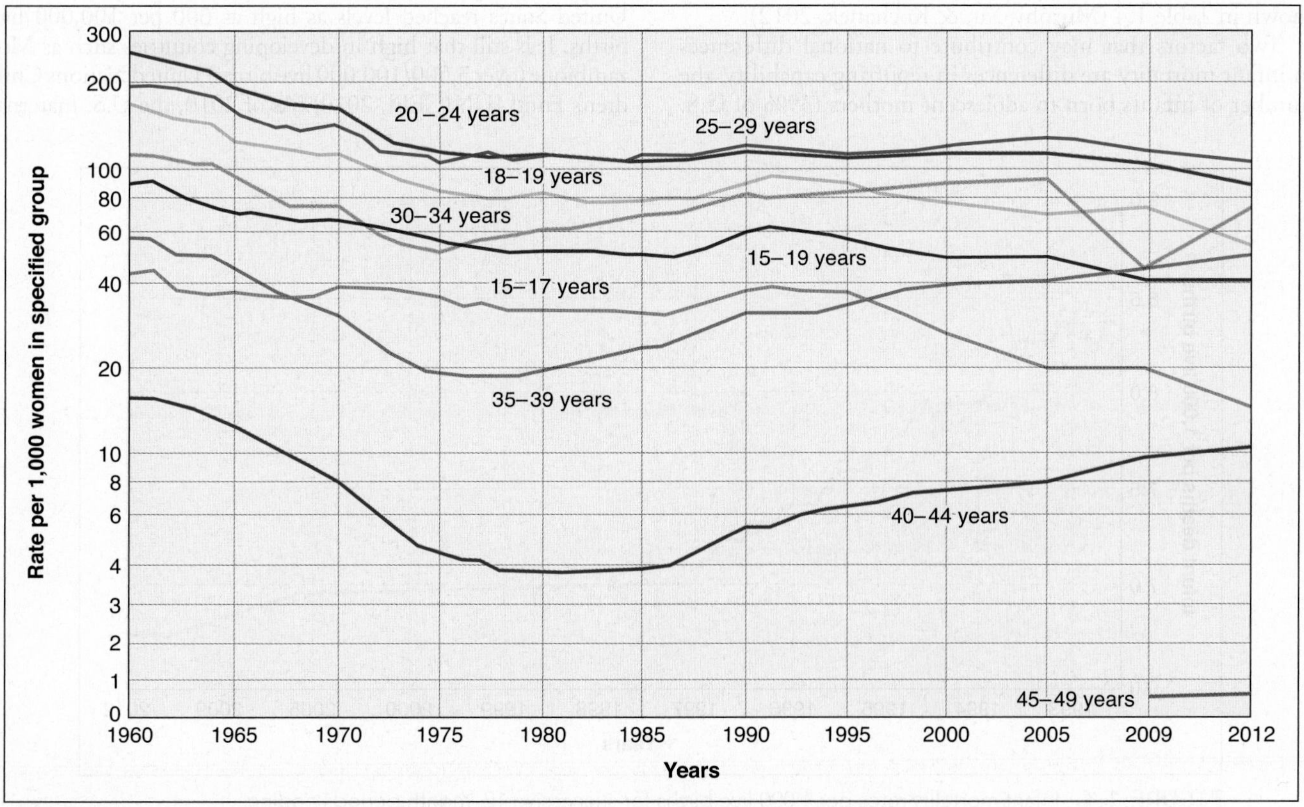

FIGURE 1.3 Birth rates by age of mother: United States, 1965–2012. (National Center for Health Statistics. [2013]. Births, marriages, divorces and deaths. *National Vital Statistics Report, 61*[5], 8.)

care, overall nutrition, and sanitation, as well as infant health and available care. This rate is the traditional standard used to compare the health of a nation with previous years or with other countries.

Thanks to the introduction of prenatal care and other community health measures (such as efforts to encourage breastfeeding, require immunizations, initiate better unintentional injury prevention measures [e.g., requiring car seats], and reduce sudden infant death syndrome [SIDS] or the sudden death of an infant less than 1 year of age that cannot be explained after a thorough investigation of the cause of death), in combination with the many technologic advances available for care, the U.S. infant mortality rate has decreased 86%, from 47.0 in 1940 to 6.7 per 1,000 live births today (Mathews & MacDorman, 2011) (Fig. 1.4).

Unfortunately, infant mortality is not equal among all American subpopulations. For example, the rate is higher among Native Alaskan, Native American, and African American infants than it is for Caucasian or non-Hispanic newborns. These differences are thought to be related to a combination of factors, including the higher proportion of births to young mothers and unequal provision of and access to health care in different communities (NCHS, 2012).

The infant mortality rate also varies greatly from state to state within the United States (Table 1.3). For example, in the District of Columbia, the area with the highest infant mortality, the rate is almost three times that of Massachusetts, the state with the lowest rate.

Worldwide, one would expect the United States, which has one of the highest gross national products in the world and is known for its technologic capabilities, to have the lowest infant mortality rate of all countries. The U.S. infant mortality rate, however, ranks higher than 29 other countries as shown in Table 1.4 (Murphy, Xu, & Kochanek, 2012).

Two factors that may contribute to national differences in infant mortality are differences in reporting capability, the number of infants born to adolescent mothers (39% of U.S. infants are born to women under 20 years of age), as well as the type of health insurance and care available. In Sweden, for example, a comprehensive health care program provides state-sponsored maternal and child health care to all residents. Women who attend prenatal clinics early in pregnancy receive a monetary award, a practice that almost guarantees women will come for prenatal care. This type of health care policy contrasts sharply with the availability of health care in an occupation-linked insurance system such as the one in the United States.

Fortunately, the proportion of pregnant women who receive prenatal care, which has the potential to identify risks and allow preventive strategies against complications of pregnancy, is increasing (about 70% of women now begin care in the first 3 months of their pregnancy).

The main causes of infant mortality in the United States are problems that occur at birth or shortly thereafter, such as prematurity, low birth weight, congenital malformations, and SIDS.

Although other factors that contribute to SIDS are yet to be identified, the recommendations made by the American Academy of Pediatrics (AAP) to place infants on their back to sleep, use room sharing but not bed sharing, avoid exposure to overheating or cigarette smoke, and possible use of pacifiers, have led to an almost 50% decrease in its incidence (AAP, 2011). Nurses have been instrumental in reducing the number of these deaths, as they are the health care professionals who most often discuss newborn care and make recommendations for new parents.

Maternal Mortality Rate

Early in the 20th century, the maternal mortality rate in the United States reached levels as high as 600 per 100,000 live births. It is still that high in developing countries such as Mozambique (over 3,500/100,000 live births) United Nations Children's Fund [UNICEF], 2010). As of 2010, the U.S. maternal

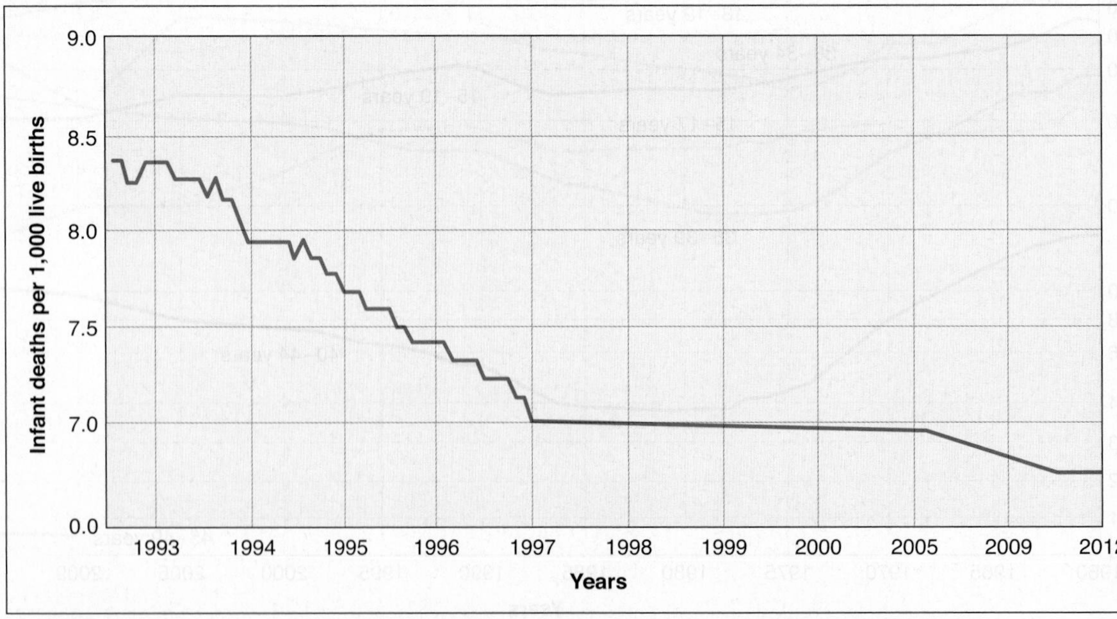

FIGURE 1.4 Infant mortality rates per 1,000 live births for successive 12–month periods ending with month indicated: United States, 2012. (National Center for Health Statistics. [2012]. Births, marriages, divorce and deaths. *National Vital Statistics Report, 61*[6], 7.)

TABLE 1.3 Infant Mortality Rate (Deaths per 1,000 Live Births) by State

State	Rate	State	Rate
Massachusetts	4.8	Kansas	7.0
New Hampshire	4.9	Nebraska	7.0
Maine	5.1	Florida	7.2
Utah	5.3	Hawaii	7.2
California	5.4	Virginia	7.2
Minnesota	5.5	Pennsylvania	7.3
Oregon	5.5	Indiana	7.7
Vermont	5.5	Maryland	7.7
Washington	5.5	Missouri	7.7
Iowa	5.8	Ohio	7.7
Texas	5.9	Illinois	7.8
Colorado	6.0	North Dakota	7.8
Nevada	6.0	West Virginia	7.9
New Jersey	6.1	Oklahoma	8.0
New York	6.1	Michigan	8.1
Connecticut	6.4	Arkansas	8.3
New Mexico	6.4	North Carolina	8.4
South Dakota	6.4	Georgia	8.7
Wyoming	6.5	South Carolina	9.0
Idaho	6.6	Tennessee	9.0
Arizona	6.7	Alabama	9.3
Kentucky	6.7	Puerto Rico	9.4
Rhode Island	6.7	Delaware	9.6
Alaska	6.8	Louisiana	9.8
Montana	6.9	Mississippi	10.5
Wisconsin	6.9	District of Columbia	11.4

(National Center for Health Statistics. [2012]. Births, marriages, divorces, and deaths. *National Vital Statistics Report, 61*(5), 8.

mortality rate was 15.2 per 100,000 live births (Fig. 1.5). This decrease can be contributed to improved preconceptual, prenatal, labor and birth, and postnatal care such as:

- Increased participation of women in prenatal care
- Greater detection of disorders such as ectopic pregnancy or placenta previa and prevention of related complications through the use of ultrasound
- Increased control of complications associated with hypertension of pregnancy
- Decreased use of anesthesia with childbirth
- Ability to better prevent or control hemorrhage and infection

This dramatic decrease is not a cause for celebration, however. Over the past few years, this rate has begun to increase

TABLE 1.4 Infant Mortality Rate (Deaths per 1,000 Live Births) for Selected Countries, 2005

Country	Rate	Country	Rate
1. Singapore	2.1	16. Austria	4.2
2. Sweden	2.4	17. Denmark	4.4
3. Hong Kong	2.4	18. Israel	4.6
4. Japan	2.8	19. Italy	4.7
5. Finland	3.0	20. Netherlands	4.9
6. Norway	3.1	21. England & Wales	5.0
7. Czech Republic	3.4	22. Australia	5.0
8. Portugal	3.5	23. New Zealand	5.1
9. France	3.6	24. Scotland	5.2
10. Belgium	3.7	25. Canada	5.4
11. Greece	3.8	26. Hungary	6.2
12. Germany	3.9	27. Cuba	6.2
13. Ireland	4.0	28. Northern Ireland	6.3
14. Spain	4.1	29. Poland	6.4
15. Switzerland	4.2	30. United States	6.5

(Murphy, S. L., Xu, J., & Kochanek, K. D. [2012]. Deaths: Preliminary data for 2010. *National Vital Statistics Reports, 60*[4], 1–69.

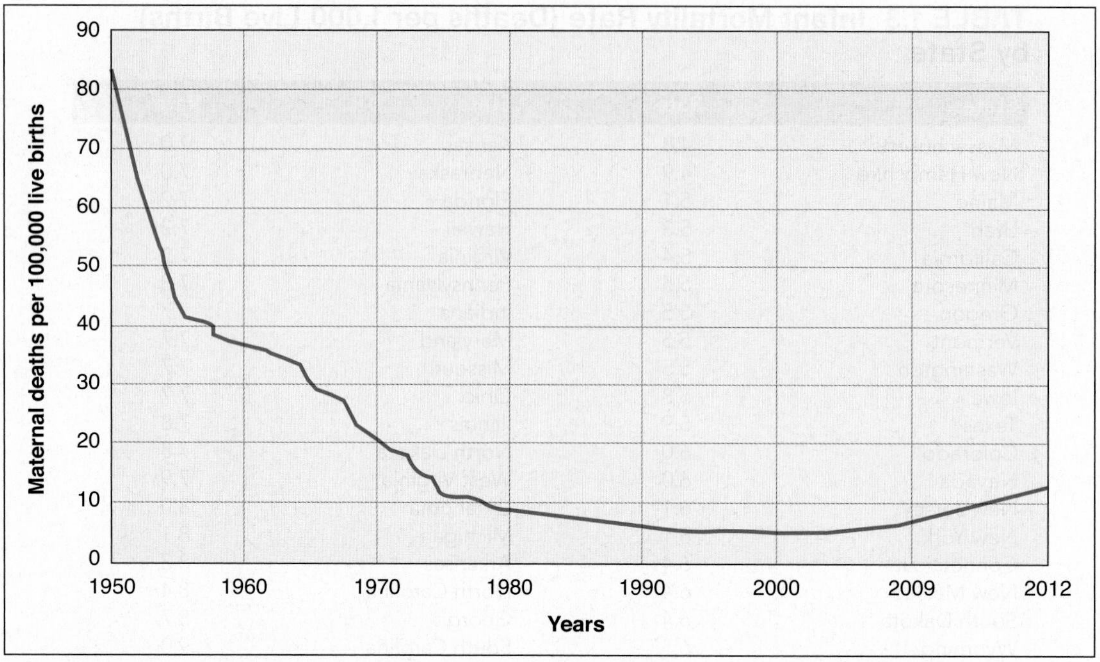

FIGURE 1.5 Maternal mortality rates. (National Center for Health Statistics. [2012]. Births, marriages, divorce and deaths. *National Vital Statistics Report, 61*[6], 7.)

again and in some areas is as high as 24 per 100,000 live births. This increasing rate is associated with more cesarean births, more gestational hypertension related to preexisting hypertensive disorders, and lack of health insurance for many Americans. Nurses who are alert to the signs and symptoms of hypertension are invaluable guardians of the health of pregnant women and newborns (Clark, 2012).

QSEN Checkpoint Question 1.2

Informatics

Mrs. Chung's doctor has told her that her baby's most dangerous time will be until the perinatal period ends. When does the perinatal period take place?

a. From the day of birth until 1 month afterward
b. During the time the infant will be on ventilator support
c. From the 20th week of pregnancy to 4 to 6 weeks after birth
d. Until the infant's body temperature stabilizes following birth

Look in Appendix A for the best answer and rationale.

Child Mortality Rate

Like the infant mortality rate, the child mortality rate in the United States is also declining, although about 20 countries have better rates (UNICEF, 2010). In 1980, for example, the mortality rate was about 6.4% for children aged 1 to 4 years; today, it is 4.7%. Children in the prepubescent period (age 5 to 14 years) have the lowest mortality rate of any child age group, 1.4%. Between 15 and 24 years, the rate increases to 6.6% (Kochanek, Xu, Murphy, et al., 2011).

The most frequent causes of childhood death are shown in Box 1.5. Notice unintentional injuries are the leading

BOX 1.5 Major Causes of Death in Childhood

Under 1 Year

1. Congenital malformations and chromosomal abnormalities
2. Disorders related to short gestation age and low birth weight
3. Sudden infant death syndrome
4. Maternal complications of pregnancy
5. Unintentional injuries (accidents)

1–4 Years

1. Unintentional injuries (accidents)
2. Congenital malformations and chromosomal abnormalities
3. Malignant neoplasms
4. Assault or homicide
5. Diseases of the heart

5–14 Years

1. Unintentional injuries (accidents)
2. Malignant neoplasms
3. Assault or homicide
4. Intentional self-harm (suicide)
5. Congenital malformations and chromosomal abnormalities

15–24 Years

1. Unintentional injuries (accidents)
2. Assault or homicide
3. Intentional self-harm (suicide)
4. Malignant neoplasm
5. Diseases of the heart

(National Center for Health Statistics. [2011]. *Trends in the health of Americans.* Hyattsville, MD: Author.)

cause of death in children, although many of these accidents are largely preventable through education about the value of car seats and seat belt use, the dangers of drinking/drug abuse and driving, and the importance of pedestrian safety.

A particularly disturbing mortality statistic is the high incidence of homicide and suicide in the 10- to 19-year-old age group (more girls than boys attempt suicide, but boys are more successful). Although school-age children and adolescents may not voice feelings of depression or anger during a health care visit, such underlying feelings may actually be a primary concern (Bridge, McBee-Strayer, Cannon, et al., 2012). Nurses who are alert to cues of depression or anger can be instrumental in detecting these emotions and lowering the risk of self-injury.

Childhood Morbidity Rate

Health problems commonly occurring in large proportions of children today include respiratory disorders (including asthma and tuberculosis), gastrointestinal disturbances, and consequences of injuries. Obesity has become such a health problem that in some communities over 20% of school-age children are categorized as obese (Centers for Disease Control and Prevention [CDC], 2012a). Obesity in school-age children can lead to cardiovascular disorders, self-esteem issues, and type 2 diabetes, so counseling children about maintaining a healthy weight is an important nursing responsibility (Junnila, Aromaa, Heinonen, et al., 2012). Morbid obesity in pregnant women can lead to complications during pregnancy, at birth, and following birth (Machado, 2012).

As more immunizations for childhood diseases become available, fewer children in the United States are affected by common childhood communicable diseases. Continued education about the benefits of immunization against rubella (German measles) is still needed because if a woman contracts this form of measles during pregnancy, her infant can be born with severe congenital malformations. The new vaccine against human papillomavirus (HPV), suggested for both prepubescent girls and boys, should help prevent HPV infections that can have the same disastrous results (Nan, 2012).

Although the decline in the overall incidence of preventable childhood diseases is encouraging, as many as 40% of children younger than 4 years of age in some communities are still not fully immunized (CDC, 2011). There is a potential for childhood infectious diseases to increase again if immunization is not maintained as a high national priority.

The advent of the human immunodeficiency virus (HIV) has changed care in all areas of nursing, but has particular implications for maternal and child health nursing. Sexually active teenagers are at risk for becoming infected with HIV through sexual contact. Infected women may transmit the virus to a fetus during pregnancy through placental exchange or at birth through body secretions (Owen, 2012).

Nurses play a vital role in helping to prevent the spread of HIV by educating adolescents and young adults about safer sexual practices (Nachman, Chernoff, Williams, et al., 2012) (see Chapter 5). Follow standard infectious precautions in all areas of nursing practice to safeguard yourself, other health care providers, and clients from the spread of this and other infections.

A number of infectious diseases that are increasing in incidence include syphilis; genital herpes; hepatitis A, B, and C; and tuberculosis. The rise in syphilis, hepatitis C, and genital herpes probably stems from an increase in nonmonogamous sexual relationships and lack of safer sex practices. The increase in hepatitis B is due largely to drug abuse and the use of infected injection equipment. One reason for the increase in hepatitis A is shared diaper-changing facilities in day care centers. Tuberculosis, once considered close to eradication, has experienced such a resurgence that one form occurs as an opportunistic disease in HIV-positive persons and is particularly resistant to usual therapy (Hesseling, Kim, Madhi, et al., 2012). Methicillin-resistant *Staphylococcus aureus* (MRSA) is an infection that occurs often in hospitals, causes skin infections or pneumonia, and is also growing in incidence (Moran, Krishnadasan, Gorwitz, et al., 2012).

The incidence of social concerns, such as intimate partner violence and child maltreatment, remain high. Part of the reason for this is more effective reporting. Both forms of violence tend to be associated with stress in a family, so when the economy becomes depressed or a natural disaster occurs, their incidence rises. As pregnancy can add stress to a family, these behaviors occur at a higher incidence in pregnant families than in others (Brownridge, Taillieu, Tyler, et al., 2011).

Also increasing in incidence is autism spectrum disorder, a range of complex neurodevelopment disorders characterized by social impairment, communication difficulty, and repetitive stereotyped patterns of behavior (Dworzynski, Ronald, Bolton, et al., 2012). Despite the lack of an identified specific cause for the spectrum, it is increasing so rapidly in incidence, it now occurs in as many as 1 in every 88 children (CDC, 2012b).

Trends in the Health Care Environment

The settings for health care as well as nursing roles are changing, with the goal of being able to better meet the needs of increasingly well-informed and vocal consumers.

Initiating Cost Containment

Cost containment refers to reducing the cost of health care by closely monitoring the costs of personnel, use and brands of supplies, length of hospital stays, number of procedures carried out, and number of referrals requested, yet maintaining quality care (Saunier, 2011). Examples of delegation responsibility or teamwork to make care more cost effective or family centered are highlighted in Interprofessional Care Maps throughout this text. Examples of effective communication are shown in Effective Communication Boxes throughout chapters.

Increasing Health Insurance Coverage Costs

The United States is unique among developed countries in that its health care system is privately financed or controlled by work sites. This contrasts with other countries where national health insurance is available to everyone and has no connection to a person's employment. Because of this unique system, the United States spends about 17% of its gross national product on health care, whereas other countries, for example Switzerland, spends less yet has healthier citizens (Zakaria, 2012). In the United States, people most apt to not have health insurance are young adults, individuals who have moved recently or are unemployed, and those who have low incomes. Nurses have important roles at health care agencies to ensure people receive comprehensive care and encourage more children and women to receive preventive care.

Increasing Alternative Settings and Styles for Health Care

The past 100 years have seen several major shifts in settings for maternity and child care. At the turn of the 20th century, for example, most births took place in the home, with only the very poor or ill giving birth in "lying-in" hospitals. By 1940, about 40% of live births occurred in hospitals. Today, the figure has risen to 95% to 99% (NCHS 2012).

This statistic is predicted to change in the future because increasing numbers of women are choosing home birth or birthing in freestanding alternative birth centers. Women who give birth in these alternative settings feel they have a greater control of their birth experience and their family can be more involved in the birth. Alternative settings also allow more practice opportunities for nurses in advanced practice roles, such as nurse-midwives (Osborne & Hanson, 2012).

An important outcome of this movement is that hospitals have responded to consumers' demands for more natural childbirth environments by refitting labor and delivery suites as homelike birthing rooms, often called labor-delivery-recovery (LDR) or labor-delivery-recovery-postpartum (LDRP) rooms (Fig. 1.6). Partners, family members, and other support people can stay with the woman in labor as if they were home and so can feel a part of the childbirth. Couplet care—care for both the mother and newborn by a primary nurse—is encouraged after the birth. Whether childbirth takes place at home, in a birthing center, or in a hospital, the goal is to keep it as natural as possible while ensuring the protection experienced health care providers offer.

Health care settings for children are also changing. Clients' homes, community centers, or school-based or retail setting emergent care clinics are examples of places in which comprehensive health care may be administered. Retail clinics or emergent care clinics located in shopping malls are often staffed by nurse practitioners, so nurses play a vital role in seeing such health care settings do not limit continuity of care (Rohrer, Garrison, & Angstman, 2012).

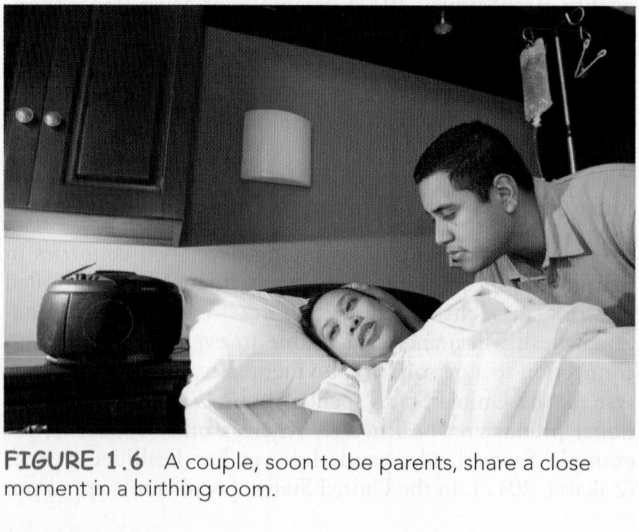

FIGURE 1.6 A couple, soon to be parents, share a close moment in a birthing room.

In ambulatory settings of this nature, a nurse practitioner may provide immunizations, screenings, health and safety education, counseling, crisis intervention, or parenting classes. This form of community-based care has the potential to provide cost-effective health promotion, disease prevention, and patient care to large numbers of children and families in an environment familiar to them.

More and more, children and women experiencing a pregnancy complication or an acute illness, who might otherwise have been admitted to a hospital, are now being cared for in ambulatory clinics or at home. Separating a child from his or her family during a long hospitalization has been shown to be potentially harmful to the child's development, so any effort to reduce the incidence of separation has a positive effect (see Chapter 36). Avoiding long hospital stays for women during pregnancy is also a preferable method of care because it helps to maintain family integrity.

Ambulatory or non–hospital-based care requires intensive health teaching by the nursing staff and follow-up by home care or community health nurses to ensure a smooth transition to and from this setting. Teaching parents of an ill child or a woman with a complication of pregnancy what danger signs to watch for that will warrant immediate attention includes not only imparting self-care information but also providing support and reassurance that the client or parents are capable of accomplishing this level of care.

Increasing Use of Technology

The use of technology is increasing in all health care settings. The field of assisted reproduction technology such as in vitro fertilization and the possibility of stem cell research are forging new pathways (Palermo, Neri, Monahan, et al., 2012). Charting by computer into electronic health records and monitoring fetal heart rates by Doppler ultrasonography are other examples (Stewart, Letourneau, Masuda, et al., 2011). Using an electronic charting system has the ability to allow different health care providers to share information (e.g., an X-ray taken at one site can be reviewed at another, a caregiver can be alerted to all the medicines a pregnant woman has been prescribed). As long as privacy is maintained, the system allows for a coordination of care never before possible.

To protect patient privacy, the DHHS has established a privacy rule (the Health Insurance Portability and Accountability Act, commonly referred to as HIPAA) that creates national standards to protect individuals' medical records and other personal health information and applies to health care providers who conduct health care transactions electronically. The rule requires appropriate safeguards be put into place to protect the privacy of personal health information and sets limits and conditions on the uses and disclosures that may be made of such information without patient authorization. The rule also gives patients rights over their health information, including the rights to examine and obtain a copy of their health record and to request corrections (DHHS, 2007).

In addition to learning these technologies and rules, maternal and child health nurses must be able to explain their use and their advantages to clients. Otherwise, clients may find new technologies more frightening than helpful to them.

QSEN Checkpoint Question 1.3

Quality Improvement

Nurses must always be aware of quality improvement because as society changes with new situations, nursing care must make responding adjustments. Which of the following is a trend that will influence the care that the Chung family's new baby is apt to receive?

a. More and more children are treated in ambulatory, not hospital, settings so nurses will be less significant in the future.
b. Immunizations are available for all childhood infectious diseases so the Chung's baby will never need treatment for these.
c. The use of multiple technologies can make parents feel overwhelmed unless they receive nursing support.
d. Prematurely born infants, assuming their mother received prenatal care, rarely need long-term or follow-up care.

Look in Appendix A for the best answer and rationale.

Meeting Work Needs of Pregnant and Breastfeeding Women

As many as 90% of women work at least part time outside their home, and many pregnant women want to continue to work during a pregnancy (in many families, women earn more than their husband, making them the primary wage earner in the family). Following the birth of their child, however, women may want or need a leave from work to care for their newborn.

The Family Medical Leave Act of 1993 is a federal law that requires employers with 50 or more employees to provide a minimum of 12 weeks of unpaid, job-protected leave to employees under four circumstances crucial to family life:

- Birth of the employee's child
- Adoption or foster placement of a child with the employee
- Need for the employee to care for a parent, spouse, or child with a serious health condition
- Inability of the employee to perform his or her functions because of a serious health condition

A serious health condition is defined as "an illness, injury, impairment, or physical or mental condition involving such circumstances as inpatient care or incapacity requiring 3 workdays' absence" (U.S. Department of Labor, 1995). Specifically mentioned in the law is any period of incapacity due to pregnancy or for prenatal care with or without treatment. Illness must be documented by a health care provider. Nurse practitioners and nurse-midwives are specifically listed as those who can document a health condition, so they have an equal role with physicians in alerting women to this benefit. Although not as generous a program as many other developed countries, paid leave helps appreciably with the care of an ill child or a woman who is ill during pregnancy.

Whether women should be able to breastfeed at work is a controversial subject for many people (Hojnacki, Bolton, Fulmer, et al., 2012). In 2010, President Obama signed into law the Patient Protection and Affordable Care Act (PPACA), which mandates work settings with more than 50 employees to provide "reasonable break time for a woman to express breast milk for her nursing child for 1 year after the child's birth each time such employee has need to express milk." Employers are also required to provide "a place, other than a bathroom, that is shielded from view and free from intrusion for a setting to express breast milk."

This law has had a major impact on allowing women to continue breastfeeding while working full time. To support the aim of the law, many employers are now also allowing women to breastfeed at work if doing so does not disrupt their work schedule or work outcome.

Regionalizing Intensive Care

To avoid duplication of care sites, communities are establishing centralized maternal or pediatric health services. Such planning creates one site that is properly staffed and equipped for potential problems rather than a number of lesser equipped sites. When a newborn, older child, or parent is hospitalized in a regional center, the family members who have been left behind need a great deal of support. They may feel they have "lost" their infant, child, or parent unless health care personnel can keep them abreast of the ill family member's progress by means of phone calls or snapshots and by encouraging the family to visit as soon as possible.

When regionalization concepts of newborn care were first introduced, transporting the ill or premature newborn to the regional care facility was the method of choice (Fig. 1.7). Today, if it is known in advance that a child may be born with a life-threatening condition, it may be safer to transport the mother to the regional center at the time of birth because the uterus has advantages as a transport incubator that far exceed those of any commercial incubator yet designed.

Important arguments against regionalization for pediatric care include children will feel homesick in strange settings, become overwhelmed by the number of sick children they see, and grow frightened because they are miles from home.

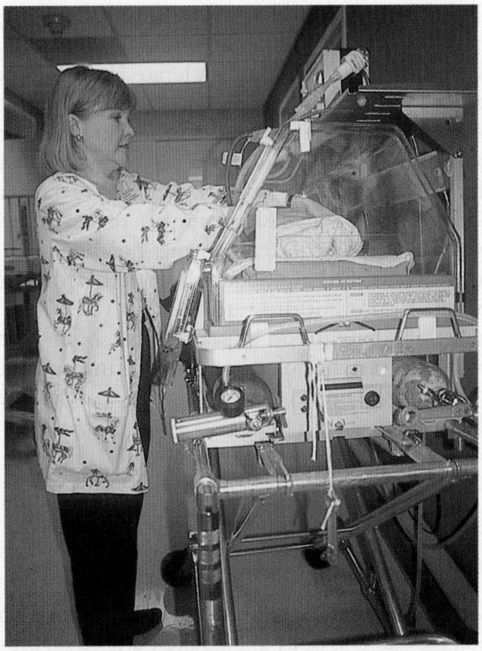

FIGURE 1.7 A nurse prepares an infant transport incubator to move a premature infant to a regional hospital. Helping with the safe movement of pregnant women and ill newborns to regional centers is an important nursing responsibility. (© Caroline Brown, RNC, MS, DEd.)

An important argument against regionalization of maternal care is that being away from her community and support network places a great deal of stress on the woman and her family and limits her primary care provider's participation in her care. These are important considerations. Because nurses more than any other health care group set the tone for hospitals, they are responsible for ensuring clients and families feel as welcome in a regional center as they would have been in a small hospital. Staffing should be adequate to allow sufficient time for nurses to comfort frightened children and prepare them for new experiences or to support a frightened pregnant woman and her family. Documenting the importance of such actions allows them to be incorporated in critical pathways and preserves the importance of the nurse's role (LeFlore, Thomas, Zielke, et al., 2011).

What if... 1.1 Melissa Chung has to remain in her local hospital after the birth of her new baby for an extended time while her baby is cared for at a regional center. If you were a nurse at the regional center, how could you help her keep in touch with her new baby?

Increasing Use of Alternative Treatment Modalities

There is a growing tendency for families to use alternative forms of therapy, such as acupuncture or therapeutic touch, in addition to or instead of traditional health care measures. Nurses have an increasing obligation to be aware of complementary or alternative therapies as they have the potential to either enhance or detract from the effectiveness of traditional therapy (D. Adams, Cheng, Jou, et al., 2011).

Health care providers who are unaware of the existence of some alternative forms of therapy may lose an important opportunity to capitalize on the positive features of that particular therapy. For instance, it would be important to know that an adolescent who is about to undergo a painful procedure is experienced at meditation because asking the adolescent if she wants to meditate before the procedure could help her relax. Not only could this increase her comfort but it could also offer her a feeling of control over a difficult situation. People are using an increasing number of herbal remedies, such as drinking herbal teas during pregnancy to relieve morning sickness. Asking about these at health assessment is important to prevent drug interactions (Dennehy, 2011). Boxes which highlight the importance of both nursing responsibility for pharmacology and respecting cultural diversity are shown in chapters throughout the text to accent these areas of care (Box 1.6).

QSEN Checkpoint Question 1.4

Evidence-Based Practice

A growing body of knowledge suggests skin-to-skin contact between mother and baby immediately after birth provides numerous benefits, including regulating heartbeat and temperature for the baby and promoting feelings of calm and well-being in both mother and baby. To see if fathers were interested in participating in this form of care (often called kangaroo care), researchers interviewed seven new fathers who had spent time in skin-to-skin interaction with their newborn. Findings showed kangaroo care allowed fathers to feel more in control and also that they were doing something good for their infant (Blomqvist, Rubertsson, Kylberg, et al., 2012).

Based on the previous study, what action would you take?

a. Assess whether Mr. Chung is willing to try skin-to-skin care.
b. Suggest neither parent use skin-to-skin care to prevent infection.
c. Encourage Mr. Chung to praise his wife when she provides skin-to-skin care.
d. Apologize to his wife because men do skin-to-skin care more effectively than women.

Look in Appendix A for the best answer and rationale.

BOX 1.6 Nursing Care Planning To Respect Cultural Diversity

The term *alternative health care practices* refers to therapy such as acupuncture, homeopathy, therapeutic touch, herbalism, and chiropractic care, or nontraditional sources of care such as tribal medicine or Hispanic herbalists such as *yerberos* or *curanderos*. Some people seek out these types of therapy or alternative providers before consulting a traditional health care provider; others consult with them after they perceive they have received inadequate care by a traditional provider. Still, others rely on these methods as their major form of health care and therapy.

Respect for these forms of care can be instrumental in showing families their sociocultural traditions are important in their plan of care. Assessing what alternative measures are being used is also important because the action of an herb can interfere with prescribed medications. For example, the consumption of traditional ethnic remedies such as *Jin Bu Huan*, a Chinese herbal medicine to relieve pain, can cause adverse effects such as life-threatening bradycardia and respiratory depression. Lead poisoning has resulted from ingestion of *greta*, a traditional Hispanic remedy used as a laxative.

Increasing Reliance on Home Care

Shortened hospital stays have resulted in transition from hospital to home of many women and children before they are optimally ready to care for themselves. In some instances, ill children and women with complications of pregnancy may choose to remain at home for care rather than be hospitalized. This has created a "second system" of care requiring many additional care providers (Turnbull & Osborn, 2012).

Nurses can be instrumental in assessing women and children at hospital discharge and help them plan the best type of continuing care, devise and modify procedures for home care, and sustain clients' morale so a transition to home is seamless. Home care as a unique and expanding area in maternal and child health nursing is discussed in Chapter 4.

What if...1.2 Melissa Chung demands her 6-year-old, diagnosed with pneumonia, be hospitalized, even though it is your clinic's policy to have such children cared for at home by their parents. Would you advocate for hospitalization?

Health Care Concerns and Attitudes

As we progress through the 21st century, there are likely to be even more changes as the United States actively works toward effective health goals and improved health care for all citizens. These steps can create new concerns.

Increasing Concern for Quality of Life

In the past, health care of women and children was focused on maintaining physical health. Today, many patients view quality of life to be as important as physical health, so the scope of health care has expanded to include the assessment of psychosocial facets of life in such areas as self-esteem and independence. Good interviewing skills are necessary to elicit this information at health care visits. Nurses can not only help obtain such information but also plan ways to improve quality of life in the areas the client considers most important.

One way in which quality of life is being improved for children with chronic illness is the national mandate to allow them to attend regular schools, guaranteeing entrance despite severe illness or use of medical equipment such as a ventilator (Public Law 99–452). Under this same law, adolescents who are pregnant cannot be excluded from school. School nurses or nurses asked to be consultants to schools play important roles in honoring these children's rights and making these changes possible.

Increasing Awareness of the Individuality and Diversity of Clients

Maternal and child clients do not fit easily into any set mold. Varying family structures, cultural backgrounds, socioeconomic levels, and individual circumstances lead to unique and diverse clients. Women having children may range in age from 12 or 13 years to women having their first pregnancy after the age of 40 (Johnson & Tough, 2012). Teenagers have high levels of complications during pregnancy related to their immature body systems; with prenatal care, a woman older than 40 years can expect to have a stress-free and healthy pregnancy.

Family structure varies; about 38% of babies are born to women outside of marriage. Gay and lesbian couples raise families alongside traditional families, conceiving children through alternative insemination or adoption. As a result of advances in research and therapy, women who were once unable to have children, such as those with cystic fibrosis, are now able to manage a full-term pregnancy. Individuals with cognitive and physical challenges who once would have been isolated from childbearing are now able to establish families and rear children.

Many families who have emigrated from other countries enter the U.S. health care system for the first time during a pregnancy or with a sick child. This requires sensitivity to sociocultural aspects of care on the part of health care providers, as people not used to nongovernment-sponsored health care can easily be lost in the U.S. system. They may have different cultural beliefs about health and illness than their health care provider. Some families may live in unsafe neighborhoods and so may not feel safe with home care. All of these concerns require increased nursing attention.

What if...1.3 Melissa Chung is concerned because she's already 42 and wants to have a third child in a few years. Are many women delaying childbirth until their 40s? Do you anticipate this trend will continue into the future?

Empowerment of Health Care Consumers

In part because of the influence of market-driven care and a strengthened focus on health promotion and disease prevention, individuals and families have recently begun to take increased responsibility for their own health. For most families, this means learning preventive measures such as following a more nutritious diet and planning regular exercise; for some families, this means adopting an entirely new lifestyle. When a family member is ill, learning more about the illness, participating in the treatment plan, and preventing the illness from returning can offer a sense of empowerment. Parents want to stay with their ill child in the hospital and are eager for information about their child's health and ways they can contribute to the decision-making process. They may question a treatment or care plan if they believe it is not in their child's best interest. If health care providers do not provide answers to a client's questions or are insensitive to needs, many health care consumers are willing to take their business to another health care setting or rely totally on therapies or information they find from Internet sites (Gallagher, Bell, Waddell, et al., 2012).

Nurses can promote empowerment of parents and children by respecting their views and concerns, regarding parents as important participants in their own or in their child's health, keeping them informed, and helping and supporting them to make decisions about care. Although a nurse may have seen 25 clients already in a particular day, he or she can make each client feel as important as the first by showing a warm manner and keen interest. Boxes on ways to help empower families at home or at health care facilities are shown in following chapters.

QSEN Checkpoint Question 1.5

Safety

Mrs. Chung waited until she was 42 to have her second baby. She asks you if that is the reason her baby was born prematurely. Which of the following would be the best reassuring statement for her?

a. "It's hard to say because so few women over 40 are having babies today."
b. "No one can say for certain. You did all you could to ensure a healthy pregnancy."
c. "It's good to see you taking responsibility for your child's prematurity."
d. "You should ideally have had your children as a teenager as that's the safest time."

Look in Appendix A for the best answer and rationale.

LEGAL CONSIDERATIONS OF MATERNAL–CHILD PRACTICE

Legal concerns arise in all areas of health care. Maternal and child health nursing carries some legal concerns above and beyond other areas of nursing because care is often given to an "unseen client"—the fetus—or to clients who are not of legal age for giving consent. New technologies (e.g., assisted reproduction, surrogate motherhood, umbilical cord sampling, safety of new medicines with children, and end-of-life decisions) can lead to potential legal action, especially if clients are uninformed about the reason or medical necessity for these procedures.

Nurses are legally responsible for protecting the rights of their clients, including confidentiality, and are accountable for the quality of their individual nursing care and that of other health care team members. New regulations on patient confidentiality guarantee patients can see their medical record if they choose, but health information must be kept confidential from others (Duffy, 2011).

Understanding the **scope of practice** (the range of services and care that may be provided by a nurse based on state requirements) and standards of care can help nurses practice within appropriate legal parameters.

Documentation is essential for justifying actions. This concern is long lasting, because children who feel they were wronged by health care personnel can bring a lawsuit at the time they reach legal age. This means a nursing note written today may need to be defended as many as 21 years into the future. The specific legal ramifications of procedures or care are discussed in later chapters as procedures or treatment modalities are described. Personal liability insurance is strongly recommended for all nurses, so they do not incur great financial losses during a malpractice or professional negligence lawsuit.

Nurses need to be conscientious about obtaining informed consent for invasive procedures in children and determining if pregnant women are aware of any risk to the fetus associated with a procedure or test. A parent can be contacted by phone or e-mail if not present with the child at the time the consent is needed.

In divorced or blended families (those in which two adults with children from previous relationships now live together), it is important to establish who has the right to give consent for health care. Adolescents who support themselves or who are pregnant are frequently termed "emancipated minors" or "mature minors" and have the right to sign for their own health care.

The term "wrongful birth" is the birth of a disabled child whose pregnancy the parents would have chosen to end if they had been informed about the disability during pregnancy. "Wrongful life" is a claim that negligent prenatal testing on the part of a health care provider resulted in the birth of a disabled child. "Wrongful conception" denotes that a contraceptive measure failed, allowing an unwanted child to be conceived and born. As many genetic disorders can be identified prenatally, the scope of both "wrongful birth" and "wrongful life" grows yearly (Whitney & Rosenbaum, 2011).

If a nurse knows the care provided by another practitioner was inappropriate or insufficient, he or she is legally responsible for reporting the incident. Failure to do so can lead to a charge of negligence or breach of duty.

✓ QSEN Checkpoint Question 1.6

Patient-Centered Care

Melissa Chung is concerned as to how she will give consent for procedures for her newborn baby because the baby is hospitalized so far away. Which statement would be best to reassure her?

a. "Informed consent is not needed for newborn care as newborns are underage."
b. "Newborn care requires parental consent only for procedures that will involve pain."
c. "Health care providers can omit informed consent if the parent is not present with the child."
d. "Consent is required: you can be contacted by telephone or e-mail for long distance consultation."

Look in Appendix A for the best answer and rationale.

ETHICAL CONSIDERATIONS OF PRACTICE

Some of the most difficult ethical quandaries in health care today are those that involve children and their families. Examples include:

- Conception issues, especially those related to in vitro fertilization, embryo transfer, ownership of frozen oocytes or sperm, and surrogate motherhood
- Abortion, particularly partial-birth abortion
- Fetal rights versus rights of the mother
- Stem cell research
- Resuscitation (for how long should it be continued?)
- Number of procedures or degree of pain a child should be asked to endure to achieve a degree of better health
- Balance between modern technology and quality of life
- Difficulty maintaining confidentiality of records when there are multiple caregivers

Legal and ethical aspects of issues are often intertwined, which makes the decision-making process in this area complex. Because maternal and child health nursing is so strongly family centered, it is common to encounter some situations in which the interests of one family member are in conflict with those of another or the goals of a health care provider are different from the family's. Maintaining privacy yet aiding problem solving in these instances can be difficult but is a central nursing role (Clemens, 2012). Nurses can help clients by providing factual information and supportive listening, and helping the family and health care providers clarify their values.

The Pregnant Woman's Bill of Rights and the United Nations Declaration of Rights of the Child (available at http://thePoint.lww.com/Pillitteri7e) provide guidelines for determining the rights of women and children with regard to maternal and child health care.

What if . . . 1.4 You are particularly interested in exploring one of the 2020 National Health Goals with respect to maternal and child health (see p. 6). What would be a possible research topic to explore, pertinent to these goals, that would be applicable to the Chung family and could also advance evidence-based practice?

Key Points for Review

- Standards of maternal and child health nursing practice have been formulated by the American Nurses Association to serve as guidelines for practice.
- QSEN competencies, combined with the nursing process, provide a sound method of care for expanding areas of practice.
- Nursing research and use of evidence-based practice are methods by which maternal and child health nursing expands and improves.
- The most meaningful and important measure of maternal and child health is the infant mortality rate, which is the number of deaths among infants from birth to 1 year of age per 1,000 live births. This rate is declining steadily, but in the United States it is still higher than in 29 other nations.
- Trends in maternal and child health nursing include changes in the settings of care, increased concern about health care costs, improved preventive care, and family-centered care.
- Practice roles in maternal and child health nursing are expanding rapidly as nurses become more versed in evidence-based practice and technologic skills.
- Maternal and child health care have both legal and ethical considerations and responsibilities over and above those in other areas of practice because of the role of the fetus and child.

Critical Thinking Care Study

Tommy is a 10-year-old who has asthma. He is home schooled after having two serious asthma attacks at school because he is allergic to the cleaning product used in his primary school classroom. His mother is pregnant with a new brother or sister but hasn't come for prenatal care because she noticed the clinic uses the same cleaning solution and doesn't want her new baby to develop an allergy to it. At the same time, she wants a sonogram so she can see if she's having a girl or boy.

1. Nurses work in a wide range of settings in maternal and child health. What actions could you take to help Tommy get back to school and his mother begin to come for prenatal care?
2. Cost containment along with limitations of health insurance make it important for nurses to be aware of the cost of supplies and procedures. Is having a sonogram just to know the sex of a fetus a good use of health care funds?
3. Homelessness is becoming an increasing concern in modern society. Suppose Tommy's family became homeless? How do you anticipate this will affect their overall health?

Patient Scenario

The Head Family

Read about the Head family, a family with health concerns, then answer the questions to further sharpen your skills and grow more familiar with NCLEX-type questions related to trends in maternal and child health care. Confirm your answers are correct by reading the rationales.

Visit http://thePoint.lww.com

Answers and Rationales

Looking for answers to the What If. . . and Critical Thinking Care Study questions?

Visit http://thePoint.lww.com

References

Adams, D., Cheng, F., Jou, H., et al. (2011). The safety of pediatric acupuncture: A systematic review. *Pediatrics, 128*(6), e1575–e1587

Adams, H. A. (2011). A perioperative education program for pediatric patients and their parents. *AORN: Association of Operating Room Nurses Journal, 93*(4), 472–481.

Alio, A. P., Mbah, A. K., Grunsten, R. S., et al. (2011). Teenage pregnancy and the influence of paternal involvement on fetal outcomes. *Journal of Pediatric & Adolescent Gynecology, 24*(6), 404–409.

American Academy of Pediatrics Task Force on Sudden Infant Death Syndrome. (2011). SIDS and other sleep-related infant deaths. *Pediatrics, 128*(5), 1030–1039.

American Nurses Credentialing Center. (2012). *Magnet Recognition Program® model.* Silver Springs, MD: Author.

Benner, P. (2011). Formation in professional education: An examination of the relationship between theories of meaning and theories of the self. *Journal of Medicine & Philosophy, 36*(4), 342–353.

Blomqvist, Y. T., Rubertsson, C., Kylberg, E., et al. (2012). Kangaroo mother care helps fathers of preterm infants gain confidence in the paternal role. *Journal of Advanced Nursing, 68*(9), 1988–1996.

Bridge, J. A., McBee-Strayer, S. M., Cannon, E. A., et al. (2012). Impaired decision making in adolescent suicide attempters. *Journal of the American Academy of Child & Adolescent Psychiatry, 51*(4), 394–403.

Brownridge, D. A., Taillieu, T. L., Tyler, K. A., et al. (2011). Pregnancy and intimate partner violence: risk factors, severity, and health effects. *Violence Against Women, 17*(7), 858–881.

Burkhard, A. (2013). A different life: Caring for an adolescent or young adult with severe cerebral palsy. *Journal of Pediatric Nursing,* Feb 9 [Epub ahead of print].

Carpenito, L. J. (2012). *Nursing diagnosis: Application to clinical practice* (14th ed.). Philadelphia, PA: Lippincott Williams & Wilkins.

Centers for Disease Control and Prevention. (2011). National and state vaccination coverage among children aged 19–35 months. *Morbidity and Mortality Weekly Report, 60*(34), 1157–1163.

Centers for Disease Control and Prevention. (2012a). *Overweight and obesity*. Atlanta, GA: Author.

Centers for Disease Control and Prevention. (2012b). *Autism spectrum disorders*. Atlanta, GA: Author.

Christian, B. J. (2012). Translating research into everyday practice—The essential role of pediatric nurses. *Journal of Pediatric Nursing, 27*(2), 184–185.

Clark, S. (2012). Strategies for reducing maternal mortality. *Seminars in Perinatology, 36*(1), 42–47.

Clemens, N. A. (2012). Privacy, consent, and the electronic mental health record: The Person vs. the System. *Journal of Psychiatric Practice, 18*(1), 46–50.

Cronenwett, L., Sherwood, G., & Gelmon, S. B. (2009). Improving quality and safety education: The QSEN Learning Collaborative. *Nursing Outlook, 57*(6), 304–312.

Dennehy, C. (2011). Omega–3 fatty acids and ginger in maternal health: Pharmacology, efficacy, and safety. *Journal of Midwifery & Women's Health, 56*(6), 584–590.

Disch, J. (2012). QSEN? What's QSEN? *Nursing Outlook, 60*(2), 58–59.

Dong, Y., Chen, S. J., & Yu, J. L. (2012). A systematic review and meta-analysis of long-term development of early term infants. *Neonatology, 102*(3), 212–221.

Duffy, M. (2011). iNurse: Patient privacy and company policy in online life. *American Journal of Nursing, 111*(9), 65–69.

Dworzynski, K., Ronald, A., Bolton, P., et al. (2012). How different are girls and boys above and below the diagnostic threshold for autism spectrum disorders? *Journal of the American Academy of Child & Adolescent Psychiatry, 51*(8), 788–797.

Falk, J., Wongsa, S., Dang, J., et al. (2012).Using an evidence-based practice process to change child visitation guidelines. *Clinical Journal of Oncology Nursing, 16*(1), 21–23.

Gallagher, F., Bell, L., Waddell, G., et al. (2012). Requesting cesareans without medical indications: An option being considered by young Canadian women. *Birth, 39*(1), 39–47.

Hamilton, B. E., Martin, J. A., & Ventura, S. J. (2011). Births: Preliminary data for 2010. *National Vital Statistics Report, 60*(2), 1–60.

Hedges, C. C., Nichols, A., & Filoteo, L. (2012). Relationship-based nursing practice: Transitioning to a new care delivery model in maternity units. *Journal of Perinatal & Neonatal Nursing, 26*(1), 27–36.

Hess, R., Desroches, C., Donelan, K., et al. (2011). Perceptions of nurses in Magnet® hospitals, non-magnet hospitals, and hospitals pursuing magnet status. *Journal of Nursing Administration, 41*(7–8), 315–323.

Hesseling, A. C., Kim, S., Madhi, S., et al. (2012). High prevalence of drug resistance amongst HIV-exposed and -infected children in a tuberculosis prevention trial. *International Journal of Tuberculosis & Lung Disease, 16*(2), 192–195.

Hojnacki, S. E., Bolton, T., Fulmer, I. S., et al. (2012). Development and piloting of an instrument that measures company support for breastfeeding. *Journal of Human Lactation, 28*(1), 20–27.

Johnson, J. A., & Tough, S. (2012). Delayed child-bearing. *Journal of Obstetrics & Gynaecology Canada, 34*(1), 80–93.

Junnila, R., Aromaa, M., Heinonen, O. J., et al. (2012). The weighty matter intervention: A family-centered way to tackle an overweight childhood. *Journal of Community Health Nursing, 29*(1), 39–52.

Kochanek, K. D., Xu, J., Murphy, S. L., et al. (2011). Deaths: Final data for 2009. *National Vital Statistics Report, 60*(3), 64.

LeFlore, J., Thomas, P. E., Zielke, M. A., et al. (2011). Educating neonatal nurse practitioners in the 21st century. *Journal of Perinatal & Neonatal Nursing, 25*(2), 200–205.

Machado, L. S. (2012). Cesarean section in morbidly obese parturients: Practical implications and complications. *North American Journal of Medical Sciences, 4*(1), 13–18.

Mathews, T. J., & MacDorman, M. F. (2011). Infant mortality statistics from the 2007 period linked birth/infant death data set. *National Vital Statistics Report, 59*(6), 1–30.

Moran, G. J., Krishnadasan, A., Gorwitz, R. J., et al. (2012). Prevalence of methicillin-resistant *Staphylococcus aureus* as an etiology of community-acquired pneumonia. *Clinical Infectious Diseases, 54*(8), 1126–1133.

Murphy, S. L., Xu, J., & Kochanek, K. D. (2012). Deaths: Preliminary data for 2010. *National Vital Statistics Reports, 60*[4], 1–69.

Nachman, S., Chernoff, M., Williams, P., et al. (2012). Human immunodeficiency virus disease severity, psychiatric symptoms, and functional outcomes in perinatally infected youth. *Archives of Pediatric & Adolescent Medicine, 166*(6), 528–535.

Nan, X. (2012). Communicating to young adults about HPV vaccination. *Health Communication, 27*(1), 10–18.

National Center for Health Statistics. (2012). *Births, marriages, divorces, and deaths*. Hyattsville, MD: Author.

Orem, D. E., & Taylor, S. G. (2011). Reflections on nursing practice science: The nature, the structure, and the foundation of nursing sciences. *Nursing Science Quarterly, 24*(1), 35–41.

Osborne, K., & Hanson, L. (2012). Directive versus supportive approaches used by midwives when providing care during the second stage of labor. *Journal of Midwifery & Women's Health, 57*(1), 3–11.

Owen, S. M. (2012). Testing for acute HIV infection: Implications for treatment as prevention. *Current Opinion in HIV AIDS, 7*(2), 125–130.

Palermo, G. D., Neri, Q. V., Monahan, D., et al. (2012). Development and current applications of assisted fertilization. *Fertility & Sterility, 97*(2), 248–259.

Papp, L. M. (2012). Longitudinal associations between parental and children's depressive symptoms in the context of interparental relationship functioning. *Journal of Child & Family Studies, 21*(2), 199–207.

Paulson, J. F., & Bazemore, S. C. (2010). Prenatal and postpartum depression in fathers and its association with maternal depression. *Journal of the American Medical Association, 303*(19), 1961–1969.

Rohrer, J. E., Garrison, G. M., & Angstman, K. B. (2012). Early return visits by pediatric primary care patients with otitis media: A retail nurse practitioner clinic versus standard medical office care. *Quality Management in Health Care, 21*(1), 44–47.

Roy, C. (2011). Research based on the Roy adaptation model: Last 25 years. *Nursing Science Quarterly, 24*(4), 312–320.

Rubin, R. (1963). Maternal touch. *Nursing Outlook, 11*(2), 828–829.

Salsman, J. M., Grunberg, S. M., Beaumont, J. L., et al. (2012). Communicating about chemotherapy-induced nausea and vomiting: A comparison of patient and provider perspectives. *Journal of National Comprehensive Cancer Network, 10*(2), 149–157.

Saunier, B. (2011). The devil is in the details: Managed care and the unforeseen costs of utilization review as a cost containment mechanism. *Issues in Law & Medicine, 27*(1), 21–48.

Stewart, M., Letourneau, N., Masuda, J. R., et al. (2011). Online solutions to support needs and preferences of parents of children with asthma and allergies. *Journal of Family Nursing, 17*(8), 357–379.

Turnbull, C., & Osborn, D. A. (2012). Home visits during pregnancy and after birth for women with an alcohol or drug problem. *Cochrane Database of Systematic Reviews,* (1), CD004456.

United Nations. (2000). *Millennium health goals, 2000–2015*. New York, NY: Author.

United Nations Children's Fund. (2010). *Official summary: The state of the world's children 2010*. New York, NY: Author.

U.S. 99th Congress. (1986). Public Law 99-452. Congressional Record, 132 (1986): 1.

U.S. Department of Health and Human Services. (2010). *Healthy people 2020*. Washington, DC: Author.

U.S. Department of Health and Human Services, Office of Civil Rights. (2007). *Medical privacy—National standards to protect the privacy of personal health information: The Health Insurance portability and Accountability Act*. Hyattsville, MD: U.S. Department of Health and Human Services.

U.S. Department of Labor. (1995). The Family and Medical Leave Act of 1993: Final rule. *Federal Register, 60*(4), 2179–2279.

Whitney, D. W., & Rosenbaum, K. N. (2011). Recovery of damages for wrongful birth. *Journal of Legal Medicine, 32*(2), 167–204.

Zakaria, F. (2012). Health Insurance is for everyone. *Time, 179*(12), 22–23.

Chapter 2

The Childbearing and Childrearing Family

KEY TERMS

- blended family
- boomerang generation
- ecomap
- family
- family-centered nursing
- family of orientation
- family of procreation
- gay
- genogram
- lesbian
- polyandry
- polygamy
- polygyny
- sandwich family

OBJECTIVES

After mastering the contents of this chapter, you should be able to:

1. Identify common family structures, functions, and roles of families and use critical thinking to analyze ways these are changing in modern society.
2. Identify 2020 National Health Goals related to the family and specific ways nurses can help the nation achieve these goals.
3. Assess a family for structure and healthy function.
4. Formulate nursing diagnoses related to family health.
5. Develop expected outcomes to help a family achieve optimal health as well as manage seamless transitions across differing health care settings.
6. Using the nursing process, plan nursing care that includes the six competencies of Quality & Safety Education for Nurses (QSEN): Patient-Centered Care, Teamwork & Collaboration, Evidence-Based Practice (EBP), Quality Improvement (QI), Safety, and Informatics.
7. Implement nursing care to teach a family more effective wellness behaviors or to help a family modify its lifestyle to adjust to a pregnancy or accommodate an ill child.
8. Evaluate outcome criteria for achievement and effectiveness of care to be certain expected outcomes have been achieved.
9. Integrate knowledge of families with the interplay of nursing process, the six competencies of QSEN, and Family Nursing to promote quality maternal and child health nursing care.

Marlo Hanovan is a 32-year-old woman with a 12-year-old child, Charles, from a first marriage. She is presently married to Stone, 35, who has two children from a first marriage: James, 17, and Brian, 2. James and Brian are both well but Charles has been sick since birth with cystic fibrosis, a genetic disease that compromises his gastrointestinal and respiratory function. Mrs. Hanovan, a full-time bookkeeper, also attends a community college to study photography. She is 4 months pregnant with a new baby. Because Stone is unemployed, she tells you on many days her income is stretched so far, she's forced to choose between routine health care for her family and groceries.

The previous chapter discussed the philosophy of maternal and child health nursing. This chapter adds information about the structure of families and how nurses can help ensure healthy family outcomes.

Are the Hanovans a well or a dysfunctional family? How typical is their structure? What are some concerns they may need help in resolving?

Humans have always tended to live in groups or families, but the types of families formed and family goals established have changed as technology has changed and life has become more complicated (Lavoie-Tremblay, Bonin, Bonneville-Roussy, et al., 2012). For example, when families lived on farms, they were extended or had a wealth of relatives or friends close by to provide both physical and psychological support. As more people moved into cities, families became typically nuclear with only two parents and children present. Less support in terms of family members was available.

Today, 24% of children younger than 18 years of age live in a single-mother family; an additional 4.8% live in a single-father family (Mather, 2010). This has important implications when planning nursing care, as parents in these types of families may not have even one other adult to offer them support. This causes families to look more and more to health care providers, especially nurses, for guidance when a problem with pregnancy or childrearing occurs.

Families are important to children's growth, as no other social group has the potential to provide the depth of support and long-lasting emotional ties as a person's own family. What people learn in their family determines how they relate to people, what moral values they follow, and the molding of their basic perspectives on both the present and the future (Parker, Mandleco, Olsen Roper, et al., 2011).

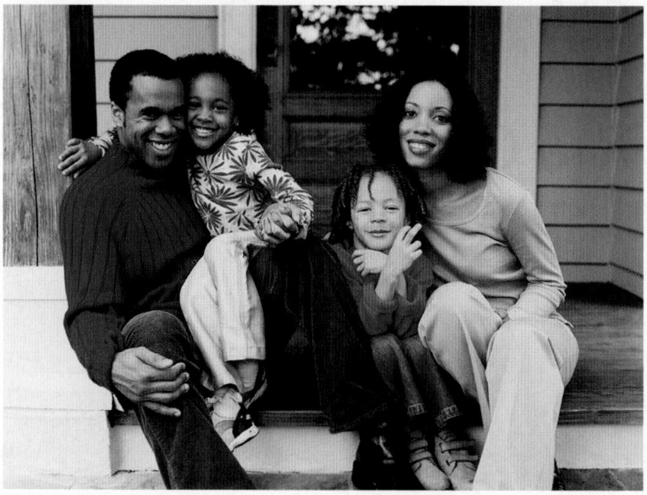

FIGURE 2.1 Families are a universal among almost all civilizations.

BOX 2.1 Nursing Care Planning Based on 2020 National Health Goals

The 2020 National Health Goals are goals set in place by the U.S. Department of Health & Human Services (DHHS) to improve the health of the nation for the next millennium and are kept current by updates every 10 years. A number of 2020 National Health Goals focus on ways to improve the quality of families or community life. Representative of these include:

- Increase the percentage of adult smokers aged 18 years and older attempting to stop smoking from 48.3% to 80%.
- Increase the proportion of young children who are screened for an autism spectrum disorder (ASD) and other developmental delays by 24 months of age from a present level of 19.5% to 21.5%.
- Reduce postpartum relapse of smoking among women who quit smoking during pregnancy.
- Increase the proportion of children with special health care needs who receive their care in family-centered, comprehensive, and coordinated environments from a present level of 20.4% to 22.4%.
- Increase the rate of infants who are breastfed until 6 months from 43.5% to 60.6%.
- Reduce physical violence directed at women by male partners to no more than 27 per 1,000 couples from a current baseline of 30 per 1,000 couples (DHHS, 2010 [see www.healthypeople.gov]).

Nurses can help the nation meet these goals for healthier family living by assessing families and their environment to identify families at risk, assisting with counseling, and maintaining contact with families to ensure that as a family grows, its changing needs can be recognized and met. Intimate partner violence and child maltreatment are further discussed in Chapter 55.

Maintaining healthy family life is so important to the health and welfare of the nation, several 2020 National Health Goals speak directly to maintaining healthy family and community life (Box 2.1). Because families have such influence on individuals and individuals on families, nursing care that considers not only a single patient but his/her family (**family-centered nursing**) has a strong focus in modern nursing practice.

For a family to adjust to a dramatic change, such as a new family member or an ill child, a family must have structure and roles flexible enough to be able to adjust to the changes pregnancy or a long-term medicine or nutrition regimen for a child bring. The roles individuals assume in the family and their ability to adjust to new roles as their family's structure or situation changes play a major factor in whether a family can adjust to and work through difficult times to achieve a positive family outcome.

Because families do not live in isolation, the family's ability to thrive in and gain strength from a community is equally important. Always consider the strengths, vulnerabilities, and patterns of both a patient's family and the surrounding community to encourage healthy coping mechanisms and to improve overall family health (Fig. 2.1).

Nursing Process Overview

For Promotion of Family Health

Assessment

Assessment of the structure and function, as well as the strengths and challenges, of families provides information on the ability of a family to remain well during either calm or stressful times. It can reveal the meaning of a current health situation for a family as well as the emotional support an individual family member can expect from other family members or the community. This can be vital to understanding what a pregnancy or childhood illness will mean to different family members, especially if not all members appear to be in agreement.

Nursing Diagnosis

Nursing diagnoses formulated for families generally relate to the family's ability to handle stress and to provide a positive environment for the growth and development of the members. Examples include:

- Impaired parenting related to unplanned pregnancy
- Parental role conflict related to prolonged separation from the child during a long hospital stay
- Interrupted family processes related to emergency hospital admission of the oldest child
- Ineffective family coping mechanisms related to an inability to adjust to the mother's illness during pregnancy
- Readiness for enhanced family coping mechanisms related to improved perceptions of the child's capabilities
- Health-seeking behaviors related to the birth of a first child

Outcome Identification and Planning

Planning for nursing care is most effective if it includes a design that is both family and community centered and also both appropriate and desired by the majority of family members; otherwise, opposing family members can resist following the plan.

It would not be helpful, for example, to suggest a mother quit work to better supervise a child's medication regimen if she is the sole wage earner for her family. Helping all family members assume a portion of the responsibility for safe medicine administration might be a more workable solution. To help parents keep up to date on health insurance issues, family leave, and family rights, an interesting Web site to recommend is The National Partnership for Women & Families (www.nationalpartnership.org). In addition, the National Safety Council (www.nsc.org) discusses what families can do to help make their home and community safer. The Nurse-Family Partnership (www.nursefamilypartnerhip.org) offers useful information on helping first-time parents effectively succeed.

Implementation

Implementations to improve family health should flow smoothly if family members have agreed on a plan of action in support of one another. It may be necessary in some instances, however, to encourage family members to agree to a plan or to abide by a chosen plan. Otherwise, they can expend needless energy carrying out activities counterproductive or in direct opposition to their major goal.

Outcome Evaluation

An evaluation should reveal not only that a goal has been achieved but also that the family feels more cohesive after working together toward the goal. If the evaluation does not reveal these two factors, reassess the goal as necessary to determine whether further interventions are required or whether the goal was inadequate. Examples of expected outcomes that might be established include:

- Family members state they are adapting well to a newborn joining the family.
- The mother states she feels prepared to manage home care for her ill child.
- Parents state they have arranged the family finances to accommodate new health care expenses for the family.
- The grandmother states she will omit trans-fatty acids from cooking to better safeguard the health of her family.

FAMILY STRUCTURES

How well a family works together when times are good and how well it can organize itself against potential threats depends on both its structure (who its members are) and its function (the activities or roles family members carry out). Recognizing different family structures can help you better focus on family-centered care as well as provide a family-friendly environment for health care.

The Concept of Family

A **family** is defined by the U.S. Census Bureau (USCB, 2010) as "a group of people related by blood, marriage, or adoption living together." This definition is workable for gathering comparative statistics but has limitations when assessing a family for its health concerns or support people available, because some families are made up of unrelated couples, and at points in life not all family members live together.

Allender (2013) defines the family in a much broader context as "two or more people who live in the same household (usually), share a common emotional bond, and perform certain interrelated social tasks." This is a better working definition for health care providers because it addresses the broad range of types of families apt to be encountered in health care settings.

Family Types

What type of family a person belongs to changes over time as a family is affected by birth, death, possibly divorce, and the growth of family members. For the purposes of assessing families, two basic family types can be described:

- **Family of orientation** (the family one is born into; or oneself, mother, father, and siblings, if any)
- **Family of procreation** (a family one establishes; or oneself, spouse or significant other, and children, if any)

Almost all families, regardless of their type, share common activities and those activities influence the health and activities of their members (Chapman, Watkins, Zappia, et al., 2012). Specific descriptions of types vary greatly depending on how many members are present, people's roles, generational issues, means of family support, and sociocultural influences (Box 2.2).

The Dyad Family

A dyad family is two people living together without children. This category usually refers to single young adults who live together in shared apartments or dormitories for companionship and financial security while completing school or beginning a career. Dyad families are generally viewed as temporary arrangements, but this could extend into a lifetime arrangement.

- **Positive aspects:** Companionship, possibly shared resources
- **Potential negative aspects:** Often a short-term arrangement so can result in a sense of loss when the relationship ends

The Cohabitation Family

Cohabitation families are composed of couples, perhaps with children, who live together but remain unmarried. Although such a relationship may be temporary, it may also be as long-lasting and as meaningful as a more traditional alliance. Many couples choose cohabitation as a way

BOX 2.2 Nursing Care Planning to Respect Cultural Diversity

Although families are more mobile today than in the past, cultural values and characteristics tend to remain constant. Knowing some of the basic norms and taboos of different cultural groups allows you to understand the differences behind varying practices, a family's value system, and the degree of support family members are able to provide.

Some cultures, for example, respect elderly family members, depend on them for advice, and ensure they receive health care; other families are more oriented to the present and so treat older family members with less respect. Some cultures have extended families; others have a high number of single-parent families. Whether families are headed by men or women is also culturally determined.

Poverty tends to be a problem for nondominant (minority) ethnic groups. Some characteristic responses sometimes described as cultural limitations are actually the consequences of poverty—for example, a mother seeking medical care for her child late in the course of an illness or late in pregnancy is just as apt to be a financial influence as a cultural one. Solving this type of problem may be a question of locating financial resources rather than modifying care to respect cultural patterns.

of getting to know a potential life partner before marriage because of the hope this will make their eventual marriage stronger. Statistically, however, couples who cohabit before marriage have a higher divorce rate than those who do not (Cherlin, 2012).

This probably happens because cohabitation couples enter the union thinking, "If this living arrangement doesn't work, I can leave with no trouble." Feeling a union can be easily broken this way may influence the couple not to work at the relationship. That is a contrast to married couples who theoretically enter a union with an "until death do I part" philosophy, prompting them to work (sometimes very hard) to make a marriage last.

Long-term cohabitation unions of this type are growing in number because of the pressure to adhere to a monogamous relationship to avoid contracting sexually transmitted infections, the advantage of shared incomes, and widespread acceptance of cohabitation by society (Henrich, Boyd, & Richerson, 2012).

- **Positive aspects:** Companionship, possibly financial security; encourages a monogamous relationship
- **Potential negative aspects:** As with dyad families, may result in a feeling of loss if only short term and the breakup isn't desired by both partners

The Nuclear Family

The traditional nuclear family is composed of a husband, wife, and children. In the past, it was the most common family structure seen worldwide. Today, however, in the United States, the number of nuclear families has declined to about 49% of families due to the increase in divorce, acceptance of single parenthood, remarriage, and a greater acceptance of same sex partnerships or marriage (National Center for Health Statistics [NCHS], 2012). The biggest advantage of a nuclear family is its ability to provide support to family members because, with its small size, people know each other well and can feel genuine affection and support for and from each other. Unfortunately, in a time of crisis, this same characteristic may become a challenge to a family because there are few family members to share the burden or look at a problem objectively. Helping nuclear families locate and reach out to support people in their extended family or community during a crisis can be an important nursing responsibility.

- **Positive aspects:** Support for family members; sense of security
- **Possible negative aspects:** May lack support people in a crisis situation

The Polygamous Family

Although **polygamy** (a marriage with multiple wives or husbands) has been illegal in the United States since 1978, such families are not an unusual arrangement worldwide, so new immigrants may report they have been raised in this type of family (or may still be living in this arrangement). This category can be further divided into **polygyny** (a family with one man and several wives) and **polyandry** (one wife with more than one husband) (Jacobson & Burton, 2011).

- **Positive aspects:** Companionship; shared resources
- **Possible negative aspects:** Not sanctioned by law; disapproval by community; decreased value of women

The Extended (Multigenerational) Family

An extended family includes not only a nuclear family but also other family members such as grandmothers, grandfathers, aunts, uncles, cousins, and grandchildren. An advantage of such a family is it contains more people to serve as resources during crises and provides more role models for behavior or values (Keene, Prokos, & Held, 2012). In a typical extended family, however, there is usually only one main income provider, a situation which can strain the family's resources, and to include all family members in shared decisions may be difficult. When assessing such families, remember that, because many members are present, a parent's strongest support person may not be their spouse, and a child's primary caregiver may not be his or her biologic parent. The grandmother, an aunt, or another sibling, for example, may provide the largest amount of support or child care, so may be the person best prepared to talk about a child's health. Helping the family maintain meaningful communication between all members is an important nursing responsibility (Box 2.3).

- **Positive aspects:** Many people for child care and member support
- **Possible negative aspects**: Resources may be stretched thin because of few wage earners

The Single-Parent Family

Single-parent families play a large role in childrearing. Unfortunately, low income is often a problem encountered

BOX 2.3 Nursing Care Planning to Empower a Family

TIPS TO IMPROVE FAMILY COMMUNICATION

Q. Suppose Mrs. Hanovan says to you, "My family doesn't communicate well. How can I improve this?"

A. Traditionally, families gathered for an evening meal, and this practice allowed a set period of time each day for interaction, problem solving, and conflict resolution while problems were still small. If sit-down-together meals aren't possible because of busy work or school schedules, suggestions for better communication could include:

- Plan a time (even 15 minutes) daily when all family members "touch base" with each other.
- Have all members check in daily by e-mail or a text message.
- Use a telephone answering machine to leave daily messages.
- Set up a bulletin or chalk board that family members can check each day for messages.
- Plan an earlier wake-up time two or three mornings per week so all family members can sit and have breakfast together.
- Reserve one night a week as "family night," when the family plans a special activity to do together such as play a board game or watch a favorite movie.
- Agree family night is off limits for cell phones, television, computers, iPods, etc., so family members are not distracted by outside sources.
- Limit the amount of time children work on their computers in their own bedrooms or spend in sedentary activities such as television watching; encourage more time in creative activities, discussing the day's events, or participating in an activity where all family members are brought together.
- Plan special activities for holidays or weekends that involve the whole family such as a hike or picnic or visiting a museum or park.
- Participate in each other's activities (e.g., if one member is playing in a ball game, all family members come and watch).

by single-parent families, especially if a woman is the head of the household. Women's incomes for the same jobs are lower than men's by about 33% (Cherlin, 2012). Single parents have difficulty working full time plus taking total care of young children. Trying to fulfill several central roles (mother and father) is not only time consuming but also mentally and physically exhausting and, in many instances, not rewarded.

Such a parent may develop low self-esteem if things are not going well, especially if a spouse left them for another or if the other parent refuses to help with child support or shared custody. Single-parent fathers may have difficulty with home management or child care if they had little experience with those roles before the separation. It's important to identify low self-esteem, as it has the potential to interfere with decision making and impede daily functioning.

Single-parent families have a special strength, however, as such a family can offer a child a rich parent–child relationship as well as increased opportunities for self-reliance and independence.

If there has been a divorce, one parent may have been given legal custody of the children or both parents may share custody (Carlsund, Eriksson, Löfstedt, et al., 2013). Either way, both parents often participate in decision making. At a time of illness, both may stay with an ill child in the hospital and be eager to receive reports of the child's progress. Identifying who is the custodial parent is especially important when consent forms for care need to be signed, so be certain this is clearly marked in the child's health care records.

- **Positive aspects:** Ability to offer a unique and strong parent–child bond
- **Possible negative aspects:** Resources may be limited

QSEN Checkpoint Question 2.1

Patient-Centered Care

It's important that care extends to include the concerns of a patient's family. Mrs. Hanovan and Charles were a single-parent family before Mrs. Hanovan remarried. What is the most common challenge among single-parent families that nurses must address when planning care?

a. Education is frequently compromised.
b. Finances can be extremely limited.
c. Communication is often limited.
d. Emotional engagement is often lacking.

Look in Appendix A for the best answer and rationale.

The Blended Family

In a blended family (a remarriage or reconstituted family), a divorced or widowed person with children marries someone who also has children. Although the arrangement is apt to be a positive one because it creates a nuclear family, childrearing problems can arise in this type of family from rivalry among the children for the attention of a parent. In addition, each spouse may encounter difficulties in helping rear the other's children if their philosophy of childrearing differs from the biologic parent's, particularly in terms of discipline. Children may not welcome a stepparent because they have not yet resolved their feelings about the separation of their biologic parents (through either divorce or death); they may believe the stepparent threatens their relationship with their biologic parent. They may become extremely distressed at seeing their other biologic parent move into another home and become a stepparent to other children.

Children also may have heard so many stories about evil stepparents from children's books they come into the new family already prejudiced against their new parent.

Although blended families usually lessen financial difficulties, finances can be severely limited, especially if one or both parents are obligated to pay child support for children from a previous relationship while supporting the children of the current marriage. If there is economic disparity between what a biologic parent earns and a stepparent earns, conflicts and distorted expectations can occur between parents. Nurses can be instrumental in offering emotional support to members of a blended family until these adjustments for mutual living can be resolved (Box 2.4).

- **Positive aspects:** Increased security and resources; exposure to different customs or culture may help children become more adaptable to new situations
- **Possible negative aspects:** Rivalry or competition among children; difficulty adjusting to a stepparent

The Gay or Lesbian Family

Gay is the socially preferred term to describe men who have sex with men; **lesbian** is used to denote women who have sex with women. Gay couples or lesbian couples live together as partners for companionship, financial security, and sexual fulfillment, or form the same structure as a nuclear family. As laws are being changed to legally sanction gay marriage, this type of family is increasing in number. Such a relationship offers support in times of crisis comparable to that offered by a nuclear or cohabitation family.

Some lesbian and gay families include children from previous heterosexual marriages or through the use of alternative insemination, adoption, or surrogate motherhood. If the marriage

BOX 2.4 Nursing Care Planning Based on Family Teaching

TIPS FOR REDUCING FAMILY STRESS

Q. Suppose Mr. Hanovan tells you he is worried because the tension level in his family is growing so bad he fears his wife will leave him. He asks you, "How can my family better manage stress?"

A. Managing stress calls for interventions specific to each family, but some general suggestions include:

- Try to describe why you and family members feel so stressed. Almost nothing limits the extent of a threat more than being able to describe it accurately (put a fence around it). Detailing a problem is the beginning of problem solving.
- Recognize stress levels differ from person to person. Because one person is not upset by some condition does not mean another person will not be. On the other hand, if a situation does not annoy a person, that person should not feel he or she has to react to it just because someone else does.
- Anticipate life events and plan for them to the extent possible. Anticipatory guidance will not totally prepare you for a coming event but will at least assist you in preparing for the event.
- Try to reduce the number of stressors coming at you by turning off television, dimming the lights, and spending time with just your inner self.
- Ask yourself if you really need to accomplish all the tasks piling up around you. Do you need to volunteer to be a schoolroom helper this month? Does the garage really need to be cleaned this week?
- Face a situation as honestly as possible. As a rule, knowing the exact nature of a threat is less stressful than a "something-is-out-there" feeling. On the other hand, do not feel compelled to face intense threats, such as a serious complication of pregnancy or a fatal illness in a child, until you have had time to mobilize your defenses, or you may feel overwhelmed.
- Learn to change those things you cannot accept and accepting those things you cannot change. Trial and error is often required to determine the difference.
- Consider that a total change may be unnecessary; a simple modification in one thing will create a cascade or be enough to make a difference.
- Reach out for support. When you are under stress, it's easy to become so involved in the problem you don't realize people around you want to help. Sometimes people closest to you are under the same threat and so are no longer able to offer support. When this happens, you might have to call on second- or third-level support people (extended family or the community) for help.
- Remind family members that unintentional injuries increase when people are under stress. A person worrying about a complication of pregnancy, for example, is more apt to have an automobile accident than a person who is stress free. Children are more apt to poison themselves when the family is under stress as parents are more apt to leave pills on counters during this time.
- Remember that action feels good during stress. Doing something brings a sense of control over feelings of helplessness and disorganization. Action often is so satisfying that people write threatening letters or shout harmful remarks they later regret. Channel your energy into therapeutic action (such as going for a long walk and quietly reflecting) instead.
- Do not rush decisions or make final adaptive outcomes to a stressful situation. As a rule, major decisions should be delayed at least 6 weeks after a stressful event; 6 months is even better.
- Reach out to give support when others are being threatened. Survival is a collaborative effort of social groups; a favor offered now can be called in when you are in need at a later date.

is not officially recognized by the state, it can affect health care planning as health insurance of one partner may not cover the other partner or a child. Lack of understanding by health care providers of the strength and richness of these unions can further impede health care response (Chapman et al., 2012).

- **Positive aspects:** Provides the advantages of a nuclear family
- **Possible negative aspects:** May suffer discrimination from neighbors who do not thoroughly approve or accept this family type

What if...2.1 The Hanovan family identifies their main family problems as a poor financial base, a serious family illness, and limited family communication. Would this change if they were an extended family? A single-parent family? A cohabitation family?

The Foster Family

Children whose parents can no longer care for them may be placed in a foster or substitute home by a child protection agency (Kubiak, Kasiborski, Karim, et al., 2012). Foster parents may have children of their own; they receive remuneration for care of the foster child. Theoretically, foster home placement is temporary until children can be returned to their own parents. Unfortunately, if return does not become possible, children may be raised to adulthood in a series of foster care families. Such children can experience a high level of insecurity, concerned that they will have to soon move again. In addition, they may have some emotional difficulties related to the reason they were removed from their original home (Taussig, Culhane, Garrido, et al., 2012).

Most foster parents are as concerned with health care as biologic parents and can be depended on to follow health care instructions conscientiously. When caring for children from foster homes, be certain to determine who has legal responsibility to sign for health care for the child (a foster parent may or may not have this responsibility).

- **Positive aspects:** Prevents children from being raised in large orphanage settings
- **Possible negative aspects:** Insecurity and inability to establish meaningful relationships because of frequent moves

The Adoptive Family

Families of a great many types (nuclear, extended, cohabitation, blended, single parent, gay, and lesbian) adopt children today. No matter what the family structure, adopting not only brings unusual joy and fulfillment to a family but can also offer a number of challenges for both the adopting parents and the child as well as for any other children in the family (Jones, 2012).

Regardless of whether the adoption was arranged privately or through an adoption agency, new parents should visit a health care facility shortly after a child is placed in their home so a baseline of health information on the child can be established, potential problems can be discussed, and solutions can be explored (Niemann & Weiss, 2012). If the birth mother of an adopted child ate inadequately or received little prenatal care, for example, the adopted child is at a higher risk for abnormal neurologic development than usual. Children from war-torn or poverty-stricken countries have a greater risk of having illnesses such as hepatitis B, intestinal parasites, and growth restriction. They may lack routine immunizations or have delayed motor development from having been raised in a restricted institutional setting (Roeber, Tober, Bolt, et al., 2012).

When assessing a family with a newly adopted child, be certain to determine the stage of parenting the parents have reached. Nonadopting parents have 9 months to prepare physically and emotionally for a coming child. Adoptive parents may be asked to make the mental steps toward parenthood in as little as 24 hours.

If partners have low self-esteem because they were unable to conceive, they may need reassurance at health care visits that they are functioning as well as other parents. With the increase in foreign adoptions, parents often express a conflict between trying to preserve the child's native culture and socializing the child into the community and so appreciate having this problem addressed as well.

Also be certain to assess siblings' responses to an adopted child. Biologic children (whether born before or after the adoption) may feel inferior to the adopted child because they were "just born," not "chosen." They may, however, feel superior because they are the "real" children of the parents. These feelings can interfere with their relationship with the adopted child as well as their parents if not discussed and resolved.

It is generally accepted that adopted children should be told as early as they can understand they are adopted (at about 2 or 3 years). Knowing this from early childhood is not nearly as stressful as accidentally stumbling onto the information when they are school aged or adolescents. At least by 4 years, children are old enough to fully understand the story of their adoption: they grew inside the body of another woman who, because she could not care for them after they were born, gave them to the adopting parent to raise and love. It's important for parents not to criticize a birth mother as part of the explanation as children need to know for their own self-esteem their birth parents were good people and they were capable of being loved by them. Things just didn't work out that way.

When children are first told they are adopted, they may exhibit "honeymoon behavior" or may try to behave perfectly for fear of being given away again. After this honeymoon period, children may deliberately test their parents to see whether, despite bad behavior such as disobeying a house rule or even shoplifting, the parents will still keep them. It helps parents to put this behavior in perspective if they are aware it may happen. Nonadopted children may also use the same testing strategies on some occasions.

Counseling an adopted child or forming a relationship with one as a health care provider carries additional responsibility: making certain the relationship is not ended abruptly or thoughtlessly. When ending a relationship, try to introduce the person who will continue health supervision to the child so the child doesn't feel abandoned for a second time.

When hospitalized, all preschoolers worry about being abandoned and left in the hospital. Preschoolers who have just been told they were adopted or were chosen by their adoptive parents "from all the babies in the hospital nursery," may be terribly afraid they are now being returned to the hospital to be given back. Parents of an adopted child may need additional help in preparing the child for the hospital experience and also should be encouraged to stay with the child in the hospital as much as possible to reduce this type of postadoption fear.

As adopted children enter puberty and begin to think about having children of their own, they may begin to worry if they will make good parents or fail at parenthood as did their birth mother. Some children of this age feel a lack of a sense of identity because they do not know who their birth parents are. It's common for them to spend time tracing records to try to locate their birth parents. Counsel adopting parents that this is not a criticism of their care, but a normal consequence of being adopted. Children seek their birth parents not because they do not love their adoptive parents, but because they need information to know where they fit into the eternal scheme of life.

- **Positive aspects**: Children grow up well cared for and experiencing a sense of love; a woman who relinquishes her child for adoption can feel a sense of relief her baby will have a lifestyle better than what she could provide
- **Possible negative aspects:** Divorce of the adopting parents can be devastating if the child views himself as the cause of the separation or as a child unable to find a secure family for a second time

FAMILY FUNCTIONS AND ROLES

A family is a small community group, and as such, works best if it can designate certain people to complete necessary tasks. Otherwise, it is easy for work in a family to be duplicated or never completed. The roles family members view as appropriate for themselves are usually ones they saw their own parents fulfilling. As each new generation takes on the values of the previous generation, family traditions and culture pass to the next generation.

Because family roles tend to be more flexible and often not as well defined as in the past, an important part of a family assessment is to identify what roles family members have assumed. Most families, for example, can identify an individual who serves as the *wage earner* or who supplies the bulk of the income for the family. In the past, this was typically the father. Today, it may just as easily be both mother and father, as in 40% of dual-earner families the mother contributes as much as 44% of the income (Mundy, 2012). Also usually identified can be the *financial manager* (the person who determines how money will be spent), the *problem solver*, the *decision maker*, the *nurturer*, the *health manager*, the *environmentalist*, the *culture bearer*, and the *gatekeeper* or the person who allows information into and out of the family (Table 2.1). Identifying what these roles consist of and who fulfills these roles in a family allows you to work with a specific person and for assessment or counseling to be most effective (Fig. 2.2).

If a hospitalized child will need continued care after he or she returns home, for example, it would be important to identify and contact the nurturing member of the family, because this person is probably the one who will supervise or give the needed care at home so it can continue seamlessly. Be careful not to make assumptions about which family members play which roles based on gender or stereotyping because every family operates differently. Although nurturing has typically been thought of as a female characteristic, many men best fill this role today.

QSEN Checkpoint Question 2.2

Teamwork & Collaboration

You notice Mrs. Hanovan serves many roles in her family. If, while you're talking to Charles, her 12-year-old son, she interrupts and says to him, "Don't tell our family secrets," you would want your team members to appreciate she is fulfilling what family role?

a. Decision maker
b. Gatekeeper
c. Problem solver
d. Safety officer

Look in Appendix A for the best answer and rationale.

Family Tasks

In addition to family roles, Duvall and Miller (1990) identified eight tasks essential for a family to perform to survive as a healthy unit. These tasks differ in degree from family to family and depend on the growth stage of the family, but they are usually present to some extent in all families. Wellness behaviors such as these may decrease during periods of heightened stress. Therefore, assessing families for these characteristics is helpful to better establish the extent of stress on a family as well as to empower the family to move toward healthier family behaviors.

- *Physical maintenance:* A healthy family provides food, shelter, clothing, and health care for its members. Being certain a family has enough resources to provide for a new or ill member is an important assessment.
- *Socialization of family members:* This task includes being certain that children feel part of the family and learning appropriate ways to interact with people outside the family such as teachers, neighbors, or police. It means the family has an open communication system among family members and outward to the community.
- *Allocation of resources:* This involves determining which family needs will be met and their order of priority, including not only material goods but also affection and space. In healthy families, there is justification, consistency, and fairness in the distribution. In many families, resources are limited, so for example, no one has new shoes. A danger sign would be a family in which one child is barefoot while the others wear $100 sneakers.
- *Maintenance of order:* This task includes establishing family values, establishing rules about expected family responsibilities and roles, and enforcing common regulations for family members such as using "time out" for toddlers. In healthy families, members know the family rules and respect and follow them; in dysfunctional families, you may see a flagrant disregard of rules.
- *Division of labor:* Healthy families not only evenly divide the workload among members but are also flexible enough to interchange workloads as needed.
- *Reproduction, recruitment, and release of family members:* Often not a great deal of thought is given to who lives in a family; membership often happens more by changing circumstances than by true choice. Having to accept a new infant into an already crowded household may make a pregnancy a less-than-welcome event; allowing a young

TABLE 2.1 Planning Nursing Care Based on Assessment

Area of Assessment	Questions to Ask
Type of family	How many family members live in the home? What are their ages and relationships?
Financial support	Who is responsible for the family's income? Are finances adequate? Is money divided evenly among family members?
Safety	Is the home safe from fire or unintentional injuries? (Are smoke alarms present and police and fire numbers posted?) If there are small children, are poisons put on high shelves or in locked cabinets? Are prescription medicines and alcohol in safe places?
Environment	Is there adequate space? Heat? Hot water? Adequate plumbing?
Health	What is a typical breakfast? Lunch? Dinner? Do members monitor the amount of saturated fat and trans-fatty acids in their diet? Do they receive adequate sleep? Do they have a primary care health provider? Are immunizations current? Is there a balance between work and recreation? Does the family feel it copes with problems adequately?
Emotional support within family	Do members eat together or spend an equal amount of time with each other daily? Do they band together to defend each other from outsiders?
Emotional support outside family	Is the family active in community organizations or activities? Do they visit (or are they visited by) friends and relatives? Can the family name at least one outside person they can always rely on for help in a time of crisis?
Cultural diversity	Are there specific customs or traditions that will affect health care? Can they obtain favorite foods locally? What holidays do they celebrate?
Religion	Does the family have a religious affiliation? Do members attend religious services? Are there foods or activities restricted in relation to this that might influence care planning?
Family roles	
Nurturer	Who is the primary caregiver to children or a physically or cognitively challenged member?
Provider	Who brings in the bulk of the family's income?
Decision maker	Who makes decisions, particularly in the area of lifestyle and how leisure time is spent?
Financial manager	Who supervises the family finances (pays the bills, provides savings for the future)?
Problem solver	Who does the family depend on to provide a solution to problems?
Health manager	Who makes health care decisions, ensures family members keep health appointments, immunizations are kept current, and preventive care such as a mammogram for the mother is scheduled?
Culture bearer	Who maintains family and community customs so children can develop a sense of where they belong in history?
Environmentalist	Who is responsible for recycling and not wasting electricity or water?
Gatekeeper	Who determines what information will be released from the family or what new information can be introduced?

adult to move to a college dorm may be viewed as abandonment by a close-knit family.

- *Placement of members into the larger society:* Healthy families realize they do not have to operate alone but can reach out to other families or their community for help as needed. They are able to select community resources, such as schools, affiliations, a place to worship, a birth setting, a hospital, hospice, or a political group, that correlates with the family's beliefs and values. A family that lives in a community with a culture or values different from its own may find this a difficult task.
- *Maintenance of motivation and morale:* Healthy families are able to maintain a sense of unity and pride in their family. When this is present, it helps members defend the family against threats as well as allows them to support each other during a crisis. It means parents are growing with and through the experience of their children the same as children grow through contact with their parents. Assessing whether a feeling of loyalty to other family members is present tells you a lot about the overall health of a family.

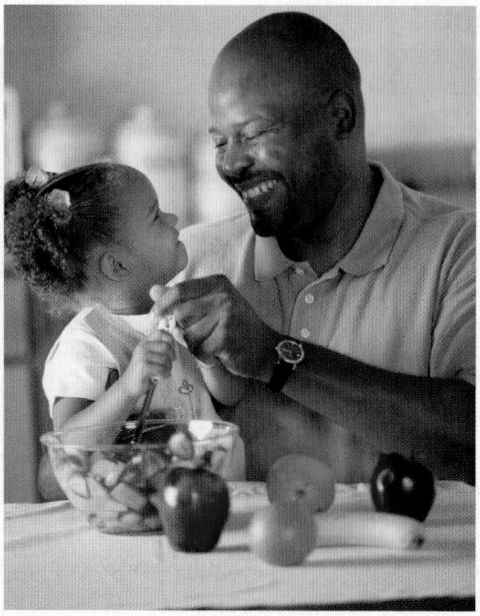

FIGURE 2.2 A healthy family supports each member and performs roles flexibly. Here, a father and daughter help fix dinner.

What if...2.2 Charles complains to you he has to do more than his share of the work in his family because he's expected to keep his own room clean and his 2-year-old brother doesn't have to do that. How would you respond to him?

Developmental Stages

Families, like individuals, not only have specific tasks to carry out but pass through predictable developmental stages (Duvall & Miller, 1990). To assess whether a family is using stage-appropriate health promotion activities, it is helpful to first determine what stage the family is experiencing. The age of the oldest child is used to mark the stage. Because families are delaying the age at which they have a first child and parents are living longer, the lengths of stages 1, 7, and 8 are growing longer, whereas stage 1 is growing shorter.

Stage 1: Marriage

Although Duvall refers to this stage as marriage, what occurs during it is also applicable to couples forming cohabitation, lesbian or gay, or dyad alliances. During this first stage of family development, members work to:

- Establish a mutually satisfying relationship
- Learn to relate well to their families of orientation
- If applicable, engage in reproductive life planning

During this stage, it's important for the couple to merge the values they brought into the relationship from their families of orientation, including not only adjusting to each other in terms of routines (such as sleeping, eating, housecleaning) but also sexual and economic aspects. The stage can be a tenuous one, as evidenced by the high rate of divorce or separation of partners during this stage. The illness of a family member or an unplanned pregnancy at this stage could be enough to destroy the still delicate bonds if the partners do not receive support from their former family members or if health care providers don't recognize that a problem exists.

Stage 2: The Early Childbearing Family

The birth or adoption of a first baby begins this stage. Important tasks of this stage include:

- Integration of the new member into the family
- Making whatever financial and social adjustments are necessary to meet the needs of the new member while continuing to meet the meets of the parents

An important nursing role during this period is health education about well-child care. Even if a family integrates a well newborn adequately, it requires a further developmental step for a family to change from being able to care for a well baby to being able to care for an ill one. One way of determining whether a parent has made this change is to ask what the new parent has tried to do to solve a childrearing or health problem (Plutzer, Spencer, & Keirse, 2011).

Even if what the person answers is not therapeutic or the best solution to the problem, as long as it is sensible (not "I don't do anything when the baby is sick; just take her right to my mother" but instead, "I've given her a little water to keep her temperature down"), it probably means the parent has mastered this developmental step. Parents who have difficulty with this step need a great deal of support and counseling from health care providers to be able to care for an ill child or to manage a difficult pregnancy.

Stage 3: The Family With a Preschool Child

A family at this stage is a busy one because preschool children have such an active imagination and they demand a great deal of supervision. Important tasks for parents include:

- Preventing unintentional injuries (accidents) such as poisoning or falls
- Beginning socialization through play dates, child care, or nursery school settings

If a child returns home for further care after a hospitalization, a family in this stage may need continued support and help (and clear and concise discharge instructions) to provide necessary health care in light of all their other responsibilities.

Stage 4: The Family With a School-Age Child

Parents of school-age children have the important responsibility of preparing their children to function in a world more complex than the one they experienced during their school-age years, while at the same time trying to meet technologic challenges of the adult world. Important family responsibilities during this stage include:

- Promoting children's health through immunizations, dental care, and routine health assessments
- Promoting child safety related to home and automobiles
- Encouraging socialization experiences outside the home such as sports participation, music lessons, or hobby activities
- Encouraging a meaningful school experience to make learning a lifetime concern, not one of merely 12 years

These responsibilities can make this a trying time for families if they grow overwhelmed by so many activities. Illness of a family member at this stage adds to the burden already present and may be enough to dissolve a family. Such a family may need to turn to a tertiary level of support, such as friends, a religious affiliation, or health care providers, for advice and help with problem solving.

Stage 5: The Family With an Adolescent

The primary goal for a family with a teenager differs considerably from the goal of the family in previous stages, which was to strengthen family ties and maintain family unity. At this stage, the family's goals include:

- Loosening ties enough to allow an adolescent more freedom while still remaining safe
- Beginning to prepare adolescents for life on their own

Because parents may not believe their adolescent is mature enough to make independent decisions as yet, this stage can be a trying one for both adolescents and adults. Violence—automobile accidents, homicide, and self-injury—occurs more often in this age group than any other and is the major cause of death (Murphy, Xu, & Kochanek, 2012). As children at this age become sexually active, they risk contracting sexually transmitted diseases and hepatitis C. If there is a large "generation gap" between the parents and an adolescent, the adolescent may not be able to talk to parents about these important problems, particularly those of a controversial nature such as sexual responsibility. In these instances, a nurse can be the neutral person needed to assist families when they are unable to clearly voice their or their family's needs (Box 2.5).

Stage 6: The Launching Stage Family: The Family With a Young Adult

For many families, the stage at which children leave to establish their own households is the most difficult stage of family life because it represents a break up of the family. Parents need to:

- Change their role from mother or father to once-removed support persons or guideposts
- Encourage independent thinking and adult-level decision skills in their child

Parents may encounter a loss of self-esteem as they feel themselves replaced by other people in their children's lives. This can make them feel old for the first time and less able to cope with responsibilities. Illness imposed on a family at this stage can be detrimental to the family structure, helping to further break up an already noncohesive group. It's important to help parents see that they have spent their lives preparing for this event and appreciate that a child leaving home is a positive, not a negative, step in family growth.

Many young adults today return home to live with their family after college or a failed relationship until they can afford their own apartment or find a new live-in partner. A term used to describe this is the "**boomerang**" generation. As a general rule, this arrangement works best if there are not young children in the home (which prevents a big gap in care needed) and if the young adult has a job to cover at least part of personal expenses. Young men who return to their family this way tend to remain home longer than young women; women are generally asked to do more work around the house and are chaperoned more closely so leave again earlier (Cherlin, 2012).

Young adults returning home can also create a "**sandwich family**" or a family that is squeezed into taking care of both aging parents and a returning young adult. Help parents to recognize their child returning home is a positive happening or proof they have provided a warm and loving atmosphere for the child during growth years; otherwise, a young adult would not choose these living arrangements.

BOX 2.5 Nursing Care Planning Based on Effective Communication

The Hanovan family consists of Mr. and Mrs. Hanovan and three children: James, 17; Charles, 12; and Brian, 2. You notice Brian has missed so many health maintenance visits, he is underimmunized.

Less Effective Communication

Nurse: It's good to see you in clinic today, Mrs. Hanovan. I know money is a problem, but you've got to start coming more until your child gets caught up with immunizations.
Mrs. Hanovan: It's hard with a 2-year-old—
Nurse: Babies, you know, have almost no natural immunity. That's why they need immunizations.
Mrs. Hanovan: It's hard—
Nurse: It's hard to understand a reason important enough not to get him immunized.
Mrs. Hanovan: I'll do better in the future. I promise.

More Effective Communication

Nurse: It's good to see you in clinic today, Mrs. Hanovan. I know money is a problem, but you've got to start coming more until Brian gets caught up with his immunizations.
Mrs. Hanovan: It's hard with a 2-year-old—
Nurse: Is there anything I could do to make coming to the clinic easier?
Mrs. Hanovan: I should never come. Brian's outgrown his car seat so it's illegal for me to drive him here.
Nurse: Let me give you the number of an agency you can call to borrow a seat, not only so you can come to the clinic more often but so you can take him out safely at other times as well.

In our zeal to educate people about good health practices, it is easy to rush in and teach without first assessing a family's needs. Unless these needs are met, people may agree to comply with a better health regimen but then be unable to do so because their original need was not met.

Stage 7: The Family of Middle Years

When all children have left home, a family returns to a two-partner or single-person unit, the same as it was before childbearing. In light of this change, partners may view this stage either as the prime time of their life (an opportunity to travel, enjoy economic independence, and spend time on hobbies) or as a period of gradual decline (longing for the constant activity and stimulation of children). Family responsibilities in this stage include:

- Adjusting to "empty nest" syndrome by reawakening their relationship with their supportive partner
- Preparing for retirement so when they reach that stage they will not be unprepared socially or financially

Unfortunately, supportive partners may realize at this stage they have grown in such different ways since they began their relationship with each other, they now have very little in common (the second highest rate of divorce occurs at this age). Both women and men tend to experience less "empty nest" feelings if they are able to value their personal worth when children are not present (Dare, 2011; Gratton & Gutmann, 2010).

Because the family has returned to being only a two-partner union, support people may not be as plentiful as they once were. Also, because women are having children later and later in life, beginning a new family at this point could be viewed as exciting or worrisome, depending on how many other things are going on in the family's life such as aging parents who also require care and concern.

Stage 8: The Family in Retirement or Older Age

Families of retirement age account for approximately 20% to 25% of the population (U.S. Social Security Administration [SSA], 2012). Common family responsibilities at this stage include:

- Maintaining heath by preventive care in light of aging
- Participating in social, political, and neighborhood activities to keep active and enjoy this stage of life

Although families at this stage are no longer having children, they remain important in maternal and child health because many grandparents care for grandchildren while parents are at work. They play important roles in health supervision and care, although it can become a strain on older adults as they struggle to meet young children's needs in light of a lesser energy level and the finances needed.

✔ QSEN Checkpoint Question 2.3

Quality Improvement

The Hanovan family consists of two parents plus James, 17; Charles, 12; and Brian, 2. Mrs. Hanovan is 4 months pregnant. When examining how to improve the quality of your health teaching with the Hanovan family, which of Duvall's family life stages would you consider the family currently experiencing?

a. Pregnancy stage
b. Preschool stage
c. Launching stage
d. Adolescent stage

Look in Appendix A for the best answer and rationale.

ASSESSMENT OF FAMILY STRUCTURE AND FUNCTION

Family characteristics can be assessed on a variety of levels and in varying degrees of detail. The type of family data collected and the method of collection should match the way in which the assessment data will be used.

General characteristics of family type and functioning can be assessed using observation and general history questions (see Table 2.1). If more detailed information about family environment and roles is required, using an assessment tool specifically developed for that purpose can be most effective.

The Well Family

Assessment of psychosocial family wellness requires a measurement of how the family relates and interacts as a unit, including communication patterns, bonding, roles and role relationships, division of tasks and activities, governance, decision making, problem solving, and leadership within the family unit. Assessment also looks at how the family relates to the outside community.

A **genogram** is a diagram that details family structure and provides information about the family's health history and the roles of various family members across several generations. It can provide a basis for discussion and analysis of family interaction at health care visits (Fig. 2.3).

Another aspect of family assessment is to document the "fit" of a family into their community. This is done by means of an **ecomap**, a diagram of family and community relationships (Fig. 2.4). To construct such a map, first draw a circle in the center to represent the family. Around the outside, draw circles that represent the family's community contacts such as church, school, neighbors, or other organizations. Families who "fit" well into their community usually have many outside circles or community contacts. A mark of families who are new to a community is they have few community contacts as they have not formed these as yet. This pattern is also the mark of an abusive or dysfunctional family if such a family deliberately keeps outside people separate from them. Constructing such a map helps you assess the emotional support that will be available to a family in a time of crisis. A family whom you assess as having few connecting lines between its members and the community may need increased nursing contact and support to remain a well family. Box 2.6 shows an interprofessional care map illustrating both nursing and team planning for the Hanovan family.

What if...2.3 You discover the Hanovan family is "out of sync" with its community (they are the only family on their block who does not work at the local factory, they attend a different church than many, they are having a new baby when many neighbors have college-age children). How could you help them fit into their community better?

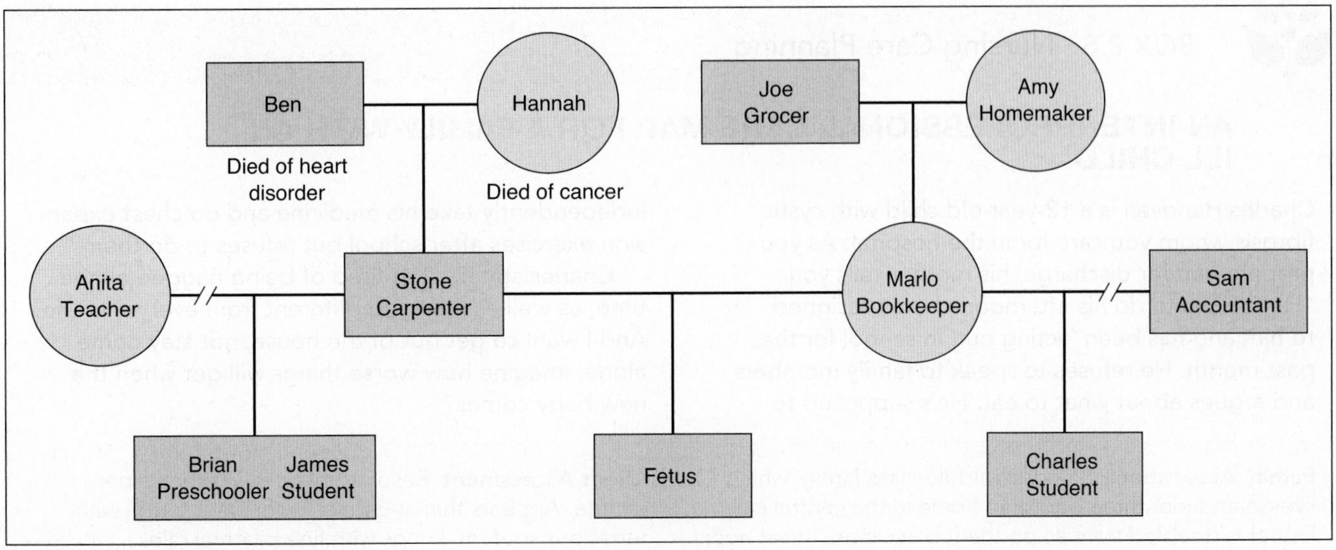

FIGURE 2.3 A genogram of the Hanovan family showing three generations. Males are shown by squares, females by circles.

Changing Patterns of Family Life

Family life has changed significantly across the world during the past 50 years due to many complex and interrelated factors, such as an increase in divorce, families in which both parents work outside the home (dual-earner families), single-parent families, and shared childrearing responsibilities. Many more couples delay marriage and childrearing today until they are completely finished with school and established in their careers. This delay has implications for fertility and the need for assisted reproduction technology.

Understanding the impact these changes have on family structure and family life can help you create care plans that are realistic and better meet the needs of today's families.

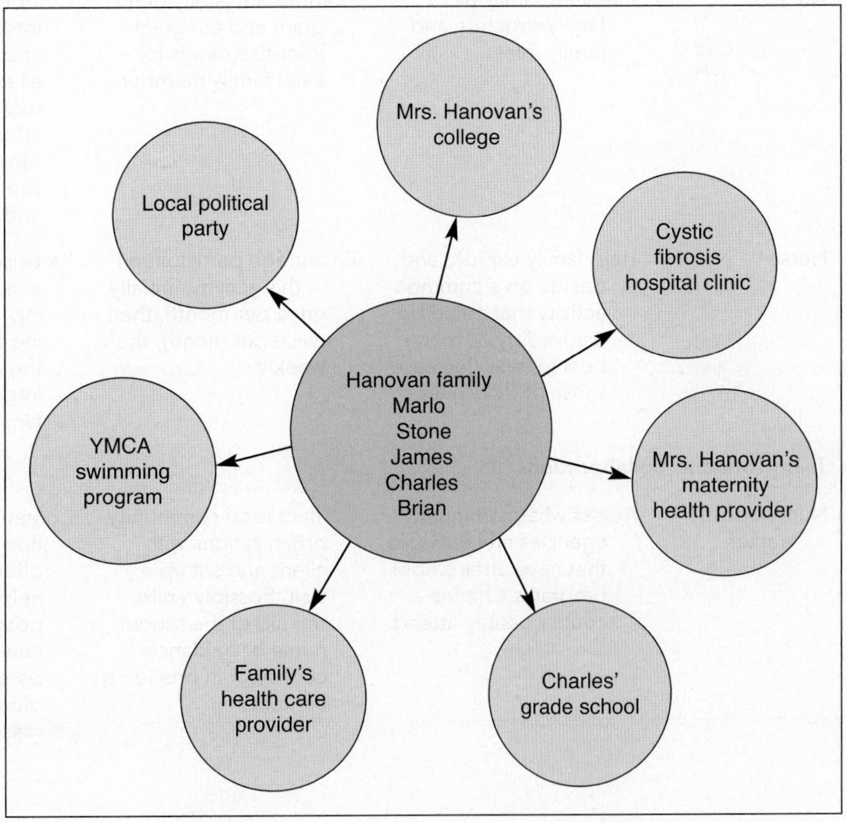

FIGURE 2.4 An ecomap of the Hanovan family's relationship to its community. The family members are shown in the center circle; the outer circles show community contacts.

BOX 2.6 Nursing Care Planning

AN INTERPROFESSIONAL CARE MAP FOR A FAMILY WITH AN ILL CHILD

Charles Hanovan is a 12-year-old child with cystic fibrosis whom you care for in the hospital. As you prepare him for discharge, his mother tells you, "He refuses to do his afternoon chores assigned to him and has been 'acting out' in school for the past month. He refuses to speak to family members and argues about what to eat. He's supposed to independently take his medicine and do chest expansion exercises after school but refuses to do them."

Charles states, "I'm tired of being nagged all the time, as well as being so different from everyone else. And I want to get out of the house, not stay home alone. Imagine how worse things will get when the new baby comes?"

Family Assessment Blended middle-class family, which lives in an older three-bedroom home in the central city. Father is disabled from an on-the-job accident 1 year ago; does not participate in any community activities. Mother works as a bookkeeper and also attends a community college; she is 4 months pregnant and active in local political party. Client is a middle child with two stepbrothers, age 17 and age 2. Mother swims weekly at the local YMCA; the rest of family refuses to go with her. Charles is responsible for homework and cleaning kitchen after school while he is home alone (father is at physical therapy visits). Admits to having few close friends. Two neighbors are available in case of emergency during his alone time.

Client Assessment Respiratory rate: 26 breaths per minute. Appears thin and pale. Productive cough with tenacious sputum. Lungs with fine bilateral rales.

Nursing Diagnosis Interrupted family processes related to effect of child's illness and situational stressors limiting communication.

Outcome Criteria Family demonstrates greater participation in family activities, interaction with ill child, and positive methods of communication by 3 months' time.

Charles states he feels more family attachment and increased self-esteem by 3 months' time.

Team Member Responsible	Assessment	Intervention	Rationale	Expected Outcome
Activities of Daily Living, Including Safety				
Nurse	Interview family as to family structure and family roles.	Complete a family genogram and ecogram. Prioritize needs for each family member.	Combining a family interview, genogram, and ecogram profile as to how family members relate and interact with each other and community should help prioritize and focus care.	Family supplies interview, genogram, and ecogram information with needs of family from their standpoint prioritized by follow-up visit.
Nurse	Help family explore and decide on a common activity that could be enjoyed by all members to help decrease sense of loneliness.	Encourage participation in this activity, initially once per month, then twice per month, then weekly.	Participation in a group activity fosters bonding. Gradually increasing the frequency of the activity promotes integration into the family routine.	Client maintains a schedule documenting his participation in the chosen family activity.
Teamwork and Collaborations				
Nurse/Social worker	Assess what community agencies are available that have after-school programs Charles could possibly attend.	Contact local community organizations with client and set up a visit. Possibly enlist the aid of the school nurse or guidance counselor in providing contacts.	Contacting the organization with the client offers support and helps reduce his possible anxiety with new situations. School personnel provide additional support and reassurance.	Client visits at least one local or school agency that could provide a community contact and support by next health care visit.

Procedures/Medications for Quality Improvement				
Nurse	Assess and list all of child's required exercises, therapy, and medications.	Demonstrate procedures, if necessary, and ask client to return demonstrations. Help client incorporate regimens into usual routine.	Review and redemonstration helps to reinforce measures and ensures client is doing them correctly. Incorporating them into client's routine helps to promote positive adjustment and decrease feelings of being different.	Client redemonstrates procedures with 90% accuracy. Combines at least one exercise or medication with usual routine. Taking more responsibility for therapy should offer a sense of "growing up" and decrease need for reminders.
Nurse/Physical or respiratory therapist	Help family assess which family member could serve as backup support for child's exercise and medication regimens.	Meet with family and plan a schedule that will allow a backup family member to participate in child's exercise and therapy regimens so he isn't alone.	Family involvement divides the responsibility and minimizes the risk of added stress on the family system.	Family members state they use a checklist to ensure one of them is available to cooperate with and encourage client to follow treatment regimen. Client states he is adhering to treatment regimen 90% of time.
Nutrition				
Nurse/ Nutritionist	Assess nutrition needs based on medical prescription.	Review special diet needed by client with client and father (food preparer). Brainstorm foods client would like to eat.	The food preparer needs to be as well informed about a special diet as the client.	Both client and father state they understand a special diet is necessary and describe an innovative breakfast, lunch, and dinner for diet.
Nurse/ Nutritionist	Assess family's eating habits.	Encourage family to eat together as a family unit at least two times per week.	Eating together should not only help client to comply with nutrition plan but provide a time for family sharing and communication.	Family reports they eat together at least one meal twice per week or, if not possible, arrange for a substitute "sharing time."
Patient-Centered Care				
Nurse	Assess client's and family's present knowledge of his illness.	Review with client and parents the cause and therapy for illness based on their present knowledge base.	Building on a client's knowledge base facilitates teaching and learning and minimizes repetition.	Client and family state they understand the underlying cause of illness and importance of treatments.
Nurse	Assess with client what a typical day consists of; how many friends he can identify.	Brainstorm with client ways he could make a new friend or "fit" in at school routine better.	A feeling of "being different" can be detrimental to high self-esteem.	Client states he has made at least one new friend by 2 months' time; feels a "better fit" at school.
Psychosocial/Spiritual/Emotional Needs				
Nurse	Help each family member identify the area of his or her greatest stress.	Help family members reduce stress by teaching better problem-solving techniques such as time or anger management.	Identifying problems is the first step in effective problem solving. Use of therapeutic measures such as time management helps meet needs and so can reduce stress.	Family members identify the greatest stressors in their family life and means they are using to decrease stress by next health care visit.

(continued on page 38)

BOX 2.6 Nursing Care Planning (continued)

Informatics for Seamless Health Care Planning

Nurse/Case manager	Assess home rules and delegation of responsibilities. Meet with family to identify areas of needed support when child returns home.	Encourage joint cooperation in household tasks so client doesn't feel so isolated when home alone.	Joint ownership of household tasks encourages a sense of family.	Family members demonstrate they have a family schedule that evens out tasks and involves all members.
Nurse/Case manager	Assess what resources are available in the Hanovan's community, such as the Cystic Fibrosis Foundation, that could be used as a support resource.	Meet with family to see if members are interested in using any identified community organizations as resources.	Community resources can provide additional support in areas of need.	Family members state they have attended at least one Parents of Cystic Fibrosis Children or similar meeting by 3 months' time.

QSEN Checkpoint Question 2.4

Safety

Because of smaller families, the supervision of children may be delegated to many different caregivers during a day's time. What age group has the most automobile-related unintentional injuries if not supervised conscientiously?

a. Infants, because child car seats are often installed incorrectly
b. Toddlers, because they walk in front of cars in parking lots
c. School-aged children, because they ride school buses almost daily
d. Adolescents, because of alcohol or distraction while driving

Look in Appendix A for the best answer and rationale.

Increased Divorce Rate

Divorce is rarely easy for either children or adults. Because parents are so emotionally entangled and their roles change so dramatically after divorce, they may be unable to give their children the support they need during this time (Vélez, Wolchik, Tein, et al., 2011). This can leave long-term, negative effects on children as the loss of a parent or favorite grandparent through divorce is little different from the loss of a parent through death.

Children react in differing ways to divorce depending on their age and understanding of what is happening and the explanations their parents give them. Divorce, as a rule, has three separate phases in which children follow a course similar to grief.

- The first phase is apt to be an antagonistic time as parents realize they are no longer compatible, marked by quarreling, hurt feelings, and whispered conversations. This phase can be particularly upsetting for children because they usually haven't been told what is happening as yet. They may assume the quarreling is their fault (i.e., if they had behaved better, this wouldn't be happening).
- The second phase is the actual separation stage. Everyone in the family is forced to take on an unfamiliar role, perhaps move to a new home, and probably realize a marked difference in finances. Although it is comforting to be free from a house filled with tension and arguing, most children wish they had their old life back as they grieve for the missing parent.
- The third phase involves reshaping lives. The family becomes a single-parent family or, if the custodial parent remarries, a blended one. Financial arrangements, whether higher or lower, stabilize. Children realize their lives are permanently changed and they cannot go back to the time before the divorce and so must move forward.

Boys generally have more emotional trauma from divorce than girls, probably because they lose their gender role model, as the mother is most apt to become the parent with custody. All children may manifest their grief with physical symptoms such as nausea or fatigue. Their school performance may suffer. Most children report that when the noncustodial parent remarries, it is one of the hardest moments for them because at that point they have no choice but to accept the finality of the divorce (Angarne-Lindberg & Wadsby, 2012).

Although all three stages of divorce are stressful for children, following a divorce, a redeeming feature may be that children may actually feel less stress than they experienced living in a home where there was a high level of conflict between parents. To help them adjust to their changing situation, children need an explanation of why the divorce occurred and assurance that it was not their fault. The parent who will now be raising them may need help in avoiding playing the role of the injured party or portraying the former partner as dishonorable, selfish, or unreliable. Although a former spouse was not a good marriage partner, he or she may have been a good parent and may be well loved and missed by the children (Sigal, Wolchik, Tein, et al., 2012).

QSEN Checkpoint Question 2.5

Evidence-Based Practice

In previous years, few parents asked for shared or joint custody of their children following a divorce. Today, this type of custody is seen in as many as 30% of custody arrangements. To investigate whether joint custody of this type—where a child spends some time in both parents' homes following a divorce—poses behavioral risks such as increased smoking or drug use, researchers interviewed a cohort of 15-year-old Swedish teenagers.

Findings revealed adolescents living in shared physical custody had higher rates of health risk behaviors such as beginning smoking or drinking alcohol compared with adolescents from two-parent families (60% and 50% higher, respectively). At the same time, adolescents in this study had significantly lower rates of these health risk behaviors than their counterparts in single-parent families (Carlsund et al., 2013).

Suppose Mr. and Mrs. Hanovan divorce. Based on this study, what would be an important responsibility when you are discharging James, an adolescent, from a hospital stay to his home care setting?

a. Suggest his mother, who will be his primary caregiver, quit work so he will be able to have a stay-at-home mother for his care.
b. Assess the parent's custodial pattern to be certain a responsible adult will be available no matter which home James returns to.
c. Assure his parents that shared custody is a common pattern today and therefore does not pose a risk to teenagers, otherwise no one would choose it.
d. Assume the parents are responsible adults and will sensibly solve any problems that arise according to their custodial agreement.

Look in Appendix A for the best answer and rationale.

Decreased Family Size

The U.S. birth rate has declined steadily from 1900 to the present, putting the United States at a rate of almost zero population growth or with fewer births each year than deaths. The average number of children in families has decreased from 4 or 5 at the beginning of the last century to 2.1 children today (NCHS, 2012). Because parents in small families spend less total time providing direct child care, this limits parents' experience in childrearing, so the amount of childrearing counseling time by nurses needed per parent increases. As children have fewer older sibling role models than before, they may need more counseling in behaviors such as how to manage stress, how to survive a failing grade at school, or how to deal with a sports team's loss.

Increased Dual-Parent Employment

As many as 60% of women of childbearing age work full-time outside their home and as many as 90% work at least part-time (Cherlin, 2012). The implication of this trend for health care providers is that health care facilities need to schedule appointments at times when parents are free to come (parents will willingly miss work if their child is sick, but not necessarily for a health maintenance or a routine prenatal visit). Instructions about how to give medication must take into account both the child's and the parents' schedules. For instance, help parents tailor administration of medicine to the times they will be with the child to supervise the administration (perhaps before breakfast, following after-school child care, and at bedtime) rather than suggesting the more traditional 10 am, 2 pm, and 6 pm schedule.

The amount of time spent watching television and what Internet sites are being visited are important for parents to monitor with self-care school-age children. It is important for children to learn to live in a fast-paced world, but parents need to be certain children understand news of world events are reported over and over. Otherwise, serial repetition of that type can frighten children as it may seem as if 100 airplanes have crashed instead of one airplane crash being reported over and over.

To avoid exposure to excessive violence on television, the American Academy of Pediatrics (AAP) recommends children's television viewing time be limited until they reach 2 years of age (AAP, 2012). Many parents restrict this through school age so children have adequate time to spend with friends and on required homework. Caution parents that they need to monitor time spent on the Internet because of the misinformation posted and the risk from Internet predators.

Dual-parent employment has increased the number of children attending day care centers or after-school programs (Copeland, Sherman, Kendeigh, et al., 2012). This high attendance rate may have an impact on health care as well because children attending day care centers have an increased incidence of infections such as acute diarrhea and upper respiratory infections. They may engage in less gross motor activities than children playing at home. Helping parents choose a quality day care center or after-school program that takes the necessary precautions against infections and includes physical as well as academic activities can be a nursing responsibility (see Chapter 31).

Dual working parents may also require school-age children to spend some time alone after school before their parents return from work. Helping parents prevent loneliness in these "latchkey" or "self-care" children as well as helping children make good use of their time alone can be another important nursing responsibility (see Chapter 32).

QSEN Checkpoint Question 2.6

Informatics

The amount of technology and media that children are exposed to increases yearly. What is the youngest age you would suggest the Hanovan family introduce their new baby to television viewing based on the recommendation of the AAP?

a. 1 year
b. 18 months
c. 2 years
d. 4 years

Look in Appendix A for the best answer and rationale.

High Levels of Violence in Families

An alarming statistic in today's families is that the incidence and reports of intimate partner violence and child maltreatment remain high (Symes, 2011). This is apparently related to high stress levels in families and better reporting of violence and maltreatment. Detecting these behaviors begins with the awareness that they occur. Both intimate partner violence and child maltreatment are discussed in detail in Chapter 55.

What if...2.4 You are particularly interested in exploring one of the 2020 National Health Goals with respect to healthy families (see Box 2.1). What would be a possible research topic to explore pertinent to this goal that would be applicable to the Hanovan family and also would advance evidence-based practice?

Key Points for Review

- A family is a group of people who share a common emotional bond and perform certain interrelated social tasks.
- Because families work as a unit, the unmet needs of any member can spread to become the unmet needs of all family members.
- Common types of families include nuclear, extended, single-parent, blended, cohabitation, gay and lesbian, foster, and adopted families.
- Common family tasks are physical maintenance, socialization of family members, allocation of resources, maintenance of order, division of labor, reproduction, recruitment and release of members, placement of members into the larger society, and maintenance of motivation and morale.
- Common life stages of families are marriage; early childbearing; families with preschool, school-age, and adolescent children; launching stage; middle-years families; and the family in retirement.
- Changes in patterns of family life that are occurring include dual-parent employment, increased divorce rates, reduced family size, and social problems such as intimate partner violence.
- Considering a family as a unit (a single client) helps in planning nursing care that not only meets QSEN competencies but also best meets the family's total needs.
- Because families exist within communities, assessment of the community and the family's place in the community yields further information on family functioning and abilities.

Critical Thinking Care Study

The Garcia family consists of Mr. Garcia, 42; Mrs. Garcia, 36; Mrs. Garcia's mother, 62; Jose, 14; Anna 12; and Carlos, 4. Mr. Garcia works as a city bus driver. All six members live in a crowded apartment in the center of the city. Mrs. Garcia recently solved the problem of someone needing to care for her mother who has Alzheimer disease by quitting her job as a secretary to care for her. She tells you she used to enjoy entertaining her children's friends but now asks them not to visit because her mother needs quiet.

1. What type of family do the Garcia's represent? Who do you think is the family problem solver? The health supervisor? The gatekeeper?
2. What is the stage of the Garcia family? Would their situation be different if the children were other ages?
3. Carlos was adopted because his mother, Mrs. Garcia's sister, died in a car accident. What are special concerns of adopted children you need to consider when giving nursing care?

Patient Scenario

The Nahid Family

Read about the Nahid family, a family with a troubled adolescent, then answer the questions to further sharpen your skills and grow more familiar with NCLEX-type questions related to family health. Confirm your answers are correct by reading the rationales.

Visit http://thePoint.lww.com

Answers and Rationales

Looking for answers to the What If… and Critical Thinking Care Study questions?

Visit http://thePoint.lww.com

References

Allender, J. A. (2013). *Community & public health nursing*. Philadelphia, PA: Lippincott Williams & Wilkins.

American Academy of Pediatrics. (2012). *Where we stand: TV viewing time*. Washington, DC: Author.

Angarne-Lindberg, T., & Wadsby, M. (2012). Psychiatric and somatic health in relation to experience of parental divorce in childhood. *International Journal of Social Psychiatry, 58*(1), 16–25.

Carlsund, A., Eriksson, U., Löfstedt, P., et al. (2013). Risk behaviour in Swedish adolescents: Is shared physical custody after divorce a risk or a protective factor? *European Journal of Public Health, 23*(1), 3–8.

Chapman, R., Watkins, R., Zappia, T., et al. (2012). Second-level hospital health professionals' attitudes to lesbian, gay, bisexual and transgender parents seeking health for their children. *Journal of Clinical Nursing, 21*(5–6), 880–887.

Cherlin, A. J. (2012). *Public and private families*. New York, NY: McGraw-Hill.

Copeland, K. A., Sherman, S. N., Kendeigh, C. A., et al. (2012). Societal values and policies may curtail preschool children's physical activity in child care centers. *Pediatrics, 129*(2), 265–274.

Dare, J. S. (2011). Transitions in midlife women's lives: Contemporary experiences. *Health Care of Women International, 32*(2), 111–133.

Duvall, E. M., & Miller, B. (1990). *Marriage and family development*. Philadelphia, PA: Lippincott Williams & Wilkins.

Gratton, B., & Gutmann, M. P. (2010). Emptying the nest: Older men in the United States, 1880–2000. *Population & Development Review, 36*(2), 331–356.

Henrich, J., Boyd, R., & Richerson, P. J. (2012). The puzzle of monogamous marriage. *Philosophical Transactions of the Royal Society of London, 367*(1589), 657–669.

Jacobson, C. K., & Burton, L. (Eds.). (2011). *Modern polygamy in the United States: Historical, cultural, and legal issues*. New York, NY: Oxford University Press.

Jones, V. F. (2012). Comprehensive health evaluation of the newly adopted child. *Pediatrics, 129*(1), e214–e223.

Keene, J. R, Prokos, A. H., & Held, B. (2012). Grandfather caregivers: Race and ethnic differences in poverty. *Sociological Inquiry, 82*(1), 49–77.

Kubiak, S. P., Kasiborski, N., Karim, N., et al. (2012). Does subsequent criminal justice involvement predict foster care and termination of parental rights for children born to incarcerated women? *Social Work in Public Health, 27*(1–2), 129–147.

Lavoie-Tremblay, M., Bonin, J. P., Bonneville-Roussy, A., et al. (2012). Families' and decision makers' experiences with mental health care reform: The challenge of collaboration. *Archives of Psychiatric Nursing, 26*(4), e41–e50.

Mather, M. (2010). *U.S. children in single-mother families*. Washington, DC: Population Reference Bureau.

Mundy, L. (2012). Women, money & power. *Time, 179*(12), 28–34.

Murphy, S. L., Xu, J., & Kochanek, K. D. (2012). Deaths: Preliminary data for 2010. *National Vital Statistics Reports, 60*(4), 1–69.

National Center for Health Statistics. (2012). Changing demographics. *National Vital Statistics Reports, 58*(1), 2–4.

Niemann, S., & Weiss, S. (2012). Factors affecting attachment in international adoptees at 6 months post adoption. *Children and Youth Services Review, 34*(1), 205–212.

Parker, J. A., Mandleco, B., Olsen Roper, S. et al. (2011). Religiosity, spirituality, and marital relationships of parents raising a typically developing child or a child with a disability. *Journal of Family Nursing, 2*(17), 82–104.

Plutzer, K., Spencer, A. J., & Keirse, M. J. (2011). How first-time mothers perceive and deal with teething symptoms: a randomized controlled trial. *Child: Care, Health and Development, 38*(2), 292–299.

Roeber, B. J., Tober, C. L., Bolt, D. M., et al. (2012). Gross motor development in children adopted from orphanage settings. *Developmental Medicine and Child Neurology, 54*(6), 527–531.

Sigal, A. B., Wolchik, S. A., Tein, J. Y., et al. (2012) Enhancing youth outcomes following parental divorce: A longitudinal study of the effects of the new beginnings program on educational and occupational goals. *Journal of Clinical Child & Adolescent Psychology, 41*(2), 150–165.

Symes, L. (2011). Abuse across the lifespan: Prevalence, risk, and protective factors. *Nursing Clinics of North America, 46*(4), 391–411.

Taussig, H. N., Culhane, S. E., Garrido, E., et al. (2012). RCT of a mentoring and skills group program: Placement and permanency outcomes for foster youth. *Pediatrics, 130*(1), e33–e39.

U.S. Census Bureau. (2010). *Statistical abstract of the United States*. Washington, DC: U.S. Department of Commerce.

U.S. Department of Health and Human Services. (2010). *Healthy people 2020*. Washington, DC: Author.

U.S. Social Security Administration. (2012). *Monthly statistical snapshot*. Washington, DC: Research, Statistics & Public Policy.

Vélez, C. E., Wolchik, S. A., Tein, J. Y., et al. (2011). Protecting children from the consequences of divorce: A longitudinal study of the effects of parenting on children's coping processes. *Child Development, 82*(1), 244–257.

Chapter 3

Cultural Diversity and Maternal and Child Health Nursing

KEY TERMS

- acculturation
- assimilation
- cultural awareness
- cultural competence
- cultural humility
- cultural values
- culture
- culture specific
- culture universal
- discrimination
- diversity
- ethnicity
- ethnocentrism
- minority
- mores
- norms
- prejudice
- stereotyping
- taboos
- transcultural nursing

OBJECTIVES

After mastering the contents of this chapter, you should be able to:

1. Identify common areas or concerns of cultural diversity and apply these to nursing practice.
2. Identify 2020 National Health Goals related to diversity considerations and specific ways nurses can help the nation achieve these goals.
3. Assess a family for aspects of cultural diversity that might influence the way the family responds to childbearing and childrearing.
4. Formulate nursing diagnoses related to culturally influenced aspects of nursing care.
5. Develop outcomes to assist families who have specific cultural needs so they can thrive in their community as well as manage seamless transitions across different health care settings.
6. Using the nursing process, plan nursing care that includes the six competencies of Quality & Safety Education for Nurses (QSEN): Patient-Centered Care, Teamwork & Collaboration, Evidence-Based Practice (EBP), Quality Improvement (QI), Safety, and Informatics.
7. Implement nursing care to assist a family adapt to today's changing sociocultural environment.
8. Evaluate expected outcomes for achievement and effectiveness of care to be certain that expected outcomes have been achieved.
9. Integrate aspects of cultural diversity with the interplay of nursing process, the six competencies of QSEN, and Family Nursing to achieve quality maternal and child health nursing care.

Maria Rodriques is a 12-year-old child who is hospitalized for surgical repair of a broken tibia, which was fractured when she rode her bicycle into a busy street.

In planning care for Maria, you assume, because her culture is Hispanic, her family orientation will be male dominant, her time focus will be on the present, and her nutrition preferences will be Mexican American.

You are surprised on the second day of her hospital stay to hear Maria tell you she feels "second class." Her father has been asked for more input about her care than she has. She hasn't been given any milk to drink so is worried her bone will not heal. She's concerned she won't be able to play soccer by next month but no one else seems worried about that.

The previous chapters described the standards and philosophy of maternal and child health nursing as well as family health. This chapter adds information on caring for families from diverse cultures. Such information can both enrich care and help improve the health of childbearing and childrearing families.

If you had really planned care in this way, of what would you have been guilty? What would have been a better approach for determining Maria's cultural preferences?

Culture is a view of the world and a set of traditions a specific social group uses and transmits to the next generation.

- **Transcultural nursing** is care guided by cultural aspects and respects individual differences (Andrews, 2011a).
- **Cultural values** are preferred ways of acting based on cultural traditions (Giger, 2012).
- **Culture-specific** values are norms and patterns of behavior unique to one particular culture.
- **Culture universal** refers to values, norms, and patterns shared across almost all cultures.
- **Ethnicity** refers to the cultural group into which a person was born, although the term is sometimes used in a narrower context to mean only race.
- **Race** refers to a category of people who share a socially recognized physical characteristic; the term is rarely used today as the research on the human genome shows no basic differences in structure among people.
- **Diversity** in a population means there is a mixture or variety of lifestyles and beliefs in the population. The United States is an example of a country with varied cultural groups and socioeconomic conditions, so you are likely to see a wide range of behaviors and family structures exhibited in any health care setting (Fig. 3.1).

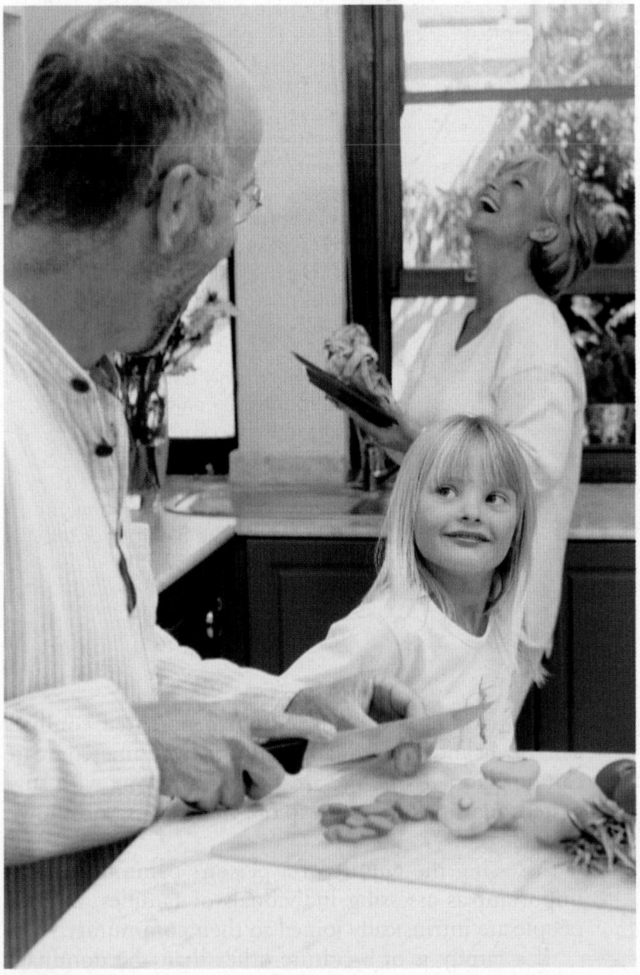

FIGURE 3.1 Various cultural preferences are evident in childrearing. Many extended family members, such as grandparents, are the primary caregivers today.

Assessing cultural diversity, ethnicity, and individual beliefs of families and clients can reveal why people take the type of preventive health measures they do or why they seek a particular type of care, because the way people react to health care is a cultural value (Chen, Wei, Yeh, et al., 2013).

Cultural values often arise from environmental conditions (in a country where water is scarce, daily bathing is not valued; in a country where meat is scarce, ethnic recipes use little meat). The usual values of a group are termed **mores** or **norms**. Expecting women to come for prenatal care and parents to bring children for immunizations are examples of norms in the United States, but these are not beliefs worldwide or even among all Americans (Diekema, 2012).

Actions not acceptable to a culture are called **taboos**. Three universal taboos are murder, incest, and cannibalism. Issues such as abortion, robbery, and lying are controversial taboos because these are taboos only to some people, not everyone.

Cultural values form early in life and strongly influence the manner in which people plan for childbearing and childrearing, as well as the way they respond to health and illness (Lewallen, 2011). When doing research, nurses need to be mindful to include all cultural groups in research samples, so more can be learned about cultural preferences in relation to nursing interventions and care.

The way people respond to pain is an example of a trait that is heavily influenced by culture. Some women and children scream with pain; others remain stoic and quiet. Both are "proper" responses, just culturally different.

Cultural differences such as drinking alcohol or smoking cigarettes occur across not only different ethnic backgrounds but also different lifestyles (Wray, Jupka, Berman, et al., 2012). Adolescents, urban youth, the hearing challenged, and gay or lesbian couples have separate cultures from the mainstream and respecting these cultures is just as important as respecting ethnic differences. A parent who has been deaf since birth, for example, expects her deaf culture to be respected by having health care professionals locate a sign language interpreter for her while she is in labor. A lesbian mother might appreciate being asked, "Is your partner here?" rather than, "Is your husband here?" at a well-child visit.

Differing cultural values can be a major source of conflict between parents and children because children learn opposing values from friends and school peers. Nurses can be instrumental in helping relieve this type of conflict by always including a cultural assessment at a health care visit (Hickling, 2012). Box 3.1 shows 2020 National Health Goals that reference cultural influences on health care.

QSEN Checkpoint Question 3.1

Evidence-Based Practice

Pregnancy is such a personal experience for women; it's important to respect family traditions or cultural beliefs. To identify what characteristics women attending two prenatal clinics preferred in their caregivers, nurse researchers interviewed 22 African American women aged between 19 and 28 years who were attending prenatal care. Characteristics woman said they wanted from care providers were (a) nurses to demonstrate quality patient–provider communication, (b) compassionate care, (c) continuity of care, and (d) respect. Most importantly, they

BOX 3.1 Nursing Care Planning Based on 2020 National Health Goals

A number of 2020 National Health Goals are directly concerned with health practices that can be influenced by cultural diversity:

- Increase the proportion of pregnant women who receive early and adequate prenatal care from a baseline of 70.5% to a target of 77.6%.
- Increase the proportion of mothers who breastfeed their babies in the early postpartum period from a baseline of 43.5% to a target of 60.6%.
- Increase the proportion of healthy full-term infants who are put down to sleep on their backs from a baseline of 69.0% to a target of 75.9%.
- Increase the proportion of young children who receive all vaccines that have been recommended for universal administration from a baseline of 68% to a target of 80% (U.S. Department of Health and Human Services [DHHS], 2010; see www.healthypeople.gov).

Nurses can help the nation achieve these goals by helping design prenatal and childcare services that take into account cultural diversity and by promoting the nutritional and immunologic advantages of breastfeeding in a culturally sensitive manner.

wanted to feel as if their nurses knew them and remembered them from visit to visit (Lori, Yi, & Martyn, 2011).

Based on this study, which form of greeting would you instruct your team members to use to greet Mrs. Rodriques at a prenatal visit?

a. "How have things been going since we last spoke?"
b. "I'm happy that you were able to come in today."
c. "It's good to see you again, Mrs. Rodriques."
d. "How do you think that your baby is doing?"

Look in Appendix A for the best answer and rationale.

Nursing Process Overview
For Care That Respects Cultural Diversity

Assessment

An assessment of cultural diversity factors is important so care can be planned based not on predetermined assumptions, but on the actual preferences of a family. Remember, poverty is a major problem for many minority ethnic groups. Many characteristic responses described as cultural limitations are actually the consequences of poverty (e.g., parents seeking medical care for their children late in the course of an illness or a woman not taking prenatal vitamins during pregnancy). Solving these problems may be a question of locating adequate financial resources rather than overcoming cultural influences.

To assess clients for aspects of diversity, assess them as individuals, not as one of a group. Note particularly any cultural characteristic that differs from the usual expectations of your care setting so potential conflicts can be acknowledged and culturally competent care can be planned. Specific areas to assess, along with suggested questions to help explore these areas, are shown in Table 3.1.

TABLE 3.1 Assessing for Cultural Values

Area of Assessment	Questions to Ask or Observations to Make
Ethnicity	Where were the parents and grandparents born? What ethnicity does the family state is theirs?
Communication	What's the main language used in the home?
Touch	Does the family typically touch or hug each other? Do they mainly use intimate or conversational space?
Time	Is being on time important? Is planning for the future important?
Occupation	Is work important? Does the family plan leisure time or leave it unstructured?
Pain	Do family members express pain or remain stoic in the face of it? What do family members believe best relieves pain?
Family structure	Is the family nuclear? Extended? Single parent? Are family roles clear?
Male and female roles	Is the family male or female dominant?
Religion	What is the family's religion? Do members actively practice? Will any of their beliefs directly affect your care or their treatment?
Health beliefs	What does the family believe makes one healthy? Causes illness? Makes illness better? Do members use alternative therapies or traditional medical practices?
Nutrition	Does the family mainly eat ethnic foods? Are the foods they enjoy easily available in their community?
Community	Is the predominant culture in the community the same as the family's? Can members name a neighbor they could call on in a crisis?

Assessing the culture of a person's community is as important as assessing individuals or families, because people are intrinsically joined to their community.

If a family is of a culture other than the dominant community one, the family may have strong ties with its members but may have difficulty making strong, effective relationships in the community. This causes the family to be more isolated than it would like to be and more dependent on health care providers. The importance of community assessment is further discussed in Chapter 4.

Nursing Diagnosis

Several nursing diagnoses speak to the consequences of ignoring cultural preferences in care, including:

- Powerlessness related to expectations of care not being respected
- Impaired verbal communication related to limited English proficiency
- Imbalanced nutrition, less than daily requirements, related to unmet cultural food preferences
- Anxiety related to a cultural preference for not wanting to bathe while ill
- Fear related to possible ethnic discrimination

Outcome Identification and Planning

Planning needs to be very specific for individual families because cultural diversity preferences tend to be very personal. You might want to begin care with an in-service education for team members who are unfamiliar with a particular cultural practice and its importance to a specific family involved. You also might want to ask if your agency could change a policy to accommodate a family's cultural preferences, such as the length of visiting hours, types of food served, or type of hospital clothing provided (e.g., women from the Middle East may only feel comfortable in long-sleeved gowns and with head scarves).

This type of planning can be beneficial not only because it makes health care more acceptable to families but also because it can motivate providers to examine policies, question the rationale behind them, and initiate more diverse care. Good Web sites to use for additional information on the importance of diversity are those of the National Association of Hispanic Nurses (www.nahnnet.org), the National Black Nurses' Association (www.nbna.org), and the Transcultural Nursing Society (www.tcns.org).

Implementation

When implementing care, be certain not to force your cultural values on others. Appreciate that such values are ingrained and usually very difficult to change (in yourself as well as in others). An example of implementing care might be to make arrangements for a new Native American mother to take home the placenta after birth of her child if that is important to her, or planning home care for a Chinese American child whose family uses herbal medicine. It might be to establish a network of health care agency personnel or personnel from a nearby university or importing firm to serve as interpreters. It might be educating a child, family, or community about the reason for a hospital practice. Don't feel that you or your health care agency are always the ones who must adapt; however, a particular situation may call for both sides to adjust (cultural negotiation).

Outcome Evaluation

Assessing whether expected outcomes have been met should reveal a family's cultural diversity preferences have been considered and respected during care. If this was not achieved, procedures or policies may need to be modified until this can be realized. Examples of expected outcomes that might be established include:

- Parents list three ways they are attempting to preserve cultural traditions in their children.
- Child states she no longer feels socially isolated because of cultural differences.
- Family members state they have learned to substitute easily purchased foods for traditional, but unavailable foods to obtain adequate nutrition.
- Child with severe hearing impairment writes that he feels communication with ambulatory care staff has been adequate.

METHODS TO RESPECT DIVERSITY IN MATERNAL AND CHILD HEALTH NURSING

Cultural differences cause behavior to vary widely from one community to another. Given the multicultural mix in large communities, almost any behavior can be considered appropriate for some individuals at some time and place.

Stereotyping is expecting a person to act in a characteristic way without regard to his or her individual traits. It is generally derogatory in nature such as, "Men never diaper babies well," or "Japanese women are never assertive." The phenomenon usually occurs because of lack of exposure to people in a particular group and, consequently, a lack of understanding of the wide range of differences among people. Traditionally, a person whose culture differs most drastically from the dominant culture suffers the greatest amount of rejection or prejudice because they are least able to assimilate (Bergsieker, Leslie, Constantine, et al., 2012). In the previous examples, the first speaker, having seen one man change diapers poorly, assumes he represents the entire male population. The second speaker demonstrates lack of knowledge of a changing culture.

It's important to avoid stereotyping as it can prevent you from planning care that is accurate, individualized, and valued. At the same time, it is important not to ignore cultural characteristics in an attempt to not stereotype, because most people take pride in their cultural heritage. You can acknowledge and celebrate a client's culture without stereotyping by such actions as admiring the way a woman cooks an ethnic meal once a week to remind her family of its ethnic roots or the way a woman recites a Hispanic lullaby to "call her child outside" while in labor.

In the past, the United States was viewed as a giant cultural "melting pot," where all new arrivals gave up their native country's traditions and values and became Americans. Today, many people question the idea America ever was a melting pot; instead, the preferred concept is of a "salad bowl," in which cultural traditions and values are tossed together, but with all their individual crispness and flavor retained. Maintaining ethnic traditions this way strengthens and enriches family life. It provides security to younger family members as they realize they are one of a continuing line of people who have a past and will have a future (Fig. 3.2) (Box 3.2).

Women are often called the "keepers of the culture" or the people most influential in passing on cultural traditions from one generation to another and in honoring the many cultural traditions of childbirth and childrearing (Lauderdale, 2011).

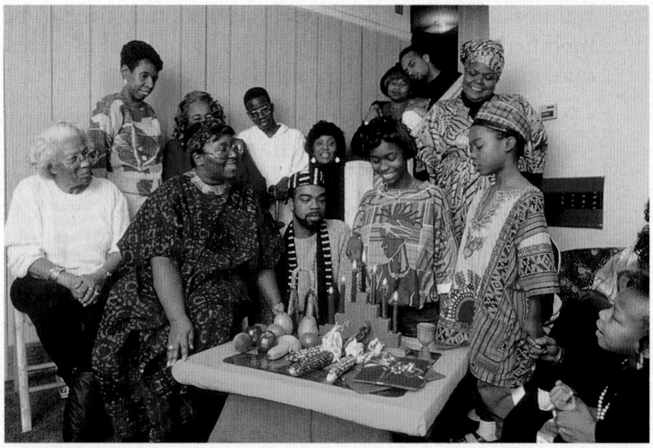

FIGURE 3.2 Cultural traditions passed from one generation to the next offer a sense of security to children.

- **Acculturation** refers to the loss of ethnic traditions because of disuse.
- Cultural **assimilation** means people blend into the general population or adopt the values of the dominant culture.
- **Ethnocentrism** is the belief one's own culture is superior to all others.

In the past, a great deal of ethnocentrism existed because many Americans were intolerant of any behavior that was not like middle-class Americans, believing the American way (which actually was the northern European way) was the "best" way. A more modern philosophy is that the world is large enough to accommodate a diversity of ideas and behaviors and that there is probably no "best" way to accomplish anything.

- **Prejudice** is a negative attitude toward members of a group or is an intellectual act.
- **Discrimination** is the action of treating people differently based on their physical or cultural traits or is a doing act.
- **Cultural awareness** is being aware cultural differences exist.
- **Cultural competence** is respecting cultural differences or diversity (Fitzpatrick, 2011).
- **Cultural humility** is a lifelong process of self-reflection and self-critique that begins, not with an assessment of a client's beliefs, but rather with an assessment of your own (Hoke & Robbins, 2011).

Learning as much as you can about different cultures by reading about or talking to members of as many different ethnic groups as possible is a good way to learn different cultural beliefs about common measures such as what makes a person well, what causes illness, how ill people should act, what ill people should eat, whether babies should wear diapers, and whether antibiotics should always be prescribed for infection. Realizing how many different opinions people hold can alert you that it may be time to begin to look at your beliefs objectively and explore whether your beliefs might need some updating (e.g., Does walking in the rain really cause colds? Does chicken soup really cure colds?)

Numerous levels of cultural intolerance or acceptance continue to persist because people continue to hold different beliefs along a cultural competence continuum (Fig. 3.3). When planning nursing care, try to not only respect these cultural differences but also help people share their cultural beliefs with health care providers so their beliefs can be considered and respected.

QSEN Checkpoint Question 3.2

Quality Improvement

While she is in the hospital, Maria Rodriques, 12 years old, makes the following statements. Which of the following most clearly suggests that she received culturally competent care?

a. "My doctor is funny; he tells jokes and makes me laugh."
b. "The nurses keep asking me who makes decisions in my family."
c. "I'm sure my leg will heal quickly; the nurse said I'm an overall healthy person."
d. "The nurse asked me what I like to eat and then brought me the taco I wanted."

Look in Appendix A for the best answer and rationale.

BOX 3.2 Nursing Care Planning Based on Family Teaching

PRESERVING A FAMILY'S CULTURAL HERITAGE

Q. Mrs. Rodriques tells you, "I'm proud of my family's ethnic traditions. What are good ways to help my family preserve these?"

A. Preserving individual heritage traditions while living in another culture calls for creative planning. Some common suggestions for doing this include:

- Plan an "ethnic night" once per week when only ethnic food is served. Encourage children to invite friends for the meal and discuss the traditions behind the various foods.
- Reserve one night per week when family members speak only the native language, if a foreign language is part of your tradition, so children come to value both languages.
- Choose books for children written by authors from your culture or that positively describe your culture. Read them together as a family and discuss the story.
- Monitor television for programs that focus positively on your culture. Watch them with your children and comment on how such traditions enrich family life.
- Speak to your children about your childhood and traditions and values at bedtime or "talk time," so they can appreciate how long these values have been revered by your family.
- Celebrate holidays in your traditional manner. Including cultural influences in holiday celebrations adds a rich ingredient and feeling of security to these occasions.

CULTURAL DESTRUCTIVENESS	CULTURAL BLINDNESS	CULTURAL AWARENESS	CULTURAL SENSITIVITY	CULTURAL COMPETENCE	CULTURAL HUMILITY
Making everyone fit the same cultural pattern, and excluding of those who don't fit—forced assimilation. Emphasis on differences as barriers.	Do not see or believe there are cultural differences among people. Everyone is the same.	Being aware that we all live and function within a culture of our own and that our identity is shaped by it.	Understanding and accepting different cultural values, attitudes, and behaviors.	The capacity to work effectively and with people, integrating elements of their culture—vocabulary, values, attitudes, rules, and norms. Translation of knowledge into action.	The lifelong process of self-reflection and self-critique that begins, not with an assessment of a client's belief, but rather an assessment of your own.

FIGURE 3.3 A cultural competence continuum.

Assessing for Diversity

Almost all nations have a set of people who are its dominant or advantaged group. They hold the greater share of wealth in the nation and hold the majority of political offices. Almost all nations also have **minority** or disadvantaged groups, groups not necessarily fewer in number, but who hold less power and wealth. When scanning a list of characteristics typically seen with people of a specific culture, remember those behaviors may not apply at all to your client. *Ask* what things are important to the individual. General categories related to the structure (composition) and function (roles and actions) of families are discussed in the following paragraphs as they may require special considerations for care.

Communication Patterns

Communication patterns (not only what people say but also how they say it) are strongly culturally influenced. People who ordinarily associate only with members of their own culture, and therefore always speak their native language, can have great difficulty detailing a health history in English when they or their child is ill because their ability to cope and to express themselves in any language when they are stressed may be at a low point (Sundararajan, Sullivan, & Chapman, 2012). Some clients prefer to consult a Chinese herbalist or a Hispanic *yerbero* or *curandero* rather than or in connection with other health care providers because they can relate health problems with no language barrier.

Children who are embarrassed or bashful about speaking another language may simply not talk at a health care visit or have a great deal of difficulty recalling the English words for symptoms such as nausea or dizziness, words not commonly taught in English as a second language class. Unless you appear receptive as a listener, a client might omit mentioning a symptom rather than try to pantomime it or describe it in a different way.

Listening to English instructions and translating them into another language is another area that can cause confusion. The statement, "I need you to wait," for example, is easy to translate as "I need your weight." The word "hallmark" translates as "mark on the hall" or graffiti.

Working with an interpreter also can cause miscommunication. General tips for working with interpreters are shown in Box 3.3. As a general rule, it is unfair to ask children to interpret for their parents because this can place a child in situations that require adult judgment and knowledge. In some cultures, it might be unacceptable for a younger person to serve as an interpreter for an older person or for a subservient woman to interpret for a dominant male because this shifts authority.

BOX 3.3 Nursing Care Planning to Empower a Family

WHEN A FAMILY HAS LIMITED ENGLISH PROFICIENCY

1. Many people can speak a second language better than they can read it. Assess each client's reading level as well as speaking level and rewrite information at an easier level if necessary.
2. Ask an interpreter to translate and copy material into the family's primary language as necessary so it can be clearly understood.
3. When using an interpreter, be certain the interpreter understands the question you are asking (e.g., Does he or she understand "malignant" and "cancer" are interchangeable words?).
4. Be certain rooms in your health care agency, such as bathrooms, are labeled with international symbols that do not require reading ability.
5. Learn a few phrases, such as "Good morning" or "This won't hurt," from other languages, and use them in interactions with clients to show you're receptive to participating in solving language difficulties.
6. Use hand gestures or draw a figure, if need be, to help ensure productive communication. Imparting health information is what is important for safe care, not worrying how you look.
7. When using an interpreter, do not ignore the person seeking health care in preference to the interpreter. Observe facial expressions for confirmation that a person understands instructions. Use short sentences; avoid slang words that don't interpret accurately.

When caring for patients who speak a different dialect or language than your own, always ask them to repeat your instruction to be certain it was interpreted correctly. Repeat what the patient said so he or she can confirm you understood correctly. Don't be reluctant to ask for an interpreter to help clarify forms, such as informed consent for surgery or wishes regarding right-to-life care, as necessary.

Communication problems arise not only from foreign languages but also from differences within a country. Some people gesture wildly to express any topic; others rarely raise their hands. Something as simple as a New Englander adding an "r" sound to the end of words (saying "idear" instead of "idea") can make an explanation difficult to follow. The slow cadence of a person from the South may seem strange to someone who is used to the rapid speech pattern of New York City residents. Inner-city residents often speak a dialect unique to their area. To care for such clients, learn their dialect's cadence and common words but don't attempt to use them yourself, unless that is your dialect. Trying to speak in a dialect not your own could be misinterpreted as mockery.

Tattoos are another cause of misunderstanding (Karacaoglan, 2012). These generally symbolize an important event in the person's life. Respecting these is yet another way to assure a person you respect them even though body adornments may not be a value you share.

Touch, such as whether to greet another person with a kiss or a hug, is a form of communication and so is culturally determined. Some people don't like to be hugged. Some prefer to bow in contrast to shaking hands. Some Asian Americans feel rumpling the hair or palpating fontanelles is an intrusive gesture because they believe the head is the seat of the body's spirit and should not be touched (Andrews, 2011b).

Whether people look at one another when talking is also culturally determined. Chinese Americans, for example, may not make eye contact during a conversation. This social custom shows respect for the position of the health care professional and is a compliment, not an avoidance issue.

Be certain cultural variations are as respected in written communications as they are in oral communications. In many instances, written communication is even more problematic than oral communication because many people can speak a second language but cannot write or read it. Using short, easy sentences and being certain not to use words with double meanings when writing instructions for patients are important techniques (Box 3.4).

What if . . . 3.1 When you talk to Mrs. Rodriques, you realize she is pregnant but hasn't gone for prenatal care as yet. She states before coming to the clinic she wants to visit a *yerbero* who will both predict her child's sex and guarantee a safe birth. Would recommending she have a sonogram (which also could predict the fetal sex) be likely as satisfying for her?

BOX 3.4 Nursing Care Planning Based on Effective Communication

Anna Rodriques, Maria's mother, brings her 4-year-old son to your pediatric clinic because she thinks he has an ear infection. Because she speaks little English, she has brought a neighbor as an interpreter.

Less Effective Communication

Nurse: What's the reason you're here today, Mrs. Rodriques?
Neighbor: She thinks her son has an ear infection.
Nurse: Is he pulling or tugging at it?
Neighbor: Not that I've seen.
Nurse: Does he have any pain?
Neighbor: She hasn't said anything about that.
Nurse: Well, I'll take his temperature, but I doubt it's an infection.

More Effective Communication

Nurse: What's the reason you're here today, Mrs. Rodriques?
Neighbor: She thinks her son has an ear infection.
Nurse: Ask if he has been pulling or tugging at it.
Neighbor: I haven't seen him doing that.
Nurse: Would you ask his mother if she has seen him doing that?

[The neighbor addresses Anna and then reports back.]

Neighbor: She says he's been pulling at it all morning.
Nurse: Would you ask Jose if he has any pain?

[The neighbor addresses the child and then reports back.]

Neighbor: He says yes. His ear hurts.
Nurse: Those are symptoms of an ear infection, all right. *To interpreter:* After the nurse practitioner sees him, I'm going to ask you to help me write out some instructions in Spanish that Jose's mother will need to follow.

Effectively using an interpreter adds additional responsibility to history taking. The nurse in the first scenario asked her first question of the mother but then directed all other questions to the interpreter. This means she secured a secondary history. When using an interpreter, be certain the interpreter is "interpreting," not giving the history.

Use of Conversational Space

People of different cultures use the space around them differently.

- *Intimate space* is the space closely surrounding a person. Physical examinations are conducted in this very tight space because palpation and auscultation are parts of the examination.
- Conversational space is usually 18 in. to 4 ft away.
- Beyond 4 ft is *business space*, as this amount of distance allows room for a desk between parties.
- *Public space* is any distance beyond business space such as shouting across a parking lot. Use of the Internet or telephone can vary from private space ("I have a secret to tell you") to public space (conversation in a chat room).

Everyone has had the uncomfortable experience of speaking to someone who moves closer to him or her than expected or invades his or her intimate space while talking. Likewise, everyone has had someone shout something he or she wanted to be kept confidential (violation of public space). Being aware that the use of space can vary from person to person helps you to respect the use of space for clients when giving health instructions.

Respect for modesty is another way to respect a client's space. Be aware that women from Middle Eastern cultures adhere to a level of modesty exceeding what you may appreciate, so it's a courtesy to add additional modesty sheets for physical examinations.

QSEN Checkpoint Question 3.3

Teamwork & Collaboration

Maria Rodriques is a 12-year-old student. What advice should you provide to an unlicensed care provider about communicating effectively with Maria?

a. "Speak in a clear and natural tone when you're talking with Maria."
b. "Maria is Hispanic, so avoid talking about current children's movies."
c. "Maria's first language is Spanish, so avoid talking about difficult topics."
d. "If possible, try to speak to Maria in an accent that's similar to hers."

Look in Appendix A for the best answer and rationale.

Time Orientation

The cultural pattern in the United States is geared toward punctuality regarding appointments. "Time is money" is an often-quoted axiom. In some South Asian cultures, however, the use of time contrasts greatly—being late for appointments is a sign of respect (giving the person you are meeting time to organize and be prepared for your arrival). Other cultures believe time is to be enjoyed. For such a person, there is no such thing as wasted time.

Women who do not have a strict time orientation may have difficulty following a strict medical regimen. If they are told, for example, to give a child a medication at 8 AM, noon, and 6 PM daily and to return for another appointment at 2 PM in a week's time, you may need to stress that the medication should be taken three times a day, not necessarily at the specific times, but returning for a checkup at a set time is important because their primary health care provider is only available at that time.

Another way time orientation differs is in whether a culture concentrates on the past, the present, or the future. The dominant U.S. culture is oriented to the present and future. People are expected to not only take care of themselves in the present but also make plans for the future. Other cultures are oriented toward the past: they carefully preserve traditions, allowing only the slightest changes or variations in practices. Still others are oriented toward the present; saving money for college (a future-oriented action) might seem important to you but would not be a high priority in these cultures.

If a family's orientation is for the present or the past, members may have difficulty accepting a long-term rehabilitation plan. They may need to be motivated by indications of progress (e.g., last week all their child could do was sit up; today, he was able to walk two or three steps).

People with strong religious convictions may be future oriented (looking forward to a future existence better than their present one on Earth). The Amish and some Native Americans are examples of past-oriented cultures: they adhere to time-honored traditions that do not include technologic advances. People from lower socioeconomic groups tend to be present oriented because the struggle just to get through each day limits them to the present. People with different time orientations tend to make different health care decisions based on their outlook (Boyle, 2011).

QSEN Checkpoint Question 3.4

Safety

Maria tells you she rates the pain she has from bruising as 5 on a 10-point scale. You offer to bring her a tablet of acetaminophen (Tylenol). Her grandmother produces a packet of herbs from her purse and tells you, "Good. I'll give her a family remedy along with that." What would be the best culturally respectful response?

a. "Wonderful. I'm sure herbs will complement what your doctor prescribed."
b. "I wouldn't bother with that. Drugs are much more likely to be effective."
c. "Good. I understand you people often use home cures for many things."
d. "Let's check first to be certain the herbs won't cause an interaction."

Look in Appendix A for the best answer and rationale.

Work and School Orientation

The predominant culture in the United States stresses that all adults should be employed productively (called the Protestant work ethic) and that work should be a pleasure and valued in itself (i.e., as important as the product of the work). Other cultures do not value work in itself but see it as only a means to an end (i.e., you work to get money or food, not satisfaction).

Suppose a pregnant woman you care for has been told she must be at home on bed rest for the remainder of her pregnancy? It's easy to think she will be most concerned about having to take a leave from her job as a grade school teacher. A woman without a strong work orientation, however, might be more distressed because she can no longer continue her favorite past time (going to baseball games). This is why asking what is important to people is necessary to appreciate this type of cultural or individual variation.

Because people in the United States are expected to work, they also are expected to finish school so they can learn an occupation and support themselves for their adult life—another value that is not stressed in all cultures. Work orientation has expanded to include using leisure time effectively, such as for exercising or learning a new skill rather than just passively watching television. An assessment can reveal differences in what people prefer to do during their leisure time and also the effect this can have on their overall health, for example, if sufficient exercise and a curb on eating saturated fats aren't included (Bloemers, Collard, Paw, et al., 2012).

✔ QSEN Checkpoint Question 3.5

Informatics

You are including Maria's nursing care plan with her discharge instructions so a visiting community nurse can make her change from reduced activity to full sports participation as seamless as possible. Which of the following aspects of her care planning could be regarded as an act of discrimination?

a. Document the fact that Maria's mother is responsible for making most of the family's decisions.
b. Caution against Maria's participation in the local soccer league because she is unlikely to fit in.
c. Add to her electronic health record a list of foods Maria does not eat because of her preference for Mexican-American dishes.
d. Document the fact that Maria's priest plays an important role in the family's spiritual life.

Look in Appendix A for the best answer and rationale.

Family Structure

The way families structure themselves and the roles family members play are yet a further area of lifestyle that is culturally determined. In most cultures, the nuclear family (mother, father, and children) is most common. In other cultures, extended families (nuclear family plus grandparents, aunts, uncles, and cousins) and single-parent families (one parent and children) may be more desired or common.

Some cultures stress that family boundaries should be carefully guarded or information about a family should not be given freely at health care visits (a way of keeping the family intact and unique and perhaps also as a reflection of mistrust of outside influences). Other families willingly share the same information. When caring for children, be certain to identify a child's primary caregiver before asking what the child likes or giving health care instructions because which family member cares for the child can vary by culture.

Male and Female Roles

In most cultures, the man is the dominant figure. In a strongly male-dominant culture, if approval for hospital admission or therapy is needed, the man would be the one to give this approval. A woman might be unable to offer an opinion of her own health or be too embarrassed to submit to a physical examination from a male health care provider unless a female nurse was also present. A woman's pregnancy may have resulted, not from a mutual decision, but from sexual relations she felt she could not refuse (Brownridge, Taillieu, Tyler, et al., 2011). The incidence of intimate partner violence may be higher in male-dominant cultures and may rise even higher with pregnancy (Weeks & Leblanc, 2011). See Chapter 55 for an in-depth discussion of intimate partner violence and how it increases with any type of stress situation.

As a contrast, in some cultures, women are the dominant person in their family. The oldest woman in the home may be the one to give consent for treatment or hospital admission.

Evaluating male and female roles this way can help you understand the impact of illness on a family. If a woman is the family's dominant person and can no longer make her usual decisions because she is ill during pregnancy, for example, the entire family can be thrown into confusion. If the woman is a nondominant member, you may have to act as an advocate for her with a more dominant partner (Luce, Redmer, Gideonsen, et al., 2011).

What if...3.2 Mr. Rodriques says he wants no role in labor when his wife has her new baby. Would you encourage him to time contractions (a typical role for fathers) or allow him to sit quietly in a corner of the room as he prefers?

Religion

There are wide variations in religious practices, and many of these are culturally determined. Because religion guides a person's overall life philosophy, it influences how people feel about health and illness, what foods they eat, and their preferences about birth and death rituals (Sternthal, Williams, Musick, et al., 2012). Knowing which religion a family practices can help you locate the correct religious support person if one is needed. It helps in planning care if you know a woman or adolescent wants a time or times set aside daily for private prayer or if they intend to fast, such as during Ramadan. It guides implementation because many practices, such as whether the family eats meat, what and when holidays are celebrated, whether ill newborns should be baptized, and what clothing is proper to wear in public are all dictated by religious beliefs. It also can have important implications for decision making during a difficult pregnancy or for childhood terminal care.

Health Beliefs

Even health beliefs are not universal. For example, most people are familiar with the current controversy about whether male circumcision is necessary. More surprising to many people is the belief that, in some cultures, female circumcision (amputation of the clitoris and perhaps a portion of the vulva) is practiced (Mswela, 2010).

The cause of illness is another area strongly culturally influenced. People in developed countries, for example, understand that illness is caused by documented factors such as bacteria, viruses, or trauma. In other cultures, illness may be viewed primarily as a punishment from God, the effect of an evil spirit, or as the work of a person who wishes harm to the sick person.

People who believe their own sins caused an illness may not be highly motivated to take medication or other measures to get well again since they do not believe penicillin can cure them. People with such beliefs may receive more comfort from a spiritualist or counselor than from their primary health care provider. Another consequence may be reluctance to ask for pain medication if they believe the pain is necessary to be rid of the illness. Understanding different beliefs of this kind allows you to better work out mutual goals even when opposing beliefs are present. Box 3.5 shows an interprofessional care map illustrating how compromise may be necessary in both nursing and team planning in order to respect cultural diversity.

Pregnancy is an area where illness concepts vary widely, as women's concepts of whether pregnancy is a time of wellness or illness and whether breastfeeding is a desired choice differ a great deal across the world (Robinson, & VandeVusse, 2011). Most American women, for example, visit health care facilities early in pregnancy, follow prenatal directives, and at birth, allow a health care provider to supervise the birth. In other cultures, pregnancy and childbearing are considered such natural processes that a health care provider is unnecessary. The woman knows the special rules and taboos she must follow to ensure a safe birth and depends on close friends rather than health care providers to guide her safely through labor and birth. She may plan to breastfeed until the next child is born, or for as long as 5 years. Unless differences such as these are respected, it is difficult to plan prenatal or newborn care that meets individual women's needs.

The type of therapy people choose to restore health is also dependent on culture. When a parent notices a child has an upper respiratory infection, for example, he or she may immediately call a health care provider for a formal prescription. Another parent will depend on an herbal or "natural" self-help method. Be aware when taking health histories that many people today from all cultures rely on complementary or alternative therapies. Knowing about these is a way to be certain a medication that has been prescribed will not counteract or be synergistic with what herbs are being used (Pilkington & Boshnakova, 2012).

What if . . . 3.3 The Rodriques family tells you they believe the accident that caused Maria's broken leg was "God's will," not Maria's fault? Would it be appropriate to educate Maria about street safety, or would doing so interfere with the family's cultural beliefs?

Nutrition Practices

Foods and their methods of preparation are yet another area strongly related to culture. In many instances, children cannot find any food on a hospital menu that appeals to them because of cultural likes or dislikes. A typical Japanese diet, for example, includes many vegetables such as bean sprouts, broccoli, mushrooms, water chestnuts, and alfalfa. Both children and adults with this preference tire quickly of the macaroni and cheese that is common to a middle-class American menu. Fortunately, in most instances, a family member can provide food that is appealing culturally and is still within prescribed dietary limitations.

When counseling a woman about nutrition during pregnancy, remember that respect for culturally preferred foods is important (Higginbottom, Vallianatos, Forgeron, et al., 2011). People from other cultures, for example, tend to eat much less meat than those from the United States. Adequate protein is ingested, however, by mixing sources of incomplete protein such as beans and rice. Some women may omit various foods during pregnancy because they believe a particular food will mark a baby (eating strawberries will cause birthmarks, eating raisins will cause brown spots), or they believe it is necessary to eat "hot" or "cold" foods to ensure optimal fetal growth. Pregnancy is usually considered a "hot" condition, so it may be difficult for a woman who is trying to eat only "cold" foods to agree to increase her intake of meat, usually considered a "hot" food. Asian women may believe in a similar pattern of required balances (yin and yang).

Before beginning nutrition counseling, try to learn what the dominant type of food that is stocked in stores in the community of your health care agency because women who cannot buy the foods you recommend in their own neighborhood may not eat well because of the inconvenience (and increased cost) involved in shopping elsewhere (Fig. 3.4).

An ethnically determined trait present in many people is lactose intolerance. This condition is the absence of lactase, the enzyme that breaks down the sugar (lactose) in milk to the state where the sugar can be used by the body. People with lactose intolerance (including many Asians and African Americans) develop diarrhea and stomach cramps when they drink milk or milk products because of the unprocessed lactose (Chong, Bunn, & Newland, 2011).

It is important for pregnant women to ingest adequate calcium, but be certain not to advise a woman who is lactose intolerant to drink milk as her main source of calcium. Women can instead obtain calcium through pills or eating other foods high in calcium, such as dark green vegetables. Buying lactose-free milk (soy based) or adding a lactase additive to milk so lactose can be utilized are yet other suggestions.

Celiac disease is a genetically acquired illness where children and adults are allergic to gluten, a protein found in wheat, barley, and rye and is seen in some populations more than others (Zannini, Jones, Renzetti, et al., 2012). Consuming a gluten-free diet is necessary for these individuals to avoid gastrointestinal symptoms such as diarrhea and intestinal pain. Gluten-free foods are not necessary for people without celiac disease, do not cause weight loss, and are not the best food choices (Pietzak, 2012).

QSEN Checkpoint Question 3.6

Patient-Centered Care

Maria, 12 years old, tells you she never eats peanut butter because her mother has warned her against it. Because peanut butter can be a good source of protein, how should you best respond to her?

a. "Almost everyone in America eats peanut butter when they're young."
b. "Your mother's wrong; at 12, you should learn the truth about foods."
c. "I understand. I don't like the taste of peanut butter either."
d. "Let's look at your menu and pick out something you would like to eat."

Look in Appendix A for the best answer and rationale.

- *Stereotyping* is expecting a person to act in a characteristic way without regard to his or her individual traits. *Prejudice* is *thinking* people are different in some way. *Discrimination* involves *treating* people differently based on their physical or cultural traits.
- Each culture differs to some degree from every other. Most people are proud of these differences or cultural traits.
- Cultural practices usually arise from environmental conditions and are transmitted by both formal and informal ways from generation to generation.
- Although cultural concepts adapt from time to time, they tend to remain constant among tight-knit populations.
- There is wide variation within a culture concerning values and actions, because individuals make up the group and individually express their cultural heritage.
- People bring cultural values and beliefs to nursing interactions, and these affect nursing and health care.
- Cultural aspects that are important to assess are communication patterns; use of conversational space; response to pain; time, work, and family orientation; and social organization including nutrition, family roles, and health beliefs.
- Considering cultural diversity when caring for a family not only meets QSEN competencies but best meets the family's total needs.

Critical Thinking Care Study

Rhea Bhaskar is a 32-year-old woman, 20 weeks pregnant, whom you meet at a prenatal clinic. She works as a computer programmer for a wicker import company. She has a 12-year-old daughter from a previous marriage. She has been married to Siddharth, who sells real estate for 6 months. Rhea is concerned because they have just moved to a new community and her daughter (whose father was African American) "hates" their new house and her new school; she also feels as if she "doesn't fit in." She no longer likes to eat at home because Rhea has begun using Indian spices, such as curry, when she cooks to please her new husband. Rhea asks you if cooking more "soul food" the way she used to would make her daughter feel more like part of her family and new community. Rhea is also not pleased with her prenatal clinic; when she said she wanted rhubarb tea as her only fluid to drink during labor, wanted silence during the birth, and to keep her placenta to be turned into capsules for her to take afterward, the charge nurse told her she could not give her the placenta as that would be against infection rules and rhubarb tea wasn't on their list of approved beverages.

1. Rhea is trying to integrate two cultures. Will changing only one thing, such as preparing food differently, make a difference in how her 12-year-old feels about fitting in with their new lifestyle? What are other suggestions you might make to help her daughter adapt to a new family lifestyle?
2. Was the nurse accurate when she said taking a placenta home would be against infection guidelines? Were Rhea's other requests so difficult to carry out that a birth center couldn't adapt to meet them?
3. Rhea's daughter feels she's different than other children at her school. What ideas could you suggest to Rhea to help her daughter better adjust to her new school and community?

Patient Scenario

The Whitefeather Family

Read about the Whitefeather family, a family with cultural concerns, then answer the questions to further sharpen your skills and grow more familiar with NCLEX-type questions related to cultural diversity. Confirm your answers are correct by reading the rationales.

Visit http://thePoint.lww.com

Answers and Rationales

Looking for answers to the What If. . . and Critical Thinking Care Study questions?

Visit http://thePoint.lww.com

References

Andrews, M. M. (2011a). Theoretical foundations of transcultural nursing. In M. M. Andrews & J. S. Boyle (Eds.), *Transcultural concepts in nursing care* (pp. 3–14). Philadelphia, PA: Lippincott Williams & Wilkins.

Andrews, M. M. (2011b). Culturally competent nursing care. In M. M. Andrews & J. S. Boyle (Eds.), *Transcultural concepts in nursing care* (pp. 15–33). Philadelphia, PA: Lippincott Williams & Wilkins.

Bergsieker, H. B., Leslie, L. M., Constantine, V. S., et al. (2012). Stereotyping by omission: Eliminate the negative, accentuate the positive. *Journal of Personality & Social Psychology, 102*(6), 1214–1238.

Bloemers, F., Collard, D., Paw, M. C., et al. (2012). Physical inactivity is a risk factor for physical activity-related injuries in children. *British Journal of Sports Medicine, 46*(9), 669–674.

Boyle, J. S. (2011). Culture, family & community. In M. M. Andrews & J. S. Boyle (Eds.), *Transcultural concepts in nursing care* (pp. 261–296). Philadelphia, PA: Lippincott Williams & Wilkins.

Brownridge, D. A., Taillieu, T. L., Tyler, K. A., et al. (2011). Pregnancy and intimate partner violence: Risk factors, severity, and health effects. *Violence Against Women, 17*(7), 858–881.

Chen, Y. C., Wei, S. H., Yeh, K. W., et al. (2013). Learning strengths from cultural differences: A comparative study of maternal health-related behaviors and infant care among Southern Asian immigrants and Taiwanese women. *BMC International Health & Human Rights, 13*(1), 5-6.

Chong, C. K., Bunn, J., & Newland, P. (2011). Lactose intolerance in infants. *Archives of Disease in Childhood, 96*(6), 611.

Diekema, D. S. (2012). Improving childhood vaccination rates. *New England Journal of Medicine, 366*(5), 391–393.

Fitzpatrick, J. J. (2011). Extending our understanding of cultural competence in nursing education. *Nursing Education Perspectives, 32*(6), 359.

Fortier, M. A., Wahi, A., Maurer, E. L., et al. (2012). Attitudes regarding analgesic use and pain expression in parents of children with cancer. *Journal of Pediatric Hematology/Oncology, 34*(4), 257–262.

Giger, J. N. (2012). *Transcultural nursing: Assessment and intervention* (6th ed.). New York, NY: Elsevier.

Hickling, F. W. (2012). Understanding patients in multicultural settings: A personal reflection on ethnicity and culture in clinical practice. *Ethnicity & Health, 17*(1–2), 203–216.

Higginbottom, G. M., Vallianatos, H., Forgeron, J., et al. (2011). Food choices and practices during pregnancy of immigrant and aboriginal women in Canada: A study protocol. *BMC Pregnancy & Childbirth, 7*(11), 100.

Hoke, M. M., & Robbins, L. K. (2011). Continuing the cultural competency journey through exploration of knowledge, attitudes, and skills with advanced practice psychiatric nursing students: An exemplar. *Nursing Clinics of North America, 46*(2), 201–205.

Karacaoglan, U. (2012). Tattoo and taboo: On the meaning of tattoos in the analytic process. *International Journal of Psychoanalysis, 93*(1), 5–28.

Lauderdale, J. (2011). Transcultural perspectives in childbearing. In M. M. Andrews & J. S. Boyle (Eds.), *Transcultural concepts in nursing care* (pp. 85–115). Philadelphia, PA: Lippincott Williams & Wilkins.

Lewallen, L. P. (2011). The importance of culture in childbearing. *Journal of Obstetrics, Gynecology & Neonatal Nursing, 40*(1), 4–8.

Lori, J. R., Yi, C. H., & Martyn, K. K. (2011). Provider characteristics desired by African American women in prenatal care. *Journal of Transcultural Nursing, 22*(1), 71–76.

Luce, H., Redmer, J., Gideonsen, M., et al. (2011). Culturally specific maternity care in Wisconsin. *Wisconsin Medical Journal, 110*(1), 32–37.

Mswela, M. (2010). Female genital mutilation: Medico-legal issues. *Medical Law Review, 29*(4), 523–536.

Pietzak, M. (2012). Celiac disease, wheat allergy, and gluten sensitivity: When gluten free is not a fad. *Journal of Parenteral & Enteral Nutrition, 36*(1, Suppl.), 68S–75S.

Pilkington, K., & Boshnakova, A. (2012). Complementary medicine and safety. *Complementary Therapeutic Medicine, 20*(1–2), 73–82.

Robinson, K. M., & VandeVusse, L. (2011). African American women's infant feeding choices: Prenatal breast-feeding self-efficacy and narratives from a black feminist perspective. *Journal of Perinatal & Neonatal Nursing, 25*(4), 320–328.

Sternthal, M. J., Williams, D. R., Musick, M. A., et al. (2012). Religious practices, beliefs, and mental health: Variations across ethnicity. *Ethnicity & Health, 17*(1–2), 171–185.

Sundararajan, K., Sullivan, T. S., & Chapman, M. (2012). Determinants of family satisfaction in the intensive care unit. *Anaesthesia and Intensive Care, 40*(1), 159–165.

U.S. Department of Health and Human Services. (2010). *Healthy people 2020.* Washington, DC: Author.

Weeks, L. E., & Leblanc, K. (2011). An ecological synthesis of research on older women's experiences of intimate partner violence. *Journal of Women Aging, 23*(4), 283–304.

Wray, R. J., Jupka, K., Berman, S., et al. (2012). Young adults' perceptions about established and emerging tobacco products. *Nicotine & Tobacco Research, 14*(2), 184–190.

Zannini, E., Jones, J. M., Renzetti, S., et al. (2012). Functional replacements for gluten. *Annual Review of Food Science & Technology, 3*(10), 227–245.

Chapter 4

The Childbearing and Childrearing Family in the Community

KEY TERMS

- community
- direct care
- home care
- hospice care
- indirect care
- skilled home nursing care

OBJECTIVES

After mastering the contents of this chapter, you should be able to:

1. Describe what constitutes a healthy community and the usual nursing and client concerns when home care is required during pregnancy or childhood.
2. Identify 2020 National Health Goals related to home care during pregnancy and childhood that nurses can help the nation achieve.
3. Assess a pregnant woman or child and their community for likely success with home care.
4. Formulate nursing diagnoses related to care of a child or pregnant client at home.
5. Identify expected outcomes for a family requiring home care as well as help manage seamless transitions across differing health care settings.
6. Using the nursing process, plan nursing care that includes the six competencies of Quality & Safety Education for Nurses (QSEN): Patient-Centered Care, Teamwork & Collaboration, Evidence-Based Practice (EBP), Quality Improvement (QI), Safety, and Informatics.
7. Implement nursing care to meet the needs of a pregnant woman or child on home care such as teaching techniques of intravenous therapy or suggesting ways to keep in contact with significant others.
8. Evaluate outcome criteria for achievement and effectiveness of nursing care to be certain expected outcomes have been achieved.
9. Integrate knowledge of home care with the interplay of nursing process, the six competencies of QSEN, and Family Nursing to promote quality maternal and child health nursing care.

Lisa Puente, a 16-year-old, is 20 weeks pregnant. She was admitted to the hospital for 3 days at 14 weeks of her pregnancy and placed on a program of gastrostomy feedings because she'd been losing weight from vomiting at least four times daily since the beginning of pregnancy. Her condition improved until last week when her blood pressure rose to 160/90 mmHg and she was diagnosed with gestational hypertension. She was placed on bed rest with fetal and uterine surveillance at home. She tells you it's impossible for her to rest at home: she's bored with school assignments and her friends (and boyfriend) no longer visit. You notice she's missed at least three doses of her hypotensive agent. She asks to be hospitalized again for care.

Previous chapters discussed common types of families and how cultural traditions affect families. This chapter adds information about families and their community as they prepare to care for an ill family member at home.

Is Lisa a good candidate for home care? What additional interventions would she need to make home care more successful?

BOX 4.1 Nursing Care Planning Based on 2020 National Health Goals

National Health Goals are concerned with eliminating common infectious diseases of childhood and reducing complications of pregnancy. These measures are important because both eliminating common infections and complications of pregnancy could reduce the hours spent in home care.

- Increase to at least 77% the proportion of all pregnant women who receive early and adequate prenatal care, from a baseline of 70.5%.
- Reduce the rate of preterm births, from a baseline of 12.7% to a target of 11.4%
- Reduce or eliminate vaccine-preventable diseases such as measles (from 115 to 30 cases per year); pertussis (from 2,777 to 2,500 cases per year); varicella (chickenpox) (from 482,535 to 100,000 cases per year); and keep poliomyelitis at zero cases per year (U.S. Department of Health and Human Services [DHHS], 2010; see www.Healthypeople.gov).

Nurses can help the nation achieve these goals by helping women better accept and adhere to home care if it is advised during pregnancy. They can remind parents how important it is to have children routinely immunized so children no longer contract "childhood infections."

Home care, as the name suggests, is care of persons in their homes, provided or supervised by a certified home health care or community health care agency. In recent years, as hospital stays have decreased in length, the periods of needing home care have grown substantially.

Postsurgical children or those recovering from an acute illness are often candidates for follow-up home care. It is well documented that women who receive prenatal care have better pregnancy outcomes than those who don't (Bernstein & VanBuren, 2013). Because home care can be a means of increasing personalized prenatal surveillance and initiating specific health teaching, pregnant women who need these added measures are also good home care candidates (Olander, Atkinson, Edmunds et al., 2012). Many children in terminal stages of disease are also cared for at home (**hospice care**).

Assessing and orienting families to home care, making home visits, supervising and coordinating home health personnel, providing health teaching, and evaluating whether home care remains appropriate are all important nursing responsibilities. Box 4.1 shows 2020 National Health Goals that speak to home care.

Nursing Process Overview

For the Pregnant Woman or Child on Home Care

Assessment

Being able to assess communities as well as families is important. Today's short hospital stays have caused both pregnant women and ill children to spend more time at home recuperating from illnesses than ever before. The average patient who will be scheduled for home care is first seen in an ambulatory or acute health care setting for initial diagnosis and then discharged with a referral to a home care program. Assessing the total family is important to be certain home care will match a family's usual self-care or childrearing practices.

Nursing Diagnosis

Nursing diagnoses for home care may address the physiologic reason for supervised home care or the effect of the experience on the family, such as:

- Deficient knowledge related to complication of pregnancy and necessary procedures and treatments needed
- Interrupted family processes related to need for home care
- Ineffective role performance related to bed rest at home
- Social isolation related to the need for home care
- Anxiety related to complication of pregnancy, which has required home care

Home care of a child can place a heavy burden on a family as the stress of being responsible for an ill child's daily health status can have a negative impact on a parent's self-esteem or a couple's marriage; it can prevent parents from spending time with their other children or each other. Examples of possible nursing diagnoses that arise out of these factors include:

- Readiness for enhanced family coping related to increased time together because of home care
- Health-seeking behaviors related to skills needed to continue home care
- Risk for delayed growth and development related to lack of usual childhood activities
- Interrupted family processes related to dependence of ill child
- Disabled family coping related to changes in family routine brought about by home care needs of ill child

Outcome Identification and Planning

Both outcome identification and planning for home care require close collaboration between the health care providers supervising care at home and the family experiencing home care. A major portion of this involves reviewing with a family exactly what their needs are, what will be expected of them, what they can expect of the nurse, and developing outcomes that address these needs and expectations. Good Internet referral sites for families regarding home care are The International Association for Hospice & Palliative Care (www.hospicecare.com), The National Association for Home Care and Hospice (www.nahc.org), and the Home Health Nurses Association (www.hhna.org). Individual cities may also provide other local organizations that can be helpful to families on home care such as Women, Infants & Children (WIC) (supplies food for qualifying children as well as women during pregnancy) and Literacy Volunteers (offers help to increase reading levels so families can better understand health care directions or increase their health literacy).

Implementation

Women and children receiving home care have the advantage over those hospitalized of being in their own environment with their families and not confined in a distant place. Because home care providers may only visit intermittently, however, there is the disadvantage of patients not being constantly supervised. Both women and children may need assurance that their condition is not changing so it is safe for them to remain at home on their present program. If changes do occur, introducing new interventions, evaluating their effectiveness, and suggesting changes will be necessary.

Interventions performed for a client at home, ranging from teaching and counseling to hands-on care, are little different from those performed in an acute care facility. In order to do all these tasks, home care nurses need to have the same background and level of expertise as acute care nurses. In addition, they need to be extremely flexible because each home visit may be very different from the one just before or after.

Nursing interventions for home care often involve not only giving care but also teaching family members how to give care. This may include encouraging members to voice the frustration they feel at being constantly confined at home or what they perceive to be a lack of progress in their child's or partner's condition. If a child has a terminal illness, parents may need support to express their grief. They can grow discouraged because the work they are accomplishing is making the child comfortable but is not preventing death.

Outcome Evaluation

Because a home setting is less structured than a health care facility, an evaluation will show some goals for care, such as bed rest, are more difficult to accomplish in the home; at the same time, because there is more individual care and room for innovation at home, goals involving patient teaching can be more easily accomplished. The evaluation may reveal circumstances, such as the client requires more monitoring than originally believed, demands are greater than the family is able to undertake, or a family's composition has changed, making a responsible caregiver no longer available.

The outcome evaluation for the pregnant woman receiving home care includes determining whether the woman and her fetus are remaining well at home and whether the woman feels comfortable and secure with the arrangement. For many women, successful home care will mean the difference between too early a birth and a successful term pregnancy.

Examples of outcome criteria for pregnant women could include:

- Client demonstrates adequate skill at performing home monitoring procedures.
- Client verbalizes changes in condition she will need to report to her health care provider.
- Client participates as a member of the family within limitations imposed by pregnancy complication.
- Family members state they have adjusted to home care of mother.
- Client states she is able to maintain contact with friends and family despite complete bed rest at home.

Examples of outcome criteria for an ill child might include:

- Parents state they have been able to make adjustments to accommodate care of an ill child at home.
- Child states he or she enjoys respite care in hospice setting one weekend per month.
- Parents state they are actively trying to supply adequate growth experiences for siblings in light of home care of oldest child.

THE FAMILY AS PART OF A COMMUNITY

Families rarely live alone on islands; instead, they are a part of and interact with their surrounding community to buy food, use transportation, and receive wages for work (Jilcott, Vu, Morgan, et al., 2012). A **community** can be defined in many ways, but it is generally accepted to refer to a group of individuals interacting within a limited geographic area (Allender, 2013). When asked what community they are from, people may mention an entire city, a school district, a geographic district (e.g., "the East Side"), a street name (e.g., "Pine Street area"), or a natural marking (e.g., "the Lower Creek area").

Because the health of individuals is influenced by the health of their community, it is important to become acquainted with the community in which you practice or where a specific client lives. A community assessment can reveal if there are aspects about the community that contributed to a person's illness (and therefore need to be corrected). It also helps determine whether a person will be able to return to their community without extra help and counseling after recovering from an illness (Fig. 4.1).

Knowing the individual aspects of a community also helps you understand why some people reach the illness level they do before they come for health care (e.g., a woman living in a rural area has no transportation to prenatal care until her husband comes home from work, a 5-year-old child develops measles because there are no free immunization services in his community).

Community assessment consists of examining the various systems that are present in almost all communities to see whether they are functioning adequately. For example, it is easier for you to prepare a woman or child for return to a

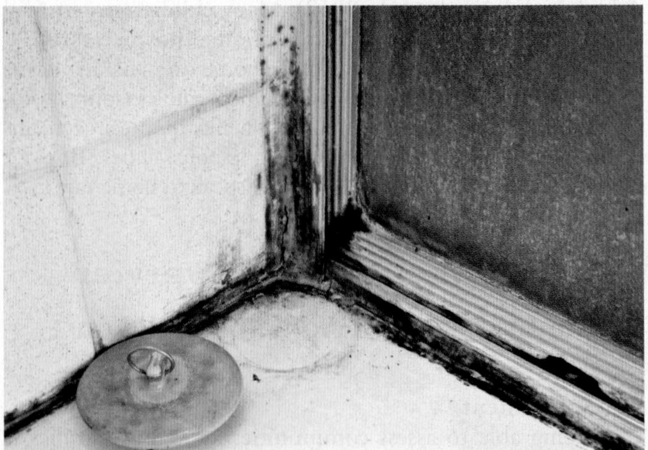

FIGURE 4.1 Community assessment reveals unsafe conditions that can lead to illness, such as mold (© fotosearch.com).

TABLE 4.1 Assessing a Community

Area of Assessment	Questions to Ask
Age span	Is the community a "young," a "settled-in," or a "retired" one? Is the family within the usual age span of residents in the community and thereby assured of support people?
Education	If the family has school-age children, are there schools nearby? Is there a public library for self-education? Is there easy access to such places if the person becomes physically challenged? If a special program such as diet counseling is needed, does it exist?
Environment	Are environmental risks present, such as air pollution? Busy highways? Train yards? Pools of water where drowning could occur? Could hypothermia be a problem?
Financial status	Is there a high rate of unemployment in the community, which could increase the crime rate? What is the average occupation? Will this family have adequate finances to manage comfortably in this neighborhood? Are supplemental aid programs available?
Health care	Is there a health care agency the family can use for comprehensive care? Is it convenient, in terms of finances, time, and transportation? Is it handicapped accessible?
Housing	Are houses mainly privately owned or apartments or condos? Are homes close enough together to afford easy contact? Are they in good repair? Will new construction or deteriorated housing be a safety problem?
Politics	Is the community active politically? Can adults reach a local polling place to vote, or do they know how to apply for absentee ballots?
Recreation	Are recreational activities of interest available? Are they economically feasible? Are there some sites that are apt to create health problems such as ski resorts (broken bones), a lake (drowning), or horse racing tracks (smoke-filled air)?
Religion	Is there a facility where the family can worship as they choose? Is there a mixture of worship centers to show the community accepts cultural diversity?
Safety	Is there adequate protection so family members can feel safe to hike or jog? Do they feel safe to remain home alone? Do they know about available hotlines and local police and fire department numbers? Do houses have smoke and carbon monoxide alarms in the bedrooms and near the kitchen?
Culture	What is the dominant culture in the community? Does the family fit into this environment? Are foods that are culturally significant available?
Transportation	Is there public transportation? Will family members have access to it if they become physically challenged?

community after childbirth or a hospital stay if you know specific features such as information about the water supply, whether the area consists of apartments or homes, or if there is public transportation.

Table 4.1 summarizes common areas to assess in relation to communities. Drawing an ecomap or a diagram of a family's relationship to its community (see Chapter 2, Fig. 2.4) can help identify what community resources are being used by a family or the family's "fit" into the community.

Nursing a Community

Nursing a community refers to nurses' ability and responsibility to help make communities safer by participating in community activities and organizations with the goal of strengthening the community. Activities originate out of the family assessment when a family mentions such things as street lights are blown so it seems unsafe to walk outside at night, two recent automobile accidents have occurred at a particular street corner because the traffic light is not working, or the duck pond in a nearby park needs better signage to show it is over 3 ft deep.

It could also mean participating in fundraising charity events such as a walkathon, encouraging a block of homeowners to form a Block Parent association (parents all come out onto their porches at the time children walk to or from school to help prevent bullying and to provide a safe passage for children), or organize adolescents from a local high school to begin a reading program at a grade school to increase interest in reading and improve the literacy rate in their neighborhood.

It is easy to think a single telephone call or an e-mail about a problem won't make a difference but if all nurses took on their neighborhoods as clients, the number of telephone calls or e-mails would become far too many to be ignored by city officials or others in charge of community design and safety.

HOME CARE

Home care is possible today because specialized therapies such as total parenteral nutrition, fetal monitoring, or laboratory analysis are available in portable versions for home care.

In addition, voluntary agencies are able to supply services, such as transportation to and from health care agency assessments, or for specialized testing, such as X-ray appointments. Home care educators are available to supply necessary individual instruction on how to perform a procedure or prepare a special diet in the home (Vivian-Taylor, Roberts, Chen, et al., 2012).

Home care visits vary in frequency depending on a client's condition and the ability of the client or family to learn and maintain specific procedures. In some settings, telephone, e-mail, and chat room contacts are set up to link health care providers with families so questions can be answered immediately even when the health care provider isn't physically present in the home.

Home care is not a level of care adequate for everyone or every situation, so evaluating whether a family is a good candidate for home care is the first assessment needed. Based on this evaluation, the number of home care visits and what provider would be best for home visits can be determined.

Care at home may include:

- **Direct care**, in which a nurse remains in continual attendance or visits frequently and actually administers care
- **Indirect care**, in which a nurse plans and supervises care given by others, such as home care assistants

Nursing care is considered **skilled home nursing care** if it includes primary health care provider–prescribed procedures such as dressing changes, administration of medication, health teaching, or observation of a woman's or child's progress or status through such activities as monitoring vital signs or fetal heart rate. Whether nursing care is categorized as skilled or not can determine whether it will be paid for by third-party reimbursement.

Frequency of visits varies with individual factors. For example:

- Those clients whose conditions are categorized as low risk probably need only weekly visits; a home health care aide may make the majority of visits.
- Those at intermediate risk need one to three visits per week; a nurse is necessary for the level of care needed.
- Those at high risk may need as many as seven visits per week; a nurse combined with other team members such as a nursing assistant, physical therapist, or a respiratory therapist will be needed for this complex level of care.

Determining family roles (see Chapter 2), such as who is the wage earner, the decision maker, the nurturer, or the problem solver, is an important part of planning. Home care is most successful when these family roles are not disrupted, but strengthened, to support whatever new activities or concerns need to be addressed (Box 4.2).

QSEN Checkpoint Question 4.1

Evidence-Based Practice

Adolescents may spend hours each day on social media Web sites or talking with friends. To determine if adolescents on home care experience depression from lack of social interaction, researchers conducted an online survey of 422 adolescents on home care. Findings from the survey revealed adolescents voiced positive aspects to solitude, but they also strongly rejected wanting or liking spending time alone. They expressed feelings such as fear, boredom, and separation anxiety. Those who reported feeling lonely were significantly less likely to enjoy being home alone during the day than those who weren't experiencing loneliness (Ruiz-Cesares, 2012).

Lisa Puente is alone all day at home because both of her parents work. Based on the study, what would you suggest to help Lisa prevent loneliness?

a. She could arrange to go on brief outings with her friends.
b. She could begin keeping a reflective diary of her thoughts and feelings.
c. She and friends could all download a book to their e-readers, then discuss it by phone or online.
d. She could keep up with her cheerleading squad by cheering along with them on Skype.

Look in Appendix A for the best answer and rationale.

BOX 4.2 Nursing Care Planning Based on Respect for Cultural Diversity

Whether home care is successful is strongly influenced by cultural expectations (Hines, 2012). This may be especially true with regard to male–female roles in a home. In a family in which men and women share responsibilities, care tasks as well as time away from the stress of home care can be distributed equally. In contrast, in cultures in which the male is dominant and child care is strictly delegated to women, a woman can become exhausted from trying to keep her house clean, prepare meals, care for her husband and other children, and also care for a medically fragile child. In male-dominant cultures, the idea of a man giving care to his wife or an ill child contradicts a usual pattern. If a woman is the dominant member of the household, becoming a passive, cared-for partner may be extremely difficult for her.

Because the structure of families is culturally determined, home care may be easier in some cultures than in others. If the family is extended, for example, a mother may be so involved in the care of other family members, such as an older adult, she is unable to rest adequately at home or add enough time to care for an ill child to her other responsibilities. In such a family, however, there may be many people to offer care and support, so home care will be ideal.

Some cultures stress women must be active during pregnancy to help ensure a small baby and therefore an easier birth. That can make bed rest difficult if a woman wants to be active rather than resting. The culture of a particular community might oppose the use of technology, so a family living there might not like having a van to supply needed oxygen or intravenous equipment parked outside. Assessing each family individually helps determine how cultural diversity may affect that particular family and how to individual plans (Andrews, 2011).

Home care works best when a family is strongly committed to home care and well prepared to cooperate with health care providers. Pregnant women with complications such as preterm labor that has been halted, hyperemesis gravidarum (excessive nausea and vomiting of pregnancy), and gestational hypertension are examples of conditions that can be managed at home with supervision and periodic visits by a community or home care nurse. Frequent home visits are also helpful to monitor the health of newborns who were born at low birth weights or who arrived prematurely (Whyte, 2010). Although it is not well documented that bed rest prolongs such pregnancies, women with multiple pregnancies may be another example (Bigelow & Stone, 2011).

Low birth weight occurs in newborns when preterm labor begins and cannot be halted. In other instances, labor can be halted, but the woman needs careful monitoring for the rest of her pregnancy to be certain her fetus is continuing to grow and labor is not beginning again. Nurses can be instrumental in ensuring women who are candidates for monitoring at home receive enough orientation and support to feel comfortable with their at-home arrangements so low birth weight can be prevented. Nurses can also be instrumental in making sure the time spent during home care is not wasted but is used as a time of preparation for birth and childrearing.

There may be an advantage of placing women with premature ruptured membranes on home care rather than hospital care because of the decreased exposure to infection in their own homes compared to hospitals. Children with chronic illnesses who need monitoring, but not critical care, are equally good candidates (Smith, 2011). It is possible that having a caring person such as a community health nurse visit frequently and take an interest in a family may have long-term effects, such as identifying or lowering the incidence of intimate partner violence or child maltreatment and injury (Wider, 2012). Being able to do these things with a high degree of autonomy also creates a satisfying nursing role (Graham, Davies, Woodend, et al., 2011).

Factors that have contributed to the success of the home as a health care setting include:

- It prevents extensive disruption of the family. For children who are acutely but not terminally ill, this extra emotional support may not be as immediately important as physical care. For those who are chronically ill or dying, being close to their family and friends may be the most important aspect of their care. For these children, home care is ideal (Ergün, Sülü, & Başbakkal, 2011).
- It is less costly for the health care delivery system. It is less costly to care for pregnant women or children at home rather than in a hospital setting largely because the number of health care personnel needed is reduced. Home care can also reduce the cost of care when monitoring is the main type of care needed.
- Technologic advances have made it possible for potentially complicated procedures, such as ventilator therapy, to be performed safely at home.
- It presents the opportunity to focus not only on a specific health problem but also on promoting healthy behaviors for the entire family. For example, to prevent a child or woman from being exposed to secondary smoke, family members should agree to establish a "smoke-free" home, allowing a family illness to improve the lifestyle of a whole family (Ashford & Westneat, 2012).
- It can increase a woman's or child's self-confidence and self-efficacy because it allows for more self-care and often more control of circumstances.
- Families can be better assessed in their own environment than in an agency environment because family interactions, values, and priorities are more obvious at home than in a health care setting.
- Home visits provide a private, one-on-one opportunity for health teaching.

Disadvantages of home care include:

- Cost containment has to be weighed against the safety and quality of care. Not all home settings are safe for care and not all families have the commitment necessary, so it is not an alternative for all families. In addition, although home care is cost-effective for health care agencies, it may not be cost-effective for the family. Costs that health insurance would have paid for had the client been hospitalized, such as dressings and medications, may no longer be covered once the person is transferred to home care. This means it can actually increase the cost for an individual family if the family's insurance does not cover the cost of nursing visits or necessary supplies.
- The physical care required (e.g., tracheal suctioning or a complicated medication regimen) can be overwhelming for family caregivers.
- A financial strain can arise if at least one parent or a spouse has to quit work and, therefore, cannot earn an income.
- Bed rest at home can cause social isolation and a disruption of normal family life.

What if...4.1 Lisa's mother is concerned she will become exhausted because of the need for Lisa's around-the-clock care. What suggestions could you offer to make home care more successful?

ASSESSING A FAMILY FOR HOME CARE

Assessment begins with an interview to determine present structure and function of the family and then identifies ways family members think the illness and care at home will change their lives. This could include a wide range of changes such as increased expenses, the need for a parent or spouse to take a leave from work, the need for family members to help with frequent ambulatory health care visits, and the need to arrange for child care for other children. Because these needs change as the course of an illness changes, assessment must be ongoing.

A first home visit usually includes a thorough health history and physical examination to document a woman's or child's current status, as well as an environmental, community, and social assessment. Other assessments focus on likely adherence to medical, preventive, or medication regimens; whether the family will be able to safely monitor the client's health at home; and what other services or resources the family will need, such as the services of a home health care assistant or further nursing visits to ensure home care is optimal. Future visits focus on continuing the assessment and evaluation of patient progress and readiness to help the woman or child move to another level of health care.

The term "resources" refers not only to material objects (such as a hospital bed, oxygen, fetal home monitor) but also

TABLE 4.2 Assessing a Home for Safe Home Care

Category of Information	Conditions to Note
Safety	Is there a smoke and carbon monoxide detector in the patient's bedroom? Do caregivers know the emergency call system procedure in their community? Does the primary caregiver know what steps to take if the patient is suddenly worse?
Oxygen therapy	If oxygen will be used, is there a sign to omit smoking in the room? Is the oxygen away from a fireplace, gas space heater, or gas stove? Does the family know not to light candles near oxygen in a power failure or for a birthday?
Space	Is there a bathroom in easy proximity to the patient's bedroom? Is there a working refrigerator if medicine needs to be kept cold? Is there adequate storage space for supplies? Does the family know how to reorder supplies?
Patient support	Is there a family member who will be the consistent caregiver? Does this person understand the importance of this role?
Electricity	Is the home well lit? Are there adequate three-pronged plugs needed for the care equipment available? Has the power company been notified if an electrical appliance is necessary for life support? What would be the caregiver's actions in a power failure? Do they need to purchase a battery power source?
Environment	Is the home a house or an apartment? Will the bedroom used for care be upstairs or downstairs? Is the home smoke free? Is there evidence of roaches, rats, mice, or fleas?
Nutrition	Are food preparation areas in the kitchen clean? If a special diet is necessary, does the person who will do the cooking have adequate knowledge of food preparation?

whether a family is ready to deal with the chronic stress of home care. For example, women may have to quit work to become home care patients. One parent of an ill child usually has to do the same. This automatically reduces a family's income, which can lead to severe financial problems.

TABLE 4.3 Assessing a Home for Home Care of Children by Age Group

Age	Points to Assess
Newborn or infant	Is there a suitable sleeping place? Do side rails of a crib lock securely? Can the infant be heard from the parents' room at night (do they need a baby monitor)? Is there a freezer if stored breast milk will be used? Is there protection from mosquitoes? Is the home free of rodents that might attack a small infant? Is the infant kept safe from secondary smoking?
Toddler and preschooler	Is there a safe area for play free from stairs and poisoning possibilities? Are there screens or locks on windows to prevent a child from crawling out onto a ledge? Is there provision for stimulation and learning activities?
School-age child and adolescent	What is the provision for schooling (possibly an intercom with a regular classroom or home tutor)? Is peer interaction possible? If adolescent is self-medicating, will reminder sheets or some other reminder system be necessary?

An assessment of the family's environment ascertains whether the home's physical surroundings will be adequate for home care (Table 4.2). Table 4.3 lists additional important assessments to make depending on the age of a child.

Typically, women receiving home care are taught how to self-assess various health parameters such as blood pressure, temperature, pulse, protein in the urine, serum glucose (with the use of a glucometer), fundal height, fetal movement, fetal heart rate, and uterine contractions. Parents or other family members of ill children invariably need to assess vital signs, comfort level, oxygenation (by means of an oximeter), and side effects of medications. When teaching these assessments, be certain to spend enough time with the woman or family so they thoroughly understand both the reason for the assessment and the procedure for doing it. At subsequent home care visits, assess not only the results of the measurements but whether they are being done correctly and consistently.

BEGINNING HOME CARE

Discharge planners in acute care settings can be instrumental in helping set the stage for home care by discussing the need for continued health supervision as well as helping clients begin to establish personal goals for home care. A number of steps are then necessary for an actual home visit to be successful. These steps can be divided into previsit, visit, and postvisit phases.

Preparing for a Home Visit

Typically, a first home visit is made within 24 hours of discharge or notice from an acute care or ambulatory care facility. Be certain to obtain a copy of the client's referral form to familiarize yourself with the client's treatment course and plan of care. Obtain any supplies that may be needed for the visit, such as a thermometer. Keep in mind you are going to be a guest in the client's home, so respect for the client's and family's privacy, beliefs, lifestyles, routines, culture, and requests is crucial.

As a part of individualizing care, telephone a client or family in advance to arrange a time for a visit so it will be convenient for the client and the family. Obtain necessary instructions to reach the home. To avoid disrupting family routines, try not to visit at prayer times or mealtimes unless observing family interaction or what a client is eating for a typical meal is necessary for an assessment. Keep in mind that the ethical and legal aspects of nursing care, such as confidentiality, informed consent, decision making, and client rights commonly associated with acute care nursing, are also applicable to home care. Remember this especially when transporting a chart or notes, electronically recording the visit, or when discussing the visit with others.

Ensuring Personal Safety

Because home care visits are often made alone, be certain to take measures to ensure your personal safety on your way to a client's home, during a visit, and afterward. Safety tips for traveling in an unfamiliar community are shown in Box 4.3.

QSEN Checkpoint Question 4.2

Patient-Centered Care

You need to make a first home visit with Lisa, 16 years old, following a hospital stay. Which of the following would be most important?

a. Telephone her home to establish a time both she and a parent will be present.

b. Drop in unannounced so you can obtain a true picture of Lisa's home conditions.

c. Visit at a time Lisa will be there by herself so she can better express her feelings.

d. E-mail Lisa you will arrive at 10 AM; you expect a parent to also be home at that time.

Look in Appendix A for the best answer and rationale.

Making the Visit

Depending on the location of a client's home, the ease of finding it may vary. Its type may vary from a house, an apartment, a mobile home, or a shelter. Upon arrival at the home, knock or ring the bell and wait for someone to physically or verbally let you enter (even though you don't want the client to get out of bed to let you in, walking in without permission could be interpreted as a home invasion). Greet the client, any other family members present, and pets if they come to greet you (but don't pet strange dogs). Dogs typically serve a guard function, and you want them to view you as a friendly, not a threatening, visitor. Sometimes special advance arrangements, such as having a neighbor let you in, may be necessary if a woman lives alone and cannot walk down a stairway or a long hallway to answer the door.

As in any health care setting, wash your hands before touching a client for assessment and follow standard precautions while giving care. Most home care nurses carry liquid

BOX 4.3 Safety Tips for Home Health Care Travel and Visits

- Plan your trip in advance using a reliable map of the area, a navigation system, or a computer mapping program so you don't become lost in a strange neighborhood.
- Let an agency member know where you are going and when you expect to return.
- Keep your automobile in good repair and filled with gasoline or electrically charged so you don't run out of gas and can avoid having to make stops at unfamiliar service stations.
- Park your car in a well-lit, busy area. Lock the car door.
- Lock any valuables in the trunk of your car before you leave the health care agency, not after you park in front of a home so no one sees you do this.
- Do not leave valuable objects such as expensive electronic equipment in your car or a briefcase on the seat that someone might think contains drugs, so the car is not a target for car thieves.
- Learn the location of public phones in the area, or keep a cellular phone with you.
- If you suspect someone is following you in your car, drive to the nearest police or fire station.
- Do not carry a purse or backpack that suggests you are carrying a large sum of money, drugs, or valuables. If you suspect someone is following you while you are walking, walk into a business establishment.
- Carry only minimal supplies so your hands are free to defend yourself. Walk determinedly, as if you have a purpose and are in charge of your environment and situation.
- Avoid shortcuts through alleys or unoccupied areas; drive or walk on main or busy streets.
- Avoid approaching homes by a dark, back alley; use the front door or a busy hallway.
- Use special caution in stairwells and elevators. Leave a stairwell or elevator if a potentially threatening person enters, with an excuse such as, "Silly me. I've forgotten my red pen."
- When you first enter a home, assess it for personal safety. Ask who is at home. If there are animals in the house, ask if they are friendly.
- If there are animals, take precautions to avoid getting bitten by fleas (sit on a kitchen chair, not an upholstered one).
- Be cautious about accepting food or drink if you are not certain about the hygiene of the dishes or food. Decline it gracefully with an excuse such as, "I'm trying to cut down on the amount of coffee I drink," or "It's against my agency's rules."
- Look under your car when approaching it and in the back seat before entering it to be certain no one is there. Relock your car door immediately once inside.
- Have your car keys in your hand when you leave the house so you can unlock and enter your car quickly.
- If either you or your client are in personal danger, call 911 for help. Leave a home immediately if you feel threatened or unsafe.

soap and paper towels or disposable wipes with them for hand washing, as these facilities in a home may not be convenient or available.

Assessing the Client

At a first home visit, you are going to be conducting a thorough health assessment, including a health history and physical examination, as well as an evaluation of the social environment, medications, nutrition, safety, and adherence to treatment thus far. In addition, consent for treatment and release of information forms may need to be signed.

Provide privacy and confidentiality when obtaining the health history and performing a physical examination. At all times, despite the informality of the setting, use your usual good interviewing and physical assessment skills (Box 4.4). Keep in mind that some homes may be too cool early in the morning for a physical assessment because the heat has been turned down during the night. Arranging for a visit later in the day alleviates this problem. If a home has few rooms, finding a private location for interviewing or for a physical examination can be difficult. Ask other family members to give you privacy as needed.

Be certain to include an assessment not only of the physical aspects of a client but also the mental or psychosocial ones to detect depression, which can occur out of worry or loneliness (Bruce, Sheeran, Raue, et al., 2011). Families receiving home care may be eager to have a nurse assess their wellness and the accuracy of their self-assessments. Throughout the assessment, evaluate the client's needs and provide instructions and reinforcement on any specific areas that are necessary.

If bed rest is required, ask how the client occupies his or her time. A woman is not really resting if she is concerned about her family or finances, is caring for older children, or is so bored that she is frequently turning or sitting up. A child is not really resting if he or she is playing active electronic games.

Before leaving the home, be certain to evaluate the family's understanding of the illness and what danger signs to report immediately if they should occur. Be certain the family has a means of obtaining refills on prescriptions and knows what measures to take if the woman's or child's condition should worsen, such as telephoning 911, the hospital, or a primary care provider. Many clients or families feel more comfortable calling the nurse's home care agency rather than the primary care provider's office. A nurse on call can then help the client determine what action would be best to take.

As a final check, be certain families know when home care personnel will visit again, any modifications of their home that need to be made, the dates and times they need to return to a health care facility, and if they have transportation for these visits.

What if . . . 4.2 Lisa's family lives in a trailer park. Their nearest neighbor stops you every time you visit to ask you how Lisa is doing. How would you answer her?

Assessing the Environment

During a visit, observe whether the house will be or is safe for home care. This means verifying that there is adequate water, electricity, heat, and refrigeration. Are there smoke detectors in the home? Are they in working order? Are there drafts or broken windows? Are there rodents, insects, or lead-based paint in the house that make the environment unsafe?

Evaluate how far the bathroom is from the client's bed to determine if a bedside commode will be necessary to avoid a

BOX 4.4 Nursing Care Planning Based on Effective Communication

Lisa is receiving home care because of hyperemesis of pregnancy and elevated blood pressure. She lost 15 lb at the beginning of pregnancy but now, at 20 weeks, has gained back the lost pounds, plus 2 lb extra, since beginning supplemental gastrostomy feedings every day. A home health care assistant visits her three times per week to supervise her nutrition. She always seems pleased to be visited by a home care nurse once per week.

Less Effective Communication

Nurse: Hello, Lisa. Is everything going all right?
Lisa: Great.
Nurse: How are your stomach feedings going?
Lisa: Great.
Nurse: Not throwing up anymore, are you?
Lisa: No.
Nurse: Good. I'm glad you're doing so well.

More Effective Communication

Nurse: Hello, Lisa. How is everything?
Lisa: Great.
Nurse: Are you doing your own gastrostomy feedings?
Lisa: Right.
Nurse: Do you have any concerns about those?
Lisa: They make me throw up once—maybe twice—a day.
Nurse: I need to do a more thorough assessment.

Because home settings are more informal than those of health care agencies, it is easy to forget a home is a health care setting and to let a relationship become more relaxed than therapeutic. In the first scenario, the nurse lapsed into using conversational or leading questions rather than structured ones for her health interview. Lisa responded to the leading questions by supplying answers it sounded like the ones the nurse wanted to hear, not necessarily the true answers.

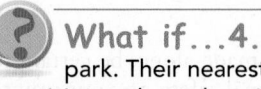

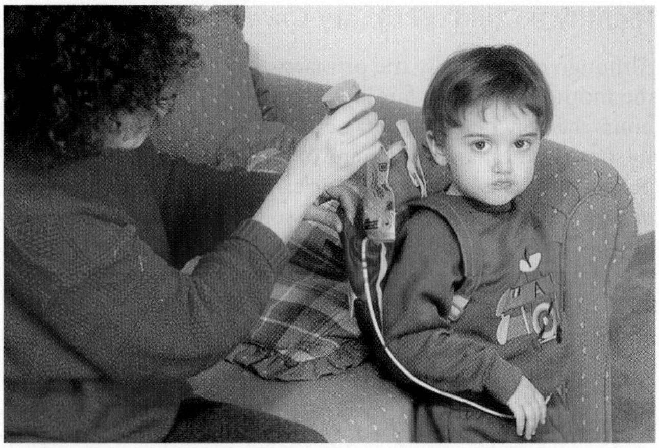

FIGURE 4.2 Procedures at home need to be modified to adjust to the setting. Here, a young boy uses a backpack to carry an ambulatory bag for his gastrostomy tube feeding. (John Meyer/Custom Medical Stock Photograph.)

long walk. Check that there is a telephone nearby or that the client has a cell phone so there is a means for calling someone, both to prevent loneliness and to secure emergency help. If a client needs assistance with personal hygiene, evaluate that the size of the bathroom is adequate if a wheelchair will be used or evaluate the need for a referral for a home health assistant.

Be certain any medical equipment needed, such as an oxygen source, can be accommodated (Fig. 4.2). Hospital beds can be rented from medical supply companies. If a family cannot afford one, they can elevate a house bed on wooden or concrete blocks to make bed care easier. Many home mattresses are not firm; a piece of plywood slid under the mattress improves firmness. A cardboard box or additional pillows can be placed under the mattress to elevate the head of a regular bed to a gatch position. Bed trays can be purchased at any department store, made from a heavy cardboard box, or rented from a medical supply house.

If the client will use a wheelchair to ambulate, family members need to consider if adaptations to their home will be necessary. A local carpenter can build a ramp across the house steps or a split-level elevation to allow wheelchair access. Unless the person will be using a motorized wheelchair, the ramp should have a railing that can be grasped to pull the chair upward or to stop the wheelchair from moving downward too fast. Wheelchair lifts or elevators can be purchased and mounted alongside house steps, but they are more expensive.

Because it is difficult to move a wheelchair across a high-pile carpet, covering the carpet with plastic is helpful. Throw rugs usually have to be removed because they may become entangled in wheelchair wheels. Placing furniture up against the walls allows for increased safe turning space for a wheelchair.

It is almost impossible to reach high shelves from a wheelchair. A pair of tongs can be helpful to use for out of reach items. Family members may have to move supplies that are used often, such as boxes of cereal, to a lower cabinet so the wheelchair-challenged family member can reach them. If a kitchen counter is too high to prepare foods, placing a cutting board across the wheelchair's arms provides a workspace.

If a stove has controls at the back, it is difficult and dangerous for a person in a wheelchair to reach across the burners. A microwave oven placed on a low table can be a solution that allows a wheelchair-challenged person to warm meals and prepare snacks independently (caution children not to place metal articles in the microwave to prevent fire). Installing a safety rail by the toilet in the bathroom helps a person transfer from a wheelchair to the toilet. A chair placed in the bathtub alongside safety rails allows the person to transfer to the bathtub. If families choose, they can contact a local contractor to install a walk-in bathtub.

QSEN Checkpoint Question 4.3

Safety

In the middle of a visit to Lisa's home, her former boyfriend arrives and threatens he will "punch" both you and Lisa if you don't leave. What would be your best action?

a. Tell him threatening someone is not mature behavior and he should stop.
b. Suggest Lisa have her parents change their locks so this man can't visit again.
c. Leave the home and notify your agency you were in unsafe circumstances.
d. Telephone 911 and report both you and your client are being threatened.

Look in Appendix A for the best answer and rationale.

Home Care Assistants

Effective home care requires a team of health care providers, including a supervising primary health care provider, home care nurses, and other persons such as health equipment suppliers and home care assistants. Home health assistants can supply the bulk of personal care services such as assisting with or providing hygiene, assisting with ambulation, or helping to feed clients. Home care assistants have varied levels of preparation depending on their home health or community health care agency policies and the level of care they are being asked to provide.

When working with unlicensed assistive personnel:

- Be certain you are familiar with their level of ability and education so you do not assign a task that is either above their ability or that prevents them from using their full potential.
- When making assignments, be certain they understand that making an assessment (such as recording a blood pressure) is not the same as evaluating the meaning of the assessment. That requires professional expertise.
- When they are in a client's house, remind them they are a guest in the house and need to respect the values and patterns of that household.
- When a client no longer needs home care and the time comes to terminate the relationship, health care assistants may need your help ending the relationship and saying good-bye because their services have been of such a personal nature.

What if...4.3 When you're visiting Lisa, you discover large mouse holes in the bedroom that will be used by her new baby. What would you do?

Postvisit Planning

Postvisit planning consists of documenting all information gained from the visit in relation to the client's condition, completing agency forms so billing for supplies and nursing time can be accurate, and evaluating a client's current status and future needs. It may include communicating a change in status to the primary health care provider, asking for a renewal of prescriptions, or updating and revising the plan of care. Although the forms may vary, the rules for accurate documentation in home care are the same as for any health care facility and just as essential. Privacy rules (Health Insurance Portability and Accountability Act [HIPAA] regulations) apply the same as in hospital or ambulatory care settings.

Follow-Up Visits

Subsequent home visits are planned depending on the client's circumstances and the amount of health education and supervision needed. A second visit could be scheduled as often as the next day or as infrequently as once per month. Frequent assessments accomplished at subsequent visits include vital signs, nutrition assessment, medication adherence, and nursing care actions such as health education.

QSEN Checkpoint Question 4.4

Informatics

Lisa says one reason she doesn't like home care is because private things about her won't be respected. You could assure her of which of the following?

a. Privacy rules (HIPAA) apply to home care health records the same as hospital records.
b. Ita is a problem but you will do your best to respect her privacy and gain her confidence.
c. You won't keep a record of home care procedures so she doesn't need to worry.
d. Electronic home care records are protected by copyright rules the same as all records.

Look in Appendix A for the best answer and rationale.

Nursing Diagnoses and Related Interventions

Nursing Diagnosis: The family process is interrupted related to the stress of caring for ill family member at home.

Outcome Evaluation: Family members state they feel able to manage home care; family meets weekly to discuss problems and share accomplishments.

Health Promotion

Nursing responsibilities for women and children receiving home care vary greatly because the reason for home care and the actions needed vary so greatly. Typical interventions carried out in homes are concerned with promoting both a healthy environment and healthy family function.

Identify a Child's Primary Caregiver

Although traditionally the primary caregiver for an ill child is the mother, in today's families, if a father works more flexible hours, he may be the parent best able to give the bulk of care. In some homes, a grandparent or an older sibling will be the person primarily responsible for care. Arrange to include this person in planning and problem solving because this person knows best what strategy of care will be most effective with the child, as well as what strategy will be most appropriate in light of the physical layout of the home and the family's financial ability and lifestyle.

Determine Knowledge (Health Literacy) Level of Family

Before anyone can be cared for at home, teaching will be required so the family understands the illness and principles of care. Include in teaching both the things that must be learned immediately and additional care measures that will need to be taught as the client's condition changes. Box 4.5 shows an interprofessional care map illustrating both nursing and team planning and education for a family cared for in their community.

Identify Available Resources

Assess where the nearest fire company is that is able to respond in case cardiopulmonary resuscitation (CPR) is necessary, whether a backup resource is available to power needed equipment if a blackout should occur, and if the client can be evacuated easily in case of a fire.

Promote Healthy Family Functioning

A family that is supportive of all family members and provides an environment conducive to each member's continued growth and development is more likely to be able to manage home care than a family with a history of ineffective or destructive coping strategies (e.g., a family in which parents have unrealistic expectations of family members, a family with a history of abusive relationships, or members who do not cope effectively with stressors). A careful assessment is necessary because even a family that appears to be functioning well may become so adversely affected by factors such as the loss of employment income, resentment over missed promotions, or cramped living space all caused by home care that its members' ability to be successful can fail. Remember, every family operates differently and handles stress in different ways. This means events that may seem overwhelming for a visiting health care provider may actually be easy for the family to handle. Conversely, problems that seem minor could be disruptive enough to affect the family's ability to continue adequate care at home.

Many women fulfill multiple roles in their family, such as financial manager, peacemaker, problem solver, nurturer, and decision maker. Even when a woman is on bed rest, help her to continue in these roles to ensure the family's usual functioning, because support people often have great difficulty assuming these roles in her place. In some families, the ill child may fill one of these roles and so needs to be encouraged to continue in the role as well.

As a general rule, support people can only be supportive if they understand the need for and importance of their role. Arranging for a homemaker service to help care for children

BOX 4.5 Nursing Care Planning

AN INTERPROFESSIONAL CARE MAP FOR A PREGNANT ADOLESCENT AT HOME ON BED REST

Lisa Puente, a 16-year-old, 20 weeks pregnant, was admitted to the hospital for 3 days at 14 weeks of pregnancy and placed on a program of gastrostomy feedings because she was losing weight and vomiting at least four times daily since the beginning of pregnancy. She managed well until last week when she was also diagnosed with gestational hypertension and placed on bed rest with fetal and uterine surveillance at home. She tells you it's impossible for her to rest at home: she's bored with school assignments and her friends (and boyfriend) no longer visit. You notice she's missed at least three doses of her hypotensive agent. She asks to be hospitalized again for care.

Family Assessment Client lives with parents in a two-story home. Client's bedroom is on second floor with bathroom located approximately 20 ft from client's bed. Client's mother is primary wage earner in the family; works full time as a travel agent. Husband drives a delivery van; is home until noon daily.

Client Assessment Vital signs: Temperature, 98.4°F; pulse, 76 beats per minute; respirations, 22 breaths per minute; blood pressure (BP), 144/94 mmHg; fetal heart rate (FHR), 148 beats per minute. Mild facial edema; +1 protein in urine; 2-lb weight gain in last week.

Nursing Diagnosis Ineffective coping related to need for bed rest secondary to nausea and gestational hypertension.

Outcome Criteria Client identifies methods to continue in school while maintaining bed rest, expresses increased satisfaction with imposed bed rest, and is able to maintain bed rest until fetal maturity. BP remains 140/80 mmHg or less; FHR within acceptable parameters; urine for protein remains +1 or less; weight gain limited to 1 lb/week; edema limited and without increase for the duration of pregnancy.

Team Member Responsible	Assessment	Intervention	Rationale	Expected Outcome
Activities of Daily Living, Including Safety				
Nurse	Assess vital signs, including heart rate, BP, and FHR at every visit.	Instruct client how to take own vital signs. Review how to do a "count-to-10" assessment daily to assess fetal movement.	Assessment of vital signs and fetal activity provides a baseline for future comparison and evidence of the client's and fetus' status.	Client demonstrates she is able to accurately obtain own pulse, BP, and fetal activity. Findings compare with nurse's weekly findings.
Teamwork and Collaboration				
Nurse/Primary health care provider	Assess what care services will be most appropriate for an adolescent client.	Arrange for home care visiting by hospital home care team. Care assistant: daily; registered nurse: once a week.	Home care functions best when it is part of a "seamless" service.	Client agrees to services of hospital home care team.
Procedures/Medications for Quality Improvement				
Nurse	Assess random urine specimen for protein at each home visit. Assess what client interprets home bed rest to mean.	Instruct client to assess urine specimen and weigh herself every day. Review concept of complete bed rest. Arrange for a bedside commode if necessary.	Proteinuria +1 suggests limited kidney function. Weight gain suggests fluid retention. Bed rest will reduce symptoms of gestational hypertension.	Client voices an understanding of need for bed rest and adheres to restriction. Demonstrates ability to carry out procedures accurately.

(continued on page 68)

BOX 4.5 Nursing Care Planning (continued)

Nutrition				
Nurse/Nutritionist	Obtain a 24-hour recall of gastrostomy feeding pattern to determine if nutritional intake is adequate.	Ensure client is using the prescribed liquid feeding; encourage additional fluid intake.	An adequate nutritional intake is needed for fetal growth.	Client describes a 24-hour intake of gastrostomy feedings adequate for pregnancy.
Patient-Centered Care				
Nurse/Social worker	Assess what client feels are her chief needs that could make her more agreeable to remaining on bed rest at home.	Assist client with planning effective bed rest; discuss possible sources of help from friends and family.	Planning concrete methods to make bed rest more tolerable alleviates stress.	Client demonstrates ways she has adapted to bed rest restrictions.
	Assess what measures would make her more agreeable to continuing school work.	Urge parents to speak to school for more creative schooling arrangements.	Collaboration with school officials should help teenager to remain in school.	Voices plan for creative measures taken so she can remain in contact with school.
Psychosocial/Spiritual/Emotional Needs				
Nurse	Discuss usual activities with client and how lack of these has led to boredom.	Encourage client to plan activities such as reading and listening to music that are both enjoyable and compatible with bed rest.	Discussion provides baseline information to identify client's needs, beliefs, and responsibilities.	Client lists at least three restful activities she can use to occupy her day so she feels less boredom.
Informatics for Seamless Health Care Planning				
Nurse	Assess for readiness to continue with home care.	Instruct client and family about increased blood pressure or sharp headache she will need to report to primary care provider.	Knowledge of danger signs allows for early identification and prompt intervention.	Client lists signs and symptoms she will report to primary care provider if any of them occur.

or an aging parent or to help with light housework may be necessary to prevent support people from feeling stretched so thin when the usual manager of the home is ill. At home visits, ask a woman how her support people are coping and if there are ways this experience could be made easier for them as well as for her. The ability to be allowed to make decisions about her own care can make a significant difference in whether a woman thinks her home care experience is satisfactory.

Health Maintenance

Health maintenance actions are a step beyond health promotion or are taken when a specific risk of ill health is present.

Maintain Skin Care

Both adults and children who are on long-term home care can develop skin ulcers the same as hospital patients if their caretakers don't use preventive measures against this (e.g., good nutrition, position changes, cleaning skin, and promoting mobility) (McCaskey, Kirk, & Gerdes, 2011).

Promote Elimination

Constipation occurs at a high rate during pregnancy and can occur in children on bed rest from lack of exercise. Encourage a diet high in fiber and fluid to minimize this problem.

Ensure Bed Rest

One solution to help both adults and children cope with the stress of bed rest is for them to keep busy in some way, such as using their time to learn a new skill. Most women can name activities they would like to do but have never had time before to begin. For example, bed rest could provide an ideal time for a woman to catch up on her reading she has been putting aside for a long time (Fig. 4.3).

Electronic readers make it possible for women and children to download reading material immediately. If a woman has children, she could spend part of her time reading to them. She could also use the time to take a home-study course, learn to knit, write a short story, or study for a certifying examination related to her work. In any event, helping

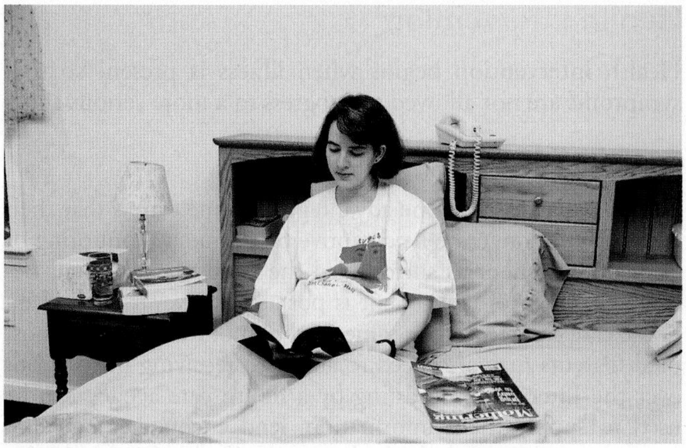

FIGURE 4.3 Bed rest can be stressful. Helping a woman who is on bed rest identify enjoyable and productive activities to pass the time can help ease stress.

her plan meaningful activities such as these can help her view home care not as wasted time, but as time invested in her family or career (Box 4.6).

Children need to involve themselves in school work or play, perhaps by learning a new game or solving Suduko or crossword puzzles. Otherwise, they may spend their time simply watching television or napping.

Although play is a universal activity of children, not all parents realize how important it is to children, so nurses can play an important role in teaching this. When a child is not proficient in English and English is the language of the health care provider, games such as stacking blocks or building with Tinkertoys can be played despite communication difficulty. Playing recordings of well-loved children's songs can also be effective, because the child doesn't need to be able to understand the words to enjoy the music or clap with the rhythm.

Teach Monitoring of Vital Signs

Monitoring vital signs in the home does not differ from monitoring them in a health care agency, except that mercury thermometers may be used in place of electronic ones. If the family will be using a mercury/glass thermometer, caution them that mercury is a toxic contaminant if the thermometer should break; also, this type of thermometer takes a full 3 minutes to register rather than the more convenient few seconds needed by electronic thermometers. To avoid risk of mercury ingestion, they shouldn't be used with children under 5 years of age.

Blood pressure is best measured on the same arm and when the person is in the same position (lying down or sitting up) each time. Using an automated cuff simplifies taking blood pressure. These can be purchased for a low cost from pharmacies or from home care agencies.

Teach Self-Monitoring of Uterine Height, Contractions, and Fetal Heart Rate

Uterine (fundal) height during pregnancy is measured by using a paper tape measure according to McDonald's rule (see Chapter 9). If a woman is asked to record weekly fundal height measurements, demonstrate the correct technique and have her give a return demonstration, as this measurement varies greatly depending on where the tape measure is placed. Be sure a woman is measuring the height in the same manner each time.

Many women conduct fetal movement counts (also called kick counts) daily (see Chapter 9) to help assess fetal well-being (Russo, Henderson, & Costigan, 2011). Fetal heart rate (FHR) is usually recorded by the home care nurse at each home visit. In addition, a client may be taught how to obtain this herself. FHR can be recorded by listening with a Doppler, a fetoscope, or an electronic monitoring device supplied as part of her home care program.

BOX 4.6 Nursing Care Planning Based on Empowering a Family

Q. Lisa tells you, "I feel like I'm wasting my time being home all the time this way. Tell me what to do to keep busy."
A. Try these suggestions:

- Concentrate on school work; make this a time to really delve into a subject.
- Ask your teacher if there is a special project you could work on from home while on bed rest for extra credit.
- Renew an old hobby or begin a new one such as solving crossword puzzles.
- Ask someone to bring you books on newborn care from the library or download them on an electronic reader (you'll be an expert on newborn care by the time your baby is born).
- Telephone your friends. Rest next to a telephone so friends know they won't be disturbing you when they return calls.
- Catch up on your correspondence. Friends and family will be surprised and delighted to receive a letter as so few people write them anymore.
- Investigate whether there is a local community project (such as telephoning for a political campaign, urging neighbors to write letters of support for a new playground) you could work on while on bed rest.
- E-mail friends or join a social media site (if you have a limited data plan, be conscious of the extra charges that might result). If you have a Skype connection, invite friends to show you what is new with them.
- Learn a second language; many books and online sites are available on this.
- Take a mail-order or Internet course on something you want to learn more about (such as creative writing, learning to be a paralegal, how to cook French sauces).
- Ask your home care nurse about preparation-for-childbirth information or download a book on this. By conscientiously practicing breathing exercises while on bed rest, you can become well prepared for labor and birth.

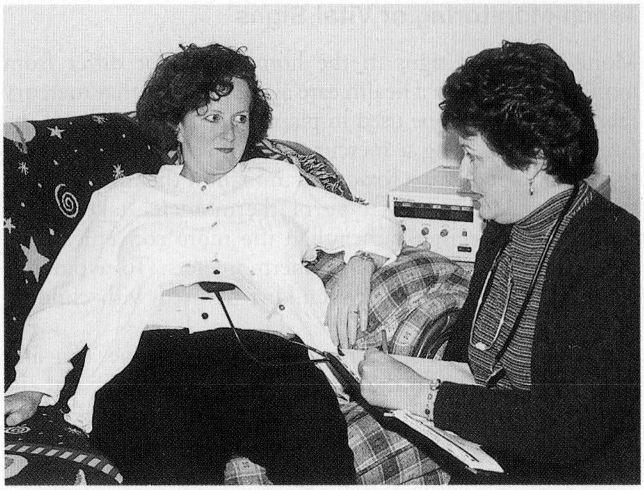

FIGURE 4.4 Fetal heart rate and uterine contractions can be recorded successfully by women at home. (Photograph by Melissa Olson, with permission of Healthy Home Coming, Inc., Bensalem, PA.)

The client can self-monitor uterine contractions using a uterine monitor, the same as in a health care facility, or by palpation (see Chapter 15). A rhythm strip or nonstress test can be conducted using a portable monitor no bigger than 3 × 4 inches in size. A woman straps this device to her abdomen for 20 to 30 minutes at a set time every day, or at any time she feels contractions or is concerned about the lack of fetal movement (Fig. 4.4). The monitor records both uterine contractions and FHR. At the conclusion of the monitoring period, the monitor is held next to a telephone and the tracing is transmitted to a central facility for evaluation.

If you discover a woman is omitting something such as counting FHR, spend some time asking why she's omitting it. It may be because she's unsure she's doing it correctly, or it may be because she's afraid it will reveal her fetus is not doing well (the philosophy of what she doesn't know won't hurt her). It's helpful to try to turn her fear into positive action; discovering an abnormal FHR will allow a health care provider to initiate an action to save her baby and so is a helpful step, not one to fear.

✔ QSEN Checkpoint Question 4.5

Teamwork & Collaboration

Since Lisa has begun eating oral food after gastrostomy feedings were discontinued, she has begun to develop constipation. What measure would you want your team members to suggest she take to help prevent this?

a. Drink more milk, as increased calcium prevents constipation.
b. Walk for at least half an hour daily to stimulate peristalsis.
c. Drink at least eight full glasses of a fluid, such as water, daily.
d. Eat more frequent small meals instead of three large ones daily.

Look in Appendix A for the best answer and rationale.

Health Intervention

Health intervention begins when illness is present so that symptoms are not allowed to progress to a more serious state.

Explain Advances in Technology

A family may assume one advantage of home care is that their child will no longer be held captive by so much monitoring or oxygen equipment as surrounded the child in a hospital. Because so much of equipment is portable, however, a child on home care can receive the same level of monitoring as in a hospital. Parents may also need to adjust to receiving instructions over the Internet. Webcasting by a health care agency can be used to supply them information, lend encouragement, and answer questions they have about care (Smith-Stoner, 2011). Caution adolescents there are some downsides to too much Internet use as there is an apparent association between depression and spending excessive amounts of time on social media chat rooms, so much so, a syndrome termed "Facebook depression" has been identified (O'Keeffe & Clarke-Pearson, 2011). Parents also need to alert children and adolescents that not all Internet sites are safe to visit because of the possibility that predators or pedophiles also visit such sites (Burgess Dowdell, 2011).

Provide Health Teaching

Because the home setting is private, a home care visit can provide many more opportunities for one-on-one health teaching than a health care agency setting. An important aspect of teaching for a pregnant woman might be providing childbirth education, because a woman on bed rest will not be able to attend formal classes. For a child, it could be teaching the whole family about the child's illness and why the current therapy is needed.

Provide for Safe Medicine Administration

Most people receiving home care are prescribed some type of medicine, such as a tocolytic for pregnant women to halt preterm labor or chemotherapy for children because of cancer (Ewen, Combs, Popelas, et al., 2012). Review the rules of safe medication administration with the family to minimize mistakes such as taking the medicine more frequently than prescribed or forgetting to take it (Box 4.7).

Provide for Adequate Nutrition and Hydration

A woman who is on home care often needs help maintaining adequate nutrition. If ordinarily she is the person who plans menus, shops for food, and cooks for the family, with her on bed rest, other family members must assume these roles. If other family members are inexperienced at cooking, the entire family, including the pregnant woman, may not eat enough healthy foods.

As ill children don't get as much activity as usual, they may not be as hungry at mealtime as usual. You may need to make suggestions for healthy snacks so a child's total daily intake is adequate even if not a lot of food is eaten at formal meals.

All women during pregnancy should drink six to eight full glasses of fluid a day to obtain adequate fluid for effective kidney function and placental exchange (Harnisch, Harnisch, & Harnisch, 2012). Be certain women on bed rest have a supply of fluid close to their bed, such as a bottle of water, so they can do this easily.

BOX 4.7 Nursing Care Planning Based on Family Teaching

SAFETY TIPS FOR SAFELY TAKING MEDICINE AT HOME

- Keep drugs in a safe place. In most homes, this is in a locked medicine cabinet or drawer above the height a child could reach.
- Keep alert that most childhood poisonings occur when a family is under stress; that is because during these times, the family can forget usual procedures such as locking away medicine. Families need to take more and more precautions the higher the stress level rises in the home.
- Never take medicine in front of children (children can imitate this action with the parent's medication).
- Don't pour or prepare medicine in the dark. Because almost all medicine bottles dispensed from local pharmacies look and feel the same, it is easy to pour the wrong liquid, extract the wrong pills, or read the bottle instructions incorrectly without adequate light.
- Read instructions as to whether medicine should be taken with food or not and whether pills can be chewed or not. Try and drink a full glass of water with pills to ensure they reach the stomach.
- Create a reminder sheet and hang it in a prominent place. Cross off each time the medication is taken.
- Purchase a medicine box with an individual compartment for each day of the week. Such boxes help to eliminate confusion over whether medicine was taken or not.

Many pregnant women or children on home care receive intravenous therapy as a route of medication or fluid administration. Women with hyperemesis gravidarum (uncontrolled vomiting during pregnancy) or oligohydramnios (less than usual amount of amniotic fluid) receive it as a means of hydration (Patrelli, Gizzo, Cosmi, et al., 2012; Tamay & Kuşçu, 2011). Women and children with blood dyscrasias may receive blood transfusions in the home (Marouf, 2011).

Because peripheral intravenous lines frequently become dislodged, in the home setting, intravenous fluid is often administered by a central line or a peripherally inserted central catheter (PICC) line threaded to a central blood vessel. Many drugs, especially antibiotics, are given through bagged "piggyback" infusions kept frozen until the time of administration. Specially pressurized fluid containers allow for fast and easy administration of special solutions. To be certain fluid infuses slowly and accurately, an intravenous infusion pump is strongly recommended. Be certain a woman or a family member knows how to operate a pump, how to monitor intravenous insertion sites for inflammation and infiltration, how to protect the site from becoming infected (e.g., cover it with plastic rather than letting it get wet), when to remind a health care provider the site should be changed, and how to monitor the amount and kind of fluid or medication infused.

Home Enteral Nutrition

Chronically ill children and women who have hyperemesis gravidarum may receive nutrition by a gastrostomy or nasogastric tube. The supplies necessary for enteral feedings, such as feeding tubes and enteral pumps, are available for rent or purchase through pharmacies, medical supply houses, or the home care agency. Such tubes are usually changed every 2 to 4 weeks. The home care nurse will most likely be the person responsible for changing the tube, but this depends on the home care agency's policies. In addition to assessing the amount of formula infused by this route, be certain the woman or a family member is familiar with all aspects of care for the tube, equipment, and administration of the feeding. Caution the family to monitor the amount of formula for the feedings they have on hand so they don't run out, especially over weekends or holidays when their supplier may be closed. Clients on enteral feedings probably will need to weigh themselves periodically and record their weight. They may need to test blood serum for glucose with a glucometer. Be certain they use the same scale, wear consistent clothing, and know when to call for advice if they are unsure if their weight is remaining adequate.

Total Parenteral Nutrition

Total parenteral nutrition (TPN) is yet another way to supply complete nutrition and fluid to clients on home care. The home care agency or a separate vendor will furnish and deliver the formula, tubing, clean dressings, and an infusion pump. The formula, which consists of amino acids, hypertonic glucose, vitamins, and minerals in solution, needs to be stored in the client's refrigerator until 1 to 2 hours before use; it is then removed from the refrigerator and allowed to warm to room temperature. Women and children requiring this type of intravenous nutritional therapy usually have a central venous access device such as a central venous catheter or PICC line inserted. The home care nurse plays a key role in teaching family members about the therapy and also in assessing the woman's or child's response to therapy.

Throughout therapy, be certain the client or a family member knows how to monitor the infusion of the solution and the patency of the tube, how to change dressings (if that will be their responsibility), how to observe the insertion site for redness or inflammation, and how to assess body temperature for a possible infection. They also must be aware of any restrictions that should be adhered to (such as no baths if the water level will rise above the catheter insertion site) and the interval at which blood should be drawn for monitoring. Because TPN solutions are hypertonic, a woman or a family member needs to obtain blood glucose levels as necessary, test them with a glucometer, and keep a record of these. Be sure the family knows what findings they should report immediately to a health care provider.

Teach Self-Monitoring by Serum or Urine Testing

Women who develop gestational diabetes will be required to self-monitor their serum glucose level using a glucometer at least once daily, some three or four times daily (Evensen, 2012). Children with diabetes need to do these actions as well (Garg & Hirsch, 2012). Both women and children need support to be conscientious about continuing to do these actions when home care extends for a long time. A nurse can be instrumental in being the person to supply this support.

Manage Pain

Children who are on home care after surgery or those with a chronic or terminal illness may need efficient pain management for long periods of time. Be certain parents understand the principles of pain management such as to give medication before pain becomes acute. A detailed discussion with other pain management philosophies is discussed in Chapter 39.

QSEN Checkpoint Question 4.6

Quality Improvement

Lisa has been on home care for a long time. Which of her following statements would worry you most about whether her home is a safe place for home care?

a. "My mother is trying to quit smoking; she usually goes outside to smoke."
b. "If the lights go out, I know the circuit breaker is located in the garage."
c. "A police report says there's never been a robbery in this neighborhood."
d. "My father had the paint in the bathroom tested last year and it is lead free."

Look in Appendix A for the best answer and rationale.

Health Rehabilitation

Health rehabilitation begins at the point complications have arisen and a patient is learning to adapt to chronic illness or take active steps toward restoring function. It can also mean accepting end of life care.

Long-Term Home Care

Although many families are good candidates for home care in the beginning, they have difficulty maintaining this high level of commitment as home care becomes long term. They may need both advice and support to continue to adapt constructively to the changing phases of an illness. They can develop low self-esteem and depression, feelings which can harm a marital relationship or prevent parents from spending time with other children (Fig. 4.5).

Help families maintain healthy functioning by promoting communication with each other and encouraging family members to identify and share their feelings about the situation at home. Encourage members to voice the frustration they can feel at being constantly confined at home or what they perceive to be a lack of progress in the ill person's condition. If a child has a terminal illness, support parents to express their grief and not grow discouraged, because the work they are accomplishing is making the child comfortable. Continued successful coping will require the family to acknowledge and take seriously the impact of home care on each family member and work together to solve identified problems. To do this effectively, they may need to renegotiate roles and responsibilities within the family or seek outside help.

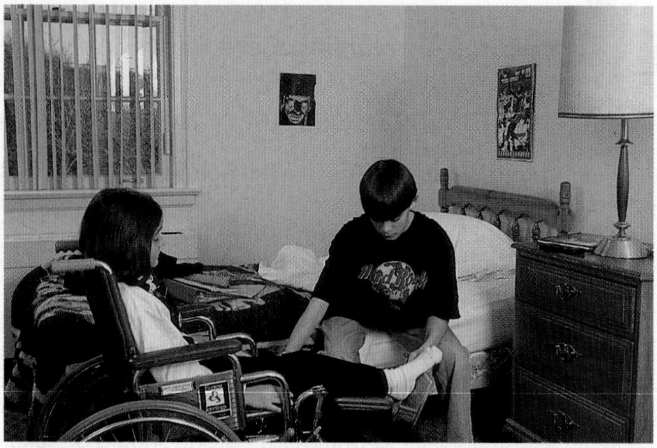

FIGURE 4.5 Home care of a child is family care. Here, a brother helps his sister transfer to a wheelchair.

Children on home care need to continue with school if at all possible so they can maintain contact with friends, so they don't fall behind a grade level, and so they can continue the stimulation of learning. This means parents should make some sort of arrangement for schooling either through their local school district (many schools can establish a telecommunication setup for children ill at home) or investigate their ability to home school.

When a family has difficulty functioning well at the beginning of home care or does not adjust readily to continued care, nursing measures to support family functioning become even more important. A family whose coping strategies are maladaptive may not be able to care for a sick family member at home for long without strong nursing and other health care professional support.

What if... 4.4 You are particularly interested in exploring one of the 2020 National Health Goals with respect to home care (see Box 4.1). What would be a possible research topic to explore pertinent to this goal that would be applicable to Lisa's family and also advance evidence-based practice?

Key Points for Review

- Families exist within communities; assessment of the community and the family's place in the community yields important information on family functioning and abilities.
- Home care is increasing as a way of providing care to chronically ill children and women with a complication of pregnancy. It has the advantages of being cost-effective and keeping families intact to provide meaningful comfort and support.

- Disadvantages of home care include that families can become fatigued, the loss of a job for the primary caregiver can cause financial hardship, and social isolation and disruption of normal home life can occur.
- Home care requires careful planning and a combined effort between health care providers and the family to ensure collaboration and continuity of care.
- Not all homes are ideal for home care. Assessing that a primary family care provider is present; that the family is knowledgeable about the care necessary; necessary resources are available; and safety features such as a smoke detector, a safe area for oxygen storage, and a working refrigerator for food or medicine are present are important nursing actions.
- Parents may need respite care to continue to be effective care providers for children just as professionals need time off. Help family members take turns giving care so each has some free time during the week.
- Considering a family as both a single client and as part of a community helps in planning nursing care that meets not only QSEN competencies but also the family's total needs.

Critical Thinking Care Study

Kimi Toi Hackett is a 23-year-old who just gave birth to a baby boy named Harding. She lives in a high-rise condo that was recently converted into apartments from an unused warehouse in the center of the city. Harding weighs 5.5 lb, has congenital heart disease, and will be cared for at home until he gains 5 more pounds and can have his heart repaired. He's being breastfed; his care instructions include never letting him cry, keeping him away from people with infections, and being certain he gets adequate sleep. Kimi Toi used to be a nanny for two school-age children before she quit work to take care of Harding. Her husband works nights at the post office. Kimi calls you for advice because she doesn't know any of her neighbors and so has no one to help her keep Harding from crying. Harding sleeps instantly if she puts him in his car seat and drives around the block, but she's afraid to go into the underground parking garage at night because there's no night guard. She feels she has moved into a totally wrong community; all of her neighbors are well-to-do businessmen or retired older adults.

1. Kimi Toi feels she and her husband have made a poor choice when they chose to move into a loft. Moving to any new community can be a major adjustment for a family. What are community features this family should have investigated before they bought a loft?
2. Kimi Toi is afraid to walk down to the parking garage at night to get her car. What suggestions could you make to help Harding stop crying in place of driving him around the block?
3. The Hackett's building was just redone so it's easy to assume their condo has all the qualities needed for home care. To be certain, what questions would you want to ask Kimi Toi about the loft?

Patient Scenario
The Breaker Family

Read about the Breaker family, a family with a mother on bed rest at home, then answer the questions to further sharpen your skills and grow more familiar with NCLEX-type questions related to family health and home care. Confirm your answers are correct by reading the rationales.

Visit http://thePoint.lww.com

Answers and Rationales

Looking for answers to the What If… and Critical Thinking Care Study questions?

Visit http://thePoint.lww.com

References

Allender, J. A. (2013). *Community & public health nursing*. Philadelphia, PA: Lippincott Williams & Wilkins.

Andrews, M. M. (2011). Culturally competent nursing care. In M. M. Andrews & J. S. Boyle (Eds.), *Transcultural concepts in nursing care* (pp. 15–33). Philadelphia, PA: Lippincott Williams & Wilkins.

Ashford, K., & Westneat, S. (2012). Prenatal hair nicotine analysis in homes with multiple smokers. *Nursing Clinics of North America, 47*(1), 13–20.

Bernstein, H. B., & VanBuren, G. (2013). Normal pregnancy. In A. H. DeCherney, L. Nathan, M. Goodwin, et al. (Eds.), *Current diagnosis & treatment in obstetrics & gynecology* (11th ed., pp. 141–153). New York, NY: McGraw-Hill.

Bigelow, C., & Stone, J. (2011). Bed rest in pregnancy. *Mt. Sinai Journal of Medicine, 78*(2), 291–302.

Bruce, M. L., Sheeran, T., Raue, P. J., et al. (2011). Depression care for patients at home. *Home Healthcare Nurse, 29*(7), 416–426.

Burgess Dowdell, E. (2011). Risky internet behaviors of middle-school students: Communication with online strangers and offline contact. *Computers, Informatics, Nursing, 29*(6), 352–359.

Ergün, S., Sülü, E., & Başbakkal, Z. (2011). Supporting the need for home care by mothers of children with hemophilia. *Home Healthcare Nurse, 29*(9), 530–538.

Evensen, A. E. (2012). Update on gestational diabetes mellitus. *Primary Care, 39*(1), 83–94.

Ewen, B. M., Combs, R., Popelas, C., et al. (2012). Chemotherapy in home care: One team's performance improvement journey toward reducing medication errors. *Home Healthcare Nurse, 30*(1), 28–37.

Garg, S. K., & Hirsch, I. B. (2012). Self-monitoring of blood glucose. *International Journal of Clinical Practice, 66*(175), 2–7.

Graham, K. R., Davies, B. L., Woodend, A. K., et al. (2011). Impacting Canadian public health nurses' job satisfaction. *Canadian Journal of Public Health, 102*(6), 427–431.

Harnisch, J. M., Harnisch, P. H., & Harnisch, D. R., Sr. (2012). Family medicine obstetrics: Pregnancy and nutrition. *Primary Care, 39*(1), 39–54.

Hines, D. (2012). Cultural competence assessment and education resources for home care and hospice clinicians. *Home Healthcare Nurse, 30*(1), 38–45.

Jilcott, S. B., Vu, M. B., Morgan, J., et al. (2012). Promoting use of nutrition and physical activity community resources among women in a family planning clinic setting. *Women's Health, 52*(1), 55–70.

Marouf, R. (2011). Blood transfusion in sickle cell disease. *Hemoglobin, 35*(5–6), 495–502.

McCaskey, M. S., Kirk, L., & Gerdes, C. (2011). Preventing skin breakdown in the immobile child in the home care setting. *Home Healthcare Nurse, 29*(4), 248–255.

O'Keeffe, G. S., & Clarke-Pearson, K. (2011). The impact of social media on children, adolescents, and families. *Pediatrics, 127*(4), 800–804.

Olander, E. K., Atkinson, L., Edmunds, J. K., et al. (2012). Promoting healthy eating in pregnancy: What kind of support services do women say they want? *Primary Health Care Research & Development, 13*(3), 237–243.

Patrelli, T. S., Gizzo, S., Cosmi, E., et al. (2012). Maternal hydration therapy improves the quantity of amniotic fluid and the pregnancy outcome in third-trimester isolated oligohydramnios. *Journal of Ultrasound Medicine, 31*(2), 239–244.

Ruiz-Cesares, M. (2012). "When it's just me at home, it hits me that I'm completely alone": An online survey of adolescents in self-care. *Journal of Psychology, 146*(1–2), 135–153.

Russo, M. L., Henderson, J., & Costigan, K. A. (2011). Fetal assessment. In K. J. Hurt, M. W. Guile, J. L. Bienstock, et al. (Eds.), *The Johns Hopkins manual of gynecology and obstetrics* (4th ed., pp. 90–98). Philadelphia, PA: Lippincott, Williams & Wilkins.

Smith, T. (2011). Bringing children home: Bridging the gap between inpatient pediatric care and home healthcare. *Home Healthcare Nurse, 29*(2), 108–117.

Smith-Stoner, M. (2011). Webcasting in home and hospice care services: Virtual communication in home care. *Home Healthcare Nurse, 29*(6), 337–341.

Tamay, A. G., & Kuşçu, N. K. (2011). Hyperemesis gravidarum: Current aspects. *Journal of Obstetrics & Gynaecology, 31*(8), 708–712.

U.S. Department of Health and Human Services. (2010). *Healthy people 2020*. Washington, DC: Author.

Vivian-Taylor, J., Roberts, C., Chen, J., et al. (2012). Motor vehicle accidents during pregnancy: A population-based study. *BJOG: British Journal of Obstetrics & Gynecology, 119*(4), 499–503.

Wider, L. C. (2012). Identifying and responding to child abuse in the home. *Home Healthcare Nurse, 30*(2), 75–81.

Whyte, R. (2010). Safe discharge of the late preterm infant. *Paediatrics & Child Health, 15*(10), 655–666.

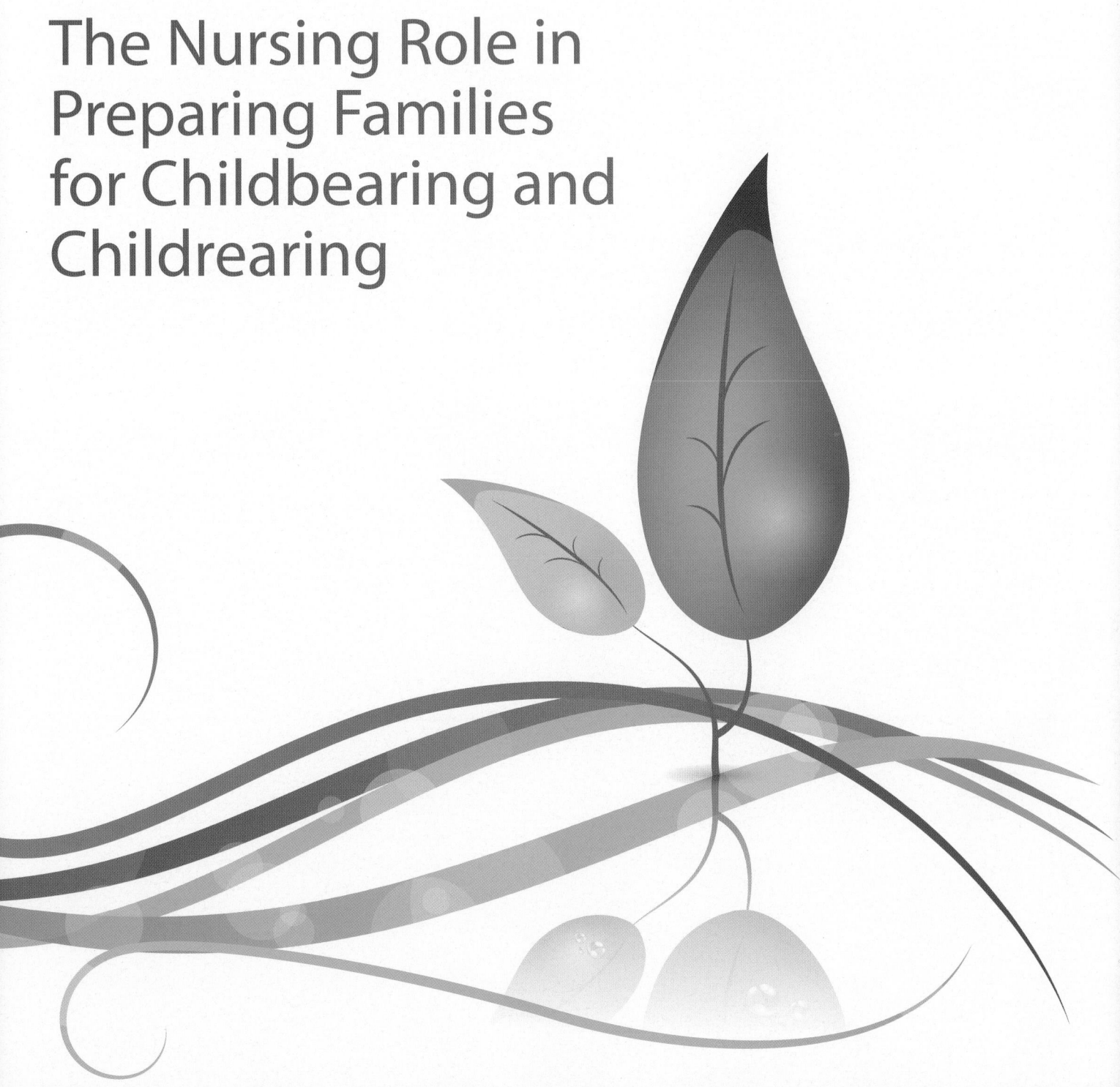

Unit 2

The Nursing Role in Preparing Families for Childbearing and Childrearing

Chapter 5

The Nursing Role in Reproductive and Sexual Health

KEY TERMS

- adrenarche
- andrology
- anteflexion
- anteversion
- aspermia
- bicornuate uterus
- biologic gender
- culdoscopy
- cystocele
- dyspareunia
- erectile dysfunction
- gender identity
- gender role
- gonad
- gynecology
- gynecomastia
- laparoscopy
- menarche
- menopause
- menorrhagia
- metrorrhagia
- oocyte
- premature ejaculation
- puberty
- rectocele
- retroflexion
- retroversion
- spermatic cord
- thelarche
- transsexual
- transvestite
- vaginismus
- voyeurism

OBJECTIVES

After mastering the contents of this chapter, you should be able to:

1. Describe anatomy and physiology pertinent to reproductive and sexual health.
2. Discuss 2020 National Health Goals related to reproductive health and sexuality that nurses can help the nation achieve.
3. Assess a couple for anatomic and physiologic health, biologic gender, gender role, gender identity, and readiness for childbearing.
4. Formulate nursing diagnoses related to reproductive and sexual health.
5. Develop expected outcomes for reproductive and sexual health education to manage seamless transitions across differing health care settings.
6. Using the nursing process, plan nursing care that includes the six competencies of Quality & Safety Education for Nurses (QSEN): Patient-Centered Care, Teamwork & Collaboration, Evidence-Based Practice (EBP), Quality Improvement (QI), Safety, and Informatics.
7. Implement nursing care related to reproductive and sexual health, such as educating middle school children about menstruation.
8. Evaluate expected outcomes for achievement and effectiveness of care.
9. Integrate knowledge of preparation for childbearing with the interplay of nursing process, the six competencies of QSEN, and Family Nursing to promote quality maternal and child health nursing care.

Suzanne and Kevin Matthews, a young adult couple, planned to have a baby as soon as they married; however, it took Suzanne 1 year before she conceived. Now, 12 weeks pregnant, she comes to your clinic for a prenatal visit. In tears, she states, "My husband isn't interested in me anymore. We haven't had sex since I became pregnant." Kevin states, "I'm afraid I'll hurt the baby."

Previous chapters presented the scope of maternal and child health nursing and how the structure, function, and culture of families can have a significant impact on health. This chapter adds information about how to educate children, women, and their partners about anatomy, physiology, and sexuality to better prepare them for childbearing and childrearing.

How would you counsel Suzanne and Kevin Matthews?

Whether or not someone is planning on childbearing, everyone is wiser for being familiar with reproductive anatomy and physiology and his or her own body's reproductive and sexual health. Women and their partners who are planning on childbearing may become curious about reproductive physiology and the changes a pregnant woman will undergo during pregnancy. Women who are pregnant are also very interested, so these are frequent times nurses are asked by both men and women about reproductive and gynecologic health (Wade, Herrman, & McBeth-Snyder, 2012).

Although the general public is becoming increasingly sophisticated about their bodies because of courses in school on sexuality, misunderstandings about sexuality, about conception (preventing or promoting), and about childbearing still abound. When caring for children of school age or adolescence, they may ask you a variety of detailed questions about sexuality or reproductive health they heard about in class but didn't really understand. For instance, many adolescents want to know more about what is a "normal" menstrual period; young adults may want to know what is the "normal" expected frequency for sexual relations.

A general rule in answering a question about sexual relations is normal sexual behavior includes any act mutually satisfying to both sexual partners. Actual frequency and type of sexual activity vary widely. According to a definition by the Centers for Disease Control and Prevention (CDC, 2010), sexual health is not just an absence of disease, dysfunction, or infirmity but a condition of physical, emotional, and psychosocial well-being.

One of the most important contributions nurses can make to the education of clients about sexual health is to encourage them to ask questions in this area. With this attitude, problems of sexuality and reproduction can be brought out to the open and made as solvable as other health concerns. If this is an area that you were raised to not discuss freely, learning to be comfortable with the topic and your own sexuality can be the first step needed (Chang & Lin, 2013).

A sample of 2020 National Health Goals that speak directly to improving reproductive or sexual health are shown in Box 5.1.

BOX 5.1 Nursing Care Planning Based on 2020 National Health Goals

A number of 2020 National Health Goals speak directly to reproductive and sexual health:

- Increase the proportion of adolescents who, by age 15, have never engaged in sexual intercourse to 80.2% of girls and 79.2% of boys from baselines 72.9% and 72.0%
- Increase to at least 91.3% the proportion of sexually active 15- to 19-year-olds at risk for unintended pregnancy who used contraception at last sexual intercourse from a baseline of 83.0%.
- Reduce deaths from cancer of the uterine cervix to no more than 2.2 per 100,000 women, from a baseline rate of 2.4 per 100,000.
- Reduce breast cancer deaths to no more than 20.6 per 100,000 women, from a baseline rate of 22.9 per 100,000.
- Improve the health, safety, and well-being of lesbian, gay, bisexual, and transgender (LGBT) individuals (developmental goal) (U.S. Department of Health and Human Services [DHHS], 2010; see www.healthypeople.gov).

Nurses can help the nation achieve these goals by educating adolescents about abstinence as well as refusal skills, safer sex practices, and the advantage of obtaining a vaccine against human papillomavirus (HPV), the virus associated with cervical cancer. The need to participate in screening activities such as vulvar and testicular self-examination are also important to teach.

Nursing Process Overview

For Promotion of Reproductive and Sexual Health

Assessment

Problems of sexuality or reproductive health may not be evident on first meeting clients because it may be difficult for people to bring up the topic until they feel more secure with your relationship. This makes good follow-through and planning important, because even if people find the courage to discuss a problem once, they may be unable to do so again. If the problem is ignored or forgotten through a change in caregivers, the problem can go unsolved.

Any change in physical appearance (such as occurs with puberty or with pregnancy) can intensify or create a sexual or reproductive concern. The person with a sexually transmitted infection (STI); excessive weight loss or gain; a disfiguring scar from surgery or an unintentional injury; hair loss such as occurs with chemotherapy; surgery, inflammation, or infection of reproductive organs; chronic fatigue or pain; spinal cord injury; or the presence of a retention catheter needs to be assessed for problems regarding sexual role as well as other important areas of reproductive functioning.

Nursing Diagnosis

Common nursing diagnoses used with regard to reproductive health include:

- Health-seeking behaviors related to reproductive functioning
- Anxiety related to inability to conceive after 6 months without contraception
- Pain related to uterine cramping from menstruation
- Disturbance in body image related to early development of secondary sex characteristics
- Risk for infection related to high-risk sexual behaviors

Diagnoses relevant to sexuality may include:

- Sexual dysfunction related to as yet unknown cause
- Altered sexuality patterns related to chronic illness
- Self-esteem disturbance related to recent reproductive tract surgery
- Altered sexuality patterns related to fear of harming a fetus
- Anxiety related to fear of contracting an STI
- Health-seeking behavior related to learning responsible sexual practices

Outcome Identification and Planning

A major part of nursing care in this area is to empower clients to feel control over their bodies. Plan health teaching to provide clients with knowledge about their reproductive system and specific information about ways to alleviate discomfort or prevent reproductive disease. It may also be important to plan individualized interventions to strengthen the person's gender identity or gender role. It is essential to design care that demonstrates acceptance of all gender-related lifestyles equally. One helpful referral organization is People with a Lesbian, Gay, Bisexual, Transgender, or Queer Parent (www.colage.org), and www.sexualityandu.ca, a Web site with helpful tips on both sexuality and reproductive life planning.

Implementation

A primary nursing role concerning reproductive anatomy and physiology is education, because both female and male clients may feel more comfortable asking questions of nurses rather than other health care providers. Men who have sex with men (MWM), women who have sex with women (WWW), or others with alternative lifestyles usually reveal their sexual orientation to health care providers because they want to be certain their lifestyle is not adding to a health concern. They may also need help or suggestions on dealing with friends or family who are having difficulty accepting their gender identity. In addition to support, providing health education that addresses potential concerns of clients of all lifestyles will enhance their sexual health. For example, include a discussion about anal or oral–genital sex practices when presenting information on safer sex.

Outcome Evaluation

The evaluation in the area of reproductive health must be ongoing, because health education needs change with circumstances and increased maturity. For example, the needs of a woman at the beginning of a pregnancy may be different from her needs at the end.

How people feel about themselves sexually also changes throughout life. Their concept of themselves may have a great deal to do with how quickly they recover from an illness, how quickly they are ready to begin self-care after childbirth, or even how motivated they are as an adolescent to accomplish activities in life phases that depend on being sure of their sexuality or gender role.

Examples of expected outcomes include:

- Client states he is taking precautions to prevent contracting an STI.
- Client states she is better able to manage symptoms of premenstrual dysphoric syndrome.
- Couple states they have achieved a mutually satisfying sexual relationship.
- Client states he is ready to tell family about MWM gender identity.

ASSESSING AND MEETING REPRODUCTIVE CONCERNS

Assessing sexuality is not appropriate as a routine part of every health assessment. However, it should be included when appropriate, such as when discussing adolescent development or before providing reproductive life planning information, during pregnancy, and after childbirth. At other times, it is wise to listen for subtle verbal or nonverbal clues that suggest a person wants to discuss a sexual or reproductive concern such as, "I guess marriage isn't for everyone," "I'm not the woman I used to be," or "Are there ever funny effects from this medicine I'm taking?" Telling a seemingly inappropriate sexual joke may be yet another clue. Nonverbal clues may include extreme modesty or obvious embarrassment in response to a question about voiding, perineal pain, or stitches.

An assessment in the area of reproductive health begins with interviewing to determine a client's knowledge level of the reproductive process, STIs, concerns about his or her reproductive functioning, or safer sex practices (Box 5.2). This area of health interviewing takes practice and the conviction that exploring sexual health is as important as exploring less emotionally involved areas of health, such as dietary intake or activity level. The 14-year-old girl, who is not yet menstruating, for instance, may be anxious about that fact but may be reluctant to say so unless asked directly.

A statement such as the following invites discussion: "Although many of your friends at school may be menstruating, it's not at all uncommon for some girls not to begin their periods until age 15 or 16 years. How do you feel about not yet having your period?" This combination of providing information and questioning may encourage an adolescent to discuss not only her possible concern about delayed **menarche** (the beginning of menstruation) but also other areas that will reveal her knowledge or lack of knowledge about reproductive health. Specific questions to include in a sexual history are shown in Box 5.3

It's important to include in a physical examination observation for normal distribution of body hair such as triangle-shaped pubic hair in women and diamond-shaped pubic hair in men, for normal genital and breast development, and for signs and symptoms of STIs. Many STIs are asymptomatic, so it is important to assess whether the client is at risk for contracting such an infection (see Chapters 33 and 47 for documentation of stages of sexual development and signs of STIs).

To help clients better understand reproductive functioning and sexual health throughout their life, specific teaching might include:

- Encouraging women over 40 years of age to have mammograms
- Explaining to a school-aged boy that nocturnal emissions are normal
- Teaching an early adolescent about normal anatomy and physiology and the process of reproduction
- Teaching a young adolescent safer sex practices
- Explaining reproductive physiology to a couple who wish to become pregnant

Teaching may be in response to a direct question posed by a parent (Box 5.4). It is often enhanced by the use of illustrations from books or journals, video clips, or models of internal and external reproductive organs. Nursing interventions in this area, however, should include much more than just distributing educational materials. You need to follow-up by asking if the education material answered the client's questions. In addition, offer empathy for a client's concerns, such as a woman's worry that increased tension before menstruation is a symptom of premenstrual dysphoric syndrome, to

BOX 5.2 Nursing Care Planning Based on Effective Communication

Kevin brings his 16-year-old nephew, Mark, into your health care clinic because Mark has had painful urination for 2 days. A culture is taken to determine whether he has contracted a sexually transmitted infection (STI).

Less Effective Communication

Nurse: Mark, because you're sexually active, your symptoms suggest you may have contracted a sexually transmitted infection.
Mark: Uh-huh.
Nurse: Do you practice safer sex?
Mark: Uh, yeah.
Nurse: I assume that means you always use a condom.
Mark: Right.
Nurse: It would be hard to contract an STI if you always do.
Mark: Guess I'm just an unlucky kid.

More Effective Communication

Nurse: Mark, because you're sexually active, your symptoms suggest you may have contracted a sexually transmitted infection.
Mark: Uh-huh.
Nurse: Do you practice safer sex?
Mark: Uh, yeah.
Nurse: What measures do you take?
Mark: My girlfriend's on the pill, so that's all we need to know, isn't it?
Nurse: Let's talk about the different kinds of protection needed to prevent pregnancy and STIs.

Adolescents are often so concerned about protecting their privacy from adults they may offer as little information as possible at a health care visit, especially in regard to sexual issues. Asking specific, open-ended questions is important to ensure a positive exchange of information and effective health teaching. As they offer details, remain nonjudgmental to encourage them to continue to elaborate.

help her validate her suspicions. Web sites set up by health professionals can be an ideal method for adolescents to learn more about their bodies and safer sex practices because they can do this in a private, nonjudgmental setting (Shoveller, Knight, David, et al., 2012). Again, follow-up is important to be certain the content was understood and the adolescent didn't also visit Internet sites with misleading information.

BOX 5.3 Interviewing for a Sexual History

Specific Questions to Include in a Sexual History

Are you sexually active?
Is your sexual partner of the same or different gender?
How many sexual partners have you had in the past 6 months?
Are you satisfied with your sex life? If not, why not?
Do you have any concerns about your sex life? If so, what are they? What would you like to change?
Do you practice "safer sex"?
Have you ever contracted a sexually transmitted infection or are you worried you have one now?
Have you ever experienced a problem such as maintaining an erection, erectile dysfunction, failure to achieve orgasm, or pain during intercourse?
If you're sexually active, are you using a method to prevent pregnancy or sexually transmitted diseases?
Are you satisfied with your current reproductive planning method, or do you have any questions about it?
For adolescents: Are you vaccinated against human papillomavirus (HPV)?

Serving as a role model for gender roles can also be a valuable intervention, particularly for young clients. Discussing the subject of reproduction in a matter-of-fact way, or treating menstruation as a positive sign of growth in a woman rather than as a burden, can help clients assume a positive attitude about these subjects.

Interventions that strengthen an individual's sense of maleness or femaleness are important to include in care. A woman who believes part of a female role is to be assertive needs opportunities in her care plan for making decisions and self-care; a hospitalized adolescent who views a male's role as being a person who watches Monday night football needs time structured for this activity at the same priority level as other activities. Unless such activities are structured, they can be easily omitted by busy health care providers.

REPRODUCTIVE DEVELOPMENT

Reproductive development begins at the moment of conception and continues through life.

Intrauterine Development

The sex of an individual is determined at the moment of conception by the chromosome information supplied by the particular ovum and sperm that join to create the new life. A **gonad** is a body organ that produces the cells necessary for reproduction (the ovary in females, the testis in males). At approximately week 5 of intrauterine life, mesonephric (wolffian) and paramesonephric (müllerian) ducts, the tissue that will become ovaries and testes, have already formed. By week 7 or 8, in chromosomal males, this early gonadal

BOX 5.4 Nursing Care Planning Based on Family Teaching

GENDER IDENTITY CONCERNS

Q. Suzanne asks you, "Is it all right to call body parts by nicknames, such as 'peter' for penis, when we talk to children? Or should we use the anatomic name?"

A. Although this decision is strictly up to parents, using anatomic names is usually advised. This prevents children from thinking of one part of their body as so different from others (and perhaps dirty or suspect) it can't be called by its real name.

Q. Kevin asks you, "Will it be important to give our child unisex toys? Can't girls play with dolls and boys play with trucks anymore?"

A. Developing a sense of gender involves more than the toys children use for play. If parents are concerned with instituting unisex roles in children, they need to begin by monitoring their own perspective. Once they project a feeling roles are interchangeable, such as both genders participate in sports and both parents cook and do dishes, the general home milieu does more than any one action to teach this principle to children.

tissue begins formation of testosterone. Under the influence of testosterone, the mesonephric duct develops into male reproductive organs and the paramesonephric duct regresses. If testosterone is not present by week 10, the paramesonephric duct becomes dominant and develops into female reproductive organs. When ovaries form, all of the **oocytes** (cells that will develop into eggs throughout the woman's mature years) are already present (Edmonds, 2012).

At about week 12 of intrauterine life, the external genitals begin to develop. In males, penile tissue elongates and the ventral surface of the penis closes to form a urethra. In females, with no testosterone present, the uterus, labia minora, and labia majora form. If, for some reason, testosterone secretion is halted in utero, a chromosomal male could be born with female-appearing genitalia (ambiguous genitalia). If a pregnant woman should be prescribed a form of testosterone or, because of a metabolic abnormality, she produce a high level of testosterone, a chromosomal female could be born with male-appearing genitalia (Kumar, 2012).

Pubertal Development

Puberty is the stage of life at which secondary sex changes begin. These changes in girls are stimulated when the hypothalamus synthesizes and releases gonadotropin-releasing hormone (GnRH), which then triggers the anterior pituitary to release follicle-stimulating hormone (FSH) and luteinizing hormone (LH). FSH and LH are termed gonadotropin (*gonad* = "ovary"; *tropin* = "growth") hormones not only because they begin the production of androgen and estrogen, which in turn initiate secondary sex characteristics, but also because they continue to cause the production of eggs and influence menstrual cycles throughout women's lives (Christensen, Bentley, Cabrera, et al., 2012).

Although the mechanism that initiates this pubertal change is not well understood, the hypothalamus apparently serves as a gonadostat or regulation mechanism to "turn on" gonad functioning. Although it is not proven, the general consensus is a girl must reach a critical weight of approximately 95 lb (43 kg) or develop a critical mass of body fat before the hypothalamus is triggered to send initial stimulation to the anterior pituitary gland to begin the formation of FSH and LH. Probably because of the combination of better nutrition and increased obesity, girls are beginning puberty at earlier ages than ever before (9 to 12 years of age) (Cheng, Buyken, Shi, et al., 2012). Studies of female athletes and girls with anorexia nervosa demonstrate that delays or halts in menstruation are related to the lack of body fat or energy expenditure (Doyle-Lucas, Akers, & Davy, 2010). The phenomenon of what triggers puberty is even less understood in boys but is probably also related to body weight.

The Role of Androgen

Androgenic hormones are the hormones responsible for muscular development, physical growth, and the increase in sebaceous gland secretions that cause typical acne in both boys and girls during adolescence. In males, androgenic hormones are produced by the adrenal cortex and the testes, and, in females, by the adrenal cortex and the ovaries.

The level of the primary androgenic hormone, testosterone, is low in males until puberty (between ages 12 and 14 years) when it rises to influence pubertal changes in the testes, scrotum, penis, prostate, and seminal vesicles; the appearance of male pubic, axillary, and facial hair; laryngeal enlargement with its accompanying voice change; maturation of spermatozoa; and closure of growth plates in long bones (termed **adrenarche**). In girls, testosterone influences enlargement of the labia majora and clitoris and formation of axillary and pubic hair.

The Role of Estrogen

When triggered at puberty by FSH, ovarian follicles in females begin to excrete a high level of the hormone estrogen. This increase influences the development of the uterus, fallopian tubes, and vagina; typical female fat distribution; hair patterns; and breast development. It also closes the epiphyses of long bones in girls the same way testosterone closes the growth plate in boys. The beginning of breast development is termed **thelarche**, which usually starts 1 to 2 years before menstruation.

Secondary Sex Characteristics

Adolescent sexual development has been categorized into stages (Tanner, 1990). There is wide variation in the time required for adolescents to move through these developmental stages; however, the sequential order is fairly constant. In girls, pubertal changes typically occur as:

- Growth spurt
- Increase in the transverse diameter of the pelvis
- Breast development
- Growth of pubic hair
- Onset of menstruation
- Growth of axillary hair
- Vaginal secretions

The average age at which menarche (the first menstrual period) occurs is 12.4 years of age (Ledger, 2012). It may occur as early as age 9 years or as late as age 17 years, however, and still be within a normal age range. Irregular menstrual periods are the rule rather than the exception for the first year or two. Menstrual periods do not become regular until ovulation occurs consistently and this does not tend to happen until 1 to 2 years after menarche (see Chapter 33 for a discussion of the use of oral estrogen–based contraceptives to help regulate menstrual periods in girls). In boys, production of spermatozoa does not begin in intrauterine life as does the production of ova in girls nor are spermatozoa produced in a cyclic pattern as are ova; rather, they are produced in a continuous process. The production of ova stops at menopause. In contrast, sperm production continues from puberty throughout the male's life.

Secondary sex characteristics of boys usually occur in the order of:

- Increase in weight
- Growth of testes
- Growth of face, axillary, and pubic hair
- Voice changes
- Penile growth
- Increase in height
- Spermatogenesis (production of sperm)

QSEN Checkpoint Question 5.1

Patient-Centered Care

Suzanne Matthews tells you she's worried she might be subfertile because both breast development and her first menstrual period occurred later than most of her friends. To increase her self-esteem and meet her learning needs, you could assure her of what fact?

a. Adrenarche, the development of breasts, typically occurs before the first menstrual period.
b. Breast development, termed mamarche, is not fully complete until about age 25 years.
c. The time for development of breasts varies a great deal and is termed thelarche.
d. Menarche, the term for breast development, typically occurs before 12 years of age.

Look in Appendix A for the best answer and rationale.

ANATOMY AND PHYSIOLOGY OF THE REPRODUCTIVE SYSTEM

Although the structures of the female and male reproductive systems differ greatly in both appearance and function, they are homologues; that is, they arise from the same or matched embryonic origin. The study of the female reproductive organs is **gynecology**. **Andrology** is the study of the male reproductive organs.

The Male Reproductive System

The male reproductive system consists of both external and internal divisions (Fig. 5.1).

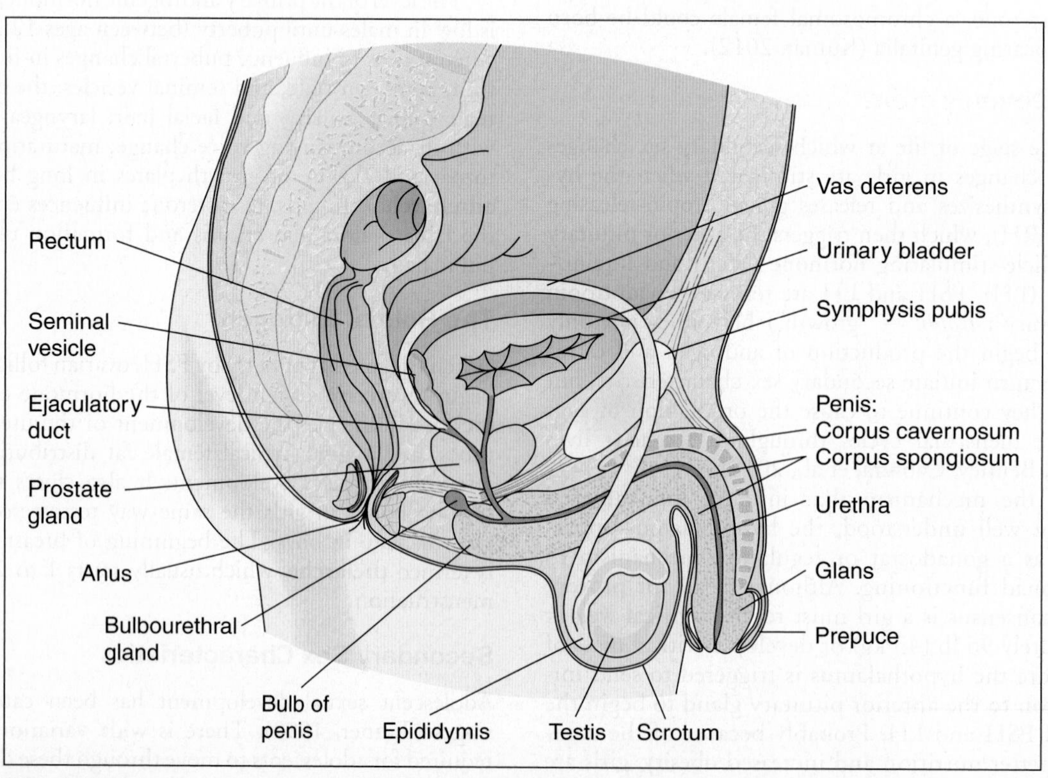

FIGURE 5.1 The male internal and external reproductive organs.

Male External Structures

External genital organs of the male include the testes (which are encased in the scrotal sac) and the penis.

The Scrotum. The scrotum is a rugated, skin-covered, muscular pouch suspended from the perineum. Its functions are to support the testes and help regulate the temperature of sperm. In very cold weather, the scrotal muscle contracts to bring the testes closer to the body. In very hot weather, or in the presence of fever, the muscle relaxes, allowing the testes to fall away from the body. In this way, the temperature of the testes can remain as even as possible to promote the production and viability of sperm.

The Testes. The testes are two ovoid glands, 2 to 3 cm wide, that rest in the scrotum. Each testis is encased by a protective white fibrous capsule and is composed of a number of lobules. Each lobule contains interstitial cells (Leydig cells) that produce testosterone and a seminiferous tubule that produces spermatozoa.

Testes in a fetus first form in the pelvic cavity then descend late in intrauterine life (about the 34th to 38th week of pregnancy) into the scrotal sac. Because this descent occurs so late in pregnancy, many male infants born preterm still have undescended testes. These infants need to be monitored closely to be certain their testes do descend at what would have been the 34th to 38th week of gestational age because testicular descent does not occur as readily in extrauterine life as it does in utero. Testes that remain in the pelvic cavity (cryptorchidism) may not produce viable sperm and have a four to seven times increased rate of testicular cancer (Ellsworth, 2012).

Although spermatozoa are produced in the testes, they reach maturity through a complex sequence of events. First, the hypothalamus releases GnRH, which in turn influences the anterior pituitary gland to release FSH and LH, the same as in women. FSH in men is responsible for the release of androgen-binding protein (ABP). LH is responsible for the release of testosterone from the testes. ABP and testosterone then combine to promote sperm formation. When the production of testosterone reaches a peak amount, a feedback effect on the hypothalamus and anterior pituitary gland is created, which slows the production of FSH and LH and ultimately decreases or regulates sperm production.

In most males, one testis is slightly larger than the other and is suspended slightly lower in the scrotum than the other (usually the left one). Because of this, testes tend to slide past each other more readily on sitting or muscular activity, and there is less possibility of trauma to them. Most body structures of importance are more protected than the testes (e.g., the heart is surrounded by ribs of hard bone). However, spermatozoa do not survive at a temperature as high as that of the internal body, so the location of the testes outside the body, where the temperature is about 1°F lower than body temperature, provides protection for sperm survival (Huether & McCance, 2012).

Normal testes feel firm and smooth, and are egg shaped. Beginning in early adolescence, boys need to learn testicular self-examination so they can detect tenderness or any abnormal growth in testes (see Chapter 34).

The Penis. The penis is composed of three cylindrical masses of erectile tissue in the penis shaft. The urethra passes through these layers of tissue, allowing the penis to serve as both the outlet for the urinary and reproductive tracts in men. With sexual excitement, nitric oxide is released from the endothelium of blood vessels. This causes dilation and an increase in blood flow to the arteries of the penis (engorgement). The ischiocavernosus muscle at the base of the penis, under stimulation of the parasympathetic nervous system, then contracts, trapping both venous and arterial blood in the three sections of erectile tissue. This leads to distention (and erection) of the penis.

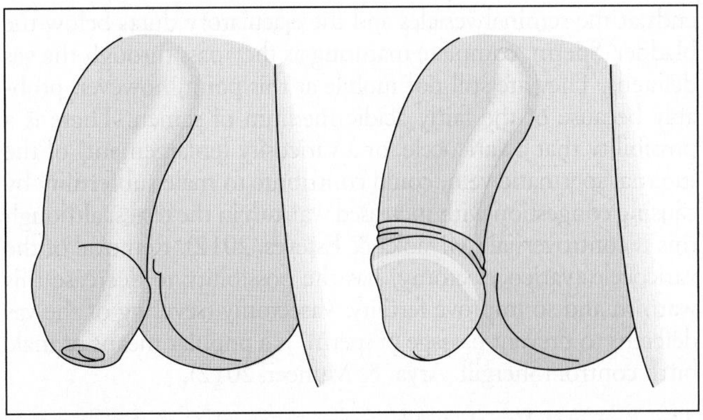

FIGURE 5.2 An uncircumcised and a circumcised penis.

At the distal end of the organ is a bulging, sensitive ridge of tissue called the glans. A retractable casing of skin, the prepuce, protects the nerve-sensitive glans at birth. Based on religious or cultural beliefs, many male infants have the prepuce tissue removed surgically (circumcision) shortly after birth (Fig. 5.2). Although controversial to some, the American Academy of Pediatrics (AAP) recommends male circumcision be done in consultation with parents for all male infants because the practice's advantages outweigh its risks. Its advantages allow for better hygiene as well as protection from HIV, STIs, and penile cancer (American Academy of Pediatrics [AAP], 2012).

Male Internal Structures

The male internal reproductive organs are the epididymis, the vas deferens, the seminal vesicles, the ejaculatory ducts, the prostate gland, the urethra, and the bulbourethral glands (see Fig. 5.1).

The Epididymis. The seminiferous tubule of each testis leads to a tightly coiled tube, the epididymis, which is responsible for conducting sperm from the tubule to the vas deferens, the next step in the passage to the outside. Because each epididymis is so tightly coiled, its length is extremely deceptive: it is actually over 20 ft long. Some sperm are stored in the epididymis, and a part of the alkaline fluid (semen, or seminal fluid that contains a basic sugar and protein) that will surround sperm at maturity is produced by the cells lining the epididymis.

Sperm are immobile and incapable of fertilization as they pass through or are stored at the epididymis level. It takes at least 12 to 20 days for them to travel the length of the tube, and a total of 65 to 75 days for them to reach full maturity. This is one reason **aspermia** (absence of sperm) and oligospermia (fewer than 20 million sperm per milliliter) are problems that do not appear to respond immediately to therapy, but do respond after 2 months of treatment (Tortora & Derrickson, 2012).

The Vas Deferens (Ductus Deferens). The vas deferens is an additional hollow tube surrounded by arteries and veins and protected by a thick fibrous coating, which, altogether, are referred to as the **spermatic cord**. It carries sperm from the epididymis through the inguinal canal into the abdominal cavity, where it ends at the seminal vesicles and the ejaculatory ducts below the bladder. Sperm complete maturing as they pass through the vas deferens. They are still not mobile at this point, however, probably because of the fairly acidic medium of semen. There is a possibility that a varicocele, or a varicosity (enlargement) of the internal spermatic vein, could contribute to male subfertility by causing congestion with increased warmth in the testes, although this is controversial (Miyaoka & Esteves, 2012). Removal of the varicocele (varicocelectomy) has the possibility to decrease this warmth and so improve fertility. Vasectomy (severing of the vas deferens to prevent passage of sperm) is a popular means of male birth control (Shergill, Arya, & Muneer, 2012).

The Seminal Vesicles. The seminal vesicles are two convoluted pouches that lie along the lower portion of the bladder and empty into the urethra by ejaculatory ducts. These glands secrete a viscous alkaline liquid with a high sugar, protein, and prostaglandin content. Sperm become increasingly motile because this added fluid surrounds them with a more favorable pH environment.

The Prostate Gland. The prostate is a chestnut-sized gland that lies just below the bladder and allows the urethra to pass through the center of it, like the hole in a doughnut. The gland's purpose is to secrete a thin, alkaline fluid, which, when added to the secretion from the seminal vesicles, further protects sperm by increasing the naturally low pH level of the urethra. In middle life, many men develop benign hypertrophy of the prostate. This swelling interferes with both fertility and urination because it reduces the lumen of the urethra. Benign prostatic hypertrophy can be relieved by medical therapy or surgery and needs to be differentiated by a health care provider from prostate cancer, which can also occur (Nickel, 2012).

The Bulbourethral Glands. Two bulbourethral, or Cowper's, glands lie beside the prostate gland and empty by short ducts into the urethra. They supply one more source of alkaline fluid to help ensure the safe passage of spermatozoa. Semen, therefore, is derived from the prostate gland (60%), the seminal vesicles (30%), the epididymis (5%), and the bulbourethral glands (5%).

The Urethra. The urethra is a hollow tube leading from the base of the bladder, which, after passing through the prostate gland, continues to the outside through the shaft and glans of the penis. It is about 8 in. (18 to 20 cm) long. Like other urinary tract structures, it is lined with mucous membrane.

✔ QSEN Checkpoint Question 5.2

Quality Improvement

Suppose Kevin Matthews tells you he is planning on having a vasectomy after the birth of his new child, but is worried about having his testes removed this way. You would want your clinic's educational material on vasectomy to clearly state that this procedure involves which of the following structures?

a. The seminal vesicles
b. The epididymis
c. The vas deferens
d. The ducts of the bulbourethral glands

Look in Appendix A for the best answer and rationale.

The Female Reproductive System

The female reproductive system, like the male, has both external and internal components.

Female External Structures

The structures that form the female external genitalia are termed the vulva (from the Latin word for "covering") and are illustrated in Figure 5.3.

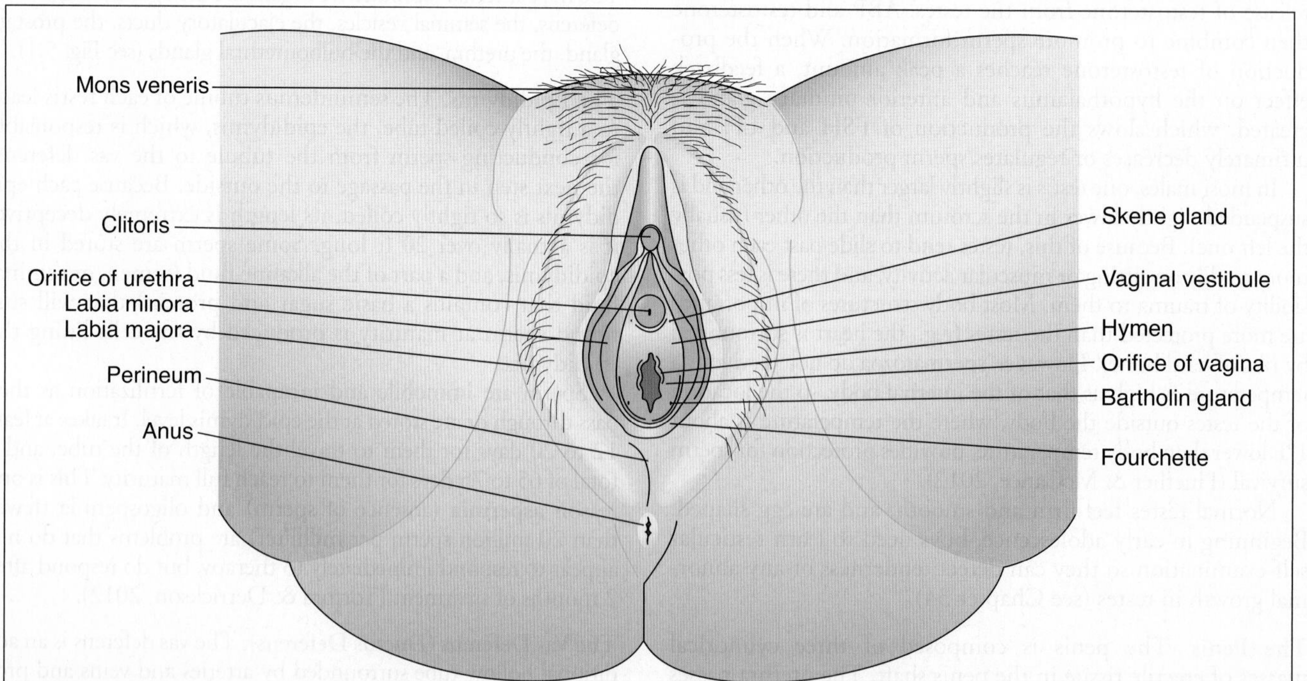

FIGURE 5.3 The female external genitalia.

The Mons Veneris. The mons veneris is a pad of adipose tissue located over the symphysis pubis, the pubic bone joint. Covered by a triangle of coarse, curly hairs, the purpose of the mons veneris is to protect the junction of the pubic bone from trauma.

The Labia Minora. Just posterior to the mons veneris spread two hairless folds of connective tissue, the labia minora. Before menarche, these folds are fairly thin; by childbearing age, they have become firm and full; and after menopause, they atrophy and again become much smaller. Normally, the folds of the labia minora are pink in color; the internal surface is covered with mucous membrane, and the external surface is covered with skin. The area is abundant with sebaceous glands, so localized sebaceous cysts may occur here. Women who perform monthly vulvar examinations are able to detect infection or other abnormalities of the vulva such as sebaceous cysts or herpes lesions.

The Labia Majora. The labia majora are two folds of tissue, fused anteriorly but separated posteriorly, which are positioned lateral to the labia minora and composed of loose connective tissue covered by epithelium and pubic hair. The labia majora serve as protection for the external genitalia; they shield the outlets to the urethra and vagina. Trauma to the area, such as occurs from childbirth or rape, can lead to extensive edema formation because of the looseness of the connective tissue base.

Other External Organs. The *vestibule* is the flattened, smooth surface inside the labia. The openings to the bladder (the urethra) and the uterus (the vagina) both arise from this space. The *clitoris* is a small (approximately 1 to 2 cm), rounded organ of erectile tissue at the forward junction of the labia minora. It's covered by a fold of skin, the prepuce; is sensitive to touch and temperature; and is the center of sexual arousal and orgasm in a woman. Arterial blood supply for the clitoris is plentiful. When the ischiocavernosus muscle surrounding it contracts with sexual arousal, the venous outflow for the clitoris is blocked and this leads to clitoral erection.

In nations which allow it, young girls approaching puberty may be circumcised or have their clitoris removed with the labia minora excised as well. Aside from being a very painful procedure, female circumcision can lead to contractions and scarring of the vulva that makes vaginal childbirth difficult because the vagina is unable to expand with birth (Mswela, 2010).

Two Skene glands (paraurethral glands) are located on each side of the urinary meatus; their ducts open into the urethra. Bartholin glands (vulvovaginal glands) are located on each side of the vaginal opening with ducts that open into the proximal vagina near the labia minora and hymen. Secretions from both of these glands help to lubricate the external genitalia during coitus. The alkaline pH of their secretions also helps to improve sperm survival in the vagina. If the Skene glands or the Bartholin glands (the most common site) become infected, they swell, feel tender, and produce a serous discharge.

The *fourchette* is the ridge of tissue formed by the posterior joining of the labia minora and the labia majora. This is the structure that sometimes tears (laceration) or is cut (episiotomy) during childbirth to enlarge the vaginal opening.

Posterior to the fourchette is the perineal muscle (often called the perineal body). Because this is a muscular area, it stretches during childbirth to allow enlargement of the vagina and passage of the fetal head. Many exercises suggested for pregnancy (such as Kegel exercises, squatting, and tailor sitting) are aimed at making the perineal muscle as flexible as it can be to allow for optimal expansion during birth and to prevent tearing of this tissue.

The *hymen* is a tough but elastic semicircle of tissue that covers the opening to the vagina during childhood. It is often torn during the time of first sexual intercourse. However, because of the use of tampons and active sports participation, many girls who have not had sexual relations can also have torn hymens at the time of their first pelvic examination. Occasionally, a girl has an imperforate hymen, or a hymen so complete that it does not allow for the passage of menstrual blood from the vagina (hematocolpometra) or for sexual relations until it is surgically incised (Poll & Flake, 2011).

The Vulvar Blood Supply. The blood supply of female external genitalia is mainly from the pudendal artery and a portion is from the inferior rectus artery. Venous return is through the pudendal vein. Pressure on this vein by the fetal head during pregnancy can cause extensive back pressure and development of varicosities (distended veins) in the labia majora and in the legs. A disadvantage of this rich blood supply is trauma to the area, such as occurs from pressure during childbirth or a bicycle seat injury, can cause large hematomas. An advantage is that it contributes to the rapid healing of any tears in the area after childbirth or other injury (Huether & McCance, 2012).

The Vulvar Nerve Supply. The anterior portion of the vulva derives its nerve supply from the ilioinguinal and genitofemoral nerves (L1 level). The posterior portions of the vulva and vagina are supplied by the pudendal nerve (S3 level). Such a rich nerve supply makes the area extremely sensitive to touch, pressure, pain, and temperature. Luckily, at the time of birth, normal stretching of the perineum causes a temporary loss of sensation to the area, limiting the amount of local pain felt during childbirth.

Female Internal Structures

Female internal reproductive organs (Fig. 5.4) are the ovaries, the fallopian tubes, the uterus, and the vagina.

The Ovaries. The ovaries are approximately 3 cm long by 2 cm in diameter and 1.5 cm thick, or the size and shape of almonds. They are grayish-white and appear pitted, with minute indentations on the surface.

The ovaries are located close to and on both sides of the uterus in the lower abdomen. Normally, they lie so low they cannot be located by abdominal palpation. Only if an abnormality exists, such as an enlarging ovarian cyst, can the resulting tenderness and enlargement be evident on lower left or lower right abdominal palpation.

The function of the two ovaries is to produce, mature, and discharge ova (the egg cells). In the process of producing ova, the ovaries also produce estrogen and progesterone and initiate and regulate menstrual cycles. If the ovaries are removed before puberty (or are nonfunctional), the resulting absence of estrogen normally produced by the ovaries prevents maturation and maintenance of secondary sex characteristics; in addition, pubic hair distribution will assume a more male than female pattern. After menopause, or cessation of ovarian

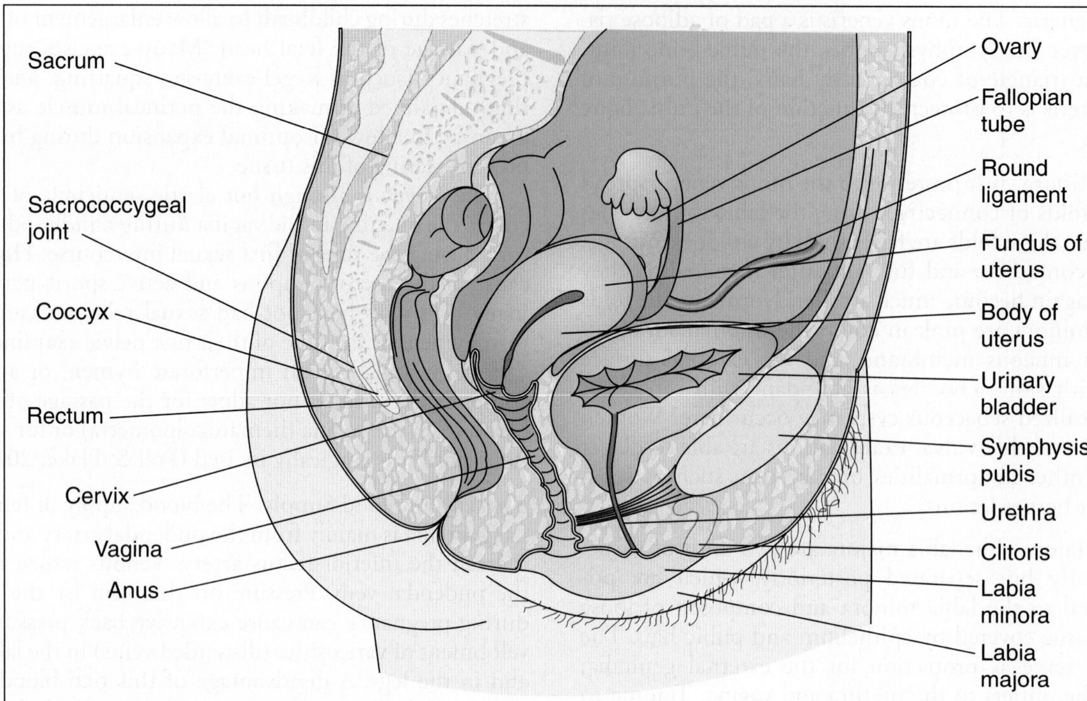

FIGURE 5.4 The female internal reproductive organs.

function, the uterus, breasts, and ovaries all undergo atrophy or a reduction in size because of a lack of estrogen.

This decrease in estrogen can lead to osteoporosis, or weakness of bones, because without estrogen, calcium tends to withdraw from the skeleton (Institute of Medicine [IOM], 2012). This can result in serious spinal, hip, and wrist fractures. Because cholesterol is incorporated into estrogen, a decrease in the production of estrogen may also allow cholesterol levels to rise and result in atherosclerosis (artery disease) in older women.

The ovaries are held suspended and in close contact with the ends of the fallopian tubes by three strong ligaments that attach both to the uterus and the pelvic wall. Ovaries are unique among pelvic structures in that they are not covered by a layer of peritoneum. Because they are not covered this way, ova can readily escape from them and enter the uterus by way of the fallopian tubes. Because they are suspended in position rather than being firmly fixed, an abnormal tumor or cyst growing on them can enlarge to a size easily twice that of the organ before pressure on surrounding organs or the ovarian blood supply leads to symptoms of compression. This is the reason ovarian cancer continues to be one of the leading causes of death from cancer in women (the tumor can grow without symptoms for an extended period) (Hunn & Rodriquez, 2012).

The Division of Reproductive Cells (Gametes). At birth, each ovary contains approximately 2 million immature ova (oocytes), which were formed during the first 5 months of intrauterine life. Although these cells have the unique ability to produce a new individual, they basically contain the usual components of cells: a cell membrane, an area of clear cytoplasm, and a nucleus that contains chromosomes.

One way they do differ from all other body cells is in the number of chromosomes their nuclei contain. All other human cells, have 46 chromosomes: 22 pair of autosomes (paired matching chromosomes) and one pair of sex chromosomes (two X sex chromosomes in the female, and an X and a Y sex chromosome pair in the male). In contrast to this, reproductive cells (both ova and spermatozoa) have only half the usual number of chromosomes. This is so that, when sperm and egg combine (fertilization), the new individual formed will not have twice the needed number, but rather, 46 chromosomes. The way reproductive cells divide is what causes this change in chromosome number.

Other cells in the body undergo cell division by *mitosis*, or daughter cell division; prior to a point of division, all the chromosomes are duplicated, leaving both new daughter cells with the right number of chromosomes.

In intrauterine life, oocytes divide by one typical mitotic division. Division activity then halts until puberty, when a second type of cell division, *meiosis* (cell reduction division), occurs. In the male, this reduction division occurs just before the spermatozoa mature. In the female, it occurs just before ovulation. After this reduction division, a typical ovum will have 22 autosomes and an X sex chromosome; a spermatozoon will have 22 autosomes and either an X or a Y sex chromosome. A new individual formed from the union of an ovum and the X-carrying spermatozoon will be female (an XX chromosome pattern); an individual formed from the union of an ovum and the Y-carrying spermatozoon will be male (an XY chromosome pattern).

The Maturation of Oocytes. Between 5 and 7 million ova form in utero. Most never develop beyond a primitive state and then atrophy, so by birth only about 2 million are still present. By age 7 years, only about 500,000 are present in each ovary; by 22 years of age, the count is down to 300,000; and by menopause, or the end of the fertile period in females, none are left (all have either matured or atrophied). "The point at which no functioning oocytes remain in the ovaries" is one definition of menopause.

The Fallopian Tubes. The fallopian tubes arise from each upper corner of the uterine body and extend outward and backward

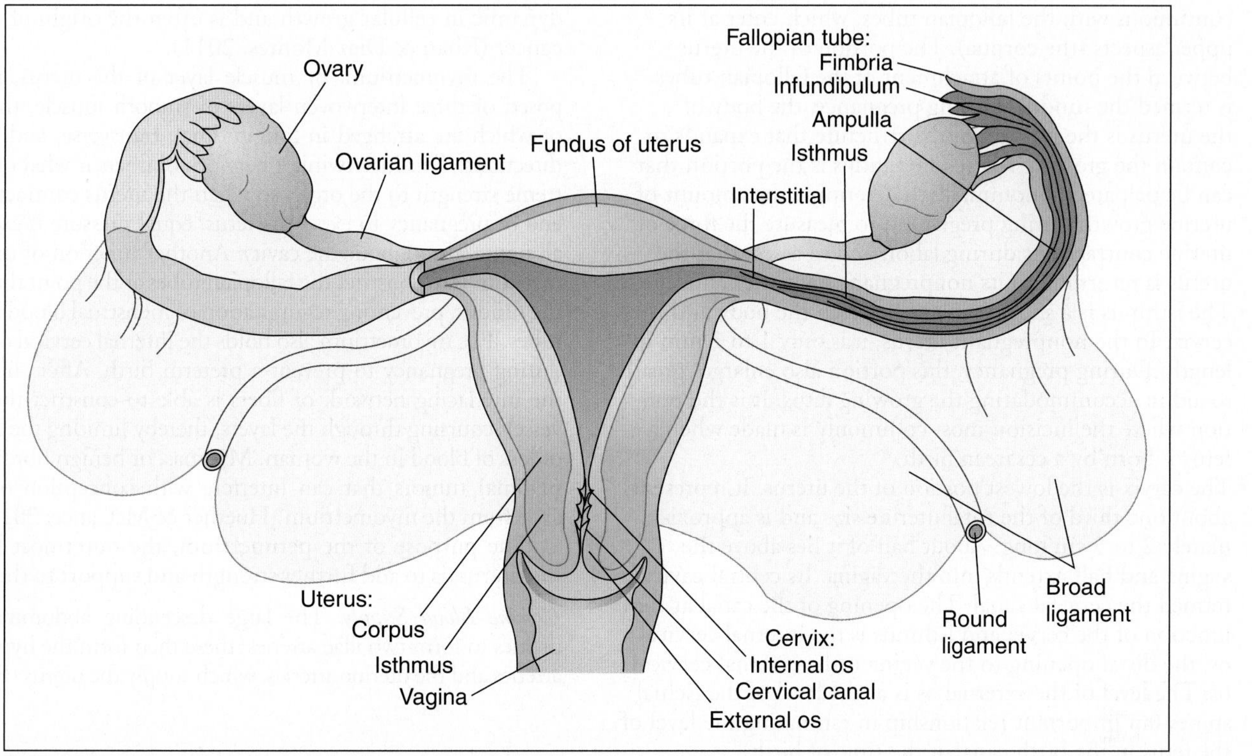

FIGURE 5.5 An anterior view of female reproductive organs showing the relationship of the fallopian tubes and body of the uterus.

until each opens at its distal end, next to an ovary. Fallopian tubes are approximately 10 cm long in a mature woman. Their function is to convey the ovum from the ovaries to the uterus and to provide a place for fertilization of the ovum by sperm.

Although a fallopian tube is a smooth, hollow tunnel, it is anatomically divided into four separate parts (Fig. 5.5).

- The most proximal division, the interstitial portion, is the part of the tube that lies within the uterine wall. This portion is only about 1 cm in length; its lumen is only 1 mm in diameter.
- The next distal portion is the isthmus. This is about 2 cm in length and like the interstitial tube, remains extremely narrow. This is the portion of the tube that is cut or sealed in a tubal ligation, or tubal sterilization procedure.
- The ampulla is the third and also the longest portion of the tube. It is about 5 cm in length and is the portion of the tube where fertilization of an ovum usually occurs.
- The infundibular portion is the most distal segment of the tube. It is about 2 cm long, funnel shaped, and covered by fimbria (small hairs) that help to guide the ovum into the fallopian tube.

The lining of the fallopian tubes is composed of a mucous membrane, which contains both mucus-secreting and ciliated (hair-covered) cells. Beneath this mucous lining are connective tissue and a circular muscle layer. The muscle layer is important because it is able to produce peristaltic motions that help conduct the ovum the length of the tube (probably also aided by the action of the ciliated lining and the mucus, which acts as a lubricant). The mucus produced may also serve as a source of nourishment for the fertilized egg, because it contains protein, water, and salts.

Because the fallopian tubes are open at their distal ends, a direct pathway exists from the external genital organs, through the vagina to the uterus and tubes, to the peritoneum. This open pathway is what makes conception possible. It also, however, can lead to infection of the peritoneum (peritonitis) if germs spread from the perineum through the uterus and tubes to the pelvic cavity. For this reason, clean technique must be used during pelvic examinations. During labor and birth, vaginal examinations are done with sterile technique to ensure no organisms can enter by this route.

The Uterus. The uterus is a hollow, muscular, pear-shaped organ located in the lower pelvis, posterior to the bladder and anterior to the rectum. During childhood, it is about the size of an olive; the cervix is the largest portion and the uterine body is the smallest part. When a girl reaches about 8 years of age, an increase in the size of the organ begins. This growth is so slow, however, the young woman is closer to 17 years old before the uterus reaches its adult size and changes its proportions so the body cavity, not the cervix, is its largest portion. Small uterine size may be a contributing factor to the number of low–birth-weight babies typically born to adolescents younger than this age (March of Dimes Foundation [MODF], 2012).

With maturity, a uterus is about 5 to 7 cm long, 5 cm wide, and, in its widest upper part, 2.5 cm deep. In a nonpregnant state, it weighs approximately 60 g. The function of the uterus is to receive the ovum from the fallopian tube; provide a place for implantation and nourishment; furnish protection to a growing fetus; and, at maturity of the fetus, expel it from a woman's body. After a pregnancy, the uterus never returns to exactly its nonpregnant size but remains approximately 9 cm long, 6 cm wide, 3 cm thick, and 80 g in weight.

Anatomically, the uterus consists of three divisions: the body or corpus, the isthmus, and the cervix.

- The body of the uterus is the uppermost part and forms the bulk of the organ. The lining of the cavity is

continuous with the fallopian tubes, which enter at its upper aspects (the cornua). The portion of the uterus between the points of attachment of the fallopian tubes is termed the fundus. During pregnancy, the body of the uterus is the portion of the structure that expands to contain the growing fetus. The fundus is the portion that can be palpated abdominally to determine the amount of uterine growth during pregnancy, to measure the force of uterine contractions during labor, and to assess that the uterus is returning to its nonpregnant state after childbirth.
- The isthmus is a short segment between the body and the cervix. In the nonpregnant uterus, it is only 1 to 2 mm in length. During pregnancy, this portion also enlarges greatly to aid in accommodating the growing fetus. It is the portion where the incision most commonly is made when a fetus is born by a cesarean birth.
- The cervix is the lowest portion of the uterus. It represents about one third of the total uterine size and is approximately 2 to 5 cm long. About half of it lies above the vagina and half extends into the vagina. Its central cavity is termed the cervical canal. The opening of the canal at the junction of the cervix and isthmus is the internal cervical os; the distal opening to the vagina is the external cervical os. The level of the external os is at the level of the ischial spines (an important relationship in estimating the level of the fetus in the birth canal at the time of birth).

Uterine and Cervical Coats. The uterine wall consists of three separate coats or layers of tissue:

- The endometrium, an inner layer of mucous membrane
- The myometrium, a middle layer of muscle fibers
- The perimetrium, an outer layer of connective tissue

The endometrium layer of the uterus is formed of two layers of cells and is the one important for menstrual function. The cell layer closest to the uterine wall, the basal layer, remains stable, uninfluenced by hormones. In contrast, the inner glandular layer is dramatically influenced by both estrogen and progesterone. It grows and becomes so thick and responsive each month under the influence of estrogen and progesterone that it becomes capable of supporting a pregnancy. If pregnancy does not occur, this is the layer that is shed as the menstrual flow.

The mucous membrane that lines the cervix is termed the endocervix. Continuous with the endometrium, these cells are also affected by hormones, although their changes are more subtle. A responsibility of such cells is to secrete mucus to provide an alkaline, lubricated surface to reduce the acidity of the upper vagina and to aid the passage of spermatozoa through the cervix; the efficiency of this lubrication increases or wanes depending on hormone stimulation. At the point in the menstrual cycle when estrogen production is at its peak, as much as 700 ml of mucus per day is produced; at the point estrogen is at its lowest level, only a few milliliters is produced. During pregnancy, so much mucus is produced, the endocervix becomes plugged with mucus, forming a seal to keep out ascending infections (the operculum).

Both the lower outer surface of the cervix and the internal cervical canal are lined not with a mucous membrane but with a stratified squamous epithelium, similar to that lining the vagina. Locating the point at which this tissue changes from epithelium to mucous membrane (squamocolumnar junction) is important when obtaining a Papanicolaou smear (a test for cervical cancer), because this tissue interface is most dynamic in cellular growth and is often the origin of cervical cancer (Khan & Diaz-Montes, 2011).

The myometrium, or muscle layer of the uterus, is composed of three interwoven layers of smooth muscle, the fibers of which are arranged in longitudinal, transverse, and oblique directions. This intertwining network of fibers is what offers extreme strength to the organ so when the uterus contracts at the end of pregnancy to expel the fetus, equal pressure is exerted at all points throughout the cavity. Another function of the myometrium is to constrict the fallopian tubes at the point they enter the fundus, preventing regurgitation of menstrual blood into the tubes. The myometrium also holds the internal cervical os closed during pregnancy to prevent a preterm birth. After childbirth, the interlacing network of fibers is able to constrict the blood vessels coursing through the layers, thereby limiting the amount of loss of blood in the woman. Myomas, or benign fibroid (leiomyoma) tumors that can interfere with conception or birth, arise from the myometrium (Huether & McCance, 2012).

The purpose of the perimetrium, the outermost layer of the uterus, is to add further strength and support to the organ.

Uterine Blood Supply. The large descending abdominal aorta divides to form two iliac arteries; these then form the hypogastric arteries and the uterine arteries, which supply the uterus (Fig. 5.6).

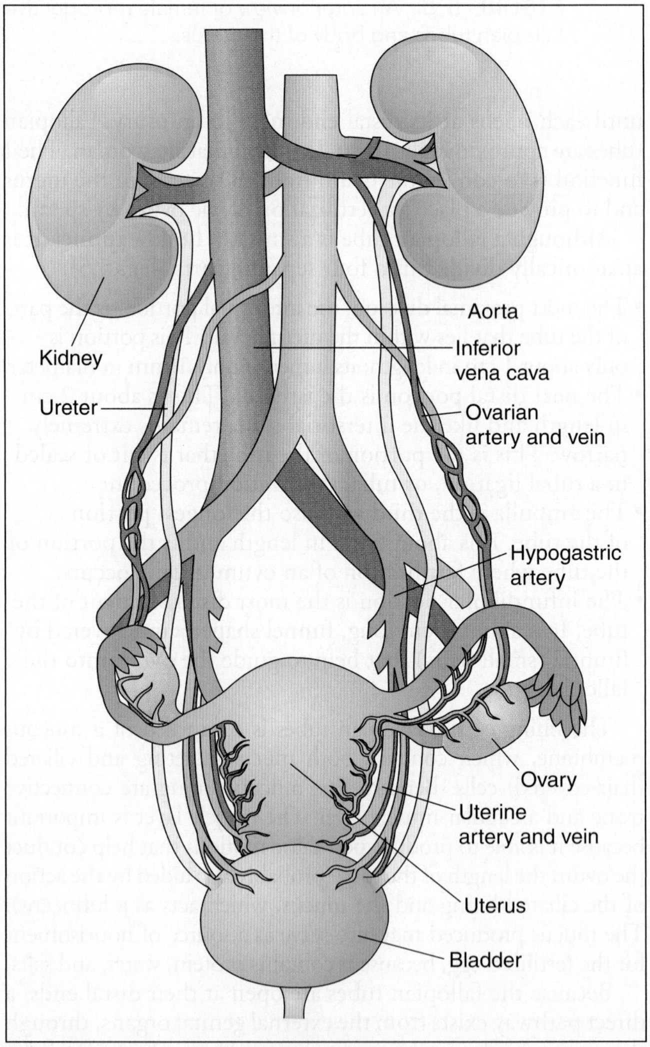

FIGURE 5.6 Blood supply to the uterus.

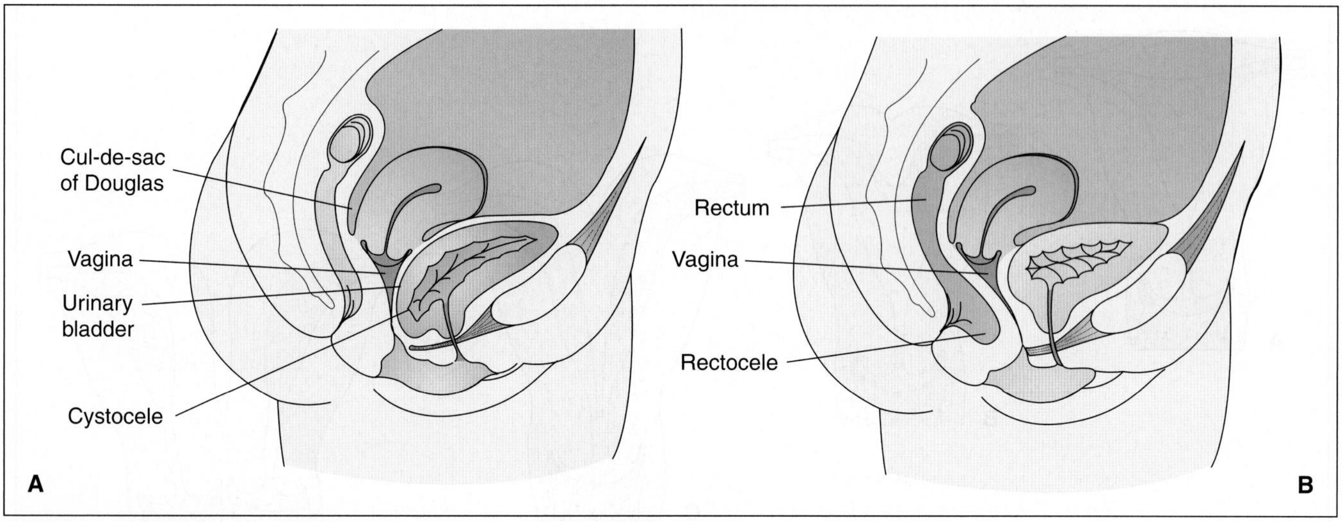

FIGURE 5.7 **(A)** A cystocele. The bladder has herniated into the anterior wall of the vagina. **(B)** A rectocele. The posterior of the vagina is herniated.

Because the uterine blood supply is not far removed from the aorta this way, it is guaranteed to be copious and adequate to supply the growing needs of a fetus. As an additional guarantee that enough blood will be available, after supplying the ovaries with blood, the ovarian artery (a direct subdivision of the aorta) joins the uterine artery and adds more blood to the uterus.

The blood vessels that supply the cells and lining of the uterus look tortuous against the sides of the uterine body in nonpregnant women. As a uterus enlarges with pregnancy, the vessels "unwind" and stretch as another guarantee that the uterus will maintain an adequate blood supply as the organ grows larger. The uterine veins follow the same twisting course as the arteries; they empty into the internal iliac veins.

An important organ relationship to be aware of is the close proximity of uterine blood vessels and ureters. Ureters pass from the kidneys on their way to the bladder directly in back of the ovarian vessels, near the fallopian tubes (see Fig. 5.5). This close anatomic relationship has implications in procedures such as tubal ligation, cesarean birth, and hysterectomy (removal of the uterus), because a ureter this close to the fallopian tubes can be injured if bleeding during surgery is controlled by clamping of the uterine or ovarian vessels. This is a reason a first voiding after uterine or tubal surgery is measured and assessed carefully for color or the presence of blood.

Uterine Nerve Supply. The uterus is supplied by both efferent (motor) and afferent (sensory) nerves. The efferent nerves arise from the T5 through T10 spinal ganglia. The afferent nerves join the hypogastric plexus and enter the spinal column at T11 and T12. The fact that sensory innervation from the uterus registers lower in the spinal column than does motor control has implications for controlling pain in labor. An anesthetic solution can be injected to stop the pain of uterine contractions at the T11 and T12 levels without stopping motor control or contractions (which are registered higher, at the T5 to T10 level). This is the principle of both epidural and spinal anesthesia (see Chapter 16).

Uterine Supports. The uterus is suspended in the pelvic cavity by a number of ligaments that also help support the bladder; it is further supported by a combination of fascia and muscle. Because the uterus is suspended this way, it is free to enlarge without discomfort during pregnancy. If its ligaments become overstretched during pregnancy, however, they may not support the bladder well afterward, and the bladder can then herniate into the anterior vagina (a **cystocele**), possibly causing frequent urinary infections from status of urine (Fig. 5.7A). If the rectum pouches into the vaginal wall, a **rectocele** (Fig. 5.7B) develops, possibly leading to constipation (Carter & Gabel, 2012).

A fold of peritoneum behind the uterus is the posterior ligament. This forms a pouch (Douglas cul-de-sac) between the rectum and uterus. Because this is the lowest point of the pelvis, any fluid (such as blood) released from a condition, such as a ruptured tubal (ectopic) pregnancy, tends to collect in this space. The space can be examined for the presence of fluid or blood to help in diagnosis by inserting a culdoscope through the posterior vaginal wall **(culdoscopy)** or a laparoscope through the abdominal wall **(laparoscopy)** (Givens & Lipscomb, 2012).

The *broad ligaments* are two folds of peritoneum that cover the uterus in the front and back and extend to the pelvic sides to help steady the uterus. The *round ligaments* are two fibrous, muscular cords that pass from the body of the uterus through the broad ligaments and down into the inguinal canal, inserting into the fascia of the vulva. The round ligaments act as additional "stays" to further steady the uterus. If a pregnant woman moves quickly, she may pull one of these ligaments, causing a quick, sharp pain of frightening intensity in one of her lower abdominal quadrants. Pain of this type calls for conscientious assessment or it can be mistaken for labor or appendicitis pain.

What if...5.1 Suzanne Matthews decides to have a tubal ligation (clamping of the fallopian tubes) after the birth of her baby. You notice the first time she voids following surgery that her urine looks blood tinged. Would you assume the urine was contaminated by vaginal secretions so its appearance is innocent? Or would you report this as a potentially serious finding (her surgery was on her reproductive, not her urinary system)?

Uterine Deviations. A number of uterine deviations (i.e., shape and position) can interfere with fertility or pregnancy and so are helpful to recognize. When a uterus first forms in intrauterine

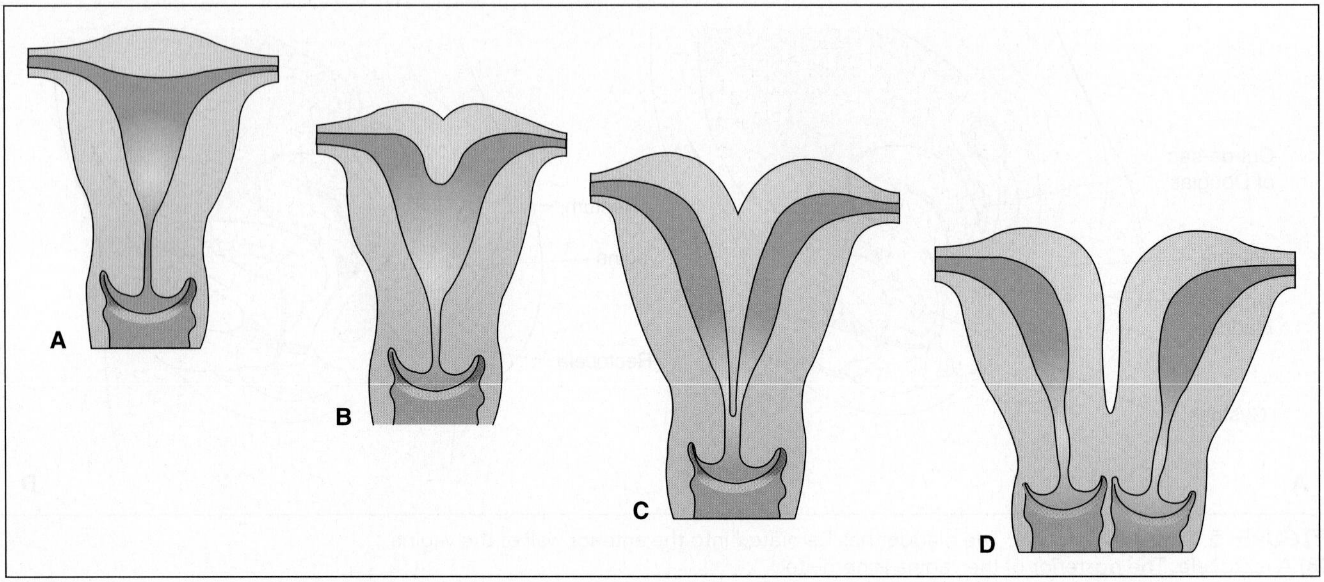

FIGURE 5.8 **(A)** A normal uterus. **(B)** A bicornuate uterus. **(C)** A septum-dividing uterus. **(D)** A double uterus. Abnormal shapes of uterus allow less placenta implantation space.

life, it is split by a longitudinal septum into two portions. As the fetus matures, this septum dissolves, so, typically at birth, no remnant of the division remains. In some women, half of the septum or even the entire septum never atrophies, so the uterus remains as two separate compartments. Still other women have oddly shaped "horns" at the junction of the fallopian tubes—a **bicornuate uterus**. Any of these malformations may decrease the ability to conceive or to carry a pregnancy to term (Grimes & Chen, 2011). Some examples of these types of uterine formation are shown in Figure 5.8. The specific effects of these deviations on fertility and pregnancy are discussed in later chapters.

Ordinarily, the body of the uterus tips slightly forward. Positional deviations of the uterus that are commonly seen include:

- **Anteversion:** the entire uterus tips far forward
- **Retroversion:** the entire uterus tips far back
- **Anteflexion:** the body of the uterus is bent sharply forward at the junction with the cervix
- **Retroflexion:** the body of the uterus is bent sharply back just above the cervix (Fig. 5.9)

Minor variations of these positions do not tend to cause reproductive problems. Extreme abnormal flexion or version positions may interfere with fertility because the sharp bend can block the deposition or migration of sperm.

The Vagina. The vagina is a hollow, musculomembranous canal located posterior to the bladder and anterior to the rectum. It extends from the cervix of the uterus to the external vulva. Its function is to act as the organ of intercourse and to convey sperm to the cervix. With childbirth, it expands to serve as the birth canal.

When a woman lies on her back, as she does for a pelvic examination, the course of the vagina is inward and downward. Because of this downward slant and the angle of the uterine cervix, the length of the anterior wall of the vagina is about 6 to 7 cm and the length of the posterior wall is 8 to 9 cm. At the cervical end of the structure, there are recesses on all sides, termed the posterior, anterior, and lateral fornices. The posterior fornix serves as a place for the pooling of semen after coitus; this allows for a large number of sperm to remain close to the cervix and encourages sperm migration into the cervix.

The vaginal wall is so thin at the fornices that an examiner can palpate the bladder through the anterior fornix, the ovaries through the lateral fornices, and the rectum through the posterior fornix.

The vagina is lined with stratified squamous epithelium similar to that covering the cervix. Under this, it has a middle connective tissue layer and a strong muscular wall. Normally, the walls contain many folds or rugae that lie in close approximation to each other. These folds make the vagina very elastic and able to expand so much that, at the end of pregnancy, a full-term baby can pass through without tearing. A circular muscle at the external opening of the vagina, called the bulbocavernosus muscle, acts as a voluntary sphincter. Relaxing and tensing this external vaginal sphincter muscle a set number of times each day (Kegel exercises) makes it more supple for birth and helps maintain tone after birth.

The blood supply to the vagina is furnished by the vaginal artery, a branch of the internal iliac artery. Vaginal tears at childbirth tend to bleed profusely because of this rich blood supply. The same rich blood supply, however, is also the reason any vaginal trauma at birth heals rapidly.

The vagina has both sympathetic and parasympathetic nerve innervations originating at the S1 to S3 levels. Despite this dual nerve supply, the vagina is not an extremely sensitive organ. Sexual excitement, often attributed to a vaginal origin, is actually mainly a clitoral function.

Mucus produced by the vaginal lining has a rich glycogen content. When this glycogen is broken down by the lactose-fermenting bacteria that frequent the vagina (Döderlein bacillus), lactic acid is formed. This causes the usual pH of the vagina to be acid, a condition detrimental to the growth of pathologic bacteria, so even though the vagina connects directly to the external surface, infection of the vagina does not readily occur. You can advise women not to use vaginal douches or sprays as a daily hygiene measure so they do not clear away this natural acid medium because this would invite

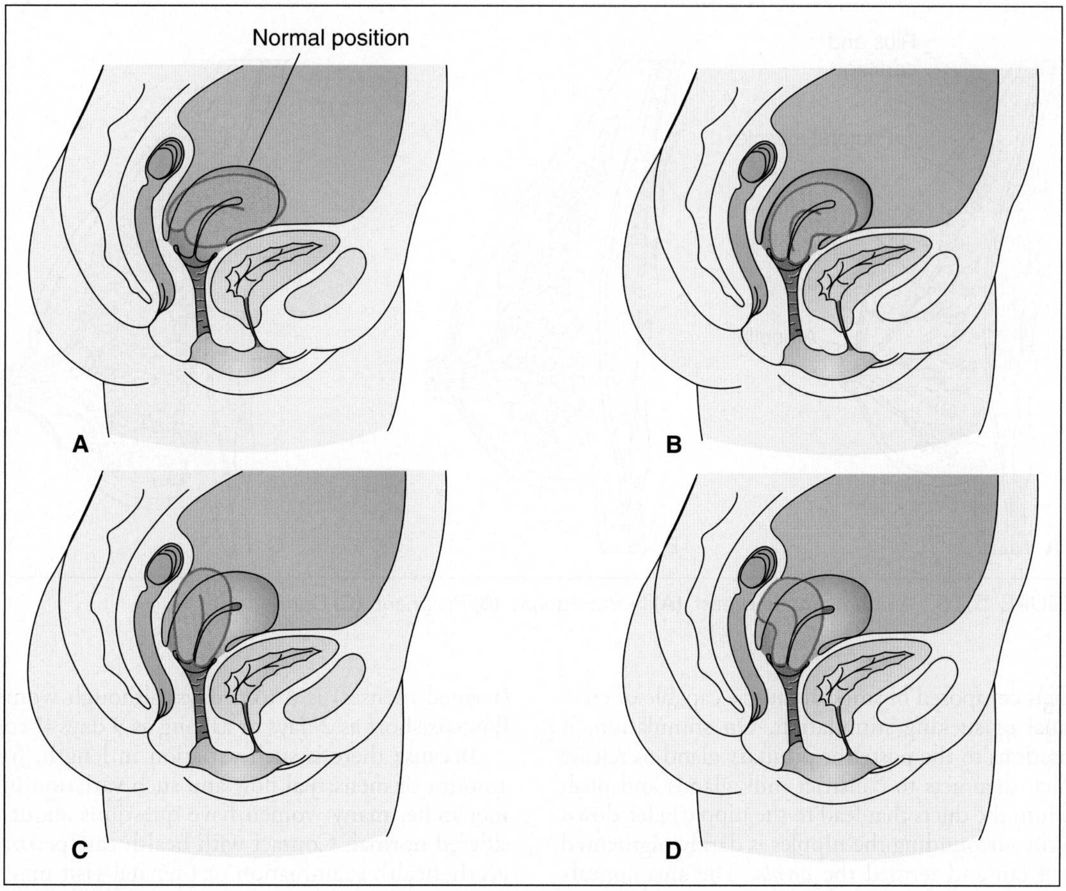

FIGURE 5.9 Uterine flexion and version. **(A)** Anteversion. **(B)** Anteflexion. **(C)** Retroversion. **(D)** Retroflexion.

infection. After menopause, the pH of the vagina changes and becomes closer to 7.5 or slightly alkaline, one reason vulvovaginitis infections occur more frequently in women in this age group (Guile & Keller, 2011).

QSEN Checkpoint Question 5.3

Teamwork & Collaboration

On physical examination, Suzanne Matthews is found to have a cystocele. You should confirm that the vocational nurse who is contributing to Suzanne's care knows that a cystocele can cause which of the following?

a. A fear of developing cancer from the sebaceous vulvar cyst that develops
b. Nagging pain from protrusion of the lower intestine into the posterior vagina
c. Bleeding from the prolapse of the uterine body and cervix into the distal vagina
d. Urinary infection from the pocket caused by pressure against the anterior vaginal wall

Look in Appendix A for the best answer and rationale.

The Breasts. The mammary glands, or breasts, form early in intrauterine life. They then remain in a halted stage of development until a rise in estrogen at puberty causes them to increase in size. This increase occurs mainly because of growth of connective tissue plus deposition of fat. The glandular tissue of the breasts, necessary for successful breastfeeding, remains undeveloped until a first pregnancy begins. Boys, especially those who are obese, may notice a temporary increase in breast size at puberty, termed **gynecomastia** (Sarwer, Spitzer, & Crerand, 2012). If boys are not prepared that this is a normal change of puberty, they may be concerned that they are developing abnormally.

Breasts are located anterior to the pectoral muscle (Fig. 5.10) and, in many women, breast tissue extends well into the axilla. When palpating for breast health, always include the axillary region in the examination, or this breast tissue can be missed. It is not uncommon for women or men to have supernumerary breast tissue along mammary lines on the front of their body. The nipple on these auxiliary sites may look like a mole, so adolescents may report this as a "mole changing in color" or be concerned they have skin cancer. You can assure them supernumerary breast tissue or nipples are not uncommon and are innocent findings.

Women should be aware of the usual appearance of their breasts (breast awareness) so they can report any change in contour or density to their health care provider.

Milk glands of the breasts are divided by connective tissue partitions into approximately 20 lobes. All of the glands in each lobe produce milk by acinar cells and deliver it to the nipple via a lactiferous duct. The nipple has approximately 20 small openings through which milk is secreted. An ampulla portion of the duct, located just posterior to the nipple, serves as a reservoir for milk before breastfeeding.

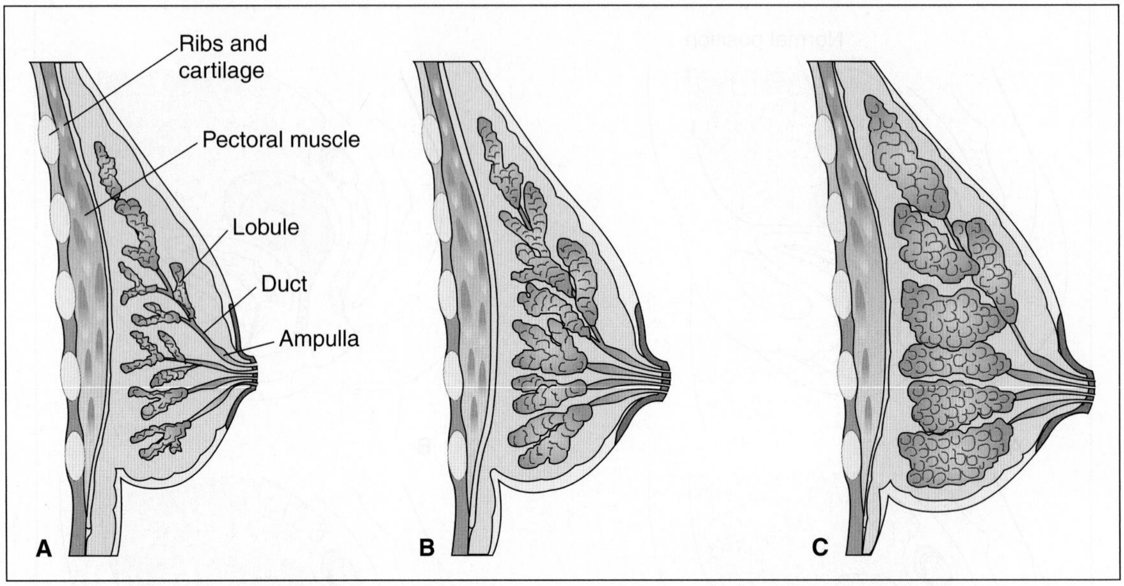

FIGURE 5.10 Anatomy of the breast. **(A)** Nonpregnant. **(B)** Pregnant. **(C)** During lactation.

The nipple is composed of smooth muscle capable of erection on manual or sucking stimulation. On stimulation, it transmits sensations to the posterior pituitary gland to release oxytocin, which then acts to constrict milk glands and push milk forward into the ducts that lead to the nipple (a let-down reflex). The skin surrounding the nipples is darkly pigmented out to about 4 cm and termed the *areola*. The area appears rough on the surface because it contains many sebaceous glands, called Montgomery tubercles. Because the milk glands are the structures important for breastfeeding and the size of breasts is associated with fat deposits, the size of breasts has no effect on whether a woman can successfully breastfeed.

The blood supply to the breasts is profuse because it is supplied by large thoracic branches of the axillary, internal mammary, and intercostal arteries. This effective blood supply is necessary so milk glands can be supplied with nutrients and fluid to make possible a plentiful supply of milk for breastfeeding. Unfortunately, this rich blood connection also aids in the metastasis of breast cancer if cancer is not discovered early (Huether & McCance, 2012).

MENSTRUATION

A menstrual cycle (the female reproductive cycle) is episodic uterine bleeding in response to cyclic hormonal changes. The purpose of a menstrual cycle is to bring an ovum to maturity and renew a uterine tissue bed that will be necessary for the ova's growth should it be fertilized. Because menarche may occur as early as 9 years of age, it is good to include health teaching information on menstruation to both school-age children and their parents as early as fourth grade as part of routine care. It is a poor introduction to sexuality and womanhood for a girl to begin menstruation unwarned and unprepared for the important internal function it represents.

The length of menstrual cycles differs from woman to woman, but the average length is 28 days (from the beginning of one menstrual flow to the beginning of the next). It is not unusual for cycles to be as short as 23 days or as long as 35 days. The length of the average menstrual flow (termed menses) is 4 to 6 days, although women may have flows as short as 2 days or as long as 9 days (Ledger, 2012).

Because there is such variation in length, frequency, and amount of menstrual flow and such variation in the onset of menarche, many women have questions about what is considered normal. Contact with health care personnel during a yearly health examination or prenatal visit may be their first opportunity to ask questions they have had for some time. Table 5.1 summarizes the normal characteristics of menstruation for quick reference.

The Physiology of Menstruation

Four body structures are involved in the physiology of the menstrual cycle: the hypothalamus, the pituitary gland, the ovaries, and the uterus. For a menstrual cycle to be complete,

TABLE 5.1 Characteristics of Normal Menstrual Cycles

Characteristic	Description
Beginning (menarche)	Average age at onset, 12.4 years; average range, 9–17 years
Interval between cycles	Average, 28 days; cycles of 23–35 days not unusual
Duration of menstrual flow	Average flow, 4–6 days; ranges of 2–9 days not abnormal
Amount of menstrual flow	Difficult to estimate; average 30–80 ml per menstrual period; saturating a pad or tampon in less than 1 hr is heavy bleeding
Color of menstrual flow	Dark red; a combination of blood, mucus, and endometrial cells
Odor	Similar to marigolds

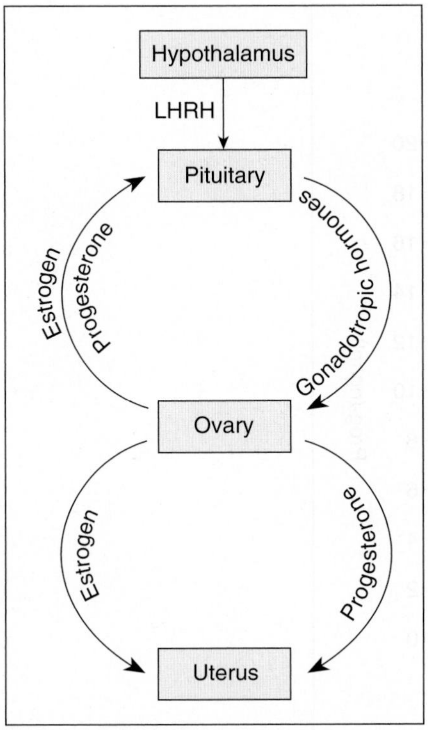

FIGURE 5.11 The interaction of pituitary–uterine–ovarian functions in a menstrual cycle.

all four organs must contribute their part; inactivity of any part results in an incomplete or ineffective cycle (Fig.5.11).

The Hypothalamus

The release of GnRH (also called luteinizing hormone-releasing hormone [LHRH]) from the hypothalamus initiates the menstrual cycle. GnRH then stimulates the pituitary gland to send gonadotropic hormone to the ovaries to produce estrogen. When the level of estrogen rises, release of GnRH is repressed and no further menstrual cycles will occur (the principle that birth control pills use to eliminate menstrual flows). Excessive levels of pituitary hormones can also inhibit release.

During childhood, the hypothalamus is apparently so sensitive to the small amount of estrogen produced by the adrenal glands, release of GnRH is suppressed. Beginning with puberty, the hypothalamus becomes less sensitive to estrogen feedback, so every month in females, the hormone is released in a cyclic pattern.

Diseases of the hypothalamus, which cause deficiency of this releasing factor, can result in delayed puberty. Likewise, a disease that causes early activation of GnRH can lead to abnormally early sexual development or precocious puberty (Kim & Lee, 2012) (see Chapter 47).

The Pituitary Gland

Under the influence of GnRH, the anterior lobe of the pituitary gland (the adenohypophysis) produces two hormones:

- FSH, a hormone active early in the cycle that is responsible for maturation of the ovum.
- LH, a hormone that becomes most active at the midpoint of the cycle and is responsible for ovulation, or release of the mature egg cell from the ovary. It also stimulates growth of the uterine lining during the second half of the menstrual cycle.

The Ovaries

FSH and LH are called gonadotropic hormones because they cause growth (trophy) in the gonads (ovaries). Every month during the fertile period of a woman's life (from menarche to menopause), one of the ovary's oocytes is activated by FSH to begin to grow and mature. As the oocyte grows, its cells produce a clear fluid (follicular fluid) that contains a high degree of estrogen and some progesterone. As the follicle surrounding the oocyte grows, it is propelled toward the surface of the ovary. At full maturity, the follicle is visible on the surface of the ovary as a clear water blister approximately 0.25 to 0.5 in. across. At this stage of maturation, the small ovum (barely visible to the naked eye, about the size of a printed period) with its surrounding follicular membrane and fluid is termed a *graafian follicle.*

By day 14 or the midpoint of a typical 28-day cycle, the ovum has divided by mitotic division into two separate bodies: a primary oocyte, which contains the bulk of the cytoplasm, and a secondary oocyte, which contains so little cytoplasm that it is not functional. The structure also has accomplished its meiotic division, reducing its number of chromosomes to the haploid (having only one member of a pair) number of 23.

After an upsurge of LH from the pituitary at about day 14, prostaglandins are released and the graafian follicle ruptures. The ovum is set free from the surface of the ovary, a process termed *ovulation.* It is swept into the open end of a fallopian tube. It is important to teach women that ovulation does not necessarily occur on the 14th day of their cycle; it occurs 14 days *from the end of their cycle.* If their menstrual cycle is only 20 days long, for example, their day of ovulation would be day 6 (14 days from the end of the cycle). If their cycle is 44 days long, ovulation would occur on day 30, not day 22.

After the ovum and the follicular fluid have been discharged from the ovary, the cells of the follicle remain in the form of a hollow, empty pit. The FSH has done its work at this point and now decreases in amount. The second pituitary hormone, LH, continues to rise in amount and directs the follicle cells left behind in the ovary to produce lutein, a bright-yellow fluid high in progesterone. With lutein production, the follicle is renamed a *corpus luteum* (yellow body).

The basal body temperature of a woman drops slightly (by 0.5° to 1°F) just before the day of ovulation because of the extremely low level of progesterone that is present at that time. It rises by 1°F on the day after ovulation because of the concentration of progesterone, which is thermogenic. The woman's temperature remains at this elevated level until approximately day 24 of the menstrual cycle, when the progesterone level again decreases (Huether & McCance, 2012). Therefore, taking body temperature daily is one method of predicting that ovulation has occurred.

If conception (fertilization by a spermatozoon) occurs as the ovum proceeds down a fallopian tube and the fertilized ovum implants on the endometrium of the uterus, the corpus luteum remains throughout the major portion of the pregnancy (to about 16 to 20 weeks). If conception does not occur, the unfertilized ovum atrophies after 4 or 5 days, and the corpus luteum (now called a "false" corpus luteum) remains for only 8 to 10 days. As the corpus luteum regresses, it is gradually replaced by white fibrous tissue, and the resulting structure is termed a corpus albicans (white body). Figure 5.12A summarizes the times when ovarian hormones are secreted at peak levels during a typical 28-day menstrual cycle to cause these changes.

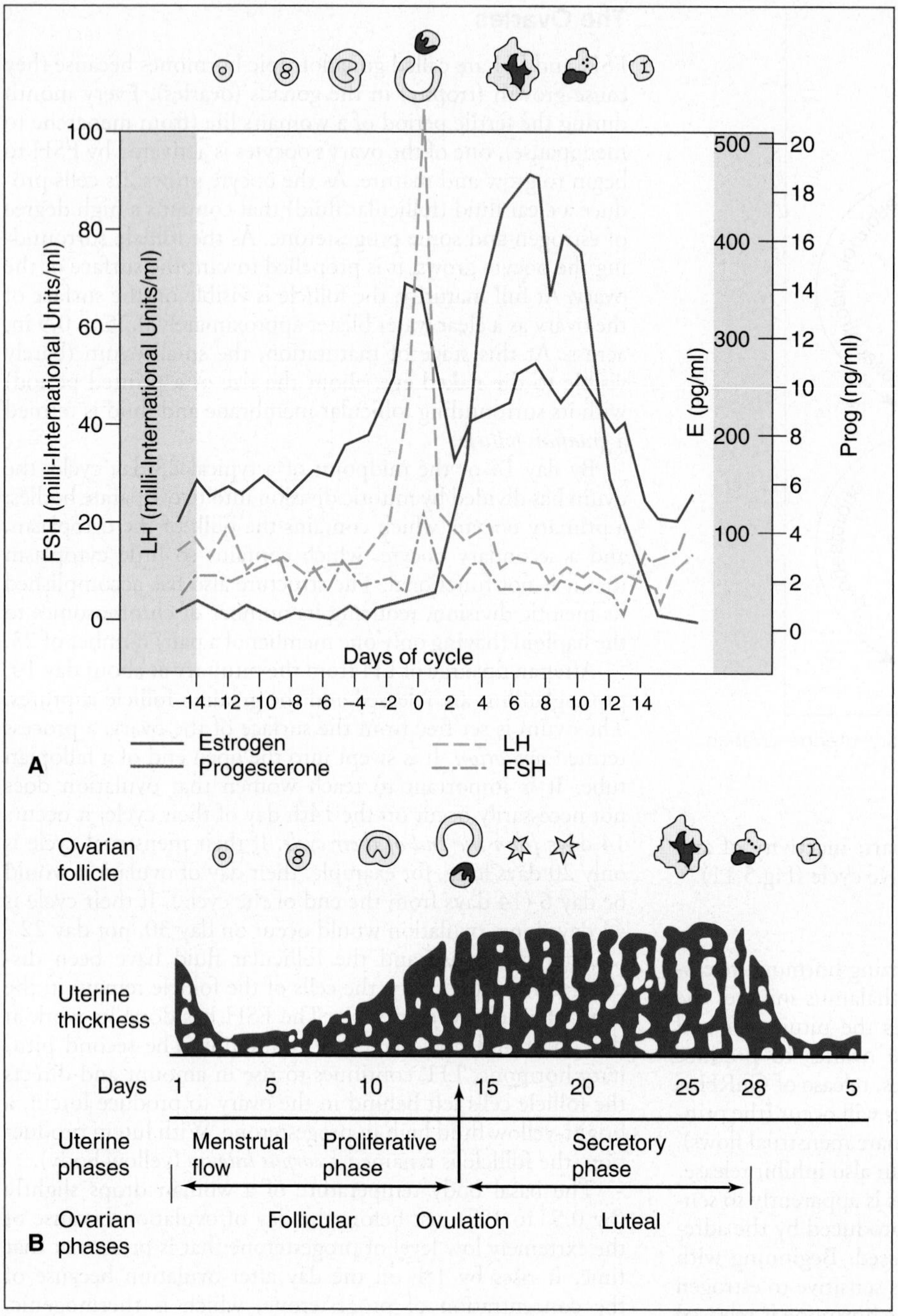

FIGURE 5.12 **(A)** Plasma hormone concentrations in the normal female reproductive cycle. **(B)** Ovarian events and uterine changes during the menstrual cycle.

The Uterus

Figure 5.12B also illustrates uterine changes that occur monthly as a result of stimulation from the estrogen and progesterone produced by the ovaries.

The First Phase of the Menstrual Cycle (Proliferative). Immediately after a menstrual flow (which occurs during the first 4 or 5 days of a cycle), the endometrium, or lining of the uterus, is very thin, approximately one cell layer in depth. As the ovary begins to produce estrogen (in the follicular fluid, under the direction of the pituitary FSH), the endometrium begins to proliferate so rapidly the thickness of the endometrium increases as much as eightfold from day 5 to day 14. This first half of a menstrual cycle is interchangeably termed the proliferative, estrogenic, follicular, or postmenstrual phase.

The Second Phase of the Menstrual Cycle (Secretory). After ovulation, the formation of progesterone in the corpus luteum (under the direction of LH) causes the glands of the uterine endometrium to become corkscrew or twisted in appearance and dilated with quantities of glycogen (an elementary sugar) and mucin (a protein). It takes on the appearance of rich, spongy velvet. This second phase of the menstrual cycle is termed the progestational, luteal, premenstrual, or secretory phase.

The Third Phase of the Menstrual Cycle (Ischemic). If fertilization does not occur, so the corpus luteum in the ovary begins to regress after 8 to 10 days, the production of progesterone decreases. With the withdrawal of progesterone, the endometrium of the uterus begins to degenerate (at about day 24 or day 25 of the cycle). The capillaries rupture, with minute hemorrhages, and the endometrium sloughs off.

The Fourth Phase of the Menstrual Cycle (Menses). Menses, or a menstrual flow, is composed of a mixture of blood from the ruptured capillaries; mucin; fragments of endometrial tissue; and the microscopic, atrophied, and unfertilized ovum.

Menses is actually the end of an arbitrarily defined menstrual cycle. Because it is the only external marker of the cycle, however, the first day of menstrual flow is used to mark the beginning day of a new menstrual cycle.

Contrary to common belief, a menstrual flow contains only 30 to 80 ml of blood; if it seems to be more, it is because of the accompanying mucus and endometrial shreds. The iron loss in a typical menstrual flow is approximately 11 mg. This is enough loss that many women need to take a daily iron supplement to prevent iron depletion during their menstruating years (Coad & Conlon, 2011).

✔ QSEN Checkpoint Question 5.4

Informatics

You document the fact that Suzanne Matthews typically has a menstrual cycle of 34 days. If she had coitus on days 8, 10, 15, and 20 of her last cycle, which is the day on which she most likely conceived?

a. The 8th day
b. The 10th day
c. Day 15
d. Day 20

Look in Appendix A for the best answer and rationale.

Cervical Changes

The mucus of the uterine cervix also changes in structure and consistency each month during a menstrual cycle. At the beginning of each cycle, when estrogen secretion from the ovary is low, cervical mucus is thick and scant. Sperm survival in this type of mucus is poor. At the time of ovulation, when the estrogen level has risen to a high point, cervical mucus becomes thin, stretchy (spinnbarkeit), and copious. Sperm penetration and survival in this thin mucus are both excellent. Because progesterone becomes the major influencing hormone during the second half of the cycle, cervical mucus again thickens and sperm survival is again poor.

Women can analyze cervical mucus changes to help plan coitus so it coincides with ovulation if they want to increase their chance of becoming pregnant or plan to avoid coitus at the time of ovulation to prevent pregnancy (natural family planning; see Chapter 6) by analyzing how thick or thin is cervical mucus. During ovulation, the body of the cervix is softer and the os is slightly open compared with the rest of the cycle when it is firm and the os is closed as another indication of ovulation.

The Fern Test

An interesting property of cervical mucus just before ovulation when estrogen levels are high is the ability to form fernlike patterns on a microscope slide when allowed to dry. This pattern is known as arborization or ferning (Fig. 5.13). When progesterone is the dominant hormone, as it is just after ovulation, this fern pattern is no longer discernible. Cervical mucus, therefore, can be examined at midcycle for ferning to detect whether a high estrogen surge is present. Women who do not ovulate usually show a ferning pattern throughout their menstrual cycle (progesterone levels never become dominant), or they never demonstrate it because their estrogen levels never rise.

A

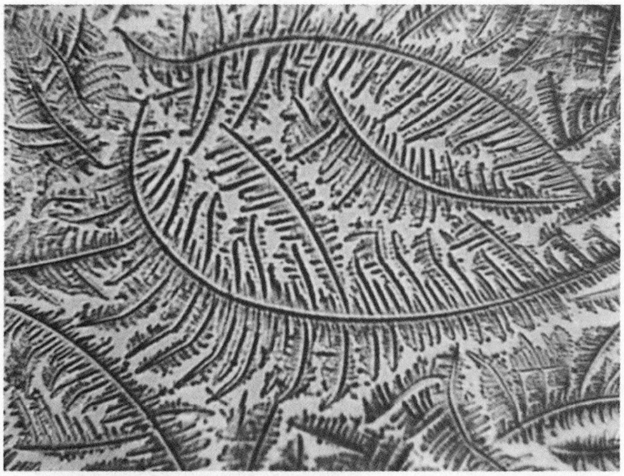

B

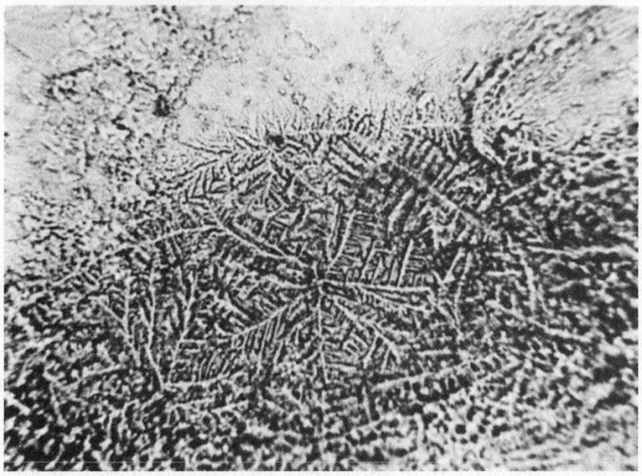

FIGURE 5.13 **(A)** A ferning pattern of cervical mucus occurs with high estrogen levels. **(B)** Incomplete ferning during secretory phase of cycle. (From Scott, J. R. [1990]. *Danforth's obstetrics and gynecology* [6th ed.]. Philadelphia, PA: J. B. Lippincott.)

The Spinnbarkeit Test

At the height of estrogen secretion, yet another property of cervical mucus is the ability to stretch into long strands, a contrast to its thick, viscous state when progesterone is the dominant hormone. That means performing this test, known as *spinnbarkeit*, at the midpoint of a menstrual cycle is another way to demonstrate high levels of estrogen are being produced and, by implication, ovulation is about to occur. A woman can do this herself by stretching a mucus sample between thumb and finger, or it can be tested in an examining room by smearing a cervical mucus specimen on a slide and stretching the mucus between the slide and cover slip (Fig. 5.14).

Education for Menstruation

Education about menstruation is an important component of comprehensive sexuality education. Many myths about menstruation still exist, such as women should not wash their hair during their menses, they should not plant vegetables or they all will die, or they should not eat sour foods as this will cause cramping. Early preparation for menstruation to dispel these myths is important to elevate a girl's concept of herself because it teaches her to trust her body or to think of menstruation

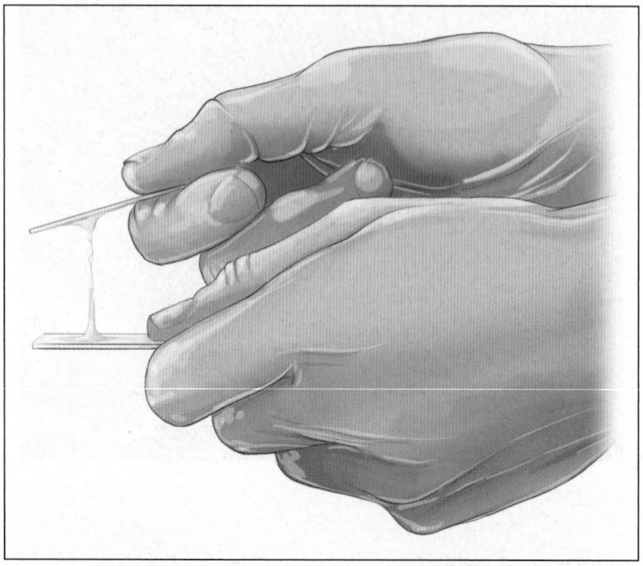

FIGURE 5.14 Spinnbarkeit is the property of cervical mucus to stretch a distance before breaking.

as a mark of pride and growing up rather than as a burden. Education regarding menstruation is equally important for boys so they can appreciate the cyclic process a woman's reproductive system activates and can be active participants in helping plan or prevent the conception of children.

Girls who are well prepared for menstruation and view it as a positive happening are more likely to cope with any menstrual discomfort effectively, so a positive attitude results in fewer missed school days than those who view menstruation as an ill time. Important teaching points for girls at menarche regarding menstruation are summarized in Table 5.2. Menstrual disorders, including dysmenorrhea (painful menstruation), **menorrhagia** (abnormally heavy menstrual flows), **metrorrhagia** (bleeding between menstrual periods), menstrual migraines, premenstrual dysphoric syndrome, and polycystic ovary syndrome (PCOS) are discussed in Chapter 47 with other reproductive system disorders.

Menopause

Menopause is the cessation of menstrual cycles. *Perimenopausal* is a term used to denote the period during which menopausal changes are occurring. *Postmenopausal* describes the period following the final menses. *Climacteric* refers to the total changes that occur at this life stage. The age range at which menopause occurs is wide, between approximately 40 and 55 years, with a mean age of 51 years (Panay, 2012).

The age at which menopause symptoms begin appears to be genetically influenced. Another influence may be nicotine because women who smoke tend to have earlier menopause than others (Lacey, 2012).

Menopause causes physical changes because, when ovaries begin to atrophy, estrogen production is reduced and "hot flashes," vaginal dryness, or osteoporosis (loss of bone mineral density) may occur. Urinary incontinence from lack of bladder support may occur. Women who notice excessive vaginal dryness can be advised to use a lubricating jelly such as K-Y Jelly prior to sexual relations. The application of estrogen cream or the insertion of a vaginal ring that dispenses low-dose estrogen are other possibilities being evaluated. Low-dose estrogen or testosterone can also be prescribed to increase sexual libido. Practicing Kegel exercises (see Chapter 11) can help strengthen bladder supports and reduce urinary incontinence (Marques, Stothers, & MacNab, 2010).

An older term to describe menopause was "change of life," because it marked the end of a woman's ability to bear children and the beginning of a new phase in her life. Such a role change can produce psychologic stress, although, through health teaching, nurses can help women appreciate that their role in life is bigger than just bearing children. If the woman know she is finished with childbearing, loss of uterine function

TABLE 5.2 Teaching About Menstrual Health

Area of Concern	Teaching Points
Exercise	Moderate exercise during menses promotes a general sense of well-being. Sustained excessive exercise, such as professional athletes maintain, can cause amenorrhea.
Sexual relations	Not contraindicated during menses although the male should wear a condom to prevent exposure to body fluid. Heightened or decreased sexual arousal may be noticed. Orgasms may increase the amount of menstrual flow. It is improbable but not impossible for conception to occur from coitus during menses.
Activities of daily life	Nothing is contraindicated (many people believe incorrectly activities such as running or bathing are harmful).
Pain relief	Prostaglandin inhibitors such as ibuprofen (Motrin) are most effective for menstrual pain because they reduce inflammation as well as relieve pain. Applying local heat may also be helpful. If a migraine headache occurs, specific drugs for this are now available, such as sumatriptan (Imitrex). Adolescents under age 18 years should not take aspirin (acetylsalicylic acid) because of the association between this and Reye syndrome.
Rest	More rest may be helpful if dysmenorrhea interferes with sleep at night.
Nutrition	Many women need iron supplementation to replace iron lost during menses. Eating pickles or cold food does not cause dysmenorrhea.

may make almost no change in her life, and for a woman who has also had dysmenorrhea (painful menstruation), menopause can be a long-awaited and welcome change.

SEXUALITY

Sexuality is a multidimensional phenomenon that includes feelings, attitudes, and actions. It has both biologic and cultural diversity components. It encompasses and gives direction to a person's physical, emotional, social, and intellectual responses throughout life.

Biologic gender is the term used to denote a person's chromosomal sex: male (XY) or female (XX). **Gender identity** or sexual identity is the inner sense a person has of being male or female, which may be the same as or different from biologic gender. **Gender role** is the male or female behavior a person exhibits, which, again, may or may not be the same as biologic gender or gender identity (Fig. 5.15).

The Human Sexual Response

Sexuality has always been a part of human life, but only in the past few decades has it been studied scientifically. One common finding of researchers has been that feelings and attitudes about sex vary widely across cultures and individuals (Box 5.5). Although the sexual experience is unique to each individual, sexual physiology (how the body responds to sexual arousal) has common features (Kimmel & Rogers, 2011).

The Sexual Response Cycle

Two of the earliest researchers of sexual response were Masters and Johnson. In 1966, they published the results of a major study based on more than 10,000 episodes of sexual activity among more than 600 men and women (Masters et al., 1998). In this study, they described the human sexual response as a cycle with four discrete stages: excitement, plateau, orgasm, and resolution. Whether stages are felt as separate steps this way or blended into one smooth process of desire, arousal, and orgasm is individualized.

Excitement. Excitement occurs with physical and psychological stimulation (sight, sound, emotion, or thought) that causes parasympathetic nerve stimulation. This leads to arterial dilation and venous constriction in the genital area. The resulting increased blood supply leads to vasocongestion and increasing muscular tension. In women, this vasocongestion causes the clitoris to increase in size and mucoid fluid to appear on vaginal walls for lubrication. The vagina widens in diameter and increases in length. Breast nipples become erect. In men, penile erection occurs, as well as scrotal thickening and elevation of the testes. In both sexes, there is an increase in heart and respiratory rate and blood pressure.

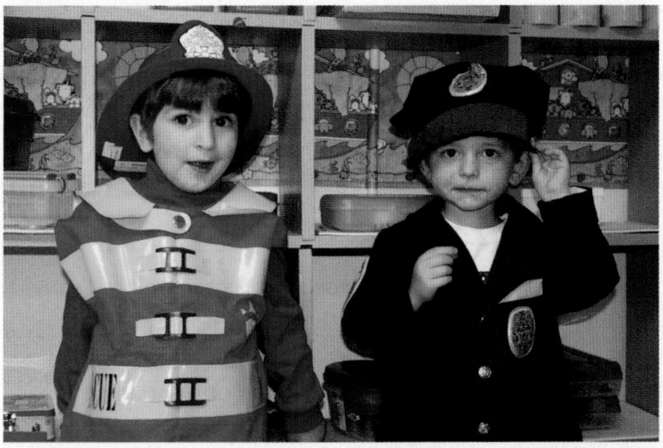

FIGURE 5.15 Early school-age children imitate adult roles to learn more about them and whether they will "fit" the role. Here, children pretend to be a fireman and a policeman.

BOX 5.5 Nursing Care Planning to Respect Cultural Diversity

How gender role is expressed by individuals is strongly culturally influenced. In almost all societies, women are viewed as having intrinsic nurturing qualities, which gives them the main responsibility for childrearing and homemaking. Men are viewed as the financial providers. A downside of having such a wide difference in roles is that intimate partner violence occurs more frequently in societies when there is a wide disparity in gender roles. Women have worked hard to see that gender roles today are viewed as more interchangeable in an attempt to reduce violence as well as increase earning capability. The success of the movement is reflected by the way women today can pursue all types of jobs and careers without loss of femininity; men participate in childrearing and household duties without loss of masculinity.

Types of sexual roles are also accepted more freely today although any community contains individuals who still hold stereotyped views. Some religions approve or don't approve of alternative life styles. A nursing role can be to help people understand the world is big enough for diverse and alternative ways of living.

Plateau. The plateau stage is reached just before orgasm. In the woman, the clitoris is drawn forward and retracts under the clitoral prepuce; the lower part of the vagina becomes extremely congested (formation of the orgasmic platform), and there is increased breast nipple elevation.

In men, vasocongestion leads to distention of the penis. Heart rate increases to 100 to 175 beats/min and respiratory rate to about 40 breaths/min.

Orgasm. Orgasm occurs when stimulation proceeds through the plateau stage to a point at which a vigorous contraction of muscles in the pelvic area expels or dissipates blood and fluid from the area of congestion. The average number of contractions for the woman is 8 to 15 contractions at intervals of 1 every 0.8 seconds. In men, muscle contractions surrounding the seminal vessels and prostate project semen into the proximal urethra. These contractions are followed immediately by three to seven propulsive ejaculatory contractions, occurring at the same time interval as in the woman, which force semen from the penis (Masters et al., 1998).

As the shortest stage in the sexual response cycle, orgasm is usually experienced as intense pleasure affecting the whole body, not just the pelvic area. It is also a highly personal experience: descriptions of orgasms vary greatly from person to person.

Resolution. The resolution is a 30-minute period during which the external and internal genital organs return to an unaroused state. For the male, a refractory period occurs during which further orgasm is impossible. Women do not go through this refractory period, so it is possible for women who are interested and properly stimulated to have additional orgasms immediately after the first.

Controversies About Female Orgasm

The female orgasm has been a topic of much controversy over the years, beginning with Freud, who deducted there were two types of female orgasms: clitoral and vaginal. He believed clitoral orgasms (originating from masturbation or other noncoital acts) represented sexual immaturity and only vaginal orgasms were the authentic, mature form of sexual behavior in women. Accordingly, he considered women to be neurotic if they did not achieve orgasm through coitus.

Masters et al. (1998) revealed that women report a difference in intensity and character between orgasms achieved through coitus and through direct stimulation of the clitoris and some prefer one to the other, but there is no physiologic difference between the two. For most women, adequate time for foreplay is essential for them to be orgasmic.

In recent years, a subject of controversy regarding female sexuality has arisen regarding the existence of a "G spot." First described in 1950 by the German physician Gräfenberg, the G spot, presumably located on the inner portion of the vaginal wall halfway between the pubic bone and the cervix, has been promoted as an area of heightened erotic sensitivity (Kimmel & Rogers, 2011). Several studies carried out in the past 10 years have not been able to verify the existence of this particular anatomic site, although some women claim to possess such an erotic trigger (Kilchevsky, Vardi, Lowenstein, et al., 2012).

The Influence of the Menstrual Cycle on Sexual Response

During the second half of the menstrual cycle—the luteal phase—there is increased fluid retention and vasocongestion in the woman's lower pelvis. Because some vasocongestion is already present at the beginning of the excitement stage of the sexual response, women appear to reach the plateau stage more quickly and achieve orgasm more readily during this time. Women also may be more interested in initiating sexual relations during this time.

The Influence of Pregnancy on Sexual Response

Pregnancy is another time in life when there is vasocongestion of the lower pelvis because of the blood supply needed by a rapidly growing fetus. This causes some women to experience their first orgasm during their first pregnancy. Following a pregnancy, many women continue to experience increased sexual interest because the new growth of blood vessels during pregnancy lasts for some time and continues to facilitate pelvic vasocongestion. These differences in response are why discussing sexual relationships is an important part of health teaching during pregnancy. At a time when a woman may want sexual contact very much, she needs to be free of myths and misconceptions, such as the notion that orgasm will cause a spontaneous miscarriage. Although the level of oxytocin, the hormone that rises with labor, does appear to rise in women after orgasm, this rise is not enough that women should worry that sexual relations will lead to premature labor in the average woman.

For some women, the increased breast engorgement that accompanies pregnancy results in extreme breast sensitivity during coitus. Foreplay that includes sucking or massaging of the breasts may also cause release of oxytocin, but it is not contraindicated unless the woman has a history of premature labor. Box 5.6 shows an interprofessional care map illustrating both nursing and team planning for reproductive and sexual health.

Types of Sexual Orientation

Sexual gratification can be experienced in a number of ways. What is considered normal varies greatly among cultures,

BOX 5.6 Nursing Care Planning

AN INTERPROFESSIONAL CARE MAP FOR A COUPLE NEEDING SEXUAL COUNSELING

Suzanne and Kevin Matthews, a young adult couple, 6 months pregnant, come to your antepartal clinic for a routine visit. Suzanne, in tears, states, "My husband isn't interested in me anymore. We haven't had sex since I became pregnant." The couple engaged in coitus two to three times per week prior to this pregnancy. Kevin states, "I'm afraid I'll hurt the baby."

Family Assessment Couple has been married for 4 years; lives in two-bedroom apartment in the central city. Husband works as a high school teacher; wife works as a baker in a local coffeehouse.

Client Assessment A previous pregnancy, 2 years ago, ended at 8 weeks with a spontaneous miscarriage. Blood pressure today is 118/70 mmHg; overall health is "good."

Nursing Diagnosis Altered sexuality pattern related to pregnancy and fear of harming fetus.

Outcome Criteria Couple states they recognize coitus is not harmful in normal pregnancy; reports engaging in sexual intercourse as well as pleasurable noncoital sexual activities by next visit if desired.

Team Member Responsible	Assessment	Intervention	Rationale	Expected Outcome
Activities of Daily Living, Including Safety				
Nurse	Assess lifestyle and sexual concerns.	Encourage couple to continue routine prenatal care. Discuss alternative sexual activities, such as cuddling or massage.	As pregnancy progresses, discomfort, fatigue, and increasing abdominal size may interfere with a satisfying sexual relationship.	Couple continues prenatal care. Describes other ways of sexual expression.
Teamwork and Collaboration				
Nurse/Primary Care Provider	Assess signs and symptoms of pregnancy; note any indication of complications.	Consult with team primary care provider to be certain the client has no contraindications to remaining sexually active during pregnancy.	In a few women who have had previous miscarriages, or if vaginal bleeding is present, sexual relations may be contraindicated or the pregnancy will be threatened.	The couple's primary care provider supplies information on ability of couple to remain sexually active throughout pregnancy.
Procedures/Medications for Quality Improvement				
Nurse	Assess whether alternative types of sexual activity would fulfill couple's needs.	Review alternative sexual positions for optimal comfort and pleasure, such as side-lying.	Alternative sexual positions may be necessary to provide comfort late in pregnancy as the woman's abdomen expands.	Couple describes alternative positions or other ways they relate to each other.
Patient-Centered Care				
Nurse/Primary Care Provider	Assess what couple understands about reproductive anatomy and usual sexual response.	Explain sexual relations are allowed during pregnancy until labor begins. Use charts and illustrations to show how the fetus is protected in utero.	Barring complications, couples can engage in sexual intercourse to the extent it is comfortable and desired. Visual aids enhance learning.	Couple states they understand sexual relations are allowed during a normal pregnancy.
Spiritual/Psychosocial/Emotional Needs				
Nurse	Assess whether couple knows hormones can change sexual desire during pregnancy.	Encourage the couple to talk openly about their feelings, concerns, desires, and changes in interest to each other throughout the pregnancy.	Physical and psychological changes occur in both the pregnant woman and her partner throughout pregnancy. Open communication enhances the relationship.	Couple reports they are able to voice their feelings and concerns during the pregnancy.
Nurse	Assess what communication pattern couple uses to share information with each other.	Teach importance for a couple of maintaining communication.	Beginning a sound communication pattern during pregnancy can lay a foundation for a sound future relationship.	Couple reports they appreciate the importance of good communication for their ongoing relationship.
Informatics for Seamless Health Care Planning				
Nurse	Assess whether couple's questions and concerns were answered satisfactorily.	Review concern about sexual relations at each visit as indicated.	Continued interest in a couple's problem allows them to continue to voice concerns.	Electronic record documents questions were asked and answered at continuing visits.

although general components of accepted sexual activity are that it is an activity of adults with privacy, consent, and lack of force included. Sexual violence or violence in general occurs when one partner does not respect these boundaries. This is a particular concern for maternal and child health nurses because intimate partner violence tends to occur at an increased frequency during pregnancy (Holden, McKenzie, Pruitt, et al., 2012). Young children and adolescents are also persons targeted for sexual maltreatment. All forms of maltreatment or partner violence are discussed in Chapter 55.

Heterosexuality

A heterosexual is a person who finds sexual fulfillment with a member of the opposite gender. Because interest in the opposite sex and sexual relationships may begin as early as the beginning of puberty, it is important to provide information on safer sex practices and planning for their use to children as young as 10 to 12 years of age. Otherwise, this knowledge comes too late to be most helpful. Safer sex suggestions are shown in Box 5.7.

What if...5.2 Kevin's adolescent nephew Mark comes into your pediatric clinic because he has symptoms of an STI? He says he doesn't think that's possible because he and his girlfriend are faithful to each other. What additional questions would you want to ask Mark? Would any advice on safer sex practices differ because he's still an adolescent, not an adult?

Homosexuality

A homosexual is a person who finds sexual fulfillment with a member of his or her own sex. Many homosexual men prefer the term "gay." "Lesbian" refers to a homosexual woman. More recent terms are "men who have sex with men" (MWM) and "women who have sex with women" (WWW).

Why homosexual gender identity develops is unknown, although there is evidence this sexual orientation is genetically

BOX 5.7 Nursing Care Planning to Empower a Family

GUIDELINES FOR SAFER SEX PRACTICES

Q. Mark, 16 years old, asks you, "What do you mean by safer sex practices?"
A. Safer sex practices can keep an individual free of infection from sexual contact.

1. Abstinence is the only 100% guarantee against not contracting a sexually transmitted infection.
2. If you do have sex, be selective in choosing sexual partners. By having sex, you are exposing yourself to the infections of everyone with whom your partner has ever had sex. The more partners you have relations with, the greater your danger of contracting a sexually transmitted infection.
3. Don't be reluctant to ask a sexual partner about his or her sexual lifestyle before engaging in sexual relations. If a partner has a history of casual contacts or unprotected sex, there is a greater hazard of infection for you than if your partner has been choosy about partners.
4. Avoid sexual relations with intravenous drug users or prostitutes (male or female) or sexual partners who have had sexual relations with such people, because such people have a greater than usual chance of carrying the human immunodeficiency virus (HIV),hepatitis B or C, or other infections.
5. Inspect your sexual partner for any lesions or abnormal drainage in the genital area. Do not engage in sexual relations with anyone who exhibits these signs.
6. The use of a condom is the best protection against infection. Condoms should be latex; the chance of the condom tearing is less if it is a prelubricated brand. Use water-based lubricants such as K-Y Jelly on condoms, because oil-based lubricants can weaken the rubber.
7. Condoms should be protected from excessive heat to avoid rubber deterioration and should be inspected to be certain they are intact before use. Do not inflate condoms before use to test for intactness, though, because this weakens the rubber.
8. Condoms should be fitted over the erect penis with a small space left at the end to accept semen. The condom should be held against the sides of the penis while the penis is withdrawn to prevent spillage of semen.
9. Void immediately after sexual relations to help wash away contaminants on the vulva or in the urinary tract.
10. Anal intercourse carries a higher risk for HIV and hepatitis A infection as well as infection from intestinal organisms. Always use a condom. Use lubricants for anal penetration to keep bleeding and condom resistance to a minimum.
11. Do not engage in oral–penile sex unless the male wears a condom, because even preejaculatory fluid may contain viruses and bacteria. For safer oral–vaginal sex, a condom split in two or a plastic dental dam (like that used for dentistry) covering the mouth should be used to protect against the exchange of body fluids.
12. Hand-to-genital contact may be hazardous if open cuts are present on hands. Use a latex glove or finger cot for protection.
13. To decrease the possibility of transferring germs, do not share sexual aids such as vibrators.
14. If you think you have contracted a sexually transmitted infection, do not engage in sexual relations until you have contacted a health care provider and are again free of infection. Alert any recent sexual partners you might have an infection so they also can receive treatment.

determined or develops because of the effect of an unusual level of estrogen or testosterone in utero. Even before puberty, most individuals who are homosexual realize they are "different" in that they are not interested in opposite-sex classmates. It is during adolescence, in seeking a sense of identity, that they realize the reason they feel "different" is because they are homosexual. This can create a stressful time for the boy who first realizes he is gay or the girl who first realizes she is lesbian because revealing this to family and friends or "coming out" may be difficult. Part of the reason for the high suicide rate in adolescence may occur because gay or lesbian teenagers don't know where to turn for help in a heterosexual-dominant culture (McKay, 2011). Although attitudes are changing, some people refuse to associate with homosexuals to such an extent that a fear termed homophobia exists (Chapman, Wardrop, Freeman, et al., 2012).

Although MWM and WWW often have demonstrated behaviors consistent with a homosexual role from early childhood, young adulthood is the time most persons begin to assume a homosexual lifestyle or are ready to reveal this to health care providers. It is important for health care providers to be extremely sensitive to needs in this area. MWM may need counseling to help them avoid acquiring HIV and other STIs because issues such as avoiding contact through anal intercourse or vaccination against hepatitis A and human papillomavirus virus (HPV) may not be routinely covered in sex education classes (Fairley & Read, 2012). If WWW cohort with bisexuals, they have the same risk of STIs as other people. If they avoid partners who are bisexual, they may be at less risk for STIs because of the low incidence of these infections in a strictly female population.

Bisexuality

People are bisexual if they achieve sexual satisfaction from both homosexual and heterosexual relationships. Gay men who have sex with bisexual men may be at a greater risk for contracting HIV and STIs than others. Female partners of bisexual men need to be aware that they are also at increased risk for HIV and other STIs.

Transsexuality

A **transsexual** or transgender person is an individual who, although of one biologic gender, feels as if he or she is of the opposite gender (Knezevich, Viereck, & Drincic, 2012). People who have this feeling may have gender affirmation surgery (previously termed sex change operations) so they appear cosmetically as the sex they feel they really are. Although capable of sexual relations in this new role (a synthetic vagina or penis is created), the person is incapable of reproduction because such operations do not change the person's chromosomal structure. The incidence of gender affirmation surgery has decreased in recent years because of disappointment after the surgery: despite a new outward appearance, the person realizes he or she is still not totally the person he or she wished to become. Children of a transsexual parent may have a great deal of difficulty understanding why their parent changed their appearance so drastically from male to female or female to male.

Types of Sexual Expression

Because people are individuals, types of sexual expression are individualized and also vary.

Sexual Abstinence

Sexual abstinence (celibacy) is separation from sexual activity. It is the avowed state of certain religious orders. It is also a way of life for many adults and one that is becoming fashionable among a growing number of young adults. It is the main point of many high school–age sex education classes (Markham, Tortolero, Peskin, et al., 2012). The theoretical advantage of sexual abstinence is the ability to concentrate on a means of giving and receiving love other than through sexual expression and, of course, is the most effective way to prevent pregnancy or an STI.

✔ QSEN Checkpoint Question 5.5

Evidence-Based Practice

Suzanne Matthews wishes she had conceived sooner in her marriage than she did. Other women have the opposite worry: they became pregnant before they intended. To identify what sociocultural factors are associated with sexual-risk behaviors that could lead to teenage pregnancy, nurse researchers interviewed 255 rural teenagers as to their lifestyles. Findings of the study revealed sexual-risk status did not differ statistically by gender or socioeconomic status.

There was, however, a correlation between sexual-risk behaviors and lower religiosity, lower parental monitoring, lower social connectedness, and higher levels of peer influence. Teenagers with high sexual-risk behaviors were also more likely to engage more in overall health-risk behaviors such as smoking and drinking alcohol (Rew, Carver, & Li, 2011).

Based on the previous study, if you were a school nurse, what would be your best action to help lower sexual-risk behaviors in Mark, Kevin Matthews' nephew?

a. Suggest he attend a church of his choice every Sunday.
b. Provide him with educational materials on smoking cessation.
c. Help him learn to make decisions without his friends' influence.
d. Teach him the negative consequences of unintended pregnancy.

Look in Appendix A for the best answer and rationale.

Masturbation

Masturbation is self-stimulation for erotic pleasure; it can also be a mutually enjoyable activity for sexual partners. It offers sexual release, which may be interpreted by the person as overall tension or anxiety relief. Masters et al. (1998) reported women may find masturbation to orgasm the most satisfying sexual expression and use it more commonly than men. Children between 2 and 6 years of age discover masturbation as an enjoyable activity as they explore their bodies. Preschoolers who are under a high level of tension may become accustomed to using masturbation as a means of falling asleep at night or at naptime. They do this without any attempt at concealment because they have not yet been affected by society's view that such activity should not be public.

School-age children and adolescents continue to use masturbation for enjoyment or to relieve tension, but they perform such activities in private. In a hospital setting, a school-age child may assume he or she has more privacy than actually exists, however. Such an assumption means you might discover a school-age child or adolescent masturbating if you walk unannounced into the room.

After reproductive tract surgery or childbirth, many adult men and women voice concern about how soon they will be able to have sexual relations without feeling pain. They may masturbate to orgasm to test whether everything in their body is still functioning, much like the preschooler does.

Autoerotic asphyxia is the extreme practice of causing oxygen deficiency (usually by hanging) during masturbation with the goal of producing a feeling of extreme sexual excitement. Adolescents need to be cautioned against this because, not aware the act can be fatal, a number of teenagers are killed by this practice each year (Byard & Winskog, 2012).

Erotic Stimulation

Erotic stimulation is the use of visual materials such as magazines or photographs for sexual arousal. Although this is thought to be mostly a male phenomenon, there is increasing interest in erotic literature, DVDs, and centerfold photographs in magazines marketed primarily to women. Some parents of adolescents may need to be assured that an interest in this type of material is developmental and normal. Respect this type of reading material when straightening patients' rooms in a health care facility.

Fetishism

Paraphilia is sexual arousal to objects, situations, or individuals. The most common form of this is fetishism, the sexual arousal from the use of certain objects perceived to have erotic qualities such as leather, rubber, shoes, or feet. The object of stimulation does not just enhance a sexual experience; rather, it becomes the focus of arousal and a person may come to require the object or situation for stimulation (Wright, 2010). Paraphilia can be viewed as an individual idiosyncrasy unless the habit is disruptive to social relationships or interferes with general health.

Transvestism

A **transvestite** is a form of fetishism in which an individual dresses in the clothes of the opposite sex. Transvestites can be heterosexual, homosexual, or bisexual. Many are married. Some transvestites, particularly married heterosexuals, may be under a great deal of strain to keep their lifestyle a secret from friends and neighbors (Zucker, Bradley, Owen-Anderson, et al., 2012).

Voyeurism

Voyeurism is obtaining sexual arousal by looking at another person's body. Almost all children and adolescents pass through a stage when voyeurism is appealing, but this passes with more active sexual expressions. That some voyeurism exists in almost everyone is illustrated by the large number of R-rated movies that are produced and by the erotic descriptions in modern novels. If voyeurism is practiced to the exclusion of other sexual experiences, such an extreme probably reflects insecurity or the inability to feel confident enough to relate to others on more personal levels. Stalking, a crime that includes elements of voyeurism, is illegal (McNamara & Marsil, 2012). It is discussed in Chapter 33.

Sadomasochism

Sadomasochism involves inflicting pain (sadism) or receiving pain (masochism) to achieve sexual satisfaction (Wright, 2010). It is a practice generally considered to be within the limits of normal sexual expression as long as the pain involved is minimal and the experience is consensual and satisfying to both sexual partners.

Additional Types of Sexual Expression

A multitude of other types of sexual expression exist such as exhibitionism, obscene phone calling, bestiality, and pedophilia (Domoney, 2012). Exhibitionism is revealing one's genitals in public. Bestiality is sexual relations with animals. Pedophiles are individuals who are interested in sexual encounters with children. They are registered as sex offenders. When they move into a new community, families are notified of the move according to Megan's Law, a national law designed to alert citizens to the presence of a sex offender in a community. Ways to keep children safe from sex offenders are discussed in Chapter 31, along with other aspects of community safety for young children.

What if...5.3 When Kevin unpacks his suitcase for a hospital admission, you discover he has brought a wardrobe of woman's clothing. What would you do?

SEXUAL HARASSMENT

Sexual harassment is unwanted, repeated sexual advances, remarks, or behavior toward another that is offensive to the recipient or interferes with job or school performance. It can involve actions as obvious as a job superior demanding sexual favors from an employee, or it could be a man or woman sending sexist jokes by e-mail to another person in the department. In school, it can refer to bullying (Marks, Mountjoy, & Marcus, 2011).

Two types exist. One is *quid pro quo* (an equal exchange), in which an employer asks for something in return for sexual favors, such as a hiring or promotion preference. The second is a *hostile work environment*, in which an employer creates an environment in which an employee feels uncomfortable and exploited (such as being addressed as "honey" or "babe," asked to wear revealing clothing, or working where walls are decorated with sexist posters).

Sexual harassment rules apply to same-gender as well as opposite-gender harassment. In addition to causing occupational disruption, sexual harassment may be so distressing that it can lead to short- or long-term psychosocial consequences for victims and their families such as emotional distress (e.g., anxiety, depression, posttraumatic stress disorder, substance abuse), interpersonal conflict, and impaired intimacy and sexual functioning (Stock & Tissot, 2012).

Sexual harassment has been illegal in the United States since 1964. Clients who report being subjected to harassment should be advised to report the situation to their personnel supervisor. Nurses should be aware of sexual harassment guidelines in their own work setting and likewise report such behavior to keep their workplace free of this type of strain.

DISORDERS OF SEXUAL FUNCTIONING

Disorders involving sexual functioning can be lifelong (primary) or acquired (secondary). They can have a psychogenic origin (produced by psychic rather than organic factors), a biogenic origin (produced by biologic processes), or both. They occur in both men and women.

Failure to Achieve Orgasm

The failure of a woman to achieve orgasm can be a result of poor sexual technique, concentrating too hard on achievement, or negative attitudes toward sexual relationships. Treatment is aimed at relieving the underlying cause. It may include instruction and counseling for the couple about sexual feelings and needs. Female Viagra (often referred to as "pink" Viagra) is not yet available in the United States. Caution women to use online prescription sites carefully to avoid purchasing inactive or possibly harmful medications advertised as pink Viagra.

Erectile Dysfunction

Erectile dysfunction (ED), formerly referred to as impotence, is the inability of a man to produce or maintain an erection long enough for penetration or partner satisfaction (Ghanem, Salonia, & Martin-Morales, 2013). It affects as many as 40% of men by age 40 years and 65% of men by age 65 years. Most causes of ED are physical, such as aging, atherosclerosis, or diabetes, all of which are conditions that limit blood supply to the penis. It may also occur as a side effect of certain drugs, such as antidepressants (Burnett, 2011) or after discontinuation of finasteride, a drug for male pattern baldness (Irwig & Kolukula, 2011).

The problem is compounded by doubt about the ability to perform and reluctance to discuss the problem with health care providers. Typical drugs prescribed today for ED are sildenafil citrate (Viagra), tadalafil (Cialis), and vardenafil (Levitra), taken up to once a day to stimulate penile erection by increasing blood flow (Karch, 2013) (Box 5.8). These are contraindicated in men with a risk of cardiovascular illness and in those who are taking medications that contain nitrates. Also helpful can be testosterone administration, intracavernosal injections of prostaglandin E1, vacuum erection devices, or surgical implants (Hamilton, 2012). Avanafil is a newer drug (a phosphodiesterase type 5 [PDE5] inhibitor), which blocks the body protein that prevents blood vessels from expanding. This allows blood to enter the penis and become trapped there, leading to an erection during times of sexual excitement (Segal & Burnett, 2012).

In all instances, frank discussion about the cause of the problem and currently available therapies is helpful. Various herbal products such as fennel extracts are available for women, which may improve sexual libido. Vibration or vacuum devices are also available to increase clitoral enlargement and sexual arousal in women.

Premature Ejaculation

Premature ejaculation is ejaculation before the sexual partner's satisfaction has been achieved (Mulhall, 2012). It applies to both same sex and opposite sex couples. Premature ejaculation can be unsatisfactory and frustrating for both partners.

The cause, like that of ED, can be psychological. Masturbating to orgasm (in which orgasm is achieved quickly because of lack of time) may play a role. Other reasons suggested are doubt about masculinity and fear of impregnating a partner, which prevent the man from sustaining an erection.

BOX 5.8 Nursing Care Planning Based on Responsibility for Pharmacology

SILDENAFIL CITRATE (VIAGRA)

Classification: A phosphodiesterase type 5 (PDE5) inhibitor. Prescribed as therapy for erectile dysfunction in males.
Action: Causes smooth muscle relaxation and inflow of blood to the corpus cavernosum of the penis achieving erection or increased sensitivity (Karch, 2013).
Dosage: 25 to 50 mg orally as needed 1 hour before sexual activity, up to one dose per day.
Possible Adverse Effects: The most common side effects are headache, facial flushing, and upset stomach. Less commonly, ventricular arrhythmia, bluish vision, blurred vision, impairment of blue/green discrimination or sensitivity to light. Advise patients not to take this drug within 4 hours of taking an alpha-blocker or the effect of the alpha-blocker will be intensified.

Nursing Implications

- Assess patient for preexisting cardiovascular risk.
- Caution patient the dose should be limited to one time per day.
- Possible severe hypotension and serious cardiac events can occur if the drug is combined with nitrates or alpha adrenergic blockers; this combination must be avoided.
- Erection lasting more than 4 hours (priapism) can occur. This condition can lead to penile tissue damage so should be reported to a health care provider.
- Caution patients this drug does not protect against sexually transmitted infections or pregnancy, so the user must continue to use safer sex practices.
- In rare instances, taking PDE5 inhibitors have led to a sudden decrease or loss of vision. Caution patients if they experience this to stop taking the medication and call their health care provider.

Sexual counseling for both partners to reduce stress as well as serotonergic antidepressants currently under study, such as mirtazapine (Remeron) or dapoxetine, a short-acting selective serotonin reuptake inhibitor (SSRI), may be helpful for alleviating the problem (McCarty & Dinsmore, 2012).

Persistent Sexual Arousal Syndrome

Persistent sexual arousal syndrome (PSAS) occurs in women and is the excessive and unrelenting sexual arousal in the absence of desire (Brotto, Bitzer, Laan, et al., 2010). It may be triggered by either medications or psychological factors and is associated with restless leg syndrome and overactive bladder. When assessing someone with the disorder, be certain to ask if the person is taking any herbal remedies such as ginkgo biloba or a partner is using a treatment for male pattern baldness as these can have arousal effects.

Pain Disorders

Because the reproductive system has a sensitive nerve supply, when pain occurs in response to sexual activities, it can be acute and severe and can impair a person's ability to enjoy this aspect of their life.

Vaginismus

Vaginismus is involuntary contraction of the muscles at the outlet of the vagina when coitus is attempted, which prohibits penile penetration (Reissing, 2012). Vaginismus may occur in women who have been raped. Other causes are unknown, but it could also be the result of early learning patterns in which sexual relations were viewed as bad or sinful. As with other sexual problems, sexual or psychological counseling to reduce this response may be necessary.

Dyspareunia

Dyspareunia is pain during coitus. Dyspareunia can occur because of endometriosis (abnormal placement of endometrial tissue), vestibulitis (inflammation of the vestibule), vaginal infection, or hormonal changes such as those that occur with menopause and cause vaginal drying. A psychological component may be present. Treatment is aimed at the underlying cause. Encouraging open communication between sexual partners can be instrumental in resolving the problem.

✔ QSEN Checkpoint Question 5.6

Safety

The Matthews' neighbor, Cindy, is a woman who has sex with women. When you see Cindy in your clinic, to help keep her safe, you would want to teach her which of the following?

a. Falling estrogen levels are apt to cause her an early menopause.
b. She doesn't need to practice safer sex because she doesn't have male partners.
c. Her risk for contracting an STI is statistically lower than if she were heterosexual.
d. Because she will never be sexually active, she needs no advice in this area.

Look in Appendix A for the best answer and rationale.

Individuals With Unique Needs or Concerns

A number of individuals have special concerns concerning reproductive health.

The Individual With a Disability

Individuals who are physically challenged have sexual desires and needs the same as all others (Meaney-Tavares & Gavidia-Payne, 2012). They may, however, have difficulty with sexual identity or sexual fulfillment because of their disability. Males with upper spinal cord injury, for example, may have difficulty with erections and ejaculation because these actions are governed at the spinal level. Manual stimulation of the penis or psychological stimulation can, however, achieve erection in most men with spinal cord lesions, allowing the man a satisfying sexual relationship with his partner. Most women with spinal cord injuries cannot experience orgasm but are able to conceive and have children.

Any person who interprets a procedure such as a colostomy as disfiguring may be reluctant to participate in sexual activities, fearing the sight of an apparatus will diminish their partner's satisfaction. People with chronic pain such as from arthritis may be too uncomfortable to enjoy sexual relations. Individuals with urinary catheters may be concerned about their ability to enjoy coitus with the catheter in place. For women, a retention catheter should not interfere with coitus. Men can be taught how to replace their own catheter, so they can remove it for sexual relations. In all instances in which one sexual partner is disabled in some way, the response of a loving partner does much to enhance body image and feelings of adequacy of a mate. Encouraging these clients to ask questions and work on specific difficulties is a nursing role.

Sexuality is a facet of rehabilitation that has not always received attention. If a person can accomplish activities of daily living such as eating, elimination, and mobility, then he or she is often considered to be leading a normal or near-normal life. However, establishing a satisfying sexual relationship is an important part of living as well and so should be included in assessments of clients in rehabilitation programs.

The Individual With a Hypoactive Sexual Desire

Lessened interest in sexual relations is normal in some circumstances, such as after the death of a family member, a divorce, or a stressful job change. The support of a caring sexual partner or relief of the tension causing the stress allows a return in sexual interest.

Decreased sexual desire can also be a side effect of many medicines. Chronic diseases, such as peptic ulcers or chronic pulmonary disorders that cause frequent pain or discomfort, may interfere with a man's or a woman's overall well-being and interest in sexual activity. Obese men and women may not feel as much satisfaction from sexual relations as others because they have difficulty achieving deep penetration due to the bulk of their abdomens. An individual with an STI such as genital herpes may choose to forgo sexual relations rather than inform a partner of the disease. Some women experience a decrease in sexual desire during perimenopause. Administration of androgen (testosterone) to both women and men may be helpful at that time, because it can improve interest in sexual activity (Shelton & Rajfer, 2012; White, Grady, Giudice, et al., 2012).

What if...5.4 You are interested in exploring one of the 2020 National Health Goals related to reproductive or sexual health (see Box 5.1). Most government-sponsored money for nursing research is allotted based on these goals. What would be a possible research topic to explore pertinent to these goals that would be applicable to the Matthews family and that would also advance evidence-based practice?

Key Points for Review

- The reproductive and sexual organs form early in intrauterine life, and full functioning occurs at puberty.
- The female internal organs of reproduction include the ovaries, the fallopian tubes, the uterus, and the vagina.
- The female external organs of reproduction include the mons veneris, the labia minora and majora, the vestibule, the clitoris, the fourchette, the perineal body, the hymen, and the Skene and the Bartholin glands.
- The male external reproductive structures are the penis, scrotum, and testes. Internal organs are the epididymis, the vas deferens, the seminal vesicles, the ejaculatory ducts, the prostate gland, the urethra, and the bulbourethral glands.
- A menstrual cycle is periodic uterine bleeding in response to cyclic hormones. Menarche is the first menstrual period. Menopause is the end of menstruation. Menstrual cycles are possible because of the interplay between the hypothalamus, the pituitary gland, the ovaries, and the uterus.
- Biologic gender is determined by a person's chromosomes (XX or XY) and is set at conception. Gender identity is a person's concept of being male or female. This develops over a lifetime. Gender role is yet a third aspect and is the behavior a person demonstrates based on his or her gender identity as male or female.
- Masters and Johnson (Masters et al., 1998) identified a sexual response cycle consisting of excitement, plateau, orgasm, and resolution stages. Disorders of sexual dysfunction include failure to achieve orgasm, vaginismus, dyspareunia, inhibited sexual desire, premature ejaculation, and erectile dysfunction.
- People assume varying sexual orientations, such as heterosexual, homosexual (WWW or MWM), or bisexual. Common sexual expressions are voyeurism, fetishism, and celibacy.
- Educating people about reproductive function is an important primary health strategy because it teaches people to better monitor their own health through vulvar or testicular self-examination.
- Considering reproductive and sexual health in a patient assessment helps in planning nursing care that not only meets QSEN competencies but also best meets a family's total needs.
- Teach adolescents that with sexual maturity comes sexual responsibility. They need to be aware of safer sex practices as protection against both an STI or an unintentional pregnancy.

Critical Thinking Care Study

Bob Anderson, who works as an accountant, and Charlie Lee, who works as a high school teacher, are a gay married couple. A female friend of theirs has volunteered to be a surrogate mother for them so they can adopt a baby. They're debating which of them should quit work to stay at home with the newborn.

1. Bob and Charlie are in the middle of making plans to become new parents. Is the idea of one of them giving up a career to become a stay-at-home parent a wise decision? Would sharing childrearing responsibilities be a better idea?
2. Suppose Bob is eager to quit work because he's subjected to sexual harassment at work. Is this a good reason to be the newborn's chief caregiver?
3. Both Bob and Charlie have practiced safer sex practices since they were teenagers. Now that they have a monogamous relationship, do they need to continue to do this?

Patient Scenario

The Snellen Family

Read about the Snellen family, a family with an adolescent who needs information about reproduction and safer sex practices, then answer the questions to further sharpen your skills and grow more familiar with NCLEX-type questions related to reproductive and sexual health. Confirm your answers are correct by reading the rationales.

Visit http://thePoint.lww.com

Answers and Rationales

Looking for answers to the What If. . . and Critical Thinking Care Study questions?

Visit http://thePoint.lww.com

References

American Academy of Pediatrics. (2012). *Where we stand: Circumcision.* Evanston, IL: Author.

Brotto, L. A., Bitzer, J., Laan, E., et al. (2010). Women's sexual desire and arousal disorders. *Journal of Sexual Medicine, 7*(1, Pt. 2), 586–614.

Burnett, A. (2011). Evaluation and management of erectile dysfunction. In W. S. McDougal, A. J. Wein, L. R. Kavoussi, et al. (Eds.), *Campbell-Walsh urology* (10th ed., pp. 126–128). Philadelphia, PA: Elsevier/Saunders.

Byard, R. W., & Winskog, C. (2012). Autoerotic death: Incidence and age of victims—A population-based study. *Journal of Forensic Science, 57*(1), 129–131.

Carter, D., & Gabel, M. B. (2012). Rectocele-does the size matter? *International Journal of Colorectal Disorders, 27*(7), 975–980.

Centers for Disease Control and Prevention. (2010). *A public health approach for advancing sexual health in the United States: Rationale and options for implementation, meeting report of an external consultation.* Atlanta, GA: Author.

Chang, Y. T., & Lin, M. L. (2013). Menarche and menstruation through the eyes of pubescent students in eastern Taiwan: Implications in sociocultural influence and gender differences issues. *Journal of Nursing Research, 21*(1), 10–18.

Chapman, R., Wardrop, J., Freeman, P., et al. (2012). A descriptive study of the experiences of lesbian, gay and transgender parents accessing health services for their children. *Journal of Clinical Nursing, 21*(7–8), 1128–1135.

Cheng, G., Buyken, A. E., Shi, L., et al. (2012). Beyond overweight: Nutrition as an important lifestyle factor influencing timing of puberty. *Nutrition Review, 70*(3), 133–152.

Christensen, A., Bentley, G. E., Cabrera, R., et al. (2012). Hormonal regulation of female reproduction. *Hormone & Metabolic Research, 44*(8), 587–591.

Coad, J., & Conlon, C. (2011). Iron deficiency in women: Assessment, causes and consequences. *Current Opinion in Clinical Nutrition & Metabolic Care, 14*(6), 625–634.

Domoney, C. (2012). Sexual dysfunction. In D. K. Edmonds (Ed.), *Dewhurst's textbook of obstetrics & gynaecology* (8th ed., pp. 785–797). Oxford, UK: John Wiley & Sons.

Doyle-Lucas, A. F., Akers, J. D., & Davy, B. M. (2010). Energetic efficiency, menstrual irregularity, and bone mineral density in elite professional female ballet dancers. *Journal of Dance Medicine & Science, 14*(4), 146–154.

Edmonds, D. K. (2012). Normal and abnormal development of the genital tract. In D. K. Edmonds (Ed.), *Dewhurst's textbook of obstetrics & gynaecology* (8th ed., pp. 421–434). Oxford, UK: John Wiley & Sons.

Ellsworth, P. I. (2012). Cryptorchidism. In F. J. Domino (Ed.), *The 5-minute clinical consult* (pp. 314–315). Philadelphia, PA: Lippincott Williams & Wilkins.

Fairley, C. K., & Read, T. R. (2012). Vaccination against sexually transmitted infections. *Current Opinion in Infectious Diseases, 25*(1), 66–72.

Ghanem, H. M., Salonia, A., & Martin-Morales, A. (2013). Physical examination and laboratory testing for men with ED. *Journal of Sexual Medicine, 10*(1), 108–111.

Givens, V. M., & Lipscomb, G. H. (2012). Diagnosis of ectopic pregnancy. *Clinical Obstetrics & Gynecology, 55*(2), 387–394.

Grimes, C. L., & Chen, C. C. G. (2011). Anatomy of the female pelvis. In K. J. Hurt, M. W. Guile, J. L. Bienstock, et al. (Eds.), *The Johns Hopkins manual of gynecology and obstetrics* (4th ed., pp. 289–305). Philadelphia, PA: Lippincott Williams & Wilkins.

Guile, M. W., & Keller, J. (2011). Infections of the genital tract. In K. J. Hurt, M. W. Guile, J. L. Bienstock, et al. (Eds.), *The Johns Hopkins manual of gynecology and obstetrics* (4th ed., pp. 322–339). Philadelphia, PA: Lippincott Williams & Wilkins.

Hamilton, M. (2012). Infertility. In D. K. Edmonds (Ed.), *Dewhurst's textbook of obstetrics & gynaecology* (8th ed., pp. 567–579). Oxford, UK: John Wiley & Sons.

Holden, K. B., McKenzie, R., Pruitt, V., et al. (2012). Depressive symptoms, substance abuse, and intimate partner violence among pregnant women of diverse ethnicities. *Journal of Health Care for the Poor & Underserved, 23*(1), 226–241.

Huether, S. E., & McCance, K. L. (2012). *Understanding pathophysiology* (5th ed.). New York, NY: Elsevier Publishing.

Hunn, J., & Rodriquez, G. (2012). Ovarian cancer: Etiology, risk factors, and epidemiology. *Clinical Obstetrics & Gynecology, 55*(1), 3–23.

Institute of Medicine. (2012). *New vitamin D and calcium recommendations.* Washington, DC: Author.

Irwig, M. S., & Kolukula, S. (2011). Persistent sexual side effects of finasteride for male pattern hair loss. *Journal of Sexual Medicine, 8*(6), 1747–1753.

Karch, A. M. (2013). *2013 Lippincott's nursing drug guide.* Philadelphia, PA: Lippincott Williams & Wilkins.

Khan, M., & Diaz-Montes, T. P. (2011). Cervical cancer. In K. J. Hurt, M. W. Guile, J. L. Bienstock, et al. (Eds.), *The Johns Hopkins manual of gynecology and obstetrics* (4th ed., pp. 541–558). Philadelphia, PA: Lippincott Williams & Wilkins.

Kilchevsky, A., Vardi, Y., Lowenstein, L., et al. (2012). Is the female g-spot truly a distinct anatomic entity? *Journal of Sexual Medicine, 9*(3), 719–726.

Kim, E. Y., & Lee, M. I. (2012). Psychosocial aspects in girls with idiopathic precocious puberty. *Psychiatry Investigation, 9*(1), 25–28.

Kimmel, M., & Rogers, L. (2011). Female sexual response and sexual dysfunction. In K. J. Hurt, M. W. Guile, J. L. Bienstock, et al. (Eds.), *The Johns Hopkins manual of gynecology and obstetrics* (4th ed., pp. 497–506). Philadelphia, PA: Lippincott Williams & Wilkins.

Knezevich, E. L., Viereck, L. K., & Drincic, A. T. (2012). Medical management of adult transsexual persons. *Pharmacotherapy, 32*(1), 54–66.

Kumar, W. (2012). Fetal anomalies. In D. K. Edmonds (Ed.), *Dewhurst's textbook of obstetrics & gynaecology* (8th ed., pp. 219–229). Oxford, UK: John Wiley & Sons.

Lacey, J. V. Jr. (2012). Smoking lowers the age at natural menopause among smokers and raises important questions. *Menopause, 19*(2), 119–120.

Ledger, W. L. (2012). The menstrual cycle. In D. K. Edmonds (Ed.), *Dewhurst's textbook of obstetrics & gynaecology* (8th ed., pp. 487–494). Oxford, UK: John Wiley & Sons.

March of Dimes Foundation. (2012). *Teenage pregnancy.* White Plains, NY: Author.

Markham, C. M., Tortolero, S. R., Peskin, M. F., et al. (2012). Sexual risk avoidance and sexual risk reduction interventions for middle school youth: A randomized controlled trial. *Journal of Adolescent Health, 50*(3), 279–288.

Marks, S., Mountjoy, M., & Marcus, M. (2011). Sexual harassment and abuse in sport. *British Journal of Sports Medicine, 46*(13), 905–908.

Marques, A., Stothers, L., & MacNab, A. (2010). The status of pelvic floor muscle training for women. *Canadian Urological Association Journal, 4*(6), 419–424.

Masters, W. H., Johnson, V. E., & Kolodny, R. C. (1998). *Heterosexuality.* New York, NY: Smithmark Publishing.

McCarty, E., & Dinsmore, W. (2012). Dapoxetine: An evidence-based review of its effectiveness in treatment of premature ejaculation. *Core Evidence, 7*(1), 1–14.

McKay, B. (2011). Lesbian, gay, bisexual, and transgender health issues, disparities, and information resources. *Medical Reference Services Quarterly, 30*(4), 393–401.

McNamara, C. L., & Marsil, D. F. (2012). The prevalence of stalking among college students: The disparity between researcher- and self-identified victimization. *Journal of American College Health, 60*(2), 168–174.

Meaney-Tavares, R., & Gavidia-Payne, S. (2012). Staff characteristics and attitudes towards the sexuality of people with intellectual disability. *Journal of Intellectual & Developmental Disability, 37*(3), 269–273.

Miyaoka, R., & Esteves, S. C. (2012). A critical appraisal on the role of varicocele in male infertility. *Advances in Urology, 5*(1), 1–9.

Mswela, M. (2010). Female genital mutilation: medico-legal issues. *Medicine & Law, 29*(4), 523–536.

Mulhall, J. P. (2012). Premature ejaculation. In W. S. McDougal, A. J. Wein, L. R. Kavoussi, et al. (Eds.), *Campbell-Walsh urology* (10th ed., pp. 1134–1135). Philadelphia, PA: Elsevier/Saunders.

Nickel, J. C. (2012). Prostatitis and related conditions. In W. S. McDougal, A. J. Wein, L. R. Kavoussi, et al. (Eds.), *Campbell-Walsh urology* (10th ed., pp. 56–60). Philadelphia, PA: Elsevier/Saunders.

Panay, N. (2012). Menopause & the postmenopausal woman. In D. K. Edmonds (Ed.), *Dewhurst's textbook of obstetrics & gynaecology* (8th ed., pp. 553–556). Oxford, UK: John Wiley & Sons.

Poll, L. W., & Flake, P. (2011). Imperforate hymen with hematocolpometra. *New England Journal of Medicine, 365*(7), 157–158.

Reissing, E. D. (2012). Consultation and treatment history and causal attributions in an online sample of women with lifelong and acquired vaginismus. *Journal of Sexual Medicine, 9*(1), 251–258.

Rew, L., Carver, T., & Li, C. C. (2011). Early and risky sexual behavior in a sample of rural adolescents. *Issues in Comprehensive Pediatric Nursing, 34*(4), 189–204.

Sarwer, D. B., Spitzer, J. C., & Crerand, C. E. (2012). The psychological burden of idiopathic adolescent gynecomastia. *Plastic Reconstructive Surgery, 129*(1), 8–9.

Segal, R., & Burnett, A. L. (2012). Avanafil for the treatment of erectile dysfunction. *Drugs Today, 48*(1), 7–15.

Shelton, J. B., & Rajfer, J. (2012). Androgen deficiency in aging and metabolically challenged men. *Urology Clinics of North America, 39*(1), 63–75.

Shergill, I., Arya, M., & Muneer, A. (2012). Vasectomy illustrated. *BJU: British Journal of Urology International, 109*(7), 1116–1127.

Shoveller, J., Knight, R., Davis, W., et al. (2012). Online sexual health services: Examining youth's perspectives. *Canadian Journal of Public Health, 103*(1), 14–18.

Stock, S. R., & Tissot, F. (2012). Are there health effects of harassment in the workplace? A gender-sensitive study of the relationships between work and neck pain. *Ergonomics, 55*(2), 147–159.

Tanner, J. M. (1990). *Fetus into man: Physical growth from conception to maturity* (2nd ed.). Cambridge, MA: Harvard University Press.

Tortora, G. J., & Derrickson, B. H. (2012). The reproductive systems. In G. J. Tortora, & B. H. Derrickson (Eds.), *Principles of anatomy and physiology* (13th ed., pp. 1129–1180). Hoboken, NJ: John Wiley & Sons.

U.S. Department of Health and Human Services. (2010). *Healthy people 2020.* Washington, DC: Author.

Wade, G. H., Herrman, J., & McBeth-Snyder, L. (2012). A preconception care program for women in a college setting. *MCN: American Journal of Maternal/Child Nursing, 37*(3), 164–170.

White, W. B., Grady, D., Giudice, L. C., et al. (2012). A cardiovascular safety study of LibiGel (testosterone gel) in postmenopausal women with elevated cardiovascular risk and hypoactive sexual desire disorder. *American Heart Journal, 163*(1), 27–32.

Wright, S. (2010). Depathologizing consensual sexual sadism, sexual masochism, transvestic fetishism, and fetishism. *Archives of Sexual Behavior, 39*(6), 1229–1230.

Zucker, K. J., Bradley, S. J., Owen-Anderson, A., et al. (2012). Demographics, behavior problems, and psychosexual characteristics of adolescents with gender identity disorder or transvestic fetishism. *Journal of Sex & Marital Therapy, 38*(2), 151–189.

Chapter 6

Nursing Care for the Family in Need of Reproductive Life Planning

KEY TERMS

- abstinence
- barrier methods
- basal body temperature
- cervical cap
- coitus
- coitus interruptus
- condom
- contraceptive
- diaphragm
- elective termination of pregnancy
- fertile days
- fertility awareness
- intrauterine device
- laparoscopy
- natural family planning
- reproductive life planning
- spermicide
- transdermal contraception
- tubal ligation
- vaginal ring
- vasectomy

OBJECTIVES

After mastering the contents of this chapter, you should be able to:

1. Describe common methods of reproductive life planning and the advantages, disadvantages, and risk factors associated with each.
2. Identify 2020 National Health Goals related to reproductive life planning that nurses can help the nation achieve.
3 Assess clients for reproductive life planning needs.
4. Formulate nursing diagnoses related to reproductive life planning concerns.
5. Identify expected outcomes for couples desiring reproductive life planning as well as manage seamless transitions across differing health care settings.
6. Using the nursing process, plan nursing care that includes the six competencies of Quality & Safety Education for Nurses (QSEN): Patient-Centered Care, Teamwork & Collaboration, Evidence-Based Practice (EBP), Quality Improvement (QI), Safety, and Informatics
7. Implement nursing care related to reproductive life planning, such as educating adolescents about the use of condoms as a safer sex practice as well as to prevent unintended pregnancy.
8. Evaluate expected outcomes for achievement and effectiveness of care.
9. Integrate knowledge of reproductive life planning with the interplay of nursing process, the six competencies of QSEN, and Family Nursing to promote quality maternal and child health nursing care.

Seventeen-year-old Dana Crews has come to your community health clinic for a pelvic examination and Papanicolaou (Pap) smear. She tells you she is sexually active and her boyfriend "sometimes" uses a condom. She trusts he will "stop in time" when they aren't using one. She doesn't want to take birth control pills because she can't afford them and also she's afraid her parents will find out she's broken her abstinence pledge if they see the pills.

The previous chapter described the anatomy and physiology of the male and female reproductive systems and the importance of practicing safer sex. This chapter adds information about ways to prevent pregnancy or to plan and space children. Such information builds a base for both care and health teaching of families.

What additional health teaching does Dana need to be well informed about reproductive life planning?

Reproductive life planning includes all the decisions an individual or couple make about whether and when to have children, how many children to have, and how they are spaced. Some couples you will meet want counseling about how to avoid conception. Others want information on increasing fertility and about their ability to conceive. Others need counseling because a **contraceptive** (a measure to halt conception) has failed (Bond, 2013).

It is important for the health of children that pregnancies should be intended because, when a pregnancy is unintended or mistimed, both short-term and long-term consequences can result. The woman may be less likely to seek prenatal care, less likely to breastfeed, and less careful to protect her fetus from harmful substances. A disproportionate share of women who bear children whose conception was unintended are adolescents; such women are less apt to complete high school or college and more likely to require public assistance and/or live in poverty than their peers who are not mothers. The child of such a pregnancy is at greater risk of low birth weight, dying in the first year of life, being maltreated, and not receiving sufficient resources for healthy development (Centers for Disease Control and Prevention [CDC], 2012).

Planning for reproductive choices is so important that several 2020 National Health Goals speak directly to this area of care (Box 6.1).

BOX 6.1 Nursing Care Planning Based on 2020 National Health Goals

A number of 2020 National Health Goals speak directly to reproductive life planning:

- Increase the proportion of adolescents who receive formal instruction on abstinence before 18 years of age from a baseline of 87.2% to a target of 95.9%.
- Increase the proportion of females less than 15 years of age who have never had sexual intercourse from a baseline of 82.9% to a target of 91.2%; of males, from 82.0% to 90.2%.
- Reduce the proportion of females experiencing pregnancy despite use of a reversible contraceptive method from a baseline of 12.4% to a target of 9.9%.
- Increase the proportion of intended pregnancies from a baseline of 51% to a target of 56%.
- Decrease the proportion of births occurring within 18 months of a previous birth from a baseline of 35.3% to a target of 31.7% (U.S. Department of Health and Human Services [DHHS], 2010; see www.healthypeople.gov).

Nurses can help the nation achieve these objectives by teaching people, especially adolescents, about contraceptive options while being cautious to avoid indirectly encouraging sexual activity among teens.

Nursing Process Overview

For Reproductive Life Planning

Assessment

As a result of changing social values and lifestyles, many people today are able to talk easily about reproductive life planning. Other people, however, may be uncomfortable with this topic and may not voice their interest in the subject independently. For this reason, at health assessments, ask clients if they want more information or need any help with reproductive life planning as part of obtaining a basic health history.

Nursing Diagnosis

Because reproductive life planning touches so many facets of life, nursing diagnoses can differ greatly depending on the circumstances and individual preferences. Examples might include:

- Readiness for enhanced knowledge regarding contraception options related to a desire to prevent pregnancy
- Deficient knowledge related to use of a diaphragm
- Spiritual distress related to partner's preferences for contraception
- Decisional conflict regarding choice of birth control because of health concerns
- Decisional conflict related to unintended pregnancy
- Powerlessness related to failure of chosen contraceptive
- Altered sexuality pattern related to fear of pregnancy
- Risk for ineffective health maintenance related to lack of knowledge about natural family planning methods

Planning and Implementation

When establishing expected outcomes for care in this area, be certain plans are realistic for each couple. If a woman has a history of poor compliance with medication, for instance, it might not be realistic for her to plan on taking an oral contraceptive every day. If she only desires temporary contraception, tubal ligation or vasectomy for her partner would certainly be inappropriate. Be certain when counseling to be sensitive to a couple's religious, cultural, and moral beliefs before suggesting possible methods. It is equally important to explore your own beliefs and values before counseling. This not only helps develop self-awareness of how these beliefs affect nursing care but it also allows you to become more sensitive to the beliefs of others.

Clients are required to provide informed consent for surgical contraceptive methods or procedures such as vasectomy or tubal ligation. The risks, benefits, alternatives, and proper use of the method and the client's understanding of his or her rights and responsibilities should be included in the consent form as this helps ensure clients have weighed their options and know the procedure may be irreversible. If you are helping to obtain a consent signature, always do so in the presence of a witness.

An organization helpful for referral so people can learn more about reproductive life planning is Planned Parenthood (www.plannedparenthood.org) and the CDC (www.cdc.gov). *Choosing Wisely*, a program available on the Web site www.SexualityandU.ca, is an interactive program to help women select their ideal birth control method. Another Web site, www.Not-2-Late.com, is dedicated to explaining emergency contraception.

Outcome Evaluation

Evaluation is important in reproductive life planning, because anything that causes clients to discontinue or misuse a particular method will leave them at risk of pregnancy. Reassess early (within 1 to 3 weeks) after a couple begins a new method of contraception, to prevent such an occurrence. Evaluate not only whether a chosen method is effective but also whether the woman and her partner are satisfied or have further questions. Examples of expected outcomes include:

- Client voices confidence in chosen contraceptive method by next visit
- Client expresses satisfaction with chosen method at follow-up visit
- Client consistently uses chosen method without pregnancy for 1 year's time

CONTRACEPTION

As many as 93% of women of childbearing age in the United States use some form of contraception (CDC, 2012). Major benefits of this increase in contraception include decreases in unintended adolescent pregnancies, the need for "morning after" or postcoital medications, and elective terminations of pregnancy (CDC, 2012).

Important things to consider when helping a couple choose a method that will be right for them include:

- Personal values
- Ability to use a method correctly
- If the method will affect sexual enjoyment
- Financial factors
- If a couple's relationship is short term or long term
- Prior experiences with contraception
- Future plans

Understanding how various methods of contraception work and how they compare in terms of benefits and disadvantages is necessary for successful counseling (Box 6.2). When counseling, in addition to assessing to determine a best contraceptive option, be certain to emphasize safer sex practices (see Box 5.7 in Chapter 5). Although there are many contraceptive options for reliable pregnancy prevention, only condoms (both male and female) provide protection against sexually transmitted infections (STIs) or HIV—an important concern if a relationship is not a monogamous one.

Many postpartum services distribute printed information on contraception packaging to women at discharge. Women are then invited to ask questions as necessary about the material. Read these materials carefully to be certain they are accurate before distributing them and, if suggestions are needed, make them to the correct health care committee. Be certain to make it clear you are available to answer questions about contraception; otherwise, women are in such a hurry to take their newborn home, they tend to postpone questions "until later," a time when the question may be too late to be effective or a health care provider is no longer available.

BOX 6.2 Nursing Care Planning Using Assessment

Assessing a Woman for Possible Contraindications to Contraceptive Use

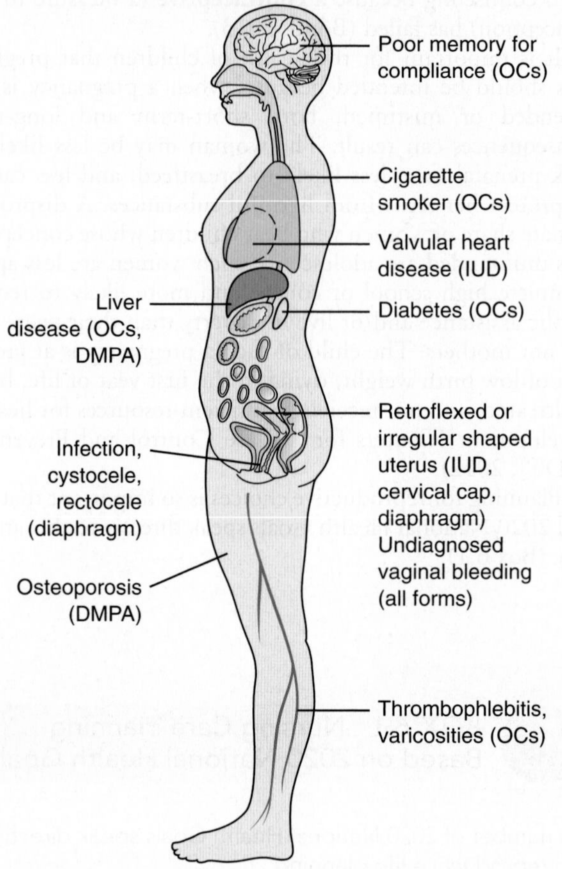

DMPA, depot medroxyprogesterone acetate; IUD, intrauterine device; OCs, oral contraceptives.

Consider each person's lifestyle and overall health, as these influence what type of conception a woman will choose (Box 6.3). Morbidly obese women, for example, may need to choose different types than women with an

BOX 6.3 Nursing Care Planning to Respect Cultural Diversity

People differ greatly in the way they desire or accept information on reproductive life planning, depending on individual preferences and sociocultural influences. For example, certain religions do not believe a method beyond abstinence or fertility awareness is right to use. People with lower incomes cannot afford surgical procedures or methods such as daily combination pills. Be certain while counseling in this area that you do not impose your own values on people, but rather, work together to identify a system that your patient will be able to follow consistently.

average body mass index (Scott-Ram, Chor, Bhogireddy, et al., 2012). Women from a male-dominant family may have little choice as to what reproductive life planning method they can choose. If their partner does not wish to participate in contraception planning, it would be inappropriate to suggest a type where male cooperation is needed, such as use of a male condom or natural family planning.

Because no method of contraception, except abstinence, offers 100% protection against pregnancy, it is important to carefully answer a patient's questions regarding methods of contraception. It is necessary to be prepared to answer questions about postcoital protection if there were unprotected sexual relations as well as elective termination of pregnancy if contraception failed. Only when couples have sufficient information in all these areas and the freedom to discuss specific concerns can they be prepared to make a decision that will be right for them (Paterno & Jordan, 2012).

An ideal contraceptive should be:

- Safe
- Effective
- Compatible with religious and cultural beliefs and personal preferences of both the user and sexual partner
- Free of bothersome side effects
- Convenient to use and easily obtainable
- Affordable and needing few instructions for effective use
- Free of effects (after discontinuation) on future pregnancies

Before a patient begins using a new method of contraception, information that should be obtained includes:

- Vital signs, possibly a Pap smear, pregnancy test, gonococcal and chlamydial screening, and perhaps hemoglobin for detection of anemia
- Obstetric history, including STIs, past pregnancies, previous elective abortions, failure of previously used methods, and compliance history with previously used methods
- Subjective assessment of the client's desires, needs, feelings, and understanding of conception (a teen may believe she is too young to get pregnant; a woman in the immediate postpartum period may believe she cannot conceive immediately, especially if she is breastfeeding)
- Sexual practices, such as frequency, number of partners, feelings about sex, and body image

How well contraceptive methods meet ideal requirements is discussed with each type. The range of effectiveness of frequently used contraceptive methods is shown in Table 6.1. This table shows the effectiveness of each method by listing the *ideal failure rate* (the number of unintended pregnancies that will occur in 1 year) for couples who use the method consistently and correctly and also the *failure rate* for routine use (less-than-perfect use). A method that shows a large difference between the ideal failure rate and the actual failure rate may not be easy and convenient to use.

Natural Family Planning

Natural family planning methods, also called periodic abstinence methods, are, as the name implies, methods that involve no introduction of chemical or foreign material into the body (Hanson & Burke, 2011).

Many people hold religious beliefs that rule out the use of birth control pills or devices; others simply believe a "natural" way of planning pregnancies that will involve no expense, does not introduce a foreign substance into their body, and has no risk to a fetus should they become pregnant is best for them. The effectiveness of these methods varies greatly from a 2% ideal failure rate to about a 25% failure rate, depending mainly on the couple's ability to refrain from having sexual relations on **fertile days** or days on which a woman has the most likely chance to become pregnant (Zinaman, Johnson, Ellis, et al., 2012).

Abstinence

Abstinence, or refraining from sexual relations, has a theoretical 0% failure rate and is also the most effective way to prevent STIs. Clients, however, particularly adolescents, may find it difficult to adhere to abstinence because of peer pressure. In a moment of passion, many otherwise responsible people may completely overlook abstinence as an option. Because it is difficult for many women to adhere to abstinence, the method has a failure rate as high as 85% (Russo & Nelson, 2010).

Many sex education classes for adolescents advocate abstinence as the only contraceptive measure, so teenagers and young adults who take these courses may know little about other options. When discussing abstinence as a contraceptive method, be certain to provide information not only on the method but suggestions of ways to comply with this method (Box 6.4). A worry is adolescents who make "abstinence pledges" to not have sexual intercourse until they are married may "tune out" not only additional information on contraception but also on safer sex practices. Then, if they break their pledge (about 50% do), that could leave them more vulnerable to STIs and pregnancy than others (Cherlin, 2012).

Lactation Amenorrhea Method

As long as a woman is breastfeeding, there is both natural suppression of ovulation and the return of menses (Baselice & Lawson, 2011). Lactation amenorrhea method (LAM) is a safe birth control method (a failure rate of about 1% to 5%) if an infant is:

- Under 6 months of age
- Being totally breastfed at least every 4 hours during the day and every 6 hours at night
- Receives no supplementary feedings, and
- Menses has not returned

After 6 months, or if the infant begins to receive supplemental feedings or isn't sucking well, the use of LAM as an effective birth control method becomes questionable and the woman probably should be advised to choose another method of contraception (Türk, Terzioğlu, & Eroğlu, 2010). A woman should also consider a different method of contraception once her baby begins sleeping through the night, even if this occurs before the child reaches 6 months of age.

Coitus Interruptus

Coitus interruptus (withdrawal) is one of the oldest known methods of contraception. The couple proceeds with coitus until the moment of ejaculation. Then the man withdraws and spermatozoa are emitted outside the vagina.

TABLE 6.1 Contraception Failure Rates

Type of Contraceptive	Ideal Failure Rate (%) Perfect Use[a]	Failure Rate (%) Typical Use	Advantages	Disadvantages
Natural Family Planning				
Abstinence	100%	85%	Acceptable to all religious groups No cost	Requires high motivation and periods of abstinence
Lactation, amenorrhea	1%–5% (under 6 months)	95% (after 6 months)	Effective while infant is totally breastfed; approved by all religions and cultures	Temporary measure Not reliable if infant takes supplemental feedings
Calendar	1%–9%	25%	No cost	Requires motivation, cooperation
Standard day method: CycleBeads©	4%–5%	12%–13%	Visual aid can improve compliance Available as iPhone app	Initial cost May need to mark on a calendar they have moved a bead rather than rely on memory
Basel body temperature (BBT)	3%	25%	Cost of thermometer	Requires motivation and cooperation by male partner
Ovulation method	3%	25%	No cost	Requires motivation and cooperation by male partner
Symptothermal	2%	25%	No cost	Requires motivation and cooperation from male partner
Two-day method	3%–4%	13%–14%	No cost	Requires motivation and cooperation from male partner
Withdrawal	4%	19%–27%	A male-controlled method	Sperm may be present in pre-ejaculatory fluid
Barrier Methods				
Spermicide	8%	25%	Easy to use Sold over the counter	May leave an annoying vaginal discharge
Male condom	2%	15%	Protects against STIs Male responsibility No prescription necessary	Requires interruption of sexual activity
Female condom	5%	15%	Protection against STIs	Insertion may be difficult
Sponge (parous woman)	20%	35%	Easy to insert No prescription	May cause leakage Necessary to take measures to avoid danger of TSS
Sponge (nulliparous woman)	9%	16%–20%	Easy to insert No prescription	May cause leakage Necessary to take measures to avoid TSS
Diaphragm	6%	18%	Easy to insert	Prescription needed Necessary to take measures to avoid TSS
Cervical cap (parous woman)	23%	35%	Can leave in place for several days if desired	May be difficult to insert Can irritate cervix Necessary to take measures to avoid TSS
Cervical cap (nulliparous woman)	9%	18%	Can leave in place for several days if desired	May be difficult to insert Can irritate cervix Necessary to take measures to avoid TSS

Type of Contraceptive	Ideal Failure Rate (%) Perfect Use[a]	Failure Rate (%) Typical Use	Advantages	Disadvantages
Hormonal Methods				
Transdermal patch	0.2%–0.3%	5%	Easy to apply	Irritation at local site
Vaginal ring	0.2%–0.3%	5%	Easy to insert	May need reminder to insert
Combination oral contraceptives (COCs)	0.2%–0.3%	5%–8%	Coitus independent	Continual cost Possible side effect of thrombophlebitis
Progestin-only pills (mini-pills)	0.5%	5%–8%	Coitus independent No side effects of COCs	Continual cost
Injectable progesterone (DMPA)	0.3%	0.3%	Coitus independent Dependable for 12 weeks	Continual cost Continual injections
Intradermal implant (Implanon)	0.05%	0.05%	Coitus independent Dependable for 5 years	Initial cost Appearance on arm
IUD (copper T)	0.1%	0.5%–0.6%	No memory or motivation needed	Cramping, bleeding Expulsion possible
Mirena IUD	0.1%	0.1%	No memory or motivation needed	Cramping, bleeding Expulsion possible
Surgical Methods				
Female sterilization	0.5%	0.5%	Permanent and highly reliable	Initial cost Irreversible
Male sterilization	0.1%	0.15%	Permanent and highly reliable	Initial cost Irreversible
Postcoital (Emergency) Methods				
Postcoital pills	1%–2%	25%	Can be purchased over the counter	May cause nausea
Postcoital IUD	0.1%	25%	Can be inserted up to 5 days after unprotected coitus Can be left in place as contraceptive measure	Visit to a health care provider is needed within 5 days (120 hr) of unprotected coitus

[a]Couples who use the method consistently and correctly during a year's time.

DMPA, depot medroxyprogesterone acetate; IUD, intrauterine device; STI, sexually transmitted infection; TSS, toxic shock syndrome.

Modified from Shoupe, D., & Kjos, S. (Eds.). (2010). *The handbook of contraception.* Totowa, NJ: Humana Press.

BOX 6.4 Nursing Care Planning to Empower a Family

SUGGESTIONS FOR PROMOTING ABSTINENCE

Q. Dana, 17 years old, asks you, "How can I avoid being pressured into unwanted sex?"

A. A few suggestions are:

- Discuss with your partner in advance which sexual activities you will permit and which you will not.
- Try to avoid high-pressure situations such as a party with known drug use, excessive alcohol consumption; for teenagers: no adult supervision.
- Be certain your partner understands when you say, "No," you mean it.
- Make it clear your partner understands you consider being forced into relations against your wishes the same as rape, not simply irresponsible conduct.
- Do not accept any drug to "help you relax" or "be cool," as such a drug could impair your judgment. The drug could also be the "date rape" drug flunitrazepam (Rohypnol), which causes loss of memory for recent events.

Unfortunately, ejaculation may occur before withdrawal is complete and, despite the caution used, some spermatozoa may be deposited in the vagina. Furthermore, because there may be a few spermatozoa present in pre-ejaculation fluid, fertilization may occur even if withdrawal seems controlled (Killick, Leary, Trussell, et al., 2011). For these reasons, coitus interruptus is only about 75% effective, and the method should be used with caution as it also can lead to STIs (Tafuri, Martinellim, Germinario, et al., 2011).

Postcoital Douching

Douching following intercourse, no matter what solution is used, is ineffective as a contraceptive measure as sperm may be present in cervical mucus as quickly as 90 seconds after ejaculation, long before douching could be accomplished.

Fertility Awareness Methods

Fertility awareness methods rely on detecting when a woman will be capable of impregnation (fertile) so she can use periods of abstinence during that time. There are a variety of ways to determine a fertile period, such as using a calendar to calculate the period of time based on a set formula, using a visual tool such as "Cyclebeads," measuring the woman's body temperature, observing the consistency of cervical mucus, or employing a combination of these methods (Taylor, Aldad, McVeigh, et al., 2012). The methods consider the typical length of sperm survival (up to 3 to 4 days) and the length of time an ova is ripe for fertilization (about 1 day). Based on this, a fertile period exists from 5 days before ovulation to 1 day after.

Calendar (Rhythm) Method

The calendar method requires a couple to abstain from coitus on the days of a menstrual cycle when the woman is most likely to conceive. To plan for this, the woman keeps a diary of about six menstrual cycles. To calculate "safe" days, she subtracts 18 from the shortest cycle she documented. This number predicts her first fertile day. She then subtracts 11 from her longest cycle. This represents her last fertile day. If she had six menstrual cycles ranging from 25 to 29 days, her fertile period would be from the 7th day (25 [the shorted cycle] – 18) to the 18th day (29 [the longest cycle] – 11). To avoid pregnancy, she would avoid coitus during those days (Fig. 6.1A).When used conscientiously, the method has a low failure rate; in typical use, however, this rate rises substantially because of irregular menstrual cycles, miscalculation, or disregard for predicted fertile days.

Basal Body Temperature Method

Just before the day of ovulation, a woman's **basal body temperature** (BBT), or the temperature of her body at rest, falls about 0.5°F. At the time of ovulation, her BBT rises a full Fahrenheit degree (0.2°C) because of the rise in progesterone with ovulation. This pattern serves as the basis for the BBT method of contraception (Taylor et al., 2012).

To use this method, the woman takes her temperature, either orally or with a tympanic thermometer, each morning immediately after waking before she rises from bed or undertakes any activity; this is her BBT. A woman who works nights should take her temperature after awakening from her longest sleep period, no matter what the time of day.

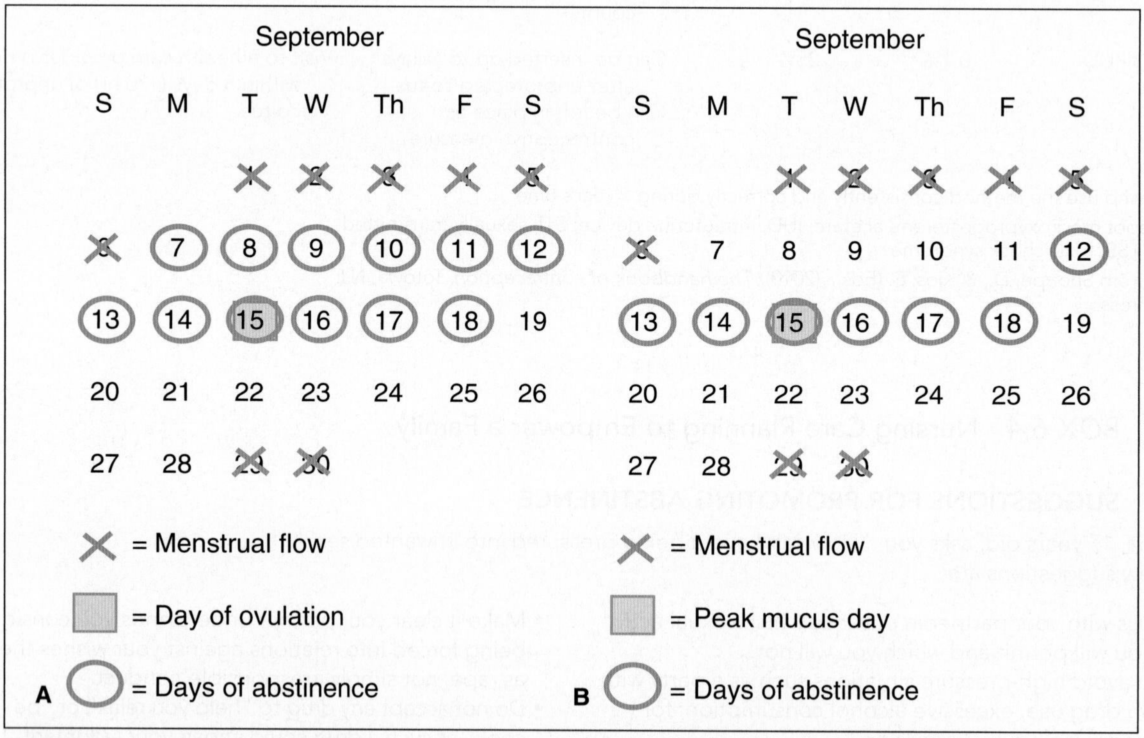

FIGURE 6.1 **(A)** A typical month showing predicted fertile days using the calendar method as a natural family planning method. **(B)** A typical month using the cervical mucus method of natural family planning. Unmarked days are those predicted to be unfertile and therefore safe for sexual relations.

As soon as a woman notices a slight dip in temperature followed by an increase, she knows she has ovulated. She refrains from having **coitus** (sexual relations) for the next 3 days (the possible life of the discharged ovum).

Because sperm can survive for at least 4 days and possibly as many as 7 days in the female reproductive tract, it is usually recommended that the couple combine this method with a calendar method, so they abstain for a few days before ovulation as well. The BBT method has an ideal failure rate as low as 3%, but a failure rate of 25% (see Table 6.1). For more information on BBT and how it also can be used to aid conception, see Chapter 8 and Figure 8.2.

A problem with assessing BBT for fertility awareness is that many factors can affect BBT. For example, a temperature rise caused by illness could be mistaken as the signal of ovulation. If this happens, a woman could mistake a fertile day for a safe one. Changes in the woman's daily schedule, such as starting an aerobic program or getting up earlier than usual, could also affect BBT.

Cervical Mucus Method (Billing's Method)

Yet another method to predict ovulation is to use the changes in cervical mucus that occur naturally with ovulation (Fig. 6.1B). Before ovulation each month, the cervical mucus is thick and does not stretch when pulled between the thumb and finger. Just before ovulation, mucus secretion increases. On the day of ovulation (the peak day), it becomes copious, thin, watery, and transparent. It feels slippery (like egg white) and stretches at least 1 inch before the strand breaks, a property known as *spinnbarkeit* (see Chapter 5, Figure 5.14). In addition, breast tenderness and an anterior tilt to the cervix occur. All the days on which cervical mucus is copious, and for at least 3 to 4 days afterward, are considered to be fertile days, or days on which the woman should abstain from coitus to avoid conception (Hanson & Burke, 2011).

A woman using this method must be conscientious about assessing her vaginal secretions every day, or she will miss the change in texture and amount. The feel of vaginal secretions after sexual relations is unreliable, because seminal fluid (the fluid containing sperm from the male) has a watery, postovulatory consistency and can be confused with ovulatory mucus. Figure 6.1B shows a hypothetical month using this method. This method has a failure rate of about 25% because of difficulty in interpreting mucus status (Shoupe & Kjos, 2010). Because sperm have a life span up to 3 to 4 days, a woman needs to abstain for 4 days prior to the appearance of estrogen-influenced mucus; therefore, this method should be combined with a calendar method for best results.

Two-Day Method

To use a two-day method, a woman assesses for vaginal secretions daily. If she feels secretions for 2 days in a row, she avoids coitus that day and the day following as the presence of secretions suggests fertility. The method requires conscientious daily assessment and results in about 12 days per month in which she should avoid coitus, the same as a calendar method (Jennings, Sinai, Sacieta, et al., 2011).

Symptothermal Method

The symptothermal method of birth control combines the cervical mucus and BBT methods (Soler & Barranco-Castillo, 2010). The woman takes her temperature daily, watching for the rise in temperature that marks ovulation. She also analyzes her cervical mucus every day and observes for other signs of ovulation such as *mittelschmerz* (midcycle abdominal pain) or if her cervix feels softer than usual. The couple then abstains from intercourse until 3 days after the rise in temperature or the fourth day after the peak of mucus change. The symptothermal method, because it assesses more clues to ovulation, is more effective than either the BBT or the cervical mucus method alone (ideal failure rate, about 2%).

Standard Days Method: CycleBeads

This method is designed for women who have menstrual cycles between 26 and 32 days (Bekele & Fantahun, 2012). A woman purchases a circle of beads that helps her predict fertile days (Fig. 6.2). The first bead on the ring is red and marks the first day of her menstrual flow; this is followed by 6 brown beads which indicate "safe" days. Twelve glow-in-the dark white beads, which mark fertile days (during which she needs to abstain from coitus), and 13 additional brown "safe" days follow. The woman advances one bead per day during the month. If she reaches a dark brown bead (appears on the 27th day) before she begins her next menses, her cycle is too short for the method to be reliable. If she reaches the end of the string of beads (32 days) before menses, she knows her cycle is too long for the method to be reliable. The system is easy to use and, if a woman wants a more technology-based system than using a circle of beads, there is an iPhone app available in place of actual beads (iCycleBeads). The system is easy to understand; most women, however, need to use a calendar to check off daily that they have moved a bead or they can lose track of the system.

Ovulation Detection

Still another method to predict ovulation is by the use of an over-the-counter ovulation detection kit. These kits detect the midcycle surge of luteinizing hormone (LH) that can be detected in urine 12 to 24 hours before ovulation. Such kits are 98% to 100% accurate in predicting ovulation. Although they are fairly expensive and not intended to be used as a contraceptive aid, combining a cervical mucus assessment and the ovulation detector to mark the peak fertile day is becoming the method of choice for many families. An ovulation detector can be used in the future to help conception when the couple is ready to have children.

Side Effects and Contraindications for Natural Family Planning

Natural family planning methods do not have side effects. If there is a contraindication to their use it would be for couples who must prevent conception (perhaps because the woman is taking a drug that would be harmful to a fetus or the couple absolutely does not want the responsibility of children), because the failure rate of all forms is about 25%.

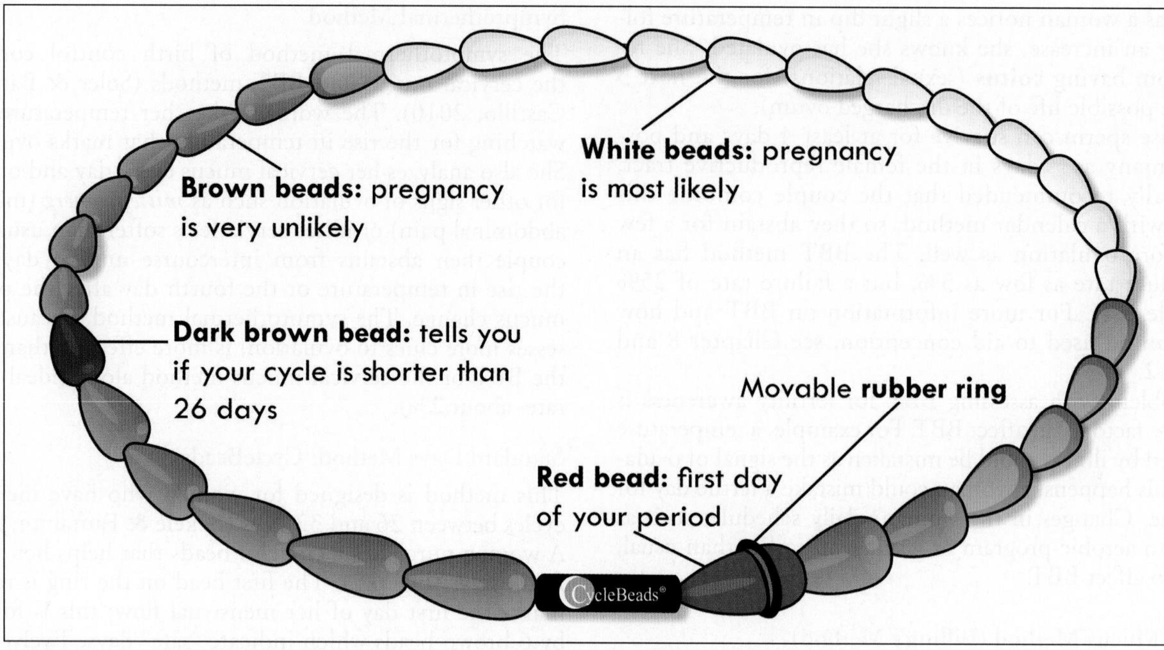

FIGURE 6.2 With CycleBeads©, a woman moves one bead every day to predict her fertile days if her menstrual cycles range from 26 to 32 days. (Courtesy of Cycle Technologies, Inc., Washington, DC.)

Natural Family Planning and Effect on Pregnancy

Natural family planning methods have no effect if a woman should get pregnant while using them as well as no effect on future pregnancies.

Natural Family Planning and Effect on Sexual Enjoyment

Once a couple is certain of a woman's nonfertile days using one of the natural planning methods, more spontaneity in sexual relations is possible than with methods that involve vaginal insertion products. However, the required days of abstinence may make a natural planning method unsatisfactory and unenjoyable for a couple. Coitus interruptus may be unenjoyable because of the need to withdraw before ejaculation.

Natural Family Planning and the Adolescent

Natural methods of family planning (with the exception of abstinence) are usually not the contraceptive method of choice for adolescents, as they require a great deal of thought and persistence. Adolescent boys may lack the control or experience to use coitus interruptus effectively. Girls tend to have occasional anovulatory menstrual cycles for several years after menarche and so may not experience definite cervical changes or an elevated body temperature each month. In addition, these methods require adolescents to say "no" to sexual intercourse on fertile days, a task that may be difficult to complete under peer pressure.

Natural Family Planning and the Perimenopausal Woman

Perimenopausal women are good candidates for natural family planning methods because they may not be able to use hormonal methods such as birth control pills because of risk to them if they have a history of high blood pressure, thromboembolic disease, or cigarette smoking. As menopause approaches, however, they may not have as much cervical mucus as previously, causing the contrast between fertile and nonfertile days more difficult to detect.

Natural Family Planning and the Postpartal Woman

After a successful pregnancy, most women are interested in delaying their next pregnancy until their new baby is older. This makes them good candidates for natural family planning as they can breastfeed with these methods without worrying about hormonal contamination or a decrease in breast milk.

QSEN Checkpoint Question 6.1

Patient-Centered Care

Suppose Dana, 17 years old, tells you she wants to use a fertility awareness method of contraception. How should you best meet Dana's learning needs?

a. You should teach her to record if she feels hot and whether she is perspiring heavily.
b. You should teach her to assess whether her cervical mucus is thin and watery.
c. You should teach her to monitor her emotions for sudden anger or crying.
d. You should teach her to assess whether her breasts feel sensitive to cool air.

Look in Appendix A for the best answer and rationale.

Barrier Methods of Contraception

Barrier methods are forms of birth control that place a chemical or latex barrier between the cervix and advancing sperm so sperm cannot reach and fertilize an ovum.

Spermicides

A **spermicide** is an agent that causes the death of spermatozoa before they can enter the cervix. Such agents are not only actively spermicidal but also change the vaginal pH to a strong acid level, a condition not conducive to sperm survival. They do not protect against STIs. In addition to the general benefits for barrier contraceptives, the advantages of spermicides include:

- They may be purchased without a prescription or an appointment with a health care provider, so they allow for greater independence and lower costs.
- When used in conjunction with another contraceptive, they increase the other method's effectiveness.
- Various preparations are available, including gels, creams, sponges, films, foams, and vaginal suppositories.

Gels or creams are easily inserted into the vagina before coitus with the provided applicator (Fig. 6.3). The woman should do this no more than 1 hour before coitus. If she chooses to douche to remove the spermicide afterward (no need to do this) she should wait 6 hours after coitus to ensure the agent has completed its spermicidal action.

Another form of spermicidal protection is a film of glycerin impregnated with a spermicidal agent that is folded and inserted vaginally. On contact with vaginal secretions or precoital penile emissions, the film dissolves and a carbon dioxide foam forms to protect the cervix against invading spermatozoa.

Still other vaginal products are cocoa butter and glycerin-based vaginal suppositories containing a spermicide. Because it takes about 15 minutes for a suppository to dissolve, it must be inserted 15 minutes before coitus.

Foam-impregnated synthetic sponges are moistened to activate the impregnated spermicide, then inserted vaginally to block sperm access. Well liked by most users, they are easy to insert and have an ideal failure rate of 9% and a typical use failure rate of about 16% to 20% (Shoupe & Kjos, 2010). Caution women preparations labeled "feminine hygiene" products are for vaginal cleanliness and are not spermicidal; therefore, they are not effective contraceptives.

Side Effects and Contraindications

Vaginally inserted spermicidal products are contraindicated in women with acute cervicitis because they might further irritate the cervix. Some women find the vaginal leakage after use of these products bothersome. Vaginal suppositories, because of the cocoa butter or glycerin base, are the most bothersome in this regard.

Male and Female Condoms

A male **condom** is a latex rubber or synthetic sheath that is placed over the erect penis before coitus to trap sperm (Fig. 6.4). Male condoms have an ideal failure rate of 2% and a true failure rate of about 15%, because breakage or spillage occurs in up to 15% of uses (see Table 6.1). A big advantage of male condoms is they are one of the few "male-responsibility" birth control measures available. In addition, no health care visit or prescription is needed. They are recommended for partners who do not maintain a monogamous relationship because, although latex condoms do not necessarily offer protection against diseases spread by skin-to-skin contact such as human papillomavirus (HPV), syphilis, or genital herpes, they do prevent the spread of STIs such as gonorrhea and chlamydia; their use has become a major part of the fight to prevent infection from HIV.

To be effective, a condom must be applied before any penile-vulvar contact as even pre-ejaculation fluid may contain some sperm. The condom should be positioned so it is loose enough at the penis tip to collect the ejaculate without placing undue pressure on the condom. The penis (with the condom held carefully in place) must be withdrawn before it begins to

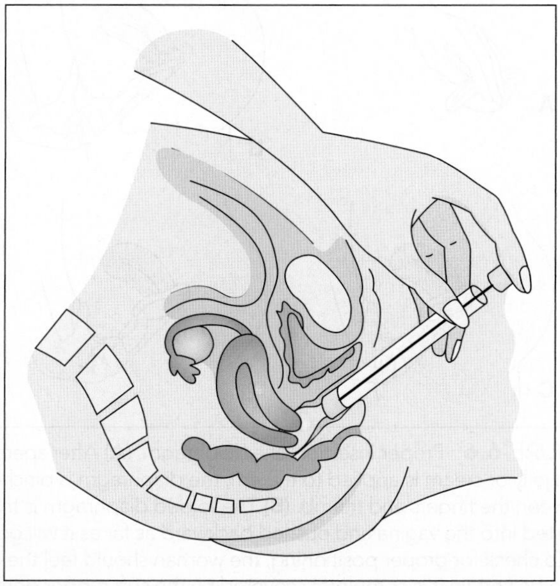

FIGURE 6.3 Vaginal insertion of a spermicidal agent.

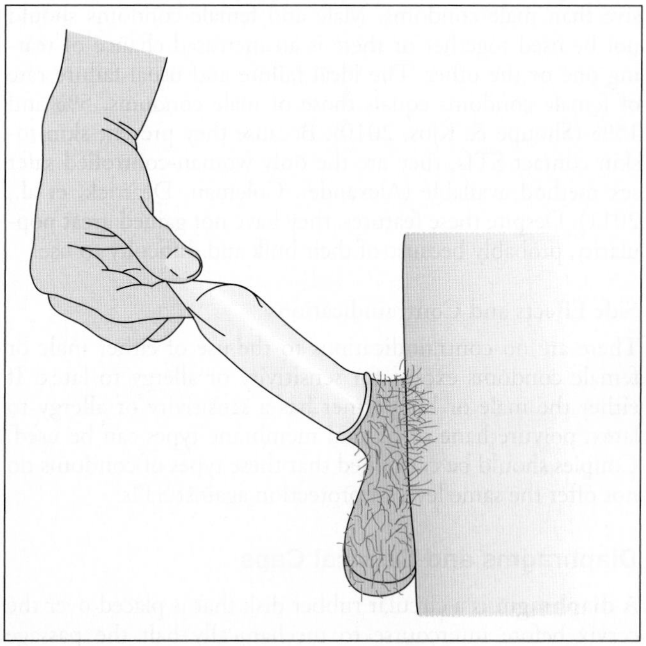

FIGURE 6.4 Proper application of a male condom. Being certain space is left at the tip helps to ensure the condom will not break with ejaculation.

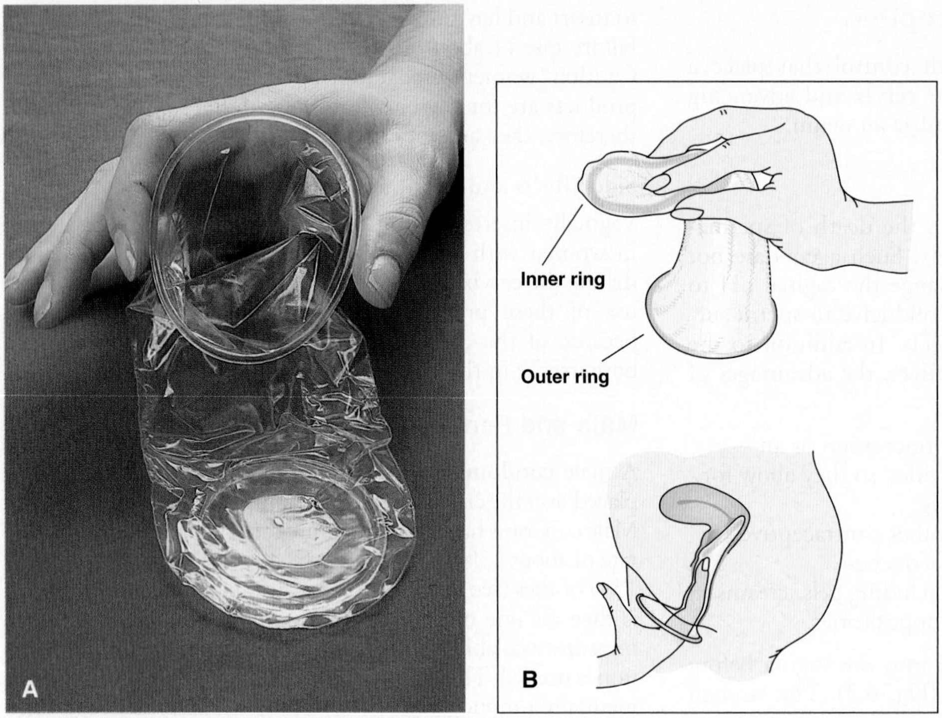

FIGURE 6.5 A female condom. Such a device is effective protection against both sexually transmitted infections and pregnancy. **(A)** The REALITY (WP-333) female condom. (© Barbara Proud.) **(B)** Insertion technique. (Courtesy of Wisconsin Pharmaceutical Company, Inc.)

become flaccid after ejaculation to prevent sperm from leaking from the now loosely fitting sheath into the vagina.

Condoms for females are sheaths made of latex or polyurethane, prelubricated with a spermicide so, the same as male condoms, they offer protection against conception as well as STIs and HIV. The inner ring (closed end) covers the cervix, and the outer ring (open end) rests against the vaginal opening. The sheath may be inserted any time before sexual activity begins and then removed after ejaculation occurs. Like male condoms, they are intended for one-time use (Fig. 6.5). They can be purchased without a prescription but are more expensive than male condoms. Male and female condoms should not be used together or there is an increased chance of tearing one or the other. The ideal failure and usual failure rate of female condoms equals those of male condoms, 5% and 15% (Shoupe & Kjos, 2010). Because they prevent skin-to-skin contact STIs, they are the only woman-controlled safer sex method available (Alexander, Coleman, Deatrick, et al., 2011). Despite these features, they have not gained great popularity, probably because of their bulk and difficulty to use.

Side Effects and Contraindications

There are no contraindications to the use of either male or female condoms except for sensitivity or allergy to latex. If either the male or his partner has a sensitivity or allergy to latex, polyurethane or natural membrane types can be used. Couples should be cautioned that these types of condoms do not offer the same level of protection against STIs.

Diaphragms and Cervical Caps

A **diaphragm** is a circular rubber disk that is placed over the cervix before intercourse to mechanically halt the passage of sperm (Fig. 6.6). Although use of a spermicide to coat a diaphragm is not required, using a spermicidal gel with one combines a barrier and a chemical method of contraception so one is usually added. With the use of a spermicide, the failure rate of the diaphragm is as low as 6% (ideal) to 18% (typical use) (see Table 6.1).

A diaphragm is prescribed and fitted initially by a health care provider to ensure a correct fit. Because the shape of a woman's cervix changes with pregnancy, miscarriage, cervical surgery (dilatation and curettage [D&C]), or elective termination of pregnancy, teach women to return for a second fitting if any of these circumstances occur. A woman should also have the fit of the diaphragm checked if she gains or loses more than 15 lb, because this could also change her pelvic and vaginal contours.

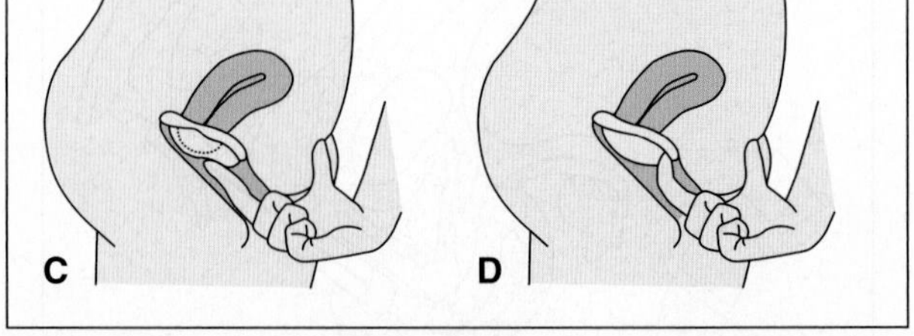

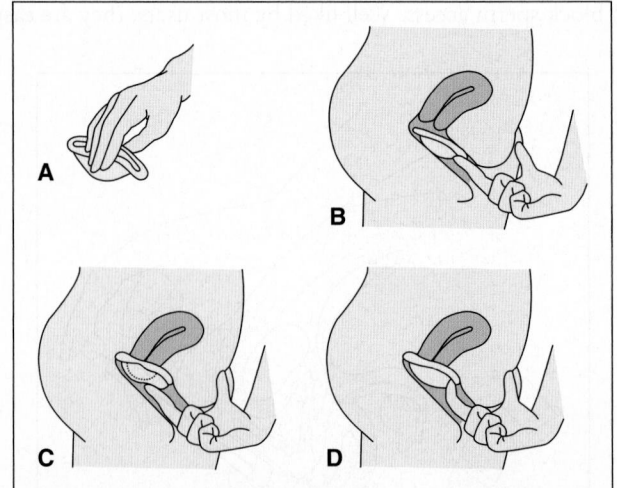

FIGURE 6.6 Proper insertion of a diaphragm. **(A)** After spermicidal jelly or cream is applied to the rim, the diaphragm is pinched between the fingers and thumb. **(B)** The folded diaphragm is then inserted into the vagina and pushed backward as far as it will go. **(C)** To check for proper positioning, the woman should feel the cervix to be certain it is completely covered by the soft rubber dome of the diaphragm. **(D)** To remove the diaphragm, a finger is hooked under the forward rim and the diaphragm is pulled down and out.

Before expected coitus, after first coating the inside rim and center portion of the diaphragm with a spermicide gel, the diaphragm is inserted into the vagina, sliding it along the posterior wall and pressing it up against the cervix so it is gripped by the vaginal fornices. A woman should check a diaphragm with a finger after insertion to be certain it is fitted well up over the cervix; she should be able to palpate the cervical os through the center of the diaphragm.

Diaphragms should remain in place for at least 6 hours after coitus, because spermatozoa remain viable in the vagina for that length of time; they may be left in place for as long as 24 hours. Leaving them in place longer than this can cause cervical inflammation (erosion) or urethral irritation from the pressure against the vaginal walls. If coitus is repeated before 6 hours, both a diaphragm or cap should not be removed and replaced; more spermicidal gel should be added to the vagina by an applicator.

A diaphragm is removed by inserting a finger into the vagina and loosening the diaphragm by pressing against the anterior rim and then withdrawing it vaginally. After use, a diaphragm should be washed in mild soap and water, dried gently, and stored it in its protective case. With this care, a diaphragm will last for 2 years, after which it should be replaced.

Side Effects and Contraindications

Diaphragms may not be effective if a uterus is prolapsed, retroflexed, or anteflexed to such a degree the cervix is also displaced in relation to the vagina. Intrusion on the vagina by a cystocele or rectocele where the walls of the vagina are displaced by bladder or bowel, may also make insertion of a diaphragm difficult. Users of diaphragms may experience a higher number of urinary tract infections (UTIs) than nonusers, probably because of pressure on the urethra. Diaphragms should not be used in the presence of acute cervicitis, herpes virus infection, or a papillomavirus infection, because the close contact of the rubber and the use of a spermicide can cause additional irritation. Other contraindications include:

- History of toxic shock syndrome (TSS; a staphylococcal infection introduced through the vagina)
- Allergy to rubber or spermicides
- History of recurrent UTIs

To prevent TSS (see Chapter 47) while using a diaphragm or cervical cap (discussed in the following), advise women to:

1. Wash their hands thoroughly with soap and water before insertion or removal.
2. Do not use a diaphragm during a menstrual period.
3. Do not leave a diaphragm in place longer than 24 hours.
4. Be aware of the symptoms of TSS, such as elevated temperature, diarrhea, vomiting, muscle aches, and a sunburn-like rash.
5. If symptoms of TSS should occur, immediately remove the diaphragm and telephone a health care provider.

Cervical Caps

A **cervical cap** is made of soft rubber shaped like a thimble, which fits snugly over the uterine cervix (Fig. 6.7). The failure rate is estimated to be as high as 23% (ideal) to 35% (typical use) because caps tend to dislodge more readily than diaphragms during coitus (see Table 6.1). The precautions for use are the same as for diaphragm use except caps can be kept in place longer (up to 48 hours) because they do not put pressure on the vaginal walls or urethra.

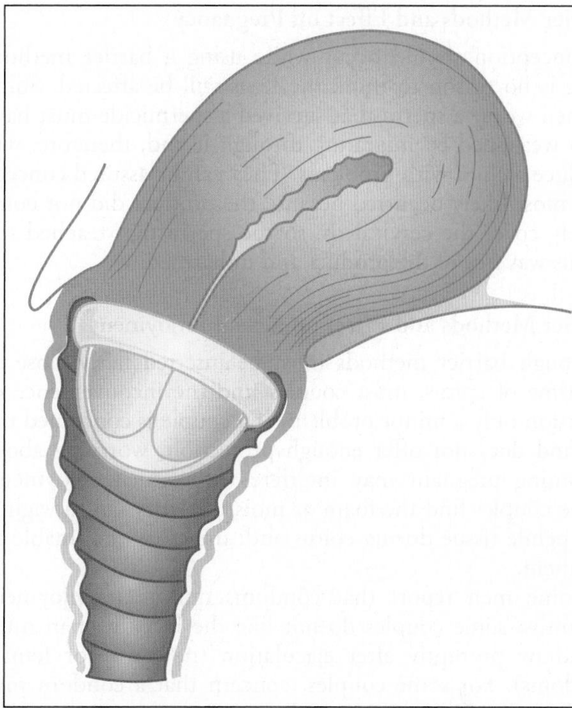

FIGURE 6.7 A cervical cap is placed over the cervix and used with a spermicidal jelly the same as a diaphragm.

Many women cannot use cervical caps because their cervix is too short for the cap to fit properly. Like diaphragms, they must be fitted individually by a health care provider. They include a small strap, which can be grasped for easy removal. They are contraindicated in any woman who has:

- An abnormally short or long cervix
- A current abnormal Pap smear
- A history of TSS
- An allergy to latex or spermicide
- A history of cervicitis or cervical infection
- A history of cervical cancer
- Undiagnosed vaginal bleeding

They may not be as effective in parous women as those who have never had children because the cervix does not conform as well to a thimble shape after childbirth.

QSEN Checkpoint Question 6.2

Quality Improvement

Dana, 17 years old, wants to try female condoms as her reproductive planning method. If you were creating a relevant educational handout, it should include which of the following directives?

a. The hormone that condom use stimulates may cause mild weight gain.

b. Female condoms should be inserted before any penile penetration.

c. Women should coat the condom with a spermicide before use.

d. Female condoms, unlike male condoms, can be reused after being washed.

Look in Appendix A for the best answer and rationale.

Barrier Methods and Effect on Pregnancy

If conception should occur while using a barrier method, there is no reason to think the fetus will be affected. Some women worry a sperm that survived a spermicide must have been weakened by migrating through it and, therefore, will produce a child with problems. They can be assured conception most likely occurred because the product did not completely cover the cervical os, so the sperm that reached the uterus was free of the product and unharmed.

Barrier Methods and Effect on Sexual Enjoyment

Although barrier methods must be inserted fairly close to the time of coitus, most couples find the inconvenience of insertion only a minor problem. If a couple is concerned the method does not offer enough protection, worrying about becoming pregnant may interfere with sexual enjoyment. Some couples find the foam or moisture irritating to vaginal and penile tissue during coitus and, therefore, are unable to use them.

Some men report that condoms dull their enjoyment of coitus; some couples do not like the fact the man must withdraw promptly after ejaculation (not true for female condoms). For some couples, concern that a condom may break or slip may inhibit sexual pleasure.

Use of a vibrator as a part of foreplay, frequent penile insertion, or the woman-superior position during coitus may dislodge a diaphragm or cap; therefore, these may not be the contraceptive of choice for some couples. Some couples may find the precaution that more spermicidal gel should be added to the vagina if coitus is repeated before 6 hours restricting. An advantage of the diaphragm or cap is they allow sexual relations during menses (although see the earlier precaution on TSS). They may also offer some protection against STIs.

What if...6.1 Dana, 17 years old, tells you she and a friend intend to share a diaphragm because they don't have enough money for each to buy one. Is this good planning?

Barrier Methods and the Adolescent

Many adolescents use spermicides as their chief method of birth control because no parental permission or extensive expense is involved. Because of the nontraditional settings in which adolescents may engage in coitus (cars or couches), some young women find inserting the product awkward and consequently may not use it, even though they have purchased it and intended to be more cautious.

Adolescents may be fitted for either diaphragms or caps. Because an adolescent girl's vagina will change in size as she matures and begins sexual relations, these devices may not remain as effective as they do with older women and so need refitting more often. Adolescents may need to be reminded that pelvic examinations will be necessary to ensure the diaphragm or cap continues to fit properly. Some adolescents may not know where their cervix is or how to feel for it when checking the placement of a diaphragm. Use an anatomic diagram or model to show them or give them a mirror to use to view their own cervix during a pelvic examination. Caution them not to accidentally tear the diaphragm with long or sharp fingernails.

Male adolescents are showing increased ability to use condoms responsibly. They may need to be cautioned that condoms should never be reused, because even a pinpoint hole can allow thousands of sperm to escape. Adolescent boys who have infrequent coitus may have condoms they have owned and stored for a long time. The effectiveness of these old condoms, especially if they are carried in a warm pocket, is questionable. For many adolescent couples, use of a dual method, such as a vaginally inserted spermicide by the girl and a condom by her partner, is a preferred method of birth control. The effectiveness of these two methods used in conjunction becomes about 95% (Higgins & Cooper, 2012).

Barrier Methods and the Perimenopausal Woman

Women older than 35 years have a higher incidence of cystocele or rectocele than younger women so diaphragms or cervical caps may not be the ideal contraceptive for them. Spermicide foam can help lubricate the vagina to increase sexual enjoyment in women nearing menopause. The use of vaginal film or suppository is not recommended as lessened vaginal secretions might prevent the film or suppository from dissolving completely.

Barrier Methods and the Postpartal Woman

Vaginal spermicides are appealing to postpartal women as they can be purchased over the counter and have no effect on breastfeeding and so can be used in the short-time period before a postpartal checkup when a more permanent form of contraception can be discussed and prescribed.

As the cervix changes considerably with childbirth, women must be refitted for diaphragms and cervical caps after childbirth. This is usually done at a 4- or 6-week checkup.

What if...6.2 Dana asks you to help her choose a barrier contraceptive method. What method of reproductive life planning would you recommend? Would your recommendation be different if she had a guaranteed monogamous relationship?

Hormonal Contraception

Hormonal contraceptives are, as the name implies, hormones that when taken orally, transdermally, intravaginally, or intramuscularly, cause such fluctuations in a normal menstrual cycle that ovulation or sperm transport does not occur.

Combination Oral Contraceptives

Oral contraceptives, commonly known as the pill, OCs (for **o**ral **c**ontraceptive), or COCs (for **c**ombination **o**ral **c**ontraceptives), are composed of varying amounts of natural estrogen (17*β*-estradiol, estradiol valerate) or synthetic estrogen (ethinyl estradiol) combined with a small amount of synthetic progesterone (progestin). The estrogen acts to suppress follicle-stimulating hormone (FSH) and LH to suppress ovulation. The progesterone action causes a decrease in the permeability of cervical mucus and so limits sperm motility and access to ova. Progesterone also interferes with tubal transport and endometrial proliferation to such an extent the possibility of implantation is significantly decreased.

Popular COCs prescribed in the United States are:

- *Monophasic* pills, which contain fixed doses of both estrogen and progestin throughout a 21-day cycle
- *Biphasic,* or preparations that deliver a constant amount of estrogen throughout the cycle but varying amounts of progestin
- *Triphasic* and *tetraphasic* preparations, which vary in both estrogen and progestin content throughout the cycle

Typical pills are supplied in 28-pill dispensers (21 active pills and 7 placebo pills) labeled with the day of the cycle they should be taken. Newer forms designed to eliminate menses are supplied in 84-day dispensers (see the following). Caution women to always take pills in the order designated by the dispenser or the progesterone level could be inaccurate and ineffective for that day (Fig. 6.8).

COCs must be prescribed by a health care provider after a pelvic examination, screening for eligibility, and usually a Pap smear. When used correctly, they are 99.9% effective. Because women occasionally forget to take them, however, and because of individual physiologic differences, the typical failure rate is closer to 5% (Shoupe & Kjos, 2010).

Oral contraceptives have benefits in addition to preventing pregnancy, such as decreasing incidences of:

- Dysmenorrhea, because of lack of ovulation
- Premenstrual dysphoric syndrome and acne, because of the increased progesterone levels
- Iron deficiency anemia, because of the reduced amount of menstrual flow
- Acute pelvic inflammatory disease (PID) and resulting tubal scarring
- Endometrial and ovarian cancer, ovarian cysts, and ectopic pregnancies
- Fibrocystic breast disease
- Possibly osteoporosis, endometriosis, uterine myomata (fibroid uterine tumors), and possibly rheumatoid arthritis
- Colon cancer (Schindler, 2010)

Because estrogen interferes with lipid metabolism, it may also lower the concentration of low-density lipoproteins (LDL) and increase the high-density lipoprotein (HDL) level.

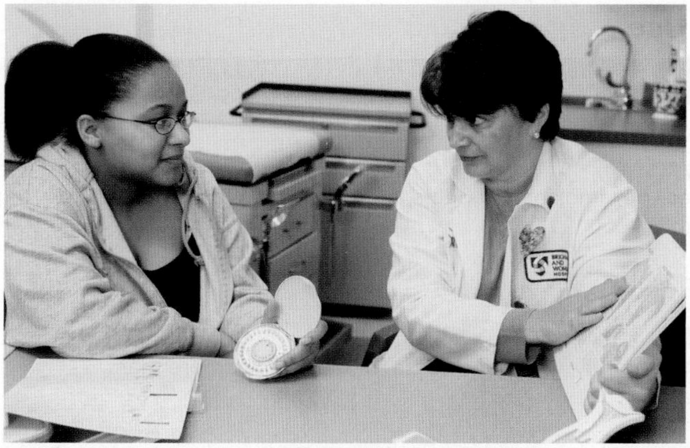

FIGURE 6.8 Counseling women on how to follow an oral contraceptive schedule and what to do if they miss a day or more is an important nursing responsibility. (© Caroline Brown, RNC, MS, DEd.)

Women can set a start date for a cycle of pills in one of four ways:

- Sunday start: Take the first pill on the first Sunday after the beginning of a menstrual flow.
- Quick start: Begin pills as soon as they are prescribed. Beginning pills immediately after a prescription is filled may increase compliance, reducing unintended pregnancies.
- First day start: Begin pills on the first day of menses.
- After childbirth, a woman should start the contraceptive on a day (or Sunday) closest to 2 weeks after birth; after an elective termination of pregnancy, she could begin on a chosen day or the first Sunday after the procedure.

Because COCs are not effective for the first 7 days, advise women to use a second form of contraception during the initial 7 days that they take pills. A woman begins a second dispenser of pills the day after finishing the first dispenser. Menstrual flow will begin during the 7 days on which she is taking the placebo tablets.

If a woman does not want to have menstrual flows, she can eliminate her period by beginning a new cycle of pills immediately after finishing the active pills in a dispenser instead of taking the placebo pills. This should not be used routinely, but to accommodate special circumstances.

With extended-use pills, pills are taken for 84 days and a woman will have a menstrual flow only every 3 months or 4 times a year. *Lybrel* is a new low-dose combination estrogen and progestin pill that is taken 365 days a year without a placebo or pill-free interval so menstrual periods are completely eliminated for 1 year. Such pills are especially attractive to physically active women or those who have long work schedules such as military deployment (Goyal, Borrero, & Schwarz, 2012). Extensive study documents that suppressing menstrual flows for long periods this way appears to have no long-term effects (Hanson & Burke, 2011).

The key to being certain ovulation suppressants are effective is for women to take them consistently and conscientiously. Some women may set an alarm on their phone to alert them it is time to take their pill. Other women may leave them in plain sight on bathroom or kitchen counters so they are reminded to take them. Caution women with young children that this is a potentially dangerous practice. Poisoning with increased blood clotting from the high estrogen content could result if a small child ingested the pills accidentally (urge the woman to use her calendar or some other method to remind her). Women who have difficulty remembering to take a contraceptive in the morning may find it easier to take a daily pill at bedtime or with a meal (the time of day makes no difference; it is the consistency that is important) (Box 6.5). Also, some women find taking pills at bedtime rather than in the morning has the advantage of eliminating any nausea they otherwise may experience.

Progestin-Only Pills (Mini-Pills)

Oral contraceptives containing only progestins are popularly called mini-pills and, like combination types, must be taken conscientiously every day. Without estrogen content, ovulation may occur, but because the progestins have not allowed the endometrium to develop fully or sperm to freely access the cervix, fertilization and implantation will not take place.

BOX 6.5 Nursing Care Planning Based on Family Teaching

SUGGESTIONS ON ORAL CONTRACEPTIVE MANAGEMENT

Q. Dana, 17 years old, asks you, "What do I do if I forget to take an oral contraceptive pill?"
A. The answer differs, depending on your situation:

1. If the pill omitted was one of the placebo ones, ignore it and just take the next pill on time the next day.
2. If you forgot to take one of the active pills, take it as soon as you remember. Continue the following day with your usual pill schedule. Doing so might mean taking two pills on one day if you don't remember until the second day, but that's all right. *Missing one pill this way should not initiate ovulation.*
3. If you miss two consecutive active pills, take two pills as soon as you remember. Then continue the following day with your usual schedule. You may experience some breakthrough bleeding (vaginal spotting) with two forgotten pills. Do not mistake this bleeding for your menstrual flow. *Missing two pills may allow ovulation to occur, so an added contraceptive such as a spermicide should be used for the remainder of the month.*
4. If you miss three or more pills in a row, throw out the rest of the pack and start a new pack of pills. *You might not have a period because of this routine and should use extra protection until 7 days after starting a new pack of pills.*
5. If you think you might be pregnant, stop taking pills and notify your health care provider.

Side Effects and Contraindications of All Oral Contraceptives

The main side effects women may experience with COCs are:

- Nausea
- Weight gain
- Headache
- Breast tenderness
- Breakthrough bleeding (spotting outside the menstrual period)
- Monilial vaginal infections
- Mild hypertension
- Depression

Side effects such as nausea and breakthrough bleeding usually subside after a few months of pill use. They may be lessened by using a different routine or brand of contraceptive.

It is no longer believed the use of COCs leads to an increased risk of myocardial infarction, and the risk of increased clotting or blood pressure elevation is low. Nevertheless, COCs are not routinely prescribed for women with a history of thromboembolic disease or a family history of cerebral or cardiovascular accident, who are over 40 years of age, or who smoke because of the increased tendency toward clotting as an effect of the increased estrogen (Karch, 2013).

Advise all women taking COCs to notify their health care provider if symptoms of myocardial or thromboembolic complications occur, such as:

- Chest pain (pulmonary embolus or myocardial infarction)
- Shortness of breath (pulmonary embolus)
- Severe headache (cerebrovascular accident)
- Severe leg pain (thrombophlebitis)
- Eye problems, such as blurred vision (hypertension, cerebrovascular accident)

It is also recognized that COCs can interfere with glucose metabolism. For this reason, women with diabetes mellitus or a history of liver disease, including hepatitis, are evaluated individually before COCs are prescribed. The World Health Organization (WHO) recommends women who experience migraines with an aura or those who take certain drugs for seizures avoid the use of oral contraceptives as these women may be at an increased risk of cerebrovascular accident (WHO, 2011). Table 6.2 lists all risk factors and contraindications the WHO has associated with COCs. Oral contraceptives

TABLE 6.2 Estrogen-Based Oral Contraceptive Use

Contraindications
• Breastfeeding and less than 6 weeks postpartum • Aged 35 years or older and smoking 15 or more cigarettes per day • Multiple risk factors for arterial cardiovascular disease, such as older age, smoking, diabetes, moderate or severe hypertension • Current or history of deep vein thrombosis or pulmonary embolism • Major surgery that requires prolonged immobilization • Current or history of ischemic heart disease or cerebrovascular accident • Complicated valvular heart disease • Migraine with focal neurologic symptoms (migraine with aura) • Current breast cancer or diabetes with nephropathy, retinopathy, neuropathy, vascular disease, or diabetes of more than 20 years' duration • Severe cirrhosis or liver tumors • Women taking certain seizure drugs such as phenobarbital or Dilantin and women taking Rifabutan for tuberculosis treatment • Women prescribed certain broad-spectrum antibiotics such as tetracycline

From World Health Organization. (2011). *Family planning: A global handbook for providers.* Geneva, Switzerland: Author.

apparently do not increase the risk of breast cancer as was once feared and actually decrease the incidence of ovarian and uterine cancer (Hanson & Burke, 2011).

COCs typically increase or strengthen the action of some drugs such as caffeine and corticosteroids. They may also interact with drugs such as acetaminophen, anticoagulants, and some anticonvulsants by reducing their therapeutic effect, so women may be advised to temporarily change their method of birth control while prescribed these drugs. Several drugs, such as barbiturates, griseofulvin, isoniazid, penicillin, and tetracycline, decrease the effectiveness of COCs, so women might want to change their contraceptive method temporarily while taking these drugs (Karch, 2013).

When discussing COCs, be certain to assess both a woman's ability to pay for them and her ability to follow instructions faithfully (Box 6.6). Women using COCs should return for a yearly follow-up visit (for a pelvic examination, Pap smear, and breast examination), as long as they continue to use this form of birth control. Women without risk factors may continue to take low-dose OCs until they reach menopause.

Progestin-only pills have the disadvantage of causing more breakthrough bleeding than combination pills, but they are just as effective and do not pose a danger of thrombophlebitis (Vaillant-Roussel, Ouchchane, Dauphin, et al., 2011). These pills are taken every day, even through the menstrual flow. Because they do not interfere with milk production, they may be taken during breastfeeding.

Hormonal Contraceptives and Effect on Sexual Enjoyment

For the most part, not having to worry about becoming pregnant because of the reliability of the contraceptive can make sexual relations more enjoyable for a couple. Some women appear to lose interest in coitus after taking COCs for about 18 months, possibly because of the long-term effect of altered hormones in their body. Sexual interest increases again after they change to another form of contraception. Some women experience nausea from COCs and find this interferes with sexual enjoyment as well as with other activities. If they are having side effects with one brand, they might be able to take another brand that has a different strength of estrogen without problems.

Estrogen/Progesterone Transdermal Patch

Transdermal contraception refers to patches that slowly but continuously release a combination of estrogen and progesterone (Fig. 6.9). Patches are applied each week for 3 weeks. No patch is applied the fourth week. During the week on which the woman is patch free, a menstrual flow will occur. After the patch-free week, a new cycle of 3 weeks on, 1 week off begins again. The efficiency of transdermal patches is equal to COCs, although they may be less effective in women who are obese. Because they contain estrogen, they have the same risk for thromboembolic symptoms as COCs. They may be particularly appealing to adolescents because they represent a "new" method of contraception and are easy to apply (Sucato, Bhatt, Murray, et al., 2011).

Patches may be applied to one of four areas: upper outer arm, upper torso (front or back, excluding the breasts), abdomen, or buttocks. They should not be placed on any area where makeup, lotions, or creams will be applied; at the waist where bending might loosen the patch; or anywhere the skin is red, irritated, or has an open lesion.

Patches can be worn in the shower, while bathing, or while swimming. If a patch does comes loose, the woman should

BOX 6.6 Nursing Care Planning Based on Effective Communication

You notice Dana, 17 years old, is reading a pamphlet on oral contraceptives while she waits to be seen by the nurse practitioner.

Less Effective Communication

Nurse: Is that pamphlet helpful? Tell you everything you need to know?
Dana: Not really. I need a way to remind me to take a pill every day.
Nurse: If you're old enough to be sexually active, don't you think you should be responsible enough to do that without a reminder?
Dana asks no more questions.

More Effective Communication

Nurse: Is that pamphlet helpful? Tell you everything you need to know?
Dana: Not really. I need a way to remind me to take a pill every day.
Nurse: Will that be a problem?
Dana: Duh. I think so.
Nurse: Your pill dispenser is meant to serve as a daily reminder. If that doesn't work for you, I could help you make out a reminder chart for your mirror. As a long-term solution, though, have you thought about using a method that doesn't require a reminder more than once a month such a vaginal ring? Or not at all such as an IUD? Why don't I discuss different types with you so you can think about some more options?

Reproductive life planning measures have to be individualized to fit a person's lifestyle; otherwise, they are quickly discontinued. Taking the time to help a woman assess how particular measures fit her lifestyle is better than just giving advice with a "one size fits all" philosophy.

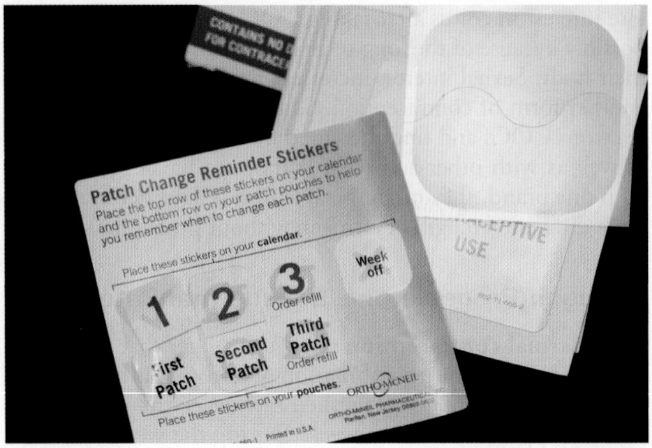

FIGURE 6.9 Estrogen/progesterone-based patches help adherence because they need attention only once a week. They may be applied on the arms, the trunk, or buttocks.

remove it and immediately replace it with a new patch. No additional contraception is needed if the woman is sure the patch has been loose for less than 24 hours. If the woman is not sure how long the patch has been loose, she should remove it and apply a new patch to start a new 4-week cycle, with a new day 1 and a new week to change the patch. She also should use a backup contraception method, such as a condom or spermicide for the first week of this new cycle.

Although mild breast discomfort as well as irritation at the application site may occur, one reason transdermal patches are so effective is the woman does not need to remember to take a daily pill.

Vaginal Estrogen/Progestin Rings (NuvaRing)

A *NuvaRing* is a flexible silicone **vaginal ring** that, when placed around the cervix, continually releases a combination of estrogen and progesterone (Fig. 6.10). The ring is inserted vaginally by the woman and left in place for 3 weeks, then removed for 1 week with menstrual bleeding occurring during the ring-free week (Bitzer, 2012). The hormones released are absorbed directly by the mucous membrane of the vagina, thereby avoiding a "first pass" through the liver, as happens with COCs; this is an advantage for women with liver disease. Rings do not need to be removed for intercourse. The effectiveness is equal to COCs. Women may need to mark a conspicuously posted calendar to remind themselves to remove and replace the ring. Some women may need to be encouraged to use vaginal rings, as introducing a ring vaginally may at first seem more complicated than taking a pill every day. Some women may experience vaginal discomfort or infection, both of which would make the ring an undesirable method of contraception. Women should be counseled that if they should take out the ring for more than 4 hours for any purpose, they should replace it with a new ring and use a form of barrier protection for the next 7 days.

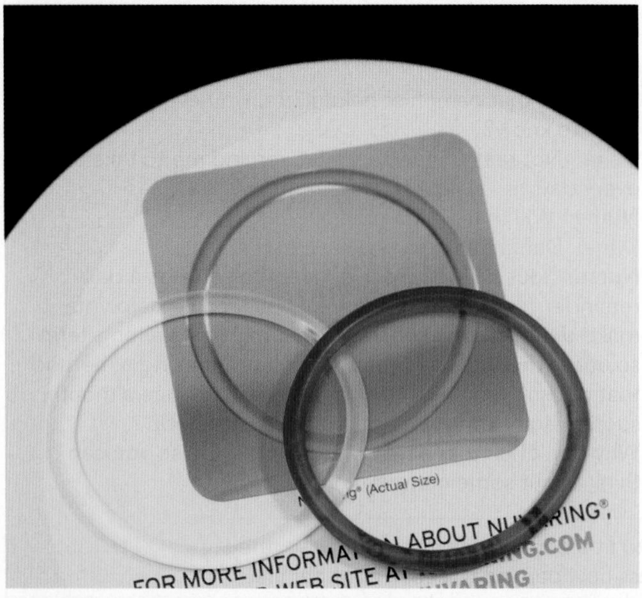

FIGURE 6.10 A vaginal ring. Progesterone is gradually released to be absorbed by the vaginal walls.

QSEN Checkpoint Question 6.3

Safety

Suppose Dana, 17 years old, chooses to use a COC as her family planning method? What is a danger sign of COCs you would ask her to report?

a. A stuffy or runny nose
b. Arthritis-like symptoms
c. Weight gain over 5 lb
d. Severe migraine headache

Look in Appendix A for the best answer and rationale.

Subdermal Hormone Implants

A progestin-filled miniature rod no bigger than a matchstick (*Implanon*) can be embedded just under the skin on the inside of the upper arm where it will slowly release progestin over a period of 5 years. Once embedded, the implant is barely noticeable; it appears as an irregular crease on the skin, simulating a small vein. As with oral progestin, the implant is able to effectively suppress ovulation, thicken cervical mucus, and change the endometrium lining, making implantation difficult.

The rod is inserted as an in-office procedure with the use of a local anesthetic during menses or no later than day 7 of a menstrual cycle to be certain a woman is not pregnant at the time of insertion. It can be placed immediately after an elective termination of pregnancy or 6 weeks after the birth of a baby. An implant is so effective, the failure rate is less than 1%, comparable to oral contraception (Shoupe & Kjos, 2010).

A major disadvantage of the implant method is its cost ($500 on average). However, a major advantage of this long-term reversible contraceptive is that compliance issues associated with COCs are eliminated. Rod insertion also offers an effective and reliable alternative to COCs' estrogen-related side effects. Sexual enjoyment is not inhibited, as may happen with condoms, spermicides, diaphragms, and natural family planning methods. An implant can be used during breastfeeding without an effect on milk production. Implants may also be used in adolescents. The rapid return to fertility after removal is an advantage for women when they become ready to begin a family.

Side Effects and Contradictions

Side effects include weight gain, irregular menstrual cycle (heavy bleeding, spotting, breakthrough bleeding, and amenorrhea), depression, scarring at the insertion site, and need for removal.

Contraindications to a subdermal rod are pregnancy, desire to be pregnant within 1 to 2 years, and undiagnosed uterine bleeding. A complication that can occur is an infection at the insertion site, although this is very rare. Most people who ask to have them removed do so because of irregular or heavy menstrual flows (Casey, Long, Marnach, et al., 2011).

Intramuscular Injections

A single intramuscular injection of depot medroxyprogesterone acetate (DMPA), a progesterone given every 12 weeks, inhibits ovulation, alters the endometrium, and thickens the cervical mucus so sperm progress is difficult (Box 6.7). The effectiveness rate of this method is almost 100%, making it an increasingly popular contraceptive method (Shoupe & Kjos, 2010). The injection is made deep into a major muscle (buttocks, deltoid, or thigh) before the fifth day after the beginning of a menstrual flow. Be sure the woman does not massage the injection site after administration so the drug can absorb slowly from the muscle.

Intramuscular injections have the advantage of long-term reliability without many of the side effects and contraindications associated with COCs. There also is no visible sign a birth control measure is being used as with a subdermal implant, making them attractive to adolescents. However, the thought of weight gain may not be appealing (Verhaeghe, 2012).

Because DMPA contains only progesterone, it can be used during breastfeeding, although women should wait about 6 weeks after birth for the first injection. Advantageous effects are reductions in ectopic pregnancy, endometrial cancer, endometriosis, and for unknown reasons, the frequency of sickle cell crises (Taylor et al., 2012).

The woman must return to a health care provider for a new injection every 12 weeks for the method to remain reliable. A reminder system, such as a postcard mailed by the prescribing agency, may be necessary to be certain women return on time for their next injection. Alternative methods of administration, such as allowing pharmacists to give the injections or selling them over the counter so women can inject themselves, are being investigated and might increase compliance.

Side Effects and Contraindications

Common side effects include headache, weight gain, and depression, irregular or heavy menstrual cycles for 1 year, no menstrual bleeding after the first year. DMPA may also impair glucose tolerance in women at risk for diabetes so it should be prescribed cautiously for this population. Because there also may be an increase in the risk for osteoporosis from a loss of bone mineral density, women need to include an adequate amount of calcium in their diet (up to 1,200 mg/day) and engage in weight-bearing exercise daily to minimize this risk.

The manufacturer of DMPA has added a "black box" warning for women not to use the method long term (not over 2 years) to protect against bone loss. For this reason, although often prescribed to adolescents, DMPA should be prescribed with caution to this age group, as this is during the time when the bulk of their calcium deposits are being laid down (Isley & Kaunitz, 2011).

Hormone Contraception and Effect on Pregnancy

Different hormonal applications have different effects on pregnancy.

- *Estrogen/progestin combination pills (COCs).* If a woman taking an estrogen/progestin combination pill suspects she is pregnant, she should discontinue taking any more pills if she intends to continue the pregnancy as high levels of estrogen might be teratogenic to a growing fetus (Karch, 2013). After women stop taking COCs, they may not be able to become pregnant for 1 or 2 months, and possibly 6 to 8 months, because the pituitary gland requires a recovery period to resume cyclic gonadotropin stimulation. If ovulation does not return spontaneously after this time, it can be stimulated by administration of FSH, LH, or clomiphene citrate (Clomid) to restore fertility.

BOX 6.7 Nursing Care Planning Based on Responsibility for Pharmacology

DEPOT MEDROXYPROGESTERONE ACETATE

Classification: Contraceptive
Action: Depot medroxyprogesterone acetate (DMPA) is a progesterone derivative that inhibits the secretion of pituitary gonadotropins, thereby altering the endometrium and preventing follicular maturation and ovulation (Karch, 2013).
Pregnancy Category: X
Dosage: 150 mg intramuscular injection every 3 months
Possible Adverse Effects: Spotting, breakthrough bleeding, amenorrhea, irregular menstrual flow, headaches, weight fluctuations, fluid retention, edema, rash or acne, abdominal discomfort, glucose intolerance, pain at injection site, or osteoporosis (loss of bone density).

Nursing Implications

- Advise client to have an annual physical examination that includes breast examination, pelvic examination, and Pap smear.
- Caution the client that potential side effects such as weight gain may occur.
- Advise client to maintain a high calcium intake to reduce development of osteoporosis.
- Advise the client to report pain or swelling of the legs, acute chest pain, or shortness of breath; tingling or numbness in the extremities; loss of vision; sudden severe headaches; dizziness; or fainting; these could be signs of potentially serious cardiovascular complications.

- *Progestin-impregnated rings or progestin patches.* If a woman using a progestin ring or patch becomes pregnant, the progestin should have no effect on a developing fetus. After discontinuing both methods, women become fertile again immediately.
- *Subdermal implants.* If a woman becomes pregnant while using a subdermal implant, the rod can be removed; although, because the implant releases only progestin, there should be no effect on the fetus. At the end of 3 years, when the implant is removed (a less than 1 minute procedure) the woman will be fertile again almost immediately.
- *DMPA.* DMPA, like other progestin products, should have no effect if a woman becomes pregnant. A worrisome postuse effect for some women, however, is that the return to fertility is often delayed by 6 to 12 months.

Hormone Contraception and the Adolescent

It is usually recommended that adolescent girls have well-established menstrual cycles for at least 2 years before beginning COCs. This reduces the chance the estrogen content will cause permanent suppression of pituitary-regulating activity. Estrogen has the side effect of causing the epiphyses of long bones to close and growth to halt; therefore, waiting at least 2 years also helps ensure the preadolescent growth spurt will not be halted. Because adolescents' compliance with most medications is low, adolescent girls may not take either combined or progestin-only pills reliably enough to make them effective. In addition, the cost of a continuing supply of pills may be prohibitive for teens. COCs have side benefits of improving facial acne in some girls because of the increased estrogen/androgen ratio created and also decreasing dysmenorrhea, both of which are appealing to most adolescents and may increase their compliance rate. The pill may be prescribed to some adolescents specifically to decrease dysmenorrhea, especially if endometriosis is present (Gordon & Pitts, 2012) (see Chapter 47).

Hormonal Contraception and the Perimenopausal Woman

As women near menopause, they are likely over the age of 35 years, and so are less likely to be good candidates for COCs than when they were younger, especially if they smoke. Help women in this age group find an alternative method that will meet their personal preferences as well as still be maximally effective for them, such as an **intrauterine device** (IUD), progestin-only patches, or vaginal rings (Beasley, 2010).

Hormonal Contraception and the Postpartal Woman

Women who are lactating should not take estrogen-based contraceptives as a small amount of the hormone will not only be excreted in breast milk but will reduce the amount of breast milk formed. Women who want hormonal contraception are, therefore, usually prescribed progestin-only pills or progesterone-activated vaginal rings until they are no longer breastfeeding (Nath & Sitruk-Ware, 2010).

Intrauterine Devices

An IUD is a small plastic device that is inserted into the uterus through the vagina. Although a popular choice worldwide because they are almost 100% effective and need no memory aide, IUDs are used by only a relatively small number of U.S. women (Cameron & Glasier, 2012).

Even though the insertion of foreign objects into the uterus for contraceptive purposes dates back thousands of years (ancient camel drivers used uterine stones for their animals), the mechanism of action for the method is still not fully understood. The method is thought, however, to prevent fertilization as well as to create a local sterile inflammatory reaction that prevents implantation. When copper is added to the device, the possibility sperm will not be able to successfully cross the uterine space and reach the ovum increases as well.

IUDs may be used by women who have never had children as well as those who have. The device must be fitted by a health care provider who first performs a Pap test and pelvic examination and, in women with high risk for STIs, a test for chlamydia. The device is inserted before a woman has had coitus after a menstrual flow, so the health care provider can be assured the woman is not pregnant at the time of insertion.

The device is inserted in a collapsed position, then enlarged to its final shape in the uterus when the inserter is withdrawn. The woman may feel a sharp cramp as the device is passed through the internal cervical os, but she will not feel the IUD after it is in place. Properly fitted, such devices are contained wholly within the uterus, although an attached string protrudes through the cervix into the vagina. Women may continue to use tampons or menstrual cups for menstrual flow with no danger of dislodging an IUD (Wiebe & Trouton, 2012).

Two common types are approved for use in the United States:

- Copper T380 (ParaGard®) is a T-shaped plastic device wound with copper. It is effective for 10 years, after which time it should be removed and replaced with a new IUD.
- Mirena IUD, which features a drug reservoir of progesterone in the stem (Fig. 6.11). The progesterone (levonorgestrel) in the drug reservoir gradually diffuses into the uterus through the plastic; it both prevents endometrium proliferation and thickens cervical mucus. Because it reduces endometrium proliferation, it also has the potential to reduce endometrial cancer (Hanson & Burke, 2011). It is effective for 5 years (possibly as long as 7 years).

QSEN Checkpoint Question 6.4

Teamwork and Collaboration

Suppose Dana, 17 years old, chooses intramuscular injections of DMPA as her method of reproductive life planning. What instructions would you want members of your care team to give her with regard to this method?

a. "Encourage Dana to limit cigarette smoking to no more than one pack per day."
b. "Encourage Dana to drink a glass of milk or take a calcium supplement daily."
c. "Teach Dana not to swim for longer than an hour at any one time."
d. "Teach Dana not to expose the injection site to direct sunlight."

Look in Appendix A for the best answer and rationale.

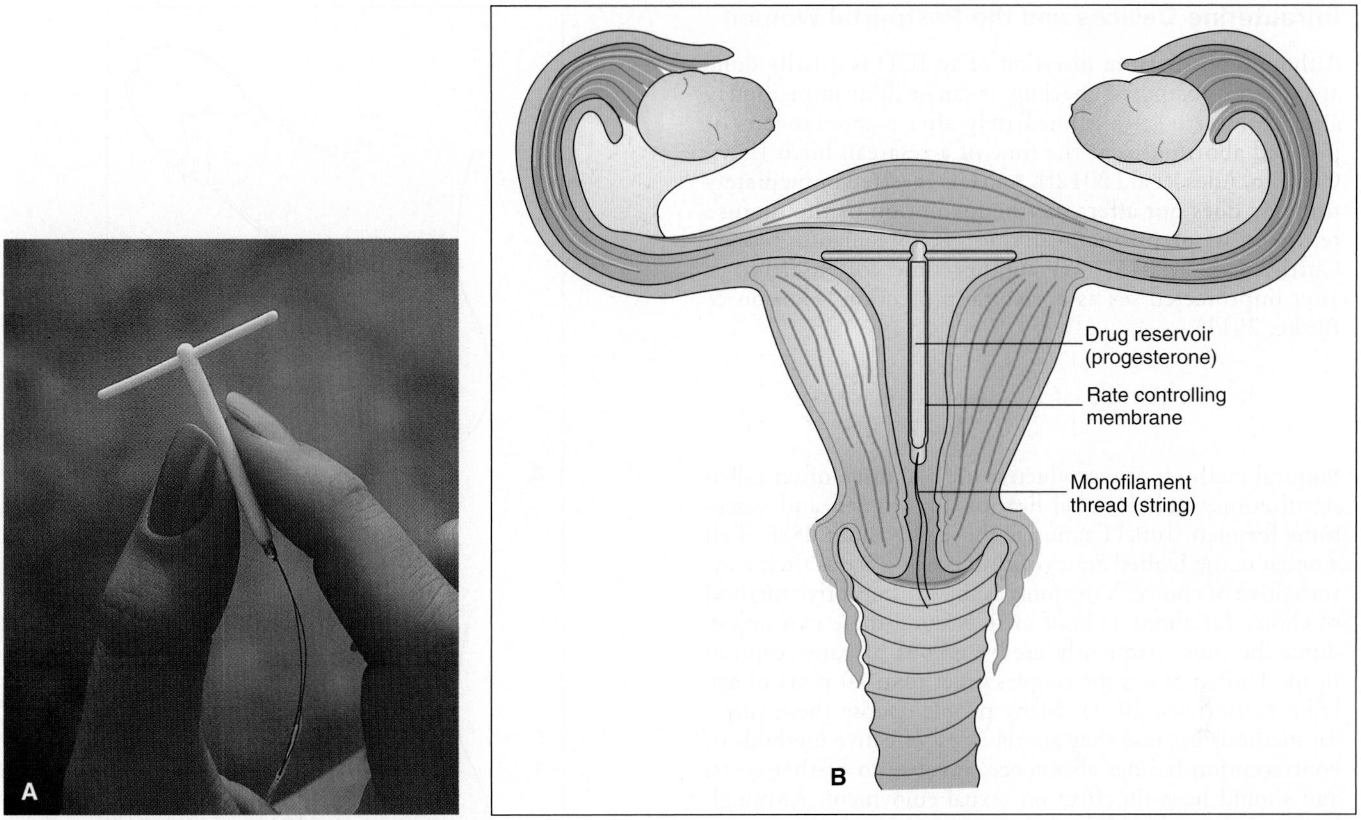

FIGURE 6.11 **(A)** An intrauterine device. **(B)** An IUD in place in the uterus. (Courtesy of ALZA Pharmaceuticals, Palo Alto, CA.)

Both IUD types have an ideal failure rate as low as 0.1% (see Table 6.1). They have several advantages over other contraceptives in that only one insertion is necessary, so there is no continuing expense. They are appropriate for women who are at risk for complications associated with estrogen-based side effects. There is little change in the timing of menstrual flows, although monthly flow may be heavier with the copper IUD. Teach women to regularly check after each menstrual flow to make sure the IUD string is in place and to obtain a yearly pelvic examination as usual.

Side Effects and Contraindications

A woman may notice some spotting or uterine cramping the first 2 or 3 weeks after IUD insertion; as long as this is present, she should use an additional form of contraception, such as a spermicide. Ibuprofen, a prostaglandin inhibitor, is helpful in relieving the pain. Occasionally, a woman continues to have cramping and spotting after insertion; in such instances, she is likely to expel the device spontaneously. If this happens she should use an alternative method of birth control until she can visit her health care provider to have a new one inserted (or choose a different type of protection). Nulliparous women may have a higher percentage of spontaneous expulsion than others.

It was once a concern nulliparous women could not be fitted with IUDs and any woman with an IUD in place might have a higher risk for PID than others. Nulliparous women can be fitted (although they may have a higher rate of expulsion); infection is no longer a concern because the vaginal string no longer conducts fluid (Hanson & Burke, 2011). The Mirena IUS may actually help resist infection because of the change created in the cervical mucus.

Use of an IUD may be contraindicated for a woman whose uterus is distorted in shape (the device might perforate the uterine wall). IUD use also is not advised for a woman with severe dysmenorrhea (painful menstruation), menorrhagia (bleeding between menstrual periods), or a history of ectopic (tubal) pregnancy because use may increase the incidence of these conditions. Because use of a copper IUD can cause heavier than usual menstrual flow, a woman with anemia also may not be considered a good candidate for an IUD.

Effect on Pregnancy

If a woman with an IUD in place suspects she is pregnant, she should alert her primary health care provider. The woman will receive an early sonogram to document placement of the IUD and rule out ectopic pregnancy. Following confirmation of the IUD's location, it may be left in place during the pregnancy, but it is usually removed vaginally to prevent the possibility of infection or spontaneous miscarriage during the pregnancy.

Intrauterine Devices and the Adolescent

IUDs are not often prescribed for very young adolescents because such teenagers may not yet have a uterus large enough for a safe insertion.

Intrauterine Devices and the Perimenopausal Woman

Women who are premenopausal are, overall, good candidates for IUDs.

Intrauterine Devices and the Postpartal Woman

Although postpartum insertion of an IUD is usually done at a 6-week postpartal checkup, it can be done immediately after childbirth (also immediately after a spontaneous or induced abortion or at the time of a cesarean birth [Levi, Cantillo, Ades, et al., 2012]). An IUD inserted immediately this way does not affect uterine involution or the uterus's return to its prepregnant uterine size (Steenland, Tepper, Curtis, et al., 2011). Yet another time for insertion is after unprotected sex as postcoital protection (Hanson & Burke, 2011).

Surgical Methods of Reproductive Life Planning

Surgical methods of reproductive life planning, often called sterilization, include tubal ligation for women and vasectomy for men. Tubal ligation is chosen by about 28% of all women in the United States of childbearing age as their contraceptive of choice. Vasectomy is the contraceptive method of choice for about 11% of men, making these two procedures the most frequently used methods of contraception in the United States for couples older than 30 years of age (Zite & Borrero, 2011). Many people choose these surgical methods because they are the most effective methods of contraception besides abstinence, involve no further costs, and should have no effect on sexual enjoyment. Although both sexes should think of these procedures as permanent before they have them, between 6% and 7% of both men and women in the United States who have had these procedures ask to have the procedures reversed (Monteith & Berger, 2012).

Reversal techniques may be much more complicated and expensive than the sterilization itself, and success rates are only 70% to 80%. For this reason, surgical methods should be chosen with great thought and care. These procedures may not be recommended for individuals whose fertility is important to their self-esteem. Counseling should be especially intensive for men and women younger than 30 years of age, because the possibility of divorce, death of a sexual partner, loss of a child, or remarriage could change a person's philosophy toward childbearing.

Vasectomy

In a **vasectomy**, a small puncture wound (referred to as "no-scalpel technique) is made on the scrotum. The vas deferens on each side are then pulled forward, cut and tied, cauterized, or plugged, blocking the passage of spermatozoa (Cameron & Glasier, 2012) (Fig. 6.12). A vasectomy can be done under local anesthesia in an ambulatory setting, such as in a primary health care provider's office or a reproductive life planning clinic. The man may experience a small amount of local pain afterward, which can be managed by taking a mild analgesic and applying ice to the site. Although the procedure is about 99.5% effective, spermatozoa, which were present in the vas deferens at the time of surgery, can remain viable for as long as 6 months. Therefore, although the man can resume sexual intercourse within 1 week, an additional birth control method should be used until two negative sperm reports at about 6 and 10 weeks have been obtained (proof all sperm in the vas deferens have been eliminated, usually requiring 10 to 20 ejaculations).

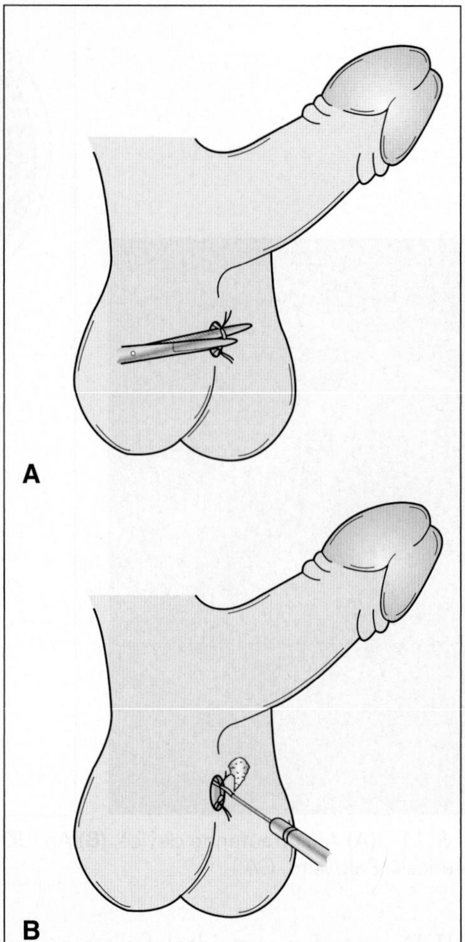

FIGURE 6.12 A vasectomy. **(A)** The left vas deferens being cut with surgical scissors. **(B)** The cut ends of the vas deferens are cauterized or clamped to completely ensure blockage of the passage of sperm.

Some men resist the concept of vasectomy because they are not sufficiently aware of their anatomy to know exactly what the procedure will involve. They can be assured a vasectomy does not interfere with the production of sperm; the testes continue to produce sperm as always, but the sperm simply do not pass beyond the plugged vas deferens and are absorbed at that point. The man will still have full erection capacity and continue to produce testosterone. Because he also continues to form seminal fluid, he will ejaculate seminal fluid; it will just not contain sperm.

There are very few complications associated with a vasectomy. A hematoma at the surgical site may occur, although this is seen less frequently with "no scalpel" or puncture incisions. The procedure may also be associated with the development of urolithiasis (kidney stones). A few men develop chronic pain after vasectomy (postvasectomy pain syndrome); having the procedure reversed relieves this pain (Horovitz, Tjong, Domes, et al., 2012).

Some men develop autoimmunity or form antibodies against sperm following a vasectomy, so even if reconstruction is successful, sperm may not have good mobility or be incapable of fertilization. Men who want their sperm to be available for the future can have it sperm banked before vasectomy.

Tubal Ligation

Sterilization of women could include removal of the uterus or ovaries (hysterectomy), but it usually refers to a minor surgical procedure, such as **tubal ligation**, where the fallopian tubes are occluded by cautery, crushed, clamped, or blocked, thereby preventing passage of both sperm and ova. A fimbriectomy, or removal of the fimbria at the distal end of the tubes, is another possible but little used technique. Tubal ligation has a 99.5% effectiveness rate (Shoupe & Kjos, 2010). It also is associated with a decreased incidence of ovarian cancer.

After a menstrual flow and before ovulation, with the woman under general or local anesthesia, an incision as small as 1 cm is made just under the woman's umbilicus by **laparoscopy** technique. A lighted laparoscope is inserted through the incision. Carbon dioxide then may be pumped into the incision to lift the abdominal wall upward and out of the line of vision. A surgeon locates the fallopian tubes by viewing the field through a laparoscope. An electrical current to coagulate tissue is then passed through the instrument for 3 to 5 seconds, or the tubes are clamped by plastic, metal, or rubber rings, then cut; they also may be filled with a silicone gel to seal them. All procedures provide immediate contraception.

The woman is discharged from the hospital a few hours after the procedure. She may notice a day or two of abdominal discomfort caused by local necrosis if clips were used and she may notice abdominal bloating for the first 24 hours, until the carbon dioxide infused at the beginning of the procedure is absorbed. The presence of carbon dioxide can also cause sharp diaphragmatic or shoulder pain if some of the carbon dioxide escapes under the diaphragm and presses on ascending nerves. Possible complications include bowel perforation, hemorrhage, and the risks of general anesthesia if this was used.

A newer system, *Essure,* consists of a spring-loaded mechanism that, when inserted through the vagina and uterus into a fallopian tube (a hysteroscopy procedure), releases a soft micro-insert into the tube (Fig. 6.13). This is done as an in-office procedure. Women must use a second form of contraception afterward until at 3 months, an infusion sonogram, hysterosalpingogram, or magnetic resonance imaging (MRI) is done to confirm the fallopian tubes are firmly blocked (Correia, Ramos, Machado, et al., 2011).

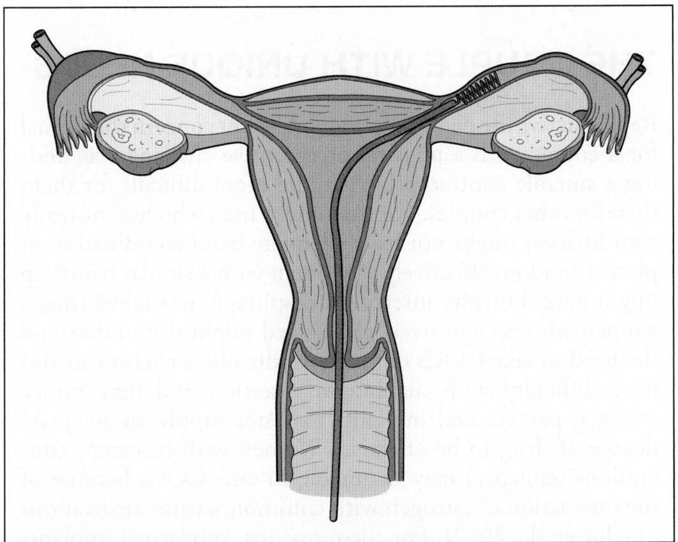

FIGURE 6.13 An Essure procedure blocks the fallopian tubes by a coiled spring introduced vaginally.

Women may return to having coitus as soon as 2 to 3 days after the procedure. Be certain they understand tubal ligation, unlike a hysterectomy, does not affect the menstrual cycle, so they will still have a monthly menstrual flow.

Side Effects and Contraindications

If tubal ligation surgery is done by laparoscopy, an umbilical hernia or ureter or bowel perforation are possible complications. Extensive obesity might require a full laparotomy to allow adequate visualization. A number of women develop vaginal spotting, intermittent vaginal bleeding, and even severe lower abdominal cramping after tubal ligation—symptoms termed *posttubal ligation syndrome*. Removal of the fallopian tubes appears to relieve these symptoms.

Not only is it difficult to reconstruct fallopian tubes after tubal ligation but there is also a possibility that, afterward, the anastomosis site could cause an ectopic (tubal) pregnancy because of its irregular surface. If a silicone gel has been instilled into the tubes as a blocking agent, this can be removed at a later date to reverse the procedure much more easily. As with a vasectomy, however, woman should view tubal ligation as a permanent, irreversible procedure as the length of their tube may be shortened afterward, interfering with fertilization (Jayakrishnan & Baheti, 2011); otherwise, they can develop postprocedural regret. However, women could turn to in vitro fertilization (IVF) as a method to have future children (see Chapter 8).

Effect on Pregnancy

Because both vasectomy and tubal ligation are nearly 100% effective, pregnancy rarely occurs. If it should, there is no effect on the fetus. If sperm were present in a woman's fallopian tube prior to ligation, an ovum could be fertilized in the blocked tube, causing an ectopic pregnancy.

Surgical Methods and Effect on Sexual Enjoyment

Both tubal ligation and vasectomy may lead to increased sexual enjoyment, because they largely eliminate the possibility of pregnancy. However, if either partner changes his or her mind about having children, the surgery may become an issue between them that interferes not only with sexual enjoyment but also with their entire relationship.

Surgical Methods and the Adolescent

As a rule, counsel adolescents to use more temporary forms of birth control because their future goals may change so drastically that what they think they want at age 16 or 18 years may not be what they desire at age 30 years. Later, if they still feel a vasectomy or tubal ligation is the method of reproductive life planning for them, the option will still be available.

Surgical Methods and the Perimenopausal Woman

When a woman realizes childbearing for her is complete, a vasectomy for her partner or tubal ligation for her are the two most frequently requested forms of contraception as they require no further expense or motivation for success.

Surgical Methods and the Postpartal Woman

Tubal ligation can be done as soon as 4 to 6 hours after the birth of a baby or after an elective termination of a pregnancy, although it may be more common at 12 to 24 hours after birth. The abdominal distention at this time may make locating the tubes difficult, so a mini-laparotomy may be used. Such procedures can be done in an ambulatory surgery department with the woman under local anesthesia.

QSEN Checkpoint Question 6.5

Informatics

Dana, 17 years old, e-mails you to ask how a tubal ligation prevents pregnancy. To be certain she's fully informed, which would be your best answer?

a. Sperm can no longer reach the ova because fallopian tubes are blocked.
b. Sperm cannot enter the uterus because the cervical entrance is blocked.
c. Prostaglandins released from the cut fallopian tubes effectively kill sperm.
d. The ovary no longer releases ova because there is nowhere for them to go.

Look in Appendix A for the best answer and rationale.

Emergency Postcoital Contraception

A number of regimens, often referred to as "morning-after pills," are available for emergency postcoital contraception (EC), which is needed after unprotected voluntary coitus or involuntary situations such as rape (Devine, 2012).

Two types are most common:

- High-dose progestin-based pills
- Insertion of a copper IUD

It may be important to explain to women postcoital methods such as Plan B One-Step and Next Choice (the most frequently used forms) do not cause abortion; the pills work by inhibiting ovulation and interfering with fertilization by slowing the transport of sperm. An IUD creates changes in the endometrium and cervical mucus to also slow or prevent sperm transport (Harper, Speidel, Drey, et al., 2012).

Plan B One-Step and Next Choice are available over the counter without a prescription by males or females. Despite their young age, studies show young adolescents are able to read the pamphlet instructions and take the pills just as independently as adults (Raine, Ricciotti, Sokoloff, et al., 2012). One or two pills, depending on the brand, containing a high dose of levonorgestrel, a progestin, are taken anytime within 72 hours (3 days) of unprotected coitus to successfully interrupt a pregnancy.

A newer form of pill, ulipristal acetate (known as ella) requires a prescription and may be taken as late as 120 hours (5 days) after unprotected intercourse (Gizzo, Fanelli, Gangi, et al., 2012). The dose is the same (one pill). Most women expect the pills will begin a menstrual flow; caution them this will not happen, although they may notice some spotting from the change of hormones in their body. Their next menstrual flow may begin either earlier or later than usual.

Overall, the rate of effectiveness for EC if taken within 72 hours is about 75% (American Congress of Obstetricians and Gynecologists [ACOG], 2011). Be certain women know the pills do not protect against STIs and they will not continue to protect against pregnancy should coitus recur. A woman needs to begin a protective measure for this or use a postcoital method again.

An ethical question that was asked when postcoital pills were first approved was whether the availability of EC would encourage risky sexual behavior; this does not seem to be so. It is important women don't think of postcoital contraception as a routine contraceptive method but as a true emergency measure (Melton, Stanford, & Dewitt, 2012). The chief side effect is nausea; if a woman notices this, she can take an over-the-counter antiemetic. Rh-negative women do not need RhoGAM® injections after postcoital pills or IUD insertion because a fetus never formed, thus negating isoimmunization (see Chapter 26 for a full discussion of Rh-negative blood, isoimmunization, and pregnancy).

Although EC pills have the potential to greatly reduce the number of unintended pregnancies and abortion, fear of side effects, reluctance to have a pelvic examination (not necessary), lack of knowledge about how to use the pills, and reluctance to ask a family pharmacist for the pills limit the number of these products being sold (Devine, 2012). Internet drug companies can serve as a resource for EC as they provide both privacy protection and competitive prices (about $35 to $50). Such sites are appreciated by young adults and also can supply education on different reproductive life planning methods for the future (Fehring, Schneider, & Raviele, 2011).

A postcoital IUD is inserted by a health care provider with the same technique as for routine use. It can then be left in place and continue as the woman's reproductive life planning method so unprotected intercourse will not happen again.

What if...6.3 Dana does not follow your advice for reproductive life planning and is prescribed Plan B One-Step for emergency postcoital contraception. Her mother asks you to give her something so painful she'll not want to engage in unprotected coitus again. Would you agree to her philosophy of care?

THE COUPLE WITH UNIQUE NEEDS

Reproductive life planning can be a greater concern than usual for a couple with a physical or cognitive challenge, as finding a suitable contraceptive may be more difficult for them than for other couples. For example, a man who has unsteady coordination might not have adequate hand coordination to place a condom effectively. A woman with a similar handicap might have difficulty inserting a diaphragm or vaginal ring; a woman who is cognitively challenged might not understand the need to take COCs daily. Morbidly obese clients can also have difficulty with diaphragm insertion and may notice estrogen patches and implants may not supply an adequate dosage of drug to be effective. Women with recurrent convulsions (epilepsy) may be unable to take COCs because of the interaction of estrogen with common seizure medications (Taylor et al., 2012). For these reasons, subdermal implants or surgical intervention may be the ideal contraceptive for many couples with a disability.

FUTURE TRENDS IN CONTRACEPTION

Although COCs contain much less estrogen today than originally, estrogen remains responsible for most of the side effects associated with COCs. Therefore, studies are being conducted using even lower doses and different forms of estrogen. Biodegradable implants that do not have to be removed or an estrogen-based gel that is rubbed onto the skin may be used in the future. A progesterone-filled vaginal ring that is permanently implanted is yet another possibility. A birth control vaccine consisting of antibodies against human chorionic gonadotropin hormone is a distant possibility. Injections of testosterone for males (which halts sperm production, just as estrogen halts ova production in women) are being tested at major centers. Hormone-related male contraception, however, has inherent problems; because sperm production is continuous, there is not just one event (ovulation) to halt. Administration of FSH and LH to men could stop sperm production through effects on the pituitary and hypothalamus. However, this approach would also decrease production of testosterone, which is necessary for male muscle strength. Until the matter of how to balance the amount of needed testosterone and excessive testosterone (which produces aggression) is solved, hormonal male contraception remains an elusive concept (Grimes, Lopez, Gallo, et al., 2012).

Until some method is found that satisfies all of the criteria for an ideal contraceptive (completely safe, no side effects, low cost, easy availability, easy reversibility, and user acceptability), both women and men need opportunities to discuss options to find the method right for them. Box 6.8 shows an interprofessional care map illustrating both nursing and team planning for reproductive life planning.

✔ QSEN Checkpoint Question 6.6

Evidence-Based Practice

"Choosing Wisely" is an interactive program on the Internet site www. SexualityandU.ca that is designed to help a woman choose a birth control method that would be right for her. To discover if there was a difference in what adolescents and adult women chose, researchers categorized the responses of 3,178 first-time adolescent users and 4,206 first-time adult women users over a 6-month period. The results showed 61% of adolescents preferred a contraceptive that halted menses; 83% thought a pregnancy would be devastating; 54% reported menstrual cramps and, of these, 29% did not believe they could reliably take a pill daily. Seventy-three percent claimed to be willing to use a contraceptive method that required interruption of intercourse (Nguyen & Jamieson, 2011).

Based on the previous study, assuming Dana, 17 years old, is a typical adolescent, she is likely to adhere to which of the following beliefs?

a. COC pills are the best birth control method to use.
b. Fertility awareness techniques prevent pregnancy most accurately.
c. No birth control method exists that is ideal for adolescents.
d. IUD insertion would be best as this eliminates monthly menses.

Look in Appendix A for the best answer and rationale.

ELECTIVE TERMINATION OF PREGNANCY

Unsupervised abortions are terminations of pregnancy performed by unskilled people, often under less than sterile conditions at any point in pregnancy. An **elective termination of pregnancy** is a procedure performed by a knowledgeable heath care provider to end a pregnancy before fetal viability. Such procedures are also referred to as therapeutic, medical, or induced abortions. At present, as many as one-third of women may have such an elective procedure in their lifetime, although this number is expected to decrease as emergency postcoital contraception becomes more widely used (Norman, 2012). Whereas unsupervised abortions carry a high risk for infection or excessive bleeding that can lead to death, the maternal mortality rate for elective terminations is only 0.6 per 100,000 procedures. This rate correlates to elective termination being about 11 times safer for women than childbirth, for which the mortality rate is closer to 6 per 100,000 births (Shoupe & Kjos, 2010).

Elective terminations of pregnancy would be unnecessary if women acted within 120 hours of unprotected coitus to take emergency postcoital contraception. Reasons that elective terminations are most often requested are for a pregnancy that:

- Threatens a woman's life, such as pregnancy in a woman with class IV heart disease
- Involves a fetus found on amniocentesis to have a chromosomal defect
- Is unwanted because it is the result of rape or incest
- Is unwanted because a woman chooses not to have a child at this time in her life for such reasons as being too young, not wanting to be a single parent, wanting no more children, having financial difficulties, or from failed contraception. The majority of pregnancy terminations are done for this last reason.

In the United States, although drugs to induce abortion safely are available, elective termination of pregnancy is still mainly a surgical procedure. Nurses employed in health care agencies where induced abortions are performed are asked to assist with such procedures as a part of their duties.

Be certain women do not view elective termination as a method of reproductive life planning but as remediation for failed contraception. In addition, be certain women are aware of all their options such as adoption or single parenthood before the procedure (Chervenak & McCullough, 2012).

In 1973, the U.S. Supreme Court ruled elective terminations must be legal in all states as long as the pregnancy is less than 12 weeks. Individual states regulate whether termination of second-trimester pregnancies are allowed and can prohibit termination of third-trimester pregnancies that are not life threatening. They can also mandate additional regulations regarding the procedures, such as requiring a 24-hour waiting period for counseling or requiring parental approval for minors. Whether a particular institution or health care provider performs elective termination services depends on the policy and choice of that institution or individual.

Medically Induced Termination

Mifepristone (RU-486) is a progesterone antagonist that blocks the effect of progesterone, preventing implantation of the fertilized ovum and therefore causing the pregnancy to be

BOX 6.8 Nursing Care Planning

AN INTERPROFESSIONAL CARE MAP FOR AN ADOLESCENT SEEKING CONTRACEPTIVE INFORMATION

Seventeen-year-old Dana Crews has come to your community health clinic for a pelvic examination and Pap smear. She is sexually active and tells you her boyfriend "sometimes" uses a condom. She trusts he will "stop in time" when they aren't using one. She doesn't want to take birth control pills because she can't afford it and she's afraid her parents will find out she's broken her abstinence pledge if they see the dispenser.

Family Assessment Client lives at home with parents and younger sister, 12 years old. Father works as Boy Scout administrator. Mother is stay-at-home-mom. Client states family finances are "good; no problem."

Client Assessment Past medical history is negative for major health problems. Menarche at age 12. Menstrual cycles range from 28 to 35 days, with a moderately heavy flow lasting 5 to 7 days. She has enough cramping monthly she "has to stay home from school for one day." Last menstrual flow was 1 week ago. Denies history of STIs or other reproductive problems. Weight is appropriate for height. Secondary sex characteristics are present. You notice her smoking a cigarette outside in the parking lot. Following her health care visit, she is prescribed Ortho-ovum 7/7/7, a 28-day-cycle triphasic oral contraceptive. Decided against DMPA because of cost.

Nursing Diagnosis Readiness for enhanced knowledge related to knowledge deficit concerning contraception

Outcome Criteria Client identifies options available to her; states valid reasons for method chosen; demonstrates correct use of and appropriate follow-up care for chosen method; voices satisfaction with method chosen by 1 month's time.

Team Member Responsible	Assessment	Intervention	Rationale	Expected Outcome
Activities of Daily Living, Including Safety				
Nurse	Assess client's lifestyle.	Discuss when she will take pill and where she will store them. Help make out a reminder sheet. Caution against smoking while taking an estrogen-based pill.	Reviewing lifestyle may provide clues to possible reasons why the method will be ineffective or not continued.	Client describes lifestyle to health care provider and actively participates in devising lifestyle changes that will add to contraceptive's effectiveness.
Teamwork and Collaboration				
Nurse/Nurse practitioner	Consult with nurse practitioner to determine whether method client chooses will be optimal, safe, and effective.	Secure prescription for medication.	Effective health care is a collaborative effort drawing on interdisciplinary expertise.	Consultation reveals the contraceptive method client has chosen will be optimal, safe, and effective; client receives prescription.
Procedures/Medications for Quality Improvement				
Nurse/Nurse practitioner	Assess what additional information client will need to use chosen form of contraception most effectively.	Help complete pre-prescription procedures such as a Pap test and pelvic examination.	Medication administration invariably requires discussion to help clients comply.	Procedures necessary for prescription are carried out safely with optimal respect for client privacy and concern.
	Determine whether client has any questions regarding pelvic examination or other procedures scheduled.	Review method of administration of prescription and steps to take if she forgets to take a pill.	Nurses can be invaluable in lending psychological and physical support during procedures.	Client states she understands the importance of prescription procedures to ensure her safety.

Nutrition				
Nurse/Nutritionist	Determine whether client commonly eats a dietary source of folic acid such as green vegetables.	Discuss with client that oral contraceptive use can lead to folic acid deficiency.	Knowledge of side effects is important to create informed consumers.	Client acknowledges she needs to be conscious of the need for folic acid; names two good sources of folic acid in food.
Patient-Centered Care				
Nurse	Determine whether client has any further questions regarding chosen contraceptive measure.	Have client repeat information for return demonstration.	Instruction provides an opportunity for learning to improve compliance.	Client describes the action of oral contraceptives and the need to take them conscientiously.
Psychosocial/Spiritual/Emotional Needs				
Nurse	Assess if client has discussed with boyfriend that contraception is different than safer sex practices.	Review and discuss the need for safer sex practices in addition to contraception.	Safer sex practices promote health, empower the client, and minimize the risk of STIs.	Client acknowledges need for safer sex practices to prevent STIs and states she will ask her partner to use a condom.
Informatics for Seamless Health Care Planning				
Nurse	Assess if client understands she will need continued health supervision while on an oral contraceptive.	Explain the need for routine follow-up in 1 month and yearly pelvic examinations.	Follow-up is essential for evaluating adherence and satisfaction and for reducing the risk of possible complications.	Client states she will return for a follow-up visit in 1 month and every year thereafter.

STI, sexually transmitted infection.

lost. Mifepristone is not solely used for induced terminations and so may also be prescribed to women for regression of uterine leiomyomas or detoxification in cocaine overdose. When used for a medical termination of pregnancy, the compound is taken as a single oral dose any time before 63 days gestational age followed by buccal or vaginal misoprostol (a prostaglandin), which causes uterine contractions (Godfrey, Bordoloi, Moorthie, et al., 2012). Some women may also be prescribed an antibiotic as prophylactic protection against infection.

Another medical regimen is methotrexate and misoprostol. Methotrexate (also used to end ectopic pregnancies or trophoblastic disease; see Chapter 21) interferes with the DNA synthesis of dividing cells and so prevents growth of the zygote. A mifepristone/misoprostol regimen is about 96% effective; methotrexate/misoprostol is slightly lower (Hanson & Burke, 2011).

Because the blood type of the conceptus is unknown with either medical or surgical termination, all women with Rh-negative blood should receive Rh_o(D) immune globulin (RhoGAM or RHIG) at the time the mifepristone is prescribed or within 72 hours after the procedure to prevent the buildup of antibodies in the event the conceptus was Rh positive (Sandler, Li, Langeberg, et al., 2012). (See Chapter 26 for a full discussion of Rh isoimmunization.)

Medically induced termination of pregnancy is contraindicated if a woman has:

- A confirmed or suspected ectopic pregnancy (only methotrexate is used and the woman needs additional follow-up)
- An IUD in place
- A serious medical condition such as chronic adrenal failure
- A history of current long-term systemic corticosteroid therapy
- A history of allergy to mifepristone, misoprostol, or other prostaglandins
- A hemorrhagic disorder or is taking concurrent anticoagulant therapy

Advantages of medically induced over surgical termination include the decreased risk of damage to the uterus through instrument insertion and decreased use of anesthesia necessary for surgically performed procedures. The complications of medically induced termination include nausea and vomiting, diarrhea, severe uterine cramping, incomplete abortion, and the possibility of prolonged bleeding.

A woman can expect to have mild vaginal spotting and perhaps cramping for 2 weeks postprocedure. Caution her to use sanitary pads rather than tampons and not to douche to help avoid infection. She should not take aspirin for discomfort as this can increase bleeding (advise acetaminophen [Tylenol] instead).

She can resume regular activities, but avoid heavy lifting or strenuous exercise for about 3 days. Her usual menstrual period will return in 2 to 4 weeks. It's best if she doesn't have sexual relations until a scheduled checkup to avoid infection, but if she does, she should advise her partner to use a condom to avoid a second pregnancy.

It's important that she notify her health care provider if she has heavy vaginal bleeding (more than two pads saturated in 1 hour), passing of clots, abdominal pain or tenderness, oral temperature over 102.4°F, or if she notices severe depression or sadness. As a last measure, she should be certain to keep her follow-up appointment in about 2 weeks for postprocedure ultrasonography or a pregnancy test to ensure the pregnancy has ended and obtain contraceptive counseling so she can avoid a repeat procedure.

Surgical Elective Termination Procedures

Elective surgical terminations involve several different techniques, depending on the gestational age at the time the termination is performed.

Menstrual extraction or suction evacuation is performed on an ambulatory basis 5 to 7 weeks after the last menstrual period. A narrow polyethylene catheter is introduced through the vagina into the cervix and uterus; the lining of the uterus that would be shed with a normal menstrual flow is suctioned and removed by the vacuum pressure of a syringe (Fig. 6.14A). The procedure causes only a minimum of discomfort (perhaps slight uterine cramping).

D&C is used when the gestational age of a pregnancy is still less than 13 weeks. This is done in an ambulatory setting using a paracervical anesthetic block that does not eliminate all pain but limits what the woman experiences to cramping and a feeling of pressure. The cervix is dilated and the uterus is scraped clean with a curette, removing the zygote and trophoblast cells with the uterine lining (Fig. 6.14B). D&C has a potential risk of uterine perforation from the instruments used and carries an increased risk of uterine infection compared with menstrual extraction because of the greater cervical dilatation.

Dilatation and vacuum extraction (D&E) is used with terminations between 12 and 16 weeks of gestation. They are done in either an inpatient or ambulatory setting. In some centers, dilatation of the cervix is begun the day before the procedure by administration of buccal misoprostol or insertion of a laminaria tent (seaweed that has been dried and sterilized) into the cervix. In a moist body part such as the cervix, the seaweed absorbs fluid and swells in size. Over a 24-hour period, gradually, painlessly, and without trauma, it dilates the cervix enough for a vacuum extraction tip to be inserted. There is some concern that if a woman needs frequent surgical dilatation of the cervix, as would occur from frequent abortion procedures, it could lead to a cervix that dilates so easily it would not remain contracted during a subsequent pregnancy. Therefore, laminaria dilatation is often chosen for young women who may have more than one pregnancy termination in their lifetime as the gradual dilation of a cervix by this method helps to safeguard their childbearing potential. Antibiotic prophylaxis may be initiated at the time of the laminaria insertion, and the woman is cautioned not to have sexual relations until the process is complete to protect against infection.

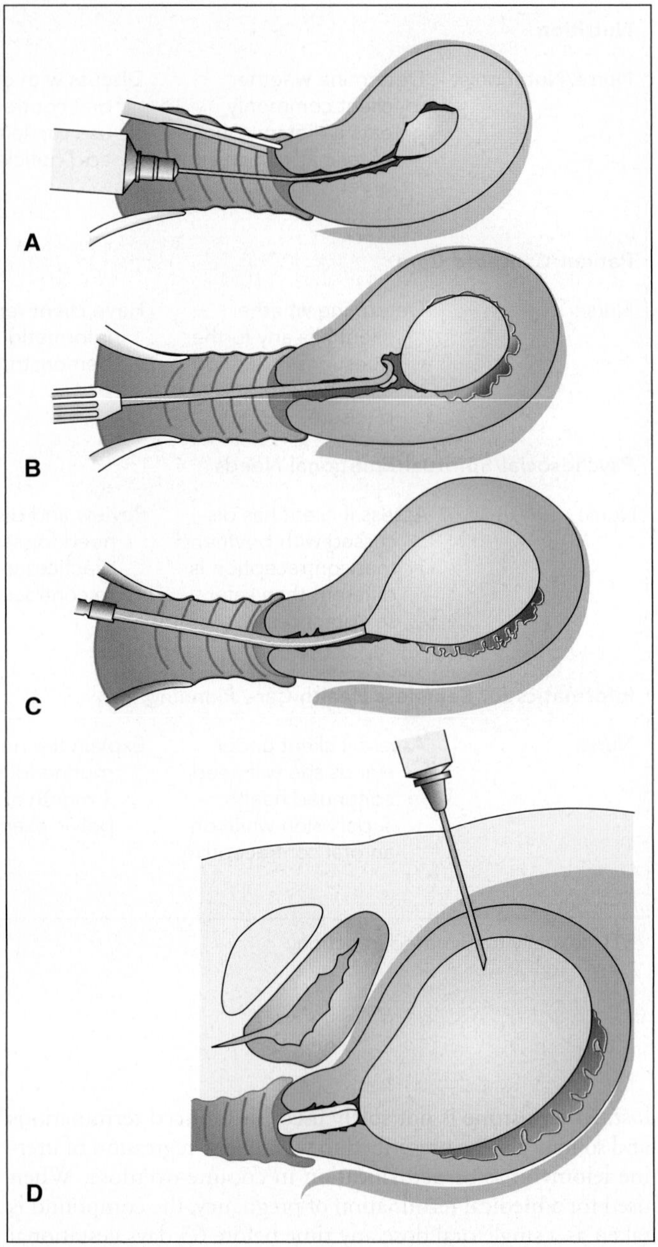

FIGURE 6.14 Techniques of surgical elective termination of pregnancy. **(A)** Menstrual extraction. **(B)** Dilatation and curettage (D&C). **(C)** Dilatation and vacuum extraction (D&E). **(D)** Saline induction.

For the actual procedure, a narrow suction tip is introduced into the cervix (Fig. 6.14C). A suction pump or vacuum container gently evacuates the uterine contents over a 15-minute period. The woman will feel pain as the cervical dilatation is performed and some pressure and cramping, similar to menstrual cramps, during suction, but it is not a markedly painful procedure.

Prostaglandin or a saline induction is used if a pregnancy is between 16 and 24 weeks (Fig. 6.14D) and is done on an inpatient or same-day surgery basis. Following oral misoprostol or vaginal laminaria to prepare the cervix for dilatation, prostaglandin F2 or E2 is administered followed by a 20% saline injection into the uterus. The saline, because it is hypertonic, causes fluid shifts and sloughing of the placenta and endometrium.

A dilute intravenous solution of oxytocin to assist the start of contractions may also be used. Pain from the procedure is similar to natural birth but can be controlled by analgesics and breathing exercises.

Oxytocin administration is discussed in Chapter 23. As with the woman receiving oxytocin for term labor, the woman needs to be observed carefully for signs of water intoxication (fluid accumulating in body tissue), such as severe headache and confusion. A serious potential complication of saline administration is hypernatremia from accidental injection of the hypertonic saline solution into a blood vessel within the uterine cavity. This could cause interstitial fluid to shift into the blood vessels in an attempt to equalize osmotic pressure and result in serious hypertension and dehydration of tissue. If an intravascular puncture should occur, the woman immediately experiences an increased pulse rate, a flushed face, and a severe headache. The injection must be stopped immediately and an intravenous solution such as 5% dextrose is begun to dilute the saline solution and restore fluid balance.

After expulsion of the products of conception after about 12 to 36 hours, all the tissue expelled should be examined to determine whether the entire conceptus (fetus and placenta and membranes) have been expelled. If a woman wishes to see the fetus, wrap it as if it were a full-term infant and allow her to do this to begin effective grieving or closure. Assess for vaginal hemorrhage following the procedure, the same as after a term birth. If a procedure is prolonged, a woman may develop disseminated intravascular coagulation (see Chapter 21), making her very susceptible to hemorrhage because her blood clotting mechanism has become compromised.

Hysterotomy, or removal of the fetus by surgical intervention, is similar to a cesarean birth (see Chapter 24) and is performed if the gestational age of the pregnancy is more than about 20 to 24 weeks. Surgery is necessary at this point because the uterus becomes resistant to the effect of oxytocin as it reaches this phase of pregnancy and so may not respond to saline induction, even with the assistance of oxytocin. Furthermore, the chance is great at this gestational age that, because the uterus is so enlarged, it will not contract well afterward, leading to hemorrhage. Because this is so late in pregnancy, fewer than 1% of surgical terminations are done using this technique.

Partial birth abortion was a surgical technique formerly used during the last 3 months of pregnancy if the fetus was discovered to have a congenital anomaly that would be incompatible with life or would result in a severely compromised child. With the advent of so many reproductive life planning methods and early fetal screening measures, this late-in-pregnancy procedure is no longer needed and is believed to be unethical by many (Wilson, 2012). For these reasons, this type of termination is no longer legal in the United States.

Psychological Aspects of Elective Termination of Pregnancy

Women of all ages request elective terminations. For such a procedure, the usual profile is a woman who:

- Is young
- Is unmarried
- Has had no previous live births
- Undergoes the procedure to end an unintended pregnancy
- Has not taken any or adequate protection against becoming pregnant
- Has become pregnant because of involuntary coitus from intimate partner violence or rape

Between 10% and 14% of women are raped at some time in their life (CDC, 2011). As many as 4% to 8% of women suffer intimate partner violence that not only leads to pregnancy but also increases in the level of violence during the pregnancy (Lee & Lee, 2011) (see Chapter 55).

Be certain to give women undergoing termination procedures the same kind of explanations and support that women in labor receive (women do not share termination experiences with each other the way they share labor experiences, so women usually have little advance education as to what to expect). Remembering that this is not a decision taken lightly helps in planning nursing care aimed at making an elective termination as nontraumatic as possible.

The majority of women report they are relieved with their decision following an elective termination of pregnancy (Foster, Gould, & Kimport, 2011). Those few who express sadness and guilt may need to be referred for professional counseling so they can integrate and accept this event in their lives.

What if...6.4 You are particularly interested in exploring one of the 2020 National Health Goals in respect to reproductive life planning (see Box 6.1). What would be a possible research topic to explore that is pertinent to this goal, that would be applicable to Dana, and that would also advance evidence-based practice?

Key Points for Review

- Reproductive life planning involves personal decisions based on each individual's background, experiences, and sociocultural beliefs. It involves thorough planning to be certain the method chosen is acceptable and can be used effectively.
- Natural family planning (periodic abstinence and fertility awareness) methods are varied but involve determining the fertile period each month and then avoiding sexual relations during that time.
- Oral contraceptives are combinations of estrogen and progesterone or progesterone-only pills. They provide one of the most reliable forms of contraception outside of abstinence. Women who are breastfeeding, are older than 40 years of age, and who smoke are not candidates for COCs, because the estrogen can reduce breast milk supply as well as lead to cardiovascular complications such as thromboembolism. Progestin-only oral contraceptives do not contain estrogen, so do not have cardiovascular risk; they can be used during breastfeeding.
- A subdermal implant (renewed every 3 to 5 years), intramuscular injections of DMPA (renewed every 3 months), transdermal patches, and vaginal rings are also effective family planning methods.
- IUDs are small plastic devices wound with copper or filled with slow-acting progesterone placed in the uterus to prevent fertilization and implantation.
- Barrier methods of contraception include the diaphragm, cervical cap, sponges, vaginal spermicides,

and condoms (male and female). Such methods are low in cost but are not as effective as ovulation suppressant methods. Use of diaphragms may be associated with UTIs.

- Postcoital or "Plan B" protection involves administration of a high dose of progesterone that prevents FSH release, which then prevents ovulation. A copper-wound IUD may also be used for postcoital protection; its insertion creates changes in the endometrium and cervical mucus to slow or prevent sperm transport.
- Surgical methods of contraception are tubal ligation in women and vasectomy in men. Counsel individuals who wish to undergo these procedures that they are largely irreversible and should not be considered lightly.
- An elective termination of pregnancy can be accomplished medically by administration of mifepristone and misoprostol or surgically by menstrual extraction, D&C, D&E, or prostaglandin or saline induction. Counsel women not to think of elective termination of pregnancy as a contraceptive method, but as a recourse to be used if preventive measures fail. Women who are Rh negative need to receive $Rh_o(D)$ immune globulin after these procedures.
- When counseling clients about reproductive life planning, nurses have the second responsibility to teach about safer sex practices. Such thoroughness not only helps in planning care that meets QSEN guidelines but also best meets the family's total needs (see Table 5.7).

Critical Thinking Care Study

Eve, 27, and Lamar, 33, are a young couple who have just gotten married. They both are heavy smokers. Eve had a miscarriage before marriage when they were using a cervical mucus method of natural planning. It's important to her now not to become pregnant again for 2 years so she can finish a master's degree in psychology. Lamar wants a contraceptive that when discontinued, will allow fertility to return immediately. He also wants a contraceptive that will prevent sexually transmitted diseases.

1. What contraceptive would you recommend as best for Eve?
2. Lamar has special requests. What contraceptive would best meet his needs?
3. Is it safe to use a contraceptive method for as long as 2 years? What if Eve has another miscarriage, making her over 30 by the time she's pregnant for the third time?

Patient Scenario

The Burrows Family

Read about the Burrows family, a family with a member in need of reproductive life counseling, then answer the questions to further sharpen your skills and grow more familiar with NCLEX-type questions related to families in need of reproductive life planning. Confirm your answers are correct by reading the rationales.

Visit http://thePoint.lww.com

Answers and Rationales

Looking for answers to the What If. . . and Critical Thinking Care Study questions?

Visit http://thePoint.lww.com

References

Alexander, K. A., Coleman, C. L., Deatrick, J. A., et al. (2011). Moving beyond safe sex to women-controlled safe sex: A concept analysis. *Journal of Advanced Nursing, 68*(8), 1858–1869.

American Congress of Obstetricians and Gynecologists. (2011). *Emergency contraception*. Washington, DC: Author.

Baselice, J., & Lawson, S. (2011). Postpartum care and breast-feeding. In K. J. Hurt, M. W. Guile, J. L. Bienstock, et al. (Eds.), *The Johns Hopkins manual of gynecology and obstetrics* (4th ed., pp. 257–264). Philadelphia, PA: Lippincott Williams & Wilkins.

Beasley, A. (2010). Contraception for specific populations. *Seminars in Reproductive Medicine, 28*(2), 147–155.

Bekele, B., & Fantahun, M. (2012). The Standard Days Method®: An addition to the arsenal of family planning method choice in Ethiopia. *Journal of Family Planning & Reproductive Health Care, 38*(3), 157–166.

Bitzer, J. (2012). The vaginal ring (NuvaRing®) for contraception in adolescent women. *Gynecology & Endocrinology, 28*(2), 125–129.

Bond, S. (2013). No-cost contraceptive reduces unintended pregnancies and abortion rates at a population level. *Journal of Midwifery & Women's Health, 58*(2), 226–227.

Cameron, S. T., & Glasier, A. (2012). Contraception and sterilization. In D. K. Edmonds (Ed.), *Dewhurst's textbook of obstetrics & gynaecology* (8th ed., pp. 495–512). Oxford, UK: John Wiley & Son.

Casey, P. M., Long, M. E., Marnach, M. L., et al. (2011). Bleeding related to etonogestrel subdermal implant in a U.S. population. *Contraception, 83*(5), 426–430.

Centers for Disease Control and Prevention. (2011). *Rape prevention and education*. Atlanta, GA: Author.

Centers for Disease Control and Prevention. (2012). *Unintended pregnancy prevention*. Washington, DC: Author.

Cherlin, A. J. (2012). *Public and private families*. New York, NY: McGraw Publishing Company.

Chervenak, F., & McCullough, L. B. (2012). Responsibly counseling women about the clinical management of pregnancies complicated by severe fetal anomalies. *Journal of Medical Ethics, 38*(7), 397–398.

Correia, L., Ramos, A. B., Machado, A. I., et al. (2011). Magnetic resonance imaging and gynecological devices. *Contraception, 85*(6), 538–543.

Devine, K. S. (2012). The underutilization of emergency contraception. *American Journal of Nursing, 112*(4):44–50.

Fehring, R. J., Schneider, M., & Raviele, K. (2011). Pilot evaluation of an internet-based natural family planning education and service program. *Journal of Obstetric, Gynecologic & Neonatal Nursing, 40*(3), 281–291.

Foster, D. G., Gould, H., & Kimport, K. (2011). How women anticipate coping after an abortion. *Contraception, 85*(3), 257–262.

Gizzo, S., Fanelli, T., Gangi, S. D., et al. (2012). Nowadays which emergency contraception? Comparison between past and present: Latest news in terms of clinical efficacy, side effects and contraindications. *Gynecological Endocrinology, 28*(10), 758–763.

Godfrey, E. M., Bordoloi, A., Moorthie, M., et al. (2012). Medication abortion within a student health care clinic: A review of the first 46 consecutive cases. *Journal of American College Health, 60*(2), 178–183.

Gordon, C. M., & Pitts, S. A. (2012). Approach to the adolescent requesting contraception. *Journal of Clinical Endocrinology & Metabolism, 97*(1), 9–15.

Goyal, V., Borrero, S., & Schwarz, E. B. (2012). Unintended pregnancy and contraception among active-duty servicewomen and veterans. *American Journal of Obstetrics & Gynecology, 206*(6), 463–469.

Grimes, D. A., Lopez, L. M., Gallo, M. F., et al. (2012). Steroid hormones for contraception in men. *Cochrane Database of Systematic Reviews*, (3), CD004316.

Hanson, S. J., & Burke, A. E. (2011). Fertility control: Contraception, sterilization, and abortion. In K. J. Hurt, M. W. Guile, J. L. Bienstock, et al. (Eds.), *The Johns Hopkins manual of gynecology and obstetrics* (4th ed., pp. 382–395). Philadelphia, PA: Lippincott Williams & Wilkins.

Harper, C. C., Speidel, J. J., Drey, E. A., et al. (2012). Copper intrauterine device for emergency contraception. *Obstetrics & Gynecology, 119*(2, Pt. 1):220–226.

Higgins, J. A., & Cooper, A. D. (2012). Dual use of condoms and contraceptives in the USA. *Sexual Health, 9*(1), 73–80.

Horovitz, D., Tjong, V., Domes, T., et al. (2012). Vasectomy reversal provides long-term pain relief for men with the post-vasectomy pain syndrome. *Journal of Urology, 187*(2), 613–617.

Isley, M. M., & Kaunitz, A. M. (2011). Update on hormonal contraception and bone density. *Review of Endocrinology Metabolic Disorders, 12*(2), 93–106.

Jayakrishnan, K., & Baheti, S. N. (2011). Laparoscopic tubal sterilization reversal and fertility outcomes. *Journal of Human Reproductive Science, 4*(3), 125–129.

Jennings, V., Sinai, I., Sacieta, L., et al. (2011). TwoDay Method: A quick-start approach. *Contraception, 84*(2), 144–149.

Karch, A. M. (2013). *2013 Lippincott's nursing drug guide.* Philadelphia, PA: Lippincott Williams & Wilkins.

Killick, S. R., Leary, C., Trussell, J., et al. (2011). Sperm content of pre-ejaculatory fluid. *Human Fertility* (Cambridge), *14*(1), 48–52.

Lee, A. S. D., & Lee, J. M. (2011). Domestic violence and sexual assault. In K. J. Hurt, M. W. Guile, J. L. Bienstock, et al. (Eds.), *The Johns Hopkins manual of gynecology and obstetrics* (4th ed., pp. 396–405). Philadelphia, PA: Lippincott Williams & Wilkins.

Levi, E., Cantillo, E., Ades, V., et al. (2012). Immediate postplacental IUD insertion at cesarean delivery: A prospective cohort study. *Contraception, 86*(2), 102–105.

Melton, L., Stanford, J. B., & Dewitt, M. J. (2012). Use of levonorgestrel emergency contraception in Utah: Is it more than "plan B"? *Perspectives on Sexual & Reproductive Health, 44*(1), 22–29.

Monteith, C. W., & Berger, G. S. (2012). Successful pregnancies after removal of intratubal microinserts. *Obstetrics & Gynecology, 119*(2, Pt. 2), 470–472.

Nath, A., & Sitruk-Ware, R. (2010). Progesterone vaginal ring for contraceptive use during lactation. *Contraception, 82*(5), 428–434.

Nguyen, L. N., & Jamieson, M. A. (2011). Adolescent users of an online contraception selection tool: How user preferences and characteristics differ from those of adults. *Journal of Pediatric & Adolescent Gynecology, 24*(5), 317–319.

Norman, W. V. (2012). Induced abortion in Canada 1974–2005: Trends over the first generation with legal access. *Contraception, 85*(2), 185–191.

Paterno, M. T., & Jordan, E. T. (2012). A review of factors associated with unprotected sex among adult women in the United States. *Journal of Obstetric, Gynecologic & Neonatal Nursing, 41*(2), 258–274.

Raine, T. R., Ricciotti, N., Sokoloff, A., et al. (2012). An over-the-counter simulation study of a single-tablet emergency contraceptive in young females. *Obstetrics & Gynecology, 119*(4), 772–779.

Russo, J. A., & Nelson, A. L. (2010). Behavior methods of contraception. In D. Shoupe & S. Kjos (Eds.), *The handbook of contraception* (pp. 179–194). Totowa, NJ: Humana Press.

Sandler, S. G., Li, W., Langeberg, A., et al. (2012). New laboratory procedures and Rh blood type changes in a pregnant woman. *Obstetrics & Gynecology, 119*(2, Pt. 2), 426–428.

Schindler, A. E. (2010). Non-contraceptive benefits of hormonal contraceptives. *Minerva Ginecologica, 62*(4), 319–329.

Scott-Ram, R., Chor, J., Bhogireddy, V., et al. (2012). Contraceptive choices of overweight and obese women in a publically funded hospital. *Contraception, 86*(2), 122–126.

Shoupe, D., & Kjos, S. L. (Eds.). (2010). *The handbook of contraception.* Totowa, NJ: Humana Press.

Soler, F., & Barranco-Castillo, E. (2010). The symptothermal (double check) method: An efficient natural method of family planning. *European Journal of Contraceptive & Reproductive Health Care, 15*(5), 379–380.

Steenland, M. W., Tepper, N. K., Curtis, K. M., et al. (2011). Intrauterine contraceptive insertion postabortion: A systematic review. *Contraception, 84*(5), 447–464.

Sucato, G. S., Bhatt, S. K., Murray, P. J., et al. (2011). Transdermal contraception as a model for adolescent use of new methods. *Journal of Adolescent Health, 49*(4), 357–362.

Tafuri, S., Martinellim, D., Germinario, C., et al. (2011). A study on the sexual and contraception behaviours of the pre-university students in Puglia (South-Italy). *Journal of Preventive Medicine & Hygiene, 52*(4), 219–223.

Taylor, H. S., Aldad, T. S., McVeigh, E., et al. (2012).*Oxford American handbook of reproductive medicine.* New York, NY: Oxford University Press.

Türk, R., Terzioğlu, F., & Eroğlu, K. (2010). The use of lactational amenorrhea as a method of family planning in eastern Turkey and influential factors. *Journal of Midwifery & Women's Health, 55*(1), e1–e7.

U.S. Department of Health and Human Services. (2010). *Healthy people 2020.* Wahington, DC: Author.

Vaillant-Roussel, H., Ouchchane, L., Dauphin, C., et al. (2011). Risk factors for recurrence of venous thromboembolism associated with the use of oral contraceptives. *Contraception, 84*(5), e23–e30.

Verhaeghe, J. (2012). Clinical practice: Contraception in adolescents. *European Journal of Pediatrics, 171*(6), 895–899.

Wiebe, E. R., & Trouton, K. J. (2012). Does using tampons or menstrual cups increase early IUD expulsion rates? *Contraception, 86*(2), 119–121.

Wilson, K. (2012). Abortion bans premised on fetal pain capacity. *Hastings Center Reports, 42*(5), 10–11.

World Health Organization. (2011). *Family planning: A global handbook for providers.* Geneva, Switzerland: Author.

Zinaman, M., Johnson, S., Ellis, J., et al. (2012). Accuracy of perception of ovulation day in women trying to conceive. *Current Medical Research & Opinion, 28*(5), 749–754.

Zite, N., & Borrero, S. (2011). Female sterilisation in the United States. *European Journal of Contraception & Reproductive Health Care, 16*(5), 336–340.

Chapter 7

The Nursing Role in Genetic Assessment and Counseling

KEY TERMS

- alleles
- chromosomes
- cytogenetics
- dermatoglyphics
- genes
- genetics
- genome
- genotype
- heterozygous
- homozygous
- imprinting
- isochromosome
- karyotype
- meiosis
- mosaicism
- nondisjunction
- phenotype

OBJECTIVES

After mastering the contents of this chapter, you should be able to:

1. Describe the nature of inheritance, patterns of recessive and dominant mendelian inheritance, and common chromosomal aberrations causing physical or cognitive disorders.
2. Identify 2020 National Health Goals related to genetic disorders that nurses can help the nation achieve.
3. Assess a family for adjustment to the probability of inheriting a genetic disorder.
4. Formulate nursing diagnoses related to genetic disorders.
5. Establish expected outcomes that meet the needs of the family undergoing genetic assessment and counseling as well as manage seamless transitions across differing health care settings.
6. Using the nursing process, plan nursing care that includes the six competencies of Quality & Safety Education for Nurses (QSEN): Patient-Centered Care, Teamwork & Collaboration, Evidence-Based Practice (EBP), Quality Improvement (QI), Safety, and Informatics.
7. Implement nursing care such as counseling a family with a genetic disorder.
8. Evaluate expected outcomes for achievement and effectiveness of care.
9. Integrate knowledge of genetic inheritance with the interplay of nursing process, the six competencies of QSEN, and Family Nursing to promote quality maternal and child health nursing care.

Amy Alvarez, 26 years old, is a woman you meet at a genetic counseling center. She was adopted as a newborn and never felt a need to locate her birth parents because her adoptive parents provided her with a "close to perfect" childhood. After college, she married the most eligible bachelor in her hometown. She is now pregnant with her first child. At 15 weeks into her pregnancy, after serum and sonography testing, she has been advised her child may have translocation Down syndrome. She asks you, "How could this happen? There's no disease like that in either of our families. Can you imagine how this will change my life?"

Previous chapters described common family types and how they are affected by sociocultural and community influences. This chapter discusses the basic principles by which disorders can be inherited and information about the necessary assessments, care, and guidelines for counseling of families if it is discovered there is a potential for a genetic disorder in the family. Such information can influence the health of a childbearing or childrearing family for generations to come.

How would you answer Amy?

As many as 1 in 20 newborns inherits a genetic disorder. As many as 70% of pediatric hospital admissions may be for genetic-influenced disorders (Simpson, Holzgreve, & Driscoll, 2012). The possibility a child could have a genetic disorder crosses the minds of most pregnant women and their partners at some point in pregnancy, whether or not there is any family history of such disorders. This causes pregnant couples to ask health care providers about their chances of having a child with a genetic disorder and about genetic testing (Tasker & McClure, 2013).

Because genetics is a constantly changing field of study, it is important for nurses to keep current with new advances so they can appreciate how a new discovery will affect a family and the child's therapy, or if it could cure the child (Duffin, 2012). Twenty years ago, for example, most children with cystic fibrosis (a disorder of lung and pancreatic dysfunction) died in early childhood. Today, with good management, such children live into adulthood because the gene mutation that causes the disorder has been identified, giving hope for an eventual cure for this puzzling illness, including a new view of counseling (Kmietowicz, 2012).

Due to the Human Genome Project and the determination of the location of specific genes in the human genome, the necessity to improve techniques of screening for genetic disorders has become such a national priority that a number of 2020 National Health Goals speak to this area of maternal and child health (Box 7.1).

BOX 7.1 Nursing Care Planning Based on 2020 National Health Goals

A number of 2020 National Health Goals speak directly to genetic diseases and screening, including:

- Increase the number of states (and the District of Columbia) that verify through linkage with vital records all newborns are screened shortly after birth for conditions mandated by their state-sponsored screening program from 21% to 45%.
- Reduce the proportion of children diagnosed with a disorder through newborn blood spot screening who experience developmental delay requiring special education services from 15.1% to 13.6%.
- Increase the proportion of screen-positive children who receive follow-up testing within the recommended time period from 98.1% to 100%.
- Increase the proportion of youth with special health care needs whose health care provider has discussed transition planning from pediatric to adult health care from 41.2% to 45.3%.
- Reduce the number of children and youth with disabilities (aged 21 years and younger) living in congregate care residences from 28,890 to 26,001 (U.S. Department of Health and Human Services [DHHS], 2010; see www.healthypeople.gov).

Nurses can help the nation achieve these goals by being sensitive to the need for and educating parents about genetic screening in preconceptual, prenatal, and birth settings.

Nursing Process Overview

For Genetic Assessment and Counseling

Assessment

Assessment measures for genetic disorders begin with a detailed family history, preferably of three generations, a physical examination of both the parents and any affected children, and an ever-growing series of laboratory assays of blood, amniotic fluid, and maternal and fetal cells. For example, women are offered a routine sonogram screening (a nuchal translucency scan) and an analysis of maternal serum levels of α-fetoprotein (MSAFP) by a quadruple screen early in pregnancy to evaluate for neural tube, abdominal wall, or chromosomal disorders in the fetus. Chorionic villi sampling (CVS) and amniocentesis are both techniques that may be offered to women who are older than 35 years of age, or to those whose MSAFP level is abnormal, to further screen for genetic disorders. Couples who already know of the existence of a genetic disorder in their family or those who have had a previous child born with a congenital anomaly can have additional, more extensive testing such as karyotyping from the maternal serum. Nurses serve as members of genetic assessment and counseling teams to help obtain the initial family history, assist with the physical examination, obtain blood serum for analysis, and assist with procedures such as amniocentesis as part of this process.

Nursing Diagnosis

Typical nursing diagnoses related to the area of genetic disorders include:

- Decisional conflict related to continuation of genetic-affected pregnancy
- Fear related to outcome of genetic screening tests
- Situational low self-esteem related to identified chromosomal disorder
- Deficient knowledge related to inheritance pattern of the family's inherited disorder
- Readiness for enhanced knowledge related to potential for genetic transmission of disease
- Altered sexuality pattern related to fear of conceiving a child with a genetic disorder

Outcome Identification and Planning

Outcome identification and planning for families undergoing a genetic assessment differ according to the types of assessments performed and the results obtained. This may include determining what information the couple needs to know before testing can proceed or helping couples arrange for further assessment measures. When counseling such families, it is helpful to guide them to concentrate on short-term goals and actions or to help them look first at the immediate needs of their family, the fetus, and the newborn, and later on at what type of continued follow-up will be necessary. For instance, after the birth, will the baby need to be hospitalized for immediate surgical correction of accompanying congenital anomalies, or will the parents be able to take the baby home? What kind of special schooling the child will need is a decision that can wait until later.

Help parents identify health care personnel with whom the parents will need to maintain contact during the next few months such as a surgeon or an orthopedist. Ensuring the parents have health care providers they know they can turn to, especially when they are moving out of the denial stage, helps them move forward to their next step in accepting their child's diagnosis faster.

It is also helpful to identify support people who can assist the parents during their time of disorganization. These people may be usual family resources, such as grandparents or other family members. In some families, however, these people are as disturbed by the diagnosis as the parents and therefore cannot offer their usual support. Helpful Web sites to use for referral are the National Human Genome Research Institute (www.genome.gov), the March of Dimes Foundation (www.marchofdimes.com), the American Association of Klinefelter Syndrome Information and Support (www.AAKSIS.org), the National Fragile X Foundation (www.NFXF.org), the National Down Syndrome Society (www.ndss.org), and the Turner Syndrome Society (www.turnersyndrome.org).

Implementation

Parental reactions to the knowledge their child has a possible genetic disorder or to the birth of a child with a genetically inherited disorder usually involves a grief reaction, similar to that experienced by parents whose child has died at birth (their "perfect" child is gone). Both parents may pass through stages of shock and denial ("This cannot be true"), anger ("It's not fair this happened to us"), and bargaining ("If only this would go away") before they reach reorganization and acceptance ("It has happened to us and it is all right"). For some couples, a genetic disorder is diagnosed during the pregnancy; for others, it may not be discovered until birth, or possibly not even until the child is of school age. For these parents, these reactions will occur at that later point of diagnosis. Reach out and support couples in whatever stage they have reached when you care for them and help them work through and adjust to their child's diagnosis.

Outcome Evaluation

Examples of expected outcomes for a family with a known genetic disorder might be:

- Couple states they feel capable of coping no matter what the outcome of genetic testing.
- Client accurately states the chances of a genetic disorder occurring in her next child.
- Couple states they have resolved their feelings of low self-esteem related to birth of a child with a genetic disorder.

A couple's decisions about genetic testing and childbearing do not necessarily remain constant. For example, a decision made at age 25 years not to have children because of a potential genetic disorder may be difficult to maintain at age 30 years as the couple sees many of their friends with growing families. Be certain such couples have the contact information of a genetic counselor. Urge them to call periodically for news of recent advances in genetic screening techniques or disease therapy so they can remain current and well informed for future planning.

GENETIC DISORDERS

Inherited or genetic disorders are disorders that can be passed from one generation to the next because they result from some disorder in the gene or chromosome structure. **Genetics** is the study of the way such disorders occur. **Cytogenetics** is the study of chromosomes by light microscopy and the method by which chromosomal aberrations are identified.

Genetic disorders occur in some ethnic groups more than others because people tend to marry within their own cultural group (Box 7.2). In addition, concern is increasing that some genetic disorders may occur due to occupational hazards, such as toxic substances in the environment of workplaces (Arbour, Beking, Le, et al., 2010).

These disorders occur at the moment an ovum and sperm fuse or even earlier, in the meiotic division phase of the ovum or sperm when the chromosome count is halved from 46 to 23. Some genetic disorders are so severe that fetal growth cannot continue past that point. This early cell division is so precarious, in fact, that up to 50% of first trimester spontaneous miscarriages may occur as the result of chromosomal disorders (McNair & Altman, 2011). Other genetic disorders do not affect life in utero, so the result of the disorder only becomes apparent at the time of fetal testing or after birth.

Women having in vitro fertilization (IVF) can have both the egg and sperm examined for genetic disorders of single gene or chromosome concerns before implantation. With ongoing stem cell research, it may be possible not only to identify aberrant genes for disorders this way but also to insert healthy genes in their place using stem cell implantation (Harper, Magli, Lundin, et al., 2012). Gene replacement therapy is encouraging in the treatment of blood, neural tube, eye, and congenital metabolic disorders as well as for cancers and immunodeficiency syndromes (Domen, Gandy, & Dalal, 2012; Mele, 2012).

Stem cells can be obtained from bone marrow (adult cells), embryos, or umbilical cord blood (embryonic stem cells). After giving birth, many women today privately bank or donate a sample of cord blood to a public stem cell bank so stem cells can be available for bone marrow or other cell transplantation procedures if someone in their community

BOX 7.2 Nursing Care Planning to Respect Cultural Diversity

Different ancestry backgrounds cause different genetic disorders to be more common in some ethnic groups than in others. The blood disorder β-thalassemia, for example, occurs most frequently in families of Greek or Mediterranean heritage, whereas α-thalassemia occurs most often in persons from the Philippines or southeast Asia. Sickle-cell anemia occurs most often in people with an African ancestry. Tay-Sachs disease, a deterioration of muscle and mental facilities, occurs most often in people of eastern Jewish ancestry.

It is important that families who are at high risk for particular genetic disorders such as these because of their ethnic heritage be informed of the incidence of these disorders and offered genetic screening as appropriate during preconceptual counseling.

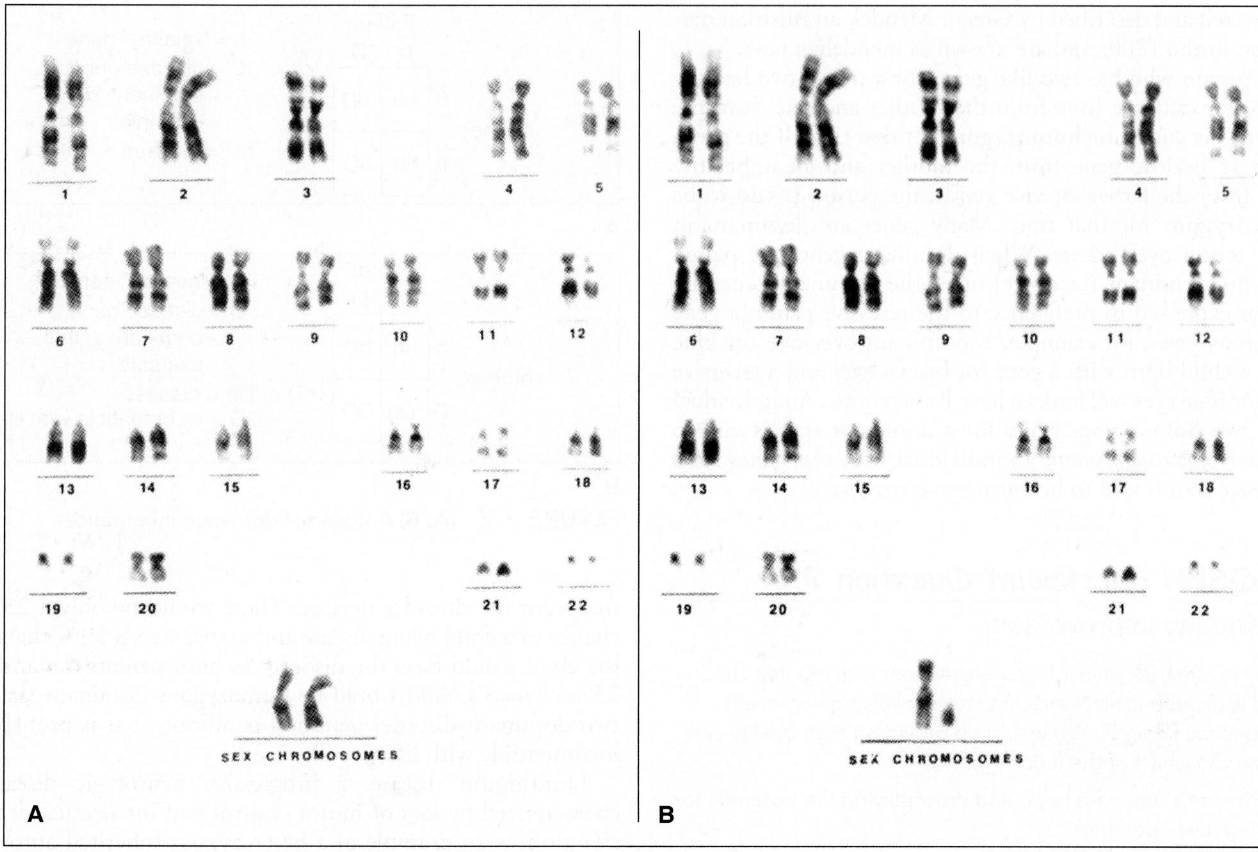

FIGURE 7.1 Photomicrographs of human chromosomes karyotypes. **(A)** A normal female karyotype. **(B)** A normal male karyotype.

needs them. A second large source of adult stem cells for replacement therapy is menstrual blood; this also may be a contribution women can make toward stem cell research (Allickson, Sanchez, Yefimenko, et al., 2011).

Neither the American Congress of Obstetricians and Gynecologists (ACOG) nor the American Academy of Pediatrics (AAP) recommends private cord blood banking unless the family has a relative with a disorder known to be treatable by a stem cell transplant because banking is costly and the length of viability of stem cells is unknown, so an infant's own stem cells might not be available if the child should develop a disease in the future (Waller-Wise, 2011).

Nature of Inheritance

Genes are the basic units of heredity that determine both the physical and cognitive characteristics of people. Composed of segments of DNA, they are woven into strands in the nucleus of all body cells to form **chromosomes.**

In humans, each cell, with the exception of the sperm and ovum, contains 46 chromosomes (44 autosomes and 2 sex chromosomes). Spermatozoa and ova each carry only half of the chromosome number (23 chromosomes). For each chromosome in a sperm cell, there is a like chromosome of similar size, shape, and function in the ovum. Because genes are always located at fixed positions on chromosomes, there are two like genes **(alleles)** on autosomes for every trait in the ovum and sperm. The one chromosome that does not have a mirror match is the chromosome for determining gender. If the sex chromosomes are both type X (large symmetric) in the zygote formed from the union of a sperm and ovum, the individual is female (Fig. 7.1A). If one sex chromosome is an X and one a Y (a smaller type), the individual is a male (see Fig. 7.1B).

A person's **phenotype** refers to his or her outward appearance or the expression of genes. A person's **genotype** refers to his or her actual gene composition. It is impossible to predict a person's genotype from the phenotype, or outward appearance.

A person's **genome** is the complete set of genes present (about 50,000 to 100,000). A normal genome is abbreviated as 46XX or 46XY (the designation of the total number of chromosomes plus a graphic description of the sex chromosomes present). If a chromosomal aberration exists, it is listed after the sex chromosome pattern. In such abbreviations, the letter *p* stands for short arm disorders and *q* stands for long arm disorders. For example, the abbreviation 46XX5p− is the abbreviation for a female with 46 total chromosomes but with the short arm of chromosome 5 missing (cri-du-chat syndrome). In Down syndrome, the person has an extra chromosome 21, so this is abbreviated as 47XX21+ or 47XY21+.

Mendelian Inheritance: Dominant and Recessive Patterns

The principles of genetic inheritance of disease are the same as those that govern genetic inheritance of other physical characteristics, such as eye or hair color. These principles were discovered and described by Gregor Mendel, an Austrian naturalist, in the 1800s and are known as mendelian laws.

A person who has two like genes for a trait—two healthy genes, for example (one from the mother and one from the father)—is said to be **homozygous** for that trait. If the genes differ (a healthy gene from the mother and an unhealthy gene from the father, or vice versa), the person is said to be **heterozygous** for that trait. Many genes are dominant in their action over others. When dominant genes are paired with nondominant (recessive) ones, the dominant genes are always expressed in preference to the recessive genes (a gene for brown eyes, for example, is dominant over one for blue eyes; a child born with a gene for brown eyes and a recessive one for blue eyes will look to have brown eyes). An individual with two homozygous genes for a dominant trait is said to be *homozygous dominant*; an individual with two genes for a recessive trait is said to be *homozygous recessive*.

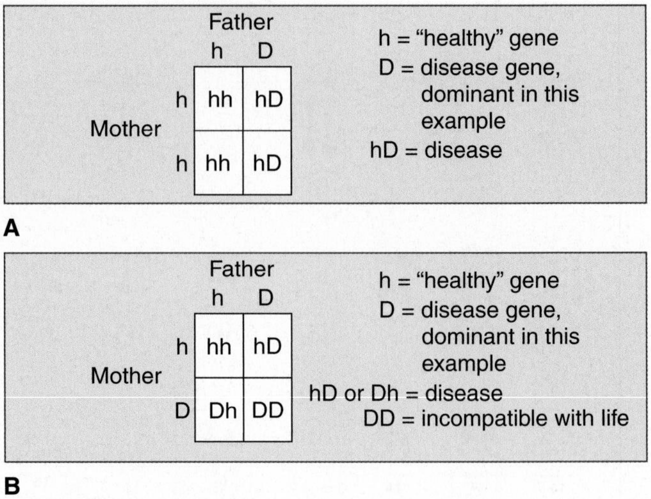

FIGURE 7.2 **(A, B)** Autosomal dominant inheritance.

QSEN Checkpoint Question 7.1

Quality Improvement

Amy Alvarez, 26 years of age, is pregnant with her first child and is experiencing significant stress following her recent diagnostic findings. You would be providing high-quality care if you did which of the following?

a. Provided Amy with hope and downplaying the potential for negative outcomes
b. Referred Amy to Web sites and journals in the field of genetics
c. Described the most serious consequences of genetic disorders
d. Described genetics in a way that directly meets her learning needs

Look in Appendix A for the best answer and rationale.

Inheritance of Disease

Since the entire human genome has been mapped, an increasing number of types of disease inheritance have been identified.

Autosomal Dominant Disorders

Although more than 3,000 autosomal dominant disorders are known, only a few are commonly seen because the majority of these are not compatible with life after birth. Most of those that do occur cause structural disorders. With an autosomal dominant condition, either a person has two unhealthy genes (is homozygous dominant) or is heterozygous, with the gene causing the disease stronger or more dominant than the corresponding healthy recessive gene for the same trait.

If a person who is heterozygous or has a dominant illness gene opposing a recessive healthy gene mates with a person who is free of the trait, as shown in Figure 7.2, the chances are even (50%) a child born to the couple would have the disorder or would be disease and carrier free (that is, carrying no affected gene for the disorder).

Two heterozygous people with the same dominantly inherited disorder are unlikely to choose each other as reproductive partners, but if they did, their chances of having children free from the disorder decline. There would be only a 25% chance of a child being disease and carrier free, a 50% chance the child would have the disorder as both parents do, and a 25% chance a child would be homozygous dominant (have two dominant disorder genes), a condition that is probably incompatible with life (see Fig. 7.2B).

Huntington disease, a progressive neurologic disease, characterized by loss of motor control and intellectual deterioration, is an example of a heterozygous inherited autosomal dominant disorder. Although the disorder is present from birth, it is unusual among diseases because the symptoms don't manifest themselves until people reach 35 to 45 years of age. Because some people who are destined to develop this disorder want to know before that age if they will develop the disease, a test is available to analyze for the specific gene on chromosome 4 that causes the disorder (Banaszkiewicz, Sitek, Rudzińska, et al., 2012). Unfortunately, there is no cure for Huntington disease, so potentially affected individuals have to make the difficult choice to decide to have the predictive analysis performed because, until gene therapy is perfected, there is nothing but palliative care available for this ultimately fatal disorder (Harrington, Smith, Zhang, et al., 2011).

Other examples of autosomal dominantly inherited disorders include facioscapulohumeral muscular dystrophy (a disorder of muscle weakness), a form of osteogenesis imperfecta (a disorder where bones are exceedingly brittle), and Marfan syndrome (a disorder of connective tissue that results in an individual being thinner and taller than usual and perhaps with associated heart and aortic defects) (Jondeau, Michel, & Boileau, 2011). The inherited breast/ovarian cancer syndromes that account for 5% to 10% of breast cancer in women also fall into this category of genetic illnesses (Liu, Yang, Sun, et al., 2012). In assessing family genograms (maps of family relationships) for the incidence of inherited disorders, a number of common findings are usually discovered when a dominantly inherited pattern is present in a family:

- One of the parents of a child with the disorder also will have the disorder (a vertical transmission picture).
- The sex of the affected individual is not important in inheritance.
- There is usually a history of the disorder in other family members.

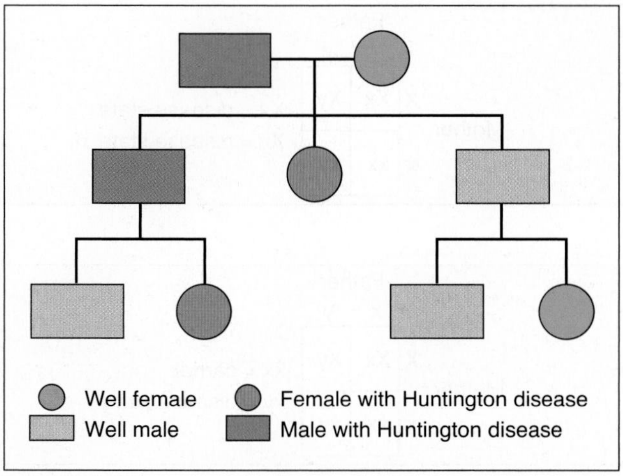

FIGURE 7.3 Family genogram: autosomal dominant inheritance.

Figure 7.3 shows a typical genogram of a family with an autosomal dominantly inherited disorder.

Autosomal Recessive Inheritance

More than 1,500 autosomal recessive disorders have been identified. In contrast to structural disorders, these tend to have a biochemical or enzymatic basis. Such diseases do not occur unless both parents have recessive genes for the disease (a homozygous recessive pattern). Examples of diseases in this category include cystic fibrosis (a disease with lung and pancreatic involvement), adrenogenital syndrome (where genital appearance can be altered), albinism (loss of skin pigment), Tay-Sachs disease and phenylketonuria (cognitively challenged syndromes), galactosemia (difficulty regulating the sugar found in milk), limb-girdle muscular dystrophy (a muscle wasting illness), and Rh-factor incompatibility (a condition where antibodies can attack Rh protein in a fetus). All of these disorders are discussed in later chapters with nursing responsibilities for care.

Figure 7.4A shows the pattern of autosomal recessive inheritance in cystic fibrosis. Both parents in this illustration are disease free of cystic fibrosis, but both are heterozygous in genotype, so each carries a recessive gene for the disease. With this genetic pattern, there is a 25% chance a child born to the couple will be disease and carrier free (homozygous dominant for the healthy gene); a 50% chance the child will be, like the parents, free of disease but carrying the unexpressed disease gene (heterozygous); and a 25% chance the child will have the disease (homozygous recessive).

Suppose a woman with the heterozygous genotype shown in Figure 7.4A mated with a man who had no trait for cystic fibrosis. If that happened, there would be a 50% chance a child born to the couple would be completely disorder and carrier free, like the father. Likewise, there is a 50% chance their child will be heterozygous (a carrier), like the mother (see Fig. 7.4B). There is no chance in this instance any of their children will have the disorder. However, the parents should be counseled that if one of their children who carries the trait has children with a partner who also has a recessive gene for the trait, grandchildren could manifest the disease. Cystic fibrosis is caused by an errant gene on the seventh chromosome. As many as 1 in every 29 Caucasian people carry the trait. Women who are concerned as to whether they may have a recessive gene that will cause the disorder in a fetus can have a DNA analysis of fetal cells in their bloodstream to reveal fetal status (Carter & Marshall, 2011).

Looking at still other possibilities, if a person with cystic fibrosis (homozygous recessive) chooses a sexual partner without the trait, none of their children will have the disorder, but all will be carriers of a recessive gene for the disorder (see Fig. 7.4C).

If the person with cystic fibrosis mated with a person with an unexpressed gene for the disease, there would be a 50% chance a child would have the disorder (be homozygous) and a 50% chance he or she would be heterozygous for the disorder (see Fig. 7.4D). If a person with the disorder mated with a person who also had the disorder, as shown in Figure 7.4E, there is a 100% chance their child would have the disorder.

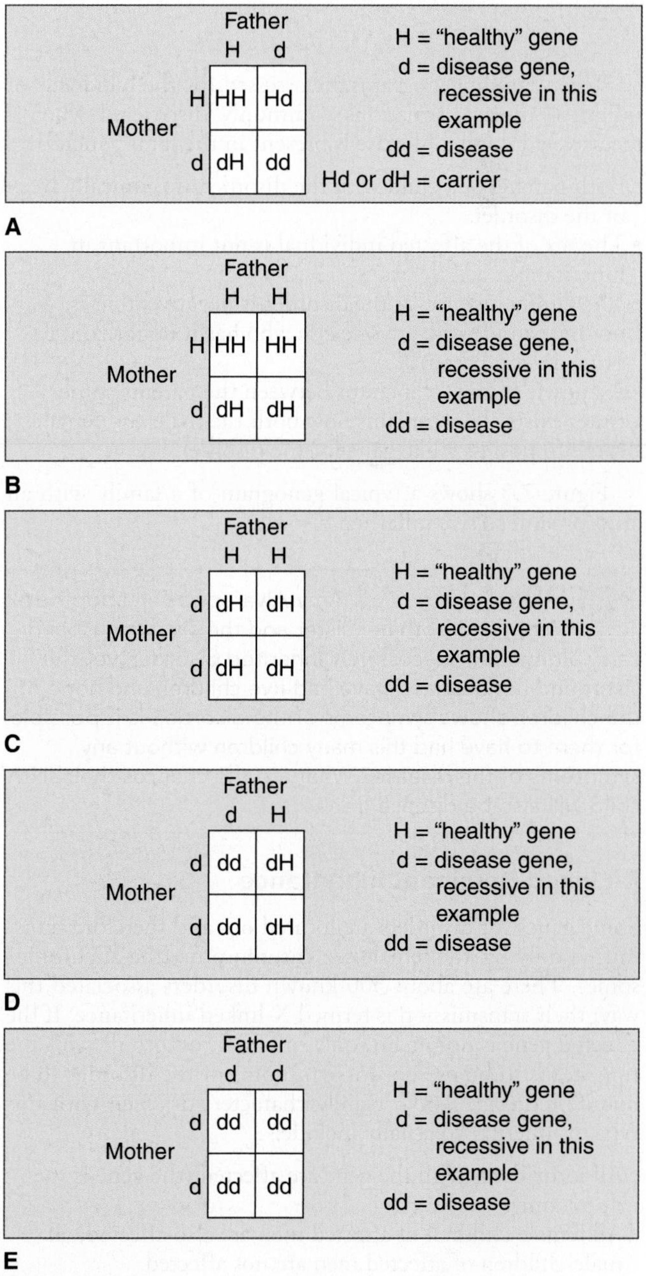

FIGURE 7.4 Autosomal recessive inheritance.

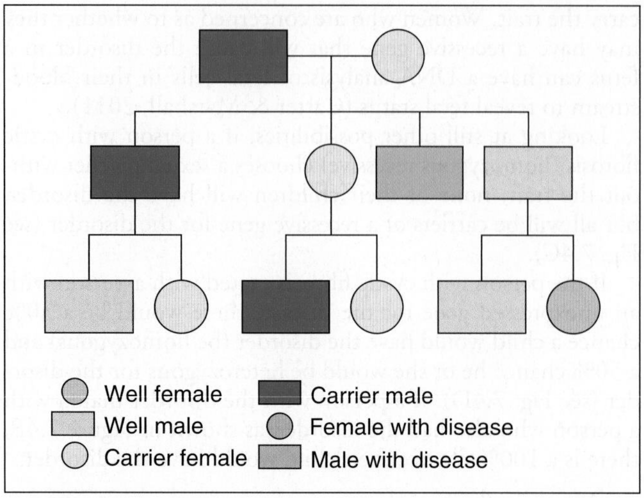

FIGURE 7.5 Family genogram: autosomal recessive inheritance.

When family genograms are assessed for the incidence of inherited disease, situations commonly discovered when a recessively inherited disease is present in the family include:

- Both parents of a child with the disorder are clinically free of the disorder.
- The sex of the affected individual is not important in inheritance.
- The family history for the disorder is negative; that is, no one can identify anyone else who has it (a horizontal transmission pattern).
- A known common ancestor between the parents sometimes exists. This explains how both the male and female came to possess a like gene for the disorder.

Figure 7.5 shows a typical genogram of a family with an autosomal recessive inherited disorder.

What if...7.1 Amy Alvarez has an adopted sister, and both her sister and the sister's husband carry a gene for a recessively inherited disorder, yet the sister and her husband have had five children and none of the children shows symptoms of the disorder. Is it possible for them to have had this many children without any symptoms of the disease? What are the chances their sixth child will also be disease free?

X-Linked Dominant Inheritance

Some genes for disorders are located on, and therefore transmitted only by, the female sex chromosome (the X chromosome). There are about 300 known disorders associated this way; their transmission is termed X-linked inheritance. If the affected gene is dominant, only one X chromosome with the trait needs to be present for symptoms of the disorder to be manifested (Fig. 7.6A). Family characteristics seen with this type of inheritance usually include:

- All individuals with the gene are affected (the gene is dominant).
- All female children of affected men are also affected; all male children of affected men are not affected.
- It appears in every generation.

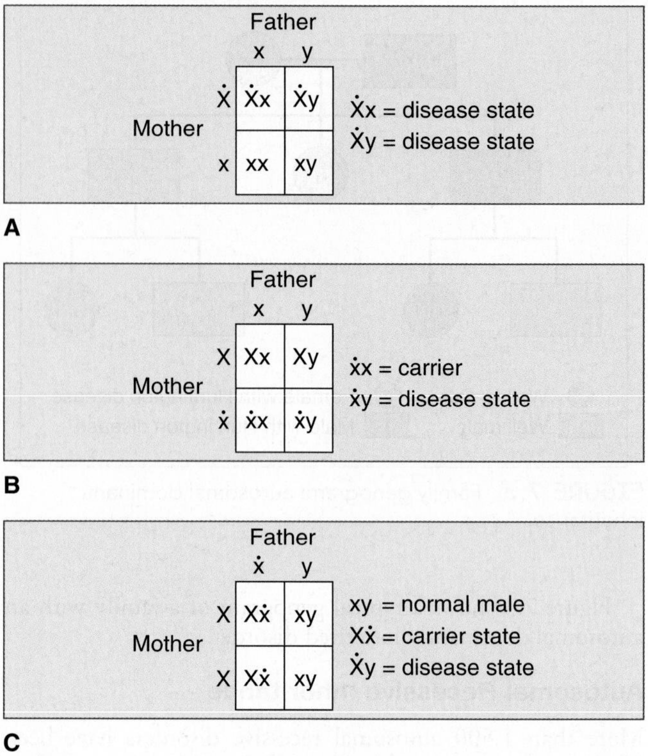

FIGURE 7.6 Sex-linked inheritance: **(A)** sex-linked dominant, **(B, C)** sex-linked recessive.

- All children of homozygous affected women are affected. Fifty percent of the children of heterozygous affected women are affected (Fig. 7.7).

An example of a disease in this group is Alport syndrome, a progressive kidney failure disorder.

X-Linked Recessive Inheritance

Most X-linked inherited disorders are not dominant, but recessive. When the inheritance of a recessive gene comes from both parents (homozygous recessive), it appears to be incompatible with life. Therefore, females who inherit the affected gene will be heterozygous, and, because a normal gene is also present, the expression of the disease will be blocked.

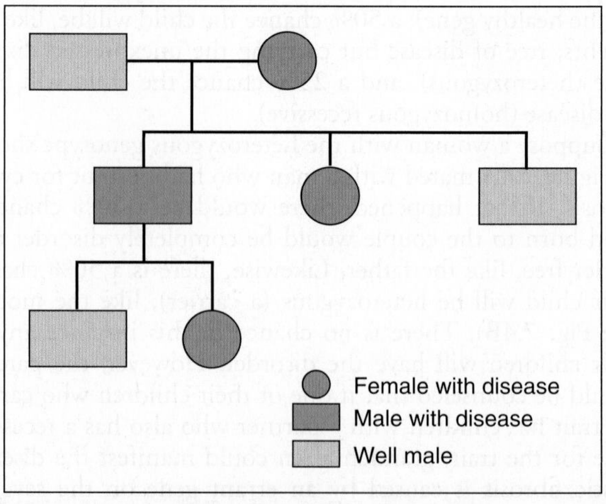

FIGURE 7.7 Family genogram: X-linked dominant inheritance.

However, because males have only one X chromosome, the disease will be manifested in any male children who receive the affected gene from their mother.

Hemophilia A and Christmas disease (blood-factor deficiencies), color blindness, Duchenne (pseudohypertrophic) muscular dystrophy, and fragile X syndrome (a cognitively challenged syndrome) are examples of this type of inheritance. Such a pattern is shown in Figure 7.6B, in which the mother has the affected gene on one of her X chromosomes and the father is disease free. In this instance, the chances are 50% that a male child will manifest the disease and 50% that a female child will carry the disease gene. If the father had the disease and chose a sexual partner who was free of the disease gene, the chances would be 100% that a daughter would have the sex-linked recessive gene, but there is no chance a son would have the disease (see Fig. 7.6C).

When X-linked recessive inheritance is present in a family, a family genogram will reveal the following:

- Only males in the family have the disorder.
- A history of girls dying at birth for unknown reasons (females who had the affected gene on both X chromosomes).
- Sons of an affected man are not affected.
- The parents of affected children do not have the disorder.

Figure 7.8 shows a typical family genogram in which there is an X-linked recessive inheritance pattern.

Y-Linked Inheritance

Although genes responsible for features such as height and tooth size are found on the Y chromosome, tall stature appears to be the only consistent phenotypic feature associated with having an extra Y chromosome (karyotype 47XYY) (Levy & Marion, 2011).

Multifactorial (Polygenic) Inheritance

Many childhood disorders such as heart disease, type 1 diabetes mellitus, pyloric stenosis, cleft lip and palate, neural tube disorders, hypertension, and mental illness tend to have a higher than usual incidence in some families and appear to occur from multiple gene combinations or disorders. Type 1 diabetes mellitus is a disease that has been extensively studied in this regard. Certain human lymphocyte antigens (HLAs) inherited from both parents appear to play a role in genetic susceptibility to the illness. Children who will develop type 1 diabetes mellitus can be shown to have an increased frequency of HLA B8, B15, DR3, and DR4 on chromosome 6. They lack DR2, an HLA that appears to be protective against diabetes mellitus (Noble & Erlich, 2012).

Diseases caused by multiple factors this way do not follow mendelian laws because more than a single gene or HLA is involved. Environmental influences may be instrumental in determining whether the disorder is expressed. It can be more difficult for parents to understand why these disorders occur because their incidence is so unpredictable. A family history, for instance, may reveal no set pattern. Some of these conditions have a predisposition to occur more frequently in one sex (cleft palate occurs more often in girls than in boys), but they can occur in either sex.

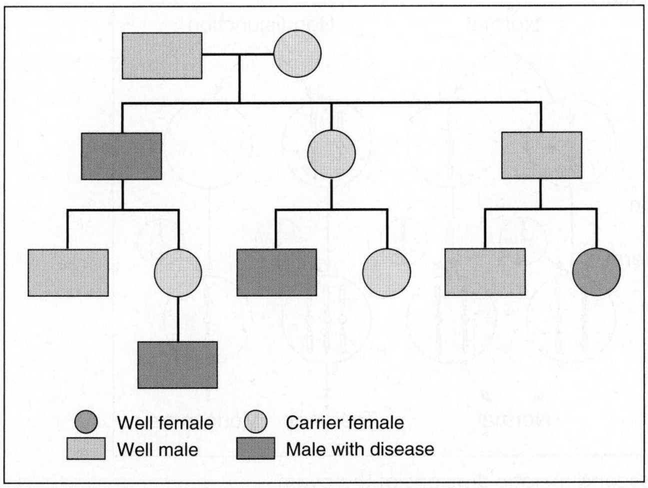

FIGURE 7.8 Family genogram: X-linked recessive inheritance.

✔ QSEN Checkpoint Question 7.2

Evidence-Based Practice

If it is predicted during a pregnancy that a couple will have a child with Down syndrome, the couple is asked to make a choice as to whether they want to continue the pregnancy or terminate it at that point. To discover how couples feel about having a child with Down syndrome, researchers surveyed 2,044 parents on the mailing lists of six nonprofit Down syndrome organizations. The majority of parents reported they are happy with their decision to have their child and find their sons and daughters great sources of love and pride. Ninety-nine percent reported they love their affected son or daughter, 97% reported being proud of them, 79% felt their outlook on life was more positive because of them, only 5% felt embarrassed by them, and only 4% regretted having them. In a following study, siblings also reported their relationship with their affected sibling as a positive one. Less than 10% felt embarrassed, and less than 5% expressed a desire to trade their sibling in for another brother or sister (Skotko, Levine, & Goldstein, 2011a; Skotko, Levine, & Goldstein, 2011b).

Based on the findings of the previous studies, how would you answer Mrs. Alvarez's question, "Can you imagine how this will change my life?"

a. "You're right. Having a genetically affected child can potentially be a serious burden."
b. "Don't worry so much about what others think; just concentrate on your own life."
c. "Change can create good things in life; I believe as a door closes, a window opens."
d. "Would it help if you talk to a family who has a child with Down syndrome?"

Look in Appendix A for the best answer and rationale.

Mitochondrial Inheritance

Mitochondria are organelles found in cells but outside the nucleus. They are responsible for converting energy obtained from food into energy for the body. They are inherited solely from the cytoplasm of the ovum. Male carriers cannot pass a disorder carried in the mitochondria to any of their children. Females, however, will pass mitochondrial disorders to 100% of their children. A number of rare myopathies (muscle diseases) and possibly Alzheimer and Parkinson diseases are inherited in this way (Menezes & Ouvrier, 2012).

Imprinting

Imprinting refers to the differential expression of genetic material and allows researchers to identify whether the chromosomal material has come from the male or female parent. In some instances, such as a disruption of placental trophoblast cells (sometimes referred to as a hydatidiform mole; see Chapter 21), it can be shown that two separate sperm fertilized a single ovum (Savage & Seckl, 2012). In Prader–Willi syndrome, a chromosome 15 abnormality in which children are severely obese and may be cognitively challenged, no paternal contribution is present at certain gene points (Cassidy, Schwartz, Miller, et al., 2012).

Chromosomal Disorders (Cytogenic Disorders)

In some instances of genetic disease, the disorder occurs not because of dominant or recessive gene patterns but through a fault in the number or structure of chromosomes, which results in missing or distorted genes. When chromosomes are photographed and displayed, the resulting arrangement is termed a **karyotype**. The number of chromosomes and specific parts of chromosomes can be identified by karyotyping or by a process termed fluorescent in situ hybridization (FISH) or 24-chromosome single nucleotide polymorphism (SNP).

Nondisjunction Disorders

Meiosis is the type of cell division in which the number of chromosomes in a cell is reduced to the haploid (half) number for reproduction (reduced to 23 rather than 46 chromosomes). All sperm and ova undergo a meiosis cell division early in formation. During this division, half of the chromosomes are attracted to one pole of the cell and half to the other pole. The cell then divides cleanly, with 23 chromosomes in the first new cell and 23 chromosomes in the second new cell. Chromosomal disorders occur if the division is uneven **(nondisjunction)**. The result may be one new sperm cell or ovum with 24 chromosomes and the other with only 22 (Fig. 7.9). If a sperm or ovum with 24 or 22 chromosomes fuses with a normal sperm or ovum, the zygote (sperm and ovum combined) will have either 47 or 45 chromosomes, not the usual 46. The presence of 45 chromosomes does not appear to be compatible with life and the embryo or fetus probably will be spontaneously miscarried. Down syndrome (trisomy 21) (47XX21+ or 47XY21+) is an example of a nondisjunction disorder in which the individual has 47 chromosomes. There are three rather than two copies of chromosome 21 (Fig. 7.10).

The incidence of Down syndrome increases with maternal age: the incidence is 1:100 in women older than 40 years of age, compared with 1:1,600 in women younger than 20 years of age (Russell, Denne, & Schwartz, 2011). It is highest if the mother is older than 35 years and the father is older than 55 years as if aging presents an obstacle to clean cell division. Other examples of cell nondisjunction include trisomy 13 (Fig. 7.11) and trisomy 18 (other cognitively challenged syndromes) in which children have an extra chromosome 13 or 18 (see Chapter 54).

If nondisjunction occurs in the sex chromosomes, still other types of disorders occur. Turner syndrome (marked by a webbed neck, short stature, sterility, and possibly cognitive

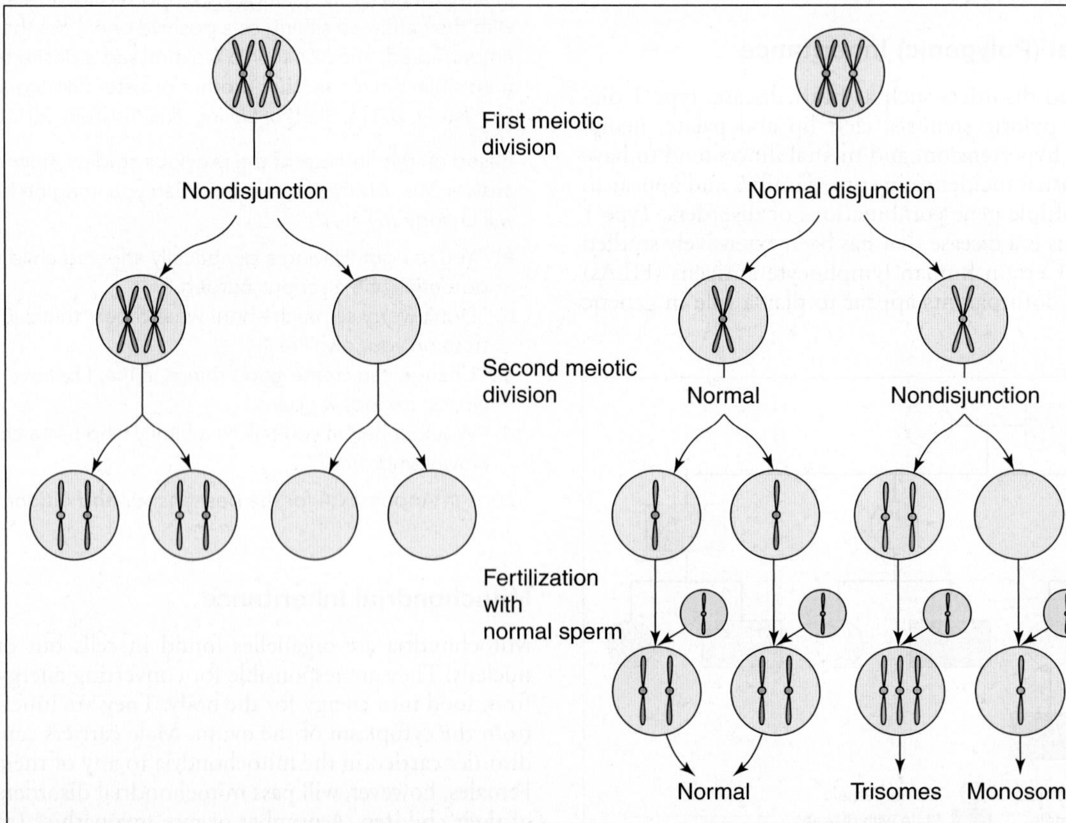

FIGURE 7.9 Process of nondisjunction at the first and second meiotic divisions of the ovum and fertilization with normal sperm.

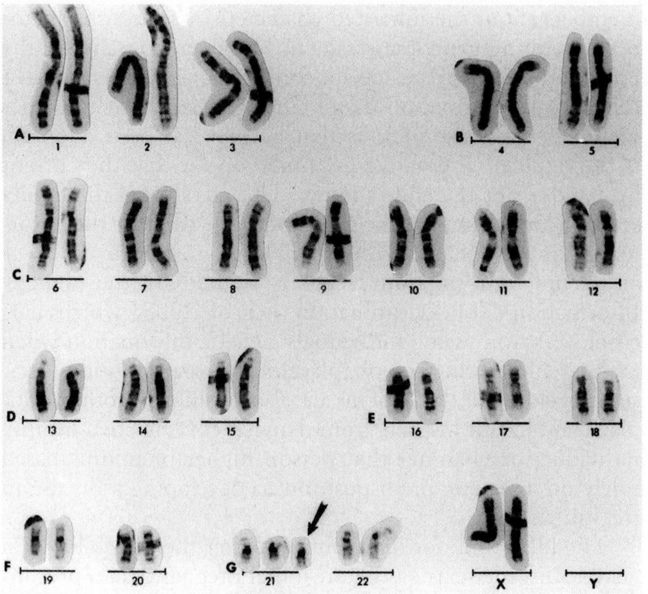

FIGURE 7.10 Karyotype of trisomy 21. (Courtesy of Dr. Kathleen Rao, Dept. of Ped., UNC.)

challenge), and Klinefelter syndrome (marked by sterility and possibly cognitive challenge) are the most common types seen. In Turner syndrome (45XO), the individual, although female, has only one X chromosome (or has two X chromosomes but one is defective). Her appearance (phenotype) will be female because of the one X chromosome. In Klinefelter syndrome, the individual has male genitalia but the sex chromosomal pattern is 47XXY, or an extra X chromosome is present.

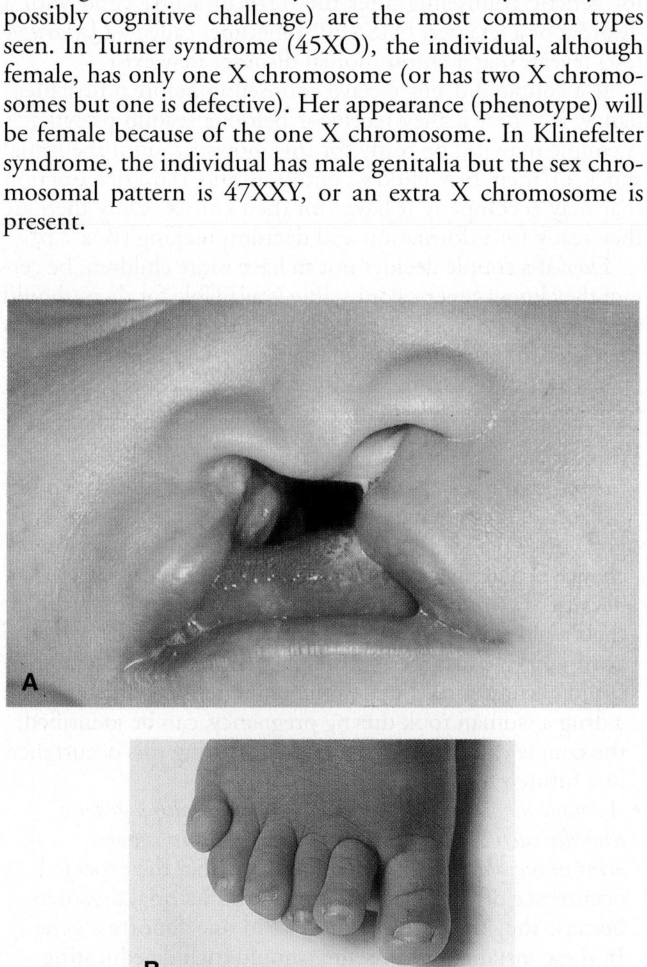

FIGURE 7.11 An infant with trisomy 13 has **(A)** a cleft lip and palate and **(B)** supernumerary digits (polydactyly). (© NMSB/Custom Medical Stock Photograph.)

Deletion Disorders

Deletion disorders are a form of chromosome disorder in which part of a chromosome breaks during cell division, causing the affected person to have the normal number of chromosomes plus or minus an extra portion of a chromosome, such as 45.75 chromosomes or 47.25. For example, in cri-du-chat syndrome, a cognitively challenged syndrome (46XY5q−), one arm of chromosome 5 is missing (Tsai, Manchester, & Elias, 2012).

Translocation Disorders

Translocation disorders are perplexing situations in which a child gains an additional chromosome through yet another route. A form of Down syndrome occurs as an example of this. In this instance, one parent of the child has the correct number of chromosomes (46), but chromosome 21 is misplaced; instead of standing alone, it is abnormally attached to another chromosome, such as chromosome 14 or 15. The parent's appearance and functioning are normal because the total chromosome count is a normal 46. He or she is termed a balanced translocation carrier.

If, during meiosis, the abnormal chromosome 14 (carrying the extra 21 chromosome) and a normal chromosome 21 from the other parent are both included in one sperm or ovum, the resulting child will have a total of 47 chromosomes because of the extra number 21. Such a child is said to have an unbalanced translocation syndrome. The phenotype (appearance) of the child will be indistinguishable from a child with the form of Down syndrome that occurs from simple nondisjunction.

About 2% to 5% of children with Down syndrome have this type of unbalanced chromosome pattern. It is important that parents who are translocation carriers are identified because their chance of having a child born with Down syndrome is higher than usual and is not associated with aging. If the father is the carrier, this risk is about 5%; if the mother is the carrier, the risk is about 15%. As many as 15% of couples who have frequent early spontaneous miscarriages may have this type of chromosomal aberration (Quenby, 2012).

Mosaicism

Usually, a nondisjunction abnormality occurs during the meiosis stage of cell division, when sperm and ova halve their number of chromosomes. **Mosaicism** is an abnormal condition that is present when the nondisjunction disorder occurs after fertilization of the ovum as the structure begins mitotic (daughter-cell) division. If this occurs, different cells in the body will have different chromosome counts. The extent of the disorder depends on the proportion of tissue with normal chromosome structure related to tissue with abnormal chromosome constitution. Children with Down syndrome who have near-normal intelligence may have this type of pattern.

The occurrence of such a phenomenon at this stage of development suggests a teratogenic (harmful to the fetus) insult, such as X-ray or drug exposure, existed at that point in growth to disturb normal cell division. The genetic pattern in a female with Down syndrome caused by mosaicism would be abbreviated as 46XX21+/47XX21+ to show some cells contain 46 and some 47 chromosomes.

Isochromosomes

If a chromosome accidentally divides not by a vertical separation but by a horizontal one, a new chromosome with mismatched long and short arms can result. This is an **isochromosome**. It has much the same effect as a translocation disorder when an entire extra chromosome exists. Some instances of Turner syndrome (45XO) may occur because of isochromosome formation.

QSEN Checkpoint Question 7.3

Informatics

Amy Alvarez has just learned she is a balanced translocation carrier for Down syndrome. As a nursing action, you would want her electronic record to show which of the following?

a. It's good she's having a girl because only males develop translocation syndromes.
b. She has a higher chance than usual for having a child with Down syndrome.
c. She must have two recessive genes for the disorder or it wouldn't have occurred.
d. Because her husband is the cause of the disorder, marital counseling may be necessary.

Look in Appendix A for the best answer and rationale.

GENETIC COUNSELING AND TESTING

It is advantageous for an individual concerned with the possibility of transmitting a disease to his or her children to ask for genetic counseling at a preconceptual health visit for advice on the inheritance of disease because counseling can serve to:

- Provide concrete, accurate information about the process of inheritance and inherited disorders
- Reassure people who are concerned their child may inherit a particular disorder that the disorder will not occur
- Allow people who are affected by inherited disorders to make informed choices about future reproduction
- Allow people to pursue potential interventions that may exist such as fetal surgery
- Allow families to begin preparation for a child with special needs

Genetic counseling can result in making individuals feel "well" or free of guilt for the first time in their lives if they discover a disorder they were worried about is not an inherited one but rather occurred by chance.

In other instances, counseling can result in informing individuals they are carriers of a trait responsible for a child's condition. Even when people understand they had no control over this, knowledge about passing a genetic disorder to a child can cause guilt and self-blame. Marriages and relationships can end unless both partners receive adequate support.

It is essential that information revealed in genetic screening be kept confidential because such information could be used to damage a person's reputation or harm a future career or relationship. This necessity to maintain confidentiality prevents health care providers from alerting other family members about the inherited characteristic unless the member requesting genetic assessment has given consent for the information to be revealed. In some instances, a genetic history reveals information that a family doesn't want the other members to know, such as that a child has been adopted, is the result of alternative insemination, or that the current husband is not the child's father. The member of the family seeking counseling has the right to decide whether this information may be shared with other family members.

Keeping information secure is assured by the Genetic Information Nondiscrimination Act of 2008, which bars employers from using individuals' genetic information when making hiring, firing, job placement, or promotion decisions (Feldman, 2012). The act also prohibits group health plans and health insurers from denying coverage to a healthy individual or charging that person higher premiums based solely on a genetic predisposition to developing a disease in the future.

The ideal time for discussing whether the possibility of a genetic disorder exists is before a first pregnancy at a preconceptual health visit (Russell et al., 2011). Some couples take this step even before committing themselves to marriage so they can offer not to involve their partner in a marriage if children of the marriage would be subject to a serious inherited disorder. Other couples first become aware of the need for genetic counseling after the birth of a first child with a disorder or a fetal test (MSAFP, sometimes called a *Quadruple* test) reveals that a chromosomal disorder may exist.

If a couple did not receive counseling before a first pregnancy, it is best if they receive it before a second pregnancy. A couple may not be ready for this, however, until the initial shock of their first child's condition and the grief reaction that may accompany it have run their course. Only then are they ready for information and decision making (Box 7.3).

Even if a couple decides not to have more children, be certain they know genetic counseling is available for them should their decision change. Also be certain they are aware that, as their children reach reproductive age, they too may benefit from genetic counseling. Couples who are most apt to benefit from a referral for genetic testing or counseling include:

- *A couple who has a child with a congenital disorder or an inborn error of metabolism.* Many congenital disorders occur because of teratogenic invasion during pregnancy that has gone unrecognized. Learning the disorder occurred by a chance occurrence rather than inheritance is important because the couple will not have to spend the remainder of their childbearing years concerned another child may be born with the disorder (although a chance circumstance could occur again). If a definite teratogenic agent, such as a drug a woman took during pregnancy, can be identified, the couple can be advised about preventing this occurrence in a future pregnancy.
- *A couple whose close relatives have a child with a genetic disorder such as a translocation disorder or an inborn error of metabolism.* It is difficult to predict the expected occurrence of many "familial" or multifactorial disorders because they may involve more than one abnormal gene. In these instances, counseling should include educating the couple about the disorder, treatment available, and the prognosis or outcome of the disorder. Based on this information, the couple can make an informed reproductive choice about children.

BOX 7.3 Nursing Care Planning Based on Family Teaching

GENETIC SCREENING

Q. Amy Alvarez is anxious to have her fetus' health confirmed. She asks you, "Why do I have to wait so late in pregnancy for genetic studies by amniocentesis?"

A. A genetic analysis is done on skin cells obtained from amniotic fluid. The test cannot be scheduled until enough amniotic fluid is present for analysis, which is about the 15th week of pregnancy. Fortunately, it is possible to do an analysis of fetal red cells circulating in maternal blood very early (at about 10 weeks) in pregnancy.

Q. Why do laboratories take so long to return karyotyping results?

A. Karyotyping has traditionally (and by necessity) been done on cells at the metaphase (center phase) of division, so the laboratory had to delay testing until the cells had grown to reach this phase. New techniques now allow an analysis to be done immediately so results are available much sooner.

Q. If there are no inherited diseases in a couple's family, should the couple have a karyotype done "just to be sure" before they have their first baby?

A. A genetic analysis is not routinely recommended unless there is evidence or suspicion of genetic disease in the family. Remember, karyotyping reveals only diseases present on chromosomes. A "perfect" karyotype, therefore, doesn't guarantee a newborn will not be ill in a noninherited way.

- *Any individual who is a known balanced translocation carrier.* Understanding his or her own chromosome structure and the process by which future children could be affected can help such individuals make an informed choice about reproduction and also alert the person to the importance of fetal karyotyping during any future pregnancy. Box 7.4 shows an interprofessional care map illustrating both nursing and team planning for a woman concerned about genetic disorders.
- *Any individual who has an inborn error of metabolism or chromosomal disorder.* Any person with a disease should know the inheritance pattern of the disease and, like those who are balanced translocation carriers, should be aware if prenatal diagnosis is possible for his or her particular disorder.
- *A consanguineous (closely related) couple.* The more closely related two people are, the more genes they have in common, so the more likely it is that a recessively inherited disease will be expressed. A brother and sister, for example, have about 50% of their genes in common; first cousins have about 12% of their genes in common.
- *Any woman older than 35 years of age and any man older than 55 years of age.* This is directly related to the association between advanced parental age and the occurrence of Down syndrome.
- *Couples of ethnic backgrounds in which specific illnesses are known to occur.* Mediterranean people, for example, have a high incidence of thalassemia, a blood disorder; those with a Chinese ancestry have a high incidence of glucose-6-phosphate dehydrogenase (G6PD) deficiency, a blood disorder where destruction of red cells can occur (Panepinto & Scott, 2011).

Nursing Responsibilities

Nurses play important roles in assessing for signs and symptoms of genetic disorders, in offering support to individuals who seek genetic counseling, and in helping with reproductive genetic testing procedures.

A great deal of time may need to be spent offering support for a grieving couple confronted with the reality of how tragically the laws of inheritance have affected their lives. Direct counseling is a role for nurses only if they are adequately prepared in the study of genetics, however, because without this background, genetic counseling can be dangerous and destructive (Box 7.5).

Whether one is acting as the nurse member of a genetic counseling team or as a genetic counselor, some common principles apply.

- The individual or couple being counseled needs a clear understanding of the information provided. People may listen to the statistics of their situation ("Your child has a 25% chance of having this disease") and construe a "25% chance" to mean if they have one child with the disease, they can then have three other children without any worry. A 25% chance, however, means *with each pregnancy* there is a 25% chance the child will have the disease (chance has no "memory" of what has already happened). It is as if the couple had four cards, all aces, with the ace of spades representing the disease. When a card is drawn from the set of four, the chance of it being the ace of spades is one in four (25%). When the couple is ready to have a second child, it is as if the card drawn during the first round is returned to the set, so the chance of drawing the ace of spades in the second draw is exactly the same as in the first draw. Similarly, the couple's chance of having a child with the disease remains one in four in each successive pregnancy.
- It is never appropriate for a health care provider to impose his or her own values or opinions on others. Individuals with known inherited diseases in their family must face difficult decisions, such as how much genetic testing to undergo or whether to terminate a pregnancy that will result in a child with a specific genetic disease. Be certain couples have been told all the options available to them, then leave them to think about the options and make their decision by themselves. Help them to understand that no one is judging their decision because they are the ones who must live with the decision in the years to come.

BOX 7.4 Nursing Care Planning

AN INTERPROFESSIONAL CARE MAP FOR A COUPLE CONCERNED ABOUT GENETIC DISORDERS IN FUTURE CHILDREN

Amy Alvarez is a woman you meet at a genetic counseling center. She was adopted as a newborn and never felt a need to locate her birth parents because her adoptive parents provided a "close to perfect" childhood for her. After college, she married the most eligible bachelor in her hometown. She is now pregnant with her first child. At 15 weeks into her pregnancy, she has been advised that her child may have translocation Down syndrome. She asks you, "Why is this happening? There's no disease like this in either of our families."

Family Assessment Client's family history is unknown because she was adopted. Husband's family has no history of Down syndrome, but does have two cousins who are cognitively challenged. Client is presently attending law school. Husband works as a county public defender. Family lives in condo by lake front. Finances rated as "good."

Client Assessment Client's and husband's past medical histories show no evidence of major health problems. Pregnancy is at 15 weeks. Maternal serum α-fetoprotein showed decreased level.

Nursing Diagnosis Readiness for enhanced knowledge related to possible genetic disorder inheritance

Outcome Criteria Couple accurately states the cause of this genetic disorder and agrees to further genetic testing to confirm fetal diagnosis and describes range of options open to them so any decision they make regarding the pregnancy is an informed one.

Team Member Responsible	Assessment	Intervention	Rationale	Expected Outcome
Activities of Daily Living, Including Safety				
Nurse/Nurse practitioner	Obtain a detailed history of the client and spouse, including information about family members and other relatives.	Perform a physical examination to document current health.	A thorough history and physical examination provide baseline information to direct need for follow-up.	Couple participates fully in health examination, so family history obtained is as complete as possible.
Teamwork and Collaboration				
Nurse/Genetic counselor	Assess whether couple would like to speak to an expert in the field of genetics to clarify their understanding.	Refer client to genetic counselor so they can be aware of exact inheritance pattern and options available.	Couples cannot make informed choices without being aware of extent of problem.	Couple meets with genetic counselor within 1 week.
Procedures/Medications for Quality Improvement				
Nurse/Primary health care provider	Perform genetic testing. Develop a family genogram for client and spouse.	Be certain couple receives written documentation of chromosome disorder to take to genetic counselor.	A family genogram may provide additional information about the client's and spouse's family histories.	Couple receives results of test in a timely and appropriate manner. A family genogram is developed and maintained with electronic health documentation.
Nutrition				
Nurse /Dietitian	Assess the couple's nutrition patterns.	Analyze whether couple maintains healthy diet during testing and consultation period.	A healthy diet during pregnancy is important if pregnancy will be continued.	Client confirms she continues to take prenatal vitamins and adequate protein intake.

Patient-Centered Care				
Nurse/Nurse practitioner	Ask couple if they have further questions about their particular inheritance pattern.	Review with the couple the mode of transmission and chances for manifesting Down syndrome in children.	Down syndrome may be inherited at a higher incidence in a balanced translocation carrier than in others.	Couple accurately describes the mode of transmission of Down syndrome.
Spiritual/Psychosocial/Emotional Needs				
Nurse	Assess whether couple would be interested in contacting the hospital's religious counselor for support or learning some activities to reduce stress.	If requested, instruct the couple in positive coping mechanisms. Include activities such as information sharing, relaxation and breathing exercises, and physical activity.	Positive coping mechanisms assist in controlling fear and minimizing its intensity, thus promoting effective problem solving.	Couple demonstrates positive coping mechanisms. Couple states the emotional support they received throughout their period of genetic screening and counseling was adequate.
Informatics for Seamless Health Care Planning				
Nurse/Social worker	Assess community for support organizations available.	If the couple chooses to continue the pregnancy, refer them to national support group (e.g., Down Syndrome Foundation) and local parents support group.	Additional counseling and support may be necessary as pregnancy progresses. Community resources can help reduce feelings of isolation and loneliness.	Couple records the names and telephone numbers of support groups as well as the genetic counseling team and states they will keep numbers available if they should need further future information.

BOX 7.5 Nursing Care Planning Based on Effective Communication

Amy Alvarez tell you her mother has advised her not to have any more children rather than risk having another child with Down syndrome.

Less Effective Communication

Nurse: Hello, Amy. What's the reason you've come to the clinic today?

Amy: I need to know more about the chance all my children will have Down syndrome.

Nurse: You're only 26, far too young to be worrying about that. Down syndrome only occurs in older women.

Amy: Wow. It's good to get good information like that.

More Effective Communication

Nurse: Hello, Amy. What's the reason you've come to the clinic today?

Amy: I need to know what is the chance all my children will have Down syndrome.

Nurse: That isn't the kind of question I can answer off the top of my head. Let me ask you some questions about your family to get started, then we can talk to a genetic counselor to get your answer.

Because we live in an age in which information can be obtained quickly, people tend to believe predictions about the inheritance of disorders can also be supplied quickly. More important than getting information to people quickly is being certain they are getting it accurately. Because Amy is a balanced translocation carrier, more aspects than her age must be considered in predicting her chance for having children with Down syndrome.

QSEN Checkpoint Question 7.4

Patient-Centered Care

Amy Alvarez is a balanced translocation carrier for Down syndrome. What would you want Amy to understand regarding this?

a. She should be certain all of her family members understand what this means.
b. She should look into the various costs of medical and surgical abortion techniques.
c. She should be able to state clearly that she knows she should not have any more children.
d. She should feel free to ask you questions after discovering this about herself.

Look in Appendix A for the best answer and rationale.

The Assessment for Genetic Disorders

A genetic assessment begins with careful study of the pattern of inheritance in a family. A history, physical examination of family members, and laboratory analysis, such as karyotyping or DNA analysis, are performed to define the extent of the problem and the chance of inheritance. Parents can obtain a DNA analysis from a profit-making private laboratory (direct-to-consumer marketing), but this is rarely advised because genetic results usually need to be accompanied by counseling to be certain parents understand the often complicated result narrative.

History

Taking a health history for a genetic diagnosis can be difficult because the facts detailed may evoke uncomfortable emotions such as sorrow, guilt, or inadequacy in parents. Try, however, to obtain information and document diseases in family members for a minimum of three generations because a history can be a chief tool in discovering transmitted disorders (American Congress of Obstetricians and Gynecologists [ACOG], 2011). Remember to include half brothers and sisters or anyone related in any way as family. Document the mother's age because some disorders increase in incidence with age. Document also whether the parents are consanguineous or related to each other.

Documenting the family's ethnic background can reveal risks for certain disorders that occur more commonly in some ethnic groups than others. If the couple seeking counseling is unfamiliar with their family history, ask them to talk to senior family members about other relatives (grandparents, aunts, uncles) before they come for an interview about such instances as spontaneous miscarriage or children in the family who died at birth. In many instances, these children died of unknown chromosomal disorders or were miscarried because of one of the 70 or more known chromosomal disorders inconsistent with life.

Many people have only sketchy information about their families, such as, "The baby had some kind of nervous disease" or "Her heart didn't work right." Attempt to obtain as much information as you can by asking the couple to describe the appearance or activities of the affected individual ("She had no left side to her heart") or asking for permission to obtain health records.

An extensive prenatal history of any affected person should be obtained to determine whether environmental conditions could account for the condition. Based on the previous information, draw a family genogram (see Fig. 7.7). Such a diagram helps to not only identify the possibility of a chromosomal disorder occurring in a particular couple's children but also helps identify other family members who might benefit from genetic counseling.

When a child is born dead, parents are advised to have a chromosomal analysis and autopsy performed on the infant. If, at some future date, they wish genetic counseling, this would allow their genetic counselor to have additional medical information.

Physical Assessment

Because genetic disorders often occur in varying degrees of expression, a careful physical assessment of any family member with a disorder, that person's siblings, and the couple seeking counseling is necessary because it is possible that another family member has such a minimal expression of the disorder it has gone previously undiagnosed. During inspection, pay particular attention to certain body areas, such as the space between the eyes; the height, contour, and shape of ears; the number of fingers and toes and the presence of webbing as these often suggest structural genetic disorders. **Dermatoglyphics** (the study of surface markings of the skin) is also helpful because unusual fingerprints, abnormal palmar creases, hair whorls, or coloring of hair are also present with some disorders.

Careful inspection of newborns is often the first time a child with a potential chromosomal disorder is identified. Infants with multiple congenital anomalies, those born at less than 35 weeks gestation, and those whose parents have had other children with chromosomal disorders need extremely close assessment. Table 7.1 lists the physical characteristics suggestive of some common inherited syndromes in children.

Diagnostic Testing

Many diagnostic tests are available to provide clues or to diagnose disorders. Before pregnancy, DNA analysis or karyotyping of both parents and an already affected child provides a picture of the family's genetic pattern and can be used for prediction in future children. Once a woman is pregnant, several other tests may be performed to help in the prenatal diagnosis of a genetic disorder. These include MSAFP or quadruple test analysis, CVS, amniocentesis, percutaneous umbilical blood sampling (PUBS), and sonography. Because some fetal cells always enter maternal serum, it is possible to obtain a fetal DNA from maternal serum (Choolani, Mahyuddin, & Hahn, 2012). All of these tests not only reveal important information but also create ethical and personal concerns for parents because, if an abnormality is discovered, parents are asked to make a decision as to whether to continue the pregnancy (Choi, Van Riper, & Thoyre, 2012).

Nuchal Translucency Screening. A number of genetic disorders such as Down syndrome and Turner syndrome can be detected on a sonogram taken during the first trimester of pregnancy (11 to 13 weeks) because of unusual fat or fluid deposits at the back of the fetal neck, which show on a sonogram as excessive thickening. Such findings are then followed by a chromosome or gene analysis to confirm the finding.

TABLE 7.1 Common Physical Characteristics of Children With Chromosomal Syndromes

Characteristic	Probable Syndrome
Late closure of fontanelles	Down syndrome
Bossing (prominent forehead)	Fragile X syndrome
Microcephaly (small head)	Trisomy 18, trisomy 13
Low-set ears	Trisomy 18, trisomy 13
Slant of eyes	Down syndrome
Epicanthal fold	Down syndrome
Abnormal iris color	Down syndrome
Large tongue	Down syndrome
Prominent jaw	Fragile X syndrome
Low-set hairline	Turner syndrome
Multiple hair whorls	Trisomy 18, trisomy 13
Webbed neck	Turner syndrome
Wide-set nipples	Trisomy 13
Heart disorders	Many syndromes
Large hands	Fragile X syndrome
Clinodactyly (curved little finger)	Down syndrome
Overriding of fingers	Trisomy 18
Rocker-bottom feet	Trisomy 13
Abnormal dermatoglyphics (fingerprints)	Down syndrome
Simian crease on palm	Down syndrome
Absence of secondary sex characteristics	Klinefelter syndrome, Turner syndrome

Nuchal translucency may also suggest congenital heart defects because it can be caused from interference of lymphatic or vascular flow (Mogra, Alabbad, & Hyett, 2012).

Karyotyping. For classical karyotyping, a sample of peripheral venous blood or a scraping of cells from the buccal membrane is taken. Lymphocytes are identified and allowed to grow until they reach metaphase or prophase, the most easily observed phases. Cells are then stained, placed under a microscope, and photographed. Chromosomes are labeled according to size, shape, and stain; cut from the photograph; and arranged as in Figure 7.1. Any additional, lacking, or abnormal chromosomes can be easily visualized by this method.

Molecular karyotyping using chromosome microarray analysis (CMA) studies individual genes rather than chromosomes and so detects even more pathogenic anomalies than classical karyotyping, making CMA likely to become a first-tier test for prenatal diagnosis; a prescription for testing may use CMA terminology instead of karyotyping (Macleod & Drexler, 2013). Newer methods of analysis, FISH and 24-chromosome SNP arrays, allow analysis to be done immediately, rather than waiting for the cells to reach metaphase. These methods also allow for a more detailed analysis. Examples of diseases that can be identified this way are cystic fibrosis, Huntington disease, fragile X syndrome, hemophilia, and Duchenne muscular dystrophy.

Maternal Serum Screening. Because a number of discarded trophoblast (placenta) cells or fetal red cells always enter the maternal bloodstream (few in number during the first and second trimesters but plentiful during the third trimester), a sample of maternal blood can be examined for a karyotype, fetal DNA, and sex of the fetus as early as 7 weeks of a pregnancy. This technique has the major advantage of being noninvasive for the fetus and so carries no risk of fetal infection or a disruption of the pregnancy (Geaghan, 2012).

During the first trimester, women can be offered a pregnancy-associated plasma protein-A (PAPP-A) in combination with a test for human chorionic gonadotropin (hCG). If a PAPP-A test is low, it suggests a trisomy disorder is present. In contrast, if an hCG level is elevated, it suggests presence of a midline closure anomaly.

Between the 15th and 20th weeks of pregnancy, a woman's blood can be obtained for a quadruple marker screen, which measures:

- α-Fetoprotein (AFP), a glycoprotein produced by the fetal liver
- Unconjugated estriol (UE), a protein produced in the placenta and in the fetal liver
- hCG, a hormone produced by the placenta
- Inhibin A, a protein produced by the placenta

AFP in maternal blood is elevated more than twice the value of the mean for that gestational age if a neural tube disorder such as myelomeningocele is present; it is decreased in amount if the fetus has a chromosomal disorder such as trisomy 21 (Bredaki, Poon, Birdir, et al., 2012). Lower than normal levels of UE may also indicate a woman is at high risk for having a baby with Down syndrome.

If the results of a quadruple screen are abnormal, amniotic fluid is then assessed. Because this is done with guided sonography, fetal neck translucency can be studied at the same time. Unfortunately, a quadruple screen has a false-positive rate as high as 30% if the date of conception is not well documented, so dating the pregnancy is important if this can be done.

Receiving a false-positive report is unfortunate because it can potentially interfere with the mother's bonding with her infant. Women may need some "debriefing" time after false-positive reports and may need to be reassured several times that the report of a possible chromosomal deviation was not true.

Chorionic Villi Sampling. CVS is a diagnostic technique that involves the retrieval and analysis of chorionic villi from the growing placenta for chromosome or DNA analysis (Katorza & Achiron, 2012). Although the test is highly accurate, it is more invasive than analyzing maternal serum or amniocentesis, and therefore, carries a higher risk for interference with the pregnancy. For that reason, it is less used today than formerly. There have been some instances of children being born with missing limbs after the procedure (limb reduction

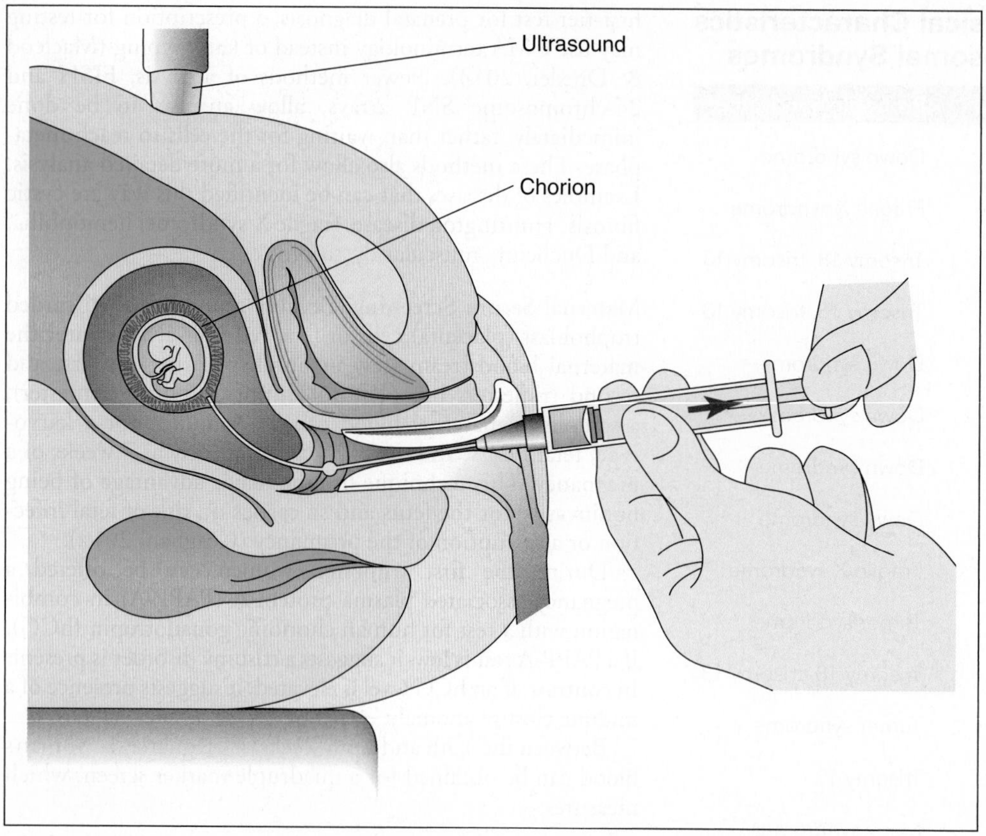

FIGURE 7.12 Chorionic villi sampling. Because the villi arise from trophoblast cells, their chromosome structure is the same as in the fetus.

syndrome) occurring at a high enough frequency that women need to be well informed of this risk beforehand.

With this technique, the chorion cells are located by ultrasound. A thin catheter is then inserted vaginally, or a biopsy needle is inserted abdominally or intravaginally, and a number of chorionic cells are removed for analysis (Fig. 7.12).

After CVS, instruct a woman to report chills or fever, suggesting (although this is rare) that she might have an infection or symptoms of threatened miscarriage (uterine contractions or vaginal bleeding). Women with an Rh-negative blood type need Rh immune globulin administration after the procedure to guard against isoimmunization in the fetus.

The cells removed in CVS are karyotyped or submitted for DNA analysis to reveal whether the fetus has a genetic disorder. Because chorionic villi cells are rapidly dividing, results are available quickly, perhaps as soon as the next day. If a twin or multiple pregnancy is present, with two or more separate placentas, cells need to be removed separately from each placenta. Because fraternal twins are derived from separate ova, one twin could have a chromosomal disorder whereas the other does not.

Be certain parents understand that not all inherited diseases can be detected by CVS, only those disorders involving abnormal chromosomes or nondisjunction, or those whose specific gene location is known. The test is not apt to reveal the existence of a neural tube disorder, for example.

What if . . . 7.2 Amy tells you, "My family will be so ashamed if a genetic defect happens in our family." What does her statement tell you about her family's knowledge of genetic disorders?

Amniocentesis. Amniocentesis is the withdrawal of amniotic fluid through the abdominal wall for analysis at the 15th to 20th week of pregnancy (Simpson et al., 2012). Because amniotic fluid has reached about 200 ml at this point, enough fluid can be withdrawn for karyotyping or molecular analysis of skin cells floating in the fluid.

For the procedure, a pocket of amniotic fluid is located by sonography. Then a needle is inserted transabdominally, and about 20 ml of fluid is aspirated. Skin cells in the fluid are analyzed for chromosomal number and structure. The level of AFP and acetylcholinesterase, a breakdown product of blood, are also analyzed. If no acetylcholinesterase is found in the specimen, it confirms an elevated AFP level is not a false-positive reading caused by blood in the fluid. Some disorders, such as Tay-Sachs disease, can be identified by the lack of a specific enzyme, such as hexosaminidase A, found in amniotic fluid (Lewis, 2011).

Amniocentesis has the advantage over CVS of carrying only a 0.5% risk of spontaneous miscarriage. Unfortunately, because it is usually not done until the 14th to 16th week of pregnancy, this may prove to be a difficult time for the couple because, by this date, a woman is beginning to accept her pregnancy and bond with the fetus. In addition, termination of pregnancy during the second trimester is more difficult than during a first trimester. Support women while they wait for test results and to make a decision about the pregnancy. As with CVS, women with an Rh-negative blood type need Rh immune globulin administration after the procedure to protect against isoimmunization in the fetus. All women need to be observed for about 30 minutes after the procedure to be certain labor contractions are not beginning and the fetal heart rate remains within normal limits. Because amniocentesis is also a common assessment for fetal maturity, it is discussed further in Chapter 9 (see also

TABLE 7.2 Common Genetic Disorders That Can Be Detected by Maternal Serum, Amniocentesis, or Chorionic Villus Sampling

Syndrome	Chromosomal Characteristics	Clinical Signs in Child
Down syndrome	Extra chromosome 21	Cognitively challenged Protruding tongue Epicanthal folds Hypotonia
Translocation Down syndrome	Translocation of a chromosome, perhaps 21/14	Same clinical signs as trisomy 21
Trisomy 18	Extra chromosome 18	Cognitively challenged Congenital malformations
Trisomy 13	Extra chromosome 13	Cognitively challenged Multiple congenital malformations Eye agenesis
Cri-du-chat syndrome	Deletion of short arm of chromosome 5	Cognitively challenged Facial structure anomalies Peculiar catlike cry
Fragile X syndrome	Distortion of the X chromosome	Cognitively challenged
Philadelphia chromosome	Deletion of one arm of chromosome 21	Chronic granulocytic leukemia
Turner syndrome	Only one X chromosome present (45XO)	Short stature Streak ovaries Infertility Webbed neck
Klinefelter syndrome	An extra X chromosome present (47XXY)	Small testes Gynecomastia Subfertility

Fig. 9.14). Table 7.2 shows common chromosomal disorders that can be diagnosed through amniocentesis. Examples of additional disorders that can be identified by DNA analysis are myotonic dystrophy, Huntington disease, sickle-cell anemia, β-thalassemia, and Duchenne muscular dystrophy.

The decision to undergo either CVS or amniocentesis is a major one for a couple because, as a rule, they are not making a decision simply for CVS or amniocentesis; if the analysis from these reveals their child has a disorder, they then have to make a second decision about the future of the pregnancy.

Deciding to terminate a pregnancy based on a laboratory finding is rarely easy. If a couple decides to terminate the pregnancy, they need support for their decision to end the pregnancy. If they decide not to terminate the pregnancy, they may need support during the remainder of the pregnancy and in the days following birth. If a couple could not believe what the test showed was true, only when they inspect the baby and see the test was accurate—the child does have a genetic disorder—do they grasp the reality of what has happened. This can result in long-lasting depression, guilt, or grief for the perfect child they had hoped for at the beginning of the pregnancy.

Percutaneous Umbilical Blood Sampling. PUBS, or cordocentesis, is the removal of blood from the fetal umbilical cord at about 17 weeks using an amniocentesis technique (Fig. 7.13). This allows for an analysis of blood components as well as more rapid analysis than is possible when only skin cells are removed. PUBS is discussed further in Chapter 9.

Fetal imaging. Magnetic resonance imaging (MRI) and ultrasonography are diagnostic tools used to assess a fetus for general size and structural disorders of the internal organs, spine, and limbs. Because some genetic disorders are associated with physical appearance, both of these methods may be helpful (Collins & Impey, 2012).

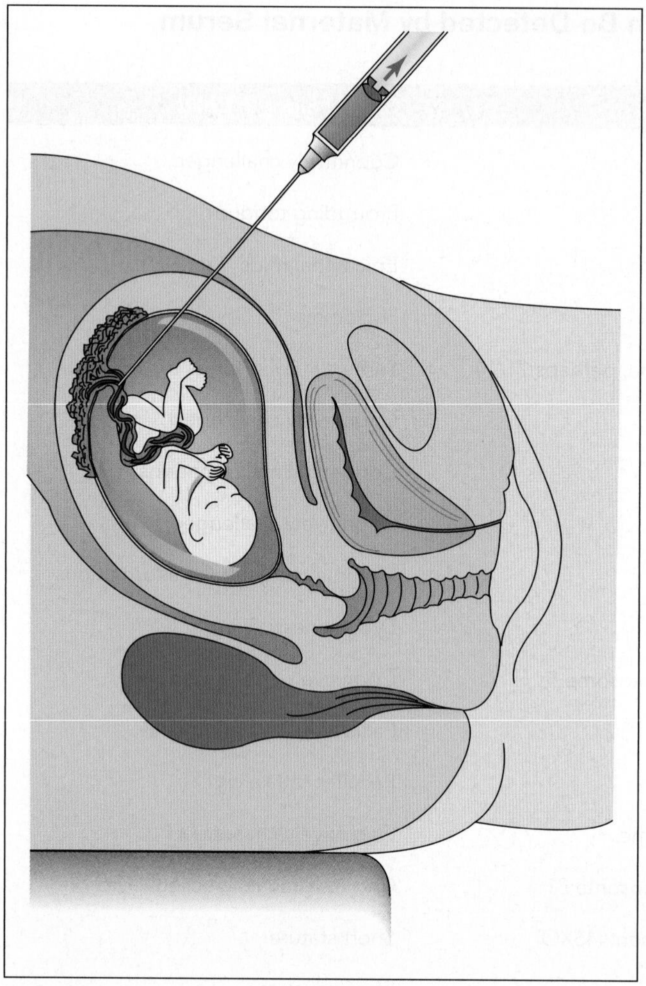

FIGURE 7.13 Percutaneous umbilical blood sampling. Blood is withdrawn from the umbilical cord using an amniocentesis technique.

Fetoscopy. Fetoscopy is the insertion of a fiber optic fetoscope through a small incision in the mother's abdomen into the uterus and membranes, usually under local anesthesia, so an examiner can visually inspect the fetus for gross disorders. It can be used to confirm a sonography finding, to remove skin cells for DNA analysis, or to perform surgery for a congenital disorder such as a stenosed (blocked) urethra or if blood vessels are unusually joined, causing twin-to-twin transfusion (Mosquera, Miller, & Simpson, 2012).

Preimplantation Diagnosis. Preimplantation diagnosis is possible for IVF procedures (both sperm and ova are assessed for DNA before implantation in the uterus or tubes) (Bodurtha & Strauss, 2012). It is conceivable that a naturally fertilized ovum could be removed from the uterus by lavage before implantation and studied for DNA or chromosome analysis this same way. Whether the ovum is reinserted would depend on the findings and the parents' wishes. Both procedures provide genetic information even before implantation or the point many people believe pregnancy begins.

Newborn Screening. Newborns are tested in all 50 states for a number of disorders, including phenylketonuria (a cognitively challenged metabolic syndrome) and congenital hypothyroidism, by heel prick analysis 24 to 48 hours after birth. Allowing newborns to be diagnosed this early in life allows for early treatment and the best chance to avoid complications.

Reproductive Alternatives

Some couples are reluctant to seek genetic counseling because they are afraid they will be told it would be unwise to have children. Helping them to realize viable alternatives for having a family exist can allow them to seek the help they need.

Alternative insemination by donor (AID) is an option for couples if the genetic disorder is one inherited by the male partner or is a recessively inherited disorder carried by both partners. AID is available in all major communities and can permit the couple to experience the satisfaction and enjoyment of a usual pregnancy (Christianson & Wallach, 2011).

If the inherited problem is one arising from the female partner, surrogate embryo transfer is an assisted reproductive technique that is a possibility (Check, Katsoff, Wilson, et al., 2012). For this, an oocyte is donated by a friend or relative or provided by an anonymous donor, which is then fertilized by the husband's sperm in the laboratory and implanted into a woman's uterus. Like AID, donor embryo transfer offers the couple a chance to experience a usual pregnancy.

Use of a surrogate mother (a woman who agrees to be alternately inseminated, typically by the male partner's sperm, and bear a child for the couple) is yet another possibility (Golombok, Readings, Blake, et al., 2011). All of these procedures are expensive and, depending on individual circumstances, may have disappointing success rates. Assisted reproductive techniques are discussed in more detail in Chapter 8.

Adoption is an alternative many couples can also find rewarding (see Chapter 2). Lastly, choosing to remain childfree should not be discounted as a viable option. Many couples who have every reason to think they will have healthy children choose this alternative because they believe their existence is full and rewarding without the presence of children.

Diagnosis of a disorder during pregnancy with prompt treatment at birth to minimize the prognosis and outcome of the disorder is another route to explore. Termination of a pregnancy that reveals a chromosomal or metabolic disorder is a final option.

Help couples decide on a solution that is correct for them, not one they sense you or a counselor feels would be best. They need to consider the ethical philosophy or beliefs of other family members when making their decision, although ultimately, they must do what they believe is best for them as a couple. A useful place to start counseling is with values clarification, to be certain a couple understands what is most important to them.

Future Possibilities

Stem cell research is looking at the possibility immature cells from a healthy embryo (stem cells) could be implanted into an embryo with a known abnormal genetic makeup, replacing the abnormal cells or righting the affected child's genetic composition (Rodts, 2012). Although presently possible, stem cell research is costly and produces some ethical questions (e.g., Is it ethical to change the life course of a fetus who has no rights? Is it ethical to use embryo cells as a source of stem cells?).

Legal and Ethical Aspects of Genetic Screening and Counseling

Nurses can be instrumental in making sure couples who seek genetic counseling receive results in a timely manner and with compassion about what the results may mean to future childbearing. Always keep in mind several legal responsibilities of genetic testing, counseling, and therapy including:

- Participation by couples or individuals in genetic screening must be elective.
- People desiring genetic screening must sign an informed consent for the procedure.
- Results must be interpreted correctly yet provided to the individuals as quickly as possible.
- The results must not be withheld from the individuals and must be given only to those persons directly involved.
- After genetic counseling, persons must not be coerced to undergo procedures such as abortion or sterilization. Any procedure must be a free and individual decision.

Failure to heed these guidelines could result in charges of invasion of privacy, breach of confidentiality, or psychological injury caused by "labeling" someone or imparting unwarranted fear and worry about the significance of a disease or carrier state. If couples are identified as being at risk for having a child with a genetic disorder and are not informed of the risk and offered an appropriate diagnostic procedure such as amniocentesis during a pregnancy, they can bring a "wrongful birth" lawsuit if their child is born with the unrevealed genetic disorder.

What if...7.3 Amy Alvarez is pregnant with twins. One twin fetus is diagnosed as having Down syndrome and the other is not. How would you counsel her if she wanted to abort the affected child when the procedure also might endanger the child without the disorder?

COMMON CHROMOSOMAL DISORDERS RESULTING IN PHYSICAL OR COGNITIVE DEVELOPMENTAL DISORDERS

A number of chromosomal disorders, particularly nondisjunction disorders, are easily detected at birth on physical examination. Many of these disorders leave children cognitively challenged (discussed in Chapter 54).

Trisomy 13 Syndrome (47XY13+ or 47XX13+)

In trisomy 13 syndrome (Patau syndrome), the child has an extra chromosome 13 and is severely cognitively challenged. The incidence of the syndrome is low, approximately 0.45 per 1,000 live births. Midline body disorders such as cleft lip and palate, heart disorders (particularly ventricular septal defects), and abnormal genitalia are present. Other common findings include microcephaly with disorders of the forebrain and forehead, eyes that are smaller than usual (microphthalmos) or absent, and low-set ears (Carey, 2012). Most of these children do not survive beyond early childhood (see Fig. 7.11).

Trisomy 18 Syndrome (47XY18+ or 47XX18+)

Children with trisomy 18 syndrome have three copies of chromosome 18. The incidence is approximately 0.23 per 1,000 live births. These children are severely cognitively challenged and tend to be small for gestational age, have markedly low-set ears, a small jaw, congenital heart defects, and usually misshapen fingers and toes (the index finger deviates or crosses over other fingers). Also, the soles of their feet are often rounded instead of flat (rocker-bottom feet). As in trisomy 13 syndrome, most of these children do not survive beyond infancy (Nelson, Hexem, & Feudtner, 2012).

Cri-du-Chat Syndrome (46XX5p− or 46XY5P−)

Cri-du-chat syndrome is the result of a missing portion of chromosome 5. In addition to an abnormal cry, which sounds much more like the sound of a cat than a human infant's cry, children with cri-du-chat syndrome tend to have a small head, wide-set eyes, a downward slant to the palpebral fissure of the eye, and a recessed mandible. They are severely cognitively challenged (Levy & Marion, 2011).

Turner Syndrome (45X0)

The child with Turner syndrome (gonadal dysgenesis) has only one functional X chromosome. The child is short in stature and has only streak (small and nonfunctional) ovaries. She is sterile and, with the exception of pubic hair, secondary sex characteristics do not develop at puberty. The hairline at the nape of the neck is low set, and the neck may appear to be webbed and short (Fig. 7.14). A newborn may have appreciable edema of the hands and feet and a number of

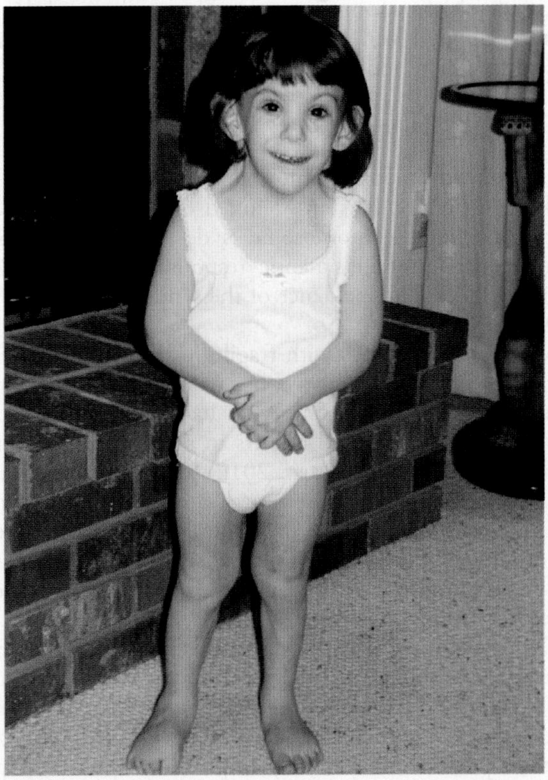

FIGURE 7.14 A 3-year-old with Turner syndrome. Note the wide neck folds.

congenital anomalies, most frequently coarctation (stricture) of the aorta, as well as kidney disorders. The incidence of the syndrome is approximately 1 per 10,000 live births. The disorder can be identified on a sonogram during pregnancy (a nuchal translucency scan) because of the extra skin at the sides of the neck (Levy & Marion, 2011).

Although children with Turner syndrome may be severely cognitively challenged, difficulty in this area is more commonly limited to learning disabilities. Socioemotional adjustment problems may accompany the syndrome because of the lack of fertility and if the nuchal folds are prominent.

Human growth hormone administration can help children with Turner syndrome achieve additional height (Knickmeyer, 2012). If treatment with estrogen is begun at approximately 13 years of age, secondary sex characteristics will appear, and osteoporosis from a lack of estrogen during growing years may be prevented. If females continue taking estrogen for 3 out of every 4 weeks, this produces withdrawal bleeding that results in a menstrual flow. This flow, however, does not correct the basic problem of sterility; ovarian tissue is scant and inadequate for ovulation because of the basic chromosomal aberration. A woman with Turner syndrome could, however, have IVF with surrogate oocyte transfer in order to become pregnant (Karnis, 2012).

Klinefelter Syndrome (47XXY)

Children with Klinefelter syndrome are males with an extra X chromosome. Characteristics of the syndrome may not be noticeable at birth. At puberty, secondary sex characteristics do not develop; the child's testes remain small and produce ineffective sperm (Jospe, 2011). Affected individuals tend to develop gynecomastia (increased breast size) and have an increased risk of male breast cancer. The incidence of the syndrome is about 1 per 1,000 live births. Karyotyping can be used to reveal the additional X chromosome.

Fragile X Syndrome (46XY23q−)

Fragile X syndrome is the most common cause of cognitive challenge in males. It is an X-linked disorder in which one long arm of an X chromosome is defective, which results in inadequate protein synaptic responses (Wang, Bray, & Warren, 2012). The incidence of the syndrome is about 1 in 4,000 males.

Before puberty, boys with fragile X syndrome may typically demonstrate maladaptive behaviors such as hyperactivity, aggression, or autism. They may have reduced intellectual functioning, with marked deficits in speech and arithmetic (Lubs, Stevenson, & Schwartz, 2012). On physical exam, frequent findings identified are a large head, a long face with a high forehead, a prominent lower jaw, large protruding ears, and obesity. Hyperextensive joints and cardiac disorders may also be present. After puberty, enlarged testicles may become evident. Affected individuals are fertile and can reproduce.

Carrier females may show some evidence of the physical and cognitive characteristics. Although intellectual function from the syndrome cannot be improved, a combination of stimulants, α agonists, atypical antipsychotics, and serotonin reuptake inhibitors may improve symptoms of poor concentration and impulsivity (McLennan, Polussa, Tassone, et al., 2011).

QSEN Checkpoint Question 7.5

Safety

Mr. Alvarez reports he has two cognitively challenged cousins who are diagnosed as having fragile X syndrome. Based on the symptoms of this syndrome, what counseling would you consider giving to a parent whose child is diagnosed with this syndrome?

a. Be aware the child will probably not live past puberty.
b. Be certain to limit how much sugar you give your child.
c. Childproof your house of breakable or sharp items.
d. His thickened neck may cause difficulty swallowing.

Look in Appendix A for the best answer and rationale.

Down Syndrome (Trisomy 21) (47XY21+ or 47XX21+)

Trisomy 21, the most frequently occurring chromosomal disorder, occurs in about 1 in 800 pregnancies. In women who are older than 35 years of age, the incidence is as high as 1 in 100 live births (Levy & Marion, 2011).

The physical features of children with Down syndrome are so marked that fetal diagnosis is possible by sonography in utero. The nose is broad and flat. The eyelids have an extra fold of tissue at the inner canthus (an epicanthal fold), and the palpebral fissure (opening between the eyelids) tends to slant laterally upward. The iris of the eye may have white specks, called Brushfield spots. The tongue is apt to protrude from the mouth because the oral cavity is smaller than usual. The back of the head is flat, the neck is short, and an extra pad of fat at the base of the head causes the skin to be so loose it can be lifted easily and so thin it can be revealed on a fetal sonogram.

The ears may be low set. Muscle tone is poor, giving the newborn a rag-doll appearance. This muscle tone can be so lax that the child's toe can be touched against the nose (not possible in the average mature newborn). The fingers of many children with Down syndrome are short and thick, and the little finger is often curved inward. There may be a wide space between the first and second toes and between the first and second fingers. The palm of the hand shows a peculiar crease (a simian line), or a single horizontal crease rather than the usual three creases in the palm (Fig. 7.15).

Children with Down syndrome are usually cognitively challenged to some degree. The challenge can range from an intelligence quotient [IQ] of 50 to 70 to a child who is profoundly affected (IQ less than 20). The extent of the cognitive challenge is not evident at birth, but the fact the brain is not developing well is usually evidenced by a head size smaller than the 10th or 20th percentile at well-child health care visits.

Internally, congenital heart disease, especially an atrioventricular defect, is common. Stenosis or atresia of the duodenum, strabismus, and cataract disorders may also be present. In addition, the child's immune function may be altered, because as these children grow, they are prone to upper respiratory tract infections. Probably due to a second gene aberration, they tend to develop acute lymphocytic leukemia about 20 times more frequently than the general population (Buitenkamp, Pieters, Gallimore, et al., 2012). Even if children are born without an accompanying disorder such as heart disease or don't develop leukemia, their life span usually

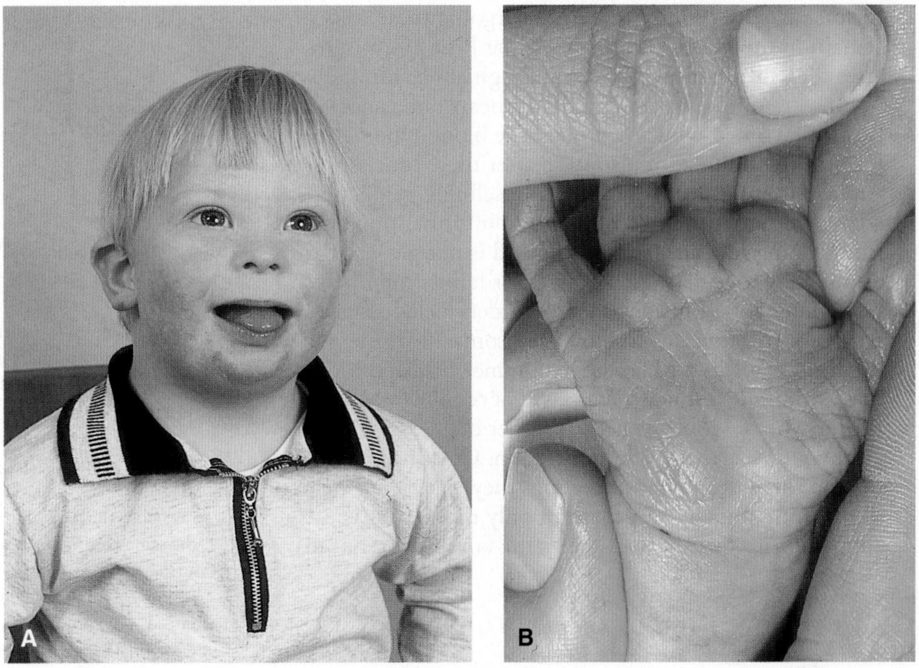

FIGURE 7.15 **(A)** Typical facial features of a child with Down syndrome. **(B)** A simian line, a horizontal crease seen in children with Down syndrome. (SPL/Custom Medical Stock Photograph.)

is limited to only 50 to 60 years, because aging seems to occur faster than usual.

It's important for children with Down syndrome to be enrolled in early educational and play programs so they can develop to their full capacity (see Chapter 54). Because they are prone to infections, sensible precautions such as using a good hand washing technique are important when caring for them. The enlarged tongue may interfere with swallowing and cause choking unless the child is fed slowly. As their neck may not be fully stable, an X-ray to ensure stability is recommended before they engage in strenuous activities such as competitive sports or Special Olympics. As with all newborns, these infants need a physical examination at birth to enable the detection of the genetic disorder and the initiation of parental counseling, support, and future planning.

QSEN Checkpoint Question 7.6

Teamwork & Collaboration

Amy Alvarez's child is born with Down syndrome. What is a common physical feature of newborns with this disorder you would want all of your team members to recognize?

a. Spastic neck muscles
b. An unusual pattern of palm creases
c. A white lock of forehead hair
d. Wrinkles on the soles of the feet

Look in Appendix A for the best answer and rationale.

Childhood Tumors

A number of cancers in children are also associated with chromosomal aberrations. Chief among these are retinoblastoma (chromosome 13), Wilms tumor (chromosome 11), and neuroblastoma (chromosome 1 or 11) (Nicholson & Cimini, 2011). Siblings of children with these cancers need to be tested to reveal if they carry the gene aberration as well and followed closely by a health care provider so early diagnosis and therapy can begin.

What if...7.4 You are particularly interested in exploring one of the 2020 National Health Goals with respect to genetic disorders (see Box 7.1). What would be a possible research topic to explore pertinent to this goal that would be applicable to Amy's family and that would also advance evidence-based practice?

Key Points for Review

- Genetic disorders are those resulting from a distortion in the structure or number of genes or chromosomes. Genetics, the study of gene variation, includes examining how and why such disorders occur.
- A phenotype is a person's outward appearance. Genotype refers to the actual gene composition. A person's genome is the complete set of genes present. A karyotype is a graphic representation of the chromosomes present.
- A person is homozygous for a trait if he or she has two like genes for the trait. A person is heterozygous if he or she has two unlike genes for the trait.
- Mendelian laws predict the likely incidence of recessive or dominant diseases. Division disorders, including nondisjunction disorders, deletion, translocation, and mosaicism, also create genetic disorders.
- Genetic counseling can be a role for nurses with advanced preparation and education. An assessment of genetic disorders consists of a health history, physical examination, and diagnostic studies such as CVS, amniocentesis, and MSAFP analysis.
- Some karyotyping tests, such as CVS and amniocentesis, introduce a risk of spontaneous or threatened

miscarriage. Be certain women undergoing these tests remain in the health care facility for at least 30 minutes after these procedure to be certain vaginal bleeding, uterine cramping, or abnormal fetal heart rate is not present. Women with an Rh-negative blood type need Rh immune globulin administration after these procedures.

- An important aspect of genetic counseling is respecting a couple's right to privacy. Be certain information gained from testing remains confidential and is not given indiscriminately to others, including other family members.
- Common nondisjunction genetic disorders include Down syndrome (trisomy 21), trisomy 13, trisomy 18, Turner syndrome (45XO), and Klinefelter syndrome (47XXY). Most of these syndromes include some degree of cognitive challenge.
- People who are told a genetic disorder does exist in their family may suffer a loss of self-esteem. Offering support to help them deal with the feelings they experience helps in planning nursing care that not only meets QSEN competencies but also best meets the family's total needs.

Critical Thinking Care Study

Gabby Castro, 24 years of age, works as a police officer; her dream is to become a homicide detective. She learned last week her brother, Alex, 26 years of age, has fragile X syndrome. She always knew he was aggressive (and now is serving a jail term for armed robbery), but she thought his aggression was because they moved a lot when they were little and so she thought he never had a chance to achieve in school. Gabby's fiancé, Stanley, 25 years of age, is a manager in his family's hardware store. He asks if the reason she enjoys being a police officer (he views this as mainly a man's occupation) could be because she's missing her X chromosomes. He wants her to have a DNA analysis before they get married to be certain a son won't have fragile X syndrome.

1. Fragile X syndrome is one of the most frequently seen chromosomal abnormalities in boys. Is it true this is associated with aggression? Could the family's frequent moves have contributed to the syndrome?
2. Is it probable that Gabby carries a gene for fragile X syndrome? Is it fair for Stanley to ask her to have a DNA analysis before he agrees to marry her?
3. Stanley asks if the reason Gabby wants to be a detective could be because her X chromosomes are missing. Is this likely? Would you recommend Gabby rethink her relationship with Stanley before agreeing to marriage?

Patient Scenario

The Summerton Family

Read about the Summerton family, a family concerned about a genetic disorder, then answer the questions to further sharpen your skills and grow more familiar with NCLEX-type questions related to genetic assessment and counseling. Confirm your answers are correct by reading the rationales.

Visit http://thePoint.lww.com

Answers and Rationales

Looking for answers to the What If. . . and Critical Thinking Care Study questions?

Visit http://thePoint.lww.com

References

Allickson, J. G., Sanchez, A., Yefimenko, N., et al. (2011). Recent studies assessing the proliferative capability of a novel adult stem cell identified in menstrual blood. *Open Stem Cell Journal, 3*(2011), 4–10.

American Congress of Obstetricians and Gynecologists. (2011). *Committee opinion: Family history as a risk assessment tool.* Washington, DC: Author.

Arbour, L. T., Beking, K., Le, N. D., et al. (2010). Rates of congenital anomalies and other adverse birth outcomes in an offspring cohort of registered nurses from British Columbia, Canada. *Canadian Journal of Public Health, 101*(3), 230–234.

Banaszkiewicz, K., Sitek, E. J., Rudzińska, M., et al. (2012). Huntington's disease from the patient, caregiver and physician's perspectives: Three sides of the same coin? *Journal of Neural Transmission, 119*(11), 1361–1365.

Bodurtha, J., & Strauss, J. F. (2012). Genomics and perinatal care. *New England Journal of Medicine, 366*(1), 64–73.

Bredaki, F. E., Poon, L. C., Birdir, C., et al. (2012). First-trimester screening for neural tube defects using alpha-fetoprotein. *Fetal Diagnostic Therapies, 31*(2), 109–114.

Buitenkamp, T. D., Pieters, R., Gallimore, N. E., et al. (2012). Outcome in children with Down syndrome and acute lymphoblastic leukemia: Role of IKZF1 deletions and CRLF2 aberrations. *Leukemia, 26*(10), 2204–2211.

Carey, J. C. (2012). Perspectives on the care and management of infants with trisomy 18 and trisomy 13: Striving for balance. *Current Opinion in Pediatrics, 24*(6), 672–678.

Carter, E. R., & Marshall, S. G. (2011). Cystic fibrosis. In K. J. Marcdante, R. M. Kliegman, H. B. Jenson, et al. (Eds.), *Nelson essentials of pediatrics* (6th ed., pp. 520–522). Philadelphia, PA: Saunders/Elsevier.

Cassidy, S. B., Schwartz, S., Miller, J. L., et al. (2012). Prader-Willi syndrome. *Genetics in Medicine, 14*(1), 10–26.

Check, J. H., Katsoff, B., Wilson, C., et al. (2012). Pregnancy outcome following fresh vs frozen embryo transfer into gestational carriers using a simplified slow freeze protocol. *Clinical & Experimental Obstetrics & Gynecology, 39*(1), 23–24.

Choi, H., Van Riper, M., & Thoyre, S. (2012). Decision making following a prenatal diagnosis of down syndrome: An integrative review. *Journal of Midwifery & Women's Health, 57*(2), 156–164.

Choolani, M., Mahyuddin, A. P., & Hahn, S. (2012). The promise of fetal cells in maternal blood. *Best Practice & Research: Clinical Obstetrics & Gynaecology, 26*(5), 655–667.

Christianson, M. S., & Wallach, E. E. (2011). Infertility and assisted reproductive technologies. In K. J. Hurt, M. W. Guile, J. L. Bienstock, et al. (Eds.), *The Johns Hopkins manual of gynecology and obstetrics* (4th ed., pp. 421–437). Philadelphia, PA: Lippincott Williams & Wilkins.

Collins, S. L., & Impey, L. (2012). Prenatal diagnosis: Types and techniques. *Early Human Development, 88*(1), 3–8.

Domen, J., Gandy, K., & Dalal, J. (2012). Emerging uses for pediatric hematopoietic stem cells. *Pediatric Research, 71*(4–2), 411–417.

Duffin, C. (2012). Nurses need to keep pace with genetics knowledge, say experts. *Nursing Standard, 26*(19), 11.

Feldman, E. A. (2012). The Genetic Information Nondiscrimination Act (GINA): Public policy and medical practice in the age of personalized medicine. *Journal of General Internal Medicine, 6*(2), 743–746.

Geaghan, S. M. (2012). Fetal laboratory medicine: On the frontier of maternal-fetal medicine. *Clinical Chemistry, 58*(2), 337–352.

Golombok, S., Readings, J., Blake, L., et al. (2011). Families created through surrogacy: Mother-child relationships and children's psychological adjustment at age 7. *Developmental Psychology, 47*(6), 1579–1588.

Harper, J., Magli, M. C., Lundin, K., et al. (2012). When and how should new technology be introduced into the IVF laboratory? *Human Reproduction, 27*(2), 303–313.

Harrington, D. L., Smith, M. M., Zhang, Y., et al. (2011). Cognitive domains that predict time to diagnosis in prodromal Huntington disease. *Journal of Neurology, Neurosurgery & Psychiatry, 83*(6), 612–619.

Jondeau, G., Michel, J. B., & Boileau, C. (2011). The translational science of Marfan syndrome. *Heart, 97*(15), 1206–1214.

Jospe, N. (2011). Disorders of puberty. In K. J. Marcdante, R. M. Kliegman, H. B. Jenson, et al. (Eds.), *Nelson essentials of pediatrics* (6th ed., pp. 645–653). Philadelphia, PA: Saunders/Elsevier.

Karnis, M. F. (2012). Fertility, pregnancy, and medical management of Turner syndrome in the reproductive years. *Fertility & Sterility, 98*(4), 787–791.

Katorza, E., & Achiron, R. (2012). Early pregnancy scanning for fetal anomalies—The new standard? *Clinical Obstetrics & Gynecology, 55*(1), 199–216.

Kmietowicz, Z. (2012). Trial is started to see whether gene therapy can improve lung function in cystic fibrosis. *BMJ: British Medical Journal, 344*(3), e2141.

Knickmeyer, R. C. (2012). Turner syndrome: Advances in understanding altered cognition, brain structure and function. *Current Opinion in Neurology, 25*(2), 144–149.

Levy, P. A., & Marion, R. W. (2011) Chromosomal disorders. In K. J. Marcdante, R. M. Kliegman, H. B. Jenson, et al. (Eds.), *Nelson essentials of pediatrics* (6th ed., pp. 179–182). Philadelphia, PA: Saunders/Elsevier.

Lewis, D. W. (2011). Neurodegenerative disorders. In K. J. Marcdante, R. M. Kliegman, H. B. Jenson, et al. (Eds.), *Nelson essentials of pediatrics* (6th ed., pp. 704–706). Philadelphia, PA: Saunders/Elsevier.

Liu, G., Yang, D., Sun, Y., et al. (2012). Differing clinical impact of BRCA1 and BRCA2 mutations in serous ovarian cancer. *Pharmacogenomics, 13*(13), 1523–1535.

Lubs, H. A., Stevenson, R. E., & Schwartz, C. E. (2012). Fragile X and X-linked intellectual disability: Four decades of discovery. *American Journal of Human Genetics, 90*(4), 579–590.

Macleod, R. A., & Drexler, H. G. (2013). Classical and molecular cytogenetic analysis. *Methods in Molecular Biology,* 946, 39–60.

McLennan, Y., Polussa, J., Tassone, F., et al. (2011). Fragile X syndrome. *Current Genomics, 12*(3), 216–224.

McNair, T., & Altman, K. (2011). Miscarriage & recurrent pregnancy loss. In K. J. Hurt, M. W. Guile, J. L. Bienstock, et al. (Eds.), *The Johns Hopkins manual of gynecology and obstetrics* (4th ed., pp. 438–447). Philadelphia, PA: Lippincott Williams & Wilkins.

Mele, C. (2012). Gene therapy: A genetic era of technological development to treat pediatric genetic disorders. *Journal of Pediatric Nursing, 27*(2), 180–183.

Menezes, M. P., & Ouvrier, R. A. (2012). Peripheral neuropathy associated with mitochondrial disease in children. *Developmental Medicine & Child Neurology, 54*(5), 407–414.

Mogra, R., Alabbad, N., & Hyett, J. (2012). Increased nuchal translucency and congenital heart disease. *Early Human Development, 88*(5), 261–267.

Mosquera, C., Miller, R. S., & Simpson, L. L. (2012). Twin-twin transfusion syndrome. *Seminars in Perinatology, 36*(3), 182–189.

Nelson, K. E., Hexem, K. R., & Feudtner, C. (2012). Inpatient hospital care of children with trisomy 13 and trisomy 18 in the United States. *Pediatrics, 129*(5), 869–876.

Nicholson, J. M., & Cimini, D. (2011). How mitotic errors contribute to karyotypic diversity in cancer. *Advances in Cancer Research, 112*(4), 43–75.

Noble, J. A., & Erlich, H. A. (2012). Genetics of type 1 diabetes. *Cold Spring Harbor Perspectives in Medicine, 2*(1), a007732.

Panepinto, J. A., & Scott, J. P. (2011). Anemia. In K. J. Marcdante, R. M. Kliegman, H. B. Jenson, et al. (Eds.), *Nelson essentials of pediatrics* (6th ed., pp. 559–572). Philadelphia, PA: Saunders/Elsevier.

Quenby, S. (2012). Recurrent miscarriage. In D. K. Edmonds (Ed.), *Dewhurst's textbook of obstetrics & gynaecology* (8th ed., pp. 60–65). Oxford, UK: John Wiley & Sons.

Rodts, M. F. (2012). Cord blood stem cells and cord tissue to aid bone regeneration. *Orthopedic Nursing, 31*(1), 35–36.

Russell, J. B., Denne, E. W., & Schwartz, D. (2011). Preconception counseling and prenatal care. In K. J. Hurt, M. W. Guile, J. L. Bienstock, et al. (Eds.), *The Johns Hopkins manual of gynecology and obstetrics* (4th ed., pp. 56–72). Philadelphia, PA: Lippincott Williams & Wilkins.

Savage, P., & Seckl, M. (2012). Gestational trophoblast tumours. In D. K. Edmonds (Ed.), *Dewhurst's textbook of obstetrics & gynaecology* (8th ed., pp. 66–75). Oxford, UK: John Wiley & Sons.

Simpson, J. L., Holzgreve, W., & Driscoll, D. A. (2012). Genetic counseling and genetic screening. In S. G. Gabbe, J. R. Niebyl, J. L. Simpson, et al. (Eds.), *Obstetrics: Normal and problem pregnancies* (6th ed., pp. 193–209). Philadelphia, PA: Elsevier/Saunders.

Skotko, B. G., Levine, S. P., & Goldstein, R. (2011a). Having a brother or sister with Down syndrome: Perspectives from siblings. *American Journal of Medical Genetics, 155*(10), 2335–2347.

Skotko, B. G., Levine, S. P., & Goldstein, R. (2011b). Having a son or daughter with Down syndrome: Perspectives from mothers and fathers. *American Journal of Medical Genetics, 155*(10), 2348–2359.

Tasker, R. C., & McClure, R. (2013). Genetics. In R. C. Tasker & R. McClure (Eds.), *Oxford handbook of paediatrics* (pp. 925–952). Oxford, UK: Oxford University Press.

Tsai, A. C., Manchester, D. K., & Elias, E. R. (2012). Genetics & dysmorphology. In W. Hay, M. Levin, R. Deterding, et al. (Eds.), *Current diagnosis & treatment pediatrics* (21st ed., pp. 1088–1122). New York, NY: McGraw-Hill/Lange.

U.S. Department of Health and Human Services. (2010). *Healthy people 2020.* Washington, DC: Author.

Waller-Wise, R. (2011). Umbilical cord blood: Information for childbirth educators. *Journal of Perinatal Education, 20*(1), 54–60.

Wang, T., Bray, S. M., & Warren, S. T. ((2012). New perspectives on the biology of fragile X syndrome. *Current Opinion in Genetics & Development, 22*(3), 256–263.

Chapter 8

Nursing Care of the Family Having Difficulty Conceiving a Child

KEY TERMS

- alternative insemination
- anovulation
- cryptorchidism
- endometriosis
- erectile dysfunction
- in vitro fertilization
- pelvic inflammatory disease
- sperm count
- sperm motility
- spermatogenesis
- sterility
- subfertility
- varicocele

OBJECTIVES

After mastering the contents of this chapter, you should be able to:

1. Describe common causes of difficulty with conception or subfertility in both men and women.
2. Identify 2020 National Health Goals related to subfertility that nurses can help the nation achieve.
3. Describe common assessments necessary to detect subfertility.
4. Formulate nursing diagnoses related to subfertility.
5. Identify expected outcomes for a subfertile couple to help them manage seamless transitions across differing health care settings.
6. Using the nursing process, plan nursing care that includes the six competencies of Quality & Safety Education for Nurses (QSEN): Patient-Centered Care, Teamwork & Collaboration, Evidence-Based Practice (EBP), Quality Improvement (QI), Safety, and Informatics.
7. Implement nursing care designed to improve subfertility and increase ability to conceive a child, such as health teaching about ovulation and conception.
8. Evaluate outcomes for achievement and effectiveness of nursing care to be certain expected outcomes have been achieved.
9. Integrate knowledge of fertility and subfertility with the interplay of nursing process, the six competencies of QSEN and Family Nursing to promote quality maternal and child health nursing care.

Cheryl and Bob Carl, married when they were both 25 years old, planned to wait 5 years before beginning their family so they could save money for a house. On the day they moved into their new home, Cheryl stopped taking her birth control pills. At the end of a year, however, she still was not pregnant so she began fertility testing. Three years later, they are now undergoing their second cycle of in vitro fertilization and embryo transfer. The Carls have applied for a second mortgage on their house to finance the fertility testing. At a health care visit, Mrs. Carl states, "This is my fault because I'm so rigid. Look how I had to buy the house before I could even consider getting pregnant, and now we'll probably lose it. I've made our whole life revolve around trying to get pregnant instead of enjoying life."

Previous chapters described normal ovulation and conception and ways to prevent pregnancy. This chapter adds information about care of the couple who is unable to conceive.

How could you best help the Carls?

Many marriage customs, such as throwing rice, originate from ancient rituals to promote fertility. The existence of such common rituals is evidence of the importance of having children for the average couple and society as a whole.

Infertility is a term used to describe the inability to conceive a child or sustain a pregnancy to birth. A couple is said to be *infertile* if they have not become pregnant after at least 1 year of unprotected sex. Because most couples have the potential to conceive, but they are just less able to conceive without additional help, the term **subfertility** is more often used today. Subfertility affects as many as 11% to 14% of couples who desire children (Sheaves, 2013).

Couples who feel they need fertility testing consist of a wide range of people: many are married couples, some are planning to marry, some desire to remain single but bear a child, and some are men who have sex with men or women who have sex with women who want to have a child through an assisted fertility method. Occasionally, others are looking for assurance they are unable to have children so they can discontinue a contraceptive method (although they'll need to be cautioned to maintain safer sex practices if their relationship isn't monogamous). People who are discontinuing using condoms so a woman can become pregnant need this same safer sex caution.

When a couple first begins fertility counseling, they usually have fears and anxieties not only about their ability to conceive but also about what an identified problem will mean to their future lifestyle and family. Without information about the cause of their subfertility, each may blame the other or carry unexpressed anger toward his or her partner. Some couples may strongly desire a child but feel anxious about impending parenthood, which would bring with it a loss of independence. For all these reasons, subfertility screening and counseling can be both an emotionally difficult and a physically demanding process, often creating a high level of strain on a couple's relationship, especially if they don't maintain open communication (Chachamovich, Chachamovich, Ezer, et al., 2010). The level of stress a couple is experiencing is important because increased family stress produces a higher than usual level of intimate partner violence (American Congress of Obstetricians and Gynecologists [ACOG], 2011). Having healthy children when they are wanted is such a priority, a 2020 National Health Goal aimed at reducing subfertility has been established (Box 8.1).

BOX 8.1 Nursing Care Planning Based on 2020 National Health Goals

One of the 2020 National Health Goals identified by *Healthy People 2020* directly addresses the problem of subfertility:

- Reduce the proportion of woman aged 18 to 44 years who have impaired fecundity (fertility) from 12% to a target of 10.8% (U.S. Department of Health and Human Services [DHHS], 2010; see www.healthypeople.gov).

To meet this health objective, nurses need to keep active in health promotion, identify and help prevent problems that could lead to subfertility such as poor nutrition early in life, and play active roles in teaching clients about safer sex practices (see Chapter 5) so the incidence of sexually transmitted infections and pelvic inflammatory disease can be reduced.

Nursing Process Overview

For a Couple With Subfertility

Assessment

Subfertility assessment used to require many months and many tests, all of which had the potential to interfere with a couple's self-image, self-esteem, and lifestyle. Today, a subfertility investigation is usually limited to only three assessments: semen analysis, ovulation monitoring, and tubal patency. Even with this more directed approach to evaluation, a nursing assessment often reveals that one or both partners feel inadequate or angry and frustrated by what has happened to them and their need to undergo testing. Questions such as, "How do you feel about what has happened?" or "How do you think your partner feels about not being able to conceive?" may be enough to encourage partners to express these concerns. Talking with both partners together may be advantageous, because they may feel more comfortable speaking about their problem together. It is important, however, to spend some time alone with each client in case there is anything a partner wishes to discuss privately. This might be the only opportunity for one of them to ask that one "silly" question or voice a fear he or she believes is too foolish to ask or bring up in front of his or her partner.

Nursing Diagnosis

Nursing diagnoses related to subfertility are likely to focus on psychosocial issues associated with the inability to conceive and the potentially nerve-wracking process of fertility testing and management. Examples of possible diagnoses include:

- Fear related to possible outcome of subfertility studies
- Situational low self-esteem related to the apparent inability to conceive
- Anxiety related to what the process of fertility testing will entail
- Deficient knowledge related to measures to promote fertility
- Anticipatory grieving related to failure to conceive or sustain a pregnancy
- Powerlessness related to repeated unsuccessful attempts at achieving conception
- Hopelessness related to perception of no viable alternatives to usual conception

If required tests interfere with a couple's relationship (including sexual patterns), "sexual dysfunction related to command performance of subfertility therapy" might be applicable.

Expected Outcomes and Planning

In establishing expected outcomes with a couple undergoing fertility testing and counseling, be certain the couple realizes even after the reason for their subfertility is identified, fertility may not be instantaneous. In some instances, a couple may need to change or modify their goals if tests begin to show what they first wanted—to have a child without medical intervention—is impossible. Participation in a support group may allow a couple to work through the stress fertility testing places on their lives. The National Infertility Association (www.resolve.org) is a helpful support group for couples with subfertility and can be helpful in offering referral sources and support. A second helpful organization is the American Society for Reproductive Medicine (www.asrm.org).

Implementation

Fertility testing can be costly for a couple because not all health insurance programs provide reimbursement for these procedures. Because of this, be certain couples are informed beforehand of specific estimates of the cost of testing or therapy so they can budget and plan their resources and the next steps they want taken.

Suggesting a couple combine involvement with fertility testing with ongoing activities or beginning new activities together, such as taking a night school course, planting a garden, or learning a new sport or hobby, is a way of helping them reduce the feeling that their entire existence revolves around the testing procedures. It also may help provide them with time for sharing experiences and increasing intimacy, helping to compensate for any decreased enjoyment that comes from "scheduled" sexual relations.

Throughout testing, couples need thorough education about the various procedures being done. Make sure to review any specific instructions about preprocedural and postprocedural care. Depending on their motivations, a couple's reaction to study results may vary from relief, to stoic acceptance, to grief for children never to be born. Each partner may wonder whether the other will be able to continue the relationship if he or she turns out to be the "subfertile" one. Couples need the active support of health care personnel from the first day they brace themselves to ask, "Exactly why are we childless?" until the end, regardless of the results.

Outcome Evaluation

Examples of expected outcomes in this area include:

- The client rearranges work plans to manage the schedule of fertility testing by 1 month's time.
- The couple verbalizes they understand their individual subfertility problem after preliminary testing.
- The couple demonstrates a high level of self-esteem after fertility studies, even in the face of disappointing study outcomes.

For a couple with a problem of subfertility, an evaluation is best if it is ongoing because, as circumstances around them change, so may their goals and desires. Until they can accept an alternative method of having children—adoption or an assisted reproductive technique such as **alternative insemination** (deposition of sperm into a woman's cervix or uterus) or **in vitro fertilization** (IVF; the union of sperm and ovum under laboratory conditions)—former plans to have children have been crushed.

Continuing or future evaluations are also important because a couple who decides at age 20 years to choose child-free living may change their minds at a later date. In the same way, a couple who chooses an assisted reproductive technique may decide after a number of unsuccessful attempts that they are no longer interested in this method of conception. Keeping the evaluation as an ongoing process allows such plans to be modified as necessary. Because establishing fertility is an ever changing field of study, encourage couples seen for subfertility who couldn't conceive but are still interested in having a child to contact their subfertility setting every 6 to 12 months to inquire about new discoveries in the field and if any of these might apply to their situation.

SUBFERTILITY

As previously mentioned, subfertility is said to exist when a pregnancy has not occurred after at least 1 year of engaging in unprotected coitus (Hamilton, 2012). In *primary subfertility*, there have been no previous conceptions; in *secondary subfertility*, there has been a previous viable pregnancy but the couple is unable to conceive at present. **Sterility** is the inability to conceive because of a known condition, such as the absence of a uterus.

In about 40% of couples with a subfertility problem, the cause of subfertility is multifactorial; in other words, more than one reason for the loss of full fertility is involved. In about 30% of couples, it is the man who is subfertile; in 70%, it is the woman. Of women seen for a fertility evaluation, 20% to 25% experience ovulatory failure; another 20% experience tubal, vaginal, cervical, or uterine problems. In about 10% of couples, no known cause for the subfertility can be discovered despite all the diagnostic tests currently available. Such couples are categorized as having unexplained subfertility (Hanson & Burke, 2011).

Some couples, because they are unaware of the average length of time it takes to achieve a pregnancy, may worry they are subfertile when they are not. On average, if they engage in coitus about four times per week, 65% to 75% of couples will conceive within 6 months; 90% within 12 months. These periods will be longer if sexual relations are less frequent (Ghadir, Ambartsumyan, & Decherny, 2013).

Couples who engage in coitus daily, hoping to cause early impregnation, may actually have more difficulty conceiving than those who space coitus every other day. This is because too-frequent coitus can lower a man's sperm count to a level below optimal fertility. All couples who focus their sexual relations on trying to increase sperm/ovum exposure by scheduling sex may find their lives governed by temperature charts and "good days" and "bad days" to such an extent that their relationship suffers.

Age is related to subfertility. Because of this gradual decline in fertility, women who defer pregnancy into their late 30s are apt to have more difficulty conceiving than their younger counterparts. Women who are using oral, injectable, or implanted hormones for contraception may have difficulty becoming pregnant for several months after discontinuing these medications because it takes that long for the body to restore normal functioning. Most couples can benefit from some practical information on how to increase the chances of achieving conception on their own (Box 8.2).

What if...8.1 You hear Cheryl Carl repeat she believes her subfertility problem is her fault because she's too rigid. Does a rigid personality affect fertility? How could you help Cheryl feel more comfortable about what has happened in her life?

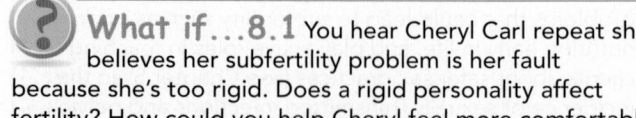

BOX 8.2 Nursing Care Planning to Empower a Family

Q. Cheryl Carl asks you, "Is there anything we can do to help increase our chances of conception?"
A. The following are time-honored suggestions to help aid conception:

- Determine the time of ovulation through the use of basal body temperature or analysis of cervical secretions, then plan sexual relations for every other day around the time of ovulation.
- Although frequent intercourse may stimulate sperm production, men need sperm recovery time after ejaculation to maintain an adequate sperm count. This is why coitus every other day, rather than every day, during the fertile period will probably yield faster results.
- The male-superior position is the best position for coitus to achieve conception because it places sperm closest to the cervical opening.
- The male should try for deep penetration so ejaculation places sperm as close as possible to the cervix. Elevating a woman's hips on a small pillow can facilitate sperm being deposited near the opening to the cervix.
- A woman should remain on her back with knees drawn up for at least 20 minutes after ejaculation to help sperm remain near the cervix.
- Don't use douching or lubricants before or after intercourse so vaginal pH is unaltered, which can interfere with sperm mobility.
- Eat a diet high in slowly digested carbohydrates, low in saturated or trans fats, and moderate in protein.
- Maintain a body weight that results in a body mass index between 18.5 and 24.9.
- Exercise about 30 minutes per day to help keep blood glucose and insulin levels stabilized.
- Choose a new activity the two of you can do together, such as learning how to bowl or ballroom dance, so you create an activity separate from planning a baby. This not only helps to pass the time in a positive way but also offers a positive outlook for a month when you don't conceive.

FERTILITY ASSESSMENT

The age of a couple and the degree of apprehension they feel about possible subfertility can make a difference in determining when they should be referred for fertility evaluation. Although some health care plans or specific settings set limits on the age range in which fertility testing can be scheduled, such as not before age 18 years and not after age 45 years, other settings do not establish such limits, allowing couples of any age to benefit from assessment.

As a rule:

- If a woman is younger than 35 years of age, it is usually suggested she have an evaluation after 1 year of subfertility.
- If a woman is older than 35 years, she should be seen after 6 months. Referral is recommended sooner because assisted reproductive strategies such as IVF, as well as common alternatives to natural childbearing such as adoption, are also limited by age. It would be doubly unfortunate if a couple delayed fertility testing so long they not only learned they could not conceive but also were considered to be "too old" to be prospective parents by alternative methods.
- If the couple is extremely apprehensive or knows of a specific problem that could be causing their difficulty in conceiving, studies should never be delayed, regardless of the couple's age (Fritz & Speroff, 2010).

Because most fertility tests are conducted in ambulatory settings, nurses play key roles on fertility teams to help achieve this goal, such as:

- Educating couples about the variety of tests and procedures that may be performed
- Helping clients identify and express their feelings about their desire to have a child
- Helping clients express how far they are willing to go in testing and procedures to achieve a child or how they might feel if, at the end of testing, it is revealed pregnancy will not be possible
- Assuming responsibility for health assessment, client education, and counseling
- Helping educate couples about advanced techniques of assisted reproduction, many of which are complex and demand knowledgeable, ongoing involvement from the couple
- Counseling clients about available alternatives when pregnancy cannot be achieved, such as adoption or child-free living

No matter what problem is suspected, basic fertility assessment begins with a health history and physical examination of both sexual partners.

QSEN Checkpoint Question 8.1

Patient-Centered Care

Cheryl is unhappy that she waited until she bought a house to plan on having a child. What fact could you cite to Cheryl?

a. She should have begun trying to conceive by age 25 years, but her outcome should still be positive.
b. She asked for testing well before the average woman, who asks at age 30 years.
c. Waiting for 1 year after being unable to conceive is the average time for seeking help.
d. We all make decisions in life that later on we wish we had not made.

Look in Appendix A for the best answer and rationale.

Health History

Nurses often assume the responsibility for the initial history taking with a subfertile couple. Because of the wide variety of factors that may be responsible for subfertility, a minimum history for the man should include:

- His general health
- A typical 24-hour food intake, including alternative therapies such as herbs and whether he ingests alcohol, uses recreational drugs, or smokes or uses tobacco
- If he had a congenital health problem, such as hypospadias or cryptorchidism (defined below) or a past illness such as mumps orchitis, urinary tract infection, or a sexually transmitted disease that could affect fertility
- If he ever had radiation to his testes because of childhood cancer, X-rays, or an industrial accident
- If he had an operation such as surgical repair of a hernia or torsion of the testes, which could have compromised the blood supply to his testes
- If he has any current illness, particularly an endocrine one or a low-grade infection
- If his job or lifestyle involves sitting all day
- What his sexual practices are, such as frequency of coitus, masturbation, coital positions used, or if he ever experiences failure to achieve ejaculation
- What past contraceptive measures, if any, he has used or if he has children from a previous relationship

Asking about alternative therapies is important because a couple who wants to have a child could be investigating nontraditional as well as traditional methods that they have heard will aid in conception (Frass, Strassl, Friehs, et al., 2012). Asking about herbs they may be using can reveal the couple is using an herb that could possibly be causing subfertility or one that would interfere with any procedure or medication prescribed for them after their subfertility investigation is complete.

Most couples assume subfertility is the woman's problem. Many women, even after a careful explanation that the problem is their male partner's and not theirs, continue to show low self-esteem, as if the fault did rest with them. For a thorough women's health history, ask about:

- Past pregnancies, miscarriages, or abortions
- History of contraceptive use
- Current or past reproductive tract problems, such as infections
- Overall health, emphasizing endocrine problems such as galactorrhea (breast nipple secretions) or symptoms of thyroid dysfunction (always tired or hyperactive)
- Abdominal or pelvic operations that could have compromised blood flow to pelvic organs
- Past history of a childhood cancer treated with radiation that might have reduced ovarian function
- The use of douches or intravaginal medications or sprays that could interfere with vaginal pH
- Exposure to occupational hazards, such as X-rays or toxic substances
- Nutrition, including an adequate source of folic acid and avoidance of trans fats
- If she can detect ovulation through such symptoms as breast tenderness, midcycle "wetness," or lower abdominal pain (*mittelschmerz*)
- If she is from a country that allows the practice, ask about female circumcision as this can leave vulvar scars that interfere with penetration and deposition of sperm close to the cervix

Also obtain a menstrual history, including age of menarche; length, regularity, and frequency of menstrual periods; amount of flow; and any difficulties the woman experiences, such as dysmenorrhea or premenstrual dysphoric disorder (PDD) (see Chapter 47).

While obtaining health histories, be certain to take time with each partner individually and as a couple to encourage questions and to discuss overall attitudes toward sexual relations, pregnancy, and parenting. A frank discussion centered on resolving the couple's fears and clearing up any long-standing confusion or misinformation will help to set a positive tone for future interactions, and hopefully, establish a feeling of trust and increased self-esteem. Talking with both partners can also help them clarify their feelings about subfertility and why they are seeking help in this area of their life (Box 8.3).

It is not unusual to see a couple move through steps of denial, anger, bargaining, and depression before they reach a level of acceptance that they are different in this one area of life from others, but that they are not limited in their ability to achieve in other areas. Acceptance in this way helps them make adjustments in their wants or plans and feel fulfilled again.

Physical Assessment

After a thorough history, both men and women need a complete physical examination. For the man, important aspects of this are whether secondary sexual characteristics, such as pubic hair, are present as well as no genital abnormalities, such as the absence of a vas deferens or the presence of undescended testes or a varicocele (enlargement of a testicular vein), are present. A hydrocele (a collection of fluid in the tunica vaginalis of the scrotum) is rarely associated with subfertility but should be documented if present.

For a woman, a thorough physical assessment, including a breast and thyroid examination, is necessary to rule out current illness. Of particular importance, again, are secondary sex characteristics, which indicate maturity and suggest good pituitary function (see Chapter 33 for a discussion of Tanner stages). A complete pelvic examination, including a Pap test (see Chapter 11), is needed to rule out anatomic disorders and infection.

Fertility Testing

Basic fertility testing is geared toward answering three questions:

1. Is there sperm of good quality and number available?
2. Are ova (eggs) available (i.e., woman is ovulating)?
3. Is it capable for the sperm and egg to meet in a receptive environment?

To answer these questions, only three tests are commonly used: semen analysis in the male and ovulation monitoring and tubal patency assessment in the female. Nurses play key roles in preparing couples for these tests, helping them schedule the studies appropriately, and supporting them while they wait for results (Eggertson, 2011).

Additional testing for men, if warranted, can include urinalysis; a complete blood count; blood typing, including Rh factor; a serologic test for syphilis; a test for the presence of

BOX 8.3 Nursing Care Planning Based on Effective Communication

Cheryl Carl has been trying to get pregnant for 4 years. She and her husband agreed to in vitro fertilization at a cost of approximately $10,000 per month, even though her religion does not approve of this technique. Every time you see her at the fertility clinic, she seems sadder than the previous time.

Less Effective Communication

Nurse: How is everything going, Mrs. Carl?
Mrs. Carl: Fine. I'm just tired of no results.
Nurse: You know that's partly your fault, Mrs. Carl. You waited 4 years before you came for an evaluation.
Mrs. Carl: I guess I don't make good decisions.
Nurse: Good parents know how to do that, so that's something you'll need to learn, assuming you do get to be a parent.

More Effective Communication

Nurse: How is everything going, Mrs. Carl?
Mrs. Carl: Fine. I'm just tired of no results.
Nurse: Considering you have been trying for such a long time, I think you're doing very well.
Mrs. Carl: Being patient is hard.
Nurse: Think of how well learning to be patient the way you're doing now will help you become a good parent.

Clients may not make the same choices about fertility testing or management you might make because such decisions are based on individual circumstances and situations. Therefore, be careful not to criticize clients for making choices that were not the same as yours would have been. A more effective technique is to support them at that point and help them find ways to continue to feel good about themselves in order to maintain self-esteem.

(HIV; erythrocyte sedimentation rate (an increased rate indicates inflammation); protein-bound iodine (a test for thyroid function); cholesterol level (arterial plaques could interfere with pelvic blood flow); and follicle-stimulating hormone (FSH), luteinizing hormone (LH), and testosterone levels (Sabanegh & Agarwal, 2012).

Advanced testing for a woman may include a rubella titer, a serologic test for syphilis, an HIV evaluation, a thyroid uptake determination, and assays for FSH, estrogen, LH, and serial progesterone levels. If a woman has a history of galactorrhea (breast milk secretions), a serum prolactin level will be obtained, as increased prolactin levels reduce the secretion of pituitary hormones. A pelvic sonogram may be performed to rule out ovarian, tubal, or uterine structural disorders.

FACTORS THAT CAUSE MALE SUBFERTILITY

The factors that most commonly lead to male subfertility include:

- Disturbance in **spermatogenesis** (production of sperm cells)
- Inadequate production of FSH and LH in the pituitary, which stimulates the production of sperm
- Obstruction in the seminiferous tubules, ducts, or vessels, which prevent the movement of spermatozoa
- Qualitative or quantitative changes in the seminal fluid, which prevent **sperm motility** (movement of sperm)
- Development of autoimmunity, which immobilizes sperm
- Problems in ejaculation or deposition, which prevents spermatozoa from being placed close enough to a woman's cervix to allow ready penetration and fertilization
- Chronic or excessive exposure to X-rays or radioactive substances, general ill health, poor diet, and stress, all of which may interfere with sperm production

Limited Sperm Count

The **sperm count** is the number of sperm in a single ejaculation or in a milliliter of semen. The minimum sperm count considered normal has:

- Thirty-three to 46 million sperm per milliliter of seminal fluid, or 50 million per ejaculation
- Fifty percent of sperm that are motile
- Thirty percent that are normal in shape and form

Spermatozoa must be produced and maintained at a temperature slightly lower than body temperature to be fully motile. This is why the testes, in which sperm are produced and stored, are suspended in the scrotal sac away from body heat. Any condition that significantly increases body temperature, such as a chronic infection from tuberculosis or recurrent sinusitis, has the potential to raise scrotal heat enough to lower a sperm count. Actions that directly increase scrotal heat, such as working at a desk job or driving a great deal every day (e.g., salesmen, motorcyclists) may have lower sperm counts compared with men whose occupations allow them to be ambulatory at least part of each day. Frequent use of hot tubs or saunas may also lower sperm counts. Maintaining an ideal body weight (body mass index [BMI] of 18.5 to 24.9) is a general health measure to maintain as excessive weight may alter testosterone production and sperm production (Fariello, Pariz, Spaine, et al., 2012).

Congenital abnormalities, such as **cryptorchidism** (undescended testes) if surgical repair of this problem was not completed until after puberty or if the spermatic cord became twisted after the surgery, is yet another reason sperm count may be lowered.

Another worry is that a **varicocele** (varicosity of the spermatic vein) could increase temperature within the testes and thus slow and disrupt spermatogenesis; although whether this actually causes much temperature difference is in doubt. In some men, surgery to repair the varicocele has the potential to increase the chance for conception (Miyaoka & Esteves, 2012).

Still other conditions that may inhibit sperm production are past trauma to the testes; surgery on or near the testicles that has resulted in impaired testicular circulation; and endocrine imbalances, particularly of the thyroid, pancreas, or pituitary glands. Drug use or excessive alcohol use and environmental factors, such as exposure to X-rays or radioactive substances, have also been found to negatively affect spermatogenesis. Men who are exposed to radioactive substances in their work environment should be provided adequate protection of the testes. When you are assisting with pelvic X-rays, be certain men and boys are furnished a protective lead shield to guard against radiation to the testes.

Testing for Sperm Number and Availability

A number of common tests, such as semen analysis and sperm motility, help to identify whether adequate sperm for conception are present.

Analysis of Pituitary Hormones. Whether adequate levels of FSH and LH are present can be determined by a blood test and analysis. In a man with typical male features, this is rarely the problem for a limited sperm count.

Semen Analysis. For a semen analysis, after 2 to 4 days of sexual abstinence, a man ejaculates by masturbation into a clean, dry specimen jar or a special condom (one without spermicide). The number of sperm in the specimen are counted and then examined under a microscope within 1 hour (Box 8.4). An average ejaculation should produce a minimum of 1.4 to 1.7 ml of semen and should contain a minimum of 33 to 46 million spermatozoa per milliliter of fluid (World Health Organization [WHO], 2010). The analysis may need to be repeated after 2 or 3 months, because spermatogenesis is an ongoing process and 30 to 90 days is needed for new sperm to reach maturity. If reluctant to have their sperm counted at a health care facility, men can test their sperm motility at home by a self-test kit such as Fertell (Kokopelli Technologies, 2012). If the man has a vas deferens obstruction, sperm can be obtained by testes biopsy.

Sperm Penetration Assay and Antisperm Antibody Testing. For impregnation to take place, sperm must be mobile enough to navigate the vagina, uterus and a fallopian tube to reach the ova. Although sperm penetration studies are rarely necessary, they may be scheduled to determine whether a man's sperm, once they reach an ovum, can penetrate it effectively. With the use of an assisted reproductive technique such as IVF, poorly mobile sperm or those with poor penetration can be injected directly into a woman's ovum under laboratory conditions (intracytoplasmic sperm injection), bypassing the need for sperm to be fully mobile.

What if...8.2 While the Carls are undergoing IVF, Cheryl's mother asks you, "How can I ever love a child created in a 'test tube'?" How would you answer her?

Therapy for Increasing Sperm Count and Motility

If sperm are present but the total count is low, a man may be advised to abstain from coitus for 7 to 10 days at a time to increase the count. Ligation of a varicocele (if present) and changes in lifestyle, such as wearing looser clothing, avoiding long periods of sitting, and avoiding prolonged hot baths, may also be helpful to reduce scrotal heat and increase the sperm count.

Obstruction or Impaired Sperm Motility

In some men, adequate sperm are manufactured, but there is obstruction at some point along the pathway spermatozoa must travel to reach the outside: the seminiferous tubules, the epididymis, the vas deferens, the ejaculatory duct, or the urethra (see Chapter 5, Fig. 5.1). Diseases such as *mumps orchitis* (testicular inflammation and scarring due to the mumps virus), epididymitis (inflammation of the epididymis), and infections such as gonorrhea or ascending urethral infection

BOX 8.4 Nursing Care Planning Based on Family Teaching

TIPS FOR ENSURING AN ACCURATE SEMEN ANALYSIS

Q. Bob Carl asks you, "What is the right way to do a semen sample?"

A. Effective guidelines include:

- Abstain from intercourse or masturbation for at about 3 days.
- Use a clean, dry plastic or glass container with a secure lid to collect the sample.
- Collect the specimen as close as possible to your usual time of sexual activity.
- Avoid using any lubricants before you collect the specimen.
- After you've collected the specimen in the container, close it securely and write down the time you collected it.
- Take the specimen to the laboratory or health care provider's office immediately so it can be analyzed within 1 hour of collection.
- Keep the specimen at body temperature while transporting it. Carrying it next to your chest is one way to do this.

can result in this type of obstruction because adhesions form and occlude sperm transport (Hedger, 2011). Congenital stricture of a spermatic duct may occasionally be seen. Benign hypertrophy of the prostate gland occurs in most men beginning at about 50 years of age. Pressure from the enlarged gland on the vas deferens can then interfere with sperm transport. Infection of the prostate, through which the sperm and seminal fluid must pass, or infection of the seminal vesicles (spread from a urinary tract infection) can change the composition of the seminal fluid enough to reduce sperm motility.

A few men who have vasectomies develop an autoimmune reaction or form antibodies that immobilize their own sperm after the procedure; they also may experience long-term pain unless the procedure is reversed (Horovitz, Tjong, Domes, et al., 2012). It is conceivable that men with obstruction in the vas deferens from other causes, such as scarring after an infection, could also develop an autoimmune reaction that immobilizes sperm the same way.

Anomalies of the penis, such as hypospadias (urethral opening on the ventral surface of the penis), epispadias (urethral opening on the dorsal surface), or Peyronie disease (a bent penis) can cause sperm to be deposited too far from the sexual partner's cervix to allow optimal cervical penetration. Extreme obesity in a male may also interfere with effective penetration and deposition (Hammoud, Meikle, Reis, et al., 2012).

Testing for Sperm Transport Disorders

Sperm transport disorders are suspected when FSH and LH hormones, which stimulate the production of sperm, are adequate but the sperm count remains limited.

Therapy for Sperm Transport Disorders

If sperm are not able to pass through the vas deferens because of obstruction, surgery to relieve the obstruction is extensive, costly, and may not have a positive outcome. A better solution can be extracting sperm from a point above the blockage and injecting it into the vagina or uterus of the man's partner by intrauterine insemination (IUI) (Akanji Tijani & Bhattacharya, 2010). If the problem appears to be that sperm are immobilized by vaginal secretions due to an immunologic factor, the response can be reduced by abstinence or condom use for about 6 months. However, to avoid this prolonged time interval (which is difficult for a couple who want to have a child immediately), washing of the sperm followed by IUI may be preferred. The administration of corticosteroids to a woman may have some effect in decreasing sperm immobilization because it reduces her immune response and antibody production.

Ejaculation Problems

Erectile dysfunction or the inability to achieve an erection (formerly called impotence), which may occur from psychological problems; diseases such as a cerebrovascular accident, diabetes, or Parkinson disease; use of certain antihypertensive agents; as well as the discontinuation of finasteride, a drug used for male pattern baldness (Irwig & Kolukula, 2011), may result in erectile dysfunction. This condition is *primary* if the man has never been able to achieve erection and ejaculation and *secondary* if the man was able to achieve ejaculation in the past but now has difficulty. Erectile dysfunction can be a difficult problem to solve if it is associated with stress, because this is not easily relieved.

Premature ejaculation (ejaculation before penetration) is another factor that may interfere with the proper deposition of sperm. It is another problem often attributed to psychological causes. Adolescents may experience it until they become more experienced in sexual techniques.

Testing for Ejaculation Concerns

Ejaculation concerns are identified by a sexual history. It may be difficult for a man to discuss this area of his life, especially if a nurse is female, so skillful patient interviewing technique is required.

Therapy for Ejaculation Concerns

Solutions for erectile dysfunction include psychological or sexual counseling as well as the use of a phosphodiesterase inhibitor, such as sildenafil (Viagra) or tadalafil (Cialis) (see Chapter 5, Box 5.8). Dapoxetine, a short-acting selective serotonin reuptake inhibitor, is a drug that has been developed especially for the treatment of premature ejaculation and shows good results when taken about 1 hour before planned coitus (Hutchinson, Cruickshank, & Wylie, 2012).

QSEN Checkpoint Question 8.2

Safety

The Carls introduce themselves to you as an "infertile" couple. As a safety measure, you would want them to understand which of the following?

a. Couples are not termed infertile until they have been trying to conceive for 2 years.
b. Infertility can cause depression, so the couple should report any feeling of sadness.
c. If their relationship is not monogamous, they still need to use safer sex practices.
d. Infertility is related to antibiotic-resistant infections, so they need to be tested for these.

Look in Appendix A for the best answer and rationale.

FACTORS THAT CAUSE FEMALE SUBFERTILITY

The factors that cause subfertility in women are analogous to those causing subfertility in men:

- Limited production of FHS or LH, which interfere with ova growth
- Anovulation (faulty or inadequate expulsion of ova)
- Problems of ova transport through the fallopian tubes to the uterus
- Uterine factors, such as tumors or poor endometrial development
- Cervical and vaginal factors, which immobilize spermatozoa
- Poor nutrition, increased body weight, and lack of exercise, which may compound these problems

Anovulation

The steps of ova formation and ovulation are described in Chapter 5. **Anovulation** (absence of ovulation or release of ova from the ovary), the most common cause of subfertility in women, may occur from a genetic abnormality such as Turner syndrome (hypogonadism), in which there is limited ovarian tissue available to produce ova. More often, it results from a hormonal imbalance caused by a condition such as hypothyroidism, which interferes with hypothalamus-pituitary-ovarian interaction. Ovarian tumors or polycystic ovary syndrome may also produce anovulation due to feedback stimulation on the pituitary. Chronic or excessive exposure to X-rays or radioactive substances, general ill health, poor diet, and stress may all contribute to poor ovarian function (Fritz & Speroff, 2010).

Nutrition, body weight, and exercise are all important for adequate ova production because they all influence the blood glucose/insulin balance (Nodine & Hastings-Tolsma, 2012). When either glucose or insulin levels are too high, they can disrupt the production of FSH and LH, leading to ovulation failure. Vitamin D may also be instrumental in maintaining pituitary hormone levels (Lerchbaum & Obermayer-Pietsch, 2012).

The ideal body weight to maintain is a BMI of 18.5 to 24.9. Eating slowly digested carbohydrate foods (e.g., brown rice, pasta, dark bread, beans) and fiber-rich vegetables (e.g., asparagus, broccoli) rather than easily digested carbohydrate foods (e.g., white bread, cold breakfast cereals) can not only increase fertility by keeping insulin levels balanced but also may prevent gestational diabetes when a woman becomes pregnant (Speroni, Earley, Seibert, et al., 2012).

To compliment healthy eating habits, exercising 30 minutes per day by walking or doing mild aerobics also helps regulate blood glucose levels and so is yet another way to increase fertility. Stress may play a role in limiting ovulation as this may lower hypothalamic secretion of gonadotropin-releasing hormone (GnRH), which then lowers the production of LH and FSH, which leads to anovulation. Decreased body weight or a body fat ratio of less than 10%, as may occur in female athletes such as competitive runners or in women who are excessively lean or anorexic, can reduce pituitary hormones such as FSH and LH and halt ovulation (termed hypogonadotrophic hypogonadism) (Fritz & Speroff, 2010).

The most frequent cause, however, for anovulation is naturally occurring variations in ovulatory patterns or polycystic ovary syndrome, a condition in which the ovaries produce excess testosterone, thus lowering FSH and LH levels, which then causes irregular and unpredictable menstrual cycles (Weiss & Bulmer, 2011).

Polycystic ovary syndrome is associated with metabolic syndrome (a waist circumference of 35 in. or more in women, a fasting blood glucose over 100 mg/dl, serum triglycerides over 150 mg/dl, blood pressure over 135/85 mmHg, and high-density lipoprotein cholesterol over 50 mg/dl, plus development of hirsutism [unwanted body hair]) (Smith & Schust, 2011). Metabolic syndrome is also associated with increased cardiac disease, so efforts to reduce weight and lower triglycerides and cholesterol can improve heart health as well. It is discussed further in Chapter 11.

Testing for Anovulation

Many tests to detect ovulation are ones women can do at home by themselves, giving them both a sense of control over what is happening and the ability to learn more about their body's functioning.

Ovulation Monitoring. The fastest way to investigate if ovulation is occurring is to measure the woman's serum progesterone level during the luteal phase of her menstrual cycle (about day 21 to day 28 of a typical cycle). If this is elevated, it implies a corpus luteum has formed or ovulation has occurred.

The least costly way to determine a woman's ovulation pattern is to ask her to record her basal body temperature (BBT) for at least 4 months. To determine this, a woman takes her temperature each morning, before getting out of bed or engaging in any activity, eating, or drinking, using a special BBT or tympanic thermometer. She plots this daily temperature on a monthly graph while noting any conditions that might affect her temperature, such as an infection or sleeplessness. At the time of ovulation, the BBT can be seen to dip slightly (about 0.5°F), it then rises to a level no higher than normal body temperature, and then stays at that level until 3 or 4 days before the next menstrual flow. This increase in BBT marks the time of ovulation, because it occurs immediately after ovulation (actually at the beginning of the luteal phase of the menstrual cycle, which can occur only if ovulation has occurred). If the temperature rise does not last at least 10 days, it suggests a woman has a luteal phase defect (progesterone is not being produced long enough in a cycle so adequate endometrium for implantation can be laid down). Typical graphs of BBT are shown in Figure 8.1.

What if...8.3 Cheryl Carl tells you she works nights as a cocktail waitress, goes to bed at 4 AM, then wakes at 6 AM to drive her husband to work. Starting at noon, she sleeps for 4 or 5 hours before getting up to go to work. When during the day should you tell her is the best time to record her BBT?

Ovulation Determination by Test Strip. Various brands of commercial kits are available for assessing the upsurge of LH that occurs just before ovulation and can be used in place of BBT monitoring. A woman dips a test strip into a midmorning urine specimen and then compares it with the kit instructions for a color change. Such kits are purchased over the counter, are easy to use, and have the advantage of marking the point just before ovulation occurs rather than just after ovulation, as is the case with BBT. They are not as economical as simple temperature recording, but they are advantageous for women with irregular work or daily activity, which can make BBT measurements inaccurate.

A new test kit (Fertell) contains materials to test both FSH on the third day of a woman's menstrual cycle (an abnormally high level is an indicator her ovaries are not responding well to ovulation) as well as a sperm motility test for the male (Kokopelli Technologies, 2012). The woman's result is available in 30 minutes; the man's result is available in 90 minutes. The kits are expensive but can be helpful to a couple as a first step in self-fertility testing. Be certain the woman realizes this is not a test of her time of ovulation but a test as to whether she has adequate FSH to stimulate egg growth; therefore, she shouldn't use the test at the midpoint of her menstrual cycle.

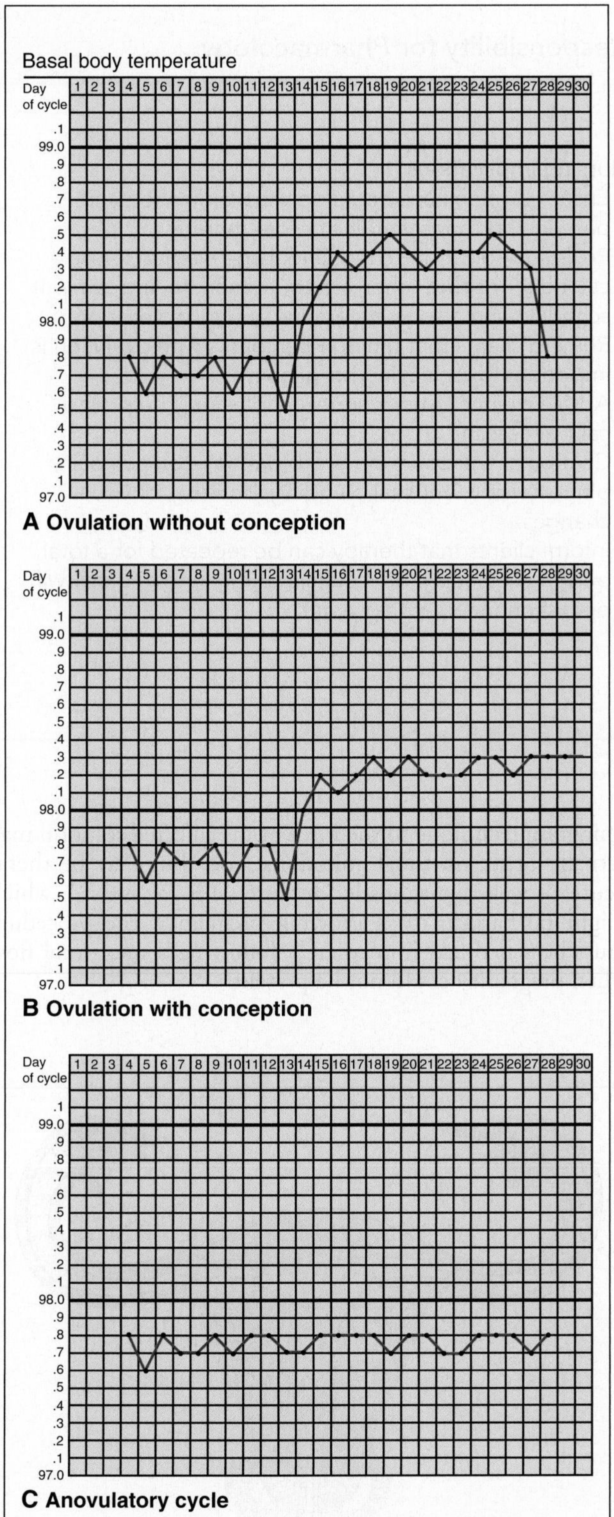

FIGURE 8.1 Basal body temperature graph. **(A)** A woman's temperature dips slightly at midpoint in the menstrual cycle, then rises sharply, which is an indication of ovulation. Toward the end of the cycle (the 24th day), her temperature begins to decline, indicating progesterone levels are falling and she did not conceive. **(B)** A woman's temperature rises at the midpoint in the cycle and remains at that elevated level past the time of her normal menstrual flow, suggesting pregnancy has occurred. **(C)** There is no preovulatory dip, and no rise of temperature anywhere during the cycle. This is the typical pattern of a woman who does not ovulate.

Polycystic ovary syndrome can be detected by examining the woman's menstrual history, but even if a woman experiences regular monthly menstruation, it does not necessarily indicate she is also ovulating on a regular basis (Balen, 2012). Fasting-glucose, testosterone, and estrogen levels are analyzed. A pelvic sonogram can be used to confirm cysts are present on the ovaries and may be the cause of subfertility (Hamilton, 2012).

Therapy for Anovulation

If a disturbance in ovulation is identified as the subfertility concern, administration of GnRH is a possibility (this will stimulate the pituitary to secrete more FSH and LH). Therapy with clomiphene citrate (Clomid, Serophene) may also be used to stimulate ovulation (Box 8.5). In other women, ovarian follicular growth can be stimulated by the administration of combinations of FSH and LH in conjunction with administration of human chorionic gonadotropin (hCG) to produce ovulation. If increased prolactin levels are identified, bromocriptine (Parlodel) is added to the medication regimen to reduce prolactin levels and allow for the rise of pituitary gonadotropins (Karch, 2013).

Administration of either clomiphene citrate or gonadotropins may overstimulate an ovary, causing multiple ova to come to maturity, and possibly resulting in multiple births. Counsel women who receive these agents that this is a possibility.

Tubal Transport Problems

Difficulty with tubal transport usually occurs because scarring has developed in the fallopian tubes, which is typically caused by chronic salpingitis (chronic pelvic inflammatory disease [PID]). This could also result from a ruptured appendix or from abdominal surgery, which involved infection that spread to the fallopian tubes and left adhesion formation in the tubes. Complete tubal obstruction is the chief problem if a woman had a tubal ligation in years past but now wants to become pregnant.

Pelvic inflammatory disease is infection of the pelvic organs: the uterus, fallopian tubes, ovaries, and their supporting structures. The initial source of the infection is usually a sexually transmitted disease such as chlamydia or gonorrhea. PID occurs at a rate of about 25 per 100 women; in other words, one-fourth of all women will experience this type of infection in a lifetime. About 12% of those who acquire PID will be left subfertile because of tubal scarring (Guile & Keller, 2011).

PID invasion of fallopian tubes is most apt to occur at the end of a menstrual period, because menstrual blood provides such an excellent growth medium for bacteria. There also is a loss of the normal cervical mucus barrier at this time, which increases the risk for initial invasion. When PID is left unrecognized and untreated, it enters a chronic phase, which causes the scarring that can lead to stricture of the fallopian tubes and the resulting fertility problem.

There is a higher incidence of PID among women who have multiple sexual partners (Hanson & Burke, 2011). Based on this, it is good advice for women to limit the number of their sexual partners or always insist on condom protection to help reduce the incidence of sexually transmitted infections and possibly subfertility.

BOX 8.5 Nursing Care Planning Based on Responsibility for Pharmacology

CLOMIPHENE CITRATE (CLOMID)

Action: Clomiphene citrate (Clomid) is an estrogen agonist commonly used to stimulate the ovary. The drug binds to estrogen receptors, decreasing the number of available estrogen receptors, which falsely signals the hypothalamus to increase follicle-stimulating hormone and luteinizing hormone secretion. This results in ovulation (Karch, 2013).
Pregnancy Category: X
Dosage: Initially, 50 mg/day orally for 5 days (started anytime if no menstrual flow has occurred recently or about the fifth day of the cycle if menstrual flow is occurring). If ovulation does not occur with this initial therapy, the drug can be followed by a prescription of 100 mg/day for 5 days started as early as 30 days after the initial course of therapy. This second course may be repeated one more time.
Possible Adverse Effects: Abdominal discomfort, distention, bloating, nausea, vomiting, breast tenderness, vasomotor flushing, ovarian enlargement, ovarian overstimulation, multiple births, and visual disturbances.

Nursing Implications
- Ensure women have had a pelvic examination and baseline hormonal studies before therapy.
- Review medication scheduling. Urge women to use a calendar or some other system to mark their treatment schedule and also to determine and plot ovulation.
- Remind clients that timing intercourse with ovulation is important for achieving pregnancy.
- Advise clients 24-hour urine samples may be periodically necessary.
- Caution clients to report any bloating, stomach pain, blurred vision, unusual bleeding, bruising, or visual changes.
- Inform clients that therapy can be repeated for a total of three courses; if no results are obtained, therapy will be discontinued at that point.

Testing for Tubal Patency

Ultrasound or X-ray imaging and direct visualization by a hysteroscope of fallopian tubes are all effective methods used to determine the patency of fallopian tubes.

Sonohysterosalpingogram. A sonohysterosalpingogram is a sonographic examination of the fallopian tubes and uterus using an ultrasound contrast agent introduced into the uterus through a narrow catheter inserted into the uterine cervix (Fig. 8.2) followed by intravaginal scanning. If the tubes are patent, they will fill with the contrast medium and be detailed on the ultrasound screen. The procedure is contraindicated if infection of the vagina, cervix, or uterus is present (infectious organisms might be forced through the tubes into the pelvic cavity); it is usually scheduled just following a menstrual flow when a woman could not be pregnant.

Although only a small amount of contrast medium is used, it does slightly distend the uterus and tubes, possibly causing momentary painful uterine cramping. After the study, the small amount of contrast medium used drains out through the vagina. Although it is possible that the procedure could be therapeutic as well as diagnostic as the pressure of the solution could break up adhesions as it passes through the fallopian tubes, this is unlikely because the amount of contrast medium used is so small. Although extremely rare, the procedure carries a small risk of infection (a chlamydia screen before the procedure is usually advised); although unlikely, an allergic reaction to the contrast medium or embolism from the medium entering a uterine blood vessel could also occur.

Hysterosalpingogram. A hysterosalpingogram is similar to a sonohysterosalpingogram except a radiopaque contrast medium is used and the fallopian tubes are revealed by X-ray. This procedure uses more contrast medium than with the sonogram technique so the force of the injected solution may actually break up tubal adhesions, and thus may be therapeutic as well as diagnostic. Because an X-ray is used, which might be harmful to a growing pregnancy, the procedure must be scheduled immediately following a menstrual flow when pregnancy could not be present.

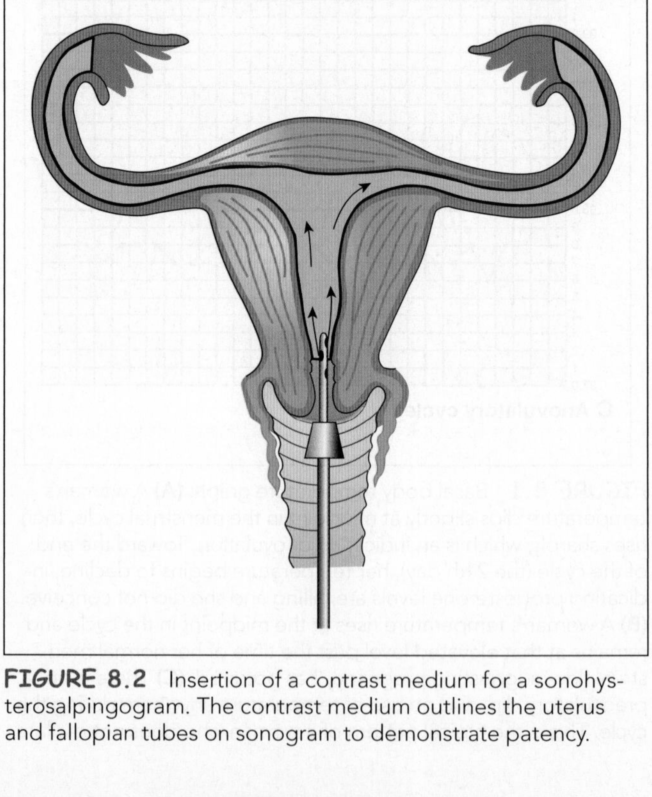

FIGURE 8.2 Insertion of a contrast medium for a sonohysterosalpingogram. The contrast medium outlines the uterus and fallopian tubes on sonogram to demonstrate patency.

Transvaginal Hydrolaparoscopy. Transvaginal hydrolaparoscopy is begun with the instillation of a paracervical local anesthetic block followed by introduction of a hysteroscope into an incision just behind the cervix through the cul-de-sac of Douglas into the peritoneal cavity. About 200 ml of normal saline is then introduced to move the bowel away from the uterus so the posterior wall of the uterus, the ovaries, and the fallopian tubes can be assessed. Tubal patency can be evaluated if, following the insertion of a small amount of dye into the cervix, it can be viewed exiting the fimbrial end of the tubes. At the end of the procedure, the fluid is drained from the peritoneal cavity; the small incision will heal without stitches (Catenacci & Goldberg, 2012).

Therapy for Lack of Tubal Patency

If the subfertility problem is identified as tubal insufficiency from inflammation, the prescription of diathermy or steroid administration may be helpful to reduce adhesions. Hysterosalpingography (instillation of a contrast dye under X-ray monitoring) can be attempted to see if the force of the dye insertion will break adhesions. Canalization of the fallopian tubes and plastic surgical repair (microsurgery) are other possible treatments. If peritoneal adhesions or nodules of endometriosis are holding the tubes fixed and away from the ovaries, these can be removed by laparoscopy or laser surgery (Magos, 2012).

It is possible for fallopian tubes, which have been ligated as a contraception procedure, to be reopened surgically but the success of the operation is not more than 70% to 80%. Also, the irregular incision line left by surgery can result in an ectopic pregnancy (i.e., a tubal pregnancy) if a fertilized ovum is stopped at the irregular point (Deffieux, Morin Surroca, Faivre, et al., 2011). IUI is more commonly used today and more apt to result in a viable pregnancy.

QSEN Checkpoint Question 8.3

Teamwork & Collaboration

Cheryl Carl is scheduled to have a sonohysterosalpingography. Which of the following instructions would you want your care team members to know so patient teaching can be consistent?

a. She may feel some mild cramping when the contrast medium is inserted.
b. The X-ray of the uterus will reveal any fibroid tumors or adhesions present.
c. She will not be able to conceive for at least 3 months after the procedure.
d. Many women experience mild bleeding for up to 2 hours as an aftereffect.

Look in Appendix A for the best answer and rationale.

Uterine Concerns

Tumors such as fibromas (leiomyomas) may be a rare cause of subfertility if they block the entrance of the fallopian tubes into the uterus or limit the space available on the uterine wall for effective implantation. A congenitally deformed uterine cavity may also limit implantation sites, but this also is rare.

Endometriosis and poor secretion of estrogen or progesterone are more common uterine reasons for subfertility as these result in inadequate endometrial formation (overproduction or underproduction), which then interferes with implantation and embryo growth.

Endometriosis refers to the implantation of uterine endometrium, or nodules, that have spread from the interior of the uterus to locations outside the uterus (Gunderson & Yates, 2011). The occurrence of endometriosis may indicate the endometrial tissue has different or more friable qualities than usual (perhaps due to a luteal phase defect) and therefore is a type of endometrium that also does not support embryo implantation as well as usual.

Endometriosis symptoms begin in adolescence, with the most common sites of endometrium spread to the fallopian tubes, the cul-de-sac of Douglas, the ovaries, the uterine ligaments, and the outer surface of the uterus and bowel (Fig. 8.3). Some evidence of endometriosis occurs in as many as 50% of women, usually from reflux through the fallopian tubes at the time of menstruation. If viable particles of endometrium, which enter a tube this way, begin to proliferate, they can cause tubal obstruction; growths on the ovaries can displace fallopian tubes away from the ovaries, preventing the entrance of ova into the tubes. Peritoneal macrophages, which are drawn to nodules of endometrium, can destroy sperm.

Testing for Uterine Concerns

Tests to determine if a uterine concern is leading to subfertility include a sonogram or hysteroscopy to view the structure of the uterus, blood work to analyze for hormones, and perhaps an endometrial biopsy.

Hysteroscopy. Hysteroscopy is visual inspection of the uterus through the insertion of a hysteroscope (a thin hollow tube) through the vagina, cervix, and into the uterus. This is helpful to further evaluate uterine adhesions, malformations, or other abnormalities such as fibroid tumors or polyps that were discovered on sonogram imaging. Women are screened for chlamydia before the examination to avoid introduction of bacteria into the uterus.

Uterine Endometrial Biopsy. Uterine endometrial biopsy may be used to reveal an endometrial problem, such as a luteal phase defect. If the endometrium sample removed by biopsy resembles a corkscrew (a typical progesterone-dominated endometrium) seen in the second half of a menstrual cycle, this suggests ovulation has occurred. Although very diagnostic of progesterone-associated concerns, endometrial biopsies are being performed less commonly than they once were, having been replaced with serum progesterone level evaluations that are simpler and also suggest ovulation has occurred.

If an endometrial biopsy is required, it is done 2 or 3 days before an expected menstrual flow (day 25 or 26 of a typical 28-day menstrual cycle). After a paracervical block and a screen for chlamydia, a thin probe and biopsy forceps are introduced through the cervix. A woman may experience mild-to-moderate discomfort from maneuvering the instruments. There may be a moment of sharp pain as the biopsy specimen is taken from the anterior or posterior uterine wall. Possible complications include pain, excessive bleeding, infection, and uterine perforation. This procedure is contraindicated if pregnancy is suspected (although the chance it would interfere with a pregnancy is probably less than 10%) or if an

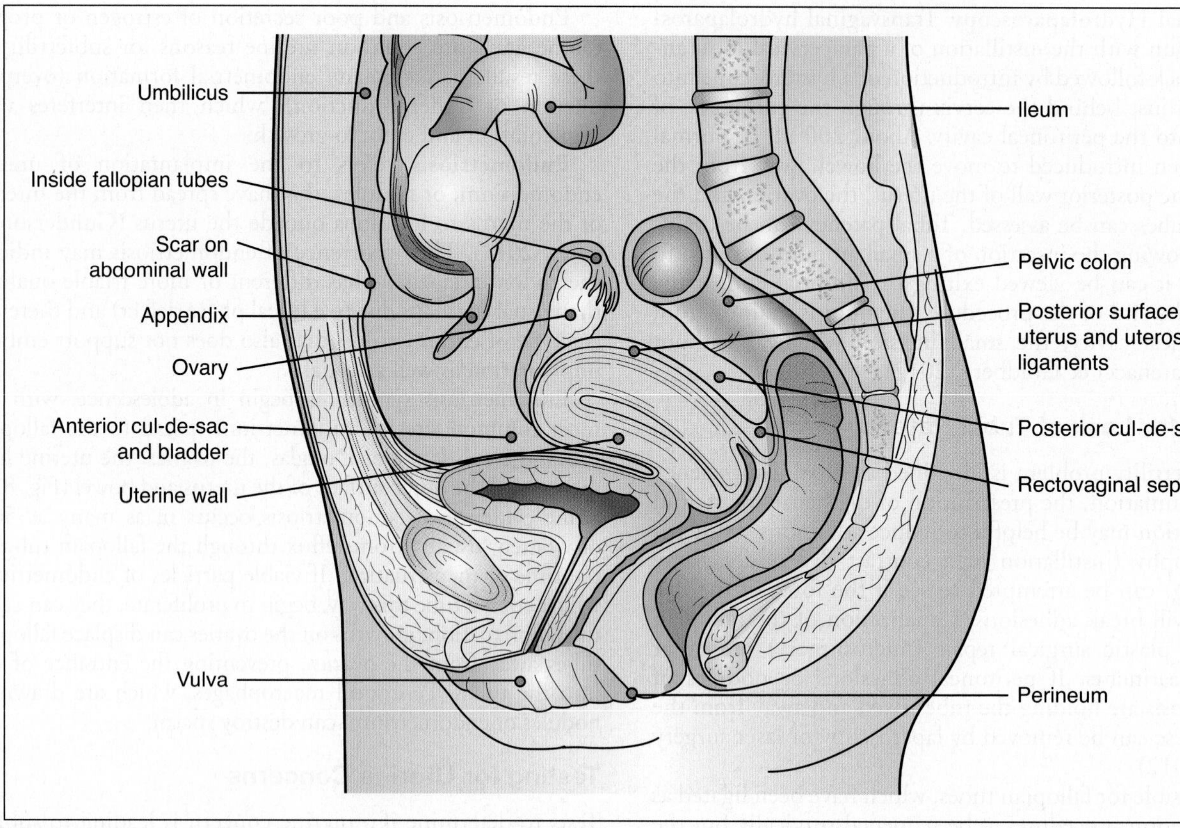

FIGURE 8.3 Common sites of endometriosis formation.

infection such as acute PID or cervicitis is present. Caution the woman that she might notice a small amount of vaginal spotting after the procedure. For follow-up, she needs to telephone her primary care provider if she develops a temperature greater than 101°F, has a large amount of bleeding, or passes clots. She needs to telephone the health care agency when she has her next menstrual flow as this helps "date" the endometrium and the accuracy of the analysis.

Laparoscopy. Laparoscopy is the introduction of a thin, hollow, lighted tube (a fiber optic telescope or laparoscope) through a small incision in the abdomen, just under the umbilicus, to examine the position and state of the fallopian tubes and ovaries. This allows an examiner to view whether the ovaries are close enough to the fallopian tubes to allow an ovum to enter. It is rarely done unless the results of a uterosalpingography are abnormal because it involves general anesthesia, which is necessary because of the pain caused by extensive maneuvering. It is scheduled during the follicular phase of a menstrual cycle. The woman is positioned in a steep Trendelenburg position (which brings the reproductive organs down out of the pelvis). Carbon dioxide is usually introduced into the abdomen to move the abdominal wall outward and to offer better visualization. Women may feel bloating of the abdomen from the infusion of the carbon dioxide after such a procedure. If some carbon dioxide escapes under the diaphragm, they may feel extremely sharp shoulder pain from the pressure of the gas on the cervical nerves.

During the procedure, a contrast medium can be injected into the uterus through a polyethylene cannula placed in the cervix to assess tubal patency (if tubes are patent, the dye will appear in the abdominal cavity). A scope may be passed directly into a fallopian tube to reveal information about the presence and condition of the fimbria and the tubal lining. If fimbria have been destroyed by PID, the chance for a normal conception is in doubt because ova seem to be unable to enter a tube if fimbrial currents are absent.

Therapy for Uterine Concerns

If the problem of subfertility appears to be a luteal phase defect, this can be corrected by progesterone vaginal suppositories begun on the third day of a woman's temperature rise and continued for the next 6 weeks (if pregnancy occurs) or until a menstrual flow begins.

If a myoma (fibroid tumor) or intrauterine adhesions are found to be interfering with fertility, a myomectomy, or surgical removal of the tumor and adhesions, can be scheduled (Gambadauro, Gudmundsson, & Torrejón, 2012). If the growth is small, this can be done by a hysteroscopic ambulatory procedure. During the procedure, an intrauterine device (IUD) may be inserted to prevent the uterine sides from touching and forming new adhesions; the woman may be prescribed estrogen for 3 months as another method to prevent adhesion formation. This treatment can be difficult for a woman to accept, because preventing pregnancy (using an IUD) is exactly what she does not want to do. Be certain she has a good explanation of the IUD's purpose and that it can be easily removed in about 1 month's time.

For problems of abnormal uterine formation, such as a septate uterus, surgery is also available. However, these defects are usually related to early pregnancy loss, not initial subfertility. Endometriosis can be treated both medically and surgically; treatment is discussed in Chapter 47 with other causes of dysmenorrhea.

Vaginal and Cervical Concerns

At the time of ovulation, the cervical mucus is thin and watery and can be easily penetrated by spermatozoa for a period of 12 to 72 hours. If coitus is not synchronized with this time, the cervical mucus may be too thick to allow spermatozoa to penetrate the cervix. Infection or inflammation of the cervix (erosion) can also cause cervical mucus to thicken so much that spermatozoa cannot penetrate it easily or survive in it. A stenotic cervical os or obstruction of the os by a polyp may further compromise sperm penetration. This is rarely enough of a problem to be the sole cause of subfertility, however. A woman who has undergone dilatation and curettage (D&C) procedures several times or cervical conization (cervical surgery) should be evaluated in light of the possibility that scar tissue and tightening of the cervical os has occurred.

Infection of the vagina can cause the pH of vaginal secretions to become acidotic, thus limiting or destroying the motility of spermatozoa. Some women appear to have sperm-immobilizing or sperm-agglutinating antibodies in their blood plasma, which act to destroy sperm cells in the vagina or cervix. Either of these immune-based problems can limit the ability of sperm to survive in the vagina and enter the uterus.

Testing and Therapy for Vaginal and Cervical Concerns

If sperm do not appear to survive in vaginal secretions because secretions are too scant or tenacious, a woman may be prescribed low-dose estrogen therapy to increase mucus production during days 5 to 10 of her cycle. Conjugated estrogen (Premarin) is a type of estrogen prescribed for this purpose.

If a vaginal infection is present, the infection will be treated according to the causative organism based on culture reports (see Chapter 47). Vaginal infections such as trichomoniasis and moniliasis tend to recur, requiring close supervision and follow-up. If the woman's sexual partner is the source of infection, and is therefore reinfecting her, the partner needs antibiotic therapy as well. Caution women who are prescribed metronidazole (Flagyl) for a *Trichomonas* infection; it may be teratogenic early in pregnancy and therefore should not be continued if the woman suspects she has become pregnant.

UNEXPLAINED SUBFERTILITY

In a small percentage of couples, no known cause for subfertility can be discovered. It may be that the problem of one partner alone is not significant, but when combined with a small problem in the other partner, together, these become sufficient to create subfertility. It is obviously discouraging for couples to complete a fertility evaluation and be told their inability to conceive cannot be explained. Offer active support to help the couple find alternative solutions at this point, such as continuing to try to conceive, using an assisted reproductive technique, choosing to adopt, or agreeing to a child-free life.

QSEN Checkpoint Question 8.4

Informatics

Cheryl Carl is diagnosed as having endometriosis as a cause of her subfertility. You would want her electronic health record to reflect the fact that this condition interferes with fertility because of which of the following?

a. The ovaries stop producing estrogen and progesterone.
b. The uterine cervix becomes very inflamed and swollen.
c. Pressure on the pituitary leads to decreased FSH levels.
d. Endometrial implants obstruct both of the fallopian tubes.

Look in Appendix A for the best answer and rationale.

ASSISTED REPRODUCTIVE TECHNIQUES

If ovulation, sperm production, or sperm mobility problems cannot be corrected, assisted reproductive strategies are the next step for a couple to consider. Before beginning any of these procedures, urge a woman to be in excellent health by discontinuing smoking or recreational drug behaviors, ingesting a diet high in protein, and having a BMI within a normal range of 18.5 to 24.9. She probably also will have, if she has not already had them, tests for HIV and hepatitis C, a hormone profile including levels of FSH, LH, estrogen, and progesterone to test for ovarian reserves (whether ovaries have the capacity to produce multiple oocytes) as well as an intravaginal sonogram to visual usual structures. Whether a woman feels comfortable choosing assisted reproduction is strongly socioculturally related, as people on a limited budget and without health insurance may not be able to afford these therapies, or their religion or cultural beliefs may make these unacceptable procedures (Box 8.6).

BOX 8.6 Nursing Care Planning to Respect Cultural Diversity

Obtaining a sexual history is often difficult because cultural taboos can make couples feel uncomfortable discussing this part of their life. Simple factors, such as how often couples engage in sexual relations, for example, are influenced by culture and religion. According to Orthodox Jewish law, a couple may not engage in sexual relations for 7 days following menstruation (the *nida* period). This practice can result in fertility problems if a woman ovulates within the 7-day period. Some cultures forbid alternative insemination because preserving male lineage is so important. The Roman Catholic Church does not approve of in vitro fertilization or any form of conception outside the body. Being aware of cultural differences can help you understand the different ways couples react to a diagnosis of subfertility and help you appreciate the full meaning of this diagnosis to an individual couple.

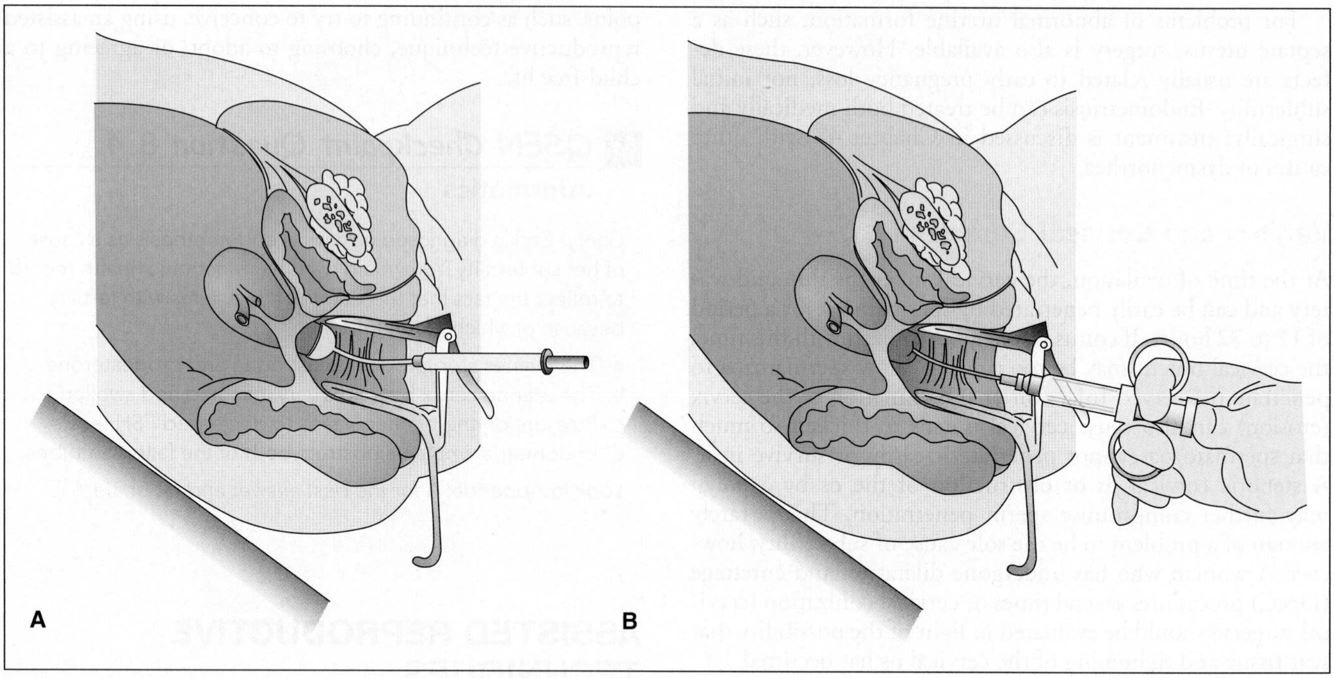

FIGURE 8.4 Alternative insemination. **(A)** Sperm are deposited next to the cervix, or **(B)** injected directly into the uterine cavity.

Alternative Insemination

Alternative or intrauterine insemination is the instillation of sperm from a masturbatory sample into the female reproductive tract by means of a cannula to aid conception at the time of ovulation (Huang, Hansen, Factor-Litvak, et al., 2012). The sperm can either be instilled into the cervix (intracervical insemination) or directly into the uterus (IUI) at the time of predicted ovulation. BBT charting, mucus analysis, or urinary test kits for LH can be used to detect the day of ovulation (Hamilton, 2012).

Either the male partner's sperm (alternative insemination by male partner) or donor sperm (alternative insemination by donor) can be used. These procedures are used if the man has none or an inadequate sperm count or if a woman has a vaginal or cervical factor that interferes with sperm motility. Donor insemination can be used if the man has a known genetic disorder he does not want transmitted to children or if a woman has no male partner. It is also a useful procedure for men who underwent a vasectomy but now wish to have children. In the past, men who underwent chemotherapy or radiation for testicular cancer had to accept being child-free afterward because they were no longer able to produce sperm. Today, sperm can be cryopreserved (frozen) in a sperm bank before radiation or chemotherapy and then used for alternative insemination afterward (Dillon & Gracia, 2012).

One disadvantage of using cryopreserved sperm is that it tends to have slower motility than unfrozen specimens. However, although the rate of conception may be lower from this source, there appears to be no increase in the incidence of congenital anomalies in children conceived by this method, and sperm remain viable even after years of storage.

To prepare for alternative insemination, a woman receives an injection of clomiphene (Clomid) or FSH 1 month prior to the insemination so follicle growth of ova is stimulated and a day of ovulation can be predicted. On the selected day of insemination (confirmed by a serum analysis of progesterone), the sperm sample is instilled next to her cervix using a device similar to a cervical cap or diaphragm, or sperm are injected directly into the uterus using a flexible catheter (Fig. 8.4).

Donors for alternative insemination are volunteers who have no history of disease and no family history of possible inheritable disorders. The blood type, or at least the Rh factor, can be matched with the woman's to prevent incompatibility. Sperm can be selected according to desired physical or mental characteristics if desired. If FSH was used to stimulate follicle growth, caution women that the chance for a multiple birth (twins or triplets) increases so she can be prepared for this (Trew & Lavery, 2012).

Because conception through alternative insemination takes an average of 6 months to achieve, and some couples may have religious or ethical beliefs that prohibit the use of sperm from either the male partner or a donor, it may not be right for every couple. Also, because it can be a discouraging process for a couple to have to wait 6 months (or longer) to see results, couples may need support to continue the technique.

QSEN Checkpoint Question 8.5

Quality Improvement

Bob Carl asks you several questions about the way in which his wife may be prepared for IUI. The clinical protocol for this procedure should include which of the following?

a. The patient would undergo genetic testing prior to the procedure.
b. The patient would wear a transdermal estrogen patch for 2 weeks prior to the procedure.
c. The patient would receive an injection of Clomid or FSH 1 month prior to the procedure.
d. The patient would be prescribed bed rest for 48 to 72 hours following the procedure.

Look in Appendix A for the best answer and rationale.

Some states have specific laws regarding inheritance, child support, and responsibility concerning children conceived by donor insemination, which may also limit whether a couple finds the technique desirable.

In Vitro Fertilization

IVF is most often used for couples who have not been able to conceive because the woman has obstructed or damaged fallopian tubes. It is also used when the man has oligospermia or a very low sperm count. IVF may also be helpful for couples when an absence of cervical mucus prevents sperm from entering the cervix, or antisperm antibodies cause immobilization of sperm. In addition, couples with unexplained subfertility of long duration may be helped by IVF.

For the procedure, one or more mature oocytes are removed from a woman's ovary by laparoscopy and fertilized by exposure to sperm in a laboratory. About 40 hours after fertilization, the laboratory-grown fertilized ova (now zygotes) are inserted into a woman's uterus, where, ideally, one or more of them will implant and grow.

A donor ovum, rather than the woman's own ovum can be used for a woman who does not ovulate or who carries a sex-linked disease she does not want to pass on to her children. Young women who had extensive ovarian radiation or ovaries removed before surgery for ovarian cancer can have oocytes cryopreserved before surgery and used for IVF (Bouchlariotou, Tsikouras, Benjamin, et al., 2012).

As with alternative insemination, 1 month before the procedure, the woman is given FSH to stimulate oocyte growth. Beginning about the 10th day of the menstrual cycle, the ovaries are examined daily by sonography to assess the number and size of developing ovarian follicles. When a follicle appears to be mature, a woman is given an injection of hCG, which causes ovulation in 38 to 42 hours.

A needle is then introduced intravaginally and guided by ultrasound, and the oocyte is aspirated from its follicle. Because of the drugs given to induce ova maturation, many oocytes may ripen at once, and perhaps as many as 3 to 12 can be removed. The oocytes chosen are incubated for at least 8 hours to ensure viability. In the meantime, the male partner or donor supplies a fresh or frozen semen specimen. The sperm cells and oocytes are mixed and allowed to incubate in a growth medium. Genetic analysis to reveal chromosomal abnormalities or the potential sex can be completed at this point.

In the past, many sperm were necessary even under laboratory conditions to allow sperm to make their way through the resistant zona pellucida surrounding the ovum. A number of techniques, such as creating passages through the resistant cells (i.e., zona drilling), have been discovered to help sperm cross the zona. In some instances, it has been possible to inject sperm directly under the zona pellucida (i.e., intracytoplasmic sperm injection). This is the technique that makes it possible for fertilization to take place with only one sperm. Worry that this technique could lead to an increased number of birth defects is unproven (Desai, Goldberg, Austin, et al., 2012).

After fertilization of the chosen oocytes occurs, the zygotes formed almost immediately begin to divide and grow. By 40 hours after fertilization, they will have undergone their first cell division. In the past, multiple eggs were chosen and implanted to ensure a pregnancy resulted, but this technique also resulted in many multiple births. Because newborns from multiple births have a much smaller chance of surviving the neonatal period than others, today if a woman is under 35 years of age, only one or two fertilized eggs are chosen and transferred back to her uterine cavity through the cervix by means of a thin catheter. In women age 40 years, up to five embryos may be transferred (Christianson & Wallach, 2011) (Fig. 8.5).

If the couple desires, any eggs that are not used can be cryopreserved for use at a later time. As with sperm cryopreservation, egg cryopreservation presents a range of ethical and religious dilemmas as to who should "own" them if the couple should divorce or disagree about their disposal at a later date.

A lack of progesterone can occur if the corpus luteum was injured by the aspiration of the follicle. Therefore, progesterone or LH may be prescribed to a woman following IVF if it is believed she will not produce enough on her own to support implantation. Proof the zygote has implanted can be demonstrated by a routine serum pregnancy test as early as 11 days after transfer. A few women develop an ovarian

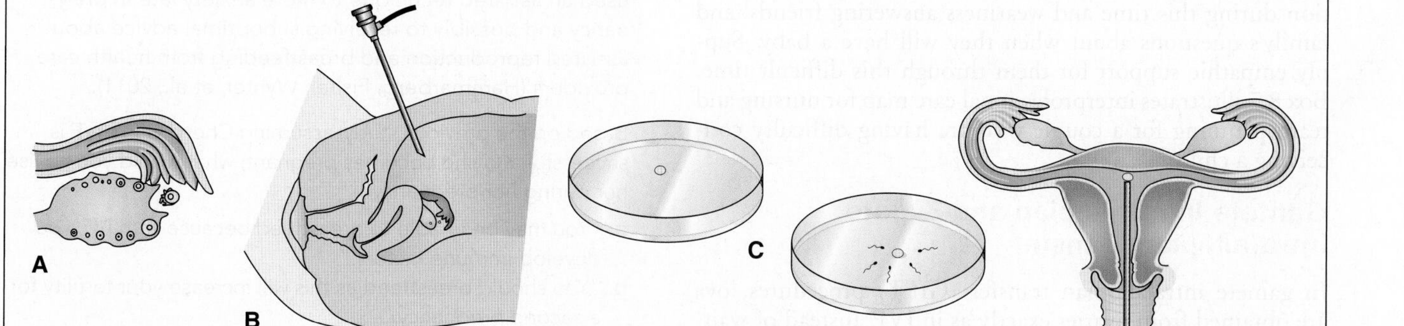

FIGURE 8.5 Steps involved in in vitro fertilization. **(A)** Ovulation. **(B)** Capture of ova (done here intra-abdominally). **(C)** Fertilization of ova and growth in culture medium. **(D)** Insertion of fertilized ova into uterus.

hyperstimulation syndrome with IVF. Their ovaries become swollen and painful and they may have accumulating abdominal and lung fluid. Women need to report these symptoms so ovarian stimulation can be halted until their ovaries return to normal; removing a number of oocytes and cryopreserving them can reduce the need for further stimulation with future procedures (Imudia, Awonuga, Kaimal, et al., 2012).

In some centers, nurse practitioners are the health care providers who complete oocyte removal and transfer. In all centers, nurses have a responsibility to supply support and counseling to help sustain a couple through the process. The recovery rate for harvesting ripened eggs is high (about 90%), as is the ability to fertilize eggs by sperm in vitro. However, the overall pregnancy rate by IVF is as low as 30% to 35% per treatment cycle for women under 35 years; it is as low as 6% to 10% for woman age 40 years (American Pregnancy Association [APA], 2012).

About 25% of pregnancies end in spontaneous miscarriage (the same rate as for natural pregnancies). Once a pregnancy has been successfully established, a woman's prenatal care is the same as for any pregnancy, although the pregnancy may be categorized as high risk because women who have IVF procedures tend to be older than average, may be obese, and may have accompanying uterine concerns (Zollner & Dietl, 2013). Because the couple was committed to the procedure, the typical couple adjusts to pregnancy and parenthood well. Encourage the woman and offer support for breastfeeding so she can be as successful with this as other women (Fisher, Rowe, & Hammarberg, 2012).

If a sonogram reveals that a multiple pregnancy of more than two zygotes has been achieved, selective termination of gestational sacs until only two remain may be recommended to help ensure the pregnancy will come to term. This is done by intraabdominal injection of potassium chloride into the gestational sacs chosen to be eliminated (Hasson, Shapira, Many, et al., 2011). This is obviously a difficult decision for a couple to agree upon, so they may need maximum support at this step.

IVF is expensive (about $10,000 per cycle) and is available only at specialized centers. A complication of maternal infection can occur if bacteria are introduced at any point in the transfer. Waiting to be accepted by a center's program and then waiting for the time to obtain the oocyte, allow for laboratory growth, and then pregnancy success is a major psychological strain. Couples report a feeling of social isolation during this time and weariness answering friends' and family's questions about when they will have a baby. Supply empathic support for them through this difficult time. Box 8.7 illustrates interprofessional care map for nursing and team planning for a couple who are having difficulty conceiving a child.

Gamete Intrafallopian and Zygote Intrafallopian Transfer

In gamete intrafallopian transfer (GIFT) procedures, ova are obtained from ovaries exactly as in IVF. Instead of waiting for fertilization to occur in the laboratory, however, both ova and sperm are instilled, within a matter of hours, using a laparoscopic technique, into the open end of a patent fallopian tube. Fertilization then occurs in the tube, and the zygote moves to the uterus for implantation. It requires at least one patent fallopian tube; it may be a preferred procedure by some couples because conception occurs in the fallopian tube and so is not contradictory to their religious beliefs.

Zygote intrafallopian transfer (ZIFT) is similar to IVF in that the egg is fertilized in the laboratory, but like GIFT, the fertilized egg is transferred by laparoscopic technique into the end of a waiting fallopian tube. Although available, this technique is little used today because of the extensive laparoscopic technique needed.

Surrogate Embryo Transfer

Surrogate embryo transfer is an assisted reproductive technique for a woman who does not produce ova. For the process, the oocyte is donated by a friend, relative, or an anonymous donor (Check, Katsoff, Brasile, et al., 2011). The menstrual cycles of the donor and recipient are synchronized by administration of gonadotropic hormones. At the time of ovulation, the donor's ovum is removed by a transvaginal, ultrasound-guided procedure. The oocyte is then fertilized in the laboratory by the recipient woman's partner's sperm (or donor sperm) and placed in the recipient woman's uterus by embryonic transfer. Once pregnancy occurs, it progresses the same as an unassisted pregnancy.

✔ QSEN Checkpoint Question 8.6

Evidence-Based Practice

It is generally agreed that breast milk is the natural and best food for babies for the entire first year or at least until 6 months. To see if women who had babies through assisted reproductive techniques such as IVF choose to breastfeed as much as women having babies without an assisted technique, researchers interviewed 183 women who conceived using an assisted technique as to whether they breastfed their baby or not. Results showed that more women who conceived with the help of an assisted technique began breastfeeding than others (89.3% versus 83.3%). By 3 months, however, a smaller number of women who had used an assisted technique were exclusively breastfeeding (46% versus 57%); at 8 months, only 23% were still breastfeeding versus 57% of nonassisted women. Researchers attributed the decline in breastfeeding among women who used an assisted technique to more anxiety late in pregnancy and possibly to receiving suboptimal advice about assisted reproduction and breastfeeding from health care providers (Hammarberg, Fisher, Wynter, et al., 2011).

Based on the previous study, assuming Cheryl Carl's IVF is successful and she becomes pregnant, what would you advise her during her pregnancy?

a. "You may be unable to breastfeed because with IVF, you develop immune factors."
b. "You should breastfeed as this will increase your fertility for a second pregnancy."
c. "After your child's birth, you should be able to begin breastfeeding effectively."
d. "Try not to worry; worry causes hormones necessary for vaginal birth to decrease."

Look in Appendix A for the best answer and rationale.

BOX 8.7 Nursing Care Planning

AN INTERPROFESSIONAL CARE MAP FOR A COUPLE SEEKING A FERTILITY EVALUATION

Cheryl and Bob Carl married when they were both 25 years old. Three years later, they are now undergoing their second cycle of in vitro fertilization (IVF) and embryo transfer. They have applied for a second mortgage on their house to finance the fertility testing.

Today, at a visit, Mrs. Carl stated, "This is my fault because I'm so rigid. Look how I had to buy the house before I could even consider getting pregnant, and now we'll probably lose it. I've made our whole life revolve around trying to get pregnant instead of enjoying life."

Family Assessment Couple live in three-bedroom, middle-income home; husband works as a bank manager; wife works as a receptionist in a medical office. Husband reports finances as "not good." Couple both appear discouraged about their apparent inability to have children.

Client Assessment Past medical history negative for any major health problems; wife reports a menstrual cycle of 5 days' duration with moderate flow every 30 to 37 days; never any dysmenorrhea. Used a combined estrogen/progestin oral contraceptive for 6 years; discontinued 3 years ago. Baseline laboratory studies and vital signs within normal limits.

Nursing Diagnosis Situational low self-esteem related to seeming inability to conceive.

Outcome Criteria Couple verbalizes feelings about subfertility and effect on self-esteem; participates actively in care and treatment decisions; states they feel some control over situation and required treatment.

Team Member Responsible	Assessment	Intervention	Rationale	Expected Outcome
Activities of Daily Living, Including Safety				
Nurse	Assess couple's lifestyle to identify areas in which they are successful.	Review and reinforce with client activities they have achieved successfully.	Identifying positive attributes can provide a foundation for rebuilding self-esteem.	Couple names at least three positive achievements, such as graduating from college or planting a garden.
Nurse	Assess if there is a common interest they could draw upon.	Ask couple to propose a new activity that would interest both of them.	Beginning a new activity can eliminate total concentration on fertility management.	Couple names and begins to participate in a new activity by 2 weeks' time.
Teamwork and Collaboration				
Nurse/Social worker	Assess the couple's community for available community resources.	Ask couple if they would like a referral to a support group, such as Resolve.	A national organization can help supply effective support during a family crisis.	Couple confirms they have contacted an outside support group and have attended at least one meeting or online chat group.
Procedures/Medications for Quality Improvement				
Nurse/Primary health care provider	Assess whether couple needs a review of IVF procedure and how their participation is important for success.	Encourage clients to ask questions about procedure; if prescribed an ovulation stimulant, review dosage and administration schedule.	Fully informed clients are better able to participate in their own care.	Clients state they understand procedure and are interested in being an active part of it by asking questions and demonstrating successful medication adherence.

(continued on page 180)

BOX 8.7 Nursing Care Planning (continued)

Nutrition				
Nurse/Nutritionist	Assess whether couple ingests a healthy diet in light of busy lifestyle.	Remind client to take prenatal vitamin (because of folic acid content) during fertility studies to be well prepared when pregnancy is achieved.	Folic acid is necessary in early pregnancy to help prevent neural tube anomalies. Overall health may contribute to fertility.	Client demonstrates she has filled her prenatal vitamin prescription and confirms she takes them daily. Client lists a healthy diet and states she does not smoke or take recreational drugs.
Patient-Centered Care				
Nurse	Assess whether couple is continuing to have a positive relationship in light of the diagnosis of unexplained subfertility.	Help partners review reasons they married, other than to have children.	Helping a couple find common interests can help them remain a couple and better prepare them for a parenting partnership.	Couple states they are taking steps to remain a close couple in light of the stress and possible negative results of assisted reproduction.
Spiritual/Psychosocial/Emotional Needs				
Nurse	Attempt to identify what it means to have unexplained subfertility for each client, individually and as a couple.	Clarify any misconceptions clients may have about unexplained subfertility.	Misconceptions can negatively affect self-esteem.	Clients accurately describe situation and manifest adequate self-esteem.
Informatics for Seamless Health Care Planning				
Nurse	Assess whether couple has any further questions about assisted reproduction and how they are active partners in the procedure Assess for intimate partner violence.	It is common for assisted reproduction to be extremely stressful. After pregnancy is achieved, waiting for a much-desired pregnancy to come to term can be just as stressful.	Identifying and describing stressful situations can help the couple prepare for them. Unresolved, stress can lead to intimate partner violence.	Couple states they feel well equipped to manage whatever changes assisted reproduction brings to their life.
Nurse	Determine who the couple has to turn to for support outside of health care providers.	Discuss possible support persons and groups.	Additional support can assist in reinforcing positive attributes, thus enhancing self-esteem.	Clients list at least two persons or groups to use for support.

Preimplantation Genetic Diagnosis

The individual retrieval of oocytes and their fertilization under laboratory conditions has led to close inspection and recognition of differences in sperm and oocytes. After the oocytes are fertilized in IVF and ZIFT procedures, the DNA of both sperm and oocytes can be examined for specific genetic abnormalities such as Down syndrome or hemophilia (Chang, Chen, Tsai, et al., 2011).

Couples participating in intrauterine transfer and alternative insemination can also have the sex of their children predetermined using these methods. Such techniques can be useful, because popular methods to influence the sex of a child (such as douching with a baking soda mixture before coitus to have a boy or with a vinegar solution to have a girl) have been proven to be more folklore than scientific fact. Allowing couples to choose the sex of children has ethical concerns because it could result in skewed male/female ratios if used by a majority of couples.

ALTERNATIVES TO CHILDBIRTH

For some couples, even treatment for subfertility with procedures such as IVF is not successful. These couples need to consider still other options.

Surrogate Mothers

A surrogate mother is a woman who agrees to carry a pregnancy to term for a subfertile couple (Jovic, 2011). The surrogate may provide the ova, which is then impregnated by the man's sperm in the laboratory. In other instances, the ova and sperm both may be donated by the subfertile couple; in a third technique, both donor ova and sperm are used. Surrogate mothers are often friends or family members who assume the role out of friendship or compassion, or they can be referred to the couple through an agency or attorney and receive monetary reimbursement for their expenses. The subfertile couple can enjoy the pregnancy as they watch it progress in the surrogate.

A number of ethical and legal problems arise if the surrogate mother decides at the end of pregnancy that she has formed an attachment to the fetus and wants to keep the baby despite the prepregnancy agreement she signed. Court decisions have been split on whether the surrogate or the subfertile couple has the right to the child. Another potential problem occurs if the child is born imperfect and the subfertile couple then no longer wants the child. Who should have responsibility in this instance? For these reasons, the couple and the surrogate mother must be certain they have given adequate thought to the process and to what will be the outcome should these problems occur before they attempt surrogate mothering.

Adoption

Adoption, once a ready alternative for subfertile couples, is still a viable alternative, although today there are fewer children available for adoption from official agencies. Urge couples to consider foreign-born or physically or cognitively challenged children or children of other cultures to make their family feel complete. The process of adoption is discussed in Chapter 2 with different types of families.

Child-Free Living

Child-free living is an alternative lifestyle available to both fertile and subfertile couples. For many subfertile couples who have been through the rigors and frustrations of subfertility testing and unsuccessful treatment regimens, child-free living may emerge as the option they finally wish to pursue. A couple in the midst of fertility testing may begin to reexamine their motives for pursuing pregnancy and may decide pregnancy and parenting are not worth the emotional or financial cost of future treatments. They may decide the additional stress of going through an adoption is not for them either, or they may simply decide children are not necessary for them to complete their family unit.

Child-free living can be as fulfilling as having children because it allows a couple more time to help other people and contribute to society through personal accomplishments. It has advantages for a couple in that it also allows time for both members to pursue careers. They can travel more or have more time and money to pursue hobbies or continue their education. If a couple still wishes to include children in their lives in some way, many opportunities are available to do this through family connections (most parents welcome offers from siblings or other family members to share in childrearing), through volunteer organizations (such as Big Brother or Big Sister programs), or through local schools and town recreational programs.

Many couples who believe overpopulation is a major concern choose child-free living even if subfertility is not present. Parents who choose child-free living typically rate their marriage as happier than for those with children probably because of the decreased expense involved and the availability of more free time, which allow them greater freedom in life (Cherlin, 2012).

What if...8.4 You are particularly interested in exploring one of the 2020 National Health Goals with respect to subfertility (see Box 8.1)? What would be a possible research topic to explore pertinent to this goal that would be applicable to the Carl family and that would also advance evidence-based practice?

Key Points for Review

- Subfertility is said to exist when a pregnancy has not occurred after 1 year of unprotected coitus. Sterility refers to the inability to conceive due to a known condition.
- About 14% of couples experience subfertility. The incidence increases with the age of the couple.
- Subfertility testing can be an intense psychological stressor for couples. Help couples to not only persist through the experience but to also maintain their relationship as a couple.
- Couples who are told a subfertility problem has been discovered are apt to suffer a loss of self-esteem. Offering support to help them recognize that they are still productive, healthy people in other aspects of their lives helps in planning nursing care that not only meets QSEN competencies but best meets the family's total needs.
- Male factors that contribute to subfertility are inadequate sperm count, obstruction or impaired sperm motility, and problems with ejaculation. Female factors that cause subfertility are problems with ovulation, cervical or tubal transport, or impaired implantation.
- Basic subfertility assessment procedures consist of a health history; a physical examination; laboratory tests to document general health; and specific tests for semen, ovulation, tubal patency, and uterine environment.
- Measures to induce fertility are aimed at improving sperm number and transport, decreasing infections, stimulating ovulation, improving nutrition, and regulating hormones.
- Alternative insemination, donor egg transfer, IVF, adoption, surrogate motherhood, and child-free living are all possible solutions for subfertility.

Critical Thinking Care Study

Josephine Rice is 26 years old, works as a nurse on an oncology service, and has been married for 6 years. Her husband, Peter, 28 years of age, is a race car driver. They have been trying to have a child for 4 years. A fertility study revealed that this is probably because Josephine doesn't ovulate every month. A specialist suggested she lose weight (her BMI is 27.5) and try IVF. She confides in you she feels the fault is not ovulation. It's because, unknown to her family, she had a Plan B abortion while in college and this is her "payback."

1. Does Josephine have risk factors because of her work? Are these more apt to be the reason for her subfertility than her former abortion?
2. Does Peter's job also create risk factors?
3. Was Josephine well advised to lose weight? How would you counsel her about the guilt she feels about having had an abortion?

Patient Scenario

The Newman Family

Read about the Newmans, a family who is having trouble conceiving a child, then answer the questions to further sharpen your skills and grow more familiar with NCLEX-type questions related to families having difficulty conceiving a child. Confirm your answers are correct by reading the rationales.

Visit http://thePoint.lww.com

Answers and Rationales

Looking for answers to the What If... and Critical Thinking Care Study questions?

Visit http://thePoint.lww.com

References

American Congress of Obstetricians and Gynecologists. (2011). *Intimate partner violence.* Washington, DC: Author.

Akanji Tijani, H., & Bhattacharya, S. (2010). The role of intrauterine insemination in male infertility. *Human Fertility, 13*(4), 226–232.

American Pregnancy Association. (2012). *In vitro fertilization.* Irving, TX: Author.

Balen, A. (2012). Polycystic ovary syndrome and secondary amenorrhea. In D. K. Edmonds (Ed.), *Dewhurst's textbook of obstetrics & gynaecology* (8th ed., pp. 513–533). Malden, MA: Blackwell Publishing.

Bouchlariotou, S., Tsikouras, P., Benjamin, R., et al. (2012). Fertility sparing in cancer patients. *Minimally Invasive Therapy & Allied Technologies, 21*(4), 282–292.

Catenacci, M., & Goldberg, J. K. (2012). Transvaginal hydrolaparoscopy technique & feasibility. *Seminars in Reproductive Medicine, 29*(2), 95–100.

Chachamovich, J. R., Chachamovich, E., Ezer, H., et al. (2010). Agreement on perceptions of quality of life in couples dealing with infertility. *Journal of Obstetric, Gynecologic, & Neonatal Nursing, 39*(5), 557–565.

Chang, L. J., Chen, S. U., Tsai, Y. Y., et al. (2011). An update of preimplantation genetic diagnosis in gene diseases, chromosomal translocation, and aneuploidy screening. *Clinical & Experimental Reproductive Medicine, 38*(3), 126–134.

Check, J. H., Katsoff, B., Brasile, D., et al. (2011). Comparison of pregnancy outcome following frozen embryo transfer (ET) in a gestational carrier program according to source of the oocytes. *Clinical & Experimental Obstetrics & Gynecology, 38*(1), 26–27.

Cherlin, A. J. (2012). *Public and private families.* New York, NY: McGraw Publishing Company.

Christianson, M. S., & Wallach, E. E. (2011). Infertility and assisted reproductive technologies. In K. J. Hurt, M. W. Guile, J. L. Bienstock, et al. (Eds.), *The Johns Hopkins manual of gynecology and obstetrics* (4th ed., pp. 421–437). Philadelphia, PA: Lippincott Williams & Wilkins.

Deffieux, X., Morin Surroca, M., Faivre, E., et al. (2011). Tubal anastomosis after tubal sterilization: A review. *Archives of Gynecology & Obstetrics, 283*(5), 1149–1158.

Desai, N., Goldberg, J., Austin, C., et al. (2012). Cryopreservation of individually selected sperm: Methodology and case report of a clinical pregnancy. *Journal of Assisted Reproduction & Genetics, 29*(5), 375–379.

Dillon, K. E., & Gracia, C. R. (2012). Pediatric and young adult patients and oncofertility. *Current Treatment Options in Oncology, 13*(2), 161–173.

Eggertson, L. (2011). Fertility nurses: Giving mother nature a helping hand. *Canadian Nurse, 107*(9), 32–36.

Fariello, R. M., Pariz, J. R., Spaine, D. M., et al. (2012). Association between obesity and alteration of sperm DNA integrity and mitochondrial activity. *British Journal of Urology, 110*(6), 863–867.

Fisher, J. R., Rowe, H., & Hammarberg, K. (2012). Admissions for early parenting difficulties among women with infants conceived by assisted reproductive technologies: A prospective cohort study. *Fertility & Sterility, 97*(6), 1410–1416.

Frass, M., Strassl, R. P., Friehs, H., et al. (2012). Use and acceptance of complementary and alternative medicine among the general population and medical personnel: A systematic review. *The Ochsner Journal, 12*(1), 45–56.

Fritz, M. A., & Speroff, L. (2010). Female infertility. In M. A. Fritz & L. Speroff (Eds.), *Clinical gynecologic endocrinology and infertility* (8th ed., pp. 1137–1191). Philadelphia, PA: Lippincott Williams & Wilkins.

Gambadauro, P., Gudmundsson, J., & Torrejón, R. (2012). Intrauterine adhesions following conservative treatment of uterine fibroids. *Obstetrics & Gynecology International, 2012,* 853269.

Ghadir, S., Ambartsumyan, G., & Decherny, A. H. (2013). Infertility. In A. H. DeCherney, L. Nathan, T. M. Goodwin, et al. (Eds.), *Current diagnosis and treatment: Obstetrics and gynecology* (11th ed., pp. 879–888). Columbus, OH: McGraw-Hill/Lange.

Guile, M. W., & Keller, J. (2011). Infections of the genital tract. In K. J. Hurt, M. W. Guile, J. L. Bienstock, et al. (Eds.), *The Johns Hopkins manual of gynecology and obstetrics* (4th ed., pp. 322–339). Philadelphia, PA: Lippincott Williams & Wilkins.

Gunderson, C., & Yates, M. (2011). Menstrual disorders: Endometriosis, dysmenorrhea & premenstrual dysphoric syndrome. In K. J. Hurt, M. W. Guile, J. L. Bienstock, et al. (Eds.), *The Johns Hopkins manual of gynecology and obstetrics* (4th ed., pp. 454–463). Philadelphia, PA: Lippincott Williams & Wilkins.

Hamilton, M. (2012). Infertility. In D. K. Edmonds (Ed.), *Dewhurst's textbook of obstetrics & gynaecology* (8th ed., pp. 567–579). Oxford, UK: John Wiley & Son.

Hammarberg, K., Fisher, J. R., Wynter, K. H., et al. (2011). Breastfeeding after assisted conception: A prospective cohort study. *Acta Paediatrica, 100*(4), 529–533.

Hammoud, A. O., Meikle, A. W., Reis, L. O., et al. (2012). Obesity and male infertility: A practical approach. *Seminars in Reproductive Medicine, 30*(6), 486–495.

Hanson, S. J., & Burke, A. E. (2011). Fertility control. In K. J. Hurt, M. W. Guile, J. L. Bienstock, et al. (Eds.), *The Johns Hopkins manual of gynecology and obstetrics* (4th ed., pp. 382–395). Philadelphia, PA: Lippincott Williams & Wilkins.

Hasson, J., Shapira, A., Many, A., et al. (2011). Reduction of twin pregnancy to singleton: Does it improve pregnancy outcome? *Journal of Maternal-Fetal, & Neonatal Medicine, 24*(11), 1362–1366.

Hedger, M. P. (2011). Immunophysiology and pathology of inflammation in the testis and epididymis. *Journal of Andrology, 32*(6), 625–640.

Horovitz, D., Tjong, V., Domes, T., et al. (2012). Vasectomy reversal provides long-term pain relief for men with the post-vasectomy pain syndrome. *Journal of Urology, 187*(2), 613–617.

Huang, H., Hansen, K. R., Factor-Litvak, P., et al. (2012). Predictors of pregnancy and live birth after insemination in couples with unexplained or male-factor infertility. *Fertility & Sterility, 97*(4), 959–967.

Hutchinson, K., Cruickshank, K., & Wylie, K. (2012). A benefit-risk assessment of dapoxetine in the treatment of premature ejaculation. *Drug Safety, 35*(5), 359–372.

Imudia, A. N., Awonuga, A. O., Kaimal, A. J., et al. (2012). Elective cryopreservation of all embryos with subsequent cryothaw embryo transfer in patients at risk for ovarian hyperstimulation syndrome reduces the risk of adverse obstetric outcomes: A preliminary study. *Fertility & Sterility, 98*(S3), S184.

Irwig, M. S., & Kolukula, S. (2011). Persistent sexual side effects of finasteride for male pattern hair loss. *Journal of Sexual Medicine, 8*(6), 1747–1753.

Jovic, O. S. (2011). Surrogate motherhood as a medical treatment procedure for women's infertility. *Medicine & Law, 30*(1), 23–37.

Karch, A. M. (2013). *2013 Lippincott's nursing drug guide.* Philadelphia, PA: Lippincott Williams & Wilkins.

Kokopelli Technologies. (2012). *Fertility for men.* Santa Fe, NM: Author.

Lerchbaum, E., & Obermayer-Pietsch, B. R. (2012). Vitamin D and fertility: A systematic review. *European Journal of Endocrinology, 166*(1), 765–778.

Magos, A. (2012). Hysteroscopy & laparoscopy. In D. K. Edmonds (Ed.), *Dewhurst's textbook of obstetrics & gynaecology* (8th ed., pp. 448–470). Oxford, UK: John Wiley & Son.

Miyaoka, R., & Esteves, S. C. (2012). A critical appraisal on the role of varicocele in male infertility. *Advances in Urology, 5*(1), 1–9.

Nodine, P. M., & Hastings-Tolsma, M. (2012). Maternal obesity: Improving pregnancy outcomes. *American Journal of Maternal Child Nursing, 37*(2), 110–115.

Sabanegh, E., & Agarwal, A. (2012). Male infertility. In W. S. McDougal, A. J. Wein, L. R. Kavoussi, et al. (Eds.), *Campbell-Walsh urology* (10th ed., pp. 106–112). Philadelphia, PA: Elsevier.

Sheaves, C. (2013). Advances in endometriosis treatment. *Nurse Practitioner, 38*(5): 42–47.

Smith, M. L., & Schust, D. J. (2011). Endocrinology and recurrent early pregnancy loss. *Seminars in Reproductive Medicine, 29*(6), 482–490.

Speroni, K. G., Earley, C., Seibert, D., et al. (2012). Effect of Nurses Living Fit™ exercise and nutrition intervention on body mass index in nurses. *Journal of Nursing Administration, 42*(4), 231–238.

Trew, G., & Lavery, S. (2012). Assisted reproduction. In D. K. Edmonds (Ed.), *Dewhurst's textbook of obstetrics & gynaecology* (8th ed., pp. 580–596). Oxford, UK: John Wiley & Son.

U.S. Department of Health and Human Services. (2010). *Healthy people 2020.* Washington, DC: Author.

Weiss, T. R., & Bulmer, S. M. (2011). Young women's experiences living with polycystic ovary syndrome. *Journal of Obstetric, Gynecologic, & Neonatal Nursing, 40*(6), 709–718.

World Health Organization. (2010). *WHO laboratory manual for the examination & processing of human semen* (5th ed.). Geneva, Switzerland: Author.

Zollner, U., & Dietl, J. (2013). Perinatal risks after IVF and ICSI. *Journal of Perinatal Medicine, 41*(1), 17–22.

Unit 3

The Nursing Role in Caring for Families During Normal Pregnancy, Birth, the Postpartum, and Newborn Period

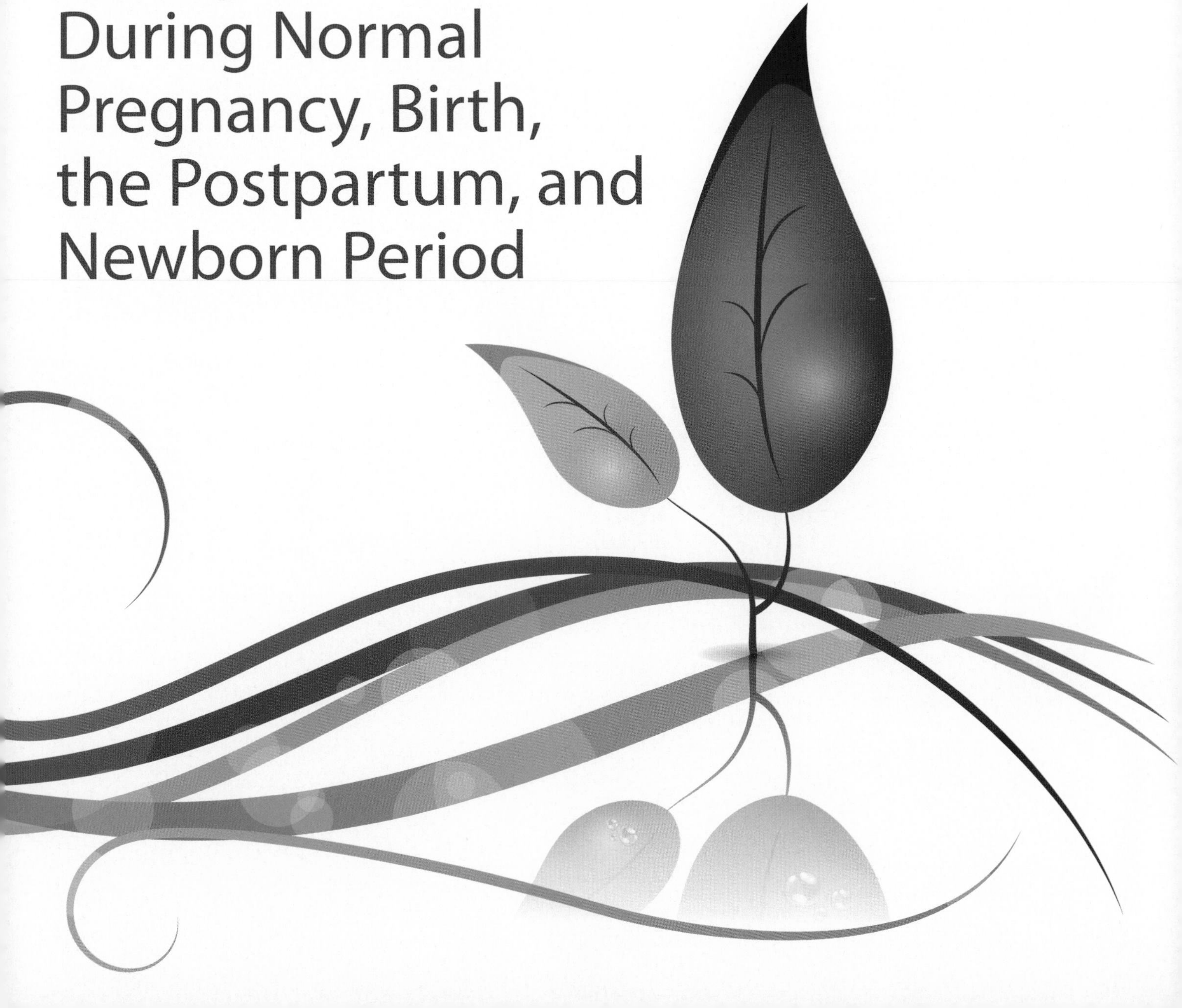

Chapter 9

Nursing Care of the Growing Fetus

KEY TERMS

- age of viability
- amniocentesis
- amniotic membrane
- cephalocaudal
- chorionic membrane
- chorionic villi
- decidua
- embryo
- estimated date of birth
- fertilization
- fetoscopy
- fetus
- foramen ovale
- hydramnios
- implantation
- McDonald's rule
- meconium
- nonstress test
- oligohydramnios
- organogenesis
- surfactant
- trophoblast
- umbilical cord
- zygote

OBJECTIVES

After mastering the contents of this chapter, you should be able to:

1. Describe the growth and development of a fetus by gestation week.
2. Identify 2020 National Health Goals related to fetal growth that nurses can help the nation achieve.
3. Assess fetal growth and development through maternal and pregnancy landmarks.
4. Formulate nursing diagnoses related to the needs of a fetus.
5. Establish expected outcomes to meet the perceived needs of a growing fetus as well as manage a seamless transition from fetus to newborn.
6. Using the nursing process, plan nursing care that includes the six competencies of Quality & Safety Education for Nurses (QSEN): Patient-Centered Care, Teamwork & Collaboration, Evidence-Based Practice (EBP), Quality Improvement (QI), Safety, and Informatics.
7. Implement nursing care to help ensure both a safe fetal environment and a safe pregnancy outcome.
8. Evaluate expected outcomes for achievement and effectiveness of care.
9. Integrate knowledge of fetal growth and development with the interplay of nursing process, the six competencies of QSEN, and Family Nursing to promote quality maternal and child health nursing care.

Liz Calhorn, an 18-year-old, is 20 weeks pregnant. Although she says she knows she should have stopped smoking before pregnancy, she has not been able to do this as yet. Twice during the pregnancy (at the 4th and 10th week), she drank beer at summer picnics. Today, at a clinic visit, she tells you she has felt her fetus move. She states, "Feeling the baby move made me realize there's someone inside me, you know what I mean? It made me realize it's time I started being more careful with what I do." Liz works at a fast food restaurant. Her boyfriend (the father of fetus) is supportive, but has no money to give her. Client states, "I'm not getting married. Just not ready for that big a commitment yet."

Feeling a fetus move is often the trigger that makes having a baby "real" for many women. The more women know about fetal development before and after this event, the easier it is for them to begin to think of the pregnancy not as something interesting happening to them, but as an act producing a separate life. A previous chapter described reproductive anatomy. This chapter adds information about fetal growth and development and assessment of fetal health.

In light of Liz's revelation, what additional health teaching does she need?

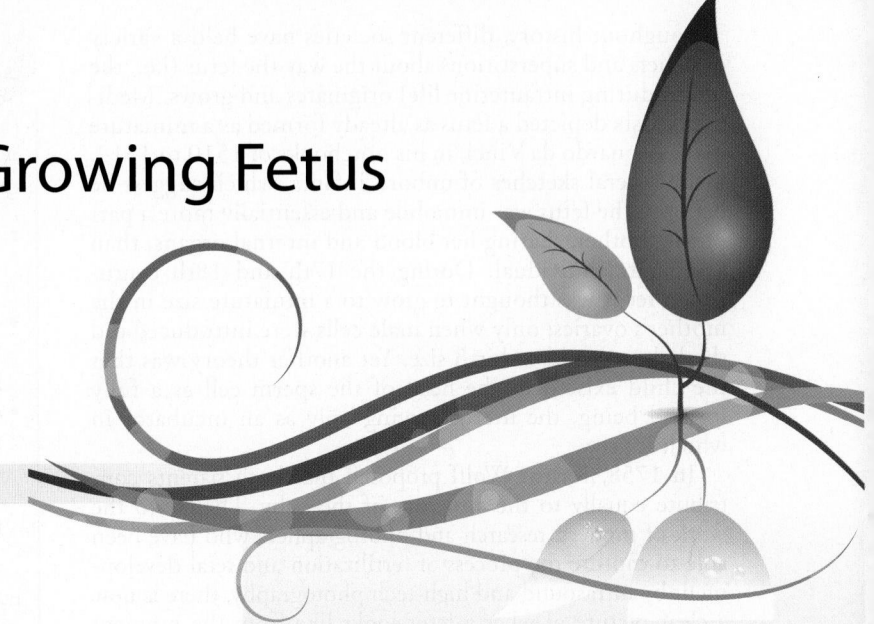

Throughout history, different societies have held a variety of beliefs and superstitions about the way the fetus (i.e., the infant during intrauterine life) originates and grows. Medieval artists depicted a fetus as already formed as a miniature man. Leonardo da Vinci, in his notebooks of 1510 to 1512, made several sketches of unborn infants, which suggest he believed the fetus was immobile and essentially more a part of the mother, sharing her blood and internal organs, than a separate individual. During the 17th and 18th centuries, a fetus was thought to grow to a miniature size in the mother's ovaries; only when male cells were introduced did the baby expand to birth size. Yet another theory was that the child existed in the head of the sperm cell as a fully formed being, the uterus serving only as an incubator in which it grew.

In 1758, Kaspar Wolff proposed that both parents contribute equally to the structure of the baby. Thanks to the work of modern research and photographers who have been able to capture the process of fertilization and fetal development by ultrasound and high-tech photography, there is now a clear picture of what a fetus looks like from the moment of conception until birth. It allows both families and health care providers to view the fetus as a patient separate from the mother (McCoyd, 2013; Miesnik, 2012).

Because you cannot have healthy children without healthy intrauterine growth, several 2020 National Health Goals speak to the importance of protecting fetal growth (Box 9.1).

BOX 9.1 Nursing Care Planning Based on 2020 National Health Goals

A number of 2020 National Health Goals address fetal growth.

- Reduce the fetal death rate (death between 20 and 40 weeks of gestation) to no more than 5.6 per 1,000 live births from a baseline of 6.2 per 1,000.
- Reduce low birth weight to an incidence of 7.8% of live births and very low birth weight to 1.4% of live births from baselines of 8.2% and 1.5%.
- Increase the proportion of women of childbearing potential with an intake of at least 400 mg of folic acid from fortified foods or dietary supplements from a baseline of 23.8% to 26.2% (U.S. Department of Health and Human Services [DHHS], 2010; see www.healthypeople.gov).

Folic acid deficiency in pregnancy can lead to midline closure defects such as neural tube disorders. Nurses can help the nation achieve these goals by urging women to plan their pregnancies so they can enter the pregnancy in good health and with an optimum folic acid level. Educating women about the importance of attending prenatal care is another important role.

Nursing Process Overview

To Help Ensure Fetal Health

Assessment

Assessing fetal growth throughout pregnancy, by such means as measuring fundal height and fetal heart rate, is important because these signs of fetal development provide guidelines for determining the well-being of a fetus. For the expectant family, knowledge about fetal growth and development can help a woman understand some of the changes going on in her body as well as allow all family members to begin thinking about and accepting a new member to their family. For this reason, not only assess fetal development at prenatal visits but also convey the findings to the family in as much detail as parents request.

Nursing Diagnosis

Common nursing diagnoses related to growth and development of the fetus focus on the mother and family as well as the fetus. Examples might include:

- Readiness for enhanced knowledge related to usual fetal development
- Anxiety related to lack of fetal movement
- Deficient knowledge related to the need for good prenatal care for healthy fetal well-being

Outcome Identification and Planning

Be certain plans for care include ways to educate potential parents about teratogens (i.e., any substance harmful to a fetus) that have the potential to interfere with fetal health. Be certain that outcome criteria established for teaching about fetal growth are realistic and based on the parents' previous knowledge and desire for information. When additional assessment measures are necessary, such as an amniocentesis or an ultrasound examination, add this information to the teaching plan, explaining why further assessment is necessary and what the parents can expect from the procedure. Interesting Web sites for parents that show fetal development in photographs are www.Babycenter.com and www.MedicineNet.com. Suspected workplace teratogens can be reported to the Occupational Safety & Health Administration at www.osha.gov.

Implementation

Most expectant parents are interested in learning about how mature their fetus is at various points in pregnancy as this helps them visualize their coming newborn. This, in turn, helps them to understand the importance of implementing healthy behaviors, such as eating well and avoiding substances that may be dangerous to a fetus such as recreational drugs. Viewing a sonogram and learning the fetal sex is a big step toward helping initiate bonding between the parents and the infant. Remember each woman's pregnancy is unique to her; be certain implementations are individualized for each woman for the best chance of outcome success.

Outcome Evaluation

An outcome evaluation related to fetal growth and development usually focuses on determining whether a woman or family has made any changes in lifestyle necessary to ensure fetal growth and whether a woman voices confidence that her baby is healthy and growing. Examples of expected outcomes include:

- Parents describe smoke-free living by next prenatal visit.
- Client records number of movements fetus makes during 1 hour daily.
- Couple attends all scheduled prenatal visits.
- Client states she is looking forward to the birth of her baby.

STAGES OF FETAL DEVELOPMENT

In just 38 weeks, a fertilized egg (ovum) matures from a single cell to a fully developed fetus ready to be born. Although different cultures or religions debate the point at which life begins, for ease of discussion, all agree fetal growth and development can be divided into three time periods:

- Pre-embryonic (first 2 weeks, beginning with fertilization)
- Embryonic (weeks 3 through 8)
- Fetal (from week 8 through birth)

Table 9.1 lists common terms used to describe the fetus at various stages in this growth.

Fertilization: The Beginning of Pregnancy

Fertilization (also referred to as conception and impregnation) is the union of an ovum and a spermatozoon. This usually occurs in the outer third of a fallopian tube, termed the ampullar portion (Taylor & Badell, 2011).

Usually, only one of a woman's ova reaches maturity each month. Once the mature ovum is released (i.e., ovulation), fertilization must occur fairly quickly because an ovum is capable of fertilization for only about 24 hours (48 hours at the most). After that time, it atrophies and becomes nonfunctional. Because the functional life of a spermatozoon is also about 48 hours, possibly as long as 72 hours, the total critical time span during which sexual relations must occur for fertilization to be successful is about 72 hours (48 hours before ovulation plus 24 hours afterward).

TABLE 9.1 Terms Used to Describe Fetal Growth

Name	Time Period
Ovum	From ovulation to fertilization.
Zygote	From fertilization to implantation.
Embryo	From implantation to 5–8 weeks.
Fetus	From 5–8 weeks until term.
Conceptus	Developing embryo and placental structures throughout pregnancy.
Age of viability	The earliest age at which fetuses survive if they are born is generally accepted as 24 weeks, or at the point a fetus weighs more than 500–600 g.

As the ovum is extruded from the graafian follicle of an ovary with ovulation, it is surrounded by a ring of mucopolysaccharide fluid (the zona pellucida) and a circle of cells (the corona radiata). The ovum and these surrounding cells (which increase the bulk of the ovum and serve as protective buffers against injury) are propelled into a nearby fallopian tube by currents initiated by the fimbriae—the fine, hairlike structures that line the openings of the tubes. A combination of peristaltic action of the tube and movements of the tube cilia help propel the ovum along the length of the tube.

Normally, an ejaculation of semen averages 2.5 ml of fluid containing 50 to 200 million spermatozoa per milliliter, or an average of 400 million sperm per ejaculation (Christianson & Wallach, 2011). At the time of ovulation, there is a reduction in the viscosity (thickness) of the woman's cervical mucus, which makes it easy for spermatozoa to penetrate it. Sperm transport is so efficient close to ovulation that spermatozoa deposited in the vagina generally reach the cervix within 90 seconds and the outer end of a fallopian tube within 5 minutes after deposition.

The mechanism whereby spermatozoa are drawn toward an ovum is probably a species-specific reaction, similar to an antibody–antigen reaction. Spermatozoa move through the cervix and the body of the uterus and into the fallopian tube, toward a waiting ovum by the combination of movement by their flagella (tails) and uterine contractions.

All of the spermatozoa that reach the ovum cluster around its protective layer of corona cells. Hyaluronidase (a proteolytic enzyme) is released by the spermatozoa and dissolves the layer of cells protecting the ovum. Under ordinary circumstances, only one spermatozoon is able to penetrate the cell membrane of the ovum. Once it penetrates the cell, the cell membrane changes composition to become impervious to other spermatozoa. An exception to this is the formation of gestational trophoblastic disease in which multiple sperm enter an ovum; this leads to abnormal zygote formation (Digiulio, Wiedaseck, & Monchek, 2012) (see Chapter 21).

Immediately after penetration of the ovum, the chromosomal material of the ovum and spermatozoon fuse to form a **zygote**. Because the spermatozoon and ovum each carried 23 chromosomes (22 autosomes and 1 sex chromosome), the fertilized ovum has 46 chromosomes. If an X-carrying spermatozoon entered the ovum, the resulting child will have two X chromosomes and will be female (XX). If a Y-carrying spermatozoon fertilized the ovum, the resulting child will have an X and a Y chromosome and will be male (XY).

Fertilization is never a certain occurrence because it depends on at least three separate factors:

- Equal maturation of both sperm and ovum
- Ability of the sperm to reach the ovum
- Ability of the sperm to penetrate the zona pellucida and cell membrane and achieve fertilization

Out of this single-cell fertilized ovum (zygote), the future child and also the accessory structures needed for support during intrauterine life (placenta, fetal membranes, amniotic fluid, and umbilical cord) will form.

Implantation

Once fertilization is complete, a zygote migrates over the next 3 to 4 days toward the body of the uterus, aided by the currents initiated by the muscular contractions of the fallopian tubes. During this time, mitotic cell division, or cleavage, begins.

loop of cord is found around the fetal neck (nuchal cord) at birth (Hoh, Sung, & Park, 2012). If this loop of cord is removed before the newborn's shoulders are born (not usually hard to do) so there is no traction on it, the oxygen supply to the fetus remains unimpaired.

The walls of the umbilical cord arteries are lined with smooth muscle. When these muscles contract after birth, the cord arteries and vein are compressed to prevent hemorrhage of the newborn through the cord. Because the umbilical cord contains no nerve supply, it can be clamped and cut at birth without discomfort to either the child or mother.

QSEN Checkpoint Question 9.2

Safety

Suppose Liz Calhorn tells you she is worried her baby will be born with a congenital heart disease. What assessment of the umbilical cord at birth would be most important to help detect congenital heart defects?

a. Assessing whether the pH of the Wharton jelly is higher than 7.2
b. Assessing whether the umbilical cord has two arteries and one vein
c. Measuring the length of the cord to be certain it is longer than 3 ft
d. Determining that the umbilical cord is neither green nor yellow stained

Look in Appendix A for the best answer and rationale.

ORIGIN AND DEVELOPMENT OF ORGAN SYSTEMS

Following the moment of fertilization, the zygote, which later becomes an embryo and then a fetus, begins to grow at an active pace.

Stem Cells

During the first 4 days of life, zygote cells are termed totipotent stem cells, or cells so undifferentiated they have the potential to grow into any cell in the human body. In another 4 days, as the structure implants and becomes an embryo, cells begin to show differentiation, or lose their ability to become any body cell. Instead, they are slated to become specific body cells, such as nerve, brain, or skin cells and are termed pluripotent stem cells. In yet another few days, the cells grow so specific they are termed multipotent, or are so specific they cannot be deterred from growing into a particular body organ such as spleen or liver or brain (Bernstein & Srivastava, 2012).

Zygote Growth

As soon as conception has taken place, development proceeds in a **cephalocaudal** (head-to-tail) direction; that is, head development occurs first and is followed by development of the middle, and finally, the lower body parts. This pattern of development continues after birth as shown by the way infants are able to lift up their heads approximately 1 year before they are able to walk.

Primary Germ Layers

As a fetus grows, body organ systems develop from specific tissue layers called germ layers. At the time of implantation, the blastocyst already has differentiated to a point at which three separate layers of these cells are present: the *ectoderm*, the *endoderm*, and the *mesoderm* (see Fig. 9.1). Each of these germ layers develops into specific body systems (Table 9.2). Knowing which structures arise from each germ layer is helpful to know because coexisting congenital disorders found in newborns usually arise from the same germ layer. For example, a fistula between the trachea and the esophagus (both of which arise from the endoderm layer) is a common birth anomaly. In contrast, it is rare to see a newborn with a malformation of the heart (which arises from the mesoderm) and also a malformation of the lower urinary tract (which arises from the endoderm). One reason rubella infection is so serious in pregnancy is because this virus is capable of infecting all three germ layers so can cause congenital anomalies in a myriad of body systems (White, Boldt, Holditch, et al., 2012).

All organ systems are complete, at least in a rudimentary form, at 8 weeks gestation (the end of the embryonic period). During this early time of **organogenesis** (organ formation), the growing structure is most vulnerable to invasion by eratogens (i.e., any factor that affects the fertilized ovum, embryo, or fetus adversely, such as a teratogenic medicine; an infection such as toxoplasmosis; cigarette smoking; or alcohol ingestion) (Box 9.2). Figure 9.4 illustrates critical periods of fetal growth when it is most important for women to minimize their exposure to teratogens. The effect of individual teratogens and how to avoid them is discussed in Chapter 12.

Cardiovascular System

The cardiovascular system is one of the first systems to become functional in intrauterine life. Simple blood cells joined

TABLE 9.2 Origin of Body Tissue

Germ Layer	Body Portions Formed
Ectoderm	Central nervous system (brain and spinal cord) Peripheral nervous system Skin, hair, nails, and tooth enamel Sense organs Mucous membranes of the anus, mouth, and nose Mammary glands
Mesoderm	Supporting structures of the body (connective tissue, bones, cartilage, muscle, ligaments, and tendons) Upper portion of the urinary system (kidneys and ureters) Reproductive system Heart, lymph, and circulatory systems and blood cells
Endoderm	Lining of pericardial, pleura, and peritoneal cavities Lining of the gastrointestinal tract, respiratory tract, tonsils, parathyroid, thyroid, and thymus glands Lower urinary system (bladder and urethra)

BOX 9.2 Nursing Care Planning Based on Family Teaching

Q. Liz Calhorn tells you, "I have to work. How can I guard against fetal teratogens at work?"

A. Here are a number of helpful tips:

- Ask your employer for a statement on hazardous substances at your work site; discuss your need to avoid these substances during pregnancy.
- Ask your employer to maintain a smoke-free site if that is not already a rule.
- Avoid any room, such as a coffee room, where smokers gather.
- Refrain from drinking alcohol, a frequent accompaniment to work lunches or social functions; ask for nonalcoholic drinks to be available at such events.
- Locate a fellow coworker who will "buddy" with you to help you avoid alcohol or tobacco at work activities.
- If quitting smoking is difficult, try a supportive telephone or Internet quitline. Ask your primary health care provider before using a nicotine patch, nicotine gum, or bupropion (Zyban), a drug to assist smokers to quit. Both nicotine and Zyban are category C drugs; Zyban is particularly contraindicated in women with symptoms of gestational hypertension as it can cause seizures in high doses.

to the walls of the yolk sac progress to become a network of blood vessels and a single heart tube, which forms as early as the 16th day of life and beats as early as the 24th day. The septum that divides the heart into chambers develops during the sixth or seventh week; heart valves develop in the seventh week. The heartbeat may be heard with a Doppler instrument as early as the 10th to 12th week of pregnancy. An electrocardiogram (ECG) may be recorded on a fetus as early as the 11th week, although the accuracy of such ECGs is in doubt until about the 20th week of pregnancy, when conduction is more regulated.

The heart rate of a fetus is affected by oxygen level, activity, and circulating blood volume, just as in adulthood. After the 28th week of pregnancy, when the sympathetic nervous system has matured, the heart rate stabilizes or begins to show a consistent beat of 110 to 160 beats/min.

Fetal Circulation

Fetal circulation (Fig. 9.5) differs from extrauterine circulation because the fetus derives oxygen and excretes carbon dioxide not from gas exchange in the lungs but from exchange in the placenta.

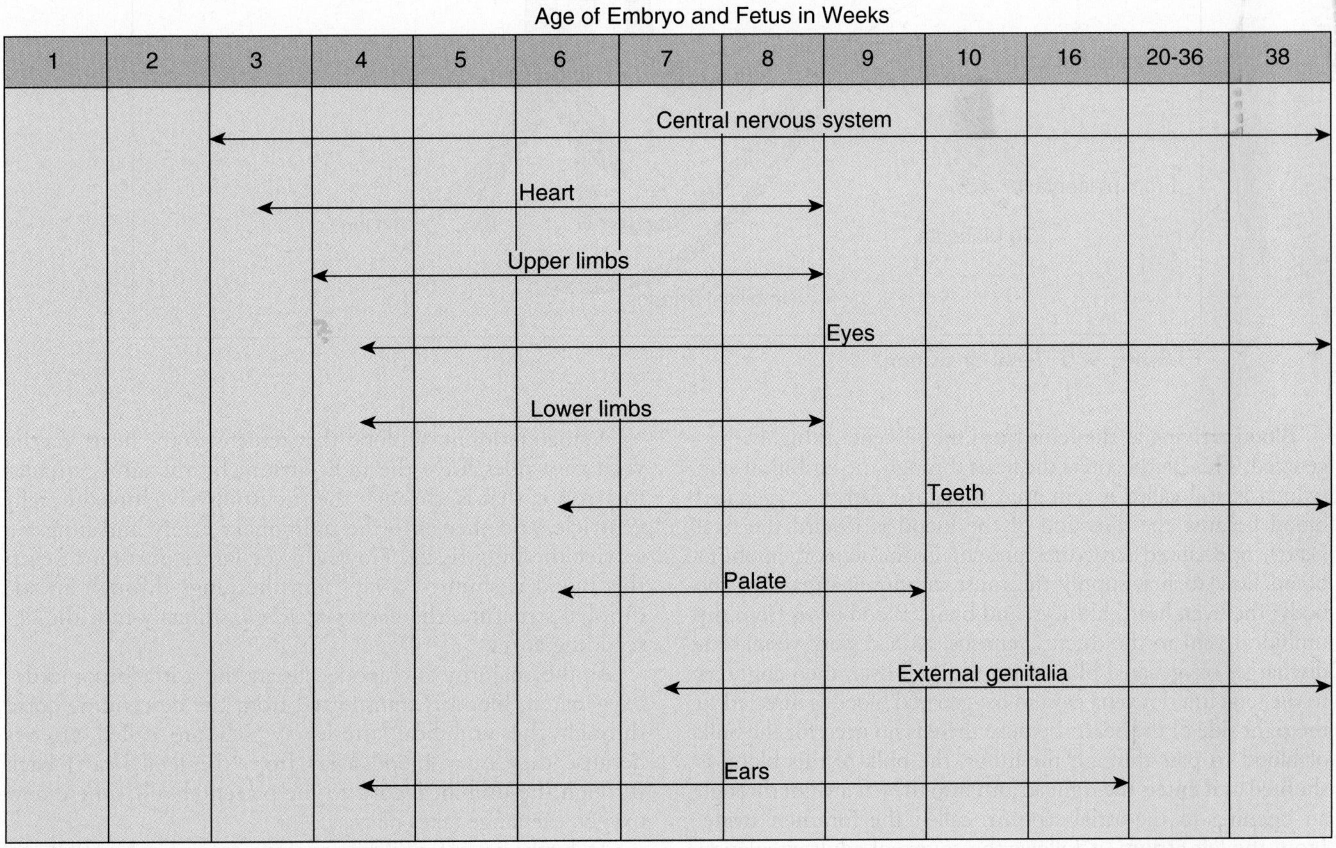

FIGURE 9.4 Critical periods of fetal growth.

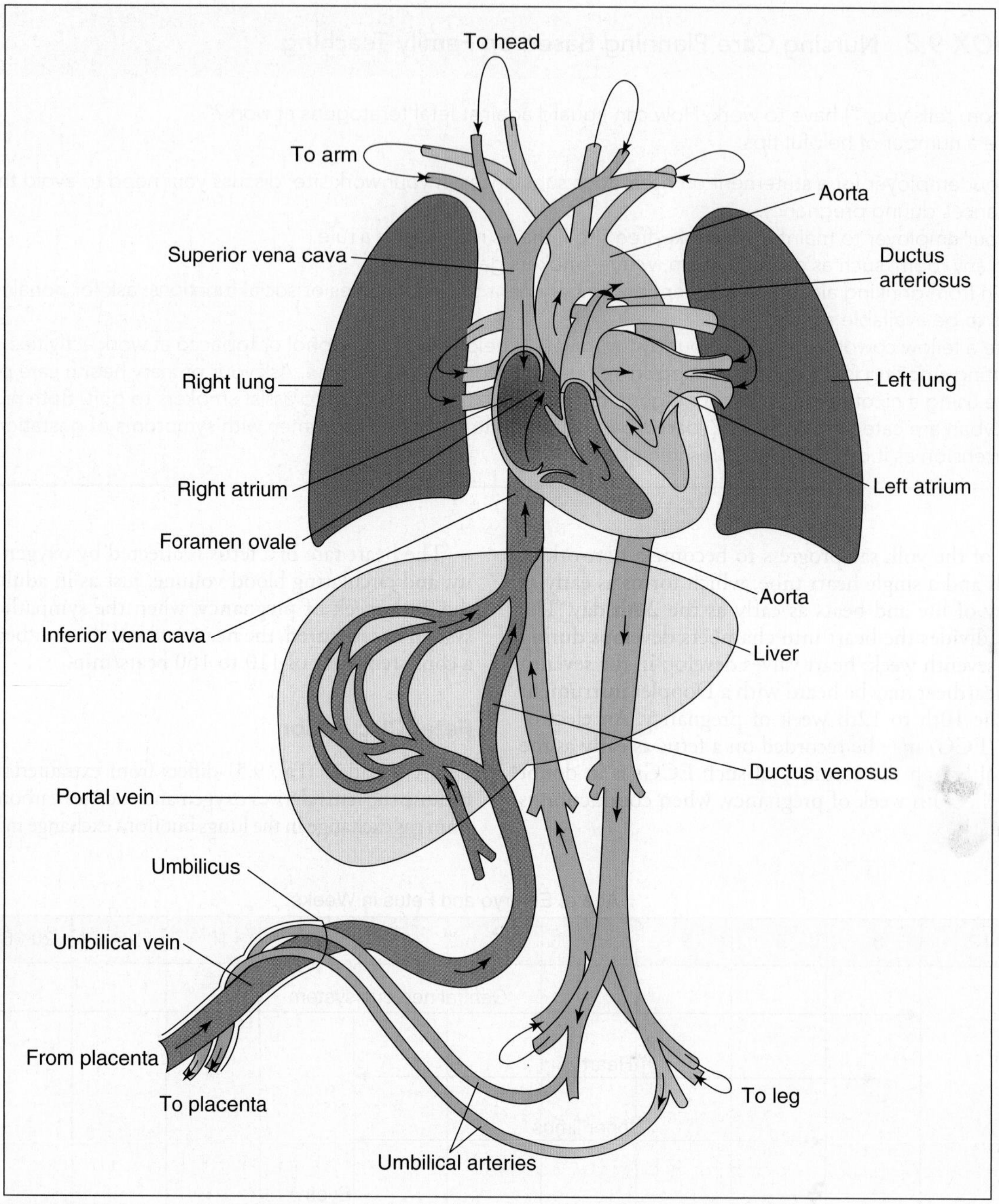

FIGURE 9.5 Fetal circulation.

Blood arriving at the fetus from the placenta is highly oxygenated. This blood enters the fetus through the umbilical vein (which is still called a vein even though it carries oxygenated blood because the direction of the blood is toward the fetal heart). Specialized structures present in the fetus then shunt blood flow to first supply the most important organs of the body: the liver, heart, kidneys, and brain. Blood flows from the umbilical vein to the ductus venosus, an accessory vessel that discharges oxygenated blood into the fetal liver, then connects to the fetal inferior vena cava so oxygenated blood is directed to the right side of the heart. Because there is no need for the bulk of blood to pass through the lungs, the bulk of this blood is shunted as it enters the right atrium into the left atrium through an opening in the atrial septum, called the **foramen ovale**. From the left atrium, it follows the course of adult circulation into the left ventricle, then into the aorta, and out to body parts.

A small amount of blood that returns to the heart via the vena cava does leave the right atrium by the adult circulatory route; that is, through the tricuspid valve into the right ventricle, and then into the pulmonary artery and lungs to service the lung tissue. However, the larger portion of even this blood is shunted away from the lungs through an additional structure, the *ductus arteriosus*, directly into the descending aorta.

As the majority of blood cells in the aorta become deoxygenated, blood is transported from the descending aorta through the umbilical arteries (which are called arteries because they carry blood away from the fetal heart) back through the umbilical cord to the placental villi, where new oxygen exchange takes place.

At birth, an infant's oxygen saturation level is 95% to 100% and pulse rate is 80 to 140 beats/min. Because there is a great deal of mixing of blood in the fetus, the oxygen saturation level of fetal blood reaches only about 80%. In light of this, the fetal heart has to beat rapidly (110 to 160 beats/min) to supply needed oxygen to cells. Even with this low blood oxygen saturation level, however, carbon dioxide does not accumulate in the fetal system because it rapidly diffuses into maternal blood across a favorable placental pressure gradient.

Fetal Hemoglobin

Fetal hemoglobin differs from adult hemoglobin in several ways. It has a different composition (two alpha and two gamma chains, compared with two alpha and two beta chains of adult hemoglobin). It is also more concentrated and has greater oxygen affinity, two features that increase its efficiency. Because hemoglobin is more concentrated, a newborn's hemoglobin level is about 17.1 g/100 ml, compared with a normal adult level of 11 g/100 ml; a newborn's hematocrit is about 53%, compared with a normal adult level of 45%.

The change from fetal to adult hemoglobin levels begins before birth (gamma cells are exchanged for beta cells) but the process is still not complete at birth. Major blood dyscrasias, such as sickle cell anemia, tend to be defects of the beta hemoglobin chain, which is why clinical symptoms of these disorders do not become apparent until the bulk of fetal hemoglobin has matured to adult hemoglobin, at about 6 months of age (Panepinto & Scott, 2011).

Respiratory System

At the third week of intrauterine life, the respiratory and digestive tracts exist as a single tube. Like all body tubes, initially this forms as a solid structure, which then canalizes (i.e., hollows out). By the end of the fourth week, a septum begins to divide the esophagus from the trachea. At the same time, lung buds appear on the trachea.

Until the seventh week of life, the diaphragm does not completely divide the thoracic cavity from the abdomen. This causes lung buds to extend down into the abdomen, re-entering the chest only as the chest's longitudinal dimension increases and the diaphragm becomes complete (at the end of the seventh week). If the diaphragm fails to close completely, the stomach, spleen, liver, or intestines may be pulled up into the thoracic cavity. This causes the child to be born with intestine present in the chest (i.e., diaphragmatic hernia), compromising the lungs and perhaps displacing the heart (Gowen, 2011).

Other important respiratory developmental milestones include:

- Spontaneous respiratory practice movements begin as early as 3 months gestation and continue throughout pregnancy.
- Specific lung fluid with a low surface tension and low viscosity forms in alveoli to aid in expansion of the alveoli at birth; it is rapidly absorbed shortly after birth.
- **Surfactant**, a phospholipid substance, is formed and excreted by the alveolar cells of the lungs beginning at about the 24th week of pregnancy. This decreases alveolar surface tension on expiration, preventing alveolar collapse and improving the infant's ability to maintain respirations in the outside environment at birth (Rojas-Reyes, Morley & Soll, 2012).

Surfactant has two components: lecithin (L) and sphingomyelin (S). Early in the formation of surfactant, sphingomyelin is the chief component. At about 35 weeks, there is a surge in the production of lecithin, which then becomes the chief component by a ratio of 2:1. As a fetus practices breathing movements, surfactant mixes with amniotic fluid. Using an amniocentesis technique, an analysis of the lecithin/sphingomyelin (L/S) ratio in surfactant (whether lecithin or sphingomyelin is the dominant component) is a primary test of fetal maturity. Respiratory distress syndrome, a severe breathing disorder, can develop if there is a lack of surfactant or it has not changed to its mature form at birth (see Chapter 26).

Any interference with the blood supply to the fetus, such as occurs with placental insufficiency or maternal hypertension, appears to raise steroid levels in the fetus and enhance surfactant development. Synthetically increasing steroid levels in the fetus (e.g., the administration of betamethasone to the mother late in pregnancy) can also hurry alveolar maturation and surfactant production without interfering with permanent lung function prior to a preterm birth (Hjalmarson & Sandberg, 2011).

✔ QSEN Checkpoint Question 9.3

Informatics

Liz Calhorn asks you why her nurse midwife is concerned whether her fetus's lungs are producing surfactant. Your best answer would be:

a. "Surfactant keeps lungs from collapsing at birth, so it aids newborn breathing."
b. "Surfactant is produced by the fetal liver, so its presence reveals liver maturity."
c. "Surfactant is necessary for antibody production, so it helps prevents infection."
d. "Surfactant reveals mature kidney function, as it is important for fetal growth."

Look in Appendix A for the best answer and rationale.

Nervous System

Like the circulatory system, the nervous system begins to develop extremely early in pregnancy.

- A neural plate (a thickened portion of the ectoderm) is apparent by the third week of gestation. The top portion differentiates into the neural tube, which will form the central nervous system (brain and spinal cord), and the neural crest, which will develop into the peripheral nervous system.
- All parts of the brain (cerebrum, cerebellum, pons, and medulla oblongata) form in utero, although none are completely mature at birth. Brain growth continues at high levels until 5 or 6 years of age.
- Brain waves can be detected on an electroencephalogram (EEG) by the eighth week.
- The eye and inner ear develop as projections of the original neural tube.
- By 24 weeks, the ear is capable of responding to sound and the eyes exhibit a pupillary reaction, indicating sight is present.

The neurologic system seems particularly prone to insult during the early weeks of the embryonic period and can result in neural tube disorders, such as a meningocele (i.e., herniation of the meninges), especially if there is lack of folic acid (which is contained in green leafy vegetables and pregnancy vitamins) (Cohen & Uddin, 2011). All during pregnancy and at birth, the system is vulnerable to damage if anoxia should occur.

Endocrine System

The function of endocrine organs begins along with neurosystem development.

- The fetal pancreas produces insulin needed by the fetus (insulin is one of the few substances that does not cross the placenta from the mother to the fetus).
- The thyroid and parathyroid glands play vital roles in fetal metabolic function and calcium balance.
- The fetal adrenal glands supply a precursor necessary for estrogen synthesis by the placenta.

Digestive System

The digestive tract separates from the respiratory tract at about the fourth week of intrauterine life and, after that, begins to grow extremely rapidly. Initially solid, the tract canalizes (hollows out) to become patent. Later in the pregnancy, the endothelial cells of the gastrointestinal tract proliferate extensively, occluding the lumen once more, and the tract must canalize again. Atresia (blockage) or stenosis (narrowing) of the track are common fetal anomalies and develop if either the first or second canalization does not occur (Lin, Munsie, Herdt-Losavio, et al., 2012). The proliferation of cells shed in the second recanalization forms the basis for meconium (see below).

Because of this rapid intestinal growth, by the sixth week of intrauterine life, the intestine becomes too large to be contained by the abdomen. A portion of the intestine, therefore, is pushed into the base of the umbilical cord, where it remains until about the 10th week of intrauterine life or until the abdominal cavity has grown large enough to accommodate the bulky intestines. As intestine returns to the abdominal cavity at this point, it must rotate 180 degrees. Failure to do so can result in inadequate mesentery attachments, possibly leading to volvulus of the intestine in the newborn.

If any intestine remains outside the abdomen in the base of the cord, a congenital anomaly, termed *omphalocele*, will be present at birth. A similar defect, *gastroschisis*, occurs when the original midline fusion that occurred at the early cell stage is incomplete (Thilo & Rosenberg, 2011).

Meconium, a collection of cellular wastes, bile, fats, mucoproteins, mucopolysaccharides, and portions of the vernix caseosa (i.e., the lubricating substance that forms on the fetal skin), accumulates in the intestines as early as the 16th week. Meconium is sticky in consistency and appears black or dark green (obtaining its color from bile pigment). An important neonatal nursing responsibility is recording that a newborn has passed meconium as this rules out a stricture (noncanalization) of the anus (Marcelis, de Blaauw, & Brunner, 2011).

The gastrointestinal tract is sterile before birth. Because vitamin K, necessary for blood clotting, is synthesized by the action of bacteria in the intestines, vitamin K levels are almost nonexistent in a fetus and are still low in a newborn (vitamin K is routinely administered intramuscularly at birth). Sucking and swallowing reflexes are not mature until the fetus is at about 32 weeks gestation, or weighs 1,500 g.

The ability of the gastrointestinal tract to secrete enzymes essential for carbohydrate and protein digestion is mature at 36 weeks. However, amylase, an enzyme found in saliva and necessary for digestion of complex starches, does not mature until 3 months after birth. Many newborns have also not yet developed lipase, an enzyme needed for fat digestion (a reason breast milk is the best food for newborns because its digestion does not depend on these enzymes).

The liver is active throughout intrauterine life, functioning as a filter between the incoming blood and the fetal circulation and as a deposit site for fetal stores such as iron and glycogen. Unfortunately, during intrauterine life, the fetal liver is unable to prevent recreational drugs or alcohol ingested by the mother from entering the fetal circulation and possibly causing birth anomalies (Singer, Moore, Fulton, et al., 2012). Newborns need careful assessment at birth for hypoglycemia (low blood sugar) and hyperbilirubinemia (excessive breakdown products from destroyed red blood cells), two serious problems that can occur in the first 24 hours after birth because, although active, liver function is still immature.

Musculoskeletal System

During the first 2 weeks of fetal life, cartilage prototypes provide position and support to the fetus. Ossification of this cartilage into bone begins at about the 12th week, continues all through fetal life and into adulthood. Carpals, tarsals, and sternal bones generally do not ossify until birth is imminent. A fetus can be seen to move on ultrasonography as early as the 11th week, although the mother usually does not feel this movement (*quickening*) until almost 20 weeks of gestation.

What if...9.1 Liz Calhorn repeats that not only have her feelings toward her baby changed since she felt the baby move but she's also more interested in how to keep him safe now. How would you modify your health teaching with her because of this?

Reproductive System

A child's sex is determined at the moment of conception by a spermatozoon carrying an X or a Y chromosome and can be ascertained as early as 8 weeks by chromosomal analysis or analysis of fetal cells in the mother's bloodstream. At about the sixth week after implantation, the gonads (i.e., ovaries or testes) form. If testes form, testosterone is secreted, apparently influencing the sexually neutral genital duct to form other male organs (i.e., maturity of the wolffian, or mesonephric, duct). In the absence of testosterone secretion, female organs will form (i.e., maturation of the müllerian, or paramesonephric, duct). This is an important phenomenon, because if a woman should unintentionally take an androgen or an androgen-like substance during this stage of pregnancy, a child who is chromosomally female could appear more male than female at birth. If deficient testosterone is secreted by the testes, both the müllerian (female) duct and the wolffian (male) duct could develop (i.e., pseudohermaphroditism, or intersex) (Douglas, Axelrad, Brandt, et al., 2012).

The testes first form in the abdominal cavity and do not descend into the scrotal sac until the 34th to 38th week of intrauterine life. Because of this, many male preterm infants are born with undescended testes. These boys need a follow-up to be certain their testes do descend when they reach what would have been the 34th to 38th week of gestational age, because testicular descent does not always occur as readily in extrauterine life as it would have in utero. Testes that do not descend (cryptorchidism) require surgery as they are associated with poor sperm production and possibly testicular cancer later in life (Zeitler, Travers, Nadaou, et al., 2011).

Urinary System

Although rudimentary kidneys are present as early as the end of the fourth week of intrauterine life, the presence of kidneys does not appear to be essential for life before birth because the placenta clears the fetus of waste products. Urine, however, is formed by the 12th week and is excreted into the amniotic fluid by the 16th week of gestation. At term, fetal urine is being excreted at a rate of up to 500 ml/day. An amount of amniotic fluid less than usual (oligohydramnios) suggests fetal kidneys are not secreting adequate urine and that there is a kidney, ureter, or bladder disorder (Kumar, 2012).

The complex structure of the kidneys gradually develops during intrauterine life and continues to mature for months afterward. The loop of Henle, for example, is not fully differentiated until the child is born. Glomerular filtration and concentration of urine in the newborn are still not efficient, because the ability to concentrate urine is still not mature at birth.

Early in the embryonic stage of urinary system development, the bladder extends as high as the umbilical region and there is an open lumen between the urinary bladder and the umbilicus. If this fails to close, (termed a patent urachus), this is revealed at birth by the persistent drainage of a clear, acid–pH fluid (urine) from the umbilicus (Samra, McGrath, & Wehbe, 2011).

Integumentary System

The skin of a fetus appears thin and almost translucent until subcutaneous fat begins to be deposited underneath it at about 36 weeks. Skin is covered by soft downy hairs (lanugo) that serve as insulation to preserve warmth in utero, as well as a cream cheese–like substance, vernix caseosa, which is important for lubrication and for keeping the skin from macerating in utero. Both lanugo and vernix are still present at birth.

Immune System

Immunoglobulin (Ig) G maternal antibodies cross the placenta into the fetus as early as the 20th week and certainly by the 24th week of intrauterine life to give a fetus temporary passive immunity against diseases for which the mother has antibodies. These often include poliomyelitis, rubella (German measles), rubeola (regular measles), diphtheria, tetanus, infectious parotitis (mumps), hepatitis B, and pertussis (whooping cough). Infants born before this antibody transfer has taken place have no natural immunity and so need more than the usual protection against infectious disease in the newborn period.

A fetus only becomes capable of active antibody production late in pregnancy. Generally, it is not necessary for a fetus to produce antibodies because they need to be manufactured only to counteract an invading antigen, and antigens rarely invade the intrauterine space. Because IgA and IgM antibodies (the types which develop to actively counteract infection) cannot cross the placenta, their presence in a newborn is proof that the fetus has been exposed to an infection.

Milestones of Fetal Growth and Development

When fetal milestones occur can be confusing because the life of the fetus is typically measured from the time of ovulation or fertilization (ovulation age), but the length of a pregnancy is more commonly measured from the first day of the last menstrual period (gestational age). Because ovulation and fertilization take place about 2 weeks after the last menstrual period, the ovulation age of the fetus is always 2 weeks less than the length of the pregnancy or the gestational age.

Both ovulation and gestational age are typically reported in lunar months (4-week periods) or in trimesters (3-month periods) rather than in weeks. In lunar months, a total pregnancy is 10 months (40 weeks, or 280 days) long; a fetus grows in utero for 9.5 lunar months or three full trimesters (38 weeks, or 266 days).

The following discussion of fetal developmental milestones is based on gestational weeks, because it is helpful when talking to expectant parents to correlate fetal development with the way they measure pregnancy—from the first day of the last menstrual period. Figure 9.6 illustrates the comparative size and appearance of human embryos and fetuses at different stages of development.

End of Fourth Gestational Week

- The length of the embryo is about 0.75 cm; weight is about 400 mg.
- The spinal cord is formed and fused at the midpoint.
- The head is large in proportion and represents about one third of the entire structure.
- The rudimentary heart appears as a prominent bulge on the anterior surface.
- Arms and legs are bud-like structures; rudimentary eyes, ears, and nose are discernible.

End of Eighth Gestational Week

- The length of the fetus is about 2.5 cm (1 in.); weight is about 20 g.
- Organogenesis is complete.
- The heart, with a septum and valves, beats rhythmically.
- Facial features are definitely discernible; arms and legs have developed.
- External genitalia are forming, but sex is not yet distinguishable by simple observation.
- The abdomen bulges forward because the fetal intestine is growing so rapidly.
- A sonogram shows a gestational sac, which is diagnostic of pregnancy (Fig. 9.7).

End of 12th Gestational Week (First Trimester)

- The length of the fetus is 7 to 8 cm; weight is about 45 g.
- Nail beds are forming on fingers and toes.
- Spontaneous movements are possible, although they are usually too faint to be felt by the mother.
- Some reflexes, such as the Babinski reflex, are present.
- Bone ossification centers begin to form.
- Tooth buds are present.
- Sex is distinguishable on outward appearance.
- Urine secretion begins but may not yet be evident in amniotic fluid.
- The heartbeat is audible through Doppler technology.

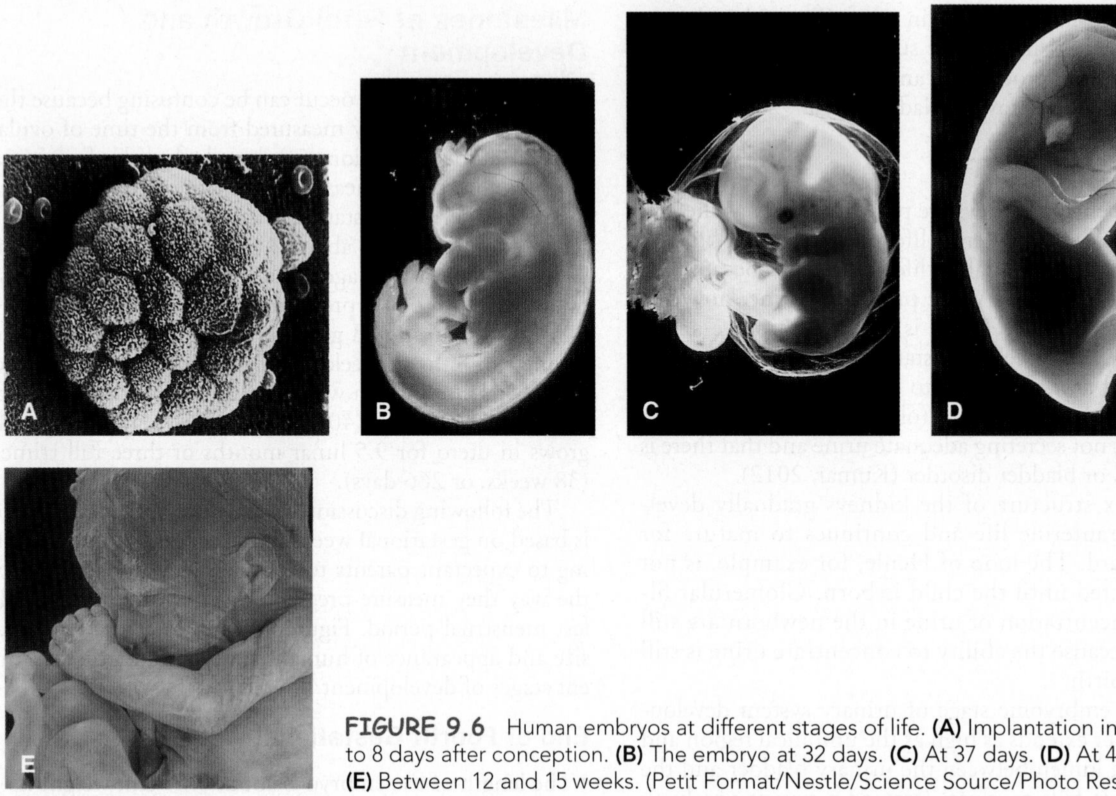

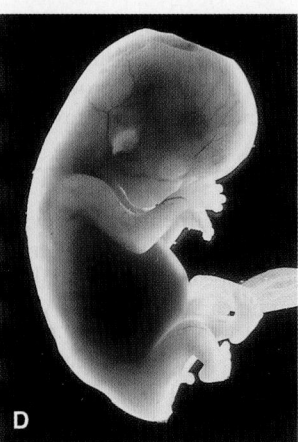

FIGURE 9.6 Human embryos at different stages of life. **(A)** Implantation in uterus 7 to 8 days after conception. **(B)** The embryo at 32 days. **(C)** At 37 days. **(D)** At 41 days. **(E)** Between 12 and 15 weeks. (Petit Format/Nestle/Science Source/Photo Researchers.)

End of 16th Gestational Week

- The length of the fetus is 10 to 17 cm; weight is 55 to 120 g.
- Fetal heart sounds are audible by an ordinary stethoscope.
- Lanugo is well formed.
- Both the liver and pancreas are functioning.
- The fetus actively swallows amniotic fluid, demonstrating an intact but uncoordinated swallowing reflex; urine is present in amniotic fluid.
- Sex can be determined by ultrasonography.

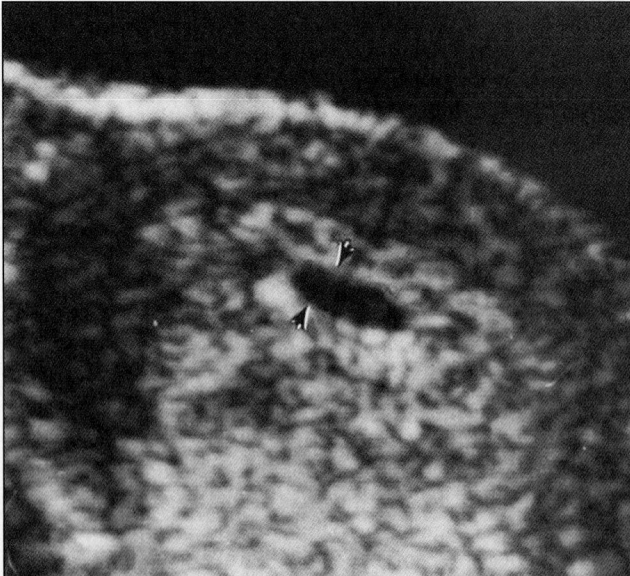

FIGURE 9.7 Sonogram showing the characteristic circle diagnostic of pregnancy (the gestational sac). (From Benson, C. B., Lavery M. J., & Platt, L. [1988]. *Atlas of obstetrical ultrasound.* Philadelphia, PA: J. B. Lippincott.)

End of 20th Gestational Week

- The length of the fetus is 25 cm; weight is 223 g.
- Spontaneous fetal movements can be sensed by the mother.
- Antibody production is possible.
- Hair, including eyebrows, forms on the head; vernix caseosa begins to cover the skin.
- Meconium is present in the upper intestine.
- Brown fat, a special fat that aides in temperature regulation, begins to form behind the kidneys, sternum, and posterior neck.
- Passive antibody transfer from mother to fetus begins.
- Definite sleeping and activity patterns are distinguishable as the fetus develops biorhythms that will guide sleep/wake patterns throughout life.

End of 24th Gestational Week (Second Trimester)

- The length of the fetus is 28 to 36 cm; weight is 550 g.
- Meconium is present as far as the rectum.
- Active production of lung surfactant begins.
- Eyelids, previously fused since the 12th week, now open; pupils react to light.
- Hearing can be demonstrated by response to sudden sound.
- When fetuses reach 24 weeks, or 500–600 g, they have achieved a practical low-end **age of viability** if they are cared for after birth in a modern intensive care nursery.

End of 28th Gestational Week

- The length of the fetus is 35 to 38 cm; weight is 1,200 g.
- Lung alveoli are almost mature; surfactant can be demonstrated in amniotic fluid.
- Testes begin to descend into the scrotal sac from the lower abdominal cavity.
- The blood vessels of the retina are formed but thin and extremely susceptible to damage from high oxygen concentrations (an important consideration when caring for preterm infants who need oxygen).

End of 32nd Gestational Week

- The length of the fetus is 38 to 43 cm; weight is 1,600 g.
- Subcutaneous fat begins to be deposited (the former stringy, "little old man" appearance is lost).
- Fetus responds by movement to sounds outside the mother's body.
- An active Moro reflex is present.
- Iron stores, which provide iron for the time during which the neonate will ingest only breast milk after birth, are beginning to be built.
- Fingernails reach the end of fingertips.

End of 36th Gestational Week

- The length of the fetus is 42 to 48 cm; weight is 1,800 to 2,700 g (5 to 6 lb).
- Body stores of glycogen, iron, carbohydrate, and calcium are deposited.
- Additional amounts of subcutaneous fat are deposited.
- Sole of the foot has only one or two crisscross creases, compared with a full crisscross pattern evident at term.
- Amount of lanugo begins to diminish.
- Most babies turn into a vertex (head down) presentation during this month.

End of 40th Gestational Week (Third Trimester)

- The length of the fetus is 48 to 52 cm (crown to rump, 35 to 37 cm); weight is 3,000 g (7 to 7.5 lb).
- Fetus kicks actively, sometimes hard enough to cause the mother considerable discomfort.
- Fetal hemoglobin begins its conversion to adult hemoglobin.
- Vernix caseosa is fully formed.
- Fingernails extend over the fingertips.
- Creases on the soles of the feet cover at least two thirds of the surface.

In primiparas (i.e., women having their first baby), the fetus often sinks into the birth canal during the last 2 weeks of pregnancy, giving the mother a feeling the load she is carrying is less. This event, termed *lightening*, is a fetal announcement the third trimester of pregnancy has ended and birth is at hand.

Determination of Estimated Birth Date

It is impossible to predict with a high degree of accuracy the exact day an infant will be born because fewer than 5% of pregnancies end exactly 280 days from the last menstrual period; fewer than half end within 1 week of the 280th day.

Traditionally, this date was referred to as the estimated date of confinement (EDC). Because women are no longer "confined" after childbirth, the acronym EDB (**estimated date of birth**) is more commonly used today.

If fertilization occurred early in a menstrual cycle, the pregnancy will probably end "early"; if ovulation and fertilization occurred later than the midpoint of the cycle, the pregnancy will end "late." Because of these normal variations, a pregnancy ending 2 weeks before or 2 weeks after the calculated EDB is considered well within the normal limit (38 to 42 weeks). Gestational age wheels and birth date calculators, which can be used to predict a birth date are available, but calculation by Naegele's rule is the standard method used to predict the length of a pregnancy (Box 9.3).

BOX 9.3 Naegele's Rule

To calculate the date of birth by this rule, count backward 3 calendar months from the first day of a woman's last menstrual period and add 7 days. For example, if the last menstrual period began May 15, you would count back 3 months (April 15, March 15, February 15) and add 7 days, to arrive at the predicted date of birth as February 22.

What if...9.2 Liz Calhorn first came to your prenatal clinic on August 5 and told you she had her last menstrual period from March 13 to March 18. What would be her child's EDB?

ASSESSMENT OF FETAL GROWTH AND DEVELOPMENT

Tests for fetal growth and development are commonly done for a variety of reasons, including to:

- Predict the outcome of the pregnancy
- Manage the remaining weeks of the pregnancy
- Plan for possible complications at birth
- Plan for problems that may occur in the newborn infant
- Decide whether to continue the pregnancy
- Find conditions that may affect future pregnancies

Both fetal growth and development can be compromised if a fetus has a metabolic or chromosomal disorder that interferes with normal growth, if the supporting structures such as the placenta or cord do not form normally, or if environmental influences such as the nicotine in cigarettes causes fetal growth restriction (including testes growth in a male fetus) (Virtanen, Sadov, & Toppari, 2012).

Nursing responsibilities for these assessment procedures include verifying that a signed consent form has been obtained as needed (which is necessary if the procedure poses any risk to the mother or fetus that would not otherwise be present), being certain the woman and her support person are aware of what the procedure will entail and any potential risks, preparing the woman physically and psychologically, providing support during the procedure, assessing both fetal and maternal responses during and after the procedure, providing any necessary follow-up care, and managing equipment

BOX 9.4 Nursing Care Planning

AN INTERPROFESSIONAL CARE MAP FOR A WOMAN UNDERGOING FETAL STUDIES

Liz Calhorn, an 18-year-old, is about 20 weeks pregnant (can't remember date of last menstrual period). Although she says she knows she should have stopped smoking before pregnancy, she has not been able to do this as yet. Twice during the pregnancy (at the 4th and 10th week), she drank beer at summer picnics. Today, at a clinic visit, she tells you she has felt her fetus move. She states, "Feeling the baby move made me realize there's someone inside me, you know what I mean? It made me realize it's time I started being more careful with what I do." Liz works at a fast food restaurant. Boyfriend (father of fetus) is supportive, but has no money to offer her for support. Client states, "I'm not getting married. Just not ready for that level of commitment yet."

Family Assessment Client lives in one-bedroom apartment; supports self by working at a fast food restaurant. States, "My parents would help out if I begged them, but I'm not going to do that."

Client Assessment Client smokes a pack of cigarettes a day. Takes aspirin, 10 g, for almost daily sinus headaches. No recreational drug use.

Nutrition: Breakfast: None, to help control her weight.
Lunch: A hotdog and salad. One diet cola.
Dinner: Macaroni and cheese; applesauce. One cup coffee.
Snack: Half bag of potato chips and cream-cheese dip.

Physical examination: Fundal height is 16 cm. Fetal heart tones by Doppler at 160 beats/min. Has been advised to have an ultrasound done to assess for fetal growth and to date pregnancy.

Nursing Diagnosis Risk for altered fetal growth related to inadequate nutrition and alcohol and nicotine consumption.

Outcome Criteria Client consents to sonogram for fetal growth assessment; reports lessened alcohol and cigarette use at the next visit.

Team Member Responsible	Assessment	Intervention	Rationale	Expected Outcome
Activities of Daily Living, Including Safety				
Nurse	Ask patient to describe a "typical day" to reveal any actions possibly detrimental to fetal growth.	Discuss common actions unsafe during pregnancy, such as smoking and drinking alcohol.	Knowing what constitutes unsafe practices during pregnancy is a woman's best safeguard against fetal harm.	Client states she will stop drinking alcohol; is using a supportive Internet quitline to help reduce smoking.
Teamwork and Collaboration				
Primary health care provider/nurse	Determine whether sonogram department has appointments free in coming week.	Schedule sonogram 1 week in advance with sonogram department.	Client believes she might be 20 weeks pregnant. Fundal height, recent fetal movements correspond more closely to 16 weeks.	Client reports for scheduled ultrasound in 1 week.
Procedures/Medications for Quality Improvement				
Nurse	Assess what prescription or over-the-counter or alternative therapies client is using.	Discuss with client inadvisability of taking aspirin during pregnancy; suggest she take acetaminophen (Tylenol) instead.	Acetylsalicylic acid (aspirin) can lead to bleeding or prolonged pregnancy.	Client reports at next prenatal visit she takes acetaminophen for any pain.
Nutrition				
Nurse/nutritionist	Ask client for a 24-hour recall nutrition history.	Discuss the advisability of eating breakfast while pregnant to help avoid hypoglycemia in fetus.	Knowing what constitutes a healthy diet helps ensure a fetus will receive adequate nutrients.	Client reports at prenatal visits she eats breakfast before leaving for work in the morning. Includes more protein in intake.

Patient-Centered Care				
Nurse	Determine whether client understands ultrasound is not an X-ray, so it is not harmful to the fetus.	Instruct client about preparation for sonogram (drink fluid; avoid emptying bladder).	A well-prepared client is more apt to result in an effective procedure and a satisfied client.	Client will describe accurate preparations for procedure. Receives printed instructions for ambulatory ultrasound.
Spiritual/Psychosocial/Emotional Needs				
Primary health care provider/nurse	Assess the extent of factors, such as alcohol and cigarette use, that could have led to intrauterine growth restriction.	Review the possibility with client that her pregnancy dating may be wrong, because fundal height is below usual. Alternate cause could be fetal growth restriction.	Understanding contributors to fetal health is necessary for women to make informed choices during pregnancy.	Client states she understands the discrepancy in fundal height and weeks gestation following explanation.
Informatics for Seamless Health Care Planning				
Nurse/Primary health care provider	Perform complete assessment to help ensure continuity of care with other services.	Mark chart as high-risk client for intrauterine growth restriction (fundal height below average for weeks gestation).	Documenting risk factors helps to safeguard the fetus.	The patient chart documents high-risk status.

and specimens. Box 9.4 shows an interprofessional care map illustrating both nursing and team planning for fetal care, including assessment procedures.

Providing follow-up care may include being certain a couple understands what the results of a test mean. When a result is good, parents feel assured their infant is growing well. When results are not encouraging, a couple can experience a mixture of feelings. On the one hand, they feel committed to the pregnancy; on the other, they want to protect their child, themselves, and their family from the burden of having a child with a severe disability. In some instances, they will be asked to make a life and death decision depending on the results. Quiet listening so a couple has time to thoroughly think through what option will be right for them may be difficult to do but is usually the soundest action for health care providers (Choi, Van Riper, & Thoyre, 2012).

Health History

Like all assessments, a fetal assessment begins with a health history. Ask the mother specifically about any prepregnancy illnesses such as gestational diabetes or heart disease as these both can interfere with fetal growth. Ask about any drugs a woman takes; for instance, common drugs taken for recurrent seizures can be teratogenic and therefore pose a risk in pregnancy (Mawhinney, Campbell, Craig, et al., 2012). Ask also about nutritional intake because if a woman is not eating a well-balanced diet, she may not be taking in enough nutrients for fetal growth (Whitney & Rolfes, 2012). Be certain to also ask about personal habits such as cigarette smoking, both prescription and recreational drug use, alcohol consumption, and exercise, because all of these may influence glucose/insulin balance and fetal growth. Most women are aware alcohol ingestion can harm a fetus (e.g., fetal alcohol spectrum disorder) but many are not yet aware of fetal tobacco syndrome (Wong, Ordean, & Kahan, 2011).This syndrome applies to the fetus of a woman who smokes more than five cigarettes a day and who is born growth restricted (i.e., birth weight under 2,500 g at term). Smoking may also be a cause of ectopic (tubal) pregnancy as fallopian tubes may become irritated (Shao, Zou, Wang, et al., 2012).

Most women instinctively protect a fetus growing inside them so pregnancy may be the push they need to improve their lifestyle (Box 9.5). Asking if a woman has had any exposure to teratogens can reveal exposure to such substances as chemicals, paint fumes, cleaning products, poor air quality, or a loud noise level (Krueger, Horesh, & Crossland, 2012). Asking about unintentional injuries or intimate partner violence can help reveal whether a fetus could have suffered any trauma from these sources (e.g., intimate partner violence tends to increase during pregnancy because of the stress a pregnancy can create; Dalton, 2012).

Physical Examination

A physical examination of the mother is the second step in evaluating fetal health. Assess maternal weight and general appearance, as both obesity and underweight are clues that the mother's nutrition may not be adequate for sound fetal growth (Warren, Rance, & Hunter, 2012). Bruises may indicate intimate partner violence that could have bruised the fetus as well. An elevated blood pressure may be the beginning of hypertension of pregnancy, which can restrict fetal growth (Vest & Cho, 2012).

BOX 9.5 Nursing Care Planning to Respect Cultural Diversity

Different cultures have different ideas as to what foods to eat, how much exercise is good during pregnancy, and whether fetal tests for well-being are ethical. Whether a woman's religion or personal beliefs allow her to use reliable conception can influence whether she is happy to discover she is pregnant, which can then influence how soon she goes for prenatal care or begins to eat a more nutritious diet. If her religion is one that mandates she have a large family to increase the number of members in her religion, she may be happy to be pregnant, but also unsure she can love this additional child.

Cultural beliefs also affect everyday things, such as believing it is wrong to have a photograph taken during pregnancy because that will alert unknown spirits that the woman is pregnant (the origin of lullabies were songs to keep away Lilith, an avenging creature in Jewish folklore who was thought to bring harm to babies). Believing photographs are harmful may make a woman reluctant to have a sonogram taken during pregnancy; unlike most women, she may not like a photograph of the ultrasound for a baby keepsake.

QSEN Checkpoint Question 9.4

Evidence-Based Practice

To investigate what the risk factors are that lead to women smoking, researchers surveyed 570 women from Appalachian Ohio as to social, demographic, and psychological factors and whether they smoked. Findings revealed women with low socioeconomic status, those who scored high on a depression assessment score, and those who had their first baby before they were 17 years of age were more likely to smoke. Almost 50% of women with both low socioeconomic status and rated as depressed smoked (Wewers, Salsberry, Ferketich, et al., 2012).

Based on the previous study, which statement by Liz Calhorn would make you most worried she might have difficulty quitting smoking during the remainder of her pregnancy?

a. "I don't have a lot of spare cash, just like everyone else in my family."
b. "When I feel tense, I like to shop. It really takes away that bad feeling."
c. "I'm trying to stop smoking so I won't have to smoke around my baby."
d. "My mother had five children with no trouble; why am I so different?"

Look in Appendix A for the best answer and rationale.

Estimating Fetal Health

A number of procedures, both noninvasive and invasive, are used to evaluate fetal health. Because there are many procedures, helping a woman with a high-risk pregnancy maintain a sense of control or empowerment as she is scheduled for them is an important nursing responsibility (Box 9.6).

Fetal Growth

As a fetus grows, the uterus expands to accommodate its size. Although not evidence grounded, typical fundal (top of the uterus) measurements are:

- Over the symphysis pubis at 12 weeks
- At the umbilicus at 20 weeks
- At the xiphoid process at 36 weeks

McDonald's rule, another symphysis–fundal height measurement (although, again, not documented to be thoroughly reliable), is an easy method of determining midpregnancy growth. Typically, tape measurement from the notch of the symphysis pubis to over the top of the uterine fundus as a woman lies supine is equal to the week of gestation in centimeters between the 20th and 31st weeks of pregnancy (e.g., in a pregnancy of 24 weeks, the fundal height should be 24 cm) (Fig. 9.8).

BOX 9.6 Nursing Care Planning to Empower a Family

Women may find the names of tests like MSAFP and substances being tested for (acetylcholinesterase) so confusing that they feel as if their life is being taken over by scheduled tests or exams. To help a woman maintain control:

- Encourage her to ask questions until her primary health care provider simplifies instructions or test results enough that she thoroughly understands them.
- Encourage her to set the time and date of appointments if possible so she can fit fetal testing in with her schedule, rather than be expected to appear "on command."
- Encourage her to bring her significant other with her for fetal testing so he/she hears the same explanation she does and so that person can also ask questions rather than hearing the information second hand.
- Don't refer to a fetus as "it" during testing because that is such an impersonal term. If the woman has chosen a name, use that while referring to her fetus; otherwise, use he or she.
- Respect modesty during exams where the woman's abdomen will be exposed. Movie stars are often pictured today with their pregnant abdomen on view, but not every woman wants her body exposed unnecessarily that way.
- Remember that late in pregnancy, women's movements can be painful and may feel awkward, so respect that asking a woman to step up and lie on an examining table is not asking her to complete an easy task. Offer help as necessary but also remember feeling independent is an empowering feeling.

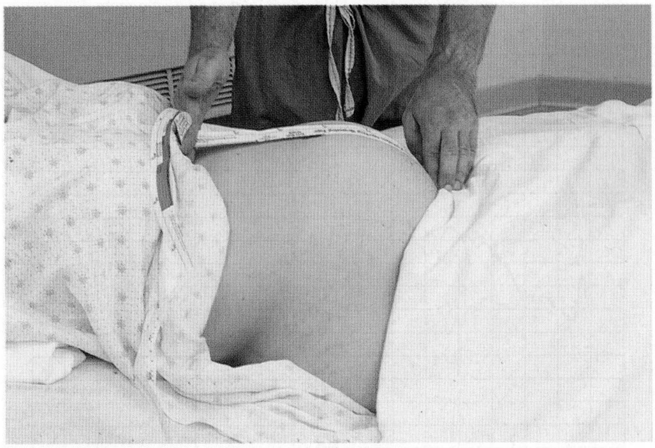

FIGURE 9.8 Measuring fundal height from the superior aspect of the pubis to the fundal crest. The tape is pressed flat against the abdomen for the measurement.

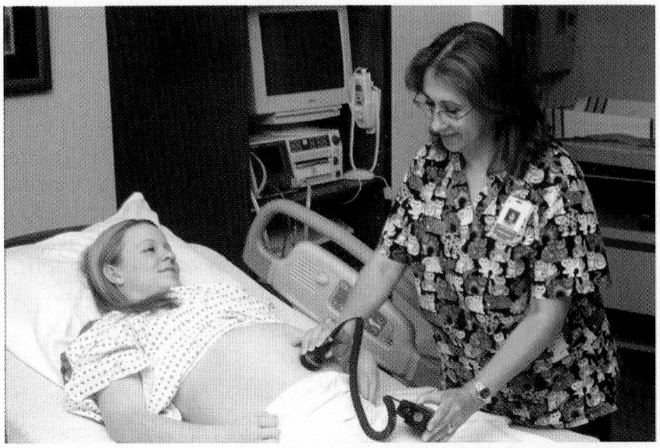

FIGURE 9.9 Measuring fetal heart rate with a Doppler transducer, which detects and broadcasts the fetal heart rate to the parents-to-be, as well as you.

A fundal height much greater than this standard suggests a multiple pregnancy, a miscalculated due date, a large-for-gestational-age (LGA) infant, hydramnios (increased amniotic fluid volume), or possibly even gestational trophoblastic disease (see Chapter 21). A fundal measurement much less than this suggests the fetus is failing to thrive (e.g., intrauterine growth restriction), the pregnancy length was miscalculated, or an anomaly interfering with growth has developed. McDonald's rule becomes inaccurate during the third trimester of pregnancy because the fetus is growing more in weight than in height during is time.

Assessing Fetal Well-being

A number of actions or procedures are helpful in detecting and documenting the fetus is not only growing but is also apparently healthy.

Fetal Heart Rate

Fetal heart sounds can be heard and counted as early as the 10th to 11th week of pregnancy by the use of an ultrasound Doppler technique (Fig. 9.9). This is done routinely at every prenatal visit past 10 weeks.

Daily Fetal Movement Count (Kick Counts)

Fetal movement that can be felt by the mother (quickening) occurs at approximately 18 to 20 weeks of pregnancy and peaks in intensity at 28 to 38 weeks. After that time, a healthy fetus moves with a degree of consistency, at about 10 times per hour. In contrast, a fetus who is not receiving enough nutrients because of poor maternal nutrition or placental insufficiency has greatly decreased movements. The technique for "kick counts" varies from institution to institution, but a typical method used is to ask women with high-risk pregnancies to:

- Lie in a left recumbent position after a meal.
- Observe and record the number of fetal movements (kicks) their fetus makes until they have counted 10 movements.
- Record the time (typically this is under an hour).
- If an hour passes without 10 movements, they should walk around a little and try a count again.
- If 10 movements (kicks) cannot be felt in a second 1-hour period, they should telephone their primary health care provider. The fetus could be healthy but sleeping during this time, so lack of typical movements may not be serious, but it is an indication for further assessment.

Kick counts are particularly useful in growth-restricted or postterm pregnancies to reveal if a fetus is still receiving adequate nutrition (Caughey, 2012). Make certain the woman knows fetal movements do vary, especially in relation to sleep cycles, her activity, and the time since she last ate. Otherwise, she can become unduly worried her fetus is in jeopardy when the fetus is asleep or just having an inactive time.

What if...9.3 You give instructions to Liz Calhorn to count fetal movements (count kicks) daily after lunch and she tells you she can't do that because she snacks all day long rather than eats at regular times. Which would be more important: that she should count kicks after meals or that she do it every day?

Rhythm Strip Testing. The term "rhythm strip testing" refers to an assessment of the fetal heart rate for whether a good baseline rate and both long- and short-term variability are present. For this, help the woman into a semi-Fowler's position (either in a comfortable lounge chair or on an examining table or bed with an elevated backrest) to prevent her uterus from compressing the vena cava and causing supine hypotension syndrome during the test. Attach an external fetal heart rate monitor abdominally (Fig. 9.10A). Record the fetal heart rate for 20 minutes.

The baseline reading refers to the average rate of the fetal heartbeat. Short-term variability (also called beat-to-beat variability) denotes the small changes in rate that occur from second to second if the fetal parasympathetic nervous system is receiving adequate oxygen and nutrients. In the rhythm strip in Figure 9.10B, for example, the baseline (average) of the fetal heartbeat is 130 beats/min. Beat-to-beat variability is present.

Long-term variability reflects the state of the fetal sympathetic nervous system. On a rhythm strip, it is the differences in heart rate that occur over the 20-minute time period. Note in Figure 9.10B how the heart rate varies from 150 to 130 beats/min. Because the average fetus moves about twice every 10 minutes, and movement causes the heart rate to increase, there will typically be two or more instances of fetal heart rate acceleration in a 20-minute rhythm strip.

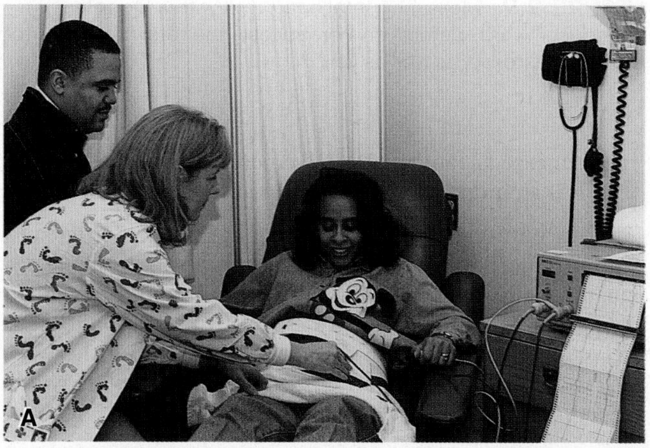

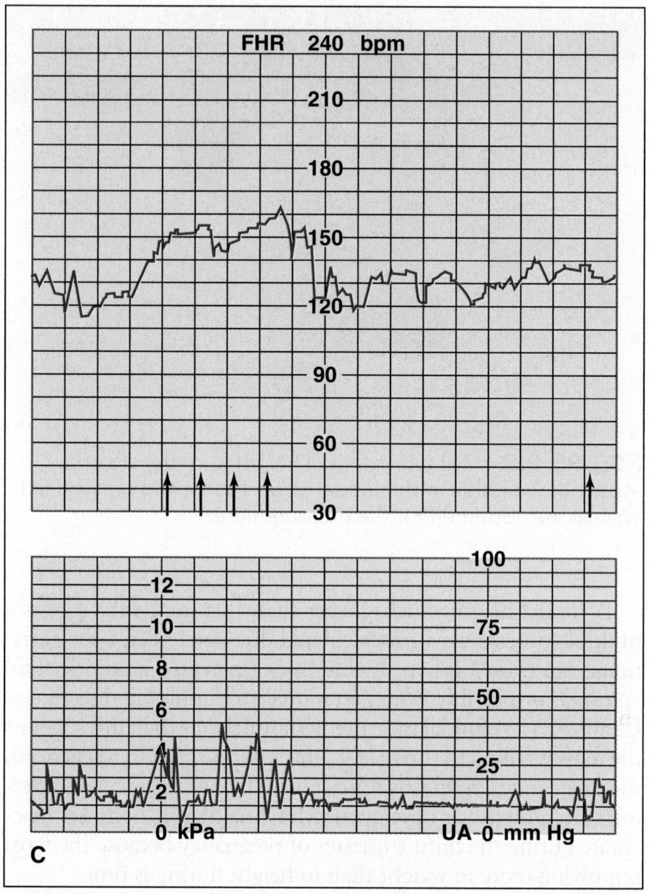

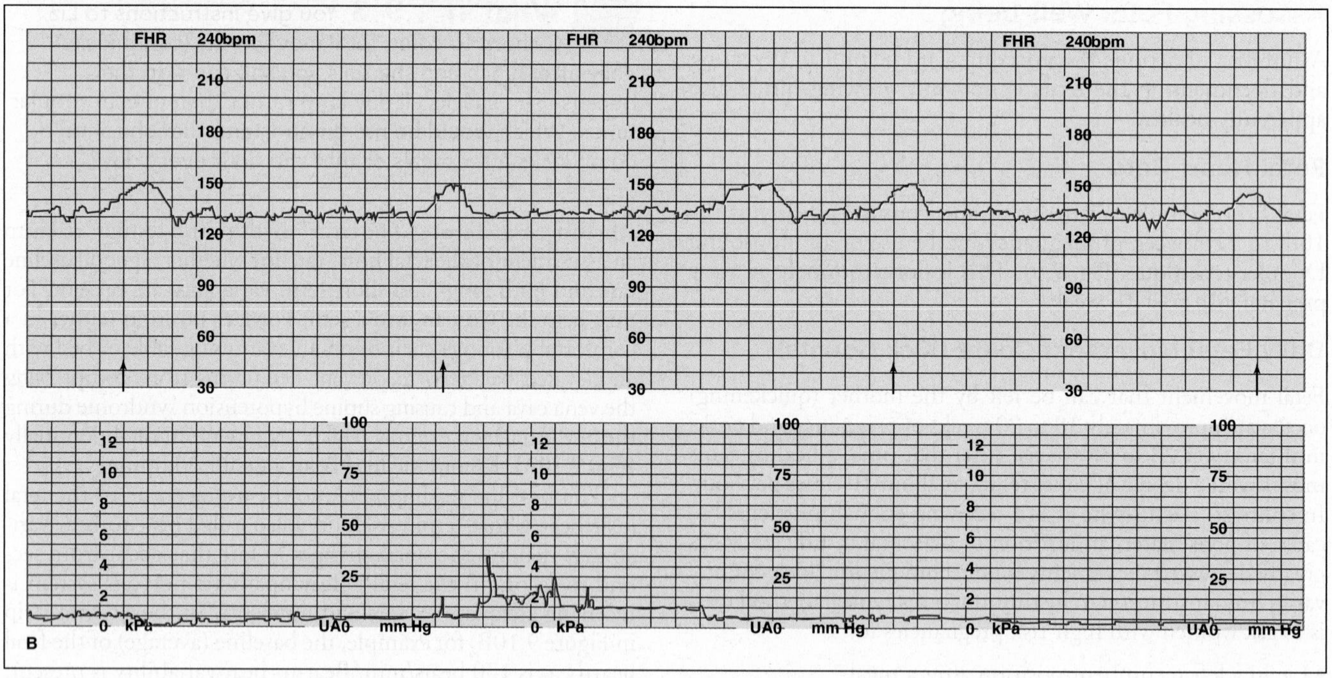

FIGURE 9.10 Rhythm strip and nonstress testing of fetal heart rate. **(A)** The woman sits in a comfortable chair to avoid supine hypotension. Both a uterine contraction monitor and fetal heart rate monitor are in place on her abdomen. (Photograph by Melissa Olson, with permission of Chestnut Hill Hospital, Philadelphia, PA.) **(B)** A rhythm strip. The upper strip signifies heart rate; the lower strip indicates uterine activity. Arrows signal fetal movement. **(C)** Baseline fetal heart rate on this strip is 130 to 132 beats/min. This strip shows fetal heart rate acceleration in response to fetal movement, shown by arrows. (Photograph by Melissa Olson, with permission of Chestnut Hill Hospital, Philadelphia, PA.)

Variability is rated as:

- Absent: No peak-to-trough range is detectable
- Minimal: An amplitude range is detectable but the rate is 5 beats/min or fewer
- Moderate or normal: An amplitude range is detectable; rate is 6 to 25 beats/min
- Marked: An amplitude range is detectable; rate is greater than 25 beats/min (American Congress of Obstetricians and Gynecologists [ACOG], 2009)

Rhythm strip testing requires a woman to remain in a fairly fixed position for 20 minutes. Keep her well informed of the importance and purpose of the test and be certain she understand the meaning of the results after the test. Electronic fetal heart rate recording is further discussed in Chapter 15 as it can also be used to assess fetal well-being at the beginning of labor.

Nonstress Testing. A **nonstress test** measures the response of the fetal heart rate to fetal movement. Position the woman and attach both a fetal heart rate and a uterine contraction monitor. Instruct the woman to push the button attached to the monitor (similar to a call bell) whenever she feels the fetus move. This will create a dark mark on the paper tracing at these times.

When the fetus moves, the fetal heart rate should increase about 15 beats/min and remain elevated for 15 seconds. It should decrease to its average rate again as the fetus quiets (Fig. 9.10C). If no increase in beats per minute is noticeable on fetal movement, poor oxygen perfusion of the fetus is suggested.

A nonstress test usually is done for 20 minutes. The test is said to be reactive (healthy) if two accelerations of fetal heart rate (by 15 beats or more) lasting for 15 seconds occur after movement within the time period. The test is nonreactive (fetal health may be affected) if no accelerations occur with the fetal movements. The results also can be interpreted as nonreactive if no fetal movement occurs or if there is low short-term fetal heart rate variability (less than 6 beats/min) throughout the testing period (Russo, Henderson, & Costigan, 2011).

If a 20-minute period passes without any fetal movement, it may only mean that the fetus is sleeping, although other reasons for lessened variability are maternal smoking, drug use, or hypoglycemia. Although not evidence based, if you give the woman an oral carbohydrate snack, such as orange juice, it can cause her blood glucose level to increase enough to cause fetal movement. The fetus also may be stimulated by a loud sound (discussed later) to cause movement.

Because both rhythm strip and nonstress testing are noninvasive procedures and cause no risk to either mother or fetus, they can be used as screening procedures in all pregnancies. They can be done at home daily as part of a home monitoring program for the woman who is having a complication of pregnancy. If a nonstress test is nonreactive, an additional fetal assessment, such as a biophysical profile test, will be scheduled.

Vibroacoustic Stimulation. For acoustic (sound) stimulation, a specially designed acoustic stimulator is applied to the mother's abdomen to produce a sharp sound of approximately 80 dB at a frequency of 80 Hz, thus startling and waking the fetus (Russo et al., 2011).

During a standard nonstress test, if a spontaneous acceleration has not occurred within 5 minutes, apply a single 1- to 2-second sound stimulation to the lower abdomen. This can be repeated again at the end of 10 minutes if no further spontaneous movement occurs, so two movements within the 20-minute window can be evaluated.

Ultrasonography

Ultrasonography, which measures the response of sound waves against solid objects, is a much-used tool for fetal health assessments. It can be used to:

- Diagnose pregnancy as early as 6 weeks gestation.
- Confirm the presence, size, and location of the placenta and amniotic fluid.
- Establish a fetus is growing and has no gross anomalies such as hydrocephalus; anencephaly; or spinal cord, heart, kidney, and bladder concerns.
- Establish the sex if a penis is revealed.
- Establish the presentation and position of the fetus.
- Predict maturity by measurement of the biparietal diameter of the head or crown-to-rump measurement.
- Discover complications of pregnancy, such as the presence of an intrauterine device, hydramnios (excessive amniotic fluid) or oligohydramnios (lessened amniotic fluid), ectopic pregnancy, missed miscarriage, abdominal pregnancy, placenta previa (a low-implanted placenta), premature separation of the placenta, coexisting uterine tumors, or multiple pregnancy. Genetic disorders such as Down syndrome and fetal anomalies such as neural tube disorders, diaphragmatic hernia, or urethral stenosis also can be diagnosed. Fetal death can be revealed by a lack of heartbeat and respiratory movement.
- After birth, a sonogram may be used to detect a retained placenta or poor uterine involution in the new mother.

For an ultrasound, intermittent sound waves of high frequency (above the audible range) are projected toward the uterus by a transducer placed on the abdomen or in the vagina. The sound frequencies that bounce back from the fetus can be displayed on an oscilloscope screen as a visual image. The frequencies returning from tissues of various thicknesses and properties present distinct appearances. A permanent record can be made of the scan for the woman's electronic health record; a copy of the scan can be offered to her as a baby book souvenir.

Images are so clear that the fetal heart as well as movement of the extremities, such as bringing a hand to the mouth to suck a thumb, can be seen. A parent who is in doubt her fetus is well or whole can be greatly reassured by viewing such a sonogram image.

Before an ultrasound examination, be certain a woman has received a good explanation of what the procedure will be like and reassurance that the process does not involve X-rays and so will be safe for the fetus (Box 9.7). This means it is also safe for the father of the child to remain in the room during the test and see the images as well.

The sound waves reflect best if the uterus can be held stable so it is helpful if the woman has a full bladder at the time of the procedure. To ensure this, ask her to drink a full glass of water every 15 minutes beginning 90 minutes before the procedure and to not void until after the procedure.

Help the woman up to an examining table and drape her for modesty, but with her abdomen exposed. To prevent supine hypotension syndrome, place a towel under her right buttock to tip her body slightly so the uterus will roll away from the vena cava. A gel is then applied to her abdomen to improve the contact of the transducer. Be certain the gel is at room temperature or even slightly warmer, or it may cause uncomfortable uterine cramping. The transducer is then applied to her abdomen and moved both horizontally and vertically until the uterus and its contents are fully scanned (Fig. 9.11). Ultrasonography also may be performed using an intravaginal technique, although this is not necessary for routine testing.

Although the long-term effects of ultrasound are not yet known, the technique appears to be safe for both mother and fetus and causes no discomfort to the fetus. Usually, the only discomfort for the woman is the messiness of the contact lubrication and a strong desire to void before the scan is

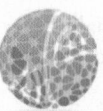

BOX 9.7 Nursing Care Planning Based on Effective Communication

Liz Calhorn is scheduled for an ultrasound.

Less Effective Communication

Nurse: Do you have any questions about what will happen, Liz?
Liz: I guess. I can't decide if I want to know my baby's sex or not.
Nurse: Most people do these days. It helps them plan better.
Liz: I think I'd rather be surprised. I know I don't want a boy.
Nurse: If it were me, I'd want to know. How else do you know what color clothes to buy?
Liz: Okay, tell me what the ultrasound shows.

More Effective Communication

Nurse: Do you have any questions about what will happen, Liz?
Liz: I guess. I can't decide if I want to know my baby's sex or not.
Nurse: That's an individual decision. What things are you thinking about?
Liz: I think I'd rather be surprised. I know I don't want a boy.
Nurse: You don't want a boy?
Liz: A guy got me into this trouble. The last thing I need is another one around the house.
Nurse: Let's talk about what it will mean if you should have a boy.

Becoming so engrossed in sharing her personal feelings, the nurse in the first example forgot to listen to exactly what the client was saying. Taking the time to discover what the client wanted, as was done in the second example, revealed the sex of the child was only a small part of what the mother was afraid to learn.

completed. Taking home a photograph of the sonographic image can enhance bonding because it is proof the pregnancy exists and the fetus appears well. As desirable as it is, however, caution women against having ultrasound images done just for the purpose of having "keepsake" photographs. Commercial firms offering these services are not well regulated and their equipment may be outdated and unsafe.

In medical practice, a number of specific features are studied by sonogram.

Biparietal Diameter. Ultrasonography may be used to predict fetal maturity by measuring the biparietal diameter (side-to-side measurement) of the fetal head. In 80% of pregnancies in which the biparietal diameter of the fetal head is 8.5 cm or greater, it can be predicted the infant will weigh more than 2,500 g (5.5 lb) at birth or is at a fetal age of 40 weeks. Figures 9.12 and 9.13 are sonograms showing the biparietal diameter of a fetus at 24 weeks and a fetus close to term.

Figure 9.12 is a sonogram showing the biparietal diameter of a fetus at 24 weeks. Figure 9.13 shows a fetus close to term.

Doppler Umbilical Velocimetry. Doppler ultrasonography measures the velocity at which red blood cells in the uterine and fetal vessels travel. Assessment of the blood flow through uterine blood vessels is helpful to determine the vascular resistance present in women with gestational diabetes or hypertension and whether resultant placental insufficiency is occurring. Decreased velocity is an important predictor that uterine growth restriction will occur because it reveals that only a limited number of nutrients are able to reach the fetus (Kaponis, Harada, Makrydimas, et al., 2011).

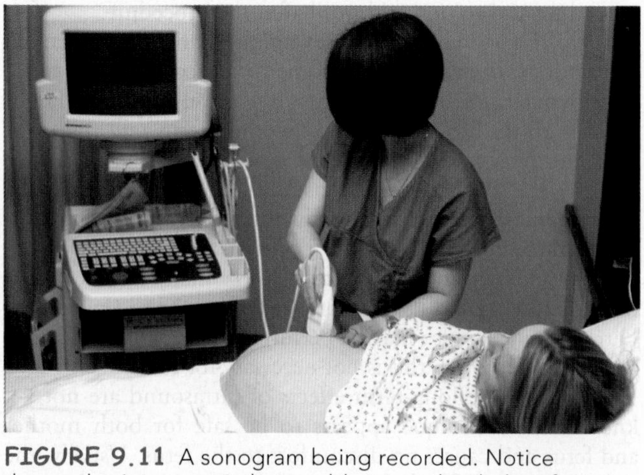

FIGURE 9.11 A sonogram being recorded. Notice the mother's interest in being able to see her baby's first photograph.

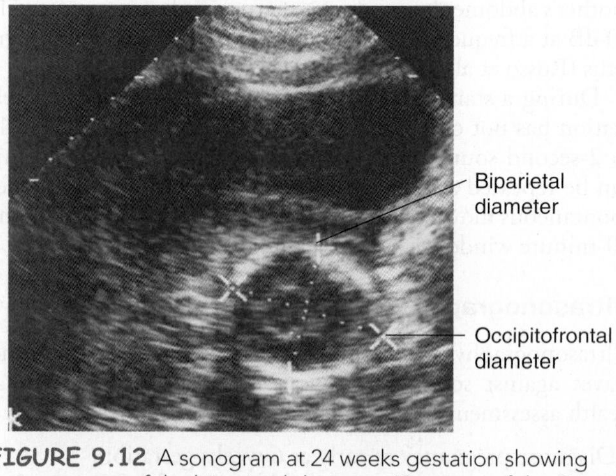

FIGURE 9.12 A sonogram at 24 weeks gestation showing measurement of the biparietal diameter. (Courtesy of the Department of Medical Photography, Children's Hospital, Buffalo, NY.)

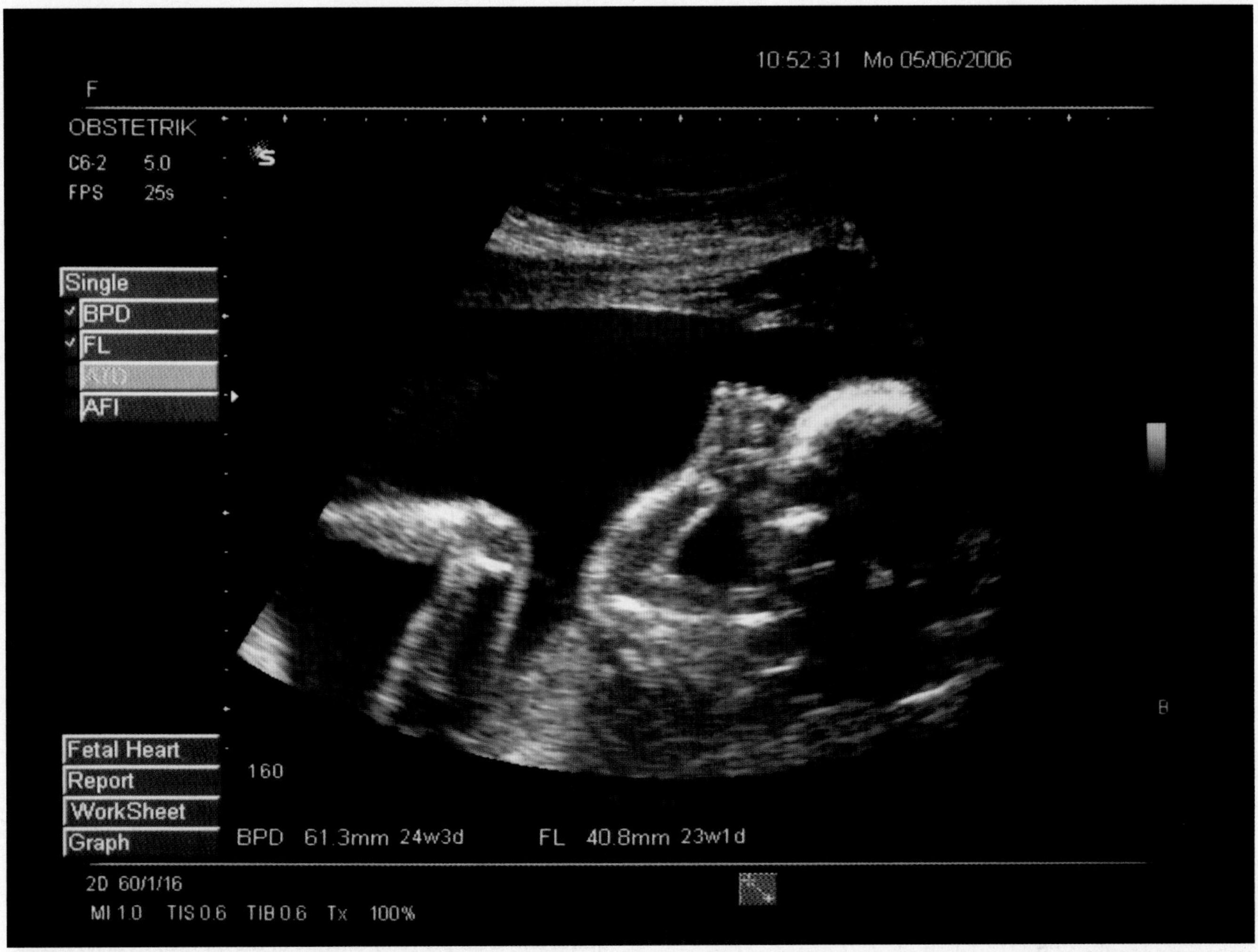

FIGURE 9.13 A sonogram showing a fetus close to term.

Placental Grading for Maturity. Placentas can be graded by ultrasound based on the particular amount of calcium deposits present in the base. Placentas are graded as:

- 0: Between 12 and 24 weeks
- 1: 30 to 32 weeks
- 2: 36 weeks
- 3: 38 weeks (Because fetal lungs are apt to be mature by 38 weeks, a grade 3 placenta suggests the fetus is mature.)

Amniotic Fluid Volume. The amount of amniotic fluid present is yet another way to estimate fetal health because a portion of the fluid is formed by fetal kidney output. If a fetus is becoming so stressed in utero that circulatory and kidney function is failing, urine output and, consequently, the volume of amniotic fluid will decrease. A decrease in amniotic fluid volume puts the fetus at risk for compression of the umbilical cord with interference of nutrition as well as lack of room to exercise and maintain muscle tone. Between 28 and 40 weeks, the total pockets of amniotic fluid revealed by sonogram average 12 to 15 cm. An amount greater than 20 to 24 cm indicates hydramnios (i.e., excessive fluid, perhaps caused by inability of the fetus to swallow). An amount less than 5 to 6 cm indicates oligohydramnios (i.e., decreased amniotic fluid, perhaps caused by poor perfusion and kidney failure).

Nuchal Translucency. Children with a number of chromosome anomalies have unusual pockets of fat or fluid present in their posterior neck, which show on sonograms as nuchal translucency. Chromosomal anomalies associated with this are discussed in Chapter 7.

QSEN Checkpoint Question 9.5

Patient-Centered Care

Liz Calhorn is scheduled to have an ultrasound examination and you want to ensure that she understands and is prepared for this procedure to mitigate her anxiety. What instruction would you give her before her examination?

a. "Use the restroom immediately before the procedure to reduce your bladder size."

b. "The intravenous fluid used to dilate your uterus does not hurt the fetus."

c. "You will need to drink at least three glasses of water before the procedure."

d. "You can have medicine for the pain of any contractions caused by the test."

Look in Appendix A for the best answer and rationale.

Biophysical Profile

A biophysical profile combines five parameters (i.e., fetal reactivity, fetal breathing movements, fetal body movement, fetal tone, and amniotic fluid volume) into one assessment. The fetal heart and breathing record measures short-term central nervous system function; the amniotic fluid volume helps measure long-term adequacy of placental function. The scoring for a complete profile is shown in Table 9.3. By this system, each item has the potential for scoring a 2, so 10 would be the highest score possible. A biophysical profile is more accurate in predicting fetal well-being than any single assessment (Oyelese & Vintzileos, 2011). Because the scoring system is similar to an Apgar score determined at birth on infants, it is popularly called a fetal Apgar score.

Biophysical profiles may be done as often as daily during a high-risk pregnancy. The fetal scores are as follows:

- A score of 8 to 10 means the fetus is considered to be doing well.
- A score of 6 is considered suspicious.
- A score of 4 denotes a fetus potentially in jeopardy.

For simplicity, some centers use only two assessments (amniotic fluid index [AFI] and a nonstress test) for the analysis. Referred to as a modified biophysical profile, this predicts short-term viability by the nonstress test and long-term viability by the AFI. A healthy fetus should show a reactive nonstress test and an AFI range between 5 and 25 cm (Russo et al., 2011). Nurses play a large role in obtaining the information for both a modified and a full biophysical profile by obtaining either the nonstress test or the sonogram reading.

Magnetic Resonance Imaging

Magnetic resonance imaging (MRI) is yet another way to assess a growing fetus. Because the technique apparently causes no harmful effects to the fetus or woman, MRI has the potential to replace or complement ultrasonography as a fetal assessment technique because it can identify structural anomalies or soft tissue disorders (O'Connor, Rooks, & Smith, 2012). An MRI may be most helpful in diagnosing complications such as ectopic pregnancy or trophoblastic disease (see Chapter 21), because later in a pregnancy, fetal movement (unless the fetus is sedated) can obscure the findings.

Maternal Serum

Because a number of trophoblast cells pass into the maternal bloodstream beginning at about the seventh week of pregnancy, maternal serum analysis can reveal information about the mother as well as the fetus.

Maternal Serum α-Fetoprotein. AFP is a substance produced by the fetal liver that can be found in both amniotic fluid and maternal serum (maternal serum α-fetoprotein [MSAFP]). The level is abnormally high if the fetus has an open spinal or abdominal wall defect, because the open defect allows more AFP to enter the mother's circulation than usual. Although the reason is unclear, the level is low if the fetus has a chromosomal defect such as Down syndrome. MSAFP levels begin to rise at 11 weeks gestation and then steadily increase until term. Traditionally assessed at the 15th week of pregnancy, between 85% and 90% of neural tube anomalies and 80% of babies with Down syndrome can be detected by this method (Rogers & Worley, 2012).

Maternal Serum for Pregnancy-Associated Plasma Protein A. Pregnancy-associated plasma protein A (PAPP-A) is a protein secreted by the placenta; low levels in maternal blood are associated with fetal chromosomal anomalies, including trisomies 13, 18, and 21 or small-for-gestational-age (SGA) babies. A high PAPP-A level may predict an LGA baby.

Quadruple Screening. Quadruple screening analyzes four indicators of fetal health: AFP, unconjugated estriol (UE; an enzyme produced by the placenta that estimates general well-being), hCG (also produced by the placenta), and inhibin A (a protein produced by the placenta and corpus luteum associated with Down syndrome).

As with the measurement of MSAFP, quadruple testing requires only a simple venipuncture of the mother. Because it measures four separate values, it the most common of the maternal serum tests used today (Manipalviratn, Trivax, & Huang, 2013).

Fetal Gender. Although fetal gender is usually determined by an ultrasound screen at about 4 months, it can be determined as early as 7 weeks by analysis of maternal serum. This early diagnosis could be helpful to a woman who has an X-carrying genetic disorder so she could discover if she has a male fetus who could inherit the disease or a female fetus who will be dis-

TABLE 9.3 Biophysical Profile Scoring

Assessment	Instrument	Criteria for a Score of 2
Fetal breathing	Sonogram	At least one episode of 30 s of sustained fetal breathing movements within 30 min of observation.
Fetal movement	Sonogram	At least three separate episodes of fetal limb or trunk movement within a 30-min observation.
Fetal tone	Sonogram	The fetus must extend and then flex the extremities or spine at least once in 30 min.
Amniotic fluid volume	Sonogram	A pocket of amniotic fluid measuring more than 2 cm in vertical diameter must be present.
Fetal heart reactivity	Nonstress test	Two or more accelerations of fetal heart rate of 15 beats/min lasting 15 s or more following fetal movements in a 20-min period.

ease free (Mortarino, Garagiola, Lotta, et al., 2011). Screening of this type has some ethical connotations, because if the fetus is determined to be the "wrong" gender, there could be serious consequences for the now unwanted child.

Invasive Fetal Testing

If a genetic or growth concern is identified by noninvasive measures, a number of invasive measures allow for more refined investigation.

Chorionic Villi Sampling. Chorionic villi sampling (CVS) is a biopsy and chromosomal analysis of chorionic villi done at 10 to 12 weeks of pregnancy. As fetal cells can be more easily obtained from the maternal blood stream for study, the method may be used for chromosomal analysis but is rarely necessary (see Chapter 7 for chromosome analysis).

Amniocentesis. **Amniocentesis** (from the Greek *amnion* for "sac" and *kentesis* for "puncture") is the aspiration of amniotic fluid from the pregnant uterus for examination. The procedure can be done in a health care office or in an ambulatory clinic. It is typically scheduled between the 14th and 16th weeks of pregnancy so a generous amount of amniotic fluid will be present. The technique can be used again near term to test for fetal maturity.

Amniocentesis is a technically easy procedure, but it can be very frightening to the woman on whom it is done. Because it involves penetration of the integrity of the amniotic sac, there also are risks to the fetus such as hemorrhage from penetration of the placenta, infection of the amniotic fluid, and puncture of the fetus, although the incidence of these is very low (less than 0.5%). If the procedure leads to irritation of the uterus, it could initiate premature labor and preterm birth (Attilakos & Overton, 2012).

In preparation for amniocentesis, ask the woman to void (to reduce the size of the bladder and prevent an inadvertent puncture). Place her in a supine position on an examining table and drape her appropriately, exposing only her abdomen. Slip a folded towel under her right buttock to tip her body slightly to the left to move her uterus off her vena cava and help prevent supine hypotension syndrome. Attach fetal heart rate and uterine contraction monitors. Take her blood pressure and measure the fetal heart rate for baseline levels.

Next, a sonogram is done to determine the position of the fetus, the location of a pocket of amniotic fluid, and the placenta. The abdomen is then swabbed with an antiseptic solution, and a local anesthetic is injected. Caution a woman she may feel a slight prick as the anesthetic is introduced and a sensation of pressure as the needle used for aspiration, a 3- or 4-in., 20- to 22-gauge spinal needle, is introduced. Do not suggest she take a deep breath and hold it as a distraction against discomfort because this lowers the diaphragm against the uterus and shifts intrauterine contents.

The needle is inserted, carefully avoiding the fetus and placenta, until it reaches a pool of amniotic fluid (Fig. 9.14). A syringe is attached, and about 15 ml of amniotic fluid is withdrawn. The needle is then removed, and the woman rests quietly for 30 minutes. During the procedure and for the 30 minutes afterward, observe the fetal heart rate monitor to be certain the rate remains normal, and observe the uterine contraction monitor to be certain no contractions begin to occur.

If the woman has Rh-negative blood, Rho(D) immune globulin (RhIG; RhoGAM) is administered after the procedure to prevent fetal isoimmunization or help ensure maternal antibodies will not form against any placental red blood cells that might have accidentally been released into the maternal bloodstream during the procedure.

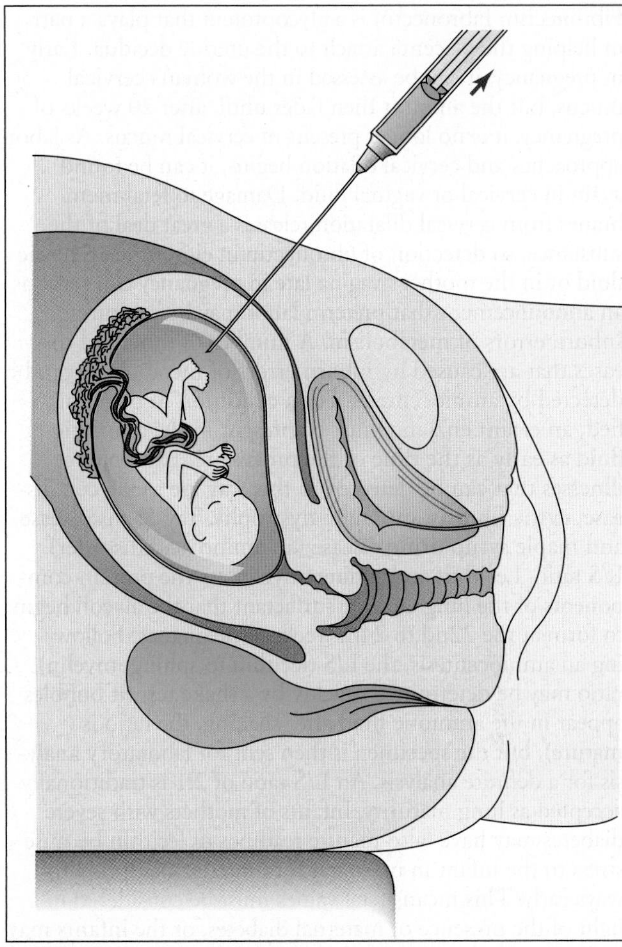

FIGURE 9.14 Amniocentesis. A pocket of amniotic fluid is located by sonogram. A small amount of fluid is removed by needle aspiration.

Amniotic fluid can be analyzed for:

- AFP.
- Acetylcholinesterase, another compound that rises to high levels if a neural tube anomaly is present.
- Bilirubin determination. The presence of bilirubin may be analyzed if a blood incompatibility is suspected. If bilirubin is going to be analyzed, the specimen must be free of blood or a false-positive reading will occur.
- Chromosome analysis. A few fetal skin cells are always present in amniotic fluid so these cells may be cultured and stained for karyotyping for genetic analysis. Examples of genetic diseases that can be detected by prenatal amniocentesis and their significance to health are discussed in Chapter 7.
- Color. Normal amniotic fluid is the color of water; late in pregnancy, it may have a slightly yellow tinge. A strong yellow color suggests a blood incompatibility (the yellow results from the presence of bilirubin released from the breakdown of red blood cells). A green color suggests meconium staining, a phenomenon associated with fetal distress.

- Fibronectin. Fibronectin is a glycoprotein that plays a part in helping the placenta attach to the uterine decidua. Early in pregnancy, it can be assessed in the woman's cervical mucus, but the amount then fades until, after 20 weeks of pregnancy, it is no longer present in cervical mucus. As labor approaches and cervical dilation begins, it can be found again in cervical or vaginal fluid. Damage to fetal membranes from cervical dilatation releases a great deal of the substance, so detection of fibronectin in either the amniotic fluid or in the mother's vagina late in pregnancy can serve as an announcement that preterm labor may be beginning.
- Inborn errors of metabolism. A number of inherited diseases that are caused by inborn errors of metabolism can be detected by amniocentesis. For a condition to be identified, an errant enzyme must be present in the amniotic fluid as early as the time of the procedure. Examples of illnesses that can be detected in this way are sickle cell disease, cystic fibrosis, muscular dystrophy, Tay-Sachs disease, and maple syrup urine disease (an amino acid disorder).
- L/S ratio. Lecithin and sphingomyelin are the protein components of the lung enzyme surfactant that the alveoli begin to form at the 22nd to 24th weeks of pregnancy. Following an amniocentesis, the L/S (lecithin to sphingomyelin) ratio may be determined quickly by a shake test (if bubbles appear in the amniotic fluid after shaking, the ratio is mature), but the specimen is then sent for laboratory analysis for a definite analysis. An L/S ratio of 2:1 is traditionally accepted as lung maturity. Infants of mothers with severe diabetes may have false-mature readings of lecithin because stress to the infant in utero tends to mature lecithin pathways early. This means fetal values must be considered in light of the presence of maternal diabetes, or the infants may be born with mature lung function but be immature overall (a fragile giant), causing them to not do well in postnatal life (Hay, 2012). Some laboratories interpret a ratio of 2.5:1 or 3:1 as a mature indicator in infants of women with diabetes.
- Phosphatidylglycerol and desaturated phosphatidylcholine. These are additional compounds, in addition to lecithin and sphingomyelin, found in surfactant. Pathways for these compounds mature at 35 to 36 weeks. Because they are present only with mature lung function, if they are present in the sample of amniotic fluid, it can be predicted with even greater confidence that respiratory distress syndrome is not likely to occur.

QSEN Checkpoint Question 9.6

Quality Improvement

Liz Calhorn is scheduled to have an amniocentesis to test for fetal maturity. To help make sure the procedure is successful, what instruction would be best to give her before this procedure?

a. "Void (pee) immediately before the procedure to reduce the size of your bladder."
b. "The X-ray used to reveal your fetus's position will have no long-term fetal effects."
c. "The IV fluid used to dilate your uterus is isotonic saline so will not hurt the fetus."
d. "Your fetus will have less amniotic fluid for the rest of pregnancy, but that's all right."

Look in Appendix A for the best answer and rationale.

Percutaneous Umbilical Blood Sampling. Percutaneous umbilical blood sampling (PUBS; also called cordocentesis or funicentesis) is the aspiration of blood from the umbilical vein for analysis. After the umbilical cord is located by sonography, a thin needle is inserted by amniocentesis technique into the uterus and is then guided by ultrasound until it pierces the umbilical vein. A sample of blood is then removed for blood studies, such as a complete blood count, direct Coombs test, blood gases, and karyotyping. To ensure the blood obtained is fetal blood, it is submitted to a Kleihauer–Betke test, which measures the difference between adult and fetal hemoglobin. If a PUBS test reveals that the fetus is anemic, blood may be transfused into the cord using this same technique. Because the umbilical vein continues to ooze for a moment after the procedure, there is a high chance fetal blood could enter the maternal circulation after the procedure, so RhIG is given to Rh-negative women to prevent sensitization. Fetal heart rate and uterine contractions need to be monitored before and after the procedure to be certain uterine contractions are not beginning and also by ultrasound to be certain no bleeding is evident. This procedure carries little additional risk to the fetus or woman over amniocentesis and can yield information not available by any other means, especially about blood dyscrasias.

Fetoscopy. The use of a **fetoscopy**, in which the fetus is visualized by inspection through a fetoscope (an extremely narrow, hollow tube inserted by amniocentesis technique), can be yet another way to assess fetal well-being. This method allows direct visualization of both the amniotic fluid and the fetus (Richter, Wergeland, Dekoninck, et al., 2012). If a photograph is taken through the fetoscope, it can document a problem or reassure parents that their infant is perfectly formed. The main reasons the procedure is used are to:

- Confirm the intactness of the spinal column.
- Obtain biopsy samples of fetal tissue and fetal blood samples.
- Determine meconium staining is not present.
- Perform elemental surgery, such as inserting a polyethylene shunt into the fetal ventricles to relieve hydrocephalus or anteriorly into the fetal bladder to relieve a stenosed urethra. It may be possible to repair a neural tube defect such as meningocele or improve the outcome of myelomeningocele by fetoscopy (Danzer, Johnson, & Adzick, 2012).

The earliest time in pregnancy a fetoscopy can be performed is about the 16th or 17th week. For the procedure, the mother is draped as for amniocentesis. A local anesthetic is injected into the abdominal skin. The fetoscope is then inserted through a minor abdominal incision. If the fetus is very active, meperidine (Demerol) may be administered to the woman to help sedate the fetus to avoid fetal injury by the scope and allow for better observation.

A fetoscopy carries a small risk of premature labor or amnionitis (infection of the amniotic fluid). To avoid infection, the woman may be prescribed antibiotic therapy after the procedure. The number of procedures performed by a fetoscopy is limited because of the manipulation involved and the ethical quandary of the mother's autonomy being compromised by fetal needs if further procedures are necessary such as asking the mother to undergo general anesthesia so the fetus can have surgery.

WOMEN WITH UNIQUE NEEDS OR CONCERNS

Fetal assessment can be more difficult in some women than others. It is more difficult to hear fetal heart sounds in a morbidly obese woman, for example. If the straps for fetal heart rate monitors are not long enough to circle a woman's abdomen, they may need to be held in place manually. If a woman is not easily mobile, she can have difficulty obtaining a clean catch urine for protein and glucose testing. Be ready to assist in these circumstances as needed.

Women who are wheelchair challenged can remain in their wheelchair for fetal heart rate monitoring. All individuals who use wheelchairs need to periodically press on the armrests with their hands and raise their buttocks off the seat of the wheelchair to help prevent pressure ulcers as the danger of ulcers increases with pregnancy because of the added weight. During a lengthy test, a woman may need to take a break to stretch; mark the break on a rhythm strip so a sudden corresponding fetal movement on the strip is not misinterpreted.

Remember that women who are hearing challenged will not be able to hear their baby's heartbeat by Doppler assessment. Observing a rhythm strip is a better method to prove to them their baby appears healthy. In contrast, a woman who is visually impaired would be most assured by listening to the beeping of a Doppler rather than the blurry outlines (for her) of a rhythm strip. Women with special needs are further discussed in Chapter 22. Assess each woman individually to be certain each has obtained and understands the results of fetal assessments accurately and doesn't have continuing questions about her baby's health.

What if...9.4 You are particularly interested in exploring one of the 2020 National Health Goals in respect to fetal health (see Box 9.1). What would be a possible research topic to explore pertinent to this goal that would be applicable to Liz and her family and also advance evidence-based practice?

KEY POINTS FOR REVIEW

- Being aware of healthy fetal growth helps in planning nursing care that not only meets QSEN competencies, but also best meets a family's need for health teaching.
- The union of a single sperm and egg (fertilization) signals the beginning of pregnancy.
- The fertilized ovum (zygote) travels by way of a fallopian tube to the uterus, where implantation takes place in about 8 days.
- From implantation to 5 to 8 weeks, the growing structure is called an embryo. The period after 8 weeks until birth is the fetal period.
- Growth of the umbilical cord, amniotic fluid, and amniotic membranes proceeds in concert with fetal growth. The placenta produces a number of important hormones: estrogen, progesterone, hPL, and hCG.
- Various methods to assess fetal growth and development include fundal height, fetal movement, fetal heart tones, ultrasonography, MRI, MSAFP, amniocentesis, PUBS, quadruple screening, and fetoscopy.
- A biophysical profile is a combination of fetal assessments that predicts fetal well-being better than measuring single parameters.

CRITICAL THINKING CARE STUDY

Maeve is a 35-year-old woman who is about 3 months pregnant. She recently broke her fibula in a touch football game and so has her leg encased in a mid-calf level cast. It's not a walking cast, so she will be using a wheelchair for the next 6 weeks. She's worried she'll gain too much weight because she's no longer active. As she's not sure of the date of her last menstrual period, she'd like a sonogram done to date her pregnancy. She asks if that can be done with her in a wheelchair.

1. How would you answer Maeve's question about using her wheelchair for a sonogram?
2. What other special considerations does Maeve need with regard to fetal health because she uses a wheelchair?
3. Maeve asks you if her baby has hair yet. That's important to her because if her baby is a boy she doesn't want him to be as bald as her husband, who at 36, has already lost most of his hair.

Patient Scenario: The Menendez Family

Read about the Menendez family, a family who has concerns about fetal health, then answer the questions to further sharpen your skills and grow more familiar with NCLEX-type questions related to fetal health. Confirm your answers are correct by reading the rationales.

Visit http://thePoint.lww.com

Answers and Rationales

Looking for answers to the What If. . . and Critical Thinking Care Study questions?

Visit http://thePoint.lww.com

References

American Congress of Obstetricians and Gynecologists. (2009). ACOG practice bulletin: Intrapartum fetal heart rate monitoring. *Obstetrics & Gynecology, 114*(1), 193–200.

Attilakos, G., & Overton, T. G. (2012). Antenatal care. In D. K. Edmonds (Ed.), *Dewhurst's textbook of obstetrics & gynaecology* (6th ed., pp. 42–52). Oxford, UK: John Wiley & Son.

Bernstein, H. S., & Srivastava, D. (2012). Stem cell therapy for cardiac disease. *Pediatric Research, 71*(4, Pt. 2), 491–499.

Caughey, A. G. (2012). Post term pregnancy. In D. K. Edmonds (Ed.), *Dewhurst's textbook of obstetrics & gynaecology* (6th ed., pp. 269–286). Oxford, UK: John Wiley & Son.

Chitra, T., Sushanth, Y. S., & Raghavan, S. (2012). Umbilical coiling index as a marker of perinatal outcome: An analytical study. *Obstetrics and Gynecology International.* Advance online publication. doi: 10.1155/2012/213689

Choi, H., Van Riper, M., & Thoyre, S. (2012). Decision making following a prenatal diagnosis of Down syndrome: An integrative review. *Journal of Midwifery & Women's Health, 57*(2), 156–164.

Christianson, M. S., & Wallach, E. E. (2011). Infertility and assisted reproductive technologies. In K. J. Hurt, M. W. Guile, J. L. Bienstock, et al. (Eds.), *The Johns Hopkins manual of gynecology and obstetrics* (4th ed., pp. 421–437). Philadelphia, PA: Lippincott, Williams & Wilkins.

Cleary, B., Eogan, M., O'Connell, M., et al. (2012). Methadone and perinatal outcomes: A prospective cohort study. *Addiction, 107*(8), 1482–1492.

Coad, J., & Dunstall, M. (2011a). Physiological adaptation to pregnancy. In J. Coad & M. Dunstall (Eds.), *Anatomy & physiology for midwives* (pp. 257–288). London, England: Elsevier/Churchill Livingstone.

Coad, J., & Dunstall, M. (2011b). The placenta. In J. Coad & M. Dunstall (Eds.), *Anatomy & physiology for midwives* (pp. 173–198). London, England: Elsevier/Churchill Livingstone.

Cohen, S., & Uddin, S. (2011). Primary and preventive care. In K. J. Hurt, M. W. Guile, J. L. Bienstock, et al. (Eds.), *The Johns Hopkins manual of gynecology and obstetrics* (4th ed., pp. 1–14). Philadelphia, PA: Lippincott, Williams & Wilkins.

Dalton, M. (2012). Domestic violence and sexual assault. In D. K. Edmonds (Ed.), *Dewhurst's textbook of obstetrics & gynaecology* (6th ed., pp. 798–804). Oxford, UK: John Wiley & Son.

Danzer, E., Johnson, M. P., & Adzick, N. S. (2012). Fetal surgery for myelomeningocele: Progress and perspectives. *Developmental Medicine & Child Neurology, 54*(1), 8–14.

Digiulio, M., Wiedaseck, S., & Monchek, R. (2012). Understanding hydatidiform mole. *American Journal of Maternal Child Nursing, 37*(1), 30–34.

Douglas, G., Axelrad, M. E., Brandt, M. L., et al. (2012). Guidelines for evaluating and managing children born with disorders of sexual development. *Pediatric Annuals, 41*(4), e1–e7.

Feng, Y. L., Zhou, C. J., Li, X. M., et al. (2012). Alpha-1-antitrypsin acts as a preeclampsia-related protein: A proteomic study. *Gynecologic & Obstetric Investigation, 73*(3), 252–259.

Gardosi, J. (2012). Normal fetal growth. In D. K. Edmonds (Ed.), *Dewhurst's textbook of obstetrics & gynaecology* (6th ed., pp. 26–34). Oxford, UK: John Wiley & Son.

Ghionzoli, M., James, C. P., David, A. L., et al. (2012). Gastroschisis with intestinal atresia—Predictive value of antenatal diagnosis and outcome of postnatal treatment. *Journal of Pediatric Surgery, 47*(2), 322–328.

Gowen, C. W., Jr. (2011). Respiratory diseases of the newborn. In K. J. Marcdante, R. M. Kliegman, H. B. Jenson, et al. (Eds.), *Nelson essentials of pediatrics* (6th ed., pp. 237–244). Philadelphia, PA: Saunders/Elsevier.

Hay, W. W., Jr. (2012). Care of the infant of the diabetic mother. *Current Diabetes Reports, 12*(1), 4–15.

Hjalmarson, O., & Sandberg, K. L. (2011). Effect of antenatal corticosteroid treatment on lung function in full-term newborn infants. *Neonatology, 100*(1), 32–36.

Hoh, J. K., Sung, Y. M., & Park, M. I. (2012). Fetal heart rate parameters and perinatal outcomes in fetuses with nuchal cords. *Journal of Obstetrics and Gynaecology Research, 38*(2), 358–363.

Huppertz, B., & Kingdom, J. C. P. (2012). The placenta and fetal membranes. In D. K. Edmonds (Ed.), *Dewhurst's textbook of obstetrics & gynaecology* (6th ed., pp. 16–25). Oxford, UK: John Wiley & Son.

Kaponis, A., Harada, T., Makrydimas, G., et al. (2011). The importance of venous Doppler velocimetry for evaluation of intrauterine growth restriction. *Journal of Ultrasound Medicine, 30*(4), 529–545.

Krueger, C., Horesh, E., & Crossland, B. A. (2012). Safe sound exposure in the fetus and preterm infant. *Journal of Obstetric, Gynecologic, & Neonatal Nursing, 41*(1), 166–170.

Kumar, S. (2012). Fetal anomalies. In D. K. Edmonds (Ed.), *Dewhurst's textbook of obstetrics & gynaecology* (6th ed., pp. 219–229). Oxford, UK: John Wiley & Son.

Lin, S., Munsie, J. P., Herdt-Losavio, M. L., et al. (2012). Maternal asthma medication use and the risk of selected birth defects. *Pediatrics, 129*(2), e317–e324.

Manipalviratn, S., Trivax, B., & Huang, A. (2013). Genetic disorders & sex chromosome disorders. In A. H. DeCherney, L. Nathan, T. M. Goodwin, et al. (Eds.), *Current diagnosis and treatment: Obstetrics and gynecology* (11th ed., pp. 67–96). Columbus, OH: McGraw-Hill/Lange.

Mawhinney, E., Campbell, J., Craig, J., et al. (2012). Valproate and the risk for congenital malformations: Is formulation and dosage regime important? *Seizure, 21*(3), 215–218.

Marcelis, C., de Blaauw, I., & Brunner, H. (2011). Chromosomal anomalies in the etiology of anorectal malformations: A review. *American Journal of Medical Genetics, 155*(11), 2692–2704.

McCoyd, J. L. (2013). Preparation for prenatal decision-making: A baseline of knowledge and reflection in women participating in prenatal screening. *Journal of Psychosomatic Obstetrics & Gynaecology, 34*(1), 3–8.

Miesnik, S. R. (2012). The fetus as patient. *Journal of Obstetric, Gynecologic, & Neonatal Nursing, 41*(3), 417–418.

Mortarino, M., Garagiola, I., Lotta, L. A., et al. (2011). Non-invasive tool for foetal sex determination in early gestational age. *Haemophilia, 17*(6), 952–956.

O'Connor, S. C., Rooks, V. J., & Smith, A. B. (2012). Magnetic resonance imaging of the fetal central nervous system, head, neck, and chest. *Seminars in Ultrasound, CT & MR, 33*(1), 86–101.

Oyelese, Y., & Vintzileos, A. M. (2011). The uses and limitations of the fetal biophysical profile. *Clinical Perinatology, 38*(1), 47–64.

Panepinto, J. A., & Scott, J. P. (2011). Hematology. In K. J. Marcdante, R. M. Kliegman, H. B. Jenson, et al. (Eds.), *Nelson essentials of pediatrics* (6th ed., pp. 555–584). Philadelphia, PA: Saunders/Elsevier.

Peroviá, M., Garalejiá, E. Gojniá, M., et al. (2011). Sensitivity and specificity of ultrasonography as a screening tool for gestational diabetes mellitus. *Journal of Maternal–Fetal & Neonatal Medicine, 25*(8), 1348–1353.

Petrozella, L. N., Dashe, J. S., McIntire, D. D., et al. (2011). Clinical significance of borderline amniotic fluid index and oligohydramnios in preterm pregnancy. *Obstetrics & Gynecology, 117*(2, Pt. 1), 338–342.

Pipkin, F. B. (2012). Maternal physiology. In D. K. Edmonds (Ed.), *Dewhurst's textbook of obstetrics & gynaecology* (6th ed., pp. 5–15). Oxford, UK: John Wiley & Son.

Richter, J., Wergeland, H., Dekoninck, P., et al. (2012). Fetoscopic release of an amniotic band with risk of amputation: Case report and review of the literature. *Fetal Diagnosis & Therapy, 31*(2), 134–137.

Rogers, V. L., & Worley, K. C. (2012). Obstetrics and obstetric disorders. In S. J. McPhee, M. A. Papadakis, & M. W. Rabow (Eds.), *Current medical diagnosis & treatment* (51st ed., pp. 760–786). Columbus, OH: McGraw-Hill.

Rojas-Reyes, M. X., Morley, C. J., & Soll, R. (2012). Prophylactic versus selective use of surfactant in preventing morbidity and mortality in preterm infants. *Cochrane Database of Systematic Reviews,* (3), CD00051.

Russo, M. L., Henderson, J., & Costigan, K. A. (2011). Fetal assessment. In K. J. Hurt, M. W. Guile, J. L. Bienstock, et al. (Eds.), *The Johns Hopkins manual of gynecology and obstetrics* (4th ed., pp. 90–98). Philadelphia, PA: Lippincott Williams & Wilkins.

Samra, H. A., McGrath, J. M., & Wehbe, M. (2011). Enhancing nurse practitioner understanding of urachal anomalies. *Journal of Obstetric, Gynecological & Neonatal Nursing, 40*(4), 399–411.

Schneider, D. S. (2011). The cardiovascular system. In K. J. Marcdante, R. M. Kliegman, H. B. Jenson, et al. (Eds.), *Nelson essentials of pediatrics* (6th ed., pp. 525–555). Philadelphia, PA: Saunders/Elsevier.

Shao, R., Zou, S., Wang, X., et al. (2012). Revealing the hidden mechanisms of smoke-induced fallopian tubal implantation. *Biology of Reproduction, 86*(4), 131–133.

Singer, L. T., Moore, D. G., Fulton, S., et al. (2012). Neurobehavioral outcomes of infants exposed to MDMA (Ecstasy) and other recreational drugs during pregnancy. *Neurotoxicology & Teratology, 34*(3), 303–310.

Stohl, H., & Satin, A. J. (2011). Perinatal infections. In K. J. Hurt, M. W. Guile, J. L. Bienstock, et al. (Eds.), *The Johns Hopkins manual of gynecology and obstetrics* (4th ed., pp. 137–153). Philadelphia, PA: Lippincott Williams & Wilkins.

Taylor, R. N., & Badell, M. L. (2011). The endocrinology of pregnancy. In D. G. Gardner & D. Shoback (Eds.), *Greenspan's basic & clinical endocrinology* (9th ed., pp. 553–572). New York, NY: McGraw-Hill.

Thilo, E. H., & Rosenberg, A. A. (2011). The newborn infant. In W. Hay, M. J. Levin, J. M. Sondheimer, et al. (Eds.), *Current diagnosis & treatment pediatrics* (20th ed., pp. 1–63). New York, NY: McGraw-Hill Publishing.

U.S. Department of Health and Human Services. (2010). *Healthy people 2020.* Washington, DC: Author.

Vest, A. R., & Cho, L. S. (2012). Hypertension in pregnancy. *Cardiology Clinics, 30*(3), 407–423.

Virtanen, H. E., Sadov, S., & Toppari, J. (2012). Prenatal exposure to smoking and male reproductive health. *Current Opinion in Endocrinology, Diabetes & Obesity, 19*(3), 228–232.

Warren, L., Rance, J., & Hunter, B. (2012). Feasibility and acceptability of a midwife-led intervention programme called 'Eat Well Keep Active' to encourage a healthy lifestyle in pregnancy. *BMC Pregnancy & Childbirth, 12*(1), 27.

Wewers, M. E., Salsberry, P. J., Ferketich, A. K., et al. (2012). Risk factors for smoking in rural women. *Journal of Women's Health, 21*(5), 548–556.

White, S. J., Boldt, K. L., Holditch, S. J., et al. (2012). Measles, mumps, and rubella. *Clinical Obstetrics & Genecology, 55*(2), 550–559.

Whitney, E. N., & Rolfes, S. R. (2012). Life cycle nutrition: Pregnancy & lactation. In E. N. Whitney & S. R. Rolfes (Eds.), *Understanding nutrition* (pp. 492–527). Belmont, CA: Wadsworth Publishing.

Wong, S., Ordean, A., & Kahan, M. (2011). Substance use in pregnancy. *Journal of Obstetrics & Gynaecology Canada, 33*(4), 367–384.

Zeitler, P. S., Travers, S. H., Nadaou, K., et al. (2011). Endocrine disorders. In W. Hay, M. J. Levin, J. M. Sondheimer, et al. (Eds.), *Current diagnosis & treatment pediatrics* (20th ed., pp. 943–983). New York, NY: McGraw-Hill Publishing.

Chapter 10

Nursing Care Related to Psychological and Physiologic Changes of Pregnancy

KEY TERMS

- ballottement
- Braxton Hicks contractions
- Chadwick's sign
- couvade syndrome
- diastasis
- Goodell's sign
- Hegar's sign
- lightening
- linea nigra
- melasma
- Montgomery's tubercles
- multipara
- operculum
- polyuria
- primigravida
- quickening
- striae gravidarum

OBJECTIVES

After mastering the contents of this chapter, you should be able to:

1. Describe common psychological and physiologic changes that occur with pregnancy and the relationship of the changes to pregnancy diagnosis.
2. Identify 2020 National Health Goals related to preconception counseling and prenatal care that nurses can help the nation achieve.
3. Assess a woman and her support team for psychological adjustment to the physiologic changes that occur with pregnancy.
4. Formulate nursing diagnoses related to adjustments necessary because of psychological and physiologic changes of pregnancy.
5. Identify expected outcomes in relation to a family's psychological and physical adaptation to pregnancy to help them manage seamless transitions across differing health care settings.
6. Using the nursing process, plan nursing care that includes the six competencies of Quality & Safety Education for Nurses (QSEN): Patient-Centered Care, Teamwork & Collaboration, Evidence-Based Practice (EBP), Quality Improvement (QI), Safety, and Informatics.
7. Implement nursing care, such as health teaching related to the expected changes of pregnancy.
8. Evaluate outcomes for achievement and effectiveness of goals to be certain expected outcomes have been achieved.
9. Integrate knowledge of psychological and physiologic changes of pregnancy with the interplay of nursing process, the six competencies of QSEN, and Family Nursing to promote quality maternal and child health nursing care.

Lauren Maxwell is a part-time model who has come to your clinic for her first prenatal visit. She has a 3-year-old at home. She tells you she missed her period 4 weeks ago and immediately took a home pregnancy test. She's happy it was positive but also sad because she had to turn down a modeling assignment in Paris for the summer. "I want to have a second child," she explains, "just not so soon." You suspect she's also anxious because she says, "I know there's no turning back but what will a second child do to my career?" She adds her husband, John, doesn't seem a bit worried. "Is that a good thing or not?" she asks. She also seems concerned about being a good parent as she says, "I'd die if I turn into the same kind of parent as my mother."

In addition to the positive home pregnancy test, Lauren presents with amenorrhea, breast tenderness, fatigue, and morning sickness. She's interested in learning when she will begin to look pregnant and what she can do for the morning sickness.

Previous chapters discussed the anatomy and physiology of women. This chapter

(Continued on next page)

(Continued from previous page)

adds information about the physiologic and psychological changes that occur in both a woman and her partner during pregnancy. Knowing such information can help you protect the health of a family and a fetus for the next 9 months.

What psychological development tasks of pregnancy does Lauren need to complete? Should you assure her that her worry about being a good parent is unfounded?

Clients are often interested in learning more about the physical or psychological changes that pregnancy brings, because these changes both verify the reality and mark the progress of pregnancy.

Physiologic changes of pregnancy occur gradually but eventually affect all of a woman's organ systems. They are necessary changes because they allow a woman's body to be able to provide oxygen and nutrients for her growing fetus as well as extra nutrients for her own increased metabolism. They also ready her body for labor and birth and for lactation (breastfeeding) once her baby is born (Bernstein & VanBuren, 2013). Despite the magnitude of these changes, such as a woman's blood volume doubling in amount, they are all extensions of normal physiology. At the end of pregnancy, her body will virtually return to its prepregnant state.

Psychological changes of pregnancy occur in response not only to the physiologic alterations happening but also to the increased responsibility associated with welcoming a new and completely dependent person to a family.

Because pregnancy changes are extensions of normal psychological and physiologic baselines, pregnancy represents a time of wellness, not of illness. A major responsibility for nurses caring for pregnant women and their families is to help the family maintain a feeling of wellness throughout the pregnancy and into early parenthood (Rogers & Worley, 2012). Box 10.1 shows 2020 National Health Goals relevant to these changes that come with pregnancy.

BOX 10.1 Nursing Care Planning Based on 2020 National Health Goals

A number of 2020 National Health Goals speak to the care necessary because of physiologic and psychological changes of pregnancy:

- Increase abstinence from alcohol, cigarettes, and illicit drugs among pregnant women from baselines of 89.4%, 89.6%, and 94.9% to target levels of 98.4%, 98.6%, and 100%.
- Reduce maternal deaths from a baseline of 12.7/100,000 live births to a target of 11.4/100,000.
- Increase the proportion of pregnant women who receive early and adequate prenatal care from a baseline of 70.5% to a target level of 77.6% (U.S. Department of Health and Human Services [DHHS], 2010; see www.healthypeople.gov).

Nurses can help the nation achieve these objectives by being certain women receive counseling in nutrition, safer sex practices, and low uses of alcohol and tobacco before pregnancy so they can enter intended pregnancies in the best health possible.

Nursing Process Overview

For Healthy Adaptation to Pregnancy

Assessment

Ideally, assessment for pregnancy begins before the pregnancy with preconception counseling. During a preconception assessment, evaluate a woman's overall health status, nutritional intake (ask specifically about sufficient intake of folic acid and protein), and lifestyle (especially drinking, smoking, and recreational drug habits); identify any potential problems (such as a risk for ectopic pregnancy because of tubal scarring); and identify a woman's understanding and expectations of conception, pregnancy, and parenthood.

In early pregnancy, be certain you establish a trusting relationship with a woman so she will see you as a person who is capable of counseling her and helping her solve problems and in whom she will be able to confide about any worries she has. Continue to assess a woman's health and nutritional status as well as the well-being of her fetus at all prenatal visits. Physical changes can be learned through health history, physical assessment, and laboratory tests. An assessment in psychological areas is obtained primarily through interviewing and should include societal, cultural, family, and personal influences as a woman adapts to pregnancy.

Nursing Diagnosis

Examples of nursing diagnoses involving the changes that occur with pregnancy include:

- Altered breathing patterns related to respiratory system changes of pregnancy
- Disturbed body image related to weight gain from pregnancy
- Deficient knowledge related to normal changes of pregnancy
- Imbalanced nutrition, less than body requirements, related to early morning nausea
- Powerlessness related to unintended pregnancy
- Possible impaired health and prenatal care behaviors associated with cultural beliefs

Outcome Identification and Planning

Planning nursing care in connection with the physiologic and psychological changes of pregnancy should involve a plan to review the common concerns women have about being pregnant before changes occur, so there are no surprises. Interesting Web sites to help women learn more about prenatal care are www.marchofdimes.com, www.babycenter.com, and www.womenshealth.gov.

Before there were sonograms and maternal serum pregnancy tests, pregnancy was diagnosed on symptoms reported by the woman and the signs elicited by a health care provider. These signs and symptoms, still important today, are traditionally divided into three classifications: presumptive (subjective symptoms); probable (objective signs); and positive (documented signs) (Table 10.2).

Presumptive (Subjective) Symptoms

Presumptive symptoms are those which, when taken as single entities, could easily indicate other conditions (Russell et al., 2011). These findings, discussed in connection with the body system in which they occur, are experienced by the woman but cannot be documented by an examiner (Box 10.6).

TABLE 10.2 Presumptive, Probable, and Positive Indications of Pregnancy

Time From Implantation (Weeks)	Presumptive Finding	Probable Finding	Positive Finding	Description
1		Maternal serum test		A venipuncture of blood serum reveals the presence of human chorionic gonadotropin hormone
2	Breast changes			Feelings of tenderness, fullness, tingling; enlargement and darkening of areola
2	Nausea, vomiting			Nausea or vomiting on arising or when fatigued
2	Amenorrhea			Absence of menstruation
3	Frequent urination			Sense of having to void more often than usual
6		Chadwick's sign		Color change of the vagina from pink to violet
6		Goodell's sign		Softening of the cervix
6		Hegar's sign		Softening of the lower uterine segment
6		Sonographic evidence of gestational sac		Characteristic ring is evident
8			Sonographic evidence of fetal outline	Fetal outline can be seen and measured by sonogram
10–12			Fetal heart audible	Doppler ultrasound reveals heartbeat
12	Fatigue			General feeling of tiredness
12	Uterine enlargement			Uterus can be palpated over symphysis pubis
16		Ballottement		When lower uterine segment is tapped on a bimanual examination, the fetus can be felt to rise against the abdominal wall
18	Quickening			Fetal movement felt by woman
20			Fetal movement felt by examiner	Fetal movement can be palpated through abdomen
20		Braxton Hicks contractions		Periodic uterine tightening occurs
20		Fetal outline felt by examiner		Fetal outline can be palpated through abdomen
24	Linea nigra			Line of dark pigment forms on the abdomen
24	Melasma			Dark pigment forms on face
24	Striae gravidarum			Red streaks form on abdomen

BOX 10.6 Nursing Care Planning Using Assessment

Assessing a Woman for Presumptive Symptoms of Pregnancy

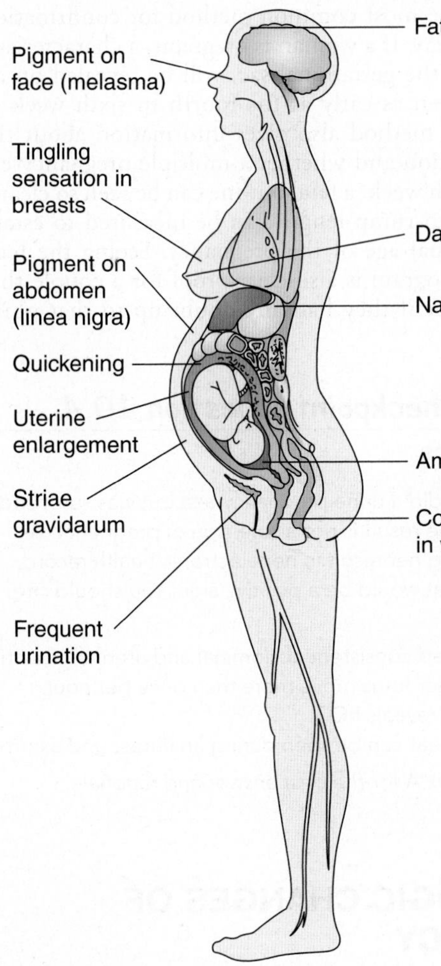

BOX 10.7 Nursing Care Planning Using Assessment

Assessing a Woman for Probable Signs of Pregnancy

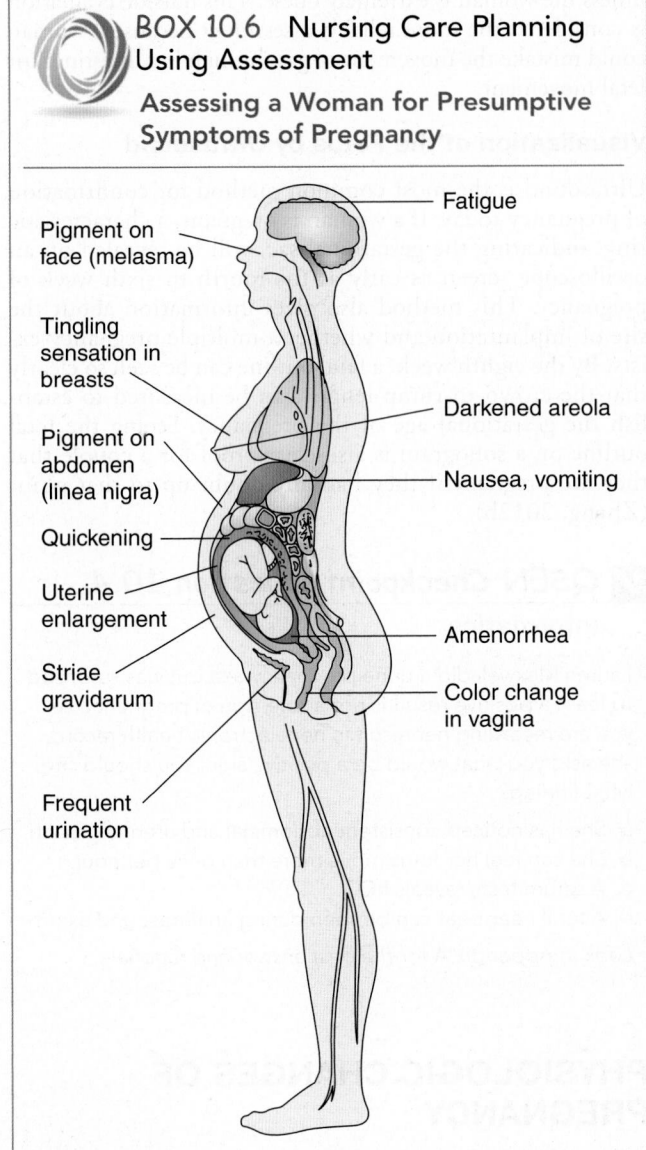

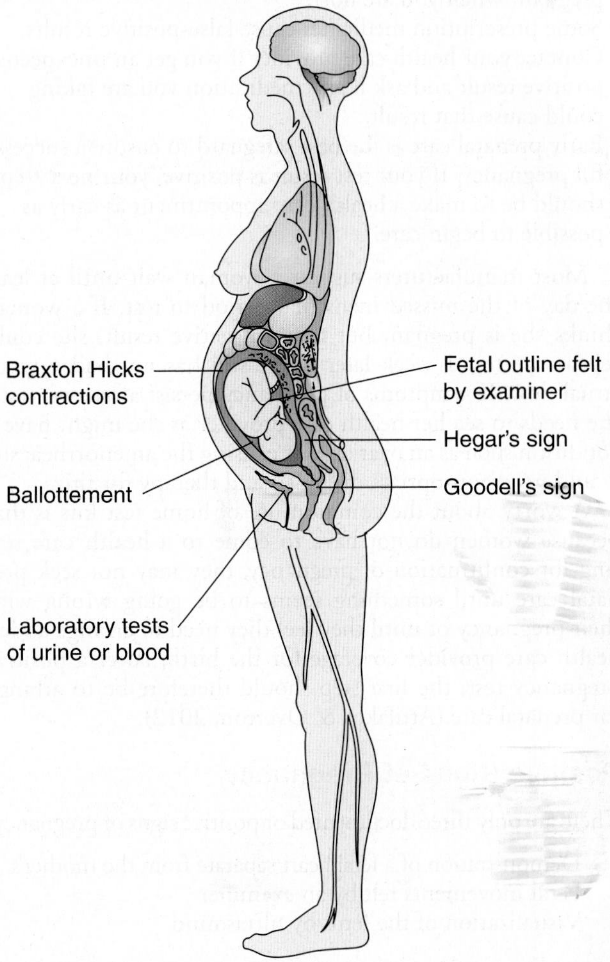

Probable Signs

In contrast to presumptive symptoms, probable signs of pregnancy are objective and so can be verified by an examiner. Although they are more reliable than presumptive symptoms, they still do not positively diagnosis a pregnancy (Box 10.7).

Laboratory Tests

The commonly used laboratory tests for pregnancy are based on the use of a venipuncture or a urine specimen to detect the presence of human chorionic gonadotropin (hCG), a hormone created by the chorionic villi of the placenta, in the urine or blood serum of the pregnant woman. Because these tests are only accurate 95% to 98% of the time, positive results from these tests are considered probable rather than positive signs.

In the nonpregnant woman, no units of hCG will be detectable because there are no trophoblast cells producing hCG. In the pregnant woman, trace amounts of hCG appear in her serum as early as 24 to 48 hours after implantation and reach a measurable level (about 50 milli-International Unit/ml 7 to 9 days after conception. Levels peak at about 100 milli-International Unit/ml between the 60th and 80th day of gestation. After that point, the concentration of hCG declines again so, at term, it is again barely detectable in serum or urine.

Home Pregnancy Tests

A number of brands for pregnancy testing are available over the counter, take only 2 to 3 minutes to complete, and have a high degree of accuracy (97% to 99%) if the instructions are followed exactly because they can detect as little as 35 milli-International Unit/ml of hCG. For the test, a woman dips a reagent strip into her stream of urine. A color change or the appearance of two bars on the strip denotes pregnancy.

Tips to give the woman for successful testing include:

- Check the expiration date on the package to be certain the kit has not expired; an outdated kit can give false-positive results.
- Read the instruction pamphlet provided with the test, noting especially the time period you should wait before reading the result, and follow this instruction carefully.

- A concentrated urine sample such as a first urine in the morning tests best. Don't drink a large quantity of water beforehand because this can dilute a urine sample.
- Read the test results at the exact time the instructions dictate. Reading the strip after the designated time can cause inaccurate results (e.g., denoting that you are pregnant when you are not).
- Some prescription medicines cause false-positive results. Contact your health care provider if you get an unexpected positive result and ask if any medication you are taking could cause that result.
- Early prenatal care is the best safeguard to ensure a successful pregnancy. If your test result is positive, your next step should be to make a health care appointment as early as possible to begin care.

Most manufacturers suggest a woman wait until at least the day of the missed menstrual period to test. If a woman thinks she is pregnant but gets a negative result, she could repeat the test 1 week later if she still has not had a menstrual flow. If symptoms of pregnancy persist after two tests, she needs to see her health care provider as she might have a condition such as an ovarian cyst causing the amenorrhea; she would need appropriate diagnosis and therapy for this.

A worry about the common use of home test kits is that because women do not have to come to a health care setting for confirmation of pregnancy, they may not seek prenatal care until something seems to be going wrong with their pregnancy or until they feel they need to arrange added health care provider coverage for the birth. After a positive pregnancy test, the first step should therefore be to arrange for prenatal care (Attilakos & Overton, 2012).

Positive Signs of Pregnancy

There are only three documented or positive signs of pregnancy:

1. Demonstration of a fetal heart separate from the mother's
2. Fetal movements felt by an examiner
3. Visualization of the fetus by ultrasound

Demonstration of a Fetal Heart Separate From the Mother's

Although a fetal heart beat cannot be heard through an ordinary stethoscope until 18 to 20 weeks of pregnancy, an echocardiography can demonstrate a heartbeat as early as 5 weeks. An ultrasound can reveal a beating fetal heart as early as the sixth to seventh week of pregnancy. Doppler instrumentation that converts ultrasonic frequencies to audible frequencies is able to detect fetal heart sounds as early as the 10th to 12th week of gestation.

The fetal heart rate ranges between 110 and 160 beats/min. Sounds are more difficult to hear if a woman's abdomen has a great deal of subcutaneous fat or if there is a larger than normal amount of amniotic fluid present (hydramnios). They are heard best when the position of the fetus is determined by palpation and the stethoscope is placed over the area of the fetal back.

Fetal Movements Felt by an Examiner

Fetal movements may be felt by a woman as early as 16 to 20 weeks of pregnancy. An objective examiner can discern fetal movements at about the 20th to 24th week of pregnancy unless the woman is extremely obese. This outside evaluation is considered the more reliable assessment because a woman could mistake the movement of gas through her intestines for fetal movement.

Visualization of the Fetus by Ultrasound

Ultrasound is the most common method for confirmation of pregnancy today. If a woman is pregnant, a characteristic ring, indicating the gestational sac, will be revealed on an oscilloscope screen as early as the fourth to sixth week of pregnancy. This method also gives information about the site of implantation and whether a multiple pregnancy exists. By the eighth week, a fetal outline can be seen so clearly that the crown-to-rump length can be measured to establish the gestational age of the pregnancy. Seeing the fetal outline on a sonogram is also clear proof for a couple that they are pregnant if they had any doubt up to that point (Zheng, 2012b).

✔ QSEN Checkpoint Question 10.4

Informatics

Lauren Maxwell did a urine pregnancy test but was surprised to learn a positive result is not a sure sign of pregnancy. As you are recording her result in her electronic health record, she asks you what would be a positive sign. You should cite what finding?

a. She has noticed consistent abdominal and uterine growth.
b. She can feel her fetus move more than once per hour.
c. A serum tests reveals hCG.
d. A fetal heartbeat can be seen during an ultrasound exam.

Look in Appendix A for the best answer and rationale.

PHYSIOLOGIC CHANGES OF PREGNANCY

Physiologic changes that occur during pregnancy are the basis for the signs and symptoms used to confirm a pregnancy. They can be categorized as local (i.e., confined to the reproductive organs) or systemic (i.e., affecting the entire body). For easy reference, Table 10.3 summarizes the changes that occur during a typical 40-week pregnancy.

Reproductive System Changes

Reproductive tract changes are those involving the uterus, ovaries, vagina, and breasts.

Uterine Changes

The most obvious alteration in a woman's body during pregnancy is the increase in size of the uterus to accommodate the growing fetus. Over the 10 lunar months of pregnancy, the uterus increases in length, depth, width, weight, wall thickness, and volume.

- Length grows from approximately 6.5 cm to 32 cm.
- Depth increases from 2.5 cm to 22 cm.
- Width expands from 4 cm to 24 cm.
- Weight increases from 50 g to 1,000 g.

TABLE 10.3 Timetable for Physiologic Changes of Pregnancy

Location of Change	First Trimester	Second Trimester	Third Trimester
Cardiovascular	Blood volume increasing Pseudoanemia may occur Clotting factors increasing	Blood pressure slightly decreased	Blood pressure returns to prepregnancy levels
Ovarian	Corpus luteum active	Corpus luteum fading	
Uterine	Steady increased growth	Placenta producing estrogen and progesterone	
Cervix	Softening begins	Softening increases	"Ripe"
Vaginal	White discharge present		Increasing in amount
Musculoskeletal		Progressive cartilage softening Lordosis increasing	
Pigmentation		Progressively increasing	
Kidney	Maternal glomerular filtration rate increasing Glycosuria begins and increases Aldosterone increased, aiding retention of sodium and fluid		
Gastrointestinal		Slowed peristalsis	
Thyroid	Increased metabolic rate		

- Early in pregnancy, the uterine wall thickens from about 1 cm to about 2 cm; toward the end of pregnancy, the wall thins to become supple and only about 0.5-cm thick.
- The volume of the uterus increases from about 2 ml to more than 1,000 ml. This makes it possible for a uterus to hold a 7-lb (3,175-g) fetus plus 1,000 ml of amniotic fluid for a total of about 4,000 g.

This great uterine growth is due partly to formation of a few new muscle fibers in the uterine myometrium but principally to the stretching of existing muscle fibers (by the end of pregnancy, muscle fibers in the uterus, because of fibroblastic tissue that forms between them, are two to seven times longer than they were before pregnancy). Because uterine fibers simply stretch during pregnancy and are not newly built, the uterus is able to return to its prepregnant state at the end of the pregnancy with little difficulty and almost no destruction of tissue (Edmonds, 2012).

By the end of the 12th week of pregnancy, the uterus is large enough that it can be palpated as a firm globe under the abdominal wall, just above the symphysis pubis. An important factor to assess regarding uterine growth at health care visits is its constant, steady, and predictable increase in size (Fig. 10.2).

- By the 20th or 22nd week of pregnancy, it typically reaches the level of the umbilicus.
- By the 36th week, it usually touches the xiphoid process and can make breathing difficult.
- About 2 weeks before term (the 38th week) for a **primigravida**, a woman in her first pregnancy, the fetal head settles into the pelvis and the uterus returns to the height it was at 36 weeks.

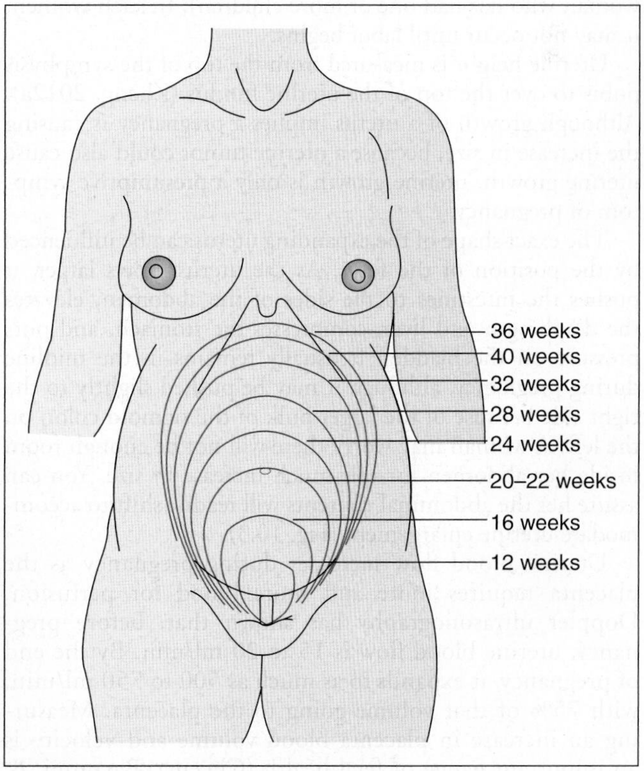

FIGURE 10.2 Fundus height at various weeks of pregnancy.

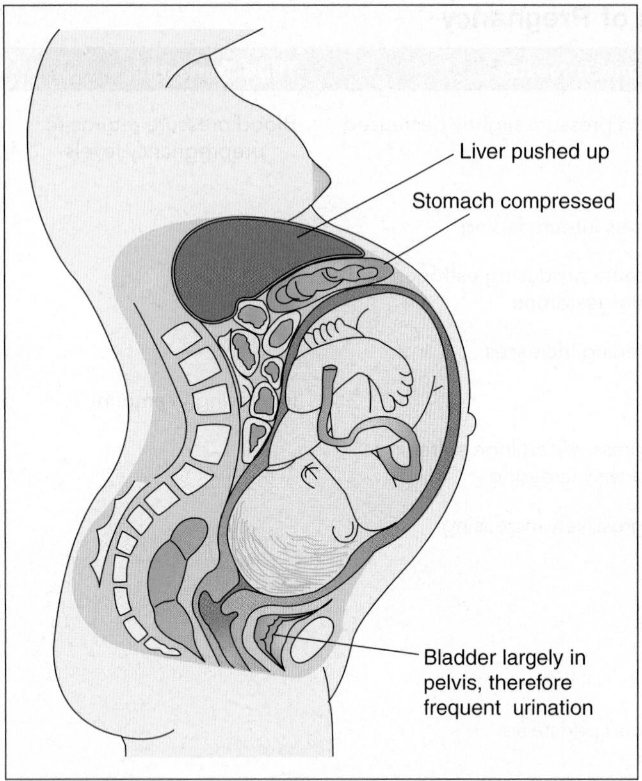

FIGURE 10.3 Crowding of abdominal contents late in pregnancy.

This settling of the fetus into the midpelvis is termed **lightening**, because a woman's breathing is so much easier that she feels as if her load is lightened. The point at which lightening will occur is not predictable in a **multipara** (a woman who has had one or more children). In such women, it may not occur until labor begins.

Uterine height is measured from the top of the symphysis pubis to over the top of the uterine fundus (Zheng, 2012a). Although growth of a uterus implies a pregnancy is causing the increase in size, because a uterine tumor could also cause uterine growth, uterine growth is only a presumptive symptom of pregnancy.

The exact shape of the expanding uterus can be influenced by the position of the fetus. As the uterus grows larger, it pushes the intestines to the sides of the abdomen, elevates the diaphragm and liver, compresses the stomach, and puts pressure on the bladder. It usually remains in the midline during pregnancy, although it may be pushed slightly to the right side because of the larger bulk of the sigmoid colon on the left. A woman may worry there will not be enough room inside her abdomen for this much increase in size. You can assure her the abdominal contents will readily shift to accommodate uterine enlargement (Fig. 10.3).

Uterine blood flow increases during pregnancy as the placenta requires more and more blood for perfusion. Doppler ultrasonography has shown that, before pregnancy, uterine blood flow is 15 to 20 ml/min. By the end of pregnancy, it expands to as much as 500 to 750 ml/min, with 75% of that volume going to the placenta. Measuring an increase in placenta blood volume and velocity is an important gauge of fetal health (Cheema, Bayoumi, & Gudmundsson, 2011).

Circulation to the uterus increases so much that, toward the end of pregnancy, one sixth of a woman's blood supply is circulating through the uterus at any given time; this means uterine bleeding in pregnancy has to always be regarded as serious because it could result in sudden and major blood loss. Caution women to contact their health care provider if any vaginal bleeding occurs during pregnancy.

A bimanual examination (one finger of an examiner is placed in the vagina, the other hand on the abdomen) can demonstrate, during a pregnancy, that the uterus feels more anteflexed, larger, and softer to the touch than usual. At about the sixth week of pregnancy (at the time of the second missed menstrual flow), the lower uterine segment just above the cervix becomes so soft when it is compressed between examining fingers on bimanual examination that the wall feels as thin as tissue paper (Russell et al., 2011). This extreme softening of the lower uterine segment is known as **Hegar's sign** (Fig. 10.4).

During the 16th to 20th week of pregnancy, when the fetus is still small in relation to the amount of amniotic fluid present, if the lower uterine segment is tapped sharply during a pelvic exam, the fetus can be felt to bounce or rise in the amniotic fluid up against a hand placed on the abdomen. This phenomenon, termed **ballottement** (from the French word *ballotter*, meaning "to quake"), may, however, also be simulated by a loosely attached uterine tumor and, therefore, is no more than a probable sign of pregnancy.

Between the 20th and 24th week of pregnancy, the uterine wall becomes thinned to such a degree a fetal outline within the uterus may be palpated by a skilled examiner. Because a tumor with calcium deposits could simulate a fetal outline, palpation of what seems to be a fetus, like other uterine assessments, does not constitute a sure confirmation of pregnancy.

Uterine contractions begin early in pregnancy, at least by the 12th week, and are present throughout the rest of pregnancy, becoming stronger and harder as the pregnancy ad-

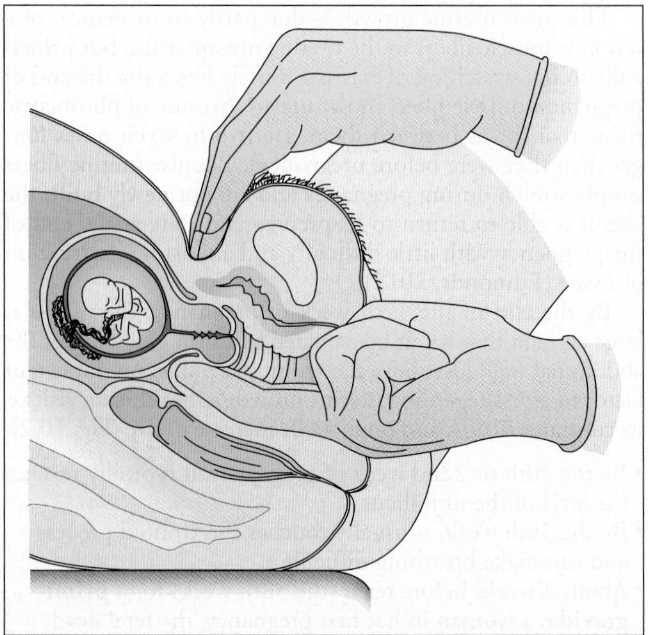

FIGURE 10.4 Examining for Hegar's sign. If the sign is present, the wall of the uterus is softer than usual.

vances. A woman experiences them as waves of hardness or tightening across her abdomen. If a hand is placed on her abdomen, an examiner may be able to feel these contractions as well; an electronic monitor can easily measure both the frequency and length of such contractions.

These "practice" contractions, termed **Braxton Hicks contractions**, serve as warm-up exercises for labor and also play a role in ensuring the placenta receives adequate blood. They may become so strong in the last month of pregnancy that a woman mistakes them for labor contractions (i.e., false labor). One way they can be differentiated from true contractions is that true contractions cause cervical dilation, and Braxton Hicks contractions do not (Attilakos & Overton, 2012). Although these contractions are always present with pregnancy, they also could accompany any growing uterine mass; so, like ballottement, they are no more than a probable sign of pregnancy.

Amenorrhea

Amenorrhea (i.e., an absence of a menstrual flow) occurs with pregnancy because of the suppression of follicle-stimulating hormone (FSH) by rising estrogen levels. In a healthy woman who has menstruated previously, the absence of a menstrual flow strongly suggests impregnation has occurred. Amenorrhea, however, also heralds the onset of menopause or could result from unrelated reasons such as uterine infection, anxiety (perhaps over becoming pregnant), a chronic illness such as severe anemia, or undue stress. It also is seen in athletes who train strenuously, especially in long-distance runners and ballet dancers if their body fat percentage drops below a critical point (Doyle-Lucas, Akers, & Davy, 2010). Amenorrhea is, therefore, only a presumptive symptom of pregnancy.

Cervical Changes

In response to the increased level of circulating estrogen produced by the placenta during pregnancy, the cervix of the uterus becomes more vascular and edematous than usual. A mucous plug, called the **operculum**, forms to seal out bacteria and help prevent infection in the fetus and membranes. Increased fluid between cells causes it to soften in consistency, and increased vascularity causes it to darken from a pale pink to a violet hue (**Goodell's sign**).

The consistency of a nonpregnant cervix can be compared with that of the nose; the consistency of a pregnant cervix more closely resembles an earlobe. Just before labor, the cervix becomes so soft it takes on the consistency of butter or is said to be "ripe" for birth (Aguirre & Chou, 2011).

Vaginal Changes

Under the influence of estrogen, the vaginal epithelium and underlying tissues increase in size as they become enriched with glycogen. Muscle fibers loosen from their connective tissue base in preparation for great distention at birth. This increase in the activity of the epithelial cells results in a slight white vaginal discharge throughout pregnancy (but this is only a presumptive symptom as vaginal infections also produce discharges).

An increase in the vascularity of the vagina parallels the vascular changes in the uterus. The resulting increase in circulation changes the color of the vaginal walls from their normal light pink to a deep violet (**Chadwick's sign**).

Vaginal secretions before pregnancy have a pH value greater than 7 (an alkaline pH). During pregnancy, the pH level falls to 4 or 5 (an acid pH), which helps make the vagina resistant to bacterial invasion for the length of the pregnancy. This occurs because of the action of *Lactobacillus acidophilus,* a bacteria that grows freely in the increased glycogen environment, which increases the lactic acid content of secretions.

Ovarian Changes

Ovulation stops with pregnancy because of the active feedback mechanism of estrogen and progesterone produced early in pregnancy by the corpus luteum and late in pregnancy by the placenta. This feedback causes the pituitary gland to halt production of FSH and luteinizing hormone (LH); without stimulation from FSH and LH, ovulation does not occur.

The corpus luteum that was created after ovulation continues to increase in size on the surface of the ovary until about the 16th week of pregnancy, by which time the placenta takes over as the chief provider of progesterone and estrogen. The corpus luteum, no longer essential for the continuation of the pregnancy, regresses in size and appears white and fibrous on the surface of the ovary (a corpus albicans).

✔ QSEN Checkpoint Question 10.5

Patient-Centered Care

Lauren Maxwell's doctor told her she had a positive Chadwick's sign. When she asks you what this means, your best answer would be which of the following?

a. "Your abdomen feels soft and tender, a normal finding."
b. "Your uterus has tipped forward, a potential complication."
c. "Your cervical mucus feels sticky, just as it should feel."
d. "Your vagina looks dark in color, a typical pregnancy sign."

Look in Appendix A for the best answer and rationale.

Changes in the Breasts

Subtle changes in the breasts may be one of the first physiologic changes of pregnancy a woman notices (at about 6 weeks) (Fig. 10.5). Typical changes are a feeling of fullness, tingling, or tenderness that occurs because of the increased stimulation of breast tissue by the high estrogen level in her body. As the pregnancy progresses, breast size increases because of growth in the mammary alveoli and in fat deposits. The areola of the nipple darkens, and its diameter increases from about 3.5 cm (1.5 in.) to 5 cm or 7.5 cm (2 or 3 in.). There is additional darkening of the skin surrounding the areola in some women, forming a secondary areola.

Early in pregnancy, the breasts begin readying themselves for the secretion of milk. By the 16th week, colostrum—the thin, watery, high-protein fluid that is the precursor of breast milk—can be expelled from the nipples. As vascularity of the breasts increases, blue veins may become prominent over the surface of the breasts. The sebaceous glands of the areola (**Montgomery's tubercles**), which keep the nipple supple and help to prevent nipples from cracking and drying during lactation, enlarge and become protuberant.

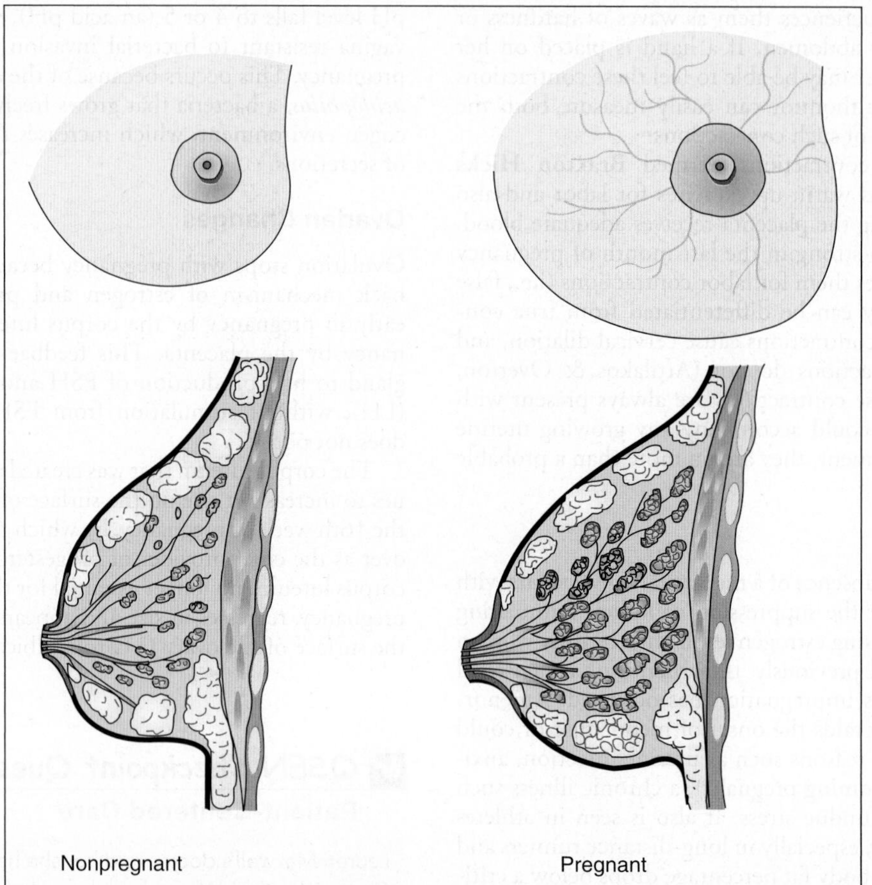

FIGURE 10.5 Comparison of nonpregnant and pregnant breasts.

Talking to women during pregnancy about breast changes and how these changes are devised to aid breastfeeding can be the trigger that alerts women to the importance of breastfeeding for their baby (Baselice & Lawson, 2011).

Systemic Changes

Although the physiologic changes first noticed by a woman are apt to be those of the reproductive system, changes also occur in almost all body systems.

Endocrine System

Almost all aspects of the endocrine system increase during pregnancy in order to support fetal growth (Smith & Schust, 2011). Important among these is the presence of a new endocrine organ, or the placenta.

Placenta. The placenta is responsible for the production of large amounts of estrogen, progesterone, hCG, human placental lactogen (hPL), relaxin, and prostaglandins during pregnancy.

- The effect of estrogen is to cause breast and uterine enlargement. Palmar erythema (i.e., redness and itching of the palms) may occur early in pregnancy as a response to this high circulating estrogen level.
- Progesterone has a major role in maintaining the endometrium, inhibiting uterine contractility, and aiding in the development of the breasts for lactation.
- hCG is secreted by the trophoblast cells beginning early in pregnancy. It stimulates progesterone and estrogen synthesis in the ovaries until the placenta can assume this role.
- hPL, also known as human chorionic somatomammotropin, serves as an antagonist to insulin, making insulin less effective, and so allows more glucose to become available for fetal growth.
- Relaxin, secreted by the corpus luteum of the ovary as well as the placenta, is responsible for helping to inhibit uterine activity and to soften the cervix and the collagen in joints. Softening of the cervix allows for dilatation at birth; softening of collagen allows for laxness in the lower spine, which helps enlarge the birth canal.
- Prostaglandins affect smooth muscle contractility to such an extent they may be the trigger that initiates labor at term.

Pituitary Gland. A major change in the pituitary gland is the halt in production of FSH and LH because of the high estrogen and progesterone levels produced by the placenta.

- At the same time, there is increased production of other pituitary hormones such as growth hormone and melanocyte-stimulating hormone, which causes skin pigment changes.
- Prolactin production begins late in pregnancy and helps breasts prepare for lactation.
- Late in pregnancy, the posterior pituitary also begins to produce oxytocin, which is needed to aid labor (Cunningham, Leveno, Bloom, et al., 2010).

Thyroid and Parathyroid Glands. The thyroid gland enlarges to produce increased levels of protein-bound iodine, butanol-extractable iodine, and thyroxine to such an extent a woman's basal body metabolic rate increases by about 20%. These thyroid changes along with emotional lability, tachycardia, palpitations, and increased perspiration may lead to a mistaken diagnosis of hyperthyroidism if pregnancy has not yet been diagnosed (Yazbeck & Sullivan, 2012).

The parathyroid glands, which are necessary for the metabolism of calcium, also increase in size during pregnancy. Because calcium is important for fetal growth, the hypertrophy and increased action is probably necessary to satisfy this increased requirement.

Adrenal Glands. Adrenal gland activity increases in pregnancy so additional levels of corticosteroids and aldosterone can be produced. These increased levels probably aid in suppressing an inflammatory reaction or help reduce the possibility of a woman's body rejecting the foreign protein of the fetus, the same as it would reject a foreign-tissue transplant. They also help to regulate the woman's glucose metabolism.

The increased level of aldosterone plays a major role in promoting sodium reabsorption and maintaining osmolarity in the amount of fluid retained, which indirectly helps to safeguard the blood volume and provide adequate perfusion pressure across the placenta.

Pancreas. The pancreas increases the production of insulin in response to the higher levels of glucocorticoid produced by the adrenal glands. Insulin is less effective than usual, however, because estrogen, progesterone, and hPL are all antagonists of insulin. Overall, this diminished action of insulin is beneficial because it ensures a ready supply of glucose for fetal growth. As a rule, to maintain a high insulin level during pregnancy, a woman who is diabetic and self-injects insulin may need to increase the amount of insulin she takes while she is pregnant. A woman who is prediabetic may develop overt diabetes for the first time and may need insulin administration during pregnancy.

The glucose level of a fetus averages about 30 mg/100 ml, lower than the maternal serum glucose level. Because the rapidly developing fetus uses so much glucose in early pregnancy, a woman's fasting blood glucose level early in pregnancy may be unusually low (80 to 85 mg/100 ml).

To prevent fetal hypoglycemia with resultant cell destruction or lack of fetal growth, maternal serum glucose usually rises to a higher than normal level as pregnancy progresses. This allows a woman to maintain a fairly steady level of serum glucose despite long intervals between meals or days of increased activity. To help ensure against hypoglycemia, a pregnant woman should keep her diet adequate in calories and should try to not go longer than 12 hours between meals.

✔ QSEN Checkpoint Question 10.6

Safety

Lauren Maxwell overheard her doctor say insulin is not as effective during pregnancy as usual. How would you explain how decreased insulin effectiveness safeguards the health of her fetus?

a. Decreased effectiveness of insulin prevents the fetus from having low blood sugar.
b. Because insulin is ineffective, it cannot cross the placenta and harm the fetus.
c. The lessened action of insulin prevents the fetus from gaining too much weight.
d. It is the mother, not the fetus, who is guarded by this decreased insulin action.

Look in Appendix A for the best answer and rationale.

Immune System

Immunologic competency during pregnancy decreases, probably to prevent a woman's body from rejecting the fetus as if it were a transplanted organ. Immunoglobulin G (IgG) production is particularly decreased, which can make a woman more prone to infection during pregnancy. A simultaneous increase in the white blood cell count may help to counteract this decrease in the IgG response.

Integumentary System

As the uterus increases in size, the abdominal wall must stretch to accommodate it. This stretching (plus possibly increased adrenal cortex activity) can cause rupture and atrophy of small segments of the connective layer of the skin, leading to pink or reddish streaks (**striae gravidarum**) on the sides of the abdominal wall and sometimes on the thighs (Fig. 10.6). During the weeks after birth, striae gravidarum lighten to a silvery color (striae albicantes or atrophicae), and, although permanent, they become barely noticeable.

Occasionally, the abdominal wall has difficulty stretching enough to accommodate the growing fetus, causing the rectus muscles underneath the skin to actually separate, a condition known as **diastasis**. If this happens, it will appear after pregnancy as a bluish groove at the site of separation.

The umbilicus is stretched by pregnancy to such an extent that by the 28th week, its depression becomes obliterated and it is pushed so far outward in most women, it appears as if it has turned inside out, protruding as a round bump at the center of the abdominal wall.

Extra pigmentation generally appears on the abdominal wall, because of melanocyte-stimulating hormone from the pituitary. A narrow, brown line (**linea nigra**) may form, running from the umbilicus to the symphysis pubis and separating the abdomen into right and left halves (see Fig. 10.6).

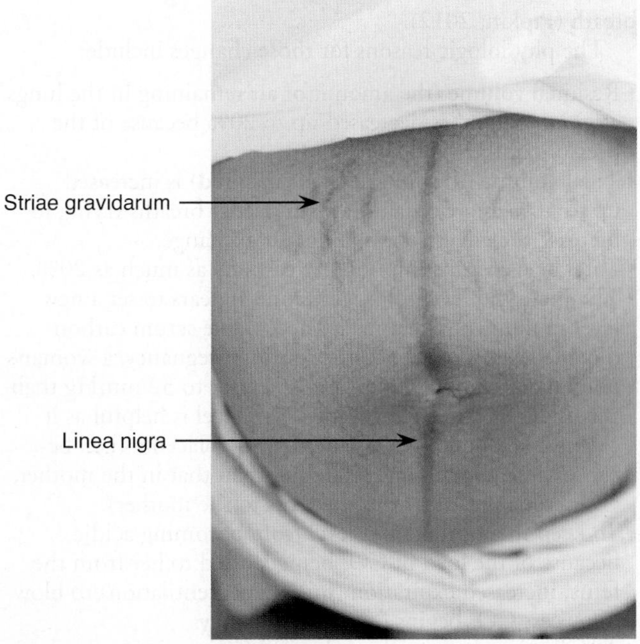

FIGURE 10.6 Skin changes in pregnancy: striae gravidarum and linea nigra. (From Klossner, N. J., & Hatfield, N. T. [2010]. *Introductory maternity & pediatric nursing*. Lippincott Williams & Wilkins.)

Darkened or reddened areas may appear on the face as well, particularly on the cheeks and across the nose. This is known as **melasma** (chloasma) or the "mask of pregnancy." With the decrease in the level of melanocyte-stimulating hormone after pregnancy, these areas lighten and disappear.

Vascular spiders or telangiectasias (small, fiery-red branching spots) sometimes develop on the skin, particularly on the thighs. Palmar erythema, as mentioned earlier, may occur on the hands. Both of these symptoms result from the increased level of estrogen in the body; telangiectasias may fade but not completely disappear after pregnancy. The activity of sweat glands increases throughout the body beginning early in pregnancy, leading to increased perspiration. Fewer hairs on the head enter a resting phase because of overall increased metabolism, so scalp hair growth is increased.

Respiratory System

A local change that often occurs in the respiratory system is marked congestion, or "stuffiness," of the nasopharynx, a response, again, to increased estrogen levels. Women may worry this stuffiness indicates an allergy or a cold. Not realizing it is a symptom of pregnancy, some women take over-the-counter cold medications or antihistamines in an effort to relieve the congestion. Ask women at prenatal visits if they are taking any kind of medicine for this to detect this possibility and to be certain the medication they are taking is safe during pregnancy.

Because the uterus enlarges so much during pregnancy, the diaphragm, and ultimately, the lungs, receive an increasing amount of pressure. Toward the end of pregnancy, this can actually displace the diaphragm by as much as 4 cm upward. Even with all this crowding, however, a woman's vital capacity (the maximum volume exhaled after a maximum inspiration) does not decrease during pregnancy because, although the lungs are crowded in the vertical dimension, they can still expand horizontally. Two major changes do occur with pregnancy: a more rapid than usual breathing rate (18 to 20 breaths/min) and a chronic feeling of shortness of breath (Pipkin, 2012).

The physiologic reasons for those changes include:

- Residual volume (the amount of air remaining in the lungs after expiration) is decreased up to 20% because of the pressure of the diaphragm.
- Tidal volume (the volume of air inspired) is increased up to 40% as a woman draws in deeper breaths trying to increase the effectiveness of her air exchange.
- Total oxygen consumption increases by as much as 20%.
- The increased level of progesterone appears to set a new level in the hypothalamus for acceptable serum carbon dioxide levels (Pco_2) because, during pregnancy, a woman's body tends to maintain a Pco_2 at closer to 32 mmHg than the usual 40 mmHg. This low Pco_2 level is helpful as it causes a favorable CO_2 gradient at the placenta (i.e., because the fetal CO_2 level is higher than that in the mother, CO_2 crosses readily from the fetus to the mother).
- To keep the mother's pH level from becoming acidic because of the load of CO_2 being shifted to her from the fetus, increased expiration (mild hyperventilation) to blow off excess CO_2 begins early in pregnancy.
- At full term, a woman's total ventilation capacity may have risen by as much as 40%. This increased ventilation may become so extreme toward the end of pregnancy that a woman develops a respiratory alkalosis or exhales more than the usual amount of CO_2. To compensate, kidneys excrete plasma bicarbonate in urine to lower this pH. This results in increased urination or **polyuria**, a sign of pregnancy.
- The slight increase in pH in serum because of the changed expiratory effort is advantageous because it slightly increases the binding capacity of maternal hemoglobin and thereby raises the oxygen content of maternal blood (Po_2), from a usual level of about 92 mmHg to about 106 mmHg. This can be advantageous to fetal growth because it helps ensure good oxygenation of the fetus.
- The total respiratory changes and the compensating mechanisms that occur in the respiratory system can be described as a chronic respiratory alkalosis fully compensated by a chronic metabolic acidosis (Hegewald & Crapo, 2011).

TABLE 10.4 Respiratory Changes During Pregnancy

Variable	Change
Vital capacity	No change
Tidal volume	Increased by 30%–40%
Respiratory rate	Increased by 1 or 2 breaths/min
Residual volume	Decreased by 20%
Plasma Pco_2	Decreased to about 27–32 mmHg
Plasma pH	Increased to 7.40–7.45
Plasma Po_2	Increased to 104–108 mmHg
Respiratory minute volume	Increased by 40%
Expiratory reserve	Decreased by 20%

Changes in respiratory function during pregnancy are summarized in Table 10.4.

Temperature

Early in pregnancy, body temperature increases slightly because of the secretion of progesterone from the corpus luteum (the temperature, which increased at ovulation, remains elevated). As the placenta takes over the function of the corpus luteum at about 16 weeks, the temperature usually decreases to normal.

Cardiovascular System

Changes in the circulatory system are extremely significant to the health of a fetus, because they determine whether there will be adequate placental and fetal circulation for oxygenation and nutrition. Table 10.5 summarizes these changes.

Blood Volume. To provide for an adequate exchange of nutrients across the placenta and for adequate blood to compensate for maternal blood loss at birth, the total circulatory blood volume of a woman's body increases by at least 30%

TABLE 10.5 Changes in the Cardiovascular System During Pregnancy

Assessment Factor	Prepregnancy	Pregnancy
Cardiac output		25%–50% increase
Heart rate (beats/min)	70–80	80–90
Blood volume (ml)	4,000	5,250
Red blood cell mass (mm^3)	4,200,000	4,650,000
Leukocytes (mm^3)	7,000	20,500
Fibrinogen (mg/dl)	300	450
Blood pressure		Decreases in second trimester, rises to prepregnancy level in third trimester

(and possibly as much as 50%) during pregnancy. This is important protection because blood loss at a normal vaginal birth is 300 to 400 ml; blood loss from a cesarean birth can be as high as 800 to 1,000 ml.

The increase in blood volume occurs gradually, beginning at the end of the first trimester. It peaks at about the 28th to the 32nd week and then continues at this high level throughout the third trimester. Because the plasma volume increases faster than red blood cell production, the concentration of hemoglobin and erythrocytes usually declines early in pregnancy, giving the woman pseudoanemia. Her body compensates for this change by producing more red blood cells, bringing the hemoglobin level back to near normal by the second trimester (Bernstein & VanBuren, 2013).

Iron, Folic Acid, and Vitamin Needs. Almost all women need some iron supplementation during pregnancy by prenatal vitamins because of a number of factors:

- The fetus requires a total of about 350 to 400 mg of iron per day to grow.
- The increases in the mother's circulatory red blood cell mass require an additional 400 mg of iron per day, which creates a total needed increase of about 800 mg.
- Iron absorption may be impaired during pregnancy as a result of decreased gastric acidity (iron is absorbed best from an acid medium) (Whitney & Rolfes, 2012).

A hemoglobin concentration of less than 11 g/100 ml, a hematocrit value below 33% in the first or third trimester of pregnancy, or a hemoglobin concentration of less than 10.5 g/dl (hematocrit <32%) in the second trimester is considered true anemia. Daily supplementation of iron for values above this level (over and above as a component of prenatal vitamins) is generally recommended as needed (Reveiz, Gyte, Cuervo, et al., 2011). If iron is prescribed, caution women that, although the prescribed dose is good for them, excess iron can lead to stomach irritation and possibly iron accumulation in body cells (see Chapter 20 for additional information on anemia in pregnancy).

The demand for folic acid increases beginning early on in pregnancy. If the intake of this is not great enough, megalohemoglobinemia (i.e., large, nonfunctioning red blood cells) can result. Inadequate folic acid levels are also linked to an increased risk of neural tube or abdominal wall disorders in fetuses (Lumley, Watson, Watson, et al., 2011). For this reason, prenatal vitamins that contain folic acid are routinely prescribed. Encourage women to eat foods that are high in folic acid such as spinach, asparagus, and legumes both during their prepregnancy period and during pregnancy so that the prenatal vitamin is truly a supplement.

You may need to remind women to be conscientious about not just buying but taking a prescribed prenatal vitamin to be certain their intake of common vitamins is adequate. Surprisingly, although other factors also come into play, an association between multivitamin supplementation during pregnancy and reduced cancers in children such as neuroblastoma, leukemia, and brain tumors can be documented (Talaulikar & Arulkumaran, 2011).

Heart. To handle the increase in blood volume in the circulatory system, a woman's heart rate increases by at least 10 beats/min, causing her cardiac output to increase as much as 25% to 50%. Some women develop audible functional (innocent) heart murmurs during pregnancy, probably because of the increased blood volume and pressure from the diaphragm shifts heart position.

The bulk of these cardiac changes occur during the second trimester, with a small increase in the third trimester. Although the average woman barely notices these circulatory system changes, the increased heart rate along with the rise in circulating blood volume can have serious implications for a woman with cardiac disease because her heart can be overwhelmed by these new requirements placed on it (Hatton, Colman, Sermer, et al., 2012).

Sudden palpitations of the heart are not uncommon during pregnancy, particularly on quick motion. You can caution women not to feel frightened if these do occur. In the early months of pregnancy, they are probably caused by sympathetic nervous system stimulation; in later months, a cause could be increased thoracic pressure from the upward pressure of the diaphragm. Either way, unless the woman has a previous heart condition or if they are caused by supine hypotension syndrome (see the following), they are innocent sensations.

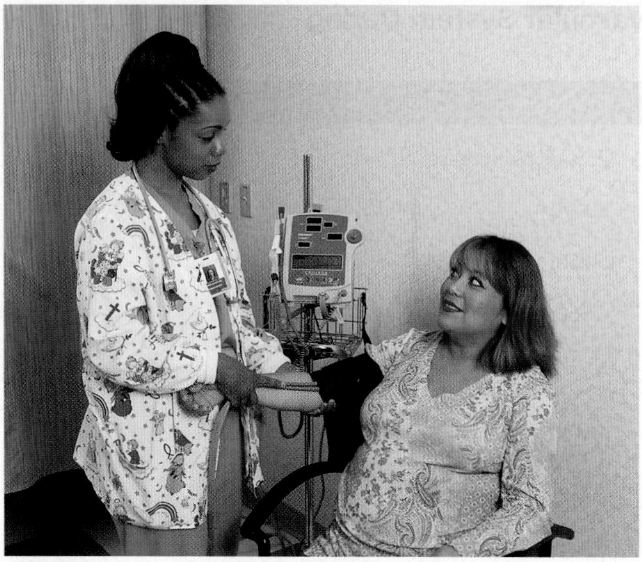

FIGURE 10.7 Blood pressure determination is an important assessment during pregnancy. Normally, this does not elevate during pregnancy.

Blood Pressure. Despite the hypervolemia of pregnancy, blood pressure in women normally does not rise because the increased heart action takes care of the greater amount of circulating blood. Average blood pressures for adult women are available at http://thePoint.lww.com/Pillitteri7e.

In some women, blood pressure actually decreases slightly during the second trimester because the expanding placenta causes peripheral resistance to circulation to lower. During the third trimester, the blood pressure rises again to first trimester levels (Fig. 10.7). A steadily increasing blood pressure is a danger sign that gestational hypertension may be developing.

Peripheral Blood Flow. During the third trimester of pregnancy, blood flow to the lower extremities is impaired by the pressure of the expanding uterus on veins and arteries. This resistance to blood flow in the venous system can lead to edema and varicosities of the vulva, rectum, and legs (Pipkin, 2012).

What if... 10.3 Lauren's husband is worried because his wife sometimes has heart palpitations and often seems short of breath. He tells you, "She eats almost nothing to stay 'model-slim.' Should she even have tried to have another child?" How would you answer him?

Supine Hypotension Syndrome. When a pregnant woman lies supine, the weight of the growing uterus presses the vena cava against the vertebrae, obstructing blood flow from the lower extremities. This causes a decrease in blood return to the heart and, consequently, decreased cardiac output and hypotension (Fig. 10.8). A woman experiences this hypotension as light-headedness, faintness, and palpitations. The condition is potentially dangerous because it can cause fetal hypoxia (Edwardson & Hueppchen, 2011).

To lessen the possibility that the syndrome will happen, women develop an increase in collateral blood circulation during pregnancy. The symptoms can be alleviated by having a woman turn onto her side (preferably the left side), so blood flow through the vena cava increases again. Teach women to always rest on the left side rather than their back, because even with additional collateral circulation, a supine position can lead to hypotension.

Blood Constitution. A variety of changes occur in the constitution of blood.

- The level of circulating fibrinogen, a constituent of the blood necessary for clotting, increases by as much as 50%, probably stimulated by the increased level of estrogen.
- Other clotting factors, such as factors VII, VIII, IX, and X, and the platelet count also increase as safeguards against major bleeding should the placenta be dislodged and the uterine arteries or veins open.
- The total white blood cell count rises significantly, both as a protective mechanism against infection and as a reflection of a woman's increased total blood volume (to about 20,000 cells/mm^3).
- The total protein level of blood decreases, perhaps indicating the amount of protein being used by the fetus.

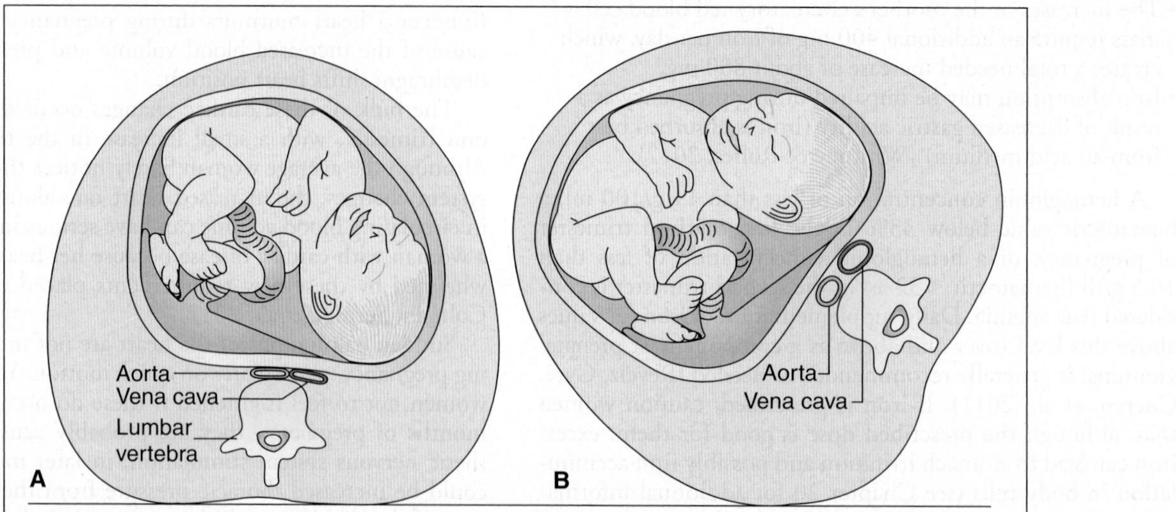

FIGURE 10.8 Supine hypotension can occur if a pregnant woman lies on her back. **(A)** The weight of the uterus compresses the vena cava, trapping blood in the lower extremities. **(B)** If a woman turns on her side, pressure is lifted off of the vena cava.

- Blood lipids increase by one third, and the cholesterol serum level increases by 90% to 100% to provide a ready supply of available energy for the fetus.

Because the circulating system has a lower total protein load, in combination with hypervolemia, fluid readily leaves the blood vessels for interstitial tissue to equalize osmotic and hydrostatic pressure. This leads to the common ankle and foot edema of pregnancy (not to be confused with nondependent or generalized edema, which is a symptom of hypertension of pregnancy (Attilakos & Overton, 2012).

Gastrointestinal System

At least 50% of women experience some nausea and vomiting early on in pregnancy. For many women, this is the first sensation a woman experiences with pregnancy (it can be noticed even before the first missed menstrual period). It is most apparent early in the morning, on rising, or if a woman becomes fatigued during the day.

Known as morning sickness, nausea and vomiting begins to be noticed at the same time levels of hCG and progesterone begin to rise so these may contribute to its cause. Another reason may be a systemic reaction to increased estrogen levels or decreased glucose levels, because glucose is being used in such great quantities by the growing fetus. Nausea usually subsides after the first 3 months, after which time a woman may have a voracious appetite (Naumann, Zelig, Napolitano, et al., 2012). Many alternate or complementary methods to help reduce nausea are available, such as acupuncture or wrist bands (discussed in Chapter 13). Box 10.8 is an interprofessional care map illustrating both nursing and team planning for a woman with nausea of pregnancy.

In addition to nausea, other gastrointestinal tract changes occur:

- Although the acidity of stomach secretions decreases during pregnancy, heartburn can readily result from reflux of stomach contents into the esophagus, caused by both the upward displacement of the stomach by the uterus, and a relaxed cardioesophageal sphincter, caused by the action of relaxin produced by the ovary. Interventions for heartburn are discussed in Chapter 13.
- As the uterus increases in size, it pushes the stomach and intestines toward the back and sides of the abdomen. At about the midpoint of pregnancy, this pressure may be sufficient to slow intestinal peristalsis and the emptying time of the stomach, leading to renewed heartburn, constipation, and flatulence.
- Pressure from the uterus on veins returning from the lower extremities can lead to hemorrhoids.
- The entire gastrointestinal tract may become less active from the combined actions of relaxin and progesterone. This natural slowing of the stomach and intestine can be helpful because the blood supply is reduced in the gastrointestinal tract as more blood is drawn to the uterus.
- Women with chronic gastric reflux usually find their condition either improved because the acidity of the stomach is decreased or worsened because of upward uterine pressure.
- Because of the gradual slowing of the gastrointestinal tract, decreased emptying of bile from the gallbladder may result. This can lead to reabsorption of bilirubin into the maternal bloodstream, giving rise to a symptom of generalized itching (subclinical jaundice). A woman who has had gallstones may have an increased tendency for stone formation during pregnancy as a result of the increased plasma cholesterol level and additional cholesterol incorporated in bile.
- Some pregnant women notice hypertrophy at their gum lines and bleeding of gingival tissue when they brush their teeth. There also may be increased saliva formation (hyperptyalism), probably as a local response to increased levels of estrogen. This is an annoying, but not a serious problem.
- A lower than normal pH of saliva may lead to increased tooth decay if tooth brushing is not done conscientiously. This can be a problem for homeless women or any women who do not have frequent access to a place to brush their teeth.

Urinary System

Like other systems, the urinary system undergoes specific physiologic changes during pregnancy, including alterations in fluid retention and renal, ureter, and bladder function. These changes, summarized in Table 10.6, result from:

- Effects of high estrogen and progesterone levels
- Compression of the bladder and ureters by the growing uterus
- Increased blood volume that increases kidney production of more urine
- Postural influences

Fluid Retention. To provide sufficient fluid volume for effective placental exchange, a woman's total body water almost doubles. Because nutrients can pass to the fetus only when dissolved in or carried by fluid, this ready fluid supply is a safeguard to ensure the fetus can be supplied with adequate nutrients. It also can provide excess fluid to replenish the mother's blood volume, should hemorrhage occur.

Under the influence of progesterone, an increased response of the angiotensin–renin system in the kidney occurs leading to an increase in aldosterone production and increased sodium reabsorption and regulation of serum osmolarity. Progesterone appears to be potassium sparing, so even with an increased urine output, potassium levels remain adequate.

Renal Function. During pregnancy, a woman's kidneys must excrete not only the waste products from her body but also those of the fetus. Also, her kidneys must be able to excrete additional fluid and manage the demands of an increased renal blood flow.

The glomerular filtration rate (GFR) and renal plasma flow both increase in pregnancy by 30% to 50% in order to meet the increased demands of the circulatory system volume. The elevation of the GFR leads to increased filtration of glucose into the renal tubules. Because reabsorption of glucose by the tubule cells occurs at a fixed rate, this causes some accidental spilling of glucose into the urine during pregnancy. Lactose, which is being produced by the mammary glands but which is not used during pregnancy, will also be spilled into the urine. Although minimal spilling of glucose into the urine normally occurs, the finding of more than a trace of glucose in a routine sample of urine from a pregnant woman is considered abnormal until proven otherwise, because this can be a sign of gestational diabetes (American Diabetes Association [ADA], 2012) (see Chapter 20).

Another tract change is that urinary output gradually increases by about 60% to 80%. In contrast, the specific gravity of urine, the blood urea nitrogen (BUN) and creatinine levels all lower.

A BUN of 15 mg/100 ml or higher, or a serum creatinine concentration greater than 1 mg/100 ml are considered abnormal values and reflect the kidneys' difficulty in handling

BOX 10.9 Nursing Care Planning to Empower a Family

Q. You notice Lauren Maxwell rubbing her back at a prenatal visit. She asks how she can keep her backache from becoming worse.

A. Backache is a common symptom of pregnancy because of the strain the extra uterine weight puts on lower vertebrae. Common measures to relieve backache in pregnancy include:

- Limit the use of high heels because they add to the natural lordosis of pregnancy.
- Try to rest daily with feet elevated.
- Walk with head high and pelvis straight.
- Pelvic rocking (see Chapter 14) at the end of the day may relieve pain for the night.

Backache should be reported if:

- It is experienced as waves of pain (i.e., could be preterm labor).
- There are accompanying urinary symptoms, such as frequency and pain on urination (i.e., could be a urinary tract infection).
- The back is tender at the point of backache (i.e., could be pyelonephritis or a kidney infection or a ruptured vertebrae).
- Rest doesn't relieve it (i.e., could be a muscle strain).

To change her center of gravity and make ambulation easier, a pregnant woman tends to stand straighter and taller than usual. This stance is sometimes referred to as the "pride of pregnancy." Standing this way, with the shoulders back and the abdomen forward, however, creates a lordosis (forward curve of the lumbar spine), which may lead to chronic backache, particularly in older women (Klemetti, Kurinczuk, & Redshaw, 2011) (Box 10.9).

WOMEN WITH UNIQUE CONCERNS IN PREGNANCY

Women with disabilities may have specific concerns about how to care for themselves during pregnancy and for their child when he or she is born, and so need a careful assessment as to their feelings about having a baby along with an assessment of special adjustments they may need to make during pregnancy (Mitra, Lu, & Diop, 2012). Assess if they are concerned their child may be born with their disability. Research or ask a knowledgeable team member to be certain your advice will be accurate before assuring women this is not apt to happen.

Two other concerns that arise more frequently in pregnant women than others are restless leg syndrome and carpal tunnel syndrome.

Carpal tunnel syndrome is named for the Greek word *karpos* meaning "wrist" and the narrow space where the median nerve passes between the bones of the wrist. Repetitive movements, such as typing or swinging a tennis racket, can irritate the nerve resulting in sensations of pain, tingling, and numbness. Probably because of the effect of the hormone relaxin secreted by the placenta, pregnant women seem to be more susceptible to this condition than others (LeBlanc & Cestia, 2011). Actions women can take to avoid the syndrome and usual therapy is discussed in Chapter 49.

Restless leg syndrome is the uncontrollable urge to move the legs, often accompanied by itching, tingling, or aching to such an extent a person has difficulty falling or staying asleep (Neau, Marion, Mathis, et al., 2010). It tends to occur more often in pregnant women and people with iron deficiency than others. Therapy for the condition is discussed in Chapter 51.

What if... 10.4 You are particularly interested in exploring one of the 2020 National Health Goals with regard to psychological or physiologic changes in pregnancy (see Box 10.1)? What would be a possible research topic to explore pertinent to this goal that would be applicable to Lauren or her family and that would also advance evidence-based practice?

KEY POINTS FOR REVIEW

- The ability of a woman to accept and enjoy a pregnancy depends on social, cultural, family, and individual influences.
- The psychological tasks of pregnancy are centered on ensuring safe passage for the fetus. They consist of, in the first trimester, accepting the pregnancy; in the second trimester, accepting the baby; and in the third trimester, preparing for parenthood.
- Common emotional responses that occur with pregnancy can include grief, narcissism, introversion or extroversion, stress, couvade syndrome, body image and boundary confusion, emotional lability, and changes in sexual desire.
- Physiologic changes that occur with pregnancy are both local, such as uterine, ovarian, and vaginal changes, as well as systemic changes such as those that occur in the endocrine, respiratory, cardiovascular, urinary, and immune systems.
- Women may have read about the expected psychological and physiologic changes of pregnancy, but once they are experiencing them may find them more intense than anticipated.
- The confirmation of pregnancy may be assisted by three levels of findings: presumptive (subjective), probable (objective), and positive (documented).
- The positive signs of pregnancy are demonstration of a fetal heartbeat separate from the mother's, fetal movement felt by an examiner, and visualization of a fetus by ultrasound.

- Although a woman may be in a prenatal health care setting for only an hour, if her pregnancy is confirmed at that visit, she invariably feels "more pregnant" when she leaves. Early diagnosis or confirmation is important so a woman can begin to change unhealthy habits or, if necessary, have adequate time to carry out a therapeutic termination of pregnancy.
- Teaching women common psychological and physiologic changes that occur with pregnancy helps to plan nursing care that not only meets QSEN competencies but also best meets a family's total needs.

Critical Thinking Care Study

Joella Sanchez is a 22-year-old woman who just realized she is pregnant. She is delighted with the news, so was surprised to hear her 4-year-old daughter, Michelle, scream that she didn't want a brother or sister. Joella and Michelle both live with Joella's mother in a two-bedroom house. Her mother's reaction to learning about the pregnancy was to ask, "How will I fit another crib in here?" Joella works nights as a nurse's assistant at a local nursing home. Her supervisor's reaction was to frown and say, "Don't ask me to change your work schedule because you're tired all the time."

1. Is Michelle's reaction to learning a new sibling is on the way unusual? What could Joella do to win her over about the new baby?
2. Both Joella's mother and her work supervisor don't sound happy about the new baby either. What could Joella do to win them over?
3. Joella is happy about her pregnancy but surrounded by a circle of negative reactions. Could this affect her acceptance of the pregnancy? Should she have expected these reactions might occur before getting pregnant?

Patient Scenario

The O'Leary Family

Read about the O'Leary family, a family with concerns about pregnancy, then answer the questions to further sharpen your skills and grow more familiar with NCLEX-type questions related to psychological and physiologic changes of pregnancy. Confirm your answers are correct by reading the rationales.

Visit http://thePoint.lww.com

Answers and Rationales

Looking for answers to the What If... and Critical Thinking Care Study questions?

Visit http://thePoint.lww.com

References

American Diabetes Association. (2012). Diagnosis and classification of diabetes mellitus. *Diabetes Care, 35*(Suppl. 1), S64–S71.

Aguirre, F., & Chou, B. (2011). Normal labor and delivery, operative delivery and malpresentations. In K. J. Hurt, M. W. Guile, J. L. Bienstock, et al. (Eds.), *The Johns Hopkins manual of gynecology and obstetrics* (4th ed., pp. 73–89). Philadelphia, PA: Lippincott Williams & Wilkins.

Attilakos, G., & Overton, T. G. (2012). Antenatal care. In D. K. Edmonds (Ed.), *Dewhurst's textbook of obstetrics & gynaecology* (6th ed., pp. 42–52). Oxford, UK: John Wiley & Son.

Baselice, J., & Lawson, S. (2011). Postpartum care & breast-feeding. In K. J. Hurt, M. W. Guile, J. L. Bienstock, et al. (Eds.), *The Johns Hopkins manual of gynecology and obstetrics* (4th ed., pp. 257–264). Philadelphia, PA: Lippincott Williams & Wilkins.

Behruzi, R., Hatem, M., Goulet, L., et al. (2011). The facilitating factors and barriers encountered in the adoption of a humanized birth care approach in a highly specialized university affiliated hospital. *BMC Women's Health, 11*(11), 53.

Bergink, V., Bouvy, P. F., Vervoort, J. S., et al. (2012). Prevention of postpartum psychosis and mania in women at high risk. *American Journal of Psychiatry, 169*(6), 609–615.

Bernstein, H. B., & VanBuren, G. (2013). Normal pregnancy. In A. H. DeCherney, L. Nathan, T. M. Goodwin, et al. (Eds.), *Current diagnosis and treatment: Obstetrics and gynecology* (11th ed., pp. 141–153). Columbus, OH: McGraw-Hill/Lange.

Bianchi, S. M. (2011). Changing families, changing workplaces. *Future Child, 21*(2), 15–36.

Bowen, A., Bowen, R., Butt, P., et al. (2012). Patterns of depression and treatment in pregnant and postpartum women. *Canadian Journal of Psychiatry, 57*(3), 161–167.

Brown, L. D., Feinberg, M. E., & Kan, M. L. (2012). Predicting engagement in a transition to parenthood program for couples. *Evaluation & Program Planning, 35*(1), 1–8.

Centers for Disease Control and Prevention. (2012). *Unintended pregnancy prevention.* Hyattsville, MD: Author.

Cheema, R., Bayoumi, M. Z., & Gudmundsson, S. (2011). Multivascular Doppler surveillance in high risk pregnancies. *Journal of Maternal–Fetal & Neonatal Medicine, 25*(7), 970–974.

Coad, J., & Dunstall, M. (2011). Sexual differentiation and behavior. In J. Coad & M. Dunstall (Eds.), *Anatomy & physiology for midwives* (pp. 99–114). London, England: Elsevier/Churchill Livingstone.

Coall, D. A., & Hertwig, R. (2010). Grandparental investment: Past, present, and future. *Behavioral & Brain Sciences, 33*(1), 1–19.

Cunningham, F., Leveno, J., Bloom, S., et al. (2010). Maternal physiology. In F. Cunningham, J. Leveno, S. Bloom, et al. (Eds.), *William's obstetrics* (23rd ed., pp. 107–135). New York, NY: McGraw-Hill.

Dennis, A. E., & Altaus, J. E. (2011). Preterm labor & premature rupture of membranes. In K. J. Hurt, M. W. Guile, J. L. Bienstock, et al. (Eds.), *The Johns Hopkins manual of gynecology and obstetrics* (4th ed., pp. 122–129). Philadelphia, PA: Lippincott Williams & Wilkins.

Doyle-Lucas, A. F., Akers, J. D., & Davy, B. M. (2010). Energetic efficiency, menstrual irregularity, and bone mineral density in elite professional female ballet dancers. *Journal of Dance Medicine & Science, 14*(4), 146–154.

Dunkel-Schetter, C., & Tanner, L. (2012). Anxiety, depression and stress in pregnancy: Implications for mothers, children, research, and practice. *Current Opinion in Psychiatry, 25*(2), 141–148.

Dunn, C., Hanieh, E., Roberts, R., et al. (2012). Mindful pregnancy and childbirth: Effects of a mindfulness-based intervention on women's psychological distress and well-being in the perinatal period. *Archives of Women's Mental Health, 15*(2), 139–143.

Edmonds, D. K. (2012). Puerperium and lactation. In D. K. Edmonds (Ed.), *Dewhurst's textbook of obstetrics & gynaecology* (6th ed., pp. 365–376). Oxford, UK: John Wiley & Son.

Edwardson, J., & Hueppchen, N. A. (2011). Surgical disease and trauma in pregnancy. In K. J. Hurt, M. W. Guile, J. L. Bienstock, et al. (Eds.), *The Johns Hopkins manual of gynecology and obstetrics* (4th ed., pp. 248–256). Philadelphia, PA: Lippincott Williams & Wilkins.

Engnes, K., Lidén, E., & Lundgren, I. (2012). Experiences of being exposed to intimate partner violence during pregnancy. *International Journal of Qualitative Studies on Health & Well-Being, 7.* Advance online publication. doi: 10.3402/qhw.v7i0.11199

Erikson, E. (1993). *Childhood and society* (3rd ed.). New York, NY: W. W. Norton.

Fenwick, J., Bayes, S., & Johansson, M. (2012). A qualitative investigation into the pregnancy experiences and childbirth expectations of Australian fathers-to-be. *Sexual & Reproductive Healthcare, 3*(1), 3–9.

Fortinash, K. M., & Holoday Worret, P. A. (2012).Therapeutic communication: Interviews and interventions. In K. M. Fortinash & P. A. Holoday Worret (Eds.), *Psychiatric mental health nursing* (5th ed., pp. 59–86). St. Louis, MO: Elsevier/Mosby.

Goecke, T. W., Voigt, F., Faschingbauer, F., et al. (2012). The association of prenatal attachment and perinatal factors with pre- and postpartum depression in first-time mothers. *Archives of Gynecology & Obstetrics, 286*(2), 309–316.

Hatton, R., Colman, J. M., Sermer, M., et al. (2012). Cardiac risks and management of complications in pregnant women with congenital heart disease. *Future Cardiology, 8*(2), 315–327.

Hayatbakhsh, M. R., Flenady, V. J., Gibbons, K. S., et al. (2012). Birth outcomes associated with cannabis use before and during pregnancy. *Pediatric Research, 71*(2), 215–219.

Hegewald, M. J., & Crapo, R. O. (2011). Respiratory physiology in pregnancy. *Clinics in Chest Medicine, 32*(1), 1–13.

Ibanez, G., Charles, M. A., Forhan, A., et al.(2012). Depression and anxiety in women during pregnancy and neonatal outcome. *Early Human Development, 88*(8), 643–649.

Klemetti, R., Kurinczuk, J. J., & Redshaw, M. (2011). Older women's pregnancy related symptoms, health and use of antenatal services. *European Journal of Obstetric & Gynecologic Reproductive Biology, 154*(2), 157–162.

Krans, E. E., & Chang, J. C. (2011). Low-income African American women's beliefs regarding exercise during pregnancy. *Maternal Child Health Journal, 16*(6), 1180–1187.

Kulier, R., Kapp, N, Gülmezoglu, A. M., et al. (2011). Medical methods for first trimester abortion. *Cochrane Database of Systematic Reviews,* (11), CD002855.

Lauderdale, J. (2011). Transcultural perspectives in childbearing. In M. M. Andrews & J. S. Boyle (Eds.), *Transcultural concepts in nursing care* (pp. 85–115). Philadelphia, PA: Lippincott Williams & Wilkins.

LeBlanc, K. E., & Cestia, W. (2011). Carpal tunnel syndrome. *American Family Physician, 83*(8), 952–958.

Lumley, J., Watson, L., Watson, M., et al. (2011). Periconceptional supplementation with folate and/or multivitamins for preventing neural tube defects. *Cochrane Database of Systematic Reviews,* (2), CD001056.

Marc, I., Toureche, N., Ernst, E., et al. (2011). Mind-body interventions during pregnancy for preventing or treating women's anxiety. *Cochrane Database of Systematic Reviews, 2011* (11), CD007559.

Mitra, M., Lu, E., & Diop, H. (2012). Smoking among pregnant women with disabilities. *Women's Health Issues, 22*(2), e233–e239.

Naumann, C. R., Zelig, C., Napolitano, P. G., et al. (2012). Nausea, vomiting, and heartburn in pregnancy: A prospective look at risk, treatment, and outcome. *Journal of Maternal–Fetal & Neonatal Medicine, 25*(8), 1488–1493.

Neau, J. P., Marion, P., Mathis, S., et al. (2010). Restless legs syndrome and pregnancy: Follow-up of pregnant women before and after delivery. *European Neurology, 64*(6), 361–366.

Ossa, X., Bustos, L., & Fernandez, L. (2011).Prenatal attachment and associated factors during the third trimester of pregnancy in Temuco, Chile. *Midwifery, 28*(5), e689–696.

Palmsten, K., Setoguchi, S., Margulis, A. V., et al. (2012). Elevated risk of preeclampsia in pregnant women with depression: Depression or antidepressants? *American Journal of Epidemiology, 175*(10), 988–997.

Pipkin, F. B. (2012). Maternal physiology. In D. K. Edmonds (Ed.), *Dewhurst's textbook of obstetrics & gynaecology* (6th ed., pp. 5–15). Oxford, UK: John Wiley & Son.

Reveiz, L., Gyte, G. M., Cuervo, L. G., et al. (2011). Treatments for iron-deficiency anaemia in pregnancy. *Cochrane Database of Systematic Reviews,* (10), CD003094.

Rilby, L., Jansson, S., Lindblom, B., et al. (2012). A qualitative study of women's feelings about future childbirth: Dread and delight. *Journal of Midwifery & Women's Health, 57*(2), 120–125.

Rogers, V. L., & Worley, K. C. (2012). Obstetrics and obstetric disorders. In S. McPhee, M. Papadakis, & M. W. Rabow (Eds.), *Current medical diagnosis & treatment* (51st ed., pp. 760–786). New York, NY: McGraw-Hill/Lange.

Russell, J. B., Denne, E. W., & Schwartz, D. (2011). Preconception counseling and prenatal care. In K. J. Hurt, M. W. Guile, J. L. Bienstock, et al. (Eds.), *The Johns Hopkins manual of gynecology and obstetrics* (4th ed., pp. 56–72). Philadelphia, PA: Lippincott Williams & Wilkins.

Sagiv-Reiss, D. M., Birnbaum, G. E., & Safir, M. P. (2011). Changes in sexual experiences and relationship quality during pregnancy. *Archives of Sexual Behavior, 41*(5), 1241–1251.

Schaffer, M. A., Goodhue, A., Stennes, K., et al. (2012). Evaluation of a public health nurse visiting program for pregnant and parenting teens. *Public Health Nursing, 29*(3), 218–231.

Smith, M. L., & Schust, D. J. (2011). Endocrinology and recurrent early pregnancy loss. *Seminars in Reproductive Medicine, 29*(6), 482–490.

Talaulikar, V. S., & Arulkumaran, S. (2011). Folic acid in obstetric practice: A review. *Obstetrical & Gynecological Survey, 66*(4), 240–247.

Urgesi, C., Romanò, M., Fornasari, L., et al. (2012). Investigating the development of temperament and character in school-aged children using a self-report measure. *Comprehensive Psychiatry, 53*(6), 875–883.

U.S. Department of Health and Human Services. (2010). *Healthy people 2020.* Washington, DC: Author.

Whitney, E. N., & Rolfes, S. R. (2012). Life cycle nutrition: Pregnancy & lactation. In E. N. Whitney & S. R. Rolfes (Eds.), *Understanding nutrition* (pp. 492–527). Belmont, CA: Wadsworth Publishing.

Yazbeck, C. F., & Sullivan, S. D. (2012). Thyroid disorders during pregnancy. *Medical Clinics of North America, 96*(2), 235–256.

Yu, C. Y., Hung, C. H., Chan, T. F., et al. (2012). Prenatal predictors for father-infant attachment after childbirth. *Journal of Clinical Nursing, 21*(11–12), 1577–1583.

Zheng, T. (2012a). Prenatal diagnosis. In T. Zheng (Ed.), *Comprehensive handbook of obstetrics & gynecology* (pp. 80–81). Paradise Valley, AZ: Phoenix Medical Press.

Zheng, T. (2012b). Ultrasound in pregnancy. In T. Zheng (Ed.), *Comprehensive handbook of obstetrics & gynecology* (pp. 85–91). Paradise Valley, AZ: Phoenix Medical Press.

Chapter 11

Nursing Care Related to Assessment of a Pregnant Family

KEY TERMS

- chloasma
- diagonal conjugate
- erosion
- gravida
- ischial tuberosity
- lithotomy position
- multigravida
- multipara
- nulligravida
- para
- primigravida
- primipara
- speculum

OBJECTIVES

After mastering the contents of this chapter, you should be able to:

1. Describe the areas of health assessment commonly included in prenatal visits.
2. Identify 2020 National Health Goals related to prenatal care that nurses can help the nation achieve.
3. Assess the readiness for parenthood and the health status of a pregnant woman and her family.
4. Formulate nursing diagnoses related to a woman's health status during pregnancy.
5. Identify expected outcomes to help ensure a safe pregnancy as well as manage seamless transitions across health care settings.
6. Using the nursing process, plan nursing care that includes the six competencies of Quality & Safety Education for Nurses (QSEN): Patient-Centered Care, Teamwork & Collaboration, Evidence-Based Practice (EBP), Quality Improvement (QI), Safety, and Informatics.
7. Implement nursing care such as establishing a risk score for a client during pregnancy.
8. Evaluate expected outcomes for the childbearing family to establish achievement and effectiveness of goals.
9. Integrate knowledge of pregnancy health assessment with the interplay of nursing process, the six competencies of QSEN, and Family Nursing to promote quality maternal and child health nursing care.

Sandra Czerinski is a 29-year-old woman, 12 weeks pregnant, who comes for a first prenatal visit. She is concerned because she did not realize she was pregnant until a week ago. As a result, she has been actively dieting (two diet drinks plus one meal of mainly vegetables daily) plus lifting weights at a health club. She has not had a pelvic examination since she was in high school, when she had a vaginal infection. She remembers that examination as being very painful. She is worried she has a urinary tract infection now because she has to "go all the time." She does not want any blood work done because she does not have health insurance.

Previous chapters described normal anatomy and physiology of the reproductive tract and the psychological and physiologic changes that occur during pregnancy. This chapter adds information about care needed during pregnancy to help ensure a healthy outcome for both the woman and her child.

What type of health teaching does Sandra need? Is Sandra a high-risk or a low-risk patient?

Prenatal care, essential for ensuring the overall health of newborns and their mothers, is a major strategy for helping to reduce complications of pregnancy such as the number of preterm or low–birth-weight babies born each year (Mehta & Sokol, 2013). Prenatal care is so important that several 2020 National Health Goals directly address it (Box 11.1).

Ideally, preparation for a healthy pregnancy begins during a woman's childhood as good preparation includes a lifetime of an adequate intake of calcium and vitamin D to prevent rickets (which can distort pelvic size), adequate immunizations against contagious diseases so a woman has protection against viral diseases such as rubella during pregnancy, and maintenance of an overall healthy lifestyle to ensure the best state of health possible for a woman and her partner when entering pregnancy. Preconceptual care and risk assessment should be provided at every health care visit throughout the childbearing years for both men and women.

Other phases of an overall healthy lifestyle are a positive attitude about sexuality, womanhood, and childbearing. Once a woman becomes sexually active, preparation for a successful pregnancy includes practicing safer sex, regular pelvic examinations, and prompt treatment of any sexually transmitted infection to prevent complications that could lead to subfertility (Ray, Shah, Gudi, et al., 2012). It also includes not smoking or using recreational drugs. Acquisition and use of reproductive life planning information can help ensure each pregnancy is intended and wanted.

BOX 11.1 Nursing Care Planning Based on 2020 National Health Goals

A number of 2020 National Health Goals speak directly to the importance of prenatal care:

- Increase the proportion of pregnant women who receive early and adequate prenatal care from a baseline of 70.5% to a target of 77.6%.
- Increase the proportion of pregnant women who attend a series of prepared childbirth classes (developmental).
- Increase the proportion of women delivering a live birth who received preconception care services and practiced key recommended preconception health behaviors (developmental).
- Increase the proportion of women of childbearing potential who have an intake of at least 400 μg of folic acid from fortified foods or dietary supplements before pregnancy from a baseline of 23.8% to a target level of 26.2%.
- Increase the proportion of mothers who achieve a recommended weight gain during their pregnancies (developmental) (U.S. Department of Health and Human Services [DHHS], 2010; see www.healthypeople.gov).

Nurses can help the nation achieve these goals by educating women and their families about the importance of both preconceptual and prenatal care as well as making sites for prenatal care "family friendly" or maximally receptive to women and families.

The initial prenatal visit is the first time many women have been to a health care facility since their routine health maintenance visits of childhood and adolescence. It also may be the first time they have had an appointment that focuses more on health promotion than on the diagnosis of disease. A woman usually comes with a specific goal in mind for the visit, such as confirming her pregnancy. However, a prenatal visit is much more than this; it is also a time for health promotion, pregnancy education, and encouraging a pattern of healthy behaviors for the family to use in the future. Individualized teaching varies depending on the lifestyle, age, and parity of a woman and her degree of family support (Kingston, Heaman, Fell, et al., 2012). Urging her to continue prenatal care is important because lack of prenatal care is associated with pregnancy complications such as preterm birth (Attilakos & Overton, 2012).

Nursing Process Overview

For Prenatal Care

Assessment

The first prenatal visit is a time to establish baseline data relevant to a woman's health and identify health-promotion strategies that will be important at every prenatal visit. This begins by obtaining a detailed health and sexual history including screening for the risk of teratogen (any factor that may adversely affect the fetus) exposure as well as any concerns a woman has about her pregnancy. Explaining why specific assessment data are important has the potential to lead to health teaching. For instance, while you are weighing a woman, discuss the importance of a healthy body mass index (BMI) and how her expected weight gain over the coming months will be calculated based on her prepregnancy value. Relating assessment information and health-promotion activities this way helps keep a woman and her family both well informed and eager to comply with further health care recommendations.

Nursing Diagnosis

Although most women probably have used a home pregnancy kit to find out if they are pregnant, the first prenatal visit officially confirms this, so nursing diagnoses usually focus on the response of a woman and her family to that information. Examples include:

- Decisional conflict related to desire to be pregnant
- Risk for ineffective coping related to confirmation of unintended pregnancy

Nursing diagnoses appropriate to prenatal care include:

- Health-seeking behaviors related to guidelines for nutrition and activity during pregnancy
- Deficient knowledge regarding exposure to teratogens during pregnancy
- Health-seeking behaviors related to strong cultural desire to have a healthy child
- Risk for injury to fetus related to lifestyle choices

Outcome Identification and Planning

Be certain to reserve sufficient time at prenatal visits so care can be thorough and there is enough time to set realistic goals and expected outcomes with both a woman and her partner, if needed. Establishing a pattern of regular appointments is crucial to the provision of effective, individualized prenatal care, so be certain a woman schedules an appointment for a following visit. Ask if she has transportation to the health care facility because lack of transportation can be a major reason women don't consistently attend prenatal care. Representative Internet sites that are helpful to refer women to for questions about preconceptual or prenatal care are the National Institute of Child Health and Human Development (www.nichd.nih.gov) and the March of Dimes (www.marchofdimes.com).

Implementation

An important nursing intervention at prenatal visits is teaching women and their families about a safe pregnancy lifestyle. Women often discount prepared lists, believing their pregnancy is too personal to be a condition for which there are routine lists of advice. Advice, therefore, needs to be individualized for each woman. For visual learners, it can be helpful to offer a woman and her partner pamphlets that cover the same topics discussed verbally. Be certain all printed materials you give to families are consistent with what you say and with the views of the woman's primary health care provider. In addition, reinforce to the woman that she should feel free to call or e-mail the health care setting between visits with any problems or questions. Some women may feel reluctant to "bother" a health care provider outside of scheduled visits unless you give them this permission.

Outcome Evaluation

Evaluation during prenatal visits should concentrate on a woman's initial understanding of the goals for care during pregnancy and assessing outcomes established for specific concerns. Examples of expected outcomes include:

- Couple states they have reached a mutual decision to both stop smoking.
- Client states she feels well informed about the common body changes of pregnancy and actions to take to relieve any discomfort these cause.
- Client lists ways to avoid exposure to teratogens at her work site during pregnancy.

HEALTH PROMOTION BEFORE AND DURING PREGNANCY

The overall purposes of prenatal care are to:

- Establish a baseline of present health
- Determine the gestational age of the fetus
- Monitor fetal development and maternal well-being
- Identify women at risk for complications
- Minimize the risk of possible complications by anticipating and preventing problems before they occur
- Provide education about pregnancy, lactation, and newborn care

The Preconceptual Visit

Preconceptual care is best if it is not provided at a single visit but included at every health care visit for all women of childbearing age. Before planning a pregnancy, a woman should schedule a specific appointment with her primary care provider to obtain accurate reproductive life planning information, receive reassurance about fertility (based on a thorough health history and physical examination), and identify any problems that may need correction to help ensure fertility (Dhanjal, 2012). At this visit, her hemoglobin level and blood type (including Rh factor) may be determined and a Papanicolaou (Pap) smear taken (a vaginal and cervical swab obtained to rule out cervical cancer) (ACOG, 2010). If a vaginal infection such as chlamydia is found to be present, this can be treated to help ensure fertility. Yeast infections do not tend to interfere with fertility, although, if present, they should be treated as well. Be certain to counsel women on the importance of a diet with adequate protein, folic acid, iron, and vitamins. A prenatal vitamin may be prescribed to ensure folic acid intake will be adequate for pregnancy. Stress the importance of early prenatal care for when pregnancy occurs. If vaccinations are not current, women can be immunized against human papillomavirus (HPV), and influenza at a preconception visit (Rogers & Worley, 2012).

Choosing a Health Care Provider for Pregnancy and Childbirth

Once a woman becomes pregnant, her next step is to choose a primary health care provider to care for her throughout the pregnancy and birth. Nurses contribute to the success of prenatal care through individualized assessment, counseling, and educating. Many clinics and group practices provide an initial educational seminar for women in the early stages of their pregnancy, often led by a nurse or nurse practitioner. Some practices form cohorts of women to meet monthly (cluster prenatal care) and discuss their concerns to be certain they will have support from others during pregnancy (Rotundo, 2012; Ruiz-Mirazo, Lopez-Yarto, & McDonald, 2012). Box 11.2 summarizes ways prenatal care can be individualized so all women feel comfortable in prenatal settings and return for continuing care.

QSEN Checkpoint Question 11.1

Evidence-Based Practice

One of the first things a woman who suspects she is pregnant must do is choose a primary health care provider to guide her through her pregnancy. Many women ask, "What type of care provider should I choose?"

To investigate whether pregnancy care and outcomes differed when women chose a nurse-midwife rather than a physician as their primary care provider, researchers interviewed a sample of 6,421 Canadian women, all 15 years of age or older, all who had given birth to a singleton baby, and all who were living with their infant. Results of the study showed women whose primary prenatal care provider was a nurse-midwife were more likely to be satisfied with their maternity experience and information provided on pregnancy and birth topics. They were prescribed fewer ultrasounds and were more likely to attend prenatal classes. They were almost half as likely to have labor induced and 7.33 times more likely to experience a medication-free birth. Postpartally, they were more likely to initiate and maintain breastfeeding at 3 and 6 months (O'Brien, Chalmers, Fell, et al., 2011).

Based on the previous study, if Sandra asks you if she should choose a nurse-midwife as her primary care provider, what would your best answer be?

a. "Of course. Nurses are always more 'patient friendly' than physicians."
b. "Who you choose is such a personal choice; I shouldn't give you any advice."
c. "Nurse-midwives tend to use less medication with birth. Is that important to you?"
d. "Nurse-midwives don't talk to women as much as doctors. Would you like that?"

Look in Appendix A for the best answer and rationale.

BOX 11.2 Suggestions to Individualize Prenatal Care

- Schedule appointments for women within 1 week after they first call the health care setting so they see the health care site as one interested in meeting their particular needs.
- Try to schedule further appointments at times convenient for a woman and her support person and with the same primary care provider to encourage a long-term relationship.
- Ask whether there are outside pressures, such as having to report for work or older children coming home from school, that make a certain time of day for appointments best.
- Try to schedule appointments so there won't be a long wait time because late in pregnancy, a woman may feel uncomfortable sitting for a long stretch of time. Almost every woman is too busy to spend unnecessary time waiting at health care facilities.
- Make waiting time at the site educational by providing materials such as pamphlets or videos on pregnancy in the waiting room.
- Provide privacy for assessments such as blood pressure and weight.
- Be certain that pregnant women meet health care providers while fully clothed and upright, not naked and in a lithotomy position on an examining table.
- Encourage women to feel responsible for their health record. If a woman's first language is not English, contact an interpreter if necessary to be certain she understands prenatal instructions and will feel free to ask questions.
- Educate pregnant women about care options and encourage them to participate in making decisions about their care.
- Encourage family members and friends to accompany a woman for prenatal care. Allow them to enter the examination room and participate in all aspects of care to the extent they and the woman desire.
- Be certain women have a specific person's name and that person's phone number or e-mail contact in case they have any pregnancy-related questions before their next visit.

HEALTH ASSESSMENT DURING THE FIRST PRENATAL VISIT

Women should schedule a first prenatal visit as soon as they suspect they are pregnant. Although evidence-based practice is investigating whether the number of prenatal visits traditionally scheduled is still needed during a usual pregnancy, after the first prenatal visit, return appointments are usually scheduled every 4 weeks through the 28th week of pregnancy, every 2 weeks through the 36th week, and then every week until birth. Women categorized as high risk are followed more closely.

An important focus of all prenatal visits, in addition to education about pregnancy and helping a woman achieve a healthy pregnancy lifestyle, is to assure women that their pregnancy is progressing well (Van Dijk, Anderko, & Stetzer, 2011). Another important action is to screen for danger signs that might reveal a complication is beginning. The major causes of serious illness or death during pregnancy for women today are ectopic pregnancy, hypertension, hemorrhage, embolism, infection, morbid obesity, and anesthesia-related complications such as intrapartum cardiac arrest (Centers for Disease Control and Prevention [CDC], 2012c).

Screening at a first prenatal visit to detect subtle signs of any of these conditions includes an extensive health history, a complete physical examination (including a pelvic examination), and obtaining blood and urine specimens for laboratory analysis. In addition, manual pelvic measurements to determine pelvic adequacy can be taken at this visit or they can be delayed until midpregnancy. Ultrasonography has decreased the need to manually measure pelvic diameters for this purpose.

QSEN Checkpoint Question 11.2

Patient-Centered Care

Sandra Czerinski feels healthy, so she asks you why she needs to bother coming for prenatal care. What benefit should you cite when responding to Sandra's statement?

a. Discovering any allergies can reduce the risk of preterm labor.
b. It allows for the collection of accurate epidemiologic and demographic data.
c. It provides time for education about pregnancy and birth.
d. It provides important time to interact with a prenatal group.

Look in Appendix A for the best answer and rationale.

The Initial Interview

Because obtaining an initial health history can be time consuming, a woman may be asked to complete some necessary forms before arrival. Appropriate interviewing techniques, however, are important to obtain a thorough and meaningful health history and the rapport established by face-to-face interviewing with health care personnel may be as much a reason a woman returns for follow-up care as her desire to be assured her pregnancy is progressing normally (Box 11.3). Some women are extremely frightened at the thought of birth and thus need education and assurance about this as well (Hildingsson, Nilsson, Karlström, et al., 2011).

BOX 11.3 Nursing Care Planning Based on Effective Communication

Sandra has come to her obstetrician's office for a first prenatal visit.

Less Effective Communication

Nurse: The first thing I'd like you to do is describe what a typical day is like for you.
Ms. Czerinski: I don't have typical ones. Or very interesting ones.
Nurse: What about yesterday? Could you describe that for me?
Ms. Czerinski: Up at 7:00, at work by 9:00. A friend picked me up after work and we celebrated his birthday. Back home and in bed by 10:00. That's it.
Nurse: You're right. It doesn't sound too interesting. Let's talk about your family medical history instead.

More Effective Communication

Nurse: The first thing I'd like you to do is describe what a typical day is like for you.
Ms. Czerinski: I don't have typical ones. Or very interesting ones.
Nurse: What about yesterday? Could you describe that to me?
Ms. Czerinski: Up at 7:00, at work by 9:00. A friend picked me up after work and we celebrated his birthday. Back home and in bed by 10:00. That's it.
Nurse: What did you have for breakfast?
Ms. Czerinski: Nothing. I was far too rushed to eat.
Nurse: Dinner?
Ms. Czerinski: We went to a bar. Cheese blintzes, I think. And beer. A lot of beer.

Most people are not aware how much information can be revealed by a day history, so they give only a scant description of their day. Asking additional questions to make them elaborate on various parts often reveals poor nutrition, poor exercise, or risky pregnancy patterns such as alcohol intake.

Remember that pregnancy symptoms are subtle, so a woman may not regard certain information as important, causing her to provide vague answers instead of specific information in these areas. She may be unaware, for example, that she is the only person who knows the answer to a question such as "How do you feel about being pregnant?" or "Have you been taking anything for your nausea in the morning?" For best success, remember the following:

- Interviewing is best accomplished in a private, quiet setting. Pregnancy is too private an affair to be discussed in a crowded hallway or a full waiting room.
- Caution a woman that a first visit may be lengthy because of all the things that need to be accomplished. This prevents a woman from trying to fit the visit in between other errands or from having to terminate the interview because of another appointment.
- Be certain to ask how a woman wants you to address her (e.g., using Mrs. or Miss, or by her first name). Make certain she also knows your name and understands your role. If she views you as someone only gathering preliminary data, she may be willing to discuss superficial facts (name, address, phone number, and the like) but will resist discussing more intimate things (her feelings toward this pregnancy, the difficulty she has reworking old fears, or how scared she is about birth).

Components of the Health History

An initial interview includes both present and past history. General principles of interviewing are discussed in Chapter 34. Included in Table 11.1 is a review of elements pertinent to a pregnancy history.

Demographic Data

Demographic data usually obtained include name, age (additional testing such as genetic screening may be necessary if she is over age 35 years), address, telephone number, e-mail address, religion, ethnicity, type and place of employment, and health insurance information.

Chief Concern

The chief concern is the reason the woman has come to the health care setting—in this instance, the fact that she is or thinks she is pregnant.

- Document the date of her last menstrual period, whether it was normal for her and whether she has used a home test pregnancy kit.
- Elicit information about the usual signs that occur with early pregnancy, such as nausea, vomiting, breast changes, or fatigue.
- Ask if she is feeling any discomfort with her pregnancy, such as constipation, backache, or frequent urination.
- Ask also about any danger signs of pregnancy, such as bleeding, abdominal pain, continuous headache, visual disturbances, or swelling of the hands and face.
- Document whether the pregnancy was intended. If you feel uncomfortable asking about this directly, use a statement such as, "All pregnancies are a bit of a surprise. Is that how it was with this one?" Another way to word such a question might be, "Some couples plan on having children right away; some plan on waiting. How was it with you?" If a woman says the pregnancy was not intended, explore with her if she has reached a decision about whether to continue with the pregnancy. A question such as, "Some women

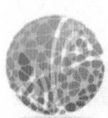

TABLE 11.1 Typical Assessments for a First Pregnancy Visit

Health History	
Demographic data	Name, address, age, ethnicity, telephone number, health insurance
Chief concern (her reason for coming for prenatal care)	Was this pregnancy intended? When was the woman's last normal menstrual period (LNMP)? Any exposure to infectious diseases or ingestion of drugs other than those prescribed since a woman thinks she has been pregnant?
Family and social profile	What is the woman's family composition? Does the woman have a support person? What is her occupation? Source of income? Level of exercise? Hobbies? Recreational drug use? Living conditions? Nutrition? Sleep pattern? Tobacco and alcohol use?
Past medical history	Any past history of abdominal surgery, kidney disease, heart disease, hypertension, sexually transmitted infections, diabetes, or allergies? What immunizations has she had?
Gynecologic history	When was menarche? What is length of menstrual cycle? Duration of menstrual flow?
Obstetric history	Any previous pregnancies? When? Type and outcome of birth? Any history of previous miscarriages or therapeutic abortions?
Review of systems	Brief review of all body systems
Physical Examination	
Baseline data	Height, weight, prepregnancy body mass index, vital signs, fundal height measurement (after 12 weeks), fetal heart sounds
System assessment	Full physical examination to confirm general health
Pelvic examination	General assessment; Pap smear and human papillomavirus (HPV) culture; additional cultures for chlamydia, gonorrhea, and group B *Streptococcus*; pelvic measurements may be taken
Laboratory Assessment	
Blood	Complete blood count, serologic test for syphilis, blood type and Rh, maternal α-fetoprotein (MAFP), pregnancy-associated plasma protein A (PAPP-A), antibody titer against Rh, hepatitis B and possibly C, rubella, and possibly varicella and HIV
Urinalysis	Clean catch for glucose, protein, and culture
Tuberculosis	Purified protein derivative (PPD; Mantoux) test or serum test
Ultrasound	To date pregnancy or confirm fetal health (if date of last menstrual period is unknown)

change their mind about wanting a baby once they realize they are pregnant; some don't. How has it been for you?" is an effective way to obtain this type of information because it indicates that either answer is possible and acceptable. You just want her to tell you which is happening.

Family Profile

Obtaining information about the woman's family structure and function early in an interview helps you get to know her, identify her important support persons, shape the nature and kind of questions you want to ask, and evaluate the possible impact of the woman's culture on care. It also lays a foundation for health teaching. Areas important to ask about include:

- Marital status and support people available and if a partner will be accompanying her for visits. As a rule, both married and unmarried women want you to know their married status because they want to alert you if they do not have a firm support person available. Box 11.4 offers suggestions to help make a partner feel like an important part of prenatal visits.
- Educational level of her and her partner (helps you estimate the level of teaching you will need to plan).
- If she works outside the home, exactly what her job consists of; for example, does it involve heavy lifting, long hours of standing in one position, or handling a toxic substance (all actions that may need to be modified during pregnancy)?
- Size and structure of the apartment or house. You'll need this information so you can talk with her in the coming months about space for a baby. If she is restricted from climbing stairs more than once or twice a day during the last part of pregnancy or after birth, knowing whether essential rooms are located on the ground floor is helpful.
- Lifestyle. Are finances a problem? Does the woman take usual safety precautions such as use of a seatbelt when in her car? Does she smoke, drink alcohol, or use recreational

BOX 11.4 Nursing Care Planning Based on Family Teaching

Q. Sandra asks you, "What can I do to make sure my boyfriend feels involved with my prenatal care?"

A. Have you tried these ideas?

- Ask for appointments to be scheduled at a time that is convenient for both of you.
- A prenatal visit can be lengthy. Be certain your partner reserves enough time so the visit doesn't become more of an inconvenience than an enjoyable event.
- Ask your partner to accompany you into the examining room at visits so you both can share your pregnancy progress or decisions.
- Be certain your partner listens to the fetal heart at visits as soon as it can be heard.
- If a sonogram is scheduled, ask your partner to view it with you (it's an exciting moment for both of you to see your fetus moving).

drugs? Does she have smoke and carbon monoxide monitors in her home?

- Document whether a woman has recently experienced any lifestyle changes such as a change in status from independence to dependence, a chronic illness, the death or loss of a significant person, a geographic move, financial hardship, or lack of support people. These are all examples of stressful situations that could hinder a woman's ability to accept her pregnancy and child.

History of Past Illnesses

Questions about a woman's past medical history are important because a past condition can become active during or immediately following pregnancy. Representative diseases that pose potential difficulty during pregnancy include kidney disease, heart disease (coarctation of the aorta and heart valve problems cause concern most often), hypertension, sexually transmitted infections (including hepatitis B and C, herpes, and HIV), diabetes, thyroid disease, recurrent seizures, gallbladder disease, urinary tract infections, varicosities, phenylketonuria, tuberculosis, and asthma.

It is also important to ask whether a woman had childhood diseases such as chickenpox (varicella), mumps (epidemic parotitis), measles (rubeola), German measles (rubella), and poliomyelitis or if she has had immunizations against these illnesses. Confirm whether a woman has had an HPV vaccine; many women are not yet aware that the vaccine has the potential not only to prevent HPV infections but also to prevent cervical cancer. It is now routinely prescribed for both male and female adolescents (CDC, 2012b).

From the information obtained about common infectious diseases and immunizations, you can estimate the degree of antibody protection a woman has against these diseases if she is exposed to them during her pregnancy. Pregnant women appear to develop more complications from influenza (the flu), for example, than others, so a woman who will be pregnant during the flu season (October through May) should receive an influenza vaccine (Fortner, Kuller, Rhee, et al., 2012). She can also be immunized against poliomyelitis by the Salk (killed virus) vaccine. She cannot be immunized with the oral Sabin poliomyelitis vaccine or with the vaccine against measles, mumps, or rubella because the vaccines for these contain live viruses that could be harmful to the fetus if the virus crossed the placenta (White, Boldt, Holditch, et al., 2012). Because many women don't know if they have ever had rubella, almost all women have blood drawn for an antibody titer against rubella at a first prenatal visit. After birth, a woman who shows a high titer could then be immunized against the disease to provide fetal protection for a following pregnancy.

Be certain to ask also about any allergies, including any drug sensitivities. Although it is controversial, encouraging women with allergies of any magnitude to breastfeed rather than bottle feed may help avoid allergy-related diseases such as atopic dermatitis in their infants (Kramer, 2011).

Any past surgical procedures are also important to document because adhesions resulting from past abdominal surgery such as a ruptured appendix could interfere with uterine growth.

History of Family Illnesses

Identifying any illnesses that occur frequently in a woman's relatives can help identify potential problems a woman or her infant could experience during pregnancy or after birth. Ask specifically about cardiovascular and renal disease, cognitive impairment, blood disorders, and any known genetically inherited diseases or congenital anomalies.

Day History/Social Profile

Information about a woman's current nutrition, elimination, sleep, recreation, and interpersonal interactions can be elicited best by asking a woman to describe what her typical day is like. If any of this information is not reported spontaneously as she describes her day, ask for additional details.

Nutrition. Information about what and how much a woman eats is important, particularly in light of the number of young adults with eating disorders (Stiles-Shields, Hoste, Doyle, et al., 2012). Asking for a "24-hour recall" is a helpful way to obtain accurate nutrition information because, by doing this, a woman is more apt to tell you what she actually ate, not what she should have eaten. In addition, questions such as, "Do you ever vomit excess food you've eaten after meals?" and "Are you happy with your weight?" help identify a woman who has anorexia nervosa or binge eating (see Chapter 54). "Are you on a diet now?" helps to identify women who are dieting (which is not advised during pregnancy to be certain a fetus receives adequate nutrients for growth).

Women need to take a prenatal vitamin that contains folic acid (600 μg/day) all during pregnancy. Although the vitamin is found in vegetable and fruit sources, women are unable to eat enough of these natural sources to achieve an adequate amount of folic acid for pregnancy. Prenatal vitamins also supply higher amounts of iron (30 mg on average).

Exercise. Daily exercise is healthy for women all through life. Suggestions for exercise that should be safe during pregnancy are provided in Chapter 12. Asking about the type, amount, and frequency of exercise a woman enjoys each week helps determine her routine pattern and whether that will be consistent with a recommended level for pregnancy (American Congress of Obstetricians and Gynecologists [ACOG], 2012).

If a woman hikes or camps, for example, this type of exercise is good for her but also can put her at risk for exposure to Lyme disease, an infection carried by deer ticks. Ask if she knows about precautions to prevent this disease (see Chapter 43).

Hobbies. Most hobbies are harmless, but certain ones, such as working with lead-based glazes and ceramics, need to be identified because it might not be wise to continue such a hobby during pregnancy because lead is a known teratogen (Couloures & Vasan, 2011).

Tobacco, Alcohol, and Drug Consumption. As many as 6 out of every 10 women of childbearing age drink alcohol; one third of this number binge drink. As many as 19% of women of childbearing age either smoke cigarettes, use oral tobacco, or are routinely exposed to secondary smoke (CDC, 2012a). Excessive alcohol intake can not only lead to poor nutrition but can also be directly responsible for the impact of fetal alcohol sequence disorders (unusual facial features and cognitive challenges) and preterm birth (Paintner, Williams, & Burd, 2012).

Because smoke, whether first-hand or second-hand, increases the rate of preterm birth and intrauterine growth restriction, obtaining information about a woman and her family's smoking habits helps to analyze whether the fetus will be at risk (Larzelere & Williams, 2012).

If a woman answers vaguely about how much she smokes or drinks ("I drink socially" or "I only smoke occasionally"), ask her to clarify exactly what she means by "socially" or "occasionally" so you can more accurately evaluate the frequency of these events.

Be sure to ask about recreational/illicit drugs as well, such as marijuana or cocaine, as these, like alcohol, are associated with preterm or low–birth-weight infants (Creanga, Sabel, Ko, et al., 2012). Ask specifically about intravenous drug use because of the increased risk for exposure to HIV and hepatitis B through the use of contaminated needles. Although this type of information under usual circumstances may not be readily revealed, most women will answer these questions honestly during pregnancy because they are concerned about protecting the health of their fetus.

Medication and Herbal Therapy. Ask whether a woman takes any medications, prescribed or over-the-counter, because their effect on a growing fetus will have to be evaluated. Tetracycline, for example, an antibiotic commonly prescribed for facial acne, causes long bone defects in the fetus and will need to be discontinued during pregnancy (Karch, 2013). Many women take herbal supplements to relieve the nausea of early pregnancy, so ask also about any herbal preparations a woman might be using because even seemingly innocent alternative therapies could be detrimental if they stimulate uterine contractions or in any other way interfere with fetal health. Ginger, for example, often suggested to relieve nausea, can cause anticoagulation, which could be fatal if a placenta loosened and a woman bled (Tiran, 2012).

Intimate Partner Violence. Women and adolescents who are trapped in a violent intimate partner relationship need to be identified because both the amount and severity of violence are apt to increase with pregnancy (Chalfin, Burke, & Tonelli, 2012). Examples of the types of question you could ask are, "Have you ever been hurt by anyone?" "Are you afraid of anyone?" or "Have you ever been forced to have sex when you didn't want to?"

Gynecologic History

In the past, most women had children early in their childbearing years, so they experienced few reproductive tract or women's health disorders, such as breast disease, before pregnancy. Today, with women delaying conception of their first child past 30 years of age, it is not unusual to discover a woman who has had a reproductive tract or breast disorder. Table 11.2 lists common gynecologic illnesses that occur and their possible significance in pregnancy.

Menstrual History. A woman's past experience with her reproductive system may have some influence on how well she accepts a pregnancy as well as whether she'll develop a complication. Information to obtain includes her age of menarche (first menstrual period) and how well she was prepared for it. Ask about her usual cycle, including the interval, duration, amount of menstrual flow, and any discomfort she feels. If she has discomfort with periods, document when the discomfort occurs, how long it lasts, and what she does to relieve it.

This is important because some women with severe dysmenorrhea can be looking forward to pregnancy because it will mean 9 months without discomfort. However, if she describes menstrual cramps as "horrible" and wonders "how I live through them some months," you can anticipate that she might need additional counseling to help her prepare for the pain of labor. Anticipate the need for counseling in the postpartum period about active ways to relieve menstrual discomfort when menstrual periods resume (see Chapter 47).

Perineal and Breast Self-Examination. Perineal self-examination is inspecting the external genitalia monthly for signs of infection or lesions (see Chapter 34 for the technique). Immigrants from other countries may have had female circumcision (clitoris removed) in childhood; this needs to be documented because scarring and strictures can limit the size of the birth canal (Box 11.5).

Breast self-examination is no longer thought to yield enough reliable information to be continued as a monthly self-care routine, but women should be alerted to normal breast changes during pregnancy and about the responsibility to begin having mammograms when they reach 40 years of age (American Cancer Society [ACS], 2012). They still should have a yearly breast examination by a health care provider, so this will be done at a first prenatal visit (Alvarez & Jacobs, 2011).

TABLE 11.2 Common Gynecologic Disorders Seen in Pregnancy

Disorder	Possible Symptoms	Significance and Suggested Therapy
Disorders of the Vulva		
Cysts or infection of Skene or Bartholin glands	Cysts appear as asymptomatic swelling at the sides of the urinary meatus or vestibule; if infected, glands appear swollen and reddened and can be painful	Such cysts are surgically incised to prevent blockage of the gland duct. Infections are treated with antibiotics.
Condylomata acuminata	Painless cauliflower-like lesion on vulva	Tends to occur in women with chronic vaginitis. Caused by the same virus that causes common warts. Removed by cryocautery or knife excision.
Lichen sclerosis	Whitish papules on the vulva; asymptomatic	No need for removal; the area is biopsied, however, because leukoplakia, a potentially cancerous condition, has an almost identical appearance.
Leukoplakia	Thick, gray, patchy epithelium that cracks; possibly a premalignant state that infects easily, accompanied by itching and pain	Therapy involves hydrocortisone and frequent return visits to health care personnel (every 6 months) for observation to detect any changes suggestive of carcinoma.
Carcinoma of the vulva	A shallow vulvar ulcer that does not heal	Vulvar cancer occurs most often in postmenopausal women; represents only 3%–4% of all reproductive tract cancers in women. Therapy is vulvectomy—vagina is left intact, and sexual relations and pregnancy, with cesarean birth to prevent tearing of fibrotic vulvar tissue, may be possible afterward.
Female circumcision	Surgical removal of the clitoris; possibly vagina is sewed closed	Illegal in United States; done as a cultural ritual in young girls from African and Middle Eastern countries. Vaginal stricture may need to be excised to allow for menstrual flow and childbirth.
Disorders of the Vagina and Cervix		
Cervical polyp	Red, vascular, protruding pedunculated tissue that bleeds readily with trauma	May be discovered because of vaginal spotting on coitus, tampon insertion, or vaginal examination. Removed vaginally by excision. Often associated with chronic cervical inflammation.
Cervicitis (erosion)	Reddened cervical tissue with a whitish exudate	Douching with a vinegar solution aids healing. May be treated with cryosurgery if extensive.
Nabothian cyst	Clear shining circles on cervix from blocked gland ducts	No therapy necessary.
Cervical carcinoma	Postcoital spotting, unexplained vaginal discharge, or spotting between menstrual periods	The most frequent type of reproductive tract malignancy seen; risk factors include coitus with multiple partners or uncircumcised males, herpes type 2 or human papillomavirus (HPV) infections. Diagnosed by Pap test or colposcopy. Therapy is conization, radiation, or surgical excision. Pregnancy is possible following cervical carcinoma; cesarean birth may be necessary because of fibrotic cervical tissue. HPV vaccine can reduce the incidence.
Disorders of the Ovaries		
Endometrial cyst	Chocolate-brown cyst on tender enlarged ovary; may cause acute pain if rupture occurs	Endometriosis is the cause; occurs in women age 20–40 years. Therapy is surgical excision; ovary may or may not be removed depending on extent of cyst.
Follicular cyst	Amenorrhea and possibly dyspareunia; ovary tender and enlarged	Cysts typically regress after 1 or 2 months; low-dose oral contraceptive may be prescribed for 6–12 weeks to suppress ovarian activity; estrogen may be continued for 6 months.

(continued on page 252)

TABLE 11.2 Common Gynecologic Disorders Seen in Pregnancy (continued)

Disorder	Possible Symptoms	Significance and Suggested Therapy
Polycystic ovary syndrome	A syndrome of chronic follicular cysts, anovulation, insulin resistance, and excess testosterone production leading to perimenopausal onset of hirsutism, obesity, subfertility, and elevated triglycerides	Excess testosterone secretion by ovaries leads to inhibition of follicle-stimulating hormone and anovulation, causing subfertility. Weight loss, reduction in triglycerides and cholesterol levels, clomiphene citrate therapy to induce ovulation, and a combination of spironolactone (Aldactone) with estrogen-progestin oral contraceptives to reduce hirsutism are all used as therapy.
Corpus luteum cyst	Delayed menstrual flow followed by prolonged bleeding; ovary enlarged and tender	A corpus luteum persists rather than atrophies. Most regress in about 2 months; a low-dose oral contraceptive may be prescribed for 6 weeks to suppress ovarian activity.
Dermoid cyst	Asymptomatic; ovary enlarged on examination	Cyst originates from embryonic tissue; may contain hair, cartilage, and fat. Most common ovarian tumor of childhood; also occurs at age 30–50 years. Therapy is surgical resection.
Serous cystadenoma	Bilateral; asymptomatic except for signs of pelvic pressure	The most common type of ovarian cyst; high malignancy rate of 20%–30%. Therapy is surgical resection.
Carcinoma	Asymptomatic; intermenstrual bleeding	Ovarian cancer originates in epithelial tissue most often in women over 50 years of age. Tendency may be inherited; environmental contamination such as use of talcum powder may play a role in development. Therapy is hysterectomy and salpingo-oophorectomy.
Disorders of the Uterus		
Endometrial polyp	Intermenstrual bleeding	Polyp is removed by dilatation and curettage.
Leiomyomas (fibroids)	Asymptomatic or with increased menstrual flow; uterus may be enlarged	Muscle and fibrous connective tissue form in response to estrogen stimulation. May increase in size during pregnancy; may cause interference with cervical dilatation and result in postpartal hemorrhage. Stress to the myometrium by uterine contractions may be the original cause of formation. Therapy is embolization (blocking the blood supply), oral contraceptives or gonadotropin-releasing hormone agonists to lower estrogen level, surgical resection (myomectomy), or hysterectomy if childbearing is complete.
Endometrial carcinoma	Vaginal bleeding between menstrual periods	Diagnosis is by endometrial washing, not Pap test. Initial therapy is hysterectomy.
Uterine prolapse	Vaginal pressure and low back pain	The uterus has descended into the vagina due to overstretching of uterine supports and trauma to the levator ani muscle. Occurs most often in women who had insufficient prenatal care, birth of a large infant, a prolonged second stage of labor, bearing-down efforts or extraction of a baby before full dilatation, instrument birth, and poor healing of perineal tissue postpartally. Therapy is surgery to repair uterine supports or placement of a pessary, a plastic uterine support. Women with pessaries in place need to return for a pelvic examination every 3 months to have the pessary removed, cleaned, and replaced and the vagina inspected; otherwise, vaginal infection or erosion of the vaginal walls can result. Surgical replacement is also possible.

Past Surgery. Any type of past surgery on the reproductive tract is important to document because it can influence a woman's ability to conceive and give birth. For example, if a woman had tubal surgery following an ectopic pregnancy, her statistical risk of another tubal pregnancy is greater than usual because of possible tubal scarring. If she had uterine surgery, a cesarean birth may be necessary because her uterus may not be able to contract as efficiently as usual because of a surgical scar. If she has undergone frequent dilatation and curettage of the uterus or cervical biopsies, her cervix may be weakened or unable to remain closed for 9 months, leading to preterm birth unless she has a surgical procedure (cerclage) to prevent premature dilation (see Chapter 21).

BOX 11.5 Nursing Care Planning to Respect Cultural Diversity

Female circumcision is the removal of a portion or all of the female genitalia done in early adolescence as a way of controlling sexual activity in girls before marriage. The practice arises from religious or cultural customs.

Both the clitoris and the labia minora may be removed; the labia majora may be stitched closed. If keloid formation or scarring occur, the vaginal opening may be so obstructed that neither menstrual flow nor childbirth may be possible; coitus can be difficult and painful. Female circumcision is seen most in women from African and Middle Eastern nations. The practice is illegal in the United States and opposed by the World Health Organization because it violates a woman's right to well health and physical integrity. It is an important assessment to make when obtaining a health history at preconceptual or first prenatal visits because it influences not just sexual health but the ability to conceive and whether vaginal childbirth will be possible.

Reproductive Planning. Ask also about what reproductive planning method, if any, a woman has been using. Occasionally, a woman may become pregnant with an intrauterine device (IUD) in place. If this occurs, it needs to be removed to prevent infection during pregnancy. Another woman, not certain she is pregnant, may be continuing to take an oral contraceptive. If a pregnancy is confirmed, you can assure her taking the pill while pregnant will not cause fetal harm but she should discontinue taking it for the remainder of pregnancy (Waller, Gallaway, Taylor, et al., 2010).

Sexual History. Be certain to obtain a sexual history, including the number of sexual partners and the use of safer sex practices, to establish a woman's risk for contracting a sexually transmitted infection such as herpes (a viral infection spread by direct contact) or hepatitis C (a viral infection spread by contact with blood or by intercourse with a partner who is infected) (Rosen, 2011).

Stress Incontinence. As part of any woman's gynecologic history, assess for the possibility of stress incontinence (incontinence of urine on laughing, coughing, deep inspiration, jogging, or running). Urinary incontinence occurs with these actions because they cause the diaphragm to descend, which then increases overall abdominal pressure and bladder tension; increased tension leads to sudden emptying if the woman lacks strength in her perineal muscles or bladder supports. Commonly, this weakness occurs from past difficult births, the birth of large infants, grand multiparity, or instrument births. During pregnancy, stress incontinence can become intensified from the increasing abdominal pressure of the growing uterus. Some women, however, accept this incontinence as a normal consequence of childbearing and may not report it unless asked.

Women can relieve stress incontinence to some degree by strengthening perineal muscles with the use of Kegel exercises (periodic tightening of the perineal muscles; see Chapter 12). Surgical correction to increase support to the bladder neck could be performed following the pregnancy.

QSEN Checkpoint Question 11.3

Informatics

You are reviewing Sandra's electronic health record. While doing so, you ask Sandra to clarify and confirm her surgical history. Why is it important to ask Sandra about past surgery during a pregnancy health history?

a. Previous use of general anesthetics is a risk factor for preterm labor.
b. Adhesions from surgery could potentially limit uterine growth.
c. Previous experience with surgery means that she will likely be comfortable in a hospital setting.
d. Abdominal incisions are associated with potential uterine rupture.

Look in Appendix A for the best answer and rationale.

Obstetric History

Do not assume the current pregnancy is a woman's first pregnancy simply because she is very young or says she has only recently been married. She may have had an adolescent pregnancy, or this could be a second marriage. For each previous pregnancy, document the newborn's sex and the place and date of birth. Review the pregnancy briefly by asking:

- Was the pregnancy intended?
- How did the pregnancy go, overall? Did she have any complications, such as vaginal spotting, swelling of her hands or feet, falls, or surgery?
- Did she take any medication? If so, what and why?
- Did she receive prenatal care? If so, when did she start?
- What was the duration of the pregnancy?
- What was the duration of labor? Was it what she expected? Worse? Better?
- What was the type of birth? Vaginal or cesarean? Vertex or breech? In a health care facility or at home? What type of anesthesia, if any, was used?
- Did she have stitches following birth?
- Did she have any complications following birth, such as excessive bleeding or infection?
- What was the infant's birth weight and sex? Did the infant cry right away? What was the infant's Apgar score? (Most mothers know this.)
- Was any special care needed for the baby, such as suctioning, oxygen, or an incubator?
- Was the baby discharged from the health care setting with her?
- What is the child's present state of health?

Ask also about any previous miscarriages or therapeutic abortions and whether she had any complications during or following those. If a woman's blood type is Rh negative, ask if she received Rh immune globulin (RhIG [RhoGAM]) after miscarriages, abortions, or previous births so you will know whether Rh sensitization could have occurred. In conjunction with that, ask if she has ever had a blood transfusion to establish possible risk of hepatitis B or HIV exposure or Rh sensitization from a blood transfusion.

After this history of previous pregnancies is obtained, rate the woman's status with respect to the number of times she has been

TABLE 11.3 Terms Related to Pregnancy Status

Term	Definition
Para	The number of pregnancies that have reached viability, regardless of whether the infants were born alive
Gravida	A woman who is or has been pregnant
Primigravida	A woman who is pregnant for the first time
Primipara	A woman who has given birth to one child past age of viability
Multigravida	A woman who has been pregnant previously
Grand multigravida	A woman who has been pregnant many times
Multipara	A woman who has carried two or more pregnancies to viability
Nulligravida	A woman who has never been and is not currently pregnant

pregnant, including the present pregnancy (her **gravida** status), and the number of children over the age of viability (20 weeks gestation) she has previously delivered (her **para** status). Table 11.3 explains these terms. For example, a woman who had two previous pregnancies that ended in miscarriages at 12 weeks (under the age of viability) and is now pregnant is a gravida 3, para 0. If she had given birth from the two previous pregnancies and is now pregnant, she would be gravida 3, para 2.

A more comprehensive system for classifying pregnancy status (GTPAL or GTPALM) provides greater detail on a woman's pregnancy history. By this system, the gravida classification remains the same, but para is broken down as follows:

T: The number of full-term infants born (infants born at 37 weeks or after)
P: The number of preterm infants born (infants born before 37 weeks)
A: The number of spontaneous miscarriages or therapeutic abortions
L: The number of living children
M: Multiple pregnancies

Using this system, a woman in the first example who is pregnant and has two children at home would be gravida 3, para 2002 (GTPAL) or gravida 3, para 20020 (GTPALM). A multigestation pregnancy is considered as one para. For example, a woman who had term twins, then one preterm infant, and is now pregnant again would be a gravida 3, para 21031 (GTPALM).

What if...11.1 A pregnant woman has the following past history: a boy born at 39 weeks gestation, alive and well; a girl born at 40 weeks gestation, alive and well; and a girl born at 33 weeks gestation, alive and well. How would you summarize her gravida and para status?

Review of Systems

A review of systems completes the subjective information of a health history. Use a systematic approach, such as head to toe, and explain what you will be doing by an explanation such as, "I'm going to start at the top of your head and go through to your toes, asking about body parts or systems and any diseases you may have had." A review of systems helps women recall concerns they forgot to mention earlier, such as a urinary tract infection, a condition that can influence the outcome of pregnancy and thus would be important to your history taking.

The following body systems and questions about conditions constitute the minimum information to be addressed in a review of systems for a first prenatal visit:

- *Head:* Headache? Head injury? Seizures? Dizziness? Fainting?
- *Eyes:* Vision? Glasses needed? Diplopia or double vision? Infection? Glaucoma? Cataract? Pain? Recent changes? Last vision examination and outcome?
- *Ears:* Infection? Discharge? Earache? Hearing loss? Tinnitus? Vertigo?
- *Nose:* Epistaxis (nose bleeds)? Discharge? How many colds a year? Allergies? Postnasal drainage? Sinus pain?
- *Mouth and pharynx:* Dentures? Condition of teeth? Toothaches? Any bleeding of gums? Hoarseness? Difficulty in swallowing? Tonsillectomy? Last dental examination and outcome?
- *Neck:* Stiffness? Masses?
- *Breasts:* Lumps? Secretion? Pain? Tenderness?
- *Respiratory system:* Cough? Wheezing? Asthma? Shortness of breath? Pain? Serious chest illness, such as tuberculosis or pneumonia?
- *Cardiovascular system:* History of heart murmur? History of heart disease such as rheumatic fever or Kawasaki disease? Hypertension? Any pain? Palpitations? Anemia? Does she know her blood pressure? Has she ever had a blood transfusion?
- *Gastrointestinal system:* What was her prepregnancy weight? Vomiting? Diarrhea? Constipation? Change in bowel habits? Rectal pruritus? Hemorrhoids? Pain? Ulcer? Gallbladder disease? Hepatitis? Appendicitis?
- *Genitourinary system:* Urinary tract infection? Hematuria? Frequent urination? Sexually transmitted infection? Pelvic inflammatory disease? Hepatitis B? HIV? Did she have a problem getting pregnant? Is subfertility a concern?
- *Extremities:* Varicose veins? Pain or stiffness of joints? Any fractures or dislocations? Carpal tunnel syndrome? Restless leg syndrome?
- *Skin:* Any rashes? Acne? Psoriasis?

Interview Conclusion

End an interview by asking if there is anything you have not covered that the woman wants to discuss; this gives her one more chance to ask any questions she has about this new life experience. Explore any further concerns she mentions because these can be equally as important as her first concern mentioned.

Support Person's Role

Both partners and young children accompany women for prenatal care (Fig. 11.1). Some women bring a female friend or a relative as their best support person. If family members are present, should they be included in an initial interview? As a whole, interviewing is most effective if it is a one-to-one

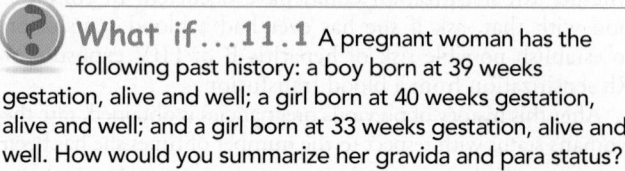

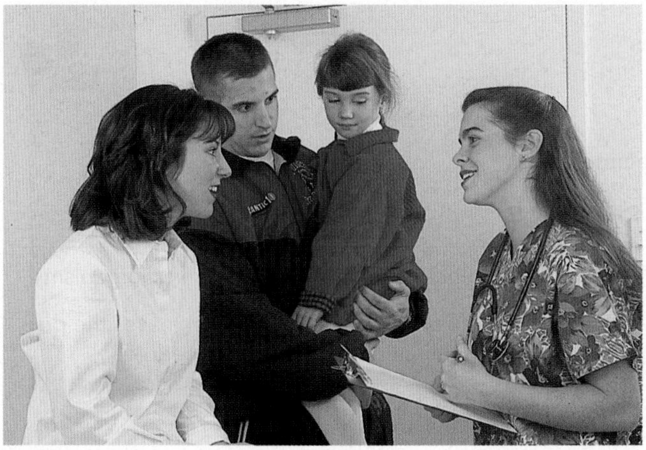

FIGURE 11.1 Include support people in a prenatal visit so visits are family centered. (© Barbara Proud.)

interaction because a woman may be unwilling to mention certain concerns when her family is present for fear of worrying them.

If childbearing is to be a family affair, however, it is important to determine a partner's degree of acceptance of the pregnancy and how well prepared he or she is of assuming a new parenting role. Including the fetus's siblings in a prenatal visit also provides them an opportunity to be involved.

Interviewing a woman alone and then inviting the support person and family to join her while you talk about pregnancy symptoms with them as a family can be an effective compromise. In addition, providing some private interview time with a partner allows the partner to express any of his or her concerns or worries.

If a woman wishes, a partner can accompany her during the physical examination. After confirmation of pregnancy, include the partner in health care information or suggestions.

Physical Examination

The next step in health assessment is physical examination. Ask a woman to void for a clean-catch urine specimen before the examination because this will provide a urine specimen for either immediate dipstick or laboratory testing of bacteria, protein, glucose, and ketone determinations. In addition, an empty bladder makes the pelvic examination more comfortable and, by reducing bladder size, allows for easier identification of pelvic organs. If you are not already familiar with obtaining a clean-catch urine specimen, Box 11.6 provides instructions.

A physical examination at a first prenatal visit typically includes inspection of major body systems, with emphasis on the changes that occur with pregnancy or that could signal a developing complication. General techniques of physical examination are discussed in Chapter 34.

Baseline Height/Weight and Vital Sign Measurement

A woman's weight and height are measured at a first prenatal visit to establish a pregnancy BMI to serve as a baseline for future comparison. Record this assessment with her prepregnancy BMI, if available, to determine how much weight she has already gained or lost (Fig. 11.2). When obtaining women's weight, be certain to convey an air of "weight gain is healthy" so a woman feels comfortable gaining 30 to 40 lb during pregnancy (many adolescents need to gain 40 lb to help ensure a healthy fetus).

Measure vital signs, including blood pressure, respiratory rate, and pulse rate, again, for baseline levels. A sudden increase in blood pressure and a sudden weight gain are both danger signs that gestational hypertension may be occurring. A sudden increase in pulse or respirations could suggest undetected bleeding. If close monitoring of blood pressure will be necessary during pregnancy, teach a support person or the woman herself how to do this so the woman can continue assessing blood pressure at home.

Assessment of Body Systems

General Appearance and Mental Status. Physical examination always begins with an inspection of general appearance to form an overall impression of a woman's health and well-being. General appearance is important because the manner in which people dress, the way they speak, and the body posture they assume all suggest how they feel about themselves. Remember that not all women are thoroughly happy about being pregnant. Closely inspect for signs such as careless hygiene, unwashed hair, inappropriate or soiled clothing, and sad facial expression that suggest fatigue or depression about their diagnosis.

If a woman has any Band-Aids or other dressings in place, remove and inspect the skin underneath because they could hide an important finding such as a malignant melanoma (skin cancer), which is an increasing problem in young adults as a result of excessive sun exposure and tanning beds (Dusza, Halpern, Satagopan, et al., 2012). Bandages could also be concealing intimate partner violence. Such violence is not only dangerous to the woman but also can lead to early pregnancy loss (Engnes, Lidén, & Lundgren, 2012).

Most marks from violence occur on the face, the ulnar surfaces of the forearms (from a woman raising her arms to defend herself), the abdomen or buttocks (from being kicked), or the upper arms (from being grabbed and held forcefully). Noting the color of any ecchymotic areas not only helps document that violence occurred but also helps to date when the violence occurred because these marks typically progress from black or blue (at 1 to 5 days), to green or dark yellow (at 5 to 10 days), to yellow and disappearing (at 10 to 15 days). A woman may have multiple areas at different stages of the healing process if she was punched or kicked on different occasions.

Head and Scalp. Examine a woman's head for symmetry, normal contour, and tenderness. Hair growth speeds up during pregnancy as a result of the overall increased metabolic rate, and women may comment they have noticed this. Assess hair for presence, distribution, thickness, excessive dryness or oiliness, cleanliness, and the use of hair dye (it is unlikely that hair dye is carcinogenic or causes fetal injury if used infrequently and according to the package instructions). Look for **chloasma** (extra pigment on the face that occurs from melanocyte-stimulating hormone), an early sign of pregnancy. Also note:

- Dryness or sparseness of hair, which suggests poor nutrition.
- Lack of cleanliness may suggest fatigue, reflecting that a woman has not felt well enough to wash it recently. It is important to urge women during pregnancy to let some other tasks go so they save energy for self-care and can continue to feel good about their appearance. Dandruff shampoos can be used during pregnancy because they are not absorbed.

BOX 11.6 Nursing Care Planning Using Procedures

OBTAINING A CLEAN-CATCH URINE SPECIMEN

Purpose: Helping a woman obtain a clean-catch urine specimen

PROCEDURE	PRINCIPLE
1. Ask the woman to wash her hands.	1. Handwashing helps prevent spread of microorganisms.
2. She then needs to open the commercial clean-catch urine specimen kit and moisten the cotton balls with the antiseptic solution or open the prepared antiseptic wipes.	2. Preparation enhances efficiency and decreases the possibility of contamination during the procedure.

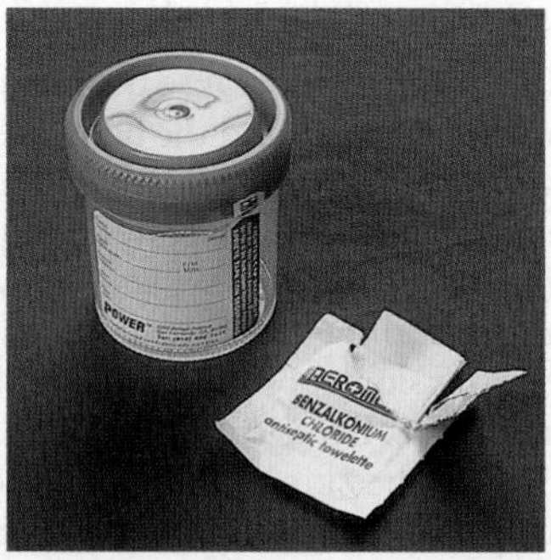

PROCEDURE	PRINCIPLE
3. a. Ask the woman to sit on the commode and separate her labia with her nondominant hand.	3. Cleansing helps prevent microorganisms from entering the urine specimen.

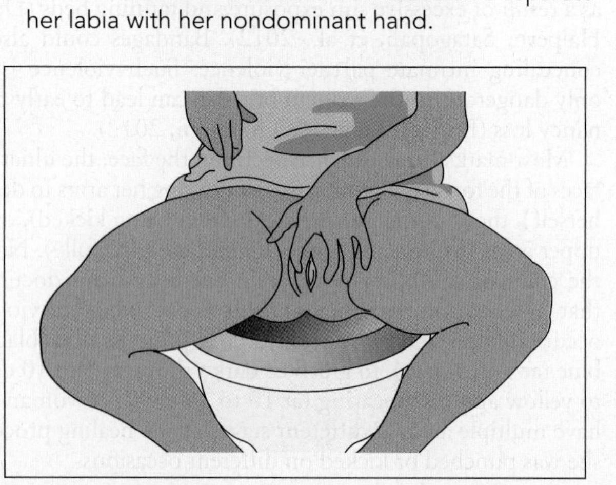

PROCEDURE	PRINCIPLE
b. She should then cleanse her perineum, washing from front to back, using a cotton ball or wipe for only one stroke and then discarding it.	Cleansing from front to back prevents bringing rectal contamination forward.

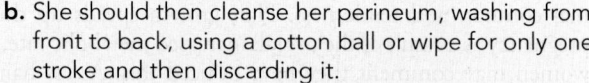

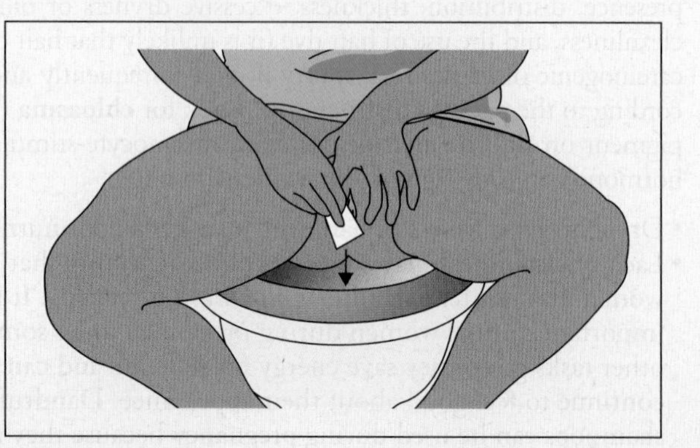

PROCEDURE	PRINCIPLE
4. Caution her to avoid touching the inside of the container or cap.	4. Careful handling of equipment prevents contamination.
5. The woman should begin urinating, allowing the first urine to flow into the toilet. Next, she should hold the container under the urine stream until approximately 10 to 20 ml has been obtained. Once the specimen is obtained, she can remove the container, release her hand from her labia, and finish voiding into the toilet.	5. The first flow of urine washes microorganisms and debris from the urinary meatus and thus shouldn't be collected. Collecting the specimen midstream helps ensures that a sterile specimen is obtained.

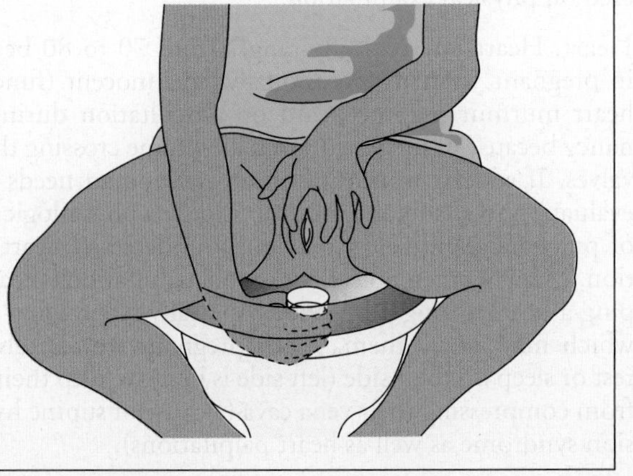

6. To finish, she should cap the specimen container, wash her hands, and bring the specimen to you. Encourage her to report whether she felt any pain on urination.	6. Capping the container prevents inadvertent spilling and possible contamination of the specimen. Pain on urination is a symptom of urinary tract infection.

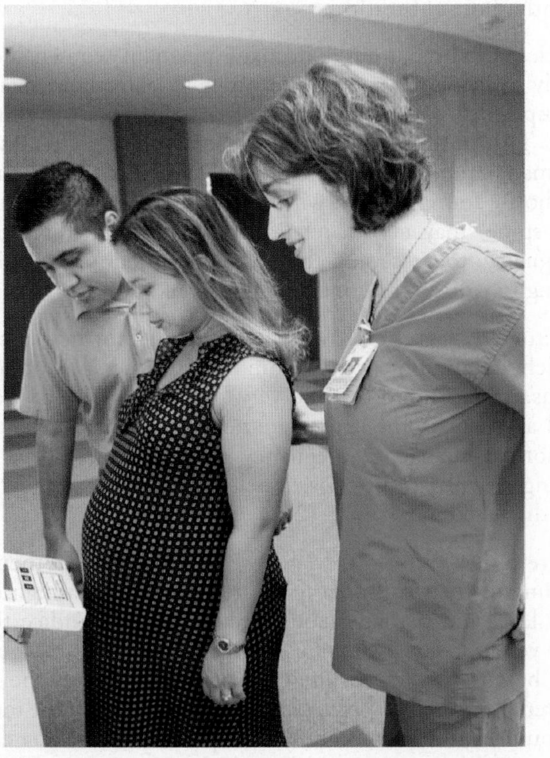

FIGURE 11.2 A woman weighs in at a prenatal visit. Pregnant women may need reassurance that gaining weight aids fetal growth. (© Barbara Proud.)

Eyes. Edema of the eyelids combined with a swollen optic disk (identified on ophthalmoscopic examination) suggests edema from gestational hypertension, a potentially dangerous condition of pregnancy. On interview, women with gestational hypertension also usually report seeing spots in their vision or diplopia (double vision). Teach pregnant women that symptoms of changing vision are a potential danger sign of pregnancy that need to be reported. If they do close desk work, caution them to take a break every hour so they do not confuse sensations of eyestrain with actual danger signs of pregnancy.

Nose. The increased level of estrogen associated with pregnancy can cause nasal congestion or the appearance of swollen nasal membranes. Even topical medicines such as nose drops or nasal sprays used to reduce this are absorbed to some degree, so advise women to avoid these during pregnancy without their primary care provider's knowledge and consent.

Ears. The nasal stuffiness that accompanies pregnancy may lead to blocked eustachian tubes and therefore a feeling of "fullness" in the ears or dampening of sound during early pregnancy. Usually this disappears as the body adjusts to a new estrogen level. Normal hearing level and normal tympanic landmarks should be present.

Sinuses. Sinuses should feel nontender. Establishing a lack of tenderness over sinuses helps to determine that a woman's report of headache during pregnancy (a danger sign until ruled otherwise) is probably not sinus related.

Mouth, Teeth, and Throat. Gingival (gum) hypertrophy may result from estrogen stimulation during pregnancy. The gums look slightly swollen and are tender to touch, but not reddened. Pregnant women are prone to vitamin deficiencies because of the rapid growth of the fetus. Assess carefully, therefore, for cracked corners of the mouth, a sign of vitamin A deficiency. Assess also for pinpoint lesions with an erythematous base on the lips that suggest a herpes infection (a herpes lesion on the gum line is more often a shallow ulcer). Because newborns are susceptible to herpes infection, lesions present at birth may necessitate a woman needing to wear a mask to breastfeed her newborn.

Teach all women not to neglect their dental hygiene or yearly dental visits while pregnant. They should maintain thorough toothbrushing (some stop thorough brushing because they notice slightly blood-tinged saliva because of gingival hypertrophy). If many dental caries are obvious, a woman should be referred to a dental health care provider early in pregnancy because carious teeth are a source of infection and should be treated before abscesses develop and cause more serious problems. Contrary to what many women believe, dental X-rays can be safely taken during pregnancy as long as a woman reminds her dentist she is pregnant and is given a lead apron to shield her abdomen. Urge her to obtain permission from her primary care provider before consenting to extensive dental work requiring anesthesia.

Neck. Slight thyroid hypertrophy may occur with pregnancy because the overall metabolic rate is increased. Suggest that all women eat a serving (preferably two servings) of seafood, such as salmon, cod, crab, or shrimp, once a week to supply enough iodine for their accompanying increased thyroxine production so they don't develop thyroid hypertrophy from the gland struggling to produce hormones dependent on iodine (Yazbeck & Sullivan, 2012). Albacore tuna, chunk white tuna, and tuna steak should be avoided because these have a potentially high mercury content (Abelsohn, Vanderlinden, Scott, et al., 2011).

Encourage a woman who uses iodized salt because she lives in an area low in iodine soil (the Great Lakes region, for example) to continue using this during pregnancy because, without a reminder, some women will think of iodine as an unnecessary additive and discontinue using it. Thyroid hypertrophy (goiter) is obvious on a physical examination as a large swelling at the midline on the front of the neck.

Lymph Nodes. No palpable lymph nodes should be present in a woman's neck or under her arms; however, because pregnant women may develop an increased number of upper respiratory infections because of reduced immunologic resistance during pregnancy, one or two pea-sized (sometimes called "shotty") cervical lymph nodes at the sides of the neck may be palpable. If a woman has a tooth abscess from bacterial growth under hypertrophied gingival tissue (periodontal disease), submaxillary (under the chin) lymph nodes may be palpable.

Breasts. Breast changes may be one of the first things women notice in pregnancy:

- Areolae darken.
- Secondary areolae develop.
- Montgomery tubercles (sebaceous glands in the areolae) become prominent.
- Overall breast size increases and the consistency firms.
- Breasts feel tender because of increasing size and hormonal changes.
- Blue streaking of veins becomes prominent.
- Colostrum may be expelled from the nipple as early as the 16th week of pregnancy.
- Any supernumerary nipples also may become darker and enlarge in size.

In addition to these healthy changes, both benign breast lesions, such as fibrocystic breast disease (discussed in Chapter 47), and malignant breast pathology may be discovered on physical examination.

Heart. Heart rate typically ranges from 70 to 80 beats/min in pregnant women. Occasionally, an innocent (functional) heart murmur may be heard on auscultation during pregnancy because of increased vascular volume crossing the heart valves. If a heart murmur is heard, a woman needs further evaluation to ensure the murmur is only a physiologic change of pregnancy and not a previously undetected heart condition. Many women notice occasional palpitations (heart skipping a beat) during pregnancy, especially when lying supine, which may worry them. Teach pregnant women always to rest or sleep on their side (left side is best) to keep their uterus from compressing their vena cava (a cause of supine hypotension syndrome as well as heart palpitations).

Lungs. Assess respiratory rate and rhythm. Rate may increase slightly because lung tissue assumes a more horizontal position during pregnancy than usual. Vital capacity, however, is not reduced. Late in pregnancy, diaphragmatic excursion (diaphragm movement) is lessened because the diaphragm cannot descend as fully as usual because of the distended uterus. This is also normal but may cause women to feel constantly short of breath.

Back. The lumbar curve in many pregnant women increasingly deepens on standing in order to help them maintain an upright body posture in the face of enlarging abdominal size. This posture can cause considerable back pain. Assess a woman's spine for any abnormal curve that would suggest scoliosis. Young women with scoliosis (sideways curvature of the spine) may need a referral to their orthopedist early in pregnancy to be certain the extra abdominal pressure is not going to worsen the condition (Fairbank, 2011).

Rectum. Assess the rectum closely for hemorrhoidal tissue, which commonly occurs from uterine pressure on pelvic veins. Hemorrhoids can be very uncomfortable for women and also worrisome if they are not assured hemorrhoids are a normal change of pregnancy and, like most pregnancy changes, will fade afterward. Self-therapies for hemorrhoids are discussed in Chapter 12.

Extremities and Skin. Many women develop erythema or itching of their palms early in pregnancy from a high estrogen level and perhaps subclinical jaundice (jaundice that is not yet apparent by a color change) from reabsorbed bilirubin because of slowed intestinal peristalsis. Assess the lower extremities carefully for varicosities, filling time of the toenails (should be under 5 seconds), and presence of edema caused by impaired venous return from the lower extremities because of uterine pressure. Any edema more than ankle swelling is a danger sign of pregnancy that needs to be investigated.

Body joints become more relaxed with pregnancy because of relaxin, a hormone produced by the placenta. As a last measure, therefore, assess the gait of pregnant women to be certain they don't have pain on walking and are keeping their pelvis tucked under the weight of their abdomen as this position prevents them from developing muscle strains from abnormal abdominal muscle tension. Many pregnant women develop a "waddling" gait late in pregnancy from relaxation of the symphysis pubis. If this is extreme, they may need to be fitted with a stabilizing belt to allow them to continue to be ambulatory for the remainder of pregnancy.

What if...11.2 Sandra's job at a commercial laundry ironing sheets keeps her on her feet for long periods. Is she apt to be exposed to toxic substances doing this work? Is there a greater opportunity than usual for her to develop upper respiratory infections? What effect might her job have on her hips and posture?

Measurement of Fundal Height and Fetal Heart Sounds

At about 12 to 14 weeks of pregnancy, the uterus becomes palpable as a firm globular sphere showing over the symphysis pubis. It grows to reach the umbilicus at 20 to 22 weeks and the xiphoid process of the sternum at 36 weeks. In primiparas, it then often returns to about 4 cm below the xiphoid process because of "lightening" for the rest of pregnancy. If a woman is past 12 weeks of a pregnancy, assess whether the fundus of the uterus is palpable, measure the fundal height (from the top notch of the symphysis pubis to the superior aspect of the fundus), and plot the height on a graph such as the one shown in Figure 11.3; plotting uterine growth at each visit this way can help detect any unusual variation in uterine or fetal growth. If an abnormality is detected, further investigation with ultrasound can be scheduled to determine the cause of the unusual increase or lack of growth.

Auscultate for fetal heart sounds (a rate of 110 to 160 beats/min is normal) by Doppler if the pregnancy is past 10 weeks (the lower limit at which they can usually be heard). Palpate for fetal outline and position after the 28th week as a further estimation of fetal size and growth.

QSEN Checkpoint Question 11.4

Quality Improvement

Sandra reports that the palms of her hands are always itchy, and you notice scratches on them when you perform a physical examination. Your plan of care should specify that this problem is most likely due to what factor in women who are pregnant?

a. Anxiety or fear about the pregnancy
b. A potential Rh incompatibility
c. Peripheral edema related to changes in fluid and electrolyte levels
d. A common reaction to increasing estrogen levels

Look in Appendix A for the best answer and rationale.

Pelvic Examination

A pelvic examination reveals information on the health of both a woman's internal and external reproductive organs. The following equipment is required:

- A **speculum** (a metal or plastic instrument with movable flat blades; Fig. 11.4)
- A spatula for cervical scraping
- Clean examining gloves
- Lubricant
- A glass slide or liquid collection device for a Pap smear
- A culture tube
- Two or three sterile cotton-tipped applicators or cytobrushes for obtaining cervical cultures
- A good examining light
- A movable stool at correct sitting height

Pelvic examinations have the reputation of being painful and causing a loss of modesty. If this is a first pregnancy, it may be the first time a woman has ever had this type of examination. Having heard stories about how painful these examinations can be may cause a woman to tense just thinking about it. When pelvic muscles are tense, however, not only can the examination become painful but also an examiner has difficulty assessing the status of pelvic organs.

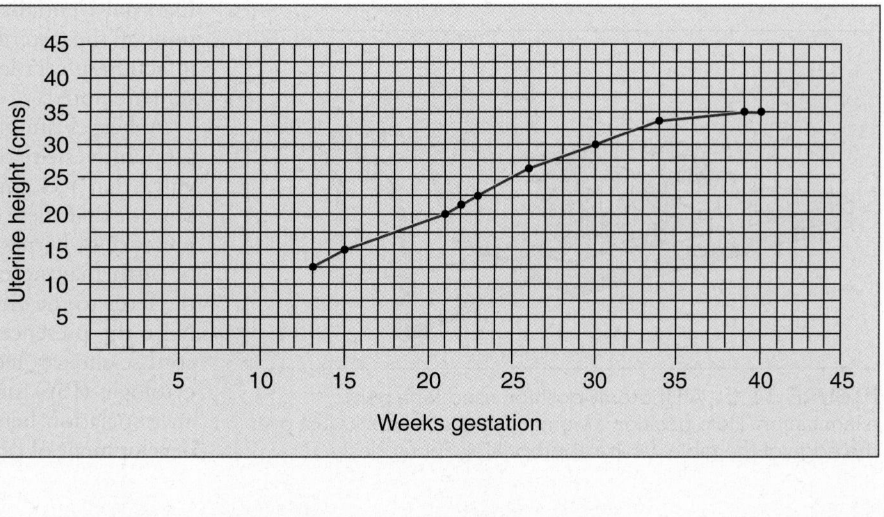

FIGURE 11.3 Plotting uterine height on a uterine height graph at prenatal visits (recorded typically after 12 weeks gestation) helps to monitor whether fundal height is increasing.

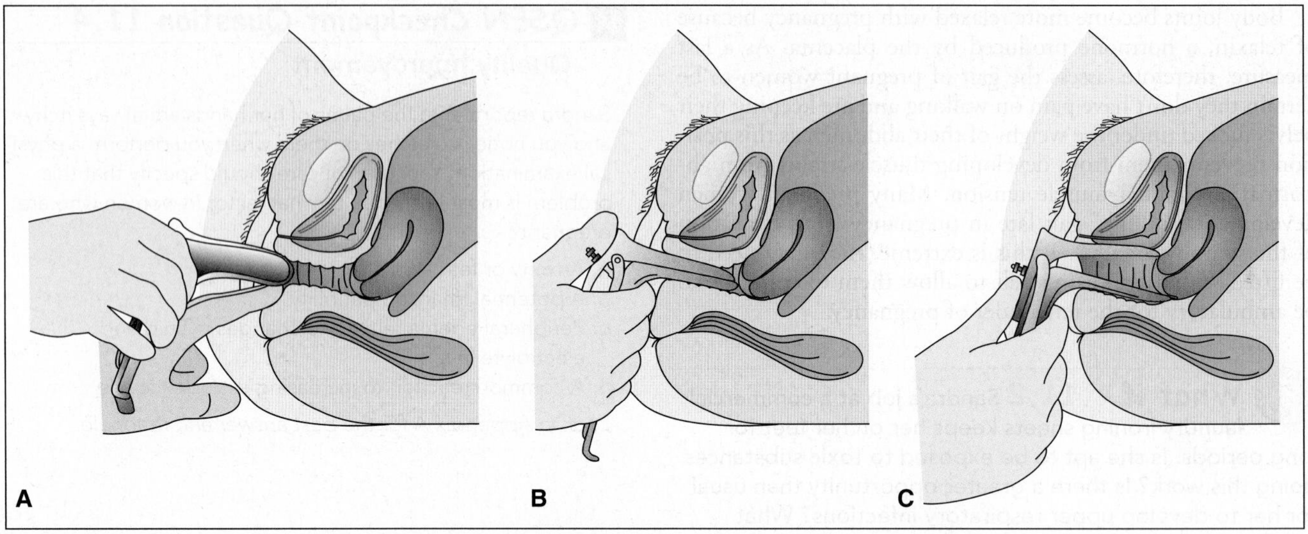

FIGURE 11.4 Insertion of a vaginal speculum. **(A)** Blades held obliquely on entering the vagina. **(B)** Blades rotated to horizontal position as they pass the introitus. **(C)** Blades separated by depressing thumbpiece and elevating handle. The position of the blades is maintained by adjusting a thumbscrew.

Allow a woman the opportunity to talk with the person performing the examination while sitting up, before being placed in a lithotomy position, because this can enhance her sense of self-esteem and control. Many women want their support person to remain with them at the head of the table during the examination. In addition, it is customary, especially on an initial visit, for a nurse or nursing assistant to be in the room with a woman for a pelvic examination to offer additional support. This is true whether the examiner is male or female.

After the woman empties her bladder, have her lie in a **lithotomy position** (on her back with her thighs flexed and her feet resting in the examining table stirrups; Fig. 11.5). If a woman is uncomfortable in a lithotomy position, the exam can be done with her lying flat on a bed or table with her knees raised. Make sure her buttocks extend slightly beyond the end of the examining table if possible. Place a pillow under her head or slightly elevate the head of the examination table to help her relax her abdominal muscles.

Properly drape her with a draw sheet over her abdomen that extends over her legs for modesty. Be sure pregnant women remain in a lithotomy position for as short a time as possible to help prevent thromboembolism (from pressure of the metal stirrups on the calves of her legs) and supine hypotension syndrome (from pressure of the uterus on the vena cava) (Edwardson & Hueppchen, 2011). Placing a firm wedge under one side of her hips to tilt her pelvis can help relieve supine hypotension symptoms.

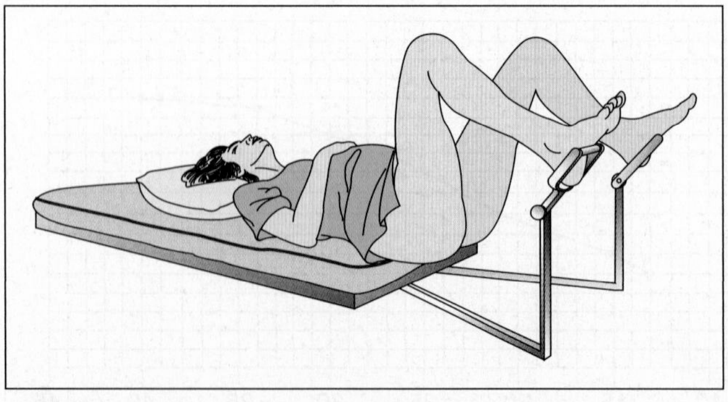

FIGURE 11.5 A lithotomy position used for a pelvic examination. Help position a woman with her buttocks just over the edge of the table. Drape appropriately for modesty.

When serving as a support person, remember to remain at the head of the table so you can hold a woman's hand or put a hand on her shoulder if she needs the support of physical contact. Give explanations of what is happening, what she might be feeling (such as pressure), and what the examiner is doing as needed. Conversation with the examiner over her head is not helpful. Suggesting a woman breathe in and out (not hold her breath as she is likely to do) is a good technique to help her relax (holding her breath pushes the diaphragm down and makes the pelvic organs tense and unyielding).

If desired, a woman may watch the pelvic examination with an overhead mirror or a mirror held by herself or the examiner. Seeing vaginal and cervical anatomy can help her understand any kind of problem she might have and the interventions necessary to improve it. The pelvic examination can be used as a teachable moment for sexually active women to learn how to do a monthly perineal examination so they can detect perineal lesions.

External Genitalia. A pelvic examination begins with inspection of the external genitalia. Any signs of inflammation, infection, ulcerations, lesions, vaginal discharge, or circumcision are noted.

A herpes simplex 2 viral infection appears as clustered, pinpoint vesicles on an erythematous (reddened) base on the vulva that feel painful when touched or irritated. It is important that these are detected during pregnancy because the presence of herpes lesions on the vulva or vagina at the time of birth may necessitate cesarean birth to prevent exposing the fetus to the virus during passage through the birth canal. Note the presence of a herpes infection in the woman's record so she can receive future follow-up care with scheduled cytologic (Pap) smears after the pregnancy because there is an association between herpes simplex 2 infections and the development of cervical cancer in later life (Zheng, 2012).

Next, the Skene glands that empty into the urethra and Bartholin glands that enter into the posterior vagina are checked for size and consistency. If they are swollen or emit a discharge, the discharge is cultured because an infection here could be caused by something as simple as streptococci; it may also be a more serious infection such as gonorrhea that could cause subfertility in the woman and conjunctivitis in her newborn.

Problems with vaginal muscle wall support, such as a rectocele (a forward pouching of the rectum into the posterior vaginal wall) or a cystocele (a pouching of the bladder into the anterior vaginal wall), are usually evaluated next. To reveal these, while the labia are gently separated to allow a view of the vaginal walls, a woman is asked to bear down as if she were moving her bowels, an action that will reveal irregular pouching on the vaginal walls.

Internal Genitalia. To view the cervix, the vagina must be opened and held open with a speculum. Use warm water to lubricate speculum blades because even a water-soluble lubricant might interfere with the interpretation of the Pap smear that will be taken. Use warm rather than cold water so a woman does not contract her vaginal muscles when she feels the cold instrument.

A speculum is introduced with the blades in a closed position and directed toward the less sensitive posterior rather than the anterior vaginal wall (see Fig. 11.4A). A speculum enters most readily if it is inserted at an oblique angle (the crease of the blades directed to 4:00 or 8:00), then rotated to a horizontal position when fully inserted (the crease of the blades pointing to a 3:00 or 9:00 position) (see Fig. 11.4B). When fully inserted and rotated to this horizontal position, the blades are opened and the cervix becomes visible. They are secured in the open position by a thumb screw (metal speculum) or sliding latch (plastic speculum) at the side (see Fig. 11.4C).

With the speculum in place, the cervix is inspected for position. Normally, the uterine cervix is centered in the vagina; the cervix of a retroverted uterus will be positioned anteriorly, and the cervix of an anteverted uterus is positioned posteriorly. The cervix color (a nonpregnant cervix is light pink; in pregnancy, it changes to almost purple) and any lesions, ulcerations, discharge, or otherwise abnormal appearance are documented.

In a **nulligravida** (a woman who is not now or never has been pregnant), the cervical os appears round and small (Fig. 11.6A1). In a woman who has had a previous vaginal birth, the cervical os has much more of a slitlike appearance (see Fig. 11.6A2). If a woman had a cervical tear during a previous birth, the cervical os may appear as a transverse crease the width of the cervix or a typical star-like (stellate) formation (see Fig. 11.6A3).

If a cervical infection is present, cervical lesions (herpes simplex 2; see Fig. 11.6B1), chancre (syphilis; see Fig. 11.6B2), or a mucus discharge may be present. With infection, the epithelium of the cervical canal often enlarges and spreads onto the area surrounding the os, giving the cervix a reddened appearance that bleeds easily (**erosion**; see Fig. 11.6B3).

Typical infections that might be found are trichomoniasis, candidal (yeast) infection, gonorrhea, and chlamydia. Trichomoniasis, a protozoal infection, if present, causes petechial spots on the vaginal walls, cervical redness, and a profuse, whitish, bubbly discharge (Gulmezoglu & Azhar, 2011). A candidal

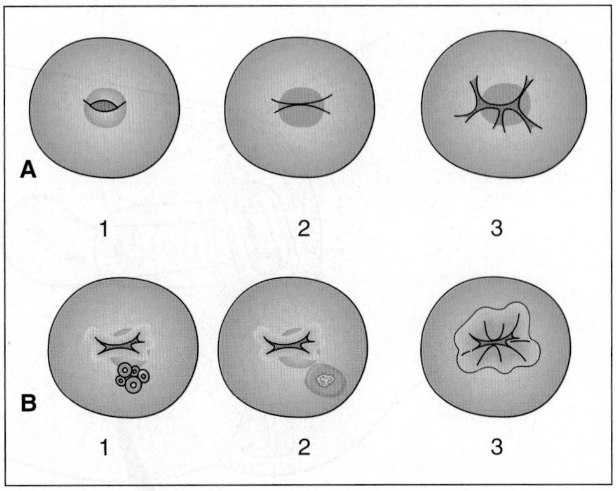

FIGURE 11.6 **(A)** Appearances of the cervix. *(1)* Nulligravida cervix. *(2)* Cervix after childbirth. *(3)* "Stellate" cervix seen after mild cervical tearing. **(B)** Possible cervical lesions. *(1)* Herpes simplex 2. *(2)* Chancre of syphilis. *(3)* Erosion or infection.

infection causes an itching and burning sensation in addition to producing a clumpy cheeselike discharge that may cause bleeding if scraped away from the vaginal walls. A gonorrhea infection presents with a thick, greenish-yellow discharge and extreme inflammation. Chlamydia is called a "silent" or "invisible" infection because it shows almost no external symptoms but internally may cause a mucopurulent cervical discharge and slight cervical redness (Mylonas, 2012).

A nonpregnant woman needs medication to relieve discomfort from these infections. A pregnant woman needs medication to not only relieve discomfort but also to prevent preterm birth or transmission of the infection to the newborn as the newborn passes through the birth canal at term (Kalkanci, Güzel, Khalil, et al., 2012). A candidal infection in the newborn, for example, causes thrush or *oral candidiasis*. A chlamydia infection can cause pneumonia or conjunctivitis in a newborn. Gonorrhea causes such a severe conjunctivitis that it can lead to blindness (Owens, 2012). Specific therapies for these infections are discussed in Chapter 47.

Carcinoma of the cervix appears as an irregular, granular growth (Tewari & Monk, 2012). Cervical polyps (red, soft, pedunculated benign protrusions) are also occasionally seen at the os to the cervix. Women should have a first Pap smear to detect cervical cancer when they reach 21 years of age and then every 3 years thereafter (Simon, 2012).

Papanicolaou Smear. A Pap smear is taken from the endocervix at a first prenatal visit to be certain a precancerous or cancerous condition of the uterine cervix, vulva, or vagina is not present (Fig. 11.7). In addition, a photograph of the cervix may be taken to document the appearance of a suspicious lesion on the cervix or confirm that a previous lesion from an infection has healed.

To obtain a specimen for a Pap smear, a small broomlike collection device is inserted into the endocervical canal and rotated to scrape cells from both the exterior and internal cervix. The cells obtained by the device are then rinsed off in a special collection vial filled with a fixative solution; the vial is then capped, labeled, and sent to the laboratory where the cells are computer analyzed.

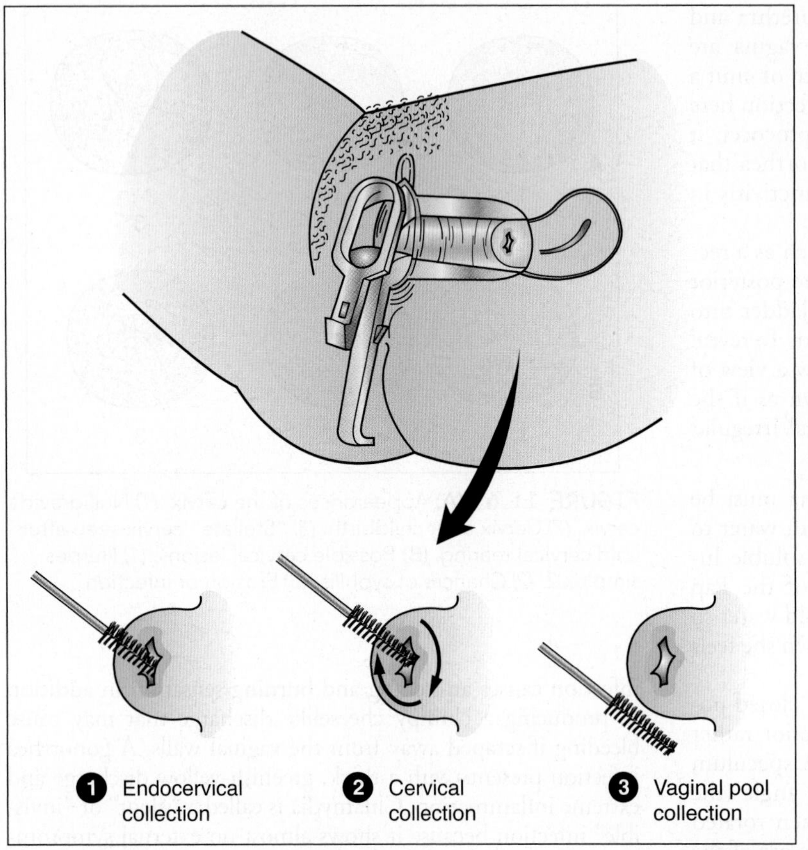

FIGURE 11.7 Obtaining a Papanicolaou smear from the cervix.

The most commonly used classification system used to interpret Pap smears is the Bethesda system shown in Table 11.4. Be certain when discussing results of Pap exams with woman that they are not overinterpreting results (Mackay, 2012). As shown in Table 11.4, the first three levels describing squamous cells reveal some abnormal cells are present, but only the last category indicates that cancer is present.

Women who engage in anal intercourse may have an anal swab taken as well as vaginal swabs to detect anal squamous neoplasms. The technique for obtaining an anal Pap smear is the same as that for vaginal specimens (a cytobrush is used). Caution the patient that she may have slight rectal bleeding following this procedure so she isn't unnecessarily concerned.

What if...11.3 The foot of an examining table in a clinic faces the room door, leaving women to feel exposed if someone should walk in unexpectedly. This saves an examiner steps, but is this the best position for the table?

Vaginal Inspection. Before the vaginal speculum is removed, a culture for trichomoniasis (microscope slide wet mount sample) or group B *Streptococcus* (done at 34 to 36 weeks gestation) may be taken. A Pap test specimen can be analyzed for gonorrhea, chlamydia, and HPV, so a separate swab for these infections is not required. Treatment to eliminate all of these infections during early pregnancy helps guard maternal, fetal, and newborn health (Edmonds, 2012).

A speculum must be unlocked and partially closed before removal; otherwise, pain from excessive stretching could

TABLE 11.4 Interpretation of Pap Smears by the Bethesda System

Finding	Interpretation
Negative	No precancerous or cancerous cells are found.
Squamous Cells	
Atypical squamous cells (ASC)	Some cells appear different than normal, but cannot be classified as precancerous.
Low-grade squamous intraepithelial lesion (LSIL)	Mild precancerous changes may have been found in some cells.
High-grade squamous intraepithelial lesion (HSIL)	Moderate to severe precancerous changes may have been found in some cells.
Squamous cell carcinoma	Cancerous cells are present.
Glandular Cells	
Atypical glandular cells	There is an increased risk of precancer or cancerous cells.
Adenocarcinoma	Cancerous cells are present.

From Mackay, H. T. (2012). Gynecologic disorders. In S. J. McPhee, M. Papadakis, & M. W. Radow (Eds.), *Current medical diagnosis and treatment* (pp. 727–759). Columbus, OH: McGraw-Hill.

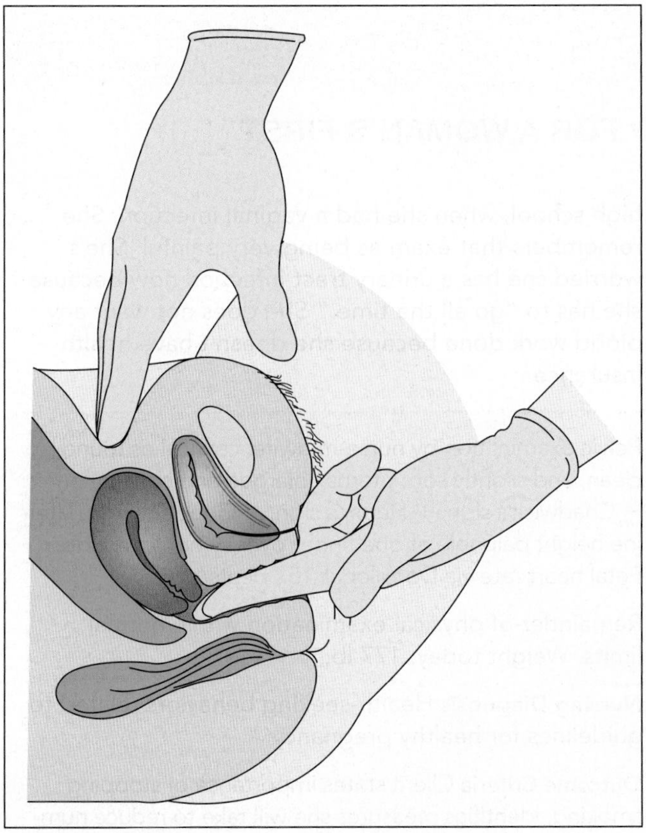

FIGURE 11.8 A bimanual examination to determine uterine size.

occur. If the speculum is kept partially open as it is removed, however, it should not cause pain, and the sides of the vagina can be inspected as it is withdrawn. In a nonpregnant woman, vaginal walls are light pink; pregnancy turns them dark blue to purple. Any areas of inflammation, ulceration, lesions, or discharge should be noted.

Examination of Pelvic Organs. Following the speculum examination, a bimanual (two-handed) examination is performed to assess the position, contour, consistency, and tenderness of pelvic organs (Fig. 11.8). The index and middle fingers of a gloved hand are lubricated and inserted into the vagina so the walls of the vagina can be palpated for abnormalities. The other hand is then placed on a woman's abdomen and pressed downward toward the hand still in the vagina until the uterus can be felt between them. Next, the right and left ovaries are identified by the same method. Ovaries are normally slightly tender, so the pressure caused by palpation may cause a woman some discomfort.

Abnormalities that can be noted by bimanual examination include ovarian cysts, enlarged fallopian tubes (perhaps from pelvic inflammatory disease), and an enlarged uterus. An early sign of pregnancy (Hegar's sign) is elicited on bimanual examination as well (see Chapter 10, Fig. 10.4).

Rectovaginal Examination. After a bimanual pelvic examination, the hand is withdrawn from the vagina. The index finger is reinserted into the vagina and the middle finger into the rectum. By palpating the tissue between the examining fingers in this way, it is possible to assess the strength and irregularity of the posterior vaginal wall. This maneuver may be slightly uncomfortable for a woman because of rectal pressure. Some examiners use a clean pair of gloves before they perform a rectovaginal examination so they will not spread an infection from the vagina to the rectum. After the rectal examination, if it is necessary to re-examine the vagina for any reason, the glove must be changed to avoid contaminating the vagina with fecal material.

After completing the examination, any excess lubricant is wiped away from the vaginal and rectal openings. Be certain to wipe front to back to prevent bringing rectal contamination forward from the rectum to the vagina. Box 11.7 shows an interprofessional care map illustrating both nursing and team planning for a first prenatal visit including support during a pelvic examination.

QSEN Checkpoint Question 11.5

Teamwork & Collaboration

Sandra has not had a pelvic examination since she was in high school. Consequently, the nurse-midwife has asked you to help make her more at ease during her first prenatal pelvic examination. What nursing action should you take?

a. Have her take a deep breath and hold it as long as she can during the examination.
b. Tell her to bear down slightly as the speculum is inserted.
c. Encourage her to moan in a low-pitched tone because this will push down the diaphragm.
d. Teach her to breathe slowly and evenly while being examined.

Look in Appendix A for the best answer and rationale.

The Pelvis: Establishing Adequacy for Childbirth

The pelvis is a bony ring formed by four united bones: the two innominate (flaring hip) bones, which form the anterior and lateral portion of the ring, and the coccyx and sacrum, which form the posterior aspect (Fig. 11.9). The pelvis serves both to support and protect pelvic organs.

- Each innominate bone is divided into three parts: *ilium*, *ischium*, and *pubis*.
- The ilium forms the upper and lateral portion. The flaring superior border forms the prominence of the hip (the crest of the ilium).
- The ischium is the inferior portion.
- At the lowest portion of the ischium are two projections: the ischial tuberosities, or the part of the bone on which a person sits. These projections are important markers used to determine lower pelvic width.
- The ischial spines are small projections that extend from the lateral aspects of the pelvis into the pelvic cavity. They mark the midpoint of the pelvis. Their location is used to assess the level to which a fetus has descended into the birth canal just before or during labor.
- Where the two anterior portions of the innominate bone meet is the symphysis pubis.
- The sacrum is the upper posterior portion of the pelvic ring. There is a marked anterior projection of this bone at the point where it touches the lower lumbar vertebrae (the sacral prominence), which is used as a landmark when securing pelvic measurements.

BOX 11.7 Nursing Care Planning

AN INTERPROFESSIONAL CARE MAP FOR A WOMAN'S FIRST PRENATAL VISIT

Sandra Czerinski is a 29-year-old woman, 12 weeks pregnant, who comes for a first prenatal visit. She's concerned because she didn't realize she was pregnant until a week ago. As a result, she has been actively dieting plus lifting weights at a health club. She hasn't had a pelvic examination since she was in high school, when she had a vaginal infection. She remembers that exam as being very painful. She's worried she has a urinary tract infection now because she has to "go all the time." She does not want any blood work done because she doesn't have health insurance.

Family Assessment Single woman; lives by self in one-bedroom apartment. Works at a laundry. Boyfriend is a roofing salesman; out of town 4 days a week.

Client Assessment Gravida 1, para 0. Last menstrual period 3 months ago. Had nausea last month but thought it was the "flu."

Menarche at age 11 years; menstrual cycle every 29 days, 6 days duration with moderate flow and mild cramps. Past history positive for sinusitis; appendectomy at age 12 years. Smokes about ½ pack per day, "more when I'm stressed at work"; denies alcohol use. "I drink club soda with lime or mineral water."

ROS: Height, 5 ft 5 in.; prepregnancy weight, 160 lb (BMI: 27.5 or overweight). Slight gingival hyperplasia; breasts full and slightly tender.

Pelvic examination by nurse-midwife: cervical os round, clean, and slightly soft; uterus enlarged and soft; + Chadwick's sign, + Hegar's sign, + Goodell's sign. Uterine height palpable at one finger over symphysis pubis. Fetal heart rate via Doppler at 152 beats/min

Remainder of physical examination within normal limits. Weight today: 177 lb.

Nursing Diagnosis Health-seeking behaviors related to guidelines for healthy pregnancy

Outcome Criteria Client states importance of stopping smoking, identifies measures she will take to reduce number of cigarettes smoked per day, and states she will no longer try to lose weight. Makes appointment for follow-up visits.

Team Member Responsible	Assessment	Intervention	Rationale	Expected Outcome
Activities of Daily Living, Including Safety				
Nurse/Nurse-midwife	Assess client's expectations about this pregnancy, including whether she expects to continue to work and continue present lifestyle.	Discuss the effect of pregnancy on her partner and any religious or cultural beliefs that would interfere with her ability to adapt to pregnancy changes.	Assessing expectations is important to assist a woman in identifying areas of need and adaptation necessary for pregnancy.	Client describes the likely effect of the pregnancy on herself and partner; identifies areas where she anticipates life changes.
Teamwork and Collaboration				
Nurse/Nurse-midwife	Fully assess symptoms of urinary frequency to rule out urinary tract infection; collect clean-catch urine specimen.	Discuss with client a few laboratory tests are necessary to ensure a safe pregnancy.	Urinary tract infections are associated with preterm birth. Client has no health insurance.	Nurse-midwife documents urinary tract infection and prescribes or give samples of appropriate antibiotic if indicated.
Procedures/Medications for Quality Improvement				
Nurse/Nurse-midwife	Establish baseline findings of present health.	Obtain initial health history and physical exam.	Initial assessment provides a baseline for future comparison and identification of factors that may place a client at risk.	Client receives a thorough initial assessment, to lay a psychological and physiologic foundation of health care information for prenatal care.

Nurse	Obtain additional measures of wellness during pregnancy.	Obtain weight, vital signs, urine and blood specimens.	A baseline weight and vital signs are necessary for future comparison.	Client's weight and vital signs are monitored and compared with previous values at each prenatal visit.
Nutrition				
Nurse/Nutritionist	Obtain a 24-hour nutrition recall.	Discuss with client her increased nutritional needs during pregnancy. Provide information about a high-protein diet with prenatal vitamin supplementation.	A well-balanced diet with adequate fluid intake and use of prenatal vitamins helps to ensure an optimal environment for fetal growth and development.	Client voices an understanding of the increased food she needs during pregnancy. Client voices she will discontinue dieting.
Patient-Centered Care				
Nurse	Assess if client is interested in decreasing smoking during pregnancy.	Instruct client in the effects of smoking on the fetus. Assist client with methods to reduce and stop, if possible.	Nicotine in cigarettes has been shown to be teratogenic to a fetus.	Based on the fetal effects of nicotine, client describes a plan to stop smoking at least until after the birth and, ideally, long term.
Nurse	Assess if client is aware of the danger signs of pregnancy she will need to report immediately should they occur.	Instruct client about possible danger signs. Emphasize that although these signs are important, they do not necessarily mean something is wrong.	Knowledge of possible danger signs allows for early detection and prompt intervention should it be necessary.	Client and partner list danger signs of pregnancy to report immediately.
Psychosocial/Spiritual/Emotional Needs				
Nurse	Assess if client has questions or concerns about success of pregnancy.	Assure client that concern during pregnancy is a normal response. Include information about physiologic and psychological changes of pregnancy.	Anxiety can interfere with ability to adjust to pregnancy. Reviewing information reinforces understanding.	Client describes any concerns about pregnancy and receives appropriate information or assurance.
Informatics for Seamless Health Care Planning				
Nurse	Assess whether client will have any difficulty continuing with prenatal care.	Assist client with setting up appointments for future visits keeping in mind that she has no health insurance.	Assisting with appointment setting helps to ensure adherence.	Client states plan for expected antepartal care visits and affirms her willingness to adhere to the plan.

- The coccyx, just below the sacrum, is composed of five very small bones fused together. Although the bone itself is stiff, there is a degree of movement possible in the joint between the sacrum and the coccyx (the sacrococcygeal joint). This movement is important during labor because it permits the coccyx to be pressed backward, allowing more room for the fetal head to pass through the bony pelvic ring at birth.

For obstetric purposes, the pelvis is further divided into the false pelvis (the superior half) and the true pelvis (the inferior half) (Fig. 11.10). The false pelvis supports the uterus during the late months of pregnancy and aids in directing the fetus into the true pelvis for birth. The false pelvis is divided from the true pelvis only by an imaginary line, the linea terminalis. This imaginary line is drawn from the sacral prominence at the back of the pelvis to the superior aspect of the symphysis pubis at the front.

Other important terms in relation to the pelvis are the inlet, the outlet, and the pelvic cavity.

- The *inlet* is the entrance to the true pelvis, or the upper ring of bone through which the fetus must pass to be born vaginally. It is at the level of the linea terminalis or is marked by the sacral prominence in the back, the ilium on the sides, and the superior aspect of the symphysis pubis in the front. If you looked down at the pelvic inlet, the passageway would appear heart-shaped because of the jutting sacral prominence. It is wider transversely (sideways) than in the anteroposterior dimension.

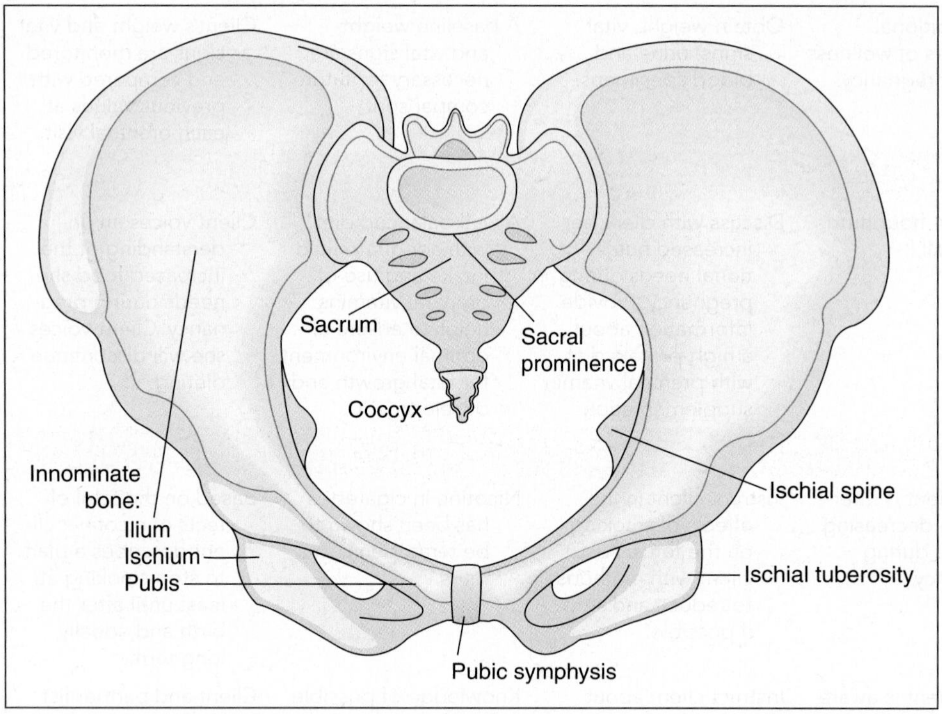

FIGURE 11.9 Structure of the pelvis.

- The *outlet* is the inferior portion of the pelvis, or that portion bounded in the back by the coccyx, on the sides by the ischial tuberosities, and in the front by the inferior aspect of the symphysis pubis. In contrast to the inlet of the pelvis, the greatest diameter of the outlet is its anteroposterior diameter.

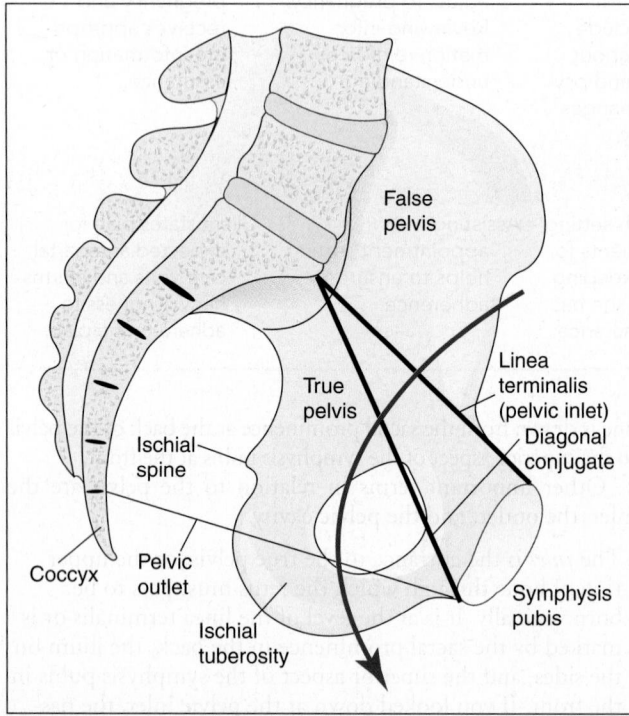

FIGURE 11.10 True and false pelvis. Portion above linea terminalis is false pelvis; portion below is true pelvis. *Arrow* shows "stovepipe" curve the fetus must follow to be born.

- The *pelvic cavity* is the space between the inlet and the outlet. This space is not a straight but a curved passage; the purpose of its curve is to slow and control the speed of birth. This helps reduce sudden pressure changes in the fetal head, lowering the danger of ruptured cerebral arteries. The snugness of the cavity also serves to compress the chest of the fetus as he or she passes through. This helps to expel lung fluid and mucus and thereby better prepare lungs for good aeration at birth.

For a baby to be born vaginally, he or she must be able to pass through the inlet, the cavity, and the outlet of the pelvic bone. This is not a problem for the average fetus; it may, however, be a problem if the mother is a young adolescent who has not yet achieved full pelvic growth (girls younger than age 14 years are most prone to this difficulty) or a woman who has had a pelvic injury from something such as an automobile accident.

Estimating Pelvic Size

It is impossible to predict from the outward appearance of a woman whether her pelvic ring will be adequate for a fetus to pass through its center without difficulty. This is because some women appear to have a wide pelvis but, in reality, have only wide iliac crests and a normal or even smaller-than-usual internal ring. Other women look as if their pelvis will be small because the iliac crests are nonflaring, but the internal pelvis, the part that must be sufficiently large for childbirth, is of average size, allowing them to give birth vaginally without difficulty.

Differences in pelvic contour occur mainly because of hereditary factors, but disease such as rickets, now rarely seen in the United States but still a concern in undeveloped countries, may cause contraction of the pelvis and severely narrow the pelvic outlet (Mughal, 2011).

If on an initial prenatal visit, the primary care provider establishes that a woman is pregnant, and if she has never given birth vaginally before, pelvic measurements may be taken. Some care providers prefer, however, to take these measurements later in pregnancy, when a woman's pelvic muscles are more relaxed, making measurement easier. Estimation of pelvic adequacy must be done at least by the 24th week of pregnancy, because by this time there is danger that the fetal head has reached a size that would interfere with safe passage and birth if the pelvic measurements are small.

Once a woman has given birth vaginally, her pelvis has been proven adequate for vaginal birth, so it is unnecessary for pelvic measurements to be repeated unless she had an intervening history or trauma to the pelvis between pregnancies.

Types of pelves found in women can be categorized into four groups (Fig. 11.11): android, anthropoid, gynecoid, and platypelloid.

- A *gynecoid*, or "female," pelvis has an inlet that is well rounded forward and backward and has a wide pubic arch. This pelvic type is ideal for childbirth.
- In an *android*, or "male," pelvis, the pubic arch forms an acute angle, making the lower dimensions of the pelvis extremely narrow. A fetus may have difficulty exiting from this type of pelvis.
- In an *anthropoid*, or "ape-like," pelvis, the transverse diameter is narrow; the anteroposterior diameter of the inlet is larger than usual. Even though the inlet is large, the shape of the pelvis does not accommodate a fetal head as well as a gynecoid pelvis.
- A *platypelloid*, or "flattened," pelvis has a smoothly curved oval inlet, but the anteroposterior diameter is shallow. A fetal head might not be able to rotate to match the curves of the pelvic cavity.

Internal pelvic measurements reveal the diameters of the inlet and outlet and can be obtained by pelvimetry at the time of a routine sonogram examination done to date a pregnancy. The following measurements are most commonly determined:

- The **diagonal conjugate** is the measurement between the anterior surface of the sacral prominence and the posterior surface of the symphysis pubis. The average measurement is 10.5 to 11 cm.
- The **ischial tuberosity** diameter is the distance between the ischial tuberosities, or the transverse diameter of the outlet (the narrowest diameter at that level, or the one most apt to cause a misfit). It is made at the medial and lowermost aspect of the ischial tuberosities at the level of the anus. A diameter of 11 cm is considered adequate because it will allow the widest diameter of the fetal head, or 9 cm, to pass freely through the outlet.

Laboratory Assessment

A number of laboratory studies are included as part of assessment at a first prenatal visit to confirm general health and rule out sexually transmitted infection that could injure a growing

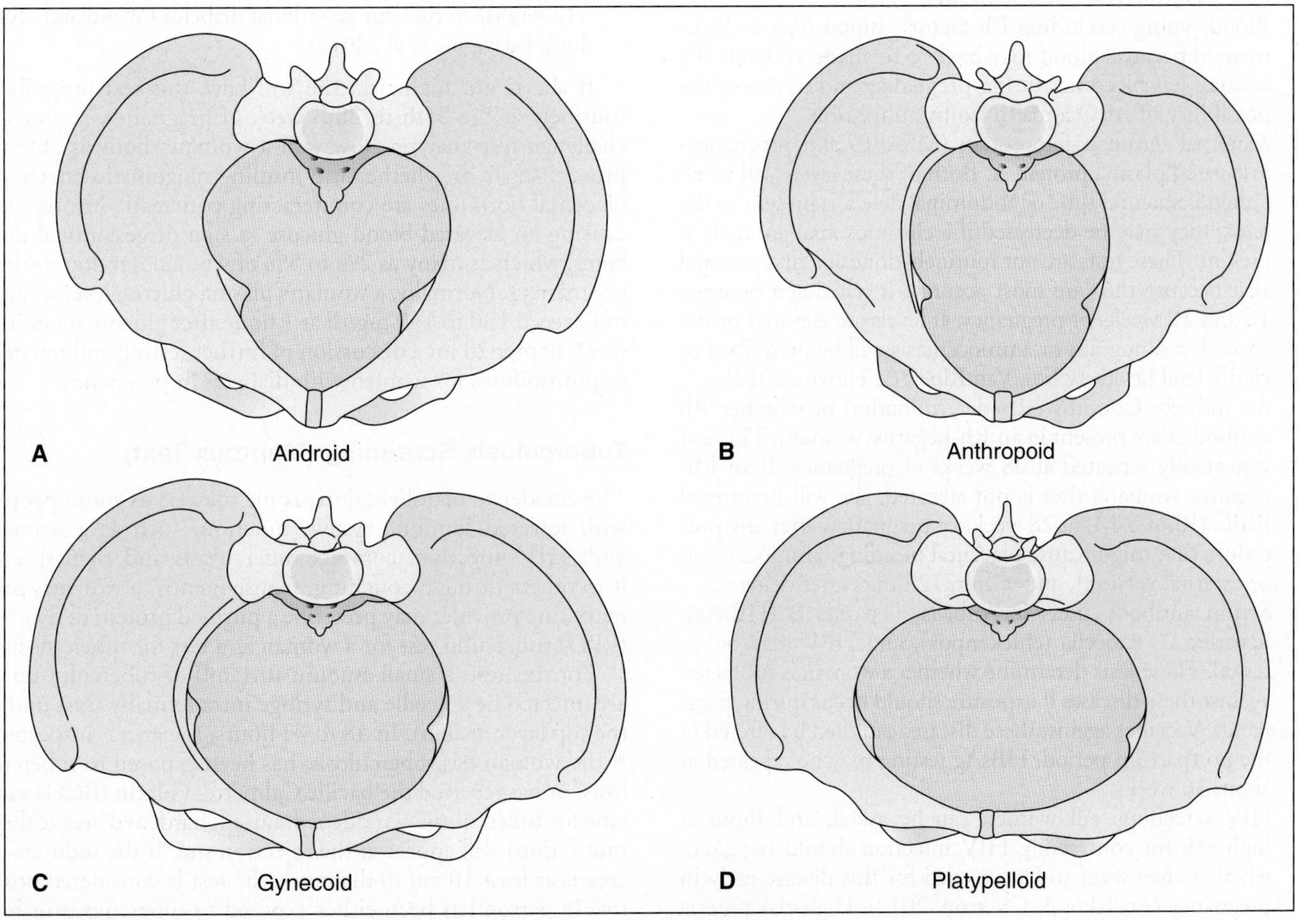

FIGURE 11.11 Types of pelves. **(A)** *Android*, or "male," pelvis. **(B)** *Anthropoid*, or "ape-like," pelvis. **(C)** *Gynecoid*, or "female," pelvis. **(D)** *Platypelloid*, or "flattened," pelvis.

fetus. Normal levels for these studies are available at http://thePoint.lww.com/Pillitteri7e.

Urinalysis

Urine is tested for proteinuria (protein in urine), glycosuria (glucose in urine), nitrites (bacteria in urine), and pyuria (white blood cells in urine suggesting an infection). All four of these can be assessed by point of care tests, or the urine can be sent for microscopic examination in a laboratory.

Blood Serum Studies

The following serum studies are usually obtained at a first prenatal visit:

1. A complete blood count, including hemoglobin or hematocrit and red cell index to determine the presence of anemia, a white blood cell count to determine infection, and a platelet count to estimate clotting ability.
2. A genetic screen for common ethnically inherited diseases. African American women, for example, may have a blood sample taken to screen for sickle-cell trait or disease and glucose-6-phosphate dehydrogenase (G6PD). Asian and Mediterranean women may have this done for beta-thalassemia, those with Jewish ancestry may have this done for Tay-Sachs disease, and Caucasian women may be tested to see if they are a carrier for cystic fibrosis.
3. A serologic test for syphilis (VDRL or rapid plasma reagin test). If syphilis is present, it must be treated early in pregnancy before fetal damage occurs.
4. Blood typing (including Rh factor). Blood type is documented because blood may have to be made available if a woman has bleeding during pregnancy and to detect the possibility of ABO and Rh isoimmunization.
5. Maternal serum α-fetoprotein (MSAFP) and pregnancy-associated plasma protein A. Both of these levels will be elevated if a neural tube or abdominal defect is present in the fetus; they may be decreased if a chromosomal anomaly is present. These tests are not routinely done at a first prenatal visit because they are most accurate if scheduled between 16 and 18 weeks of pregnancy. If levels are elevated or decreased, a sonogram or amniocentesis will be prescribed to clarify fetal health (Choi, Van Riper, & Thoyre, 2012).
6. An indirect Coombs test (determination of whether Rh antibodies are present in an Rh-negative woman). This test is generally repeated at 28 weeks of pregnancy. If an Rh-negative woman's titer is not elevated, she will be offered RhIG (RhoGAM) at 28 weeks of pregnancy, after any procedure that might cause placental bleeding (amniocentesis or external version), and within 72 hours after delivery.
7. Serum antibody titers for rubella, hepatitis B (HBsAg), hepatitis C, varicella (chickenpox), and HPV may be assessed. These tests determine whether a woman is protected against these diseases if exposure should occur during pregnancy. Vaccines against these diseases can then be offered in the postpartum period. HBsAg testing may be repeated at about 36 weeks.
8. HIV screening. All women can be asked, and those at high risk for contracting HIV infection should be asked, whether they want to be screened for this disease early in pregnancy (Attilakos & Overton, 2012). High-risk criteria include women who have used or are using intravenous drugs; have engaged in sex with multiple partners; have had sexual partners who are infected or are at risk because they are bisexual, intravenous drug users, or hemophiliac; or received a blood transfusion between 1977 and 1985.

   Screening for HIV is done by an enzyme-linked immunosorbent assay (ELISA) on a blood sample. If this is positive, the finding is confirmed by a second test (a Western blot). Testing for HIV early in pregnancy allows a woman who is found to be HIV antibody positive the opportunity to begin therapy with zidovudine (AZT), which can decrease the risk of her infant acquiring the virus. It also allows a woman the option of choosing to terminate a pregnancy to avoid giving birth to an infant who has a high risk of HIV infection if she chooses.

   Because there is still no cure for HIV infection, some women may choose not to have a blood titer taken because they would rather not know they have the illness. Screening is not mandatory, so this is their option. Because HIV testing is controversial, be certain the information given about test results is relayed accurately and with tact and compassion (a high blood antibody titer means the woman has been exposed to the virus, not that she is necessarily infected). The result of HIV testing, like all patient information, is confidential; be certain not to report this information to anyone other than the woman.
9. If a woman has a history of previously unexplained fetal loss, has a family history of diabetes, has had babies who were large for gestational age (9 lb or more at term), is obese, or has glycosuria, she will need to be scheduled for a 50-g oral 1-hour glucose loading or tolerance test (sometimes called a glucose challenge test) toward the end of the first trimester (12 weeks) to rule out gestational diabetes (Wendland, Torloni, Falavigna, et al., 2012).

If she is not high risk, she will have this test prescribed routinely at the 24th to 28th week of pregnancy. A glucose challenge test analyzes how well a woman's body is able to process sugar or whether the insulin-antagonistic effects of placental hormones are counteracting pancreatic insulin and causing an elevated blood glucose (a sign of gestational diabetes, which as many as 2% to 5% of woman develop during pregnancy). Normally, a woman's plasma glucose level should not exceed 130 to 140 mg/dl at 1 hour after glucose ingestion (see Chapter 20 for a discussion of further testing and nursing responsibilities for women with diabetes in pregnancy).

Tuberculosis Screening (Mantoux Test)

The incidence of tuberculosis is on the rise as more people with lowered immune system function, such as a woman with HIV infection, contract tuberculosis and then spread it to others through coughing. Consequently, a woman's primary care provider may prescribe a purified protein derivative (PPD) tuberculin test for a woman as a test for tuberculosis.

For this test, a small amount (0.1 ml) of tuberculin units are injected by a needle and syringe intradermally (just under the top layer of skin). In 48 to 72 hours, the area is inspected. If the woman has tuberculosis, has been exposed to tuberculosis, or has received the bacille Calmette–Guérin (BCG) vaccine for tuberculosis, a reddened, raised, hardened area (called induration) will appear at the injection site. If the induration area is at least 10 cm in diameter, the test is considered positive (a person has been either exposed to tuberculosis or has tuberculosis); in a person with a lowered immune response, 5 cm can be considered a positive result.

If a woman has a positive result, a chest X-ray will be prescribed to assess her current disease status. Women are often reluctant to have X-rays done during pregnancy because they know radiation is harmful to a growing fetus. You can assure her that her fetus will be protected as long as she is given a lead apron to cover her abdomen.

Tuberculosis screening may also be done by a blood serum test called an interferon-gamma release assay (IGRA). IGRA testing is the preferred method because:

- In a woman who has a history of tuberculosis or who has received the BCG vaccine, a PPD test can cause an extreme reaction. BCG vaccine is not administered to people in the United States, but women from other countries may have received it.
- It can offer results for a woman who states it will be difficult for her to return for a follow-up appointment for a PPD test to be read and interpreted.

Screening for tuberculosis early in pregnancy is important because it is a chronic and debilitating disease that increases the risk of miscarriage. Further, the change in the shape of the maternal lung tissue as the growing uterus presses on the lungs may reactivate already healed lesions, thus worsening the disease (McCarthy, 2012).

Ultrasonography

If the date of the last menstrual period is unknown, a woman will be scheduled for a sonogram to confirm the pregnancy length and document healthy fetal growth at 7 to 11 weeks of pregnancy. A sonogram can also be scheduled between 16 and 20 weeks gestation to verify healthy fetal structures and gender. Be certain women know that a sonogram done under 8 weeks will show only the presence of a gestation sac, not a moving, kicking fetus, so their expectations of what they will see are not disappointing (Russell, Denne, & Schwartz, 2011).

Risk Assessment

Following information gathering at a first prenatal visit, findings are analyzed to determine whether a pregnancy is apt to continue with a good outcome or there is likely to be some risk that it will end before term or with an unfavorable fetal or maternal outcome (a high-risk pregnancy).

Table 11.5 lists a minimum of factors that would identify a pregnancy as high risk. A woman identified as high risk will need close observation during prenatal visits to be certain the pregnancy is progressing well; the infant born of a woman identified this way needs close observation in the neonatal period until it is confirmed the newborn is responding well to postuterine life.

Risk assessment should be updated at each prenatal visit because events can cause a pregnancy first rated as low risk to change to high risk. Chapters 20 through 22 discuss specific conditions that cause high-risk pregnancy and nursing for these responsibilities.

SIGNS INDICATING POSSIBLE COMPLICATIONS OF PREGNANCY

Although most signs that suggest a complication may be occurring appear toward the end of pregnancy, women need to be aware of what these are from the beginning. To introduce the topic of danger signs, assure a woman you have every reason to believe she is going to have a normal, uncomplicated pregnancy (assuming that is true) but, if any danger signs do occur, you want her to be informed as to what they are so she can inform her health care provider by telephone or e-mail immediately. Be certain you give her an alternate contact number to call if the health care facility is closed. Assure her as well that if one of these danger signs should occur, it serves merely as a signal of the possibility that something may be happening, not that something serious has already happened. It is important for her to report a danger sign immediately, though, so it can be dealt with before something harmful does occur. A pregnant woman should report the following signs or symptoms immediately:

- Vaginal bleeding. A woman should report vaginal bleeding, no matter how slight, because some of the serious bleeding complications of pregnancy begin with only slight spotting. If a woman reports bleeding, ask her how she discovered the blood. If she found it on toilet paper following a bowel movement, she's probably reporting spotting from hemorrhoids. Until the bleeding is found to be innocent this way, however, all women with spotting need further evaluation.
- Persistent vomiting. Once- or twice-daily vomiting is not uncommon during the first trimester of pregnancy. Persistent, frequent vomiting is not normal nor is vomiting that continues past the 12th week of pregnancy. Persistent or extended vomiting depletes the nutritional supply available to a fetus and thus is a danger to the pregnancy. (See Chapter 13 for an in-depth discussion of persistent vomiting [hyperemesis gravidarum].)
- Chills and fever or pain on urination. Chills and fever may be symptoms of a relatively benign gastroenteritis, but they also may indicate an intrauterine infection, a potentially serious complication for both a woman and a fetus. Pain on urination is a symptom of a urinary infection, which is potentially serious because these infections are associated with preterm birth. Because a woman cannot make a definite determination about the cause of a fever herself, further evaluation by a health care provider is necessary.
- Sudden escape of clear fluid from the vagina. When a gush of clear fluid is discharged suddenly from the vagina, it means the membranes have ruptured and mother and fetus are now both threatened because the uterine cavity is no longer sealed against infection. If a fetus is small so the head does not fit snugly into the cervix, the umbilical cord may prolapse. If the fetal head then presses on the misplaced cord, oxygenation can be compromised and the fetus will be in immediate and grave danger. Alerting a health care provider to any sudden escape of fluid is crucial so a safe and controlled birth can be planned.

Occasionally, a woman confuses stress incontinence (involuntary loss of urine on coughing or sneezing or lifting a heavy object) for membranes breaking. In this situation, vaginal examination typically reveals that the membranes are still intact and the pregnancy is not in danger. Urine can be identified by nitrazine paper as urine is acidotic (the test strip turns yellow), whereas amniotic fluid is alkaline (the strip turns blue).

- Abdominal or chest pain. Abdominal or chest pain at any time is a signal something is abnormal, so a woman should also report these immediately. Some women may think abdominal pain is normal because the growing uterus is

TABLE 11.5 Assessments That Might Categorize a Pregnancy as At Risk

Assessment	Risk Factors
Obstetric history	Existing uterine or cervical anomaly History of subfertility, recurrent miscarriages, or grand multiparity Last pregnancy less than 1 year previous History of abnormal Pap smear Previous premature cervical dilatation, preterm labor, preterm birth, low–birth-weight infant, or cesarean birth Previous macrosomic infant or multiple gestation Previous abnormal gestational trophoblastic disease Previous ectopic pregnancy or stillborn/neonatal death Previous infant with neurologic deficit, birth injury, or congenital anomaly
Past illness history	A chronic disease such as diabetes mellitus, heart disease, renal disease, or chronic hypertension Emotional disorder or cognitive challenge Family history of severe inherited disorders Fibroid tumors or previous surgeries on reproductive organs Maternal reproductive tract anomalies or malignancy Seizure disorders Sexually transmitted infections Surgery required during pregnancy
Current obstetric status	Abnormal fetal surveillance tests Abnormal presentation; fetal version necessary Premature separation of the placenta or placenta previa Cervical cerclage Limited prenatal care Maternal weight loss or weight gain less than 10 lb by midpregnancy Multiple gestation or hydramnios (excessive amniotic fluid) Gestational hypertension or preeclampsia Premature rupture of membranes or preterm labor Rh sensitization Sexually transmitted infection
Psychosocial factors	Attempt or ideation of self-injury Dangerous occupation Lack of support people Inadequate finances; inadequate nutrition or poor housing Lack of acceptance of pregnancy
Demographic factors	Maternal age under 16 or over 40 years
Lifestyle	Alcohol use during pregnancy Smoking greater than 10 cigarettes a day or living with a person who smokes this much Heavy lifting or long periods of standing Recreational drug use Unusual stress

deflecting other organs from their usual alignment, but a pregnant uterus normally expands painlessly. Abdominal pain is therefore a sign of some other problem, such as a tubal (ectopic) pregnancy, separation of the placenta, preterm labor, or something unrelated to the pregnancy but perhaps equally serious, such as appendicitis, ulcer, or pancreatitis. Chest pain and shortness of breath may indicate a pulmonary embolus, a complication that can follow thrombophlebitis.

- Gestational hypertension. Gestational hypertension refers to a potentially severe and even fatal elevation of blood pressure that occurs during pregnancy usually after 20 weeks of pregnancy. A number of symptoms signal that gestational hypertension is developing:
  - Rapid weight gain (over 2 lb/week in the second trimester, over 1 lb/week in the third trimester)
  - Swelling of the face or fingers
  - Flashes of light or dots before the eyes
  - Dimness or blurring of vision
  - Severe, continuous headache
  - Decreased urine output
  - Blood pressure increased above 160/90 mmHg

One by one, these are vague symptoms, so a woman may need some help appreciating they are important enough to report during pregnancy. Some edema of the ankles during pregnancy is normal, for example, particularly if it occurs after a woman has been on her feet all day. Swelling of the hands (ask if she has noticed if her rings are tight) or face (difficulty opening eyes in the morning because of edema of the eyelids), however, indicates edema that is more extensive than usual. Visual disturbances or a continuous headache may signal cerebral edema or acute hypertension.

BOX 11.8 Nursing Care Planning to Empower a Family

ASSESSMENTS AND INTERVENTIONS A WOMAN CAN EXPECT AT CONTINUING PRENATAL VISITS

Health Interview

Interim history or new personal or family developments since last visit (every visit)
Review of danger signs of pregnancy (every visit)
Review of symptoms of beginning labor (every visit)
Any new concerns with pregnancy or family since last visit (every visit)

Physical Examination

Blood pressure (every visit)
Clean-catch urine for glucose, protein, and leukocytes (every visit)
Blood serum level for maternal serum α-fetoprotein (MSAFP) and pregnancy-associated plasma protein A (PAPP-A) (at 16 weeks)
VDRL test for syphilis if possibility of new exposure
Glucose screen (24 to 28 weeks)
Glucose challenge (24 to 28 weeks), if warranted
Anti-Rh titer (28 weeks)
Group B *Streptococcus* (GBS) screen (35 to 37 weeks)

Fetal Health

Fetal heart rate counted (every visit)
Fundal height measured (every visit)
Questions about quickening (first fetal movement, which occurs at 16 to 20 weeks) or continuing fetal movement (every visit)
Ultrasound dating of pregnancy (if necessary)
Ultrasound evaluation for fetal health (about 20 weeks)

Be certain a woman is not reporting symptoms such as visual difficulties and headaches she had before she became pregnant. If she had the same symptoms before pregnancy as she is reporting now, she may need to see an ophthalmologist rather than her obstetrician for help with the problem. (See Chapter 21 for an in-depth discussion of gestational hypertension.)

- Increase or decrease in fetal movement. Because a fetus normally moves more or less the same amount every day, an unusual increase or decrease in movement suggests a fetus responding to a need for more oxygen. Be certain to ask a woman about typical fetal movements and whether she has noticed any increase or decrease in this rate. If there has been a change, she is a candidate for further testing such as a fetal "kick count" or a nonstress test. Common tests of fetal movement and health of this type are discussed in Chapter 9.
- Uterine contractions before 37 weeks of pregnancy. Women do have faint and irregular Braxton Hicks contractions prior to this point, but regular rhythmic contractions before 37 weeks suggest preterm birth is beginning. A woman needs to lie down, drink a glass of water to ensure she is well hydrated, and telephone her primary care provider. Such contractions may be innocent, but it is better to report them than to ignore them and allow a preterm birth to continue.

QSEN Checkpoint Question 11.6

Safety

You are reviewing danger signs of pregnancy with Sandra. In the interests of safety, which of the following would you tell her to report if it should occur?

a. Her uterus becomes palpable over the symphysis pubis before 12 weeks.
b. Blue veins appear and can be readily observed on both of her breasts.
c. She gains more than 3 lb a week beginning at 20 weeks.
d. She tends to lose her balance when she wears high-heeled shoes.

Look in Appendix A for the best answer and rationale.

Be certain that after a first prenatal visit, a woman understands she needs to continue with spaced prenatal care. No one likes surprises, so reviewing with a woman what she can expect at future visits can help her understand the importance of keeping them. Box 11.8 lists components of assessments and care important for these continuing prenatal visits.

What if...11.4 You are interested in exploring one of the 2020 National Health Goals related to prenatal care (see Box 11.1). Most government-sponsored money for nursing research is allotted based on these goals. What would be a possible research topic to explore pertinent to these goals that would be applicable to Sandra or her family and also advance evidence-based practice?

Key Points for Review

- The purpose of prenatal care is to establish a baseline of present health, determine the gestational age of the fetus, monitor fetal development, identify women at risk for complications, and minimize the risk of possible complications of pregnancy by anticipating and preventing problems before they occur, as well as providing time for education about pregnancy and possible dangers. Planning nursing care that includes these things and not only meets QSEN competencies but also best meets the family's total needs.
- Prenatal care has the potential to reduce the incidence of preterm birth and the infant mortality rate.
- A first prenatal visit confirms a pregnancy, but it is also a time for important assessments such as a health history, physical examination, and laboratory tests. The physical examination includes measurement of fundal height and assessment of fetal heart sounds if the pregnancy is beyond 12 weeks, a pelvic examination (including a Pap smear and HPV test), and possibly an estimation of pelvic size.
- A first prenatal visit sets the tone for visits to follow. Maintaining a supportive manner is helpful to establish

rapport and allow a woman to feel comfortable returning for future care.

- Common pelvic types include gynecoid (well-rounded with a wide pubic arch), anthropoid (narrow), platypelloid (flattened), and android (male or with a sharp pubic arch). A gynecoid pelvis is ideal for childbearing.
- For a pelvic examination, pregnant women should remain in a lithotomy or supine position for as short a time as possible to help prevent thromboembolism and supine hypotension syndrome.
- Danger signs for women to report during pregnancy are vaginal bleeding, persistent vomiting, chills and fever, escape of fluid from the vagina, abdominal or chest pain, swelling of the face and fingers, vision changes or continuous headache, rhythmic cramping, burning with urination, and a pronounced decrease in fetal movement.
- Remember that a family, not a woman alone, is having a baby, and include family members in procedures and health teaching as desired.

Critical Thinking Care Study

Macie is a 40-year-old, G5 T3 P0 A1 L2 woman pregnant with her fifth child. She had a miscarriage with her second pregnancy, and her last child died at 3 months from sudden infant death syndrome (SIDS). Her other two children are healthy, ages 5 and 3 years. She has heard that using pacifiers and putting babies to sleep on their backs decreases the chance of SIDS and is worried she caused her baby girl's death.

1. Pregnancy creates a vulnerable period for Macie because she may be dealing with both losses from her previous pregnancies. What actions can you take to ensure that Macie will discuss openly her fears and concerns about this pregnancy?
2. Macie works as a cheerleading coach. Her husband works at adding insulation to homes. What special questions would you want to ask her about her job to see if it poses some concerns during pregnancy? About her husband's job?
3. How could grieving for the loss of her children affect Macie's adaptation to this pregnancy?

Patient Scenario
The Newman Family

Read about the Newman family, a family who comes for a first prenatal visit, then answer the questions to further sharpen your skills and grow more familiar with NCLEX-type questions related to prenatal assessment. Confirm your answers are correct by reading the rationales.

Visit http://thePoint.lww.com

Answers and Rationales

Looking for answers to the What if . . . and Critical Thinking Care Study questions?

Visit http://thePoint.lww.com

References

Abelsohn, A., Vanderlinden, L. D., Scott, F., et al. (2011). Healthy fish consumption and reduced mercury exposure: Counseling women in their reproductive years. *Canadian Family Physician, 57*(1), 26–30.

Alvarez, A., & Jacobs, L. J. (2011). Breast diseases. In K. J. Hurt, M. W. Guile, J. L. Bienstock, et al. (Eds.), *The Johns Hopkins manual of gynecology and obstetrics* (4th ed., pp. 15–32). Philadelphia, PA: Lippincott Williams & Wilkins.

American Cancer Society. (2012). *Breast cancer: Early detection.* Atlanta, GA: Author.

American Congress of Obstetricians and Gynecologists. (2010). *The Pap test: Committee opinion.* Washington, DC: Author.

American Congress of Obstetricians and Gynecologists. (2012). *Exercise and fitness.* Washington, DC: Author.

Attilakos, G., & Overton, T. G. (2012). Antenatal care. In D. K. Edmonds (Ed.), *Dewhurst's textbook of obstetrics & gynaecology* (8th ed., pp. 42–52). Oxford, UK: John Wiley & Sons.

Centers for Disease Control and Prevention. (2012a). *Alcohol and public health.* Washington, DC: Author.

Centers for Disease Control and Prevention. (2012b). Human papillomavirus-associated cancers: United States, 2004–2008. *MMWR: Morbidity & Mortality Weekly Report, 20*(61), 258–261.

Centers for Disease Control and Prevention. (2012c). Pregnancy-related mortality in the United States. *Reproductive Health.* Washington, DC: Author.

Chalfin, S. F., Burke, P., & Tonelli, M. (2012). Intimate partner violence and adolescent mothers. *Journal of Pediatric & Adolescent Gynecology, 25*(2), 158–159.

Choi, H., Van Riper, M., & Thoyre, S. (2012). Decision making following a prenatal diagnosis of Down syndrome: An integrative review. *Journal of Midwifery & Women's Health, 57*(2), 156–164.

Couloures, K., & Vasan, R. (2011). Prenatal lead poisoning due to maternal exposure results in developmental delay. *Pediatrics International, 53*(2), 242–244.

Creanga, A. A., Sabel, J. C., Ko, J. Y., et al. (2012). Maternal drug use and its effect on neonates: A population-based study in Washington state. *Obstetrics & Gynecology, 119*(5), 924–933.

Dhanjal, M. K. (2012). Preconception counseling. In D. K. Edmonds (Ed.), *Dewhurst's textbook of obstetrics & gynaecology* (8th ed., pp. 35–41). Oxford, UK: John Wiley & Sons.

Dusza, S. W., Halpern, A. C., Satagopan, J. M., et al. (2012). Prospective study of sunburn and sun behavior patterns during adolescence. *Pediatrics, 129*(2), 309–317.

Edmonds, D. K. (2012). Benign diseases of the vagina, cervix and ovary. In D. K. Edmonds (Ed.), *Dewhurst's textbook of obstetrics & gynaecology* (8th ed., pp. 706–714). Oxford, UK: John Wiley & Sons.

Edwardson, J., & Hueppchen, N. A. (2011). Surgical disease and trauma in pregnancy. In K. J. Hurt, M. W. Guile, J. L. Bienstock, et al. (Eds.), *The Johns Hopkins manual of gynecology and obstetrics* (4th ed., pp. 248–256). Philadelphia, PA: Lippincott Williams & Wilkins.

Engnes, K., Lidén, E., & Lundgren, I. (2012). Experiences of being exposed to intimate partner violence during pregnancy. *International Journal of Quality Studies on Health & Well-Being,* 7, ID11199.

Fairbank, J. (2011). Idiopathic scoliosis. In C. Bulstrode, J. Wilson-MacDonald, D. Eastwood, et al. (Eds.), *Oxford textbook of trauma & orthopaedics* (2nd ed., pp. 206–213). Oxford, NY: Oxford University Press.

Fortner, K. B., Kuller, J. A., Rhee, E. J., et al. (2012). Influenza and tetanus, diphtheria, and acellular pertussis vaccinations during pregnancy. *Obstetrical & Gynecology Survey, 67*(4), 251–257.

Gulmezoglu, A. M., & Azhar, O. (2011). Interventions for trichomoniasis in pregnancy. *Cochrane Database of Systematic Reviews,* (3), CD000220.

Hildingsson, I., Nilsson, C., Karlström, A., et al. (2011). A longitudinal survey of childbirth-related fear and associated factors. *JOGNN: Journal of Obstetric, Gynecology & Neonatal Nursing, 40*(5), 532–543.

Kalkanci, A., Güzel, A. B., Khalil, I. I., et al. (2012). Yeast vaginitis during pregnancy: Susceptibility testing of 13 antifungal drugs and boric acid and the detection of four virulence factors. *Medical Mycology, 50*(6), 585–593.

Karch, A. M. (2013). *2013 Lippincott's nursing drug guide*. Philadelphia, PA: Lippincott Williams & Wilkins.

Kingston, D., Heaman, M., Fell, D., et al. (2012). Comparison of adolescent, young adult, and adult women's maternity experiences and practices. *Pediatrics, 129*(5), e1228–e1237.

Kramer, M. S. (2011). Breastfeeding and allergy: The evidence. *Annals of Nutrition & Metabolism, 59*(Suppl. 1), 20–26.

Larzelere, M. M., & Williams, D. E. (2012). Promoting smoking cessation. *American Family Physician, 85*(6), 591–598.

Mackay, H. T. (2012). Gynecologic disorders. In S. J. McPhee, M. Papadakis, & M. W. Radow (Eds.), *Current medical diagnosis & treatment* (pp. 727–759). Columbus, OH: McGraw-Hill.

McCarthy, A. (2012). Miscellaneous medical disorders. In D. K. Edmonds (Ed.), *Dewhurst's textbook of obstetrics & gynaecology* (8th ed., pp. 173–184). Oxford, UK: John Wiley & Sons.

Mehta, S. H., & Sokol, R. J. (2013). Assessment of at-risk pregnancy. In A. H. DeCherney, L. Nathan, N. Laufer, et al. (Eds.), *Current diagnosis and treatment: Obstetrics and gynecology* (11th ed., pp. 223–233). Columbus, OH: McGraw-Hill/Lange.

Mughal, M. Z. (2011). Rickets. *Current Osteoporosis Reports, 9*(4), 291–299.

Mylonas, I. (2012). Female genital *Chlamydia trachomatis* infection: Where are we heading? *Archives of Gynecology & Obstetrics, 285*(5), 1271–1285.

O'Brien, B., Chalmers, B., Fell, D., et al. (2011). The experience of pregnancy and birth with midwives: Results from the Canadian maternity experiences survey. *Birth, 38*(3), 207–215.

Owens, L. K. W. (2012). Postpartum & newborn drugs. In J. L. Kee, E. R. Hayes, & L. E. McCuistion (Eds.), *Pharmacology: A nursing process approach* (pp. 848–866). St. Louis, MO: Elsevier/Saunders.

Paintner, A., Williams, A. D., & Burd, L. (2012). Fetal alcohol spectrum disorders: Implications for child neurology. *Journal of Child Neurology, 27*(2), 258–263.

Ray, A., Shah, A., Gudi, A., et al. (2012). Unexplained infertility: An update and review of practice. *Reproductive Biomedicine Online, 24*(6), 591–602.

Rogers, V. L., & Worley, K. C. (2012). Obstetrics & obstetric disorders. In S. J. McPhee, M. A. Papadakis, & M. W. Rabow (Eds.), *Current Medical Diagnosis & Treatment* (pp. 760–786). Columbus, OH: McGraw-Hill.

Rosen, H. R. (2011). Clinical practice: Chronic hepatitis C infection. *New England Journal of Medicine, 364*(25), 2429–2438.

Rotundo, G. (2012). Centering pregnancy: The benefits of group prenatal care. *Nursing for Women's Health, 15*(6), 508–517.

Ruiz-Mirazo, E., Lopez-Yarto, M., & McDonald, S. D. (2012). Group prenatal care versus individual prenatal care: A systematic review and meta-analyses. *Journal of Obstetrics & Gynaecology Canada, 34*(3), 223–229.

Russell, J. B., Denne, E. W., & Schwartz, D. (2011). Preconception counseling and prenatal care. In K. J. Hurt, M. W. Guile, J. L. Bienstock, et al. (Eds.), *The Johns Hopkins manual of gynecology and obstetrics* (4th ed., pp. 56–72). Philadelphia, PA: Lippincott Williams & Wilkins.

Simon, S. (2012). *New cervical cancer screening guidelines*. Atlanta, GA: American Cancer Society.

Stiles-Shields, C., Hoste, R. R., Doyle, P. M., et al. (2012). A review of family-based treatment for adolescents with eating disorders. *Reviews of Recent Clinical Trials, 7*(2), 133–140.

Tewari, K. S., & Monk, B. J. (2012). Management of diseases of the cervix. In P. J. DiSaia & G. Chaudhuri (Eds.), *Women's health review* (pp. 327–333). Philadelphia, PA: Elsevier/Saunders.

Tiran, D. (2012). Ginger to reduce nausea and vomiting during pregnancy: Evidence of effectiveness is not the same as proof of safety. *Complementary Therapies in Clinical Practice, 18*(1), 22–25.

U.S. Department of Health and Human Services. (2010). *Healthy people 2020.* Washington, DC: Author.

Van Dijk, J. W., Anderko, L., & Stetzer, F. (2011). The impact of prenatal care coordination on birth outcomes. *JOGNN: Journal of Obstetric, Gynecology & Neonatal Nursing, 40*(1), 98–108.

Waller, D. K., Gallaway, M. S., Taylor, L. G., et al. (2010) Use of oral contraceptives in pregnancy and major structural birth defects in offspring. *Epidemiology, 21*(2), 232–239.

Wendland, E. M., Torloni, M. R., Falavigna, M., et al. (2012). Gestational diabetes and pregnancy outcomes. *BMC Pregnancy & Childbirth, 12* (1), 23.

White, S. J., Boldt, K. L., Holditch, S. J., et al. (2012). Measles, mumps, and rubella. *Clinical Obstetrics & Gynecology, 55*(2), 550–559.

Yazbeck, C. F., & Sullivan, S. D. (2012). Thyroid disorders during pregnancy. *Medical Clinics of North America, 96*(2), 235–256.

Zheng, T. (2012). Cervical cancer. In T. Zheng (Ed.), *Comprehensive handbook of obstetrics & gynecology* (pp. 320–323). Paradise Valley, AZ: Phoenix Medical Press.

Chapter 12

Nursing Care to Promote Fetal and Maternal Health

KEY TERMS

- cytomegalovirus
- fetal alcohol spectrum
- Herpes simplex virus type 2 (HSV2)
- leukorrhea
- Sims position
- teratogen
- toxoplasmosis

OBJECTIVES

After mastering the contents of this chapter, you should be able to:

1. Describe common lifestyle behaviors important for a healthy pregnancy outcome.
2. Identify 2020 National Health Goals related to a healthy pregnancy lifestyle that nurses can help the nation achieve.
3. Assess a woman for minor discomforts of pregnancy and corresponding measures to counteract such discomforts as well as healthy lifestyle practices and concerns during pregnancy.
4. Formulate nursing diagnoses concerned with a healthy pregnancy.
5. Identify expected outcomes to promote a healthy pregnancy, such as limiting exposure to teratogens, as well as manage seamless transitions across differing health care settings.
6. Using the nursing process, plan nursing care that includes the six competencies of Quality & Safety Education for Nurses (QSEN): Patient-Centered Care, Teamwork & Collaboration, Evidence-Based Practice (EBP), Quality Improvement (QI), Safety, and Informatics.
7. Implement nursing care to promote healthy practices during pregnancy.
8. Evaluate outcomes for achievement and effectiveness of care.
9. Incorporate knowledge of a healthy lifestyle with the interplay of the nursing process, the six competencies of QSEN, and Family Nursing to promote quality maternal and child health nursing care.

Julberry Adams, a single, 30-year-old woman, is 4 months pregnant when you first see her in a prenatal clinic. She works as a curator for an art gallery but has missed work this past week because of nausea. She is worried she will not be able to work past 6 months of her pregnancy because her job involves a great deal of walking. She has already stopped her volunteer work teaching children's swimming at the YMCA. She wants to travel to see her sister in St. Louis because her sister is very ill but has heard pregnant women should not drive more than 100 miles at a time. She asks you if marijuana would help reduce her early pregnancy nausea.

Previous chapters discussed normal anatomy and physiology and the changes that occur with pregnancy. This chapter adds information about the usual health teaching women need during pregnancy to ensure a healthy outcome for themselves and their child.

What additional health teaching does Ms. Adams need?

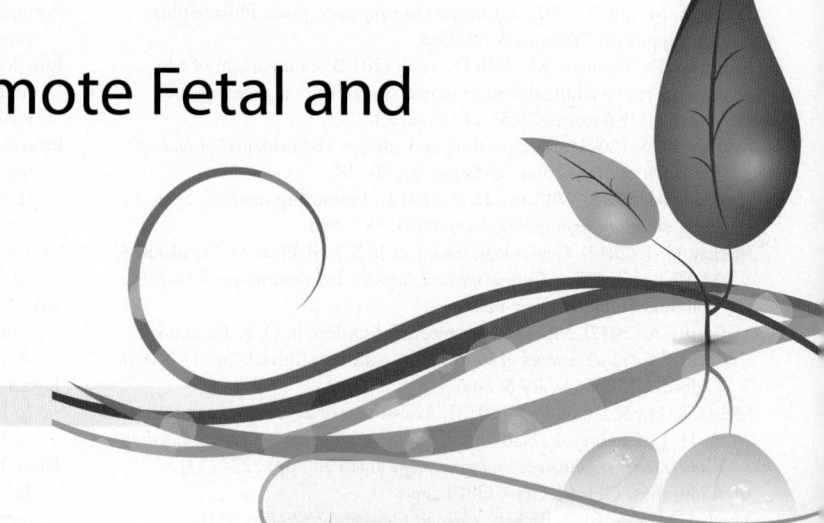

The health of a fetus and the health of a mother are inextricably linked. Generally, a woman who eats well and takes care of her own health during pregnancy provides a healthy environment for fetal growth and development. However, a woman may need instructions on exactly what constitutes a healthy lifestyle during pregnancy. Most women have questions regarding how much extra rest they need, what type of exercise they can continue, and whether all the changes going on in their bodies, some of which bring them at least slight daily discomfort, are normal. Because of this, a major role in promoting maternal and fetal health is education about these subjects. Providing empathetic advice about ways to prevent or alleviate minor discomforts of pregnancy and keeping abreast of the latest evidence-based practice studies on maternal exposure to **teratogens** (factors detrimental to fetal health) are all part of this role. Because the health of women is so important to a nation, the United Nations (UN) lists "improve maternal health" and "reduce child mortality" as Millennium Global Health Goals (UN, 2000). Because effective prenatal care is such an important means to improve women's health, the 2020 National Health Goals speak to the importance of all pregnant women receiving counseling and prenatal care (Box 12.1).

BOX 12.1 Nursing Care Planning Based on 2020 National Health Goals

A number of 2020 National Health goals speak to the importance of women maintaining a healthy lifestyle during pregnancy:

- Increase the proportion of pregnant women who receive early and adequate prenatal care from a baseline of 70.5% to a target of 77.6%.
- Increase to 100% from a baseline of 94.9% the proportion of pregnant women who abstain from illicit drugs during pregnancy.
- Increase to 98.5% from a baseline of 89.6% the proportion of pregnant women who abstain from cigarette smoking during pregnancy.
- Increase to 95% from a baseline of 90% the proportion of pregnant women who abstain from alcohol during pregnancy.
- Increase to 100% from a baseline of 95% the proportion of pregnant women who abstain from binge drinking (i.e., drinking a large amount of alcohol over a short time with the primary intention of becoming intoxicated) during pregnancy (U.S. Department of Health and Human Services [DHHS], 2010; see www.healthypeople.gov).

Because nurses are important members of prenatal health care teams, they play an important role in ensuring women are aware that preconceptual and early pregnancy care are important. Evidence-based practice and nursing research to answer such questions as to which aspects of preconceptual care are most important in reducing pregnancy complications and which are effective incentives to make women come in early for prenatal care would be important to help the nation meet these goals.

Nursing Process Overview

For Health Promotion of a Fetus and Mother

Assessment

A thorough health history, physical evaluation, and initial laboratory data are obtained at a first prenatal visit. A continuing assessment concentrates on screening for any abnormalities in physical or emotional health that might be occurring and for the possibility of teratogens in the pregnant woman's environment. Encourage the woman to discuss whatever concerns she is having during all visits. Although some of these concerns may represent minor common body changes associated with a normal pregnancy, others may be early indicators of potential problems such as gestational hypertension or gestational diabetes. Knowing what is happening as soon as possible allows you to provide information and guidance on ways to alleviate any discomforts of pregnancy and also allows you to alert a woman's primary health care provider of your findings as soon as they appear.

Nursing Diagnosis

Examples of nursing diagnoses related to health promotion of the pregnant woman and fetus include:

- Health-seeking behaviors related to interest in maintaining optimal health during pregnancy
- Anxiety related to minor body changes of pregnancy
- Risk of deficient fluid volume related to gestational nausea and vomiting
- Disturbed body image related to changes in appearance with pregnancy
- Risk of altered sexual patterns related to fear of harming fetus during pregnancy
- Disturbed sleep pattern related to frequent need to empty bladder during night
- Risk for fetal injury related to intimate partner violence

Outcome Identification and Planning

When establishing goals and outcomes, be certain that plans are individualized and realistic for a woman's situation and lifestyle. Try to turn long-term goals into more manageable, short-term ones if possible. For example, a goal of reducing smoking during pregnancy may be more realistic than a goal of stopping smoking forever. Eliminating the pressure of making a major permanent lifestyle change this way can help a woman concentrate her efforts on herself and her fetus over the next several months. Continued reinforcement of her progress could then help her to continue reducing the number of cigarettes smoked or to quit smoking altogether after the baby is born so she can provide a smoke-free environment for her child. Similarly, you cannot set a goal for a woman to be free of the nausea of early pregnancy. The best you can expect to accomplish is to be certain she maintains good nutrition and adequate weight gain in the face of it.

Often, helping a woman plan to avoid teratogens is difficult because a total change in lifestyle and environment, such as not smoking, not drinking alcohol, or changing a work environment, may be impossible. Fortunately, most women are highly motivated to complete a pregnancy satisfactorily. With this level of motivation, planning becomes the task of determining the best route to achieve a goal rather than educating about the need for goal achievement. Additional information on specific teratogenic chemicals can be obtained from the National Institute for Occupational Safety and Health (NIOSH) (www.cdc.gov/NIOSH). The National Center for Complementary and Alternative Medicine (NCCAM) maintains a Web site (www.NCCAM.NIH.gov) to evaluate if specific alternative therapies, such as herbs, are safe during pregnancy. A good site for referral of prenatal care in general is The March of Dimes Web site (www.marchofdimes.com). Be certain women do not consult "chat rooms," as these may contain anecdotal information that is often misleading or incorrect.

Implementation

The major intervention associated with health promotion during pregnancy is education. Although the average woman is aware minor body changes will occur with pregnancy, these changes may seem extreme when they are happening to *her*. Often, adolescent girls are uninformed about common minor body changes during pregnancy because they lack a set of peers with pregnancy experience and so are surprised by them. Even an adolescent who knows it is normal for breast tenderness to occur during pregnancy may not be sure the amount she is feeling is normal. A woman who had a mental image of herself as someone who would not gain much weight during pregnancy may be very concerned because she is, in fact, gaining a great deal of weight. Education about minor body changes can switch this type of worry situation into a pleasant reminder that the pregnancy is progressing as expected.

Outcome Evaluation

An evaluation is an ongoing process at prenatal health care visits. Expected outcomes developed with a woman at one prenatal visit need to be assessed at the next. Examples of expected outcomes include:

- Client states measures she will use to manage increased discomfort from hemorrhoids formed during pregnancy.
- Client reports she is resting for a half-hour twice a day.
- Client verbalizes positive statements about her appearance.
- Client and her partner both state they have stopped smoking.
- Client expresses positive feelings about the manner in which her prenatal care providers accommodated her cultural needs.
- Client documents by use of a pedometer that she walks the length of a city block daily.

HEALTH PROMOTION DURING PREGNANCY

Women in prenatal care settings create an ideal teaching audience because the average woman is eager to learn more about her pregnancy and the steps she can take to maintain health during pregnancy. In addition to general health teaching, good role modeling, such as not smoking in prenatal settings and exhibiting a healthy lifestyle including sound nutrition and exercise, is important (Power, Wilson, Hogan, et al., 2013).

When planning teaching strategies, a woman's receptiveness to instruction is key. Regardless of how excited and pleased a woman is about being pregnant, she can assimilate only so much information at one time. It is important, therefore, to be selective about the health information you provide and include those points most relevant to the individual woman. For example, you would want to discuss varicosity prevention more for a woman with a history of varicosities in a former pregnancy than for one who is pregnant for the first time and is athletic. Keep in mind that health measures taught must be maintained for an extended time—40 weeks. To help a woman follow changes for this long, choose individualized priorities so health advice is specific and meaningful (Box 12.2).

BOX 12.2 Nursing Care Planning to Respect Cultural Diversity

What people do to keep well is culturally influenced. Some women, for example, may rely on herbs and folk remedies for minor discomforts of pregnancy; others feel a need to rely on only medical management.

Implementing prenatal care to meet the needs of all of the different cultures represented in the United States includes careful assessment to identify individual needs. It then may include providing special classes in prenatal health, exploring how health-promotion regimens fit with women's cultural belief systems, and maintaining an attitude of advocacy to help women adjust to a more formal health care system than they are used to.

Also remember the basic tenet of teaching and learning: learning is enhanced when the information has direct and immediate application to that person. This principle means devising a plan that spaces out health-promotion and health-maintenance information into two sections. The first should include teaching those measures that are immediately applicable; the second should come later and include those measures that have relevance only toward the end of pregnancy.

Remind the woman at every visit to bring problems to her health care provider's attention as soon as she becomes worried; otherwise, a provider has no opportunity to take the necessary measures to prevent long-term discomfort or symptoms. For example, common minor body changes associated with early pregnancy are shown in Box 12.3. Many women, however, do not mention these discomforts or body changes unless specifically asked because they may not be aware of their significance to a pregnancy or because they are reluctant to take up a busy health care provider's time for little things. To illustrate, a woman experiencing constipation may not mention it early enough to take preventive measures against the occurrence of hemorrhoids, which can become a long-term problem not only throughout the pregnancy but afterward as well.

Self-Care Needs

Because pregnancy is a state of wellness, few special care measures or advice other than common sense measures about

BOX 12.3 Nursing Care Planning Using Assessment

Assessing a Woman for Minor Body Changes of Pregnancy

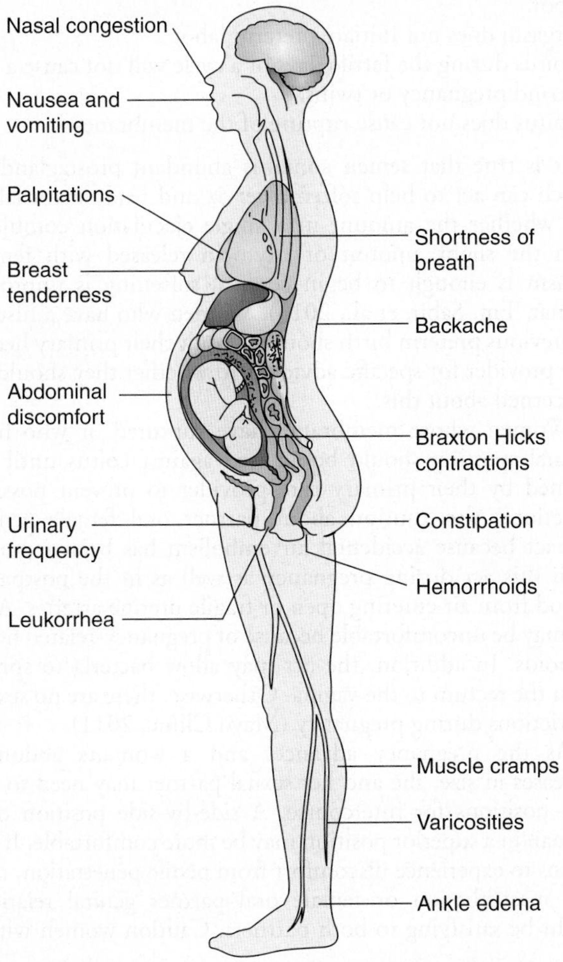

self-care are needed. Many women, however, have heard different warnings about what they should or should not do during pregnancy, which makes them need some help separating fact from fiction. Doing so may enable the woman to enjoy her pregnancy unhampered by unnecessary restrictions. In no other area of nursing, except possibly infant feeding, does there seem to be as many misconceptions or inappropriate information available to women.

Bathing

During pregnancy, sweating tends to increase because a woman excretes waste products for both herself and the fetus. She also has an increase in vaginal discharge. For these reasons, daily tub baths or showers are recommended. Women should not soak for long periods in extremely hot water or in hot tubs, however, as heat exposure for a lengthy time could lead to hyperthermia in the fetus and birth defects, specifically esophageal atresia, omphalocele, and gastroschisis (Duong, Shahrukh-Hashmi, Ramadhani, et al., 2011).

As pregnancy advances, a woman may have difficulty maintaining her balance when getting in and out of a bathtub. If so, she should change to showering or sponge bathing for her own safety. If membranes rupture or vaginal bleeding is present, tub baths become contraindicated because there might be a danger of contamination of uterine contents. During the last month of pregnancy, when the cervix may begin to dilate, some health care providers restrict tub bathing for the same reason.

Breast Care

Women need to make few changes related to breast care during pregnancy. A general rule is: as her breast size increases, a woman should be certain to wear a firm, supportive bra with wide straps to spread breast weight across the shoulders. Interestingly, evidence shows that a woman's breasts enlarge more if the fetus she carries is female than if the fetus is male (Galbarczyk, 2011). Regardless of fetal sex, women may need to buy a larger bra size halfway through pregnancy to accommodate breast changes. Assuming a woman plans on breastfeeding, recommend she choose bras suitable for this (open in the front) so she can continue to use them after the baby's birth.

At about the 16th week of pregnancy, colostrum secretion begins in the breasts. The sensation of a fluid discharge from the breasts can be frightening unless a woman has been cautioned of this possibility. Teach her to wash her breasts with clear tap water (no soap, because that could be drying and cause her nipples to crack) daily to remove the colostrum and reduce the risk of infection. After washing, she should dry her nipples well by patting them with a soft towel.

If colostrum secretion is profuse, a woman may need to place gauze squares or breast pads inside her bra, changing them frequently to maintain dryness. Otherwise, constant moisture next to the breast nipples can cause nipple excoriation, pain, and fissuring. Asking about colostrum at prenatal visits provides a good time to also discuss the benefits of breastfeeding for both a woman and her child (see Chapter 19).

Dental Care

There is a strong correlation between poor oral health and preterm birth, so maintaining good oral health during pregnancy is important (Horton & Boggess, 2012). Without adequate brushing, gingival tissue tends to hypertrophy and, unless a pregnant woman brushes her teeth well, pockets of plaque form readily between the swollen gum line and teeth, possibly leading to periodontal diseases (Lachat, Solnik, Nana, et al., 2011).

When bacteria in the mouth interact with sugar, this lowers the pH of the mouth, creating an acid medium that can lead to etching or destruction of the enamel of teeth (i.e., tooth decay). Because 9 months is a fairly long time to be without preventive dental care, in addition to stressing brushing on arising, after meals, and at bedtime, encourage pregnant women to see their dentists regularly for routine examination and cleaning. Encourage women to snack on nutritious foods, such as fresh fruits and vegetables, rather than sugar-rich snacks to reduce the amount of sugar in contact with their teeth. If a woman has trouble avoiding sweet snacks such as candy, suggest eating snacks that dissolve easily (like a chocolate bar) rather than one that remains in the mouth a long time (like chewy caramel). This helps to minimize the level of sugar in the mouth and its long-term contact with teeth.

Women should question the need for X-rays during pregnancy; although, if these are necessary for dental health, they can be done safely as long as a woman's abdomen is shielded with a lead apron.

Perineal Hygiene

Women have increased vaginal discharge during pregnancy and so need to maintain good perineal hygiene. Caution them to always wipe front to back after voiding to prevent bringing contamination forward from the rectum. Even if the vaginal discharge seems excessive, douching is contraindicated because the force of the irrigating fluid could cause the solution to enter the cervix, leading to a uterine infection. In addition, douching alters the pH of the vagina, leading to an increased risk of vaginal bacterial growth (Guile & Keller, 2011).

Clothing

Maternity clothing should be comfortable. Women should be cautioned to avoid garters, extremely firm girdles with panty legs, and knee-high stockings during pregnancy because these may impede lower extremity circulation. Suggest wearing shoes with a moderate-to-low heel to minimize pelvic tilt and possible backache as well as to reduce the risk of falling.

Sexual Activity

Some women feel lessened sexual desire in early pregnancy probably because of the combination of increased estrogen and a tendency to guard the body, which comes from an awareness that they are pregnant (Corbacioglu, Bakir, Akbayir, et al., 2012). Breast tenderness may limit a usual pattern of sexual arousal. As pelvic congestion increases from the additional uterine blood supply at midpregnancy, most women notice increased clitoral sensation. Some women may experience orgasm for the first time during pregnancy because of this. Asking a woman at a prenatal visit if she has any questions about sexual activity allows her to voice concerns about coitus (Box 12.4). This conversation allows a woman to feel more comfortable and secure that coitus is not harming her fetus. You may need to replace myths with facts, such as:

- Coitus on the expected date of her period does not initiate labor.
- Orgasm does not initiate preterm labor.
- Coitus during the fertile days of a cycle will not cause a second pregnancy or twins.
- Coitus does not cause rupture of the membranes.

It is true that semen contains abundant prostaglandins, which can act to help soften a cervix and ready it for labor, but whether the amount in a single ejaculation combined with the slight amount of oxytocin released with female orgasm is enough to begin cervical softening is unproven (Omar, Tan, Sabir, et al., 2013). Women who have a history of previous preterm birth should consult their primary health care provider for specific advice as to whether they should be concerned about this.

Women whose membranes have ruptured or who have vaginal spotting should be advised against coitus until examined by their primary care provider to prevent possible infection. Also caution about partner oral–female genital contact because accidental air embolism has been reported from this act during pregnancy as well as in the postpartal period from air entering open or fragile uterine arteries. Anal sex may be uncomfortable because of pregnancy-related hemorrhoids. In addition, the act may allow bacteria to spread from the rectum to the vagina. Otherwise, there are no sexual restrictions during pregnancy (Mayo Clinic, 2011).

As the pregnancy advances and a woman's abdomen increases in size, she and her sexual partner may need to use new positions for intercourse. A side-by-side position or a woman in a superior position may be more comfortable. If she begins to experience discomfort from penile penetration, mutual masturbation or female oral–partner genital relations might be satisfying to both partners. Caution women with a

BOX 12.4 Nursing Care Planning Based on Effective Communication

Julberry Adams is 4 months pregnant and no longer lives with the father of her baby.

Less Effective Communication

Nurse: Do you have any questions, Mrs. Adams?
Julberry: I'm not Mrs. Adams.
Nurse: I'm sorry, Ms. Adams. Do you have any questions?
Julberry: How long into pregnancy can I have sex?
Nurse: Well, since you're single, you don't really need that kind of advice. Let's talk about exercise and nutrition instead.

More Effective Communication

Nurse: Do you have any questions, Mrs. Adams?
Julberry: I'm not Mrs. Adams.
Nurse: I'm sorry, Ms. Adams. Do you have any questions?
Julberry: How long into pregnancy can I have sex?
Nurse: Basically, as long as you're comfortable and you don't have any complications.
Julberry: Good. My new boyfriend made me promise to ask today.

Health teaching is an art separate from teaching morality. In the first scenario, the nurse cuts off communication by making a judgment and a choice to supply only information the nurse thinks her client needs. In the second scenario, the nurse actively listens to the client, focuses on the client's needs and concerns, and supplies the information the client has requested.

nonmonogamous male sexual partner that the partner needs to use a condom to prevent transmission of a sexually transmitted infection during pregnancy (Marrazzo & Cates, 2011). Women may use female condoms throughout pregnancy.

QSEN Checkpoint Question 12.1

Teamwork & Collaboration

A member of your care team is relating some statements made by Julberry Adams. Which statement would alert you and your care team that there is a need to review self-care practices during pregnancy with her?

a. "I take either a shower or tub bath because I know both are safe."
b. "I wash my breasts with clear water, not with soap, every day."
c. "I know if my partner uses a condom it can tear fetal membranes."
d. "I'm wearing low-heeled shoes to try to avoid backache."

Look in Appendix A for the best answer and rationale.

Exercise

Extreme exercise in women has been associated with difficulty conceiving but after pregnancy occurs, moderate exercise is healthy (Szymanski & Satin, 2012). During pregnancy, exercise can offer a general sense of well-being. It also helps prevent circulatory stasis in the lower extremities. For some women, teaching about exercise focuses on both helping them realize the need for exercise and urging them to get enough. Others may need to be cautioned to restrict exercise, such as for those who participate in contact sports like touch football or unrefereed soccer.

As a rule, average, well-nourished women should exercise during pregnancy about three times weekly for 30 consecutive minutes (Russell, Denne, & Schwartz, 2011). Their exercise program should consist of 5 minutes of warm-up exercises, an active "stimulus" phase of 20 minutes, and then 5 minutes of cool-down exercises. Movements that exercise large muscle groups rhythmically, such as walking, are best but the type of activity chosen should depend on their interests. Advise women to eat a protein and a complex carbohydrate such as peanut butter and whole wheat bread at least 15 minutes before exercise to keep blood sugar from falling during exercise, and to drink water before and after to prevent dehydration.

As a rule, a woman can continue any sport she participated in before pregnancy unless it was one that involved body contact, such as soccer. If a woman is a competent horsewoman, for example, there is little reason for her to discontinue riding until it becomes uncomfortable. Pregnancy is not the time to learn to ride, however, because a beginning rider is at greater risk for being thrown than an experienced one. The same principle applies to skiing and bicycling. An accomplished skier or bicyclist may continue the activity in moderation until balance becomes a problem. Pregnancy is not the time to learn to ski or ride a bicycle, however, because the lack of skill could result in many falls.

The intensity of the exercise program depends on cardiopulmonary fitness. Both pregnant and nonpregnant women should exercise at 70% to 85% of their maximum heart rate. The easiest way to calculate this is for women to subtract their age from 220, then calculate 70% or 85% of that number. For example, after exercise, a 23-year-old woman should have a pulse range of 137 to 167 beats/min (220 – 23 [= 197] × 70% [= 137.90] or 85% [= 167.4]). For a woman of 35 years, this target range would be 129 to 157 beats/min. An additional way for women to assess if they are exercising too strenuously is to evaluate their ability to continue talking while exercising. If a woman is too short of breath to do this, she is exercising beyond her target heart rate.

Because walking is the best exercise during pregnancy, women should be encouraged to take a walk daily unless inclement weather, many levels of stairs, or an unsafe neighborhood are contraindications. Yoga is also a good exercise as long as positions are limited to those in which pregnant women are able to maintain balance (Babbar, Parks-Savage, & Chauhan, 2012). Jogging, in contrast, is questioned because of the strain the extra weight of pregnancy places on the knees. Late in pregnancy, jogging can also cause pelvic pain from relaxed symphysis pubis movement.

Swimming is a good activity for pregnant women and, like bathing, is not contraindicated as long as membranes are intact. It not only increases muscle tone but may help relieve backache. Diving, long-distance swimming, or any other activity carried out to a point of extreme fatigue should be avoided. A moderate-impact aerobic program such as dancing is well tolerated during pregnancy, but a high-impact aerobics program is usually contraindicated because it can be strenuous on both pelvic and knee joints (Kramer & McDonald, 2010).

An epidemiologic study suggests an elevation of maternal body temperature by 2°C for at least 24 hours can cause a range of fetal defects, but there is little information on thresholds for shorter exposures such as occur with exercise. Use of hot tubs and saunas after workouts, similar to a hot bath, should be limited to no longer than 15 minutes, again on the chance these can lead to hyperthermia in the fetus and birth defects, specifically esophageal atresia, omphalocele, and gastroschisis (Duong et al., 2011).

General guidelines for exercise during pregnancy are highlighted in Box 12.5. Beginning an exercise program during pregnancy not only offers the advantage of being healthy during pregnancy but also provides long-term benefits such as:

- Lowering cholesterol levels
- Reducing the risk of osteoporosis
- Increasing energy levels
- Maintaining a healthy body weight
- Decreasing the risk of heart disease
- Increasing self-esteem and well-being

Women who know they have an incompetent cervix or have had cerclage to correct this and women who develop any complication of pregnancy such as bleeding, gestational hypertension, preterm rupture of membranes, preterm labor, or whose fetus is growth restricted should consult with their primary health care provider before beginning or continuing an exercise program.

Sleep

The optimal condition for body growth occurs when growth hormone secretion is at its highest level—that is, during sleep.

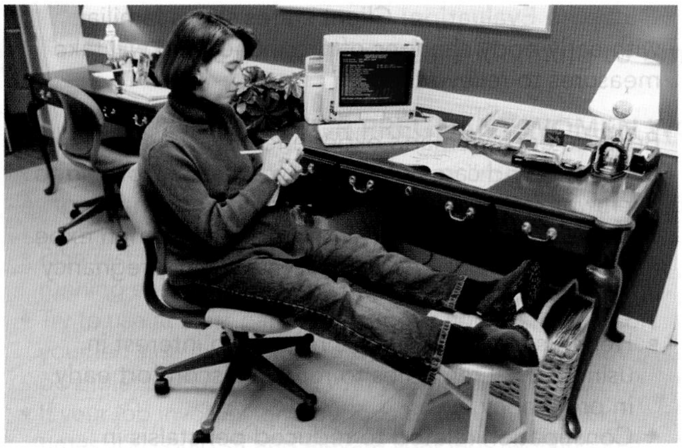

FIGURE 12.3 A "feet-up" break during a workday helps prevent ankle edema. (© Caroline Brown, RNC, MS, DEd.)

pregnancy is not an illness and so they proceed as if nothing is happening to them. Rarely is there justification during a normal pregnancy for women to take extra days off from work because of their condition, but it is also unrealistic to proceed as if nothing is happening. Fatigue can increase the amount of morning nausea a woman experiences. If she becomes too tired, she may not eat properly and nutrition can suffer. If she remains on her feet without at least one break during a day, the risk for varicosities and the danger of thromboembolic complications increase.

For all these reasons, ask women at prenatal visits whether they manage to have at least one short rest period every day. A woman who works outside her home at a job that requires her to be on her feet most of the day might use part of her lunch hour to sit with her feet elevated (Fig. 12.3). After she returns home from work in the evening, she may need to modify her customary routine from typical activities such as cooking dinner or watching a child's soccer game to resting, then cooking dinner or going to the soccer game, or resting while her partner cooks dinner.

QSEN Checkpoint Question 12.3

Evidence-Based Practice

Almost all women experience a number of minor discomforts during pregnancy. To investigate whether these symptoms are serious enough to lead to depression, researchers scored 1,507 Australian women during their first pregnancy on a depression inventory questionnaire. The women were also asked what minor body changes they were experiencing. The most frequent body changes reported were exhaustion (86.9%), morning nausea (64.3%), back pain (45.6%), constipation (43.5%), and severe headache or migraine (29.5%). Women who reported five or more physical health problems were three times more likely to also report depressive symptoms (Perlen et al., 2013).

Based on the previous study, which statement by Julberry would give you the most concern that she should be assessed at her next prenatal visit as to whether she could be depressed?

a. "I wake up every morning with backache. Do I need a new mattress?"
b. "I like the job I do, although I come home exhausted almost every day."
c. "Between the headache, the backache, and the nausea, pregnancy isn't fun."
d. "The amount of constipation I have is a surprise; I don't usually get that."

Look in Appendix A for the best answer and rationale.

Muscle Cramps

Decreased serum calcium levels, increased serum phosphorus levels, and, possibly, interference with circulation commonly cause muscle cramps of the lower extremities during pregnancy. This problem is best relieved if a woman lies on her back momentarily and extends the involved leg while keeping her knee straight and dorsiflexing the foot until the pain disappears (Fig. 12.4).

Taking a calcium supplement, which would lower the phosphorus level, does not seem to be helpful. If a woman is experiencing frequent leg cramps, she may be advised to take magnesium lactate or citrate once in the morning and again in the evening as these bind phosphorus in the intestinal tract and thereby lower its circulating level (Young & Jewell, 2011). Elevating lower extremities frequently during the day to improve circulation and avoiding full leg extension, such as stretching with the toes pointed, may also be helpful. Typically, muscle cramps are a minor symptom of pregnancy, but the pain is extreme and the intensity of the contraction can be frightening. Always ask at prenatal visits if this is a problem. Otherwise, women may not realize cramping is pregnancy related and so fail to report it.

Hypotension

Supine hypotension is a symptom that occurs when a woman lies on her back and the uterus presses on the vena cava, impairing blood return to her heart (Pipkin, 2012). A woman experiences an irregular heart rate and a feeling of apprehension. Relieving the problem is simple: if a woman turns or is turned onto her side, pressure is removed from the vena cava, blood flow is restored, and the symptoms quickly fade.

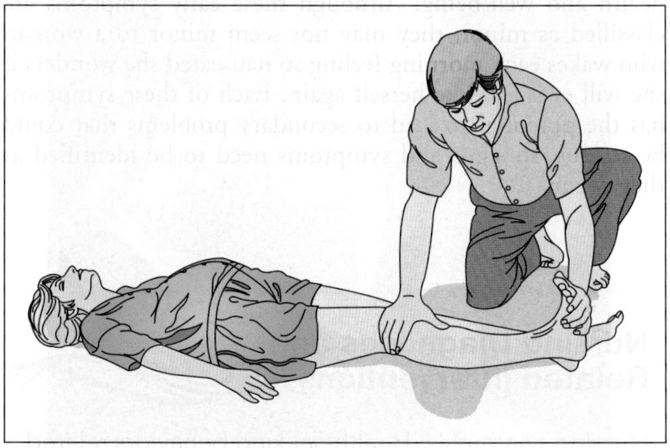

FIGURE 12.4 Relieving a leg cramp in pregnancy. Pressing down on the knee and pressing the toes backward (dorsiflexion) relieves most cramps. Here, a woman's partner helps.

To prevent the syndrome, advise pregnant women to always rest or sleep on their side, not their back. If they can only fall asleep on their back, they should insert a small firm pillow under their right hip to cause the weight of their uterus to shift off their vena cava.

If a woman rises suddenly from a lying or sitting position or stands for an extended time in a warm or crowded area, she may faint from the same phenomenon (blood pooling in the pelvic area or lower extremities). Rising slowly and avoiding extended periods of standing prevents this problem. If a woman should feel faint, sitting with her head lowered—the same action as for any person who feels faint—alleviates the problem.

Varicosities

Varicosities, or the development of tortuous leg veins, commonly form in pregnancy because the weight of the distended uterus puts pressure on the veins returning blood from the lower extremities (Attilakos & Overton, 2012). This causes blood pooling and vessel distention. The veins become enlarged, inflamed, and painful. Although usually confined to the lower extremities, varicosities can extend up to and including the vulva. They occur most frequently in women with a family history of varicose veins, those who are obese, and those who have a large fetus or a multiple pregnancy. Urge such women to take active measures to prevent varicosities beginning in early pregnancy; if left until late in pregnancy, the best they will be able to accomplish is relief of pain from already formed varicosities.

Resting in a Sims position or on the back with the legs raised against the wall (with a small firm pillow under their right hip) or elevated on a footstool for 15 to 20 minutes twice a day is a good precaution (Fig. 12.5). Caution women not to sit with their legs crossed or their knees bent and to avoid constrictive knee-high hose or garters.

Some women who developed varicosities during a previous pregnancy may need elastic support stockings for relief of varicosities in a second pregnancy. If a woman needs to wear these, urge her to put them on before she arises in the morning because once she is on her feet, blood pooling begins, and the stockings will be less effective. When applied properly, the stockings should reach an area above the point of distention.

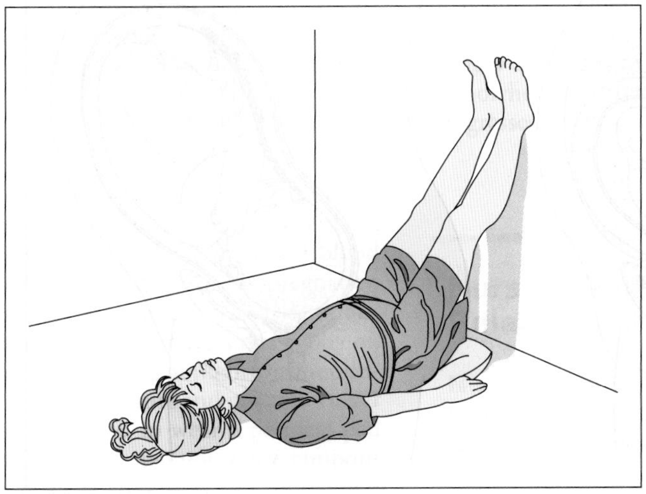

FIGURE 12.5 Position to relieve varicosities. The mother keeps a pad under her right hip to prevent supine hypotensive syndrome.

Be certain a woman understands the stockings she buys should be labeled "medical support hose." Otherwise, as many pantyhose manufacturers advertise their stockings as giving "firm support," she may assume erroneously this is sufficient for her.

Because it stimulates venous return, exercise is as effective as rest periods for alleviating varicosities. Most women assume they do not need set exercise periods during pregnancy because they work hard at other activities. If they analyze the type of work they do, however, they may realize a great deal of their work leads to venous stasis of their lower extremities. Women stand in one position to wash dishes, run a copying machine, defend a client in court, process a part on an assembly line, or teach a class. Sitting at a desk for prolonged periods of time with legs bent at the knee also encourages venous stasis.

To increase circulation, advise women to break up these long periods of sitting or standing with a "walk break" at least twice a day. As a rule, their families or fellow workers will benefit by accompanying them on such walks as partners may discover that when they analyze their day, they, too, sit more than walk during their workday.

Vitamins C, A, and B complex are all important for circulatory health. Vitamin C appears to be most important as it is necessary for the formation of blood vessel collagen and endothelium. Ask at prenatal visits if women are taking a daily prenatal vitamin as well as including fresh fruit or juice in their diet every day as yet another measure to help prevent varicosities.

What if...12.2 Julberry knows taking a prenatal vitamin every day is important but is having trouble remembering to take one. What are some suggestions you could make to help her remember to take this daily?

Hemorrhoids

Hemorrhoids (i.e., varicosities of the rectal veins) occur commonly in pregnancy because of pressure on these veins from the bulk of the growing uterus (Klemetti, Kurinczuk, & Redshaw, 2011). Daily bowel evacuation to prevent constipation, drinking adequate fluid, eating adequate fiber, and resting in a modified Sims position are all helpful measures to both prevent these and relieve pain. At day's end, assuming a knee–chest position (Fig. 12.6) for 10 to 15 minutes is an excellent way to reduce the pressure on rectal veins. A knee–chest position may initially make a woman feel light-headed. If this happens, advise her to remain in this position for only a few minutes at first, and then gradually increase the time until she can maintain the position comfortably for about 15 minutes.

In addition to the previous measures, a stool softener such as docusate sodium (Colace) may be recommended if a woman already has hemorrhoids when she enters pregnancy. Replacing external hemorrhoids with gentle finger pressure and applying witch hazel, a cold compress, or over-the-counter hemorrhoid cream are other helpful measures to relieve pain. Hydrocortisone-pramoxine (Proctofoam-HC) is a prescription medication that is also helpful and is safe for the fetus (Ebrahimi, Vohra, Gedeon, et al., 2011). As with varicosities, think prevention, not just providing help for already established hemorrhoids.

to TORCH screening, ask women if it is all right to screen them for human immunodeficiency virus (HIV); you must obtain separate permission for this test (Whitmore, Taylor, Espinoza, et al., 2012).

Malaria

Malaria in humans is caused by intraerythrocytic protozoa of the genus *Plasmodium* transmitted to humans by the bite of an infected female *Anopheles* mosquito. Health care providers can contact it from infected blood products. During pregnancy, women can transmit malaria to a fetus. Most malaria infections in the United States occur among people who have traveled to areas where malaria is epidemic, such as Africa or South America.

A number of drugs, such as chloroquine or artesunate in the first trimester and mefloquine in the second or third trimesters, are helpful. Women who will be visiting in an area known to be epidemic for malaria can begin treatment as prophylaxis up to 2 weeks before travel (Mali, Kachur, & Arguin, 2012).

Toxoplasmosis

Toxoplasmosis, a protozoan infection, is spread most commonly through contact with uncooked meat, although it may also be contracted through handling cat stool in soil or cat litter (Gülmezoglu & Azhar, 2011).

As many as 1 in 900 pregnancies may be affected by toxoplasmosis. Prepregnancy serum analysis can be done to identify women who have never had the disease and so are susceptible (about 50% of women). Removing a cat from the home during pregnancy as a means of prevention is not necessary as long as the cat is healthy. However, taking in a new cat, which could be infected, is unwise. Instruct pregnant women to avoid undercooked meat and also not to change a cat litter box or garden in soil in an area where cats may defecate to avoid exposure to the disease. Also, reinforce proper hand washing after handling uncooked meat.

Rubella (German Measles)

The rubella virus usually causes only a mild rash and mild systemic illness in a woman, but the teratogenic effects on a fetus can be devastating, such as hearing impairment, cognitive and motor challenges, cataracts, cardiac defects (most commonly patent ductus arteriosus and pulmonary stenosis), restricted intrauterine growth (i.e., small for gestational age), thrombocytopenic purpura, and dental and facial clefts, such as cleft lip and palate (White, Boldt, Holditch, et al., 2012).

Typically, a rubella titer from a pregnant woman to estimate whether a woman is susceptible to rubella is obtained on the first prenatal visit. A titer greater than 1:8 suggests immunity to the disease. A titer of less than 1:8 suggests a woman is susceptible to viral invasion. A titer that is greatly increased over a previous reading or is initially extremely high suggests a recent infection has occurred.

A woman who is not immunized before pregnancy cannot be immunized during pregnancy because the vaccine contains a live virus that would have effects similar to those occurring with a subclinical case of rubella. After rubella immunization, a woman is advised not to become pregnant for about 3 months, until the rubella virus is no longer active. Immediately after a pregnancy, assess whether a woman who has a low rubella titer would like to be immunized to provide protection against rubella in future pregnancies.

An increasing concern is women who demonstrate antibodies against rubella yet still become reinfected during pregnancy. Because of this, all pregnant women should avoid contact with children with rashes. Infants who are born to mothers who had rubella during pregnancy may be capable of transmitting the disease for a time after birth. Because of this, such an infant is isolated from other newborns during the newborn period. Be certain a woman is aware her infant might infect others, including pregnant women. Nurses who care for pregnant women or newborns should receive immunization against rubella to ensure they neither spread nor contract the disease (Marcdante, Kliegman, Jenson, et al., 2011).

Herpes Simplex Virus Type 2 (Genital Herpes Infection)

Herpes simplex virus type 2 (HSV2) is a sexually transmitted infection spread by intimate contact. The first time a woman contracts an HSV2 infection, systemic involvement occurs. The virus spreads into the bloodstream (viremia) and, if a woman is pregnant, can cross the placenta to a fetus, thus posing substantial fetal risk (Jaiyeoba, Amaya, Soper, et al., 2012).

If the infection takes place in the first trimester, severe congenital anomalies or spontaneous miscarriage can occur. If the infection invades during the second or third trimester, there is a high incidence of premature birth, intrauterine growth restriction, neurologic disease, and continuing infection of the newborn at birth. Mortality may be as high as 60% (Stohl & Satin, 2011).

If a woman has had herpes simplex virus type 1 (HSV1) infections (popularly called cold sores) before the genital invasion or if the HSV2 infection is a recurrence, antibodies to the virus in her system apparently prevent spread of the virus to the fetus across the placenta.

If genital lesions are present at the time of birth, however, a fetus may contract the virus from direct exposure during birth. For this reason, if a woman has existing genital lesions at the time of birth, cesarean birth is usually advised to reduce the risk of this route of infection. This awareness of the placental spread of HSV2 has increased the importance of obtaining information about exposure to HSV2 or any painful perineal or vaginal lesions that might indicate this infection at prenatal visits through conscientious history taking.

Intravenous acyclovir (Zovirax) or valacyclovir (Valtrex) can both be safety administered to women who develop lesions after the first trimester of pregnancy as well as to their newborns at birth (Walsh, 2012). The primary mechanism for protecting a fetus, however, is disease prevention. Urging women to practice safer sex is important to lessen their exposure to this and other sexually transmitted infections.

Cytomegalovirus

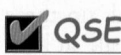

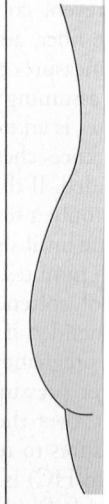

Cytomegalovirus (CMV), a member of the HSV family, is another teratogen that can cause extensive damage to a fetus while causing few symptoms in a woman (Stohl & Satin, 2011). It is not sexually transmitted but spreads from person to person by droplet infection such as occurs with sneezing. If a woman acquires a primary CMV infection during pregnancy and the virus crosses the placenta, the infant may be born with severe neurologic challenges (e.g., hydrocephalus, microcephaly, or spasticity) or with eye damage (e.g., optic atrophy or chorioretinitis), hearing impairment, or chronic liver disease. The newborn's skin may be covered with large petechiae (i.e., "blueberry-muffin" lesions). Because a woman has almost no symptoms, she may not even be aware she contracted an infection. Diagnosis in the mother or infant can be established by the isolation of CMV antibodies in blood serum. Unfortunately, there is no treatment for the infection even if it presents in the mother with enough symptoms to allow detection. Because there is no treatment or vaccine for the disease, routine screening for CMV during pregnancy is not recommended. Advise women to wash hands thoroughly before eating and to avoid crowds of young children at daycare or nursery school settings to help prevent exposure (Johnson, Anderson, & Pass, 2012).

Like HSV, a primary CMV infection may become latent, reactivating periodically. These recurrences are not thought to have a teratogenic effect on a fetus, but they can cause infection of a newborn during birth from genital secretions or postpartum from exposure to CMV-infected breast milk. CMV infection contracted at or shortly after birth is not associated with serious adverse effects except in babies of very low birth weight.

Other Viral Diseases

It is difficult to detect other viral teratogens, but rubeola (measles), coxsackievirus, infectious parotitis (mumps), varicella (chickenpox), poliomyelitis, influenza, and viral hepatitis all may be teratogenic. Women are advised to be vaccinated against influenza before pregnancy. If contracted during pregnancy, parvovirus B19, the causative agent of erythema infectiosum (also called fifth disease) and a common viral disease in school age children, can cross the placenta and attack the red blood cells of the fetus. Infection with the virus during early pregnancy is associated with fetal death. If the infection occurs late in pregnancy, the infant may be born with severe anemia and congenital heart disease (Dijkmans, de Jong, Dijkmans, et al., 2012).

Syphilis. Syphilis, a sexually transmitted infection, is of great concern for the maternal–fetal population. Despite the availability of accurate screening tests and proven medical treatment, it is growing in incidence; it places a fetus at risk for intrauterine or congenital syphilis (Walker, 2010). Early in pregnancy, when the cytotrophoblast layer of the chorionic villi is still intact, the causative spirochete of syphilis, *Treponema pallidum*, apparently cannot cross the placenta and damage the fetus. When this layer atrophies at about the 16th to 18th week of pregnancy, however, the spirochete can cross and cause extensive fetal damage. If syphilis is detected in the mother and treated with an antibiotic such as intramuscular benzathine penicillin in the first trimester, a fetus is rarely affected. If left untreated beyond the 18th week of gestation, hearing impairment, cognitive challenge, osteochondritis, and fetal death are possible.

For these reasons, serologic screening (either by a venereal disease research laboratory [VDRL] or a rapid plasma reagin [RPR] test) is done at a first prenatal visit; the test may then be repeated again close to term (the eighth month) if recent exposure is a concern. Even when a woman has been treated with antibiotics, the serum titer remains high up to 200 days; an increasing titer, however, suggests reinfection has occurred. In an infant born to a woman with syphilis, the serologic test for syphilis may remain positive for up to 3 months even though the disease was treated during pregnancy.

The newborn with congenital syphilis may have congenital anomalies, extreme rhinitis (sniffles), and a characteristic syphilitic rash, all of which identify the baby as high risk at birth (Follett & Clarke, 2011). When the baby's primary teeth come in, they are often oddly shaped (i.e., Hutchinson teeth). As the infant requires long-term follow-up, medical and nursing care of the newborn with congenital syphilis is discussed in Chapter 47. As with all sexually transmitted infections, prevention through safer sex practices is key.

Infections That Cause Illness at Birth. A number of infections are not teratogenic to a fetus during pregnancy but are harmful if they are present at the time of birth. Gonorrhea, candidiasis, chlamydia, streptococcus B, and hepatitis B infections are examples of these. Chapters 45 and 47 discuss the effects of these infections on maternal, fetal, and neonatal health.

Potentially Teratogenic Vaccines

Live virus vaccines, such as measles, HPV, mumps, rubella, and poliomyelitis (Sabin type), are contraindicated during pregnancy because they may transmit a viral infection to a fetus (Russell et al., 2011). Care must be taken in routine immunization programs at high schools to be certain adolescents about to be vaccinated are not pregnant. Women who work in biologic laboratories where vaccines are manufactured are well advised to use protective gear or not to work with live virus products during pregnancy.

Teratogenic Drugs

Many women assume the rule of being cautious with drugs during pregnancy applies only to prescription drugs and continue to take over-the-counter drugs or herbal supplements freely during pregnancy. Although not all drugs cross the placenta (heparin, for example, does not because of its large molecular size), most do (Fig. 12.8).

To help ensure the safety of drugs during pregnancy, the U.S. Food and Drug Administration (FDA, n.d.) rates drugs according to five categories in relation to pregnancy

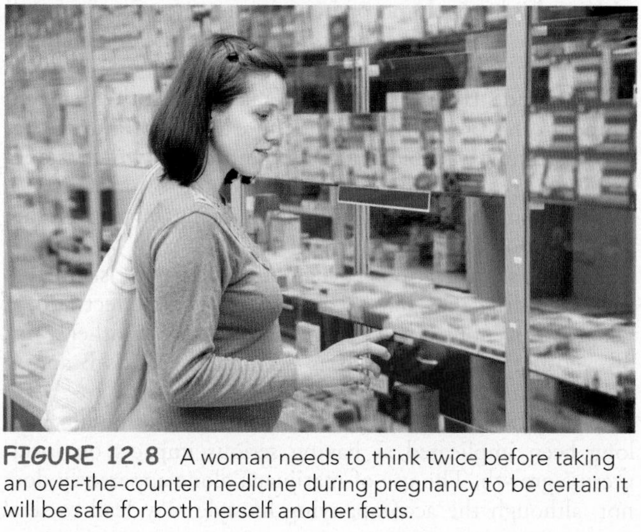

FIGURE 12.8 A woman needs to think twice before taking an over-the-counter medicine during pregnancy to be certain it will be safe for both herself and her fetus.

TABLE 12.1 FDA Pregnancy Risk Categories of Drugs

Category	Description	Example
A	No risk to fetus. Studies have not shown risk of fetal harm.	Thyroid hormone
B	No risk in animal studies. Well-controlled studies in pregnant women are not available. It is assumed there is little to no risk in pregnant women.	Insulin
C	Animal studies indicate risk to the fetus. Controlled studies on pregnant women are not available. Risk versus benefit of the drug must be determined.	Docusate sodium (Colace)
D	Risk to the human fetus has been proven. Risk versus benefit of the drug must be determined. Could be used in lifesaving situations.	Lithium citrate
X	Risk to the human fetus has been proven. Risk outweighs the benefit so the drug should be avoided during pregnancy.	Thalidomide

From U.S. Food and Drug Administration. (n.d.). *FDA pregnancy categories*. Washington, DC: Author.

(Table 12.1). Always look for a drug's listed category before administering it to a pregnant woman to be certain it will be safe to administer. In addition, two principles always govern drug intake during pregnancy:

- Any drug or herbal supplement, under certain circumstances, may be detrimental to fetal welfare. Therefore, during pregnancy, women should not take any drug or supplement not specifically prescribed or approved by their primary health care provider.
- A woman of childbearing age should not take any drug other than one prescribed by a primary health care provider to avoid exposure to a drug should she become pregnant.

The classic example of a drug that can cause harm in pregnancy is thalidomide, which was once liberally prescribed for morning nausea in Europe. Never approved for use in the United States, thalidomide caused amelia or phocomelia (i.e., total or partial absence of extremities) in 100% of instances when taken between the 34th and 45th day of pregnancy. Thalidomide is again available as it is effective as an anticancer drug, specifically for patients with multiple myeloma or hepatic cancer, so women still need to be cautioned about its detrimental fetal effects (Chen, Yen, Chou, et al., 2012).

Finasteride (Propecia), a drug taken by both men and women to restore hair growth, is an example of a drug that may be readily available in a modern home but which is documented to cause fetal deformities (Stout & Stumpf, 2010). Other examples of drugs capable of being teratogenic are shown in Box 12.8.

Almost all recreational drugs put a fetus at risk in two ways: the drug may have a direct teratogenic effect and, if taken intravenously, the drug increases the mother's risk of exposure to diseases such as HIV and hepatitis B and C (Milloy, Marshall, Kerr, et al., 2012).

Narcotics such as meperidine (Demerol) and heroin have long been implicated as having serious impacts on intrauterine growth. The use of marijuana alone apparently does not, although the accompanying lifestyle may lead to fetal growth restriction and preterm birth (Hayatbakhsh, Flenady, Gibbons, et al., 2012).

Cocaine, particularly in crack form, is potentially harmful to a fetus because it causes severe vasoconstriction in the mother, thus compromising placental blood flow and perhaps dislodging the placenta. Its use is associated with spontaneous miscarriage, preterm labor, meconium staining, and intrauterine growth restriction (Russell et al., 2011). Whether cocaine causes long-term effects in the infant remains controversial (Shankaran, Das, Bauer, et al., 2011). See Chapter 22 for more information on the potential hazards of cocaine or heroin use during pregnancy.

An area of recreational drug use rising in incidence is that of inhalant abuse ("huffing"). Substances frequently used as inhalants include gasoline, butane lighter fluid, Freon, glue, and nitrous oxide (NIOSH, 2010). Although the teratogenic properties of these inhalants are not well studied, they all carry the possibility of a respiratory distress effect on the mother, which could limit the oxygen supply to a fetus. They are used most often by adolescents as they are easy to obtain on a limited budget.

Herbs

Herbs are not regulated by the FDA in the same way as medications; therefore, they are not rated with regard to their safety in pregnancy. Even though most are safe, American ginseng, used to improve general well-being, has been associated with birth defects; and St. John's wort, an herb taken as a mood enhancer, can interfere with the action of seizure-control drugs, such as dilantin and phenobarbital, and so should be avoided by women prescribed such drugs (NCCAM, 2010).

Green tea, a common breakfast drink, may interfere with the absorption of folic acid. As folic acid is needed in pregnancy to help prevent birth defects, this should be avoided in pregnancy or in women hoping to soon become pregnant (Shiraishi, Haruna, Matsuzaki, et al., 2010). As with medicine, women should not take herbs in pregnancy until they discuss the herbs' safety with their primary care provider.

BOX 12.8 Nursing Care Planning Based on Responsibility for Pharmacology

SOME POTENTIALLY OR POSITIVELY TERATOGENIC DRUGS

CATEGORY	EXAMPLE	DRUG USE	TERATOGENIC EFFECT
Alcohol (ethanol)	Wine, whiskey	Social use	Fetal alcohol spectrum disorder
Analgesics	Acetylsalicylic acid (aspirin)	Minor pain relief	Prolonged pregnancy; maternal bleeding
	Nonsteroidal anti-inflammatory drugs (NSAIDs)		Patent ductus arteriosus
Antineoplastics	Methotrexate	Chemotherapy	Multiple anomalies
	Cyclophosphamide (Cytoxan)	Chemotherapy	Multiple anomalies
Androgens	Danazol	Endometriosis	Masculinization of female fetus
Anticonvulsants	Phenytoin (Dilantin)	Seizures	Fetal hydantoin syndrome
	Valproic acid		Neural tube defects
	Carbamazepine		Neural tube defects
	Lamotrigine		Possibly fetal anomalies
Anticoagulants	Warfarin (Coumadin)	Anticoagulation	Fetal bleeding or anomalies
Antidepressants	Imipramine (Tofranil)	Elevate mood	Cardiovascular anomalies
Antidiabetic agents	Chlorpropamide	Lower blood glucose	Neonatal hypoglycemia
Antischizophrenic	Lithium	Schizophrenia	Hydramnios
Antithyroid	Methimazole	Hypothyroidism	Hypothyroidism in fetus
Antibiotics	Ribavirin	Respiratory infection	Multiple anomalies
	Sulfonamides	Infection	Hyperbilirubinemia in newborn
	Tetracycline	Infection	Teeth and bone deformities
Antihelmintics	Lindane	Eradication of lice	Manufacturer recommends limiting exposure to two dosages
Angiotensin-converting enzyme inhibitors	Enalapril (Vasotec)	Reduce hypertension	Oligohydramnios (reduced amount of amniotic fluid
	Captopril (Capoten)		
Caffeine	Coffee, soft drinks, chocolate	Social use	Low birth weight
Hypoglycemics	Tolbutamide (Orinase)	Type 2 diabetes	Profound hypoglycemia in newborn
Nicotine	Tobacco	Relaxation	Growth restriction
Radiopharmaceuticals	Iodide-131	Diagnostic studies	May destroy thyroid of fetus
Narcotics	Cocaine	Social pleasure	Dysmorphic and central nervous system (CNS) anomalies
	Heroin		Growth restriction; narcotic abstinence in newborn
Tranquilizers	Benzodiazepine (diazepam)	Reduce anxiety	Growth restriction; CNS dysfunction
			Hypotonia, respiratory depression
Vaccines (live)	Rubella	Provide immunity	Possible infection in fetus
Vitamin A derivatives	Etretinate (Tegison)	Psoriasis	Craniofacial, cardiac, CNS anomalies

From Koren, G. (2012). Special aspects of perinatal & pediatric pharmacology. In B. G. Katzung, S. B. Masters, & A. J. Trevor (Eds.), *Basic & clinical pharmacology* (11th ed., pp. 1039–1050). Columbus, OH: McGraw-Hill/Lange.

Teratogenicity of Alcohol

Evidence confirms that when women consume a large quantity of alcohol during pregnancy, their babies demonstrate a high incidence of characteristic congenital craniofacial deformities including short palpebral fissures, a thin upper lip, an upturned nose, as well as cognitive impairment (**fetal alcohol spectrum**; Paintner, Williams, & Burd, 2012). Fetuses cannot remove the breakdown products of alcohol from their body. The large buildup of these leads to vitamin B deficiency and accompanying neurologic damage.

Because of individual variations in metabolism, it is impossible to define a safe level of alcohol consumption. Women, therefore, should be screened for alcohol use at a first prenatal visit and are best advised to abstain from alcohol completely for the remainder of their pregnancy. Be certain to ask about binge drinking (e.g., consuming more than four alcoholic drinks in an evening with the intention of becoming intoxicated) because women may refer to this as only "occasional drinking." If necessary, refer women with alcohol addiction to an alcohol treatment program as early in pregnancy as possible to help them reduce their alcohol intake.

Teratogenicity of Tobacco

Cigarette smoking is associated with infertility in women. If used by a pregnant woman, it has been shown to cause fetal growth restriction. In addition, a fetus may be at greater risk for being stillborn and, after birth, may be at a greater risk than others for sudden infant death syndrome (Treyster & Gitterman, 2011).

Low birth weights in infants of smoking mothers result from vasoconstriction of the uterine vessels, an effect of nicotine. This limits the blood supply to a fetus. Another contributory effect may be related to inhaled carbon monoxide. Secondary smoke, or inhaling the smoke of another person's cigarettes, may be as harmful as actually smoking because of inhaled carbon monoxide. All prenatal health care settings should be smoke-free environments for this reason.

If a woman cannot stop smoking during pregnancy (and, realistically, many women cannot), reducing the number of cigarettes smoked per day should help diminish adverse effects on a fetus as well as also protect a woman's own health from long-term illnesses, such as chronic respiratory diseases, in the future.

The best way to urge women to discontinue smoking is to educate them about the risks to themselves and their fetus at the first prenatal visit and then offer a support program to help them throughout the pregnancy. It may be effective to encourage women to sign a contract with their health care provider to try to stop or to join a smoking-cessation program. Be certain pregnant women know it would be best if they didn't enter a stop-smoking program that uses drug therapy such as nicotine patches until it is clear if such patches are not harmful to a fetus (Coleman, Cooper, Thornton, et al., 2012). Box 12.9 shows an interprofessional care map illustrating both nursing and team planning to address decreasing alcohol and tobacco use during pregnancy.

Environmental Teratogens

Teratogens such as impure air or water can be as damaging to a fetus as those that are directly or deliberately ingested. Women are exposed to these through contact at home or at work sites. Breathing air filled with pollutants, for example, has been shown to lead to fetal growth restriction (Lee, Roberts, Catov, et al., 2013).

Metal and Chemical Hazards

Pesticides and carbon monoxide, such as from automobile exhaust, should be avoided as these are examples of chemical teratogens. Arsenic, a byproduct of copper and lead smelting, used in pesticides, paints, and leather processing; formaldehyde, used in paper manufacturing; and mercury, used in the manufacture of electrical apparatuses and found in high proportions in swordfish and tuna, are all teratogens that can be found at work sites.

Lead poisoning generally is considered a problem of young children who eat lead-based paint chips, but it can be a fetal hazard as well. Women may ingest lead by drinking water that travels through old pipes that are leaking lead, by "sniffing" lead-based gasoline, or eating paint chips (paint tastes sweet and may be eaten as a symptom of pica). Lead ingestion during pregnancy may lead to a newborn who is both cognitively and neurologically challenged (Couloures & Vasan, 2011).

Radiation

Rapidly growing cells are extremely vulnerable to destruction by radiation. This makes radiation a potent teratogen to unborn children because they have such a high proportion of rapidly growing cells. Radiation produces a range of malformations depending on the stage of development of the embryo or fetus and the strength and length of exposure. If the exposure occurs before implantation, for example, the growing zygote apparently is killed. If the zygote is not killed, it survives apparently unharmed. The most damaging time for exposure and subsequent damage is from implantation to 6 weeks after conception (a time when many women are not yet aware they are pregnant). The nervous system, brain, and the retinal innervation are growing rapidly at this time and so are most affected (CDC, 2012).

Even with this danger of radiation, X-rays to maternal parts other than the pelvis, including computerized tomography (CT) can be performed safely during pregnancy as long as a lead pelvic shield is provided (Nelson-Piercy, 2012). If a woman of childbearing age requires a pelvic X-ray for any reason, this should be scheduled during the first 10 days of a menstrual cycle (when pregnancy is unlikely because ovulation has not yet occurred); during pregnancy, X-rays of the pelvis should be avoided except in emergency situations. Even fluoroscopy, which uses lower radiation doses than regular X-ray photography, should also be avoided during pregnancy—again, except in an emergency. A serum pregnancy test to rule out pregnancy can be completed on women who have reason to believe they might be pregnant before diagnostic tests involving X-rays are scheduled.

X-rays should be taken at term only if the data obtained are vitally important for birth and cannot be obtained by any other means. Sonography and magnetic resonance imaging can be used for confirmation of situations such as a multiple pregnancy because these do not appear to be teratogenic (Nemec, Nemec, Brugger, et al., 2012). Although still being investigated, long-term use of slight radiation sources, such as a computer, microwave oven, or cellular phone, also do not appear to be teratogenic (Feychting, 2011).

BOX 12.9 Nursing Care Planning

AN INTERPROFESSIONAL CARE MAP FOR A PREGNANT WOMAN WITH THREATS TO FETAL HEALTH

Julberry Adams, a single 30-year-old woman, is 4 months pregnant when you first see her in a prenatal clinic. She works as a curator for an art gallery but has missed work this past week because of nausea. She's worried she will not be able to work past 6 months of her pregnancy because her job involves a great deal of walking. She has already stopped her volunteer work of teaching children's swimming at the YMCA. She wants to travel to see her sister in St. Louis because her sister is very ill but has heard pregnant women should not drive more than 100 miles. She asks you if marijuana would help reduce her early pregnancy nausea.

Family Assessment Client lives by herself in one-bedroom apartment. Rates finances as "Good, unless I have to quit work because of pregnancy." She asks you, "Will I have to have an ultrasound? I'm worried about that."

Client Assessment Gravida 1, para 0. Unsure of date of last menstrual period, but it was about 11 weeks ago. Uterine height barely above symphysis. Fetal heart rate at 148 beats/min by Doppler. History of frequent sinus headaches. "I use Sudafed (pseudoephedrine) at least three to four times a week; sometimes other things." Smokes one-half pack of cigarettes "some days." Drinks two to three glasses of wine per week at art gallery functions. Denies history of marijuana or other recreational drug use.

Nursing Diagnosis Risk for fetal injury related to knowledge deficit concerning possible fetal exposure to teratogens.

Outcome Criteria Client reports a decrease in smoking to less than 10 cigarettes per day and no alcohol consumption by next prenatal visit; verbalizes no use of recreational drugs, including marijuana.

Client states she has contacted health care provider about whether she should continue to use sinus medications.

Team Member Responsible	Assessment	Intervention	Rationale	Expected Outcome
Activities of Daily Living, Including Safety				
Nurse	Assess what activities client wants to participate in during pregnancy.	Discuss desired activities and any modification necessary for pregnancy with client.	Finding a match between desired activities and necessary modifications will help with adherence.	Client discusses what activities she intends to continue during pregnancy and ways to modify them as necessary.
Nurse/Primary health care provider	Assess what work or travel plans entail.	Assure client she can continue work, travel to sister's home.	Reassurance helps client maintain usual lifestyle.	Client states she will continue work, maintain contact with sister.
Teamwork and Collaboration				
Nurse/Primary health care provider	Assess what medications client is currently taking.	Consult with health care provider about safety of over-the-counter (OTC) sinus medications.	Not all OTC medications are safe during pregnancy.	Client states she will follow recommendations of primary health care provider regarding medications.
Procedures/Medications for Quality Improvement				
Nurse/Primary health care provider	Anticipate the need for follow-up ultrasound examination to date pregnancy.	Explain the need for ultrasound exam to assess dating and possible fetal growth restriction because of alcohol and cigarette smoking habits.	Teratogen exposure may have slowed fetal growth, which will be revealed by ultrasound exam. Date of last menstrual period is unknown.	Client states she is aware of purpose of ultrasound exam and will allow exam to be scheduled.

(continued on page 296)

BOX 12.9 Nursing Care Planning (continued)

Nutrition				
Nurse/Nutritionist	Assess client's lifestyle to see what beverages she could substitute for alcohol, what measures she could use best for nausea.	Suggest client replace alcohol consumption with caffeine-free beverages. Suggest measures to combat nausea and vomiting, such as dry crackers or acupuncture band.	Alcohol consumption during pregnancy is associated with fetal alcohol spectrum. Decreasing nausea to increase food intake aids fetal growth and development.	Client voices intent to replace alcohol consumption with caffeine-free beverages. Client suggests measures that appeal to her to reduce nausea and vomiting.
Patient-Centered Care				
Nurse/Primary health care provider	Assess whether client has tried any nonmedicinal measures to relieve sinus headaches.	Discuss with client possible nonmedicinal measures to assist with sinus headache relief, such as saline nasal sprays, humidification, and warm compresses to nasal area.	Complementary comfort measures may provide symptomatic relief without danger to the fetus.	Client describes two complementary therapies she will at least try to relieve sinus congestion.
Psychosocial/Spiritual/Emotional Needs				
Nurse/Social worker	Discuss with client whether her current support system is adequate.	Help client locate at least one person she can depend on if a pregnancy emergency should arise.	Pregnancy can be a very stressful time for a woman who has an insecure support system.	Client telephones or e-mails the health care facility with questions rather than relying on nonexperienced friends for information; names one reliable support person.
Informatics for Seamless Health Care Planning				
Nurse	Assess extent of cigarette smoking.	Encourage the client to decrease smoking and quit if possible. Offer suggestions to accomplish this goal, including use of sugar-free gums or candies, distraction, and activity. Refer to a smoking-cessation group if appropriate.	Cigarette use during pregnancy can lead to fetal growth restriction. Support and suggestions provide concrete measures to assist client with cutting down and quitting.	Client voices intention to decrease smoking and, if possible, quit smoking during pregnancy.

In addition to immediate fetal damage, evidence demonstrates that radiation can have long-lasting effects on the health of a child. There appears to be an increased risk of cancer in children who are exposed to radiation in utero. Exposure of the fetal gonads could lead to a genetic mutation that will not be evident until the next generation (Wang, Chong, Kielar, et al., 2012).

Hyperthermia and Hypothermia

Hyperthermia to a fetus can be detrimental to growth because it interferes with cell metabolism. This can occur from the use of saunas, hot tubs, or tanning beds; from a work environment next to a furnace, such as in welding or steel making; or from a high maternal fever early in pregnancy (4 to 6 weeks). For this reason, advise pregnant women not to use hot tubs, saunas, or tanning beds during pregnancy.

The effect of hypothermia on pregnancy is not well known. Because the uterus is an internal organ, a woman's body temperature would have to be lowered significantly before a great deal of fetal temperature change would result.

Teratogenic Maternal Stress

There is some evidence that a pregnancy filled with anxiety and worry beyond the usual amount could produce physiologic changes through their effects on the sympathetic division of the autonomic nervous system. The primary change this would cause includes constriction of the peripheral blood vessels (i.e., a fight-or-flight syndrome). If the anxiety is prolonged, the constriction of uterine vessels (the uterus is a peripheral organ) could substantially interfere with the blood and nutrient supply to a fetus (Alderdice, Lynn, & Lobel, 2012).

It is important to remember these phenomena are characteristic only of long-term, extreme stress, not the normal anxiety of pregnancy. Personal tragedies such as a house fire, illness or death of one's partner, difficulty with relatives, marital discord, living in a war zone, and illness or death of another child are examples of stressful situations that might provoke this excessive level of anxiety.

It's not easy to help a woman resolve complex problems of this type during pregnancy because they are complicated. To prevent maternal stress from becoming severe, advise counseling for women with low stress levels at prenatal care visits before the levels become extreme.

QSEN Checkpoint Question 12.6

Safety

Julberry Adams makes the following statements. Which one would you rate as the safest practice?

a. "My brother takes medicine for heartburn; if I think of it, I'll borrow his."
b. "I'm going to get a measles shot; I don't want measles while I'm pregnant."
c. "There are so many medicines for headache; I'll ask my doctor what to take."
d. "I know all over-the-counter medicine is safe; that's why it's over the counter."

Look in Appendix A for the best answer and rationale.

PREPARATION FOR LABOR

At about the midpoint of pregnancy, along with cautioning women about new minor body changes and possible teratogenic threats, it is a good time to review the signs or symptoms that signal the beginning of labor so women will not be surprised by these happenings or dismiss them as something other than the important events that they are. These are discussed in the following sections and summarized in Table 12.2.

Preliminary Signs of Labor

In the days or hours before labor begins, a woman often experiences subtle signs or symptoms that signal labor is imminent. Because these signs and symptoms are subtle, they are easily missed if a woman is not informed of them in advance.

Lightening

In primiparas, *lightening*, or descent of the fetal presenting part (usually the fetal head) into the pelvis, occurs approximately 10 to 14 days before labor begins. This fetal descent changes a woman's abdominal contour because it positions the uterus lower and more anterior in the abdomen. Lightening gives a woman relief from the diaphragmatic pressure and shortness of breath she has been experiencing and in this way "lightens" her load. Lightening probably occurs early in primiparas this way because of tight abdominal muscles. In multiparas, it is not as dramatic and usually occurs on the day of labor or even after labor has begun. As the fetus sinks lower into the pelvis, a woman may experience shooting leg pains from the increased pressure on a sciatic nerve, increased amounts of vaginal discharge, and urinary frequency from pressure on her bladder.

TABLE 12.2 Beginning Signs and Symptoms of Labor

Sign or Symptom	Cause
Lightening	Sinking of the fetal head into the true pelvis
Slight loss of weight	As progesterone level falls, more fluid is excreted, slightly lowering body weight
Excess energy	Burst of adrenaline to provide energy for labor
Backache	Beginning but unrecognized uterine contractions
Ripening of the cervix	Prostaglandins soften the cervix to allow for shortening and dilatation
Rupture of membranes	Membranes have ruptured with release of amniotic fluid
Show	Internal cervical mucus plug has been released
Uterine contractions	True beginning of labor

Increase in Energy

A woman may awaken on the morning of labor full of energy, in contrast to the feeling of chronic fatigue that she has been feeling for the previous month. This increase in activity is related to a boost in epinephrine release, which is initiated by a decrease in progesterone production by the placenta. This additional epinephrine prepares a woman's body for the work of labor ahead. It's important that the woman recognizes this sensation for what it is or she may use this burst of energy to clean her house or finish paperwork at the office and exhaust herself before labor begins. If she can recognize this symptom as an initial sign of labor, she can conserve her energy in preparation for labor.

Slight Loss of Weight

As progesterone level falls, body fluid is more easily excreted from the body. This increase in urine production can lead to a weight loss between 1 and 3 lb.

Backache

Because labor contractions begin in the back, an intermittent backache stronger than usual may be the first symptom a woman notices.

Braxton Hicks Contractions

In the last week or days before labor begins, a woman usually notices extremely strong Braxton Hicks contractions. A woman having her first child may have such difficulty distinguishing between these and true contractions that she may come to the labor unit of a hospital or birthing center believing she is in labor. It is discouraging for a woman when this happens (strong Braxton Hicks contractions cause true discomfort) to be told she is not in true labor and should return home. When this happens, you can assure the woman that misinterpreting labor signals is common. Remind her that if contractions have become strong enough to be mistaken for true labor, true labor is not far away.

Ripening of the Cervix

Ripening of the cervix is an internal sign seen only on pelvic examination. Throughout pregnancy, the cervix feels softer than usual to palpation, similar to the consistency of an earlobe (Goodell's sign). At term, the cervix becomes still softer (described as "butter soft"), and it tips forward. Cervical ripening this way is an internal announcement that labor is very close at hand.

Signs of True Labor

Signs of true labor involve both uterine and cervical changes. The contrast between true and false labor is summarized in Chapter 15, Table 15.3.

Uterine Contractions

True labor contractions usually begin in the back and sweep forward across the abdomen similar to the tightening of a rubber band. They gradually increase in frequency and intensity over a period of hours. Because contractions are involuntary and come without warning, their intensity can be frightening in early labor. Helping a woman appreciate that she can predict when her next one will occur and therefore can control the degree of discomfort she feels by using breathing exercises offers her a sense of control.

Advise a woman to telephone her primary care provider when contractions begin to alert health care personnel that she is in labor. Her health care provider will advise her as to what point in labor she should come to the health care facility she has chosen or when to begin preparations for home birth if that is her choice. The typical time for this is when contractions are 5 minutes apart, but this will vary depending on a woman's past and present pregnancy history. In all instances, if a woman should become exceptionally anxious, be home alone, or have a long drive, she should be given options as to when it would be best for her to leave home.

Show

As the cervix softens and ripens, the mucus plug that filled the cervical canal during pregnancy is expelled. The exposed cervical capillaries seep blood as a result of pressure exerted by the fetus. This blood, mixed with mucus, takes on a pink tinge and is referred to as "show" or "bloody show." Women need to be aware of this event so they do not think they are bleeding abnormally.

Rupture of the Membranes

Labor may begin with rupture of the membranes, experienced either as a sudden gush or as a scanty, slow seeping of clear fluid from the vagina. Some women may worry if their labor begins with a rupture of the membranes because they have heard labor will then be "dry" and this will cause it to be difficult and long. Actually, amniotic fluid continues to be produced until delivery of the membranes after the birth of their child, so no labor is ever "dry." Early rupture of the membranes can actually be advantageous as it can cause the fetal head to settle snugly into the pelvis, aiding cervical dilation and shortening labor.

A woman should telephone her primary health care provider immediately when her membranes rupture as two risks are associated with ruptured membranes: intrauterine infection and prolapse of the umbilical cord (which could cut off the oxygen supply to the fetus) (Brailovschi, Sheiner, Wiznitzer, et al., 2012). In most instances, the fetal head is already snugly fitting the cervix, so prolapse is not a concern. If labor does not spontaneously begin by 24 hours after membrane rupture and the pregnancy is at term, labor will likely be induced to help reduce the risk of infection.

What if... 12.4 You are particularly interested in exploring one of the 2020 National Health Goals with respect to fetal and maternal health (see Box 12.1). What would be a possible research topic to explore pertinent to this goal that would be applicable to Julberry or her family and that would also advance evidence-based practice?

Key Points for Review

- Prenatal education is an important part of prenatal care. The more women know about measures they should take during pregnancy to safeguard their health, the more likely they will be to avoid substances or activities harmful to fetal growth.
- Urge women to find the best way for them to modify their individual lifestyle for pregnancy as this helps in planning nursing care that not only meets QSEN competencies but also best meets the family's total needs. Remember, pregnancy is 9 months long, so modifications must be agreeable to the woman or she will not maintain them over such a long time.
- Women need to make provisions for rest periods during their day and to be aware of any potential teratogens at a work site, such as exposure to radiation or heavy metals.
- Women who travel should plan for break periods to avoid congestion in their lower extremities. Seat belts should be used when traveling by car. On an airplane, a woman may need to ask for an extension seatbelt.
- Common minor body changes of early pregnancy include breast tenderness, constipation, palmar erythema, nausea and vomiting, fatigue, muscle cramps, pain from varicosities or hemorrhoids, heart palpitations, frequency of urination, and leukorrhea. If women know these symptoms may occur, they will not interpret them as complications but usual events.

- Minor body changes of middle or late pregnancy include backache, dyspnea, ankle edema, Braxton Hicks contractions, sleep disturbance, restless leg syndrome, and carpal tunnel syndrome. Caution women that contractions could be a sign of labor.
- Women should take active measures to avoid exposure to infectious diseases such as rubella, HIV, hepatitis B and C, cytomegalovirus, herpes simplex virus, syphilis, and toxoplasmosis during pregnancy.
- Counsel pregnant women about the necessity to avoid the use of any drug or herbal supplement not specifically approved by their primary health care provider as well as alcohol and tobacco.
- It is almost impossible for a woman to modify a behavior, such as smoking, if her support person does not agree to change also. Including a woman's family in care is an important way to help support persons understand the need for the modification and increasing cooperation.
- Beginning signs of labor for which a pregnant woman should be alert include lightening, show, excess energy, rupture of membranes, and uterine contractions.

CRITICAL THINKING CARE STUDY

Emma Hennigan is a 34-year-old woman who is 3 months pregnant with her second pregnancy. She has a 2-year-old son at home. She tells you this pregnancy has not "been fun" because it is so different from her first pregnancy. She has had nausea, fatigue, and frequent urination 24/7 for the last 3 months. She wants to quit her job as a short-order cook so she can feel better, but her boyfriend won't let her "even consider this" as they need the money. The only thing she does all week to feel "like her old self" or to make the pregnancy "bearable" is to jog around a neighborhood park two times a day.

1. Emma wants to quit work so she feels better. Would you recommend she do this?
2. Emma needs to use a restroom often at work because she has the symptom of frequent urination. This is difficult, however, because this involves a long walk and time away from cooking. She asks if drinking less fluid will help relieve this symptom. How would you advise her?
3. Emma finds two breaks during the day during which she jogs—the only activity that is making her pregnancy "bearable." Would you encourage her to continue doing this for the remainder of her pregnancy?

Patient Scenario:

The Harper Family

Read about the Harper family, a family experiencing a first pregnancy, then answer the questions to further sharpen your skills and grow more familiar with NCLEX-type questions related to minor changes of pregnancy and prenatal care. Confirm your answers are correct by reading the rationales.

Visit http://thePoint.lww.com

Answers and Rationales

Looking for answers to the What If. . . and Critical Thinking Care Study questions?

Visit http://thePoint.lww.com

References

ADA Amendments Act of 2008, Pub. L. 110–325, S. 3406 (2008).

Alderdice, F., Lynn, F., & Lobel, M. (2012). A review and psychometric evaluation of pregnancy-specific stress measures. *Journal of Psychosomatic Obstetrics & Gynaecology, 33*(2), 62–77.

Allahdin, S., & Kambhampati, L. (2012). Stress urinary incontinence in continent primigravidas. *Journal of Obstetrics & Gynaecology,* 32(1), 2–5.

Amant, F., Brepoels, L., Halaska, M. J., et al. (2010). Gynaecologic cancer complicating pregnancy: An overview. *Best Practice & Research: Clinical Obstetrics & Gynaecology, 24,* 61–79.

Attilakos, G., & Overton, T. G. (2012). Antenatal care. In D. K. Edmonds (Ed.), *Dewhurst's textbook of obstetrics & gynaecology* (6th ed., pp. 42–52). Oxford, UK: John Wiley & Son.

Babbar, S., Parks-Savage, A. C., & Chauhan, S. P. (2012). Yoga during pregnancy: A review. *American Journal of Perinatology, 29*(6), 459–464.

Brailovschi, Y., Sheiner, E., Wiznitzer, A., et al. (2012). Risk factors for intrapartum fetal death and trends over the years. *Archives of Gynecology & Obstetrics, 285*(2), 323–329.

Centers for Disease Control and Prevention. (2011). *Traveler's health.* Washington, DC: Author.

Centers for Disease Control and Prevention. (2012). *Radiation and pregnancy*. Washington, DC: Author.

Chen, Y. Y., Yen, H. H., Chou, K. C., et al. (2012). Thalidomide-based multidisciplinary treatment for patients with advanced hepatocellular carcinoma: A retrospective analysis. *World Journal of Gastroenterology, 18*(5), 466–471.

Coad, J., & Dunstall, M. (2011). Physiological adaptation to pregnancy. In J. Coad & M. Dunstall (Eds.), *Anatomy & physiology for midwives* (pp. 257–288). London, England: Elsevier/Churchill Livingstone.

Coleman, T., Cooper, S., Thornton, J. G., et al. (2012). A randomized trial of nicotine-replacement therapy patches in pregnancy. *New England Journal of Medicine, 366*(9), 808–818.

Corbacioglu, A., Bakir, V. L., Akbayir, O., et al. (2012). The role of pregnancy awareness on female sexual function in early gestation. *Journal of Sexual Medicine, 9*(7), 1897–1903.

Couloures, K., & Vasan, R. (2011). Prenatal lead poisoning due to maternal exposure results in developmental delay. *Pediatrics International, 53*(2), 242–244

Dijkmans, A. C., de Jong, E. P., Dijkmans, B. A., et al. (2012). Parvovirus B19 in pregnancy: Prenatal diagnosis and management of fetal complications. *Current Opinion in Obstetrics & Gynecology, 24*(2), 95–101.

Dixit, A., Bhardwaj, M., & Sharma, B. (2012). Headache in pregnancy: A nuisance or a new sense? *Obstetrics and Gynecology International.* Advance online publication. doi: 10.1155/2012/697697

Duong, H. T., Shahrukh-Hashmi, S., Ramadhani, T., et al. (2011). Maternal use of hot tub and major structural birth defects. *Birth Defects Research, 91*(9), 836–841.

Ebrahimi, N., Vohra, S., Gedeon, C., et al. (2011). The fetal safety of hydrocortisone-pramoxine (Proctofoam-HC) for the treatment of hemorrhoids in late pregnancy. *Journal of Obstetrics & Gynaecology Canada, 33*(2), 153–158.

Family and Medical Leave Act of 1993, Pub. L. No. 103-3, 107 Stat. 6 (1993).

Fantasia, H. C., Sutherland, M. A., Fontenot, H. B., et al. (2012). Chronicity of partner violence, contraceptive patterns and pregnancy risk. *Contraception, 86*(5), 530–535.

Feychting, M. (2011). Mobile phones, radiofrequency fields, and health effects in children—Epidemiological studies. *Progress in Biophysics & Molecular Biology, 107*(3), 343–348.

Follett, T., & Clarke, D. F. (2011). Resurgence of congenital syphilis: Diagnosis and treatment. *Neonatal Network, 30*(5), 320–328.

Fortner, K. B., Kuller, J. A., Rhee, E. J., et al. (2012). Influenza and tetanus, diphtheria, and acellular pertussis vaccinations during pregnancy. *Obstetrical & Gynecology Survey, 67*(4), 251–257.

Fung, A. M., Wilson, D. L., Barnes, M., et al. (2012). Obstructive sleep apnea and pregnancy: The effect on perinatal outcomes. *Journal of Perinatology, 32*(6), 399–406.

Galbarczyk, A. (2011). Unexpected changes in maternal breast size during pregnancy in relation to infant sex: An evolutionary interpretation. *American Journal of Human Biology, 23*(4), 560–562.

Guile, M. W., & Keller, J. (2011). Infections of the genital tract. In K. J. Hurt, M. W. Guile, J. L. Bienstock, et al. (Eds.), *The Johns Hopkins manual of gynecology and obstetrics* (4th ed., pp. 322–348). Philadelphia, PA: Lippincott Williams & Wilkins.

Gülmezoglu, A. M., & Azhar, M. (2011). Interventions for trichomoniasis in pregnancy. *Cochrane Database of Systematic Reviews,* (5), CD000220.

Hayatbakhsh, M. R., Flenady, V. J., Gibbons, K. S., et al. (2012). Birth outcomes associated with cannabis use before and during pregnancy. *Pediatric Research, 71*(2), 215–219.

Hezelgrave, N. L., Whitty, C. J., Shennan, A. H., et al. (2011). Advising on travel during pregnancy. *British Medical Journal, 342*(4), d2506.

Horton, A. L., & Boggess, K. A. (2012). Periodontal disease and preterm birth. *Obstetrics & Gynecological Clinics of North America, 39*(1), 17–23.

Ishaque, S., Yakoob, M. Y., Imdad, A., et al. (2011). Effectiveness of interventions to screen and manage infections during pregnancy on reducing stillbirths: A review. *BMC Public Health, 11*(Suppl. 3), S3.

Jaiyeoba, O., Amaya, M. I., Soper, D. E., et al. (2012). Preventing neonatal transmission of herpes simplex virus. *Clinical Obstetrics & Gynecology, 55*(2), 510–520.

Johnson, J., Anderson, B., & Pass, R. F. (2012). Prevention of maternal and congenital cytomegalovirus infection. *Clinical Obstetrics & Gynecology, 55*(2), 521–530.

Jones, L., Othman, M., Dowswell, T., et al. (2012). Pain management for women in labour: An overview of systematic reviews. *Cochrane Database of Systematic Reviews,* (3), CD009234.

Karch, A. M. (2012). *2013 Lippincott's nursing drug guide.* Philadelphia, PA: Lippincott Williams & Wilkins.

Klemetti, R., Kurinczuk, J. J., & Redshaw, M. (2011). Older women's pregnancy related symptoms, health and use of antenatal services. *European Journal of Obstetrics, Gynecology & Reproductive Biology, 154*(2), 157–162.

Koren, G. (2012). Special aspects of perinatal & pediatric pharmacology. In B. G. Katzung, S. B. Masters, & A. J. Trevor (Eds.), *Basic & clinical pharmacology* (11th ed., pp. 1039–1050). Columbus, OH: McGraw-Hill/Lange.

Kovacs, F. M., Garcia, E., Royuela, A., et al. (2012). Prevalence and factors associated with low back pain and pelvic girdle pain during pregnancy. *Spine, 37*(17), 1516–1533.

Kramer, M. S., & McDonald, S. W. (2010). Aerobic exercise for women during pregnancy. *Cochrane Database of Systematic Reviews,* (6), CD000180.

Lachat, M. F., Solnik, A. L., Nana, A. D., et al. (2011). Periodontal disease in pregnancy: Review of the evidence and prevention strategies. *Journal of Perinatal & Neonatal Nursing, 25*(4), 312–319.

Lee, P., Roberts, J. M., Catov, J. M., et al. (2013). First trimester exposure to ambient air pollution, pregnancy complications and adverse birth outcomes in Allegheny County, PA. *Maternal and Child Health Journal, 17*(3), 545–555

Lyberg, A., Viken, B., Haruna, M., et al. (2012). Diversity and challenges in the management of maternity care for migrant women. *Journal of Nursing Management, 20*(2), 287–295.

Mali, S., Kachur, S. P., & Arguin, P. M. (2012). Malaria surveillance—United States, 2010. *Morbidity & Mortality Weekly Report, 61*(2), 1–17.

Marcdante, K. J., Kliegman, R. M., Jenson, H. B., et al. (2011). Congenital infections. In K. J. Marcdante, R. M. Kliegman, H. B. Jenson, et al. (Eds.), *Nelson essentials of pediatrics* (6th ed., pp. 258–264). Philadelphia, PA: Saunders/Elsevier.

Marrazzo, J. M., & Cates, W. (2011). Interventions to prevent sexually transmitted infections, including HIV infection. *Clinical Infectious Diseases, 53* (Suppl. 3), S64–S78.

Mayo Clinic. (2011). *Mayo Clinic guide to a healthy pregnancy.* Rochester, MN: Author.

Milloy, M. J., Marshall, B., Kerr, T., et al. (2012). Social and structural factors associated with HIV disease progression among illicit drug users: A systematic review. *AIDS, 26*(9), 1049–1063.

National Center for Complementary and Alternative Medicine. (2010). *Herbs at a glance.* Washington, DC: Author.

National Institute of Occupational Safety and Health. (2010). *Pocket guide to chemical hazards.* Washington, DC: DHHS.

Nelson-Piercy, C. (2012). Heart disease in pregnancy. In D. K. Edmonds (Ed.), *Dewhurst's textbook of obstetrics & gynaecology* (6th ed., pp. 111–120). Oxford, UK: John Wiley & Son.

Nemec, S. F., Nemec, U., Brugger, P. C., et al. (2012). MR imaging of the fetal musculoskeletal system. *Prenatal Diagnosis, 32*(3), 205–213.

Omar, N. S., Tan, P. C., Sabir, N., et al. (2013). Coitus to expedite the onset of labour: A randomised trial. *BJOG: An international journal of obstetrics and gynaecology, 120*(3), 338–345.

Paintner, A., Williams, A. D., & Burd, L. (2012). Fetal alcohol spectrum disorders—Implications for child neurology. *Journal of Child Neurology, 27*(2), 258–263.

Pavlova, M., & Sheikh, L. S. (2011). Sleep in women. *Seminars in Neurology, 31*(4), 397–403.

Perlen, S., Woolhouse, H., Gartland, D., et al. (2013). Maternal depression and physical health problems in early pregnancy: Findings of an Australian nulliparous pregnancy cohort study. *Midwifery,* 29(3), 233–239.

Pipkin, F. P. (2012). Maternal physiology. In D. K. Edmonds (Ed.), *Dewhurst's textbook of obstetrics & gynaecology* (6th ed., pp. 5–15). Oxford, UK: John Wiley & Son.

Power, M. L., Wilson, E. K, Hogan, S.O., et al. (2013). Patterns of preconception, prenatal and postnatal care for diabetic women by obstetrician-gynecologists. *Journal of Reproductive Medicine, 58*(1–2), 7–14.

Rasmussen, S. A. (2012). Human teratogens update 2011: Can we ensure safety during pregnancy? *Birth Defects Research, 94*(3), 123–128.

Rogers, V. L., & Worley, K. C. (2011). Obstetrics & obstetric disorders. In S. J. McPhee, M. A. Papadakis, & M. W. Rabow (Eds.), *Current medical diagnosis & treatment* (51st ed., pp. 760–787). Columbus, OH: McGraw-Hill.

Russell, J. B., Denne, E. W., & Schwartz, D. (2011). Preconception counseling and prenatal care. In K. J. Hurt, M. W. Guile, J. L. Bienstock, et al. (Eds.), *The Johns Hopkins manual of gynecology and obstetrics* (4th ed., pp. 56–72). Philadelphia, PA: Lippincott Williams & Wilkins.

Salihu, H. M., Myers, J., & August, E. M. (2012). Pregnancy in the workplace. *Occupational Medicine (London), 62*(2), 88–97.

Sanders, A. P., Flood, K., Chiang, S., et al. (2012). Towards prenatal biomonitoring in North Carolina: Assessing arsenic, cadmium, mercury, and lead levels in pregnant women. *PLoS One, 7*(3), e31354.

Shankaran, S., Das, A., Bauer, C. R., et al. (2011). Prenatal cocaine exposure and small-for-gestational-age status: Effects on growth at 6 years of age. *Neurotoxicology & Teratology, 33*(5), 575–581.

Shiraishi, M., Haruna, M., Matsuzaki, M., et al. (2010). Association between the serum folate levels and tea consumption during pregnancy. *Bioscience Trends, 4*(5), 225–230.

Sibai, B. M. (2011). Evaluation and management of severe preeclampsia before 34 weeks' gestation. *American Journal of Obstetrics & Gynecology, 205*(3), 191–198.

Stohl, H., & Satin, A. J. (2011). Perinatal infections. In K. J. Hurt, M. W. Guile, J. L. Bienstock, et al. (Eds.), *The Johns Hopkins manual of gynecology and obstetrics* (4th ed., pp. 137–153). Philadelphia, PA: Lippincott Williams & Wilkins.

Stout, S. M., & Stumpf, J. L. (2010). Finasteride treatment of hair loss in women. *Annals of Pharmacotherapy, 44*(6), 1090–1097

Szymanski, L. M., & Satin, A. J. (2012). Exercise during pregnancy: Fetal responses to current public health guidelines. *Obstetrics & Gynecology, 119*(3), 603–610.

Treyster, Z., & Gitterman, B. (2011). Second hand smoke exposure in children: Environmental factors, physiological effects, and interventions within pediatrics. *Reviews on Environmental Health, 26*(3), 187–195.

Tsai, S. Y., Kuo, L. T., Lai, Y. H., et al. (2011). Factors associated with sleep quality in pregnant women: A prospective observational study. *Nursing Research, 60*(6), 405–412.

United Nations. (2000). *Millennium Health Goals, 2000-2015.* New York, NY: Author.

U.S. Department of Health and Human Services. (2010). *Healthy people 2020.* Washington, DC: Author.

U.S. Food and Drug Administration. (n.d.). *FDA pregnancy categories.* Washington, DC: Author.

U.S. Senate Committee on Labor and Human Resources. (1980). *Legislative history of the Pregnancy Discrimination Act of 1978.* Washington, DC: Government Printing Office.

Walker, G. J. A. (2010). Antibiotics for syphilis diagnosed during pregnancy. *Cochrane Database of Systematic Reviews,* (1), CD001143.

Walsh, M. (2012). Drugs for disorders in women's health. In J. L. Kee, E. R. Hayes, & L. E. McCuistion (Eds.), *Pharmacology: A nursing process approach* (pp. 903–921). St. Louis, MO: Elsevier/Saunders.

Wang, P. I., Chong, S. T., Kielar, A. Z., et al. (2012). Imaging of pregnant and lactating patients. *American Journal of Roentgenology, 198*(4), 778–784.

White, S. J., Boldt, K. L., Holditch, S. J., et al. (2012). Measles, mumps, and rubella. *Clinical Obstetrics & Gynecology, 55*(2), 550–559.

Whitmore, S. K., Taylor, A. W., Espinoza, L., et al. (2012). Correlates of mother-to-child transmission of HIV in the United States and Puerto Rico. *Pediatrics, 129*(1), e74–e81.

Young, G. L., & Jewell, D. (2011). Interventions for leg cramps in pregnancy. *Cochrane Database of Systematic Reviews,* (11), CD000121.

Chapter 13

The Nursing Role in Promoting Nutritional Health During Pregnancy

KEY TERMS

- bariatric surgery
- body mass index
- complete protein
- Hawthorne effect
- hypercholesterolemia
- hyperplasia
- hypertrophy
- incomplete protein
- lactase
- obese
- overweight
- pica
- pyrosis
- underweight

OBJECTIVES

After mastering the contents of this chapter, you should be able to:

1. Discuss recommendations for healthy nutrition during pregnancy.
2. Identify 2020 National Health Goals related to pregnancy nutrition that nurses can help the nation achieve.
3. Assess a woman for nutritional adequacy during pregnancy.
4. Formulate nursing diagnoses related to nutritional concerns during pregnancy.
5. Develop expected outcomes to assist a pregnant woman to achieve optimal nutrition during pregnancy as well as manage seamless transitions across differing health care settings.
6. Using the nursing process, plan nursing care that includes the six competencies of Quality & Safety Education for Nurses (QSEN): Patient-Centered Care, Teamwork & Collaboration, Evidence-Based Practice (EPB), Quality Improvement (QI), Safety, and Informatics.
7. Implement nursing care that encourages healthy nutritional practices during pregnancy.
8. Evaluate outcomes for achievement and effectiveness of nursing care to be certain expected outcomes have been achieved.
9. Integrate knowledge of nutrition and pregnancy with the interplay of nursing process, the six competencies of QSEN, and Family Nursing to promote quality maternal and child health nursing care.

Tori Alarino, 19 years old, is 4 months pregnant. She works at a fast-food restaurant and eats breakfast and lunch at the restaurant. Her partner, Alessa, works four evenings a week, so Tori cooks for herself on those evenings. She dislikes milk, so she drinks milkshakes as a source of calcium. She is concerned because she has already gained 23 lb. She craves oranges, eating six to eight of them a day. She tells you, "I thought pregnant women always craved pickles and ice cream. What's wrong with me?"

Previous chapters described normal anatomy and physiology, the changes associated with pregnancy, and common discomforts and danger signs of pregnancy. This chapter adds information about prenatal nutrition, an important aspect to help ensure a healthy outcome for both a woman and her child.

What nutritional counseling does Ms. Alarino need?

BOX 13.1 Nursing Care Planning Based on 2020 National Health Goals

A number of 2020 National Health Goals speak to nutrition in pregnancy. These include:

- Reduce iron deficiency among pregnant women from a baseline of 16.1% to 14.5%.
- Increase the proportion of women of childbearing potential with intake of at least 400 μg of folic acid from fortified foods or dietary supplements from a baseline of 23.8% to a target of 26.2%.
- Increase the proportion of women who achieve a recommended weight gain during their pregnancies (developmental) (U.S. Department of Health and Human Services [DHHS], 2010; see www.healthypeople.gov).

Nurses can help the nation achieve these goals by stressing the importance of balanced nutrition for all people so women enter pregnancy with adequate nutritional stores, especially of folic acid. They can help pregnant women plan ways to ingest adequate iron daily and to remember to take their prenatal vitamin (which contains an iron and folic acid supplement) daily.

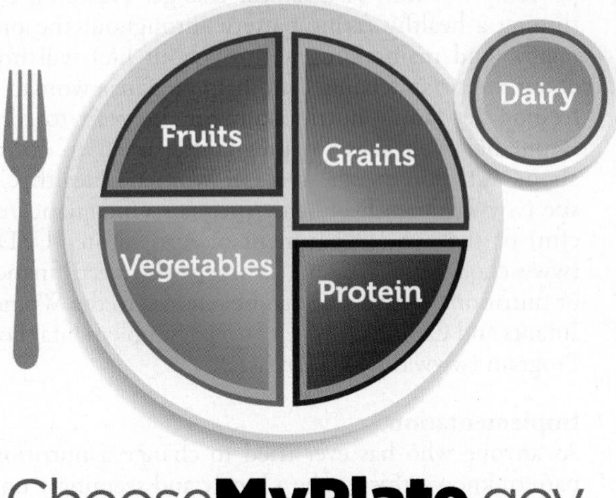

FIGURE 13.1 The Choose MyPlate guide to healthy eating. Note that the word protein is substituted for meat; vegetables occupy the largest portion on the plate. (From U.S. Department of Agriculture. [2012a]. *Choose my plate: A guide to daily food choices.* Washington, DC: Author.)

Although adequate nutrition during pregnancy cannot guarantee a good pregnancy outcome, it does make an important contribution because both the nutritional state a woman brings into pregnancy and her nutrition during pregnancy have a direct bearing on her health and on fetal growth and development. A poor diet, such as one deficient in folic acid before and during pregnancy, for example, is associated with fetal growth restriction or birth anomalies such as neural tube defects (Branum, Bailey, & Singer, 2013).

Good nutrition during pregnancy is recognized as so important that the subject is addressed in 2020 National Health Goals (Box 13.1).

Nursing Process Overview

For Promoting Nutritional Health During Pregnancy

Assessment

An assessment begins with a woman's preconceptual nutrition patterns. From this assessment, determine whether a client is eating healthy food sources and healthy proportions of food (Fig. 13.1). Also, evaluate any cultural, environmental, or social lifestyles that could affect eating habits. A 24-hour recall history followed by a physical examination to document weight and vitality are the best ways to secure necessary information, confirm well-balanced nutrition, and identify areas for teaching and learning.

Nursing Diagnosis

Nursing diagnoses related to nutritional status of a pregnant woman consider the desired health and growth of both the fetus and the woman. A woman who is eating large amounts of nutritionally inferior food and a woman who has a problem eating because of fatigue or nausea both may be at risk for the same problem: fetal growth restriction. Being sensitive to a woman's concern about maintaining her own appearance in light of her need to gain sufficient weight helps her keep a healthy perspective on "eating for two." Examples of nursing diagnoses include:

- Imbalanced nutrition, less than body requirements, related to increased physiologic needs
- Imbalanced nutrition, less than body requirements, related to nausea every morning
- Health-seeking behaviors related to determining best food choices in pregnancy
- Imbalanced nutrition, more than body requirements, related to chronic poor eating habits
- Deficient knowledge related to need for increased intake of nutrients and calories during pregnancy

Outcome Identification and Planning

In large health centers, nutritionists are available to meet with women prenatally and help them plan nutrition during pregnancy. In other settings, a nutritionist may be available only for women with special needs, so the responsibility for nutrition advice falls directly on nurses. When helping a woman set expected outcomes for improving her nutrition, be certain to consider all the cultural and lifestyle factors that give different meanings to food. Because food is an expensive commodity, consider financial resources as well. Teaching about long-term outcomes such as building iron stores or bone mass is as important as short-term goals, such as to eat better for a week. Eating more nutritious foods for a week will probably not lead to a radical change. However, continuing a healthy eating pattern throughout the pregnancy (and maintaining it throughout life) will bring about important changes and help prepare a woman for feeding her family nutritionally for the years to come. Reputable Web sites for pregnant woman to consult about nutrition are the DHHS Women's Health Care site (www.womenshealth.gov/pregnancy/pregnancy/eat.cfm) or the U.S. Department of Agriculture (USDA) (www.choosemyplate.gov). Women who need financial or nutritional counseling can be referred to the Women, Infants and Children (WIC) Special Supplemental Food Program (www.fns.usda.gov/wic).

Implementation

As anyone who has ever tried to change a nutritional pattern knows, this can be a lonely and seemingly unrewarding endeavor as results occur slowly. Begin by emphasizing the physiologic basis for nutritional needs in pregnancy (a woman is building a whole new person). Based on this, explain what nutritional deficits you have identified, and then show the woman how to change her nutritional pattern to improve this situation.

Pregnant women are usually highly motivated to adopt healthy behaviors for the sake of their baby's health; although they still need support and encouragement because this can involve a major life change, such as eating a different lunch than everyone around them is eating, getting up 15 minutes earlier to prepare breakfast rather than just dashing to work with only coffee, or resisting having a soft drink with dinner and drinking milk instead.

Asking women to list what foods they eat daily and to bring in a chart to show you at a prenatal visit is an effective motivating technique. In research studies, this is called a **Hawthorne effect**, or a positive change in behavior that occurs because of the attention received. Because of this effect, the average woman will eat better than she usually does so her list of food looks better when she presents it. As soon as she realizes these better eating patterns are making her feel better, she will hopefully continue them indefinitely.

Outcome Evaluation

When evaluating whether a woman's nutritional pattern has been improved, rely on the most important assessments: weight, energy level, general appearance, bowel function, and when available, hemoglobin and urinalysis findings. Urge women to be honest about whether they are actually following a nutrition plan. If they are not, it probably means the plan did not fit their lifestyle or degree of motivation. Examples of outcomes that would demonstrate improved nutrition include:

- Client demonstrates weekly menus that include three main meals and two snacks per day.
- By next prenatal visit, client demonstrates knowledge of meat and nonmeat sources of protein by providing menus of meals eaten in the last week that include fish, eggs, beans, or peanut butter.
- Client verbalizes correct information about calcium needs during pregnancy.
- Client states she is able to make up later in the day meals missed because of nausea.
- Client's food lists for 1 week include three sources of calcium per day.
- Client describes pattern she is using to increase fluid intake to eight glasses of fluid daily.

RELATIONSHIP OF MATERNAL NUTRITION AND FETAL HEALTH

During pregnancy, a woman must eat adequately to not only support her own nutrition but also to supply enough nutrients so the fetus can grow. Adequate protein and calcium intake is vital because so much of these are needed by the fetus to build a strong body framework. Adequate protein may also help prevent complications of pregnancy such as gestational hypertension or preterm birth. Either deficiencies or overuse of vitamins may contribute to poor intrauterine growth (Harnisch, Harnisch, & Harnisch, 2012). Therefore, a pregnant woman should be counseled to consult her primary care provider prior to taking any new vitamin or herbal supplement aside from her prescribed prenatal vitamin.

Early in pregnancy, fetal growth occurs largely by an increase in the number of cells formed **(hyperplasia)**; late in pregnancy, it occurs mainly by enlargement of existing cells **(hypertrophy)**. This means a fetus deprived of adequate nutrition early in pregnancy could be small for gestational age because of an inadequate number of cells formed in the body. Later on, although the number of cells may be normal, restricted growth can occur because cells cannot grow to their full potential. To ensure early pregnancy deficiencies do not occur, encourage women of childbearing age to follow a healthy nutrition plan before pregnancy (preconceptual care) that specifically supplies adequate folic acid (400 μg/day) (Russell, Denne, & Schwartz, 2011). Otherwise, in the time before a woman recognizes she is pregnant (about 6 weeks), her poor diet and lack of important nutrient stores could already have seriously impaired fetal growth (Lumley, Watson, Watson, et al., 2011).

Pregnancy provides opportune nutrition "teaching moments" as a woman finds herself suddenly more interested in her weight and well-being than usual (Monte, Valenti, Giorgio, et al., 2011). Always comment on the things a woman is doing correctly rather than what she is doing wrong. Positive reinforcement, a basic rule of teaching, enhances learning, self-esteem, and compliance more than criticism. Remember, women will have some degree of nutritional "backsliding" on holidays and special events. To help prevent this, a woman needs to make definite, concrete plans for what foods to avoid as well as how to substitute healthy foods for them.

Be careful when nutrition counseling not to make general statements such as, "Eat high-protein foods." Food in the supermarket, after all, is not labeled "high protein"; it's labeled meat, cheese, etc. Based on this, provide advice whenever possible in more specific terms such as, "Eat three servings of some type of meat or fish every day." An effective counseling session should also include teaching the patient how to read a food label and adequately measure serving size.

The word "diet" has come to mean a form of unpleasant food denial for most women. Rather than talk about a "pregnancy diet," therefore, talk about "foods that are best for you during pregnancy" or "pregnancy nutrition." These terms not only sound more positive but also refer more closely to what you are encouraging a woman to do: eat healthy meals.

Giving a woman a clearly written list of suggested foods may be a help to some women. Be certain a list of that type is short, clear, and specific. Complicated lists of foods or a list of don'ts tend to be overwhelming and, therefore, ignored.

Recommended Weight Gain During Pregnancy

One of the things women begin to wonder about when they first realize they are pregnant is how much weight they will gain during pregnancy. As a rule, the average woman should gain 11.3 to 15.8 kg (25 to 35 lb) during pregnancy. To predict individual weight gain, first calculate a woman's **body mass index** (BMI) or the ratio of body fat to weight and height. This can be done most easily by visiting a Web site such as the National Heart, Lung and Blood Institute (www.nhlbisupport.com/bmi). A BMI calculator for children and teenagers can be found at www.apps.nccd.cdc.gov/dnpabmi.

Women whose weight falls into the normal BMI category (18.5 to 24.9) should aim to gain 25 to 35 lb; underweight women or those whose BMI is less than 18.5 should gain 28 to 40 lb; overweight women (a BMI over 25 to 29.9) should gain 15 to 25 lb; and obese women (a BMI over 30) should gain 11 to 20 lb (Institute of Medicine [IOM], 2009).

Weight gain in pregnancy occurs from both fetal growth and an accumulation of maternal stores (Box 13.2) and increases by approximately 0.8 kg (1.5 lb) per month during the first trimester and then 0.4 kg (1 lb) per week during the last two trimesters (a trimester minimum weight gain of 4.5 lb, 12 lb, and 12 lb, respectively). Although this may seem to be a lot of weight gain, women can be assured most of the weight gained with pregnancy is easily lost afterward.

- To ensure adequate fetal nutrition, advise women not to diet to lose weight during pregnancy.
- A woman who reaches the midpoint of pregnancy and has gained less than 10 lb needs to have her daily nutrition intake reevaluated as low weight gain is associated with fetal growth restriction.
- Even obese women need to gain a minimum of 0.5 lb per week or 11 to 15 lb total to help ensure adequate fetal growth.
- Weight gain will be higher for a multiple pregnancy than for a single pregnancy (Table 13.1). You can encourage women who are pregnant with multiple fetuses to gain at least 1 lb per week for a total of 37 to 54 lb.
- Sudden increases in weight suggest fluid retention or hydramnios (excessive amniotic fluid); a loss of weight suggests illness and should also be carefully evaluated at prenatal visits.

BOX 13.2 Nursing Care Planning Using Assessment

Assessing Maternal Weight Gain

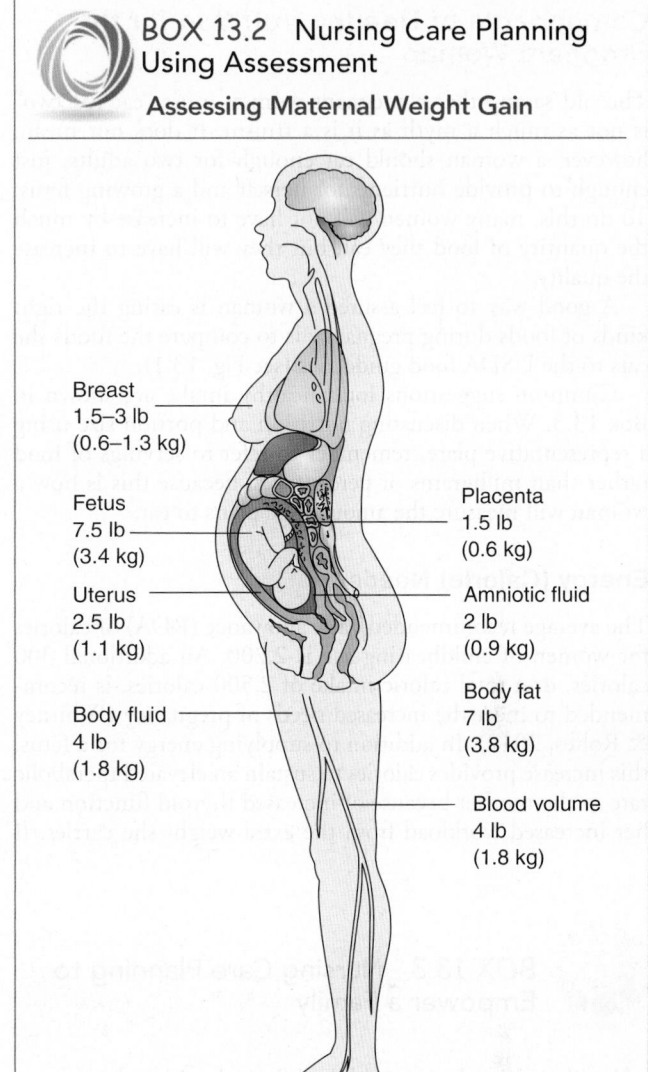

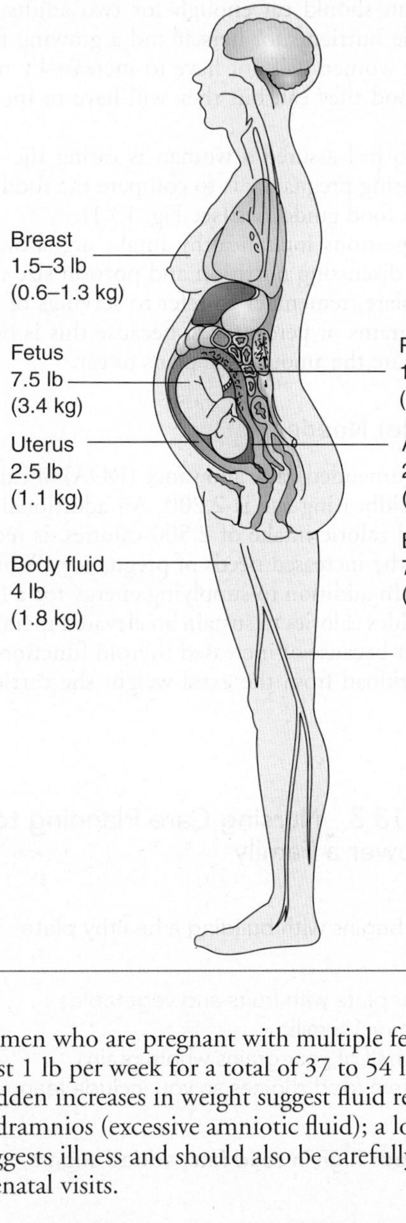

TABLE 13.1 Total Weight Gain During Pregnancy, by Prepregnancy Body Mass Index (BMI)

Prepregnancy BMI	BMI+ (kg/m²) (WHO)	Total Weight Gain Range (lb) Single Fetus	Total Weight Gain Range (lb) Multiple Fetuses[a]
Underweight	<18.5	28–40	
Normal weight	18.5–24.9	25–35	37–54
Overweight	25.0–29.9	15–25	31–50
Obese (includes all classes)	≥30.0	11–20	25–42

[a]Weight gain recommendations for multiple fetuses are provisional.

Institute of Medicine (IOM) and NRC (National Research Council). 2009. *Weight Gain During Pregnancy Reexamining the Guidelines.* Rasmussen, K. M., Yaktine, A. L, eds. Washington, DC: National Academies Press.

Components of Healthy Nutrition for the Pregnant Woman

The old saying that a pregnant woman must "eat for two" is not as much a myth as it is a truism. It does not mean, however, a woman should eat enough for two adults, just enough to provide nutrients for herself and a growing fetus. To do this, many women will not have to increase by much the quantity of food they eat, but they will have to increase the quality.

A good way to feel assured a woman is eating the right kinds of foods during pregnancy is to compare the foods she eats to the USDA food guidelines (see Fig. 13.1).

Common suggestions for a healthy intake are shown in Box 13.3. When discussing nutrition and portion size using a representative plate, remember to refer to servings of food rather than milligrams or percentages, because this is how a woman will measure the amount she plans to eat.

Energy (Calorie) Needs

The average recommended daily allowance (RDA) of calories for women of childbearing age is 2,200. An additional 300 calories, or a total caloric intake of 2,500 calories, is recommended to meet the increased needs of pregnancy (Whitney & Rolfes, 2012). In addition to supplying energy for a fetus, this increase provides calories to sustain an elevated metabolic rate in the mother because of increased thyroid function and her increased workload from the extra weight she carries. If a woman should begin restricting her carbohydrate intake so her calorie intake is below this in order to avoid gaining weight, her body will begin to break down protein to supply energy, depriving a fetus of essential protein, and possibly resulting in ketoacidosis, a possible cause of fetal growth restriction and newborn neurologic disorders.

Advise women to obtain their carbohydrate calories from complex carbohydrates (cereals and grains) rather than simple carbohydrates (sugar and fruits) because complex carbohydrates are more slowly digested. Doing so will help regulate glucose and insulin levels more consistently. Do not recommend sugar substitutes for women during pregnancy, because a pregnant woman needs sugar to maintain glucose levels. Even obese women should never consume fewer than 1,500 calories per day (Whitney & Rolfes, 2012).

When helping a woman plan an increased caloric intake, consider her lifestyle. For example, many women commonly skip meals, have erratic eating patterns, or rely on fast and convenience foods. During pregnancy, in addition to carbohydrate calories, a woman needs protein calories furnished by eating foods rich not only in protein but also in iron and other essential nutrients. Suggest preparing snacks such as carrot sticks or cheese and crackers early in the day, when fatigue is usually less, and keeping them readily available in the refrigerator. Otherwise, later in the day when she is tired, a woman may snack on empty-calorie foods such as pretzels and doughnuts simply because they require no preparation.

Measuring fundal height at prenatal visits is an indirect way to assess if a woman's nutrition intake is adequate. The easiest method for determining if a woman's caloric intake is adequate is assessing if she is gaining weight. Keep in mind a woman's weight gain pattern is as important as the total weight gain. Even if a woman has surpassed her target weight before the end of the third trimester, encourage her not to restrict her caloric intake. She should continue to gain weight because a fetus grows rapidly during these final weeks.

Protein Needs

The RDA for protein in women is 34 to 46 g. During pregnancy, the need for protein increases to 71 g daily. If protein needs are met, overall nutritional needs are likely to be met as well (with the possible exceptions of vitamins A, C, and D) because of the high incorporation of other nutrients with protein foods. If protein intake is inadequate, iron, B vitamins, calcium, and phosphorus also will probably be inadequate. Vitamin B_{12} is found almost exclusively in animal protein, so if animal protein is excluded from the diet, vitamin B_{12} deficiency can occur unless this is supplemented. This is why it is important to ascertain whether your patient follows a vegetarian or vegan diet during your initial assessment. Such a diet may lead to serious vitamin deficiencies that can affect both the mother and fetus unless supplements are added.

Meat, poultry, fish, yogurt, eggs, and milk best supply extra protein because the protein in these forms contains all nine essential amino acids required **(complete proteins)**. The protein in nonanimal sources does not contain all essential amino acids (and so is an **incomplete protein** source). It is possible to provide all amino acids by combining nonanimal or incomplete proteins. Proteins that when cooked together provide all essential amino acids are termed *complementary proteins*. Examples are beans and rice, legumes and rice, or beans and wheat.

BOX 13.3 Nursing Care Planning to Empower a Family

Healthy eating begins with building a healthy plate of food.

- Fill half of your plate with fruits and vegetables.
- Switch to skim or 1% milk.
- Make at least half of your grains whole grains.
- Vary your protein food choices so you include lean sources.

Cut back on foods high in solid fats, added sugars, and salt.

- Read food labels and eliminate foods high in sodium.
- Try to eliminate foods high in solid (saturated) fat.

Eat the right amount of calories for you.

- Enjoy your food, but eat less.
- Cook more often at home, where you are in control of what's in your food.
- When eating out, choose lower calorie menu options.

Model good nutrition.

- Provide healthy snacks as well as healthy meals.
- Remember that you are your children's most important role model.
- Don't just tell children to eat their vegetables—show them that you eat and enjoy vegetables every day.

A woman with a family history of high cholesterol levels **(hypercholesterolemia)** probably should not eat more than two or three eggs per week. She also should monitor her intake of red meat because of the high cholesterol content. Encourage such women to eat lean meat, to cook with olive oil instead of lard or butter, and to remove the skin from poultry to reduce its fat content. She also should not eat lunch meats such as bologna or salami as food staples, because their protein content may not be high, their fat content is invariably exceptionally high, and they may be a source of *Listeria*, a bacteria harmful to fetal growth (Goulet, Hebert, Hedberg, et al., 2012).

Milk is another rich source of protein. Unfortunately, some women resist drinking it because it can be high in calories and fat. Others cannot drink it because of lactose intolerance. Women who are lactose intolerant can add a lactase supplement to milk (which predigests milk and makes it possible for them to drink it without discomfort) or substitute soy milk (Siddiqui & Osayande, 2011). Nonfat milk supplies the same amount of protein as regular milk with half the calories of regular milk, and so can be recommended. Buttermilk, although it contains a large amount of sodium, can also be substituted for milk; chocolate or another flavoring can be added to make milk palatable. Yogurt, cheese, cream soup, custards, and eggnogs are yet other good substitutes for milk.

QSEN Checkpoint Question 13.1

Teamwork & Collaboration

Tori Alarino has a BMI of 25 so is considered to be slightly overweight. The interprofessional team should recommend what range of weight gain during her pregnancy?

a. 10–12 lb
b. 15–25 lb
c. 30–35 lb
d. 40–60 lb

Look in Appendix A for the best answer and rationale.

Fat Needs

Omega-3 fatty acids, particularly linoleic acid, are fats that are essential for new cell growth but that cannot be manufactured by the body. Vegetable oils such as safflower, corn, olive, peanut, and cottonseed; fatty fish; omega-3–infused eggs; and omega-3–infused spreads are all good sources (Mozurkewich & Klemens, 2012). Pregnant women should ingest 200 and 300 mg of omega-3 fatty acids daily. An added advantage of using vegetable oils rather than animal-based oils (butter) is that they have low cholesterol contents. For this reason, they are recommended for all adults as a means of preventing hypercholesterolemia and coronary heart disease. Because some fish may be contaminated by mercury, alert women that the American Pregnancy Association (APA) recommends that marlin, orange roughy, tilefish, swordfish, shark, king mackerel, and bigeye and yellowfin tuna should be avoided during pregnancy. For information regarding other types of fish, the Natural Resources Defense Council has a list of fish and their mercury levels all women can assess to be informed on what they are consuming (APA, 2011).

Vitamin Needs

The intake of vitamins as a daily dietary supplement has become so common that their importance may be underestimated by some women. A supplement is necessary during pregnancy, however, because requirements for both fat- and water-soluble vitamins increase to support the growth of new fetal cells.

Deficiency of vitamins can result in several common problems. Vitamin D, for example, found in fortified milk, cheese, eggs, and salmon is essential for calcium absorption, formation of bones and teeth, and possibly for immune system functioning. A lack of the vitamin may lead to speech and language delays in a newborn (Whitehouse, Holt, Serralha, et al., 2012). A deficiency can also lead to decreased fetal and maternal mineral bone density (Thandrayen & Pettifor, 2012). For all these reasons, a vitamin D supplement of 600 International Units is recommended for women during pregnancy.

When vitamin A—a substance necessary for new cell growth, healthy skin, oral health, and vision in dim light—is deficient, this results in tender gums or tongues, cracks at the corner of the mouth, and poor night vision. Vitamin A is found in dark green and yellow vegetables and fruits and in animal sources such as liver, milk, butter, cheese, and eggs.

Vitamin C is an antioxidant vitamin needed for the formation of collagen in both the mother and fetus; it also improves iron absorption from the woman's stomach and increases her resistance to infection. It is found in many fresh vegetables and fruits.

Although folic acid (folate or folacin) belongs to the B-vitamin group, its importance during pregnancy warrants a separate discussion. Found predominately in fresh fruits and vegetables, folic acid is necessary for red blood cell formation and to prevent neural tube defects. As a woman's blood volume doubles during pregnancy, this makes her folic acid needs increase substantially. Without adequate folic acid, megaloblastic anemia (large but ineffective red blood cells) may develop. If a woman has this blood pattern at the time of birth, the infant may be affected as well (Clark, Thomson, & Greer, 2012). For these reasons, pregnant women should eat foods high in folic acid, such as vegetables and fruit, as well as take a prenatal vitamin that contains a folic acid supplement of 0.4 to 0.6 mg (Sizer & Whitney, 2011).

Although almost all vitamin needs increase during pregnancy, most of the requirements can be easily met by eating a healthy, varied diet with plenty of fruits and vegetables plus a daily prenatal vitamin supplement. Women who were taking oral contraceptives before they became pregnant should be certain to include good sources of vitamins A and B and folic acid in early pregnancy because oral contraceptives may deplete stores of these vitamins (newer forms of contraceptives are being manufactured with folic acid added to eliminate this problem) (Kennedy & Koren, 2012). If women are constipated, counsel them not to use mineral oil as a laxative because it can prevent absorption of fat-soluble vitamins such as vitamins A and D from the gastrointestinal tract, thus limiting their availability to the body.

BOX 13.4 Nursing Care Planning Based on Responsibility for Pharmacology

PRENATAL VITAMINS (MATERNA)

Action: A vitamin and mineral combination used to treat or prevent a lack of vitamins or minerals before, during, and after pregnancy and during breastfeeding. The folic acid content helps prevent megaloblastic anemia in the mother and neural tube defects in the fetus.

Ingredients: Selected ingredients are vitamin A (1,000 International Units), vitamin D (400 Units), vitamin E (30 International Units), vitamin C (85 mg), vitamin B_1 (1.4 mg), vitamin B_2 (1.4 mg), vitamin B_6 (1.9 mg), vitamin B_{12} (2.6 μg), niacin (18 mg), folic acid (1.0 mg), pantothenic acid (6 mg), calcium (250 mg), iron (27 mg), copper (1 mg), zinc (7.5 mg), and magnesium (50 mg) (Wyeth Ayerst Pharmaceuticals, 2012)

Dosage: One tablet daily prior to conception, during pregnancy, and when breastfeeding

Possible Side Effects: Nausea, bloating

Possible Adverse Effects: Folic acid may mask the signs of pernicious anemia.

Nursing Implications

- A woman should start taking a prenatal multivitamin at least 10 weeks prior to conception (when she is trying to conceive or planning a pregnancy). She should continue to take this until she stops breastfeeding.
- Tablets are best taken with a meal to help the tablet disintegrate and to maximize nutrient absorption as well as to minimize the potential for gastrointestinal upset among women sensitive to iron.
- If a woman has difficulty swallowing a tablet, she can crush it and mix the crushed tablet in a liquid such as milk or fruit juice.
- Materna can be purchased without a prescription so women can begin taking the medication preconceptually or before they have made a prenatal health care visit.
- Encourage women to take the medication exactly as prescribed; caution women not to exceed the recommended dosage.
- Assist with ways to remind women to take the medication, such as a note on the refrigerator.
- Advise women to keep prenatal vitamins, like all medications, out of the reach of small children to prevent accidental poisoning from the high folate level.

Multivitamin supplements are especially designed for pregnancy and the preconceptual period to be certain pregnant women do take in enough vitamins (Box 13.4). Caution women that it is important to take a prescribed prenatal vitamin, not an over-the-counter one, because of the specific additives and not to leave prescribed vitamins within reach of small children as the excessive folic acid and iron content in them can cause poisoning in small children.

In addition, caution women that even though a supplemental vitamin compound is good for them during pregnancy, megadoses are not. The efficiency of placental transfer of water-soluble vitamins regularly makes fetal blood levels of vitamins higher than maternal blood levels, so a maternal overdose could cause extreme fetal toxicity. Fat-soluble vitamins are stored in the body rather than excreted and so can reach toxic levels even more easily. Megadoses of vitamin C, for example, may cause withdrawal scurvy in a newborn if the fetus received an overdose. There is an association between excessive vitamin A intake and fetal malformation in animals so excessive vitamin A may have human fetal effects as well (Karch, 2012).

Mineral Needs

Minerals are necessary for building new cells in a fetus. Because they are found in so many foods and because mineral absorption appears to improve during pregnancy, mineral deficiency, with the exceptions of calcium, iodine, and iron, is rare.

Calcium and Phosphorus. Calcium and phosphorus are both necessary for calcification of fetal bones beginning at about week 12 of pregnancy. Because tooth growth begins as early as 8 weeks in utero, these minerals also contribute to this formation (Gardosi, 2012).

To supply the large amount of calcium and phosphorus required, pregnant women need to eat foods high in calcium and vitamin D (vitamin D is necessary for calcium to be absorbed from the gastrointestinal tract and to enter bones). The recommended amount of calcium during pregnancy in adolescents is 1,300 mg; in women older than 18 years, it is 1,000 mg. A cup of milk supplies about 300 mg of calcium so drinking four glasses (a quart) daily easily supplies enough calcium. The type of milk (whole, 2%, nonfat, or soy) does not matter as to calcium value; whole milk as well as milkshakes and many "smoothies" add a lot of unnecessary saturated fat along with the calcium, however. If a woman cannot drink milk or eat milk products such as cheese, she can be prescribed a daily calcium supplement. There is little concern a woman will not receive enough phosphorus as most foods high in protein are also high in phosphorus; by eating high-protein foods, women receive enough of both.

Before nutrition counseling in pregnancy became common, women expected to lose "a tooth a child"—or believed a fetus, as he or she grew, drained enough calcium from their system to destroy their teeth. In actuality, the calcium in teeth is not as readily absorbed as that of bone so it is more likely inadequate calcium intake will result in diminished maternal bone density rather than weakened teeth. With an adequate calcium intake, however, neither will happen and a fetus will receive needed calcium for growth and mineralization of the fetal skeleton as well.

What if...13.1 Tori Alarino insists drinking milkshakes is a good source of calcium. How would you advise her?

Iodine. Iodine is essential for the thyroid gland to be able to produce thyroxine (which is necessary for overall body metabolism). As thyroid function increases during pregnancy, a woman needs to be certain to ingest more iodine than usual to supply this increased need. If iodine intake is inadequate, hypothyroidism (poorly functioning thyroid gland) and thyroid enlargement (goiter) can occur. In extreme instances, these same symptoms can occur in a fetus. Thyroid enlargement in a newborn is potentially serious because the increased pressure of the enlarged gland against the airway could lead to early respiratory distress. If not discovered at birth, hypothyroidism can lead to the infant being cognitively challenged (De Groot, Abalovich, Alexander, et al., 2012). The RDA for iodine is 250 μg daily during pregnancy. Seafood is the best dietary source of this.

In areas where the water and soil are known to be deficient in iodine, women may be prescribed an iodine supplement. It is suggested that women from these areas also use iodized salt and be certain to include a serving of seafood in their diet at least once per week (Whitney & Rolfes, 2012).

Iron. Because of low oxygen levels during intrauterine life, a fetus at term has a hemoglobin level of 17 to 21 g/100 ml of blood (compared with a usual adult level of 11 g/100 ml). An increased iron intake is necessary to build this necessary elevated level of hemoglobin. After week 20, a fetus needs even more iron as he or she begins to store enough iron in the liver to last through the first 3 months of life, when intake will consist mainly of milk, a fluid typically low in iron. In addition to supplying these high fetal needs, a woman needs iron to build an increased red cell volume for herself and to protect against iron lost in blood at birth.

The RDA for iron for pregnant women is 27 mg. An average diet supplies about 6 mg iron per 1,000 calories. If a woman eats a 2,200-calorie diet daily, her daily intake, therefore, is about 15 mg iron. Because only 10% to 20% of dietary iron is absorbed, she is actually taking in less than this amount (closer to 1.5 mg to 3 mg). Therefore, dietary supplementation per day during pregnancy helps ensure adequate iron is ingested and absorbed. Stress to women that iron supplementation is intended as a supplement, not a replacement for iron-rich foods.

Women with low incomes may find it difficult to eat adequate iron-rich foods, because the foods richest in iron, such as organ meats; eggs; green, leafy vegetables; whole grains; enriched breads; or dried fruits, are also expensive. Iron absorption increases in an acid environment, so eating iron-rich foods or swallowing iron pills with orange juice may increase absorption. Caution women that iron compounds will turn stools black, can be irritating to the stomach, and cause constipation. If these happen, urge women not to stop taking the iron compound but to take the iron pills with food and increase fluid intake or fiber to relieve the constipation. Some women may need a prescribed stool softener such as docusate sodium (Colace); this stool softener is not associated with teratogenic action, so it can be taken safely during pregnancy. A health care provider may also prescribe a prenatal vitamin that contains a stool softener to help combat constipation.

QSEN Checkpoint Question 13.2

Informatics

You are helping Tori evaluate some of the claims on a Web site that is aimed at pregnant women. Which statement from the Web site is most accurate?

a. "It's best to take your iron pills with milk."
b. "If you prefer, you can crush your iron pills to disguise the taste."
c. "Iron pills are most effective if taken with a carbonated beverage."
d. "Orange juice is an acceptable beverage to take with your iron pills."

Look in Appendix A for the best answer and rationale.

Fluoride. Because fluoride aids in the formation of strong teeth, a pregnant woman should drink fluoridated water. In an area where the water is not fluoridated either naturally or artificially, supplemental fluoride is recommended. Fluoride in large amounts causes brown-stained teeth, however, so a woman should not take a supplement more often than prescribed and not if tap water in her area is already fluoridated. Many women, worried about added chemicals in their city water supply, switch to bottled water during pregnancy. If they do this, advise them to buy a fluoridated type or alert their health care provider that they may need a fluoride supplement.

Sodium. Sodium is the major electrolyte that acts to maintain fluid in the body: when sodium is retained rather than excreted by the kidneys, an equal or balancing amount of fluid is also retained (Huether & McCance, 2011). Retaining enough fluid in the maternal circulation this way during pregnancy is important to ensure a pressure gradient to allow optimal exchange of nutrients across the placenta.

As with everyone, to help prevent hypertension later in life, women should use moderation with foods that are extremely salty, such as potato chips, or foods with the additive monosodium glutamate. Too much salt could result in retention of excessive amounts of fluid, putting a strain on her heart as blood volume doubles.

Zinc. Zinc is necessary for the synthesis of DNA and RNA and so is important for fetal growth. The RDA for zinc during pregnancy is 12 mg, or an increase of 3 to 4 mg over prepregnancy needs. Most people who take in adequate protein also take in adequate zinc because zinc is contained in foods such as meat, liver, eggs, and seafood. It is also a component of prenatal vitamins to help ensure an adequate intake (Karch, 2012).

Fiber Needs

Constipation can occur during pregnancy because bowel peristalsis slows due to the effect of progesterone and pressure of the uterus on the intestine. Eating fiber-rich foods (i.e., foods consisting of parts of the plant cell wall resistant to normal digestive enzymes such as fruit, broccoli, and asparagus) is a natural way to prevent constipation, because the bulk of the fiber left in the intestine aids evacuation. Fiber also has the advantage of lowering cholesterol levels and may remove carcinogenic contaminants from the intestine. Eating fiber-rich foods this way is a better choice for preventing constipation than taking a fiber laxative as it allows a woman to receive nutrients from the food as well as prevents constipation (Kee, Hayes, & McCuistion, 2011).

Fluid Needs

Extra amounts of water are needed during pregnancy to promote kidney function because a woman must excrete waste products for two. Eight glasses of fluid daily (e.g., two glasses of fluid over and above a daily quart of milk) is a common recommendation.

QSEN Checkpoint Question 13.3

Evidence-Based Practice

Gaining too much weight in pregnancy can lead to complications in the mother such as gestational diabetes; in addition, the fetus can gain excess weight with possible long-term weight problems. To see how much weight gain women perceived they needed in pregnancy, nurse researchers surveyed 54 women who were less than 20 weeks pregnant. Results of the questionnaire showed 39% of the women were overweight or obese before pregnancy. Daily caloric intake ranged from 599 to 5,856 calories. Women in all racial/ethnic groups were taking in less than recommended amounts of protein, carbohydrates, calcium, iron, folate, and fiber. Central American Hispanic women were the group who perceived they needed to gain the most weight for a healthy pregnancy; Caribbean black women, as a group, perceived they needed to gain the least weight (Brooten, Youngblut, Golembeski, et al., 2012).

Based on the previous study, which showed the average woman was taking in less nutrients than required during pregnancy, how would you advise Tori about what foods she should eat during pregnancy?

a. "Protein makes you gain weight too rapidly so keep all your meat portions small."
b. "Eat as much as you like all during pregnancy; you can always diet close to term."
c. "Make sure that you work plenty of leafy green vegetables into your diet."
d. "Iron causes constipation so limit your intake of iron-rich foods any way you can."

Look in Appendix A for the best answer and rationale.

Foods to Avoid or Limit in Pregnancy

Foods to avoid during pregnancy include those that are known to be teratogenic and, because a woman's immunologic resistance is lowered, those that may spread bacteria, such as:

- Raw eggs and undercooked chicken (danger of salmonella)
- Soft unpasteurized cheese (can harbor *Listeria* bacteria)
- Raw milk
- Raw seafood and sushi (can harbor hepatitis A virus)
- Cold cuts (deli meats should be heated until steaming to kill any bacteria)
- Alcoholic beverages (known to cause fetal alcohol spectrum disorder)
- Saccharin (has a long half-life and so can reach toxic levels in a fetus)
- Fish with high mercury content such as mackerel and swordfish
- Weight loss diets or supplements (women need additional nutrients, not less in pregnancy)
- Caffeine (excessive amounts may be a cause of miscarriage, although research is still ongoing)

Foods with Caffeine

Caffeine is thought of by many women as just an incidental ingredient in beverages. Actually, it is a central nervous system stimulant capable of increasing heart rate, urine production in the kidneys, and secretion of acid in the stomach.

A daily intake of over three cups of coffee per day may interfere with fertility (Hatch, Wise, Mikkelsen, et al., 2012). Whether caffeine increases the risk of miscarriage is controversial as it is difficult to separate the intake of caffeine from other lifestyle factors (Brent, Christian, & Diener, 2011; Stefanidou, Caramellino, Patriarca, et al., 2011).

Women who want to limit their caffeine intake need to limit not only the amount of coffee they drink but also other sources of caffeine such as chocolate, soft drinks, and tea. If a woman has difficulty omitting these common foods from her diet, she can still reduce the amount of caffeine she ingests by modifying food preparation. For example, instant coffee has less caffeine than brewed coffee. Decaffeinated coffee, as the name implies, contains almost no caffeine.

Tea, like coffee, varies in caffeine content depending on the type and time of brewing, as the longer tea brews, the greater the caffeine content. Both herbal teas that do not contain caffeine and decaffeinated teas are readily available. Green or oolong tea should both be avoided not because of their caffeine content but because they tend to lower a woman's level of folic acid, which is necessary for healthy fetal growth (Shiraishi, Haruna, Matsuzaki, et al., 2010).

Soft drinks do not naturally contain caffeine; it is added to them by their manufacturer to improve their flavor. To limit the amount of caffeine consumed, encourage pregnant women to choose from the many caffeine-free types available or, better, to drink fruit juice, which not only provides benefit from the fluid intake but nutrients as well.

Artificial Sweeteners

Artificial sweeteners are used to improve the taste and to limit the caloric content of foods. It is probably safest for pregnant women to reduce their intake of these because they need the glucose of regular sugar to help supply daily energy. Both sucralose (Splenda) and aspartame (NutraSweet) are approved by the U.S. Food and Drug Administration (FDA) as safe for pregnancy, but large amounts of the aspartame compound should probably be avoided until its safety in pregnancy is thoroughly confirmed. The use of saccharin is not recommended during pregnancy because it is eliminated so slowly from the fetal bloodstream that it could rise to toxic amounts (FDA, 2012).

What if...13.2 Tori Alarino states, "I love coffee. There's always a pot brewing where I work and everyone drinks it on morning breaks." What suggestions could you make to help her reduce her caffeine intake?

Weight Loss Diets

As a rule, measures to protect against excessive weight gain during pregnancy are wise because excessive weight gain is difficult for women to lose after pregnancy and is part of the reason for the present obesity epidemic (Tanentsapf, Heitmann, & Adegboye, 2011). In contrast, weight reduction is not wise. Liquid diets and/or diets that are combined with weight-reducing drugs are particularly contraindicated because they may lead to fetal ketoacidosis and poor growth. If women have been following such diets before becoming pregnant, they may enter pregnancy with so few nutritional stores that additional vitamin and mineral supplementation may be necessary.

ASSESSING NUTRITIONAL HEALTH

Women who follow good nutrition practices before pregnancy come into pregnancy in better health and are best prepared to avoid pregnancy complications (Riedijk, Oudesluijs, & Tibben, 2012). The best method for assessing a woman's nutritional intake before pregnancy or during pregnancy is to ask a woman to describe a "typical day," or a 24-hour nutrition recall, to isolate usual patterns and possible nutritional risk factors (Table 13.2). First, ask if yesterday was a typical day. If it was, ask a woman to list all the food she ate within the past 24 hours, starting with when she awakened until she went to sleep. Be certain she includes all snack foods as well as sit-down meals. This method of history taking yields much more accurate information than asking a woman how often she eats specific foods.

In addition to actual food intake, ask if a woman thinks she has any problem with nutrition (such as cravings). Also, assess the circumstances of eating, such as cultural preferences, who prepares food in the family, and how many meals are eaten outside the home weekly, as these are important to form a total nutrition picture (Table 13.3).

To strengthen history findings, assess a woman's prepregnancy weight and calculate her BMI. People with poor nutrition are typically overweight or underweight and show typical physical signs. Table 13.4 lists important physical examination assessments that suggest a good nutritional intake or evidence of poor nutrition.

After obtaining a full nutritional pattern, compare the types and amounts of food the woman eats with those shown in Figure 13.1 to see if all food groups and adequate amounts are included. Comparing foods from the person's 24-hour recall with a food guide is helpful because it shows clients that what they thought was a "perfect" intake is imperfect, or what they thought was a "little" problem actually involves the loss of an entire food group. Once a woman sees such a deficit exists, she may be more motivated to improve her nutrition. Such a picture also offers an instant reward for a woman who is including all food groups every day.

TABLE 13.2 Common Nutritional Risk Factors During Pregnancy

Risk	Rationale
Adolescent (less than 18 years old)	Adolescents require nutrition for both their own growth and fetal growth.
Short intervals between pregnancies	A woman's body has not had time to replace nutritional stores depleted during a previous pregnancy.
Low income	Family may not have resources to purchase iron-rich foods to meet pregnancy nutritional needs.
Food fads or dieting	Foods eaten may not be those adequate for pregnancy.
Drug use (including cigarettes and alcohol)	Drugs may be ingested in preference to healthy foods as well as cause teratogenic effects.
Existence of a chronic illness requiring a special diet	Intake may be low in an essential substance such as carbohydrates or protein.
Underweight or overweight	Underweight and overweight status may indicate chronic inadequate nutrition.
Multiple pregnancy	A woman must supply enough nutrition for multiple fetal development.
Anemic at conception	A woman has no iron stores for fetal growth.
Lactose intolerance	A woman may not be ingesting adequate calcium for fetal skeletal growth.
Post–bariatric surgery	A woman may not be able to eat large enough portions to meet pregnancy nutritional needs.

PROMOTING NUTRITIONAL HEALTH DURING PREGNANCY

Be certain plans made for improving nutritional patterns take into account a woman's lifestyle, family preferences, financial resources, customs, and cultural desires because she and her family must follow them for 9 months for them to be successful (Fig. 13.2).

Family Considerations

Meal planning is best if it involves the entire family because even if a woman is receptive to changing her eating habits, she may have difficulty carrying out recommendations if her family resists the change. In families where a member has a special nutritional need, such as restricted sodium, change may be even more difficult. You may need to speak with the person who prepares meals for a pregnant adolescent as well as the adolescent to be certain recommended changes will be carried out.

Financial Considerations

Food is costly, so to provide the extra servings required during pregnancy, a woman must spend more on food for herself

TABLE 13.3 Areas to Assess for a Total Nutrition History

Area of Assessment	Pertinent Questions
Food preparation	Who does the cooking at your house? Do you cook for people besides yourself? How do you usually prepare food (fried or baked)? What spices or condiments do you commonly use? What type of oil do you use for frying (saturated or unsaturated)?
Food pattern	How many meals do you eat on a typical day? Which is your biggest meal? How many snacks do you eat a day? What are they? How many meals do you eat outside your home? Where do you eat them? Cafeteria? Fast-food store? Restaurant? Bagged lunch? Are there any foods you cannot or will not eat? Why?
Financial concerns	Does your family have enough money for food? Who does the food shopping? Would you eat differently if more money were available? Do you use any supplementary financial programs such as the SNAP or WIC programs?
Activity level	Are you normally active or sedentary? (An active lifestyle increases calorie need.)
Lifestyle	Were you dieting before you became pregnant? Were you taking oral contraceptives before pregnancy? Do you take supplemental vitamins? What type? How many? Do you drink alcohol? What type? How much? Do you smoke cigarettes? How many?
Health	Do you have any allergies to food? Do you have any trouble with chewing or digestion? What is your bowel movement frequency? What is your stress level? Does stress affect your appetite? Are you ill in any way, such as with heart disease or inflammatory bowel disease? If you have a secondary illness? Are there foods you cannot eat?
Personal food preferences	Are you always hungry for a particular food? Do you ever eat nonfoods or ice chips? Are there any foods you particularly enjoy or dislike? Are there any foods you feel are harmful or particularly beneficial during pregnancy? Do you have any cultural or religious preferences that influence what you eat?
Family dietary patterns	Is anyone in your family on a special diet? Is anyone obviously overweight or underweight? Does your family eat meals together? Is mealtime a social time?

per week than she was spending previously. Women generally view this increased expense as an investment in their child's health and do not regard it as a burden. A woman on a marginal income, however, although she understands the importance of this, may have difficulty actually doing it. If this occurs, review what foods the woman is eating to be certain she is not filling her plate with less expensive starchy foods, such as pasta, in preference to higher protein foods such as meat. Help her secure available financial assistance such as from the Supplemental Nutrition Assistance Program (SNAP) or the Women, Infants and Children (WIC) Special Supplemental Food Program if needed.

Since 1939, under the SNAP program, a family with a low income can be issued an Electronic Benefit Transfer (EBT) or debit card that can be used to buy food items. SNAP cards cannot be used to buy hot and prepared food, cigarettes, alcohol, personal care items, paper commodities, pet food, household supplies, or medication. The amount of the debit card varies depending on the needs of the family. In general, a family of four whose monthly income is under $2,000 can increase their monthly food buying power by as much as $650 per month (U.S. Department of Agriculture [USDA], 2012b).

The advantage of this type of supplemental program is to help provide money for food but that places almost no restrictions on what foods, except for those mentioned previously. For a low-income family, it can make the difference between a healthy intake and a low-nutrient one.

WIC is a federal program that provides nutritional support for low-income women and children not only to reduce the risk of low birth weight but also to aid with the cost of newborn nutrition. Established in 1972, WIC is funded by the Food and Nutrition Service of the U.S. Department of

TABLE 13.4 Physical Signs and Symptoms of Adequate Pregnancy Nutrition

Assessment Area	Signs of Good Nutrition	Signs of Poor Nutrition
Hair	Shiny; strong, with good body	Hair dull and lifeless (possible protein deficit)
Eyes	Good eyesight, particularly at night; conjunctiva moist and not pale	Pale and dry conjunctiva (iron and fluid deficit); difficulty with night vision (vitamin A deficit)
Mouth	No cavities in teeth; no swollen or inflamed gum line; no cracks or fissures at corners of mouth; mucous membrane moist and pink; tongue smooth and nontender	Fissures at corners of mouth; tongue rough and tender (vitamin A deficit); mucous membrane pale (iron deficit)
Neck	Normal contour of thyroid gland	Thyroid gland enlarged (iodine deficit)
Skin	Smooth, with normal color and turgor; no ecchymotic or petechial areas present	Rough texture; poor turgor (fluid deficit) Vitamin K deficiency leads to petechia
Extremities	Normal muscle mass and circumference; normal strength and mobility; edema limited to slight ankle involvement; normal reflexes	Poor muscle tone; diminished reflexes (protein deficit)
Fingernails and toenails	Smooth; pink; normal contour	Pale; break easily; little growth (protein deficit)
Weight	Within normal limits of ideal weight before pregnancy; following normal pattern of pregnancy weight gain	Overweight or underweight; unusually slow or rapid weight gain (inadequate or excessive carbohydrate)
Blood pressure	Within normal limits for length of pregnancy	Decreased from anemia (iron deficit); increased from hypertension

Agriculture. The program supplies supplemental foods and nutrition education for:

- Pregnant women
- Postpartum women up to 6 months
- Nursing mothers up to 1 year
- Children from birth to age 5

Each state defines the income eligibility level for its citizens, but the eligibility for all programs is based on three criteria: income level, geographic area, and nutritional risk. To receive food, clients must live in an area that has been designated as a funding area. The nurse or nutritionist in the health care facility determines possible risk and nutritional need and helps enroll a family in the program. Factors considered that put pregnant women at nutritional risk include age (an adolescent or woman over age 40 years), poor obstetric history such as previous spontaneous miscarriage, a short period between pregnancies, having given birth to a previous low–birth-weight infant, gestational diabetes, anemia, poor weight gain, or inadequate consumption of food by nutrition history.

For the pregnant woman, foods typically offered by the program include those with high-quality protein, iron, calcium, and vitamins A and C, such as fresh fruits and vegetables, eggs, milk, legumes, whole grain cereals and breads, and canned fish. Vegetarian families or those with allergies can receive tofu and soy-based beverages or foods. At predetermined intervals, WIC clients are reevaluated to see if the program supplements are helpful or still necessary. WIC has been successful at improving nutrition during pregnancy because it not only supplies additional food to recipients but also provides periodic evaluations for nutritional counseling (Whaley, Ritchie, Spector, et al., 2012).

The school lunch program is yet another federal program that can furnish some pregnant adolescents with nutritional help. Millions of schoolchildren qualify for free or reduced-price school breakfasts or lunches designed to provide one third of requirements for protein, vitamin A, vitamin C, iron, calcium, and calories. Communities are working hard

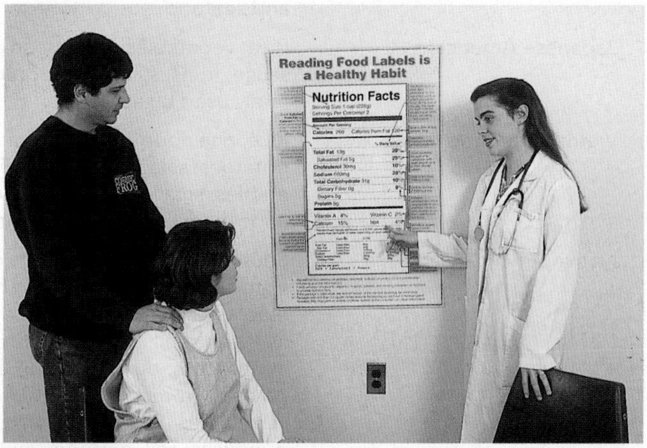

FIGURE 13.2 Encourage pregnant women and their partners to eat a varied diet with a high iron and protein content. This may be difficult for a woman early in pregnancy because of nausea and late in pregnancy because of fatigue. (© Barbara Proud.)

to replace burgers, fries, and burritos with salads, fresh fruits, simply prepared meats, and whole grain breads in schools. Soft drinks are being replaced with fat-free milk or water.

For many adolescents, this improved menu may represent the most nutritious meal they eat all day. Because there is a selection of food choices that can be made, a pregnant adolescent or one with other special needs may need some individual counseling to allow her to choose foods best for her, not those her friends are eating (HEALTHY Study Group, Mobley, Stadler, et al., 2012).

Cultural Considerations

When helping plan nutrition during pregnancy, try to suggest foods that are individually or culturally favored, as these are the foods women tend to enjoy most and so will eat most consistently. Common cultural differences to be aware of during nutritional counseling are shown in Box 13.5. Remember when counseling using such a table, not to stereotype women into cultural boxes. "Americanized" women may prepare few foods from their ethnic background because their spouse or significant other is of a contrasting culture with differing preferences.

BOX 13.5 Nursing Care Planning to Respect Cultural Diversity

CHARACTERISTICS OF CERTAIN ETHNIC DIETS

Group and Place of Origin	Staple Foods	Common Customs
Hispanic Americans from Puerto Rico	Steamed white rice; many varieties of beans; starchy vegetables, such as cassavas or yams; salted fish or pork; sugared fruit juices; cafe con leche (coffee and hot milk)	Milk is rarely consumed as a beverage. Most foods are cooked for long periods of time or fried. Malt beer is believed to be nutritious and may be given to children and breastfeeding mothers.
Hispanic Americans from Mexico, Central America	Many varieties of beans; steamed rice; corn products such as tortillas; chili peppers, fresh fruit, potatoes; meat; fish; poultry; eggs; milk cheeses; milk custards and bread puddings	Most vegetables are cooked for a long time so they lose most of their nutritional value. Diet is high in fiber and starch. Animal fat is frequently added during food preparation. Diet may be inadequate in calcium, iron, vitamin A, and vitamin C.
Hispanic Americans from Cuba	Stews and casseroles; soup is served daily; fried foods, especially fish, poultry, and eggs; rice; many varieties of beans	Fruits and vegetables are not eaten on a regular basis. Main meal is usually served at lunch.
Southern African Americans from West Africa	Hominy grits; biscuits; corn bread; rice; legumes; sweet potatoes; okra; green leafy vegetables cooked in salt pork; pork, poultry, and fish; thick stews; bread puddings; pies and sweets	African American food patterns are similar to Caucasians in same region. Northern African Americans may be unfamiliar with "soul food." Frying is common; diet tends to be high in fat and salt, low in calcium.
Chinese Americans (diets vary sometimes with region)	Rice; wheat noodles; many seasonal cooked vegetables and fruits; various shoots; soybean products such as tofu, soy sauces, and soy milk; small portions of meat, fish, poultry, and seafood	Yin (feminine)–yang (masculine) concept of balancing intake; moderation is valued. Diet is high in fiber and many nutrients, is low in fat, and may be low in protein.
Japanese Americans	Rice; vegetables; tofu, bean paste, and soy sauce; fruits; salads; fish, green tea; milk is rarely used by adults	Foods are broiled, steamed, boiled, and stir fried. Meat portions are small. Diet is low in fat, rich in nutrients, high in sodium.
Vietnamese Americans	Rice, rice noodles; curries of asparagus and potatoes; salads; tropical fruits and vegetables; small portions of poultry; eggs; fish; nuoc mam (a strong, fermented fish sauce)	Rice may be eaten at every meal. Lactose intolerance is common. Little fat is used in preparation. Diet may be low in iron and calcium.
Native Americans	Southeast: corn; cornmeal; coontie (flour from a palmlike plant); fried breads; vegetables; alligator, snake, wild hog, duck, fish, and shellfish; Northeast: many berries, beans; corn; pumpkins; fish, lobster, and wild game; Midwest: bison; beans; corn; fruits and vegetables; Southwest: corn, beans, squash, pumpkins, chili peppers, melons, cactus; Northwest: salmon, other fish, bear, elk, wild fruits, nuts, wild greens.	Food has great religious and social significance. Corn is a status food for most tribes. Milk is seldom used; calcium intake may be low.

From Dudek, S. (2010). *Nutrition essentials for nursing practice* (6th ed.). Philadelphia, PA: Lippincott Williams & Wilkins.

QSEN Checkpoint Question 13.4

Quality Improvement

A health history document is being modified by an interprofessional group. To obtain the most accurate nutrition history from a pregnant client such as Tori, what should the assessment document specify?

a. Ask the client to tell you how much protein she eats daily.
b. Assess whether the client feels satisfied with her nutrition.
c. Ask the client to describe what she ate in the last 24 hours.
d. Prompt the client to describe her concept of ideal nutrition.

Look in Appendix A for the best answer and rationale.

Managing Common Problems Affecting Nutritional Health

Specific nutrition problems may result from a number of factors or circumstances during pregnancy.

Nausea and Vomiting

As many as three fourths of pregnant women report nausea and vomiting in early pregnancy (Rogers & Worley, 2012). No definite cause has been established for this symptom of early pregnancy, but it may be related to:

- Sensitivity to the high level of chorionic gonadotropin hormone produced by the trophoblast cells
- High estrogen or progesterone levels
- Lowered maternal blood sugar caused by the needs of the developing embryo
- Lack of pyridoxine (vitamin B_6)
- Diminished gastric motility

Nausea is aggravated by fatigue and possibly by emotional disturbances. Most women notice the sensation as early as the first missed menstrual period and experience it through the first 3 months of pregnancy. The sensation is usually most intense on rising but may occur from smelling certain foods or while a woman is preparing meals. Vomiting at least once daily is common. Women who work nights and sleep days often experience "evening sickness," because that is the time when they arise.

The traditional solution for preventing nausea is for women to keep dry crackers, such as saltines, by their bedside and eat a few before rising because increasing carbohydrate intake seems to relieve nausea better than any other nutrition remedy. Sucking on sour candies may serve the same purpose. A woman may then eat a light breakfast or delay breakfast until 10 AM or 11 AM, or past the time her nausea seems to persist. To be certain she maintains good food intake during pregnancy even in the face of nausea, urge her to be certain to compensate for any missed meals later in the day. If preparing food for others makes her feel queasy, she might try to give this responsibility to another family member, at least through the worst phase of this symptom. Preparing and freezing meals ahead of time, perhaps at night when the nausea is less bothersome, may also help.

Other therapy such as acupressure, anti–motion sickness wrist bands, and avoiding fluid with meals are other measures effective for many women. It is a good rule for women not to go longer than 12 hours between meals during pregnancy to prevent hypoglycemia. To prevent this from happening, women may need to eat a snack before bedtime to compensate for a late breakfast. Some women are able to tolerate fruit and raw vegetables during the morning before other food. Urge a woman to experiment with soups or vegetable drinks she may not usually think of as breakfast foods but that can give her early-morning calories.

Common measures to take to relieve nausea are summarized in Box 13.6. Caution women against self-medicating for nausea by using a scopolamine patch, a drug used for motion sickness. Although it has not been proven unsafe for pregnancy, it is not intended for long-term use. Also caution against taking excessive amounts of antacids containing sodium bicarbonate as their sodium content could cause fluid retention.

About 10% of women have nausea and vomiting that are so acute they need additional measures to feel comfortable and to prevent fluid and nutrient shortages. Pyridoxine HCl or a combination of pyridoxine HCl plus doxylamine succinate (Unisom) can be prescribed. Dimenhydrinate (Dramamine) is an H_1 receptor antagonist that also can be helpful (Clark, Costantine, & Hankins, 2012). Fortunately, nausea usually disappears spontaneously as women enter their fourth month of pregnancy. If it persists beyond this month or is so extreme in early pregnancy that it interferes with nutrition, it may indicate the development of hyperemesis gravidarum, a serious complication of pregnancy and a complication for which the woman needs additional therapy (Kuru, Sen, Akbayır, et al., 2011).

Cravings

Cravings for food or aversions to certain foods during pregnancy are so common they are considered a normal part of adaptation to pregnancy.

When taking a nutrition history, ask if a woman notices any particular cravings. As long as this is a healthy type of food, help her plan an intake that includes the food, at least in moderation, to help her enjoy her pregnancy without feeling guilty.

Some women report a craving for foods such as oranges or chocolate. Others, however, crave a nonfood substance (termed **pica**, from the Latin for magpie, a bird that is an indiscriminate eater). The most common form of pica in the past was a craving for laundry starch. Today, women are more apt to report cravings for clay, dirt, cornstarch, or ice cubes (Young, 2010).

Although some of these items do no harm in themselves, the ingestion of large quantities of nonfood substances can leave a woman deficient in nutrients essential for a healthy pregnancy outcome (Box 13.7).

Always ask women at prenatal visits if they crave any nonfood items, as most women do not supply this information unless asked directly. They worry you will find their behavior odd, or they may not realize their habit is pregnancy related as much as being a nervous habit.

Stopping the woman from eating the nonfood substance may be difficult because the habit may be deeply ingrained. Because pica is a symptom that often accompanies iron-deficiency anemia, suggest that her primary care provider assess her serum iron levels as correcting this underlying problem with an iron supplement may correct the pica. At subsequent visits, be certain to assess if a woman's hemoglobin is increasing and ask if she has noticed any difference in her cravings.

BOX 13.6 Nursing Care Planning Based on Family Teaching

MEASURES TO REDUCE AND EVALUATE NAUSEA DURING PREGNANCY

Q. Tori Alarino tells you, "I've been nauseated ever since I became pregnant. What can I do to make this better?"

A. Common nonpharmacologic measures you can take to *prevent* nausea include:

- Be aware between 50% and 90% of women experience nausea during pregnancy, so what you are experiencing is absolutely normal.
- Eat a few dry crackers, toast, or a sour ball before you get out of bed in the morning to increase your carbohydrate intake.
- Eat small but frequent meals rather than large infrequent ones.
- Avoid greasy or highly seasoned food.
- Delay breakfast until nausea passes (or dinner if it is evening nausea).
- Make up missed meals at some other time of the day to maintain nutrition.
- Avoid sudden movements and fatigue because these may increase or cause nausea.
- Eat a snack before bedtime so delaying breakfast won't cause you to go a long time between meals.
- Purchase a wrist acupressure band (purchased in travel stores for motion sickness) or schedule an acupuncture visit.

If nausea is present:

- Try sipping a carbonated beverage.
- Try a walk outside in the fresh air or take deep breaths through an open window.

Notify your health care provider if:

- You vomit more than once daily.
- You are losing weight rather than gaining it.
- You have not gained the projected amount of weight for your week of pregnancy.
- You are unable to make up for lost meals some other time of the day.
- You have signs of dehydration such as little urine output.
- Nausea has lasted past 12 weeks of pregnancy.
- The amount of nausea you are feeling is interfering with what you want to do in a day's time.

Diminished Gastric Mobility

As peristalsis slows from the effect of progesterone and the weight of a growing uterus presses against her bowel, constipation occurs in nearly 50% of pregnant women (Perlen, Woolhouse, Gartland, et al., 2013). Discuss preventive measures with women early in pregnancy to help them avoid this problem. Encourage them to evacuate their bowels regularly (many women neglect this first simple rule); increase the amount of roughage in their diet by eating raw fruits, bran, and vegetables; and drink at least eight 8-oz glasses of water daily.

Some women find that prescribed oral iron supplements contribute to constipation. Because this supplement is necessary to build fetal iron stores, help a woman find a method to relieve or prevent constipation other than omitting taking the supplement.

Women should not use mineral oil to relieve constipation as it can prevent absorption of fat-soluble vitamins A, D, K, and E, vitamins necessary for both good fetal and maternal health. Enemas also should be avoided because their action might initiate labor. Over-the-counter laxatives are also contraindicated, as are all nonessential drugs during pregnancy, unless specifically prescribed or sanctioned by a woman's primary health care provider. If dietary measures and attempts at regular bowel evacuation fail, a stool softener such as docusate sodium (Colace), or evacuation suppositories such as glycerin may be helpful.

Some women have extensive flatulence accompanying constipation. Recommend avoiding gas-forming foods, such as cabbage or beans, to help control this problem.

Pyrosis

Pyrosis (heartburn) is a burning sensation along the esophagus caused by regurgitation of gastric contents into the lower esophagus (Naumann, Zelig, & Napolitano, 2012). In pregnancy, it may accompany early nausea; it may also persist beyond the resolution of nausea and even increase in severity as pregnancy advances.

Pyrosis is probably caused by decreased gastric motility (an effect of progesterone, which slows gastric emptying) as well as the effect of pressure from the expanding uterus pushing up against the stomach. Common suggestions to help prevent reflux into the esophagus and relieve pain are:

- Eat small meals frequently rather than large meals.
- Sleep on the left side with two pillows to elevate the upper torso.
- Do not lie down immediately after eating; try to wait at least 2 hours.

BOX 13.7 Nursing Care Planning Based on Effective Communication

Tori comes to your prenatal clinic, and you want to obtain her nutrition history.

Less Effective Communication

Nurse: Hi, Tori. Are you eating a nutritious diet?
Tori: I eat everything in sight. No problem.
Nurse: Have you ever compared what you eat to a food guide to see if you're eating all the different types of food it shows?
Tori: Sure. Grain is on one side; meat is on the other. I eat both of those.
Nurse: It's important to drink at least a quart of milk a day. Are you doing that?
Tori: I'm drinking milkshakes so I not only get calcium but extra calories.
Nurse: That's great. I'm glad you're so aware of good nutrition.

More Effective Communication

Nurse: Hi, Tori. Are you eating a nutritious diet?
Tori: I eat everything in sight. No problem.
Nurse: Tell me what you ate yesterday.
Tori: A muffin and coffee for breakfast, a milkshake for lunch, a hamburger and fries for supper. A soft drink before bed. And ice cubes. I suck on them all day like candy.
Nurse: Let's talk about ways you might get some fruit and vegetables into your day.

Most people believe they eat well, so if just asked general questions about nutrition, they respond that their nutrition is adequate. Only when they are asked to actually describe what they ate during one day is the truth revealed. Eating ice cubes may reflect iron deficiency anemia.

- Avoid fatty and fried foods, coffee, carbonated beverages, tomato products, and citrus juices.

Aluminum hydroxide (Amphojel, pregnancy class N or not classified) or a combination of aluminum and magnesium hydroxide (Maalox, class B) may be prescribed for relief. If these do not relieve the discomfort, an H_2 receptor antagonist such as cimetidine (Tagamet, class B) or ranitidine (Zantac, class B) may be prescribed (Attilakos & Overton, 2012). Be certain a woman understands this "chest" pain is from her gastrointestinal tract and, although it is called heartburn, it has nothing to do with her heart.

Hypercholesterolemia

Women with a family history of hypercholesterolemia may enter pregnancy with already elevated cholesterol levels. During pregnancy, increasing progesterone levels cause a further elevation. Combined with intrahepatic cholestasis, this can lead to an increased risk for gallstone formation (cholelithiasis) and cardiovascular disease during pregnancy. Preventing cholelithiasis is important because gallstones can cause extremely sharp pain. Fortunately, surgery to remove gallstones during pregnancy is possible with new ambulatory laparotomy techniques.

A woman who has had difficulty with hypercholesterolemia before pregnancy may need to continue to eat only moderate amounts of fat during pregnancy to prevent any increase in cholesterol. Helpful ways to reduce cholesterol include:

- Exercising daily
- Eating oat cereal
- Broiling, grilling, or baking meat rather than frying it
- Using a minimum of salad oils
- Substituting new omega-3 products in place of butter
- Eating fish high in omega-3 oil, such as salmon or trout

Although tuna is also high in omega-3 oil, current recommendations are for pregnant women to limit their intake of tuna, swordfish, and mackerel because of their potentially high mercury content (Abelsohn, Vanderlinden, Scott, et al., 2011). Eating raw fish is also not advised because of the danger of parasitic contamination.

Urge women to check with their health care provider about the wisdom of continuing to take cholesterol-lowering drugs (statins such as Lipitor, class X) during pregnancy, because these drugs are proven to be teratogenic (Lecarpentier, Morel, Fournier, et al., 2012). A low-cholesterol diet will automatically be lower in calories than the average diet because oils and fats add many calories. Therefore, be certain women watching their fat intake are taking in enough calories for adequate weight gain during pregnancy. Also make certain a woman includes some oil daily (perhaps as olive oil on a salad) so she has included a source of omega-3 oil in her daily intake.

✔ QSEN Checkpoint Question 13.5

Patient-Centered Care

Which statement by Tori would best suggest she has developed pica?

a. "I eat the erasers off pencils. It helps relieve my heartburn."
b. "I can't eat a thing before eleven o'clock every morning."
c. "I notice I've been hungry for lemon cookies lately."
d. "I crave oranges; can't get enough of them every day."

Look in Appendix A for the best answer and rationale.

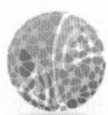

WOMEN WITH UNIQUE NEEDS

A number of lifestyles make it difficult for women to enter pregnancy with sound nutrition stores or to make the healthiest nutrition choices during pregnancy. Such women need careful assessments and counseling during pregnancy to help them modify their lifestyle enough so they can meet nutritional needs.

The Adolescent

A pregnant adolescent needs a higher caloric intake (2,400 calories per day) than a mature woman to supply energy because of the dual demand of consuming enough food to provide for fetal growth and for her own continuing growth. The nutrients most often lacking from a typical adolescent diet tend to be calcium, iron, folic acid, and total calories. Look for sources of these when analyzing a teenager's pregnancy intake.

An adolescent who is trying to hide an unintended pregnancy may eat very little to keep her abdomen from growing or eat a lot hoping the overall weight she gains will hide the size of her abdomen. She may have been on a diet before pregnancy and want to continue this to "not get fat." Because she's not meeting nutritional needs with any of these eating patterns, she runs a high risk of developing anemia, which can lead to fetal growth restriction and possibly preterm birth (Barroso, Allard, Kahan, et al., 2011).

In their search for identity, adolescents may avoid foods their parents see as important, such as milk, warm cereal, vegetables, or fruit, and indulge instead in foods such as soft drinks, potato chips, and French fries. If they eat lunch or breakfast at a school cafeteria, finding healthy food choices may be difficult.

To help an adolescent plan nutritional intake for pregnancy, respect her right to reject traditional foods as long as what she does eat includes sufficient nutrients. A cheese and sausage pizza, a glass of milk, and an apple compose a lunch that provides all basic food groups (meat: sausage; bread: pizza crust; vegetable: tomato sauce; dairy: cheese and milk; fruit: apple). A fish or hamburger taco (fish or hamburger, salsa, sour cream, and taco shell) plus a mango or tangerine provides the same.

Most adolescents snack frequently during the day. Toward the end of pregnancy, when preparing nutritious snacks becomes more difficult because of fatigue, you may notice they list more and more "junk food" when detailing what they eat. Advising them to prepare nutritious snacks such as carrot sticks or cheese bites early each day when they have more energy might be helpful. This way, if they are tired later in the day, eating a nutritious snack will not involve so much effort.

Because adolescents often do not prepare the foods they eat, you may need to speak to a parent or a support person (with permission) who does prepare foods to alter the adolescent's nutrition pattern. Encourage the food preparer to suggest a number of foods that would fill a deficit and let the adolescent choose from them to provide a sense of control.

Adolescents with eating disorders (bulimia or anorexia nervosa) enter pregnancy with major nutrient deficiencies. It is important to identify these girls at the first pregnancy visit so they can receive close supervision and supplementation of specific nutrients as needed (Zauderer, 2012).

The Woman Older Than 40 Years of Age

Today, many women are older than 40 by the time they have their first child, and many more are older than 40 when they have their second or third child (Cooke, Mills, & Lavender, 2012). The nutritional needs of women in this age group are not well studied, but it is obvious women in this age group should maintain the same careful pregnancy nutrition as younger women. Because women in this age group may have slightly decreased kidney function, they should be certain to maintain a high fluid intake to remove waste products for themselves and for their fetus. They need adequate calcium to prevent bone density loss. Many women at this point in life may also be caring for elderly parents and/or have delayed childbearing to establish a career; this means they may eat whatever they are preparing for elderly parents or depend on packed or fast-food lunches for at least part of their nutrition. Focus your nutrition counseling on maintaining adequate nutrition during pregnancy, based on these changing lifestyles.

The Woman With a Stressful Lifestyle

A stressful lifestyle can interfere with pregnancy nutrition as such women may simply have too many other stresses in their lives to concentrate on eating healthy meals. Examples of women who have this problem might be a busy executive trying to meet project time lines; one taking care of an ill child, partner, or aging parents; or one who is homeless or lacking enough money to purchase adequate food. Women who live in a situation with intimate partner violence may not have enough freedom to select what foods they prepare or serve to include all food groups every day. A conscientious assessment of women at first prenatal visits (hopefully at preconceptual visits) can help identify women in this group and provide the additional support they need to achieve adequate nutrition and a safe pregnancy outcome.

The Woman With Decreased Nutritional Stores

A woman with high parity or a short interval between pregnancies or one who has been dieting rigorously to lose weight before pregnancy may enter pregnancy with such depleted nutritional reserves she has little to draw on during the first part of pregnancy. If her folic acid intake has been inadequate, her fetus is susceptible to neural tube defects (Fehr, Fehr, & Protudjer, 2011). This shortage of nutrients may become critical during the time she is unable to eat well because of the usual nausea and vomiting of pregnancy. Be alert for:

- Women from low-income families, who may enter pregnancy with anemia because they haven't been able to purchase iron-rich foods
- Women who used diuretics for a dieting program, who may be deficient in potassium as this can be removed in urine by some diuretics
- Women who have been taking oral contraceptives, who may have decreased folate stores
- Women who were using intrauterine devices or who have menorrhagia (heavy menstrual flow), who may be deficient in iron from excessive blood loss with menstrual flows
- Women who drink alcohol excessively, who may be deficient in thiamine

Women with these decreased nutritional stores need to be identified early in pregnancy through history taking so they can be referred to a nutritionist for specific nutritional counseling. They may need additional supplements during pregnancy to help restore a particular nutrient.

The Woman Who Has Been Dieting or Following a Food Fad

Women who have been dieting and those who have been following a food fad such as eating nothing but cabbage soup are another group who may enter pregnancy with nutrient deficiencies. Be certain to ask if a woman has been dieting at a first prenatal visit.

The Woman Who Cannot Obtain Culturally Preferred Foods

Because the United States is such a blend of different cultures and people move rapidly from place to place for various reasons, a pregnant woman may find herself living in a community where grocery stores do not stock the foods she is most comfortable eating. If she lives in an apartment, she also has no opportunity to grow any favorites. This situation presents a good opportunity to discuss what she can find as substitutes. Fortunately, most major stores carry a wide range of ethnic foods. Support a woman's efforts to speak to her grocery store manager to stock an item she prefers as practice for motherhood when she will need to learn to serve as a strong supporter or advocate for her child.

The Woman Who Is Underweight

Today's emphasis on slim, model-like female figures makes it easy to admire rather than appreciate the health problems of a woman who is underweight. A woman who enters a pregnancy underweight, however, needs nutritional counseling just as much as an overweight woman.

Underweight is defined as a state in which a woman's weight is 10% to 15% less than the ideal weight for her height, or a BMI of less than 18.5. Most women who are underweight tire easily because they have an accompanying iron-deficiency anemia. Even when underweight women gain more weight than usual during a pregnancy, they still tend to have a higher than usual incidence of low–birth-weight infants and preterm birth (Taylor-Robinson, Agarwal, Diggle, et al., 2011). This is one reason why preconceptual health care visits and assessments are so important.

Being underweight may occur for a variety of reasons:

- Dieting for weight loss
- Poverty and the inability to buy adequate food (however, many poor women are obese, not underweight, because starchy foods are less expensive than those that have a higher protein content, such as meat and eggs)
- Excessive worry or stress, which can lead to a loss of appetite
- Depression, which causes a chronic loss of appetite
- An eating disorder, such as anorexia nervosa or bulimia, in which a woman has developed a revulsion to food (Eagles, Lee, Raja, et al., 2012) (see Chapter 54)

The major reason for being underweight, however, is insufficient intake of food because of chronic poor nutritional habits.

Convincing women who are underweight to eat more may be difficult because you are asking women to change lifelong eating habits. Counseling also can be challenging because, during the first trimester of pregnancy when fetal need is greatest and a woman has nausea and vomiting, you are asking her to take in additional food.

Begin counseling by asking a woman for a 24-hour nutrition recall. Total daily caloric intake for the underweight woman may need to be as high as 3,200 calories (500 to 1,000 calories more than the usual specified daily amount). Work with women to develop menus based on well-planned meals rather than on quick take-out foods. Suggest additional calories in the form of a concentrated formula such as an instant liquid breakfast drink. Be certain a woman understands that this should not be a high-protein drink used for high-protein dieting regimens. Such diet drinks deliver a concentrated solute load (breakdown products of protein) to the kidneys (already working to capacity because of the pregnancy) and provide so little carbohydrates in proportion to protein that they encourage the breakdown of protein for body energy, a process that results in acidosis. High-protein diets of this nature are not recommended for long-term use by anyone, but they should be totally avoided by women during pregnancy.

A 500-calorie increase over normal requirements should result in a weight gain of an additional pound per week. Be certain to plan for this additional gain when the total weight gain during pregnancy is calculated at each office visit. Otherwise, the total weight gain of a woman may seem excessive when it is actually healthy.

If a lack of nutritional stores makes a woman feel tired, urge her to schedule adequate rest periods daily so she can feel sufficiently energetic to prepare nutritious meals. Be certain she is taking her prescribed vitamin and iron supplements. Additional nutritional counseling in the postpartum period may be necessary so she can maintain better nutrition throughout her life and enter a subsequent pregnancy (if she desires one) in a state of nutritional health.

The Woman Who Is Overweight

A woman is considered **overweight** if she is 20% above ideal weight or has a BMI over 25. She is considered **obese** if she weighs more than 200 lb, she is 50% above ideal body weight for height, or her BMI is above 30. As many as 60% of women in the United States are overweight; 35% are obese (Centers for Disease Control and Prevention [CDC], 2012). Less-educated women and those living in poverty tend to be more overweight than others. Obesity in pregnancy is serious because it is associated with an increased incidence of gestational diabetes and gestational hypertension (Nodine & Hastings-Tolsma, 2012).

Although obesity may occur from hypothyroidism, it most often occurs as a result of excessive caloric intake and decreased energy expenditure. It becomes a problem during pregnancy because:

- Pregnancy causes circulatory volume to increase by 20% to 50% and metabolism to increase to meet the demands of the pregnancy, placing additional stress on a possibly already overworked body.
- It is often difficult to hear fetal heart tones in an obese woman; palpating for position and size of a fetus at birth is also difficult.

- Obese women are at increased risk for giving birth to infants with macrosomia (excessive fetal growth); this increases the incidence of cesarean births in this population (Machado, 2012).
- Performing a cesarean birth, if necessary, may be difficult because of the excessive adipose tissue that must be incised to reach the uterus.
- The pregnancies of obese women are more apt to be prolonged, leading to postmature infants.
- Ambulating during pregnancy and immediately afterward is more difficult because of the increased energy expenditure necessary, increasing the risk for complications such as thrombophlebitis and pneumonia.
- Many overweight women are hypertensive when they enter pregnancy and develop severe gestational hypertension (Sohlberg, Stephansson, Cnattingius, et al., 2012).

Most obesity is caused by overeating, but the habit of overeating has many causes. For some women, overeating is a habit learned in childhood when they were told to "clean their plate"; for others, it is a coping mechanism for stress. When they feel tense or worried, they help themselves to a "comforting" food. Because pregnancy can be stressful, it may be a particularly difficult time for a woman to change her food intake pattern. If a woman has been serving her family, as well as herself, an excessive amount of calories, then the entire family may have to change their eating pattern to bring about a change in a woman's intake. The children of obese women also tend to be obese, probably because of excessive food served to them combined with the lack of physical exercise (Hernandez, Thompson, Cheng, et al., 2012).

Dieting to reduce weight is not recommended during pregnancy because if carbohydrates are reduced too much, the body will use protein and fat for energy, thus depriving the fetus of protein for growth (Muktabhant, Lumbiganon, Ngamjarus, et al., 2012). This can also lead to ketoacidosis, and although the long-term effects of mild ketoacidosis on a fetus are not well studied, it can be avoided if the daily caloric intake, even in the most obese woman, does not go below 1,500 to 1,800 per day.

Overweight women tend to exercise less than women of normal weight. Exercising is more awkward and more tiring, and they may feel self-conscious wearing exercise clothing. Try to encourage them, however, to engage in at least a minimum activity program, such as walking around the block once a day, in conjunction with lessened carbohydrate intake.

Helping a woman look at her nutrition in terms of empty-calorie versus nutritious foods may help her to eat less fat and more protein foods. Early in pregnancy, when she is eager to appear pregnant, may be the most difficult time to limit intake. Stress that a fetus grows best on nutritious foods, not necessarily those with the most calories. Provide additional nutritional counseling in the postpartum period so she can prepare more nutritious meals in the future for herself and her growing family. If successful, she will not enter another pregnancy severely overweight.

The Woman Who Is Morbidly Obese

When a woman weighs over 300 lb or has a BMI over 40, she is classified as *morbidly obese*. During a pregnancy, she presents with a series of special care problems because she is even more prone to complications of pregnancy, such as:

- Gestational or type 2 diabetes
- Hypertension
- Back pain
- Thrombophlebitis or thromboembolism, for which she may be prescribed support hose to aid lower leg circulation
- Difficulty sleeping or sleep apnea, which may make her feel tired over and above normal pregnancy fatigue
- Difficulty hearing fetal heart sounds and palpating for fetal position
- Difficulty exercising
- Prolonged pregnancy with a high rate of cesarean birth (Machado, 2012)

Children born of an obese mother may develop obesity, diabetes, and cardiovascular diseases later in life at a higher proportion than usual weight women (Aviram, Hod, & Yogev, 2011).

At a prenatal visit, morbidly obese women may need special care equipment furnished for them such as a wider examining table, a larger examining gown, a wider wheelchair, and longer straps for fetal monitoring equipment than usual. Be discrete when arranging for this type of equipment for a woman as she may be sensitive to her appearance and weight.

Although women with morbid obesity generally eat large amounts of food, take a nutrition history to be assured their large intake includes protein-rich, not empty-calorie, foods.

The Woman Who Has Had Bariatric Surgery

Bariatric surgery is a weight-control method to reduce overeating by surgically reducing stomach size from about 30 to 40 oz to 3 to 4 oz. For gastric bypass surgery, the smaller, upper part of the stomach is stapled to separate it from the rest of the stomach, thereby reducing the amount of food a woman can eat. Next, the small intestine is rerouted and connected to the smaller stomach pouch, lessening the amount of nutrient absorption possible. In Lap-Band surgery, a silicone rubber band is placed around the top of the stomach, creating a small stomach pouch and reducing the amount of food a woman can eat at any one time. A sleeve gastrectomy is a laparoscopic procedure where the greater curve of the stomach is removed, again, reducing the size of the stomach and the amount that can be eaten at any one meal. A sleeve gastrectomy has the advantage of being a laparoscopy procedure and so requires only a small incision and, like Lab-Band surgery, the pyloric value to the small intestine is left intact.

Gastric bypass surgery results in an average of 60% to 80% loss in presurgery weight; banding and sleeve gastrectomy result in a 45% to 50% weight loss (Chopra, Chao, Etkin, et al., 2012). Although once limited to mature women, the number of adolescents who are having these types of surgeries is increasing so ask about bariatric surgery in teenagers as well as mature women (Nguyen, Karipineni, Masoomi, et al., 2011).

Both women and adolescents are advised not to become pregnant for about 18 months after a gastric bypass and for 6 months after banding or sleeve gastrectomy. This is the period of greatest weight loss, during which it would be difficult to supply enough nutrients for sound fetal growth.

After surgery, all women are required to maintain a conscientious diet of small but healthy portions as well as to take daily a chewable or liquid multivitamin supplement that includes iron, folate, vitamin B_{12}, vitamin A, vitamin B_1 (thiamine), and zinc. Ask if women have been taking their supplement to establish whether they are entering pregnancy with vitamin deficits. Urge them to eat their protein source first in a meal so they are certain to ingest enough protein.

If a woman does neglect eating a small meal and eats a large one or one extremely rich in calories (e.g., birthday cake with butter cream frosting, ham with buttered sweet potatoes), this can cause a "dumping syndrome" or sudden symptoms of nausea, bloating, and diarrhea. Be certain to mark the chart of a woman who has had bariatric surgery so her primary health care provider can decide if a 50-g glucose tolerance test will be safe or stimulate acute dumping symptoms. Because a woman who has undergone bariatric surgery will have an overall small intake during pregnancy, her weight gain will be less than others; she is prone to develop iron, protein, folic acid, and vitamin B_{12} deficiencies. Women who have had a gastric bypass are also prone to fat-soluble vitamin deficiencies because fat is no longer well absorbed.

Women may ask if bariatric surgery was a wise choice for them. You can assure them that following their surgery and subsequent weight loss, they are better candidates for pregnancy than they were when they were morbidly obese. They also have a lesser chance of developing gestational hypertension and gestational diabetes, both serious complications of pregnancy (Lesko & Peaceman, 2012).

The Woman Who Is Vegetarian

Some women are vegetarians because of religious guidelines or moral conviction. Others turn to vegetarianism to both maintain healthy nutrition and avoid excess fat and food contaminants. Vegetarian diets are consistent with the Dietary Guidelines for Americans so are safe during pregnancy (DOA, 2012a).

Most women vegetarians are closer to their ideal weight and have lower serum cholesterol and blood pressure levels than women who eat a more typical American diet. Nurses may find many pregnant women, therefore, who want to exclude meat from their intake (Conway & Cullum, 2010). Vegetarians vary as to what they can eat:

- Lacto-ovo vegetarians eat no animal flesh or fish, but dairy products and eggs are allowed.
- Lacto-vegetarians eat no meat, fish, or eggs, but dairy products are allowed.
- Vegans eat nothing derived from an animal, including butter and eggs.
- Semi-vegetarians usually restrict meat, fish, and poultry.
- Macrobiotics eat whole grains such as brown rice and vegetables; they avoid meat, eggs, milk, and cheese.

To replace meat, fish, and poultry at meals, women need to eat three or more servings a day of both fruits and vegetables, six or more servings per day of grains, and two or more servings per day of legumes such as kidney, black, or lima beans. Most vegetarians are knowledgeable about nutrients needed and can discuss what foods are high in various nutrients and how they incorporate such foods into their daily intake.

Special concerns during pregnancy are that vegetarians may lack vitamin B_{12} (meat is the chief source of this), an adequate intake of calcium because milk is a prime source of this (recommend dark green vegetables or soy milk to supplement this), and vitamin D (fortified soy milk and sunlight are good sources of this). Urge women who are vegetarians to remember to take their daily prenatal supplement, like all women, to ensure adequate iron and folic acid. Vegetarian nutrition for their new infant is discussed in Chapter 29.

The Woman With Phenylketonuria

Phenylketonuria (PKU) is an inherited disorder in which a person cannot convert phenylalanine, an essential amino acid, into tyrosine. Without conversion, phenylalanine accumulates in the person's blood serum, eventually leaving the bloodstream to invade body cells. When brain cells are invaded, severe cognitive challenge and accompanying neurologic damage, such as recurrent seizures, develop (see Chapter 48). A fetus of a woman with uncontrolled PKU can develop a cognitive challenge, microcephaly, intrauterine growth restriction, and neurologic damage from exposure to excessive phenylalanine levels (Marcdante & Kliegman, 2011).

Woman with the disorder need to avoid foods high in phenylalanine, which are those high in protein such as meat and legumes; examples of foods low in phenylalanine are fruits and vegetables such as orange juice, bananas, squash, spinach, and peas. Children with PKU follow a diet with restricted phenylalanine intake until at least past adolescence. A woman with PKU should consult her internist when she is planning to become pregnant and if she is not following a restricted intake should return to a low-phenylalanine diet for at least 3 months before she becomes pregnant. She then follows this low-phenylalanine diet during the pregnancy and as long as she is breastfeeding. A woman needs to discuss with her primary health care provider if she should continue to take sapropterin dihydrochloride (Kuvan), a drug to lower phenylalanine serum levels, during pregnancy as it is a class C category drug (its safety during pregnancy is unproven) (Karch, 2012).

Because a PKU diet is restrictive, a woman needs support during pregnancy to adhere to such restricted intake. It is particularly disappointing to have to follow the diet if a woman does not become pregnant immediately because each month she is "prepregnant" extends the period she has to follow the restrictions. Woman with PKU are usually well informed about their particular nutritional needs. Although they may wish they could eat more liberally, they are aware phenylalanine is destructive to developing brain cells, and not following a restricted plan could leave their future child severely cognitively challenged (Prick, Hop, & Duvekot, 2012).

The Woman With a Multiple Pregnancy

Twinning occurs naturally at about 4 in every 1,000 births, but the increased use of intrauterine fertilization has caused the number of multiple births to increase to as high as 15 per 1,000 births (Kilby & Oepkes, 2012). A woman with a multiple pregnancy tends to gain more weight overall and at a faster pace than a woman carrying a single child because of the increased fetal weight.

- A woman with a normal BMI should gain 37 to 54 lb.
- A woman with an overweight BMI, 31 to 50 lb.
- A woman with an obese BMI, 25 to 42 lb (IOM, 2009).

To sustain her own nutrition stores, a woman with a multiple pregnancy must ingest high levels of protein and carbohydrate as well as iron and folic acid. For this reason, a multiple pregnancy needs to be recognized early so nutritional supplements as well as overall close supervision can be added as needed (Kilby & Oepkes, 2012) (see Chapter 21).

What if...13.3 Tori Alarino is pregnant with a multiple pregnancy and tells you she is "eating for three." You notice on her list of foods that she lists three desserts every day for lunch. Will this hurt her or just add a few extra pounds?

The Woman Who Smokes or Uses Drugs or Alcohol

The specific effects of alcohol, cigarette smoking, and recreational drug use on fetal growth are discussed in Chapter 22. In addition to specific teratogenic fetal effects, these substances can lead to general nutrition problems because a woman is ingesting these substances rather than eating nutritious foods.

The Woman With a Concurrent Health Problem

Any health concern that requires rigid salt, protein, or carbohydrate restriction poses a potential threat to fetal nutrition. That means women who have medical problems such as kidney disease, diabetes, tuberculosis, bulimia, inflammatory bowel disease, celiac disease, or anorexia nervosa should consult their primary care provider before pregnancy because of the specific metabolic disorders involved with these illnesses. Women who develop gestational diabetes need the same type of nutrition counseling. Nursing interventions and nutrition concerns for women with major health problems such as these are discussed in Chapter 20.

The Woman Who Eats Many Fast-Food Meals

As many as 90% of women of childbearing age work at least part-time outside their homes (Cherlin, 2012). This means nutritional counseling for pregnancy must include helping women who rely on packed lunches or fast-food meals to ingest adequate pregnancy nutrition. One big difficulty with fast-food restaurants is the limited choice of food available. This can cause a woman to grow tired of the same thing and so eat little or have little choice but to eat foods with more empty calories than nutritionally effective ones. Unless there is a salad bar, the menu is apt to be particularly limited in fruits and vegetables, so advising her to carry an apple or other fruit to eat with what she selects from the menu can help her achieve a better food balance.

Caution women that fast-food restaurants have been associated with outbreaks of infection due to undercooked hamburger (*Escherichia coli*) or contaminated salad bars (*Salmonella*). Along these lines, caution women to inspect a salad bar for cleanliness and order hamburgers well done to help prevent gastrointestinal upsets of severe vomiting and diarrhea, which could lead to a serious fluid and electrolyte imbalance (Taylor, Holt, Mahon, et al., 2012).

A packed lunch poses few problems in pregnancy as long as a woman uses creativity in preparation so she does not grow so tired of packed lunches that she reduces her noontime intake or substitutes fast food in their place. Packing her lunch at bedtime rather than in the morning, when she may feel nauseated (and therefore packs little because nothing looks good), is a good recommendation early in pregnancy. Late in pregnancy, a woman may feel too tired at bedtime to do this so could change back to preparing it in the morning when she has more energy. Including a thermos with a cream soup is a good way to add milk and calcium to her diet. Packing sliced oranges or cucumbers, tomatoes, or apples helps to make a lunch nutritious and also makes food available for a midmorning or midafternoon snack. Having these snacks available prevents her from having long stretches of time without eating or eating empty-calorie foods from vending machines. Box 13.8 shows an interprofessional care map illustrating both nursing and team planning for sound nutrition for a woman who works outside her home during pregnancy.

The Woman With Lactose Intolerance

The sugar in milk is called lactose. In the intestines, lactose is broken down into glucose and galactose by the enzyme **lactase**. Most of the world's population has sufficient lactase as an infant to make this conversion but the amount of lactase available fades by school age. After this point, people can have difficulty digesting lactose or become lactose intolerant. African Americans, Native Americans, and Asians tend to have the highest percentage of lactose intolerance (approximately 70% of African American adults cannot drink milk). Those most able to tolerate milk are Northern Europeans and their descendants (Fox & Kelly, 2012; Mattar, de Campos Mazo, & Carrilho, 2012).

When people who are lactose intolerant drink milk, they experience nausea, diarrhea, cramps, gas, and a general feeling of bloating. For these women, fortified soy milk is a good substitute; it is rich in protein, calcium, and vitamin D and is easily digestible. Women who don't like the taste of soy milk may be able to eat cheese because the processing of cheese changes its lactose content; yogurt may also be tolerated. Lactase tablets to be chewed before ingesting milk products can be prescribed to supplement absent lactase, although the woman needs to consult with her primary health care provider before taking these as they are a class N drug (not assigned a pregnancy category of safety). Even if a woman does take lactase tablets, a calcium supplement (1,200 mg daily) and a vitamin D supplement (400 International Units) may also be prescribed. This is because the amount of cheese or yogurt needed to replace the calcium of milk is too large to be practical. Because milk is also a good source of protein, be sure to assess whether, without milk, a woman's intake of protein is adequate.

Because many baby magazines, television advertisements, and government pamphlets on pregnancy repeatedly mention that it is important to drink milk during pregnancy, you may need to explain to a woman with lactose intolerance as long as she ingests the same nutrients from other foods, the actual drinking of milk is not important.

BOX 13.8 Nursing Care Planning

AN INTERPROFESSIONAL CARE MAP FOR A PREGNANT WOMAN WITH AN INADEQUATE NUTRITIONAL PATTERN

Tori Alarino, 19 years of age, is 4 months pregnant. She works at a fast-food restaurant and eats breakfast and lunch at the restaurant. Her partner, Alessa, works four evenings a week, so Tori cooks for herself on those evenings. She dislikes milk, so she drinks milkshakes as a source of calcium. She is concerned because she has already gained 23 lb. She craves oranges, eating six to eight of them a day. She tells you, "I thought pregnant women always craved pickles and ice cream. What's wrong with me?"

Family Assessment Client lives with her partner in a four-bedroom home; partner works as an electrician. Client's father (aged 58) lives with them since recent divorce.

Client Assessment Primigravida; last menstrual period (LMP) 16 weeks ago. Height 5′6″. Prepregnancy weight: 110 lb (10 lb under desirable weight for height); BMI 17.8 (underweight). Weight today: 116 lb (minimum weight gain for first trimester). History of weight problem during adolescence; usually controls weight by eating only one main meal per day. Reports feeling tired and "rundown." 24-hour dietary recall: Breakfast: 1 cup coffee with muffin; lunch: 1 milkshake; dinner: 1 hamburger with French fries and 1 milkshake; snacks: 8-oz soft drink.

Nursing Diagnosis Imbalanced nutrition, less than body requirements, related to desire to control weight

Outcome Criteria Client reports increased intake of foods adequate in calories, high in iron, calcium, and protein by next prenatal visit.

Demonstrates weight gain appropriate for stage of pregnancy and prepregnancy weight.

Team Member Responsible	Assessment	Intervention	Rationale	Expected Outcome
Activities of Daily Living, Including Safety				
Nurse	Assess if the fatigue client reports is interfering with adequate food preparation.	If fatigue is a problem, recommend preparing food early in day when less fatigued.	Fatigue can increase nausea/vomiting in early pregnancy and can interfere with food preparation all throughout pregnancy.	Client states she is willing to cook and realizes eating fast food at all meals may not be her best action.
Teamwork and Collaboration				
Nurse/Primary health care provider/ Nutritionist	Assess nutrition requirements based on client's BMI and individual preferences.	Consult with nutritionist about recommended caloric and mineral requirements.	Caloric recommendations may need to be increased in light of client's BMI and prepregnancy and current weight.	An ideal nutrition plan is created with client's input.
Procedures/Medications for Quality Improvement				
Nurse	Assess if client has experience with keeping a journal.	Ask if client will record all food and fluid intake for 1 week; review with client at next visit.	Keeping a journal provides concrete evidence of client's adherence to nutritional plan.	Client brings log to next prenatal visit and reviews it with prenatal staff.
Nutrition				
Nurse/Nutritionist	Assess if client could eat more food prepared at home.	Give suggestions as to foods client's father or partner could prepare. Provide written information as needed.	Involving other family members could improve nutrition for entire family. Printed information enhances learning.	Client and nutritionist prepare a schedule in which all family members participate in food preparation.

(continued on page 324)

BOX 13.8 Nursing Care Planning (continued)

Patient-Centered Care				
Nurse/Nutritionist	Assess if there are other food choices client could make at the fast food restaurant that are more nutritious.	Discuss other possible food choices with client.	Knowledgeable clients can best follow a nutritious meal plan.	Client lists foods she will include for healthy pregnancy nutrition; if none available, pack own lunch.
Psychosocial/Spiritual/Emotional Needs				
Nurse	Question client about food likes and dislikes. Investigate any cultural influences on food choices.	Ask client to list foods in each food group that are her favorites and she enjoys cooking or eating.	Ascertaining food preferences and cultural influences provides a baseline for future food selections and suggestions.	Client lists foods she prefers and knows she can eat consistently.
Informatics for Seamless Health Care Planning				
Nurse	Assess best times for client to return for prenatal appointments based on work/family obligations.	Schedule a follow-up nurse appointment in 1 week if possible.	Changing nutritional habits and behaviors can be difficult. Scheduling close follow-up provides an opportunity for evaluation and instruction.	Client states she will return for follow-up nutritional counseling.

✔ QSEN Checkpoint Question 13.6
Safety

Tori described what foods she eats daily. What is apt to be her greatest nutritional risk if she is a vegetarian?

a. Lack of iron
b. Lack of vitamin C
c. Lack of folic acid
d. Lack of vitamin B_{12}

Look in Appendix A for the best answer and rationale.

The Woman With Hyperemesis Gravidarum

Hyperemesis gravidarum (sometimes called pernicious or persistent vomiting) is nausea and vomiting of pregnancy prolonged past week 16 of pregnancy or that is so severe that dehydration, ketonuria, and significant weight loss occur within the first 12 weeks of pregnancy (Kuru et al., 2011). It occurs at an incidence of 2% in pregnant women. The cause is unknown, but women with the disorder may have increased thyroid function because of the thyroid-stimulating properties of human chorionic gonadotropin. Some studies reveal it is associated with *Helicobacter pylori*, the same bacteria that causes peptic ulcers (Mansour & Nashaat, 2011).

With hyperemesis gravidarum, weight loss can be severe because, with so much nausea and vomiting, a woman cannot maintain her usual nutrition. Urine may test positive for ketones, evidence the woman's body is breaking down stored fat and protein for cell growth. An elevated hematocrit concentration may be detected at a monthly prenatal visit because the inability to retain fluid has resulted in hemoconcentration (which is dangerous because it can lead to thromboembolism). In contrast, concentrations of sodium, potassium, and chloride may be reduced because of a woman's low intake; hypokalemic alkalosis may develop from loss of hydrochloric acid from the stomach. In some women, ataxia and confusion, caused by deficiency of vitamin B_1 (thiamine), develops. If left untreated, a woman with hyperemesis may become so dehydrated she can no longer provide a fetus with essential nutrients for growth, and intrauterine growth restriction or preterm birth can result (McCarthy, 2012).

Assessment. Always try to determine exactly how much nausea and vomiting women are having during pregnancy. Ask each to describe the events of the day before. How late into the day did the nausea last? How many times did she vomit and how much? What was the total amount of food she was able to eat?

Therapeutic Management. Women with hyperemesis gravidarum may need to be hospitalized for about 24 hours to document and monitor their intake, output, and blood chemistries and to restore hydration.

All oral food and fluids are usually withheld for the first 24 hours. Intravenous fluid (e.g., 3,000 ml Ringer's lactate with added vitamin B_1) may be administered to increase hydration. An antiemetic, such as metoclopramide (Reglan, pregnancy class B), may be prescribed to control vomiting. Throughout this period, carefully measure intake and output, including the amount of vomitus, so the degree of hydration can best be evaluated.

If there is no vomiting after the first 24 hours of oral restriction, small amounts of clear fluid can be started and the woman discharged home, usually with a referral for home care. If she can continue to take clear fluid without vomiting, small quantities of dry toast, crackers, or cereal can be added every 2 or 3 hours, after which the woman may be gradually advanced to a soft diet, then to a regular diet. If vomiting returns at any point, enteral or total parenteral nutrition may be prescribed to ensure she receives adequate nutrition (Tan & Omar, 2012).

Nursing Diagnoses and Related Interventions

The main challenge in the beginning of excessive vomiting is fluid deficiency. As hyperemesis of pregnancy continues, lack of total nutrition becomes a concern. A woman with hyperemesis gravidarum needs the opportunity to express how she feels about this strange phenomenon that is happening to her and how it feels to live with ever present nausea. Some women are under such psychosocial stress from this they appreciate counseling to help them decide whether to terminate a pregnancy or allow it to go to completion.

Nursing Diagnosis: Imbalanced nutrition, less than body requirements, related to prolonged vomiting

Outcome Evaluation: Client ingests 2,200 calories daily or receives supplemental nutrition intravenously or enterally.

Like the typical nausea and vomiting of pregnancy, the vomiting of hyperemesis gravidarum may be precipitated by fatigue and the smell of cooking. Encourage a woman to serve herself small portions so the amount on her plate does not appear overwhelming. If she is hospitalized, try to limit her exposure to food odors. Be certain hot foods are served hot, and cold foods are served cold. Check to be certain food carts smelling of food such as fish, bacon, or coffee are not parked outside her room door.

An emesis basin is an important piece of equipment for a woman who is vomiting. Put it out of sight, though, and not on a bedside table, so a woman is not constantly reminded of vomiting. Do not urge a woman who is already struggling to eat to "Eat just a little more. You don't want to hurt your baby." Urging women to eat in this way may cause them to feel guilty on top of feeling so nauseated.

If a woman is receiving total parenteral nutrition, she needs her blood tested for glucose about twice daily. If this is elevated, it suggests the infusion solution contains more glucose than her body's metabolism can process. In contrast, if ketones are present in her urine, it means her body is not receiving enough nutrients and is breaking down protein. If either of these findings is positive, she needs a nutrition reassessment to see if she needs a change in her prescription for the enteral or total parenteral therapy.

Fortunately, despite its extreme symptoms, if hyperemesis is identified early in pregnancy and managed, it will not lead to pregnancy loss or low birth weight, but rather, to a healthy pregnancy.

What if... 13.4 You are particularly interested in exploring one of the 2020 National Health Goals with respect to nutrition and pregnancy (see Box 13.1). What would be a possible research topic to explore pertinent to this goal that would be applicable to the Alarino family and also advance evidence-based practice?

KEY POINTS FOR REVIEW

- Assessment of nutritional health should include a health history (24-hour recall) and physical examination.
- Aiding women to include about 300 additional calories daily to provide energy, spare protein, and provide for fetal growth requirements not only helps meet QSEN competencies but also best meets a woman's pregnancy needs.
- Important minerals necessary for pregnancy include iron, iodine, calcium, fluoride, sodium, and zinc. Most women need to take an iron supplement to prevent iron-deficiency anemia and may need additional calcium and vitamin D supplementation as well.
- Women should monitor their intake of caffeine and artificial sweeteners during pregnancy and should restrict alcohol and tobacco to the lowest amounts possible.
- Remind women to use prescribed prenatal vitamins rather than over-the-counter ones during pregnancy because prescribed vitamins contain additional folic acid, calcium, and iron supplements. Be certain women regard pregnancy vitamins as medication and follow the medication rule: take nothing other than medications specifically recommended by their primary care providers, or else toxicity could result.
- Advise pregnant women not to go longer than 12 hours between meals to avoid hypoglycemia.
- Common nutrition concerns associated with pregnancy include nausea and vomiting, constipation, cravings (including pica), and pyrosis.
- Women who are at high risk for inadequate nutrition include those who are adolescent or over age 40 years; those who have decreased nutrition stores; and women with a multiple pregnancy or who are lactose intolerant, underweight, or overweight. Others at high risk are those with a secondary health concern; who are on a special diet; who use recreational drugs, including alcohol or cigarettes; and those who experience hyperemesis gravidarum (extreme nausea and vomiting).
- Hyperemesis gravidarum is nausea and vomiting of pregnancy that extends past 16 weeks of pregnancy or that is too extreme to allow for adequate nutrition. Women with this condition may need antiemetic medication or nutrition supplemented by total parenteral nutrition or enteral feedings.

CRITICAL THINKING CARE STUDY

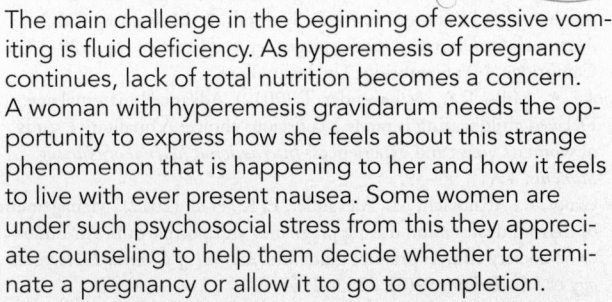

Annette Milano is 26 years old and 5 months pregnant. She has a PhD in psychology and lives alone in an apartment near the university where she teaches. She tells you she "didn't mean" to get pregnant, and also that she is afraid to go outside at night because gangs "own" her neighborhood. She began feeling nauseated early in pregnancy and has continued to feel this way into her fifth month. She vomits three or four times a day.

24-hour nutrition recall:
Breakfast: None
Lunch: 1 cup of tea, a few dry crackers
Dinner: 1 slice pizza, 1 glass chocolate milk
Snack: 1 apple

Annette knows she is eating very little but tells you, "I have a PhD so I'm not stupid. You can trust me the amount is what I've always eaten so is all right for me."

1. Is Annette's food intake adequate for pregnancy? How would you respond to her admonition she is not stupid?
2. Suppose Annette is hospitalized so she can receive total parental nutrition. What common steps would you want to take to try to decrease her feeling of nausea?
3. You want to assess Annette daily for dehydration. What would be important factors to assess to see if she is well hydrated?

Patient Scenario:

The Malu Family

Read about the Malu Family, a family with a concern about pregnancy nutrition, then answer the questions to further sharpen your skills and grow more familiar with NCLEX-type questions related to nutrition and pregnancy. Confirm your answers are correct by reading the rationales.

Visit http://thePoint.lww.com

Answers and Rationales

Looking for answers to the What If . . . and Critical Thinking Care Study questions?

Visit http://thePoint.lww.com

References

Abelsohn, A., Vanderlinden, L. D., Scott, F., et al. (2011). Healthy fish consumption and reduced mercury exposure: Counseling women in their reproductive years. *Canadian Family Physician, 57*(1), 26–30.

American Pregnancy Association. (2011). *Mercury levels in fish.* Irving, Texas: Author.

Attilakos, G., & Overton, T. G. (2012). Antenatal care. In D. K. Edmonds (Ed.), *Dewhurst's textbook of obstetrics & gynaecology* (6th ed., pp. 42–52). Oxford, UK: John Wiley & Son.

Aviram, A., Hod, M., & Yogev, Y. (2011). Maternal obesity: Implications for pregnancy outcome and long-term risks—A link to maternal nutrition. *International Journal of Gynaecology & Obstetrics, 115*(Suppl. 1), S6–S10.

Barroso, F., Allard, S., Kahan, B. C., et al. (2011). Prevalence of maternal anaemia and its predictors: A multi-centre study. *European Journal of Obstetrics, Gynecology & Reproductive Biology, 159*(1), 99–105.

Branum, A. M., Bailey, R., & Singer, B. J. (2013). Dietary Supplement Use and Folate Status during Pregnancy in the United States. *Journal of Nutrition, 143*(4), 486–492.

Brent, R. L., Christian, M. S., & Diener, R. M. (2011). Evaluation of the reproductive and developmental risks of caffeine. *Birth Defects Research: Developmental and Reproductive Toxicology, 92*(2), 152–187.

Brooten, D., Youngblut, J. M., Golembeski, S., et al. (2012). Perceived weight gain, risk, and nutrition in pregnancy in five racial groups. *Journal of the American Academy of Nurse Practitioners, 24*(1), 32–42.

Centers for Disease Control and Prevention. (2012). *Defining overweight & obesity.* Washington, DC: Author.

Cherlin, A. J. (2012). *Public and private families.* New York, NY: McGraw-Hill.

Chopra, A., Chao, E., Etkin, Y., et al. (2012). Laparoscopic sleeve gastrectomy for obesity: Can it be considered a definitive procedure? *Surgical Endoscopy, 26*(3), 831–837.

Clark, S. M., Costantine, M. M., & Hankins, G. D. (2012). Review of NVP and HG and early pharmacotherapeutic intervention. *Obstetrics and Gynecology International.* Advance online publication. doi: 10.1155/2012/252676.

Clark, P., Thomson, A. J., & Greer, I. A. (2012). Haematological problems in pregnancy. In D. K. Edmonds (Ed.), *Dewhurst's textbook of obstetrics & gynaecology* (6th ed., pp. 151–172). Oxford, UK: John Wiley & Son.

Conway, R., & Cullum, A. (2010). Vegetarians and vegans during pregnancy and lactation. In M. E. Symonds, & M. Ramsay (Eds.), *Maternal–fetal nutrition during pregnancy and lactation* (pp. 129–137). Cambridge, NY: Cambridge University Press.

Cooke, A., Mills, T. A., & Lavender, T. (2012). Advanced maternal age: Delayed childbearing is rarely a conscious choice: A qualitative study of women's views and experiences. *International Journal of Nursing Students, 49*(1), 30–39.

De Groot, L., Abalovich, M., Alexander, E. K., et al. (2012). Management of thyroid dysfunction during pregnancy and postpartum: An Endocrine Society clinical practice guideline. *Journal of Clinical Endocrinology & Metabolism, 97*(8), 2543–2565.

Eagles, J. M., Lee, A. J., Raja, E. A., et al. (2012). Pregnancy outcomes of women with and without a history of anorexia nervosa. *Psychological Medicine, 22*(3), 1–10.

Fehr, K. R., Fehr, K. D., & Protudjer, J. L. (2011). Knowledge and use of folic acid in women of reproductive age. *Canadian Journal of Dietetic Practice & Research, 72*(4), 197–200.

Fox, P. F., & Kelly, A. L. (2012). Biochemistry of milk processing. In B. K. Simpson (Ed.), *Food biochemistry & food processing* (pp. 465–490). Ames, IA: John Wiley & Sons.

Gardosi, J. (2012). Normal fetal growth. In D. K. Edmonds (Ed.), *Dewhurst's textbook of obstetrics & gynaecology* (6th ed., pp. 26–34). Oxford, UK: John Wiley & Son.

Goulet, V., Hebert, M., Hedberg, C., et al. (2012). Incidence of listeriosis and related mortality among groups at risk of acquiring listeriosis. *Clinical Infectious Diseases, 54*(5), 652–660.

Harnisch, J. M., Harnisch, P. H., & Harnisch, D. R. Sr. (2012). Family medicine obstetrics: Pregnancy and nutrition. *Primary Care, 39*(1), 39–54.

Hatch, E. E., Wise, L. A., Mikkelsen, E. M., et al. (2012). Caffeinated beverage and soda consumption and time to pregnancy. *Epidemiology, 23*(3), 393–401.

HEALTHY Study Group, Mobley, C. C., Stadler, D. D., et al. (2012). Effect of nutrition changes on foods selected by students in a middle school-based diabetes prevention intervention program: The HEALTHY experience. *Journal of School Health, 82*(2), 82–90.

Hernandez, R. G., Thompson, D. A., Cheng, T. L., et al. (2012). Early-childhood obesity: How do low-income parents of preschoolers rank known risk factors? *Clinical Pediatrics, 51*(7), 663–670.

Huether, S. E., & McCance, K. L. (2011). *Understanding pathophysiology* (5th ed., 98–109). New York, NY: Elsevier Publishing.

Institute of Medicine & National Research Council. (2009). *Weight gain during pregnancy: Reexamining the guidelines.* Rasmussen, K. M., Yaktine, A. L., Eds. Washington, DC: The National Academies Press.

Karch, A. M. (2012). *2013 Lippincott's nursing drug guide.* Philadelphia, PA: Lippincott Williams & Wilkins.

Kee, J. L., Hayes, E. R., & McCuistion, L. E. (2011). Drugs for gastrointestinal tract disorders. In J. L. Kee, E. R. Hayes, & L. E. McCuistion (Eds.), *Pharmacology: A nursing process approach* (pp. 695–712). St. Louis, MO: Elsevier/Saunders.

Kennedy, D., & Koren, G. (2012). Identifying women who might benefit from higher doses of folic acid in pregnancy. *Canadian Family Physician, 58*(4), 394–397.

Kilby, M. D., & Oepkes, P. (2012). Multiple pregnancy. In D. K. Edmonds (Ed.), *Dewhurst's textbook of obstetrics & gynaecology* (6th ed., pp. 230–246). Oxford, UK: John Wiley & Son.

Kuru, O., Sen, S., Akbayır, O., et al. (2011). Outcomes of pregnancies complicated by hyperemesis gravidarum. *Archives of Gynecology & Obstetrics, 285*(6), 1517–1521.

Lecarpentier, E., Morel, O., Fournier, T., et al. (2012). Statins and pregnancy: Between supposed risks and theoretical benefits. *Drugs, 72*(6), 773–788.

Lesko, J., & Peaceman, A. (2012). Pregnancy outcomes in women after bariatric surgery compared with obese and morbidly obese controls. *Obstetrics & Gynecology, 119*(3), 547–554.

Lumley, J., Watson, L., Watson, M., et al. (2011). Periconceptional supplementation with folate and/or multivitamins for preventing neural tube defects. *Cochrane Database of Systematic Reviews,* (4), CD001056.

Machado, L. S. (2012). Cesarean section in morbidly obese parturients: Practical implications and complications. *North American Journal of Medicine & Science, 4*(1), 13–18.

Mansour, G. M., & Nashaat, E. H. (2011). Role of *Helicobacter pylori* in the pathogenesis of hyperemesis gravidarum. *Archives of Gynecology & Obstetrics, 284*(4), 843–847.

Marcdante, K. J., & Kliegman, R. M. (2011). Amino acid disorders. In K. J. Marcdante & R. M. Kliegman (Eds.), *Nelson essentials of pediatrics* (6th ed., pp. 197–200). Philadelphia, PA: Saunders/Elsevier.

Mattar, R., de Campos Mazo, D. F., & Carrilho, F. J. (2012). Lactose intolerance: Diagnosis, genetic, and clinical factors. *Clinical & Experimental Gastroenterology,* (5), 113–121.

McCarthy, A. (2012). Miscellaneous medical disorders. In D. K. Edmonds (Ed.), *Dewhurst's textbook of obstetrics & gynaecology* (6th ed., pp. 173–184). Oxford, UK: John Wiley & Son.

Monte, S., Valenti, O., Giorgio, E., et al. (2011). Maternal weight gain during pregnancy and neonatal birth weight: A review of the literature. *Journal of Prenatal Medicine, 5*(2), 27–30.

Mozurkewich, E. L., & Klemens, C. (2012). Omega-3 fatty acids and pregnancy: Current implications for practice. *Current Opinion in Obstetrics & Gynecology, 24*(2), 72–77.

Muktabhant, B., Lumbiganon, P., Ngamjarus, C., et al. (2012). Interventions for preventing excessive weight gain during pregnancy. *Cochrane Database of Systematic Reviews,* (4), CD007145.

Naumann, C. R., Zelig, C., Napolitano, P. G., et al. (2012). Nausea, vomiting, and heartburn in pregnancy: A prospective look at risk, treatment, and outcome. *Journal of Maternal-Fetal & Neonatal Medicine, 25*(8), 1488–1493.

Nguyen, N. T., Karipineni, F., Masoomi, H., et al. (2011). Increasing utilization of laparoscopic gastric banding in the adolescent: Data from academic medical centers, 2002–2009. *American Surgery, 77*(11), 1510–1514.

Nodine, P. M., & Hastings-Tolsma, M. (2012). Maternal obesity: Improving pregnancy outcomes. *American Journal of Maternal Child Nursing, 37*(2), 110–115.

Perlen, S., Woolhouse, H., Gartland, D., et al. (2013). Maternal depression and physical health problems in early pregnancy. *Midwifery, 29*(3), 233–239.

Prick, B. W., Hop, W. C., & Duvekot, J. J. (2012). Maternal phenylketonuria and hyperphenylalaninemia in pregnancy. *American Journal of Clinical Nutrition, 95*(2), 374–382.

Riedijk, S., Oudesluijs, G., & Tibben, A. (2012). Psychosocial aspects of preconception consultation in primary care. *Journal of Community Genetics, 3*(3), 213–219.

Rogers, V. L., & Worley, K. C. (2012). Obstetrics and obstetric disorders. In S. J. McPhee, M. A. Papadakis, & M. W. Rabow (Eds.), *Current medical diagnosis & treatment* (51st ed., pp. 760–786). Columbus, OH: McGraw-Hill.

Russell, J. B., Denne, E. W., & Schwartz, D. (2011). Preconception counseling and prenatal care. In K. J. Hurt, M. W. Guile, J. L. Bienstock, et al. (Eds.), *The Johns Hopkins manual of gynecology and obstetrics* (4th ed., pp. 56–72). Philadelphia, PA: Lippincott Williams & Wilkins.

Shiraishi, M., Haruna, M., Matsuzaki, M., et al. (2010). Association between the serum folate levels and tea consumption during pregnancy. *Bioscience Trends, 4*(5), 225–230.

Siddiqui, Z., & Osayande, A. S. (2011). Selected disorders of malabsorption. *Primary Care, 38*(3), 395–414.

Sizer, F., & Whitney, E. (2011). Pregnancy: The impact of nutrition on the future. In F. Sizer & E. Whitney (Eds.), *Nutrition: Concepts & controversies* (pp. 491–531). Belmont, CA: Wadsworth/CINGAGE.

Sohlberg, S., Stephansson, O., Cnattingius, S., et al. (2012). Maternal body mass index, height, and risks of preeclampsia. *American Journal of Hypertension, 25*(1), 120–125.

Stefanidou, E. M., Caramellino, L., Patriarca, A., et al. (2011). Maternal caffeine consumption and sine causa recurrent miscarriage. *European Journal of Obstetrics, Gynecology & Reproductive Biology, 158*(2), 220–224.

Tan, P. C., & Omar, S. Z. (2011). Contemporary approaches to hyperemesis during pregnancy. *Current Opinion in Obstetrics & Gynecology, 23*(2), 87–93.

Tanentsapf, I., Heitmann, B. L., & Adegboye, A. R. (2011). Systematic review of clinical trials on dietary interventions to prevent excessive weight gain during pregnancy among normal weight, overweight and obese women. *BMC Pregnancy & Childbirth, 11*(10), 81.

Taylor, E. V., Holt, K. G., Mahon, B. E., et al. (2012). Ground beef consumption patterns in the United States. *Journal of Food Protection, 75*(2), 341–346.

Taylor-Robinson, D., Agarwal, U., Diggle, P. J., et al. (2011). Quantifying the impact of deprivation on preterm births: A retrospective cohort study. *PLoS One: Public Library of Science, 6*(8), e23163.

Thandrayen, K., & Pettifor, J. M. (2012). Maternal vitamin D status: Implications for the development of infantile nutritional rickets. *Rheumatic Diseases Clinics of North America, 38*(1), 61–79.

U.S. Department of Agriculture. (2012a). *Choose my plate: A guide to daily food choices*. Washington, DC: Author.

U.S. Department of Agriculture. (2012b). *Food stamp program.* Washington, DC: Author.

U.S. Department of Health and Human Services. (2010). *Healthy people 2020.* Washington, DC: Author.

U.S. Food and Drug Administration. (2012). *Sugar alternatives.* Washington, DC: Author.

Whaley, S. E., Ritchie, L. D., Spector, P., et al. (2012). Revised WIC food package improves diets of WIC families. *Journal of Nutrition, Education & Behavior, 44*(3), 204–209.

Whitehouse, A. J., Holt, B. J., Serralha, M., et al. (2012). Maternal serum vitamin D levels during pregnancy and offspring neurocognitive development. *Pediatrics, 129*(3), 485–493.

Whitney, E. N., & Rolfes, S. R. (2012). Life cycle nutrition: Pregnancy & lactation. In E. N. Whitney & S. R. Rolfes (Eds.), *Understanding nutrition* (pp. 492–527). Belmont, CA: Wadsworth Publishing.

Wyeth Ayerst Pharmaceuticals. (2012). *Product information*. Philadelphia, PA: Author.

Young, S. L. (2010). Pica in pregnancy: New ideas about an old condition. *Annual Review of Nutrition, 30*(8), 403–422.

Zauderer, C. R. (2012). Eating disorders and pregnancy: Supporting the anorexic or bulimic expectant mother. *American Journal of Maternal Child Nursing, 37*(1), 48–55.

Chapter 14

Preparing a Family for Childbirth and Parenting

KEY TERMS

- alternative birthing centers (ABCs)
- birthing bed
- birthing chair
- birthing room
- cleansing breath
- conditioned reflexes
- conscious relaxation
- consciously controlled breathing
- distraction
- doula
- effleurage
- gating control theory of pain perception
- labor-birth-recovery-postpartum room (LBRP)
- Leboyer method
- psychoprophylactic
- vaginal birth after cesarean birth (VBAC)

OBJECTIVES

After mastering the contents of this chapter, you should be able to:

1. Describe common preparations for childbirth and parenting, including common settings for birth.
2. Identify 2020 National Health Goals related to preparation for parenthood and how nurses can help the nation achieve these goals.
3. Assess the readiness of a couple for childbirth with regard to choice of birth attendant, preparation for labor, and birth setting.
4. Formulate nursing diagnoses related to preparation for childbirth and parenting.
5. Identify expected outcomes for a couple preparing for childbirth and parenting while helping them manage seamless transitions across differing health care settings.
6. Using the nursing process, plan nursing care that includes the six competencies of Quality & Safety Education for Nurses (QSEN): Patient-Centered Care, Teamwork & Collaboration, Evidence-Based Practice (EBP), Quality Improvement (QI), Safety, and Informatics.
7. Implement nursing care to assist a couple in selecting and preparing for an alternative birth setting such as a free standing clinic or their home as well as support a woman during labor by controlled breathing.
8. Evaluate outcome criteria for achievement and effectiveness of care.
9. Integrate knowledge of prepared childbirth with the interplay of nursing process, the six competencies of QSEN, and Family Nursing to promote quality maternal and child health nursing care.

Elena Garza is a 30-year-old woman who is pregnant with her second child. During her first pregnancy, she did not attend any childbirth classes and received an epidural for the birth. During a prenatal visit for her current pregnancy, Elena tells you she would now like to have a more natural birth in a birthing center. She asks you for information on childbirth education classes. Her partner, Joe, a Navy Seal, wants Elena to go to the hospital and have an epidural like the last time. He says, "The doctors know what they're doing. Just let them do their job." After further speaking with Joe, you discover he doesn't want Elena to go through the pain of natural childbirth because he fears he may be out of town when she's in labor.

Previous chapters discussed normal anatomy and physiology, and nursing care necessary during pregnancy. This chapter adds information about ways couples can make labor and birth a more satisfying experience. The information helps protect the mental as well as the physical health of both women and children throughout the continuum of pregnancy, birth, and childrearing.

How can you help alleviate some of Joe's concerns and best advise the Garzas on preparations for childbirth?

BOX 14.1 Nursing Care Planning Based on 2020 National Health Goals

Preparation-for-childbirth classes supply information not only on how to prepare for childbirth but also on how to parent. A number of 2020 National Health Goals that speak directly to such classes or counseling include:

- Increase the proportion of pregnant women who attend a series of prepared childbirth classes (Developmental).
- Increase the proportion of pregnant women who receive early and adequate prenatal care from a baseline of 70.5% to a target of 77.6%.
- Increase the proportion of women delivering a live birth who received preconception care services and practiced key recommended preconception health behaviors (Developmental) (U.S. Department of Health and Human Services [DHHS], 2010; see www.healthypeople.gov).

Nurses have a direct role in helping the nation achieve these objectives by participating as instructors in preparation for childbirth and parenting classes as well as teaching and supervising prenatal care.

As active consumers of health care, expectant families can find themselves faced with a wide array of choices for a childbirth experience and preparation for parenting. Three important decisions families need to make before labor include:

- Choice of birth attendant
- Choice of setting
- How much and what type of analgesic they want to use in labor

For example, a woman may elect to have her family doctor, an obstetrician, or a nurse-midwife as her birth attendant. She may choose to be supported by her intimate partner, other family members, friends, or a **doula** (a woman experienced in childbirth who provides continuous emotional and physical support). She may choose to give birth in a birthing center or a hospital with specially equipped birthing rooms (MacDorman, Mathews, & Declercq, 2012).

No matter what setting the woman or couple choose, expectant parents are well advised to be as prepared as possible for the physical and emotional aspects of childbirth (Kemp, Kingswood, Kibuka, et al., 2013). Box 14.1 shows 2020 National Health Goals related to preparation for childbirth and parenting.

Nursing Process Overview

For Childbirth and Parenting Education

Assessment

Assessing each woman's or couple's readiness for decision making about childbirth, as well as providing foundation information early in the process can help a woman or couple make plans for childbirth. Some couples have a clear idea of where and how they wish their child's birth to occur from the moment they realize they are pregnant. Others cannot even consider the actual birth until they have adjusted to the idea of pregnancy.

Childbirth education is not just for primiparas because if a woman expecting her second or third child has waited several years between children, she usually appreciates refresher information as much as a primipara hungers for new information. Whether a woman is a primipara or multipara, ask whether either she or her support person wants to attend childbirth or parenting courses. Provide appropriate information on what classes are available and how and when they should enroll.

Nursing Diagnosis

Nursing diagnoses tend to cluster around whether the woman or couple is sure of their decision about the birth setting and childbirth preparation. Examples include:

- Health-seeking behaviors related to learning more about childbirth and newborn care.
- If there is a lack of a support person, the following diagnoses might apply:
  - Ineffective coping related to lack of a support person
  - Anxiety related to absence of significant other
- For a couple unable to make a decision about a childbirth setting, an appropriate diagnosis might be decisional conflict related to lack of information about advantages and disadvantages of various childbirth settings.
- If there are older children in the family, a nursing diagnosis might be anxiety related to sibling role in pending birth event and sibling ability to welcome a new family member.

Outcome Identification and Planning

When planning with couples for labor and birth, goals that are set should seem both realistic and flexible. For example, the goal of preparation is to help couples make informed choices, rather than to follow a rigid plan.

Not all women want to go through labor without analgesia, so setting a goal to do so would be unrealistic for such a woman. The majority of women, however, want to participate as fully as possible in their labor and birth experience, so setting a goal for them to do that would be very realistic. Some women may be reluctant to attend a childbirth preparation course because of fear attending will mean they are committing themselves to a medication-free birth. You can assure them that learning about medications or other methods to reduce the pain of childbirth does not mean they have to use one or the other of these methods. In the same way, women who are certain they want medication before having taken a class will not be held to this afterward.

Helpful Internet referral sources for couples making childbirth plans are Childbirth Connection (www.childbirthconnection.org), Lamaze International (www.lamaze.org), International Childbirth Education Association (www.icea.org), La Leche League International (www.llli.org), and the Coalition for Improving Maternity Services (www.motherfriendly.org).

Implementation

Be certain to provide a woman and her partner with information on the benefits and drawbacks of birthing options without influencing them in a particular direction. To remain objective, examine your own attitudes, cultural influences, and values related to childbirth and explore how these beliefs might differ from those of your clients (Box 14.2). Referring couples to a childbirth preparation course can provide many answers for them in a sympathetic group setting, where feelings and anxieties can be shared. Be familiar with the content of courses available in your community so you can be certain the courses you suggest are appropriate for individual couples and present adequate and accurate information.

Review the arrangements a woman needs to make for labor and birth at the midpoint of pregnancy. No matter how calm a woman seems when discussing these details, many women experience some fear at the last minute and will forget what they need to do when labor begins. Be certain a woman has thought through arrangements for transportation to the hospital or birthing center and for child care if she has other children at home. Be certain a woman who anticipates a home birth has organized her home and purchased supplies for birth well in advance of her expected due date.

Outcome Evaluation

Evaluate whether expected outcomes for childbirth education have been achieved during the last few prenatal visits. By this time, a woman or couple should know where the baby will be born and should have worked out transportation and child care details. Encourage women who will be coached through childbirth by their partners or another support person to continue practicing breathing and relaxation techniques together up to the time of birth so they do not lose these skills. A final evaluation as to whether the couple was satisfied with their birth setting or preparation choices takes place after the birth. Examples of expected outcomes that would demonstrate the success of interventions include:

- The couple states they feel prepared for childbirth.
- The client states she feels confident she can use breathing exercises for contractions as long as 70 seconds.
- The client has made preparations for a doula to support her during labor.
- The sibling states she is ready to welcome a new brother or sister into the family.
- The couple states they were well prepared for birth and that it was both a satisfying and a growth experience for them.

CHILDBIRTH EDUCATION

Although parenting is unarguably an important occupation, it is one of the few occupations that requires no formal education, no examination to test a person's ability to take on such a role, and no refresher course to ensure a parent is following healthy standards of childrearing. Assessing whether couples need preparation for childbirth or parenting classes or encouraging them to take one can therefore be extremely important to make childbirth a satisfying experience, to help a family bond with its new member, and to help couples become effective parents (Box 14.3).

BOX 14.2 Nursing Care Planning to Respect Cultural Diversity

Whether women want or are able to take a childbirth and parenting preparation course depends a great deal on cultural and socioeconomic factors and individual choices. In some cultures, for example, the advice of a friend or family member carries more weight than the advice of a professional health care practitioner. A very old cross-cultural belief is a knife placed under the mattress will "cut the pain" better than a Lamaze program, so you may need to advocate to allow this type of pain relief. Asking each woman separately whether she is interested in a course and being certain women are fully informed about the options available are two ways to be certain all women receive as much advice and knowledge as they wish about childbirth.

Who women choose as a support person or coach in labor also differs depending on one's cultural background. Some women would not think of choosing anyone but their male partner; whereas others' first choice would be a female relative or friend. Assess each couple individually to be certain cultural preferences such as these are respected.

BOX 14.3 Nursing Care Planning Using Assessment

Assessing a Woman's Preparation for Labor

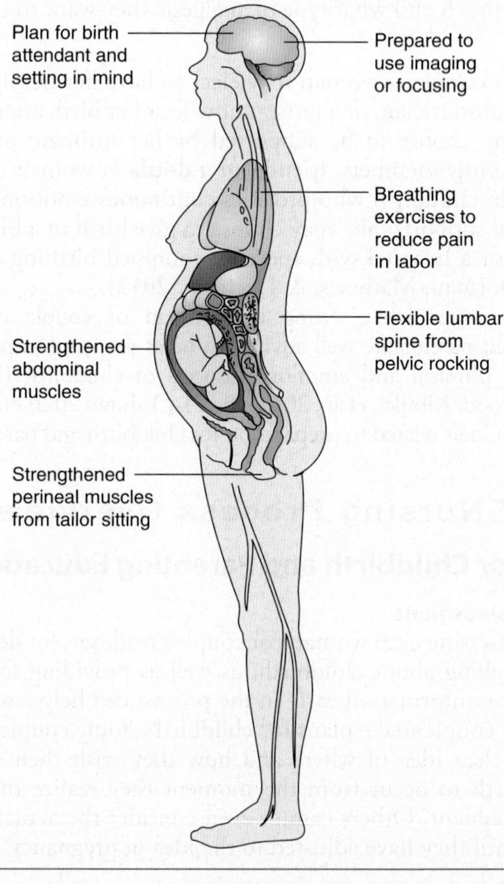

Preparation for childbirth courses that teach this material should be individualized to meet the parents' needs. Classes should be personalized and structured for women with special needs such as adolescents, career women, women who are physically challenged, or those experiencing a high-risk pregnancy. There also are classes available to help prepare siblings or grandparents learn more about their role. Women having a **vaginal birth after cesarean (VBAC)** or women who are having a scheduled cesarean birth can attend classes specially designed for them (Horey, Weaver, & Russell, 2011).

Preparation for childbirth courses initially began in the early 1900s to encourage women to come for prenatal care (Kiely & Kogan, 2012). Classes continue today because, with all the birth choices available, they fulfill an important need for education about labor and childbirth. As many as 15% of women express fear or anxiety about what will happen in labor, so counseling can be very important to alleviate this fear (Alder, Breitinger, Granado, et al., 2011).

The overall goals of childbirth education are to prepare expectant parents emotionally and physically for childbirth while promoting wellness behaviors that can be used by parents and families for life. Women usually enjoy such classes because they offer them a sense of "family" if their intimate partner also attends as well as create a sense of empowerment or confidence that they will be knowledgeable enough to participate fully in their birth experience.

Childbirth Educators and Methods of Teaching

Childbirth educators are usually health care providers who have a professional degree in the helping professions as well as a certificate from a course on childbirth education. They teach expectant parents about the physical and emotional aspects of pregnancy, childbirth, and early parenthood as well as present coping skills and labor support techniques. Although childbirth education is an interdisciplinary field, it has historically been associated with nursing, and nurses play major roles in designing and teaching such courses. Most classes are taught in a group format, incorporating a variety of teaching techniques such as DVD or PowerPoint presentations, lectures, and demonstrations (especially for content on relaxation and breathing techniques). One of the most important aspects of these courses, however, is group interaction. Women and their partners enjoy the opportunity to share their fears and hopes about their pregnancy and upcoming birth with others as they learn together (Box 14.4).

Efficacy of Childbirth Education Courses

Many studies have been done to determine just how effective childbirth courses are at reducing the pain of childbirth, shortening the length of labor, decreasing the amount of medication used, and increasing overall enjoyment of the experience. Because of the variability in courses offered and the variability in women's reactions to childbirth, however, it is often difficult to compare results of attending childbirth classes versus not attending them. This is also partly because people who volunteer to attend classes already have a high degree of positive motivation, which may skew the results. Despite these difficulties with measurement, it is generally accepted that preparation courses can increase satisfaction, reduce the amount of reported pain, decrease risky behaviors such as smoking, and increase feelings of control during childbirth (Al-Sahab, Saqib, Hauser, et al., 2010; Records & Wilson, 2011). It is documented that by attendance in discussions of breastfeeding, the proportion of new mothers who breastfeed can be increased (Johnson & Strube, 2011).

BOX 14.4 Nursing Care Planning Based on Effective Communication

You care for Elena at a prenatal clinic visit. She is in the 24th week of an uncomplicated pregnancy.

Less Effective Communication

Nurse: Have you signed up for a childbirth preparation class yet, Elena?
Elena: No.
Nurse: Don't wait too much longer. You're already in your sixth month.
Elena: I don't really need to go to one.
Nurse: Okay. You know best.

More Effective Communication

Nurse: Have you signed up for a childbirth preparation class yet, Elena?
Elena: No.
Nurse: Don't wait too much longer. You're already in your sixth month.
Elena: I don't really need to go to one.
Nurse: Why is that?
Elena: Classes are at the wrong time. And cost too much.
Nurse: Let's work together to find a course that's right for you. We can use the Internet to find out what options are available.

Because women should have input into how much preparation they want to do for childbirth, it is easy to take a woman's answer at face value for not wanting to attend a class. Careful listening often reveals time or money concerns are the real reason why couples choose not to attend a course. Helping to investigate the many options is the beginning of problem solving.

THE CHILDBIRTH PLAN

Most classes for expectant parents urge couples to make a written childbirth plan to include information such as their choice of setting, birth attendant, special needs such as the extent of family participation they wish during labor, birthing positions, medication options, plans for the immediate postpartum period, baby care, and family visitation—all measures to give them a better sense of control (Kuo, Lin, Hsu, et al., 2010).

Urge couples to make these decisions at least 1 month before the expected day of birth. This way, if an expectant couple has a strong desire in a certain area, this gives them time to communicate their wish so it can be accommodated if possible. If plans are left to the last minute, the couple may find decisions determined by agency policy or the circumstances at the moment rather than by their input.

When talking to couples about their birth plan, be certain it includes flexibility as well as is centered on the ultimate goal of childbirth: a healthy baby and healthy parents rather than concentration on a limited goal, such as not having fetal monitoring or using a particular birthing position. This is because, in the event of a complication that requires an emergency cesarean birth, their preference to have the baby without anesthesia will need to be modified. Making a birth plan in a group setting has the advantage of allowing a couple to sort out their questions and feelings about what they want to consider in their plan as they share information with others. Box 14.5 is a sample birth plan.

PRECONCEPTION CLASSES

Preconception classes are held for couples who plan to get pregnant within a short time and want to know more about what they can expect pregnancy to be like and what birth setting and procedure choices exist. These classes stress that pregnancy brings with it psychological as well as physical changes and include recommended preconception nutrition modifications such as a good intake of folic acid (e.g., green leafy vegetables) and protein (e.g., meat, tofu, beans) and perhaps a prenatal vitamin during the time waiting to get pregnant to ensure a healthy fetus (Saravelos & Regan, 2011). Box 14.6 lists questions a couple might want to discuss about birth.

QSEN Checkpoint Question 14.1

Patient-Centered Care

Elena, 30 years of age, shows you the birth plan that she has drafted. Which statement by her would help assure you that she has a workable plan?

a. "I've written down everything I have to have to make labor a success."
b. "I didn't include anything my boyfriend wanted; I'm the one having the baby."
c. "My mother strongly suggested I ask for morphine like she did, so I'm going to add that."
d. "I've tried to keep it flexible because I know circumstances can change."

Look in Appendix A for the best answer and rationale.

BOX 14.5 Birth Plan: Elena Garza

Birth Attendants:
Alexander Coppin, MD, and nurse-midwife Kaitlin Brandywine, or whoever is on call for the big day.

Birth Setting
Room Number 1 at Huntington Alternative Birth Center

Support Persons
My boyfriend Joe and my sister Adrienne. Adrienne will serve as my doula.

Activities During Labor
I want to walk around or rock in the rocking chair or play Monopoly.
I want to use breathing exercises with contractions.
I want to wear my own nightgown and listen to Lady Antebellum's CD *Own the Night*
I want to wear my glasses, not my contact lenses.
I want to eat "anything chocolate" during labor.
I want to drink raspberry-flavored water to stay hydrated (partner will supply).
I want a walking epidural for pain as soon as I'm far enough dilated to have it.

Birth
Position for birth: on my side (no stirrups, please).
No episiotomy please.
Joe wants to cut the cord.
I want my older son to watch if he wants to (my mother will babysit).
I want to cord bank a sample of my baby's blood.
I'm okay with circumcision.
I want the first voice my baby hears to be my voice so no talking please while he's born.

Postpartum
I want to breastfeed immediately and exclusively (will probably need some help).
I want to use skin-to-skin care to keep the baby warm.
I want to room-in constantly.
Joe wants to sleep over on bedside cot.

EXPECTANT PARENTING CLASSES

Expectant parenting classes are designed for couples to attend early in pregnancy. They focus on the woman's health during a pregnancy by covering such topics as the psychological and physical changes of pregnancy, pregnancy nutrition, routine health care such as dental checkups, and newborn care. A typical course plan for 8 weeks is shown in Box 14.7.

Both the woman and her support person are invited to classes; the curriculum is individualized for the group members and their needs such as women in the military, sibling preparation, refresher classes for grandparents, classes for expectant adoptive parents, pregnant adolescents, or women with physical disabilities. If all the women in the group

BOX 14.6 Nursing Care Planning Based on Family Teaching

CHOOSING A BIRTH SETTING

Q. Elena and her partner Joe ask you, "There are so many options available for a birth setting. How do we decide which one to choose?"

A. Choosing a birth setting is a personal decision. Some questions you might want to ask to help with the decision include:

- What type of health care provider do I want to supervise my prenatal care and labor and birth? Nurse-midwife? Family doctor? Obstetrician?
- What settings does a particular childbirth provider let me choose from? A birthing room? An alternative birthing center? My home?
- Will the same person be present at prenatal visits as for the birth? Does the setting offer preparation for childbirth or childrearing classes?
- Will I be allowed to choose a birth position? Will I have input into the amount of anesthesia used? Can a doula be with me in labor? Can administration of ophthalmic ointment for the baby's eyes be delayed so it doesn't interrupt bonding? Can I begin breastfeeding immediately? Will nurses who are supportive and informed about breastfeeding be available if I have a problem?
- Will the setting allow my support person to participate? Will he or she be allowed to stay with me throughout labor and birth? Could he or she cut the cord or help with the birth? Can older children participate? Can I record the birth on video or by photographs?
- Is early discharge available? Will a follow-up home visit be included in care?
- If I should have a complication during labor or birth, is there adequate equipment and personnel available for emergency care? If our baby should have a complication, is there provision for immediate emergency care or transport to a high-risk facility? Will my partner be able to go with the baby?

already have children, for example, they may not need a tour of a maternity unit as part of the program; instead, they may want to learn what is new in baby food or child care. If all the women in the class work at least part time, discussion of "brown bag nutrition" and how to include rest periods during work hours might be most useful. If all the women are teenagers, they may be most interested in what is going to happen to their bodies during pregnancy, or what sports are safe to continue. They may also need extended information on how to care for a newborn. They probably will also want a tour of the maternity unit (Fig. 14.1).

BOX 14.7 Sample Outline for Weekly Expectant Parents Classes

Lesson 1: Review of Physiologic Changes of Pregnancy and Fetal Growth
Lesson 2: Personal Care During Pregnancy
  Nutrition, hygiene such as bathing, dental care, exercise, and rest
Lesson 3: Emotional Changes During Pregnancy
Lesson 4: Labor and Birth
  The process of birth, exercises, and breathing techniques, and medication in labor
Lesson 5: Plans for Birth
  Birth settings available, supplies to take to birth settings, tour or film of a typical birth
Lesson 6: The Postpartum Period
Lesson 7: Infant Care
  Nutrition and hygiene
Lesson 8: Reproductive Life Planning

Sibling Education Classes

Sibling classes are organized to acquaint older brothers and sisters with what happens during birth and what they can expect a newborn to look and act like. The classes review how babies grow and things children can do to help their mother during a pregnancy, such as eating healthy foods with her and not leaving toys on the floor that need to be picked up.

If the classes are held at a hospital, a tour of a newborn nursery is included so children can see how small their new sibling will be (otherwise they may envision the new baby as

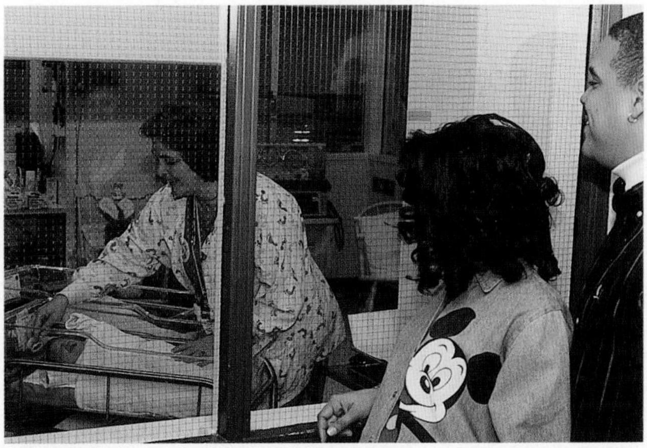

FIGURE 14.1 An enjoyable part of a preparation-for-parenthood class is touring a maternity service. Here, although they will be rooming-in with their newborn, parents-to-be view a newborn nursery.

big enough to play with them). A hospital room like the one their mother will occupy may also be visited.

To be certain sibling classes are successful, be certain the information presented is age appropriate. Chapters 29 through 33 discuss growth and development expectations by age group and when children are ready for formal instruction. Younger children in a group may need assurance their parents will continue to love them after the new baby arrives. Older children may be interested in learning about newborn care and receiving assurance their life will not be totally changed after the arrival of the new family member (Gabriel, 2011).

Breastfeeding Classes

Breastfeeding classes are designed to help women learn more about breastfeeding so they not only choose breastfeeding over bottle feeding but also so they continue with breastfeeding for at least 6 months following their child's birth. Such classes cover the physiology of breastfeeding as well as the psychological aspects. Classes are often taught by a certified La Leche League instructor who is an expert on what problems new mothers are apt to encounter (see Chapter 19 for breastfeeding techniques) (Monica & du Plessis, 2011).

What if... 14.1 Elena tells you her partner won't be coming to childbirth classes with her because, as a Navy Seal, he may be out of town when she's in labor. She asks you if it is really important to have someone with her. How would you advise her?

Preparation for Childbirth Classes

Preparation for childbirth classes focus mainly on explaining the psychological and physiologic changes that occur with childbirth and ways to prevent or reduce the pain of childbirth.

Common areas taught include:

- Preparing the expectant woman and her support person for the childbirth experience
- Helping women become more informed about the options available for childbirth
- Explaining the role of both pharmacologic and nonpharmacologic methods of pain control that are useful for labor
- Helping increase the couple's overall enjoyment of and satisfaction with the childbirth experience

In addition to teaching about normal labor and pain relief, classes also include a number of exercises to ready the body for labor.

Exercise During Pregnancy

Encourage women to maintain an active exercise program during pregnancy overall because such a program will both increase blood circulation to the fetus and help prevent excessive weight gain in the mother (Szymanski & Satin, 2012).

Women should not, however, enroll or participate in a formal exercise program without their primary health care provider's approval. They should also not attempt to exercise if any of the danger signs of pregnancy are present and should never exercise to a point of fatigue (Box 14.8).

Prenatal Yoga

Prenatal yoga classes are aimed at helping a woman relax and manage stress better for all times in her life, not just pregnancy. Yoga exercises help a woman stay overall fit by their focus on gentle stretching and deep breathing. They can also help a woman experience high self-esteem as she masters difficult levels or positions. Yoga breathing techniques are also useful in labor to help both relaxation and pain management (Smith, Levett, Collins, et al., 2011).

Caution women that, as pregnancy progresses, it will become difficult to maintain yoga positions that involve balancing. Urge women to use a chair or a wall for stabilization and to avoid twisting exercises late in pregnancy because, when joints soften in preparation for labor, muscle or joint strain could occur.

Perineal and Abdominal Exercises

Women can practice specific exercises to strengthen pelvic and abdominal muscles to make these muscles stronger and more supple for labor. If perineal muscles are supple, this allows for stretching during birth, reduces discomfort, and

BOX 14.8 Nursing Care Planning to Empower a Family

EXERCISE GUIDELINES FOR LABOR PREPARATION

Q. Elena asks you, "How can I be sure the exercises I'm doing to be ready for birth won't hurt me or my baby?"
A. Good rules to follow include:

- Always rise from the floor slowly to prevent feeling dizzy from orthostatic hypotension.
- To rise from the floor, roll over to the side first and then push up to avoid strain on the abdominal muscles or round ligaments because this can cause intense pain.
- To prevent leg cramps when doing leg exercises, never point the toes (extend the heel instead).
- To prevent back pain, do not attempt exercises that hyperextend the lower back.
- Do not hold your breath while exercising, because this increases intra-abdominal and intrauterine pressure.
- Do not continue with exercises if any danger signal of pregnancy occurs.
- Never exercise to a point of fatigue.
- Never practice second-stage pushing. Pushing increases intrauterine pressure and could rupture membranes.

helps perineal muscles function more efficiently after childbirth, which helps reduce the possibility of urinary incontinence (Hay-Smith, Herderschee, Dumoulin, et al., 2011).

A woman may begin exercises as early in pregnancy as she likes. Many exercises can be incorporated into daily activities so they take little time from a busy day. It is best, however, for a woman to set aside a specific time each day for practicing exercises; otherwise, her participation may be sporadic. Initially, women should do each exercise only a few times, and gradually increase the number with each session.

Tailor Sitting

Although many women may be familiar with tailor sitting, they may have to be retaught the position so it is done in a way that stretches perineal muscles without occluding blood supply to the lower legs. A woman should put one leg in front of the other, not put one ankle on top of the other to avoid interfering with leg circulation (Fig. 14.2). As she sits in this position, she should then gently push on her knees toward the floor until she feels her perineum stretch. This is a good position to use to watch television, read, talk to friends on the phone, or file papers in a lower cabinet at work. If a woman sits in this position for at least 15 minutes every day, by the end of pregnancy, her perineum should be so supple when she tailor sits, her knees will almost touch the floor if pushed.

Squatting

Squatting (Fig. 14.3) also stretches the perineal muscles and can be a useful position for second-stage labor as well, and, like tailor sitting, should be practiced for about 15 minutes a day. For pelvic muscles to stretch, a woman should keep her feet flat on the floor and not raise on her tiptoes. Incorporating squatting into daily activities such as picking up toys from the floor reduces the amount of time a woman must devote to daily exercises.

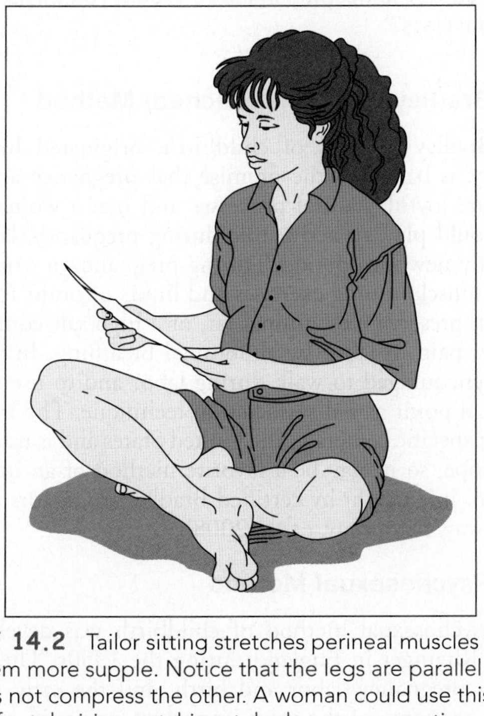

FIGURE 14.2 Tailor sitting stretches perineal muscles to make them more supple. Notice that the legs are parallel so one does not compress the other. A woman could use this position for television watching, telephone conversations, or playing with an older child.

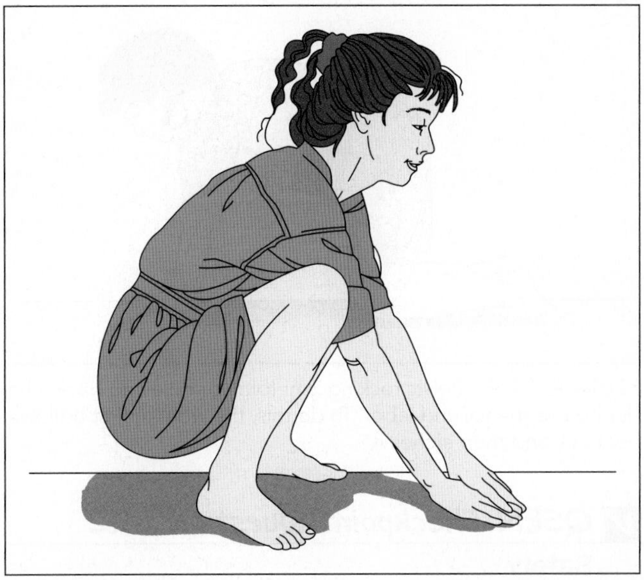

FIGURE 14.3 Squatting helps to stretch the muscles of the pelvic floor. Notice the feet are flat on the floor for optimal perineal stretching.

Pelvic Floor Contractions (Kegel Exercises)

Pelvic floor contractions can be done easily during daily activities. While sitting at her desk or working around the house, a woman can tighten the muscles of her perineum by doing Kegel exercises (see Chapter 12, Box 12.7). Such perineal muscle-strengthening exercises are helpful in the postpartum period to reduce pain and promote perineal healing. They also have long-term effects of increasing sexual responsiveness and helping prevent stress incontinence (Allahdin & Kambhampati, 2012).

Abdominal Muscle Contractions

Abdominal muscle contractions may help strengthen abdominal muscles during pregnancy, help prevent constipation, and help restore abdominal tone after pregnancy. Strong abdominal muscles can also contribute to effective second-stage pushing during labor. Abdominal contractions can be done in a standing or lying position. A woman merely tightens her abdominal muscles, then relaxes them. She can repeat the exercise as often as she wishes during the day.

Another way to do the same thing is to practice "blowing out a candle." A woman takes a fairly deep inspiration, then exhales normally. Holding her finger about 6 in. in front of herself, as if it were a candle, she then exhales forcibly, pushing out residual air from her lungs as if her finger were a lit candle. She can feel her abdominal muscles contract as she reaches the end of a forcible exhalation.

Pelvic Rocking

Pelvic rocking (Fig. 14.4) helps relieve backache during pregnancy and early labor by making the lumbar spine more flexible. It can be done in a variety of positions: on hands and knees, lying down, sitting, or standing. A woman arches her back, trying to lengthen or stretch her spine. She holds the position for 1 minute, then hollows her back. If a woman does this at the end of the day about five times, it not only increases her flexibility but also helps relieve back pain and make her more comfortable during the night.

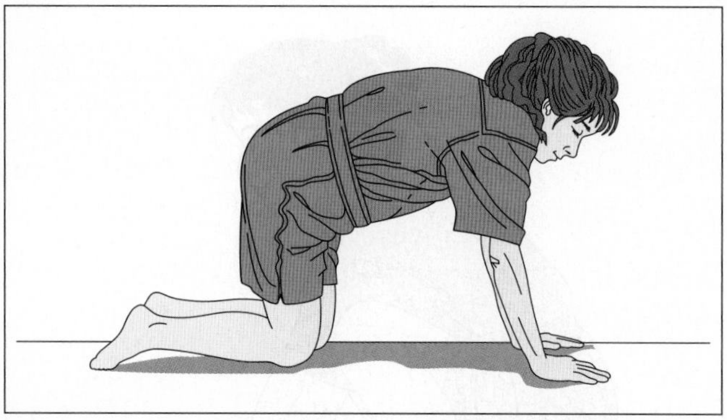

FIGURE 14.4 Pelvic rocking is helpful for relieving backache during pregnancy and labor. To do this, the woman first hollows her back and then arches it.

QSEN Checkpoint Question 14.2

Safety

Elena asks you which type of exercise is best to strengthen her perineal muscles in anticipation of birth. Which of the following recommendations is safest and most effective?

a. Walk or jog 20 minutes daily at a fairly rapid pace.
b. Squat or tailor sit for 15 minutes out of every day.
c. Periodically bear down as hard as possible while holding her breath.
d. Lift both of her legs into the air while she lies on her back.

Look in Appendix A for the best answer and rationale.

Birthing Slings

A birthing sling is a rectangular piece of material often called a *rebozo* (Mexico), a *manta* (Peru), a *kanga* (Africa), or a *selendang* (Indonesia) that is slipped under a woman's back as she lies supine, then held by one or two assistants who gently sway the woman's body back and forth sideways, causing the fetus to rock in the amniotic fluid. The rocking technique is advocated by doulas to relieve uterine ligament tension during pregnancy; this technique as well as "dangling" from a sling can be used to facilitate fetal rotation and descent during labor as this enlarges the pelvic outlet (Simkin, Bolding, Keppler, et al., 2010).

It is difficult to find evidence-based documentation for the use of birthing slings during pregnancy so, although you will see them in use, women should check with their primary care provider before using them during pregnancy and labor to be certain they are safe for them.

Birthing Aids

During early labor, a woman needs to discover what activities she could use for **distraction** that would be unique for her such as playing cards or listening to specific music; further into labor, she should plan what she could use as a greater distraction for even stronger contractions such as singing out loud, having her partner massage her back, or center intently on breathing exercises. Caution her partner that by mid-labor, women become so intent on the process of birthing that they no longer want to talk or joke. Remind women that they probably can't use cell phones because these interfere with monitoring equipment.

In order to help fetal descent and help relieve pain, women can use an exercise ball, a Jacuzzi tub, or change of position such as squatting, swaying with a partner, or rocking in a chair. These alternative pain and descent methods are discussed in Chapter 16 with other measures that are useful in labor but don't involve practice during pregnancy.

METHODS TO MANAGE PAIN IN CHILDBIRTH

Beginning in the late 1950s, many specific methods for non-pharmacologic pain reduction during labor were developed. These included the Lamaze, Dick-Read, Kitzinger, and Bradley methods, all named after the professionals who developed them. More recently, childbirth education has moved away from a strict method approach like these to more eclectic ones. Many educators teach a variety of approaches, including the use of complementary or herbal therapies.

Most approaches to reducing discomfort in labor are based on the following three principles:

1. A woman needs to come into labor informed about what causes labor pain and prepared with breathing exercises to use to minimize pain during contractions.
2. A woman experiences less pain if her abdomen is relaxed and the uterus is allowed to rise freely against the abdominal wall with contractions.
3. Using the **gating control theory of pain perception**, distraction techniques can be employed to alter how pain is received (Box 14.9).

What if . . . 14.2 Elena tells you she does not intend to take a preparation for labor class because she wants to have epidural anesthesia as soon as she is admitted to the hospital in labor. Would you advise her to attend a class?

The Bradley (Partner-Coached) Method

The Bradley method of childbirth, originated by Robert Bradley, is based on the premise that pregnancy and childbirth are joyful, natural processes and that a woman's partner should play an active role during pregnancy, labor, and the early newborn period. During pregnancy, a woman performs muscle-toning exercises and limits or omits foods that contain preservatives, animal fat, or a high salt content. She reduces pain in labor by abdominal breathing. In addition, she is encouraged to walk during labor and to use an internal focal point as a disassociation technique. The method is used at specific centers in the United States and is used widely in Europe, so it may be a favorite method of an immigrant woman. It is taught by certified Bradley instructors (Bradley, Hathaway, Hathaway, et al., 2008).

The Psychosexual Method

The psychosexual method of childbirth was developed by Sheila Kitzinger in England during the 1950s. The method stresses pregnancy, labor and birth, and the early newborn period are some of the most important points in a woman's life. It includes a program of conscious relaxation and levels of

BOX 14.9 Gating Control Mechanisms to Reduce Pain

Pain flows through pathways because:

1. The endings of small peripheral nerve fibers detect a stimulus.
2. Small nerve fibers transmit the sensation of pain to cells in the dorsal horn of the spinal cord.
3. Impulses pass through a dense, interfacing network of cells in the spinal cord (the substantia gelatinosa).
4. Immediately, a synapse occurs in a motor nerve that initiates a response at the peripheral site. For example, a woman touches a hot stove, the impulse travels to the spinal cord, immediately returns to her fingers, and the woman jerks her hand away from the stove burner.
5. After this short-circuit synapse, the impulse then continues in the spinal cord to reach the hypothalamus and cortex of the brain.
6. The impulse is interpreted (e.g., the burner is hot) and is perceived as pain.

Gating Theory of Pain Control

The gating theory of pain perception refers to gate control mechanisms in the substantia gelatinosa that are capable of halting an impulse at the level of the spinal cord so the impulse is never perceived at the brain level as pain—a process similar to closing a gate. Techniques that can assist gating mechanisms include:

- *Cutaneous stimulation.* If large peripheral nerves next to an injury site are stimulated, the ability of the small nerve fibers at the injury site to transmit pain impulses appears to decrease. Therefore, rubbing an injured part or applying transcutaneous electrical nerve stimulation (TENS) or heat or cold to the site (cutaneous stimulation) are effective maneuvers to suppress pain. Effleurage, or light massage used in the Lamaze method, also accomplishes this.
- *Distraction.* If the cells in the brain cortex that will register an impulse as pain are preoccupied with other stimuli, a pain impulse cannot register. Different childbirth classes use different breathing, vocalization, or focusing techniques such as imaging to accomplish this. Breathing techniques not only furnish distraction but can increase oxygenation to the mother and fetus.
- *Reduction of anxiety.* Pain impulses are perceived more quickly if a woman is anxious. The third technique of gating, therefore, is to reduce patient anxiety as much as possible. Teaching a woman what to expect during labor is a means of achieving this.

progressive breathing that encourage a woman to "flow with" rather than struggle against contractions (Kitzinger, 2011).

The Dick-Read Method

The Dick-Read method is based on an approach proposed by Grantly Dick-Read, an English physician. The premise is that fear leads to tension, which leads to pain. If a woman can prevent fear from occurring or can break the chain between fear and tension or tension and pain, then she can reduce the pain of labor contractions. A woman achieves lack of fear through education about childbirth, and she achieves reduced pain by focusing on abdominal breathing during contractions (Dick-Read & Gaskin, 2013).

The Lamaze Philosophy

The Lamaze method of prepared childbirth, a philosophy based on the gating control theory of pain relief, is the one most often taught in the United States today (Amis, 2010). The method is based on the theory that through stimulus-response conditioning, women can learn to use controlled breathing to reduce pain during labor. It was originally termed the **psychoprophylactic** method because it focuses on preventing pain in labor (prophylaxis) by use of the mind (psyche). The method was developed in Russia based on Pavlov's conditioning studies but was popularized by a French physician, Ferdinand Lamaze. Formal classes are organized by Lamaze International and the International Childbirth Education Association.

Lamaze preparation is not so much a method to help a woman cope with labor as it is a total philosophy of how to enjoy a safe and satisfying childbirth experience. Information to guide a woman and her coach through pregnancy such as prenatal nutrition, exercises, and common discomforts of pregnancy are discussed in classes along with information to prepare couples for unexpected circumstances of birth, such as malpresentation, cesarean birth, or the need for analgesia or anesthesia. Suggestions for supplies a woman or couple might want to pack in advance and bring to the hospital for labor and birth are shown in Table 14.1.

TABLE 14.1 Supplies to Use During Labor

Item	Purpose
Lip balm	To prevent dry lips
Mouthwash	For rinsing dry mouth
Toothbrush and toothpaste	To prevent dry mouth
Warm socks	Comfort
Small rolling pin covered with soft cloth	Back massage
Tennis ball	Back massage
Focal point	To increase concentration
Busy work such as knitting or magazines	To pass time
Paper bag	To correct hyperventilation
Extra pillow	For semi-Fowler's position in labor
Wristwatch	For timing contractions
Scented oil	For reducing friction of effleurage
Lollipops or hard candy	For energy and dry mouth
Bottled water	To keep well hydrated
Music and music player	To increase relaxation
Snacks such as apples or potato chips	For coach's comfort

Throughout the program, the following six major concepts are stressed:

1. Labor should begin on its own, not be induced.
2. Women should walk, move around, and change positions throughout labor.
3. Women should bring a loved one, friend, or doula for continuous support.
4. Interventions that are not medically necessary should be avoided.
5. Women should be allowed to give birth in other positions than on their back and should follow their body's urges to push.
6. Mother and baby should be kept together after birth; it is best for the mother, baby, and for breastfeeding (Amis, 2010).

In addition, the following three main principles are taught in the prenatal period related to the gating control method of pain relief:

1. If a couple understands the process of labor and birth, they can enter labor with decreased tension.
2. Concentrating on breathing patterns or imagery or focusing can block incoming pain sensations.
3. **Conditioned reflexes**, or reflexes that automatically occur in response to a stimulus, can also be used to displace pain during labor. For example, a woman is conditioned to relax automatically on hearing a command ("contraction beginning") or at the feel of a contraction beginning. The responses to contractions must be recently conditioned to be effective (because conditioned responses fade if not reinforced). This is the reason it is generally recommended that women attend Lamaze classes in the last trimester of pregnancy. A disadvantage of enrolling so late is that it limits the total amount of time directed to perineal exercises. If labor begins early, a woman may have had little or no practice with this type of exercise.

Lamaze classes are kept small so there is time for individual instruction and attention to each couple (Fig. 14.5). Advise a woman to bring the support person who will serve as her coach in labor to class with her to practice breathing exercises. Exercises taught vary from teacher to teacher, especially in terms of complexity, but have common features, which are discussed as follows.

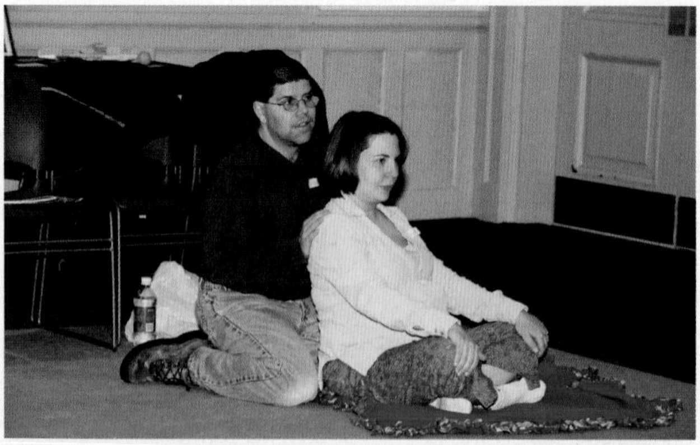

FIGURE 14.5 Every woman needs to be well prepared for birth. Here, a partner practices a position for pushing. Caution women not to actually push to avoid rupturing membranes.

Conscious Relaxation. This is learning to relax body parts so, unknowingly, a woman does not remain tense and cause unnecessary muscle strain and fatigue during labor. She practices **conscious relaxation** by deliberately relaxing one set of muscles, then another, and another until her body is completely relaxed. Her support person concentrates on noticing symptoms of tension such as a wrinkled brow, clenched fists, or a stiffly held arm. By either placing a comforting hand on the tense body area or telling a woman to relax that area, the support person can help her to achieve complete relaxation.

The Cleansing Breath. To begin all breathing exercises, a woman breathes in deeply and then exhales deeply **(cleansing breath)**. To end each exercise, she repeats this step. It is an important step to take because it limits the possibility of either hyperventilation (blowing off too much carbon dioxide) or hypoventilation (not exhaling enough carbon dioxide), both of which could happen with rapid breathing patterns and can interfere with an adequate fetal oxygen supply. If women do become light-headed during labor from hyperventilation (i.e., develop respiratory alkalosis), breathing into a paper bag can help because it causes rebreathing of exhaled carbon dioxide. The cleansing breath also signals to the woman's partner a contraction is about to begin or has ended.

QSEN Checkpoint Question 14.3

Evidence-Based Practice

One of the most controversial aspects of childbirth addresses the question of the best birth position for women to use. To evaluate the impact of birth position on maternal and newborn well-being, researchers reviewed 40 studies on birth position published over the past 15 years.

The results showed both physical and psychological benefits for women when they are able to adopt positions other than on their back for labor. Women allowed to birth in an upright position had a shorter duration of the first and second stages of labor, experienced less medical intervention, and reported less severe pain; they also had an increased rate of satisfaction with their childbirth experience than women who gave birth in a semi-recumbent or supine/lithotomy position. The only disadvantage identified of an upright position was increased blood loss during the third stage of labor, which may be due to increased perineal edema caused by the upright position (Priddis, Dahlen, & Schmied, 2011).

Based on the previous study, what would you like to see included in Elena's birth plan?

a. "I don't want any medical interventions in labor, like an IV."
b. "I want to labor the same way that you see women do it on TV and in movies."
c. "I'm willing to try anything safe that will make my labor shorter."
d. "I'm afraid I'll get dizzy if I try to sit up or stand during labor."

Look in Appendix A for the best answer and rationale.

Consciously Controlled Breathing. Using **consciously controlled breathing**, or set breathing patterns at specific rates, provides distraction as well as prevents the diaphragm from descending fully and putting pressure on the expanding uterus. To practice, after a cleansing breath, a woman inhales comfortably but fully, then exhales, with her exhalation a little stronger than her inhalation (to help prevent hypoventilation). She practices breathing in this manner at a controlled pace, depending on the intensity of contractions through the following various levels of breathing:

- *Level 1.* Slow deep chest breathing of comfortable but full respirations at a rate of 6 to 12 breaths/min. This level is used for early contractions in labor when the cervical dilation is between 0 and 3 cm.
- *Level 2.* Lighter and more rapid breathing than level 1. The rib cage should expand but be so light that the diaphragm barely moves. The rate of respirations is up to 40 breaths/min. This is a good level of breathing for contractions when cervical dilation is between 4 and 6 cm.
- *Level 3.* Even more shallow and more rapid breathing. The rate is 50 to 70 breaths/min. As the respirations become faster, the exhalation must be a little stronger than the inhalation to allow good air exchange and to prevent hypoventilation. If a woman practices saying "out" with each exhalation, she almost inevitably will make exhalation stronger than inhalation. A woman uses this level for transition contractions when cervical dilation is between 7 and 10 cm. Keeping the tip of her tongue against the roof of her mouth helps prevent her oral mucosa from drying out during such rapid breathing.
- *Level 4.* Another pattern effective for transition contractions is a "pant-blow" pattern, or taking three or four quick breaths (in and out), then a forceful exhalation. Because this type of breathing sounds like a train (breath-breath-breath-huff), it is sometimes referred to as "choo-choo" or "hee-hee-hee-hoo" breathing.
- *Level 5.* Quiet, continuous, very shallow panting at about 60 breaths/min. This can be used during strong contractions or during the second stage of labor to prevent a woman from pushing before full dilatation.

Some courses stop teaching at the point a woman has mastered these levels of breathing; others have her learn to shift from one level to the other on command or at the point she feels a need for more pain relief.

Figure 14.6 illustrates the use of levels of breathing. At the beginning of a mild, early labor contraction, a woman's coach says, "Contraction beginning." A woman takes a cleansing breath, then breathes at level 1; she feels no bite from the contraction and so does not need to change to a more involved breathing pattern. Later in labor, contractions are stronger and longer. Now, at the sound of "Contraction beginning," a woman takes a cleansing breath, then begins level 1 breathing (3 breaths), shifts to level 2 (4 to 6 breaths), and then shifts to level 3 (10 breaths). The contraction is lessening. She shifts down to level 2 (4 to 6 breaths), then to level 1 (3 or 4 breaths). The contraction is gone. She takes a final cleansing breath.

During actual labor, her coach can tell the strength of contractions by resting a hand on her abdomen or observing a uterine contraction monitor. A coach can tell a woman when to shift breathing levels depending on the coach's estimation of the strength of the contraction with words such as, "contraction beginning, getting stronger, now getting weaker, gone." In the time before transition to the second stage of labor, when contractions are longest and strongest, a woman may need to use her level 4 breathing or continuous light panting as well. A woman who can perform all five levels of breathing and maintain relaxation can be assured she is prepared to handle all labor contractions up to the second stage of labor (Lothian, 2011).

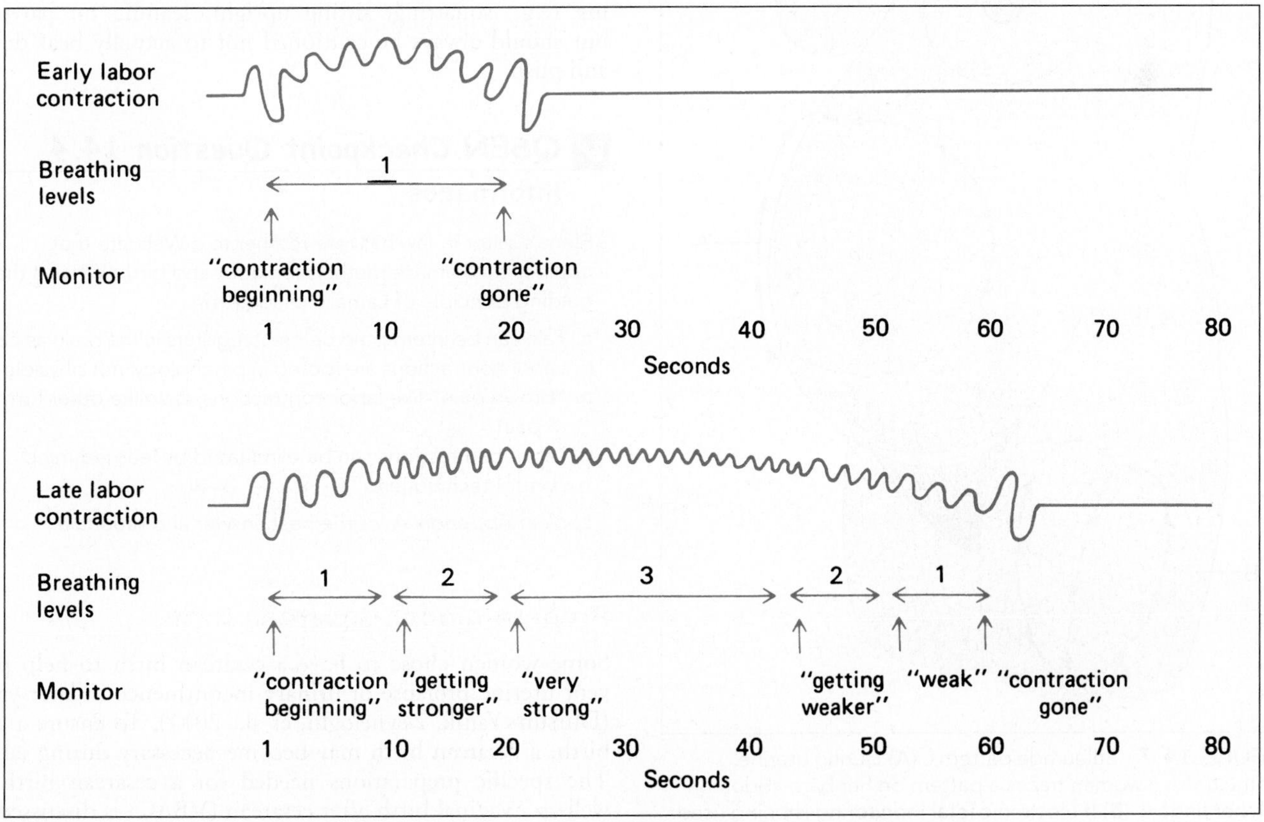

FIGURE 14.6 An example of differing breathing patterns during a single contraction. 1, 2, and 3 are levels of breathing. A cleansing breath is taken at the beginning and end of the contraction.

Effleurage. One additional technique to encourage relaxation and displace pain in the Lamaze method is **effleurage**, which is French for "light abdominal massage"; it is done with just enough pressure to avoid tickling. To do this, a woman traces a pattern on her abdomen with her fingertips (Fig. 14.7). The rate of effleurage should remain constant even though breathing rates change. Effleurage serves as a distraction technique and decreases sensory stimuli transmission from the abdominal wall, helping limit local discomfort. If an external electronic monitor is in place on the abdomen, effleurage can be done superior or inferior to it or even on the thighs. Effleurage can also be done by the support person.

Focusing or Imagery. Focusing intently on an object (sometimes called "sensate focus") is another method of keeping sensory input from reaching the cortex of the brain (Marc, Toureche, Ernst, et al., 2011). For example, a woman brings into labor a photograph of her partner or children, a graphic design, or just something that appeals to her like an ocean scene she can concentrate on during contractions (Fig. 14.8). Other women use imagery by imagining they are in a calm place such as on a beach watching waves rolling in to them or relaxing on a porch swing. Be careful not to step into a woman's line of vision during a contraction to break her concentration on an object; also, don't ask questions or try to talk to women while they are focused and breathing or you will break their concentration.

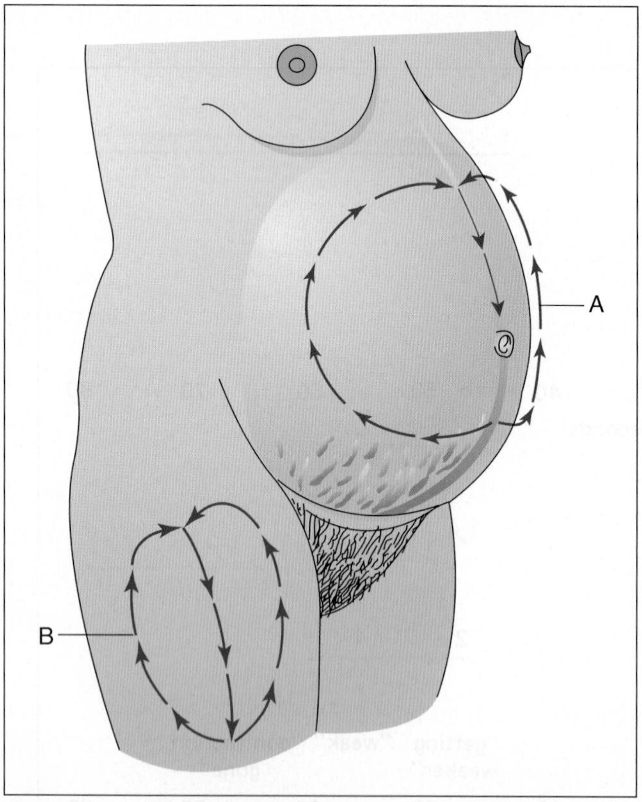

FIGURE 14.7 Effleurage patterns. **(A)** During uterine contractions, a woman traces a pattern on her bare abdomen with her fingers. **(B)** If electronic fetal monitoring is being used, effleurage may be performed on the thigh.

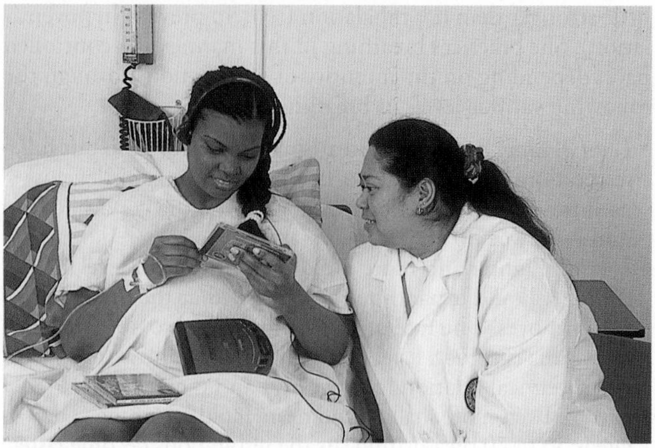

FIGURE 14.8 A woman chooses what object she wishes to focus on during labor. Here, a woman and nurse listen to the music the woman will focus on during contractions. (© Barbara Proud.)

Second-Stage Breathing. During the second stage of labor, when the baby is pushed down the birth canal, the type of breathing that is best to use is controversial. In the past, women were told to hold their breath while they pushed. Now it is believed holding the breath for a prolonged time impairs blood return from the vena cava (a Valsalva maneuver), so this practice is now discouraged. Based on this, suggest women breathe any way that is natural for them, except holding their breath during this stage of labor.

Women should not practice pushing during pregnancy or if in labor before the end of the first stage because the possibility they could rupture membranes by doing this is too great. They can practice assuming a good position for pushing (e.g., squatting, sitting upright, leaning on partner) but should always be cautioned not to actually bear down and push.

QSEN Checkpoint Question 14.4

Informatics

Elena's sister-in-law has referred her to a Web site that outlines the Lamaze method for labor and birth. What is the guiding principle of Lamaze childbirth?

a. Pain can be interrupted before it registers in the brain as pain.
b. Labor contractions are rooted in psychology, not physiology.
c. "Brown pain" like labor contractions, is unlike other forms of pain.
d. Labor contractions can be eliminated by learned mind control techniques.

Look in Appendix A for the best answer and rationale.

Preparation for Cesarean Birth

Some women chose to have a cesarean birth to help prevent uterine prolapse or urinary incontinence in later years (Dursun, Yanik, Zeyneloglu, et al., 2011). To ensure a safe birth, a cesarean birth may become necessary during labor. The specific preparations needed for a cesarean birth as well as a vaginal birth after cesarean (VBAC) is discussed in Chapter 24.

THE BIRTH SETTING

Besides how to best prepare for labor, choosing a birth setting is another important decision that a couple needs to make during pregnancy (Hodnett, Downe, Walsh, et al., 2010). This decision depends on a woman's health and that of her fetus, the couple's preferences, and on how much and what kind of supervision they want for the birth. Although hospitals are the usual site for birth today in the United States, that has not always been true. Up until the late 1800s, childbirth was conducted in the home setting with little pain relief. Analgesia or anesthesia for childbirth first became popular when Queen Victoria birthed Prince Leopold under chloroform in 1853. Although chloroform relieved pain, it also complicated birth because not only were women asleep for one of the most memorable moments of their life but it also caused them to not be able to push effectively during the second stage of labor, thus making it necessary to use a lithotomy position, an episiotomy, and forceps for birth.

Part of the reason for giving so much anesthesia during birth can be attributed to health care providers misinterpreting the moment of birth as the time that produces the greatest degree of discomfort. As a result, women were allowed to labor without pain medication and then were given anesthesia or analgesia right before the baby was born. Although the pain felt at birth is intense, it is also only a hot flash and over quickly, unlike the hours of labor that precede it, making women not as uncomfortable during the actual birth as they are during labor. Birth is also such an exhilarating time that the excitement of the moment and natural perineal anesthesia can mask pain.

Fortunately, based on women's descriptions of the pain of childbirth, birthing practices have changed to better meet women's needs (Gabriel, 2011). Nurses are in a strong position to advocate for making childbirth as "natural" a process as possible and conducted in the least restrictive setting possible. At the same time, nurses have a strong responsibility to encourage parents to respect any restriction that will allow the birth to remain safe.

Choosing a Birth Attendant and Support Person

In the United States, most births are supervised by an obstetrician, a physician specializing in labor and birth; a family practitioner; or a nurse-midwife (Hodnett, Gates, Hofmeyr, et al., 2011). In addition to selecting who will medically supervise her baby's birth, many women choose a doula, or a person specially prepared to assist with birth. Doulas can be especially helpful as support people because having such a person present frees the father to enjoy the birth rather than feel occupied with coaching instructions. Although research in the subject is not extensive, there are suggestions that rates of oxytocin augmentation, epidural anesthesia, and cesarean birth can all be reduced by doula support (Gilliland, 2011). With specific education, many nurses are participating as either a doula or special support nurse to women in labor.

Choosing a Birth Setting

Women who are low risk for complications may choose hospitals, birthing centers, or their homes as settings for birth. Women who might have a complication are advised to give birth at birthing centers or hospitals. Women with high-risk pregnancies are advised to give birth in hospitals where more immediate emergency care is available.

The Hospital Birth

The maternity services of hospitals have changed a great deal in recent years, having been influenced by the Coalition for Improving Maternity Services (CIMS). This organization rates hospitals as to whether they are mother friendly or not based on if a woman has the opportunity for any of the following:

- Experience a healthy and joyous birth experience, regardless of her age or circumstances
- Give birth as she wishes in an environment in which she feels nurtured and secure
- Have access to the full range of options for pregnancy, birth, and nurturing her baby
- Receive accurate and up-to-date information about the benefits and risks of all procedures, drugs, and tests suggested for use during pregnancy, birth, and the postpartum period, with the right to informed consent and informed refusal
- Receive support for making informed choices about what is best for her and her baby based on her individual values and beliefs (CIMS, 2012)

To qualify as a mother-friendly hospital, a hospital should not have routine policies that include practices for such things as perineal shaving, admission enemas, withholding food or fluid during labor, rupturing membranes to hurry labor, or the use of continuous intravenous lines or constant fetal monitoring. It also should have low rates of episiotomies, induction for labor, and cesarean births. In contrast, it should also have a high VBAC rate (60% or more [CIMS, 2012]). Urge women to ask their primary care provider if the hospital they recommend is rated as mother friendly because this should influence both a couple's choice of a hospital and their birth attendant.

The major advantage of a hospital birth is that equipment and expert personnel are readily available if the mother, fetus, or newborn should have a complication. When hospital birth is compared to births at alternative settings as to how many complications occur, women who give birth in hospitals invariably have more complications. Remember, though, that women at high risk for complications choose to give birth at hospitals so, of course, more complication will occur there.

A woman usually comes to the hospital when her contractions are approximately 5 minutes apart and regular in pattern. If she has preregistered at the hospital, she is admitted to a **birthing room** without any separation time from her support person. Birthing rooms are also called labor-birth-recovery rooms (LBRs) or **labor-birth-recovery-postpartum rooms (LBRPs)**. Such rooms are decorated in a homelike way, and couples can bring favorite music or reading materials with them to use during labor (Fig. 14.9).

Women are expected to use a prepared method of childbirth with a minimum of analgesia and anesthesia (although an advantage of a hospital birth is that anesthesia such as an epidural is readily available if needed). The woman's partner or other family members can stay with her throughout labor and birth, allowing a couple and their families to feel they have control over and can share in the birth experience. The bed is used as a labor bed until birth, when it is

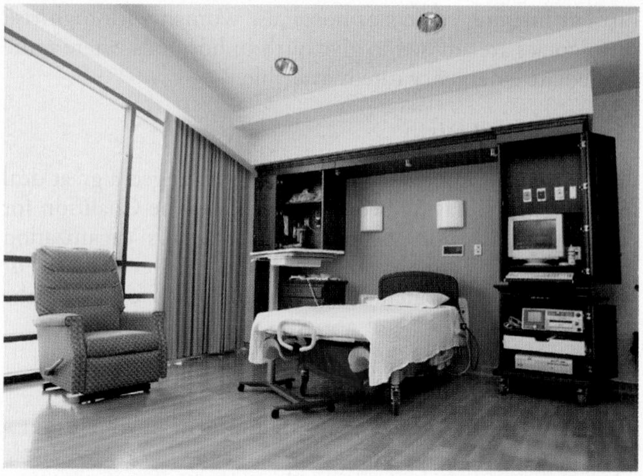

FIGURE 14.9 A birthing (labor-birth-recovery) room designed to maintain a homelike atmosphere in a hospital setting.

then converted into a **birthing bed**. Women can choose a birthing position: squatting, supine with head raised, or side-lying. Woman can choose to use a supine recumbent position (on her back with knees flexed) rather than a lithotomy position (legs elevated into stirrups) because such a position reduces tension on the perineum and is not only more comfortable but also may result in fewer perineal tears than with a lithotomy position.

Following birth, additional cabinets in the room are opened and converted into a space for baby care. A support person can cut the umbilical cord if desired. Women can choose whether to have their male infant circumcised. The mother is encouraged to breastfeed immediately.

Some hospitals screen women in early labor with an external monitor to evaluate both fetal heart rate and uterine contractions. If the fetal heart rate is good, monitors are then removed and a simple Doppler monitor is used if any periodic screening is needed as labor progresses.

A **birthing chair**, a comfortable reclining chair with a slide-away seat that allows a woman to assume a comfortable position during labor and also furnishes perineal exposure so a birth attendant can assist with the birth, could also be used (Fig. 14.10). The chair has the advantage of maintaining a woman in a semi-Fowler's position, a position that acts with gravity and so may speed the second stage of labor.

Postpartum Care

Women giving birth in LBRPs remain in the room with their families for the rest of their hospital stay. Women giving birth in birthing rooms may be transferred to a postpartum unit after birth where they remain for the length of their hospital stay. Both LBRPs and postpartum units serve as "rooming-in" units in which the infant remains in the mother's room either constantly or for most of the day, whichever is her choice. Urge a couple to keep their newborn with them as much as possible so they have ample time to become acquainted and learn their baby's cues for hunger. Mothers can then breastfeed when the infant is hungry, not according to any schedule. There should be no restrictions on visiting for the primary support person; in many institutions, a rollaway bed can be provided so that the partner can remain constantly. Siblings and friends of the newborn should be allowed to visit as much as the mother chooses. Mother and infant remain in the hospital up to 48 hours and are then discharged home.

✔ QSEN Checkpoint Question 14.5

Teamwork & Collaboration

Elena wants to use controlled breathing for early labor and you are reviewing with her doula the actions that Elena will take. What should you review with Elena's doula about controlled breathing early in labor?

a. She should try to breathe exclusively through her nose.
b. She should breathe as rapidly as possible to distract from early contractions.
c. If hypoventilation occurs, she should begin to sip on ice water.
d. She should breathe at a rate of 6 to 12 breaths/min for mild contractions.

Look in Appendix A for the best answer and rationale.

A

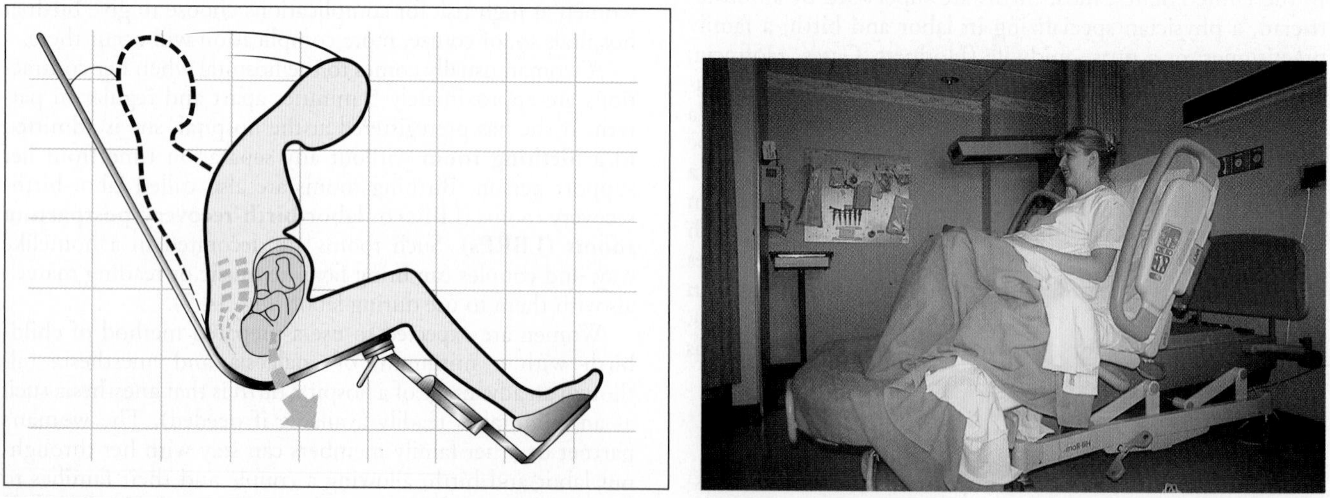

B

FIGURE 14.10 **(A)** A birthing chair allows a woman to maintain a semi-Fowler's position. **(B)** A birthing chair used during labor. (© Caroline Brown, RNC, MS, DEd.)

Alternative Birthing Centers

Alternative birthing centers (ABCs) are wellness-oriented childbirth facilities designed to remove childbirth from the acute care hospital setting while still providing medical resources for emergency care should a complication of labor or birth arise. These settings are established inside, next door, or at least within an easy distance to a hospital. The primary birth attendants tend to be nurse-midwives. Because the facility is located outside an acute care setting, where infections abound, the risk of hospital-acquired infection to a woman is thought to be reduced. Women who deliver in ABCs are screened for potential complications before being rated as eligible for admittance. Because of this, the mortality rate of mothers and infants is no higher and may be lower in these out-of-hospital settings than in hospital settings.

Like hospitals, ABCs have LBRP rooms where a woman and her support person can invite friends and siblings to participate in the birth. In some centers, a central play area for siblings and cooking facilities are also available. ABCs encourage a woman to express her own needs and wishes during the labor process. A minimum of analgesia and anesthesia is provided, and she can choose a birth position. She can bring her own music or distraction objects, and the partner can perform such tasks as cutting the umbilical cord if he or she chooses.

Women remain in an ABC from 4 to 24 hours after birth. Because minimum analgesia or anesthesia is used, a woman recovers quickly after birth and is ready to be discharged early. Box 14.10 shows an interprofessional care map illustrating both nursing and team planning for a birthing center experience.

QSEN Checkpoint Question 14.6

Quality Improvement

Suppose Elena follows her boyfriend's wishes and decides on a hospital birth. What would be an advantage of hospital birth that can be cited to women considering this birth setting?

a. She can give birth in a sterile environment.
b. Both labor and childbirth can generally be pain free.
c. Extended high-risk newborn care is available.
d. Hospital care costs are lower than other settings.

Look in Appendix A for the best answer and rationale.

Home Birth

Home birth is the usual mode of birth in developing countries and is also a popular choice for birth in Europe; however, only about 1% of women in the United States choose this method (MacDorman et al., 2012). Home birth may be supervised by a physician, but nurse-midwives are the more likely choice as a birth attendant in this setting. The Frontier Nursing Service of Kentucky is an example of an organization in the United States that maintains an active and well-accepted program of home birth.

Most women who choose home birth are well educated and from middle-income families. They choose home birth so they are not separated from their family for even a short time, they can have their baby close by after birth to help integrate the child into the family, they can have more control over their childbirth experience, and they can give birth in familiar, low-cost surroundings.

Home birth can have a disadvantage in that it puts responsibility on a woman to prepare her home for the birth and to give full care to the infant after birth. Some women, however willing, may be unable to take on these roles because, passing through their first postpartum or "taking-in" phase, they may feel more comfortable maintaining a dependent-passive role than immediately taking responsibility for the infant's care. They also may feel exhausted from their last weeks of pregnancy or they don't know the best recourse in a crisis situation.

To be a candidate for a home birth, a woman:

- Should be in good overall health
- Must be able to adjust to changing circumstances
- Must have adequate support people to sustain her during labor and to assist her for the first few days after birth

Women with any complication of pregnancy are not good candidates for home birth. Be certain women planning home birth know the following:

- Adequate equipment other than first-line emergency equipment will not be available.
- An abrupt change of goals may be necessary if a complication occurs.
- Both she and her support person may become exhausted because of the responsibility placed on them during labor or the postpartum period.
- She must be prepared to independently monitor her postpartal status.
- Interference with the "taking-in phase" may occur postpartally because she must "take hold" rather than allow herself a rest phase.

Children Attending Birth

Most birthing centers and some hospitals allow children to view the birth of a sibling. It is good advice to suggest that parents and siblings attend a class designed to prepare children to witness a birth beforehand to keep the event from becoming overwhelming. If children will be present, a person separate from the main support person needs to be designated to provide entertainment, explanations, food, and a place for them to nap. This prevents the likelihood that a child who is without supervision during this time will remember the experience as one of rejection rather than an exciting, happy experience. The mother should not be expected to provide such supervision during labor because she will want to concentrate on distraction or breathing techniques (Babycenter Medical Advisory Board [BMAB], 2012).

Help couples to consider whether the birth experience will be a positive and enjoyable one for the family based on the sibling's developmental level and stage. Allowing a child to witness the birth of kittens or puppies might be an alternative way to expose the child to birth.

ALTERNATIVE METHODS OF BIRTH

In addition to varied settings, several methods of childbirth are popular. These include alternative birth methods such as the Leboyer method of birth, birth under water, and unassisted birthing.

expel feces from pushing in the second stage of labor, the water bath may become contaminated. Most women who choose underwater birth, however, enjoy the experience and are pleased that they chose this method (Jones, Othman, Dowswell, et al., 2012).

UNASSISTED BIRTHING

Unassisted birthing, freebirthing, or couples birth refers to women giving birth without health care provider supervision (Dahlen, Jackson, & Stevens, 2011). It differs from home birth because, using this technique, a woman learns pregnancy care from reading books or articles found on the Internet and then arranges to have her child birth at home, perhaps accompanied by her family or friends, but without health care supervision.

Some women choose this method of birth because they believe birth is such a natural process that no medical supervision is necessary. Others choose it because they have no health insurance and so can't afford either a hospital or alternative birth setting (Dahlen et al., 2011). Unassisted birthing is potentially dangerous because, if a complication should occur, the woman may not recognize that what is happening is serious until damage to her child or herself results. Even if she recognizes that a problem is occurring, there is a gap of time before emergency help can arrive to assist her, which puts her at risk for harm. Unassisted birthing is particularly dangerous if a woman avoids prenatal care or depends solely on online information because she may be high risk for a complication but not know it. Educating women that not all online information is reliable and that supervised birth does not mean they have no choice in their care decisions, such as whether they want pain relief or to use a special position for birth, is an effective way to help women make safer choices about birth.

WOMEN WITH UNIQUE NEEDS

There are a number of women who have special needs related to preparations for childbirth.

The Woman With a Disability

Care of women with disabilities during pregnancy is discussed in Chapter 22. Women with these special circumstances may need additional help to prepare for labor and birth based on their unique concern. It may not be realistic, for example, for a woman who has chronic back pain to practice pelvic rocking; a woman with poor balance may not be able to practice squatting safely. A woman who is immobile or in a wheelchair may have difficulty attending a preparation class if the classroom is not located in a handicapped-accessible building. Women with vision or hearing disabilities can have difficulty following classroom content. A highly stressed woman may not have the patience to concentrate on learning controlled breathing.

Encourage women with special needs to think through any circumstance that will require special adaptation and be certain they include this requirement in their birth plan.

The Woman With Cultural Concerns

Because the United States has such a diverse mixture of cultures, a preparation for labor and birth class can include women from a diverse mix of cultures. Urging women to share cultural traditions enriches discussions at such classes. Be certain to encourage women who are worried that their cultural preferences will not be respected when they are in labor to discuss their concerns with their primary care provider at their next visit. A woman who believes in circumcision as a religious necessity, for example, does not want to listen to a discussion on the pros and cons of circumcision. A woman who wants to be fully clothed during labor may need to plan on bringing her own nonrevealing gown to a birthing center, and she may not want to be offered showering or tub bathing as pain management because these will not respect modesty. Be certain women include these special needs in their written birth plan so they are not overlooked by busy labor service personnel.

The Woman Who Is Morbidly Obese

Women with a body mass index over 30 may have difficulty practicing exercises such as squatting or tailor sitting because not only do these positions require balance but they also may tire easily. Overweight women should, however, have no difficulty preparing for labor by practicing controlled breathing or doing abdominal and perineal strengthening by doing exercises such as Kegel or abdominal contractions. Urge women to think through what pain management measures they think may cause a problem for them in labor such as leaning forward against a birthing bar or a birthing ball or bathing in warm water (the bar or ball or a plastic tub might not support their weight). For modesty, they may also need to bring their own gown to their birthing center. Encourage women to add what will be important for them to do or not to do on their birthing plan so they remain active participants in the experience.

What if... 14.4 You are particularly interested in exploring one of the 2020 National Health Goals with respect to preparation for labor (see Box 14.1). What would be a possible research topic to explore pertinent to this goal that would be applicable to Joe and Elena and that would also advance evidence-based practice?

KEY POINTS FOR REVIEW

- Couples should be encouraged to make a flexible childbirth plan early in pregnancy, which includes a birth attendant, setting, desired method of pain management, and any special wishes.
- Common exercises taught in pregnancy to strengthen perineal muscles are tailor sitting, squatting, and Kegel exercises. Abdominal muscle contraction and pelvic rocking exercises both strengthen the abdominal muscles and help relieve backache.
- Types of childbirth preparations include the Bradley (partner coached), Kitzinger (psychosexual), Dick-Read, and Lamaze methods. Lamaze is the most common method used in the United States.

- Commonly used nonpharmacologic techniques for pain relief in labor are conscious relaxation, consciously controlled breathing, effleurage, focusing, imagery, and hydrotherapy.
- Classes for expectant parents provide information on pregnancy, birth, and child care.
- Common sites for childbirth include hospitals, ABCs, and home settings.
- Couples should determine if their preferred birth setting is rated as mother friendly before choosing a birth site.
- Considering childbirth as one of the biggest events in a woman's life should help in planning nursing care that not only meets QSEN competencies but also best meets the family's total needs.

Critical Thinking Care Study

Brooke is a 28-year-old woman having her first baby. She has worked as a nurse on a labor and delivery service for the past 3 years. She didn't take a preparation for childbirth class because she felt no material would be presented she didn't already know. She doesn't feel she needs a doula because she has had so much experience with women in labor. Her husband will be with her during labor.

1. Brooke's husband asks you at a prenatal visit if he should time contractions in labor with his watch or by the wall clock. Also, he asks if it will be all right if Brooke drinks coffee during labor. Why do you think he's asking so many basic questions?
2. Brooke's mother tells you she knows she can't be with Brooke in labor but she wants special permission to hold her new grandson before he's taken away to a nursery. She also wants to make it clear she needs to do that before her ex-husband or his "fluffy" girlfriend have a chance to hold the baby. Does Brooke's mother understand the options available to her in a mother-friendly hospital?
3. Brooke doesn't seem to have shared much information about labor with her family. Can you assume this is because she's so independent she wants to manage her labor by herself, or would you worry she doesn't have a strong support system?

Patient Scenario

The Jackson Family

Read about the Jackson family, a family making plans for childbirth, then answer the questions to further sharpen your skills and grow more familiar with NCLEX-type questions related to preparing a family for childbirth and parenting. Confirm your answers are correct by reading the rationales.

Visit http://thePoint.lww.com

Answers and Rationales

Looking for answers to the What If. . . and Critical Thinking Care Study questions?

Visit http://thePoint.lww.com

References

Alder, J., Breitinger, G., Granado, C., et al. (2011). Antenatal psychobiological predictors of psychological response to childbirth. *Journal of the American Psychiatric Nurses Association, 17*(6), 417–425.

Allahdin, S., & Kambhampati, L. (2012). Stress urinary incontinence in continent primigravidas. *Journal of Obstetrics & Gynaecology, 32*(1), 2–5.

Al-Sahab, B., Saqib, M., Hauser, G., et al. (2010). Prevalence of smoking during pregnancy and associated risk factors among Canadian women: A national survey. *BMC Pregnancy & Childbirth, 10*(5), 24–25.

Amis, D. (2010). *Prepared childbirth: The family way.* New York, NY: Lamaze International.

Babycenter Medical Advisory Board. (2012). *Preparing your child to attend a sibling's birth.* Retrieved from http://www.babycenter.com/0_preparing-your-child-to-attend-a-siblings-birth_176.bc

Bradley, R., Hathaway, M., Hathaway, J., et al. (2008). *Husband-coached childbirth* (5th ed.). New York, NY: Bantam Books.

Coalition for Improving Maternity Services. (2012). *The mother-friendly childbirth initiative.* Retrieved from http://www.mother-friendly.org/MFCI

Cluett, E. R., & Burns, E., (2012). Immersion in water in pregnancy, labour and birth. *Cochrane Database of Systematic Reviews,* (7), CD000111.

Dahlen, H. G., Jackson, M., & Stevens, J. (2011). Homebirth, freebirth and doulas: Casualty and consequences of a broken maternity system. *Women & Birth, 24*(1), 47–50.

Dick-Read, G., & Gaskin, I. M. (2013). *Childbirth without fear: The principles & practice of natural childbirth.* London, UK: Pinter & Martin, LTD.

Dursun, P., Yanik, F. B., Zeyneloglu, H. B., et al. (2011). Why women request cesarean section without medical indication? *Journal of Maternal-Fetal & Neonatal Medicine, 24*(9), 1133–1137.

Gabriel, C. (2011). *Natural hospital birth: The best of both worlds.* Boston, MA: Harvard Common Press.

Gilliland, A. L. (2011). After praise and encouragement: Emotional support strategies used by birth doulas in the USA and Canada. *Midwifery, 27*(4), 525–531.

Hay-Smith, J. C., Herderschee, R., Dumoulin, C., et al. (2011). Comparisons of approaches to pelvic floor muscle training for urinary incontinence in women. *Cochrane Database of Systematic Reviews,* (12), CD009508.

Hodnett, E. D., Downe, S., Walsh, D., et al. (2010). Alternative versus conventional institutional settings for birth. *Cochrane Database of Systematic Reviews,* (7), CD000012.

Hodnett, E. D., Gates, S., Hofmeyr, G. J., et al. (2011). Continuous support for women during childbirth. *Cochrane Database of Systematic Reviews,* (2), CD003766.

Horey, D., Weaver, J., & Russell, H. (2011). Information for pregnant women about caesarean birth. *Cochrane Database of Systematic Reviews,* (3), CD003858

Johnson, T. S., & Strube, K. (2011). Breast care during pregnancy. *Journal of Obstetric, Gynecologic & Neonatal Nursing, 40*(2), 144–148.

Jones, L., Othman, M., Dowswell, T., et al. (2012). Pain management for women in labour: An overview of systematic reviews. *Cochrane Database of Systematic Reviews,* (3), CD009234.

Kemp, E., Kingswood, C. J., Kibuka, M., et al. (2013). Position in the second stage of labour for women with epidural anaesthesia. *Cochrane Database of Systematic Reviews, 2013*(1):CD008070.

Kiely, J. L., & Kogan, M. D. (2012). *Reproductive health of women: Prenatal care.* Atlanta, GA: Centers for Disease Control and Prevention.

Kitzinger, S. (2011). *The new pregnancy & childbirth.* London, England: Penguin/Dorling Kindersley.

Kuo, S. C., Lin, K. C., Hsu, C. H., et al. (2010). Evaluation of the effects of a birth plan on Taiwanese women's childbirth experiences, control and expectations fulfillment: A randomised controlled trial. *International Journal of Nursing Students, 47*(7), 806–814.

Leboyer, F. (2009). *Birth without violence.* Rochester, VT: Healing Arts Press.

Lothian, J. A. (2011). Lamaze breathing: What every pregnant woman needs to know. *Journal of Perinatal Education, 20*(2), 118–120.

MacDorman, M. F., Mathews, T. J., & Declercq, E. (2012). Home births in the United States, 1990–2009. *NCHS Data Brief,* (84), 1–8.

Marc, I., Toureche, N., Ernst, E., et al. (2011). Mind-body interventions during pregnancy for preventing or treating women's anxiety. *Cochrane Database of Systematic Reviews,* (7), CD007559.

Monica, K. C., & du Plessis, R. A. (2011). Discussion of the health benefits of breastfeeding within small groups. *Community Practice, 84*(1), 31–34.

Priddis, H., Dahlen, H., & Schmied, V. (2011). What are the facilitators, inhibitors, and implications of birth positioning? *Women & Birth, 25*(3), 100–106.

Records, K., & Wilson, B. L. (2011). Reflections on meeting women's childbirth expectations. *Journal of Obstetric, Gynecologic & Neonatal Nursing, 40*(4), 394–398.

Saravelos, S. H., & Regan, L. (2011). The importance of preconception counseling and early pregnancy monitoring. *Seminars in Reproductive Medicine, 29*(6), 557–568.

Simkin, P., Bolding, A., Keppler, A., et al. (2010). Movement and positions for labor. In P. Simkin, A. Bolding, A. Keppler, et al. (Eds.), *Pregnancy, childbirth & the newborn: The complete guide* (4th ed., pp. 220–222). Minnetonka, MN: Meadowbrook Press.

Smith, C. A., Levett, K. M., Collins, C. T., et al. (2011). Relaxation techniques for pain management in labour. *Cochrane Database of Systematic Reviews,* (12), CD009514.

Szymanski, L. M., & Satin, A. J. (2012). Exercise during pregnancy: Fetal responses to current public health guidelines. *Obstetrics & Gynecology, 119*(3), 603–610.

U.S. Department of Health and Human Services. (2010). *Healthy people 2020.* Washington, DC: Author.

Chapter 15

Nursing Care of a Family During Labor and Birth

KEY TERMS

- attitude
- breech presentation
- cardinal movements of labor
- cephalic presentation
- crowning
- dilatation
- doula
- effacement
- engagement
- fetal descent
- fetal position
- Leopold maneuvers
- lie
- molding
- ripening
- station
- transition

OBJECTIVES

After mastering the contents of this chapter, you should be able to:

1. Describe common theories explaining the onset of labor and the role of passenger, passage, powers, and psyche in labor.
2. Identify 2020 National Health Goals related to safe labor and birth that nurses can help the nation achieve.
3. Assess a family in labor and birth and identify the woman's readiness, stage, and progression.
4. Formulate nursing diagnoses related to the physiologic and psychological aspects of labor and birth.
5. Develop expected outcomes to meet the needs of a family throughout the labor process as well as manage seamless transitions across differing health care settings.
6. Using the nursing process, plan nursing care that includes the six competencies of Quality & Safety Education for Nurses (QSEN): Patient-Centered Care, Teamwork & Collaboration, Evidence-Based Practice (EBP), Quality Improvement (QI), Safety, and Informatics.
7. Implement nursing care for a family during labor such as teaching about the stages of labor.
8. Evaluate expected outcomes for achievement and effectiveness of care.
9. Integrate knowledge of labor and birth with the interplay of nursing process, the six competencies of QSEN, and Family Nursing to promote quality maternal and child health nursing care.

Celeste Bailey is a 26-year-old woman having her first baby whom you admit to a birthing room. She has been having labor contractions for 6 hours; her contractions are now 45 seconds long and 3 minutes apart. She tells you she wants to have her baby "naturally" without any analgesia or anesthesia. Her husband, a long distance truck driver, is on his way home but has not arrived yet. Her teenage sister who is with her states she has no idea how to coach her, except to pray. As you finish assessing contractions, Celeste grips her abdomen, screams, and shouts, "I'm breathing just like I'm supposed to do! Why does this hurt so bad?"

Previous chapters discussed the anatomic and physiologic changes that occur in pregnancy as well as effective steps women can take to prepare for labor. This chapter adds information about the process of labor and how to offer effective support and education to a woman in labor. Without this type of support, labor can be a frightening rather than an enjoyable event.

What additional teaching and support does Celeste need so her labor and birth are memorable experiences for her?

Labor is the series of events by which uterine contractions and abdominal pressure expel a fetus and placenta from the uterus. Regular contractions cause progressive dilatation of the cervix and create sufficient muscular uterine force to allow a baby to be pushed out into the extrauterine world. Labor represents a time of change as it is both an ending and a beginning for the woman, her fetus, and her family (Archie & Roman, 2013).

Labor and birth are unique events, requiring a woman to employ all the psychological and physical coping methods she has available. Regardless of the amount of childbirth preparation or the number of times a woman has been through the birth experience, family-centered nursing care is the approach that best supports the woman as she focuses on the beginning of her new family. This goal for nursing is further emphasized by 2020 National Health Goals (Box 15.1).

BOX 15.1 Nursing Care Planning Based on 2020 National Health Goals

Because labor and birth are potentially high-risk times for both a fetus and a mother, a number of 2020 National Health Goals speak directly to these:

- Reduce the rate of maternal deaths to no more than 11.4 out of 100,000 live births, from a baseline of 12.7 out of 100,000 live births.
- Reduce maternal illness due to pregnancy complications developed during hospitalized labor and delivery from a baseline of 31.1% to a target level of 28.0%.
- Reduce cesarean births among low-risk (full-term, singleton, vertex presentation) women from a baseline of 26.5% to a target of 23.9%.
- Reduce the rate of fetal deaths at 20 or more weeks gestation to no more than 5.6 out of 1,000 live births, from a baseline of 6.2 out of 1,000.
- Reduce the rate of fetal and infant deaths during the perinatal period (28 weeks gestation to 7 days after birth) to no more than 5.9 out of 1,000 live births, from a baseline of 6.6 out of 1,000 live births (U.S. Department of Health and Human Services [DHHS], 2010; see www.healthypeople.gov).

Nurses can help the nation achieve these goals by closely monitoring women during labor and birth and by teaching women as much as possible about labor so they are able to use as little analgesia and anesthesia as possible. The less anesthesia and analgesia used, the fewer complications that occur, resulting in reduced fetal or maternal death.

Nursing Process Overview

For the Woman in Labor

Assessment

A woman in labor is keenly aware of both nonverbal and verbal expressions around her (i.e., not only words spoken but gestures such as eye rolling or sighing). Because of this sensitivity, an assessment must be done quickly yet thoroughly and gently because she may have difficulty being patient, for example, while admission information is obtained or relaxing for a vaginal examination.

Remember that pain is a subjective symptom. Only the woman can evaluate how much she is experiencing or how much she wants to endure. Assess how much discomfort she is experiencing and how she feels about her labor not only by what she scores on a pain scale but also by subtle signs of pain such as facial tenseness, flushing or paleness of the face, hands clenched in a fist, rapid breathing, or rapid pulse rate. Appreciate that the fetus as well as the mother is under stress from the process of labor, so both need vital sign assessments.

Nursing Diagnosis

Nursing diagnoses in labor generally relate to a woman's reaction to labor. Common nursing diagnoses include:

- Pain related to labor contractions
- Anxiety related to process of labor and birth
- Health-seeking behaviors related to management of discomfort of labor
- Situational low self-esteem related to inability to use planned childbirth method

Although the discomfort of labor contractions is commonly referred to as "contractions" rather than "pain," do not omit the word "pain" from a nursing diagnosis because the term strengthens an understanding of the problem as well as alerts a woman she should feel free to ask for something for pain at the point she feels she needs additional help.

Outcome Identification and Planning

When establishing expected outcomes for a woman in labor and her partner, be certain they are realistic and that they can be met. Although labor usually takes place over a relatively short time frame (average, 12 hours), it is important not to project a definite time limit for labor to be completed because the length of labor can vary greatly from woman to woman and still be within normal limits. It is necessary also to appreciate the magnitude of labor. It is unlikely all the fear or anxiety experienced during a woman's labor can be completely alleviated. Often, because it is such an unusual and significant experience, the average couple may need guidance in order to be able to employ additional coping measures.

Be certain to incorporate a support person as well as the woman in planning so the experience is a shared one. Although a couple may have learned about the stages of labor and what to expect at each stage during pregnancy, the reality of labor may seem very different from what they imagined. Be certain also that planning is flexible and individualized, allowing the woman to experience the full significance of the event. Helpful Web sites to recommend to women to learn more about birth are the Baby Center (www.Babycenter.com) and the Natural Birth Center & Women's Wellness (www.naturalbirthcenter.com).

Implementation

As much as possible, interventions during labor should always be carried out between contractions so the woman can use a prepared childbirth technique to limit the discomfort of contractions. This calls for good coordination of care among health care providers and the woman and her support person. The person a woman chooses to stay with her during childbirth is often culturally determined and varies from being a husband, a significant other or partner, the father of the child, a sister, a parent, or a close friend.

Outcome Evaluation

An evaluation during labor should be ongoing to preserve the safety of the woman and her newborn. After birth, an evaluation helps to determine the woman's opinion of her experience with labor and birth. Ideally, the experience should not only be one she was able to endure but also one that allowed her self-esteem to grow and the family bond to intensify through a shared experience. It is advantageous to talk to women following birth about their labor experience because doing so serves as a means of evaluating nursing care during labor. It also provides a woman the chance to "work through" the experience and incorporate it into her self-image. Possible outcome criteria include:

- Client states pain during labor was tolerable because of her advance preparation.
- Client verbalizes that her need for nonpharmacologic comfort measures was met.
- Client and family members state the labor and birth experience was a positive growth experience for them, both individually and as a family.

THEORIES OF WHY LABOR BEGINS

Labor normally begins between 37 and 42 weeks of pregnancy, when a fetus is sufficiently mature to adapt to extrauterine life, yet not too large to cause mechanical difficulty with birth. In some instances, labor begins before a fetus is mature (preterm birth). In others, labor is delayed until the fetus and the placenta have both passed beyond the optimal point for birth (postterm birth).

Although in animals it has been shown that progesterone withdrawal is the trigger that stimulates labor, the association that converts the random, painless Braxton Hicks contractions of pregnancy into strong, coordinated, productive labor contractions in women is still largely undocumented (Bernal & Norwitz, 2012).

A number of theories, including a combination of factors originating from both the woman and fetus, have been proposed to explain why progesterone withdrawal begins. Some of the theories include:

- The uterine muscle stretches from the increasing size of the fetus, which results in release of prostaglandins.
- The fetus presses on the cervix, which stimulates the release of oxytocin from the posterior pituitary.
- Oxytocin stimulation works together with prostaglandins to initiate contractions.
- Changes in the ratio of estrogen to progesterone occurs, increasing estrogen in relation to progesterone, which is interpreted as progesterone withdrawal.
- The placenta reaches a set age, which triggers contractions.
- Rising fetal cortisol levels reduce progesterone formation and increase prostaglandin formation.
- The fetal membrane begins to produce prostaglandins, which stimulate contractions (Impey & Child, 2012).

The role of prostaglandins answers the often asked question: Does coitus help induce labor? Semen does contain prostaglandins, which can be helpful in softening, also known as "**ripening**" of the cervix; if a cervix is ready to ripen, semen prostaglandins could possibly stimulate the beginning of contractions. Rhythmical contractions brought on by a woman's orgasm can conceivably help as well, although, again, not until a uterus is prepared and ready for labor.

THE COMPONENTS OF LABOR

A successful labor depends on four integrated concepts, often referred to as the four P's:

1. The *passage* (a woman's pelvis) is of adequate size and contour.
2. The *passenger* (the fetus) is of appropriate size and in an advantageous position and presentation.
3. The *powers* of labor (uterine factors) are adequate.
4. A woman's *psychological outlook* is preserved, so afterward, labor can be viewed as a positive experience.

The Passage

The passage refers to the route a fetus must travel from the uterus through the cervix and vagina to the external perineum. Because the cervix and vagina are contained inside the boney pelvis, the fetus must also pass through the bony pelvic ring. (Pelvic anatomy is illustrated in Chapter 11; see Figs. 11.9 and 11.11). The two pelvic measurements that are important to determine the adequacy of the pelvis are the *diagonal conjugate* (the anteroposterior diameter of the inlet) and the *transverse diameter* of the outlet. At the pelvic inlet, the anteroposterior diameter is the narrowest diameter; at the outlet, the transverse diameter is the narrowest (Fig. 15.1).

In most instances, if a disproportion between fetus and pelvis occurs, the pelvis is the structure at fault. If the fetus is the cause of the disproportion, it is often not because the fetal head is too large, but because it is presenting to the birth canal at less than its narrowest diameter. Keep this in mind when discussing with parents why an infant may not be able to be born vaginally. It can be upsetting for parents to learn that a child cannot be born vaginally because the mother's pelvis is too small. It can be much more upsetting to think their infant's head is too large because it implies something may be seriously wrong with their baby (and that is rarely true). Avoiding this type of negative thought helps promote good parent–child bonding.

The Passenger

The passenger is the fetus. The body part of the fetus that has the widest diameter is the head, so this is the part least likely to be able to pass through the pelvic ring. Whether a fetal skull can pass depends on both its structure (bones, fontanelles, and suture lines) and its alignment with the pelvis.

Structure of the Fetal Skull

The cranium, the uppermost portion of the skull, is composed of eight bones. The four superior bones—the frontal (actually two fused bones), the two parietal, and the occipital—are the bones important in childbirth. The other four bones of the skull (sphenoid, ethmoid, and two temporal bones) lie at the base of the cranium and so are of little significance in

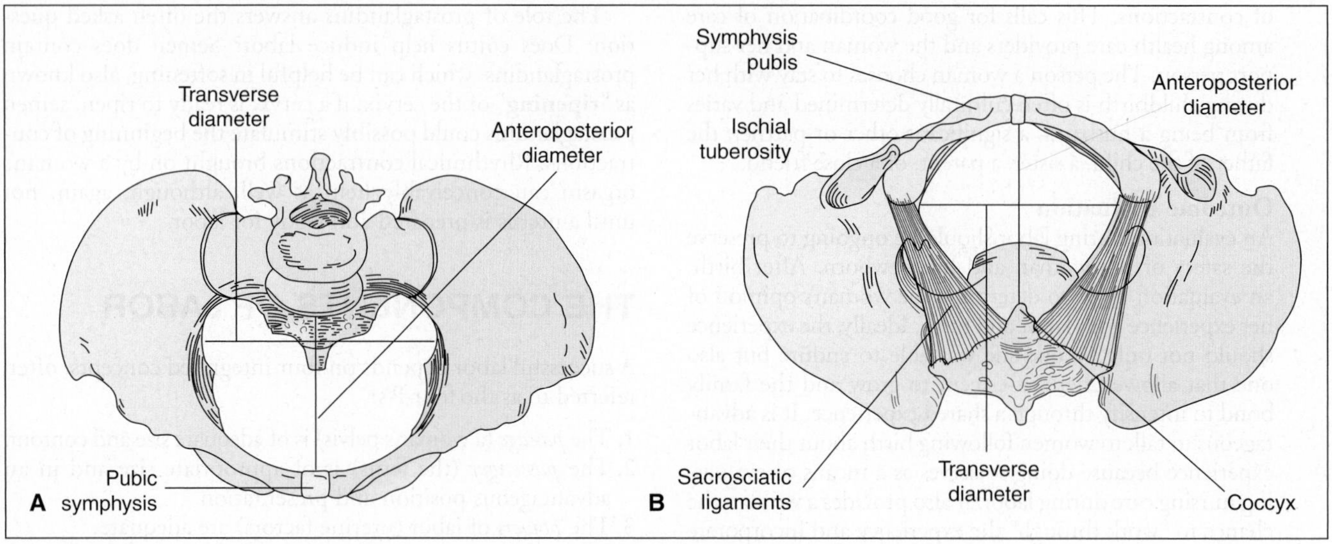

FIGURE 15.1 Views of the pelvic inlet and outlet: **(A)** the pelvic inlet, **(B)** the pelvic outlet.

childbirth because they are never presenting parts. The chin, referred to by its Latin name *mentum*, can be a presenting part.

The bones of the skull join together at suture lines. The sagittal suture joins the two parietal bones at the top of the skull. The coronal suture is the line of juncture between the frontal bones and the two parietal bones. The lambdoid suture is the line of juncture between the occipital bone and the two parietal bones. The suture lines are important in birth because, as membranous interspaces, they allow the cranial bones to move and overlap, causing cranial molding or a diminishing size of the skull so it is able to pass through the birth canal more readily.

Significant membrane-covered spaces called the fontanelles are found at the junction of the main suture lines. The anterior fontanelle (sometimes referred to as the bregma) lies at the frontal junction of the coronal and sagittal sutures. Because the frontal bone consists of two fused bones, four bones (counting the two parietal bones) are actually involved at this junction so the anterior fontanelle has four sides, or is diamond-shaped. Its anteroposterior diameter measures approximately 3 to 4 cm; its transverse diameter, 2 to 3 cm. It closes and can no longer be felt when the infant reaches 12 to 18 months of age.

The posterior fontanelle lies at the rear of the skull at the junction of the lambdoidal and sagittal sutures. Because three bones—the two parietal bones and the occipital bone—are involved at this junction, the posterior fontanelle is triangular shaped. It is smaller than the anterior fontanelle, measuring only 2 cm across its widest part. Because of its small size, it closes when an infant is about 2 months of age.

The space between the two fontanelles is referred to as the vertex. The area over the frontal bone is referred to as the sinciput. The area over the occipital bone is referred to as the occiput (Fig. 15.2).

Fontanelle spaces compress during birth to aid in molding of the fetal head. Their presence can be assessed manually through the cervix after the cervix has dilated during labor. Palpating for fontanelle spaces during a pelvic examination helps to establish the position of the fetal head and whether it is in a favorable position for birth.

Diameters of the Fetal Skull

The shape of a fetal skull causes it to be wider in its anteroposterior diameter than in its transverse diameter. To fit through the inlet of the birth canal best, a fetus must present the smaller diameter (the transverse diameter) of the head to the smaller diameter of the maternal pelvis (the diagonal conjugate); otherwise, progress can be halted and vaginal birth may not be possible. The diameters of the fetal skull vary depending on where the measurement is taken (Fig. 15.2A).

- The smallest diameter of the fetal skull is the biparetal diameter or the transverse diameter, which measures about 9.25 cm.
- The smallest anteroposterior diameter is the suboccipitobregmatic measurement (approximately 9.5 cm) and is measured from the inferior aspect of the occiput to the center of the anterior fontanelle.
- The occipitofrontal diameter, measured from the occipital prominence to the bridge of the nose, is approximately 12 cm.
- The occipitomental diameter, which is the widest anteroposterior diameter (approximately 13.5 cm), is measured from the posterior fontanelle to the chin.

The anteroposterior diameter of the pelvis, a space approximately 11 cm wide, is the narrowest diameter at the pelvic inlet, and so the best presentation for birth is when the fetus presents a biparietal diameter (the narrowest fetal head diameter) to this (see Fig. 15.2B). At the outlet, the fetus must rotate to present this narrowest fetal head diameter (the biparietal diameter) to the maternal transverse diameter, a space, again, approximately 11 cm wide.

- If a fetus presents one of the anteroposterior diameters of the skull to the anteroposterior diameter of the inlet, **engagement**, or the settling of the fetal head into the pelvis, may not occur.
- If the fetus does not rotate, leaving the anteroposterior diameter of the skull presenting to the transverse diameter of the outlet, an arrest of progress may occur.

Which anteroposterior diameter that presents to the birth canal is determined not only by rotation but also by the degree of flexion of the fetal head (Fig. 15.3).

- In full flexion, the fetal head flexes so sharply that the chin rests on the chest, and the smallest anteroposterior diameter, the suboccipitobregmatic, presents to the birth canal.

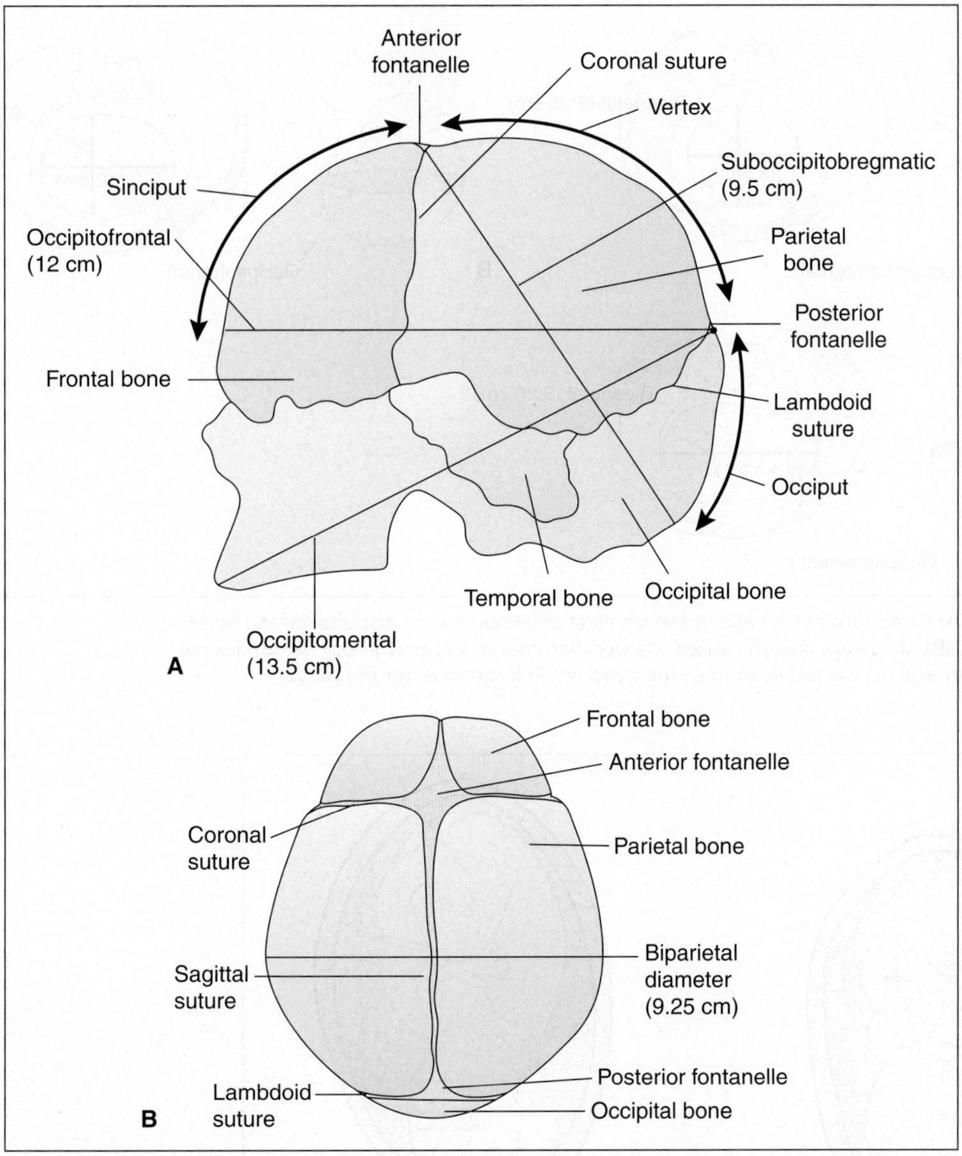

FIGURE 15.2 The fetal skull: **(A)** the lateral view, **(B)** the vertex view.

- If the head is held in moderate flexion, the occipitofrontal diameter presents.
- In poor flexion (the head is hyperextended), the largest diameter (the occipitomental) will present.

It follows that full head flexion is an important aspect of labor because a fetal head presenting a diameter of 9.5 cm will fit through a pelvis much more readily than if the diameter is 12.0 or 13.5 cm.

Molding

Molding is overlapping of skull bones along the suture lines, which causes a change in the shape of the fetal skull to one long and narrow, a shape that facilitates passage through the rigid pelvis. Molding is caused by the force of uterine contractions as the vertex of the head is pressed against the not yet dilated cervix. The overlapping that occurs in the sagittal suture line and, generally, the coronal suture line can be easily palpated on the newborn skull. Parents can be reassured that molding only lasts a day or two and will not be a permanent condition. There is little molding when the brow is the presenting part (described later), because frontal bones are fused. No skull molding occurs when a fetus is breech, because the buttocks, not the head, present first. Babies born by cesarean birth when there is no preprocedure labor also typically have no molding.

Fetal Presentation and Position

Other factors that play a part in whether a fetus is properly aligned in the pelvis and is in the best position to be born are fetal attitude, fetal lie, fetal presentation, and fetal position.

Fetal Attitude. **Attitude** describes the degree of flexion a fetus assumes during labor or the relation of the fetal parts to each other (Fig. 15.4).

- A fetus in *good* attitude is in complete flexion: the spinal column is bowed forward, the head is flexed forward so much that the chin touches the sternum, the arms are flexed and folded on the chest, the thighs are flexed onto the abdomen, and the calves are pressed against the posterior aspect of the thighs (see Fig. 15.4A). This usual

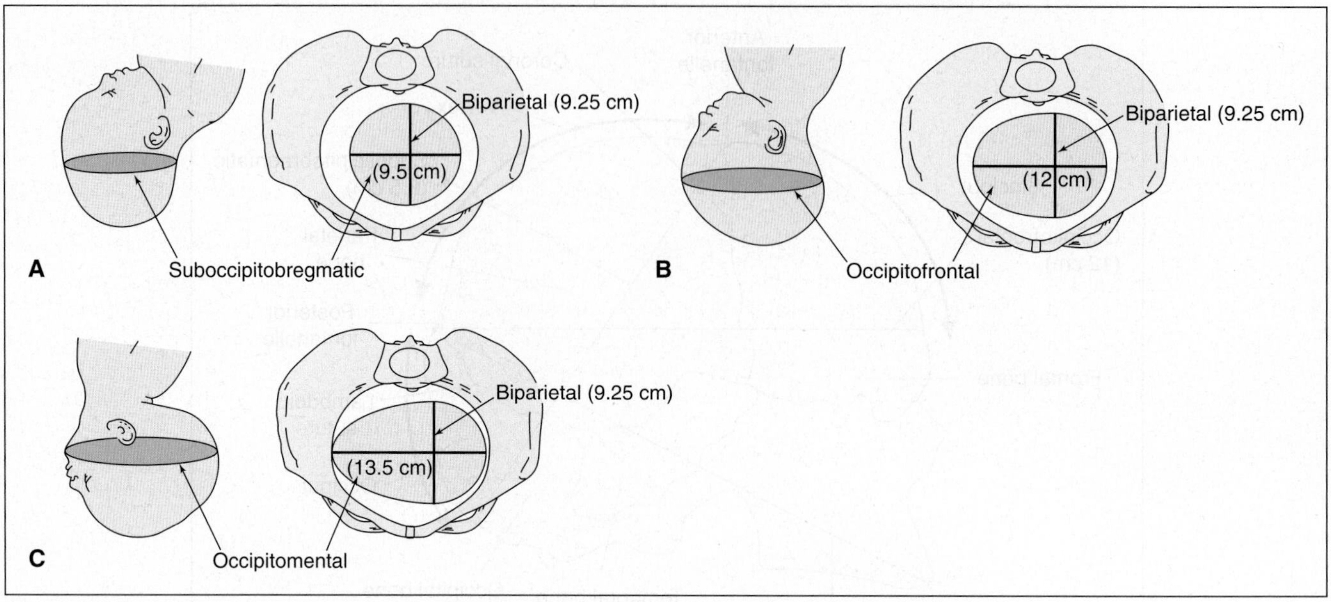

FIGURE 15.3 **(A)** Complete flexion allows the smallest anteroposterior diameter of the head to enter the pelvis. **(B)** Moderate flexion causes a larger diameter to enter. **(C)** Poor flexion forces the largest diameter against the pelvic brim so the head is too large to enter the pelvis.

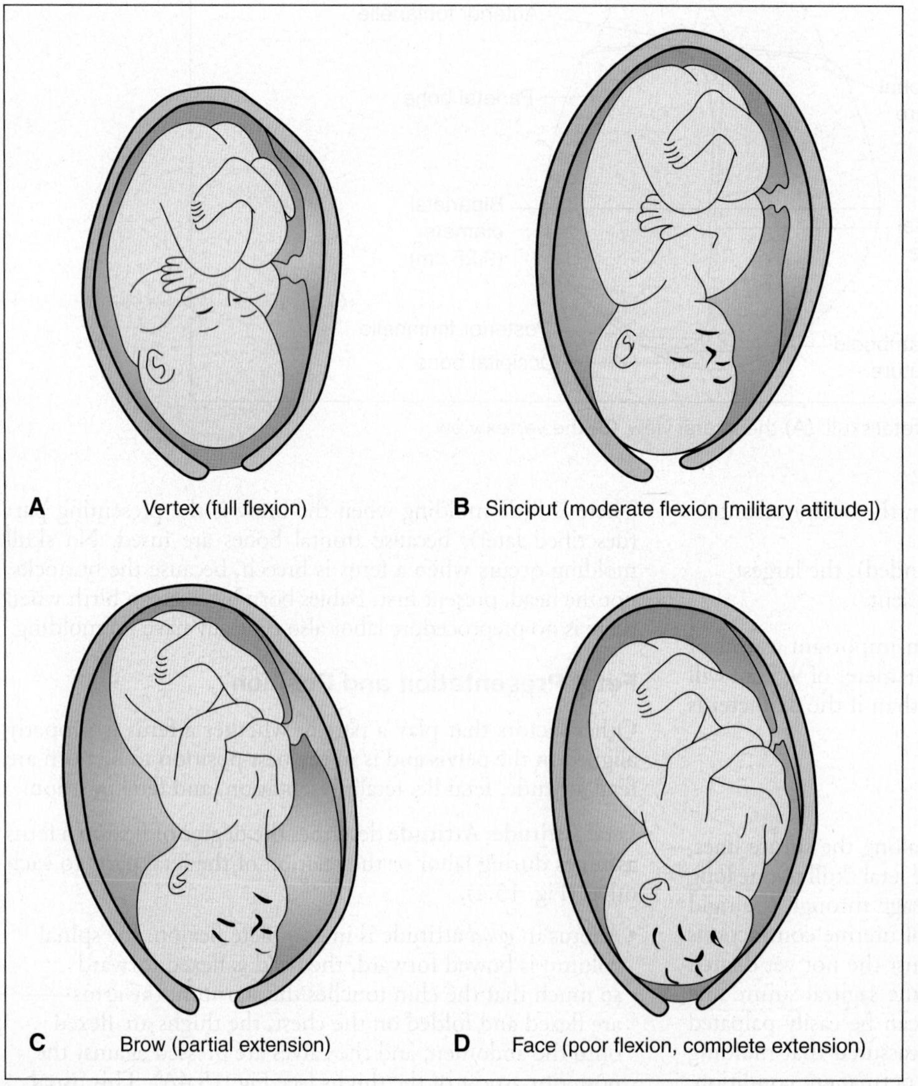

FIGURE 15.4 Fetal attitude. **(A)** The fetus in full flexion presents the smallest anteroposterior diameter (suboccipitobregmatic) of the skull to the inlet in this good attitude (vertex presentation). **(B)** The fetus is not as well flexed (military attitude) and presents the occipitofrontal diameter to the inlet (sinciput presentation). **(C)** The fetus in partial extension (brow presentation). **(D)** The fetus in complete extension presents a wide (occipitomental) diameter (face presentation).

TABLE 15.1 Types of Cephalic Presentations

Type	Lie	Attitude	Description
Vertex	Longitudinal	Good (full flexion)	The head is sharply flexed, making the parietal bones or the space between the fontanelles (the vertex) the presenting part. This is the most common presentation and allows the suboccipitobregmatic diameter to present to the cervix.
Brow	Longitudinal	Moderate (military)	Because the head is only moderately flexed, the brow or sinciput becomes the presenting part.
Face	Longitudinal	Poor	The fetus has extended the head to make the face the presenting part. From this position, extreme edema and distortion of the face may occur.
Mentum	Longitudinal	Very poor	The fetus has completely hyperextended the head to present the chin, causing the presenting diameter (the occipitomental) to be so wide that vaginal birth may not be possible.

"fetal position" is advantageous for birth because it helps a fetus present the smallest anteroposterior diameter of the skull to the pelvis and also because it puts the whole body into an ovoid shape, occupying the smallest space possible.

- A fetus is in *moderate* flexion if the chin is not touching the chest but is in an alert or "military position" (see Fig. 15.4B). This position causes the next widest anteroposterior diameter, the occipitofrontal diameter, to present to the birth canal. A fair number of fetuses assume a military position early in labor. This does not usually interfere with labor, however, because later mechanisms of labor (descent and flexion) force the fetal head to fully flex.
- A fetus in partial extension presents the "brow" of the head to the birth canal (see Fig. 15.4C).
- If a fetus is in complete extension, the back is arched and the neck is extended, presenting the occipitomental diameter of the head to the birth canal (a face presentation; see Fig. 15.4D). This unusual position usually presents too wide a skull diameter to the birth canal for vaginal birth. Such a position may occur in an otherwise healthy fetus or may be an indication there is less than the usual amount of amniotic fluid present (oligohydramnios), which is not allowing the fetus adequate movement space. It also may reflect a neurologic abnormality in the fetus causing spasticity.

Fetal Lie. **Lie** is the relationship between the long (cephalocaudal) axis of the fetal body and the long (cephalocaudal) axis of a woman's body—in other words, whether the fetus is lying in a horizontal (transverse) or a vertical (longitudinal) position. Approximately 99% of fetuses assume a longitudinal lie (with their long axis parallel to the long axis of the woman) (Coad & Dunstall, 2011).

Longitudinal lies are further classified as cephalic, which means the fetal head will be the first part to contact the cervix, or breech, with a foot or the buttocks as the first portion to contact the cervix.

Fetal Presentation

Fetal presentation denotes the body part that will first contact the cervix or be born first and is determined by the combination of fetal lie and the degree of fetal flexion (attitude).

Cephalic Presentation. A **cephalic presentation** is the most frequent type of presentation, occurring as often as 95% of the time. With this type of presentation, the fetal head is the body part that first contacts the cervix. The four types of cephalic presentation (vertex, brow, face, and mentum) are described in Table 15.1. The vertex is the ideal presenting part because the skull bones are capable of effectively molding to accommodate the cervix. This exact fit may actually aid in cervical dilatation as well as prevent complications such as a prolapsed cord (a portion of the cord passes between the presenting part and the cervix and enters the vagina before the fetus) (Zheng, 2012).

During labor, the area of the fetal skull that contacts the cervix often becomes edematous from the continued pressure against it. This edema is called a *caput succedaneum.* In the newborn, what was the point of presentation can be analyzed from the location of the caput.

Breech Presentation. A **breech presentation** means either the buttocks or the feet are the first body parts that will contact the cervix. Breech presentations occur in approximately 3% of births and are affected by fetal attitude the same as vertex presentations (Aguirre & Chou, 2011).

- A good attitude brings the fetal knees up against the fetal abdomen.
- A poor attitude means the knees and legs are extended.

Breech presentation can cause a difficult birth, with the presenting point influencing the degree of difficulty. Three types of breech presentation (complete, frank, and footling) are possible and described in Table 15.2.

Shoulder Presentation. In a transverse lie, a fetus lies horizontally in the pelvis so the longest fetal axis is perpendicular to that of the mother. The presenting part is usually one of the shoulders (acromion process), an iliac crest, a hand, or an elbow (Fig. 15.5). The usual contour of the mother's abdomen at term may appear fuller side to side rather than top to bottom.

Fewer than 1% of fetuses lie transversely. This presentation may be caused by pelvic contractions, in which the horizontal space is greater than the vertical space or by the presence of a placenta previa (the placenta is located low in the uterus, obscuring some of the vertical space). It also can be caused by relaxed abdominal walls from grand multiparity, which allow the unsupported uterus to fall forward (Al, 2012).

If an infant is preterm and smaller than usual, an attempt to turn the fetus to a horizontal lie (external fetal

TABLE 15.2 Types of Breech Presentations

Type	Lie	Attitude	Description
Complete	Longitudinal	Good (full flexion)	The fetus has the thighs tightly flexed on the abdomen; both the buttocks and the tightly flexed feet present to the cervix.
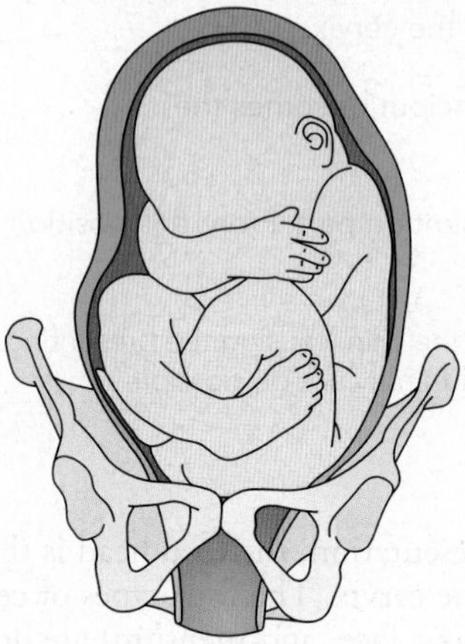			
Frank	Longitudinal	Moderate	Attitude is moderate because the hips are flexed, but the knees are extended to rest on the chest. The buttocks alone present to the cervix.
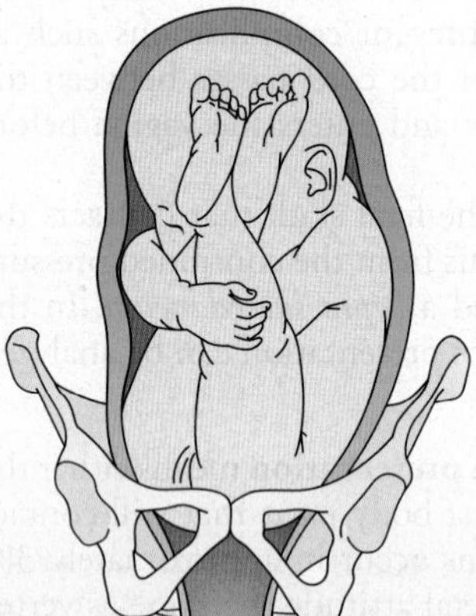			
Footling	Longitudinal	Poor	Neither the thighs nor lower legs are flexed. If one foot presents, it is a single-footling breech; if both present, it is a double-footling breech.
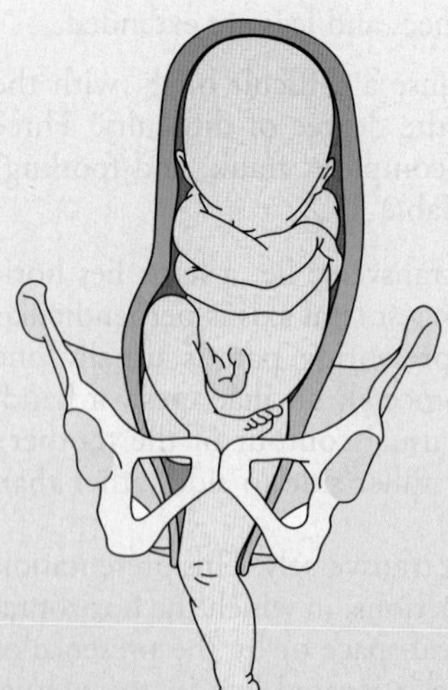			

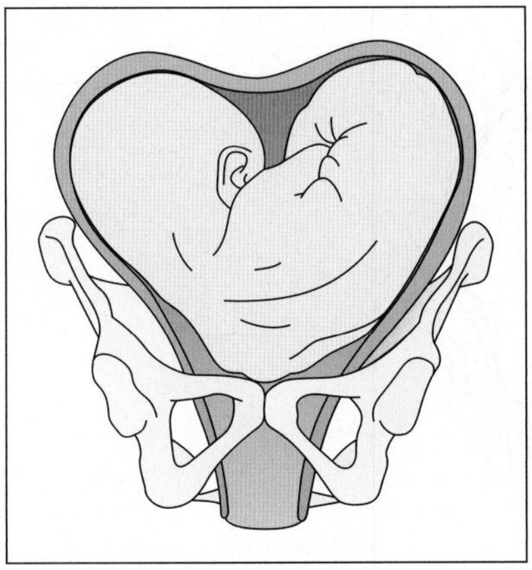

FIGURE 15.5 A transverse or shoulder presentation.

version) may be made. Most infants in a transverse lie must be born by cesarean birth, however, because they can neither be turned or born vaginally due to this "wedged" position. Discovering a shoulder presentation during labor is an important assessment because it almost always identifies a birth position that puts both mother and child in jeopardy unless skilled health care personnel are available to complete a cesarean birth.

Fetal Position

Fetal position is the relationship of the presenting part to a specific quadrant and side of a woman's pelvis. For convenience, the maternal pelvis is divided into four quadrants according to the mother's right and left: (a) right anterior, (b) left anterior, (c) right posterior, and (d) left posterior. Four parts of a fetus are typically chosen as landmarks to describe the relationship of the presenting part to one of the pelvic quadrants.

- In a vertex presentation, the occiput (O) is the chosen point.
- In a face presentation, it is the chin (mentum [M]).
- In a breech presentation, it is the sacrum (Sa).
- In a shoulder presentation, it is the scapula or the acromion process (A).

Position is indicated by an abbreviation of three letters. The middle letter denotes the fetal landmark (O for occiput, M for mentum, Sa for sacrum, and A for acromion process). The first letter defines whether the landmark is pointing to the mother's right (R) or left (L). The last letter defines whether the landmark points anteriorly (A), posteriorly (P), or transversely (T).

If the occiput of a fetus points to the left anterior quadrant in a vertex position, for example, this is a left occipitoanterior (LOA) position. If the occiput points to the right posterior quadrant, the position is right occipitoposterior (ROP). LOA is the most common fetal position, and right occipitoanterior (ROA) is the second most frequent. Box 15.2 summarizes possible positions. Six common positions in cephalic presentations are illustrated in Figure 15.6.

Position is important because it can influence both the process and efficiency of labor. Typically, a fetus is born fastest from an ROA or LOA position. Labor can be considerably extended if the position is posterior (ROP or LOP) and may be more painful for a woman because the rotation of the fetal head puts pressure on sacral nerves. Encouraging a woman to rest in a Sims position on the same side as the fetal spine or use a hands and knees position may encourage rotation from an occipitoposterior to an occipitoanterior position prior to and during labor (Simkin, 2010).

Engagement. Engagement refers to the settling of the presenting part of a fetus far enough into the pelvis that it rests at the level of the ischial spines, the midpoint of the pelvis. Descent to this point means the widest part of the fetus (the presenting skull diameter in a cephalic presentation, or the intertrochanteric diameter in a breech presentation) has passed through the pelvis or the pelvic inlet has been proven adequate for birth. In a primipara, nonengagement of the head at the beginning of labor suggests that a possible complication such as an abnormal presentation or position, abnormality of the fetal head, or cephalopelvic disproportion exists. In multiparas, engagement may or may not be present at the beginning of labor. The degree of engagement is established by a vaginal and cervical examination.

- A presenting part that is not engaged is said to be "floating."
- One that is descending but has not yet reached the ischial spines may be referred to as "dipping."

Station. **Station** refers to the relationship of the presenting part of the fetus to the level of the ischial spines (Fig. 15.7).

- When the presenting fetal part is at the level of the ischial spines, it is at a 0 station (synonymous with engagement).
- If the presenting part is above the spines, the distance is measured and described as minus stations, which range from –1 to –4 cm.
- If the presenting part is below the ischial spines, the distance is stated as plus stations (+1 to +4 cm).
- At a +3 or +4 station, the presenting part is at the perineum and can be seen if the vulva is separated (i.e., it is crowning).

BOX 15.2 Examples of Possible Fetal Positions

Vertex Presentation (Occiput)	Breech Presentation (Sacrum)	Shoulder Presentation (Acromion process)
LOA, left occipitoanterior	LSaA, left sacroanterior	LAA, left scapuloanterior
LOP, left occipitoposterior	LSaP, left sacroposterior	LAP, left scapuloposterior
LOT, left occipitotransverse	LSaT, left sacrotransverse	RAA, right scapuloanterior
ROA, right occipitoanterior	RSaA, right sacroanterior	RAP, right scapuloposterior
ROP, right occipitoposterior	RSaP, right sacroposterior	
ROT, right occipitotransverse	RSaT, right sacrotransverse	

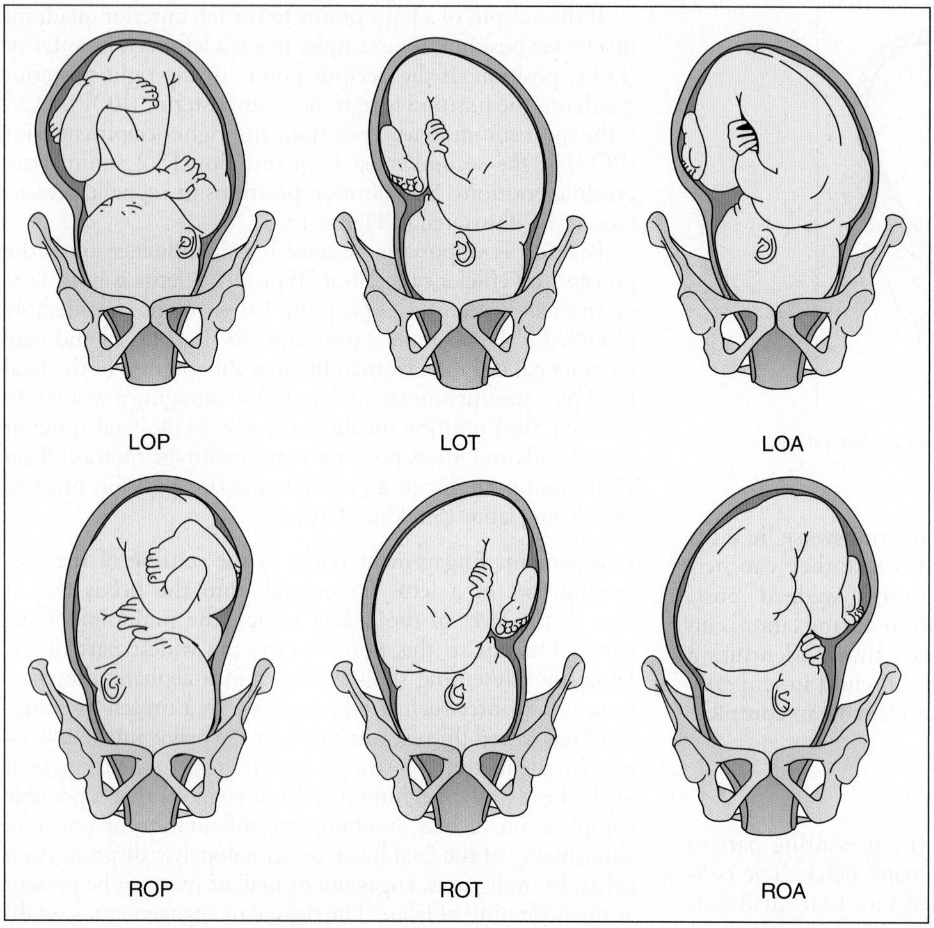

FIGURE 15.6 The fetal position. All are vertex presentations. A, anterior; L, left; O, occiput; P, posterior; R, right; T, transverse.

QSEN Checkpoint Question 15.1

Teamwork & Collaboration

You are collaborating with Celeste Bailey's obstetrician and you are planning possible interventions in light of fetal position. Which of the following fetal positions is considered ideal and is most conducive to a birth that requires few interventions by the obstetrician?

a. Right occipitoanterior with full flexion
b. Left transverse anterior in moderate flexion
c. Right occipitoposterior with no flexion
d. Left sacroanterior with full flexion

Look in Appendix A for the best answer and rationale.

Mechanisms (Cardinal Movements) of Labor

Effective passage of a fetus through the birth canal involves not only position and presentation but also a number of different position changes in order to keep the smallest diameter of the fetal head (in cephalic presentations) always presenting to the smallest diameter of the pelvis. These position changes are termed the **cardinal movements of labor**: descent, flexion, internal rotation, extension, external rotation, and expulsion (Fig. 15.8).

Descent. Descent is the downward movement of the biparietal diameter of the fetal head within the pelvic inlet. Full descent occurs when the fetal head protrudes beyond the dilated cervix and touches the posterior vaginal floor. Descent occurs because of pressure on the fetus by the uterine fundus. As the pressure of the fetal head presses on the sacral nerves at the pelvic floor, the mother will experience the typical "pushing sensation," which occurs with labor. As a woman contracts her abdominal muscles with pushing, this aids descent.

Flexion. As descent is completed and the fetal head touches the pelvic floor, the head bends forward onto the chest, causing the smallest anteroposterior diameter (the suboccipitobregmatic diameter) to present to the birth canal. Flexion is also aided by abdominal muscle contraction during pushing.

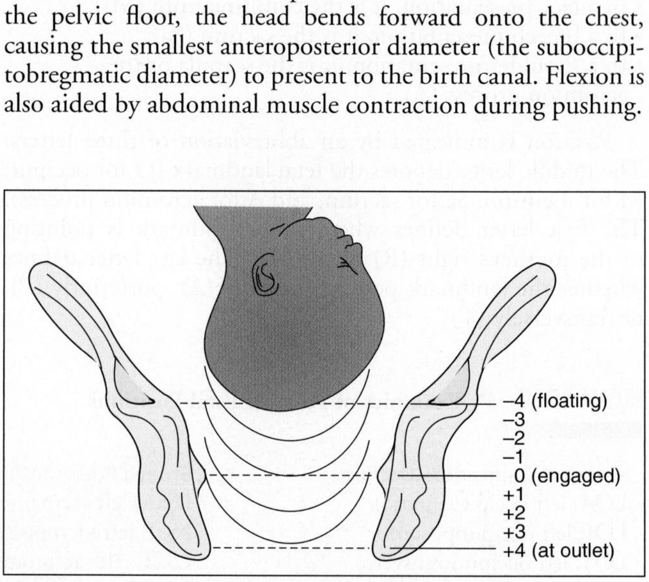

FIGURE 15.7 The station (anteroposterior view). The station, or degree of engagement, of the fetal head is designated by centimeters above or below the ischial spines. At –4 station, the head is "floating." At 0 station, the head is "engaged." At +4 station, the head is "at outlet."

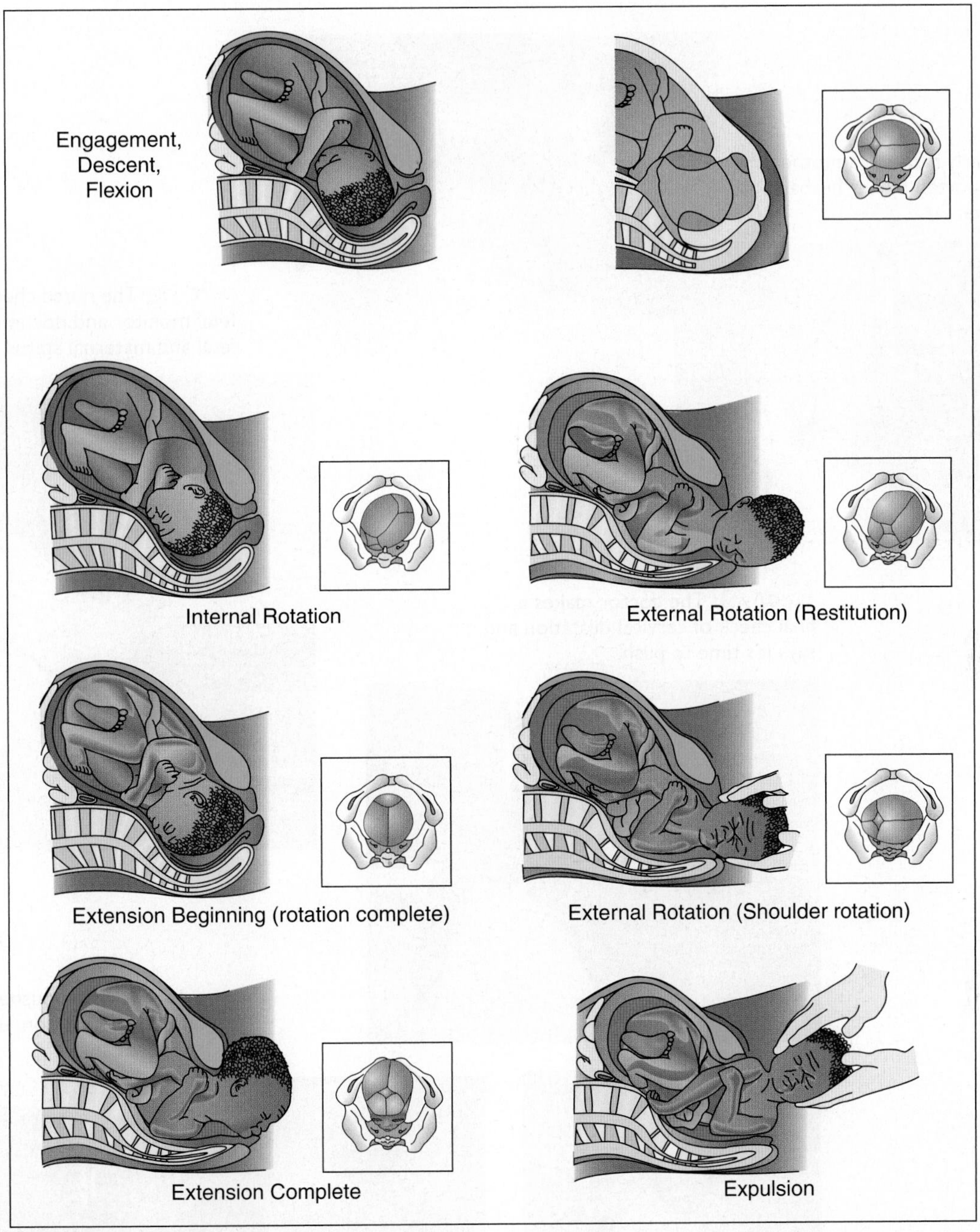

FIGURE 15.8 The mechanism of normal labor and cardinal positions of the fetus from a left occipitoanterior position.

Internal Rotation. During descent, the biparietal diameter of the fetal skull was aligned to fit through the anteroposterior diameter of the mother's pelvis. As the head flexes at the end of descent, the occiput rotates so the head is brought into the best relationship to the outlet of the pelvis, or the anteroposterior diameter is now in the anteroposterior plane of the pelvis. This movement brings the shoulders, coming next, into the optimal position to enter the inlet, or puts the widest diameter of the shoulders (a transverse one) in line with the wide transverse diameter of the inlet.

Extension. As the occiput of the fetal head is born, the back of the neck stops beneath the pubic arch and acts as a pivot for the rest of the head. The head extends, and the foremost parts of the head, the face and chin, are born.

External Rotation. In external rotation, almost immediately after the head of the infant is born, the head rotates a final time (from the anteroposterior position it assumed to enter the outlet) back to the diagonal or transverse position of the early part of labor. This brings the aftercoming shoulders into an anteroposterior position, which is best for entering the outlet. The anterior shoulder is born first, assisted perhaps by downward flexion of the infant's head.

Expulsion. Once the shoulders are born, the rest of the baby is born easily and smoothly because of its smaller size. This movement, called expulsion, is the end of the pelvic division of labor. For a view of the complete birth sequence, see Figure 15.9.

(text continues on page 362)

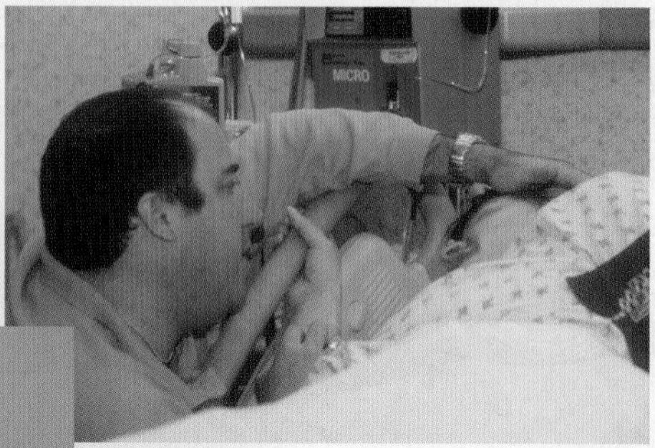

6:00 AM: Early in labor, a mother-to-be is supported by her husband and her sister.

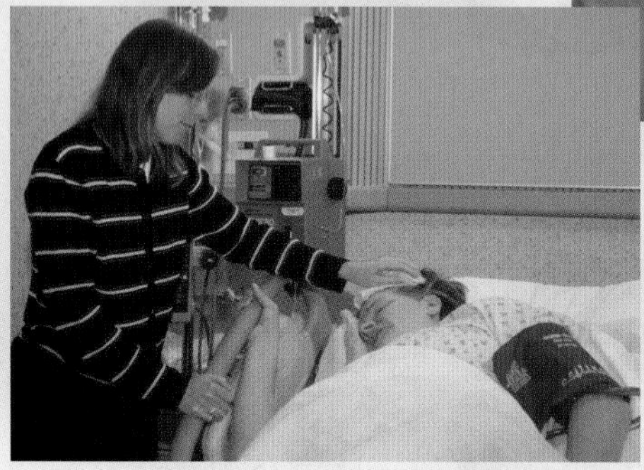

9:00 AM: The nurse checks the fetal monitor and documents fetal and maternal status.

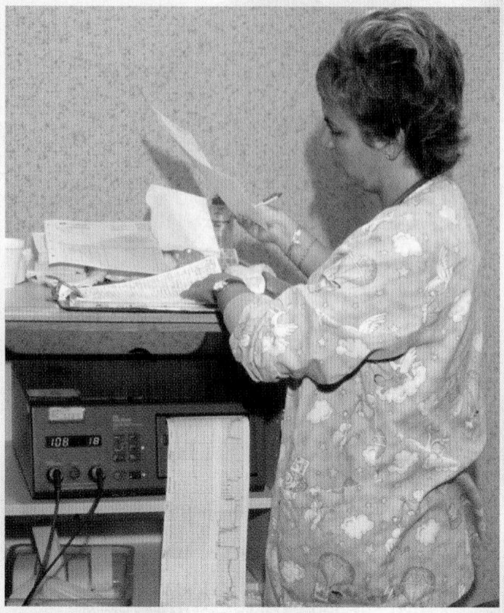

10:00 AM: The doctor makes a final check of cervical dilatation and says it's time to push.

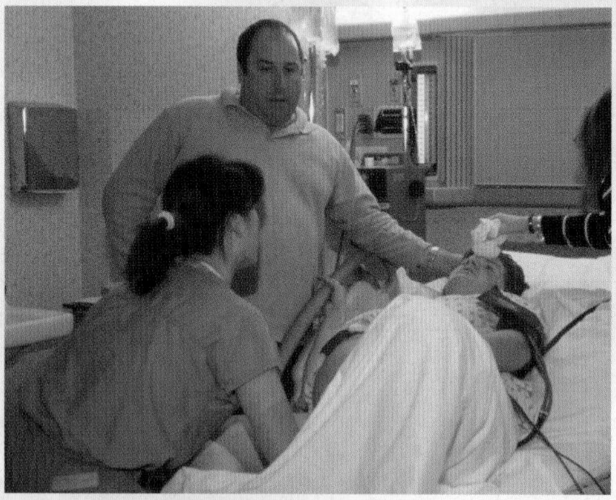

11:15 AM: She pushes from an alternative position, using a support bar.

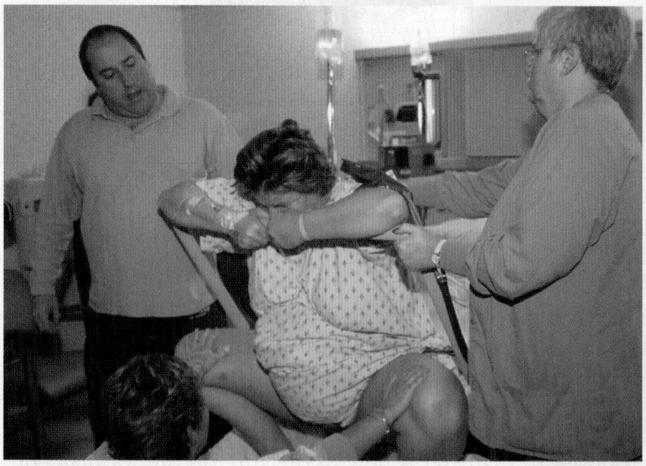

10:30 AM: The mother pushes in the dorsal recumbent position with her coach.

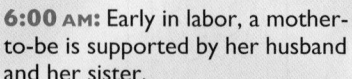

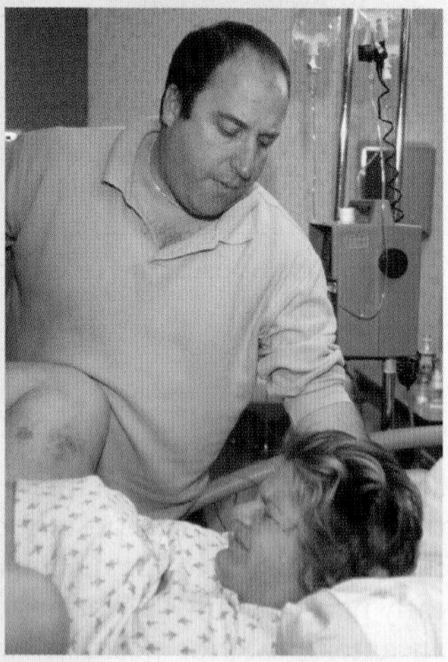

FIGURE 15.9 A day in the life of a new family.

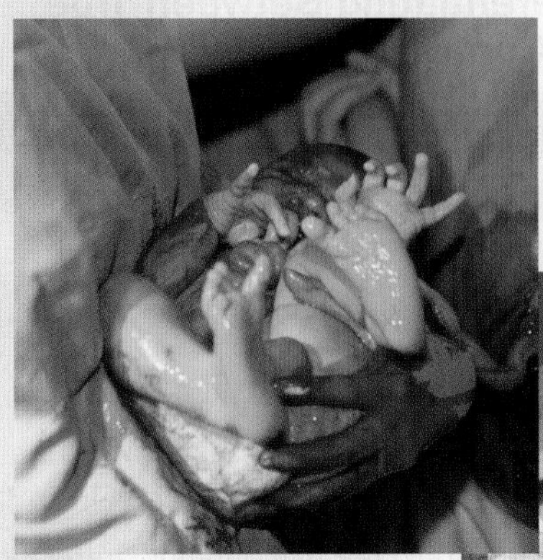

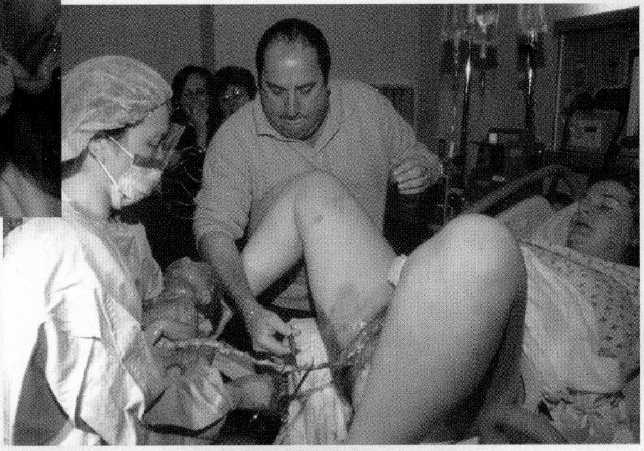

12:12 PM: Welcome to the world! Dad cuts the cord.

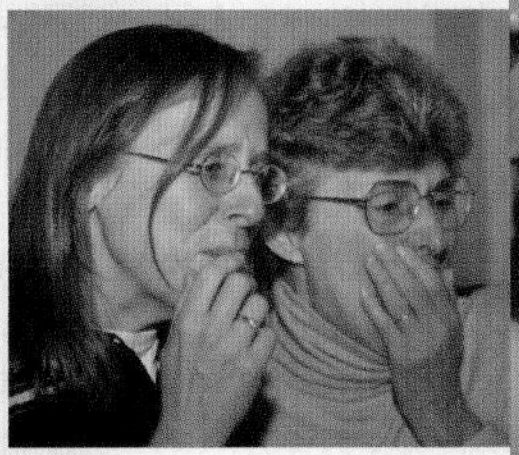

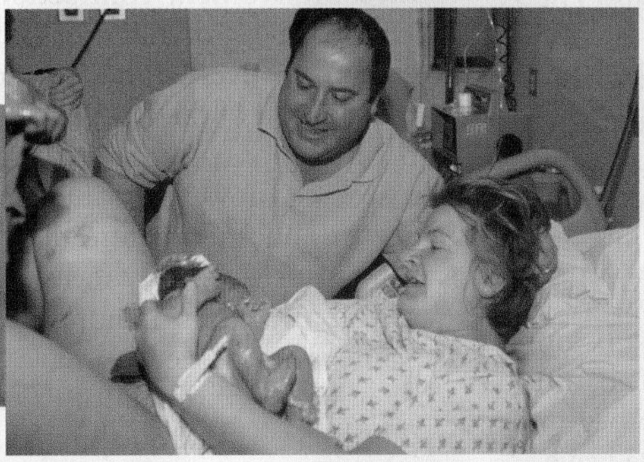

12:15 PM: Mom holds her son for the first time. Her mother and sister (now a grand-mother and aunt!) look on.

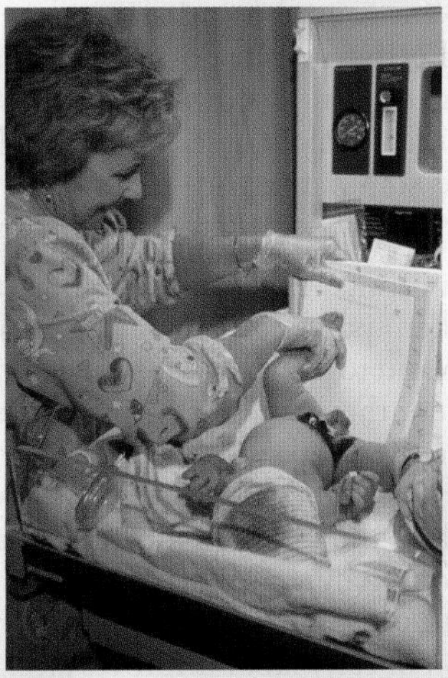

12:30 PM: The nurse takes the baby's footprints.

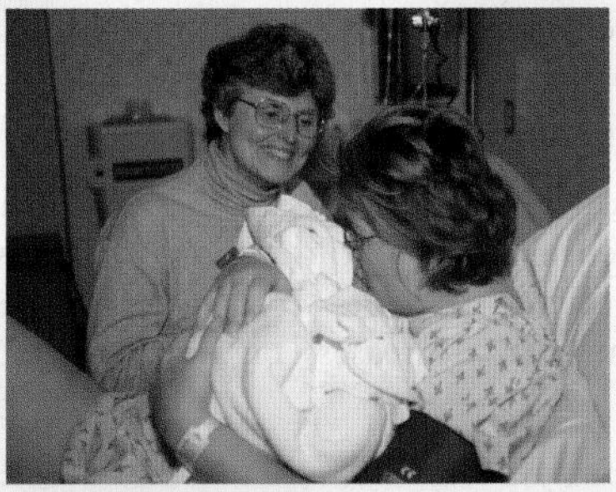

1:15 PM: Cleaned and swaddled, the newborn gets a kiss from Mom.

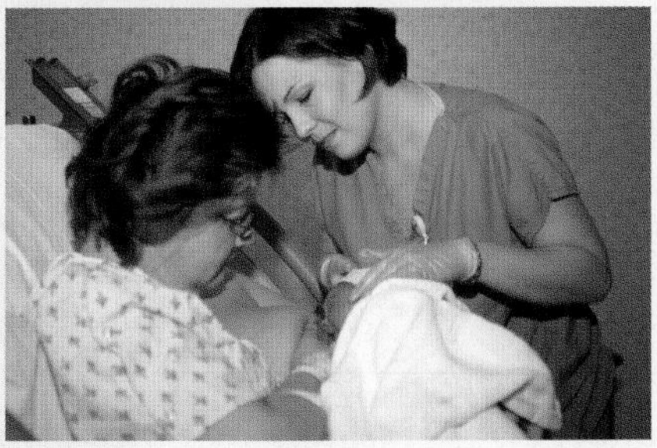

3:00 PM: The new mom gives Stephen his first feeding, with support from the nurse.

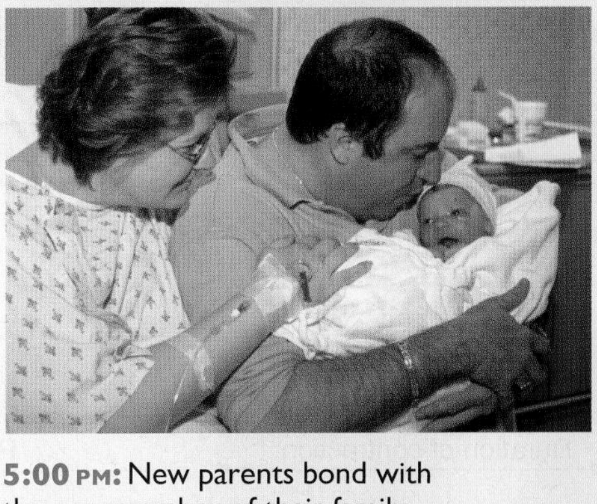

5:00 PM: New parents bond with the new member of their family.

FIGURE 15.9 *(continued)*

The Powers of Labor

The third important requirement for a successful labor is effective powers of labor. This is the force supplied by the fundus of the uterus and implemented by uterine contractions, which causes cervical dilatation and then expulsion of the fetus from the uterus. After full dilatation of the cervix, the primary power is supplemented by use of a secondary power source, the abdominal muscles. It is important for women to understand that they should not bear down with their abdominal muscles to push until the cervix is fully dilated. Doing so impedes the primary force and could cause fetal and cervical damage.

Uterine Contractions

During pregnancy, the uterus begins to contract and relax periodically as if it is rehearsing for labor (Braxton Hicks contractions, or false labor). These contractions are usually mild but can be so strong that a woman mistakes them for true labor. As a rule, even if a woman thinks what she is feeling cannot be true labor, she needs to phone or e-mail her primary care provider to have the contractions further evaluated in case she is mistaking preterm labor for practice contractions. The mark of Braxton Hicks contractions is that they are usually irregular and are painful but do not cause cervical dilation. In contrast, effective uterine contractions have rhythmicity, a progressive increase in length and intensity, and accompany dilatation of the cervix. These differences between false and true labor are summarized in Table 15.3. Contractions are assessed according to frequency, duration, and strength.

Origins. Like cardiac contractions, labor contractions begin at a "pacemaker" point located in the uterine myometrium near one of the uterotubal junctions. Each contraction begins at that point and then sweeps down over the uterus as a wave. After a short rest period, another contraction is initiated and the downward sweep begins again.

In early labor, the uterotubal pacemaker may not operate in a synchronous manner. This makes contractions sometimes strong, sometimes weak, and somewhat irregular. This mild incoordination of early labor improves after a few hours as the pacemaker becomes more attuned to calcium concentrations in the myometrium and begins to function effectively.

TABLE 15.3 Differentiating Between True and False Labor Contractions

False Contractions	True Contractions
Begin and remain irregular	Begin irregularly but become regular and predictable
Felt first abdominally and remain confined to the abdomen and groin	Felt first in lower back and sweep around to the abdomen in a wave
Often disappear with ambulation or sleep	Continue no matter what the woman's level of activity
Do not increase in duration, frequency, or intensity	Increase in duration, frequency, and intensity
Do not achieve cervical dilatation	Achieve cervical dilatation

In some women, contractions appear to originate in the lower uterine segment rather than in the fundus. These are reversed and ineffective and may actually cause tightening rather than dilatation of the cervix. It is difficult to tell from palpation that contractions are being initiated in a reverse pattern. It can be suspected, however, if the woman tells you she feels pain in her lower abdomen before the contraction is readily palpated at the fundus. It is truly revealed only when apparently strong uterine contractions do not cause cervical dilatation.

Some women seem to have additional pacemaker sites in other portions of the uterus. If this is so, contractions can be uncoordinated. Uncoordinated contractions may slow labor and can lead to failure to progress and fetal distress because they may not allow for adequate placental filling. All of these possibilities make evaluating the rate, intensity, and pattern of uterine contractions an important nursing responsibility.

Phases. A contraction consists of three phases: the increment, when the intensity of the contraction increases; the acme, when the contraction is at its strongest; and the decrement, when the intensity decreases (Fig. 15.10). Between

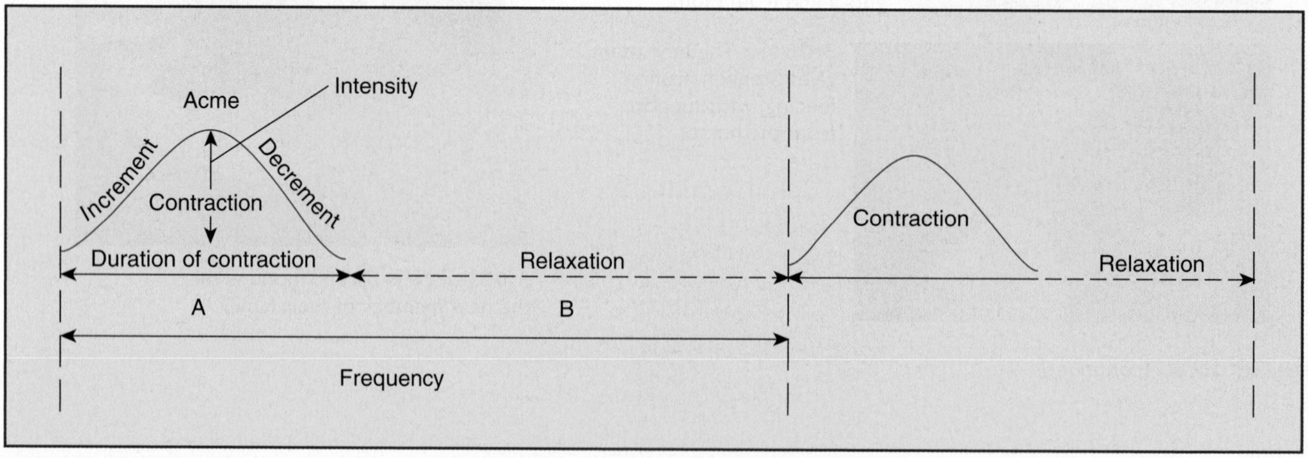

FIGURE 15.10 The interval and duration of uterine contractions. The frequency of contractions is the time from the beginning of one contraction to the beginning of the next. It consists of two parts: **(A)** the duration of the contraction and **(B)** the period of relaxation. The broken line indicates an indeterminate period because the relaxation time **(B)** is usually of longer duration than the actual contraction **(A)**.

contractions, the uterus relaxes. As labor progresses, the relaxation intervals decrease from 10 minutes early in labor to only 2 to 3 minutes. The duration of contractions also changes, increasing from 20 to 30 seconds at the beginning to a range of 60 to 70 seconds by the end of the first stage (Bernal & Norwitz, 2012).

Contour Changes. As labor contractions progress and become regular and strong, the uterus gradually differentiates itself into two distinct functioning areas: an upper portion, which thickens, and a lower segment, which becomes thin-walled, supple, and passive so the fetus can be pushed out of the uterus easily. The contour of the overall uterus also changes from a round, ovoid structure to an elongated one with a vertical diameter markedly greater than the horizontal diameter. This lengthening straightens the body of the fetus, bringing it into better alignment with the cervix and pelvis. The elongation of the uterus can cause pressure against the diaphragm and causes the often expressed sensation that a uterus is "taking control" of a woman's body.

Cervical Changes

Even more marked than the changes in the body of the uterus are two changes that occur in the cervix: effacement and dilatation.

Effacement. **Effacement** is shortening and thinning of the cervical canal. All during pregnancy, the canal is approximately 1 to 2 cm long. During labor, the longitudinal traction from the contracting uterus shortens the cervix so much that the cervix virtually disappears (Fig. 15.11).

In primiparas, effacement is accomplished before dilatation begins. Be sure to inform women of both effacement and dilation following a pelvic examination. If a woman is told at noon, for example, she is 3 cm dilated and then at 4 PM she is told she is still 3 cm dilated, it is a discouraging report because it seems as if absolutely nothing has happened in 4 hours. Effacement, however, will have been occurring; telling her about this can be the encouragement she needs to continue breathing or working with contractions.

In multiparas, dilatation may proceed before effacement is complete. Effacement must occur by the end of dilatation, however, before the fetus can be safely pushed through the cervical canal; otherwise, cervical tearing can result.

Dilatation. **Dilatation** refers to the enlargement or widening of the cervical canal from an opening a few millimeters wide to one large enough (approximately 10 cm) to permit passage of a fetus (see Fig. 15.11).

Dilatation occurs first because uterine contractions gradually increase the diameter of the cervical canal lumen by pulling the cervix up over the presenting part of the fetus. Secondly, the fluid-filled membranes push ahead of the fetus and serve as an opening wedge. If they are ruptured, the presenting part will serve this same function, although maybe not as effectively.

As dilatation begins, there is an increase in the amount of vaginal secretions (show), because minute capillaries in the cervix rupture and the last of the mucus plug that has sealed the cervix since early pregnancy is released.

QSEN Checkpoint Question 15.2

Quality Improvement

Celeste Bailey didn't recognize for over an hour that she was in labor. During her prenatal education, Celeste should have been taught to recognize which sign of true labor?

a. Sudden loss of energy from epinephrine release
b. "Nagging" but constant pain in the lower back
c. Urinary urgency from increased bladder pressure
d. "Show" or release of the cervical mucus plug

Look in Appendix A for the best answer and rationale.

The Psyche

The fourth "P," or a woman's psychological outlook, refers to the psychological state or feelings a woman brings into labor. For many women, this is a feeling of apprehension or fright. For almost everyone, it includes a sense of excitement or awe.

Women who manage best in labor typically are those who have a strong sense of self-esteem and a meaningful support person with them. These factors allow women to feel in control of sensations and circumstances they have never experienced before and which may not be what they pictured (Hodnett, Gates, Hofmeyr, et al., 2011). Women without adequate support can have a labor experience so frightening

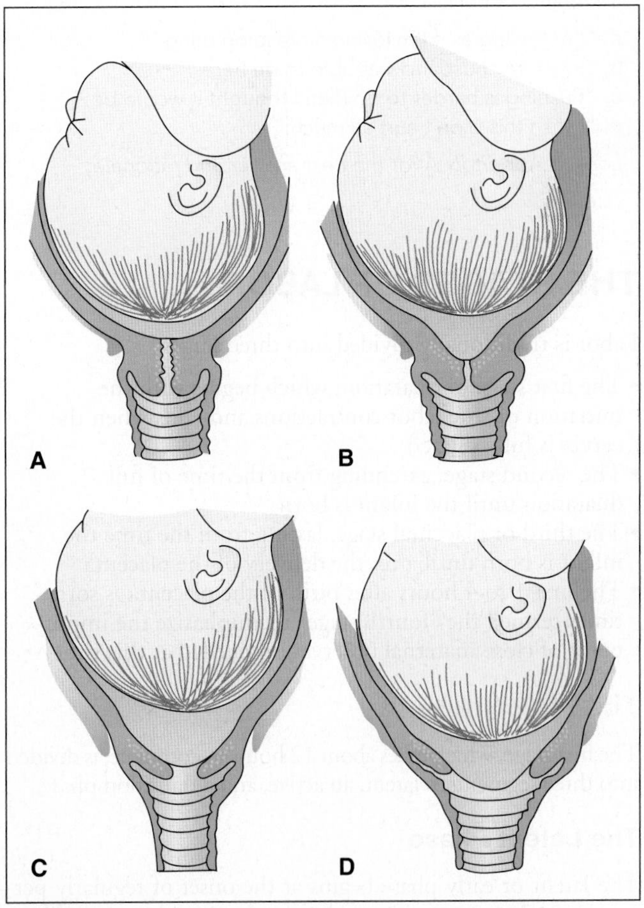

FIGURE 15.11 Effacement and dilation of the cervix. **(A)** The beginning of labor. **(B)** Effacement is beginning; dilation is not apparent yet. **(C)** Effacement is almost complete. **(D)** After complete effacement, dilation proceeds rapidly.

and stressful that they develop symptoms of posttraumatic stress disorder (PTSD) (Beck, Gable, Sakala, et al., 2011).

Encourage women to ask questions at prenatal visits and to attend preparation for childbirth classes so they are as well prepared for labor as possible. Encourage them after birth to talk about and share their experience because a "debriefing time" can be an important way to help them appreciate everything that happened and integrate the experience into their total life.

QSEN Checkpoint Question 15.3

Evidence-Based Practice

Labor and birth can be such overwhelming events that between 1% and 6% of women develop PTSD after childbirth. "Hotspots" are moments of extreme distress that strongly influence the development of PTSD. To find what are the hotspots in labor, researchers asked 675 women who experienced a difficult or traumatic birth to complete a questionnaire describing their labor and birth experience. Of the women, 67% reported at least one hotspot during birth and 52.9% had reexperiencing anxiety of these hotspots. Women were more likely to have PTSD if hotspots involved fear and lack of control or if the hotspots concerned interpersonal difficulties or maternal complications compared to complications with the baby (Harris & Ayers, 2012).

Based on the previous study, which statement by Celeste would worry you most that labor could be becoming traumatic for her?

a. "I'm feeling as if I'm losing a grasp on things."
b. "I wish my husband was able to be here."
c. "Pushing is harder to do than I thought it would be."
d. "I wish this didn't hurt so much."

Look in Appendix A for the best answer and rationale.

THE STAGES OF LABOR

Labor is traditionally divided into three stages:

- The first stage of dilatation, which begins with the initiation of true labor contractions and ends when the cervix is fully dilated
- The second stage, extending from the time of full dilatation until the infant is born
- The third or placental stage, lasting from the time the infant is born until after the delivery of the placenta
- The first 1 to 4 hours after birth of the placenta is sometimes termed the "fourth stage" to emphasize the importance of close maternal observation needed at this time.

The First Stage

The first stage, which takes about 12 hours to complete, is divided into three segments: a latent, an active, and a transition phase.

The Latent Phase

The latent or early phase begins at the onset of regularly perceived uterine contractions and ends when rapid cervical dilatation begins. Contractions during this phase are mild and short, lasting 20 to 40 seconds. Cervical effacement occurs, and the cervix dilates from 0 to about 3 cm. The phase averages 6 hours in a nullipara and 4.5 hours in a multipara. A woman who enters labor with a "nonripe" cervix will probably have a longer than average latent phase. If a woman wants analgesia at this point, she shouldn't be denied of it, but analgesia given too early in labor is a factor that tends to prolong this phase. Measuring the length of the latent phase is important because a reason for a prolonged latent phase could be cephalopelvic disproportion (a disproportion between the size of the fetal head and pelvis), which could require a cesarean birth (Maharaj, 2010).

In a woman who is psychologically prepared for labor and who does not tense at each tightening sensation in her abdomen, latent phase contractions cause only minimal discomfort and can be managed by controlled breathing. During this phase, encourage women to continue to walk about and make preparations for birth, such as doing last-minute packing for her stay at the hospital or birthing center, preparing older children for her departure and the upcoming birth, or giving instructions to the person who will take care of them while she is away. If desired, she could begin alternative methods of pain relief such as aromatherapy, distraction, or acupressure (Smith, Collins, Crowther, et al., 2011). If the woman should come to a birthing setting this early, encourage her to continue to be active and to use any nonpharmacotherapeutic measures she finds effective.

The Active Phase

During the active phase of labor, cervical dilatation occurs more rapidly, increasing from 4 to 7 cm at a rate of about 1 cm per hour in nulliparas and 2 cm per hour in multiparas. Contractions grow stronger, lasting 40 to 60 seconds, and occur approximately every 3 to 5 minutes. This phase averages 3 hours in a nullipara and 2 hours in a multipara. Show (increased vaginal secretions) and perhaps spontaneous rupture of the membranes may occur during this time. Encourage women to be active participants in labor by keeping active and assuming whatever position is most comfortable for them during this time, except flat on their back (Downe, 2011).

This phase can be difficult for a woman because contractions grow so much stronger and last so much longer than they did in the latent phase that she begins to experience true discomfort. It is also both an exciting and a frightening time because it is obvious something dramatic is definitely happening. In a few hours, a woman will have a new baby. Her life will never be the same again.

The Transition Phase

During the **transition** phase, contractions reach their peak of intensity, occurring every 2 to 3 minutes with a duration of 60 to 70 seconds, and a maximum cervical dilatation of 8 to 10 cm occurs. If it has not previously occurred, show will occur as the last of the mucus plug from the cervix is released. If the membranes have not previously ruptured, they will usually rupture at full dilatation (10 cm). By the end of this phase, both full dilatation (10 cm) and complete cervical effacement (obliteration of the cervix) have occurred.

During this phase, a woman may experience intense discomfort that is so strong, it might be accompanied by nausea and vomiting. She may also experience a feeling of loss of control, anxiety, panic, and/or irritability. Because of the intensity and duration of the contractions, it may seem as though labor has taken charge of her. A few minutes before, she may have enjoyed having her forehead wiped with a cool cloth or her back rubbed. Now she may knock a partner's hand away from her. Her focus turns entirely inward to the task of birthing her baby. As a woman reaches the end of this stage at 10 cm of dilatation, unless she has been administered epidural anesthesia, a new sensation, the irresistible urge to push, usually begins.

What if...15.1 Celeste tells you she is certain her labor is going wrong because it has lasted over 6 hours. Is this an unusually long time for a first stage of labor for a woman having her first child? Do you think she would be comforted by learning the usual length?

The Second Stage

The second stage of labor is the time span from full dilatation and cervical effacement to birth of the infant. With uncomplicated birth and without epidural anesthesia this stage takes about 1 hour (Friedman, 1978). A woman typically feels contractions change from the characteristic crescendo–decrescendo pattern to an uncontrollable urge to push or bear down with each contraction as if to move her bowels. She may experience momentary nausea or vomiting because pressure is no longer exerted on her stomach as the fetus descends into the pelvis. She pushes with such force that she perspires and the blood vessels in her neck become distended.

The fetus begins descent and, as the fetal head touches the internal perineum to begin internal rotation, her perineum begins to bulge and appear tense. The anus may become everted, and stool may be expelled. As the fetal head pushes against the vaginal introitus, this opens and the fetal scalp appears at the opening to the vagina and enlarges from the size of a dime, to a quarter, then a half-dollar. This is termed **crowning**.

It takes a few contractions of this new type for a woman to realize everything is all right, just different, and to appreciate it feels satisfying, not frightening, to push with contractions. As she concentrates on pushing, she may become unaware of the conversation in the room. Pain may disappear as all of her energy and thoughts are directed toward giving birth. As the fetal head is pushed out of the birth canal, it extends, then rotates to bring the shoulders into the best line with the pelvis. The body of the baby is then born.

The Third Stage

The third stage of labor, the placental stage, begins with the birth of the infant and ends with the delivery of the placenta. Two separate phases are involved: *placental separation* and *placental expulsion.*

After the birth of the infant, the uterus can be palpated as a firm, round mass just below the level of the umbilicus. After a few minutes of rest, uterine contractions begin again, and the organ assumes a discoid shape. It retains this new shape until the placenta has separated, approximately 5 minutes after the birth of the infant.

Placental Separation

As the uterus contracts down on an almost empty interior, there is such a disproportion between the placenta and the contracting wall of the uterus, that folding and separation of the placenta occur. Active bleeding on the maternal surface of the placenta begins with separation, which helps to separate the placenta still further by pushing it away from its attachment site. As separation is completed, the placenta sinks to the lower uterine segment or the upper vagina.

The placenta has loosened and is ready to deliver when:

- There is lengthening of the umbilical cord.
- A sudden gush of vaginal blood occurs.
- The placenta is visible at the vaginal opening.
- The uterus contracts and feels firm again.

If the placenta separates first at its center and lastly at its edges, it tends to fold on itself like an umbrella and presents at the vaginal opening with the fetal surface evident. Approximately 80% of placentas separate and present in this way. Appearing shiny and glistening from the fetal membranes, this is called a *Schultze* presentation. If, however, the placenta separates first at its edges, it slides along the uterine surface and presents at the vagina with the maternal surface evident. It looks raw, red, and irregular, with the ridges or cotyledons that separate blood collection spaces evident; this is called a *Duncan* presentation. Although there is no difference in the outcome, record which way the placenta presented. A simple trick of remembering the presentations is remembering that, if the placenta appears shiny, it is a Schultze presentation. If it looks "dirty" (the irregular maternal surface shows), it is a Duncan presentation (Fig. 15.12).

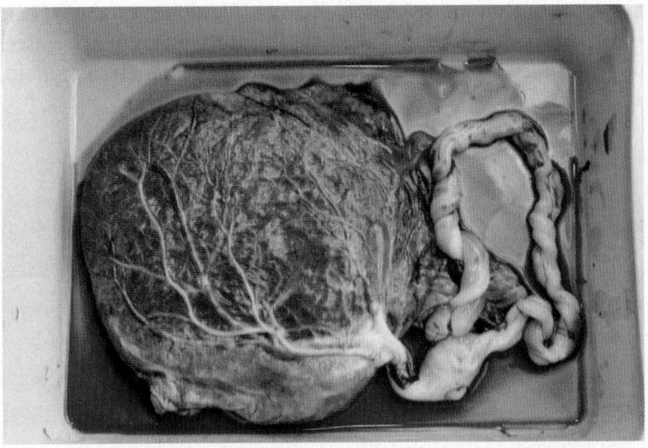

A

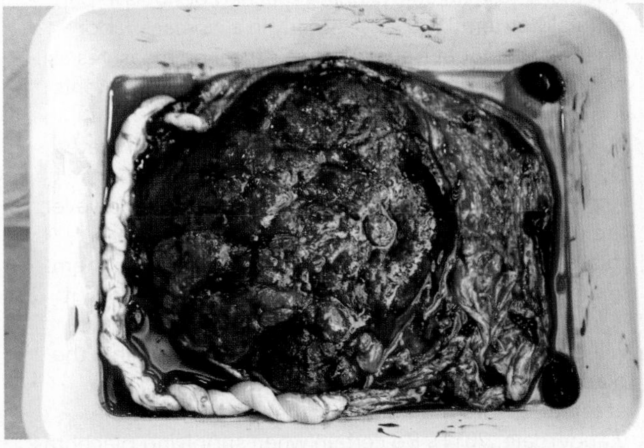

B

FIGURE 15.12 The fetal **(A)** and maternal **(B)** surfaces of the placenta. (Photos by Joe Mitchell.)

This stage takes a total of about 15 minutes. Because bleeding occurs as the placenta separates, before the uterus contracts sufficiently to seal maternal capillaries, there is a blood loss of about 300 to 500 ml, not a great amount in relation to the extra blood volume that was formed during pregnancy.

Placental Expulsion

Once separation has occurred, the placenta delivers either by the natural bearing-down effort of the mother or by gentle pressure on the contracted uterine fundus by the primary health care provider (a Credé maneuver). Pressure should never be applied to a uterus in a noncontracted state, because doing so could cause the uterus to evert (turn inside out), accompanied by massive hemorrhage (Stevens & Wittich, 2011). If the placenta does not deliver spontaneously, it can be removed manually. It needs to be inspected after delivery to be certain it is intact and part of it was not retained (which could prevent the uterus from fully contracting and lead to postpartal hemorrhage). In recognition of cultural preferences, be certain to ask if a woman wants to take home the placenta because this can be a strong cultural tradition you don't want to break (Box 15.3).

Some women choose to have a cord blood sample withdrawn from the cord to be banked for stem cell transplantation in the future. In some major health centers, women may be asked to donate a placental blood sample for a community stem cell banking program (Arrojo, Lamas, Verdugo, et al., 2012). The placenta and membranes may also be reserved to be used as temporary coverings for burns (Bárcena, Muench, Kapidzic, et al., 2011).

BOX 15.3 Nursing Care Planning to Respect Cultural Diversity

It is important for women to understand what is happening to them during labor so they can make informed decisions as to their care. If a woman is not proficient in English, make arrangements to locate an interpreter. If she is hearing challenged, it is the health care facility's responsibility to provide an interpreter for her so she can receive adequate explanations of her progress. Remember, whether a woman enjoys being touched or not is in part culturally determined. Assess early in a woman's labor whether she might benefit from such caring measures as having her hand held or her back rubbed or if she wants this only from her support person.

For most health care providers in the United States, a placenta has little importance or meaning after its work of fetal oxygenation is done. Worldwide, however, the placenta has continuing importance. Based on this, ask women if they want to take it home with them. In a number of Asian and Native American cultures, it is important to bury the placenta to ensure the child will continue to be healthy. In some parts of China, the placenta is cooked then ground into a powder and eaten to ensure the continued health of the mother (Lauderdale, 2011). Be certain when supplying placentas to women to take home that you respect standard infection precautions and hospital policy.

QSEN Checkpoint Question 15.4

Patient-Centered Care

Celeste is anxious for her placenta to deliver so she can move to a rocking chair and help relieve her back pain. In order to best facilitate Celeste's wishes, which action would be best to do?

a. Tug gently on the umbilical cord until the placenta comes loose.
b. Ask Celeste to continue hard pushing as she did to birth her baby.
c. Push on the lax fundus of her uterus to cause the placenta to loosen.
d. Assure her that a placenta loosens quickly so the waiting time will not be long.

Look in Appendix A for the best answer and rationale.

MATERNAL AND FETAL RESPONSES TO LABOR

Labor is a local process that involves the abdomen and reproductive organs, but because it is such an intense process, it has systemic physiologic effects on both a woman and her fetus. Its intensity is so great that almost all body systems are affected by it.

The Physiologic Effects on a Woman

The Cardiovascular System

Labor involves strenuous work and effort and so requires a response from the cardiovascular system.

Cardiac Output. Each uterine contraction greatly decreases blood flow to the uterus because the contracting uterine wall puts pressure on the uterine arteries. This pressure increases the amount of blood that remains in a woman's general circulation, leading to an increase in peripheral resistance, which in turn results in an increase in systolic and diastolic blood pressure. In addition, the work of pushing during labor may increase cardiac output by as much as 40% to 50% above the prelabor level.

The average blood loss with birth (300 to 500 ml) is not detrimental to most women because of the blood volume increase that occurred during pregnancy and may actually play an advantageous role by reducing blood volume to prepregnancy levels. Immediately after birth, with the weight and pressure of the fetus removed from the pelvis, blood from the peripheral circulation floods into the pelvic vasculature, momentarily dropping blood pressure in the vena cava. The body quickly compensates for this by sending a heavy bolus of blood to the heart, raising cardiac output to about 80% above prelabor levels. Cardiac output then gradually decreases from this high level back to a prepregnancy level within the first hour after birth. An average woman's heart adjusts well to these sudden changes. If she has a cardiac problem, however, these sudden hemodynamic changes can have implications for her health and make the time of these sudden shifts a hazardous time for her (see Chapter 25) (Opotowsky, Siddiqi, D'Souza, et al., 2012). The amount of blood that is lost with birth is estimated and recorded postbirth; an amount over 500 ml is documented as postpartal hemorrhage.

Blood Pressure. With the increased cardiac output caused by contractions during labor, systolic blood pressure rises an average of 15 mmHg with each contraction. Higher increases should be noted because they could be a sign of pathology. If a woman lies in a supine position and pushes during the second stage of labor, pressure of the uterus on the vena cava causes her blood pressure to drop precipitously, leading to hypotension. An upright or side-lying position during the second stage of labor not only makes pushing more effective but also can help avoid such a problem (Layer, 2011). One of the potential side effects of epidural anesthesia is hypotension, so women who receive this need to be well hydrated before the anesthetic is administered and monitored carefully afterward to detect this complication (see Chapter 16).

The Hematopoietic System

The major change in the blood-forming system that occurs during labor is the development of leukocytosis, or a sharp increase in the number of circulating white blood cells, possibly as a result of stress and heavy exertion. At the end of labor, the average woman has a white blood cell count of 25,000 to 30,000 cells/mm^3, compared with a usual count of 5,000 to 10,000 cells/mm^3.

The Respiratory System

Whenever there is an increase in cardiovascular parameters, the body responds by increasing the respiratory rate to supply additional oxygen. Total oxygen consumption increases, therefore, by about 100% during the second stage of labor. Women adjust well to this change because it is comparable to that of a person performing a strenuous exercise such as running. Because a woman is breathing rapidly, however, hyperventilation can result. Using appropriate breathing patterns during labor can help avoid severe hyperventilation and the associated feeling of dizziness that comes with it. Rebreathing into a paper bag can also be helpful.

Temperature Regulation

The increased muscular activity associated with labor can cause a slight elevation (1°F) in temperature. Diaphoresis occurs with accompanying evaporation to cool and limit excessive warming.

Fluid Balance

Insensible water loss increases during labor due to diaphoresis and the increase in rate and depth of respirations (which causes moisture to be lost with each breath), both of which help keep maternal temperature from rising. Encourage women to sip fluid during labor the same as they would if they were exercising to keep hydrated (labor is called "labor" because it is physical hard work). If a woman is nauseated by labor, encourage sips of fluid, ice chips, or hard candy to supply some extra fluid.

The Urinary System

Pressure of the fetal head as it descends in the birth canal against the anterior bladder reduces bladder tone or the ability of the bladder to sense filling. It's important, therefore, to ask a woman to void approximately every 2 hours during labor to avoid overfilling because overfilling can decrease postpartal bladder tone. With a decrease in fluid intake during labor combined with the increased insensible water loss, kidneys begin to concentrate urine to preserve both fluid and electrolytes. This causes specific gravity to rise to a high normal level of 1.020 to 1.030. It is not unusual for protein (trace to 1+) to be evident in urine because of the breakdown of protein caused by the increased muscle activity. This fades almost immediately as a woman rests after labor.

The Musculoskeletal System

Throughout the pregnancy, *relaxin*, a hormone released from the ovary, has acted to soften the cartilage between bones and make joints more flexible. In the week before labor, considerable additional release and softening causes the symphysis pubis and the sacral/coccyx joints to become even more movable, allowing them to stretch apart to increase the size of the pelvic ring by as much as 2 cm. A woman may report this increased pubic flexibility as increased back pain or irritating, nagging pain at the pubis as she walks or turns in labor (Nitsche & Howell, 2011).

The Gastrointestinal System

The gastrointestinal system becomes fairly inactive during labor, probably because blood shunts to more life-sustaining organs and also because of pressure on the stomach and intestines from the contracting uterus. Digestive and emptying time of the stomach becomes lengthened. Some women experience a loose bowel movement as contractions grow strong, similar to what they might experience with menstrual cramps. Even if women don't feel hungry during labor, they can usually eat small but high calorie snacks (chocolate bars, sports drinks, or yogurt) to supply energy.

Neurologic and Sensory Responses

The neurologic responses that occur during labor are those which typically occur with pain, such as increased pulse and respiratory rate. Early in labor, the contraction of the uterus and dilatation of the cervix are the cause of the discomfort. Pain from contractions is registered at uterine and cervical nerve plexuses (at the level of the 11th and 12th thoracic nerves). At the moment of birth, the pain is centered on the perineum and registered at S2 to S4 as it stretches to allow the fetus to move past it. Where pain registers is important in appreciating why epidural anesthesia is effective. For early labor, the anesthetic block needs to suppress the lower thoracic synapses; for birth, it needs to block sacral nerves.

The Psychological Responses of a Woman to Labor

Labor can lead to emotional distress because it is not only painful and fatiguing but it also represents the beginning of a major life change for a woman and her partner. Even for the most organized woman, the level of pain experienced can reduce her ability to cope. It can cause her to be short tempered or quick to criticize things around her. Admitting her quickly to a birthing room, an environment free from outside interference, and individualizing her care can help her begin to control her breathing patterns and reduce the pain of early contractions, as well as allow her to begin to organize coping strategies. "Admit" the woman's support person as well and encourage this person to give continuous support because it is well documented that individualized psychological support greatly influences birth satisfaction as well as possibly shortens labor and decreases the amount of analgesia needed (Gilliland, 2011).

The Response to Pain

Cultural factors can strongly influence a woman's experience and satisfaction with labor. In the past, American women were accustomed to expecting hospital procedures and a medical model of care; based on this, they followed instructions with few questions. Today, women are encouraged to help plan their care. In addition, every woman responds to cultural cues in some way. This makes her response to pain, her choice of nourishment, her preferred birthing position, the proximity and involvement of a support person, and customs related to the immediate postpartal period highly individualized.

To make labor a positive experience, be prepared to adapt care to the woman's specific needs. If a woman has traditions that run counter to hospital protocols, address these differences and make arrangements to accommodate her desires, beliefs or customs, if possible, such as advocating for special foods to eat, ballroom dancing in order to remain upright, or saving the placenta for the mother to take home.

The Response to Fatigue

By the time the date of birth approaches, a woman is generally tired from the burden of carrying so much extra weight and has not slept well for the past month (Facco, 2011). For example, a side-lying position caused backache; when she turned onto her back, her fetus kicked and wakened her; when she turned back to her side, her back ached again. Sleep hunger from this type of discomfort can make it difficult for a woman to perceive situations clearly or to adjust rapidly to new situations. It can make a small deficiency such as a wrinkled sheet appear as a major threatening discrepancy in her care. It can make the process of labor loom as an overwhelming, unendurable experience unless she has competent people with her to offer support, reassurance, and comfort.

The Response to Fear

Women appreciate a review of the labor process early in labor as a reminder that childbirth is not a strange, bewildering event but a predictable and well-documented one. Being taken by surprise—labor moving faster or slower than the woman thought it would or contractions harder and longer than she remembers from last time—can lead a woman to feel out of control and increase the level of pain she experiences. This sense of lack of control combined with pain may cause her to begin to worry for her infant and may make her afraid she will not meet her own behavioral expectations. Explain and repeat as necessary that labor is predictable, but also variable. Contractions last a certain length and reach a certain intensity, but always have a rest period in between so she can have a break from pain. Fear of labor this way releases adrenaline, and adrenaline interferes with oxytocin release and so can limit the effectiveness of uterine contractions (Aguirre & Chou, 2011).

Fetal Responses to Labor

The pressure and circulatory changes that occur with contractions not only affect the mother but also can cause detectable physiologic changes in the fetus as well.

The Neurologic System

Uterine contractions exert pressure on the fetal head, so the same response that is involved with any instance of increased intracranial pressure occurs. The fetal heart rate (FHR) decreases by as much as 5 beats/min during a contraction, as soon as contraction strength reaches 40 mmHg; although not measurable, fetal blood pressure also rises. The decrease in FHR appears on a fetal heart monitor as a normal or early deceleration pattern.

The Cardiovascular System

A sufficiently mature fetus is unaffected by the continual variations of heart rate that occur with labor contractions. During a contraction, as the arteries of the uterus become sharply constricted, and the filling of cotyledons almost completely halts, the amount of nutrients, including oxygen, exchanged during this time is greatly reduced, causing a slight but inconsequential fetal hypoxia. The increase in blood pressure caused by increased intracranial pressure raises blood pressure and keeps circulation from falling below normal for the duration of a contraction.

The Integumentary System

The pressure involved in the birth process is often reflected in minimal petechiae or ecchymotic areas on a fetus (particularly the presenting part). There may also be edema of the presenting part (caput succedaneum) from this pressure.

The Musculoskeletal System

The force of uterine contractions tends to push a fetus into a position of full flexion or with the head bent forward, which is the most advantageous position for birth.

The Respiratory System

The process of labor appears to aid in the maturation of surfactant production by alveoli in the fetal lung. Both the pressure applied to the chest from contractions and passage through the birth canal help to clear the respiratory tract of lung fluid. For this reason, an infant born vaginally is usually able to establish respirations more easily than a fetus born by cesarean birth.

MEASURING PROGRESS IN LABOR

A woman's progress in labor is recorded on a labor record (a Partogram) devised by the World Health Organization, or a like form on which vital signs, FHR, cervical dilation, descent of the fetal head, urine tests, and any drugs administered can be recorded.

Remember, when using such forms, how much and what type of analgesia a woman receives in labor can influence the length of labor. Because "norms" on such a record refer to averages, an individual woman's labor can vary greatly from the ideal projected course of labor and still be normal for that woman.

After each cervical examination, cervical dilatation and **fetal descent** (which may be referred to as "moulding") are plotted on the graph. The pattern of cervical dilatation usually plots as a rising S-shaped curve. You may need to remind women that assessments of cervical dilation are subjective, so one examiner may report a different finding from another (Archie & Roman, 2013). At the end of the latent phase of the first stage of labor, cervical dilatation is 3 to 4 cm. As a woman enters the active phase of the first stage, cervical dilation proceeds at a minimum of 1 cm/hr, or about 7 additional hours to reach full dilation (10 cm). The form shows an "alert" line, which marks when 4 hours has passed. Four hours beyond that, an "action" line advises a primary care provider that cervical dilation is taking longer than usual and that an intervention may be necessary to make the labor safe and effective. Maintaining an ongoing record and alerting the care provider that the alert line or action line is approaching are important nursing responsibilities.

Maternal Danger Signs of Labor

Wide variation exists among individuals in their response to labor and their pattern of labor contractions. Certain signs, however, indicate that the course of events is deviating from usual. These signs, both fetal and maternal, are described in Box 15.4. Nursing care of a woman who is experiencing these signs and so may be developing a complication during labor or birth is addressed in Chapter 23. In addition to problems of cervical dilation or contractions, other symptoms suggest augmentation or intervention of labor are necessary.

High or Low Blood Pressure

Normally, a woman's blood pressure rises slightly in the second (pelvic) stage of labor because of her pushing effort. A systolic pressure greater than 140 mmHg and a diastolic pressure greater than 90 mmHg, or an increase in the systolic pressure of more than 30 mmHg or in the diastolic pressure of more than 15 mmHg (the basic criteria for gestational hypertension), should be reported. Just as important to report is a falling blood pressure because it may be the first sign of intrauterine hemorrhage, although a falling blood pressure from hemorrhage is often associated with other clinical signs of hypovolemic shock, such as apprehension, increased pulse rate, and pallor.

Abnormal Pulse

Most women during pregnancy have a pulse rate of 70 to 80 beats/min. This rate normally increases slightly during the second stage of labor because of the exertion involved. A maternal pulse rate greater than 100 beats/min during labor is unusual and should be reported because it may be another indication of hemorrhage.

Inadequate or Prolonged Contractions

Uterine contractions normally become more frequent, intense, and longer as labor progresses. If they become less frequent, less intense, or shorter in duration, this may indicate uterine exhaustion (inertia). This problem may be correctable but needs augmentation or other interventions to accomplish this.

Observe also if there is a period of relaxation between contractions so the intervillous spaces of the uterus can fill and maintain an adequate supply of oxygen and nutrients for the fetus. As a rule, uterine contractions lasting longer than 70 seconds are becoming long enough to compromise fetal well-being because this interferes with adequate uterine artery filling.

Abnormal Lower Abdominal Contour

If a woman has a full bladder during labor, a round bulge appears on her lower anterior abdomen. This is a danger signal for two reasons: first, the bladder may be injured by the pressure of the fetal head pressing against it; and second, the pressure of the full bladder may not allow the fetal head to descend. To avoid a full bladder, ask women to try to void about every 2 hours during labor.

Increasing Apprehension

Warnings of psychological danger during labor are as important to consider in assessing maternal well-being as are physical signs. As she approaches the second stage of labor, a woman who is becoming increasingly apprehensive despite clear explanations of unfolding events may not be "hearing" because she has a concern that has not been met. Using an approach such as, "You seem more and more concerned. Could you tell me what is worrying you?" may be helpful. Increasing apprehension also needs to be investigated for physical reasons, because it can be a sign of oxygen deprivation or internal hemorrhage.

Fetal Danger Signs of Labor

As well as observing for a woman's danger signs of pregnancy, observing fetal danger signs is equally important. These fetal danger signs include the following.

BOX 15.4 Nursing Care Planning Using Assessment

Assessing for Danger Signs of Labor

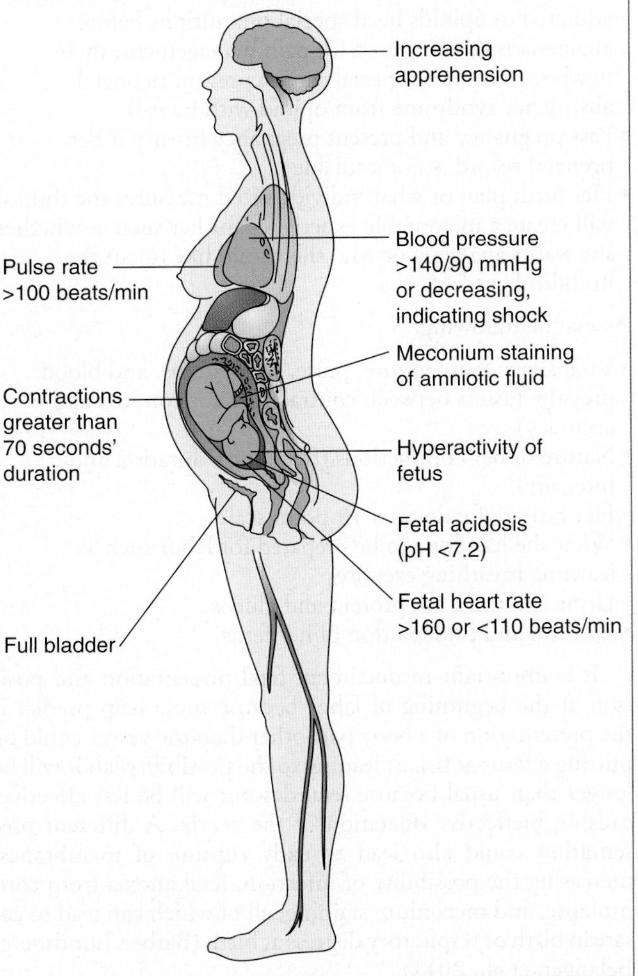

High or Low Fetal Heart Rate

As a rule, an FHR of more than 160 beats/min (fetal tachycardia) or less than 110 beats/min (fetal bradycardia) is a sign of possible fetal distress. An equally important sign is a late or variable deceleration pattern revealed on a fetal monitor (described later in this chapter). Frequent monitoring by a fetoscope, Doppler, or a monitor is necessary to detect these changes as they first occur.

Meconium Staining

This is not always a sign of fetal distress but is highly correlated with its occurrence. Meconium staining, a green color in the amniotic fluid, reveals the fetus has had a loss of rectal sphincter control, allowing meconium to pass into the amniotic fluid. It may indicate a fetus has or is experiencing hypoxia, which stimulates the vagal reflex and leads to increased bowel motility. Although meconium staining may be usual in a breech presentation because pressure on the buttocks causes meconium loss, it should always be reported immediately even with breech presentations so its cause can be investigated.

Hyperactivity

Ordinarily, a fetus remains quiet and barely moves during labor. Fetal hyperactivity may be a subtle sign that hypoxia is occurring because frantic motion is a common reaction to the need for oxygen.

Low Oxygen Saturation

Oxygen saturation in a fetus is normally 40% to 70%. A fetus can be assessed for this by a catheter inserted next to the cheek (under 40% oxygenation needs further assessment). If fetal blood is obtained by scalp puncture, the finding of acidosis (blood pH lower than 7.2) suggests fetal well-being is becoming compromised and that further investigation is also necessary.

✔ QSEN Checkpoint Question 15.5

Safety

Suppose Celeste is having long and hard uterine contractions. What length of contraction would you report as indicative of a potential safety risk?

a. Any length of contraction over 30 seconds
b. A contraction over 70 seconds in length
c. A contraction that peaks at 20 seconds
d. A contraction that appears intensely painful

Look in Appendix A for the best answer and rationale.

MATERNAL AND FETAL ASSESSMENTS DURING LABOR

Women are invariably nervous when they arrive at a hospital or birth center. Nursing assessment is important to detect how they are managing physically and emotionally to this intense event in their life (Nyman, Downe, & Berg, 2011).

The Immediate Assessment of a Woman in First Stage of Labor

A number of immediate assessment measures are necessary to safeguard maternal and fetal health when a woman first arrives at a birthing facility. After she and her support person are oriented to the area, focus on obtaining this vital assessment data.

The Initial Interview and Physical Examination

Information about the woman's pregnancy can be gained from her prenatal record electronically on admission or if a paper copy has been forwarded to the birth setting beforehand. Additional important data that needs to be obtained includes a description of her labor thus far, her general physical condition, and her preparedness and plans for labor and birth. This amount of information is scant but helps to establish whether the woman is in active labor and needs immediate preparation for birth or whether she has arrived at the birthing setting at an early stage of labor and therefore will benefit most from paced interventions.

Ask about the following:

- Her baby's expected date of birth (EDB)
- When her contractions began
- Amount and character of any show
- Whether rupture of membranes has occurred
- Any known drug allergies
- If she uses any recreational or prescription drugs (women addicted to opioids need special precautions before analgesia is administered for pain management; their newborn may need special care to prevent neonatal abstinence syndrome from opioid withdrawal)
- Past pregnancy and present pregnancy history if her prenatal record is not available
- Her birth plan or what individualized measures she thinks will create a memorable experience for her such as whether she wants analgesia or who she would like to cut the umbilical cord

Assess the following:

- Vital signs: temperature, pulse, respirations, and blood pressure (assess between contractions for comfort and accuracy)
- Nature of her contractions (frequency, duration and intensity)
- Her rating of pain on a 10-point scale
- What she has done to be prepared for labor such as learning breathing exercises
- Urine specimen for protein and glucose
- Position and presentation of her fetus

It is important to document fetal presentation and position at the beginning of labor because these help predict if the presentation of a body part other than the vertex could be putting a fetus at risk or leading to the possibility labor will be longer than usual because fetal descent will be less effective, causing ineffective dilatation of the cervix. A different presentation could also lead to early rupture of membranes, increasing the possibility of infection, fetal anoxia from cord prolapse, and meconium staining, all of which can lead to cesarean birth or respiratory distress at birth (Barber, Lundsberg, Belanger, et al., 2011).

The Detailed Assessment During the First Stage of Labor

If the woman is in active labor, the history taken on arrival may be the only history obtained until after her baby is born. If birth is not imminent, both a more extensive history and a physical examination can be obtained.

The History

Performing a detailed interview of a woman in labor can be difficult because of the constant interruptions labor contractions cause. Be patient until a contraction ends so you don't interrupt any form of controlled breathing a woman is using. Remember, the longest contraction is rarely more than 60 seconds. If a woman concentrates so intently on a breathing exercise she completely forgets a question asked just before a contraction, repeat the question as the contraction subsides, as if it had not been asked before, or as if it is no trouble to ask it again.

Current Pregnancy History. Important information needed for a complete history includes: documentation of gravida and parity status, a description of this pregnancy (e.g., intended or not, place and pattern of prenatal care, adequacy of nutrition, whether any complications such as spotting, falls, hypertension of pregnancy, infection, alcohol or drug ingestion occurred during pregnancy), plans for labor (e.g., Does she want to have the baby naturally? Will she use breathing exercises? Will her support person be able to remain with her continuously?), and plans for child care (e.g., Will she breastfeed? Has she chosen a primary health care provider for the baby? If she's having a boy, does she want him circumcised?).

Past Pregnancy History. Document prior pregnancies, abortions, or miscarriages, including number, dates, types of birth, any complications, and outcomes, including health, sex, and birth weights of previous children.

Past Health History. Document any previous surgeries (abdominal surgical adhesions might interfere with fetal passage), heart disease or diabetes (special precautions will be required during labor and birth), anemia (blood loss at birth may be more important than usual), tuberculosis (she'll need testing after birth to be certain healed lung lesions weren't reactivated by birth), kidney disease or hypertension (blood pressure must be monitored even more carefully than usual), or if she has ever had a sexually transmitted infection such as herpes (the infant may be exposed to the disease by vaginal contact if the disease is active). Determine also whether a woman's lifestyle places her at high risk for prescription or nonprescription drug abuse or HIV exposure.

Family Medical History. Ask if any family member has a condition that could be inherited such as a cognitive challenge, heart disease, blood dyscrasia, diabetes, kidney disease, allergies, seizures, hearing loss, or malignant hyperthermia (a dominantly inherited disorder that causes a dangerous increase in temperature in response to certain anesthetics). If any of these are present, adequate preparation can then be made for a child who might have special needs at birth.

The Physical Examination

After history taking, a woman needs a physical examination, including a pelvic examination, to confirm her general health, the presentation and position of the fetus, and the stage of cervical dilatation. In order to have an HIV test, a woman must sign additional informed consent over and above her usual health facility consent.

The physical assessment during labor begins, as does all physical assessments, with the woman's overall appearance: Does she appear tired? Pale? Ill? Frightened? Are there signs of edema or dehydration? Does she have open lesions anywhere? Be prepared to adapt further examination techniques with regard to a woman's stage of labor, frequency of contractions, and labor progression.

Be certain to palpate for enlargement of neck lymph nodes to detect the possibility of a respiratory infection. Inspect the mucous membrane of her mouth and the conjunctiva of her eyes for color to see if paleness suggests anemia. Examine her teeth for caries or abscesses because an oral infection might account for a postpartal fever. Examine the outer and inner surfaces of her lips carefully to detect herpes lesions (pinpoint vesicles on an erythematous base). Report to her primary care provider if herpetic lesions are present anywhere because, although oral lesions are invariably a type 1 herpes virus (common cold sores), type 2 (genital) herpes virus needs to be identified because this can be lethal to newborns; a woman's primary health care provider may suggest that the woman with oral herpes lesions take isolation precautions such as not kissing her newborn until the lesions crust.

Auscultate the woman's lungs to be certain they are clear of rales. Listen for normal heart sounds and rhythms as well. Many pregnant women at term have a grade 2 to 3 systolic ejection murmur because of the extra volume of blood that must cross their heart valves. Document if this is noticeable. Next, inspect and palpate her breasts. Are they free of cysts and lumps? Mark the chart of a woman who has a palpable mass in her breasts for reexamination after labor and birth. This is probably an enlarged milk gland, but needs further evaluation to be certain it is not something more serious such as a breast malignancy.

Abdominal and Lower Leg Assessment. Assessing a woman's abdomen is important to estimate fetal size by fundal height (which should be at the level of the xiphoid process at term). Palpate and percuss the bladder area (over the symphysis pubis) to detect a full bladder. Assess for abdominal scars to reveal previous abdominal or pelvic surgery that could have left adhesions.

Finally, inspect lower extremities for skin turgor to assess hydration, and also for edema and varicose veins. Women with large varicosities are more prone to thrombophlebitis after birth than other women. Severe edema suggests hypertension of pregnancy. A blood pressure 140/90 mmHg or higher can confirm this.

Determining Fetal Position, Presentation, and Lie. Four methods can be used to determine if the fetus is in an optimal position for birth:

- Determining the place on the woman's abdomen where fetal heart tones are heard strongest
- Abdominal inspection and palpation, called Leopold maneuvers
- Vaginal examination
- Sonography

Leopold Maneuvers

Leopold maneuvers are a systematic method of observation and palpation to determine fetal presentation and position and are done as part of a physical examination. Steps for this are described in Box 15.5.

BOX 15.5 Nursing Care Planning Using Procedures

LEOPOLD MANEUVERS

Purpose: Systematically observe and palpate the abdomen to determine fetal presentation and position.

PROCEDURE	PRINCIPLE
1. Explain the procedure and instruct the woman to void to empty her bladder.	1. Explanation reduces anxiety and enhances cooperation. An empty bladder promotes comfort and allows for more productive palpation because fetal contour will not be obscured by a distended bladder.
2. Wash your hands using warm water. Provide privacy.	2. Hand washing prevents the spread of possible infection. Using warm water aids in client comfort and prevents tightening of abdominal muscles during palpation.
3. Position the woman supine with knees slightly flexed. Place a small pillow or rolled towel under her left side.	3. Flexing the knees relaxes the abdominal muscles. Using a pillow or towel tilts the uterus off the vena cava, preventing supine hypotension syndrome.
4. Observe the woman's abdomen as to which is the longest diameter and where fetal movement is apparent.	4. The longest diameter (axis) is the length of the fetus. The location of activity most likely reflects the position of the feet.
5. First maneuver: Stand at the foot of the woman, facing her, and place both hands flat on her abdomen. Palpate the superior surface of the fundus. Determine consistency, shape, and mobility.	5. This maneuver determines whether the fetal head or breech is in the fundus. A head feels more firm than a breech, is round and hard, and moves independently of the body; the breech feels softer and moves only in conjunction with the body).

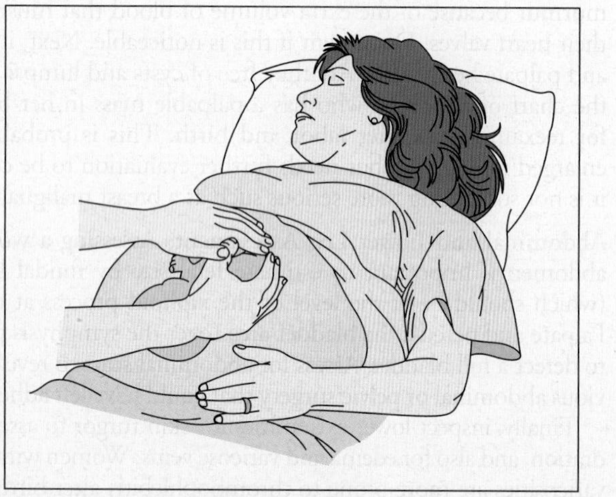

PROCEDURE	PRINCIPLE
6. Second maneuver: Face the woman, hold the left hand stationary on the left side of the uterus while you palpate with the right hand on the opposite side of the uterus from top to bottom. Repeat palpation using the opposite side.	6. This maneuver locates the back of the fetus. The fetal back feels like a smooth, hard, and resistant surface; the knees and elbows of the fetus on the opposite side feel more like a number of angular bumps or nodules.

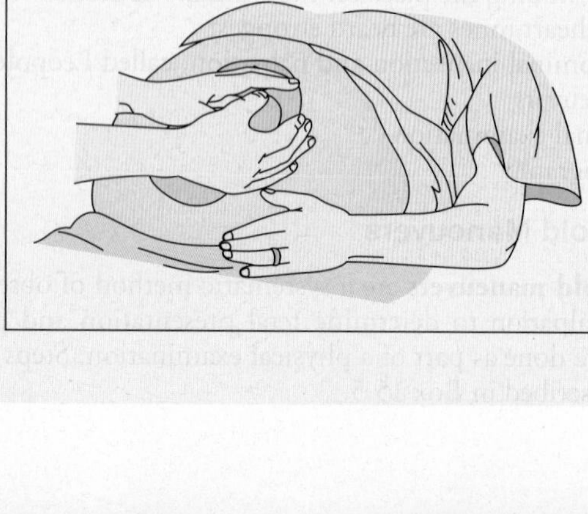

PROCEDURE	PRINCIPLE
7. Third maneuver: Gently grasp the lower portion of the abdomen just above the symphysis pubis between the thumb and fingers and try to press the thumb and finger together. Determine any movement and whether the part feels firm or soft. 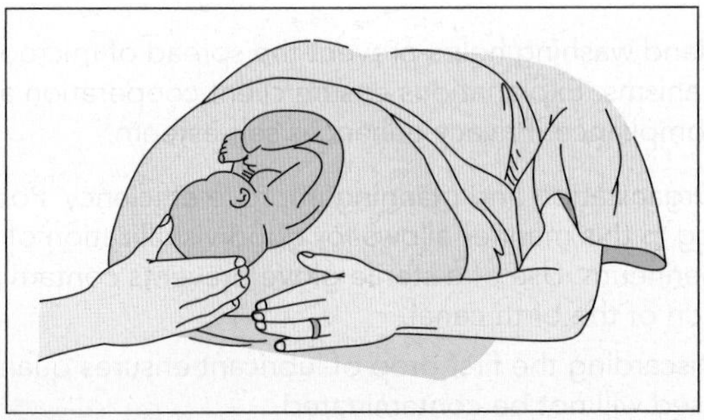	7. This maneuver determines which part of the fetus is at the inlet and its mobility. If the presenting part moves upward so your fingers and thumb can be pressed together, the presenting part is not engaged (not firmly settled into the pelvis). If the part is firm, it is the head; if soft, then it is the breech.
8. Fourth maneuver: Place fingers on both sides of the uterus approximately 2 inches above the inguinal ligaments, pressing downward and inward in the direction of the birth canal. Allow fingers to be carried downward. 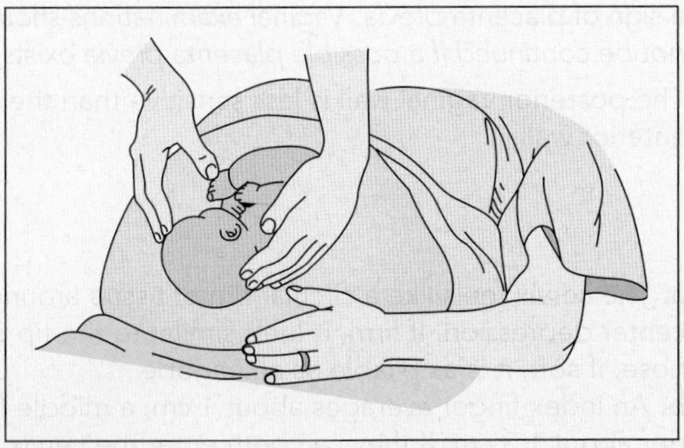	8. This maneuver is only done if the fetus is in a cephalic presentation because it determines fetal attitude and degree of fetal extension into the pelvis. The fingers of one hand will slide along the uterine contour and meet no obstruction, indicating the back of the fetal neck. The other hand will meet an obstruction an inch or so above the ligament—this is the fetal brow. The position of the fetal brow should correspond to the side of the uterus that contained the elbows and knees of the fetus. If the fetus is in a poor attitude, the examining fingers will meet an obstruction on the same side as the fetal back; that is, the fingers will touch the hyperextended head. If the brow is very easily palpated (as if it lies just under the skin), the fetus is probably in a posterior position (the occiput is pointing toward the woman's back).

The Vaginal Examination

A vaginal examination is necessary to determine the extent of cervical softening, effacement, and dilatation and to confirm the fetal presentation, position, and degree of descent. These are traditionally done by the primary care provider, but, if not available, can be done by a nurse skilled in the technique. Responsibilities for helping with a vaginal examination during labor are shown in Box 15.6.

Vaginal examinations are best done between contractions. Although more of the fetal skull can be palpated during a contraction, because the cervix retracts more at that time, an examination during a contraction is more uncomfortable and rarely is justified by the additional amount of information gained. A palpation of membranes during a contraction, when they are under pressure, also can cause them to rupture.

Women are anxious to have frequent reports during labor to reassure them that everything is progressing well, but vaginal exams should be kept to a minimum to prevent infection. The woman's primary care provider will tell a woman immediately after an examination about her progress. If giving a progress report, remember that most women are aware of the word dilatation but not effacement. Just saying, "no further dilatation," therefore, is a depressing report. "You're not dilated a lot more, but a lot of thinning is happening and that's just as important" is the same report given in a positive manner. After a vaginal examination, plot the new degree of dilatation and descent of the presenting part on a labor progress graph, as described earlier.

Vaginal examinations should not be done in the presence of fresh bleeding, because fresh bleeding may indicate that a placenta previa (implantation of the placenta so low in the uterus that it is encroaching on the cervical os) is present. Performing a vaginal examination in this instance might tear the placenta and cause hemorrhage, resulting in danger to both the mother and fetus. Make certain a primary care provider knows about the fresh bleeding before attempting a vaginal examination.

Women from cultures where female circumcision is allowed may have tightened or obstructed vaginal openings from scarring, which can make a vaginal exam painful. Note this because it also indicates a woman may need a cesarean birth to prevent perineal tearing if her vagina cannot dilate adequately.

BOX 15.6 Nursing Care Planning Using Procedures

ASSISTING WITH A VAGINAL EXAMINATION

Purpose: Determine cervical readiness for labor and fetal position and presentation.

PROCEDURE	PRINCIPLE
1. Wash your hands, and explain the procedure to the client. Provide privacy.	1. Hand washing helps prevent the spread of microorganisms. Explanations ensure client cooperation and compliance. Privacy enhances self-esteem.
2. Assemble equipment, including sterile examining gloves, sterile lubricant, and gauze squares. Ask the woman to turn onto her back with knees flexed (a dorsal recumbent position).	2. Organization and planning improve efficiency. Positioning in this manner allows for good visualization of the perineum. Use of a sterile glove prevents contamination of the birth canal.
3. Discard one drop of clean lubricating solution and drop an ample supply on tips of gloved fingers of examiner.	3. Discarding the first drop of lubricant ensures quantity used will not be contaminated.
4. The examiner places a hand on the outer edges of the woman's vulva and spread her labia while inspecting for lesions. Help look for red, irritated mucous membranes; open, ulcerated sores; and clustered, pinpoint vesicles.	4. Presence of any lesions may indicate an infection and may possibly preclude vaginal birth.
5. Note any fluid escaping from the vagina that could be amniotic fluid, in addition to the presence of the umbilical cord or bleeding.	5. Amniotic fluid implies membranes have ruptured and the umbilical cord may have prolapsed. Bleeding may be a sign of placenta previa. *Vaginal examinations should not be continued if a possible placenta previa exists.*
6. If there is no bleeding or cord visible, the examiner stabilizes the uterus by placing a hand on the woman's abdomen, then introducing the index and middle fingers of the other hand into the vagina, directing them toward the posterior vaginal wall.	6. The posterior vaginal wall is less sensitive than the anterior wall.
7. The examiner touches the cervix with gloved fingers to assess: **a.** Cervical consistency, position, and rate if *firm* or *soft*. **b.** Extent of dilatation and whether an anterior rim or lip of cervix is present. 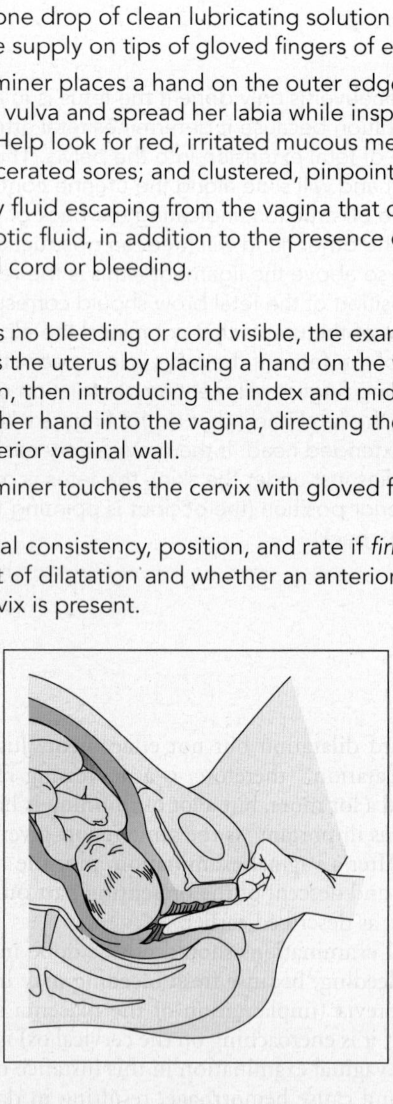 **c.** Estimate the degree of effacement. **d.** Estimate whether membranes are intact.	7. **a.** The cervix feels like a circular rim of tissue around a center depression. If firm, it feels similar to the tip of a nose; if soft, it is as pliable as an earlobe. **b.** An index finger averages about 1 cm; a middle finger about 1.5 cm. If they can both enter the cervix, the cervix is dilated 2.5 to 3 cm. If there would be room for double the width of two fingers, the dilatation is about 5 to 6 cm. When the space is four times the width of two fingertips, dilatation is complete at 10 cm. **c.** Effacement is estimated in a percentage depending on thickness. A cervix before labor is 2 to 2.5 cm thick. If it is only 1 cm thick, it is 50% effaced. If it is tissue paper thin, it is 100% effaced. With a 100% effaced cervix, dilatation is difficult to feel because the edges of the cervix are so thin. **d.** The membranes (with a slight amount of amniotic fluid in front of the presenting part) assume the shape of a watch crystal. With a contraction, they bulge forward, become prominent, and can be felt much more readily.

PROCEDURE	PRINCIPLE
8. Next, the examiner locates the ischial spines, identifies the presenting part, and rates the station of the fetus.	8. Ischial spines are palpated as notches at the 4 and 8 o'clock positions of the pelvic outlet. Station is the number of centimeters above or below the spines the presenting fetal part has reached. Identifying the presenting part confirms findings obtained with Leopold maneuvers. The vertex has a hard, smooth feel. Fetal hair may be palpable but massed together and wet, and it may be difficult to appreciate through gloves. Palpating the two fontanelles, one diamond-shaped and one triangular, helps identification. Buttocks feel softer and give under fingertip pressure. Identifying the anus may be possible because the sphincter action will "trap" an examining finger.
9. Next is establishment of the fetal position.	9. The fontanelle palpated is invariably the posterior one because the fetus maintains a flexed position, presenting the posterior not the anterior fontanelle. If it points toward an anterior quadrant, the position is ROA or LOA. In a breech presentation, the anus can serve as a marker for position.
10. Upon withdrawal of the examining hand, help wipe the perineum front to back to remove secretions or examining lubricant. Help client return to side or sit up.	10. Wiping front to back prevents moving rectal contamination forward to the vagina. Side lying or sitting helps prevent supine hypotension syndrome.
11. Document procedure, assessment findings, and how client tolerated procedure.	11. Documentation provides a means for communication and evaluation of care and client outcomes.

Sonography

Although not routine, sonography may be used to determine the diameters of the fetal skull and to determine presentation, position, flexion, and degree of descent of a fetus at the beginning of labor. This is usually done by a portable unit, but if it's necessary for a woman to be transported to another department to have this done, be certain someone accompanies her, so, if labor should become more active, she can be returned quickly to the labor or birth service for needed care.

Assessing Rupture of Membranes

One out of every four labors begins with spontaneous rupture of the fetal membranes. When this occurs, a woman feels a sudden gush or a slow trickle of amniotic fluid from her vagina. This is a startling sensation for most women because it feels as if she has lost bladder control. She may feel embarrassed before she realizes the warm fluid on her perineum and legs is not urine but an unexpected announcement that labor is beginning. If the fluid expelled was only a small amount, there may be a question as to whether the membranes have ruptured.

A sterile vaginal examination using a sterile speculum usually reveals whether amniotic fluid is present in the vagina. After vaginal secretions are obtained with a sterile, cotton-tipped applicator, test them with a strip of Nitrazine paper. Vaginal secretions are usually acid; amniotic fluid, in contrast, is alkaline. If amniotic fluid has passed through the vagina recently, the pH of the vaginal fluid will probably be alkaline (greater than 6.5) when tested by Nitrazine paper (appears blue-green or gray to deep blue). A false blue reading may occur in a woman with intact membranes who has a heavy, bloody show because blood is also alkaline. An additional test that can be done is a fern test (examination of vaginal secretions under a microscope). Because of its high estrogen content, amniotic fluid will show a fern pattern (see Chapter 5, Fig. 5.13A) when dried and examined in this way; urine will not.

If the woman's membranes ruptured at home, ask her to describe the color of the amniotic fluid, the amount, the odor, and the approximate time of rupture. Amniotic fluid should be clear as water. Yellow-stained fluid suggests a blood incompatibility between the mother and fetus (the amniotic fluid is bilirubin stained from the breakdown of red blood cells). Green fluid suggests meconium staining. Although meconium staining is normal in breech births because of compression of the buttocks, in a vertex presentation, it may indicate fetal anoxia. Either way, a fetus with meconium staining needs immediate assessment. After birth, the infant continues to need close assessment at birth to rule out possible meconium aspiration (Swarnam, Soraisham, & Sivanandan, 2012). If the fluid is malodorous, there could be an infection. If membranes rupture during labor, assess FHR immediately to be certain the umbilical cord hasn't prolapsed and is now being compressed against the cervix by the fetal head. The time of rupture is important because the potential time clock for an infection begins with ruptured membranes. It's preferable if the baby is born within 24 hours of rupture to reduce the risk of infection.

Assessment of Pelvic Adequacy

Evaluating pelvic adequacy using internal conjugate and ischial tuberosity diameters is generally done during pregnancy either manually or by sonogram, so, by weeks 32 to 36 of pregnancy, a primary care provider can be alerted that cephalopelvic disproportion could occur. Because the diameters obtained during pregnancy have not changed, they are not retaken if already obtained.

Vital Signs

Vital signs are taken at the beginning and then periodically during labor, as summarized in Table 15.4.

TABLE 15.4 Typical Time Intervals for Nursing Interventions During the First Stage of Labor

Intervention	Assessment on Admission	Latent Phase (0–3 cm)	Active Phase (4–7 cm)	Transition Phase (8–10 cm)
Assess and Record				
Temperature	X	q4h (unless membranes are ruptured, then q2h)	q4h (unless membranes are ruptured, then q2h)	q4h (unless membranes are ruptured, then q2h)
Pulse	X	q30–60 min	q30–60 min	q15–30 min
Respirations	X	q30–60 min	q30–60 min	q15–30 min
Blood pressure	X	q30–60 min	q30–60 min	q15–30 min
Voiding	X	q2h	q2h	q2h
Fetal heart rate	X	q30–60 min	q15–30 min	q15–30 min
Contractions	X	q30–60 min	q15–30 min	q10–15 min
Perineum	X	q30–60 min	q30 min	q15 min
Provide				
Ambulation and change of position	X	Continuously; question if membranes rupture	Continuously; question if membranes rupture	Continuously
Support	X	Continuously	Continuously	Continuously

Temperature. Temperature is usually obtained every 4 hours during labor. Report a temperature greater than 99°F (37.2°C) because it may indicate the development of infection. Unless there are accompanying symptoms, however, temperature elevation in a woman who has taken little fluid by mouth usually reflects dehydration (urge her to drink at least sips of water to maintain hydration). After rupture of the membranes, temperature should be taken every 2 hours because the possibility for infection markedly increases after that time.

Pulse and Respiration. The pulse and respiration rate should be measured and recorded at the same time intervals as temperature. A woman's pulse may be rapid on admission because she is nervous and anxious. After she has become better acquainted with her surroundings and has been assured everything is going well, her pulse usually falls in a range between 70 and 80 beats/min. A persistent pulse rate of more than 100 beats/min could be tachycardia from dehydration or hemorrhage and so needs investigation. Respiratory rate during labor is usually 18 to 20 breaths/min. Do not count respirations during contractions because women tend to breathe rapidly from pain. Conversely, if a woman is using controlled breathing to decrease pain in labor, her respiration rate during contractions can be abnormally slow.

Observe for hyperventilation (rapid, deep respirations) because prolonged hyperventilation can cause a "blowing off" of carbon dioxide and accompanying symptoms of dizziness and tingling of hands and feet. Rebreathing into a paper bag and reassurance the feeling is normal help to reverse this process.

Blood Pressure. Blood pressure is usually measured and recorded every 4 hours as well. As with pulse and respirations, measure blood pressure between contractions, both for a woman's comfort and for accuracy, because maternal blood pressure tends to rise 5 to 15 mmHg during a contraction. An increase in blood pressure at other times is potentially dangerous because it may indicate the development of hypertension of pregnancy. A decrease in blood pressure or a decrease in the pulse pressure (the difference between the systolic and diastolic pressures) may indicate hemorrhage. If a woman received an analgesic agent (such as meperidine), which tends to cause hypotension, check her blood pressure approximately 15 minutes after administration to be certain extreme hypotension did not occur.

Laboratory Analysis

Most women have some preliminary laboratory studies done in early labor.

Blood. Blood is drawn for hemoglobin and hematocrit, a serologic test for syphilis (Venereal Disease Research Laboratory [VDRL] test), hepatitis B antibodies, and blood typing to determine whether a blood incompatibility is likely to exist in the newborn and what type of blood will need to be supplied if the woman should have an acute blood loss. If a woman gives permission for HIV testing, blood for this will be drawn as well.

Urine. Obtain a clean-catch urine specimen and test it at the point of care for protein and glucose, then send it to the laboratory for a complete urinalysis. If a woman reports any symptoms that suggest a urinary tract infection such as burning on urination, blood in urine, extreme frequency, or flank pain, obtain a clean-catch specimen for culture. A woman in labor is able to void most easily if she is allowed to use a bathroom. However, if a woman has ruptured membranes, check whether she should ambulate to a bathroom until it is confirmed the fetal head is well engaged so gravity does not cause a prolapsed cord. Use a bedpan or receptacle placed on a commode to collect any material passed from the vagina so this can be assessed as well.

The Assessment of Uterine Contractions

Depending on the hospital or birthing center policy, most women are monitored by an external contraction monitor for about 10 minutes in early labor. The monitor is then removed and contractions are assessed intermittently by Doppler because extensive electronic monitoring has not shown to lower fetal mortality with low-risk women, limits mobility, and can lead to an increase in cesarean birth (Barber et al., 2011). The use of internal fetal monitoring is reserved for high-risk pregnancies and is described in Chapter 24.

Length of Contractions. To determine the length of a contraction with a monitor in place, simply observe the rhythm strip and, using the time line, count the number of seconds the contraction lasted. To determine the beginning of a contraction without a monitor, rest a hand on a woman's abdomen at the fundus of the uterus very gently until you sense the gradual tensing and upward rising of the fundus that accompanies a contraction (Fig. 15.13). Time the duration of the contraction from the moment the uterus first tenses until it has relaxed again. It is possible to palpate this tensing approximately 5 seconds before the woman is able to feel the contraction because contractions become palpable when the intrauterine pressure reaches approximately 20 mmHg. However, the pain of a contraction is not usually felt until pressure reaches approximately 25 mmHg.

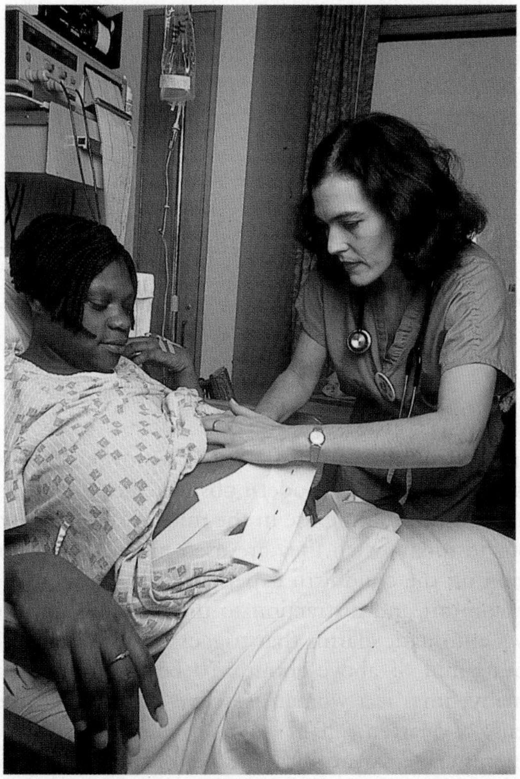

FIGURE 15.13 Contractions can be assessed by very gently placing a hand over the fundus of the uterus.

Intensity of Contractions. The intensity of a contraction refers to its strength. On a monitor, this is the height of the waveform. If you are assessing manually, rate a contraction according to:

- Mild, if the uterus does not feel more than minimally tense
- Moderate, if the uterus feels firm
- Strong, if the uterus feels as hard as a wooden board or you are unable to indent the uterus with your fingertips at the peak of the contraction

After estimating either the intensity or duration of a contraction, recheck the fundus at the conclusion of the contraction to be certain it does relax and becomes soft to the touch again. This demonstrates that the uterus is not in continuous contraction but is providing a relaxation time, during which placental blood vessels can fill to supply the fetus with adequate oxygen.

Frequency of Contractions. Lastly, time the frequency of contractions or how often they are occurring. Frequency is timed from the beginning of one contraction to the beginning of the next (see Fig. 15.10).

Use as light a touch as possible on a woman's abdomen while evaluating contractions or estimating their strength manually. Otherwise, the uterine fundus can become tender if it has to push against the extra weight of a hand with each contraction, creating unnecessary discomfort for a woman in labor.

What if...15.2 Celeste Bailey refuses to have any electronic fetal monitoring. Would this worry you? Would you try to convince her she needs this?

The Initial Fetal Assessment

Although fairly passive in labor, a fetus is subjected to extreme pressure by uterine contractions and passage through the birth canal, so it is important to ascertain that the FHR remains within normal limits despite these pressures.

Auscultation of Fetal Heart Sounds

Fetal heart sounds are transmitted best through the convex portion of a fetus because that is the part that lies in closest contact with the uterine wall.

- In a vertex or breech presentation, fetal heart sounds are usually best heard through the fetal back.
- In a face presentation, the back becomes concave so the sounds are best heard through the more convex thorax.
- In breech presentations, fetal heart sounds are heard most clearly high in the uterus, at a woman's umbilicus or above.
- In cephalic presentations, they are heard loudest low in a woman's abdomen.
- In an ROA position, sounds are heard best in the right lower quadrant.
- In an LOA position, sounds are heard best in the left lower quadrant.
- In posterior positions (LOP or ROP), heart sounds may be loudest at a woman's side.

Figure 15.14 illustrates where fetal heart sounds radiate best from various fetal positions.

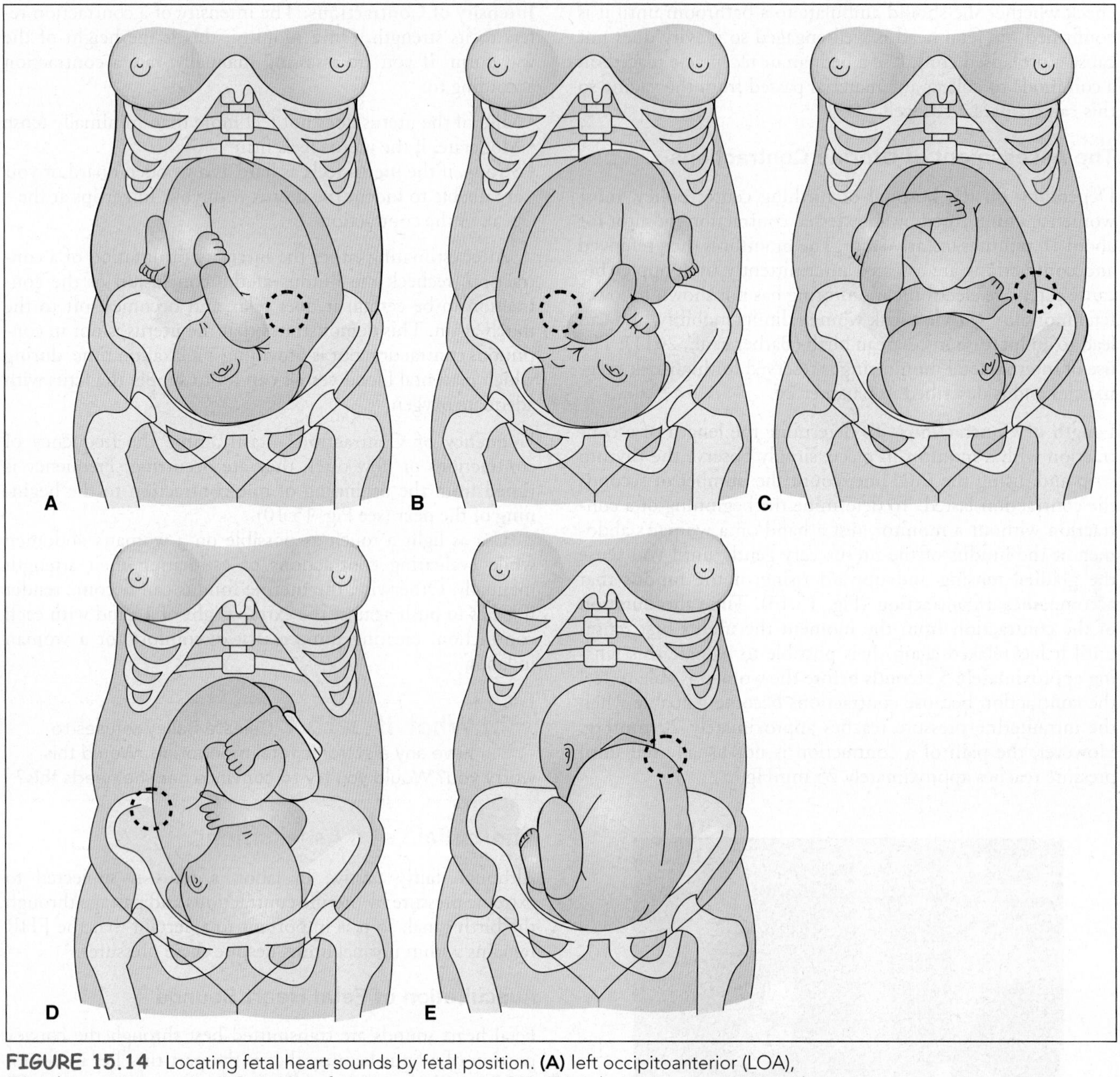

FIGURE 15.14 Locating fetal heart sounds by fetal position. **(A)** left occipitoanterior (LOA), **(B)** right occipitoanterior (ROA), **(C)** Left occipitoposterior (LOP), **(D)** right occipitoposterior, and **(E)** left sacroanterior (LSaA).

Hearing fetal heart sounds in these positions not only confirms that the fetus is responding well to labor but also provides confirmatory information about fetal position. Conversely, recognizing fetal position aids in locating fetal heart sounds.

As a rule, determine the FHR every 30 minutes during beginning latent labor, every 15 minutes during active first stage labor, and every 5 minutes during the second stage of labor. This can be done by inspecting an FHR monitoring strip or by periodic auscultation by a fetoscope (a modified stethoscope attached to a headpiece), a Pinard stethoscope (a hollow tube that directs sound into the ear), or a Doppler unit (which uses ultrasound waves that bounce off the fetal heart to produce echoes or clicking noises, which reflect the fetal heart beat [Fig. 15.15]) as labor progresses.

Electronic Monitoring

The use of fetal monitors in labor has provoked one of the biggest controversies in modern obstetric health care as their use moved from routine use in the mid-1970s for all women in labor to today when they are used judiciously to prevent intrusion on the childbirth experience and to prevent needless discomfort and distraction to the mother. Monitors are set with automatic alarms that trigger if an FHR goes below 110 beats/min or above about 170 beats/min and so may ring many times if a woman is active in labor (Jacquemyn, Martens, & Martens, 2012). This causes their use to result in unnecessary cesarean births as well as frightened parents (which could adversely affect early parent–infant bonding).

Monitoring does offer advantages from a health care provider's standpoint because observing the FHR on a monitor

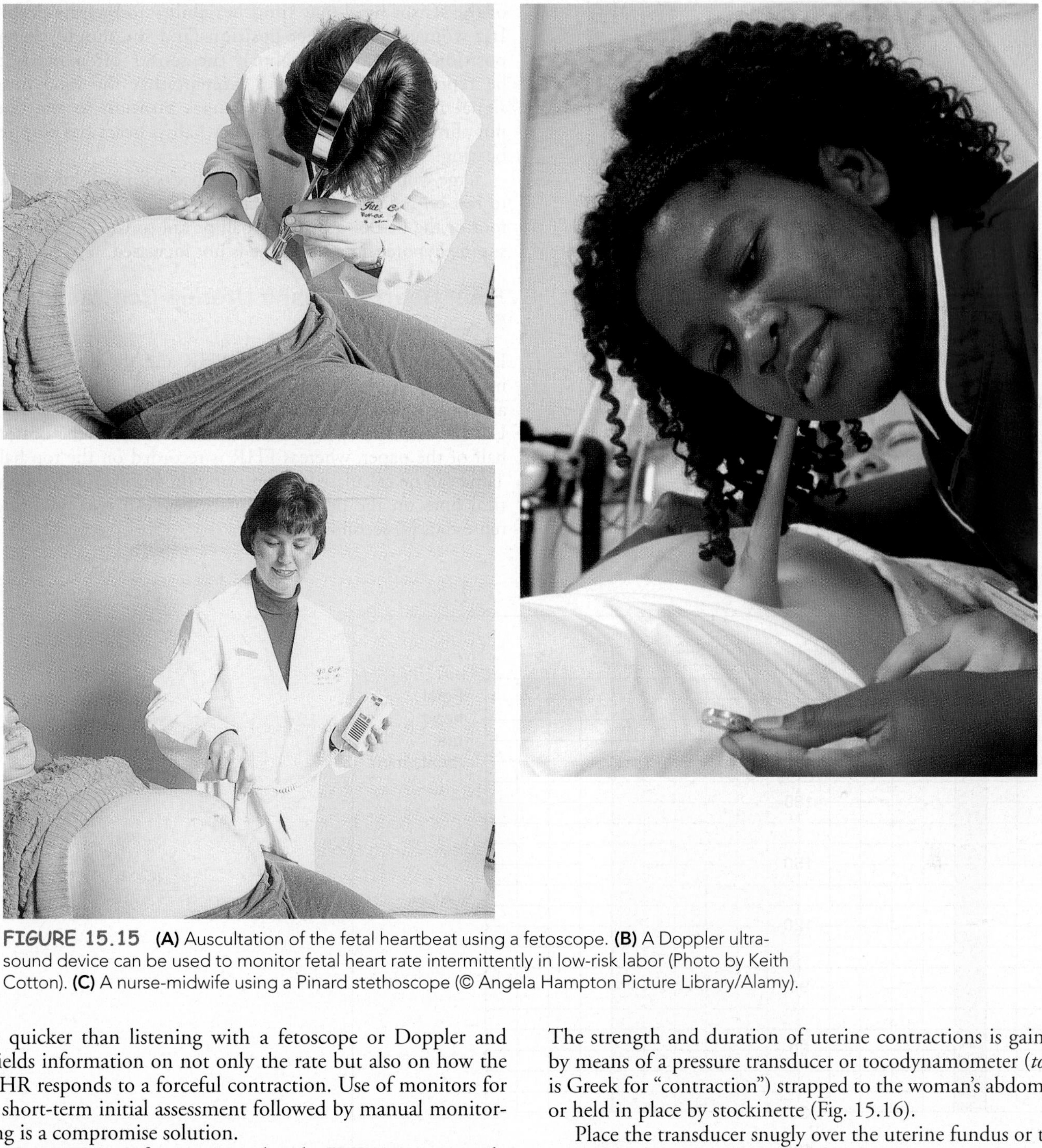

A

B

C

FIGURE 15.15 **(A)** Auscultation of the fetal heartbeat using a fetoscope. **(B)** A Doppler ultrasound device can be used to monitor fetal heart rate intermittently in low-risk labor (Photo by Keith Cotton). **(C)** A nurse-midwife using a Pinard stethoscope (© Angela Hampton Picture Library/Alamy).

is quicker than listening with a fetoscope or Doppler and yields information on not only the rate but also on how the FHR responds to a forceful contraction. Use of monitors for a short-term initial assessment followed by manual monitoring is a compromise solution.

Be certain to inform parents that the FHR can vary greatly during labor so they're not surprised when they see this, and also that a monitor is only an aid and should not be the focus of their attention. Otherwise, a couple can become so focused on a monitor screen or paper strip that they lose the ability to concentrate on previously learned relaxation and breathing techniques. When giving care, be sure not to focus solely on the equipment, continue to communicate to the couple, not the machine, and offer support to the woman and her partner as needed.

Initial Electronic Monitoring

Electronic monitoring is noninvasive, easily applied, and does not require cervical dilatation or fetal descent before it can be used, so it can be introduced at any time during labor. The strength and duration of uterine contractions is gained by means of a pressure transducer or tocodynamometer (*toko* is Greek for "contraction") strapped to the woman's abdomen or held in place by stockinette (Fig. 15.16).

Place the transducer snugly over the uterine fundus or the area where contractions are most easily felt. The transducer works to convert the pressure originated by the contraction into an electronic signal that is then recorded on graph paper.

The FHR is monitored with the use of an ultrasonic sensor or monitor (see Fig. 15.16) also strapped against a woman's abdomen at the level of the fetal chest. The small Doppler unit converts fetal heart movements into audible beeping sounds and also records them on graph paper.

A woman who is worried something will happen to her child during labor can find it reassuring to listen to the regular beeping sound of an undistressed fetal heartbeat from a fetal heart transducer. Many women ask for and can have a short graph tracing to save for their baby book.

A disadvantage is the woman may feel discomfort from the straps holding the monitors in place, and the snugness

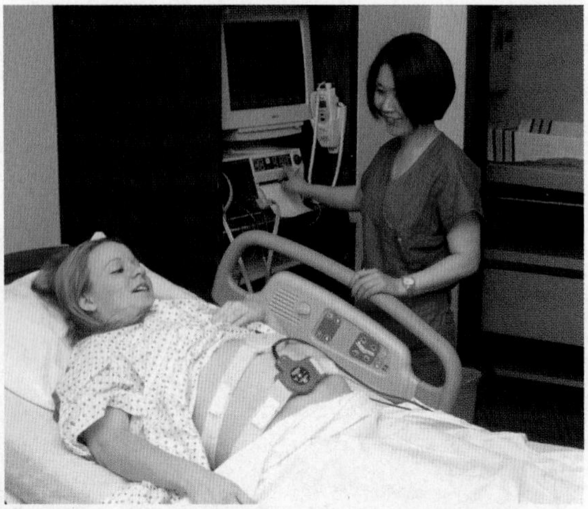

FIGURE 15.16 External electronic monitoring in place. Two devices (a transducer for the uterus and an ultrasound sensor for the fetus) are strapped to the woman's abdomen.

of the sensor head may limit her ability to breathe deeply. If a woman changes her position (and she should change position often during labor), the sensor often needs to be repositioned. Remind a woman that the fetal heart signal may stop when she changes position so she does not think by the silence that her baby's heart has stopped beating.

Urge women not to lie on their backs for monitoring but to rest on their side, sit in a chair, or bend forward over the foot of the bed or a birthing ball or rail so the likelihood of supine hypotension syndrome is not increased.

Fetal Heart Rate and Uterine Contraction Records

Labor monitors trace both the FHR and the duration and interval of uterine contractions onto an oscilloscope screen and produce a permanent record on paper rolls (Fig. 15.17). Uterine contraction information is recorded on the bottom half of the paper, whereas FHR is recorded on the top half. Time can be calculated by counting the number of bold vertical lines on the paper (the space between two bold lines represents 60 seconds).

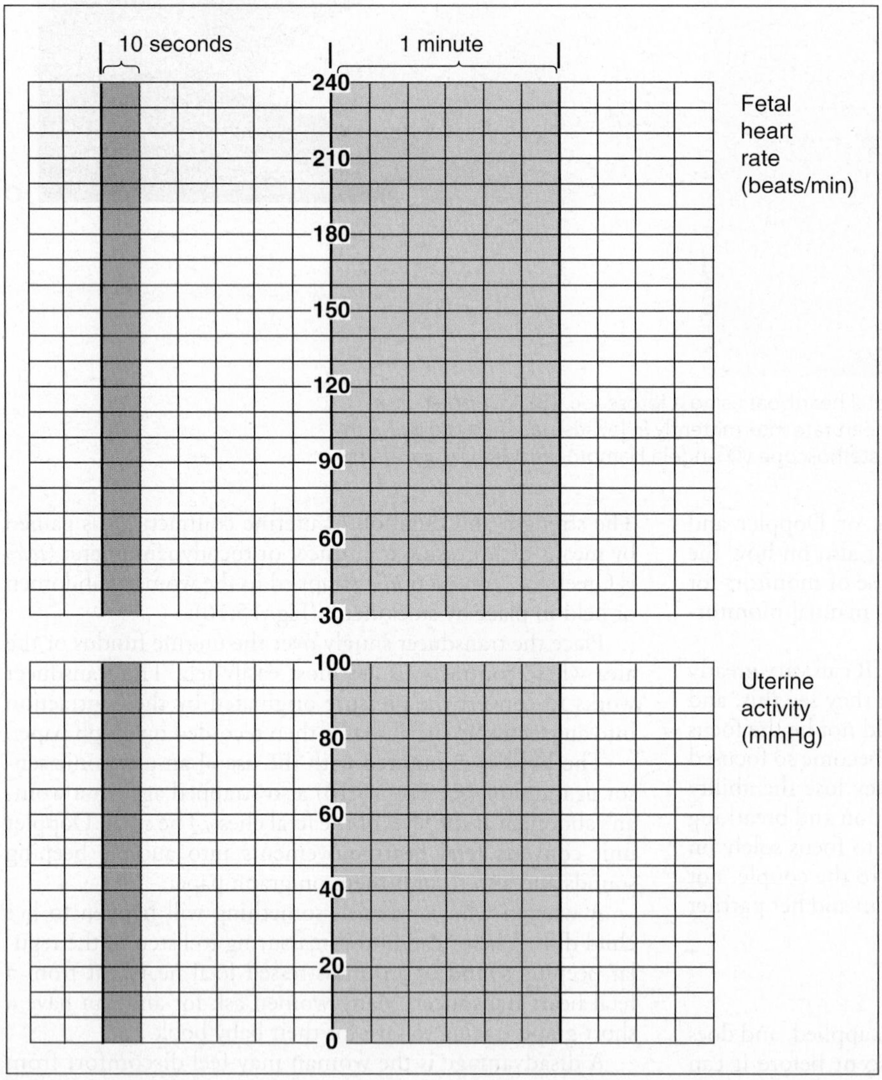

FIGURE 15.17 A paper strip for recording electronic fetal monitoring data.

Fetal Heart Rate Parameters

Assessing and interpreting FHR patterns involves evaluating three parameters: the baseline rate, variabilities in the baseline rate, and periodic changes in the rate (acceleration and deceleration) (Penna, 2011).

The Baseline Fetal Heart Rate

A baseline FHR is determined by analyzing the pace of fetal heartbeats recorded in a minimum of 2 minutes obtained between contractions. A normal rate is 110 to 160 beats/min.

Variability

FHR variability or the difference between the highest and lowest heart rates shown on a strip is one of the most reliable indicators of fetal well-being. Variability is reflected on an FHR tracing as a slight irregularity or "jitter" to the wave. The degree of baseline variability increases (5 to 15 beats/min) when a fetus moves; it slows if a fetus sleeps. If no variability is present, it indicates the natural pacemaker activity of the fetal heart (effects of the sympathetic and parasympathetic nervous systems) may be affected. This may occur as a response to narcotics or barbiturates administered to a woman in labor, but the possibility of fetal hypoxia and acidosis must also be considered and investigated. Very immature fetuses show diminished baseline variability because of a reduced nervous system response to stimulation and immature cardiac node function.

Variability should be recorded as:

- Absent: No amplitude range is detectable.
- Minimal: Amplitude range is detectable but is 5 beats/min or fewer.
- Moderate (normal): Amplitude range is 6 to 25 beats/min.
- Marked: Amplitude range is greater than 25 beats/min.

Other patterns in the baseline rate that can be detected include fetal bradycardia (FHR is lower than 110 beats/min for 10 minutes) and fetal tachycardia (FHR is faster than 160 beats/min for a 10-minute period).

- Moderate bradycardia is 100 to 109 beats/min and is not considered serious, probably due to a vagal response elicited by compression of the fetal head during labor.
- Marked bradycardia (less than 100 beats/min) is a sign of possible hypoxia and is potentially dangerous.
- Moderate tachycardia is 161 to 180 beats/min.
- Marked tachycardia is a rate greater than 180 beats/min. Marked fetal tachycardia may be caused by fetal hypoxia, maternal fever, an effect of maternal drugs, fetal arrhythmia, or maternal anemia or hyperthyroidism. In all instances, the cause needs to be investigated to ensure the fetus does not become exhausted by maintaining this rapid heart rate.

Periodic Changes

Periodic changes or fluctuations in FHR occur in response to contractions and fetal movement and are described in terms of *accelerations* or *decelerations*. Periodic changes are short-term changes in rate other than baseline; they last from a few seconds to 1 or 2 minutes.

Accelerations. Nonperiodic accelerations are temporary normal increases in FHR caused by fetal movement, a change in maternal position, or administration of an analgesic.

- An acceleration is a visually apparent abrupt increase (onset to peak in less than 30 seconds) in the FHR.
- At 32 weeks of gestation and beyond, an acceleration has a peak of 15 beats/min or more above baseline with a duration of 15 seconds or more but less than 2 minutes from onset to return.
- Before 32 weeks of gestation, an acceleration has a peak of 10 beats/min or more above baseline, with a duration of 10 seconds or more but less than 2 minutes from onset to return.
- Prolonged acceleration lasts 2 minutes or more but less than 10 minutes in duration.
- If an acceleration lasts 10 minutes or longer, it is a baseline change or a new baseline is established.

Decelerations. Decelerations are visually apparent, usually symmetrical, periodic decreases in FHR resulting from pressure on the fetal head during contractions as parasympathetic stimulation in response to vagal nerve compression brings about a slowing of FHR. Early deceleration follows the pattern of the contraction, beginning when the contraction begins and ending when the contraction ends. However, the waveform of the FHR change is the inverse of the contraction waveform, or the lowest point of the deceleration occurs with the peak of the contraction (a mirror image of the contraction). The rate rarely falls below 100 beats/min, and it returns quickly to between 110 and 160 beats/min at the end of the contraction (Fig. 15.18).

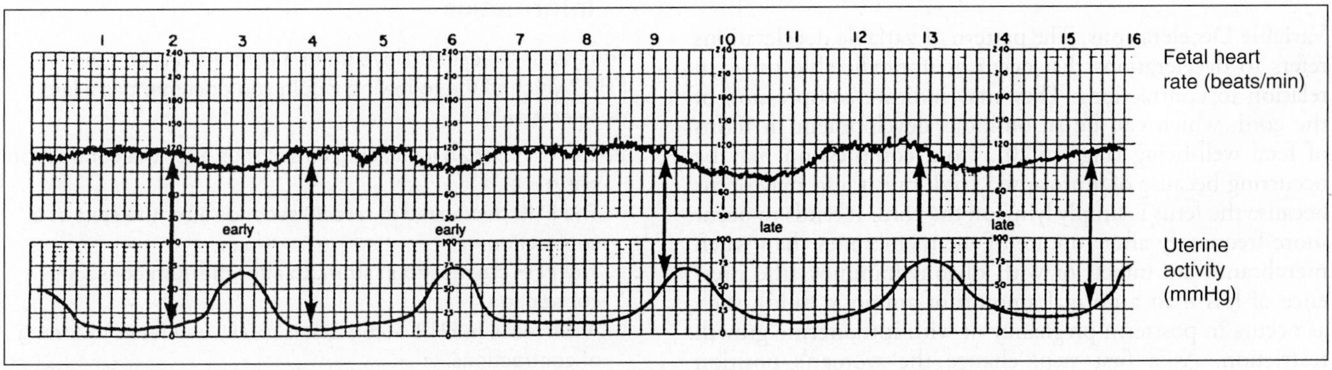

FIGURE 15.18 Early fetal heart rate deceleration (the time between 2 and 4 seconds) follows the pattern of the contraction starting when the contraction begins and ending when the contraction subsides. This is a normal pattern of a healthy fetus.

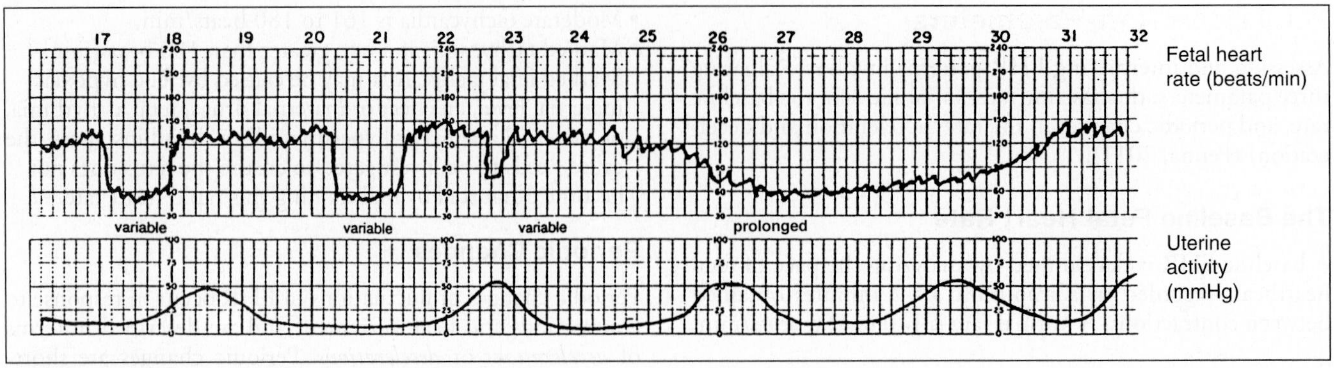

FIGURE 15.19 Late deceleration (the time between 20 and 22 seconds) occurs after the peak of a contraction and continues beyond the end of the contraction. This is an ominous pattern in labor because it suggests the fetus is growing short of oxygen. The prolonged deceleration (between 26 and 31 seconds) is also ominous.

Early decelerations normally occur late in labor, when the head has descended fairly low; they are viewed as innocent. If they occur early in labor, before the head has fully descended, the head compression causing the waveform change could be the result of cephalopelvic disproportion and is a cause to investigate.

Late Decelerations. Late decelerations are those that are delayed until 30 to 40 seconds after the onset of a contraction and continue beyond the end of a contraction (see Fig. 15.9). This is an ominous pattern in labor, because it suggests uteroplacental insufficiency or decreased blood flow through the intervillous spaces of the uterus during uterine contractions. This pattern may occur with marked hypertonia or increased uterine tone. Immediately change the woman's position from supine if she is lying down to lateral to relieve pressure on the vena cava and supply more blood to the uterus and fetus. Intravenous fluid or oxygen may be prescribed. Prepare for a prompt cesarean birth of the infant if the late decelerations persist or if FHR variability becomes abnormal (absent or decreased).

Prolonged Decelerations. Prolonged decelerations are decelerations that are a decrease from the FHR baseline of 15 beats/min or more and last longer than 2 to 3 minutes but less than 10 minutes. They generally reflect an isolated occurrence, but they may signify a significant event, such as cord compression or maternal hypotension. For this reason, they must be reported and documented. If a deceleration lasts longer than 10 minutes, it is considered a baseline change.

Variable Decelerations. The pattern of variable decelerations refers to decelerations that occur at unpredictable times in relation to contractions. They may indicate compression of the cord, which can be an ominous development in terms of fetal well-being (Fig. 15.20). Cord compression may be occurring because of a prolapsed cord, but it also may occur because the fetus is simply lying on the cord. It tends to occur more frequently after rupture of the membranes than when membranes are intact, or with oligohydramnios (the presence of less than a normal amount of amniotic fluid), such as occurs in postterm pregnancy or with intrauterine growth restriction. As a first step, change the woman's position from supine to lateral if she is not already lying on her side. If a prolapsed cord is diagnosed as the cause of the variable decelerations, oxygen will be prescribed as well as changing her position to a knee-to-chest one to help relieve pressure on the cord. Because a prolapsed cord is a potential serious complication of labor, nursing care and outcomes are further discussed in Chapter 23.

The Sinusoidal Pattern

In a fetus who is severely anemic or hypoxic, central nervous system control of heart pacing may be so impaired that the FHR pattern resembles a smooth, frequently undulating wave with a cycle frequency of 3 to 5 per minute and persisting 20 minutes or more. Although the cause of this pattern is poorly understood, it is recognized to be as ominous as a late deceleration or variable deceleration pattern and so needs to be reported. For unknown reasons, on occasion, especially after administration of a narcotic to the mother, a *pseudo*sinusoidal or false sinusoidal pattern may appear. These are usually transient, resolve spontaneously without intervention, and are associated with a good fetal outcome. The pattern may show some variability and perhaps an FHR acceleration. Identifying these is equally important so they can be differentiated from a true sinusoidal pattern.

FHR baseline, variability, and patterns are categorized from 1 to 3 to help establish if a deviation is serious. Knowing these helps you to understand why interventions are initiated at certain points (Table 15.5).

QSEN Checkpoint Question 15.6

Informatics

You assess Celeste Bailey's uterine contractions and the FHR. Which of the following would you document as a late deceleration?

a. The FHR began increasing 45 seconds after the contraction was over.
b. The FHR decreased in rate 30 seconds after the start of a contraction.
c. The FHR decreased in strength after the 10th consecutive contraction.
d. A decrease in FHR occurs but is totally unrelated to timing of contractions.

Look in Appendix A for the best answer and rationale.

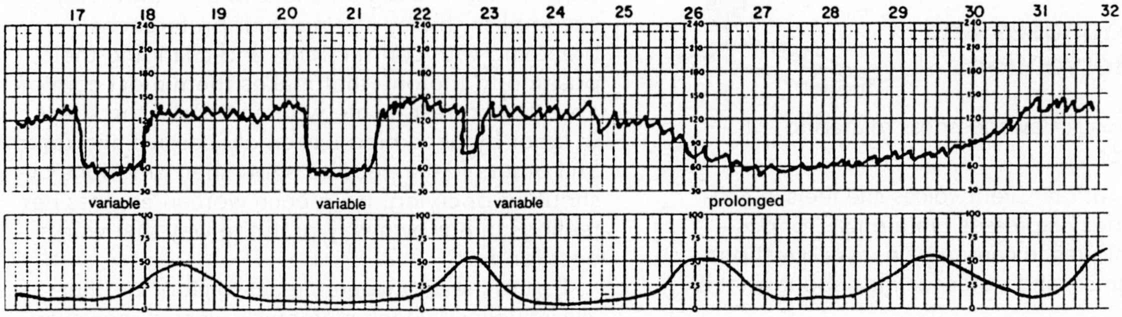

FIGURE 15.20 A fetal heart rate (FHR) showing variable and prolonged decelerations. Note the abrupt drop in FHR in both types of decelerations. The variable decelerations return to baseline more quickly than the prolonged deceleration at 26 to 31 minutes, however.

THE CARE OF A WOMAN DURING THE FIRST STAGE OF LABOR

Labor and birth are natural processes, so the average woman should be able to complete labor and birth without assistance from medical interventions. Nurses can be instrumental in keeping labor as free of unnecessary interventions as possible so it remains not only safe but also a joyful and memorable experience (Association of Women's Health, Obstetric and Neonatal Nurses [AWHONN], 2011). Six major concepts that make labor and birth as natural as possible include the following:

- Labor should begin on its own, not be artificially induced.
- Women should be able to move about freely throughout labor, not be confined to bed.
- Women should receive continuous support from a caring support person during labor.
- No interventions such as intravenous fluid should be used routinely.
- Women should be allowed to assume a nonsupine position such as upright and side lying for birth.
- Mother and baby should be housed together after the birth, with unlimited opportunity for breastfeeding (Amis, 2010).

Because the first stage of labor begins with the start of uterine contractions and takes hours to complete, most women have been having labor contractions for hours before they arrive at a birthing center or hospital. This means, most likely, that they have been experiencing pain and relying on their own or their partner's judgment that everything is going well for a long time. One of their chief needs when they arrive at a birthing setting, therefore, is reassurance their judgment has been correct—everything is going well and the exhaustion and increasing pain they feel is part of usual labor.

TABLE 15.5 The American Congress of Obstetricians and Gynecologists Categories of Fetal Heart Rate Monitoring

Category	Importance	Recommended Action
Category I	FHR factors (baseline and variability) are normal.	Continue routine monitoring; no specific action needed.
Category II	FHR factors are indeterminate.	Continue surveillance and reevaluation.
Category III	FHR tracings are abnormal.	Prompt evaluation is required. Expedite action to determine the cause and resolve the situation is required. This may include but is not limited to provision of maternal oxygen, change in maternal position, discontinuation of labor stimulation, treatment of maternal hypotension, and treatment of tachysystole with FHR changes. If category III tracing does not resolve with these measures, birth should be undertaken.

FHR, fetal heart rate.
From American Congress of Obstetricians and Gynecologists. (2009). ACOG practice bulletin: Intrapartum fetal heart rate monitoring. *Obstetrics & Gynecology, 114*(1), 193–200.

Nursing Diagnoses and Related Interventions

Nursing Diagnosis: Powerlessness related to duration of labor

Outcome Evaluation: Client voices she feels in control of happenings, expresses preferences for positions and techniques to control pain, asks questions about her progress, and states feelings about what is happening.

After admission, care during the first stage of labor centers on helping a woman feel confident in her ability to control pain and maintain physiologic stability in the face of it. At first, it is exciting for a woman to feel labor contractions. They are little more than menstrual cramps and project a "this-is-really-happening" sensation. Soon, however, if a woman is not concentrating on controlled breathing, the contractions become biting in their intensity. Despite the fact she is becoming more and more uncomfortable, however, nothing seems to be happening. This can cause a couple to begin to worry something is going wrong—to think because the 9 months are over, that victory should be near, yet it is eluding them. Give couples frequent progress reports during labor, so they do not become discouraged or fearful this way at this seeming lack of progress (Box 15.7).

Help Empower Women

Most women want to feel in control of what is happening to them during labor in order to be able to face this big an event in their life. They accomplish this by stating their preferences, breathing with contractions, and changing their position to the one that makes them most comfortable. In contrast, some women handle the stress of labor by becoming extremely passive and quiet. Still others feel a need to show their emotions by shouting or crying. Help each woman express her feelings in her own way or in the way that works best for her.

Part of the way women react to labor is culturally influenced. Don't stereotype women, however, by studying a list of how a typical Hispanic, Middle Eastern, or Asian woman is most apt to react in labor. Instead, ask each woman what will make her feel most comfortable and able to feel in control. A list of expected behaviors may not apply to some women at all.

Respect Contraction Time

Do not interrupt a woman who is in the middle of breathing exercises during labor to perform a procedure or ask questions because, once her concentration is disrupted, she will feel the pain of the contraction and, if she has been successfully using breathing exercises to reduce pain, suddenly feeling the full force of a contraction can be extremely frightening. She tenses and the pain becomes worse, causing her to doubt her ability to breathe constructively in the face of the next contraction. Instead of interrupting, allow her to finish breathing with her contraction, then ask questions or announce what procedure needs to be done next. (See Chapter 16 for a discussion of pain management techniques during labor.)

BOX 15.7 Nursing Care Planning Based on Effective Communication

Celeste Bailey is having a great deal of back pain as well as strong uterine contractions.

Less Effective Communication

Nurse: You don't look very comfortable, Mrs. Bailey. Would you feel better if you sat in the rocking chair rather than stay in bed?
Celeste: Can I do that?
Nurse: I told you on admission you can do whatever is most comfortable for you.
Celeste: Can I walk over to the window?
Nurse: How many times do you want me to repeat instructions? Do whatever is most comfortable for you.
Celeste: I guess I'm not being a very good patient.

More Effective Communication

Nurse: You don't look very comfortable, Mrs. Bailey. Would you feel better if you sat in the rocking chair rather than stay in bed?
Celeste: Can I do that?
Nurse: You can use any position comfortable for you.
Celeste: Can I walk over to the window?
Nurse: Whatever is most comfortable.
Celeste: Thank you. You're very understanding.

Women in labor may be enduring so much pain and are under so much stress that they don't hear or process instructions well. Reminding them they have not processed information well is not therapeutic because it can lower self-esteem and a sense of self-control. Be prepared to repeat instructions as necessary to keep a woman from becoming confused and feeling she is being unfairly criticized.

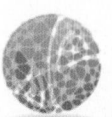

Promote Change of Positions

Because the bed is the main piece of furniture in a birthing room, many women assume they are expected to lie quietly in bed during labor. In early labor, however, a woman should be out of bed walking or sitting in a chair, kneeling, squatting, on all fours, or in whatever position she prefers because active movement can shorten the beginning stage of labor (Selby, Valencia, Garcia, et al., 2012) (Fig. 15.21). Ballroom dancing or swaying with her partner to music they have brought with them can be a helpful activity. Soaking in a tub of warm water (98.6°F [37°C]) or taking a warm shower with the water directed on the abdomen both feel relaxing and so may also help. Water tubs give a woman buoyancy and so make it easier for her to change position. Remember, they also can make a woman feel drowsy, so never leave a woman alone in a tub. Be certain the tub is kept clean of feces so a vaginal examination can be done with the woman in the tub without worry of vaginal contamination.

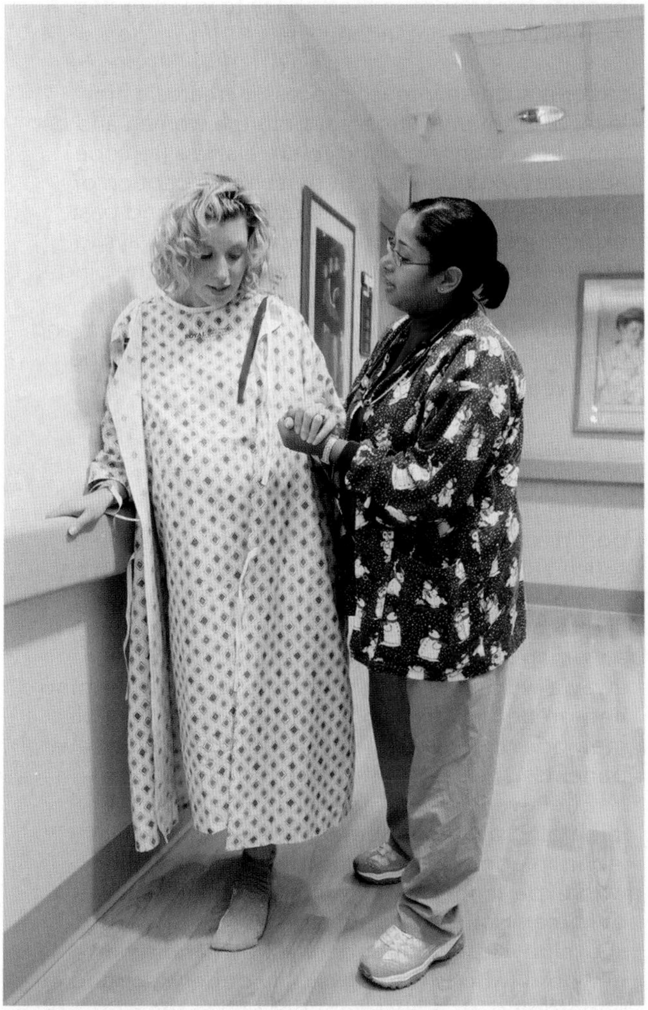

FIGURE 15.21 Finding a comfortable position during early labor is important. Here, a nurse assists a woman with walking during labor.

The exception to being active in labor is a woman whose membranes have ruptured in early labor. She should lie on her side until it is established the FHR is stable or she has had a vaginal examination by her primary care provider to rule out the umbilical cord has not prolapsed into the vagina and would be compressed if she walked.

If a woman receives medication for pain such as a narcotic, she may need to remain in bed for about 15 minutes afterward to avoid a fall if she should become dizzy from the medication. While she is in bed, encourage her to lie on her left side so the heavy uterus tips forward, away from the vena cava, allowing free blood return from the lower extremities and adequate placental filling and circulation. Most women are comfortable in this position and adjust to it readily. Position the chair for the support person facing her so she doesn't keep turning onto her back to talk.

Some women have practiced breathing exercises in a supine position while at home and may need additional coaching to do them in a sitting or dancing position. If a woman feels she must lie on her back during a contraction to make her breathing exercises effective, place a folded towel under her left hip to tilt her uterus to the side. Remind her to return to her side or sit up between contractions.

Help With Fetal Alignment

A baby's birth is easiest from an ROA or LOA position because a fetus that presents in an LOP or ROP position needs to rotate into an anterior position to be born. Either squatting or an "all fours" position may help the fetus turn and shorten labor. A birthing sling is a long piece of fabric that can be slipped under a woman's back as she lies supine or over the abdomen if she is in a hands-and-knees position (Simkin, 2010). A support person uses the sling to gently rock the mother's abdomen, a technique which is advocated as also helping a fetus move into good alignment with the pelvis. It is difficult to find evidence-based practice that birthing slings accomplish this, so they should be used with caution until their worth is more firmly established. There is little need for them with the fetus who is already in good alignment.

Promote Voiding and Provide Bladder Care

A full bladder or bowel can impede fetal descent, so encourage a woman to void, if possible, at least every 2 to 4 hours during labor. The way a full bladder can impede descent of a fetus is illustrated in Figure 15.22. The reason you need to remind a woman to void during labor is because she may mistakenly interpret the discomfort of a full bladder as part of the sensations of labor. You can assess for a full bladder by percussion (an empty bladder sounds dull; a full one sounds resonant). If a woman cannot void and the bladder becomes distended, she may need to be catheterized. Catheterizing a woman in labor is uncomfortable for her and difficult

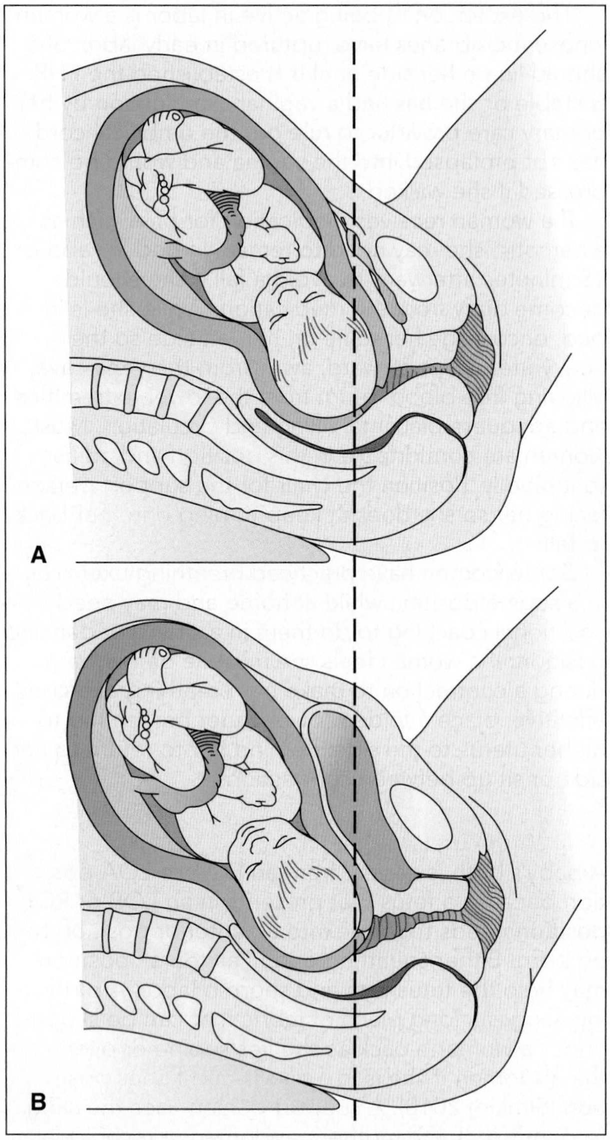

FIGURE 15.22 The effect of a full bladder on fetal descent. **(A)** The bladder is empty. **(B)** A full bladder impedes fetal progress.

for you: the vulva is edematous from the pressure of the fetal presenting part, stretching the urethral canal downward and making the urethra difficult to locate. For best results, use a small catheter (No. 12 to 14F), and insert it between contractions. Use extremely careful aseptic technique to avoid introducing any microorganisms that might result in a urinary tract infection.

Nursing Diagnosis: Risk for ineffective breathing pattern related to breathing exercises

Outcome Evaluation: Client's respiratory rate returns to normal limits after a contraction; skin is her usual color, cool, and dry. No reports of light-headedness or tingling/numbness in extremities.

Hyperventilation (an accelerated rate of respiration) occurs when a woman exhales more deeply than she inhales. As a result, extra carbon dioxide is blown off and respiratory alkalosis results. This can occur when a woman is practicing breathing exercises in preparation for labor, but it is most apt to occur during actual labor. The woman feels lightheaded and may have tingling or numbness in her toes and fingertips. If allowed to progress, hyperventilation can lead to loss of consciousness.

The best way to manage hyperventilation is to prevent it. Be certain that when a woman is breathing rapidly, she ends all breathing sessions with a long cleansing breath to help restore carbon dioxide balance. If hyperventilation begins, ask her to breathe in and out into a paper bag, so she rebreathes the carbon dioxide she has exhaled. If a paper bag is unavailable, a woman can use her cupped hands or those of her partner.

Nursing Diagnosis: Anxiety related to stress of labor

Outcome Evaluation: Client states she feels in control of her situation; she and her support person express confidence in their ability to weather this extraordinary event in their life.

Labor is such an intense process it creates a high level of emotional stress for both the woman and her support person. Ability to tolerate stress (to cope adequately) depends on a person's perception of the event, the support people available, and past experience in using coping mechanisms. Ways to reduce stress in labor, therefore, center on helping a woman to perceive labor clearly, providing opportunities for her partner to provide support, and helping her gain confidence that she can manage this event.

Offer Support

Support needs to come from health care personnel as well as a woman's individual support person. There is no substitute for personal touch and contact as a way to provide support during labor (unless she's a person who doesn't like to be touched). Patting an arm while telling a woman she is progressing in labor, brushing away a wisp of hair from her forehead, and wiping her forehead with a cool cloth are indispensable methods of conveying support and produce several benefits.

Effective support can make the difference in helping a woman feel able to continue with labor. In addition, a woman who is touched, who experiences the warmth and friendliness of human contact during labor—a time when she is physically dependent—may handle her newborn (who is also physically dependent and undergoing an adjustment not unlike the one she has just gone through) more warmly and affectionately.

Respect and Promote the Support Person

Be certain to admit a woman's support person to the birthing area along with the woman and encourage him or her to remain with the woman throughout the birth because having someone familiar with her during labor helps to counteract the sensation everything is new and unexpected. Acquaint the support person with the physical layout of the birthing room and point out where supplies such as towels, washcloths, and ice chips are stored, so he or she can get them as necessary. Be certain that all health care personnel are aware of who the support person is and the importance of making him or her feel welcome.

If the support person will be acting as a labor coach, ask whether he or she has attended a prepared childbirth class and exactly how the support person wants to help the woman manage the pain of contractions. If a support person is hesitant to give coaching instructions, it's better to review techniques than to take over. Offer praise not only for the woman but also for the support person as well because watching a birth is often as totally a new experience for this person as for the woman. Relieve the support person as necessary, so he or she can take a break and get something to eat or visit with older children (Fig. 15.23). If older children will view the birth, be certain they are oriented and have a child care provider to entertain them during the long hours of labor.

In addition to having a support person, many women choose a **doula** or an expert support person to be with them in labor. Having such a person present frees the woman's partner to enjoy the birth rather than feel occupied with coaching instructions. Although research in the subject is not extensive, there are suggestions that rates of oxytocin augmentation, the need for epidural anesthesia, and cesarean birth rates can be reduced through doula support (Gilliland, 2011).

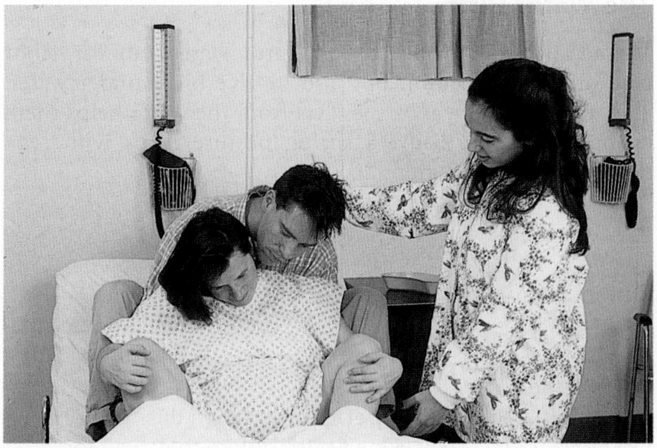

FIGURE 15.23 Encouraging a support person so he can continue to give support is an important nursing role. (© Barbara Proud.)

Support a Woman's Pain Management Needs

Many women plan on using nonpharmacologic pain relief measures such as hydrotherapy (soaking in a tub of warm water or taking a warm shower), aromatherapy, or acupuncture during labor; ask if the woman has planned any of these and what you could do to help her make these effective (Smith, Levett, Collins, et al., 2011). Other women want pharmacologic help in labor. Support whichever decision a woman has made coming into labor as well as any change she decides on as labor progresses (see Chapter 16 for a discussion of common nonpharmacologic as well as pharmacologic measures for labor).

Some health care providers are reluctant to suggest to a woman that pharmacologic pain relief is available as this might influence her to accept an analgesic rather than continue to use nonpharmacologic methods. Part of being in control, however, is knowing your options and feeling free to elect the one most appropriate at that time. Because pain is subjective, only the woman knows how much pain she can endure and whether she needs some supplemental help to make childbirth the experience she planned.

What if . . . 15.3 Celeste's doula and Celeste's teenage sister disagree on whether Celeste needs medication for pain during labor. Whose suggestion would you pay most attention to? How could you resolve the issue?

Nursing Diagnosis: Risk for fluid volume deficit related to prolonged lack of oral intake and diaphoresis from the effort of labor

Outcome Evaluation: Client drinks at least one glass of selected beverage every hour, states she does not feel thirsty; voids at least 30 ml/hr every 2 to 4 hours.

Women need to remain well hydrated during labor so urge them to drink at least a glass of fluid every hour. Sucking on ice chips, popsicles, or lollipops can help supply additional fluid. Some women need isotonic sports drinks to prevent secondary uterine inertia (a cessation of labor contractions) as well as to combat generalized dehydration and exhaustion. Even with an adequate fluid intake, a woman's mouth and lips can become uncomfortably dry because of mouth breathing. Applying lip balm to prevent or relieve this discomfort can be helpful.

THE CARE OF A WOMAN DURING THE SECOND STAGE OF LABOR

The second stage of labor is the time from full cervical dilatation to birth of the newborn. Even women who have taken childbirth education classes and who believe they are well prepared for any length or type of contractions are surprised at the intensity of the pushing sensation they feel in this stage of labor. Because the feeling to push becomes so strong, some women react to this by growing argumentative and angry, or by crying and screaming. Other women react by tensing their abdominal muscles and trying to resist pushing, thus making the sensation even more painful and frightening. If the woman has not received an epidural for pain management, she should push with contractions and rest in between. In the past, women were told to hold their breath while they did this. Holding the breath for a prolonged time, however, impairs blood return from the vena cava (a Valsalva maneuver), so this should be discouraged. Instead, encourage women to assume any position that is comfortable for them and breathe any way that is natural for them, except by holding their breath while they push (Plaat, 2012) (Box 15.8).

A support person plays a vital role during this time because all of the preparations done up to this point may still not be enough to sustain a woman during these final contractions unless she feels well supported. This participation also creates an important sharing time later after the birth and can give a couple a sense of family for the first time.

Women also need to have an experienced health care person with them as they enter this stage of labor to reassure them that the change in contractions is normal and to give knowledgeable support everything is all right. Box 15.9 shows an interprofessional care map illustrating both nursing and team planning for labor.

A general timetable for second-stage care is shown in Table 15.6. Be certain to assess fetal heart sounds at the beginning of the second stage to be certain the start of the baby's passage into the birth canal is not occluding the cord and interfering with fetal circulation. Assisting a woman into whatever position she feels will be most effective for pushing (e.g., squatting, sitting upright, leaning forward against her partner) is important to help align the fetal presenting part with the cervix, increase the pelvic diameters, and use the fetal weight to help descent so that a prolonged second stage (over 2 hours) does not occur. A danger of a prolonged second stage is chorioamionitis (membrane infection), an increased rate of cesarean birth, and future urinary incontinence (Brown, Gartland, Donath, et al., 2011).

Preparing the Place of Birth

For a multipara, convert a birthing room into a birth room by opening the sterile packs of supplies on waiting tables when the cervix has dilated to 7 to 8 cm. For a primipara, this can be delayed until the head has crowned to the size of a quarter or half-dollar (full dilatation and descent). Be certain drapes and materials used for birth are sterile so no microorganisms can be accidentally introduced into the uterus. A table arranged with equipment such as sponges, drapes, scissors, basins, clamps, vaginal packing, and sterile gowns, gloves, and towels can be left, if covered, for up to 8 hours.

A birthing bed is "broken" or the foot folded down to allow the primary care provider ready access to support a crowning newborn head. Be certain that once a bed is broken, someone remains continuously at the foot of the bed so if the fetus is born suddenly, the head and body can be supported and born safely.

To provide for baby care, open the partition at the end of the room to reveal the "baby island," or newborn care area. Such areas include a radiant heat warmer, equipment for suction and resuscitation, and supplies for eye care and identification of the newborn. Turn on the radiant heat warmer in advance, so the bottom mattress is pleasantly warm to the touch at the time of birth. Place sterile towels and a blanket on the warmer so they will also be warm when used to dry and cover the infant to help prevent hypothermia.

Positioning for Birth

Women can choose a variety of positions for birth. In the past, a lithotomy position was the preferred position for birth because it offers a clear view of the perineum, but it is no longer a position of choice as a woman lying flat on her back may slow, not help, fetal descent, and lying longer than 1 hour in a lithotomy position can lead to intense pelvic congestion and possibly thrombophlebitis. More effective birth positions include the lateral or Sims position, a dorsal recumbent position (on the back with knees flexed), semi-sitting, or squatting. Using these positions plus warm compresses to the perineum place less tension on the perineum and result in fewer perineal tears (Aasheim, Nilsen, Lukasse, et al., 2011).

The Water Birth

Women may not only use a warm water tub for labor comfort and relaxation but also to give birth under water. The increased buoyancy they feel from the water helps them change positions easily; a sitting posture helps with fetal descent (Impey & Child, 2012).

BOX 15.8 Nursing Care Planning to Empower a Family

Q. Celeste asks you, "How will I know when I should begin to push with labor?"

A. After full cervical dilatation, the baby's head descends in the pelvis to the level of the pelvic floor. When this happens, you'll realize a strong feeling you have to push as if you need to move your bowels. Don't push before that; wait for the natural signal. Pushing is a great moment in labor because as you push (remember not to hold your breath), you no longer feel pain, just a wonderful awareness your baby is about to be born.

BOX 15.9 Nursing Care Planning

AN INTERPROFESSIONAL CARE MAP FOR A WOMAN DURING LABOR AND BIRTH

Celeste Bailey is a 26-year-old woman you admit to a birthing room. She tells you she wants to have her baby "naturally," without any analgesia or anesthesia. Her husband, a long distant truck driver, is on his way home but hasn't arrived as of yet. Her teenage sister is with her. She states she has no idea how to coach her except to pray. As you finish assessing contractions, Celeste grips her abdomen, screams, and shouts, "I'm breathing just like I'm supposed to do! Why does this hurt so bad?"

Family Assessment Client lives with husband in fixed rent housing project. Finances rated as "horrible." She says, "If you want to be rich, don't marry a truck driver." Her sister and parents live nearby.

Client Assessment Gravida 1, para 0. Contractions of moderate intensity, 45 seconds in duration, 3 minutes apart. Cervix dilated 3 cm, 60% effaced. Membranes intact. Fetal heart rate (FHR), 148 beats/min; fetus in right occipitoanterior (ROA) position. Attended childbirth education classes, but appears to be using breathing exercises ineffectively without her coach. Brought a red rose to use as a focusing object. Has not voided for past 4 hours.

Nursing Diagnosis Pain related to uterine contractions and pressure on pelvic structures from labor

Outcome Criteria Client manages her discomfort in labor with nonpharmacologic methods, identifies additional pain relief measures if needed, responds to questions and instructions; states labor and birth were a positive experience for her.

Team Member Responsible	Assessment	Intervention	Rationale	Expected Outcome
Activities of Daily Living, Including Safety				
Nurse	Inspect the client's suprapubic area and palpate for bladder distention because she has not voided for 4 hours.	Encourage client to void every 2 hours.	A full bladder contributes to the client's discomfort and impedes fetal descent, possibly prolonging labor.	Client has no signs of bladder distention and voids every 2 hours during labor.
Nurse	Assess level of pain from uterine contractions and pelvic pressure by both verbal and nonverbal indicators; use 1 to 10 pain score.	Review and observe breathing patterns with client and teenage sister to be certain she is obtaining maximum relief.	Pain is a subjective symptom, so only the client can determine her degree of pain or what is most helpful to relieve it.	Client rates her level of pain from labor contractions as good to tolerable. Teenage sister offers effective support.
Teamwork and Collaboration				
Nurse/Primary care provider	Ask sister if she will serve as labor coach until husband arrives. Determine if a nurse anesthetist is available in case the client changes mind about analgesia because husband is not with her.	Demonstrate to sister how to serve as coach. Consult with nurse anesthetist about client's wish to not receive any pharmacologic pain relief.	Respecting client's wishes is a prime mode of encouraging self-efficacy. A support person can play a major role in making labor a tolerable experience.	Sister serves as effective labor coach. Pain management team supports client's wish for no pharmacologic interventions, but will be prepared to administer pain relief if client's wishes change or an emergency should change the client's goal.

(continued on page 390)

BOX 15.9 Nursing Care Planning (continued)

Procedures/Medications for Quality Improvement				
Nurse	Assess what particular care measures, if any, client desires during labor such as walking or using a water tub.	Establish a birth plan with client so all staff members can be aware of her individual preferences.	Respecting a client's choice helps to maintain self-esteem and a feeling of control.	Client expresses her preferences during labor.
Nutrition				
Nurse	Assess when client last ate. Ask about preferences for fluid during labor.	Provide client with ice chips, hard candy, or other fluid as desired.	Ice chips or hard candy can relieve mouth dryness from breathing exercises, and fluid is important to prevent dehydration.	Client states she has no mouth discomfort and does not feel hungry. Drinks at least a glass of fluid every hour.
Patient-Centered Care				
Nurse	Assess what client knows about the usual process and time intervals of labor.	Provide information to supplement client's knowledge of labor; and update client frequently on labor progress.	Frequent updates about client's progress help to alleviate anxiety.	Client states she understands the process of usual labor and indicates progress reports are helpful.
Psychosocial/Spiritual/Emotional Needs				
Nurse	Assess if physical environment seems conducive to labor.	Provide a comfortable environment. Encourage client to assume different positions and to change them regularly. Respect the need for focusing during contractions.	A comfortable environment aids in relaxation and minimizes distractions. Position changes promote fetal descent. Interrupting focusing can lessen effectiveness of the technique.	Client reports environment is comfortable and she feels secure. She assumes a variety of positions during labor as desired. She expresses she is able to use a rose for focus during contractions unimpaired by health care providers.
Informatics for Seamless Health Care Planning				
Nurse	Assess how client evaluates her labor experience.	Help client voice her satisfaction or dissatisfaction with her labor experience.	Reviewing a possibly traumatic experience helps debrief (put it into perspective among life events).	Client states labor and birth were at worst a tolerable experience, and at best, a highlight of her life.

As women begin to push with contractions, they also often move their bowels so the water can become contaminated with feces. Keep the bath water as free as possible by lifting any feces out with a plastic scoop so, if the infant is born in the tub, he or she will be born into as clean an environment as possible.

The baby is born underwater and then immediately brought to the surface for a first breath. A potential difficulty is contamination of the bath water with feces, which could lead to uterine infection or aspiration of contaminated bath water by a newborn, which could lead to pneumonia. Newborns, however, have a dive reflex, which alerts them not to breathe while under water, so this is not usually a problem. A dive reflex may not be operative if the baby's head is brought to the surface before the entire baby is born so the timing of this is important. Maternal chilling when a woman leaves the water is another factor to consider and prevent. Yet another concern is that a short umbilical cord could tear as the baby is brought to the surface. To help prevent this, limit the amount of water in the tub to about 12 inches.

Tub bathing can effectively shorten the second stage of labor and so result in less pain, but it also may lead to increased perineal tearing as the perineum cannot be massaged as readily. Be certain to observe for perineal bleeding afterward to detect this potential complication (Cortes, Basra, & Kelleher, 2011). Be certain tubs are cleaned with the agency-designated solution at the finish of labor so it will be clean for the next couple.

TABLE 15.6 Time Intervals for Nursing Interventions During the Second Stage of Labor

Intervention	Beginning of Second Stage	Continued Frequency	After Birth of Infant	After Delivery of Placenta
Assess and Record				
Temperature	X	q2h	X	q1h
Pulse	X	q1h	X	q15 min
Respirations	X	q5–30 min	X	q15 min
Blood pressure	X	q5–30 min	X	X
Fetal heart rate	X	q5 min		
Contractions	X	q5 min		
Perineum	X	q15 min	X	q15 min
Provide				
Support	X	Continuously	Continuously	Continuously

Promoting Effective Second-Stage Pushing

For the most effective pushing during the second stage of labor, a woman should wait to feel the urge to push even though a pelvic exam has revealed she is fully dilated (Osborne & Hanson, 2012). Pushing is usually best done from a semi-Fowler's position with legs raised against the abdomen, squatting, or on all-fours rather than lying flat to allow gravity to aid the effort (Fig. 15.24). Make sure the woman pushes with contractions and rests between them. She can use short pushes or long, sustained ones, whichever feels more comfortable. Holding the breath

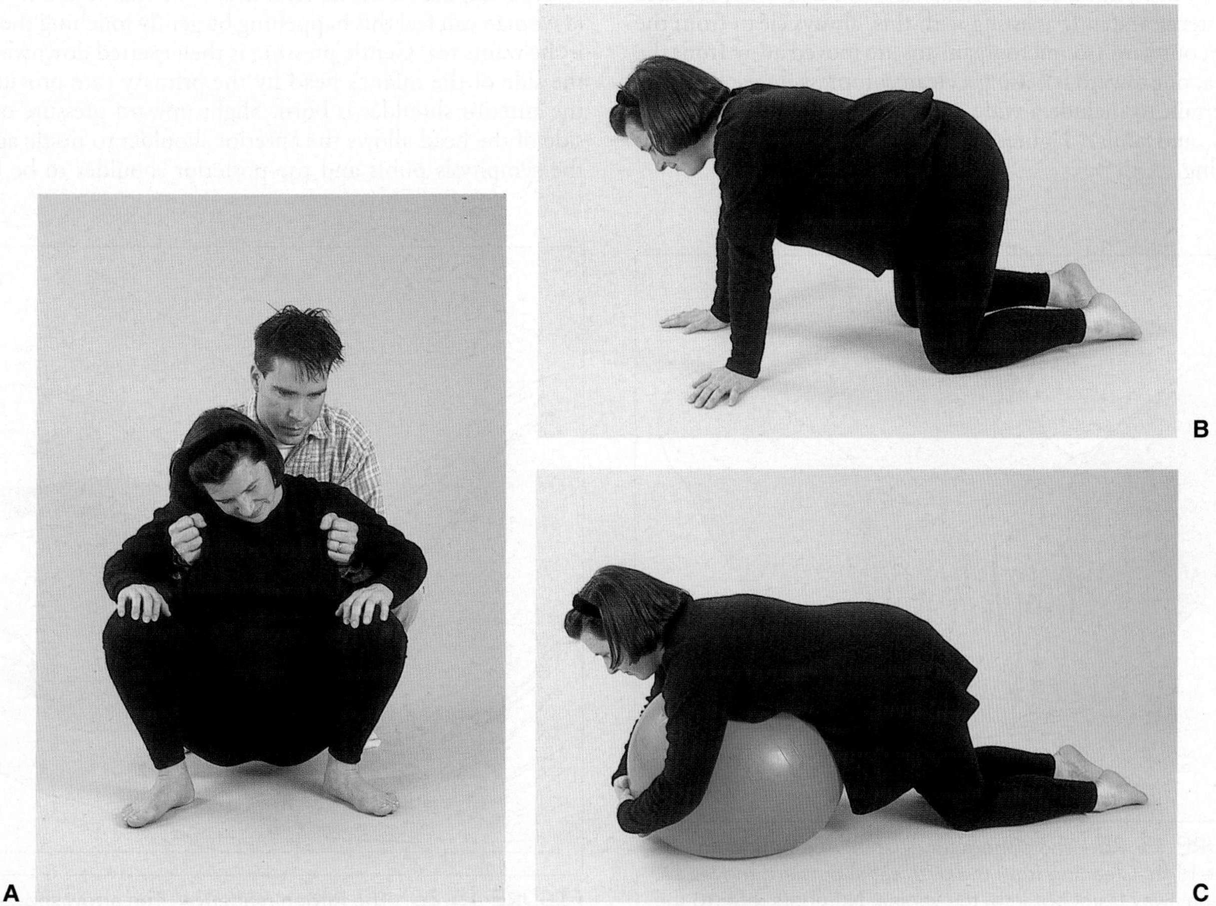

FIGURE 15.24 Positions for pushing during second stage labor: **(A)** squatting with support person, **(B)** on all fours, and **(C)** on all fours with chest support. (© Barbara Proud.)

during a contraction could cause a Valsalva maneuver or temporarily impede blood return to her heart because of increased intrathoracic pressure, which could then also interfere with blood supply to the uterus. To prevent her from holding her breath during pushing, urge her to grunt or breathe out during a pushing effort (as tennis players do).

If there is a reason such as a nuchal cord (cord located around the baby's neck), which must be removed before the infant is fully born, it may be necessary to prevent a woman from pushing at some point. To help her do this, ask her to pant with contractions. Because it is difficult to push effectively when she is using her diaphragm for panting, this limits pushing. Remember, however, that pushing is involuntary. Regardless of how much a woman wants to cooperate, stopping this overwhelming urge to push is almost beyond her power. Demonstrating "panting like a puppy" and panting with her may be most effective. Be sure she is inhaling adequately with panting. Otherwise, she might hyperventilate and become lightheaded. Have her take deep cleansing breaths between contractions to prevent this.

Perineal Cleaning and Massage

Massaging the perineum as the fetal head enlarges the vaginal opening helps to keep it supple and prevent tearing. To remove vaginal or rectal secretions and prepare the cleanest environment for the birth of the baby, the care provider may clean the perineum with a warmed antiseptic such as Iodaphor (cold solution causes cramping), and then rinse the area with sterile water. If assisting with this, always clean from the vagina outward (so microorganisms are moved away from the vagina, not toward it), using a clean compress for each stroke. Be certain to include a wide area (vulva, upper inner thighs, pubis, and anus). Figure 15.25 shows a typical pattern for cleaning.

The Birth

As soon as the head of a fetus is prominent (approximately 8 cm across) at the vaginal opening, one technique to help the fetus achieve extension and allow the smallest head diameter to present is for the care provider to place a sterile towel over the rectum and press forward on the fetal chin while the other hand presses downward on the occiput (a Ritgen maneuver) (Fig. 15.26). This also influences the rate at which the head is born. Pressure should never be applied to the fundus of the uterus to effect birth because uterine rupture could occur.

The woman is asked to continue pushing until the occiput of the fetal head is firmly at the pubic arch. The head is then gently born between contractions. This helps to prevent the head from being expelled too rapidly, creating a major pressure change in the skull, which might then rupture cerebral blood vessels. It also reduces the possibility of a perineal tear. A woman who has not had anesthesia experiences the birth of the head as a flash of pain or a burning sensation, as if someone had momentarily poured hot water on her perineum. It is a fleeting sensation and is not particularly uncomfortable.

Immediately after birth of the baby's head, the primary care provider passes his or her fingers around the newborn's neck to determine whether a loop of umbilical cord is encircling the neck. It is not uncommon for a single loop of cord to be positioned this way (termed a nuchal cord). If such a loop is felt, it is gently loosened and drawn down over the fetal head. If it is too tightly coiled to allow this, it is clamped and cut before the shoulders are born. Otherwise, it could tear and interfere with the fetal oxygen supply.

After expulsion of the fetal head, external rotation occurs (a woman can feel this happening by gently touching the head if she wants to). Gentle pressure is then exerted downward on the side of the infant's head by the primary care provider so the anterior shoulder is born. Slight upward pressure on the side of the head allows the anterior shoulder to nestle against the symphysis pubis and the posterior shoulder to be born.

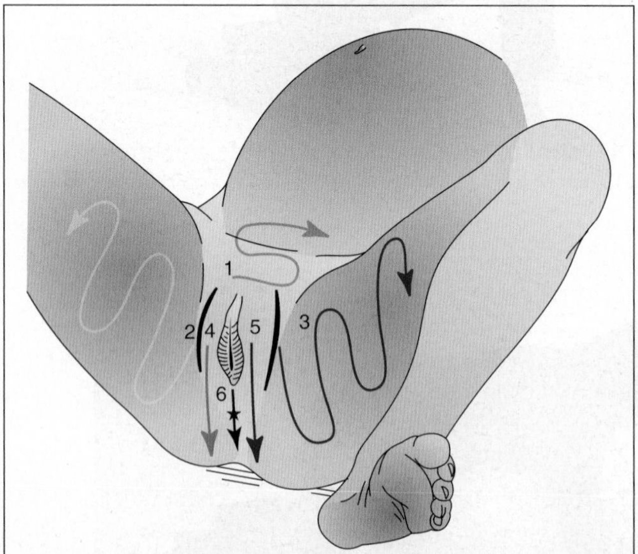

FIGURE 15.25 The pattern for cleaning the perineum before birth. Cleaning from the birth canal outward moves bacteria away from, not into, the vagina. Numbers refer to the steps of the procedure.

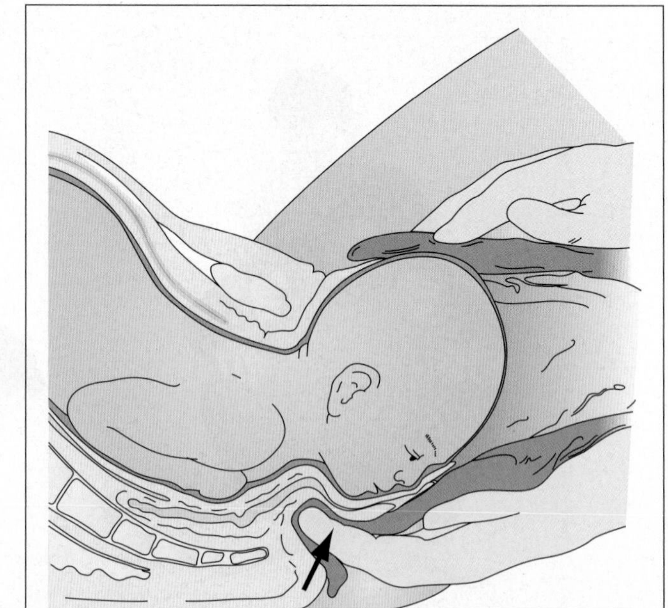

FIGURE 15.26 The Ritgen maneuver. The arrow shows direction of pressure.

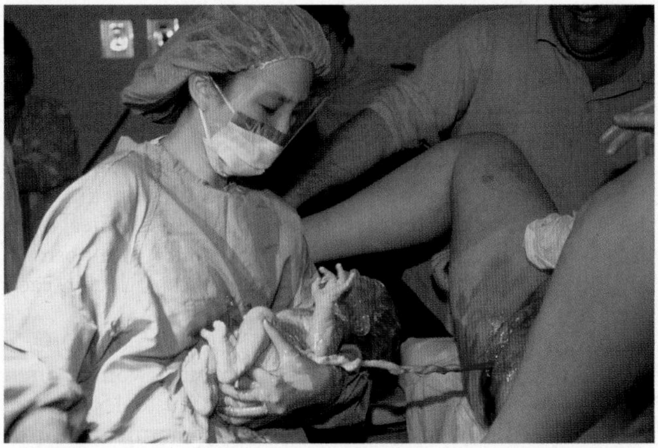

FIGURE 15.27 A child is considered born when the whole body is born. (© Barbara Proud.)

The remainder of the body then slides free without any further difficulty.

A child is considered born when the whole body is born. This is the time that should be noted and recorded as the time of birth, which is a nursing responsibility (most primary care providers regard it as their responsibility or pleasure to announce the sex of the infant). The newborn is immediately laid on the mother's naked abdomen and covered with a warmed blanket and cap to conserve heat and encourage mother–infant bonding (Moore, Anderson, Bergman, et al., 2012). With this, the second stage of labor is complete (Fig. 15.27).

Cutting and Clamping the Cord

Cutting the cord is part of the stimulus that initiates a first breath or marks the newborn's most important transition into the outside world, the establishment of independent respirations. The timing of cord clamping, however, varies depending on the parent's preference and the maturity of the infant.

The umbilical cord continues to pulsate for a few minutes after birth, and then the pulsation ceases. Delaying cutting (also called physiologic clamping) until pulsation ceases and maintaining the infant at a uterine level allows as much as 100 ml more of blood to pass from the placenta into the fetus than if the infant were held in a superior position or the cord was immediately cut. Delaying cutting, therefore, helps ensure an adequate red blood cell and white cell count in the newborn (Main, 2012). The timing of cord clamping, however, is individualized because late clamping of the cord this way could cause overinfusion with placental blood and the possibility of polycythemia and hyperbilirubinemia in a susceptible newborn, a particular concern if the infant is preterm.

Before cutting, the cord is clamped with two hemostats placed 8 to 10 inches from the infant's umbilicus. The woman's partner or support person may then have the privilege of cutting the cord between the hemostats. A cord blood sample is obtained to provide a ready source of infant blood if blood typing or other emergency measures, such as establishing whether fetal acidosis was present, needs to be done. Blood may also be taken for cord blood banking so the family has stem cells available if needed in the future.

The vessels in the cord are then counted to be certain three are present and an umbilical clamp is applied to replace the forceps (Fig. 15.28). Some umbilical clamps in hospitals have

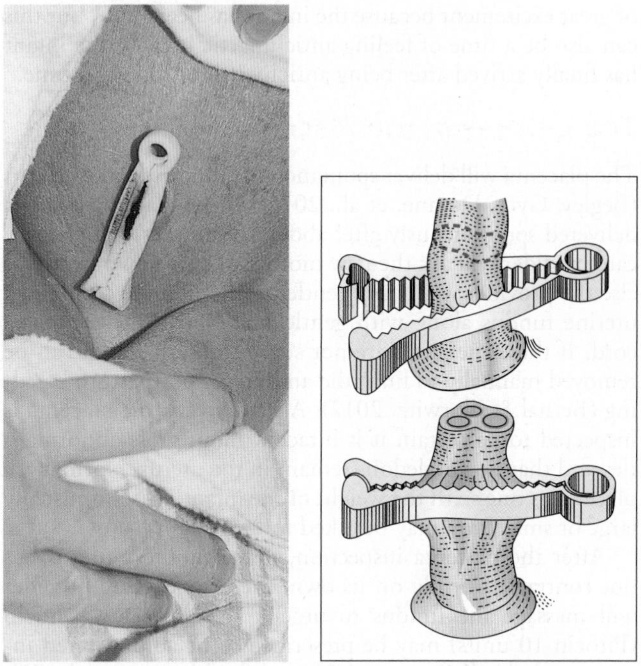

A B

FIGURE 15.28 **(A)** An umbilical clamp applied to the cord. (© Caroline Brown, RNC, MC, DEd.) **(B)** Placing clamp, and locking the clamp.

an alarm attached that will ring if the infant is taken further than set hospital boundaries, a precaution against newborn abduction.

Introducing the Infant

After the cord is cut, it is time for the new parents to spend quality time with their newborn. The infant can remain on the mother's abdomen for skin-to-skin contact. If the woman's partner or support person wants to hold the infant, dry the infant well with a warmed towel, wrap him or her in a sterile blanket, and cover the head with a wrapped towel or cap. Be certain to handle newborns gently but firmly as they are slippery from amniotic fluid and vernix.

Most newborns receive prophylactic eye ointment against the possibility of a chlamydia infection. Don't administer this until after the parents have had this chance to see their infant for the first time (and the infant has had a chance to see them) (see Chapter 18 for continuing infant care such as weighing and measuring). This initial newborn visit is also the optimal time for a mother to begin breastfeeding because an infant seems to be hungry at birth and sucking at the breasts stimulates the release of endogenous oxytocin, encouraging uterine contraction and involution, or the return of the uterus to its prepregnant state (Baselice & Lawson, 2011).

THE CARE OF A WOMAN DURING THE THIRD AND FOURTH STAGES OF LABOR

The third stage of labor is the time from the birth of the baby until the placenta is delivered. For most women, this is a time of great excitement because the infant has been born, but this can also be a time of feeling anticlimactic because the infant has finally arrived after being anticipated for so long a time.

The Delivery of the Placenta

The placenta will deliver spontaneously following most births (Begley, Gyte, Devane, et al., 2011). If the placenta has not delivered spontaneously after about 10 minutes, the primary care provider will ask the new mother to bear down gently or else the provider will apply gentle pressure on the contracted uterine fundus along with gentle traction on the umbilical cord. If these measures are not successful, a placenta can be removed manually to limit the amount of postpartum bleeding (Bernal & Norwitz, 2012). After delivery, the placenta is inspected to be certain it is intact without gross abnormalities and that no cotyledons remain in the uterus. Normally, a placenta is one sixth the weight of the infant. If it is unusually large or small, you may be asked to weigh it.

After the placenta inspection, if the mother's uterus has not contracted firmly on its own, the primary care provider will massage the fundus to urge it to contract. Oxytocin (Pitocin 10 units) may be prescribed to be administered intramuscularly (IM) or per 1,000 ml fluid intravenously (IV) to also help contraction (Karch, 2013). If excessive bleeding with poor uterine contraction remains, an injection of carboprost tromethamine (Hemabate) is yet another solution to increase uterine contraction and to guard against hemorrhage.

The administration of these drugs is a nursing responsibility in most health care facilities. Because Pitocin causes hypertension by vasoconstriction, be certain to obtain a baseline blood pressure measurement before administration. Question the use of such a drug if the woman had an elevated blood pressure during pregnancy that is still present.

The fourth stage of labor includes the first few hours after birth (discussed in Chapter 17). It signals the beginning of dramatic changes because it marks the beginning of both a new life and a new family.

The Perineal Inspection

To be certain a woman's perineum did not tear from the pressure of the fetal head, the perineum is carefully inspected after birth. About 3% of women do have a small tear extending backward from the vagina. Perineal tears are rated grade 1 to grade 4, grade 1 being minimal and grade 4 extending to and including the rectum (see Chapter 25 for grading definitions and care).

Most are small enough that no suturing is needed (Elharmeel, Chaudhary, Tan, et al., 2011). If a tear is large enough to require suturing, a woman usually has enough natural perineal anesthesia from pressure of the fetal head or enough effect from epidural anesthesia, she will not feel pain from the suturing. If she does have pain, a local anesthetic can be given to make the process pain free.

The Immediate Postpartum Assessment and Nursing Care

This is the beginning of the postpartal period or the fourth stage of labor. Because the uterus may be so exhausted from labor that it cannot maintain contraction, there is a high risk for hemorrhage during this time (it is the most dangerous time of birth for the mother). Obtain vital signs (pulse, respirations, and blood pressure) every 15 minutes for the first hour and then according to agency policy or the woman's condition. Pulse and respirations may be fairly rapid immediately after birth (80 to 90 beats/min and 20 to 24 breaths/min), and blood pressure may be slightly elevated due to exertion and excitement of the moment or recent oxytocin administration. Wash the perineum with the agency-designated solution and apply a perineal pad. Palpate a woman's fundus for size, consistency, and position and observe the amount and characteristics of lochia each time you record vital signs.

Return the birthing bed to its original position. Offer a clean gown and a warmed blanket, because a woman often experiences chills and a shaking sensation 10 to 15 minutes after birth. This may be due to the low temperature of a birthing room, but may also be a result of the sudden release of pressure on pelvic nerves or of excess epinephrine production during labor. In any event, it is a normal phenomenon but can be frightening to the mother if she associates the chills with fever or infection and worry she will be ill at a time when she most wants to be well to care for her new child. You can reassure her this is a transitory sensation, is very common, and passes quickly. Continuing assessments are discussed in Chapter 17 with care of a postpartal family.

THE WOMAN WITH UNIQUE CONCERNS IN LABOR

The Woman Without a Support Person

Some women choose to labor without their partner—the usual support person—during labor. Other times, a partner is not available due to work or other commitments. Such women then ask a family member or close friend to act as their support person. A woman who brings no support person with her needs a supportive nurse to remain with her continuously during labor.

A woman whose acceptance of her pregnancy was slow to develop due to lack of adequate support people may not have completed the psychological tasks of pregnancy by the time she is in labor. This could make her more apprehensive about being alone and being asked to begin a new life role. Increased assessment of parent–child bonding may be necessary in the immediate postpartal period to be certain her loneliness does not affect her relationship with her child.

The Woman Who Will Be Placing Her Baby for Adoption

Even if a woman has decided to place her baby for adoption during pregnancy, she needs to be an active participant in her labor and the baby's birth and be allowed to hold her child afterward. Each state has a set number of days in which a mother must decide whether she wants to keep her baby or decide on adoption. Although this decision may have seemed easier to make during pregnancy, once a woman holds the baby in her arms, the prospect of giving up the child may be more painful than she realized. Offer support no matter what decision she eventually makes; also offer support as to whether she wants to hold the child or begin breastfeeding. Be certain you do not offer influencing advice, because the woman is the only person who knows whether keeping this child will be right for her or for the child in the future.

The Woman With Cultural Concerns

A number of women from countries where female circumcision is allowed may have difficulty with a successful second stage of labor because their perineum has so much scar tissue that their vagina cannot dilate adequately for a fetal head to pass. They may need an episiotomy (discussed in Chapter 24) to avoid extensive perineal tearing. Some women are scheduled for cesarean births because their perineum is so strictured. Help a woman accept these surgical interventions as necessary in order to preserve her own health and limit pressure on the fetal head.

The Woman Who Is Morbidly Obese

The incidence of morbidly obese women seen in birth settings is growing yearly (Oteng-Ntim, Varma, Croker, et al., 2012). Care of women with a high body mass index (BMI) requires a number of special interventions in labor and birth.

On admission, a woman may be unusually fatigued from her efforts to keep active in early labor. Because many overweight women have elevated blood pressure, be certain to assess this on admission (but then repeat it about 15 minutes later when she is more rested to be certain an elevated pressure was not from anxiety). Assess her ankles carefully for edema because this is common from overworked circulation in her lower extremities. Be certain to assess her urine for protein and glucose because gestational diabetes occurs more often in obese women than in others (Ovadia & Dixit, 2012). Fetal heart sounds may be difficult to auscultate in obese women. Electronic monitors may not have straps long enough to hold the sensors snugly in place, so they may have to be handheld or attached by wrapped gauze or stockinette.

It's important for all women to remain active in labor. The typical rocking chair provided in the birthing room may not be wide enough for the woman to sit in comfortably. Because birthing room beds are constructed to be narrow enough to fit through the average doorway, they are very narrow in relation to the girth of an obese woman's abdomen. Be certain that when she turns from side to side, she isn't in danger of not having enough space to do this on a narrow bed.

Some women who are obese are very self-conscious about their size. Be certain to respect modesty while helping her change from a soiled gown to a clean one or that she is adequately covered if she plans to walk in the birthing center or hospital hallway.

Morbidly obese women tend to have infants with larger than usual shoulders (macrosomia), which can slow or even halt fetal descent. Be certain to particularly monitor the length of the second stage of labor (the average time is 1 hour; 2 hours is time for care providers to be alerted that a complication may be occurring) because this is when the lack of descent becomes most apparent.

Again, be aware that a birthing bed is narrow in relation to her body when she holds her newborn and begins breastfeeding after birth. Praise her for her work well done in giving birth. Birth is such a dramatic experience that it may be the motivation that allows her to improve her own health in the year to come so she can enter a second pregnancy in better health (Garabedian, Williams, Pearce, et al., 2011).

What if...15.4 You are interested in exploring one of the 2020 National Health Goals related to labor and birth (see Box 15.1). Most government-sponsored money for nursing research is allotted based on these goals. What would be a possible research topic to explore pertinent to these goals that would be applicable to Celeste and her family and that would also advance evidence-based practice?

KEY POINTS FOR REVIEW

- Labor is the series of events by which uterine contractions expel a fetus and placenta from a woman's body.
- The exact reason why labor begins is unknown. It most likely occurs because of an interplay between fetal and uterine factors that registers as progesterone withdrawal.
- Effective labor depends on interactions between the passage, the passenger, the power of contractions, and a woman's psychological readiness.
- Labor is an almost overwhelming experience because it involves intense sensations and emotions never felt before. Urge women to bring a support person with them to help cope with the experience. Orient and explain what is happening to this person as well as the woman in labor.
- The fetal presentation (the fetal body part that will initially contact the cervix), the position (the relationship of the fetal presenting part to a specific quadrant of the woman's pelvis), and the lie (whether the fetus is presenting the head or breech to the birth canal) are important determinants of the success of labor.
- The first stage of labor lasts from the onset of cervical dilatation until dilatation is complete (10 cm). The second stage extends from the time of full dilatation until the infant is born. A third or placental stage lasts from the time the infant is born until after delivery of the placenta. A fourth stage comprises the first few hours after birth.
- Danger signs of labor include an abnormal FHR, meconium staining of amniotic fluid, abnormal maternal pulse or blood pressure, inadequate or prolonged contractions, development of an abnormal lower abdomen contour, or increasing apprehension.
- Monitoring of uterine contractions and FHR is an important nursing responsibility. Fetal bradycardia, tachycardia, and FHR variability are important observations to make.
- Interventions such as keeping a woman active during labor and promoting voiding help to strengthen contractions and make labor more effective.
- Offering psychological support is crucial to maternal well-being and helps in planning nursing care that not only meets QSEN competencies but also best meets the family's total needs.
- Pushing during the second stage of labor should be guided by the woman's need to push. Urge her to breathe out while pushing, if possible.
- The placental stage follows birth and consists of both placental separation and expulsion. Observe for excessive bleeding during this time. Do not pull on the cord to hasten separation because this can lead to uterine inversion.
- A fetus is in potential danger when the membranes rupture because of the possibility of cord prolapse. Always assess FHR at this point to safeguard the fetus.

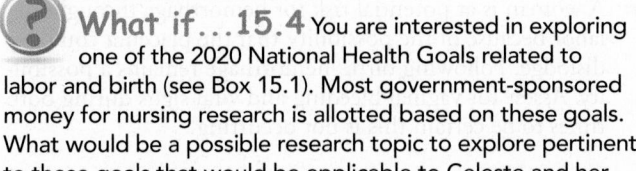

- A woman is at potential risk for hemorrhage throughout labor because of the possibility that the placenta could dislodge. Following birth, hemorrhage remains a possibility. Assess for vaginal bleeding and vital signs during both times to be certain this is not occurring.

Critical Thinking Care Study

Gail Taylor is an obese-appearing 16-year-old whom you meet as she is admitted to your labor service. Her cervix is fully effaced, 10 cm dilated, and she is pushing. Her mother tells you she didn't know Gail was pregnant because she's been living at her boyfriend's apartment for 8 months. She didn't realize she was in labor until an hour ago when she dropped by the apartment and found the living room set up for a home birth. She pulled Gail into her car and drove her to the hospital, which took over an hour because of early morning freeway traffic. Gail's mother tells you the boyfriend (a 20-year-old college student) is waiting downstairs in the parking lot; she threatened she'd charge him with rape if he came any further inside than the front door of the hospital. Gail received no prenatal care or preparation for labor; when you ask her if she's happy she's having a baby, her mother interrupts and says, "I don't want her to even see it. We'll give it away for adoption."

1. This is a family with a multitude of problems. Did the mother make a good decision when she brought Gail to the hospital in her car rather than dial for emergency help if she was worried about her? Which would have been the best place for Gail to give birth: at an apartment arranged for home birth or in a car on a busy freeway?
2. Gail is automatically a high-risk patient because of her age. What other factors make her high risk?
3. Gail's mother seems to be making decisions for everyone here. Does she have any right to make an adoption decision for Gail?

Patient Scenario: The Hudson Family

Read about the Hudson family, a family about to have a new family member, then answer the questions to further sharpen your skills and grow more familiar with NCLEX-type questions related to labor and birth. Confirm your answers are correct by reading the rationales.

Visit http://thePoint.lww.com

Answers and Rationales

Looking for answers to the What If. . . and Critical Thinking Care Study questions?

Visit http://thePoint.lww.com

References

Aasheim, V., Nilsen, A. B., Lukasse, M., et al. (2011). Perineal techniques during the second stage of labour for reducing perineal trauma. *Cochrane Database of Systematic Reviews,* (12), CD006672.

Aguirre, F., & Chou, B. (2011). Normal labor & delivery, operative delivery & malpresentations. In K. J. Hurt, M. W. Guile, J. L. Bienstock, et al. (Eds.), *The Johns Hopkins manual of gynecology and obstetrics* (4th ed., pp. 73–89). Philadelphia, PA: Lippincott Williams & Wilkins.

Al, J. F. (2012). Grandmultiparity: A potential risk factor for adverse pregnancy outcomes. *Journal of Reproductive Medicine, 57*(1–2), 53–57.

American Congress of Obstetricians & Gynecologists. (2009). ACOG practice bulletin: Intrapartum fetal heart rate monitoring. *Obstetrics & Gynecology, 114*(1), 193–200.

Amis, D. (2010). *Prepared childbirth: The family way.* New York, NY: Lamaze International.

Archie, C., & Roman, A. S. (2013). Normal & abnormal labor & delivery. In A. H. DeCherney, L. Nathan, T. M. Goodwin, et al. (Eds.), *Current diagnosis and treatment: Obstetrics and gynecology* (11th ed., pp. 154–162). Columbus, OH: McGraw-Hill/Lange.

Arrojo, I. P., Lamas, M. C, Verdugo, L. P., et al. (2012). Trends in cord blood banking. *Blood Transfusion, 10*(1), 95–100.

Association of Women's Health, Obstetric and Neonatal Nurses. (2011). Nursing support of laboring women. *Journal of Obstetric, Gynecologic & Neonatal Nursing, 40*(5), 665–666.

Barber, E. L., Lundsberg, L. S., Belanger, K., et al. (2011). Indications contributing to the increasing cesarean delivery rate. *Obstetrics & Gynecology, 118*(1), 29–38.

Bárcena, A., Muench, M. O., Kapidzic, M., et al. (2011). Human placenta and chorion: Potential additional sources of hematopoietic stem cells for transplantation. *Transfusion, 51*(Suppl. 4), 94S–105S.

Baselice, J., & Lawson, S. (2011). Postpartum care and breastfeeding. In K. J. Hurt, M. W. Guile, J. L. Bienstock, et al. (Eds.), *The Johns Hopkins manual of gynecology and obstetrics* (4th ed., pp. 257–264). Philadelphia, PA: Lippincott Williams & Wilkins.

Beck, C. T., Gable, R. K., Sakala, C., et al. (2011). Posttraumatic stress disorder in new mothers: Results from a two-stage U.S. national survey. *Birth, 38*(3), 216–227.

Begley, C. M., Gyte, G. M., Devane, D., et al. (2011). Active versus expectant management for women in the third stage of labour. *Cochrane Database of Systematic Reviews,* (11), CD007412.

Bernal, A. L., & Norwitz, E. R. (2012). The normal mechanisms of labor. In D. K. Edmonds (Ed.), *Dewhurst's textbook of obstetrics & gynaecology* (8th ed., pp. 247–268). Oxford, UK: John Wiley & Sons.

Brown, S. J., Gartland, D., Donath, S., et al. (2011). Effects of prolonged second stage. *BJOG: International Journal of Obstetrics & Gynaecology, 118*(8), 991–1000.

Coad, J., & Dunstall, M. (2011). Physiology of parturition. In J. Coad & M. Dunstall (Eds.), *Anatomy & physiology for midwives* (pp. 317–362). London, UK: Elsevier/Churchill Livingstone.

Cortes, E., Basra, R., & Kelleher, C. J. (2011). Waterbirth and pelvic floor injury: A retrospective study and postal survey using ICIQ modular long form questionnaires. *European Journal of Obstetrics, Gynecology & Reproductive Biology, 155*(1), 27–30.

Downe, S. (2011). Care in the second stage of labor. In S. MacDonald & J. Magill-Cuerden (Eds.), *Mayes midwifery* (14th ed., pp. 509–520). London, UK: Bailliere Tindall/Elsevier.

Elharmeel, S., Chaudhary, Y., Tan, S., et al. (2011). Surgical repair of spontaneous perineal tears that occur during childbirth versus no intervention. *Cochrane Database of Systematic Reviews,* (8), CD008534.

Facco, F. L. (2011). Sleep-disordered breathing and pregnancy. *Seminars in Perinatology, 35*(6), 335–339.

Friedman, E. (1978). *Labor, clinical evaluation and management* (2nd ed.). New York, NY: Appleton-Century-Crofts.

Garabedian, M. J., Williams, C. M., Pearce, C. F., et al. (2011). Extreme morbid obesity and labor outcome in nulliparous women at term. *American Journal of Perinatology, 28*(9), 729–734.

Gilliland, A. L. (2011). After praise and encouragement: Emotional support strategies used by birth doulas in the USA and Canada. *Midwifery, 27*(4), 525–531.

Harris, R., & Ayers, S. (2012). What makes labour and birth traumatic? *Psychology & Health, 27*(10), 1166–1177.

Hodnett, E. D., Gates, S. Hofmeyr, G. J., et al. (2011). Continuous support for women during childbirth. *Cochrane Database of Systematic Reviews,* (2), CD003766.

Impey, L., & Child, T. (2012). Labour 1: Mechanism: Anatomy and physiology. In L. Impey & T. Child (Eds.), *Obstetrics & gynaecology* (4th ed., pp. 239–245) West Sussex, UK: John Wiley & Sons.

Jacquemyn, Y., Martens, E., & Martens, G. (2012). Foetal monitoring during labour: Practice versus theory in a region-wide analysis. *Clinical & Experimental Obstetrics & Gynecology, 39*(3), 307–309.

Karch, A. M. (2013). *2013 Lippincott's nursing drug guide.* Philadelphia, PA: Lippincott Williams & Wilkins.

Lauderdale, J. (2011). Transcultural perspectives in childbearing. In M. M. Andrews & J. S. Boyle (Eds.), *Transcultural concepts in nursing care* (pp. 85–115). Philadelphia, PA: Lippincott Williams & Wilkins.

Layer, J. (2011). An overview of upright positions during second stage labor. *Midwifery Today with International Midwife,* (98), 36–39.

Maharaj, D. (2010). Assessing cephalopelvic disproportion: Back to the basics. *Obstetrical & Gynecological Survey, 65*(6), 387–395.

Main, C. (2012). Changing practice: Physiological cord clamping. *Practicing Midwife, 15*(1), 30–31.

Moore, E. R., Anderson, G. C., Bergman, N., et al. (2012). Early skin-to-skin contact for mothers and their healthy newborn infants. *Cochrane Database of Systematic Reviews,* (5), CD003519.

Nitsche, J. F., & Howell, T. (2011). Peripartum pubic symphysis separation: A case report and review of the literature. *Obstetrical & Gynecological Survey, 66*(3), 153–158.

Nyman, V., Downe, S., & Berg, M. (2011). Waiting for permission to enter the labour ward world: First time parents' experiences of the first encounter on a labour ward. *Sexual & Reproductive Healthcare, 2*(3), 129–134.

Opotowsky, A. R., Siddiqi, O. K., D'Souza, B., et al. (2012). Maternal cardiovascular events during childbirth among women with congenital heart disease. *Heart, 98*(2), 145–151.

Osborne, K., & Hanson, L. (2012). Directive versus supportive approaches used by midwives when providing care during the second stage of labor. *Journal of Midwifery & Women's Health, 57*(1), 3–11.

Oteng-Ntim, E., Varma, R., Croker, H., et al. (2012). Lifestyle interventions for overweight and obese pregnant women to improve pregnancy outcome: Systematic review and meta-analysis. *BMC Medicine, 10*(1), 47–48.

Ovadia, C., & Dixit, A. (2012). The management of gestational diabetes. *Current Diabetes Reviews, 8*(4), 247–256.

Penna, L. (2011). Fetal surveillance in labor. In S. Arulkumaran, L. Regan, A. Papageorghiou, et al. (Eds.), *Oxford desk reference: Obstetrics & gynaecology* (pp. 378–383). Oxford, UK: Oxford University Press.

Plaat, F. (2012). Analgesia, anaesthesia & induction. In D. K. Edmonds (Ed.), *Dewhurst's textbook of obstetrics & gynaecology* (8th ed., pp. 356–363). Oxford, UK: John Wiley & Son.

Selby, C., Valencia, S., Garcia, L., et al. (2012). Activity level during a one-hour labor check evaluation: Walking versus bed rest. *MCN: American Journal of Maternal Child Nursing, 37*(2), 101–107.

Simkin, P. (2010). The fetal occiput posterior position: State of the science and a new perspective. *Birth, 37*(1), 61–71.

Smith, C. A., Collins, C. T., Crowther, C. A., et al. (2011). Acupuncture or acupressure for pain management in labour. *Cochrane Database of Systematic Reviews,* (7), CD009232.

Smith, C. A., Levett, K. M., Collins, C. T., et al. (2011). Relaxation techniques for pain management in labour. *Cochrane Database of Systematic Reviews,* (12), CD009514.

Stevens, J. R., & Wittich, A. C. (2011). A rare case of occult uterine inversion at an Army community hospital: A case report. *Military Medicine, 176*(12), 1450–1452.

Swarnam, K., Soraisham, A. S., & Sivanandan, S. (2012). Advances in the management of meconium aspiration syndrome. *International Journal of Pediatrics, 2012,* 359571.

U.S. Department of Health and Human Services. (2010). *Healthy people 2020.* Washington, DC: Author.

Zheng, T. (2012). Normal labor & delivery. In T. Zheng (Ed.), *Comprehensive handbook of obstetrics & gynecology* (pp. 320–323). Paradise Valley, AZ: Phoenix Medical Press.

Chapter 16

The Nursing Role in Providing Comfort During Labor and Birth

KEY TERMS

- analgesia
- anesthesia
- doula
- endorphins
- epidural anesthesia
- pain
- pressure anesthesia
- pudendal nerve block
- reflexology

OBJECTIVES

After mastering the contents of this chapter, you should be able to:

1. Describe the physiologic basis of contractions during labor and how nonpharmacologic therapies, as well as analgesia and anesthesia, can be used to promote a woman's comfort during labor and birth.
2. Identify 2020 National Health Goals related to comfort and drug-free pain management measures effective in childbirth that nurses can help the nation achieve.
3. Assess the degree and type of discomfort a woman is experiencing during labor and birth, including her ability to cope with pain effectively and the maternal and fetal impact of pain management, including side effects and safety.
4. Formulate nursing diagnoses related to the effect of pain or pain management during labor and birth.
5. Establish expected outcomes to meet the needs of a woman experiencing discomfort during labor and birth and manage seamless transitions across differing health care settings.
6. Using the nursing process, plan nursing care that includes the six competencies of Quality & Safety Education for Nurses (QSEN): Patient-Centered Care, Teamwork & Collaboration, Evidence-Based Practice (EPB), Quality Improvement (QI), Safety, and Informatics.
7. Implement common complementary and pharmacologic measures for pain management during labor and birth.
8. Evaluate expected outcomes for effectiveness and achievement of care.
9. Integrate knowledge of pain management during labor and birth with the interplay of nursing process, the six competencies of QSEN, and Family Nursing to promote quality maternal and child health nursing care.

Jonny Baranca is a primipara in early labor whom you admit to a birthing unit. Her cervix is 3 cm dilated. She tells you her sister had epidural anesthesia that completely obliterated her pain in labor for the birth of her baby 3 months ago. Based on her sister's experience, Jonny expected to be given epidural anesthesia as soon as she arrived at the hospital as she "is in early labor." Her physician, however, asked her to wait until she is 4 cm dilated. When you enter her room, you find her lying on her back in a birthing bed, crying. Her husband shouts his "wife deserves better care than this."

The previous chapter discussed the process of labor and birth and nursing care responsibilities. This chapter adds information to your knowledge base about how to promote comfort during labor. Effective pain management in labor can change labor from an experience so negative it can result in a posttraumatic stress syndrome to a positive, forward-moving experience.

Was the information Jonny received from her sister realistic? What are some immediate interventions you could do to help Jonny better cope with her pain?

Concerns about the discomfort and pain that accompany labor and birth can dominate a pregnant woman's or couple's thoughts during pregnancy; these can become particularly strong as the baby's due date approaches. As discussed in Chapter 14, prepared childbirth classes provide couples with an opportunity to learn and practice a variety of pain management techniques, such as breathing patterns, to help reduce pain in labor.

Often, however, the labor experience is so intense it becomes overwhelming, so administration of an analgesic or a regional anesthetic may be necessary to reduce discomfort sufficiently to allow a woman to regain control over herself and use breathing patterns. If the use of regional anesthesia makes labor a satisfying, positive experience, the intervention can ultimately promote the entire family's health. Some women, however, may feel they have let down themselves, a partner, or childbirth educator by asking for anesthesia; if this happens, asking for pain medication can make labor a negative experience.

You can alert women that labor can be exceedingly painful and is not a contest with winners and losers. Using medication or not using medication are both routes to the same end: a woman becoming a new parent with both a healthy mother and healthy newborn (Kemp et al., 2013).

Much has been written in nursing literature about using the neutral term *contraction* instead of *labor pain* to keep from reminding a woman contractions are painful. The theory is a sound one, not only because a woman is experiencing a *contracting* sensation but also because calling it *pain* could magnify fear and tension; tension, in turn, magnifies pain. Remember, however, renaming it will not change its basic nature. Discomfort accompanies labor regardless of what term is used for it. Fortunately, many nursing interventions can help reduce pain, so labor is as fulfilling and rewarding an experience as a woman hoped it would be.

Making labor and birth a memorable experience for families is so important that 2020 National Health Goals have been established to address this topic. These are shown in Box 16.1.

BOX 16.1 Nursing Care Planning Based on 2020 National Health Goals

Because administration of either analgesia or anesthesia during labor can prolong labor and can possibly increase the number of instruments used or risk for cesarean birth, several 2020 National Health Goals are related to the types of pain relief used in labor. Examples include:

- Reduce the maternal mortality rate to no more than 11.4 deaths per 100,000 live births from a baseline of 12.7 per 100,000.
- Reduce the fetal/newborn death rate during the perinatal period (28 weeks of gestation to 7 days after birth) to no more than 5.9 per 1,000 live births from a baseline of 6.6 per 1,000 live births (U.S. Department of Health and Human Services [DHHS], 2010; see www.healthypeople.gov).

Nurses can help the nation achieve these goals by educating women about the advantages of preparing for childbirth, helping them to use breathing patterns or other complementary and alternative therapies and techniques during labor so they need a minimum of analgesia and anesthesia, and conscientiously monitoring women who receive analgesics and anesthesia.

Nursing Process Overview

For Pain Relief During Labor and Childbirth

Assessment

Pain, the sensation of discomfort, is a subjective, personal symptom; it is what the experiencing person says it is and present when the experiencing person says it is present (McCaffery, 1972). It is unique to each individual, so a woman is the only person who can describe or know the extent of her pain. To assess the amount of discomfort a woman is having in labor, listen carefully to not only what she says but also how she rates her discomfort level on a pain assessment scale. Also look for subtle signs such as facial tenseness, flushing or paleness, hands clenched in fists, rapid breathing, or rapid pulse rate.

Nursing Diagnosis

Although pain related to labor contractions is the most obvious nursing diagnosis applicable to labor, it is not the only relevant one because pain can create other problems for the laboring woman that can negatively affect the childbirth experience. If not resolved, these problems can intensify pain. Some women, for example, may become more concerned with their reaction to the pain than to the pain itself. Because of this, applicable nursing diagnoses might include:

- Pain related to labor contractions
- Powerlessness related to the duration and intensity of labor
- Anxiety related to lack of knowledge about "normal" labor process
- Risk for situational low self-esteem related to ineffectiveness of prepared childbirth breathing exercises
- Decisional conflict related to use of analgesia or anesthesia during labor

Outcome Identification and Planning

When developing realistic outcomes and planning interventions to manage discomfort during labor, consider the woman's perceptions about childbirth, her past childbirth experiences (if any), and the amount and type of childbirth preparation she and her partner have made. For example, if a woman is using breathing exercises well, expecting she will need medication late in labor is probably not realistic. However, if a woman has not made any preparation as to how she will manage labor contractions, expecting that no medication will be used might be inappropriate.

Be aware that pharmacologic agents used during labor and birth may pose risks for both the woman, such as hypotension, as well as the fetus, such as bradycardia. Therefore, when considering use of pharmacologic intervention, the benefit to the woman and the fetus must outweigh the risks of medication use. In addition, a decision to use analgesia or anesthesia may also affect family functioning if the method chosen limits the partner's participation in the birth. Two good Internet sites to refer women who need help making a decision as to what type of pain relief they want in labor are the Mayo Clinic site (www.mayoclinic.com) and the Childbirth Connection site (www.childbirthconnection.org).

Implementation

Keeping a woman and her support person informed about their options and how they differ as labor progresses is important. For instance, simply knowing that birth is getting closer can make the next few contractions easier to withstand. Supporting and encouraging a woman to use methods of complementary and alternative therapies for pain management, such as a birthing ball, ambulation, relaxation, and controlled breathing, also are helpful. Offering analgesia or assisting with anesthesia administration during labor or birth requires nursing judgment and a caring presence to help one woman accept analgesia when she needs it and to encourage another to experience childbirth without pharmacologic intervention when that is what she desires.

Outcome Evaluation

Evaluations are ongoing and typically must occur within a short time frame. Examples of short-term expected outcomes that would indicate successful achievement during labor are:

- Client states pain during labor is within a tolerable level for her.
- Couple reports they feel control throughout the labor process.
- Client and fetus remain physiologically stable with use of pharmacologic interventions.
- Client verbalizes satisfaction with current pain control measures.

A long-term evaluation should reveal a woman found labor and birth to be an experience not only endurable but also that it allowed her to grow in self-esteem and the family to grow through a shared experience. Asking a woman to describe her labor experience afterward in relation to pain not only aids an evaluation of whether pain management was adequate but also helps her work through this emotional period of life and integrate it into her previous experiences as well.

BOX 16.2 Nursing Care Planning Using Assessment

Assessing a Woman for Symptoms of Pain During Labor and Childbirth

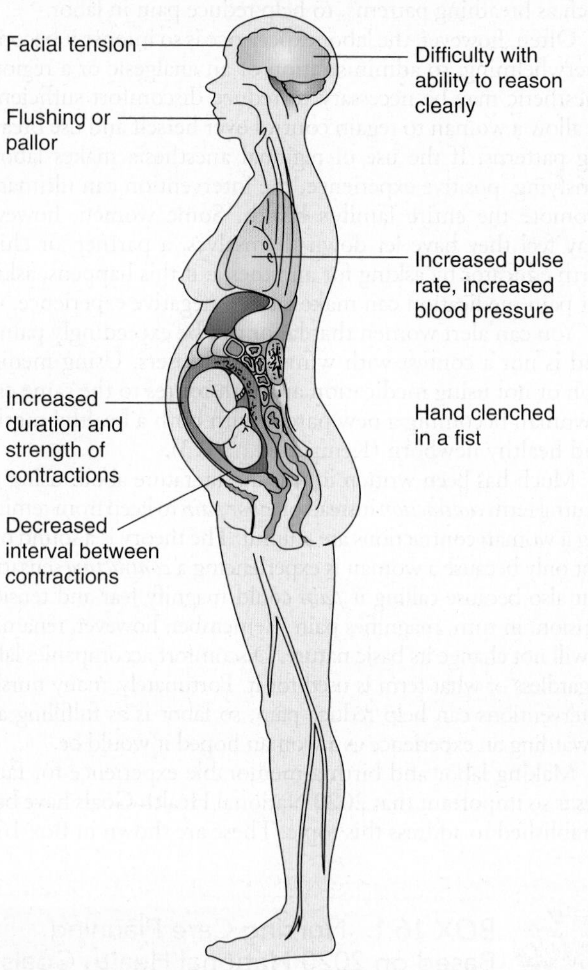

EXPERIENCE OF PAIN DURING CHILDBIRTH

Pain accompanies labor contractions for several different reasons and manifests itself in different ways for each woman (Box 16.2).

Etiology of Pain During Labor and Birth

Normally, contractions of involuntary muscles, such as the heart, stomach, and intestine, do not cause pain. This concept makes uterine contractions unique because they do cause pain. Several explanations exist for why this happens. During contractions, blood vessels constrict, reducing the blood supply to uterine and cervical cells, resulting in anoxia to muscle fibers. This anoxia can cause pain in the same way blockage of the cardiac arteries causes the pain of a heart attack. As labor progresses and contractions become longer and more intense, the ischemia to cells increases, the anoxia increases, and the pain intensifies.

Pain also probably results from stretching of the cervix and perineum. This phenomenon is the same as the intestinal pain that results when accumulating gas stretches the intestines. At the end of the transitional phase in labor, when stretching of the cervix is complete and the woman feels she has to push, pain from the contractions often disappears as long as the woman is pushing, until the fetal presenting part causes a final stretching of the perineum (Tocher, 2011).

Additional discomfort in labor may stem from the pressure of the fetal presenting part on tissues, including pressure on surrounding organs, such as the bladder, the urethra, and the lower colon. In addition to these factors, cultural expectations effect how pain is perceived (Box 16.3). All these factors make nursing support, in addition to a doula or a partner, important as it can have a positive influence on pain relief in all situations of labor.

Physiology of Pain

Pain is a basic protective mechanism that alerts a person that something threatening is happening somewhere in the body.

BOX 16.3 Nursing Care Planning to Respect Cultural Diversity

Some women believe their expected role during labor is to be stoic and nonverbal even in the face of intense pain. Others believe expressing their discomfort by screaming or verbalizing their discomfort is what is expected. If a woman is not proficient in English, it may be particularly difficult for her to describe her level of discomfort and that she needs some assistance. Assess each woman individually to determine not only what level of comfort she feels is right for her during labor but also the manner in which she feels most able to express discomfort. Assessing individuals in this way rather than relying on a list of "typical" ways Hispanic women, Asian women, and so forth, react to pain achieves better individual care. Because of Americanization, a woman's surname or her appearance may be not be indicative at all of how she wants to manage pain.

The amount of analgesia women desire or will accept is dependent both on the situation and her culture. In a culture in which birth is seen as a "natural" process or if a woman has attended a class to prepare for birth, the less analgesia is generally desired. Any woman who has an effective support person with her generally needs less pharmacologic pain relief than one who does not.

The sensation begins in nociceptors, the end points of afferent nerves, when they are activated by mechanical, chemical, or thermal stimuli. Nociceptors are located predominantly in the skin, bone periosteum, joint surfaces, and arterial walls. When these end terminals are stimulated, chemical mediators such as prostaglandins, histamine, bradykinin, and serotonin are synthesized and help transmit the pain impulse along small, unmyelinated C fibers and large, myelinated A-delta fibers to the spinal cord. The more numerous C fibers conduct slowly and apparently carry dull, low-level pain; the fewer A-delta fibers apparently carry sharp, well-localized pain such as labor contractions (Euliano, Gravenstein, Gravenstein, et al., 2011).

In the dorsal horn of the spinal cord, somatostatin, cholecystokinin, and substance P serve as neurotransmitters or assist the pain impulse across the synapse between the peripheral nerve and the spinal nerve. The pain impulse then ascends the spinal cord to the brain cortex, where it is interpreted as pain.

The Melzack–Wall gate control theory of pain (Melzack & Wall, 1965), the most widely accepted theory of pain response, proposes pain can be halted at three points:

- The peripheral end terminals
- The synapse points in the dorsal horn of the spinal cord
- The point at which the impulse is interpreted as pain in the brain cortex

Pain in peripheral terminals is automatically reduced by the production of endorphins and encephalins, naturally occurring opiates that limit transmission of pain from the end terminals. Pain can be reduced further at these end points by mechanically irritating nerve fibers through an action such as rubbing the skin, which blocks nerve transmission.

A major way to block spinal cord neurotransmitters (i.e., never allowing the pain impulse to cross to a spinal nerve) is by the administration of pain medications. In addition, the brain cortex can be distracted from sensing impulses as pain by such techniques as imagery, thought stopping, and perhaps aromatherapy or yoga.

Sensory impulses of pain from the uterus and cervix synapse at the spinal column at the level of T10 through L1, whereas motor impulses register higher in the cord at T5 through T10. Anesthetic pain relief measures for the first stage of labor, therefore, are designed to stop pain by blocking the lower sensory sites, but not the upper motor sites, so strong contractions can continue.

Sensory impulses from the perineum, which is involved in the second stage of labor, are carried by the pudendal nerve to join the spinal column at S2, S3, and S4. When the perineum is initiating the pain, anesthetic pain relief must block these lower receptor sites. This is an important point to remember when talking to a woman in labor about pain relief. Some interventions relieve pain for both the first and second stages of labor, whereas others work for one stage but not both.

Perception of Pain

The amount of discomfort a woman experiences during contractions differs according to her expectations of and preparation for labor; the length of her labor; the position of her fetus; the presence of fear, anxiety, worry, body image, and self-efficacy; and the availability of meaningful people around her to offer support (Fig. 16.1). As a rule, women who believe

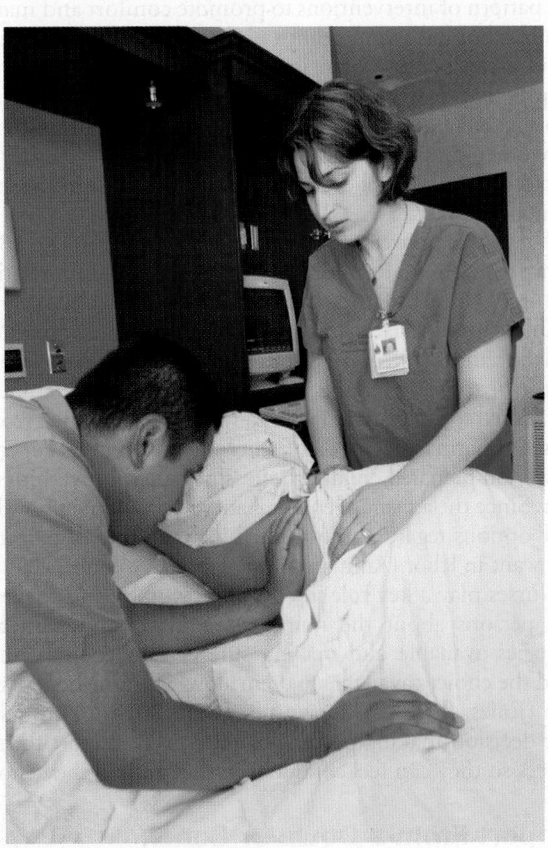

FIGURE 16.1 The discomfort a woman experiences during childbirth is related to the amount of support she receives from her family and health care providers. Here, the woman's support person uses the palm of his hand to apply counter pressure to her lower back, helping to ease back pain.

they can control their situation (have self-efficacy) are more apt to report a satisfactory birth experience than those who do not feel in control (Howarth, Swain, & Treharne, 2011).

Fetal position is a physical variable that influences the degree of pain a woman experiences because if the fetus is in an occiput posterior position, the woman often reports intense or nagging back pain, even between contractions, much more than if a fetus is in an occipitoanterior position (Impey & Child, 2012).

Pain is perceived differently by different individuals because of psychosocial, physiologic, and cultural responses. The body's ability to produce and maintain **endorphins** (naturally occurring opiate-like substances) may influence a person's overall pain threshold and the amount of pain a person perceives at any given time. Women who come into the labor experience believing the pain will be horrible are usually surprised afterward to realize the agony they expected never materialized. However, women who thought pain would be minimal can be overwhelmed by its intensity. Unrealistic expectations of labor pain can make a woman so tense during labor her pain feels worse than it would have if she had been relaxed. A woman cannot relax simply because she is instructed to do so by another person, however. Some additional interventions must be used.

COMFORT AND PAIN RELIEF MEASURES

The pattern of interventions to promote comfort and manage pain in labor has swung from a philosophy of no intervention (none given because pain in labor was expected), to a philosophy that drug intervention was always required (excessive amounts were given), to the modern approach of empowering women and their partners with information so they can choose how to best relieve pain during labor within the limits of medical safety.

With the discovery of ether and chloroform in the 1800s, it was realized that childbirth could be managed relatively pain free. Unfortunately, this goal was achieved by means of complete anesthesia or unconsciousness for the woman during labor and birth. Women, afterward, had difficulty believing the birth was over and that the infant was their child.

This led to an era (late 1960s to the 1980s) in which women refused pharmacologic pain relief in labor and depended entirely on prepared childbirth measures such as breathing patterns. Since the advent of epidural anesthesia, women now have more options regarding how much or what kind of pain relief they want in labor (Anim-Somuah, Smyth, & Jones, 2011).

Nurses play a key role in educating women and their support persons about the numerous comfort and pain relief strategies available and making sure certain couples understand the choices available to them along with the benefits and risks (Jones, Othman, Dowswell, et al., 2012). Throughout their decision-making process, couples need support for their choices so they can feel confident in the method they choose.

Support From a Doula or Coach

Although, historically, women have always attended other women in childbirth, in the past 40 years or so, the father or partner of a woman's child has traditionally served as her chief support person in labor. Some partners or fathers, however, find it difficult to serve as effective coaches because they are so emotionally involved in the birth. Some women prefer to ask a sister, mother, or friend to serve as a coach.

A **doula** is a woman who is experienced in childbirth and postpartum support. These support persons (who may hold certificates as birth or postpartum doulas) provide physical, emotional, and informational support prenatally, during labor and birth, and even at home in the postnatal period (DONA International, 2012), Having an effective doula can increase a woman's self-esteem, speed the labor process, and improve breastfeeding success, as well as decrease rates of oxytocin augmentation, epidural anesthesia, cesarean birth, and postpartum complications (Gilliland, 2011).

✔ QSEN Checkpoint Question 16.1

Patient-Centered Care

Jonny Baranca is having a painful labor. She asks you if she should have hired a doula. Your best answer would be which of the following?

a. "Definitely. Doulas time contractions and perform many tasks, taking the burden off you."
b. "Maybe. Doulas are good at telling you if you are doing everything correctly."
c. "That's an individual choice, but a doula can serve as an important support person."
d. "No. A second person giving advice is apt to cause conflict."

Look in Appendix A for the best answer and rationale.

Complementary and Alternative Therapies for Pain Relief

Complementary and alternative therapies for pain relief involve nonpharmacologic measures that may be used either as a woman's total pain management program or to complement pharmacologic interventions. Most of these interventions are based on the gate control theory concept that distraction can be effective at preventing the brain from processing pain sensations coming into the cortex. Many of the same techniques may help the descent of a fetus.

Relaxation

The technique of relaxation, as discussed in Chapter 14, is taught in most preparation for childbirth classes but can be taught in early labor as well. Relaxation keeps the abdominal wall from becoming tense, allowing the uterus to rise with contractions without pressing against the hard abdominal wall. It also serves as a distraction technique because, while concentrating on relaxing, a woman cannot concentrate on pain. Asking a woman to bring favorite music or aromatherapy with her to enjoy in the birthing room, although not evidence based, can help with relaxation (Smith, Collins, & Crowther, 2011). Remember, no aromatic candles should be used because of nearby oxygen outlets.

Focusing and Imagery

Concentrating intently on an object is another method of distraction, or another method of keeping sensory input from reaching the cortex of the brain (Smith, Levett, Collins, et al.,

2011). For this technique, a woman uses a photograph of someone important to her or some setting she finds appealing such as a beautiful sunset. She concentrates on the photo during contractions (focusing). A woman can also concentrate on a mental image, such as waves rolling onto a beach (imagery), or chant a word or phrase such as the new baby's name during contractions, all of which help prevent her from concentrating on the pain of contractions. If a woman has never used these techniques before, she may question how effective they are. Urge her to try one of them at least for a few contractions before she dismisses them entirely, as evidence supports their efficacy (Gedde-Dahl & Fors, 2012). Do not ask questions or talk while a woman is using focusing, imagery, or chanting because that is apt to break her concentration and let the sensation of pain break through.

QSEN Checkpoint Question 16.2

Evidence-Based Practice

To investigate if listening to music can help women feel less pain and anxiety in labor, researchers assigned 30 primiparas expected to have normal spontaneous births to either an experimental group that received routine labor care or a control group that received routine care plus music therapy. Both women and their nurses assessed the degree of pain experienced during labor. Results of the study revealed women who listened to music had significantly lower pain during the latent phase of labor. No significant differences were found between the two groups during the active phase of labor (Liu, Chang, & Chen, 2010).

Based on this study, which statement by Jonny represents the best way to use music therapy in labor?

a. "I've brought techno music to play during the second stage so I can push to a rhythm."
b. "I'll need distraction most just before I have to push. I'll save my music until then."
c. "I know music probably won't make a difference but I'll enjoy listening to it anyway."
d. "I brought some romantic music to play during early labor to help me relax."

Look in Appendix A for the best answer and rationale.

Prayer

For many women, prayer may be the first measure they use to relieve a stress they are facing (Marc, Toureche, Ernst, et al., 2011). Provide uninterrupted time as needed. Women may bring helpful worship objects such as a Bible or Qur'an into their birthing setting to use during prayer. Remember, these are sacred objects; be careful when changing sheets that you do not accidentally throw such important objects away or let them fall to the floor.

Breathing Techniques

Breathing patterns are taught in most preparation for childbirth classes and are well documented to decrease pain in labor (Dick-Read & Gaskin, 2013). They are largely distraction techniques because a woman concentrating on slow-paced breathing cannot concentrate on pain. Breathing strategies can be taught to a woman in labor if she is not familiar with their advantages before labor (see Chapter 14). Stay with her until she appreciates how useful slow spaced breathing can be and feels comfortable using this technique independently.

Herbal Preparations

Several herbal preparations have traditionally been used to reduce pain with dysmenorrhea or labor, although there is little evidence-based support for their effectiveness. Examples include chamomile tea for its relaxing properties; raspberry leaf tea (women freeze it into ice cubes to suck on), which is thought to strengthen uterine contractions; skullcap; and catnip, which are thought to help with pain. Jasmine and lavender may both be mixed into oils and rubbed on the perineum before and during labor to soften the muscle and help prevent perineal tears (Jones, 2011). Black cohosh (squaw root), an herb that induces uterine contractions, is not recommended because of the risk of acute toxic effects such as cerebrovascular accident to the mother or fetus (Chillemi & Chillemi, 2012).

Aromatherapy and Essential Oils

Aromatherapy is the use of aromatic oils to complement emotional and physical well-being. Their use is based on the principle that the sense of smell plays a significant role in overall health. When an essential oil is inhaled, its molecules are transported via the olfactory system to the limbic system in the brain. The brain then responds to particular aromas with emotional responses such as relaxation. These oils should not be applied directly to the skin to avoid irritation but are used in a mister so they are inhaled, then carried throughout the body. The oils may be able to penetrate cell walls and transport nutrients or oxygen to the inside of cells. The use of aromatherapy, although pleasant, has little evidence-based support and so should be recommended with that in mind (Smith, Collins, et al., 2011).

QSEN Checkpoint Question 16.3

Informatics

You offer to teach Jonny controlled breathing to help with pain management until she can receive her epidural. Which would be the best instruction?

a. "Lie on your back and breathe in slowly while repeating, 'I can do this.'"
b. "Hold your breath as long as you possibly can before exhaling."
c. "Breathe in as slowly as you can, then breathe out just as slowly."
d. "Pant rapidly as this best lifts your abdominal wall off your expanding uterus."

Look in Appendix A for the best answer and rationale.

Heat or Cold Application

The application of heat and cold has always been used for pain relief after injuries such as minor burns or strained muscles. It is only lately that their use has been investigated as effective ways to help relieve the pain of labor. Women who are having back pain may find the application of heat to the lower back by a heating pad, instant hot pack, or warm moist compress extremely comforting. Heat applied to the

(*tsubos*) located along meridians that course throughout the body to supply the organs of the body with energy. Activation of these points (which are not necessarily near the affected organ) results in a release of endorphins, which makes this system helpful, especially in the first stage of labor (Hamidzadeh, Shahpourian, Orak, et al., 2012).

Acupressure is the application of pressure or massage at these same points (Robinson, Lorenc, & Liao, 2011). It seems to be most effective for low back pain. A common point used for women in labor is Co4 (Hoku or Hegu point), which is located between the first finger and thumb on the back of the hand. Women may report their contractions feel lighter when a support person holds and squeezes their hand because the support person is accidentally triggering this point.

What if...16.1 You had met Jonny during pregnancy and discovered she did not attend any preparation for childbirth classes because she planned to rely totally on epidural anesthesia for pain relief. Would you have supported her plan? Now that she is in early labor, what are some complementary and alternative therapies you could teach her to use while she waits for anesthesia?

Pharmacologic Measures for Pain Relief During Labor

Pharmacologic management of pain during labor and birth includes **analgesia**, which reduces or decreases awareness of pain, and **anesthesia**, which causes partial or complete loss of pain sensation. For the best results, be certain women are included in the selection of these methods and understand any fetal effects or maternal side effects that might occur.

Virtually all medications given during labor cross the placenta and have some effect on the fetus, which makes it important to do regular assessments of maternal and fetal responses to the administration of systemic medication. However, labor should not test a woman to the limit of her endurance because both analgesia and anesthesia are available. Be sure to caution women not to take acetylsalicylic acid (aspirin) for pain in labor as aspirin interferes with blood coagulation, increasing the risk for bleeding in the newborn or herself. In addition, the manufacturers of pain relief patches such as Salonpas, Absorbine Jr., and Icy Hot caution women not to use these in labor because of the potentially teratogenic effect of the menthol ingredient.

Goals of Pharmacologic Management of Pain During Labor

The ideal or goal of medications used during labor is to relax a woman and relieve her discomfort, yet have minimal systemic effects on uterine contractions, her pushing effort, or the fetus (Box 16.4). Whether a drug affects a fetus depends on its ability to cross the placenta and that depends on its molecular weight. Drugs with a molecular weight of less than 600 Daltons (Da) cross very readily; drugs with a molecular weight of more than 1,000 Da cross poorly. Drugs with highly charged molecules or molecules strongly bound to protein also tend to cross more slowly than others. Fat-soluble drugs cross the easiest.

If a drug causes a systemic response, such as hypotension in a woman, it can result in a decreased oxygen (Po_2) gradient across the placenta, causing the indirect result of fetal hypoxia. If a drug causes confusion or disorientation, a woman may be unable to work effectively with contractions, thus prolonging labor and increasing discomfort for her. A preterm fetus, which has an immature liver and is unable to metabolize or inactivate drugs, is generally more affected by drugs than a term fetus. If a medication causes changes in a fetus, such as a decreased heart rate or central nervous system (CNS) depression, it may be difficult for the newborn infant to initiate respirations at birth, severely compromising the infant in the important first minutes of life. In addition, if a drug reduces or eliminates the bearing down reflex, a woman may have difficulty pushing effectively, which may prolong the second stage and increase the risk for a cesarean birth.

Lastly, because pain is a subjective sensation, some women are most aware of pain early in labor, whereas some report the second stage of labor as the most difficult. The point at which pain medication is needed, therefore, differs from one individual to another and should be given at whatever point an individual woman feels she needs it. When labor is in the active phase of the first stage, medication to relieve discomfort tends to speed labor progress because, with the pain gone, a woman can relax and work with, not against, her contractions. In contrast, at the second stage, epidural anesthesia or a drug that disorients a woman can slow progress and may result in more instrumentation or cesarean births. For

BOX 16.4 Nursing Care Planning Based on Family Teaching

Q. Jonny asks you, "Can I choose what medicine I want to use in labor for pain or do I have to do whatever my doctor says?"

A. A number of helpful rules about pain in labor are:

- You have the right to choose how much pharmacologic pain relief you want to use.
- It's best if analgesia and anesthesia are begun after labor is well established, although this should be balanced against the need for pain relief.
- Any drug used should provide maximum relief for you and have minimal effect on your fetus.
- Constant fetal and maternal monitoring should be available, although periodic monitoring is acceptable.
- Any medicine given should not interfere with the ability of your uterus to contract during labor or interfere with contraction after labor to prevent uterine hemorrhage.

all these reasons, no perfect analgesic agent exists for labor or birth that has no effect on labor, the mother, or the fetus.

Preparation for Medication Administration

The type of medication used during labor varies among different health care providers and also changes based on new research as the effectiveness and safety of new drugs for use during labor are tested. To be safe, follow the Joint Commission's 2012 National Patient Safety Goals (The Joint Commission, 2012) and remember the criteria a drug must fulfill to be used in pregnancy at any point. Never give a drug to a pregnant woman unless you know the benefit outweighs the risk for both of your clients: the mother and the fetus. Be certain to ask about allergies to all medications before administering them during labor as women in distress from pain can be too distracted to mention this unless directly asked.

Prepare a woman for the type of agent prescribed, how it will be administered with an explanation such as "You'll need to lie on your side" as well as what she can expect to happen after administration ("I'll be taking your blood pressure frequently"). Women in labor are under a lot of stress. That can make experiencing surprising body sensations from a drug without preparation about the effects that may occur so frightening it can defeat their individual coping ability and any relaxation potential associated with it.

Opioid (Narcotic) Analgesics

Narcotics may be given during labor because of their potent effect, but all drugs in this category cause maternal respiratory depression as well as fetal CNS depression to some extent and so should be used cautiously (Koren, 2012).

Timing the administration of narcotics during labor is especially important as, if given too early (before 3 cm cervical dilatation), they tend to slow labor. If given close to birth, because the fetal liver takes 2 to 3 hours to activate a drug, the effect will not be registered in the fetus for 2 to 3 hours after birth. For this reason, narcotics are preferably given when the mother is more than 3 hours away from birth. This allows the peak action of the drug in the fetus to have passed by the time of birth so the newborn breathes easily.

It can be puzzling to see a sleepy baby born to a woman who was given butorphanol tartrate 2 hours before birth, for example, and an alert baby delivered to a woman who had the same drug within 1 hour of birth. In the second instance, the peak action or peak effect has not yet occurred in the infant. This newborn needs careful assessment for the next 4 hours until the drug does reach its peak.

Common opioid analgesics used in labor traditionally include butorphanol tartrate (Stadol), morphine sulfate, nalbuphine (Nubain), meperidine (Demerol), and fentanyl (Sublimaze). None of these drugs completely eliminate the pain of contractions, but they do reduce pain sensation to a level where other nonpharmacologic methods of pain relief can begin to be effective. They all begin to work 15 to 30 minutes after intramuscular administration or about 5 minutes after intravenous administration. A drawback to all these opioids is they may cause nausea and vomiting in some women (Ullman, Smith, Burns, et al., 2011). They also produce a feeling of euphoria, so women often report they feel as if they are "floating"; because of this sensation, they may feel they have lost control or are unable to breathe effectively with contractions. Routes of administration and common side effects are shown in Table 16.1.

Two narcotics being added to the traditionally used ones are remifentanil (Ultiva) and oxycodone. Remifentanil is potent yet short acting and has been found to be superior in pain relief to meperidine in clinical trials (Leong, Sng, & Sia, 2011).

Because of the fetal effects, whenever a narcotic is given during labor, a narcotic antagonist such as naloxone hydrochloride (Narcan) should be available for administration to the infant at birth if needed (Box 16.5). Carefully observe any infant who received naloxone hydrochloride in the immediate postpartum period, because the infant's respirations may become severely depressed again when the drug's effect wears off (Karch, 2012). If severe infant respiratory depression is anticipated, naloxone hydrochloride can be given to a woman just before birth. It readily crosses the placenta and, because it interferes with or competes for narcotic binding sites, may increase the chance for spontaneous respiratory activity in the newborn.

What if... 16.2 Jonny receives no narcotics during labor, yet her newborn is born very sleepy. Would you administer naloxone hydrochloride? Would asking Jonny if she uses recreational drugs be warranted in order to discover the cause of newborn respiratory depression?

Additional Drugs

Additional drugs, such as tranquilizers, may be administered during labor to reduce anxiety or potentiate the action of a narcotic. An example of such a drug is hydroxyzine hydrochloride (Vistaril). These drugs do not relieve pain, so the woman in labor needs pain management measures in addition to these drugs.

Regional (Local) Anesthesia

Regional anesthesia is the injection of a local anesthetic such as chloroprocaine (Nesacaine) or bupivacaine (Marcaine) to block specific nerve pathways (Anim-Somuah et al., 2011). This achieves pain relief by blocking sodium and potassium transport in the nerve membrane, thereby stabilizing the nerve in a polarized resting state so the nerve is unable to conduct sensations.

Various regional anesthetic injection sites are shown in Figure 16.3. Any woman with a bleeding defect, such as those that may occur with preeclampsia, need to be assessed carefully before regional anesthesia is administered to prevent bleeding at the injection site.

Because regional anesthetics are not introduced into the maternal circulation, it was once believed they had no effect on a fetus. However, research has demonstrated there is some uptake of these drugs by a fetus, possibly resulting in transient fetal heart rate variations (Wolfler, Salvo, Sortino, et al., 2010). Effects are minimal when compared with those of systemic anesthetic agents, however, and have no effect on breastfeeding (Gizzo, Di Gangi, Saccardi, et al., 2012).

Most importantly, regional anesthesia is able to completely eliminate pain yet allow a woman to be completely awake and aware of what is happening during birth. It can make pushing with second stage labor more difficult, but it does not depress uterine tone, so the uterus remains capable of optimal contraction after birth, thereby helping to prevent postpartal hemorrhage.

In the rare event an infant is born with symptoms of toxicity from a regional anesthetic, an exchange transfusion at

TABLE 16.1 Analgesics and Anesthetics Commonly Used in Labor and Birth

Type	Drug	Method of Administration	Effect on Mother	Effect on Labor Progress	Effect on Fetus or Newborn
Narcotic analgesic	Butorphanol tartrate (Stadol)	Intramuscular or intravenous	Effective analgesic; withdrawal symptoms if woman is opiate dependent	Possible slowing of labor if given early	Results in some respiratory depression
	Nalbuphine (Nubain)	Intramuscular or intravenous	Effective analgesic; slowing of respiratory rate	Mild maternal sedation	Results in some respiratory depression
	Morphine sulfate	Intrathecal prior to epidural anesthesia	Pruritus; effective analgesia	Possible slowing of labor contractions	Some respiratory depression
	Fentanyl (Sublimaze)	Intravenous	Hypotension; respiratory depression	Slowing of labor if given early	May result in respiratory depression
Lumbar epidural block	Local anesthetic Bupivacaine (Marcaine) Ropivacaine (Naropin)	Injected by anesthesiologist or nurse anesthetist at L3–L4 for first stage of labor; with continuous block, anesthesia will last through birth; fentanyl or morphine possibly added to cerebral spinal fluid first	Rapid onset in minutes lasting 60–90 min; loss of pain perception for labor contractions and birth; possible maternal hypotension	Slowing of labor if given too early; pushing feeling is obliterated, resulting in possible prolonged second stage	May be some differences in response in first few days of life
Pudendal block	Local anesthetic Lidocaine (Xylocaine)	Administered just before birth for perineal anesthesia; injected through vagina	Rapid anesthesia of perineum	None apparent	None apparent
Local infiltration of perineum	Local anesthetic Lidocaine (Xylocaine)	Injected just before episiotomy incision	Anesthesia of perineum almost immediately	None apparent	None apparent
General anesthetic	Thiopental sodium	Intravenous by anesthesiologist or nurse-anesthetist	Rapid anesthesia; also rapid recovery	Forceps required because abdominal pushing is no longer possible	Results in infant being born with central nervous system depression

From Karch, A. M. (2013). *2013 Lippincott's nursing drug guide*. Philadelphia, PA: Lippincott Williams & Wilkins.

BOX 16.5 Nursing Care Planning Based on Responsibility for Pharmacology

NALOXONE HYDROCHLORIDE (NARCAN)

Action: Naloxone hydrochloride is a narcotic antagonist that counteracts the effect of narcotic analgesics (Karch, 2012). It is used to counteract respiratory depression in newborns when a woman has received a narcotic analgesic during labor.

Pregnancy Risk Category: B

Dosage: 0.01 mg/kg, administered either intravenously via umbilical vein, subcutaneously, or intramuscularly; repeated at 2- to 3-minute intervals until a response is obtained

Possible Adverse Effects: Hypotension, hypertension, tachycardia, diaphoresis, tremulousness

Nursing Implications

- Anticipate the need for newborn resuscitative measures including the use of naloxone hydrochloride; have resuscitative equipment and emergency drugs readily available.
- If no intravenous access is available, prepare for possible administration via endotracheal tube.
- If no response is seen after two or three doses, question whether the respiratory depression is caused by maternal narcotic administration.
- Continuously monitor all vital signs for changes.
- Remember that the pain-relieving effect of a narcotic will be reversed as the narcotic is cleared from the baby's system; assess for pain in the neonate if a narcotic was given for pain relief.

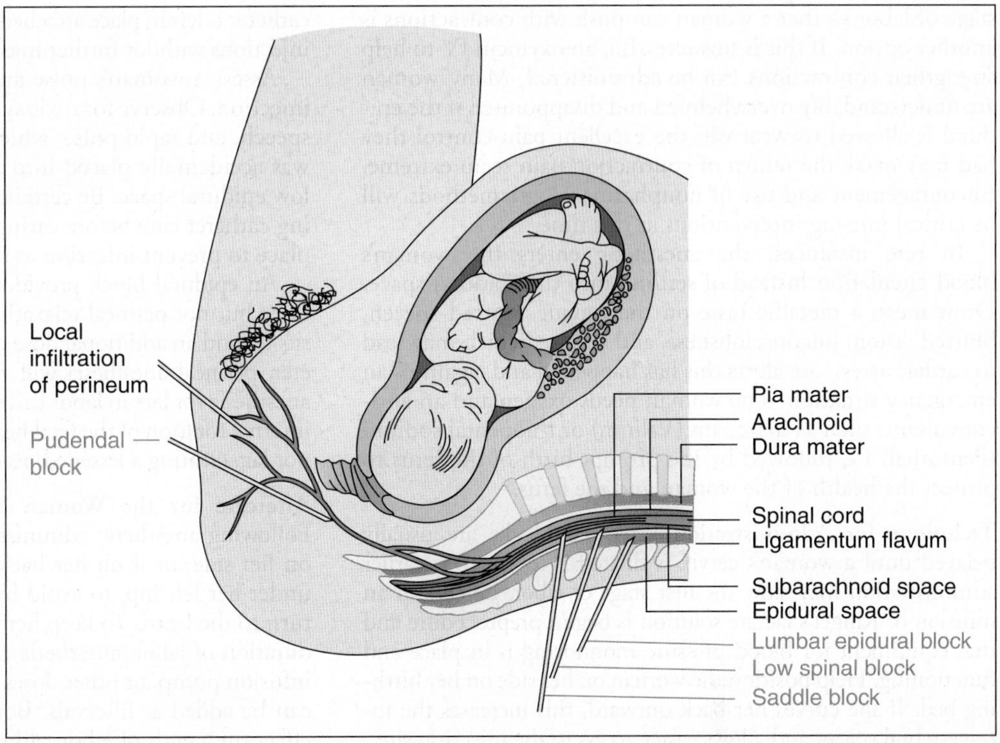

FIGURE 16.3 Anatomy of the spinal canal and sites of injection for regional anesthesia.

birth will remove the anesthetic from the infant's bloodstream. Gastric lavage also will remove a great deal of anesthetic, because anesthetics have a strong affinity for acid media, such as stomach acid.

Epidural Anesthesia. The nerves in the spinal cord are protected by several tissue layers.

- The *pia mater* is the membrane adhering to the nerve fibers.
- Surrounding this is the *cerebrospinal fluid* (CSF).
- Next comes the arachnoid membrane, and outside that, the *dura mater*.
- Outside the dura mater is a vacant space (the *epidural space*).
- Beyond it is the *ligamentum flavum*, yet another protective shield for the vulnerable spinal cord (see Fig. 16.3).

An anesthetic agent introduced into the CSF in the subarachnoid space is *spinal injection* or *spinal anesthesia*. An anesthetic agent placed just inside the ligamentum flavum in the epidural space is called **epidural anesthesia**. Anesthetic agents placed in the epidural space at the L4–L5, L3–L4, or L2–L3 interspace block not only spinal nerve roots in the space but also the sympathetic nerve fibers that travel with them. Therefore, these blocks can provide pain relief during both labor and birth. Because a woman no longer experiences pain, the release of catecholamines (epinephrine) with a β-blocking effect from a pain response is decreased, making this a very effective pain relief measure for labor (Impey & Child, 2012).

Epidural blocks are suitable for almost all women. They are advantageous for women with heart disease, pulmonary disease, diabetes, and sometimes severe gestational hypertension because they make labor virtually pain free and thereby reduce stress from the discomfort of labor. Because the woman does not feel contractions, her physical energy is preserved. Epidural blocks are acceptable for use in preterm labor because the drug has scant effect on a fetus and allows for a controlled and gentle birth with lessened trauma to an immature fetal skull. Because the woman receives no systemic medication, the infant responds more quickly after birth than if systemic narcotic analgesics were used.

The chief concern with epidural anesthesia is its tendency to cause hypotension because of its blocking effect on the sympathetic nerve fibers in the epidural space. This blocking leads to decreased peripheral resistance in the woman's circulatory system. Decreased peripheral resistance causes blood to flow freely into peripheral vessels, and a pseudohypovolemia develops, which registers as hypotension. This risk can be reduced by being certain a woman is well hydrated with 500 to 1,000 ml of intravenous (IV) fluid, such as Ringer's lactate, before the anesthetic is administered. Ringer's lactate is preferable to a glucose solution, because too much maternal glucose can cause hyperglycemia with rebound hypoglycemia in the newborn. Be certain a woman does not lie supine after an epidural block, but remains on her side to help prevent supine hypotension syndrome.

If hypotension should occur, raising the woman's legs and administering oxygen and additional IV fluid along with an antihypotensive agent such as ephedrine to elevate blood pressure may be necessary to stabilize cardiovascular status. This is an emergency because if the woman is severely hypotensive, blood is shunted away from the uterus and leads to poor perfusion of the placenta, eventually causing fetal distress.

A disadvantage of epidural anesthesia is that the bearing down reflex may be reduced or absent, making it difficult for a woman to push effectively. This may delay fetal descent, thus prolonging the second stage of labor and leading to an increased number of instrument-assisted births (Schrock & Harraway-Smith, 2012). A second stage delay this way occurs primarily when the fetus is in an occipitoposterior position. Changing the woman's position (e.g., to all fours) to help fetal rotation can be helpful to aid descent. For both of these situations, allowing an epidural to wear off by the second stage of labor so that a woman can push with contractions is another option. If this is unsuccessful, an oxytocin IV to help strengthen contractions can be administered. Many women are understandably overwhelmed and disappointed if the epidural is allowed to wear off; the excellent pain control they had may make the return of contraction pain seem extreme. Encouragement and use of nonpharmacologic methods will be critical nursing interventions at this time.

In rare instances, the anesthetic enters the woman's blood circulation instead of settling into the epidural space. Drowsiness, a metallic taste on the tongue, slurred speech, blurred vision, unconsciousness, and seizure, which may lead to cardiac arrest, are alerts this has happened and, again, is an emergency situation. The woman needs oxygen and an anticonvulsant, such as diazepam (Valium) or thiopental sodium (Pentothal) IV, followed by the prompt birth of the fetus to protect the health of the woman and the fetus.

Technique for Administration. Epidural blocks are usually delayed until a woman's cervix is dilated 3 to 5 cm as earlier administration may slow the first stage of labor. Be certain an infusion of Ringer's lactate solution is begun preprocedure and that equipment for blood pressure monitoring is in place and functioning. Help position the woman on her side on her birthing bed. If she curves her back outward, this increases the intravertebral spaces and allows easier access to the injection site.

An epidural block may consist of only an anesthetic injection into the epidural space or a combined method where a low-dose anesthetic is injected into the epidural space and a small dose of an analgesic such as fentanyl is also injected into the cerebral spinal fluid space. This combination of drugs and technique is advantageous because it results in a "walking" or "mobile" block, which produces anesthesia up to the level of the umbilicus in 10 to 15 minutes that will last for 40 minutes to 2 hours (Drasner & Larson, 2011). Its second advantage is that it allows a woman to move about and walk while anesthesia is in effect. A catheter is left in place attached to a syringe to allow for repeated injections without further injection pain (Fig. 16.4).

Assess a woman's pulse and blood pressure following the injection. Observe for toxic symptoms of hypotension, slurred speech, and rapid pulse, which would occur if the anesthetic was accidentally placed into a blood vessel and not the hollow epidural space. Be certain to review agency policy regarding catheter care before caring for a person with a catheter in place to prevent infection at the site (Horlocker, 2011).

An epidural block provides anesthesia for uterine contractions but not perineal relaxation. Close to birth, if the woman sits up and an additional dose of anesthesia is added to the catheter, perineal anesthesia will result as well. Leaving the lower anesthesia for late in labor this way is thought to allow for better internal rotation of the fetal head, because the perineal muscle is not lax, creating a lessened need for forceps for rotation.

Aftercare for the Woman With an Epidural Anesthesia. Following anesthetic administration, be certain a woman lies on her side, or if on her back, she should place a firm towel under her left hip, to avoid hypotension from poor blood return to the heart. To keep her free from discomfort during the duration of labor, anesthetic can be continually infused by an infusion pump, or other doses of anesthetic, termed "top-ups," can be added at intervals. Both techniques are equal in their effect on length of labor, although continuous administration may result in more cesarean births because of difficulty pushing and fetal descent (Skrablin, Grgic, Mihaljevic, et al., 2011).

Each time, before an additional top-up dose is administered, ask the woman to say out loud a phrase such as "I can do it" three times. If she is unable to do this, question the dose; lack of fine motor coordination and slurred speech can indicate a slowly occurring toxic reaction.

Yet another technique used to maintain epidural anesthesia is self-administration or patient-controlled epidural analgesia (PCEA). With this technique, following a lockout

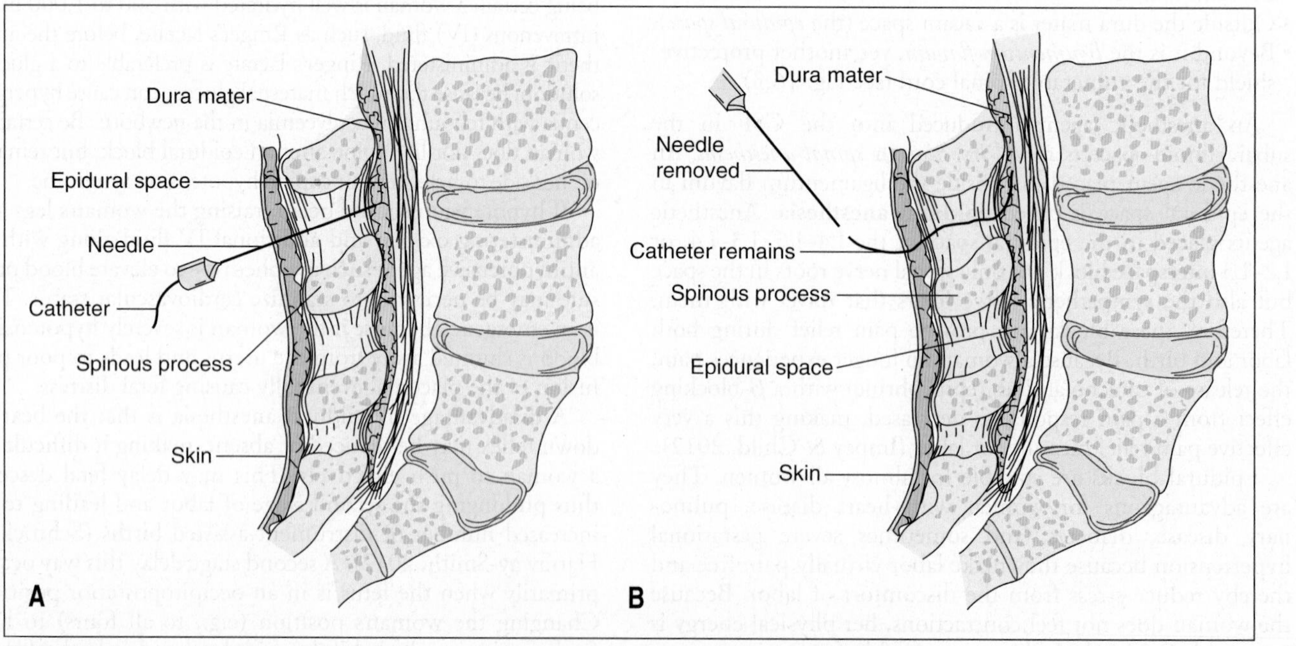

FIGURE 16.4 Epidural anesthesia. **(A)** A needle is inserted into the epidural space. **(B)** A catheter is threaded into the space; the needle is then removed. The catheter allows medication to be administered intermittently or continuously to relieve pain during labor and childbirth.

period when no more anesthetic can be administered to avoid overdosing, an analgesic mixture is delivered whenever the client presses a button on a PCEA pump (Loubert, Hinova, & Fernando, 2011). This method of administration is advantageous because less anesthetic is required compared with continuous epidural infusion (CEI) and can give the woman a feeling of empowerment as she controls her own pain management (Haydon, Larson, Reed, et al., 2011).

A nurse should be in continuous attendance as long as epidural anesthesia is being used. When recording vital signs, be aware epidural anesthesia can cause a temporary elevation in temperature, which is not serious unless it rises above 101°F (Greenwell, Wyshak, Ringer, et al., 2012).

Possible complications that can occur from epidural blocks include hypotension, pruritus (especially if morphine was used), urinary retention, nausea and vomiting, and rarely, a postpartal dural puncture headache (PDPH) (because the subarachnoid space was entered for the analgesic injection).

To detect if hypotension is occurring, continuously monitor blood pressure for the first 20 minutes after each new injection of anesthetic. Continue to periodically monitor blood pressure throughout the time the anesthetic is in effect to be certain the woman's systolic pressure does not fall to less than 100 mmHg or decrease by 20 mmHg or more in a hypertensive woman. A drop greater than this could be life threatening to a fetus unless prompt and effective corrective measures are taken, such as repositioning and administering an antihypotensive agent (e.g., ephedrine) to ensure the fetal outcome will not be compromised.

After an epidural block, a woman loses sensation of bladder filling. Remind her to void every 2 hours, monitor intake and output, and observe and palpate for bladder distention to avoid overfilling, especially if labor is prolonged. Be aware of the standards and policies of the health care agency related to who may add additional anesthesia or remove the catheter. To assess after birth whether the anesthesia is wearing off, touch a woman's leg and ask if she can feel your touch. Ask her to raise her knees and observe whether she can do this easily. Even after feeling in her legs returns, walking may be difficult for her. Be certain to stay with the woman the first time she is out of bed following regional block anesthesia to prevent her from falling.

Spinal (Subarachnoid) Anesthesia. Spinal anesthesia is not used frequently in preference to epidural blocks, but it may be used in an emergency or for a cesarean birth because the administration technique is simpler than that of an epidural and can be accomplished more rapidly.

Before spinal anesthesia, as a guard against hypotension, an IV fluid such as Ringer's lactate solution is usually begun to ensure good hydration. Be certain the fluid is infusing well before the anesthesia is administered.

For spinal anesthesia, a local anesthetic agent such as bupivacaine (Marcaine) is injected using lumbar puncture technique into the subarachnoid space (into the CSF) at the L3 and L4 interspace. A narcotic agonist such as morphine or fentanyl may be added for additional pain relief. For administration, the woman is usually asked to sit on the side of the bed with legs dangling and head bent. Ask her to bend her head forward so her back curves and the intravertebral spaces open. Be sure either you or her support person steadies her in this sitting position because she is very "front heavy" as a result of her pregnancy and could easily fall forward if not well supported.

After injection, the anesthetic normally rises to the level of T10. Anesthesia up to the umbilicus and including both legs will be achieved. Spinal anesthetic agents may be "loaded" or "weighted" with glucose to make them heavier than CSF. This helps prevent them from rising too high in the spinal canal and interfering with the motor control of the uterus or with respiratory muscles (Drasner & Larson, 2011).

Following the anesthetic injection, if the woman was sitting, the anesthesiologist will ask the woman to lie down. It's important a woman lies down at this time, because if she continues to sit upright, the anesthetic will not rise high enough in the canal to achieve pain relief. She must not lie down before this time, however, or the anesthetic could rise too high in the canal. Lying with a pillow under the head is another method to help ensure the anesthesia will be confined to the lower spinal canal.

As mentioned, hypotension from sympathetic blockage in the lower extremities may occur immediately after spinal anesthetic administration. This leads to vasodilation and a decrease in central blood pressure. If hypotension occurs, placental blood perfusion can be compromised. Turn the woman to her left side to reduce vena cava compression. Expect the anesthesiologist to quickly increase the rate of IV fluid administration to increase blood volume; ephedrine to increase blood pressure and oxygen also may be administered. Never place a woman in a Trendelenburg position (head lower than her body) to help restore blood pressure after spinal anesthesia. This could make the anesthetic rise high in her spinal column, causing uterine or respiratory function to cease. A late complication of spinal anesthesia is a PDPH or "spinal headache." This occurs because of CSF leakage from the needle insertion site and also possibly from the irritation of a small amount of air that entered at the injection site. The shift in pressure of the CSF causes strain on the cerebral meninges, initiating the pain. The incidence of such headaches is reduced if a woman is well hydrated before injection and a small-gauge needle is used for the injection. If a headache occurs, the postpartum woman can be encouraged to drink a large quantity of fluid because a high fluid intake rapidly provides replacement of spinal fluid.

A spinal headache can be relieved by the administration of hydrocortisone to reduce inflammation (Alam, Rahman, & Ershad, 2012). Having the woman lie flat and administering an analgesic also helps. Some women find a cold cloth applied to their forehead helpful. If a headache is incapacitating, it can be treated with a blood patch technique. For this, 10 to 20 ml of blood is withdrawn from an accessible vein and then immediately injected into the epidural space over the spinal injection site. The injected blood clots and seals off any further leakage of CSF (Paech, Doherty, Christmas, et al., 2011).

✔ QSEN Checkpoint Question 16.5

Teamwork & Collaboration

Jonny has chosen to have epidural anesthesia and you have consequently informed the anesthesiologist. What are two risks that are potentially associated with this form of anesthesia?

a. Hypotension and a prolonged second stage of labor can occur.
b. Severe headache and peripheral cyanosis can occur.
c. Women have increased back pain and abrupt transitions between stages of labor.
d. Maternal hypertension and a reduced red blood cell count can occur.

Look in Appendix A for the best answer and rationale.

Medication for Pain Relief During Birth

Stretching of the perineum causes pain that occurs during the birth. The simplest form of relief for this type of pain is the natural **pressure anesthesia** that results from the fetal head pressing against the stretched perineum. This natural anesthesia is often adequate to allow the fetal head to be born with only momentary pain, which, although intense and hot, occurs suddenly and is over quickly. Often, after the hours of hard contractions a woman has come through, this flash of pain seems insignificant. For some women, however, additional medication is needed to reduce the pain of birth.

Local Anesthetics

Local anesthesia reduces the ability of local nerve fibers to conduct pain.

Local Infiltration. Local infiltration is the injection of an anesthetic such as lidocaine (Xylocaine) into the superficial nerves of the perineum along the vulva. The effect lasts for approximately 1 hour, allowing for a less painful birth and suturing of an episiotomy (a cut to enlarge the vagina opening; discussed in Chapter 24).

Pudendal Nerve Block. A **pudendal nerve block** is the injection of a local anesthetic such as bupivacaine (Marcaine) through the vagina to anesthetize the pudendal nerve. It is used for a woman who has not had an epidural to provide a pain-free birth and, if the woman should have an episiotomy, painless surgical suturing and repair. Although a pudendal nerve block is local, assess the fetal heart rate and the mother's blood pressure immediately after the injection to be certain maternal hypotension does not occur.

General Anesthesia

General anesthesia is never preferred for childbirth because it carries the dangers of hypoxia and possible inhalation of vomitus during administration. Because it is used so rarely, you probably will not see this used; if it is used, there are special precautions you need to be aware of. Pregnant women are particularly prone to gastric reflux and aspiration because of increased stomach pressure from the weight of the full uterus beneath it. The gastroesophageal valve at the top of the stomach also may be displaced and possibly functioning improperly. Despite these risks, general anesthesia may be necessary in emergency situations, such as if the placenta loosens before the fetus is born (placental abruption), spinal anesthesia is contraindicated, or an immediate cesarean birth is required.

For complete and rapid anesthesia during childbirth, thiopental sodium (Pentothal), a short-acting barbiturate, is usually the drug of choice. It causes rapid induction of anesthesia and, because it has a short half-life, allows for good uterine contraction afterward and so prevents postpartal hemorrhage. All women who receive a general anesthetic, however, must be observed closely in the postpartal period for uterine relaxation and the risk of uterine atony and postpartal hemorrhage.

For the procedure, after induction with thiopental sodium, the woman is intubated, and anesthesia is then maintained by administration of nitrous oxide and oxygen. Thiopental sodium crosses the placenta rapidly, so an infant born to a woman anesthetized by this method may be slow to respond at birth and may need resuscitation.

Some women comment that their throat feels raw or sore after general anesthesia administration; this is from the insertion and maintenance of an endotracheal tube. Using an anesthetic throat spray or gargle, sipping cold liquids, or sucking on ice chips (as soon as this is safe after general anesthesia) can help to relieve the discomfort.

Preparation for the Safe Administration of General Anesthesia. To ensure safe general anesthesia administration, an anesthesiologist or nurse anesthetist needs a minimum of six drugs readily available:

- Ephedrine to use in the event blood pressure falls
- Atropine sulfate to dry oral and respiratory secretions to prevent aspiration
- Thiopental sodium (Pentothal) for rapid induction
- Succinylcholine (Anectine) to achieve laryngeal relaxation for intubation
- Diazepam (Valium) to control seizures, a possible reaction to anesthetics
- Isoproterenol (Isuprel) to reduce bronchospasm, should aspiration occur

In addition to these medications, an adult laryngoscope, an endotracheal tube, a breathing bag with a source of 100% oxygen, and a suction catheter and suction source should be at hand.

Aspiration of Vomitus. There is a danger of vomiting with a general anesthetic; this can be fatal if a woman's airway becomes occluded by foreign matter. In addition, stomach contents have an acid pH that can cause chemical pneumonitis and secondary infection of the respiratory tract.

Some anesthesiologists may prescribe IV ranitidine (Zantac) or an oral antacid such as sodium citrate to be given before general anesthesia is administered to reduce the level of acid in stomach contents should aspiration occur. Metoclopramide (Reglan) increases gastric emptying and may also be prescribed.

For general anesthesia administration, the woman is asked to lie on her back with a wedge under her left hip to displace the uterus from the vena cava. To reduce the occurrence of hypotension and to establish a line for emergency medications, IV fluid administration is begun. The woman is then given a rapid-induction IV agent, followed by intubation with a cuffed endotracheal tube. To prevent gastric reflux and aspiration before intubation is achieved, cricoid pressure, which seals off the esophagus by compressing it between the cricoid cartilage and the cervical vertebrae (Fig. 16.5), must be applied as soon as the IV agent is begun until the cuff on the tube is inflated and firmly in place.

The moments of induction of general anesthesia before the endotracheal tube is safely in place are critical ones for the anesthesiologist. Respect his or her need to concentrate by not talking until the task is achieved.

If aspiration of vomitus should occur following administration, prompt attention is essential. The anesthesiologist suctions the woman's trachea to remove as much foreign material as possible. The woman is intubated, if she was not previously, and given 100% oxygen. IV isoproterenol to reduce bronchospasm and a corticosteroid to reduce inflammation may be given. Positive-pressure ventilation may be initiated. Blood gas analysis and a chest X-ray usually are obtained to determine how much aeration the woman is still capable of achieving.

The woman may receive mechanical ventilation until her overall clinical condition improves, as shown by X-ray films and blood gas concentrations. She may be critically ill at the time of aspiration and, after the cesarean birth, often will be transferred to an intensive care unit for the special care she needs to survive this emergency.

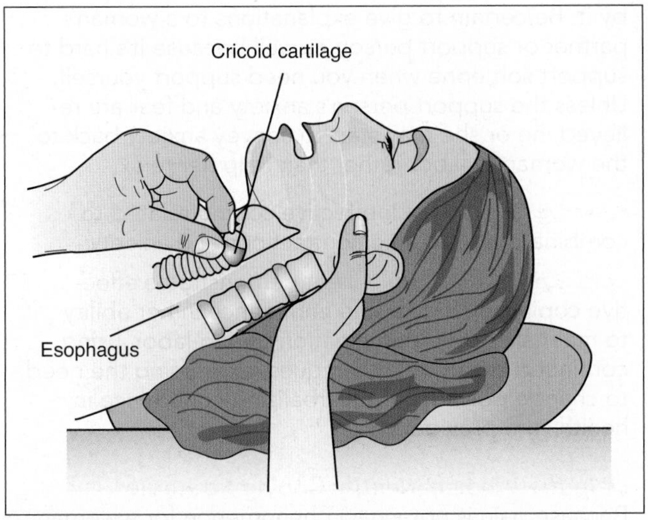

FIGURE 16.5 Cricoid pressure. The cricoid cartilage is located at the top of the tracheal rings and compresses easily with finger and thumb pressure.

QSEN Checkpoint Question 16.6

Quality Improvement

There is no reason to think Jonny will need a general anesthetic. But if she did, what type of drug would you want to ensure is readily available on a birthing unit to help minimize the risk of aspiration of vomitus?

a. An anticonvulsant such as diazepam (Valium)
b. A nerve relaxant such as phenobarbital
c. Metoclopramide (Reglan) to speed gastric emptying
d. Oxytocin to increase the effectiveness of labor

Look in Appendix A for the best answer and rationale.

NURSING CARE TO PROMOTE THE COMFORT OF A WOMAN DURING LABOR

The best approach to pain management for women in labor is to always aid any pharmacologic intervention with a complementary or alternative therapy measure. For example, an intramuscular analgesic can be linked with breathing exercises to make both more effective.

Nursing Diagnoses and Related Interventions

Nursing Diagnosis: Anxiety related to more pain than expected from labor contractions

Outcome Evaluation: Client identifies beginning and end of contractions, expresses confidence rather than confusion about ongoing process, states she feels less anxious, and is able to concentrate on controlled breathing.

In addition to causing local discomfort, pain can evoke a general stress response (fight-or-flight syndrome). This releases epinephrine, which causes peripheral and uterine vasoconstriction. This can increase the degree of pain experienced because of the resulting increase in tissue anoxia. Reducing anxiety through relaxation techniques such as spaced breathing exercises or through administration of medication to reduce anxiety can reduce vasoconstriction and help reduce pain.

Reduce Anxiety With Explanations of the Labor Process. Planning with women their options for pain relief during labor should begin prenatally (Box 16.6).

BOX 16.6 Nursing Care Planning to Empower a Family

PAIN RELIEF DURING LABOR

Q. Jonny tells you, "I know my friends have told me pain during labor would be horrible, but what can I do so I won't hurt so much?"

A. Here are some common suggestions to help with pain relief:

- Ask your primary health care provider early in pregnancy about pain management options for labor. The options your care provider suggests may actually influence your decision as to whether this is the optimal care provider for you.
- Attend childbirth preparation classes during pregnancy and conscientiously practice breathing or other relaxation exercises. These measures can be adequate all by themselves; if not, they may complement pharmacologic methods of pain relief.
- Make a birth plan detailing what position you choose for labor and other options you want to use. This helps give you a greater sense of control in the face of pain.
- Be certain a support person will be with you during labor. Name a second person or investigate using a doula if you are uncertain whether your usual support person will be available or can fill this role.
- Late in pregnancy, if you are still concerned, let your primary health care provider know. In addition to medication for pain relief during labor, medication to reduce anxiety is also available.
- On admission to the hospital, let the medical and nursing staff know you are concerned so they can work with you to find satisfactory pain management.
- The most commonly used options today are oral, intramuscular, or intravenous administration of narcotics or injection of regional anesthesia by epidural block. Ask questions about any method suggested if necessary so you're aware of action and side effects.
- Be aware the choice of receiving analgesia or anesthesia is yours. However, if a complication occurs, be ready to compromise in the interest of safety for yourself and your child.

During labor, use a standard method of pain assessment, such as asking a woman to rate her pain level on a scale of 1 to 10 or show her a paper with a line marked 1 to 10 if she's more visually oriented so she can rate her pain. Based on her response, evaluate whether pain relief is adequate and effective.

Introduce natural methods based on the gate control theory of pain relief such as chanting or effleurage (see Chapter 14). Be sure to offer careful explanations of what is happening or what will happen during labor, because this can help alleviate anxiety and thereby reduce some discomfort.

Be certain to explain the characteristics of contractions (e.g., labor contractions are rhythmic and come and go repeatedly), and reinstruct as necessary. Do not assume a woman is aware of this simply because she is experiencing the contractions. Her pain may be so intense and the intensity so unexpected that she is unaware of any relief between contractions (Box 16.7).

This on/off effect of labor contractions differentiates the pain from that of a toothache or headache, which is continuous. Sometimes, just knowing this can help a woman tolerate the pain even as it increases in intensity.

Do not assume a woman knows such things like when membranes rupture it is painless, that a pink-stained show is normal, or that contractions change in character during labor. A woman having her first child may not know these things. A woman having her second child may not remember what her labor was like the last time, or she may find this time so different (even if it is well within usual limits) she is frightened by it. Be certain to give explanations to a woman's partner or support person as well because it's hard to support someone when you need support yourself. Unless the support person's anxiety and fear are relieved, he or she may start to convey anxiety back to the woman in labor rather than help her relax.

Nursing Diagnosis: Ineffective coping related to combination of uterine contractions and anxiety

Outcome Evaluation: Client demonstrates effective coping by expressing confidence in her ability to maintain active participation during labor, using continued breathing techniques, expressing the need to change position, and verbalizing confidence in health care providers.

Help the Woman Identify Coping Strategies. Because pain is not a new phenomenon for a woman of childbearing age, it can be helpful to ask her to recall methods she usually uses to combat pain or anxiety, such as meditation or applying a cool cloth. Associating labor pain with usual circumstances can go a long way toward helping her collect her resources and decide on a workable pain relief strategy. Box 16.8 shows an interprofessional care map illustrating both nursing and team planning for helping reduce anxiety to manage discomfort during labor.

Provide Comfort Measures. Usually, anyone can tolerate a little discomfort from a backache, being thirsty, having dry lips, or having a leg cramp.

BOX 16.7 Nursing Care Planning Based on Effective Communication

Suppose Jonny stated early in labor that she didn't want to use any medication for pain relief. As soon as her contractions became 30 seconds in length, however, she requested some analgesia. Her physician prescribed intramuscular butorphanol tartrate (Stadol). Her contractions are now 40 seconds in duration and only moderately strong. She looks increasingly uncomfortable with each contraction.

Less Effective Communication

Nurse: How are you feeling, Jonny? Is there anything I can do for you?
Jonny: I need something stronger for pain.
Nurse: Didn't the medicine I gave you work at all?
Jonny: It's working for now, but it won't be enough by another half hour. I'll need something else by then.
Nurse: You won't be able to get anything for another 2 hours. I'm sorry.

More Effective Communication

Nurse: How are you feeling, Jonny? Is there anything I can do for you?
Jonny: I need something stronger for pain.
Nurse: On a scale of 1 to 10, with 1 being little pain and 10 being the worst pain ever, how would you rate the pain you're having?
Jonny: Two, but I know it'll be 10 in another half hour when my contractions get so strong that they're constant.
Nurse: I'm sorry. I must not have explained contractions always have a space in between them. Let's talk about that and how you always have a chance to catch your breath and relax in between them.

Because women in labor are under stress, they may not hear instructions when they are given. Asking a woman to rate her pain on a scale of 1 to 10 is more effective than just asking how she feels. Assessing whether a woman has a clear understanding of the nature of labor contractions is another way to make it easier for her to manage them.

BOX 16.8 Nursing Care Planning

AN INTERPROFESSIONAL CARE MAP FOR A WOMAN REQUIRING COMFORT MEASURES DURING LABOR AND BIRTH

Jonny Baranca is a primipara in early labor whom you admit to a birthing unit. Her contractions are 7 minutes apart and her cervix is 3 cm dilated. She tells you her sister had epidural anesthesia that completely obliterated her pain in labor for the birth of her baby 3 months ago. Based on her sister's experience, Jonny expected to be given epidural anesthesia as soon as she arrived at the hospital. As she is in early labor, her physician asked her to wait until she is 4 cm dilated. When you enter her room, you find her lying on her back in a birthing bed, crying from pain. Her husband shouts at you that his "wife deserves better care than this."

Family Assessment Gravida 1, para 0; accompanied by husband who will act as support person and coach. Client works as clerk in clothing store; husband is physical education major at local university.

Client Assessment Contractions are of moderate intensity, every 6 to 7 minutes, with a duration of 35 seconds. Cervix dilated 3 cm, 80% effaced, −1 station. Membranes intact. Fetal heart rate (FHR), 148 beats/min; fetus in ROA position. Attended childbirth education classes but did not practice breathing exercises. Last meal: 3 hours ago; last voided, 2 hours ago.

Nursing Diagnosis Pain related to effects of uterine contractions and pressure on pelvic structures

Outcome Criteria Client confirms discomfort is controlled (pain is a 3 or less on a 1 to 10 pain scale) with either nonpharmacologic or pharmacologic methods; responds to questions and instructions; identifies need for additional pain relief measures if required.

Team Member Responsible	Assessment	Intervention	Rationale	Expected Outcome
Activities of Daily Living, Including Safety				
Nurse	Assess what birth plan the woman wants to follow. Inspect her suprapubic area and palpate for bladder distention.	Remind client she does not need to remain in bed. Encourage her to void every 2 hours.	Ambulation can increase comfort and progress. A full bladder contributes to discomfort and may impede fetal descent, possibly prolonging labor.	Client ambulates in early labor. Has no signs of bladder distention; voids every 2 hours during labor.
Teamwork and Collaboration				
Nurse/Primary health care provider	Locate which health care provider is on call to provide anesthetic pain relief in labor at the point it will be opportune to give.	Notify nurse-anesthetist concerning client's wish to receive an epidural block as soon as possible.	Respecting client's wishes is a prime method of encouraging self-efficacy.	Pain management team supports client's wish for pharmacologic intervention; encourages nonpharmacologic measures until epidural anesthetic is appropriate.
Procedures/Medications for Quality Improvement				
Nurse	Assess how client's husband views his role in labor. Assess if client will try controlled breathing exercises learned in preparation for labor class.	Refresh controlled breathing and imagery with support of husband. Allow husband occasional breaks. Stay with the client during this time to provide support.	A support person increases satisfaction with labor; controlled breathing and imagery can be learned during labor.	Support person helps client with imagery and controlled breathing. Client allows health care providers to substitute for husband so husband can take occasional breaks.
Nutrition				
Nurse	Determine what client would like to eat or drink while in labor.	Provide client with a beverage at least every hour; food as desired.	Fluid maintains hydration; ice chips or hard candy can relieve mouth dryness from breathing exercises.	Client states she has no mouth discomfort from breathing; drinks fluid every hour.

(continued on page 416)

BOX 16.8 Nursing Care Planning (continued)

Patient-Centered Care				
Nurse/Nurse anesthetist	Assess if epidural anesthesia is still the client's chief choice for a method of pain management.	Provide information on epidural anesthesia as needed; update the couple on labor progress.	Frequent updates on progress help alleviate anxiety and fears that may exacerbate pain.	Couple confirm they are certain epidural anesthesia is their method of choice; receive frequent updates on labor progress.
Psychosocial/Spiritual/Emotional Needs				
Nurse	Assess level of client's pain by verbal, pain scale, and nonverbal indicators. Use 1 to 10 scale and evaluate response to techniques used.	Support client in her ability to manage pain until her epidural can be given.	Praise can instill a sense of control and motivation to continue to use alternative methods of pain control.	Client rates her level of pain from labor contractions not above 3 on a 1 to 10 scale.
Nurse	Assess what nonpharmacologic measures (such as music, touch, environmental calm) client thinks would help complement epidural block and aid comfort once this is given.	Provide a comfortable environment: clean sheets, cool washcloth to forehead, closed room door. Refrain from intervening with client during a contraction.	A comfortable environment aids in relaxation, promoting effective coping. Interrupting the client's breathing can make the technique ineffective as a pain relief measure.	Client reports she feels environment is comfortable and complements other pain relief measures.
Informatics for Seamless Health Care Planning				
Nurse	Ask client and husband to evaluate their labor experience.	Review with client pain relief measures used and determine which were most effective.	Reviewing a possibly traumatic experience helps to put it into perspective among life events.	Client and support person state labor and birth were, at worst, a tolerable experience and, at best, a highlight of their lives.

However, few people can tolerate having all of these discomforts simultaneously or feeling even one of them while experiencing a labor contraction.

Assist the woman's support person to provide the usual comfort measures that are helpful for anyone with pain, such as reassurance, massage, or a change in position. For dry lips, ice chips to suck on, moistening the lips with a wet cloth, or using a moisturizing jelly or balm can be helpful. A cool cloth to wipe perspiration from the forehead, neck, and chest can keep a woman from feeling overheated.

A woman's sheets and clothing may wrinkle rapidly and stick to her skin if she is perspiring. The waterproof pad under her buttocks will become soiled with vaginal secretions and will begin to feel hot and sticky. Never apply sanitary pads in labor because, although they absorb vaginal secretions well, they also tend to slip out of place, possibly carrying pathogens from the rectal area forward to the vaginal opening. Instead, change waterproof pads frequently. At least halfway through the first stage of labor, or more frequently as indicated by the woman's condition, change her sheets, offer her a clean gown, and ask if she'd like to bathe or take a shower. These measures can help her feel clean and refreshed, with a ready-to-go-again feeling.

Think of comfort measures for the woman's support person as well. Is the chair by the side of the bed comfortable? Does he or she need to stretch or take a beverage or bathroom break? Could you serve as the coach while the support person makes some phone calls? Breaks such as these allow a partner to come back rested and ready to give support again.

Nursing Diagnosis: Pain related to labor contractions

Outcome Evaluation: Client states pain is reduced to a tolerable level with techniques used so she is able to handle or "work with" contractions and demonstrates ability to listen and respond to questions and instructions.

Assist the Woman With Prepared Childbirth Method. Depending on the type of childbirth preparation a woman and her support person have had, the method used may include breathing exercises, distraction by focusing on an external object, acupressure, therapeutic touch, music therapy, guided imagery, self-hypnosis, or a combination of these methods (see Chapter 14). The use of biofeedback is not well documented in labor but may also be effective.

Even though a woman conscientiously practiced breathing or focusing in a relaxed, fun setting of an antepartal class, the discomfort and stress of labor may make it easy for her to forget what she learned. As necessary, review previously learned breathing techniques with her. Urge her to begin using these early in labor, before contractions become strong, so she gains confidence that they can be effective at diminishing pain. If a woman has had no prior training in breathing exercises, sit with her and teach her a simple breathing pattern so she can begin to utilize this to relieve some of her pain.

Massage is another pain relief method that can be taught to a woman and her support person during labor. This may be especially useful if a woman is experiencing back pain, because rubbing or massaging the sacral area often alleviates that. Firm massage on her shoulders can provide a relaxing distraction from the sensation of internal pressure and pain.

Encourage Comfortable Positioning. An upright position, sitting, walking, or swaying with a partner may be most comfortable for a woman in early labor and aids contractions and descent through gravity (see Chapter 15). If a woman wants to walk and has no support person, walk with her as she may need support during a contraction. Leaning forward against a birthing ball or pelvic rocking between contractions may relieve tense back muscles. If a woman must remain in bed because of a situation such as her membranes have ruptured and the fetal head is not engaged, urge her to keep active within the limits of bed rest and especially not to lie on her back to avoid supine hypotension syndrome. Move bedclothes or monitor leads, if any are attached, as needed to allow her to be able to turn and remain active.

Position changes during the second stage of labor help fetal descent and may shorten labor. Urge a woman to sit, stand, kneel on hands and knees, lie in a lateral recumbent position, squat, or use whatever position she prefers (see Chapter 15). Keep in mind that maintaining these positions often requires assistance from one or two support people to keep an unbalanced woman from falling.

Provide Pharmacologic Pain Relief. Helping a woman decide if and when medication for pain relief should be used requires an in-depth understanding of the available drugs, their effects on the mother and the fetus, and their mechanism and duration of action. It also requires sympathetic listening and counseling skills. Many women come into labor wishing to avoid drugs entirely. Once in labor, they may change their minds but hesitate to say so, especially if their partners also believe a birth without the use of drugs is ideal. Other women come into labor asking to receive something immediately to avoid experiencing any pain. In both instances, provide information about the use of drugs and their ultimate effects. Maintain a supportive presence to help a woman make the best decision for herself and her baby. Some women require analgesia or anesthesia because of a complication. Helping these women and their support persons understand why the medication is necessary calls for equal care and skill. As a rule, record a baseline fetal heart rate and maternal blood pressure and pulse before administering medication; reassess 15 minutes later for fetal and maternal safety.

What if... 16.3 **Jonny, who is still in early labor, tells you if she can't have an epidural immediately, she wants a general anesthetic. If she can't have that, she will leave the hospital. Her physician has said she cannot justify a general anesthetic for uncomplicated labor. You find Jonny crying because her doctor won't give her anything for pain. How would you handle this situation?**

THE WOMAN WITH UNIQUE NEEDS

The Morbidly Obese Woman

Morbidly obese women may have more difficulty using some nonpharmacologic measures for pain relief than other women. For example, be certain a portable birthing tub (looks like a child's plastic pool) will be sturdy enough to support her weight as she leans against the side. Check to be certain the labor room shower is wide enough if she wishes to use warm water sprays for pain management. Remember, birthing beds are not very wide; be cautious when you ask her to turn that she has adequate space to do that. Straddling a chair and leaning against the back may be unsafe if the chair is not strong enough to support her weight.

Analgesic administration may also pose a problem as a usual dose may not be as effective in extremely obese women. Question doses for women who might need a larger amount so they can achieve pain relief. Anesthetic administration may also cause concern as it may be more difficult for an anesthetist to identify the L3 to L4 intravertebral space for injection. They also experience more hypotension and variability on fetal heart rate tracings than other women (Vricella, Louis, Mercer, et al., 2011).

The Woman With Cultural Concerns

Because of cultural traditions, some women are very opposed to the use of analgesia or anesthesia in labor. Be certain to respect this concern by aiding women in any way possible to use the methods they have chosen for pain control and to not interrupt distraction techniques such as controlled breathing, meditation, or chanting. Mark a nursing care plan as to the woman's preference so other team members don't suggest analgesia. Caution other team members as well to remain quiet while the baby is born if there is a special prayer a partner or the woman wants to say at this time.

In many cultures, childbearing is a woman's field of expertise so male partners may have large gaps of knowledge about what is expected of them during birth. Be certain to explain the purpose of procedures, and assist the partner to help with breathing exercises, warming hot pads, making tea, or other comfort measures if he wants to help in other ways.

If analgesia or anesthesia becomes necessary because of an unanticipated emergency, talk to the woman and her partner afterward to be certain they understand why the additional pain management method was necessary. Stress that the overriding aim of labor is a healthy mother and healthy baby; using analgesia or anesthesia or using none at all are only different means to achieve that end.

The Woman Addicted to Illicit or Prescription Drugs

The incidence of women who are addicted to illicit or prescribed drugs is rising, so the number of women seen in labor with these concerns is also increasing. Include a question on the use of recreational and prescription drugs when history taking at a woman's admittance to a birthing center. Concern about their baby's health, the possibility of overdosing from an analgesic administered to them during labor, or their newborn acquiring neonatal abstinence syndrome from opioid withdrawal all encourage women to answer a question about illicit drug use honestly. Women addicted to prescription drugs may not realize they are using more of a drug than is healthy for them or their fetus and so may not mention this unless asked directly.

If a woman states she uses illicit drugs, ask what drug she uses and when was the last time she used to prevent administering an analgesic overdose. Be certain the anesthetist who will administer a regional block has this same information. Marijuana is a drug frequently smoked at the beginning of labor by users because it offers such a relaxed feeling. There is little evidence that marijuana has immediate effects on a newborn, but to be cautious and because a marijuana user may also be a polydrug user, a woman needs to alert her primary health care provider she used it as an alternative pain measure. Cocaine is also a frequent choice for women beginning labor because, again, it has such a euphoric effect. Cocaine use during pregnancy is associated with loosening of the placenta (placenta abruption) so a woman who has taken this drug needs to be observed closely for signs of poor fetal circulation, such as a decreasing heart rate (Mbah, Alio, Fombo, et al., 2011).

Women who consistently use opioids may not receive the same pain relief from an analgesic such as butorphanol tartrate (Stadol) as nonusers, so be prepared to suggest alternative measures of pain relief as well. Their newborn may need special care at birth as many newborns of consistent users are small for gestational age and need observation for opioid withdrawal or neonatal abstinence signs (Creanga, Sabel, Ko, et al., 2012).

Many women who are addicted to opioids are identified during pregnancy and prescribed methadone to substitute for their drug of addiction. Methadone has the same effect on a newborn as all opioids, so it is equally important that these women identify themselves in labor so their newborn can be closely monitored (Peles, Schreiber, Bloch, et al., 2012).

A typical prescription drug abused by women is hydrocodone-acetaminophen as this is frequently prescribed for chronic pain such as carpal tunnel syndrome or back pain. The half-life of this drug is about 2 hours in addicted women (Kokki, Franco, Raatikainen, et al., 2012). It appears to have little effect on newborns; however, because the compound contains an adult dosage of acetaminophen, the newborn needs to be observed for both withdrawal and liver effects.

The Woman Who Uses Tobacco

Women who smoke cigarettes typically turn to them when they are stressed, so it may be very difficult for a tobacco user to go without a cigarette if her labor lasts more than 4 hours (and labor typically does). A woman needs to ask her primary health care provider if she could use nicotine gum or a patch during labor; nicotine is a pregnancy category C drug, so she needs to alert the team that she is a tobacco user as her infant may have a low birth weight and may need special care (Quesada, Gotman, Howell, et al., 2012).

What if...16.4 You are particularly interested in exploring one of the 2020 National Health Goals with respect to analgesia in labor (see Box 16.1). What would be a possible research topic to explore pertinent to this goal that would be applicable to Jonny Baranca's family and that would also advance evidence-based practice?

KEY POINTS FOR REVIEW

- Pain in labor occurs because of anoxia to uterine cells, stretching of the cervix and perineum, and pressure of the presenting part of the fetus on maternal tissues.
- Each person perceives pain differently. Only a woman herself can describe the type or extent of her pain.
- Usually, the better prepared a woman is for childbirth and the more effective her support person is, the less there is a need for analgesia and anesthesia.
- Encourage complementary and alternative therapies such as reducing anxiety, providing changes in position, increasing knowledge, supporting prepared childbirth exercises, and prescribed analgesics or anesthesia as this helps in planning/implementing nursing care that not only meets QSEN competencies but best meets a family's total needs.
- Be certain to ask about allergies to medications before administering them. Women under stress from pain may be too concerned to mention this unless directly asked.
- Women may lose their ability to use controlled breathing after systemic opioid administration because of a light-headed feeling. They may need additional support during this time to be able to continue with a breathing technique until this feeling passes and the analgesic agent begins to have an effect.
- Regional anesthesia, such as epidural anesthesia, is extremely effective at relieving labor pain. Be certain the woman is well hydrated with IV fluid and her blood pressure is within normal limits before assisting with administration of the anesthetic agent.

- Remind all women to lie on their side or place a firm towel under their right hip while in labor to help avoid supine hypotension. During general anesthesia administration, if a woman must lie supine, position a wedge under her right buttock to help prevent hypotension. If hypotension should occur after epidural anesthesia administration, elevating a woman's legs and administering an antihypotensive agent such as ephedrine are emergency measures to help relieve hypotension.
- If an opioid analgesic is used, naloxone hydrochloride (Narcan) must be available to use for possible newborn resuscitation.
- General anesthesia is not administered for an uncomplicated labor because it has risks for both the mother and the infant, but it may still be used in an emergency.

Critical Thinking Care Study

Bailey is a 32-year-old gravida 1, para 0 woman in active labor. She is 6 cm dilated, 40% effaced, and having moderate-to-strong intensity contractions. She has brought some rock-and-roll music with her to play during labor. Her support person is her apartment roommate Cheryl rather than her boyfriend because he "hates hospitals."

1. What is the chance an apartment roommate will make as good a support person in labor for Bailey as the father of her baby? Should she have insisted he come to be with her?
2. Bailey has brought music that is not at all relaxing. It is loud and boisterous. Should you suggest she play music you supply with sounds of the ocean to help her relax?
3. Bailey is using controlled breathing and you hear her roommate say "push" with each contraction as well. What additional information do you need to know if her support person is giving her good advice in labor?

Patient Scenario
The Mazjewski Family

Read about the Mazjewski family, a family who needs pain relief in labor, then answer the questions to further sharpen your skills and grow more familiar with NCLEX-type questions related to pain management for labor. Confirm your answers are correct by reading the rationales.

Visit http://thePoint.lww.com

Answers and Rationales

Looking for answers to the What If. . . and Critical Thinking Care Study questions?

Visit http://thePoint.lww.com

References

Aasheim, V., Nilsen, A. B., Lukasse, M., et al. (2011). Perineal techniques during the second stage of labour for reducing perineal trauma. *Cochrane Database of Systematic Reviews,* (12), CD006672.

Alam, M. R., Rahman, M. A., & Ershad, R. (2012). Role of very short-term intravenous hydrocortisone in reducing postdural puncture headache. *Journal of Anaesthesiology & Clinical Pharmacology, 28*(2), 190–193.

Anim-Somuah, M., Smyth, R. M., & Jones, L. (2011). Epidural versus non-epidural or no analgesia in labour. *Cochrane Database of Systematic Reviews,* (12), CD000331.

Chillemi, S., & Chillemi, M. (2012). *The complete herbal guide: A natural approach to healing the body.* Morrisville, SC: Lulu Publishing.

Cluett, E. R., & Burns, E. (2012). Immersion in water in labour and birth. *Cochrane Database of Systematic Reviews,* (2), CD000111.

Creanga, A. A., Sabel, J. C., Ko, J. Y., et al. (2012). Maternal drug use and its effect on neonates: A population-based study in Washington State. *Obstetrics & Gynecology, 119*(5), 924–933.

Cushman, A., Doe, M., Leif, J., et al. (2012). *The mindful way through pregnancy.* Boston, MA: Shambhala Publications Inc.

Derry, S., Straube, S., Moore, R. A., et al. (2012). Intracutaneous or subcutaneous sterile water injection compared with blinded controls for pain management in labour. *Cochrane Database of Systematic Reviews,* (1), CD009107.

Dick-Read, G., & Gaskin, I. M. (2013). *Childbirth without fear: The principles & practice of natural childbirth.* London, UK: Pinter & Martin, LTD.

DONA International. (2012). *Position paper: Birth doulas make a difference.* Aurora, CO: Author.

Dowswell, T., Bedwell, C., Lavender, T., et al. (2011). Transcutaneous electrical nerve stimulation (TENS) for pain management in labour. *Cochrane Database of Systematic Reviews,* (9), CD007214.

Drasner, K., & Larson, M. D. (2011). Spinal and epidural anesthesia. In R. D. Miller & M. Pardo (Eds.), *Basics of anesthesia* (pp. 252–283). Philadelphia, PA: Elsevier/Saunders.

East, C. E., Begg, L., Henshall, N. E., et al. (2012). Local cooling for relieving pain from perineal trauma sustained during childbirth. *Cochrane Database of Systematic Reviews,* (5), CD006304.

Euliano, T. Y., Gravenstein, J. S., Gravenstein, N., et al. (2011). *Essential anesthesia: Science to practice* (2nd ed.). New York, NY: Cambridge University Press.

Gedde-Dahl, M., & Fors, E. A. (2012). Impact of self-administered relaxation and guided imagery techniques during final trimester and birth. *Complementary Therapies in Clinical Practice, 18*(1), 60–65.

Gilliland, A. L. (2011). After praise and encouragement: Emotional support strategies used by birth doulas in the USA and Canada. *Midwifery, 27*(4), 525–531.

Gizzo, S., Di Gangi, S., Saccardi, C., et al. (2012). Epidural analgesia during labor: Impact on delivery outcome, neonatal well-being, and early breastfeeding. *Breastfeeding Medicine, 7*(4), 262–268.

Greenwell, E. A., Wyshak, G., Ringer, S. A., et al. (2012). Intrapartum temperature elevation, epidural use, and adverse outcome in term infants. *Pediatrics, 129*(2), e447–e454.

Hamidzadeh, A., Shahpourian, F., Orak, R. J., et al. (2012). Effects of LI4 acupressure on labor pain in the first stage of labor. *Journal of Midwifery & Women's Health, 57*(2), 133–138.

Haydon, M. L., Larson, D., Reed, E., et al. (2011). Obstetric outcomes and maternal satisfaction in nulliparous women using patient-controlled epidural analgesia. *American Journal of Obstetrics & Gynecology, 205*(3), 271–276.

Horlocker, T. T. (2011). Complications of regional anesthesia and acute pain management. *Anesthesiology Clinics, 29*(2), 257–278.

Howarth, A. M., Swain, N., & Treharne, G. J. (2011). Taking personal responsibility for well-being increases birth satisfaction of first time mothers. *Journal of Health Psychology, 16*(8), 1221–1230.

Impey, L., & Child, T. (2012). Labour 2: Management. *Obstetrics & gynaecology* (4th ed., pp. 246–265). West Sussex, UK: John Wiley & Sons.

The Joint Commission. (2012). *2012 National patient safety goals.* Oakbrook Terrace, IL: Author.

Jones, C. (2011). The efficacy of lavender oil on perineal trauma: A review of the evidence. *Complementary Therapies in Clinical Practice, 17*(4), 215–220.

Jones, L., Othman, M., Dowswell, T., et al. (2012). Pain management for women in labour: An overview of systematic reviews. *Cochrane Database of Systematic Reviews,* (3), CD009234.

Karch, A. M. (2013). *2013 Lippincott's nursing drug guide.* Philadelphia, PA: Lippincott Williams & Wilkins.

Kemp, E., Kingswood, C. J., Kibuka, M., et al. (2013). Position in the second stage of labour for women with epidural anaesthesia. *Cochrane Database of Systematic Reviews,* (1):CD008070.

Kokki, M., Franco, M. G., Raatikainen, K., et al. (2012). Intravenous oxycodone for pain relief in the first stage of labour—Maternal pharmacokinetics and neonatal exposure. *Basic Clinical Pharmacology & Toxicology, 110*(3), 1742–1744.

Koren, G. (2012). Special aspects of perinatal & pediatric pharmacology. In B. Katsung & S. Masters (Eds.), *Basic and clinical pharmacology* (12th ed., pp. 1039–1050). New York, NY: McGraw Hill Companies.

Krieger, D. (1990). Therapeutic touch: Two decades of research, teaching, and clinical practice. *Imprint, 37*(3), 83–89.

Landolt, A. S., & Milling, L. S. (2011). The efficacy of hypnosis as an intervention for labor and delivery pain: A comprehensive methodological review. *Clinical Psychology Review, 31*(6), 1022–1031.

Leong, W. L., Sng, B. L., & Sia, A. T. (2011). A comparison between remifentanil and meperidine for labor analgesia: A systematic review. *Anesthesia & Analgesia, 113*(4), 818–825.

Liu, Y. H., Chang, M. Y., & Chen, C. H. (2010). Effects of music therapy on labour pain and anxiety in Taiwanese first-time mothers. *Journal of Clinical Nursing, 19*(7–8), 1065–1072.

Loayza, I. M. B., Solà, I., & Prats C. J. (2011). Biofeedback for pain management during labour. *Cochrane Database of Systematic Reviews,* (6), CD006168.

Loubert, C., Hinova, A., & Fernando, R. (2011). Update on modern neuraxial analgesia in labour: A review of the literature of the last 5 years. *Anaesthesia, 66*(3), 191–212.

Marc, I., Toureche, N., Ernst, E., et al. (2011). Mind-body interventions during pregnancy for preventing or treating women's anxiety. *Cochrane Database of Systematic Reviews,* (7), CD007559.

Mbah, A. K., Alio, A. P., Fombo, D. W., et al. (2011). Association between cocaine abuse in pregnancy and placenta-associated syndromes using propensity score matching approach. *Early Human Development, 88*(6), 333–337.

McCaffery, M. (1972). *Nursing management of the patient with pain.* Philadelphia, PA: Lippincott Williams & Wilkins.

Melzack, R., & Wall, P. (1965). Pain mechanisms: A new theory. *Science, 150*(2), 971–982.

Paech, M. J., Doherty, D. A., Christmas, T., et al. (2011). The volume of blood for epidural blood patch in obstetrics: A randomized, blinded clinical trial. *Anesthesia & Analgesia, 113*(1), 126–133.

Peles, E., Schreiber, S., Bloch, M., et al. (2012). Duration of methadone maintenance treatment during pregnancy and pregnancy outcome parameters in women with opiate addiction. *Journal of Addiction Medicine, 6*(1), 18–23.

Quesada, O., Gotman, N., Howell, H. B., et al. (2012). Prenatal hazardous substance use and adverse birth outcomes. *Journal of Maternal-Fetal & Neonatal Medicine, 25*(8), 1222–1227.

Rakestraw, T. (2010). Reiki: The energy doula. *Midwifery Today with International Midwife, 92*(1): 16–17.

Robinson, N., Lorenc, A., & Liao, X. (2011). The evidence for Shiatsu: A systematic review of Shiatsu and acupressure. *BMC Complementary & Alternative Medicine, 11*(10), 88–89.

Schrock, S. D., & Harraway-Smith, C. (2012). Labor analgesia. *American Family Physician, 85*(5), 447–454.

Simpkins, A. M., & Simpkins, C. A. (2011). *Meditation and yoga in psychotherapy.* Hoboken, NJ: John Wiley & Sons.

Skrablin, S., Grgic, O., Mihaljevic, S., et al. (2011). Comparison of intermittent and continuous epidural analgesia on delivery and progression of labour. *Journal of Obstetrics & Gynaecology, 31*(2), 134–138.

Smith, C. A., Collins, C. T., & Crowther, C. A. (2011). Aromatherapy for pain management in labour. *Cochrane Database of Systematic Reviews,* (7), CD009215.

Smith, C. A., Levett, K. M., Collins, C. T., et al. (2011). Relaxation techniques for pain management in labour. *Cochrane Database of Systematic Reviews,* (12), CD000111.

Smith, C. A., Levett, K. M., Collins, C. T., et al. (2012). Massage, reflexology and other manual methods for pain management in labour. *Cochrane Database of Systematic Reviews,* (2), CD009290.

Tocher, J. M. (2011). Physiology of pain in labor. In R. Mander (Eds.), *Pain in childbearing and it's control* (2nd ed., pp. 51–60). Oxford, UK: John Wiley & Son.

Ullman, R., Smith, L. A., Burns, E., et al. (2011). Parenteral opioids for maternal pain management in labour. *Cochrane Database of Systematic Reviews,* (10), CD007396l.

U.S. Department of Health and Human Services. (2010). *Healthy people 2020.* Washington, DC: Author.

Vricella, L. K., Louis, J. M., Mercer, B. M., et al. (2011). Impact of morbid obesity on epidural anesthesia complications in labor. *American Journal of Obstetrics & Gynecology, 205*(4), 370–376.

Wolfler, A., Salvo, I., Sortino, G., et al. (2010). Epidural analgesia with ropivacaine and sufentanil is associated with transient fetal heart rate changes. *Minerva Anesthesiology, 76*(5), 340–345.

Wright, A. (2012). Exploring the evidence for using TENS to relieve pain. *Nursing Times, 108*(11), 20–23.The Nursing Role in Providing Comfort During Labor and Birth

Chapter 17

Nursing Care of a Postpartal Family

KEY TERMS

- afterpains
- attachment
- bonding
- diastasis recti
- en face position
- engorgement
- engrossment
- Homans sign
- involution
- letting-go phase
- lochia
- rooming-in
- taking-hold phase
- taking-in phase
- uterine atony

OBJECTIVES

After mastering the contents of this chapter, you should be able to:

1. Describe the psychological and physiologic changes that occur in a postpartal woman and her family.
2. Identify 2020 National Health Goals related to the postpartal period that nurses can help the nation achieve.
3. Assess the physiologic and psychological changes of the postpartal woman and her family.
4. Formulate nursing diagnoses related to physiologic and psychological transitions of the postpartal period.
5. Develop expected outcomes for a postpartal woman and family related to the changes during this period as well as manage seamless transitions across differing health care settings.
6. Using the nursing process, plan nursing care that includes the six competencies of Quality & Safety Education for Nurses (QSEN): Patient-Centered Care, Teamwork & Collaboration, Evidence-Based Practice (EBP), Quality Improvement (QI), Safety, and Informatics.
7. Implement nursing care to aid the progression of physiologic and psychological transitions occurring in a postpartal woman and family.
8. Evaluate outcome criteria for achievement and effectiveness of care.
9. Integrate knowledge of postpartal women and families with the interplay of nursing process, the six competencies of QSEN, and Family Nursing to promote quality maternal and child health nursing care.

As the nurse working on a postpartum unit, you care for Leana Cooper, who gave birth to a healthy 8-lb 2-oz baby girl 6 hours ago. She is on maternity leave from her job as a court reporter. Her husband, Mike, plans to take a week off from work to help take care of the baby.

Leana has not voided since she gave birth. Although her baby sucks well, Leana is worried she's not getting enough milk. She tells you, "I haven't smoked in 9 months. Can't wait to go home so I can light up." Mike pulls you aside and says, "Sometimes, I see my wife crying for no reason. Why does she get so upset over little things? Isn't she as happy as I am?"

Previous chapters discussed caring for the pregnant woman and her family during the antepartal and intrapartal periods. This chapter adds information about caring for a postpartal woman and family. Nurses are able to play major roles in assessment, promotion of comfort, and education during this period as they help a new family adjust to the many physiologic and psychological changes that occur during this period.

What additional postpartal health care teaching does the Cooper family need?

The postpartal period, or *puerperium* (from the Latin *puer*, for "child," and *parere*, for "to bring forth"), refers to the 6-week period after childbirth. It is a time of maternal changes that are both retrogressive (involution of the uterus and vagina) and progressive (production of milk for lactation, restoration of the normal menstrual cycle, and beginning of a parenting role). Protecting a woman's health as these changes occur is important for preserving her future childbearing function and for ensuring she is physically well enough to incorporate her new child into her family (Souza, Gülmezoglu, Vogel, et al., 2013). The period is also popularly termed the *fourth trimester of pregnancy*.

The physical care a woman receives during the postpartal period can influence her health for the rest of her life. The emotional support she receives can influence the emotional health of her child and family so much that it can be felt into the next generation (Newton, 2012). Box 17.1 shows 2020 National Health Goals related to the postpartal period that nurses can help the nation achieve.

BOX 17.1 Nursing Care Planning Based on 2020 National Health Goals

The postpartal period is an extremely important one because of the possibility of uterine hemorrhage and because it is the optimal period for parent–child bonding. 2020 National Health Goals that involve this time period include:

- Reduce the maternal mortality rate to no more than 11.4/100,000 live births from a baseline of 12.7/100,000.
- Increase to at least 82% the proportion of mothers who breastfeed their babies in the early postpartum period from a baseline of 74% and increase the proportion of mothers who still breastfeed at 6 months to 60.6% from a baseline of 43.5%.
- Increase the proportion of live births that occur in facilities that provide care for lactating mothers and their babies from 2.9% to 8.1%.
- Reduce postpartum relapse of smoking among women who quit smoking during pregnancy (developmental).
- Increase the proportion of women who used contraception to plan their pregnancy (developmental) (U.S. Department of Health and Human Services [DHHS], 2010; see www.healthypeople.gov).

Nurses can help the nation achieve these goals by maintaining close observation in the immediate postpartal period to detect maternal hemorrhage, encouraging and supporting women as they begin breastfeeding, and ensuring women receive reproductive life planning information if desired.

Nursing Process Overview

For a Postpartal Woman and Family

Assessment

During the puerperium, assessment of a woman is accomplished by health interview, physical examination, and analysis of laboratory data. It is important to ensure that physical changes, such as uterine involution, are occurring by evaluating uterine size and consistency and the amount of lochia flow.

Assessment of a woman's psychological adjustment begins with her reaction to her baby at birth (Was she disappointed or happy with the appearance of her baby? Is she glad to be through with the pregnancy or still longing to be back in it?) and continues with every contact made with the family during and after a hospital stay. Assess the extent and quality of the woman's interaction with her child (Does she hold and talk to the infant?), her overall mood (Do you observe her crying? Does she have long periods of staring into space or not talking?), and her ability to begin infant and self-care. A woman who feels good about herself, even though she is exhausted from childbirth, usually will try to maintain her appearance. If she is depressed, however, she probably has little energy to do things such as comb her hair or worry about her appearance.

Nursing Diagnosis

Nursing diagnoses during the postpartal period are often "risk for" diagnoses and concerned with a family's ability to accept and bond with a new child or with physiologic considerations. Examples include:

- Health-seeking behaviors related to care of newborn
- Risk for impaired parenting related to disappointment in the sex of the child
- Fear related to lack of preparation for child care
- Risk for deficient fluid volume related to postpartal hemorrhage
- Risk for altered family coping related to an additional family member

Outcome Identification and Planning

Be certain that outcomes established during this time are realistic in light of a woman's changed life pattern. Most postpartal families remain in the hospital for a relatively short time, only 48 to 72 hours. The postpartum stay in an alternative birth center can be as short as 4 hours. That means outcomes must be devised that can be accomplished and evaluated during this short period of client contact. If an outcome cannot be evaluated within this short time frame, follow-up home care, ambulatory visits, or phone calls may be necessary.

When planning care in the postpartal period, try to arrange procedures to allow optimal time for family–infant interaction and yet provide adequate time for a woman to rest to prevent exhaustion, because this can improve her coping ability and plans for self-care. After adequate instruction, a woman should be prepared to monitor her own health after she returns home.

Planning should also include ample time for health teaching such as care of the newborn and the need for flexibility in care, because the parents do not yet know what their new life will be like or how tired they will become after being awakened frequently during the night. Brainstorming with the parents—practicing to produce at least three different methods of reaching a particular goal—is excellent practice for parenting because giving advice only solves an immediate problem; helping parents learn good problem-solving techniques improves their ability to handle the many challenges that will arise with childrearing. Helpful Internet sites to recommend to parents who feel a need for additional support during this time are the Mayo Clinic Newborn Care Web site (www.mayoclinic.com) and the Postpartal Support International Web site (www.postpartum.net), a site that helps women dealing with postpartal depression.

Implementation

All interventions in the postpartal period should be family centered, to enhance family functioning and bonding, and geared toward increasing a woman's self-esteem, allowing her to view herself as a new mother, and helping her view her new infant as part of her family.

Outcome Evaluation

If a woman fails to make an adequate adjustment to her new life changes, she may have difficulty integrating an infant into the family. This could affect a child's physical and mental health, self-esteem, and ability to form a sense of trust.

Evaluation in the postpartal period, then, involves not only being certain a woman and her baby are safe but also that the woman knows how to maintain her own and her infant's health. Such follow-up evaluation can be done by telephone, during home visits, or during postpartal and well-child assessments. Examples of expected outcomes include:

- The parents spontaneously verbalize at least one positive comment about their child's characteristics before hospital discharge.
- The client states she believes she will be able to manage newborn care with the support of her significant other.
- The client's lochial flow is no more than one saturated perineal pad (50 ml) every 3 hours.
- The client states she is tired but feels able to manage her newborn and family care.

PSYCHOLOGICAL CHANGES OF THE POSTPARTAL PERIOD

A *transition* is a movement or passage from one position or concept to another or a pause between what was and what is to be.

People move through several predictable stages during transition: first is the act of ending old ways of thinking or believing; next, there is a neutral zone, during which the old way is gone but the new way is not yet comfortable; and finally, there is a new beginning, during which new ideas and concepts are put into action (Bridges, 1994). The postpartum period is a time of transition, during which a couple gives up concepts such as "childless" or "parents of one" and moves to not only trying out their new role but also determining whether they "fit" the new role. Nurses can help couples acknowledge the extent of the change, so that they can gain closure on their previous lifestyle. Opening channels for communication, anticipating new needs, and highlighting potential gains that will occur because of the change are important actions.

Behavioral Adjustment: Phases of the Puerperium

In her classic work on maternal behavior, Reva Rubin, a nurse, divided the puerperium into three separate phases (Rubin, 1977). The first of these is the **taking-in phase**, or the time when the new parents review their pregnancy and the labor and birth. The subsequent phases, called the **taking-hold** and **letting-go phases**, are times of renewed action and forward movement. At the time these phases of the puerperium were identified, women were hospitalized for 5 to 7 days after childbirth and moved in a paced manner from one step to the next. Today, with a stay in a health care facility as short as a few hours, women appear to move through these phases much more quickly and may even experience two different phases at once.

Taking-In Phase

The taking-in phase is largely a time of reflection. During this 1- to 3-day period, a woman is largely passive. She prefers having a nurse attend to her needs and make decisions for her, rather than do these things herself. This dependence results partly from her physical discomfort because of afterpains or hemorrhoids, partly from her uncertainty in caring for her newborn, and partly from the exhaustion that follows childbirth.

As part of thinking and pondering about her new role, the woman usually wants to talk about her pregnancy, especially about her labor and birth. She holds her new child with a sense of wonder and asks: Is birth really over? Could this child really have been inside me? She wants to rest to regain her physical strength and experience a calm atmosphere around her to quiet and contain her swirling thoughts. Encouraging her to talk about the birth is an important way to help her integrate the experience into her total life experiences (Box 17.2).

Taking-Hold Phase

After a time of passive dependence, a woman begins to initiate action. She prefers to get her own washcloth or to make her own decisions. Women who give birth without any anesthesia may reach this second phase in a matter of hours after birth.

During the taking-in period, a woman may have been too tired to care for her child. Now, she begins to take a stronger interest in her infant and begins maternal role behaviors. As a rule, it is usually best to give a woman a brief demonstration of baby care and then allow her to care for her child herself—with watchful guidance—as she enters this phase.

Although a woman's actions suggest greater independence during this time, she often still feels insecure about her ability to care for her new child. She needs praise for the things she does well, such as supporting the baby's head or beginning breastfeeding, to give her confidence. This positive reinforcement begins in the health care facility and continues after discharge, at home and at postpartum and well-baby visits.

Do not rush a woman through the phase of taking-in or prevent her from taking hold when she reaches this point. For many young mothers, learning to make decisions about their child's welfare is one of the most difficult phases of motherhood. It helps if a woman has practice in making such decisions in a sheltered setting, such as a hospital, rather than first taking on that level of responsibility after she is home alone.

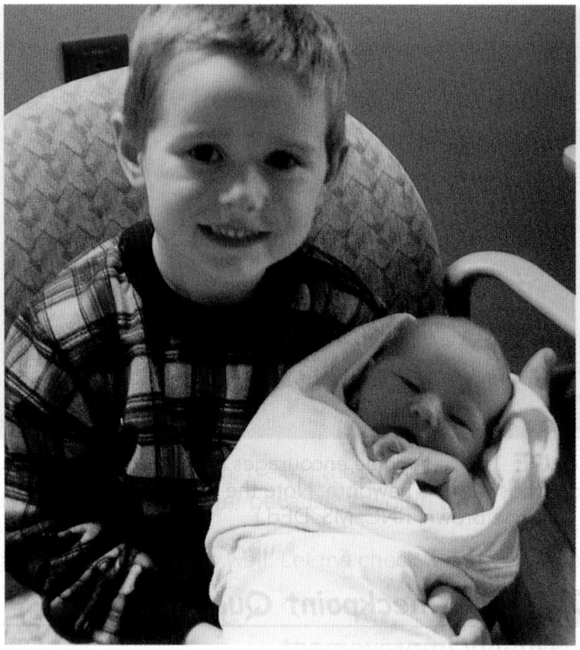

FIGURE 17.3 Sibling visiting is important to bring a family together.

The visit can help to relieve some of the impact of separation and also help to make the baby a part of the family (Fig. 17.3). Assess to be certain siblings are free of contagious diseases such as upper respiratory tract illnesses or recent exposure to chickenpox before they visit. Then, have them wash their hands and, if they choose, hold or touch the newborn with parental assistance.

Encourage the success of a family visit by suggesting the woman take her pain medication before the visit. If she had a cesarean birth, protecting her abdomen with padding can decrease anxiety of the siblings about the condition of their mother.

You may need to caution a woman that the opinions of a new brother or sister expressed by her older children may not be complimentary; for example, this baby with little hair may not be their idea of a "pretty baby." If they thought the new baby would be big enough to play with, they may not agree that he is a "big baby."

Maternal Concerns and Feelings in the Postpartal Period

Traditionally, it is assumed the bulk of a woman's concerns in the postpartal period center on the care of her new infant. As a result, classes in the postpartal period have traditionally focused on teaching how to breastfeed and bathe infants. Many women, however, are not as concerned about infant care as they are about their adjustment to a new role change.

Typical issues identified by postpartal women that they would like to hear discussed are breast soreness; regaining their figure; regulating the demands of a job, housework, their partner, and their children; coping with emotional tension and sibling jealousy; and how to combat fatigue.

Abandonment

Many mothers, if given the opportunity, admit to feeling abandoned and less important after giving birth than they did during pregnancy or labor. Only hours before, after all, they were the center of attention, with everyone asking about their health and well-being. Now, suddenly, the baby is everyone's chief interest. Relatives ask about the baby's health; the gifts are all for the baby. Even a woman's primary health care provider, who has made her feel so important for the last 9 months, may ask during a visit, "How's that healthy 8-pound boy?" Comments such as this can make a woman experience a sensation very close to jealousy. And how can a good mother be jealous of her own baby?

You can help a woman move past these feelings by verbalizing the problem: "How things have changed! Everyone's asking about the baby today and not about you, aren't they?" These are reassuring words for a woman and help her realize that, although uncomfortable, the feeling she is experiencing is normal.

When a newborn comes home, a father or partner may express much the same feelings as he or she feels resentful of the time the mother spends with the infant. Examination of these competitive feelings can help a couple realize that parenthood involves some compromise in favor of the baby's interests. Making infant care a shared responsibility can help alleviate these feelings and make both partners feel equally involved in the baby's care. You can help parents or partners move past this competitive stage by pointing out positive parenting behaviors, positive self-care behaviors, and the warm infant response to their behaviors.

Disappointment

Another common feeling parents or partners may experience is disappointment in the baby. All during pregnancy, they pictured a chubby-cheeked, curly-haired, smiling girl or boy. They have instead a skinny baby, without any hair, who seems to cry constantly. This can make it difficult to feel positive immediately toward a child who does not meet their expectations. It can cause parents to remember their adolescence, when they felt gangly and unattractive, or to experience feelings of inadequacy all over again.

You can never change the sex, size, or look of a child, but in the short time you care for a postpartal family, it is possible for a key person such as a nurse to tip a scale toward acceptance or at least help a person involved to take a clearer look at his or her situation and begin to cope with the new circumstances. As an example, handle the child warmly, to show you find the infant satisfactory or even special. Comment on the child's good points, such as long fingers, lovely eyes, and healthy appetite. Be aware, however, that, culturally, some groups are fearful for the baby if these types of comments are made because they could draw evil influences toward the child.

Postpartal Blues

During the postpartal period, as many as 50% of women experience some feelings of overwhelming sadness or "baby blues" (Baselice, 2011). They may burst into tears easily or feel let down and irritable. This phenomenon may be caused by hormonal changes, particularly the decrease in estrogen and progesterone that occurred with delivery of the placenta. For some women, it may be a response to dependence and low self-esteem caused by exhaustion, being away from home, physical discomfort, and the tension engendered by assuming a new role, especially if a woman is not receiving support from her partner. In addition to crying, the syndrome is evidenced by feelings of inadequacy, mood lability, anorexia, and sleep disturbance.

Anticipatory guidance and individualized support from health care personnel are important to help the parents understand that this unexpected response is normal. Be certain support persons also receive assurance of this type, or they can think the woman is unhappy with them or the new baby or is keeping some terrible news about the baby secret.

Give the woman a chance to verbalize her feelings and make as many decisions as she wants to help her gain a sense of control and move past this strange postpartal emotion.

Remember, however, not all postpartal women you see crying are doing so because they have baby blues. Perhaps problems at home have become overwhelming. A partner may have been laid off from a job just at this time when they most need money. One of her parents may be ill, or her house may have been damaged by a disaster such as a flood. Encouraging women to talk about their postpartal feelings helps to differentiate between problems that can be handled best with discussion and concerned understanding and those that should be referred to a social service department or a community health agency for additional support.

Women are at greater risk (19% to 48%) for moderate to severe depression after childbirth requiring formal counseling, especially if they are economically stressed or have a comorbid condition such as diabetes (Farr, Dietz, Williams, et al., 2011). Severe psychosis also can occur in women during this time (Heron, Gilbert, Dolman, et al., 2012). Because these are deeper level concerns, postpartal depression beyond the scope of "baby blues" and psychosis are discussed in Chapter 25.

PHYSIOLOGIC CHANGES OF THE POSTPARTAL PERIOD

Retrogressive physiologic changes that occur during the postpartal period include those related specifically to the reproductive system as well as other systemic changes (Box 17.4).

Reproductive System Changes

Involution is the process whereby the reproductive organs return to their nonpregnant state. A woman is in danger of hemorrhage from the denuded surface of the uterus until involution is complete (Katz, 2012).

The Uterus

Involution of the uterus involves two processes. First, the area where the placenta was implanted is sealed off to prevent bleeding. Second, the organ is reduced to its approximate pregestational size.

The sealing of the placenta site is accomplished by rapid contraction of the uterus immediately after delivery of the placenta. This contraction pinches the blood vessels entering the 7-cm-wide area left denuded by the placenta and halts bleeding. With time, thrombi form within the uterine sinuses and permanently seal the area. Eventually, endometrial tissue undermines the site and obliterates the organized thrombi, covering and healing the area so completely the process leaves no scar tissue within the uterus so does not compromise future implantation sites.

BOX 17.4 Nursing Care Planning Using Assessment

Assessing the Postpartal Woman

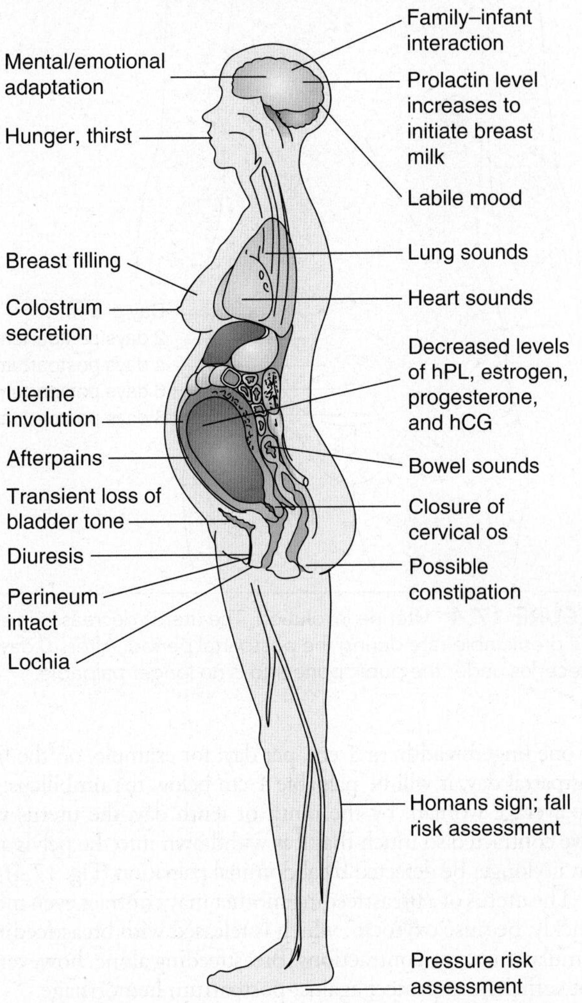

The same contraction process reduces the bulk of the uterus. Devoid of the placenta and the membranes, the walls of the uterus thicken and contract, gradually reducing the uterus from a container large enough to hold a full-term fetus to one the size of a grapefruit, a phenomenon that can be compared with a rubber band that has been stretched for many months and now is regaining its normal contour. None of the rubber band is destroyed; the shape is simply altered. For this reason, the postpartal period, like pregnancy, is not a period of illness, of necrosing cells being evacuated, but primarily a period of healthy change (Edmonds, 2012).

Immediately after birth, the uterus weighs about 1,000 g. At the end of the first week, it weighs 500 g. By the time involution is complete (6 weeks), it weighs approximately 50 g, similar to its prepregnancy weight. Because uterine contraction begins immediately after placental delivery, the fundus of the uterus is palpable through the abdominal wall, halfway between the umbilicus and the symphysis pubis, within a few minutes after birth. One hour later, it will rise to the level of the umbilicus, where it remains for approximately the next 24 hours. From then on, it decreases

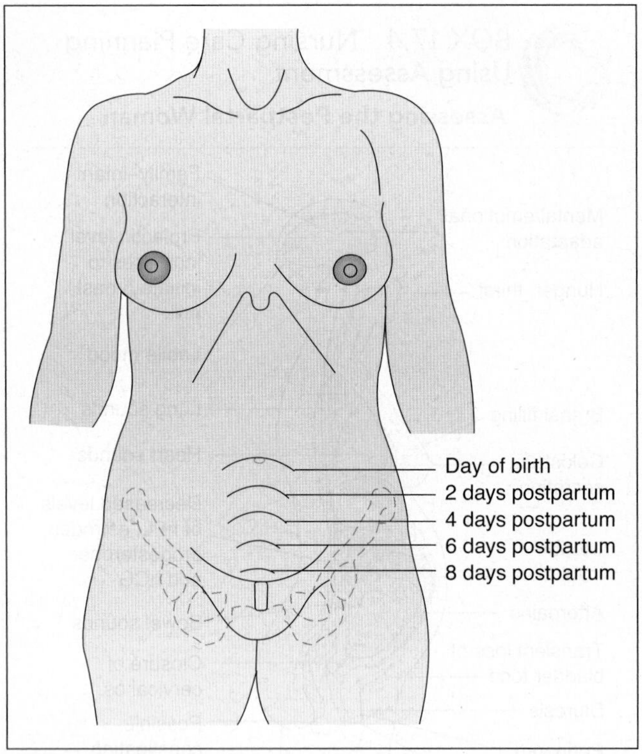

FIGURE 17.4 Uterine involution. The uterus decreases in size at a predictable rate during the postpartal period. After 10 days, it recedes under the pubic bone and is no longer palpable.

by one fingerbreadth, or 1 cm, per day; for example, on the first postpartal day, it will be palpable 1 cm below the umbilicus. In the average woman, by the ninth or tenth day, the uterus will have contracted so much that it is withdrawn into the pelvis and can no longer be detected by abdominal palpation (Fig. 17.4).

The uterus of a breastfeeding mother may contract even more quickly, because oxytocin, which is released with breastfeeding, stimulates uterine contractions. Breastfeeding alone, however, is not sufficient to protect against postpartum hemorrhage.

The fundus is normally located in the midline of the abdomen. Occasionally, it can be felt slightly to the right, because the bulk of the sigmoid colon forced it to that side during pregnancy and it tends to remain in that position. Assess fundal height shortly after a woman has emptied her bladder for most accurate results, because a full bladder can keep the uterus from contracting, pushing it upward and increasing the risk of excess bleeding and blood clot formation in the uterus.

Involution will occur most dependably in a woman who is well nourished and who ambulates early after birth as gravity may play a role. Involution may be delayed by a condition such as the birth of multiple fetuses, hydramnios, exhaustion from prolonged labor, grand multiparity, or physiologic effects of excessive analgesia. Contraction may be ineffective if there is retained placenta or membranes (Samanta, Roy, Mistri, et al., 2013).

An estimation of the consistency of the postpartal uterus is as important as measurement of its height. A well-contracted fundus feels so firm it can be compared with a grapefruit in both size and tenseness. Whenever the fundus feels boggy (soft or flabby), it is not as contracted as it should be, despite its position in the abdomen.

The first hour after birth is potentially the most dangerous time for a woman. If her uterus should become relaxed during this time (**uterine atony**), she will lose blood very rapidly, because no permanent thrombi have yet formed at the placental site.

In some women, contraction of the uterus after birth causes intermittent cramping termed **afterpains**, similar to that accompanying a menstrual period. Afterpains tend to be noticed most by multiparas than by primiparas and by women who have given birth to large babies or multiple births. In these situations, the uterus must contract more forcefully to regain its prepregnancy size. These sensations are noticed most intensely with breastfeeding, when the infant's sucking causes a release of oxytocin from the posterior pituitary, increasing the strength of the contractions.

Lochia

The separation of the placenta and membranes occurs in the spongy layer or outer portion of the decidua basalis of the uterus. By the second day after birth, the layer of decidua remaining under the placental site (an area 7 cm wide) and throughout the uterus differentiates into two distinct layers. The inner layer attached to the muscular wall of the uterus remains, serving as the foundation from which a new layer of endometrium will be formed. The layer adjacent to the uterine cavity becomes necrotic and is cast off as a vaginal discharge similar to a menstrual flow. This flow, consisting of blood, fragments of decidua, white blood cells, mucus, and some bacteria, is termed **lochia** (Chi, Bapir, Lee, et al., 2010).

The portion of the uterus where the placenta was not attached is so fully cleansed by this sloughing process it will be in a reproductive state in about 3 weeks' time; it takes approximately 6 weeks (the entire postpartal period) for the placental implantation site to be healed.

For the first 3 days after birth, a lochia discharge consists almost entirely of blood, with only small particles of decidua and mucus. Because of its mainly red color, it is termed *lochia rubra.* As the amount of blood involved in the cast-off tissue decreases (about the fourth day) and leukocytes begin to invade the area, as they do with any healing surface, the flow becomes pink or brownish (*lochia serosa*). On about the 10th day, the amount of the flow decreases and becomes colorless or white with streaks of brownish mucus (*lochia alba*). Lochia alba is present in most women until the third week after birth, although it is not unusual for a lochia flow to last the entire 6 weeks of the puerperium. Characteristics of lochia are summarized in Table 17.1. Several rules for judging whether lochia flow is normal are summarized in Box 17.5.

TABLE 17.1 Characteristics of Lochia

Type of Lochia	Color	Postpartal Day	Composition
Lochia rubra	Red	1–3	Blood, fragments of decidua, and mucus
Lochia serosa	Pink	3–10	Blood, mucus, and invading leukocytes
Lochia alba	White	10–14 (may last 6 weeks)	Largely mucus; leukocyte count high

BOX 17.5 Nursing Care Planning Based on Family Teaching

EVALUATING LOCHIA FLOW

Q. Leana Cooper asks you, "How do I know if my lochia is normal?"
A. Several guidelines are helpful for evaluating lochia flow:

Amount: Lochia amount varies greatly from woman to woman. Mothers who breastfeed tend to have less lochial discharge than those who do not, because the natural release of the hormone oxytocin during breastfeeding strengthens uterine contractions. Lochial flow increases on exertion, especially the first few times a woman is out of bed, but decreases again with rest. Saturating a perineal pad in less than 1 hour is considered an abnormally heavy flow and should be reported. Don't use tampons to halt the flow or this could lead to infection.

Consistency: Lochia should contain no exceedingly large clots as these may indicate a portion of the placenta has been retained and is preventing closure of the maternal uterine blood sinuses. In any event, large clots denote poor uterine contraction, which needs to be corrected.

Pattern: Lochia is red for the first 1 to 3 days (lochia rubra), pinkish-brown from days 4 to 10 (lochia serosa), and then white (lochia alba) for as long as 6 weeks after birth. The pattern of lochia (rubra to serosa to alba) should not reverse as this suggests a placental fragment has been retained or uterine contraction is decreasing and new bleeding is beginning.

Odor: Lochia should not have an offensive odor as this suggests the uterus has become infected. Immediate intervention is needed to halt postpartal infection.

Absence: Lochia should never be absent during the first 1 to 3 weeks as absence of lochia, like presence of an offensive odor, may indicate postpartal infection. Lochia may be scant in amount after cesarean birth, but it is never altogether absent.

The Cervix

Immediately after birth, a uterine cervix feels soft and malleable to palpation. Both the internal and external os are open. Like contraction of the uterus, contraction of the cervix toward its prepregnant state begins at once. By the end of 7 days, the external os has narrowed to the size of a pencil opening; the cervix feels firm and nongravid again.

In contrast to the process of uterine involution, in which the changes consist primarily of old cells being returned to their former position by contraction, the process in the cervix does involve the formation of new muscle cells. Because of this, the cervix does not return exactly to its prepregnancy state. The internal os closes as before, but after a vaginal birth, the external os usually remains slightly open and appears slitlike or stellate (star shaped), whereas previously it was round. Finding this pattern on pelvic examination suggests that childbearing has taken place.

The Vagina

After a vaginal birth, the vagina feels soft, with few rugae, and its diameter is considerably greater than normal. The hymen is permanently torn and heals with small, separate tags of tissue. It takes the entire postpartal period for the vagina to involute (by contraction, as with the uterus) until it gradually returns to its approximate prepregnancy state. Thickening of the walls appears to depend on renewed estrogen stimulation from the ovaries. Because a woman who is breastfeeding may have delayed ovulation, she may continue to have thin-walled or fragile vaginal cells that cause slight vaginal bleeding during sexual intercourse until about 6 weeks' time. If a woman practices Kegel exercises, the strength and tone of the vagina will increase more rapidly (see Chapter 12). This may be important for the sexual enjoyment of both a woman and her partner.

✔ QSEN Checkpoint Question 17.3

Safety

You want to prepare Leana to assess her own health after discharge. Which statement by her would make you worry that she needs added information?

a. "I know about lochia; I'll use tampons just like I do for my periods."
b. "I admit I don't like having lochia, but I understand its purpose."
c. "I know to wash my hands after I change perineal pads and before handling the baby."
d. "I'll look for the color of my lochia to change from red to pink."

Look in Appendix A for best answer and rationale.

The Perineum

Because of the great amount of pressure experienced during birth, the perineum is edematous and tender immediately after birth. Ecchymosis patches from ruptured capillaries may show on the surface. The labia majora and labia minora typically remain atrophic and softened after birth, never returning to their prepregnancy state.

Systemic Changes

The same body systems that were involved in pregnancy are also involved in postpartal changes as the body returns to its prepregnancy state.

The Hormonal System

Pregnancy hormones begin to decrease as soon as the placenta is no longer present. Levels of human chorionic gonadotropin (hCG) and human placental lactogen (hPL) are almost negligible by 24 hours. By week 1, progestin, estrone, and estradiol are all at prepregnancy levels (estriol may take an additional week before it reaches prepregnancy levels). Follicle-stimulating hormone (FSH) remains low for about 12 days and then begins to rise as a new menstrual cycle is initiated.

The Urinary System

During pregnancy, as much as 2,000 to 3,000 ml of excess fluid accumulates in the body so extensive diaphoresis (excessive sweating) and diuresis (excess urine production) begin almost immediately after birth to rid the body of this fluid. This easily increases the daily urine output of a postpartal woman from a normal level of 1,500 ml to as much as 3,000 ml/day during the second to fifth day after birth. This marked increase in urine production causes the bladder to fill rapidly.

Because during a vaginal birth, the fetal head exerts a great deal of pressure on the bladder and urethra as it passes on the bladder's underside, this may leave the bladder with a transient loss of tone that, together with the edema surrounding the urethra, decreases a woman's ability to sense when she has to void. A woman who has had epidural anesthesia can feel no sensation in the bladder area until the anesthetic has worn off.

To prevent permanent damage to the bladder from overdistention, assess a woman's abdomen frequently in the immediate postpartal period. On palpation, a full bladder is felt as a hard or firm area just above the symphysis pubis. On percussion (placing one finger flat on the woman's abdomen over the bladder and tapping it with the middle finger of the other hand), a full bladder sounds resonant, in contrast to the dull, thudding sound of non–fluid-filled tissue. Pressure on this area may make a woman feel as if she has to void, but she is then unable to do so. As the bladder fills, it displaces the uterus; uterine position and lack of contraction are, therefore, a second good gauge of whether a bladder is full or empty (Mulder, Schoffelmeer, Hakvoort, et al., 2012).

The hydronephrosis or increased size of ureters that occurred during pregnancy remains present for about 4 weeks after birth. The increased size of these structures, in conjunction with reduced bladder sensitivity, increases the possibility of urinary stasis and urinary tract infection in the postpartal period.

The Circulatory System

The diuresis that is evident between the second and fifth days after birth, as well as the blood loss at birth, acts to reduce the added blood volume a woman accumulated during pregnancy. This reduction occurs so rapidly, in fact, that the blood volume returns to its normal prepregnancy level by the first or second week after birth.

The usual blood loss with a vaginal birth is 300 to 500 ml. With a cesarean birth, it is 500 to 1,000 ml. A 4-point decrease in hematocrit (proportion of red blood cells to circulating plasma) and a 1-g decrease in hemoglobin value occur with each 250 ml of blood lost. For example, if an average woman enters labor with a hematocrit of 37%, it will be about 33% on the first postpartal day, and hemoglobin will fall from 11 to 10 g/dl. If the woman was anemic during pregnancy, she can expect to continue to be anemic afterward. As excess fluid is excreted, the hematocrit gradually rises (because of hemoconcentration), reaching prepregnancy levels by 6 weeks after birth.

Women usually continue to have the same high level of plasma fibrinogen during the first postpartal weeks as they did during pregnancy. This is a protective measure against hemorrhage. However, this high level also increases the risk of thrombus formation. There is also an increase in the number of leukocytes in the blood. The white blood cell count may be as high as 30,000 cells/mm^3 (mainly granulocytes) compared to a normal level of 5,000 to 10,000 cells/mm^3, particularly if labor was long or difficult. This, too, is part of the body's defense system, a defense against infection and an aid to healing.

Any varicosities that are present from pregnancy will recede, but they rarely return to a completely prepregnant appearance. Although vascular blemishes, such as spider angiomas, fade slightly, they may not disappear completely either. Bilateral ankle edema is not uncommon but should not progress above the knees. This decreases over time as fluid shifts and returns to the circulatory system.

The Gastrointestinal System

Digestion and absorption begin to be active again soon after birth unless a woman has had a cesarean birth. Almost immediately, the woman feels hungry and thirsty, and she can eat without difficulty from nausea or vomiting during this time.

Hemorrhoids (distended rectal veins) that have been pushed out of the rectum because of the effort of pelvic-stage pushing often are present. Bowel sounds are active, but passage of stool through the bowel may be slow because of the still-present effect of relaxin on the bowel. Bowel evacuation may be difficult because of pain if a woman has episiotomy sutures or from hemorrhoids.

The Integumentary System

After birth, the stretch marks on a woman's abdomen (striae gravidarum) still appear reddened and may be even more prominent than during pregnancy, when they were tightly stretched. Typically, in a Caucasian woman, these will fade to a pale white over the next 3 to 6 months; in an African American woman, they may remain as areas of slightly darker pigment. Excessive pigment on the face and neck (chloasma) and on the abdomen (linea nigra) will become barely detectable by 6 weeks' time. If **diastasis recti** (overstretching and separation of the abdominal musculature) occurred, the area will appear as a slightly indented bluish streak in the abdominal midline. Modified sit-ups help to strengthen abdominal muscles and return abdominal support to its prepregnant level. Diastasis recti, however, may require surgery to correct (Hickey, Finch, & Khanna, 2011).

Retrogressive Changes of the Puerperium

The overall effects of postpartal retrogressive changes are exhaustion and weight loss.

Exhaustion

As soon as birth is completed, a woman experiences total exhaustion. For the last several months of pregnancy, she probably experienced some difficulty sleeping. All during labor, she worked hard with little or no sleep. Now she has "sleep hunger," which may make it difficult for her to cope with new experiences and stressful situations until she has enjoyed a sustained period of sleep.

Weight Loss

The rapid diuresis and diaphoresis during the second to fifth days after birth usually result in a weight loss of 5 lb (2 to 4 kg), in addition to the approximately 12 lb (5.8 kg) lost at birth.

Lochia flow causes an additional 2- to 3-lb (1-kg) loss, for a total weight loss of about 19 lb. Additional weight loss is dependent on the amount of pregnancy weight gain and on whether a woman continues active measures to lose weight (Cahill, Freeland-Graves, Shah, et al., 2012). It is also influenced by nutrition, exercise, and breastfeeding. The weight a woman reaches at 6 weeks after birth becomes her baseline postpartal weight unless she continues active measures to lose the weight. In many women, this baseline is higher than their prepregnancy weight and one of the reasons that obesity has become a national health concern (Lipsky, Strawderman, & Olson, 2012).

Vital Sign Changes

Vital sign changes in the postpartum period reflect the internal adjustments that occur as a woman's body returns to its prepregnant state.

Temperature. Temperature is always taken orally or tympanically (never rectally) during the puerperium, because of the danger of vaginal contamination and the discomfort involved in rectal intrusion.

A woman may show a slight increase in temperature during the first 24 hours after birth because of dehydration that occurred during labor. If she takes in adequate fluid during the first 24 hours, this temperature elevation will return to normal. Most women are thirsty immediately after birth and are eager to take in fluid, so drinking a large quantity of fluid is not a problem unless the woman is nauseated from a birth analgesic.

Any woman whose oral temperature rises above 100.4°F (38°C), excluding the first 24-hour period, is considered by criteria of the Joint Commission on Maternal Welfare to be febrile, and such a high temperature may indicate that a postpartal infection is present (Johnson, Thakar, & Sultan, 2012). Occasionally, when a woman's breasts fill with milk on the third or fourth postpartum day, her temperature will rise for a period of hours because of the increased vascular activity involved. If the elevation in temperature lasts longer than a few hours, however, infection is a more likely reason. Because infection is a major cause of postpartal mortality and morbidity, nurses have the important role of being the health care providers who may first detect the problem.

Pulse. A woman's pulse rate during the postpartal period is usually slightly slower than usual. During pregnancy, the distended uterus obstructed the amount of venous blood returning to the heart; after birth, to accommodate the increased blood volume returning to the heart, stroke volume increases. This increased stroke volume reduces the pulse rate to between 60 and 70 beats/min. As diuresis diminishes the blood volume and causes blood pressure to fall, the pulse rate increases accordingly. By the end of the first week, the pulse rate will have returned to normal.

Evaluate pulse rate conscientiously in the postpartal period, because a rapid and thready pulse during this time could be a sign of hemorrhage.

Blood Pressure. Blood pressure should also be monitored carefully during the postpartal period, because a decrease in this can also indicate bleeding. In contrast, an elevation above 140 mmHg systolic or 90 mmHg diastolic may indicate the development of postpartal hypertension of pregnancy, an unusual but serious complication of the puerperium (Chhabra, Tyagi, Bhavani, et al., 2012) (see Chapter 21).

To evaluate blood pressure, compare a woman's pressure with her prepregnancy level if possible, rather than with standard blood pressure ranges; otherwise, if her blood pressure rose during pregnancy, a significant postpartal decrease in pressure could be missed.

Oxytocics, drugs frequently administered during the postpartal period to achieve uterine contraction, cause contraction of all smooth muscle, including blood vessels (Karch, 2013). Consequently, these drugs can increase blood pressure. Always measure blood pressure before administering one of these agents; if blood pressure is greater than 140/90 mmHg, withhold the agent and notify the woman's primary care provider to prevent hypertension and, possibly, a cerebrovascular accident.

A major complication in women who have lost an appreciable amount of blood with birth is orthostatic hypotension, or dizziness that occurs on standing because of the lack of adequate blood volume to maintain nourishment of brain cells. To test whether a woman will be susceptible to this, assess her blood pressure and pulse while she is lying supine. Next, raise the head of the bed fully upright, wait 2 or 3 minutes, and reassess these values. If the pulse rate is increased by more than 20 beats/min and blood pressure is 15 to 20 mmHg lower than formerly, the woman might be susceptible to dizziness and fainting when she ambulates. Inform the woman's primary care provider of these findings. Advise her to always sit up slowly and "dangle" on the side of her bed before attempting to walk. If she notices obvious dizziness on sitting upright, support her during ambulation to avoid the possibility of a fall. Caution her not to attempt to walk carrying her newborn until her cardiovascular status adjusts to her blood loss.

What if...17.1 Leana Cooper, now 12 hours postpartum, has an oral temperature of 99°F (37.2°C) and is uncomfortable from profuse diaphoresis and extreme fatigue. What actions would you take?

Progressive Changes of the Puerperium

Two physiologic changes that occur during the puerperium involve progressive changes, or the building of new tissue. Because this requires good nutrition, caution women against strict dieting that would limit cell-building ability during the first 6 weeks after childbirth (Whitney & Rolfes, 2012).

Lactation

The formation of breast milk (lactation) begins in a postpartal woman whether or not she plans to breastfeed (Stuebe, 2012). Early in pregnancy, the increased estrogen level produced by the placenta stimulated the growth of milk glands; breasts increased in size because of these larger glands, accumulated fluid, and some extra adipose tissue. For the first 2 days after birth, an average woman notices little change in her breasts from the way they were during pregnancy because, since midway through pregnancy, she has been secreting colostrum, a thin, watery, prelactation secretion. On the third day after birth, her breasts become full and feel tense or tender as milk forms within breast ducts and replaces colostrum.

Breast milk forms in response to the decrease in estrogen and progesterone levels that follows delivery of the placenta (which stimulates prolactin production and, consequently, milk production). A woman's breasts become fuller, larger, and firmer as blood and lymph enter the area to contribute fluid to the formation of milk. In many women, breast distention becomes so marked it is accompanied by a feeling of heat or throbbing pain, or breast tissue may appear reddened as if an acute inflammatory or infectious process were present. This feeling of tension in the breasts on the third or fourth day after birth is termed primary **engorgement**. It fades as the infant begins effective sucking and empties the breasts of milk. Whether milk production continues depends on whether an infant can suck effectively as this releases oxytocin and causes new milk to form. Whether women continue to breastfeed after hospital discharge is influenced by such factors as employment, personal habits, and how important they view breastfeeding to be for themselves and their newborn (Gage, Williams, Von Rosen-Von Hoewel, et al., 2012; McCarter-Spaulding, Lucas, & Gore, 2011). While breastfeeding, women must be certain to drink adequate fluid daily, eat a nutritious diet, and check with their health care provider before ingesting medicine or alternative therapies such as herbs because most of these can be found in breast milk and their use may not be evidence based (Schaffir & Czapla, 2012). Breastfeeding techniques are discussed in Chapter 19.

Return of Menstrual Flow

With the delivery of the placenta, the production of placental estrogen and progesterone ends. The resulting decrease in hormone concentrations causes a rise in production of FSH by the pituitary, which leads, with only a slight delay, to the return of ovulation. This initiates the return of normal menstrual cycles.

A woman who is not breastfeeding can expect her menstrual flow to return in 6 to 10 weeks after birth. If she is breastfeeding, a menstrual flow may not return for 3 or 4 months (*lactational amenorrhea*) or, in some women, for the entire lactation period. However, the absence of a menstrual flow does not guarantee that a woman will not conceive during this time, because she may ovulate well before menstruation returns (Kramer & Kakuma, 2012).

NURSING CARE OF A WOMAN AND FAMILY DURING THE FIRST 24 HOURS AFTER BIRTH

A woman remains in a birthing room for at least the first hour after birth so she has time to become acquainted with her newborn and to provide for careful health care team observation. She then remains in the room as a postpartal patient or is transferred to a separate postpartal room. With this, the most dangerous hour in childbearing—the first hour after birth—has passed.

Hemorrhage is still a possibility for the first 2 or 3 days after birth, until the myometrial vessels have sclerosed. One of the worries for a woman giving birth at home is that she will not appreciate how dangerous a time this is. With attention focused more on the newborn than on her, postpartal hemorrhage could occur. In the hospital, various health care personnel may be involved in caring for a woman: be certain all members of your health care team are knowledgeable about this danger.

Assessment

Assessment of a postpartal woman includes history, physical examination, and analysis of laboratory findings.

Health History

The technical aspects of a woman's pregnancy, labor, and birth can be learned from her electronic record. Most of this information is best obtained from a woman herself, however, because this supplies not only information on the events of her pregnancy and labor but also her emotions and impressions about them.

Family Profile. Information for a family profile includes age, support persons, other children, type of housing and community setting, occupation, education and socioeconomic level, or that information necessary to evaluate the impact a new child will have on the woman and her family. This information also lays a foundation for teaching self-care and child care specific to the woman's knowledge level and needs.

Pregnancy History. Information for a pregnancy history includes para and gravida status (and the reason for any discrepancy), expected date of birth, whether the pregnancy was intended, and any problems or complications such as spotting or gestational hypertension that occurred during pregnancy. This information helps you gauge a woman's potential for bonding, because an unplanned pregnancy or complications arising during pregnancy can interfere greatly with bonding.

Labor and Birth History. It's important to gather information on the length of labor, position of the fetus, type of birth, any analgesia or anesthesia used, problems during labor such as fetal distress, supine hypotension syndrome, and the presence of perineal sutures because this information helps in planning necessary procedures. In addition, explore the mother's thoughts and feelings about labor and birth and whether this was a positive experience for her.

Infant Data. The sex and weight of the infant, any difficulty at birth such as the need for resuscitation, plans to breastfeed or formula feed, and any congenital anomalies present are the major facts to obtain, because, again, this information helps in planning care for the infant and promoting bonding with the parents.

Postpartal Course. To assess a woman's postpartal course and plan anticipatory guidance needed, ask about her general health; her activity level since the birth; a description of lochia; the presence of perineal, abdominal, or breast pain; difficulty with elimination; success with infant feeding; and response of her support person to parenting.

Laboratory Data

Women who had a cesarean birth, prenatal anemia, or an excessive blood loss will routinely have their hemoglobin and hematocrit levels measured 12 to 24 hours after birth, to determine whether blood loss at birth has left them anemic. If the hemoglobin finding is lower than 10.5 g/100 ml, supplemental iron is usually prescribed. It's important that postpartal anemia be detected because the responsibilities of being a new mother, coupled with the additional burden of an undetected low hemoglobin level, can severely tax a woman's energy levels and increase her risk for postpartum depression (East, 2012).

Physical Assessment

During early labor, a woman is given a fairly complete physical examination. During the immediate postpartal period, therefore, repetition of a complete examination is not usually necessary. However, crucial assessments examining particular aspects of health, such as an estimation of nutrition and fluid state, energy level, presence or absence of pain, breast health, fundal height and consistency, lochia amount and character, perineal integrity, and circulatory adequacy, are required.

General Appearance. A woman's general appearance in the postpartal period reveals a great deal about her energy level, her self-esteem, and whether she is moving into a taking-hold phase. Before beginning assessment, ask a woman to void so she has an empty bladder. Observe how much energy she uses when reaching for her robe or walking to the bathroom—does she struggle or move listlessly, or does she accomplish this task quickly? Observe for a cringing expression or hand pressure against her abdomen that suggests pain on movement. Observe whether she has combed her hair and put on her own clothing. Many women choose to sleep in an agency gown to prevent lochia stains on their own clothing, but a woman who is pleased with herself, her pregnancy, and her birth experience is usually anxious to wear her own clothing and "fuss" with her appearance within an hour after birth. In contrast, a woman who is extremely exhausted or depressed probably will not bother with her appearance this way. Keep in mind, however, a woman whose labor progressed so rapidly she came to a health care agency as an emergency admission may not have had time to pack a comb and brush or her own clothing. Cultural variations also affect appearance and actions.

Hair. Palpate the woman's hair to determine its firmness and strength; whenever a diet is full of nutrients, hair is firm and crisp, whereas if a woman's intake during pregnancy was deficient in nutrients, her hair feels listless and "stringy." Many women begin to lose a quantity of hair in the postpartal period because, during pregnancy, their increased metabolism caused hair to grow rapidly and many hairs to reach maturity at the same time. As the woman's body returns to a normal metabolism level following birth, this rapid-growth hair will be lost. You may need to reassure a woman that hair loss is not a sign of illness but just another aspect of return to her prepregnant state.

Face. Assess the woman's face for evidence of edema such as puffy eyelids or a prominent fold of tissue inferior to the lower eyelid. Normally, this should be negligible. However, in a woman who had gestational hypertension and thus accumulated excessive fluid, it will be evident. It also will become evident in a woman who is developing postpartal hypertension (although this condition is rare). Facial edema is most apparent early in the morning because the woman has been lying flat with her head level during the night.

Eyes. Inspect the color and texture of the inner conjunctiva. If a woman is dehydrated, the area appears dry. The conjunctiva of a woman who is anemic from poor pregnancy nutrition or excessive blood loss is pale. Be alert to possible variations because of skin color, however, as dark-skinned women may have a ruddy conjunctiva appearance even with anemia. Check the electronic record of any woman with paler than usual conjunctivae to determine whether anemia (revealed by a low hemoglobin level) is present.

Breasts. Breast tissue increases in size as breast milk forms. To assess breasts, ask a woman to remove her bra and cover her breasts with a towel or folded sheet to protect modesty. Ask her to raise her hands and tuck them under her head, because this stretches and thins breast tissue. Inspect and then palpate for breast size, shape, and color.

Breast tissue should feel soft on palpation on the first and second postpartal day. On the third day, it should begin to feel firm and warm (described as *filling*). On the third or fourth day, breasts appear large and reddened, with taut, shiny skin (engorgement) and, on palpation, feel hard and tense and painful. Because, normally, engorgement causes the entire breast to feel warm or appear reddened, if only one portion of a breast appears this way, inflammation or, possibly, infection of glands or milk ducts (mastitis) is suggested (Katz, 2012).

Occasionally, a firm nodule is detected on palpation. Usually, this is only a temporarily blocked milk duct preventing milk from flowing forward to the nipple. Note the location of the nodule and report its presence to the woman's primary care provider so that it can be thoroughly reassessed to ascertain whether a fibrocystic or malignant growth unrelated to the pregnancy is present.

Note also whether the breast nipples are normally erect and not inverted. Assess for any cracks, fissures, or the presence of caked milk. Avoid squeezing the nipples, because this can be painful. Unnecessary nipple manipulation also may increase the risk of mastitis by providing a portal for infection.

Uterus. For uterine assessment, position the woman supine so the height of the uterus is not influenced by an elevated position. Observe her abdomen for contour, to detect distention, and for the appearance of striae or a diastasis. If a diastasis is present (a slightly indented, possibly bluish-tinged groove in the midline of the abdomen), measure the width and length by fingerbreadths.

Palpate the fundus of the uterus by placing one hand on the base of the uterus, just above the symphysis pubis, and the other at the umbilicus. Press in and downward with the hand at the umbilicus until you "bump" against a firm globular mass in the abdomen: the uterine fundus (Fig. 17.5). Assess consistency (firm, soft, or boggy), location (midline), and height. For the first hour after birth, the height of the fundus is at the umbilicus or even slightly above it; it then decreases one fingerbreadth in size daily. Measure the distance under the umbilicus in fingerbreadths, such as "2 F↓" or 2 cm beneath the umbilicus. Although this measurement seems less scientific than a measurement of the height of the uterus from the pubis, it is a more certain measurement and demonstrates the gradual decline in size of the uterus.

Never palpate a uterus without supporting the lower segment, because the uterus potentially could invert (turn inside out) if not stabilized, resulting in a massive hemorrhage.

Palpation of a fundus should not cause pain as long as the action is done gently. If the uterus is not firm on palpation, massage it gently with the examining hand; this usually causes the fundus to contract and immediately become firm. Use a gentle rotating motion, never a hard or forceful touch, so that you do not cause pain or cause the uterus to expend excess energy in contracting. If the uterine fundus does not grow firm with massage, extreme atony, possibly retained placenta fragments, or an excess amount of blood loss may be occurring. Notify the woman's primary care provider. Administer oxytocin as prescribed. In addition, placing the woman's infant at her breast will cause endogenous release of oxytocin and achieve the same effect as oxytocin administration.

If massage appears ineffective, the cause of this may be a clot present in the cavity of the uterus. This may be expressed

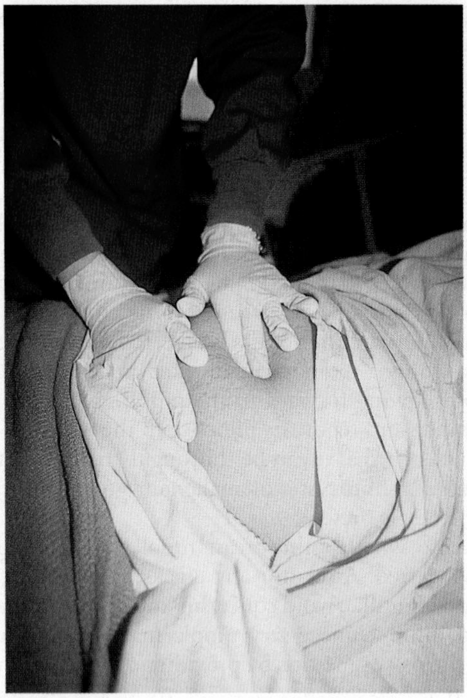

FIGURE 17.5 To palpate a uterus, be certain to place one hand at the base of the uterus. This fundus measures about two fingerbreadths below the umbilicus.

from the uterus by gentle pressure on the fundus, but only after the uterus has been massaged and is fairly firm. As mentioned earlier, if fundal pressure is applied with the uterus totally relaxed, fundal pressure could cause inversion of the uterus, an extremely serious complication that leads to rapid hemorrhage. Another reason the uterus may not be well contracted is that a rapidly filling bladder is preventing contraction. If contraction remains inadequate, a lower abdominal ultrasound may be prescribed to help detect an abnormality.

A woman who received no oxytocin after birth to help her uterus contract is at greater risk for poor uterine contraction than is a woman who did receive oxytocin and thus needs frequent uterine assessment (about every 10 to 15 minutes for the first hour).

Once this first hour has passed, height and consistency can be assessed less frequently, depending on institutional policy. By the 9th or 10th day after delivery, the uterus will have become so small that it is no longer palpable above the symphysis pubis.

✔ QSEN Checkpoint Question 17.4

Teamwork & Collaboration

You are performing massage of Leana's fundus 2 days postpartum. What assessment finding should prompt you to contact Leana's primary care provider immediately?

a. Leana's fundal height is two fingerbreadths below her umbilicus.
b. Leana's uterus does not become firm when massaged.
c. Firm massage of Leana's fundus results in pain.
d. The fundus is located midline on Leana's abdomen.

Look in Appendix A for best answer and rationale.

Lochia. A woman can expect to have lochia for 2 to 6 weeks. Characteristics of normal lochia and the change in pattern from red to pink to white were described in Table 17.1.

During the first hour after birth, when the fundus is checked every 15 minutes, also remove the mother's perineal pad and evaluate lochia character, amount, color (rubra, serosa, or alba), odor, and the presence of any clots. If the woman has perineal stitches, be certain the pad is not adhering to those before removing it.

Ask the woman to turn so you can inspect under her buttocks to be certain blood is not pooling beneath her. If you observe a constant trickle of vaginal flow or a woman is soaking through a pad every 60 minutes, she is losing more than the average amount of blood. She needs to be examined by her primary care provider to be certain there is no cervical or vaginal tear or that poor uterine contraction is not causing excessive bleeding.

While a woman is at the health care facility, inspect her lochia discharge once every 15 minutes for the first hour, and then according to the institution's policy (usually hourly for the next 4 hours, then every 8 hours after that). Make certain a woman understands that she should wash her hands after handling pads and must use only her own personal care equipment so that she does not contract or spread infection. Demonstrate good role modeling for hand washing and nonsharing of equipment. Encourage a woman to change perineal pads frequently as she begins self-care, because lochia is an excellent medium for bacterial growth that could spread through the vagina to the uterus. The presence of constantly wet pads against an episiotomy suture line also slows healing. Be certain she knows not to use tampons until after she returns for her postpartal checkup, to diminish the risk for infection and possibly toxic shock syndrome (see Chapter 47). Ensure women are familiar with the criteria for judging the amount and type of normal lochia (see Box 17.5), so they can do this accurately when they return home.

Perineum. While asking a woman to turn on her side to evaluate whether lochia is pooling, also inspect her perineum. If a woman has no episiotomy or a midline one, which side she turns to does not matter. If she has a mediolateral incision, ask her to turn so the incision is on the bottom buttock because this tends to cause less pain and offers better visibility. Gently lift the upper buttock and inspect for ecchymosis, a hematoma, erythema, edema, intactness, and presence of drainage or bleeding from any episiotomy stitches.

Episiotomies are rarely done today because they may increase the risk for extended perineal lacerations. If stitches are present, the suture line is 1 or 2 in. long. If a laceration extends beyond the episiotomy incision, stitches may extend from the vagina back to the rectum or go into the muscle and tissues surrounding the perineal area. The incision line is usually fused (edges sealed) by 24 hours after birth; if it is a midline incision, it may be almost invisible to see because the perineal fold obscures it. If there is clotted lochia along the incision line, review postpartal perineal care so that this does not continue to occur. Before discharge, teach a woman who has stitches how to lie on her back and view her perineum with a handheld mirror, so that, once a day while at home, she can inspect her perineum for redness, sloughing of sutures, pus formation, drainage at the suture line, or development of a hematoma. A hematoma is a collection of blood in the subcutaneous space from bleeding from the episiotomy incision that can become so extensive it causes intense pain and disrupts the suture line (see Chapter 25).

Following perineal assessment, assess the rectal area for the presence of hemorrhoids. If any are present, document their number, appearance, and size in centimeters. Because postpartum women are not on bed rest unless they have a serious complication, assess risk of skin breakdown as per facility protocol using an assessment scale such as the Braden Assessment Scale (Tescher, Branda, Byrne, et al., 2012).

What if... 17.2 Leana Cooper, at 18 hours postpartum, tells you she has had to change her perineal pads twice in the last 30 minutes because they were saturated. In addition, she noticed two large clots on her last pad. To guard her safety, what should be your first action?

Nursing Diagnoses and Related Interventions

Nursing Diagnosis: Risk for fluid volume deficit related to uterine atony

Outcome Evaluation: Client maintains vital signs within normal range; fundus is firm to palpation; lochia discharge is small to moderate with a minimum of clot formation.

In order to assess if uterine atony is present, frequently assess vital signs, lochia amount, and fundal height. Teach client the usual involution process and how to check her fundus and evaluate lochia so she can do this after she returns home.

Nursing Diagnosis: Pain related to perineal discomfort, uterine cramping (afterpains), or muscular aches

Outcome Evaluation: Client states that degree of pain is tolerable; client demonstrates knowledge of measures for adequate pain relief.

Women experience pain postpartally as a result of uterine contraction as well as from the aftereffects of pushing during labor.

Provide Pain Relief for Afterpains. Pain from uterine contractions is similar to pain from menstrual cramps and can be intense. It's usually helpful to assure a woman that this type of discomfort, although painful, is normal and rarely lasts longer than 3 days. If necessary, either ibuprofen (such as Motrin), which has anti-inflammatory and antiprostaglandin properties, or a common analgesic such as acetaminophen (such as Tylenol) is effective for pain relief. As with any abdominal pain, heat to the abdomen should be avoided, because it could cause relaxation of the uterus and subsequent uterine bleeding. Remind the woman that the total 24-hour dose for acetaminophen is 3,000 mg so she does not take an excessive amount after returning home (Karch, 2013).

Relieve Muscular Aches. Many women feel so sore and achy after labor and birth that they describe feeling as if they have "run for miles." A backrub is usually effective for relieving an aching back or shoulders, but some woman may appreciate a mild analgesic such as acetaminophen for the pain. Carefully assess a woman who states she has pain in the calf of her leg on standing because pain in the calf on standing (a position that dorsiflexes the foot) is Homans sign and could indicate that thrombophlebitis is present (see later discussion).

Administer Cold and Hot Therapy. Applying an ice or cold pack to the perineum during the first 24 hours reduces perineal edema and the possibility of hematoma formation, and also reduces pain and promotes healing and comfort. Be certain not to place ice or plastic directly on the woman's perineum. Use a commercial cold pack, or wrap an ice bag first in a towel or disposable pad, to decrease the chance of a thermal burn (risk of injury increases because the perineum has decreased sensation from edema after birth).

Ice to the perineum after the first 24 hours is no longer therapeutic because, after this time, healing increases best if circulation to the area is encouraged by the use of heat. Dry heat in the form of a perineal hot pack or moist heat with a sitz bath are both effective ways to increase circulation to the perineum, provide comfort, reduce edema, and promote healing.

Commercial hot packs grow warm after they are "cracked" and the chemicals in them combine. Caution women to use a washcloth or gauze square between the pack and their skin, to prevent a possible burn.

Promote Perineal Exercises. Some women find that carrying out perineal exercises three or four times a day can greatly relieve perineal edema. The most effective exercise consists of contracting and relaxing the muscles of the perineum 5 to 10 times in succession, as if trying to stop voiding (Kegel exercises). This aids comfort by improving circulation to the area and decreasing edema. When repeated frequently, Kegel exercises can also help a woman regain her prepregnant muscle tone and help prevent urinary incontinence (Boyle, Hay-Smith, Cody, et al., 2012).

Give Suture Line Care for Women With an Episiotomy. Although relatively small in size, episiotomy sutures can cause considerable discomfort, because the perineum is an extremely sensitive area and the muscles of the perineum are involved in so many activities such as sitting, walking, stooping, squatting, bending, urinating, and defecating.

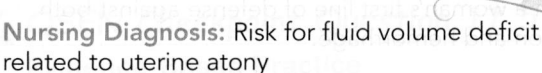

Because the perineal area heals rapidly, you can assure a woman that discomfort is normal and does not usually last longer than 5 or 6 days. Most primary care providers prescribe a soothing anesthetic cream or spray to be applied to the suture line to reduce discomfort. A cortisone-based cream or warm sitz bath helps to decrease inflammation and relieve tension in the area. Because of their cooling effect, witch hazel–impregnated pads

care provider for an examination at 2 to 4 weeks of age. If a woman does not have an adequate rubella antibody titer and anticipates further pregnancies, she should be asked if she wants a rubella immunization before discharge. Women who are Rh negative and who have had an Rh-positive infant will receive RhIG or Rh antibodies to prevent isoimmunization concerns in a future pregnancy (Kline, 2012).

Be certain that home care instructions for the family are given both verbally and in writing. Getting ready to go home, dressing the baby, seeing him or her in new clothes for the first time, and experiencing the thrill of realizing the baby is really theirs to take home is so exciting that it is easy for oral instructions to go unheard.

Many health care agencies have a community liaison person, ideally a nurse, who calls or makes a home visit to women after discharge. This person helps the new mother assess her own health and that of her baby and answers questions from families who lose their instructions or are unable to interpret them after they have returned home.

Making a telephone call to or visiting a family 24 hours after discharge is another way to evaluate whether the family is able to continue self-evaluation and infant care and is able to integrate the new infant into the family. Such calls or visits also have the potential to reduce the number of acute care visits and rehospitalizations for newborns.

Postpartal Examination

Every woman should have a checkup by her primary care provider at 4 to 6 weeks after birth (the end of the postpartal period) to assure herself and her health care provider that she is in good health and has no residual problems from her pregnancy.

During this examination, the woman's abdominal wall is inspected for tone and to determine that her uterus involution is so complete that the uterus is no longer palpable abdominally. Her breasts are inspected to see whether they have returned to their nonpregnant state if she is not breastfeeding or whether they are unfissured and free of complications if she is breastfeeding. Most important, a thorough internal examination is performed to be certain involution is complete, the ligaments and the pelvic muscle supports have returned to functional alignment, and any lacerations sustained during birth have healed (Table 17.4).

If a woman has hemorrhoids or varicosities as a result of the pregnancy, her primary care provider will discuss with her whether further management of these conditions is necessary. Always ask about the possibility of intimate partner violence, because this can increase during the postpartal period because of the added stress of adding a new family member (Malta, McDonald, Hegadoren, et al., 2012). Review the necessity of having a breast examination, Papanicolaou (Pap) smear, and pelvic examination every year as a means of screening for breast, cervical, and uterine cancer. If a woman is older than 40 years, include a discussion about the need for mammogram examinations. Encourage women who have stopped smoking during pregnancy to continue to be smoke free as yet another good health measure for both themselves and their new child.

If reproductive life planning was not discussed immediately after birth, this visit is the opportune time for such a discussion. If a woman desires to use a diaphragm or a cervical cap, these can be fitted during this examination. Injectable progesterone (depot medroxyprogesterone acetate) also can be begun at this time. Women who are breastfeeding can begin on progesterone-only birth control pills (Costa, Cecatti, Krupa, et al., 2012).

✔ QSEN Checkpoint Question 17.6

Informatics

You care for Leana Cooper at a 6-week postpartum visit. You read in her electronic health record that her fundal height has been progressing in a healthy and predicted manner. What should her fundal height be during this current visit?

a. At least six fingerbreadths below the umbilicus
b. No longer palpable over the symphysis pubis
c. Four centimeters below the top of the iliac crest
d. Still palpable above her pubic hair line

Look in Appendix A for best answer and rationale.

NURSING CARE OF A POSTPARTAL WOMAN AND FAMILY WITH UNIQUE NEEDS

A Woman Who Chooses Not to Keep Her Child

Although the availability of birth control information and the availability of post-coital pregnancy protection have reduced the number of unwanted or unintended pregnancies, some women still may complete a pregnancy and then give up their child for adoption immediately after birth. There are numerous reasons for a decision such as this: a woman may be unmarried, or her marriage may be failing and she does not want to raise a child alone. She may feel that her family is already complete. She may want to finish school before having a child, or she may want to pursue a career.

During pregnancy, most women decide whether they will keep their child. During labor, they express confidence in their decision, but with the actual birth of their child, they may find their resolve wavers. A woman who was certain she was going to surrender her child for adoption may realize she wants to keep the child. A woman who was certain she was going to keep her child could become aware for the first time of the responsibility involved and decide that the best course for the child is adoption. In either event, a woman's feelings can become confused.

For a woman who chooses not to keep her child, the wait in the birthing room for preparations to transfer the baby to a nursery may seem unusually long. She may also be alone, with no partner or support person with her during this time. Every woman has a right to see, hold, and feed her child if she wishes. A woman who is not going to keep her child may feel proud that she has produced a healthy baby. The realization that the baby is well can provide a foundation on which to build a sounder future so she does not have to make this choice again.

Do not attempt to change a woman's mind about keeping her child or placing the child for adoption during the postpartal period because she is extremely vulnerable to suggestion at this time, and such decisions are too long range and

TABLE 17.4 Six-Week Physical Assessment

Area of Assessment	Data Collection
History	Assess chief concern, family profile (support system, bonding, self-esteem, family integrity), interval history, and review of systems (urinary system for pain, frequency, or stress incontinence along with gastrointestinal tract and reproductive tract in particular). Assess maternal intake because some new mothers are too fatigued to eat well.
Physical Examination	Expected Findings
General appearance	Alert; positive mood. If not, woman is probably still extremely fatigued.
Weight	Achievement of prepregnant weight; if not, this will be her baseline postpregnant weight.
Hair	Healthy, firm hair; excess loss of hair from early postpartal period has halted.
Eyes	Pink and moist conjunctiva; if pallor persists, diet may be inadequate in iron.
Breasts	
Breastfeeding woman	Full and firm to palpation; blue veins prominent under skin. No palpable nodules or lumps. If erythematous or extremely tender, mastitis or nipple fissure may be present. An occasional filled milk gland may present as a lump; re-examine after breastfeeding.
Nonbreastfeeding woman	Return to prepregnant size; no palpable nodules or lumps.
Abdomen	Striae less prominent; linea nigra fading, muscle tone improving. No distended bowel from constipation. No distended bladder from retention. No history of pain, frequency, or blood on urination. Urinary symptoms probably reflect urinary infection that needs specific treatment.
Perineum and uterus	Lochia no longer present; cervix closed; uterus has returned to prepregnant size. Pap test is normal. Ask woman to bear down during pelvic examination to observe for uterine prolapse, rectocele, or cystocele. If involution is not complete, reason for subinvolution must be investigated.
Lower extremities	Varicosities barely noticeable.
Rectum	Hemorrhoids receded to prepregnant size or are no longer observable.
Mental	Positive interaction with infant, appropriate personal hygiene (clean hair, etc.). No indication of postpartal depression or psychosis is present.
Laboratory Reports	
Laboratory values	Hct: 37%; Hgb: 11–12 g/100 ml. If these are low, reassess diet; possibly iron supplement may be needed. Rubella antibody titer: 1:8; if low, additional immunization is recommended before a second pregnancy.
Immunization status	Assess need for human papillomavirus (HPV) [Gardasil] or rubella vaccine.

Hct, hematocrit; Hgb, hemoglobin.

too important to be made at such an emotional time. Her earlier conclusion may be the sound one. Instead, offer nonjudgmental support. Be especially aware of your own feelings about this issue, to avoid influencing a woman's decision making unnecessarily.

During the taking-in phase of the puerperium, be especially careful that you do not "lead" the woman's thinking. Women enjoy having decisions made for them during this time and may ask what you think is best. An answer such as, "You're the one who has to make this decision. What are your thoughts about it?" can help her begin to think through the problem.

It is not uncommon for women who surrender their infants for adoption to experience grief reactions, the same as those of women whose children have died. If a woman decides to surrender her child for adoption, refer her to an official adoption agency, if she has not contacted one already, because an official agency gives a woman the best assurance the parents chosen for her child will be appropriate. This assurance can help relieve any misgivings or guilt she may feel in future years about surrendering the child, such as wondering whether the child is well cared for and is getting everything the mother could have given her.

Some women do not openly voice a wish to give up their child, but their actions demonstrate they feel little attachment to their newborn. A woman who wants to keep her baby has a tentative but eager approach to her newborn, whereas a woman who has doubts is slow to make contact, barely touching the baby even by the time of discharge, and asking few questions about newborn care. When this happens, the hospital social service department can be of assistance in helping the woman plan the child's future.

It is a fallacy to assume that everything will work out once the woman and infant arrive home. The number of children who experience intrafamily maltreatment seen in hospital emergency departments is proof of the harm that can follow when assessment to detect poor parent–child bonding is inadequate in the first few days of life (Louwers, Korfage, Affourtit, et al., 2012).

A Woman Who Is Discharged but Whose Child Remains Hospitalized

Newborns who are ill at birth often are transported to a regional center or to a neonatal intensive care nursery for care, a move that automatically separates them from their parents. Encourage parents to take photographs of the baby on their phone or using a camera before transport and to be certain they have the nursery telephone number and the name of a nurse to contact for questions or information. Most transport teams call the parents after they arrive at the distant hospital to assure them their infant managed the stress of transport well.

Maintaining communication with the nursery is important so parents can begin to bond with their child despite the imposed separation. Urge them to call the nursery at least once daily to ask about their infant. If the infant is hospitalized in the same hospital, help transport the mother to the nursery, so that she can see and, ideally, hold her child daily. Without this assistance, some women will be so overwhelmed by the technology in the nursery, they are reluctant to call or visit. Assure a mother her telephone calls and visits are expected and valued. Visiting in an intensive care nursery is further discussed in Chapter 26.

It is easy for a woman who is separated from her newborn to feel despondent. Be certain to evaluate whether a woman seems depressed or needs additional support to overcome this unexpected outcome to her pregnancy.

A Family Who Is Adopting a Child

A family who is adopting an infant may come into the hospital or birthing center to meet their new infant for the first time. Such a couple needs the same introduction to newborn care as biologic parents. Additional needs of adopting parents are discussed in Chapter 2.

What if...17.4 You are interested in exploring one of the 2020 National Health Goals related to postpartal care (see Box 17.1). Most government-sponsored money for nursing research is allotted based on these goals. What would be a possible research topic to explore pertinent to these goals that would be applicable to the Cooper family and also advance evidence-based practice?

KEY POINTS FOR REVIEW

- The postpartal period (puerperium) is the 6-week period after childbirth. Women move through an initial "taking-in" phase, in which they are dependent; a "taking-hold" phase, in which they manifest independence; and a "letting-go" phase, in which the mother role is finally defined.
- Rooming-in is the preferred health care agency arrangement for postpartal families, because it allows a new family the best chance for quality interaction. The more time new parents spend with a newborn, the more likely it is that effective bonding will occur. Help parents to feel comfortable with their newborn by offering anticipatory guidance and role modeling infant care, as this not only helps in planning nursing care that meets QSEN competencies but also best meets the family's total needs.
- "Postpartal blues" are a normal accompaniment to childbirth. You can assure a woman that such feelings are normal and offer supportive care until the emotion passes.
- Uterine involution is the process whereby the uterus returns to its prepregnant state. A uterus decreases in size one fingerbreadth (1 cm) a day until it disappears under the pubic bone at about day 10. Lochia is the name of the vaginal flow after childbirth: the flow is lochia rubra (red) for the first 1 to 3 days, lochia serosa (pink to brown) on days 4 through 10, and lochia alba (white) until 2 to 6 weeks after the birth.
- A woman is at great risk for hemorrhage in the postpartal period, so assessments done to reveal this are some of the most critical assessments made in nursing. Do not discount the importance of these assessments because the overall content of the postpartal period is so focused on wellness.
- Lactation is the production of breast milk. Colostrum is present immediately after birth; milk forms on the third to fourth postpartal day. A feeling of fullness and firmness on this day is termed *filling*; if warmth and discomfort occur, it is termed *engorgement.*
- Women may need various comfort measures to alleviate pain from uterine pain (afterpains) and breast tenderness. Application of cold or heat and administration of analgesics are important nursing interventions.
- Women need to learn about self-care before health care agency discharge, so they can maintain self-care at home. A follow-up telephone call or home visit can be helpful to answer questions. All women should conscientiously return for a health assessment visit at 6 weeks after childbirth to be certain their reproductive organs have returned to their nonpregnant state. Menstrual flow should return within 6 to 10 weeks in the nonbreastfeeding mother or after 3 to 4 months in the breastfeeding mother.

CRITICAL THINKING CARE STUDY

Katie is a 30-year-old primigravida. She is being discharged with her healthy daughter Sarah this evening. Katie delivered vaginally 50 hours ago without complications and is breastfeeding without difficulty. You chart evidence of positive bonding behaviors. Her postdelivery hemoglobin is 9.5 mg/dl. She has a history of depression during high school. Her mother is planning to help for the next few weeks until Katie and Sarah get settled at home.

1. While preparing for Katie's discharge, you would anticipate teaching about which factors that are most concerning to you?
2. Katie's mother is a support person for her, so how can you include her family in the education?
3. What parenting behaviors would indicate positive bonding between Katie and Sarah?

Patient Scenario

The Chang Family

Read about the Chang family, a postpartal family with a newborn, then answer the questions to further sharpen your skills and grow more familiar with NCLEX-type questions related to nursing care of a postpartal family. Confirm your answers are correct by reading the rationales.

Visit http://thePoint.lww.com

Answers and Rationales

Looking for answers to the What if . . . and Critical Thinking Care Study questions?

Visit http://thePoint.lww.com

References

Avsar, A. F., & Keskin, H. L. (2010). Haemorrhoids during pregnancy. *Journal of Obstetrics & Gynaecology, 30*(3), 231–237.

Baselice, J. (2011). Postpartal care and breast-feeding. In K. J. Hurt, M. W. Guile, J. L. Bienstock, et al. (Eds.), *The Johns Hopkins manual of gynecology and obstetrics* (4th ed., pp. 257–264). Philadelphia: Lippincott, Williams & Wilkins.

Boyle, R., Hay-Smith, E. J., Cody, J. D., et al. (2012). Pelvic floor muscle training for prevention and treatment of urinary and faecal incontinence in antenatal and postnatal women. *Cochrane Database of Systematic Reviews,*(10), CD007471.

Bridges, W. (1994). *Job shift: How to prosper in a workplace without jobs.* Menlo Park, CA: Addison-Wesley.

Cahill, J. M., Freeland-Graves, J. H., Shah, B. S., et al. (2012). Determinants of weight loss after an intervention in low-income women in early postpartum. *Journal of the American College of Nutrition, 31*(2), 133–143.

Chhabra, S., Tyagi, S., Bhavani, M., et al. (2012). Late postpartum eclampsia. *Journal of Obstetrics & Gynaecology, 32*(3), 264–266.

Chi, C., Bapir, M., Lee, C. A., et al. (2010). Puerperal loss (lochia) in women with or without inherited bleeding disorders. *American Journal of Obstetrics & Gynecology, 203*(1), 56.e1–56.e2

Costa, M. L., Cecatti, J. G., Krupa, F. G., et al. (2012). Progestin-only contraception prevents bone loss in postpartum breastfeeding women. *Contraception, 85*(4), 374–380.

Dale-Hewitt, V., Slade, P., Wright, I., et al. (2012). Patterns of attention and experiences of post-traumatic stress symptoms following childbirth: An experimental study. *Archives of Women's Mental Health, 15*(4), 289–296.

East, M. (2012). Postpartum anaemia. Are we vigilant enough? *Practicing Midwife, 15*(6), 37–39.

Edmonds, D. K. (2012). Puerperium and lactation. In D. K. Edmonds (Ed.), *Dewhurst's textbook of obstetrics & gynaecology* (8th ed., pp. 365–376). Oxford, UK: John Wiley & Sons.

Elliott-Carter, N., & Harper, J. (2012). Keeping mothers and newborns together after cesarean: How one hospital made the change. *Nursing for Women's Health, 16*(4), 290–295.

Farr, S. L., Dietz, P. M., Williams, J. R., et al. (2011). Depression screening and treatment among nonpregnant women of reproductive age in the United States, 1990-2010. *Preventing Chronic Disease, 8*(6), A122.

Gage, H., Williams, P., Von Rosen-Von Hoewel, J., et al. (2012). Influences on infant feeding decisions of first-time mothers in five European countries. *European Journal of Clinical Nutrition, 66*(8), 914–919.

Granek, L., & Fergus, K. (2012). Resistance, agency, and liminality in women's accounts of symptom appraisal and help-seeking upon discovery of a breast irregularity. *Social Science & Medicine, 75*(10), 1753–1761.

Gross, S. M., Resnik, A. K., Nanda, J. P., et al. (2011). Early postpartum: A critical period in setting the path for breastfeeding success. *Breastfeeding Medicine, 6*(6), 407–412.

Heron, J., Gilbert, N., Dolman, C., et al. (2012). Information and support needs during recovery from postpartum psychosis. *Archives of Women's Mental Health, 15*(3), 155–165.

Hickey, F., Finch, J. G., & Khanna, A. (2011). A systematic review on the outcomes of correction of diastasis of the recti. *Hernia, 15*(6), 607–614.

Johnson, A., Thakar, R., & Sultan, A. H. (2012). Obstetric perineal wound infection: Is there underreporting? *British Journal of Nursing, 21*(5), S28–S32.

Karch, A. M. (2013). *2013 Lippincott's nursing drug guide.* Philadelphia, PA: Lippincott Williams & Wilkins.

Katz, V. L. (2012). Postpartum care. In S. G. Gabbe, J. R. Niebyl, J. L. Simpson, et al. (Eds.), *Obstetrics: Normal and problem pregnancies* (6th ed., pp. 517–532). Philadelphia, PA: Elsevier/Saunders.

Kline, N. E. (2012). Alterations of hematologic function in children. In S. E. Huether & K. L. McCance (Eds.), *Understanding pathophysiology* (5th ed., pp. 535–551). New York, NY: Elsevier Publishing.

Kramer, M. S., & Kakuma, R. (2012). Optimal duration of exclusive breastfeeding. *Cochrane Database of Systematic Reviews,* (8), CD003517.

Kurth, E., Kennedy, H. P., Spichiger, E., et al. (2011). Crying babies, tired mothers: What do we know? A systematic review. *Midwifery, 27*(2), 187–194.

Lipsky, L. M., Strawderman, M. S., & Olson, C. M. (2012). Maternal weight change between 1 and 2 years postpartum: The importance of 1 year weight retention. *Obesity, 20*(7), 1496–1502.

Louwers, E. C., Korfage, I. J., Affourtit, M. J., et al. (2012). Effects of systematic screening and detection of child abuse in emergency departments. *Pediatrics, 130*(3), 457–464.

Malta, L. A., McDonald, S. W., Hegadoren, K. M., et al. (2012). Influence of interpersonal violence on maternal anxiety, depression, stress and parenting morale in the early postpartum: A community based pregnancy cohort study. *BMC Pregnancy & Childbirth, 12*(1), 153–154.

McCarter-Spaulding, D., Lucas, J., & Gore, R. (2011). Employment and breastfeeding outcomes in a sample of black women in the United States. *Journal of the National Black Nurses Association, 22*(2), 38–45.

Meadows-Oliver, M. (2012). Screening for postpartum depression at pediatric visits. *Journal of Psychosocial Nursing & Mental Health Services, 50*(9), 4–5.

Milman, N. (2012). Postpartum anemia: Prevention and treatment. *Annals of Hematology, 91*(2), 143–154.

Mulder, F. E., Schoffelmeer, M. A., Hakvoort, R. A., et al. (2012). Risk factors for postpartum urinary retention: A systematic review and meta-analysis. *BJOG: International Journal of Obstetrics & Gynaecology, 119*(12), 1440–1446.

Newton, E. R. (2012). Lactation & breastfeeding. In S. G. Gabbe, J. R. Niebyl, J. L. Simpson, et al. (Eds.), *Obstetrics: Normal and problem pregnancies* (6th ed., pp. 533–564). Philadelphia, PA: Elsevier/Saunders.

Rubin, R. (1977). Binding-in in the postpartum period. *Maternal Child Nursing Journal, 6*(2), 67–69.

Samanta, A., Roy, S. G., Mistri, P. K., et al. (2013). Efficacy of intra-umbilical oxytocin in the management of retained placenta: A randomized controlled trial. *Journal of Obstetrics & Gynaecology Research, 39*(1), 75–82.

Schaffir, J., & Czapla, C. (2012). Survey of lactation instructors on folk traditions in breastfeeding. *Breastfeeding Medicine, 7*(8), 230–233.

Smith, P. B., Moorem, K., & Peters, L. (2012). Implementing baby-friendly practices: Strategies for success. *MCN: American Journal of Maternal Child Nursing, 37*(4), 228–233.

Souza, J. P., Gülmezoglu, A. M., Vogel, J., et al. (2013). Moving beyond essential interventions for reduction of maternal mortality: A cross-sectional study. *Lancet, 381*(9879), 1747–1755.

Stuebe, A. M. (2012). Postpartum care. In V. Berghella (Ed.), *Obstetric evidence-based guidelines* (2nd ed., pp. 242–249). New York, NY: Informa Healthcare.

Tescher, A. N., Branda, M. E., Byrne, T. J., et al. (2012). All at-risk patients are not created equal: Analysis of Braden pressure ulcer risk scores to identify specific risks. *Journal of Wound, Ostomy & Continence Nursing, 39*(3), 282–291.

U.S. Department of Health and Human Services. (2010). *Healthy people 2020.* Washington, DC: Author.

Whitney, E., & Rolfes, S. R. (2012). Life cycle nutrition: Pregnancy & lactation. In E. Whitney & S. R. Rolfes (Eds.), *Understanding nutrition* (pp. 508–545). Belmont, CA: Wadsworth Publishing.

Chapter 18

Nursing Care of a Family With a Newborn

KEY TERMS

- acrocyanosis
- acute bilirubin encephalopathy
- caput succedaneum
- cavernous hemangioma
- central cyanosis
- cephalohematoma
- conduction
- convection
- erythema toxicum
- evaporation
- hemangioma
- jaundice
- lanugo
- meconium
- milia
- mongolian spot
- natal teeth
- neonatal period
- neonate
- nevus flammeus
- physiologic jaundice
- pseudomenstruation
- radiation
- strawberry hemangioma
- subconjunctival hemorrhage
- thrush
- transitional stool
- vernix caseosa

OBJECTIVES

After mastering the contents of this chapter, you should be able to:

1. Describe the normal characteristics of a term newborn.
2. Identify 2020 National Health Goals related to newborn care that nurses could help the nation achieve.
3. Assess a newborn for normal growth and development.
4. Formulate nursing diagnoses related to a newborn or the family of a newborn.
5. Identify expected outcomes for a newborn and family during the first 4 weeks of life to help them manage seamless transitions across differing health care settings.
6. Using the nursing process, plan nursing care that includes the six competencies of Quality & Safety Education for Nurses (QSEN): Patient-Centered Care, Teamwork & Collaboration, Evidence-Based Practice (EBP), Quality Improvement (QI), Safety, and Informatics.
7. Implement nursing care for a normal newborn, such as instructing parents on care of their newborn.
8. Evaluate outcome criteria for the achievement and effectiveness of care.
9. Integrate knowledge of newborn growth and development with the interplay of nursing process, the six competencies of QSEN, and Family Nursing to promote quality maternal and child health nursing care.

Carlotta Ruiz, a 29-year-old woman, has just given birth to her second child, a 39 weeks and 2 days, 6-lb, 5-oz baby girl named Beth. Apgar scores at 1 and 5 minutes were 6 and 8, respectively. Vital signs are temperature (axillary), 98.2°F (36.8°C); heart rate, 136 beats/min; respirations, 74 breaths/min. Beth is 18.5 in. long, with a head circumference of 34 cm and a chest circumference of 32 cm. She has a small port-wine birthmark on her right thigh.

While Jose, Carlotta's husband, is in the room, Carlotta tells you she is a "veteran" at baby care. Jose adds, "Little Joe [their 3-year-old] will be so excited to see his new sister. That's all he's been talking about."

When Carlotta is alone, you notice she seems apprehensive about caring for her new daughter. She tells you, "She's so much smaller than Joe was. And why does it sound like she has a cold? Or have this rash all over her? Isn't it bad enough she has a birthmark?"

Previous chapters described the care of a pregnant woman and family during the

(Continued on next page)

(Continued from previous page)

antepartal, intrapartal, and postpartal periods. This chapter adds information about caring for the family with a newborn. The newborn period is a critical one for a family because it lays the foundation for the rest of the family's childrearing years.

Does Carlotta know as much about newborns as she thought? What additional teaching does this family need?

Newborns undergo profound physiologic changes at the moment of birth (and, probably, psychological changes as well) as they are released from a warm, snug, dark, liquid-filled environment that has met all of their basic needs into a chilly, unbounded, brightly lit, gravity-based, outside world. Within minutes after being plunged into this strange environment, a newborn has to initiate respirations and adapt a circulatory system to extrauterine oxygenation. Within 24 hours, neurologic, renal, endocrine, gastrointestinal, and metabolic functions must be operating competently for life to be sustained.

How well a newborn makes these major adjustments depends on his or her genetic composition, the competency of the recent intrauterine environment, the care received during labor and birth, and the care received during the newborn or **neonatal period** (the time from birth through the first 28 days of life) (Walsh & Goser, 2013). One half of all deaths that occur during the first year of life occur in the neonatal period. More than half occur in the first 24 hours after birth—an indication of how hazardous a time this is for an infant (World Health Organization [WHO], 2012).

Newborn health is so important to families that 2020 National Health Goals related to newborn health have been devised (Box 18.1). Nurses play a major role in achieving these goals because nurses are the heath care providers who give care to newborns and newborn instructions to new parents.

BOX 18.1 Nursing Care Planning Based on 2020 National Health Goals

A number of 2020 National Health Goals speak directly to the newborn period:

- Increase the proportion of mothers who breastfeed their babies in the early postpartal period from a baseline of 74% to 81.9%.
- Increase the proportion of mothers who continue exclusive breastfeeding until their babies are 3 months old from a baseline of 33.6% to 46.2%.
- Increase the percentage of healthy full-term infants who are put to sleep on their backs from a baseline of 69% to 75.9%.
- Reduce the proportion of young children aged 3 to 5 years with dental caries in their primary teeth (which could originate from nighttime bottle feeding) from a baseline of 33.3% to 30%.
- Reduce the perinatal mortality rate to no more than 5.9 per 1,000 live births from a baseline of 6.6 per 1,000 live births (U.S. Department of Health and Human Services [DHHS], 2010; see www.healthypeople.gov).

Nurses can help the nation achieve these goals by encouraging women to not only begin breastfeeding but to also continue breastfeeding through the first 6 months of life, by advising parents of the advantage of placing infants on their backs to sleep, and advising parents of the danger of tooth decay from allowing a baby to drink from a bottle of milk or juice while falling asleep. By discussing early signs and symptoms of illness in a newborn, parents can learn to better evaluate their newborn's health and ask for their primary care provider's opinion before their infant becomes seriously ill.

Nursing Process Overview

For Health Promotion of the Term Newborn

Assessment

The assessment of a newborn or **neonate** (a baby in the neonatal period) includes a review of the mother's pregnancy history, a physical examination of the infant, an analysis of laboratory reports such as hematocrit and blood type, and an assessment of parent–child interactions to be certain bonding is beginning. This assessment begins immediately after birth and is continued at every contact during a newborn's birthing center stay, at early home visits, and at well-baby visits. Teaching new mothers and their partners to make assessments concerning their infant's temperature, respiratory rate, and overall health is crucial so they can continue to monitor their infant's health at home.

Nursing Diagnosis

Nursing diagnoses associated with newborns center on the difficulty of establishing respirations, beginning nutrition, and assisting with parent–newborn bonding. Examples include:

- Ineffective airway clearance related to mucus in the airway
- Ineffective thermoregulation related to heat loss from exposure in the birthing room
- Imbalanced nutrition, less than body requirements, related to poor sucking reflex
- Readiness for enhanced family coping related to birth of planned infant
- Health-seeking behaviors related to newborn needs

If a minor deviation from the normal is present, such as a birthmark, a diagnosis such as "Parental fear related to hemangioma on left thigh of newborn" might be relevant.

Outcome Identification and Planning

Nursing care planning should take into account both the newborn's needs during this transition period, a mother's need for adequate rest during the postpartal period, and the necessity for parents to become acquainted with their new child. Try to adapt teaching time to the schedules of the mother, her partner, and the newborn. Although the woman must learn as much as possible about newborn care, she also must go home from the health care setting with enough energy to practice what she has learned. Important planning measures for newborns include helping them regulate their temperature and helping them grow accustomed to feeding. Helpful Internet sites to recommend to women or their partner include BabyCenter (www.BabyCenter.com) and the Mayo Clinic site (www.MayoClinic.com). For questions about car seats, parents can consult the Centers for Disease Control and Prevention (CDC) (www.cdc.gov/MotorVehicleSafety/Child_Passenger_Safety/CPS-Factsheet.html). To check if an infant product has been recalled, parents can consult the Web site of the U.S. Consumer Product Safety Commission (www.CPSC.gov).

Implementation

A major portion of implementation in the newborn period is role modeling to help new parents grow confident with their newborn. Be aware how closely parents observe you for guidance in newborn care. Conserving newborn warmth and energy, to help prevent hypoglycemia and respiratory distress, should be an important consideration to accompany all interventions.

Outcome Evaluation

An evaluation of expected outcomes should reveal that a baby's primary caregiver is able to give beginning newborn care with confidence. Be certain a woman and her partner make arrangements for continued health supervision for their newborn, so the evaluation can be continued and the family's long-term health needs can be met. Examples indicating achievement of outcomes concerning newborns include:

- Infant establishes respirations of 30 to 60 breaths/min.
- Infant maintains temperature at 97.8° to 98.6°F (36.5° to 37°C).
- Mother demonstrates competence in caring for newborn.
- Infant breastfeeds well with a strong sucking reflex.

THE PROFILE OF A NEWBORN

It is not unusual to hear the comment "all newborns look alike" from people viewing a nursery full of babies. In actuality, every child is born with individual physical and personality characteristics that make him or her unique right from the start (Fig. 18.1).

Some newborns are born stocky and short, some are large and bony, and some are thin and rangy. Some have a temperament that causes them to feed greedily, protest procedures loudly, and respond to their parent's inexperienced handling with restlessness and spitting up. Other newborns sleep soundly, make no protest over procedures or diaper changes, and seem passive in accepting this new step in life. With experience in working with newborns, it becomes easier to differentiate newborns who are merely demonstrating these extremes of normal behavior from those whose behavior or appearance indicates a need for more skilled care as their adjustment to independent life is not progressing smoothly (Box 18.2).

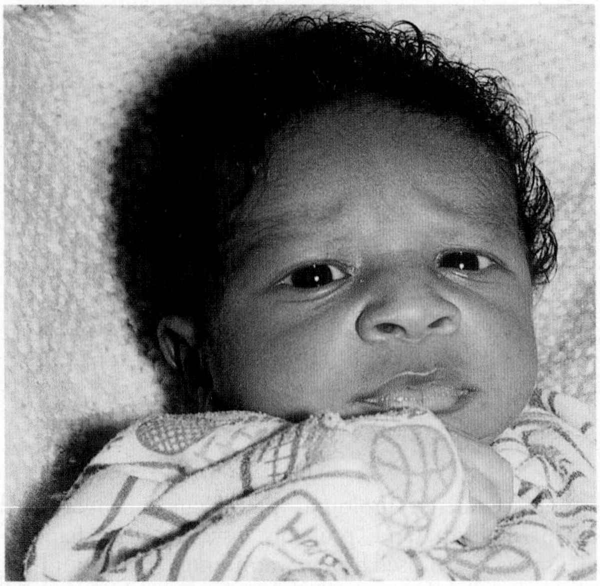

FIGURE 18.1 Personality is apparent in a newborn from the start. Note the alert, searching interest.

Vital Statistics

Vital statistics measured for a newborn usually consist of the baby's weight, length, and head and chest circumferences. The technique for obtaining these is shown in Chapter 34, along with other aspects of health assessment. Be certain all health care providers who care for newborns are aware of safety issues specific to newborn care when taking these measurements, such as not leaving a newborn unattended on a bed or scale and protecting against hypothermia.

BOX 18.2 Nursing Care Planning Using Assessment

Assessing the Average Newborn

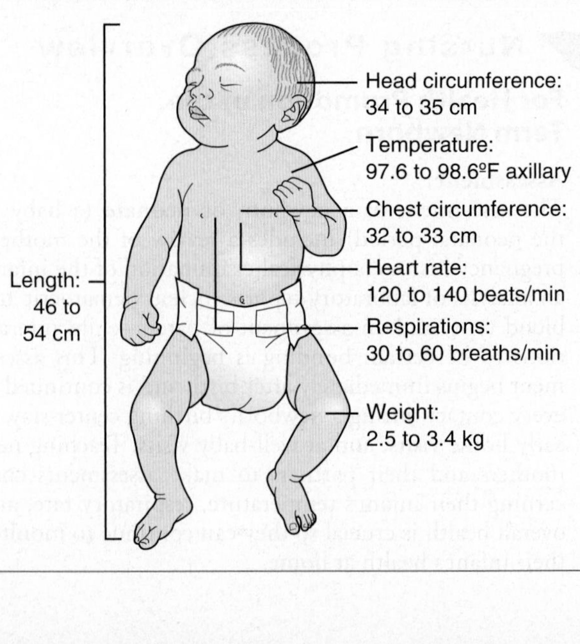

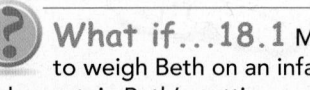

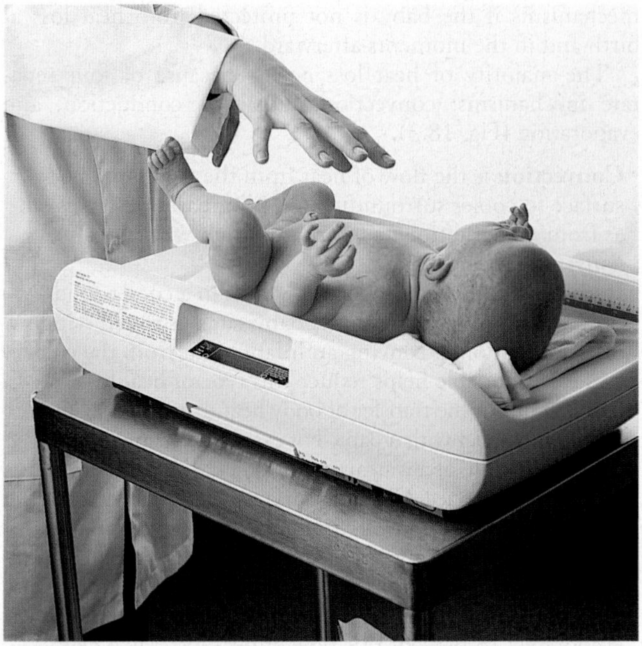

FIGURE 18.2 Weighing a newborn. Notice the protective hand held over the infant.

Weight

As long as newborns are breathing well, they are weighed nude and without a blanket soon after birth in the birthing room (Fig. 18.2). Measurements such as body length and head, chest, and abdominal circumferences are also done but can be obtained later because performing these measurements while an infant is still damp exposes the newborn unnecessarily to chilling.

A newborn's weight is important because it helps to determine maturity as well as establish a baseline against which all other weights can be compared. Following this initial weight, an infant is weighed nude once a day, at approximately the same time every day, during a hospital or birthing center stay.

The birth weight of newborns varies depending on the racial, nutritional, intrauterine, and genetic factors that were present during conception and pregnancy. The weight in relation to the gestational age should be plotted on a standard neonatal graph, such as the one available at http://thePoint.lww.com/Pillitteri7e. Plotting weight this way helps identify newborns who are at risk because they are less than usual weight. This information also separates those who are small for their gestational age (newborns who have suffered intrauterine growth restriction) from preterm infants (infants who are healthy but small in weight only because they were born early).

Plotting weight in conjunction with height and head circumference is also helpful because it highlights disproportionate measurements. All three of these measurements should fall near the same percentile in an individual child. For example, a newborn who falls within the 50th percentile for height and weight but whose head circumference is in the 90th percentile may have abnormal head growth. A newborn who is in the 50th percentile for weight and head circumference but in the 3rd percentile for height may have a growth problem.

According to CDC (2010) Growth Chart data, the average birth weight (50th percentile) for a white, mature female newborn is 3.4 kg (7.4 lb) and for a white, mature male newborn is 3.6 kg (7.9 lb). Newborns from other backgrounds weigh approximately 0.5 lb less. The arbitrary lower limit of expected birth weight for all newborns is 2.5 kg (5.5 lb). Birth weight exceeding 4.7 kg (10 lb) is unusual, but weights as high as 7.7 kg (17 lb) have been documented (CDC, 2010).

If a term newborn weighs more than 4.7 kg, the baby is said to be macrosomic, a condition that usually occurs in conjunction with a maternal illness, such as gestational diabetes (Song, Zhang, & Song, 2012). Second-born children usually weigh more than first-born ones. Birth weight continues to increase with each succeeding child in a family.

During the first few days after birth, a newborn loses 5% to 10% of birth weight (6 to 10 oz) (Smith, 2011). This weight loss occurs because a newborn is no longer under the influence of salt- and fluid-retaining maternal hormones. This causes diuresis to begin to remove a part of the infant's high fluid load; in addition, the newborn voids and passes stool. Breastfed newborns have a limited intake until about the third day of life because of the relatively low caloric content and small amount of colostrum they ingest; formula-fed newborns need time to establish effective sucking. This lack of intake also plays a part in weight loss.

After this initial loss of weight, a newborn has about 1 day of stable weight, then begins to gain weight. The breastfed newborn recaptures birth weight within 10 days; a formula-fed infant accomplishes this gain within 7 days. After this, all infants begin to gain about 2 lb per month (6 to 8 oz per week) for the first 6 months of life.

While the newborn is still in the birthing center, compare the weight obtained each day with that of the preceding day to be certain an infant is not losing more than 5% to 10% of birth weight because abnormal loss of weight may be the first indication that a newborn has an inborn error of metabolism, such as adrenocortical insufficiency (salt-dumping type), or is becoming dehydrated.

What if...18.1 Mrs. Ruiz tells you she wants to weigh Beth on an infant scale after each feeding to be certain Beth's getting enough breast milk. Would you agree that is a good idea? What would you want Mrs. Ruiz to know before she does this?

Length

A newborn's length at birth in relation to weight is a second important determinant used to confirm that a newborn is healthy.

- The average birth length (50th percentile) of a mature female newborn is 49 cm (19.2 in.).
- For mature males, the average birth length is 50 cm (19.6 in.).
- The lower limit of expected birth length is arbitrarily set at 46 cm (18 in.).
- Although rare, babies with lengths as great as 57.5 cm (24 in.) have been reported.

Head Circumference

Head circumference is measured with a tape measure drawn across the center of the forehead and then around the most prominent portion of the posterior head (the occiput) (see Chapter 34, Fig. 34.5).

- In a mature newborn, the head circumference is usually 34 to 35 cm (13.5 to 14 in.).
- A mature newborn with a head circumference greater than 37 cm (14.8 in.) or less than 33 cm (13.2 in.) should be carefully assessed for neurologic involvement, although occasionally a well newborn falls within these limits.

Chest Circumference

Chest circumference is measured at the level of the nipples. If a large amount of breast tissue or edema of the breasts is present, this measurement will not be accurate until the edema has subsided. The chest circumference in a term newborn is about 2 cm (0.75 to 1 in.) less than head circumference.

Vital Signs

Vital sign measurements begin to change from those present in intrauterine life at the moment of birth.

Temperature

The temperature of newborns is about 99°F (37.2°C) at birth because they have been confined in their mother's warm and supportive uterus. Temperature will fall almost immediately to below normal because of heat loss, the temperature of birthing rooms (approximately 68° to 72°F [21° to 22°C]), and the infant's immature temperature-regulating mechanisms if the baby is not protected from heat loss at birth and in the moments afterward.

The majority of heat loss occurs because of four separate mechanisms: convection, radiation, conduction, and evaporation (Fig. 18.3).

- **Convection** is the flow of heat from the newborn's body surface to cooler surrounding air. Eliminating drafts, such as from air conditioners, is an important way to reduce convection heat loss.
- **Radiation** is the transfer of body heat to a cooler solid object not in contact with the baby, such as a cold window or air conditioner. Moving an infant as far from the cold surface as possible helps reduce this type of heat loss.
- **Conduction** is the transfer of body heat to a cooler solid object in contact with a baby. For example, a baby placed on the cold base of a warming unit quickly loses heat to the colder metal surface. Covering surfaces with a warmed blanket or towel is necessary to help minimize conduction heat loss.
- **Evaporation** is loss of heat through conversion of a liquid to a vapor. Newborns are wet when born, so they can lose a great deal of heat as the amniotic fluid on their skin evaporates. To prevent this type of heat loss, lay a newborn on the mother's abdomen immediately after birth and cover with a warm blanket for skin-to-skin contact (Moore, Anderson, Bergman, et al., 2012). In addition, drying the infant—especially the face and hair—also effectively reduces evaporation because the head, which is a large surface area in a newborn, can be responsible for

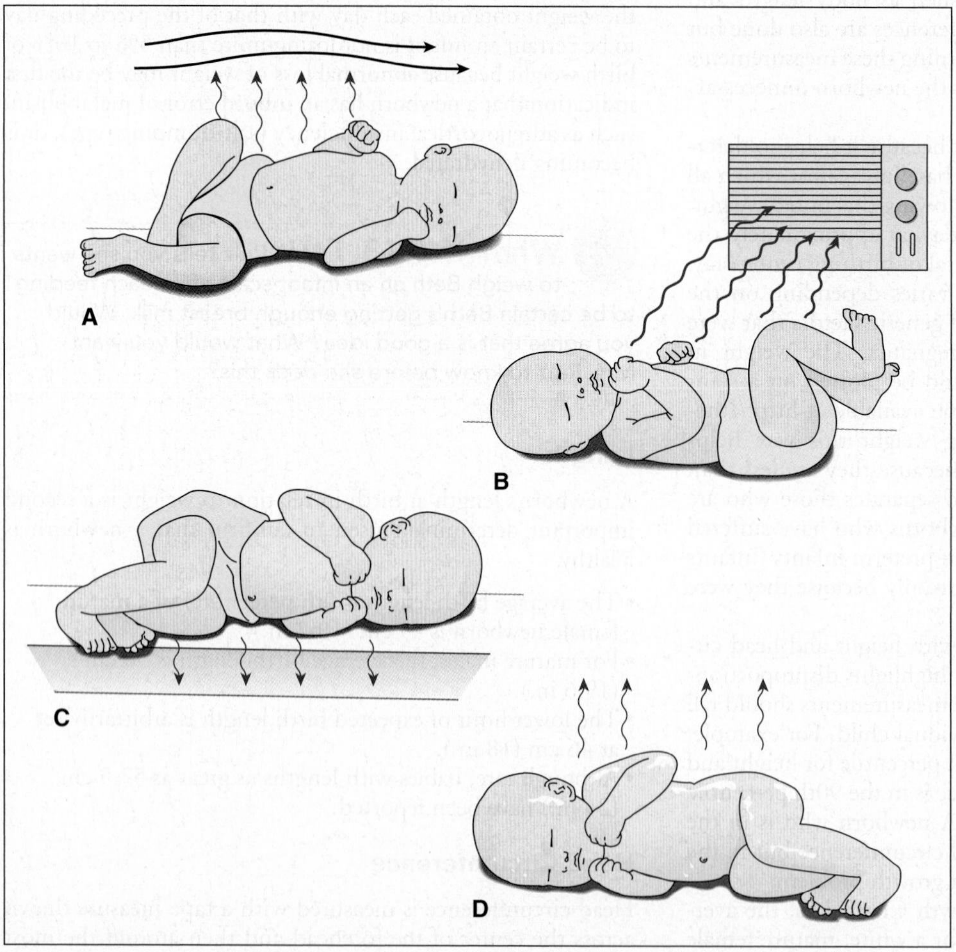

FIGURE 18.3 Heat loss in the newborn. **(A)** Convection. **(B)** Radiation. **(C)** Conduction. **(D)** Evaporation.

a great amount of heat loss. Covering the hair with a cap after drying further reduces the possibility of evaporation cooling (Lunze & Hamer, 2012).

A newborn not only loses heat easily by the means just described but also has difficulty conserving heat under any circumstance. Insulation, an efficient means of conserving heat in adults, is not as effective in newborns because they have little subcutaneous fat to provide insulation. Shivering, a means of increasing metabolism and thereby providing heat in adults, is also rarely seen in newborns.

Newborns can conserve heat by constricting blood vessels and moving blood away from the skin. *Brown fat*, a special tissue found in mature newborns, apparently helps to conserve or produce body heat by increasing metabolism as well as regulating body temperature similar to that of a hibernating animal. The greatest amounts of brown fat are found in the intrascapular region, the thorax, and behind the kidneys. In later life, brown fat may influence the proportion of body fat a person retains.

Other ways newborns are able to increase their metabolic rate and produce more heat include kicking and crying. This reaction, however, also forces them to increase their respiratory rate to allow them to take in more oxygen. All newborns can easily become fatigued from this extra exertion, thus placing additional strain on an already stressed cardiovascular system. An immature newborn with poor lung development may have extreme difficulty making such an adjustment and may fail to deliver sufficient oxygen to body systems.

In addition, as muscles become overstressed, they release lactic acid. Every newborn is born slightly acidotic. Any new buildup of acid created by cold exposure may be the straw that leads to severe, life-threatening acidosis.

Drying and placing newborns on their mother's abdomen (covered by a warm blanket), drying and wrapping them and placing them in warmed cribs, or drying and placing them under a radiant heat source are all excellent mechanical measures to help conserve heat or prevent heat loss. One more method is to be certain all early newborn care is done speedily and exposes the newborn to cool air as little as possible. Be certain that any procedure during which a newborn must be uncovered such as resuscitation or circumcision is done under a radiant heat source.

If chilling is prevented by these methods, a newborn's temperature stabilizes at 98.6°F (37°C) within 4 hours after birth. In contrast to an adult who typically runs an increased temperature with an infection, a newborn may run a subnormal temperature. Based on this, if a newborn's temperature does not stabilize shortly after birth, the cause needs to be investigated to rule out an infection (Hofer, Müller, & Resch, 2012).

Pulse

The heart rate of a fetus in utero averages 110 to 160 beats/min. Immediately after birth, as the newborn struggles to initiate respirations, the heart rate may be as rapid as 180 beats/min. Within 1 hour after birth, as the newborn settles down to sleep, the heart rate stabilizes to an average of 120 to 140 beats/min.

The heart rate of a newborn often remains slightly irregular because of immaturity of the cardiac regulatory center in the medulla, and transient murmurs may result from the incomplete closure of fetal circulation shunts. During crying, the rate may rise again to 180 beats/min. In addition, heart rate can decrease during sleep, ranging from 90 to 110 beats/min.

You should be able to palpate femoral pulses in a newborn, but the radial and temporal pulses are more difficult to palpate with any degree of accuracy. Therefore, a newborn's heart rate is best determined by listening for an apical heartbeat for a full minute, rather than assessing a pulse in an extremity or over the carotid artery. Always palpate for femoral pulses, however, and document that they are present because their absence suggests possible coarctation (narrowing) of the aorta, which is a possible cardiovascular abnormality (Schneider, 2011).

Respiration

The respiratory rate of a newborn in the first few minutes of life may be as high as 90 breaths/min. As respiratory activity is established and maintained over the next hour, this rate will settle to an average of 30 to 60 breaths/min. Respiratory depth, rate, and rhythm are likely to be irregular, and short periods of apnea (without cyanosis), sometimes called *periodic respirations*, are also common and normal during this time. Respiratory rate can be observed most easily by watching the movement of a newborn's abdomen, because breathing primarily involves the use of the diaphragm and abdominal muscles.

Coughing and sneezing reflexes are present at birth to clear the airway. Newborns are obligate nose breathers, however, and show signs of acute distress if their nostrils become obstructed. Short periods of crying, which increase the depth of respirations and aid in aerating deep portions of the lungs, may be beneficial to a newborn. Long periods of crying, however, exhaust the cardiovascular system, become fatiguing, and serve no purpose.

Blood Pressure

The blood pressure of a newborn is approximately 80/46 mmHg at birth. By the 10th day, it rises to about 100/50 mmHg and remains at that level for the infant year. Because measurement of blood pressure in newborns is somewhat inaccurate due to the small size of their arms, it is not routinely measured unless a cardiac anomaly is suspected. For an accurate reading, the cuff width used must be no more than two thirds the length of the upper arm or thigh.

Blood pressure tends to increase with crying (and a newborn cries when disturbed and manipulated by such procedures such as taking blood pressure) so a Doppler method may achieve better results (see Chapters 34 and 36). Hemodynamic monitoring is helpful when a continuous assessment is necessary.

QSEN Checkpoint Question 18.1

Patient-Centered Care

Beth Ruiz, like all newborns, is in danger of losing body heat by conduction. You are taking action to ensure that Beth's body temperature is maintained in order to protect her health and comfort. Under which condition is heat loss by conduction most apt to occur?

a. A fan is operating in the room.
b. Beth is wet from amniotic fluid at birth.
c. She pulls off the cap you put on her head.
d. You place her on a scale that has not been prewarmed.

Look in Appendix A for the best answer and rationale.

Physiologic Functions

Just as changes occur in vital signs after birth, so do changes in all major body systems occur.

Cardiovascular System

Changes in the cardiovascular system are necessary after birth because now the lungs are responsible for oxygenating blood that was formerly oxygenated by the placenta. As soon as the umbilical cord is clamped, which stimulates a neonate to take in oxygen through the lungs, fetal cardiovascular shunts begin to close.

With the first breath, blood pressure decreases in the pulmonary artery (the artery leading from the heart to the lungs). As this pressure decreases, the ductus arteriosus, the fetal shunt between the pulmonary artery and aorta, begins to close. At the same time, increased blood flow to the left side of the heart causes the foramen ovale (the opening between the right and left atria) to close because of the pressure against the lip of the structure (permanent closure does not occur for weeks). With the remaining fetal circulatory structures (umbilical vein, two umbilical arteries, and ductus venosus) no longer receiving blood from the placenta, the blood within them clots and closes them, and the vessels atrophy over the next few weeks.

Figure 18.4 summarizes these respiratory and cardiovascular changes that occur at birth. The peripheral circulation of a newborn remains sluggish for at least the first 24 hours. Because of this slowed peripheral blood flow, it is common to observe cyanosis in the infant's feet and hands **(acrocyanosis)** and for a newborn's feet to feel cold to the touch.

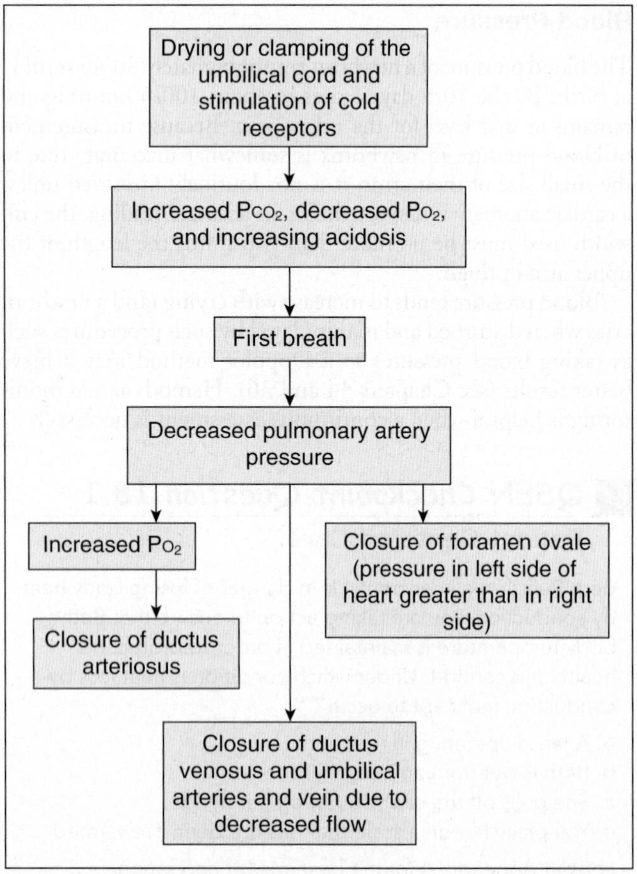

FIGURE 18.4 Circulatory events at birth.

Blood Values. A newborn's blood volume is 80 to 110 ml/kg of body weight, or about 300 ml total. Because a newborn has more red blood cells than the average adult, the hemoglobin level averages 17 to 18 g/100 ml of blood (the average for an adult is 11 to 12 g/ml). A newborn's hematocrit is between 45% and 50% (for an adult, 36% to 45%). A newborn's red blood cell count is about 6 million cells/mm^3 (for an adult, 3.5 to 5.5 million cells/mm^3).

Capillary heel sticks may reveal a falsely high hematocrit or hemoglobin value because of the sluggish peripheral circulation. Before obtaining a blood specimen from a heel, warm the foot by wrapping it in a warm cloth to increase circulation and improve the accuracy of this value.

Once proper lung oxygenation has been established, the need for the high red cell count diminishes so, within a matter of days, red cells begin to be destroyed. As these cells are broken down, bilirubin is released and the serum indirect bilirubin level rises. At birth, the indirect bilirubin level is between 1 and 4 mg/100 ml. Any increase over this amount reflects that excessive red blood cells have begun their breakdown (Brashers & McCance, 2012).

A newborn has a corresponding high white blood cell count, about 15,000 to 30,000 cells/mm^3 at birth (40,000 cells/mm^3 if the birth was stressful). Seeing the count increased, therefore, is not evidence of infection but reflects how stressful an event birth is for a fetus. However, although the high white blood cell count makes infection difficult to prove in a newborn, infection must not be dismissed as a possibility if other signs of infection such as pallor, respiratory difficulty, or cyanosis are present. Usual blood values in a newborn are available at http://thePoint.lww.com/Pillitteri7e.

Blood Coagulation. Vitamin K, synthesized through the action of intestinal flora, is responsible for the formation of factor II (prothrombin), factor VII (proconvertin), factor IX (plasma thromboplastin component), and factor X (Stuart-Prower factor) in the clotting sequence. Because a newborn's intestine is sterile at birth unless membranes were ruptured more than 24 hours, it will take about 24 hours for flora to accumulate and for ongoing vitamin K to be synthesized. This causes most newborns to be born with a lower than usual level of vitamin K, leading to a prolonged coagulation or prothrombin time.

Because almost all newborns can be predicted to have this diminished blood coagulation ability, vitamin K (AquaMEPHYTON) is usually administered intramuscularly into the lateral anterior thigh, the preferred site for all injections in newborns, immediately after birth (Box 18.3). If parents object to an injection, vitamin K can be administered orally, although the efficiency of this is not rated as high (Karch, 2013). Whether giving this orally or by injection, be certain the administration doesn't interfere with parent bonding or beginning breastfeeding as these are also vitally important in the first hours after birth (Rossman & Ayoola, 2012).

The Respiratory System

A first breath is a major undertaking because it requires a tremendous amount of pressure (about 40 to 70 cm H_2O) for a newborn to be able to inflate alveoli for the first time.

BOX 18.3 Nursing Care Planning Based on Responsibility for Pharmacology

VITAMIN K (PHYTONADIONE, AQUAMEPHYTON)

Action: Vitamin K is used to prevent and treat hemorrhagic disease in newborns. It is a necessary component for the production of certain coagulation factors (II, VII, IX, and X) and is produced by microorganisms in the intestinal tract (Karch, 2013).

Pregnancy Risk Category: C

Dosage: Prophylaxis: 0.5 to 1.0 mg intramuscularly (IM) one time in the first hour after birth; treatment of hemorrhagic disease: 1 to 2 mg IM or subcutaneously (SC) daily.

Possible Adverse Reactions: Local irritation, such as pain and swelling at the site of injection.

Nursing Implications

- Anticipate the need for injection within an hour after birth.
- Administer IM injection into a large muscle, such as the anterolateral muscle of a newborn's thigh.
- Be certain to administer the injection at a time it doesn't interrupt parent–child bonding or beginning breastfeeding.
- If giving vitamin K for treatment, obtain prothrombin time before administration (the single best indicator of vitamin K–dependent clotting factors).
- Assess for signs of bleeding in the infant, such as black, tarry stools (different from meconium stools, which have a greenish shade), hematuria (blood in urine), decreased hemoglobin and hematocrit levels, and bleeding from any open wound or at the base of the cord. (These signs would indicate more vitamin K is necessary because bleeding control has not been achieved.)

The reflex to breathe is initiated by a combination of cold receptors; a lowered partial pressure of oxygen (Po_2), which falls from 80 mmHg to as low as 15 mmHg before a first breath; and an increased partial carbon dioxide pressure (Pco_2), which rises as high as 70 mmHg before a first breath.

Some fluid present in the lungs from intrauterine life makes a newborn's first breath possible, because fluid eases surface tension on alveolar walls and allows alveoli to inflate more easily than if the lung walls were dry. About one third of this fluid is forced out of the lungs by the pressure of vaginal birth. The rest of the fluid is quickly absorbed by lung blood vessels and lymphatics after the first breath.

Once the alveoli have been inflated this first time, breathing becomes much easier for a baby, requiring only about 6 to 8 cm H_2O pressure. Within 10 minutes after birth, most newborns have established easy respirations as well as a good residual volume. By 10 to 12 hours of age, vital capacity is established at newborn proportions (the heart in a newborn takes up proportionately more space than in an adult, so the amount of lung expansion space available for a large vital capacity is limited).

A baby born by cesarean birth does not have as much lung fluid expelled at birth as one born vaginally and so typically has more difficulty establishing effective respirations, because the excessive fluid blocks air exchange space. In newborns who are born preterm, their alveoli may collapse each time they exhale (because of the lack of pulmonary surfactant). They, therefore, also have difficulty establishing effective residual capacity and respirations. In these infants, because alveoli do not open well, the foramen ovale and ductus arteriosus may also not close as usual. This results because their closure depends on free blood flow through the pulmonary artery and good oxygenation of blood.

Because of the association between ineffective respirations and heart disease, any newborn who had difficulty establishing respirations at birth needs to be examined closely in the postpartal period for a cardiac murmur or any other indication that he or she still has patent cardiac structures, especially a patent ductus arteriosus (Schneider, 2012).

The Gastrointestinal System

Although the gastrointestinal tract is usually sterile at birth, bacteria may be cultured from the tract in most babies within 5 hours after birth and from all babies at 24 hours of life. Most of these bacteria enter the tract through the newborn's mouth from airborne sources. Others may come from vaginal secretions at birth, from hospital bedding, and from contact at the breast. That bacteria begin to accumulate is helpful because bacteria in the gastrointestinal tract are necessary for digestion through probiotics and for the synthesis of vitamin K.

Although a newborn stomach holds about 60 to 90 ml, a newborn has limited ability to digest everything taken in, especially fat and starch because the pancreatic enzymes, lipase and amylase, remain deficient for the first few months of life. Also, because the cardiac sphincter between the stomach and esophagus is immature, a newborn tends to regurgitate easily. Immature liver function can lead to a tendency toward lowered glucose and protein serum levels.

Stools. The first stool of a newborn is usually passed within 24 hours after birth. It consists of **meconium**, a sticky, tarlike, blackish-green, odorless material formed from mucus, vernix, lanugo, hormones, and carbohydrates that accumulated in the bowel during intrauterine life. If a newborn does not pass a meconium stool by 24 to 48 hours after birth, the possibility of some factor such as meconium ileus, imperforate anus, or volvulus, which is causing blockage of the bowel, should be suspected.

About the second or third day of life, newborn stool changes in color and consistency. Termed a **transitional stool**, bowel contents appear both loose and green; they may resemble diarrhea to the untrained eye.

- By the fourth day of life, breastfed babies pass three or four light yellow stools per day. They are sweet smelling, because breast milk is high in lactic acid, which reduces the amount of putrefactive organisms in the stool.
- A newborn who receives formula usually passes two or three bright yellow stools a day. These have a slightly more noticeable odor, compared with the stools of breastfed babies.

- A newborn placed under phototherapy lights as therapy for jaundice will have bright green stools because of increased bilirubin excretion.
- Newborns with bile duct obstruction have clay-colored (gray) stools, because bile pigments cannot enter the intestinal tract.
- Blood-flecked stools usually indicate an anal fissure.
- Occasionally, a newborn has swallowed some maternal blood during birth and either vomits fresh blood immediately after birth or passes a black tarry stool after two or more days. Whether bleeding is caused by ingestion of maternal blood at birth or newborn bleeding may be differentiated by a dipstick Apt test. If stools remain black or tarry, this suggests newborn intestinal bleeding rather than swallowed blood.
- If mucus is mixed with stool or the stool is watery and loose, a milk allergy, lactose intolerance, or some other condition interfering with digestion or absorption should be suspected.

The Urinary System

The average newborn voids within 24 hours after birth. A newborn who does not take in much fluid for the first 24 hours may void later than this, but the 24-hour point is a good general "alert" rule. Newborns who do not void within this time need to be assessed for the possibility of urethral stenosis or absent kidneys or ureters.

The kidneys of newborns do not concentrate urine well, making newborn urine usually light colored and odorless. The infant is about 6 weeks of age before much control over reabsorption of fluid in tubules and concentration of urine becomes evident.

A single voiding in a newborn is only about 15 ml and may be easily missed in a thick diaper. Specific gravity ranges from 1.008 to 1.010. The daily urinary output for the first 1 or 2 days is about 30 to 60 ml total. By week 1, total daily volume rises to about 300 ml. The first voiding may be pink or dusky because of uric acid crystals that were formed in the bladder in utero; this looks a lot like blood in urine but is an innocent finding. If tested for protein, a small amount may be normally present in voidings for the first few days of life until the kidney glomeruli are more fully mature. Diapers can be weighed to determine the amount and timing of voiding if there is a concern the newborn is voiding an adequate amount.

The possibility of obstruction in the urinary tract can also be assessed by observing the force of the urinary stream in both male and female infants. Males should void with enough force to produce a small projected arc; females should produce a steady stream, not just continuous dribbling. Projecting urine farther than normal may signal urethral obstruction because it indicates urine is being forced through a narrow channel.

The Immune System

Newborns have limited immunologic protection at birth because they are not able to produce antibodies until about 2 months (the reason most immunizations are not administered until 2 months of age). Newborns are, however, born with passive antibodies (immunoglobulin G) passed to them from their mother that crossed the placenta. In most instances, these include antibodies against poliomyelitis, measles, diphtheria, pertussis, chickenpox, rubella, and tetanus. Newborns are routinely administered hepatitis B vaccine before they leave their birth setting to promote antibody formation against this disease (American Academy of Pediatrics [AAP], 2012b). Because the newborn has little natural immunity against herpes simplex, health care personnel with herpes simplex eruptions (cold sores) should not care for newborns until the lesions have crusted. Without antibody protection, herpes simplex type 2 infections can become systemic or create a rapidly fatal form of the disease in a newborn (Shah, Aronson, Mohama, et al., 2011).

The Neuromuscular System

Term newborns demonstrate neuromuscular function by moving their extremities, attempting to control head movement, exhibiting a strong cry, and demonstrating newborn reflexes. Limpness or total absence of a muscular response to manipulation is never normal and suggests narcosis, shock, or cerebral injury. A newborn occasionally makes twitching or flailing movements of the extremities in the absence of a stimulus because of the immaturity of the nervous system; these are common and normal. Newborn reflexes can be tested with consistency by using a number of simple maneuvers.

The Blink Reflex. A blink reflex in a newborn serves the same purpose as it does in an adult—to protect the eye from any object coming near it by rapid eyelid closure. It may be elicited by shining a strong light such as a flashlight or otoscope light into an eye. A sudden movement toward the eye sometimes can elicit the blink reflex, but this is not as reliable.

The Rooting Reflex. If a newborn's cheek is brushed or stroked near the corner of the mouth, the infant will turn the head in that direction. This reflex serves to help a newborn find food; when a mother holds the child and allows her breast to brush the newborn's cheek, the reflex causes the baby to turn toward the breast. The reflex disappears at about the sixth week of life, not coincidentally at the same time a newborn's eyes focus steadily so a food source can be seen.

The Sucking Reflex. When a newborn's lips are touched, the baby makes a sucking motion. Like the rooting reflex, this reflex also helps a newborn find food as when the newborn's lips touch the mother's breast or a bottle, the baby sucks and takes in food. The sucking reflex begins to diminish at about 6 months of age. It disappears immediately if it is never stimulated such as in a newborn with a tracheoesophageal fistula who cannot take in oral fluids. It can be maintained in such an infant by offering the child a nonnutritive sucking object such as a pacifier (after the fistula has been corrected by surgery and until oral feedings can be given).

The Swallowing Reflex. The swallowing reflex in a newborn is the same as in the adult. Food that reaches the posterior portion of the tongue is automatically swallowed. Gag, cough, and sneeze reflexes also are present in newborns to maintain a clear airway in the event that normal swallowing does not keep the pharynx free of obstructing mucus.

The Extrusion Reflex. In order to prevent the swallowing of inedible substances, a newborn extrudes any substance that is placed on the anterior portion of the tongue. If newborns are offered solid food before this reflex fades at 4 months, it seems as if they are spitting out any type of food offered. Be certain parents are aware of this reflex so they preferably don't offer solid food this early (or if they do, they don't erroneously label their child a "picky" eater).

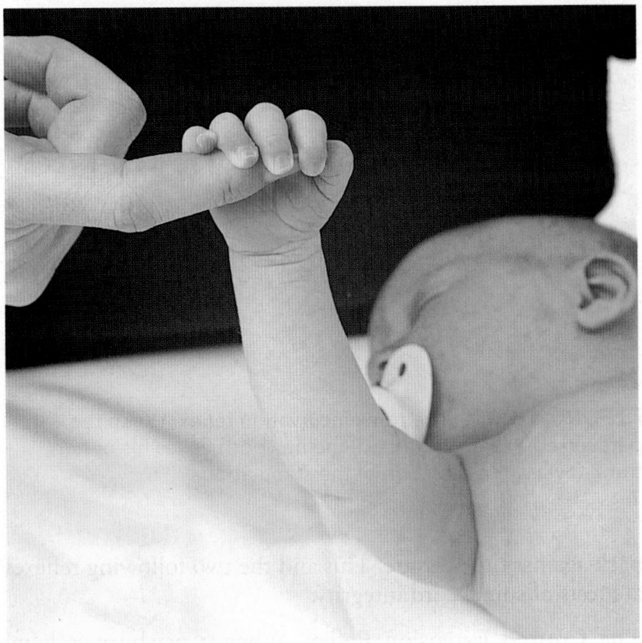

FIGURE 18.5 The palmar grasp reflex.

The Palmar Grasp Reflex. Newborns grasp an object placed in their palm by quickly closing their fingers on it (Fig. 18.5). Mature newborns grasp so strongly they can be raised from a supine position and suspended momentarily from an examiner's fingers. This reflex disappears at about 6 weeks to 3 months of age; after it fades, a baby begins to grasp meaningfully.

The Step (Walk)-In-Place Reflex. Newborns who are held in a vertical position with their feet touching a hard surface will take a few quick, alternating steps (Fig. 18.6). This reflex disappears by 3 months of age so that by 4 months, babies can bear a good portion of their weight unhindered by this reflex.

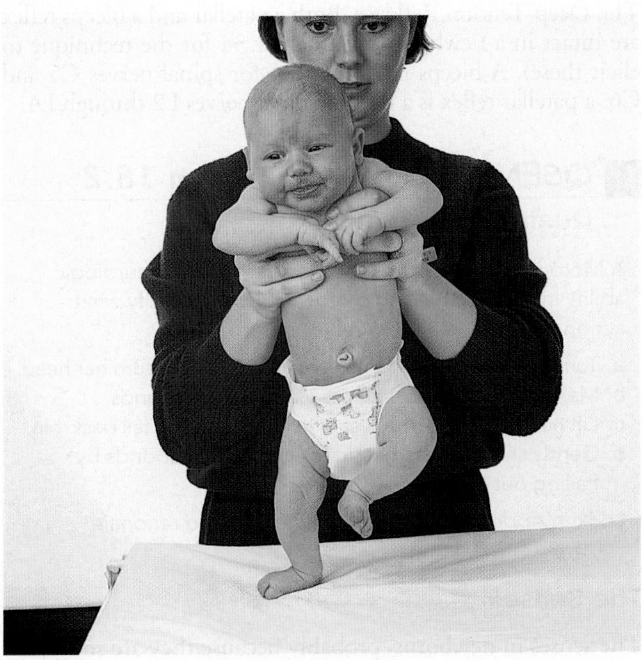

FIGURE 18.6 The step-in-place reflex.

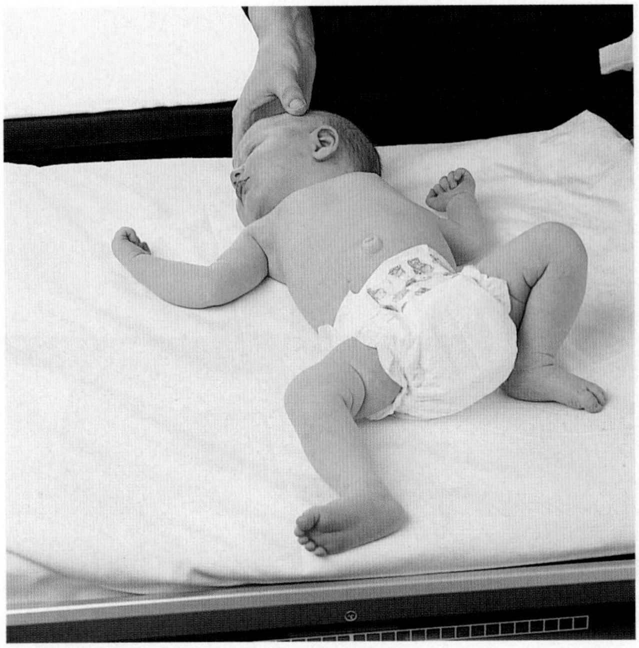

FIGURE 18.7 The tonic neck reflex.

The Placing Reflex. The placing reflex is similar to the step-in-place reflex, except it is elicited by touching the anterior surface of the lower part of a newborn's leg against a hard surface such as the edge of a bassinet or table. The newborn makes a few quick lifting motions, as if to step onto the table.

The Plantar Grasp Reflex. When an object touches the sole of a newborn's foot at the base of the toes, the toes grasp in the same manner as the fingers. This reflex disappears at about 8 to 9 months of age in preparation for walking. However, it may be present during sleep for a longer period of time.

The Tonic Neck Reflex. When newborns lie on their backs, their heads usually turn to one side or the other. The arm and the leg on the side toward which the head turns extend, and the opposite arm and leg contract (Fig. 18.7). This posture is most evident in the arms but should not be totally absent in the legs. If you turn a newborn's head to the opposite side, he or she will often change the extension and contraction of legs and arms accordingly. This is sometimes called a "boxer" or "fencing reflex," because the position simulates someone preparing to box or stab with a sword. Unlike other reflexes, it is difficult to see this reflex's function or purpose. It may play a role in stimulating eye coordination, because the extended arm moves in front of the face. Another possibility is it signifies handedness. The reflex typically disappears between the second and third months of life.

The Moro Reflex. A Moro (startle) reflex (Fig. 18.8) can be initiated by startling a newborn with a loud noise or by jarring the bassinet. The most accurate method of eliciting the reflex, however, is to hold a newborn in a supine position and then allow the head to drop backward about 1 in. In response to this sudden backward head movement, the newborn abducts and extend arms and legs, then swings the arms into an embrace position and pulls up the legs against the abdomen (Gowen, 2011). The reflex simulates the action of someone trying to ward off an attacker, then covering up to protect the body. It is strong for the first 8 weeks of life

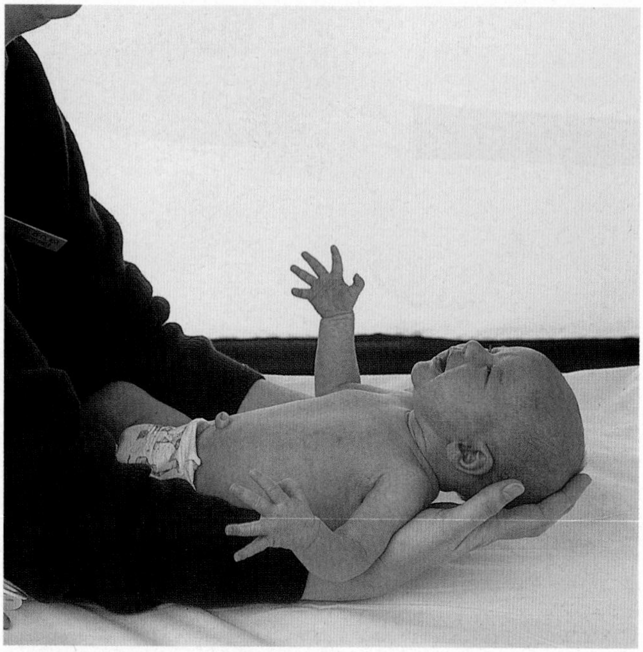

FIGURE 18.8 The Moro reflex.

and then fades by the end of the fourth or fifth month, at the same time an infant can roll away from danger.

The Babinski Reflex. When the sole of a newborn's foot is stroked in an inverted "J" curve from the heel upward, a newborn fans the toes (positive Babinski sign) (Fig. 18.9). This is in contrast to the adult, who flexes the toes if the foot is stroked this way. The reflex remains positive (toes fan) until at least 3 months of age, when it is supplanted by the downturning or adult flexion response.

The Magnet Reflex. If pressure is applied to the soles of the feet of a newborn lying in a supine position, he or she pushes back against the pressure. This and the two following reflexes are tests of spinal cord integrity.

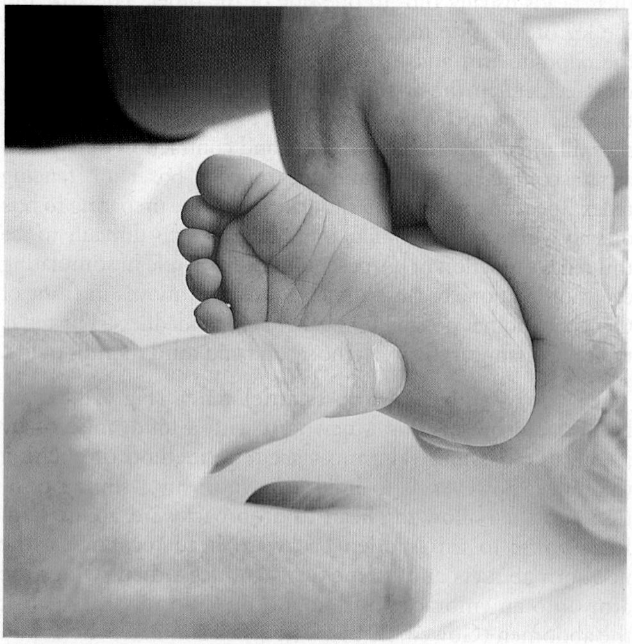

FIGURE 18.9 The Babinski reflex. When the examiner moves her finger upward, the newborn's toes will fan outward.

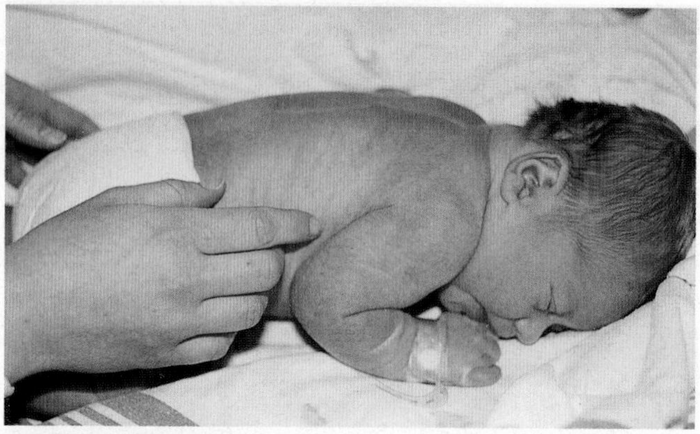

FIGURE 18.10 The trunk incurvation reflex. When the paravertebral area is stroked, the newborn flexes his or her trunk toward the direction of the stimulation.

The Crossed Extension Reflex. When a newborn is lying supine, if one leg is extended and the sole of that foot is irritated by being rubbed with a sharp object, such as a thumbnail, the infant raises the other leg and extends it as if trying to push away the hand irritating the first leg.

The Trunk Incurvation Reflex. When a newborn lies in a prone position and is touched along the paravertebral area on the back by a probing finger, the newborn flexes the trunk and swings the pelvis toward the touch (Fig. 18.10).

The Landau Reflex. When a newborn is supported in a prone position by a hand, the newborn should demonstrate some muscle tone. A baby may not be able to lift the head or arch the back in this position (as will be possible at 3 months of age), but neither should the infant sag into an inverted "U" position. The latter response indicates extremely poor muscle tone, the cause of which needs to be investigated.

The Deep Tendon Reflexes. Both a patellar and a biceps reflex are intact in a newborn (see Chapter 34 for the technique to elicit these). A biceps reflex is a test for spinal nerves C5 and C6; a patellar reflex is a test for spinal nerves L2 through L4.

✔ QSEN Checkpoint Question 18.2

Quality Improvement

A Moro reflex is the single best assessment of neurologic ability in a newborn. Unit protocols should specify what action for eliciting a Moro reflex in Beth?

a. Turn her onto her abdomen and see if she can turn her head.
b. Make a sharp noise, such as clapping your hands.
c. Lift her head while she is supine and allow it to fall back 1 in.
d. Gently shake Beth's bassinette until she responds by flailing out her arms.

Look in Appendix A for the best answer and rationale.

The Senses

The senses in newborns, probably because they are so important for survival, are already fully developed at birth.

TABLE 18.1 Periods of Reactivity: Normal Adjustment to Extrauterine Life

Assessment	First Period (First 15–30 min)	Resting Period (30–120 min)	Second Period (2–6 hr)
Color	Acrocyanosis is present.	Color begins to stabilize.	Quick color changes occur with movement or crying.
Temperature	Temperature begins to fall from intrauterine temperature of about 100.6°F (38.1°C).	Temperature stabilizes at about 99°F (37.2°C).	Temperature increases to 99.8°F (37.6°C).
Heart rate	Heart rate is rapid, as much as 180 beats/min while crying.	Heart rate slows to 120–140 beats/min.	Wide swings in rate occur with activity but stabilize at 120–140 beats/min.
Respirations	Breathing is irregular; 30–90 breaths/min while crying; some nasal flaring and occasional retraction may be present.	Breathing slows to 30–50 breaths/min; barreling of chest may occur.	Breathing rate becomes irregular with activity but stabilizes at 30–60 breaths/min.
Activity	Alert; watching.	Sleeping.	Awakening.
Ability to respond to stimulation	Vigorous reaction.	Difficult to arouse.	Becoming responsive again.
Mucus	Visible in mouth.	Small amount present while sleeping.	Mouth full of mucus, possibly causing gagging.
Bowel sounds	Can be heard after first 15 min.	Present.	Often passage of first meconium stool.

From Desmond, M. M., Franklin, R. R., Vallvona, C., et al. (1963). The clinical behavior of the newly born: The term infant. *Journal of Pediatrics, 62*(3), 307–309.

Hearing. Acoustic stimulation reveals a fetus is able to hear in utero by the infant's response to loud sound (Russo, Henderson, & Costigan, 2011). As soon as amniotic fluid drains or is absorbed from the middle ear by way of the eustachian tube within hours after birth, hearing becomes acute. Newborns respond with generalized activity to a sound such as a bell; they appear to have difficulty locating where a sound is coming from, however, and so do not turn toward it consistently. Similarly, newborns appear to recognize their mother's voice almost immediately and calm to the sound of it as if they have heard it in utero.

Vision. A pupillary reflex or ability to contract the pupil is present from birth. Newborns demonstrate they can see by blinking at a strong light (blink reflex) or by following a bright light or toy a short distance with their eyes as soon as they are born; possibly, they have been "seeing" light and dark in utero for the last few months of pregnancy as the uterus and the abdominal wall were stretched thin (Graven, 2011). Be certain parents know their newborn cannot follow an object past the midline or appears to lose track of objects easily so they don't worry there is something wrong with their child's eyesight. Teach also that newborns focus best on black and white objects at a distance of 9 to 12 in.

Touch. The sense of touch is also well developed at birth. Newborns demonstrate this by quieting at a soothing touch, crying at painful stimuli, and by showing sucking and rooting reflexes, which are elicited by touch.

Taste. A newborn has the ability to discriminate taste because taste buds are developed and functioning even before birth. A fetus in utero, for example, will swallow amniotic fluid more rapidly than usual if glucose is added to sweeten its taste. The swallowing decreases if a bitter flavor is added. After birth, a baby turns away from a bitter taste such as salt but readily accepts the sweet taste of milk or glucose water.

Smell. The sense of smell is present in newborns as soon as the nose is clear of lung and amniotic fluid. Newborns probably turn toward their mothers' breasts partly out of recognition of the smell of breast milk and partly as a manifestation of the rooting reflex.

The Physiologic Adjustment to Extrauterine Life

All newborns appear to move through periods of irregular adjustment in the first 6 hours of life, until, at that point, their body systems stabilize. These periods were first described by Desmond in 1963 and are termed three periods of reactivity (Desmond, Franklin, Vallvona, et al., 1963) (Table 18.1). Newborns who are ill or who had difficulty in utero or at birth may not pass through these typical stages or, for example, they may never have periods of alertness or periods of quiet, their vital signs may not fall and rise again but remain rapid, or their temperature may remain subnormal. Demonstration of these typical reactivity patterns, therefore, is an indication a newborn's neurologic system is intact and healthy and the newborn is adjusting well to extrauterine life. Explain these periods to new mothers because the alert periods are ideal periods for parent–infant bonding to begin.

ASSESSMENTS FOR WELL-BEING

A number of traditional standardized assessments as well as a history and physical examination are done at birth to evaluate a newborn for maturity and general well-being.

TABLE 18.2 Apgar Scoring Chart

	Score		
Sign to Assess	*0*	*1*	*2*
Heart rate	Absent	Slow (<100 beats/min)	>100 beats/min
Respiratory effort	Absent	Slow, irregular; weak cry	Good; strong cry
Muscle tone	Flaccid	Some flexion of extremities	Well flexed
Reflex irritability:			
Response to catheter in nostril, *or*	No response	Grimace	Cough or sneeze
Slap to sole of foot	No response	Grimace	Cry and withdrawal of foot
Color	Blue, pale	Body normal pigment; extremities blue	Normal skin coloring

Total score:
- Score of <4 indicates serious danger of respiratory or cardiovascular failure; newborn needs resuscitation.
- Score of 4–6 indicates a guarded condition; newborn may need clearing of the airway and supplementary oxygen.
- Score of 7–10 indicates the infant scored as high as 70%–90% of all infants at 1 and 5 min after birth or is adjusting well to extrauterine life.

From Apgar, V., Holaday, D. A., James, L. S., et al. (1958). Evaluation of the newborn infant: Second report. *JAMA: Journal of the American Medical Association, 168*(15), 1985–1988. Copyright 1958, American Medical Association.

Apgar Scoring

At 1 minute and 5 minutes after birth, newborns are observed and rated according to an Apgar score, an assessment scale used as a standard for newborn evaluation since 1958 (Apgar, Holaday, James, et al., 1958). As shown in Table 18.2, heart rate, respiratory effort, muscle tone, reflex irritability, and color of the infant are each rated 0, 1, or 2. There is a high correlation between low 5-minute Apgar scores and neurologic illness (Gowen, 2011). The following points should be considered in obtaining the rating (Rubarth, 2012).

Heart Rate. Auscultating a newborn heart with a stethoscope is the best way to determine heart rate; however, heart rate also may be obtained by observing and counting the pulsations of the umbilical cord at the abdomen if the cord is still uncut.

Respiratory Effort. Respirations are counted by observing chest movements. A mature newborn usually cries and aerates the lungs spontaneously at about 30 seconds after birth. By 1 minute, he or she is maintaining regular, although rapid, respirations. Difficulty with breathing might be anticipated in a newborn whose mother received large amounts of analgesia or a general anesthetic during labor or birth.

Muscle Tone. Term newborns hold their extremities tightly flexed, simulating their intrauterine position. Muscle tone is tested by observing their resistance to any effort to extend their extremities.

Reflex Irritability. One of two possible cues is used to evaluate reflex irritability: response to a suction catheter in the nostrils or response to having the soles of the feet slapped. A baby whose mother was heavily sedated for birth will probably demonstrate a low score in this category.

Color. All infants appear cyanotic at the moment of birth. They grow pink with or shortly after the first breath, which makes the color of newborns correspond to how well they are breathing. Acrocyanosis (cyanosis of the hands and feet) is so common in newborns that a score of 1 in this category can be thought of as normal.

The Respiratory Evaluation

Good respiratory function obviously has the highest priority in newborn care, so the assessment for it is ongoing at every newborn contact. The Silverman-Andersen index, originally devised in 1956 (Silverman & Andersen, 1956) is a standard method, which can be used to estimate degrees of respiratory distress in newborns. For this assessment, a newborn is observed and then scored on each of five criteria (Fig. 18.11).

✔ QSEN Checkpoint Question 18.3

Informatics

Beth Ruiz had Apgar scores of 6 at 1 minute and 8 at 5 minutes after birth. Which of the following are the five areas assessed with Apgar scoring?

a. Heart rate, respiratory effort, muscle tone, reflex irritability, and color
b. Respiratory rate, abdominal tone, reflexes, color, and head circumference
c. Color, breathing rate, cry, amount of brown fat, and response to loud noise
d. Abdominal tone, persistence, reflexes, blood pressure, and response to pain

Look in Appendix A for the best answer and rationale.

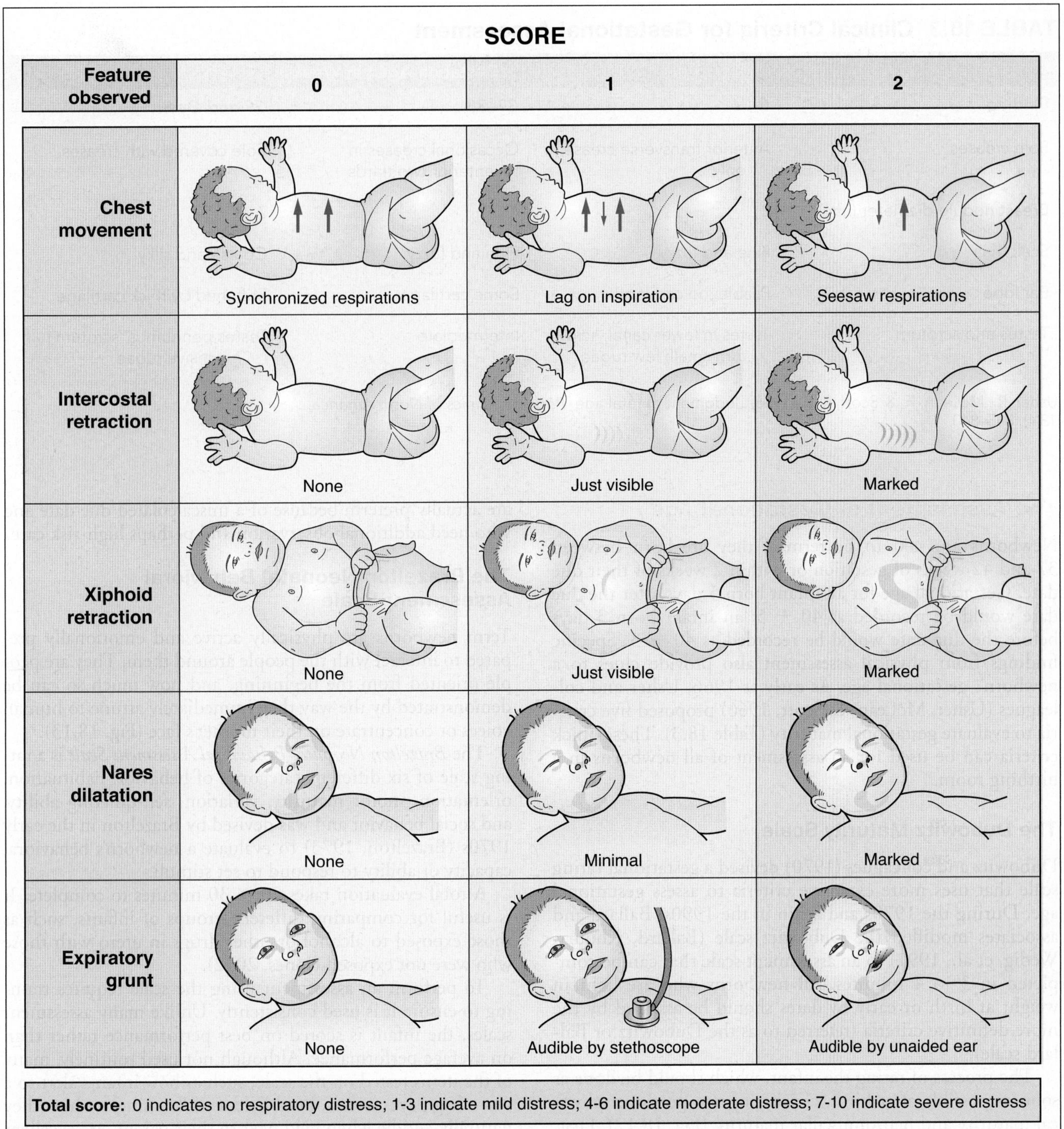

SCORE
Feature observed
0
1
2
Chest movement
Synchronized respirations
Lag on inspiration
Seesaw respirations
Intercostal retraction
None
Just visible
Marked
Xiphoid retraction
None
Just visible
Marked
Nares dilatation
None
Minimal
Marked
Expiratory grunt
None
Audible by stethoscope
Audible by unaided ear
Total score: 0 indicates no respiratory distress; 1-3 indicate mild distress; 4-6 indicate moderate distress; 7-10 indicate severe distress

FIGURE 18.11 Grading of neonatal respiratory distress based on the Silverman–Andersen index. (Silverman, W. A., & Andersen, D. H. [1956]. A controlled clinical trial of effects of water mist on obstructive respiratory signs, death rate and necroscopy findings among premature infants. *Pediatrics, 17*[4]: 1–9.)

TABLE 18.3 Clinical Criteria for Gestational Assessment

	Gestation Age (in Weeks)		
Finding	***0–36***	***37–38***	***39 and Over***
Sole creases	Anterior transverse crease only	Occasional creases in anterior two thirds	Sole covered with creases
Breast nodule diameter (mm)	2	4	7
Scalp hair	Fine and fuzzy	Fine and fuzzy	Coarse and silky
Ear lobe	Pliable; no cartilage	Some cartilage	Stiffened by thick cartilage
Testes and scrotum	Testes in lower canal; scrotum small; few rugae	Intermediate	Testes pendulous, scrotum full; extensive rugae

Usher, R., McLean, F., & Scott, K. E. (1966). Judgment of fetal age. *Pediatric Clinics of North America, 13*(4), 835–840.

The Assessment of Gestational Age

Newborns are said to be term if they are born between 37 and 42 weeks of gestation or within 2 weeks of their due date. Gestational age for an infant born 5 days after the due date would be recorded as 40 + 5; an infant born 3 days before the due date would be recorded as 40 − 3. Specific findings from physical assessment also provide clues to a newborn's gestational age. As early as 1966, Usher and colleagues (Usher, McLean, & Scott, 1966) proposed five criteria to evaluate gestational maturity (Table 18.3). These quick criteria can be used for an assessment of all newborns in a birthing room.

The Dubowitz Maturity Scale

Dubowitz and colleagues (1970) devised a gestational rating scale that uses more extensive criteria to assess gestational age. During the 1970s and again in the 1990s, Ballard and associates modified the Dubowitz scale (Ballard, Khoury, Wedig, et al., 1991) to an assessment scale that can be completed in 3 to 4 minutes. All newborns who are light in weight at birth or early by dates should be assessed by the more definitive criteria (referred to as the Dubowitz or Ballard scale).

The process of rating the infant, which should be done as soon as possible after birth, consists of two portions: physical maturity and neuromuscular maturity (Fig. 18.12). First, skin, lanugo, foot creases, breast maturity, eyes and ears, and genitalia are observed and given a score of −1 to +5, as described in Figure 18.12A. Illustrations of mature and immature body features for the scale are shown in Chapter 26 as part of the discussion of the preterm infant.

To complete the second half of the examination, observe or position a newborn as shown in Figure 18.12B. Again, score the child's response numerically from −1 to +5. To establish a baby's gestational age, the total score obtained (on both sections) is compared with the rating scale in Figure 18.12C. For example, an infant with a total score of 5 is rated as having a gestational age of 26 weeks; a total score of 50 points indicates an infant is term or 40 weeks gestation.

Using such a standard method to rate maturity is helpful in detecting infants who were thought to be term but instead are actually preterm because of a miscalculated due date and who need additional observation and perhaps high-risk care.

The Brazelton Neonatal Behavioral Assessment Scale

Term newborns are physically active and emotionally prepared to interact with the people around them. They are people oriented from the beginning, and how much so can be demonstrated by the way they immediately attune to human voices or concentrate on their mother's face (Fig. 18.13).

The *Brazelton Neonatal Behavioral Assessment Scale* is a rating scale of six different categories of behavior: habituation, orientation, motor maturity, variation, self-quieting ability, and social behavior and was devised by Brazelton in the early 1970s (Brazelton, 1973) to evaluate a newborn's behavioral capacity or ability to respond to set stimuli.

A total evaluation takes 20 to 30 minutes to complete. It is useful for comparing different groups of infants, such as those exposed to alcohol or other drugs in utero with those who were not exposed (Jones, 2012).

To perform an assessment using the scale requires training to ensure it is used consistently. Unlike many assessment scales, the infant is scored on best performance rather than on average performance. Although not used routinely, many of the items tested on the scale, such as how infants alert to a voice (e.g., eyes widen, head held as if listening) or how they naturally cuddle when held next to their parent, are excellent examples of newborn behavior to point out to parents to help them increase interactions with their newborn.

The Health History

The history of a newborn is obtained from examination of the mother's pregnancy record if this is available, her labor and birth record, and an interview with the mother. Important information to gather includes:

- Any complications of pregnancy such as gestational diabetes, hypertension, premature rupture of membranes, serious falls, or other injuries
- Length of pregnancy and length of labor
- Type of birth (vaginal or cesarean) and whether the infant breathed spontaneously or needed assistance at birth

SIGN	SCORE −1	0	1	2	3	4	5
Skin	Sticky, friable, transparent	Gelatinous, red, translucent	Smooth pink, visible veins	Superficial peeling and/or rash, few veins	Cracking, pale areas, rare veins	Parchment, deep cracking, no vessels	Leathery, cracked, wrinkled
Lanugo	None	Sparse	Abundant	Thinning	Bald areas	Mostly bald	
Plantar Surface	Heel-toe 40–50mm: –1 <40 mm: –2	>50 mm, no crease	Faint red marks	Anterior transverse crease only	Creases ant. 2/3	Creases over entire sole	
Breast	Imperceptible	Barely perceptible	Flat areola, no bud	Stippled areola, 1–2 mm bud	Raised areola, 3–4 mm bud	Full areola, 5–10 mm bud	
Eye / Ear	Lids fused loosely: –1 tightly: –2	Lids open; pinna flat stays folded	Sl. curved pinna; soft; slow recoil	Well-curved pinna; soft but ready recoil	Formed and firm instant recoil	Thick cartilage; ear stiff	
Genitals (Male)	Scrotum flat, smooth	Scrotum empty; faint rugae	Testes in upper canal; rare rugae	Testes descend-ing; few rugae	Testes down; good rugae	Testes pendulous; deep rugae	
Genitals (Female)	Clitoris prominent and labia flat	Prominent clitoris and small labia minora	Prominent clitoris and enlarging minora	Majora and minora equally prominent	Majora large, minora small	Majora cover clitoris and minora	

A

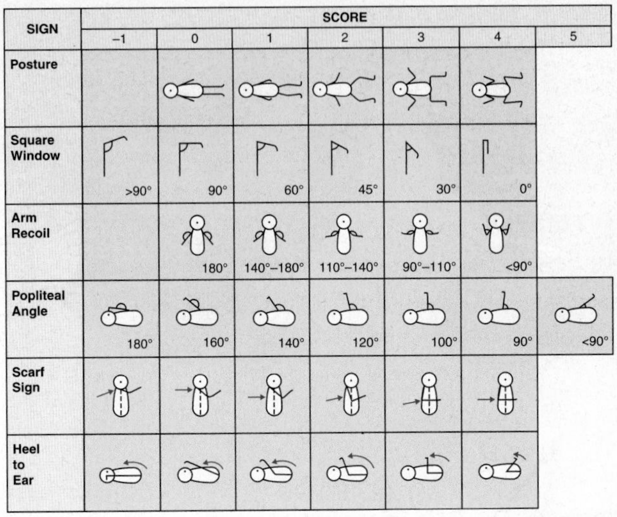
SIGN
SCORE
−1
0
1
2
3
4
5
Posture
Square Window
>90°
90°
60°
45°
30°
0°
Arm Recoil
180°
140°–180°
110°–140°
90°–110°
<90°
Popliteal Angle
180°
160°
140°
120°
100°
90°
<90°
Scarf Sign
Heel to Ear

B

TOTAL SCORE (NEUROMUSCULAR + PHYSICAL)	Weeks
−10	20
−5	22
0	24
5	26
10	28
15	30
20	32
25	34
30	36
35	38
40	40
45	42
50	44

C

FIGURE 18.12 Ballard assessment of gestational age criteria. **(A)** Physical maturity assessment criteria. **(B)** Neuromuscular maturity assessment criteria. *Posture:* With infant supine and quiet, score as follows: arms and legs extended = 0; slight or moderate flexion of hips and knees = 2; legs flexed and abducted, arms slightly flexed = 3; full flexion of arms and legs = 4. *Square window:* Flex hand at the wrist. Exert pressure sufficient to get as much flexion as possible. The angle between hypothenar eminence and anterior aspect of forearm is measured and scored. Do not rotate wrist. *Arm recoil:* With infant supine, fully flex forearm for 5 seconds, then fully extend by pulling the hands and release. Score as follows: remain extended or random movements = 0; incomplete or partial flexion = 2; brisk return to full flexion = 4. *Popliteal angle:* With infant supine and pelvis flat on examining surface, flex leg on thigh and fully flex thigh with one hand. With the other hand, extend leg and score the angle attained according to the chart. *Scarf sign:* With infant supine, draw infant's hand across the neck and as far across the opposite shoulder as possible. Assistance to elbow is permissible by lifting it across the body. Score according to location of the elbow: elbow reaches opposite anterior axillary line = 0; elbow between opposite anterior axillary line and midline of the thorax = 1; elbow at midline of thorax = 2; elbow does not reach midline of thorax = 3; elbow at proximal axillary line = 4. *Heel to ear:* With infant supine, hold infant's foot with one hand and move it as near to the head as possible without forcing it. Keep pelvis flat on examining surface. **(C)** Scoring for the Ballard assessment scale. The point total from assessment is compared to the left column. The matching number in the right column reveals the infant's age in gestation weeks. (From Ballard, J. L., Khoury, J. C., Wedig, K., et al. [1991]. New Ballard Score, expanded to include extremely premature infants. *Journal of Pediatrics, 119*[3]: 417–424.)

The Physical Examination

A newborn is given a preliminary physical examination as soon as parents have had an initial time to spend with their new child in addition to height and weight determinations, to establish gestational age and to detect any observable condition such as difficulty breathing, a congenital heart anomaly, or any birthmarks (Table 18.4). This assessment may be the responsibility of the primary care provider or a nurse depending on the facility and circumstances of birth. Always complete such assessments quickly to prevent exposing a newborn to chilling, yet not so swiftly that important findings are overlooked. About 20 hours after birth, when the baby's systems have had time to stabilize, a more thorough and detailed examination is performed (Xu, Yolton, & Khoury, 2011).

The Appearance of a Newborn

Although all newborns have similar physical findings, each is unique and has individual differences from all others.

The Skin

General inspection of a newborn's skin includes color, any birthmarks, and general appearance.

The Color

Most term newborns have a ruddier complexion for their first month than they will have later in life because of the increased concentration of red blood cells in their blood vessels and a decrease in the amount of subcutaneous fat, which makes blood vessels more visible. Infants with poor central nervous system control or respiratory difficulty may appear pale and cyanotic. Twins may be born with a twin transfusion phenomenon, in which one twin is larger and has good color and the smaller twin has pallor (Gandhi, Papanna, Teach, et al., 2012).

Cyanosis. Generalized mottling of the skin is a common finding in newborns. The lips, hands, and feet are likely to appear blue from immature peripheral circulation (termed

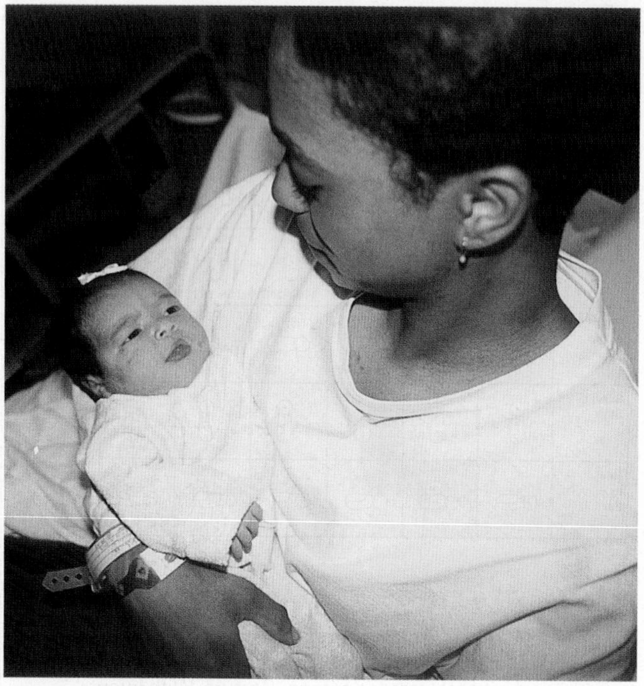

FIGURE 18.13 A newborn alerts at the sight of her parent's face and sound of her voice.

acrocyanosis). This can be so prominent in some newborns that the infant's hands appear as if a stricture at the wrist must be cutting off circulation because there is usual skin color on one side and blue on the other. Acrocyanosis this way is a normal finding at birth through the first 24 to 48 hours after birth.

In contrast, **central cyanosis**, or cyanosis of the trunk, is always a cause for concern. Central cyanosis indicates decreased oxygenation that could be occurring as the result of a temporary respiratory obstruction, and also could reflect a serious underlying respiratory or cardiac disease. Mucus obstructing a newborn's respiratory tract causes sudden cyanosis and apnea, but this can be relieved by suctioning of the mucus from the mouth and nose. In newborns, always suction the mouth before the nose, because suctioning the nose first may trigger a reflex gasp, possibly leading to aspiration if there is mucus in the posterior throat. Follow mouth suctioning with suction to the nose, because the nose is the chief conduit for air in newborns.

Hyperbilirubinemia. Hyperbilirubinemia is caused by the accumulation of excess bilirubin in blood serum. In the average newborn, the skin and sclera of the eyes begin to appear noticeably yellow on the second or third day of life as a result of a breakdown of fetal red blood cells (called **physiologic jaundice**), happening because, as the high red blood cell count built up in utero is being reduced, heme and globin are released.

- Heme is further broken down into iron (which is reused and not involved in the jaundice) and protoporphyrin.
- Protoporphyrin is then broken down into indirect bilirubin, a compound which is fat soluble and so cannot be excreted by the kidneys. In order to be removed from the body, it must be converted by the liver enzyme glucuronyl transferase into direct bilirubin, which is water soluble, and is then incorporated into the stool and excreted as feces.

Newborns can have difficulty with this process because their immature liver function prevents indirect bilirubin from being converted to direct bilirubin. As long as the buildup of indirect bilirubin that occurs remains in the circulatory system, the red coloring of the blood cells covers the yellow tint of the bilirubin. After the level of this indirect bilirubin rises to more than 7 mg/100 ml, however, bilirubin permeates through the blood vessels to tissue outside the circulatory system and the infant begins to appear jaundiced (Baston, 2012).

TABLE 18.4 Congenital Anomaly Appraisal

Procedure	Abnormalities Considered
Inquire for hydramnios or oligohydramnios	Presence of hydramnios (excessive amount of amniotic fluid) suggests congenital gastrointestinal obstruction. Oligohydramnios (lessened amount of amniotic fluid) suggests genitourinary obstruction or extreme prematurity.
Appearance of abdomen	Distended abdomen suggests ascites or tumor. Empty abdomen suggests diaphragmatic hernia.
Passage of nasogastric tube (#8 feeding catheter) through nares into stomach	Failure to pass nasogastric tube through nares on either side establishes choanal atresia. Failure to pass it into the stomach confirms presence of esophageal atresia.
Aspiration of stomach contents from feeding tube with recording of color and amount of fluid obtained.	With excess of 20 ml of fluid or yellow fluid, duodenal or ileal atresia is suspected.
Insertion of feeding tube into rectum	Failure to pass or obtain meconium on tip suggests imperforate anus or higher obstruction.
Counting of umbilical arteries	The presence of one artery suggests possible congenital urinary or cardiac anomalies or chromosomal trisomy (if other portions of examination are consistent).

Van Leeuwen, G., & Glenn, L. (1968). Screening for hidden congenital anomalies. *Pediatrics, 41*(6): 147–152. Copyright 1968, American Academy of Pediatrics.

Carefully observe infants who are prone to extensive bruising (large, breech, or preterm babies) for beginning jaundice because bruising leads to hemorrhage of blood into the subcutaneous tissue or skin; this blood then has to be broken down so can add to the amount of indirect bilirubin accumulating. A **cephalohematoma** is a collection of blood under the periosteum of the skull bone caused by pressure at birth. As the red blood cells in this type of lesion are hemolyzed, additional indirect bilirubin is also released and so can be yet another cause of jaundice (Nelson, Doering, Anderson, et al., 2012).

Another reason indirect bilirubin levels can increase is if a newborn has an intestinal obstruction because, with this, stool cannot be evacuated. Intestinal flora in the bowel then breaks down bile into its basic components, one of which is indirect bilirubin. Early feeding of newborns promotes intestinal movement and excretion of meconium and helps prevent indirect bilirubin buildup from this source.

Above normal indirect bilirubin levels are potentially dangerous because, if enough indirect bilirubin (about 20 mg/100 ml) leaves the bloodstream, it can interfere with the chemical synthesis of brain cells, resulting in permanent cell damage, a condition termed **acute bilirubin encephalopathy** or *kernicterus*. If this occurs, permanent neurologic damage, including cognitive challenge and vision and hearing disorders, may result.

The level of jaundice developing in newborns can be grossly judged by estimating the extent to which it has progressed on the surface of the infant's body because it is noticed first in the head and then spreads downward onto the body and legs.

Various commercial devices (transcutaneous bilirubinometry devices) are available to measure skin tone and help in estimating the level of bilirubin present. Although use of these devices rarely replaces serum measurements, they can be used to identify infants who need serum bilirubin determinations.

Treatment for physiologic jaundice or the routine rise in indirect bilirubin in newborns is rarely necessary, except for preventive measures such as early feeding to speed the passage of meconium.

There is no set level at which indirect serum bilirubin requires treatment because other factors, such as age, maturity, and breastfeeding status, affect this determination. If the level rises to more than 10 to 12 mg/100 ml, treatment is usually considered. Phototherapy (exposure of the infant to light to initiate maturation of liver enzymes) is common therapy (see Chapter 26). If this is necessary, the incubator and light source can be moved to the mother's room so the mother is not separated from her baby. Some infants need continued therapy after discharge and receive phototherapy at home either by a light-emitting diode (LED) or fluorescent lights over their crib or a phototherapy blanket (Baston, 2012).

Compared with formula-fed babies, a small proportion of breastfed babies may have more difficulty converting indirect bilirubin to direct bilirubin because breast milk contains pregnanediol (a metabolite of progesterone), which depresses the action of glucuronyl transferase. However, breastfeeding alone rarely causes enough jaundice to warrant therapy (Thilo & Rosenberg, 2011). The decision to stop nursing in the first 2 weeks of life because of jaundice must never be made lightly because it could interfere with breast filling and breast milk supply.

Pallor. Pallor in newborns is potentially serious because it usually occurs as the result of anemia, which may be caused by a number of circumstances such as:

- Low iron stores caused by poor maternal nutrition during pregnancy.
- Blood incompatibility in which a large number of red blood cells were hemolyzed in utero.
- Fetal–maternal transfusion.
- Inadequate flow of blood from the cord into the infant before the cord was cut.
- Excessive blood loss when the cord was cut.
- Internal bleeding. To detect this, a baby who appears pale should be watched closely for signs of blood in the stool or vomitus.

Newborns identified as having anemia need therapy such as supplemental iron or a packed red cell transfusion to restore their blood volume.

The Harlequin Sign. Occasionally, because of immature blood circulation, a newborn who has been lying on his or her side appears red on the dependent side of the body and pale on the upper side, as if a line had been drawn down the center of the body. This is a transient phenomenon and, although startling, is of no clinical significance. The odd coloring fades immediately if the infant's position is changed or the baby kicks or cries.

Birthmarks

Several common types of birthmarks occur in newborns. It is important to be able to differentiate the various types of hemangiomas that occur because some are more serious than others, and you do not want to give family members false reassurance nor worry them unnecessarily about these lesions.

Hemangiomas. The **hemangiomas** are vascular tumors of the skin and occur in three distinct types.

Nevus Flammeus. A **nevus flammeus** (Fig. 18.14A) is a macular purple or dark-red lesion (sometimes called a *port-wine stain* because its color is the same as that of red wine). These lesions are present at birth and typically appear either on the face or a thigh. Those present above the bridge of the nose tend to fade; others are less likely to do so. Because the lesion is level with the skin surface (macular), it can be covered by a cosmetic preparation later in life or, if large, removed by laser therapy (Faurschou, Olesen, Leonardi-Bee, et al., 2011).

Nevus flammeus lesions also occur as lighter, pink patches at the nape of the neck, known as *stork beak marks* or *telangiectasia* (see Fig. 18.14B). These occur more often in females than in males and do not fade, but because they are covered by the hairline, are of little consequence.

Strawberry Hemangioma. **Strawberry hemangiomas** are elevated areas formed by a combination of immature capillaries and endothelial cells (see Fig. 18.14C). Typically, these are not seen in preterm infants because of the immaturity of their epidermis. In term infants, most are present at the time of birth, although they may first appear up to 2 weeks after birth and continue to enlarge from their original size up to 1 year of age. After that, they tend to be absorbed and shrink in size. By the time the child is 7 years old, 50% to 75% of these lesions have disappeared, although a child may be 10 years old before the absorption is complete (Lyon, 2011).

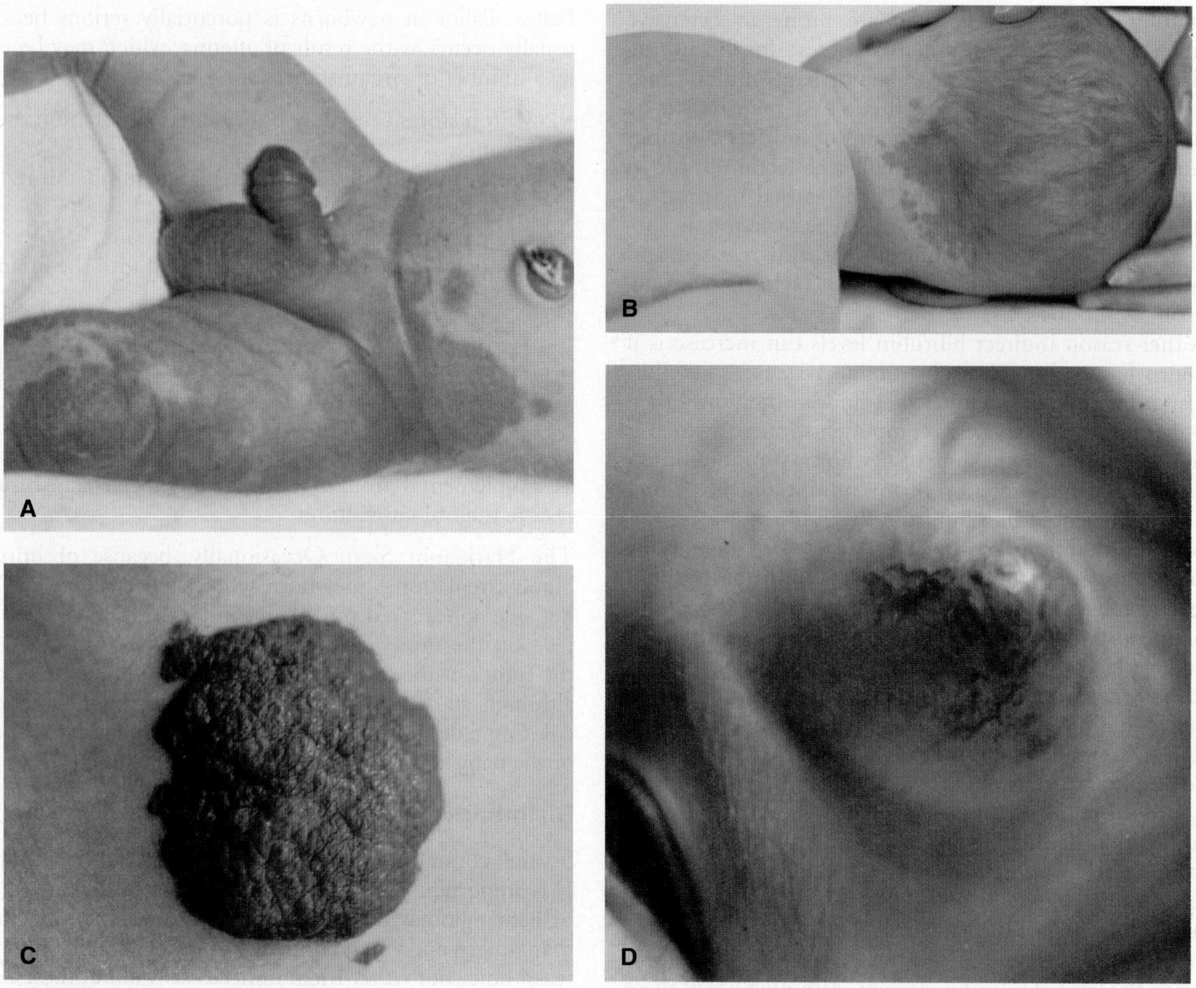

FIGURE 18.14 Types of hemangiomas found on a newborn. **(A)** Nevus flammeus (port-wine stain) formed of a plexus of newly formed capillaries in the papillary layer of the corium. It is deep red to purple, does not blanch on pressure, and does not fade with age. **(B)** A telangiectasia or stork beak mark, commonly occurring on nape of neck. It blanches on pressure; although it does not fade, it is not noticeable as it becomes covered by hair. **(C)** Strawberry hemangiomas consist of dilated capillaries in entire dermal and subdermal layers. They continue to enlarge after birth but usually disappear by age 10 years. **(D)** Cavernous hemangiomas consist of a communicating network of venules in subcutaneous tissue and do not fade with age.

Be certain parents understand that strawberry hemangiomas usually increase in size during their child's early years. Otherwise, they can worry their child has skin cancer (a skin lesion increasing in size is one of the seven danger signals of cancer). Be certain they also understand that the birthmark will eventually disappear, so they do not think of their child as imperfect. Surgery to remove strawberry hemangiomas is rarely recommended because this could lead to secondary infection with scarring and permanent disfigurement. A number of studies show the administration of propranolol (Inderal), administration of steroids, and pulsed laser therapy may be effective in speeding involution (Kroshinsky, Alper, & Holmes, 2011; Leonardi-Bee, Batta, O'Brien, et al., 2011).

Cavernous Hemangioma. **Cavernous hemangiomas** (see Fig. 18.14D) are caused by dilated vascular spaces. These are raised and irregular in shape and so resemble a strawberry hemangioma in appearance. They do not disappear with time, however, so will be permanent marks. They can be removed surgically, although because the lesion is deep, the place where it was removed may be evident afterward. Additional therapies such as administration of steroids, interferon alfa-2a, vincristine, or radiation to reduce these lesions in size may also be prescribed, although all of these therapies must be weighed in light of the serious effects these potent agents could create.

Children who have this type of skin lesion may have additional lesions on internal organs such as the spleen or liver (Sogawa, Fukuda, Tayama, et al., 2012). If these are present, blows to the abdomen, such as from a childhood game, could cause internal bleeding. For this reason, children with cavernous hemangiomas usually have their hematocrit levels assessed at health maintenance visits to evaluate for possible internal blood loss.

Mongolian Spots. **Mongolian spots** are collections of pigment cells (melanocytes) that appear as slate-gray patches across the sacrum or buttocks and possibly on the arms and legs of newborns. They tend to occur most often in children of

Asian, Southern European, or African ethnicity and disappear by school age without treatment (Thilo & Rosenberg, 2011). Be sure to inform parents that, although these look like bruises on a newborn, they are not. Otherwise, they may worry their baby sustained a birth injury from improper handling.

What if...18.2 Beth's father tells you he's not worried about the port-wine stain on his baby's thigh because he knows all birthmarks fade by school age. As a nurse, how would you respond to him?

Vernix Caseosa

Vernix caseosa is the white, cream cheese–like substance that serves as a skin lubricant in utero. Some of it is invariably noticeable on a term newborn's skin, at least in the skin folds, at birth. Document the color of any vernix present, because it takes on the color of the amniotic fluid (yellow vernix implies the amniotic fluid was stained from excessive bilirubin or a blood dyscrasia may be present; green vernix suggests meconium was present in the amniotic fluid).

Until the first bath, when vernix is washed away, handle newborns with gloves to protect yourself from exposure to this body fluid. Never rub it away harshly because newborn skin is tender and breaks in the skin caused by too vigorous attempts at removal could open portals of entry for bacteria.

Lanugo

Lanugo is the fine, downy hair that covers a term newborn's shoulders, back, upper arms, and possibly also the forehead and ears. Postterm infants (born after more than 42 weeks of gestation) rarely have lanugo. Babies born at 37 to 39 weeks, in contrast, have a generous supply of lanugo. Following birth, lanugo is rubbed away by the friction of bedding and clothes against the newborn's skin. By 2 weeks of age, it has usually totally disappeared.

Desquamation

Within 24 hours after birth, the skin of most newborns begins to dry. The dryness is particularly evident on the palms of the hands and soles of the feet and results in areas of peeling similar to those caused by sunburn. This is a temporary reaction to suddenly living in an air-filled rather than a liquid-filled environment and so needs no treatment. Parents may apply hand lotion to prevent excessive dryness if they wish.

Newborns who are postterm and have suffered intrauterine malnutrition may have such extremely dry skin that it has a leathery appearance and there are actual cracks in the skin folds. This should be differentiated from normal desquamation because it helps to diagnose the newborn as postterm.

Milia

Sebaceous glands in a newborn are immature, so at least one pinpoint white papule (a plugged or unopened sebaceous gland) is usually found on a cheek or across the bridge of the nose of every newborn. Such lesions, termed **milia** (Fig. 18.15), disappear by 2 to 4 weeks of age as the sebaceous glands mature and the plugged ones drain. Caution parents to avoid scratching or squeezing the papule while they wait for this to clear to prevent secondary infection.

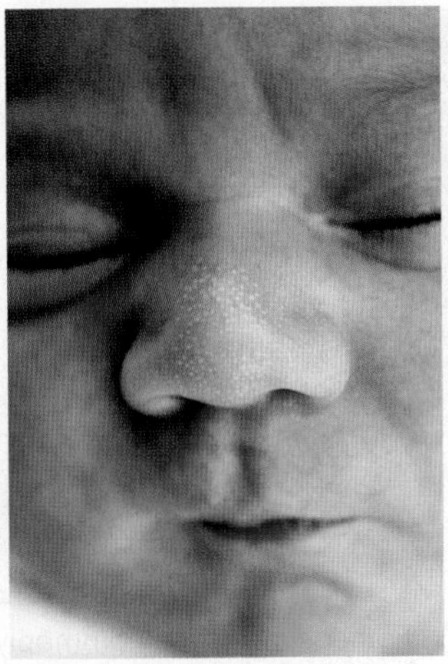

FIGURE 18.15 Milia are unopened sebaceous glands frequently found on the nose, chin, or cheeks of a newborn.

Erythema Toxicum

In most term newborns, some degree of a rash, called **erythema toxicum**, is present (Fig. 18.16). The rash usually appears in the first to fourth day of life, but may appear as late as 2 weeks of age. It begins with small papules, increases in severity to become erythematous by the second day, and then disappears by the third day. It is sometimes called a *flea-bite rash* because the lesions are so minuscule. One of the chief characteristics of the rash, aside from the pinpoint lesions, is its lack of pattern. It occurs sporadically and unpredictably and may last hours rather than days. It is probably caused by the newborn's eosinophils reacting to the rough environment of sheets and clothing rather than a smooth liquid against the skin. It requires no treatment. It is

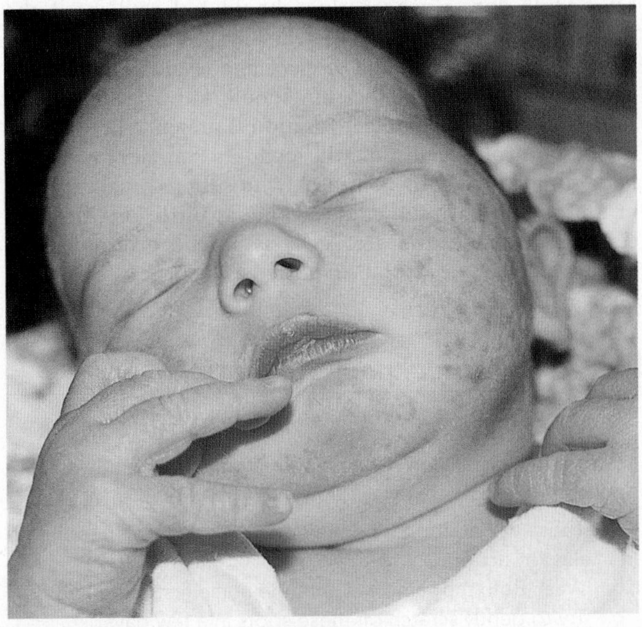

FIGURE 18.16 Erythema toxicum is found on almost all newborns. The reddish rash consists of sporadic pinpoint papules on an erythematous base. It fades spontaneously in a few days.

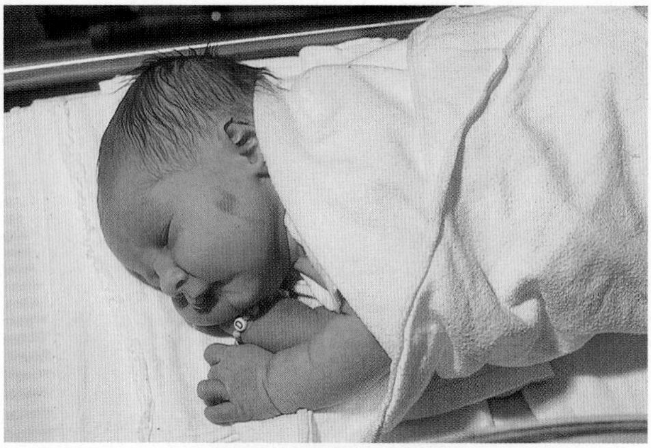

FIGURE 18.17 Forceps marks are commonly found in newborns born by forceps. Such marks are transient and disappear in a day or two.

important it be differentiated from lesions of herpes simplex (clustered vesicles) because herpes simplex is a serious finding in a newborn (Paul, 2011).

Forceps Marks

Forceps are rarely used for birth today, but if they are used (see Chapter 23), they may leave a circular or linear contusion matching the rim of the forceps blade on the infant's cheek (Fig. 18.17). The mark is the result of normal forceps use and does not denote unskilled or too vigorous application of forceps. The mark disappears in 1 to 2 days, along with the edema that accompanies it. Closely assess the face of a newborn with a forceps mark especially during a crying episode to be certain the infant's mouth is symmetrical, to detect any potential facial nerve injury requiring further evaluation.

Skin Turgor

Like adult skin, newborn skin should feel resilient if the underlying tissue is well hydrated. Grasp a fold of the skin between your thumb and fingers and evaluate if it feels elastic. When released, the skin should fall back to form a smooth surface. If severe dehydration is present, the skin will not smooth out again but will remain as an elevated ridge. Poor turgor is seen in newborns who suffered malnutrition in utero, who have difficulty sucking at birth, or who have certain metabolic disorders such as adrenocortical insufficiency. It always needs to be reported as it suggests extremely poor hydration.

QSEN Checkpoint Question 18.4

Safety

Beth Ruiz has milia on her nose. What teaching point would constitute a safety risk?

a. "These will disappear on their own, so you don't need to take any action."
b. "Wash Beth the same way that the nurse first taught you."
c. "Try to gently scratch off these spots in a few days."
d. "Make sure that you keep Beth bundled warmly."

Look in Appendix A for the best answer and rationale.

The Head

A newborn's head usually appears disproportionately large because it is about one fourth of the total body length compared with an adult, whose head is one eighth of total height. Other features include:

- The forehead of a newborn appears large and prominent.
- The chin appears to be receding, and it quivers easily if the infant is startled or cries.
- If a newborn has hair, the hair should look full bodied; both poorly nourished and preterm infants have thin, lifeless hair.
- If internal fetal monitoring was used during labor (see Chapter 24), a newborn may have a pinpoint ulcer at the point where the monitor was attached.

Fontanelles

The fontanelles are the spaces or openings where the skull bones join. The anterior fontanelle is located at the junction of the two parietal bones and the two fused frontal bones. It is diamond shaped and measures 2 to 3 cm (0.8 to 1.2 in.) in width and 3 to 4 cm (1.2 to 1.6 in.) in length. The posterior fontanelle is located at the junction of the parietal bones and the occipital bone. It is triangular and measures about 1–2 cm (0.4–0.7 in.) in length.

The anterior fontanelle can be felt as a soft spot. It should not appear indented (a sign of dehydration) or bulging (a sign of increased intracranial pressure) when the infant is held upright. The fontanelle may bulge if the newborn strains to pass a stool, cries vigorously, or is lying supine. The anterior fontanelle normally closes at 12 to 18 months of age. In some newborns, the posterior fontanelle is so small that it cannot be palpated readily. It closes by the end of the second month.

Sutures

The skull *sutures*, the separating lines of the skull, may override at birth because of the extreme pressure exerted on the head during passage through the birth canal. If the sagittal suture between the parietal bones overrides, the fontanelles are less perceptible than usual. The overriding subsides in 24 to 48 hours.

Suture lines should never appear widely separated in newborns. Wide separation suggests increased intracranial pressure because of abnormal brain formation, abnormal accumulation of cerebrospinal fluid in the cranium (hydrocephalus), or an accumulation of blood from a birth injury such as subdural hemorrhage. Fused suture lines also are abnormal; they require X-ray confirmation and further evaluation because this will prevent the head from expanding with brain growth.

Molding

The part of the infant's head that engaged the cervix (usually the vertex) molds to fit the cervix contours during labor. After birth, this area appears prominent and asymmetric (Fig. 18.18). You can assure parents the head will restore to its normal shape within a few days after birth.

Caput Succedaneum

Caput succedaneum (Fig. 18.19A) is edema of the scalp that forms on the presenting part of the head. It occurs in about

30% of cephalic births and can either involve wide areas of the head, or be so confined that it's the size of a large egg. The edema, which crosses the suture lines, is gradually absorbed and disappears at about the third day of life with no treatment needed (Wisser, Rothschild, Schmolling, et al., 2012).

Cephalohematoma

A *cephalohematoma*, a collection of blood between the periosteum of a skull bone and the bone itself, is caused by rupture of a periosteal capillary because of the pressure of birth (see Fig. 18.19B). Although the blood loss is negligible, edema, which appears by 24 hours after birth, appears severe and is well outlined as an egg shape. It may be discolored (black and blue) because of the presence of coagulated blood underneath the periosteum. Unlike a caput, a cephalohematoma is confined to an individual bone, so the associated swelling stops at the bone's suture line.

It often takes weeks for the blood under the periosteum to be absorbed, so it seems as if the blood could be aspirated to relieve the condition. However, such a procedure would introduce the risk of infection and is unnecessary because the condition will subside by itself. As the blood captured in the space is broken down, however, the infant needs to be observed for jaundice, which can occur from the great amount of indirect bilirubin that may be released (Watchko, 2011).

Craniotabes

Craniotabes is a localized softening of the cranial bones probably caused by pressure of the fetal skull against the mother's pelvic bone in utero. It is more common in first-born infants than in infants born later because of the lower position of the fetal head in the pelvis during the last 2 weeks of pregnancy in primiparous women. With craniotabes, the skull is

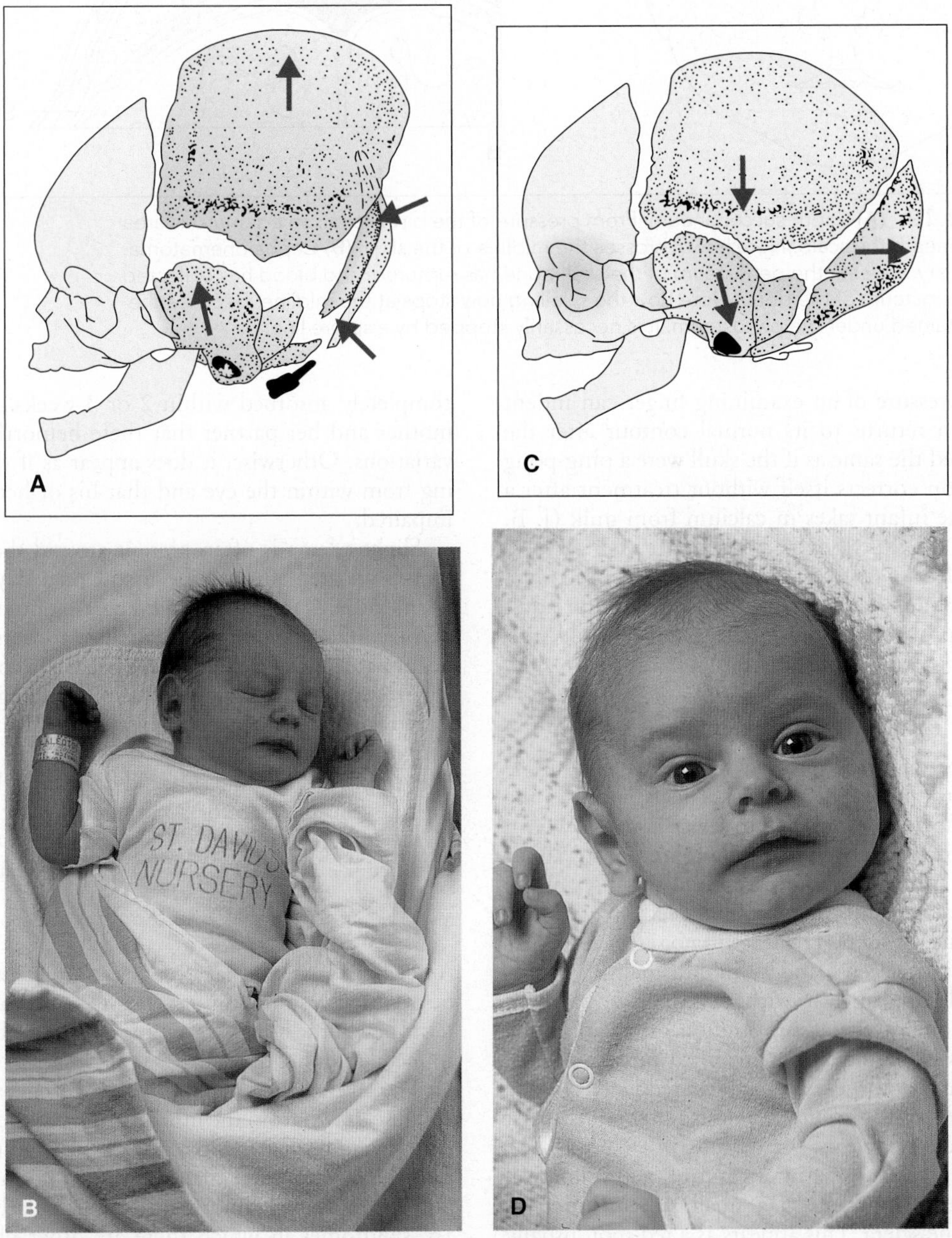

FIGURE 18.18 Molding. **(A,B)** The infant head molds to fit the birth canal more easily. On palpation, the skull sutures will be felt to be overriding. **(C,D)** The head shape returns to normal within 1 week.

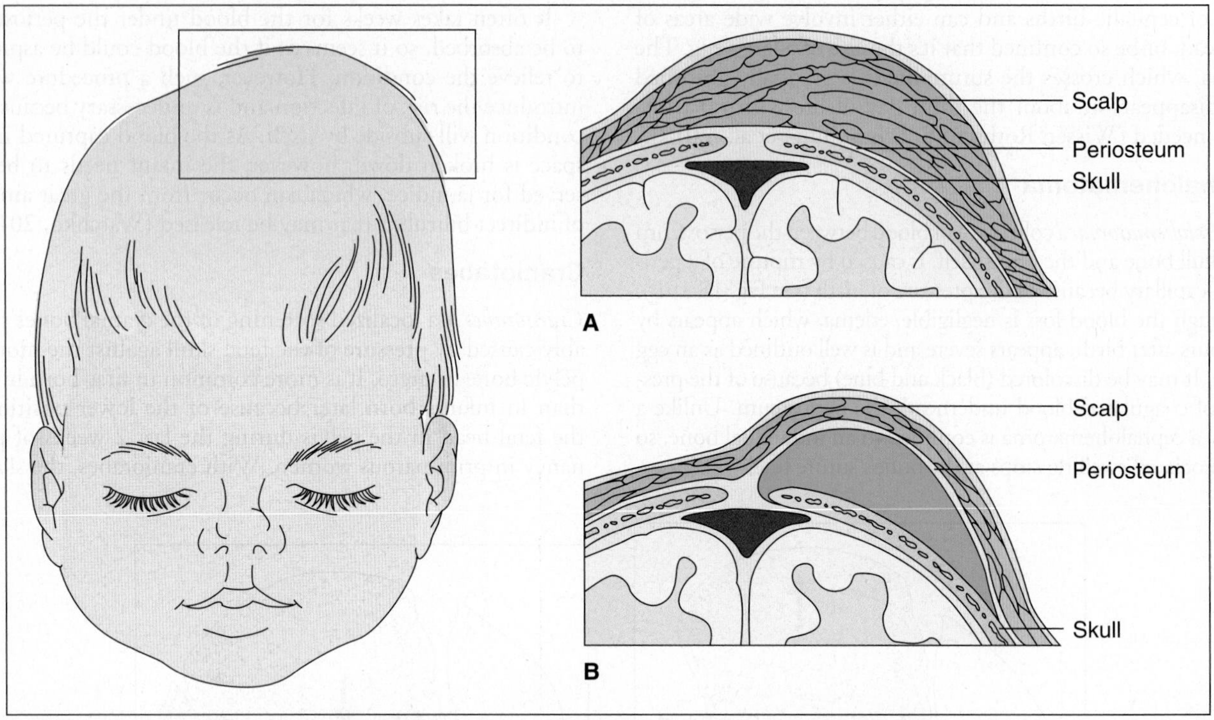

FIGURE 18.19 **(A)** Caput succedaneum. From pressure of the birth canal, an edematous area is present beneath the scalp. Note how it crosses the midline of the skull. **(B)** Cephalohematoma. A small capillary beneath the periosteum of the skull bone has ruptured, and blood has collected under the periosteum of the bone. Note how the swelling now stops at the midline. Because the blood is contained under the periosteum, it is necessarily stopped by a suture line.

so soft that the pressure of an examining finger can indent it. The bone then returns to its normal contour after the pressure is removed the same as if the skull were a ping-pong ball. The condition corrects itself without treatment after a few months as the infant takes in calcium from milk (J. B. Smith, 2011).

It is an example of a condition that is normal if seen in a newborn but would be pathologic in an older child or adult (because then it probably would be the result of faulty calcium metabolism or kidney dysfunction).

The Eyes

To inspect the eyes of a newborn, lay the infant in a supine position and lift the head; this maneuver usually causes the baby to open his or her eyes. It's rare to see tears in a newborn because their lacrimal ducts do not fully mature until about 3 months of age. Almost without exception, the irises of the eyes look gray or blue; the surrounding sclera may appear light blue due to its thinness. The iris will not assume its permanent color until between 3 and 12 months of age.

The eyes should appear clear, without redness or purulent discharge. Occasionally, the administration of an antibiotic ointment such as erythromycin at birth, to protect against chlamydia has caused the eyes to appear reddened with a slight discharge; if this has occurred, it lasts for about the first 24 hours of life before it clears.

Pressure during birth sometimes ruptures a conjunctival capillary of the eye, resulting in a small **subconjunctival hemorrhage** on the sclera. This appears as a red spot, usually on the inner aspect of the eye, or as a red ring around the cornea. The bleeding is slight, requires no treatment, and is completely absorbed within 2 or 3 weeks. You can assure a mother and her partner that these hemorrhages are normal variations. Otherwise, it does appear as if the baby is bleeding from within the eye and that his or her vision might be impaired.

Slight edema is often present around the orbit or on the eyelids and remains for the first 2 or 3 days until the newborn's kidneys are capable of evacuating fluid more efficiently.

Be certain the cornea of each eye appears round and proportionate in size to an adult eye because a cornea that appears larger than usual may be the result of congenital glaucoma. An irregularly shaped pupil or discolored iris may denote a congenital formation such as a coloboma (see Chapter 50). The pupil, as in adults, should appear dark. A white pupil suggests the presence of a congenital cataract or distortion of the retina (retinopathy of prematurity) (Rivera, Sapieha, Joyal, et al., 2011) (see Chapter 50 and Chapter 26).

The Ears

A newborn's external ear is not as completely formed as it will be eventually, so the pinna tends to bend forward easily. In a term newborn, however, the pinna should be strong enough to recoil after bending.

The level of the top part of the external ear should be even to a line drawn from the inner canthus to the outer canthus of the eye and back across the side of the head (see Chapter 34). Ears that are set lower than this are found in infants with certain chromosomal abnormalities, particularly trisomy 18 and 13, syndromes in which there are other physical variations coupled with varying degrees of cognitive challenge (Tsai, Manchester, & Elias, 2011) (see Chapters 7 and 54).

A small tag of skin is sometimes found just in front of an ear. Although these tags may be associated with chromosomal abnormalities or kidney disease, they usually are isolated findings of no consequence. They can be removed by ligation immediately or when the child is closer to 1 week old. Always inspect closely in front of newborns' ears for pinpoint-size openings that lead down to a hollow sinus because an open track under the skin lined with squamous epithelium may also be present at these sites. The sinus itself is usually small and inconsequential, but caution parents the closed space can become infected. If this occurs, the site will appear red and swollen and the infant will need an antibiotic ointment for this. The parents can have the tract removed surgically to prevent further infection.

Amniotic fluid and flecks of vernix usually still fill the ear canal, obliterating the tympanic membrane and its accompanying landmarks; therefore, visualization of the membrane is usually not attempted.

The AAP recommends all newborns be tested by a commercial standardized response to sound or confirmation they can hear before discharge from their birth setting (AAP, 2011). While waiting for a hearing examiner, infants can be tested by ringing a small bell held about 6 in. from each ear. A hearing infant will blink, attend to the bell's sound, and possibly startle.

The Nose

A newborn's nose usually has milia present and tends to appear large for the face. Always test for choanal atresia (blockage at the rear of the nose) when examining a newborn by closing the infant's mouth while compressing one naris at a time with your fingers. Note any discomfort or distress with breathing while one side of the nose is blocked this way.

The Mouth

A newborn's mouth should open evenly when he or she cries. If one side of the mouth curves more than the other, facial nerve injury is suggested. The tongue may appear short or "tongue tied" because the frenulum membrane is attached close to the tip. At one time, it was almost routine to snip a newborn's frenulum membrane to lengthen it. Now this procedure is regarded as harmful, because it leaves a portal of entry for infection, risks hemorrhage because of the low level of vitamin K in most newborns, and causes feeding difficulties by making the tongue sore and irritated. This procedure is also unnecessary because, as the tongue grows, the frenulum recedes to its adult placement.

Inspect the palate of a newborn to be certain it is intact. Occasionally, one or two small round, glistening, well-circumscribed cysts (Epstein pearls) can be seen on the palate from extra calcium having been deposited in utero. Be sure to inform parents that these pearl-like cysts are insignificant, require no treatment, and will disappear spontaneously within a week. Otherwise, a parent may mistake them for **thrush**, a *Candida* infection, which usually appears on the tongue and sides of the cheeks as white or gray patches and needs therapy with an antifungal drug such as nystatin (S. Smith, 2011).

Small, white epithelial pearls (benign inclusion cysts) may be noticed on the gum margins. Like Epstein pearls, no therapy is necessary for these. It is highly unusual for a newborn to have teeth, but sometimes one or two (called **natal teeth**) will have erupted. Any teeth that are present must be evaluated for stability. If loose, they are usually extracted (they remove easily) to prevent possible aspiration during feeding (Basavanthappa, Kagathur, Basavanthappa, et al., 2011).

It is rare to see a newborn without some mucus in the mouth. Newborns born by cesarean birth usually have an increased amount over vaginal birth infants. If a newborn is placed on the side, the mucus drains from the mouth and results in no distress. If the mouth is filled with so much mucus that the neonate seems to be blowing bubbles, suspect a tracheoesophageal fistula or a connection between the trachea and esophagus. It's important that this be confirmed or ruled out before the newborn is fed; otherwise, formula could be aspirated into the lungs from the inadequately formed esophagus (see Chapter 45 for a discussion of such fistulas).

The Neck

The neck of a newborn appears short and often chubby, with creased skin folds. The head should rotate or turn freely on it. If there is rigidity of the neck, congenital torticollis, caused by injury to the sternocleidomastoid muscle during birth, might be present (see Chapter 27). In newborns whose membranes were ruptured more than 24 hours before birth, there is a possibility nuchal rigidity could be a beginning sign of meningitis.

The neck of a newborn is not strong enough to support the total weight of the head but in a sitting position, a newborn should make a momentary effort at head control. When lying prone, newborns can raise the head slightly, usually enough to lift the nose out of mucus or spit-up milk. If they are pulled into a sitting position from a supine position, the head will lag behind considerably. Again, however, they should make some effort to control and steady the head as they reach a sitting position.

The trachea usually appears prominent on the front of the neck. The thymus gland also appears enlarged because of the rapid growth of glandular tissue (in comparison with other body tissue) early in life. Even though the thymus appears to be enlarged and bulging, it is rarely a cause of respiratory difficulty; in addition, it plays too critical a role in providing immunity to be removed (Rote, 2012).

The Chest

The chest in most newborns looks small because the head is so large in proportion to it (an important finding at birth so the largest diameter of the baby is born first). The chest averages 2 cm (0.75 to 1 in.) smaller in circumference than the head and is as wide in the anteroposterior diameter as it is across. Both right and left sides should appear symmetric. Not until a child is 2 years of age does the chest measurement exceed that of the head.

The clavicles should appear straight and feel smooth. A *crepitus* (crackling) or an actual separation of one or the other clavicle suggests a fracture occurred during birth (which occurs most often in large infants) and calcium is now being deposited at that point (Lurie, Wand, Golan, et al., 2011).

A supernumerary nipple (usually found below and in line with the normal nipples) may be present. In both female and male infants, the breasts may be engorged because of the influence of maternal hormones during pregnancy. Occasionally, the breasts of newborn babies secrete a thin, watery fluid popularly termed *witch's milk.* As soon as the hormones are cleared from the infant's system (about 1 week), the engorgement and

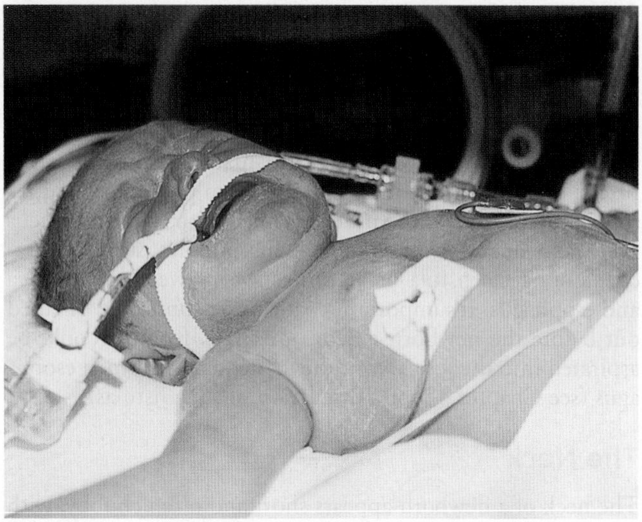

FIGURE 18.20 Sternal retractions are a sign of respiratory distress requiring immediate intervention, such as mechanical ventilation or increased oxygen.

any fluid that is present will subside. Fluid should never be expressed from infants' breasts, because the manipulation could introduce bacteria and lead to *mastitis* (infection of the breast).

Respirations are normally rapid (30 to 60 breaths/min) but not distressed. *Retraction* (drawing in of the chest wall with inspiration) should not be present. An infant who is breathing with retractions (Fig. 18.20) is using such a strong force to pull air into the respiratory tract that he or she is pulling in the anterior chest muscle as well. Newborns do not have the strength to breathe this way for a long period of time, and so need immediate help such as oxygen therapy before respirations fail.

Because a newborn's lung alveoli open slowly over the first 24 to 48 hours and the baby invariably has mucus in the back of the throat, listening to lung sounds often reveals the sounds of rhonchi—the harsh, innocent sound of air passing over mucus. An abnormal sound, such as grunting, suggests *respiratory distress syndrome*, and a high, crowing sound on inspiration suggests stridor or immature tracheal development, both conditions, again, that need immediate consultation (see Chapter 40).

The Abdomen

The contour of a newborn abdomen looks slightly protuberant. A scaphoid or sunken appearance suggests missing abdominal contents or a diaphragmatic hernia (bowel positioned in the chest instead of the abdomen). Bowel sounds or proof the bowel is beginning peristalsis should be present within 1 hour after birth. On the right side, the edge of the liver is usually palpable 1 to 2 cm below the costal margin. On the left side, the edge of the spleen may be palpable 1 to 2 cm below the left costal margin. It is difficult to determine if the newborn feels tenderness in the abdomen. If sensitivity is extreme, however, palpation will cause the infant to cry, thrash about, or tense the abdominal muscles to protect against any more pressure on the abdomen.

For the first hour after birth, the stump of the umbilical cord appears as a white, gelatinous structure marked with the blue and red streaks of the one umbilical vein and the two arteries. Any child with a single umbilical artery needs close observation and assessment until anomalies are ruled out because these are frequently associated with the lack of an umbilical artery (Kondi-Pafiti, Kleanthis, Mavrigiannaki, et al., 2011).

Always inspect the cord clamp to be certain it is secure. After the first hour of life, the cord will begin to dry, shrink, and turn brown as if it were the dead end of a vine. By the second or third day, it will have turned black. On day 6 to 10, it breaks free, leaving a granulating area a few centimeters wide that will heal during the following week.

There should be no bleeding at the base of the cord because this suggests the cord clamp has become loosened or the cord has been tugged loose by the friction of bedclothes. In addition, the base of the cord should not appear wet. A moist or odorous cord suggests infection, a situation that requires immediate antibiotic therapy to prevent the infectious organisms from entering the newborn's bloodstream and causing septicemia. Moistness at the base of the cord also may indicate a patent urachus (a narrow opening that connects the bladder and the umbilicus), which will drain urine at the cord site until it is surgically repaired (Tsai & Yeh, 2011).

As a last assessment, inspect the base of the cord to be certain no abdominal wall defect such as an umbilical hernia is present. If there is a fascial (abdominal wall) defect smaller than 2 cm in diameter, this will usually close on its own by school age; if the defect is larger than this, it will probably require surgical correction. Taping or putting buttons or coins on the cord are home remedies often suggested to help fascial defects to close. In truth, heavy taping may worsen the condition by preventing the development of good muscle tone in the abdominal wall. Tape also tends to keep the cord moist, making an infection more likely than when it is dry.

When a newborn voids, it only demonstrates there is one kidney functioning (but not two); therefore, attempt to verify the presence of kidneys by deep palpation of the right and left abdomen within the first few hours after birth because, after this time, the intestines fill with air, thus making palpation more difficult (see Chapter 34). A small kidney suggests decreased function; an enlarged kidney suggests a polycystic kidney or pooling of urine from a urethral obstruction.

To finish an abdominal assessment, elicit an abdominal reflex. Stroking each quadrant of the abdomen with a finger should cause the umbilicus to move or "wink" in that direction. This superficial abdominal reflex, a test of spinal nerves T8 through T10, although usually present at birth, may not be observable until it is stronger at about the 10th day of life.

✔ QSEN Checkpoint Question 18.5

Teamwork & Collaboration

Mrs. Ruiz is preparing to take her new daughter home and has asked an unlicensed care provider when Beth's dried umbilical cord will fall off. You should confirm that the care provider has stated what time?

a. Day 1
b. Days 2 to 3
c. Days 6 to 10
d. Day 30

Look in Appendix A for the best answer and rationale.

The Anogenital Area

Examine the anus of a newborn to be certain the structure is present. Test for anal patency and that the anus is not covered by a membrane (imperforate anus) by gently inserting the tip of your gloved and lubricated little finger. Also note the time after birth at which the infant first passes meconium. If a newborn does not do so in the first 24 hours, suspect an imperforate anus or meconium ileus (Zderic & Lambert, 2012).

The Male Genitalia

The scrotum in most male newborns is edematous and has rough rugae on the surface. It may be deeply pigmented in dark-skinned newborns. Both testes should be palpable in the scrotum. If one or both testicles are not present (cryptorchidism), referral is needed to establish the extent of the problem. This condition could be caused by agenesis (absence of the testes), ectopic testes (the testes are present in the abdomen but cannot enter the scrotum because the opening to the scrotal sac is closed), or undescended testes (the vas deferens or artery is too short to allow the testes to descend). Make a practice of pressing your nondominant hand against the inguinal ring before palpating for testes, so they do not slip upward and out of the scrotal sac as you palpate (Fig. 18.21). Newborns with agenesis of the testes are usually referred for investigation of kidney anomalies, because the testes arise from the same germ tissue as the kidneys (Tasian, Copp, & Baskin, 2011).

Always elicit a cremasteric reflex by stroking the internal side of the thigh while inspecting testes (as the skin on the thigh is stroked, the testis on that side moves perceptibly upward). The response is indication that spinal nerves T8 through T10 are intact, although it may be absent before 10 days of age when nerve stabilization is complete.

The penis of newborns appears small, approximately 2 cm long. If it is less than this, the newborn should be referred for evaluation by an endocrinologist to be certain there aren't other occurring anomalies. Inspect the tip of the penis to be certain the urethral opening is at the tip of the glans, not on the dorsal surface (epispadias) or on the ventral surface (hypospadias). In most newborns, the prepuce (foreskin) slides back poorly from the meatal opening, so don't try to retract it.

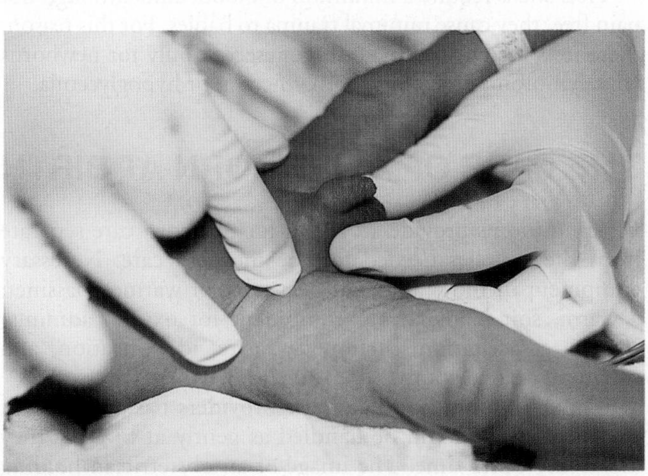

FIGURE 18.21 Press the nondominant hand against the inguinal ring when palpating the testes.

The Female Genitalia

The vulva in female newborns may appear swollen because of the effect of maternal hormones during intrauterine life. Some female newborns also have a mucus vaginal secretion, sometimes blood tinged **(pseudomenstruation)**, which is caused, again, by the action of maternal hormones. The discharge disappears in 1 or 2 days and should not be mistaken for an infection or taken as an indication that trauma has occurred.

The Back

A newborn normally assumes the position maintained in utero for days after birth, so the back is held rounded with the arms and legs flexed across the abdomen and chest. A child who was born in a frank breech position tends to straighten the legs at the knee and bring them up next to the face. The position of a baby with a face presentation sometimes simulates opisthotonos (backward arching of the spine) for the first week, because the curve of the back is deeply concave.

The spine of a newborn typically appears flat in the lumbar and sacral areas because the curves seen in an adult appear only after a child is able to sit and walk. Inspect the base of a newborn's spine carefully to be certain there is no pinpoint opening, dimpling, or sinus tract in the skin, because this is a common place for these to occur and would suggest a dermal sinus or spina bifida occulta (see Chapter 27) (Paneth, 2011).

The Extremities

The arms and legs of a newborn appear short in proportion to the trunk. The hands may seem plump and are typically held clenched into fists. Newborn fingernails feel soft and smooth, and are usually long enough to extend over the fingertips. Test the upper extremities for muscle tone by unflexing the arms for approximately 5 seconds then letting them return to their flexed position (which typically occurs immediately if muscle tone is good). Next, hold the arms down by the sides and note their length. The fingertips on both sides should reach as far as the mid-thigh. Unusually short arms may signify achondroplasia (dwarfism) and so needs documented.

Observe also for unusual curvature of the little finger, and inspect the palm for a simian crease (a single palmar crease, in contrast to the three creases normally seen in a palm). Although curved fingers and simian creases can occur normally, they are a mark of Down syndrome (Haldeman-Englert, Saitta, & Zackai, 2011).

When a newborn moves, the arms and legs should move symmetrically (unless the infant is demonstrating a tonic neck reflex). If one arm hangs limp and unmoving, it suggests possible birth injury, such as injury to a clavicle or to the brachial or cervical plexus or fracture of a long bone. Assess for webbing (syndactyly) between fingers as well as missing or extra fingers (polydactyly). Test to see whether the fingernails fill immediately after blanching from pressure to test for adequate blood circulation in the arms.

Newborn legs appear bowed as well as short. The sole of the foot is flat because of an extra pad of fat in the longitudinal arch. The foot of a term newborn has many crisscrossed lines on the sole, covering approximately two thirds of the foot. If these creases cover less than two thirds of the foot or are absent, it suggests the infant is preterm.

Move the ankle through a range of motion to evaluate that the heel cord is not unusually tight. Check for ankle clonus by supporting the lower leg in one hand and dorsiflexing the foot sharply two or three times by pressure on the sole of the foot with the other hand. After the dorsiflexion, one or two continued movements are normal. Rapid alternating contraction and relaxation (clonus) is not and suggests neurologic or calcium insufficiency involvement. The feet of many newborns turn in (varus deviation) because of their former intrauterine position. This simple deviation needs no correction if the feet can be brought into the midline position by easy manipulation. When the infant begins to bear weight, the feet will align themselves without treatment.

If a foot does not align readily or will not turn to a definite midline position, a talipes deformity (clubfoot) may be present. This condition needs further investigation because congenital problems of this kind are best treated in the immediate newborn period.

To test if the femur is situated comfortably in the hip socket, with a newborn in a supine position, flex both hips and abduct the legs as far as they will go (typically 180 degrees or the knees touch or nearly touch the surface of the bed) (Fig. 18.22). If the hip joint seems to lock short of this distance (160 to 170 degrees), hip subluxation (a shallow and poorly formed acetabulum) is suggested (Walter, 2011). Confirm subluxation by holding the infant's legs with the fingers on the greater and lesser trochanters and then abduct the hips; if subluxation is present, a "clunk" of the femur head striking the shallow acetabulum can be heard (Ortolani sign). If the femur can be felt to actually slip in and out of the socket, this is a Barlow sign. A subluxated hip may be bilateral but is usually unilateral. Like talipes disorders, it is important that a hip subluxation be discovered as early as possible because correction is most successful if it is initiated early.

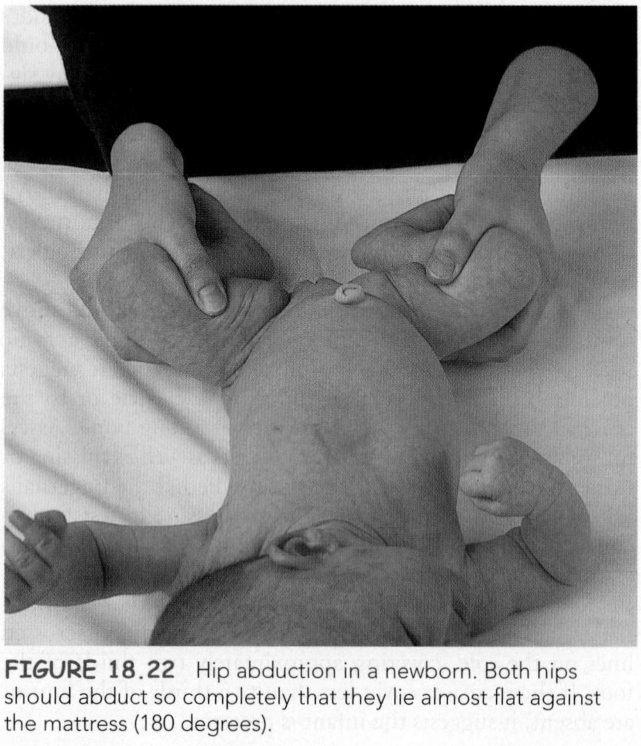

FIGURE 18.22 Hip abduction in a newborn. Both hips should abduct so completely that they lie almost flat against the mattress (180 degrees).

Lastly, inspect the feet for missing or extra toes or unusual spacing of toes, particularly between the big toe and the others; although this finding can be a normal finding in some families, it is also present in certain chromosomal disorders. When placed on their abdomen, newborns should be capable of bringing their arms and legs underneath them and raising their stomach off the bed high enough for a hand to be slipped underneath. The ability to do this helps to prevent pressure or rubbing at the cord site, because in this position, the cord does not actually touch the bedding. The preterm newborn is not able to do this, so raising the stomach this way is an indication of a term infant.

Laboratory Studies

After the first hour of undisturbed rest, depending on health agency policy, newborns may have a heel-stick test for hematocrit, hemoglobin, and hypoglycemia determinations. Hemoglobin is assessed to detect newborn anemia that could have been caused by hypovolemia because of bleeding from placenta previa or abruptio placentae or by a cesarean birth that involved incision into the placenta. Another condition as dangerous as anemia is the presence of an excess of red blood cells (polycythemia), probably caused by excessive flow of blood into an infant from the umbilical cord. A heel-stick hematocrit reveals both hypovolemia and hypervolemia if they are present; treatment can then be instituted. A normal hematocrit level at 1 hour of life is about 50% to 55%.

Hypoglycemia, like anemia, produces few symptoms in newborns, therefore the heel capillary blood sample is necessary to determine if it is present. If the serum glucose reading is found to be less than 40 mg/100 ml of blood (30 mg/100 ml in the first 3 days of life), hypoglycemia is said to be present. To correct this condition, the infant is prescribed oral glucose or is breastfed immediately because either of these therapies will elevate the infant's blood sugar to a safe level. It is important to treat hypoglycemia quickly this way because, if brain cells become completely depleted of glucose, brain damage can result. If a newborn exhibits symptoms of hypoglycemia (e.g., jitteriness, lethargy, seizures) in addition to the low laboratory test results, intravenous glucose probably will be prescribed. A continuous intravenous infusion of glucose may be necessary if the newborn is unable to maintain glucose levels higher than 40 mg/100 ml.

Heel sticks require a minimum of blood, and, although not pain free, they cause minimal trauma to babies. For this reason, these tests are not routine but are reserved only for newborns with symptoms of anemia, polycythemia, or hypoglycemia.

THE CARE OF A NEWBORN AT BIRTH

Birthing rooms provide an island for newborn care separate from the supplies needed for the mother's care. Necessary equipment includes a radiant heat table or warmed bassinet; a warm, soft blanket; and equipment for oxygen administration, resuscitation, suction, eye care, identification, and weighing of a newborn.

The philosophy of health care providers has always been that newborns should be handled as gently at birth as they are at any other time. The image of an obstetrician holding a newborn up by the heels and spanking to stimulate breathing exists only in movies because holding a baby by the feet and letting the back extend fully is probably painful after the months spent in a flexed position in utero. In addition, a measure such as spanking is not as effective in helping a newborn breathe as is gentle stimulation, such as rubbing the back.

Newborn Identification and Registration

Because newborns have no way of identifying themselves, an important nursing responsibility is to be certain they have an identification band in place, so medicine administration or performing procedures can be done safely.

Identification Banding

One traditional form of identification used with newborns is a plastic bracelet with a permanent lock that requires cutting to be removed. A number that corresponds to the mother's hospital number; the mother's name; and the sex, date, and time of the infant's birth are printed on the band. If an identification band is attached to a newborn's arm or leg, two bands should be used because a newborn's wrist and hand, as well as the ankle and foot, are not very different in width, so bands can slide off easily. A newer form of identification band has a built-in sensor unit that sounds an alarm—similar to those attached to clothing in department stores to stop shoplifting—if a baby is transported beyond set hospital boundaries (Fig. 18.23).

After identification bands are attached, an infant's footprints may be taken (Fig. 18.24A) and thereafter kept with the baby's electronic record for permanent identification (see Fig. 18.24B). Babies who are born elsewhere and then admitted to the hospital should have bands applied and their footprints taken on admission.

Infant Abduction. Another reason that infant identification is important is because there exists the possibility that a newborn may be handed to the wrong mother or be switched or abducted from a health care facility. The profile of someone who might abduct a newborn is a woman who has recently lost a pregnancy or had an infant stillborn and therefore desires an infant very much. She often is someone familiar with hospitals; she may pretend to be a volunteer or an unlicensed health care worker and says she needs to take a baby out of the nursery or the mother's room for a procedure. Although this is rare, all health care agency personnel need to be alert to the potential danger of newborn abduction and not only take measures to prevent this from happening but also alert parents to the danger so they can take measures as well (Box 18.4).

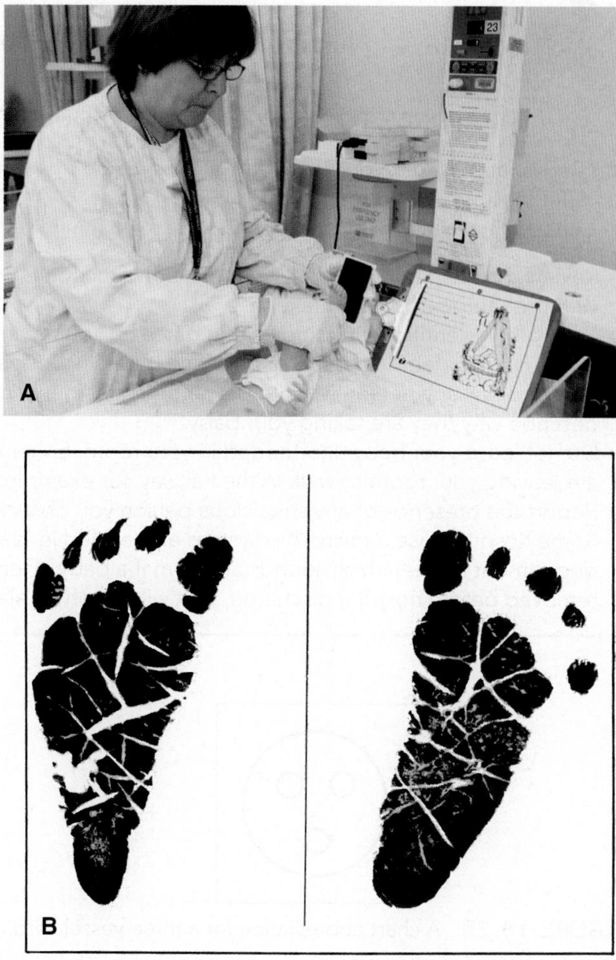

FIGURE 18.24 **(A)** Footprinting a newborn for identification. **(B)** Newborn footprints.

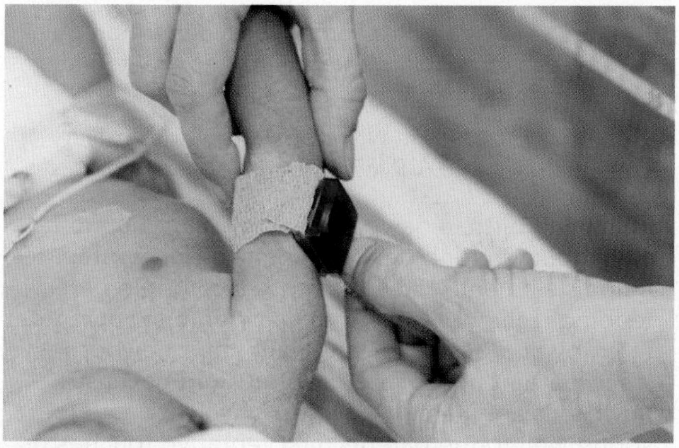

FIGURE 18.23 This newborn is wearing a security band, which sets off an alarm and locks exits if an infant is taken off the unit.

Birth Registration

The primary care provider who supervised a newborn's birth has the responsibility to be certain a birth registration is filed with the Bureau of Vital Statistics for the state in which the infant was born. The infant's name, the mother's name, the father's name (if the mother chooses to reveal this), and the birth date and place are recorded. Official birth information such as this is important for proving eligibility for school and, later, for voting, passports, and Social Security benefits.

Birth Record Documentation. The infant's chart is also a vital piece of documentation because it serves as a baseline indicating whether the infant was well at birth. Be certain a newborn chart contains the following:

- Time of birth
- Time the infant breastfed
- Whether respirations were spontaneous or aided
- Apgar score at 1 minute and at 5 minutes of life
- Whether eye prophylaxis was given

BOX 18.4 Nursing Care Planning Based on Family Teaching

MEASURES TO HELP PREVENT ABDUCTION FROM A BIRTH SETTING UNIT

Q. Beth's mother tells you, "I've read babies are being kidnapped from hospitals. How can we make sure that doesn't happen to us?"

A. Although abduction is rare, it can happen. To minimize the risk, use the following guidelines:

- Review the hospital's newborn identification procedure with a nurse so you are familiar with it and can feel comfortable with the safeguards being taken.
- Check that identification bands are in place on your infant as you care for her because these can slide off easily over small hands or feet. If a band or necklace is missing, ask a nurse to replace it immediately.
- Do not allow any person without proper hospital identification to remove your baby from your room. Be certain they describe why they are taking your baby.
- Do not leave your baby unattended in your room. Either return the baby to the nursery or take your baby with you if you are leaving your room to walk in the hallway, for example.
- Report the presence of any suspicious person you observe in the unit.
- Some hospitals use a microchip system embedded in identification bands, similar to the tag used to thwart shoplifting in department stores, which sounds an alarm if a baby is removed from the unit. If this type of band is used, be certain it is removed before hospital discharge, or it will set off an alarm as you leave.

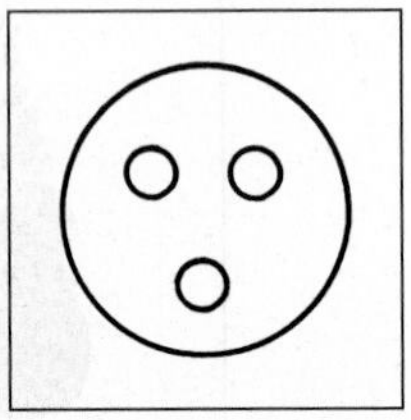

FIGURE 18.25 A chart abbreviation for a three-vessel cord.

BOX 18.5 Nursing Care Planning to Respect Cultural Diversity

What new parents believe is usual newborn care is not consistent across cultures and actually varies a great deal. Although it is enjoyable to point out the positive aspects of their new child to parents in order to aid parent–child bonding, in some areas of the world, such as Cambodia and Laos, newborns are not given compliments this way because it is believed compliments could leave them vulnerable to invading spirits. In other cultures, it is vitally important for a newborn to have an amulet (good-luck charm) tied around the neck or wrist to ward off danger. Respect these as important items and leave them in place when caring for the infant.

In the traditional Haitian culture and some Native American cultures, infants are not named immediately, but only after a set period of time (to be certain the name will truly reflect the child's personality). Oiling the infant's body and placing a belly band over the umbilical cord (thought to reduce the incidence of umbilical hernias) also are common care practices. Being aware of cultural variations in newborn care such as these helps you plan care specific and meaningful to individual parents and can aid parent–child bonding as well as parent–nurse relationships.

- Whether vitamin K was administered
- General condition of the infant
- Number of vessels in the umbilical cord
- Whether cultures were taken (they are taken if at some point a sterile birth technique was broken or if the mother has a history of vaginal or uterine infection)
- Whether the infant voided and whether he or she passed a stool (this information is helpful if, later on, the diagnosis of bowel obstruction or the absence of a kidney is considered)

Many nurses indicate a three-vessel cord with the symbol shown in Figure 18.25. Do not mistake this drawing for a "smiling face" and assume it is not important in a health record.

Nursing Diagnoses and Related Interventions

Nursing Diagnosis: Risk for ineffective thermoregulation related to newborn's transition to extrauterine environment

Outcome Evaluation: Newborn establishes axillary temperature of 98.6°F (37°C) by 1 hour after birth.

Following birth, a newborn is placed on the mother's abdomen for a period of skin-to-skin contact to help retain heat. Allow the mother to begin breastfeeding if she wishes and to allow time for parents to enjoy and get acquainted with their newborn. It's important not to interrupt this time because newborns are alert (first period of activity) and respond well to the parents' first tentative touches or interactions with them during this time (Box 18.5).

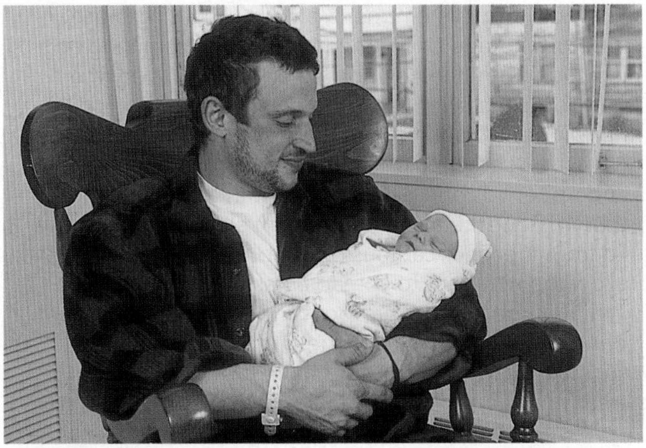

FIGURE 18.26 A newborn wrapped and capped to conserve body heat.

After about a half hour, is a good time to begin routine care such as footprinting and administering eye drops if the parents want eye drops administered. Be certain to adhere to standard infection precautions, such as wearing gloves, when caring for newborns. Grasp a newborn firmly when lifting him or her off the mother's abdomen. Newborn skin is slippery because of amniotic fluid and vernix caseosa, which means they can slip through your hands easily.

All of the measures mentioned previously such as skin-to-skin contact, gently rubbing a newborn dry, swaddling the infant with a blanket, and placing a cap on the infant's head (Fig. 18.26) not only help to prevent heat loss but also help to mimic the tight confines of the uterus, which can offer a sense of security and comfort (Pillai-Riddell, Racine, Turcotte, et al., 2011).

Although the temperature of newborns who are dried, wrapped, and then held by their parents immediately after birth apparently falls slightly lower than that of infants placed in heated cribs, their core temperature does not fall below safe limits.

At the end of the first hour of life, a newborn can be bathed quickly to remove excess vernix caseosa and blood, then dressed in a shirt and diaper, reswaddled in a snug blanket, and placed in a bassinet or returned to one or the other of the parents.

During the first day of life, a newborn's temperature is usually taken and recorded every 4 to 8 hours. After that, unless the infant's temperature is elevated or subnormal or the infant appears to be in distress, temperature measurement once a day while in the health care facility is enough. If an infant has difficulty maintaining temperature, place him or her in a warmed incubator or on a radiant heat warmer and notify the primary care provider because the infant may be more immature than was estimated or is ill in some way.

Nursing Diagnosis: Risk for ineffective airway clearance related to presence of mucus in mouth and nose at birth

Outcome Evaluation: Neonate maintains a respiratory rate of 30 to 60 breaths/min without evidence of retraction or grunting by 5 minutes after birth.

A number of measures help ensure a newborn is breathing effectively.

Record the First Cry: A crying infant is a breathing infant because the sound of crying is made by a current of air passing over the larynx. The more lusty the cry, the greater the assurance the newborn is breathing deeply and forcefully. Vigorous crying may also help blow off the extra carbon dioxide that makes all newborns slightly acidotic, and so helps to correct this condition. Although gentleness is necessary to make an infant's transition from intrauterine life to extrauterine life as nontraumatic as possible for these reasons, there is no need to completely halt the initial crying of a newborn.

A newborn who does not breathe spontaneously at birth or who takes a few quick, gasping breaths but then is unable to maintain respirations needs resuscitation as an emergency measure. An infant with grunting respirations needs careful observation for respiratory distress syndrome (see Chapter 26).

Promote Adequate Breathing Pattern and Prevent Aspiration: Although not done routinely, if a newborn appears to have a great deal of mucus in the mouth following birth, the primary care provider can suction this from the infant's mouth by a bulb syringe before the infant is laid on the mother's abdomen in order to prevent aspiration of the secretions. If the infant continues to have an accumulation of mucus in the mouth or nose after these first steps, you may need to suction further after the baby is placed under a warmer. Use a bulb syringe or a soft, small (#10 or 12) catheter. Never suction vigorously, because this irritates the mucous membrane and could leave a portal of entry for infection. Brisk suctioning also has been associated with bradycardia in newborns because of vagal nerve stimulation. If you use a bulb syringe, decompress the bulb before inserting it into the infant's mouth or nose; otherwise, the force of decompression of the bulb will push secretions back into the pharynx or bronchi rather than remove them. Although the use of the procedure is not standardized, when an infant is born with meconium-stained amniotic fluid, intubation may be performed so deep tracheal suction can be accomplished before the first breath to help prevent meconium aspiration into the lungs (Leone & Finer, 2011). The use of surfactant and inhaled nitric oxide may also be helpful to assist breathing if meconium aspiration has occurred (discussed in Chapter 26) (Swarnam, Soraisham, & Sivanandan, 2012).

Nursing Diagnosis: Risk for infection related to newly clamped umbilical cord and exposure of eyes to vaginal secretions

Outcome Evaluation: Area around cord is dry and free of erythema. Eyes are free of inflammation and drainage. Axillary temperature is maintained between 97.6°F and 98.6°F (36.5°C and 37°C).

Inspect and Care for the Umbilical Cord: The umbilical cord pulsates for a moment after an infant is born as a last flow of blood passes from the placenta into the infant. Two clamps are then applied to the cord about 8 inches from the infant's abdomen, and the cord is cut between the clamps. The woman's partner may choose to cut the cord as his or her responsibility. The infant cord is then reclamped by a permanent cord clamp, such as a Hazeltine or a Kane clamp (see Chapter 15, Fig. 15.28).

Every time you handle a newborn, inspect the cord to be certain it is clamped securely, because if a clamp should loosen before thrombosis obliterates the umbilical vessels, hemorrhage could result. As previously mentioned, the number of cord vessels should be counted and noted immediately after the cord is cut because they are most visible before drying begins. Until the cord falls off, at about 7 to 10 days later, be certain diapers are folded below the level of the umbilical cord, so, when the diaper becomes wet, the cord does not become wet also.

Remind parents to continue to keep the cord dry until it falls off after they return home. Discourage the use of creams, lotions, and oils near the cord because these tend to slow drying of the cord as well as invite infection. Remind them to use sponge baths rather than immerse the infant in a tub of water. Some health care agencies recommend that parents apply rubbing alcohol to the cord site once or twice a day to hasten drying. Others prefer that the cord be strictly left alone, because manipulation of this type could invite infection. Follow the policy of the agency where you work.

After the cord falls off, a small, pink, granulating area about a quarter of an inch in diameter may remain. This should also be left clean and dry until it has healed (about 24 to 48 more hours). If the ulcerous area is still present after a week, it may require cautery with silver nitrate (a simple and quick office procedure) to speed healing.

Administer Eye Care: Although the practice may shortly become obsolete (as it is in Europe), most birth settings in the United States and Canada still administer prophylactic eye treatment (erythromycin ointment) to help prevent gonorrheal and chlamydia conjunctivitis. Such infections are usually acquired from the mother as the infant passes through the birth canal; therefore, if a mother is certain she does not have either of these diseases, she can request eye drops not be given. In the past, eye prophylaxis was applied immediately after birth. If it is given, it is better, however, to allow parents to interact with their infant before the procedure to be certain their newborn can focus on them without blurry vision caused by the ointment (Zuppa, D'Andrea, Catenazzi, et al., 2011).

If applying eye ointment, always use a single-use tube or package of ointment to avoid transmitting an infection from one newborn to another. First dry the newborn's face with a soft gauze square so the skin is not slippery. Open the newborn's eyes by shading them from the overhead light, then press on both the lower and upper lids one eye at a time with a finger and your thumb. Squeeze a line of ointment along the lower eyelid from the inner canthus outward. Let the eye close to allow the ointment to spread across the conjunctiva.

If it is the health care policy to instill eye ointment, babies born at home or in less orthodox settings such as a car or taxi should have the prophylactic treatment administered on admission to the hospital unless the parents are certain they are both free of gonorrheal and chlamydial infections.

General Infection Precautions: Each newborn should have his or her own private bassinet so the infant has a place to sleep in a mother's postpartal room. Compartments in the bassinet should hold an individual supply of diapers, shirts, gowns, and individual equipment for bathing and temperature taking. Avoid sharing of these items because this could lead to the spread of infection.

Health care workers caring for newborns should thoroughly wash their hands and arms to the elbows with an antiseptic soap before handling infants. Although not proven to reduce infections, agency personnel are usually required to wear cover gowns or nursery uniforms when directly caring for infants (Webster & Pritchard, 2011).

Staff members with infections (particularly sore throats, upper respiratory tract infections, or herpes lesions) should be excluded from caring for mothers or infants until the condition has completely cleared. If a mother might have a contagious illness, her newborn should be excluded from her room until there is no longer a possibility of contagion. A photograph taken daily either by a digital camera or a phone can be shown to the mother so she can follow the baby's progress. The mother should manually express breast milk during the time the infant is excluded from her room to maintain her milk supply. The mother can resume breastfeeding as soon as it is both possible and safe for her infant.

Any baby born outside a hospital or under circumstances conducive to infection, such as rupture of membranes more than 24 hours before birth, should be kept in the mother's room (not brought into a central nursery) until negative cultures show the newborn is free of infection. Likewise, any newborn in whom symptoms of infection develop should be housed in the mother's room or an isolation nursery to prevent the spread of infection to babies in a common nursery. There is no reason for parents not to visit a baby housed in isolation care. In fact, they may have more of a need to hold a baby who is isolated than average parents because they have an extra reason to be worried that something could be permanently wrong with their child. To visit in isolation nurseries, parents should be required to use the same infection control techniques staff members use such as masks or gowns.

NURSING CARE OF A NEWBORN AND FAMILY IN THE POSTPARTAL PERIOD

Newborns are cared for in either a birthing room or a transitional nursery for optimal safety in the first few hours of life. Box 18.6 shows an interprofessional care map illustrating both nursing and team planning for newborn care during a health care agency stay.

The Initial Feeding

The Baby-Friendly Hospital Initiative (BFHI) is a global program sponsored by the World Health Organization (WHO) and the United Nations Children's Fund (UNICEF) to encourage and recognize hospitals and birthing centers that offer an optimal level of care for breastfeeding.

To qualify as a Baby-Friendly–designated facility, a setting must:

- Maintain a written breastfeeding policy that is routinely communicated to all health care staff.
- Educate all health care staff in skills necessary to implement the written policy.
- Inform all pregnant women about the benefits and management of breastfeeding.
- Help mothers initiate breastfeeding within 1 hour of birth.
- Show mothers how to breastfeed and how to maintain their milk supply, even if they are separated from their infants.
- Offer breastfed newborns no pacifiers, food, or drink other than breast milk unless medically indicated.
- Practice "rooming in" or allow mothers and infants to remain together 24 hours a day.
- Encourage unrestricted or "on-demand" breastfeeding.
- Foster the establishment of breastfeeding support groups and refer mothers to them on discharge from the birth setting (Goodman & DiFrisco, 2012).

After a first feeding in the birthing room, both formula-fed and breastfed infants do best with an "on-demand" schedule (i.e., are fed when they are hungry), not at a set 3-hour or 4-hour interval. Many need to be fed as often as every 2 hours in the first few days of life. Chapter 19 discusses techniques of both breastfeeding and formula feeding.

Bathing

In most hospitals, newborns receive a complete sponge bath to wash away vernix caseosa within an hour after birth. Babies of mothers with HIV infection should have a thorough bath immediately to decrease the possibility of HIV transmission. Thereafter, all babies are sponge bathed once a day, although the procedure may be limited to washing only the baby's face, diaper area, and skin folds. Wear gloves when handling newborns until the first bath to avoid exposing your hands to body secretions such as the vernix caseosa.

Plan to help a mother give a first bath before (not after) a feeding to prevent spitting up or vomiting and possible aspiration. Check to be certain the mother's room is warm (about 75°F [24°C]), to prevent chilling. Supply bath water at 98° to 100°F (37° to 38°C), a temperature that feels pleasantly warm to the elbow or wrist, plus a washcloth, towel, comb, and clean diaper and shirt.

As a rule, bathing should proceed from the cleanest parts of the body to the most soiled areas—that is, from the eyes and face to the trunk and extremities and, last, to the diaper area. Wipe a newborn's eyes with clear water from the inner canthus outward, using a clean portion of the washcloth for each eye to prevent spread of infection to the other eye. Remind the mother to wash around the cord with care so she doesn't soak the cord and to give particular care to the creases of skin where milk tends to collect if the child spits up after feedings. If the mother wants to use soap for sponging, be sure she rinses well so no soap is left on the skin (soap is drying and newborns are susceptible to desquamation), and also to dry well. It's good for parents to wash the infant's hair daily

BOX 18.6 Nursing Care Planning

AN INTERPROFESSIONAL CARE MAP FOR A TERM NEWBORN

Carlotta Ruiz has just given birth to her second child, a 39 weeks and 2 days, 6-lb, 5-oz baby girl. While Jose, Carlotta's husband, is in the room, Carlotta tells you she is a "veteran" at baby care. When Carlotta is alone, however, you notice she seems apprehensive about caring for her new daughter.

Family Assessment Family is composed of two parents, a 3-year-old sibling, and newborn. They live in a three-bedroom flat over a dry cleaning store. Father clerks in a grocery store; mother works as a school bus driver. Finances rated as "hanging in there."

Client Assessment Birth from left occipitoanterior (LOA) position. Apgar score: 6 at 1 minute; 8 at 5 minutes after administration of blow-by oxygen. Respirations are 74 breaths/min. She has a 2 × 3 cm red pigmented area on outer right thigh. Mother attempted breastfeeding in birthing room, but newborn had difficulty sucking because of rapid respirations. Remainder of physical examination within acceptable parameters.

Nursing Diagnosis Risk for ineffective parenting related to infant's smaller than expected size and birthmark.

Outcome Criteria Respiratory rate is decreased to 30 to 50 breaths/min, infant sucks well at breast every 2 to 3 hours, and mother voices she is pleased with infant's appearance and progress.

(continued on page 480)

and are then put back into the infant's mouth. Clipping the pacifier onto the infant's shirt helps prevent this problem. If parents use pacifiers, be certain they are of one-piece construction, so loose parts cannot be aspirated. Mothers who are breastfeeding should use pacifiers sparingly until breastfeeding is well established because sucking on a pacifier takes less effort than sucking at a breast (Nelson, 2012).

QSEN Checkpoint Question 18.6

Evidence-Based Practice

Shaken baby syndrome, or abusive head trauma caused by a parent or caregiver shaking an infant in anger or frustration, creates a potentially lethal situation because forceful shaking can lead to subdural bleeding. To investigate whether a nurse-initiated program could reduce the incidence of abusive head trauma by shaking, nurse researchers offered an educational program including a leaflet explaining abusive head trauma, helpful ways to cope safely with an infant's crying, and an 8-minute video on the subject given to all new mothers at their hospital. Results of the study showed a decrease from 2.8 injuries per year (14 cases in 5 years prior to the intervention) to 0.7 injuries per year (2 cases in 3 years) or a 75% reduction in injuries following the intervention (Altman, Canter, Patrick, et al., 2011).

You notice Mrs. Ruiz grows irritated with Beth when Beth doesn't suck readily when she begins to breastfeed. Based on the previous study, what action would be best to take?

a. Evaluate whether Beth can hear because this may be the underlying problem.
b. List the dangers of shaken baby syndrome for Mrs. Ruiz.
c. Discuss the fact that breastfeeding is a new skill, so infants take time to learn this.
d. Suggest that Mrs. Ruiz ask the physician for a sedative so she can better tolerate newborn crying.

Look in Appendix A for the best answer and rationale.

Car Safety: Automobile accidents are a safety problem all during childhood, beginning with the newborn period. For protection while in automobiles, newborns should always be transported in rear facing car seats placed in the back seat, not the front seat (Durbin, 2011). Without this protection, if a car should stop suddenly, an infant could be thrown onto the floor or, in a collision, thrown out of the car or through the windshield. At a speed of only 30 mph, an infant may hit the dashboard with a force equal to a fall from a three-story building. If an adult holding the infant is not wearing a seat belt, the adult can be thrown against the infant, causing even more damage.

When purchasing a car seat, caution parents to look at the brand and style to be certain the seat meets current federal guidelines. The AAP Web site (www.aap.org) lists current recommendations and types of seats to purchase (Fig. 18.29). Some hospitals and Red Cross chapters loan infant car seats for temporary use, such as when visiting out of state with grandparents or when first coming home from the hospital. New cars are mandated to be equipped with lower anchors and tethers for safe use of car seats. A mirror can be positioned in the back seat so a parent can observe the infant from the front seat while driving.

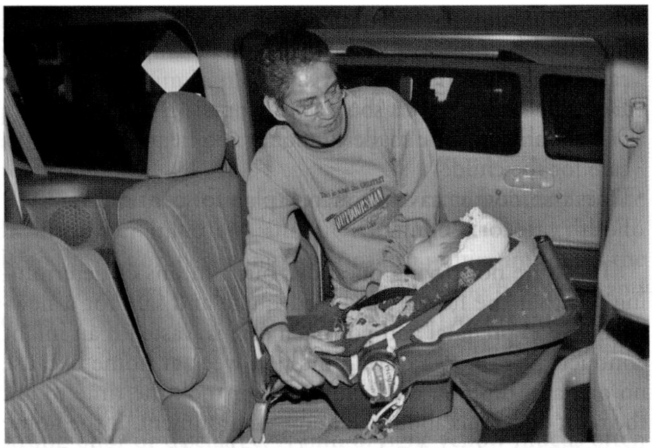

FIGURE 18.29 To be safe, newborns need to ride in an appropriately sized backward facing car set while in an automobile. Be sure every family leaving the health care facility is properly equipped.

The ideal model has a five-point harness with broad straps, which helps spread the force of a collision over the chest and hips, and a shield, which cushions the head. Advise parents not to use a sack sleeper or papoose bunting nor should they wrap the baby in a bulky blanket so the straps will securely fashion the infant into the seat. To provide extra warmth, a blanket can be draped over the child and straps as needed. To support the baby's head, parents can use a rolled-up receiving blanket, towel, or diaper on each side of the head or purchase commercial head supports.

Caution parents that plastic car seats grow extremely hot in the summer, so they should test the temperature of the surface before placing their infant into the seat. Stress also that it is as dangerous to not use a car seat as it is to use a car seat improperly, such as not fastening the harness or not securing the seat belt.

What if . . . 18.3 You notice the Ruiz family does not have a car seat to transport Beth home. As their discharge nurse, would you insist they will have to stay in the hospital until they purchase a car seat?

Continued Health Maintenance for a Newborn: Parents do not need to continue to weigh a newborn or take an infant's temperature at home because these practices only cause worry, as weight fluctuates day by day, and infant activity and clothing can influence temperature. Instead, teach parents to judge their infant's state of health by the child's overall appearance, eagerness to eat, general activity, and disposition, as well as weight gain assessed at health care visits.

Make certain parents make and keep their health care appointment for a first newborn assessment according to their primary care provider's schedule (2 to 6 weeks). The mother was conscientious throughout pregnancy to bring a well child into the world. Parents must now begin a health care program to keep the child well.

What if...18.4 You are particularly interested in exploring one of the 2020 National Health Goals with respect to newborn care (see Box 18.1). What would be a possible research topic to explore pertinent to this goal that would be applicable to both Beth and her family and that would also advance evidence-based practice?

Key Points for Review

- A newborn history and physical examination yields important information not only on the infant's appearance but also on gestational age and any factors that suggest additional care is needed.
- Using a standardized method of assessment such as an Apgar score, a Dubowitz/Ballard scale, or a Silverman-Andersen scale are important measures to help document that an infant is adjusting well to extrauterine life.
- Converting from fetal to newborn respiratory function is a major step in extrauterine adaptation. Newborns need particularly close observation during the first few hours of life to determine if this adaptation occurs.
- Maintaining body heat is a second major problem of newborns. When a procedure requires undressing an infant for an extended period of time, the procedure should be done under a radiant heat source to guard against chilling and hypothermia.
- Newborns may suffer hypoglycemia in the first few hours of life because they use so much energy to establish respirations and maintain heat. Signs of jitteriness and a blood glucose level of less than 40 mg/100 ml by heel stick help to identify hypoglycemia.
- A great deal of nurses' responsibility for newborns is being certain a mother and her partner spend enough time and give enough care to their newborn at the birth setting that they feel confident in giving care at home. Be certain they are well informed about controversial topics such as circumcision, common screening measures, or prophylactic antibiotic eye drops because this helps in planning nursing care that not only meets QSEN competencies but also best meets a family's total needs.
- Assess that identification bands are securely attached while a newborn is hospitalized; assess these one last time compared to the mother's before birth setting discharge. To help prevent the possibility of infant abduction, be certain of the identification of anyone to whom you give a newborn.
- Be certain that caregivers have a car seat to use at discharge for their infant and that they know to schedule a well-child visit at 2 to 6 weeks of age.

Critical Thinking Care Study

U2 is a 7-lb, 5-oz neonate born in the "dirty backseat" of a taxi because her 16-year-old mother, Debbie Tillerman, didn't realize she was in labor. The baby's grandparents are angry with Debbie because, although grounded for breaking a house rule, she took the bus to visit her boyfriend out of town and was there when her labor started. Apgar scores were not recorded. The grandparents want the baby moved to the neonatal intensive care unit because, although the baby's weight is that of a term newborn, they are concerned the baby is preterm. "Don't trust anything Debbie tells you about her due date," they tell you. "She lies all of the time."

1. What standardized assessment would you want to do on U2 to assess if she best resembles a preterm or a term newborn? Who would you ask to obtain a pregnancy history: Debbie or the grandparents?
2. Debbie is going to call her baby U2 rather than a typical name. Would you be concerned about this? Would you perhaps talk to her about changing it before the birth certificate is filed?
3. What special care will U2 need because she was born in the "dirty backseat" of a taxi cab? Are there any special instructions Debbie will need to know to care for her?

Patient Scenario

The Farmer Family

Read about the Farmer family, a family with an infant born breech, then answer the questions to further sharpen your skills and grow more familiar with NCLEX-type questions related to nursing care of a family with a newborn. Confirm your answers are correct by reading the rationales.

Visit http://thePoint.lww.com

Answers and Rationales

Looking for answers to the What If . . . and Critical Thinking Care Study questions?

Visit http://thePoint.lww.com

References

Altman, R. L., Canter, J., Patrick, P. A., et al. (2011). Parent education by maternity nurses and prevention of abusive head trauma. *Pediatrics, 128*(5), e1164–e1172.

American Academy of Pediatrics. (2011). *Newborn hearing screening and your baby.* Elk Grove Village, IL: Author.

American Academy of Pediatrics. (2012a). *Male circumcision*. Elk Grove Village, IL: Author.

American Academy of Pediatrics. (2012b). *Recommended immunization schedule for persons aged 0 through 6 years*. Elk Grove Village, IL: Author.

Apgar, V., Holaday, D. A., James, L. S., et al. (1958). Evaluation of a newborn infant: Second report. *JAMA: Journal of the American Medical Association, 168*(15), 1985–1988.

Ballard, J. L., Khoury, J. C., Wedig, K., et al. (1991). New Ballard Score, expanded to include extremely premature infants. *Journal of Pediatrics, 119*(3), 417–424.

Basavanthappa, N. N., Kagathur, U., Basavanthappa, R. N., et al. (2011). Natal and neonatal teeth: A retrospective study of 15 cases. *European Journal of Dentistry, 5*(2), 168–172.

Baston, H. (2012). Use of technology in childbirth: Phototherapy. *The Practicing Midwife, 15*(3), 36–39.

Bechtel, K., Le, K., Martin, K. D., et al. (2011). Impact of an educational intervention on caregivers' beliefs about infant crying and knowledge of shaken baby syndrome. *Academic Pediatrics, 11*(6), 481–486.

Brashers, V. L., & McCance, K. L. (2012). Cardiovascular and lymphatic systems. In S. E. Huether & K. L. McCance (Eds.), *Understanding pathophysiology* (5th ed., pp. 551–668). New York, NY: Elsevier Publishing.

Brazelton, T. B. (1973). Neonatal behavior assessment scale. *Clinics in Developmental Medicine, 50*(5), 1–15.

Centers for Disease Control and Prevention. (2010). *Growth charts.* Atlanta, GA: Author.

Chaux, A., & Cubilla, A. L. (2012). Advances in the pathology of penile carcinomas. *Human Pathology, 43*(6), 771–789.

Dawrant, J. M., Pacaud, D., Wade, A., et al. (2011). Informatics of newborn screening for congenital hypothyroidism in Alberta 2005–08. *Canadian Journal of Public Health, 102*(1), 64–67.

Desmond, M. M., Franklin, R. R., Vallvona, C., et al. (1963). The clinical behavior of the newly born: The term infant. *Journal of Pediatrics, 62*(3), 307–325.

Dubowitz, L. M., Dubowitz, V., & Goldberg, C. (1970). Clinical assessment of gestational age in a newborn infant. *Journal of Pediatrics, 77*(1), 1–12.

Durbin, D. R. (2011). Child passenger safety. *Pediatrics, 127*(4), 788–793.

Faurschou, A., Olesen, A. B., Leonardi-Bee, J., et al. (2011). Lasers or light sources for treating port-wine stains. *Cochrane Database of Systematic Reviews,* (11), CD007152.

Gandhi, M., Papanna, R., Teach, M., et al. (2012). Suspected twin-twin transfusion syndrome: How often is the diagnosis correct and referral timely? *Journal of Ultrasound Medicine, 31*(6), 941–945.

Goodman, K., & DiFrisco, E. (2012). Achieving Baby-Friendly designation: Step-by-step. *MCN: American Journal of Maternal Child Nursing, 37*(3), 146–152.

Gowen, C. W. (2011). Assessment of the mother, fetus & newborn. In K. J. Marcdante, R. M. Kliegman, H. B. Jenson, et al. (Eds.), *Nelson essentials of pediatrics* (6th ed., pp. 213–231). Philadelphia: Saunders/Elsevier.

Graven, S. N. (2011). Early visual development: Implications for the neonatal intensive care unit and care. *Clinical Perinatology, 38*(4), 671–683.

Haldeman-Englert, C. R., Saitta, S. C., & Zackai, E. H. (2011). Specific chromosome disorders in newborns. In C. A. Gleason & S. U. Devaskar (Eds.), *Avery's diseases of the newborn* (9th ed., pp. 196–208). Philadelphia, PA: Elsevier/Saunders.

Heimall, L. M., Storey, B., Stellar, J. J., et al. (2012). Beginning at the bottom: Evidence-based care of diaper dermatitis. *MCN: American Journal of Maternal Child Nursing, 37*(1), 10–16.

Hofer, N., Müller, W., & Resch, B. (2012). Neonates presenting with temperature symptoms: Role in the diagnosis of early onset sepsis. *Pediatrics International, 54*(4), 486–490.

Ipema, H. J. (2012). Use of oral vitamin k for prevention of late vitamin k deficiency bleeding in neonates when injectable vitamin k is not available. *Annals of Pharmacotherapy, 46*(6), 879–883.

Jones, N. A. (2012). Delayed reactive cries demonstrate emotional and physiological dysregulation in newborns of depressed mothers. *Biological Psychology, 89*(2), 374–381.

Karch, A. M. (2013). *2013 Lippincott's nursing drug guide.* Philadelphia, PA: Lippincott Williams & Wilkins.

Kondi-Pafiti, A., Kleanthis, K. C., Mavrigiannaki, P., et al. (2011). Single umbilical artery: Fetal and placental histopathological analysis of 24 cases. *Clinical & Experimental Obstetrics & Gynecology, 38*(3), 214–216.

Kroshinsky, D., Alper, J. C., & Holmes, L. B. (2011). Birthmarks. In L. B. Holmes (Ed.), *Common malformations* (pp. 395–426). New York, NY: Oxford University Press.

Leonardi-Bee, J., Batta, K., O'Brien, C., et al. (2011). Interventions for infantile haemangiomas (strawberry birthmarks) of the skin. *Cochrane Database of Systematic Reviews,* (5), CD006545.

Leone, T. A., & Finer, N. N. (2011). Resuscitation in the delivery room. In C. A. Gleason & S. U. Devaskar (Eds.), *Avery's diseases of the newborn* (9th ed., pp. 328–340). Philadelphia, PA: Elsevier/Saunders.

Lönnqvist, P. A. (2010). Regional anaesthesia and analgesia in the neonate. *Best Practice & Research: Clinical Anaesthesiology, 24*(3), 309–321.

Lunze, K., & Hamer, D. H. (2012). Thermal protection of the newborn in resource-limited environments. *Journal of Perinatology, 32*(5), 317–324.

Lurie, S., Wand, S., Golan, A., et al. (2011). Risk factors for fractured clavicle in the newborn. *Journal of Obstetrics & Gynaecology Research, 37*(11), 1572–1574.

Lyon, V. B. (2011). Dermatology. In K. J. Marcdante, R. M. Kliegman, H. B. Jenson, et al. (Eds.), *Nelson essentials of pediatrics* (6th ed., pp. 713–734). Philadelphia, PA: Saunders/Elsevier.

Moon, R. Y. (2011). SIDS and other sleep-related infant deaths: Expansion of recommendations for a safe infant sleeping environment. *Pediatrics, 128*(5), 1030–1039.

Moore, E. R., Anderson, G. C., Bergman, N., et al. (2012). Early skin-to-skin contact for mothers and their healthy newborn infants. *Cochrane Database of Systematic Reviews,* (5), CD003519.

Nelson, A. M. (2012). A comprehensive review of evidence and current recommendations related to pacifier usage. *Journal of Pediatric Nursing, 27*(6), 690–699.

Nelson, L., Doering, J. J., Anderson, M., et al. (2012). Outcome of clinical nurse specialist-led hyperbilirubinemia screening of late preterm newborns. *Clinical Nurse Specialist, 26*(3), 164–168.

Paneth, N. (2011). Neonatal and perinatal epidemiology. In C. A. Gleason & S. U. Devaskar (Eds.), *Avery's diseases of the newborn* (9th ed., pp. 1–9). Philadelphia, PA: Elsevier/Saunders.

Paul, S. P. (2011). Infantile vesicular rash. *Practicing Midwife, 14*(11), 11–14.

Pillai-Riddell, R. R., Racine, N. M., Turcotte, K., et al. (2011). Non-pharmacological management of infant and young child procedural pain. *Cochrane Database of Systematic Reviews,* (10), CD006275.

Rivera, J. C., Sapieha, P., Joyal, J. S., et al. (2011). Understanding retinopathy of prematurity: Update on pathogenesis. *Neonatology, 100*(4), 343–353.

Rossman, C. L., & Ayoola, A. B. (2012). Promoting individualized breastfeeding experiences. *MCN: American Journal of Maternal Child Nursing, 37*(3), 193–199.

Rote, N. S. (2012). Adaptive immunity. In S. E. Huether & K. L. McCance (Eds.), *Understanding pathophysiology* (5th ed., pp. 142–164). New York, NY: Elsevier Publishing.

Rubarth, L. (2012). Back to basics: The Apgar score: Simple yet complex. *Neonatal Network, 31*(3), 169–177.

Russo, M. L., Henderson, J., & Costigan, K. A. (2011). Fetal assessment. In K. J. Hurt, M. W. Guile, J. L. Bienstock, et al. (Eds.), *The Johns Hopkins manual of gynecology and obstetrics* (4th ed., pp. 90–98). Philadelphia, PA: Lippincott Williams & Wilkins.

Scheiwe, A., Hardy, R., & Watt, R. G. (2010). Four-year follow-up of a randomized controlled trial of a social support intervention on infant feeding practices. *Maternal & Child Nutrition, 6*(4), 328–337.

Schneider, D. [Daniel]. (2011). The cardiovascular system. In K. J. Marcdante, R. M. Kliegman, H. B. Jenson, et al. (Eds.), *Nelson essentials of pediatrics* (6th ed., pp. 525–554). Philadelphia, PA: Saunders/Elsevier.

Schneider, D. [Douglas]. (2012). The patent ductus arteriosus in term infants, children, and adults. *Seminars in Perinatology, 36*(2), 146–153.

Shah, S. S., Aronson, P. L., Mohama, Z., et al. (2011). Delayed acyclovir therapy and death among neonates with herpes simplex virus infection. *Pediatrics, 128*(6), 1153–1160.

Silverman, W. A., & Andersen, H. (1956). A controlled clinical trial of effects of water mist on obstructive respiratory signs, death rate and necroscopy findings among premature infants. *Pediatrics, 17*(4), 1–9.

Smith, J. B. (2011). Initial evaluation: History and physical examination of the newborn. In C. A. Gleason & S. U. Devaskar (Eds.), *Avery's diseases of the newborn* (9th ed., pp. 277–299). Philadelphia, PA: Elsevier/Saunders.

Smith, S. (2011). Cutaneous infections. In K. J. Marcdante, R. M. Kliegman, H. B. Jenson, et al. (Eds.), *Nelson essentials of pediatrics* (6th ed., pp. 374–376). Philadelphia, PA: Saunders/Elsevier.

Sogawa, M., Fukuda, T., Tayama, M., et al. (2012). Reconstruction of the right ventricular outflow tract after surgical removal of a cardiac hemangioma. *General Thoracic & Cardiovascular Surgery, 60*(10), 661–663.

Song, Y., Zhang, S., & Song, W. (2012). Significance of neonatal body indices in identifying fetal macrosomia. *Journal of Perinatology, 33*(2), 103–106.

Swarnam, K., Soraisham, A. S., & Sivanandan, S. (2012). Advances in the management of meconium aspiration syndrome. *International Journal of Pediatrics,* 2012, 359571.

Tasian, G. E., Copp, H. L., & Baskin, L. S. (2011). Diagnostic imaging in cryptorchidism: Utility, indications, and effectiveness. *Journal of Pediatric Surgery, 46*(12), 2406–2413.

Thilo, E. H., & Rosenberg, A. A. (2011). The newborn infant. In W. W. Hay, M. J. Levin, J. M. Sondheimer, et al. (Eds.) *Current diagnosis & treatment: Pediatrics* (20th ed., pp. 1–63). Columbus, OH: McGraw-Hill.

Tsai, A. C., Manchester, D. K., & Elias, E. R. (2011). Genetics & dysmorphology. In W. W. Hay, J. M. Levin, J. M. Sondheimer, et al. (Eds.). *Current diagnosis and treatment: Pediatrics* (20th ed., pp. 1020–1054). Columbus, OH: McGraw-Hill.

Tsai, M. S., & Yeh, M. L. (2011). Images in clinical medicine. Patent urachus. *New England Journal of Medicine, 365*(14), 1328.

U.S. Department of Health and Human Services. (2010). *Healthy people 2020.* Washington, DC: Author.

Usher, R., McLean, F., & Scott, K. E. (1966). Judgment of fetal age. *Pediatric Clinics of North America, 13*(4), 835–840.

Van Leeuwen, G., & Glenn, L. (1968). Screening for hidden congenital anomalies. *Pediatrics, 41*(6), 147–152.

Walter, K. E. (2011). The hip. In K. J. Marcdante, R. M. Kliegman, H. B. Jenson, et al. (Eds.), *Nelson essentials of pediatrics* (6th ed., pp. 741–744). Philadelphia, PA: Saunders/Elsevier.

Walsh, J., & Goser, L. (2013). Development of an innovative NICU teen parent support program: One unit's experience. *Journal of Perinatal & Neonatal Nursing, 27*(2), 176–183.

Watchko, K. F. (2011). Neonatal indirect hyperbilirubinemia & kernicterus. In C. A. Gleason & S. U. Devaskar (Eds.), *Avery's diseases of the newborn* (9th ed., pp. 1123–1164). Philadelphia, PA: Elsevier/Saunders.

Webster, J., & Pritchard, M. A. (2011). Gowning by attendants and visitors in newborn nurseries for prevention of neonatal morbidity and mortality. *Cochrane Database of Systematic Reviews,* (3), CD003670.

Wisser, M., Rothschild, M. A., Schmolling, J. C., et al. (2012). Caput succedaneum and facial petechiae-birth-associated injuries in healthy newborns under forensic aspects. *International Journal of Legal Medicine,126*(3), 385–390.

World Health Organization. (2012). *Neonatal mortality levels for 193 countries in 2009 with trends since 1990.* Geneva, Switzerland: Author.

Xu, Y., Yolton, K., & Khoury, J. (2011). Earliest appropriate time for administering neurobehavioral assessment in newborn infants. *Pediatrics, 127*(1), e69–e75.

Zderic, S. A., & Lambert, S. M. (2012). Developmental abnormalities of the genitourinary system. In C. A. Gleason & S. U. Devaskar (Eds.), *Avery's diseases of the newborn* (9th ed., pp. 1191–1205). Philadelphia, PA: Elsevier/Saunders.

Zuppa, A. A., D'Andrea, V., Catenazzi, P., et al. (2011). Ophthalmia neonatorum: What kind of prophylaxis? *Journal of Maternal-Fetal & Neonatal Medicine, 24*(6), 769–773.

Chapter 19

Nutritional Needs of a Newborn

KEY TERMS

- areola
- bifidus factor
- colostrum
- engorgement
- fore milk
- hind milk
- interferon
- lactiferous sinuses
- lactoferrin
- let-down reflex
- lysozyme
- prolactin

OBJECTIVES

After mastering the contents of this chapter, you should be able to:

1. Describe nutritional requirements for a term newborn.
2. Identify 2020 National Health Goals related to newborn nutrition that nurses can help the nation achieve.
3. Assess the nutritional intake and feeding method of a newborn to determine if the infant has an adequate nutritional status.
4. Formulate nursing diagnoses related to newborn nutrition.
5. Establish expected outcomes for a newborn and parents related to nutrition as well as help parents manage seamless transitions across differing health care settings.
6. Using the nursing process, plan nursing care that includes the six competencies of Quality & Safety Education for Nurses (QSEN): Patient-Centered Care, Teamwork & Collaboration, Evidence-Based Practice (EBP), Quality Improvement (QI), Safety, and Informatics.
7. Implement nursing care, such as supporting a new mother while beginning breastfeeding.
8. Evaluate expected outcomes for achievement and effectiveness of care.
9. Integrate knowledge of newborn nutrition with the interplay of nursing process, the six competencies of QSEN, and Family Nursing to promote quality maternal and child health nursing care.

Linda Satir is a new mother of a 7-lb term baby girl. During the pregnancy, she and her husband, Paul, both agreed Linda would breastfeed. Linda will be returning to work as an executive assistant after her 6-week maternity leave. She attempted to breastfeed her newborn in the birthing room with minimal success. As you offer to help her feed her baby for the second time, she says, "Did I make the right choice? Maybe I should formula feed her. Paul could help that way and I won't have to worry about what to do when I'm back at work."

Previous chapters described the care of a woman and family during the antepartal, intrapartal, postpartal, and newborn periods. This chapter adds information about the nutritional needs of a newborn. A newborn's nutritional needs are high during this time because of a rapid rate of both growth and development. Knowing these needs enables you to play a key role in educating parents on how to provide adequate nutrition to meet both physiologic and psychological needs of their newborn.

How would you answer Linda?

Proper nutrition is essential for optimal growth and development, especially in the first few months of life, because brain growth proceeds at such a rapid rate during this time. Feeding for a newborn extends beyond the physiologic need of adequate nutrition, however; it also fulfills important psychological needs. During feeding, a parent is close to the infant, and a baby is apt to be particularly sensitive to the parent's demonstration of affection or lack of warmth. The feeding experience, therefore, enables an emotional bond between infant and caregiver and helps provide an environment that enhances the psychosocial development of the infant as well as aids physical growth (Lutter & Morrow, 2013). Box 19.1 shows 2020 National Health Goals related to newborn nutrition.

Nursing Process Overview

For Promoting Nutritional Health in a Newborn

Assessment

An assessment of infant nutrition begins during pregnancy with an assessment of the mother's and her partner's attitudes and choices about infant feeding. Breastfeeding is widely accepted as the preferred method of human newborn nutrition and should be recommended. However, if a mother chooses not to breastfeed because of her individual circumstances, it is important she not be made to feel guilty for her choice, because formula feeding can be substituted. Most importantly, parents need to feel comfortable with and confident about the feeding method they choose.

Part of assessment includes recognizing signs of hunger in the newborn. Ask parents if they can identify restlessness, tense body posture, smacking lips, and tongue thrusting as signs of hunger in their infant. Otherwise, they may wait for their infant to cry, and this is actually a late sign of newborn hunger. Once infant feeding begins, assess whether the parents know how to judge the amount the infant is receiving is adequate, which is not by how long the newborn breastfeeds at one time or by how much formula is taken at a feeding, but by a larger measure, such as whether the newborn is voiding, growing, and is alert (Box 19.2). A formula-fed newborn regains birth weight at about 10 days; a breastfed infant does so at about 14 days.

Nursing Diagnosis

Nursing diagnoses in relation to nutrition usually center on a woman's choice regarding the method of feeding or a newborn's nutritional intake and feeding patterns. It may be difficult to establish diagnoses during the first part of the newborn period, because the mother and infant are still getting used to each other. Examples of nursing diagnoses include:

- Effective breastfeeding related to a well-prepared mother and a healthy newborn
- Risk for ineffective breastfeeding related to nipple soreness
- Imbalanced nutrition, less than body requirements, related to poor newborn sucking response
- Risk for impaired parenting related to a need to formula feed the newborn

BOX 19.1 Nursing Care Planning Based on 2020 National Health Goals

The number of 2020 National Health Goals that address the nutrition of a newborn was increased in the 2010 update to include two that speak to exclusive breastfeeding.

- Increase to at least 81.9% the proportion of infants who are breastfed from a baseline of 74.0%.
- Increase to at least 60.6% the proportion of mothers who continue breastfeeding until their babies are 6 months old from a baseline of 43.5%.
- Increase to 34.1% the proportion of mothers who continue breastfeeding until 1 year of age from a baseline of 22.7%.
- Increase to at least 46.2% the proportion of mothers who breastfeed exclusively through 3 months from a baseline of 33.6%.
- Increase to 25.5% the proportion of mothers who breastfeed exclusively through 6 months from a baseline of 14.1%.
- Increase to 38% the proportion of employers that have work site lactation support programs from a baseline of 25%.
- Increase to 8.1% the proportion of live births that occur in facilities that provide recommended care for lactating mothers from a baseline of 2.9% (U.S. Department of Health and Human Services [DHHS], 2010; see www.healthypeople.gov).

Nurses can help the nation achieve these goals by educating women while they are pregnant about the importance of breastfeeding as well as by supporting a family during the subsequent year while a woman is breastfeeding. Home visits with families and well-child health assessments provide opportunities to advocate for continued and exclusive breastfeeding.

Outcome Identification and Planning

Because breastfeeding is best for newborns, planning begins while a woman is still pregnant, focusing on providing her with the information necessary to allow her to become familiar and comfortable with breastfeeding. After birth, a teaching plan addressing the nutritional needs of both the woman and her newborn should be developed. Helpful Internet sites for referral are La Leche League International (www.llli.org) and the International Lactation Consultant Association (www.ilca.org). Despite the advantages of breastfeeding, some parents still choose formula feeding because of their individual preferences. Parents who choose formula feeding need to plan ways to make feeding time an intimate or special one for both themselves and the baby. An Internet site that discusses formula feeding is www.keepkidshealthy.com.

Implementation

A major intervention related to newborn nutrition is supporting a mother's choice of feeding method and helping her to trust her judgment as to whether her infant is full and content and the feeding method is as natural as possible. In addition to sponsoring classes on

BOX 19.2 Nursing Care Planning Using Assessment

Assessing the Newborn for Adequate Nutrition

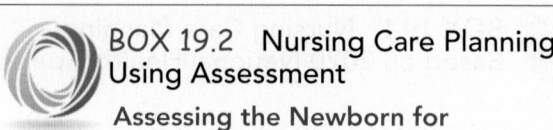

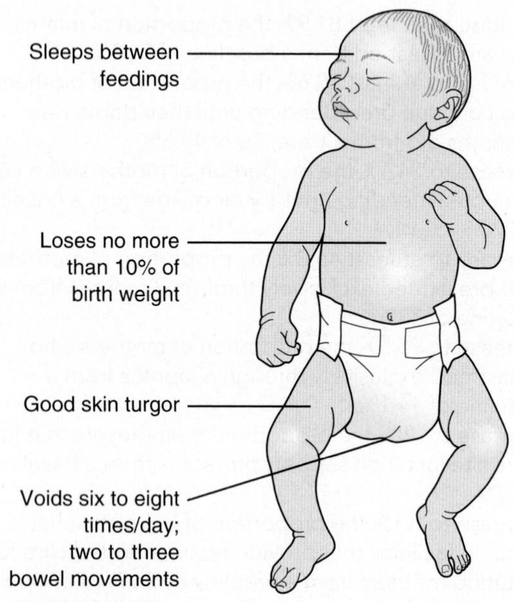

breastfeeding, a helpful service of La Leche League is its hotline, through which a breastfeeding woman who is discouraged or is having difficulty can contact a member and ask for advice. *The Womanly Art of Breastfeeding*, published by La Leche League International (2010), is a comprehensive and informative book to recommend to both new mothers and fathers.

When assisting a new mother with breastfeeding, remember that breast milk can carry the human immunodeficiency virus (HIV). Adhere to standard infection precautions, therefore, when helping with manual expression of milk or when disposing of soiled breast pads.

Outcome Evaluation

The evaluation is an important final step to ensure a newborn receives adequate nutrition because unforeseen circumstances, such as an unsuspected milk allergy or mastitis (breast infection), may interfere with and require drastic changes to reach desired outcomes. Help parents appreciate the fact that newborns are very adaptive and can adjust to another feeding method if necessary. Examples suggesting successful expected outcomes related to newborn feeding include:

- Infant breastfeeds every 2 to 3 hours, is content, and sleeps between feedings.
- Newborn ingests a total of 12 oz of formula with iron every 24 hours.
- Mother states she feels satisfied with chosen method of infant feeding.
- Infant voids six times daily as a measure of adequate hydration by 1 week.

NUTRITIONAL ALLOWANCES FOR A NEWBORN

Nutritional allowances for a newborn need to take into account total calories, protein, vitamins, minerals, and fluid.

Calories

Growth in the neonatal period and early infancy is more rapid than at any other period of life (Krebs & Primak, 2011); therefore, the caloric requirements exceed those at any other age. For example, an infant up to 2 months of age requires 110 to 120 calories per kilogram of body weight (50 to 55 kcal/lb) every 24 hours to provide an adequate amount for maintenance and growth. After 2 months of age, this amount gradually declines until the requirement at 1 year is 100 kcal/kg (45 kcal/lb) per day. In contrast, the adult caloric requirement is 42 kcal/kg (20 kcal/lb) per day (U.S. Department of Agriculture [USDA], 2011).

The actual caloric requirement, of course, depends on an infant's individual activity level and growth rate. For example, an active infant, one who cries frequently and squirms constantly, needs more calories than one who is more passive, who is content to spend long hours playing quietly or just studying the environment. During growth spurts, more calories are needed to supply additional energy.

Commercial infant formulas are designed to simulate breast milk and so have the same number of calories per ounce as breast milk. They contain about 9% to 12% of their calories as protein and 45% to 55% of calories as lactose carbohydrate. The balance (34% to 46%) is fat, of which linoleic acid accounts for about 4%.

Protein

The newborn has a high requirement of protein, which is necessary for the formation of new cells, during this period to provide for a rapid growth of new cells as well as maintenance of existing cells. The nutritional allowance of protein for the first 2 months of life is 2.2 g per kilogram of body weight. Both human milk and commercial formulas provide all the essential amino acids necessary to form protein. Histidine, an amino acid that appears to be essential for infant growth but is not necessary for adult growth, is found in both milk forms.

Unaltered cow's milk is not recommended for newborns because it contains about 16% of its calories as protein, whereas human milk contains about 8%. This means cow's milk can create such a rich solute load (i.e., the amount of urea and electrolytes that must be excreted in the urine) that a newborn's kidneys could be overwhelmed. In addition, cow's milk can cause microscopic bleeding of the gastrointestinal tract, leading to blood loss and anemia. These problems occur because the protein in cow's milk, *casein*, differs from that in human milk, *lactalbumin*, both in composition and in amount. This is important because the amount of casein present in milk determines its curd tension. Because of the increased amount of casein in cow's milk, the curd is large, tough, and difficult to digest, whereas in human milk the curd is softer and digests easily. This is the rationale behind recommending formula-fed infants be given a commercial formula containing albumin rather than cow's milk. Cow's milk products, such as yogurt and cottage cheese, should not be introduced until 9 to 12 months of age because of this same reason.

Fat

Linoleic acid, an essential fatty acid, is necessary for brain growth and skin integrity in infants. When the amount of linoleic acid is sufficient, the infant can then manufacture docosahexaenoic acid (DHA), an omega-3 fatty acid, and arachidonic acid (ARA), an omega-6 fatty acid, both of which are important for brain growth. Breast milk contains a generous supply of all three of these fatty acids. Commercial formulas contain varying amounts depending on the brand and type of fats included in the formula.

Because fat is so important for brain and nerve growth, use of fat-free milk for long periods in newborns and infants (when other sources of food are not being offered) can result in linoleic acid deficiency. Therefore, parents should not feed fat-free milk as a means of preventing obesity in newborns or young infants. In addition, fat-free milk does not contain sufficient calories for a newborn; it only has about half as many calories as commercial formulas or breast milk.

Carbohydrate

Lactose, the disaccharide found in human milk and added to commercial formulas, appears to be the most easily digested of the carbohydrates. Lactose also improves calcium absorption and aids in nitrogen retention. It produces stools consisting predominantly of gram-positive rather than gram-negative bacteria and therefore decreases the possibility of gastrointestinal illness (which usually results from gram-negative organisms). Adequate lactose also allows protein to be used for building new cells rather than for calories, encouraging normal water balance and preventing abnormal metabolism of fat. Lactose intolerance, which can occur in older children, is rarely present in newborns; they typically use the calories provided by lactose well.

Fluid

It is important to maintain a sufficient fluid intake in newborns because their metabolic rate is so high (and metabolism requires water). In addition, a newborn's body surface area is large in relation to body mass. This means a baby loses water by evaporation much more readily than does an adult and, because the kidneys of a newborn are not yet capable of fully concentrating urine, a newborn cannot conserve body water by this mechanism to prevent dehydration.

Another difference between newborns and adults is that body water is distributed differently. In a newborn, 30% to 35% of body weight is extracellular fluid; in an adult, this proportion is only 20%. Consequently, if a newborn's extracellular fluid store is depleted through loss of fluid or inadequate fluid intake, as much as 35% of a newborn's fluid component may be lost.

Because of all these factors, a newborn needs 150 to 200 ml/kg (2.5 to 3.0 oz/lb) of water intake every 24 hours (adults require 2,400 ml per day or less than 1 oz/lb). This requirement can be supplied completely by breastfeeding or formula feeding. Fruit juice is not recommended for infants younger than 6 months because it supplies no protein and, if not pasteurized, can carry infectious organisms (American Academy of Pediatrics [AAP], 2012d).

✔ QSEN Checkpoint Question 19.1

Patient-Centered Care

A nursing assessment of Linda Satir's plan for her infant's nutrition should begin with which of the following?

a. An assessment of Linda's beliefs and attitudes about breastfeeding
b. An assessment of the infant's body mass index and glucose levels
c. An assessment of Linda's education level and reading ability
d. An assessment of the infant's ability to suck and swallow

Look in Appendix A for the best answer and rationale.

Minerals

A number of minerals are particularly important to early growth.

Calcium.

Calcium is important to the newborn because a newborn's skeleton grows so rapidly. Because milk is high in calcium, tetany resulting from a low calcium level seldom occurs in infants who suck well, regardless of whether they are fed human milk or commercial formula.

Iron.

The term newborn of a mother who had adequate iron intake during pregnancy will be born with iron stores that, theoretically, will last for the first 3 months of life, until the newborn begins to produce adult hemoglobin. Because not all mothers eat an iron-rich diet during pregnancy (and socioeconomic level is not a good criterion for judging the quality of a diet), the American Academy of Pediatrics (AAP) recommends infants who are formula fed ingest an iron-enriched formula for the entire first year of life (Szymlek-Gay, Lonnerdal, Abrams, et al., 2012). Some women who breastfeed are also advised to supplement iron to ensure their infant does not develop iron-deficiency anemia (Ziegler, Nelson, & Jeter, 2011).

Fluoride.

Fluoride is essential for building sound teeth and for preventing tooth decay. Because teeth are already set in their primary form during pregnancy, it is important for women to drink fluoridated water during pregnancy. A lactating mother should continue drinking fluoridated water (although only a small amount of fluoride passes into breast milk), and formulas should be prepared with fluoridated water. This is an essential point to remember, because a mother may think she is helping her child by using bottled, "natural" water in formula rather than chlorinated (and fluoridated) water from a tap.

If a mother is breastfeeding and a source of fluoridated water is not available (the family drinks well, spring, or bottled water, or the tap water is not fluoridated), a fluoride supplement, 0.25 mg daily, may be given to the infant beginning at 6 months of age. Remind parents that too much fluoride can be detrimental or cause staining of the teeth to prevent them from giving additional but unnecessary fluoride supplements. Fluoride toothpaste should not be used with children under 2 years of age as they tend to swallow toothpaste (AAP, 2012b).

Vitamins

Although both breast milk and commercial formulas contain sufficient vitamins for growth, the AAP now recommends that breastfed babies be given a supplement of 400 International Units per day of vitamin D, beginning in the first few days of life. Babies who are fully or partially formula fed but drink less than 32 oz of formula a day also benefit from a daily 400 International Units vitamin D supplement (AAP, 2012c). Additional vitamins are not usually begun until the infant approaches 6 months of age.

BREASTFEEDING

It is universally agreed that breast milk is the preferred method of feeding for newborns because it provides numerous health benefits to both a mother and an infant; it remains the ideal nutritional source for infants through the first year of life (AAP, 2012a). Nurses are prime health care professionals to teach women about the benefits of breastfeeding and provide anticipatory guidance for problems that may occur (Rempel & McCleary, 2012; Tengir & Centinkaya, 2011). You can also help create an atmosphere conducive to breastfeeding success in health care facilities by implementing steps, such as:

- Educating all pregnant women about the benefits and management of breastfeeding.
- Helping women initiate breastfeeding within half an hour after birth.
- Assisting mothers to breastfeed and maintain lactation even if they should be separated from their infant.
- Not giving newborns food or drink other than breast milk unless medically indicated, so they are hungry to breastfeed. Advise women they need not introduce solid food until at least 4 months.
- Not giving newborns pacifiers to quiet them as this can reduce the sucking initiative.
- Supporting rooming-in (such as allowing mothers and infants to remain together) 24 hours a day.
- Encouraging breastfeeding on demand.
- Fostering the establishment of breastfeeding support groups and referring mothers to them on discharge from the birthing center or hospital.

Physiology of Breast Milk Production

Breast milk is formed in the acinar or alveolar cells of the mammary glands (Fig. 19.1). With the delivery of the placenta following birth, the level of progesterone in a woman's body falls dramatically, stimulating the production of **prolactin**, an anterior pituitary hormone. Prolactin acts on the acinar cells of the mammary glands to stimulate the production of milk. In addition, when an infant sucks at a breast, nerve impulses travel from the nipple to the hypothalamus to stimulate the production of prolactin-releasing factor. This factor stimulates further active production of prolactin. Other anterior pituitary hormones, such as adrenocorticotropic hormone, thyroid-stimulating hormone, and growth hormone, probably also play a role in growth of the mammary glands and their ability to secrete milk.

Colostrum, a thin, watery, yellow fluid composed of protein, sugar, fat, water, minerals, vitamins, and maternal antibodies, is secreted by the acinar breast cells starting in the fourth month of pregnancy. For the first 3 or 4 days after birth,

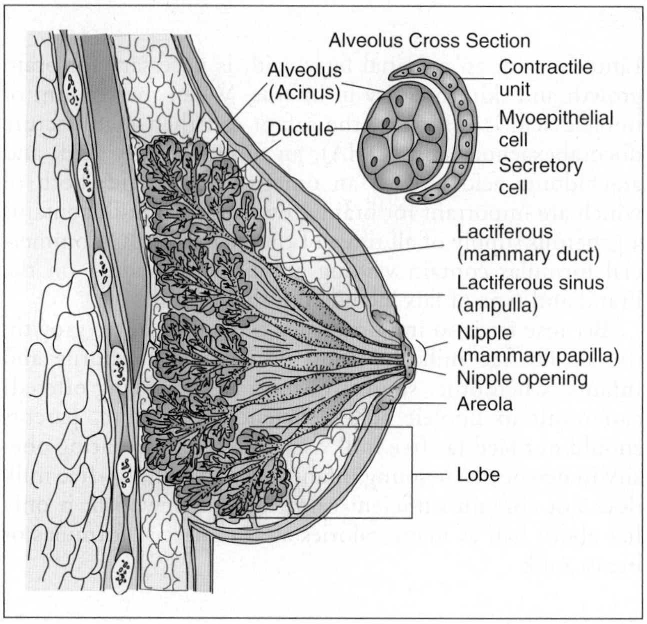

FIGURE 19.1 Anatomy of the breast.

colostrum production continues. Because it is high in protein and fairly low in sugar and fat, colostrum is easy to digest and capable of providing adequate nutrition for a newborn until it is replaced by transitional breast milk on the second to fourth day. True or mature breast milk is produced by the 10th day.

Milk flows from the alveolar cells, where it is produced, through small tubules to reservoirs for milk, the **lactiferous sinuses**, located behind the nipple. This constantly forming milk is called **fore milk**. Its availability depends very little on the infant's sucking at the breast. As the infant sucks at the breast, oxytocin, released from the posterior pituitary, causes the collecting sinuses of the mammary glands to contract, forcing milk forward through the nipples, making it available for the baby. This action is called a **let-down reflex**. A let-down reflex may also be triggered by the sound of a baby crying or by thinking about the baby. New milk, called **hind milk**, is formed after the let-down reflex. Hind milk, which is higher in fat than fore milk, is the milk that makes a breastfed infant grow most rapidly. The release of oxytocin has a second advantage in that, by causing smooth muscle contraction, it helps contract the uterus. As a result, a woman may feel a small tugging or cramping in her lower pelvis during the first few days of breastfeeding (i.e., afterpains) (Edmonds, 2012).

The average mother of a term infant is able to produce an adequate supply of breast milk for her infant without additional stimulation. Mothers of preterm infants, however, may need a milk production stimulant such as domperidone (Motilium), which increases prolactin production by the pituitary gland because their breasts were not fully ready for milk production at the time of their child's birth (Knoppert, Page, Warren, et al., 2013).

Advantages of Breastfeeding

Little controversy exists that breastfeeding is the best nutrition for human infants and is contraindicated in only a few circumstances, such as:

- An infant with galactosemia (such infants cannot digest the lactose in milk).

- Herpes lesions on a mother's nipples.
- Maternal diet is nutrient restricted, preventing quality milk production.
- Maternal exposure to radioactive compounds (such as occurs with thyroid testing).
- Mothers receiving antimetabolites or chemotherapeutic agents.
- Mothers receiving prescribed medications that would be harmful to an infant, such as lithium or methotrexate.
- Mothers who live in an area where environmental contaminants can be carried via breast milk to the infant.
- Women with maternal active, untreated tuberculosis, who need to be evaluated individually depending on the stage of their disease.
- Women who are positive for HIV, who are advised not to breastfeed in the United States until further studies confirm the risk of not being breastfed outweighs the risk of breast milk transmission of the virus (AAP, 2012a). In developing countries, HIV-positive women may be advised to breastfeed because commercial formula is not available.
- Women who are addicted to drugs, who also must be evaluated individually as to the drug, the half-life of the drug, and if drinking breast milk might actually aid drug withdrawal symptoms in the newborn.

A number of situations call for individual planning such as a mother or an infant too ill for breastfeeding or a mother who has undergone breast-reduction surgery where the nipples were detached during surgery. Cigarette smoking is not a contraindication to breastfeeding, but women should be aware some nicotine is carried in breast milk. The milk of mothers who smoke also tends to be lower in protein and may be less in amount (Bachour, Yafawi, Jaber, et al., 2012). In addition, the infant is exposed to secondhand smoke, which could lead to an increase in respiratory illnesses.

Advantages of Breastfeeding for Women.

A woman gains several physiologic benefits from breastfeeding:

- The release of oxytocin from the posterior pituitary gland aids in uterine involution.
- Breastfeeding may serve a protective function in preventing breast cancer and possibly ovarian cancer.
- A woman may return to her prepregnant weight sooner and, if menstruation is delayed, this may serve as a temporary family planning method.
- Successful breastfeeding can have an empowering effect because it is a skill only a woman can master.
- Breastfeeding reduces the cost of feeding and preparation time for infant feeding.
- A long-term effect may include a decreased risk of hip fractures and osteoporosis in the postmenopausal period for the woman (AAP, 2012a).
- Breastfeeding provides an excellent opportunity to enhance a true symbiotic bond between mother and child. Although this does readily occur with breastfeeding, a woman who holds her baby to formula feed can form this bond as well.

Common reasons women give for not exclusively breastfeeding include (a) insufficient milk supply, (b) feeling very tired, (c) having trouble with the infant latching to breast, and (d) wanting to allow their partner to feed the infant (DeFrisco, Goodman, Budin, et al., 2011).

Some women are reluctant to breastfeed because they fear having to be available to feed their baby every 3 or 4 hours will tie them down. Like mothers who formula feed, however, they can leave a bottle with expressed breast milk with a caregiver if they need to be away from their baby at the time of a feeding.

QSEN Checkpoint Question 19.2

Evidence-Based Practice

The AAP recommends infants be exclusively breastfed for 4 months. To discover the characteristics of women who were exclusively breastfeeding at the time of hospital discharge, researchers studied all term hospital births in the province of Ontario, Canada for a year. From this pool of over 90,000 infants, 56,865 were identified as still being exclusively breastfed at discharge. Characteristics of women who were exclusively breastfeeding were older age, nonsmoking, higher income, and no pregnancy complications or reproductive assistance. They also had a single rather than twin infants and had attended prenatal classes. Patients of obstetricians were less likely to exclusively breastfeed than those cared for by midwives or family physicians. Women who had a planned cesarean birth were more apt to breastfeed than those who had an unplanned cesarean birth.

Based on the previous findings, which statement by Linda would be the best indicator that she will be successful at exclusive breastfeeding?

a. "I enjoyed going for prenatal visits."
b. "I wish my husband earned more money."
c. "I can't wait until discharge when I can have a cigarette."
d. "I like having my first baby at 23; I'm young enough to adjust."

Look in Appendix A for the best answer and rationale.

Advantages for Infants.

Breastfeeding has major physiologic advantages for infants as well as it does for women. Breast milk contains secretory immunoglobulin A (IgA), which binds large molecules of foreign proteins, including viruses and bacteria, thus keeping them from being absorbed from the gastrointestinal tract.

Lactoferrin is an iron-binding protein in breast milk that interferes with the growth of pathogenic bacteria. The enzyme **lysozyme** in breast milk apparently actively destroys bacteria by lysing (dissolving) their cell membranes, possibly increasing the effectiveness of antibodies. Leukocytes in breast milk provide protection against common respiratory infectious invaders. Macrophages, responsible for producing **interferon** (a protein that protects against viruses), help interfere with virus growth. The **bifidus factor** is a specific growth-promoting factor for the beneficial bacteria *Lactobacillus bifidus*. The presence of *L. bifidus* in breast milk interferes with the colonization of pathogenic bacteria in the gastrointestinal tract, thus reducing the incidence of diarrhea (Whitney & Rolfes, 2012).

In addition to these anti-infective properties, breast milk contains the ideal electrolyte and mineral composition for human infant growth. It is high in lactose, an easily digested sugar that provides ready glucose for rapid brain growth. The protein in breast milk is easily digested, and the ratio of cysteine to methionine (two amino acids) in breast milk favors rapid brain growth in the early months. It contains nitrogen in compounds other than protein, so an infant can receive cell-building materials from sources other than just protein.

Breast milk contains more linoleic acid, an essential fatty acid for skin integrity, and less sodium, potassium, calcium, and phosphorus than do many formulas. Breast milk also has a better balance of trace elements, such as zinc. These levels of nutrients are enough to supply the infant's needs, yet they spare the infant's kidneys from having to process a high renal solute load of unused nutrients. Exclusively breastfeeding for at least 3 to 4 months or longer was found to reduce the incidence of certain allergies in 42% of infants where there was a family history of allergies (AAP, 2012a).

Yet another advantage of breastfeeding is that breastfed newborns appear to be able to regulate their calcium/phosphorus levels better than infants who are formula fed. Decreased calcium levels in a newborn can lead to tetany (muscle spasm). The increased concentration of fatty acid in commercial formulas may bind calcium in the gastrointestinal tract, also increasing the danger of tetany. Breastfeeding may also help prevent excessive weight gain in infants. It has been shown that exclusive breastfeeding into the infant's fourth month of life can decrease obesity as late as adolescence (Chivers, Hands, Parker, et al., 2010).

In addition, a great deal of discussion about the benefits of breastfeeding has centered on the effects of breastfeeding on the formation of the dental arch, because babies suck differently from a breast than from a bottle (Fig. 19.2). Babies pull their tongue backward as they suck from a breast. They thrust their tongue forward to suck from a rubber nipple. That may make breastfeeding the best preparation for forming common speech sounds (Diouf, Ngom, Badiane, et al., 2010).

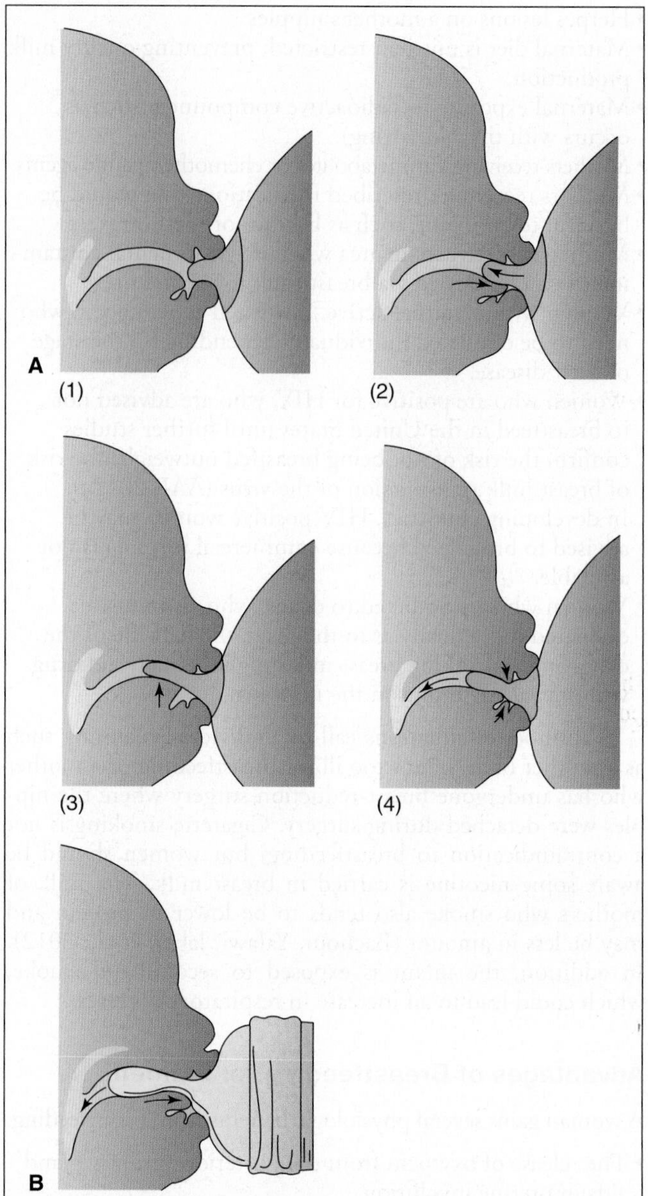

FIGURE 19.2 Differences in the sucking mechanism. **(A)** Breastfeeding. *(1)* Lips of the infant clamp in a C shape. The cheek muscles contract. *(2)* The tongue thrusts forward to grasp the nipple and areola. *(3)* The nipple is brought against the hard palate as the tongue pulls backward, bringing the areola into the mouth. *(4)* The gums compress the areola, squeezing milk into the back of the throat. **(B)** Formula feeding. The large rubber nipple of a bottle strikes the soft palate and interferes with the action of the tongue. The tongue moves forward against the gums to control the overflow of milk into the esophagus.

QSEN Checkpoint Question 19.3

Informatics

Linda asks you why breastfeeding is so beneficial for her newborn. You would want her to know breast milk has which of the following characteristics?

a. It is more nutritious than formula because it never needs to be warmed.
b. It will provide immunity as well as nutrients for her newborn.
c. It will protect her child from gastrointestinal cancer.
d. It will ensure her baby will never be obese as an adult.

Look in Appendix A for the best answer and rationale.

Techniques of Breastfeeding

Ask all women during pregnancy whether they plan to breastfeed their newborns because thinking about feeding in advance allows a woman and her partner to make an informed choice. If a partner expresses jealousy at the thought of breastfeeding, early discussion can help work through this natural sensation, with the eventual realization that parenting will involve many other opportunities for interaction with their child.

Physical preparation, such as nipple rolling, which was advised in the past as a way of making a woman's nipples more protuberant, is not necessary because few women have inverted or nonprotuberant nipples. In addition, oxytocin, which is released by this maneuver, could lead to preterm labor (nipple rolling is used to create uterine contractions for stress tests). The occasional woman who has inverted nipples may need to wear a nipple shield (a plastic shell) to help her nipples become more protuberant (Hanna, Wilson, & Norwood, 2012).

Beginning Breastfeeding

Breastfeeding should begin as soon after birth as possible, ideally while the woman is still in the birthing room and while the infant is in the first reactivity period (Perrine, Scanlon, Li, et al., 2012). The release of oxytocin by breastfeeding at this time begins the let-down of milk and also stimulates uterine contraction. However, if the woman is overly fatigued or extremely modest, trying to learn this new skill at this time may only convince her breastfeeding is not for her, so care must be individualized.

Most women enjoy having an experienced nurse with them for a first feeding to offer guidance. Be certain that infants open their mouths wide enough to grasp both the nipple and the **areola** (the pigmented circle surrounding the nipple) when sucking. This gives them effective sucking action and helps to empty the collecting sinuses completely.

An important principle for women to learn is that milk forms in response to being used. If breasts are completely emptied, they completely fill again. If half emptied, they only half fill, and after a time, milk production will become insufficient for proper nourishment. Urge women to always place their infant first at the breast at which the infant fed last in the previous feeding, to help ensure each breast is completely emptied at every other feeding. Box 19.3 shows an interprofessional care map illustrating both nursing and team planning for a woman who is breastfeeding for the first time.

Manual expression of breast milk is a means of completely emptying breasts or supplying milk to infants when the mother and baby are separated. This consists of supporting the breast firmly, then placing the thumb and forefinger on the opposite sides of the breast just behind the areolar margin, and first pushing backward toward the chest wall and then downward until secretions begins to flow (Box 19.4). Teach women to wash their breasts with clear water before beginning because soap tends to dry and crack nipples.

Because it takes less energy for an infant to suck at a bottle, urge parents not to offer bottles of breast milk until 4 to 6 weeks of age, or after the infant is thoroughly accustomed to breastfeeding. The AAP (2011) recommends not only preventing overheating and placing infants on their backs to sleep but also offering them pacifiers for the full first year of life to help prevent sudden infant death syndrome (SIDS). Offering a pacifier, however, can be delayed until about 1 month of age in breastfed infants or until breastfeeding is well established.

What if...19.1 Linda told you she doesn't really want to breastfeed but her husband is insisting she do so? What would you do?

Prolonged Jaundice in Breastfed Infants

Jaundice, or yellowing of the skin, occurs in as many as 15% of breastfed infants because pregnanediol (a breakdown product of progesterone) in breast milk depresses the action of glucuronyl transferase, the enzyme that converts indirect bilirubin (which cannot be excreted) to the direct form, which is then readily excreted in bile (Huether & McCance, 2011). To prevent this excess buildup of bilirubin (i.e., hyperbilirubinemia) in their infant, women should feed frequently in the immediate postbirth period because colostrum is a natural laxative and helps promote passage of both meconium and bile. Newborns who are discharged early from their birth setting or born at home need to be observed carefully for jaundice. Breastfeeding rarely results in a serum bilirubin level high enough to warrant therapy or to require discontinuation of breastfeeding, however, because pregnanediol remains in breast milk for only 24 to 48 hours (Thilo & Rosenberg, 2011).

BOX 19.3 Nursing Care Planning

AN INTERPROFESSIONAL CARE MAP FOR A WOMAN WHO IS BREASTFEEDING FOR THE FIRST TIME

Linda Satir is a new mother of a term baby girl. During the pregnancy, she and her husband, Paul, both agreed Linda would breastfeed. She attempted to breastfeed her newborn in the birthing room, with minimal success. As you offer to help her feed her baby for the second time, she says, "Do you think I made the right choice? Maybe I should formula feed her. Paul could help that way and I won't have to worry about what to do when I go back to work."

Family Assessment Client lives with husband in two-bedroom trailer in suburban trailer park. Husband works as an interpreter for local Chamber of Commerce. Linda will be returning to work as an executive assistant at an advertising agency after her 6-week maternity leave.

Client Assessment Mother is 2 hours postpartum. Newborn had difficulty latching onto breasts immediately after birth. Nipples without signs of redness or irritation. Breasts slightly firm. Colostrum present. Client discouraged with first breastfeeding attempt.

Nursing Diagnosis Risk for ineffective breastfeeding related to anxiety and inexperience

Outcome Criteria Client describes ways to properly position a newborn at the breast; states newborn is latching on and sucking; verbalizes increasing satisfaction and confidence with each feeding session.

(continued on page 496)

(Continued from previous page)

pregnancy with a preexisting disorder, such as cardiac or respiratory illness, that can complicate pregnancy.

How would you answer Angelina? Do you think she realizes pregnancy often becomes high risk not because of any one factor, but an accumulation of them?

When a woman enters pregnancy with a chronic condition such as cardiovascular or kidney disease, or if she experiences an unintentional injury or develops a chronic illness during pregnancy, both she and the fetus can be at risk for complications. Either the pregnancy can complicate the disease or the disease can complicate the pregnancy, affecting the fetus or leaving the woman less equipped to function in the future or undergo a future pregnancy. Nursing care needs to include close observation of both maternal health and fetal well-being, education for the woman and her family about special danger signs to watch for during pregnancy, and actions to minimize complications whenever possible, including:

- Preventing disorders from affecting the health of the fetus
- Helping a woman regain her health as quickly as possible so she can continue a healthy pregnancy and prepare herself psychologically and physically for labor, birth, and the arrival of her newborn
- Helping a woman learn more about her illness so she can continue to safeguard her health during her childrearing years

Conditions that cause severe symptoms such as a marked change in fluid and electrolyte balance, altered cardiovascular or respiratory function, or severe blood loss are especially dangerous to a fetus (Gregory, Korst, Lu, et al., 2013). Because of this danger, 2020 National Health Goals related to complications of pregnancy have been established (Box 20.1).

Although pregnancy can be a stressful time, generally, women experience overall good health during pregnancy, perhaps in part because of their extra care and concern in keeping healthy for two. This extra motivation also encourages a woman with a high-risk pregnancy to carefully follow a therapeutic regimen established for her to keep herself and her fetus safe.

BOX 20.1 Nursing Care Planning Based on 2020 National Health Goals

Several National Health Goals are aimed at reducing complications of pregnancy that arise from existing or newly acquired disorders.

- Reduce the rate of fetal deaths to 5.6 per 1,000 live births from a baseline of 6.2 per 1,000 live births.
- Reduce the rate of maternal deaths to 11.4 per 100,000 live births from a baseline of 12.7 per 100,000 live births.
- Reduce the rate of maternal illness and complications during pregnancy to 28 per 100 births from a baseline of 31.1 per 100 births (U.S. Department of Health and Human Services [DHHS], 2010; see www.healthypeople.gov).

Nurses can help the nation reach these goals by educating women about the importance of entering pregnancy in the best state of health possible. Helping women who have diabetes mellitus understand the importance of prepregnancy care so they enter pregnancy without hyperglycemia is an important step toward reducing congenital anomalies in newborns. Supporting women with kidney, heart, or respiratory disease during pregnancy to continue to follow their medical regimen is yet another way.

Nursing Process Overview

For Care of a Woman With a Preexisting or Newly Acquired Illness

Assessment

An accurate prenatal assessment of a woman with a preexisting or newly acquired illness requires a thorough understanding of the signs and symptoms of the illness in addition to an understanding of the course of a normal pregnancy (Fig. 20.1). Assessment techniques include objective measures such as establishing baseline vital signs as well as subjective factors such as the extent of edema or level of exhaustion a woman is experiencing. Such assessment is best made by health care personnel who care for a woman consistently throughout the pregnancy so that subtle changes can be recognized. It's also important to teach a woman how to assess her own health in relation to objective parameters. She could report exhaustion, for example, in relation to daily activity such as, "Two weeks ago I could walk a block without being short of breath. Today I could walk only half a block" or "The last time I was in for a checkup, edema didn't occur until bedtime. Now I notice it every afternoon by the time my son comes home from school."

Nursing Diagnosis

Nursing diagnoses developed for a woman with a high-risk pregnancy address her specific, disease-related condition as well as any therapeutic restrictions her condition might require. Examples of possible nursing diagnoses include:

- Ineffective tissue perfusion (cardiopulmonary) related to poor heart function secondary to mitral valve prolapse during pregnancy
- Pain related to pyelonephritis secondary to uterine pressure on ureters
- Social isolation related to prescribed bed rest during pregnancy secondary to concurrent illness
- Ineffective role performance related to increasing level of daily restrictions secondary to chronic illness and pregnancy
- Knowledge deficit related to normal changes of pregnancy versus illness complications
- Fear regarding pregnancy outcome related to chronic illness
- Health-seeking behaviors related to the effects of illness on pregnancy
- Situational low self-esteem related to illness during pregnancy

Outcome Identification and Planning

Be certain that expected outcomes are realistic in light of a woman's pregnancy and the restrictions placed on her

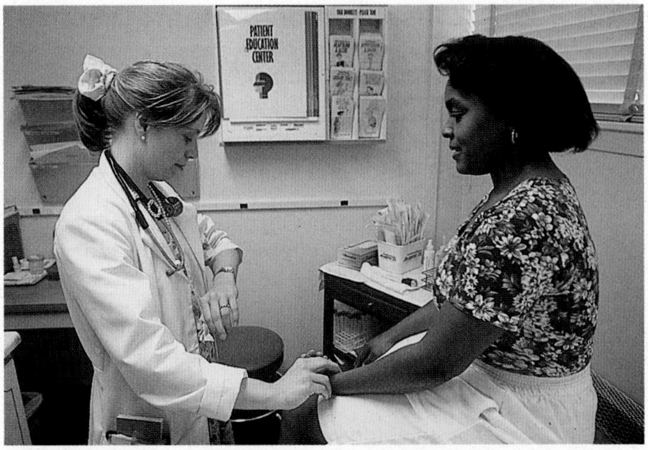

FIGURE 20.1 It is important to establish baseline vital signs to later identify a complication related to a preexisting condition. (© Bob Kramer.)

by her health. Remember that one family member with illness affects all family members; therefore, outcomes should relate to the entire family's health.

When making plans with a woman who has a preexisting medical condition, base them on the pattern of her life before the pregnancy. For example, to ensure a pregnant woman receives enough rest during pregnancy, planning for an afternoon rest period each day is usually adequate. However, for a woman with cardiac disease who took two rest periods a day before pregnancy, this would be ineffective because now she probably needs four rest periods. A primary goal for a woman with a severe chronic condition might be to maintain her health during pregnancy so she can remain at home as long as possible, thereby minimizing hospitalization and family disruptions.

Planning for a new illness may be difficult for a woman because of the shock of the diagnosis. Be careful, however, not to make plans for her such as, "Your best plan would be to begin strict bed rest." Instead, give a woman the available alternatives such as, "There are two possible therapies. Let me review with you the advantages and disadvantages of each one." Allowing a woman to choose among alternatives in this way helps her to participate in her own care and also maintain self-esteem as well as helps her move a step toward parenthood and assuming care for her family. Web sites that can be helpful to recommend to families are those of the American Heart Association (www.americanheart.org), the National Kidney Foundation (www.kidney.org), the American Diabetes Association (www.diabetes.org), and the Sickle Cell Disease Association of America (www.sicklecelldisease.org).

Implementation

Nursing interventions for a pregnant woman with a chronic illness may focus on teaching her new or additional measures to maintain health during the pregnancy. Imaginative solutions to problems may need to be created because, otherwise, a woman may be unable to adjust to the extent of changes she must make.

Outcome Evaluation

If an evaluation of outcomes at health care visits reveals that an expected outcome is not being met, a new assessment, analysis, and planning need to be done. In some instances, an outcome is not met because a woman did not understand the need for an additional pregnancy measure. At other times, a woman may need better psychological support to continue to follow a health care routine consistently because 9 months is a long time to adhere to restrictions. Make evaluation ongoing to ensure that you know throughout the pregnancy whether interventions are successful. Some examples of outcomes that might be established include:

- Client states she rests for 2 hours morning and afternoon; dependent edema remains at 1+ or less at next prenatal visit.
- Family members state they are all participating in an exercise program since mother developed gestational diabetes.
- Client reports no burning on urination or flank pain at next prenatal visit.
- Client states she understands the importance of taking daily thyroid medicine for total length of pregnancy.

IDENTIFYING A HIGH-RISK PREGNANCY

A **high-risk pregnancy** is one in which a concurrent disorder, pregnancy-related complication, or external factor jeopardizes the health of the woman, the fetus, or both.

It's important that women with such pregnancies be identified because illness during pregnancy can complicate not only the pregnancy but also a woman's entire lifestyle and that of her family. In most instances, more than one factor contributes to the classification of a pregnancy as high risk. The pregnancy of a woman with diabetes, for example, is automatically considered as having a greater than normal risk because it forces a fetus to grow in an environment in which **hyperglycemia** (increased serum glucose levels) becomes the rule. During such a pregnancy, a woman, worrying that something will happen to her baby, may fail to begin the "pregnancy work" that she must do so bonding can take place. At birth, her child is in double jeopardy: not only is the baby born with altered glucose metabolism but he or she also is at high risk for poor maternal–child or parent–child attachment.

Remembering that the term "high risk" rarely refers to just one causative factor but includes psychological and social as well as physical aspects helps in the planning of holistic, and ultimately effective, nursing care. Preexisting or newly acquired maternal illnesses that can make a pregnancy high risk are discussed in this chapter. Chapter 21 discusses conditions directly related to pregnancy that can make a pregnancy high risk. Chapter 22 covers populations that are at high risk because of age (younger than 18 years or older than 40 years), the presence of a disability or trauma, or drug abuse.

CARDIOVASCULAR DISORDERS AND PREGNANCY

The number of women of childbearing age who have heart disease is diminishing as more and more congenital heart anomalies (discussed in Chapter 41) are corrected in early infancy. Also, rheumatic fever is being more actively prevented and treated so that cardiac damage from this disorder is also reduced. For these reasons, cardiovascular disease (even with hypertension included), which was once a major threat to pregnancy, now complicates only approximately 1% of all pregnancies. Cardiovascular disease is still a concern in pregnancy, however, because it can lead to such serious complications. It is responsible for 5% of maternal deaths during pregnancy (Cunningham, Leveno, Bloom, et al., 2010).

The cardiovascular disorders that most commonly cause difficulty during pregnancy are valve damage concerns caused by rheumatic fever or Kawasaki disease and congenital anomalies such as atrial septal defect or uncorrected coarctation of the aorta (Kuo, Yang, Chang, et al., 2012). Aortic dilatation may occur from Marfan syndrome and is also a concern (Easterling & Stout, 2012). As the number of women delaying their first pregnancy until later in life increases, there is a corresponding increase in the incidence of coronary artery disease and varicosities during pregnancy. In contrast, heart disease that occurs specifically with pregnancy (peripartum heart disease) still only rarely occurs as it is apparently unrelated to age. With improved management of women with cardiac disorders, women who might never have risked pregnancy in the past are able to complete pregnancies successfully today.

A woman with cardiovascular disease needs an interprofessional team approach to care during pregnancy. Ideally, she should visit her pregnancy care provider for preconception care so her state of health and baseline data when she is not pregnant can be established. She should begin prenatal care as soon as she suspects she is pregnant (1 week after the first missed menstrual period or as soon as she has a positive home pregnancy test) so her general condition and circulatory system can be monitored from the beginning of pregnancy.

Pregnancy taxes the circulatory system of every woman, even those without cardiac disease, because both the blood volume and cardiac output increase approximately 30% (and up to as much as 50%) during pregnancy. Half of this increase occurs by 8 weeks; it is maximized by midpregnancy (Gilbert, 2011).

Because of the increased blood flow past valves, functional (innocent) or transient murmurs can be heard in many women without heart disease during pregnancy. Heart palpitations on sudden exertion are also usual.

The danger of pregnancy in a woman with cardiac disease occurs primarily because of this increase in circulatory volume. The most dangerous time for her is in weeks 28 to 32, just after the blood volume peaks. However, if heart disease is severe, symptoms can occur at the very beginning of pregnancy. Toward the end of pregnancy, her heart may become so overwhelmed by the increase in blood volume that her cardiac output falls to the point vital organs (including the placenta) can no longer be perfused adequately. When this happens, the oxygen and nutritional requirements of her cells and those of the fetus are not met.

The estimation of whether a woman with cardiovascular disease can complete a pregnancy successfully depends on the type and extent of her disease. As a rule, a woman with an artificial but well-functioning heart valve, a woman with a pacemaker implant, and even a woman who has had a heart transplant can expect to have successful pregnancies as long as they have effective prenatal and postnatal care (Humphreys, Wong, Milner, et al., 2012).

TABLE 20.1 Classification of Heart Disease

Class	Description
I	Uncompromised. Ordinary physical activity causes no discomfort. No symptoms of cardiac insufficiency and no anginal pain.
II	Slightly compromised. Ordinary physical activity causes excessive fatigue, palpitation, and dyspnea or anginal pain.
III	Markedly compromised. During less than ordinary activity, woman experiences excessive fatigue, palpitations, dyspnea, or anginal pain.
IV	Severely compromised. Woman is unable to carry out any physical activity without experiencing discomfort. Even at rest, symptoms of cardiac insufficiency or anginal pain are present.

From Criteria Committee of the New York Heart Association. (1994). *Nomenclature and criteria for diagnosis of diseases of the heart and great vessels* (9th ed.). Boston, MA: Little, Brown & Co.

To predict a pregnancy outcome, heart disease is divided into four categories based on criteria established by the New York Heart Association (Table 20.1). A woman with class I or II heart disease can expect to experience a normal pregnancy and birth. Women with class III can complete a pregnancy by maintaining special interventions such as bed rest. Women with class IV heart disease are usually advised to avoid pregnancy because they are in cardiac failure even at rest and when they are not pregnant.

A Woman With Cardiac Disease

Cardiac disease can affect pregnancy in different ways depending on whether it involves the left or the right side of the heart.

A Woman With Left-Sided Heart Failure

Left-sided heart failure occurs in conditions such as mitral stenosis, mitral insufficiency, and aortic coarctation. In these instances, the left ventricle cannot move the large volume of blood forward that it has received by the left atrium from the pulmonary circulation. This causes back pressure—the left side of the heart becomes distended, systemic blood pressure decreases in the face of lowered cardiac output, and pulmonary hypertension occurs. When pressure in the pulmonary vein reaches a point of about 25 mmHg, fluid begins to pass from the pulmonary capillary membranes into the interstitial spaces surrounding the lung alveoli and then into the alveoli themselves (pulmonary edema). Pulmonary edema produces profound shortness of breath as it interferes with oxygen–carbon dioxide exchange (Brushers, 2012). If pulmonary capillaries rupture under the pressure, small amounts of blood leak into the alveoli and the woman develops a productive cough with blood-speckled sputum. Because of the limited oxygen exchange, a woman with left-sided heart failure is at an extremely high risk for spontaneous miscarriage, preterm labor, or even maternal death.

As the oxygen saturation of the blood decreases from dysfunction of the alveoli, chemoreceptors stimulate the respiratory center to increase respiratory rate. At first, this is noticeable only on exertion, then finally with rest also. As the systemic decrease in blood pressure registers on the pressoreceptors in the aorta, the heart rate increases and peripheral vasoconstriction occurs in an attempt to increase the systemic blood pressure. As the fall in blood pressure is registered with the renin-angiotensin system, retention of both sodium and water occurs. A woman experiences increased fatigue, weakness, and dizziness. The placenta may not receive adequate blood because of the decreased peripheral circulation.

As pulmonary edema becomes severe, a woman cannot sleep in any position except with her chest and head elevated **(orthopnea)**, as elevating her chest this way allows fluid to settle to the bottom of her lungs and frees space for gas exchange. She may also notice **paroxysmal nocturnal dyspnea**—suddenly waking at night with shortness of breath. This occurs because heart action is more effective when she is at rest. With the more effective heart action, interstitial fluid returns to the circulation. This overburdens her circulation, causing increased left-side failure and increased pulmonary edema.

If mitral stenosis is present, it is so difficult for blood to leave the left atrium that a secondary problem of thrombus formation can occur from noncirculating blood. If coarctation of the aorta is causing the difficulty, dissection of the aorta from high blood pressure from trying to push blood past the constriction can occur. To prevent thrombus formation, a woman may be prescribed an anticoagulant. To decrease the strain on the aorta, antihypertensives may be prescribed to control blood pressure, diuretics to reduce blood volume, and β-blockers to improve ventricular filling. A woman will be scheduled for serial ultrasound and nonstress tests after weeks 30 to 32 of pregnancy to monitor fetal health and to rule out poor placental perfusion. A balloon valve angioplasty to loosen mitral valve adhesions and improve valve function can be performed safely during pregnancy (Traill, 2012).

If an anticoagulant is required, low-molecular-weight heparin is the drug of choice for early pregnancy because it does not cross the placenta and so does not have teratogenic effects.

A Woman With Right-Sided Heart Failure

Right-sided heart failure occurs when the right ventricle is overwhelmed by the amount of blood received by the right atrium from the vena cava. It can be caused by an unrepaired congenital heart defect such as pulmonary valve stenosis, but the anomaly most apt to cause right-sided heart failure in women of reproductive age is Eisenmenger syndrome, a right-to-left atrial or ventricular septal defect with an accompanying pulmonary valve stenosis (Wolff & Weitzel, 2011).

With this, congestion of the systemic venous circulation and decreased cardiac output to the lungs occurs. Blood pressure decreases in the aorta because less blood is able to reach it; in contrast, pressure is high in the vena cava from back pressure of blood. Both jugular venous distention and increased portal circulation are evident. The liver and spleen both become distended. Extreme liver enlargement can cause dyspnea and pain in a pregnant woman because the enlarged liver, as it is pressed upward by the enlarged uterus, puts extreme pressure on the diaphragm. Distention of abdominal and lower extremity vessels can lead to exudate of fluid from the vessels into the peritoneal cavity (i.e., ascites) or peripheral edema.

Women who have an uncorrected anomaly of this type may be advised not to become pregnant. If they do plan a pregnancy, because they need oxygen administration and frequent arterial blood gas assessments to ensure fetal growth, they can expect to be hospitalized for at least some days during the last part of pregnancy. During labor, they may need a pulmonary artery catheter inserted to monitor pulmonary pressure. Women with this condition also need extremely close monitoring after epidural anesthesia to minimize the risk of hypotension.

A Woman With Peripartum Heart Disease

An extremely rare condition, **peripartal cardiomyopathy** can originate in pregnancy in women with no previous history of heart disease (Hess & Weinland, 2012). Although the cause is unknown, this apparently occurs because of the stress of the pregnancy on the circulatory system. The mortality rate can be as high as 50%. It occurs most often in African American multiparas in conjunction with gestational hypertension. A woman develops signs of myocardial failure such as shortness of breath, chest pain, and nondependent edema. Her heart increases in size (i.e., cardiomegaly). For therapy, she must sharply reduce her physical activity; many women also need a diuretic, an arrhythmia agent, and digitalis therapy to maintain heart function. Low–molecular-weight heparin may be administered to decrease the risk of thromboembolism. Immunosuppressive therapy is yet another possibility to improve symptoms.

If the cardiomegaly persists past the postpartum period, it is generally suggested a woman not attempt any further pregnancies because the condition tends to recur or worsen in additional pregnancies. At the same time, oral contraceptives are contraindicated because of the danger of thromboembolism that these can create. Some women's disease progresses so much that following pregnancy, a woman may need a heart transplant (Dalzell, Jackson, & Gardner, 2011).

Assessment of a Woman With Cardiac Disease

Nurses play a major role in the care of pregnant women with cardiovascular disease because continuous assessment of women's health status, health education, and health-promotion activities are so essential. Assessment begins with a thorough health history to document prepregnancy cardiac status (Box 20.2). Document a woman's level of exercise performance (i.e., what level she can do before growing short of breath and what physical symptoms she experiences, such as cyanosis of the lips or nail beds). Ask if she normally has a cough or edema (it's important that women with cardiac disease always report coughing during pregnancy because pulmonary edema from heart failure may first manifest itself as a simple cough).

Documenting edema is also important because the usual innocent edema of pregnancy must be distinguished from the beginning of edema from heart failure (serious). An important difference is the usual edema of pregnancy involves only the feet and ankles but becomes systemic with heart failure. It can begin as early as the first trimester, and other symptoms such as irregular pulse, rapid or difficult respirations, and perhaps chest pain on exertion will probably also be present. Be certain to record a baseline blood pressure, pulse rate, and respiratory rate in either a sitting or lying position

BOX 20.2 Nursing Care Planning Using Assessment

Assessing a Pregnant Woman With Cardiac Disease

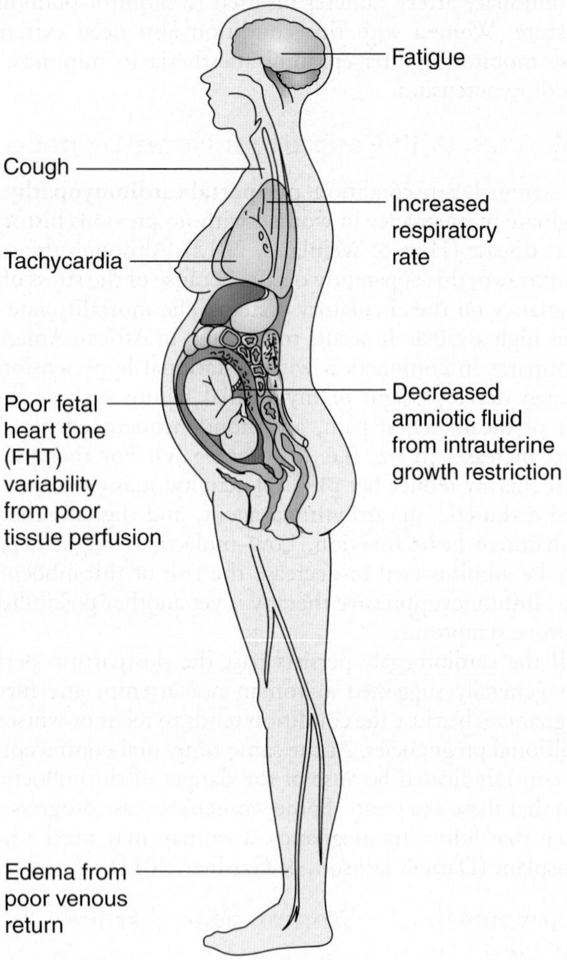

at the first prenatal visit; at future health visits, always obtain these in the same position for the most accurate comparison. Making comparison assessments for nail bed filling (should be <5 seconds) and jugular venous distention can also be helpful throughout pregnancy.

If a woman's heart disease involves right-sided heart failure, assess liver size at prenatal visits. Keep in mind that liver assessments can become difficult and probably inaccurate late in pregnancy because the enlarged uterus presses the liver upward under the ribs and makes it difficult to palpate.

For an additional cardiac status assessment, an electrocardiogram (ECG) or an echocardiogram may be done at periodic points in pregnancy. Assure the woman that an ECG merely measures cardiac electrical discharge and so cannot harm her fetus in any way. Echocardiography uses ultrasound and, likewise, will not harm her fetus.

Fetal Assessment

At the point that maternal blood pressure becomes insufficient to provide an adequate supply of blood and nutrients to the placenta, fetal health can be compromised. For this reason, the infants of women with severe heart disease tend to have low birth weights or be small for gestational age because of acidosis, which develops due to poor oxygen/carbon dioxide exchange or not being furnished with enough nutrients. This can result in preterm labor, which exposes the newborn to the hazards of immaturity as well as low birth weight. If the placenta is not filling well, a fetus may not respond well to labor (evidenced by late deceleration patterns on a fetal heart monitor), and a cesarean birth may be necessary (an increased risk for both the mother and fetus).

Nursing Diagnoses and Related Interventions

Nursing Diagnosis: Deficient knowledge regarding steps to take to reduce the effects of maternal cardiovascular disease on the pregnancy and fetus

Outcome Evaluation: Client identifies danger signs such as angina pain and steps to take when they occur; maternal blood pressure is maintained above 100/60 mmHg and fetal heart rate at 110 to 160 beats/min.

Be certain that goals and outcomes established with a woman with heart disease are realistic. Not all women with heart disease, for example, will be able to complete a pregnancy successfully; some infants of women with severe involvement will be born with the effects of placental insufficiency, such as neurologic involvement or cognitive challenge. However, there are positive actions a woman with heart disease can take to reduce or eliminate complications during pregnancy, such as increasing periods of rest to strengthen heart action.

Promote Rest. As a rule, women with cardiac disease need two rest periods a day (fully resting, not getting up frequently) and a full night's sleep (not tossing and turning) to obtain adequate rest. Rest should be in the left lateral recumbent position to prevent supine hypotension syndrome and increased heart effort.

Women should plan activities so they stop exercising before the point when cardiac output becomes insufficient to meet systemic body demands causing peripheral and uterine/placental constriction. Be certain they know exactly how much they should limit their exercise. Some women, for example, may need to discontinue employment early in pregnancy rather than work until the end. A prescription to allow "normally heavy" housework may mean nothing more strenuous than dusting to some women. To others, it may mean washing windows, turning mattresses, and shoveling snow. Ask enough questions, therefore, to make certain a woman's definition of "heavy work" is the same as yours and her primary care provider's.

Promote Healthy Nutrition. A woman with cardiac disease may need closer supervision of nutrition during pregnancy than the average woman because she must gain enough weight to ensure a healthy pregnancy and a healthy baby, but she must not gain so much weight that her heart and circulatory system become overburdened.

Be certain she is remembering to take her prenatal vitamins. These contain an iron supplement to help prevent anemia. Anemia is important to prevent because it places an extra burden on the heart because her circulatory system must circulate blood more vigorously than usual to distribute oxygen to all body cells. If a woman was following a sodium-restricted diet before pregnancy, this may be continued during pregnancy; although typically, a woman's sodium intake is only limited, not severely restricted, during pregnancy because it's important to obtain enough sodium to maintain fluid volume and balance as well as furnish an adequate supply of blood to the fetus.

What if...20.1 Angelina is diagnosed as having class II heart disease. Because of her work as a fundraiser, she is on her feet all day. What suggestions could you make to help her incorporate more rest into each day?

Educate Regarding Medication. Women taking cardiac medication, such as digoxin, before pregnancy may need to increase their maintenance dose because of their expanded blood volume during pregnancy. A woman who was not digoxin dependent before pregnancy may need such therapy prescribed as pregnancy advances and her cardiac output has to be increased or strengthened. To aid a woman in continuing to think of herself as basically a well person, help her to understand this does not mean her heart function is weakening, but rather it is only temporarily being stressed by the increased circulatory load of pregnancy. Digoxin also has a unique use during pregnancy as it can be administered to the woman to slow the fetal heart if fetal tachycardia is present. Arrhythmia agents such as adenosine, β-blockers, and angiotensin-converting enzyme (ACE) inhibitors to reduce hypertension are safe to use during pregnancy and are also frequently prescribed. Nitroglycerin, a compound often prescribed for angina, although not well studied during pregnancy (a category C drug), is also considered safe (Karch, 2013).

A woman who was taking penicillin prophylactically because she had rheumatic fever as a child (which is often taken for 10 years after the occurrence of rheumatic fever, or at least until age 18 years) should continue to take this drug during pregnancy because penicillin is not known to be a teratogen (a category B drug). Close to the anticipated day of birth, some primary care providers prescribe an additional course of ampicillin, amoxicillin (Amoxil), or clindamycin (Cleocin) to prevent streptococci bacteria from invading the denuded placental site on the uterus and creating a subacute bacterial endocarditis.

It is often difficult to keep healthy women from taking over-the-counter medicines during pregnancy; conversely, it can be just as difficult to encourage women to take medicine prescribed during pregnancy. Help women with heart disease to understand there are valid exceptions to the rule of "no medicine during pregnancy" so they make out reminders to adhere to their prescribed regimen.

Educate Regarding Avoidance of Infection. A systemic infection almost automatically increases body temperature, forcing a woman to expend more energy and increase her cardiac output as her metabolism increases, an effect that could be too extreme for a woman with heart disease to withstand. Caution women with heart disease, therefore, to avoid visiting or being visited by people with infections and to alert health care personnel at the first indication of an upper respiratory tract infection or urinary tract infection (UTI) so that, if warranted, antibiotic therapy can begin early in the course of the infection. Monthly screening for bacteriuria with a clean-catch urine test at prenatal visits should help detect UTIs.

Be Prepared for Emergency Actions. If women with heart disease overexert during a prenatal visit, they may need supplemental oxygen or cardiac resuscitation. The rules for cardiac resuscitation for women who are pregnant do not differ from the usual technique (Box 20.3).

What if...20.2 Angelina tells you she has abruptly discontinued taking the daily penicillin she has been prescribed for her heart disease since childhood. As it has been a long time since she had rheumatic fever, would you recommend she could omit taking this during pregnancy?

Nursing Interventions During Labor and Birth

Frequently assess a woman's blood pressure, pulse, and respirations and monitor fetal heart rate and uterine contractions during labor for women with heart disease to be certain their circulatory system is not failing and the placenta is filling adequately. A rapidly increasing pulse rate (>100 beats/min) is an indication a heart is pumping ineffectively and so has increased its rate in an effort to compensate. Normally, it's good to advise a woman to assume a side-lying position during labor to reduce the possibility of supine hypotension syndrome. If a woman has some pulmonary edema, however, it may be necessary for her to elevate her head and chest (a semi-Fowler's position) to ease the work of breathing. If this is necessary, be certain to place a towel under her right hip to shift the uterus off the vena cava, the same as would happen with a side-lying position. Remember, fatigue is a symptom of heart decompensation. Evaluate women carefully, therefore, to determine whether the fatigue a woman reports is heart or labor related.

Women with extreme heart disease may need oxygen administered during labor because of the need for extra oxygen due to the exertion of labor; continuous hemodynamic monitoring such as by a Swan-Ganz catheter to monitor heart

BOX 20.3 Nursing Care Planning Using Procedures

CARDIOPULMONARY RESUSCITATION DURING PREGNANCY

Purpose: To restore cardiac and respiratory function.

PLAN	PRINCIPLE
1. Determine the woman is unconscious and not breathing by shaking and shouting her name.	1. Shaking the shoulders and shouting are effective actions to determine unconsciousness and rouse a woman who may have fainted or is asleep.
2. Call for emergency help and have them bring a cardiac defibrillator.	2. The woman may need more than simple resuscitation.
3. Begin chest compressions. Place both hands on the lower sternum just above the xiphoid process and compress the chest a distance of 2 in. at a rate of 100 times a minute.	3. External chest compressions stimulate the action of the heart to maintain tissue perfusion. Allow chest recoil after each compression.
4. A second rescuer can deliver respiratory ventilations at a rate of 1 breath every 6 to 8 seconds (8 to 10 breaths/min).	4. Ventilation improves oxygenation.
5. If an automated external defibrillator (AED) is necessary, remove any fetal or uterine monitors if these are in place. Follow standard application and procedure according to agency protocol.	5. AED is effective at stimulating heart action and is not detrimental to pregnancy or a fetus.
6. When the emergency rescue team has arrived and relieved you as a first responder, place a rolled or folded towel under the woman's right hip.	6. A towel placed under one hip helps to prevent uterine compression on the vena cava and helps prevent supine hypotension syndrome.

function may be prescribed. Many women with heart disease should not push with contractions, as pushing requires more effort than they should expend. That makes epidural anesthesia the anesthetic of choice for women with heart disease because this decreases the sensation of pushing and can make both labor and birth less taxing. Because of the lack of pushing, low forceps or a vacuum extractor may be used for birth. A woman may be disappointed during labor to learn her labor is not going to be "natural." Stress that these measures may not be what she anticipated, but they can help her achieve her ultimate goal, a healthy newborn and a mother able to care for her new baby.

Postpartum Nursing Interventions

The period immediately after birth is a critical time for a woman with heart disease because, with delivery of the placenta, the blood that supplied the placenta is released into her general circulation, increasing her blood volume by 20% to 40%. During pregnancy, the increase in blood volume that occurred did so over a 6-month period, so her heart had time to gradually adjust to this change. After birth, the increase in pressure takes place within 5 minutes, so the heart must make a rapid and major adjustment (Easterling & Stout, 2012).

To compensate for these circulatory changes, a woman may need a program of decreased activity and possibly anticoagulant and digoxin therapy until her circulation stabilizes. Antiembolic stockings or intermittent pneumatic compression (IPC) boots may be prescribed to increase venous return from the legs. If prophylactic antibiotics had not been started prior to birth, they should be started immediately after birth to discourage subacute bacterial endocarditis caused by the introduction of microorganisms through the placental site.

A woman with heart disease is often interested in close inspection of her baby immediately after birth because she wants to know if her infant has a heart defect or was harmed by any medication she took during pregnancy. Be certain to point out that acrocyanosis is normal in newborns so she does not interpret her baby's peripheral cyanosis as cardiac inadequacy.

In the postpartum period, a stool softener can be prescribed to prevent straining with bowel movements. Agents to encourage uterine involution, such as oxytocin (Pitocin), should be used with caution because they tend to increase blood pressure, which necessitates increased heart action. As a rule, women with heart disease can breastfeed without difficulty. Kegel exercises are acceptable for perineal strengthening immediately, but the woman should not begin postpartum exercises to improve abdominal tone until her primary care provider approves them. Before discharge, be certain a woman has thought through if she will need help at home so she can continue getting periods of rest. Also ensure that she schedules a return appointment for a postpartum checkup for both her gynecologic health and her cardiac status.

A Woman With an Artificial Valve Prosthesis

In the past, women with heart valve prostheses were advised not to become pregnant for fear the increased blood volume gained during pregnancy would overwhelm the artificial valve. Today, evidence shows women with a valve prosthesis can complete a pregnancy safely (Suri, Keepanasseril, Aggarwal, et al., 2011). One potential problem involves the use of oral anticoagulants women take to prevent the formation of blood clots at the valve site. Because the usual maintenance drug for this, sodium warfarin (Coumadin), increases the risk of congenital anomalies in infants (pregnancy risk category D), women are usually placed on low–molecular-weight heparin therapy (category C) before becoming pregnant and during pregnancy. Subclinical bleeding from continuous anticoagulant therapy has the potential to cause placental dislodgement. Therefore, observe a woman who is taking an anticoagulant for signs of petechiae and premature separation of the placenta during both pregnancy and labor.

A Woman With Chronic Hypertensive Vascular Disease

Women with chronic hypertensive disease enter pregnancy with an elevated blood pressure (140/90 mmHg or above). Hypertension of this kind is usually associated with arteriosclerosis or renal disease, making it a problem for the older pregnant woman. Chronic hypertension can be serious because it places both the woman and fetus at high risk because of poor heart, kidney, and/or placental perfusion during the pregnancy (Gelson, Curry, Gatzoulis, et al., 2011). Management includes a prescription of β-blockers and ACE inhibitors to reduce blood pressure by peripheral dilation to a safe level, but not to reduce it below the threshold that allows for good placenta circulation. Methyldopa (Aldomet) is a typical drug that may be prescribed.

A Woman With Venous Thromboembolic Disease

The incidence of venous thromboembolic disease increases during pregnancy because of a combination of stasis of blood in the lower extremities from uterine pressure and hypercoagulability (the effect of elevated estrogen; Box 20.4). When the pressure of the fetal head at birth puts additional pressure on lower extremity veins, damage can occur to the walls of the veins. With this triad of effects in place (stasis, vessel damage, and hypercoagulation), the stage is set for thrombus formation in the lower extremities. The likelihood of **deep vein thrombosis (DVT)** leading to pulmonary emboli is highest in women 30 years of age or older because increased age is yet another risk factor for thrombosis formation (Sorensen, Horvath-Puho, Lash, et al., 2011).

The risk of thrombus formation can be reduced through common-sense measures such as avoiding the use of constrictive knee-high stockings, not sitting with legs crossed at the knee, and avoiding standing in one position for a long period. If a thrombus does occur during pregnancy, a woman will notice pain and redness usually in the calf of a leg. It is diagnosed by a woman's history and Doppler ultrasonography. In order to keep the thrombus from moving and becoming a pulmonary embolus, a woman will be treated with bed rest and intravenous heparin for 24 to 48 hours. After this, she may be prescribed subcutaneous heparin she can self-inject every 12 or 24 hours for the duration of the pregnancy. It is generally recommended the lower abdomen be used for rotating sites for subcutaneous heparin administration. With pregnancy, however, this site is usually avoided and the injection sites are limited to the arms and thighs. Heparin dosage is regulated by the anti-Xa test, the most accurate assay for monitoring unfractionated heparin and low–molecular-weight heparin (Schulman, 2012).

BOX 20.4 Nursing Care Planning Using Assessment

Assessing a Pregnant Woman With Venous Thromboembolic Disease

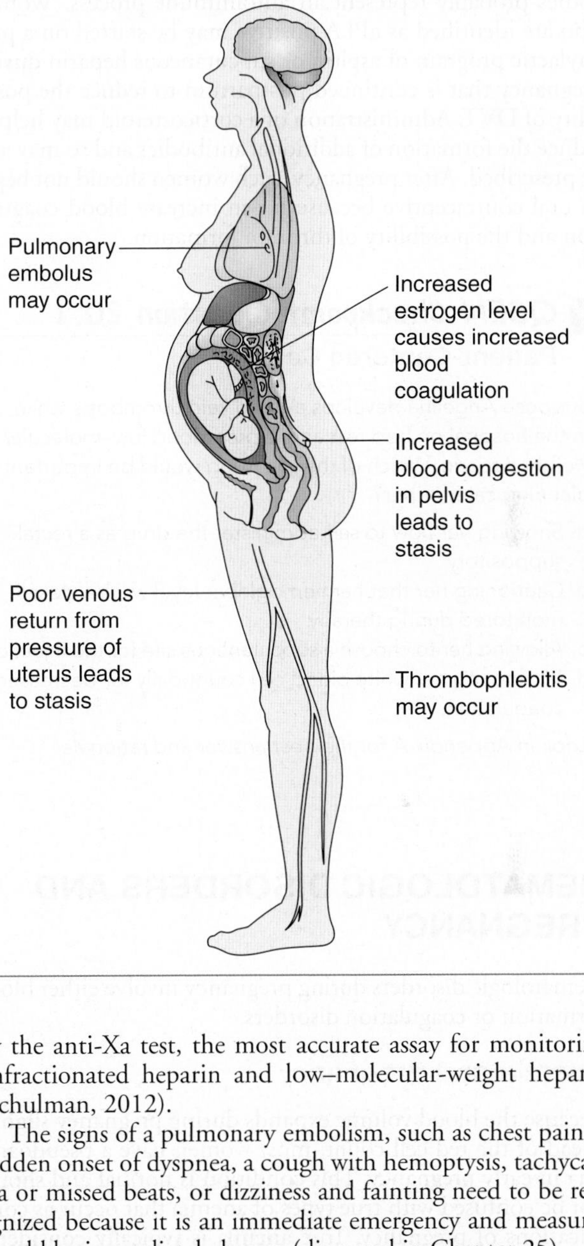

The signs of a pulmonary embolism, such as chest pain, a sudden onset of dyspnea, a cough with hemoptysis, tachycardia or missed beats, or dizziness and fainting need to be recognized because it is an immediate emergency and measures should be immediately begun (discussed in Chapter 25).

Caution women taking heparin during pregnancy not to take any additional injections once labor begins to help reduce the possibility of hemorrhage at birth. Women taking heparin are not candidates for routine episiotomy or epidural anesthesia for this same reason unless at least 4 hours has passed since the last heparin dose was given. Either heparin or sodium warfarin (Coumadin) can be prescribed after birth if a woman is not breastfeeding; however, Coumadin should be used cautiously while breastfeeding. The majority of thromboses that occur with pregnancy occur in the postpartum period; additional measures of care for a woman with DVT, such as heat, elevation, and bed rest are discussed in Chapter 25.

A particular group of women has been identified as being more susceptible to thrombi formation, spontaneous miscarriage, fetal death, and hypertension of pregnancy than others. They include: women with antiphospholipid antibodies (aPLAs) (Danza, Ruiz-Irastorza, & Khamashta, 2012). It is not known why aPLAs occur in some women, but these antibodies probably represent an autoimmune process. Women who are identified as aPLA positive may be started on a prophylactic program of aspirin or subcutaneous heparin during pregnancy that is continued postpartum to reduce the possibility of DVT. Administration of a corticosteroid may help to reduce the formation of additional antibodies and so may also be prescribed. After pregnancy, such women should not begin an oral contraceptive because it can increase blood coagulation and the possibility of thrombi formation.

QSEN Checkpoint Question 20.1

Patient-Centered Care

Suppose Angelina develops a deep vein thrombosis while in the hospital on bed rest and is prescribed low–molecular-weight heparin. Which of the following would be important in planning care for her?

a. Showing her how to self-administer the drug as a rectal suppository.
b. Cautioning her that her hemoglobin level will be closely monitored during therapy.
c. Allowing her to choose a subcutaneous site for the injection.
d. Monitoring her white blood cell count daily for decreased coagulation.

Look in Appendix A for the best answer and rationale.

HEMATOLOGIC DISORDERS AND PREGNANCY

Hematologic disorders during pregnancy involve either blood formation or coagulation disorders.

Anemia and Pregnancy

Because the blood volume expands during pregnancy slightly ahead of the red cell count, most women have a pseudoanemia in early pregnancy. This condition is normal and should not be confused with true types of anemia that occur as complications of pregnancy. True anemia is typically considered to be present when a woman's hemoglobin concentration is less than 11 g/dl (hematocrit <33%) in the first or third trimester of pregnancy or when the hemoglobin concentration is less than 10.5 g/dl (hematocrit <32%) in the second trimester (Samuels, 2012).

A Woman With Iron-Deficiency Anemia

Iron-deficiency anemia is the most common anemia of pregnancy, complicating as many as 15% to 25% of all pregnancies (Imdad & Bhutta, 2012). Many women enter pregnancy with a deficiency of iron stores resulting from a combination of a diet low in iron, heavy menstrual periods, or unwise weight-reducing programs. Iron stores are also apt to be low in women who were pregnant less than 2 years before the current pregnancy or those from low socioeconomic levels who have not had iron-rich diets. Iron-deficiency anemia is confirmed by a corresponding low serum iron level (under 30 μg/dl) and an increased iron-binding capacity (over 400 μg/dl).

Iron is made available to the body by absorption from the duodenum into the bloodstream after it has been ingested. In the bloodstream, it is bound to transferrin for transport to the liver, spleen, and bone marrow. At these sites, it is incorporated into hemoglobin or stored as ferritin.

The type of anemia is characteristically a microcytic (i.e., small red blood cell) and hypochromic (i.e., less hemoglobin than the average red cell) anemia, which occurs when such an inadequate supply of iron is ingested that iron is not available for incorporation into red blood cells. A woman experiences extreme fatigue and poor exercise tolerance because she cannot transport oxygen effectively. The condition is mildly associated with low birth weight and preterm birth. Because the body recognizes that it needs increased nutrients, some women with this condition develop pica, or the craving and eating of substances such as ice or starch (Khan & Tisman, 2010). It is also associated with restless leg syndrome (Sethi & Mehta, 2012).

To prevent this common anemia, women should take prenatal vitamins containing 27 mg of iron as prophylactic therapy during pregnancy. In addition, they need to eat a diet high in iron and vitamins (e.g., green leafy vegetables, meat, and legumes) so the supplement is truly a supplement. Women who develop iron-deficiency anemia will be prescribed therapeutic levels of medication (120 to 200 mg elemental iron per day), usually in the form of ferrous sulfate or ferrous gluconate.

Iron is absorbed best in an acid medium. Advise women, therefore, to take iron supplements with orange juice or a vitamin C supplement, which supplies ascorbic acid. If they are not already enrolled in the Special Supplemental Nutrition Program for Women, Infants, and Children (WIC) but are eligible (www.fns.usda.gov/wic), making a referral could help ensure a better diet. When women begin to take a prescribed iron supplement, new red blood cells should begin to increase almost immediately, or their reticulocyte count should rise from a range of between 0.5% and 1.5% to 3% to 4% by 2 weeks. Some women report constipation or gastric irritation when taking oral iron supplements. Increasing roughage in the diet and always taking the pills with food can help reduce these symptoms. Ferrous sulfate turns stools black, so caution women about this to prevent them from worrying that they are bleeding internally. If iron-deficiency anemia is severe and a woman has difficulty with oral iron therapy, intravenous iron can be prescribed.

A Woman With Folic Acid–Deficiency Anemia

Folic acid, or folacin, one of the B vitamins, is necessary for the normal formation of red blood cells in the woman as well as being associated with preventing neural tube and abdominal wall defects in the fetus. Folic acid–deficiency anemia occurs most often in multiple pregnancies because of the increased fetal demand; in women with a secondary hemolytic illness in which there is rapid destruction and production of new red blood cells; in women who are taking hydantoin, an anticonvulsant agent that interferes with folate absorption; in women who have been taking oral contraceptives; and in women who have poor gastric absorption, such as in those who have had a gastric bypass for morbid obesity (Greenberg, Bell, Guan, et al., 2011).

The anemia that develops is a **megaloblastic anemia** (enlarged red blood cells). Because of the size of the cells, the mean corpuscular volume will be elevated in contrast to the lowered level seen with iron-deficiency anemia. Slow to progress, the deficiency may take several weeks to develop or may not be apparent until the second trimester of pregnancy. Full blown, it may be a contributory factor in early miscarriage or premature separation of the placenta.

All women expecting to become pregnant are advised to begin a supplement of 400 μg folic acid daily in addition to eating folacin-rich foods (e.g., green leafy vegetables, oranges, dried beans). Over-the-counter multivitamin preparations generally do not contain adequate folic acid for pregnancy so be certain women are specifically taking a prenatal one. Women who develop folic acid–deficiency anemia are prescribed even higher or therapeutic levels of folic acid (Clark, Thomson, & Greer, 2012).

A Woman With Sickle-Cell Anemia

Sickle-cell anemia is a recessively inherited hemolytic anemia caused by an abnormal amino acid in the beta chain of hemoglobin. If the abnormal amino acid replaces the amino acid valine, sickling hemoglobin (HbS) results; if it is substituted for the amino acid lysine, nonsickling hemoglobin (HbC) results. An individual who is heterozygous (i.e., has only one gene in which the abnormal substitution has occurred) has the sickle-cell trait (HbAS). If the person is homozygous (i.e., has two genes in which the substitution has occurred), sickle-cell disease (HbSS) results (Rote & McCance, 2012).

With the disease, the majority of red blood cells are irregular or sickle shaped, so they cannot carry as much hemoglobin as normally shaped red blood cells can. When oxygen tension becomes reduced, as occurs at high altitudes, or blood becomes more viscid than usual, such as occurs with dehydration, the cells clump together because of their irregular shape, resulting in vessel blockage with reduced blood flow to organs. The cells then will hemolyse (i.e., be destroyed), thus reducing the number available and causing a severe anemia.

Approximately 1 in every 10 African Americans has the sickle-cell trait or carries a recessive gene for S hemoglobin but is asymptomatic; theoretically, 1 in every 400 African Americans has the disease, although with interracial marriages increasing, the disease is no longer confined to one ethnic group (MacMullen & Dulski, 2011).

Although the sickle-cell trait does not appear to directly influence the course of pregnancy, preterm birth, growth restriction, miscarriage, or perinatal mortality rates tend to be higher for women with the homozygous disease. At any time in life, sickle-cell anemia is a threat to life if vital blood vessels such as those to the liver, kidneys, heart, lungs, or brain become blocked. In pregnancy, blockage to the placental circulation can directly compromise the fetus, causing low birth weight and possibly fetal death.

Assessment

All African American women who have not been previously tested should be screened for sickle-cell anemia at a first prenatal visit. Hemoglobin levels for all women with sickle-cell disease should then be obtained throughout pregnancy. A woman with sickle-cell disease may normally have a hemoglobin level of 6 to 8 mg/100 ml. Unless she receives active interventions to raise this level, she will maintain it during pregnancy, potentially reducing oxygen to the fetus. If a hemolytic sickle-cell crisis occurs, a woman's hemoglobin level can fall to 5 or 6 mg/100 ml in a few hours, causing an accompanying rise in indirect bilirubin because the woman cannot conjugate the bilirubin released from so many destroyed red blood cells.

Because a pregnant woman with sickle-cell anemia has vascular stasis, they are more susceptible to bacteriuria than other women; periodically collect a clean-catch urine sample during pregnancy to detect developing bacteriuria while a woman is still asymptomatic.

Throughout pregnancy, monitor a woman's nutritional intake to be certain she is consuming sufficient amounts of folic acid and possibly an additional folic acid supplement, which is necessary for replacing red blood cells that have been destroyed. Women should *not* take a routine iron supplement as sickled cells cannot incorporate iron in the same manner as non-sickled cells. Ensure the woman is drinking at least eight glasses of fluid daily to be certain she is guarding against dehydration. Early in pregnancy, when she may be nauseated, it is easy for her fluid intake to decrease, causing dehydration and a subsequent sickle-cell crisis.

Assess a woman's lower extremities at prenatal visits for varicosities or pooling of blood in leg veins, which can lead to red cell destruction. Standing for long periods during the day increases this pressure, whereas sitting on a chair with the legs elevated or lying on the side in a modified Sims position encourages venous return from the lower extremities. Help a woman plan her day so she has limited long periods of standing and adequate rest periods.

Fetal health is usually monitored during pregnancy by an ultrasound examination at 16 to 24 weeks to assess for intrauterine growth restriction and by weekly nonstress or ultrasound examinations beginning at about 30 weeks. Blood flow through the uterus and placenta may be measured by blood flow velocity. If blood flow velocity is reduced, the chance of intrauterine growth restriction increases.

Therapeutic Management

Interventions to prevent a sickle-cell crisis can include periodic exchange or blood transfusions throughout pregnancy to replace sickled cells with non-sickled cells. An exchange transfusion serves a secondary purpose of removing a quantity of the increased bilirubin resulting from the breakdown of red blood cells as well as restoring the hemoglobin level (Ngô, Kayem, Habibi, et al., 2010). If a crisis occurs, controlling pain, administering oxygen as needed, and increasing the fluid volume of the circulatory system to lower viscosity are important interventions (see Chapter 44 for a further discussion of therapy for sickle-cell anemia).

If a woman develops an infection that raises her temperature and causes her to perspire more than usual (which creates dehydration) or contracts a respiratory infection that compromises air exchange so that her Po_2 is lowered, hospitalization for observation may be necessary to rule out the development of a sickle-cell crisis and subsequent hemolysis of crowded cells (Howard & Oteng-Ntim, 2012).

When the fetus is mature, the time and method of birth are individualized. Be certain to keep a woman in labor well hydrated and help her resist strenuous exertion. If an operative birth is necessary, epidural anesthesia is the method of choice because general anesthesia poses a possible risk of hypoxia. In the postpartal period, early ambulation and wearing pressure stockings or IPC boots can help reduce the risk of thromboembolism from stasis in lower extremities.

Women are generally interested in determining at birth whether their child has inherited the disease. Because the disorder is recessively inherited, if one of the parents has the disease and the other is free of the disease and trait, the chance the child will inherit the disease is zero. If a woman has the disease and her partner has the trait, the chance the child will be born with the disease is 50%. If both parents have the disease, all their children will also have the disease (see Chapter 7).

Electrophoresis of red blood cells obtained from maternal serum or by amniocentesis during pregnancy can reveal the presence of the disease on the few β-hemoglobin chains already present in fetal life. If not assessed during pregnancy, although the symptoms of sickle-cell disease do not become clinically apparent until 3 to 6 months of age, a routine newborn serum screening at birth will also reveal the disease.

✔ QSEN Checkpoint Question 20.2

Safety

Angelina is friends with a woman in your clinic who has sickle-cell anemia and they often talk together about their care. Which statement by her friend would alert you that she may need further instruction on prenatal care?

a. "I understand why folic acid is important for red cell formation."
b. "I'm careful to drink at least eight glasses of fluid every day."
c. "I take an iron pill every day to help grow new red blood cells."
d. "I've temporarily stopped jogging so I don't risk becoming dehydrated."

Look in Appendix A for the best answer and rationale.

The Woman With Thalassemia

The thalassemias are a group of autosomal recessively inherited blood disorders that lead to poor hemoglobin formation and severe anemia. They occur most frequently in Mediterranean, African, and Asian populations (Leung & Lao, 2012). Symptoms first appear in childhood. Treatment focuses on combating anemia through such measures as folic acid supplementation and perhaps blood transfusion to infuse hemoglobin-rich red blood cells. Women with thalassemia do not usually take an iron supplement during pregnancy because they could receive an iron overload because iron is infused with blood transfusions. Care of a child with both forms of thalassemia, alpha and beta, is discussed in Chapter 44.

The Woman With Malaria

Malaria is a protozoan infection that is transmitted to people by *Anopheles* mosquitoes (Fried, Muchlenbacks, & Duffy, 2012). The infection causes red blood cells to stick to the surface of capillaries causing obstruction of these vessels and resulting in end-organ anoxia and blood not reaching organs effectively.

Although the disorder does not have a high incidence in the United States, newly immigrated women may be infected with it. It's important to consider during pregnancy as it can not only make women high risk for blood clotting during pregnancy but also, if untreated, can be transmitted to a fetus by mother-to-fetus transmission.

The incubation period for the most frequently occurring type is 12 to 14 days. The most noticeable symptoms are elevated liver function tests accompanying fever, malaise, and headache. Because of the altered blood cells, thrombocytopenia (i.e., low platelet count), anemia, and renal failure can develop.

Malaria can be prevented by wearing clothing that covers most of the body as well as using an insect repellent when in an area infested with mosquitoes, sleeping at night with a mosquito net, or keeping windows closed to prevent mosquitoes from entering. As further prevention, urge women to delay travel to endemic areas until after pregnancy if possible.

Treatment is with a combination of antimalarial drugs, which will both stop the course of the disease and help reduce the incidence of low birth weight and preterm birth. Sulfadoxine/pyrimethamine is safe to administer during the last trimester of pregnancy. Chloroquine is safe to administer all during pregnancy and so is the drug of choice (Irvine, Einarson, & Bozzo, 2011). Quinine, Malarone, or tetracyclines, although effective against the disease, should not be used at any point in pregnancy or with women who are breastfeeding as they are teratogenic.

Coagulation Disorders and Pregnancy

Most coagulation disorders are sex linked or occur only in males and so have little effect on pregnancies. However, one of them, von Willebrand disease, is a coagulation disorder inherited as an autosomal dominant trait and so does occur in women (Shahbazi, Moghaddam-Banaem, Ekhtesari, et al., 2012). Women will have normal platelet counts, but bleeding time is prolonged. Levels of factor VIII–related antigen (VIII-R) and factor VIII coagulation activity (VIII-C) are both reduced. From the time she was a child, a woman with the disorder might have noticed menorrhagia or frequent episodes of epistaxis. If these symptoms were not severe, however, the condition can go undiagnosed until pregnancy when a woman experiences a spontaneous miscarriage or postpartum hemorrhage. Replacement of the missing coagulation factors by infusion of cryoprecipitate or fresh frozen plasma may be necessary before labor to prevent excessive bleeding with birth.

Hemophilia B (Christmas disease, factor IX deficiency) is a sex-linked disorder, so the actual disease occurs only in males. However, female carriers may have such a reduced level of factor IX (only 33% of normal) that hemorrhage with labor or a spontaneous miscarriage can be a serious complication. As with von Willebrand disease, carriers of the disorder need to be identified before pregnancy. Restoration of factor IX levels can be quickly restored by infusion of factor IX concentrate or fresh frozen plasma.

Maternal serum analysis can be used to detect whether a fetus has a coagulation disorder during pregnancy. If there is a family history of a coagulation disorder, before an internal fetal heart rate monitor is attached or fetal scalp blood sampling is done, it should be determined if the fetus has a coagulation defect. If one is present, these procedures are contraindicated because they could result in extensive fetal blood loss.

Idiopathic thrombocytopenic purpura (ITP), which is a decreased number of platelets, is not inherited, can occur at any time in life, and so occasionally occurs during pregnancy. The cause of the condition is unknown, but because symptoms usually occur shortly after a viral invasion such as an upper respiratory tract infection, it is assumed to be an autoimmune reaction (an antiplatelet antibody that destroys platelets is apparently released) (Gasim, 2011).

Laboratory studies reveal a marked thrombocytopenia (platelet count may be as low as 20,000/mm^3 from a usual count of 150,000/mm^3). Without an adequate level of platelets, the woman is prone to frequent nosebleeds and minute petechiae or large ecchymoses appear on her body.

The illness typically runs a 1- to 3-month limited course, but because a low platelet count also appears with hypertension of pregnancy with HELLP (**h**emolysis, **e**levated **l**iver enzymes, **l**ow **p**latelet count) syndrome, a serious complication of pregnancy (see Chapter 21), the condition is frightening until it is differentiated as ITP. Oral prednisone or a platelet transfusion or plasmapheresis may be administered to temporarily increase the platelet count to prevent increased bleeding at birth. The antiplatelet factor can cross the placenta and cause accompanying platelet destruction in the newborn or allow a newborn to be born with the illness, so a careful assessment of the baby is necessary at birth (see Chapter 44 for care of the child with ITP).

RENAL AND URINARY DISORDERS AND PREGNANCY

Adequate kidney function is important for a successful pregnancy outcome because a woman is excreting waste products not only for herself but also for the fetus. This dual function makes any condition that interferes with kidney or urinary function always potentially serious.

A Woman With a Urinary Tract Infection

As many as 4% to 10% of nonpregnant women have asymptomatic bacteriuria (i.e., organisms are present in the urine without symptoms of infection). In a pregnant woman, because the ureters dilate from the effect of progesterone, stasis of urine can occur. The minimal presence of abnormal amounts of glucose **(glycosuria)** that also occurs with pregnancy provides an ideal medium for growth for any organisms present. Combined, these factors cause asymptomatic urinary tract infections (UTIs) in as many as 10% to 15% of pregnant women (Trautner, 2012). Asymptomatic infections are potentially dangerous because they can progress to pyelonephritis (i.e., infection of the pelvis of the kidney) and are associated with preterm labor and premature rupture of membranes. Women with known vesicoureteral reflux (i.e., backflow of urine into the ureters) tend to develop UTIs or pyelonephritis more often than others. The organism most commonly responsible for UTI is *Escherichia coli* from an ascending infection. A UTI can also occur as a descending infection or can begin in the kidneys from the filtration of organisms present from other body infections. If the infectious organism is determined to be *Streptococcus* B, vaginal cultures should be obtained because streptococcal B infection of the genital tract is associated with pneumonia in newborns.

Assessment

A UTI typically manifests as frequency and pain on urination. With pyelonephritis, a woman develops pain in the lumbar region (usually on the right side) that radiates downward. The area feels tender to palpation. She may have accompanying nausea and vomiting, malaise, pain, and frequency of urination. Her temperature may be elevated only slightly or may be as high as 103° to 104°F (39° to 40°C). The infection usually occurs on the right side because there is greater compression and urinary stasis on the right ureter from the uterus being pushed that way by the large bulk of the intestine on the left side. A urine culture will reveal over 100,000 organisms per milliliter of urine, a level diagnostic of infection.

Therapeutic Management

Obtain a clean-catch urine sample for culture and sensitivity to assess for asymptomatic bacteriuria or symptoms of UTI (see Chapter 11). A sensitivity test will then determine which antibiotic will best combat the infection. Amoxicillin, ampicillin, and cephalosporins are effective against most organisms causing UTIs and are safe antibiotics during pregnancy. The sulfonamides can be used early in pregnancy but not near term because they can interfere with protein binding of bilirubin, which then leads to hyperbilirubinemia in the newborn. Tetracyclines are contraindicated during pregnancy as they cause retardation of bone growth and staining of the deciduous teeth (Karch, 2013).

Nursing Diagnoses and Related Interventions

Nursing Diagnosis: Risk for infection related to stasis of urine with pregnancy

Outcome Evaluation: Oral temperature is below 100.4°F (38°C), and a clean-catch urine specimen has a bacteria count below 100,000 colonies per milliliter.

As part of prenatal education, remind all women during pregnancy of common measures to prevent UTIs, such as:

- Voiding frequently (at least every 2 hours)
- Developing a habit of urinating as soon as the need is felt and emptying the bladder completely when urinating
- Wiping front to back after voiding and bowel movements
- Wearing cotton, not synthetic fiber, underwear
- Voiding immediately after sexual intercourse
- Drinking a glass of cranberry juice daily

The pregnant woman with a UTI needs to take the additional measure of drinking an increased amount of fluid to flush out the infection from the urinary tract. To be most effective, do not simply tell her to "push fluids" or "drink lots of water." Give her a specific amount to drink every day (up to 3 to 4 L per 24 hours) to make certain she increases her fluid intake sufficiently.

A woman can promote urine drainage by assuming a knee–chest position for 15 minutes morning and evening. In this position, the weight of the uterus is shifted forward, releasing the pressure on the ureters and allowing urine to drain more freely.

If a woman has one UTI during pregnancy, the chances are high she will develop another late in pregnancy, when urinary stasis tends to grow even greater. She may, therefore, be kept on prophylactic antibiotics throughout the remainder of the pregnancy. Ask at prenatal visits whether she is continuing to take this type of prophylactic medicine. When women have pain and symptoms of urinary frequency, they usually take medication consistently. When they no longer have any clinical evidence they are ill, their compliance rate may begin to fall dramatically. Urge a woman to post a chart on her refrigerator door or in her bathroom as a reminder to take the medication. Encourage her not to leave the medication on the counter as a reminder because she needs to begin to childproof her home.

Pyelonephritis occurs as an extension of a UTI or infection that originated in or spread to the kidney (Schneeberger, Geerlings, Middleton, et al., 2012). If this develops, a woman may be hospitalized for 24 to 48 hours while she is treated with intravenous antibiotics. After this acute episode, she will be maintained on a drug such as oral nitrofurantoin (Macrodantin) for the remainder of the pregnancy. Acidifying urine by the use of ascorbic acid (vitamin C), which is often recommended in nonpregnant women, is not usually recommended during pregnancy because a newborn can develop scurvy in the immediate neonatal period from vitamin C withdrawal.

After birth, a woman who developed more than one UTI may have an ultrasound scheduled to detect any urinary tract abnormality that might be present, such as vesicoureteral reflux, to help prevent future infections.

✔ QSEN Checkpoint Question 20.3

Quality Improvement

Suppose you are the charge nurse of a prenatal clinic and, when reviewing antenatal electronic records, you note that a high number of pregnant women seen in the clinic, including Angelina Gomez, have developed UTIs during their pregnancies. You should emphasize the need for your staff nurses to do which of the following?

a. Ensure that the housekeeping department is adequately cleaning the toilets.
b. Suggest all women be prescribed a prophylactic antibiotic during their first trimester.
c. Educate women on the need for sound perineal care during pregnancy.
d. Urge women to restrict fluid to keep their urine acidic and concentrated.

Look in Appendix A for the best answer and rationale.

A Woman With a Hyperactive Bladder

A hyperactive bladder refers to a bladder that contracts more frequently than usual, causing symptoms of frequency, urgency, and incontinence. During pregnancy, these symptoms can increase greatly because of the additional pressure from the uterus on the bladder. Fesoterodine (Toviaz; pregnancy category C), an antispasmodic drug frequently prescribed for the disorder should be used during pregnancy and breastfeeding only if the risk outweighs the benefit until it is proven not to be teratogenic (Armstrong, Malone, & Bui, 2012).

A Woman With Chronic Renal Disease

In the past, females with chronic renal disease did not reach childbearing age or were advised not to have children because of their automatic high-risk status during pregnancy. Today, with conscientious prenatal care, women with chronic renal disease and even women who have had renal transplants, can expect to have healthy pregnancies and healthy children (Fontana, Santori, Fazio, et al., 2012).

Women with chronic renal disease need to be monitored carefully during pregnancy because their diseased kidneys may not produce erythropoietin, a glycoprotein necessary for red cell formation and so they may develop a severe anemia (Box 20.5). Fortunately, synthetic erythropoietin is now available and is safe to take during pregnancy (Jelkmann, 2011).

Because the glomerular filtration rate normally increases during pregnancy, a woman's serum creatinine level (a measure of kidney function that elevates when kidneys are under stress) may be actually slightly below normal during pregnancy or may fall from a usual level of 0.7 mg/100 ml to about 0.5 mg/100 ml. Women with kidney disease who normally have a serum creatinine level greater than 2.0 mg/dl may be advised not to undertake a pregnancy in case the increased strain on already damaged kidneys leads to kidney failure.

Many women with renal disease routinely take a corticosteroid such as oral prednisone at a maintenance level. This drug therapy typically is continued throughout pregnancy. Although animal studies have shown an increased incidence of cleft palate from corticosteroid use during pregnancy, this does not appear to be true in humans. The infant may be hyperglycemic at birth, however, because of the suppression of insulin activity by the corticosteroid.

Women with severe renal disease may require dialysis to aid kidney function during pregnancy (Piccoli, Conijn, Consiglio, et al., 2010). With dialysis, there is a risk of preterm labor, perhaps because progesterone is removed with the dialysis. To prevent this complication, progesterone may be administered intramuscularly before the procedure. If hemodialysis is used, it should be scheduled frequently and for short durations to avoid acute fluid shifts. The heparin administered in connection with hemodialysis is safe during pregnancy because it does not cross the placenta. Even in light of the expanding uterine size, peritoneal dialysis is actually preferred over hemodialysis because it normally causes less drastic fluid shifts. This can be accomplished on an ambulatory basis (continuous ambulatory peritoneal dialysis) throughout pregnancy.

If a woman is on a low potassium diet to avoid a buildup of potassium that accumulates because their diseased kidneys do not evacuate it well, they may need a nutrition consultation

BOX 20.5 Nursing Care Planning Using Assessment

Assessing a Pregnant Woman With Renal Disease

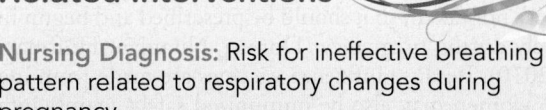

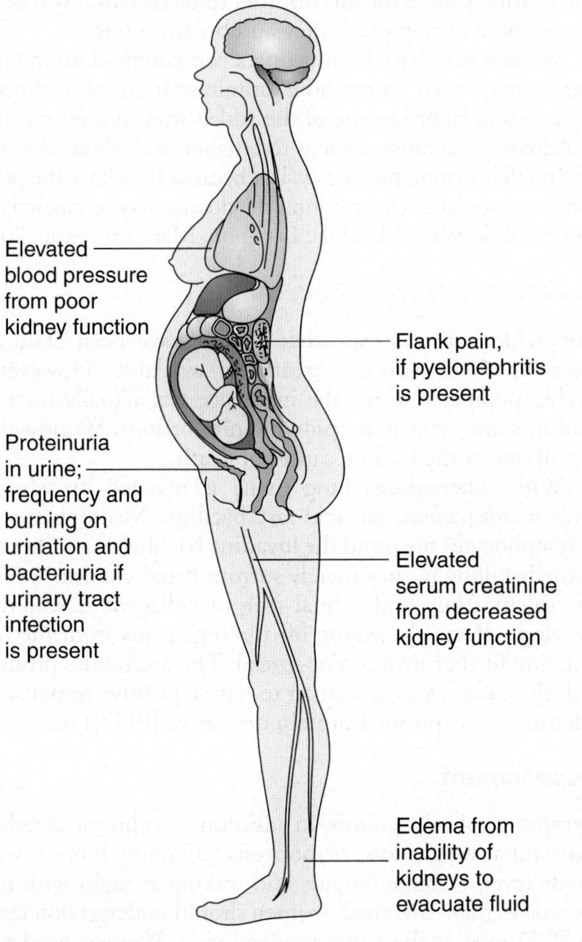

to be certain they can continue to avoid potassium yet also eat a healthy pregnancy diet. They also may need a great deal of emotional support during pregnancy since they are aware of the stress of pregnancy on damaged kidneys. By being pregnant, they are risking not only the life of the child growing inside them but also their own life. They may also need extra time with their infant at birth for bonding because they may have been too concerned during pregnancy to begin this process.

Although successful pregnancies in women with kidney transplants are to be expected, women should be considered individually to determine whether they will be able to carry a pregnancy to term before a pregnancy is initiated (Lopez, Martinez, Vinolo, et al., 2011). Criteria to be evaluated include:

- A woman's general health and the time since the transplant (preferably >2 years)
- A woman's serum creatinine level
- The presence of proteinuria or hypertension or signs of graft rejection
- Medications the woman is taking to reduce graft rejection

It is helpful if the drugs a woman is taking are limited to prednisone to ensure fetal safety during pregnancy.

RESPIRATORY DISORDERS AND PREGNANCY

Respiratory diseases have a wide range from mild (e.g., the common cold) to severe (e.g., pneumonia) to chronic (e.g., tuberculosis or chronic obstructive pulmonary disease [COPD]). Any respiratory condition can worsen in pregnancy because the rising uterus compresses the diaphragm, thus reducing the size of the thoracic cavity and available lung space. Any respiratory disorder can also pose serious hazards to the fetus if allowed to progress to the point where the mother's oxygen–carbon dioxide exchange is altered or the mother or fetus cannot receive enough oxygen.

Nursing Diagnoses and Related Interventions

Nursing Diagnosis: Risk for ineffective breathing pattern related to respiratory changes during pregnancy

Outcome Evaluation: Respiratory rate is 16 to 20 breaths/min, Po_2 is above 80 mmHg, Pco_2 is below 40 mmHg, and fetal heart rate is 110 to 160 beats/min with good variability.

Respiratory illnesses in women who are pregnant can become extremely serious and may require therapy such as oxygen and medication to help increase oxygenation in both the woman and her fetus.

A Woman With Acute Nasopharyngitis

Acute nasopharyngitis (i.e., the common cold) tends to be more severe during pregnancy than at other times because, during pregnancy, estrogen stimulation normally causes some degree of nasal congestion. This means that even with a minor cold, a woman can find it difficult to breathe. Women should not take aspirin as a remedy for a headache, which commonly accompanies an upper respiratory infection, because this can interfere with blood clotting in both the mother and fetus and the possibility of prolonged pregnancy at term (Karch, 2013). Because common colds are invariably caused by a virus, antibiotic therapy is unnecessary except to prevent a secondary infection. And although most simple cough syrups don't contain ingredients that would make them unsafe for use during pregnancy, women should check with their health care provider before taking any over-the-counter medication other than honey and lemon lozenges. Urge women to use simple measures to combat a cold, such as:

- Be sure to get extra rest and sleep and eat a diet high in vitamin C (e.g., orange juice and fruit) to help boost the immune system.
- Take acetaminophen (Tylenol) every 4 hours for aches and pains (up to 3,000 mg/day). Do not take acetylsalicylic acid (Aspirin) during pregnancy because it can interfere with blood clotting.

- Use a room humidifier or apply a medicated vapor rub to the chest, especially at night, to moisten nasal secretions and help mucus drain.
- Use cool or warm compresses to relieve sinus headaches.

A Woman With Influenza

Influenza is caused by a virus, identified as type A, B, or C. The disease spreads in epidemic form and is accompanied by high fever, extreme prostration, aching pains in the back and extremities, and generally, a sore, raw throat. Contrary to early reports, influenza infection has not been clearly correlated with congenital anomalies in newborns, although it can be a cause of preterm labor. For unknown reasons, some studies have shown a link between influenza during pregnancy and schizophrenia in children born of that pregnancy (Moreno, Kurita, Holloway, et al., 2011). Treatment includes an antipyretic such as acetaminophen (Tylenol) to control fever. The risk for the woman of not taking oseltamivir (Tamiflu), an oral antiviral drug that is category C, is greater than if it's not taken, so it should be prescribed and begun immediately during pregnancy (Donner, Niranjan, Hoffmann, et al., 2010). Because influenza vaccines are made from inert viruses, women may also be immunized safely against influenza during pregnancy (Gorman, Brewer, Wang, et al., 2012).

A Woman With Pneumonia

Pneumonia is the bacterial or viral invasion of lung tissue by pathogens such as *S. pneumoniae*, *Haemophilus influenzae*, and *Mycoplasma pneumoniae*. After the invasion, an acute inflammatory response occurs in the lung alveoli, causing an exudate of red blood cells, fibrin, and polymorphonuclear leukocytes to flood into the alveoli. This process has the helpful effect of confining the bacteria or virus within segments of the lobes of the lungs, but it also has a less helpful effect of filling alveoli with fluid, blocking off breathing space. If the collection of fluid becomes extreme, it can limit the oxygen available not only to the woman but also to the fetus. Therapy involves the use of an appropriate antibiotic and perhaps oxygen administration. With severe disease, ventilation support may be necessary. Pneumonia during pregnancy is associated with fetal growth restriction and preterm birth because of the oxygen deficit (Chen, Keller, Wang, et al., 2012). If pneumonia is present during labor, oxygen should be administered so the fetus has adequate oxygen resources during contractions.

A Woman With Asthma

Asthma is a disorder marked by reversible airflow obstruction, airway hyperreactivity, and airway inflammation. Symptoms are often triggered by an inhaled allergen such as pollen or cigarette smoke. With inhalation of the allergen, there is an immediate release of bioactive mediators such as histamine and leukotrienes from an immunoglobulin interaction. This results in constriction of the bronchial smooth muscle, marked mucosal inflammation and swelling, and the production of thick bronchial secretions. These three processes cause a woman to have difficulty pulling in air; on exhalation, she has so much difficulty releasing air she makes a high-pitched whistling sound (i.e., bronchial wheezing) from air being pushed past the bronchial narrowing. Asthma has the potential of reducing the oxygen supply to a fetus leading to preterm birth or fetal growth restriction if a major attack should occur during pregnancy; however, this is less of a threat with well-managed asthma (Dombrowski & Schatz, 2010). Some women find that their asthma actually improves during pregnancy because of the high circulating levels of corticosteroids present. A woman should check with her primary care provider before pregnancy about the safety of the medications she routinely takes for this disorder to be certain it will be safe to continue during pregnancy and breastfeeding.

Women who have been taking a corticosteroid during pregnancy may need intravenous administration of hydrocortisone during labor because of the added stress during this time. β-Adrenergic agonists such as terbutaline and albuterol may be taken safely during pregnancy, but because they have the potential to reduce labor contractions, the dosage may be tapered close to term if possible (Mendola, Laughon, Männistö, et al., 2013).

A Woman With Tuberculosis

Tuberculosis is a disease that should have been eradicated because of the effective treatment available. However, in highly populated areas, the incidence has actually increased and in some areas is at epidemic proportions. Worldwide, it is still one of the leading causes of death.

With tuberculosis, lung tissue is invaded by *Mycobacterium tuberculosis*, an acid-fast bacillus. Macrophages and T lymphocytes surround the invading bacillus, but rather than actually killing it, they merely surround and confine it. Fibrosis, calcification, and a final ring of collagenous scar tissue develop, effectively sealing off the organisms from the body and any further invasion or spread. The antibodies produced will thereafter cause a woman to have a positive response to a Mantoux test (purified protein derivative [PPD]) test.

Assessment

Symptoms of tuberculosis, in addition to a chronic cough, are substantial weight loss, hemoptysis (coughing blood), a low-grade fever, extreme fatigue, and waking at night with night sweats. In high-risk areas, women should undergo skin testing (a PPD test) at their first prenatal visit. Women need to be cautioned that a positive reaction does not necessarily mean they have the disease; it can only mean they have at some time been exposed to tuberculosis and so have antibodies in their system. If a woman has a positive reaction, a chest X-ray (which is safe during pregnancy as long as her abdomen is lead shielded) or a sputum culture for acid-fast bacillus to confirm the diagnosis will be scheduled.

Therapeutic Management

Women with active tuberculosis need treatment during pregnancy (Nhan-Chang & Jones, 2010). Isoniazid (INH), rifampin (RIF), and ethambutol hydrochloride (Myambutol)—the drugs of choice for tuberculosis—may be given without apparent teratogenic effects. INH, however, may result in a peripheral neuritis if a woman does not also take supplemental pyridoxine (vitamin B_6). Ethambutol has the side effect of causing optic atrophy and loss of green color recognition in the woman. To detect this, test the woman's ability to recognize green at prenatal visits using the color section of a Snellen (eye test) chart. If symptoms develop, inform her health provider about possibly discontinuing the drug.

A woman who had tuberculosis earlier in life must be especially careful to maintain an adequate level of calcium during pregnancy to ensure the calcium tuberculosis pockets in her lungs are not broken down and the disease is not reactivated. A woman is usually advised to wait 1 to 2 years after the infection becomes inactive before attempting to conceive as pressure on the diaphragm from the enlarging uterus changes the shape of the lung and can break open recently calcified pockets more readily than well-calcified lesions. Pockets may also break open during labor from the increased intrapulmonary pressure of pushing. Recent inactive tuberculosis may also become active during the postpartum period as the lung returns to its more vertical prepregnant position following birth.

Although tuberculosis can be spread by the placenta to the fetus, if it is active, it usually is spread to the infant after birth by the mother's coughing. Obtaining a negative sputum culture after birth rules out active tuberculosis. Urge the woman to continue taking her tuberculosis medications as prescribed during breastfeeding as only small amounts of these are secreted in breast milk and so are safe for her infant.

A Woman With Chronic Obstructive Pulmonary Disease

COPD is constriction of the airway associated most often with long-term cigarette smoking. When women had their children between 20 and 30 years of age, COPD was rarely associated with pregnancy. Now that more and more women are waiting until age 35 to 40 years to have children, it is now possible to see the condition with pregnancy. Constrictive air disease limits the amount of oxygen that can reach the lungs, so the condition is associated with fetal growth restriction and preterm birth. Women may need additional rest during pregnancy because of fatigue and may need continuous supplemental oxygen during the day. If they experience sleep apnea, they may be prescribed continuous positive airway pressure (CPAP) at night (Bourjeily, Barbara, Larson, et al., 2012). During labor, a woman might grow so short of breath from the exertion needed for pushing that she may be advised to have a cesarean birth.

Pregnancy may be the time a woman with COPD realizes she needs to stop smoking not only to preserve her own health but also to be able to supply a smoke-free environment for her baby. Offer support at prenatal visits for her attempt to do this, but caution her it is difficult to stop smoking unless her entire family takes this same step toward wellness.

A Woman With Cystic Fibrosis

Cystic fibrosis is a recessively inherited disease in which there is generalized dysfunction of the exocrine glands (Thorpe-Beeston, Madge, Gyi, et al., 2013). This dysfunction leads to mucous secretions, particularly in the pancreas and lungs, which become so viscid that normal lung and pancreatic functions become compromised.

Many men with cystic fibrosis are subfertile because their semen is so thick that sperm cannot be motile. Fertility may be lessened in women with the disorder because sperm cannot migrate through viscid cervical mucus. This can make reproductive technologies such as alternative insemination or in vitro fertilization necessary for conception.

Persons with the disease typically show symptoms of chronic respiratory infection and overinflation of their lungs from the thickened mucus present; they have difficulty digesting fat and protein because the pancreas cannot release amylase. During a pregnancy, poor pulmonary function can result in inadequate oxygen supply to the fetus, resulting in an increased risk for growth restriction, preterm labor, and perinatal death. Identifying whether the fetus also has the disease can be done by chorionic villi sampling, amniocentesis, or identification of the abnormal gene on chromosome 7 in fetal cells obtained from the woman's blood serum. Screening for the disorder is included in routine neonatal screening programs after birth (American Congress of Obstetricians and Gynecologists [ACOG], 2012).

Therapy for the illness consists of administration of pancrelipase (Pancrease) to supplement pancreatic enzymes. Although pancrelipase is a pregnancy risk category C drug (i.e., teratogenic effects are unknown), it does not appear to affect the fetus, so caution women to continue to take this even with nausea of early pregnancy. Women are often also prescribed a bronchodilator or antibiotic to reduce pulmonary symptoms. They should schedule a preconception meeting with their health care provider to discuss whether all of these will be safe during pregnancy. In addition to pharmacologic measures, women with cystic fibrosis must perform chest physiotherapy daily to reduce the buildup of lung secretions; this should continue during pregnancy. As women with the disorder excrete a higher level of sodium in perspiration than others, monitor them carefully during labor to be certain they do not become dehydrated.

Modifications for Pregnancy

Because pancrelipase may interfere with iron absorption, a woman is at greater risk for iron-deficiency anemia during pregnancy than others. Therefore, an iron supplement usually is prescribed. They also have a higher than usual incidence of developing diabetes mellitus because of pancreas involvement; therefore, women also need close monitoring of serum glucose levels at prenatal visits to detect the development of gestational diabetes.

Chest physiotherapy can become difficult late in pregnancy because the process is exhausting, moving to new positions is difficult, and lying prone, a position used frequently in postural drainage, is contraindicated in late pregnancy. To continue this effectively, therefore, a woman may need to plan more frequent and shorter sessions in modified positions (other than prone) during pregnancy (Fig. 20.2). Fetal

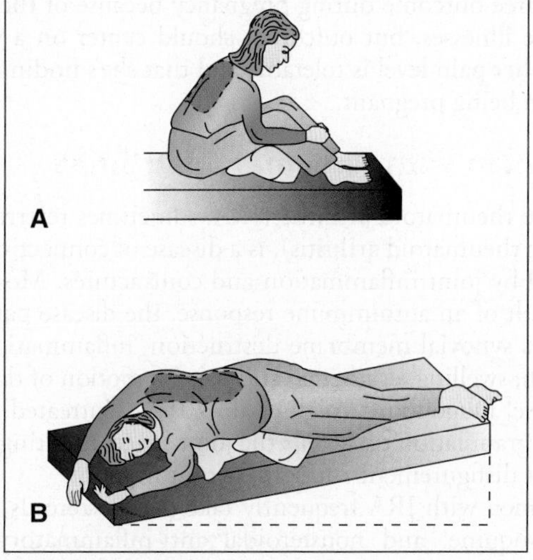

FIGURE 20.2 Modified positions for chest physiotherapy during pregnancy: (A) chest physiotherapy for the upper lobes; (B) chest physiotherapy for the lower lobes.

health will be monitored by ultrasound and nonstress tests to identify intrauterine growth restriction.

Modifications for the Postpartum Period

Help a woman plan how to conserve her energy for infant care in the immediate postpartum period so she does not become exhausted and can enjoy her newborn. The milk of a nursing mother with cystic fibrosis is high in sodium, and potentially places the infant at risk for hypernatremia, so women with cystic fibrosis are usually advised not to breastfeed (Chetty, Shaffer, & Norton, 2011). Although not their first choice for infant care, you can assure mothers that their infant will do well on formula.

✔ QSEN Checkpoint Question 20.4

Teamwork & Collaboration

Suppose Angelina had tuberculosis as a teenager and her primary care provider orders a chest X-ray during pregnancy. You would want your care team members to know that this is necessary because of which danger of tuberculosis during pregnancy?

a. Calcium deposits that wall off old tuberculosis lesions can break down.
b. Latent tuberculosis can turn to pneumonia if a woman has a folic acid deficit.
c. PPD tests are always negative during pregnancy so tuberculosis often goes undetected.
d. The disease can result in neural tube defects in the fetus.

Look in Appendix A for the best answer and rationale.

RHEUMATIC DISORDERS AND PREGNANCY

Several rheumatic disorders that occur in young adult women can be seen during pregnancy. Because most of these illnesses result in discomfort, the most common primary nursing diagnosis for these is pain. Women may not be able to achieve a pain-free outcome during pregnancy because of the nature of these illnesses, but outcomes should center on a woman stating her pain level is tolerable and that she's finding enjoyment in being pregnant.

A Woman With Rheumatoid Arthritis

Juvenile rheumatoid arthritis (JRA; sometimes referred to as chronic rheumatoid arthritis), is a disease of connective tissue marked by joint inflammation and contractures. Most likely the result of an autoimmune response, the disease pathology involves synovial membrane destruction, inflammation with effusion, swelling, erythema, and painful motion of the joints (Guthrie, Dugowson, Voigt, et al., 2010). Untreated, formation of granulation tissue fills the joint space, resulting in permanent disfigurement and loss of joint motion.

Women with JRA frequently take corticosteroids, hydroxychloroquine, and nonsteroidal anti-inflammatory drugs (NSAIDs) to prevent joint pain and loss of mobility. Some women may be taking oral aspirin therapy. Although they should continue to take these medications during pregnancy to prevent joint damage, large amounts of salicylates have the potential to lead to increased bleeding at birth or prolonged pregnancy (salicylate interferes with prostaglandin synthesis, so labor contractions are not initiated) (Karch, 2013). The infant may be born with a bleeding defect and may also experience premature closure of the ductus arteriosus because of the drug's effects. For this reason, the woman is asked to decrease her intake of salicylates approximately 2 weeks before term. A number of women also take low-dose methotrexate, a carcinogen (pregnancy risk category X). As a rule, they should stop taking this prepregnancy because of the danger of head and neck defects in the fetus.

Joint symptoms of the disease may improve during pregnancy because of the naturally increased circulating level of corticosteroids in the maternal bloodstream during pregnancy. During the postpartum period, when a woman's corticosteroid levels fall to prepregnancy levels, arthritis symptoms will probably recur (Guthrie et al., 2010).

In the postpartum period, the determination as to the safety of breastfeeding must be individualized based on the medication each woman is taking. Those taking NSAIDs, such as ibuprofen, can breastfeed. Those taking methotrexate or large doses of aspirin may be advised not to breastfeed because of the danger to the infant.

A Woman With Systemic Lupus Erythematosus

Systemic lupus erythematosus (SLE) is a multisystem chronic disease of connective tissue that occurs most frequently in woman 20 to 40 years of age (Lateef & Petri, 2012). Widespread degeneration of connective tissue (especially of the heart, kidneys, blood vessels, spleen, skin, and retroperitoneal tissue) occurs with onset of the illness. A marked skin change is a characteristic erythematous butterfly-shaped rash on the face. In the kidneys, fibrin deposits develop, plugging and blocking the glomeruli and leading to necrosis and scarring. The thickening of collagen tissue in the blood vessels can cause vessel obstruction. This obstruction can be life-threatening to a woman if blood flow to vital organs becomes compromised and life-threatening to a fetus if blood flow to the placenta is obstructed. Many women with SLE have antiphospholipid antibodies, which increase the tendency for thrombi to form (Baer & Petri, 2011). In contrast, marked thrombocytopenia (i.e., decreased platelet count) may be present, so clotting may be deficient. Prior to pregnancy, a woman may be taking a combination of NSAIDs, low–molecular-weight heparin, salicylates, hydroxychloroquine, low-dose prednisone, or azathioprine (an immunosuppressant) to reduce disease symptoms. She can continue these during pregnancy if used with caution but may be asked to reduce the dose of salicylates 2 weeks prior to labor to prevent bleeding in the newborn.

The naturally increased circulation of corticosteroids during pregnancy may lessen symptoms in some women. In others, the chief complication of the disorder—acute nephritis with glomerular destruction—may occur for the first time during pregnancy. With associated nephritis, a woman's blood pressure will rise sharply and she will develop hematuria, proteinuria with decreased urine output, and edema. It is difficult to differentiate these symptoms from the symptoms of gestational hypertension, except that with gestational hypertension, there is no hematuria. Frequent monitoring of serum creatinine levels will be necessary to assess if kidney function is adequate. If this value is over 1.5 mg/dl and proteinuria and a decreased creatinine clearance value are also present, the fetus is seriously threatened with growth restriction and the pregnancy is also threatened to be preterm. Dialysis to remove excess creatinine or plasmapheresis to replace platelets may be necessary to guard against hemorrhage in the woman at birth.

During labor, intravenous hydrocortisone may be administered to help a woman adjust to stress at this time. During the postpartum period, there may be an acute exacerbation of symptoms as corticosteroid levels again fall to normal. Infants of women with SLE may be born with a lupus-like rash, anemia, thrombocytopenia (low platelet count), and neonatal heart block. Such newborn symptoms last about 6 months and then fade. If congenital heart block occurs, a newborn pacemaker may be necessary. Screening for the exact type of autoantibodies present may be helpful in predicting which newborns will be susceptible to this.

GASTROINTESTINAL DISORDERS AND PREGNANCY

Although minor gastrointestinal discomforts (such as nausea, heartburn, and constipation) are common during pregnancy, acute abdominal pain and protracted vomiting are causes for concern because complications such as premature separation of the placenta or ectopic pregnancy often manifest with acute abdominal pain and protracted vomiting can lead to dehydration. In some women, sudden abdominal pain is caused by a condition completely unrelated to the pregnancy, such as ulcerative colitis, hepatitis, hiatal hernia, or cholecystitis, conditions that may be known to a woman before she becomes pregnant or that may develop or be discovered during her pregnancy. In either event, they need a clear assessment and therapy to maintain the woman's overall health. Women who have colostomies may ask if they can complete a pregnancy without difficulty; the answer is yes. Even a previous liver transplant is not a contraindication to pregnancy (Parhar, Gibson, & Coffin, 2012).

Nursing Diagnoses and Related Interventions

Nursing Diagnosis: Imbalanced nutrition, less than body requirements, related to a gastrointestinal disorder during pregnancy

Outcome Evaluation: Client's weight gain amounts to 25 to 30 lb during pregnancy, hemoglobin is above 11 mg/dl, and specific gravity of urine is below 1.030.

Because most gastrointestinal disorders interfere with nutrition or fluid/electrolyte balance, a major intervention with all of these disorders is to ensure women are taking in adequate food and fluid for their well-being and that of their fetus, and to assess that their disease process is resolving.

A Woman With Appendicitis

The incidence of appendicitis, or inflammation of the appendix, is high in young adults and occurs as frequently as 1 in 1,500 to 2,000 pregnancies (Miloudi, Brahem, Ben Abid, et al., 2012).

Assessment

History taking is important. Appendicitis usually begins with a few hours of nausea, and then an hour or two of generalized abdominal discomfort. Then comes the typical sharp, peristaltic, lower right quadrant pain of acute appendicitis.

Pain from an overstretched round ligament or a ruptured ectopic pregnancy may both cause sharp lower quadrant pain, so the pain from these needs to be differentiated from that of appendicitis. The major difference is that the pain of an overstretched round ligament fades almost instantly; appendicitis pain not only continues, but grows more intense. With an ectopic pregnancy, a woman may experience morning sickness, and the pain she feels is either diffuse or sharp. With appendicitis, the nausea and vomiting is much more intense and the pain is sharp and localized at McBurney point (a point halfway between the umbilicus and the iliac crest on the lower right abdomen). In the pregnant woman, this can shift higher in the abdomen because the appendix is often displaced so far up in the abdomen by the uterus that the pain may resemble the pain of gallbladder disease (Fig. 20.3).

The woman's temperature is usually elevated, a urine sample reveals ketones, and a complete blood count reveals leukocytosis. Because pregnant women typically have an elevated white blood cell (WBC) count, however, an elevated WBC is not as diagnostic in pregnancy as it might be otherwise. An ultrasound or magnetic resonance imaging (MRI) scan will confirm the inflamed appendix.

Advise a woman in an emergency room that while she is waiting to be evaluated for possible appendicitis not to eat any food, drink any liquid, or consume any laxatives because increasing peristalsis could cause an inflamed appendix to rupture.

Therapeutic Management

If a woman is near term (past 37 weeks) and the fetus is believed to be mature, a cesarean birth may be performed along with removal of the inflamed appendix at the same time. If appendicitis occurs early in pregnancy, the inflamed appendix is usually removed by laparoscopy. As long as the anesthesiologist is aware the woman is pregnant and carefully controls oxygen levels during anesthesia administration, the outcome of both the surgery and the pregnancy will be good.

If the appendix ruptures before surgery, the risk to both mother and fetus increases dramatically. This occurs because, with rupture, infected fecal material escapes into the peritoneum and could spread by the fallopian tubes to the fetus. Also, generalized peritonitis is such an overwhelming infection that it would be difficult for a woman's body to combat it effectively and also maintain the pregnancy. As a third concern, peritoneal adhesions may develop after an appendix ruptures, resulting in future subfertility because of changes in the placement of fallopian tubes (Edwardson & Hueppchen, 2011).

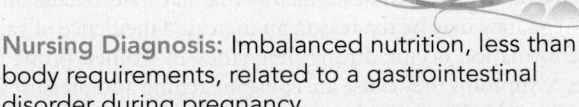

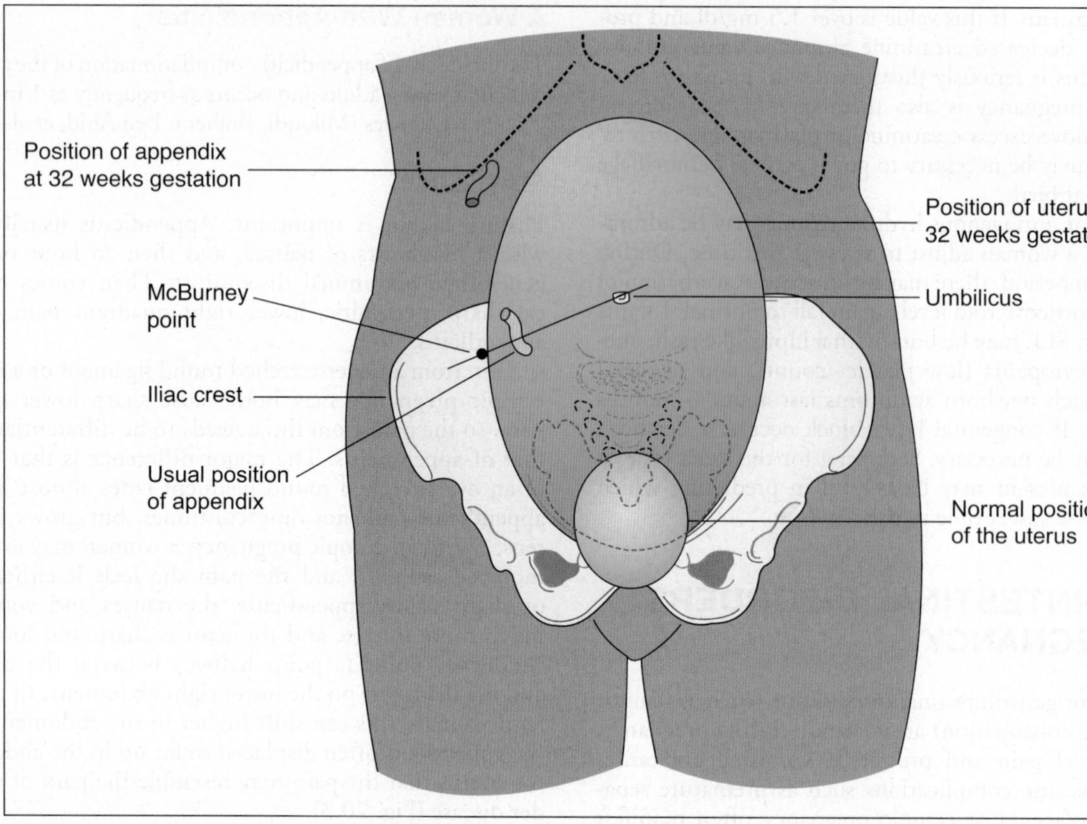

FIGURE 20.3 The change in position of appendix during pregnancy.

A Woman With Gastroesophageal Reflux Disease or Hiatal Hernia

Gastroesophageal reflux disease (GERD) refers to the reflux of acid stomach secretions into the esophagus (Fill Malfertheiner, Malfertheiner, Kropf, et al., 2012). Hiatal hernia is a condition in which a portion of the stomach extends and protrudes up through the diaphragm into the esophagus, trapping stomach acid and causing it to reflux into the esophagus. Although these conditions can be present constantly, symptoms most often occur only sporadically after increased peristaltic action. Both conditions may generate symptoms for the first time during pregnancy as the uterus pushes the stomach up against the esophageal valve and increases the reflux of acid or the extent of the hernia. Symptoms include:

- Heartburn, which is particularly extreme when lying supine after a full meal
- Gastric regurgitation
- Dysphagia (difficulty swallowing)
- Possible weight loss because of the stomach pain
- Hematemesis (i.e., vomiting of blood) if extreme esophageal irritation occurs

During pregnancy, these conditions are usually diagnosed by ultrasound, although direct endoscopy could be used. In most women, an over-the-counter antacid or a prescription for a proton pump inhibitor such as esomeprazole magnesium (Nexium; pregnancy category B) will effectively dilute or inhibit gastric acid production and so relieve symptoms. As additional measures, advise a woman to wear clothing that is loose around her waist and to sleep with her head elevated on two or more pillows to help confine stomach secretions.

Esomeprazole magnesium has not been studied as to its safety during breastfeeding, but as the uterine pressure is eliminated following birth, the symptoms generally become less noticeable or disappear and the woman no longer needs the drug. Some women may continue to have pain post birth and so need to take an acid inhibitor for several months until their irritated esophagus is completely healed.

A Woman With Cholecystitis and Cholelithiasis

Cholecystitis (i.e., gallbladder inflammation) and cholelithiasis (i.e., gallstone formation) are most frequently associated with women older than 40 years of age, who are obese, are multiparas, and ingest a high-fat diet. Because gallstones form from cholesterol, the hypercholesterolemia that naturally occurs during pregnancy may be the reason an increased incidence of gallstone formation occurs during pregnancy in women prone to these. Symptoms they cause are constant aching and pressure in the right epigastrium, perhaps accompanied by jaundice.

Medical therapy to prevent both conditions is to lower fat intake; however, during pregnancy, women should not eliminate it entirely because of the importance of linoleic acid for fetal brain growth. If symptoms of acute cholecystitis occur during pregnancy, the condition can be diagnosed by ultrasound. It can generally be managed by temporarily halting oral intake to rest the gastrointestinal tract and administering intravenous fluids to provide fluid and nutrients as well as analgesics for pain. Surgery for gallbladder removal by laparoscopic technique may be done during pregnancy if a woman's symptoms cannot be controlled by conservative management (Othman, Stone, Hashimi, et al., 2012).

A Woman With Pancreatitis

Pancreatitis (i.e., inflammation of the pancreas) is a rare disorder that tends to occur in young adults and so may occur during pregnancy (Tang, Rodriguez-Frias, Singh, et al., 2010). The woman experiences severe epigastric pain, nausea, vomiting, anorexia, and fever. Diagnosis may be difficult as serum amylase, which rises with pancreatitis, is also normally elevated during pregnancy. If serum amylase levels are greater than two times above normal, however, pancreatitis should be suspected. The disorder is treated the same during pregnancy as in nonpregnant women: nasogastric suction, bowel rest, analgesia (because pancreatic pain is sharp), and intravenous hydration through parenteral nutritional supplementation (Lau, 2011). The inflammation usually subsides within a week. Pregnancy loss, however, can occur from acidosis, hypovolemia, and fetal hypoxia (Igbinosa, Poddar, & Pitchumoni, 2013).

A Woman With Hepatitis

Hepatitis is a liver disease that occurs from invasion of the hepatitis A, B, C, D, or E virus. Hepatitis A is spread mainly by fecal–oral contact (children in day-care settings have a high incidence) or by ingestion of fecally contaminated water or shellfish. It has an incubation period of 2 to 6 weeks. Pregnant women exposed to hepatitis A may be given prophylactic γ-globulin to try to prevent the disease after exposure. This form follows a rather benign course and is not thought to be transmitted to the fetus (Panda, Panda, & Riley, 2010).

Hepatitis B and C are spread by exposure to contaminated blood or blood products or by contact with contaminated semen or vaginal secretions (and so are considered sexually transmitted infections [STIs]). These can be transmitted to the fetus across the placenta. Hepatitis D and E are apparently spread by the same methods as hepatitis B and C, but are rarely seen in pregnant women.

Hepatitis C demonstrates few symptoms, and these may not be present for 12 months after exposure. It is, however, the most common cause of chronic liver disease and liver transplantation in the United States (Murphy, Fang, Tu, et al., 2010).

Hepatitis B occurs about 1 in every 2,000 pregnancies (Salihu, Connell, Salemi, et al., 2012). It has an incubation period of 6 weeks to 6 months. It occurs in both an acute and chronic form, leading to liver cell necrosis with scarring and an inability to convert indirect to direct bilirubin or to excrete direct bilirubin. Women exposed to the virus receive immune globulin for prophylaxis; a hepatitis B vaccine can be administered to those who are at high risk, such as women who handle blood products, to prevent the illness.

Assessment

With all forms of hepatitis, a woman experiences nausea and vomiting. Her liver area may feel tender to palpation. Urine will turn dark yellow from excretion of bilirubin; stools will be light-colored from lack of bilirubin. Jaundice occurs as a late symptom. On physical examination, hepatomegaly (i.e., enlargement of the liver) is noted. The serum bilirubin level is elevated. Levels of liver enzymes, such as transaminase, are increased. Specific antibodies against the virus can be detected in the blood serum, so women at high risk may be routinely screened for this during pregnancy. If a liver biopsy is necessary for diagnosis, this can be performed safely during pregnancy as this is done under local anesthesia.

Therapeutic Management

A woman is usually prescribed bed rest and encouraged to eat a high-calorie diet because her liver has difficulty converting stored glycogen into glucose in its diseased state and so hypoglycemia can result. A cesarean birth may be planned at term to reduce the possibility of blood exchange between mother and fetus. Follow standard infection precautions when you give care to avoid contact with body fluids.

Hepatitis during pregnancy may lead to spontaneous miscarriage or preterm labor. Unlike most other diseases that cause maximum fetal threat in the first trimester, the later in pregnancy a woman contracts hepatitis B infection, the greater the risk the infant will be affected or develop hepatitis B. If this should occur, it is a serious consequence because a proportion of hepatitis B Ag-positive infants will develop liver cirrhosis or carcinoma later in life (Han, Xu, Zhao, et al., 2012). Use precautions during birth to avoid exposure to maternal body fluids. After birth, a woman may breastfeed as the infection is apparently not transmitted by breast milk. The infant should be washed well to remove any maternal blood; hepatitis B immune globulin (HBIG) and the first dose of hepatitis B should be administered (see Chapter 34 for the full immunization series). The infant then needs to be observed carefully for symptoms of infection during the first few months of life and for chronic liver disease as he or she grows older.

A Woman With Inflammatory Bowel Disease

Crohn disease (i.e., inflammation of the terminal ileus) and ulcerative colitis (i.e., inflammation of the distal colon) occur most often in young adults between ages 12 and 30 years. The cause of these diseases is unknown, but an autoimmune process is thought to be responsible. They are also associated with passive and active smoking (van der Heide, Nolte, Kleibeuker, et al., 2010). In both diseases, the bowel develops shallow ulcers. A woman experiences chronic diarrhea, weight loss, occult blood in stool, and nausea and vomiting. If extreme, obstruction and fistula formation with peritonitis can occur. With Crohn disease, malabsorption, particularly of vitamin B (the absorption of which occurs almost entirely in the ileum), can occur. Because of the potential difficulty with absorbing nutrients in both disorders, women with these disorders need careful monitoring for weight gain during pregnancy. There is a potential for fetal growth restriction if extreme malabsorption occurs. Therapy for the disorders is rest for the gastrointestinal tract by administration of total parenteral nutrition. Sulfasalazine (Azulfidine), an anti-inflammatory and a mainstay of therapy, may be continued during pregnancy without fetal injury. Close to birth, the dosage of sulfasalazine, because of its sulfa base, is reduced because it may interfere with bilirubin binding sites and cause neonatal jaundice (Karch, 2013). Infliximab (IFX) and adalimumab (ADA) are other attractive treatment options, but there is still limited data on the benefit/risk profile during pregnancy (Schnitzler, Fidder, Ferrante, et al., 2011).

NEUROLOGIC DISORDERS AND PREGNANCY

Neurologic illness, as a whole, does not occur at a high incidence in women of childbearing age. However, any neurologic disease with symptoms of seizures must be carefully managed during pregnancy because the anoxia that could be caused by severe seizures could deprive a fetus of oxygen.

A Woman With a Seizure Disorder

Recurrent seizures have several causes, such as head trauma or meningitis. However, the causes of most recurrent seizures, such as epilepsy, are unknown (i.e., are idiopathic). Recurrent seizures are seen in about 3 to 5 women per 1,000 births.

Therapeutic Management

The goal of care is to establish the best seizure control with the fewest possible number of antiseizure drugs prior to pregnancy. During pregnancy, because almost all antiseizure drugs are at least mildly teratogenic, dosages may have to be decreased even further to protect the fetus, which unfortunately then increases the risk of seizures (Burakgazi, Pollard, & Harden, 2011). Be certain women understand the rule "Do not take medication during pregnancy" does not apply to antiseizure medications, so that they continue to conscientiously take them despite the nausea or vomiting of early pregnancy. It is important the levels of antiseizure drugs be monitored and the doses adjusted routinely during pregnancy and again after birth. As blood volume increases with pregnancy, some women may need their dosage increased or their serum level will be diluted. Common drugs prescribed to control seizures are trimethadione (Tridione; pregnancy risk category D); valproic acid (sodium valproate and divalproex sodium; pregnancy risk category D); carbamazepine (Tegretol; pregnancy risk category C); ethosuximide (Zarontin; pregnancy risk category C), a drug often used to control absence seizures; and phenytoin sodium (Dilantin; pregnancy risk category D).

Women who have been taking phenytoin (Dilantin) for some time may have developed chronic hypertension, so a baseline blood pressure should be established early in pregnancy so any changes that occur with pregnancy can be interpreted correctly. Dilantin is recognized as the cause of a fetal syndrome, including cognitive impairment, vitamin K deficiency, and a peculiar facial proportion not unlike that of fetal alcohol sequence. To counteract the vitamin K deficiency and prevent hemorrhage in the newborn, women may be prescribed vitamin K during labor or the last 4 weeks of gestation.

Nursing Diagnoses and Related Interventions

Nursing Diagnosis: Risk for ineffective tissue (placental) perfusion related to hypoxia resulting from maternal seizure

Outcome Evaluation: Client informs health care personnel about history of seizures; states importance of immediate care and oxygen therapy should she begin a seizure. Apgar score of infant is 7 to 10, with no apparent birth anomalies.

Absence seizures (often just a rapid fluttering of the eyelids or a moment's staring into space) should have no effect on a woman or fetus. Tonic–clonic seizures (sustained, full-body involvement) could affect a fetus because spasm of the woman's chest muscles could lead to hypoxia. If a seizure should occur during pregnancy, a woman must be evaluated to be certain the cause of the seizure was the underlying seizure disorder, not a beginning sign of gestational hypertension. Nonpregnant women experiencing tonic–clonic seizures do not need oxygen administered during a seizure, but in pregnancy, administering oxygen by mask is a good prophylaxis to ensure adequate fetal oxygenation.

Woman who have recurrent seizures may worry their children will develop seizures as they grow older. If a woman's seizures were the result of an acquired disorder such as meningitis or head trauma, you can assure her that her child's risk for seizures is no greater than that for any other child. If the etiology of her seizures is unknown, the chance her child also will develop them is slightly higher than in the rest of the population. This prediction is only theoretical, however, and cannot be made without a thorough review of the onset and nature of the woman's disorder. Be certain a woman spends enough time with her newborn so she can become acquainted with the sudden jerking motions that occur in newborns such as when a newborn is startled (Moro reflex) or the jaw quivers after prolonged crying so she doesn't interpret these normal movements as seizure activity.

A Woman With Myasthenia Gravis

Myasthenia gravis is an autoimmune disorder characterized by the presence of an IgG antibody against acetylcholine receptors in striated muscle. The presence of the antibody causes failure of the striated muscles to contract, particularly those of the oropharyngeal, facial, and extraocular groups. The disorder usually occurs in 20 to 30 year olds, although it also is seen in young children. Women with the disorder need to be carefully monitored during pregnancy as pregnancy can cause major exacerbations of the disease (De Baets, 2010).

The disorder is treated with anticholinesterase drugs such as pyridostigmine (Mestinon) or neostigmine (Prostigmin) and possibly a corticosteroid such as prednisone. These medications may be continued during pregnancy, as the fetus will experience no effects from them. Be certain a woman understands atropine is the lifesaving antidote for neostigmine if an overdose should occur. Plasmapheresis (i.e., removal of and replacement of plasma) to remove immune complexes from the bloodstream may be prescribed to reduce symptoms. It must be carried out gradually during pregnancy, however, to reduce the risk of fluid overload or hypotension. Because smooth muscle is not affected by the disease, labor should occur without complications. Magnesium sulfate (administered to halt preterm labor or treat hypertension of pregnancy) should be avoided at any point in pregnancy because it can diminish the acetylcholine effect and therefore increase disease symptoms.

An infant born to a woman with myasthenia gravis may demonstrate disease symptoms at birth because of the transfer of antibodies (see Chapter 51).

A Woman With Multiple Sclerosis

Multiple sclerosis (MS) occurs predominantly in women of childbearing age, usually between 20 and 40 years of age (Finkelsztejn, Brooks, Paschoal, et al., 2011). With MS, nerve fibers become demyelinated and therefore lose function. Women develop symptoms of fatigue, numbness, blurred vision, and loss of coordination. ACTH (adrenocorticotropic hormone) or a corticosteroid is commonly given to strengthen nerve conduction and both can be administered safely during pregnancy. In contrast, immunosuppressants such as cyclosporine (Sandimmune), azathioprine (Imuran), and cyclophosphamide (Cytoxan), which are also frequently prescribed, should be used cautiously during pregnancy. Women may continue with plasmapheresis (i.e., withdrawal and replacement of plasma), another treatment regimen, during pregnancy as long as the volume of exchange is well controlled to prevent hypotension. Although women with the disorder may grow increasingly fatigued as pregnancy progresses, pregnancy does not affect the long-term course of MS. In some women, symptoms may actually improve during pregnancy because of the increased circulating corticosteroid levels. Monitor for UTIs at prenatal visits as these tend to occur as a poorly defined consequence of the illness.

MUSCULOSKELETAL DISORDERS AND PREGNANCY

Falls or other unintentional injuries that may lead to bone fractures or muscle sprains in women of childbearing age are discussed in Chapter 22. A chronic musculoskeletal disorder that is first identified during adolescence and so may play a role in childbearing is scoliosis.

A Woman With Scoliosis

Scoliosis (i.e., lateral curvature of the spine) begins to be noticed first in girls between 12 and 14 years of age. If it is uncorrected at this time, the curvature progresses until it can interfere with respiration and heart action because of chest compression. Pelvic distortion can interfere with childbirth, especially at the pelvic inlet. If a woman's spine is extremely curved, epidural anesthesia may be difficult to administer for pain management in labor.

Girls with scoliosis may wear a body brace during their adolescent years to maintain an erect posture. Although these braces are not as bulky as they once were, unless they are modified, they cannot be worn during the last half of pregnancy. For surgical correction, girls have stainless steel rods surgically implanted on both sides of their vertebrae to strengthen and straighten their spine. Such rod implantations do not interfere with pregnancy; a woman may notice more than usual back pain, however, from increased tension on back muscles. If a woman's pelvis is distorted, a cesarean birth may be scheduled to ensure a safe birth. Vaginal birth, if permitted, requires the same management as for any woman. With the improved management of scoliosis, the high maternal and perinatal risks associated with the disorder reported in earlier literature no longer exist (Chopra, Adhikari, Agarwal, et al., 2011). Plot the course of labor on a labor graph so an unusually long first stage, suggesting cephalopelvic disproportion, can be recognized. Chapter 51 discusses in detail the nursing care of adolescents following surgery to have rods inserted.

ENDOCRINE DISORDERS AND PREGNANCY

Endocrine disorders have the potential to be serious complications of pregnancy because enzymes and hormones control so many specific body functions (Amin, Robinson, & Teoh, 2011).

A Woman With a Thyroid Dysfunction

As a normal effect of pregnancy, the thyroid gland enlarges (i.e., hypertrophies) slightly because of increased vascularity and blood flow. A woman with a preexisting thyroid illness may have difficulty making this pregnancy transition.

Nursing Diagnoses and Related Interventions

Nursing Diagnosis: Risk for maternal and fetal injury related to preexisting thyroid disorder during pregnancy

Outcome Evaluation: No congenital anomalies are present in infant at birth; Apgar score is 7 to 10. Mother continues prepregnancy level of activities.

Thyroid function is necessary for the regulation of almost all body functions. Problems that affect pregnancy are either those of too little thyroid response (i.e., hypothyroidism) or too great a response (i.e., hyperthyroidism).

A Woman With Hypothyroidism

Hypothyroidism, or underproduction of the thyroid hormone, is a rare condition in young adults and especially rare in pregnancy because women with symptoms of untreated hypothyroidism are often anovulatory and unable to conceive. A woman who does conceive can then face another obstacle in that she can have difficulty increasing thyroid functioning to a necessary pregnancy level, which can then lead to early spontaneous miscarriage. Women with hypothyroidism fatigue easily, tend to be obese, their skin is dry (myxedema), and they have little tolerance for cold. It may be associated with an increased incidence of extreme nausea and vomiting (i.e., hyperemesis gravidarum).

Most women with hypothyroidism take levothyroxine (Synthroid) to supplement their lack of thyroid hormone. A woman who is taking levothyroxine needs to consult with her primary care provider when she is planning on becoming pregnant to be certain her dose of this will be high enough to sustain a pregnancy. She needs to come for an early diagnosis and close follow-up as soon as she suspects she is pregnant (1 week past her missed menstrual period). As a rule, her dose of levothyroxine will need to be increased as much as 20% to 30% for the duration of the pregnancy to simulate the increase that would normally occur in pregnancy (Stagnaro-Green & Pearce, 2012). Be certain a woman realizes the importance of taking this increased dose. Also caution women that they should take thyroxine at a different time from any medication containing iron, calcium, or any soy product by about 4 hours to be certain there is no problem with the absorption of thyroxine (Karch, 2013).

After the pregnancy, the dose of levothyroxine prescribed for pregnancy must be gradually tapered back to the prepregnancy level for both her health and so she can breastfeed safely. Be certain a woman does not continue to take her pregnancy dose (e.g., in trying to be economical and use up her higher dose pills), or she could pass beyond normal thyroid function and develop hyperthyroidism.

A Woman With Hyperthyroidism

Hyperthyroidism, or overproduction of thyroid hormone, causes symptoms such as a rapid heart rate, exophthalmos (i.e., protruding eyeballs), heat intolerance, heart palpitations, and weight loss. Sometimes called Graves disease, it is more apt to be seen in pregnancy than is hypothyroidism. If undiagnosed, a woman may develop heart failure because her heart, already stressed, cannot manage the increasing blood volume that occurs with pregnancy. She is also more prone than the average woman to symptoms of gestational hypertension, fetal growth restriction, and preterm labor.

Hyperthyroidism is normally diagnosed by a nuclear medicine imaging study involving the radioactive uptake of ^{131}I subtype. This diagnostic procedure should not be used during pregnancy because the fetal thyroid would also incorporate this drug, possibly resulting in destruction of the fetal thyroid. Treatment for hyperthyroidism is with thioamides (methimazole [Tapazole] or propylthiouracil [PTU]), which reduce thyroid activity. These drugs, unfortunately, cross the placenta and can lead to congenital hypothyroidism and, consequently, an enlarged thyroid gland (i.e., a goiter) in the fetus. Women should be regulated on the lowest possible dose of the drug and cautioned to keep a careful record of doses taken so they do not forget or unintentionally duplicate a dose, because if a goiter in the fetus enlarges enough, it can obstruct the airway and make resuscitation difficult at birth. Methimazole is the preferred drug for pregnant women as it appears to cross the placenta less easily (Chen, Xirasagar, Lin, et al., 2011).

If hyperthyroidism is not regulated during pregnancy, an infant may be born with symptoms of hyperthyroidism because of the excess stimulation he or she receives in utero. The newborn may appear jittery with tachypnea and tachycardia. An assay of fetal cord blood will reveal the level of T_4 and thyroid-stimulating hormone and the need for therapy in the infant. Women receiving smaller or minimal doses of antithyroid drugs may breastfeed, although women receiving large doses of these drugs may be advised not to breastfeed because they are excreted in breast milk (Karras, Tzotzas, & Kaltsas, 2010).

Surgical treatment to reduce the functioning of the maternal thyroid gland can be accomplished, but this is generally not the treatment of choice during pregnancy because of the need for general anesthesia. After a pregnancy, if a woman desires other children, the procedure might be suggested as an interpregnancy procedure so she does not enter a second pregnancy with hyperthyroidism.

A Woman With Diabetes Mellitus

Diabetes mellitus is an endocrine disorder in which the pancreas cannot produce adequate insulin to regulate body glucose levels. The disorder affects 3% to 5% of all pregnancies and is the most frequently seen medical condition in pregnancy (Ringholm, Mathiesen, Kelstrup, et al., 2012). It is increasing in incidence as more and more obese adolescents develop type 2 diabetes (Dea, 2011).

Before insulin was produced synthetically in 1921, women with type 1 diabetes (i.e., diabetes acquired in childhood) died before reaching childbearing age, were subfertile, or had spontaneous miscarriages early in pregnancy. Now that both type 1 and type 2 diabetes can be well managed, three new challenges have developed:

- How to manage both type 1 and type 2 diabetes during pregnancy to achieve a healthy glucose/insulin balance during pregnancy
- How to protect an infant in utero from the adverse effects of increased glucose levels
- How to care for the infant in the first 24 hours after birth until the infant's insulin–glucose regulatory mechanism stabilizes

Reproductive planning may be a fourth concern, as women with diabetes may not be good candidates for oral contraceptives because progesterone interferes with insulin activity and therefore increases blood glucose levels.

Pathophysiology and Clinical Manifestations

The possible etiology and pathology of diabetes mellitus are discussed in detail in Chapter 48. The primary concern for any woman with this disorder is controlling the balance between insulin and blood glucose levels to prevent hyperglycemia or hypoglycemia. Both of these conditions are dangerous during pregnancy not only because of long-term effects on the woman's health but also because of the threat to normal fetal growth. Infants of women with unregulated diabetes are five times more apt to be born large for gestational age or with birth anomalies (Garne, Loane, Dolk, et al., 2012).

If a woman's insulin production is insufficient, glucose cannot be used by body cells. The cells register the need for glucose, and the liver quickly converts stored glycogen to glucose to increase the serum glucose level. Because insulin is still not available, however, the body cells still cannot use the glucose, so the serum glucose levels rise (i.e., hyperglycemia). When the level of blood glucose reaches 150 mg/100 ml (normal level is 80 to 120 mg/dl), the kidneys begin to excrete quantities of glucose in the urine (i.e., glycosuria) in an attempt to lower the level. This causes large quantities of fluid to be excreted with urine (i.e., polyuria).

As dehydration begins to occur, the blood serum becomes concentrated and the total blood volume decreases. With the reduced blood flow, cells do not receive adequate oxygen, and anaerobic metabolic reactions cause large stores of lactic acid to pour out of muscles into the bloodstream. To replace needed glucose, fat is mobilized from fat stores and metabolized for energy, pouring large amounts of acidic ketone bodies into the bloodstream.

As the process continues, protein stores are tapped in a final attempt to find a source of energy. Utilizing protein for energy this way reduces the supply of protein to body cells. As cells die, they release potassium and sodium, which is lost from the body in the extensive polyuria. These factors combined create an immediate severe metabolic acidosis. Long-term effects are vascular narrowing that leads to kidney, heart, and retinal dysfunction.

Diabetes During Pregnancy

In type 1 diabetes, which, although unproven, is probably an autoimmune disorder because marker antibodies are present, the pancreas fails to produce adequate insulin for body requirements (Brezar, Carel, Boitard, et al., 2011). In type 2 diabetes, there is a gradual loss of insulin production, but some ability to produce insulin will still be present.

Women with either type 1 or type 2 diabetes who have successful regulation of glucose and insulin metabolism before pregnancy are apt to develop less-than-optimal control during pregnancy because all women experience several changes in the glucose–insulin regulatory system as pregnancy progresses. In all pregnancies, the glomerular filtration of glucose is increased (the glomerular excretion threshold is lowered), causing slight glycosuria. The rate of insulin secretion is increased, and the fasting blood sugar level is lowered. All women appear to develop an insulin resistance as pregnancy progresses or insulin does not seem as effective during pregnancy, a phenomenon that is probably caused by the presence of the hormone human placental lactogen (i.e., chorionic somatomammotropin) and high levels of cortisol, estrogen, progesterone, and catecholamines. This resistance to or destruction of insulin is helpful in a healthy pregnancy because it prevents the maternal blood glucose from falling to dangerous limits. It causes difficulty for a pregnant woman with diabetes because she must then increase her insulin dosage beginning at about week 24 of pregnancy to prevent hyperglycemia.

At the same time, she must guard against **hypoglycemia** (i.e., lowered serum glucose levels) and ketoacidosis caused by the constant use of glucose by the fetus. If a woman has preexisting kidney disease (revealed by proteinuria, decreased creatinine clearance, and hypertension), the risk of hypertension of pregnancy rises markedly (Negrato, Mattar, & Gomes, 2012).

Infants of women with poorly controlled diabetes tend to be large (>10 lb) because the increased insulin the fetus must produce to counteract the overload of glucose he or she receives acts as a growth stimulant. Hydramnios may develop because a high glucose concentration causes extra fluid to shift and enlarge the amount of amniotic fluid. A macrosomic infant may create birth problems at the end of the pregnancy because of cephalopelvic disproportion. This, combined with an increased risk for shoulder dystocia, may make it necessary for infants of women with diabetes to be born by cesarean birth.

There is also a high incidence of congenital anomaly, especially caudal regression syndrome (failure of the lower extremities to develop), spontaneous miscarriage, and stillbirth in women with uncontrolled diabetes. At birth, neonates are more prone to hypoglycemia, respiratory distress syndrome, hypocalcemia, and hyperbilirubinemia. The first trimester of pregnancy is the most important time for fetal development; if a woman can be kept from becoming hyperglycemic during this time, the chances of a congenital anomaly are greatly lessened (Box 20.6) (Ballas, Moore, & Ramos, 2012).

BOX 20.6 Nursing Care Planning Using Assessment

Assessing a Pregnant Woman With Diabetes Mellitus

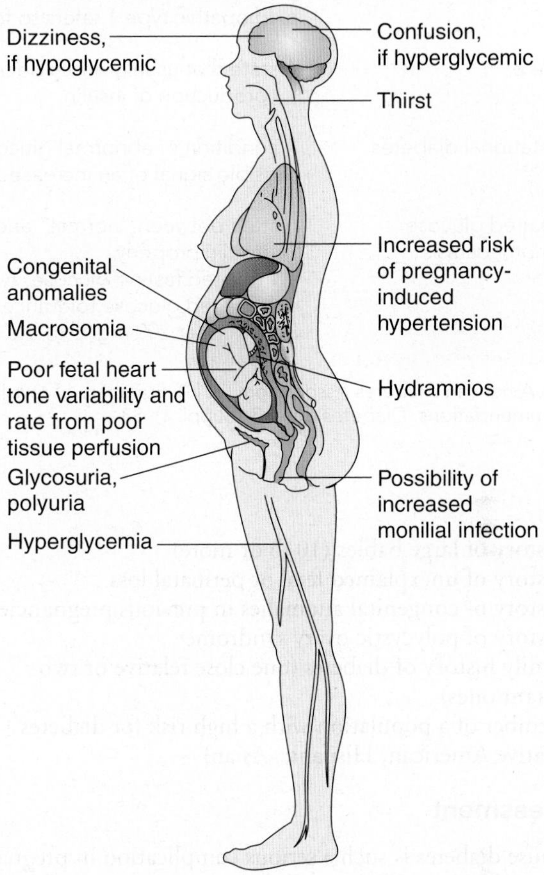

Classification of Diabetes Mellitus

Diabetes is divided into various categories that can be used to predict a pregnancy outcome (Table 20.2). Approximately 2% to 3% of all women who do not begin a pregnancy with diabetes develop the condition during pregnancy, usually at the midpoint of pregnancy when insulin resistance becomes most noticeable. This is termed gestational diabetes mellitus (Landon, Catalano, & Gabbe, 2012). The symptoms fade again at the completion of pregnancy, but the risk of developing type 2 diabetes later in life may be as high as 50% to 60%. It is unknown whether gestational diabetes results from inadequate insulin response to carbohydrate, from excessive resistance to insulin, or from a combination of both. Risk factors for developing gestational diabetes include:

- Obesity
- Age over 25 years

TABLE 20.2 Classification of Diabetes Mellitus

Class	Description
Type 1	A state characterized by the destruction of the beta cells in the pancreas that usually leads to absolute insulin deficiency. a. Immune-mediated diabetes mellitus results from autoimmune destruction of the beta cells. b. Idiopathic type 1 refers to forms that have no known cause.
Type 2	A state that usually arises because of insulin resistance combined with a relative deficiency in the production of insulin.
Gestational diabetes	A condition of abnormal glucose metabolism that arises during pregnancy. Possible signal of an increased risk for type 2 diabetes later in life.
Impaired glucose homeostasis	A state between "normal" and "diabetes" in which the body is no longer using and/or secreting insulin properly. a. Impaired fasting glucose: A state when fasting plasma glucose is at least 110 but under 126 mg/dl. b. Impaired glucose tolerance: A state when results of the oral glucose tolerance test are at least 140 but under 200 mg/dl in the 2-hour sample.

From American Diabetes Association. (2011). Summary of revisions to the 2011 clinical practice recommendations. *Diabetes Care, 34*(Suppl. 1), S3.

- History of large babies (10 lb or more)
- History of unexplained fetal or perinatal loss
- History of congenital anomalies in previous pregnancies
- History of polycystic ovary syndrome
- Family history of diabetes (one close relative or two distant ones)
- Member of a population with a high risk for diabetes (Native American, Hispanic, Asian)

Assessment

Because diabetes is such a serious complication in pregnancy, all women should be screened during pregnancy for gestational diabetes. A fasting plasma glucose greater than or equal to 126 mg/dl or a nonfasting plasma glucose greater than or equal to 200 mg/dl meets the threshold for the diagnosis of diabetes and needs to be confirmed on a subsequent test as soon as possible. This is usually done using a 75-g oral **glucose challenge test.**

For this, after a fasting glucose sample is obtained, the woman drinks an oral 75-g glucose solution; a venous blood sample is then taken for glucose determination at 1, 2, and 3 hours later. If two of the four blood samples collected for this test are abnormal or the fasting value is above 95 mg/dl, a diagnosis of diabetes is made. The values that confirm diabetes are reviewed in Table 20.3.

TABLE 20.3 Oral Glucose Challenge Test Values (Fasting Plasma Glucose Values) for Pregnancy Following a 75-g Glucose Solution

Test Type	Pregnant Glucose Level (mg/dl)
Fasting	95
1 hr	180
2 hr	155
3 hr	140

Monitoring a Woman With Diabetes

A woman with diabetes (type 1 or type 2) before preganancy should meet with her primary health care provider prior to becoming pregnant; during this period, her condition can be well regulated so that hyperglycemia does not develop during the early weeks of pregnancy, when the tendency for congenital anomalies in the fetus is highest. A woman should use a home test kit to determine she is pregnant so she knows this at the earliest possible time. The best insulin control program for her during pregnancy can then be determined. The measurement of **glycosylated hemoglobin**, a measure of the amount of glucose attached to hemoglobin, is used to detect the degree of hyperglycemia present. Measuring glycosylated hemoglobin is advantageous not just because it offers a present value of glucose, but because it reflects the average blood glucose level over the past 4 to 6 weeks (i.e., the time the hemoglobin in red blood cells were picking up the glucose). The upper normal level of HbA1c is 6% of total hemoglobin.

A urine culture may be done each trimester to detect asymptomatic UTIs as the increased glucose concentration in urine may lead to increased infection. An ophthalmic examination should be done once during the pregnancy for a woman with gestational diabetes and at each trimester for women with known diabetes because common background retinal changes that are common in diabetes, such as increased exudate (Fig. 20.4), dot hemorrhage, and macular edema, can progress or originate during pregnancy. Laser therapy to halt these changes can be done during pregnancy without risk to the fetus.

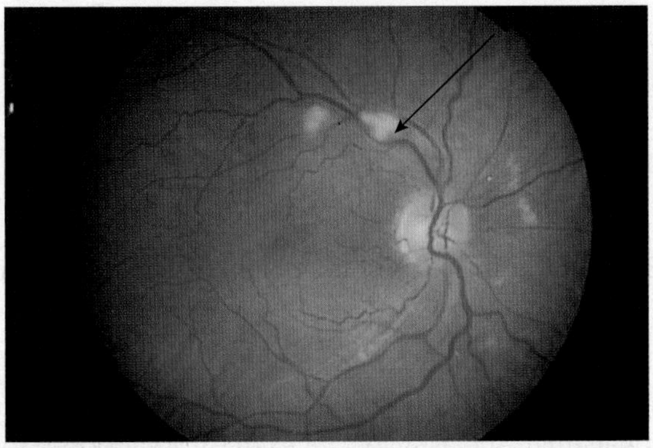

FIGURE 20.4 Increased exudate in the retina can occur with progressing diabetes during pregnancy. It appears as a "cloud-like" finding obscuring a retinal vessel.

Nursing Diagnoses and Related Interventions

Because diabetes is such a complex disorder, associated nursing diagnoses are many and varied. Examples include:

- Risk for ineffective tissue perfusion related to reduced vascular flow
- Imbalanced nutrition, less than body requirements, related to inability to use glucose
- Risk for ineffective coping related to required change in lifestyle
- Risk for infection related to impaired healing accompanying condition
- Deficient fluid volume related to polyuria accompanying the disorder
- Deficient knowledge related to complex health problem
- Health-seeking behaviors related to voiced need to learn home glucose monitoring

The following nursing diagnosis and related interventions illustrate one of the most important facets of the nurse's role in caring for the pregnant woman with diabetes: health teaching. Important topics include nutrition, exercise, insulin administration, blood glucose monitoring, and explanations of the various fetal assessment tests that will be done. Box 20.7 shows an interprofessional care map illustrating both nursing and team planning for a woman with diabetes.

Nursing Diagnosis: Deficient knowledge related to a therapeutic regimen necessary during pregnancy

Outcome Evaluation: Client states importance of careful attention to nutrition, exercise, and home monitoring of glucose levels during pregnancy; describes nutrition and exercise program; states intention to keep nutrition and exercise constant.

Education Regarding Nutrition During Pregnancy. Women need to be aware of how much carbohydrate they eat daily by estimating the total carbohydrate each anticipated meal will contain, then administer a number of units of insulin prior to that based on a predetermined insulin-to-carbohydrate ratio. As children also need to adjust insulin amounts to carbohydrate ratios, carbohydrate counting is discussed in Chapter 48.

Dietary control, or maintaining an adequate glucose intake so hypoglycemia does not occur, may be extremely difficult early in pregnancy because of nausea and vomiting. An 1,800- to 2,400-calorie diet (or one calculated at 30 kcal/kg of ideal weight), divided into three meals and three snacks to try and keep carbohydrate evenly distributed during the day so the glucose level remains constant, is a typical nutrition regimen during pregnancy. Ideally, 20% of dietary calories should be from protein, 40% to 50% from carbohydrate, and up to 30% from fat (Dornhorst & Williamson, 2012).

In addition, a woman's diet should be certain to include a reduced amount of saturated fats and cholesterol and an increased amount of dietary fiber. Increasing fiber decreases postprandial hyperglycemia and so lowers insulin requirements. Women are extremely vulnerable to hypoglycemia at night during pregnancy because of the continuous fetal use of glucose during the time they sleep. Urge a woman to make her final snack of the day one of protein and a complex carbohydrate (e.g., an egg and whole grain toast, hummus and whole grain crackers) to allow slow digestion during the night. If a woman cannot eat because of vomiting or nausea early in pregnancy or heartburn in later pregnancy, she should immediately notify her health care provider as she may need temporary intravenous fluid and glucose supplementation. Later in pregnancy, she must be extremely nutrition conscious to maintain good control of glucose levels and to keep her weight gain to a suitable amount (approximately 25 to 30 lb) in the hope of limiting the size of her infant and making a vaginal birth possible. Urge women, however, not to reduce their intake to below 1,800 calories during pregnancy as an intake this low in carbohydrates can lead to fat breakdown and acidosis.

What if...20.3 Angelina develops gestational diabetes. She's resistant to learn much about her condition, though, because she knows her symptoms are only temporary and will fade at the end of pregnancy. What type of teaching plan would you devise to help her learn in the face of this attitude?

Education Regarding Exercise During Pregnancy. Exercise is another mechanism that lowers serum glucose levels and, therefore, the need for insulin.

BOX 20.7 Nursing Care Planning

AN INTERPROFESSIONAL CARE MAP FOR A WOMAN WITH MULTIPLE THREATS TO PREGNANCY

Angelina Gomez, 22 years old, is pregnant with her first child. She fainted this afternoon while participating in an aerobic class.

Family Assessment Client lives with 30-year-old Josh, the father of her child. She works as a fundraiser for a movie producer. Josh works as an animation artist. Finances are rated as "workable." She fainted this afternoon while participating in her weekly hour-long aerobic class.

Client Assessment Client had rheumatic fever with mitral stenosis as a child. She developed gestational diabetes early in this pregnancy (her serum glucose level is 207 mg/dl; her blood pressure (BP) is 100/60 mmHg. A uterine monitor shows moderate-strength uterine contractions 7 minutes apart; fetal heart rate (FHR) is 167 beats/min. She asks you, "If exercise is supposed to be good for you, why did this happen?"

Nursing Diagnosis Risk for ineffective tissue perfusion (peripheral) related to lowered blood pressure secondary to mitral stenosis and gestational diabetes.

Outcome Criteria BP returns to 120/70 mmHg; pulse rate at 70 to 90 beats/min; fetal heart rate at 110 to 160 beats/min. Serum glucose is less than 126 mg/dl; labor is halted.

Team Member Responsible	Assessment	Intervention	Rationale	Expected Outcome
Activities of Daily Living, Including Safety				
Nurse/Primary care provider	Assess whether client understands it is healthy for her to exercise regularly.	Review with client the need to regulate glucose during pregnancy by consistent diet and exercise.	Strenuous exercise increases cardiac output, placing additional workload on the heart.	Client describes a more consistent exercise program to use during pregnancy rather than an aerobic class once a week.
Teamwork and Collaboration				
Nurse/Emergency room medical care provider	Telephone pregnancy and cardiac care providers and alert them to client's admission.	Coordinate care with pregnancy and cardiac health care providers who know client best.	Collaboration with pregnancy and cardiac health care providers helps ensure a healthy outcome for the woman and fetus.	Both pregnancy and cardiac care providers contact emergency staff to coordinate care.
Procedures/Medications for Quality Improvement				
Nurse/Emergency room medical care provider	Monitor client's BP, pulse rate, FHR, and uterine contractions by continuous monitoring.	Determine client progress by monitor and physical exam. Inform client of signs of beginning labor.	Increased FHR (tachycardia) is a sign of possible fetal distress. Uterine contractions could mark the beginning of preterm labor.	Client voices an understanding labor may be beginning; has confidence in emergency room (ER) staff to manage her condition until her primary care provider arrives.
Nurse/Cardiac ultrasound technician/ Consulting medical care provider	Explain process of echocardiogram to document mitral valve function.	Assure client echocardiogram is safe during pregnancy. Assist as necessary.	Mitral stenosis can lower blood pressure by not allowing adequate blood flow to aorta.	Echocardiogram is recorded in an expedient manner.

Nutrition				
Nurse	Assess serum glucose every 15 minutes by finger stick.	Document pattern of blood glucose. Administer intravenous (IV) fluid, insulin additive as prescribed.	Correcting blood glucose is vital to both maternal and fetal well-being.	Client's serum glucose maintained within normal level within 45 minutes.
Patient-Centered Care				
Nurse	Assess client's understanding that her complex situation (both cardiac and diabetes disorders) could be compromising her pregnancy.	Educate client about need for rest in lateral recumbent position until condition is stabilized.	Activity restriction can help prevent uteroplacental insufficiency and supine hypotension syndrome.	Client voices she understands need for continuous monitoring and rest. Complies with position for rest.
Psychosocial/Spiritual/Emotional Needs				
Nurse	Assess who is client's main support person and ask if she would like him notified.	Locate support person and invite him to join client in emergency department.	Anxiety and stressors can increase the workload of the heart. Support person can be instrumental in reducing stress.	Support person arrives and works with staff to alleviate anxiety.
Informatics for Seamless Health Care Planning				
Nurse/Primary care provider	Assess if client is aware of need for admittance to hospital to continue monitoring.	Assist client in transfer to hospital unit.	Continuous monitoring is necessary to detect if uterine contractions and preterm birth were halted.	Client is satisfactorily transferred to hospital unit for further monitoring and care.

If a woman begins an exercise program for the first time during pregnancy, she may notice excessive glucose fluctuations at first. Therefore, it's best if she begins her exercise program before pregnancy, when glucose fluctuation can be evaluated and food and snacks adjusted accordingly before a fetus is involved.

With exercise, blood glucose levels decrease because the muscles increase their need for glucose, an effect which lasts for at least 12 hours after exercise. If the arm in which a woman injected insulin is actively exercised, the insulin is released so quickly that it can cause hypoglycemia. To avoid this phenomenon, a woman should eat a snack consisting of a protein or complex carbohydrate before exercise and should maintain a consistent exercise program—she should not do aerobic exercises one day and then none the next, but rather, do 30 minutes of walking every day. In a woman with poor blood glucose control, extreme exercise will cause hyperglycemia and ketoacidosis as the liver both releases glucose and breaks down fatty acids in an attempt to supply enough energy for the exercise, yet the body cannot use them because of inadequate insulin.

Therapeutic Management

As keeping blood glucose levels near normal helps minimize the risk of maternal and fetal complications, both women with gestational diabetes and those with overt diabetes need more frequent prenatal visits than usual to ensure close monitoring of their condition and that of the fetus.

Insulin. Early in pregnancy, a woman with diabetes may need less insulin than before pregnancy because the fetus is using so much glucose for rapid cell growth. Later in pregnancy, she will need an increased amount because her metabolic rate and need increase. If she has been taking one particular kind of insulin and a specified dosage for a long time before the pregnancy, changing the type and dosage may be unnerving to her. Be certain she understands that re-regulation is a necessity because of the changes in her metabolism. Women with gestational diabetes will be started on insulin therapy if diet alone is unsuccessful in regulating glucose values.

The type of insulin chosen is usually a short-acting insulin (regular) combined with an intermediate type. Two thirds of the total amount of the day's insulin is given in the morning; the other third is given in the evening. This is self-administered 30 minutes before breakfast in a ratio of 2:1 (intermediate to regular) and again just before dinner in a ratio of 1:1. Use of a very short-acting insulin such as Lispro or insulin aspart, which have a 1-hour peak time, can lead to more fluctuations in blood glucose levels than regular insulin but are ideal for some women. Caution women to eat almost immediately after injecting these short-acting insulins to prevent hypoglycemia before mealtimes. Oral hypoglycemia agents are not used for regulation during pregnancy because, unlike insulin, they cross the placenta and are potentially teratogenic to a fetus.

For best control, help a woman plan her day based on the time interval her insulin takes to reach its peak. For example, an intermediate insulin given before breakfast reaches its peak after lunch or late in the afternoon just before dinner. Regular insulin given before breakfast reaches its peak just after breakfast. An intermediate insulin given in the evening reaches its peak into the next day before breakfast; the evening regular insulin injection peaks after dinner or at bedtime. Knowing when insulin reaches its peak level makes serum glucose monitoring meaningful and alerts women to the time of the day when they are most apt to be hypoglycemic (see Chapter 48).

Insulin is adjusted to keep a fasting blood glucose level below 95 to 100 mg/dl and a 2-hour postprandial level below 120 mg/dl. Be certain a woman is using an injection technique for insulin of stretching the skin taut and injecting at a 90-degree angle. Although this is normally intramuscular injection technique, insulin syringes have such short needles (5/8 in.) that this places the insulin in the subcutaneous tissue. During pregnancy, most women prefer to use thigh and upper arm sites rather than abdominal ones. Because insulin is absorbed differently from different sites, a woman should maintain a consistent rotating injection routine to maintain as consistent a level of absorption as possible.

Blood Glucose Monitoring. All women with diabetes need to do blood glucose monitoring to determine whether hyperglycemia or hypoglycemia exists. For this, a woman typically uses one of her fingertips as the site of lancet puncture. She places a drop of blood on a test strip. The strip is then inserted into a glucose meter that determines and prints out the glucose level.

If a woman discovers hypoglycemia is present, she should drink fluid with some form of sustained carbohydrate such as a glass of milk and some crackers. Taking a less-concentrated fluid such as milk rather than orange juice and including a complex carbohydrate helps prevent a rebound phenomenon in which a high glucose level is created, which would produce even more pronounced hypoglycemia.

If a woman discovers an elevated blood glucose level, she should assess her urine for ketones. If she finds ketones in two separate specimens, she should inform her health care provider because this suggests she is acidic. The most common time during pregnancy for hypoglycemia to occur is the second and third months, before insulin resistance peaks; for hyperglycemia, it is the sixth month, or the time insulin resistance is becoming most pronounced.

Insulin Pump Therapy (Continuous Subcutaneous Insulin Infusion). Because a woman will have some periods of relative hyperglycemia and hypoglycemia no matter how carefully she maintains her diet and balances her exercise levels, an effective method to keep serum glucose constant is to administer insulin by a continuous pump during pregnancy (de Valk & Visser, 2011). An insulin pump is an automatic pump about the size of a cell phone. A syringe of regular insulin is placed in the pump chamber and a small-gauge needle is attached to a length of thin polyethylene tubing, which is then implanted into the subcutaneous tissue of a woman's abdomen or thigh (Fig. 20.5). Day and night, at a continuous rate of about 1 unit per hour, the pump edges the syringe barrel forward, infusing insulin continually into the subcutaneous tissue. Depending on the individual prescription, before a snack and before a meal, a woman can dial or press a button on the pump; the pump then pushes the syringe barrel forward to administer a bolus of additional insulin. A woman should clean the site of the pump insertion daily and cover it with sterile gauze; she should also change the site every 24 to 48 hours to ensure absorption remains optimal and to decrease the possibility of infection.

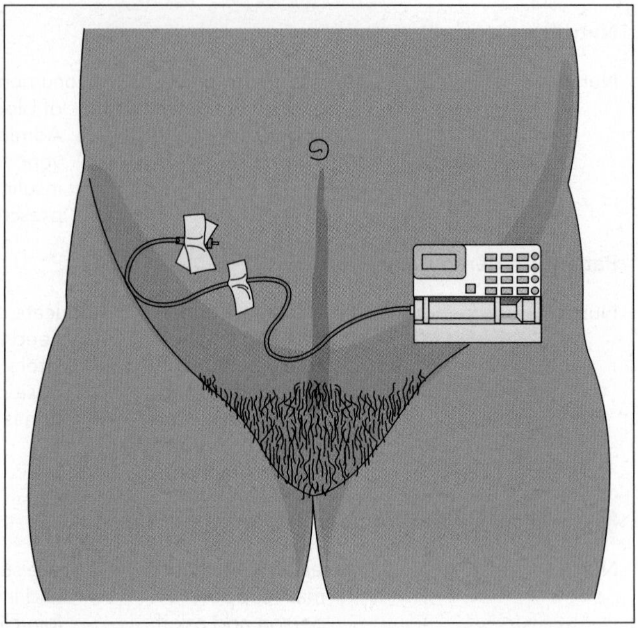

FIGURE 20.5 Using an insulin pump during pregnancy is the best assurance that insulin levels will remain constant.

Women who use insulin pumps should be aware of the following precautions. She should remove the pump (not the syringe and tubing) when showering, and she should remove the complete apparatus (pump, syringe, and tubing) to bathe or swim (but caution her not to leave it disconnected for more than 1 hour). A woman can wear clothing that hides the pump's outline if she wishes (it can either be held against her abdomen by an over-the-shoulder sling or hung from a belt around her waist). To assess whether the pump is delivering insulin at the designated rate, she needs to do blood glucose determinations about four times throughout the day (fasting and 1 hour after each meal). When pump therapy first begins, she must wake at night and do a 2:00 AM blood glucose determination because this is a time when she is most vulnerable for hypoglycemia and her pattern of insulin release may not be well regulated as yet.

Tests for Placental Function and Fetal Well-Being

Monitoring of fetal well-being will be individualized depending on the woman's overall health. Because women with diabetes tend to have infants with a higher than normal incidence of birth anomalies, a woman will have a serum α-fetoprotein level obtained at 15 to 17 weeks to assess for a neural tube defect and an ultrasound examination performed at approximately 18 to 20 weeks to detect gross abnormalities. A creatinine clearance test may be ordered each trimester. A normal creatinine clearance rate suggests a woman's vascular system is intact because kidney function is normal. By default, this also implies uterine perfusion is also adequate. Placental functioning may also be assessed by a weekly nonstress test or biophysical profile during the last trimester of pregnancy (see Chapter 9) if a woman is in good control, or a daily nonstress test if her regulation is poor.

In addition, a woman may be asked to self-monitor fetal well-being by recording how many movements occur an hour (usually about 10 fetal kicks) (see Chapter 9). Be certain she understands that fetal activity varies depending on her activity and meal patterns to prevent her from becoming frightened by normal variations. An ultrasound examination may be taken at week 28 and then again at week 36 to 38 to determine fetal growth, amniotic fluid volume, placental location, and biparietal diameter. Oligohydramnios (i.e., a small amount of amniotic fluid) may indicate fetal growth restriction or a fetal renal abnormality, whereas hydramnios (i.e., an excessive amount of amniotic fluid) may indicate gastrointestinal malformation or poorly controlled disease. A lecithin/sphingomyelin ratio by amniocentesis is usually performed by week 36 of pregnancy to assess fetal maturity. In pregnancies complicated by diabetes, this ratio tends not to show maturity as early as in other pregnancies probably because the synthesis of phosphatidylglycerol, the compound that stabilizes surfactant, is delayed if hyperglycemia is present.

Because lung surfactant does not appear to form as early in these fetuses as in others, the presence of phosphatidylglycerol, an ingredient of surfactant, at amniocentesis is used to indicate lung maturity for these infants. Although it is known that administering corticosteroids to the mother during the last week of pregnancy can hasten lung maturity, corticosteroids may also impair fetal insulin release and perhaps fetal pancreatic islet development. Therefore, with a fetus who already has a risk at birth from poor glucose control, corticosteroid use to improve lung maturity is not usually recommended.

Fetal surveillance can be both difficult and time consuming for a woman. Having to wait during each weekly test to hear how her fetus is doing is emotionally draining, especially for a woman who believes it is somehow her fault all the tests are necessary (it is, after all, her diabetes). She needs support people with her to minimize the feeling she is alone and without support in this crisis.

Timing for Birth

Among the most hazardous times for a fetus during a diabetes-involved pregnancy are weeks 36 to 40 of pregnancy, when the fetus is drawing large stores of maternal nutrients because of his or her large size. In the past, many infants were birthed early by routine cesarean birth at 37 weeks gestation to prevent fetal loss from placental insufficiency during these final weeks; unfortunately, if the fetus was still immature, this relieved one concern but created another, such as respiratory distress syndrome in the infant (infants of women with diabetes may be more prone to this than usual because surfactant is not as mature).

Cesarean birth was chosen because it is difficult to induce labor this early in pregnancy because the cervix is not yet ripe or responsive to labor contractions; babies of women with diabetes are large, making vaginal birth difficult; and a fetus suffering placental dysfunction or insufficiency did not do well in labor.

Today, when an accurate assessment of fetal age is available by amniocentesis and the pregnancy can be maintained within safe limits by the use of nonstress testing for a longer period, the last weeks of pregnancy are not as hazardous as before, and the timing and type of birth is much more individualized.

If at all possible, vaginal birth is preferred. Labor may be induced by rupture of the membranes or an oxytocin infusion after measures to induce cervical ripening (see Chapter 23). Both labor contractions and fetal heart sounds need to be consciously monitored during labor to ensure early detection of placental dysfunction. A woman's glucose level is regulated during labor by an intravenous infusion of short-acting or regular insulin with frequent blood glucose assays to prevent hypoglycemia in the mother or rebound hypoglycemia in the newborn (see Chapter 26 for care of the infant of a woman with diabetes at birth).

If a woman will be given an epidural anesthetic, use of an intravenous glucose solution as a plasma volume expander should be avoided to prevent hyperglycemia from developing; Ringer's lactate or 0.9% saline is infused instead.

Postpartum Adjustment

During the postpartum period, a woman who came into pregnancy with diabetes must undergo yet another readjustment to insulin regulation. With insulin resistance gone, often she needs no insulin during the immediate postpartum period; in another few days, however, she will return to her prepregnant insulin requirements. One- or 2-hour postprandial blood glucose determinations help to regulate how much insulin she needs during this adjustment period. A woman with gestational diabetes usually demonstrates normal glucose values by 24 hours after birth and then will need no further diet or insulin therapy. She requires careful observation, however, during the immediate postpartum period because if hydramnios was present during pregnancy, she is at risk of hemorrhage from poor uterine contraction. Women with diabetes may breastfeed because insulin is one of the few substances that does not pass into breast milk from the bloodstream (de Valk & Visser, 2011).

Because a woman who has had gestational diabetes is at risk for developing type 2 diabetes later in life, she should have glucose testing done during health maintenance visits throughout life. Be certain that women receive contraceptive information as appropriate. Remind women with ongoing diabetes before they plan a second pregnancy that they will need to be certain their disease is stabilized and in good control.

QSEN Checkpoint Question 20.5

Informatics

Angelina is prescribed an insulin pump to administer insulin for her gestational diabetes. Which of the following would you want to teach her as to why nighttime is a particularly hazardous time for her fetus during pump therapy?

a. The fetus can develop hyperglycemia from excessive insulin administration.
b. Continuous insulin administration with no food intake can lead to hypoglycemia.
c. Her lack of exercise at night tends to lead to hypercalcemia from muscle disuse.
d. Her lack of fluid intake during the night causes a relative increase in serum insulin levels.

Look in Appendix A for the best answer and rationale.

MENTAL ILLNESS AND PREGNANCY

Mental illness may precede or occur with pregnancy the same as it can at any point in life. Schizophrenia tends to have its highest incidence in adolescents and young adults and so may occur in young pregnant women. Depression occurs almost four times more commonly in women than in men, and often in young adults, making it the most common mental illness seen in pregnant women.

Even normal levels of stress make it difficult to use effective coping mechanisms, so pregnancy or childbirth may be the additional stress that reveals mental illness for the first time. Because of this, a woman with a psychiatric disorder is best cared for by a team approach, including both a psychiatric care team and a prenatal care group, to ensure the stress of pregnancy is not exacerbating the mental illness and that distorted perceptions or depression do not complicate the pregnancy. Any psychotropic medication taken by a pregnant woman should be evaluated before pregnancy for possible fetal harm (Galbally, Snellen, & Lewis, 2011). For example, lithium, a mainstay of therapy for mood disorders such as bipolar disorder, and serotonin-reuptake inhibitors used to counteract depression, are potentially teratogenic (Karch, 2013).

As the care of a newborn requires such a major life change, mental illness may also occur in the postpartum period (postpartum depression or psychosis are discussed in Chapter 25).

QSEN Checkpoint Question 20.6

Evidence-Based Practice

Women who have had a complication of pregnancy have the potential to develop depression in the postpartal period because their pregnancy did not go the way they wanted or imagined. To see what factors tend to be associated with depression in women who develop gestational diabetes, researchers administered a questionnaire to 71 women at 4 to 15 weeks postpartum. Results of the study showed that 34% of the women who developed gestational diabetes showed depressive symptoms; factors most associated with depression were cesarean birth and more weight gain than expected during pregnancy (Nicklas, Miller, Zera, et al., 2012).

Based on the previous study, which statement by Angelina would worry you most that she might develop postpartum depression?

a. "I want to shed some pounds so I'll fit into the new dress I bought for New Year's Eve."
b. "I hated giving insulin to myself; I'm relieved to not be doing that anymore."
c. "My baby is bigger than I expected, but his eyes are beautiful and he's cute."
d. "I think my husband adjusted better to my having diabetes than I did."

Look in Appendix A for the best answer and rationale.

CANCER AND PREGNANCY

The malignancies most commonly seen with pregnancy are those that occur most frequently in women during childbearing years such as ovarian cancer, uterine cancer, cervical cancer, breast cancer, thyroid cancer, leukemia, melanoma, and Hodgkin lymphoma (Han, Kesic, Van Calsteren, et al., 2013). Although immunologic mechanisms are altered during pregnancy, there is no evidence that pregnant women are more prone to cancer or that pregnancy changes the course of an existing disease.

If a woman is in the first trimester of pregnancy when a malignancy is diagnosed, she and her partner are asked to make a difficult decision: to delay treatment to avoid teratogenic risks to a fetus from treatment (possibly increasing a woman's risk), to end the pregnancy to allow chemotherapy or radiation treatment to be initiated, or to choose chemotherapy or radiation treatment with the knowledge they may cause birth anomalies in the fetus (Lataifeh, Al Masri, Barahmeh, et al., 2011).

As a rule, women can receive chemotherapy in the second and third trimesters without adverse fetal effects. In contrast, radiation therapy, another modality that is a mainstay of cancer therapy, puts the fetus at risk throughout pregnancy if the fetus is directly exposed.

A biopsy to confirm the diagnosis or surgery to remove a tumor can be completed during pregnancy with the understanding the fetus is at some risk for anoxia if a general anesthesia is used. Cervical conization for cervical cancer has a particularly high fetal risk because the surgery may directly disrupt the pregnancy. With a vaccine against human papillomavirus (HPV) now available, cervical cancer incidence should be seen much less in the future (Anttila, Kotaniemi-Talonen, Leinonen, et al., 2010). Following surgery of any kind, a woman is at a higher risk of thrombus formation because of the increased coagulation process accompanying pregnancy.

Cancer in a woman does not appear to metastasize to the fetus. This is because the placenta serves as a barrier against this spread and also because the fetus may be capable of resisting the invasion of the foreign cells. Melanoma is the exception to this, as this does seem capable of spreading to the fetus (Raso, Mascelli, Nozza, et al., 2010).

What if . . . 20.4 You are interested in exploring one of the 2020 National Health Goals related to acquired health disorders and pregnancy (see Box 20.1). Most government-sponsored money for nursing research is allotted based on these goals. What would be a possible research topic to explore pertinent to these goals that would be applicable to Angelina's family and that would also advance evidence-based practice?

KEY POINTS FOR REVIEW

- When women with a preexisting disease become pregnant, it is crucial to obtain a thorough history and physical examination at the first prenatal visit to establish a baseline of information on the condition. Documentation by a medication reconciliation form of any medication being taken is important to protect against adverse drug interactions and the possibility of teratogenic effects on the fetus.
- Teaching is an important nursing intervention because a woman with a preexisting illness must modify her usual therapy to adjust to pregnancy. Health teaching and how it affects women's overall health helps in planning nursing

care that not only meets QSEN competencies but also best meets the family's total needs.

- Because blood volume increases by as much as 50% during pregnancy, cardiac function may become inadequate if cardiovascular disease is present. Cardiac illnesses that cause difficulty can be either acquired disorders such as Kawasaki disease and rheumatic fever or congenital disorders such as mitral valve stenosis and coarctation of the aorta.
- Iron-deficiency anemia, sickle-cell anemia, and folic acid–deficiency anemia are examples of various forms of anemia that can also cause complications of pregnancy. Such anemias can result in fetal distress because of inadequate oxygen transport.
- Urinary tract disorders can lead to pregnancy complications because pregnancy increases the workload of the kidneys. UTIs and chronic renal disease are two disorders that may lead to early pregnancy loss.
- Acute nasopharyngitis, asthma, pneumonia, influenza, and tuberculosis are common respiratory disorders seen in pregnancy. The incidence of tuberculosis is on the increase and special assessments and care are needed for these women.
- Juvenile rheumatoid arthritis and systemic lupus erythematosus are examples of rheumatic disorders seen in pregnancy. These disorders generally require large doses of NSAIDs for therapy. Women taking salicylates are advised to decrease use 2 weeks before birth to avoid bleeding disorders in the newborn.
- Some gastrointestinal illnesses that occur with pregnancy are hiatal hernia, cholecystitis, viral hepatitis, inflammatory bowel disease, and appendicitis. If surgery is necessary for conditions such as cholecystitis or appendicitis, it can be performed by laparoscopic technique during pregnancy, but this may result in preterm labor.
- Recurrent seizures are the most frequently seen neurologic condition during pregnancy. Many drugs used to control seizures are teratogenic. Women need to have their medical regimen evaluated before pregnancy to be certain they are regulated on the fewest medications and the lowest dosages possible.
- The major endocrine disorder seen during pregnancy is diabetes mellitus. Gestational diabetes is diabetes that occurs only during pregnancy.

CRITICAL THINKING CARE STUDY

Tawnlee Pawlinsky is a 37-year-old G40030, 30-week pregnant woman who comes to your high-risk prenatal clinic for care. She has chronic hypertension and mitral valve insufficiency, which cause her to be short of breath if she hurries up a ladder at her job as a roofer or runs to catch a bus after work. When you talk about pregnancy nutrition with her, she makes a point that she is a vegan. Her hemoglobin is 9 g/ml; her red blood cells are microcytic and microchromic.

1. Tawnlee is diagnosed as having iron-deficiency anemia. Because she is a vegan, in addition to taking the iron supplement prescribed for her, what foods would you suggest she include daily in meals? Would you suggest she change her eating philosophy for the remainder of pregnancy to include meat?
2. Suppose Tawnlee ran from the bus stop into the clinic to avoid being late for her appointment. As soon as she reached the reception desk, she fell to the floor. You realize she needs cardiopulmonary resuscitation (CPR). What rate of respiratory/cardiac ratio would you use because she is 30 weeks pregnant?
3. Tawnlee is concerned because she was prescribed enalapril for hypertension before pregnancy but was changed to methyldopa at her prepregnancy consultation. She doesn't feel confident methyldopa will work as well and she fears she will grow dizzy working on a roof and fall. Would you assure her the medication change was a good one, or urge her to ask her primary care provider to change the prescription back to enalapril so she feels more secure at work?

Patient Scenario
The Taylor Family

Read about the Taylor family, a family with a pregnant woman who comes to a high-risk clinic for follow-up care, then answer the questions to further sharpen your skills and grow more familiar with NCLEX-type questions related to caring for a family experiencing a pregnancy complication from a preexisting or newly acquired illness. Confirm your answers are correct by reading the rationales.

Visit http://thePoint.lww.com

Answers and Rationales

Looking for answers to the What If. . . and Critical Thinking Care Study questions?

Visit http://thePoint.lww.com

References

American Congress of Obstetricians and Gynecologists. (2012). ACOG Committee Opinion No. 486: Update on carrier screening for cystic fibrosis. *Obstetrics & Gynecology, 117*(4), 1028–1031.

Amin, A., Robinson, S., & Teoh, T. G. (2011). Endocrine problems in pregnancy. *Postgraduate Medical Journal, 87*(1024), 116–124.

Anttila, A., Kotaniemi-Talonen, L., Leinonen, M., et al. (2010). Rate of cervical cancer, severe intraepithelial neoplasia, and adenocarcinoma in situ in primary HPV DNA screening with cytology triage: Randomised study within organised screening programme. *BMJ: British Medical Journal, 340*, c1804.

Armstrong, E .P., Malone, D. C., & Bui, C. N. (2012). Cost-effectiveness analysis of anti-muscarinic agents for the treatment of overactive bladder. *Journal of Medical Economics, 15*(Suppl. 1), 35–44.

Baer, A. N., & Petri, M. (2011). Lupus and pregnancy. *Obstetrics and Gynecology Survey, 66*(10), 639–653.

Ballas, J., Moore, T. R., & Ramos, G. A. (2012). Management of diabetes in pregnancy. *Current Diabetic Reports, 12*(1), 33–42.

Bourjeily, G., Barbara, N., Larson, L., et al. (2012). Clinical manifestations of obstructive sleep apnoea in pregnancy: More than snoring and witnessed apnoeas. *Journal of Obstetrics & Gynaecology, 32*(5), 434–438.

Brezar, V., Carel, J. C., Boitard, C., et al. (2011). Beyond the hormone: Insulin as an autoimmune target in type 1 diabetes. *Endocrine Reviews, 32*(5), 623–669.

Brushers, V. L. (2012). Alterations of pulmonary function. In S. E. Huether & K. L. McCance (Eds.), *Understanding pathophysiology* (5th ed., pp. 678–706). St. Louis, MO: Elsevier Mosby.

Burakgazi, E. P., Pollard, J., & Harden, C. (2011). The effect of pregnancy on seizure control and antiepileptic drugs in women with epilepsy. *Reviews in Neurological Diseases, 8*(1–2), 16–22.

Chen, C. H., Xirasagar, S., Lin, C. C., et al. (2011). Risk of adverse perinatal outcomes with antithyroid treatment during pregnancy: A nationwide population-based study. *International Journal of Obstetrics & Gynaecology 118*(11), 1365–1373.

Chen, Y. H., Keller, J., Wang, I. T., et al. (2012). Pneumonia and pregnancy outcomes: A nationwide population-based study. *American Journal of Obstetrics & Gynecology, 207*(4), 288.e1–288.e7.

Chetty, S. P., Shaffer, B. L., & Norton, M. (2011). Management of pregnancy in women with genetic disorders: Inborn errors of metabolism, cystic fibrosis, neurofibromatosis type 1, and Turner syndrome in pregnancy. *Obstetrical Gynecology Survey, 66*(12), 765–776.

Chopra, S., Adhikari, K., Agarwal, N., et al. (2011). Kyphoscoliosis complicating pregnancy: Maternal and neonatal outcome. *Archives of Gynecology & Obstetrics, 284*(2), 295–297.

Clark, P., Thomson, A. J., & Greer, I. A. (2012). Haematological problems in pregnancy. In D. K. Edmonds (Ed.), *Dewhurst's textbook of obstetrics & gynaecology* (8th ed., pp. 151–172). Oxford, UK: John Wiley & Son.

Cunningham, F. G., Leveno, K., Bloom, S. L., et al. (2010). Cardiovascular disease. In F. G. Cunninghan, K. Leveno, S. L. Bloom, et al. (Eds). *Williams obstetrics* (23rd ed., pp. 958–983). New York, NY: McGraw-Hill Companies.

Dalzell, J. J., Jackson, C. E., & Gardner, R. S. (2011). An update on peripartum cardiomyopathy. *Expert Review of Cardiovascular Therapies, 9*(9), 1155–1160.

Danza, A., Ruiz-Irastorza, G., & Khamashta, M. (2012). Antiphospholipid syndrome in obstetrics. *Best Practice & Research in Clinical Obstetrics & Gynecology, 26*(1), 65–76.

Dea, T. L. (2011). Pediatric obesity & type 2 diabetes. *MCN: American Journal of Maternal Child Nursing, 36*(1), 42–48.

De Baets, M. (2010). Insights in the autoimmunity of myasthenia gravis. *Autoimmunity, 43*(5–6), 341–343.

de Valk, H. W., & Visser, G. H. (2011). Insulin during pregnancy, labour and delivery. *Best Practice & Research in Clinical Obstetrics and Gynaecology, 25*(1), 65–76.

Dombrowski, M. P., & Schatz, M. (2010). Asthma in pregnancy. *Clinical Obstetrics & Gynecology, 53*(2), 301–310.

Donner, B. N., Niranjan, V., & Hoffmann, G. (2010). Safety of oseltamivir in pregnancy: A review of preclinical and clinical data. *Drug Safety, 33*(8), 631–642.

Dornhorst, A., & Williamson, C. (2012). Diabetes & endocrine disease in pregnancy. In D. K. Edmonds (Ed.), *Dewhurst's textbook of obstetrics & gynaecology* (6th ed., pp. 121–136). Oxford, UK: John Wiley & Son.

Easterling, T. R., & Stout, K. (2012). Heart disease. In S. G. Gabbe, J. R. Niebyl, J. L. Simpson, et al. (Eds.), *Obstetrics: Normal and problem pregnancies* (8th ed., pp. 825–850).Philadelphia, PA: Elsevier/Saunders.

Edwardson, J., & Hueppchen, N. A. (2011). Surgical disease & trauma. In K. J. Hurt, M. W. Guile, J. L. Bienstock, et al. (Eds.), *The Johns Hopkins manual of gynecology and obstetrics* (4th ed., pp. 248–256). Philadelphia, PA: Lippincott Williams & Wilkins.

Fill Malfertheiner, S., Malfertheiner, M. V., Mönkemüller, K., et al. (2012). A prospective longitudinal cohort study: Evolution of GERD symptoms during the course of pregnancy. *BMC Gastroenterology, 12*(9), 131.

Finkelsztejn, A., Brooks, J. B., Paschoal, F. M., et al. (2011). What can we really tell women with multiple sclerosis regarding pregnancy? A systematic review and meta-analysis of the literature. *British Journal of Obstetrics and Gynecology, 118*(7), 790–797.

Fontana, I., Santori, G., Fazio, F., et al. (2012). The pregnancy rate and live birth rate after kidney transplantation: A single-center experience. *Transplantation Proceedings, 44*(7), 1910–1911.

Fried, M., Muehlenbachs, A., & Duffy, P. E. (2012). Diagnosing malaria in pregnancy: An update. *Expert Review of Anti-Infective Therapy, 10*(10), 1177–1187.

Galbally, M., Snellen, M., & Lewis, A. J. (2011). A review of the use of psychotropic medication in pregnancy. *Current Opinion in Obstetrics & Gynecology, 23*(6), 408–414.

Garne, E., Loane, M., Dolk, H., et al. (2012). Spectrum of congenital anomalies in pregnancies with pregestational diabetes. *Birth Defects Research, 94*(3), 134–140.

Gasim, T. (2011). Immune thrombocytopenic purpura in pregnancy: A reappraisal of obstetric management and outcome. *Journal of Reproductive Medicine, 56*(3–4), 163–168.

Gelson, E., Curry, R., Gatzoulis, M. A., et al. (2011). Effect of maternal heart disease on fetal growth. *Obstetrics and Gynecology, 117*(4), 886–891.

Gilbert, E. S. (2011). Cardiac disease. In E. S. Gilbert (Ed.), *Manual of high risk pregnancy & delivery* (5th ed., pp. 243–257). St. Louis, MO: Mosby/Elsevier.

Gorman, J. R., Brewer, N. T., Wang, J. B., et al. (2012). Theory-based predictors of influenza vaccination among pregnant women. *Vaccine, 31*(1), 213–218.

Greenberg, J. A., Bell, S. J., Guan, Y., et al. (2011). Folic acid supplementation and pregnancy: More than just neural tube defect prevention. *Reviews in Obstetrics & Gynecology, 4*(2), 52–59.

Gregory, K. D., Korst, L. M., Lu, M. C., et al. (2013). AHRQ patient safety indicators: Time to include hemorrhage and infection during childbirth. *Joint Commission Journal of Quality Patient Safety, 39*(3):114–122.

Guthrie, K. A., Dugowson, C. E., Voigt, L. F., et al. (2010). Does pregnancy provide vaccine-like protection against rheumatoid arthritis? *Arthritis & Rheumatism, 62*(7), 1842–1848.

Han, G. R., Xu, C. L., Zhao, W., et al. (2012). Management of chronic hepatitis B in pregnancy. *World Journal of Gastroenterology, 18*(33), 4517–4521.

Han, S. N., Kesic, V. I., Van Calsteren, K., et al. (2013). Cancer in pregnancy: A survey of current clinical practice. *European Journal of Obstetrics & Gynecology & Reproductive Biology, 167*(1), 18–23.

Hess, R. F., & Weinland, J. A. (2012). The life-changing impact of peripartum cardiomyopathy: An analysis of online postings. *American Journal of Maternal Child Nursing, 37*(4), 241–246.

Howard, J., & Oteng-Ntim, E. (2012). Management of sickle-cell disease. *Best Practice & Research: Clinical Obstetrics & Gynaecology, 26*(1), 25–36.

Humphreys, R. A., Wong, H. H., Milner, R., et al. (2012). Pregnancy outcomes among solid organ transplant recipients in British Columbia. *Journal of Obstetrics & Gynecology Canada, 34*(5), 416–424.

Igbinosa, O., Poddar, S., & Pitchumoni, C. (2013). Pregnancy associated pancreatitis revisited. *Clinics and Research in Hepatology and Gastroenterology, 37*(2), 177–181.

Imdad, A., & Bhutta, Z. A. (2012). Routine iron/folate supplementation during pregnancy: Effect on maternal anaemia and birth outcomes. *Paediatric & Perinatal Epidemiology, 26*(Suppl. 1), 168–177.

Irvine, M. H., Einarson, A., & Bozzo, P. (2011). Prophylactic use of antimalarials during pregnancy. *Canadian Family Physician, 57*(11), 1279–1281.

Jelkmann, W. (2011). Regulation of erythropoietin production. *Journal of Physiology, 589*(Pt. 6), 1251–1258.

Karch, A. M. (2013). *2013 Lippincott's nursing drug guide*. Philadelphia, PA: Lippincott Williams & Wilkins.

Karras, S., Tzotzas, T., Kaltsas, T., et al. (2010). Pharmacological treatment of hyperthyroidism during lactation: Review of the literature and novel data. *Pediatric Endocrinology Reviews, 8*(1), 25–33.

Khan, Y., & Tisman, G. (2010). Pica in iron deficiency: A case series. *Journal of Medical Case Reports, 12*(4), 86.

Kuo, H. C., Yang, K. D., Chang, W. C., et al. (2012). Kawasaki disease: An update on diagnosis and treatment. *Pediatric Neonatology, 53*(1), 4–11.

Landon, M. B., Catalano, P. M., & Gabbe, S. G. (2012). Diabetes mellitus complicating pregnancy. In S. G. Gabbe, J. R. Niebyl, J. L. Simpson, et al. (Eds.), *Obstetrics: Normal and problem pregnancies* (6th ed., pp. 581–591). Philadelphia, PA: Elsevier/Saunders.

Lataifeh, I. M., Al Masri, M., Barameh, S., et al. (2011). Management of cancer during pregnancy: Obstetric and neonatal outcomes. *International Journal of Gynecology Cancer, 21*(6), 1159–1166.

Lateef, A., & Petri, M. (2012). Management of pregnancy in systemic lupus erythematosus. *Nature Reviews Rheumatology, 8*(12), 710–718.

Lau, M. T. (2011). Parenteral nutrition in the malnourished: Dialysis, cancer, obese, and hyperemesis gravidarum patients. *Journal of Infusion Nursing, 34*(5), 315–318.

Leung, T. Y., & Lao, T. T. (2012). Thalassaemia in pregnancy. *Best Practice & Research in Clinical Obstetrics & Gynaecology, 26*(1), 37–51.

Lopez, V., Martinez, D., Vinolo, C., et al. (2011). Pregnancy in kidney transplant recipients: Effects on mother and newborn. *Transplantation Proceedings, 43*(6), 2177–2178.

MacMullen, N. J., & Dulski, L. A. (2011). Perinatal implications of sickle cell disease. *MCN: American Journal of Maternal Child Nursing, 36*(4), 232–238.

Mendola, P., Laughon, S. K., Männistö, T. I., et al. (2013). Obstetric complications among U.S. women with asthma. *American Journal of Obstetrics & Gynecology, 208*(2), 127.e1–127.e8.

Miloudi, N., Brahem, M., Ben Abid, S., et al. (2012). Acute appendicitis in pregnancy: Specific features of diagnosis and treatment. *Journal of Visceral Surgery, 149*(4), e275–279.

Moreno, J. L., Kurita, M., Holloway, T., et al. (2011). Maternal influenza viral infection causes schizophrenia-like alterations of 5-HT. *Journal of Neuroscience, 31*(5), 1863–1872.

Murphy, E. L., Fang, J., Tu, Y., et al. (2010). Hepatitis C virus prevalence and clearance among U.S. blood donors, 2006–2007: Associations with birth cohort, multiple pregnancies, and body mass index. *Journal of Infectious Diseases, 202*(4), 576–584.

Negrato, C. A., Mattar, R., & Gomes, M. B. (2012). Adverse pregnancy outcomes in women with diabetes. *Diabetology & Metabolic Syndrome, 4*(1), 41.

Ngô, C., Kayem, G., Habibi, A., et al. (2010). Pregnancy in sickle cell disease: Maternal and fetal outcomes in a population receiving prophylactic partial exchange transfusions. *European Journal of Obstetrics, Gynecology & Reproductive Biology, 152*(2), 138–142.

Nhan-Chang, C. L., & Jones, T. B. (2010). Tuberculosis in pregnancy. *Clinical Obstetrics & Gynecology, 53*(2), 311–321.

Nicklas, J. M., Miller, L. J., Zera, C. A., et al. (2012). Factors associated with depressive symptoms in the early postpartum period among women with recent gestational diabetes mellitus. *Maternal Child Health Journal, 2012.*

Othman, M. O., Stone, E., Hashimi, M., et al. (2012). Conservative management of cholelithiasis and its complications in pregnancy is associated with recurrent symptoms and more emergency department visits. *Gastrointestinal Endoscopy, 760*(3), 564–569.

Panda, B., Panda, A., Riley, L. E. (2010). Selected viral infections in pregnancy. *Obstetrics & Gynecology Clinics of North America, 37*(2), 321–331.

Parhar, K. S., Gibson, P. S., & Coffin, C. S. (2012). Pregnancy following liver transplantation: Review of outcomes and recommendations for management. *Canadian Journal of Gastroenterology, 26*(9), 621–626.

Piccoli, G. B., Conijn, A., Consiglio, V., et al. (2010). Pregnancy in dialysis patients: Is the evidence strong enough to lead us to change our counseling policy? *Clinical Journal of The American Society of Nephrology, 5*(1), 62–71.

Raso, A., Mascelli, S., Nozza, P., et al. (2010). Detection of transplacental melanoma metastasis using quantitative PCR. *Diagnostic Molecular Pathology, 19*(2), 78–82.

Ringholm, L., Mathiesen, E. R., Kelstrup, L., et al. (2012). Managing type 1 diabetes mellitus in pregnancy-from planning to breastfeeding. *Nature Reviews Endocrinology, 8*(11), 659–667.

Rote, N. S., & McCance, K. L. (2012). Structure and function of the hematologic system. In S. E. Huether, & K. L. .McCance, *Understanding pathophysiology* (5th ed., pp. 481–507). New York: Elsevier Publishing.

Salihu, H. M., Connell, L., Salemi, J. L., et al. (2012). Prevalence and temporal trends of hepatitis B, hepatitis C, and HIV/AIDS co-infection during pregnancy across the decade, 1998–2007. *Journal of Women's Health, 21*(1), 66–72.

Samuels, P. (2012). Hematologic complications of pregnancy. In S. G. Gabbe, J. R. Niebyl, J. L. Simpson, et al. (Eds.), *Obstetrics: Normal and problem pregnancies* (6th ed., pp. 659–672). Philadelphia, PA: Elsevier/Saunders.

Schneeberger, C., Geerlings, S. E., Middleton, P., et al. (2012). Interventions for preventing recurrent urinary tract infection during pregnancy. *Cochrane Database of Systematic Reviews,* (11), CD009279.

Schnitzler, F., Fidder, H., Ferrante, M., et al. (2011). Outcome of pregnancy in women with inflammatory bowel disease treated with antitumor necrosis factor therapy. *Inflammatory Bowel Disease, 17*(9), 1846–1854.

Schulman, S. (2012). Advances in the management of venous thromboembolism. *Best Practice & Research: Clinical Haematology, 25*(3), 361–377.

Sethi, K. D., & Mehta, S. H. (2012). A clinical primer on restless legs syndrome: What we know, and what we don't know. *American Journal of Managed Care, 18*(5, Suppl.), S83–S88.

Shahbazi, S., Moghaddam-Banaem, L., Ekhtesari, F., et al. (2012). Impact of inherited bleeding disorders on pregnancy and postpartum hemorrhage. *Blood Coagulation & Fibrinolysis, 23*(7), 603–607.

Sorensen, H. T., Horvath-Puho, E., Lash, T. L., et al. (2011). Heart disease may be a risk factor for pulmonary embolism without peripheral deep venous thrombosis. *Circulation, 124*(13), 1435–1441.

Stagnaro-Green, A., & Pearce, E. (2012). Thyroid disorders in pregnancy. *Nature Reviews Endocrinology, 8*(11), 650–658.

Suri, V., Keepanasseril, A., Aggarwal, N., et al. (2011). Mechanical valve prosthesis and anticoagulation regimens in pregnancy: A tertiary center experience. *European Journal of Obstetrics & Gynecology and Reproductive Biology, 159*(2), 320–323.

Tang, S. J., Rodriguez-Frias, E., Singh, S., et al. (2010). Acute pancreatitis during pregnancy. *Clinical Gastroenterology and Hepatology, 8*(1), 85–90.

Thorpe-Beeston, J., Madge, S., Gyi, K., et al. (2013). The outcome of pregnancies in women with cystic fibrosis-single centre experience 1998–2011. *BJOG: International Journal of Obstetrics & Gynaecology, 120*(3), 354–361.

Traill, T. A. (2012). Valvular heart disease and pregnancy. *Cardiology Clinics, 30*(3), 369–381.

Trautner, B. W. (2012). Asymptomatic bacteriuria: When the treatment is worse than the disease. *Nature Reviews Urology, 9*(2), 85–89.

United States Department of Health and Human Services. (2010). *Healthy people 2020.* Washington, DC: DHHS.

van der Heide, F., Nolte, I. M., Kleibeuker, J. H., et al. (2010). Differences in genetic background between active smokers, passive smokers, and non-smokers with Crohn's disease. *American Journal of Gastroenterology, 105*(5), 1165–1172.

Wolff, G. A., & Weitzel, N. S. (2011). Management of acquired cardiac disease in the obstetric patient. *Seminars in Cardiothoracic and Vascular Anesthesia, 15*(3), 85–97

Chapter 21

Nursing Care of a Family Experiencing a Sudden Pregnancy Complication

KEY TERMS

- abortion
- ankle clonus
- antiphospholipid antibodies
- cervical cerclage
- chorioamnionitis
- Couvelaire uterus
- early pregnancy failure
- eclampsia
- ectopic pregnancy
- erythroblastosis fetalis
- gestational trophoblastic disease
- HELLP syndrome
- hemolytic disease of the newborn
- hydramnios
- isoimmunization
- miscarriage
- oligohydramnios
- placenta previa
- postterm pregnancy
- preeclampsia
- premature cervical dilatation
- premature separation of the placenta
- preterm labor
- preterm rupture of membranes
- pseudocyesis
- recurrent pregnancy loss
- Rh incompatibility
- tocolytic agent

OBJECTIVES

After mastering the contents of this chapter, you should be able to:

1. Describe sudden complications of pregnancy that place a pregnant woman and her fetus at high risk.
2. Identify 2020 National Health Goals related to complications of pregnancy that nurses can help the nation achieve.
3. Assess a woman who is experiencing a complication of pregnancy.
4. Formulate nursing diagnoses that address the needs of a woman and her family experiencing a complication of pregnancy.
5. Identify expected outcomes to minimize the risks to a pregnant woman and her fetus when a sudden complication of pregnancy occurs as well as manage seamless transitions across differing health care settings.
6. Using the nursing process, plan nursing care that includes the six competencies of Quality & Safety Education for Nurses (QSEN): Patient-Centered Care, Teamwork & Collaboration, Evidence-Based Practice (EBP), Quality Improvement (QI), Safety, and Informatics.
7. Implement nursing care specific to a woman who has developed a sudden complication of pregnancy, such as teaching her how to recognize the symptoms of preterm labor.
8. Evaluate expected outcomes for effectiveness and achievement of care.
9. Integrate knowledge of complications of pregnancy with the interplay of nursing process, the six competencies of QSEN, and Family Nursing to promote quality maternal and child health nursing care.

Beverly Muzuki, a 20-year-old gravida 2, para 0, 30-weeks pregnant woman, noticed some mild lower abdominal pain but thought it was irritation from a bladder infection and waited to get help until she went to her scheduled appointment at the hospital. During the night, she woke up twice because of a nagging lower backache. This morning, she has intermittent sharp uterine contractions. "Why am I starting labor so early?" she asks you. "Is it because I'm Rh negative?"

Previous chapters described normal pregnancies and preexisting and newly acquired conditions that can complicate pregnancies. This chapter adds knowledge about complications directly related to the pregnancy.

Were Beverly's actions as informed as they could have been? What additional health teaching might have helped her recognize the signs of preterm labor earlier?

BOX 21.1 Nursing Care Planning Based on 2020 National Health Goals

Preventing complications of pregnancy is viewed as so important this issue is included in the 2020 National Health Goals.

- Reduce the rate of maternal deaths to 11.4 maternal deaths per 100,000 live births from a baseline of 12.7 per 100,000 live births.
- Reduce the rate of maternal illness and complications because of pregnancy to 28 per 100 births from a baseline of 31.1 per 100 births.
- Reduce the proportion of total preterm births to 11.4% from a baseline of 12.7%.
- Reduce the incidence of low birth weight to 7.1% of live births from a baseline of 8.2% of live births (U.S. Department of Health and Human Services [DHHS], 2010; see www.healthypeople.gov).

Encouraging all women to come for prenatal care is the best preventive measure for eliminating complications of pregnancy. Nurses working in prenatal settings can help to ensure women are well informed about the normal course of pregnancy so they can actively participate in risk assessment at prenatal visits and also recognize and alert health care providers if a complication begins.

Most women who enter pregnancy in good health expect to complete a pregnancy and birth without complications. In a few women, however, unexpected deviations or complications from the course of normal pregnancy occur, which place a severe burden on a woman and her family and her health care providers. All families benefit from the support and skill of a professional nurse who helps them work through the stages of pregnancy and prepares them to become new parents. For a family who must take special care to ensure the continuation of pregnancy, the support and skills of a professional nurse are essential to help them carry the baby to term. Hospitalization may be necessary. Once stabilized, a woman has to be monitored carefully until the pregnancy reaches term. As this is done on an ambulatory basis, nurses continue to be instrumental in care (Evans, 2012).

The leading complications related directly to pregnancy are thromboembolism, hemorrhage, infection, hypertension of pregnancy, and ectopic pregnancy (Mehta & Sokol, 2013). All of these have the potential to threaten both the life of the mother and the fetus. National Health Goals established to help reduce poor outcomes of complications of pregnancy such as these are shown in Box 21.1.

Nursing Process Overview

For a Woman Who Develops a Complication of Pregnancy

Assessment

Nurses often are the first health care providers to discover a complication of pregnancy. Always ask women at prenatal visits about any symptoms that might indicate a complication such as pain or vaginal symptoms (e.g., leaking of fluid or bleeding). Provide enough time for a thorough health history so more subtle problems such as headache, blurred vision, or back pains can be discovered and investigated thoroughly. In addition, review the danger signs of pregnancy with women and, if appropriate, significant family members or other support people so potential problems can be recognized early and a health care provider can be contacted. Assure women they are free to call whenever they are concerned. Otherwise, they may wait until symptoms become acute rather than call when a symptom is first noticed.

Nursing Diagnosis

Nursing diagnoses pertaining to a woman with a pregnancy complication should reflect both the physical problem and the woman's or family's concern. Some examples include:

- Anxiety related to guarded pregnancy outcome
- Fear of preterm labor ending the pregnancy
- Anticipatory grieving related to uncertain pregnancy outcome
- Deficient knowledge related to signs and symptoms of possible complications
- Risk for infection related to incomplete miscarriage
- Deficient fluid volume related to third-trimester bleeding
- Risk for ineffective tissue perfusion related to gestational hypertension

Outcome Identification and Planning

Complications of pregnancy produce emergency situations. Be sure outcomes address both fetal and maternal welfare and often total family welfare. Treatment protocols should be regularly updated and maintained so they are current. Be certain they reflect a current nursing management level, so nurses can act swiftly and independently as needed with life-saving measures. Once a woman's condition stabilizes, outcome identification can then focus on long-term objectives.

Many women who develop a pregnancy complication may spend a few days in the hospital for therapy and monitoring followed by discharge to their homes. Waiting for a pregnancy that has been threatened this way to come to term can be difficult and fraught with anxiety. Readmission to the health care facility, especially when a new complication occurs, compounds these feelings. Be certain planning considers the many feelings this experience can cause. Offer referrals for counseling and/or community support groups for both the woman and her family as needed. Internet sites that discuss complications of pregnancy that can be helpful to women are the American Pregnancy Association (www.americanpregnancy.org) and the Centers for Disease Control and Prevention (www.cdc.gov).

Implementation

Interventions for a woman experiencing a complication of pregnancy require an interprofessional approach that speaks to several different areas:

- Continued both healthy maternal and fetal physical growth
- A woman's and family's psychological health
- Continuation of the pregnancy for as long as possible

Maintaining an optimistic attitude of fetal progress is important so a woman does not begin anticipatory grieving for her fetus, which could halt the growth of bonding. If the complication can be contained and the pregnancy continues uninterrupted, this can help protect the mental health of the whole family. If the pregnancy cannot be continued, be available to offer support as the family grieves for the loss of an unborn child and, in rare instances, the loss of future childbearing potential or the woman herself.

Outcome Evaluation

After a pregnancy with complications, a woman has reason to be especially worried about her infant's health at the time of birth. Even though the woman may still be ill herself, help her spend enough time with her child to see that, although perhaps born before term, her infant is well and healthy. Pointing out the infant's ability to follow a light and respond to a voice can help her begin to view the baby as the healthy one she anticipated having. And even though the success or failure of some nursing interventions cannot be fully evaluated until a child is born or into the postnatal period, outcomes should be evaluated throughout the pregnancy if possible. Be aware that after a complication of early pregnancy, a woman cannot help but worry for the remainder of the pregnancy the complication will recur or the original insult to the fetus was severe enough to cause long-term effects. Evaluate the woman and her family's attitude and the woman's physical status at each health care visit to be certain she and her family are coping with the situation and adjusting psychosocially.

Unfortunately, even with sustained care, not all fetal outcomes will be optimal. Evaluation will then include the ability of the family to care for an ill infant or grieve because a newborn dies. Examples of expected outcomes include:

- Client's blood pressure is maintained within acceptable parameters for remainder of pregnancy.
- Couple states they feel able to cope with anxiety associated with the pregnancy complication.
- Client's signs and symptoms of hypertension of pregnancy do not progress to eclampsia.
- Client accurately verbalizes crucial signs and symptoms she should immediately report to her primary health care provider.
- Couple expresses feelings of sadness over pregnancy loss.
- Client is able to adhere to the medical treatment regimen and experiences no adverse effects from the treatment.

BLEEDING DURING PREGNANCY

Vaginal bleeding during pregnancy is always a deviation from the normal, is always potentially serious, may occur at any point during pregnancy, and is always frightening. It must always be carefully investigated because it can impair both the outcome of the pregnancy and the woman's health or life. The primary causes of bleeding during pregnancy are summarized in Table 21.1.

Although vaginal bleeding may be innocent, any degree of this during pregnancy is a potential emergency because it may mean the placenta has loosened and cut off nourishment to the fetus. Also, the amount of blood visualized may be only a fraction of the blood actually being lost because an undilated cervix and intact membranes contain blood within the uterus. A woman with any degree of bleeding, therefore, needs to be evaluated for the possibility she is experiencing a significant blood loss or is developing hypovolemic shock.

The process of shock due to blood loss is shown in Figure 21.1. Because the uterus is a nonessential body organ, danger to the fetal blood supply occurs when a woman's body begins to decrease blood flow to peripheral organs (although the increased blood volume of pregnancy allows more than normal blood loss before hypovolemic shock processes begin). Signs of hypovolemic shock (Table 21.2) occur when 10% of blood volume, or approximately 2 units of blood, have been lost; fetal distress occurs when 25% of blood volume is lost (Box 21.2). Because "normal" blood pressure varies from woman to woman, it is important to know the baseline blood pressure for a pregnant woman when evaluating for hypovolemic shock.

Nursing Diagnoses and Related Interventions

Nursing Diagnosis: Risk for deficient fluid volume related to bleeding during pregnancy

Outcome Evaluation: Client's blood pressure is maintained at above 100/60 mmHg; pulse rate is below 100 beats/min; only minimal bleeding is apparent; fetal heart rate is maintained at 110 to 160 beats/min with adequate short-term and long-term variability; maternal urine output is greater than 30 ml/hr.

Therapy for hypovolemic shock is aimed at restoring blood volume and halting the source of hemorrhage as quickly as possible (Table 21.3). Monitoring urine output is a good gauge of blood loss because kidneys need sufficient arterial blood flow and pressure to function. If they are not producing urine, it suggests the kidneys are not obtaining adequate blood. If the blood deficit continues so blood cannot reach other major organs, multiorgan failure can result (Stalder, 2012). Obtaining hemoglobin and hematocrit levels and securing a blood sample for typing or cross-matching are essential not only to help predict the extent of blood loss but also to prepare for blood replacement. A woman suspected of having serious bleeding will need intravenous fluid replacement, such as Ringer's lactate, as an early intervention. Use a large-gauge angiocath (16 or 18) for rapid fluid expansion as this will also allow a blood transfusion to be administered through the same site as soon as blood is available. If respirations are rapid, administer oxygen by mask and monitor oxygen saturation levels by pulse oximetry. A woman needs frequent assessments of vital signs and continuous fetal monitoring; therefore, an external monitoring device should be started.

Urge the woman to rest in a side-lying position (left lateral is preferred) to help prevent vena cava compression. If this is not possible, position her on her back, with a wedge under one hip to minimize uterine pressure on the vena cava and prevent blood from being trapped in the lower extremities (supine hypotension syndrome). Continue to provide information about care and emotional support to her and her family members.

A woman may have a central venous pressure catheter (measures the right atrial pressure or the pressure of blood within the vena cava) or a pulmonary capillary wedge catheter (measures the pressure in the left atrium or the filling pressure in the

TABLE 21.1 Summary of Primary Causes of Bleeding During Pregnancy

Time	Type	Cause	Assessment	Cautions
First and second trimester	Threatened spontaneous miscarriage (early: under 16 weeks; late: 16 to 24 weeks)	Unknown; possibly chromosomal or uterine abnormalities	Vaginal spotting, perhaps slight cramping	Caution women not to use tampons to halt bleeding as this can lead to infection.
	Imminent (inevitable) miscarriage	Unknown reasons but possibly poor placental attachment	Vaginal spotting, cramping, cervical dilatation	
	Missed miscarriage	Unknown	Vaginal spotting, perhaps slight cramping; no apparent loss of pregnancy	Disseminated intravascular coagulation is associated with missed miscarriage.
	Incomplete spontaneous miscarriage	Unknown; possibly chromosomal or uterine abnormalities	Vaginal spotting, cramping, cervical dilatation, but incomplete expulsion of uterine contents	High risk for uterine infection
	Complete spontaneous miscarriage	Unknown but possibly chromosomal or uterine abnormalities	Vaginal spotting, cramping, cervical dilatation, and complete expulsion of uterine contents	
	Ectopic (tubal) pregnancy	Implantation of zygote at site other than in uterus associated with tubal constrictures	Sudden unilateral lower abdominal quadrant pain; minimal vaginal bleeding, possible signs of hypovolemic shock or hemorrhage	May have repeat ectopic pregnancy in future if tubal scarring is bilateral.
Second trimester	Gestational trophoblastic disease (hydatidiform mole)	Abnormal proliferation of trophoblast cells; fertilization or division defect	Overgrowth of uterus; highly positive human chorionic gonadotropin (hCG) test; no fetus present on ultrasound; bleeding from vagina of old or fresh blood accompanied by cyst formation	Retained trophoblast tissue may become malignant (choriocarcinoma); follow for 6 months to 1 year with hCG testing.
	Premature cervical dilatation	Cervix begins to dilate and pregnancy is lost at about 20 weeks; unknown cause, but cervical trauma from dilatation and curettage (D&C) may be associated	Painless bleeding leading to expulsion of fetus	Can have cervical sutures placed to ensure a second pregnancy.
Third trimester	Placenta previa	Low implantation of placenta possibly because of uterine abnormality	Painless bleeding at beginning of cervical dilatation	Don't allow a vaginal examination to minimize placental trauma.
	Premature separation of the placenta (abruptio placentae)	Unknown cause; associated with hypertension; placenta separates from uterus before birth of fetus	Sharp abdominal pain followed by uterine tenderness; vaginal bleeding; signs of maternal hypovolemic shock, fetal distress	Disseminated intravascular coagulation is associated with condition.
	Preterm labor	Many possible etiologic factors such as trauma, substance abuse, hypertension of pregnancy, or cervicitis; increased chance in multiple gestation, maternal illness	Show (pink-stained vaginal discharge) accompanied by uterine contractions becoming regular and effective	Preterm labor may be halted if the cervix is less than 4 cm dilated and the membranes are intact. Corticosteroids are administered to aid fetal lung maturity.

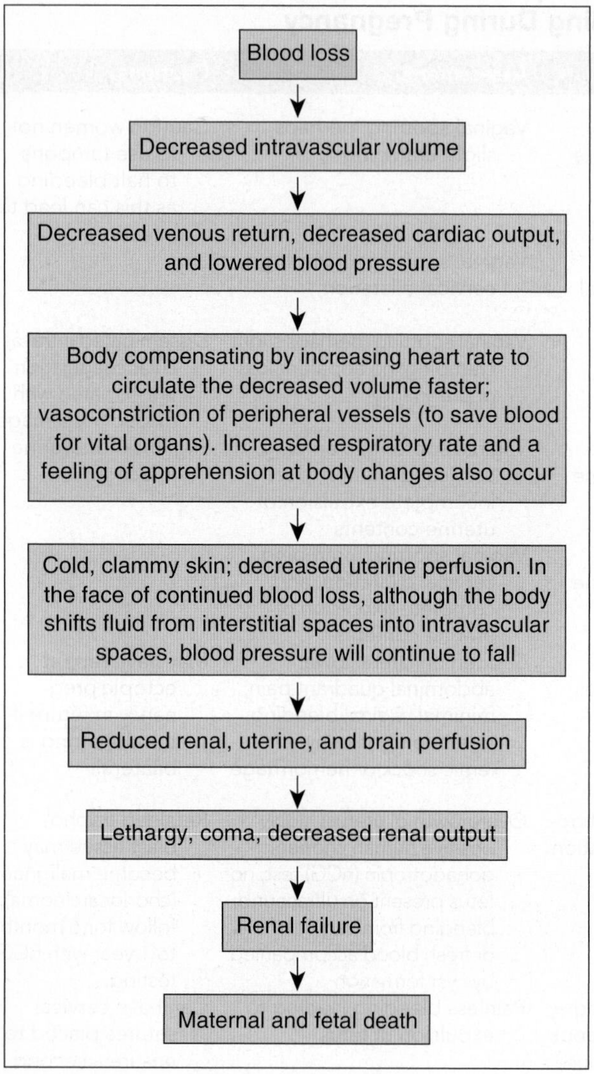

FIGURE 21.1 The process of shock because of blood loss (hypovolemia).

BOX 21.2 Nursing Care Planning Using Assessment

Assessing a Pregnant Woman With Hypovolemic Shock

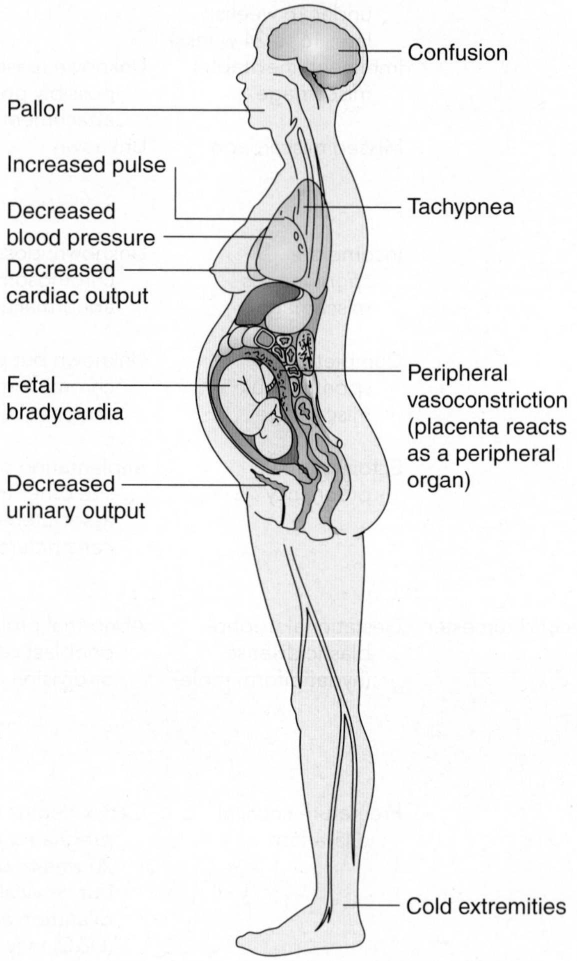

TABLE 21.2 Signs and Symptoms of Hypovolemic Shock

Assessment	Significance
Increased pulse rate	Heart attempts to circulate decreased blood volume.
Decreased blood pressure	Less peripheral resistance is present because of decreased blood volume.
Increased respiratory rate	Respiratory system attempts to increase gas exchange to better oxygenate decreased red blood cell volume.
Cold, clammy skin	Vasoconstriction occurs to maintain blood volume in central body core.
Decreased urine output	Inadequate blood is entering kidneys because of decreased blood volume.
Dizziness or decreased level of consciousness	Inadequate blood is reaching cerebrum because of decreased blood volume.
Decreased central venous pressure	Decreased blood is returning to heart because of reduced blood volume.

TABLE 21.3 Emergency Interventions for Bleeding in Pregnancy

Intervention	Rationale
Alert health care team of emergency situation.	Provides maximum coordination of care
Place woman flat in bed on her side.	Maintains optimal placental and renal function
Begin intravenous fluid such as Ringer's lactate with a 16- or 18-gauge angiocath.	Replaces intravascular fluid volume; intravenous line is established if blood replacement will be needed
Administer oxygen as necessary at 6–10 L/min by face mask.	Provides adequate fetal oxygenation despite lowered maternal circulating blood volume
Monitor uterine contractions and fetal heart rate by external monitor.	Assesses whether labor is present and fetal status; external system avoids cervical trauma
Omit vaginal examination.	Prevents tearing of placenta if placenta previa is cause of bleeding
Withhold oral fluid.	Anticipates need for emergency surgery
Order type and cross-match of 2 units of whole blood.	Allows for restoring circulating maternal blood volume if needed
Measure intake and output.	Enables assessment of renal function (will decrease to under 30 ml/hr with massive circulating volume loss)
Assess vital signs (pulse, respirations, and blood pressure every 15 min; apply pulse oximeter and automatic blood pressure cuff as necessary).	Provides baseline data on maternal response to blood loss
Assist with placement of central venous pressure or pulmonary artery catheter and blood determinations.	Provides more accurate data on maternal hemodynamic state
Measure maternal blood loss by weighing perineal pads; save any tissue passed.	Provides objective evidence of amount of bleeding; saturating a sanitary pad in less than 1 hr is heavy blood loss; tissue may be abnormal trophoblast tissue
Assist with ultrasound examination.	Supplies information on placental and fetal well-being
Maintain a positive attitude about fetal outcome.	Supports mother–child bonding
Support woman's self-esteem; provide emotional support to woman and her support person.	Assists problem solving, which is lessened by poor self-esteem.

left ventricle) inserted after bleeding is halted (see Chapter 41). During pregnancy, usual values of these measures differ from the average, so they need to be evaluated in light of the pregnancy. Central venous pressure during pregnancy is 1 to 6 mmHg and pulmonary capillary wedge pressure during pregnancy is 6 to 12 mmHg (Watson & Wilkinson, 2012).

Spontaneous Miscarriage

Abortion is a medical term for any interruption of a pregnancy before a fetus is viable (i.e., able to survive outside the uterus if born at that time), but it is better to speak of these early pregnancy losses as spontaneous miscarriages to avoid confusion with intentional terminations of pregnancies. A viable fetus is usually defined as a fetus of more than 20 to 24 weeks of gestation or one that weighs at least 500 g. A fetus born before this point is considered a **miscarriage** or is termed a premature or immature birth (Gilbert, 2011).

Spontaneous miscarriage occurs in 15% to 30% of all pregnancies and arises from natural causes (McNair & Altman, 2011). A miscarriage is an early miscarriage if it occurs before week 16 of pregnancy and a late miscarriage if it occurs between weeks 16 and 24. For the first 6 weeks of pregnancy, the developing placenta is tentatively attached to the decidua of the uterus; during weeks 6 to 12, it is moderately attached. After week 12, the attachment is penetrating and deep. Because of these degrees of attachment achieved at different weeks of pregnancy, it is important to attempt to establish the week of the pregnancy at which bleeding has become apparent. Bleeding before week 6 is rarely severe; bleeding after week 12 can be profuse because the placenta is implanted so deeply. Fortunately, at this time, with such deep placental implantation, the fetus tends to be expelled as in natural childbirth before the placenta separates. Uterine contractions, however, then help to control placental bleeding as they do postpartally. For some women, then, the stage of attachment between weeks 6 and 12 can lead to the most severe, even life-threatening bleeding.

BOX 21.3 Nursing Care Planning to Empower a Family

COPING WITH A SPONTANEOUS MISCARRIAGE

Q. Beverly Muzuki had a spontaneous miscarriage when she was younger. She asks you, "What did I do wrong that time?"

A. Early miscarriage is largely not preventable, because it is caused by such things as abnormal chromosome formation or poor uterine implantation—things over which you have no control. Eating a nutritious diet, so you enter a pregnancy in good health and avoiding cigarette smoking or drinking alcohol are sensible recommendations to reduce your risk of miscarriage. If you had extensive blood loss with your miscarriage, be certain to eat iron-rich foods (such as meat and green vegetables) to help restore red blood cells for a second pregnancy.

Causes of Spontaneous Miscarriage

The most frequent cause of miscarriage in the first trimester of pregnancy is abnormal fetal development, due either to a teratogenic factor or to a chromosomal aberration. In other miscarriages, immunologic factors may be present or rejection of the embryo through an immune response may occur (Surette & Dunham, 2013). Another common cause of early miscarriage involves implantation abnormalities, as up to 50% of zygotes probably never implant securely because of inadequate endometrial formation or from an inappropriate site of implantation. With inadequate implantation, the placental circulation does not develop adequately enough to support the pregnancy. Miscarriage may also occur if the corpus luteum on the ovary fails to produce enough progesterone to maintain the decidua basalis. Progesterone therapy may be attempted to prevent this if this cause is documented (Hızlı, Köşüş, Köşüş, et al., 2012).

Ingestion of alcohol at the time of conception or during early pregnancy can contribute to pregnancy loss because of abnormal fetal growth (Andersen, Andersen, Olsen, et al., 2012). Urinary tract infections may be a cause but are more strongly associated with preterm birth. Systemic infections such as rubella, syphilis, poliomyelitis, cytomegalovirus, and toxoplasmosis readily cross the placenta and so may also be responsible. With an infection, if the fetus fails to grow, estrogen and progesterone production by the placenta falls and leads to endometrial sloughing. With the sloughing, prostaglandins are released; uterine contractions and cervical dilatation along with expulsion of the products of the pregnancy begin.

Because miscarriage can occur from so many causes and, because the cause is often difficult to determine, couples may have difficulty understanding why it happened to them (Box 21.3).

Assessment

The presenting symptom of spontaneous miscarriage is almost always vaginal spotting. At the first indication of this, a woman should telephone her health care provider and describe how much spotting she is having and its appearance (e.g., dark or fresh blood). Because a nurse often takes this initial call, guidelines to help assess vaginal bleeding quickly are shown in Table 21.4.

TABLE 21.4 Immediate Assessment of Vaginal Bleeding During Pregnancy

Assessment Factor	Specific Questions to Ask
Confirmation of pregnancy	Does the woman know for certain she is pregnant (positive pregnancy test or health care provider confirmation)? A woman who has been pregnant before and states she is certain she is pregnant is probably right, even if she has not yet had her pregnancy confirmed.
Pregnancy length	What is the length of the pregnancy in weeks?
Duration	How long did the bleeding episode last? Is it continuing?
Intensity	How much bleeding occurred? (Ask the woman to compare it to a common measure such as a tablespoon or a cup.)
Description	Was blood mixed with amniotic fluid or mucus? Was it bright red (fresh blood) or dark (old blood)? Was it accompanied by tissue fragments? Was it odorous?
Frequency	Steady spotting? A single episode?
Associated symptoms	Cramping? Sharp pain? Dull pain? Has she ever had cervical surgery (to alert health care providers the woman may have cervical sutures in place?)
Action	What was happening at the time the bleeding started? What has she done (if anything) to control bleeding? (Caution her not to insert a tampon so the true extent of the bleeding shows.)
Blood type	Does she know this? (Rh-negative women will need Rh immune globulin to prevent Rh isoimmunization.)

The history of the episode is important to help diagnose the cause. Knowledge of a woman's actions is important to ensure she did not attempt to self-abort. Asking what she has done, if anything, to halt the bleeding may reveal she inserted a tampon, for example. If she did, although reporting only slight spotting, she actually has an unknown amount of blood loss and might be bleeding much more heavily than she first reported.

Therapeutic Management

Depending on the symptoms and the description of the bleeding, a woman's primary health care provider will decide whether she needs to be seen, and, if so, whether she should be seen in an ambulatory setting or the hospital.

Threatened Miscarriage

Symptoms of a threatened miscarriage begin as vaginal bleeding, initially only scant and usually bright red. A woman may notice slight cramping, but no cervical dilatation is present on vaginal examination. A woman with an apparent threatened miscarriage may be asked to come to the clinic or office to have fetal heart sounds assessed or an ultrasound performed to evaluate the viability of the fetus. Blood may be drawn to test for human chorionic gonadotropin (hCG) hormone at the start of bleeding and again in 48 hours (if the placenta is still intact, the level in the bloodstream should double in this time). If it does not double, poor placental function is suspected and the pregnancy probably will be lost. Avoidance of strenuous activity for 24 to 48 hours is the key intervention, assuming the threatened miscarriage involves a live fetus and presumed placental bleeding. Complete bed rest is usually not necessary as this may appear to stop the vaginal bleeding but only because blood pools vaginally. When a woman does ambulate again, the vaginal blood collection will drain and bleeding will reappear.

Women are apt to be extremely worried at the sight of bleeding. They need to talk with a sympathetic, supportive person about how distressed they are feeling. Women with threatened miscarriages often look for reasons why this could have happened, such as running up a flight of stairs, forgetting to take an iron pill, or getting angry with an older child. Being assured that none of these events causes miscarriage can help to minimize the guilt a woman may feel.

If the spotting with a threatened miscarriage is going to stop, it usually does so within 24 to 48 hours after a woman reduces her activity. Once bleeding stops, she can gradually resume normal activities. Coitus may be restricted for 2 weeks, however, to prevent infection and to avoid inducing further bleeding. As many as 50% of women with a threatened miscarriage continue the pregnancy; for the other 50%, unfortunately, the threatened miscarriage changes to imminent, or inevitable, miscarriage and the pregnancy ends (Huancahuari, 2012).

Imminent (Inevitable) Miscarriage

A threatened miscarriage becomes an imminent (i.e., inevitable) miscarriage if uterine contractions and cervical dilation occur as, with cervical dilation, the loss of the products of conception cannot be halted. A woman who reports cramping or uterine contractions is usually asked to come to the hospital or office, where she is examined. She should save any tissue fragments she has passed and bring them with her so they can be analyzed for an abnormality such as gestational trophoblastic disease (hydatidiform mole; see later). If no fetal heart sounds are detected and an ultrasound reveals an empty uterus or nonviable fetus, her primary health care provider may perform a dilatation and curettage (D&C) or a dilation and evacuation (D&E) to ensure all the products of conception are removed (Gilbert, 2011). Be certain the woman has been told the pregnancy was already lost and that all procedures, such as suction curettage, are to clean the uterus and prevent further complications such as infection and not to end the pregnancy. Save any tissue fragments passed in the labor room, along with any brought from home, so it can be established that all the products of conception have been removed from the uterus. After a woman is discharged, the woman should assess the amount of vaginal bleeding she is having by recording the number of pads she uses; saturating more than one pad per hour is abnormally heavy bleeding.

Complete Miscarriage

In a complete miscarriage, the entire products of conception (fetus, membranes, and placenta) are expelled spontaneously without any assistance. The bleeding usually slows within 2 hours and then ceases within a few days after passage of the products of conception. Because the process is complete, no therapy other than advising the woman to report heavy bleeding is needed.

Incomplete Miscarriage

In an incomplete miscarriage, part of the conceptus (usually the fetus) is expelled, but the membranes or placenta are retained in the uterus. The term "incomplete" can be confusing for women as they may interpret it to mean that, because the miscarriage was incomplete, it means the pregnancy will continue. With an incomplete miscarriage, there is a danger of maternal hemorrhage as long as part of the conceptus is retained in the uterus because the uterus cannot contract effectively under this condition. The woman will usually have a D&C or suction curettage to evacuate the remainder of the pregnancy. Again, be certain the woman knows the pregnancy is already lost and that these procedures are being done to protect her from hemorrhage and infection, not to end the pregnancy.

Missed Miscarriage

In a missed miscarriage, also commonly referred to as **early pregnancy failure**, the fetus dies in utero but is not expelled. Women can also find this term misleading because it suggests that if a miscarriage was "missed," then the pregnancy can continue. A missed miscarriage is usually discovered at a prenatal examination when the fundal height is measured and no increase in size can be demonstrated or when previously heard fetal heart sounds can no longer be heard. A woman may have had symptoms of a threatened miscarriage (e.g., painless vaginal bleeding), or she may have had no prior clinical symptoms.

After an ultrasound establishes the fetus has died, a D&C or D&E may be done to evacuate the pregnancy. If the pregnancy is over 14 weeks in length and therefore these procedures are no longer possible, labor can be induced by a prostaglandin suppository or misoprostol (Cytotec) introduced into the cervix to cause dilatation, followed by oxytocin stimulation

BOX 21.4 Nursing Care Planning Based on Effective Communication

Beverly's neighbor noticed some vaginal spotting at 10 weeks into her pregnancy. The bleeding stopped spontaneously but her health care provider was unable to hear fetal heart tones. An ultrasound revealed a missed miscarriage. You talk to her neighbor after she has received this news.

Less Effective Communication

Nurse: Hello, Vivian. How are you feeling?
Vivian: Fine. I guess this was a small thing.
Nurse: I'm sorry it happened. It must be upsetting.
Vivian: The bleeding was scary. Made me really nervous something was going wrong with the baby.
Nurse: Bleeding is always scary. I hate to see it, too.
Vivian: As long as the baby is fine, that's all that counts.
Nurse: That's the advantage of being young. There's lots of time for babies.

More Effective Communication

Nurse: Hello, Vivian. How are you feeling?
Vivian: Fine. I guess this was a small thing.
Nurse: I'm sorry it happened. It must be upsetting.
Vivian: The bleeding was scary. Made me really nervous something was going wrong with the baby.
Nurse: With the baby?
Vivian: Yes. I'm really lucky I missed having a miscarriage.
Nurse: Let me ask your doctor to re-explain what she meant by a missed miscarriage. That's a term that can be confusing.

Because many women want so badly to be pregnant, it can be easy for them to "miss" bad news about a pregnancy. In the previous scenario, the nurse was so intent on chatting she failed to realize her client was misinformed. Better listening skills in the second example revealed a serious misunderstanding of what "missed miscarriage" means.

or administration of mifepristone techniques used for elective termination of pregnancy, which cause contractions and birth (Hanson & Burke, 2011). If the pregnancy is not actively terminated this way, miscarriage usually occurs spontaneously within 2 weeks. There is a danger of allowing this normal course to happen, however, because disseminated intravascular coagulation (DIC), a coagulation defect, may develop if the dead (and possibly toxic) fetus remains too long in utero (Zheng, 2012b).

Most women hope, until the moment the ultrasound shows their fetus is dead, that their baby is alive. They may need support in accepting the reality of the situation (Box 21.4) and need counseling to begin a future pregnancy because of fears they may never be able to carry a baby to full term.

Recurrent Pregnancy Loss

In the past, women who had three spontaneous miscarriages that occurred at the same gestational age were called "habitual aborters." They were advised they were apparently too "nervous" or that something was so wrong with their hormones that childbearing was not for them. Today, the term **recurrent pregnancy loss** is used to describe this miscarriage pattern, and a thorough investigation is done to discover the cause of the loss and to help ensure the outcome of a future pregnancy. Recurrent pregnancy loss occurs in about 1% of women who want to be pregnant. Although many of these losses occur for unknown reasons, possible causes include:

- Defective spermatozoa or ova
- Endocrine factors such as lowered levels of protein-bound iodine (PBI), butanol-extractable iodine (BEI), and globulin-bound iodine (GBI); poor thyroid function; or a luteal phase defect
- Deviations of the uterus, such as septate or bicornuate uterus
- Resistance to uterine artery blood flow
- **Chorioamnionitis** or uterine infection
- Autoimmune disorders such as those involving lupus anticoagulant and **antiphospholipid antibodies** (Tsokos, 2011)

Antiphospholipid Antibody Syndrome

Antiphospholipid antibody syndrome (APS) is an autoimmune disease that occurs more frequently in women than in men. Abnormal proteins (antiphospholipid autoantibodies) initiate coagulation and so lead to clotting in arteries and veins. If this occurs in placental vessels, it can block placenta growth, and thrombi that form can loosen the placenta and interfere with oxygen and nutrient exchange. The result of this is recurrent miscarriages and hypertension of pregnancy; postpartally, it can lead to deep vein thrombosis. Clotting episodes increase with reduced activity such as would occur with bed rest, smoking, obesity, and use of estrogen-based birth control pills (Mehta & Sokol, 2013).

Prophylaxis therapy to prevent miscarriages is oral low-dose aspirin and subcutaneous injections of heparin started at the beginning of pregnancy and continued for several weeks after birth. Alternative therapies, such as intravenous immunoglobulin infusions or administration of a corticosteroid such as prednisone, can be added if heparin and aspirin alone are not adequate to prevent hypertension or pregnancy loss.

Women can be taught to administer their own heparin injections; caution them that, although low-dose aspirin may not seem important to most people, it is important for them.

Observe the woman closely postpartum for deep vein thrombosis in her legs. At the end of the postpartal period, the woman needs to be reevaluated to see if she will need continued therapy to help prevent pulmonary emboli or other thrombi consequences.

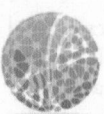

Complications of Miscarriage

As with full-term childbirth, hemorrhage and infection are two of the most likely complications after miscarriage. The risk for Rh isoimmunization and a woman's psychological state also need to be considered.

Hemorrhage. With a complete spontaneous miscarriage, serious or fatal hemorrhage is rare. With an incomplete miscarriage or in a woman who develops an accompanying coagulation defect (usually DIC), major hemorrhage becomes a possibility. Monitor vital signs for any changes to detect possible hypovolemic shock. If excessive vaginal bleeding occurs, immediately position a woman flat and massage the uterine fundus to try to aid contraction, although this may be impossible with an early pregnancy because the small uterus is not palpable above the symphysis pubis (see Chapter 17). Applying pneumatic antishock garments can help maintain blood pressure (Kausar, Morris, Fathalla, et al., 2012).

If bleeding doesn't halt, a woman may need a D&C or suction curettage to empty the uterus of the material that is preventing it from contracting and achieving hemostasis. A transfusion may be necessary to replace blood loss. Direct replacement of fibrinogen or another clotting factor may be used to increase coagulation ability.

After a self-limiting complete miscarriage, a woman needs clear instructions on how much bleeding is abnormal (more than one sanitary pad per hour is excessive) and what color changes she should expect in bleeding (gradually changing to a dark color and then to the color of serous fluid as it does with the postpartum woman). Be certain she is aware any unusual odor or passing of large clots is also abnormal. If her primary health care provider has prescribed an oral medication such as methylergonovine maleate (Methergine) to aid uterine contraction, review with her why it is being prescribed and the importance of taking it. Some women repress their feelings following a miscarriage, anxious to forget the experience as quickly as possible. Short-term repression this way can be helpful if it helps them with their anger or grief at the loss of the pregnancy. Be careful, however, in repressing the experience a woman does not also repress the memory of her medication and leave herself open to hemorrhage.

QSEN Checkpoint Question 21.1

Patient-Centered Care

Beverly Muzuki, whom you met at the beginning of the chapter, had a miscarriage when she was younger. After addressing her immediate psychosocial needs, what would be the best advice to give a woman who tells you she is miscarrying?

a. Lie down and remain on bed rest for 24 hours to stop the bleeding.
b. Continue light activity as usual because most spotting during pregnancy is harmless.
c. Save any clots or material passed for your health care provider to examine.
d. Use a tampon to put pressure on your cervix and stop the bleeding.

Look in Appendix A for the best answer and rationale.

Infection. The possibility of infection is minimal when pregnancy loss occurs over a short time, bleeding is self-limiting, and instrumentation is limited. However, there is always a possibility it may occur. It tends to develop most often in women who have lost an appreciable amount of blood. Observe such women closely to rule out this second and possibly fatal complication. Be certain the woman is familiar with common danger signs of infection, such as fever higher than 100.4°F (38.0°C), abdominal pain or tenderness, and a foul-smelling vaginal discharge. Usually, fever is the most important sign of infection, but it can also be a transient reaction to the period of decreased fluid intake that preceded or shortly followed the miscarriage. Don't dismiss any degree of elevated temperature, however, to avoid overlooking the possibility infection is developing.

The organisms responsible for infection after miscarriage are usually *Escherichia coli* (spread from the rectum forward into the vagina) or group A streptococcus (Rimawi, Soper, & Eschenbach, 2012). Caution women to always wipe their perineal area from front to back after voiding and particularly after defecation to prevent the spread of bacteria from the rectal area and to decrease the possibility of this source of infection. Be certain to advise the woman not to use tampons (stasis of any body fluid increases the risk of infection).

Infection usually involves the inner lining of the uterus (endometritis), but it may be more extensive and lead to parametritis, peritonitis, thrombophlebitis, or septicemia. The management of these infections is the same as if they were occurring after the safe birth of a child, and so are discussed in Chapter 25.

Septic Abortion. A septic abortion is an abortion complicated by infection (Barton & Sibai, 2012). Infection can occur after a spontaneous miscarriage, but more frequently it occurs in women who have tried to self-abort or whose pregnancy was aborted illegally using a nonsterile instrument such as a knitting needle. Because the uterus is a warm, moist, dark cavity, once infectious organisms are introduced, they grow rapidly in this environment, particularly if products of conception such as necrotic membranes are still present.

The woman will have symptoms of fever and crampy abdominal pain; her uterus will feel tender to palpation. Left untreated, such an infection can lead to toxic shock syndrome, septicemia, kidney failure, and death (Cappiello, Beal, & Simmonds, 2011).

Women with a septic abortion need immediate, intensive assessment and therapy. Typically, complete blood count; serum electrolytes; serum creatinine; blood type and cross-match; and cervical, vaginal, and urine cultures are obtained. An indwelling urinary (Foley) catheter may be inserted to monitor urine output hourly to assess kidney function. Intravenous fluid to restore fluid volume and to provide a route for high-dose, broad-spectrum antibiotic therapy is begun. A combination of penicillin (gram-positive coverage), gentamicin (gram-negative aerobic coverage), and clindamycin (gram-negative anaerobic coverage) is commonly prescribed to combat the infection.

A central venous pressure or pulmonary artery catheter may be inserted to monitor left atrial filling pressure and hemodynamic status. The removal of all infected or necrotic tissue from the uterus is important, so a D&C or D&E will be performed. A tetanus toxoid given subcutaneously or a tetanus immune globulin given intramuscularly will be prescribed for prophylaxis against tetanus.

Infection following a septic abortion can be so severe that a woman needs to be admitted to an intensive care setting for continuing care. Dopamine and digitalis may be necessary to maintain sufficient cardiac output. Oxygen and perhaps ventilatory support may be necessary to maintain respiratory function.

Assuming a woman recovers from such an intense episode, a final result may be infertility because of uterine scarring or fibrotic scarring of the fallopian tubes. If a woman caused the infection by trying to self-abort, she needs follow-up counseling to assist her to learn better problem-solving methods for the future.

Isoimmunization. Whenever a placenta is dislodged at any point in pregnancy, either by spontaneous birth or by a D&C/D&E, some blood from the placental villi (the fetal blood) is apt to enter the maternal circulation. If the fetus was Rh positive and the woman is Rh negative, enough Rh-positive fetal blood may enter the maternal circulation to cause **isoimmunization**, or the production of antibodies against Rh-positive blood. If the woman's next child should have Rh-positive blood, these antibodies would attempt to destroy the red blood cells of this infant during the months that infant is in utero (Kaplan, Bromiker, & Hammerman, 2011). Therefore, after a miscarriage, because the blood type of the conceptus is unknown, all women with Rh-negative blood should receive Rh (D antigen) immune globulin (RhIG) to prevent the buildup of antibodies in the event the conceptus was Rh positive.

Powerlessness or Anxiety. As with pregnancy loss for any reason, assess a woman's adjustment to a spontaneous miscarriage. Sadness and grief over the loss or the feeling that a woman has lost control of her life is to be expected. Do not forget to assess a partner's or the extended family's feelings as well, or the potential impact of their grief and possible lack of support for the woman over the pregnancy loss can be missed. Spontaneous miscarriage can be particularly heartbreaking for an older woman, because she realizes her window of childbearing is limited.

✔ QSEN Checkpoint Question 21.2

Quality Improvement

Beverly Muzuki has an Rh-negative blood type. Her electronic record shows she had a previous miscarriage at 16 weeks into her last pregnancy. What medication should the care team want to see if she received following the miscarriage to minimize isoimmunization?

a. Misoprostol (Cytotec)
b. RhIG (RhoGAM)
c. Ferrous sulfate
d. Packed red blood cell transfusion

Look in Appendix A for the best answer and rationale.

Ectopic Pregnancy

An **ectopic pregnancy** is one in which implantation occurred outside the uterine cavity. The most common site (in approximately 95% of such pregnancies) is in the fallopian tube (Fig. 21.2). Of these fallopian tube sites, approximately 80% occur in the ampullar portion, 12% occur in the isthmus, and 8% are interstitial or fimbrial (Jurkovic, 2012).

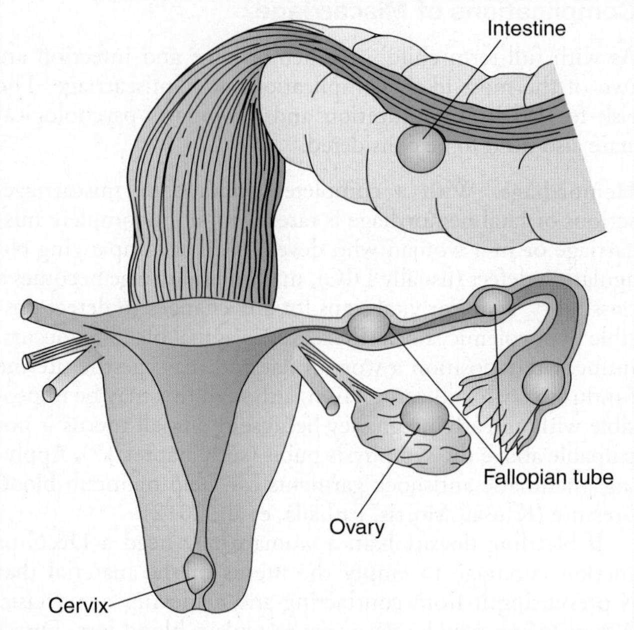

FIGURE 21.2 The sites at which an ectopic pregnancy may occur.

With ectopic pregnancy, fertilization occurs as usual in the distal third of the fallopian tube. Unfortunately, because an obstruction is present, such as an adhesion of the fallopian tube from a previous infection (chronic salpingitis or pelvic inflammatory disease), congenital malformations, scars from tubal surgery, or a uterine tumor pressing on the proximal end of the tube, the zygote cannot travel the length of the tube. It lodges at a strictured site along the tube and implants there instead of in the uterus.

Approximately 2% of pregnancies are ectopic, and because at least minimal bleeding occurs, it is the second most frequent cause of bleeding early in pregnancy. The incidence of ectopic pregnancy appears to be increasing, possibly because of the increasing rate of pelvic inflammatory disease, which can lead to tubal scarring. The incidence is also increased following in vitro fertilization (a woman might be having the in vitro fertilization because she has tubal scarring) and also in women who smoke.

Women who have one ectopic pregnancy have a higher chance of having a subsequent ectopic pregnancy. This is because salpingitis generally leaves scarring, which is bilateral. Congenital anomalies such as webbing (fibrous bands) that block a fallopian tube may also occur in both tubes. For unknown reasons, oral contraceptives used before pregnancy reduce the incidence of ectopic pregnancy (Abatangelo, Okereke, Parham-Foster, et al., 2010).

Assessment

With an ectopic pregnancy, there are no unusual symptoms at the time of implantation. The corpus luteum of the ovary continues to function as if the implantation were in the uterus so no menstrual flow occurs. A woman begins to experience the usual nausea and vomiting of early pregnancy and a pregnancy test for hCG will be positive. Many ectopic pregnancies are diagnosed because a woman has an early pregnancy ultrasound to date the pregnancy. Magnetic resonance imaging (MRI) is also effective to use for this. If not revealed by an ultrasound, at weeks 6 to 12 of pregnancy (2 to 8 weeks after a missed menstrual period), the zygote grows large enough that it ruptures the slender fallopian tube. Tearing and destruction of blood vessels and bleeding result. If implantation was in the interstitial portion of the tube (where the tube joins the uterus), rupture can cause severe intraperitoneal bleeding because of the large blood vessels in that part of the tube. Fortunately, the incidence of tubal pregnancies is highest in the ampullar area (the distal third), where the blood vessels are smaller and profuse hemorrhage is less likely. Constant, continued bleeding from this area, however, may result in a large amount of blood loss over time. Therefore, a ruptured ectopic pregnancy is serious regardless of the site of implantation.

A woman usually experiences a sharp, stabbing pain in one of her lower abdominal quadrants at the time of rupture, followed by scant vaginal spotting. The amount of bleeding evident with a ruptured ectopic pregnancy usually does not reveal the actual amount present, however, because the products of conception from the ruptured tube and the accompanying blood may be expelled into the pelvic cavity rather than into the uterus. Blood does not reach the vagina to become evident. At the point the placenta dislodges, progesterone secretion will stop and the uterine decidua will begin to slough, causing additional vaginal bleeding. As soon as the woman becomes hypotensive from blood loss, she will experience light-headedness and a rapid pulse, signs of hypovolemic shock.

Because of these symptoms, any woman with sharp abdominal pain and vaginal spotting needs to be evaluated by her health care provider to rule out the possibility of ectopic pregnancy. When helping determine whether an ectopic pregnancy is present, ask a woman what she was doing when she felt the pain, if she had pain but no vaginal bleeding. Occasionally, a woman will move suddenly and pull one of her round ligaments, the anterior uterine supports, which causes a sharp but momentary lower quadrant pain, so this must be ruled out. Vaginal spotting or bleeding does rule out ectopic pregnancy as it would be rare for this phenomenon to be reported in connection with vaginal spotting.

By the time a woman arrives at the hospital or primary health care provider's office, she may already be in severe shock, as evidenced by a rapid, thready pulse; rapid respirations; and falling blood pressure. Leukocytosis may be present, not from infection but from the trauma. Temperature is usually normal. A transvaginal ultrasound will demonstrate the ruptured tube and blood collecting in the peritoneum. Either a falling hCG or serum progesterone level suggests the pregnancy has ended. If the diagnosis of ectopic pregnancy is in doubt, a primary health care provider may insert a needle through the posterior vaginal fornix into the cul-de-sac under sterile conditions to see whether blood can be aspirated. A laparoscopy or culdoscopy can also be used to visualize the fallopian tube if the symptoms alone do not reveal a clear picture of what has happened. However, ultrasonography alone usually reveals a clear-cut diagnostic picture (Hsu & Euerle, 2012).

If a woman waits for a time before seeking help, her abdomen gradually becomes rigid from peritoneal irritation. Her umbilicus may develop a bluish-tinged hue (Cullen sign). She may have continuing extensive or dull vaginal and abdominal pain; movement of the cervix on pelvic examination can cause excruciating pain. She may feel pain in her shoulders as well from blood in the peritoneal cavity causing irritation to the phrenic nerve. A tender mass is usually palpable in Douglas cul-de-sac on vaginal examination.

Therapeutic Management

Some ectopic pregnancies spontaneously end before they rupture and are reabsorbed over the next few days, requiring no treatment. It is difficult to predict when or if this will happen, however, so when an ectopic pregnancy is revealed by an early ultrasound, the woman is shown the sonogram, and after her agreement that therapy could be lifesaving, she is usually medically treated by the oral administration of methotrexate (Beall & Decherney, 2012) (see Chapter 53 for a general discussion of chemotherapy agents of this type). The advantage of this therapy is that the tube is left intact, with no surgical scarring that could cause a second ectopic implantation. Women are treated until a negative hCG titer is achieved. A hysterosalpingogram or ultrasound is usually performed after this to assess that the pregnancy is no longer present and also whether the tube appears fully patent. If an ectopic pregnancy is not discovered early, but rather, only when it ruptures, it creates an emergency situation (Marion & Meeks, 2012).

Keep in mind the amount of blood evident with a ruptured ectopic pregnancy is a poor estimate of the actual blood loss. A blood sample needs to be drawn immediately for hemoglobin level, typing and cross-matching, and possibly the hCG level for immediate pregnancy testing, if pregnancy has not yet been confirmed. Intravenous fluid using a large-gauge catheter to restore intravascular volume will be prescribed. Blood then can be administered through this same line as soon as it is matched.

The therapy for ruptured ectopic pregnancy is laparoscopy to ligate the bleeding vessels and to remove or repair the damaged fallopian tube. A rough suture line on a fallopian tube may lead to another tubal pregnancy, so either the tube will be removed or suturing on the tube will be done with microsurgical technique. If a tube is removed, a woman is theoretically only 50% fertile, because every other month, when she ovulates from the ovary next to the removed tube, sperm should not be able to reach the ovum on that side. This cannot be used as a reliable contraceptive measure, however, as translocation of ova can occur—that is, an ovum released from the right ovary can pass through the pelvic cavity to the opposite (left) fallopian tube and become fertilized, and vice versa. As with miscarriage, women with Rh-negative blood should receive Rh (D) immune globulin (RhIG)/RoGAM after an ectopic pregnancy for isoimmunization protection in future childbearing.

Nursing Diagnoses and Related Interventions

Nursing Diagnosis: Powerlessness related to early loss of pregnancy secondary to ectopic pregnancy

Outcome Evaluation: Client states she feels sad at pregnancy loss but is able to deal with situation; has returned to previous level of activities and has forward-thinking plans.

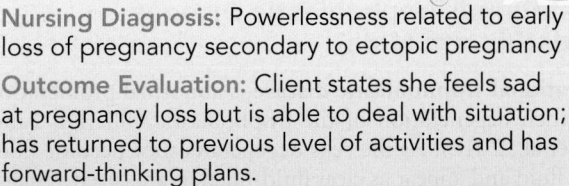

A woman who has had an ectopic pregnancy not only has grief stages to work through (she has lost a child) but also may have problems of diminished self-image and a sense of powerlessness if surgery included removal of a

fallopian tube. Encourage her to verbalize her concerns about this and her possibly reduced potential for future childbearing. This process of working through grief and role image may take weeks to months, but should begin in the hospital, where a woman has professional people to help her through the first days and to determine whether she will need further counseling.

Abdominal Pregnancy

Very rarely after an ectopic pregnancy ruptures—so rarely the instances are difficult to document—the products of conception are expelled into the pelvic cavity with a minimum of bleeding. The placenta continues to grow in the fallopian tube, spreading perhaps into the uterus for a better blood supply; or it may escape into the pelvic cavity and implant on an organ such as an intestine. The fetus will grow in the pelvic cavity (an abdominal pregnancy). This can also occur if a uterus ruptures because an old uterine scar ruptures during pregnancy (Kim, Bae, Seong, et al., 2012).

In an abdominal pregnancy, the fetal outline is usually easily palpable through the abdomen because it is directly below the abdominal wall, not inside the uterus. A woman may either not be as aware of movements as she would be normally or she may experience painful fetal movements and abdominal cramping with fetal movements. She may report she noticed sudden lower quadrant pain earlier in the pregnancy, but because there was no external bleeding, didn't report it. An ultrasound or MRI will reveal the fetus outside the uterus.

The danger of abdominal pregnancy is that the placenta could infiltrate and erode a major blood vessel in the abdomen, leading to hemorrhage. If implanted on the intestine, it may erode so deeply it causes bowel perforation, leaking of intestinal contents, and peritonitis. The fetus is also at high risk (only about 60% come to term) because without a good uterine blood supply, nutrients may not reach the fetus in adequate amounts leading to the threat of fetal deformity or growth restriction.

At term, the infant must be born through laparotomy. The placenta is often difficult to remove after birth if it has implanted onto an abdominal organ such as the intestine. It may, therefore, be left in place and allowed to absorb spontaneously in 2 or 3 months. A follow-up ultrasound can be used to detect whether this has occurred. If not, a woman can be treated with methotrexate to help the placenta absorb, although this therapy may not be effective because the remaining trophoblasts are no longer fast growing (Demendi, Langmár, Bánhidy, et al., 2011).

Gestational Trophoblastic Disease (Hydatidiform Mole)

Gestational trophoblastic disease is abnormal proliferation and then degeneration of the trophoblastic villi (Fu, Fang, Xie, et al., 2012). As the cells degenerate, they become filled with fluid and appear as clear fluid-filled, grape-sized vesicles. The embryo fails to develop beyond a primitive start. Abnormal trophoblast cells must be identified because they are associated with choriocarcinoma, a rapidly metastasizing malignancy (Fig. 21.3).

The incidence of gestational trophoblastic disease is approximately 1 in every 1,500 pregnancies. The condition tends to occur most often in women who have a low protein intake, in women older than 35 years of age, in women of Asian heritage, and in blood group A women who marry blood group O men (Lurain, 2010).

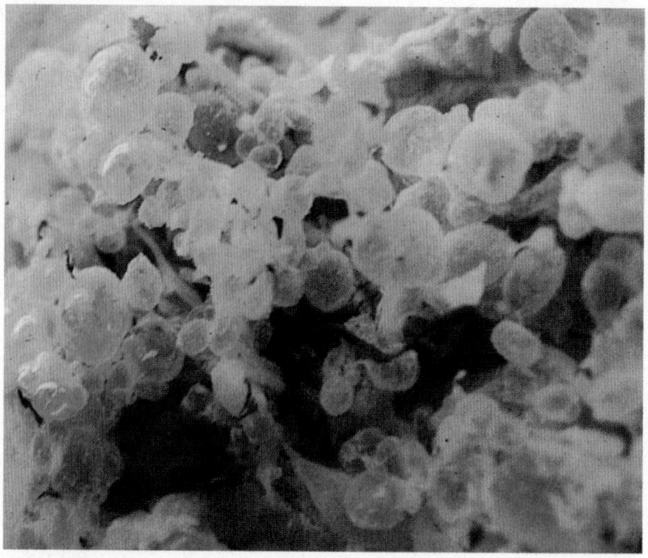

FIGURE 21.3 Gestational trophoblastic disease (hydatidiform mole). (From Rubin, E., & Farber, J. L. [1994]. *Pathology* [2nd ed.]. Philadelphia, PA: JB Lippincott.)

Two types of molar growth can be identified by chromosome analysis. With a complete mole, all trophoblastic villi swell and become cystic. If an embryo forms, it dies early at only 1 to 2 mm in size, with no fetal blood present in the villi. On chromosomal analysis, although the karyotype is a normal 46XX or 46XY, this chromosome component was contributed only by the father, or an "empty ovum" was fertilized and the chromosome material was duplicated (Fig. 21.4A).

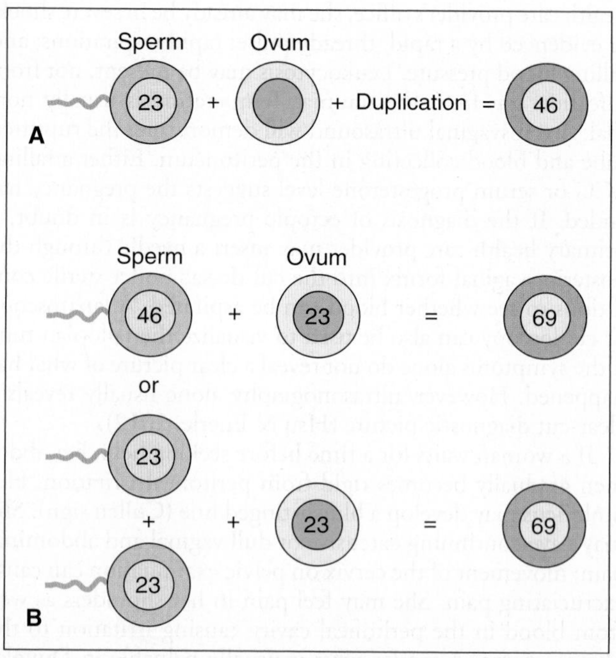

FIGURE 21.4 Formation of gestational trophoblastic disease (hydatidiform mole). **(A)** A complete mole. **(B)** A partial mole.

With a partial mole, some of the villi form normally. The syncytiotrophoblastic layer of villi, however, appears swollen and misshapen. The embryo may grow for about 9 weeks but then macerates; some fetal blood may be present in the villi. A partial mole has 69 chromosomes (69XX or 69XY) (a triploid formation in which there are three chromosomes instead of two for every pair: one set supplied by an ovum that apparently was fertilized by two sperm or an ovum fertilized by one sperm in which meiosis or reduction division did not occur). This could also occur if one set of 23 chromosomes was supplied by one sperm and an ovum that did not undergo reduction division supplied 46 (see Fig. 21.4B).

In contrast to complete moles, partial moles rarely lead to choriocarcinoma. Although still above average, hCG titers are lower in partial than in complete moles; titers also return to normal faster after gestational trophoblast evacuation (Savage & Seckl, 2012).

Assessment

Because proliferation of the abnormal trophoblast cells grow so rapidly, the uterus tends to expand faster than usual or the uterus reaches its landmarks (just over the symphysis brim at 12 weeks, at the umbilicus at 20 to 24 weeks) before the usual time. This rapid development is also diagnostic of multiple pregnancy or a miscalculated due date, however, so this finding must be evaluated carefully. Because hCG is produced by the trophoblast cells that are overgrowing, a serum or urine test of hCG for pregnancy will be strongly positive (1 to 2 million International Units compared with a normal pregnancy level of 400,000 International Units).

Results continue to be strongly positive after day 100 of pregnancy, when the level of hCG normally begins to decline. This fact must be evaluated carefully also, however, because highly positive test results can be characteristic of multiple pregnancies with more than one placenta or a miscalculated due date. The nausea and vomiting of early pregnancy is usually marked, probably because of the high hCG level present. Symptoms of gestational hypertension, such as increased blood pressure, edema, and proteinuria, are ordinarily not present before week 20 of pregnancy. With gestational trophoblastic disease, they may appear before this time. An ultrasound will show dense growth (typically a snowflake pattern) but no fetal growth in the uterus. No fetal heart sounds can be heard because there is no viable fetus.

At approximately week 16 of pregnancy, if the structure was not identified earlier by ultrasound, it will identify itself with vaginal bleeding. This may begin as spotting of dark-brown blood resembling prune juice or as a profuse fresh flow. As the bleeding progresses, it is accompanied by discharge of the clear fluid-filled vesicles. This is why it is important for any woman who begins to miscarry at home to bring any clots or tissue passed to the hospital with her. The presence of clear fluid-filled cysts changes the diagnosis from a simple miscarriage to gestational trophoblastic disease.

Therapeutic Management

Therapy for gestational trophoblastic disease is suction curettage to evacuate the abnormal trophoblast cells. Following extraction, women should have a baseline pelvic examination and a serum test for the beta subunit of hCG. The hCG is then analyzed every 2 weeks until levels are again normal. The serum hCG level is then assessed every 4 weeks for the next 6 to 12 months to see if it is declining (half of women will still have a positive reading at 3 weeks; one-fourth still have a positive test result at 40 days).

If the level plateaus or increases, it suggests a malignant transformation (i.e., choriocarcinoma) is occurring. During the waiting time for the hCG level to decline, a woman should use a reliable contraceptive such as oral estrogen/progesterone so that a positive pregnancy test (the presence of hCG) resulting from a new pregnancy will not be confused with the increasing level that occurs with a developing malignancy. After 6 months, if hCG levels are still negative, a woman is theoretically free of the risk of a malignancy. By 12 months, she could begin to plan a second pregnancy. Although the development of gestational trophoblastic disease means a pregnancy never materialized and a fetus never formed, a woman may experience the same feeling of loss after evacuation that she would have experienced after the loss of a true pregnancy—she did, after all, believe she was pregnant. In addition, she is faced with the possibility a malignancy may develop as well as also delay her childbearing plans for a year. If she had already put off having a child for some time, this may seem to be an unbearably long time.

Some primary health care providers give women who have had gestational trophoblastic disease a prophylactic course of methotrexate. However, because the drug interferes with white blood cell formation (i.e., leukopenia), prophylactic use must be weighed carefully (Fu et al., 2012). If malignancy should occur, it can be treated effectively in most instances with methotrexate at that time (Hanna & Soper, 2010). A second agent such as dactinomycin can be added to the regimen if metastasis occurs.

Women need the opportunity to express their anger and sense of unfairness at this type of event. They may feel inadequate because something went wrong with the pregnancy. They may wonder whether it will happen again in a future pregnancy or whether they will ever be able to have children. Unfortunately, women who have one incidence of gestational trophoblastic disease do have an increased risk of a second molar pregnancy (Lurain, 2010). They need early screening with ultrasound during a second pregnancy to be certain this irregular trophoblastic growth is not happening again.

What if . . . 21.1 After having had a gestational trophoblastic disorder, Beverly Muzuki told you she did not believe in birth control because of religious convictions, and so she did not intend to take the oral contraceptives prescribed following her mole evacuation. How would you advise her?

Cervical Insufficiency (Premature Cervical Dilatation)

Premature cervical dilatation, previously termed an incompetent cervix, refers to a cervix that dilates prematurely and therefore cannot retain a fetus until term (Roman, 2013). It occurs in about 1% of women. The dilatation usually occurs painlessly, so often the first symptom is show (a pink-stained vaginal discharge) or increased pelvic pressure, which then is followed by rupture of the membranes and discharge of the amniotic fluid. Uterine contractions begin and, after a short labor, the fetus is born. Unfortunately, this commonly occurs at approximately week 20 of pregnancy, when the fetus is still too immature to survive.

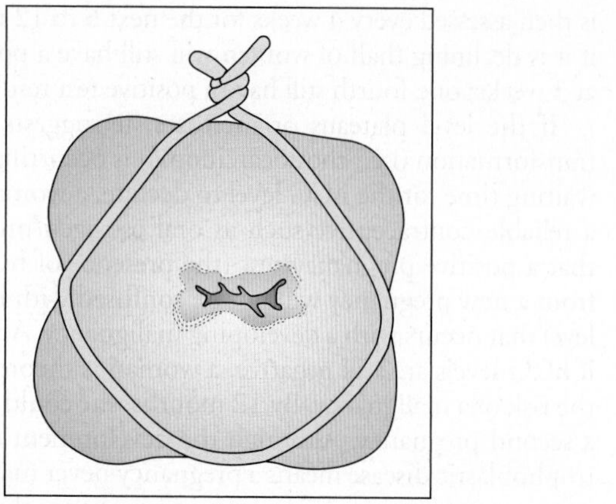

FIGURE 21.5 Shirodkar suture for cervical cerclage.

It is often difficult to explain in a particular instance what caused premature dilatation, although it is associated with increased maternal age, congenital structural defects, and trauma to the cervix, such as might have occurred with a cone biopsy or repeated D&Cs. Although it may be diagnosed by an early ultrasound before symptoms occur, it is usually diagnosed only after the pregnancy is lost.

After the loss of one child because of premature cervical dilatation, a surgical operation termed **cervical cerclage** can be performed to prevent this from happening in a second pregnancy (Alfirevic, Stampalija, Roberts, et al., 2012).

As soon as an ultrasound confirms that the fetus of a second pregnancy is healthy at approximately weeks 12 to 14, purse-string sutures are placed in the cervix by the vaginal route under regional anesthesia. This procedure is called a McDonald or a Shirodkar procedure after the surgeons who perfected the technique. The sutures serve to strengthen the cervix and prevent it from dilating until the end of pregnancy (Fig. 21.5). Still newer techniques allow purse-string sutures to be set before a woman becomes pregnant, providing added assurance she will not begin miscarrying before week 14 of pregnancy. In a McDonald procedure, nylon sutures are placed horizontally and vertically across the cervix and pulled tight to reduce the cervical canal to a few millimeters in diameter. With a Shirodkar technique, sterile tape is threaded in a purse-string manner under the submucous layer of the cervix and sutured in place to achieve a closed cervix. Although routinely accomplished by a vaginal route, sutures may be placed by a transabdominal route.

After cerclage surgery, women remain on bed rest (perhaps in a slight or modified Trendelenburg position) for a few days to decrease pressure on the new sutures. Usual activity and sexual relations can be resumed in most instances after this rest period.

With these procedures, the sutures are removed at weeks 37 to 38 of pregnancy so the fetus can be born vaginally. When a transabdominal approach is used, the sutures may be left in place and a cesarean birth performed.

Women who are discovered to have cervical dilatation but with membranes still intact at a prenatal visit may have emergent cerclage sutures placed in the cervix even at that point as prophylaxis against preterm birth. The success of this procedure is limited, however, compared to preventive suturing (Owen & Mancuso, 2012).

Be certain to ask women who are reporting painless bleeding (also the symptoms of spontaneous miscarriage) whether they have had past cervical operations to remind them they may have sutures in place. Currently, the prognosis for a successful pregnancy after surgical correction for premature cervical dilatation is very favorable. The success rate with both types of cerclage techniques averages 80% to 90% (McNair & Altman, 2011).

Placenta Previa

Placenta previa, a condition of pregnancy in which the placenta is implanted abnormally in the lower part of the uterus, is the most common cause of painless bleeding in the third trimester of pregnancy (Rao, Belogolovkin, Yankowitz, et al., 2012) (Fig. 21.6). It occurs in four degrees: implantation in the lower rather than in the upper portion of the uterus (low-lying placenta), marginal implantation (the placenta edge approaches that of the cervical os), implantation that occludes a portion of the cervical os (partial placenta previa), and implantation that totally obstructs the cervical os (total placenta previa). The degree to which the placenta covers the internal cervical os is generally estimated in percentages: 100%, 75%, 30%, and so forth.

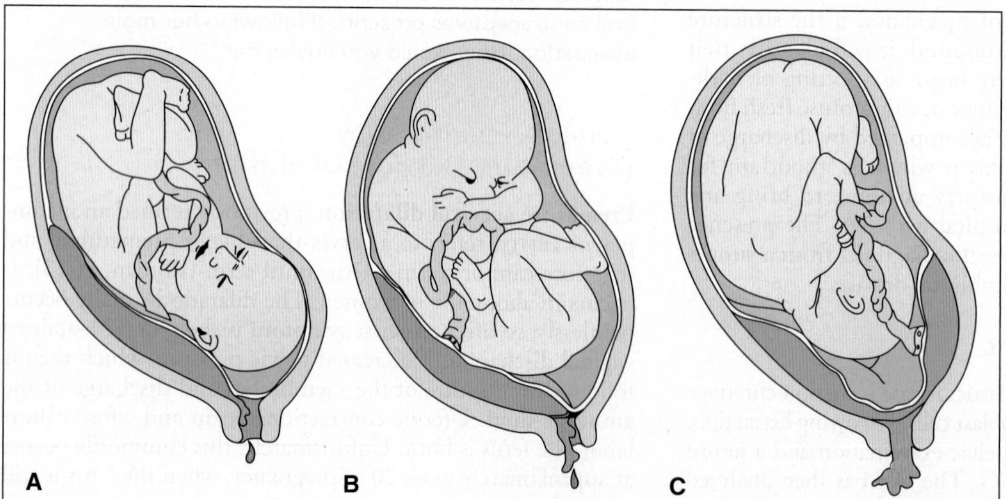

FIGURE 21.6 Degrees of placenta previa: **(A)** low implantation, **(B)** partial placenta previa, and **(C)** total placenta previa.

Increased parity, advanced maternal age, past cesarean births, past uterine curettage, multiple gestation, and perhaps a male fetus are all associated with placenta previa. The incidence is approximately 5 per 1,000 pregnancies; it is thought to occur whenever the placenta is forced to spread to find an adequate exchange surface. There is a possibility an increase in congenital fetal anomalies or fetal restricted growth could occur if the low implantation does not allow optimal fetal nutrition or oxygenation, but in actual practice, this rarely happens (Yeniel, Ergenoglu, Itil, et al., 2012).

Assessment

Placenta previa is often detected during pregnancy through a routine sonogram done to date the pregnancy. Although many low-lying placentas detected on early ultrasounds migrate upward to a noncervical position, the condition is explained to the woman and she is cautioned to call her health care provider at any sign of vaginal bleeding. The bleeding with placenta previa doesn't usually begin, however, until the lower uterine segment starts to differentiate from the upper segment late in pregnancy (approximately week 30) and the cervix begins to dilate. At that point, because the placenta is unable to stretch to accommodate the differing shape of the lower uterine segment or the cervix, a small portion loosens and damaged blood vessels begin to bleed. The bleeding is usually abrupt, painless, bright red, and sudden enough to frighten a woman. It is not associated with increased activity or participation in sports and may stop as abruptly as it began, so that, by the time a woman is seen at the health care setting, she is no longer bleeding. In other women, it may slow after the initial hemorrhage but linger as continuous spotting.

Therapeutic Management

The bleeding of placenta previa, like that of ectopic pregnancy, creates an emergency situation as the open vessels of the uterine decidua (maternal blood) place the mother at risk for hemorrhage. Because the placenta is loosened, the fetal oxygen and nutrient supply may also be compromised, placing the fetus at risk as well. With the placental loosening, **preterm labor** (labor that occurs before the end of week 37 of gestation) may begin, posing the additional threat of preterm birth to the fetus.

Immediate Care Measures. To ensure an adequate blood supply to a woman and fetus, place the woman immediately on bed rest in a side-lying position. Be certain to assess:

- Duration of the pregnancy
- Time the bleeding began
- Woman's estimation of the amount of blood—ask her to estimate in terms of cups or tablespoons (a cup is 240 ml; a tablespoon is 15 ml)
- Whether there was accompanying pain
- Color of the blood (red blood indicates bleeding is fresh or is continuing)
- What she has done, if anything, for the bleeding (if she inserted a tampon to halt the bleeding, there may be hidden bleeding)
- Whether there were prior episodes of bleeding during the pregnancy
- Whether she had prior cervical surgery for premature cervical dilatation

Inspect the perineum for bleeding and estimate the present rate of blood loss. Weighing perineal pads before and after use and calculating the difference by subtraction is a good method to determine vaginal blood loss. An Apt or Kleihauer–Betke test (test strip procedures) can be used to detect whether the blood is of fetal or maternal origin. Obtain baseline vital signs to determine whether symptoms of hypovolemic shock are present. Continue to assess blood pressure every 5 to 15 minutes or continuously with an electronic cuff. Never attempt a pelvic or rectal examination with painless bleeding late in pregnancy because any agitation of the cervix when there is a placenta previa might tear the placenta further and initiate massive hemorrhage, possibly fatal to both mother and child.

Attach external monitoring equipment to record fetal heart sounds and uterine contractions (an internal monitor for either fetal or uterine assessment is contraindicated). Hemoglobin, hematocrit, prothrombin time, partial thromboplastin time, fibrinogen, platelet count, type and cross-match, and antibody screen will be assessed to establish baselines, detect a possible clotting disorder, and ready blood for replacement if necessary. Monitor urine output frequently, as often as every hour, as an indicator her blood volume is remaining adequate to perfuse her kidneys. Administer intravenous fluid as prescribed, preferably with a large-gauge catheter to allow for blood replacement through the same line.

A vaginal birth is always safest for an infant. It is essential, therefore, to determine the placenta's location as accurately as possible in the hope that its position will make vaginal birth feasible. If the previa is under 30% by abdominal or intravaginal ultrasound, it may be possible for the fetus to be born past it. If over 30%, and the fetus is mature, the safest birth method for both mother and baby is often a cesarean birth (Bedoya-Ronga & Currie, 2012).

If only a minimum previa is detected by sonogram, the primary health care provider may attempt a careful speculum examination of the vagina and cervix to establish the degree of fetal engagement and to rule out another cause for bleeding, such as ruptured varices or cervical trauma. This should be done in an operating room or a fully equipped birthing room so that if hemorrhage does occur with cervical manipulation, an immediate cesarean birth can be carried out to remove the child and the bleeding placenta and contract the uterus. Have oxygen equipment available in case the fetal heart sounds indicate fetal distress, such as bradycardia or tachycardia, late deceleration, or variable decelerations during the exam.

Continuing Care Measures. The point at which a diagnosis of placenta previa is made and the age of the gestation dictate the final management. If labor has begun, bleeding is continuing, or the fetus is being compromised (measured by the response of the fetal heart rate to contractions), birth must be accomplished regardless of gestational age. If the bleeding has stopped, the fetal heart sounds are of good quality, maternal vital signs are good, and the fetus is not yet 36 weeks of age, a woman is usually managed by expectant watching. Typically, a woman remains in the hospital on bed rest for close observation for 24 to 48 hours. If the bleeding stops, she can be sent home with a referral for bed rest and home care. Assessments of fetal heart sounds and laboratory tests, such as hemoglobin or hematocrit, are obtained frequently. Betamethasone, a steroid that hastens fetal lung maturity, may be prescribed for the mother to encourage the maturity of fetal lungs if the fetus is less than 34 weeks gestation (Box 21.5).

BOX 21.5 Nursing Care Planning Based on Responsibility for Pharmacology

BETAMETHASONE (CELESTONE)

Action: Betamethasone is a corticosteroid that acts as an anti-inflammatory and immunosuppressive agent. It is given to pregnant women 12 to 24 hours before birth to hasten fetal lung maturity if a fetus is less than 34 weeks gestation and help prevent respiratory distress syndrome in the newborn (Karch, 2013).

Pregnancy Risk Category: C

Dosage: 12 to 12.5 mg intramuscularly (IM) initially; may be repeated in 24 hours and again in 1 to 2 weeks

Possible Adverse Effects: Burning, itching, and irritation at the injection site; swelling, tachycardia, headache, dizziness, weight gain, sodium, and fluid retention; and increased risk of infection if used long term.

Nursing Implications

- Explain the purpose of the drug to the client.
- Administer the initial dose IM. Anticipate the need for repeat dosing within 24 hours and again in 1 to 2 weeks.
- Assist with measures to halt preterm labor if indicated.
- Continue to monitor client's vital signs and fetal heart rate for changes.
- If client is also receiving a tocolytic agent, be alert for possible cardiac decompensation as a result of a drug–drug interaction. Observe for signs such as increased pulse, decreased blood pressure, and presence of edema.
- Assess for signs and symptoms of possible infection with long-term use.
- Instruct client about the possibility that a repeat dose may be necessary.

Nursing Diagnoses and Related Interventions

Because the diagnosis of placenta previa with bleeding is an emergency, all goals should reflect the short time frame of the emergency condition.

Nursing Diagnosis: Fear related to outcome of pregnancy after episode of placenta previa bleeding

Outcome Evaluation: Client discusses concerns with nurse and other health care providers; states hearing fetal heartbeat helps to reassure her about baby's health.

Often, it is difficult for a woman who has experienced bleeding late in a pregnancy to wait for the baby to come to term because she wonders whether her infant will be all right. Regardless of her outward appearance, most likely she is experiencing severe emotional stress. She cannot help but wonder if the next bleeding she experiences will kill her, the infant, or both. Listening to fetal heart sounds and being reassured they are in a healthy range is helpful, as is having a listening ear she can talk to about her fears for both the pregnancy and herself.

Birth

If the pregnancy was past 37 weeks at the time of the initial bleeding, and an amniocentesis analysis for lung maturity shows a positive result (a favorable lecithin/sphingomyelin ratio), a birth decision will generally be made immediately as it is important birth be in a controlled setting in case more than the usual blood loss occurs with birth. If the fetus is not mature, the pregnancy will be allowed to continue to the point bleeding occurs again, labor begins, the fetus shows symptoms of distress, or the fetus is mature. Offer firm support if the birth will be an emergency situation.

If the placenta previa is found to be total, birth through the placenta is impossible and the baby must be born by cesarean birth. If the placenta previa is partial, the amount of the blood loss, the condition of the fetus, and a woman's parity will influence the birth decision. For cesarean birth, if an ultrasound clearly reveals the placental location, a transverse uterine incision may still be possible, although the uterine cut must be made high, possibly vertically above the low implantation site of the placenta.

After birth, most women inspect their child carefully. They may be worried that because of the problem with placental implantation, there might be something wrong with the baby. During the postpartum period, be sure a woman has adequate time with her child to be certain she feels comfortable giving care before she leaves the health care facility.

Any woman who has had a placenta previa is more prone than normal to postpartum hemorrhage because the placental site is in the lower uterine segment, which does not contract as efficiently as the upper segment. Also, because the uterine blood supply is less in the lower segment, the placenta tends to grow larger than it would normally, leaving a larger denuded surface area when it is removed. As a second complication, a woman is more likely to develop endometritis because the placental site is close to the cervix, the portal of entry for pathogens.

✔ QSEN Checkpoint Question 21.3

Safety

Suppose a sonogram shows Beverly, who is beginning preterm labor, has a placenta previa. What would be the priority measure to take in order to ensure her safety?

a. Keep her physically active to avoid a deep vein thrombosis.
b. Perform a daily vaginal exam to assess the extent of the previa.

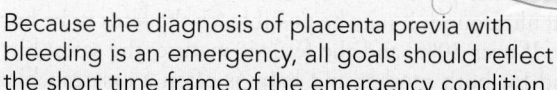

c. Assess for vaginal bleeding and clear fluid leakage every shift.
d. Keep her nothing by mouth (NPO) as she will need an emergency cesarean birth.

Look in Appendix A for the best answer and rationale.

Premature Separation of the Placenta (Abruptio Placentae)

Unlike placenta previa, in **premature separation of the placenta** (also called abruptio placentae; Fig. 21.7), the placenta appears to have been implanted correctly. Suddenly, however, it begins to separate and bleeding results. This occurs in about 10% of pregnancies and, because it can lead to extensive bleeding, is the most frequent cause of perinatal death (Pariente, Wiznitzer, Sergienko, et al., 2011). The separation generally occurs late in pregnancy; even as late as during the first or second stage of labor. Because premature separation of the placenta may occur during an otherwise normal labor, it is important to always be alert to both the amount and kind of pain and vaginal bleeding a woman is having in labor.

The primary cause of premature separation is unknown, but certain predisposing factors are high parity, advanced maternal age, a short umbilical cord, chronic hypertensive disease, hypertension of pregnancy, direct trauma (as from an automobile accident or intimate partner violence), vasoconstriction from cocaine or cigarette use, and thrombophilitic conditions that lead to thrombosis formation (Ananth, Nath, & Philipp, 2010). It also may be caused by chorioamnionitis or infection of the fetal membranes and fluid (Matsuda, Hayashi, Shiozaki, et al., 2011).

Yet another possible cause is a rapid decrease in uterine volume, such as occurs with sudden release of amniotic fluid. Usually, the fetal head is low enough in the pelvis that when membranes rupture, this prevents loss of the total volume of the amniotic fluid at one time, so normally a rapid reduction in amniotic fluid does not occur.

Assessment

A woman experiences a sharp, stabbing pain high in the uterine fundus as the initial separation occurs. If labor begins with the separation, each contraction will be accompanied by pain over and above the pain of the contraction. Tenderness can be felt on uterine palpation.

Heavy bleeding usually accompanies premature separation of the placenta, although it may not be readily apparent. External bleeding will only be evident if the placenta separates first at the edges, so blood escapes freely into the uterus and then the cervix. In contrast, if the center of the placenta separates first, blood can pool under the placenta, and although bleeding is just as intense, it will be hidden from view. Whether blood is evident or not, signs of hypovolemic shock usually follow quickly. The uterus becomes tense and feels rigid to the touch. If blood infiltrates the uterine musculature, **Couvelaire uterus** or uteroplacental apoplexy, forming a hard, boardlike uterus occurs. As bleeding progresses, a woman's reserve of blood fibrinogen becomes diminished as her body attempts to accomplish effective clot formation, and DIC syndrome can occur (see later).

If a woman is being admitted to the hospital after experiencing symptoms at home, assess when the time the bleeding began, whether pain accompanied it, the amount and kind of bleeding, and her actions to detect if trauma could have led to the placental separation. Initial blood work should include hemoglobin level, typing and cross-matching, and a fibrinogen level and fibrin breakdown products to detect DIC.

Therapeutic Management

Because of the threat to both the woman and the fetus, separation of the placenta is immediately an emergency situation (Newfield, 2012). A woman needs a large-gauge intravenous catheter inserted for fluid replacement and oxygen by mask to limit fetal anoxia. Monitor fetal heart sounds externally and record maternal vital signs every 5 to 15 minutes to establish baselines and observe progress. The baseline fibrinogen determination will be followed by additional determinations up to the time of birth. Keep a woman in a lateral, not supine, position to prevent pressure on the vena cava and additional

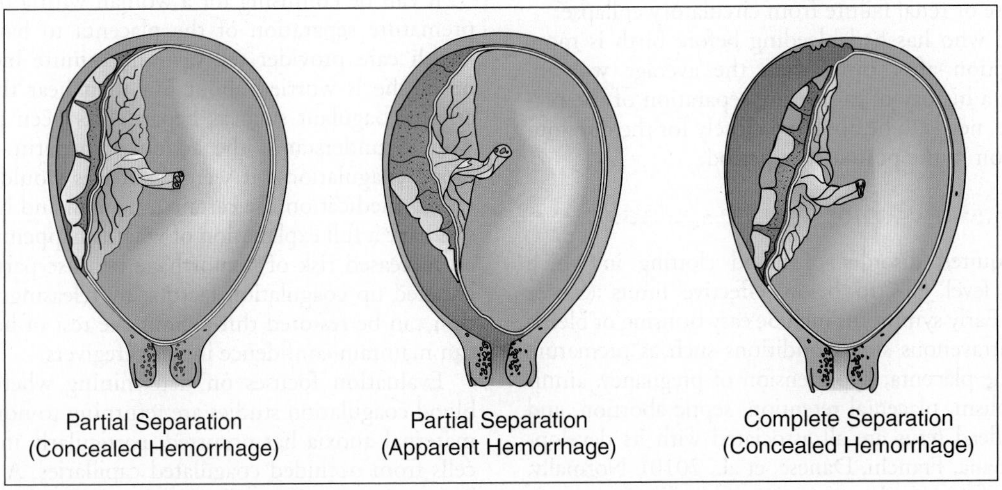

FIGURE 21.7 Premature separation of the placenta.

TABLE 21.5 Premature Separation of the Placenta: Degrees of Separation

Grade	Criteria
0	No symptoms of separation are apparent from maternal or fetal signs; the diagnosis is made after birth, when the placenta is examined and a segment of the placenta shows a recent adherent clot on the maternal surface.
1	Minimal separation, but enough to cause vaginal bleeding and changes in the maternal vital signs; no fetal distress or hemorrhagic shock occurs, however.
2	Moderate separation; there is evidence of fetal distress; the uterus is tense and painful on palpation.
3	Extreme separation; without immediate interventions, maternal hypovolemic shock and fetal death will result.

interference with fetal circulation. It is important not to disturb the injured placenta any further. Therefore, do not perform any abdominal, vaginal, or pelvic examination on a woman with a diagnosed or suspected placental separation.

For better prediction of fetal and maternal outcomes, the degrees of placental separation can be graded (Table 21.5). Unless the separation is minimal (grades 0 and 1), the pregnancy must be terminated because the fetus cannot obtain adequate oxygen and nutrients. If vaginal birth does not seem imminent, cesarean birth is the birth method of choice. If DIC has developed, cesarean birth may pose a grave risk because of the possibility of hemorrhage during the surgery and later from the surgical incision. Intravenous administration of fibrinogen or cryoprecipitate (which contains fibrinogen) can be used to elevate a woman's fibrinogen level prior to and concurrently with surgery. With the worst outcome, a hysterectomy might be necessary to prevent exsanguination.

Fetal prognosis depends on the extent of the placental separation and the degree of fetal hypoxia. Maternal prognosis depends on how promptly treatment can be instituted. Death can occur from massive hemorrhage leading to shock and circulatory collapse or renal failure from circulatory collapse.

Any woman who has had bleeding before birth is more prone to infection after birth than the average woman. A woman with a history of premature separation of the placenta, therefore, needs to be observed closely for the development of infection in the postpartum period.

Disseminated Intravascular Coagulation

DIC is an acquired disorder of blood clotting in which the fibrinogen level falls to below effective limits (Su & Chong, 2012). Early symptoms include easy bruising or bleeding from an intravenous site. Conditions such as premature separation of the placenta, hypertension of pregnancy, amniotic fluid embolism, placental retention, septic abortion, and retention of a dead fetus are all associated with its development (Montagnana, Franchi, Danese, et al., 2010). Normally, platelets quickly form a seal over a point of bleeding to prevent further loss of blood. Intrinsic and extrinsic clotting pathways then activate and strengthen this plug with fibrin threads to produce a firm, fixed structure. To prevent too much clotting from occurring, at the same time the clot is being formed, thrombin activates fibrinolysin, a proteolytic enzyme, which begins digestion of excess fibrin threads (anticoagulation). This lysis results in the release of fibrin degradation products.

DIC occurs when there is such extreme bleeding and so many platelets and fibrin from the general circulation rush to the site that there is not enough left in the rest of the body. This results in a paradox: at one point in the circulatory system, the person has increased coagulation, but throughout the rest of the system, a bleeding defect exists. DIC is an emergency because it can result in extreme blood loss. Goals for care should reflect the presence of the emergency.

Blood needs to be drawn for a platelet count (will be decreased to $\leq$100,000/μl), prothrombin (will be low because it depends on the conversion of fibrinogen to fibrin), thrombin time (will be elevated because it measures the time necessary for conversion of fibrinogen to fibrin), fibrinogen (will be decreased to $<$150 mg/dl because fibrinogen is not available), and fibrin split products (will be $>$40 μg/ml reflecting the destruction of fibrinogen or fibrin). A D-dimer analysis is specific for fibrin (not fibrinogen) degradation products and will be abnormal in 90% of patients with DIC (Tripodi, 2011).

To stop the process of DIC, the underlying insult that began the phenomenon must be halted. When the insult was a complication of pregnancy, such as premature separation of the placenta, ending the pregnancy by birthing the fetus and delivering the placenta is part of the solution. Next, the marked coagulation must be stopped so that coagulation factors can be freed and normal clotting function can be restored. This is accomplished by the administration of heparin to halt the clotting cascade, first intravenously, then by subcutaneous injection. Heparin must be cautiously given close to birth, however, or postpartum hemorrhage could occur from poor clotting after delivery of the placenta. A blood or platelet transfusion may be necessary to replace blood or platelet loss but this is usually delayed until after heparin therapy so the new blood factors are also not consumed by the coagulation process. Antithrombin III factor, fibrinogen, or cryoprecipitate (which contains fibrinogen) can all be used in place of whole blood for transfusion. If these are not available, fresh frozen plasma or platelets can also aid in restoring clotting function.

It can be confusing for a woman with a disorder such as premature separation of the placenta to have her primary health care provider tell her one minute bleeding is what he or she is worried about but then hear the next minute an anticoagulant such as heparin has been prescribed. If a woman understands the action of heparin—to discourage blood coagulation—it seems as if this would be exactly the wrong medication. Be certain a woman and her support person have a full explanation of what is happening (i.e., she has an increased risk of hemorrhage because part of her system has tied up coagulation factors; by releasing them, coagulation can be restored throughout the rest of her body) so she can maintain confidence in her caregivers.

Evaluation focuses on determining whether a woman's blood coagulation studies are returning to normal and if any maternal anoxia has occurred, particularly in renal or brain cells from occluded coagulated capillaries. A fetal and newborn assessment is equally important to evaluate the efficiency of the placental circulation in light of the increased clotting (heparin does not cross the placenta so a newborn will not be born with decreased clotting ability).

PRETERM LABOR

Preterm labor is labor that occurs before the end of week 37 of gestation. It occurs in approximately 9% to 11% of all pregnancies. It is always potentially serious, because if it results in the infant's birth, the infant will be immature. Because of this, it is responsible for almost two-thirds of all infant deaths in the neonatal period (Meguerdichian, 2012). Any woman having persistent uterine contractions, even if they are mild and widely spaced, should be considered to be in labor. A woman is documented as being in actual labor rather than having false labor contractions if contractions have caused cervical effacement over 80% or dilation over 1 cm.

Maintaining general health during pregnancy is the best preventive measure to avoid preterm birth. Other measures can help prevent an occurrence of preterm birth (Box 21.6). Knowing the signs of labor can help women identify if preterm birth is beginning because some women wait before they seek help for preterm labor because they diagnose back pain or contractions as nothing more than extremely hard Braxton Hicks contractions. Currently, when there is treatment available to delay labor for at least a few days or until a fetus reaches a level of maturity that will allow the newborn to survive in the outside environment, evaluation and the institution of therapy before membranes rupture become vital, as ruptured membranes make it that much more difficult to halt labor.

Why labor begins before a fetus is mature is usually unclear. It is associated, however, with dehydration, urinary tract infection, periodontal disease, chorioamnionitis, and perhaps large fetal size. African American women, adolescents, and those who receive inadequate prenatal care are most susceptible (Pereira, Reddy, Alexander, et al., 2010). Women who continue to work at strenuous jobs during pregnancy or perform shift work that leads to extreme fatigue may have a higher incidence than others (Bonzini, Palmer, Coggon, et al., 2011). Intimate partner violence and the trauma this causes may be yet another cause (Sanchez, Alva, Diez Chang, et al., 2012).

Common symptoms of early preterm labor women need to identify include a persistent, dull, and low backache; vaginal spotting; a feeling of pelvic pressure or abdominal tightening; menstrual-like cramping; increased vaginal discharge; uterine contractions; and intestinal cramping. Listen carefully to any woman who has these symptoms or believes she is in preterm labor because beginning symptoms of labor are subtle and best recognized by the woman herself.

It is possible to predict which pregnancies will end early by analyzing changes in the length of the cervix by ultrasound exam and analysis of vaginal mucus for the presence of fetal fibronectin, a protein produced by trophoblast cells (Sayres, 2010; Wiegerinck, Vis, & Mol, 2010). If this is present in vaginal mucus, it predicts that preterm contractions are ready to occur; absence of the protein predicts that labor will not occur for at least 14 days.

Therapeutic Management

Medical attempts can be made to stop labor if the fetal membranes have not ruptured, fetal distress is absent, there is no evidence that bleeding is occurring, the cervix is not dilated more than 4 to 5 cm, and effacement is not more than 50%.

A woman who is in preterm labor is usually first admitted to the hospital and placed on bed rest to relieve the pressure of the fetus on the cervix. External fetal and uterine contraction monitors are attached to monitor fetal heart rate and the intensity of contractions. Intravenous fluid therapy to keep her well hydrated is begun because, although not well documented, hydration may help stop contractions. This is thought to be effective because, if a woman is dehydrated,

BOX 21.6 Nursing Care Planning Based on Family Teaching

MEASURES TO HELP PREVENT A RECURRENCE OF PRETERM LABOR FOR WOMEN ON BED REST

Q. Beverly Muzuki has started preterm labor and so is prescribed bed rest on home care. She asks you, "What else can I do to help prevent having this baby early?"

A. Although there are no guarantees, several actions can be helpful to prevent a recurrence of preterm labor:

- Remain on bed rest (a lounge or couch) except to use the bathroom.
- Drink 8 to 10 glasses of fluids daily (keep a pitcher by your bed so you do not have to get up).
- Keep mentally active by reading or working on a project to prevent boredom.
- Avoid activities that could stimulate labor, such as nipple stimulation.
- Consult your primary care provider regarding whether sexual relations should be restricted.
- Immediately report signs of ruptured membranes (sudden gush of vaginal fluid) or vaginal bleeding.
- Report signs of urinary tract or vaginal infection (e.g., burning or frequency of urination, vaginal itching or pain).
- Keep appointments for prenatal care.

If uterine contractions recur:

- Empty your bladder to relieve pressure on the uterus.
- Lie down on your left or right side to encourage blood return to the uterus.
- Drink two or three glasses of fluid to increase hydration.
- Telephone your health care provider to report the incident and ask for further care measures.

the pituitary gland will be activated to secrete antidiuretic hormone, which might cause the pituitary gland to release oxytocin as well, strengthening uterine contractions.

Vaginal and cervical cultures and a clean-catch urine sample are prescribed to rule out infection. If a urinary tract infection is present, the woman will be prescribed an antibiotic that is especially effective for group B streptococcus as this infection can be fatal in a newborn.

Drug Administration

Terbutaline is a drug approved to prevent and treat bronchospasm (i.e., narrowing of airways) but may be used, off-label, as a **tocolytic agent** (i.e., an agent to halt labor). Terbutaline carries a "black box" warning, however, that it should not be used for over 48 to 72 hours of therapy because of a potential for serious maternal heart problems and death. It should not be used in an outpatient or home setting because its administration requires constant professional assessment (Roman, 2013).

Magnesium sulfate is a drug that halts calcium uptake by muscles. It is the drug of choice to manage gestational hypertension. Although not proven to have either short- or long-term effectiveness with preterm labor, its potential to reduce the ability of the uterus to contract has made it the most common drug prescribed for preterm labor as an unlabeled use of the medicine (Hunter & Gibbins, 2011). It is administered intravenously until contractions have slowed and the mother's cervix has stopped effacing or dilating or birth is imminent. There is a thin line between a therapeutic amount of magnesium sulfate and a toxic level that leads to respiratory depression. Women receiving magnesium sulfate as a tocolytic, therefore, need the same conscientious assessments as the woman who is receiving this for gestational hypertension (see below).

For reasons not clearly understood, if, in the time between when preterm contractions begin and preterm birth occurs, a woman is administered a corticosteroid such as betamethasone the formation of lung surfactant appears to accelerate, thus reducing the possibility of respiratory distress syndrome or bronchopulmonary dysplasia (Riley, Boozer, & King, 2011). During the time labor is being chemically halted, therefore, if the pregnancy is under 34 weeks, a woman may be given two doses of 12 mg betamethasone intramuscularly 24 hours apart, or four doses of 6 mg dexamethasone intramuscularly 12 hours apart.

Although the effect of betamethasone lasts for about 7 days, it takes about 24 hours for the drug to begin its effect, so it is important labor be halted for at least 24 hours. If the fetus is not born within the 7-day time span, the dose of betamethasone may be repeated, but this is controversial because any corticosteroid can interfere with glucose regulation in the woman and potentially in the fetus.

What if...21.2 You overhear Beverly tell her mother not to come to the hospital to be with her because her baby is so small, her labor should be quick and easy. Would you investigate further or assume Beverly knows what will be best for herself?

Fetal Assessment

In addition to supervising tocolytic therapy, be certain to assess overall fetal welfare in the woman who is trying to delay or prevent preterm labor by assessing the fetal heart rate and activity (Box 21.7, an interprofessional care map for a woman in preterm labor).

Following this initial therapy and if contractions have ceased and there is evidence of fetal well-being, women with arrested preterm labor can be safely cared for at home as long as they can dependably drink enough fluid to remain well hydrated and, although there is little evidence that strict bed rest prevents preterm labor, a woman limits strenuous activities (Chawanpaiboon, Pimol, & Sirisomboon, 2011; Hennessy, Volpe, Sammel, et al., 2010). It is also important for women to maintain adequate nutrition and to not smoke cigarettes as both poor nutrition and smoking are risks for preterm birth (Khader, Al-Akour, Alzubi, et al., 2011). To help with fetal assessment, a woman may be asked to record a daily fetal "kick" count or "count to 10" test (see Chapter 9 for this technique and Chapter 4 for a discussion of home care).

Labor That Cannot Be Halted

In some women, preterm labor is too far advanced (e.g., membranes have ruptured or the cervix is more than 50% effaced and more than 3 to 4 cm dilated) when they are first seen in a health care facility for it to be halted. The rupture of membranes, especially, can be thought of as a "point of no return" in stopping or delaying labor because of the increased risk of infection that begins at that point.

If the fetus is very immature at the time labor cannot be halted, a cesarean birth may be planned to reduce pressure on the fetal head and reduce the possibility of subdural or intraventricular hemorrhage from a vaginal birth, although this is controversial because infants born by cesarean birth have a higher incidence of respiratory difficulty, which is already a high risk for a very preterm infant.

Most women assume that if a fetus is preterm, labor for a vaginal birth will be shorter than normal because the infant is still so small. This is not necessarily true, however, because the first stage of labor, the longest stage, proceeds exactly as it would with a term pregnancy. The second stage of labor may be shorter because a small infant can be pushed through the dilated cervix and the birth canal more easily. Because the second stage takes, at most, 1 hour, this means the difference will not be more than 30 minutes to 1 hour. Unless a woman is given this explanation, she may worry not only that her labor is preterm but also that something is going wrong because it is lasting so long. Because of the increased risk for prolapse of the cord around a small head, artificial rupture of the membranes is not done as a rule in preterm labor until the fetal head is firmly engaged.

Analgesic agents are administered with caution because an immature infant will have enough difficulty breathing at birth without the additional burden of being sedated from a drug such as meperidine (Demerol). If a woman wants pharmaceutical pain management for labor, an epidural is preferable.

A woman may feel reassured by having an external fetal monitor during labor because the monitor screen shows evidence that, although her infant is going to be small, heart tones seem to be of good quality and the infant is reacting well to labor. Be certain that if a monitor is attached, the woman rests on her side to help prevent supine hypotension syndrome or an interference with uterine circulation.

Although an episiotomy is not routinely used because the head of a preterm infant is more fragile than that of a mature infant, one may be done to relieve excessive pressure on

BOX 21.7 Nursing Care Planning

AN INTERPROFESSIONAL CARE MAP FOR A WOMAN IN PRETERM LABOR

Beverly Muzuki is a 20-year-old gravida 2, para 0, 30 weeks pregnant, whom you see in a prenatal clinic. She has had symptoms of a urinary tract infection for the past few days but didn't call the clinic because she knew she had an appointment today and thought getting some help for it could wait until she came in. Yesterday she noticed some mild lower abdominal pain but thought it was irritation from the bladder infection. During the night, she woke twice because of a nagging lower backache. This morning, she has intermittent sharp uterine contractions. *"Why am I starting labor so early?"* she asks you. "Is it because I'm Rh negative?"

Family Assessment Client, 20 years old, lives in a two-bedroom, third-floor apartment and works as a secretary for local construction firm; husband, 26 years old, is a payroll supervisor at the same firm. Finances rated as, "Who couldn't use more money?".

Client Assessment Gravida 2, para 0, 30-week pregnancy. Heart rate, 88 beats/min; respirations, 22 breaths/min; blood pressure, 130/78 mmHg. Fetal heart rate (FHR), 142 beats/min; reports positive fetal movements. Uterine contractions every 7 minutes lasting 40 seconds. Cervical effacement 30%; dilation: 2 to 3 cm. Intravenous (IV) therapy with magnesium sulfate and IM corticosteroid prescribed.

Nursing Diagnosis Risk for injury (maternal and fetal) related to preterm labor and tocolytic therapy

Outcome Criteria Contractions halt after treatment with tocolytic; FHR remains within acceptable parameters; client remains free of signs and symptoms of adverse effects of tocolytic therapy. Client verbalizes concerns and fears; participates in decision making and relaxation measures.

Team Member Responsible	Assessment	Intervention	Rationale	Expected Outcome
Activities of Daily Living, Including Safety				
Nurse/ Primary health care provider	Attach contraction and FHR monitors for continuous evaluation of contractions and fetal response.	Institute bed rest with client in side-lying position.	Bed rest relieves pressure of the fetus on the cervix. Side-lying position enhances uterine perfusion. Uterine and fetal monitoring provides evidence of fetal well-being.	Client will remain on bed rest until labor contractions halt or further action becomes necessary.
Teamwork and Collaboration				
Nurse/Primary health care provider	Contact ultrasound personnel.	Obtain client consent for ultrasound. Arrange for ultrasound to establish fetal health and cervical length.	An ultrasound can document fetal health and cervical dilation.	Client agrees to procedure. Completes preprocedure readiness actions.
Procedures/Medications for Quality Improvement				
Nurse	Assess vital signs of client. Obtain history of events leading up to beginning of labor.	Obtain laboratory studies, including complete blood count, hemoglobin and hematocrit, and serum electrolytes. Obtain clean-catch urine for culture, vaginal and cervical cultures, and fibronectin as ordered.	Assessment provides a baseline for future comparisons. Urine, vaginal, and cervical cultures help to rule out infection as a causative factor for preterm labor. Fibronectin can help predict whether labor can be halted.	Specimens are collected and sent to lab promptly to ensure rapid assessment.

(continued on page 570)

BOX 21.7 Nursing Care Planning (continued)

Procedures/Medications for Quality Improvement				
Nurse/ Primary health care provider	Assess for contraindications to betamethasone administration. Obtain reports of urine and cervical cultures and fibronectin.	Administer betamethasone to aid fetal lung maturity and an antibiotic for urinary tract infection as prescribed.	Betamethasone, a steroid, helps to decrease the risk of respiratory distress syndrome should birth of the fetus become necessary. An antibiotic decreases urinary tract infection.	Client agrees to betamethasone and antibiotic administration.
Nurse	Establish strength, duration, and frequency of baseline uterine contractions.	Administer magnesium sulfate as prescribed as an IV piggyback with infusion pump. Continue infusion for 12 to 24 hours after cessation of contractions.	Magnesium sulfate affects the action of calcium in muscles, which must be present for the muscles of the uterus to contract, and so helps halt preterm contractions.	Uterine contractions halt within 1 hour of magnesium sulfate therapy.
Nurse	Continue maternal and fetal vital sign assessment.	Monitor client's vital signs and neurologic status closely. Respirations should be at least 12 breaths/min before each magnesium sulfate dose; FHR, 110 to 160 beats/min; maternal reflexes, 1+ to 2+.	Decreasing urine output, neurologic changes, or decreased respiration or pulse rate are major indicators of magnesium sulfate toxicity. Decreasing FHR can indicate fetal distress.	Client's and fetal vital signs, neurologic status, intake and output (renal status), and laboratory values remain within normal parameters during infusion.
Nurse	Assess if calcium gluconate is available.	Keep calcium gluconate available at the bedside.	Calcium gluconate is the antidote for magnesium sulfate toxicity.	Calcium gluconate is prepared by the pharmacy and is readily available.
Nutrition				
Nurse	Obtain hematocrit and serum electrolyte levels every 4 hours or as ordered.	Assist with or insert an IV line. Begin IV fluid therapy as prescribed.	Hematocrit, electrolyte levels, and IV intake measures the client's fluid volume status.	IV fluid improves hydration, which may help to minimize contractions.
Patient-Centered Care				
Nurse	Assess client's knowledge of preterm labor.	Instruct client about preterm labor and about steps to be taken to counteract the process.	A well-informed client can participate more fully in her own care.	Client states the cause of preterm labor cannot always be identified; describes the part she can play in halting process.
Psychosocial/Spiritual/Emotional Needs				
Nurse	Assess anxiety level of client over preterm labor. Assess for possible feelings of guilt related to cause of preterm labor.	Assist client with using relaxation techniques, such as muscle relaxation, breathing, and music. Provide frequent updates about progress. Allow client to verbalize feelings and concerns.	Relaxation techniques help to decrease anxiety and fear, enhancing feelings of control. Frequent updates about progress help to minimize fear about the unknown.	Client verbalizes her feelings about this crisis in her life. Demonstrates anxiety but at a level that allows her to cooperate with caregivers.
Nurse	Determine whether client wants a support person to be with her.	Contact support person as necessary.	The presence of a support person can offer additional comfort to a client.	Client names a support person she wants notified about hospital admission.

Informatics for Seamless Health Care Planning

Nurse	Assess client's home surroundings to determine whether they are appropriate for bed rest and continuing monitoring at home.	Contact home care nurse service to provide monitoring at home.	Monitoring to see if contractions return can safely be done at home with a conscientious and well-informed client.	Client states she feels her home and support system will be adequate for home care with self-monitoring. Agrees on appointment for first home visit with home care nurse service.

the head and hopefully reduce the possibility of a subdural or intraventricular hemorrhage. Following birth, the cord of the preterm infant is usually not clamped immediately because this extra amount of blood can help reduce the possibility of preterm anemia and the need for postbirth transfusion (Rabe, Diaz-Rossello, Duley, et al., 2012).

Nursing Diagnoses and Related Interventions

Nursing diagnoses for the woman in preterm labor whose labor cannot be halted center around fear for the uncertain outcome of the pregnancy and risk for fetal or newborn injury related to the preterm birth. Be certain these and outcomes for care are realistic in light of the threat to fetal and newborn health. Although many measures are available to help the preterm baby adjust to the outside world, a baby born preterm will be at risk for a variety of health problems, especially difficulty with respirations (see Chapter 26).

Nursing Diagnosis: Situational low self-esteem related to feelings of responsibility for preterm labor

Outcome Evaluation: Client expresses feelings and worries to nurse; states she knows she is not responsible for her labor beginning prematurely.

A woman in preterm labor is undergoing an extreme crisis situation. She cannot help asking herself, "What did I do to cause this?" Time spent taking the initial history or timing contractions presents an opportunity to not only bring that concern out in the open but any others she may have as well. She needs a strong support person with her during labor because if she has not yet taken a preparation for labor class, she may be more concerned than the average woman. Offer frequent assurance during labor that she is breathing well with contractions or just is "doing well." During the postpartum period, she may need continued reassurance as she is being asked to care for a very small and vulnerable-appearing infant. Helping rebuild self-esteem this way, therefore, not only prepares her better for the stress of labor but also to be a parent to her preterm infant.

QSEN Checkpoint Question 21.4

Teamwork & Collaboration

Beverly's husband drove her to the emergency room because she was having symptoms of preterm labor. What would you have wanted the admitting staff in the emergency department to do as their priority action?

a. Encourage her to carefully walk so the fetal head maintains pressure on her cervix.
b. Position her in a side-lying position and assess fetal heart rate and contractions.
c. Obtain blood for an hCG hormone assessment.
d. Ensure no one initiates intravenous fluid infusion because hypervolemia exacerbates preterm labor.

Look in Appendix A for the best answer and rationale.

PRETERM RUPTURE OF MEMBRANES

Preterm rupture of membranes is rupture of fetal membranes with loss of amniotic fluid before 37 weeks of pregnancy (Mercer, 2011). This occurs in 5% to 10% of pregnancies. The cause of preterm rupture is unknown, but it is strongly associated with infection of the membranes (i.e., chorioamnionitis). If rupture occurs early in pregnancy this way, it poses a major threat to the fetus as, after a rupture, the seal to the fetus is lost and uterine and fetal infections may occur. A second complication that can result is increased pressure on the umbilical cord from the loss of amniotic fluid (thus, inhibiting the fetal nutrient supply) or cord prolapse (extension of the cord out of the uterine cavity into the vagina past the small fetus), a condition that could also interfere with fetal circulation. Yet another risk to the fetus of remaining in a non–fluid-filled environment is the development of a Potter-like syndrome (i.e., distorted facial features and pulmonary hypoplasia from uterine pressure). In many instances, preterm labor follows rupture of the membranes and ends the pregnancy. If neither labor nor an infection begins, the greater the amount of amniotic fluid that remains (revealed by a sonogram), the better will be the pregnancy outcome (Storness-Bliss, Metcalfe, Simrose, et al., 2012).

Assessment

Rupture of the membranes is suggested by the history. A woman usually describes a sudden gush of clear fluid from her vagina, with continued minimal leakage. Occasionally, a woman mistakes urinary incontinence caused by exertion for rupture of membranes. Amniotic fluid cannot be differentiated from urine by appearance, so a sterile vaginal speculum examination is done to observe for vaginal pooling of fluid. If the fluid is tested with Nitrazine paper, amniotic fluid causes an alkaline reaction on the paper (appears blue) and urine causes an acidic reaction (remains yellow). The fluid can also be tested for ferning, or the typical appearance of a high-estrogen fluid on microscopic examination (amniotic fluid shows this; urine does not). The presence of a high level of α-fetoprotein (AFP) in the vagina is also diagnostic (van der Ham, van Melick, Smits, et al., 2011). If there is still a question regarding whether the membranes have ruptured, an ultrasound can be used to assess the amniotic fluid index. Because preterm rupture of membranes is associated with vaginal infection, cultures for *Neisseria gonorrhoeae*, group B streptococcus, and chlamydia are usually obtained. Blood is drawn for white blood cell count and C-reactive protein, both of which increase with membrane rupture. Avoid doing routine vaginal examinations because the risk of infection rises significantly when digital examinations are performed after preterm rupture of membranes.

Therapeutic Management

A future hope is that, by stem cell engineering, ruptured membranes can be repaired. Currently, however, if labor does not begin within 24 hours and the fetus is estimated to be mature enough by amniocentesis to survive in an extrauterine environment, labor contractions may be induced by intravenous administration of oxytocin so the infant can be born before infection can occur.

If the fetus is not at a point of viability, a woman is placed on bed rest either in the hospital or at home and administered a corticosteroid to hasten fetal lung maturity. Prophylactic administration of broad-spectrum antibiotics effective against group B streptococcus during this period may both delay the onset of labor and reduce the risk of infection in the newborn sufficiently to allow the corticosteroid to have its effect.

A woman with no signs of infection may be administered a tocolytic agent if labor contractions begin. Although its effectiveness is not well documented, a woman might be given an amnioinfusion (see Chapter 23) to reduce pressure on the fetus or cord and to allow a safer term birth (Mercer, 2011).

Nursing Diagnoses and Related Interventions

Nursing Diagnosis: Risk for infection related to preterm rupture of membranes without accompanying labor

Outcome Evaluation: Maternal white blood cell count remains below 20,000/mm^3; maternal temperature is less than 100.4°F (38.0°C) while awaiting fetal maturity.

An infection can be dangerous for both the mother and fetus; so, if at home, a woman is asked to take her temperature about twice a day and to report a fever (a temperature greater than 100.4°F [38.0°C]), uterine tenderness, or odorous vaginal discharge. She should refrain from tub bathing, douching, and coitus because of the danger of introducing infection. The white blood cell count will need to be assessed frequently. A count of more than 18,000 to 20,000/mm^3 suggests infection.

Before a woman is discharged to home care, be certain to ask if she has a thermometer, and provide her with specific instructions regarding what degree of temperature she should report, and if she understands the level of bed rest expected of her. Help her make arrangements for a daily white blood cell count through a laboratory service or home care nurse.

Many misconceptions about the difficulty of labor after preterm rupture of the membranes (i.e., "dry labor") exist. You can assure a woman that, because amniotic fluid is always being formed, there is no such thing as a dry labor.

What if . . . 21.3 Beverly is prescribed bed rest for 24 hours because of preterm contractions, but she tells you she's too busy to "waste time" on bed rest. What suggestions would you give her so she could best achieve bed rest? Does she have an ethical obligation to her fetus to rest? What about a legal obligation?

GESTATIONAL HYPERTENSION

Gestational hypertension is a condition in which vasospasm occurs in both small and large arteries during pregnancy, causing signs of increased blood pressure, proteinuria, and edema. An older term for the condition was toxemia of pregnancy because researchers pictured the symptoms as being caused by women producing a toxin of some kind in response to the foreign protein of the growing fetus. The condition occurs in 5% to 7% of pregnancies. The cause of the disorder is unknown, although it is highly correlated with the antiphospholipid syndrome or the presence of antiphospholipid antibodies in maternal blood (Danza, Ruiz-Irastorza, & Khamashta, 2012). The condition tends to occur most frequently in women of color, those with a multiple pregnancy, primiparas younger than 20 years or older than 40 years of age, women from low socioeconomic backgrounds (perhaps because of poor nutrition), those who have had five or more pregnancies, those who have **hydramnios** (i.e., overproduction of amniotic fluid; refer to discussion later), or those who have an underlying disease such as heart disease, diabetes with vessel or renal involvement, and essential hypertension (Miller, 2012).

Pathophysiologic Events

The symptoms of gestational hypertension affect almost all organs. The vascular spasm that occurs may be caused by the increased cardiac output required by pregnancy, which injures the endothelial cells of the arteries and reduces the action of prostacyclin—a prostaglandin vasodilator—and excess production of thromboxane—a prostaglandin vasoconstrictor and stimulant of platelet aggregation. Usually

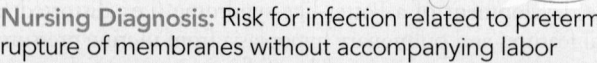

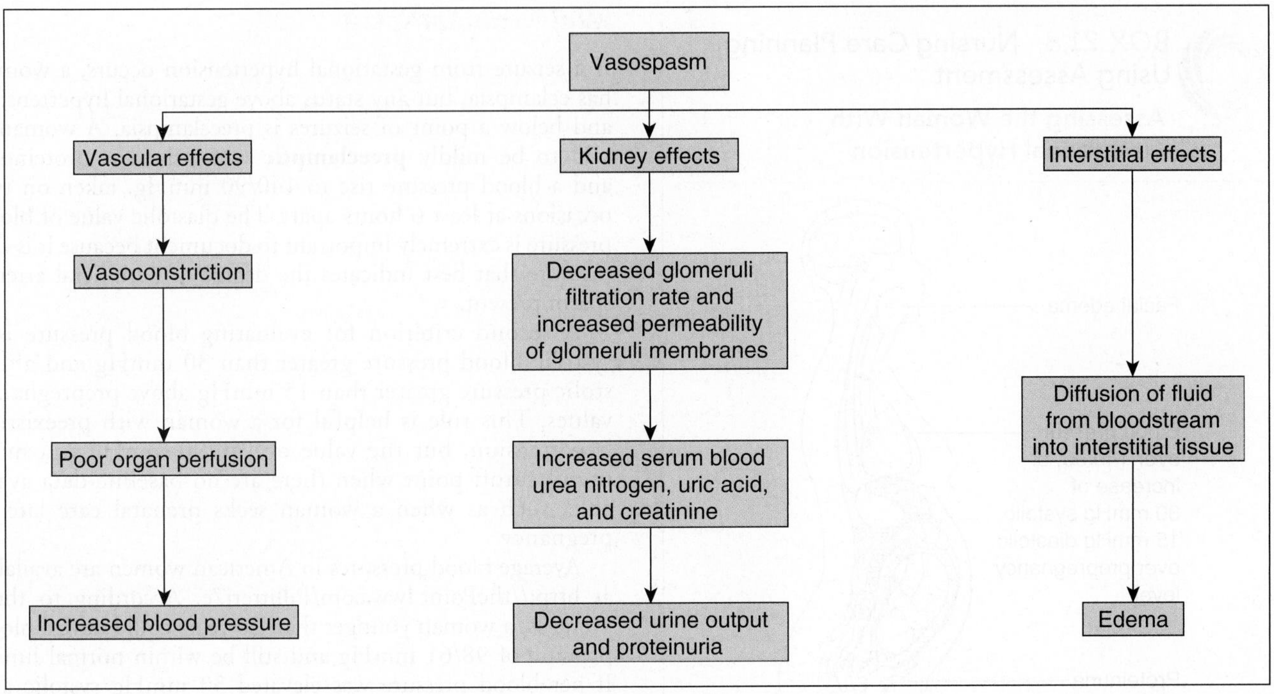

FIGURE 21.8 Physiologic changes with gestational hypertension.

during pregnancy, blood vessels are resistant to the effects of pressor substances such as angiotensin and norepinephrine, so even with the increased blood supply, blood pressure remains normal during pregnancy. With gestational hypertension, this reduced responsiveness to blood pressure changes appears to be lost because of the prostaglandin release. Vasoconstriction occurs and blood pressure increases dramatically.

Beginning about the 20th week of pregnancy, almost all body systems begin to be affected. The cardiac system, for example, can easily become overwhelmed because the heart is forced to pump against rising peripheral resistance. This causes a reduced blood supply to organs, most markedly the kidney, pancreas, liver, brain, and placenta. Poor placental perfusion reduces the fetal nutrient and oxygen supply. Ischemia in the pancreas can result in epigastric pain and an elevated amylase–creatinine ratio. If spasm occurs in the arteries of the retina, vision changes can occur. If this results in retinal hemorrhage, blindness can result.

Vasospasm in the kidney increases blood flow resistance. Degenerative changes then develop in the kidney glomeruli because of back pressure. This leads to increased permeability of the glomerular membrane, allowing the serum proteins albumin and globulin to escape into the urine (i.e., proteinuria). The degenerative changes also result in decreased glomerular filtration, so there is lowered urine output and clearance of creatinine. If increased kidney tubular reabsorption occurs, retention of sodium begins. As sodium retains fluid, edema results. Edema is further increased because, as more protein is lost, the osmotic pressure of the circulating blood falls and fluid diffuses from the circulatory system into the denser interstitial spaces to equalize the pressure (Fig. 21.8). Extreme edema can lead to maternal cerebral and pulmonary edema and seizures (**eclampsia**).

Yet another effect of the condition is that arterial spasm causes the bulk of the blood volume in the maternal circulation to be pooled in the venous circulation, so on assessment, a woman has a deceptively low arterial intravascular volume. In addition, thrombocytopenia or a lowered platelet count occurs as platelets cluster at the sites of endothelial damage. Measuring hematocrit levels helps to assess the extent of plasma loss to the interstitial space or the extent of the edema (the higher the hematocrit, the more is being lost). A hematocrit level above 40% suggests significant fluid loss into interstitial spaces.

Assessment

Although women may have additional symptoms such as vision changes, typically hypertension, proteinuria, and edema are considered the classic signs of gestational hypertension. Of the three, hypertension and proteinuria are the most significant because extensive edema occurs only after the other two are present (Box 21.8).

Gestational hypertension is classified as mild **preeclampsia**, severe preeclampsia, and eclampsia, depending on how far development of the syndrome has advanced (Table 21.6). Any woman with a high risk for gestational hypertension should be observed carefully for symptoms at prenatal visits. She needs instructions about what symptoms to watch for so she can alert her health care provider if symptoms begin to occur between visits.

Gestational Hypertension

A woman is said to have gestational hypertension when she develops an elevated blood pressure (140/90 mmHg) but has no proteinuria or edema. Perinatal mortality is not increased with simple gestational hypertension, so careful observation but no drug therapy is necessary.

BOX 21.8 Nursing Care Planning Using Assessment

Assessing the Woman With Gestational Hypertension

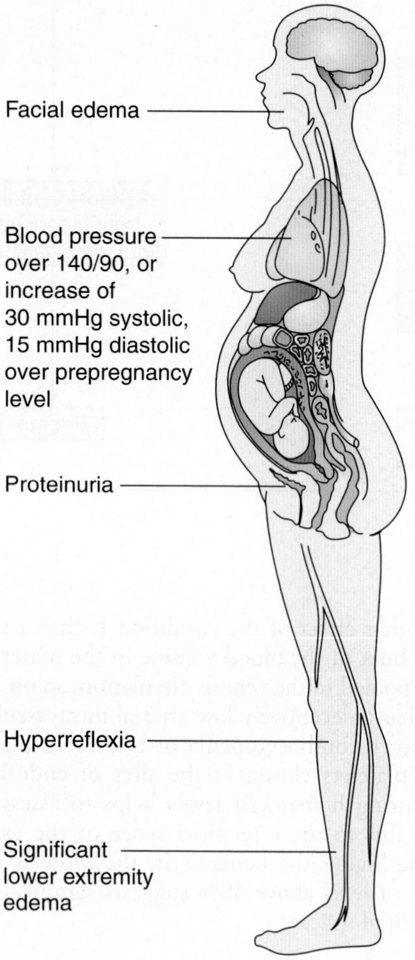

Mild Preeclampsia

If a seizure from gestational hypertension occurs, a woman has eclampsia, but any status above gestational hypertension and below a point of seizures is preeclampsia. A woman is said to be mildly **preeclamptic** when she has proteinuria and a blood pressure rise to 140/90 mmHg, taken on two occasions at least 6 hours apart. The diastolic value of blood pressure is extremely important to document because it is this pressure that best indicates the degree of peripheral arterial spasm present.

A second criterion for evaluating blood pressure is a systolic blood pressure greater than 30 mmHg and a diastolic pressure greater than 15 mmHg above prepregnancy values. This rule is helpful for a woman with preexisting hypertension, but the value of 140/90 mmHg is a more useful cutoff point when there are no baseline data available, such as when a woman seeks prenatal care late in pregnancy.

Average blood pressures in American women are available at http://thePoint.lww.com/Pillitteri7e. According to these averages, a woman younger than 20 years could have a blood pressure of 98/61 mmHg and still be within normal limits. If her blood pressure was elevated 30 mmHg systolic and 15 mmHg diastolic, it would be only 128/76 mmHg. This is well beneath the traditional warning point of 140/90 mmHg, but would represent hypertension for her.

Many women show a trace of protein during pregnancy. Actual proteinuria is said to exist when it registers as 1+ or more (this represents a loss of 1 g/L). A woman with preeclampsia will begin to show proteinuria of 1+ or 2+ on a reagent test strip on a random sample.

Occasionally, women have orthostatic proteinuria (i.e., on long periods of standing, they excrete protein; on bed rest, they do not). If proteinuria is present without other signs of gestational hypertension (no hypertension and no edema), check to see when the specimen was obtained. Ask her to bring in a first morning urine sample next time as that may reveal that orthostatic proteinuria, not preeclampsia, is the cause of protein in her urine.

Edema develops, as mentioned, because of the protein loss, sodium retention, and lowered glomerular filtration rate. The

TABLE 21.6 Symptoms of Gestational Hypertension

Hypertension Type	Symptoms
Gestational hypertension	Blood pressure is 140/90 mmHg or systolic pressure elevated 30 mmHg or diastolic pressure elevated 15 mmHg above prepregnancy level; no proteinuria or edema; blood pressure returns to normal after birth.
Mild preeclampsia	Blood pressure is 140/90 mmHg or systolic pressure elevated 30 mmHg or diastolic pressure elevated 15 mmHg above prepregnancy level; proteinuria of 1+–2+ on a random sample; weight gain over 2 lb/wk in second trimester and 1 lb/wk in third trimester; mild edema in upper extremities or face.
Severe preeclampsia	Blood pressure is 160/110 mmHg; proteinuria 3+–4+ on a random sample and 5 g on a 24-hr sample; oliguria (500 ml or less in 24 hr or altered renal function tests; elevated serum creatinine more than 1.2 mg/dl); cerebral or visual disturbances (headache, blurred vision); pulmonary or cardiac involvement; extensive peripheral edema; hepatic dysfunction; thrombocytopenia; epigastric pain.
Eclampsia	Either seizure or coma accompanied by signs and symptoms of preeclampsia are present.

edema can be separated from the typical ankle edema of pregnancy because it begins to accumulate in the upper part of the body as well. A weight gain of more than 2 lb/wk in the second trimester or 1 lb/wk in the third trimester usually indicates abnormal tissue fluid retention is occurring. No noticeable edema may be present when this sudden increase in weight first occurs or it will be the first symptom a woman notices.

Severe Preeclampsia

A woman has passed from mild-to-severe preeclampsia when her blood pressure rises to 160 mmHg systolic and 110 mmHg diastolic or above on at least two occasions 6 hours apart at bed rest (the position in which blood pressure is lowest) or her diastolic pressure is 30 mmHg above her prepregnancy level. Marked proteinuria, 3+ or 4+ on a random urine sample or more than 5 g in a 24-hour sample, and extensive edema are also present (Brown & Garovic, 2011).

With severe preeclampsia, the extreme edema is most readily palpated over bony surfaces, such as over the tibia on the anterior leg, the ulnar surface of the forearm, and the cheekbones, where the sponginess of fluid-filled tissue can be palpated against bone. If there is swelling or puffiness at these points to a palpating finger but the swelling cannot be indented with finger pressure, the edema is described as nonpitting. If the tissue can be indented slightly, this is 1+ pitting edema; moderate indentation is 2+; deep indentation is 3+; and indentation so deep it remains after removal of the finger is 4+ pitting edema. This accumulating edema will reduce a woman's urine output to approximately 400 to 600 ml per 24 hours.

It's helpful to further assess edema by asking a woman if she has noticed any swelling anywhere in her body. Women commonly report upper extremity edema as "my rings are so tight I can't get them off" and facial edema as "when I wake in the morning, my eyes are swollen shut" or "My tongue is so swollen I can't talk until I walk around awhile."

Some women report severe epigastric pain and nausea or vomiting, possibly because abdominal edema or ischemia to the pancreas and liver has occurred. If pulmonary edema has developed, a woman may report feeling short of breath. If cerebral edema has occurred, reports of visual disturbances such as blurred vision or seeing spots before the eyes may be reported. Cerebral edema also produces symptoms of severe headache and marked hyperreflexia and perhaps **ankle clonus** (i.e., a continued motion of the foot) (Box 21.9).

BOX 21.9 Nursing Care Planning Using Procedures

ELICITING A PATELLAR REFLEX AND ANKLE CLONUS

PATELLAR REFLEX

With the woman in a supine position, ask her to bend her knee slightly. Place your hand under her knee to support the leg. Locate the patellar tendon in the midline of the anterior leg just below the kneecap. Strike it firmly and quickly with a reflex hammer or the side of your hand. If the leg and foot move, a patellar reflex is present. The reflex is scored as:

0	=	No response; hypoactive; abnormal
1+	=	Somewhat diminished response but not abnormal
2+	=	Average response
3+	=	Brisker than average but not abnormal
4+	=	Hyperactive; very brisk; abnormal

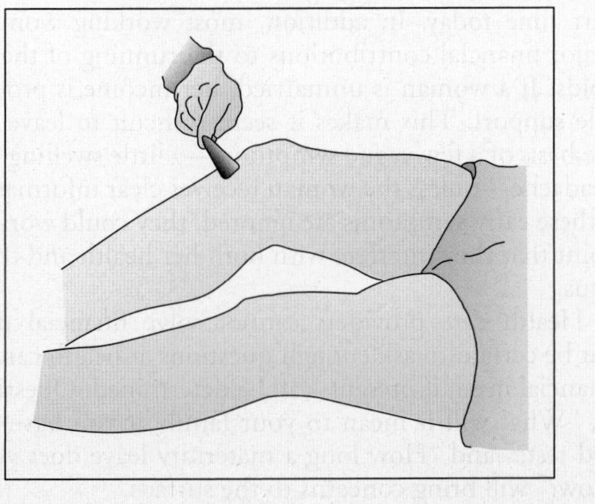

ANKLE CLONUS

To elicit ankle clonus, dorsiflex the woman's foot three times in rapid succession. As you take your hand away, observe the foot. If no further motion is present, no ankle clonus is present. If the foot continues to move involuntarily, clonus is present. Although usually just rated as present or absent, it can be rated as:

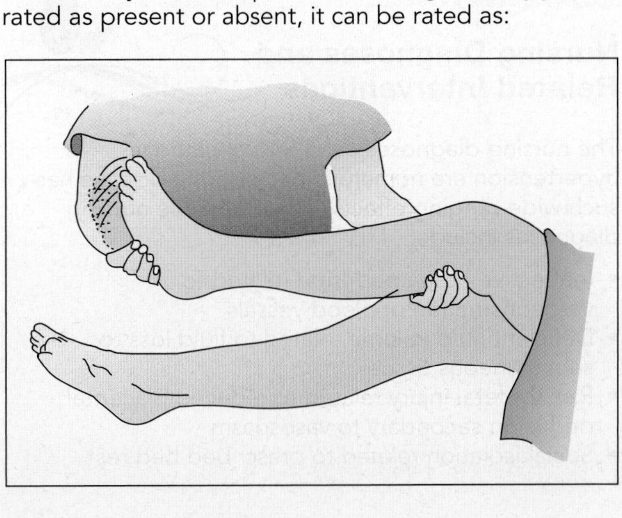

Mild = 2 movements
Moderate = 3–5 movements
Severe = Over 6 movements

Eclampsia

This is the most severe classification of gestational hypertension. A woman has passed into this stage when cerebral edema is so acute a grand mal (tonic–clonic) seizure or coma has occurred. With eclampsia, the maternal mortality can be as high as 20% from causes such as cerebral hemorrhage, circulatory collapse, or renal failure (Liu, Joseph, Liston, et al., 2011).

The fetal prognosis with eclampsia is also poor because of hypoxia, possibly caused by the seizure, with consequent fetal acidosis. If premature separation of the placenta from extreme vasospasm occurs, the fetal prognosis becomes even graver. If a fetus must be born before term, all the risks of immaturity will be faced.

QSEN Checkpoint Question 21.5

Informatics

You routinely assess all pregnant women for signs of hypertension as you interview them at your prenatal clinic and then document the findings in their electronic health record. Which statement by Beverly would you document as possible evidence that she might be developing gestational hypertension?

a. "My feet are so swollen at night I can't put on my bedroom slippers."
b. "I never guessed I would feel as tired as I do just from being pregnant."
c. "My abdomen feels firm, as if I had a blown-up balloon inside me."
d. "I can live with my puffy feet, but now it's also my hands and wrists."

Look in Appendix A for the best answer and rationale.

Nursing Diagnoses and Related Interventions

The nursing diagnoses used with gestational hypertension are numerous because the disease has such wide-ranging effects. Some possible nursing diagnoses include:

- Ineffective tissue perfusion related to vasoconstriction of blood vessels
- Deficient fluid volume related to fluid loss to subcutaneous tissue
- Risk for fetal injury related to reduced placental perfusion secondary to vasospasm
- Social isolation related to prescribed bed rest

Nursing Interventions for a Woman With Mild Gestational Hypertension

Clients with mild gestational hypertension levels can be managed at home with frequent follow-up care.

Monitor Antiplatelet Therapy

Because of the increased tendency for platelets to cluster along arterial walls, a mild antiplatelet agent, such as low-dose aspirin, may prevent or delay the development of preeclampsia (Roberge, Villa, Nicolaides, et al., 2012). Because aspirin is such a common, over-the-counter drug, be certain women appreciate that this is not something to be taken lightly but a serious drug prescription for them. Be certain they purchase low-dose aspirin (50 to 80 mg, sold as baby aspirin) as excessive salicylic levels can cause maternal bleeding at the time of birth.

Promote Bed Rest

When the body is in a recumbent position, sodium tends to be excreted at a faster rate than during activity. Bed rest, therefore, is the best method of aiding increased evacuation of sodium and encouraging diuresis of edema fluid. Be certain women know to rest in a lateral recumbent position to avoid uterine pressure on the vena cava and prevent supine hypotension syndrome.

Promote Good Nutrition

A woman needs to continue her usual pregnancy nutrition while on bed rest. At one time, stringent restriction of salt was advised in order to reduce edema. This is no longer true because stringent sodium restriction may activate the renin-angiotensin-aldosterone system and actually result in increased blood pressure, thus compounding the problem.

Assess if a woman has someone to help her prepare food, or either bed rest or nutrition may be compromised.

Provide Emotional Support

It is difficult for a woman with preeclampsia to appreciate the potential seriousness of symptoms because they are so vague; neither high blood pressure nor protein in urine is something she can see or feel. She is aware edema is present, but it seems unrelated to the pregnancy; after all, it is in her hands and face, not a body area near her growing child.

Women are also used to having severe disorders treated with some form of medication. If no other medicine than low-dose aspirin is prescribed, this can make a woman underestimate the severity of her situation, causing her to take instructions such as getting rest lightly. Almost 90% of women of childbearing age work outside their home at least part time today. In addition, most working women make major financial contributions to the running of their households. If a woman is unmarried, her income is probably her sole support. This makes it seem difficult to leave work on the basis of a few vague symptoms—a little swelling or a little headache—unless the woman receives clear information that, if these early symptoms are ignored, they could worsen to the point that they interfere with both her health and that of her fetus.

Health care providers cannot solve financial problems, but be certain to ask enough questions at health care visits so financial need, if present, can be determined. Questions such as, "What will it mean to your family if you have to be on bed rest?" and "How long a maternity leave does your work allow?" will bring concerns to the surface.

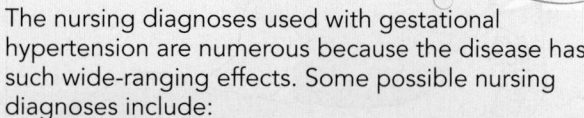

Ask if a woman with small children will need to make child care arrangements so she can get sufficient rest. The woman who spends considerable time chauffeuring school-age children to activities may need to investigate carpooling as an alternative. Ask, "What will it mean to your other children or your husband if you have to rest?" to allow her to begin to examine these problems. Remember, having a wife or mother on bed rest is a stress on the total family, so other family members may need support as well.

Women with beginning signs of hypertension will be seen approximately weekly or more frequently for the remainder of pregnancy. Be certain a woman understands that if symptoms worsen before her next health care visit, she should report them immediately.

Nursing Interventions for a Woman With Severe Gestational Hypertension

If a woman's preeclampsia is severe (systolic blood pressure of more than 160 mmHg, diastolic blood pressure of more than 110 mmHg after a woman has been on bed rest; extensive edema; marked proteinuria [3+ to 4+]; cerebral or visual disturbances; marked hyperreflexia; or oliguria [500 ml per 24 hours or less]), a woman may be admitted to a health care facility for care. If the pregnancy is 39 weeks and fetal lung maturity can be confirmed by amniocentesis, labor can be induced or a cesarean birth performed to end the pregnancy at that point. If the pregnancy is less than 39 weeks or amniocentesis reveals immature lung function, interventions will be instituted to attempt to alleviate the severe symptoms and allow the fetus to come to term.

Support Bed Rest

With severe preeclampsia, most women are hospitalized, so that bed rest can be enforced and a woman can be observed more closely than she can be on home care. Visitors are usually restricted to support people such as a partner, father of the child, mother, or older children. Because a loud noise such as a crying baby or a dropped tray of equipment can be sufficient to trigger a seizure that initiates eclampsia, a woman with severe preeclampsia is admitted to a private room so she can rest as undisturbed as possible. Raise side rails to help prevent injury if a seizure should occur.

Darken the room if possible because a bright light can also trigger seizures. However, the room should not be so dark that caregivers need to use a flashlight to make assessments. Shining a flashlight beam into a woman's eyes is the kind of sudden stimulation to be avoided.

Stress is another stimulus capable of increasing blood pressure and evoking seizures in a woman with severe preeclampsia. Be certain, therefore, the woman receives clear explanations of what is happening and what is planned, especially about the need for visitor restrictions and not to "cheat" on bed rest. Allow her opportunities to express her feelings about what is happening or how bewildered she is because the few simple symptoms she noticed 2 weeks ago (e.g., increase in weight, increasing edema) have now developed into a syndrome that may be lethal to her baby and possibly to herself.

Monitor Maternal Well-being

Take blood pressure frequently (at least every 4 hours) or with a continuous monitoring device to detect any increase, which is a warning that a woman's condition is worsening. Obtain blood studies such as a complete blood count, platelet count, liver function, blood urea nitrogen, and creatine and fibrin degradation products as prescribed to assess renal and liver function and the development of DIC, which often accompanies severe vasospasm, as well as plasma estriol levels (a test of placenta function), and electrolyte levels. Because a woman is at high risk for premature separation of the placenta and resulting hemorrhage, a blood sample for type and cross-match is usually also obtained.

Daily hematocrit levels are used to monitor blood concentration (this level will rise if increased fluid is leaving the bloodstream for interstitial tissue [edema]). A woman's optic fundus should be assessed daily for signs of arterial spasm, edema, or hemorrhage.

Obtain daily weights at the same time each day as another evaluation of fluid retention. Ensure a woman is wearing the same amount of clothing at each weighing so any change in weight is not influenced by a change in the weight of her clothing.

An indwelling urinary catheter may be inserted to allow accurate recording of output and comparison with intake. Urinary output should be more than 30 ml/hr; an output lower than this suggests oliguria. Urinary proteins and specific gravity are measured and recorded with voiding or hourly if an indwelling catheter is present. A 24-hour urine sample may be collected for protein and creatinine clearance determinations to evaluate kidney function. A woman with mild preeclampsia spills between 0.5 and 1 g of protein every 24 hours (1+ on a random sample); a woman with severe preeclampsia spills approximately 5 g per 24 hours (3+ to 4+ on an individual specimen).

Monitor Fetal Well-being

Generally, single Doppler auscultation at approximately 4-hour intervals is sufficient at this stage of management. A woman may have a nonstress test or biophysical profile done daily to assess uteroplacental sufficiency (see Chapter 9). If fetal bradycardia occurs, oxygen administration to the mother may be necessary to maintain adequate fetal oxygenation.

Support a Nutritious Intake

A woman needs a diet moderate to high in protein and moderate in sodium to compensate for the protein she is losing in urine. An intravenous fluid line is usually initiated and maintained to serve as an emergency route for drug administration as well as to administer fluid to reduce hemoconcentration and hypovolemia.

Administer Medications to Prevent Eclampsia

A hypotensive drug such as hydralazine (Apresoline), labetalol (Normodyne), or nifedipine may be prescribed to reduce hypertension. These drugs act to lower blood pressure by peripheral dilatation and thus do not interfere with placental circulation. They can, however, cause maternal tachycardia, so assess pulse and blood pressure before and after administration. Diastolic pressure should not be lowered below 80 to 90 mmHg or inadequate placental perfusion could occur. Even with these new drugs, magnesium sulfate (Table 21.7) still remains the drug of choice to prevent eclampsia (Hunter & Gibbins, 2011). This drug, classified as a cathartic, reduces

TABLE 21.7 Drugs Used in Gestational Hypertension

Drug	Indication	Dosage	Comments
Magnesium sulfate (Pregnancy risk category B)	Muscle relaxant; prevents seizures	Loading dose 4–6 g Maintenance dose 1–2 g/h IV	Infuse loading dose slowly over 15–30 min. Always administer as a piggyback infusion. Assess respiratory rate, urine output, deep tendon reflexes, and clonus every hour. Urine output should be over 30 ml/hr and respiratory rate over 12 breaths/min. Serum magnesium level should remain below 7.5 mEq/l. Observe for central nervous system (CNS) depression and hypotonia in infant at birth and calcium deficit in the mother.
Hydralazine (Apresoline) (Pregnancy risk category C)	Antihypertensive (peripheral vasodilator); used to decrease hypertension	5–10 mg IV	Administer slowly to avoid sudden fall in blood pressure. Maintain diastolic pressure over 90 mmHg to ensure adequate placental filling.
Diazepam (Valium) (Pregnancy risk category D)	Halt seizures	5–10 mg IV	Administer slowly. Dose may be repeated q 5–10 min (up to 30 mg/hr). Observe for respiratory depression or hypotension in mother and respiratory depression and hypotonia in infant at birth.
Calcium gluconate (Pregnancy risk category C)	Antidote for magnesium intoxication	1 g IV (10 ml of a 10% solution)	Have prepared at bedside as the antidote when administering magnesium sulfate. Administer at 5 ml/min.

From: Karch, A. M. (2013). *2013 Lippincott's nursing drug guide*. Philadelphia, PA: Lippincott Williams & Wilkins.

edema by causing a shift in fluid from the extracellular spaces into the intestine. It also has a central nervous system depressant action (it blocks peripheral neuromuscular transmissions), which lessens the possibility of seizures (Karch, 2013). To achieve an immediate reduction of blood pressure, magnesium sulfate may first be given intravenously in a loading or bolus dose. The drug begins to act almost immediately; unfortunately, the effect lasts only 30 to 60 minutes, so administration must be continuous.

The importance of different serum levels of magnesium sulfate is shown in Box 21.10. For the drug to act as an anticonvulsant, blood serum levels must be maintained at 5 to 8 mg per 100 ml. If the blood serum level rises above this, respiratory depression, cardiac arrhythmias, and cardiac arrest can occur.

The most evident symptoms of overdose from magnesium sulfate administration include decreased urine output, depressed respirations, reduced consciousness, and decreased deep tendon reflexes. Because magnesium is excreted from the body almost entirely through the urine, urine output must be monitored closely to ensure adequate elimination. If severe oliguria should occur (less than 100 ml in 4 hours), excessively high serum levels of magnesium can result. Before you administer further magnesium sulfate, therefore, ensure that urine output is above 25 to 30 ml/hr, with a specific gravity of 1.010 or lower. Respirations should be above 12 breaths/min, a woman should be able to answer questions asked of her such as her name or address, ankle clonus should be minimal, and deep tendon reflexes should be present. Make these assessments every hour if a continuous intravenous infusion is being used.

The easiest deep tendon reflex to assess is the patellar reflex (i.e., knee jerk). Instructions for initiating this reflex and ankle clonus are shown in Box 21.9. If an epidural block has been given for labor anesthesia, assess the biceps or triceps reflex (see Chapter 34).

In addition to making the previous assessments when magnesium sulfate is being given, a solution of 10 ml of a 10% calcium gluconate solution (1 g) should be kept ready nearby for immediate intravenous administration should a woman develop signs and symptoms of magnesium toxicity, as calcium is the specific antidote for magnesium toxicity. Severe oliguria may be treated by the intravenous infusion of salt-poor albumin. This high-colloid solution will call fluid into the bloodstream from interstitial tissue by osmotic pressure; the kidneys will then excrete the extra fluid along with magnesium sulfate levels.

A fetal heart rate monitor during pregnancy may show loss of variability of the heartbeat immediately after magnesium therapy; an ultrasound may reveal reduced fetal breathing movements. Observe carefully for other signs of fetal effects, such as late deceleration with labor contractions. Magnesium sulfate is continued for 12 to 24 hours in the woman after birth to prevent eclampsia during this period. The dose is then tapered and discontinued. Breastfeeding usually is delayed until the medication is discontinued. A long-term effect of magnesium sulfate therapy is osteoporosis. A woman may be started on a course of calcium postpartally to decrease this problem. On the planned day of birth, the baby's primary care provider should be alerted that the woman has been receiving magnesium sulfate. This is because if magnesium sulfate, which crosses the placenta, is given intravenously within 2 hours of a baby's birth, the baby may be born with severe respiratory depression.

BOX 21.10 Nursing Care Planning Based on Responsibility for Pharmacology

MAGNESIUM SULFATE

Action: Magnesium sulfate is a central nervous system depressant that acts to block neuromuscular transmission of acetylcholine to halt convulsions. It also halts premature labor, as it relaxes smooth muscle (Karch, 2013).

Pregnancy Risk Category: A

Dosage: Initially, 2 to 6 g IV administered in a 250-ml solution over a 20-minute period, followed by individually calculated IV infusion at a rate to maintain designated serum levels

- Therapeutic range: 5 to 8 mg/100 ml
- Patellar reflex disappears: 8 to 10 mg/100 ml
- Respiratory depression occurs: 15 to 20 mg/100 ml
- Cardiac conduction defects occur: More than 20 mg/100 ml

Possible Adverse Effects: Flushing, thirst; with toxicity, absence of deep tendon reflexes, respiratory depression, cardiac arrhythmias, cardiac arrest, and decreased urine output

Nursing Implications

- Administer continuous infusion piggybacked into a main IV line so it can be discontinued immediately without interfering with fluid administration.
- Always use an infusion control device to maintain a regular flow rate.
- Assess maternal blood pressure and fetal heart rate continuously with bolus IV administration.
- Assess deep tendon reflexes every 1 to 4 hours during continuous infusion. Use the patellar reflex. If patient has received epidural anesthesia, use the biceps reflex.
- Monitor intake and output every hour during continuous infusion. Urine output should be 30 ml/hr or greater.
- Assess client's level of consciousness, including ability to respond to questions, every hour.
- Obtain serum magnesium levels as indicated, usually every 6 to 8 hours.
- Keep calcium gluconate, the antidote for toxicity, readily available at the bedside.
- Maintain serum blood levels (for anticonvulsant use) at 5 to 8 mg/100 ml. If blood serum levels rise above this, respiratory depression, cardiac arrhythmias, and cardiac arrest can occur.
- Do not administer additional doses and stop infusion if deep tendon reflexes are absent or if respiratory rate is less than 12–14 breaths/min or urine output is less than 30 ml/hr.
- This drug may cause respiratory depression in the newborn if administered close to birth. Alert neonatal care personnel about this possibility.
- Magnesium sulfate may cause osteoporosis in the mother if given over a long time.

Nursing Interventions for a Woman With Eclampsia

Degeneration of a woman's condition from severe preeclampsia to eclampsia occurs when cerebral irritation from increasing cerebral edema becomes so acute that a seizure occurs. This usually happens late in pregnancy but can happen up to 48 hours after childbirth. Immediately before a seizure, a woman's blood pressure rises suddenly from additional vasospasm. The increased cerebral pressure causes her temperature to rise sharply to 103° to 104°F (39.4° to 40°C). She notices blurring of vision or severe headache (from the increased cerebral edema), and her reflexes become hyperactive. She may experience a premonition or aura that "something is happening." Vascular congestion of the liver or pancreas can lead to severe epigastric pain and nausea or vomiting. Urinary output may decrease abruptly to less than 30 ml/hr. However, eclampsia has actually occurred, by definition, only when a woman experiences a seizure.

Tonic–Clonic Seizures

An eclamptic seizure is a tonic–clonic type that occurs in stages. After the preliminary signal or aura that something is happening, all the muscles of the woman's body contract. Her back arches, her arms and legs stiffen, and her jaw closes so abruptly she may bite her tongue. Respirations halt because her thoracic muscles are held in contraction. This phase of the seizure, called the tonic phase, lasts approximately 20 seconds. It may seem longer because a woman may grow slightly cyanotic from the cessation of respirations.

During the second (clonic) stage, the woman's bladder and bowel muscles contract and relax; incontinence of urine and feces may occur. Although a woman begins to breathe during this stage, the breathing is not entirely effective so she may remain cyanotic. The clonic stage of a seizure lasts up to 1 minute. Following this she will enter an hour long postictal stage, during which she is unconscious.

The priority care for a woman with a tonic–clonic seizure is to maintain a patent airway. To prevent aspiration, turn her onto her side to allow secretions to drain from her mouth. Magnesium sulfate or diazepam (Valium) may be administered intravenously as emergency measures. Assess oxygen saturation via a pulse oximeter. Administer oxygen by face mask as needed to protect fetal oxygenation. Apply an external fetal heart monitor if one is not already in place to assess the fetal heart rate. The seizure may announce the beginning of labor, so assess as well for uterine contractions. Check for vaginal bleeding to detect placental separation, although evidence placental separation has occurred will probably appear first on the fetal heart record; vaginal bleeding will strengthen the presumption.

During the postictal stage, a woman cannot be roused except by painful stimuli for 1 to 4 hours. Extremely close observation is therefore as important during this third stage as it was during the first two stages. Be certain to assess for uterine contractions during this stage because, if labor begins during this period, the woman will be unable to report the sensation of contractions. Also, the painful stimulus of contractions may initiate another seizure. Be certain to keep the woman on her side so secretions can drain from her mouth.

Give her nothing to eat or drink. Remember that with coma, hearing is not necessarily lost, so be certain conversation is limited to those things you would say if she were awake. Continue to check for vaginal bleeding every 15 minutes.

Birth

If the fetus has reached a point of viability, a decision about birth will be made as soon as a woman's condition stabilizes, usually 12 to 24 hours after the seizure. Probably because of the increased stress that has occurred, fetal lung maturity appears to advance rapidly with gestational hypertension, so even though the fetus is younger than 37 weeks, the lecithin/sphingomyelin ratio may indicate fetal lung maturity.

Cesarean birth is always more hazardous for the fetus than vaginal birth because of the association of retained lung fluid (see Chapter 26). Further, a woman with severe high blood pressure is not a good candidate for surgery. An additional problem arises: because her vascular system is low in volume, she may become hypotensive with regional anesthesia, such as an epidural block. The preferred method for birth, therefore, is vaginal with a minimum of anesthesia. If labor does not begin spontaneously, rupture of the membranes or induction of labor with intravenous oxytocin may be instituted. If this is ineffective and the fetus appears to be in imminent danger, cesarean birth becomes the birth method of choice.

Nursing Interventions During the Postpartum Period

Postpartum hypertension may occur up to 10 to 14 days after birth, although it usually occurs within 48 hours after birth. Therefore, monitoring blood pressure in the postpartum period and at health care visits and being alert for eclampsia, which can occur as late as 2 weeks postbirth, are essential to detect this residual hypertension (Al-Safi, Imudia, Filetti, et al., 2011).

QSEN Checkpoint Question 21.6

Evidence-Based Practice

Because so many women of childbearing age work at physically demanding occupations, researchers studied the work requirements of 4,465 pregnant woman and then analyzed if there was an association between their work characteristics and the development of gestational hypertension. Results of the study showed no consistent association between any of the work-related risk factors studied, such as long periods of standing or walking, heavy lifting, night shifts, and long working hours with hypertensive disorders during pregnancy (Nugteren, Snijder, Hofman, et al., 2012).

Based on the previous study, which statement by Beverly about her job as a secretary at a construction site would give you the most concern regarding fetal health?

a. "I think I likely walk at least a mile every work day."
b. "I rarely have time to eat when I'm at work because I get so busy."
c. "Sometimes I have to move boxes of files around the office."
d. "I usually help my colleague bring boxes of paper up to the office for the photocopier."

Look in Appendix A for the best answer and rationale.

HELLP SYNDROME

HELLP syndrome is a variation of gestational hypertension that is named for the common symptoms that occur: **h**emolysis that leads to anemia, **e**levated **l**iver enzymes that lead to epigastric pain, **l**ow platelets that lead to abnormal bleeding/clotting, and **p**etechia (Abildgaard & Heimdal, 2013). The syndrome occurs in 4% to 12% of patients who have elevated blood pressure during pregnancy. It is a serious syndrome because it results in a maternal mortality rate as high as 24% and an infant mortality rate as high as 35%.

Why some women with elevated blood pressure also develop the HELLP syndrome is unknown. It occurs in both primigravidas and multigravidas and is associated with antiphospholipid syndrome or the presence of antiphospholipid antibodies (Mineo & Shaul, 2011).

In addition to proteinuria, edema, and increased blood pressure, additional symptoms of nausea, epigastric pain, general malaise, and right upper quadrant tenderness from liver inflammation occur. Laboratory studies reveal hemolysis of red blood cells (they appear fragmented on a peripheral blood smear), thrombocytopenia (a platelet count $<100,000/mm^3$), and elevated liver enzyme levels (alanine aminotransferase [ALT] and serum aspartate aminotransferase [AST]), which are all effects of hemorrhage and necrosis of the liver. Because of the low platelet count, women with the HELLP syndrome need extremely close observation for bleeding, in addition to the observations necessary for preeclampsia. Complications associated with the syndrome are subcapsular liver hematoma, hyponatremia, renal failure, and hypoglycemia from poor liver function. Mothers are also at risk for cerebral hemorrhages, aspiration pneumonia, and hypoxic encephalopathy. Fetal complications can include growth restriction and preterm birth (Iwashita, Kan'o, Hattori, et al., 2012).

Therapy for the condition is transfusion of fresh frozen plasma or platelets in order to improve the platelet count. If hypoglycemia is present, this is corrected by an intravenous glucose infusion. The infant is born as soon as feasible by either vaginal or cesarean birth. Be alert that maternal hemorrhage may occur at birth because of poor clotting ability. Epidural anesthesia may not be possible because of the low platelet count and the high possibility of bleeding at the epidural site. Laboratory results return to normal after birth, the same as preeclamptic symptoms, but the experience of developing the HELLP syndrome is frightening. Women need assurance afterward that symptoms were pregnancy related and so will not return.

MULTIPLE PREGNANCY

Multiple gestation is considered a complication of pregnancy because a woman's body must adjust to the effects of more than one fetus. The incidence of multiple births has increased dramatically because of the use of in vitro fertilization, but still only occurs in 2% to 3% of all births (Bush & Pernoll, 2012).

Identical (i.e., monozygotic) twins begin with a single ovum and spermatozoon. In the process of fusion, or in one of the first cell divisions, the zygote divides into two identical individuals. Single-ovum twins usually have one placenta, one chorion, two amnions, and two umbilical cords. The twins are always of the same sex; they account for one

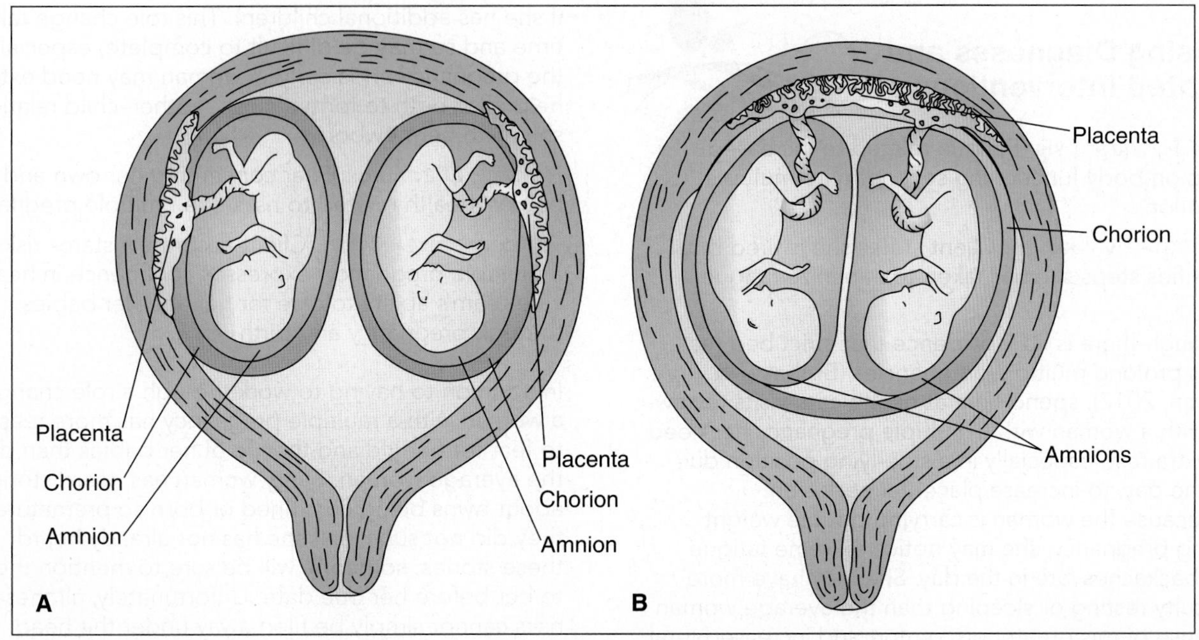

FIGURE 21.9 Multiple gestations. **(A)** Dizygotic twins showing two placentas, two chorions, and two amnions. **(B)** Monozygotic twins with one placenta, one chorion, and two amnions.

third of twin births. The other two thirds of twins are fraternal (i.e., dizygotic, nonidentical), the result of the fertilization of two separate ova by two separate spermatozoa (possibly not from the same sexual partner). Double-ova twins have two placentas, two chorions, two amnions, and two umbilical cords. The twins may be of the same or a different sex (Fig. 21.9). It is sometimes difficult to determine by ultrasound or at birth whether twins are identical or fraternal because the two fraternal placentas may fuse and appear as one large placenta.

Multiple pregnancies of two to eight children may be single-ovum conceptions, multiple-ova conceptions, or a combination of the two types. Most multiple pregnancies today occur from multiple ova being implanted as an in vitro fertility process. Naturally occurring multiple pregnancies are more frequent in blacks and Hispanics than Caucasians. The higher a woman's parity and age, the more likely she is to have a multiple gestation. Inheritance appears to play a role in natural dizygotic twinning; this has a familial maternal pattern of occurrence.

Assessment

Multiple gestation is suspected early in pregnancy, when the uterus begins to increase in size at a rate faster than usual. AFP levels will also be elevated. At the time of quickening, a woman may report flurries of action at different portions of her abdomen rather than at one consistent spot (e.g., where the feet are located). On auscultation of the abdomen, multiple sets of fetal heart sounds can be heard; although if one or more fetus has his or her back positioned toward a woman's back, only one fetal heart sound may be heard.

An ultrasound can reveal multiple gestation sacs early in pregnancy. In some instances, early ultrasound examinations reveal multiple amniotic sacs but then later in pregnancy, in as many as 30% of women, only one fetus remains (i.e., vanishing twin syndrome) (Sankaran, Rozette, Dean, et al., 2011). Women who were told they were having twins but then later in pregnancy find out they are having only one child may grieve for a vanished twin as much as if the baby had died at birth. This emotional response is important in an assessment because it could disrupt pregnancy bonding work.

Therapeutic Management

Women with a multiple gestation are more susceptible to complications of pregnancy such as gestational hypertension, hydramnios, placenta previa, preterm labor, and anemia than are women carrying one fetus. Following birth, they are more prone to postpartum bleeding because of the additional uterine stretching that occurred. Because a multiple pregnancy usually ends before term, 25% of low–birth-weight babies are from multiple pregnancies. There is a higher incidence of velamentous cord insertion (the cord inserted into the fetal membranes) with twins than with single births, so the risk of bleeding at the time of birth from a torn cord is increased. If monozygotic twins share a common vascular communication, it can lead to overgrowth of one fetus and undergrowth of the second (a twin-to-twin transfusion), resulting in discordant infants (Corsello & Piro, 2010) (see Chapter 26). If a single amnion is present, there can be knotting and twisting of umbilical cords, causing fetal distress or difficulty with birth. Because of the possibility of these complications, a woman with a twin pregnancy needs closer prenatal supervision than a woman with a single gestation to detect these problems as early as possible. A woman carrying more than two fetuses is at greatest risk.

Nursing Diagnoses and Related Interventions

Nursing Diagnosis: Fatigue related to increased stress on body functioning secondary to multiple gestation

Outcome Evaluation: Client states she is tired but identifies steps she has taken to minimize fatigue.

Although there is little evidence that strict bed rest helps prolong multiple pregnancies (Brubaker & Gyamfi, 2012), spend time at health care visits reviewing with a woman with a multiple pregnancy her need for extra rest, especially in a side-lying position during the day, to increase placental perfusion.

Because the woman is carrying double weight during pregnancy, she may notice extreme fatigue and backaches late in the day. She may have more difficulty resting or sleeping than the average woman because of this greater discomfort and increased fetal activity. As the growing uterus compresses her stomach, she may find her appetite decreasing and her intake falling. To compensate and maintain nutrition, a woman may need to eat six small meals a day rather than three large ones. She must also be sure to take her iron, folic acid, and vitamin supplements.

Toward the end of pregnancy, a woman may have extreme difficulty ambulating because of her excess weight. Her abdomen may become so stretched she feels as if she is going to burst.

Beginning with week 28 of pregnancy, a woman may be asked to come to a health care facility for monthly ultrasound examinations or weekly nonstress tests to document normal fetal growth, although this may not be necessary if the pregnancy is going well and the fetuses are growing consistently. If these tests are necessary, be certain that appointments are scheduled to conserve her energy as much as possible.

Nursing Diagnosis: Parental role conflict related to recent discovery of multiple (as opposed to single) pregnancy

Outcome Evaluation: Client states she is looking forward to caring for multiple infants (or may express concern about her ability to manage their arrival); client identifies changes she is making in preparation now that more than one baby is expected.

A woman with a multiple pregnancy has to work through an additional role change during pregnancy. First, she must accept that she is pregnant, then accept that she is having a baby. Then suddenly, at a routine office visit, two or more gestational sacs are seen on ultrasound or two or more sets of heart sounds are heard on auscultation. She is told she is going to have more than one child. Now she has to work through a second role change—for example, becoming a mother of two, not just of one (or more if she has additional children). This role change takes time and so may be difficult to complete, especially if the pregnancy ends early. A woman may need extra help after birth to form a close mother–child relationship with her newborns.

Nursing Diagnosis: Fear concerning her own and the babies' health related to risks of a multiple pregnancy

Outcome Evaluation: Client accurately states risks of a multiple pregnancy; expresses confidence in health care team's ability to care for her and her babies through pregnancy and birth.

In addition to having to work through a role change, a woman with a multiple pregnancy has more reason to fear for her life and the life of her babies than does the average woman. Every woman has heard stories about twins being conjoined or born so prematurely they did not survive. If she has not already heard these stories, someone will be sure to mention them to her before her due date. Unfortunately, all these risks cannot simply be filed away under the heading of untrue stories: both prematurity and high risk status are real hazards in multiple gestation. Help a woman deal with her fears as positively as possible. It can be helpful to tell her there is no indication so far that her babies are in any danger, so right now it is best to continue doing the things that have to be done; if any problems arise, the health care team and the woman's family will be there to support her.

Sometimes a woman is so fearful that her infants will be born too small to survive that she makes no preparations for them. She so lacks confidence in herself she cannot imagine she will be lucky enough or "good" enough to be able to carry a multiple pregnancy to term. Give her assurance during prenatal visits she is managing well, so her self-esteem is maintained at as high a level as possible. When her babies are born and all are healthy, the proof she needs she "deserved" this or was capable of it will be present in her arms. Nursing care at the birth of multiple infants is discussed in Chapter 23.

HYDRAMNIOS

Usually, the amniotic fluid volume at term is 500 to 1,000 ml. Hydramnios occurs when there is excess fluid of more than 2,000 ml or an amniotic fluid index above 24 cm (Juang & Snyder, 2012).

Hydramnios can cause fetal malpresentation because the additional uterine space can allow the fetus to turn to a transverse lie. It also can lead to premature rupture of the membranes from the increased pressure, which then leads to the additional risks of infection, prolapsed cord, and preterm birth.

Assessment

Amniotic fluid is formed by a combination of the cells of the amniotic membrane and from fetal urine. It is evacuated by being swallowed by the fetus, absorbed across the intestinal membrane into the fetal bloodstream, and transferred across the placenta. Although hydramnios can occur separate from fetal involvement, accumulation of amniotic fluid suggests difficulty with the fetus' ability to swallow or absorb, or excessive urine production. Inability to swallow occurs in infants who are anencephalic, who have tracheoesophageal fistula with stenosis, or who have intestinal obstruction (Bishop, 2011). Excessive urine output occurs in the fetuses of diabetic women (hyperglycemia in the fetus causes increased urine production).

The first sign of hydramnios may be unusually rapid enlargement of the uterus. The small parts of the fetus become difficult to palpate because the uterus is unusually tense. Auscultating the fetal heart rate can be difficult because of the depth of the increased amount of fluid surrounding the fetus. A woman may begin to notice extreme shortness of breath as the overly distended uterus pushes up against her diaphragm. She may develop lower extremity varicosities and hemorrhoids because good venous return from the lower extremities is blocked by extensive uterine pressure. The increased amount of fluid will cause increased weight gain. Generally, an ultrasound is done to document the presence of hydramnios and to discover a reason for the excessive amount of fluid.

Therapeutic Management

Women with severe hydramnios may be admitted to a hospital for bed rest and further evaluation or may be cared for at home. Regardless of the setting, maintaining bed rest helps to increase uteroplacental circulation and reduces pressure on the cervix, which may help prevent preterm labor. Teach a woman that it is vitally important to report any sign of ruptured membranes or uterine contractions. Although not common, there is a possibility that straining to defecate could increase uterine pressure and cause a rupture of membranes. Help her, therefore, avoid constipation by encouraging her to eat a high-fiber diet. Suggest a stool softener if diet alone is ineffective.

Assess vital signs as well as lower extremity edema frequently (the extremely tense uterus puts unusual pressure on both the diaphragm and the vessels of the pelvis). Amniocentesis can be performed to remove some of the extra fluid. Because amniotic fluid is replaced rapidly, however, this has to be repeated almost daily to be effective. Hydramnios can also lead to placental separation or rupture of membranes (Zheng, 2012a). If contractions begin, tocolysis may be necessary to prevent or halt preterm labor.

Even with these precautions, in most instances of hydramnios, there will be preterm rupture of the membranes because of excessive pressure, followed by preterm birth. To prevent the sudden loss of fluid and the accompanying danger of a prolapsed cord during labor, membranes can be "needled" (a thin needle is inserted vaginally to pierce them) to allow a slow, controlled release of fluid. After birth, the infant must be assessed carefully for factors that may have interfered with the ability to swallow in utero, such as a gastrointestinal blockage.

OLIGOHYDRAMNIOS

Oligohydramnios refers to a pregnancy with less than the average amount of amniotic fluid (Kumar, 2012). Because part of the volume of amniotic fluid is formed by the addition of fetal urine, this reduced amount of fluid is usually caused by a bladder or renal disorder in the fetus that is interfering with voiding. It also can occur from severe growth restriction (because of the small size, a fetus is not voiding as much as usual). Because the fetus is so cramped for space, muscles are left weak at birth, lungs can fail to develop (hypoplastic lungs), possibly leading to severe difficulty breathing after birth, and distorted features of the face occur (termed Potter syndrome).

Oligohydramnios is suspected during pregnancy when the uterus fails to meet its expected growth rate. It is confirmed by ultrasound when the pockets of amniotic fluid are less than average. Infants need careful inspection at birth to rule out kidney disease and compromised lung development.

POSTTERM PREGNANCY

A term pregnancy is 38 to 42 weeks long. A pregnancy that exceeds these limits is prolonged (i.e., **postterm pregnancy**, postmature, or postdate). The infant of such a pregnancy is considered postmature, or dysmature, if there is evidence that placental insufficiency has occurred and interfered with fetal growth. Postterm pregnancy occurs in 3% to 12% of all pregnancies (Gülmezoglu, Crowther, Middleton, et al., 2012).

Included in this group are some pregnancies that appear to extend beyond the due date set for them because of a faulty due date. Women who have long menstrual cycles (e.g., 40 to 45 days) do not ovulate on day 14 as in a typical menstrual cycle. Because they ovulate 14 days from the end of their cycle, or on day 26 or 31, their children will be considered "late" by 12 to 17 days.

In other instances, the pregnancy is truly overdue. For some reason, the trigger that initiates labor did not turn on. Such pregnancies can occur in women receiving a high dose of salicylates (for severe sinus headaches or rheumatoid arthritis) that interferes with the synthesis of prostaglandins, which may be responsible for the initiation of labor. It is also associated with myometrial quiescence, or a uterus that (for unknown reasons) does not respond to normal labor stimulation.

Remaining in utero for longer than 2 weeks beyond term creates a danger to a fetus for several reasons. Meconium aspiration is more apt to occur as fetal intestinal contents are more likely to reach the rectum. If the fetus continues to grow, macrosomia could create a birth problem. However, the usual effect of being postterm is lack of growth because a placenta seems to have adequate functioning ability for only 40 to 42 weeks. After that time, it acquires calcium deposits (becomes grade 3). This exposes a fetus to decreased blood perfusion and a lack of oxygen, fluid, and nutrients (Halloran, Cheng, Wall, et al., 2012). If oligohydramnios (a decreased amount of amniotic fluid from lessened urine production in the fetus) occurs, it can lead to variable decelerations in the FHR from cord compression.

If labor has not begun by 41 weeks, a maternal vaginal fibronectin level, a nonstress test, and/or a biophysical profile may be done to document the state of placental perfusion and the amount of amniotic fluid present. If these are normal, it suggests the due date was miscalculated. If the test results are abnormal or the physical examination or biparietal diameter measured on ultrasound suggests the fetus is term size, labor will be induced. Prostaglandin gel or misoprostol (Cytotec) applied to the cervix to initiate ripening followed by an oxytocin infusion are common methods used to begin labor. If oxytocin is ineffective, cesarean birth may be necessary. Monitor the fetal heart rate closely during labor to be certain placental insufficiency is not occurring from aging of the placenta. Nursing care for the postterm infant at birth is discussed in Chapter 26.

PSEUDOCYESIS

In **pseudocyesis** (false pregnancy), nausea and vomiting, amenorrhea, and enlargement of the abdomen occur in either a nonpregnant woman or a man (Del Pizzo, Posey-Bahar, & Jimenez, 2011). There are several theories regarding why the phenomenon occurs: wish-fulfillment theory suggests a woman's desire to be pregnant actually causes physiologic changes to occur, conflict theory suggests a desire for and fear of pregnancy create an internal conflict leading to physiologic changes, and depression theory attributes the cause to major depression. In any event, a woman's body responds with physiologic symptoms such as breast tenderness and an abdomen that enlarges so much she appears to be 7 or 8 months pregnant. On physical examination, however, it is obvious that only the abdomen, not the uterus, is enlarged. Ultrasound imaging will rule out pregnancy. Both men and women with the disorder need psychological counseling to help them better handle their needs.

ISOIMMUNIZATION (Rh INCOMPATIBILITY)

Approximately 15% of Caucasians and 10% of African Americans in the United States are missing the Rh (D) factor in their blood or have an Rh-negative blood type. **Rh incompatibility** occurs when an Rh-negative mother (one negative for a D antigen or one with a dd genotype) carries a fetus with an Rh-positive blood type (DD or Dd genotype). For such a situation to occur, the father of the child must either be homozygous (DD) or heterozygous (Dd) Rh positive. If the father of the child is homozygous (DD) for the factor, 100% of the couple's children will be Rh positive (Dd). If the father is heterozygous for the trait, 50% of their children can be expected to be Rh positive (Dd). Although blood incompatibility is basically a problem that affects the fetus, it can cause such concern and apprehension in a woman during pregnancy that it becomes a maternal problem as well.

Because people who have Rh-positive blood have a protein factor (the D antigen) that Rh-negative people do not, when an Rh-positive fetus begins to grow inside an Rh-negative mother who is sensitized, her body reacts in the same manner it would if the invading factor were a substance such as a virus—she forms antibodies against the invading substance. The Rh factor exists as a portion of the red blood cell, so these maternal antibodies cross the placenta and cause destruction (i.e., hemolysis) of fetal red blood cells (Fig. 21.10). A fetus can become so deficient in red blood cells from this that a sufficient oxygen transport to body cells cannot be maintained. This condition is termed **hemolytic disease of the newborn** or **erythroblastosis fetalis**. Management of the infant born with this condition is discussed in Chapter 26.

Theoretically, there is no connection between fetal blood and maternal blood during pregnancy, so the mother should not be exposed to fetal blood. In reality, a small amount of fetal blood does enter maternal circulation (Kim & Makar, 2012). Procedures such as amniocentesis or percutaneous umbilical blood sampling can allow this to occur. During a first pregnancy, this effect is small. As the placenta separates after birth of the first child, however, there is an active exchange of fetal and maternal blood from damaged villi. This causes most of the maternal antibodies formed against the Rh-positive blood to be formed in the first 72 hours after birth. These become a threat in a second pregnancy.

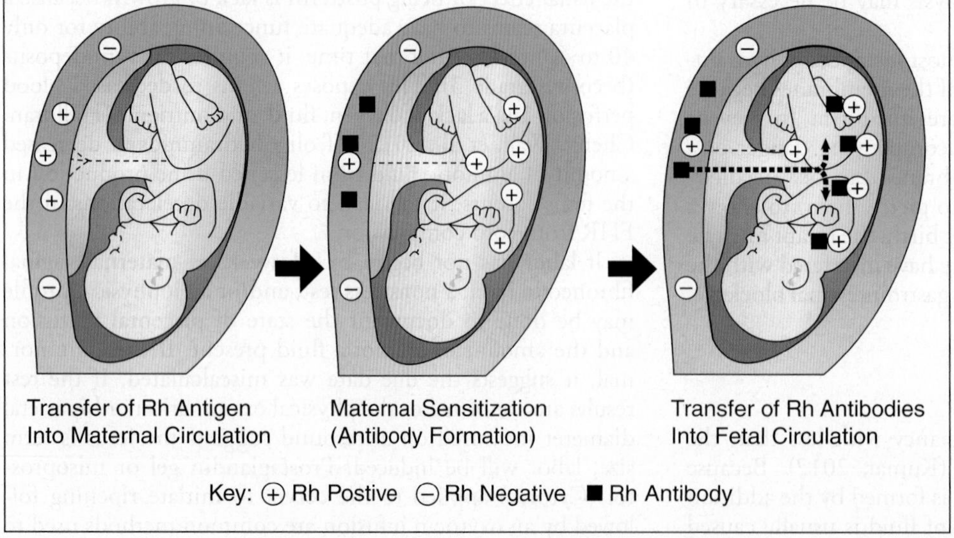

FIGURE 21.10 Maternal antibody formation against the Rh antigen.

Assessment

All women with Rh-negative blood should have an anti-D antibody titer done at a first pregnancy visit. If the results are normal or the titer is minimal (normal is 0; a ratio below 1:8 is minimal), the test is repeated at week 28 of pregnancy. If this is also normal, no therapy is needed.

If a woman's anti-D antibody titer is elevated at a first assessment (1:16 or greater), showing Rh sensitization, the well-being of the fetus in this potentially toxic environment will be monitored every 2 weeks (or more often) by Doppler velocity of the fetal middle cerebral artery, a technique that can predict when anemia is present or fetal red cells are being destroyed (Moise & Argoti, 2012).

If the artery velocity remains high, a fetus is not developing anemia and most likely is an Rh-negative fetus. If the reading is low, it means a fetus is in danger, and immediate birth will be carried out providing the fetus is near term. If the fetus is not near term, efforts to reduce the number of antibodies in the woman or replace damaged red cells in the fetus are begun.

Therapeutic Management

To reduce the number of maternal Rh (D) antibodies being formed, RhIG, a commercial preparation of passive Rh (D) antibodies against the Rh factor, is administered to women who are Rh negative at 28 weeks of pregnancy. These cannot cross the placenta and destroy fetal red blood cells because the antibodies are not the IgG class, the only type that crosses the placenta. RhIG (RhoGAM) is given again by injection to the mother in the first 72 hours after birth of an Rh-positive child to further prevent the woman from forming natural antibodies. Because RhIG is passive antibody protection, it is transient, and in 2 weeks to 2 months, the passive antibodies are destroyed. Only those few antibodies that were formed during pregnancy are left. For this reason, every pregnancy is like a first pregnancy in terms of the number of antibodies present, ensuring a safe intrauterine environment for any future pregnancies.

After birth, the infant's blood type will be determined from a sample of the cord blood. If it is Rh positive (i.e., Coombs test negative, indicating a large number of antibodies are not present in the mother), the mother will receive the RhIG injection. If the newborn's blood type is Rh negative, no antibodies have been formed in the mother's circulation during pregnancy and none will form, so passive antibody injection is unnecessary.

Although in future years, the problem of Rh sensitization will be greatly reduced, it currently remains a complication of pregnancy, particularly in women who gave birth to a first child in an undeveloped nation where they did not receive passive anti-D antibodies. Other women become sensitized because they did not receive an RhIG injection after an induced abortion, miscarriage, ectopic pregnancy, or amniocentesis.

Intrauterine Transfusion

To restore fetal red blood cells, blood transfusion can be performed on the fetus in utero. This is done by injecting red blood cells by amniocentesis technique directly into a vessel in the fetal cord or depositing them in the fetal abdomen where they migrate into the fetal circulation.

Blood used for transfusion in utero is either the fetus's own type (determined by percutaneous blood sampling) or group O negative if the fetal blood type is unknown. From 75 to 150 ml of washed red cells are used, depending on the age of the fetus. After deposition of the blood in the cord or abdomen, the cannula is withdrawn and a woman is urged to rest for approximately 30 minutes while fetal heart sounds and uterine activity are monitored.

Intrauterine transfusion is not without risk. A cord blood vessel could be lacerated by the needle, or the uterus could be so irritated by the invasive procedure labor contractions begin. For the fetus who is severely affected by isoimmunization, however, such a risk is no greater than that of being left untreated in a destructive intrauterine environment. The mother receives an RhIG injection after the transfusion to help reduce increased sensitization from any blood that might have been exchanged. Transfusion is sometimes done only once during pregnancy, or it may be repeated as often as every 2 weeks. As soon as fetal maturity is reached, as shown by a mature lecithin/sphingomyelin ratio, birth will be induced.

After birth, the infant may require therapy with phototherapy lights to reduce the level of bilirubin released from destroyed red blood cells or an exchange transfusion to remove hemolyzed red blood cells and replace them with healthy blood cells (see Chapter 26). A woman needs to discuss her plans for further childbearing with her health care provider and should be provided with contraceptive information if she does not want to undergo the strain of another pregnancy, because the constant feeling of wishing that everything was all right but never being certain it was, is more than she wants to endure again.

FETAL DEATH

Obviously, one of the most severe complications of pregnancy is fetal death. The most likely causes of this include chromosomal abnormalities, congenital malformations, infections such as hepatitis B, immunologic causes, and complications of maternal disease. If fetal death occurs before the time of quickening, a woman will not be aware the fetus has died because she is not able to feel fetal movements. This type of fetal death may be discovered at a routine prenatal visit when no fetal heartbeat can be heard. An ultrasound will reveal that no fetal heartbeat is present.

That a fetus has died early in intrauterine life may also be revealed first by the miscarriage that occurs. With this, a woman begins painless spotting, gradually accompanied by uterine contractions with cervical effacement and dilatation. The fetus is born lifeless and emaciated. Carefully observe all women who give birth to a fetus who has died for excess bleeding because if the fetus has been dead in utero for any length of time, the risk for the development of DIC increases.

If a fetus dies in utero past the point of quickening, a woman will be very aware that fetal movements are suddenly absent. She may lie down or sit in a position that she knows usually causes fetal movement. Unable to believe something could have happened, she may attribute the lack of movement to "sleeping" or "saving enough strength to be born." Because she is denying what is happening, it may be a full 24 hours before she calls her health care facility to report the apparent lack of fetal movement. On assessment, no fetal heartbeat can be heard. An ultrasound will confirm the absence of a fetal heartbeat.

If labor does not begin spontaneously once the fetal death is confirmed, it will be induced through a combination of prostaglandin gel such as misoprostol (Cytotec) applied to the cervix to effect cervical ripening and oxytocin administration to begin uterine contractions (Rattray, O'Connell, & Baskett, 2012). Blood for coagulation studies to detect DIC must be obtained to rule out the possibility of this developing.

Nursing Diagnoses and Related Interventions

Nursing Diagnosis: Powerlessness related to fetal death

Outcome Evaluation: Client and support person express meaning of pregnancy loss; identify support people/family with whom they can share grief.

Going through labor knowing a fetus is dead is difficult. A woman grieves for both her dead child and her inability to carry a pregnancy to term. She may wonder what she had done to cause this, such as forgetting to take an iron supplement, or may worry she is not as good a woman as others. Give her opportunities to express how she feels about this loss. "This must be a very difficult day for you" is the kind of statement that opens up the topic for discussion. If there are older children, it might be a help to explore how a woman plans to explain the fetal death to them.

Ask a couple about their desire for clergy or religious rites, such as baptism. Encourage a support person to remain with a woman during labor, but remember that the support person is grieving too. Although this is a difficult time, encouraging them to express their grief can help to make the fact the pregnancy has ended and allows the couple to begin rebuilding their life.

Labor involving a dead fetus is the same as for a live fetus because every fetus is basically a passive participant during labor. It may be difficult for a woman to use controlled breathing exercises, although encouraging her to use them is helpful in making the experience one of controllable pain. If a woman wishes a high level of analgesia, there is no contraindication to this because there is no living fetus to protect from narcotic effects. An epidural is also an option, as this will guard against poor uterine involution in the postpartum period from heavy analgesic sedation.

Ask if the parents wish to see the child after birth. If they do, wash away obvious blood, swaddle the baby as if he or she were a well newborn, and bring the baby to them. Point out particularly endearing features of the child as these can provide a focus for memories. Some parents may want to keep a lock of the child's hair. Others may want to keep the hospital identification bracelet or take a photograph. Parents may want to name the child. All of these measures are usual responses to grief and help to make the death real to parents, thus letting them begin the healthy process of grieving (Cacciatore, 2010).

If the child has a congenital anomaly that led to the death, prepare them for this before bringing the child to them and explain how the anomaly affected the child. Explain hospital procedures such as when the body will be released or what additional permission for autopsy is needed. Different communities have different laws concerning whether burial for an immature fetus is necessary. Consult local health department regulations so you can serve as a resource person for parents about this.

A woman needs to remain for only a few hours in the hospital, assuming no complications with labor developed. Many couples ask how soon it will be safe for them to have another child. They will need to consult with their primary care provider with regard to this, because it depends on why the fetal death occurred and whether the birth was cesarean. For some couples, beginning a second pregnancy immediately is a good recommendation. For others, waiting for an interval of time (perhaps 6 months) is better as this gives them more time to work through their grief before starting a new pregnancy. This helps prevent the new baby from becoming a "replacement baby" or someone to take the place of the dead infant rather than a unique individual in his or her own right. This is important in years to come because replacement children are rarely able to live up to the image of what the deceased baby would have been if only that baby had lived.

Prepare the couple for the possibility that they may feel sad on the day the infant would have been born if the pregnancy had been carried to term, or if they visit a friend's child of the age their child would have been. Be certain before a woman is discharged from the health care facility that she has a support person she can rely on during the following week or month, when the full impact of the fetal loss registers with her. Be certain she has a return appointment for a postpartal checkup so her physiologic and psychological health can be evaluated at that time.

What if... 21.4 You are interested in exploring one of the 2020 National Health Goals related to complications of pregnancy (see Box 21.1). Most government-sponsored money for nursing research is allotted based on these goals. What would be a possible research topic to explore pertinent to these goals that would be applicable to the Muzuki family and that would also advance evidence-based practice?

Key Points for Review

- Vaginal bleeding during pregnancy is always serious until ruled otherwise because it has the potential to diminish the blood supply to both the mother and fetus.
- The amount of bleeding that is evident may not be truly indicative of the amount of bleeding occurring because hidden, internal bleeding may also be happening.

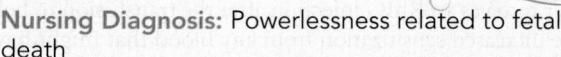

As a rule, position women with bleeding during pregnancy on their side to improve placental circulation and prevent supine hypotension syndrome.

- Spontaneous miscarriage is the loss of a pregnancy before viability of the fetus (20 to 24 weeks). The majority of these early pregnancy losses are attributed to chromosomal abnormalities. They are classified as threatened, imminent, complete, incomplete, missed, or recurrent pregnancy loss. Women who have a spontaneous miscarriage at home should bring any tissue passed to the hospital for an analysis for gestational trophoblastic disease. APS is an autoimmune disease that may contribute to recurrent miscarriages; therapy is subcutaneous (SQ) heparin and low-dose aspirin.
- Ectopic pregnancy is implantation outside the uterus, usually in a fallopian tube. If discovered before the tube ruptures, methotrexate can be administered to cause the conceptus to be reabsorbed. If not discovered early, sharp lower quadrant pain occurs at about 6 to 12 weeks as the tube ruptures. A laparoscopy is necessary to remove the conceptus and repair the tube to halt bleeding.
- Gestational trophoblastic disease is abnormal overgrowth of trophoblast cells. If not discovered by an ultrasound early in pregnancy, bleeding and expulsion of the abnormal growth occur at about the 16th week of pregnancy. Women need close follow-up after this because it can lead to choriocarcinoma, a malignancy.
- Premature cervical dilatation occurs when the cervix dilates early in pregnancy, before viability of the fetus. Sutures (cervical cerclage) can be placed to prevent the cervix from dilating prematurely this way again in a second pregnancy.
- Placenta previa is low implantation of the placenta so that it crosses the cervical os. If this is not discovered before labor, cervical dilatation may cause the placenta to tear, causing severe blood loss. Women who have symptoms of placenta previa (i.e., painless vaginal bleeding in the third trimester) should not have vaginal examinations done to prevent disruption of the low-implanted placenta.
- Premature separation of the placenta (i.e., abruptio placentae) or placental separation from the uterus before the fetus is born usually occurs late in pregnancy and cuts off blood supply to the fetus. Women with increased parity, those with previous uterine surgery, and those who are cocaine dependent are at highest risk for this. Often, it is manifested by sudden, sharp fundal pain, then a continuing dull pain and vaginal bleeding.
- DIC is a blood disorder that may occur with any trauma, so it can accompany such conditions as premature separation of the placenta and hypertension of pregnancy. Blood coagulation is so extreme at one point in the circulatory system that clotting factors become diminished, resulting in their absence in the remainder of the system. Beginning symptoms of this include easy bruising, petechiae, and oozing from intravenous sites. Heparin is used to stop the local coagulation and free up clotting factors for systemic use.
- Preterm labor is labor that occurs after 20 weeks and before the end of the 37th week of pregnancy. A woman is said to be in preterm labor when she has had uterine contractions every 10 minutes for 1 hour and cervical dilatation begins. Magnesium sulfate, parentally administered, is the drug of choice to halt preterm labor.
- A corticosteroid is also used in preterm labor management because it appears to accelerate the formation of lung surfactant in the fetus.
- Preterm rupture of the membranes is tearing of the fetal membranes with loss of amniotic fluid before the pregnancy is at term. After rupture, there is a high risk of fetal and uterine infection (i.e., chorioamnionitis) and preterm birth.
- Gestational hypertension is a unique disorder that occurs with three classic symptoms: hypertension, edema, and proteinuria. It is categorized as gestational hypertension: preeclampsia or eclampsia. If mild (blood pressure not over 140/90 mmHg), treatment is bed rest and perhaps low-dose aspirin. If severe (blood pressure over 160/110 mmHg), bed rest plus administration of magnesium sulfate will be prescribed. If a seizure occurs, the condition becomes eclampsia. Helping prevent the disease from progressing to this stage not only meets QSEN competencies but also can best meet the family's total needs.
- The HELLP syndrome is a unique form of gestational hypertension marked by hemolysis of red blood cells, elevated liver enzymes, and a low platelet count.
- Multiple gestation puts an additional strain on a woman's physical resources and may lead to preterm birth with immaturity of her infants. Helping a woman plan adequate nutrition and rest during pregnancy are nursing responsibilities.
- Postterm pregnancy is pregnancy that extends beyond 42 weeks. Because the placenta deteriorates at this time, it can cause a fetus to receive decreased nutrients.
- Hydramnios is overproduction of amniotic fluid (above 2,000 ml) and is a condition that can lead to ruptured membranes and premature birth because of increased intrauterine pressure. Oligohydramnios is the lessened amount of fluid and suggests a renal disorder exists in the fetus.
- Isoimmunization (Rh incompatibility) is a possibility when a woman who is Rh negative is sensitized and carries a fetus who is Rh positive. Maternal antibodies form and destroy fetal red blood cells, leading to anemia, edema, and jaundice in the newborn. Being certain that women are screened for blood type and antibody titer early in pregnancy is a nursing responsibility.

Critical Thinking Care Study

Maria Maya is a 37-year-old woman who works part time in the personnel office at your school. She felt nauseated after receiving the flu vaccine in the health center. Last night, she experienced right-sided lower abdominal pain with scant vaginal spotting. Today, she appears pale. She is diagnosed as having a ruptured ectopic pregnancy. She is scheduled for an emergency laparotomy.

1. Maria questions her diagnosis because she had no idea she was pregnant. How would you respond if she asks you, "Why didn't I have any pregnancy symptoms if I'm really pregnant?"
2. Maria's blood pressure is 90/60 mmHg and she appears very pale. She is refusing, however, to have surgery to end the pregnancy in case there is any chance her baby is still alive. Would you support her decision?

3. Maria's left fallopian tube was so damaged that it was removed in surgery. A week later, she quits her job, sets fire to her apartment, and swallows drain cleaner in a self-injury attempt because "I'm never going to be able to have children, now, am I?" Did Maria receive sound information about what her surgery consisted of?

Patient Scenario

The Holloman Family

Read about the Holloman family, a family with a woman experiencing placenta previa, then answer the questions to further sharpen your skills and grow more familiar with NCLEX-type questions related to a sudden pregnancy complication. Confirm your answers are correct by reading the rationales.

Visit http://thePoint.lww.com

Answers and Rationales

Looking for answers to the What If... and Critical Thinking Care Study questions?

Visit http://thePoint.lww.com

References

Abatangelo, L., Okereke, L., Parham-Foster, C., et al. (2010). If pelvic inflammatory disease is suspected empiric treatment should be initiated. *Journal of American Nurse Practitioner, 22*(2), 117–122.

Abildgaard, U., & Heimdal, K. (2013). Pathogenesis of the syndrome of hemolysis, elevated liver enzymes, and low platelet count (HELLP): A review. *European Journal of Obstetrics, Gynecology & Reproductive Biology, 166*(2), 117–123.

Alfirevic, Z., Stampalija, T., Roberts, D., et al. (2012). Cervical stitch (cerclage) for preventing preterm birth in singleton pregnancy. *Cochrane Database of Systemic Reviews,* (4), CD008991.

Al-Safi, Z., Imudia, A., Filetti, L., et al. (2011). Delayed postpartum preeclampsia and eclampsia: Demographics, clinical course, and complications. *Obstetrics & Gynecology, 118*(5), 1102–1107.

Ananth, C., Nath, C., & Philipp, C. (2010). The normal anticoagulant system and risk of placental abruption: Protein C, protein S and resistance to activated protein C. *Fetal Neonatal Medicine, 23*(12), 1377–1383.

Andersen, A., Andersen, P., Olsen, J., et al. (2012). Moderate alcohol intake during pregnancy and risk of fetal death. *International Journal of Epidemiology, 41*(2), 405–413.

Barton, J. R., & Sibai, B. M. (2012). Severe sepsis and septic shock in pregnancy. *Obstetrics & Gynecology, 120*(3), 689–706.

Beall, S., & Decherney, A. H. (2012). Management of tubal ectopic pregnancy: Methotrexate and salpingostomy are preferred to preserve fertility. *Fertility & Sterility, 98*(5), 1118–1120.

Bedoya-Ronga, A., & Currie, I. (2012). Which patients should be offered caesarean section? *Practitioner, 256*(1749), 16–18.

Bishop, W. P. (2011). The digestive system. In K. J. Marcdante, R. M. Kliegman, H. B. Jenson, et al. (Eds.), *Nelson essentials of pediatrics* (6th ed., pp. 463–498). Philadelphia, PA: Saunders/Elsevier.

Bonzini, M., Palmer, K., Coggon, D., et al. (2011). Shift work and pregnancy outcomes: A systematic review with meta-analysis of currently available epidemiological studies. *British Journal of Gynecology, 118*(12), 1429–1437.

Brown, C., & Garovic, V. (2011). Mechanisms and management of hypertension in pregnant women. *Current Hypertension Reports, 13*(5), 338–346.

Brubaker, S. G., & Gyamfi, C. (2012). Prediction and prevention of spontaneous preterm birth in twin gestations. *Seminars in Perinatology, 36*(3), 190–194.

Bush, M. C., & Pernoll, M. L. (2012). Multiple gestation. In D. K. Edmonds (Ed.), *Dewhurst's textbook of obstetrics & gynaecology* (8th ed., pp. 301–309). Oxford, UK: John Wiley & Son.

Cacciatore, J. (2010). Stillbirth: Patient-centered psychosocial care. *Clinical Obstetrics & Gynecology, 53*(3), 691–699.

Cappiello, J., Beal, M., & Simmonds, K. (2011). Clinical issues in post-abortion care. *Nurse Practitioner, 36*(5), 35–40.

Chawanpaiboon, S., Pimol, K., & Sirisomboon, R. (2011). Comparison of success rate of nifedipine, progesterone, and bed rest for inhibiting uterine contraction in threatened preterm labor. *Journal of Obstetrics & Gynaecology Research, 37*(7), 787–791.

Corsello, G., & Piro, E. (2010). The world of twins: An update. *Journal of Maternal–Fetal & Neonatal Medicine, 23*(Suppl. 3), 59–62.

Danza, A., Ruiz-Irastorza, G., & Khamashta, M. (2012). Antiphospholipid syndrome in obstetrics. *Best Practice & Research in Clinical Obstetrics & Gynaecology, 26*(1), 65–76.

Del Pizzo, J., Posey-Bahar, L., & Jimenez, R. (2011). Pseudocyesis in a teenager with bipolar disorder. *Clinical Pediatrics, 50*(2), 169–171.

Demendi, C., Langmár, Z., Bánhidy, F., et al. (2011). Successful operative management of an intact second trimester abdominal pregnancy with additional preoperative selective catheter embolization and postoperative methotrexate therapy. *Medical Science Monitor, 17*(5), CS53–CS55.

Evans, R. (2012). Emotional care for women who experience miscarriage. *Nursing Standard, 26*(42), 35–41.

Fu, J., Fang, F., Xie, L., et al. (2012). Prophylactic chemotherapy for hydatidiform mole to prevent gestational trophoblastic neoplasia. *Cochrane Database of Systematic Reviews,* (10), CD007289.

Gilbert, E. S. (2011). Spontaneous abortion. In *Manual of high risk pregnancy & delivery* (5th ed., pp. 311–330). St. Louis, MO: Mosby Elsevier.

Gülmezoglu, A. M., Crowther, C. A., Middleton, P., et al. (2012). Induction of labour for improving birth outcomes for women at or beyond term. *Cochrane Database of Systematic Reviews,* (6), CD004945.

Halloran, D. R., Cheng, Y. W., Wall, T. C., et al. (2012). Effect of maternal weight on postterm delivery. *Journal of Perinatology, 32*(2), 85–90.

Hanna, R., & Soper, J. (2010). The role of surgery and radiation therapy in the management of gestational trophoblastic disease. *Oncologist, 15*(6), 593–600.

Hanson, S. J., & Burke, A. E. (2011). Fertility control: Conception, sterilization & abortion. In K. J. Hurt, M. W. Guile, J. L. Bienstock, et al. (Eds.), *The Johns Hopkins manual of gynecology and obstetrics* (4th ed., pp. 382–295). Philadelphia, PA: Lippincott Williams & Wilkins.

Hennessy, M., Volpe, S., Sammel, M., et al. (2010). Skipping meals and less walking among African Americans diagnosed with preterm labor. *Journal of Nursing Scholarship, 42*(2), 147–155.

Hızlı, D., Köşüş, N., Köşüş, A., et al. (2012). First-trimester reference ranges for decidual thickness and its relation to progesterone levels. *Journal of Perinatal Medicine, 40*(5), 521–525.

Hsu, S., & Euerle, B. D. (2012). Ultrasound in pregnancy. *Emergency Medicine Clinics of North America, 30*(4), 849–867.

Hunter, L., & Gibbins, K. (2011). Magnesium sulfate: Past, present, and future. *Journal of Midwifery & Women's Health, 56*(6), 566–574.

Iwashita, Y., Kan'o, T., Hattori, J., et al. (2012). A case of HELLP syndrome with multiple complications. *Internal Medicine, 51*(16), 2227–2230.

Juang, D., & Snyder, C. L. (2012). Neonatal bowel obstruction. *Surgical Clinics of North America, 92*(3), 685–711.

Jurkovic, D. (2012). Ectopic pregnancy. In D. K. Edmonds (Ed.), *Dewhurst's textbook of obstetrics & gynaecology* (8th ed., pp. 77–87). Oxford, UK: John Wiley & Son.

Karch, A. M. (2012). *2013 Lippincott's nursing drug guide.* Philadelphia, PA: Lippincott Williams & Wilkins.

Kausar, F., Morris, J. L., Fathalla, M., et al. (2012). Nurses in low resource settings save mothers' lives with non-pneumatic anti-shock garment. *MCN: American Journal of Maternal Child Nursing, 37*(5), 308–316.

Khader, Y., Al-Akour, N., Alzubi, I., et al. (2011). The association between second hand smoke and low birth weight and preterm delivery. *Maternal & Child Health Journal, 15*(4), 453–459.

Kim, M. J., Bae, J. Y., Seong, W. J., et al. (2012). Sonographic diagnosis of a viable abdominal pregnancy with planned delivery after fetal lung maturation. *Journal of Clinical Ultrasound.* Advance online publication.

Kim, Y. A., & Makar, R. S. (2012). Detection of fetomaternal hemorrhage. *American Journal of Hematology, 87*(4), 417–423.

Kumar, S. (2012). Fetal anomalies. In D. K. Edmonds (Ed.), *Dewhurst's textbook of obstetrics & gynaecology* (8th ed., pp. 219–229). Oxford, UK: John Wiley & Son.

Liu, S., Joseph, K., Liston, R., et al. (2011). Incidence, risk factors, and associated complications of eclampsia. *Obstetrics & Gynecology, 118*(5), 987–994.

Lurain, J. R. (2010). Gestational trophoblastic disease I: Epidemiology, pathology, clinical presentation and diagnosis of gestational trophoblastic disease, and management of hydatidiform mole. *American Journal of Obstetrics & Gynecology, 203*(6), 531–539.

Marion, L. L., & Meeks, G. R. (2012). Ectopic pregnancy: History, incidence, epidemiology, and risk factors. *Clinical Obstetrics & Gynecology, 55*(2), 376–386.

Matsuda, Y., Hayashi, K., Shiozaki, A., et al. (2011). Comparison of risk factors for placental abruption and placenta previa: Case-cohort study. *Journal of Obstetrics & Gynaecology Research, 37*(6), 538–546.

McNair, T., & Altman, K. (2011). Miscarriage and recurrent pregnancy loss. In K. J. Hurt, M. W. Guile, J. L. Bienstock, et al. (Eds.), *The Johns Hopkins manual of gynecology and obstetrics* (4th ed., pp. 438–447). Philadelphia, PA: Lippincott Williams & Wilkins.

Meguerdichian, D. (2012). Complications in late pregnancy. *Emergency Medical Clinics of North America, 30*(4), 919–936.

Mehta, S. H., & Sokol, R. J. (2013). Assessment of high-risk pregnancy. In A. H. DeCherney, L. Nathan, T. M. Goodwin, et al. (Eds.), *Current diagnosis and treatment: Obstetrics and gynecology* (11th ed., pp. 223–233). Columbus, OH: McGraw-Hill/Lange.

Mercer, B. (2011). Premature rupture of the membranes. *Clinical Obstetrics & Gynecology, 54*(2), 305–306.

Miller, D. A. (2012). Hypertension in pregnancy. In D. K. Edmonds (Ed.), *Dewhurst's textbook of obstetrics & gynaecology* (8th ed., pp. 454–464). Oxford, UK: John Wiley & Son.

Mineo, C., & Shaul, P. W. (2011). New insights into the molecular basis of the antiphospholipid syndrome. *Drug Discovery Today: Disease Mechanisms, 8*(1–2), e47–e52.

Moise, K. J. Jr., & Argoti, P. S. (2012). Management and prevention of red cell alloimmunization in pregnancy: A systematic review. *Obstetrics & Gynecology, 120*(5), 1132–1139.

Montagnana, M., Franchi, M., Danese, E., et al. (2010). Disseminated intravascular coagulation in obstetric and gynecologic disorders. *Seminars in Thrombosis & Hemostasis, 36*(4), 404–418.

Newfield, E. (2012). Third-trimester pregnancy complications. *Primary Care, 39*(1), 95–113.

Nugteren, J. J., Snijder, A. A., Hofman, A., et al. (2012). Work-related maternal risk factors and the risk of pregnancy induced hypertension and preeclampsia during pregnancy. *PLoS One, 7*(6): e39263

Owen, J., & Mancuso, M. (2012). Cervical cerclage for the prevention of preterm birth. *Obstetrics & Gynecology Clinics of North America, 39*(1), 25–33.

Pariente, G., Wiznitzer, A., Sergienko, R., et al. (2011). Placental abruption: Critical analysis of risk factors and perinatal outcomes. *Journal of Maternal–Fetal & Neonatal Medicine, 24*(5), 698–702.

Pereira, L., Reddy, A., Alexander, A., et al. (2010). Insights into the multifactorial nature of preterm birth: Proteomic profiling of the maternal serum glycoproteome and maternal serum peptidome among women in preterm labor. *American Journal of Obstetrics & Gynecology, 202*(6), 555.e1–555.e10.

Rabe, H., Diaz-Rossello, J. L., Duley, L., et al. (2012). Effect of timing of umbilical cord clamping and other strategies to influence placental transfusion at preterm birth on maternal and infant outcomes. *Cochrane Database of Systematic Reviews,* (8), CD003248.

Rao, K. P., Belogolovkin, V., Yankowitz, J., et al. (2012). Abnormal placentation: Evidence-based diagnosis and management of placenta previa, placenta accreta, and vasa previa. *Obstetrical & Gynecological Survey, 67*(8), 503–519.

Rattray, D. D., O'Connell, C. M., & Baskett, T. F. (2012). Acute disseminated intravascular coagulation in obstetrics: A tertiary centre population review. *Journal of Obstetrics & Gynaecology Canada, 34*(4), 341–347.

Riley, C., Boozer, K., & King, T.(2011). Antenatal corticosteroids at the beginning of the 21st century. *Journal of Midwifery & Women's Health, 56*(6), 591–597.

Rimawi, B. H., Soper, D. E., & Eschenbach, D. A. (2012). Group a streptococcal infections in obstetrics and gynecology. *Clinical Obstetrics & Gynecology, 55*(4), 864–874.

Roberge, S., Villa, P., Nicolaides, K., et al. (2012). Early administration of low-dose aspirin for the prevention of preterm and term preeclampsia: A systematic review and meta-analysis. *Fetal Diagnosis & Therapy, 31*(3), 141–146.

Roman, A. S. (2013). Late pregnancy complications. In A. H. DeCherney, L. Nathan, T. M. Goodwin, et al. (Eds.), *Current diagnosis and treatment: Obstetrics and gynecology* (11th ed., pp. 250–266). Columbus, OH: McGraw-Hill/Lange.

Sanchez, S., Alva, A., Diez Chang, G., et al. (2012). Risk of spontaneous preterm birth in relation to maternal exposure to intimate partner violence during pregnancy in Peru. *Maternal Child Health Journal, 17*(S1), 573–628.

Sankaran, S., Rozette, C., Dean, J., et al. (2011). Screening in the presence of a vanished twin: Nuchal translucency or combined screening test? *Prenatal Diagnosis, 31*(6), 600–601.

Savage, P., & Seckl, M. (2012). Gestational trophoblast tumours. In D. K. Edmonds (Ed.), *Dewhurst's textbook of obstetrics & gynaecology* (8th ed., pp. 88–100). Oxford, UK: John Wiley & Son.

Sayres, W. (2010). Preterm labor. *American Family Physician, 81*(4), 477–484.

Storness-Bliss, C., Metcalfe, A., Simrose, R., et al. (2012). Correlation of residual amniotic fluid and perinatal outcomes in periviable preterm premature rupture of membranes. *Journal of Obstetrics & Gynaecology Canada, 34*(2), 154–158.

Su, L. L., & Chong, Y. S. (2012). Massive obstetric haemorrhage with disseminated intravascular coagulopathy. *Best Practice & Research: Clinical Obstetrics & Gynaecology, 26*(1), 77–90.

Surette, A., & Dunham, S. M. (2013). Early pregnancy risks. In A. H. DeCherney, L. Nathan, T. M. Goodwin, et al. (Eds.), *Current diagnosis and treatment: Obstetrics and gynecology* (11th ed., pp. 234–249). Columbus, OH: McGraw-Hill/Lange.

Tripodi, A. (2011). D-dimer testing in laboratory practice. *Clinical Chemistry, 57*(9), 1256–1262.

Tsokos, G. C. (2011). Systemic lupus erythematosus. *New England Journal of Medicine, 365*(22), 2110–2121.

U.S. Department of Health and Human Services. (2010). *Healthy people 2020.* Washington, DC: Author.

van der Ham, D., van Melick, M., Smits, L., et al. (2011). Methods for the diagnosis of rupture of the fetal membranes in equivocal cases: A systematic review. *European Journal of Obstetrics, Gynecology & Reproductive Biology, 157*(2), 123–127.

Watson, C. A., & Wilkinson, M. (2012). Monitoring central venous pressure, arterial pressure and pulmonary wedge pressure. *Anaesthesia & Intensive Care Medicine, 13*(3), 116–120.

Wiegerinck, M., Vis, J., & Mol, B. (2010). Transvaginal cervical length measurement for prediction of preterm birth in women with threatened preterm labor: A meta-analysis. *Ultrasound in Obstetrics & Gynecology, 35*(6), 756–757.

Yeniel, A. O., Ergenoglu, A. M., Itil, I. M., et al. (2012). Effect of placenta previa on fetal growth restriction and stillbirth. *Archives of Gynecology & Obstetrics, 286*(2), 295–298.

Zheng, T. (2012a). Antepartum testing. In T. Zheng (Ed.), *Comprehensive handbook of obstetrics & gynecology* (2nd ed., pp. 92–95). Paradise Valley, AZ: Phoenix Medical Press.

Zheng, T. (2012b). Spontaneous abortion. In T. Zheng (Ed.), *Comprehensive handbook of obstetrics & gynecology* (2nd ed., pp. 230–233). Paradise Valley, AZ: Phoenix Medical Press.

Chapter 22

Nursing Care of a Pregnant Family With Special Needs

KEY TERMS

- autonomic dysreflexia
- emancipated minor
- substance dependent

OBJECTIVES

After mastering the contents of this chapter, you should be able to:

1. Identify the characteristics and the risks of pregnancy for a pregnant woman who has special needs, such as one who has been injured, an adolescent, a woman over age 40 years, one who is physically or cognitively challenged, or a woman who is drug dependent.
2. Identify 2020 National Health Goals related to women with special needs that nurses can help the nation achieve.
3. Assess a woman with special needs during pregnancy.
4. Formulate nursing diagnoses related to pregnancy for a woman with special needs.
5. Identify expected outcomes for a pregnant woman with special needs to help her manage seamless transitions across differing health care settings.
6. Using the nursing process, plan nursing care that includes the six competencies of Quality & Safety Education for Nurses (QSEN): Patient-Centered Care, Teamwork & Collaboration, Evidence-Based Practice (EBP), Quality Improvement (QI), Safety, and Informatics.
7. Implement nursing care for a woman with special needs, such as encouraging her to remain ambulatory during pregnancy.
8. Evaluate outcomes for effectiveness and achievement of care.
9. Integrate knowledge of the risks of pregnancy for women with special needs with the interplay of nursing process, the six competencies of QSEN, and Family Nursing to promote quality maternal and child health nursing care.

*M*indy Carson, 16 years old and 15 weeks pregnant, received a 4-in. laceration on her leg when she was in an automobile accident on her way into prenatal clinic this morning. The father of Mindy's baby, Carlos, does not want Mindy to keep her baby after the birth because he does not want to get married until he finishes graduate school. Mindy insists she is old enough to be a parent and wants to keep her baby. Mindy's mother has accused Carlos of sharing methamphetamine with Mindy. She's worried Mindy has been working as a prostitute to support a drug habit. Mindy turns to you and asks you what you would recommend she do.

Previous chapters discussed high-risk pregnancies for women who are ill when they become pregnant and for those who develop an illness while pregnant. This chapter presents information about women who do not fit the description of the average pregnant woman—a well adult who maintains a healthy lifestyle. Representative of such women who do not fit the description of average pregnant women are very young

(Continued on next page)

(Continued from previous page)

adolescents, women who have waited until midlife to have their first child, those who are physically or cognitively challenged, those who are unintentionally injured, and those who are drug dependent.

What type of immediate assessment does Mindy need? What qualities would you look for to decide if she is ready to be a parent?

The National Center for Health Statistics reported in 2010 that 367,752 infants were born to women aged 15 to 19 years in the United States, for a live birth rate of 34.3 per 1,000 women in this age group. Birth rates fell 12% for women aged 15 to 17 years, and 9% for women aged 18 to 19 years. In addition, teen birth rates declined for all races and for Hispanics (National Center for Health Statistics, 2012). Although reasons for the declines are not clear, younger teens appear to be less sexually active, and more of those who are sexually active may be using contraception more so than in previous years. In contrast, as more and more women delay beginning a family until their 30s, birth rates continue to rise for women aged 40 to 44 years (Hamilton, Martin, & Ventura, 2011; Martinez, Copen, & Abma, 2011).

Adolescents require special consideration during pregnancy because they are physically and psychosocially immature. Women over age 40 years may need special consideration also because they can have difficulty adjusting psychosocially to a first pregnancy and the physical changes that are required (Carolan, Davey, Biro, et al., 2013).

The pregnancy rate is increasing as well among women who are physically or cognitively challenged, including those with conditions such as cerebral palsy, which might have precluded pregnancy a few years ago. Physical and cognitive conditions present a challenge to childbearing and childrearing, but do not necessarily prevent women from establishing their own families. Supportive nursing care that considers the limitations imposed by a particular disability while focusing on the normal aspects of childbearing and childrearing combined with a woman's strengths helps to make these pregnancies successful (Lu, Zhao, Zhu, et al., 2013).

Women who are drug dependent or who are injured are other high-risk women who require a great deal of nursing support and care. Ideally, a woman should give up substance abuse for the health of a fetus, but that may not be possible. When substance abuse continues, every effort must be made to provide enough prenatal care and attention to protect the fetus in other ways. Women who are injured in automobile accidents or from intimate partner violence can have substantial blood loss that threatens the health of the fetus. They need rapid emergency department assessment and care to be certain fetal health is protected.

Women with special needs have become such a large population of pregnant women that several 2020 National Health Goals have been established in relation to them (Box 22.1).

BOX 22.1 Nursing Care Planning Based on 2020 National Health Goals

Several National Health Goals have been formulated to improve the health of women with special needs during pregnancy. These include:

- Reduce the pregnancy rate among adolescent females to no more than 105.9 per 1,000 adolescents from a baseline of 117.7 per 1,000 adolescents.
- Increase abstinence from alcohol, cigarettes, and illicit drugs among pregnant women to 98.3% from a baselines of 89.4% (alcohol), 100% from a baseline of 95% (binge drinking), 100% from a baseline of 94.9% (illicit drugs), and 98.6% from a baseline of 89.6% (cigarette smoking) (U.S. Department of Health and Human Services [DHHS], 2010; see www.healthypeople.gov).

Nurses can help the nation achieve these goals by teaching unintentional injury prevention, the dangers and complications of substance dependency, and both the psychological and physical concerns of teenage pregnancy.

Nursing Process Overview

For Care of a Pregnant Woman With Special Needs

Assessment

Assessing the strengths and weaknesses of individual women is always crucial to establish accurate nursing diagnoses and realistic outcomes as well as planning effective nursing care. When a woman has a special need, assessment becomes even more important. Establishing as thorough a database as possible early in pregnancy helps to predict the risks a woman may be exposed to when pregnancy is affected by age extremes, physical or cognitive challenges, an unintentional injury, or an unhealthy lifestyle.

The capacity of a woman with special needs to adapt to pregnancy depends both on her physical capabilities and on her ability to persevere against odds to overcome obstacles. When caring for a woman who is physically challenged, keep in mind physical disabilities occur in degrees; therefore, first establish the impact of the disability on a woman's lifestyle before beginning to offer guidance for care measures during pregnancy. Be certain to assess physical strengths as well as limitations and psychosocial strengths as well as challenges. A woman with a spinal cord injury, for example, is likely to have developed ways of coping in daily life that may never occur to someone who has not experienced that disability.

For some drug-dependent women, pregnancy may be the impetus they need to break a drug habit. Others may only be able to reduce their drug use. In both instances, encourage a woman to keep coming for prenatal care. As long as she feels comfortable with you during regular visits, you may be able to establish a trusting relationship that will eventually provide her with the confidence to try a more healthful pattern of living.

Nursing Diagnosis

Nursing diagnoses established for pregnant women with special needs differ in degree, but not in substance, from the nursing diagnoses established for all pregnant women. For example, if a pregnant adolescent is still growing, sound nutrition is an extremely important issue for both her and her fetus. Examples of nursing diagnoses for women with special needs include:

- Risk for imbalanced nutrition related to combined needs of adolescent and pregnancy
- Risk for fetal injury related to drug and alcohol use
- Impaired physical mobility related to physical disability
- Risk for injury related to unstable balance
- Risk of injury related to potential for unintentional injuries
- Impaired verbal communication related to spastic muscle functioning
- Impaired home maintenance related to a sensory challenge
- Risk for social isolation related to bed rest at home
- Risk for disruption of social interactions related to unclear speech
- Disruption in family dynamics related to serious illness of family's main provider
- Readiness for enhanced family coping related to commitment to have a child in the face of a disabling condition

Outcome Identification and Planning

Be especially careful to establish realistic outcomes given a woman's particular condition or situation. An adolescent, for instance, cannot achieve independent decision making if she is not mature enough to do this. A woman who is visually challenged may not be able to read a digital display on a glucometer or use a wall clock to time contractions no matter how much she would like to do these things.

Often, a pregnant woman with a special need already has significant stressors to deal with in her life. Adolescence, for example, is a period of growth and change that can be stressful for both the teenager and her family. The physically challenged woman constantly copes with a condition that must be considered in all activities, even if she has adjusted completely to the limitations the disability imposes. The drug-dependent woman is confined by a life-threatening habit. A woman who has an unintentional injury may have to temporarily restructure her life to accommodate a hospital admission. Pregnancy brings with it a whole new set of stressors that can be overwhelming if a woman has no outside support. Planning for a pregnant woman with special needs, therefore, often involves identifying support people to help with this added stress. This support can come from family, friends, a professional organization, or health care providers. If a woman is not totally independent in her care, some planning may be required with her support person, who may be the person who actually carries out the proposed action. At the same time, be certain to not ignore a woman and plan around her. Only if she approves of the plan can pregnancy be the enjoyable experience it should be. This principle applies to any woman, but especially one with special needs.

Plans should also include ways to strengthen confidence and self-esteem, crucial attributes for a new mother. These also are areas in which a woman with a special need, especially one who perceives herself as too young or too old or who has experienced a physical dysfunction, may not have developed fully. Drug dependence may also be related to feelings of lowered self-worth, which may have been intensified if the drug-dependent woman has tried unsuccessfully to limit her drug intake in the past.

Being certain that plans are established in a wide range of areas helps to ensure planning is comprehensive. Remember to include safe care of the newborn in plans as well, because once an infant is born, it may be too late to make these plans in a comprehensive manner. The U.S. Department of Health and Human Services (DHHS) has initiated a special program to help reduce teenage pregnancy (www.girlshealth.gov), which is helpful to use for referral, along with the Substance Abuse & Mental Health Services (www.samhsa.gov). Narcotics Anonymous (www.na.org) can be helpful to women who are drug dependent. Alcoholics Anonymous (www.aa.org) is the standby for women with alcohol dependence. Women who feel they will be injured by an intimate partner can locate a shelter by calling their local police department.

Implementation

Interventions for the high-risk pregnant woman include promoting a healthy pregnancy and preventing pregnancy complications. Care focuses on teaching and encouraging a woman with any special needs to determine how best to manage her pregnancy according to her particular situation.

A high proportion of adolescents do not seek prenatal care early in pregnancy because they deny they are pregnant. Others may not feel comfortable in a health care facility that sees mainly adults. The same may be true of a woman with drug dependency, who fears discrimination from health care providers regarding her drug use. A nonjudgmental, welcoming attitude that focuses on the pregnancy and the baby, while avoiding recriminations about a woman's youth or circumstances, is essential to attracting such women to prenatal care and keeping them coming for regular visits. If they hear from a friend that the staff members at the clinic are helpful and not judgmental, they then take the first step into the facility.

Outcome Evaluation

An evaluation of nursing interventions for the care of a pregnant woman with special needs often focuses on a woman's physical and emotional readiness for childbearing, maintenance of fetal health, and a woman's ability to provide a safe and healthy environment for her newborn. Some examples include:

- Client states she will use walker to maintain balance during pregnancy.
- Adolescent lists a weekly intake of adequate calories, even with frequent meals at fast-food restaurants.
- Family members state they have been able to adjust to changing demands of pregnancy in a mother who is physically challenged.
- Client reports to methadone maintenance clinic daily and reports no other drug use.
- Client states she is able to manage a daily rest period even in light of a busy work and travel schedule.
- Client states she is able to carry out usual lifestyle activities in spite of cast on injured arm.

THE PREGNANT ADOLESCENT

Adolescent pregnancy is not a new phenomenon. Historically, it was common for women to marry as early as age 12 or 13 years and have their first baby at age 15 years. In today's society, however, marriage and childbearing are life situations thought of as belonging to later years. Reasons for the high number of teenage pregnancies that still continue include:

- Earlier age of menarche in girls (the average age is 12.4 years; many girls begin menstruating at age 9 years and so are ovulating and able to conceive by age 11 years)
- Increase in the rate of sexual activity among teenagers
- Lack of knowledge about (or failure to use) contraceptives or abstinence
- Desire by young girls to have a baby

Having an equally young sexual partner can contribute to pregnancy incidence because, in this situation, neither partner may be well versed in contraceptive options (Centers for Disease Control and Prevention [CDC], 2012b). In addition, some adolescents become pregnant as the result of rape or incest (Young, Deardorff, Ozer, et al., 2011).

Failure of adolescents to obtain adequate knowledge of contraceptive measures or abstinence is an issue that can be addressed by health care providers. As protective measures are easy to use, the average adolescent should not have difficulty following instructions. Adolescents are also capable of using emergency contraceptive measures correctly and safely. Access to emergency contraception is not associated with increased rates of unprotected intercourse or with higher rates of pregnancy or sexually transmitted infections (Beasley, 2010; Wilkinson, Fahey, Suther, et al., 2012). Unfortunately, providing this type of information does not always resolve the problem because adolescents may lack money to purchase protection such as birth control pills or a diaphragm. In addition, the egocentric phenomenon of adolescence makes a sexually active teenager believe she will not become pregnant (i.e., "It won't happen to me"). Some adolescent girls actually plan pregnancy because they believe being pregnant will free them from an intolerable school or home situation or give them someone to love who will also love them back. It puts a tremendous responsibility on a newborn to furnish love and change a girl's life; child maltreatment can occur when the newborn cannot meet such expectations (Valentino, Nuttall, Comas, et al., 2012).

At one time, many pregnant unmarried girls were sent to a "secret" home or shelter where they would stay throughout their pregnancy, give birth, place the child for adoption, and then return home as if nothing had happened to them. Today, pregnant teenagers typically remain at home, attend prenatal care, and are seen in maternity care facilities the same as older women do. They give birth in birthing rooms at hospitals, and as many as 90% keep their babies (Martin, Hamilton, Ventura, et al., 2011). Few give birth in alternative birth centers because the risk of cephalopelvic disproportion makes adolescent pregnancies high risk. Home birth is not recommended for the same reason. Offering increased guidance during pregnancy and for child care during the following years for adolescents can be an important nursing role.

Developmental Tasks of Adolescence

Adolescence is a vulnerable time for pregnancy because the developmental tasks of pregnancy are superimposed on those of adolescence. The developmental tasks of the average adolescent are fourfold: to establish a sense of self-worth or a value system, to emancipate from parents, to adjust to a new body image, and to choose a vocation (Erikson, 1963). A girl in the process of separating from her parents may be devastated by the reality that a baby will soon be dependent on her. She may need her parents' financial help to obtain prenatal care or buy clothing for her new baby. If she must depend on her parents' health insurance, she may feel virtually trapped into dependence. Helping adolescents to make their own health care decisions at health care visits helps to foster a sense of independence in the middle of this forced dependency. Consider, for example, the decision the adolescent must make about where to place a medication reminder chart: if it hangs in the kitchen, her mother may monitor it; in her bedroom or in her school locker, she alone will monitor it. An adolescent may not be able to choose when she comes for care (her mother has the car to drive her only on Tuesday afternoons), but during a visit, she can do many things to feel independent, such as weigh herself, hold a mirror to view her pelvic examination, or be interviewed apart from her parents.

Parents may have difficulty allowing a daughter to make her own health care decisions. Soon, however, she will be caring for an infant, so she needs this practice in independence and responsibility. You may need to remind parents that a pregnant adolescent is regarded as an **emancipated minor** or a *mature minor*—a person capable of making health care decisions—and so may sign permission for her own care. In some states, emancipated minors can qualify and are eligible for special health insurance coverage, so issues with privacy, parental permission, and parental notification are avoided. In August 2002, a new federal rule that is based on requirements contained in the Health Insurance Portability and Accountability Act of 1996 (HIPAA), embodies important protections for minors, along with a significant degree of deference to other laws (both state and federal) and to the judgment of health care providers. These provisions represent a compromise between competing viewpoints about the importance of parental access to minors' health information and the availability of confidential adolescent health care services (DHHS, 2012). The protection of confidentiality for adolescents is based on recognition that some minors would not seek needed health care for such concerns as sexual activity, pregnancy, HIV, sexually transmitted infections (STIs), substance abuse, or mental health if they could not receive it confidentially. Forgoing care because of this would have negative health implications for them as well as society. Maintaining privacy for adolescents needs to be especially respected with the introduction of electronic health records (Polito, 2012).

Pregnancy may interfere with the development of a healthy sexual relationship and cause difficulty in establishing future intimate relationships if a girl realizes her current relationship has led to a situation detrimental to her. To prevent this, it is useful to help her view the pregnancy as a growth-producing experience. Most people can point to a day in their life when they "grew up" (perhaps a day a parent became ill or the day they left home for college). This pregnancy can be that "growing up" revelation for a pregnant adolescent.

Establishing a value system or sense of identity can be difficult if health care personnel treat a pregnant adolescent as though she is irresponsible. Encouraging her to continue school is crucial to her self-esteem and to her future as well as to the financial future of her unborn child. Many schools have special programs for pregnant adolescents that include aspects of prenatal care to help ensure pregnant adolescents can stay in school.

Prenatal Assessment

Adolescents are considered high-risk clients because they have a high incidence of gestational hypertension, iron-deficiency anemia, and premature labor (Box 22.2). They also have a higher incidence of low–birth-weight infants, a disproportion between fetal and pelvic size, and a high rate of intimate partner violence (Derbyshire, 2012; Shrim, Ates, Mallozzi, et al., 2011). Early and consistent prenatal care is essential to their health and the health of their baby.

Unfortunately, many adolescents do not seek prenatal care until late in their pregnancies because they may view not seeking prenatal care as a way of protecting the pregnancy—if they don't tell anyone, no one can suggest they terminate the pregnancy. After the sixth month, abortion is no longer a possibility, so a girl can feel free to come for care without being subjected to this pressure.

Other factors contributing to the lack of prenatal care include:

- Denial she is pregnant
- Lack of knowledge of the importance of prenatal care
- Dependence on others for transportation
- Feeling awkward in a prenatal setting (an adult setting)
- Fear of a first pelvic examination
- Difficulty relating to authority figures

A primary nursing or case management approach that minimizes the number of health care providers a teenager is exposed to may be the most effective method for providing care during the prenatal period. Some adolescents do well in group prenatal care because it allows them to interact with peers the same as they do at school.

Health History

Take a detailed health history of an adolescent at the first prenatal visit to establish individual risks. This is best done without a parent present. The girl needs practice in being responsible for her own health, and having to account for her health practices can help her do this. It also helps prevent her from fabricating an answer to please a parent.

Some adolescents come to a facility with concerns such as "weight gain" or "feeling tired all the time" rather than saying they are pregnant, hoping health care providers will think of pregnancy as a possible reason for their symptoms. This is part denial and part pregnancy protection. Always be alert to the possibility of pregnancy when an adolescent describes symptoms that are vague and hard to define. If the importance of what she is saying when she mentions feeling "tired" or "nauseated" is dismissed, she may ask if someone will feel her stomach. If told this is not necessary for any of the symptoms she has mentioned, she may describe bigger symptoms, such as "terrible stomach pain." Think of possible pregnancy when you hear such a "growing" history.

Many adolescents want to keep their world totally separate from the adult world and, to do so, they do not voluntarily share information with adults. When interviewing adolescents, be certain to press for the responses needed to allow you to assess her safely. Do not accept statements such as "I eat okay" as a nutrition history or "I'm a very active person" as a history of rest and activity. Ask for details.

If an adolescent delayed seeking health care, ask for the reason for this at her first prenatal visit. Acknowledge that "protecting" the pregnancy is a desirable motive, but continuing with prenatal care will be much more beneficial.

If a parent accompanies a girl, ask the parent separately what, if any, concerns he or she wishes to discuss. A young adolescent is still a daughter, and a parent may be very concerned about her health during this pregnancy, as the parent was at health visits when the girl was being seen for a cold or a sports injury. If the baby's father attends prenatal care, help him to feel welcome. Because he is not married, he does not have a legal right to participate in decisions concerning the pregnancy, abortion, or adoption, but he may not be devoid of feelings for the girl or the baby (Davies, 2011). If he is an adolescent, he may feel sorrow that, because of his age, he cannot provide adequately. If a complication occurs, he may feel genuine grief things are not going well. Allowing him to offer support in the current pregnancy can help him learn more about himself as well as better define his role. In addi-

BOX 22.2 Nursing Care Planning Using Assessment

Assessing the Pregnant Adolescent for Complication Risk

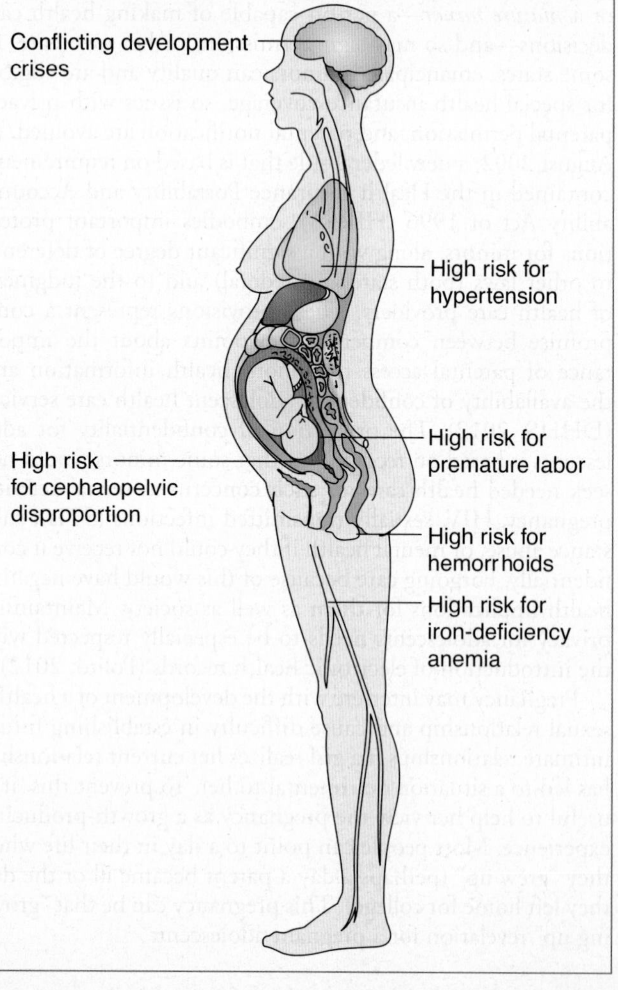

tion, be sure he receives compassionate education on preventing further pregnancies until he is more mature.

Often, adolescent girls have not talked to other pregnant women, so they may need extra teaching about common pregnancy symptoms such as urinary frequency, fatigue, and breast tenderness. Asking what symptoms an adolescent is having and reassuring her they are part of a normal pregnancy can help prevent her from attempting to treat them with potentially teratogenic over-the-counter medications.

As pregnancy progresses, listen for signs of "nest-building" behavior. An adolescent girl may not have the financial resources to buy clothing or a crib, but she may reveal nest-building feelings by asking an increasing number of questions about newborns or saving money to buy a simple baby article such as a pair of booties. This may seem like small involvement, but for a young girl without financial means, a dollar a week is actually large involvement.

Some adolescents have difficulty telling their parents about the pregnancy. Role-playing or simulation may be an effective technique to help them prepare to do this. Some girls report on a second visit their parents were not nearly as angry as they had anticipated. Instead, their parents reacted as if they had been waiting to hear this news, having accepted it as inevitable months before.

Family Profile. Adolescents may leave home if their family disapproves of their pregnancy, thus joining the ranks of homeless or adolescent runaways. Others do not leave home, but separate themselves emotionally from their family. Trying to manage by themselves leaves adolescents with a tremendous financial strain and a devastating sense of loneliness. Be sure to ask a girl at prenatal visits where she is living, what the source of her income is, and whom she would call if she suddenly became ill.

Asking about home life may reveal a dysfunctional family or an incest relationship as the cause of the pregnancy. If the girl is under legal age, incest is considered child maltreatment. Know your local and state laws on this topic and make the necessary report.

Because of family relationship problems, a girl may need help in making arrangements for the next few months of her pregnancy and for child care afterward. If she can no longer live at home, is there a relative she may live with? What kind of financial support does she need? Family and social supports for pregnant adolescents have been shown to be important influences on the maintenance of a healthy pregnancy lifestyle and to help prevent low birth weight in their children (Hodnett, Fredericks, & Weston, 2010; Jutte, Roos, & Brownell, 2010).

Be certain to ask if the girl is planning to continue with school because pregnancy is an egocentric time when outside interests do not always seem important. Help her to see that the months of pregnancy will go by faster if she keeps busy and remaining in school will be a way of doing this. It also is important in preparing for her future, because a high school education will be necessary to obtain enough marketable skills to support herself and her baby. Once she has given birth, returning to school may be difficult because she may have child care problems and because she may feel more mature than her classmates (or her classmates may make her feel this way). Any school that obtains federal money cannot discriminate against students because they are physically challenged. Many states interpret pregnancy as physically challenging, so in those states, a girl cannot be forced to leave school (or even asked to go to an alternate school) because of pregnancy. For some girls, you may need to advocate with a school committee for a proper school placement. Box 22.3 shows an interprofessional care map illustrating both nursing and team planning for a pregnant adolescent.

Day History. Adolescents may be unwilling to provide a detailed day history unless its purpose is well explained. Assure a pregnant teenager the purpose of the history is to learn more

BOX 22.3 Nursing Care Planning

AN INTERPROFESSIONAL CARE MAP FOR A PREGNANT ADOLESCENT

Mindy Carson, 16 years old and 15 weeks pregnant, received a 4-in. laceration on her leg when she was in an automobile accident on her way to the prenatal clinic this morning. The father of Mindy's baby, Carlos, is a college student who does not want Mindy to keep her baby after the birth because he does not want to get married until he finishes graduate school. Mindy insists she is old enough to be a parent and wants to keep her baby. Mindy's mother has accused Carlos of sharing methamphetamine with Mindy. She's also worried Mindy has been working as a prostitute to support a drug habit.

Family Assessment Lives with family in second-floor apartment above convenience store, which parents own and operate. Is a junior in high school but is "ready to drop out." Cares for 5-year-old sister after school while parents work downstairs.

Client Assessment Pale, tired-appearing adolescent female. Failed to come for two previous appointments. Admits to methamphetamine use since becoming pregnant. Hinted she might be using prostitution as income source. Parents want her to end pregnancy; client wants to continue pregnancy because "Now I can eat anything I want since I'm eating for two." Unhappy with arguing between parents and boyfriend. States, "I'm coming apart at the seams."

Nursing Diagnosis Altered family processes related to the stress of adolescent pregnancy

Outcome Criteria Client and family members demonstrate positive coping mechanisms by communicating effectively; client identifies plans for self and infant; clarifies relationship desired with father of child. Baby's father (Carlos) participates in pregnancy activities as desired; client halts risky, unhealthy practices.

(continued on page 596)

BOX 22.3 Nursing Care Planning (continued)

Team Member Responsible	Assessment	Intervention	Rationale	Expected Outcome
Activities of Daily Living, Including Safety				
Nurse	Assess the reason client states she is ready to drop out of school.	Discuss with client advantages of staying in school during pregnancy.	It is difficult for young women to support themselves and an infant without at least a high school education.	Client contracts to stay in school through graduation if academically possible.
Teamwork and Collaboration				
Nurse/Social worker	Investigate client's options for schooling if she no longer feels comfortable in her local public school.	Contact the client's school (with her permission) to explore options for her continued school attendance.	Discussion promotes active problem solving and positive adaptation.	Client and school personnel agree on a course of action that will optimally benefit the client.
Nurse/Social worker	Assess what community resources are available for withdrawal from methamphetamine.	Discuss the advantages of a withdrawal program during pregnancy.	Almost all substances cross the placenta and reach the fetus.	Client attends sessions for withdrawal from methamphetamine.
Procedures/Medications for Quality Improvement				
Nurse	Assess what client expects from prenatal care and if she understands the importance of regular attendance.	Discuss that prenatal care is especially important for adolescents as they are prone to complications because of immature body development.	Prenatal care is the best safeguard against complications of pregnancy and early, effective intervention if a complication occurs.	Client attends all future prenatal care appointments; participates in discussions at these times.
Nutrition				
Nurse/ Nutritionist	Assess 24-hour dietary recall with client.	Examine food intake to see if it contains all essential nutrients for pregnancy.	"Eating for two" does not mean eating more; it means eating more nutritious foods.	Client's 24-hour recall history at next visit shows improvement in necessary pregnancy nutrients.
Patient-Centered Care				
Nurse	Assess what client means by "I'm coming apart at the seams" in reference to her lack of support.	Meet with family members (with client's permission) to see if they could offer more emotional support.	Additional emotional help may be required to cope with the added demands of a teenage pregnancy.	Client states she is receiving adequate support from a combination of her family, her boyfriend, or health care providers.
Psychosocial/Spiritual/Emotional Needs				
Nurse	Assess if client's disagreement with family over continuing pregnancy is a major stressor.	Assist client with ways to adapt to changes of pregnancy and responsibility for fetal safety. Support client's decision to continue pregnancy.	Adolescence is a highly stressful time, especially without parental support, so change can be difficult if not anticipated.	Client states she is open to changes she knows will occur with pregnancy; will ask health care providers for additional suggestions to handle stress as needed.
Informatics for Seamless Health Care Planning				
Nurse	Assess what would be the best days for client and boyfriend to attend prenatal care.	Set up follow-up visits with client and support person; plan teaching strategies and discussion of all parties' needs and concerns as appropriate.	Prenatal care can help detect and prevent complications of pregnancy.	Client attends prenatal care regularly during remainder of pregnancy.

about her as a whole person, not to discover if she is doing things during the day she should not be doing. Adolescents are private people so to allow you to walk through their adolescent world for a day is a breach of adolescent philosophy. Ask in particular about nutritional practices, sleep, daily activities, use of drugs, and whether she has friends who can support her throughout this experience.

Be certain to include questions about her medication history. Ask if she is taking anything over the counter such as cold remedies or herbal supplements. Impress upon a girl the importance of not taking any medication—even nonprescription medication—without prior approval from her health care provider. It's possible for pregnancy to become an important growth experience if it provides the motivation some adolescents need to withdraw from recreational drug use.

Physical Examination

Physical examination procedures with pertinent adolescent findings are discussed in Chapter 34. Be certain to explain procedures as you do an examination. A statement such as "Oh, you're starting to have colostrum," a positive finding of pregnancy, may be frightening to an adolescent who does not know what colostrum is. A better way to phrase such a finding might be, "Your breasts are not only healthy but already beginning to produce early breast milk. Later on we'll talk about the importance of that for newborns." This kind of feedback makes a health examination both a learning experience and relieves anxiety for adolescents, who tend to be very concerned about body appearance.

Adolescents are at an increased risk for gestational hypertension, probably because of immature blood vessels or an immune response to the foreign protein of their fetus (Waugh & Smith, 2012). Few adolescents know what their blood pressure was prior to pregnancy, so they do not know their nonpregnant pressure. Obtain a baseline pressure at the first prenatal visit and make a point of informing the girl of her reading to encourage active health care participation in the future. Adolescents are often active in a waiting room (e.g., walking to get a magazine, returning it, or looking out the window); be certain the girl has 15 minutes of rest before you take a blood pressure or the recording may be falsely high.

Use a Doppler technique to obtain fetal heart tones, if possible, because hearing the fetal heart helps an adolescent acknowledge the reality of her pregnancy. For the same reason, make a point of assessing fundal height from visit to visit to show the baby is growing.

Adolescents with a substance dependency may be reluctant to supply a urine specimen for testing because they are worried you are secretly looking for evidence of drug use. In these instances, you may receive a cupful of water in place of a urine specimen. If in doubt regarding the substance you are testing, check the specific gravity. The specific gravity of water is 1.000, whereas urine specific gravity ranges from 1.003 to 1.030. Most adolescents like to weigh themselves at prenatal visits because weight gain in early pregnancy is proof they are pregnant. It is good practice to make a note of the clothing a girl is wearing the first time she is weighed, such as jeans and a T-shirt, so later weight determinations can be compared accurately. Be certain teenagers know a healthy weight gain is important for fetal growth and that this weight can be lost afterward.

QSEN Checkpoint Question 22.1

Evidence-Based Practice

To broaden understanding of the reproductive health education needs of adolescent girls, researchers conducted in-depth interviews with 12 adolescent mothers. Participants reported they perceived that becoming a mother at a young age was meaningful. They expressed a need to be addressed as adult parents who want the best for their child. Social isolation was found to be an important factor of vulnerability. The researchers recommended adolescent mothers receive counseling over and above the decision to continue or terminate pregnancy as well as subsequent information on contraception methods to avoid further pregnancies. Special care should be provided to girls who are socially isolated (Aujoulat, Libion, Berrewaerts, et al., 2010).

Based on the previous study, if Mindy comes to clinic and tells you her mother will not allow her to make independent decisions about her care, what would be your best action?

a. Avoid interfering because the mother is providing helpful input.
b. Tactfully ask the mother to leave the room, then interview Mindy privately.
c. Support Mindy in her attempts to take responsibility for her own care.
d. Supplant Mindy's mother's advice with your own suggestions that are in Mindy's best interests.

Look in Appendix A for the best answer and rationale.

Nursing Diagnoses and Related Interventions

Nursing Diagnosis: Health-seeking behaviors related to special care necessary for healthy adolescent pregnancy

Outcome Evaluation: Client states she feels confident in her ability to follow healthy prenatal guidelines to avoid pregnancy complications; asks questions as needed about her pregnancy.

Pregnancy Education

Adolescents usually need a great deal of health teaching during pregnancy because they do not know many of the common measures of care older women have learned from experience. They are also often unwilling to follow health care advice that makes them feel different in any way from their peers. However, as adolescents often do not have well-established health practices, they may be extremely adaptable and ready to change health habits for a pregnancy.

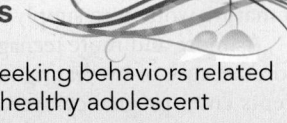

Adolescent girls may respond to health teaching that is directed to their own health more than to that of a fetus. A statement such as, "Eat a high-protein diet because protein makes your hair shiny (or prevents split fingernails)" often leads to better adherence than a reminder that protein is good for the baby. "Taking the iron supplement should make you feel less tired" might be better than, "It will help build the baby's blood supply," for the same reason. These are truthful statements and they appeal to an adolescent's preoccupation with self. In addition, this type of health teaching is the only form to which an adolescent who is denying her pregnancy can respond.

Adolescents also need instructions about possible discomforts and changes associated with pregnancy, and measures to relieve them (see Chapter 12 for a complete discussion). Many pregnant adolescents, for example, develop hemorrhoids because the disproportion of their body size to a fetus puts extra pressure on pelvic vessels, causing blood to pool in rectal veins. You can assure girls this is a pregnancy-related phenomenon that will resolve when the pregnancy is over.

Adolescents may also develop many striae across the sides of their abdomens because so much stretching of the abdominal skin occurs. Assure them, because of skin elasticity, these marks will probably fade after pregnancy. Chloasma, excess pigment deposition on the face and neck, appears at the same rate in adolescents as in older women. Adolescents, however, may be more conscious of this pigment because, overall, they are more conscious and concerned about their facial appearance. Suggesting a cover makeup and offering reassurance the pigmentation will fade after pregnancy may help.

Nutrition. Good nutrition can be a major problem during an adolescent pregnancy because many girls enter pregnancy with poor nutritional stores from years of eating a less-than-optimal diet. This lack of nutritional stores is serious because, especially in very young adolescents, it can result in preterm births and low–birth-weight newborns. To prevent these complications, a girl should have an intake that both allows for growth of the fetus and also provides for the needs of her own growing body. Otherwise, protein; iron; folic acid; and vitamins A, C, and D deficiencies may become acute. In order to compensate, she may need to gain more weight than a mature woman to supply adequate pregnancy nutrients.

As more and more teenagers are obese today than ever before because of overeating and lack of exercise, many adolescents enter pregnancy overweight or obese. This can lead to macrosomia or overgrowth in a fetus, a situation that leads to an increase in the number of cesarean births (Alexandra, Vassilios, Alexandra, et al., 2011). Such adolescents should not actively restrict nutrients during pregnancy; although they are obese, their body may be deficient in protein and vitamins.

Many adolescent girls do not eat well during pregnancy because they simply do not know what constitutes good nutrition. Some girls have little choice in what foods are prepared at home. To change a dietary pattern for these girls, you may have to talk to the person who does the cooking in the family. Besides eating the right amount of food, a pregnant adolescent may need to abandon a food fad she has been following, such as drinking soda, for a glass of orange juice (difficult to do if no one she knows drinks orange juice). The best you may be able to accomplish in this situation is to secure her agreement to switch to noncaffeinated soft drinks.

Remember, if a girl is attending school, she probably eats at least one meal away from home each day, so be certain nutrition education includes how to "brown bag" or buy a nutritious cafeteria lunch (type A school lunches are discussed in Chapter 32). If she travels by school bus, she may leave home by 6:00 AM or 7:00 AM, so she needs suggestions on how to construct a quick but healthy breakfast. Leaving so early creates a second problem of having to wait a long space of time until lunchtime. Suggest midmorning snacks, such as fruit, that also supply vitamins, not just empty calories.

Adolescents traditionally do not take medicine conscientiously, so they may need frequent reminders to take their vitamin or iron supplement. Stress that these are intended to complement nutrition during pregnancy so must not only be purchased but also must be swallowed. For a reminder system, girls may need to post a medication reminder chart at home or in her school locker or to set a reminder on her phone in order to increase adherence.

What if...22.1 Mindy tells you her daily nutrition consists of a liquid diet beverage for breakfast, a salad for lunch, and then cheese pizza for dinner. Will this typical teenage diet be adequate for her during pregnancy?

Activity and Rest. Adolescents vary greatly in their levels of activity. Assess a girl's participation in sports and determine which ones (if any), such as diving, gymnastics, or touch football, may need to be discontinued during pregnancy. Many girls practice sports for the feeling of belonging to a group or for companionship. To prevent her from feeling "shut out" by her friends, you may need to suggest alternative activities such as joining the drama or language club or perhaps inviting friends over once a week to watch a movie so she does not suffer from the loss of companionship.

Planning enough rest time during pregnancy can be yet another area of concern, especially if a girl is acting as if nothing different than usual is happening to her (Box 22.4). If this is so, it may help to explore a typical day and suggest ways to rest without compromising social relationships (e.g., sitting and talking after school rather than walking through the mall).

Physiologic Changes. A young girl may have little knowledge about body functions, so as a rule, all adolescent girls need substantial education on the physiologic changes that will occur during pregnancy. Despite all the health information given to children in school, it is not uncommon to find an adolescent who thinks her baby is growing in her stomach and so is unable to eat large meals for fear of suffocating or drowning her fetus. In addition, specific information about labor and delivery is essential to counteract all the "scare stories" girls may be hearing from their peers. Gaining this type of knowledge is another way pregnancy can be a growth experience. At the end of the pregnancy, this adolescent will know a great deal more about her body and her ability to monitor her health than her average classmate.

Childbirth Preparation. Peer companionship is a strong need for most adolescents. When girls become pregnant, because they are suddenly so different, they may find themselves cut off from fellow classmates. This can make them more inclined, therefore, to join a class of other adolescents in preparation for childbirth. Because being a student is so age appropriate for them, they usually are excellent students in a class. In addition, they have enough childish magical belief operating that they are not skeptical about whether prepared childbirth will work for them. In fact, believing prepared childbirth will work is an important component in a successful prepared childbirth experience, so this becomes a self-fulfilling prophecy.

BOX 22.4 Nursing Care Planning Based on Effective Communication

You talk to Mindy at a prenatal clinic.

Less Effective Communication	More Effective Communication
Nurse: Hello, Mindy. How are you feeling? **Mindy:** Good, but always tired. You know. **Nurse:** You should try and rest more. **Mindy:** Right. **Nurse:** Why don't you ask your boyfriend to help you more? **Mindy:** I'll do that. **Nurse:** Or stop working at the fast food restaurant. That'll leave you time to rest more. **Mindy:** Right. Great solution. **Nurse:** Glad I could be of help.	**Nurse:** Hello, Mindy. How are you feeling? **Mindy:** Good, but always tired. You know. **Nurse:** Are you getting enough sleep? **Mindy:** How can I? I work every day after school. **Nurse:** Is there anyone who could help you out more? Your boyfriend? A friend? **Mindy:** I'm pretty much alone since I got pregnant. **Nurse:** As long as you're coming to this clinic, you're not alone. Tell me about a typical day and let's investigate together ways you could get more rest.

In the first scenario, the nurse was so intent on giving advice, she forgot the first step of effective problem solving—identify the exact problem that needs solving. In the second scenario, when the nurse continues to assess rather than offer advice, she is able to identify the problem and, hopefully, work through a solution acceptable to Mindy.

Birth Decisions. Pelvic measurements should be taken early and carefully in adolescent girls because cephalopelvic disproportion is a real possibility because of the girl's incomplete pelvic growth (Malabarey, Balayla, & Abenhaim, 2012). Most girls who are told their baby will have to be born by cesarean birth respond well to the news, and some are actually relieved, because surgery seems controlled and simple compared with the agonies of labor they may imagine. Be certain the information a cesarean birth must be scheduled is shared with the girl and her parents as soon as possible as adolescents want to know the truth. They can regard the withholding of information not as protection but as an indication they are being treated as children.

Plans for the Baby. Adolescents may need additional time at prenatal visits to talk to a good listener about how they feel about being pregnant and becoming a mother. Scared? Bewildered? Numb? Happy? Be certain they know all the options available to them when their baby is born (e.g., keeping the baby, placing the baby in a temporary foster home, adoption). Adolescents, like all women, should be encouraged to breastfeed (Grassley, 2010). Breast tissue matures with pregnancy, so even very young adolescents are physically capable of breastfeeding.

Complications of Adolescent Pregnancy

As mentioned earlier, adolescent pregnancy carries the increased incidence of gestational hypertension, iron-deficiency anemia, preterm labor, and cephalopelvic disproportion (see Box 22.2). Fortunately, with conscientious prenatal care, these complications can be minimized.

Gestational Hypertension

Because adolescents are more prone to gestational hypertension than the average woman, establishing a baseline blood pressure for them is important. This is particularly important if an adolescent has not had her blood pressure measured since a preschool or school-age checkup, which may have been as many as 10 years earlier, and so has little idea what is her usual blood pressure.

The best intervention for reducing an increasing blood pressure during pregnancy is bed rest, preferably in a side-lying position. Like so many other things, bed rest may be difficult for a teenager to achieve because she may easily grow bored, and being confined to bed limits her interactions with peers and school activities. Many girls on bed rest at home may rest better if they are lying on the living room couch, where they can be aware of household activities, rather than in an upstairs bedroom, where they get up time and again to see what is happening. Also, it is easier for a parent to encourage bed rest if a girl is within eyesight. If called too many times to the distant bedroom for small tasks, a parent tends to say, "Get up and get it yourself this time," and bed rest is interrupted. Help to establish exactly what the health care provider means by bed rest—does it mean strict confinement in bed or could she sit up part of every day in a lounge chair with legs elevated? Can she take a shower? Can she walk up stairs to use the bathroom? Knowing the exact rules from the beginning helps prevent misunderstandings and hurt feelings.

Girls on bed rest usually need activities to keep them busy, such as homework, listening to music, Internet activities, or interactive games. If the bed rest period will last longer than 2 weeks, a girl needs to make arrangements for how to continue in school, perhaps through home tutoring. You may need to advocate for her with her school system for tutoring services (remembering that only rarely can this be denied on the basis of pregnancy). "Assignments" from the health care agency, such as reading about appropriate pregnancy topics or frequent telephone calls not only help to occupy time but also demonstrate concern and an opportunity to enforce health teaching points.

Although its effect is controversial, low-dose aspirin therapy may be prescribed to help reduce symptoms of gestational hypertension (Rossi & Mullin, 2011). Keep in mind adolescents often are not reliable with taking daily medicine, particularly if it seems as unimportant as aspirin, and so they may need a medicine reminder chart to be successful with taking this.

If the hypertension continues after a period of bed rest at home (or if the symptoms of gestational hypertension are advanced when they are first discovered), a girl may be admitted to the hospital so bed rest can be better enforced. As soon as the fetus is mature, labor will be induced or a cesarean birth scheduled.

Iron-Deficiency Anemia

Many adolescent girls are deficient in iron because their low intake cannot balance the amount of iron lost with menstrual flows. Deficiency is revealed by chronic fatigue, pale mucous membranes, and a hemoglobin level less than 11 g/dl. Iron-deficiency anemia is associated with pica, or the ingestion of inedible substances such as blackboard chalk (López, Marigual, Martín, et al., 2012).

A pregnancy compounds iron-deficiency anemia because a girl must now supply enough iron for fetal growth and her increasing blood volume. All pregnant women should take an iron and folic acid supplement (folic acid is important for red blood cell growth and prevention of neural tube defects), but these are especially important for the adolescent (Obican, Finnell, Mills, et al., 2010). Like any other medication prescribed for pregnancy, help an adolescent plan a time each day to take her iron supplement. Review with her how many iron-rich foods she needs to eat daily in addition to this. An iron supplement is not a supplement until her dietary intake is already strong in iron-rich foods.

As soon as her body recognizes it has additional iron, she will begin rapidly forming immature red blood cells. To measure whether the supplemental iron is causing this effect, a reticulocyte count may be scheduled after 2 weeks; if the reticulocyte count is not elevated at this time, it implies a secondary problem exists or, more likely, the girl has not been taking the supplement. Taking a stool swab and assessing it for the black tinge of an iron supplement or reassessing her serum iron level are other methods of assessing for adherence.

Preterm Labor

Adolescents are at high risk for preterm labor, probably because their uteruses are not fully grown (Khashan, Baker, & Kenny, 2010). For this reason, review the signs of labor with them by the third month of pregnancy. Stress labor contractions usually begin as only a sweeping contraction no more intense than menstrual cramps. Any vaginal bleeding is suspicious of labor and needs to be reported. Adolescent girls have gained much of their knowledge of labor from television (where a woman suddenly announces she is in labor and within 15 minutes gives birth). Therefore, they may dismiss light contractions as simple discomfort, not realizing they might be the start of labor. If they can recognize labor contractions early, it is more likely premature labor can be halted.

Complications of Adolescent Labor, Birth, and the Postpartum Period

Cephalopelvic Disproportion

Adolescent labor does not differ from labor in the older woman if cephalopelvic disproportion is absent. The presence of cephalopelvic disproportion is suggested by a lack of engagement at the beginning of labor, a prolonged first stage of labor, and poor fetal descent. Graphing labor progress is an effective way to detect labor that is becoming abnormal or prolonged. Be certain an adolescent has a support person with her in labor so she can relax and breathe effectively with contractions. If this person is also an adolescent, you may need to serve as the true support person, or at least spend considerable time coaching so this person can effectively support the girl in labor.

Postpartum Hemorrhage

Young adolescents are more prone to postpartum hemorrhage than the average woman because, if a girl's uterus is not yet fully developed, it becomes overdistended by pregnancy. An overdistended uterus is more likely not to contract as readily as a normally distended uterus in the postpartum period, thus allowing bleeding to occur (Simpson, 2010). Adolescents also may have more frequent or deeper perineal and cervical lacerations than older women because of the size of the infant in relation to their body. Young adolescents, however, are generally healthy and have supple body tissue that allows for adequate perineal stretching. If a laceration does occur, it usually heals readily without complication.

Inability to Adapt Postpartally

Giving birth is such a stress and a major crisis that almost all women have difficulty integrating it into their life. This can make the immediate postpartum period almost an unreal time for an adolescent. A girl may "block out" the hours of labor as if they did not happen. If she was particularly frightened or she received a narcotic for pain, her memory of the labor hours may not be clear. Urge her to talk about labor and birth to make the happening real to her; otherwise, postpartum depression is more apt to occur (Patel & Wisner, 2011).

Lack of Knowledge About Infant Care

Adolescents show the same positive bonding behavior with their infants as their more mature counterparts (Fig. 22.1). Although they may consider themselves to be knowledgeable in child care because they have babysat for a neighbor's child or a younger sibling, they may lack knowledge of newborn care. They can be overwhelmed in the postpartum period when realizing the baby is their own, and child care is not as simple as it seemed. When the child cries, they cannot hand it to someone else; at the end of 4 hours, when they are tired of caring for the baby, they cannot leave and walk away. Although these things were most likely discussed with an adolescent during pregnancy, these feelings may not become prominent until the child is actually born. Spend time with a girl, observing how she handles her infant. Demonstrate bathing and changing the baby as appropriate. Model good parenting behaviors whenever possible by being aware of how you hold and care for the child.

Unfortunately, most adolescent mothers choose not to breastfeed. This is probably related to a lack of understanding about the importance of breastfeeding, their perception of breastfeeding as something that will "tie them down," and anticipating that this will create a time management conflict when returning to school (Smith, Coley, Labbok, et al., 2012). Education about the importance of breastfeeding and tips for how to incorporate it into a busy lifestyle can increase the number of adolescents who breastfeed (see Chapter 19). Help young mothers who do not choose to breastfeed to select a feeding method that is satisfying to them and safe for the infant as part of the process of becoming a young, but effective, new mother.

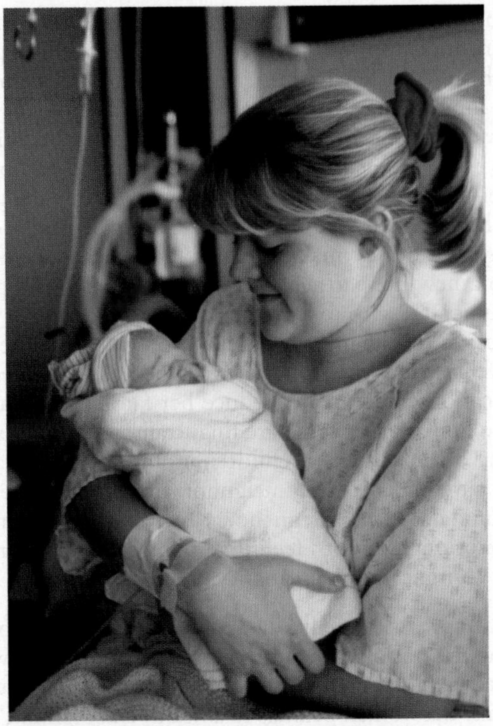

FIGURE 22.1 A new adolescent mother begins to bond with her infant (© Photo Network/Alamy).

QSEN Checkpoint Question 22.2

Informatics

Mindy was placed on an iron supplement because her hemoglobin level was below normal. What would be the best way to determine if Mindy is taking her iron supplement?

a. Perform a physical assessment noting if her nail beds have deepened in color.
b. Ask her to describe in her own words why she has been prescribed an iron supplement.
c. Look up her laboratory results to see if her reticulocyte count has increased since her last visit.
d. Analyze her urine for color that would reveal the presence of iron deposits.

Look in Appendix A for the best answer and rationale.

THE PREGNANT WOMAN OVER AGE 40 YEARS

The incidence of women delaying their first pregnancy until their late 30s or early 40s is increasing so much that 12% of births in the United States today are to women over age 35 years and 3% to 4% are to women over age 40 years (NCHS, 2012). In the past, it was assumed a woman of this age was past the optimal age for childbearing and so was at risk for many complications. Today, with the exception of a greater incidence of chromosomal abnormality, there is little evidence of serious complications in women older than age 40 years as long as prenatal care is begun early in the pregnancy.

BOX 22.5 Nursing Care Planning to Respect Cultural Diversity

What is perceived as the best time in life to have children is strongly culturally influenced. In developing countries, for example, many people believe having children while young allows parents to grow with children. In other cultures, such as the United States, many believe delaying childbirth until a family is financially secure is best. Because of these various beliefs, what you believe about the perfect time to have a baby may not be the belief of a family for whom you provide care. What may seem like a catastrophe in timing to you may seem like a blessing to someone else (and vice versa). Assess couples by history and observation to determine if childbearing appears to be timed correctly for them. If not, they may need extra time to accept a pregnancy and adapt to becoming parents.

A woman over age 40 years is more likely than a younger woman to enter pregnancy with a previously diagnosed condition, such as hypertension, varicosities, or hemorrhoids. In addition, by age 40 years, a woman usually has a major role change she must undertake during pregnancy, especially if she is well established in a career or has an accustomed routine at home or in her community. During pregnancy, she will need to think through how the pregnancy and childrearing are going to fit into and change her life. Although she may feel rich in the number of support people she perceives around her, she may discover she actually has few "pregnancy support" people because she does not have many friends her age who are also having babies, some even may be close to becoming grandparents. Many of the things these friends remember of pregnancy and labor were their particular highs and lows; the care they received may not reflect current practice. This can leave a woman without access to the daily "shop talk" of other pregnant women or someone to turn to with questions such as whether the backache she is experiencing or frequent need to urinate is normal. On the other hand, because many women delay childbearing today, she may be one of a sizable group of women in her community experiencing pregnancy at this stage of life. For this reason, be certain to assess each woman individually (Box 22.5).

Developmental Tasks and Pregnancy

The developmental challenge of the over 40 years age group is to expand their awareness or develop generativity—that is, a sense of moving away from themselves and becoming involved with the world or community (Erikson, 1963). Some people assume that once they reach adulthood, the way they are is the way they will always be. They are amazed to find not only do their bodies change (men may lose their hair; women and men both gain weight) but so do their interests. They may now find themselves joining committees and clubs, coaching Little League teams, or organizing fundraising or community events—activities they shunned when younger.

This can cause a woman in this age group who is pregnant to begin to feel ambivalent during the pregnancy because she may want to continue with community activities, yet also want to concentrate on the baby growing inside her.

Encouraging her to discuss how this conflict feels can help her balance her life and manage two life phases this way.

Women who are having a child after age 40 years tend to fall into one of two groups: those who are having their final child and those who have delayed childbearing because of education or a career and are having their first child. Many adults over the age of 40 years care for aging parents and so may also be dealing with the issues of older adults. These additional responsibilities and obligations can make it difficult for a woman to complete the psychological work of pregnancy. It also may create extra strain on her finances and time and it creates a "sandwich generation," or one pressured by responsibilities by both older and younger family members. Important worries include having enough energy, arranging for child care, and financial and space strains.

Prenatal Assessment

A woman over age 40 years, like all women, should begin prenatal care early in pregnancy. A few mistakenly believe their lack of menstruation is the result of early menopause and so do not seek an early health care consultation. Fortunately, most women of this age group recognize what is happening, are well informed about the advisability of early prenatal care, and also have adequate health insurance, so they do seek an early appointment.

Health History

Ask women in this age group to document their symptoms of pregnancy, how they feel about the pregnancy, and how it fits into their lifestyle. If a woman did not realize she was pregnant, she may have self-medicated. Ask if she has been taking any medication or herbal remedies to relieve symptoms such as nausea or fatigue. Because a woman is functioning well in a business world does not mean she follows a healthy pregnancy lifestyle. Do not accept answers such as "I drink socially" or "I take the usual drugs" without exploring what those phrases specifically mean.

Family Profile. Some women over age 40 years who are pregnant for the first time have recently changed their life pattern (e.g., become married or became involved in a long-term sexual relationship) or have decided to have a child, perhaps through in vitro fertilization, without a spouse before they are no longer able to conceive. Whereas a younger woman often waits a while after marrying or beginning a relationship with a new partner to become pregnant, a woman over age 40 often plans to become pregnant immediately because she senses her reproductive time clock ticking. Because of this, she may find herself making many adjustments at once (not only to a new life partner, house or apartment, and perhaps community, but also to a pregnancy).

Be certain to identify a woman's source of income. If she has a well-paying job, stopping work because of a pregnancy complication could greatly reduce her family's income. Also evaluate how many people are financially or emotionally dependent on her, such as children from a former marriage, elderly parents, an elderly neighbor, or fellow workers who count on her. During pregnancy, when a woman often needs extra emotional support, feeling responsible for so many people can complicate the pregnancy.

Day History. Ask specifically about a woman's type of work or home responsibilities and estimate the amount of walking or back strain those entail. Ask about recent diet or exercise programs. If a woman belongs to a health club, remind her the use of saunas and hot tubs for longer than 10 minutes at a time is contraindicated during pregnancy because of possible hyperthermia and teratogenic effects of extreme heat on a developing fetus (Duong, Shahrukh-Hashmi, Ramadhani, et al., 2011). Identify personal habits, such as cigarette smoking and alcohol consumption, that could be detrimental to a fetus to determine if counseling to halt or decrease these habits is needed.

Physical Examination

A woman over age 40 years needs a thorough physical examination at her first prenatal visit to establish her general health and to identify any problems, particularly circulatory disturbances, she may have. Inspect her lower extremities thoroughly for varicosities, because these are more common in women over age 40 years (Box 22.6). Obtain a urine

BOX 22.6 Nursing Care Planning Based on Family Teaching

TIPS ON PREVENTING VARICOSE VEINS

Q. Mindy says to you, "My mother was old when she had me so developed terrible varicose veins. How can I stop that from happening to me?"

A. Although the following activities are not foolproof, incorporating them into your day helps prevent the development of varicose veins.

- Find opportunities, such as a class or lunch break, to elevate your legs on a foot stool.
- Be certain your diet includes vitamin C every day, because this is important to strengthen vein walls.
- Rest in a side-lying position with your body tipped slightly forward (Sims position) as this allows leg veins to drain and empty.
- Avoid long periods of standing in one place; take "walk breaks" as active muscle contraction help venous return.
- Avoid sitting with your legs crossed.
- Do not wear anything constricting on your lower legs, such as knee-high stockings.
- If you're prescribed support hose, put them on before you get out of bed in the morning, before veins become swollen, for best results. Don't be fooled into thinking panty hose marked "strong support" are the same as medically prescribed support stockings.

specimen and test it for specific gravity, glucose, and protein to evaluate overall renal function and the possibility of gestational or type 2 diabetes, because older women are more prone than younger women to develop these conditions.

Assess a woman's breasts for any abnormalities, as women over age 40 years are in a higher risk group for breast cancer than are younger women. Ask if she has scheduled yearly mammograms. In addition, as gestational trophoblastic disease (hydatidiform mole) is also more common in women over age 40 years (see Chapter 21), assess carefully for fundal height and fetal movement at prenatal visits.

Chromosomal Assessment

Because the risk for Down syndrome is higher in older women than in younger women, an incidence of about 1 in 1,000 compared to 1 in 1,500 women over 35, a quad screen or integrated screen are offered (sometimes referred to as a sequential screen) in order to detect if an open spinal cord or chromosomal defect could be present in the fetus. These tests include an ultrasound to examine for nuchal translucency (seen in Down syndrome) done at 10 to 13 weeks of pregnancy as well as laboratory analysis for α-fetoprotein (AFP), a protein produced by the fetus; human chorionic gonadotropin (hCG), a hormone produced by the placenta; estriol, an estrogen produced by both the fetus and the placenta; and inhibin A, a protein produced by the placenta and ovaries, done at 15 to 16 weeks of pregnancy. These substances will be elevated in maternal serum if the fetus has an open spinal defect; they will be lower than usual if a chromosomal anomaly is present (Alldred, Deeks, Guo, et al., 2012).

Be certain a woman is prepared for these studies and receives support during them. Alert her that false-positive results can occur; to limit these, positive reports will be confirmed through a chromosomal analysis obtained by amniocentesis. Some women of this age group do not begin nest building until these tests are completed and they've been assured their child will be healthy.

Nursing Diagnoses and Related Interventions

Nursing Diagnosis: Health-seeking behaviors related to special care necessary for healthy pregnancy

Outcome Evaluation: Client states she feels confident in self-care and her ability to decrease possible complications of pregnancy.

Be certain to adapt prenatal teaching to fit an older woman's lifestyle. If she had not planned on ever being pregnant, she may have isolated herself through the years from "mothering" activities and so, despite her years, may know little about pregnancy and newborn care. Others may have read so extensively that they may know more theoretical information than a woman who has already given birth. Be certain to review information about possible discomforts of pregnancy (see Chapter 12). A pregnant woman over age 40, for example, is prone to hemorrhoids because she may have some rectal varicosities present at the beginning of pregnancy. Pain from rectal distention may, in fact, be one of the primary symptoms she reports at a first visit. Review measures to increase comfort from these (see Chapter 12).

Varicosities, like hemorrhoids, develop readily in a woman over age 40 because she may have had some tendency toward these even before the pregnancy. As with hemorrhoids, her best approach during pregnancy is to prevent formation of these. At the time of birth, be certain to document any degree of varicosity formation so nurses caring for her during the postpartum period can take special precautions to prevent thrombophlebitis because, as with venous stasis present after birth, a woman with varicosities is prone to develop this complication immediately postpartum.

Nutrition

Assess the number of meals a woman eats outside her home each week, including those she packs for lunch or eats in restaurants. If she enjoys many of these, she may need tips on how to obtain the same nutrition whether she prepares meals at home or eats them at an office or community function. Urge her to substitute a caffeine-free soft drink in place of an alcoholic beverage at social events. In the same way, substitute milk or juice or decaffeinated coffee for regular coffee. Some women this age normally drink little milk. Rather than getting used to milk again, a woman might appreciate suggestions on other ways to ingest calcium, such as puddings or yogurt or ask her health care provider for a calcium supplement.

Prenatal Classes

Because a pregnant woman over age 40 years may be unique in her circle of friends, she may be very interested in joining a childbirth preparation or prenatal exercise class where she is "one of the group" (Fig. 22.2).

Such classes for this age group often center on how to avoid complications such as varicosities, how to integrate pregnancy with a full-time work position, and supplying

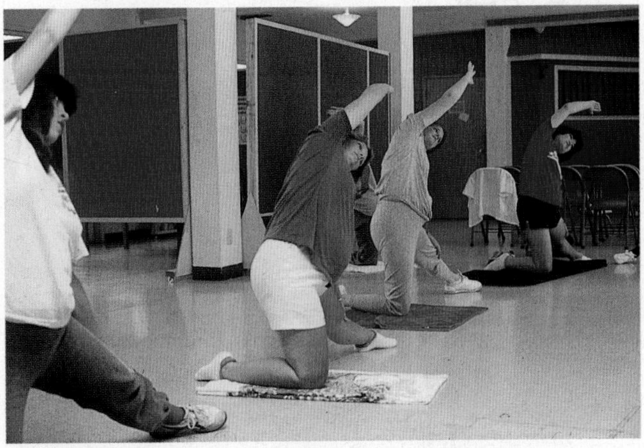

FIGURE 22.2 Exercise classes during pregnancy can provide women with an opportunity to interact with others like themselves while benefiting from a carefully monitored workout. (© Kathy Sloane.)

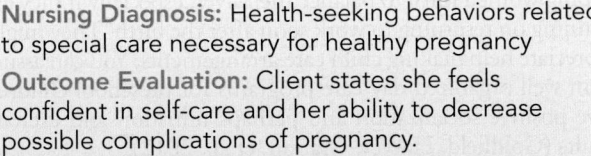

discussion time on how women are reacting to this dramatic life change. Be certain a woman or couple plan to set aside a specific time every day to do breathing exercises to be prepared for labor. Otherwise, a busy woman may never find time to get to them and will find herself unprepared in labor.

Complications of Pregnancy for a Woman Over Age 40 Years

The complications of pregnancy most likely to occur in a woman over age 40 years—gestational hypertension, preterm or postterm birth, and cesarean birth—are related to the fact that the woman's circulatory system may not be as competent as when she was younger, or her body tissues may not be as elastic as they were once (Box 22.7).

Gestational Hypertension

A woman over age 40 years has a higher risk for gestational hypertension than a younger woman because of blood vessel inelasticity, because hypertension tends to occur more frequently in nulliparas than in multiparas, and because some degree of hypertension may already exist before pregnancy (Gaillard, Bakker, Steegers, et al., 2011). At any age, the best way to reduce the symptoms of gestational hypertension is for women to take in an adequate supply of protein and obtain adequate rest each day. If a woman works full time, stopping work to obtain more rest may be difficult not only because she believes she may miss out on a promotion or risk losing her job, but also because her income is important to her family; she also is used to being productive, not merely resting all day. To allow her to rest effectively, you may need to help her plan activities she can accomplish on bed rest, such as reworking a school course outline or restructuring her office filing system.

BOX 22.7 Nursing Care Planning Using Assessment

Assessing the Pregnant Woman Over 40 Years of Age for Complications

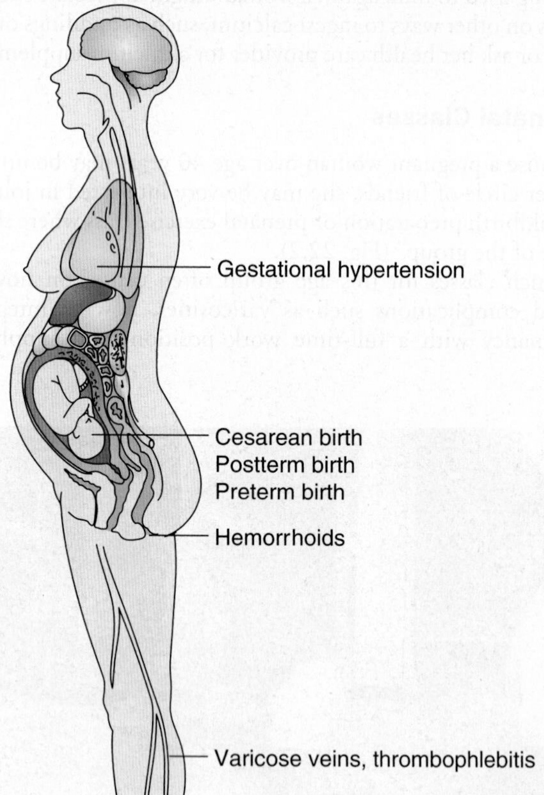

Complications of Labor, Birth, and the Postpartum Period for a Woman Over Age 40 Years

Complications that occur with a woman over age 40 years related to birth or the immediate period after birth also may be due to the body, which may not be as elastic as it once was.

Failure to Progress in Labor

Labor in an older primipara may be prolonged because cervical dilatation does not seem to occur as spontaneously as it does in younger women. Graphing labor progress is a good method to use to determine when labor is becoming prolonged. Many women this age may need a cesarean birth if labor becomes so overly prolonged it begins to place a fetus at risk. Encourage a woman to verbalize how she is feeling about her progress throughout labor to allow for reassurance and prompt intervention should problems arise. Keep in mind some older men may not be as comfortable in a birthing room as their younger counterparts because when they were young, men were excluded from watching births. You may need to spend time assuring them their presence is important so they can continue to offer active support.

Difficulty Accepting the Event

Women over age 40 years may begin to have second thoughts about childbearing this late in life as the reality of a new baby registers with them during the intrapartal and postpartum periods. Although they may have read a great deal about babies during pregnancy, they may state they wish they had read more or felt as confident with this phase of their life as they are about other areas such as their home, office, or classroom. Review plans for child care and postpartum rest, with an emphasis on helping women learn to balance their lives, especially if they are planning on returning to work soon after the birth. They might appreciate help making child care arrangements. You can assure them well organized day care programs for preschool children have positive socialization and perhaps nutrition and exercise results (Goldfield, Harvey, Grattan, et al., 2012).

Postpartum Hemorrhage

Just as the cervix may not dilate as readily during labor due to inelasticity, the uterus may not contract as readily in the postpartum period. The result of this puts women over 40 years of age at higher risk for postpartum hemorrhage (Yogev, Melamed, Bardin et al., 2010). She also may be more prone to perineal–anal tears because her perineum is less supple (Lyndon, Lee, Gilbert, et al., 2012). Because a woman over age 40 years may be an independent woman who is interested in self-care, she may ask for little help. Respect her need for independence, but at the same time, don't neglect assessing the amount of lochial flow or potential perineal bleeding to be certain these complications are detected.

QSEN Checkpoint Question 22.3

Quality Improvement

Both adolescents like Mindy and women over the age of 40 years are at increased risk for developing gestational hypertension. As a result, routine screenings for this health problem have been emphasized on the maternal unit for older mothers. What is the rationale for this change in nursing practice?

a. Many women over 40 years are underweight before they begin pregnancy.
b. Older women tend to have a higher fluid intake than do younger women.
c. Many older women are prone to edema due to their lower activity levels.
d. The blood vessels of older women may not be as elastic as those of younger women.

Look in Appendix A for the best answer and rationale.

THE PREGNANT WOMAN WHO IS PHYSICALLY OR COGNITIVELY CHALLENGED

In the past, women with conditions such as vision, hearing, cognitive, neurologic, or orthopedic challenges were sheltered by their families to such an extent women with even moderately physically challenging conditions could not meet potential sexual or marriage partners and so didn't become pregnant. In addition, many people believed this was right or that these individuals should not become pregnant. Today, women with varying degrees of disability attend public school, work in offices, join community organizations, establish sexual relationships, and plan pregnancies just like everyone else.

It's important to urge women with physical or cognitive disabilities to begin with preconceptual care so medicines they are taking can be evaluated, and careful planning for safe pregnancy care can be started early (Signore, Spong, & Krotoski, 2011). Because these women (and in some instances also their support persons) face special problems related to their conditions, nursing care during pregnancy must be designed with these special concerns in mind so the woman's and her family's challenges and needs can be addressed and met (Walsh-Gallagher, Sinclair, & McConkey, 2012).

Table 22.1 lists general areas of care that are important in planning for the physically or cognitively challenged woman who is pregnant.

Rights of the Physically or Cognitively Challenged Person

There are ethical and legal considerations related to women with disabilities. By federal law, physically disabled persons must have freedom of access to public buildings by means of ramps or handrails (U.S. Equal Employment Opportunity Commission [USEEOC], 1990). All public health care facilities must be in compliance with these laws both in terms of physical facilities and in the true spirit of the law; that is, people should be made to feel psychologically welcome as well as physically able to access the inside of the building. Under the same law, a hospital cannot deny care to a person with a disability even though the disabling condition complicates treatment considerably, possibly requiring extra personnel and time. A woman with a disability has full rights to her child, so the baby cannot be taken from her at birth without her full consent. Likewise, she cannot be forced to terminate a pregnancy or undergo sterilization unless that is her informed decision.

TABLE 22.1 Areas of Planning With Physically or Cognitively Challenged Women During Pregnancy

Area	Assessment and Planning Guidelines
Transportation	Ask if a woman has access to transportation for prenatal care and for emergencies.
Pregnancy counseling	Assess the special modifications of care that will need to be made depending on a woman's special challenge. Use additional visual or auditory aids to make your teaching points clear.
Support person	Determine who is the woman's main support person. In some instances, a woman's condition requires so much assistance during pregnancy you may need to contact community agencies to lend additional support (with her permission).
Health	Do not lose track of a woman's primary health problem. For example, a woman with cerebral palsy may need to continue an active muscle exercise program during pregnancy; a woman with multiple sclerosis may need to change her medication to avoid teratogenic effects.
Work	Assess whether a woman works outside her home and, if work is discontinued during pregnancy, what she could substitute for social contacts.
Recreation	Assess whether a woman's level of activity is adequate, and make concrete suggestions within her limitations if it needs to be increased.
Self-esteem	Assess a woman's level of self-esteem. If it is low, give praise at prenatal visits and help her make pregnancy a growth experience.

Modifications for Pregnancy

Explore with women with a disability at a first prenatal visit the exact nature of their disability and their general self-image to identify what modifications they may need you to plan for care during pregnancy. Some women who are physically or cognitively challenged maintain high self-esteem despite severe limitations and are able to modify and grow with a pregnancy, whereas others have a poor sense of self-esteem that could make change particularly difficult for them. However, for most women, pregnancy will become a special event, a 9-month announcement to everyone that, despite their seeming limitations, they are equal to other women and so are capable of participating in one of life's miracles. If a woman is housebound, be certain she is prescribed a prenatal vitamin containing vitamin D and can obtain refills because she is probably not receiving as much sun exposure as those who spend some time outside (Whitehouse, Holt, Serralha, et al., 2012).

Safety Measures to Explore

Safety is a key area of concern for a pregnant woman who is physically or cognitively challenged. Be certain to assess areas such as if she has emergency contact persons, suppliers of transportation, and individual considerations such as mobility, elimination, and possible autonomic responses. Be certain a woman reviews any medicine she is taking for her primary condition with her pregnancy care provider to be certain this will continue to be safe during pregnancy. Women with recurrent seizures, for example, may need to have their dose of antiseizure medicine reduced during pregnancy because some of these are teratogenic (Burakgazi, Pollard, & Harden, 2011).

Emergency Contacts. Evaluate the client's ability to contact someone in case of a pregnancy-related emergency. Does she have a telephone she can reach readily? Does she know how to activate the emergency medical system (911) in her community? If a woman's speech is not clear, evaluate whether she will be understood while using a telephone to call for help in an emergency. Some women with limited mobility, such as those with a spinal cord injury or cerebral palsy, have a specially designed telephone contact system in their home that connects to a paramedic or hospital emergency service through a beeper system. Check that they intend to maintain this throughout pregnancy. Some women who are hearing challenged use a specially equipped telephone (a telecommunications device for the deaf [TDD]) that prints out messages for them.

Transportation. Assess a client's ability to come for prenatal care. If a woman depends on a support person for transportation to a health care facility, you may have to arrange appointments according to that person's schedule to prevent missed appointments. Ask the woman, in an emergency, if that person is not available, how could she come for care? Women with cognitive or vision challenges, for example, may not qualify for a driver's license and so may need someone, such as a family member or friend, to drive. Women with a mobility challenge may have difficulty transferring into the specially equipped, hand-controlled car they usually drive as pregnancy progresses.

Mobility. All women who use wheelchairs are taught to press with their hands against the armrests and lift their buttocks up off the wheelchair seat for 5 seconds every hour to prevent the formation of pressure ulcers on the buttocks and posterior thighs. Encourage pregnant women to continue to perform this maneuver during pregnancy as the increased weight of a fetus increases her risk for pressure ulcer formation from additional compression. In addition, severe hip flexion from sitting in a wheelchair limits venous return from the lower extremities. For at least 1 hour every morning and afternoon, encourage women who ambulate by wheelchair to decrease the sharp bend at their knees and hips that results from sitting in the chair, to promote venous return and help prevent varicosities and thrombi formation. Resting on a couch for a time or adjusting the footrests of the wheelchair so her legs are not as sharply bent accomplishes this.

If maintaining balance is a problem, a woman may need reevaluation at the midpoint of pregnancy because as the weight of her abdomen increases, she becomes less stable. She may need to use crutches if she did not use them before, or use a wheelchair if she was ambulatory with crutches or a walker before pregnancy. Keep in mind a woman who is physically challenged achieved the degree of ambulation with which she first presents usually only after years of physical therapy and strengthening of leg and arm muscles. Help her see that reducing her degree of independence during pregnancy is not a step backward for her but a step forward, allowing her to have a safe pregnancy without the danger of falling (Fig. 22.3).

Elimination. When mobility is an effort, a woman may not drink as much as usual or use a bathroom as frequently as she would if those actions were effortless. Encourage a high fluid intake and frequent voiding, however, to prevent urinary tract infections. Women who use an indwelling catheter are at especially high risk for contracting urinary tract infections at any time and especially during pregnancy. Women who perform self-catheterization or change their own indwelling catheter may be unable to continue to do this late in pregnancy because the increasing size of their abdomen interferes with their ability to see or reach their perineum comfortably. If this happens, it may be necessary for a woman to arrange for a support person, a home care nurse, or a home health aide to do this for her.

Autonomic Responses. In a woman who has a high spinal cord injury (cervical or high thoracic), observe for **autonomic dysreflexia** during pregnancy, labor, and the immediate postpartum period. This is an exaggerated autonomic response to stimuli. Any irritating condition, such as a distended bladder,

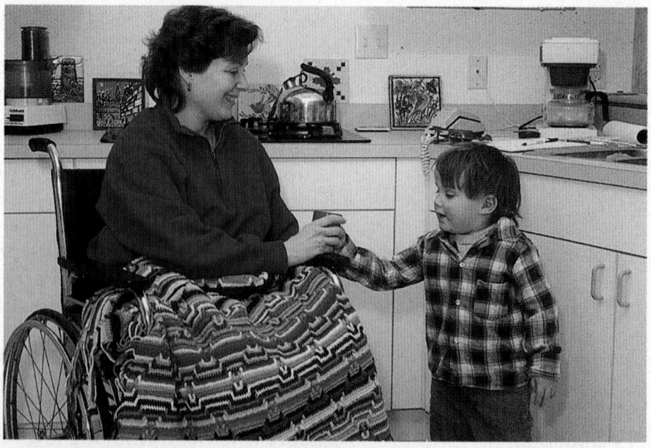

FIGURE 22.3 During pregnancy, a woman who is physically challenged may need to use a wheelchair to help safeguard herself against injury. Assure her that she may still enjoy her independence and daily activities, such as caring for an older child. (© Keith/Custom Medical Stock Photograph.)

increasing uterine size, labor contractions, or breastfeeding, may initiate the response (Rabchevsky & Kitzman, 2011). Without upper motor neuron control to reverse the phenomenon, extreme symptoms such as severe hypertension (300/160 mmHg), throbbing headache, flushing of the skin and profuse diaphoresis above the level of the spinal lesion, nausea, and bradycardia may occur. Immediate action is necessary to protect against a cerebrovascular accident or intraocular damage. Elevate a woman's head to reduce cerebral pressure and locate the irritating stimulus (usually a distended bladder or bowel). If bladder distention is the cause, the woman needs bladder pressure relieved by catheterization if an indwelling catheter is not in place. If a catheter is in place, check to see why it is not draining, then encourage it to drain by unkinking or flushing to allow urine to flow freely again. Anticipate the need for an antihypertensive agent to alleviate the extreme hypertension, although as soon as the source of irritation is removed, symptoms typically fade quickly.

Prenatal Care Modifications to Meet Specific Needs

Physical examination may need to be modified depending on individual circumstances for women with disabilities (Bates, Carroll, & Potter, 2011; Sudduth & Linton, 2011). Although women with disabilities have been followed by health care providers most of their lives, they may never have had a pelvic examination before and so need clear instructions about why it is needed and what it will consist of. Many obstetric examining tables are built for the comfort of the examiner and are too high for a woman to transfer to from a wheelchair by simply sliding onto the table. You may need to secure a ramp from the physical therapy department so the wheelchair can be elevated to the level of the table. Woman with a spinal cord injury or cerebral palsy may be unable to maintain their legs in a lithotomy position because of either hip flexion contracture or laxness of leg support. This means a dorsal recumbent position, rather than a lithotomy position, may be required for a pelvic examination.

Women who are cognitively challenged may not be aware of how they became pregnant. If a woman became pregnant because she was taken advantage of sexually, she may need some time to talk and work through this experience before she can agree to a pelvic examination.

If a visually challenged woman brings a guide dog with her to a health care visit, remember that although the dog's chief function is to offer direction, its instinct causes it to become a woman's protector. Resist petting guide dogs as this may be interpreted by the dog as a threat because it creates a distraction from safeguarding its owner.

When interviewing or teaching visually challenged women, be certain not to use your hands to illustrate points ("I'll need a urine sample of at least this much urine [measured with your fingers]"). Do not use colors as descriptions of objects ("put on the blue gown"). Use demonstration aids that allow a woman to feel or touch instead. When helping with or performing a physical assessment, let a woman know you are closing the door or drawing a curtain to ensure privacy. Always alert a woman when you are going to touch her, so as not to startle her. Otherwise, you may find yourself facing a growling guide dog that rises to protect her.

If a woman is hearing impaired, she may not be able to see the examiner's face during a pelvic examination. This means any question asked of her during this time will not be understood because she cannot see the examiner's lips to lip read (Middleton, Turner, Bitner-Glindzicz, et al., 2010). Stand by the head of the table and repeat instructions or questions as necessary.

Pregnancy Education

Try to modify health teaching to meet each woman's specific needs. For a woman who is cognitively challenged, for example, instructions about pregnancy may need to be given to her care provider. Those specifically for her might be limited to those few items crucial for safety, such as "do not drink alcohol or take any medicines except your vitamin pill."

If a woman and her support person are both visually challenged, pamphlets about pregnancy care will not be useful. If the support person can see, offer the pamphlets to him or her, suggesting the support person read them to the pregnant woman as a shared activity. This will not only be helpful to her but will also make the partner a more informed support person. Many visually challenged women have assistive technology devises such as special audio apps that record and play audio files. Nurses can contact the local branch of the national nonprofit organization Learning Ally (formerly Recording for the Blind and Dyslexic; http://www.learningally.org/) and ask if they have any material already recorded on pregnancy or breastfeeding they can supply. If not, you may be able make an audio file on the assistive technology device, including any information you particularly want a woman to remember or that she seems concerned about. Supply the health care facility telephone number at the beginning of the recording as an easy reminder for an emergency and perhaps the date of her next visit as well.

Nutritional education is another area that should be designed based on each client's specific challenges and usual routine. For example, a woman may only be able to prepare meals that do not require a stove unless her support person is with her. Nutrition counseling, therefore, needs to center on foods that can be prepared without cooking or only microwave warmed.

Activity and exercise, important for any pregnant woman, are just as crucial for a woman who is physically challenged. If exercise is likely to be very reduced in bad weather because she cannot walk safely on slippery snowy sidewalks, be certain a woman understands walking around her home or apartment can provide the same level of exercise as if she were walking around the block or exercising at a health club. Although labor and her child's birth may be modified somewhat because of a physical condition, gaining general knowledge about labor and birth and participating in a shared experience with her partner in a childbirth preparation class are still valuable. If a woman does not have many outside contacts, she may be the person in the class who has the most time to practice breathing exercises and is able to be the most adept at using such a method to control pain in labor.

The woman who is severely hearing challenged usually has heard the many television announcements on not smoking or drinking alcohol during pregnancy because she uses closed captioning. Be certain, however, that she is as aware of this as others. Likewise, if the woman depends on lip reading, be certain she is deciphering new words such as amniotic, gestation, or edema. It often helps to show her the printed words so she can see what your lip motion represents when presenting new pregnancy terms. If a woman speaks with sign language and brings an interpreter with her to translate, be certain to talk to her, not the interpreter, when interviewing.

Modifications for Labor and Birth

Women who are physically or cognitively challenged usually need a few adaptations in preparation for labor and birth. Helpful suggestions include:

- A woman with a spinal cord injury may not be able to feel uterine contractions. Late in pregnancy, she will need to palpate her abdomen periodically for tightening or the presence of contractions so she is aware of beginning labor.
- Women with muscle spasticity or spinal cord injury may not be able to push effectively for the second stage of labor and so may need a cesarean or forceps birth.
- Birth from a Sims or dorsal recumbent position is usually best as this avoids a lithotomy position (true for all women).
- Braille watches used by visually challenged persons may not have second hands. This means they may need to time the length of contractions by counting their length rather than timing them by a watch.
- During labor, the hearing-challenged woman cannot hear information on how she is progressing if you are not directly facing her. If she needs to communicate with her support person in sign language, act as an advocate to keep her hands unencumbered by equipment such as an intravenous line. Remember she cannot hear her infant cry at birth. Hand the infant to her as soon as possible after birth so she can see and feel the baby is crying and breathing well.
- Be certain to identify the usual sounds of birthing rooms (the beeping of a monitor, the swish of a central supply routing system, and so forth) for the visually challenged woman as hearing sounds and not being able to identify them can be frightening.

Modifications for Postpartum Care

After birth, be certain to assess and teach:

- Whether a woman needs additional support to be successful at breastfeeding.
- Whether she has a return appointment for both herself and her infant for follow-up care; also that the arrangements are within her capabilities, transportation, and understanding.
- Whether she desires contraceptive information and what would be best for her individual circumstances.

Women with disabilities generally feel a need to space pregnancies, but their choices of contraceptive methods can vary widely (Grover, 2011; Rowlands, 2011). A woman with poor hand control, for example, might not be able to effectively insert a diaphragm; a woman who is cognitively challenged might not understand the importance of taking an oral contraceptive every day.

Modifications for Planning Child Care

Allow ample time during the first days after birth for mother–child interaction. For example, after birth, a woman who is cognitively challenged may need extra time to understand the transition from "being pregnant" to "having a baby." She may have difficulty learning to judge when her infant is hungry. She may need extra supervision to be certain she does not leave the baby unprotected on a bed. A woman with a spinal cord disability may be particularly interested in inspecting her baby's back. A visually challenged woman will probably want to reassure herself her baby can see. Provide generous time during which she can touch her baby and feel for intact body parts. In contrast, a hearing-challenged couple may not be pleased to learn their baby can hear as they want the child to be as comfortable as they are in their nonhearing world (Lee, 2012). Point out other features such as pretty eyes or long hair to help with bonding.

Breastfeeding has special advantages for women who are physically or cognitively challenged because it is the method of feeding that is not only best for the baby but also requires the least preparation effort on a mother's part. For a woman who is visually challenged and unable to read printed instructions, breastfeeding eliminates formula errors. For a woman who is mobility challenged, it eliminates trips to the refrigerator. Breastfeeding may not be possible for a woman with muscle spasticity, however, because the let-down reflex, which depends on muscle relaxation, may not occur. Be certain women who are cognitively challenged understand they need to feed until the infant is satisfied, not until they are tired of feeding.

Some women will need a referral for home care follow-up and possibly the use of a home health aide to ensure safe child care. Encourage them to think through what baby care equipment will be best for them. Some crib rails lower by pressure on a foot pedal, for example. Others are activated by a waist-high lever. A woman who ambulates by wheelchair usually finds the waist-high lever most convenient because she can reach this most easily. A woman who is hearing impaired needs a flashing rather than a buzzing baby care monitor.

If a woman has difficulty with mobility, ask how she anticipates carrying her infant. Using an anterior baby sling usually works well for the mother who uses a wheelchair. Women who are mobile by crutches or a walker can place the baby in a small wagon and pull it if a sling makes their balance unstable. Some women lie on their back on the floor, place the baby on their chest, and scoot across the floor. The important point is not how a woman carries her baby but that she has thought through a safe and comfortable way to do this.

All parents need to make eye contact with newborns, so urge a visually challenged woman to remember to do this when talking to her infant. If she ordinarily doesn't turn on the lights in her home, encourage her to develop a habit of doing that after dinner because her infant will need light to develop vision. If her support person is also visually challenged, suggest she check with a close friend or neighbor monthly to ensure that light bulbs have not burned out.

One of the biggest worries for the hearing-impaired woman is she will not be able to hear her baby crying. Help her plan to bring the infant's crib or bassinet close to her bed so she can feel the vibration of the baby's stirring and waking. If the baby hears, urge her to talk to her infant as she gives care so the baby is introduced to sounds and words. A woman whose speech is severely affected by her hearing disorder may be reluctant to speak to strangers. Assure her that her infant welcomes the sound of her voice and will quiet readily to the sound. The child may develop her speech pattern because of this. Being spoken to and sung to during the first year is important for overall development, however, so this is still preferable to living in a world of silence.

Some women who are cognitively challenged may have been raised in a group home and only recently moved to their own apartment. Unlike those raised at home, they may have unusual difficulty making plans for child care because they have never seen the care of young children. You have a legal obligation to investigate whether a newborn will receive safe care before hospital discharge. Be certain to ask enough questions so you are sure a woman who is severely cognitively challenged, for example, has a responsible friend or partner to help her with child care.

QSEN Checkpoint Question 22.4

Patient-Centered Care

Mindy makes friends with another adolescent at the prenatal clinic: a 19-year old who has a cognitive deficit. When planning care for this patient, what would be the best way to meet this woman's educational needs?

a. Provide simple, written materials rather than providing verbal instructions.
b. Provide education to the woman's partner or another person with full cognitive function.
c. Ensure that teaching is appropriate to the woman's level of cognition.
d. Enlist the help of a social worker when teaching the woman.

Look in Appendix A for the best answer and rationale.

A WOMAN WHO IS SUBSTANCE DEPENDENT

Substance dependence is a growing health problem in women of childbearing age, so its incidence during pregnancy is also increasing. The number of women who use illicit drugs during pregnancy is unknown, but as many as 375,000 infants may be affected yearly. As many as 10% to 20% of pregnant women admit using illicit drugs during pregnancy (NCHS, 2012). Drugs frequently used are marijuana, cocaine, and methamphetamine. Adolescents have an increased rate of inhalant abuse and binge drinking.

Substance abuse is defined as the inability to meet major role obligations, an increase in legal problems or risk-taking behavior, or exposure to hazardous situations because of an addicting substance. A person is **substance dependent** when he or she has withdrawal symptoms following discontinuation of the substance, combined with abandonment of important activities, spending increased time in activities related to the substance use, using substances for a longer time than planned, or continued use despite worsening problems because of substance use. Typically, substance-dependent women are young adults as the overall incidence of drug use is highest in this group. Any woman could be substance dependent, however, so all pregnant women need to be assessed for the possibility of substance abuse and dependency.

Many women with substance dependency come late in their pregnancy for prenatal care because they are worried their drug use will be discovered and they will be reported to authorities. If a woman is using a drug that has a short-acting effect, she can have difficulty waiting a long time to be seen for an appointment at a health care facility. She may also have difficulty following prenatal instructions for proper nutrition because, although she may desire to eat well, if she only has enough money to buy either drugs or food, she may choose drugs over food as her choice. She may not have money for supplemental vitamins or iron preparations for the same reason.

Illicit drugs tend to be of small molecular weight and, therefore, readily cross the placenta. As a result, these drugs can lead to fetal effects, and drug dependency can be responsible for fetal abnormalities or preterm birth (Sithisarn, Granger, & Bada, 2011). If a woman uses injected drugs, the risk for hepatitis B or HIV infection increases. Additionally, if a woman earns money to buy drugs through prostitution, this increases the risk for STI and poses yet another threat to a fetus.

Nursing Diagnoses and Related Interventions

Nursing Diagnosis: Risk for injury to self and fetus related to chronic substance dependency

Outcome Evaluation: Client states she has enrolled in a substance-dependency treatment program and consequently has reduced or is no longer abusing drugs.

Women who are substance dependent need anticipatory guidance and nursing support all during pregnancy because this is a long time to remain drug free. Many women who are substance dependent have few effective support people outside their drug culture with whom they feel free to discuss problems or concerns or who could answer their questions about pregnancy. Because of their numerous needs, they require an interprofessional team approach involving both pregnancy health care providers and substance-dependency treatment providers. Fortunately, with good support and active participation in a drug-treatment program, pregnancy can become a stimulus for drug withdrawal and a maturing and growth experience for a woman.

If a woman is still abusing a drug by the time she begins labor, her infant may experience drug withdrawal symptoms (i.e., neonatal abstinence syndrome) shortly after birth (usually marked by nervousness, irritability or lethargy, and possibly seizures; see Chapter 26). Although it varies depending on the drug, breastfeeding is usually not encouraged for women with substance dependency because, just as all drugs cross the placenta to some extent, they also are all excreted into breast milk. Women receiving methadone as part of their drug treatment can breastfeed because only a small amount of this drug is excreted in breast milk (Isemann, Meinzen-Derr, & Akinbi, 2011). In some states, because drug dependency has the potential to seriously affect fetal health, women who test positive for drug dependency, either during pregnancy or at the time of birth, must be reported to state child protective agencies; they may be accused of child maltreatment and jailed, with their infant placed in foster care. Be certain you are familiar with agency and state policy concerning these directives (Moller, Gareri, & Koren, 2010).

What if...22.2 Mindy tells you she is not using drugs anymore during pregnancy, but when she opens her purse, you notice several packets of white powder inside. What would you do?

Common Substances Abused During Pregnancy

Recreational drugs commonly used in pregnancy are those commonly used by women in their childbearing years, such as cocaine, amphetamines, marijuana, phencyclidine, inhalants, opiates, and alcohol.

Cocaine

Cocaine is derived from *Erythroxylum coca,* a plant grown almost exclusively in South America. When sniffed into the nose or smoked in a pipe, cocaine is absorbed across the mucous membranes and affects the central nervous system. As a result, sudden vasoconstriction occurs. Respiratory and cardiac rates and blood pressure all increase rapidly in response to the vasoconstriction. Alkaloidal cocaine (i.e., crack), a concentrated mixture, produces an even more rapid and intense high when inhaled—so dramatic, in fact, that immediate death may result from cardiac failure.

Cocaine is exceptionally harmful during pregnancy because the extreme vasoconstriction can severely compromise placental circulation, leading to premature separation of the placenta, which then results in preterm labor or fetal death (Box 22.8). Infants born to cocaine-dependent women can suffer the immediate effects of intracranial hemorrhage and an abstinence syndrome of tremulousness, irritability, and muscle rigidity. Long-term effects are not well documented, but learning and social interaction defects are suspected (Accornero, Anthony, Morrow, et al., 2011).

BOX 22.8 Nursing Care Planning Using Assessment

Assessing the Pregnant Woman Who Abuses Cocaine

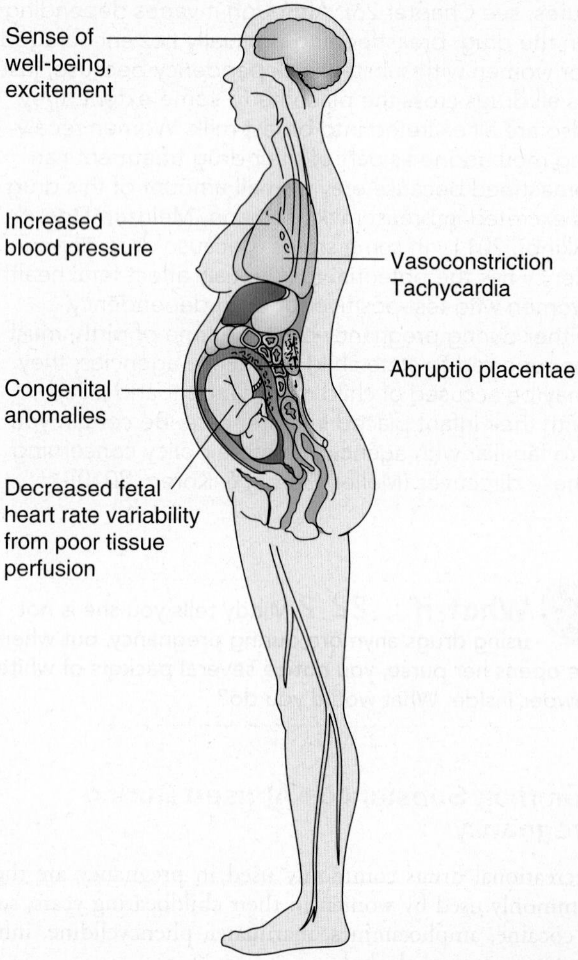

Because the effects of the drug are so intense, counseling women to discontinue cocaine use during pregnancy is often disappointing. Cocaine use can be detected by urinalysis because the metabolites of cocaine can be detected in urine up to 1 week after use.

Amphetamines

Methamphetamine (i.e., speed) is a neurostimulant and neurotoxin that has a pharmacologic effect similar to cocaine, and in some communities, because it is easily and cheaply manufactured in home labs, can be more commonly used than cocaine (Oei, Kingsbury, Dhawan, et al., 2012). Ice, a rock type of methamphetamine that is smoked, can produce high concentrations of the drug in the maternal circulation. Women develop blackened and infected teeth. Newborns whose mothers used the drug show jitteriness and poor feeding at birth and may be growth restricted (Terplan & Wright, 2011).

QSEN Checkpoint Question 22.5

Teamwork & Collaboration

Mindy tells you she uses methamphetamine almost daily. What priority nursing intervention should you perform?

a. Obtain a urine or serum sample for toxicology.
b. Emphasize the fact that meth is not good for her.
c. Advise her to stop taking the drug immediately.
d. Refer Mindy to addictions support services.

Look in Appendix A for the best answer and rationale.

Marijuana and Hashish

Both marijuana and hashish are obtained from the hemp plant, cannabis. When smoked, they produce tachycardia and a sense of well-being. Although not advised, some women use marijuana to counteract nausea in early pregnancy. The drugs' effect on fetal development is not well documented because these drugs are frequently part of polydrug abuse (Minnes, Lang, Singer, et al., 2011). They are associated with loss of short-term memory and an increased incidence of respiratory infection in adults. A frequent user may be advised not to breastfeed because of reduced milk production and the risk to the newborn from excretion of the drug in breast milk.

Phencyclidine

Phencyclidine (PCP) was developed in the 1950s as an intravenous anesthetic; it is no longer used that way because, although it creates a sense of euphoria, it also causes irritation and possibly long-term hallucinations (i.e., flashback episodes), and it is now seen most frequently as part of polydrug use by the "rave" culture. Because the drug tends to leave the maternal circulation and concentrate in fetal cells, it may be particularly injurious to a fetus.

Narcotic Agonists

Narcotic agonists (i.e., opiates), used for the relief of pain, such as morphine, oxycodone, meperidine (Demerol), and codeine, are widely abused drugs because they can be obtained by prescription and they have a dramatic euphoric effect. Heroin is a raw illicit opiate that is also increasing in incidence in young adults. It may be administered intradermally (i.e., "skin popping"), through inhalation (i.e., "snorting"), or intravenously (i.e., "shooting"). It produces an immediate and short-lived feeling of euphoria immediately followed by sedation. Pregnancy complications related to its use include gestational hypertension and—because the drug is often injected with shared needles—phlebitis, subacute bacterial endocarditis, and hepatitis B and HIV infection may occur.

Abstinence symptoms include nausea, vomiting, diarrhea, abdominal pain, shivering, insomnia, body aches, and muscle jerks. Abstinence symptoms may begin as soon as 6 hours after the last drug dose and can continue for several days. Their severity and duration depend on the amount of drug used daily and the length of the dependence period.

Heroin dependency in the pregnant woman is dangerous because it can result in fetal opiate dependence and severe abstinence symptoms in the infant after birth. Infants tend to be small for gestational age and have an increased incidence of fetal distress and meconium aspiration. They will demonstrate the same abstinence symptoms after birth as the woman would if she abruptly stopped taking the drug.

Because the fetus is exposed to drugs that must be processed by the liver, the fetal liver may mature faster than usual. For this reason, newborns of substance-abusing women can seem better able to cope with bilirubin at birth than other babies. Fetal lung tissue also appears to mature more rapidly than in other infants, apparently from the stress of the intrauterine drug exposure. This means that, although an infant is born preterm, the chance he or she will develop a condition such as respiratory distress syndrome is less than average.

If possible, an opiate-dependent woman should be enrolled in a methadone maintenance program during pregnancy (Nosyk, Marsh, Sun, et al., 2010). Infants of women taking methadone do not escape abstinence symptoms at birth, and some infants appear to have more severe reactions to methadone abstinence than to heroin. Because a woman is being provided an oral drug legally, however, a fetus is at least ensured better nutrition, better prenatal care, and less exposure to pathogens such as hepatitis B and HIV (Devarajah, Sullivan, Purcell, et al., 2012). If a methadone program is not available, women may be treated with buprenorphine. Suboxone is a combination of naloxone and buprenorphine, which also may be prescribed. Drug abstinence symptoms in the newborn and accompanying nursing care are discussed in Chapter 26.

Inhalants

Inhalant abuse refers to the "sniffing" or "huffing" of aerosol drugs. Frequently abused by adolescents, inhalants include model airplane glue, cooking sprays, and computer keyboard cleaner. Most of these substances seem innocent; however, they contain freon as a propellant, which can lead to severe respiratory and cardiac irregularities. The effect of these drugs during pregnancy is not well documented, but they appear to have effects similar to alcohol dependency (Reid, Glass, Bailey, et al., 2011). The respiratory depression they can cause could be enough to limit fetal oxygen supply to a serious level.

Alcohol

Although alcohol can be legally purchased and is served at social functions, it is just as detrimental to fetal growth as illicit drugs. There is little documentation regarding how much alcohol must be ingested before fetal alcohol spectrum disorder, a syndrome with recognizable facial features, possible cognitive challenges, and memory deficits, occurs; therefore, women are advised to drink no alcohol during pregnancy (Feldman, Jones, Lindsay, et al., 2011). When discussing alcohol ingestion with young adults, be certain to mention binge drinking (five or more alcohol drinks on one occasion) to be sure they do not believe this type of occasional drinking is safe during pregnancy.

TRAUMA AND PREGNANCY

Trauma (i.e., injury by force) is a phenomenon that seems remote from pregnancy because pregnant women usually take extra care to protect their body. Even with this, however, trauma in women does occur because the incidence of this is high during the childbearing years. Automobile accidents, homicide, and suicide attempts are among the leading causes of death. During pregnancy, the incidence of trauma is 6% to 7% (as many as 250,000 pregnant women experience trauma per year) (NCHS, 2012). Higher incidences of trauma may occur during the last trimester because of poor balance and fainting from hyperventilation. Orthopedic injuries such as broken wrists or sprained ankles occur because a pregnant woman's sense of balance is altered and she can fall easily (Box 22.9). In an automobile accident, a pregnant woman is often the front-seat passenger and, in most instances, is also the passenger who receives the most severe injury. Other women seen in emergency departments have suffered intimate partner violence, which increases in pregnancy (Bhandari, Sprague, Dosanjh, et al., 2011; Shay-Zapien & Bullock, 2010).

Preventing Unintentional Injuries

Unintentional injuries occur more frequently in people under stress than in those with little stress because, in these situations, people concentrate on the stressor, not their immediate surroundings. Because pregnancy is a life event that may cause stress in a family, a woman and her family should take extra precautions for safety. Pregnancy counseling should include education about ways to avoid unintentional injuries by means such as using automobile seat belts (Motozawa, Hitosugi, Abe, et al., 2010).

Physiologic Changes in Pregnancy That Affect Trauma Care

In an emergency situation, for a physical assessment to be meaningful, consider the physiologic changes that normally occur with pregnancy. A primary rule to remember is that after a traumatic injury, a woman's body will maintain her own homeostasis at the expense of the fetus. To maintain blood pressure in the face of hemorrhage, for example, a woman's body will use peripheral vasoconstriction. Because the uterus is a peripheral organ in a shock response, the blood supply to the uterus can be greatly diminished and the nutrient supply to the fetus can be greatly compromised when this happens (see Chapter 21, Fig. 21.1).

A woman's total plasma volume increases during pregnancy from approximately 2,600 to 4,000 ml at term. This increase serves as a safeguard to a woman if trauma with bleeding should occur because a woman can lose more blood than usual (up to 30% of her blood volume) before hypovolemia

BOX 22.9 Nursing Care Planning to Empower a Family

PREVENTIVE MEASURES TO REDUCE UNINTENTIONAL INJURY DURING PREGNANCY

Q. Mindy tells you, "I feel so clumsy since I'm pregnant. What can I do to make sure I don't hurt my baby?"
A. The following guidelines can be helpful:

- Do not stand on stepstools or stepladders (it is difficult to maintain balance on a narrow base).
- Keep small items such as footstools out of pathways (late in pregnancy, it's difficult to see your feet).
- Avoid throw rugs without a nonskid backing so you don't slip on these.
- Use caution stepping in and out of a bathtub.
- Do not overload electrical circuits (it is difficult for a pregnant woman to escape a fire because of poor mobility).
- Do not smoke, so falling asleep with a cigarette will not be a concern.
- Do not take medicine in the dark, so you can clearly read the label.
- Avoid working to a point of fatigue, as fatigue lowers judgment.
- Avoid long periods of standing, because this can lead to a drop in your blood pressure, causing you to feel dizzy and faint.
- Always use a seat belt while driving or as a passenger in an automobile.
- Refuse to ride with anyone in an automobile who has been drinking alcohol or whose judgment might be impaired in some other way.

becomes clinically evident. This also means, however, that fluid replacement volume will undoubtedly have to be higher because a pregnant woman needs more fluid than a nonpregnant woman to restore her circulatory volume. Central venous pressure (normal is 0 to 5 cm H_2O in a nonpregnant state) is increased to 2 to 7 cm H_2O during pregnancy. Although a woman needs a large amount of replacement fluid, this increased venous pressure means it must not be given too rapidly because her circulation can be overwhelmed more easily than usual by a rapid fluid infusion.

To accommodate the increased vascular load of pregnancy, cardiac output increases from 1 L/min early in pregnancy to 6 to 7 L/min in the second trimester. This volume circulates through the placenta at a rapid rate—approximately one sixth of the total blood volume is present in the placenta at all times. This fact makes a uterine laceration always potentially serious because up to one sixth of a woman's blood volume can be quickly lost.

To move this increased blood volume adequately through the body, a woman's heart rate increases 15 to 20 beats above normal, so a pulse rate of 80 to 95 beats/min is not unusual. Based on this, do not assume a rapid pulse rate indicates hemorrhage following an unintentional injury during pregnancy. In addition, since the heart is displaced by the elevated diaphragm, an electrocardiogram may show a left-axis deviation or the pattern may look distorted from the usual during pregnancy.

Peripheral venous pressure in the pregnant woman is unchanged. However, it tends to be higher in the lower extremities because of compression by the uterus on the vena cava, which causes back pressure. As a result, lacerations of the legs or perineum bleed much more profusely in the pregnant woman. In general, peripheral blood flow is increased because of decreased peripheral vascular resistance (the effect of estrogen and decreased sympathetic activity all through pregnancy). As a result, the pregnant woman can be in severe shock, yet her extremities will still not feel cold and clammy.

During pregnancy, the leukocyte count rises to 20,000 cells/mm^3 at term, so using this measure as a sign of infection after an open wound is yet another way an assessment can be problematic. The serum albumin level decreases during pregnancy, making the large loss that normally occurs with burnsa more serious response than usual. Serum liver enzyme levels such as aspartate aminotransferase, alanine aminotransferase, and lactate dehydrogenase, remain the same during pregnancy. This means, that if these are elevated after an injury, liver trauma can still be detected. Since alkaline phosphatase, a substance also usually helpful in detecting liver trauma, is three to four times greater in the pregnant woman at term than usual (from placental origin), this marker loses its importance. Pancreatic amylase levels remain unchanged during pregnancy, so the pancreas can be evaluated as usual.

Abdominal pain is difficult to localize during pregnancy because organs are pushed aside by the growing uterus. The abdomen often feels tense during pregnancy, so the important findings of guarding and rigidity of the abdominal wall may be lost. Bleeding into the abdominal cavity with an abdominal injury is apt to be forceful and extreme because of the increased pressure in the pelvic vessels. A procedure such as a needle paracentesis to assess for bleeding into the abdominal cavity must be done carefully because the bowel, dislocated from its usual position, can be easily punctured. Culdocentesis, or needle aspiration through the posterior vaginal fornix into the peritoneal cavity, may be done instead. Peritoneal lavage (the process of inserting a peritoneal dialysis catheter into the abdominal cavity, adding a quantity of an isotonic solution, aspirating it again, and analyzing it for blood or urine) may reveal bleeding or bladder rupture best.

The bladder of a pregnant woman is extremely susceptible to rupture because it is the most anterior organ and is elevated abnormally (Dorairaj, Sagili, Rani, et al., 2012). After abdominal trauma, an indwelling bladder catheter is often inserted to assess for blood in the urine (Box 22.10).

Psychosocial Considerations

When a pregnant woman is seen at a health care facility after any type of unintentional injury, she is apt to be apprehensive and frightened, both for herself and for her fetus. She worries not only about what has happened to her but also about what

BOX 22.10 Nursing Care Planning Using Assessment

Assessing the Effects of Trauma in the Pregnant Woman

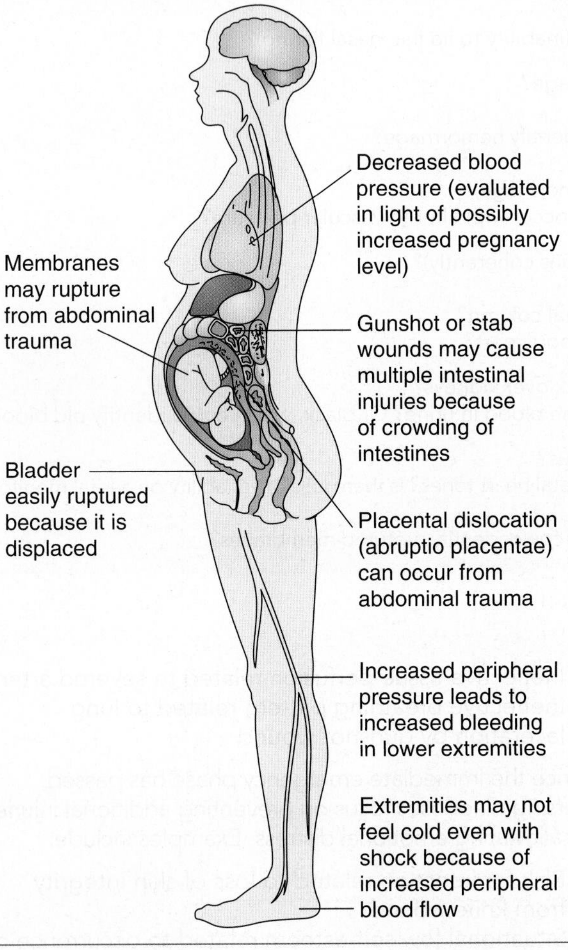
Decreased blood pressure (evaluated in light of possibly increased pregnancy level)
Membranes may rupture from abdominal trauma
Gunshot or stab wounds may cause multiple intestinal injuries because of crowding of intestines
Bladder easily ruptured because it is displaced
Placental dislocation (abruptio placentae) can occur from abdominal trauma
Increased peripheral pressure leads to increased bleeding in lower extremities
Extremities may not feel cold even with shock because of increased peripheral blood flow

could have happened (if the knife had slipped an inch farther, if the automobile had been moving faster, if she had fallen from further up the stepladder) as well as what medical care will be required (Does she need an X-ray? Will this be safe for the fetus?).

A second emotion she may feel is guilt about her carelessness (e.g., if she were really a good mother, she would have had her seat belt fastened or would not have tried to stand on a stepladder to hang drapes alone). A feeling of guilt lowers her self-esteem and can increase her level of stress. Remember, people under stress do not process information well and may not perceive correctly the information given to them. Always try to review information with a woman before discharge from an emergency department to be certain she has the facts of her injury and understands the necessary follow-up.

Assessment

Assessment of an injured pregnant woman must be done quickly yet thoroughly and should include both her psychological and physical status. Some women are so concerned with their fetus they do not realize they are injured. Other women might not even consider the possibility that the fetus could be injured until someone asks if she has felt the fetus move since the injury. Assessment, therefore, should be done concurrently with supportive reassurance (e.g., "Your blood pressure is low, but the fetal heartbeat sounds good") to try to relieve her fear of fetal damage. Use a Doppler to assess fetal heart tones if possible to demonstrate to a woman as well as to yourself that the fetus still appears to be well. Attaching an external monitor to record the fetal heart rate and uterine contractions may be the best way to rule out fetal distress or preterm labor.

Following a serious injury, a woman needs her support people around her. Locate them as necessary and assess their reaction to the trauma as well.

Health History

In an emergency situation, a few minutes spent attempting to calm a woman and move her past her initial fright is time well spent because reducing a woman's level of anxiety can enhance her ability to cooperate with a history and physical assessment. This is true unless symptoms of major body system disturbances require immediate efforts to be directed elsewhere.

Take a brief pregnancy history as well as a trauma history, such as the length of pregnancy or any complications. Ask specifically if fetal heart tones have been heard by an examiner during the pregnancy, if she has felt the fetus move since her injury, if she has any sensation of tightening or pain in her abdomen or back that could be uterine contractions, and if she knows what her prepregnancy and pregnancy blood pressures have been to help evaluate the extent of blood loss from the trauma.

Document the circumstances of the trauma: what happened, the time of the injury, signs and symptoms of injury she is experiencing, and actions she has taken to counteract these. If a woman fell, for example, how far was the fall? (A fall from the top of a stepladder is more likely to be serious than a fall from a low rung.) What body part did she land on? (Striking her abdomen may be very serious, although she may be in less pain than if she injured a wrist in the fall.) For an automobile accident, ask how fast the car was traveling, if she was thrown from the car, or if the windshield broke (windshields are usually broken from the impact of a head striking the windshield so the woman will need to be assessed for a head injury).

As a final measure, evaluate whether a woman's degree of injury is in proportion to the history. Injuries out of proportion (e.g., a woman states she tripped on her front steps, but you notice all her extremities are ecchymotic and her jaw is broken) suggest intimate partner violence, which is known to increase in pregnancy rather than a simple unintentional injury (Brownridge, Taillieu, Tyler, et al., 2011). It is important to identify such women not only to stop the abuse but also because they can have an increased incidence of postpartal depression and perhaps an increased risk of wanting to harm themselves (Cerulli, Talbot, Tang, et al., 2011) (see Chapter 55). Also analyze whether a woman seemed to be using a sensible degree of caution for the circumstances. If not, assess how aware she is of common safety measures. In rare situations, such questions may reveal a woman who self-inflicted an injury in an attempt to end an unwanted pregnancy. A naive adolescent, for example, may attempt to fall down a flight of stairs or to poison herself, which she then reports as an unintentional injury.

Physical Examination

Unintentional injuries become fatal when lung, heart, kidney, or brain function fail. Fetal health falls into jeopardy

TABLE 22.2 Initial Assessments Necessary After Trauma During Pregnancy

Body System	Assessment
Respiratory system	What is the quality of respirations (labored or even)? What is the respiration rate? Are there sounds of obstruction (wheezing, retractions, coughing)? Does the woman have cyanosis? Does the woman demonstrate oxygen hunger (inability to lie flat, nasal flaring)?
Cardiovascular system	Is her color pale, which could be from hemorrhage? Is there gross bleeding? What is the pulse rate? Increased, which could identify hemorrhage? Or absent, which identifies heart failure? What is the blood pressure (decreases with hemorrhage)? Does the woman feel apprehensive, which can occur with altered vascular pressure?
Neurologic system	Is the woman conscious (able to answer questions coherently)? Are pupils equal and react to light? Are there bruises or bumps on the head or spinal column? Is there loss of motion or sensory function in a body part?
Renal system	Is there bruising over the bladder or on the back over kidneys? Is the urine pink or red, which could identify fresh blood in urine? Or black, which could identify old blood?
Uterine–fetal system	Is there bruising on the abdomen over the uterus? Is there bradycardia, tachycardia, or absence of fetal heart tones? Is there loss of variability on a fetal monitor? Is there evidence of vaginal bleeding? Is there clear fluid leaking from the vagina, which could identify ruptured membranes?

when uteroplacental function becomes impaired. Following trauma, therefore, it's important to evaluate these body systems first (Table 22.2). All women who receive a blow to their abdomen need to be evaluated for direct insults to fetal health, such as premature separation of the placenta, although the incidence of this occurring from abdominal injury is actually small (Mirza, Devine, & Gaddipati, 2010; Petrone, Talving, Browder, et al., 2011).

With multiple trauma, a nasogastric tube is usually passed to empty the stomach. A Foley catheter is inserted to assess urine output and to rule out a ruptured bladder (blood would return or urine would be blood-tinged if bleeding were occurring).

To prevent supine hypotension syndrome, be certain a woman does not lie supine for an examination. If she must lie on her back, place a rolled towel or blanket under her right side to tip her body approximately 15 degrees to the side and manually displace her uterus off the vena cava. If surgery is necessary, the operating room table can be tipped to achieve this same effect.

Nursing Diagnoses and Related Interventions

Planning in an emergency always involves two phases: planning for immediate care to stabilize body systems and protect the fetus and planning for ongoing care to bring the woman back to wellness. Examples of nursing diagnoses include:

- Fear related to threat of injury to the fetus
- Risk for fetal injury related to apparent self-harm attempt
- Ineffective tissue perfusion related to severed artery
- Ineffective breathing pattern related to lung laceration by gunshot wound

Once the immediate emergency phase has passed, nursing diagnoses focus on preventing additional injuries or alleviating emotional distress. Examples include:

- Risk for infection related to loss of skin integrity from knife wound
- Situational low self-esteem related to occurrence of unintentional injury
- Powerlessness related to seriousness of the injury sustained or inability to prevent an unintentional injury from occurring

Therapeutic Management

Implementations in emergency situations must be done quickly while always remembering a woman's primary health condition is that she is pregnant.

- For "hands only" cardiopulmonary resuscitation (CPR): Check for unresponsiveness. If the woman is not responsive and not breathing, call for help or dial 911.
- Begin heart compressions at a rate of at least 100 per minute, depressing the chest at least 2 in. each time. Cardiac massage this way may be awkward late in pregnancy because of the size of the uterus, but undue pressure should not be necessary to create heart action.
- Continue chest compressions at this rate until additional help arrives (American Heart Association [AHA], 2012).

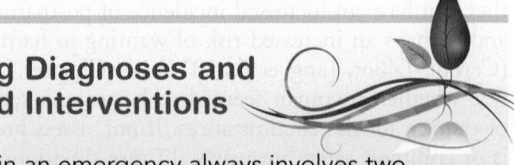

- When help arrives, ask a person to place a rolled towel or blanket under the woman's right side to relieve uterine pressure on the vena cava and help prevent supine hypotension syndrome.

In a health agency setting, cardiopulmonary resuscitation should follow agency guidelines. If there has been blood loss, a central line may need to be inserted and lactated Ringer's or another isotonic solution infused to restore fluid volume as well as to provide an open line for emergency medication.

If hypotension is present, it must be corrected quickly to maintain a pressure gradient across the placenta. However, any antihypotensive agent that achieves increased blood pressure by causing peripheral vasoconstriction is contraindicated (vessels in the uterus would constrict and cut off the fetal blood supply). Ephedrine is the drug of choice for a pregnant woman to restore blood pressure because it has a minimal peripheral vasoconstrictive effect. Following emergency interventions, care depends on the specific injury or trauma present (Farinelli & Hameed, 2012).

Nursing Diagnoses and Related Interventions

Nursing Diagnosis: Risk for ineffective tissue perfusion related to blood loss from trauma

Outcome Evaluation: Client's blood pressure remains above 100/60 mmHg, pulse rate below 100 beats/min, fetal heart rate is 120 to 160 beats/min; nonstress test shows good variability; no signs of labor contractions are present.

Open Wounds

Open wounds vary from simple lacerations to more serious puncture wounds. Because the white blood cell count is normally elevated during pregnancy, a single count is a poor indicator of the presence or extent of infection for these injuries. Serial measurements can be used, however, to assess if infection is occurring.

Lacerations. A laceration (e.g., a jagged cut) may involve only the skin layer or may penetrate to deeper subcutaneous tissue and even tendons. Lacerations generally bleed profusely. Halt bleeding by putting pressure on the edges of the laceration; this may be difficult to achieve in the lower extremities because venous pressure is so greatly increased in the legs during pregnancy. After cleaning, the area is then sutured through each layer of tissue involved to approximate the edges. A local anesthetic such as lidocaine (Xylocaine) is necessary for suturing. Because this has only a local effect, you can assure a woman that this will be safe to use during pregnancy. If the laceration is superficial and a woman is worried about the use of an anesthetic, the edges can be approximated with a butterfly strip. This will allow it to heal, although with a slightly more noticeable scar.

QSEN Checkpoint Question 22.6

Safety

Mindy has a laceration on her leg from her automobile accident. What priority nursing action should you initiate?

a. Keep the laceration clean by irrigating it with hydrogen peroxide.
b. Control bleeding by applying a pressure dressing to the wound.
c. Administer a nonsteroidal anti-inflammatory drug for pain relief.
d. Obtain written consent for surgery from Mindy.

Look in Appendix A for the best answer and rationale.

Puncture Wounds. A puncture wound results from the penetration of a sharp object such as a nail, splinter, nail file, or knife. Puncture wounds bleed little—an advantage in terms of minimizing blood loss but not in terms of wound cleaning. A puncture wound is usually not sutured because suturing would create a sealed, unoxygenated cavity below the sutures or a space where a tetanus bacilli infection could grow. If a woman has had a tetanus immunization within the past 10 years, tetanus toxoid (Tdap) is administered. If a woman has not had a tetanus immunization within 10 years (the usual condition), both tetanus toxoid (Tdap) and immune tetanus globulin (Tig) are administered. Both of these are safe to administer during pregnancy (CDC, 2012a).

Puncture wounds are usually frightening because it's difficult to tell how deep they are. They also usually occur with the added association of violence. Knife wounds cause deep penetration puncture wounds and are often directed into the abdomen. Even a paring knife may easily reach the depth of the uterus, possibly directly cutting the fetus. Most stab wounds of the abdomen, however, occur in the upper quadrants of the abdomen, above the uterus, and are more apt to strike the liver or pancreas. To determine the depth and extent of a wound, a fistulogram may be done. This is done by inserting a thin catheter into the wound and filling the wound with a radiopaque solution that outlines the depth of the wound on x-ray. If the peritoneal cavity was perforated, dye will be shown outlining the intestines. If there is a suspicion of bleeding into the abdominal cavity, a laparoscopy or celiotomy (exploratory surgical procedures into the abdominal cavity) may be performed. Although a frightening procedure for the woman, surgery this close to the uterus usually does not result in disruption of the pregnancy.

If the diaphragm was cut, the intestines may herniate into the chest cavity (diaphragmatic hernia) because of the increased abdominal pressure from the enlarged uterus, causing acute shortness of breath. After surgical repair of an injured diaphragm, cesarean birth is usually planned to avoid strain on the newly repaired diaphragm during labor. The uterus appears to have a natural resistance to infection, so even if it is punctured, infection in the uterus rarely occurs.

Animal or Snake Bites. Pregnant women are occasionally bitten by venomous snakes but are rarely bitten by any animal but a dog. Animal bites produce a form of puncture wound, so if the rabies immunization status of the dog is known to be up to date, the wound is washed and treated as a puncture wound. If the dog cannot be located or is proved to be rabid after 48 hours of observation, a woman must be administered rabies immune globulin and vaccine. Pregnancy is not a contraindication to rabies immunization because contracting the disease would be fatal (CDC, 2012a). The same is true of antivenom serum for snake bites (Lin, Lin, & Lee, 2011).

To prevent bites, caution pregnant women to avoid contact with unfamiliar dogs. If she will be camping in a remote location, caution her to avoid feeding any wild animals such as squirrels and raccoons for the same reason.

Blunt Abdominal Trauma

Blunt trauma generally occurs from automobile accidents, when a woman's abdomen strikes the steering wheel or dashboard, or occurs from someone kicking or punching her abdomen. No visible break is present in the skin. Following the injury, however, the underlying tissue becomes edematous; broken underlying blood vessels ooze and form ecchymoses or a hematoma at the site. If the bruise is over the abdomen, to assess if there is internal bleeding, a diagnostic peritoneal lavage may be done by introducing a small amount of normal saline by a syringe into the peritoneum and then withdrawing it to see if blood is evident. Ultrasound may also be used to detect this.

Careful assessment that the pregnancy has not been harmed must be made following blunt trauma because a forceful blow to the abdomen could dislodge the placenta (i.e., abruptio placentae), which would then begin preterm labor. Palpate the uterus for any abnormal contours that would suggest edema or internal bleeding; listen and record fetal heart tones. Use a Doppler not only for easy assessment but also to help assure a woman the fetal heartbeat is good. Real-time ultrasound may also be helpful in showing that the uterus and placenta are intact. A pelvic examination is usually performed to assess for vaginal bleeding or seepage of clear fluid that would suggest rupture of the amniotic membranes. If a woman reports uterine contractions, attach uterine and fetal monitors so you can estimate the strength and effect of contractions on the fetal heart rate and determine if preterm labor has begun. A tocolytic such as terbulaline will probably be prescribed to halt preterm labor once it is established the uterine environment is still intact (see Chapter 21 for a full discussion of tocolysis).

The possibility some placental blood will enter the maternal circulation with uterine trauma is a real possibility. Rh-negative women, therefore, are typically administered Rh immune globulin after abdominal trauma. That fetal blood cells are present in the maternal bloodstream can be documented by a Kleihauer–Betke test (in a sample of maternal blood, maternal cells remain colorless on staining, whereas fetal cells turn purple-pink).

Gunshot Wounds

A woman may receive a gunshot wound because she was an intended victim or because she was an innocent bystander. Occasionally, a woman attempts to harm herself by a gunshot wound. Assessment of the wound includes inspection for the point where the bullet entered the body as well as the point where it exited (the entry wound is smaller than the exit wound because, as a bullet slows, it begins to tumble, enlarging the space it occupies). The uterine wall is so thick during pregnancy that it may trap a bullet, so there may be no exit point from a woman's body if the uterus was punctured. If the bullet entered high in the abdomen, the intestines will surely be injured because so many loops of these are compressed above the uterus.

Gunshot wounds are surgically cleaned and debrided, and a woman is prescribed a high dose of an antibiotic such as ampicillin. If the bullet entered the uterus, the incidence of fetal mortality is high, especially if the placenta was torn by the bullet. After providing emergency care to a woman for the injury, remember to carefully investigate the circumstances of the injury. Since President Lincoln's assassination, gunshot wounds in the United States must be reported to the police. Stay with a woman as necessary while she recounts her history of the incident for law enforcement officers.

Poisoning

Pregnant women are not apt to swallow a poison, although poisoning can occur unintentionally, for instance, from inadequately refrigerated or undercooked foods or if a woman wakes at night and attempts to take medicine in the dark. There is also the possibility a woman might poison herself as a self-harm attempt.

Poisoning in the pregnant woman is managed the same as in a nonpregnant woman. The woman should telephone the National Poison Control Center (1-800-222-1222), state she is pregnant and what she unintentionally swallowed, then follow the specific recommendation of personnel at the poison control center. When seen in an emergency department, oral activated charcoal is safe during pregnancy and so is the drug of choice to neutralize stomach poison (Karch, 2012).

After a woman has been treated and the emergency of the poisoning is over, carefully investigate the circumstances of the poisoning to help a woman learn about safety with medications or food.

Choking

If a pregnant woman chokes on a piece of food or a foreign object blocks her airway, attempting to dislodge the object with a sudden upward thrust to the upper abdomen can be difficult because there is a lack of space between the uterus and the end of the sternum. Also, the average person may not be able to reach around a woman's enlarged abdomen to perform a usual chest thrust. Box 22.11 describes how to perform chest thrusts for a pregnant woman.

Orthopedic Injuries

Because women have poor balance late in pregnancy, it is easy for them to trip; when they fall, they almost automatically reach out a hand to prevent landing on their abdomen. Because of extra pregnancy weight, this can cause a serious wrist injury (a Colles fracture). Apply ice to the area to decrease swelling as an immediate first-aid measure. If limited motion is present, an X-ray may be necessary to determine whether a fracture is present. Assure a woman an X-ray of an extremity is safe during pregnancy as long as her abdomen is shielded during the procedure. Be certain to delegate someone to accompany her to the X-ray department and remain with her (outside the actual X-ray room) to ensure lead protection is offered and to remain alert for signs of preterm labor that could suddenly develop as a result of a yet undetected injury.

Because women of childbearing age are usually healthy, fractures or torn ligaments generally heal rapidly without

BOX 22.11 Nursing Care Planning Using Procedures

CHEST THRUSTS FOR A PREGNANT WOMAN

Purpose: To relieve tracheal aspiration

PLAN	PRINCIPLE
For Conscious Victim in Standing Position	
1. Stand behind the woman and encircle her chest with your arms.	1. Proper positioning ensures proper placement for chest pressure and prevents inadvertent injury to underlying body structures.

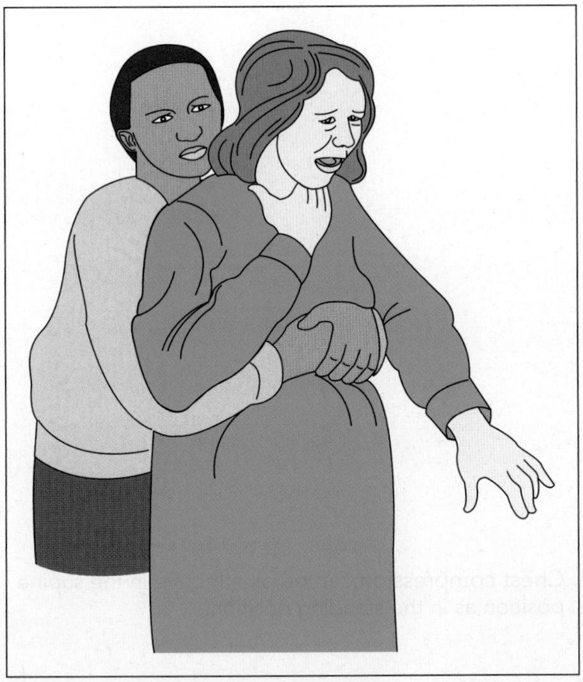

PLAN	PRINCIPLE
2. Place the thumb side of your fist on the middle of the woman's sternum.	2. Placement of fist against the chest ensures a solid structure for compression.

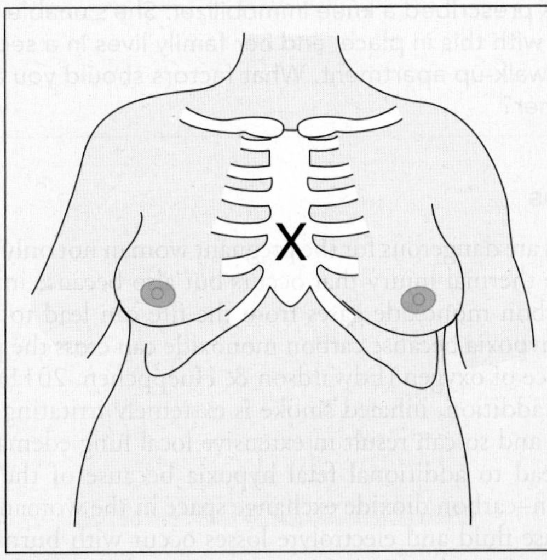

PLAN	PRINCIPLE
3. Grab the fist with the other hand and perform backward thrusts until the foreign body is expelled.	3. Pressure on the chest compresses the ribs, increasing chest and lung pressure. This increased pressure forces an object lodged in the airway to move upward.

(continued on page 618)

BOX 22.11 Nursing Care Planning Using Procedures (continued)

CHEST THRUSTS FOR A PREGNANT WOMAN

PLAN	PRINCIPLE
For Unconscious Victim in Supine Position	
1. Place the woman in the same position as for external heart compressions (heel of the hand on the lower sternum).	1. Loss of consciousness interferes with the woman's ability to maintain an upright position.
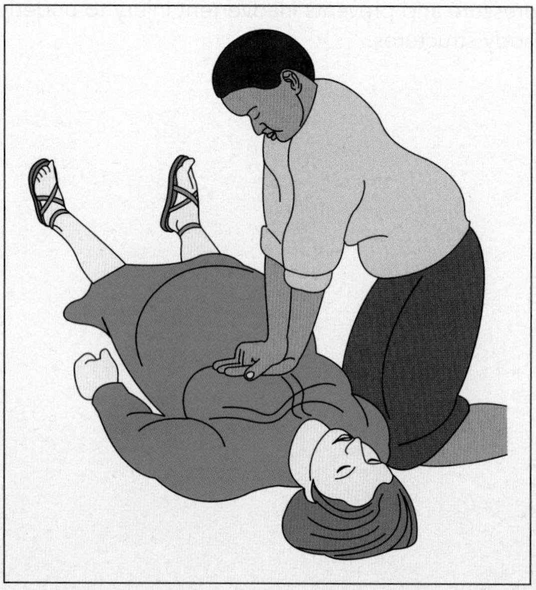	
2. Follow steps 2 and 3 as with a conscious victim.	2. Chest compression can be as effective in the supine position as in the standing position.

complications. Be certain a woman can identify good calcium food sources if she has a fracture so both she and the fetus can obtain adequate calcium for new bone growth.

Because many more adolescent girls and young adult women participate in sports today than ever before, combined with the cartilage softening and extra weight caused by pregnancy, an increasing number of pregnant women suffer knee cartilage or knee ligament injuries.

Any woman who has had a previous knee injury should have it reevaluated early in the pregnancy because a support device such as a knee immobilizer may be required for the last 3 months of pregnancy to keep the joint from dislocating or the ligament from tearing again. You can assure her having a knee immobilizer in place at the time of birth will not interfere with birth.

The laxness of body cartilage may also cause separation of the symphysis pubis if a woman falls with her legs outspread. Many women experience some nagging suprapubic joint pain during pregnancy. A suture separation is very painful, especially when walking or turning. To avoid pain and allow the cartilage to heal, a woman is usually advised to remain on bed rest at home for 4 to 6 weeks. If separation of the symphysis pubis is still present at the time of birth, this can make labor very painful, especially during the pelvic division of labor as the fetus is pushed through the pelvic ring. She may need additional analgesia at this time.

What if...22.3 **Mindy tore her anterior cruciate ligament (ACL) in an automobile accident and is prescribed a knee immobilizer. She's unable to drive with this in place, and her family lives in a second floor walk-up apartment. What factors should you assess with her?**

Burns

Burns are dangerous for the pregnant woman not only because of the thermal injury that occurs but also because inhalation of carbon monoxide gases from the fire can lead to extreme fetal hypoxia because carbon monoxide can cross the placenta in place of oxygen (Edwardson & Hueppchen, 2011).

In addition, inhaled smoke is extremely irritating to lung tissue and so can result in extensive local lung edema, which can lead to additional fetal hypoxia because of the lack of oxygen–carbon dioxide exchange space in the woman's lungs. Because fluid and electrolyte losses occur with burns, hypotension from hypovolemia or an electrolyte imbalance can occur. Yet another concern, in response to a severe trauma such as a burn, is that prostaglandins are produced, possibly causing preterm labor. The more extensive the burned area, the poorer the prognosis for both the woman and fetus. Interestingly, burn tissue heals more quickly than usual during pregnancy, probably related to the overall increased metabolism and the increased corticosteroid serum level, which prevents inflammation and damage to tissue from the pressure of edema. Care of burns is discussed in Chapter 52.

Postmortem Cesarean Birth

If a pregnant woman does not survive serious trauma, it may still be possible for her child to be born safely by a postmortem cesarean birth (Katz, 2012). This is usually attempted if the fetus is past 24 weeks and less than 20 minutes has passed since the mother died (preferably 5 minutes). By general practice, no consent is necessary for the procedure because the fetus is assumed to want to live but cannot give consent. A classic cesarean incision is used. Personnel should be available to resuscitate the newborn immediately.

What if...22.4 You are particularly interested in exploring one of the 2020 National Health Goals with respect to women with special needs during pregnancy (see Box 22.1). Most government-sponsored money for nursing research is allotted based on these goals. What would be a possible research topic to explore pertinent to these goals that would be applicable to the Carson family and that would also advance evidence-based practice?

Key Points for Review

- Adolescent pregnancy is a major concern, because although it is decreasing in incidence, it still occurs at a high rate and can interfere with the development of both an adolescent and fetus. Nursing care needs to be individualized to meet the prepartal, intrapartal, and postpartum needs of this age group. Planning nursing care that helps adolescents view a pregnancy as a growth experience not only meets QSEN competencies but can also best help a girl mature to be an effective parent.
- Women who delay childbearing until age 40 years may need additional discussion time at prenatal visits to help them incorporate a pregnancy into their lifestyle. They may need reminders to save time during the day for rest, particularly if at risk for gestational hypertension or varicosities.
- Women who are physically, cognitively, visually, mobility, or hearing challenged are apt to have special needs during pregnancy that must be addressed by health care providers so adjustments to ensure a safe outcome can be made during pregnancy. Providing time for discussion early in pregnancy so these needs can be identified and anticipated is an important role for nurses.
- Women who are physically or cognitively challenged may need help adjusting their usual regimen to pregnancy. Be certain they are aware of how to contact help in an emergency. Ensure all medications they are taking for their primary disorder are safe for use during pregnancy.
- A woman who is substance dependent presents a unique challenge for health care providers during pregnancy. Encouraging her to decrease or halt her drug intake to safeguard the health of a fetus is a short-term goal. Addressing her need to decrease her drug intake for the remainder of her life so she can be a quality parent is a long-term goal.
- The fetus of a woman who is substance dependent is at high risk because of the direct effects of the drug and the indirect effects of an unhealthy lifestyle. Women should be encouraged to join drug reduction/maintenance programs if possible to reduce fetal risk.
- Trauma in pregnancy results from sources such as violence, automobile accidents, and falls. Women with traumatic injuries need to be carefully assessed to be certain their fetus is unhurt and to determine if intimate partner violence could have been the cause of the trauma.

Critical Thinking Care Study

Anifisa Alkaev is a 42-year-old Russian Catholic woman who, after several fertility treatments, is 10 weeks pregnant. She lived with her parents in Russia until 1 year ago, and she speaks almost no English. She met her American partner online approximately 1 year ago. She began living with him 6 months ago in a conservative Jewish community. In Russia, Anifisa was a lawyer but is currently not working because of her language barrier. Her partner's 90-year-old mother has just moved in with them. A 15-year-old niece whom Anfisa does not know well will also be staying with them until she finishes high school. You notice Anifisa is both hypertensive and overweight.

1. Analyzing Anifisa's situation, what needs would you identify?
2. What nursing interventions would you implement?
3. What complications of pregnancy could Anifisa be at a high risk for that you would want to especially assess for during her pregnancy?

Patient Scenario

The Drew Family

Read about the Drew family, a family with a teenager who is substance dependent, then answer the questions to further sharpen your skills and grow more familiar with NCLEX-type questions related to pregnant women with special needs. Confirm your answers are correct by reading the rationales.

Visit http://thePoint.lww.com

Answers and Rationales

Looking for answers to the What If. . . and Critical Thinking Care Study questions?

Visit http://thePoint.lww.com

REFERENCES

Accornero, V. H., Anthony, J. C., Morrow, C. E., et al. (2011). Estimated effect of prenatal cocaine exposure on examiner-rated behavior at age 7 years. *Neurotoxicology & Teratology, 33*(3), 370–378.

Alexandra, P., Vassilios, B., Alexandra, V., et al. (2011). Population-based trends of pregnancy outcome in obese mothers: What has changed over 15 years? *Obesity, 19*(9), 1861–1865.

Alldred, S. K., Deeks, J. J., Guo, B., et al. (2012). Second trimester serum tests for Down's syndrome screening. *Cochrane Database of Systematic Reviews,* (6), CD009925.

American Heart Association. (2012). *Hands-Only CPR fact sheet.* Irving, TX: Author.

Aujoulat, I., Libion, F., Berrewaerts, J., et al. (2010). Adolescent mothers' perspectives regarding their own psychosocial and health needs: A qualitative exploratory study in Belgium. *Patient Education and Counseling, 81*(3), 448–453.

Bates, C. K., Carroll, N., & Potter, J. (2011). The challenging pelvic examination. *Journal of General Internal Medicine, 26*(6), 651–657.

Beasley, A. (2010). Contraception for specific populations. *Seminars in Reproductive Medicine, 28*(2), 147–155.

Bhandari, M., Sprague, S., Dosanjh, S., et al. (2011). The prevalence of intimate partner violence across orthopaedic fracture clinics in Ontario. *Journal of Bone & Joint Surgery, 93*(2), 132–141.

Brownridge, D. A., Taillieu, T. L., Tyler, K., et al. (2011). Pregnancy and intimate partner violence: Risk factors, severity, and health effects. *Violence Against Women, 17*(7), 858–881.

Burakgazi, E., Pollard, J., & Harden, C. (2011). The effect of pregnancy on seizure control and antiepileptic drugs in women with epilepsy. *Reviews in Neurological Diseases, 8*(1–2), 16–22.

Carolan, M. C., Davey, M. A., Biro, M., et al. (2013). Very advanced maternal age and morbidity in Victoria, Australia: A population based study. *BMC Pregnancy Childbirth, 13*(1),80–81.

Centers for Disease Control and Prevention. (2012a). General recommendations on immunization: Recommendations of the Advisory Committee on Immunization Practices (ACIP). *MMWR: Morbidity and Mortality Weekly Report, 60*(2), 26.

Centers for Disease Control and Prevention. (2012b). Prepregnancy contraceptive use among teens with unintended pregnancies resulting in live births. *MMWR: Morbidity and Mortality Weekly Report, 61*(2), 25–29.

Cerulli, C., Talbot, N. L., Tang, W., et al. (2011). Co-occurring intimate partner violence and mental health diagnoses in perinatal women. *Journal of Women's Health, 20*(12), 1797–1803.

Davies, J. (2011). Why young dads matter. . .and how to reach them. *Practicing Midwife, 14*(7), 22–24.

Derbyshire, E. (2012). Strategies to improve iron status in women at risk of developing anaemia. *Nursing Standard, 26*(20), 51–57.

Devarajah, S., Sullivan, J. V., Purcell, A., et al. (2012). Methadone use in pregnancy: Evidence of progression in the severity of addiction. *Journal of Obstetrics & Gynaecology, 32*(8), 753–755.

Dorairaj, J., Sagili, H., Rani, R., et al. (2012). Delayed presentation of intraperitoneal bladder rupture following domestic violence in pregnancy. *Journal of Obstetrics & Gynaecology Research, 38*(4), 753–756.

Duong, H. T., Shahrukh-Hashmi, S., Ramadhani, T., et al. (2011). Maternal use of hot tub and major structural birth defects. *Birth Defects Research, 91*(9), 836–841.

Edwardson, J., & Hueppchen, N. A. (2011). Surgical disease & trauma in pregnancy. In K. J. Hurt, M. W. Guile, J. L. Bienstock, et al. (Eds.), *The Johns Hopkins manual of gynecology and obstetrics* (4th ed., pp. 248–256). Philadelphia, PA: Lippincott Williams & Wilkins.

Erikson, E. (1963). *Childhood and society.* New York, NY: Norton.

Farinelli, C. K., & Hameed, A. B. (2012). Cardiopulmonary resuscitation in pregnancy. *Cardiology Clinics, 30*(3), 453–461.

Feldman, H. S., Jones, K. L., Lindsay, S., et al. (2011). Patterns of prenatal alcohol exposure and associated non-characteristic minor structural malformations: A prospective study. *American Journal of Medical Genetics, 155*(12), 2949–2955.

Gaillard, R., Bakker, R., Steegers, E. A., et al. (2011). Maternal age during pregnancy is associated with third trimester blood pressure level: The generation R study. *American Journal of Hypertension, 24*(9), 1046–1053.

Goldfield, G. S., Harvey, A., Grattan, K., et al. (2012). Physical activity promotion in the preschool years: A critical period to intervene. *International Journal of Environmental Research & Public Health, 9*(4), 1326–1342.

Grassley, J. (2010). Adolescent mothers' breastfeeding social support needs. *Journal of Obstetric, Gynecologic, & Neonatal Nursing, 39*(6), 713–722.

Grover, S. R. (2011). Gynaecological issues in adolescents with disability. *Journal of Pediatrics & Child Health, 47*(9), 610–613.

Hamilton, B., Martin, J., & Ventura, S. (2011). Births: Preliminary data for 2010. *National Vital Statistics Reports, 60*(2), 1–6.

Hodnett, E. D., Fredericks, S., & Weston, J. (2010). Support during pregnancy for women at increased risk of low birthweight babies. *Cochrane Database of Systematic Reviews,* (6), CD000198.

Isemann, B., Meinzen-Derr, J., & Akinbi, H. (2011). Maternal and neonatal factors impacting response to methadone therapy in infants treated for neonatal abstinence syndrome. *Journal of Perinatology, 31*(1), 25–29.

Jutte, D., Roos, N., Brownell, M., et al. (2010). The ripples of adolescent motherhood: Social, educational, and medical outcomes for children of teen and prior teen mothers. *Academic Pediatrics, 10*(5), 293–301.

Karch, A. M. (2012). *2013 Lippincott's nursing drug guide.* Philadelphia, PA: Lippincott Williams & Wilkins.

Katz, V. L. (2012). Perimortem cesarean delivery: Its role in maternal mortality. *Seminars in Perinatology, 36*(1), 68–72.

Khashan, A., Baker, P., & Kenny, L. (2010). Preterm birth and reduced birthweight in first and second teenage pregnancies: A register-based cohort study. *BMC Pregnancy & Childbirth, 10*(7), 36.

Lee, C. (2012). Deafness and cochlear implants: A deaf scholar's perspective. *Journal of Child Neurology, 27*(6), 821–823.

Lin, H. L., Lin, T. Y., & Lee, W. C. (2011). Snakebite: Use of antivenom in a pregnant woman. *American Journal of Emergency Medicine, 29*(4), 457.

López, L. B., Marigual, M., Martín, N., et al. (2012). Characteristics of pica practice during pregnancy in a sample of Argentine women. *Journal of Obstetrics & Gynaecology, 32*(2), 150–153.

Lu, E., Zhao, Y., Zhu, F., et al. (2013). Birth hospitalization in mothers with multiple sclerosis and their newborns. *Neurology, 80*(5), 447–452.

Lyndon, A., Lee, H. C., Gilbert, W. M., et al. (2012). Maternal morbidity during childbirth hospitalization in California. *Journal of Maternal-Fetal & Neonatal Medicine, 25*(12), 2529–2535.

Malabarey, O. T., Balayla, J., & Abenhaim, H. A. (2012). The effect of pelvic size on cesarean delivery rates: Using adolescent maternal age as an unbiased proxy for pelvic size. *Journal of Pediatric & Adolescent Gynecology, 25*(3), 190–194.

Martin, J., Hamilton, B., Ventura, S., et al. (2011). Births: Final data for 2009. *National Vital Statistics Reports, 60*(1), 1–4.

Martinez, G., Copen, C. E., & Abma, J. C. (2011). Teenagers in the United States: Sexual activity, contraceptive use, and childbearing, 2006–2010. *National Vital Health Statistics, 23*(31), 1–3.

Middleton, A., Turner, G. H., Bitner-Glindzicz, M., et al. (2010). Preferences for communication in clinic from deaf people: A cross-sectional study. *Journal of Evaluation in Clinical Practice, 16*(4), 811–817.

Minnes, S., Lang, A., & Singer, L. (2011). Prenatal tobacco, marijuana, stimulant, and opiate exposure: Outcomes and practice implications. *Addiction Science & Clinical Practice, 6*(1), 57–70.

Mirza, F. G., Devine, P. C., & Gaddipati, S. (2010). Trauma in pregnancy: A systematic approach. *American Journal of Perinatology, 27*(7), 579–586.

Moller, M., Gareri, J., & Koren, G. (2010). A review of substance abuse monitoring in a social services context: A primer for child protection workers. *Journal of Clinical Pharmacology, 17*(1), 177–193.

Motozawa, Y., Hitosugi, M., Abe, T., et al. (2010). Effects of seat belts worn by pregnant drivers during low-impact collisions. *American Journal of Obstetrics & Gynecology, 203*(1), e1–e8.

National Center for Health Statistics. (2012). *Trends in the health of Americans.* Hyattsville, MD: Author.

Nosyk, B., Marsh, D. C., Sun, H., et al. (2010). Trends in methadone maintenance treatment participation, retention, and compliance to dosing guidelines in British Columbia, Canada: 1996–2006. *Journal of Substance Abuse & Treatment, 39*(1), 22–31.

Obican, S., Finnell, R., Mills, J., et al. (2010). Folic acid in early pregnancy: A public health success story. *Federation of American Societies for Experimental Biology, 24*(11), 4167–4174.

Oei, J. L., Kingsbury, A., Dhawan, A., et al. (2012). Amphetamines, the pregnant woman and her children: A review. *Journal of Perinatology, 32*(10), 737–747.

Patel, S. R., & Wisner, K. L. (2011). Decision making for depression treatment during pregnancy and the postpartum period. *Depression and Anxiety, 28*(7), 589–595.

Petrone, P., Talving, P., Browder, T., et al. (2011). Abdominal injuries in pregnancy: A 155-month study at two level 1 trauma centers. *Injury, 42*(1), 47–49.

Polito, J. M. (2012). Ethical considerations in internet use of electronic protected health information. *Neurodiagnostic Journal, 52*(1), 34–41.

Rabchevsky, A. G., & Kitzman, P. H. (2011). Latest approaches for the treatment of spasticity and autonomic dysreflexia in chronic spinal cord injury. *Neurotherapeutics, 8*(2), 274–282.

Reid, A., Glass, D. C., Bailey, H. D., et al. (2011). Parental occupational exposure to exhausts, solvents, glues and paints, and risk of childhood leukemia. *Cancer Causes & Control, 22*(11), 1575–1585.

Rossi, A. C., & Mullin, P. M. (2011). Prevention of pre-eclampsia with low-dose aspirin or vitamins C and E in women at high or low risk: A systematic review with meta-analysis. *European Journal of Obstetrics, Gynecology & Reproductive Biology, 158*(1), 9–16.

Rowlands, S. (2011). Learning disability and contraceptive decision-making. *Journal of Family Planning & Reproductive Health Care, 37*(3), 173–178.

Shay-Zapien, G., & Bullock, L. (2010). Impact of intimate partner violence on maternal child health. *American Journal of Maternal-Child Nursing, 35*(4), 206–212.

Shrim, A., Ates, S., Mallozzi, A., et al. (2011). Is young maternal age really a risk factor for adverse pregnancy outcome in a Canadian tertiary referral hospital? *Journal of Pediatric and Adolescent Gynecology, 24*(4), 218–222.

Signore, C., Spong, C. Y., Krotoski, D., et al. (2011). Pregnancy in women with physical disabilities. *Obstetrics and Gynecology, 117*(4), 935–947.

Simpson, K. R. (2010). Postpartum hemorrhage. *MCN:American Journal of Maternal/Child Nursing, 35*(2), 124.

Sithisarn, T., Granger, D. T., & Bada, H. S. (2011). Consequences of prenatal substance use. *International Journal of Adolescent Medicine & Health, 24*(2), 105–112.

Smith, P. H., Coley, S. L., Labbok, M. H., et al. (2012). Early breastfeeding experiences of adolescent mothers: A qualitative prospective study. *International Breastfeeding Journal, 7*(1), 13.

Sudduth, A., & Linton, D. (2011). Gynecologic care of women with disabilities: Implications for nurses. *Nursing for Women's Health, 15*(2), 138–147.

Terplan, M., & Wright, T. (2011). The effects of cocaine and amphetamine use during pregnancy on the newborn: Myth versus reality. *Journal of Addictive Diseases, 30*(1), 1–5.

U.S. Department of Health and Human Services. (2010). *Healthy people 2020.* Washington, DC: Author.

U.S. Equal Employment Opportunity Commission. (1990). *The American Disabilities Act.* Washington, DC: Author.

Valentino, K., Nuttall, A. K., Comas, M., et al. (2012). Intergenerational continuity of child abuse among adolescent mothers. *Child Maltreatment, 17*(2), 72–181.

Walsh-Gallagher, D., Sinclair, M., & McConkey, R. (2012). The ambiguity of disabled women's experiences of pregnancy, childbirth and motherhood. *Midwifery, 28*(2), 156–162.

Waugh, J. S., & Smith, M. C. (2012). Hypertensive disorders. In D. K. Edmonds (Ed.), *Dewhurst's textbook of obstetrics & gynaecology* (8th ed., pp. 101–110). Oxford, UK: John Wiley & Son.

Whitehouse, A. J., Holt, B. J., Serralha, M., et al. (2012). Maternal serum vitamin D levels during pregnancy and offspring neurocognitive development. *Pediatrics, 129*(3), 485–493.

Wilkinson, T., Fahey, N., Suther, E., et al. (2012). Access to emergency contraception for adolescents. *Journal of the American Medical Association, 307*(4), 362–363.

Yogev, Y., Melamed, N., Bardin, R., et al. (2010). Pregnancy outcome at extremely advanced maternal age. *American Journal of Obstetrics & Gynecology, 203*(6), e1–e7.

Young, M., Deardorff, J., Ozer, E., et al. (2011). Sexual abuse in childhood and adolescence and the risk of early pregnancy among women ages 18–22. *Journal of Adolescent Health, 49*(3), 287–293.

Chapter 23

Nursing Care of a Family Experiencing a Complication of Labor or Birth

KEY TERMS

- amnioinfusion
- amniotic fluid embolism
- augmentation of labor
- battledore placenta
- dysfunctional labor
- dystocia
- external cephalic version
- hypertonic uterine contraction
- hypotonic uterine contraction
- induction of labor
- oxytocin
- placenta accreta
- placenta circumvallata
- placenta marginata
- placenta succenturiata
- precipitate labor
- umbilical cord prolapse
- uterine inversion
- vacuum extraction

OBJECTIVES

After mastering the contents of this chapter, you should be able to:

1. Describe the common deviations in the power (i.e., force of labor), the passage, or the passenger that can cause complications during labor or birth.
2. Identify the 2020 National Health Goals related to complications of labor that nurses can help the nation achieve.
3. Assess a woman in labor and during birth for deviations from the usual labor process.
4. Formulate nursing diagnoses related to deviations in labor and birth.
5. Identify expected outcomes associated with deviations from usual labor and birth such as induction of labor as well as help couples manage seamless transitions across differing health care settings.
6. Using the nursing process, plan nursing care that includes the six competencies of Quality & Safety Education for Nurses (QSEN): Patient-Centered Care, Teamwork & Collaboration, Evidence-Based Practice (EBP), Quality Improvement (QI), Safety, and Informatics.
7. Implement nursing care related to complications of labor or birth, such as preparing the family for a cesarean birth.
8. Evaluate expected outcomes for achievement and effectiveness of care.
9. Integrate knowledge of deviations from normal labor and birth with the interplay of nursing process, the six competencies of QSEN, and Family Nursing to promote quality maternal and child health nursing care.

You admit Rosann Bigalow, a 28-year-old woman about to give birth to her first baby, to a birthing room. Her contractions have been 5 minutes apart for 10 hours. She feels more pain in her back than in her abdomen, saying it feels "like my spine is tearing apart." A contraction monitor shows contractions are hypotonic. A sonogram shows her fetus is "borderline" large for gestation and in an occipitoposterior position. Her husband asks you if the reason Rosann's labor is taking so long is because she's overweight.

Previous chapters discussed uncomplicated pregnancy and labor and birth. This chapter adds information about what happens when complications of labor occur. Nurses play a vital role in making any labor safe. They play an even greater role when a complication arises. The sooner a complication in labor is recognized, the better the chance the situation can be corrected, the concern resolved, and both fetal and maternal health can be protected.

How would you answer Mr. Bigalow?

Although labor often proceeds without any deviation from the normal, many potential complications can occur. A difficult labor—**dystocia**—can arise from any of the four main components of the labor process: (a) the power, or the force that propels the fetus (uterine contractions); (b) the passenger (the fetus); (c) the passageway (the birth canal); or (d) the psyche (the woman's and family's perception of the event) (Lanni & Seeds, 2013).

Because complications can occur at any point in labor, a continuous assessment of a laboring woman and her fetus as well as providing emotional support for her and her family are essential. The hours of labor are stressful even when everything is proceeding normally. Be certain to reassure all women in labor that everything is going smoothly and both she and her fetus appear to be doing well. If a complication arises and assurances cannot be given as freely, it is doubly important that a woman has someone who is both knowledgeable about the deviation and what measures need to be taken as well as able to feel empathetic to her sense of helplessness and the necessary change in her birth plan (Anderson & Kilpatrick, 2012). Nurses are able to play a key role in providing this type of care because they are skilled practitioners of both physical and emotional care.

The National 2020 Health Goals that relate to attempts to decrease maternal complications and prevent infant injury related to birth are shown in Box 23.1.

BOX 23.1 Nursing Care Planning Based on 2020 National Health Goals

A number of 2020 National Health Goals speak directly to complications of labor.

- Reduce the number of cesarean births among low-risk women to no more than 23.9 per 100 births from a baseline of 26.5 per 100 births.
- Reduce the number of cesarean births among women who have had a previous cesarean birth to no more than 61.7 per 100 births from a baseline of 90.8 per 100 births.
- Reduce the maternal mortality rate to no more than 11.4 per 100,000 live births from a baseline of 12.7 per 100,000 live births.
- Reduce the rate of maternal complications during hospitalized labor and birth to no more than 28 per 100 births from a baseline of 31.1 per 100 births (U.S. Department of Health and Human Services [DHHS], 2010; see www.healthypeople.gov).

Nurses can help the nation achieve these goals by helping identify women in labor who are developing a complication; by assisting with cesarean births and careful assessment during labor; and by being alert to the preliminary symptoms of uterine rupture, which accounts for a substantial number of maternal deaths during labor.

Nursing Process Overview

For a Woman With a Labor or Birth Complication

Assessment

One of the major nursing roles with a woman who is having a variation in labor is a conscientious assessment of labor progress. One of the major assessment tools used to detect deviations is a fetal and uterine monitor. Because such equipment can limit a woman's ability to walk about or even turn freely, thus making labor different than anticipated, a woman in labor may not be totally accepting of technologic or pharmacologic intervention. This calls for frequent adjustment of the equipment to achieve a clear tracing. Caring for a woman with such an apparatus in place involves explaining its importance to both a woman and her partner, winning their cooperation, and using judgment in reading the various patterns.

Nursing Diagnosis

Common nursing diagnoses specific to a woman experiencing a complication during labor or birth refer to specific problems. Some examples might include:

- Pain related to induction and labor procedures
- Fear related to uncertainty of pregnancy outcome
- Anxiety related to medical procedures and apparatus necessary to ensure health of woman and fetus
- Fatigue related to loss of glucose stores through work and duration of labor
- Ineffective coping related to lack of knowledge or lack of preparation for labor
- Fatigue related to prolonged labor
- Risk for ineffective tissue perfusion related to excessive loss of blood with complication of labor
- Risk for injury (maternal or fetal) related to effect on woman and fetus of a labor complication and treatment required
- Risk for injury (maternal or fetal) related to labor involving a multiple gestation pregnancy
- Anticipatory grieving related to nonviable monitoring pattern of fetus

Outcome Identification and Planning

If a complication of labor or childbirth occurs, identification of expected outcomes can be difficult because an outcome that must be included in planning may not be what the woman desires. Encouraging a couple to clarify their priorities when a complication occurs is helpful. For example, early in labor, a woman's birth plan might state her chief goal is to avoid monitoring equipment or any analgesia. If fetal bradycardia occurs, however, monitoring and a cesarean birth may become necessary. If this happens, reminding the woman her primary goal is really to have a healthy baby, not to avoid specific interventions can help her accept these changes. Helpful Internet Web sites for referral about complications of childbirth are The Childbirth Organization (www.childbirth.org) and the Centers for Disease Promotion and Prevention (www.cdc.gov).

Implementation

If a woman develops a complication of labor or birth, actions to increase the fetal heart rate (FHR) or to strengthen uterine contractions are a priority and possibly an emergency.

Interventions must be planned and performed efficiently and effectively, based on the individual circumstances. Be certain to provide psychological reassurance to accompany actions to fully safeguard both the woman and her fetus.

Outcome Evaluation

An evaluation of proposed outcomes may reveal unhappiness because not every woman who experiences a deviation from the normal in labor and birth will be able to give birth to a healthy child. Some deviations will be too great; some interventions will not be maximally effective because of individual circumstances. Some infants will die; a few women may be left unable to bear future children. An evaluation may lead to a new analysis that the couple's chief need at that point is to grieve for the child or for a lifestyle that can no longer be theirs. If the outcome is more positive, evaluate the couple for signs that they are able to begin interacting with their child after their harrowing experience.

Examples of outcome achievement might include:

- Client voices confidence she can cope with the fear she feels about her fetus' welfare.
- Client demonstrates adequate energy during course of labor to maintain effective breathing patterns.
- Client's blood pressure remains higher than 110/60 mmHg despite excessive blood loss with delivery of the placenta.
- Client begins positive grieving behaviors in response to loss of newborn.

COMPLICATIONS WITH THE POWER (THE FORCE OF LABOR)

Inertia is a time-honored term to denote sluggishness of contractions, or that the force of labor, is less than usual. A more current term is **dysfunctional labor** (Sandström, Cnattingius, Wikström, et al., 2012). Dysfunction can occur at any point in labor, but it is generally classified as primary (i.e., occurring at the onset of labor) or secondary (i.e., occurring later in labor). The risk of maternal postpartal infection, hemorrhage, and infant mortality is higher in women who have a prolonged labor than in those who do not. Therefore, it is vital to recognize and prevent dysfunctional labor to the extent possible (Le Ray, Fraser, Rozenberg, et al., 2011).

Prolonged labor appears to result from several factors but is most likely to occur if a fetus is large or hypotonic, hypertonic, or uncoordinated contractions occur (Box 23.2).

Ineffective Uterine Force

Uterine contractions are the basic force that moves the fetus through the birth canal. They occur because of the interplay of the contractile enzyme adenosine triphosphate and the influence of major electrolytes such as calcium, sodium, and potassium, specific contractile proteins (actin and myosin), epinephrine and norepinephrine, **oxytocin** (a posterior pituitary hormone), estrogen, progesterone, and prostaglandins. In about 95% of labors, contractions follow a predictable, efficient course. When they have less strength than usual or are rapid but ineffective, dysfunctional labor occurs (Kish, 2013).

BOX 23.2 Common Causes of Dysfunctional Labor

- Primigravida status
- Pelvic bone contraction that has narrowed the pelvic diameter so a fetus cannot pass (cephalopelvic disproportion [CPD]) such as could occur in a woman with rickets
- Posterior rather than anterior fetal position or extension rather than flexion of the fetal head
- Failure of the uterine muscle to contract properly or overdistention of the uterus, as with a multiple pregnancy, hydramnios, or an excessively oversized fetus
- A nonripe cervix
- Presence of a full rectum or urinary bladder that impedes fetal descent
- A woman becoming exhausted from labor
- Inappropriate use of analgesia (excessive or too early administration)

Hypotonic Contractions

Figure 23.1A illustrates the appearance of normal uterine contractions recorded on a uterine contraction monitor. With **hypotonic uterine contractions**, the number of contractions is unusually infrequent (not more than two or three occurring in a 10-minute period). The resting tone of the uterus remains less than 10 mmHg, and the strength of contractions does not rise above 25 mmHg (Fig. 23.1B). Hypotonic contractions occur during the active phase of labor and tend to occur after the administration of analgesia, especially if the cervix is not dilated to 3 to 4 cm or if bowel or bladder distention is preventing descent or firm engagement. They also may occur in a uterus that is overstretched by a multiple gestation, a larger than usual single fetus, hydramnios, or in a uterus that is lax from grand multiparity. Such contractions are not exceedingly painful because of their lack of intensity. Keep in mind, however, that pain is a subjective symptom. Some women, therefore, may interpret these contractions as very painful.

Hypotonic contractions will increase the length of labor because more of them are necessary to achieve cervical dilatation. If the uterus becomes exhausted, this can cause it to not contract as effectively during the postpartal period, thus increasing a woman's chance for postpartal hemorrhage. In the first hour after birth following a labor of hypotonic contractions, it is very important to palpate the uterine fundus, obtain the woman's blood pressure, and assess the amount of lochia every 15 minutes for the first hour to ensure postpartal contractions are not also hypotonic and therefore not adequate to halt postpartal hemorrhage.

Hypertonic Contractions

Hypertonic uterine contractions are marked by an increase in resting tone to more than 15 mmHg (Fig. 23.1C). However, the intensity of the contraction may be no stronger than that associated with hypotonic contractions. In contrast to hypotonic contractions, these occur frequently and are most commonly seen in the latent phase of labor. Hypertonic

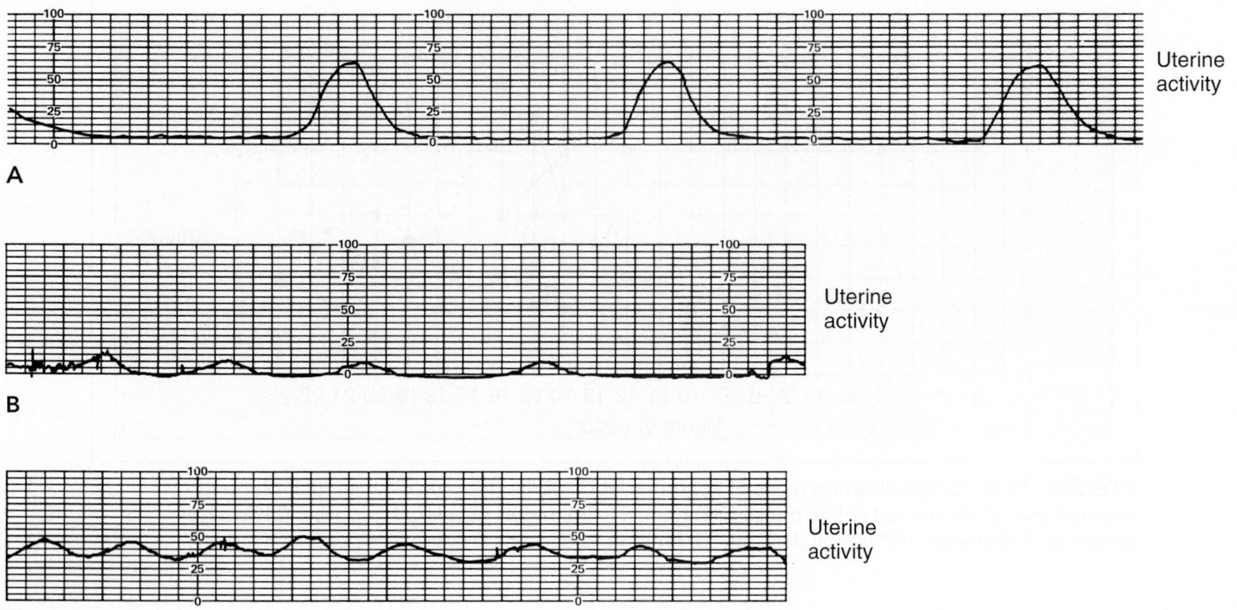

FIGURE 23.1 **(A)** Normal uterine contractions. **(B)** Hypotonic contractions; notice that the rise in pressure is no more than 10 mmHg. **(C)** Hypertonic contractions; notice the high resting pressure (35–40 mmHg).

contractions may occur because more than one uterine pacemaker is stimulating contractions or because the muscle fibers of the myometrium do not repolarize or relax after a contraction, thereby "wiping it clean" to accept a new pacemaker stimulus. They tend to be more painful than usual, because the myometrium becomes tender from constant lack of relaxation and the anoxia of uterine cells that results.

A danger of hypertonic contractions is that the lack of relaxation between contractions may not allow optimal uterine artery filling; this can lead to fetal anoxia early in the latent phase of labor. Applying a uterine and a fetal external monitor to any woman whose pain seems out of proportion to the quality of her contractions will help identify that the resting phase between contractions is adequate and that the FHR is not showing late deceleration.

If deceleration in the FHR, an abnormally long first stage of labor or lack of progress with pushing (i.e., "second-stage arrest") occurs, cesarean birth may be necessary. Although this is disappointing, be certain the woman and her support person understand that, although contractions are strong, they are ineffective and are not achieving cervical dilatation. To help identify the difference, hypotonic and hypertonic contractions are compared in Table 23.1.

TABLE 23.1 Comparison of Hypotonic and Hypertonic Contractions

Criteria	Hypertonic	Hypotonic
Most common phase of occurrence	Latent	Active
Symptoms	Painful	Limited pain
Medications used		
Oxytocin	Unfavorable reaction	Favorable reaction
Sedation	Helpful	Little value

Uncoordinated Contractions

Normally, all contractions are initiated at one pacemaker point high in the uterus. A contraction sweeps down over the organ, encircling it; repolarization occurs; relaxation or a low resting tone is achieved; and another pacemaker-activated contraction begins. With uncoordinated contractions, more than one pacemaker may be initiating contractions, or receptor points in the myometrium may be acting independently of the pacemaker. Uncoordinated contractions can occur so closely together that they can interfere with the blood supply to the placenta. Because they occur so erratically, such as one on top of another and then a long period without any, it may be difficult for a woman to rest between contractions or to breathe effectively with contractions.

Applying a fetal and a uterine external monitor and assessing the rate, pattern, resting tone, and fetal response to contractions for 15 minutes (or longer if necessary in early labor) reveals the abnormal pattern. Oxytocin administration may be helpful in uncoordinated labor to stimulate a more effective and consistent pattern of contractions with a better, lower resting tone.

Dysfunctional Labor and Associated Stages of Labor

For a graphic illustration of the most frequent times dysfunctional labor is apt to occur, see Figure 23.2. Regardless of when dysfunctional labor occurs, the effect on a woman and her support person will be the same: anxiety, fear, or

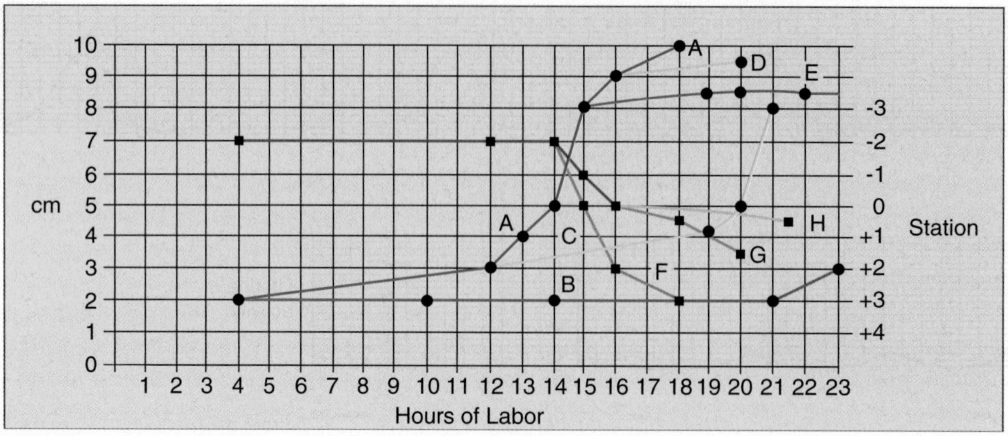

FIGURE 23.2 Graph showing types of abnormal labor. *(A)* Normal labor curve. *(B)* Prolonged latent phase. *(C)* Protracted active-phase dilatation. *(D)* Prolonged deceleration phase. *(E)* Secondary arrest of dilatation. *(F)* Normal descent. *(G)* Prolonged descent. *(H)* Arrest of descent.

discouragement. A woman needs good explanations of what is happening: "We're going to take an ultrasound to check the baby's position." "This is a drug to make your contractions stronger." "I know resting is the last thing you feel like doing, but that is what I want you to try to do."

Dysfunction at the First Stage of Labor

Dysfunction that occurs with the first stage of labor involves a prolonged latent phase, protracted active phase, prolonged deceleration phase, and secondary arrest of dilatation.

Prolonged Latent Phase. When contractions become ineffective during the first stage of labor, a prolonged latent phase can develop. How long the stages of labor take is affected by individual circumstances and whether a woman has received analgesia or an epidural anesthesia (El-Sayed, 2012). Usual parameters for the stages of labor that can be expected are highlighted in Table 23.2. A prolonged latent phase, as defined by Friedman (1978), is a latent phase that lasts longer than 20 hours in a nullipara or 14 hours in a multipara. This may occur if the cervix is not "ripe" at the beginning of labor. It may occur if there is excessive use of an analgesic early in labor. With a prolonged latent phase, the uterus tends to be in a hypertonic state. Relaxation between contractions is inadequate, and the contractions are only mild (less than 15 mmHg on a monitor printout) and, therefore, ineffective. One segment of the uterus may be contracting with more force than another segment.

Management of a prolonged latent phase in labor that has been caused by hypertonic contractions involves helping the uterus to rest, providing adequate fluid for hydration, and pain relief with a drug such as morphine sulfate. Changing the linen and the woman's gown, darkening room lights, and decreasing noise and stimulation can also be helpful. These measures usually combine to allow labor to become effective and begin to progress. If it does not, a cesarean birth or

TABLE 23.2 Lengths of Phases and Stages of Normal Labor in Hours

	Nullipara		Multipara	
Phase	***Average***	***Upper Normal***	***Average***	***Upper Normal***
First stage: Time span from beginning of regular contractions to complete cervical dilation				
Latent phase: Onset of labor to 4 cm dilation	8.6 hr	20.0 hr	5.3 hr	14.0 hr
Active phase: 4 cm to complete dilatation	4.9 hr; minimum rate of dilation 1.2 cm/hr	12.0 hr	2.5 hr; minimum rate of dilation 1.5 cm/hr	6.0 hr
Second stage: From full dilatation to birth of infant	1 hr	Under 2 hr without epidural; under 3 hr with epidural	0.5 hr	Under 1 hr without epidural; under 2 hr with epidural
Placenta stage	30 min		30 min	

amniotomy (i.e., artificial rupture of membranes) and oxytocin infusion to assist labor may be necessary.

Protracted Active Phase. A protracted active phase is usually associated with fetal malposition or cephalopelvic disproportion (CPD) (the diameter of the fetal head is larger than the woman's pelvic diameters), although it may reflect ineffective myometrial activity. This phase is prolonged if cervical dilatation does not occur at a rate of at least 1.2 cm/hr in a nullipara or 1.5 cm/hr in a multipara, or if the active phase lasts longer than 12 hours in a primigravida or 6 hours in a multigravida (see Table 23.2). If the cause of the delay in dilatation is fetal malposition or CPD, cesarean birth may be necessary. Dysfunctional labor during the dilatational division of labor tends to be hypotonic, in contrast to the hypertonic action at the beginning of labor. After an ultrasound to show CPD is not present, oxytocin may be prescribed to augment labor (see later discussion on augmentation by oxytocin).

Prolonged Deceleration Phase. A deceleration phase has become prolonged when it extends beyond 3 hours in a nullipara or 1 hour in a multipara. A prolonged deceleration phase most often results from abnormal fetal head position. A cesarean birth is frequently required.

Secondary Arrest of Dilatation. A secondary arrest of dilatation has occurred if there is no progress in cervical dilatation for longer than 2 hours. Again, cesarean birth may be necessary (Torkildsen, Salvesen, & Eggebø, 2012).

Dysfunction at the Second Stage of Labor

Dysfunction that occurs with the second stage of labor involves prolonged descent and arrest of descent.

Prolonged Descent. Prolonged descent of the fetus occurs if the rate of descent is less than 1.0 cm/hr in a nullipara or 2.0 cm/hr in a multipara. It can be suspected if the second stage lasts over 2 hours in a multipara (Zheng, 2012).

With both a prolonged active phase of dilatation and prolonged descent, contractions have been of good quality and duration, effacement and beginning dilatation have occurred, but then the contractions become infrequent and of poor quality, and dilatation stops. If everything else is within normal limits except for the suddenly faulty contractions and CPD and poor fetal presentation have been ruled out by ultrasound, then rest and fluid intake, as advocated for hypertonic contractions, also applies. If the membranes have not ruptured, rupturing them at this point may be helpful. Intravenous (IV) oxytocin may be used to induce the uterus to contract effectively (see later discussion on induction of labor by oxytocin). A semi-Fowler's position, squatting, kneeling, or more effective pushing may speed descent.

Arrest of Descent. *Arrest* of descent results when no descent has occurred for 2 hours in a nullipara or 1 hour in a multipara. *Failure* of descent occurs when expected descent of the fetus does not begin or engagement or movement beyond 0 station does not occur. The most likely cause for arrest of descent during the second stage is CPD. Cesarean birth usually is necessary. If there is no contraindication to vaginal birth, oxytocin may be used to assist labor (Purcell & Bienstock, 2011).

Nursing Diagnoses and Related Interventions

It is impossible to prevent all dysfunctional labor, just as it is impossible to predict the functioning of any woman's hormonal system or individual response to labor. However, a number of nursing interventions can contribute to the progression of normal labor and help change a dysfunctional labor to a functional one.

Nursing Diagnosis: Fatigue and anxiety related to prolonged labor

Outcome Evaluation: Client states she is able to continue active participation in labor; maintains effective breathing with contractions.

Because labor is work, a woman's glucose stores can deplete over hours of labor. On a woman's admission to a birthing room, assess the likelihood of glucose depletion by asking when she ate her last meal. If she ate breakfast at 8:00 AM and then began labor by 2:00 PM, it has only been 6 hours since her last full meal. However, if she last ate at 5:00 PM the preceding evening and did not eat breakfast because she awoke with labor this morning, it has been 11 hours since a full meal. Alert her primary care provider to this situation. If the woman is still in early labor, she may be encouraged to drink a high-carbohydrate fluid such as a sports drink or to eat a light meal. Sucking on a lollipop or hard candy are enjoyable ways to supply additional glucose.

Although the effect of emotion on labor is difficult to document, for many women, the cervix seems to dilate more rapidly and therefore labor is shortened if the woman is neither tense nor frightened. To try to identify stress, ask at a health care facility admission if a woman has any special concerns. Offer explanations of all procedures. Help her support person feel welcome and comfortable as well. Allow the woman and her support person as many choices as possible to give them a sense of control. Asking a question such as, "Is labor what you thought it would be?" to both the woman and her support person often helps them express their concerns.

Remember that long-term pain is both depressing and exhausting. Encourage a partner to use nonpharmacologic comfort measures such as breathing with the woman, offering a back rub, changing sheets, using cool washcloths, or whatever else seems comforting. An individual woman may find a complementary therapy such as aromatherapy, acupressure, or music helpful for relaxation (Smith, Collins, Crowther, 2011; Smith, Levett, Collins, et al., 2011; Jones, Othman, Dowswell, et al., 2012).

Be certain that if a woman is in bed to urge her to lie on her side so that the uterus is lifted off the vena cava (to prevent hypotension syndrome). If a woman insists on lying supine, place a hip roll under one or the other of her buttocks to cause her pelvis to "tip" and, at least to some extent, move the uterus to the side.

A full bladder can slow descent of the fetus and may also impede uterine contractions. Urge a woman in labor, therefore, to void every 2 hours to keep the bladder empty so this does not add to the slow progress caused by hypotensive or hypertensive contractions.

Nursing Diagnosis: Risk for deficient fluid volume related to length and work of labor

Outcome Evaluation: Urine is free of ketones; specific gravity is between 1.003 and 1.030; skin turgor and serum electrolyte levels are within acceptable parameters.

Low levels of serum electrolytes or body fluid can occur in labor for the same reason as a decreased glucose level—there has been a long interval between eating and the end of labor. Additionally, vomiting and diarrhea occasionally accompany labor; if these occur, they can add to fluid and electrolyte losses. Ask if a woman has had any vomiting or diarrhea to determine the possible extent of these because extended vomiting or diarrhea can lead to serious dehydration and electrolyte imbalance. Profuse diaphoresis and hyperventilation that occur with labor are also factors that can further increase fluid and electrolyte loss through insensible water loss.

Test urine each time a woman voids during labor for glucose, protein, ketones, and specific gravity. Ketones in the urine suggest starvation ketosis. A concentrated specific gravity suggests a lack of fluid. Extreme dehydration not only may slow labor but also can lead to increased blood viscosity, possibly increasing the risk for thrombophlebitis during the postpartal period.

Many women react negatively to the idea of IV fluid therapy during labor to restore body fluid, possibly perceiving it as loss of control over their bodies or removal of the "naturalness" of labor and birth. Introduce the idea that IV fluid therapy has been prescribed because of her particular complication before arriving with the bag of fluid and tubing. When inserting the IV catheter, try to use an insertion site in a woman's nondominant hand and, if necessary, only a small "reminder" hand board. Use long tubing or attach extensions so that the woman can move about freely and her mobility is not limited or restricted by the short length of IV tubing. Assure a woman that being out of bed and walking, turning freely, squatting, sitting, or using whatever position she prefers during labor will not disrupt the IV line or the infusion (Fig. 23.3).

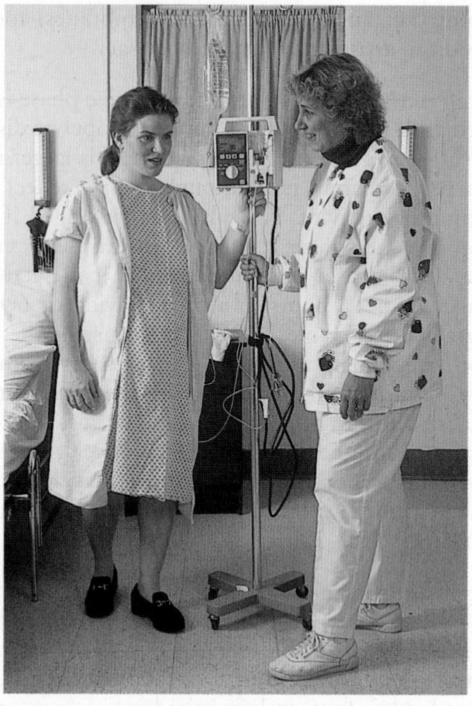

FIGURE 23.3 If intravenous fluid is used for women in labor, it does not need to limit mobility.

✔ QSEN Checkpoint Question 23.1

Patient-Centered Care

Rosann Bigalow states that her contractions are irregular in frequency and short in duration. She screams in pain, however, every time she has a contraction. What would be your best action?

a. Recognize that this is a usual response to labor and offer her a back rub.
b. Notify the anesthesiologist that Rosann needs to have epidural anesthesia.
c. Obtain a prescription from her primary care provider for an analgesic.
d. Document/report frequency and duration of contractions plus facilitate pain relief.

Look in Appendix A for the best answer and rationale.

Precipitate Labor

Precipitate dilatation is cervical dilatation that occurs at a rate of 5 cm or more per hour in a primipara or 10 cm or more per hour in a multipara. *Precipitate birth* occurs when uterine contractions are so strong a woman gives birth with only a few, rapidly occurring contractions, often defined as a labor that is completed in fewer than 3 hours (Silver & Sabatino, 2012). Such rapid labor is likely to occur with grand multiparity, or it may occur after induction of labor by oxytocin. Contractions can be so forceful they lead to premature separation of the placenta or lacerations of the perineum, placing the woman at risk for hemorrhage (Melamed, Gavish, Eisner, et al., 2013). Rapid labor also poses a risk to the fetus, because subdural hemorrhage may result from the rapid release of pressure on the head. The woman and her support person can feel overwhelmed by the speed of labor.

A **precipitate labor** can be predicted from a labor graph if, during the active phase of dilatation, the rate is greater than 5 cm/hr (1 cm every 12 minutes) in a nullipara or 10 cm/hr (1 cm every 6 minutes) in a multipara.

Caution a multiparous woman by week 28 of pregnancy that, because a past labor was so brief, her labor this time also may be brief so that she has time to plan for adequate transportation to the hospital or alternative birthing center. Both grand multiparas and women with histories of precipitate labor should have the birthing room converted to birth readiness before full dilatation is obtained. Then, even if a sudden birth should occur, it can be accomplished in a controlled surrounding.

What if...23.1 Rosann tells you her sister was only in labor 1 hour when she had her baby. Rosann is planning to spend the last days of this pregnancy camping in a mountain cabin 60 miles from the hospital. Would you advise her not to go camping?

Induction and Augmentation of Labor

When labor contractions are ineffective, several interventions, such as induction and augmentation of labor with oxytocin or amniotomy (artificial rupture of the membranes), may be initiated to strengthen them (Mozurkewich, Chilimigras, Berman, et al., 2011).

Induction of labor means labor is started artificially. **Augmentation of labor** refers to assisting labor that has started spontaneously but is not effective. Although induction may be necessary to initiate labor before the time when it would have occurred spontaneously because a fetus is in danger, it is not used as an elective procedure until the fetus is at term (over 39 weeks) or is proven to have adequate lung surfactant by amniocentesis to avoid preterm birth (Moore & Low, 2012). Conditions that might make induction necessary before that time include preeclampsia, eclampsia, severe hypertension, diabetes, Rh sensitization, prolonged rupture of the membranes, and intrauterine growth restriction. Postmaturity (a pregnancy lasting beyond 42 weeks) is yet another situation that makes it more potentially dangerous for a fetus to remain in utero than to be born.

Because either augmentation or initiation of labor carries a risk of uterine rupture or premature separation of the placenta, it must be used cautiously in women with multiple gestation, hydramnios, grand parity, who are older than 40 years, or have previous uterine scars (Norman, 2012).

Oxytocin is an effective uterine stimulant, but there is a thin line between adequate stimulation and hyperstimulation, so careful observation during the entire infusion time is an important nursing responsibility (Krening, Rehling-Anthony, & Garko, 2012). Before induction of labor is begun in term and postterm pregnancies, the following conditions should be present:

- The fetus is in a longitudinal lie.
- The cervix is ripe, or ready for birth.
- A presenting part is engaged.
- There is no CPD.
- The fetus is estimated to be mature by date (over 39 weeks) or demonstrated by a lecithin/sphingomyelin ratio or ultrasound biparietal diameter to rule out preterm birth.

Cervical Ripening

Cervical ripening, or a change in the cervical consistency from firm to soft, is the first change of the uterus in early labor because, until this has happened, dilatation and coordination of uterine contractions will not occur. To determine whether a cervix is "ripe," or ready for dilatation, Bishop (1964) established criteria for scoring the cervix (Table 23.3). Using this scale, if a woman's total score is 8 or greater, the cervix is ready for birth and should respond to induction. To help a cervix "ripen," a number of methods can be instituted. The simplest method is known as "stripping the membranes," or separating the membranes from the lower uterine segment manually, using a gloved finger in the cervix. This is an easy procedure performed during an office visit. Possible complications of this mechanical method include bleeding from an undetected low-lying placenta, inadvertent rupture of membranes, and the possibility of infection if membranes should rupture.

For a second method, the use of hygroscopic suppositories (suppositories of seaweed that swell on contact with cervical secretions), which gradually and gently urge dilatation (laminaria technique), can be inserted. They can be held in place by gauze sponges saturated with povidone-iodine or an antifungal cream. If sponges are used, documentation of how many were placed is important so it can be documented afterward that none remain.

The most common method used to promote cervical ripening, however, is the insertion of a prostaglandin such as dinoprostone (Prepidil, Cervidil) into the cervix (Khan, Abdul, & Majoko, 2011). If the prostaglandin is put in place in the evening, cervical ripening will usually have begun by morning. It's best if women remain in bed in a side-lying position to prevent loss or leakage of the medication. Monitor the FHR after each application and for side effects such as vomiting, fever, diarrhea, and hypertension in the mother. Oxytocin induction can be started 12 hours after

TABLE 23.3 Scoring of the Cervix for Readiness for Elective Induction

	Score			
Rating Factor	*0*	*1*	*2*	*3*
Dilatation (cm)	0	1–2	3–4	5–6
Effacement (%)	0–30	40–50	60–70	80
Station	−3	−2	−1–0	+1–+2
Consistency	Firm	Medium	Soft	
Position	Posterior	Midposition	Anterior	

A total score of 8 or higher indicates that the cervix is considered ready for birth and should respond to induction.

Adapted with permission from Bishop, E. H. (1964). Pelvic scoring for elective induction. *Obstetrics and Gynecology, 24*(2), 266.

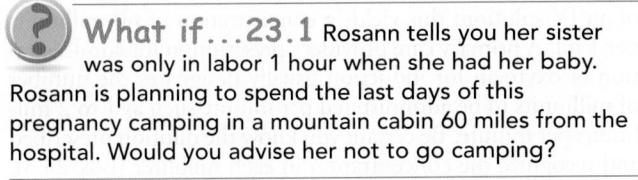

the prostaglandin dose; beginning it sooner might lead to hyperstimulation of the uterus. Even with these side effects, prostaglandins are well accepted by most women as a way to aid cervical ripening (Taher, Inder, Soltan, et al., 2011). They should be used with caution in women with asthma, renal or cardiovascular disease, glaucoma, or in those who have had past cesarean births because of the danger of side effects and hyperstimulation (Karch, 2013).

Although not approved for obstetric use by the U.S. Food and Drug Administration (FDA), misoprostol is a drug you may see used off label to assist in cervical ripening. It is as effective as dinoprostone and requires the same precautions of FHR and maternal vital sign assessments.

Induction of Labor by Oxytocin

After a cervix is "ripe," administration of oxytocin (a synthetic form of naturally occurring pituitary hormone) can be used to initiate labor contractions if a pregnancy is at term (Zheng, 2012). Oxytocin is always administered intravenously, so that, if uterine hyperstimulation should occur, it can be quickly discontinued. Because the half-life of oxytocin is approximately 3 minutes, the falling serum level and effects are apparent almost immediately after discontinuation of IV administration.

The danger of hyperstimulation is that a fetus needs 60 to 90 seconds between contractions in order to receive adequate oxygenation from placenta blood vessels. Hyperstimulation (i.e., tachysystole) is usually defined as four or more contractions in a 10-minute period or contractions lasting more than 2 minutes in duration or occurring within 60 seconds of each other, situations that have the potential to interfere with placenta filling and fetal oxygenation. If uterine hyperstimulation should occur, several interventions such as asking the woman to turn onto her left side to improve blood flow to the uterus, administering an IV fluid bolus to dilute the level of oxytocin in the maternal blood stream, and administering oxygen by mask at 8 to 10 L are all helpful. In addition, a primary care provider may prescribe magnesium sulfate to relax the uterus. The surest method to relieve tachysystole, however, is to immediately discontinue the oxytocin infusion. If in doubt, err on the side of stopping the infusion when the action isn't needed (it can easily be restarted) rather than delaying stopping it so that fetal or maternal harm results.

For administration, oxytocin (Pitocin), is commonly mixed in the proportion of 30 International Units in 1,000 ml of Ringer's lactate. Ten International Units of oxytocin is the same as 10,000 milliunits, so each milliliter of this solution contains 10 milliunits of oxytocin. An alternative dilution method is to add 15 International Units of oxytocin to 250 ml of an IV solution; this yields a concentration of 60 milliunits per 1 ml. A primary care provider's prescription for administration of oxytocin for induction usually designates the number of milliunits to be administered per minute such as 1 to 2 milliunits per minute. Be certain you know the dilution prescribed and recognize the concentration in each milliliter (Box 23.3). Don't increase the rate by more than 2 milliunits at a time.

When administering the infusion, "piggyback" the oxytocin solution to a maintenance IV solution such as Ringer's lactate and add the piggyback to the main infusion at the port closest to the woman. Then, if the oxytocin needs to be discontinued quickly during the induction, little solution remains in the tubing to still infuse and the main IV line can still be maintained. Use an infusion pump to regulate the infusion rate, so the rate will not change even if a woman changes position. In addition, a primary care provider should be immediately available during the entire procedure to ensure safety (Wing & Farinelli, 2012).

BOX 23.3 Nursing Care Planning Based on Responsibility for Pharmacology

OXYTOCIN FOR LABOR INDUCTION

Classification: Oxytocin is a synthetic form of the naturally occurring posterior pituitary hormone.

Action: Used to initiate uterine contractions in a term pregnancy (over 39 weeks)

Pregnancy Risk Category: C

Dosage: Initially 1 to 2 milliunits/min by intravenous (IV) infusion, increased at a rate no more than 1 to 2 milliunits/min at 30- to 60-minute intervals until a contraction pattern similar to normal labor is achieved

Possible Adverse Effects: Nausea, vomiting, cardiac arrhythmias, uterine hypertonicity, tetanic contractions, uterine rupture (with excessive dosages), severe water intoxication, and fetal bradycardia

Nursing Implications

- Prepare IV solution by adding 1 ml (10 International Units) to 1,000 ml of designated IV fluid (resulting solution contains 10 milliunits/ml). Obtain an oxytocin infusion solution from pharmacy (30 units/500 ml fluid).
- Use an infusion pump to ensure accurate control of infusion rate.
- Regulate infusion rate to establish uterine contractions similar to a normal labor pattern.
- Monitor frequency, duration, and strength of contractions during infusion.
- Assess maternal pulse and blood pressure, and watch for possible hypotension. If hypotension occurs, discontinue drug and notify primary care provider.
- Continuously monitor fetal heart rate for signs of fetal distress.
- Monitor intake and output and watch for signs of possible water intoxication, such as headache or vomiting. Limit IV fluids to 150 ml/hr.
- Prepare the woman for birth (Karch, 2013)

BOX 23.4 Nursing Care Planning Using Assessment

Assessing the Pregnant Woman for Danger Signs of Oxytocin Administration

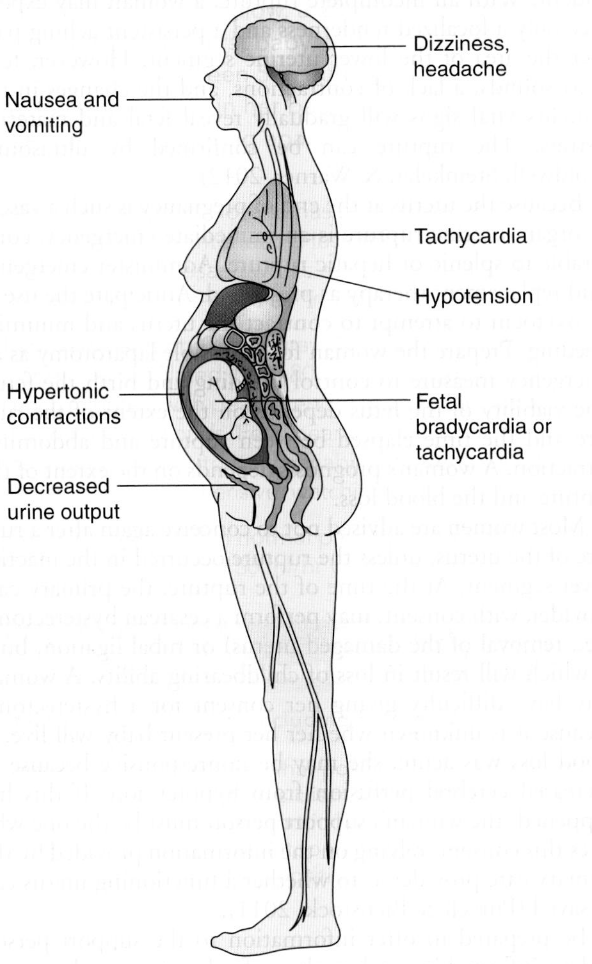

Infusions are usually begun at a rate of 1 to 2 milliunits/min. If there is no response, the infusion is gradually increased every 30 to 60 minutes by small increments of 1 to 2 milliunits/min until contractions begin. Many women respond with as little as 4 milliunits/min, and most women respond at 16 milliunits/min. Do not increase the rate to more than 20 milliunits/min without checking for further instructions because an administration rate greater than this is likely to cause tetanic contractions.

After cervical dilatation reaches 4 cm, artificial rupture of the membranes may be performed to further induce labor, and the infusion may be discontinued at that point. For other women, the infusion is continued through full dilatation.

A side effect of oxytocin is that it causes peripheral vessel dilatation, and peripheral dilation can lead to extreme hypotension. To ensure safe induction, therefore, take the woman's pulse and blood pressure every 15 minutes. Monitor uterine contractions and FHR conscientiously. (See Box 23.4 for additional assessments for danger signs of oxytocin administration.)

A second side effect of oxytocin is that it can result in decreased urine flow, possibly leading to water intoxication. This is first manifested by headache and vomiting. If you observe these danger signs in a woman during induction of labor, report them immediately and halt the infusion. Water intoxication in its most severe form can lead to seizures, coma, and death because of the large shift in interstitial tissue fluid. Keep an accurate intake and output record, and test and record urine specific gravity throughout oxytocin administration to detect fluid retention. Limit the amount of IV fluid being given to that prescribed (usually 150 ml/hr by ensuring the main IV fluid line is infusing at a rate not greater than 2.5 ml/min).

Contractions should occur no more often than every 2 minutes, should not be stronger than 50 mmHg pressure, and should last no longer than 70 seconds. The resting pressure between contractions should not exceed 15 mmHg by monitor (Fig. 23.4). If contractions become more frequent or longer in duration than these safe limits, or if signs of fetal distress occur, stop the IV infusion and seek help immediately. Anticipate oxygen administration may be needed to maintain fetal oxygenation. If stopping the oxytocin infusion does not

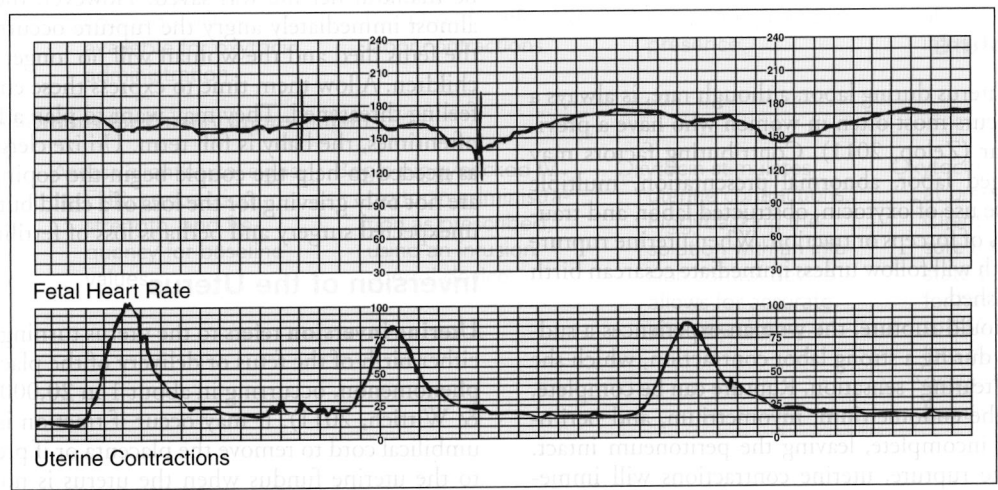

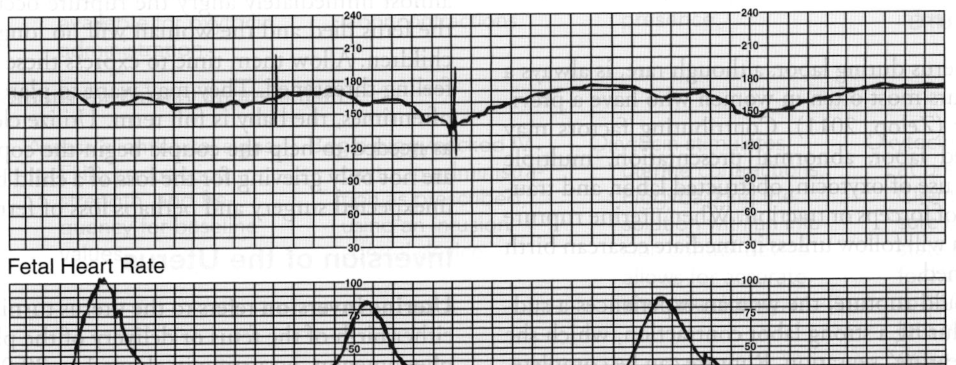

FIGURE 23.4 Hypertonic uterine contractions caused by an oxytocin infusion. Contractions are as high as 100 mmHg in intensity. Late decelerations and a fetal heart rate (FHR) of 170 beats/min baseline are present.

BOX 23.5 Nursing Care Planning (continued)

Nutrition				
Nurse	Assess amount of intake and output and test urine for specific gravity.	Monitor the IV fluid infusion and adjust rate as prescribed. Monitor amount of oral fluid to help prevent water intoxication.	Intake and output and urine specific gravity are indicators of fluid volume status. Inadvertent administration of too great an amount of IV or oral fluid can increase the risk of fluid overload.	Client shows no water intoxication symptoms: headache, lethargy, confusion, or a change in level of consciousness.
Patient-Centered Care				
Nurse	Explore the meaning of prolonged labor with the couple.	Encourage couple to verbalize feelings and concerns.	Exploration, verbalization, and active questioning provide an outlet for awareness of needs and open lines of communication.	Client and partner are able to discuss their feelings with caregivers.
Psychosocial/Spiritual/Emotional Needs				
Nurse	Assess what the couple thought labor would be like.	Include couple in the treatment process; provide frequent updates about labor progress.	Frequent updates about progress help to minimize the feelings of fear about the unknown.	Couple state they feel well informed about progress in labor.
Informatics for Seamless Health Care Planning				
Nurse	Assess whether labor experience was tolerable for couple in light of a complication.	Provide time for couple to "debrief" their labor experience.	Discussing or "putting a fence around" an experience helps to integrate it into other life events.	Couple state they feel comfortable with labor outcome.

Because inversion occurs in various degrees, the inverted fundus may lie within the uterine cavity or the vagina, or in total inversion, it may protrude from the vagina. When an inversion occurs, a large amount of blood suddenly gushes from the vagina. The fundus is no longer palpable in the abdomen. The woman begins to show signs of blood loss: hypotension, dizziness, paleness, or diaphoresis. Because the uterus is not able to contract in this position, bleeding cannot be halted or will continue to such an extent exsanguination could occur within 10 minutes.

Never attempt to replace an inversion, because handling of the uterus could increase the bleeding. Never attempt to remove the placenta if it is still attached, because this would create a larger surface area for bleeding. Oxytocin, if being used, should be discontinued because it makes the uterus more tense and difficult to replace. An IV fluid line should be inserted if one is not already present (use a large-gauge needle, because blood will need to be replaced). If a line is already in place, open it to achieve optimal flow of fluid to restore fluid volume. Administer oxygen by mask, and assess vital signs. Be prepared to perform cardiopulmonary resuscitation (CPR) if the woman's heart should fail from the sudden blood loss. The woman will immediately be given general anesthesia or possibly nitroglycerin or a tocolytic drug by IV to relax the uterus. The primary care provider then replaces the fundus manually. Administration of oxytocin *after* manual replacement helps the uterus to contract and remain in its natural place. Because the uterine endometrium was exposed, a woman will need antibiotic therapy to prevent infection. She needs to be informed that cesarean birth will probably be necessary in any future pregnancy to prevent the possibility of repeat inversion.

QSEN Checkpoint Question 23.3

Safety

Suppose when you assess the frequency of Rosann's contractions after she receives oxytocin, you notice her contractions are 70 seconds long and occur every 90 seconds. What would be your first action?

a. Ask Rosann to turn onto her left side and breathe deeply.
b. Increase the rate of Rosann's IV fluid infusion.
c. Discontinue the administration of the oxytocin infusion.
d. Give an emergency bolus of oxytocin to relax the uterus.

Look in Appendix A for the best answer and rationale.

Amniotic Fluid Embolism

Amniotic fluid embolism occurs when amniotic fluid is forced into an open maternal uterine blood sinus after a membrane rupture or partial premature separation of the placenta (Sahni, 2012).

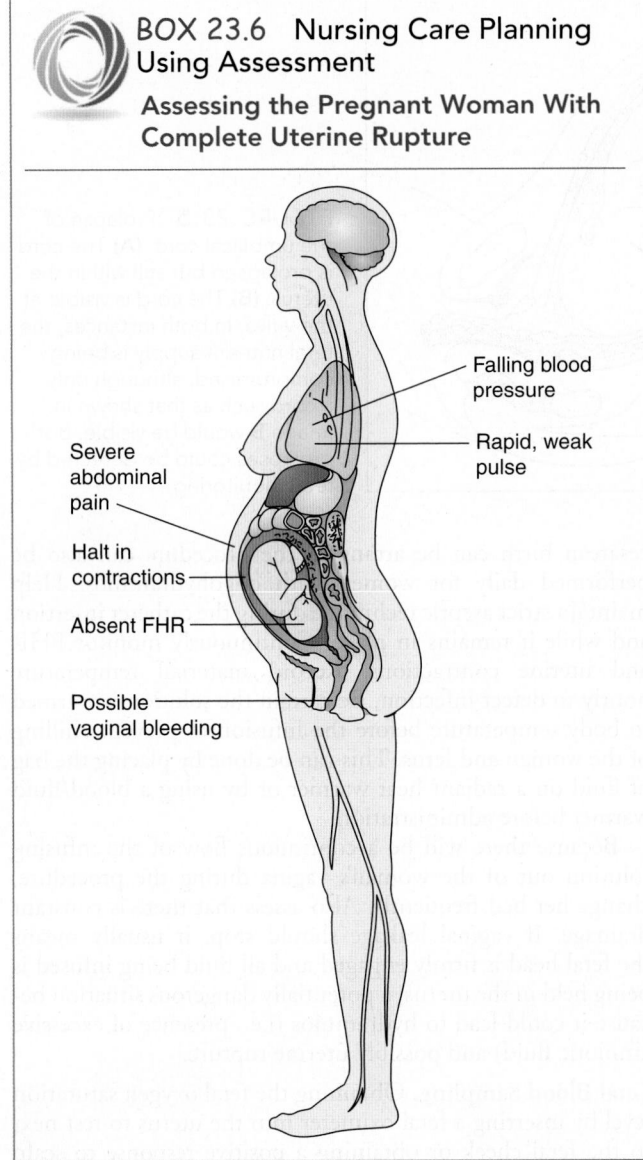

BOX 23.6 Nursing Care Planning Using Assessment

Assessing the Pregnant Woman With Complete Uterine Rupture

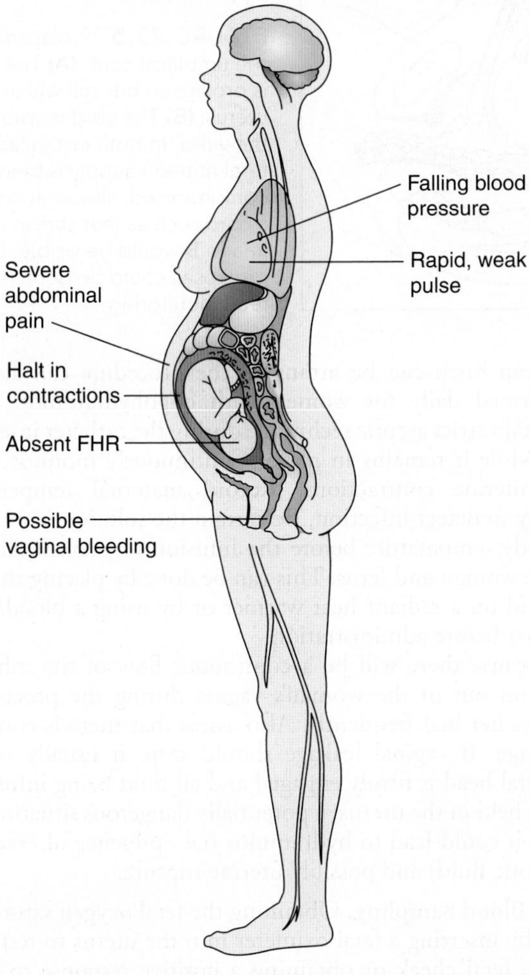

Previously, it was thought particles such as meconium or shed fetal skin cells in the amniotic fluid entered the maternal circulation and reached the lungs as small emboli. A more likely cause of symptoms is a humoral or anaphylactoid response to amniotic fluid in the maternal circulation. This condition may occur during labor or in the postpartal period. The incidence is about 1 in 20,000 births, and it accounts for at least 10% of maternal deaths in the United States (Knight, Tuffnell, Brocklehurst, et al., 2010). Although it is associated with induction of labor, multiple pregnancy, and perhaps hydramnios (i.e., excess amniotic fluid), it is not preventable because it cannot be predicted.

The clinical picture is dramatic. A woman, usually in the active phase of labor, sits up suddenly and grasps her chest because of sharp pain and inability to breathe as pulmonary artery constriction occurs. She becomes pale and then turns the typical bluish gray associated with a pulmonary embolism and lack of blood flow to the lungs. Within minutes, she could be unconscious, and her fetus is put in danger as placenta blood circulation halts. The immediate management is oxygen administration by face mask or cannula. Within minutes, she will need CPR; however, CPR may be ineffective because these procedures (inflating the lungs and massaging the heart) do not relieve the pulmonary constriction. Blood still cannot circulate to the lungs. Death may occur within minutes.

A woman's prognosis depends on the size of the embolism, the speed with which the emergency condition was detected, and the skill and speed of emergency interventions. Even if the woman survives the initial insult, the risk for disseminated intravascular coagulation (DIC) is high, further compounding her condition. In this event, she will need continued management, which includes endotracheal intubation to maintain pulmonary function and therapy with fibrinogen to counteract DIC. Most likely, she will be transferred to an intensive care unit (ICU). The prognosis for the fetus is guarded unless the fetus is born immediately by cesarean birth.

PROBLEMS WITH THE PASSENGER

Although the fetus is basically passive during birth, complications may arise if an infant is immature or preterm or if the maternal pelvis is so undersized that its diameters are smaller than the fetal skull, such as occurs in early adolescence or in women with altered bone growth from a disease such as rickets. It also can occur if the umbilical cord prolapses, if more than one fetus is present, or if a fetus is malpositioned or too large for the birth canal.

Prolapse of the Umbilical Cord

In **umbilical cord prolapse**, a loop of the umbilical cord slips down in front of the presenting fetal part (Fig. 23.5). Prolapse may occur at any time after the membranes rupture if the presenting fetal part is not fitted firmly into the cervix. It tends to occur most often with:

- Premature rupture of membranes
- Fetal presentation other than cephalic
- Placenta previa
- Intrauterine tumors preventing the presenting part from engaging
- A small fetus
- CPD preventing firm engagement
- Hydramnios
- Multiple gestation

The incidence is about 0.5% of cephalic births, but can rise as high as 15% to 20% with breech or transverse lies (Lanni & Seeds, 2013).

Assessment

In rare instances, the cord may be felt as the presenting part on an initial vaginal examination during labor or can be visualized on ultrasound if one of these is taken during labor. More often, however, cord prolapse is first discovered only after the membranes have ruptured, when the FHR is discovered to be unusually slow or a variable deceleration FHR pattern suddenly becomes apparent on a fetal monitor. On inspection, the cord may be visible at the vulva.

To rule out cord prolapse, always assess fetal heart sounds immediately after rupture of the membranes, whether this occurs spontaneously or by amniotomy.

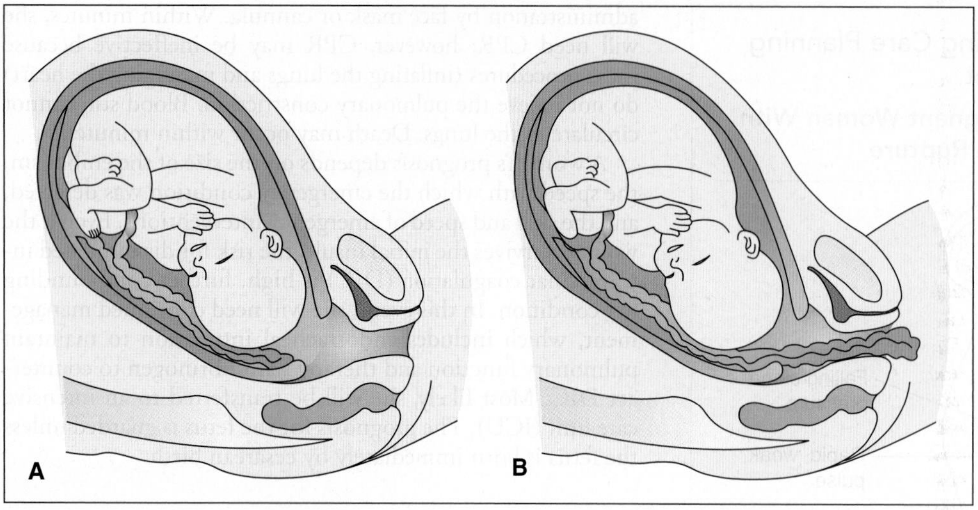

FIGURE 23.5 Prolapse of the umbilical cord. **(A)** The cord is prolapsed but still within the uterus. **(B)** The cord is visible at the vulva. In both instances, the fetal nutrient supply is being compromised, although only a cord such as that shown in image **B** would be visible. Both prolapses could be detected by fetal monitoring.

Therapeutic Management

A prolapsed cord is always an emergency situation, because the pressure of the fetal head against the cord at the pelvic brim leads to cord compression and decreased oxygenation to the fetus. Management is aimed, therefore, at relieving pressure on the cord, thereby relieving the compression and the resulting fetal anoxia. This may be done by placing a gloved hand in the vagina and manually elevating the fetal head off the cord, or by placing the woman in a knee–chest or Trendelenburg position, to cause the fetal head to fall back from the cord. Administering oxygen at 10 l/min by face mask to the woman is also helpful to improve oxygenation to the fetus. A tocolytic agent may be prescribed to reduce uterine activity and pressure on the fetus. Amnioinfusion (see later) is yet another way to relieve pressure on the cord (Hofmeyr & Lawrie, 2012).

If the cord has prolapsed to the extent it is exposed to room air, drying will begin, leading to constriction and atrophy of the umbilical vessels. Do not attempt to push any exposed cord back into the vagina because this could add to the compression by causing knotting or kinking. Instead, cover any exposed portion with a sterile saline compress to prevent drying.

Because cervical dilatation is usually incomplete at the point where the cord prolapse occurred, the birth method of choice is upward pressure on the presenting part, applied by a practitioner's hand in the woman's vagina, to keep pressure off the cord until the baby can be born by cesarean birth.

Amnioinfusion. **Amnioinfusion** is the addition of a sterile fluid into the uterus to supplement the amniotic fluid and reduce compression on the cord. For this, a sterile double-lumen catheter is introduced through the cervix into the uterus. It is then attached to IV tubing, and a solution of warmed normal saline or lactated Ringer's solution is rapidly infused. Initially, approximately 500 ml is infused, and then the rate is adjusted to infuse the least amount necessary to maintain an FHR monitor pattern without variable decelerations. Throughout the procedure, urge a woman to lie in a lateral recumbent position to prevent supine hypotension syndrome.

With cord compression, although amnioinfusion is used for only a short time until the cervix is fully dilated or a cesarean birth can be arranged, the procedure can also be performed daily for women with oligohydramnios. Help maintain strict aseptic technique during the catheter insertion and while it remains in place. Continuously monitor FHR and uterine contractions. Record maternal temperature hourly to detect infection. Be certain the solution is warmed to body temperature before the infusion to prevent chilling of the woman and fetus. This can be done by placing the bag of fluid on a radiant heat warmer or by using a blood/fluid warmer before administration.

Because there will be a continuous flow of the infusing solution out of the woman's vagina during the procedure, change her bed frequently. Also assess that there is constant drainage. If vaginal leakage should stop, it usually means the fetal head is firmly engaged and all fluid being infused is being held in the uterus, a potentially dangerous situation because it could lead to hydramnios (i.e., presence of excessive amniotic fluid) and possibly uterine rupture.

Fetal Blood Sampling. Obtaining the fetal oxygen saturation level by inserting a fetal oximeter into the uterus to rest next to the fetal cheek or obtaining a positive response to scalp stimulation usually supplies the information as to whether a fetus is becoming acidotic (see Chapter 24); however, this information can also be obtained by scalp blood or fetal blood sampling (Mahendru & Lees, 2011).

The oxygen saturation, partial pressure of oxygen (Po_2) and carbon dioxide (Pco_2), pH, bicarbonate excess, and hematocrit of fetal blood may all be determined during labor if a sample of capillary blood is taken from the fetal scalp as it presents at the dilated cervix. After cervical dilatation of 3 to 4 cm and rupture of the membranes, the fetal head is visualized by the use of an amnioscope, a small, cone-shaped instrument with a light source at the far end. The scalp is cleaned with povidone-iodine and sprayed with silicon. A small scalpel is introduced vaginally into the cervix, and the fetal scalp is nicked. The silicon causes blood to form in beads, which are caught by a capillary tube. The incision is then compressed until the bleeding has stopped. After the procedure, the woman must be observed after two or three contractions to be certain that no new fetal scalp bleeding occurs.

Although a blood sample obtained in this way may be analyzed for many parameters, usually only the pH results are necessary. If the fetus is hypoxic, the pH will fall (i.e., become acidotic). A scalp blood pH greater than 7.25 is considered normal for a fetus during labor. A pH between 7.21 and 7.25 should be measured again after 30 minutes. A scalp blood pH lower than 7.20 is acidotic and signifies a level of fetal distress. This technique may be used to verify that an ominous heart rate pattern on a monitor truly reflects anoxia or that no acidosis is occurring, even if a monitor rate is showing decreased variability.

Fetal blood sampling involves no pain for the woman, but it may involve an uncomfortable sensation of pressure because of the examining hand in the vagina. Infants who have had internal scalp blood samples taken should not have a vacuum applied to facilitate birth, because this procedure can lead to renewed bleeding at the puncture site. After birth, the small incision on the infant scalp needs to be observed to be certain it is healing and infection is not present.

QSEN Checkpoint Question 23.4

Informatics

Rosann's fetus is going to have fetal blood sampling performed. What would be your priority assessment before the procedure?

a. Determine if Rosann's membranes have already ruptured.
b. Determine if her fetus has rotated to an anterior position.
c. Determine if Rosann's diastolic blood pressure is within reference ranges.
d. Determine if Rosann knows her fetus' head will be shaved.

Look in Appendix A for the best answer and rationale.

Multiple Gestation

Multiple gestations (i.e., pregnancies with two or more fetuses) have increased substantially over the last 10 years as in vitro fertilization has become more popular and often produces a multiple pregnancy (Tiitinen, 2012). When a woman with a multiple gestation is admitted to a birthing room, it usually causes a flurry of excitement as additional personnel are needed for the birth, including as many nurses to attend to possibly immature infants as there are infants, plus additional persons skilled in newborn resuscitation. In the middle of all the preparatory activity, it is easy to forget a woman having a multiple birth may be more frightened than excited. Be certain to focus on her needs as well as those of her babies so she isn't neglected. Twins may be born by cesarean birth to decrease the risk the second fetus will experience anoxia; often, this is also the situation in multiple gestations of three or more because of the increased incidence of cord entanglement and premature separation of the placenta (Tul, Verdenik, Trojner-Bregar, et al., 2012). Anemia and gestational hypertension occur at higher than usual incidences during multiple gestations. To detect these, be certain to assess the woman's hematocrit level and blood pressure closely during labor or while waiting for cesarean arrangements.

If a woman with a multiple gestation will be giving birth vaginally, she is usually instructed to come to the hospital early in labor. The first stage of labor does not differ greatly from that of a woman with a single gestation pregnancy. Coming to a hospital this early in labor, however, will make labor seem long. Urge the woman to spend the early hours of labor engaged in an activity such as playing cards or reading to make the time pass more quickly. Multiple pregnancies often end before full term, so the woman may not yet have practiced breathing exercises. The early hours of labor can be used for this as well. During labor, support the woman's breathing exercises to minimize the need for analgesia or anesthesia; this helps to minimize any respiratory difficulties the infants may have at birth because of their immaturity.

Be certain that, when taking FHRs by Doppler or a fetal monitor, you are definitely hearing two separate beats as proof each infant is doing well. Because of the multiple fetuses, abnormal fetal presentation may occur. Also, because the babies are usually small, firm head engagement may not occur, thus increasing the risk for cord prolapse after rupture of the membranes. Uterine dysfunction from a long labor, an overstretched uterus, unusual presentation, and premature separation of the placenta after the birth of the first child may also be more common.

Most twin pregnancies present with both twins vertex. This is followed in frequency by vertex and breech, breech and vertex, and then breech and breech (Fig. 23.6). Multiple gestations of three or more fetuses have extremely varied presentations. After the first infant is born, both ends of the baby's cord are tied or clamped permanently, rather than with cord clamps, which could slip. This prevents hemorrhage through an open cord end if additional infants have shared the placenta. The first infant is identified as *A*, and newborn care is begun. In singleton pregnancies, oxytocin usually is given immediately to contract the uterus and minimize bleeding after an infant is born; with a multiple gestation woman, however, it will not be given to avoid compromising the circulation of the infants not yet born (Norwitz, Belfort, Saade, et al., 2010).

After the birth of the first child, the lie of the second fetus is determined by external abdominal palpation or ultrasound. Sublingual nitroglycerin may be prescribed to relax the uterus and make external version possible (Hofmeyr & Kulier, 2012). If version is not successful, a decision for breech birth or a cesarean birth must be made (Hehir, O'Connor, Kent, et al., 2012).

Parents usually want to inspect multiple gestation infants thoroughly after birth. The time allowed for this inspection depends on the infants' weights and conditions because, if preterm, cold hypothermia is a concern. Some parents worry the hospital will confuse their infants through improper identification. Review with them the measures used, such as armbands, to ensure this will not happen.

The infants need careful assessment to determine their true gestational age and whether a phenomenon such as twin-to-twin transfusion could have occurred (see Chapter 26). Even though women have known for months they are having multiple infants, many have difficulty believing it has really happened. They feel a need to recount over and over their surprise and to view their infants together to prove to themselves it is true. If parents are unable to inspect their infants thoroughly immediately after birth because of the infants' low birth weights and the danger of chilling, be certain they have an opportunity to do so as soon as possible to dispel any fears they had throughout pregnancy the babies would be born less than perfect.

Assess the woman carefully in the immediate postpartal period because a uterus that was overly distended because of the multiple gestation may have more difficulty contracting than usual, thus placing her at risk for hemorrhage from

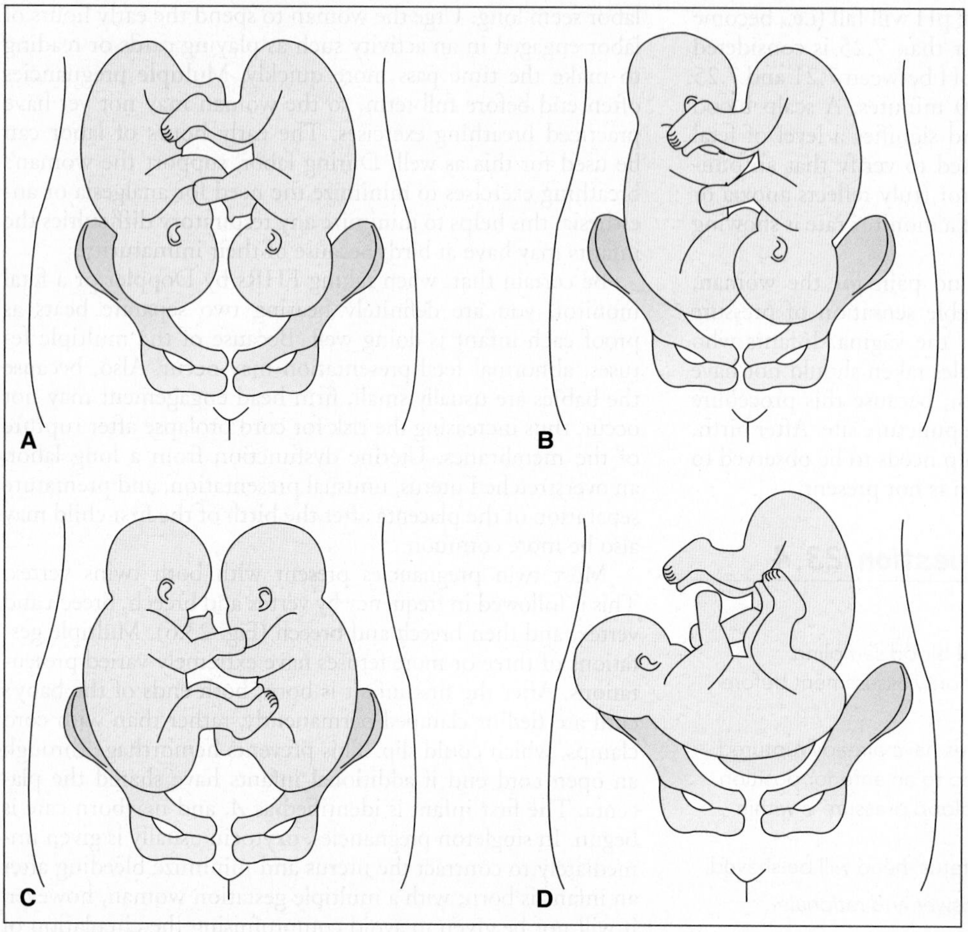

FIGURE 23.6 Four different twin presentations. **(A)** Both infants vertex. **(B)** One infant vertex and one breech. **(C)** Both infants breech. **(D)** One infant vertex and one in a transverse lie.

uterine atony (i.e., lacking normal tone). In addition, the risk for uterine infection increases if labor or birth was prolonged.

Problems With Fetal Position, Presentation, or Size

Occipitoposterior Position

In approximately one tenth of all labors, the fetal position is posterior rather than anterior. That is, the occiput (assuming the presentation is vertex) is directed diagonally and posteriorly, either to the right (ROP) or to the left (LOP). In these positions, during internal rotation, the fetal head must rotate not through a 90-degree arc (Fig. 23.7), but through an arc of approximately 135 degrees (Fig. 23.8). Rotation from a posterior position can be aided by having the woman assume a hands-and-knees position, squatting, or lying on her side (on her left side if the fetus is right occiput posterior, or on her right side if the fetus is left occiput posterior). Theoretically, shifting the weight from right to left or "lunging" or swinging her body right to left while elevating her left foot on a chair widens the pelvic path and makes fetal rotation easier. This is not evidence based, however, is not proven to be effective, and is tiring for women in labor (Desbriere, Blanc, Le Dû, et al., 2013).

Posterior positions tend to occur in women with android, anthropoid, or contracted pelves. It is suggested by a dysfunctional labor pattern such as a prolonged active phase, arrested descent, or fetal heart sounds heard best at the lateral sides of the abdomen.

A posteriorly presenting head does not fit the cervix as snugly as one in an anterior position. Because this increases the risk of umbilical cord prolapse, the position of the fetus is confirmed by vaginal examination or ultrasound. The majority of fetuses presenting in posterior positions, if they are of average size, in good flexion, and aided by forceful uterine contractions, rotate through the large arc, arrive at a good birth position for the pelvic outlet, and are born satisfactorily with only increased molding and caput formation. However, it is not unusual for the labor to be somewhat prolonged because the arc of rotation is greater (Gilbert, 2011).

Because the fetal head rotates against the sacrum, a woman may experience pressure and pain in her lower back because of sacral nerve compression. These sensations may be so intense she asks for medication for relief, not for her contractions but for the intense back pressure and pain. Applying counterpressure on the sacrum by a back rub may be helpful in relieving a portion of the pain (Fig. 23.9). Applying heat or cold, whichever feels best, and maintaining a hands-and-knees position or leaning forward over a birthing ball may help the fetus rotate (Simkin, 2010). During a long labor of this type, be certain a woman voids approximately every 2 hours to keep her bladder empty, because a full bladder could further impede descent of the fetus. Be aware of how long it has been since the woman last ate because she may need an oral sports drink or IV glucose solution to replace glucose stores she is using to keep active in labor.

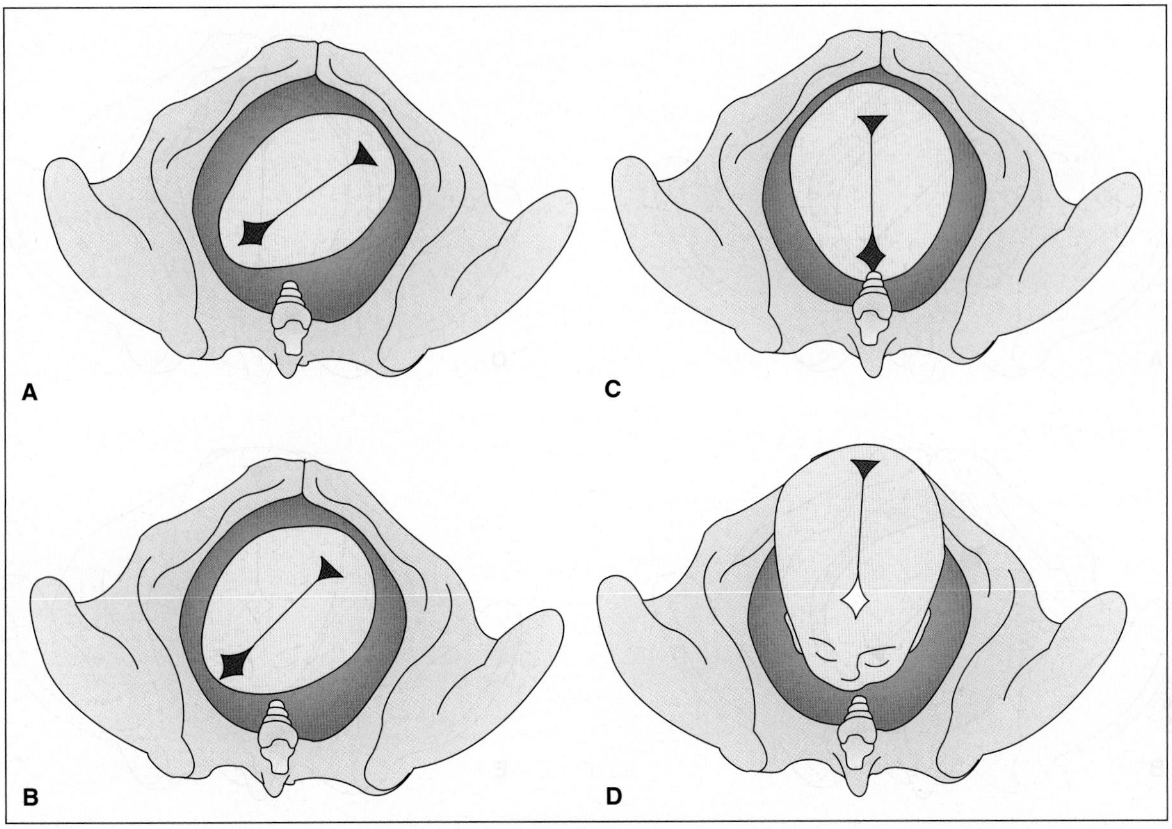

FIGURE 23.7 Left occipitoanterior (LOA) rotation. **(A)** A fetus in a cephalic presentation, LOA position. View is from the outlet. The fetus rotates 90 degrees from this position. **(B)** Descent and flexion. **(C)** Internal rotation complete. **(D)** Extension; the face and chin are born.

If contractions are not effective, or if the fetus is larger than average or not in good flexion, rotation through the 135-degree arc may not be possible. The woman may become exhausted. The fetal head may arrest in the transverse position (i.e., transverse arrest), or rotation may not occur at all (i.e., persistent occipitoposterior position). In these instances, the fetus must be born by cesarean birth.

Most women need a great deal of support during such a long labor to prevent them from becoming worried about the length of labor or that things are not going "by the book." Provide frequent reassurance that, although their pattern of labor is not "textbook," it is within safe, controlled limits. Although rare, if forceps are used to help the fetus rotate, observe a woman closely for hemorrhage from cervical lacerations or infection in the postpartum period.

QSEN Checkpoint Question 23.5

Quality Improvement

Rosann's baby is not only large but also in an occipitoposterior position. Which of the following would you want your team members to know is the best position for a woman whose baby is in this position during labor?

a. On her right side to stretch the pelvic inlet
b. Walking about to encourage fetal descent
c. Sitting in a rocking chair to aid presentation
d. On her hands and knees to help fetal rotation

Look in Appendix A for the best answer and rationale.

Breech Presentation

Most fetuses are in a breech presentation early in pregnancy. By week 38, however, in approximately 97% of all pregnancies, a fetus turns to a cephalic presentation (i.e., head down). This probably happens because, although the fetal head is the widest single diameter, the buttocks (breech) plus the legs of the fetus actually take up more space. As the fundus is the largest part of the uterus, this places the bulkiest parts of the fetus in the fundus.

There are several types of breech presentations: complete, frank, and footling (see Chapter 15). Examples of why such presentations occur are shown in Box 23.7. Overall, a breech presentation is more hazardous to a fetus than a cephalic presentation because there is a higher risk of the following:

- Developing dysplasia of the hip
- Anoxia from a prolapsed cord
- Traumatic injury to the after-coming head (possibility of intracranial hemorrhage or anoxia)
- Fracture of the spine or arm
- Dysfunctional labor
- Early rupture of the membranes because of the poor fit of the presenting part
- Meconium staining

Meconium staining occurs because of cervical pressure on the buttocks and rectum, not because of fetal anoxia and so is not a sign of fetal distress. Meconium excretion can, however, lead to meconium aspiration if the infant inhales amniotic fluid.

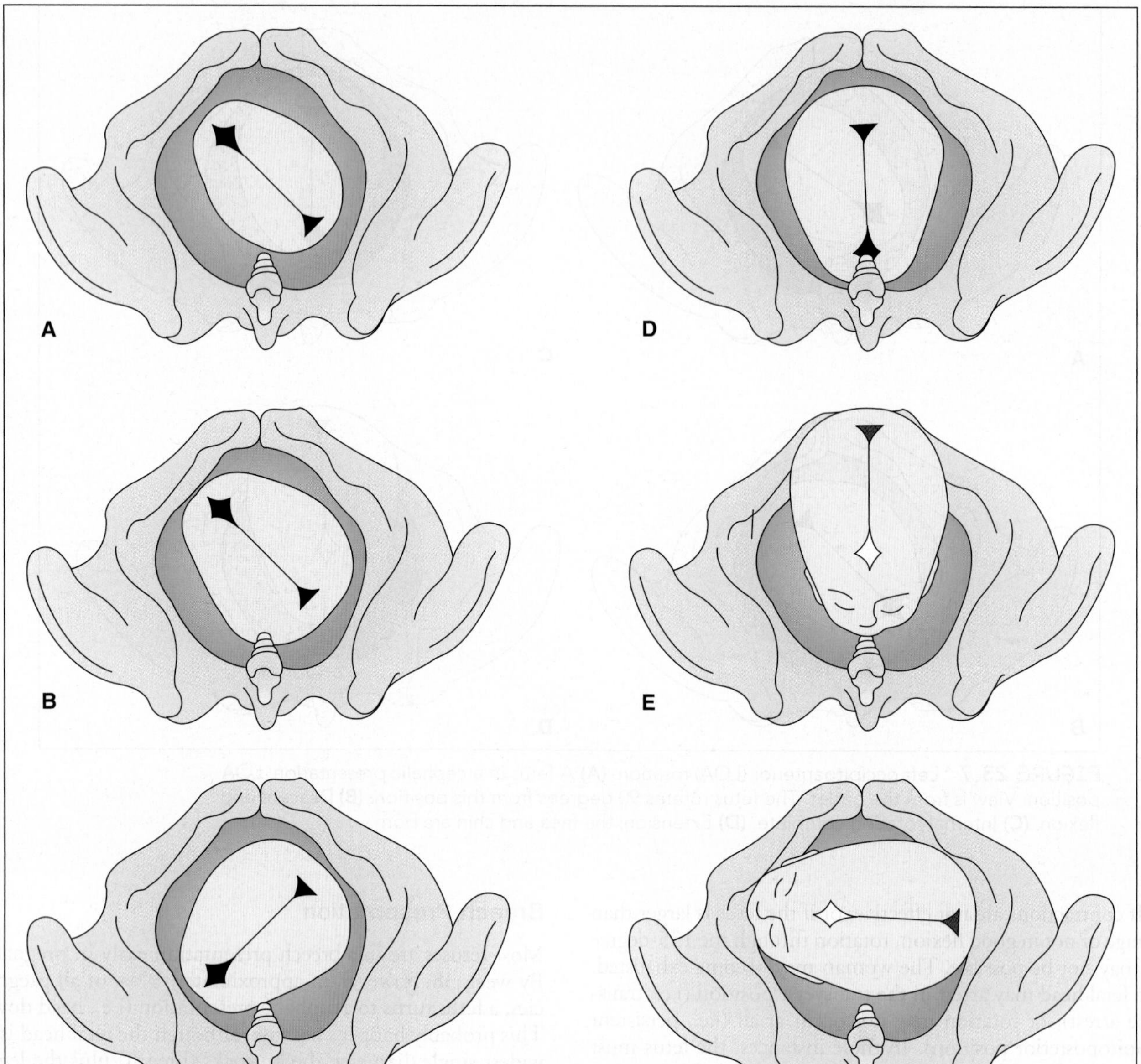

FIGURE 23.8 Left occipitoposterior (LOP) rotation. **(A)** Fetus in a cephalic presentation, LOP position. View is from outlet. The fetus rotates 135 degrees from this position. **(B)** Descent and flexion. **(C)** Internal rotation beginning. Because of the posterior position, the head will rotate in a longer arc than if it were in an anterior position. **(D)** Internal rotation complete. **(E)** Extension; the face and chin are born. **(F)** External rotation; the fetus rotates to place the shoulders in an anteroposterior position.

Assessment. With a breech presentation, fetal heart sounds usually are heard high in the abdomen. Leopold maneuvers and a vaginal examination usually reveal the presentation. If the breech is complete and firmly engaged, the tightly stretched gluteal muscles of the fetus may be mistaken on vaginal examination for a head and the cleft between the buttocks may be mistaken for the sagittal suture line. If the presentation is unclear, ultrasound clearly confirms a breech presentation. Such a study also gives information on pelvic diameters, fetal skull diameters, and evidence of possible placenta previa causing the breech presentation.

In a breech birth, the same stages of flexion, descent, internal rotation, expulsion, and external rotation occur as in a vertex birth. Always monitor FHR and uterine contractions frequently because this allows for early detection of fetal distress from a complication such as prolapsed cord or arrest of descent.

Birth Technique. If the infant will be born vaginally, a woman is allowed to push after full dilatation is achieved, and the breech, trunk, and shoulders are born (Fig. 23.10A,B). As the breech spontaneously emerges from the birth canal, it is steadied and supported by a sterile towel held against the infant's inferior surface (Fig. 23.10C). The shoulders present to the outlet with their widest diameter anteroposterior. If they are not born readily, the arm of the posterior shoulder

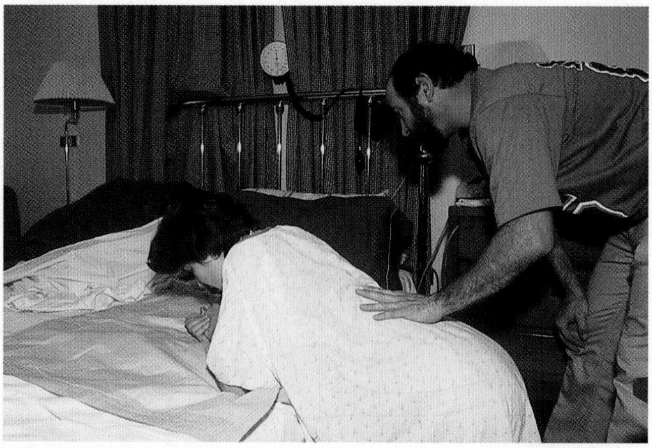

FIGURE 23.9 With a posterior fetal position, a woman may feel extensive back pressure. Pressure on her lower back by her support person may help relieve this problem. (© Kathy Sloane.)

BOX 23.7 Causes of Breech Presentation

- Gestational age less than 40 weeks
- Abnormality in a fetus, such as anencephaly, hydrocephalus, or meningocele (in a fetus with hydrocephalus, the widest fetal diameter is the head, so it retains the most "comfortable" position)
- Hydramnios that allows for free fetal movement, so the fetus fits within the uterus in any position
- Congenital anomaly of the uterus, such as a midseptum, that traps the fetus in a breech position
- Any space-occupying mass in the pelvis, such as a fibroid tumor of the uterus or a placenta previa, that does not allow the head to present
- Pendulous abdomen (if the abdominal muscles are lax, the uterus may fall so far forward that the fetal head comes to lie outside the pelvic brim, causing a breech presentation)
- Multiple gestation (the presenting infant cannot turn to a vertex position)

may be drawn downward by passing two fingers over the infant's shoulder and down the arm to the elbow, then sweeping the flexed arm across the infant's face and chest and out. The other arm is delivered in the same way. External rotation is then allowed to occur to bring the head into the best outlet diameter.

Birth of the head is the most hazardous part of a breech birth. Because the umbilicus precedes the head, a loop of cord passes down alongside the head. The pressure of the head against the pelvic brim automatically causes compression on this loop of cord.

A second danger of a breech birth is intracranial hemorrhage. With a cephalic presentation, molding to the confines of the birth canal occurs over hours. With a breech birth, pressure changes occur instantaneously, a situation that can result in tentorial tears leading to gross motor and mental incapacity or lethal damage to the fetus. A danger to the infant who is born gradually to reduce the possibility of intracranial injury is hypoxia. In contrast, the infant who is born suddenly to reduce the duration of cord compression may suffer an intracranial hemorrhage.

To aid in birth of the head, the trunk of the infant is usually straddled over the primary care provider's right forearm (Fig. 23.10D). Two fingers of the right hand are then placed in the infant's mouth. The left hand is slid into the woman's vagina, palm down, along the infant's back and pressure is applied to the occiput to flex the head fully. Gentle traction applied to the shoulders (upward and outward) delivers the head. Because of these difficulties with birth of the head is the reason why planned cesarean birth is the usual method of birth for many infants in breech presentation (Socol, 2012).

Parents of a breech baby can be worried about their baby's outcome all during labor (Guittier, Bonnet, Jarabo, et al., 2011). They usually inspect their child a little more closely after birth than do parents whose babies were not breech. They, as well as the person who makes the initial physical assessment of the infant, are looking for a possible reason for the breech presentation. An infant who was born from a frank breech position tends to keep his or her legs extended and at the level of the face for the first 2 or 3 days of life. The infant who was a footling breech may tend to keep the legs extended in a footling position for the first few days. Be sure to point out to the parents that this is normal so that they do not misinterpret the unusual posture of their infant.

What if...23.2 Rosann's baby was presenting as breech and you noticed that when her membranes ruptured, the amniotic fluid was green stained. Is this an emergency situation?

Face Presentation

A fetal head presenting at a different angle than expected is termed *asynclitism*. Face and brow presentations are examples. Face (chin, or mentum) presentation is rare, but when it does occur, the head diameter the fetus presents to the pelvis is often too large for birth to proceed. A head that feels more prominent than normal, with no engagement apparent on Leopold maneuvers, suggests a face presentation. It is also suggested when the head and back are both felt on the same side of the uterus with Leopold maneuvers. The back is difficult to outline in this presentation because it is concave. If the back is extremely concave, fetal heart tones may be transmitted to the forward-thrust chest and heard on the side of the fetus where feet and arms can be palpated. A face presentation is confirmed by vaginal examination when the nose, mouth, or chin can be felt as the presenting part.

A fetus in a posterior position, instead of flexing the head as labor proceeds, may extend the head, resulting in a face presentation; this usually occurs in a woman with a contracted pelvis or placenta previa. It also may occur in the relaxed uterus of a multipara or with prematurity, hydramnios, or fetal malformation. It is a warning signal. Something abnormal is usually causing the face presentation.

When a face presentation is suspected, an ultrasound is done to confirm it; if indicated, the pelvic diameters are measured. If the chin is anterior and the pelvic diameters are within normal limits, it may be possible for the infant to be born without difficulty (perhaps after a long first stage of labor

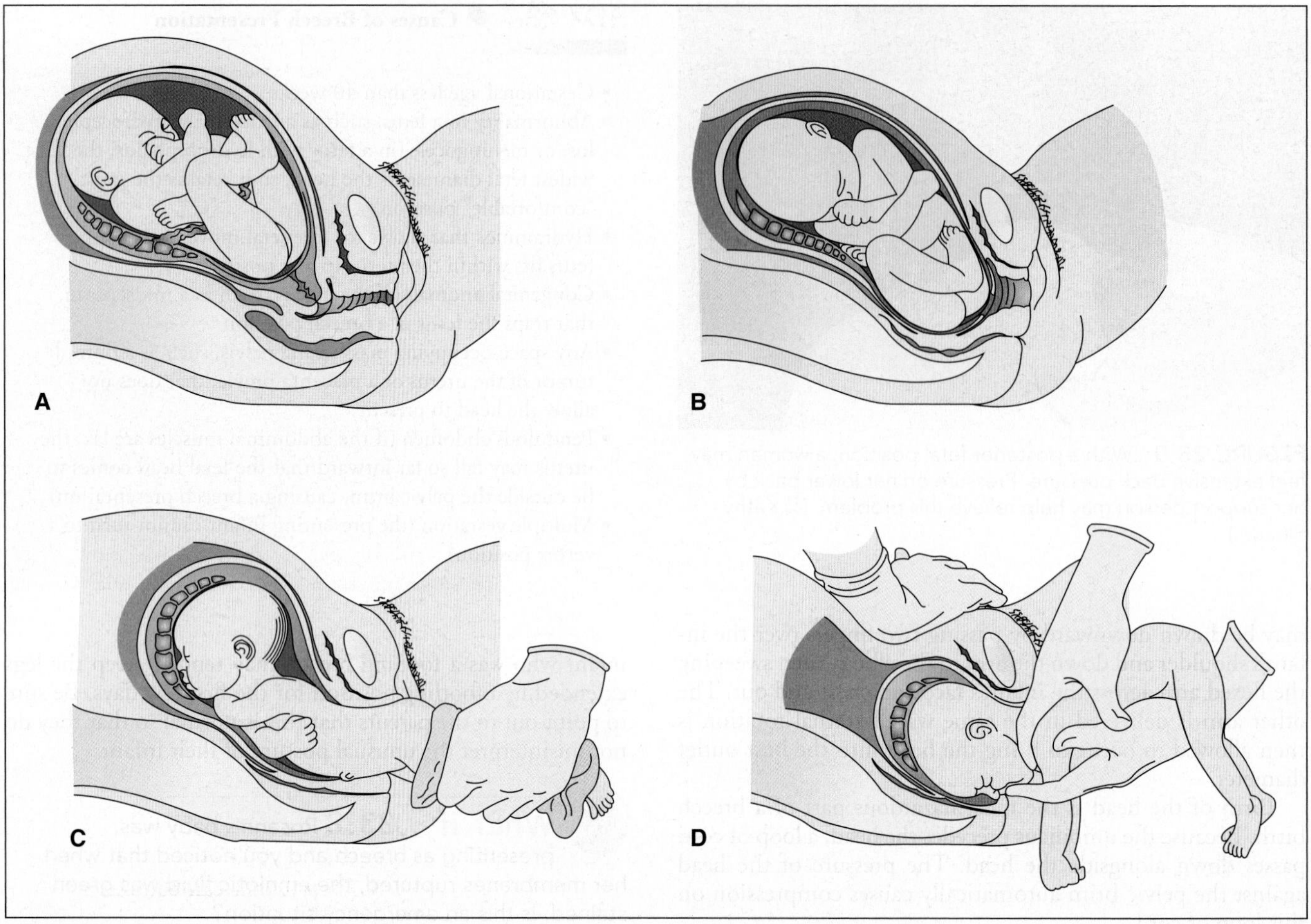

FIGURE 23.10 Breech birth. **(A)** Position before labor; left sacroposterior. **(B)** Descent and internal rotation. **(C)** Legs being born; the shoulders turn to present to the anteroposterior diameter. **(D)** The head is born. External rotation has put the anteroposterior diameter of the head in line with the anteroposterior diameter of the woman's pelvis. The head is born by gentle pressure to flex the head fully and by gentle traction to the shoulders upward and outward. Additional pressure might be applied by an assistant to the abdominal wall to ensure head flexion.

because the face does not mold well to make a firm engaging part). If the chin is posterior, cesarean birth is usually the method of choice; otherwise, it would be necessary to wait for a long posterior-to-anterior rotation to occur. Such rotation could result in uterine dysfunction or a transverse arrest.

Babies born after a face presentation have a great deal of facial edema and may be purple from ecchymotic bruising. Observe the infant closely for a patent airway. In some infants, lip edema is so severe that they are unable to suck for a day or two. Gavage feedings may be necessary to allow them to obtain enough fluid until they can suck effectively. They may be transferred to a neonatal intensive care unit (NICU) for 24 hours. Reassure the parents that the edema is transient and will disappear in a few days with no aftermath.

Brow Presentation

A brow presentation is the rarest of the presentations. It occurs in a multipara or a woman with relaxed abdominal muscles. It almost invariably results in obstructed labor, because the head becomes jammed in the brim of the pelvis as the occipitomental diameter presents. Unless the presentation spontaneously corrects, cesarean birth will be necessary to birth the infant safely. Brow presentations also leave an infant with extreme ecchymotic bruising on the face. On seeing this bruising over the same area as the anterior fontanelle, or "soft spot," parents may need additional reassurance that the child is well after birth.

Transverse Lie

Transverse lie occurs in women with pendulous abdomens, with uterine fibroid tumors that obstruct the lower uterine segment, with contraction of the pelvic brim, with congenital abnormalities of the uterus, or with hydramnios. It may occur in infants with hydrocephalus or another abnormality that prevents the head from engaging. It may also occur in prematurity if the infant has room for free movement, in multiple gestations (particularly in a second twin), or if there is a short umbilical cord.

A transverse lie usually is obvious on inspection, because the ovoid of the uterus is found to be more horizontal than vertical. The abnormal presentation can be confirmed by Leopold maneuvers. An ultrasound may be taken to further confirm the abnormal lie and to provide information on pelvic size.

A mature fetus cannot be born vaginally from this presentation. Often, the membranes rupture at the beginning of labor. Because there is no firm presenting part, the cord or an arm may prolapse, or the shoulder may obstruct the cervix. Cesarean birth is necessary.

Oversized Fetus (Macrosomia)

Size may become a problem in a fetus who weighs more than 4,000 to 4,500 g (approximately 9 to 10 lb). Babies of this size complicate up to 10% of all births and are most frequently born to women who enter pregnancy with diabetes or who develop gestational diabetes (Ouzounian, Hernandez, Korst, et al., 2011). Large babies are also associated with multiparity, because each infant born to a woman tends to be slightly heavier and larger than the one born just before.

An oversized infant may cause uterine dysfunction during labor or at birth because of overstretching of the fibers of the myometrium. The wide shoulders may pose a problem at birth, because they can cause fetal pelvic disproportion or even uterine rupture from obstruction. A woman may be left with perineal lacerations (Best, Drutz, & Alarab, 2012).

If the infant is so oversized that he or she cannot be born vaginally, a cesarean birth becomes the birth method of choice. The large size of a fetus may be missed in an obese woman, because the fetal contours are difficult to palpate and obesity does not necessarily indicate a larger than usual pelvis. Pelvimetry or ultrasound can be used to compare the size of the fetus with the woman's pelvic capacity.

The perinatal mortality rate of larger infants is substantially increased to about 15%, compared with the normal 4%. In addition, a large infant born vaginally has a higher than normal risk of cervical nerve palsy, diaphragmatic nerve injury, or a fractured clavicle because of shoulder dystocia. Postpartally, the woman has an increased risk of hemorrhage because the overdistended uterus may not contract as readily as usual.

Shoulder Dystocia

Shoulder dystocia is a birth problem that is increasing in incidence because the weight and therefore the size of newborns is increasing (Cha, Kim, Choi, et al., 2012). The problem occurs at the second stage of labor, when the fetal head is born but the shoulders are too broad to enter and be born through the pelvic outlet. This is hazardous to the woman because it can result in vaginal or cervical tears. It is hazardous to the fetus if the cord is compressed between the fetal body and the bony pelvis. In addition, the force of birth can result in a fractured clavicle or a brachial plexus injury for the fetus.

Shoulder dystocia is most apt to occur in women with diabetes, in multiparas, and in postdate pregnancies. The condition may be suspected earlier if the second stage of labor is prolonged, if there is arrest of descent, or if, when the head appears on the perineum (crowning), it retracts instead of protruding with each contraction (a turtle sign). The problem often is not identified, however, until the head has already been born and the wide anterior shoulder locks beneath the symphysis pubis.

Although not evidence based, asking a woman to flex her thighs sharply on her abdomen (McRoberts maneuver) may widen the pelvic outlet and allow the anterior shoulder to be born. Applying suprapubic pressure may also help the shoulder escape from beneath the symphysis pubis and be born (Hoffman, Bailit, Branch, et al., 2011).

QSEN Checkpoint Question 23.6

Evidence-Based Practice

To determine if there is a greater risk of complications at birth for extremely large fetuses, researchers compared a cohort of 343 extremely large babies (>5,000 g) to a cohort of 679 usual birth weight infants. The results of the study found an increased incidence of shoulder dystocia, emergency cesarean birth, and failed labor induction. Minor congenital malformations were also more frequent, as were birth injuries and minor metabolic disturbances, although not asphyxial births (Vidarsdottir, Geirsson, Hardardottir, et al., 2011).

Based on this study and the fact that a sonogram has shown Rosann's fetus to be extremely large, what assessment would you want to prioritize for Rosann's baby after birth?

a. If his abdominal wall appears to be ruptured
b. If his arms feel warm and are the same length
c. If his buttocks or back have extensive bruising
d. If his eyes can focus steadily on a nearby object

Look in Appendix A for the best answer and rationale.

Fetal Anomalies

Fetal anomalies of the head such as hydrocephalus (i.e., fluid-filled ventricles) or anencephaly (i.e., absence of the cranium) are a final category of fetal factors that can complicate birth because the fetal presenting part does not engage the cervix well (see Chapter 27).

PROBLEMS WITH THE PASSAGE

Aside from a concern with the power of labor and the passenger, the third reason dystocia can occur is a contraction or narrowing of the passageway or birth canal. This can happen at the inlet, at the midpelvis, or at the outlet. The narrowing causes CPD, or a disproportion between the size of the fetal head and the pelvic diameters, which then results in failure to progress in labor.

Inlet Contraction

Inlet contraction is narrowing of the anteroposterior diameter of the pelvis to less than 11 cm, or of the transverse diameter to 12 cm or less. It usually is caused by rickets in early life or by an inherited small pelvis. Rickets is caused by a lack of calcium, and is therefore rare in developed countries but can occur among immigrants who were raised where milk supplies were not plentiful. In primigravidas, the fetal head normally engages between weeks 36 to 38 of pregnancy. If this occurs any time before labor begins, it is proof the pelvic inlet is adequate as lightening, by definition, means the fetal head has sunk below the inlet. Following the general rule that "what goes in, comes out," a head that engages or proves it fits into the pelvic brim will probably also be able to pass through the midpelvis and through the outlet.

If engagement does not occur in a primigravida, then either a fetal abnormality (larger than usual head) or a pelvic abnormality (smaller than usual pelvis) should be suspected. As a rule, engagement does not occur in multigravidas until labor begins. For these women, previous vaginal birth of a full-term infant without problems is proof their birth canal is adequate.

Every primigravida should have pelvic measurements taken and recorded before week 24 of pregnancy so, based on these measurements and the assumption the fetus will be of average size, a birth decision can be made.

If CPD exists, because the fetus may not engage but instead remains "floating," the possibility of cord prolapse can lead to a secondary concern.

Outlet Contraction

Outlet contraction is a narrowing of the transverse diameter, the distance between the ischial tuberosities at the outlet, to less than 11 cm. This measurement is made by sonogram during pregnancy, but can also easily be made manually at a prenatal visit or at the beginning of labor.

Trial Labor

If a woman has a borderline (just adequate) inlet measurement and the fetal lie and position are good, her primary care provider may allow her a "trial" labor to determine whether labor will progress normally. The trial labor continues as long as descent of the presenting part and dilatation of the cervix continue to occur. With a trial labor, monitor fetal heart sounds and uterine contractions frequently. Urge the woman to void every 2 hours so her urinary bladder is as empty as possible, allowing the fetal head to use all the space available. If, after a definite period (6 to 12 hours), adequate progress in labor cannot be documented, or if at any time fetal distress occurs, the trial labor will be discontinued and the woman will be scheduled for a cesarean birth.

It may be difficult for women to undertake labor they know they may not be able to complete, because the effort subjects them needlessly to pain. Emphasize, but do not overstress, that it is best for their baby to be born vaginally. If the trial labor fails and cesarean birth is scheduled, provide an explanation as to why cesarean birth is necessary and why it has become the best route for the birth of their baby (Box 23.8).

Some women undergoing a trial labor feel as if they themselves are on trial. When dilatation does not occur, they begin to feel discouraged and inadequate, as if they are at fault. A woman may not be aware of how much she wanted the trial labor to work until she is told it is not working. The support person may be as frightened and feel as helpless as she does and so momentarily stops being a support person. You can assure a woman and her support person that a cesarean birth is just an alternative, not an inferior, method of birth for them. Because labor is not progressing, it is the method of choice to allow them to achieve their goal of a healthy mother and healthy child.

External Cephalic Version

External cephalic version is the turning of a fetus from a breech to a cephalic position before birth. It may be done as early as 34 to 35 weeks, although the usual time is by 37 to 38 weeks of pregnancy (Hofmeyr & Kulier, 2012). For the procedure, FHR and possibly ultrasound are recorded continuously.

BOX 23.8 Nursing Care Planning Based on Effective Communication

Rosann Bigalow is having her first baby. Her primary care provider has told her she has a borderline pelvis but she wants her to try a trial labor.

Less Effective Communication

Nurse: Hello, Rosann. Is it all right if I attach a fetal heart rate and uterine contraction monitor so we can observe you closely during labor?

Rosann: Sure. Although I should be having this baby any minute. It's already been 10 hours.

Nurse: I thought I heard your doctor say she's thinking of this as a trial labor.

Rosann: Whatever. I told her anything but surgery would be all right.

Nurse: I'm glad you have a positive outlook. That always makes labor seem to go faster.

More Effective Communication

Nurse: Hello, Rosann. Is it all right if I attach a fetal heart rate and uterine contraction monitor so we can observe you closely during labor?

Rosann: Sure. Although I should be having this baby any minute. It's already been 10 hours.

Nurse: I thought I heard your doctor say she's thinking of this as a trial labor.

Rosann: Whatever. I told her anything but surgery would be all right.

Nurse: Let's talk about what a trial labor means.

If a woman develops a complication of pregnancy, which is referred to by a Latin name, it is generally expected that the couple will not understand the term and so will need to have the complication thoroughly explained. If a condition has a common name, such as protracted pelvis or trial labor, however, it is easy to assume little explanation of the condition is necessary. In reality, couples need explanations about all conditions, because what is common to health care personnel may not be common to everyone. In the first scenario, the nurse assumed she and the woman were talking about the same thing. In the second scenario, the nurse explored a little further and discovered Rosann was not aware a trial labor might mean she would need surgery.

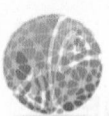

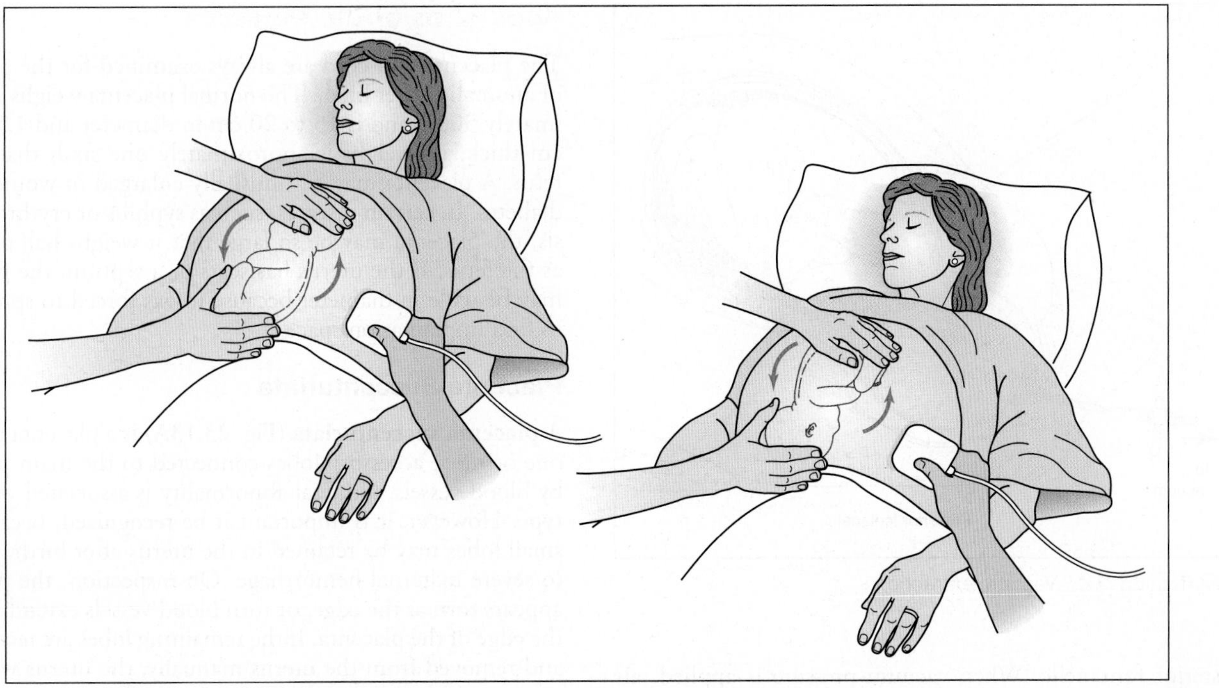

FIGURE 23.11 External cephalic version. The fetus is rotated by external pressure to a cephalic lie. An ultrasound helps guide a safe result.

A tocolytic agent may be administered to help relax the uterus. The breech and vertex of the fetus are located and grasped transabdominally by the examiner's hands on the woman's abdomen. Gentle pressure is then exerted to rotate the fetus in a forward direction to a cephalic lie (Fig. 23.11). Although not always successful, the use of external version can decrease the number of cesarean births necessary from breech presentations (Rijnders, Offerhaus, van Dommelen, et al., 2010). Contraindications to the procedure include multiple gestation, severe oligohydramnios, small pelvic diameters, a cord that wraps around the fetal neck, and unexplained third-trimester bleeding, which might be a placenta previa. External version can be uncomfortable for a woman because of the feeling of pressure. Women who are Rh negative should receive Rh immunoglobulin after the procedure in case minimal bleeding occurs.

Forceps Birth

Obstetrical forceps are steel instruments constructed of two blades that slide together at their shaft to form a handle. One blade is slipped into the woman's vagina next to the fetal head and the other is slipped into place on the other side of the head. Next, the shafts of the instrument are brought together in the midline to form the handle. The primary care provider then applies pressure on the handle to manually extract the fetus from the birth canal.

In years past, babies were routinely born with forceps. Today, the technique is rarely used (in only about 4% to 8% of births) because it can lead to rectal sphincter tears in the woman, which can lead to dyspareunia, anal incontinence, or increased urinary stress incontinence (Murphy, Macleod, Bahl, et al., 2011). Although no longer used routinely, forceps may be necessary with any of the following conditions:

- A woman is unable to push with contractions in the pelvic division of labor such as might happen with a woman who received regional anesthesia or who has a spinal cord injury.
- Cessation of descent in the second stage of labor occurs.
- A fetus is in an abnormal position.
- A fetus is in distress from a complication such as a prolapsed cord.

Although forceps appear as if they would put forceful pressure on the fetal head, the pressure registers on the steel blades rather than the head so they can actually reduce pressure, thus avoiding a complication such as subdural hemorrhage (Werner, Janevic, Illuzzi, et al., 2011).

Before forceps are applied:

- Membranes must be ruptured.
- CPD must not be present.
- The cervix must be fully dilated.
- The woman's bladder must be empty.

Record the FHR before forceps application. Because there is a danger that the cord could be compressed between the forceps blade and the fetal head, assess FHR again immediately after application. The woman's cervix needs to be carefully assessed after forceps birth to be certain no lacerations have occurred. To rule out bladder injury, record the time and amount of the first voiding. In addition, assess the newborn to be certain no facial palsy exists from pressure. A forceps birth may leave a transient erythematous mark on the newborn's cheek (see Chapter 18). This mark will fade in 1 to 2 days with no long-term effects.

Vacuum Extraction

A fetus, if positioned far enough down the birth canal, may be born by **vacuum extraction** (Schuller, Känel, Müller, et al., 2012). With the fetal head at the perineum, a soft, disk-shaped cup is pressed against the fetal scalp and over the

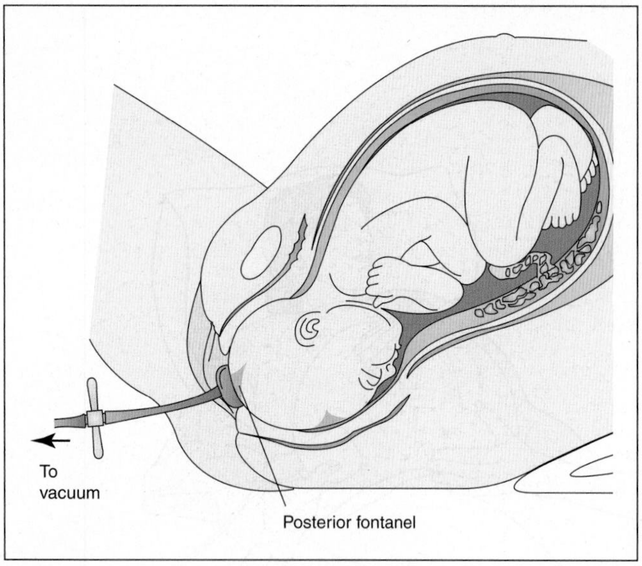

FIGURE 23.12 Vacuum extraction.

posterior fontanelle. When vacuum pressure is applied, air beneath the cup is suctioned out and the cup then adheres so tightly to the fetal scalp that traction on the vacuum cord leading to the cup extracts the fetus (Fig. 23.12).

Vacuum extraction has advantages over forceps birth in that little anesthesia is necessary, thus leaving the fetus with less respiratory depression at birth. One disadvantage over natural birth is that more perineal lacerations may occur (Melamed et al., 2012). Its major disadvantage is that it causes a marked caput on the newborn head that may be noticeable as long as 7 days after birth. Tentorial tears from extreme pressure also have occurred. A woman may need reassurance that the caput swelling is harmless for her infant and will decrease rapidly. Vacuum extraction should not be used as a method of birth if fetal scalp blood sampling was used, because the suction pressure can cause severe bleeding at the sampling site. Moreover, vacuum extraction is not advantageous for preterm infants because of the softness of the preterm skull.

ANOMALIES OF THE PLACENTA AND CORD

The third stage of labor (i.e., delivery of the placenta) can also result in complications; therefore, continued careful observation of the mother is important (Burke, 2010).

Anomalies of the Placenta

The placenta and cord are always examined for the presence of anomalies after birth. The normal placenta weighs approximately 500 g and is 15 to 20 cm in diameter and 1.5 to 3.0 cm thick. Its weight is approximately one sixth that of the fetus. A placenta may be unusually enlarged in women with diabetes. In certain diseases, such as syphilis or erythroblastosis, the placenta may be so large that it weighs half as much as the fetus. If the uterus has scars or a septum, the placenta may be wide in diameter because it was forced to spread out to find implantation space.

Placenta Succenturiata

A **placenta succenturiata** (Fig. 23.13A) is a placenta that has one or more accessory lobes connected to the main placenta by blood vessels. No fetal abnormality is associated with this type. However, it is important it be recognized, because the small lobes may be retained in the uterus after birth, leading to severe maternal hemorrhage. On inspection, the placenta appears torn at the edge, or torn blood vessels extend beyond the edge of the placenta. If the remaining lobes are recognized and removed from the uterus manually, the uterus will contract as usual with no adverse maternal effects.

Placenta Circumvallata

Ordinarily, the chorion membrane begins at the edge of the placenta and spreads to envelop the fetus; no chorion covers the fetal side of the placenta. In **placenta circumvallata**, the fetal side of the placenta is covered to some extent with chorion (Fig. 23.13B). The umbilical cord enters the placenta at the usual midpoint, and large vessels spread out from there. However, they end abruptly at the point where the chorion folds back onto the surface. (In **placenta marginata**, the fold of chorion reaches just to the edge of the placenta.) Although no abnormalities are associated with this type of placenta, its presence should be noted.

Battledore Placenta

In a **battledore placenta**, the cord is inserted marginally rather than centrally (Fig. 23.13C). This anomaly is rare and has no known clinical significance either.

Velamentous Insertion of the Cord

Velamentous insertion of the cord is a situation in which the cord, instead of entering the placenta directly, separates into small vessels that reach the placenta by spreading across a fold of amnion (Fig. 23.13D). This form of cord insertion

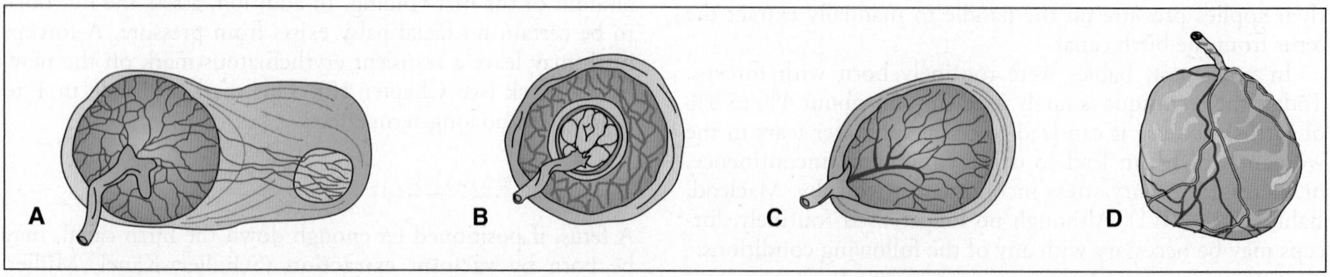

FIGURE 23.13 Abnormal placental formation. **(A)** Placenta succenturiata. **(B)** Placenta circumvallata. **(C)** Battledore placenta. **(D)** Velamentous cord insertion.

is most frequently found with multiple gestations. Because the fetal blood supply may not be as generous as usual, this type of placenta is associated with fetal anomalies. An infant born with this type of placenta needs to be examined carefully at birth.

Vasa Previa

In vasa previa, the umbilical vessels of a velamentous cord insertion cross the cervical os and therefore deliver before the fetus (Robinson & Grobman, 2011). The vessels may tear with cervical dilatation, just as a placenta previa may tear. Before inserting any instrument such as an internal fetal monitor, be certain to identify structures to prevent accidental tearing of a vasa previa because tearing would result in sudden fetal blood loss. If sudden, painless bleeding occurs with the beginning of cervical dilatation, either placenta previa or vasa previa is suspected. It can be confirmed by ultrasound. If vasa previa is identified, the infant needs to be born by cesarean birth.

Placenta Accreta

Placenta accreta is an unusually deep attachment of the placenta to the uterine myometrium, so deep that the placenta will not loosen and deliver (Kazandi, 2010). Attempts to remove it manually may lead to extreme hemorrhage because of the deep attachment. Hysterectomy to remove the uterus or treatment with methotrexate to destroy the still-attached tissue may be necessary.

What if...23.3 While inspecting the placenta, you observe one edge appears torn with torn blood vessels extending beyond its edge. Would you rate the placenta as normal or report its appearance as potentially serious?

Anomalies of the Cord

Two-Vessel Cord

A normal cord contains one vein and two arteries. The absence of one of the umbilical arteries is associated with congenital heart and kidney anomalies, because the insult that caused the loss of the vessel may have also affected other mesoderm germ layer structures. Inspection of the cord as to how many vessels are present must be made immediately after birth, before the cord begins to dry, because drying distorts the appearance of the vessels. Document the number of vessels present conscientiously because an infant with only two vessels needs to be observed carefully for other anomalies during the newborn period.

Unusual Cord Length

Although the length of the umbilical cord rarely varies, some abnormal lengths may occur. An unusually short umbilical cord can result in premature separation of the placenta or an abnormal fetal lie. An unusually long cord may be easily compromised because of its tendency to twist or knot. Occasionally, a cord actually forms a knot, but the natural pulsations of the blood through the vessels and the muscular vessel walls usually keep the blood flow adequate. It is not unusual for a cord to wrap once around the fetal neck (nuchal cord) but, again, with no interference to fetal circulation (Cohain, 2010).

What if...23.4 You are particularly interested in exploring one of the 2020 National Health Goals with respect to complications of labor. What would be a possible research topic to explore pertinent to this goal that would be applicable to the Bigalow family and that would also advance evidence-based practice?

KEY POINTS FOR REVIEW

- Complications of labor can arise from problems with the force of labor, the passage, the passenger (the fetus), or the woman's reaction to the experience (the psyche). Hypotonic, hypertonic, and uncoordinated contractions all can occur, resulting in ineffective first or second stages of labor.
- Supporting families who experience a complication of labor is important to not only plan nursing care that meets QSEN competencies but also that best meets a family's total needs.
- Precipitate labor is birth that is completed in less than 3 hours. It can be responsible for subdural hemorrhage in the fetus and cervical or perineal lacerations in the woman.
- Be certain a woman meets the criteria for labor induction before preparing an oxytocin solution. These criteria include engagement of the fetal head, a "ripe" cervix, and absence of CPD. Question if oxytocin should be used if these criteria are not met.
- Always prepare oxytocin as a "piggyback" solution, being extremely careful of the dose used. Both a uterine monitor and an FHR monitor should be used during labor induction to be certain uterine overstimulation does not occur. Observe that contractions occur no less than 2 minutes apart and are no longer than 70 seconds in duration.
- Uterine rupture, although rare, is a complication that is an immediate emergency because of blood loss to the mother and potential anoxia for the fetus.
- Uterine inversion is another rare but grave complication because it leads to inability to control hemorrhage. If the situation is not immediately corrected, emergency hysterectomy may be necessary to save the woman's life. Almost all occurrences of uterine inversion can be avoided by two axioms of care: (a) *do not put pressure on a noncontracted fundus immediately after birth* (massage it first to cause it to contract), and (b) *do not exert pressure on an umbilical cord to achieve placental delivery.*
- Amniotic fluid embolism occurs when amniotic fluid is forced into an open maternal uterine blood sinus. A woman will notice chest pain and dyspnea. Administer oxygen and notify the woman's primary care provider of this emergency.
- Prolapse of the umbilical cord is an emergency situation that requires prompt action. Position a woman quickly into either a Trendelenburg or a knee–chest position to relieve cord compression, or apply manual pressure vaginally to lift the fetal head away from the cord. Notify the woman's primary caregiver of the emergency.

- A multiple gestation can complicate birth. Many infants of multiple gestations are born by cesarean birth to avoid entangled cords or arrest of descent.
- Abnormal position, presentation, or size of the fetus (such as occipitoposterior position; breech, face, or brow presentation; transverse lie), as well as problems of the passage such as inlet and outlet contraction can lead to labor complications.
- Vacuum extraction and forceps are methods that can be used to assist birth. The woman as well as the infant needs special observation after these procedures to detect head trauma or cervical or vaginal tearing.
- Anomalies of the placenta and cord (such as placenta succenturiata, velamentous cord insertion, vasa previa, and two-vessel cord) can lead to birth complications.

Critical Thinking Care Study

Debbie and Craig O'Hara are a married couple having their first baby. Craig works as a football coach; Debbie is a telemarketer. When you admit them to a birthing room, Debbie tells you, "I'm going to have a terrible labor because something's wrong with my baby." On examination, her cervix is 4 cm dilated, 75% effaced; contraction duration is 30 seconds; and frequency is every 5 minutes. Her fetus is in an occipitoposterior position.

1. Would you assume when Debbie said "something's wrong with my baby" she meant the posterior position? Would you assure her the baby will be fine?
2. Debbie's husband tells you he's proud he's having a boy. You notice he talks to his son all during labor with comments such as, "Why aren't you following the playbook?" or "Put your head down and push. The clock is running." Would you be concerned he's coaching his son and not his wife?
3. Debbie's primary care provider wants Debbie to rest between contractions on her hands and knees in the hope that will help her fetus rotate more efficiently and avoid a cesarean birth. Craig tells you he'd rather Debbie have a cesarean than spend so long in labor. How would you respond to him?

Patient Scenario

The Sandoval Family

Read about the Sandoval family, a family with a complication of labor, then answer the questions to further sharpen your skills and grow more familiar with NCLEX-type questions related to labor complications. Confirm your answers are correct by reading the rationales.

Visit http://thePoint.lww.com

Answers and Rationales

Looking for answers to the What If. . . and Critical Thinking Care Study questions?

Visit http://thePoint.lww.com

References

Anderson, C. J. & Kilpatrick, C. (2012). Supporting patients' birth plans: Theories, strategies & implications for nurses. *Nursing & Women's Health, 16*(3), 210–218.

Best, C., Drutz, H. P., & Alarab, M. (2012). Obstetric anal sphincter injuries: A survey of clinical practice among Canadian obstetricians. *Journal of Obstetrics & Gynaecology Canada, 34*(8), 747–754.

Bishop, E. H. (1964). Pelvic scoring for elective induction. *Obstetrics and Gynecology, 24*(2), 266.

Burke, C. (2010). Active versus expectant management of the third stage of labor and implementation of a protocol. *Journal of Perinatal & Neonatal Nursing, 24*(3), 215–228.

Cha, H. H., Kim, J. Y., Choi, S. J., et al. (2012). Can a customized standard for large for gestational age identify women at risk of operative delivery and shoulder dystocia? *Journal of Perinatal Medicine, 40*(5), 483–488.

Cohain, J. S. (2010). Nuchal cords are necklaces, not nooses. *Midwifery Today With International Midwife,* (93), 46–48.

Coldwell, B. J., Steinkeler, J., & Warner, M. A. (2012). Ultrasound of the gravid uterus. *Ultrasound Quarterly, 28*(2), 87–95.

Desbriere, R., Blanc, J., Le Dû, R., et al. (2013). Is maternal posturing during labor efficient in preventing persistent occiput posterior position? A randomized controlled trial. *American Journal of Obstetrics & Gynecology*, 208(1): 60e1–8.

El-Sayed, Y. Y. (2012). Diagnosis and management of arrest disorders: Duration to wait. *Seminars in Perinatology, 36*(5), 374–378.

Friedman, E. (1978). *Labor, clinical evaluation and management* (2nd ed.). New York, NY: Appleton-Century-Crofts.

Gilbert, E. S. (2011). Dysfunctional labor. In E. S. Gilbert (Ed.), *Manual of high risk pregnancy & delivery* (5th ed., pp. 610–659). St. Louis, MO: Mosby Elsevier.

Guittier, M. J., Bonnet, J., Jarabo, G., et al. (2011). Breech presentation and choice of mode of childbirth: A qualitative study of women's experiences. *Midwifery, 27*(6), e208–e213.

Hehir, M. P., O'Connor, H. D., Kent, E. M., et al. (2012). Changes in vaginal breech delivery rates in a single large metropolitan area. *American Journal of Obstetrics & Gynecology, 206*(6), 498.e1–498.e4.

Hoffman, M. K., Bailit, J. L., Branch, D. W., et al. (2011). A comparison of obstetric maneuvers for the acute management of shoulder dystocia. *Obstetrics & Gynecology, 117*(6), 1272–1278.

Hofmeyr, G. J., & Kulier, R. (2012). External cephalic version for breech presentation at term. *Cochrane Database of Systematic Reviews,* (10), CD000083.

Hofmeyr, G. J., & Lawrie, T. A. (2012). Amnioinfusion for potential or suspected umbilical cord compression in labour. *Cochrane Database of Systematic Reviews,* (1), CD000013.

Jones, L., Othman, M., Dowswell, T., et al. (2012). Pain management for women in labour: An overview of systematic reviews. *Cochrane Database of Systematic Reviews,* (3), CD009234.

Karch, A. M. (2013). *2013 Lippincott's nursing drug guide.* Philadelphia, PA: Lippincott Williams & Wilkins.

Kazandi, M. (2010). Conservative and surgical treatment of abnormal placentation: Report of five cases and review of the literature. *Clinical & Experimental Obstetrics & Gynecology, 37*(4), 310–312.

Khan, Z. A., Abdul, B., & Majoko, F. (2011). Induction of labour with vaginal prostaglandin tablet vs gel. *Journal of Obstetrics & Gynaecology, 31*(6), 492–494.

Kish, K. (2013). Malpresentation & cord prolapse. In A. H. DeCherney, L. Nathan, N. Laufer, et al. (Eds.), *Current diagnosis and treatment: Obstetrics and gynecology* (11th ed., pp. 317–333). Columbus, OH: McGraw-Hill/Lange.

Knight, M., Tuffnell, D., Brocklehurst, P., et al. (2010). Incidence and risk factors for amniotic-fluid embolism. *Obstetrics & Gynecology, 115*(5), 910–917.

Krening, C. F., Rehling-Anthony, K., & Garko, C. (2012). Oxytocin administration: The transition to a safer model of care. *Journal of Perinatal & Neonatal Nursing, 26*(1), 15–24.

Lanni, S. M., & Seeds, G. W. (2013). Malpresentations and shoulder dystocia. In S. G. Gabbe, J. R. Niebyl, J. L. Simpson, et al. (Eds.),

Obstetrics: Normal and problem pregnancies (6th ed., pp. 388–414). Philadelphia, PA: Elsevier/Saunders.

Le Ray, C., Fraser, W., Rozenberg, P., et al. (2011). Duration of passive and active phases of the second stage of labour and risk of severe postpartum haemorrhage in low-risk nulliparous women. *European Journal of Obstetrics, Gynecology & Reproductive Biology, 158*(2), 167–172.

Mahendru, A. A., & Lees, C. C. (2011). Is intrapartum fetal blood sampling a gold standard diagnostic tool for fetal distress? *European Journal of Obstetric, Gynecology & Reproductive Biology, 156*(2), 137–139.

Melamed, N., Gavish, O., Eisner, M., et al. (2013). Third- and fourth-degree perineal tears—Incidence and risk factors. *Journal of Maternal-Fetal & Neonatal Medicine, 26*(7), 660–664.

Moore, J., & Low, L. K. (2012). Factors that influence the practice of elective induction of labor: What does the evidence tell us? *Journal of Perinatal & Neonatal Nursing, 26*(3), 242–250.

Mozurkewich, E. L., Chilimigras, J. L., Berman, D. R., et al. (2011). Methods of induction of labour, a systematic review. *Obstetrics and Gynecology, 24*(2), 266.

Murphy, D. J., Macleod, M., Bahl, R. , et al. (2011). A cohort study of maternal and neonatal morbidity in relation to use of sequential instruments at operative vaginal delivery. *European Journal of Obstetrics, Gynecology, and Reproductive Biology, 156*(1):41–45.

Norman, J. E. (2012). Induction and augmentation of labour. In D. K. Edmonds (Ed.), *Dewhurst's textbook of obstetrics & gynaecology* (8th ed., pp. 287–295). Oxford, UK: John Wiley & Son.

Norwitz, E. R., Belfort, M. A., Saade, G. R. et al. (2010). Intrapartum management in a twin pregnancy. In E. R. Norwitz, M. A. Belfort, G. R. Saade, et al. (Eds.), *Obstetric clinical algorithms: Management & evidence* (pp. 132–133). Hoboken, NJ: Wiley-Blackwell.

Ouzounian, J. G., Hernandez, G. D., Korst, L. M., et al. (2011). Pre-pregnancy weight and excess weight gain are risk factors for macrosomia in women with gestational diabetes. *Journal of Perinatology, 31*(11), 717–721.

Purcell, E., & Bienstock, J. L. (2011). Complications of labor & delivery. In K. J. Hurt, M. W. Guile, J. L. Bienstock, et al. (Eds.), *The Johns Hopkins manual of gynecology and obstetrics* (4th ed., pp. 99–109). Philadelphia, PA: Lippincott Williams & Wilkins.

Rijnders, M., Offerhaus, P., van Dommelen, P., et al. (2010). Prevalence, outcome, and women's experiences of external cephalic version in a low-risk population. *Birth, 37*(2), 124–133.

Robinson, B. K., & Grobman, W. A. (2011). Effectiveness of timing strategies for delivery of individuals with vasa previa. *Obstetrics & Gynecology, 117*(3), 542–549.

Sahni, G. (2012). Chest pain syndromes in pregnancy. *Cardiology Clinics, 30*(3), 343–367.

Sandström, A., Cnattingius, S., Wikström, A., et al. (2012). Labour dystocia-risk of recurrence and instrumental delivery in following labour-a population-based cohort study. *BJOG: An International Journal of Obstetrics and Gynaecology, 119*(13), 1648–1656.

Schuller, C., Känel, N., Müller, O., et al. (2012). Stress and pain response of neonates after spontaneous birth and vacuum-assisted and cesarean delivery. *American Journal of Obstetrics & Gynecology, 207*(5), 416.e1–416.e6.

Silver, D. W., & Sabatino, F. (2012). Precipitous and difficult deliveries. *Emergency Medical Clinics of North America, 30*(4), 961–975.

Simkin, P. (2010). The fetal occiput posterior position, state of the science and a new perspective. *Birth, 37*(1), 61–71.

Smith, C. A., Collins, C. T., & Crowther, C. A. (2011). Acupuncture or acupressure for pain management in labour. *Cochrane Database of Systematic Reviews,* (7), CD009232.

Smith, C. A., Levett, K. M., Collins, C. T., et al. (2011). Relaxation techniques for pain management in labour. *Cochrane Database of Systematic Reviews,* (12), CD009514.

Socol, M. L. (2012). The influence of practice management on primary cesarean birth. *Seminars in Perinatology, 36*(5), 399–402.

Stevens, J. R., & Wittich, A. C. (2011). A rare case of occult uterine inversion at an Army community hospital, a case report. *Military Medicine, 176*(12), 1450–1452.

Taher, S. E., Inder, J. W., Soltan, S. A., et al. (2011). Prostaglandin E2 vaginal gel or tablets for the induction of labour at term, a randomised controlled trial. *International Journal of Obstetrics and Gynecology, 118*(6), 719–725.

Tiitinen, A. (2012). Prevention of multiple pregnancies in infertility treatment. *Best Practice & Research: Clinical Obstetrics & Gynaecology, 26*(6), 829–840.

Torkildsen, E. A., Salvesen, K. Å., & Eggebø, T. M. (2012). Agreement between two- and three-dimensional transperineal ultrasound methods in assessing fetal head descent in the first stage of labor. *Ultrasound in Obstetrics & Gynecology, 39*(3), 310–315.

Tul, N., Verdenik, I., Trojner-Bregar, A., et al. (2012). Correlates of the trend of cesarean section rates in twin pregnancies. *Journal of Perinatal Medicine, 40*(3), 241–243.

U.S. Department of Health and Human Services. (2010). *Healthy people 2020.* Washington, DC: Author.

Vidarsdottir, H., Geirsson, R. T., Hardardottir, H., et al. (2011). Obstetric and neonatal risks among extremely macrosomic babies and their mothers. *American Journal of Obstetrics & Gynecology, 204*(5), 423.e1–423.e6.

Wei, S., Wo, B. L., Qi, H. P., et al. (2012). Early amniotomy and early oxytocin for prevention of, or therapy for, delay in first stage spontaneous labour compared with routine care. *Cochrane Database of Systematic Reviews,* (9), CD006794.

Werner, E. F., Janevic, T. M., Illuzzi, J., et al. (2011). Mode of delivery in nulliparous women and neonatal intracranial injury. *Obstetrics and Gynecology, 118*(6), 1239–1246.

Wing, D. A., & Farinelli, C. K. (2012). Abnormal labor & induction of labor. In S. G. Gabbe, J. R. Niebyl, J. L. Simpson, et al. (Eds.), *Obstetrics: Normal and problem pregnancies* (6th ed., pp. 99–100). Philadelphia, PA: Elsevier/Saunders.

Zelop, C. (2011). Uterine rupture during a trial of labor after previous cesarean delivery. *Clinics in Perinatology, 38*(2), 277–284.

Zheng, T. (2012). Labor & delivery. In T. Zheng, *Comprehensive handbook of obstetrics and gynecology* (2nd ed., pp. 16–58). Phoenix, AZ: Phoenix Medical Press.

Chapter 24

Nursing Care of a Family During a Surgical Intervention for Birth

KEY TERMS

- amniotomy
- cesarean birth
- classic cesarean incision
- dehiscence
- elective cesarean birth
- episiotomy
- low segment incision
- vaginal birth after cesarean (VBAC)

OBJECTIVES

After mastering the contents of this chapter, you should be able to:

1. Describe the usual indications for surgical interventions such as amniotomy, episiotomy, and cesarean birth.
2. Identify the 2020 National Health Goals related to cesarean birth that nurses can help the nation achieve.
3. Assess a woman scheduled for a surgical intervention for preoperative, intraoperative, and postoperative needs.
4. Formulate nursing diagnoses related to the family experiencing a surgical intervention for birth.
5. Establish outcomes that meet the needs of a woman requiring a surgical intervention for birth as well as help her manage seamless transitions across different health care settings.
6. Using the nursing process, plan nursing care that includes the six competencies of Quality & Safety Education for Nurses (QSEN): Patient-Centered Care, Teamwork & Collaboration, Evidence-Based Practice (EBP), Quality Improvement (QI), Safety, and Informatics.
7. Implement common preoperative and postoperative care for surgical interventions for birth.
8. Evaluate expected outcomes for achievement and effectiveness of care to be certain expected outcomes have been achieved.
9. Integrate knowledge of surgical birth interventions with the interplay of nursing process, the six competencies of QSEN, and Family Nursing to achieve quality maternal and child health nursing care.

Moja Hamma is a 29-year-old woman pregnant with her first baby. Her labor began with ruptured membranes and dark green meconium-stained amniotic fluid. Moja called her nurse-midwife, who instructed her to come to the hospital immediately. Moja drove herself and arrived in 20 minutes. Fetal heart rate (FHR) was 100 beats/min. An obstetrician was consulted, and she scheduled Moja for an immediate cesarean birth. Moja reacted calmly to the news that she needed surgery until she realized her boyfriend would not be able to get to the hospital in time to be with her in surgery. At that point, she refused to sign permission for surgery, saying, "I can't. I just can't go through this alone."

Previous chapters described the physiology of labor and the sequence of usual birth. This chapter adds information about surgical interventions for those women who must have a surgical procedure to ensure a safe outcome for themselves or their child.

Is Moja's response typical of a woman who is told she needs a surgical procedure for the birth of her baby? What would be your best action to help her accept this procedure?

BOX 24.1 Nursing Care Planning Based on 2020 National Health Goals

Two National Health Goals speak directly to cesarean birth:

- Reduce the rate of cesarean births among low-risk (full-term, singleton, vertex presentation) women having their first child to 23.9% of live births from a baseline of 26.5%.
- Reduce the rate of cesarean births among women who have had a prior cesarean birth to 81.7% of live births from a baseline of 90.8% (U.S. Department of Health and Human Services [DHHS], 2010; see www.healthypeople.gov.

Nurses can help the nation achieve these goals by exploring with women who choose elective cesarean birth whether their goals are sound and by encouraging women who fulfill the criteria for vaginal birth after cesarean (VBAC) to attempt a vaginal birth with a second child.

Cesarean birth, or birth accomplished through an abdominal incision into the uterus, is slightly more hazardous than vaginal birth, but compared with other surgical procedures, it is one of the safest types of surgeries and one with few complications (Speichinger & Holschneider, 2013).

The term *cesarean birth*, rather than *cesarean delivery*, is used in nursing literature to accentuate that this is a birth more than it is a surgical procedure. The 2020 National Health Goals related to cesarean birth are shown in Box 24.1.

Nursing Process Overview

For a Woman Having a Surgical Intervention for Birth

Assessment

Some women elect cesarean rather than vaginal birth. Women with smaller than usual pelvic diameters may be informed during pregnancy a cesarean birth will be necessary. Others learn only during labor that a cesarean birth will be necessary because a complication is developing. Surgical interventions such as episiotomy and amniotomy are not usually anticipated before labor. Assessment as to whether a woman will be a good candidate for surgery must include both physiologic and psychological status and the woman's preparedness for the procedure.

Nursing Diagnosis

Nursing diagnoses specific to surgical interventions are often related to the prevention of common complications or patient/family concerns about the procedure. Specific examples might include:

- Fear related to impending surgery
- Pain related to a surgical incision
- Deficient fluid volume related to blood loss from surgery
- Powerlessness related to medical need for episiotomy or cesarean birth
- Risk for anxiety related to unanticipated circumstances surrounding birth
- Risk for infection related to a surgical incision
- Risk for hemorrhage related to surgical procedure
- Risk for impaired parent–infant attachment related to unplanned method of birth

Outcome Identification and Planning

The same important outcome applies to a woman having a cesarean birth as to a woman giving birth vaginally: a healthy mother and a healthy baby. In either instance, decisions for a method of birth can be made so suddenly, planning is limited to only a few minutes. This means you have only a very short time to organize presurgical steps such as gastrointestinal or anesthesia preparation or to check off a presurgical checklist. Be certain plans afterward include discharge or home care instructions because a woman will remain in the health care facility only 2 to 4 days. For a woman who knows in advance she will have a cesarean birth, helpful Web sites to use for referral are the March of Dimes Association (http://www.marchofdimes.com) and the International Cesarean Awareness Network (http://www.ican-online.org).

Implementation

Every woman is aware childbirth poses some risk to health. When major surgery is superimposed on top of this, it is imperative that a woman and her support person feel confidence in the health care personnel who will care for them. When giving care to any woman during labor, be certain to establish early on a helping relationship with both the woman and her support person as this relationship becomes especially advantageous should the birth method need to be altered.

An important intervention includes coordination of health care team members such as an anesthesiologist, surgeon, pediatrician or neonatologist, and recovery room or high-risk nursery personnel.

Many interventions focus on teaching and support, because the more a woman understands what is happening, the more she can accept and cooperate. After surgery, be certain to provide adequate "talk time" to allow a woman time to review what has happened and integrate the experience with what she and her partner expected would happen.

Outcome Evaluation

Evaluation of expected outcomes is important in the care of a woman after a surgical intervention to ensure she is not developing a complication and is developing a positive mother–infant (or parent–infant or family–infant) relationship. Examples that would demonstrate successful achievement of outcomes include:

- Patient states she understands the reason for her cesarean birth.
- Patient states she felt well prepared for cesarean birth even in light of an emergency.
- Couple states they feel able to cope with newborn care even with mother recovering from surgery.
- Patient remains free of signs and symptoms of infection after an episiotomy.
- Patient states her incisional pain is controlled and tolerable.
- Patient states birth was a fulfilling experience even in light of the unplanned cesarean birth.

SURGICAL INTERVENTIONS

Amniotomy

Amniotomy is the artificial rupturing of membranes during labor if they do not rupture spontaneously to allow the fetal head to contact the cervix more directly, which supposedly increases the efficiency of contractions and therefore increases the speed of labor. As there is little evidence amniotomy actually achieves these goals, the procedure is now only rarely used (Smyth, Alldred, & Markham, 2011). If the procedure is scheduled, a woman is asked to assume a dorsal recumbent position; an amniohook (a long, thin crochet-like instrument) or a hemostat is passed vaginally. The membranes are torn, and amniotic fluid is allowed to escape. A disadvantage of amniotomy is it puts a fetus momentarily at risk for cord prolapse if a loop of cord escapes into the vagina with the fluid. Always measure the FHR immediately after the rupture of membranes to determine this did not happen (Paterson-Brown, 2012).

QSEN Checkpoint Question 24.1

Safety

Suppose Moja had an amniotomy during her labor. Immediately after this procedure, which would be the most important nursing assessment for you to make?

a. Ask her to rate her pain level after the procedure.
b. Assess maternal heart rate to detect possible bleeding.
c. Assess FHR to detect possible cord prolapse.
d. Document the amount of amniotic fluid that has been lost.

Look in Appendix A for the best answer and rationale.

Episiotomy

An **episiotomy** is a surgical incision of the perineum made to prevent tearing of the perineum, release pressure on the fetal head with birth, and possibly shorten the last portion of the second stage of labor (da Silva, de Oliveira, Bick, et al., 2012).

An episiotomy incision is made with blunt-tipped scissors in the midline of the perineum (i.e., a midline episiotomy) or is begun in the midline but directed laterally away from the rectum (i.e., a mediolateral episiotomy) (Fig. 24.1). Mediolateral incisions have the advantage over midline cuts in that, if tearing occurs beyond the incision, the tear will not be directed toward the rectum, thus creating less danger of a rectal mucosal tear, which can result in loss of sphincter function and fecal incontinence later in life (Valsky, Cohen, Lipschuetz, et al., 2012). Midline episiotomies, however, heal more easily, cause less blood loss, and result in less postpartal discomfort. The pressure of the fetal head against the perineum as a woman pushes just prior to birth is so intense the nerve endings in the perineum are momentarily deadened, allowing an episiotomy to be done without anesthesia. There is a slight loss of blood, but the pressure of the presenting part immediately seals the cut edges and minimizes bleeding. Episiotomies are sutured after birth.

Theoretically, if this is done immediately, a woman will still have so much natural-pressure anesthesia of the perineum that she will not require an anesthetic for the repair. In actuality, by the time the placenta is delivered (approximately 5 minutes), enough sensation has returned to the perineum that most women need an injection of a local anesthetic for comfort. Women who received epidural anesthesia will probably not need additional medication.

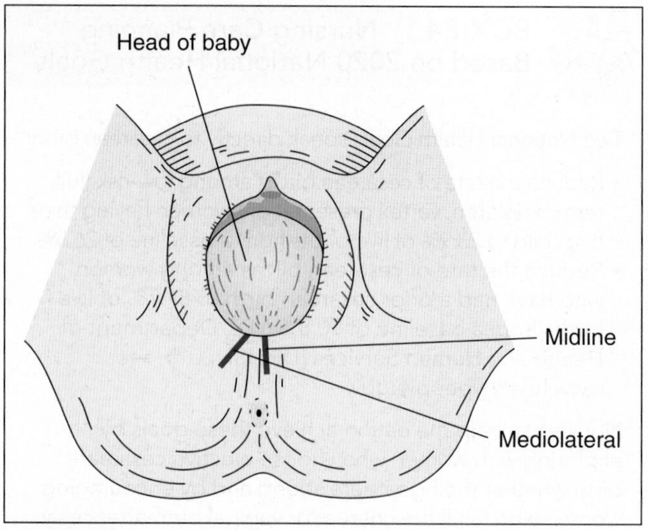

FIGURE 24.1 An episiotomy incision.

One instance in which episiotomy (defibulation) may be necessary is in women who have had female circumcision with perineal scarring because their perineum is unable to stretch to allow the vaginal outlet to open for birth (Rouzi, Al-Sibiani, Al-Mansouri, et al., 2012).

Procedures for High-Risk Pregnancies

If a woman or fetus is found to be high risk during labor, a number of procedures over and above a usual assessment can become necessary. All these procedures cause increased anxiety for the woman and her family and so need special instructions and supportive reassurance.

Internal Electronic Monitoring

Internal electronic monitoring is the most precise method for assessing FHR and uterine contractions. This can be done by wireless telemetry but is usually managed by a pressure-sensing catheter passed through the vagina after the membranes have ruptured and the cervix has dilated to at least 3 cm. It is then passed into the uterine cavity and alongside the fetus (Fig. 24.2). The end of the catheter extending from the vagina is attached to a pressure recorder. As each uterine contraction puts pressure on the uterine contents, the pressure exerted on the catheter is recorded. When contractions are monitored by an internal pressure gauge in this way, the frequency, duration, baseline strength, and peak strength of contractions can all be evaluated. Contraction strength is evaluated by the height of the peak of the contraction on the tracing. Equally important to evaluate is the return of the uterine tone to baseline strength between contractions. This ensures there is placental filling between contractions.

With contractions during the latent phase of labor, the baseline level is usually less than 5 mmHg; with active contractions, it is about 12 mmHg. During the second stage of labor, the baseline may be as high as 20 mmHg. Baseline readings that do not return to 20 mmHg or less following a contraction suggest uterine hypertonia and a possible compromise of fetal well-being.

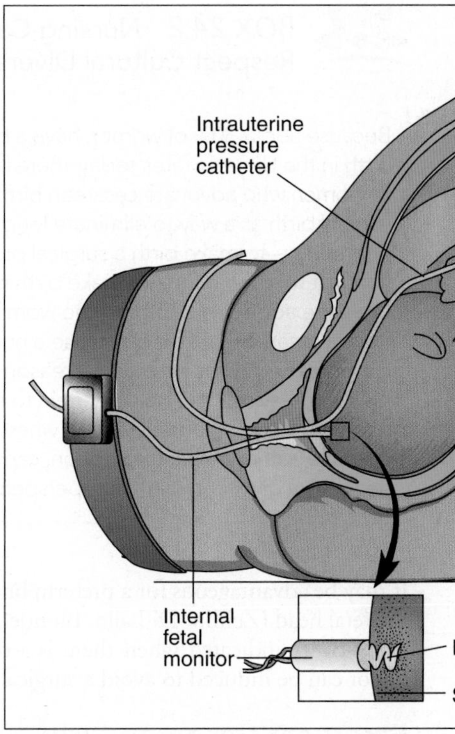

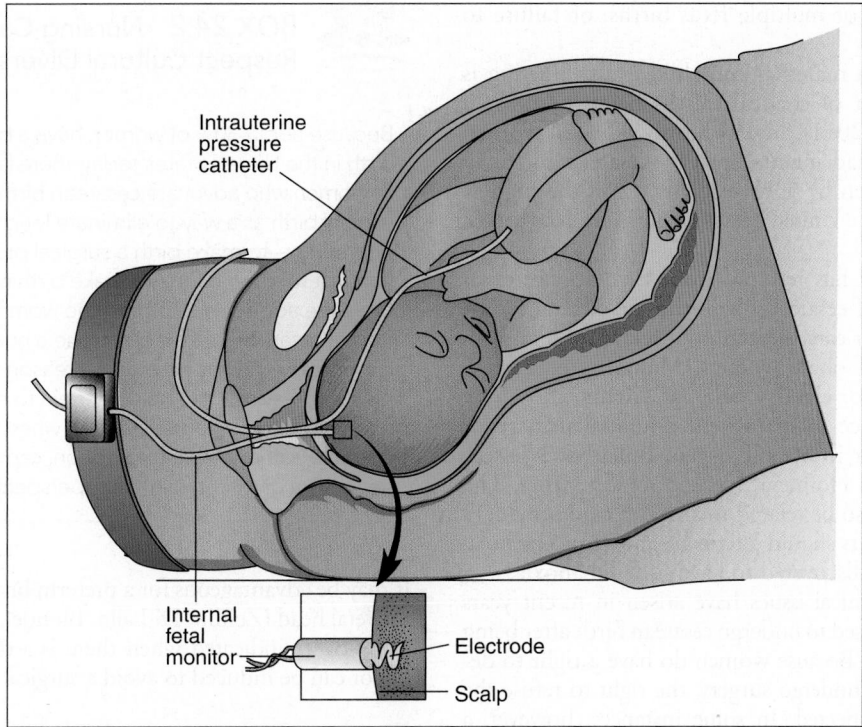

FIGURE 24.2 Internal fetal monitoring.

The FHR recording is obtained from a fetal scalp electrode. Once the fetal head is engaged, the electrode is inserted vaginally and attached to the fetal scalp with a small puncture of the skin. A fetal electrocardiograph signal is obtained, amplified, and then fed into a cardiotachometer. The output from the cardiotachometer is recorded on permanent graph paper.

Although internal monitoring produces clear details of fetal heartbeats, it is invasive, carries the risk of uterine infection, and limits a woman's movement. It is, therefore, reserved for women whose fetus is at high risk during labor.

Scalp Stimulation

Although not well studied, if a fetus shows an unresponsive heartbeat during labor, vibroacoustic stimulation can be used the same as is done for nonstress tests during pregnancy to be certain a fetus is responding well to labor (Tan & Smyth, 2010). If FHR variability appears to be depressed during labor, the welfare of a fetus can be assessed by scalp stimulation. This is done by applying pressure with the fingers to the fetal scalp through the dilated cervix (Fig. 24.3). This causes a tactile response in the fetus that momentarily increases the FHR. If the fetus is in distress and becoming acidotic, FHR acceleration will not occur. Scalp stimulation, therefore, is an assessment of acid–base balance in a fetus in labor.

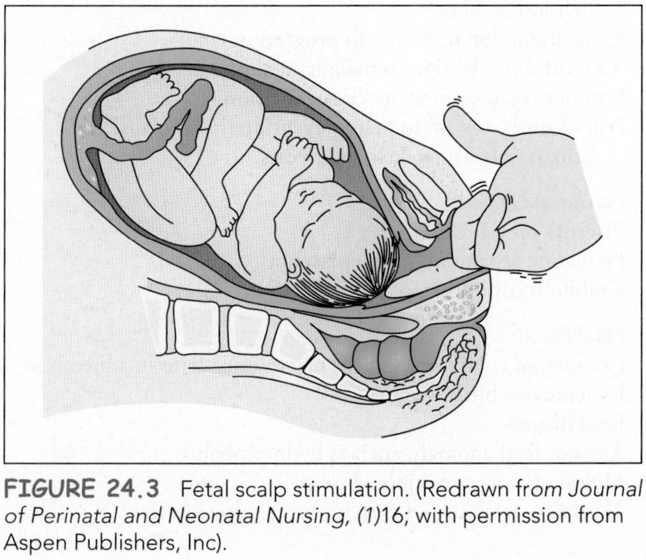

FIGURE 24.3 Fetal scalp stimulation. (Redrawn from *Journal of Perinatal and Neonatal Nursing, (1)16*; with permission from Aspen Publishers, Inc).

Fetal Oxygen Saturation Level

Fetal oxygen saturation may be measured by an oxygen saturation sensor introduced into the uterus and placed beside the fetus's cheek after membranes have ruptured. Because the procedure creates a small chance of uterine infection, this is generally reserved for women who already have an internal contraction or fetal monitor in place.

Fetal Blood Sampling

Monitoring of the fetal blood composition, obtained from the fetal scalp following cervical dilatation during labor, can reveal hypoxia in a fetus before this becomes apparent on an electrocardiogram or external monitoring system (Heazell, Riches, Hopkins, et al., 2011). A small laceration will be present on the newborn scalp from this, which needs to be observed for bleeding or signs of infection following birth.

CESAREAN BIRTH

Although cesarean birth may be elected by some women, the procedure is used most often as a prophylactic measure to alleviate problems of birth such as cephalopelvic disproportion, breech or multiple fetus births, or failure to progress in labor.

A major concern in maternal and child health nursing is the increasing number of cesarean births being performed annually (Blanchette, 2011). In 1970, only 5.5% of women in the United States had infants born by cesarean birth. In 2010, the rate had risen by 53% reaching 32%, the highest rate ever reported in the United States (Hamilton, Martin, & Ventura, 2011).

This increased rate has resulted from a combination of the increasing safety of cesarean birth, the use of fetal monitors (which provide for early detection of fetal problems), an increased incidence of obese women (Mantakas & Farrell, 2010), and scheduled or **elective cesarean births**, chosen by women for convenience or to prevent potential urinary or anal incontinence later in life (Gyhagen, Bullarbo, Nielsen, et al., 2012; Lavender, Hofmeyr, Neilson, et al., 2012). The increase in rate may also be related to a health care provider's fears of malpractice suits should a fetus be allowed to be born vaginally and then be discovered to have suffered anoxia.

Several legal and ethical issues have arisen in recent years when women have refused to undergo cesarean birth after being advised they need one. Because women do have a right to decide whether they will undergo surgery, the right to refuse the procedure must be respected. In some instances, however, a court order for the procedure has been obtained to save a fetus. Be certain you are aware of the opinion of your agency's ethics committee on this issue.

As a rule, nurse-midwifery or interprofessional birthing services have a lower incidence of cesarean births than hospital services because of the higher incidence of low-risk women in these settings (Liva, Hall, Klein, et al., 2012). Continuous support during labor by a concerned health care provider (such as a nurse) appears to decrease the incidence (Hodnett, Gates, Hofmeyr, et al., 2012).

Scheduled Cesarean Birth

Scheduled cesarean births are planned, which means there is time for thorough preparation for the experience throughout the antepartal period. Some women are even able to take a childbirth preparation class specifically for cesarean birth. Women who plan these need to be aware they will need epidural anesthesia, and the risk of injury to them from cesarean birth is higher than that from vaginal birth. Scheduling cesarean births this freely also can result in preterm birth with the accompanying threats to the fetus or newborn (Box 24.2).

In the past, many cesarean births were performed because the woman had undergone a cesarean birth with a previous child; with new surgical techniques, particularly the use of a low cervical incision, "once a cesarean, always a cesarean" no longer applies. The majority of women who have had a cesarean birth within the past 10 years are eligible to give birth vaginally in subsequent pregnancies if the circumstances are appropriate for vaginal birth (Eden, Denman, Emeis, et al., 2012).

Yet other reasons for scheduled cesarean births are when there is a physical indication such as transverse presentation, an infection that could be contacted by the fetus if born vaginally, or cephalopelvic disproportion (Box 24.3). For instance, cesarean birth reduces the transfer of the herpes type 2 from mother to newborn, so it is recommended for women who have this infection (Tita, 2012). It also can reduce mortality among infants presenting breech (Cunningham, Leveno, Bloom, et al., 2010).

BOX 24.2 Nursing Care Planning to Respect Cultural Diversity

Because about 30% of women have a baby by cesarean birth in the United States today, there is an emerging culture of women who advocate cesarean birth as superior to vaginal birth as a way to eliminate long hours of labor pain. This effect—to make birth a surgical procedure—is in sharp contrast to other efforts to make birth more natural. Because there are added risks to both the woman and her fetus from a cesarean birth, it can cause a nursing care problem if a woman who has no medical reason for a cesarean birth insists on having one. Being certain to explain that a cesarean birth is a method to be used when vaginal birth is not possible, rather than a true option, can help a woman put her choice of type of birth into perspective.

It may be advantageous for a preterm birth to avoid pressure on the fetal head (Zeitlin, Di Lallo, Blondel, et al., 2010). It is generally contraindicated when there is a documented dead fetus (labor can be induced to avoid a surgical procedure).

Emergent Cesarean Birth

Emergent cesarean births are done for reasons that arise suddenly in labor, such as placenta previa, premature separation of the placenta, fetal distress, or failure to progress. With this second type of cesarean birth, preparation must be done rapidly but with the same concern for fully informing a woman and her support person about what circumstances created the

BOX 24.3 Selected Indications for Cesarean Birth

Maternal Factors

Active genital herpes or (perhaps) human papillomavirus
AIDS or (perhaps) HIV-positive status
Cephalopelvic disproportion
Cervical cerclage
Disabling conditions, such as severe gestational hypertension, that would prevent pushing to accomplish the pelvic division of labor
Failed induction or failure to progress in labor
An obstructive benign or malignant tumor
Previous cesarean birth by classic incision
Fear of birth or wish to help prevent uterine prolapse or urinary incontinence in later years

Placental Factors

Placenta previa
Premature separation of the placenta
Umbilical cord prolapse

Fetal Factors

Compound conditions such as macrosomic fetus in a breech lie
Extreme low birth weight
Fetal distress
A major fetal anomaly, such as hydrocephalus
Multigestation or conjoined twins
Transverse fetal lie and perhaps breech presentation

need for the cesarean birth and how the birth will proceed. Cesarean birth is mentioned in most childbirth classes, so any woman who has taken such a class may at least understand that cesarean births are sometimes necessary.

An emergent cesarean birth carries with it the same risks of any emergent surgery: the woman may not be a prime candidate for anesthesia and may be psychologically unprepared for the experience. In addition, the woman may have a fluid and electrolyte imbalance and be both physically and emotionally exhausted from a long labor.

EFFECTS OF SURGERY ON A WOMAN

Like any surgical procedure, cesarean birth has systemic effects.

Stress Response

Whenever the body is subjected to stress, either physical or psychosocial, it responds with measures to preserve the function of major body systems. This results in a release of epinephrine and norepinephrine from the adrenal medulla. Epinephrine increases the heart rate, causes bronchial dilatation, and elevates the blood glucose level. It also leads to peripheral vasoconstriction, which forces blood to the central circulation and increases blood pressure. In the pregnant woman, such responses may minimize blood supply to the lower extremities. Pregnant women are already prone to thrombophlebitis from stasis of blood flow, so these responses compound or greatly increase thrombophlebitis risk.

Interference With Body Defenses

The skin serves as the primary line of defense against bacterial invasion, so when skin is incised for a surgical procedure, this important line of defense is lost. Strict adherence to aseptic techniques during surgery and in the days following the procedure are necessary to compensate for this impaired defense. If the cesarean birth is performed hours after the membranes rupture, a woman's risk for infection will be higher than if the membranes were still intact. Many women receive prophylactic antibiotics, such as ampicillin (Omnipen) or a cephalosporin, such as Ancef, to ensure protection against postsurgical endometritis, even if the membranes remained intact (Alfirevic, Gyte, & Dou, 2010).

Interference With Circulatory Function

Although vessels that must be cut for surgery are immediately clamped and ligated, some blood loss occurs with surgery. Compared to other surgeries, the amount of blood lost in a cesarean birth is comparatively high, caused by the fact abdominal and pelvic vessels are congested with blood waiting to supply the placenta. During a vaginal birth, a woman loses 300 to 500 ml of blood. This loss increases to 500 to 1,000 ml with a cesarean birth (Arulkumaran, 2011).

Interference With Body Organ Function

When any body organ is handled, cut, or repaired in surgery, it may respond with a temporary disruption in function. Therefore, close postoperative assessment, not only of the primary organ involved but also of total body function, is necessary to determine the total degree of disruption present.

Because the uterus is handled during cesarean birth, it may not contract well afterward, which can lead to postpartum hemorrhage. For a health care provider to reach the uterus, the bladder must be displaced anteriorly. As a result of this handling, the bladder may not sense filling as well as usual after the procedure (Gungorduk, Asicioglu, Celikkol, et al., 2010). During surgery, pressure is also felt by the intestine, so a paralytic ileus or halting of intestinal function with obstruction may occur (Harma, Harma, Karadeniz, et al., 2011). As mentioned previously, thrombophlebitis from impaired lower extremity blood flow is yet another possibility. After a cesarean birth, therefore, uterine, bladder, intestinal, and lower extremity circulatory function must all be carefully assessed.

Interference With Self-Image or Self-Esteem

Surgery always leaves an incisional scar that is noticeable to some extent afterward, and its appearance may cause a woman to feel self-conscious. Although most women accept cesarean birth well, a woman who was intent on having a vaginal birth may feel a loss of self-esteem and depression if she believes the procedure marks her as a woman less capable than others because she was unable to give vaginal birth (Barbadoro, Cotichelli, Chiatti, et al., 2012).

NURSING CARE FOR A WOMAN ANTICIPATING A CESAREAN BIRTH

A woman who is admitted to the hospital for an anticipated cesarean birth may be more worried about the procedure (because she has had more time to worry) than a woman who is told during labor an emergent cesarean is necessary. After the woman is admitted, allow her time to talk about any fears she has. Encourage her to do as much as possible for herself preoperatively to help her feel in control and to diminish her fear (Wang, Zhou, Coulter, et al., 2010).

Be aware that it is difficult for a woman undergoing surgery to relax as long as her support person remains nervous and worried. Make a point of including this person in all explanations and admission routines to keep his or her anxiety under control as well.

What if . . . 24.1 After learning that Moja wanted to wait for her cesarean birth to begin until her boyfriend arrives, you learn the boyfriend has telephoned to say he cannot possibly stay with Moja in the operating room; he'll feel so nauseated he'll probably faint. Would it be best to plan on supporting Moja yourself or to try to involve the boyfriend?

Preoperative Interview

Both a woman's primary care provider and the team member who will be administering the anesthesia interview a woman preoperatively to obtain a health history and to make assessments and decisions for safety of the procedure and the use of anesthesia. In addition to these, a nursing assessment is also essential. Be certain to ask about any past surgeries, secondary illnesses, allergies to foods or drugs, reactions to anesthesia, bleeding problems, or current medications to help establish surgical risk, and any body piercings that need to be removed because of the use of electrosurgery or an arterial cauterizing machine. In addition, include questions to discover the woman's knowledge about:

- What the procedure will entail
- Length of hospitalization anticipated
- If she's been told about any postsurgical equipment to be used, such as an indwelling catheter or intravenous (IV) fluid line
- Any special precautions that are being planned for her infant such as high-risk nursery care

Operative Risk for a Woman

Women who are in less than optimal physical or psychological health are at risk for a complicated surgical outcome unless the risk factor is identified and special precautions are taken.

Poor Nutritional Status

A woman who is obese because of poor nutrition is at added risk from surgery because tissue that contains an abundance of fatty cells is difficult to suture, thus causing the surgical incision to take longer to heal. A prolonged healing period increases the risk for infection and rupture of the incision (**dehiscence**) (Gilead, Salem, Sergienko, et al., 2012).

Because an obese woman's heart has an increased workload, the physiologic shock of surgery may place greater stress on the already overworked organ. In addition, an obese woman often has more difficulty turning and ambulating postoperatively than does a woman with a lower body mass index (BMI) and therefore has an increased risk for developing respiratory or circulatory complications such as pneumonia or thrombophlebitis (Marshall, Guild, Cheng, et al., 2012).

A woman with a protein or vitamin deficiency is also at risk for poorer healing because protein and vitamins C and D are necessary for new cell formation at the incision site. Vitamin K is necessary to ensure blood clotting after surgery. Pregnant women who are iron deficient (in particular, women with a multiple gestation or women who have not taken supplements), coupled with the blood loss from surgery, are at high risk for extreme fatigue after surgery, which could interfere with parent–child bonding (Milman, 2012).

Age Variations

Age affects surgical risk because it can cause both decreased circulatory and renal function. Fortunately, most pregnant women fall within the young adult age group, so are excellent candidates for surgery. A woman older than 40 years falls into a category of slightly higher risk, not because of surgery itself, but because of associated conditions such gestational diabetes (Berggren, Mele, Landon, et al., 2012).

Altered General Health

A woman who has a secondary illness such as cardiac disease, diabetes mellitus, anemia, kidney, or liver disease is at greater than usual surgical risk, depending on the extent of her primary disease, because the pathology from the secondary illness may interfere with her ability to physically adjust to the demands of surgery.

Therefore, asking if the woman has a secondary illness is an essential component of a preoperative nursing history.

A general medication history also is important, because some drugs increase surgical risk by interfering with the effect of an anesthetic or with healing of tissue. Examples of drugs that pregnant women might be taking and their potential complications are shown in Box 24.4.

Fluid and Electrolyte Imbalance

A woman who enters surgery with a lower than usual blood volume will experience the effect of surgical blood loss more than a woman who has a normal blood volume. A woman who has had a long labor before a cesarean birth is scheduled may fall into this category, because she may have had little to eat or drink for almost 24 hours. Recent vomiting, diarrhea, or a chronic poor fluid intake compound her risk. IV fluid replacement may need to be initiated preoperatively and continued postoperatively to prevent a serious fluid or electrolyte imbalance.

Fear

Women who are extremely worried about surgery need a very detailed explanation of the procedure in order to reduce their anxiety to a tolerable level. If a woman seems particularly anxious, inform the team member who will administer the

BOX 24.4 Nursing Care Planning Based on Responsibility for Pharmacology

DRUGS THAT MAY RESULT IN COMPLICATIONS OF CESAREAN BIRTH

Type of Drug	Action
Antibiotics	Specific antibiotics may predispose one to renal insufficiency or increase neuromuscular blockage; can lead to opportunistic infections
Anticoagulants	May cause hemorrhage due to lack of hemostasis during surgery
Anticonvulsants	May increase liver action and metabolism of anesthetic agent
Antihypertensives	May result in hypotension after anesthesia
Corticosteroids	May block body's response to shock and so lead to lack of adrenal function
Insulin	May lead to hypoglycemia during labor or hyperglycemia if a dextrose solution is administered
Antianxiety agents	May cause hypotension after anesthesia

anesthesia so that an antianxiety drug can be administered, if necessary, to make the experience less frightening for her.

In many instances, just helping a woman acknowledge that her fear of surgery is a normal reaction can be helpful. This does not make the procedure any less traumatic, but the woman may then view her feelings as expected, which can help to enhance her self-esteem and lower anxiety (Adams, Eberhard-Gran, & Eskild, 2012).

Operative Risk to the Newborn

Cesarean birth places a newborn at a greater risk than does a vaginal birth. When a fetus is pushed through the birth canal, pressure on the chest helps rid the newborn's lungs of fluid, making it easier for the baby to take a first breath. For this reason, more infants born by cesarean birth develop some degree of respiratory difficulty for a day or two after birth than those born vaginally (Abenhaim & Benjamin, 2011; Patel & Jain, 2010). See Chapter 26 for a discussion of this condition, which is often referred to as transient tachypnea of the newborn.

Preoperative Diagnostic Procedures

Preoperative assessment procedures for a woman who is to have a cesarean birth include documentation of fetal status, and presentation and maturity by ultrasound assessment. In addition, assessments also include circulatory and renal function and those for all presurgery patients, including:

- Vital sign determination
- Urinalysis
- Complete blood count
- Coagulation profile (prothrombin time [PT], partial thromboplastin time [PTT])
- Serum electrolytes and pH
- Blood typing and cross-matching

Remember blood values need to be evaluated in light of the changes that occur with pregnancy. During pregnancy, for example, a woman (particularly one who was in prolonged labor) can have an elevated leukocyte count (up to 20,000 cells/mm^3), so this finding is not as helpful an indicator for the presence of infection in the pregnant woman as it is in others.

Preoperative Teaching

Preoperative teaching is aimed at acquainting a woman with the cesarean procedure and any special equipment to be used so she is as informed as possible.

Before beginning teaching, assess how much a woman knows about her surgery. A woman who has had a cesarean birth for her first child and now is being admitted for a second procedure, for example, already knows many details. Even so, she will undoubtedly appreciate having her memory refreshed and recall confirmed. Answer all specific questions she has and fill in gaps in knowledge as necessary. Be certain all information you offer is accurate. Be certain not to use hospital jargon such as "NPO." People under stress do not process new information well. They cannot process information at all if they do not understand the terminology.

Be certain to explain the immediate preoperative measures that will be necessary, such as surgical skin preparation, eating nothing before the time of surgery, premedication (if this will be used), and method of transport to surgery. Review the necessity for an indwelling bladder catheter, IV fluid administration, and placement of an epidural catheter (if this will be used for postprocedure pain relief).

For scheduled cesarean births, an explanation of not only what is going to happen immediately but also what activities should be performed to help maintain respiratory and skeletal muscle function and to prevent postsurgical complications (e.g., early ambulation) should also be included in teaching. Women who practice exercises to maintain good respiratory and circulatory function postoperatively tend to experience fewer postoperative respiratory and circulatory complications than those who do not. These preventive exercises are best taught during the preoperative period, when the woman is free of pain and can concentrate on learning. Such teaching also gives a woman a positive outlook on surgery and a sense of control over her situation.

Throughout teaching, use visual aids as necessary. Draw pictures or show illustrations of anatomy, as needed. Be careful, however, not to leave textbooks about cesarean procedure techniques with a woman. Typically, these books also describe complications, and, although knowledge of possible complications is necessary for informed consent, reading about complications complete with color illustrations can be overwhelming.

Deep Breathing

Periodic deep breathing exercises fully aerate the lungs and help prevent stasis of lung mucus from the prolonged time spent in the supine position during surgery. Because stasis always has the potential to cause infection, preventing this helps prevent lung infection such as pneumonia.

A typical exercise is to take 5 to 10 deep breaths every hour. The woman simply inhales as deeply as possible, holds her breath for a second or two, and then exhales as deeply as possible. Be certain she both inhales and exhales fully. Otherwise, she might experience light-headedness from hyperventilation.

Incentive Spirometry

A common device used three to four times a day postoperatively to encourage deep breathing is an incentive spirometer. These devices, which cause a small Ping–Pong-like ball to rise in a narrow tube or cause lights to flash, are both easy and fun to operate and give a woman a sense of reward for her effort. The initial impression of most people is that the device works by blowing into it. Because its purpose is to fully aerate lung spaces, however, most models are triggered by *inhalation*, not exhalation. A gauge can be set to monitor levels and tabs to set goals.

Turning

Be certain women understand that turning postoperatively is important to prevent both respiratory and circulatory stasis.

Ambulation

The most effective way to stimulate lower extremity circulation after a cesarean birth is by early ambulation. For this reason, most primary health care providers prefer a woman to be out of bed and walking as soon as the effect of the epidural anesthesia has worn off. Helping a woman ambulate this early can be difficult because she is both fatigued and has pain from her incision. Help her to understand ambulation is extremely important after cesarean birth because the edema from the low pelvic surgery compresses circulation to the lower extremities, thus increasing the risk for lower extremity circulatory stasis. Some women may be prescribed sequential compression devices (SCDs) or antiembolic stockings (TEDS) to support and encourage venous return in addition to ambulation.

Immediate Preoperative Care Measures

A number of measures must be taken immediately before surgery to help ensure a safe outcome.

Informed Consent

Obtaining operative consent is the primary health care provider's responsibility, but being certain it is obtained prior to surgery is everyone's responsibility. You may be asked to witness a woman's signature on such a form. Before signing as a witness, be certain that it was *informed* consent, or one in which the risks and benefits of the procedure were explained in terms the woman could easily understand.

The law differs from state to state with regard to who qualifies to be considered an emancipated or mature minor. Emancipated minors can sign their own permission for a cesarean birth, even though they are legally underage.

Overall Hygiene

On admission, provide a clean hospital gown. If a woman's hair is long, encourage her to braid it or put it into a ponytail so it will more easily fit under the surgical cap she will wear; hair contained by a cap is less likely to spread microorganisms during surgery. Follow your institution's procedures with regard to removing nail polish, jewelry, contact lenses, lip or mouth piercings, or hair ornaments before surgery. A growing number of women wear acrylic fingernails and are reluctant to remove them for surgery. If this is the case, ensure that the woman's toenails are free of polish so that toenails can be used to assess capillary refill if this assessment is needed.

What if...24.2 Moja, who will have epidural anesthesia for her cesarean birth, refuses to remove her contact lenses for surgery even though it is hospital policy for anyone receiving anesthesia to do so. She tells you, "I won't be able to see my baby afterward without them." Would you insist she take them out or ask your anesthesia team member if she could be an exception to a rule?

Gastrointestinal Tract Preparation

A gastric emptying agent, such as metoclopramide (Reglan), to speed stomach emptying or a histamine blocker, such as ranitidine (Zantac), to decrease stomach secretions may be prescribed prior to surgery. Yet another possibility is an oral antacid such as citric acid and sodium citrate (Bicitra), which acts to neutralize acid stomach secretions. These precautions are necessary because the woman will be lying on her back during the procedure, making esophageal reflux and aspiration highly possible.

Baseline Intake and Output Determinations

To reduce bladder size and keep the bladder away from the surgical field, an indwelling urinary catheter may be prescribed before transport for surgery or after arrival in the surgical suite. Use good lighting so that the woman's perineum is clearly revealed. After catheter insertion, be certain urine drains freely, because fetal pressure on the urethra may considerably reduce the flow of urine. During transport, be certain to keep the drainage bag below the level of the woman's bladder to prevent urine backflow and the possible introduction of microorganisms into the bladder.

If catheterization is difficult before surgery, do not traumatize the urethra by repeated attempts as catheterization can be done in the operating room (OR) after the anesthetic agent is given. If there will be a delay between the time the catheter is inserted and the time of surgery, mark the level of drainage in the bag just before surgery or empty it, so that presurgery urine output can be differentiated from postsurgery urine output. This is because one of the gravest dangers of any surgical procedure is kidney failure from the physiologic stress of surgery or lack of blood flow to the kidneys due to decreased blood pressure. All reproductive tract surgery puts ureter flow at risk as well because the edema that collects in the surgery area can press on the ureters.

Hydration

Most women have an IV fluid line begun before surgery with a fluid such as lactated Ringer's solution. Doing so helps to ensure a woman will be fully hydrated and will not experience hypotension from epidural anesthesia administration, temporary use of a supine position, or blood loss at birth. Be certain this line is begun in the woman's nondominant hand if possible so she can hold her newborn after surgery without interference. Use a large-size catheter or needle (18 or 20 gauge), so that blood replacement therapy can be administered by the same line if needed.

QSEN Checkpoint Question 24.2

Teamwork & Collaboration

You are giving a report to an OR nurse prior to a cesarean birth and describing actions you took to reduce the size of the patient's bladder and keep it away from the surgical field during the procedure. Which action should you describe to your colleague?

a. Inserting a Foley catheter to drain the bladder and decrease its size
b. Administering an oxytocic drug to cause the bladder to forcefully contract
c. Restricting the woman's fluids for at least 16 hours before surgery
d. Administering the woman a diuretic to reduce bladder volume

Look in Appendix A for the best answer and rationale.

Preoperative Medication

A minimum of preoperative medication is used with a woman having a cesarean birth to prevent compromising the fetal blood supply and to ensure that the newborn is wide awake at birth and can initiate respirations spontaneously. Be aware if a woman has been in labor, what medications, if any, she has already received to help prevent a drug interaction.

Patient Chart and Presurgery Checklist

Documentation of nursing care up until the time a woman leaves the nursing care unit or labor room must be completed before a woman leaves for the surgical suite. Many hospitals

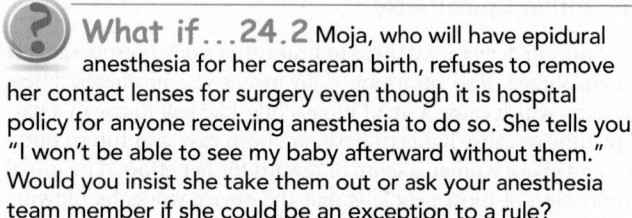

	Completed
Patient concerns	
Skin preparation	______
Identification in place	______
Temperature, pulse, respiration ______	______
Blood pressure ______	______
Height ______ Weight ______	______
Voided ______ Time ______ Amount ______	______
NPO after ______	______
Hospital gown	______
Hairpins removed	______
Nail polish removed	______
Jewelry removed	______
Preoperative medication ______	______
Dentures removed ______ In place ______	______
Contact lenses removed ______	______
Prosthetic devices removed ______	______
Abdominal piercing removed ______	______
Chart concerns	
Addressograph plate attached	______
Operative permit obtained	______
Urinalysis	______
Hematocrit or CBC	______
Blood order of ______	______
Signature ______ R.N.	

FIGURE 24.4 A preoperative checklist for cesarean birth. Checklists vary from hospital to hospital.

use an electronic preoperative checklist, such as that shown in Figure 24.4, as a reminder of all necessary measures to be taken. Checking and signing such a form indicates that the specific measures were completed.

Transport to Surgery

A woman may be transferred to surgery in her bed, or she may be helped to move to a stretcher. Urge her to lie on her left side during transport to prevent supine hypotension syndrome. Ensure additional safety by raising the side rails. Cover her with a blanket or sheet to avoid her feeling chilled. Check that her identification is secure before she leaves the patient unit. Make certain, even though steps are being completed rapidly, that her chart or electronic record remains secure and will be available to OR personnel.

QSEN Checkpoint Question 24.3

Patient-Centered Care

Moja Hamma needs to have an IV infusion started prior to her cesarean procedure. Which would be the best course of action?

a. Introduce the cannula into the back of either hand.
b. Begin the IV infusion in the hand nearest to you.
c. Ask Moja which hand she would prefer you to use.
d. Explain that IVs are typically started in the right hand.

Look in Appendix A for the best answer and rationale.

Role of the Support Person

In most instances, a woman's family can be as involved in a cesarean birth as they would be for a vaginal birth. A support person may need more encouragement to watch a cesarean than a vaginal birth because he or she may believe the surgery will be much bloodier than it actually is. Helping family members realize cesarean birth is little different from vaginal birth not only allows them to stay with a woman during the procedure but also helps them progress to bonding with the infant and incorporating the new member into their family more easily.

NURSING CARE FOR A WOMAN HAVING AN EMERGENT CESAREAN BIRTH

Many women who will have a cesarean birth have no warning during pregnancy that a cesarean birth will be necessary. Suddenly, during labor, they develop a complication such as prolapsed cord or fetal distress, and surgery becomes necessary.

A woman who has severe pain with labor and is told an emergent procedure is necessary actually may be relieved surgery has been suggested, because the surgery will alleviate the pain. In contrast, another woman might feel great disappointment when told her baby must be born by cesarean birth. In many women, both emotions intertwine.

Surgical risk in an emergent situation is determined from the baseline history and physical examination information previously obtained at the beginning of labor. Preoperative preparation measures such as vital signs, urinalysis, and blood work have also already been obtained. An immediate preparation, therefore, involves gaining an informed consent, application of SCDs or elastic stockings (if appropriate), preparing the gastrointestinal tract, adding bladder catheterization, and establishing an IV line. Because, ideally, a cesarean birth should be completed within 30 minutes from the time the procedure was documented to be necessary, teaching about postoperative measures needs to be delayed until after surgery (Lipman, Carvalho, Cohen, et al., 2013).

Available time before the surgery must be spent explaining the immediate procedures to the woman such as transfer, abdominal preparation, and anesthesia. Document carefully what was taught, so that the nurse caring for the woman postoperatively will be aware of the need for additional teaching. At birth, at least one person whose sole responsibility is neonatal resuscitation needs to be present to care for the baby. Approximately 10% of babies born by cesarean birth need assistance to begin breathing at birth; about 1% of babies need extensive resuscitation to survive (Gilbert, 2011).

✔ QSEN Checkpoint Question 24.4

Informatics

You notice that your colleague who was helping to prepare Moja has left her room to liaise with the OR in anticipation of her cesarean birth. You also notice that your colleague left Moja's electronic health record open and in view of her support people. Which of the following would be the best course of action?

a. Immediately close the record even though all care may not yet be recorded.
b. Locate the nurse and ask her to come back so she can close the record.
c. Minimize the record and wait for the nurse to come back and close it.
d. Report the nurse to the nurse manager for violating confidentiality.

Look in Appendix A for the best answer and rationale.

INTRAOPERATIVE CARE MEASURES

Cesarean birth is most similar to vaginal birth if the woman is awake during the surgery; therefore, after discussion with a woman, the anesthesia of choice is usually a regional block, such as epidural anesthesia (Box 24.5).

Administration of Anesthesia

A surgical nurse will assist a woman to move from the transport stretcher or bed to the OR table and will remain with her while anesthesia is administered. If the woman has an epidural catheter in place from labor, be careful not to dislodge it while she is being moved. During transport and while in surgery, encourage the woman to remain on her side, or place a pillow under her right hip to keep her body slightly tilted to the side, to prevent supine hypotension syndrome. If a spinal anesthetic (which may be used in an emergency) is to be administered, the anesthesiologist usually will do this with the woman sitting up. The anesthesiologist may then ask you to help the woman curve her back to separate the vertebrae and facilitate entry of the spinal needle. Remember, though, that it is difficult for a woman having uterine contractions to remain in this position for long. Talking to her while letting her lean against you is the most effective means of helping her maintain this position. Epidural anesthesia is usually administered with the woman lying on her side. Duramorph is a form of morphine commonly used in addition to a local anesthesia in epidurals. Its effect lasts up to 24 hours, but because it can cause late occurring respiratory depression, respirations should be assessed every 2 hours postsurgery. Continuous pulse oximetry must be used for 24 hours (Mancuso, De Vivo, Giacobbe, et al., 2010).

BOX 24.5 Nursing Care Planning Based on Effective Communication

Moja Hamma has been told she will need a cesarean birth because of fetal distress that has led to meconium staining.

Less Effective Communication

Nurse: Moja, can I answer any questions for you?
Moja: I want something to put me to sleep so I won't know what's happening.
Nurse: Most women want an epidural.
Moja: I have to be so sound asleep I won't know what's happening.
Nurse: Most people . . .
Moja: . . . don't have cesarean births, so what applies to them doesn't apply to me.
Nurse: I'll tell the anesthesiologist you want general anesthesia.

More Effective Communication

Nurse: Moja, can I answer any questions for you?
Moja: I want something to put me to sleep so I won't know what's happening.
Nurse: Most women want an epidural.
Moja: I have to be so sound asleep I won't know what's happening.
Nurse: You're not interested in seeing your baby born?
Moja: I'm not interested in seeing him born dead.
Nurse: Let me find your doctor to explain to you again that you need surgery to prevent something from going wrong, not because something is wrong.

Most women appreciate that cesarean births are done to prevent their infant from being harmed. Others interpret a cesarean birth as being done because the harm has already occurred. Some women interpret a cesarean birth as an announcement they are somehow not as competent as other women. Still others are relieved labor is being interrupted. Be certain to ask enough questions so you can learn the importance or meaning of the event to an individual woman.

Skin Preparation

Reducing the number of bacteria on the skin before surgery automatically reduces the possibility of bacteria entering the incision at the time of surgery. Shaving away abdominal hair, if indicated, and washing the skin area over the incision site with soap and water accomplishes this.

The skin preparation area for a cesarean birth varies among agencies. Be certain to follow agency policy. To avoid being shaved, some women who are scheduled for a planned cesarean birth have a bikini wax done 3 or 4 days before surgery.

Surgical Incision

After the anesthetic administration, a woman is positioned with a towel under her right hip to move abdominal contents away from the surgical field and to lift her uterus off the vena cava. Be sure the support person is positioned at the woman's head to provide support. Next, a screen is placed at her shoulder level and covered with a sterile drape to block the flow of bacteria from her respiratory tract to the incision site. This also helps block the woman's and the support person's lines of vision, thus preventing additional anxiety caused by the sight of the incision.

The incision area on the woman's abdomen is then scrubbed with an antiseptic such as iodine, and appropriate drapes are placed around the area so that only a small area of skin is left exposed. Sponge and instrument counts are simplified by the use of prepackaged cesarean birth components. Watching a cesarean birth is usually the first time a father or support person has ever witnessed surgery. Because of this, the person may be too overwhelmed by and interested in the procedure to be of optimum support. Prepare the woman and support person for the sights they might see, or help talk them through them as they occur.

Types of Cesarean Incision

There are two types of cesarean incisions. The type chosen depends on the presentation of the fetus and the speed with which the procedure will be performed (Fig. 24.5).

In a **classic cesarean incision**, the incision is made vertically through both the abdominal skin and the uterus. The incision is made high on the uterus so that it avoids cutting a possible placenta previa. A disadvantage of this type of incision is that it leaves a wide skin scar and also runs through the active contractile portion of the uterus. Because this type of scar could rupture during labor, if this type of incision is used, it is likely that a woman will not be able to have a subsequent vaginal birth.

A **low segment incision** (commonly referred to as a low transverse or Pfannenstiel incision) is one made horizontally across the abdomen just over the symphysis pubis and also horizontally across the uterus just over the cervix. This is the most common type of cesarean incision used today. It is also referred to as a Misgav-Ladach or a "bikini" incision, because even a low-cut bathing suit will cover the scar. Because this type of incision is through the nonactive portion of the uterus (the part that contracts minimally with labor), it is less likely to rupture in subsequent labors, making it possible for a woman to have a **vaginal birth after cesarean (VBAC)** with a future pregnancy (Aguirre & Chou, 2011). It also results in less blood loss, is easier to suture, decreases postpartal uterine infections, and is less likely to cause postpartum gastrointestinal complications (Gilbert, 2011). The major disadvantage of this incision is that it takes longer to perform, possibly making it impractical for an emergent cesarean birth. In a few instances, the skin incision is made horizontally and then the uterine incision is made vertically, or vice versa. For this reason, during a future pregnancy, do not assume a woman who has a small skin incision also has had a small uterine incision.

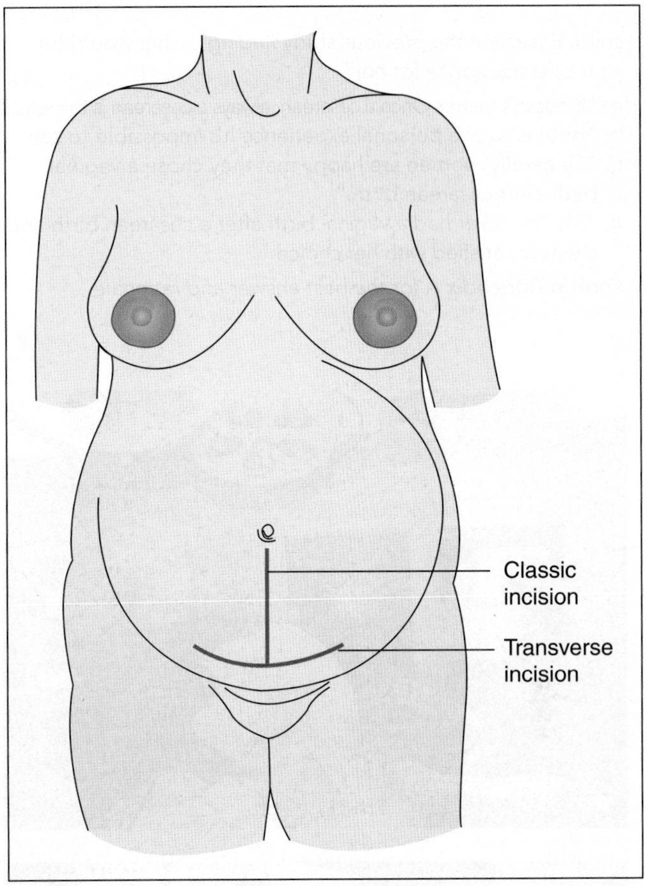

FIGURE 24.5 Types of cesarean incisions.

QSEN Checkpoint Question 24.5

Evidence-Based Practice

The majority of women who have a cesarean birth are physically eligible to have any further births vaginally. To investigate what method of birth women find most satisfying, nurse researchers asked 165 women who have had a previous cesarean birth to rate their satisfaction with their second birth 6 to 8 weeks after the birth on a 10-point scale. Results showed satisfaction scores ranged for different types of birth from 8.86 for spontaneous vaginal birth, 7.86 for elective repeat cesarean, to 6.71 for emergency cesarean birth, to 6.15 for instrumental vaginal birth. The mean score for spontaneous vaginal birth and elective repeat cesarean birth were statistically higher than the mean score for instrumental vaginal birth and emergency cesarean birth. Women who experienced instrumental vaginal birth and emergency cesarean birth also reported a higher number of postnatal health-related problems and were least likely to agree they would make the same birth choice again (Shorten & Shorten, 2012).

Moja tells you, although she knows she will be eligible, she isn't certain if she wants to have a vaginal birth for her next child. Based on the previous study findings, what would be your best assurance for her?

a. "It doesn't matter. Once a ceserean, always a ceserean is the rule."
b. "Birth is such a personal experience it's impossible to say."
c. "Generally, women are happy that they chose a vaginal birth after cesarean birth."
d. "My coworker had a vaginal birth after a cesarean birth and she was satisfied with her choice."

Look in Appendix A for the best answer and rationale.

Birth of the Infant

Once the surgical incision is complete, the uterus is then cut and the child's head is born manually (Fig. 24.6). The mouth and nose of the baby may be suctioned by a bulb syringe, before the remainder of the child is born. Oxytocin is administered via IV by the anesthesiologist as the child or placenta is delivered, to increase uterine contraction and reduce blood loss. In many instances, a woman's partner may be allowed to cut the umbilical cord the same as in a vaginal birth. After full birth, the uterus is pulled forward onto the abdomen and

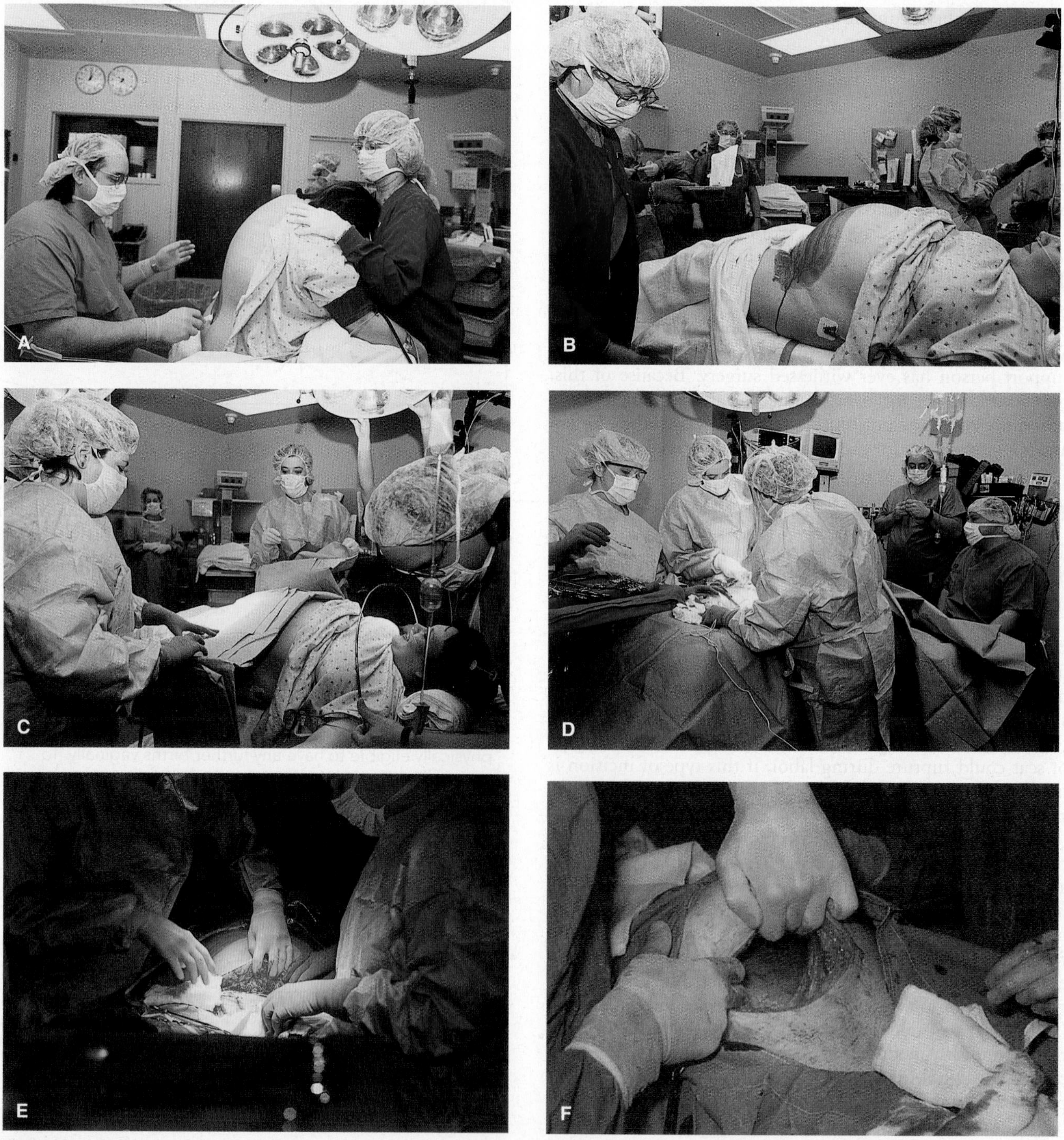

FIGURE 24.6 A cesarean birth. **(A)** Preparation for anesthesia. **(B)** Abdominal skin preparation. **(C)** Draping of operative site. **(D)** Preparation for initial incision. **(E)** The initial incision. **(F)** Opening of the peritoneum. *(continued)*

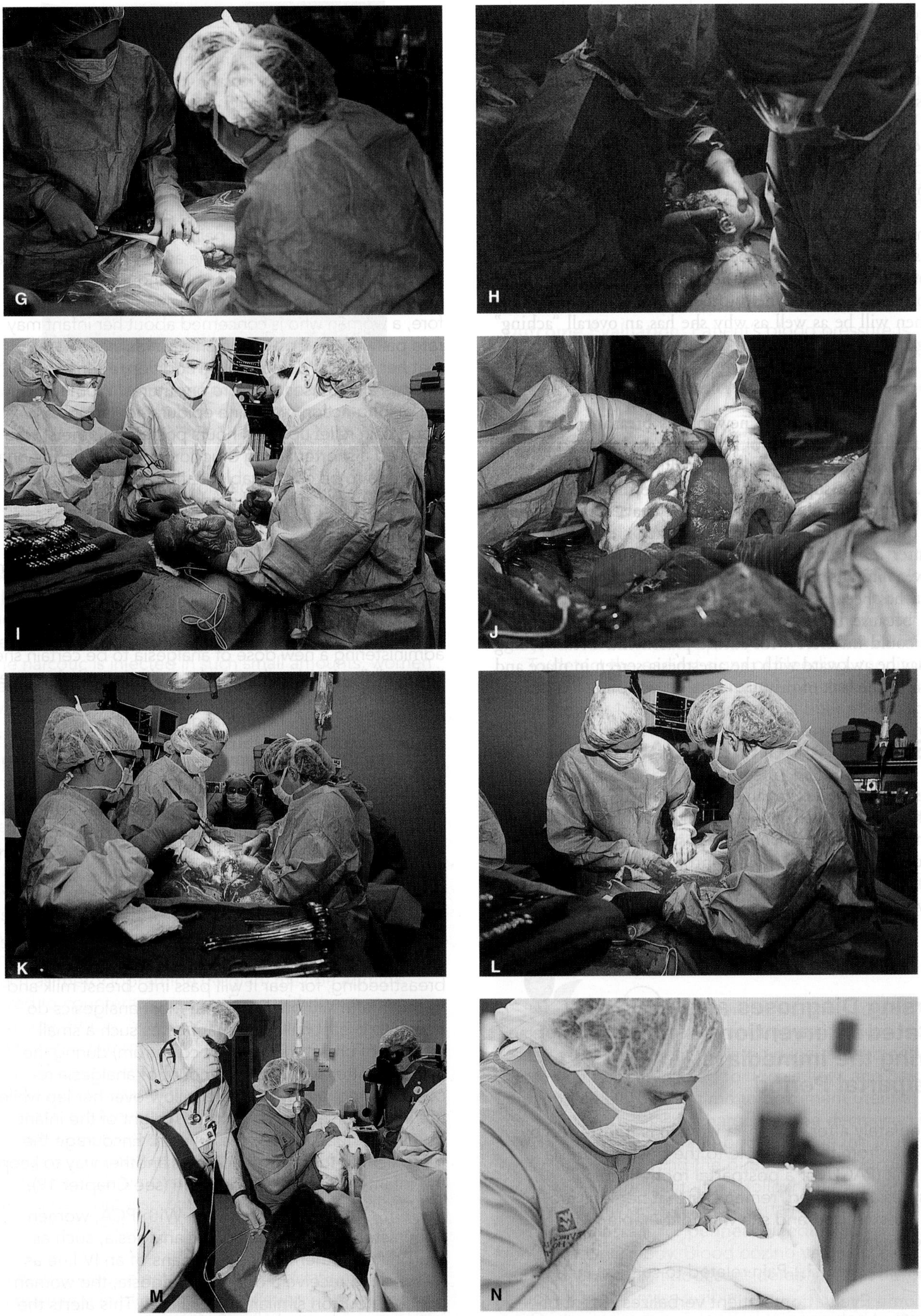

FIGURE 24.6 *(continued)* **(G)** Retractors in place. **(H)** Birth of head and posterior shoulder. **(I)** The infant is born. **(J)** Suturing of the uterus is complete. **(K)** Suturing of the abdominal layers. **(L)** Skin closure. **(M)** Family bonding with mother's first touch. **(N)** Father bonding with newborn. (© Caroline Brown, RNC, MS, DEd.)

BOX 24.7 Nursing Care Planning

AN INTERPROFESSIONAL CARE MAP FOR A WOMAN FOLLOWING AN EMERGENT CESAREAN BIRTH

Moja Hamma is a 29-year-old primigravida who underwent an emergent cesarean birth with epidural anesthesia for fetal distress. She gave birth to a healthy 8-lb 2-oz baby girl who breathed immediately. She tells you, "My mouth is dry and my stomach hurts so much I can't move. Don't ask me to hold or feed my baby until the pain goes away."

Family Assessment Client lives with boyfriend in a westside apartment. Works as a sales clerk in a bridal salon. Boyfriend is currently unemployed. Borrowed money from a friend for hospital bill because Moja has no health insurance.

Client Assessment Postcesarean birth 4 hours ago. Estimated blood loss of 700 ml. Abdomen soft but tender with low transverse incision. No bowel sounds present. Incisional dressing clean, dry, and intact. Fundus of uterus firm, one fingerbreadth below umbilicus. Minimal lochia rubra vaginal drainage present. Urine output 100 ml in last hour. Skin pink, warm, and dry with good skin turgor. Ringer's lactate infusing at 100 ml/hr. Intravenous site clean, dry, without signs of infiltration. Vital signs slightly elevated above baseline: temperature, 98.4°F; pulse rate, 78 beats/min; respirations, 23 breaths/min and shallow; blood pressure, 130/76 mmHg. States she has abdominal pain, especially at incisional area. Holding hands over abdomen; barely moving in bed. Client's mother at bedside holding her hand and stroking her forehead. Patient-controlled epidural analgesia (PCEA) pump in place but not being used by client. When asked why she wasn't using the PCEA pump, she answered, "I don't want to take the chance of being paralyzed forever."

Nursing Diagnosis Pain related to tissue trauma from abdominal incision of cesarean birth

Outcome Criteria Client identifies pain management measure of choice; reports a decrease in pain with analgesic administration; pulse, respirations, and blood pressure return to baseline.

Client holds infant warmly; maintains eye contact with infant; makes positive statements about the newborn prior to discharge.

Team Member Responsible	Assessment	Intervention	Rationale	Expected Outcome
Activities of Daily Living, Including Safety				
Nurse	Assess extent of client's ability to move in bed and breastfeed infant.	Explain the importance of getting out of bed and caring for infant.	Early ambulation helps prevent thrombophlebitis; early breastfeeding helps establish an adequate milk supply.	Client walks to chair in room and feeds infant by 4 hours' time; states chosen pain relief method is effective.
Teamwork and Collaboration				
Nurse/Pain management team	Investigate whether pain management team is available for consultation.	Ask pain management team to consult with client on a more suitable pain relief measure.	Other pain relief measures are available that would be more suitable for client.	Pain management team discusses options for pain relief with client; client chooses a suitable procedure by 2 hours' time.
Procedures/Medications for Quality Improvement				
Nurse/Pain management team	Assess what measures client feels would make her most comfortable.	Institute additional comfort measures, such as changing position, splinting incision, using pillows for support.	Comfort measures help reduce stress and anxiety, elevate mood, and raise the pain threshold, thus enhancing the therapeutic effectiveness of analgesics.	Client reports additional comfort measures aid pain relief effectively.
Nurse/Lactation consultant	Assess what measures client thinks would help her be more successful with breastfeeding.	Assist client with handling newborn. Support breastfeeding efforts.	Breastfeeding is a new skill for a first-time mother.	Client breastfeeds her infant successfully with support from health care providers.

Nutrition				
Nurse	Assess bowel sounds to determine when oral fluid can be safely offered.	Offer ice cubes for dry mouth as soon as bowel sounds are present.	Client should not drink full liquids or eat solid foods until bowel sounds return.	Client states mouth discomfort is reduced by 1 hour after first fluid consumed.
Patient-Centered Care				
Nurse/Pain management team	Assess client's expectations of pain relief measures and safety of PCEA administration.	Review PCEA pump and technique with client.	Client cannot have realistic expectations or feel safe with system unless she understands the technique.	Client states she will use PCEA pump on trial basis for 4 hours. Reevaluate pain relief at that time.
Psychosocial/Spiritual/Emotional Needs				
Nurse	Assess what additional measures client needs to feel secure after frightening experience of emergent cesarean birth.	Provide reinforcement for positive coping mechanisms that client demonstrates.	Positive reinforcement enhances self-esteem and control. Praise promotes self-esteem and confidence to manage new situations.	Client states she feels health care providers are providing her support equal to her level of pain and fatigue.
Nurse	Assess client's expectations of a newborn.	Praise client for positive behaviors and interactions with the child in light of pain and fatigue level. Encourage client to keep newborn in the room with her for extended periods as she is able.	Extended contact within the client's ability to tolerate the activity encourages bonding while minimizing the risk for additional fatigue.	Client keeps newborn with her in room for the majority of daylight hours. Feeds and interacts actively with child.
Informatics for Seamless Health Care Planning				
Nurse	Assess the level of support client will have after she returns home.	Review with client importance of maintaining a level of pain relief at home so she can ambulate and care for new child.	Ambulation and child care are important for both maternal and child health. Keeping pain to a minimum helps the client achieve these activities.	Client states she will take enough pain relief at home to allow her to be active and care for newborn. Names at least one person who will serve as her support person.
Nurse	Assess whether client understands signs and symptoms, such as pain on urination, she will need to report after discharge.	Teach signs of all complications she should report to her primary health care provider.	Knowing signs and symptoms of complications allows client to be an informed health care consumer.	Client repeats danger signs she will report to her primary health care provider.

What if...24.4 You are interested in exploring one of the 2020 National Health Goals related to cesarean birth (see Box 24.1). Most government-sponsored money for nursing research is allotted based on these goals. What would be a possible research topic to explore, pertinent to these goals, that would be applicable to Moja and her family and that would also advance evidence-based practice?

Key Points for Review

- The term *cesarean birth* is preferred to *cesarean section* or *delivery*, because it puts the focus on the childbirth rather than surgical elements of the procedure.
- Cesarean birth may be either a scheduled or an emergent procedure. Because it carries more risk for the woman and infant than does vaginal birth, it is usually undertaken only when medically necessary, although a current trend allows for elective procedures.
- The skin incision may be vertical (i.e., a classic incision), although it is usually a horizontal one just above the pubic hair. The internal incision into the uterus is also usually a horizontal incision into the lower uterine segment.
- Establishing surgical risk, including an assessment of nutritional status, age, general health, fluid and electrolyte balance, and psychological condition, not only meets QSEN competencies for safety but also best meets a woman's total needs.
- Assessment measures before surgery usually include vital sign determination; urinalysis; blood studies such as complete blood count, electrolytes, blood typing, and cross-matching; and ultrasound.
- Support people can lose a great deal of their ability to support if they feel intimidated, overwhelmed, and out of place in an OR; offer them support as needed to make this a positive experience for them as well.
- Cesarean birth is one of the safest types of surgery performed. To keep a woman safe after the procedure, remember that she is both a postsurgical and a postpartum patient. Make assessments to ensure that neither postpartum nor postsurgical complications occur.
- Adequate pain management is important to allow a woman a sense of control and comfort and bonding with her newborn.
- Women are physically exhausted after cesarean birth and may be psychologically exhausted because of the emergent nature of the experience. Provide rest time to relieve the physical strain and a chance to verbalize the experience to help relieve the psychological strain.
- A major intervention after cesarean birth is early ambulation to prevent complications. Incisional pain may make this difficult, so strong nursing support and adequate pain management are necessary.
- The old saying, "Once a cesarean, always a cesarean," is no longer true as long as cephalopelvic disproportion does not exist and the previous incision was a low transverse one.

Critical Thinking Care Study

Amy Whithaven is a 38-year-old gravida 4, para 3, who wants to have her fourth child as naturally as possible, the same as she did for her other three children. Her husband Paul, the chief executive of a public relations firm, is with her in a birthing room as her support person. He assures you Amy is a "veteran" at labor, will use controlled breathing as pain management, and will have no problems. He adds they are especially looking forward to this baby because she will be their first girl. Four hours into labor, Amy experiences sharp abdominal pain and begins to have fresh vaginal bleeding. Amy's blood pressure falls to 100/55 mmHg; the FHR decreases to 80 beats/min. Amy's obstetrician diagnoses placental abruption and asks you to prepare her for an emergent cesarean birth.

1. Because having a cesarean birth is so opposite from what the couple planned for labor, Paul says he wants to investigate Amy's symptoms on the Internet using his laptop or else secure a second opinion from another doctor before surgery can proceed. Would you support him in asking for this?
2. Amy realizes immediately that something is wrong. She asks you if this has something to do with the fact she is having her first girl. Are more girl infants born by cesarean than male infants?
3. Amy is transported to surgery and, within 20 minutes, a 7-lb 3-oz girl is born. Named Honor, she needs resuscitation to breathe and is transferred immediately afterward to the neonatal intensive care nursery for care. Paul declines to visit Honor in the nursery. He says he'll wait until Amy can be "disappointed" along with him. What actions could you take to help this couple begin bonding with their new daughter?

Patient Scenario
The Okparo Family

Read about the Okparo family, a family with a woman having a cesarean birth, then answer the questions to further sharpen your skills and grow more familiar with NCLEX-type questions related to surgical interventions for birth. Confirm your answers are correct by reading the rationales.

Visit http://thePoint.lww.com

Answers and Rationales

Looking for answers to the What If. . . and Critical Thinking Care Study questions?

Visit http://thePoint.lww.com

References

Abenhaim, H. A., & Benjamin, A. (2011). Effect of prior cesarean delivery on neonatal outcomes. *Journal of Perinatal Medicine, 39*(3), 241–244.

Adams, S. S., Eberhard-Gran, M., & Eskild, A. (2012). Fear of childbirth and duration of labour: A study of 2206 women with intended vaginal delivery. *BJOG: International Journal of Obstetrics & Gynaecology, 119*(10), 1238–1246.

Aguirre, F., & Chou, B. (2011). Normal labor & delivery, operative delivery & malpresentations. In K. J. Hurt, M. W. Guile, J. L. Bienstock, et al. (Eds.), *The Johns Hopkins manual of gynecology and obstetrics* (4th ed., pp. 73–89). Philadelphia, PA: Lippincott Williams & Wilkins.

Alfirevic, Z., Gyte, G. M., & Dou, L. (2010). Different classes of antibiotics given to women routinely for preventing infection at caesarean section. *Cochrane Database of Systematic Reviews,* (10), CD008726.

Arulkumaran, S. (2012). Malpresentation, malposition, cephalopelvic disproportion & obstetric procedures. In D. K. Edmonds (Ed.), *Dewhurst's textbook of obstetrics & gynaecology* (8th ed., pp. 311–325). Oxford, UK: John Wiley & Sons.

Baldwin, M. K., Rodriguez, M. I., & Edelman, A. B. (2012). Lack of insurance and parity influence choice between long-acting reversible contraception and sterilization in women postpregnancy. *Contraception, 86*(1), 42–47.

Barbadoro, P., Cotichelli, G., Chiatti, C., et al. (2012). Socio-economic determinants and self-reported depressive symptoms during postpartum period. *Women & Health, 52*(4), 352–368.

Berggren, E. K., Mele, L., Landon, M. B., et al. (2012). Perinatal outcomes in Hispanic and non-Hispanic white women with mild gestational diabetes. *Obstetrics & Gynecology, 120*(5), 1099–1104.

Binder, P., Gustafsson, A., Uvnas-Moberg, K., et al. (2011). Hi-TENS combined with PCA-morphine as post caesarean pain relief. *Midwifery, 27*(4), 547–552.

Blanchette, H. (2011). The rising cesarean delivery rate in America: What are the consequences? *Obstetrics and Gynecology, 118*(3), 687–690.

Centers for Disease Control and Prevention, National Vital Statistics System. (2012). Birth data. Retrieved from http://www.cdc.gov/nchs/births.htm

Cunningham, F. G., Leveno, K., Bloom, S. L., et al. (2010). Breech presentation and delivery. In F. G. Cunningham, K. Leveno, S. L. Bloom, et al. (Eds.), *Williams obstetrics* (23rd ed., pp. 527–543). New York, NY: McGraw-Hill Companies, Inc.

da Silva, F. M., de Oliveira, S. M., Bick, D., et al. (2012). Risk factors for birth-related perineal trauma: A cross-sectional study in a birth centre. *Journal of Clinical Nursing, 21*(15–16), 2209–2218.

Eden, K. B., Denman, M. A., Emeis, C. L., et al. (2012). Trial of labor and vaginal delivery rates in women with a prior cesarean. *Journal of Obstetric, Gynecology & Neonatal Nursing, 41*(5), 583–598.

Elliott-Carter, N., & Harper, J. (2012). Keeping mothers and newborns together after cesarean: how one hospital made the change. *Nursing & Women's Health, 16*(4), 290–295.

Gilbert, E. S. (2011). *Manual of high risk pregnancy & delivery* (5th ed.). St. Louis, MO: Mosby Elsevier.

Gilead, R., Salem, S. Y., Sergienko, R., et al. (2012). Maternal "isolated" obesity and obstetric complications. *Journal of Maternal-Fetal & Neonatal Medicine, 25*(12), 2579–2582.

Gungorduk, K., Asicioglu, O., Celikkol, O., et al. (2010). Iatrogenic bladder injuries during caesarean delivery: A case control study. *Journal of Obstetrics and Gynaecology, 30*(7), 667.

Gyhagen, M., Bullarbo, M., Nielsen, T., et al. (2012). The prevalence of urinary incontinence 20 years after childbirth: A national cohort study in singleton primiparae after vaginal or caesarean delivery. *BJOG: International Journal of Obstetrics and Gynaecology, 119*(12), 1471–1782.

Hamilton, B. E., Martin, J. A., & Ventura, S. J. (2011). Births: Preliminary data for 2010. *National Vital Statistics Reports, 60*(2), 1–25.

Harma, M., Harma, M. I., Karadeniz, G., et al. (2011). Idiopathic ileoileal invagination two days after cesarean section. *Journal of Obstetric & Gynaecology Research, 37*(2), 160–162.

Heazell, A. E., Riches, J., Hopkins, L., et al. (2011). Fetal blood sampling in early labour: Is there an increased risk of operative delivery and fetal morbidity? *BJOG: International Journal of Obstetrics & Gynaecology, 118*(7), 849–855.

Hodnett, E. D., Gates, S., Hofmeyr, G. J., et al. (2012). Continuous support for women during childbirth. *Cochrane Database of Systematic Reviews,* (2), CD003766.

Lavender, T., Hofmeyr, G. J., Neilson, J. P., et al. (2012). Caesarean section for non-medical reasons at term. *Cochrane Database of Systematic Reviews,* (3), CD004660.

Levi, E., Cantillo, E., Ades, V., et al. (2012). Immediate postplacental IUD insertion at cesarean delivery: A prospective cohort study. *Contraception, 86*(2), 102–105.

Lipman, S. S., Carvalho, B., Cohen, S. E., et al. (2013). Response times for emergency cesarean delivery: Use of simulation drills to assess and improve obstetric team performance. *Journal of Perinatology, 33*(4), 259–263.

Liva, S. J., Hall, W. A., Klein, M. C., et al. (2012). Factors associated with differences in Canadian perinatal nurses' attitudes toward birth practices. *Journal of Obstetric, Gynecology & Neonatal Nursing, 41*(6), 761–773.

Mancuso, A., De Vivo, D., Giacobbe, A., et al. (2010). General versus spinal anesthesia for elective caesarean sections: Effects on neonatal short-term outcome. *Journal of Maternal-Fetal and Neonatal Medicine, 23*(10), 1114–1118.

Mantakas, A., & Farrell, T. (2010). The influence of increasing BMI in nulliparous women on pregnancy outcome. *European Journal of Obstetrics, Gynecology & Reproductive Biology, 153*(1), 43–46.

Marshall, N. E., Guild, C., Cheng, Y. W., et al. (2012). Maternal superobesity and perinatal outcomes. *American Journal of Obstetrics & Gynecology, 206*(5), e1–e6.

Milman, N. (2012). Postpartum anemia II: Prevention and treatment. *Annals of Hematology, 91*(2), 143–154.

Ozyer, S., Moraloğlu, O., Gülerman, C., et al. (2012). Tubal sterilization during cesarean section or as an elective procedure? Effect on the ovarian reserve. *Contraception, 86*(5), 488–493.

Patel, R. M., & Jain, L. (2010). Delivery after previous cesarean: Short-term perinatal outcomes. *Seminars in Perinatology, 34*(4), 272–280.

Paterson-Brown, A. (2012). Obstetric emergencies. In D. K. Edmonds (Ed.), *Dewhurst's textbook of obstetrics & gynaecology* (8th ed., pp. 296–310). Oxford, UK: John Wiley & Son.

Rouzi, A. A., Al-Sibiani, S. A., Al-Mansouri, N. M., et al. (2012). Defibulation during vaginal delivery for women with type III female genital mutilation. *Obstetrics & Gynecology, 120*(1), 98–103.

Shorten, A., & Shorten, B. (2012). The importance of mode of birth after previous cesarean: Success, satisfaction, and postnatal health. *Journal of Midwifery & Women's Health, 57*(2), 126–132.

Smyth, R., Alldred, S. K., & Markham, C. (2011). Amniotomy for shortening spontaneous labour. *Cochrane Database for Systematic Reviews,* (5), CD006167.

Speichinger, E., & Holschneider, C. H. (2013). Surgical disorders in pregnancy. In A. H. DeCherney, L. Nathan, T. M. Goodwin, et al. (Eds.), *Current diagnosis and treatment: obstetrics and gynecology* (11th ed, pp. 433–453). Columbus, OH: McGraw-Hill/Lange.

Tan, K. H., & Smyth, R. (2010). Fetal vibroacoustic stimulation for facilitation of tests of fetal wellbeing. *Cochrane Database of Systematic Reviews,* (1), CD002963.

Tita, A. T. (2012). When is primary cesarean appropriate: Maternal and obstetrical indications. *Seminars in Perinatology, 36*(5), 324–327.

U.S. Department of Health and Human Services. (2010). *Healthy people 2020.* Washington, DC: Author.

Valsky, D. V., Cohen, S. M., Lipschuetz, M., et al. (2012). Three-dimensional transperineal ultrasound findings associated with anal incontinence after intrapartum sphincter tears in primiparous women. *Ultrasound in Obstetrics & Gynecology, 39*(1), 83–90.

Wang, B. S., Zhou, L. F., Coulte, D., et al. (2010). Effects of caesarean section on maternal health in low risk nulliparous women. *BMC Pregnancy and Childbirth, 10*(12), 78.

Woods, A. B., Crist, B., Kowalewski, S., et al. (2012). A cross-sectional analysis of the effect of patient-controlled epidural analgesia versus patient controlled analgesia on postcesarean pain and breastfeeding. *Journal of Obstetric, Gynecology & Neonatal Nursing, 41*(3), 339–346.

Zeitlin, J., Di Lallo, D., Blondel, B., et al. (2010).Variability in caesarean section rates for very preterm births at 28–31 weeks of gestation in 10 European regions. *European Journal of Obstetrics, Gynecology & Reproductive Biology, 149*(2), 147–152.

Chapter 25

Nursing Care of a Family Experiencing a Postpartum Complication

KEY TERMS

- endometritis
- mastitis
- peritonitis
- postpartum depression
- postpartal psychosis
- puerperal infection
- subinvolution
- thrombophlebitis
- uterine atony
- uterine inversion

OBJECTIVES

After mastering the contents of this chapter, you should be able to:

1. Describe a woman at risk for common deviations from the normal that can occur during the puerperium.
2. Identify 2020 National Health Goals related to deviations from the normal in the postpartal period that nurses can help the nation achieve.
3. Assess a woman and her family for deviations from the normal during the puerperium.
4. Formulate nursing diagnoses related to postpartum complications.
5. Establish expected outcomes for a woman and her family experiencing a postpartum complication.
6. Using the nursing process, plan nursing care that includes the six competencies of Quality & Safety Education for Nurses (QSEN): Patient-Centered Care, Teamwork & Collaboration, Evidence-Based Practice (EBP), Quality Improvement (QI), Safety, and Informatics.
7. Implement evidence-based nursing care when a woman and her family experience a postpartum complication.
8. Evaluate expected outcomes for achievement and effectiveness of care.
9. Integrate knowledge of postpartum complications with the interplay of nursing process, the six competencies of QSEN, and Family Nursing to promote quality maternal and child health nursing care.

Bailey Cheshire is a 26-year-old woman who teaches chemistry at a local university. You enter her room 2 hours after she gave birth to an 8-lb girl and find her just finishing breastfeeding. Her face appears abnormally pale. You obtain her vital signs and document her pulse as 90 beats/min and her blood pressure as 90/50 mmHg. When you fold back her bedclothes, you discover her perineal pad is saturated. The capillary refill in her fingers is sluggish. You suspect she is experiencing one of the most serious complications of pregnancy: postpartum hemorrhage.

Previous chapters discussed the nursing care for a woman during the typical postpartum period. This chapter contributes information about how to care for a woman and her family when there is a deviation from normal. Comprehensive and recurring nursing care is essential when a postpartum complication develops because it can provide an early alert to conditions that can impact the health of not only the woman but also her child and family.

What immediate measures does Ms. Cheshire need? What would be your first action?

Although the puerperium is usually a period of health, complications can occur. It's important to be knowledgeable about predisposing factors and clinical manifestations of postpartum complications to ensure the prompt initiation of corrective measures in order to prevent long-term consequences to a woman and her family (Furuta, Sandall, & Bick, 2012).

Postpartum complications are always potentially serious because they can impact so many people. A complication may be so serious it could cause a personal injury, leave a woman with her future fertility impaired, or even result in death. Any complication that affects the health of the mother can also affect her interactions with her newborn, such as causing her to discontinue breastfeeding (Brown & Jordan, 2012). Her family can be disrupted because of an extended hospital stay or from an impairment that prevents her from performing her normal family responsibilities. Financial difficulties may arise because of her inability to maintain employment and the need for additional child and health care. Fortunately, most postpartum complications are preventable, and if they do occur, the majority can be treated effectively without long-term complications. Because the health of women and newborns is so important to a nation's health, Box 25.1 describes 2020 National Health Goals that speak to possible puerperium complications (Andrighetti, 2013).

Nursing Process Overview

For a Woman Experiencing a Postpartum Complication

Assessment

Women who assume they will immediately return to an active lifestyle after birth of their child may view an extended hospitalization for a postpartum complication as more unsettling than women who view the postpartum period as one in which they are expected to rest. Assess each woman holistically, therefore, to determine how the health problem a woman is experiencing is impacting her and her family.

Assessment findings associated with a postpartum complication may be subtle, such as tenderness in the calf of a leg, an increase in uterine or perineal pain, a slight elevation in temperature, or a small increase in the amount of lochia flow (Box 25.2). Because the average woman usually has no postpartum complications and the length of stay in the hospital is short, it is easy to overlook these subtle signs, but it is important to be alert to any findings that are unusual because they may be the beginning of a serious concern. To be certain, do not rely solely on a woman's report of perineal healing or amount of lochia; always inspect her perineum and lochia yourself because the report of "I feel fine" or "my bleeding was just a small amount" may be deceptive if she has no familiarity with "normal" lochia, perineal healing, or fundal height against which to accurately compare her own condition.

BOX 25.1 Nursing Care Planning Based on 2020 National Health Goals

The postpartal period is a time when women are very susceptible to hemorrhage and thrombophlebitis and, when these complications develop, women may choose not to breastfeed because of them. The 2020 National Health Goals that speak to this include:

- Reduce the maternal mortality rate to no more than 11.4 per 100,000 live births from a baseline of 12.7 per 100,000.
- Increase the proportion of infants who are breastfed to at least 81.9% from a baseline of 74%.
- Increase the proportion of infants who are breastfed at 6 months from a baseline of 43.5% to 60.6% (U.S. Department of Health and Human Services [DHHS], 2010; see www.healthypeople.gov).

Nurses can help the nation achieve these goals by carefully monitoring uterine involution in the postpartal period and by encouraging women to breastfeed even in the face of a postpartal complication.

BOX 25.2 Nursing Care Planning Using Assessment

Assessing the Postpartal Woman With Complications

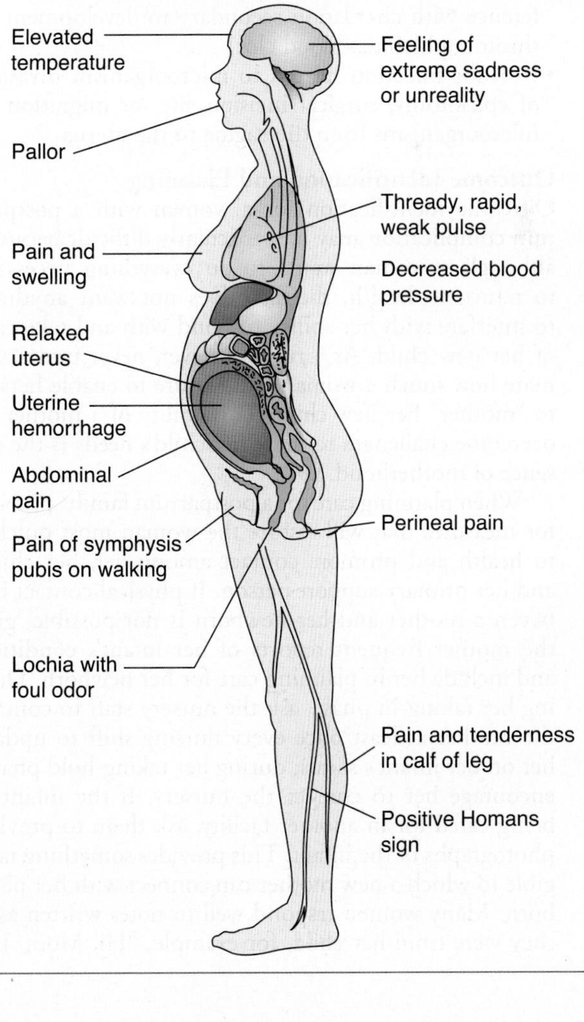

An increased temperature except during the first 24 hours after birth is a potentially extremely serious finding. Women may try to "explain away" an increased temperature because they know if they have an elevated temperature, they may not be allowed to feed their infant. Do not be tempted to rationalize such a finding with explanations such as, "The room was warm," or "She just drank some hot coffee." Although these factors may make a slight difference in body temperature, they do not affect it enough to account for an oral temperature greater than 100.4°F (38.0°C).

Nursing Diagnosis

Nursing diagnoses during this time vary depending on the postpartal complication. Some examples include:

- Deficient fluid volume related to blood loss
- Ineffective breastfeeding related to the development of mastitis
- Risk for impaired parenting related to postpartum depression
- Risk for injury to self and newborn related to postpartal psychosis
- Acute pain related to a collection of blood in traumatized tissue (hematoma) secondary to birth trauma
- Situational low self-esteem related to inability to perform regular tasks
- Social isolation related to precautions necessary to protect infant and others from infection transmission
- Ineffective peripheral tissue perfusion related to interference with circulation secondary to development of thrombophlebitis (blood clot)
- Risk for infection related to microorganism invasion of episiotomy, surgical incision site, or migration of microorganisms from the vagina to the uterus

Outcome Identification and Planning

Outcome identification for a woman with a postpartum complication may be particularly difficult because, although a woman wants to do everything necessary to return to health, she also does not want anything to interfere with her ability to bond with and take care of her new child. As a rule, however, never underestimate how much a woman will endure to enable herself to "mother" her new child. This ability of a mother to overcome challenges to meet her child's needs is the essence of motherhood.

When planning care for a postpartum family, provide for measures that will restore the woman most quickly to health and promote contact among her, her child, and her primary support person. If physical contact between a mother and her newborn is not possible, give the mother frequent reports of her infant's condition and include her in planning care for her newborn. During her taking-in phase, ask the nursery staff to contact the mother at least once every nursing shift to update her on her infant's status; during her taking-hold phase, encourage her to contact the nursery. If the infant is being cared for in another facility, ask them to provide photographs of the infant. This provides something tangible to which a new mother can connect with her newborn. Many women respond well to notes written as if they were from her child, for example, "Hi, Mom. I'm drinking well but I miss you and can't wait for you to get better and take care of me. Love, Kelsey." Such a note serves to lessen a woman's concern for her child (because she is doing well) and also helps to promote mother–infant attachment. Because childbirth is generally seen as a happy time, being faced with a postpartal complication can cause a great deal of emotional stress. The risk of both postpartal depression and postpartal psychosis increases when a complication develops. A helpful national volunteer support group for women who are depressed after childbirth can be found at the Postpartal Support International Web site (www.postpartum.net).

Implementation

Interventions for a woman with a postpartum complication should include instruction for both self-care and child care (if appropriate) because continuing to review these measures helps a woman accept her situation as temporary, thus reinforcing the idea she will be able to care for herself and her infant when she is healthy again.

Outcome Evaluation

An evaluation of a woman with a postpartal complication should address both her and her family's health as well as her family's ability to integrate the new child into the family. The evaluation may suggest the need for home care follow-up to assist a woman in coping with both old and new responsibilities in the face of reduced energy from an illness.

Examples of expected outcomes include:

- Lochia is free of foul odor.
- Fundus remains firm and midline with progressive descent.
- Client maintains a urinary output greater than 30 ml/hr.
- Lochia discharge amount is 6 in. or less on a perineal pad in 1 hour.
- Client maintains vital signs and oxygen saturation within defined normal limits.
- Client identifies signs and symptoms that should be reported.
- Client demonstrates attachment behaviors with infant despite separation or activity restrictions.

POSTPARTUM HEMORRHAGES

Hemorrhage, one of the primary causes of maternal mortality associated with childbearing, is a major threat during pregnancy, throughout labor, and continuing into the postpartum period. Traditionally, postpartum hemorrhage is defined as blood loss of 500 ml or more following a vaginal birth; this occurs in as many as 5% to 8% of postpartal women (Poggi, 2012). With a cesarean birth, hemorrhage is present when there is a 1,000 ml blood loss or a 10% decrease in the hematocrit level (Jones & Henderson, 2011). Although hemorrhage may occur either early (within the first 24 hours following birth) or late (from 24 hours to 6 weeks after birth), the greatest danger is in the first 24 hours because of the grossly denuded and unprotected uterine area left after detachment of the placenta.

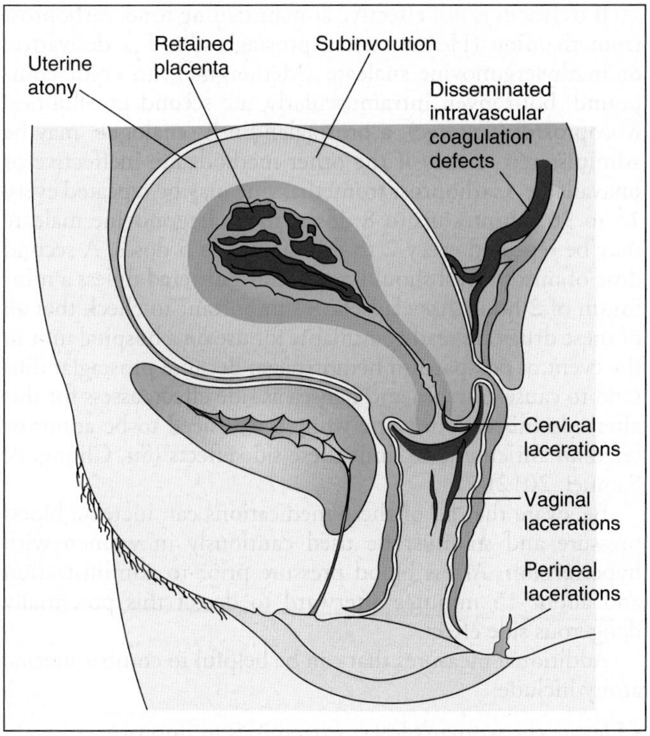

FIGURE 25.1 The common causes of a postpartal hemorrhage.

The four main reasons for postpartum hemorrhage are uterine atony, trauma (lacerations, hematomas, uterine inversion, or uterine rupture), retained placental fragments, and the development of disseminated intravascular coagulation (DIC). These causes are generally referred to as the *four T's* of postpartum hemorrhage: tone, trauma, tissue, and thrombin—a common mnemonic for the etiology of hemorrhage experienced in the puerperium (Fig. 25.1).

Uterine Atony

Uterine atony, or relaxation of the uterus, is the most frequent cause of postpartum hemorrhage; it tends to occur most often in Asian or Hispanic woman (Bryant, Mhyre, Leffert, et al., 2012). Factors that predispose a woman to poor uterine tone or the inability of her uterus to maintain a contracted state are summarized in Box 25.3. When caring for a woman in whom any of these conditions are present, be especially conscientious in your observations and be on guard for signs of uterine bleeding.

BOX 25.3 Conditions That Increase a Woman's Risk for a Postpartal Hemorrhage

Conditions that distend the uterus beyond average capacity	Multiple gestation Hydramnios (excessive amount of amniotic fluid) A large baby (>9 lb) The presence of uterine myomas (fibroid tumors)
Conditions that could have caused cervical or uterine lacerations	An operative birth A rapid birth
Conditions with varied placental site or attachment	Placenta previa Placenta accreta Premature separation of the placenta Retained placental fragments
Conditions that leave the uterus unable to contract readily	Deep anesthesia or analgesia Labor initiated or assisted with an oxytocin agent High parity or maternal age over 35 years of age Previous uterine surgery Prolonged and difficult labor Chorioamnionitis or endometritis Secondary maternal illness such as anemia Prior history of postpartum hemorrhage Prolonged use of magnesium sulfate or other tocolytic therapy
Conditions that lead to inadequate blood coagulation	Fetal death Disseminated intravascular coagulation (DIC)

Nursing Diagnoses and Related Interventions

Nursing Diagnosis: Deficient fluid volume related to excessive blood loss after birth.

Outcome Evaluation: Client's blood pressure and heart rate remains within usual defined limits; lochia flow is less than one saturated perineal pad per hour.

If the uterus suddenly relaxes, there will be an abrupt gush of blood vaginally from the placental site. This can occur immediately after birth but is more likely to occur gradually, over the first postpartum hour, as the uterus slowly loses its tone. If the loss of blood is extremely copious, a woman will quickly begin to exhibit symptoms of hypovolemic shock such as a falling blood pressure; a rapid, weak, or thready pulse; increased and shallow respirations; pale, clammy skin; and increasing anxiety. If the blood loss is unnoticed seepage, there is little change in pulse and blood pressure at first because of circulatory compensation. Suddenly, however, the system is able to compensate no more, and the pulse rate rises rapidly and becomes weak. Blood pressure then drops abruptly. With slow bleeding, a woman develops these symptoms over a period of hours; the end result of continued seepage, however, can be as life threatening as a sudden profuse loss of blood (Andrighetti, 2013).

It is difficult to estimate the amount of blood a postpartal woman is losing because it is difficult to estimate the amount of blood it takes to saturate a perineal pad (between 25 and 50 ml). By counting the number of perineal pads saturated in given lengths of time, such as half-hour intervals, a rough estimate of the amount of blood loss can be formed. Five pads saturated in half an hour is obviously a different situation from five pads saturated in 8 hours. In either situation, however, a woman will have lost approximately 250 ml of blood, and if either scenario is allowed to continue unattended, she will be in grave danger of hypovolemia. Be certain that when you are counting perineal pads, you differentiate between *saturated* and *used*. Weighing perineal pads before and after use and then subtracting the difference is an accurate technique to measure vaginal discharge: 1 g of weight is comparable to 1 ml of blood volume, so if a pad weights 50 g more after use, the woman has lost 50 ml of blood. Always be sure to turn a woman on her side when inspecting for blood loss to be certain a large amount of blood is not pooling undetected beneath her.

The best safeguard against uterine atony is to palpate a woman's fundus at frequent intervals to be assured her uterus is remaining contracted. Under usual circumstances, a well-contracted uterus feels firm and is easily recognized because it feels like no other abdominal organ. If you are unsure whether you have located a woman's fundus on palpation, it means the uterus is probably in a state of relaxation. Frequent assessments of lochia (to be certain the amount of the flow is under a saturated pad per hour and that any clots are small), as well as vital signs, particularly pulse and blood pressure, are equally important determinations.

Therapeutic Management

In the event of uterine atony, the first step in controlling hemorrhage is to attempt fundal massage to encourage contraction (Box 25.4). Unless the uterus is extremely lacking in tone, this procedure is usually effective in causing contraction, and, after a few seconds, the uterus assumes its healthy, grapefruitlike feel (Chelmow, 2011).

With uterine atony, even if the uterus responds well to massage, the problem may not be completely resolved because, as soon as you remove your hand from the fundus, the uterus may relax and the lethal seepage will begin again. To prevent this, remain with a woman after massaging her fundus and assess to be certain her uterus is not relaxing again. Continue to assess carefully for the next 4 hours.

If a woman's uterus does not remain contracted, contact her primary care provider so interventions to increase contraction such as administering a bolus or a dilute intravenous infusion of oxytocin (Pitocin) can be prescribed to help the uterus maintain tone (Roach, Abramovici, & Tita, 2012).

When oxytocin is given intravenously (IV), its action on the uterus is immediate. Be aware, however, that oxytocin has a short duration of action, approximately 1 hour, so symptoms of uterine atony can recur quickly if it is administered only as a single dose (see Chapter 23, Box 23.3 for cautions to be aware of with an oxytocin infusion).

If oxytocin is not effective at maintaining tone, carboprost tromethamine (Hemabate), a prostaglandin F_2a derivative, or methylergonovine maleate (Methergine), an ergot compound, both given intramuscularly, are second possibilities. Misoprostol (Cytotec), a prostaglandin E_1 analogue, may be administered rectally if the other methods are ineffective or unavailable. Carboprost tromethamine may be repeated every 15 to 90 minutes up to 8 doses; methylergonovine maleate may be repeated every 2 to 4 hours up to 5 doses. A second dose of misoprostol should not be administered unless a minimum of 2 hours has elapsed. It's important to check that all of these drugs are readily available for use on a hospital unit in the event of postpartum hemorrhage. Because prostaglandins tend to cause diarrhea and nausea as side effect, assess for this after administration; some women will need to be administered an antiemetic to limit these side effects (Su, Chong, & Samuel, 2012).

Be aware that all of these medications can increase blood pressure and so must be used cautiously in women with hypertension. Assess blood pressure prior to administration and about 15 minutes afterward to detect this potentially dangerous side effect.

Additional measures that can be helpful to combat uterine atony include:

- Elevate the woman's lower extremities to improve circulation to essential organs.
- Offer a bedpan or assist the woman to the bathroom at least every 4 hours to be certain her bladder is emptying because a full bladder predisposes a woman to uterine atony. To reduce the possibility of bladder pressure, insertion of a urinary catheter may be prescribed.
- Administer oxygen by face mask at a rate of about 10 to 12 L/min if the woman is experiencing respiratory distress from decreasing blood volume. Position her supine (flat) to allow adequate blood flow to her brain and kidneys.
- Obtain vital signs frequently and assess them for trends such as a continually decreasing blood pressure with a continuously rising pulse rate.

When planning continuing care after sudden blood loss, remember that a woman may be so exhausted from labor and the effect of the blood loss that she resents frequent uterine and blood pressure assessments. Explain that you realize these measures are disturbing, but that they are important for her welfare. Obtain measurements as quickly and gently as possible to cause a minimum of discomfort and disruption, allowing the woman time to rest.

Bimanual Compression. If fundal massage and administration of oxytocin or methylergonovine are not effective at stopping uterine bleeding, a sonogram may be done to detect possible retained placental fragments. The woman's primary care provider may attempt bimanual compression (Andreatta, Perosky, & Johnson, 2012). With this procedure, the primary care provider inserts one hand into a woman's vagina while pushing against the fundus through the abdominal wall with the other hand. If this is ineffective, the woman may be returned to the birthing room so that her uterine cavity can be explored manually. Under sonogram visualization, a balloon catheter may be introduced vaginally and inflated with sterile water until it puts pressure against the bleeding site. Vaginal packing is inserted during this procedure to stabilize the

BOX 25.4 Nursing Care Planning Using Procedures

FUNDAL MASSAGE

Purpose: To stimulate uterine contraction, promote uterine tone and consistency, and minimize the risk of hemorrhage.

PROCEDURE	PRINCIPLE
1. Explain the necessity for the procedure and provide privacy.	1. Explanations help to decrease anxiety, and providing privacy enhances self-esteem.
2. Ask client to void (unless bleeding is extensive and more rapid action seems necessary). Ask her to lie supine with knees flexed.	2. An empty bladder prevents displacement of the uterus and ensures accurate assessment of uterine tone. Proper positioning enhances visualization and effectiveness of procedure.
3. Put on gloves. Place one hand on the abdomen just above the symphysis pubis. Place the other hand around the top of the fundus (Fig. A).	3. This anchors the lower uterine segment and allows you to locate and assess the fundus.

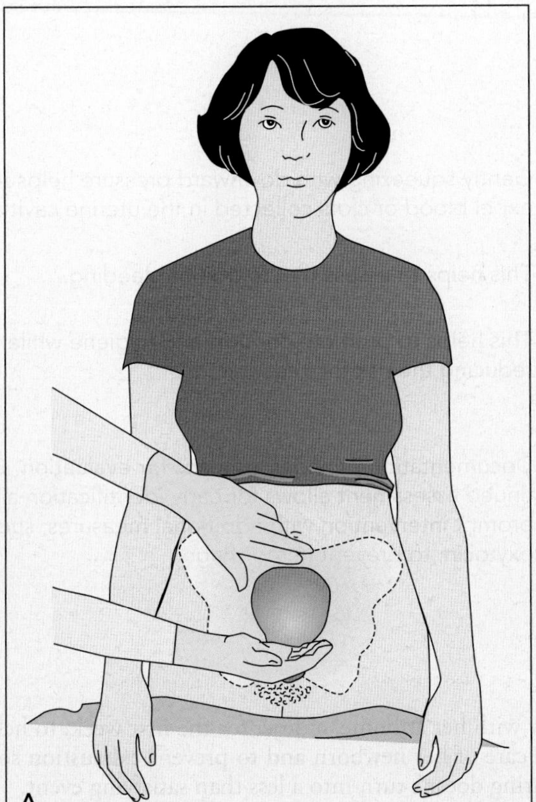

A

(continued on page 680)

BOX 25.4 Nursing Care Planning Using Procedures (continued)

FUNDAL MASSAGE

PROCEDURE	PRINCIPLE
4. Rotate the upper hand to massage the uterus until it is firm, being careful not to overmassage (Fig. B).	4. Massage should be done only when the uterus is not firm, and aggressive massage may lead to a partial or complete uterine prolapse.

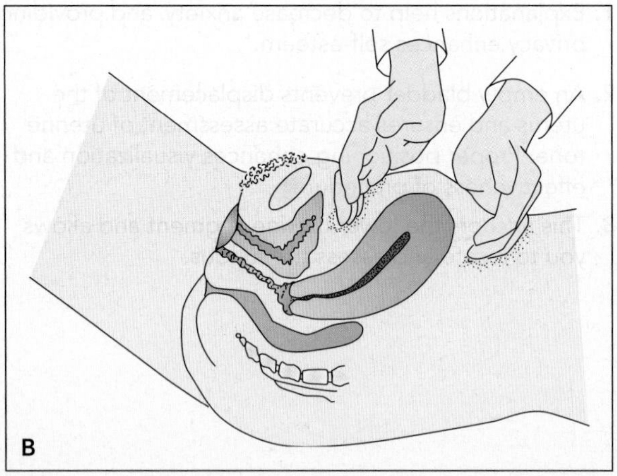

PROCEDURE	PRINCIPLE
5. When the uterus is firm, press the fundus between the hands using slight downward pressure against the lower hand.	5. Gently squeezing with downward pressure helps to expel blood or clots collected in the uterine cavity.
6. Remove and observe the woman's perineum for the passage of clots and the amount of bleeding.	6. This helps to assess the degree of bleeding.
7. Massage the uterus one more time to be certain it remains firm, cleanse the perineum, and apply a clean perineal pad. Discard gloves and soiled pads according to agency policy.	7. This helps to promote comfort and hygiene while reducing the risk for infection.
8. Document the results of the procedure. Continue to assess the fundus and lochia according to agency policy. Notify the primary care provider if the fundus does not remain firm or if bleeding continues.	8. Documentation provides a means for evaluation. Continued assessment allows for early identification and prompt intervention with additional measures, such as oxytocin, to prevent hemorrhage.

placement of the balloon. Be certain to document the presence of the packing so it can be removed before agency discharge because retained packing serves as a growth medium for microorganisms that could lead to postpartal infection (Laas, Bui, Popowski, et al., 2012).

Blood Replacement. Blood transfusion to replace blood loss with postpartal hemorrhage is often necessary. In most agencies, blood typing and crossmatching is done when a woman is admitted to the labor service so blood can be rapidly crossmatched.

Under usual circumstances, the average woman takes the full postpartal period to regain her strength. Women who experience postpartal hemorrhage tend to have an even longer recovery period because the physiologic exhaustion of body systems can interfere with recovery. Iron therapy may be prescribed to ensure good hemoglobin formation. Activity level, exertion, and postpartal exercise may be somewhat restricted. Discuss with the woman the possibility of having someone stay with her at home, at least for the first week, to help with the care of her newborn and to prevent exhaustion so childbearing doesn't turn into a less than satisfying event.

Extensive blood loss is one of the precursors of postpartal infection because of the general debilitation that results. Therefore, observe any woman who has experienced more than a normal loss of blood for changes such as scant or odorous lochia discharge. Monitor her temperature closely in the postpartal period to detect the earliest signs of developing infection. Make certain the woman knows how to assess for normal lochia and temperature once she is discharged.

Hysterectomy or Suturing. Usually, uterine massage and administration of a drug to contract the uterus are effective to halt bleeding. With extreme bleeding, embolization of pelvic and uterine vessels by angiographic techniques may be necessary. As a last resort, ligation of the uterine arteries or a hysterectomy (removal of the uterus) may be necessary (Omole-Ohonsi & Olayinka, 2012). In this totally unexpected outcome of childbearing, provide comfort and support to both the woman and her support person.

After a hysterectomy, a woman usually wants to talk about what happened, why surgery was necessary, or how she feels now that she can no longer bear children so she can sort through her feelings of "Why me?" She may reveal ambiguous feelings: she wanted to have more children (or at least have the ability to have more), but she is also grateful to be alive. She is both thankful her life has been saved, but she may also feel resentful you couldn't have done more to protect her future childbearing. She may grieve for children who will not be born. If her child was born outside the hospital (although postpartum hemorrhage is lower during home births than hospital births), she may have a need to talk about her choice of location for childbirth and that she did not choose a more controlled place for childbirth (Nove, Berrington, & Matthews, 2012).

Open lines of communication between the couple and health care providers that allow a family to vent their feelings are most helpful to a couple in this crisis. Referral to a grief counselor may be necessary because grieving for future children who will not be born can interfere with bonding with the present child.

✔ QSEN Checkpoint Question 25.1

Informatics

All postpartum women are at risk for uterine hemorrhage. What assessment data should you first collect when appraising Ms. Cheshire's risk for hemorrhage?

a. Ask her to describe her perineal care.
b. Assess the skin integrity of her abdomen.
c. Assess her oxygen saturation level.
d. Assess her uterus for height and tone.

Look in Appendix A for the best answer and rationale.

Lacerations

Small lacerations or tears of the birth canal are common and may be considered a normal consequence of childbearing. Large lacerations, however, can be sources of infection or hemorrhage. They occur most often:

- With difficult or precipitate births
- In primigravidas
- With the birth of a large infant (>9 lb)
- With the use of a lithotomy position and instruments (e.g., forceps, vacuum extraction)

Lacerations may occur in the cervix, the vagina, or the perineum. After birth, anytime a uterus feels firm but bleeding persists, suspect a laceration at one of these three sites is causing the bleeding.

Cervical Lacerations

Lacerations of the cervix are usually found on the sides of the cervix, near the branches of the uterine artery. If the artery is torn, the blood loss may be so great that blood gushes from the vaginal opening. Because this is arterial bleeding, it is a brighter red than the venous blood lost with uterine atony. Fortunately, this bleeding ordinarily occurs immediately after detachment of the placenta, when the primary care provider is still in attendance.

Therapeutic Management. The repair of a cervical laceration usually requires sutures and can be difficult because, if the bleeding is intense, this obstructs visualization of the area. A woman is not always aware of what is happening at this point, but she quickly senses something is seriously wrong. Try to maintain an air of calm and, if possible, stand beside the woman at the head of the table. She may be worried that the extra activity in the room has something to do with her baby. Assure her of her baby's condition and inform her about the need to stay in the birthing room a little longer than expected while the primary care provider places sutures or packing. Remember, the protective attitude a woman has felt toward her body all during pregnancy now turns toward her baby, so she usually is relieved to learn any problem that may be occurring is hers, not her infant's.

If the cervical laceration appears to be extensive or difficult to repair, it may be necessary for the woman to be given a regional anesthetic to relax the uterine muscle and to prevent pain. Explain the need for an anesthetic and the procedures being carried out. Be certain the primary care provider has adequate space to work, adequate sponges and suture supplies, and a good light source.

Vaginal Lacerations

Vaginal lacerations are easier to locate and assess than cervical lacerations because they are so much easier to view.

Therapeutic Management. Unfortunately, vaginal tissue is friable, making vaginal lacerations difficult to suture. A balloon tapenade similar to the type used with a uterine hemorrhage may be effective if suturing does not achieve hemostasis (Ghirardina, Alboni, & Mabrouk, 2012). Some oozing often occurs after a vaginal repair, so the vagina may be packed to maintain pressure on the suture line. An indwelling urinary catheter (Foley catheter) may be placed following the repair because the packing causes such pressure on the urethra that it can interfere with voiding. Be certain to document in the woman's electronic record when and where packing was placed so you can be certain it is removed after 24 to 48 hours or before hospital discharge to prevent infection.

Perineal Lacerations

Lacerations of the perineum are more apt to occur when a woman is placed in a lithotomy position for birth rather than a supine position, because a lithotomy position increases tension on the perineum. Perineal lacerations are classified by four categories, depending on the extent and depth of the tissue involved. These categories are shown in Table 25.1.

TABLE 25.1 Classification of Perineal Lacerations

Classification	Description of Involvement
First degree	Vaginal mucous membrane and skin of the perineum to the fourchette
Second degree	Vagina, perineal skin, fascia, levator ani muscle, and perineal body
Third degree	Entire perineum, extending to reach the external sphincter of the rectum
Fourth degree	Entire perineum, rectal sphincter, and some of the mucous membrane of the rectum

Therapeutic Management. Perineal lacerations are sutured and treated the same as an episiotomy repair. Make certain the degree of the laceration is documented because women with fourth-degree lacerations need extra precautions to avoid having sutures loosened or infected. Both sutured lacerations and episiotomy incisions tend to heal in the same length of time. A diet high in fluid and a stool softener may be prescribed for the first week after birth to prevent constipation and hard stools, which could break the new sutures. Any woman who has a third- or fourth-degree laceration should not have an enema or a rectal suppository prescribed or have her temperature taken rectally because the hard tips of equipment could open sutures near to or including those of the rectal sphincter. Although fourth-degree lacerations can lead to long-term dyspareunia, rectal incontinence, or sexual dissatisfaction, they usually heal without further complications.

Retained Placental Fragments

Occasionally, a placenta does not detach in its entirety; fragments of it separate and are left still attached to the uterus. Because the portion retained keeps the uterus from contracting fully, uterine bleeding occurs. Although this is most likely to happen with a succenturiate placenta—a placenta with an accessory lobe (see Chapter 23)—it can happen in any instance. Placenta accreta—a placenta that fuses with the myometrium because of an abnormal decidua basalis layer—may also be retained. This is associated with previous cesarean birth and in vitro fertilization and occurs at an incidence of about 1 out of 3,000 births; it can be identified by an ultrasound exam during pregnancy. Removing such a deeply embedded placenta can lead to severe postpartal hemorrhage (Balayla & Bondarenko, 2012). To identify the complication of a retained placenta, every placenta should be inspected carefully after birth to be certain it is complete. Retained placental fragments may also be detected by ultrasound. A blood serum sample that contains human chorionic gonadotropin (hCG) hormone also reveals that part of a placenta is still present.

Assessment

If an undetected retained fragment is large, bleeding will be apparent in the immediate postpartal period because the uterus cannot contract with the fragment in place. If the fragment is small, bleeding may not be detected until postpartum day 6 to 10, when the woman notices an abrupt discharge and a large amount of vaginal bleeding. On examination, usually the uterus is found to not be fully contracted.

Therapeutic Management

Removal of the retained placental fragment is necessary to stop the bleeding and can usually be accomplished by a dilatation and curettage (D&C). If it cannot be removed, methotrexate may be prescribed to destroy the retained fragment. Because the hemorrhage from retained fragments may be delayed until after a woman is at home, be certain women know to continue to observe the color of lochia and to report any tendency for the discharge to change from lochia serosa or alba back to rubra. In some instances, placenta accreta is so deeply attached that balloon occlusion and embolization of the internal iliac arteries may be necessary to minimize blood loss. In others, a hysterectomy must be performed (ACOG, 2012).

QSEN Checkpoint Question 25.2

Teamwork & Collaboration

Suppose Bailey Cheshire has a retained placental fragment that is causing extensive postpartal bleeding. Which test prescribed by her primary care provider would best reveal a retained fragment is present?

a. Placental and cord blood estrogen
b. Progesterone
c. Human chorionic gonadotropin hormone
d. Oxytocin

Look in Appendix A for the best answer and rationale.

Uterine Inversion

Uterine inversion is a prolapse of the fundus of the uterus through the cervix so that the uterus turns inside out. This usually occurs immediately after birth and so is discussed in Chapter 23.

Disseminated Intravascular Coagulation

DIC is a deficiency in clotting ability caused by vascular injury. It may occur in any woman in the postpartal period, but it is usually associated with premature separation of the placenta, a missed early miscarriage, or fetal death in utero. DIC is discussed in Chapter 21 along with these disorders.

Subinvolution

Subinvolution is the incomplete return of the uterus to its prepregnant size and shape. With subinvolution, at a 4- or 6-week postpartal visit, the uterus is still enlarged and soft. Lochial discharge usually is still present. Subinvolution may result from a small retained placental fragment, a mild **endometritis** (infection of the endometrium), or an accompanying problem such as a uterine myoma that is interfering with complete contraction.

Therapeutic Management

Oral administration of methylergonovine, 0.2 mg four times daily, is the usual prescription to improve uterine tone and complete involution. If the uterus feels tender to palpation, suggesting endometritis is present, an oral antibiotic also will be prescribed. Being certain women are able to recognize the normal process of involution and lochia discharge before hospital discharge helps women to be able to identify subinvolution and seek early care if it occurs. A chronic loss of blood from subinvolution will result in anemia and a lack of energy, conditions that possibly could interfere with infant bonding or lead to infection.

What if... 25.1 Ms. Cheshire tells you she has a PhD in chemistry and assures you from her background she knows she is having a normal amount of lochia flow, so there is no need for you to assess her perineum or perineal pad. Would you respect her privacy or insist you need to assess the amount of her lochia flow?

Perineal Hematomas

A perineal hematoma is a collection of blood in the subcutaneous layer of tissue of the perineum. The overlying skin, as a rule, is intact with no noticeable trauma. Blood accumulates underneath, however, from injury to blood vessels in the perineum during birth. Hematomas are most likely to occur after rapid, spontaneous births and in women who have perineal varicosities. They may occur at the site of an episiotomy or laceration repair if a vein was punctured during suturing. Although these can cause a woman acute discomfort and concern, they usually represent only minor bleeding.

Assessment

Perineal sutures almost always give a postpartal woman some discomfort. If a woman reports severe pain in the perineal area or a feeling of pressure between her legs, inspect the perineal area to see if a hematoma could be causing this. If a hematoma is present, it appears as an area of purplish discoloration with obvious swelling. It could be as small as 2 cm or as large as 8 cm in diameter (Fig. 25.2). At first it may feel fluctuant, but as seepage into the area continues and tissue is drawn taut, it palpates as a firm globe and feels tender.

Therapeutic Management

Report the presence of a hematoma, its estimated size, and the degree of the woman's discomfort to her primary care provider. Describe a definite size such as "5 centimeters" or the size of a quarter or a half dollar rather than documenting it as "large" or "small" as this best establishes a baseline and will enable you to assess if it is growing larger.

Administer a mild analgesic as prescribed for pain relief. Applying an ice pack (covered with a towel to prevent thermal injury to the skin) may prevent further bleeding. Usually, a hematoma is absorbed over the next 3 or 4 days. If one is large when discovered or continues to increase in size, the woman may have to be returned to the birthing room to have the site incised and the bleeding vessel ligated under local anesthesia.

You can assure the woman that, even though the hematoma is causing her considerable discomfort, it is not a serious complication and will slowly reabsorb over the next 6 weeks, causing no further difficulty. If an episiotomy incision line was opened to drain a hematoma, it may be left open and packed with gauze rather than resutured. Be certain to record this packing was placed so it can be removed in 24 to 48 hours. A suture line opened this way heals by tertiary intention or from the bottom to the top, rather than side to side, so healing will occur more slowly than a usual primary intention suture line. Be certain the woman has clear instructions before discharge regarding necessary suture line care she will need to do at home, such as keeping it clean and dry and perhaps using a sitz bath once or twice a day.

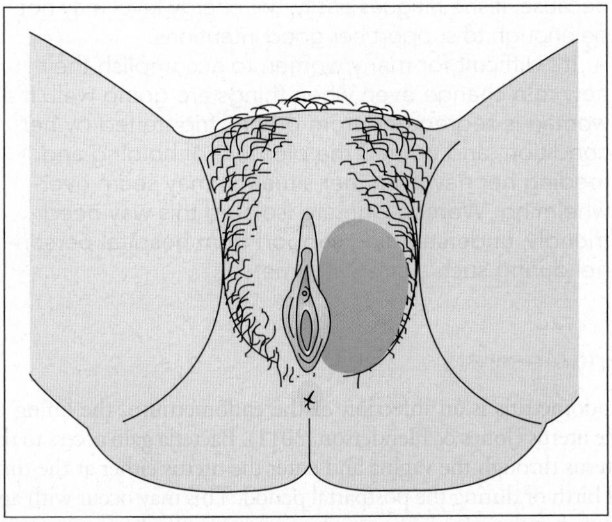

FIGURE 25.2 The appearance of a perineal hematoma from a bleeding subcutaneous vessel.

PUERPERAL INFECTIONS

Infection of the reproductive tract in the postpartal period is another major cause of maternal mortality (Edmonds, 2012). Factors that predispose women to infection during this time are shown in Box 25.5. When caring for a woman who has any of these circumstances, be aware that the risk for postpartal infection is greatly increased.

Theoretically, the uterus is sterile during pregnancy and up until the membranes rupture. After rupture, pathogens can begin to invade; the risk of infection grows even greater if tissue edema and trauma are present. If infection should occur, the prognosis for complete recovery depends on such factors as the woman's general health, virulence of the invading organism and portal of entry, the degree of uterine involution at the time of the invasion, and the presence of lacerations in the reproductive tract.

BOX 25.5 Conditions That Increase a Woman's Risk for Postpartal Infection

Risk Factor	Basis for Risk
Rupture of the membranes more than 24 hours before birth	Bacteria may have started to invade the uterus while the fetus was still in utero.
Retained placental fragments within the uterus	The tissue necroses and serves as an excellent bed for bacterial growth.
Postpartal hemorrhage	The woman's general condition is weakened.
Preexisting anemia	The woman's general condition is weakened.
Prolonged and difficult labor, particularly with instrument births	Trauma to the tissue may leave lacerations or fissures for easy portals of entry for infection.
Internal fetal heart monitoring electrode	Contamination may have been introduced with placement of the scalp electrodes.
Local vaginal infection present at the time of birth	A direct spread of infection has occurred.
Uterus explored after birth for a retained placenta or abnormal bleeding site	The infection was introduced with exploration.

A **puerperal infection** is always potentially serious, because, although it usually begins as only a local infection, it has the potential to spread to the peritoneum (peritonitis) or the circulatory system (septicemia), conditions that can be fatal in a woman whose body is already stressed from childbirth.

Organisms commonly cultured postpartally include group B streptococci, staphylococci, and aerobic gram-negative bacilli such as *Escherichia coli*. The management for puerperal infection focuses on the use of an appropriate antibiotic after culture and sensitivity testing of the isolated organism.

Nursing Diagnoses and Related Interventions

Nursing Diagnosis: Risk for infection related to loss of uterine sterility with childbirth

Outcome Evaluation: Client's temperature remains below 100.4°F [38°C] orally, excluding the first 24 hours after birth; and lochia is present without foul odor.

To help prevent an infection, any articles such as gloves or instruments that are introduced into the birth canal during labor, birth, and the postpartal period should be sterile. In addition, adherence to standard infection precautions is essential.

Be certain to instruct a postpartal woman in proper perineal care, including wiping from front to back so that she does not bring *E. coli* organisms forward from the rectum. Use good hand washing technique before, during, and after any client care to prevent cross-contamination. When giving perineal care, both wash your hands and wear gloves. Each postpartal woman should have her own perineal supplies and should not share them to prevent the transfer of pathogens from one woman to another.

Intravenous antibiotics usually are prescribed for a postpartal infection. Frequently used antibiotics include ampicillin, gentamicin, and third-generation cephalosporins such as cefixime (Suprax). If the woman will be continuing drug therapy at home, stress that she must take the full course to prevent the infection from recurring. Be certain women who are breastfeeding are not prescribed antibiotics incompatible with breastfeeding. Alert them to observe for problems in their infant, such as white plaques or thrush (oral candidiasis) in their infant's mouth that can occur when a portion of the maternal antibiotic passes into breast milk and causes an overgrowth of fungal organisms (i.e., an opportunistic infection) in the infant. The infant also should be assessed for easy bruising because a decrease in microorganisms in the bowel caused by an antibiotic passed in breast milk may lead to insufficient vitamin K formation and, consequently, decreased blood-clotting ability.

Nursing Diagnosis: Social isolation related to precautions necessary to protect baby and others from exposure to infectious microorganisms

Outcome Evaluation: Client acknowledges agency policy regarding precautions and a willingness to comply with policies. States plans for diversional activities to pass the time if separated from her newborn; demonstrates bonding behaviors, such as asking about newborn and expressing desire to see infant.

Health care agencies have well-defined guidelines on whether a woman who has an infection should be separated from other women or her newborn. As a general rule, the baby of a mother with an increased temperature (100.4°F [38°C]) for two consecutive 24-hour periods exclusive of the first 24 hours is kept in a closed incubator in her room until the cause of the infection is determined because she may have an upper respiratory or gastrointestinal tract infection unrelated to childbearing that is transmittable to a newborn.

If the cause of the fever is found to be related to childbirth but involves a closed infection, such as thrombophlebitis, there is no danger of the baby contracting the disease so the woman may care for her child as long as she maintains the degree of prescribed bed rest necessary for her primary condition. If the infection involves drainage such as can occur with endometritis or a perineal abscess, the mother should wash her hands thoroughly before holding her infant and avoid placing her baby on the bottom bed sheet, where there may be some infected drainage from her perineal pad. Instead, furnish a clean sheet for her to spread over the covers.

If the woman develops a high fever, breast milk may become deficient. Fortunately, with modern antimicrobial therapy, the period of high fever usually is transient. If the mother is too ill to nurse her baby during this time or if she is receiving an anticoagulant or antibiotic that would be harmful to the baby, the infant should be fed by a supplementary milk formula. Urge her to manually express or pump breast milk during this time to maintain the production of milk. She may need support to do this because, if she fatigues easily, her energy level may not be enough to support her good intentions.

It's difficult for many women to accomplish their new role change even when things are going well. If a woman is segregated from others, frightened by her condition, and denied the pleasure of holding and feeding her newborn, her situation may seem overwhelming. Women who are isolated this way need friendly, understanding support from hospital personnel during such a stressful time.

Endometritis

Endometritis is an infection of the endometrium, the lining of the uterus (Jones & Henderson, 2011). Bacteria gain access to the uterus through the vagina and enter the uterus either at the time of birth or during the postpartal period. This may occur with any birth, but the infection is usually associated with chorioamnionitis and a cesarean birth (Black, Hinson, & Duff, 2012).

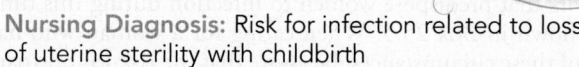

Assessment

A benign temperature elevation may occur on the first postpartal day, particularly if a woman is not drinking enough fluid. In contrast, the fever of endometritis usually manifests itself on the third or fourth postpartal day, suggesting that much of the invasion occurred during labor or birth (consistent with the time it takes for infectious organisms to grow).

Normally, the white blood cell count of a postpartal woman is increased to 20,000 to 30,000 cells/mm^3 due to the stress of labor. Because of this increase, the conventional method of detecting infection (elevated white blood cell count) is not of great value in the puerperium. Infection is suspected, instead, in postpartal women who have a temperature over 100.4°F (38°C) for two consecutive 24-hour periods. Because women may be at home when this elevated temperature occurs, be certain they know to take their temperature if they feel it is increased and to notify their primary care provider if it is elevated.

A rise in temperature that occurs on the third or fourth day postpartum occurs coincidentally at the same time as breast filling occurs. Do not be led astray by attributing an elevated temperature at this time to breast filling. Suspect fever on the third or fourth day postpartum as possible endometritis until proven otherwise.

Depending on the severity of the infection, a woman may have accompanying chills, loss of appetite, and general malaise. Her uterus usually is not well contracted and is painful to the touch. She may feel strong afterpains. Lochia usually is dark brown and has a foul odor. It may be increased in amount because of poor uterine involution, but if the infection is accompanied by high fever, lochia may, in contrast, be scant or absent. A sonogram may be prescribed to confirm the presence of placental fragments that could be a possible cause of the infection.

Therapeutic Management

When taking a culture to identify the offending organism, be certain to obtain fluid from the vagina using a sterile swab rather than from a perineal pad to ensure you are culturing the endometrial infectious organism and not an unrelated one from the pad. Treatment will consist of the administration of an appropriate antibiotic, such as clindamycin (Cleocin), as determined by the culture. An oxytocic agent such as methylergonovine may also be prescribed to encourage uterine contraction. Urge the woman to drink additional fluid to combat the fever. If strong afterpains and abdominal discomfort are present, ask if she needs an analgesic for pain relief.

Sitting in a semi-Fowler position or walking encourages lochia drainage by gravity and helps prevent pooling of infected secretions. Because any drainage on perineal pads or bed linens is contaminated, be certain to wear gloves when helping a woman change her perineal pads and changing bed linen. In addition, be certain both you and the woman use good hand washing techniques before and after handling pads.

As with any infection, endometritis can be controlled best if it is discovered early. If you can interpret the normal color, quantity, and odor of lochia discharge and the size, consistency, and tenderness of a normal postpartal uterus, you can be the first person to recognize that an infection is present. Because a woman may be at home when signs of infection occur, be certain you've taught about the signs and symptoms of endometritis before health care agency discharge.

If the infection is limited to the endometrium, the course of infection will be about 7 to 10 days. If this occurs while a woman is hospitalized, she may have to make arrangements for her baby's discharge before her own or arrange for help with newborn care when she is discharged. Be certain she knows to take the full course of antibiotics prescribed so the infection is completely eradicated and does not return.

An added danger of endometritis is that it can lead to tubal scarring and interference with future fertility. At a future time, if the woman desires more children, she may need a fertility assessment (including a sonohysterosalpingogram) to determine tubal patency. With mild endometritis, this is usually not a problem, but a woman should be forewarned that it could occur.

What if... 25.2 Just before hospital discharge on her third postpartal day, Bailey Cheshire develops a shaking chill and a fever of 101.5°F (38.6°C). She's already dressed to go home and assures you the temperature elevation is inaccurate because she just drank some hot coffee. On palpation, you notice her abdomen is tender. Would you agree with her that it's safe to be discharged?

Infection of the Perineum

If a woman has a suture line on her perineum from an episiotomy or a laceration repair, a ready portal of entry exists for bacterial invasion.

Assessment

Infections of the perineum usually remain localized. They are revealed by symptoms similar to those of any suture-line infection, such as pain, heat, and a feeling of pressure. The woman may or may not have an elevated temperature depending on the systemic effect and spread of the infection.

Inspection of the suture line will reveal inflammation. One or two stitches may have sloughed away, so an area of the suture line is open with purulent drainage present (Fig. 25.3). Notify the woman's primary care provider of the localized symptoms, and culture the discharge using a sterile cotton-tipped applicator touched to the secretions.

Therapeutic Management

Typically, either a systemic or topical antibiotic is ordered even before the culture report is returned. An analgesic may be prescribed to alleviate discomfort. It may be necessary to remove perineal sutures to open the area and allow for drainage. Sitz baths, moist warm compresses, or Hubbard tank treatments may be prescribed to hasten drainage and cleanse the area. Remind the woman to change perineal pads frequently. Because they are contaminated by drainage, if left in place too long, they might cause vaginal contamination or reinfection. Repeat again that the woman should wipe front to back after urinating or a bowel movement to prevent bringing contamination forward from the rectum onto the healing area.

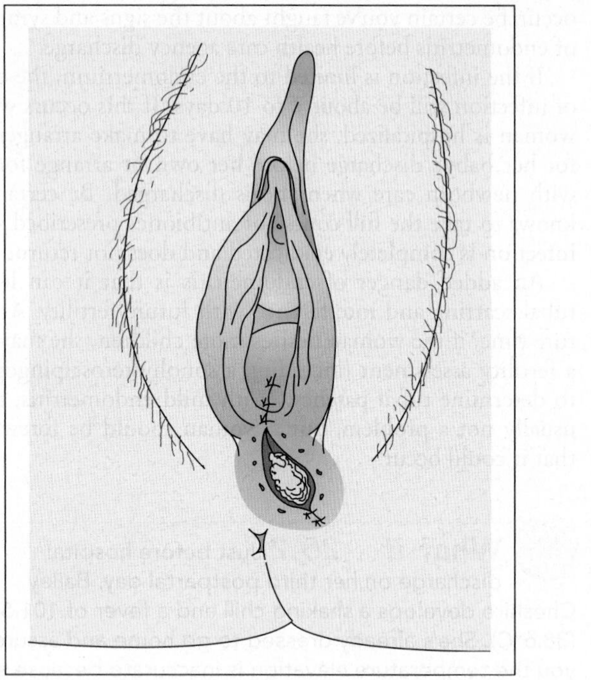

FIGURE 25.3 An infected suture line appears reddened and edematous and often contains infected secretions.

With a local infection of this nature, a woman is usually discharged with a referral for home care follow-up because the incision site, once opened, must heal by tertiary rather than by primary intention. Infections of this nature are annoying and painful, but fortunately, with improved techniques during birth and the puerperium, perineal infections occur only rarely. Because they are localized, there is no need to restrict the woman from caring for her infant as long as she washes her hands well before holding her newborn. Be certain not to place the infant on the bottom bed sheet of the woman's bed where the baby could contact pathogenic bacteria. Encourage the woman to ambulate and ask for analgesia as needed. Often, the pain from an infected suture line is severe, and the woman may decrease ambulation unless she is urged to continue.

Peritonitis

Peritonitis, or infection of the peritoneal cavity, usually occurs as an extension of endometritis. It is one of the gravest complications of childbearing and is a major cause of death from puerperal infection. The infection spreads from the uterus through the lymphatic system or directly through the fallopian tubes or uterine wall to the peritoneal cavity. An abscess may form in the cul-de-sac of Douglas because this is the lowest point of the peritoneal cavity and gravity causes infected material to localize there.

Assessment

Symptoms are the same as those of a surgical patient in whom a peritoneal infection develops: rigid abdomen, abdominal pain, high fever, rapid pulse, vomiting, and the appearance of being acutely ill. When assessing the abdomen of a postpartal woman, be sure to note not only that her uterus is well contracted but also that the remainder of her abdomen is soft because the occurrence of a rigid abdomen (i.e., guarding) is one of the first symptoms of peritonitis.

Therapeutic Management

Peritonitis is often accompanied by a paralytic ileus (a blockage of inflamed intestines). This requires insertion of a nasogastric tube to prevent vomiting and to rest the bowel. Intravenous fluid or total parenteral nutrition will then be necessary. A woman will need analgesics for pain relief and intravenous antibiotics to treat the infection. Her hospital stay will be extended, but with effective antibiotic therapy, the outcome should be good. Peritonitis can interfere with future fertility because it can leave scarring and adhesions in the peritoneum, which separate the fallopian tubes from the ovaries to the extent that ova can no longer easily enter the tubes.

QSEN Checkpoint Question 25.3

Quality Improvement

Bailey Cheshire develops endometritis. When planning nursing care, which activity would be best to advise for Bailey?

a. Walking around her room listening to music
b. Lying supine with a cold cloth on her forehead
c. Reading while resting in a slight Trendelenburg position
d. Alternating between prone and supine positions

THROMBOPHLEBITIS

Phlebitis is inflammation of the lining of a blood vessel. **Thrombophlebitis** is inflammation with the formation of blood clots. Thrombophlebitis is classified as either superficial vein disease (SVD) or deep vein thrombosis (DVT). When either type occurs in the postpartum period, it tends to occur because:

- A woman's fibrinogen level is still elevated from pregnancy, leading to increased blood clotting.
- Dilatation of lower extremity veins is still present as a result of pressure of the fetal head during pregnancy and birth so blood circulation is sluggish.

It tends to occur most often in women who:

- Are relatively inactive in labor and during the early puerperium because this increases the risk of blood clot formation
- Have spent prolonged time in a birthing room with their legs positioned in stirrups
- Have preexistent obesity and a pregnancy weight gain greater than the recommended weight gain, which can lead to inactivity and lack of exercise
- Have preexisting varicose veins
- Develop a postpartal infection
- Have a history of a previous thrombophlebitis
- Are older than age 35 years or have increased parity
- Have a high incidence of thrombophlebitis in their family
- Smoke cigarettes because nicotine causes vasoconstriction and reduces blood flow

Femoral Thrombophlebitis

With femoral thrombophlebitis, the femoral, saphenous, or popliteal veins are involved. Although the inflammation site in thrombophlebitis is a vein, an accompanying arterial spasm often occurs, diminishing arterial circulation to the leg as well. This decreased circulation, along with edema, gives the leg a white or drained appearance. It was formerly believed that breast milk drained into the leg, giving it its white appearance. The condition was, therefore, formerly called *milk leg* or *phlegmasia alba dolens* ("white inflammation").

Ambulation and limiting the time a woman remains in obstetric stirrups encourages circulation in the lower extremities, promotes venous return, and decreases the possibility of clot formation, thus helping to prevent thrombophlebitis. If stirrups on examining tables or birthing rooms are used, be certain that they are well padded to prevent any sharp pressure against the calves of the legs and that the woman remains in a lithotomy position for as short a period of time as possible. If a woman had varicose veins before or during pregnancy, wearing support stockings for the first 2 weeks after birth can help increase venous circulation and prevent stasis. If these are prescribed, be certain the woman knows to buy medical support stockings, not panty hose advertised as offering support, and to put them on before she rises in the morning. If she waits until she is already up and walking, venous congestion will have already occurred and the stockings will be less effective. Encourage her to remove the support stockings twice daily and assess her skin underneath for mottling or inflammation that would suggest inflammation of her veins.

Women are not normally prescribed acetylsalicylic acid (aspirin) for pain because aspirin is a mild anticoagulant, which interferes with blood clotting by preventing platelet aggregation and clot formation. However, women who are high risk for thrombophlebitis may be prescribed aspirin every 4 hours as a preventive measure. If this is so, be certain to not interpret aspirin used this way as an as needed (PRN) analgesic order and withhold it depending on the woman's level of pain. Other measures for preventing thrombophlebitis are summarized in Box 25.6.

Assessment

If a pelvic thrombophlebitis develops, a woman will generally have an elevated temperature, a systemic fever, chills, and pain. Comparatively, a woman experiencing a femoral thrombophlebitis will usually have unilateral localized symptoms such as redness, swelling, warmth, and a hard inflamed vessel in the affected leg. Symptoms for thrombophlebitis usually present about 10 days after birth. The woman's leg begins to swell below the lesion at the point at which venous circulation is blocked. Her skin may become so stretched from swelling that it appears shiny and white. A Homans sign (pain in the calf of the leg on dorsiflexion of the foot) may be positive; however, a negative Homans sign does not rule out obstruction. The diameter of the leg at thigh or calf level may be increased compared with the other leg. Doppler ultrasound or contrast venography will be prescribed to confirm the diagnosis (O'Connor, Scher, Gargiulo, et al., 2011).

Therapeutic Management

Treatment consists of the administration of anticoagulants, the application of moist heat (to decrease inflammation), and bed rest with the affected leg elevated. A bed cradle over the leg can lift the pressure of the bedclothes off the affected leg and can both decrease the sensitivity of the leg and improve circulation. Assess the woman for risk of a pressure ulcer and provide good back, buttocks, and heel care for as long as she is on bed rest.

Although simple in theory, application of moist compresses is, unfortunately, one of the most technically difficult treatments to carry out, because dressings invariably dry or become cold and dampen bed clothes after only a short time. Compresses and water used in this way do not have to be sterile because, with thrombophlebitis, there is no break in the skin. Because of edema in the area, be certain to test

---

BOX 25.6 Nursing Care Planning Based on Family Teaching

PREVENTING THROMBOPHLEBITIS

Q. Bailey Cheshire tells you, "My sister developed a thrombophlebitis after the birth of her first baby. How can I prevent that from happening to me?"

A. Here are a few helpful hints:

- Ask your primary care provider if you can use a side-lying or back-lying (supine recumbent) position for birth rather than a lithotomy position because a lithotomy position can increase the tendency for pooling of blood in the lower extremities.
- If you will be using a lithotomy position, ask for padding on the stirrups to prevent pressure on the calf of your legs.
- Drink adequate fluids to be certain you're not dehydrated (6–8 glasses of fluid per day).
- Do not sit with your knees crossed or bent sharply, and avoid wearing constricting clothing such as knee-high stockings.
- Ambulate as soon after birth as possible because walking is the best preventive measure. When resting in bed, wiggle your toes or do leg lifts to improve venous return.
- Ask your primary care provider if he or she recommends support stockings in the immediate postpartal period. Be certain to put these on before ambulating in the morning, before leg veins fill.
- Quit smoking, because this is associated with the development of thrombophlebitis.

water temperature by dipping your inner wrist into it before soaking a dressing to be sure it is not so warm it could cause a burn. Cover wet, warm dressings with a plastic pad to hold in heat and moisture. In addition, position a commercial pad with circulating heating coils or chemical hot packs over the plastic to ensure soaks stay warm. Be certain the weight of a hot pack or pad does not rest on the leg, causing an obstruction to flow of blood.

Never massage the skin over the clotted area because this could loosen the clot, causing a pulmonary or cerebral embolism. Check the woman's bed frequently to be certain the mattress does not become wet from seeping water. For compresses to stay in place, a woman must lay with her leg fairly immobile. However, be certain she does not interpret this as meaning she cannot turn or move about. Help her select activities to exercise the other parts of her body or stimulate her mind such as reading a good book or information on newborn care. Women who have been discharged from the hospital may be cared for at home on bed rest or may need to return to the hospital so strict bed rest can be enforced. If infection was the underlying cause of the condition, an antibiotic to treat the initial infection will be prescribed. In order to prevent further blood clotting, an anticoagulant such as unfractionated heparin (given IV) or low–molecular-weight heparin (given subcutaneously) will be prescribed. Thrombolytics (medications that dissolve clots) may also be prescribed; these should be initiated within the first 24 hours for best results. With the use of anticoagulants, a blood coagulation study will be necessary to establish a baseline value followed by sequential tests to determine the effectiveness of the drug therapy. Heparin therapy is usually continued until symptoms resolve and the international normalized ratio (INR) is >2 for at least 24 hours (Box 25.7). Be certain that protamine sulfate, the antagonist for heparin, and vitamin K, the antagonist for warfarin, are both readily available until the woman's anticoagulation therapy is stabilized.

Following this initial treatment with heparin, a woman will be discharged on subcutaneous heparin or oral anticoagulation therapy such as warfarin (Coumadin). If she will be doing her own subcutaneous injections at home, be certain she demonstrates good injection technique before discharge, is aware of complications associated with anticoagulant therapy, and understands the importance of required blood work so she schedules these appropriately.

The woman can continue to breastfeed while receiving heparin. She has to discontinue breastfeeding during therapy with Coumadin, because Coumadin-derived anticoagulants are passed in breast milk. If the thrombophlebitis does not seem to be severe and the woman wants to restart breastfeeding after the course of Coumadin (about 10 days), encourage her to manually express breast milk at the time of normal feedings so she maintains a good milk supply.

Lochia usually increases in amount in a woman who is receiving an anticoagulant. Be sure to keep a meaningful record of the amount of this discharge so that it can be estimated; "lochia serosa with scattered pinpoint clots; three perineal pads saturated in 8 hours," for example, is far more meaningful than "large amount of lochia." Also assess for other possible signs of bleeding, such as bleeding gums, ecchymotic spots on the skin, or oozing from an episiotomy suture line.

With proper treatment, the acute symptoms of femoral thrombophlebitis last only a few days, but the full course

BOX 25.7 Nursing Care Planning Based on Responsibility for Pharmacology

LOW–MOLECULAR-WEIGHT HEPARIN

Classification: Heparin is a common anticoagulant.

Action: Heparin blocks the conversion of prothrombin to thrombin and of fibrinogen to fibrin, decreasing clotting ability and resulting in the inhibition of thrombus and clot formation. It is used to prevent and treat thrombosis and pulmonary embolism (Karch, 2013).

Pregnancy Risk Category: B

Dosage: Dosage is dependent on coagulation studies. Dosage is considered therapeutic when the activated partial thromboplastin time (aPTT) is 1.5 to 3 times the control value. The drug is given by subcutaneous injection.

Possible Adverse Effects: Hemorrhage, bruising, thrombocytopenia (lowered platelet count), urticaria (hives and itching)

Nursing Implications

- Obtain coagulation studies as prescribed; *adjust dosage as necessary.*
- Heparin is usually injected into subcutaneous tissue of the abdomen. For best absorption, rotate injection sites. Do not aspirate for blood return or massage the injection site afterward to avoid bruising or hematoma formation.
- Avoid any intramuscular injection of other medications because a hematoma may form at the injection site.
- Assess a woman and alert her to self-assess for signs and symptoms of bleeding, such as oozing from the gums, nosebleeds, hematuria, or frank or occult blood in stool.
- Closely monitor client's lochia, including amount and color. Assess pad count to determine extent of vaginal bleeding.
- Keep protamine sulfate, the antidote, readily available in case of overdose.
- Instruct the woman about antibleeding precautions such as using a soft toothbrush to minimize the risk of bleeding and in the correct injection technique, and allow her to demonstrate this before health agency discharge.

of the disease takes 4 to 6 weeks before it is fully resolved. Anticoagulant therapy may need to be continued for as long as 3 to 6 months. The affected leg may never return to its former size and may always cause discomfort after long periods of standing.

Pelvic Thrombophlebitis

Pelvic thrombophlebitis involves the ovarian, uterine, or hypogastric veins. It usually follows a mild endometritis and occurs later than femoral thrombophlebitis, often around the 14th or 15th day of the puerperium. Inflammation of the blood vessels in the pelvic area causes a partial obstruction, which leads to slowed blood flow and clots in the stagnate blood in the vessel. Risk factors are the same as for femoral thrombophlebitis. The prevention of endometritis by the use of good aseptic technique during and after birth is important to help prevent the disorder (Jaiyeoba, 2012).

Assessment

With pelvic thrombophlebitis, a woman suddenly becomes extremely ill, with a high fever, chills, abdominal pain, weakness, and general malaise. Her infection can be so severe it necroses the vein and results in a pelvic abscess. In severe instances, it can become systemic and result in a lung, kidney, or heart valve abscess.

Therapeutic Management

As with femoral thrombophlebitis, therapy involves total bed rest and the administration of analgesics, antibiotics, and anticoagulants.

The disease runs a long course of 6 to 8 weeks. If an abscess forms, it can be located by sonogram and incised by laparotomy. A woman may need surgery to remove the affected vessel before she attempts to become pregnant again.

Regardless of the type of thrombophlebitis, teach women preventive measures to reduce the risk of recurrence with future pregnancies such as wearing nonconstricting clothing on their lower extremities, resting with the feet elevated, and ambulating daily. Caution a woman to tell her primary care provider before her next pregnancy of the difficulty she experienced at this time, so that extra prophylactic precautions can be taken to prevent thrombophlebitis in a future pregnancy.

✔ QSEN Checkpoint Question 25.4

Safety

Ms. Cheshire has a risk for DVT during the postpartal period. What would be the best suggestion you could make to help prevent this?

a. Rest in bed as much as possible for the first several days.
b. Assume a knee–chest position for 15 minutes every day.
c. Increase fluid intake to reduce blood viscosity.
d. Ambulate early and consistently to improve circulation.

Look in Appendix A for the best answer and rationale.

Pulmonary Embolus

A pulmonary embolus is obstruction of the pulmonary artery by a blood clot; it usually occurs as a complication of thrombophlebitis when a blood clot moves from a leg vein to the pulmonary artery (Henzler, Schoenberg, Schoepf, et al., 2012). The signs of pulmonary embolus are sudden, sharp chest pain; tachypnea; tachycardia; orthopnea (inability to breathe except in an upright position); and cyanosis (the blood clot is blocking both blood flow to the lungs and return to the heart). This is an emergency. A woman needs oxygen administered immediately and is at high risk for cardiopulmonary arrest. Her condition is extremely guarded until the clot can be lysed or adheres to the pulmonary artery wall and is reabsorbed. Because of the seriousness of this condition, a woman with a pulmonary embolism commonly is transferred to an intensive care unit for continuing care.

MASTITIS

Mastitis (infection of the breast) may occur as early as the seventh postpartal day or not until the baby is weeks or months old (Crepinsek, Crowe, Michener, et al., 2012). The organism causing the infection usually enters through cracked and fissured nipples. Therefore, to prevent mastitis, it's important to prevent nipples from cracking through measures such as:

- Making certain the baby is positioned correctly and grasps the nipple properly, including both the nipple and areola
- Helping a baby release a grasp on the nipple before removing the baby from the breast
- Washing hands between handling perineal pads and touching breasts
- Exposing nipples to air for at least part of every day
- Possibly using a vitamin E ointment daily to soften nipples
- Encouraging women to begin breastfeeding (when the infant sucks most forcefully) on an unaffected nipple (if a woman has one cracked nipple and one well nipple)

Occasionally, the organism that causes mastitis comes from the nasal–oral cavity of the infant. In these instances, the infant has usually acquired *Staphylococcus aureus*, a methicillin-resistant *Staphylococcus aureus* infection (MRSA), or candidiasis while in the hospital. The infant introduces the organisms into the milk ducts by sucking, where they proliferate (breast milk is an excellent medium for bacterial growth). Because this spreads from one person to another, this is termed epidemic mastitis or *epidemic breast abscess*. When it occurs, it is usually discovered that several women discharged from the hospital at the same time have similar infections.

Assessment

Mastitis is usually unilateral, although epidemic mastitis, because it originates with the infant, may be bilateral. The affected breast feels painful and appears swollen and reddened. Fever accompanies these first symptoms within hours, and breast milk becomes scant. If the diagnosis is not clear from the typical symptoms, the woman may have a sonogram prescribed to be certain a deep lying breast abscess isn't also present (Trop, Dugas, David, et al., 2012).

Therapeutic Management

Treatment consists of antibiotics effective against penicillin-resistant staphylococci such as dicloxacillin or a cephalosporin and, because symptoms often appear after a hospital discharge, it is treated on an outpatient basis (Summers, 2011). Breastfeeding should be continued if possible because keeping the breast emptied of milk helps to prevent the growth of bacteria. Some women find an infected breast too painful to allow their infant to suck, however, and prefer to express milk manually from the affected breast until their antibiotic has taken effect and the mastitis has diminished (about 3 days). Cold or ice compresses and a good supportive bra help with pain relief until the process improves, although warm, wet compresses can also be helpful because this reduces inflammation and edema.

If therapy is started as soon as symptoms appear, the condition runs a short course of about 2 or 3 days. If left untreated, a breast infection can become a localized abscess. If unrecognized, this can spread to involve a large portion of the breast and even rupture through the skin, with thick, purulent drainage. If an abscess forms, breastfeeding on that breast is discontinued as the abscess may need incision and drainage. Encourage women to continue to pump breast milk, if possible, until the abscess has resolved in order to preserve breastfeeding. Many women find a breast this infected too tender to do this, however, so instead choose to bottle-feed their infant. Although this is not the outcome she hoped for, you can assure a woman that formula feeding will be an acceptable alternative for this child.

Neither mastitis nor a breast abscess leaves any permanent breast disease. A woman can be assured that such an incident is not associated with the development of breast cancer and does not interfere with future breastfeeding potential. Box 25.8 shows an interprofessional care map illustrating both nursing and team planning for a woman with mastitis.

URINARY SYSTEM DISORDERS

Because a woman's bladder is compressed by the infant's head during birth, several urinary tract disorders can occur.

Urinary Retention

Urinary retention occurs when the bladder is unable to empty completely (Mulder, Schoffelmeer, Hakvoort, et al., 2012). After childbirth, bladder sensation for voiding is decreased because of bladder edema caused by the pressure of birth. This concern is compounded during prolonged labor, perineal lacerations, and the use of epidural anesthesia. Unable to empty, the bladder fills to overdistention. When the woman does void, instead of emptying completely, the bladder empties only a small portion of its contents (retention with overflow). As a result, it quickly becomes overdistended again. If it is allowed to continue, bladder overdistention can cause permanent damage to bladder tone, leading to permanent incontinence (Humburg, Troeger, Holzgreve, et al., 2011).

Assessment

In a postpartal woman, urinary retention with overflow may be more difficult to detect than primary or simple overdistention. With primary overdistention, a woman does not void at all. A longer than usual time (>8 hours) passes after birth or between voids. Assessment by percussion or palpation of the bladder reveals bladder distention.

With urinary retention and overflow, a woman is able to void. Voiding is very frequent, however, and in very small amounts, so her overall output is inadequate. Always measure the amount of a woman's first voiding after birth because, with diuresis occurring, this should be large. As a rule, if this first voiding is less than 100 ml, suspect urinary retention.

Urinary retention is confirmed by catheterizing a woman immediately after she voids. If the amount of urine left in the bladder after voiding (termed *residual*) is greater than 100 ml, the woman is retaining more than the usual amount of urine. Typically, the prescription for catheterization is written as: "Catheterize for residual urine. If this is greater than 100 ml, leave indwelling catheter in place." Always use an indwelling (Foley) catheter, rather than a temporary one (straight catheter), therefore, to catheterize for residual urine so this can be inflated and left in place. Use strict antiseptic technique to prevent introducing pathogenic bacteria into the sterile urinary tract and causing a urinary tract infection.

Catheterizing a woman during the early postpartal period can be more difficult than usual because vulvar edema often distorts the position and appearance of the urinary meatus. Use a gentle technique, remembering that a woman's perineum is apt to feel tender to the touch.

Therapeutic Management

The amount of urine to remove from an overdistended bladder is controversial. There is a suggestion that removing more than 750 to 1,000 ml of urine at any one time may create such an extreme pressure change in the lower abdomen that it causes blood to flow into the area, causing supine hypotension. There is little evidence of this actually happening, however, and particularly not in the postpartal period, when a bladder is easily distended and the uterus is larger than normal. Although this shift in pressure may not be as important as usual, follow your health care agency's policy concerning how much urine to remove from a full bladder at catheterization.

If an indwelling catheter will be left in place, be certain to explain the rationale for its insertion and how the inflated balloon will hold it in place so the woman does not limit activity and leave herself open to other complications, such as thrombophlebitis.

After 24 hours, the indwelling catheter is usually clamped for a short time, and then removed. Encourage a woman to void by the end of 6 hours after removal of the catheter by offering fluid, administering an analgesic so she can relax, assisting her to the bathroom as necessary, and trying time-tested solutions such as running water at the sink or letting her hold her hand under warm running water. In most women, bladder and vulvar edema have decreased so much by this time that they are able to void without further difficulty. If a woman has not voided by 8 hours after catheter removal, she may need reinsertion of the indwelling catheter for an additional 24 hours.

Difficulty with bladder function after childbirth is becoming less of a problem because less anesthesia and fewer forceps are used at birth, thus decreasing bladder and vulvar pressure. If problems do arise, they may be difficult for a woman to accept, because bladder elimination is a basic step of self-care and discouraging for a woman who wants to be able not only to care for herself but also a new infant. You can assure the woman that bladder complications are not uncommon after childbirth. Fortunately, they are usually present for no longer than 48 hours and most likely do not recur.

BOX 25.8 Nursing Care Planning

AN INTERPROFESSIONAL CARE MAP FOR A WOMAN WITH MASTITIS

Bailey Cheshire calls your clinic 3 weeks after childbirth because she has a fever and swelling and pain in her right breast. She comes into the clinic for an evaluation.

Family Assessment Client lives in three-bedroom apartment with boyfriend. Employed as a chemistry teacher but has not returned to work. Boyfriend is a short-order cook but is currently unemployed. Wants her to stop breastfeeding because of her infection.

Client Assessment A 30-year-old primipara woman who gave birth vaginally 3 weeks ago and is breastfeeding exclusively. Temperature 101.1°F (38.4°C). Other vital signs within acceptable parameters. Right breast reddened and edematous, tender and warm to touch. Slight fissure noted on right nipple. States, "I hurt too much to breastfeed any longer. How can I be a good mother if I don't breastfeed my baby?"

Nursing Diagnosis Pain related to development of mastitis

Outcome Criteria Client states amount of pain is decreasing with prescribed therapy; describes measures used to promote comfort. Breast swelling, redness, fever, and tenderness decrease.

Team Member Responsible	Assessment	Intervention	Rationale	Expected Outcome
Activities of Daily Living, Including Safety				
Nurse/Primary care provider	Assess extent of mastitis and whether client could continue breastfeeding with additional support.	Encourage client to continue breastfeeding on left breast. Recommend client try continuing to breastfeed on right breast.	Milk provides a medium for bacterial growth. Emptying breasts prevents stasis of milk and reduces further infection and pain.	Client states she will try to continue breastfeeding even though infection is present.
Teamwork and Collaboration				
Nurse/Lactation specialist	Assess whether client has a support person she uses for breastfeeding advice or if she would like one.	Suggest client contact the local La Leche League chapter hotline for consultation and support.	Support from experts in the technique of breastfeeding can offer helpful tips to ensure success.	Client states she will contact a support service for additional information within 2 days.
Procedures/Medications for Quality Improvement				
Nurse/Primary care provider	Assess what actions client feels will help relieve her pain best.	Instruct client in ways to apply warm moist heat, such as with a shower or warm packs, at home.	Moist heat promotes circulation to the area, decreasing inflammation, edema, and pain.	Client states she understands purpose and techniques of warm, moist heat.
Nurse	Review modifying breastfeeding strategies with mastitis.	Encourage client to nurse every 2 to 3 hours, wear a support bra, and start each infant feeding on the unaffected breast.	Beginning feeding on the unaffected breast reduces discomfort on infected breast, because infant will not suck as hard on affected breast.	Client states she will try suggested techniques.
Nutrition				
Nurse	Assess whether client understands the importance of good fluid intake for breastfeeding success.	Advise client to drink at least 8 glasses of fluid daily.	Fluid is important for breast milk formation and to prevent dehydration with fever.	Client states she has access to fluid and understands the importance of fluid intake.

(continued on page 692)

BOX 25.8 Nursing Care Planning (continued)

Patient-Centered Care				
Nurse/Nurse-midwife	Assess client's knowledge of the cause and therapy for mastitis.	Explain mastitis is not unusual postpartum and should not interfere with continued breastfeeding.	Misconceptions can negatively affect success with breastfeeding.	Client states the infection is not her fault, and she is not a "bad mother" because of it.
Psychosocial/Spiritual/Emotional Needs				
Nurse	Attempt to identify the meaning of breastfeeding to client.	Encourage client to express feelings about continuing or not continuing breastfeeding because of mastitis.	Identifying the meaning of breastfeeding assists in determining the effect a diagnosis of mastitis may have on client.	Client states she views this event as only a minor setback to her childrearing plans.
Informatics for Seamless Health Care Planning				
Nurse	Determine whether client has appointment for follow-up care.	Praise for decision-making ability to foster self-esteem. Urge boyfriend to provide breastfeeding support.	Adequate self-esteem is important to make effective childrearing decisions.	Client will discuss lack of breastfeeding support with boyfriend and keep follow-up appointment.

Urinary Tract Infections

A woman who is catheterized at the time of childbirth or during the postpartal period is prone to the development of a urinary tract infection, because bacteria may be introduced into the bladder at the time of catheterization. Pushing with labor may also have allowed some secretions to enter the urinary urethra.

Assessment

If a urinary tract infection develops, the woman notices symptoms of burning on urination, possibly blood in the urine (hematuria), and a feeling of frequency or that she always has to void. The pain feels so sharp on voiding she may resist voiding, further compounding the problem of urinary stasis. She may also have a low-grade fever and discomfort from lower abdominal pain.

Obtain a clean-catch urine specimen from any woman with symptoms of a urinary tract infection as an independent nursing action (see Nursing Care Planning Using Procedures in Chapter 11, Box 11.6). To make sure lochial discharge does not contaminate the specimen, provide a sterile cotton ball for the woman to tuck into her vagina after perineal cleansing. Be certain to ask if she removed the cotton ball after the procedure; otherwise, it could cause stasis of vaginal secretions and increase the possibility of endometritis. Mark the specimen "possibly contaminated by lochia," so that any blood in the specimen will not be overly interpreted by the laboratory technician.

Therapeutic Management

Although sulfa drugs are usually prescribed for a urinary tract infection, they are contraindicated for breastfeeding women because they can cause neonatal jaundice. Typically, therefore, a broad-spectrum antibiotic such as amoxicillin or ampicillin will be prescribed to treat a postpartal urinary tract infection. If an antibiotic contraindicated during breastfeeding is prescribed, check with a woman's primary care provider about possibly changing the antibiotic to one that is safe for breastfeeding. Otherwise, once she is home, in order to breastfeed, the woman will not take the prescribed antibiotic.

In addition to the antibiotic, encourage a woman to drink large amounts of fluid (a glass every hour) to help flush the infection from her bladder. She may need an oral analgesic, such as acetaminophen (Tylenol), to reduce the pain of urination for the next few times she voids until the antibiotic begins to have an effect and the burning sensation disappears. Otherwise, because voiding is painful, she may not drink the fluid you suggest, knowing it will increase the number of times she needs to void.

Although symptoms of a urinary tract infection decrease quickly, be certain the woman understands the importance of continuing to take the prescribed antibiotic for the full 5 to 7 days to eradicate the infection completely. Plan with the woman what will be an effective reminder system for her to use, such as a chart on her refrigerator door or a reminder signal on her smartphone, because when women are busy—and a woman caring for a newborn is busy—forgetting to take medicine is easy to do. If she stops taking the antibiotic, however, bacteria in the urine will begin to multiply again and, in another week, symptoms and the active infection will recur. Discuss with the woman common methods that all women should use to prevent urinary tract infections such as voiding after intercourse as more assurance that she can remain infection free (see Chapter 46).

What if...25.3 Eight hours after birth, Ms. Cheshire tells you that she has frequency and burning on urination. She had a urinary tract infection during pregnancy, so she recognizes the symptoms. Because she has some medicine left from pregnancy, she tells you there's no need to report her symptoms because she will take her unused medicine to cure the infection. What advice would you give her?

CARDIOVASCULAR SYSTEM DISORDERS

Because pregnancy requires major changes in the volume of blood and gestational hypertension may occur, some excess volume and pressure changes can still be present in the postpartal period.

Postpartal Gestational Hypertension

Because gestational hypertension usually develops during pregnancy, it is discussed in Chapter 21. Mild preexisting hypertension from this may increase in severity during the first few hours or days after birth. Rarely, it develops for the first time in a woman who has had no prenatal or intranatal symptoms. When this happens, the cardinal symptoms are the same as those of prenatal gestational hypertension: proteinuria, edema, and increased blood pressure (Larsen, Strong, & Farley, 2012).

The reason the condition occurs is usually retention of some placental material. The woman may be taken to surgery to have a D&C to be certain all placental fragments have been removed from her uterus. After the D&C, blood pressure often falls dramatically to normal. If not, continued treatment measures are the same as for antepartal gestational hypertension: bed rest, a quiet atmosphere, frequent monitoring of vital signs and urine output, and the administration of magnesium sulfate or an antihypertensive agent. Antihypertensive therapy can be administered in higher doses than during pregnancy because there is no longer any risk of injury to a fetus.

Seizures, if they occur postpartally as a symptom of gestational hypertension, typically develop 6 to 24 hours after birth. Seizures occurring more than 72 hours after birth are probably not the result of gestational hypertension but the result of some cause unrelated to childbearing.

Women in whom postpartal gestational hypertension develops may be bewildered by what has happened to them. If seizures occur, they are frightened to discover how little control they have over their body. They worry they will have a seizure after they are at home while holding their baby. You can assure them that gestational hypertension, although it appears late, is a condition of pregnancy, so the symptoms will fade quickly. Women with chronic hypertension need frequent monitoring during a future pregnancy to help detect gestational hypertension symptoms should these occur (Sak, Evsen, Soydinc, et al., 2012).

REPRODUCTIVE SYSTEM DISORDERS

Pregnancy has the potential to leave reproductive system organs weakened or displaced, especially in women with grand multiparity or who had an instrument birth.

Reproductive Tract Displacement

If the ligaments of the uterus are weakened because of pregnancy, they may no longer be able to maintain the uterus in its usual position or level after pregnancy, thus creating concerns such as retroflexion, anteflexion, retroversion, and anteversion or prolapse of the uterus. These uterine displacement disorders can interfere with future childbearing and fertility and may cause continued pain or a feeling of lower abdominal heaviness or discomfort.

If the walls of the vagina are weakened, a cystocele (outpouching of the bladder into the vaginal wall) or a rectocele (outpouching of the rectum into the vaginal wall) may occur (see Chapter 5, Fig. 5.7A and B). These are identified on pelvic exam or by sonogram (Chantarasorn & Dietz, 2012). If extensive, surgery to repair such conditions may be necessary. If stress incontinence (involuntary voiding on exertion) occurs, Kegel exercises to strengthen perineal muscles, injection of bulking agents, or Botox may be helpful (Elser, 2012).

Separation of the Symphysis Pubis

During pregnancy, many women feel some discomfort at the symphysis pubis because of relaxation of the joint preparatory for birth. If a fetus is unusually large or the fetal position is not optimal, the ligaments of the symphysis pubis may be so stretched by birth they actually tear. After birth, the woman experiences acute pain on turning or walking; her legs tend to rotate externally, giving her a waddling gait. A defect over the symphysis pubis can be palpated: the area is swollen and feels tender to touch (Nitsche & Howell, 2011).

Bed rest and the application of a snug pelvic binder to immobilize the joint may be necessary to relieve pain and allow healing. As with all ligament injuries, a 4- to 6-week period is necessary for healing to be complete. During this time, a woman should avoid heavy lifting; she may need to arrange for a person to help her with child care at home. She may be advised to consider a cesarean birth for any future pregnancy.

EMOTIONAL AND PSYCHOLOGICAL COMPLICATIONS OF THE PUERPERIUM

Any woman who is extremely stressed or who gives birth to an infant who in any way does not meet her expectations such as being the wrong sex, being physically or cognitively challenged, or being ill may become so depressed she has difficulty bonding with her infant. Both depression and an inability to bond is a postpartal complication with far-reaching implications, possibly affecting the future health of the entire family.

Postpartal Depression

Almost every woman notices some immediate (1 to 10 days postpartum) feelings of sadness (postpartal "blues") after childbirth. This probably occurs as a response to the anticlimactic feeling after birth and also probably is related to hormonal shifts as the levels of estrogen, progesterone, and gonadotropin-releasing hormone in her body decline.

In as many as 20% of women, however, especially in women who are disappointed in some aspect of their newborn or who have poor family support, these normal feelings continue beyond the immediate postpartal period (possibly as long as 1 year) or reflect a more serious problem than usual "baby blues." They become **postpartum depression** (Box 25.9). Depression of this type, manifested by overwhelming sadness, can occur in both new mothers and fathers (Letourneau, Tryphonopoulos, Duffett-Leger, et al., 2012). The syndrome can interfere with breastfeeding,

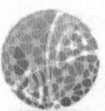

BOX 25.9 Nursing Care Planning Based on Effective Communication

Bailey Cheshire is about to be discharged from the hospital 72 hours after childbirth. You notice that, although her boyfriend visited with her, left some baby clothes, and then went downstairs to complete the discharge papers, Bailey has made no attempt to change to street clothes or dress her new baby in the baseball jersey her boyfriend left for the baby.

Less Effective Communication

Nurse: Bailey? Are you ready to leave?
Bailey: I feel too tired to go home. Are you sure I can't stay?
Nurse: Your insurance won't pay if you stay.
Bailey: How can this be right?
Nurse: What you're feeling is baby blues. Let me dress your baby so you're ready to go when your boyfriend gets back.

More Effective Communication

Nurse: Bailey? Are you ready to leave?
Bailey: I feel too tired to go home. Are you sure I can't stay?
Nurse: Tell me more about that.
Bailey: I'm so tired it feels easier for me to sit here and cry than go home, work full time, and take care of this baby.
Nurse: Is that different from how you thought things would be?
Bailey: I thought he'd ask me to marry him if I had a baby. Bet he would have if I'd had a boy instead of a girl.
Nurse: I'm worried about you going home, too.

Almost all women experience some fatigue after childbirth. As many as 70% experience a temporary feeling of sadness (baby blues). About 10%, however, develop depression severe enough to need therapy. Be sure to ask enough questions to be certain a woman's sadness is not something more serious than simple "baby blues" before she is discharged from the health care facility so she can be referred to the proper professional for help and support.

child care, and returning to a career. Both women and men may notice extreme fatigue, an inability to stop crying, increased anxiety about their own or their infant's health, insecurity (unwillingness to be left alone or inability to make decisions), psychosomatic symptoms (nausea and vomiting, diarrhea), and either depressive or extreme mood fluctuations (Meadows-Oliver, 2012) (Table 25.2). Risk factors for postpartal depression include a history of depression, a troubled childhood, low self-esteem, stress in the home or at work, a lack of effective support, different expectations between partners (e.g., if a woman wants a child and her partner does not), or disappointment in the child (e.g., a boy instead of a girl).

It is difficult to predict which women will develop postpartal depression before birth because childbirth can result in so many varied reactions. In the postpartal period, discovery of the problem as soon as symptoms develop is a nursing priority. A number of depression scales to help detect postpartum depression are available, but conscientious observation and discussion with women can reveal symptoms as well. The woman may need counseling and possibly antidepressant therapy to

TABLE 25.2 Comparing Postpartal Blues, Depression, and Psychosis

	Postpartal Blues	Postpartal Depression	Postpartal Psychosis
Onset	1–10 days after birth	1–12 months after birth	Within first year after birth
Symptoms	Sadness, tears	Anxiety, feeling of loss, sadness	Delusions or hallucinations of harming infant or self
Incidence	70% of all births	10% of all births	1%–2% of all births
Etiology (possible)	Probable hormonal changes, stress of life changes	History of previous depression, hormonal response, lack of social support	Possible activation of previous mental illness, hormonal changes, family history of bipolar disorder
Therapy	Support, empathy	Counseling, possibly drug therapy	Psychotherapy, drug therapy
Nursing role	Offer compassion and understanding	Refer to counseling	Refer to psychiatric care, safeguarding mother from injury to self and newborn

American Psychiatric Association. (2000). *Diagnostic and statistical manual of mental disorders* (4th ed.). Washington, DC: Author; Feingold, S. B. (2013). The postpartum continuum. In S. B. Feingold (Ed.), *Navigating postpartum disorders* (pp. 9–20). Far Hill, NJ: New Horizon Press.

BOX 25.10 Nursing Care Planning to Empower a Family

Q. Bailey asks you, "How can I avoid becoming depressed after I return home with my new baby?"
A. Some helpful guidelines include:

- Plan a balanced program of nutrition, exercise, and sleep. Plan meals that are easy to prepare, sleep whenever your baby sleeps, and begin a program of walking daily with your baby.
- Share your feelings with a support person. Many communities have postpartum support groups to help with this.
- Take some time every day to do something for yourself (e.g., work on a scrapbook, go shopping) so you have a break from baby care.
- Do not try to be perfect. Analyze what are the important things to do and get them done. Let unimportant things go for another day.
- Do not let yourself be isolated by baby care. Use the Internet or your cell phone to keep in contact with your friends so you are not lonely.

integrate the experience of childbirth into her life (Kurzweil, 2012). This is crucial to the development of a healthy maternal–infant bond, to the health of any other children in the family, and to overall family functioning. Ask at postpartal return visits and well-child visits about symptoms that would suggest depression, and recommend an appropriate referral. Measures to help prevent depression are shown in Box 25.10.

QSEN Checkpoint Question 25.5

Evidence-Based Practice

Postpartal depression affects not only the postpartum woman but also her entire family because fathers can become depressed during this time as well. To discover if one reason usual functioning is impaired with postpartum depression is that short-term memory is altered, researchers administered the Edinburg Postnatal Depression Scale to 395 new fathers and mothers during home visits. Results of the study revealed the prevalence of depression was 16.2% among mothers and 5.2% among fathers. Both mothers and fathers demonstrated lessened short-term memory (Pio de Almeida, Jansen, Köhler, et al., 2012). Based on the above study, which statement by Bailey's boyfriend would concern you he might be depressed the same as she seems to be?

a. "I never guessed I'd ever really be lucky enough to be a father."
b. "I call the baby 'Honey' because I keep forgetting her name."
c. "I didn't really understand the reason that Bailey bled after the baby was born."
d. "No one told me women could become depressed after birth."

Look in Appendix A for the best answer and rationale.

Postpartal Psychosis

As many as 1 woman in 500 has enough symptoms during the year after the birth of a child to be considered psychiatrically ill (this statistic seems high, but represents the current rate of overall mental illness in woman (American Psychiatric Association [APA], 2000). When the illness coincides with the postpartal period or occurs during the following year, it is termed **postpartal psychosis**. Rather than being a response to the physical aspects of childbearing, it is probably a response to the crisis of childbearing. The majority of these women have had symptoms of mental illness before pregnancy. If the pregnancy had not precipitated the illness, a death in the family, loss of a job or income, divorce, or some other major life crisis might have precipitated the same recurrence.

A woman with **postpartal psychosis** usually appears exceptionally sad. By definition, psychosis exists when a person has lost contact with reality. Because of this break with reality, the woman may deny she has had a child and, when the child is brought to her, insist she was never pregnant. She may voice thoughts of infanticide or that her infant is possessed. If observation tells you a woman is not functioning in reality, you cannot improve her concept of reality by simple measures such as explaining what her correct perception should be because her sensory input is too disturbed to comprehend this. In addition, she may interpret your contrasting opinion as threatening and respond with anger or threats. Instead, the woman needs referral to a professional psychiatric counselor and probably antipsychotic medication (Heron, Gilbert, Dolman, et al., 2012).

While waiting for such a skilled professional to arrive, do not leave the woman alone because her distorted perception might lead her to harm herself. In addition, don't leave her alone with her infant because she could harm the infant as well.

Always keep in mind when evaluating women during pregnancy or the puerperium that postpartal psychosis, although rare, does exist. Remembering childbearing can lead to this degree of mental illness helps you to put childbearing into perspective. Because it can cause such a crisis in a woman's life, it cannot be considered an everyday incident in anyone's life.

QSEN Checkpoint Question 25.6

Patient-Centered Care

You are making an effort to address Bailey Cheshire's psychosocial health in addition to her physiologic well-being. Which of her statements would be most suggestive of possible postpartal psychosis?

a. "I wish my baby had longer hair."
b. "I've felt exhausted ever since birth."
c. "I'm happy not to have any children."
d. "Breastfeeding is way harder than I thought."

Look in Appendix A for the best answer and rationale.

Women With Unique Postpartal Care Needs

A number of women have unique postpartal needs because of unexpected circumstances

The Woman Whose Child Is Born With an Illness or a Physical Challenge

Immediately after birth, the average woman often has momentary difficulty believing that her pregnancy is finally over and her child has been born. This difficulty can be compounded for a woman whose child is challenged in some way because she must not only grasp the fact that her baby has been born but also that her baby is different from the one she envisioned (Snodgrass, 2012).

During pregnancy, most women say they do not care about the sex of their child as long as the child is born healthy. This can make them feel cheated or disappointed when this one requirement is not met. They may experience a loss of self-esteem: they have given birth to an imperfect child and so they see themselves as imperfect. A woman sometimes responds with a grief reaction, as if her child had died because the image of the "perfect" child she thought she was carrying *has* died.

Parents should be shown their child moments after birth so if a condition or problem exists, the newborn's condition, prognosis, and usual plans for care can be immediately explained to them. Although hearing such an explanation is a shock to couples, it allows them to face the problem as early as possible and while they are surrounded by professional support people. The primary care provider usually makes it her or his responsibility to tell the parents about the infant's concern. Be prepared to reinforce this information or review the explanation during the postpartum period because people who are under stress are not good listeners and may need repeated explanations before they completely understand the problem.

Encourage the parents to care for the child during the postpartal period, so they can touch, relate to, and "claim" the infant in as nearly normal a manner as possible. Many women wait until their support person is present to visit an intensive care nursery so that visiting with their ill newborn is a family activity.

Open lines of communication between the parents and the hospital staff, which allow for free discussion of feelings and fears, will do much to strengthen parent–child relationships and prepare for future hospitalizations or care of the child.

The Woman Whose Newborn Has Died

A woman whose newborn dies at birth always has questions about what happened. She is likely to feel bewildered, perhaps bitter, and perhaps resentful that, despite emergency interventions, the hospital staff was not able to save her child. She asks, "Why me? Of all the women here, why was my baby the one who died?" She and her family need concerned support from health care personnel to help them cope with such a devastating loss (Avelin, Erlandsson, Hildingsson, et al., 2011).

Most women are interested in seeing the baby. This is generally therapeutic because it helps them begin grieving. Clean the baby, wrap the baby in an infant blanket, and bring him or her to the parents. Remain with them, but give them time to handle and inspect the child as they wish. Parents may want to take a photograph or a lock of hair for a memory book. Be familiar with the forms the mother or father have to sign when a baby dies or is born dead. Know whether your state requires stillborn infants to be given a name and a burial.

Other women on the unit tend to stay away from a woman whose child has died, as if what happened to her baby is contagious. Friends and relatives may be equally unable to talk about the situation. Most women, therefore, are anxious to have a nurse approach them and say, "Do you want to talk about what's happened?" Be careful not to use trite sympathy phrases such as, "One door closes, another one opens" or "God must have another purpose for you" because, although these may be your beliefs, they may not be the woman's beliefs.

Provide a private room for the family to allow them an opportunity to grieve and visit freely as they begin to work through this potentially devastating event in their life. The process of grieving and the support a woman requires at this time is further discussed in Chapter 56.

What if...25.4 You are particularly interested in exploring one of the 2020 National Health Goals with respect to complications of the puerperium (see Box 25.1). What would be a possible research topic to explore pertinent to this goal that would be applicable to Bailey's family and that would also advance evidence-based practice?

KEY POINTS FOR REVIEW

- Hemorrhage (defined as a loss of blood greater than 500 ml within a 24-hour period) is a major potential danger in the immediate postpartal period. The most frequent causes of postpartal hemorrhage are uterine atony or a retained placental fragment. Continuous limited blood loss can be as important as sudden, intense bleeding. Administration of oxytocin or carboprost tromethamine may be necessary to initiate uterine tone and halt the bleeding.
- Other causes of hemorrhage include lacerations (vaginal, cervical, or perineal) and DIC. Lacerations are most apt to occur with an instrument birth or with the birth of a large infant.
- Puerperal infection (a temperature greater than 100.4°F [38.0°C]) after the first 24 hours is a potential complication after any birth until the denuded placental surface has healed. Retained placental fragments and the use of internal fetal monitoring leads are potential sources of infection.
- Thrombophlebitis, an inflammation of the lining of a blood vessel, occurs most often as an extension of an endometrial infection. Therapy includes bed rest with moist heat applications and anticoagulant therapy. *Never massage the leg of a woman with thrombophlebitis.* Doing so can cause the clot to move and become a pulmonary embolus, which is a possibly fatal complication.
- Mastitis is an infection of the breast. The symptoms include pain, swelling, and redness. Antibiotic therapy is necessary to promote healing.
- Postpartal "blues" are a normal accompaniment to birth. Postpartal depression (a feeling of extreme sadness) and postpartal psychosis (an actual separation from reality) are not normal and need accurate assessment so a woman can receive adequate therapy for these conditions.

- A woman whose child dies at birth or is born with a physical or cognitive challenge needs special consideration after birth. This obviously creates a time of stress, and a woman needs supportive nursing care.
- Establishing a firm family–newborn relationship may be difficult when a woman has a postpartal complication. Planning nursing care that allows a woman to care for her baby and begin her new family role not only meets QSEN competencies but also best meets a family's total needs.

Critical Thinking Care Study

Jonella is a 37-year-old gravida 5, para 5 who gave birth to a boy (8 lb, 6 oz) last night. You enter her postpartum room because you've noticed her newborn has been crying for some time. You find Jonella lying in bed reading from an electronic reader, seemingly unaware that her baby, swaddled in a bassinette at the foot of the bed, is crying. When you ask her if she would like some help with her newborn, she sighs as if exhausted, slowly puts down her reader, and says, "I'm waiting for someone to bring him a bottle." Jonella's chart shows she's not going to breastfeed because she has four other children (10, 8, 5, and 2 years of age) at home. Her husband's occupation is listed as a maintenance man on a Gulf of Mexico oil rig. Because her labor only lasted 6 hours, he wasn't able to get home in time to be with her in labor. Her mother also couldn't come because she is watching Jonella's other children.

1. Jonella seems less than pleased to have had a new baby. Is her attitude typical for a mother having her fifth child or would you want to investigate mother–newborn bonding further?
2. Jonella had an episiotomy for birth and so has painful perineal stitches. She's had urinary retention since birth and has a Foley catheter inserted. When her husband arrives, you notice he is enthusiastic about having a boy because now he has a "basketball team of boys." He confides to you the only reason his wife consented to have another child was because she was certain this one would be the girl she always wanted. He tells you, "Guess she's pretty depressed." Could Jonella's lack of interest in her baby be the beginning of postpartal depression? What risk factors does she have for developing this?
3. Jonella will be discharged tomorrow. Her husband will be back at work in 3 days, and her mother has arthritis and so is "little help." In addition to developing postpartal depression, for what other postpartal complications is Jonella high risk?

Patient Scenario

The Barth Family

Read about the Barth family, a family with an adolescent who is experiencing a postpartal complication, then answer the questions to further sharpen your skills and grow more familiar with NCLEX-type questions related to postpartal complications. Confirm your answers are correct by reading the rationales.

Visit http://thePoint.lww.com

Answers and Rationales

Looking for answers to the What If. . . and Critical Thinking Care Study questions?

Visit http://thePoint.lww.com

References

American Congress of Obstetricians & Gynecologists: Committee on Obstetric Practice. (2012). Committee opinion no. 529: Placenta accreta. *Obstetrics & Gynecology, 120*(1), 207–211.

American Psychiatric Association. (2000). *Diagnostic and statistical manual of mental disorders* (4th ed.). Washington, DC: Author.

Andreatta, P., Perosky, J., & Johnson, T. R. (2012). Two-provider technique for bimanual uterine compression to control postpartum hemorrhage. *Journal of Midwifery & Women's Health, 57*(4), 371–375.

Andrighetti, T. (2013). Postpartum hemorrhage: Best practices in management. In B. A. Anderson & S. Stone (Eds.), *Best practices in midwifery* (pp. 243–256). New York, NY: Springer Publishing.

Avelin, P., Erlandsson, K., Hildingsson, I., et al. (2011). Swedish parents' experiences of parenthood and the need for support to siblings when a baby is stillborn. *Birth, 38*(2), 150–158.

Balayla, J., & Bondarenko, H. D. (2012). Placenta accreta and the risk of adverse maternal and neonatal outcomes. *Journal of Perinatal Medicine, 15*(12), 1–9.

Black, L. P., Hinson, L., & Duff, P. (2012). Limited course of antibiotic treatment for chorioamnionitis. *Obstetrics & Gynecology, 119*(6), 1102–1105.

Brown, A., & Jordan, S. (2012). Impact of birth complications on breastfeeding duration: An internet survey. *Journal of Advanced Nursing, 69*(4), 828–839.

Bryant, A., Mhyre, J. M., Leffert, L. R., et al. (2012). The association of maternal race and ethnicity and the risk of postpartum hemorrhage. *Anesthesia & Analgesia, 115*(5), 1127–1136.

Chantarasorn, V., & Dietz, H. P. (2012). Diagnosis of cystocele type by clinical examination and pelvic floor ultrasound. *Ultrasound in Obstetrics & Gynecology, 39*(6), 710–714.

Chelmow, D. (2011). Postpartum haemorrhage: Prevention. *Clinical Evidence, 4*(4), 2011–2012.

Crepinsek, M. A., Crowe, L., Michener, K., et al. (2012). Interventions for preventing mastitis after childbirth. *Cochrane Database of Systemic Reviews*, (10), CD007239.

Edmonds, D. K. (2012). Puerperium and lactation. In D. K. Edmonds (Ed.) *Dewhurst's textbook of obstetrics & gynaecology* (8th ed., pp. 365–376). Oxford: John Wiley & Son.

Elser, D. M. (2012). Stress urinary incontinence and overactive bladder syndrome: Current options and new targets for management. *Postgraduate Medicine, 124*(3):42–49.

Feingold, S. B. (2013). The postpartum continuum. In S. B. Feingold, *Navigating postpartum disorders* (pp 9–20). Far Hill, NJ: New Horizon Press.

Furuta, M., Sandall, J. & Bick, D. (2012). A systematic review of the relationship between severe maternal morbidity and post-traumatic stress disorder. *BMC Pregnancy & Childbirth, 12*(1):125.

Ghirardini, G., Alboni, C. & Mabrouk, M. (2012). Use of balloon tamponade in management of severe vaginal postpartum hemorrhage and vaginal hematoma: A case series. *Gynecology & Obstetric Investigation, 74*(4):320–323.

Henzler, T., Schoenberg, S. O., Schoepf, U. J., et al. (2012). Diagnosing acute pulmonary embolism: Systematic review of evidence base and cost-effectiveness of imaging tests. *Journal of Thoracic Imaging, 27*(5):304–314.

Heron, J., Gilbert, N., Dolman, C., et al. (2012). Information and support needs during recovery from postpartum psychosis. *Archives of Women's Mental Health, 15*(3):155–165.

Humburg, J., Troeger, C., Holzgreve, W., et al. (2011). Risk factors in prolonged postpartum urinary retention. *Archives of Gynecology & Obstetrics, 283*(2):179–183.

Jaiyeoba, O. (2012). Postoperative infections in obstetrics and gynecology. *Clinical Obstetrics & Gynecology, 5*(4):904–913.

Jones, V. A. & Henderson, J. (2011). Gestational Complications. In K. J. Hurt, M. W. Guile, J. L. Bienstock, et al. (Eds.). *The Johns Hopkins Manual of Gynecology and Obstetrics* (4th ed., pp. 110–121). Philadelphia: Lippincott Williams & Wilkins.

Karch, A. M. (2013). 2013 *Lippincott's nursing drug guide.* Philadelphia, PA: Lippincott Williams & Wilkins.

Kurzweil, S. (2012). Psychodynamic therapy for depression in women with infants and young children. *American Journal of Psychotherapy, 66*(2), 181–199.

Laas, E., Bui, C., Popowski, T., et al. (2012). Trends in the rate of invasive procedures after the addition of the intrauterine tamponade test to a protocol for management of severe postpartum hemorrhage. *American Journal of Obstetrics & Gynecology, 207*(4), 281.e1–281.e7.

Larsen, W. I., Strong, J. E., & Farley, J. H. (2012). Risk factors for late postpartum preeclampsia. *Journal of Reproductive Medicine, 57*(1–2), 35–38.

Letourneau, N., Tryphonopoulos, P. D., Duffett-Leger, L., et al. (2012). Support intervention needs and preferences of fathers affected by postpartum depression. *Journal of Perinatal & Neonatal Nursing, 26*(1), 69–80.

Meadows-Oliver, M. (2012). Screening for postpartum depression at pediatric visits. *Journal of Psychosocial Nursing & Mental Health Services, 50*(9), 4–5.

Mulder, F. E., Schoffelmeer, M. A., Hakvoort, R. A., et al. (2012). Risk factors for postpartum urinary retention: A systematic review and meta-analysis. *BJOG: International Journal of Obstetrics & Gynaecology, 119*(12), 1440–1446.

Nitsche, J. F., & Howell, T. (2011). Peripartum pubic symphysis separation: A case report and review of the literature. *Obstetrics & Gynecology Survey, 66*(3), 153–158.

Nove, A., Berrington, A., & Matthews, Z. (2012). Comparing the odds of postpartum haemorrhage in planned home birth against planned hospital birth: Results of an observational study of over 500,000 maternities in the UK. *BMC Pregnancy & Childbirth, 12*(1), 130.

O'Connor, D. J., Scher, L. A., Gargiulo, N. J. 3rd, et al. (2011). Incidence and characteristics of venous thromboembolic disease during pregnancy and the postnatal period: A contemporary series. *Annals of Vascular Surgery, 25*(1):9–14.

Omole-Ohonsi, A., & Olayinka, H. T. (2012). Emergency peripartum hysterectomy in a developing country. *Journal of Obstetrics & Gynaecology Canada, 34*(10), 954–960.

Pio de Almeida, L. S., Jansen, K., Köhler, C. A., et al. (2012). Working and short-term memories are impaired in postpartum depression. *Journal of Affective Disorders, 136*(3), 1238–1242.

Poggi, S. B. H. (2012). Postpartum hemorrhage & the abnormal puerperium. In A. H. DeCherney, L. Nathan, T. M. Goodwin, et al., (Eds.). *Current diagnosis and treatment: Obstetrics and gynecology* (11th ed., pp. 349–368). Columbus, OH: McGraw-Hill/Lange.

Roach, M. K., Abramovici, A., & Tita, A. T. (2012). Dose and duration of oxytocin to prevent postpartum hemorrhage. *American Journal of Perinatology.* Advance online publication.

Sak, M. E., Evsen, M. S., Soydinc, H. E., et al. (2012). Risk factors for maternal mortality in eclampsia: Analysis of 167 eclamptic cases. *European Review for Medical & Pharmacological Sciences, 16*(10), 1399–1403.

Snodgrass, J. L. (2012). A psychospiritual, family-centered theory of care for mothers in the NICU. *Journal of Pastoral Care & Counseling, 66*(1), 1–11.

Su, L. L., Chong, Y. S., & Samuel, M. (2012). Carbetocin for preventing postpartum haemorrhage. *Cochrane Database of Systematic Reviews,* (4), CD005457.

Summers, A. (2011). Managing mastitis in the emergency department. *Emergency Nurse, 19*(6), 22–25.

Trop, I., Dugas, A., David, J., et al. (2012). Breast abscesses: Evidence-based algorithms for diagnosis, management, and follow-up. *Radiographics, 31*(6), 1683–1699.

U.S. Department of Health and Human Services. (2010). *Healthy people 2020.* Washington, DC: Author.

Chapter 26

Nursing Care of a Family With a High-Risk Newborn

KEY TERMS

- acute bilirubin encephalopathy (ABE)
- apnea
- apparent life-threatening event
- appropriate for gestational age (AGA)
- brown fat
- caudal regression syndrome
- developmental care
- dysmature
- extracorporeal membrane oxygenation (ECMO)
- fetal alcohol spectrum disorder
- gestational age
- hemorrhagic disease of the newborn
- hydrops fetalis
- hyperbilirubinemia
- intrauterine growth restriction (IUGR)
- large for gestational age (LGA)
- low–birth-weight infant (LBW)
- macrosomia
- ophthalmia neonatorum
- periodic respirations
- periventricular leukomalacia (PVL)
- postterm infant
- postterm syndrome
- preterm infants
- retinopathy of prematurity (ROP)
- shoulder dystocia
- small for gestational age (SGA)
- term infants
- very-low-birth-weight infant (VLBW)

OBJECTIVES

After mastering the contents of this chapter, you should be able to:

1. Define the common classifications of high-risk infants and describe common illnesses that occur in these classifications of newborns.
2. Identify 2020 National Health Goals related to high-risk newborns that nurses can help the nation achieve.
3. Assess a high-risk newborn to determine whether safe transition to extrauterine life has occurred.
4. Formulate nursing diagnoses related to a high-risk newborn and family.
5. Identify expected outcomes for a high-risk newborn and family to help parents manage seamless transitions across differing health care settings.
6. Using the nursing process, plan nursing care that includes the six competencies of Quality & Safety Education for Nurses (QSEN): Patient-Centered Care, Teamwork & Collaboration, Evidence-Based Practice (EBP), Quality Improvement (QI), Safety, and Informatics.
7. Implement nursing care for a high-risk newborn, such as monitoring body temperature.
8. Evaluate expected outcomes for achievement and effectiveness of care.
9. Integrate knowledge of the needs of a high-risk newborn with the interplay of nursing process, the six competencies of QSEN, and Family Nursing to promote quality maternal and child health nursing care.

Mr. and Mrs. Atkins are the parents of a 30-week-gestation, 2-lb baby boy born last night after a short, 4-hour labor. Their baby took a few gasping respirations at birth but then stopped breathing. He was resuscitated by the neonatal nurse practitioner and respiratory therapist and then transported to the intensive care nursery. Mr. Atkins was not present for the birth because he was out of town on business. You notice Mrs. Atkins has not visited the intensive care nursery to see her son. She has also refused to fill in the birth certificate because she tells you, "I don't want to give him our favorite name because he might die." Mr. Atkins called early this morning and acted more upset that the baby was born than relieved the baby was receiving intensive care. You hear him ask his wife, "Did you do something to cause this?"

Previous chapters described the birth and care of well newborns. This chapter adds information on the care of newborns who are ill or who are born with a significant variation in gestational age or weight. Learning to recognize these infants at birth

(Continued on next page)

(Continued from previous page)

and organizing care for them can be instrumental in helping protect both their present and future health.

What type of help does the Atkins family need to better accept what has happened to them?

During pregnancy, screening women for risk factors such as younger or older than average maternal age, having concurrent disease conditions such as diabetes or HIV infection, experiencing pregnancy complications such as placenta previa, or an unhealthy maternal lifestyle such as drug abuse—all of which could lead to illness in a newborn—is essential to identify infants who may need greater than usual care at birth (Alves, Cisneiros, Dutra, et al., 2012; Hoppe, 2013).

Unfortunately, not all instances of high risk can be predicted during pregnancy or birth, because even a newborn from a "perfect" pregnancy may require specialized care or may develop a problem over the first few days of life, necessitating special interventions. Any infant, especially one who is born **dysmature**, whether preterm, term, or postterm, is at risk for complications at birth or in the first few days of life. Parents need a thorough explanation of their baby's health because these problems may require rehospitalization or additional follow-up at home. Because preterm birth, in particular, has the potential for leading to high-risk newborns, several 2020 National Health Goals directly concern preterm births (Box 26.1).

Being able to predict if an infant is at high risk allows for advanced preparation so that specialized, skilled health care personnel can be present at the child's birth to perform necessary interventions, such as resuscitating a newborn who has difficulty establishing respirations. Immediate, skilled handling of any problems that occur may help to save the newborn's life and also prevent future problems, such as neurologic disorders (Doyle & Bradshaw, 2012).

BOX 26.1 Nursing Care Planning Based on 2020 National Health Goals

A preterm birth has the potential for leading to so many complications in newborns that several 2020 National Health Goals were written specifically concerning preterm birth:

- Reduce low birth weight (LBW) to an incidence of no more than 7.8% of live births and very low birth weight (VLBW) to an incidence of no more than 1.4% of live births from baselines of 8.2% and 1.5%, respectively.
- Increase the proportion of VLBW infants born at level III hospitals or subspecialty perinatal centers from a baseline of 76.1% to a target level of 83.7%.
- Reduce the rate of fetal and infant deaths during the perinatal period (28 weeks of gestation to 7 days or more after birth) to 5.9 per 1,000 live births from a baseline of 6.6 per 1,000 live births.
- Reduce the rate of deaths from sudden infant death syndrome (SIDS) to 0.5 per 1,000 live births from a baseline of 0.55 per 1,000 live births (U.S. Department of Health and Human Services [DHHS], 2010; see www.healthypeople.gov).

Nurses can help the nation achieve these goals by teaching women the symptoms of preterm labor so that, ideally, birth can be delayed until infants reach term. Nurses also need to be prepared for resuscitation at birth for high-risk infants and to plan developmental care that can help prevent conditions such as apnea, intraventricular hemorrhage, and periventricular leukomalacia.

Nursing Process Overview

Assessment

All infants need to be assessed at birth for obvious congenital anomalies and **gestational age** (number of weeks they remained in utero). Both determinations can be done by the nurse who first examines an infant. Be certain such a first assessment is done under a prewarmed radiant heat warmer to guard against heat loss.

Continuing assessment of high-risk infants involves the use of instrumentation such as cardiac, apnea, oxygen saturation, and blood pressure monitoring. No matter how many monitors are used, however, they never replace the role of frequent, close, common sense observations by a nurse who knows an infant well from having cared for the baby consistently over time because such a nurse often senses changes before a monitor or other equipment begins to put a quantitative measurement on the factor. Carefully evaluate comments from fellow nurses such as an infant "isn't himself" or "breathes oddly." These comments, although not evidence based, are the same observations that parents who know their baby well report at health care visits.

Nursing Diagnosis

To establish nursing diagnoses for high-risk infants, it is important to be aware of the usual parameters of newborns. Examples of nursing diagnoses that center on the priority areas of care for all newborns include:

- Ineffective airway clearance related to the presence of mucus or amniotic fluid in the airway
- Ineffective tissue oxygenation related to breathing difficulty
- Ineffective thermoregulation related to immature status
- Risk for deficient fluid volume related to insensible water loss
- Risk for imbalanced nutrition, less than body requirements, related to the lack of strength for effective sucking

- Risk for infection related to lowered immune response due to prematurity
- Risk for impaired parenting related to illness in newborn at birth
- Deficient diversional activity (lack of stimulation) related to illness at birth
- Readiness for developmental care to decrease overstimulation easily caused by necessary lifesaving procedures

Outcome Identification and Planning

Be certain when establishing expected outcomes that they are consistent with a newborn's potential. A goal that implies complete recovery from a major illness, for example, may be unrealistic for one newborn but completely appropriate for another. Be certain plans for care are individualized considering a newborn's developmental as well as physiologic strengths, weaknesses, and needs. Many families of high-risk newborns will need continued support to care for their infants at home and so need referral to a home health care or other agency. Helpful Internet sites to use for referring parents are the March of Dimes (www.marchofdimes.com), the American Sudden Infant Death Syndrome (SIDS) Institute (www.sids.org), and the Newborn Individualized Developmental Care and Assistance Program (NIDCAP) Federation International (www.nidcap.org).

Implementation

Interventions for any high-risk newborn are best carried out by a consistent caregiver and should focus on conserving the baby's energy and providing a thermoneutral environment to prevent exhaustion and chilling. Painful procedures should be kept to a minimum to help the infant achieve a sense of comfort and balance. Assisting parents to participate in care such as bathing or feeding their infant can help make the child real to them for the first time and can set the stage for effective bonding.

Outcome Evaluation

High-risk newborns need long-term follow-up so any consequences of their birth status, such as minimal neurologic injury, can be identified, and arrangements for special schooling or counseling can be made. Examples of expected outcomes include:

- Infant maintains a patent airway.
- Infant demonstrates an ability to suck effectively.
- Infant tolerates procedures without accompanying apnea, bradycardia, or oxygen desaturation.
- Infant demonstrates growth and development appropriate for gestational age, birth weight, and condition.
- Infant maintains a body temperature of 98.6°F (37.0°C) in an open crib with one added blanket.
- Parents visit at least once and make three telephone calls to the neonatal nursery weekly.
- Parents demonstrate positive coping skills and behaviors in response to the newborn's condition and ability to care for their newborn.

NEWBORN PRIORITIES IN THE FIRST DAYS OF LIFE

All newborns have a number of needs in the first few days of life that take priority. They include:

1. Initiation and maintenance of respirations
2. Establishment of extrauterine circulation
3. Maintenance of fluid and electrolyte balance
4. Control of body temperature
5. Intake of adequate nourishment
6. Establishment of waste elimination
7. Prevention of infection
8. Establishment of an infant–parent/caregiver relationship
9. Institution of developmental care, or care that balances physiologic needs and stimulation for best development

These same needs are also the primary needs of high-risk newborns. Because of small size or immaturity or illness, however, fulfilling these needs may require special equipment or care measures. Not all newborns will be able to achieve full wellness because of extreme insults to their health during pregnancy or at birth or difficulty adjusting to extrauterine life. Indications a newborn is having difficulty making the immediate transition from intrauterine to extrauterine life may be first apparent by a low Apgar score rating (see Chapter 18).

Initiating and Maintaining Respirations

Ultimately, the prognosis of a high-risk newborn depends primarily on how the first moments of life are managed because most deaths occurring during the first 48 hours after birth result from the newborn's inability to establish or maintain adequate respirations (National Vital Statistics Service [NVSS], 2011). An infant who has difficulty accomplishing effective respiratory action this way and yet survives may experience residual neurologic difficulties because of cerebral hypoxia. Therefore, prompt, thorough, and immediate care is necessary for the best outcome.

Most infants are born with some degree of respiratory acidosis. However, this initial acidosis is rapidly corrected by the spontaneous onset of respirations. If respiratory activity does not begin immediately, respiratory acidosis not only doesn't fade but also increases in amount so much that the blood pH and bicarbonate buffer system can fail. Newborn defense mechanisms then become inadequate to reverse the process. This means the effort to establish respirations must be started immediately after birth because, by 2 minutes, the development of severe acidosis is already well under way (Thilo & Rosenberg, 2012).

Any infant who sustains any degree of asphyxia in utero, such as could occur from cord compression, maternal anesthesia, placenta previa, intrauterine growth restriction, or preterm separation of the placenta, may already be experiencing acidosis at birth and may have difficulty before the first 2 minutes of life.

An additional concern that ineffective respirations creates is the failure of fetal circulatory shunts, particularly the ductus arteriosus, to close. Because left-side heart pressure is stronger than right-side pressure, blood then circulates through the patent ductus arteriosus from the left to right or from the aorta to the pulmonary artery, thus creating ineffective pump action in the heart. Struggling to breathe and circulate blood, the infant is forced to use available serum glucose quickly and so may become hypoglycemic, compounding the initial problem even further.

BOX 26.2 Factors Predisposing Infants to Respiratory Difficulty in the First Few Days of Life

- Low birth weight
- Intrauterine growth restriction
- Maternal history of diabetes
- Premature rupture of membranes
- Maternal use of barbiturates or narcotics close to birth
- Meconium staining
- Irregularities detected by fetal heart monitor during labor
- Cord prolapse
- Lowered Apgar score (<7) at 1 or 5 minutes
- Postmaturity (postterm)
- Small for gestational age
- Breech birth
- Multiple birth
- Chest, heart, or respiratory tract anomalies

For all these reasons, resuscitation is important for both infants who fail to take a first breath and for those who have difficulty maintaining adequate respiratory movements on their own (Raab & Kelly, 2013). Common factors that predispose infants to respiratory difficulty and so may require resuscitation are shown in Box 26.2.

Resuscitation

Between 5% and 10% of newborns require some assistance to begin breathing at birth, but less than 1% require extensive resuscitative measures (Leone & Finer, 2012). In order that newborn resuscitation can be consistent from infant to infant and one facility to the next, the American Academy of Pediatrics (AAP) has instituted a Neonatal Resuscitation Program updated at intervals that lists steps and rationales for newborn resuscitation (McGowan, 2012).

Based on these recommendations, resuscitation should follow an organized process: (a) establish an airway, (b) expand the lungs, and (c) initiate and maintain effective ventilation. If respiratory depression becomes so severe that a newborn's heart begins to fail (heart rate is under 100 beats/min), resuscitation should then also include cardiac massage (Kattwinkel, Perlman, Azia, et al., 2010).

Airway

For a well, term newborn, usually warming, drying, and stimulating the baby by rubbing the back is enough to initiate respirations. A rubber bulb syringe is a standard piece of equipment in most birthing rooms and was often used in the past to suction infants' noses and mouths, but because bradycardia can be associated with bulb suctioning, routine suctioning of the nose and mouth is no longer recommended (Perlman, Wyllie, Kattwinkel, et al., 2010).

If a newborn does not draw in a first breath spontaneously following gentle stimulation, place the infant under a radiant heat warmer in a "sniffing" position (head slightly tipped back) and rub and dry his or her back and hair again to see if this additional stimulation initiates respirations. Assess a precordial pulse over the heart and attach a pulse oximeter to monitor heart rate and oxygen saturation.

A newborn whose amniotic fluid was meconium stained at birth but is breathing does not need suctioning to clear the airway. You may need to place an infant with meconium staining who is not breathing on the back and slide a folded towel or pad under the shoulders to raise the infant slightly so the head is in a neutral position. Slide a catheter (#8F to 12F) over the infant's tongue to the back of the throat and suction using low pressure (Fig. 26.1). Do not suction for longer than 10 seconds at a time (count seconds as you suction) to avoid removing excessive air from an infant's lungs. Be gentle because bradycardia or cardiac arrhythmias can occur from vagus stimulation (at the posterior oropharynx). In most newborns, this degree of resuscitation will initiate responsive respirations and a strong heartbeat (over 100 beats/min). Color, muscle response, and reflexes will all improve.

As a rule, do not administer air under pressure to an infant born with meconium-stained amniotic fluid because, in these infants, assuming they may have aspirated some amniotic fluid, air under pressure could push meconium down into the trachea and create a blockage. Wait for a laryngoscope to be inserted and the trachea deep suctioned to remove any meconium; at that point, air under pressure is safe to administer.

An infant who still makes no effort at spontaneous respirations after these initial steps requires immediate ventilation with air to open the airway. An endotracheal tube may need to be inserted to be certain the airway is not obstructed so air can be effectively administered. If the heart rate or oxygen saturation levels remain low with air, oxygen may be administered. In the preterm infant, however, don't use 100% oxygen; use 90%. In an infant below 32 weeks of gestation, use 30% oxygen. If only 100% oxygen is available, it is safer to administer only air (Perlman et al., 2010).

In the first few seconds of life, a newborn this severely depressed may take several weak gasps of air and then almost immediately stop breathing; the heart rate begins to fall. This period of halted respirations is termed *primary apnea*. After 1 or 2 minutes of **apnea** (defined as a pause in respirations longer than 20 seconds with accompanying bradycardia), an infant

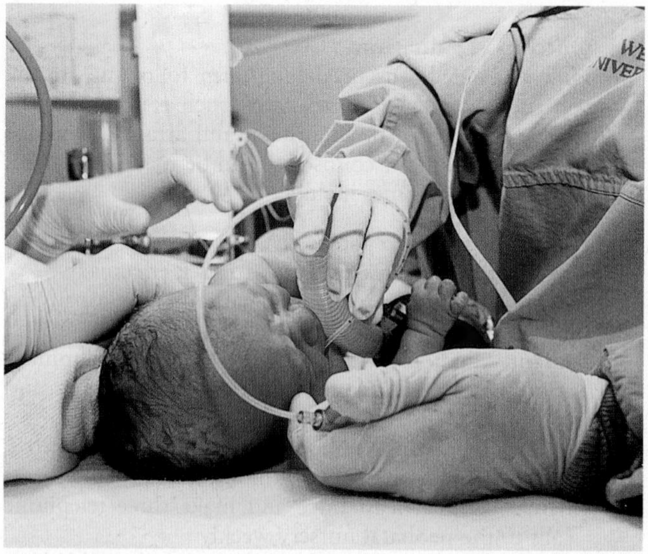

FIGURE 26.1 Suctioning a newborn with mechanical suction controlled by a finger valve. The suction is applied as the catheter is withdrawn. If the catheter is rotated as it is withdrawn, the risk of traumatizing the membrane is reduced.

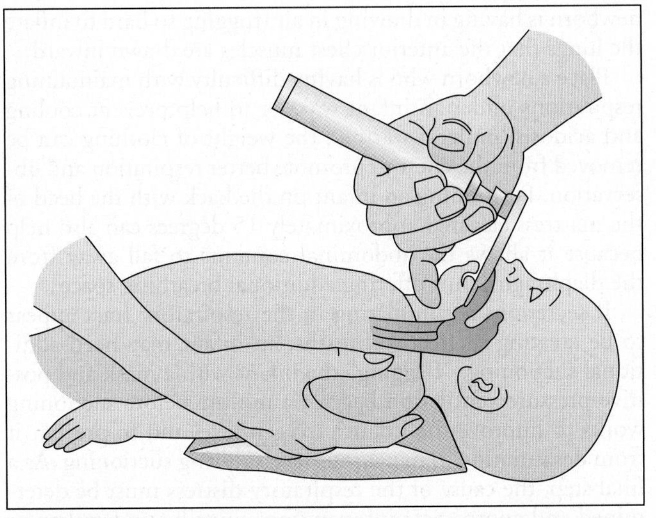

FIGURE 26.2 Intubation. Place the head in a neutral position with a towel under the shoulders. The blade of the laryngoscope is inserted to reveal the vocal cords. An endotracheal tube for ventilation is then passed into the trachea, past the laryngoscope.

again tries to initiate respirations with a few strong gasps. Most newborns, however, cannot maintain this effort longer than 4 or 5 minutes. After this, the respiratory effort will become weaker again and the heart rate will fall further until the newborn stops the gasping effort altogether. The infant then enters a period of *secondary apnea*. Although usually a phenomenon that occurs after birth, both types of apnea may occur in utero.

During the period of first gasps, resuscitation attempts are generally successful. Once a newborn is allowed to enter a secondary apnea period, however, resuscitation becomes difficult and may be ineffective. Because it is impossible to distinguish between the two periods simply by observation, resuscitation must always be started as if secondary apnea is the phase occurring.

A health care provider skilled in laryngoscope and endotracheal tube insertion should be present at the birth of all infants identified as high risk so a laryngoscope can be quickly inserted into the airway as necessary (Raghuveer & Cox, 2011). Laryngoscope insertion is easy in theory; in practice, the wide variation in the size of infants' posterior pharynges and tracheas and the emergency conditions present under which it is attempted, make it an often difficult procedure (Fig. 26.2).

Laryngoscopes are equipped with different-size blades; a size 0 or 1 should be available for newborns. Following insertion of the laryngoscope, an endotracheal tube is slid through the laryngoscope down into the trachea. Infants under 1,000 g need a 2.5-mm endotracheal tube (think of a thin coffee straw); those over 3,000 g need a 4.0-mm tube. Because preterm infants are prone to hemorrhage because of capillary fragility, gentle care during insertion is crucial.

Lung Expansion

Once an airway has been established, a newborn's lungs need to be expanded. Well newborns inflate their lungs adequately independently with a first breath. The sound of the baby crying loudly is proof that lung expansion is good because the vocal sounds are produced by a free flow of air over the vocal cords.

If an infant needs air or oxygen by bag and mask to aid lung expansion, be certain the mask covers both the mouth and the nose. On the other hand, be certain it doesn't cover the eyes because eye injury could occur from either pressure of the mask on the eyes or from drying of the cornea from air or oxygen administration. Air (or oxygen if needed) should be administered at a rate of 40 to 60 ventilations per minute. To prevent unnecessary cooling or drying, oxygen should be administered both warmed (between 89.6° and 93.2°F [32° and 34°C]) and humidified (60% to 80%).

The pressure needed to open lung alveoli for the first time can be as high as 40 cm H_2O. After that, pressures of 15 to 20 cm H_2O are generally adequate to continue inflating alveoli (Thilo & Rosenberg, 2012). The pressure from anesthesia bags is controlled solely by the pressure of a hand against the bag. Other types of bags such as the self-inflating (Ambu) bag can be set with a blow-off valve that limits the pressure in the apparatus to be certain only gentle pressure is applied (Fig. 26.3).

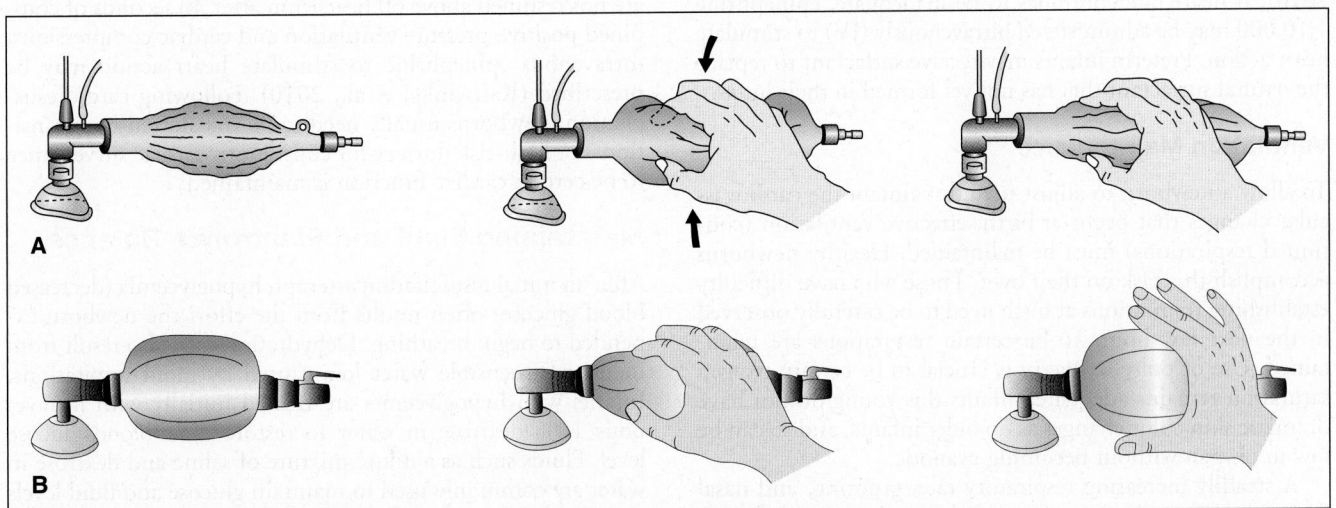

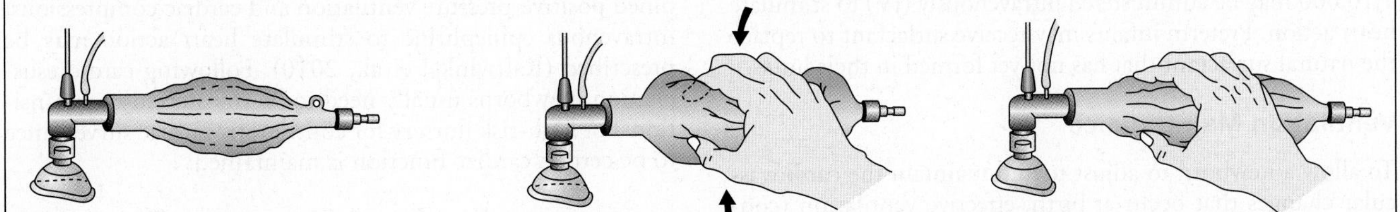

FIGURE 26.3 Types of ventilation bags used in neonatal resuscitation. **(A)** The flow-inflating (anesthesia) bag requires a compressed gas source for inflation but is able to deliver 100% oxygen. **(B)** The self-inflating (Ambu) bag remains inflated at all times and is not dependent on a compressed gas source. It is limited to delivering oxygen concentration to about 40%.

It is important not to let oxygen levels in a newborn fluctuate greatly because fluctuation can cause bleeding from immature cranial vessels. In addition, applying pressure above what is necessary could rupture lung alveoli. If adequate ventilation is not achieved, however, a newborn stands little chance of survival. To be certain air is reaching the lungs with resuscitation, monitor the newborn's oxygen saturation with pulse oximetry in addition to auscultating the chest for the sounds of air movement (Lee & Marcdante, 2011).

Be certain to listen to both lungs to verify both lungs are being aerated. If air can be heard on only one side or sounds are not symmetric, the endotracheal tube is probably at or below the bifurcation of the trachea (where the trachea splits into the left and right main-stem bronchi) and the tube is likely blocking the air from entering one of the main-stem bronchi. Drawing the tube back half a centimeter will usually free it and allow oxygen to flow to both lungs. That the tube is correctly placed in the trachea and not the esophagus can be confirmed by a CO_2 monitor (no CO_2 will return if the tube is in the esophagus) and an X-ray confirms proper depth in the trachea.

When air is given under pressure to a newborn this way, the stomach also quickly fills with air. If the resuscitation has continued for over 2 minutes, insert an orogastric tube (through the mouth to the stomach instead of through the nose to the stomach because babies are obligate nose breathers). Leaving the distal end open helps deflate the stomach and decreases the possibility that vomiting and aspiration of stomach contents from overdistention will occur.

Drug Therapy

Few medications are necessary for newborn resuscitation. Even if an infant's respiratory depression appears to be related to the administration of a narcotic such as morphine or meperidine (Demerol) to the mother during labor, naloxone (Narcan), a drug to reverse the action of narcotics, should not be routinely administered because it has little effect and may cause seizures in a newborn (Leone & Finer, 2012). Instead, resuscitation efforts should focus on effective ventilation and airway support for the persistently apneic newborn (Kattwinkel et al., 2010). If heart rate continues to be inadequate, epinephrine 1:10,000 may be administered intravenously (IV) to stimulate heart action. Preterm infants may receive surfactant to replace the natural surfactant that has not yet formed in their lungs.

Ventilation Maintenance

To allow a newborn to adjust to and maintain the cardiovascular changes that occur at birth, effective ventilation (continued respirations) must be maintained. Healthy newborns accomplish this task on their own. Those who have difficulty establishing respirations at birth need to be carefully observed in the next few hours to be certain respirations are maintained. Use of pulse oximetry is crucial to be certain oxygen saturation remains adequate; infants this young do not have dramatic skin color changes as do older infants, and so can be low in oxygen without becoming cyanotic.

A steadily increasing respiratory rate, grunting, and nasal flaring are often the first signs of obstruction or respiratory compromise in newborns. If these are present, undress the baby's chest and look for intercostal retractions (inward sucking of the anterior chest wall on inspiration). Pulling in the chest muscle this way reflects the degree of difficulty the newborn is having in drawing in air (tugging so hard to inflate the lungs that the anterior chest muscles are drawn inward).

Place a newborn who is having difficulty with maintaining respirations under an infant warmer to help prevent cooling and acidosis; under a warmer, the weight of clothing can be removed from the chest to promote better respiration and observation. Positioning an infant on the back with the head of the mattress elevated approximately 15 degrees can also help because it allows the abdominal contents to fall away from the diaphragm, thus offering additional breathing space.

If secretions accumulating in the respiratory tract appear to be creating ineffective breaths, an infant may need additional suctioning. "Bagging" the infant with a mask and positive-pressure ventilation bag for a minute before suctioning works to improve the infant's oxygen level and to prevent it from desaturating to dangerous levels during suctioning. As a final step, the cause of the respiratory distress must be determined and appropriate interventions must be undertaken to correct the difficulty (see Chapter 40).

Establishing Extrauterine Circulation

Although establishing respirations is the first priority at a high-risk infant's birth, lack of cardiac function may be present concurrently or may develop if respiratory function cannot be quickly initiated and maintained. If an infant has no audible heartbeat, or if the cardiac rate is below 60 beats/min, closed-chest massage should be started. Hold the infant with fingers encircling the chest and wrapped around the back and depress the sternum with both your thumbs on the lower third of the sternum, approximately one third of its depth (1 or 2 cm) at a rate of 100 times per minute (Perlman et al., 2010). Lung ventilation at a rate of 30 times per minute should be continued and interspersed with the cardiac massage at a ratio of 1:3. If a newborn's heart rate is between 60 and 100 beats/min, ensuring adequate ventilation is the major priority and should assist with elevation of the heart rate.

Continue to monitor pulse oximetry to evaluate respiratory function and cardiac efficiency. If the pressure and the rate of cardiac massage used are adequate, it should be possible, in addition, to palpate a femoral pulse. If heart sounds are not resumed above 60 beats/min after 30 seconds of combined positive-pressure ventilation and cardiac compressions, intravenous epinephrine to stimulate heart action may be prescribed (Kattwinkel et al., 2010). Following cardioresuscitation, newborns usually need to be transferred to a transitional or high-risk nursery for continuous cardiac surveillance to be certain cardiac function is maintained.

Maintaining Fluid and Electrolyte Balance

After an initial resuscitation attempt, hypoglycemia (decreased blood glucose) often results from the effort the newborn expended to begin breathing. Dehydration may also result from increased insensible water loss caused by rapid respirations. Infants with hypoglycemia are treated initially with intravenous 10% dextrose in water to restore their blood glucose level. Fluids such as a dilute mixture of saline and dextrose in water are commonly used to maintain glucose and fluid levels and electrolytes. Sodium, additional glucose, and potassium are added as needed according to electrolyte laboratory results.

Be certain to monitor the rate of fluid administration conscientiously in high-risk newborns because a high fluid intake can lead to fluid overload, resulting in patent ductus arteriosus or heart failure. When using a radiant warmer, remember there is a tendency for water loss from either convection or radiation. A newborn on a warmer, therefore, may require more fluid than if he or she were placed in a double-walled incubator.

Monitor fluid status both by urine output and urine specific gravity values. An output less than 2 ml/kg/hr or a specific gravity greater than 1.015 to 1.020 suggests inadequate fluid intake.

If hypovolemia is present immediately after birth, the cause is usually fetal blood loss from a condition such as placenta previa (see Chapter 21) or twin-to-twin transfusion. With hypovolemia, typically tachypnea, pallor, tachycardia, decreased arterial blood pressure, decreased central venous pressure, and decreased tissue perfusion of peripheral tissue, with a progressively developing metabolic acidosis, will develop. The hematocrit may be normal for some time after acute blood loss, however, because blood cells present are in proportion to plasma. An isotonic solution (usually normal saline) may be administered to increase blood volume. A vasopressor such as dopamine may be given to increase blood pressure and improve cell perfusion.

Regulating Temperature

All high-risk infants may have difficulty maintaining temperature because, in addition to stress from an illness or immaturity, the infant's body is often exposed for long periods during procedures such as resuscitation.

It's important to keep newborns in a neutral-temperature environment, one that is neither too hot nor too cold because doing so places less demand on them to maintain a minimal metabolic rate necessary for effective body functioning. If their environment becomes too hot, they are forced to decrease metabolism to cool their body. If it becomes too cold, they must increase their metabolism to warm body cells. Increased metabolism can be destructive because it calls for increased oxygen, and without this oxygen available because of respiratory difficulty, body cells become hypoxic. To spare oxygen for essential body functions, vasoconstriction of peripheral blood vessels occurs so blood can be pushed into the central torso. If this process continues for too long a time, pulmonary vessels become lax and pulmonary perfusion decreases. The infant's Po_2 level will fall and Pco_2 will increase. As mentioned previously, a lowered Po_2 level causes fetal shunts such as the ductus arteriosus to remain open. Surfactant production in the lungs can halt as well, further interfering with lung function. To supply glucose to maintain increased metabolism, an infant has to resort to anaerobic glycolysis, which pours acid into the bloodstream. As the infant becomes more and more acidotic, the risk of acute bilirubin encephalopathy or *kernicterus* (the accumulation of unconjugated bilirubin into brain cells) increases as more bilirubin-binding sites are lost and more bilirubin is free to pass out of the bloodstream in brain cells. In short, because of becoming chilled, heart action, breathing, electrolytic balance, and possibly brain function all become compromised.

In addition to covering the newborn with an infant cap, wiping the body and head dry, and using a radiant warmer or prewarmed incubator (Fig. 26.4), suggest skin-to-skin

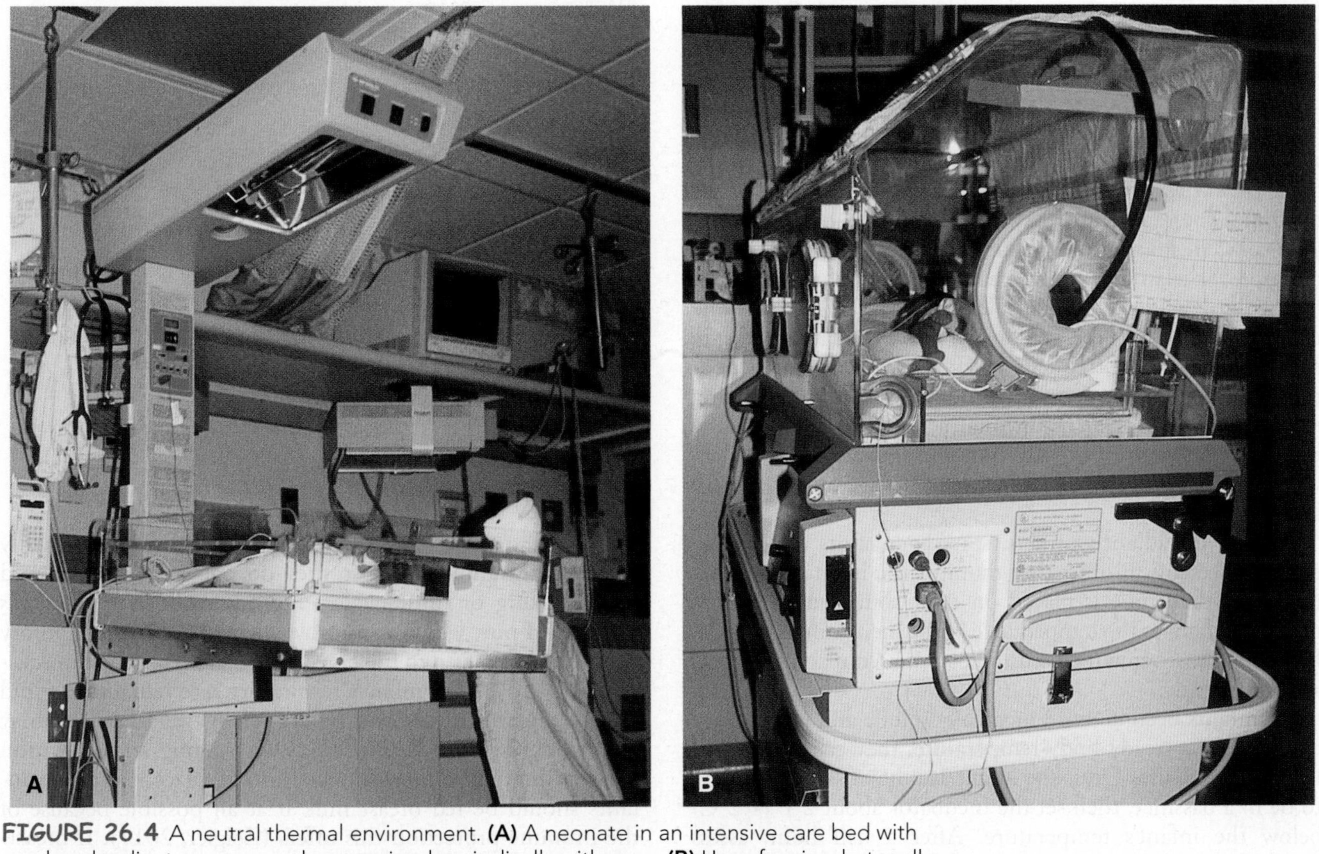

FIGURE 26.4 A neutral thermal environment. **(A)** A neonate in an intensive care bed with overhead radiant warmer can be examined periodically with ease. **(B)** Use of an incubator allows maintenance of a neutral thermal environment for neonates not requiring minute-to-minute interventions.

contact with one of the parents. Additional measures that can be used to ensure temperature stays at 97.8°F (36.5°C) axillary are plastic wrap, plastic shields, or a warmed mattresses. Also to prevent heat loss, be certain during any procedure that the infant is not placed on a cool X-ray table or scale.

Radiant Heat Sources

Radiant heat warmers are open beds that have an attached overhead source of radiant heat and so provide both warmth and visibility for observation. Such units have small probes, covered by a small shield, often silver metallic, which when placed on the baby's skin, register the baby's temperature. Abdominal skin temperature, when measured this way, should be 95.9° to 97.7°F (35.5° to 36.5°C). If an infant's temperature falls below this level, an alarm on the unit can be set to sound. Be certain, with the infant laying on his or her back, you tape the probe or disk onto the infant's abdomen between the umbilicus and the xiphoid process. Do not tape it on the underside of an infant or it will register a falsely high reading. Be certain as well it is not over the liver, because the heat generated by the liver can lead to false high readings, or over the rib cage where the thin subcutaneous tissue is also apt to yield an inaccurate reading. When performing care or leaning over the infant, be careful your head does not block the heat from the overhead source so it no longer reaches the baby. An additional warming pad placed under an infant may be necessary for very preterm infants or for lengthy procedures to maintain body heat.

Incubators

Newborns needing both warmth and visual observation may also be cared for in incubators. By placing the baby in such a steady, warm environment, the need for clothing can be eliminated, so the observation for any respiratory difficulty, possible color changes, or unusual movements (such as seizures) can be readily observed. The temperature of incubators varies with the amount of time portholes remain open and the temperature of the area in which the incubator is placed. Placing one in direct sunlight or near a warm radiator, for example, can increase the internal temperature markedly. Placing it near a cold window can decrease the temperature. For these reasons, a newborn's temperature must be assessed at frequent intervals when in an incubator to be certain the temperature level designated is being maintained. Use of an additional acrylic shield inside the incubator helps prevent radiation and convection heat loss when portholes are opened and may be necessary for very immature infants.

Similar to radiant warmers, some incubators have servo-control mechanism units that monitor the infant's temperature once the probe is placed on their abdomen and automatically changes the temperature of the incubator as needed. Portholes must remain closed to keep the servo control operating efficiently.

As infants become both medically stabile and old enough to maintain a steady body temperature, they can be weaned from an incubator. Dress the infant as if he or she were going to be in a bassinet, then set the incubator about 2°F (1.2°C) below the infant's temperature. After a half hour, assess whether the infant is able to maintain body temperature. If so, lower the incubator temperature another 2°F and continue until room temperature is reached. If an infant cannot maintain adequate temperature as the incubator temperature level is lowered, it suggests the infant is not yet ready for room-temperature air, and the weaning process should be slowed or stopped until the baby is more mature or better able to self-regulate temperature.

Skin-to-Skin Care

Originally referred to as kangaroo care, skin-to-skin care is the use of skin-to-skin contact with a parent to maintain body heat. Provide a quiet setting with lights dimmed. Undress the infant except for a diaper and perhaps a cap. Assist the parent to sit comfortably in a chair and hold the infant snugly against his or her chest, skin to skin. Place a blanket over the infant for added warmth. This method of care not only supplies heat but also encourages parent–child bonding (Moore, Anderson, Bergman, et al., 2012).

✔ QSEN Checkpoint Question 26.1

Evidence-Based Practice

To investigate whether the simple act of covering the heads of preterm or LBW infants is enough protection against evaporation and heat loss to prevent hypothermia, researchers reviewed six studies (including a total of 304 infants), which compared different methods of guarding against newborn cooling. Results of a meta-analysis revealed plastic wraps or bags, skin-to-skin care, and warmed mattresses all kept preterm infants warm. Stockinette caps alone did not provide this same protection (McCall, Alderdice, Halliday, et al., 2010).

Based on the previous study, which response by Mrs. Atkins, whose infant was born prematurely, would alert you she may need further teaching?

a. "Holding my baby directly on my chest will help with warmth and temperature stability."
b. "I like singing to him and notice that helps his temperature stay even."
c. "I'll use this adorable little hat I was given to help him stay warm."
d. "I'm afraid he'll suffocate if he sleeps on a warmed mattress."

Look in Appendix A for the best answer and rationale.

Establishing Adequate Nutritional Intake

Infants who experienced severe asphyxia at birth usually receive intravenous fluids so they do not become exhausted from sucking or until necrotizing enterocolitis (NEC) has been ruled out, which can result when there is a temporary reduction of oxygen to the bowel (see Chapter 45 for a discussion of NEC). If an infant's respiratory rate remains so rapid that the infant cannot suck effectively, gavage feedings may be introduced (Fig. 26.5). Others with a long-term nutrition concern may have gastrostomy buttons placed. Preterm infants should be fed breast milk if at all possible because of the immune protection this offers (Zeigler, 2011). If breastfeeding is not possible because the infant is too immature to suck effectively, a mother can manually express breast milk or

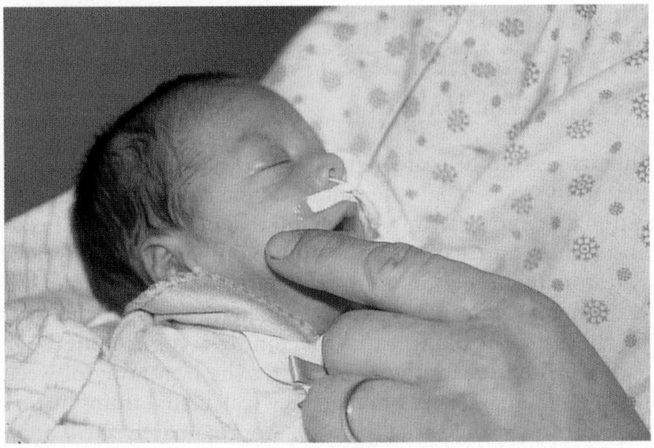

FIGURE 26.5 Infants who are ill at birth often need supplemental feedings by nasogastric or gastrostomy tube.

use a breast pump to initiate and continue her milk supply until the time the infant is mature enough or otherwise ready for effective sucking. Her expressed breast milk can then be used in the infant's gavage feeding (Black, 2012). Be certain when bottled breast milk is supplied by parents that it is well marked with the infant's name and medical record number or breast milk errors can occur the same as medication errors (Centers for Disease Control and Prevention [CDC], 2010). It should be stored in plastic bags or bottles labeled to be free of polycarbonate (bisphenol A), which can leech into stored milk and possibly lead to endocrine disruptions (Rasmussen & Geraghty, 2011).

Preterm infants reveal hunger by the same signs as term infants, such as rooting, crying, and sucking motions. All babies who are gavage or gastrostomy fed need oral stimulation from nonnutritive sucking and so seem to enjoy a pacifier at feeding times. In immature infants, this may actually help them develop an effective sucking reflex. In mature infants, pacifier use has also been shown to be a deterrent to sudden infant death syndrome (SIDS) (American Academy of Pediatrics [AAP], 2011b). Exceptions to pacifier use are for infants too immature to have a sucking reflex; infants who must not swallow air, such as those with a tracheoesophageal fistula awaiting surgery; or infants mature enough to breastfeed. The techniques of gavage feeding and gastrostomy feeding are both discussed in Chapter 37.

Establishing Waste Elimination

Although most immature infants void within 24 hours of birth, they may void later than term newborns because, as a result of all the procedures for resuscitation, their blood pressure may not be adequate to optimally supply their kidneys. Carefully document any voidings that occur during resuscitation because this is proof that hypotension is improving and the kidneys are being perfused. Immature infants also may pass stool later than the term infant because meconium has not yet reached the end of the intestine at birth.

Preventing Infections

Infections in high-risk newborns may occur from prenatal, perinatal, or postnatal causes. In some instances, such as preterm premature rupture of the membranes, the risk of adverse neurodevelopmental outcomes from the infection is what places the infant in a high-risk category (Clark & Varner, 2011). Contracting an infection has the potential to drastically complicate a high-risk newborn's ability to adjust to extrauterine life, another reason breastfeeding is good for such infants because, beginning with colostrum, it supplies important immune protection (Kim & Froh, 2012).

Infection, like chilling, has the detrimental effect of increasing metabolic oxygen demands as well as stressing an immature immune system, thus lowering defense mechanism protection.

Common viruses that affect infants during intrauterine life are cytomegalovirus and toxoplasmosis virus. An infant born after contracting either of these infections may be born with congenital anomalies from the virus invasion (see Chapter 12). The most prevalent perinatal infections are those contracted from the vagina during birth such as herpes simplex 2 and hepatitis B. Early-onset sepsis is most commonly caused by group B streptococcus, *Escherichia coli*, *Klebsiella* (a gram-negative rod that causes pneumonia), and *Listeria monocytogenes* (a gram-positive bacteria associated with nausea, vomiting, and possibly meningitis). Late-onset, or hospital-acquired infections are more commonly caused by *Staphylococcus aureus*, *Enterobacter*, and *Candida*. Late-onset infections are probably most commonly spread to newborns from health care personnel, which is the reason all persons coming in contact with or caring for infants must observe good hand washing techniques and standard precautions to reduce the risk of infection transmission. Health care personnel with infections have a professional and moral obligation to refrain from caring for newborns or wear protective measures such as a face mask to avoid spreading infections.

Establishing Parent–Infant Bonding

It is helpful if all women who are diagnosed as having a high-risk pregnancy are offered a tour of a neonatal intensive care unit (NICU) during pregnancy, so if their infant should be admitted to a NICU, they will be more comfortable in the high-tech environment.

Be certain the parents of a high-risk newborn are kept informed of what is happening during resuscitation at birth. They should be able to visit the special nursing unit to which the child is admitted as soon and as often as they choose, and, after washing and gowning, hold and touch their child, both of which are actions that help make the child's birth more real to them. Should a child not survive an initial illness, these interactions can also help make the death more real and can help parents work through their feelings to accept this event.

Most parents handle newborn babies tentatively until they have "claimed" them or have become firmly acquainted. If a child was ill at birth, it may take days or weeks before the parents are able to handle their baby comfortably and confidently because of the number of tubes involved in care and their fear of doing something that could hurt the infant. Urge parents to spend as much time with their infant in the intensive care nursery as possible, especially as the infant is improving and is able to begin interacting with them. Be certain parents have continuing access to health care personnel after discharge so they can care confidently for the child at home.

If an infant dies despite newborn resuscitation attempts, parents need to see the infant without being covered by myriad equipment. Viewing the baby can help reassure them the baby was a perfect newborn in every other way except lung function or whatever was the infant's specific fatal disorder. Believing this is one way they may be able to develop confidence to plan for other children or simply to continue their lives after such a devastating experience.

Anticipating Developmental Needs

High-risk newborns need special care to ensure the amount of pain they experience during procedures is limited to the least amount possible and that they also receive adequate stimulation for growth. Most high-risk infants enjoy "catch-up" growth once they stabilize from the trauma of birth or whatever caused them to be classified as high risk. They quickly move to playing with age-appropriate toys and interacting with parents. Some parents may need support before and after their infants are discharged home so they can begin to view their child as well and capable of doing all the things the infant is now capable of doing. Discussing usual growth and development of infants can help them be ready and looking forward to the next developmental step.

Follow-Up of High-Risk Infants at Home

Each time parents visit a high-risk nursery, assess their level of knowledge about their child's condition and development. For parents whose child has a complex concern, additional education and referral to a home care agency may be necessary to help them continue with the level of care required when the infant is discharged home (see Chapter 4). Before discharge, the safety of their home for the care of such a small or ill infant needs to be evaluated. Transporting a preterm infant in a car, for example, will require special measures, including a blanket or commercial head support, because a very small infant does not fit securely into a standard infant car seat.

Although not well documented regarding when or why it occurs, some preterm infants experience episodes of oxygen desaturation, apnea, or bradycardia when seated in standard car safety seats (DeGrazia, Chao-Yu, Wilkinson, et al., 2010). To detect if this will occur, the AAP recommends all preterm infants be assessed for cardiorespiratory stability in their car seat prior to discharge from the health care facility—the "car seat challenge" (AAP, 2012).

High-Risk Infants and Child Maltreatment

When a child is born ill or preterm, the expected reaction of parents would be to protect the child even more than the average child so no further harm could result. In actuality, particularly in reference to preterm children, the opposite may occur. Probably related to the feeling they are "different" or because they were separated from the parents for a long time following birth, preterm children are at high risk for maltreatment (see Chapter 55) (Chiesa & Sirotnak, 2012).

What if . . . 26.1 You hear Mr. Atkins repeat the question he first asked his wife when he heard his baby had been born prematurely, "What did you do to cause this?" Would you try to intervene or allow the Atkins to work out their feelings as a couple?

THE NEWBORN AT RISK BECAUSE OF ALTERED GESTATIONAL AGE OR BIRTH WEIGHT

Infants need to be evaluated as soon as possible after birth to determine their weight, height, head circumference, and gestational age to determine their immediate health care needs and to help anticipate possible future problems. Birth weight is normally plotted on a growth chart such as the Colorado (Lubchenco) Intrauterine Growth Chart, a special chart for newborns (available at http://thePoint.lww.com/Pillitteri7e).

Term infants are those born after the beginning of week 38 and before week 42 of pregnancy (calculated from the first day of the last menstrual period). Approximately 90% of all live births fall into this category. Infants born before term (before the beginning of the 38th week of pregnancy) account for approximately 12.18% of all births and are classified as **preterm infants**, regardless of their birth weight (Martin, Hamilton, Ventura, et al., 2011). Infants born after the end of week 41 of pregnancy are classified as postterm infants or postmature (Gowen, 2011).

Normally, birth weight increases for each additional gestational week of age. Infants who fall between the 10th and 90th percentiles of weight for their gestational age, whether they are preterm, term, or postterm, are considered **appropriate for gestational age (AGA)**. Infants who fall below the 10th percentile of weight for their age are considered **small for gestational age (SGA)**. Those who fall above the 90th percentile in weight are considered **large for gestational age (LGA)**. Still another term used is **low–birth-weight (LBW)** infant (one weighing under 2,500 g at birth). Those weighing 1,000 to 1,500 g are **very-low-birth-weight infants (VLBW)** infants. Those born weighing 500 to 1,000 g are considered *extremely very-low-birth-weight (EVLBW) infants.* Infants may be AGA, SGA, or LGA, as well as LBW, VLBW, or EVLBW.

Infants in all of these classifications have immediate needs that are different from or are more pronounced than the needs of AGA term newborns. Each of these categories also carries its own set of potential risks.

The Preterm Infant

A preterm infant is traditionally defined as a live-born infant born before the end of week 37 of gestation. In terms of the degree of care needed, they are further divided into *late preterm* (born between 34 and 37 weeks) and *early preterm* (born between 24 and 34 weeks). Neonatal assessments such as inspection for sole creases, skull firmness, ear cartilage, and neurologic development plus the mother's report of the date of her last menstrual period along with a sonographic estimation of age all can be helpful to determine gestational age. Preterm birth occurs in approximately 10% of live births of non–Hispanic White infants. In African American infants, the rate is approximately 17.47% (Martin et al., 2011).

All preterm infants need intensive care from the moment of birth to give them their best chance of survival without neurologic aftereffects because they are more prone than others to hypoglycemia and intracranial hemorrhage. Lack of lung surfactant, because this does not form until about the 34th week of pregnancy, makes them extremely vulnerable to respiratory distress syndrome (RDS) (Landry & Menzies, 2012).

TABLE 26.1 Contrasts Between Small-for-Gestational-Age and Preterm Infants

Characteristic	Small-for-Gestational-Age Infant	Preterm Infant
Gestational age	24–44 weeks	<37 weeks
Birth weight	<10th percentile	Normal for age
Congenital malformations	Strong possibility	Possibility
Pulmonary problems most apt to occur	Meconium aspiration, pulmonary hemorrhage, pneumothorax	Respiratory distress syndrome
Hyperbilirubinemia	Possibility	Very strong possibility
Hypoglycemia	Very strong possibility	Possibility
Intracranial hemorrhage	Strong possibility	Possibility
Apnea episodes	Possibility	Very strong possibility
Feeding problems	Most likely because of accompanying problem such as hypoglycemia	Small stomach capacity; immature sucking reflex
Weight gain in nursery	Rapid	Slow
Future restricted growth	Possibly always be <10th percentile because of poor organ development	Not likely to be restricted in growth because "catch-up" growth occurs

No matter what their weight, the initial assessment needs to differentiate healthy preterm babies from SGA babies (who also may have a low birth weight but have more possibility of being unhealthy and so require more help to adjust to extrauterine life). In contrast to an SGA infant, a preterm infant appears immature and has a low birth weight but is well proportioned for age because the baby appears to have been doing well in utero. For an unexplained reason, however, the trigger that initiates labor was activated too early and birth resulted even though the baby was not yet mature. Characteristics of SGA and preterm infants are compared in Table 26.1.

Etiology

Because preterm infant deaths account for 80% to 90% of infant mortality in the first year of life (NVSS, 2011), infant mortality could be reduced dramatically if the causes of preterm birth could be discovered and corrected and all pregnancies could be brought to term. However, even with the examples of possible causes listed in the following, the exact cause of premature labor and early birth is rarely exactly known.

Box 26.3 summarizes factors associated with preterm birth. Important among these is a high correlation between low socioeconomic level and early birth. In women from middle and upper socioeconomic groups, for example, only 4% to 8% of pregnancies are not carried to term. In women from low socioeconomic levels, as many as 10% to 20% end before term (Whitehead, 2012). The major influencing factor in these instances appears to be inadequate nutrition before and during pregnancy, as a result of either lack of money for or lack of knowledge about good nutrition. The increasing use of assisted fertility methods that result in multiple births, such as in vitro fertilization, is another reason preterm births can occur because more multiple pregnancies result in preterm birth than term pregnancies (Beck, Wojdyla, Say, et al., 2010). Iatrogenic (health care–caused) issues, such as elective cesarean birth or inducing labor before 39 weeks of pregnancy (which is not recommended but sometimes necessary because of maternal illness), also result in early births.

Assessment

Although a detailed pregnancy history may sometimes reveal the reason for a preterm birth, the pregnancy history is often normal up to the beginning of labor. When interviewing

BOX 26.3 Common Factors Associated With Preterm Birth

- Low socioeconomic level
- Poor nutritional status
- Lack of prenatal care
- Multiple pregnancy
- Previous early birth
- Race (nonwhites have a higher incidence of prematurity than whites)
- Cigarette smoking
- Age of the mother (highest incidence is in mothers younger than age 20 years)
- Order of birth (early birth is highest in first pregnancies and in those beyond the fourth pregnancy)
- Closely spaced pregnancies
- Abnormalities of the mother's reproductive system, such as intrauterine septum
- Infections (especially urinary tract infections)
- Pregnancy complications, such as premature rupture of membranes or premature separation of the placenta
- Early induction of labor
- Elective cesarean birth

parents of a preterm infant, be careful not to convey disapproval of reported pregnancy behaviors such as cigarette smoking that may have contributed to preterm birth. Once an infant is born, a new mother needs a high level of self-esteem and all of her inner resources to sustain her through this crisis and not be burdened by guilt over what should or could have been. An accurate but comforting answer to a direct inquiry about why preterm birth occurs is, "No one really knows what causes prematurity."

On the other hand, once preterm labor began, it might have been halted had a woman been able to recognize she was in labor. In a first labor, this occurs easily because television shows typically depict women in labor as having agonizingly painful contractions or the opposite, simply announcing, "This is it," and then proceeding to give birth within the 30-minute time limit of the show, making it difficult for women to appreciate that labor usually begins with subtle signs and mild contractions, not with a dramatic announcement. With preterm labor, many women report they thought all they were having was Braxton Hicks contractions or even just intestinal cramps. Because each labor proceeds differently, even a multipara may miss a sign of early labor such as backache until labor is too far advanced to be reversed. Take the time to reassure a woman that it is understandable and usual that she did not realize what was happening until cervical dilatation had occurred and labor could not be reversed (Bennett, 2012). Educate her, however, about early signs of labor so in a future pregnancy she'll be better prepared to recognize true from false labor.

Observing a number of physical findings and reflex testing are used to differentiate between term and preterm newborns at birth (Figs. 26.6 and 26.7). On gross inspection, a preterm infant's head appears disproportionately large (≥3 cm greater than chest size). The skin is generally unusually ruddy because there is so little subcutaneous fat beneath it that veins are easily noticeable; a high degree of acrocyanosis may be present. A 24- to 36-week-old infant is typically covered with thick vernix caseosa. In very preterm newborns, however (less than 25 weeks of gestation), the vernix will be absent because it has not formed yet. Lanugo is usually scant the same way in very low gestation infants, but will be extensive, covering the back, forearms, forehead, and sides of the face in late preterm babies. Both anterior and posterior fontanelles will be small. There are few or no creases on the soles of the feet (Gowen, 2011).

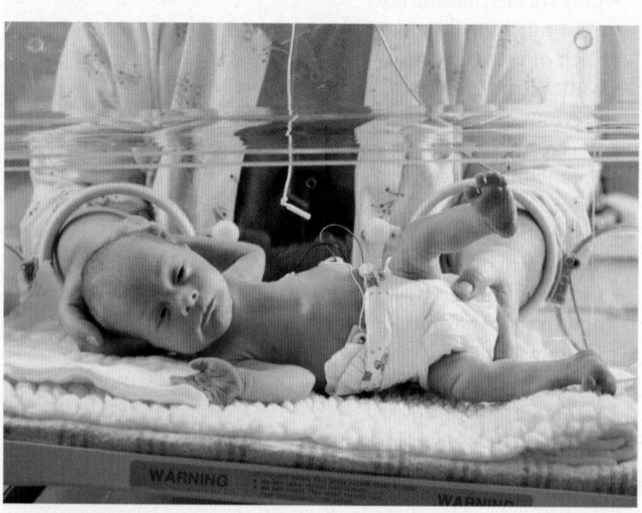

FIGURE 26.6 An immature infant. Immature infants on monitors have their position rotated frequently to allow equal pressure and growth for all areas of the body (Photodisc/PunchStock).

The eyes of most preterm infants appear small in relation to term infants. Although difficult to elicit, a pupillary reaction is present. An ophthalmoscopic examination is extremely difficult and often uninformative because the vitreous humor may be hazy. A preterm infant has varying degrees of myopia (nearsightedness) because of a lack of eye globe depth.

The ears appear large in relation to the head. The cartilage of the ear is immature and allows the pinna to fall forward. The level of the ears should be carefully inspected to rule out chromosomal abnormalities (see Chapter 7).

Neurologic function in the preterm infant is often difficult to evaluate because the neurologic system is still so immature. Observing the infant make spontaneous or provoked muscle movements can be as important as formal reflex testing. If they are tested, reflexes such as sucking and swallowing will be absent if an infant's age is below 33 weeks; deep tendon reflexes such as the Achilles tendon reflex will also be markedly diminished. During an examination, a preterm infant is much less active than a mature infant and rarely cries. If the infant does cry, the cry is weak and high pitched.

Laboratory values for a preterm infant are compared with those of the term infant at http://thePoint.lww.com/Pillitteri7e.

Potential Complications

Because of immaturity, preterm infants are prone to several specific conditions.

Anemia of Prematurity. Many preterm infants develop a normochromic, normocytic anemia (normal cells, just few in number), which can make infants appear pale, lethargic, and anorectic. Anemia occurs from a combination of immaturity of the hematopoietic system (the effective production of red cells with an elevated reticulocyte count may not begin until 32 weeks of pregnancy) combined with the destruction of red blood cells because of low levels of vitamin E, a substance that normally protects red blood cells against oxidation. Excessive blood drawing for electrolyte or blood gas analysis after birth can potentiate the problem. For this reason, it's important to see that blood draws in preterm infants are coordinated to the fewest possible and a record of the blood loss for these tallied. Delaying cord clamping at birth to allow a little more blood from the placenta to enter the infant may also help reduce the development of anemia (Rabe, Diaz-Rossello, Duley, et al., 2012).

Some infants may need supplemental blood transfusions to supply needed red blood cells as well as vitamin E and iron. Red blood cell production can be stimulated by the administration of DNA recombinant erythropoietin, but because this appears to be associated with an increased incidence of retinopathy of prematurity (ROP), administration of this would be a last, not a first, resort (Aher & Ohlsson, 2012).

Acute Bilirubin Encephalopathy. **Acute bilirubin encephalopathy (ABE)** is the destruction of brain cells by invasion of indirect bilirubin (Hansen, 2011). This invasion results from the high concentration of indirect bilirubin that forms in the bloodstream from an excessive breakdown of red blood cells at birth. Preterm infants are more prone to this condition than term infants because, with the acidosis that occurs from poor respiratory exchange, brain cells appear to be more susceptible to the effect of indirect bilirubin than usual. Preterm infants also have less serum albumin available to bind indirect bilirubin and inactivate its effect. Because of this, ABE may occur at lower levels in these infants than in term newborns (Thilo & Rosenberg, 2012). At the point that indirect bilirubin levels rise and jaundice occurs, phototherapy or exchange transfusion can be initiated to prevent excessively high indirect bilirubin levels.

Persistent Patent Ductus Arteriosus. Because preterm infants may lack surfactant, their lungs are noncompliant, so it is more difficult for them to move blood from the pulmonary artery into the lungs. This condition leads to pulmonary artery hypertension, which then interferes with closure of the ductus arteriosus. Always administer intravenous therapy cautiously to preterm infants, therefore, because increasing blood pressure could further compound this problem. In term infants, indomethacin or ibuprofen may be used to cause closure of a patent ductus arteriosus, making ventilation more efficient; however, indomethacin is given cautiously to preterm infants because it has been associated with adverse effects such as decreased renal function, decreased platelet count, and gastric irritation (Rao, Bryowsky, Mao, et al., 2011). Carefully monitor urine output and observe for bleeding, especially at injection sites, if this is prescribed.

Periventricular/Intraventricular Hemorrhage. Preterm infants are prone to periventricular hemorrhage (bleeding into the tissue surrounding the ventricles) or intraventricular hemorrhage (bleeding into the ventricles) because of fragile capillaries and immature cerebral vascular development. When there is a rapid change in cerebral blood pressure, such as could occur with hypoxia, intravenous infusion, ventilation, or pneumothorax (lung collapse), capillary rupture could occur; brain anoxia then occurs distal to the rupture.

Intraventricular hemorrhage occurs most often in VLBW infants and is classified as: grade 1, bleeding occurred in just

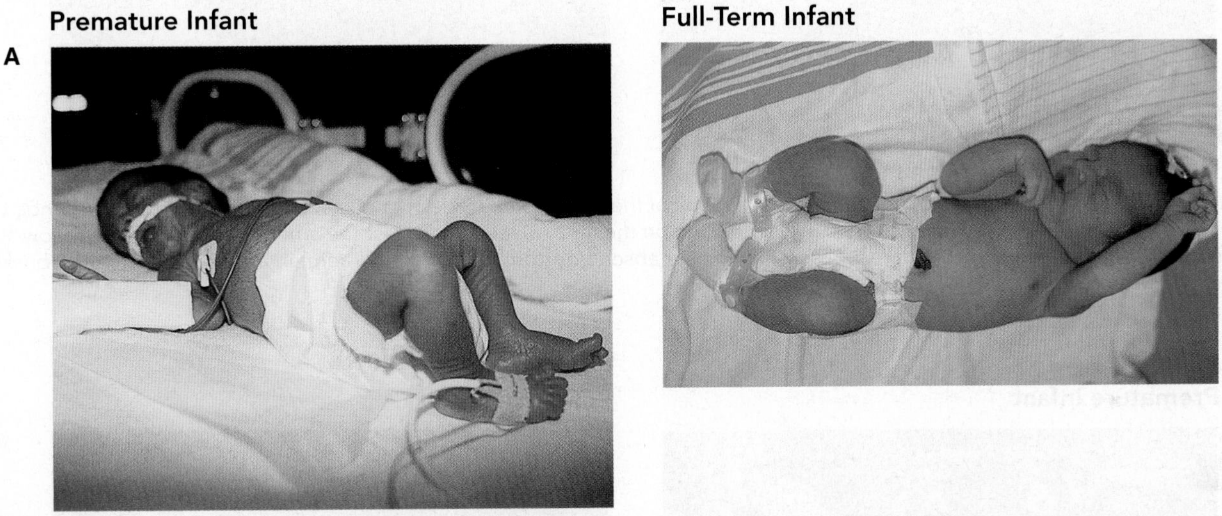

RESTING POSTURE *The premature infant is characterized by very little, if any, flexion in the upper extremities and only partial flexion of the lower extremities. The full-term infant exhibits flexion in all four extremities.*

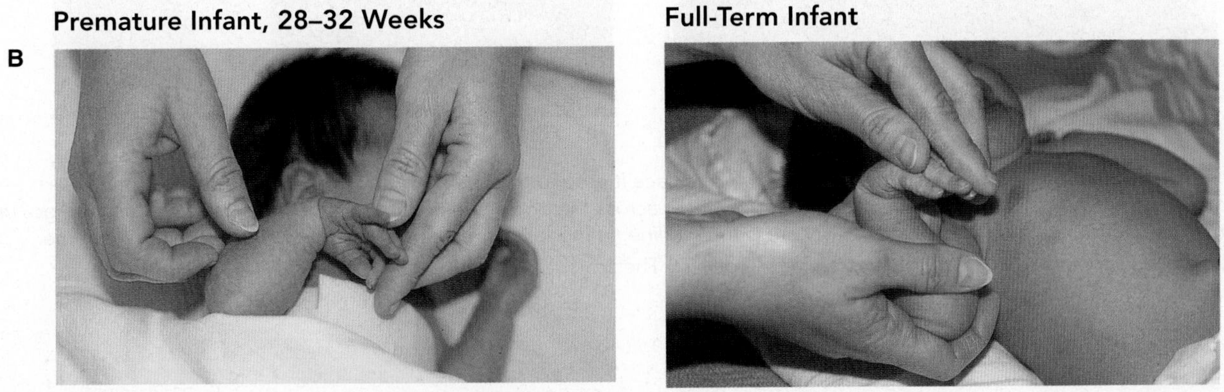

WRIST FLEXION *The wrist is flexed, applying enough pressure to get the hand as close to the forearm as possible. The angle between the hypothenar eminence and the ventral aspect of the forearm is measured. (Care must be taken not to rotate an infant's wrist.) The premature infant at 28–32 weeks gestation will exhibit a 90-degree angle. With the fullterm infant it is possible to flex the hand onto the arm.*

FIGURE 26.7 Examples of physical examination findings and reflex tests used to judge gestational age. **(A)** A resting posture. **(B)** Wrist flexion. *(continued)*

C

Premature Infant

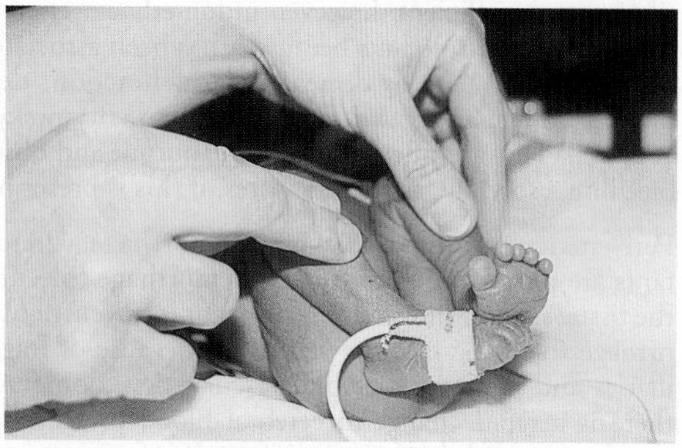

Full-Term Infant

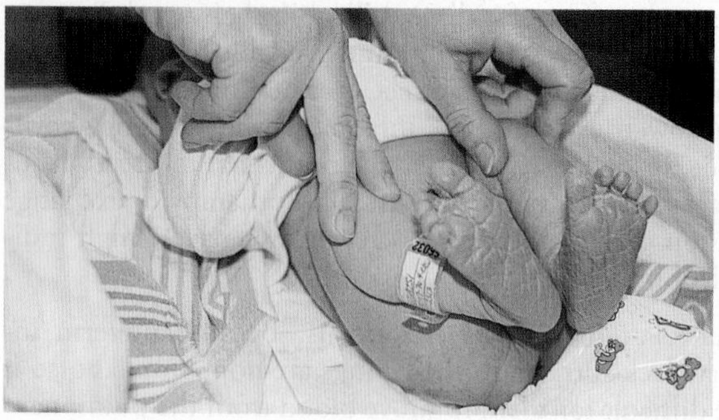

Response in Premature Infant

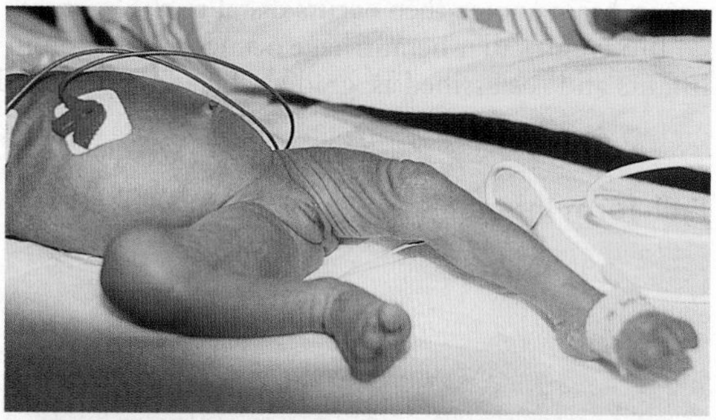

Response in Full-Term Infant

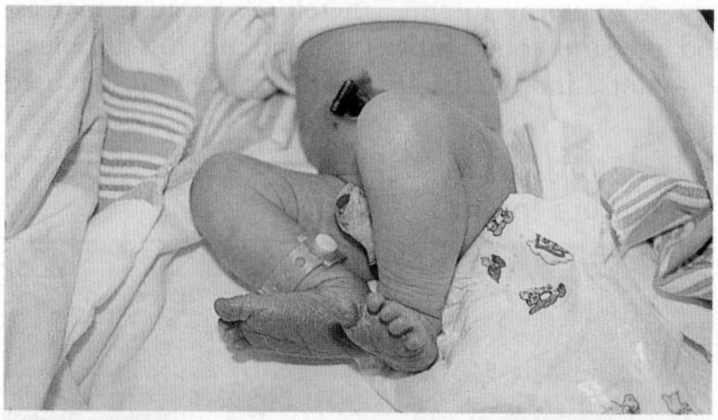

RECOIL OF EXTREMITIES *Place an infant supine. To test recoil of the legs (1) flex the legs and knees fully and hold for 5 seconds (shown in top photographs), (2) extend the legs fully by pulling on the feet, (3) release. To test the arms, flex forearms and follow same procedure. In the premature infant response is minimal or absent (bottom left); in the full-term infant extremities return briskly to full flexion (bottom right).*

D

Premature Infant

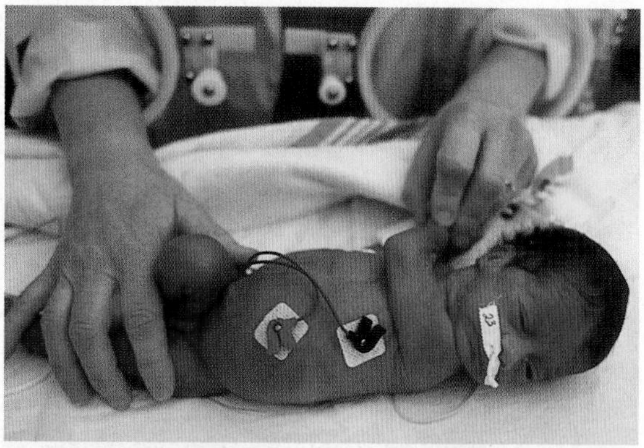

Full-Term Infant

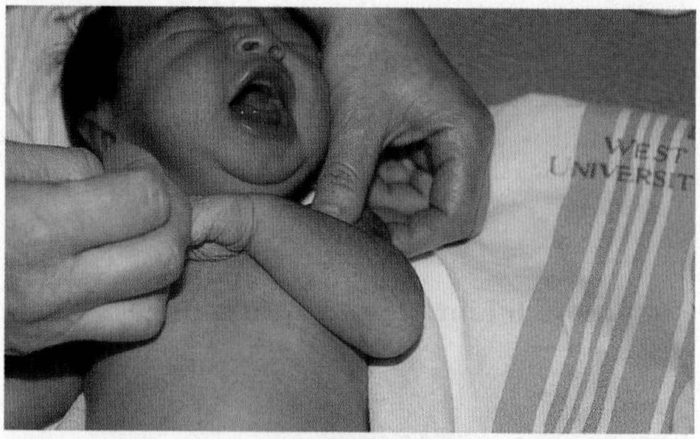

SCARF SIGN *Hold the baby supine, take the hand, and try to place it around the neck and above the opposite shoulder as far posteriorly as possible. Assist this maneuver by lifting the elbow across the body. See how far across the chest the elbow will go. In the premature infant the elbow will reach near or across the midline. In the full-term infant the elbow will not reach the midline.*

FIGURE 26.7 *(continued)* **(C)** Recoil of extremities (legs). **(D)** The scarf sign. *(continued)*

E

Premature Infant

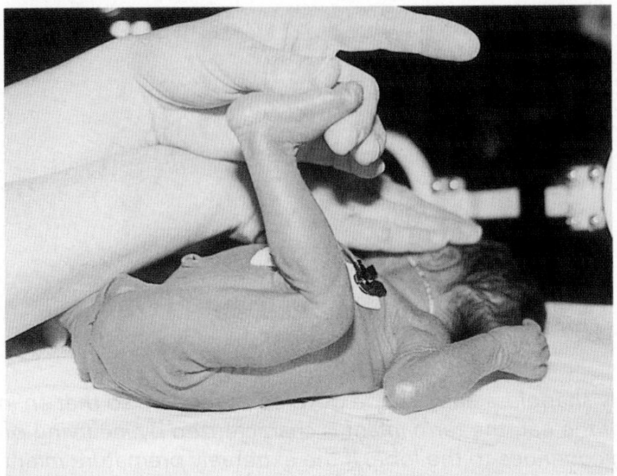

Full-Term Infant

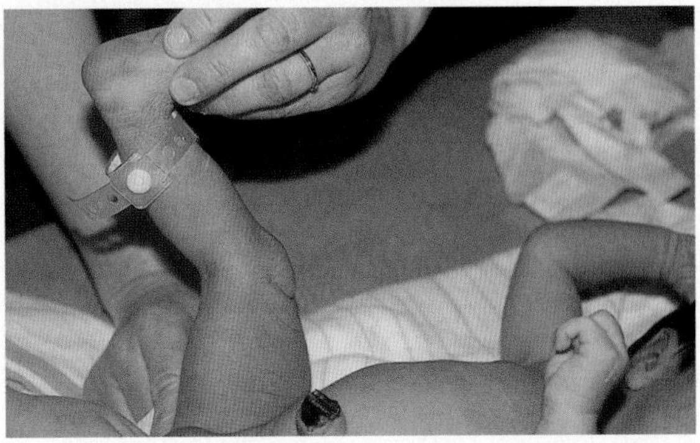

HEEL TO EAR *With the baby supine and the hips positioned flat on the bed, draw the baby's foot as near to the ear as it will go without forcing it. Observe the distance between the foot and head as well as the degree of extension at the knee. In the premature infant, very little resistance will be met. In the full-term infant there will be marked resistance; it will be impossible to draw the baby's foot to the ear.*

F

Premature Infant

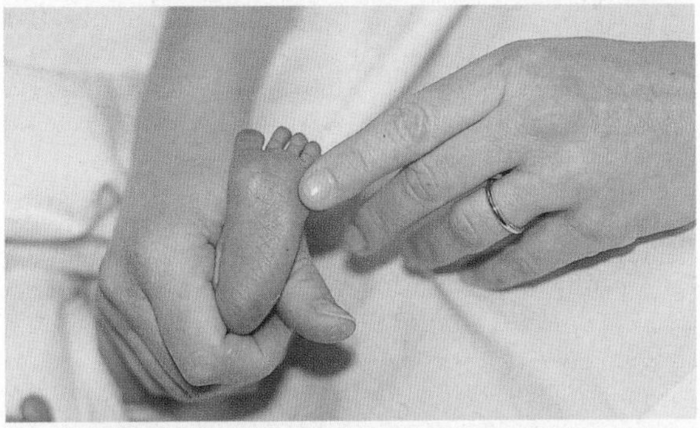

Full-Term Infant

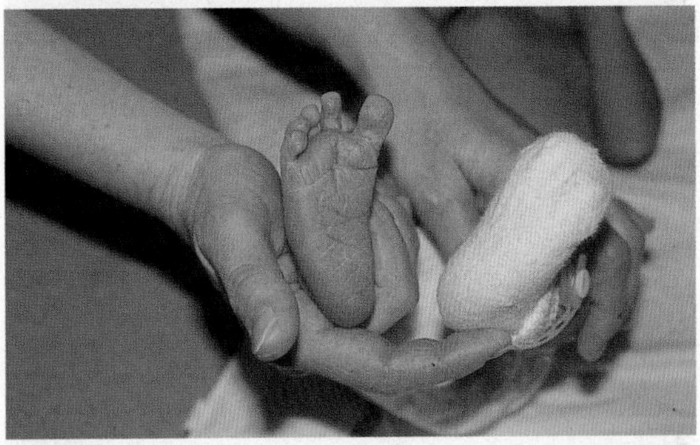

SOLE (PLANTAR) CREASES *The sole of the premature infant has very few or no creases. With the increasing gestation age, the number and depth of sole creases multiply, so that the full-term baby has creases involving the heel. (Wrinkles that occur after 24 hours of age can sometimes be confused with true creases.)*

G

Premature Infant

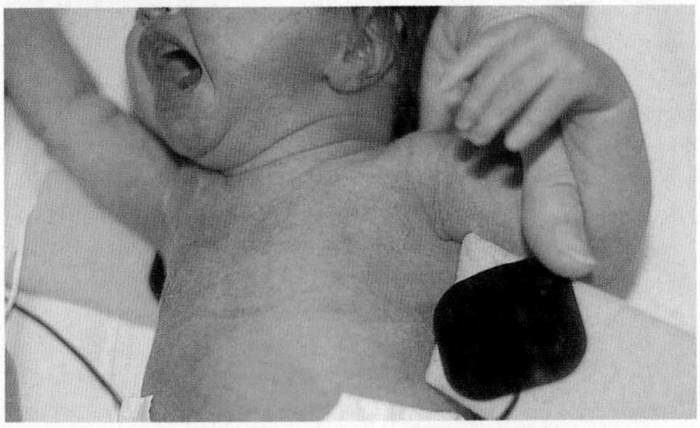

Full-Term Infant

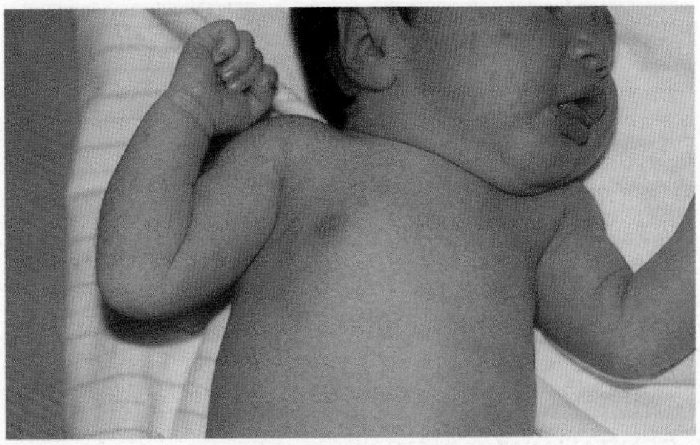

BREAST TISSUE *In infants younger than 34 weeks gestation the areola and nipple are barely visible. After 34 weeks, the areola becomes raised. Also, an infant of less than 36 weeks gestation has no breast tissue. Breast tissue arises with increasing gestational age because of maternal hormonal stimulation. Thus, an infant of 39–40 weeks will have 5–6 mm of breast tissue, and this amount will increase with age.*

FIGURE 26.7 *(continued)* **(E)** Heel to ear. **(F)** Plantar creases. **(G)** Breast tissue. *(continued)*

Premature Infant, 34–36 Weeks | **Full-Term Infant**

H

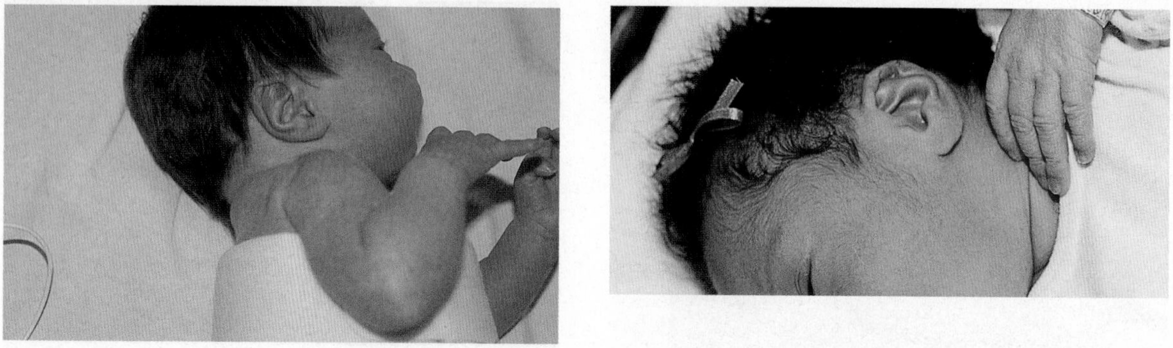

EARS *At fewer than 34 weeks gestation infants have very flat, relatively shapeless ears. Shape develops over time so that an infant between 34 and 36 weeks has a slight incurving of the superior part of the ear; the term infant is characterized by incurving of two thirds of the pinna; and in an infant older than 39 weeks the incurving continues to the lobe. If the extremely premature infant's ear is folded over, it will stay folded. Cartilage begins to appear at approximately 32 weeks so that the ear returns slowly to its original position. In an infant of more than 40 weeks gestation, there is enough ear cartilage so that the ear stands erect away from the head and returns quickly when folded. (When folding the ear over during examination, be certain that the surrounding area is wiped clean or the ear may adhere to the vernix.)*

Premature Male | **Full-Term Male**

I

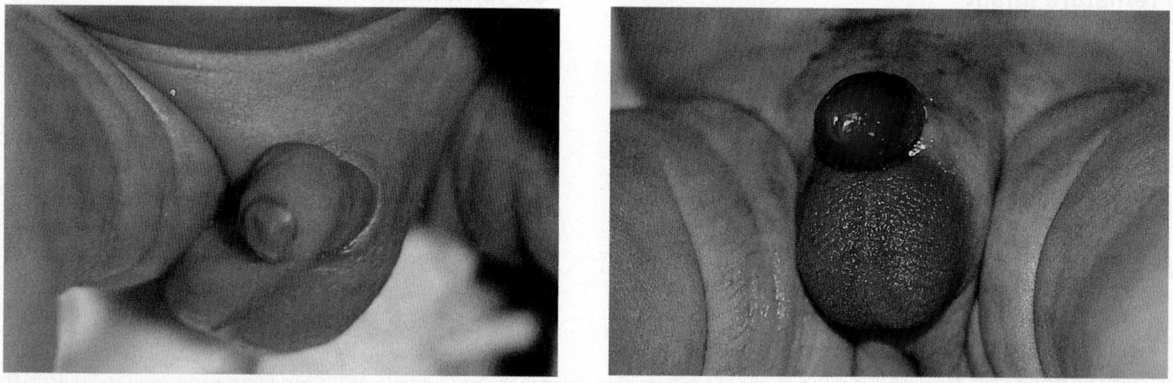

MALE GENITALIA *In the premature male, the testes are very high in the inguinal canal and there are very few rugae on the scrotum. The full-term infant's testes are lower in the scrotum and many rugae have developed.*

Premature Female | **Full-Term Female**

J

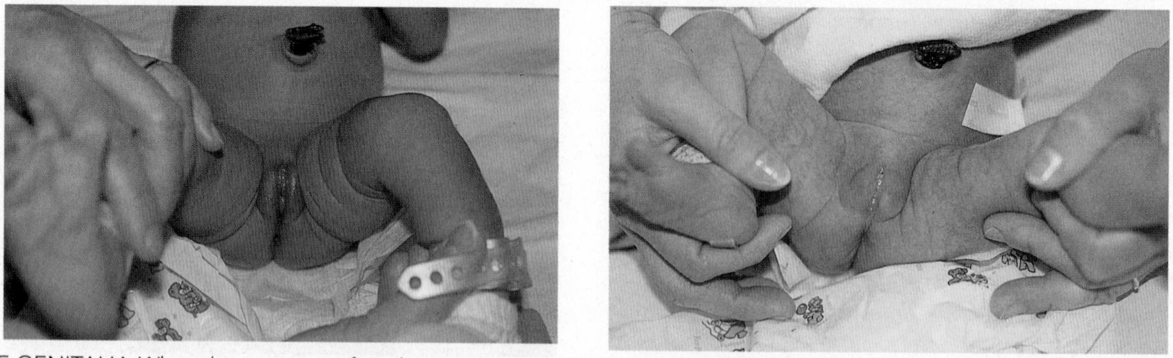

FEMALE GENITALIA *When the premature female is positioned on her back with hips abducted, the clitoris is very prominent and the labia majora are very small and widely separated. The labia minora and the clitoris are covered by the labia majora in the full-term infant.*

FIGURE 26.7 *(continued)* **(H)** Ears. **(I)** Male genitalia. **(J)** Female genitalia. (© Caroline Brown, RNC, MS, DEd.)

a small area of one ventricle; grade 2, a greater amount of bleeding occurred and multiple ventricles may be involved; grade 3, bleeding is so extensive the ventricles enlarge; and grade 4, there is bleeding into brain tissue surrounding the ventricles (Teune, Bakhuizen, Gyamfi Bannerman, et al., 2011). Infants with grade 1 or 2 bleeds have a good long-term prognosis; the prognosis of those with more intense bleeds is guarded until further complications are ruled out.

A long-term effect of hemorrhage may be the development of hydrocephalus if there was bleeding into the narrow aqueduct of Sylvius (Robinson, 2012). Preterm infants usually have a cranial ultrasound performed after the first few days of life and again just prior to discharge from the health care facility to detect if a hemorrhage has occurred.

Other Potential Complications. Preterm infants are also particularly susceptible to several illnesses in the early postnatal period, which can also occur in term infants, including RDS, apnea, and ROP (all discussed later in this chapter), as well as NEC (discussed in Chapter 45).

Nursing Diagnoses and Related Interventions

Because a preterm infant has few body resources, both physiologic and psychological stress must be reduced as much as possible and interventions should be initiated gently to prevent the depletion of available resources. Close observation and an analysis of findings are essential so concerns can be managed quickly.

Nursing Diagnosis: Impaired gas exchange related to immature pulmonary functioning

Outcome Evaluation: Newborn initiates breathing at birth after resuscitation, maintains normal newborn respirations of 30 to 60 breaths/min free of assisted ventilation; exhibits oxygen saturation levels of at least 95% as evidenced by pulse oximetry.

Preterm infants have great difficulty initiating respirations at birth because pulmonary capillaries are still so immature, and lung surfactant, which does not form in adequate amounts until about the 34th to 35th week of pregnancy, may not be present. Inadequate lung surfactant leads to alveolar collapse with each expiration. This collapse forces the infant to use maximum strength to inflate lung alveoli each time. Because this is so tiring, it becomes very difficult for infants to maintain effective inspirations under these stressful conditions. In addition, because a fetus usually turns to a vertex presentation late in pregnancy, a preterm infant may be born from a breech position. Because breech positions can result in the expulsion of meconium into the amniotic fluid, which can then be aspirated, the respiratory tract becomes aggravated by inflammation or pneumonia.

Cesarean birth, although it has the advantage of reducing pressure on the immature head, may be elected with preterm birth but also may lead to additional respiratory complications because infants born by cesarean birth retain more lung fluid than those born by vaginal birth. Giving the mother oxygen by mask during the birth can help provide a preterm infant with optimal oxygen saturation at birth (85% to 90%). Keeping maternal analgesia and anesthesia to a minimum also offers a preterm infant the best chance of initiating effective respirations.

Even term infants experience temporary respiratory acidosis until they take a first breath. Once respirations are established, however, this condition quickly clears. Because preterm infants cannot initiate effective respirations as quickly as mature infants, they are susceptible to irreversible acidosis. Birthing room teams need to be prepared with preterm-size laryngoscopes, endotracheal tubes, suction catheters, and synthetic surfactant to be administered by the endotracheal tube so resuscitation can be accomplished immediately. Be certain infants are kept warm during resuscitation so they do not have to expend extra energy to increase metabolic rate to maintain body temperature. Be certain as well that all procedures are carried out gently; a preterm infant's tissues are extremely sensitive to trauma and can be damaged or bruised easily by an oxygen mask. When blood from bruising is reabsorbed, this could yet lead to the addition problem of hyperbilirubinemia.

Many preterm babies, particularly those under 32 weeks of age, continue to have an irregular respiratory pattern (a few quick breaths, a period of 5 to 10 seconds without respiratory effort, a few quick breaths again, and so on). There is no bradycardia with this irregular pattern (sometimes termed **periodic respirations**). Although the pattern is seen in term infants as well, it seems to be intensified by immaturity. If true apnea, which needs immediate attention, is occurring, the pause in respirations is more than 20 seconds and bradycardia does occur.

The soft rib cartilage of a preterm infant is yet another source of respiratory problems because it causes ribs to collapse on expiration. The accessory muscles of respiration may be underdeveloped as well, leaving preterm infants with no backup muscles to use when they become fatigued. Because of this, preterm infants may need continued oxygen administration after resuscitation to allow them to effectively maintain respirations.

Giving a high level of oxygen to preterm infants during resuscitation or to maintain respirations presents two additional dangers: pulmonary edema and ROP (blindness of prematurity). The development of both of these conditions depends on saturation of the blood with oxygen (Po_2 of more than 100 mmHg, which usually occurs when oxygen is administered at a concentration over 70% (de Alba Campomanes, Binenbaum, & Quinn, 2012).

Nursing Diagnosis: Risk for deficient fluid volume related to insensible water loss at birth and small stomach capacity

Outcome Evaluation: Plasma glucose is between 40 and 60 mg per 100 ml; specific gravity of urine is maintained at 1.003 to 1.020; urine output is maintained at a minimum of 1 ml/kg/hr; electrolyte levels are within normal limits.

A preterm newborn experiences a high insensible water loss because of a large body surface relative to total body weight. Preterm infants also cannot concentrate urine well because of immature kidney function. Because of this, a high proportion of body fluid is excreted. All these factors may make a preterm baby need a higher percentage of fluid daily than a term infant (Mohan & Jain, 2012).

Intravenous fluid should be given via a continuous infusion pump to ensure a constant infusion rate and to prevent accidental overload. Assess intravenous sites conscientiously because, if infiltration should occur, the lack of subcutaneous tissue places a preterm newborn at risk for damaged tissue. Specially designed 27-gauge needles are available for use on small veins. However, many preterm infants lack adequately sized peripheral veins for even this small of a needle. Therefore, they need to receive intravenous fluid by an umbilical or central venous catheter.

Monitor the baby's weight, urine output and specific gravity, and serum electrolytes to ensure adequate fluid intake because too little fluid and calories can lead to weight loss, dehydration and starvation, and increased acidosis. Overhydration may lead to nonnutritional weight gain, pulmonary edema, and heart failure.

Most preterm infants void and pass meconium within 24 hours after birth, although this is delayed in very small infants. Measure urine output by weighing diapers rather than using urine collection bags because disposable collection bags can lead to skin irritation and breakdown from frequent changing and leaking.

The amount of urine output for the first few days of life in preterm babies is high in comparison with that of the term baby because of poor urine concentration: 40 to 100 ml/kg per 24 hours, compared with 10 to 20 ml/kg per 24 hours, respectively. The specific gravity is low, rarely more than 1.012 (normal term babies may concentrate urine up to 1.030). Test urine as well for glucose and ketones because these can reveal hyperglycemia caused by the glucose infusion, which then can lead to diuresis and extreme fluid loss. If too little glucose is being supplied and body cells are using protein for metabolism, ketone bodies will appear in the urine.

Blood glucose determinations should range between 40 and 60 mg/dl. Check for blood in stools to evaluate possible bleeding from the intestinal tract because this can help determine a cause of hypovolemia if this occurs.

Nursing Diagnosis: Risk for imbalanced nutrition, less than body requirements, related to additional nutrients needed for maintenance of rapid growth, possible sucking difficulty, and small stomach

Outcome Evaluation: Infant's weight follows percentile growth curve, skin turgor is good, specific gravity of urine is maintained between 1.003 and 1.020; the infant has no more than 15% weight loss in the first 3 days of life and continues to gain weight after this point.

Nutrition problems can arise with a preterm infant because the infant's body is attempting to continue to maintain the rapid rate of intrauterine growth appropriate for the gestational age. Because of this, a preterm newborn requires a relatively larger amount of nutrients than the mature infant, 115 to 140 calories per kilogram of body weight per day compared with 100 to 110 calories per kilogram of body weight per day needed by a term infant. Protein requirements are 3 to 3.5 g per kilogram of body weight, compared with 2.0 to 2.5 g per kilogram for a term newborn. Because preterm infants have a smaller stomach capacity than term neonates, as a rule, they must be fed more frequently with smaller amounts than term infants, perhaps as small as 1 or 2 ml every 2 to 3 hours.

If these nutrients are not supplied, an infant can develop hypocalcemia (decreased serum calcium) or azotemia (low protein level in the blood). Delayed feeding and a resultant decrease in intestinal motility may also add to hyperbilirubinemia, a problem infants already are at high risk of developing when fetal red blood cells begin to be destroyed.

Digestion and absorption of nutrients in a preterm infant's stomach and intestine may be immature, making the digestion of milk difficult. Nutrition problems are further compounded by a preterm infant's immature reflexes, which make swallowing and sucking difficult. Increased activity that occurs from ineffective sucking may increase the metabolic rate and oxygen requirements; if this happens, it increases the caloric requirements even more. In addition, the preterm infant's stomach capacity is so small that feedings quickly fill the stomach. If a small stomach is distended from a full feeding, this puts pressure on the diaphragm and can lead to respiratory distress. An immature cardiac sphincter (between the stomach and esophagus) allows regurgitation to occur readily. The lack of a cough reflex may lead an infant to aspirate regurgitated formula.

Feeding Schedule: With the early administration of intravenous fluid to prevent hypoglycemia and supply fluid, feedings may be safely delayed until an infant has stabilized his or her respiratory effort from birth. Very preterm infants may be fed by total parenteral nutrition until they are stable enough for other means. Breast, gavage, or bottle feedings are then begun as soon as the infant is able to tolerate them to prevent the deterioration of the intestinal villi. Preterm infants may have a chest X-ray taken before a first feeding. The presence of air in the stomach shows that the route to the stomach is clear or that no anomaly such as a tracheoesophageal fistula exists.

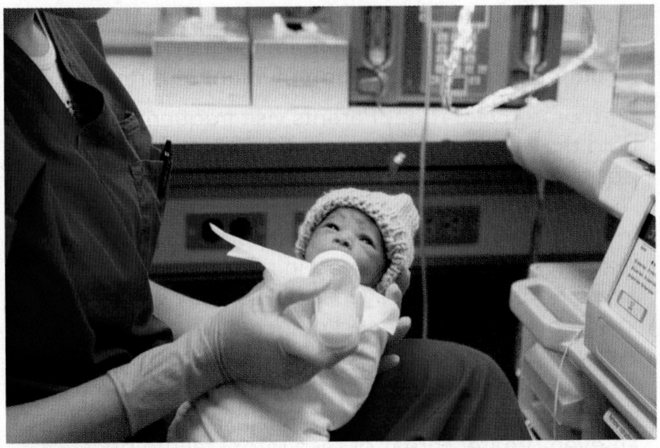

FIGURE 26.8 Feeding a preterm infant. Notice the small bottle used (Fuse/PunchStock).

Gavage Feeding: Although a sucking reflex is present earlier, the ability to coordinate sucking and swallowing is inconsistent until approximately 34 weeks of gestation. A gag reflex is not intact until 32 weeks of gestation. For this reason, for infants who are ill or experiencing respiratory distress may be started on gavage feedings; bottle feeding or breastfeeding will then be gradually introduced as the infant matures and begins to demonstrate feeding behaviors such as being awake, moving, or fussing as if hungry (Fig. 26.8). To avoid tiring, preterm nipples that are softer than regular nipples are used for bottle feedings.

Observe preterm infants closely after both oral or gavage feeding to be certain their filled stomach is not causing respiratory distress. Offering a pacifier during gavage feeding can help strengthen the sucking reflex, better prepare an infant for bottle feeding or breastfeeding, and provide oral satisfaction.

Gavage feedings may be given intermittently every few hours or continuously via tubes passed into the stomach or intestine through the mouth or nose. Infants may be fed by continuous drip feedings at about 1 ml/hr. This can be helpful for infants on ventilators or those who experience oxygen deprivation with handling. If feedings are given intermittently, stomach secretions are usually aspirated, measured, and replaced before each feeding. An infant who has a stomach content of more than 2 ml just before a feeding is receiving more formula than he or she can digest in the time allowed. Feedings should not be increased and possibly even cut back to ensure better digestion and to decrease the possibility of regurgitation and aspiration. An inability to digest in this way is also a sign that NEC, a destructive intestinal disorder that often occurs in preterm babies, may be developing (Smith, 2011) (see Chapter 45).

Breast Milk: There is increasing evidence that although preterm infants grow well on commercial formulas, the best milk for them, the same as with term infants, is breast milk (Furman & Schanler, 2012). The immunologic properties of breast milk apparently play a major role in preventing neonatal NEC, as well as an increase in immune defenses.

Mothers can express breast milk manually or with a breast pump for their infant's gavage feedings. If a woman cannot bring this in daily, she can freeze it for safe transport and storage. The sodium content of breast milk in a mother whose infant was born preterm is higher than that of milk in a mother whose infant has been born at term. Therefore, it is better for infants to receive their own mother's breast milk rather than banked milk if possible. This high level of sodium seems to be necessary for fluid retention in the preterm infant. Breast milk is 20 calories per ounce, so parents may be advised to add a human milk fortifier to supplemental bottles of breast milk to supply additional calories, protein, vitamins, and minerals (Zeigler, 2011). Urge mothers to continue to breastfeed their preterm infants after hospital discharge (Ahmed & Sands, 2010).

Formula: The caloric concentration of formulas used for preterm infants is usually 22 calories per ounce compared with 20 calories per ounce for a term baby (Mohan & Jain, 2012). Supplementing additional minerals such as iron, calcium, and phosphorus and electrolytes such as sodium, potassium, and chloride may be necessary, depending on the newborn's blood studies. Vitamin A is important in improving healing and possibly reducing the incidence of lung disease. Vitamin E seems to be important in preventing hemolytic anemia in preterm infants (Kositamongkol, Suthutvoravut, Chongviriyaphan, et al., 2011).

Nursing Diagnosis: Ineffective thermoregulation related to immaturity

Outcome Evaluation: Infant's temperature is maintained at 97.6°F (36.5°C) axillary.

Preterm newborns have a great deal of difficulty maintaining body temperature because they have a relatively large surface area per kilogram of body weight. In addition, because they do not flex their body well but remain in an extended position, rapid cooling from evaporation is more likely to occur (Gray & Flenady, 2011).

A preterm infant has little subcutaneous fat for insulation and poor muscular development and so cannot move as actively as an older infant to produce body heat. A preterm infant also has a limited amount of **brown fat**, the special tissue present in newborns that helps maintain body temperature. Preterm infants also cannot shiver, a useful mechanism to increase body temperature, nor can they sweat and thereby reduce body temperature because of their immature central nervous system and hypothalamic control. This makes preterm infants dependent on the environmental temperature provided to keep warm. In a birthing room, typically kept at 62° to 68°F (16.6° to 20°C), a 1,500-g infant exposed to this low a temperature loses 1°C of body heat every 3 minutes if left unprotected. Keeping preterm infants under radiant heat warmers, in incubators, or warmed by skin-to-skin contact helps to counteract this natural cooling.

Be certain a radiant heat warmer is prewarmed before the infant is born. Unless there are obvious abnormalities noted, a physical assessment of a preterm infant, even weighing, can be delayed until the infant can be placed in the warmth of an incubator or under a radiant warmer with a servo control.

If an infant is going to be transported to a department within the hospital, such as the X-ray department, or to a regional center for specialized care, keeping the newborn warm during transport is crucial. Remember that infants lose heat by radiation as well as conduction. If a warmed incubator is placed in a cold transport ambulance, for example, the infant will lose heat to the distant source. An additional heat shield or plastic wrap may need to be placed over an infant to help conserve heat during transport.

Nursing Diagnosis: Risk for infection related to immature immune defenses in the preterm infant

Outcome Evaluation: Temperature is maintained at 97.6°F (36.5°C) axillary; further signs and symptoms of infection such as poor growth or a reduced temperature are absent.

The skin of a preterm baby is easily traumatized and therefore offers less resistance to infection than the skin and mucous membrane of a mature baby. In addition, preterm infants have a lowered resistance to infection because they have difficulty producing phagocytes to localize infection as well as a deficiency of immune globulin (Ig)M antibodies because of insufficient production. To help prevent infection, linen and equipment used with preterm infants must not be shared with other infants. Staff members must be free of infection, and hand washing and gowning regulations should be strictly enforced.

Nursing Diagnosis: Risk for impaired parenting related to interference with parent–infant attachment resulting from hospitalization of infant at birth

Outcome Evaluation: Parents visit frequently and hold the infant; parents speak of their child in positive terms.

In a preterm infant, the first and second periods of reactivity normally observed in newborns at 1 hour and 4 hours of life (see Chapter 18) may be delayed. In some infants, no period of increased activity or tachycardia may appear until 12 to 18 hours of age. If the purpose of a period of reactivity is to stimulate respiratory function, this places a preterm infant at an even greater threat of respiratory failure because respiratory efforts may not be stimulated. A second consequence of a delayed period of reactivity is the loss of an opportunity for interaction between parents and the newborn in the early postpartum period.

Although it is extremely important to conserve a preterm infant's strength by reducing sensory stimulation as much as possible and handling an infant gently, preterm infants appear to need as much loving attention as term newborns. Rocking, singing and talking to them, and gentle holding them are measures to help preterm infants develop a sense of trust in people, which will enable them to relate satisfactorily to people in the future. Encourage parents to begin interacting with their infant as soon as possible (Box 26.4). Holding an infant with skin-to-skin contact is an effective way to begin this interaction.

BOX 26.4 Nursing Care Planning to Empower a Family

GUIDELINES FOR PARENTS OF A NEWBORN IN INTENSIVE CARE

Q. Mrs. Atkins tells you, "I'm always afraid I'll touch the wrong thing when I visit our son in the neonatal intensive care unit. What can I do to feel more comfortable there?"

A. Here are some guidelines that should be helpful:

- Learn the name of your child's primary health care provider and primary nurse or care manager. Make a point of talking to them when you visit so the information you receive is consistent and so these important people can get to know you.
- Discuss with your child's primary nurse the time you will usually visit so she or he can schedule your baby's procedures and rest times other than when you visit so there is time for you to hold your child and interact with him uninterrupted.
- Ask for explanations of any equipment or medications being used with your child so you understand the plan of care. Insist on being included in care decisions. The nurses are always nearby and will be happy to explain what can be touched and moved and what should be left alone for now.
- Any day you are unable to visit, call the nursery and ask to talk to your child's primary care nurse. Such telephone calls are not viewed as a bother but are welcomed as the mark of a concerned parent.
- Ask if you can supply expressed breast milk for your infant as soon as feedings are started so you can feel you're having a greater part in your baby's care.
- You might supply a tape recording of your voice so your baby can learn to recognize it, as well as supply a small toy for your baby's bed. These actions not only supply auditory and visual stimulation for your child but also help to give you a more "normal" feeling toward infant care.
- Use your baby's name when you talk about him (not "the baby") to help you gain a firm feeling that this is your baby, not the nursery's.
- If your child is hospitalized a distance from home, ask if transfer to a local hospital in a less technical environment will be possible as soon as he's not so ill.

Before effective bonding can be established, parents may need time to come to terms with their feelings of disappointment that the infant is so small or guilt that they were not able to prevent the preterm birth. Helping them air these feelings and develop a more positive attitude toward their preterm infant is an important nursing responsibility.

Because parents may not be psychologically ready for birth when a preterm baby is born, it may be more difficult for them to believe they have a child and to begin interacting than if the baby had been born at term. Even if an infant cannot be removed from an incubator or a radiant heat warmer, parents can still handle and stroke the infant in the incubator or warmer for interaction. Encourage women to come to the nursery and hold the baby before and after gavage feedings and to breast or bottle feed as soon as the baby is ready for this. By feeding her baby or expressing milk for feedings, a woman is directly participating in care and learning the first steps of her new role.

If the baby is going to be transferred to a regional center, make sure the parents have an opportunity to see the baby before the transfer. A photograph of the baby for them to keep is helpful in making the birth more real. Encourage them to visit the distant site as often as possible. Sending them photos snapped with a cell phone or pasting notes as if they're messages from the baby taped to the incubator or warmer ("Hi, Mom & Dad. I'm doing well") for them to see when they visit can not only keep parents involved but also help with bonding.

On days they cannot visit, parents can still stay in touch by telephone or nursery e-mail. By these means, by the time a baby is ready for discharge, the parents should be able to feel they are taking home "their" baby, one whom they know and have already begun to love.

Parents visiting a high-risk nursery often need a great deal of support from nursing personnel. Remember that, although radiant warmers, incubators, ventilators, and monitors become familiar equipment to nurses, they are unusual and frightening to parents (Box 26.5). In such a high-tech setting, a parent may want very much to touch an infant but be so afraid touching might set off an alarm that he or she stands with arms folded (Fig. 26.9).

Because preterm infants can be hospitalized for long periods, parents can feel baffled by receiving information from a parade of different health care providers or a different person every time they visit. Primary nursing or case management with one nurse as the consistent caregiver helps to reduce the number of people who contact the parents and who communicate the parents' needs to the rest of the staff.

Try to make a baby's siblings as welcome in a high-risk nursery as the baby's parents in order to build

BOX 26.5 Nursing Care Planning Based on Effective Communication

Mrs. Atkins gave birth 2 days ago to a 2-lb boy at 30 weeks of pregnancy who has been classified as a small-for-gestational-age preterm infant. Although you have told Mrs. Atkins twice she is welcome to visit the neonatal intensive care unit (NICU) as much as she'd like, you notice her electronic record indicates she has done so only once.

Less Effective Communication

Nurse: Mrs. Atkins, I've noticed you haven't been to the nursery to see your son yet.
Mrs. Atkins: I'm waiting for my husband to get here.
Nurse: Will that be today?
Mrs. Atkins: Tomorrow. He's still out of town on business.
Nurse: Have you called the nursery and asked about your son?
Mrs. Atkins: I'll wait for my husband. We'll do it together.
Nurse: Okay. Let me know if there is anything else you need.

More Effective Communication

Nurse: Mrs. Atkins, I've noticed you haven't been to the nursery to see your son yet.
Mrs. Atkins: I'm waiting for my husband to get here.
Nurse: Will that be today?
Mrs. Atkins: Tomorrow. He's still out of town on business.
Nurse: Have you called the nursery and asked about your son?
Mrs. Atkins: I'm waiting for my husband. We'll do it together.
Nurse: I know it seems important for you to go as a family, but I hate to see you miss these first few days with your son. What if I go with you?
Mrs. Atkins: Could you? I absolutely can't go up there alone.

Visiting a NICU can be intimidating for parents, not only because of the high-tech equipment that surrounds their baby but also because their baby often appears much smaller or sicker than they imagined.
In the first scenario, the nurse assumed waiting for the husband to come to the hospital was what was important. In the second scenario, the nurse asked enough questions to realize that having another person accompany her to the nursery was what the woman wanted most—a need the nurse could meet.

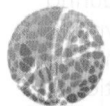

QSEN Checkpoint Question 26.2

Teamwork & Collaboration

Baby Atkin's father plays in a garage band for a hobby, and his mother enjoys knitting. Your care team has agreed to design a developmental care environment for Baby Atkins that will both make him feel secure and help his parents interact more with him. Which would be the best action for your team to take?

a. Turn up the lights in his part of the nursery so he can see his parents better.
b. Ask the father to bring in a CD recording of his band to play for the baby.
c. Arrange a blanket Mrs. Atkins has knit into a circle or "nest" for the baby.
d. Remind the parents that he must stay awake for extended periods for his eyes to fully develop.

Look in Appendix A for the best answer and rationale.

The Small-for-Gestational-Age Infant

An infant is SGA (also called microsomia) if the birth weight is below the 10th percentile on an intrauterine growth curve for that age. Such infants may be born preterm (before week 38 of gestation), term (between weeks 38 and 42), or postterm (past 42 weeks). SGA infants are small for their age because they have experienced **intrauterine growth restriction (IUGR)** or failed to grow at the expected rate in utero (Rahimian, 2013). This characteristic makes them distinctly different from infants who are born with a less weight than usual but their low weight is consistent for their gestational age.

Etiology

A woman's nutrition during pregnancy plays a major role in fetal growth, so a lack of adequate nutrition may be a major contributor to IUGR (Ota, Tobe-Gai, Mori, et al., 2012).

Adolescents are prone to having a high incidence of SGA infants because, if they eat only enough to meet their own nutritional and growth needs, the needs of a growing fetus can be compromised. In still other instances, the placental supply of nutrients is adequate but an infant cannot use them because of a chromosomal abnormality or an intrauterine infection such as rubella or toxoplasmosis.

Even in light of these nutritional influences, the most common cause of IUGR is a placental anomaly: either the placenta did not obtain sufficient nutrients from the uterine arteries or it was inefficient at transporting nutrients to the fetus. Placental underdevelopment or damage, such as partial placental separation with bleeding is an example of a situation that would limit placental function because the area of placenta that separated infarcted and fibrosed, reducing the placental surface available for nutrient exchange. Women with systemic diseases that decrease blood flow to the placenta, such as severe diabetes mellitus or gestational hypertension (diseases in which blood vessel lumens are narrowed), are at higher risk for birthing SGA babies than others. Women who smoke heavily or use opiates also tend to have SGA infants (Ortigosa, Friguls, Joya, et al., 2012).

Assessment

The SGA infant may be detected in utero when fundal height during pregnancy becomes progressively less than expected. However, if a woman is unsure of the date of her last menstrual period, this discrepancy can be hard to substantiate; a sonogram can then demonstrate the decreased size. A biophysical profile including a nonstress test, placental grading, amniotic fluid amount, and an ultrasound examination documents additional information on placental function and fetal growth. If poor placental function is apparent from such determinations, it can be predicted that the infant will do poorly during labor during the periods of relative hypoxia, which occur during contractions. Cesarean birth, therefore, is the birth method of choice in such circumstances.

Appearance. Generally, an infant who suffers nutritional deprivation early in pregnancy, when fetal growth consists primarily of an increase in the number of body cells, is below average in weight, length, and head circumference. An infant who suffers deprivation late in pregnancy, when growth consists primarily of an increase in cell size, may have only a reduction in weight. Regardless of when deprivation occurs, the infant tends to have an overall wasted appearance. The infant may have poor skin turgor and generally appears to have a large head because the rest of the body is so small. Skull sutures may be widely separated. Hair may be dull and lusterless. The child may have a small liver, which can cause difficulty regulating glucose, protein, and bilirubin levels after birth. The abdomen may be sunken. The umbilical cord often appears dry and may be stained yellow.

In contrast, because an infant's age is more advanced than the weight implies, a child may have better developed neurologic responses, sole creases, and ear cartilage than expected for a baby of that weight. The infant may also seem unusually alert and active. As a first assessment, the SGA infant needs to be examined carefully for possible congenital anomalies that occurred because of the poor nutritional intrauterine environment.

Laboratory Findings. Blood studies at birth usually show a high hematocrit level (less than normal amounts of plasma in proportion to red blood cells are present because of a lack of fluid) and an increase in the total number of red blood cells (polycythemia). The increase in red blood cells occurs because anoxia during intrauterine life stimulated excess development of them. An immediate effect of polycythemia is to cause increased blood viscosity, a condition that puts extra work on the infant's heart because it is more difficult to effectively circulate thick blood. As a consequence, acrocyanosis (blueness of the hands and feet) may be prolonged and persistently more marked than usual. If the polycythemia is extreme, vessels may actually become blocked and thrombus formation can result. If the hematocrit level is more than 65% to 70%, an exchange transfusion to dilute the blood may be necessary.

A second problem of polycythemia is hyperbilirubinemia because so many extra red blood cells break down and release bilirubin.

Because SGA infants have decreased glycogen stores, still another common problem that develops is hypoglycemia (decreased blood glucose, or a level below 45 mg/dl). Such infants may need intravenous glucose to sustain blood sugar until they are able to suck vigorously enough to take sufficient oral feedings.

Nursing Diagnoses and Related Interventions

Nursing Diagnosis: Ineffective breathing pattern related to underdeveloped body systems at birth

Outcome Evaluation: Newborn maintains respirations at a rate of 30 to 60 breaths/min after resuscitation at birth.

Birth asphyxia is a common problem for SGA infants, both because they have underdeveloped chest muscles and because they are at risk for developing meconium aspiration syndrome (MAS) as a result of meconium release, which occurs when fetal anoxia develops during labor to cause reflex relaxation of the anal sphincter. When gasping for breath in utero, the fetus draws meconium discharged from the intestine into the amniotic fluid down into the trachea and bronchi. Acting as a foreign substance, this blocks airflow into the alveoli and causes the SGA infant to need resuscitation at birth. Closely observe both respiratory rate and character in the first few hours of life as underdeveloped chest muscles not only make drawing in a first breath difficult but can make SGA infants unable to sustain an adequate newborn respiratory rate.

Nursing Diagnosis: Risk for ineffective thermoregulation related to lack of subcutaneous fat

Outcome Evaluation: Infant's temperature is maintained at 36.5°C (97.8°F) axillary.

SGA infants are less able to control body temperature than other newborns because they lack subcutaneous fat. A carefully controlled environment is essential to keep the infant's body temperature in a neutral zone (see Chapter 18).

Nursing Diagnosis: Risk for impaired parenting related to child's high-risk status and possible cognitive or neurologic impairment from lack of nutrients in utero

Outcome Evaluation: Parents express interest in infant and ask questions about what the child's care needs will be at home; parents hold infant warmly.

Although SGA infants may gain weight and appear to thrive in the first few days of life, their cognitive development may have been impaired because of lack of oxygen and nourishment in utero. Babies who were growing normally in utero but whose gestation was interrupted (true preterm, AGA babies) usually gain weight and height so rapidly that by the end of the first year of life they are near the 50th percentile on growth charts. SGA infants, in contrast, may always be below the usual height on standard growth charts. This inability to reach normal levels of growth and development can interfere with bonding if a child does not meet the parents' expectations. Eventually, it can interfere with the child's self-esteem if the child is never able to meet parental expectations or reach full height.

Yet another need of an SGA infant is adequate stimulation during the infant period in order to reach normal growth and developmental milestones. Encourage parents to provide toys suitable for their child's chronologic age, not physical size. Because an infant tires easily in the first few weeks of life, urge them to space play periods with rest periods or hypoglycemia or apnea can occur. All infants with IUGR need continued follow-up after hospital discharge because they may have neurologic deficits that will interfere with learning at preschool age (Dall'Oglio, Rosseillo, Coletti, et al., 2010).

The Large-for-Gestational-Age Infant

An infant is LGA (also termed **macrosomia**) if the birth weight is above the 90th percentile on an intrauterine growth chart for that gestational age. Such a baby appears deceptively healthy at birth because of the weight, but a gestational age examination often reveals immature development. It is important that LGA infants be identified immediately so they can be given care appropriate to their gestational age rather than being treated as term newborns (Ouzounian & Goodwin, 2010).

Etiology

Infants who are LGA have been subjected to an overproduction of nutrients and growth hormone in utero. This happens most often to infants of women who are obese or who have diabetes mellitus (Miller & Morris, 2011). Multiparous women may also have large babies because with each succeeding pregnancy, babies tend to grow larger. Beckwith–Wiedemann syndrome, a rare condition characterized by general body overgrowth and congenital anomalies such as omphalocele, may also be a cause.

Assessment

A fetus is suspected of being LGA when a woman's uterus appears to be unusually large for the date of pregnancy. Abdominal size can be deceptive, however. Because a fetus lies in a flexed fetal position, he or she does not occupy significantly more space at 10 lb than at 7 lb. If a fetus does seem to be growing at an abnormally rapid rate, a sonogram can confirm the suspicion. A nonstress test to assess the placenta's ability to sustain a large fetus during labor may be prescribed. Lung maturity may be assessed by amniocentesis.

If an infant's large size was not detected during pregnancy, it may be first recognized during labor when the baby appears too large to descend through the pelvic rim. If this happens, a cesarean birth may be necessary because **shoulder dystocia** (the wide fetal shoulders cannot pass through the outlet of the pelvis) would halt vaginal birth at that point.

- Distorted familial breathing patterns
- Decreased arousal responses
- Possible lack of surfactant in alveoli
- Sleeping in a room without moving air currents (the infant rebreathes expired carbon dioxide)

Typically, affected infants are well nourished. Parents may report an infant had a slight head cold. After being put to bed at night or for a nap, the infant is then found dead a few hours later. Infants who die this way do not appear to make any sound as they die, which indicates they die with laryngospasm. Although many infants are found with blood-flecked sputum or vomitus in their mouths or on the bedclothes, this seems to occur as the result of death, not as its cause. An autopsy often reveals petechiae in the lungs and mild inflammation and congestion in the respiratory tract. However, these symptoms are not severe enough to cause sudden death. It is clear these infants do not suffocate from bedclothes or choke from overfeeding, underfeeding, or crying. Since the AAP made its recommendation to put newborns to sleep on their back, the incidence of SIDS has declined almost 50% to 60%. Other recommendations include the use of a firm sleep surface; breastfeeding; room sharing without bed sharing; routine immunizations; consideration of using a pacifier; and avoidance of soft bedding, overheating, and exposure to tobacco smoke, alcohol, and illicit drugs (Moon & Fu, 2012). Although it was once thought having infants sleep with a fan in their room to keep air moving might decrease the incidence of SIDS, the AAP has noted that, currently, there is insufficient evidence to recommend the use of a fan as a SIDS risk-reduction strategy (AAP, 2011b).

Parents have a difficult time accepting the death of any child. This can be especially difficult when it happens so suddenly and to an infant. In discussing the child, they often use both the past and present tense as if they are not yet aware of the death. Many parents experience a period of somatic symptoms that occur with acute grief, such as nausea, stomach pain, or vertigo. Parents should be counseled by a nurse or someone else trained in counseling at the time of the infant's death; it helps if they can talk to this same person periodically for however long it takes to resolve their grief. The American Sudden Infant Death Syndrome Institute, listed at the beginning of the chapter, offers suggestions for counseling.

Autopsy reports should be given to parents as soon as they are available (if toxicology tests are included in the autopsy, results will not be available for weeks). Reading that their child's death was unexplained can help to reassure parents the death was not their fault. They need this assurance if they are to plan for other children. If there are older children in the family, they also need assurance SIDS is a disease of infants and the strange phenomenon that invaded their home and killed a younger brother or sister will not also kill them. If they wished the infant dead, as all children wish siblings were dead on some days, they need reassurance their wishes did not cause the baby's death.

When another child is born, parents can be expected to become extremely frightened at any sign of illness in their child. They need support to see them through the first few months of the second child's life, particularly until past the point at which the first child died. Some parents may need support to view a second child as an individual child and not as a replacement for the first child.

A new baby born to a family in which a SIDS infant died can be screened using a sleep assessment as a precaution within the first 2 weeks of life or, if the parents' level of anxiety is acute, before hospital discharge. The baby may then be placed on continuous apnea monitoring pending the results of the sleep assessment.

Apparent Life-Threatening Event

Some infants have been discovered cyanotic and limp in their beds but have survived after mouth-to-mouth resuscitation by parents. An episode of this kind is called an **apparent life-threatening event** (Scollan-Koliopoulos & Koliopoulos, 2010). For these infants, as well as for preterm infants with a tendency toward apnea, or new babies born to a family whose child died from SIDS, apnea monitoring may be prescribed. With apnea monitoring in place, an alarm sounds when the neonate experiences a period of apnea of 20 seconds or longer or a decreased heart rate below 80 beats/min (Fig. 26.10). If parents are going to use an apnea monitor at home, make certain they will be able to hear it in all parts of the house or apartment. Usually, for example, the alarm is not loud enough to be heard in the basement from an upstairs bedroom. Caution parents about household noises such as a loud television, radio, vacuum cleaner, or hair dryer that may interfere with hearing the alarm. Be certain they know how to apply and reposition the apnea leads and that they are comfortable enough with the monitor to see past it to the child. In addition, parents should be taught infant cardiopulmonary resuscitation before their infant is discharged from the hospital; reviewing the technique of this at health care visits is helpful (Fig. 26.11).

Caring for a child at home on an apnea monitor may be extremely stressful because parents are often reluctant to leave the baby in someone else's care for even a short time or they have difficulty finding a competent babysitter. These parents can benefit from a community or home care referral so they have a second opinion regarding how well they are managing, as well as a listening ear to discuss the strain of having to be constantly alert for a sound that means their infant has stopped breathing. Having someone periodically review with them what steps to take should the alarm sound (e.g., jiggle the baby, begin mouth-to-mouth resuscitation, call emergency response personnel) can be very comforting.

✔ QSEN Checkpoint Question 26.4

Safety

Baby Atkins is at risk for having apnea and bradycardia. What initial nursing intervention should you initiate during these events to maintain his vital signs in a safe range?

a. Administer 2 drops (gtts) of oral theophylline by a small syringe into his mouth.
b. Gently flick the sole of his foot to stimulate the baby to breathe again.
c. Monitor rectal temperatures to prevent him from becoming cold or hot.
d. Vigorously suction him every 2 hours to keep airway clear of secretions.

Look in Appendix A for the best answer and rationale.

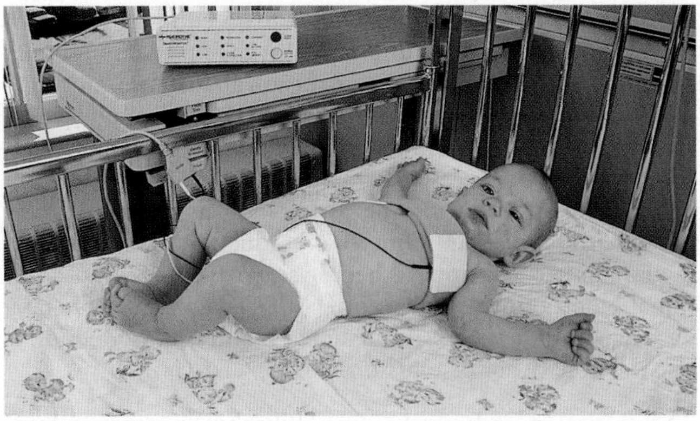

FIGURE 26.10 A home apnea monitor uses a soft belt with a Velcro attachment to hold two leads in the appropriate position on the chest.

Periventricular Leukomalacia

Periventricular leukomalacia (PVL) is the abnormal formation of the white matter of the brain (Horbar, Carpenter, Badger, et al., 2012). It is caused by an anoxic episode that interferes with circulation to a portion of the brain. Phagocytes and macrophages invade the area to clear away necrotic tissue. What is left is an abnormality in the white matter of the brain, which is revealed on a sonogram as a hollow space. PVL occurs most frequently in preterm infants who experience cerebral ischemia. Once the condition has occurred, there is no therapy. Infants may die of the original insult; they may be left with long-term effects such as learning disabilities or cerebral palsy. Any action to reduce environmental stimuli or sudden shifts in cerebral blood flow, such as avoiding rapid fluid infusions or reducing pain, is important for preventing PVL and limiting this long-term effect of prematurity (Stoll, Hansen, Bell, et al., 2010).

Hemolytic Disease of the Newborn (Hyperbilirubinemia)

The term "hemolytic" is Latin for "destruction" (lysis) of red blood cells. A certain degree of lysis of red blood cells in the newborn results from the destruction of red blood cells by a normal

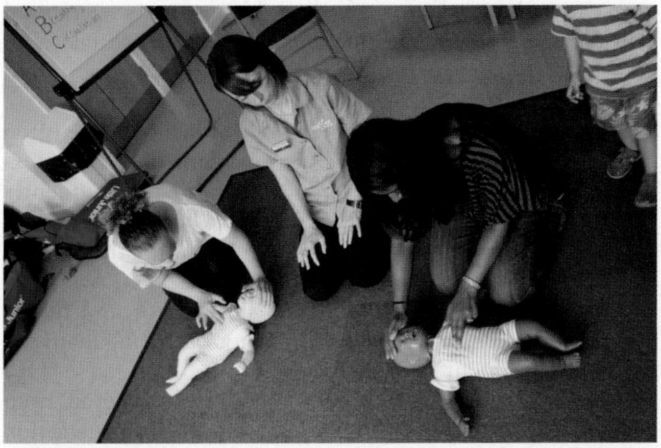

FIGURE 26.11 Parents of infants with respiratory disorders need to learn cardiac massage before their infant is discharged from the hospital. Here, parents learn the technique using specialized dolls (Ian Miles, Flashpoint Pictures/Alamy).

physiologic process as the newborn breaks down excess red blood cells formed in utero (see Chapter 18). Hemolytic disease is present when there is excessive destruction of red blood cells, which leads to elevated bilirubin levels **(hyperbilirubinemia)**. In the past, hemolytic disease of the newborn was most often caused by an Rh blood type incompatibility. Because the prevention of Rh antibody formation has been available for almost 50 years, the disorder is now most often caused by an ABO incompatibility. In both instances, because the fetus has a different blood type than the mother, the mother builds antibodies against the fetal red blood cells, leading to hemolysis of the cells, severe anemia, and hyperbilirubinemia.

Rh Incompatibility

In every pregnancy, a few red blood cells enter the maternal circulation. If the mother's blood type is Rh (D) negative and the fetal blood type is Rh positive (contains the D antigen), this introduction of fetal blood causes sensitization to occur and the woman to begin to form antibodies against the D antigen. Few antibodies actually form this way during pregnancy, however. Most form in the woman's bloodstream in the first 72 hours after birth because there is an active exchange of fetal–maternal blood as placental villi loosen and the placenta is delivered. Because of this surge in antibody formation after a pregnancy, in a second pregnancy there will be a high level of antibody D already circulating in the woman's bloodstream. This will then act to destroy the fetal red blood cells beginning early in the next pregnancy if the new fetus is Rh positive, leading to the fetus being severely compromised by the end of that pregnancy.

Rh incompatibility is little seen today because if Rh- women receive Rho immune globulin (RHIG or RhoGAM) (passive Rh antibodies) within 72 hours after birth of an Rh+ child, the process of antibody formation will be halted and sensitization will not occur. The possibility Rh incompatibility could exist, however, must be assessed for during pregnancy and again at birth because some women (especially those who received prenatal care in another country) may not have received RHIG following the birth or miscarriage of a former Rh+ fetus.

ABO Incompatibility

In most instances of ABO incompatibility, the maternal blood type is O and the fetal blood type is A; it may also occur when the fetus has type B or AB blood. A reaction in an infant with type B blood is often the most marked.

Hemolysis can become a problem with a first pregnancy in which there is an ABO incompatibility because the antibodies to A and B cell types are naturally occurring antibodies or are present from birth in anyone whose red cells lack these antigens. Fortunately, unlike the antibodies formed against the Rh D factor, these antibodies are of the large (immune globulin [Ig]M) class and so do not cross the placenta. An infant of an ABO incompatibility, therefore, is not born anemic, as the Rh-sensitized child could be. Hemolysis of the blood begins with birth, when blood and antibodies are exchanged during the mixing of maternal and fetal blood as the placenta is loosened; destruction may continue as long as 2 weeks. Interestingly, preterm infants do not seem to be affected by ABO incompatibility. This may be because the receptor sites for anti-A or anti-B antibodies do not appear on red cells until late in fetal life. Even in the mature newborn, a direct Coombs test may be only weakly positive because of the few anti-A or anti-B sites present. The reticulocyte count (immature or newly formed red blood cells) is usually elevated as the infant attempts to replace destroyed cells.

Assessment

Rh incompatibility of the newborn can be predicted by finding a rising anti-Rh titer or a rising level of antibodies (indirect Coombs test) in a woman during pregnancy. It can be confirmed by detecting antibodies on the fetal erythrocytes in cord blood (positive direct Coombs test) by percutaneous umbilical blood sampling (see Chapter 9) or at birth. The mother in this situation will always have Rh-negative blood (*dd*), and the baby will be Rh positive (*DD* or *Dd*).

With Rh incompatibility, an infant may not appear pale at birth despite the red cell destruction that occurred in utero because the accelerated production of red cells during the last few months in utero compensates to some degree for the destruction. The liver and spleen may be enlarged from attempts to destroy damaged blood cells. If the number of red cells has significantly decreased, the blood in the vascular circulation may be hypotonic to interstitial fluid, causing fluid to shift from the lower to higher isotonic pressure by osmosis, resulting in extreme edema. Finally, the severe anemia can result in heart failure as the heart has to beat so fast to push the diluted blood forward. **Hydrops fetalis** is an old term for the appearance of a severely involved infant at birth; hydrops refers to the edema and fetalis refers to the lethal state.

Most infants do not appear jaundiced at birth because the maternal circulation has evacuated the rising indirect bilirubin level. With birth, progressive jaundice, usually occurring within the first 24 hours of life, will begin, indicating in both Rh and ABO incompatibility that a hemolytic process is at work. The jaundice occurs because, as red blood cells are destroyed, indirect bilirubin is released. Indirect bilirubin is fat soluble and cannot be excreted from the body. Under usual circumstances, the liver enzyme glucuronyl transferase converts indirect bilirubin to direct bilirubin. Direct bilirubin is water soluble and combines with bile for excretion from the body with feces. In preterm infants or those with extreme hemolysis, the liver cannot convert all of the indirect bilirubin produced to direct bilirubin, so jaundice becomes extreme.

Normally, cord blood has a total serum bilirubin (TsB) level of 0 to 3 mg/100 ml. An increasing bilirubin level becomes dangerous if the level rises above 20 mg/dl in a term infant and perhaps as low as 12 mg/dl in a preterm infant because brain damage from bilirubin-induced neurologic dysfunction (BIND), a wide spectrum of disorders caused by increasingly severe hyperbilirubinemia ranging from mild dysfunction to ABE (invasion of bilirubin into brain cells), can occur. A second concern that arises from excessive red blood cell destruction is that an infant is forced to use glucose stores to maintain metabolism in the presence of anemia. This can cause a progressive hypoglycemia, compounding the initial problem. A decrease in hemoglobin during the first week of life to a level less than that of the cord blood is a later indication of blood loss or hemolysis.

Therapeutic Management

Bilirubin levels in blood may be measured by either a blood draw (total serum bilirubin [TsB]) or by holding a transcutaneous meter against the infant's skin (transcutaneous bilirubin [TcB]). The initiation of early feeding (urge mothers to breastfeed 8 to 10 times a day for the first 2 days), use of phototherapy, and exchange transfusion all may be immediate measures necessary to reduce the total serum bilirubin level in an infant affected by a blood incompatibility. In infants with severe hemolytic disease, the hemoglobin concentration can continue to drop during the first 6 months of life, or their bone marrow may fail to increase production of erythrocytes in response to continuing hemolysis so they need an additional blood transfusion to correct this late anemia. Therapy with erythropoietin to stimulate red blood cell production is also possible (Aher & Ohlsson, 2012).

The Initiation of Early Feeding. Bilirubin is removed from the body by being incorporated into feces. Therefore, the sooner bowel elimination begins, the sooner bilirubin removal begins. Early feeding (either breast milk or formula), therefore, stimulates bowel peristalsis and helps to accomplish this.

Phototherapy. An infant's liver processes little bilirubin in utero because the mother's circulation does this for an infant. With birth, exposure to light apparently triggers the liver to assume this function. Additional light supplied by phototherapy appears to speed the conversion potential of the liver. In phototherapy, an infant is continuously exposed to specialized light such as quartz halogen, cool white daylight, or special blue fluorescent light. The lights are placed 12 to 30 in. above the newborn's bassinet or incubator.

Term newborns are generally scheduled for phototherapy when the total serum bilirubin level rises to 10 to 12 mg/dl at 24 hours of age; preterm infants may have treatment begun at levels lower than this (Symons & Mahoney, 2011). Although the results of the therapy are mixed, the administration of intravenous immunoglobulin (IVIG) has been used in neonates with hemolytic disease in combination with phototherapy, especially in ABO incompatibility to try and extenuate the effect of phototherapy (Demirel, Akar, Celik, et al., 2011).

Continuous exposure to bright lights by phototherapy may be harmful to a newborn's retina, so the infant's eyes must always be covered while under bilirubin lights. Eye dressings or cotton balls can be firmly secured in place by an infant mask. Check the dressings frequently to be certain they have not slipped or are causing corneal irritation. The point at which infants are most apt to dislodge eye patches is when they cry as they wake for a feeding. Urge parents to respond quickly, therefore, if the infant is in their postpartal room to avoid eye damage and possible suffocation by the infant pushing the eye patches down over the nose (Fig. 26.12).

The stools of an infant under bilirubin lights are often bright green because of the excessive bilirubin being excreted as the result of the therapy. They are also frequently loose and may be irritating to the skin. Urine may be dark colored from urobilinogen formation. Monitor the infant's axillary temperature to prevent him or her from overheating under the bright lights. Assess skin turgor and intake and output to ensure dehydration is not occurring from the warm environment.

Infants receiving phototherapy should be removed from under the lights for feeding so they continue to have interaction with their mother. Remove the eye patches while the infant is out from under the lights for a period of visual stimulation. To prevent a lengthy hospital stay, infants may be discharged and continue therapy at home. Specialized fiber optic light systems incorporated into a fiber optic blanket also have been developed and are ideal for home care. The light generated by the blanket has the same effect on bilirubin levels as banks of overhead lights. The infant is undressed except for a diaper to protect the ovaries or testes and so as much skin surface as possible is exposed to the light. Two big advantages are that an infant can be held for long periods without interrupting the phototherapy, and eye patches are unnecessary.

Parents need an explanation of the rationale for phototherapy and why their infant needs it. Although phototherapy has not been used long enough that long-term effects can be studied, there appears to be minimal risk to an infant from the procedure, provided the infant's eyes remain covered and dehydration from increased insensitive water loss does not occur. Even though there is no evidence so far that infants who received phototherapy are at greater risk for developing skin cancer, all infants who receive phototherapy should (as should all infants) have sunscreen applied when they are in the sun and follow-up assessments in coming years to detect skin cancer that possibly could occur from the therapy (Brewster, Tucker, Fleming, et al., 2010).

Exchange Transfusion. The use of intensive phototherapy in conjunction with hydration and close monitoring of serum bilirubin levels has greatly reduced the need for exchange transfusions. If this is done, small amounts (2 to 10 ml) of the infant's blood are drawn from the infant's umbilical vein and then replaced with equal amounts of donor blood. The therapy may be used for any condition that leads to hyperbilirubinemia or polycythemia. When used as therapy for blood incompatibility, it removes approximately 85% of sensitized red cells. It reduces the serum concentration of indirect bilirubin and can prevent heart failure in infants with severe anemia or polycythemia.

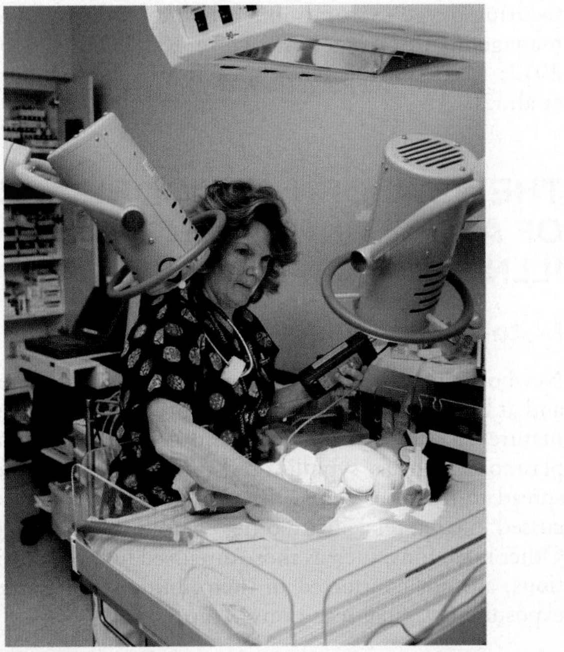

FIGURE 26.12 A newborn receiving phototherapy is undressed except for a diaper so he receives maximum exposure to the lights. His eyes are covered snugly to protect them from the ultraviolet light.

A transfusion should be done under a radiant heat warmer to keep the infant warm during what can be a lengthy procedure to prevent energy expenditure from having to maintain body temperature. Donor blood must be maintained at room temperature, or hypothermia from the cold insult could result. Use only commercial blood warmers to warm blood, not hot towels or a radiant heat warmer, to avoid destroying red cells.

The type of blood used for transfusion is O Rh-negative blood, even if an infant's blood type is positive; if Rh-positive or type A or B blood were given, the maternal antibodies that entered the infant's circulation would destroy this blood also, and the transfusion would be ineffective. If the baby will be transported to a regional center for the exchange transfusion, a sample of the mother's blood should accompany the infant, so cross-matching on the mother's serum can be done there.

After a transfusion, closely observe the infant to be certain vital signs are stable and there is no umbilical vessel bleeding or inflammation of the cord if this was the transfusion site, which would suggest infection. Report any changes in vital signs. Monitor bilirubin levels for 2 or 3 days after the transfusion to ensure the level of indirect bilirubin is not rising again and that no further phototherapy or transfusion is necessary.

Hemorrhagic Disease of the Newborn

Hemorrhagic disease of the newborn results from a deficiency of vitamin K, the vitamin essential for the formation of prothrombin by the liver (Young, 2012). Lack of vitamin K causes decreased prothrombin function and, therefore, impaired blood coagulation. Vitamin K is formed by the action of bacteria in the intestine. Because the intestinal tract of a newborn is sterile at birth, an infant forms minimal amounts of vitamin K until normal intestinal tract flora are established at about 24 hours of age. Babies born to women receiving antiseizure medication are at high risk for the condition because many of these medications also interfere with vitamin K formation. Administering vitamin K intramuscularly to these women before birth can help to protect the newborn.

Shortly after birth, newborns with vitamin K deficiency show petechiae from superficial bleeding into the skin. They may have conjunctival, mucous membrane, or retinal hemorrhages. They may vomit fresh blood or pass black, tarry stools because of bleeding into the gastrointestinal tract. Distinguishing between tarry stools and normal meconium stools can be difficult in the first 1 or 2 days of life by simple observation. However, if an infant's stool does not change as it should from greenish-black (meconium) to the yellow color of a bottle-fed or breastfed baby, or if the stool changes to yellow, then back to black, gastrointestinal bleeding should be suspected. You can check for the presence of blood in the stool using a guaiac test strip.

Vitamin K deficiency bleeding usually occurs on day 2 to day 5 of life, when the available prothrombin is at its lowest level. On laboratory analysis, the prothrombin time will be prolonged, and the coagulation time may be normal or prolonged.

Hemorrhagic disease of the newborn can be prevented by the intramuscular administration of 1 mg of vitamin K to all newborns as soon as they have had time for an initial interaction with their parents after birth. Make certain infants who were born in unusual circumstances, such as those born outside the hospital, are given vitamin K on their admission to the hospital. Also double-check that infants whose birth involved an emergency, such as maternal hemorrhage or failure of the newborn to breathe spontaneously, have received it.

An infant who develops hemorrhagic disease of the newborn is treated with additional vitamin K, given intravenously or intramuscularly. If bleeding is severe, an infant may need a transfusion of fresh, whole blood to increase the prothrombin level immediately.

Handle infants with this disease extremely gently to prevent further bleeding, because they bruise easily from heavy pressure. A subdural hemorrhage may occur, making hemorrhagic disease an easy condition to prevent, yet also a serious and potentially fatal disorder.

Twin-to-Twin Transfusion

Twin-to-twin transfusion is a phenomenon that can occur if twins are monozygotic (identical; share the same placenta) and abnormal arteriovenous shunts occur that direct more blood to one twin than the other (Swiatkowska-Freund, Pankrac, & Preis, 2012). The process occurs in as many as one third of all identical twin pregnancies, although enough blood is exchanged to be clinically important in only about 15% of such pregnancies. The result of this shift of blood leads to anemia in the donor twin and polycythemia in the receiving twin. The anemic twin may also be pale and SGA because of the lack of nutrients or oxygen for growth as well as hypoglycemic from lack of glucose stores. The polycythemic twin is prone to hyperbilirubinemia as the excessive red blood cell level is broken down.

Twin-to-twin transfusion can be identified in utero by a sonogram because one twin is noticeably larger than the other. All identical twins should have hemoglobin determinations done at birth and the results should be compared. A hemoglobin difference of more than 5.0 g/100 ml is enough to suggest a transfusion between the twins has occurred. Each twin needs therapy as indicated by the extent of the blood distribution. The donor twin may need a transfusion to establish a functioning blood cell level, and the recipient twin may need an exchange transfusion to reduce the polycythemia and viscosity of the blood.

✔ QSEN Checkpoint Question 26.5

Quality Improvement

You are concerned that Baby Atkins will develop hyperbilirubinemia because of his immaturity. Because the prevention of jaundice is one of your NICU's quality indicators, what priority nursing intervention would you initiate to best prevent hyperbilirubinemia in Baby Atkins?

a. Administer phenobarbital to all infants to help prevent jaundice.
b. Urge all mothers to breastfeed early to promote infants' bowel motility.
c. Place all preterm and SGA infants in warm, dark, comforting environments.
d. Immediately place all infants under phototherapy following birth.

Look in Appendix A for the best answer and rationale.

Necrotizing Enterocolitis

NEC is an intestinal dysfunction that develops in approximately 5% of all infants in intensive care nurseries (Bingham, 2012). The bowel develops necrotic patches, interfering with digestion and possibly leading to a paralytic ileus, perforation, and peritonitis. It occurs because of anoxia to the bowel and so may result as a complication of exchange transfusion or an episode of breathing difficulty. Because it shares common features with other gastrointestinal disorders, it is discussed in Chapter 45.

Retinopathy of Prematurity

Retinopathy of prematurity (ROP), an acquired ocular disease that leads to partial or total blindness in children, is caused by vasoconstriction of immature retinal blood vessels. It was first recognized as an eye disorder in 1942, but only later was a high concentration of oxygen established as the causative agent (Stoll et al., 2010). Immature retinal blood vessels constrict when exposed to high oxygen concentrations; endothelial cells in the periphery of the retina then proliferate, causing retinal detachment and possible blindness. Infants who are most immature and most ill (and consequently receive the most oxygen) are at the highest risk of developing ROP.

When blood Po_2 levels rise to higher than 100 mmHg, the risk of the disease increases greatly. Based on this, all preterm infants who receive oxygen must have blood oxygen levels monitored by pulse oximeter or blood gas monitoring so the blood Po_2 level can be regulated within normal limits.

In the past, once ROP occurred, there was no reversing it. Today, cryosurgery or laser therapy may be effective at preserving sight. A person experienced in recognizing ROP should examine the eyes of all babies who have received oxygen (especially LBW newborns) before discharge from a hospital nursery and again at 4 to 6 weeks of age to detect any occurrence of the syndrome. Nurses can be instrumental in limiting the occurrence of ROP by securing oxygen saturation levels and by the conscientious management of oxygen (Di Fiore, Kaffashi, Loparo, et al., 2012; Martínez-Castellanos, Schwartz, Hernández-Rojas, et al., 2013).

THE NEWBORN AT RISK BECAUSE OF A MATERNAL INFECTION OR ILLNESS

Maternal Infections

Newborns are susceptible to infections during pregnancy and at birth because their ability to produce antibodies is immature. A number of infections in newborns, such as toxoplasmosis, rubella, syphilis, and cytomegalovirus infections, spread to the fetus across the placenta in utero and are discussed in Chapter 12 with other complications of pregnancy. Other infections, such as those discussed in the following sections, are not contracted in utero, but are contracted from exposure to vaginal secretions at birth.

β-Hemolytic, Group B Streptococcal Infection

A serious cause of infection in newborns is the gram-positive β-hemolytic, group B streptococcal (GBS) organism, a natural inhabitant of the female genital tract. Between 50 and 300 infants out of every 1,000 live births display a positive culture for the organism (AAP, 2011a). It also may be spread from baby to baby if good hand washing technique is not used in caring for newborns. If a woman is found to be positive for GBS during late pregnancy (see Chapter 21), ampicillin administered intravenously during pregnancy and again during labor helps to reduce the possibility of newborn exposure.

Assessment. Universal screening is recommended for pregnant women at 35 to 37 weeks of gestation to see if they have GBS organisms in their vaginal secretions (Cagno, Pettit, & Weiss, 2012). Typically, a newborn at risk, such as one born after prolonged rupture of membranes or if the woman's vaginal culture is positive for GBS, will be screened at birth for infection by a specialized GBS blood culture.

Colonization by GBS can result in either an early-onset or a late-onset illness. With the early-onset form, signs of pneumonia such as tachypnea, apnea, extreme paleness, hypotension, or hypotonia become apparent within the first day of life. Decreased urine output can occur from the hypotension. A chest X-ray may not be diagnostic because the changes seen are almost indistinguishable from those of RDS (a ground-glass appearance). Without therapy, the disease progresses so rapidly, as many as 20% of infants who contract the infection die within 24 hours of birth.

A late-onset type occurs at 2 to 4 weeks of age. With this, instead of pneumonia being the infection focus, meningitis tends to occur. Typical signs include lethargy, fever, loss of appetite, and bulging fontanelles from increased intracranial pressure. Mortality from the late-onset type is not as high as that from the early-onset form (15% versus 20%), but neurologic consequences can occur in up to 50% of infants who survive.

Therapeutic Management. If a newborn displays signs of infection or a blood screening test is positive, antibiotics such as penicillin, cefazolin, clindamycin, or vancomycin are all effective against the GBS organism.

Parents may have difficulty understanding how their infant could suddenly have become this ill, and they may need a great deal of support to care for their infant. This is even more important if the newborn survives the infection but is left neurologically challenged. In the future, immunization of all women of childbearing age against streptococcal B organisms could decrease the incidence of newborns infected at birth.

Ophthalmia Neonatorum

Ophthalmia neonatorum is an eye infection that occurs at birth or during the first month of life (Gold, 2011). The most common causative organisms are *Neisseria gonorrhoeae* and *Chlamydia trachomatis*, which are contracted from vaginal secretions. An *N. gonorrhoeae* infection is an extremely serious form of infection because, if left untreated, the infection progresses to corneal ulceration and destruction, resulting in opacity of the cornea and severe vision impairment.

Assessment. Ophthalmia neonatorum is generally bilateral. The conjunctivae become fiery red and covered with thick pus. The eyelids appear edematous. Although this usually occurs on day 1 to day 4 of life, it should be considered as a possibility when conjunctivitis occurs in any infant younger than 30 days of age.

Prevention. The prophylactic instillation of erythromycin ointment into the eyes of newborns prevents both gonococcal and chlamydial conjunctivitis. In the past, eye prophylaxis was given immediately after birth so it was never forgotten. Now it is more customary to delay the administration of the ointment until after the first reactivity period so the newborn can clearly see the parents during this important attachment period. This makes it easy for administration to be forgotten, so use some type of a checklist as a reminder of this important prophylaxis. Infants born outside the hospital also need prophylaxis to prevent ophthalmia neonatorum, the same as for infants born in a birthing room.

Therapeutic Management. If conjunctivitis occurs, therapy is individualized depending on the organism cultured from the exudate. If gonococci are identified, intravenous ceftriaxone (Rocephin) and penicillin are effective drugs. If *Chlamydia* is identified, an ophthalmic solution of erythromycin is commonly used.

Use standard and contact infection precautions when caring for this newborn. In addition to systemic antibiotic therapy, sterile saline solution lavage to clear the copious discharge from the eyes may be prescribed. When irrigating eyes, use a sterile medicine dropper or bulb syringe and use barrier protection, including goggles to avoid splashing any solution into your own eye. The solution should be at room temperature. Direct the stream of the irrigation fluid laterally so it does not enter and contaminate the other eye.

The mother of the infected infant needs treatment for gonorrhea or chlamydia, before fallopian tube sterility or pelvic inflammatory disease can result. Sexual contacts of the mother should be treated also so the spread of the disease can be halted. With either infection, parents can be assured with early diagnosis and treatment that the prognosis for normal eyesight in their child is good.

Hepatitis B Virus Infection

Hepatitis B virus (HBV) can be transmitted to the newborn through contact with infected vaginal blood at birth when the mother is positive for the virus (positive for the surface antigen of the hepatitis B virus [HBsAg+]). Hepatitis B is a destructive illness with greater than 90% of infected infants becoming chronic carriers of the virus as well as the risk of developing liver cancer later in life (Ni, 2011). To reduce the possibility of HBsAg being spread to newborns in the future, parents are asked if they would like their infant vaccinated against hepatitis B at birth (Schleiss & Patterson, 2012).

If the mother is identified as HBsAg+, her infant should be bathed as soon as possible after birth to remove HBV-infected blood and secretions. Gentle suctioning is necessary to avoid trauma to the mucous membrane, which could allow HBV invasion. To further protect against infection, the infant is administered serum immune globulin (HBIG) in addition to the HBV vaccination. Although the virus is transmitted in breast milk, once immune globulin has been administered, women may breastfeed without risk to an infant. Hepatitis B is further discussed in Chapter 45 because it shares common symptoms with other liver disorders and also occurs in older children.

Generalized Herpesvirus Infection

A herpes simplex virus type 2 (HSV-2) infection, which is most prevalent among women with multiple sexual partners, can be contracted by a fetus across the placenta if the mother has a primary infection during pregnancy. More often, however, the virus is contracted from the vaginal secretions of a mother who has active herpetic vulvovaginitis at the time of birth. Between 15% and 30% of women of childbearing age demonstrate antibodies to this virus or have the potential to have active lesions during labor (Westhoff, Little, & Caughey, 2011).

Assessment. If the infection was acquired during pregnancy, an infant may be born with vesicles covering the skin. The long-term prognosis of the child is guarded because severe neurologic damage may have occurred simultaneously with the development of the lesions. If infants don't acquire the infection until birth, by day 4 to day 7 of life they show a loss of appetite, perhaps a low-grade fever, and lethargy. Stomatitis (ulcers of the mouth) or a few vesicles on the skin appear. Herpes vesicles always cluster, are pinpoint in size, and are surrounded by a reddened base. After the vesicles appear, infants become extremely ill. They develop dyspnea, jaundice, purpura, convulsions, and hypotension. Death may occur within hours or days. Between 25% and 70% of newborns who survive generalized herpesvirus infections have permanent central nervous system sequelae (Kimberlin, Whitley, Wan, et al., 2011).

To confirm the diagnosis, cultures are obtained from representative vesicles as well as from the nose, throat, anus, and umbilical cord. Blood serum is analyzed for IgM antibodies.

Therapeutic Management. An antiviral drug such as acyclovir (Zovirax), a drug that inhibits viral DNA synthesis, is effective in combating this overwhelming infection. Prevention, however, is the newborn's best protection. Antenatal antiviral prophylaxis reduces viral shedding and recurrences at birth and reduces the need for cesarean birth (Westhoff et al., 2011). Women with active herpetic vulvar lesions are advised to have cesarean birth rather than vaginal birth to minimize the newborn's exposure. Infants with an infection should be separated from other infants in a nursery. Although transmission from this source is rare, women with herpes lesions on their face (herpes simplex I, or cold sores) need to be assessed before they hold their newborns to be sure lesions are crusted and, therefore, are no longer contagious. Health care personnel who have herpes simplex infections should not care for newborns until the lesions are crusted. Although facial herpes simplex lesions are probably caused by herpesvirus type 1, limiting contact does not seem excessive in light of the severity of HSV-2 disease. Urge a woman who is separated from her newborn at birth to view her infant from the nursery window and participate in planning care to aid bonding.

HIV Infection

HIV infection and AIDS can be caused by placental transfer or direct contact with maternal blood during birth. Because older children can also be exposed to this disease, the care of children with this infection is discussed in Chapter 42.

Maternal Conditions Which Cause Illnesses in Newborns

A number of concerns occur in newborns during intrauterine life or at birth because of a maternal illness.

An Infant of a Woman Who Has Diabetes Mellitus

Infants of women who have diabetes mellitus whose illness was poorly controlled during pregnancy are typically longer and weigh more than other babies (macrosomia). The baby also has a greater chance of having a congenital anomaly such as a cardiac anomaly because hyperglycemia is teratogenic to a rapidly growing fetus. **Caudal regression syndrome** (hypoplasia of the lower extremities) is a syndrome that occurs almost exclusively in such infants (Hay, 2012).

Most such babies have a cushingoid (i.e., fat and puffy) appearance. They tend to be lethargic or limp in the first days of life as a result of hyperglycemia. The macrosomia results from overstimulation of pituitary growth hormone and extra fat deposits created by high levels of insulin during pregnancy. This infant's large size is deceptive, however, because, like all LGA babies, they are often immature. RDS occurs at a higher rate than usual in these infants because they may be born preterm or, if born at term, lecithin pathways may not be mature. High fetal insulin secretion during pregnancy to counteract the hyperglycemia can interfere with cortisol release. This could block the formation of lecithin and further prevent lung maturity (Murphy, Janzen, Strehlow, et al., 2013). A term frequently used for these infants is "fragile giant."

An infant of a diabetic woman loses a greater proportion of weight in the first few days of life than does the average newborn because of the loss of extra fluid accumulated. Observe such an infant closely to be certain this weight loss actually represents a loss of extra fluid and that dehydration is not occurring.

Complications. A macrosomic infant has a greater chance of birth injury, especially shoulder and neck injury. A cesarean birth may be necessary to avoid cephalopelvic disproportion. Immediately after birth, the infant tends to be hyperglycemic because the mother was at least slightly hyperglycemic during pregnancy and excess glucose transfused across the placenta. During pregnancy, the fetal pancreas responded to this high glucose level with islet cell hypertrophy, resulting in matching high insulin levels. After birth, as an infant's glucose level begins to fall because the mother's circulation is no longer supplying glucose, the overproduction of insulin will cause the development of severe hypoglycemia. Hyperbilirubinemia also may occur in these infants because, if immature, they cannot effectively clear bilirubin from their system. Hypocalcemia also frequently develops because parathyroid hormone levels are lower in these infants due to hypomagnesemia from excessive renal losses of magnesium.

Although infants of diabetic women are usually LGA, an infant born to a woman with extensive blood vessel involvement may be SGA because of poor placental perfusion. The problems of hypoglycemia, hypocalcemia, and hyperbilirubinemia remain the same.

Therapeutic Management. In a newborn, hypoglycemia is defined as a serum glucose level of less than 45 mg/dl. To avoid a serum glucose level from falling this low, infants of diabetic women need to be fed early; if they are unable to suck, a continuous infusion of glucose can be prescribed. It is important the infant not be given only a bolus of glucose, otherwise, rebound hypoglycemia (accentuating the problem) can occur. Some infants of diabetic women have a smaller than usual left colon, apparently another effect of intrauterine hyperglycemia, which can limit the amount of oral feedings they can take in their first days of life. Signs of an inadequate colon include vomiting or abdominal distention after the first few feedings. Careful monitoring for any vomiting and normal bowel movements can help identify this condition.

QSEN Checkpoint Question 26.6

Patient-Centered Care

Mrs. Atkins asks you why the baby in the incubator next to her baby whose mother has diabetes mellitus was fed so soon after birth. Why is it important for infants of diabetic women to be fed early?

a. Their stomach is larger than usual due to overgrowth.
b. This helps prevent rebound hypoglycemia from occurring.
c. The mother probably didn't eat much during her labor.
d. This helps clear thick mucus from the lower intestinal tract.

Look in Appendix A for the best answer and rationale.

An Infant of a Drug-Dependent Mother

Infants of drug-dependent women tend to be SGA. If the woman took a drug close to birth, her infant may show withdrawal symptoms (neonatal abstinence syndrome) shortly after birth (Box 26.9). These include such signs as:

- Irritability
- Disturbed sleep pattern
- Constant movement, possibly leading to abrasions on the elbows, knees, or nose
- Tremors
- Frequent sneezing
- Shrill, high-pitched cry
- Possible hyperreflexia and clonus (neuromuscular irritability)
- Convulsions
- Tachypnea (rapid respirations), possibly so severe that it leads to hyperventilation and alkalosis
- Vomiting and diarrhea, leading to large fluid losses and secondary dehydration

Specific neonatal abstinence scoring tools can be used to quantify and assess an infant's status. When symptoms begin to appear and when they fade varies with the drug involved, but, on average, symptoms occur in 24 to 48 hours and last about 2 weeks. The infants of women who were on methadone maintenance during pregnancy will show the same beginning and length of symptoms. The abstinence sequence for the cocaine-addicted neonate is usually more mild, but factors such as maladaptive coping behaviors may be present in such newborns into preschool (Lambert & Bauer, 2012).

Narcotic metabolites or quinine (heroin is often mixed with quinine) may be obtained from an infant's urine or meconium in the first hour after birth to establish that the drug was transferred into the infant before birth. These products are quickly cleared from the body, however, so by the time symptoms become severe, detection of narcotic substances may no longer be possible. Cocaine, in contrast, may be detected in infants' hair samples for an extended time.

BOX 26.9 Nursing Care Planning Using Assessment

Assessing the Newborn of a Drug-Dependent Mother

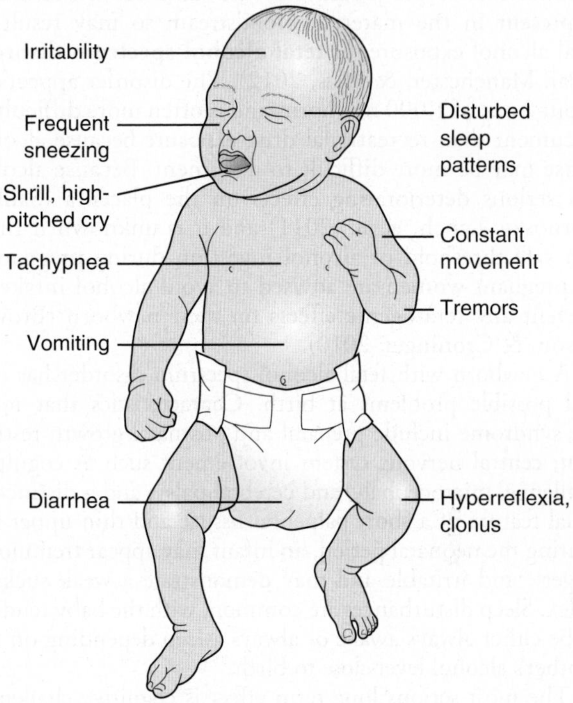

Infants of drug-dependent women usually seem most comfortable when firmly swaddled. Keep them in an environment free from excessive stimuli (a small isolation nursery or the mother's room, not a large, open nursery). Some quiet best if the room is darkened. Some may suck vigorously and continuously and seem to find comfort and quiet if given a pacifier. In contrast, infants of methadone- and cocaine-addicted women may have extremely poor sucking ability and may have difficulty achieving sufficient fluid intake unless gavage fed. Unless a woman intends to remain drug free, she is usually advised not to breastfeed to avoid passing narcotics in breast milk to the child.

Specific therapy for an infant has to be individualized according to the nature and severity of the signs. If an infant has vomiting or diarrhea, intravenous administration of fluid may be indicated. The most common drugs used to counteract abstinence symptoms are morphine and phenobarbital (Kelly, Minty, Madden, et al., 2011). Other drugs that may be used include methadone, chlorpromazine (Thorazine), and diazepam (Valium). These are typically used if the neonatal abstinence scoring system average score is elevated on three successive occasions and other nursing interventions do not reduce the score.

Once an infant has been identified as having been exposed to drugs in utero, the mother needs treatment for withdrawal symptoms and follow-up care as much as the infant. In addition, an evaluation is necessary to determine before discharge from the health care facility whether an environment that allowed for drug abuse will be safe for an infant at home (Kelly et al., 2011). Infants also need long-term follow-up because long-term neurologic problems may develop.

An Infant With Fetal Alcohol Exposure

Alcohol crosses the placenta in the same concentration as is present in the maternal bloodstream so may result in fetal alcohol exposure, or **fetal alcohol spectrum disorder** (Tsai, Manchester, & Elias, 2012). The disorder appears in about 2 out of 1,000 newborns and is often more difficult to document than recreational drug exposure because alcohol abuse may be more difficult to document. Because alcohol has serious deteriorating effects on the placenta (Salihu, Kornosky, Lynch, et al., 2011) and it is unknown if there is a safe threshold of alcohol ingestion during pregnancy, all pregnant women are advised to avoid alcohol intake to prevent any teratogenic effects on their newborn (Brown, Olson, & Croninger, 2010).

A newborn with fetal alcohol spectrum disorder has several possible problems at birth. Characteristics that mark the syndrome include prenatal and postnatal growth restriction; central nervous system involvement such as cognitive challenge, microcephaly, and cerebral palsy; and a distinctive facial feature of a short palpebral fissure and thin upper lip. During the neonatal period, an infant may appear tremulous, fidgety, and irritable and may demonstrate a weak sucking reflex. Sleep disturbances are common, with the baby tending to be either always awake or always asleep depending on the mother's alcohol level close to birth.

The most serious long-term effect is cognitive challenge. Behavior problems such as hyperactivity may occur in school-age children. Growth deficiencies may remain throughout life. An infant needs conscientious follow-up so any future problems can be discovered. The mother needs a follow-up to see if she can reduce her alcohol intake for better overall health (Eckstrand, Ding, Dodge, et al., 2012).

What if... 26.4 You are interested in exploring one of the 2020 National Health Goals with respect to high-risk newborns (see Box 26.1). Most government-sponsored money for nursing research is allotted based on these goals. What would be a possible research topic to explore pertinent to these goals that would be applicable to the Atkins family and that would also advance evidence-based practice?

KEY POINTS FOR REVIEW

- Priorities for infants born with special needs, such as preterm or postterm infants, are the same as for term infants: initiation and maintenance of respirations, establishment of extrauterine circulation, control of body temperature, intake of adequate nourishment, establishment of waste elimination, establishment of an infant–parent relationship, prevention of infection, and provision of developmental care for mental and social development.
- Many high-risk infants need resuscitation at birth. Prompt action with such measures as warmth, oxygen, intubation, and suctioning are needed.
- An SGA infant is one whose birth weight is below the 10th percentile on an intrauterine growth curve for that gestational age infant. An infant could be born preterm, term, or postterm. They typically have difficulty maintaining body warmth because of low fat stores and may develop hypoglycemia from low glucose stores.
- An LGA infant is one whose birth weight is above the 90th percentile on an intrauterine growth chart for that gestational age. The infant could be born preterm, term, or postterm. They tend to be infants of diabetic women, and they are particularly prone to hypoglycemia or birth trauma.
- An early preterm infant is one born between 24 and 34 weeks of gestation; a late preterm infant is one born between 34 and 37 weeks of gestation. Preterm infants have particular problems with respiratory function, anemia, jaundice, persistent patent ductus arteriosus, and intracranial hemorrhage.
- Infants who are born weighing 1,500 to 2,500 g are termed low–birth-weight infants; those born weighing 1,000 to 1,500 g are termed very-low-birth-weight infants; those born weighing between 500 and 1,000 g are extremely very-low-birth-weight infants. All of these infants need intensive care from the moment of birth to give them their best chance of survival without neurologic aftereffects caused by their being so close to the age of viability.
- A postterm infant is one who has remained in utero past week 42 of pregnancy. Postterm infants have particular problems with establishing respirations, meconium aspiration, hypoglycemia, temperature regulation, and polycythemia.
- RDS commonly occurs in preterm infants from a deficiency or lack of surfactant in the alveoli. Without surfactant, the alveoli collapse on expiration and require extreme force for reinflation. Primary therapy is synthetic surfactant replacement at birth, followed by oxygen and ventilatory support.
- TTN is a temporary condition caused by the slow absorption of lung fluid at birth. It is seen most often in infants born by cesarean birth. Close observation of the infant is necessary until the fluid is absorbed and respirations slow to a usual rate.
- MAS occurs when an infant aspirates meconium-stained amniotic fluid before or during birth. Meconium is irritating to the airway and so leads to both airway spasm and pneumonia. Infants need oxygen, ventilatory support, and possibly an antibiotic until the effects of the insult to the airway subside. If obvious meconium staining is present, infants may need to be suctioned before oxygen administration under pressure to prevent meconium from being forced further into their lungs.
- Apnea is a pause in respirations longer than 20 seconds with accompanying bradycardia. It tends to occur in preterm infants who have secondary stresses such as an infection, hyperbilirubinemia, hypoglycemia, or hypothermia. Apnea monitors are used to detect this, and infants who are at high risk for apnea may be discharged with a home monitoring program.
- SIDS is the sudden, unexplained death of an infant. It is associated with infants sleeping on their stomachs (prone) and infants born preterm. An important preventive

measure is advising parents to position their infant on the back and possibly use a pacifier for sleeping.

- Hyperbilirubinemia results from the destruction of red blood cells, owing either to a usual physiologic response or an abnormal destruction of red blood cells. Hemolytic disease of the newborn occurs from destruction of red blood cells from Rh or ABO incompatibility. The administration of RHIG (Rh antibodies) to Rh-negative mothers during pregnancy and after the birth of an Rh-positive infant to an Rh-negative mother has greatly reduced the incidence of the condition. Affected infants appear jaundiced from the release of bilirubin from injured red blood cells. Phototherapy and an exchange transfusion are used to prevent ABE (the deposition of bilirubin in brain cells, causing destruction of the cells).
- Hemorrhagic disease of the newborn is a lack of clotting ability resulting from a deficiency of vitamin K at birth. This disorder is prevented by administering vitamin K to infants following birth.
- ROP is destruction of the retina caused by exposure of immature retinal capillaries to high levels of oxygen. Monitoring oxygen saturation by pulse oximetry or ABGs are important preventive measures and help in planning nursing care that not only meets QSEN competencies but that also best meets a family's total needs.
- Severe infections acquired by infants at birth include streptococcal group B pneumonia, hepatitis B infection, ophthalmia neonatorum (gonococcal and chlamydial conjunctivitis), and herpesvirus infections. Assessing newborns for symptoms of these infections is an important nursing responsibility.
- Infants of women with diabetes and those of drug-abusing women are at high risk at birth for further complications. Both need a careful assessment for respiratory distress and hypoglycemia.

Critical Thinking Care Study

Priscilla Angelini is an unmarried 17-year-old who has just given birth via cesarean birth to her first baby, a girl, at 37 weeks of gestation because of a breech presentation. Priscilla did not receive any prenatal care. At birth, she tests positive for group B streptococcal infection. When assessing her newborn, you conclude she is SGA. At 6 hours of age, Priscilla calls you and explains her baby seems to be struggling to breathe. She wants to know if this is normal. When you assess the newborn, you find a respiratory rate of 70 breaths/min and mild subcostal retractions.

1. What possible risk factors should you look for in Baby Angelini?
2. What is the most likely explanation for Baby Angelini's respiratory rate and the subcostal retractions? What priority nursing intervention should you initiate? What should you tell Priscilla about the situation?
3. Does Priscilla's infection put Baby Angelini at risk? What nursing interventions should be in the newborn's care plan to prevent infection and what signs and symptoms of infection should you look for in the newborn?

Patient Scenario

The Anorak Family

Read about the Anorak family, a family with a preterm infant with respiratory distress syndrome, then answer the questions to further sharpen your skills and grow more familiar with NCLEX-type questions related to caring for a family with a high-risk newborn. Confirm your answers are correct by reading the rationales.

Visit http://thePoint.lww.com

Answers and Rationales

Looking for answers to the What if. . . and Critical Thinking Care Study questions?

Visit http://thePoint.lww.com

References

Aher, S. M., & Ohlsson, A. (2012). Early versus late erythropoietin for preventing red blood cell transfusion in preterm and/or low birth weight infants. *Cochrane Database of Systematic Reviews,*(10), CD004865.

Ahmed, A. H., & Sands, L. P. (2010). Effect of pre- and postdischarge interventions on breastfeeding outcomes and weight gain among premature infants. *JOGNN: Journal of Obstetric, Gynecologic, and Neonatal Nursing, 39*(1), 53–63.

Alves, J. G., Cisneiros, R. M., Dutra, L. P., et al. (2012). Perinatal characteristics among early (10–14 years old) and late (15–19 years old) pregnant adolescents. *BMC Research Notes, 5*(1), 531.

American Academy of Pediatrics. (2011a). Policy statement—Recommendations for the prevention of perinatal group B streptococcal (GBS) disease. *Pediatrics, 128*(3), 611–616.

American Academy of Pediatrics. (2011b). SIDS and other sleep-related infant deaths: Expansion of recommendations for a safe infant sleeping environment. *Pediatrics, 128*(5), e1341–e1367.

American Academy of Pediatrics. (2012). *Where we stand: Car seats for children.* Washington, DC: Author.

Attar, M., & Donn, S. M. (2010). Pulmonary support strategies and options for improving lung function in term neonates: Warning signs of damage. *Pediatric Health, 4*(3), 277–286.

Beck, S., Wojdyla, D., Say, L., et al. (2010). The worldwide incidence of preterm birth: A systematic review of maternal mortality and morbidity. *World Health Organization: Bulletin of the World Health Organization, 88*(1), 31–38.

Bennett, P. (2012). Preterm labour. In D. K. Edmonds (Ed.), *Dewhurst's textbook of obstetrics & gynaecology* (8th ed., pp. 338–355). Oxford, UK: John Wiley & Son.

Bingham, E. M. (2012). Optimizing nutrition in the neonatal intensive care unit: A look at enteral nutrition and the prevention of necrotizing enterocolitis. *Topics in Clinical Nutrition, 27*(3), 250–259.

Black, A. (2012). Breastfeeding the premature infant and nursing implications. *Advances in Neonatal Care, 12*(1), 10–11.

Brewster, D. H., Tucker, J. S., Fleming, M., et al. (2010). Risk of skin cancer after neonatal phototherapy: Retrospective cohort study. *Archives of Disease in Childhood, 95*(10), 826–831.

Brown, C. W., Olson, H. C., Croninger, R. G. (2010). Maternal alcohol consumption during pregnancy and infant social, mental, and motor development. *Journal of Early Intervention, 32*(2), 110–126.

Cagno, C. K., Pettit, J. M., & Weiss, B. D. (2012). Prevention of perinatal group B streptococcal disease: Updated CDC guideline. *American Family Physician, 86*(1), 59–65.

Centers for Disease Control and Prevention (2010). *Proper handling and storage of breast milk.* Atlanta, GA: Author.

Chiesa, A., & Sirotnak, A. P. (2012). Child abuse and neglect. In W. Hay, M. Levin, R. Deterding, et al. (Eds.), *Current diagnosis & treatment. Pediatrics* (21st ed., pp. 223–230). New York, NY: McGraw-Hill/Lange.

Choi, H. J., Hahn, S., Lee, J., et al. (2012). Surfactant lavage therapy for meconium aspiration syndrome: A systematic review and meta-analysis. *Neonatology, 101*(3), 183–191.

Choudhary, D., Bano, I., & Ali, S. M. (2010). Does amnioinfusion reduce caesarean section rate in meconium-stained amniotic fluid. *Archives of Gynecology and Obstetrics, 282*(1), 17–22.

Clark, E. A., & Varner, M. (2011). Impact of preterm PROM and its complications on long-term infant outcomes. *Clinical Obstetrics and Gynecology, 54*(2), 358–369.

Dall'Oglio, A. M., Rosseillo, B., Coletti, M. F., et al. (2010). Do healthy preterm children need neuropsychological follow-up? Preschool outcomes compared with term peers. *Developmental Medicine & Child Neurology, 52*(10), 955–961.

Dargaville, P. A. (2012). Respiratory support in meconium aspiration syndrome: A practical guide. *International Journal of Pediatrics, 2012,* 965159.

de Alba Campomanes, A. G., Binenbaum, G., & Quinn, G. E. (2012). Disorders of the eye. In C. A. Gleason & S. U. Devaskar (Eds.), *Avery's diseases of the newborn* (9th ed., pp. 1423–1441). Philadelphia, PA: Elsevier/Saunders.

DeGrazia, M., Chao-Yu, G., Wilkinson, A. A., et al. (2010). Weight and age as predictors for passing the infant car seat challenge. *Pediatrics, 125*(3), 526–531.

Demirel, G., Akar, M., Celik, I. H., et al. (2011). Single versus multiple dose intravenous immunoglobulin in combination with LED phototherapy in the treatment of ABO hemolytic disease in neonates. *International Journal of Hematology, 93*(6), 700–703.

Di Fiore, J. M., Kaffashi, F., Loparo, K., et al. (2012). Relationship between patterns of intermittent hypoxia and retinopathy of prematurity in preterm infants. *Pediatric Research, 72*(6), 606–612.

Doyle, K. J., & Bradshaw, W. T. (2012). Sixty golden minutes. *Neonatal Network, 31*(5), 289–294.

Dukhovny, D., Lorch, S. A., Schmidt, B., et al. (2011). Economic evaluation of caffeine for apnea of prematurity. *Pediatrics, 127*(1), e146–e155.

Eckstrand, K. L., Ding, Z., Dodge, N. C., et al. (2012). Persistent dose-dependent changes in brain structure in young adults with low-to-moderate alcohol exposure in utero. *Alcoholism: Clinical and Experimental Research, 36*(11), 1892–1902.

Furman, L., & Schanler, R. J. (2012). Breastfeeding. In C. A. Gleason & S. U. Devaskar (Eds.), *Avery's diseases of the newborn* (9th ed., pp. 937–972). Philadelphia, PA: Elsevier/Saunders.

Gold, R. S. (2011). Treatment of bacterial conjunctivitis in children. *Pediatric Annals, 40*(2), 95–105.

González, A., Fabres, J., D'Apremont, I., et al. (2010). Randomized controlled trial of early compared with delayed use of inhaled nitric oxide in newborns with a moderate respiratory failure and pulmonary hypertension. *Journal of Perinatology, 30*(6), 420–424.

Gowen, C. W. (2011). Fetal & neonatal medicine. In K. J. Marcdante, R. M. Kliegman, H. B. Jenson, et al. (Eds.), *Nelson essentials of pediatrics* (6th ed., pp. 213–264). Philadelphia, PA: Saunders/Elsevier.

Gray, P. H., & Flenady, V. (2011). Cot-nursing versus incubator care for preterm infants. *Cochrane Database of Systematic Reviews,* (8), CD003062.

Gülmezoglu, A. M., Crowther, C. A., Middleton, P., et al. (2012). Induction of labour for improving birth outcomes for women at or beyond term. *Cochrane Database of Systematic Reviews,* (6), CD004945.

Hansen, T. W. (2011). Prevention of neurodevelopmental sequelae of jaundice in the newborn. *Developmental Medicine & Child Neurology, 53*(4), 24–28.

Hay, W. W., Jr. (2012). Care of the infant of the diabetic mother. *Current Diabetic Reports, 12*(1), 4–15.

Hermansen, C. L. (2010). Transient tachypnea of the newborn: Common in the nursery, implications for beyond. *Pediatric Health, 4*(4), 427–431.

Hoppe, C. C. (2013). Prenatal and newborn screening for hemoglobinopathies. *International Journal of Laboratory Hematology, 35*(3), 297–305.

Horbar, J. D., Carpenter, J. H., Badger, G. J., et al. (2012). Mortality and neonatal morbidity among infants 501 to 1500 grams from 2000 to 2009. *Pediatrics, 129*(6), 1019–1026.

Jane-Pillow, J. (2012). Which continuous positive airway pressure system is best for the preterm infant with respiratory distress syndrome? *Clinics in Perinatology, 39*(3), 483–496.

Johnson, P. N., Miller, J., & Gormley, A. K. (2011). Continuous-infusion neuromuscular blocking agents in critically ill neonates and children. *Pharmacotherapy, 31*(6), 609–620.

Kattwinkel, J., Perlman, J. M., Azia, K., et al. (2010). Neonatal resuscitation: 2010 American Heart Association guidelines for cardiopulmonary resuscitation and emergency cardiovascular care. *Circulation, 122*(18, Suppl. 3), S909–S919.

Karch, A. M. (2013). *2013: Lippincott's nursing drug guide.* Philadelphia, PA: Lippincott Williams & Wilkins.

Kelly, L., Minty, B., Madden, S., et al. (2011). The occasional management of narcotic exposure in neonates. *Canadian Journal of Rural Medicine, 16*(3), 98–101.

Kim, J. H., & Froh, E. B. (2012). What nurses need to know regarding nutritional and immunobiological properties of human milk. *Journal of Obstetric, Gynecologic & Neonatal Nursing, 41*(1), 122–137.

Kimberlin, D. W., Whitley, R. J., Wan, W., et al. (2011). Oral acyclovir suppression and neurodevelopment after neonatal herpes. *New England Journal of Medicine, 365*(14), 1284–1292.

Kitsommart, R., Martins, B., Bottino, M. N., et al. (2012). Expectant management of pneumothorax in preterm infants receiving assisted ventilation: Report of 4 cases and review of the literature. *Respiratory Care, 57*(5), 789–793.

Kositamongkol, S., Suthutvoravut, U., Chongviriyaphan, N., et al. (2011). Vitamin A and E status in very low birth weight infants. *Journal of Perinatology, 31*(7), 471–476.

Lambert, B. L., & Bauer, C. R. (2012). Developmental and behavioral consequences of prenatal cocaine exposure: A review. *Journal of Perinatology, 32*(7), 819–828.

Landry, J. S., & Menzies, D. (2012). Occurrence and severity of bronchopulmonary dysplasia and respiratory distress syndrome after a preterm birth. *Paediatrics & Child Health, 16*(7), 399–403.

Lee, K. J., & Marcdante, K. J. (2011). Assessment & resuscitation. In K. J. Marcdante, R. M. Kliegman, H. B. Jenson, et al. (Eds.), *Nelson essentials of pediatrics* (6th ed., pp. 141–144). Philadelphia, PA: Saunders/Elsevier.

Leone, T. A., & Finer, N. N. (2012). Resuscitation in the delivery room. In C. A. Gleason & S. Devaskar (Eds.), *Avery's diseases of the newborn* (9th ed., pp. 328–340). Philadelphia, PA: Elsevier/Saunders.

Marik, P. E., Fuller, C., Levitov, A., et al. (2012). Neonatal incubators: A toxic sound environment for the preterm infant? *Pediatric Critical Care Medicine, 13*(6), 685–689.

Martin, J. A., Hamilton, B. E., Ventura, S. J., et al. (2011). Births: Final data for 2009. *National Vital Statistics Reports, 60*(1), 1–5.

Martínez-Castellanos, M. A., Schwartz, S., Hernández-Rojas, M. L., et al. (2013). Long-term effect of antiangiogenic therapy for retinopathy of prematurity. *Retina, 33*(2), 329–338.

McCall, E. M., Alderdice, F. A., Halliday, H. L., et al. (2010). Interventions to prevent hypothermia at birth in preterm and/or low birth weight infants. *Cochrane Database of Systematic Reviews,* (3), CD004210.

McGowan, J. E. (2012). Neonatal resuscitation science, education, and practice: The role of the Neonatal Resuscitation Program. *Journal of Perinatology & Neonatal Nursing, 26*(2), 158–163.

McGowan, J. E., Alderdice, F. A., Doran, J., et al. (2012). Impact of neonatal intensive care on late preterm infants: Developmental outcomes at 3 years. *Pediatrics, 130*(5), e1105–1112.

Miller, M. Q., & Morris, L. A. (2011). Development considerations in working with newborn infants of mothers with diabetes. *Neonatal Network, 30*(1), 37–45.

Mohan, S. S., & Jain, L. (2012). Care of the late preterm infant. In C. A. Gleason & S. U. Devaskar (Eds.), *Avery's diseases of the newborn* (9th ed., pp. 405–416). Philadelphia, PA: Elsevier/Saunders.

Moon, R. Y., & Fu, L. (2012). Sudden infant death syndrome: An update. *Pediatric Reviews, 33*(7), 314–320.

Moore, E. R., Anderson, G. C., Bergman, N., et al. (2012). Early skin-to-skin contact for mothers and their healthy newborn infants. *Cochrane Database of Systematic Reviews,* (5), CD003519.

Murphy, A., Janzen, C., Strehlow, S. L., et al. (2013). Diabetes mellitus and pregnancy. In A. H. DeCherney, L. Nathan, T. M. Goodwin, et al. (Eds.), *Current diagnosis and treatment: obstetrics and gynecology* (11th ed., pp. 509–518). Columbus, OH: McGraw-Hill/Lange.

Ni, Y. H. (2011). Natural history of hepatitis B virus infection: Pediatric perspective. *Journal of Gastroenterology, 46*(1), 1–8.

National Vital Statistics Service. (2011). *Trends in the health of Americans.* Hyattsville, MD: Author.

Ortigosa, S., Friguls, B., Joya, X., et al. (2012). Feto-placental morphological effects of prenatal exposure to drugs of abuse. *Reproductive Toxicology, 34*(1), 73–79.

Ota, E., Tobe-Gai, R., Mori, R., et al. (2012). Antenatal dietary advice and supplementation to increase energy and protein intake. *Cochrane Database of Systematic Reviews,* (9), CD000032.

Ouzounian, J. G., & Goodwin, T. M. (2010). Diagnosis and management of macrosomia. In T. M. Goodwin, M. N. Montoro, L. Muderspach, et al. (Eds.), *Management of common problems in obstetrics and gynecology* (5th ed., pp. 30–32). Oxford, UK: Wiley/Blackwell.

Perlman, J. M., Wyllie, J., Kattwinkel, J., et al. (2010). Neonatal resuscitation: 2010 international consensus on cardiopulmonary resuscitation and emergency cardiovascular care science with treatment recommendations. *Circulation, 122*(16, Suppl. 2), S516–S538.

Raab, E. L., & Kelly, L. K. (2013). Newborn resuscitation. In A. H. DeCherney, L. Nathan, T. M. Goodwin, et al. (Eds.), *Current diagnosis and treatment: Obstetrics and gynecology* (11th ed., pp. 369–387). Columbus, OH: McGraw-Hill/Lange.

Rabe, H., Diaz-Rossello, J. L., Duley, L., et al. (2012). Effect of timing of umbilical cord clamping and other strategies to influence placental transfusion at preterm birth on maternal and infant outcomes. *Cochrane Database of Systematic Reviews,* (8), CD003248.

Raffay, T. M., Martin, R. J., & Reynolds, J. D. (2012). Can nitric oxide-based therapy prevent bronchopulmonary dysplasia? *Clinics in Perinatology, 39*(3), 613–638.

Raghuveer, T. S., & Cox, A. J. (2011). Neonatal resuscitation: An update. *American Family Physician, 83*(8), 911–918.

Rahimian, J. (2013). Disproportionate fetal growth. In A. H. DeCherney, L. Nathan, T. M. Goodwin, et al. (Eds.), *Current diagnosis and treatment: Obstetrics and gynecology* (11th ed., pp. 290–300). Columbus, OH: McGraw-Hill/Lange.

Rao, R., Bryowsky, K., Mao, J., et al. (2011). Gastrointestinal complications associated with ibuprofen therapy for patent ductus arteriosus. *Journal of Perinatology, 31*(7), 465–470.

Rasmussen, K. M., & Geraghty, S. R. (2011). The quiet revolution: Breastfeeding transformed with the use of breast pumps. *American Journal of Public Health, 101*(8), 1356–1359.

Robinson, S. (2012). Neonatal posthemorrhagic hydrocephalus from prematurity: Pathophysiology and current treatment concepts. *Journal of Neurosurgery Pediatrics, 9*(3), 242–258.

Salihu, H. M., Kornosky, J. L., Lynch, O., et al. (2011). Impact of prenatal alcohol consumption on placenta-associated syndromes. *Alcohol, 45*(1), 73–79.

Samra, H. A., McGrath, J. M., Wehbe, M., et al. (2012). Epigenetics and family-centered developmental care for the preterm infant. *Advances in Neonatal Care, 12*(Suppl. 5), S2–S9.

Schleiss, M. R., & Patterson, J. C. (2012). Viral infections of the fetus and newborn and immunodeficiency virus infection during pregnancy. In C. A. Gleason & S. U. Devaskar (Eds.), *Avery's diseases of the newborn* (9th ed., pp. 468–512). Philadelphia, PA: Elsevier/Saunders.

Scollan-Koliopoulos, M., & Koliopoulos, J. S. (2010). Evaluation and management of apparent life-threatening events in infants. *Pediatric Nursing, 36*(2), 77–83.

Smith, C. G. (2011). In the critically ill, nothing-by-mouth infant, would enteral administration of simulated amniotic fluid improve feeding tolerance compared with the current practice of no therapy? An evidence-based review. *Neonatal Network, 30*(2), 105–115.

Soll, R. F. (2012). Inhaled nitric oxide for respiratory failure in preterm infants. *Neonatology, 102*(4), 251–253.

Stoll, B. J., Hansen, N. I., Bell, E. F., et al. (2010). Neonatal outcomes of extremely preterm infants from the NICHD neonatal research network. *Pediatrics, 126*(3), 443–456.

Swarnam, K., Soraisham, A. S., & Sivanandan, S. (2011). Advances in the management of meconium aspiration syndrome. *International Journal of Pediatrics, 2012*, 359571.

Swiatkowska-Freund, M., Pankrac, Z., & Preis, K. (2012). Results of laser therapy in twin-to-twin transfusion syndrome: Our experience. *Journal of Maternal-Fetal & Neonatal Medicine, 25*(10), 1917–1920.

Symons, A. B., & Mahoney, M. C. (2011). Neonatal hyperbilirubinemia. In J. E. South-Paul, S. C. Matheny, & E. L. Lewis (Eds.), *Current diagnosis and treatment in family medicine* (3rd ed., pp. 20–27). Columbus, OH: McGraw-Hill.

Teune, M. J., Bakhuizen, S., Gyamfi Bannerman, C., et al. (2011). A systematic review of severe morbidity in infants born late preterm. *American Journal of Obstetrics & Gynecology, 205*(4), 374.e1–374.e9.

Thilo, E. H., & Rosenberg, A. A. (2012). The newborn infant. In W. Hay, M. Levin, R. Deterding, et al. (Eds.), *Current diagnosis & treatment pediatrics* (21st ed., pp. 9–72). New York, NY: McGraw-Hill/Lange.

Tsai, A., Manchester, D. K., & Elias, E. R. (2012). Genetics and dysmorphology. In W. Hay, M. Levin, R. Deterding, et al. (Eds.), *Current diagnosis & treatment pediatrics* (21st ed., pp. 1088–1123). New York, NY: McGraw-Hill/Lange.

Udry-Jorgensen, L., Pierrehumbert, B., Borghini, A., et al. (2011). Quality of attachment, perinatal risk and mother-infant interaction in a high-risk premature sample. *Infant Mental Health Journal, 32*(3), 305–318.

U.S. Department of Health and Human Services. (2010). *Healthy people 2020.* Washington, DC: Author.

Waller, S. A., Gopalani, S., & Benedetti, T. J. (2012). Complicated deliveries: Overview. In C. A. Gleason & S. U. Devaskar (Eds.), *Avery's diseases of the newborn* (9th ed., pp. 146–158). Philadelphia, PA: Elsevier/Saunders.

Westhoff, G. L., Little, S. E., & Caughey, A. B. (2011). Herpes simplex virus and pregnancy: A review of the management of antenatal and peripartum herpes infections. *Obstetrical & Gynecological Survey, 66*(10), 629–638.

Whitehead, N. S. (2012). The relationship of economic status to preterm contractions and preterm delivery. *Journal of Maternal Child Health, 16*(8), 1645–1656.

Young, G. (2012). Hemostatic disorders of the newborn. In C. A. Gleason & S. U. Devaskar (Eds.), *Avery's diseases of the newborn* (9th ed., pp. 1056–1079). Philadelphia, PA: Elsevier/Saunders.

Yurdakok, M., & Ozek, E. (2012). Transient tachypnea of the newborn: the treatment strategies. *Current Pharmaceutical Design, 18*(21), 3046–3049.

Zeigler, E. E. (2011). Meeting the nutritional needs of the low-birth-weight infant. *Annals of Nutrition & Metabolism, 58*(1), 8–13.

Chapter 27

Nursing Care of the Child Born With a Physical or Developmental Challenge

KEY TERMS

- ankyloglossia
- atresia
- cleft lip
- cleft palate
- developmental hip dysplasia
- fistula
- frenulum
- gastroschisis
- hydrocephalus
- meconium plug
- omphalocele
- polydactyly
- spina bifida
- stenosis
- syndactyly
- transillumination
- volvulus

OBJECTIVES

After mastering the contents of this chapter, you should be able to:

1. Describe common physical and developmental disorders that occur in newborns.
2. Identify 2020 National Health Goals related to infants born physically or developmentally challenged that nurses can help the nation achieve.
3. Assess an infant who is born physically or developmentally challenged.
4. Formulate nursing diagnoses for infants born with a physical or developmental challenge.
5. Establish expected outcomes to meet the needs of a child with a physical or developmental challenge and help parents manage seamless transitions across differing health care settings.
6. Using the nursing process, plan nursing care that includes the six competencies of Quality & Safety Education for Nurses (QSEN): Patient-Centered Care, Teamwork & Collaboration, Evidence-Based Practice (EBP), Quality Improvement (QI), Safety, and Informatics.
7. Implement nursing interventions for care of an infant born with a physical or developmental challenge, such as preventing infection in a child with a neural tube disorder.
8. Evaluate expected outcomes to determine achievement and effectiveness of care.
9. Integrate knowledge of congenital physical or developmental challenges with the interplay of nursing process, the six competencies of QSEN, and Family Nursing to promote quality maternal and child health nursing care.

Bobby Jo Sparrow, age 16 years, is a new mother whose newborn has been admitted to the neonatal intensive care unit because of a neural tube disorder and congenital hip dysplasia. Ms. Sparrow is obviously upset over the diagnosis. She has not named the baby, and her parents have not visited. She says to you, "I'm a good person. The only thing I did wrong during pregnancy was to take some cough medicine. How could this have happened to me?"

Previous chapters described the importance of assessing all infants at birth. This chapter adds information about common congenital anomalies or structural disorders that may occur in newborns. This information serves as a basis for a newborn assessment and for health teaching for parents.

How would you answer this mother? What type of advice and support does she need?

Few things can change the usually joyous tone of a birthing room faster than the birth of a baby with a physical or developmental challenge. Primary care providers who are used to saying "perfect boy" or "beautiful girl" find themselves without words. The usual congratulatory remarks hang unsaid in the air.

When a child is born with an apparent physical or developmental challenge, nurses must play a major role in supporting and educating the parents so they can move forward from this point. With some infants, their congenital disorder will require surgery but the prognosis is overall good, so this will be only a temporary concern (Hedricks, 2013). Other infants, however, have serious, life-threatening concerns and their parents will have financially draining long-term responsibilities for continued care. This chapter covers physical disorders of the skeletal, gastrointestinal, and neurologic systems that are apparent at birth or recognized soon after. Congenital disorders of the cardiovascular system, which also represent life-threatening problems for an infant, are addressed in Chapter 41.

Children born with a congenital anomaly need skin-to-skin contact with parents if at all possible, the same as all newborns (Mangan & Mosher, 2012). They also need effective long-term care and consideration to be certain they are able to adjust to any residual effects of their birth disorder (Ballantyne, Stevens, Guttmann, et al., 2012). Remember, any child who is "different" in some way is more prone to child maltreatment and also more bullying in school than others (Turner, Vanderminden, Finkelhor, et al., 2011). Because their handicap will extend into adulthood, they need nursing support to transition to adult care health care providers (Davies, Rennick, & Majnemer, 2011). Box 27.1 shows 2020 National Health Goals related to decreasing the number of children born with congenital anomalies.

BOX 27.1 Nursing Care Planning Based on 2020 National Health Goals

Many congenital anomalies, such as a cleft lip, an omphalocele, and neural tube disorders, can be detected by sonogram during intrauterine life. The following 2020 National Health Goals address the importance of prevention and therapy postbirth:

- Increase the proportion of women delivering a live birth who took multivitamins/folic acid prior to pregnancy from a baseline of 30.1% to 33.1%.
- Reduce the occurrence of spina bifida from 34.2 per 100,000 live births to 30.8 per 100,000 live births per year.
- Reduce the occurrence of anencephaly from 24.6 per 100,000 live births to 22.1 per 100,000 live births per year.
- Increase the proportion of children with special health care needs who have access to a medical home from 47.1% to 51.8%.
- Increase the proportion of children aged 0 to 11 years with special health care needs who receive their care in family-centered, comprehensive, and coordinated systems from a baseline of 20.4% to 22.4%; and in children aged 12 to 17 years from 13.7% to 15.1% (U.S. Department of Health and Human Services [DHHS], 2010; see www.healthypeople.gov).

Nurses can help the nation achieve these goals by urging women to enter pregnancy with an adequate folic acid level, ensuring women obtain prenatal care, and receive comprehensive advice and support after diagnosis of a fetal or newborn disorder.

Nursing Process Overview

For Care of a Physically or Developmentally Challenged Child

Assessment

The nursing assessment of a physically or developmentally challenged newborn focuses on determining the infant's immediate physiologic needs required to sustain life and the parents' immediate emotional needs to promote bonding. The following eight primary needs of newborns should be assessed for signs that they are being established:

- Adequate respiration
- Extrauterine circulation
- Body temperature
- Prevention of infection
- An infant–parent bond
- Adequate stimulation
- Ability to take in adequate nourishment
- Ability to achieve waste elimination

Anomalies that affect a child's appearance may have the most immediate effect on the parents' ability to establish a positive bond with their child. It is important, however, not to jump to conclusions about what will be the parents' response. An assessment of the family's verbal and nonverbal responses may reveal that parents are prepared and agreeable to meet this infant's special needs.

Nursing Diagnosis

Many nursing diagnoses established for children who are physically or developmentally challenged address the effect of the disorder on body function, including the child's primary needs, and also on family interaction. Examples of possible diagnoses include:

- Imbalanced nutrition, less than body requirements, related to inability to take in adequate nutrition secondary to a physical challenge
- Impaired physical mobility related to congenital anomaly
- Risk for impaired parenting related to the birth of child with a congenital anomaly
- Anticipatory grieving (parental) related to loss of the idea of the "perfect" child

Outcome Identification and Planning

Nurses play an important role in providing immediate care to high-risk infants at birth as well as guarding their health until a child care team arrives to assume care or transport the infant to a high-risk nursery. When establishing expected outcomes and planning care, be certain to consider both the short- and long-term needs of the newborn and how these needs may affect the family. Be certain to consider the family's resources, both emotional and financial, so a plan can be devised with these in mind. Parents with supportive family members are often more able to accept the limits of a child's challenge and turn their attention to the planned treatment regimen or care priorities sooner than those without close friends or relatives to whom they can turn for comfort and support. For the latter, you may need to act not only as a source of information and support but also as a sounding board and advocate until the parents can begin to develop positive coping mechanisms to help them come to terms with this unexpected event. The following organizations can be beneficial sources of support for parents to let them know they are not alone in their situation: the Easter Seals Disability Services (www.easterseals.com), the Spina Bifida Association (www.sbaa.org), the March of Dimes Foundation (www.marchofdimes.com), and the Cleft Palate Foundation (www.cleftline.org).

Implementation

Nursing interventions for a baby born physically challenged include immediate life-sustaining measures such as providing oxygen or adequate intake of nutrients when a disorder prevents the infant from establishing respirations or sucking. Educating the parents about pretreatment and posttreatment procedures and encouraging them to hold, touch, and talk with their baby are especially important to the future emotional well-being of the child and family.

Parents may suffer a loss of self-esteem with the child's birth, feeling as if the baby is proof that something in the combination of their genes or in the prenatal environment they provided was inadequate. They may need to hear positive comments about themselves and the infant and be given support until they can realize that by caring for the child they are accomplishing more, not less, than other couples.

You can expect parents to move through the same stages of grief such as denial, anger, and bargaining as those whose child has died at birth (see Chapter 56). Most parents closely watch how nurses and other health care providers handle their baby to see if they are giving as much attention to their baby as others. Be certain to treat the child in the same manner as any other, therefore, such as rocking the baby after a feeding or cooing and talking to the baby the same as you might do with other babies. Through positive role modeling of this type, you help set the stage for healthy parent–child interactions every time you handle an infant born with a physical or developmental challenge.

Outcome Evaluation

An evaluation should focus on expected outcomes established for a child's physical health and developmental needs, as well as the family's ability to cope with whatever special care and growth needs the child may have in the future. Be certain parents have numbers to call for questions, follow-up care, and support before discharge from the health care facility.

Examples of expected outcomes may include:

- Parent describes positive features of child by 2 weeks.
- Parents state they are comfortable with enteral feeding by 1 month.
- Child is ambulatory with walker or wheelchair by 2 years of age.

CARE AT THE BIRTH OF AN INFANT BORN PHYSICALLY OR DEVELOPMENTALLY CHALLENGED

Most primary care providers believe relating the news of congenital physical or developmental anomalies to parents is their responsibility. Because this person is involved with the final stage of birth and if a neonatal specialist is not immediately available, many minutes may pass before there is time for a thorough inspection of the baby, and the parents can be told about the baby's condition and prognosis. This delay has the potential to affect parents in two ways: either leaving them to believe they have just given birth to a perfect child among very unsupportive people or they have just given birth to a child so deformed that none of the professionals feel able to describe the condition. Because of the changed atmosphere in the birthing room, the second response is by far more likely. This can cause parents to begin anticipatory grieving for what they believe is a severely deformed child. Even when they are told later that the disorder is not extensive and is easily correctable, the anticipatory grief reaction may continue and cut them off emotionally from their child (Box 27.2).

For this reason, nurses need to be familiar with the most frequently encountered physical or developmental anomalies that are present at birth so, as the person who at that moment in the birth process is most available for patient education, they can explain the problem to parents. In other instances, nurses must be ready to serve as back-up informants to answer parents' questions after they have been told by a primary care provider their child has been born less than perfect, support the parents as they seek to understand the condition, and provide information for the best way for parents to seek additional information. Many parents or family members will search the Internet for information. Guide them to reputable .edu or .gov sites for reliable information concerning their baby's condition, as well as encourage them to bring the information with them when they ask questions (Wool, 2011).

It is a good rule to explain to parents what the disorder consists of and what the usual prognosis is before showing the baby to them because parents may find it hard to look at an infant with

BOX 27.2 Nursing Care Planning to Respect Cultural Diversity

The causes of most congenital anomalies are unknown, although they probably arise from a combination of environmental and genetic factors. Despite this evidence, many people persist in believing infants with congenital anomalies are born to people less deserving than others. Common beliefs that are prevalent include myths such as being looked on by an evil eye (*mal de ojo* in Spanish) can cause a deformity, eating raisins causes brown birth marks, and eating strawberries causes red hemangiomas. New parents need an explanation of their child's disorder and a chance to talk about why they believe their child's disorder occurred to relieve any guilt that they were the cause of the anomaly so they can regain sufficient self-esteem to be able to raise a child with a congenital disorder.

a cleft lip or palate or exposed abdominal contents, for example, and listen at the same time. A typical explanation for Bobby Jo, for example, might be, "As you noticed when your doctor placed your baby on your abdomen, your baby's spinal cord isn't completely formed, something called a meningocele. Although that could be more extensive, at first inspection, it seems to be a problem that can be repaired. Her hips may also need some treatment. I'll bring the baby's incubator over so you can see her again. Notice how bright eyes and alert she is for just being born."

These are the sort of statements that define and limit the problem for parents. They also give them direction about where and how they should proceed in beginning to seek help for their child. Because most congenital abnormalities involve surgery, be certain plans are made for adequate pain assessment and management postoperatively to make the experience of surgery this early in life not an unbearable procedure for a neonate (Harrison, Yamada, & Stevens, 2010).

What if...27.1 You notice that Bobby Jo remains obviously upset at her child's appearance. She doesn't want to feed him and tells you she'd like to place him for adoption. In contrast, the child's father, also a teenager, handles the baby warmly and asks questions about surgery. No grandparents visit. What interventions would you want to begin with this family?

PHYSICAL AND DEVELOPMENTAL DISORDERS OF THE SKELETAL SYSTEM

Either genetic or environmental factors can compromise fetal physical growth to such an extent that they result in skeletal disorders in the newborn.

Absent or Malformed Extremities

Congenital skeletal disorders result from reasons such as maternal drug ingestion or virus invasion or amniotic band formation in utero. In most instances, however, the cause of the anomaly cannot be established. Children born without an extremity or with a malformed extremity can be fitted with a prosthesis as early in life as about 6 months so the infant can learn to stand at the normal time or handle and explore objects readily. Introducing a prosthesis early also prevents a child from adjusting to a missing extremity, for example, by writing with the feet or sliding across the floor rather than walking. If this happens, children can become so proficient at these adjustments that later in life they do not see the advantage of a prosthesis and may limit their potential by refusing to use one.

Depending on the condition, in many children, there is a potential for better function if the malformed portion of an extremity is amputated before a prosthesis is fitted. This creates a difficult decision for parents because it is one they cannot undo later. They need assurance that hands with malformed fingers, for example, will not later grow to become normal and that a well-fitted prosthesis will allow their child a more usual childhood and adult life than if the original disorder was left unchanged (Fig. 27.1).

Learning to use a hand prosthesis takes weeks to months. It helps if parents can think of interesting activities when introducing the prosthesis so the child can immediately see how useful it will be to use. Gait training for the use of lower extremity prostheses begins with the use of parallel bars and proceeds to independent walking and mastery of steps. Again, suggesting activities the child needs to walk to do offers motivation for trying to use the prosthesis.

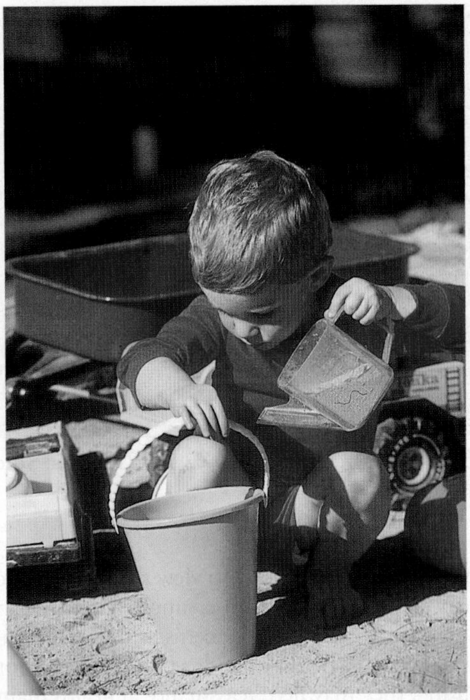

FIGURE 27.1 A young child learns to use a hand prosthesis during play. (M. Grecco/Stock Boston.)

Children who are born with an absent extremity may need help not only in mastering the use of a prosthesis but also in forming a positive body image of themselves as whole. If possible, in the newborn period, introduce parents to the rehabilitation team who will be following their child. Further steps will then be outlined to help them move past the helplessness they may be feeling to more positive actions. Visiting with a child who uses a prosthesis well can be a great help in convincing parents that their child can lead a normal life. Young children with a congenital extremity loss apparently do not grieve over the lost extremity as do adults or older children, which means they are often better prepared to move on quickly to rehabilitation.

Finger and Toe Conditions

Finger or hand deformities occur in about 3% of all births. **Polydactyly** is the presence of one or more additional fingers or toes. When an entire extra finger or toe forms, the supernumerary digit is usually amputated in infancy or early childhood. These extra fingers are often just cartilage or skin tags, and removal is simple and cosmetically sound. In **syndactyly** (two fingers or toes are fused), the fusion is usually caused by a simple webbing (Fig. 27.2); separation of the digits into two sound and cosmetically appealing ones is usually successful. In other instances, the bones of the fingers or toes are also fused, and cosmetic appearance and function cannot be fully reconstructed (Walter, 2011).

These digit anomalies are always upsetting to parents (one of the first things new parents do is count the fingers and toes of

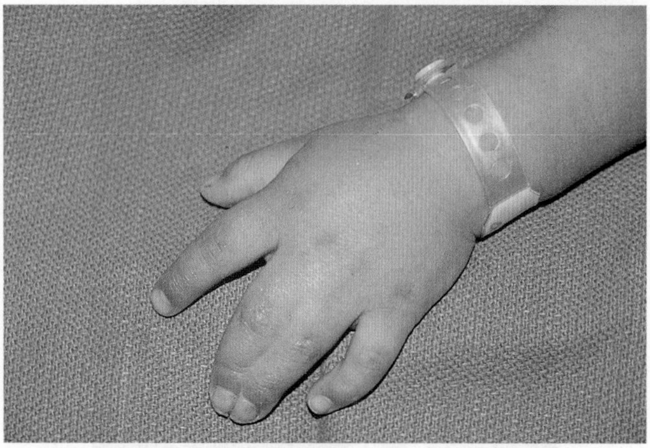

FIGURE 27.2 Syndactyly. (JPD/Custom Medical Stock Photograph.)

newborns) and may cause them to view their infant as defective rather than being an infant with a simple anomaly. Encourage them to air their feelings and concerns as they deliver the news to family and friends. Because hands are so important for writing or computing, they may need reassurance at health maintenance visits for the first few years of their child's life that the child is perfect in other ways so they can accept and help the child develop self-esteem. Children may need this same type of assurance as they grow older so they can think of themselves as well people.

Chest Deviations

Pectus excavatum, or "funnel chest," is an indentation of the lower portion of the sternum. It is the most common congenital deformity of the anterior chest, occurs in about 1 out of 500 live births, and affects boys four times more often than girls. The concern may not be present at birth, but becomes more obvious as the child grows to school age or adolescence. As a result of the deformity, lung volume is apt to be decreased and the heart is displaced to the left. The condition can be repaired, for either cosmetic reasons or physiologic reasons, such as to expand lung volume (Dean, Etienne, Hindson, et al., 2012). With *pectus carinatum*, the sternum is displaced anteriorly, increasing the anteroposterior diameter of the chest. This can be surgically corrected.

Torticollis (Wry Neck)

Torticollis is a term derived from the terms *tortus* ("twisted") and *collum* ("neck"). Torticollis (wry neck) occurs as a congenital anomaly when the sternocleidomastoid muscle is injured and bleeds during birth (S. J. Lee, Han, Lee, et al., 2011). This tends to occur in newborns with wide shoulders when pressure is exerted on the head to deliver the shoulder either with a vaginal or cesarean birth. The infant holds the head tilted to the same side as the muscle that is involved; the chin rotates to the opposite side. The injury may not be noticeable in the newborn and may become evident only as the original hemorrhage recedes and fibrous contraction occurs at 1 to 2 months of age. A thick mass over the muscle can usually be palpated at that time.

To relieve torticollis, parents need to begin a program of passive stretching exercises, lying the infant on a flat surface and rotating the head through a full range of motion. In addition, parents should always encourage the infant to look in the direction of the affected muscle. They can encourage this by holding the child to feed in such a position that the child must look in the desired direction. Placing a mobile on the child's crib can encourage the child to look toward the affected side. Speaking to and handing the child objects from the affected side is another helpful exercise.

If manual stretching is begun early and performed consistently by parents, further treatment usually is not necessary. If extreme injury to the muscle occurred, torticollis can lead to the continued elevation of one shoulder. Although a rare complication, this has the potential to lead to scoliosis later in life. Therefore, help parents to understand that their actions are important therapy, not just games. Otherwise, the exercises seem so simple parents may not take them seriously. In the few instances in which simple exercises are not effective and the condition still exists at 1 year of age, surgical correction followed by a neck immobilizer may be necessary.

Parents may ask if their child should have botulism (Botox) injections because adolescents or adults who develop spastic torticollis or who have unsuccessfully treated congenital torticollis may receive this type of treatment (Bouchard, Chouinard, & Suchowersky, 2010). Botox, however, is not recommended or necessary for most infants.

QSEN Checkpoint Question 27.1

Patient-Centered Care

Suppose Bobby Jo's baby develops a torticollis and she is distraught by her baby's appearance. What care measure would best relieve the infant's physical anomaly and Bobby Jo's distress?

a. Teach Bobby Jo how to perform her baby's neck stretching exercises.
b. Wrap the infant's neck in a warm towel for 15 minutes twice daily.
c. Assure Bobby Jo that the anomaly will resolve spontaneously.
d. Administer 80 mg of aspirin with each of his bottle feedings.

Look in Appendix A for the best answer and rationale.

Craniosynostosis

Craniosynostosis is the premature closure of the sutures of the skull. This may occur in utero or early in infancy because of rickets or irregularities of calcium or phosphate metabolism; it also occurs as a dominantly inherited trait and occurs more often in boys than in girls (Roder, 2010).

This condition needs to be detected early because premature closure of the suture line will close the fontanelles, seal the skull closed, and compromise brain growth. If the sagittal suture line is the one that closes prematurely, the child's head tends to grow anteriorly and posteriorly. If the coronal suture line fuses early, the orbits of the eyes become misshapen and the increased intracranial pressure may lead to eye disorders such as exophthalmos, nystagmus, papilledema, strabismus, and atrophy of the optic nerve with consequent loss of vision. Premature closure of the coronal suture line is associated with syndactyly. Therefore, make a point at well-child assessments to closely observe all infants with syndactyly for head circumference. Cardiac anomalies, choanal atresias, or disorders of elbows and knee joints can also be associated.

Craniosynostosis is diagnosed by X-ray or ultrasound, which reveals the fused suture line. If the suture line involved is the sagittal, treatment may involve only careful observation; if the coronal suture line is involved, it will need to be surgically opened to prevent brain compression and an abnormally shaped head by 9 to 12 months (Okada & Gosain, 2012).

Achondroplasia

Achondroplasia (chondrodystrophia) is a failure of bone growth inherited as a dominant trait, which causes a disorder in cartilage production in utero. The epiphyseal plate of long bones cannot produce adequate cartilage for longitudinal bone growth; this results in both arms and legs becoming stunted (Ireland, Donaghey, McGill, et al., 2012).

Because the bones of the cranium are of membranous origin, the head continues to grow normally, causing children's heads to appear unusually large in contrast to their extremities. The forehead is particularly prominent and the bridge of the nose becomes flattened. Children's trunks are of near-normal size, but a thoracic kyphosis (outward curve) and lumbar lordosis (inward curve) of the spine may develop. Because this is a cartilage, not a brain growth concern, gross motor development may be slowed, but intelligence is not affected.

Achondroplasia can be diagnosed in utero by ultrasound or at birth by X-ray by comparing the length of extremities to the usual length (in the average child, the arms can be extended to the distance of the midthigh). An X-ray will also reveal characteristic abnormally flaring epiphyseal lines. Children with achondroplasia rarely reach a height of more than 4 ft 6 in. (140 cm). Women with this condition may have difficulty with childbearing because of a small pelvis, generally necessitating a cesarean birth.

Children with achondroplasia become aware of their appearance as early as the preschool years. They are apt to become acutely aware of their appearance during school age, when they realize they look so different from other children. In order to help them grow, they may be prescribed growth hormone or, although controversial, leg lengthening may be possible (Singh, Song, Venkatesh, et al., 2010). Ideally, such children have parents who have helped them adjust well to their short stature as well as help them develop good self-esteem so they can be happy in their body, no matter what is their final height.

Children need to be informed as they reach adolescence that, as with all dominantly inherited disorders, there is a high probability their children will inherit the disorder. This can make adolescence a particularly difficult time for these children as they realize both some occupational and reproductive options may be limited for them. Continued guidance or counseling can help them to emerge from this period with feelings of high self-esteem as adults.

Talipes Disorders

The word *talipes* is formed from the Latin *talus* ("ankle") and *pes* ("foot"). The talipes deformities, therefore, are ankle–foot disorders, popularly called clubfoot. The term "clubfoot" implies permanent crippling to many people, and because this is no longer true with effective surgery, avoid using the term when discussing talipes disorders with parents. Concerns that may remain after surgery include that the child's right and left shoe size may vary and the child may have asymmetry of leg length.

Approximately 1 child in every 1,000 is born with a talipes disorder and it occurs more often in boys than in girls. It probably is inherited as a polygenic pattern, and it usually occurs as a unilateral problem (Pietrucin-Materek, van Teijlingen, Barker, et al., 2011).

Some newborns who appear to have a talipes disorder actually have only an unusual foot position (a pseudotalipes) that developed because of their cramped intrauterine position. In these infants, the foot can be brought into a straight position by manual manipulation. In a true disorder, the foot cannot be properly aligned without further intervention. Be certain to demonstrate to parents that, if a pseudodisorder is present, the foot can easily be brought into line or is not deformed. Otherwise, the first-time parents fit booties or shoes on the infant, they may notice this odd position and worry the foot is misshapen when it is not. Stretching the foot into line every day will solve the problem in a short time.

A true talipes disorder can be one of four separate types: plantar flexion (an equinus or "horse foot" position, with the forefoot lower than the heel); dorsiflexion (the heel is held lower than the forefoot or the anterior foot is flexed toward the anterior leg); varus deviation (the foot turns in); or valgus deviation (the foot turns out). Most children with talipes deformities have a combination of these conditions or have an equinovarus (Fig. 27.3A) or a calcaneovalgus disorder (a child walks on the heel with the foot everted).

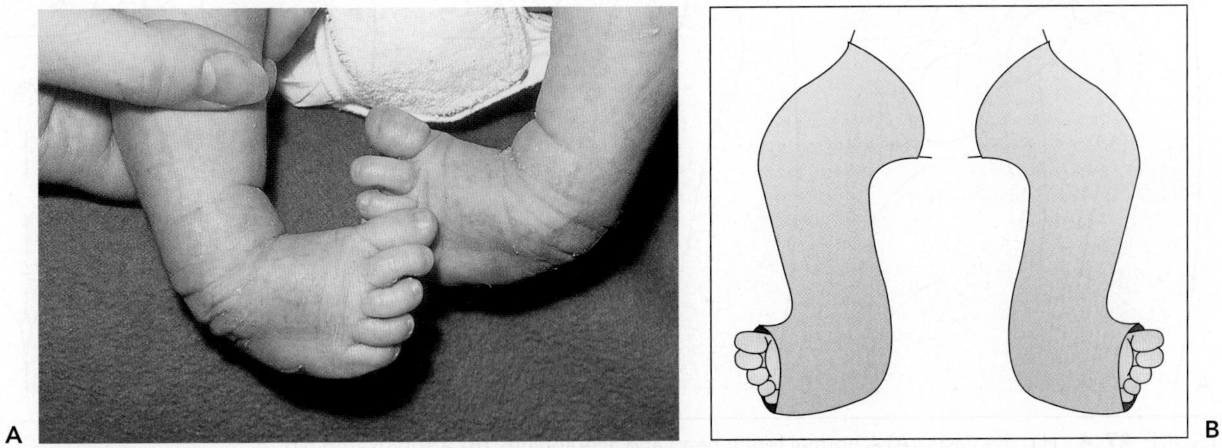

FIGURE 27.3 **(A)** Talipes equinovarus. (SPL/Photo Researchers, Inc.) **(B)** Casts for bilateral equinovarus.

Assessment

The earlier a true disorder is recognized, the better will be the correction. Make a habit, therefore, of straightening all newborn feet to the midline as part of the initial assessment to detect this disorder.

Therapeutic Management

Correction is achieved best if it is begun in the newborn period. For correction, a series of casts or braces are applied to gradually mold the foot into good alignment (a Ponseti method) (Linehan & O'Sullivan, 2011). Although the disorder involves the ankle, the cast or brace extends above the knee to ensure a firm correction (see Fig. 27.3B). (Care of the child in a cast is discussed in Chapter 51.) Because talipes casts are high on the leg, change diapers frequently to prevent a wet diaper from touching the cast and causing it to become soaked with urine or meconium. Review with parents how to check the infant's toes for coldness or blueness and how to blanch a toenail bed and watch it turn pink to assess for good circulation. Because a newborn cannot report pain except by generalized crying, they must evaluate crying episodes in the infant carefully. Such crying may be because of colic, hunger, or wet diapers, or it might also be because of the tingling feeling of circulatory compression (as when a foot is "asleep") from too tight a cast.

Infants grow so rapidly in the neonatal period that casts or braces for talipes deformities must be changed or adjusted almost every 1 or 2 weeks. If a mother has a complication or is exhausted from childbirth, be certain she will be able to make arrangements for another family member or friend to bring the infant to the hospital for frequent cast changes or brace adjustments.

After approximately 6 weeks (the time varies depending on the extent of the problem), the final cast will be removed. Following this, the infant may have to sleep in Denis Browne splints (shoes attached to a metal bar to maintain position) or high-top shoes at night for a few more months to ensure an effective correction. Parents may need to perform passive foot exercises such as putting the infant's foot and ankle through a full range of motion several times a day for several months. These seem to be simple maneuvers, so be certain to stress their importance to the parents; otherwise, they are easy exercises to omit when people's lives are busy.

Although a successful correction cannot be guaranteed, the prognosis for a full correction is good. For children who do not achieve correction by casting, additional surgery is yet another option to achieve a final correction.

Developmental Hip Dysplasia

Developmental hip dysplasia (often referred to as congenital hip dysplasia) is improper formation and function of the hip socket. It affects 1% to 2% of newborns and is a leading cause of orthopedic disability in childhood and adult life because it can lead to premature arthritis requiring hip replacement (the disorder is responsible for up to 28% of hip replacements in people under 60 years of age) (Sewell & Eastwood, 2011). The disorder may be evident as either subluxation or dislocation of the head of the femur (Fig. 27.4).

With the disorder, the acetabulum of the pelvis is unusually flattened or shallow. This prevents the head of the femur from remaining in the acetabulum and rotating adequately. In a subluxated hip, the femur "rides up" because of the flat acetabulum; in a dislocated hip, the femur rides so far up it actually leaves the acetabulum. Why the disorder occurs is unknown, but it may be from a polygenic inheritance pattern. It may also occur from a uterine position that causes less-than-usual pressure of the femur head on the acetabulum.

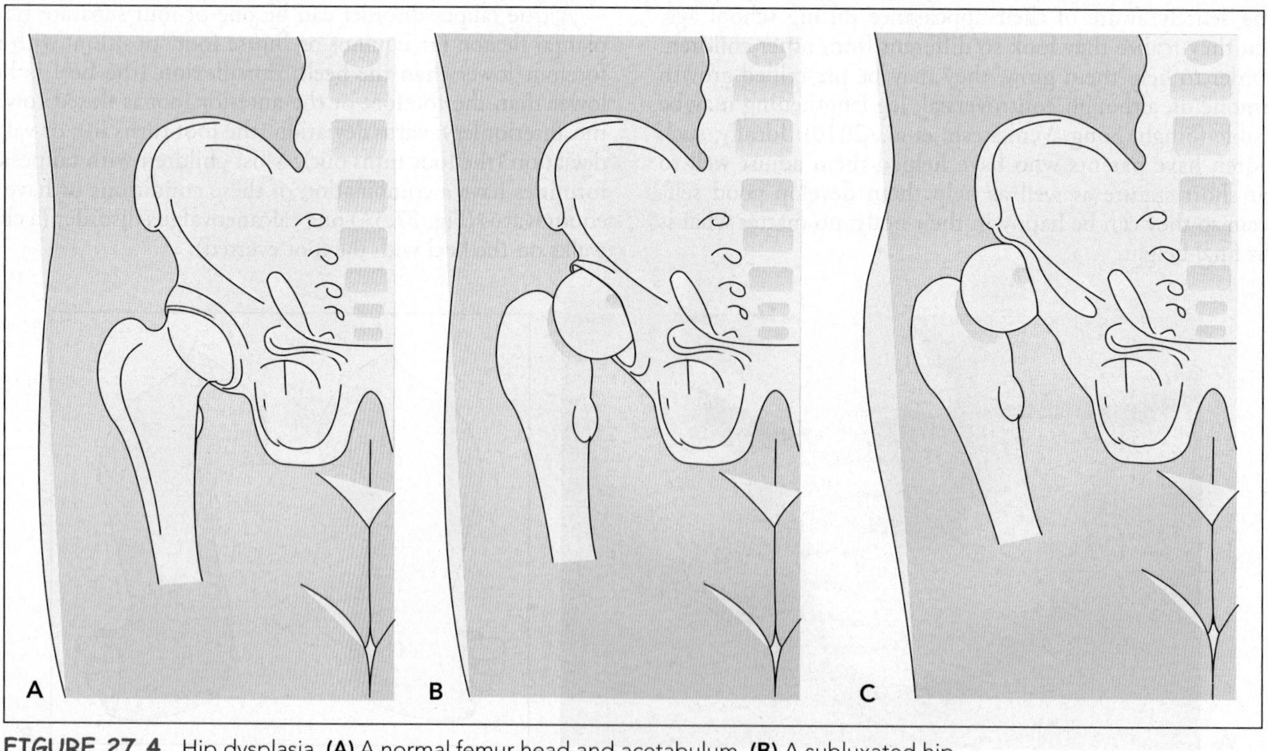

FIGURE 27.4 Hip dysplasia. **(A)** A normal femur head and acetabulum. **(B)** A subluxated hip. The femur head is "riding high" in the shallow acetabulum. **(C)** A dislocated hip. The femur head is not engaged in the shallow acetabulum.

Developmental hip dysplasia occurs most often in children of Mediterranean ancestry. It is usually unilateral and found six times more frequently in girls than in boys, possibly because the hips are normally more flaring in females and possibly because the maternal hormone relaxin causes the pelvic ligaments to be more relaxed during pregnancy, which causes the femur to not press as effectively into the acetabulum during intrauterine life, thus deepening the space. Sociocultural methods of carrying infants such as using a sling, placing them in a backpack, or carrying them on the hip may promote or decrease the extent of the involvement after birth.

Assessment

Detecting developmental hip dysplasia in the newborn is important because the longer the condition goes undetected, the more difficult it is to correct. On inspection, the affected leg may appear slightly shorter than the other because the femur head rides so high in the socket. This is most noticeable when the child is lying supine and the thighs are flexed to a 90-degree angle toward the abdomen, causing one knee to be lower than the other (a Galeazzi sign; Fig. 27.5A). An unequal number of skin folds may also be present on the posterior thighs (see Fig. 27.5B). This finding is unreliable, however, because some infants with normal hips have an uneven number of posterior thigh skin folds. Subluxated or dislocated hips are best assessed by noting whether the hips abduct (Box 27.3).

In some infants, the hip abducts properly at a newborn assessment, but at the time of a health maintenance visit at 4 to 6 weeks, a secondary shortening of the adductor muscles will have occurred, and the disorder will be first evident. Hip dysplasia may also be difficult to detect at birth in an infant who was born from a breech presentation because the knees tend to be stiff and not flex readily. Because tight adductor muscles occur in children with cerebral palsy, these children also need careful assessment. An X-ray, ultrasound, or magnetic resonance imaging (MRI) will definitely reveal the shallow acetabulum and a more lateral placement of the femur head for diagnosis.

Therapeutic Management

Correction of subluxated and dislocated hips involves positioning the hip into a flexed, abducted (externally rotated) position in order to press the femur head against the acetabulum and cause the acetabulum to deepen its contour from the pressure. A combination of splints, halters, or casts may be used. The small number of children who do not achieve correction by these noninvasive methods will have surgery and a pin inserted to stabilize the hip.

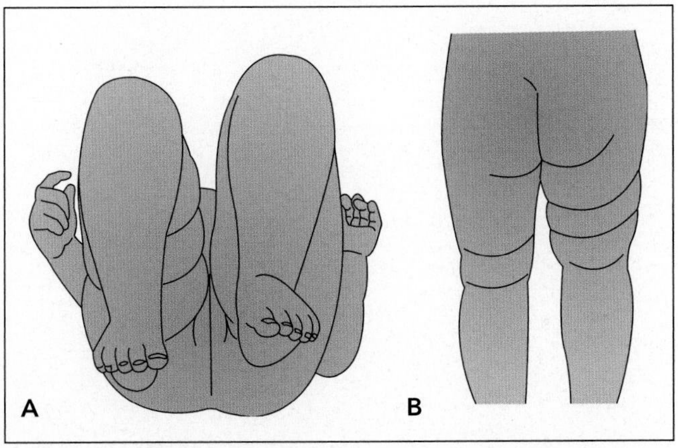

FIGURE 27.5 Signs of developmental hip dysplasia. **(A)** With the child in a supine position, the right knee on the side of the subluxation appears lower than the left because of malposition of the femur head. **(B)** Asymmetry of skin folds and prominence of the trochanter on the right side.

Nursing Diagnoses and Related Interventions

Nursing Diagnosis: Deficient parental knowledge related to splint, halter, or cast correction for hip dysplasia

Outcome Evaluation: Parents verbalize correct technique for and correctly demonstrate application and removal of splint or halter device and care of device or cast.

Multiple Diapers or Splints: Often, splint correction (to hold the legs in a frog-leg or abducted, externally rotated position) is begun during the newborn's initial hospital stay by placing two or three diapers on the infant. The extra bulk of diaper material between the child's legs effectively separates and spreads them. Many brands of disposable diapers are cut narrow between the legs so they do not offer this much bulk and so do not achieve this position as well as cloth diapers.

A Pavlik Harness: A Pavlik harness is an adjustable chest halter that abducts the legs. It is the method of choice for therapy because it reduces the time interval for therapy to 3 to 4 weeks and simplifies care (Fig. 27.6A). Soft plastic stirrups (booties) with quick-fastening closures attach to leg extension straps and hold the hips flexed, abducted, and externally rotated. Instruct parents how to lay the infant supine, grasp the infant's thighs and abduct them to place the femoral head into the acetabulum, and then apply the harness. The harness is then worn under clothing continually except for bathing. Advise parents to assess the skin under the straps daily for irritation or redness. Caution them also that the harness achieves its effect by gentle continual pressure; it will be ineffective if parents remove it frequently or forget to put it in place.

✔ QSEN Checkpoint Question 27.2

Informatics

Because Bobby Jo's baby was born with developmental hip dysplasia, he has a Pavlik harness prescribed. What information would you want Bobby Jo to know about his care?

a. The harness may not be effective, but she should trial it before surgery.
b. She should keep the harness on her baby for 12 hours a day.
c. Her baby should wear the harness at all times except while bathing.
d. For more advice she should look at mothers' blogs online.

Look in Appendix A for the best answer and rationale.

BOX 27.3 Nursing Care Planning Using Procedures

ASSESSING ORTOLANI AND BARLOW SIGNS

Purpose: To assist in detecting developmental hip dysplasia

PROCEDURE	PRINCIPLE
1. Lay the infant supine and flex the knees to 90 degrees at the hips.	1. Proper positioning helps ensure accurate results.
2. Place your middle fingers over the greater trochanter of the femur and your thumb on the internal side of the thigh over the lesser trochanter (Fig. A).	2. Placing your fingers in this way allows for abduction of the hips.

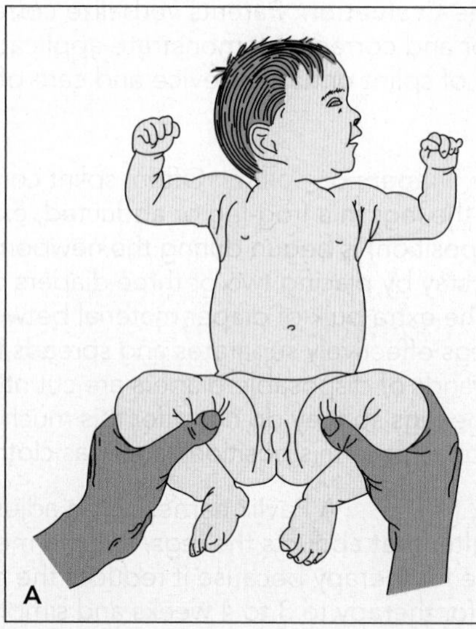

A

3. Abduct the hips while applying upward pressure over the greater trochanter, and listen for a clicking sound.	3. Normally, no sound is heard. A clicking or clunking sound is a positive Ortolani sign as it occurs when a displaced femoral head reenters the acetabulum.
4. Next, with your fingers in the same position and holding the hips and knees at 90-degree flexion, apply a backward pressure (down and laterally) and adduct the hips. Note any feeling of the femoral head slipping (Fig. B).	4. Normally, the hip joint is stable. A feeling of the femur head slipping out of the socket posterolaterally is a positive Barlow sign, which is indicative of hip instability associated with the developmental hip dysplasia.

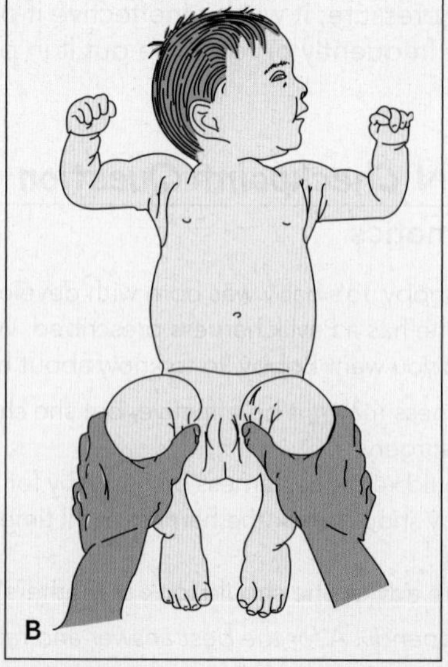

B

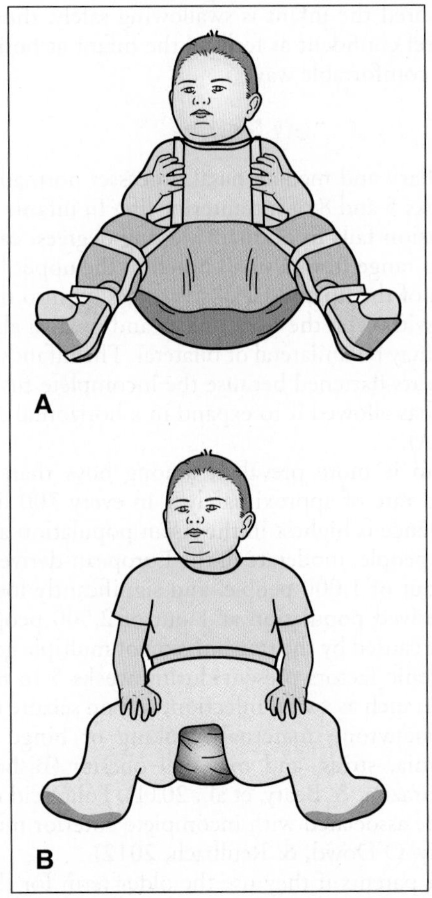

FIGURE 27.6 **(A)** A Pavlik harness (shown over clothing for illustrative purposes). **(B)** A hip abduction cast for correction of subluxation of the hip.

A Spica Cast: If a hip is fully dislocated or the subluxation is severe, an infant may be placed immediately in a frog-leg, A-line cast, or a spica cast to maintain an externally rotated hip position (see Fig. 27.6B). These casts are heavy and are so wide that dressing infants or sitting them in an infant car seat or using a bassinet can be difficult. Be certain parents have a car seat that can be modified to accommodate a large cast. Like babies with a talipes, these infants are unable to report a cast is causing circulatory constriction, so they need to be assessed hourly for circulation to the extremities for the first 24 hours the cast is in place and daily thereafter. Teach parents how to do this type of neurovascular assessment (check temperature and circulation in toes) before they take an infant home from the hospital so they can prevent circulatory compression from a rapidly growing leg outgrowing the cast. Casts will be changed as growth and casting therapy require but maintained for 6 to 9 months. Casting is a second line of correction because the child is much harder to care for because of the weight of the cast. If the reduction maneuver causes tension in the soft tissues around the hip, the resulting compression of the joint may cause transient blockage of the blood supply to the femoral head or avascular necrosis. In its severest form, this can lead to femoral head death and loss of future growth at the proximal growth plate, causing unequal leg lengths.

General Care Guidelines: No matter what type of therapy is used—double-diapering, harness, or cast—surgery may still be necessary for a final correction. Making parents aware of this from the start prevents them from thinking their child's condition is so serious that the usual methods of treatment failed. It also helps them accept from the beginning that this condition will be a long-term care concern. With severe hip involvement, some children will be 2 years old before the final cast is removed.

The child and parents will be visiting their orthopedist frequently during these early years. Assess that they also schedule general health maintenance visits for routine immunizations and overall growth and development assessment. Spend time during health maintenance visits talking with them about infant stimulation. Teach parents to hold their child for feeding and to rock and cuddle the infant, even though a large cast or a brace may be bulky and awkward. Discuss how to bring experiences to the infant because the child cannot crawl and walk toward interesting objects in the environment. A child's wagon can supply convenient and fun transportation. The child may also be able to lie prone and move about on a large skateboard. Many parents worry the child who is still in a large cast at the normal age for walking (12 months) will never learn to walk. They can be assured that this is not a problem; when the cast is removed, the child will quickly catch up with this developmental step.

PHYSICAL AND DEVELOPMENTAL DISORDERS OF THE GASTROINTESTINAL SYSTEM

Many of the most common congenital anomalies of the gastrointestinal system, such as cleft lip and cleft palate, occur because of midline closure failure extremely early in intrauterine life. Others occur because the tract first forms as a solid tube, then undergoes canalization (hollowing out). At any site where this hollowing out does not occur, a partial or complete blockage or obstruction will be present. All gastrointestinal disorders can interfere with an infant's ability to take in nourishment to some degree at birth. You may need to reinforce a mother's resolve to breastfeed in light of the disorder so she can be successful at this (Bessell, Hooper, Shaw, et al., 2011).

Ankyloglossia (Tongue-Tie)

Ankyloglossia is an abnormal restriction of the tongue occurring in a small number of newborns caused by an abnormally tight **frenulum**, the membrane attached to the lower anterior tip of the tongue (Kline, 2012). Normally, the frenulum appears short and is positioned near the tip of the tongue. As the anterior portion of the infant's tongue grows, the frenulum becomes located farther back. In most instances, therefore, an infant suspected of being tongue-tied has a normal tongue at birth; it just seems short to parents who are unaware of a newborn's appearance. This condition may rarely cause difficulty with breastfeeding or unclear speech. If it does, then surgical release can be performed in the newborn period or at about 4 years of age.

Showing parents other newborns or photographs of normal tongues is helpful to convince them that, assuming the infant is sucking well, a short newborn frenulum does not need to be corrected. Explore with them if there is a child in the family with a speech disorder or a cleft lip and palate. Do the parents need assurance in any other way their child is all right?

Thyroglossal Cysts

A thyroglossal cyst arises from an embryogenic fault that leaves a cyst formed at the base of the tongue, which then drains through a **fistula** (opening) to the anterior surface of the neck (D. Lee, Lim, & Lee, 2011). This condition may occur as a dominantly inherited trait. The cyst may involve the hyoid bone (the bone at the anterior surface of the neck at the root of the tongue) and may contain aberrant thyroid gland tissue. As the cyst fills with fluid, swelling and obstruction can lead to respiratory difficulty from pressure on the trachea. If infected, the cyst often appears swollen and reddened, with drainage of mucus or pus from the anterior neck.

The cyst is surgically removed to avoid future infection of the space and, if thyroid tissue is present, the possibility of developing thyroid carcinoma later in life. Observe infants closely in the immediate postoperative period for respiratory distress because the operative area will develop at least minimum edema from surgical trauma. Position infants on their sides so secretions drain freely from their mouths. Intravenous (IV) fluid therapy is given after surgery until the edema at the incision recedes somewhat and swallowing is safe once more (approximately 24 hours). If the mother is breastfeeding, encourage her to express her milk manually during this time to preserve her milk supply. Observe infants closely the first time they take fluid orally to be certain they do not aspirate. Be certain parents have a chance to feed their infant before the infant is discharged from the surgical unit so they can be assured the infant is swallowing safely, thus allowing them to feel confident at feeding the infant at home in a relaxed and comfortable way.

Cleft Lip and Cleft Palate

The maxillary and median nasal processes normally fuse between weeks 5 and 8 of intrauterine life. In infants with **cleft lip**, the fusion fails to occur in varying degrees, causing this disorder to range from a small notch in the upper lip to total separation of the lip and facial structures up into the floor of the nose, with even the upper teeth and gingiva absent. The deviation may be unilateral or bilateral. The infant's nose generally appears flattened because the incomplete fusion of the upper lip has allowed it to expand in a horizontal dimension (Fig. 27.7A).

Cleft lip is more prevalent among boys than girls and occurs at a rate of approximately 1 in every 700 live births. This incidence is highest in the Asian population at 1 out of every 500 people, moderate in the European-derived population at 1 out of 1,000 people, and significantly lower in the African-derived population at 1 out of 2,500 people. It appears to be caused by the transmission of multiple genes aided by teratogenic factors present during weeks 5 to 8 of intrauterine life, such as a viral infection, certain seizure medicines such as phenytoin, maternal smoking or binge drinking, hyperthermia, stress, and maternal obesity (Bishop, 2011; Dixon, Marazita, & Beaty, et al., 2011). Folic acid deficiency may also be associated with incomplete anterior midline closures (Kelly, O'Dowd, & Reulbach, 2012).

Correct parents if they use the older term for this condition, *harelip*, when talking about their child's condition. This term was used when children were left with large lip scars and possibly gross speech impediments because modern surgical techniques were not yet available. Now with current surgery, there is no need to associate the condition with negative outcomes rather than with the current positive results.

Because of the genetic influence, parents of a child with a cleft lip should be referred for genetic counseling to ensure they understand they have a small increased chance of having another child with a cleft lip or palate and that any future children are at a greater risk than usual for this problem.

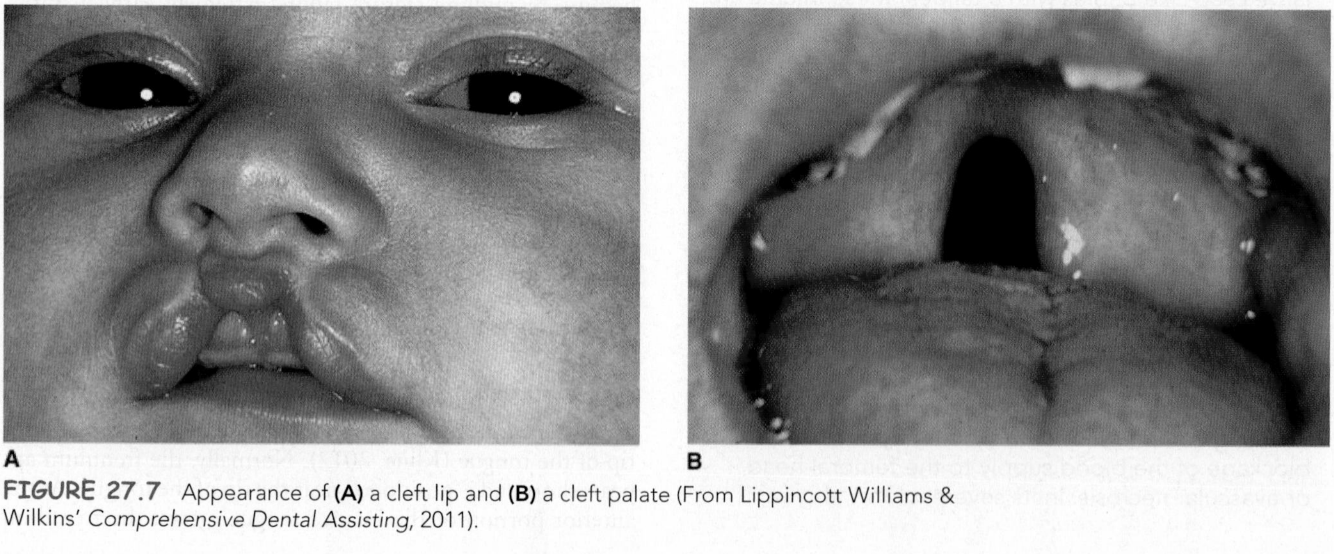

FIGURE 27.7 Appearance of **(A)** a cleft lip and **(B)** a cleft palate (From Lippincott Williams & Wilkins' *Comprehensive Dental Assisting*, 2011).

A **cleft palate** is an opening of the palate and occurs when the palatal process does not close as usual at approximately weeks 9 to 12 of intrauterine life. The incomplete closure is usually on the midline and may involve the anterior hard palate, the posterior soft palate, or both (see Fig. 27.7B). It may occur as a separate anomaly, or in conjunction with a cleft lip. As a single entity, in contrast to cleft lip, it tends to occur more frequently in girls than boys. Like cleft lip, it appears to be the result of polygenic inheritance or environmental influences. In connection with cleft lip, the incidence is approximately 1 out of every 1,000 births. As a single entity, it occurs in approximately 1 out of every 2,000 births. Almost 30% of children with both cleft lip and palate have associated birth defects, or the cleft palate occurs as only a portion of a larger syndrome (Dixon et al., 2011).

Assessment

Cleft lip may be detected by a sonogram while an infant is in utero. If not detected then, it is readily apparent on inspection of the mouth at birth. When assessing newborns, be sure you have good lighting so you can visualize the palate clearly. Because cleft palate is a component of many syndromes, assess the child for other congenital anomalies as well.

Therapeutic Management

If a cleft lip is discovered while the infant is still in utero, fetal surgery can repair the condition, although this procedure is not usually attempted. If the disorder is discovered at birth, a cleft lip can be repaired surgically shortly thereafter, often at the time of the initial hospital stay or between 2 and 12 weeks of age. Because the deviation of the lip interferes with sucking, infants may be a better surgical risk as newborns than they are after a month or more of poor nourishment. Early repair also helps infants experience the pleasure of sucking as soon as possible. It is equally important from a psychological standpoint as a parent may need caring support to bond with an infant whose face is deformed in this way. Because facial contours change as a child grows, a revision of the original repair or a nasal rhinoplasty to straighten a deviated nasal septum may be necessary when the child reaches 4 to 6 years of age. Some infants may have a nasal mold apparatus applied before surgery to shape a better nostril (Garfinkle, King, Grayson, et al., 2011).

The optimal time for repair of a cleft palate is controversial because early repair increases speech development but may result in a necessary second-stage repair as the child's palate arch expands with growth (Liao, Yang, Wang, et al., 2010). Surgery may be recommended as a two-stage palate repair, with soft palate repair at 3 months of age and hard palate repair at 6 months of age, called the Malek protocol. This type of repair results in less need for future surgery and better facial results (Broome, Herzog, Hohlfeld, et al., 2010). Using infant orthodontic devices and delaying hard palate closure until later has not been shown to increase speech clarity or overall wellness (Bartzela, Katsaros, Shaw, et al., 2010).

Currently, the results of surgical repair of cleft lip and cleft palate are excellent (Fig. 27.8). It is helpful to show parents photographs of babies with good repairs to assure them their child's outcome can also be as successful.

One problem that may remain is that, because palate repair narrows the upper dental arch, a child may be left with less space in the upper jaw for the eruption of teeth, creating poor teeth alignment. All children born with a cleft palate, therefore, need follow-up treatment by a pediatric dentist skilled in children's dental problems, so that as the child grows, extractions or realignment of teeth can be done as indicated. Children also need follow-up to detect if hearing or speech difficulty occurs; because the slant of the eustachian tube may be changed in surgery, a child may develop more ear infections than usual, possibly leading to some hearing impairment. Children with cleft problems tend to receive better, more frequent, and well-coordinated care when seen in an interprofessional team setting including pediatric dentists, audiologists, speech pathologists, geneticists, and craniofacial surgeons, so referring parents to an appropriate interprofessional center before discharge is critical for these infants and their families (Austin, Druschel, Tyler, et al., 2010).

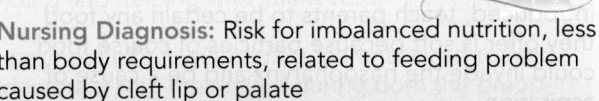

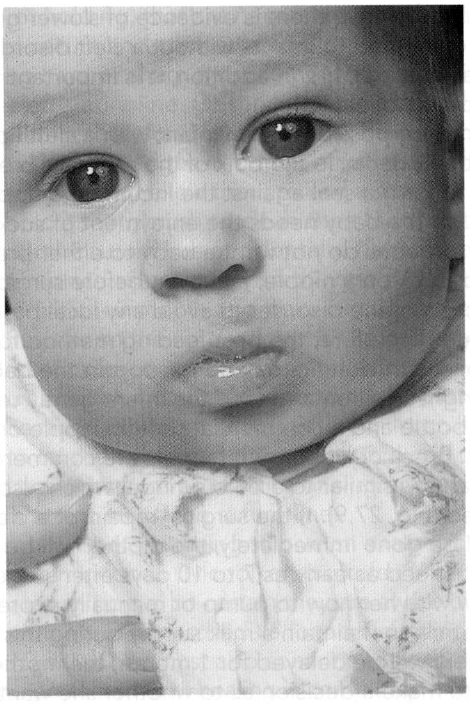

FIGURE 27.8 An infant showing surgical repair of cleft lip. Parents can be encouraged that the results of cleft lip repair are generally excellent. (Photo Researchers, Inc.)

Nursing Diagnoses and Related Interventions

Nursing Diagnosis: Risk for imbalanced nutrition, less than body requirements, related to feeding problem caused by cleft lip or palate

Outcome Evaluation: Newborn ingests an adequate diet of 110 kcal/kg (50 kcal/lb) in 24 hours; weight is maintained within 10% of birth weight.

Preoperative Period: Before a cleft lip or palate is repaired, feeding the infant becomes a concern because the infant has difficulty maintaining suction with

umbilical cord (Wiler, 2012). This creates a bulging protrusion under the skin at the umbilicus. It is rarely noticeable at birth while the cord is still present but becomes increasingly noticeable at health care visits during the first year.

Umbilical hernias occur most frequently in African American children and more often in girls than in boys. The structure is generally 1 to 2 cm (0.5 to 1 in.) in diameter but may be as large as an orange when children cry or strain. The size of the protruding mass is not as important as the size of the fascial ring through which the intestine protrudes. If this fascial ring is less than 2 cm, closure will usually occur spontaneously after the child begins to walk, so no repair of the disorder will be necessary. If the fascial ring is larger than 2 cm, ambulatory surgery for repair is generally indicated to prevent herniation and intestinal obstruction or bowel strangulation. This is usually done at 1 to 2 years of age. If the small umbilical hernia has not closed by preschool age, a repair will often be done when the child is 4 to 5 years old.

Some parents believe holding an umbilical hernia in place by using "belly bands" or taping a silver dollar over the area will help reduce the hernia. These actions can actually lead to bowel strangulation and so should be avoided.

The child returns from surgery with a dressing, which remains in place until the sutures are well healed. Remind parents to sponge bathe the child until they return for a postoperative visit when the dressing is removed. If the child is not yet toilet trained, caution parents to keep diapers folded well below the dressing to prevent contaminating the suture line with stool.

Omphaloceles

An **omphalocele** is a protrusion (herniation) of abdominal contents through the abdominal wall at the point of the junction of the umbilical cord and abdomen (Fig. 27.12). The herniated organs involved are usually the intestines, but they may include the stomach and liver. Occurring about 1 out of 5,000 live births, the organs are usually covered and contained by a thin transparent layer of amnion and chorion with the umbilical cord protruding from the exposed sac. This condition occurs because, at approximately weeks 6 to 8 of intrauterine life, the fetal abdominal contents, which grow faster than the fetal abdomen, are pushed out from

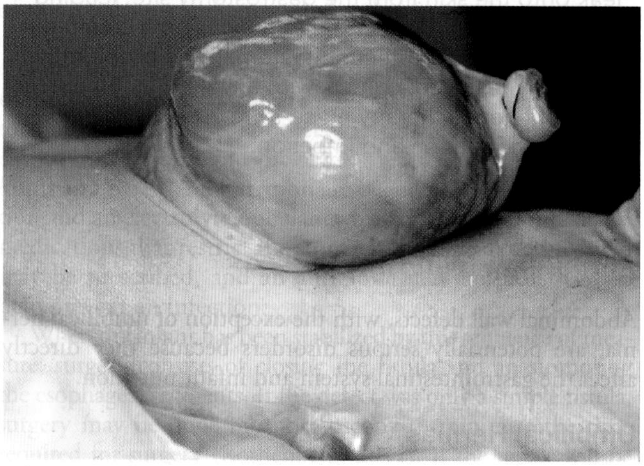

FIGURE 27.12 An omphalocele with a membrane sac covering the organs.

the abdomen into the base of the umbilical cord. At 7 to 10 weeks, when the fetal abdomen has enlarged sufficiently, the intestine normally returns to the abdomen. An omphalocele occurs when abdominal contents fail to return in the usual way. The occurrence may be associated with other congenital disorders such as heart anomalies.

Gastroschisis

Gastroschisis, a term derived from the Greek word for "stomach cleft" or "fissure," is a condition similar to an omphalocele, except the abdominal wall disorder is a distance from the umbilicus, usually to the right, and abdominal organs are not contained by a membrane but rather spill freely from the abdominal wall (Ledbetter, 2012). Also, a greater amount of intestinal contents tends to herniate, increasing the potential for volvulus and obstruction. The condition occurs because of failure of the abdominal wall to close, usually during the fourth week of development, and its incidence is about 4 to 5 per 10,000 live births. The disorder is similar to a neural tube defect (covered later in this chapter), because both are a failure to close at about the same gestational time. Children with gastroschisis often have decreased bowel motility and, even after surgical correction, may have difficulty with absorption of nutrients and passage of stool. Long-term follow-up may be necessary to ensure that nutrition and elimination are adequate (Holland, Walker, & Badawi, 2010).

Assessment. The incidence of omphalocele remains steady, whereas the incidence of gastroschisis is steadily rising, perhaps associated with maternal obesity (Blomberg & Källén, 2010). The wall defect with the herniated organs may be identified by sonogram during intrauterine life (Zamurovic, Jurisic, & Brankovic, 2012). These may also be revealed by an elevated maternal serum α-fetoprotein (MAFP) examination during pregnancy, which is done at the 15th week of pregnancy; the level of MAFP will be abnormally increased if there is an open spinal or abdominal lesion. If the result is elevated, an amniocentesis is then done to assess the level of AFP in amniotic fluid. A prenatal sonogram is also helpful to determine the presence of both abdominal wall or spinal disorders (see Chapter 11 for further discussion of these prenatal assessments). If an omphalocele or gastroschisis is not identified during pregnancy, their presence is obvious on inspection at birth. When an omphalocele or gastroschisis is identified in utero, a cesarean birth may be performed to protect the exposed intestine. If this is the only disorder identified, however, a vaginal birth may be preferred. Be certain to document the general appearance of the defect and its size in centimeters at birth to serve as a baseline assessment.

Therapeutic Management. With both omphalocele and gastroschisis, until surgery and the bowel is effectively returned to the abdomen, the infant will be fed by TPN to supply nutrients and keep the bowel from filling with air or stool. Most infants with gastroschisis will have surgery within 24 hours to replace the bowel before the blood supply becomes hampered, the intestinal membranes dry, bowel volvulus occurs, or the bowel becomes infected. It is often difficult to replace the entire bowel with immediate surgery because the infant's abdomen, which did not need to grow to accommodate the abdominal contents, is smaller at birth than usual. Replacing the total bowel into this small abdomen could result in respiratory distress from the pressure of the visceral bulk on the diaphragm and lungs. Also, the bowel might not have room for effective peristalsis. If a gastroschisis is small, a one-stage repair may be possible. If large, one surgical approach is the use of a prosthetic patch repair that bridges the unformed gap on the abdomen with a synthetic material; the skin is then drawn tight and closed over the patch. A second approach is to replace only a portion of the bowel at one time. The remainder is contained by a Silastic pouch termed a "silo" that is suspended over the infant's bed. Over the next 5 to 7 days, the bowel is gradually returned to the abdomen by multiple surgical procedures (Weil, Leys, & Rescorla, 2012).

For an omphalocele, if the sac is ruptured, the defect is treated like gastroschisis because of the potential for infection. If unruptured, an external dressing producing mild pressure may be used over the intact membrane. This gradually compresses the abdominal contents, allows the skin to stretch between treatments, and does not appear to be a painful procedure.

Nursing Diagnoses and Related Interventions

Both nursing diagnosis and outcomes established for the infant with gastroschisis or an omphalocele, like those with esophageal disorders, must be realistic in terms of the extent of the disorder, the timing of anticipated surgery, and the stage of grief or readiness for decision making and planning the parents have reached. Gastroschisis and omphalocele defects can be an extreme shock to parents because they are conditions that are obviously severe yet also generally unknown.

Nursing Diagnosis: Risk for infection related to exposed abdominal contents

Outcome Evaluation: Child's temperature remains below 98.6°F (37°C) axillary; skin surrounding omphalocele remains clean, dry, and intact, without erythema or foul drainage.

Before surgery, it is important that the lining of the peritoneum covering an omphalocele not be ruptured or allowed to dry and crack; if this happens, infection and malrotation of the uncontained intestine can then occur, thus complicating the surgical repair. Exposure of the intestine to air also causes a rapid loss of body heat. Therefore, be certain not to leave an infant with either gastroschisis or an omphalocele under a radiant heat source in the birthing room because this will quickly dry the exposed bowel. Place the baby in a warmed incubator instead. In both instances, also cover the herniated bowel with either sterile, warm, saline-soaked gauze or a sterile plastic bowel bag until surgery can be scheduled. Because of the large amount of exposed intestinal surface, be certain the saline is at body temperature to prevent lowering the baby's body temperature.

The prognosis for a final successful surgical repair with both these conditions is good (Emil, Canvasser, Chen, et al., 2012). Except for a large abdominal scar, following surgery, the child who had gastroschisis or an omphalocele will be the child originally envisioned by parents. If the size of the scar is a problem for the child in later life, cosmetic surgery can reduce its appearance.

Nursing Diagnosis: Risk for imbalanced nutrition, less than body requirements, related to exposed abdominal contents

Outcome Evaluation: Child's weight remains within 10% of birth weight; skin turgor is good; specific gravity of urine is 1.003 to 1.030.

Infants are maintained on TPN prior to surgery. A nasogastric tube for decompression is inserted at birth to prevent intestinal distention, which would enlarge the bowel lumen and make it even more difficult to replace. Do not feed the infant orally or allow the infant to suck on a pacifier until the bowel repair is complete because doing so would distend the exposed bowel with food or air and would also make its return to the abdomen more difficult. Some infants have an accompanying **volvulus** (a twisting of the bowel causing obstruction), which is another reason to omit oral feedings. After surgery, the infant continues to be maintained on TPN until the final stage of bowel repair is complete and breastfeedings or formula feedings can be gradually introduced. Assess infants carefully for signs of obstruction such as abdominal distention, constipation, diarrhea, or vomiting when they begin oral feedings to be certain a bowel obstruction or volvulus is not present.

Infants with extensive repairs can be hospitalized for as long as 1 or 2 months until second-stage or even a third-stage operation is complete (an average is about 30 days). Encourage parents to room-in or visit frequently because this is a critical adjustment period for both the infant and parents. Be sure the infant has age-appropriate toys available for stimulation.

Parents may voice frustration because their child's treatment is being done in such small stages. Offer support to help them accept this treatment method as the best way to manage this type of intestinal disorder and to protect the safety and long-term function of the bowel.

✔ QSEN Checkpoint Question 27.4

Safety

Bobby Jo tells you her baby was born on an unlucky day because the baby born before hers had his bowel outside his body. What is the most important nursing consideration at birth in the care of a baby with gastroschisis?

a. Position the infant on his or her stomach so the intestine is well contained.
b. Wrap the intestines with chilled gauze to prevent intestinal swelling.
c. Keep the infant seated upright under a radiant warmer for warmth.
d. Contain the intestine in a warmed, sterile saline–lined bowel bag.

Look in Appendix A for the best answer and rationale.

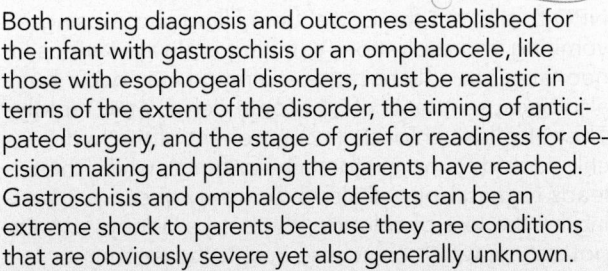

Intestinal Obstructions

If canalization of the intestine does not occur in utero at any point, an **atresia** (complete closure) or **stenosis** (narrowing) of the fetal bowel can develop, although the most common site is the duodenum.

Obstruction may also occur because the mesentery of the bowel twisted as the bowel reentered the abdomen after being contained in the base of the umbilical cord early in intrauterine life or from looseness of the intestine in the abdomen after it was returned (Juang & Snyder, 2012). This twisting pattern is termed a *volvulus* and continues to be a potential problem for the first 6 months of life until the infant develops firmer intestinal supports. Yet another reason obstruction can occur is because of thicker than usual meconium formation, blocking the lumen (meconium plug or meconium ileus).

Assessment. Intestinal obstruction may be anticipated if the mother had hydramnios during pregnancy (i.e., swallowed amniotic fluid could not be absorbed effectively by the fetus) or if more than 30 ml of stomach contents can be aspirated from the newborn stomach by catheter and syringe at birth (fluid is not passing freely through the tract). If the obstruction is not revealed by either of these findings, then symptoms of intestinal obstruction in the neonate are the same as at any other time in life: the infant passes no meconium or may pass one stool (meconium that formed below the obstruction) and then not pass any more; the abdomen becomes distended and tender. As the effect of the obstruction progresses, the infant will vomit. Remember, many neonates spit up feedings when burped. This rapid ejection of milk smells barely sour. True vomiting from intestinal obstruction is usually sour smelling (stomach acid has acted on it), includes bile, and occurs spontaneously without coughing or back patting. Vomitus may also be black from the color of meconium.

Bowel sounds will begin to increase in number as the bowel increases peristaltic action in an effort to push stool past the point of obstruction. Waves of peristalsis may be observable across the abdomen. The infant may reveal that abdominal pain is developing by crying—hard, forceful, indignant crying—and by pulling the legs up against the abdomen. Lastly, the child's respiratory rate will increase as the intestine fills, the diaphragm is pushed up harder and harder against the lungs, and lung capacity decreases. An abdominal X-ray, sonogram, MRI, or barium enema will reveal no air below the level of obstruction in the intestine or isolate the level of the obstruction.

Therapeutic Management. As soon as a bowel obstruction is confirmed, an orogastric or nasogastric tube is inserted and then attached to low suction or left open to the air to prevent further gastrointestinal distention (see Chapter 37). Always use low intermittent suction with decompression tubes in neonates because pressure greater than this can irritate and ulcerate their sensitive stomach lining.

IV therapy is begun to restore fluid and electrolyte balance; immediate surgery is scheduled to relieve the obstruction before pressure on the bowel causes death of the involved intestinal lining (Sundaram, Hoffenberg, Kramer, et al., 2012).

Repair of the obstruction (with the exception of meconium plug syndrome) can usually be accomplished by laparoscopy, although full abdominal surgery may be necessary. The area of stenosis or atresia is removed, and the bowel is anastomosed. If the repair is anatomically difficult or the infant has other anomalies that interfere with overall health, a temporary colostomy may have to be constructed and the infant discharged to home care with follow-up surgery rescheduled at 3 to 6 months of age (see Chapter 37 for care of a child with a colostomy). If a large portion of the bowel has to be removed, this can have an impact on nutrient absorption (called short bowel syndrome) as the child grows older.

Nursing Diagnoses and Related Interventions

Nursing Diagnosis: Risk for deficient fluid volume related to vomiting

Outcome Evaluation: Child's skin turgor is good; capillary refill is 1 to 2 seconds; pulse rate is at least 100 to 120 beats/min; no further vomiting occurs; urine output is at least 1 to 2 ml/kg/hour.

Once an obstruction is suspected, keep an infant NPO to prevent the bowel from filling and causing vomiting and aspiration. Vomiting is always serious in neonates not only because aspiration may occur but also because infants can become dehydrated rapidly. They also lose chloride (a component of the hydrochloric acid found in stomach contents), which then leads to metabolic alkalosis. As a way of compensating for the loss of chloride, the baby's kidneys excrete potassium, which can cause infants to become hypokalemic. Keeping an infant NPO, restoring fluid by IV therapy, and monitoring laboratory values for electrolyte balance until surgery, therefore, are crucial actions to prevent all these events. Following surgery, TPN or IV fluid will be continued until bowel sounds return; after a short postoperative course, assuming no other bowel condition such as short bowel syndrome is present, an infant should have no further problems.

Meconium Plug Syndrome

A **meconium plug** is an extremely hard portion of meconium that has completely blocked the intestinal lumen, causing bowel obstruction. The cause is unknown but probably reflects normal variations of meconium consistency. Meconium plugs usually form in the lower end of the bowel because this meconium formed early in intrauterine life and has the best chance to become dry and obstructive. The condition is associated with Hirschsprung disease, cystic fibrosis, hypothyroidism, and magnesium sulfate administration to halt preterm labor (Cuenca, Ali, Kays, et al., 2012).

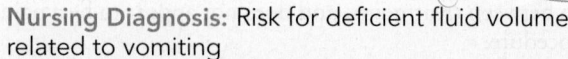

Assessment. Because the obstruction is low in the intestinal tract, signs of obstruction such as abdominal distention and vomiting may not occur for at least 24 hours. Typically, the

infant will be identified first as an infant who has had no meconium passage in the first 24 hours postbirth. A gentle rectal examination may reveal the presence of hardened stool, although the plug may be too high up in the bowel to be palpated. An X-ray or sonogram may reveal distended air-filled loops of bowel up to the point of obstruction. A barium enema not only reveals the level of obstruction but also may be therapeutic in loosening the plug.

Therapeutic Management. The administration of a small (about 5 ml) saline enema (never use tap water in newborns, infants, and young children because it can lead to water intoxication) may cause enough peristalsis to expel the plug. Instillation of acetylcysteine (Mucomyst) rectally may be prescribed to soften stool. Gastrografin, a highly osmotic radiographic substance, administered as an enema, is yet another solution. Because it is hyperosmotic, the substance pulls fluid into the bowel, allowing the stool to soften and the plug to pass. Assess that the infant is well hydrated before and after the procedure because an infant can become hypovolemic from the effect of such a strong-acting medium.

Once the thickened portion of meconium has been passed, the infant should have no further difficulty and, over the next several hours, may pass a great amount of stool. Observe the infant for further passage of meconium (which should occur at least once daily) over the next 3 days, however, to be certain additional plugs do not exist farther up in the bowel. If an infant is going to be discharged before this time, instruct parents on the importance of observing for meconium and also about phoning their primary care provider should the infant have no further bowel movements while at home.

Occasionally, a neonate passes a small plug of hardened meconium—hard enough it would have caused an obstruction except it is so small—in the first 1 or 2 days of life. Be certain to record and report such a finding because the infant will need close observation for continued defecation, the same as for the infant who actually had an obstruction, to be certain there is not a larger and truly obstructing plug higher in the bowel.

Assess the family history of a newborn who has a meconium plug for cystic fibrosis, a recessively inherited disorder (see Chapter 40), or aganglionic megacolon (Hirschsprung disease), a polygenic inherited disorder (see Chapter 45), because, if there is a family history, the infant will need observation for these disorders. Hypothyroidism can also present with constipation or hardened stool in newborns along with signs such as a large protruding tongue, lethargy, and subnormal body temperature. Both hypothyroidism and cystic fibrosis screening are done along with phenylketonuria screening in newborns. Be certain this blood test is obtained in any newborn with a meconium plug (Levy, 2010). Infants born at home, especially, may not have had this done.

Meconium Ileus

Meconium ileus (obstruction of the intestinal lumen by hardened meconium) is a specific phenomenon that occurs almost exclusively in infants with cystic fibrosis (see Chapter 40) and reflects extreme meconium plugging (Efrati, Nir, Fraser, et al., 2010). The usual symptoms of bowel obstruction occur: no meconium passage, abdominal distention, and vomiting of bile-stained fluid. Unlike simple meconium plugging, the obstruction point may be too high in the intestine for enemas to reduce it; instead, the bowel must be incised and the hardened meconium removed by laparotomy. Meconium ileus is so strongly associated with cystic fibrosis, the infant needs close follow-up by an interprofessional cystic fibrosis team in the following months.

What if...27.2 On the second day of life you notice Bobby Jo Sparrow's baby, who was born with meconium staining, is spitting up green mucus. Would it be safe to assume this is just more meconium-stained mucus? Should you consider the baby might be vomiting bile-stained vomitus?

Diaphragmatic Hernias

A diaphragmatic hernia is an opening in the diaphragm that allows for the protrusion of an abdominal organ (usually the stomach or intestine) to herniate into the chest cavity. This usually occurs on the left side, causing cardiac displacement to the right side of the chest and collapse of the left lung. It occurs in 1 to 5 per 10,000 live births, with slight increased frequency in boys and a decreased frequency in African Americans (Tovar, 2012).

The defect is caused because, early in intrauterine life, the chest and abdominal cavity are one; at approximately week 8 of intrauterine growth, the diaphragm forms and divides them. If the diaphragm does not form completely, the intestines can herniate through the diaphragm opening into the chest cavity as a diaphragmatic hernia (Fig. 27.13).

Assessment. Diaphragmatic hernia is frequently detected in utero by routine sonogram (Kotecha, Barbato, Bush, et al., 2012). If not, it is apparent at birth when the newborn has extreme difficulty establishing effective respirations. Surgeons have tried fetal surgery to correct or lessen the lung compromise from this diagnosis, but multiple randomized trials comparing prenatal surgical intervention to postnatal intervention show no benefit to prenatal intervention (Hedrick, 2013).

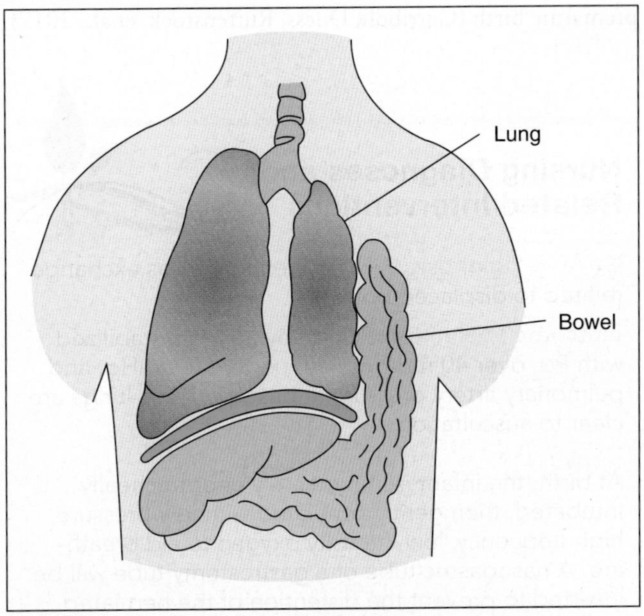

FIGURE 27.13 A diaphragmatic hernia. The bowel loop in the chest compresses the heart and lung on that side.

At birth, breath sounds are usually absent on the affected side of the chest cavity because at least one of the lobes of the lungs on that side cannot expand completely (and may not have fully formed). The infant may be cyanotic with intercostal or subcostal retractions. The abdomen generally appears sunken because it is not as filled with intestine as usual. These infants have a potential for developing persistent pulmonary hypertension because blood cannot perfuse readily through the unexpanded lung. This can lead to right-to-left shunting through the foramen ovale in the heart and also causes the ductus arteriosus to remain patent. One condition, then, has led to another until heart involvement complicates an already serious lung picture. The mechanics of right-to-left heart shunts are further discussed in Chapter 41.

Therapeutic Management. Although surgical repair may be done as an imminent surgical procedure, it is usually delayed until cardiorespiratory status has been stabilized as much as possible and the baby can be transported to a high-acuity nursery for care. Surgery includes repair of the diaphragm and replacement of the herniated intestine and organs back into the abdomen, possibly requiring both thoracic and abdominal incisions. If the disorder of the diaphragm is large, an insoluble polymer (Teflon) patch may be used to reconstruct a better diaphragm shape.

The repair can be complicated if there is not enough room in the abdomen for the intestine to be returned. In these infants, the abdominal incision may not be closed. The intestine is covered by silicone elastomer (Silastic) and left to be closed at a later date after the abdomen has grown, the same as gastroschisis surgery.

If the lung that was compressed in utero is truly hypoplastic and so cannot function, it will be removed at the time of surgery. If it is developed but just deflated, over the next week after surgery, the lung will gradually expand and begin to function. Chest tubes may not be used to avoid increased respiratory work and overdistention of the compromised lung. The mortality rate of children with diaphragmatic hernia is about 40%, with death often occurring because of associated anomalies of the heart, lung, and intestine and because of premature birth (Garriboli, Duess, Ruttenstock, et al., 2012).

Nursing Diagnoses and Related Interventions

Nursing Diagnosis: Risk for ineffective gas exchange related to displaced bowel

Outcome Evaluation: The baby appears stabilized with Po_2 over 40 mmHg, Pco_2 under 60 mmHg, and pulmonary artery pressure at baseline level; lungs are clear to auscultation.

At birth, the infant is immediately endotracheally intubated, then gently ventilated with low pressure, high frequency, low intensity oxygen to aid breathing. A nasogastric tube or a gastrostomy tube will be inserted to prevent the distention of the herniated intestine and to avoid further respiratory difficulty. Keep the infant NPO to prevent the bowel from filling and becoming distended. Be certain the suction is attached to only low intermittent suction to avoid injuring the lining of the newborn's stomach.

While they wait for surgery, infants breathe better if they are turned on their side with the compressed lung down and their head elevated because this allows the herniated intestine to fall back as far as possible into the abdomen and allows the unaffected lung to expand more completely.

Following surgery, maintain the infant in a head elevated position to keep the pressure of the replaced intestine off the repaired diaphragm. Suction the airway as necessary and keep the infant in a warmed, humidified environment to encourage lung fluid drainage from the now uncompromised lungs. Chest physiotherapy may be prescribed to ensure lung secretions do not pool and cause pneumonia. Positive-pressure ventilation may be ordered to increase lung expansion, although this pressure is kept to a minimum to prevent tearing the undeveloped or previously unopened lung tissue. Maintaining arterial oxygen (Po_2) at a lower level of 60 mmHg and permitting Pco_2 to rise to a higher level of up to 60 mmHg may help prevent damage to the immature lung, thereby improving lung function (Thilo & Rosenberg, 2012). In addition, inhaled nitric oxide, or extracorporeal membrane oxygenation (ECMO) may be used as other ways to aid respirations and increase oxygenation.

Nursing Diagnosis: Risk for imbalanced nutrition, less than body requirements, related to NPO status

Outcome Evaluation: Child's skin turgor remains good; weight is maintained within 10% of birth weight or between a percentile curve on growth chart.

After surgery, to prevent pressure on the suture line in the diaphragm by a full stomach and bowel, nutrition will be supplied with TPN. When oral feedings are started, be certain to burp the infant frequently during and after feedings to reduce the amount of swallowed air and limit bowel pressure against the diaphragm.

QSEN Checkpoint Question 27.5

Quality Improvement

You position Bobby Jo's baby on his side to keep pressure off his back. She asks you why you're not positioning a baby with diaphragmatic hernia in the same way. Before surgery, what would be the best position for a newborn with left-sided diaphragmatic hernia?

a. On his left side to support his left lung
b. On his stomach with his head turned sideways
c. On his left side elevated in an infant chair
d. On his right side so his left lung can expand

Look in Appendix A for the best answer and rationale.

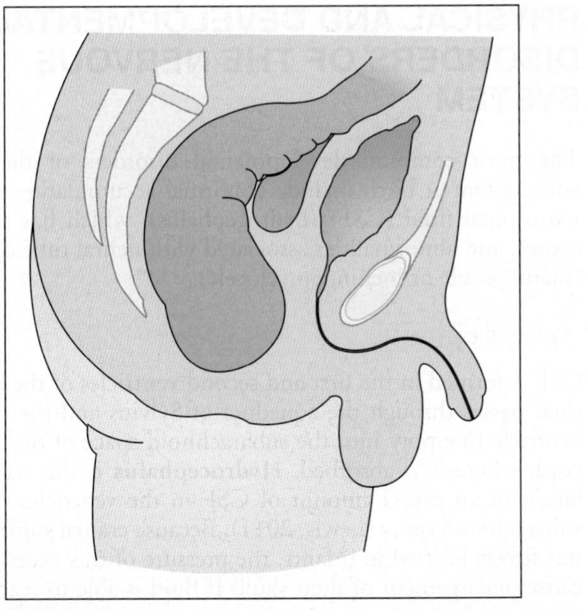

FIGURE 27.14 An imperforate anus. The lower bowel ends in a blind pouch.

An Imperforate Anus

An imperforate anus (Fig. 27.14) is a stricture or the absence of the anus (Gourlay, 2013). In week 7 of intrauterine life, the upper bowel elongates to pouch and combine with a pouch invaginating from the perineum. These two sections of bowel meet, the membranes between them are absorbed, and the bowel is then patent to the outside. If this motion toward each other does not occur or if the membrane between the two surfaces does not dissolve, an imperforate anus occurs. The disorder can be relatively minor, requiring just surgical incision of the persistent membrane, or much more severe, involving sections of the bowel that are many inches apart with no anus. There may be an accompanying fistula to the bladder in boys and to the vagina in girls, further complicating a surgical repair. The problem occurs in approximately 1 in 5,000 live births, more commonly in boys than in girls. It may occur as an additional complication of spinal cord disorders, because both the external anal canal and the spinal cord arise from the same germ tissue layer.

Assessment. The condition may be detected by a prenatal sonogram. It is discovered at birth when inspection of a newborn's anal region reveals no anus, a membrane filled with black meconium protrudes from the anus, or if it is impossible to insert a rubber catheter into the rectum. A "wink" reflex (touching the skin near the rectum should make the anus contract) cannot be elicited if sensory nerve endings in the rectum are not intact. Even with all these methods, some instances of the stricture will not be detected at birth because the anus appears as usual and the stricture exists so far inside that it can't be seen. By 24 hours, no stool will be passed, and abdominal distention will become evident. An X-ray or sonogram will reveal the disorder if the infant is held in a slightly head-down position to allow swallowed air to rise to the end of the blind pouch of the bowel. This method is also helpful to estimate the distance the intestine is separated from the perineum or the extent of the correction that will be necessary.

Because newborns are discharged at 2 or 3 days or even a few hours after birth, it's important that follow-up care by parents includes an assessment of whether the infant is defecating. If not, they may be asked to collect a urine specimen so it can be examined for the presence of meconium to help determine whether the infant has a rectal–bladder fistula. Placing a urine collector bag over the vagina in girls may reveal a meconium-stained discharge or that a rectovaginal fistula is present.

Therapeutic Management. The degree of difficulty in repairing an imperforate anus depends on the extent of the problem. If the rectum ends close to the perineum (at or below the level of the levator ani muscle) and the anal sphincter is formed, repair involves simple laparoscopy with anastomosis of the separated bowel segments (Bischoff, Levitt, & Peña, 2011). A repair becomes complicated if the end of the rectum is at a distance from the perineum (above the levator ani muscle), the anal sphincter exists only in an underdeveloped form, or a fistula to the bladder or vagina is present. If the repair is estimated to be extensive, the child may be given a temporary colostomy and the final repair performed when the infant is somewhat older (6 to 12 months).

Nursing Diagnoses and Related Interventions

Nursing Diagnosis: Imbalanced nutrition, less than body requirements, related to bowel obstruction and inability to take in oral fluid.

Outcome Evaluation: Child's weight remains within 10% of birth weight or is maintained on a percentile curve on a growth chart; skin turgor is good; urine output is 1 to 2 ml/kg/hr.

Preoperative Care: Before surgery, keep the infant NPO to avoid further bowel distention. A nasogastric tube attached to low intermittent suction for decompression will be inserted to relieve vomiting and prevent pressure on other abdominal organs or the diaphragm from the distended intestine. IV therapy or TPN will be started to maintain fluid and electrolyte balance.

Postoperative Care: The newborn will return from surgery with the nasogastric tube still in place. When bowel sounds can be heard so the nasogastric tube can be removed, small oral feedings of glucose water, formula, or breast milk can be started.

Infants who are scheduled for repair in a second-stage operation and who have a temporary colostomy are not permitted high-residue foods to lessen the bulk of stools. Although this is rarely a problem with infants because their diet naturally is a low-residue one, do not assume parents know what low residue means. Examples include rice cereal and strained fruits and vegetables. They should avoid unrefined rice and grains, vegetables with fibers, or fruits with peels.

Nursing Diagnosis: Impaired tissue integrity at rectum related to surgical incision

Outcome Evaluation: Incision line remains free of erythema or drainage until it heals by about day 7 after surgery.

If a rectal repair was completed, remember there is a fresh suture line at the rectum. Take axillary or tympanic temperatures rather than rectal temperatures to avoid loosening a suture. The infant also should have no enemas, suppositories, or any other intrusive rectal procedures (it might be helpful to hang a sign above the infant's crib cautioning against these). Infants may be prescribed a stool softener daily to keep stool from becoming hard and tearing the healing suture line. Placing a diaper under, not on, the infant may be helpful so bowel movements can be cleansed away as soon as they occur. Clean the suture line well after each bowel movement by irrigating it with normal saline or other prescribed solution to help guard against infections. Do not place the infant on the abdomen because, in this position, newborns tend to pull their knees under them, causing tension in the perineal area and the suture line. A side-lying or supine position is best.

Some infants may need rectal dilatation done once or twice a day for a few months after surgery to ensure proper patency of the rectal sphincter. Review this technique (gently inserting a lubricated cot-covered finger into the rectum) with the parents and document they are able to perform this procedure before the child is discharged from the hospital. Be certain they also understand the importance of the procedure (the best surgical repair could end in failure if constriction occurs because parents do not follow up with this procedure). If infants are to be discharged with a prescription for a daily stool softener, be certain parents understand how important it is to give this and have a plan for remembering the correct times and dosage.

Nursing Diagnosis: Risk for impaired parenting related to difficulty in bonding with infant ill from birth

Outcome Evaluation: Parents hold and comfort infant; and describe positive characteristics of infant.

An imperforate anus may be a difficult anomaly for a parent to accept because it deals with a body area that they may not feel comfortable discussing. If it involves a temporary (or permanent) colostomy, learning to care for their infant can be difficult. For these reasons, parents need a great deal of support following the diagnosis. If a final surgical repair can be completed, they can be assured their child will have relatively normal bowel function thereafter. If a final repair could not be surgically achieved, they have the task of caring for a child with a permanent ostomy. You can assure them children who always have ostomies accept these well as they grow older because they have never known any other method of defecation (see Chapter 37 for a discussion of care priorities for the child with an ostomy).

PHYSICAL AND DEVELOPMENTAL DISORDERS OF THE NERVOUS SYSTEM

The most common developmental disorders of the nervous system at birth include abnormal accumulation of cerebrospinal fluid (CSF) (hydrocephalus), which has several causes, and abnormalities associated with neural tube closure (meningocele or meningomyelocele).

Hydrocephalus

CSF is formed in the first and second ventricles of the brain, then passes through the aqueduct of Sylvius and the fourth ventricle to empty into the subarachnoid space of the spinal cord, where it is absorbed. **Hydrocephalus** is the accumulation of an excess amount of CSF in the ventricles or the subarachnoid space (Lewis, 2011). Because cranial sutures are not firmly knitted in infants, the pressure of this excess fluid causes enlargement of their skull. If fluid is able to reach the spinal cord, the disorder is called a communicating or extraventricular hydrocephalus. If there is a block to CSF so it cannot circulate into the subarachnoid space, the disorder is termed obstructive or intraventricular hydrocephalus.

Hydrocephalus is also classified regarding whether it occurs at birth (congenital) or from an incident later in life (acquired). Although the increased fluid may occur as a single concern, 90% of babies with congenital hydrocephalus also have a meningomyelocele (discussed in the following paragraphs) (Sinha, Dhua, Mathur, et al., 2012). Acquired hydrocephalus is common in the very preterm infant who has had an intraventricular hemorrhage with the degree of blockage directly related to the quantity of intraventricular blood, which then was able to block the passage of CSF (Aquilina, 2011).

Three main reasons explain why CSF accumulates:

- Overproduction of fluid by the choroid plexus in the first or second ventricle as could occur from a growing tumor (rare).
- Obstruction of the passage of fluid in the narrow aqueduct of Sylvius (the most common cause) or the foramina of Magendie and Luschka, the openings that allow fluid to leave the fourth ventricle. Hemorrhage from trauma, a growing tumor, or infections such as toxoplasmosis, meningitis, or encephalitis may leave adhesions behind that block fluid flow at these points. Arnold–Chiari disorder (elongation of the lower brain stem and displacement of the fourth ventricle into the upper cervical canal) or a Dandy–Walker cyst (a fluid-filled sack by one of the ventricles in the brain) are still other causes.
- Interference with the absorption of CSF from the subarachnoid space if a portion of the subarachnoid membrane has been removed, as occurs with surgery for a meningocele or after extensive subarachnoid hemorrhage, when portions of the membrane absorption surface become obscured.

Assessment

With an obstruction present, excessive fluid accumulates and dilates the system forward of the point of obstruction. If the atresia is in the aqueduct of Sylvius, the first, second, and third ventricles will dilate. If it is at the exit from the fourth ventricle, all ventricles will dilate. Symptoms may develop rapidly or slowly depending on the extent of the atresia.

If a hydrocephalus is present prenatally, it can sometimes be detected on a prenatal sonogram and then can even be shunted in utero, particularly if it is associated with a meningomyelocele (Danzer, Johnson, & Adzick, 2012). Although the condition occurs in approximately 3 to 4 out of 1,000 live births, it is only overtly evident during pregnancy or at birth in 15% of newborns with the disorder because intrauterine pressure prohibits skull expansion (Sinha et al., 2012). During the first few weeks of life, the infant's fontanelles widen and appear tense, the suture lines on the skull separate, and the head diameter enlarges. As the fluid accumulation continues, the scalp becomes shiny and scalp veins become prominent. The brow bulges forward (bossing), and the eyes become "sunset eyes" (the sclera shows above the iris because of upper lid retraction). Infants begin to show symptoms of increased intracranial pressure, such as decreased pulse and respirations, increased temperature and blood pressure, hyperactive reflexes, strabismus, and optic atrophy. They may become either irritable or lethargic with a typical shrill, high-pitched cry (Box 27.4).

Treatment is most effective when the disorder is recognized early, because once intracranial pressure becomes so acute that brain tissue is damaged and motor or mental deterioration results, even the best shunting procedure cannot replace and repair this damage to brain cells. To best detect hydrocephalus, measure the head circumference of all newborns within an hour of birth and again before discharge from the health care facility to establish a baseline. All children under 2 years of age should then have their head circumference recorded and plotted on an appropriate growth chart at all health care visits so the child whose head is growing abnormally can be detected (Sniderman, 2010).

Because it is possible for infants to develop hydrocephalus following head trauma, all infants who have suffered head trauma severe enough to be seen in a medical facility should have their head circumference noted at the time of the accident so, if other symptoms of increased intracranial pressure appear, this head circumference measurement can be a meaningful part of the store of information available concerning the child's condition (Ghosh & Ghosh, 2011).

In addition to the general enlargement of the head, note any asymmetry that is occurring because this may suggest the point of obstruction. A skull that is enlarging anteriorly with a shallow posterior fossa, for example, suggests the obstruction is in the aqueduct or third ventricle.

As the head continues to enlarge, the infant's motor function becomes impaired because of both neurologic impairment and atrophy caused by the inability to move such a heavy head. However, as long as a child has more than 1 cm of cerebral tissue present, motor function often is not impaired. Even with an extremely enlarged head, therefore, children's intelligence may also remain normal, although fine motor development may be affected.

Hydrocephalus can be demonstrated by ultrasound, computed tomography (CT), or MRI. A skull X-ray film will reveal the separating sutures and thinning of the skull. **Transillumination** (holding a bright light such as a flashlight or a specialized light [a Chun gun] against the skull with the child in a darkened room) will reveal that the skull is filled with fluid rather than solid brain tissue (Fig. 27.15). Assessing ventricular pressure will document the increased tension and presence of additional fluid.

BOX 27.4 Nursing Care Planning Using Assessment

Assessing an Infant With Hydrocephalus

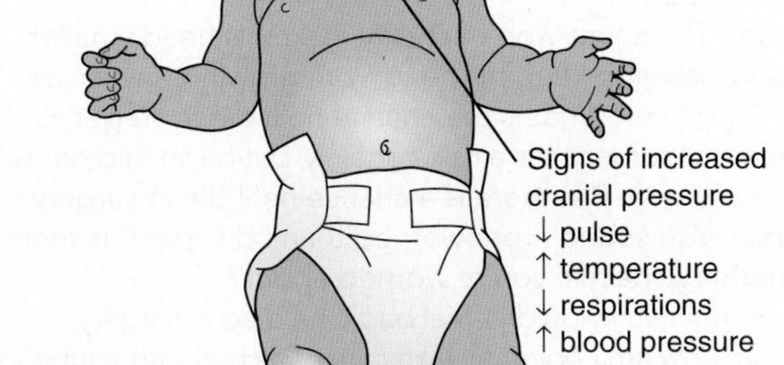

Therapeutic Management

The treatment for hydrocephalus depends on its cause and extent. If it is caused by overproduction of fluid, acetazolamide (Diamox), a diuretic, may be prescribed to promote the excretion of this excess fluid. Destruction of a portion of

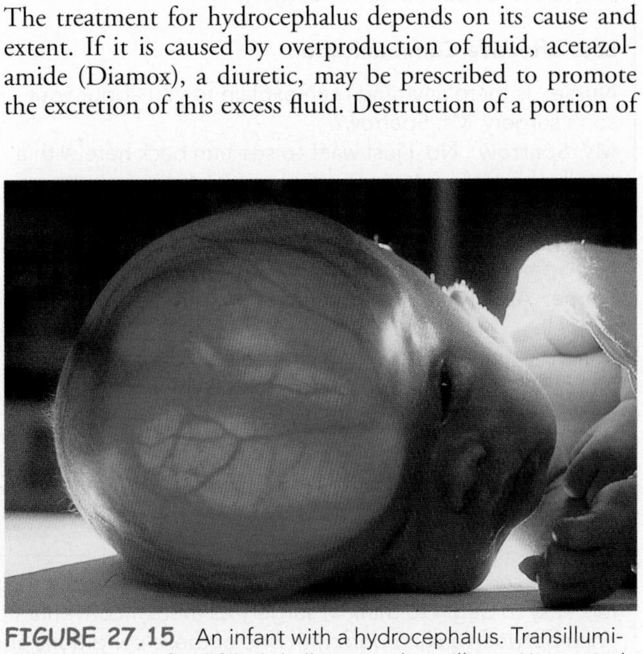

FIGURE 27.15 An infant with a hydrocephalus. Transillumination reveals a fluid-filled skull. (© Southern Illinois University/Photo Researchers, Inc.)

the choroid plexus may be attempted by ventricular endoscopy; if a tumor in that area is responsible for the overproduction of fluid, removal of the tumor should provide a solution. Hydrocephalus is usually caused by obstruction, however, so the treatment for children that do not have other neural tube involvement (such as a meningomyelocele) usually involves laser surgery to reopen the route of flow or bypassing the point of obstruction by shunting the fluid to another point of absorption. As more and more obstructions in the third or fourth ventricles are relieved by endoscopy, the next generation of children with isolated hydrocephalus may not need artificial shunting. Children today with hydrocephalus occurring with a meningomyelocele may still undergo a shunting procedure, however, and you may care for many older children or adults who have shunts in place.

A shunting procedure involves threading a thin polyethylene catheter under the skin from the ventricles to the peritoneum (a ventriculoperitoneal shunt) (Fig. 27.16). Fluid drains by this route into the peritoneum, where it is absorbed across the peritoneal membrane into the body circulation. The shunt usually has to be replaced as the child grows or it will become too short. As another complication, it could become enclosed in a fold of peritoneum and become obstructed or it could become infected.

The ultimate prognosis for a child with hydrocephalus depends on whether brain damage occurred before shunting, whether the child develops a cerebral infection, and whether the parents can accept and recognize when a shunt needs to be replaced to prevent increased intracranial pressure (Box 27.5).

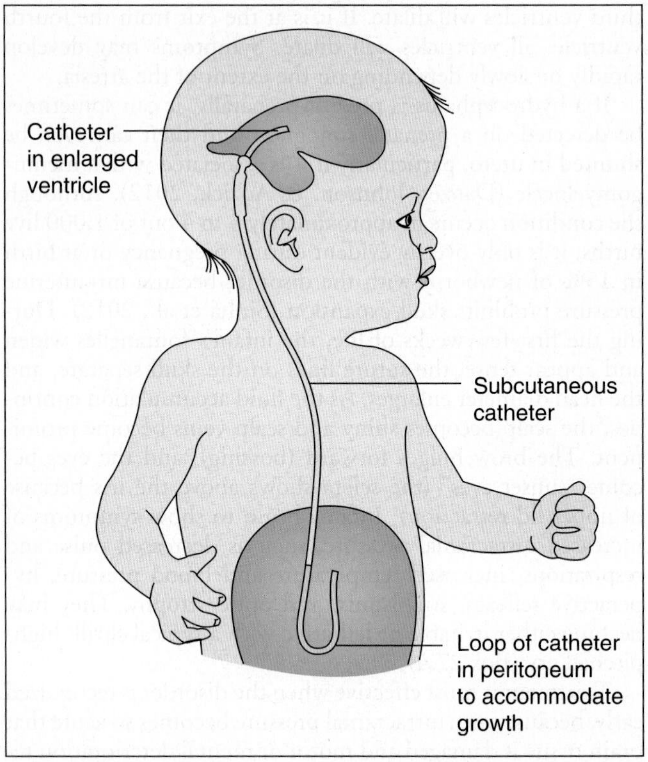

FIGURE 27.16 A ventriculoperitoneal shunt removes excessive cerebrospinal fluid from the ventricles and shunts it to the peritoneum. A one-way valve is present in the tubing behind the ear.

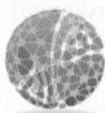

BOX 27.5 Nursing Care Planning Based on Effective Communication

Bobby Jo's baby is scheduled to have a ventriculoperitoneal shunt inserted this afternoon. You talk to Bobby Jo before surgery.

Less Effective Communication

Nurse: Is there anything I can explain to you about your son's surgery, Ms. Sparrow?
Ms. Sparrow: No. I just want to see him back here with a smaller head.
Nurse: The shunt won't actually make his head smaller. Its purpose is to keep his head from growing any larger.
Ms. Sparrow: What's the chance he'll die in surgery?
Nurse: All surgery has a risk, certainly, but he should do well.
Ms. Sparrow: But there is a chance he'll die?
Nurse: You're worrying unnecessarily. Why don't you relax, maybe go get something to drink until he's back from surgery?
Ms. Sparrow: Good idea. I'll do that.

More Effective Communication

Nurse: Is there anything I can explain to you about your son's surgery, Ms. Sparrow?
Ms. Sparrow: No. I just want to see him back here with a smaller head.
Nurse: The shunt won't actually make his head smaller. Its purpose is to keep his head from growing any larger.
Ms. Sparrow: What is the chance he'll die in surgery?
Nurse: All surgery has a risk, certainly, but he should do well.
Ms. Sparrow: But there is a chance he'll die in surgery?
Nurse: You sound more worried than I'd expect. Is there something specific you're worried about?
Ms. Sparrow: I wouldn't feel bad if he died in surgery. I mean, how am I going to take care of a child with a tube in his head?
Nurse: Let's sit down and talk about this some more.

Because surgical procedures are so safe today and the results of surgery for newborns are so successful, it is easy to begin to think of surgery as more inconvenient than serious. To a parent, however, the difference between a child born with one of these conditions and the "perfect" child the parent envisioned can be great. Handling the problem by giving quick reassurance, as in the first scenario here, can lead to missing a parent's concern. Better listening, as in the second example, revealed the true problem.

Nursing Diagnoses and Related Interventions

Nutrition and parent–child bonding are two major concerns for the infant with hydrocephalus. Box 27.6 shows an interprofessional care map illustrating both nursing and team planning for an infant with the concern.

Nursing Diagnosis: Risk for ineffective cerebral tissue perfusion related to increased intracranial pressure

Outcome Evaluation: Child shows no increased temperature or blood pressure, decreased pulse or respiratory rate or level of consciousness; PERLA (pupils equal and reactive to light and accommodation) is present; muscle strength is equal and strong bilaterally; head circumference is maintained at age-appropriate level.

Following the surgery for the initial shunt insertion, infants may have three incisions: one just behind the ear, one in the neck (done to help thread the catheter), and one in the abdomen where the end of the shunt is embedded. Their bed should be left flat or raised only about 10 degrees so their head remains level with the body so CSF does not flow too rapidly, possibly leading to tearing of cerebral arteries or signs of too rapid decompression.

A one-way valve, which is inserted into the shunt and can be palpated just behind the ear, opens when CSF has accumulated to the extent cerebral pressure has increased. It closes when enough fluid has drained to reduce the pressure. The surgeon who performed the shunting procedure prescribes how often the infant is to be turned and to what side after surgery. Often, infants are not turned to lie on the side with the shunt to prevent putting pressure on the valve, which might cause it to open and rapidly decompress CSF.

Formerly, shunts had fixed valves that allowed a set amount of CSF to be drained daily. Today, they are fitted with adjustable pressure valves. Because the value contains a magnet, it can be readjusted to regulate the amount of CSF flow by manipulation of an external magnet, thus avoiding the problem of repeat surgery for readjustment (because shunts contain a magnet, remind parents to ask their primary care provider if it would be safe for their child to have an MRI, and also to keep toys containing magnets or electronic devices such as tablet computers away from the child) (Strahle, Selzer, Muraszko, et al., 2012).

Continue to assess for signs of increased intracranial pressure after surgery such as tense fontanelles, increasing head circumference, irritability or lethargy, decreased level of consciousness, poor sucking ability, vomiting, an increase in blood pressure (difficult to measure accurately in infants unless arterial or umbilical lines are used with Doppler instrumentation), increasing temperature, and a decrease in pulse and respiratory rates (see Chapter 49 for tips on a complete neurologic assessment). Also assess for symptoms of infection such as increased temperature, increased pulse rate, general malaise, and signs of meningitis such as a stiff neck and marked irritability (Box 27.7). Be certain a child receives adequate pain management not only for comfort but also because crying elevates CSF pressure.

Nursing Diagnosis: Risk for imbalanced nutrition, less than body requirements, related to increased intracranial pressure

Outcome Evaluation: Child's weight remains within 5th to 95th percentile on height and weight chart; no vomiting occurs.

Because an abdominal incision is involved to thread the catheter into the peritoneum, an infant may be prescribed to be kept NPO until bowel sounds return. Introduce fluid gradually in small quantities because vomiting that results from the introduction of fluid too soon after any surgery causes increased intracranial pressure.

Like all infants, those with hydrocephalus should be held when being fed if possible. Be certain to support their heads well when moving them to avoid strain on their neck if their head appears enlarged. Help breastfeeding mothers to find a comfortable way to support the infant's head as needed.

Document whether the child sucks well because increasing intracranial pressure may be noted first because of poor or ineffective sucking. Vomiting after feeding without nausea (difficult to detect in a small infant) is also a common first sign of increased intracranial pressure.

Also observe whether constipation exists, because straining while passing stool is another cause of increased intracranial pressure. This is not usually a problem with infants who are totally breastfed or formula fed. It can be a problem when children return for shunt replacement at an older age. Urge parents to offer adequate fluid and roughage in their child's diet as a preventive measure as the child grows.

Nursing Diagnosis: Risk for impaired skin integrity related to extra weight and immobility of the head

Outcome Evaluation: Child's skin remains clean, dry, and intact and without signs of erythema or ulceration.

If the infant's head has enlarged, it may be difficult for the infant to move it freely because of the extra weight. As the skin of the head stretches thin, skin breakdown can occur at the pressure point. Wash the child's head daily and change the position of the head approximately every 2 hours so no portion of the head rests against the mattress for a long period. A synthetic sheepskin or silicon pad or an air, water, or alternating air mattress may help to reduce pressure points. If a Kling or stockinette bandage is used to hold a surgical head dressing in place, place a piece of gauze or cotton behind the child's ear before the bandage is applied to prevent skin surfaces from touching and becoming excoriated. Make certain the bandage does not become wet from backward-draining oral secretions or drainage from the shunt insertion site.

BOX 27.6 Nursing Care Planning

AN INTERPROFESSIONAL CARE MAP FOR A CHILD WITH HYDROCEPHALUS

At 1 month of age, Bobby Jo's baby, still not named, has a ventriculoperitoneal shunt inserted for developing hydrocephalus.

Family Assessment Child lives with 16-year-old mother, her parents, and four of mother's siblings. Child's father works as motorcycle mechanic; visits infant frequently. Mother no longer attending school because of child care. Mother asking many questions about the surgery. "This'll fix everything, right? I want a healthy baby."

Client Assessment One-month-old infant whose head circumference has continued to increase since meningomyelocele surgery at birth. Head circumference at birth was at 40th percentile, now is at 60th percentile. Mother noted infant has had increasing irritability and difficulty swallowing formula over the last few weeks.

Anterior fontanelle 4 × 4 cm; posterior fontanelle 3 × 1 cm. Sagittal suture line separated 0.25 in. Scalp veins prominent. No upward gaze. Parents report two episodes of forceful vomiting yesterday. Also, "His cry is so high pitched it hurts your ears." Cerebral perfusion pressure, 55 mmHg. Blood pressure, 100/40 mmHg; pulse, 100 beats/min; respirations, 16 breaths/min. Afebrile.

Nursing Diagnosis Risk for ineffective cerebral tissue perfusion related to increased intracranial pressure from hydrocephalus

Outcome Criteria Infant's vital signs are within age-appropriate parameters; head circumference is maintained at current level; infant responds to auditory stimuli; cerebral perfusion pressure remains above 50 mmHg.

Team Member Responsible	Assessment	Intervention	Rationale	Expected Outcome
Activities of Daily Living, Including Safety				
Nurse	Assess if infant is able to turn freely because of increased head size.	Provide an environment for child that is stimulating yet not tiring (e.g., mobile, soft toys). Urge parent to interact with child.	Lack of mobility can lead to pressure ulcers on head as well as insufficient 1-month development.	Child's parent plays with and feeds infant. Infant appears interested in age-appropriate toys. No irritated areas present on head.
Teamwork and Collaboration				
Nurse/Primary health care provider	Assess if neurosurgeon is available to answer mother's questions.	Arrange for consultation for mother with neurosurgeon to discuss surgery and child's prognosis.	Viewing a child as totally disabled can cause a parent to not appreciate the child's capabilities.	Neurosurgeon meets with mother to discuss that child's IQ appears normal, and that shunting will halt head growth.
Procedures/Medications for Quality Improvement				
Nurse	Assess infant's neurologic status postoperatively, including response to sound, pupillary response, increasing irritability, or lethargy.	Position infant with head of bed slightly elevated; prevent flexion, hyperextension, or rotation of the head. Record cerebral perfusion pressure as prescribed.	Elevating head of bed aids shunt functioning, helping to reduce intracranial pressure. Cerebral perfusion pressure reveals the extent of intracranial pressure.	Child's cerebral perfusion pressure remains greater than established parameter. Infant responds to sound; with no increasing irritability or lethargy.

Nurse	Assess head circumference and anterior fontanelle for tenseness every 4 hours as prescribed.	Document head circumference and appearance of anterior fontanelle.	A tense, bulging fontanelle or increasing head circumference indicates accumulating cerebrospinal fluid (CSF).	Child's head circumference does not increase in size; fontanelles no longer feel tense.
Nutrition				
Nurse/Nutritionist	Observe mother feeding the infant.	Assist mother with positioning as necessary; and avoid flexion or hyperextension of head during feeding.	Proper positioning is important to avoid pressure on the shunt, which could increase intracranial pressure.	Mother states she is comfortable feeding infant following surgery.
Nurse	Monitor intake and output closely.	Administer osmotic diuretic and corticosteroids as prescribed.	Adequate hydration is necessary to ensure renal function. Osmotic diuretics decrease intracranial pressure. Corticosteroids reduce inflammation.	Child's output remains over set parameter. Diuretic and corticosteroids are administered as necessary.
Patient-Centered Care				
Nurse/Nurse practitioner	Assess the parents' understanding of a hydrocephalus and treatment measures.	Review the structure and function of the brain and explain how a hydrocephalus develops. Clarify any misconceptions.	Reviewing and clarifying aid in learning and strengthen understanding.	Mother states she understands the purpose of the shunt to relieve excess CSF.
Psychosocial/Spiritual/Emotional Needs				
Nurse/Nurse practitioner	Assess mother's acceptance of child in light of congenital disorders and no name for baby as yet.	Observe mother's interaction with infant; and remind her that congenital disorders occur in a proportion of all births for unknown reasons.	Young mother may have had little experience with life crises. Needs support from health care providers to master this crisis.	Mother states she understands child's condition is neither hers nor the child's fault and states she will be able to work through the present crisis.
Informatics for Seamless Health Care Planning				
Nurse	Assess if child's parents have adequate psychological support from family members or questions about care child will need for shunt care. Explore why child has not been named as yet.	Review care of child, and assure parents health care providers can be contacted any time if they have questions. Establish a convenient follow-up care appointment.	In crisis situations, parents may need additional support to continue care of child and form a strong parent–infant bond. Positive reinforcement enhances self-esteem and aids in coping.	Mother states the grandmother is supportive. Together, they understand future care necessary, and will contact primary care provider for any questions. Mother keeps postsurgery appointment; and states she has plans to name the child.
Nurse	Assess if parent would like home care follow-up.	Make referral for home care if needed. Also refer parents to support group of other parents of children with hydrocephalus.	Support groups can decrease feelings of isolation and provide opportunities for further learning. Follow-up home care provides continuing support, guidance, and education.	Mother and grandmother state they will attend a support group at least once to evaluate benefit for them. Agree to at least one home visit for follow-up care.

BOX 27.7 Nursing Care Planning Based on Family Teaching

CARING FOR A CHILD WITH A VENTRICULOPERITONEAL SHUNT

Q. Following her child's ventriculoperitoneal shunt surgery, Bobby Jo asks you, "What do I need to do to care for him as he grows older?"

A. Here are some helpful things to remember:

- Be aware of the signs of increased intracranial pressure, such as drowsiness, vomiting, headache, irritability, and lack of appetite.
- Observe the site of the pump daily for any sign of swelling or redness.
- Don't allow your baby to fall asleep with his head hanging over the side of a couch or bed or in a position that could bend the shunt at the neck.
- Offer sufficient fruit, vegetables, cereal, and a generous amount of fluid so he doesn't become constipated; hard stool might press against the shunt in the abdomen and obstruct the flow of fluid. In addition, straining to pass a hard stool can increase intracranial pressure.
- Do not call attention to the pump behind your child's ear; teach him not to touch the pump when he's nervous or as an attention-getting action.
- Be certain your child wears a helmet for tricycle and bicycle riding (as all children should) to avoid injury to the shunt. Monitor his participation in roughhousing or school sports to avoid head trauma.
- If your child develops signs of infection such as an increased temperature, phone your primary care provider. This could be a simple respiratory infection but could also indicate an infected shunt that needs immediate treatment.
- Be certain to keep your regularly scheduled health assessment visits. As your child grows taller, the shunt will eventually need to be replaced for proper functioning.

The infant is also at risk for developing a flattened surface on the side or back of the head (nonsynostotic plagiocephaly) because of the inability to freely move the head, so awareness of position also becomes important from a cosmetic craniofacial aspect (Lennartson, 2011).

Nursing Diagnosis: Deficient knowledge related to home care needs of child with hydrocephalus

Outcome Evaluation: Parents state fears regarding ability to provide care but voice they are able to manage this; state signs of increased intracranial pressure for which they should watch; demonstrate competence in shunt care.

Caring for a child with a shunt in place is an ongoing responsibility for parents because most children will have a shunt in place for the rest of their life. If parents do not seem to be asking many questions about the child's care after surgery, do not assume this is because they are taking the child's care in stride. They may be too frightened or not understand neuroanatomy enough to know what questions to ask. An opening question such as, "Most parents are a little nervous when they think about taking a child home with a shunt in place; do you feel that way?" gives them an opportunity to discuss how they feel, and hopefully, bring their anxiety down to a manageable level. It also offers assurance that health care providers are interested in helping and supporting them.

As their child grows older, remind parents to stress to their child that the strange object that can be felt behind the ear should not be continually touched. A child nervously fidgeting with a pressure pump can inadvertently evacuate CSF from the ventricles at a dangerously rapid rate.

Before an infant with a shunt in place is discharged from the hospital after surgery, be certain the parents have ample opportunity to feed and provide care so they can feel comfortable and confident they "know" their infant. Because irritability, lethargy, vomiting, and a change in the baby's cry are signs of increased intracranial pressure, be certain parents have the telephone number of their primary health care provider so they can report these findings immediately. A referral for home care follow-up may be appropriate to offer further support.

Parents need an appointment for the child's first checkup or who to call to make an appointment. Be certain they understand an infection of the shunt is not just a possibility but a severe complication because it can lead to meningitis; this means they need to report ear or pharyngeal infections at the first sign of illness. If meningitis should develop, in addition to being rehospitalized and receiving the usual treatment for meningitis (see Chapter 49), the child may have an extraventricular shunt placed to promote drainage and allow antibiotics to be administered directly into the CSF to prevent infected CSF from draining into the peritoneal cavity, where it could cause peritonitis.

Nursing Diagnosis: Risk for delayed growth and development related to potential neurologic challenge

Outcome Evaluation: Child demonstrates regular observable growth and achieves age-appropriate developmental milestones.

Like all children, children with hydrocephalus need intellectual and emotional stimulation such as being talked to, smiled at, and played with. Always role-model talking and singing to the child to help parents include these actions in their care. As necessary, reposition mobiles or pictures over a crib so the child can receive adequate visual stimulation without turning a heavier than usual head.

As the child reaches preschool and school age, parents need to confer with their primary health care provider as to what sports will be safe. Usually, contact sports are contraindicated although may be allowed with helmet head protection. Carrying a heavy backpack or purse on the side of the shunt is also not advised to avoid breaking the shunt. Helmet use should be enforced with tricycle or bicycle riding.

QSEN Checkpoint Question 27.6

Teamwork & Collaboration

The primary health care provider for Bobby Jo's baby asks you to observe him for signs that he is developing increased intracranial pressure while he waits for surgery. What vital sign changes should most prompt you to report the findings to the primary care provider?

a. Decreased temperature and increased blood pressure
b. Increased respirations and decreased pulse rate
c. Increased temperature and decreased pulse rate
d. Decreased blood pressure and increased temperature

Look in Appendix A for the best answer and rationale.

Neural Tube Disorders

Because the neural tube forms in utero first as a flat plate and then molds to form the brain and spinal cord, it is susceptible to malformation. The term **spina bifida** (Latin for "divided spine") is most often used as a collective term for all spinal cord disorders, but there are well-defined degrees of spina bifida involvement, and not all neural tube disorders even involve the spinal cord. All of these disorders, however, occur because of a lack of fusion of the posterior surface of the embryo in early intrauterine life. They can be compared with cleft palate or cleft lip, which are also midline closure disorders.

The worldwide incidence of neural tube defects ranges from 1 to 10 per 1,000 births. The incidence of neural tube disorders has fallen dramatically in the United States since the inclusion of 600 μg of folic acid in prenatal vitamins and the mandatory inclusion of folic acid in all cereal and grain products, reducing the rate to 2 in 10,000 live births. In addition to folic acid deficiency, other risks identified are maternal age under 20 years or over 40 years, maternal education below 12th grade level, and low socioeconomic status (Au, Ashley-Koch, & Northrup, 2010). All women, especially those who have given birth to a first child with a spinal cord disorder, are advised to have maternal serum assay MAFP levels during a second pregnancy to determine if such a disorder could be present.

Types of Disorders

Anencephaly. Anencephaly is the absence of the cerebral hemispheres. It occurs when the upper end of the neural tube fails to close in early intrauterine life. It is revealed by an elevated level of MAFP, amniocentesis, or a prenatal sonogram.

Labor with an infant with anencephaly may be prolonged because the infant may present in a breech position or the underdeveloped head may not engage the cervix well. On visual inspection at birth, the disorder is obvious (Fig. 27.17). Because the respiratory and cardiac centers are located in the intact medulla, infants may survive for several days after birth but cannot survive further because they have little or no cerebral function.

When the condition is discovered prenatally, parents are offered the option of pregnancy termination. If they elect to carry the pregnancy to term, they will need concerned support in the first few days of life as they realize the baby is as ill and incomplete as predicted.

Microcephaly. Microcephaly is a disorder in which the fetal brain grows so slowly that it falls more than three standard deviations below normal on a growth chart at birth. The cause might be a disorder in brain development associated with an intrauterine infection such as rubella, cytomegalovirus, or toxoplasmosis (Bernard, Knupp, Yang, et al., 2012). Microcephaly may also result from severe malnutrition or anoxia following birth or in early infancy.

The prognosis for a normal life is guarded in children with microcephaly and depends on the extent of restriction of brain growth and on the cause. Generally, the infant is cognitively challenged because of the lack of functioning brain tissue. True microcephaly must be differentiated from *craniosynostosis* (normal brain growth but premature fusion of the cranial sutures), which also causes decreased head circumference but is curable.

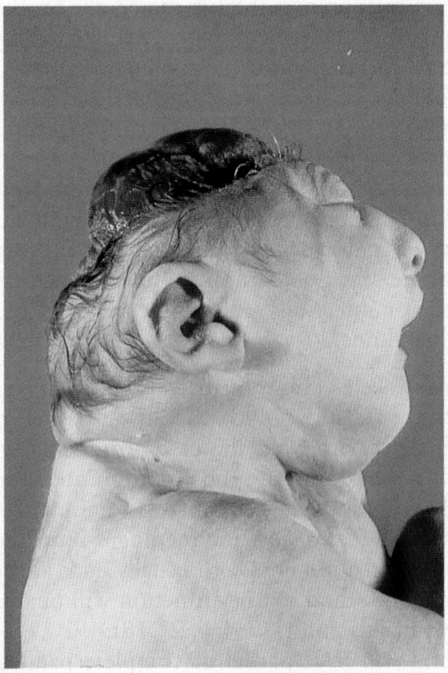

FIGURE 27.17 An infant with anencephaly. (© Joseph R. Siebert, PhD/Custom Medical Stock Photograph.)

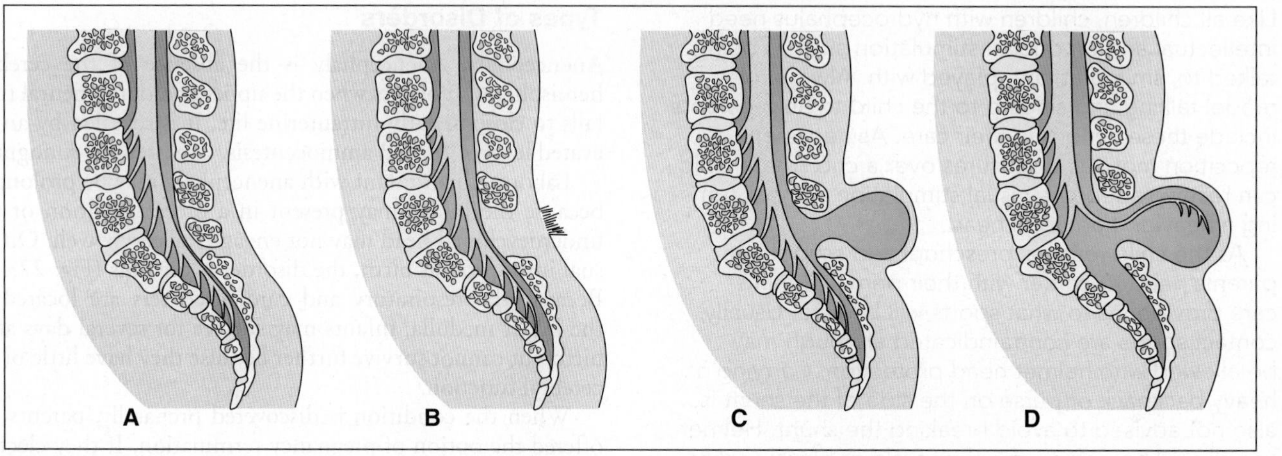

FIGURE 27.18 Degrees of spinal cord anomalies. **(A)** A normal spinal cord. **(B)** Spina bifida occulta. **(C)** A meningocele. **(D)** A meningomyelocele.

Spina Bifida Occulta. Spina bifida occulta occurs when the posterior laminae of the vertebrae fail to fuse. This occurs most commonly at the fifth lumbar or first sacral level but may occur at any point along the spinal canal. The appearance of a normal spinal cord is shown in Figure 27.18A. Spina bifida occulta may be first noticed as a dimpling at the point of poor fusion; abnormal tufts of hair or discolored skin may also be present (Fletcher & Brei, 2010). Simple spina bifida occulta is a benign disorder, and it can occur as frequently as in one out of every four children (see Fig. 27.18B).

Because the term "spina bifida" is commonly used to denote all spinal cord anomalies, parents, when told their child has a spina bifida occulta, may interpret this as meaning their child has an extremely serious disorder. Help clarify the degree of this defect for them: it simply means a surface of bone is missing, and the spinal cord is intact.

Meningocele. The spinal cord is protected by three layers of meninges or membranes: the pia mater, the arachnoid, and the dura mater. If these membranes herniate through an unformed vertebrae, they protrude as a circular mass, about the size of an orange, at the center of the back and is termed a *meningocele* (see Fig. 27.18C). The protrusion generally occurs in the lumbar region, although it might be present anywhere along the spinal canal. The protrusion is either covered by a layer of skin or, more frequently, only the clear dura mater. No sensory or motor deficits accompany the disorder unless the membrane sac should rupture, but damage to the cord could occur or infection could enter the now unprotected cerebrospinal fluid.

Meningomyelocele. This is the defect that most people think of when they say "spina bifida" because it is the most common birth defect affecting the central nervous system and is frequently viewed as the most complicated birth defect compatible with survival (Liptak & El Samra, 2010). In a meningomyelocele, not just the meninges protrude through the vertebrae, but the spinal cord usually ends at the point of protrusion. Motor and sensory function will be decreased or absent beyond this point (see Fig. 27.18D).

The child will have partial or complete paralysis, partial or complete lack of sensation of the lower extremities, as well as loss of bowel and bladder control. The infant's legs may appear lax because the infant cannot move them; urine and stools continually dribble because of a lack of sphincter control. Children may have an accompanying talipes (clubfoot) disorder and developmental hip dysplasia. A hydrocephalus develops in as many as 90% of these infants because of the lack of an adequate subarachnoid membrane for CSF absorption and obstruction of CSF circulation from the spinal deformity; the higher the meningomyelocele occurs on the cord, the more likely it is that a hydrocephalus will accompany it. Simultaneous shunting during a primary meningomyelocele repair during the first 72 hours of life has been shown to decrease hospital stay length, decrease loss of and infection rates of CSF, and lessen damage from progressive ventricular dilation (Sinha et al., 2012).

Encephalocele. An encephalocele is a cranial meningocele. These occur most often in the occipital area of the skull but may occur as a nasal or nasopharyngeal disorder. Encephaloceles generally are covered fully by skin, although they may be open or covered only by the dura. It is difficult to tell from the size of the encephalocele if only CSF is trapped in the protruding meninges or whether brain tissue could also be involved. Transillumination of the sac will reveal whether brain tissue is in the sac. A CT, MRI, or ultrasound will reveal the size of the skull disorder and help predict the extent of surgery, which will be needed.

Assessment. Neural tube disorders may be discovered during intrauterine life by prenatal ultrasound, fetoscopy, amniocentesis (discovery of increased AFP in amniotic fluid), or analysis of MAFP. If the condition is discovered in utero, it may be possible to close the lesion by fetoscopic surgery. An infant may be born by cesarean birth to avoid pressure and injury to the spinal cord. It is generally difficult to tell from visual appearance whether the disorder is a meningomyelocele (Fig. 27.19) or the simpler meningocele. Observe and record whether an infant born with a neural tube disorder has spontaneous movement of the lower extremities to assess if the child has lower motor function. Also assess the nature and pattern of voiding and defecation. The usual newborn appears to be "always wet" from voiding but actually voids in amounts of approximately 30 ml and then is dry for 2 or 3 hours before voiding again. An infant without motor or sphincter control voids continually. This pattern is the same

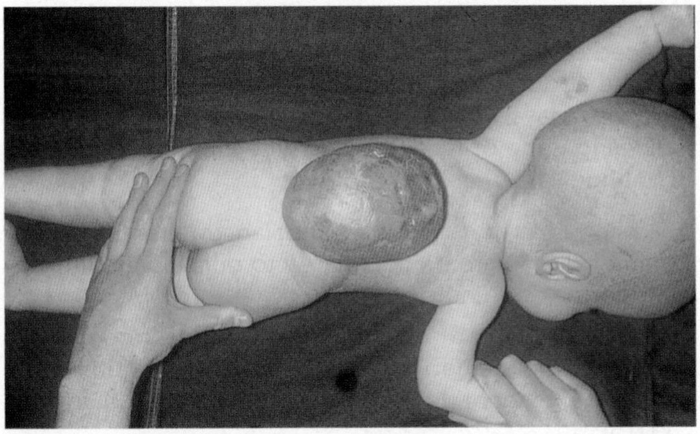

FIGURE 27.19 A meningomyelocele. The infant also has hydrocephalus and a subluxated hip. (NMSB/Custom Medical Stock Photograph.)

for defecation. Observing these features aids in differentiating between a meningocele and a meningomyelocele. Differentiation will be further established by CT, ultrasound, or MRI.

Therapeutic Management. Children with spina bifida occulta need no surgical correction because there is no tissue extruding from the vertebrae. The parents should be made aware of the defect, however, so they are not surprised if it is revealed on a spinal X-ray taken for some reason later in life, as well as know to watch for more serious symptoms as the child grows such as numbness, weakness, or pain, which might indicate a need for reevaluation. Some children may eventually need surgery to prevent vertebral deterioration because of the unbalanced spinal column.

Treatment for a meningocele or encephalocele involves immediate surgery to replace the meninges and to close the gap in the skin to prevent infection. This is done as soon after birth as possible (usually within 24 to 48 hours) so an infection through the exposed meninges does not occur. The surgery is not without risk, and if a brain disorder accompanies an encephalocele, the child's cognitive potential may be impaired. If a large portion of meninges have to be removed by surgery, this can limit the rate of absorption of CSF, which can lead to a buildup of CSF and hydrocephalus.

Children with a meningomyelocele have the same surgery to return the meninges to the spinal cord and close the gap in the skin surface. The child will continue to have partial or complete paralysis of the lower extremities and loss of bowel and bladder function because, although the lesion on the back can be repaired, the absent lower cord cannot be replaced. There also is the same risk of hydrocephalus. Table 27.1 provides a classification of motor function ability, which can be anticipated according to the location of a spinal cord disruption.

Nursing Diagnoses and Related Interventions: Immediate Concerns

Although parents of an infant with a meningomyelocele were told before surgery that their child's spinal disorder is a type that means motor and sensory function are absent in the child's lower extremities, they do not necessarily "hear" this information. It is only after surgery that they begin to comprehend the extent of physical challenges their child will face. Before the child is discharged from the hospital, be certain the parents are linked with an interprofessional care team specializing in neural tube disorders to prevent them from feeling deserted when they most need support—the time when they first begin to appreciate what this problem will mean to them in the coming years, and what it will mean to their child throughout life.

Nursing Diagnosis: Risk for infection related to rupture or bacterial invasion of the meningeal sac

Outcome Evaluation: Neural tube sac remains intact; axillary temperature remains below 98.6°F (37°C).

If the exposed meningeal sac is allowed to dry, it can crack, allowing CSF to drain and microorganisms to enter. Pressure on the protruding mass is a prime

TABLE 27.1 Motor Function Ability in Children With Meningomyelocele

Spinal Cord Lesion	Resultant Effects
T6–T12	Complete flaccid paralysis of the lower extremities; weakened abdominal and trunk musculature in higher lesions; kyphosis and scoliosis common; ambulation with maximal support
L1–L2	Hip flexion present; paraplegia; ambulation with maximal support
L3–L4	Hip flexion, adduction, and knee extension present; hip dislocation common; some control of hip and knee movement possible; ambulation with moderate support
L5	Hip flexion, adduction, and varying degrees of abduction; knee extension and weak knee flexion; paralysis of the lower legs and feet; ambulation with moderate support
S1–S2	As previous, with preservation of some foot and ankle movement; ambulation with minimal support
S3	Mild loss of intrinsic foot muscular function possible; ambulation without support

reason why the sac ruptures. When this happens, it can lead to an infection such as meningitis as well as quick decompression of the CSF. Sudden compression can lead to herniation of the brain stem into the spinal cord and interference with respiratory and cardiac centers. Such pressure may also force CSF from the sac into the spinal column, thus increasing intracranial pressure. It is crucial, therefore, to prevent the drying of and pressure on the exposed membrane.

Preoperative Positioning: Before surgery, use sterile gloves and sterile linens when caring for an infant with either a meningocele or meningomyelocele. Use a sterile, wet, warm compress of saline, antiseptic, or antibiotic gauze over the lesion to keep the sac moist. Rather than remove this to wet it again and risk rupturing the sac, merely add additional warm fluid as needed.

Position infants carefully to prevent pressure on the exposed meninges, either in a prone position or supported on their side. When they are on their side, use a rolled blanket or diaper placed behind their upper back (above the disorder) and a separate one behind their lower back (below the disorder) so no pressure will be exerted on the lesion and the infant will be protected from rolling backward onto it. Placing a folded diaper between the legs prevents skin surfaces from touching and rubbing in this position as well as helps to keep the hips from internally rotating. Positioning infants on their abdomen has the added advantage of keeping the flow of feces and urine away from the spinal defect as well as keeping the protruding meninges free from pressure (infants at home should sleep on their back but in an acute care setting with monitoring available, you can assure parents infants can be safely positioned on their abdomen). Placing a piece of plastic or sturdy plastic wrap below the protruding membranes on the child's back and taping it in place as an apron is another method of preventing feces from touching the open lesion.

A folded towel under the abdomen helps to flex the infant's hips in a prone position, reduce pressure on the sac, and ensure good leg position. Always notice if the position of the infant's legs appears comfortable because, if the infant lacks motor control, he or she cannot move them to a more comfortable position independently.

Although no pressure should be exerted on the open lesion by a top sheet or swaddling blanket, make certain the child is adequately warm. The presence of the sac adds to the amount of body surface area exposed, so heat loss will be greater than usual. Don't place the infant under a radiant heat source for warmth because the radiant heat can dry the lesion and cause cracking. An incubator both supplies a better heat source and also allows you to constantly assess and monitor the lesion. Any seepage of clear fluid from the defect should be reported promptly, because this is probably escaping CSF. If you are in doubt whether the fluid is urine or CSF, check it against a glucose test strip: CSF will test positive for glucose, whereas urine or mucus will not.

Postoperative Care: After surgery, a baby is again placed on a cardiorespiratory monitor and positioned on the abdomen until the skin incision has healed (about 7 days). The same careful precautions against allowing urine or feces to touch the incision area continue.

Nursing Diagnosis: Risk for imbalanced nutrition, less than body requirements, related to difficulty assuming normal feeding position

Outcome Evaluation: Child's skin turgor is good; weight is maintained within 10% of birth weight; specific gravity of urine remains between 1.003 and 1.015.

If the defect repair was large and the risk of picking up the infant is too great, the infant may be fed while lying on the side in an incubator or prone on a specialized bed frame. Raise the infant's head slightly by slipping a folded diaper under it. Make certain your supporting arm does not press against the lesion. Remember (and remind parents) that, when burping the infant, not to pat the infant's back over the defect. Stroke the head, arms, or upper back while the infant sucks to try to give the child the same comfort and assurance at feeding time as a baby would receive if being held. Infants may enjoy a pacifier after feeding because they do not experience the same enjoyment of sucking while feeding that would be experienced if they could be held and cuddled. If a mother plans to breastfeed, urge her to pump and freeze breast milk for the infant; as soon as the infant can be held, she can breastfeed in the nursery (which will be as early as 3 to 4 days).

Nursing Diagnosis: Risk for ineffective cerebral tissue perfusion related to increased intracranial pressure

Outcome Evaluation: Child's head circumference remains within present percentile on growth chart; signs and symptoms of increased intracranial pressure are absent.

Preoperative Care: Increasing head size from poor absorption of CSF (hydrocephalus) is a common complication of both meningocele and meningomyelocele surgical repairs. To detect increased head size, measure head circumference as prescribed in the preoperative period to set a baseline. Head circumference measurements done by various caregivers are accurate only if the tape measure is placed on the same points of the child's head each time. Placing an indelible pen mark on the scalp above and below the tape measure over both ears and on the back of the scalp allows different people to measure the head at the same point while not leaving such a large mark that it interferes with facial features.

Postoperative Care: Head circumference measurement needs to be continued after surgery because this is the time when an increase in size most often occurs. Continue to observe the child as well for signs of increased intracranial pressure such as bulging fontanelles, vital change variations, neurologic signs such as pupillary changes, or behavioral changes such as irritability or lethargy to help detect if this is happening.

Nursing Diagnosis: Risk for impaired skin integrity related to required prone positioning

Outcome Evaluation: Infant's skin on knees remains intact, without erythema or ulceration.

Preserving skin integrity is a major problem before surgery because the constant prone position puts pressure on the infant's knees and elbows. If a hydrocephalus has developed, pressure areas at the temples can occur if the head is not repositioned about every 2 hours. Laying the infant on a synthetic sheepskin helps reduce friction; continue to use this after surgery plus use paper tape or a stockinette for dressing changes or place a protective dressing such as Stomahesive on the skin under the area where the tape will touch. Change diapers frequently to prevent excessive contact of acidic urine with skin.

Nursing Diagnoses and Related Interventions: Long-Term Concerns

Nursing Diagnosis: Impaired physical mobility related to neural tube disorder

Outcome Evaluation: Child ambulates with the least amount of accessory equipment possible.

Parents need to begin to plan stimulation activities that their infant can accomplish with limited mobility as soon as surgery is completed. Encourage them to take the infant to the places children normally accompany parents, such as relatives' homes, shopping, or the zoo, because encouraging children to be as independent as possible as they grow helps them lead as active a life as possible (Fig. 27.20) (O'Mahar, Holmbeck, Jandasek, et al., 2010).

Parents will need to perform passive exercises to prevent muscle atrophy and formation of contractures if a child has impaired lower extremity motor control. The child may need leg braces to help maintain good alignment and enable walking with crutches. Parents are generally anxious to do something for their child and follow routines of passive exercises well if they are given sufficient support for their accomplishments at health care visits. As the child grows older, tendon transplants or an osteotomy may be necessary to prevent contractures and poor bone alignment. Because children with meningomyeloceles have no sensation in their lower extremities, parents should make a routine of daily inspections of the child's lower extremities and buttocks for any area of irritation or possible infection. Teach children as they grow older to do this themselves. When children are using a wheelchair, be certain they press with their arms on the armrests to raise their buttocks off the wheelchair seat at least once every hour to help provide adequate circulation to lower extremities.

Nursing Diagnosis: Risk for impaired elimination related to a neural tube disorder

Outcome Evaluation: Child demonstrates ability to independently manage bowel and bladder elimination by school age.

To ensure bladder emptying, an intermittent clean urinary catheterization technique may be taught to parents (inserting a clean catheter through the urethra into the bladder every 4 hours to drain urine from the bladder; Box 27.8). An advantage of this is children who are begun on intermittent clean catheterization from birth require fewer bladder augmentation procedures as they grow older. As they reach early school age, they can learn this technique for themselves. In addition to self-catheterization, a drug such as oxybutynin chloride (Ditropan) may improve bladder capacity and allow a child to need less frequent catheterizations (Box 27.9) (Karch, 2013). In some children, it is possible to place artificial bladder sphincters to help establish continence. In other children, a continent urinary reservoir or a ureterosigmoidostomy (see Chapter 46) can be constructed to bypass the nonfunctioning bladder.

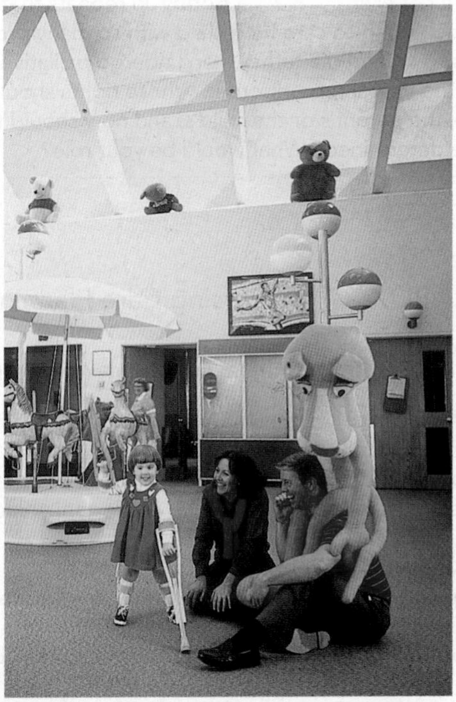

FIGURE 27.20 A child born with a neural tube disorder demonstrates her ability to walk using braces and a crutch. (Alexander Tsiara/Photo Researchers, Inc.)

BOX 27.8 Nursing Care Planning to Empower a Family

TECHNIQUE FOR CLEAN INTERMITTENT CATHETERIZATION

Q. Bobby Jo needs to learn clean intermittent catheterization for her son (now named Robert Joseph). She asks you, "How do I do this?"

A. Here are some helpful guidelines to follow:

1. The purpose of intermittent catheterization is to keep the bladder empty by using a clean technique and frequent emptying so microorganisms do not have time to grow in urine or the bladder. Always use clean equipment and catheterize at least every 4 hours.
2. Always carry catheterization equipment with you when away from home (e.g., a plastic bag containing a new catheter and a water-soluble lubricant). If you will be using a public lavatory, you might want to include a presoaped washcloth rather than have to use rough paper towels.
3. To begin catheterization, wash your hands well in warm, soapy water. This reduces the chance you will introduce germs from your hands into your child's bladder.
4. Next, wash around your child's urinary meatus with a clean washcloth or paper towel and warm, soapy water. Rinse the washcloth and wash again with clear water. This reduces the chance that germs on the child's skin will be pushed into the bladder.
5. Coat the tip of the catheter with a water-soluble lubricant. This reduces friction and allows the catheter to slide into the bladder easily.
6. Quickly but gently insert the catheter into the urinary meatus approximately 3 in. Urine should begin to flow immediately through the catheter. Let this drain into a collecting bag.
7. When urine stops flowing, gently remove the catheter. Most health insurance plans furnish enough clean catheters that you don't ever have to reuse one. If you should need to do this, clean the catheter with soap and water, rinse with clear water, and replace in the plastic bag with the lubricant.
8. Be certain that on special days such as family celebrations or while on vacation, you do not forget the importance of catheterization.
9. As your child reaches school age, you can teach him how to do this himself. He will need to insert the catheter about 6 in. Be certain he will be able to have access to a school bathroom every 4 hours during the day so he can successfully do this.
10. Phone your health care provider if urine is ever blood tinged, smells foul, or is cloudy rather than clear or if your child appears to have pain in his abdomen or lower back or has an elevated temperature. These may be symptoms of a urinary tract infection, which will need treatment.

What if...27.3 Bobby Jo repeats that she's too young to care for a child with so many problems so wants to let him die rather than undergo palliative surgery to close the neural tube disorder. Whose rights should be honored, the parent's or the child's, and how should these rights be determined? What would be your role?

Arnold–Chiari (Chiari II) Malformation

An Arnold–Chiari malformation is categorized as Chiari I, Chiari II, or Chiari III. Children with Chiari I typically show symptoms in the second or third decade of life, so it is referred to as an "adult type," although current sonogram scan capabilities have allowed for earlier incidental diagnosis. Chiari II and

BOX 27.9 Nursing Care Planning Based on Responsibility for Pharmacology

OXYBUTYNIN CHLORIDE (DITROPAN)

Classification: Oxybutynin is an anticholinergic, urinary antispasmodic.

Action: Relaxes smooth muscle to relieve symptoms of bladder instability associated with neurogenic bladder (Karch, 2013).

Pregnancy Risk Category: C

Dosage: Individually prescribed depending on weight of child.

Possible Adverse Effects: Drowsiness, dizziness, blurred vision, decreased sweating

Nursing Implications

- Advise parents to give or have the child take the medication exactly as prescribed.
- Alert parents about the need for frequent health care visits during treatment to document the drug's effect.
- Ask the child to report drowsiness or blurred vision. Caution the child to not attempt activities that require balance until they adjust to taking the drug.
- Caution the child and parents that the drug causes decreased sweating, which can cause body temperature to rise. Encourage parents to keep the child's environment cool and to avoid extreme, high temperatures.

the very rare Chiari III types are present at birth and so are considered primary neural tube abnormalities. The Chiari II disorder is caused by overgrowth of the neural tube in weeks 16 to 20 of fetal life. The cerebellum, medulla oblongata, and fourth ventricle project into the spinal canal at the cervical level, causing the upper cervical spinal cord to jackknife backward, obstructing CSF flow and causing hydrocephalus. An accompanying lumbosacral meningomyelocele is also present in about 50% of children with this anomaly (Bernard et al., 2012).

The prognosis for the child with an Arnold–Chiari malformation depends on the extent of the disorder and the surgical repair procedure possible. Because of the upper motor neuron involvement, gagging and swallowing reflexes may be absent, increasing the risk for tracheal aspiration. Serious levels of sleep apnea may also occur (Tran & Hukins, 2011), which require surgical intervention. Overall prognosis is encouraging.

What if... 27.4 You are interested in exploring one of the 2020 National Health Goals related to infants born with physical or developmental disorders (see Box 27.1). Most government-sponsored money for nursing research is allotted based on these goals. What would be a possible research topic to explore pertinent to these goals that would be applicable to the Sparrow family and that would also advance evidence-based practice?

KEY POINTS FOR REVIEW

- Learning about the way a child will be physically challenged immediately after birth helps parents adjust most easily. Advocate for parents by helping them obtain as much information as they need about their child's condition in order to help them manage seamless transitions across different health care settings.
- Parent–infant bonding can be difficult to establish when a child is hospitalized at birth. Assess family relationships at health maintenance visits to see that bonding is occurring.
- Absent or malformed extremities may range from absence of a finger to absence of an entire limb. Children may need physical therapy and teaching on how to use a prosthesis to gain full mobility and function.
- Developmental hip dysplasia is the improper formation and function of the hip socket; talipes deformities are foot and ankle deformities. Children may need extensive bracing and casting to correct these disorders.
- Cleft lips and cleft palates result from the failure of the maxillary process to fuse in intrauterine life. Surgical repair is possible early in life, with a good prognosis for both of these conditions.
- Esophageal atresias and tracheoesophageal fistulas occur from failure of the trachea and esophagus to completely divide and fully form independently in intrauterine life. Surgical intervention begins immediately but often needs to be performed in several stages.
- Omphaloceles are protrusions of abdominal contents through the abdominal wall at birth, protected only by a peritoneal membrane. When the membrane is not present, this is called gastroschisis. Although several stages of repair are often necessary, surgical correction has a good outcome.
- Intestinal obstructions can result from atresia (complete closure) or stenosis (narrowing) of a part of the bowel. Correction is surgical removal of the narrowed bowel portion.
- Meconium plugs occur when an extremely hard portion of meconium blocks the lumen of the intestine. Infants with meconium plug syndrome need to be observed for continuing bowel function and assessed for cystic fibrosis because a meconium plug is often the first symptom of this illness.
- Diaphragmatic hernias occur when the abdominal organs protrude through a defect in the diaphragm into the chest cavity. This prevents the lungs from fully forming in utero or expanding at birth. These infants are critically ill at birth and need extensive surgical correction.
- An imperforate anus is the incomplete formation of the anus, resulting in an inability to pass stool. The infant may have a temporary colostomy created before a final surgical correction can be completed.
- Physical developmental disorders of the nervous system include hydrocephalus (excess CSF in the ventricles) and neural tube disorders (incomplete closure of the vertebrae). Infants with hydrocephalus need surgery to relieve a ventricular obstruction or have a shunt implanted from their ventricles to the peritoneal cavity to remove excess CSF. Children with meningomyeloceles, the most severe form of neural tube disorder, face a permanent full or partial loss of lower neuron function and require continued rehabilitation.
- Planning nursing care that includes assurance not only meets QSEN guidelines but best meets the family's total needs.

CRITICAL THINKING CARE STUDY

Cecelia Dove is a 7-lb baby born by vaginal birth to a 25-year-old mother. At birth, she appeared healthy and cried lustfully. An hour after birth, however, the first time her mother tried to breastfeed her, she coughed and choked 5 minutes into the feeding. Her primary care provider suspects Cecelia may have esophageal atresia.

1. What steps should you immediately take because of this diagnosis while you wait for diagnostic tests to be scheduled?
2. After a barium swallow is completed, Cecelia's mother is told her infant has an isolated esophageal atresia without a fistula. The mother exclaims, "I can't take home a baby who isn't normal. My mother will say it's my fault because I never should have gotten pregnant. My boyfriend will be so embarrassed, he'll leave me." How could you help this mother gain a better insight into her child's condition?
3. Cecelia returns from the operating room after successful surgery. She has a temporary gastrostomy tube in place for decompression and feedings of breast milk. When the mother asks you, "What now?" what would be your best answer?

Patient Scenario

The Suderman Family

Read about the Suderman family, a family with a physically challenged newborn, then answer the questions to further sharpen your skills and grow more familiar with NCLEX-type questions related to infants with physical and developmental challenges. Confirm your answers are correct by reading the rationales.

Visit http://thePoint.lww.com

Answers and Rationales

Looking answers to the What If. . . and Critical Thinking Care Study questions?

Visit http://thePoint.lww.com

References

Abel, F., Bajaj, Y., Wyatt, M., et al. (2012). The successful use of the nasopharyngeal airway in Pierre Robin sequence: An 11 year experience. *Archives of Disease in Childhood, 97*(4), 331–334.

Aquilina, K. (2011). Intraventricular haemorrhage of the newborn. *Advances in Clinical Neuroscience and Rehabilitation, 11*(5), 22–24.

Au, K. S., Ashley-Koch, A., & Northrup, H. (2010). Epidemiologic and genetic aspects of spina bifida and other neural tube defects. *Developmental Disabilities Research Reviews, 16*(1), 6–15.

Austin, A. A., Druschel, C. M., Tyler, M. C., et al. (2010). Interdisciplinary craniofacial teams compared with individual providers: Is orofacial cleft care more comprehensive and do parents perceive better outcome? *Cleft Palate-Craniofacial Journal, 47*(1), 1–8.

Ballantyne, M., Stevens, B., Guttmann, A., et al. (2012). Transition to neonatal follow-up programs: Is attendance a problem? *Journal of Perinatal & Neonatal Nursing, 26*(1), 90–98.

Bartels, E., Jenetzky, E., Solomon, B. D., et al. (2012). Inheritance of the VATER/VACTERL association. *Pediatric Surgery International, 28*(7), 681–685.

Bartzela, T., Katsaros, C., Shaw, W. C., et al. (2010). A longitudinal three-center study of dental arch relationship in patients with bilateral cleft lip and palate. *Cleft Palate-Craniofacial Journal, 47*(2), 167–174.

Bernard, B. J., Knupp, K., Yang, M. L., et al. (2012). Neurologic & muscular disorders. In W. Hay, M. Levin, R. Deterding, et al. (Eds.), *Current diagnosis & treatment pediatrics* (21st ed., pp. 740–829). New York, NY: McGraw-Hill/Lange.

Bessell, A., Hooper, L., Shaw, W. C., et al. (2011). Feeding interventions for growth and development in infants with cleft lip, cleft palate or cleft lip and palate. *Cochrane Database of Systematic Reviews,* (1), CD003315.

Bischoff, A., Levitt, M. A., & Peña, A. (2011). Laparoscopy and its use in the repair of anorectal malformations. *Journal of Pediatric Surgery, 46*(8), 1609–1617.

Bishop, W. P. (2011). Oral cavity. In K. J. Marcdante, R. M. Kliegman, H. B. Jenson, et al. (Eds.), *Nelson essentials of pediatrics* (6th ed., pp. 475–476). Philadelphia, PA: Saunders/Elsevier.

Blomberg, M. I., & Källén, B. (2010). Maternal obesity and morbid obesity: The risk for birth defects in the offspring. *Birth Defects Research, 88*(1), 35–40.

Bouchard, M., Chouinard, S., & Suchowersky, O. (2010). Adult cases of congenital muscular torticollis successfully treated with botulisum toxin. *Movement Disorders, 25*(14), 2453–2456.

Broome, M., Herzog, G., Hohlfeld, J., et al. (2010). Influence of primary cleft palate surgery on the future need for orthodontic surgery in unilateral cleft lip and palate patients. *Journal of Craniofacial Surgery, 21*(5), 1615–1618.

Catalano, P., Di Pace, M. R., Caruso, A. M., et al. (2011). Gastroesophageal reflux in young children treated for esophageal atresia. *Journal of Pediatric Gastroenterology & Nutrition, 52*(6), 686–690.

Cuenca, A. G., Ali, A. S., Kays, D. W., et al. (2012). "Pulling the plug"—Management of meconium plug syndrome in neonates. *Journal of Surgical Research, 175*(2), e43–e46.

Danzer, E., Johnson, M. P., & Adzick, N. S. (2012). Fetal surgery for meningomyelocele: Progress and perspectives. *Developmental Medicine & Child Neurology, 54*(1), 8–14.

Davies, H., Rennick, J., & Majnemer, A. (2011). Transition from pediatric to adult health care for young adults with neurological disorders: Parental perspectives. *Canadian Journal of Neuroscience Nursing, 33*(2), 32–39.

Dean, C., Etienne, D., Hindson, D., et al. (2012) Pectus excavatum (funnel chest): A historical and current prospective. *Surgical & Radiologic Anatomy, 34*(7), 573–579.

Dixon, M., Marazita, M., Beaty, T., et al. (2011). Cleft lip and palate: Synthesizing genetic and environmental influences. *Nature Reviews: Genetics, 12*(3), 167–178.

Efrati, O., Nir, J., Fraser, D., et al. (2010). Meconium ileus in patients with cystic fibrosis is not a risk factor for clinical deterioration and survival. *Journal of Pediatric Gastroenterology and Nutrition, 50*(2), 173–178.

Emil, S., Canvasser, N., Chen, T., et al. (2012). Contemporary 2-year outcomes of complex gastroschisis. *Journal of Pediatric Surgery, 47*(8), 1521–1528.

Evans, K. N., Sie, K. C., Hopper, R. A., et al. (2011). Robin sequence: From diagnosis to development of an effective management plan. *Pediatrics, 127*(5), 936–948.

Fletcher, J. M., & Brei, T. J. (2010). Spina bifida—A multidisciplinary perspective. *Developmental Disabilities Research Reviews, 16*(1), 1–5.

Garfinkle, J. S., King, T. W., Grayson, B. H., et al. (2011) A 21-year anthropometric evaluation of the nose in bilateral cleft lip-cleft palate patients following nasoalveolar molding and cutting bilateral cleft lip and nose reconstruction. *Plastic and Reconstructive Surgery, 127*(4), 1659–1667.

Garriboli, M., Duess, J. W., Ruttenstock, E., et al. (2012). Trends in the treatment and outcome of congenital diaphragmatic hernia over the last decade. *Pediatric Surgery International, 28*(12), 1177–1181.

Ghosh, P. S., & Ghosh, D. (2011). Subdural hematoma in infants without accidental or nonaccidental injury: Benign external hydrocephalus, a risk factor. *Clinical Pediatrics, 50*(10), 897–903.

Gourlay, D. M. (2013). Colorectal considerations in pediatric patients. *Surgical Clinics of North America, 93*(1), 251–272.

Harrison, D., Yamada, J., & Stevens, B. (2010). Strategies for the prevention and management of neonatal and infant pain. *Current Pain and Headache Reports, 14*(2), 113–123.

Hayashi, T., Inuzuka, R., Shiozawa, Y., et al. (2012). Treatment strategy and long-term prognosis for patients with esophageal atresia and congenital heart diseases. *Pediatric Cardiology, 34*(1), 64–69.

Hedrick, H. L. (2013). Management of prenatally diagnosed congenital diaphragmatic hernia. *Seminars in Pediatric Surgery, 22*(1), 37–43.

Holland, A. J. A., Walker, K., & Badawi, N. (2010). Gastroschisis: An update. *Pediatric Surgery International, 26*(9), 871–878.

Ireland, P. J., Donaghey, S., McGill, J., et al. (2012). Development in children with achondroplasia: A prospective clinical cohort study. *Developmental Medicine & Child Neurology, 54*(6), 532–537.

Juang, D., & Snyder, C. L. (2012). Neonatal bowel obstruction. *Surgical Clinics of North America, 92*(3), 685–711.

Karch, A. M. (2013). *2013 Lippincott's nursing drug guide.* Philadelphia, PA: Lippincott Williams & Wilkins.

Kelly, D., O'Dowd, T., & Reulbach, U. (2012). Use of folic acid supplements and risk of cleft lip and palate in infants: A population-based cohort study. *British Journal of General Practice, 62*(600), e466–e472.

Kline, U. (2012). Oral medicine & dentistry. In W. Hay, M. Levin, R. Deterding, et al. (Eds.), *Current diagnosis & treatment pediatrics* (21st ed., pp. 470–471). New York, NY: McGraw-Hill/Lange.

Kotecha, S., Barbato, A., Bush, A., et al. (2012). Congenital diaphragmatic hernia. *European Respiratory Journal, 39*(4), 820–829.

Ledbetter, D. J. (2012). Congenital abdominal wall defects and reconstruction in pediatric surgery: Gastroschisis and omphalocele. *Surgical Clinics of North America, 92*(3), 713–727.

Lee, S. J., Han, J. D., Lee, H. B., et al. (2011). Comparison of clinical severity of congenital muscular torticollis based on the method of child birth. *Annals of Rehabilitation Medicine, 35*(5), 641–647.

Lee, D., Lim, S., & Lee, J. K. (2011). Thyroglossal duct cyst presenting with airway obstruction in a neonate. *Otolaryngology: Head and Neck Surgery, 144*(1), 127–128.

Lennartson, F. (2011). Developing guidelines for child health care nurses to prevent nonsynostotic plagiocephaly: Searching for the evidence. *Journal of Pediatric Nursing, 26*(5), 348–358.

Levy, P. (2010). An overview of newborn screening. *Journal of Developmental and Behavioral Pediatrics, 31*(7), 622–631.

Lewis, D. W. (2011). Neurology. In K. J. Marcdante, R. M. Kliegman, H. B. Jenson, et al. (Eds.), *Nelson essentials of pediatrics* (6th ed., pp. 671–712). Philadelphia, PA: Saunders/Elsevier.

Liao, Y., Yang, I., Wang, R., et al. (2010). Two-stage palate repair with delayed hard palate closure is related to favorable maxillary growth in unilateral cleft lip and palate. *Plastic & Reconstructive Surgery, 125*(5), 1505–1510.

Linehan, K., & O'Sullivan, M. K. (2011). The non-surgical management of congenital talipes equino varus (CTEV) in the first year of life: An Irish perspective. *International Journal of Orthopaedic & Trauma Nursing, 15*(2), 71–75.

Liptak, G. S., & El Samra, A. (2010). Optimizing health care for children with spina bifida. *Developmental Disabilities Research Reviews, 16*(1), 66–75.

Mangan, S., & Mosher, S. (2012). Challenges to skin-to-skin kangaroo care: Cesarean delivery and critically ill NICU patients. *Neonatal Network, 31*(4), 259–261.

Mildinhall, S. (2012). Speech and language in the patient with cleft palate. In M. T. Cobourne (Ed.), *Cleft lip and palate: Epidemiology, aetiology and treatment* (pp. 137–148). Unionville, CT: Karger.

Miller, S. D., Glynn, S. F., Kiely, J. L., et al. (2010). The role of nasal CPAP in obstructive sleep apnea syndrome due to mandibular hypoplasia. *Respirology, 15*(2), 377–379.

Montirosso, R., Fedeli, C., Murray, L., et al. (2012). The role of negative maternal affective states and infant temperament in early interactions between infants with cleft lip and their mothers. *Journal of Pediatric Psychology, 37*(2), 241–250.

Okada, H., & Gosain, A. K. (2012). Current approaches to management of nonsyndromic craniosynostosis. *Current Opinion in Otolaryngology & Head Neck Surgery, 20*(4), 310–317.

O'Mahar, K., Holmbeck, G. N., Jandasek, B., et al. (2010). A camp-based intervention targeting independence among individuals with spina bifida. *Journal of Pediatric Psychology, 35*(8), 848–856.

Pietrucin-Materek, M., van Teijlingen, E. R., Barker, S., et al. (2011). Parenting a child with clubfoot: A qualitative study. *The International Journal of Orthopaedic & Trauma Nursing, 15*(4), 176–184.

Roder, M. (2010). A primer on craniosynostosis. *Midwifery Today with International Midwife,* 2010–2011 Winter (96), 43–45.

Rothenberg, S. S. (2012). Thoracoscopic repair of esophageal atresia and tracheo-esophageal fistula in neonates: Evolution of a technique. *Journal of Laparoendoscopic & Advanced Surgery Technique, 22*(2), 195–199.

Sewell, M. D., & Eastwood, D. M. (2011). Screening and treatment in developmental dysplasia of the hip—Where do we go from here? *International Orthopaedics, 35*(9), 1359–1367.

Singh, S., Song, H. R., Venkatesh, K. P., et al. (2010). Analysis of callus pattern of tibia lengthening in achondroplasia and a novel method of regeneration assessment using pixel values. *Skeletal Radiology, 39*(3), 261–266.

Sinha, S. K., Dhua, A., Mathur, M. K., et al. (2012). Neural tube defect repair and ventriculoperitoneal shunting: Indications and outcome. *Journal of Neonatal Surgery, 1*(2), 21.

Sniderman, A. (2010). Abnormal head growth. *Pediatrics in Review, 31*(9), 382–384.

Strahle, J., Selzer, B. J., Muraszko, K. M., et al. (2012). Programmable shunt valve affected by exposure to a tablet computer. *Journal of Neurosurgery: Pediatrics, 10*(2), 118–120.

Sundaram, S. S., Hoffenberg, E. J., Kramer, R. E., et al. (2012). Gastrointestinal tract. In W. Hay, M. Levin, R. Deterding, et al. (Eds.), *Current diagnosis & treatment pediatrics* (21st ed., pp. 624–662). New York, NY: McGraw-Hill/Lange.

Thilo, E. H., & Rosenberg, A. A. (2012). The newborn infant. In W. Hay, M. Levin, R. Deterding, et al. (Eds.), *Current diagnosis & treatment pediatrics* (21st ed., pp. 9–72). New York, NY: McGraw-Hill/Lange.

Tovar, J. A. (2012). Congenital diaphragmatic hernia. *Orphanet Journal of Rare Diseases, 7*(1), 1–17.

Tran, K., & Hukins, C. A. (2011). Obstructive and central sleep apnea in Arnold-Chiari malformation: Resolution following surgical decompression. *Sleep and Breathing, 15*(3), 611–613.

Turner, H. A., Vanderminden, J., Finkelhor, D., et al. (2011). Disability and victimization in a national sample of children and youth. *Child Maltreatment, 16*(4), 275–286.

U.S. Department of Health and Human Services. (2010). *Healthy people 2020.* Washington, DC: Author.

Walter, K. D. (2011). Orthopedics. In K. J. Marcdante, R. M. Kliegman, H. B. Jenson, et al. (Eds.), *Nelson essentials of pediatrics* (6th ed., pp. 735–762). Philadelphia, PA: Saunders/Elsevier.

Weil, B. R., Leys, C. M., & Rescorla, F. J. (2012). The jury is still out: Changes in gastroschisis management over the last decade are associated with both benefits and shortcomings. *Journal of Pediatric Surgery, 47*(1), 119–124.

Wiler, J. L. (2012). Symptoms: Hernia with acute pain and swelling. *Emergency Medicine News, 34*(1), 18–21.

Wool, A. C. C. (2011). Systematic review of the literature: Parental outcomes after diagnosis of fetal anomaly. *Advances in Neonatal Care, 11*(3), 182–192.

Zamurovic, M., Jurisic, A., & Brankovic, S. (2012). Giant omphalocele-prenatal diagnostics, pregnancy evaluation and postnatal treatment. *Clinical Experience in Obstetrics & Gynecology, 39*(2), 258–261.

Unit 5

The Nursing Role in Health Promotion for a Childrearing Family

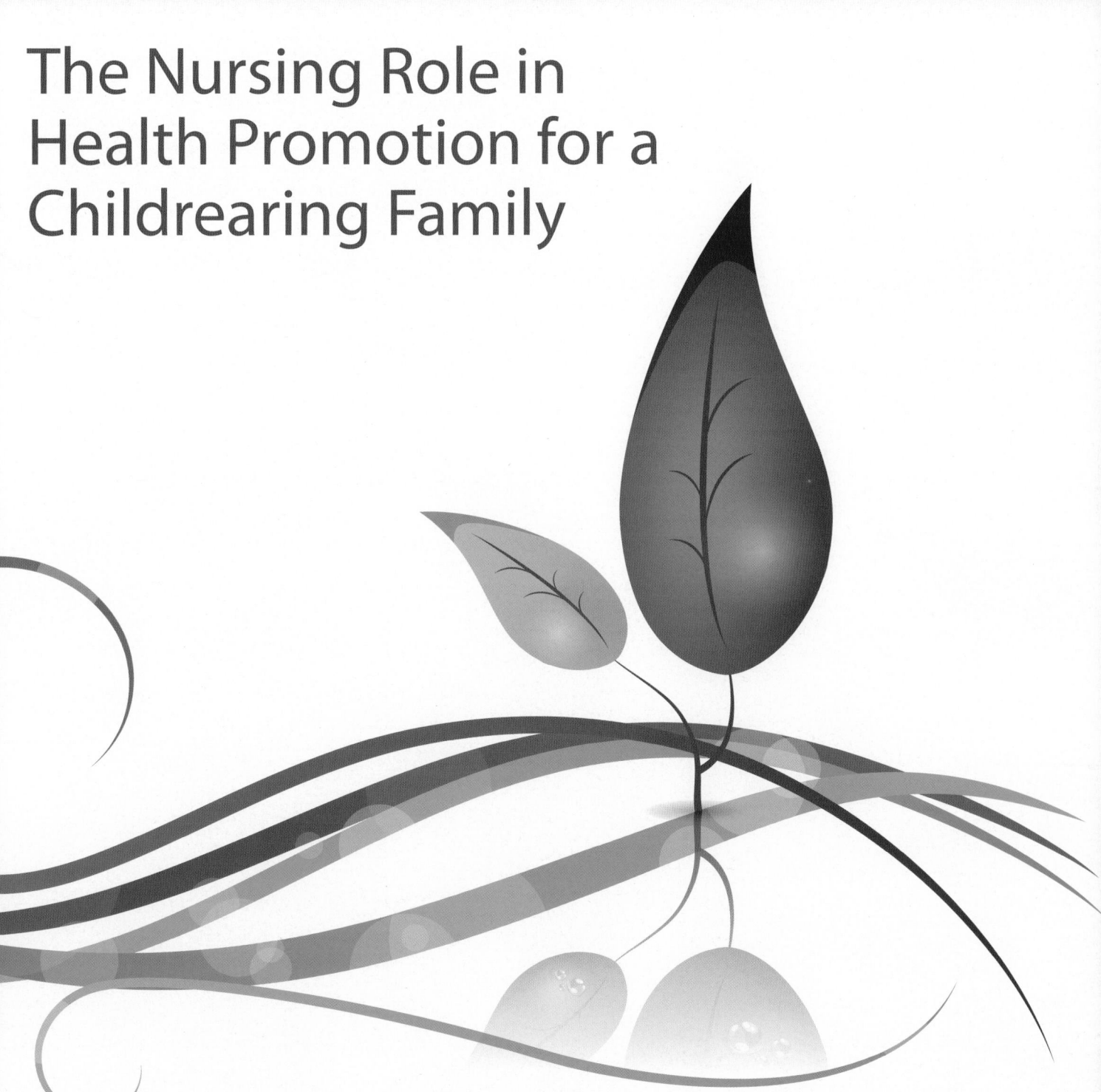

Chapter 28

Principles of Growth and Development

KEY TERMS

- abstract thought
- accommodation
- assimilation
- autonomy versus shame or doubt
- centering
- cognitive development
- conservation
- development
- developmental milestones
- developmental task
- egocentrism
- generativity versus stagnation
- growth
- identity versus role confusion
- industry versus inferiority
- initiative versus guilt
- integrity versus despair
- intimacy versus isolation
- maturation
- permanence
- reversibility
- role fantasy
- schemas
- sensorimotor stage
- temperament
- trust versus mistrust

OBJECTIVES

After mastering the contents of this chapter, you should be able to:

1. Describe principles of growth and development and developmental stages according to major theorists.
2. Identify 2020 National Health Goals related to growth and development that nurses can help the nation achieve.
3. Assess a child to determine if a stage of development has been achieved.
4. Formulate nursing diagnoses that address wellness as well as both a potential for and an actual delay in growth and development.
5. Identify expected outcomes for a growing child as well as how to manage seamless transitions across differing health care settings.
6. Using the nursing process, plan nursing care that includes the six competencies of Quality & Safety Education for Nurses (QSEN): Patient-Centered Care, Teamwork & Collaboration, Evidence-Based Practice (EBP), Quality Improvement (QI), Safety, and Informatics.
7. Implement nursing care, such as suggesting age-appropriate play materials to support normal growth and development.
8. Evaluate outcome criteria for achievement and effectiveness of care.
9. Integrate knowledge of the principles of growth and development with the interplay of nursing process, the six competencies of QSEN, and Family Nursing to promote quality maternal and child health nursing care.

John Olson is a 6-year-old, mildly overweight boy brought into an emergency department because his leg is broken from a bicycle accident. At 4 months of age, John was placed in foster care because his mother was not caring for him adequately. He was then moved back and forth among 12 different foster homes until he was finally adopted at age 3.5 years. His adoptive parents now have 3-year-old twins of their own in addition to John. They tell you that, although John has lived with them for 3 years, they find him cold and unloving. They ask you what they can do to change this.

Nurses are directly responsible for assessing the growth and development of children in many health care settings. Previous chapters discussed childbearing and what an important time the first weeks after birth can be in a child's life. This chapter adds information about growth and development that are important for a child's continuing life.

How has John's background contributed to his behavior? What stage of psychosocial development does he not seem to have achieved? How could his adoptive parents help him at this point?

BOX 28.1 Nursing Care Planning Based on 2020 National Health Goals

A number of 2020 National Health Goals speak to growth or development of children. They include:

- Increase the proportion of children with special health care needs who receive their care in family-centered, comprehensive, coordinated systems from 20.4% to a target level of 22.4%.
- Reduce the proportion of children diagnosed with a disorder through newborn blood spot screening who experience a developmental delay requiring special education services from 15.1% to a target level of 13.6%.
- Increase the proportion of young children who are screened for an autism spectrum disorder (ASD) and other developmental delays by 24 months of age from 19.5% to a target level of 21.5%.
- (Developmental) Increase the proportion of children with a developmental delay who have a first evaluation by 36 months of age.
- Reduce the proportion of children 2 to 5 years of age who are considered obese from 10.7% to a target level of 9.6%; for children 6 to 11 years, from 17.4% to 15.7%; and for adolescents, from 17.9% to 16.1% (U.S. Department of Health and Human Services [DHHS], 2010; see www.healthypeople.gov).

Recognizing normal growth and development patterns of children helps to determine if children are following normal development and when referrals are needed. Nurses are the health care providers who interact with children as they weigh and measure them or help with interviewing or examinations and so are prime people to recognize developmental delays.

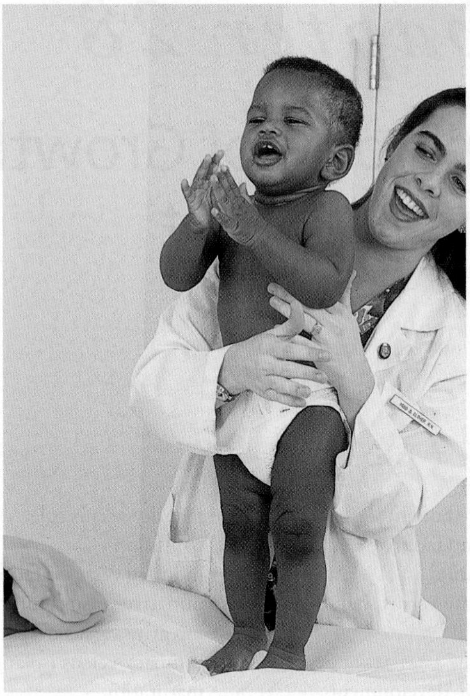
FIGURE 28.1 Growth and development are assessed by both observation and specific testing. Here, a 12-month-old demonstrates mastery of well-coordinated and intentional hand movements.

All children pass through predictable stages of growth and development as they mature. Parents often ask what to expect from their children regarding their developmental progress at health care visits. Such visits provide opportunities for you not only to assess present growth and development but also to supply anticipatory guidance on the topic (Butterworth & Kovas, 2013).

For these reasons, including growth and development is essential to establish complete and effective nursing care plans for children. This chapter addresses the most important factors to assess for each age group. Later chapters supply detailed descriptions of individual age groups. Box 28.1 shows 2020 National Health Goals that speak directly to aspects of growth and development.

Nursing Process Overview

For Promotion of Normal Growth and Development

Assessment

To assess growth and development, measure and plot height and weight on a standard growth chart for children at all health care visits to document that growth is occurring and a child's growth is remaining within a constant percentile. Take a health history from both parents and the child and observe what specific activities the child can accomplish to establish whether **developmental milestones** (major markers of normal development) are being met (Fig. 28.1). Document a 24-hour recall history for nutritional intake, sleep, and a description of school and play behaviors (see Chapter 34). Periodic screening tests such as the Denver II Tests, vision tests, and audiometry screenings should be scheduled at standard times as well. For the most accurate assessments, be certain to account for illness, sleepiness, fatigue, or "bad days" (a day on which a child did not test well).

Nursing Diagnosis

When an assessment is completed, a child profile can be devised and needs and problems can be identified. Examples of nursing diagnoses applicable to this area include:

- Risk for delayed growth and development related to lack of age-appropriate toys and activities
- Delayed growth and development related to prolonged illness
- Readiness for enhanced family coping related to parent's seeking information about child's growth and development
- Health-seeking behaviors related to appropriate stimulation for infants
- Imbalanced nutrition, less than body requirements, related to parental knowledge deficit regarding child's protein need
- Deficient knowledge related to potential long-term effects of obesity in school-age child

Outcome Identification and Planning

To provide holistic nursing care, consider all aspects of a child's health (physical, emotional, cultural, cognitive, spiritual, nutritional, and social), remembering that each child's developmental progress is unique. Children cannot be forced to achieve milestones faster than their own timetable will allow; however, through anticipatory guidance, children can be encouraged to reach maximum developmental potential. Nurses can play important roles in suggesting expected outcomes and guidance to both a child and family on ways to encourage child development and preparing children for new experiences.

Planning should include a child's family as growth and development proceed within a family context. To develop psychosocially, children need emotional support from loved ones, just as they need nutritional support to grow physically. Parents of a child with a developmental delay may use denial as a protective mechanism for a long time. This means planning may have to be centered first on helping parents accept what is happening; actual plans for a child may have to be delayed until the parents are convinced a problem exists. Helpful Web sites to use for parent referral are KidsHealth from the Nemours Foundation (www. KidsHealth.org) and the BabyCenter (www.BabyCenter.com).

Implementation

Interventions to foster growth and development include encouraging age-appropriate self-care in a child and suggesting age-appropriate toys or activities to parents. Role modeling is an important ongoing intervention to help parents accept a child's delayed growth or appreciate a child who is scoring extremely high on standard scales and needs increased stimulation. Modeling, for example, can demonstrate that problem solving is a more effective approach to life's challenges than "acting out" behaviors.

Outcome Evaluation

An evaluation for specific growth and developmental milestones (see Chapters 29 through 33) must be ongoing to be accurate and useful because changes not only happen rapidly but also many children do not test well on any given day. An ongoing evaluation is also necessary because it provides an opportunity for the early detection of various problems and for helpful anticipatory guidance. If a child has difficulty achieving one developmental task, for example, the next one may be more difficult and frustrating to achieve. An evaluation must also be comprehensive. If a developmental task involves only gross motor function, for example, it may not reveal that a child's fine motor function is also affected. In some children, fine motor function deficits are not detected until the child is asked to perform tasks such as writing in school. Examples of expected outcomes include:

- Child, 5 years of age, expresses less negativism at next clinic visit.
- At the 9-month checkup, parents describe how they have made a safe space in their home for their infant to crawl so he is not confined to a playpen.
- Parents list household tasks they believe are appropriate for a 6-year-old child by the next office visit.
- Parents describe the pattern they are using to phase out high-carbohydrate, nonnutritive snacks for their preschooler.
- Parents express confidence that they will be able to guide their toddler past the stage of the "terrible twos."

GROWTH AND DEVELOPMENT AND THE ROLE OF THE NURSE

Assessing for growth and development milestones is a nursing role in the care of both well and ill children.

Health Promotion and Illness Prevention

Determining a child's developmental stage is often the primary focus of a well-child health interview and examination. For instance, during her child's 24-month checkup, a mother might ask if it is normal that her child cannot yet pedal a tricycle, a question that cannot be answered without a full understanding of average ranges of motor coordination.

Parenting style and competence are major influences on the behavioral and mental health of children (Barton & Kirtley, 2012). In addition to reassuring parents that their child is doing well, parents also need periodic anticipatory guidance regarding their child's development. For example, it would be important to discuss additional home safety with a parent when a child is approaching the age for crawling. Parents should be cautioned to think about fencing open stairways and clearing cleaning compounds out of bottom cupboards. Parents of a child who is almost 1 year old will appreciate being cautioned that their child's appetite may decrease during the coming year; armed with this knowledge, they will not interpret a child's rejection of food as the beginning of a feeding problem but will see it as a usual step in development. The parent of a child approaching puberty generally welcomes a discussion on how to prepare a child for this challenging growth phase.

If anticipatory guidance is not offered at appropriate times, it's easy for it to be ignored. Information given too early is forgotten by the time it is needed. Given too late, parents may have already addressed the issue, possibly not in the most growth-enhancing way for their child. To be able to supply anticipatory guidance this way at the appropriate time or to plan nursing care to meet the needs of children and families, you must be able to recognize the predictable stages of growth and development, from newborn to young adult, through which each child passes (Halfon, Stevens, Larson, et al., 2011).

Health Restoration and Maintenance

It is equally essential to consider developmental stages when caring for a sick child or one having surgery. Preparing a 5-year-old child for surgery, for example, would be ineffective unless you know how much a 5-year-old child will be able to understand about such things as an anesthetic is a gas, some body parts are necessary for life and some are not, or stitches will not stay in permanently. During the postsurgical period, you need growth and development knowledge to assess whether a child is old enough to swallow pills, whether a child will be able to accurately rate a degree of pain on a standard scale, and how to approach a child who says "no" to every suggestion.

Physical growth is another important factor to consider, because disease affects children differently at various stages of growth. A 12-year-old child who has fractured a long bone, for example, has a potentially more serious fracture than an 8-year-old child who fractures the identical bone. This is because the 8-year-old must metabolize enough calcium to meet two major needs: healing the fracture site and maintaining healthy bone cells. The 12-year-old child, who is undergoing a period of rapid growth, must meet three needs: calcium for healing, maintaining existing healthy bone cells, and an additional amount for rapid bone growth. If a child does not take in adequate calcium during the healing period to supply the extra amount for growth, the affected limb could be left shorter than its mate. Recommending ways to ingest extra calcium that a 12-year-old child would like could help ensure no permanent disability results.

PRINCIPLES OF GROWTH AND DEVELOPMENT

Growing up is a complex phenomenon because of the many interrelated facets involved. Children do not merely grow taller and heavier as they get older; maturing also involves growth in their ability to perform skills, to think, to relate to people, and to trust or have confidence in themselves.

The terms "growth" and "development" are sometimes used interchangeably, but they are actually different terms.

- **Growth** is used to denote an increase in physical size or a *quantitative* change. Growth in weight, for example, is measured in pounds or kilograms; growth in height is measured in inches or centimeters.
- **Development** indicates an increase in skill or the ability to function (a *qualitative* change). Development is measured by observing a child's ability to perform specific tasks such as how well a child picks up small objects, by recording the parent's description of a child's progress, or by using standardized tests such as the Denver II Test. **Maturation** is a synonym for development.

Psychosexual development is a specific type of development that refers to developing instincts or sensual pleasure (Freudian theory). Psychosocial development refers to Erikson's stages of personality development. Kohlberg's theory of moral development is the ability to know right from wrong and to apply these to real-life situations.

Cognitive development refers to the ability to learn or understand from experience, to acquire and retain knowledge, to respond to a new situation, and to solve problems (see the section that follows on Piaget's theory of cognitive development). It is measured by intelligence tests and by observing children's ability to function effectively in different environments.

Patterns

Neither physical growth nor aspects of maturation occur haphazardly but in typical patterns governed by several principles (Box 28.2). As shown in Figure 28.2, the pattern for general growth, such as respiratory, digestive, renal, musculoskeletal, and circulatory tissue, proceeds fairly smoothly during childhood. Certain body tissues, however, mature in spurts. Neurologic tissue (spinal cord and brain) grows so rapidly during the first 2 years that the brain reaches mature proportions by 2 to 5 years of age. Lymphoid tissue (spleen, thymus, lymph nodes, and tonsillar tissue) also grows rapidly during infancy and childhood to provide young children early protection against infection. In 5-year-olds, for example, tonsillar tissue has already reached its peak size (about twice that of an adult). On assessment, the back of the throat of young school-age children appears to be "all tonsils." Although the spleen is not usually palpable in adults, the spleen is palpable 1 or 2 cm below the left ribs in preschool children as another example of this rapid immune tissue growth. In contrast, reproductive organs (genital tissue) show little growth until puberty (Levine, 2011).

✔ QSEN Checkpoint Question 28.1

Informatics

John is 6 years old. You should teach his parents that which of his body systems should be reaching its peak point of development at this time?

a. His neurologic system
b. His lymphatic system
c. His respiratory system
d. His musculoskeletal system

Look in Appendix A for the best answer and rationale.

FACTORS INFLUENCING GROWTH AND DEVELOPMENT

Genetic inheritance, or whether a child receives healthy genes or genes that will lead to an illness, influences how much a child will grow. Environmental influences are primary factors in determining if a child will be able to reach his or her genetic potential.

Temperament—the typical way a child reacts to situations—is an example of genetic influence. Whether a fetus enjoyed a healthy uterine existence or whether the child was born into a family with sufficient funds to supply adequate health care are examples of environmental influences (Pike, Jane-Pillow, & Lucas, 2012). Whether a child receives good nutrition, beginning with being breastfed, is yet another (Johnston, Landers, Noble, et al., 2012). It is the intertwining of these or a combination of these factors that determines how each child grows and matures.

Genetics

From the moment of conception when a sperm and ovum fuse, the basic genetic makeup of an individual is cast. In addition to physical characteristics such as eye color and height potential, inheritance determines characteristics such as learning style. A child may also inherit a genetic abnormality, which could result in disability or illness at birth or later in life and so prevent optimal growth.

Gender

On average, girls are born lighter (by an ounce or two) and shorter (by an inch or two) than boys. Boys tend to keep this height and weight advantage until prepuberty, at which time girls surge ahead as they begin their puberty growth spurt 6 months to 1 year earlier than boys. By the end of puberty (age 14 to 16 years), boys again tend to be taller and heavier than girls.

BOX 28.2 Nursing Care Planning Based on Family Teaching

Q. John's mother asks you, "Are there principles of growth and development I should know to be a better mother?"

A. Aspects of growth and development are well studied. General principles include:

- ***Growth and development are continuous processes from conception until death.*** Although there are highs and lows in terms of the rate at which growth and development proceed, a child is growing new cells and learning new skills at all times. An example of how the rate of growth changes is a comparison between that of the first year and later in life. An infant triples in birth weight and increases height by 50% during the first year of life. If this tremendous growth rate were to continue, a 5-year-old child, ready to begin school, would weigh 1,600 lb and be 12.5 ft tall.
- ***Growth and development proceed in an orderly sequence.*** Growth in height occurs in only one sequence—from smaller to larger. Development also proceeds in a predictable order. For example, the majority of children sit before they crawl, crawl before they stand, stand before they walk, and walk before they run. Occasionally, a child will skip a stage (or pass through it so quickly the parents do not observe the stage). Occasionally, a child will progress in a different order, but most children follow a predictable sequence of growth and development.
- ***Children pass through the predictable stages at different rates.*** All stages of development have a range of time rather than a certain point at which they are usually accomplished. Two children may pass through the motor sequence at such different rates, for example, that one begins walking at 9 months, whereas another starts at 14 months. They are both following the predictable sequence and are developing normally; they are merely developing at different rates.
- ***All body systems do not develop at the same rate.*** Certain body tissues mature more rapidly than others. For example, neurologic tissue experiences its peak growth during the first year of life, whereas genital tissue grows little until puberty.
- ***Development is cephalocaudal.*** *Cephalo* is a Greek word meaning "head"; *caudal* means "tail." Development proceeds from head to tail. Newborns can lift only their head off the bed when they lie in a prone position. By age 2 months, infants can lift both the head and chest off the bed; by 4 months, the head, chest, and part of the abdomen; by 5 months, infants have enough control to turn over; by 9 months, they can control legs enough to crawl; and by 1 year, children can stand upright and perhaps walk. Motor development has proceeded in a cephalocaudal order—from the head to the lower extremities.
- ***Development proceeds from proximal to distal body parts.*** This principle is closely related to cephalocaudal development. It can best be illustrated by tracing the progress of upper extremity development. A newborn makes little use of the arms or hands. Any movement, except to put a thumb in the mouth, is a flailing motion. By age 3 or 4 months, the infant has enough arm control to support the upper body weight on the forearms, and can coordinate the hand to scoop up objects. By 10 months, the infant can coordinate the arm and thumb and index fingers sufficiently to use a pincerlike grasp or to be able to pick up an object as fine as a piece of breakfast cereal on a high chair tray.
- ***Development proceeds from gross to refined skills.*** This principle parallels the preceding one. Once children are able to control distal body parts such as fingers, they are able to perform fine motor skills (e.g., a 3-year-old colors best with a large crayon; a 12-year-old can write with a fine pen).
- ***There is an optimum time for initiation of experiences or learning.*** Children cannot learn tasks until their nervous system is mature enough to allow that particular learning. A child cannot learn to sit, for example, no matter how much the child's parents have him or her practice, until the nervous system has matured enough to allow for back control. Children who are not given the opportunity to learn developmental tasks at the appropriate or "target" times for a task may have more difficulty than the usual child learning the task later on. A child who is confined to a body cast at 12 months, the time the child would normally learn to walk, may take a long time to learn this skill once free of the cast at, say, age 2 years. The child has passed the time of optimal learning for that particular skill.
- ***Neonatal reflexes must be lost before development can proceed.*** An infant cannot grasp an item with skill until the grasp reflex has faded nor can the infant stand steadily until the walking reflex has faded. Neonatal reflexes are replaced by purposeful movements.
- ***A great deal of skill and behavior is learned by practice.*** Infants practice over and over taking a first step before they accomplish this securely. If children fall behind in growth and development because of an illness, they are capable of "catch-up" growth to bring them equal again with their age group.

This difference in growth patterns is why different growth charts are used for boys than for girls (available at http://thePoint.lww.com/Pillitteri7e) (Pastor & Reuben, 2011).

Health

A child who inherits a genetically transmitted disease may not grow as rapidly or develop as fully as a healthy child depending on the type of illness and the therapy or care available for the disease. Before insulin was discovered in 1922, for example, many children with type 1 diabetes mellitus died in early childhood; those who lived were left physically challenged. Currently, with good health supervision and insulin therapy, the effects of type 1 diabetes can be so minimized that children with diabetes both grow and thrive. Diabetes is still a major factor in the health of children, however. As more and more children become obese because of fast food diets and lack of an exercise program, type 2 diabetes now has begun to occur in children as young as school age (Dea, 2011; Morgan, 2012).

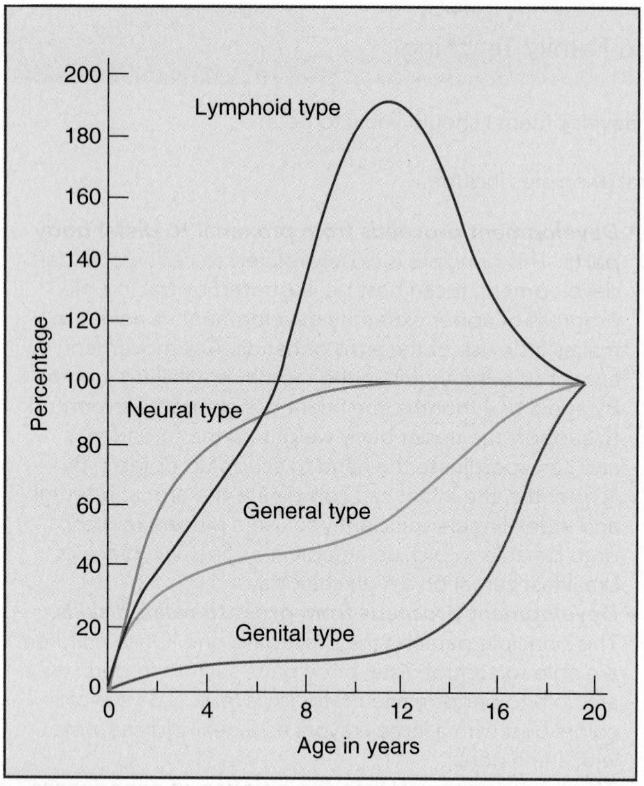

FIGURE 28.2 The main types of postnatal growth of various body tissue types. (Redrawn from Scammon, R. E. [1930]. The measurement of the body in childhood. In J. A. Harris, C. M. Jackson, D. G. Paterson, et al. [Eds.], *The measurement of man* [pp. 214–226]. Minneapolis, MN: University of Minnesota Press, with permission.)

Intelligence

Children with high intelligence do not generally grow faster physically than other children, but they do tend to advance faster in skills. Occasionally, children of high intelligence actually fall behind in physical skills because they spend their time with books or mental games rather than with games that develop motor skills. Intelligence begins to make major differences as children become adolescents and begin to plan future careers (Viner, Ozer, Denny, et al., 2012).

Temperament

Temperament is the usual reaction pattern of an individual, or an individual's characteristic manner of thinking, behaving, or reacting to stimuli in the environment (Chess & Thomas, 1985). Unlike cognitive or moral development, temperament is not developed in stages but is an inborn characteristic set at birth. Understanding that children are not all alike (e.g., some adapt quickly to new situations, others adapt slowly, some react intensely, some react passively based on an inborn disposition) helps parents better understand why their children are different from one another and help them plan individualized care for each child.

Reaction Patterns

Chess and Thomas (1985) are the researchers who identified nine separate characteristics that define temperament, or how children react to common situations. Each child's pattern is made up of a combination of these individual elements.

Activity Level. The level of activity among children differs widely right from birth. Some babies seem to be constantly on the go and rarely quiet. They wiggle and squirm in their crib as early as 2 weeks of age. Parents put such children to sleep in one end of a crib and find them in the other end an hour later; such children will not stay seated in bathtubs and refuse to be confined in playpens. Other babies, by contrast, move little, stay where they are placed, and appear to take in their environment in a quieter, more docile way. Both patterns are normal; they merely reflect the extremes of *activity level*, one characteristic of temperament.

Rhythmicity. A child who has *rhythmicity* manifests a regular rhythm in physiologic functions. Even as infants, such children tend to wake up at the same time each morning, are hungry at regular 4-hour periods, nap the same time every day, and have a bowel movement at the same time every day. They are predictable and easy to care for because their parents learn early on what to expect from them. On the other end of the scale are infants who rarely awaken at the same time 2 days in a row. They may go a long time without eating one day and the next day appear hungry almost immediately after a feeding. Such children are typically more difficult to care for because it is difficult to anticipate a schedule for them. Parents must constantly adapt their own routine to the child's routine.

Approach. *Approach* refers to a child's response on initial contact with a new stimulus. When introduced to a new situation, some children approach the challenge in an unruffled manner. They smile and "talk" to strangers and accept a first feeding or a new food without spitting up or fussing. They explore new toys without apprehension. Other children demonstrate withdrawal rather than approach. They cry at the sight of strangers, new toys, and new foods; they fuss the first time they are placed in a bathtub. They are difficult to take on vacation or to meet a new child care provider because they react so fearfully to new situations.

Adaptability. *Adaptability* is the ability to change one's reaction to stimuli over time. Infants who are adaptable can change their first reaction to a situation without exhibiting extreme distress. The first time such children are placed in a bathtub, they might protest loudly, for example, but by the third time they sit splashing happily. This is in contrast to infants who cry for months whenever they are put into a bathtub or who cannot seem to accustom themselves to a new bed, new car seat, or new caregiver.

Intensity of Reaction. A child who has an *intensity of reaction* meets new situations with their whole being. They cry loudly, thrash their arms, and begin temper tantrums when their diapers are wet, when they are hungry, and when their parents leave them. Other children, probably equally frustrated or angry, rarely demonstrate such overt symptoms or have a mild- or low-intensity reaction to stress.

Distractibility. Children who are easily distracted or who can easily shift their attention to a new situation (*distractibility*) are easy to care for. If they are crying over the loss of a toy, they can be appeased by the offer of a different one. If children cannot be distracted this way, their parents may describe them as stubborn, willful, or unwilling to compromise because they persistently return to an activity or refuse to adapt or change.

BOX 28.3 Nursing Care Planning to Empower a Family

CATEGORIES OF TEMPERAMENT

Q. Mrs. Olson asks you why her children solve problems so differently.
A. Children's temperament can be a reason they approach problems differently.

The Easy Child
Children are rated as "easy to care for" if they have a predictable rhythmicity, approach and adapt to new situations readily, have a mild-to-moderate intensity of reaction, and have an overall positive mood quality. Most children are rated by their parents as being in this category.

The Intermediate Child
Some characteristics of both easy and difficult groups are present.

The Difficult Child
Children are "difficult" if they are irregular in habits, have a negative mood quality, and withdraw rather than approach new situations. Only about 10% of children fall into this category.

The Slow-to-Warm-Up Child
Children fall into this category if, overall, they are fairly inactive, respond only mildly and adapt slowly to new situations, and have a general negative mood. About 15% of children display this pattern. When discussing this temperament with parents, try to use positive terms such as "ways to find a healthy fit for your child" rather than stressing ways the child is hard to manage.

Attention Span and Persistence. *Attention span* is the ability to remain interested in a project or activity for an average length of time. Like other aspects of temperament, this can vary a great deal among children. Some play by themselves with one toy for an hour; others spend no more than 1 or 2 minutes with each toy. The degree of *persistence* also varies. Some infants keep trying to perform an activity even when they fail time after time; others stop trying after one unsuccessful attempt.

Threshold of Response. The *threshold of response* is the intensity level of stimulation necessary to evoke a reaction. Children with a low threshold need to meet little frustration before they react; those with a high threshold need intense frustration before they become upset over a situation or with a person.

Mood Quality. A child who is always happy and laughing is said to have a positive *mood quality*. Obviously, this can make a major difference in the parents' enjoyment of a child; parents tend to spend more time with a child with a positive mood quality than with a child who seems always unhappy and whining or has a negative mood quality.

Nursing Implications and Temperament

Four categories or levels of temperament are shown in Box 28.3. Children who have a usual activity level and regular rhythmicity, who approach and adapt to new situations easily, and who have a long attention span, a high level of persistence, and a positive mood quality are "ideal" or "easy" children to care for from a parent's point of view. Highly active infants are much more difficult for parents to care for, especially if they demonstrate irregular physiologic rhythms, withdrawal rather than approach, and little ability to adapt. Such children require more planning and creative distraction measures.

Bringing characteristics of temperament to parents' attention helps them better understand their child and lays the foundation for beginning to accept and respect the child as an individual, which is essential for successful childrearing (Hudson, Dodd, Lyneham, et al., 2011).

Noticing children's temperament as they are admitted to a hospital can help you anticipate their probable reactions to precedures or pain. For example, a child with an intense reactivity pattern may voice even a minor discomfort loudly; a child with a less intense pattern may barely react. Both situations make it difficult to evaluate the true level of pain the children are experiencing unless temperament is considered.

What if... 28.1 John's mother describes her 3-year-old twins as being "totally different" from each other. One is shy and quiet; the other is aggressive and persistent. Which child does she probably view as easier to care for? As a nurse, what anticipatory guidance could you give her to help her better understand these differences in temperament in her children?

Environment

Although children cannot grow taller than their genetically programmed height potential allows, their adult height can be considerably less than their genetic potential if their environment hinders their growth. For example, a child could receive inadequate nutrition because of a family's low socioeconomic status, a parent could lack child care skills or not give a child enough attention or stimulation, or a child could contact an infectious disease and be left with a long-term disability. Illness can lower children's appetites, thus interfering with growth; others, such as certain endocrine disorders, directly alter growth rate. Having a parent who abuses alcohol or other substances can cause such inconsistency in care that it can affect mental health (Rossow & Moan, 2012).

Environmental influences, however, like genetic ones, are not always detrimental. For example, children with phenylketonuria, an inherited metabolic disease that leads to poor growth and cognitive challenge, can achieve normal growth and development in spite of their genetic makeup if their diet (a part of the environment) is properly regulated. The following environmental influences are those most likely to affect growth and development.

Socioeconomic Level

Because health care and good nutrition both cost money, children born into families of low socioeconomic means may suffer from a lack of both of these. Poor health supervision can leave them without immunization against measles or other childhood illnesses and therefore vulnerable to permanent neurologic damage (Mulholland, Griffiths, & Biellik, 2012). Poor nutrition can also leave them vulnerable to disease because antibody formation depends on a good protein intake (Whitney & Rolfes, 2012).

The Parent–Child Relationship

What a parent expects a child to become as an adult varies from culture to culture and family to family but plays a role in how much a child is guided to try to achieve in life. Cultural norms also play a role because some cultures value education and contribution to society as more important than do others (Box 28.4). Children who are loved and are paid attention to by their parents thrive better than those who are not (Feigelman, 2012). Luckily, for parents and children, either parent or even a nonparent may form this primary parent–child love relationship. When assessing families, don't just examine how much time parents spend with children; examine the quality of that time because it is the quality, not the quantity, that is most important (Box 28.5). Loss of love from a primary caregiver, as might occur with the death of a parent, or interruption of parental contact through hospitalization, imprisonment, or divorce can have such an effect on a child that it interferes with a desire to eat, improve, and advance. Supporting parents to be actively involved in their child's care so a parent–child relationship is strengthened is important in all health care and child care settings (Vicedo, 2011).

Ordinal Position in the Family

The position of a child in the family (e.g., first-born child, middle child, youngest child, only child) and the size of the family also have some bearing on a child's growth and development. An only child or the oldest child in a family, for example, generally excels in language development because conversations are mainly with adults. Youngest children, in contrast, may develop language more slowly, especially if older children talk "baby talk" with them. Children learn by watching other children, however, so a youngest child who has many examples to watch may excel in other skills, such as toilet training or writing at an early age.

Health

Diseases that come from environmental sources can have as strong an influence on growth and development as genetically inherited diseases. Infants cared for in neonatal intensive care units, for example, may develop some decrease in hearing because of the overstimulation of sound, an example of health being directly influenced by the environment (Matook, Sullivan, Salisbury, et al., 2010). Children who have residual heart impairment as a result of contracting rheumatic fever might be limited in their ability to play an active sport. The eventual degree of disability will depend, however, not only on the damage caused by the actual disease but also on the attitudes of the people around the child (i.e., how disabled they believe the child to be) (Russell, Sinclair, Poteat, et al., 2012). When parents treat children differently after they have been critically ill (i.e., don't react warmly to them), the children are referred to as "vulnerable children" (Green & Solnit, 1964). Fortunately, if an illness does not last long and leaves no permanent disability, most children achieve "catch-up" growth and score well on growth measures after an illness.

Nutrition

In the past 20 years, nutrition has become a major focus of health promotion and disease prevention because the quality of a child's nutrition during the growing years (and prenatally) has such a major influence on health, weight, and stature (Whitney & Rolfes, 2012). Poor maternal nutrition may limit the growth and intelligence potential of a child by furnishing a less than desired prenatal environment. In some communities, poor nutrition has such an effect that children begin to show inadequate physical growth as early as infancy.

BOX 28.4 Nursing Care Planning to Respect Cultural Diversity

Not all nations foster the growth and development of children in the same manner, in part because of cultural variations. Childhood in the United States covers a relatively long period. In other countries, childhood is short because girls are asked to assume domestic responsibilities early in life and outside or farm work is required early for boys. In some countries, the predominant theory of childrearing is protective nurturing. Children are not rushed into new experiences like toilet training or beginning school. In others, it is customary to treat children in a harsh, strict manner, using shame or corporal punishment for discipline. Praising children for learning a new skill may be viewed as unnecessary or actually harmful, because this could result in a child being subject to evil forces. In some Asian cultures, an infant's personality is thought to depend not so much on genetic or environmental influences but on the year and time of birth.

What foods children receive also varies with culture. Vegetables such as jicama and chayote, for example, may not even be recognized by children in the Northeast United States but may be popular with those in the Southwest.

Asking a parent questions such as, "What do you do when your baby cries?" "What kind of things do you think a 2-year-old should be able to do?" and "What do you do when your 4-year-old misbehaves?" can help you to isolate and better understand cultural differences. Recognizing cultural variations this way helps to plan care individualized to a particular child and family.

BOX 28.5 Nursing Care Planning Based on Effective Communication

You see John's mother in clinic for a follow-up visit.

Less Effective Communication

Nurse: How are you today, Mrs. Olson? How is John?
Mrs. Olson: I'm good.
Nurse: Is your family eating more meals together? Does John seem to enjoy that?
Mrs. Olson: We eat together for sure three nights a week.
Nurse: Wonderful. It's good to see John is adjusting better.

More Effective Communication

Nurse: How are you today, Mrs. Olson? How is John?
Mrs. Olson: I'm good.
Nurse: And John?
Mrs. Olson: He's the same.
Nurse: Is your family eating more meals together?
Mrs. Olson: We eat together for sure three nights a week.
Nurse: Does John seem to enjoy that?
Mrs. Olson: He never talks at the table. It's as if he isn't there.
Nurse: Let's talk about other ways you could bring John into the family.

This is a good example of what happens when you ask multiple or compound questions. The mother here always answers her half of the question, but because she doesn't continue and answer about John, the nurse actually learns nothing about him. Only when she asks individual questions does she obtain the information she needs.

A lack of energy and stamina prevents children from learning at their best intellectual level, which causes them to fall behind in school. In contrast, in other communities, eating too much food (or the wrong kinds of food) causes as many as 20% of children to be obese (Centers for Disease Control and Prevention [CDC], 2012).

Children who become obese may develop motor skills more slowly than other children because physical movement is more tiring for them. Obese children are also likely targets of taunting by playmates and so run a risk of lacking a strong and supportive group of friends. Lack of a strong support system can lead to depression as the child reaches adolescence (Ting, Huang, Tu, et al., 2012).

Nutrition also plays a vital role in the body's susceptibility to disease because poor nutrition limits the body's ability to resist infection. Lack of calcium could leave a child prone to rickets, a disease that affects growth by causing shortening or bowing of long bones. Lack of vitamins can lead to visual impairments, poor healing, and poor bone growth. Excessive obesity is linked with the development of type 2 diabetes in children as young as 6 years of age (Sizer & Whitney, 2011) as well as being linked to hypertension and heart disease.

QSEN Checkpoint Question 28.2

Evidence-Based Practice

Preventing obesity is a major health care goal worldwide. To determine if preschoolers are aware of what an average weight child looks like in contrast to one who is overweight, nurse researchers recruited 17 children between 4 and 5 years of age from preschool settings; each child was weighed and measured for height so their body mass index (BMI) could be calculated, then shown images of children of various body shapes and sizes. All the children were able to correctly identify the body shape that depicted an overweight child as if they understood the concept of overweight. When asked if they liked their own body shape, however, even those who were overweight, answered, "yes" or apparently had difficulty applying the concept of overweight to themselves (Burgess & Broome, 2012).

Based on the study, which statement by John, who is overweight (as is his mother), would be typical?

a. "No one looks fat in my family."
b. "I like the way I look in my uniform."
c. "We look like the people in these pictures."
d. "People shouldn't worry about what they look like."

Look in Appendix A for the best answer and rationale.

Nutrition Guidelines for a Healthy Diet. Basic guidelines for a healthy diet have been outlined by a variety of governmental groups, including the U.S. Department of Agriculture (DOA) and the DHHS. In 1992, a food guide pyramid was developed to illustrate these guidelines. In 2010, this was updated and changed to the photo of a plate of food to better illustrate what a plate of healthy food looks like along with emphasizing the importance of variety, moderation, and balance (DOA, 2012). Figure 13.1 in Chapter 13 shows the MyPlate diagram. Table 28.1 lists recommended servings for children from the five food groups that MyPlate features. In addition, good nutrition in children should follow a number of "healthy eating" guidelines, including the following:

- **Eat a variety of foods.** Choices from all food groups—dairy, protein, fruits, vegetables, cereals, and grains—should be included in meals every day. It is also important to vary choices within each food group, because not all foods within a group are nutritionally equivalent.

TABLE 28.1 Servings of the Five MyPlate Food Groups for Children

Group	Examples of Foods	Recommended Daily Amounts: Children 2–6 Years of Age	Recommended Daily Amounts: Older Children	Major Nutrients Provided By the Food Group
Grains	Cereals, rice, pasta (best if whole-grain and enriched)	6 servings	6–11 servings	Thiamine, niacin, riboflavin (if enriched), iron (if enriched), incomplete protein, carbohydrates
Vegetables	Vegetables (yellow and green)	3 servings	3–5 servings	Vitamin A, iron, calcium, carbohydrates (include vitamin A source at least every other day)
Fruit	Oranges, apples, lemons	2 servings	2–4 servings	Vitamin C (include vitamin C daily), carbohydrates
Dairy	Whole milk and other milk products such as yogurt and cheese	2 servings	2–3 servings	Calcium, phosphorus, complete protein, riboflavin, niacin, vitamin D (if vitamin D–fortified milk used), fats
Protein	Muscle meats (veal, beef, pork) dry beans, eggs, fish, poultry	2 servings	2–3 servings	Complete protein, iron, thiamine, riboflavin, niacin, vitamin B_{12}, fats

Data from U. S. Department of Agriculture. (2012). *Choose MyPlate: A guide to daily food choices.* Washington, DC: Author.

- **Balance the food you eat with physical activity, and maintain or improve your weight.** Although the tendency for obesity may be inherited, being overweight in early life also appears to play a long-term role. Urge parents to be certain their infants receive all the nutrients they need for the substantial growth they are undergoing (including a percentage of fat, because this is important for myelination of nerves); at the same time, it is important that infants not be overfed so they do not become obese (Kmietowicz, 2012). Physical activity, balanced with calcium intake, is the secret to strong bones and the reduction of osteoporosis (Jones, 2011).
- **Choose a diet with plenty of grain products, vegetables, and fruits.** Foods with starch and fiber are more beneficial for gastrointestinal function than more processed foods. Fiber, in particular, has been linked to the lowered incidence of a variety of illnesses such as constipation and perhaps colon cancer in later life (Brownawell, Caers, Gibson, et al., 2012). Fiber can be included as early as during preschool years in the form of whole-grain cereals and raw fruits such as apples.
- **Choose a diet low in fat, saturated fat, and cholesterol.** The American diet has changed substantially over the past 10 years to reflect this important goal. Many families now consume low-fat diets, substituting nonfat milk for whole milk, decreasing their consumption of eggs and other high-cholesterol sources, and reducing their consumption of red meat. For children, fat intake does not need to be restricted for the first 2 years of life because fat is necessary for myelination of spinal nerves. Thereafter, fat intake can be tailored to meet the guidelines of 30% of total intake (saturated fat should be less than 7% of total intake) for both children and adults.
- **Choose a diet moderate in sugars.** Too much sugar in a diet can contribute to both dental caries and obesity (Danyliw, Vatanparast, Nikpartow, et al., 2012). In addition, refined sugar such as is used in soft drinks, prepared foods, candy, and chocolate represents "empty" calories, or is high in calories yet provides no essential nutrients. Although children need adequate carbohydrates for energy, parents can give their children a good start by preventing excessive sugar intake.
- **Choose a diet moderate in salt and sodium.** The taste for salt is acquired and plays a role in both heart disease and hypertension. If unsalted or only lightly salted solid food is offered to infants from the time they begin solid food, they do not develop a desire for heavily salted foods. It is helpful to assess the diet of school-age children and check whether they are eating a diet heavier in salt than necessary because of the availability of many salty after-school snacks.
- **If drinking alcoholic beverages, do so in moderation.** Adolescents are at increased risk for establishing unhealthy patterns of alcohol use, particularly binge drinking, as they begin to explore adult life. Educating them about the long-term consequences, such as liver disease, from long-term alcohol use is as important as educating them on the importance of healthy nutrition to help ensure proper growth (see Chapter 33 for a discussion of adolescents).

Components of a Healthy Diet. Eating a variety of foods from all five MyPlate food groups in moderation is a way of guaranteeing the intake of a balanced diet of proteins, carbohydrates, fats, vitamins, and minerals (Fig. 28.3).

Protein. Protein is the major component of bones, skin, hair, and muscle and is responsible for a wide variety of essential functions in the body. Because it is essential for growth, protein intake is crucial for children. Complete proteins contain all amino acids; incomplete proteins do not, but combining two types of incomplete proteins (e.g., pasta and beans) allows the body to construct complete proteins.

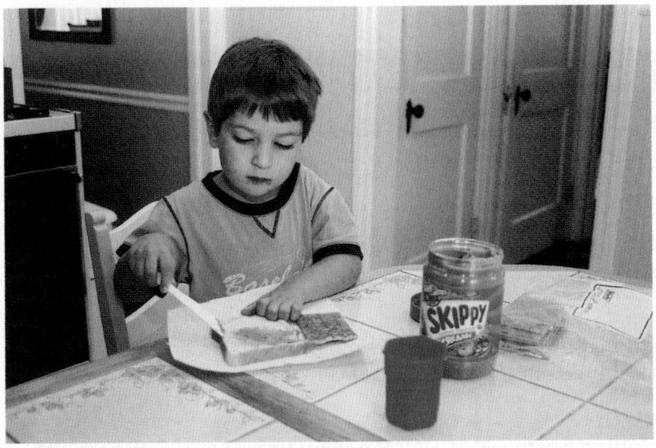

FIGURE 28.3 Good nutritional habits developed early in life provide a child with a health advantage.

Carbohydrate. Carbohydrates are the main and preferred fuel of the body to supply energy, so they are essential to the functioning of body systems and the neurologic system, in particular. This makes carbohydrates vitally important to infants and toddlers, because their brain cells are actively growing. As all athletes learn, sugar supplies an immediate but short-term source of energy; starches, as a rule, supply sustained energy.

Fat. Dietary fat is a second source of energy for the body. It can be an immediate energy source or can be stored if not used, then released when energy is required. Some fat deposits also serve as insulating material for subcutaneous tissues; in infants, fats are necessary to ensure myelination of nerve fibers.

Vitamins. Vitamins are organic compounds essential for specific metabolic actions in cells. They do not produce energy but are needed by cells to produce energy. For children, fat-soluble vitamins (A, D, K, and E) are mainly supplied by fortified dairy products, fortified cereals, and plant or fish oils. Such vitamins are not absorbed from the gastrointestinal tract by themselves but only if accompanied by fat molecules, which is why fish and plant oils are such good sources of these. Once absorbed, they are used by the cells for growth and function or are stored in the liver or fat cells for later use. Because fat-soluble vitamins can be stored by the body this way, an infant or child can ingest too many of them, although overdosing usually occurs from overuse of supplements rather than from dietary sources.

Water-soluble vitamins (B complex and C) do not need fat for absorption and are not stored well in the body, so they must be taken daily to maintain effective levels in the body. They are found most abundantly in fruits and vegetables. Sources and functions of all the essential vitamins and results of their deficiencies are summarized in Table 28.2.

Minerals. Minerals are necessary for building new cells as well as for the regulation of body processes such as fluid and electrolyte balance, nerve transmission, and muscle contractions, making them vital for optimal health in a growing infant or child. Minerals are classified according to the amounts needed daily. If more than 100 mg is needed daily, a mineral is a *macronutrient* (a major mineral). If the amount needed is less than 100 mg, it is a minor mineral or *micronutrient.* Trace minerals refer to those needed in only extremely small amounts. Sources and functions of various minerals and results of their deficiencies are shown in Table 28.3.

Promoting Adequate Nutritional Intake in Vegetarian Diets. Increasing numbers of adults of childrearing age are vegetarians; therefore, many women during pregnancy and children during their years of most rapid growth eat such diets (Krebs & Primak, 2011). Families select vegetarian diets for many reasons, including:

- Ecologic: If everyone ate lower on the food chain, world hunger could be reduced.
- Medical or health related: Avoiding animal foods stops the ingestion of hormones and chemicals used in meat and poultry production as well as lowers serum cholesterol and saturated fat, thereby reducing the frequency of atherosclerosis and obesity.
- Philosophical: They may hold a belief that killing animals for food is unnecessary or wrong.
- Religious: Religions such as Hinduism and Seventh-Day Adventist promote a vegetarian lifestyle. Islam and Judaism also have some restrictions on what meat can be eaten.
- Economic: Vegetables and grains are less expensive than animal-based food.

Although a balanced vegetarian diet is sufficient during childhood, careful assessment and family education may be necessary to ensure a child's intake is adequate for growth. Urge parents to become knowledgeable about good nutrition so they are aware of ways to include essential nutrients in vegetarian diets for growing children, particularly if their children participate in active sports.

Five main types of vegetarian diets commonly seen include:

- The lacto-ovo-vegetarian diet, which includes dairy products ("lacto"), eggs ("ovo"), and plants (vegetables, fruits, and grains).
- The ovovegetarian diet, which includes eggs but excludes dairy products.
- The lacto-vegetarian diet, which includes dairy products but excludes eggs.
- The vegan diet, which excludes all animal products and consists of only vegetables, fruits, and grains.
- The macrobiotic diet, which is a primarily vegetarian diet. Its main sources of protein are grains, seeds, and nuts, but small quantities of egg, fish, and wild game can be added.

The vegan diet is obviously the most restrictive of these diets, so it is usually recommended that parents be extremely conscientious about including a variety of foods to help ensure their children are receiving adequate nutrients. All families who eat vegetarian diets need to be conscientious that their children receive adequate amounts of several specific nutrients.

Protein. Lacto-ovo-vegetarian, ovovegetarian, and lacto-vegetarian diets provide all of the essential amino acids for growth (both eggs and dairy products provide complete proteins). Vegan diets can also supply essential amino acids by cereal and legume combinations such as peanut butter and wheat bread, corn and lima beans, pasta and beans, corn tortillas and beans, or chickpeas and sesame seeds. Complementary proteins do not have to be eaten at the same meal to be effective, as long as varied plant proteins are consumed over the course of a day.

Calcium. Dairy products such as milk and cheese supply the usual source of calcium for children. When dairy products are not eaten, calcium must be obtained from other sources such as green leafy vegetables (broccoli, spinach, or grain products) or calcium-fortified tofu or soy flour.

TABLE 28.2 Vitamins Essential for Health

Vitamin	Selected Dietary Sources	Function in Body	Results of Deficiency
Fat Soluble			
A (retinol)	Liver, carrots, spinach	Important for night vision and corneal integrity and growth	Keratinization of the eye (xerophthalmia) and blindness
D	Egg yolk, margarine, salmon, fortified milk, fortified cereals	Regulates absorption of calcium and phosphorus for bone growth	Rickets (bone deformity) in growing children
E	Margarine, corn oil, peanuts	An antioxidant that protects red blood cells from destruction by oxygen	In immature infants, severe anemia from destruction of red blood cells
K	Cabbage, spinach, pork, best source: green leafy vegetables	Aids blood clotting (synthesis of prothrombin)	Bleeding from lack of sufficient clotting action
Water Soluble			
B complex:			
Thiamine	Wheat germ, yeast, pork	Important for use of glucose in cells	Beriberi, a disease that causes nerve paralysis
Riboflavin	Beef, chicken, liver, avocados, milk	Breaks down fatty acids and amino acids for energy	Red swollen tongue, inflamed eyes, fissures of lips
Niacin	Peanuts, rice bran, liver	Converts glucose to energy; involved in carbohydrate, protein, and fat metabolism	Pellagra (diarrhea, mental confusion, dermatitis, death)
B_6 (pyridoxine)	Liver, herring, salmon, chicken, fish, pork, eggs	Metabolizes amino acids and glucose	Neuritis, depression, nausea, vomiting
B_{12} (cobalamin)	Lamb, beef kidney, egg yolk, animal products	Blood formation; DNA and RNA synthesis; myelin formation; carbohydrate, protein, and fat metabolism	Macrocytic, megaloblastic anemia (large, nonfunctioning red blood cells)
Folic acid (folacin)	Liver, asparagus, bran	Red and white blood cell structure	Poor red blood cell formation
C (ascorbic acid)	Broccoli, collards, citrus fruit	Collagen structure, antioxidant	Scurvy (weakness, easy bleeding, joint pain)

All fat-soluble vitamins can be absorbed only in the presence of lipids and can be transported only in the presence of protein.

Iron. Because there may be an association between iron-deficiency anemia and learning deficits, children need to consume good sources of iron (Black, Quigg, Hurley, et al., 2011). Meat is the richest source of iron. With meat omitted from a diet, parents should include this from foods such as legumes, whole grains, fortified cereals, dark-green leafy vegetables, or dried fruits. Vitamin C enhances the duodenal absorption of iron found in plants, so eating fruits and vegetables rich in vitamin C such as oranges or broccoli aids iron absorption.

Vitamins. Vitamin B_{12} is unique among vitamins because it is present only in animal products (Whitney & Rolfes, 2012). This includes eggs and milk. Children who totally omit animal sources, therefore, need to have this vitamin supplemented daily. Reliable supplements of B_{12} include vitamin B_{12} tablets or fortified foods such as commercial breakfast cereals, soy beverages, and some brands of nutritional yeast.

Riboflavin is a B vitamin normally supplied by fortified milk. When dairy products are not eaten, it can be supplied by soy milk, vegetables, or brewer's yeast, all of which contain all the B vitamins except B_{12}. Good sources of riboflavin in vegan diets are whole and enriched grains and cereals, nuts, and dark-green leafy vegetables.

Vitamin D is necessary for calcium and phosphorus metabolism and is normally supplied in fortified milk. It is not present in plant foods and therefore must be supplemented in a vegan or ovovegetarian diet by vitamin D drops or tablets. Exposure to sunshine also supplies vitamin D but is generally an inadequate source (Whitney & Rolfes, 2012).

Minerals. Zinc is present primarily in animal foods but is also present in brewer's yeast, nuts, and wheat germ; therefore, zinc deficiency is not a problem with vegetarian diets. Iodine is supplied normally by seafood. In a vegan or vegetarian diet,

TABLE 28.3 Minerals Essential for Health

Mineral	Selected Dietary Sources	Function in Body	Results of Deficiency or Excess
Macronutrients			
Calcium	Milk, hard cheese	Formation of bone and teeth, muscle contractility	Improper bone growth and maintenance shown by diseases such as rickets in children
Phosphorus	Milk, meats	Formation of bone and teeth, used in cell structure, aids use of glucose	Deficiency unlikely as long as calcium and protein needs are met
Sodium	Table salt	Regulates fluid volume and pH	Deficiency rare but excess leads to hypertension in genetically determined individuals
Chloride	Table salt	Formation of hydrochloric acid, regulates body fluid with sodium	Deficiency rare except with vomiting, which causes loss of hydrochloric acid
Potassium	Meats, dried fruits	Major cation of cells, essential for electrical conduction in muscle and therefore in heart action	Deficiency leading to muscle weakness and heart irritability, occurs in people taking diuretics because potassium is excreted with urine
Sulfur	Milk, meat, eggs	Essential for protein formation and cell growth	Deficiency rare as long as protein intake is adequate
Magnesium	Cocoa, nuts, green leafy vegetables	Relaxation of muscles after contraction	Deficiency leads to muscle contraction
Micronutrients			
Iodine	Seafood, dairy, iodized salt	Formation of thyroxine and regulation of metabolic rate	Reduced basal metabolic rate, goiter (enlarged thyroid gland)
Iron	Meats, fish, dried fruits, nuts, fortified cereals	Formation of hemoglobin, transport of oxygen to body cells	Deficiency leads to microcytic (small) and hypochromic (pale) red blood cells (iron-deficiency anemia); excess leads to infiltration of tissue (hemosiderosis)
Copper	Nuts, raisins, legumes	Formation of collagen and nerve fibers	Anemia, neutropenia, and severe bone demineralization
Fluoride	Fluoridated water	Reduces dental caries and demineralization from bone	Dental caries
Zinc	Meat, eggs, seafood	Formation of eyes, male reproductive organs, insulin, and taste sensation	Diabetes-like symptoms because of decreased insulin production, poor taste sensation leading to poor food intake
Manganese	Nuts, grains, legumes	Formation of enzymes	Deficiency unlikely
Molybdenum	Organ meats, grains	Mobilizes iron in body	Deficiency apparently unknown
Cobalt	Many sources	Formation of red blood cells in bone marrow	Deficiency rare as long as animal food sources are ingested
Selenium	Seafood, kidney, liver	Immunoglobulin formation and prevention of oxidation of cells	Deficiency unknown
Chromium	Meat, cheese, grains	Glucose metabolism	Deficiency seen only in severe malnutrition
Silicon	Many sources	Aids growth of connective tissue and bone	Retarded growth and bone deformity
Nickel	Many sources	Duplication of growth of cells	Has not been determined to be essential for health in humans
Vanadium	Many sources	Lipid metabolism	Has not been determined to be essential for health in humans
Tin	Many sources	Blood formation	Has not been determined to be essential for health in humans

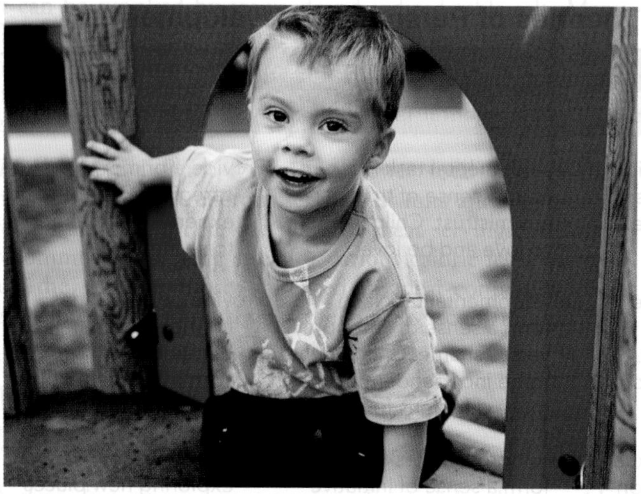

FIGURE 28.4 A toddler enjoys active, independent exploration as part of building a sense of autonomy. Here, a boy plays outdoors on playground equipment, a setting that allows for independent decision making.

however, this enforces a sense of shame and doubt. The more children are not allowed to do things they want to do, the more they begin to doubt their ability to do them, and eventually, they will stop trying to accomplish. If children leave this stage with less autonomy than shame or doubt, they can be disabled in their attempts to achieve independence and can lack confidence in their abilities to achieve well into adolescence and adulthood (Fig. 28.4).

What if... 28.2 John's parents repeat that they find him cold and unloving. You know he lived in a series of foster homes before he was adopted into their family. What developmental task has John been unable to complete? Could it be related to the frequent moves? What actions could you recommend his new parents take to try to strengthen his unfulfilled developmental task at this point?

The Preschooler

The developmental task of the preschool period is learning **initiative versus guilt**, or learning how to do things. Children initiate motor activities of various sorts on their own, or no longer merely respond to or imitate the actions of other children or their parents. The same is true for language and fantasy activities.

Another word for initiative is creativity. Whether children leave this stage with a sense of initiative outweighing a sense of guilt depends largely on how parents respond to self-initiated activities. When children are given much freedom and opportunity to initiate motor play such as running, bike riding, sliding, and wrestling or are exposed to such play materials as finger paints, sand, water, and modeling clay, their sense of initiative is reinforced. Initiative is also encouraged when parents answer a child's questions (intellectual initiative) and do not inhibit fantasy or play activity. In contrast, if children are made to feel their motor activity is bad (perhaps in a small apartment or in a hospital), their questions are a nuisance, or their play is silly, they can develop a sense of guilt over self-initiated activities that will persist in later life. Those who do not develop initiative have limited brainstorming and problem-solving skills later in life; instead, they wait for clues or guidance from others before acting. They may also be unable to use simulated learning effectively (Rutherford-Hemming, 2012).

The School-Age Child

Erikson viewed the developmental task of the school-age period as developing **industry versus inferiority**, or accomplishment rather than inferiority. During the preschool period, children learned initiative (i.e., how to do things). During school age, children learn how to do things *well.* A school-age child, while doing a project, will ask, "Am I doing this right? Is it okay to use blue?" When they are encouraged in their efforts to do practical tasks or make practical things and are praised and rewarded for the finished results, their sense of industry grows (Fig. 28.5). Parents who see their children's efforts at making and doing things as merely "busy work" or who do not show appreciation for their children's efforts may cause them to develop a sense of inferiority rather than pride and accomplishment.

During this stage of life, a child's world grows to include the school and community; success or failure in those settings can have as lasting an impact as experiences at home. Children with an intelligence quotient of 80 or 90 (slightly below normal), for example, may have a learning style so different from the average child's that they have difficulty competing. This leads to repeated failures in their efforts to learn and reinforces a sense of inferiority even when their sense of industry has been rewarded and encouraged at home. However, children whose sense of industry has not been supported at home may have it revitalized at school through the efforts of a committed teacher. A nurse during a hospitalization could also fulfill this role.

What if... 28.3 John's father does not allow his 3-year-old twins to play with finger paints. If they play with crayons, he insists they color between the lines. According to Erikson, which is more important for preschoolers: allowing free play or teaching children that neatness and accuracy count?

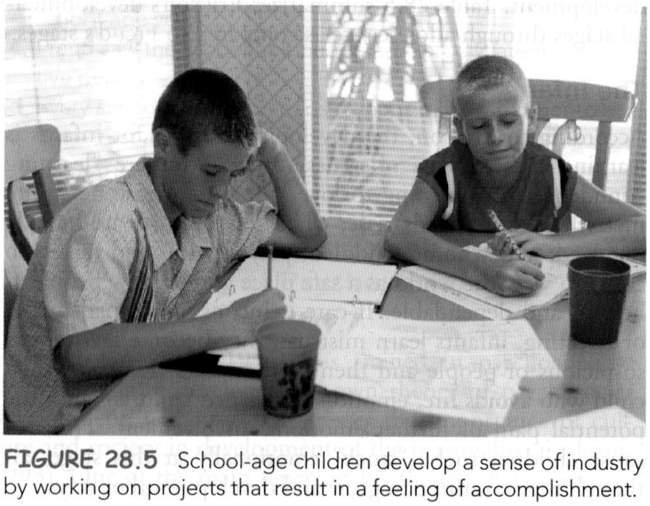

FIGURE 28.5 School-age children develop a sense of industry by working on projects that result in a feeling of accomplishment.

The Adolescent

The new interpersonal dimension that emerges during adolescence is the development of a sense of **identity versus role confusion**. To achieve this, adolescents must bring together everything they have learned about themselves as a son or daughter, an athlete, a friend, a fast-food cook, a student, a garage band musician, and so on, and integrate these different images into a whole that makes sense. If adolescents cannot do so, they are left with role confusion, or are left unsure of what kind of person they are or what kind of person they want to become. Some adolescents may seek a negative identity: being identified as a drug abuser or runaway is not a positive identification but may be preferable to seemingly having no identity at all. Body piercing and tattooing are ways adolescents can help establish their identity because they are outward expressions of who adolescents think they are (Fig. 28.6).

The Young Adult

The developmental crisis of the young adult is achieving a sense of **intimacy versus isolation**. Intimacy is the ability to relate well with other people, not only with members of the opposite sex but also with one's own sex to form long-lasting friendships.

A sense of intimacy grows out of earlier developmental tasks because people need a strong sense of identity before they can reach out fully and offer deep friendship or love to others. Because there is always the risk of being rejected or hurt when offering love or friendship, individuals cannot offer it if they do not have confidence that they can cope with rejection or if they did not develop a sense of trust as an infant or autonomy as a toddler. This is important for maternal and child health nursing because parents without a sense of intimacy may have more difficulty than others accepting a pregnancy and beginning to love a new child.

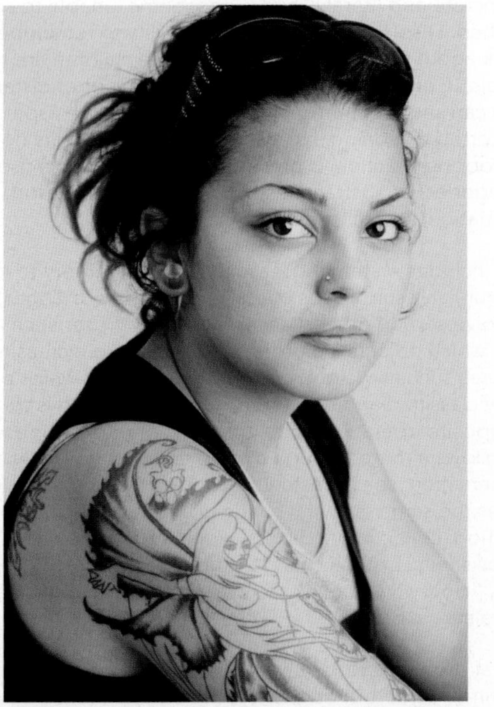

FIGURE 28.6 Adolescents express their identity in different ways. Body piercing and tattoos makes a strong statement.

QSEN Checkpoint Question 28.4

Quality Improvement

John, 6 years old, is a school-age child. According to Erikson, health promotion activities should integrate what developmental task of this period?

a. How to be creative
b. How to think abstractly
c. How to trust others
d. How to do things well

Look in Appendix A for the best answer and rationale.

The Middle-Aged Adult

The developmental task of middle age is to establish a sense of **generativity versus stagnation**. During this time, people extend their concern from just themselves and their families to the community and the world. They may become politically active, work to solve environmental concerns, or participate in far-reaching community or world-based decisions.

People with a sense of generativity are self-confident and better able to juggle their various lives (e.g., mother, soccer coach, church member, teacher, political party chairperson, gourmet cook). People without this sense become stagnated or self-absorbed. Those who have devoted themselves to only one role are more likely to find themselves at the end of middle age with a narrow perspective and lack of ability to cope with change. Women without a sense of generativity may have more difficulty than others accepting life changes such as a late-in-life pregnancy or a rebellious adolescent.

The Older Adult

Older adults play a role in childrearing because many of them give child care to grandchildren while the parents work. The developmental task of older adults is **integrity versus despair**. Older adults with integrity feel good about the life choices they have made; those with a feeling of despair wish life could begin over again so things could turn out differently. A sense of integrity is helpful in a grandparent, because it helps children to develop a sense of trust and to learn initiative (Newman & Newman, 2011).

A Criticism of Erikson's Theory

Erikson's main contribution to human development was the creation of stages, so that development can be broken down into separate phases for study. A criticism of his theory is that life does not occur in easily divided stages, and trying to divide it that way can create superficial divisions.

Piaget's Theory of Cognitive Development

Jean Piaget (1896–1980), a Swiss psychologist, introduced concepts of cognitive development, or the way children learn and think. The theory has roots similar to those of both Freud and Erikson, but with differing aspects (Piaget, 1961). Piaget defined four stages of cognitive development, within the stages of growth, then finer units or **schemas**. To progress from one period to the next, children reorganize their thinking processes to bring them closer to adult thinking. These stages of cognitive development are summarized in Table 28.6.

The Infant

Piaget referred to the infant stage as the **sensorimotor stage**. Sensorimotor intelligence is practical intelligence because an infant is not yet able to use words and symbols for thinking and problem solving at this early age. At the beginning of life, babies relate to the world through their senses, using only reflex behavior. During this stage, infants learn objects in the environment—their bottle, blocks, their bed, or even a parent—are permanent and continue to exist even though they are out of sight or changed in some way. For example:

- Infants will search for a block hidden by a blanket, knowing the block still exists.

TABLE 28.6 Piaget's Stages of Cognitive Development

Stage of Development	Age Span	Nursing Implications
Sensorimotor		
Neonatal reflex	1 month	Stimuli are assimilated into beginning mental images. Behavior entirely reflexive.
Primary circular reaction	1–4 months	Hand–mouth and ear–eye coordination develop. Enjoyable activity for this period: a rattle or tape of parent's voice.
Secondary circular reaction	4–8 months	Infant learns to initiate, recognize, and repeat pleasurable experiences from environment. Good toy for this period: mirror; good game: peek-a-boo.
Coordination of secondary reactions	8–12 months	Infant can plan activities to attain specific goals. Good toy for this period: nesting toys (i.e., colored boxes).
Tertiary circular reaction	12–18 months	Child is able to experiment to discover new properties of objects and events. Good game for this period: throw and retrieve.
Invention of new means through mental combinations	18–24 months	Transitional phase to the preoperational thought period. Good toys for this period: those with several uses, such as blocks or colored plastic rings.
Preoperational thought	2–7 years	Thought becomes more symbolic; can arrive at answers mentally instead of through physical attempt. Comprehends simple abstractions but thinking is basically concrete and literal. Child is egocentric (unable to see the viewpoint of another). Displays static thinking (inability to remember what they started to talk about so at the end of a sentence children are talking about another topic). Concept of time is now, and concept of distance is only as far as they can see. Centering or focusing on a single aspect of an object causes distorted reasoning. No awareness of reversibility (for every action there is an opposite action) is present. Unable to state cause–effect relationships, categories, or abstractions. Good toy for this period: items that require imagination, such as modeling clay.
Concrete operational thought	7–12 years	Concrete operations includes systematic reasoning. Uses memory to learn broad concepts (fruit) and subgroups of concepts (apples, oranges). Classifications involve sorting objects according to attributes such as color; seriation, in which objects are ordered according to increasing or decreasing measures such as weight; and multiplication, in which objects are simultaneously classified and seriated using weight. Child is aware of reversibility, an opposite operation or continuation of reasoning back to a starting point (follows a route through a maze and then reverses steps). Understands conservation, sees constancy despite transformation (mass or quantity remains the same even if it changes shape or position). Good activity for this period: collecting and classifying natural objects such as native plants or sea shells. Expose child to other viewpoints by asking questions such as, "How do you think you'd feel if you were a nurse and had to tell a boy to stay in bed?"
Formal operational thought	12 years	Can solve hypothetical problems with scientific reasoning. Good activity for this period: "talk time" to sort through attitudes and opinions.

From Piaget, J. (1961). *The growth of logical thinking from childhood to adolescence.* New York, NY: Basic Books, with permission.

- Infants can recognize a parent remains the same person whether dressed in a robe and slippers or pants and a T-shirt.
- Infants are only ready to play peek-a-boo when they've mastered permanence because only then do they realize the person playing with them exists behind his or her hands.
- Infants identify that they are a separate entity from objects. They learn where their body stops and their bed, playthings, or parent begins.

A great deal of the mouthing and handling of objects by infants and the delight of watching a caregiver appear is part of discovering **permanence**. The world begins to make sense and the developmental task of achieving trust falls into place when the concept of permanence has been learned (i.e., infants know their parents exist and will return to them). Gaining a concept of permanence also contributes to "eighth-month anxiety," a stage in which infants continue to cry for their parents because they know their parents still exist even when out of sight.

The Toddler

The toddler period is one of transition as children complete the final stages of the sensorimotor period and begin to develop some cognitive skills of the *preoperative* period, such as symbolic thought and egocentric thinking. Children use trial and error to discover new characteristics of objects and events. A toddler sitting in a high chair who keeps dropping objects over the edge of the tray is exploring both permanence and the different actions of toys. A toddler following a ball that has rolled under a coffee table no longer has to follow the ball's path to retrieve it but can project where it will have rolled and walk around the coffee table to find it again.

Children begin to be able to use symbols to represent objects. They may have difficulty viewing one object as being different from another, however. On a walk through a department store decorated with teddy bears, for example, children are not sure whether they are seeing a succession of bears or if the same bear keeps reappearing as if it is following them through the store, asking to be taken home.

Because toddlers' thinking is limited, they draw conclusions only from obvious facts they see: Daddy is shaving; therefore he must be going to work, because he went to work after he shaved yesterday. This type of faulty reasoning (prelogical reasoning) can lead children to wrong conclusions and faulty judgment. If you made a toddler's bed yesterday and then he was taken to surgery, he may cry at the sight of you approaching his crib with clean sheets today, thinking he will have to go to surgery again.

The Preschooler

Preschool children move on to a substage of preoperational thought termed *intuitive thinking*. During this period, when young children look at an object, they are able to see only one of its characteristics (referred to as **centering**). For example, they see a banana is yellow but do not notice that it is also long. Centering is noticeable when children are learning about medicine (they observe it tastes bitter but cannot understand it is also good for them).

Centering contributes to the preschooler's lack of **conservation** (the ability to discern truth, even though physical properties change) or **reversibility** (ability to retrace steps). For example, if preschoolers see water poured from a short fat glass into a tall, thin one, they will notice only one changing characteristic. They might say there is now more water in the second glass (because the level has risen) or there is less water in the second glass (because the second glass is thinner). When the water is poured back into the first glass, they still will not understand the amount of water is unchanged, only its appearance. This immature perception leads children, as it did during the toddler period, to make faulty conclusions. It takes more years of development and practice for children to learn that when thought processes, such as knowing the amount of water did not change, and perceptions conflict, thought processes are more trustworthy.

Preschool thinking is also strongly influenced by **role fantasy**, or how children would like something to turn out. Children use **assimilation** (taking in information and changing it to fit their existing ideas) as a part of this. For example, because a child wants to go outside and play, he says the outside is calling him to come and play. Children believe their wishes are as real as facts and dreams are as real as daytime happenings during this stage. They perceive animals and even inanimate objects as being capable of thought and feelings (e.g., a dog took their doll because the dog was feeling sad, a footstool meant to trip them). This phenomenon is often called "magical thinking." Magical thinking fades as, later on, children learn **accommodation** (they change their ideas to fit reality rather than the reverse).

Egocentrism, or perceiving that one's thoughts and needs are better or more important than those of others, is also strong during the preschool period. Preschoolers cannot believe that not everyone knows facts they know; if asked, "What is your name?" they may reply, "Don't you know it?" As a part of egocentrism, preschoolers define objects mainly in relation to themselves, so a spoon is "what I eat with," not a curved metal object; a crayon is "what I write with," not an orange wax object.

QSEN Checkpoint Question 28.5

Patient-Centered Care

Suppose John, 6 years old, tells you his broken leg wants to get better. When you are choosing an accurate and empathic response, you should be aware that he is using what form of cognition?

a. Magical thinking
b. Deductive reasoning
c. Concrete operational thinking
d. Sensorial thought

Look in Appendix A for the best answer and rationale.

The School-Age Child

Piaget viewed school age as a period during which *concrete operational thought* begins because school-age children can be seen using practical solutions to everyday problems as well as begin to recognize cause-and-effect relationships. A child who understands water does not change in amount just because it is poured from one glass to another has grasped the concept of conservation. Conservation of numbers is learned as early as age 7 years, conservation of quantity at age 7 or 8 years, conservation of weight at age 9 years, and conservation of volume at age 11 years (Wadsworth, 2003). Reasoning during school age tends to be inductive or proceeds from specific to general: a school-age child holding a broken toy reasons the toy is made of plastic, and therefore all plastic toys break easily.

The Adolescent

Adolescence is the time when cognition achieves its final form, or when formal operational thought begins. When this stage is reached, adolescents are capable of thinking in terms of possibility—what could be (**abstract thought**)—rather than being limited to thinking about what already is (concrete thought). This makes it possible for adolescents to use scientific reasoning. They can use deductive reasoning in addition to the induction reasoning they used during school age or can move from the general to the specific (e.g., plastic toys break easily, the toy they are holding is plastic, therefore it will break easily).

A Criticism of Piaget's Theory

Piaget is criticized because he used only a small sample of subjects to establish his theory (his own children). Because children today begin activities to learn counting and identifying color or reading much earlier than they did at the time the theory was devised, the age groups and "norms" may no longer be accurate. Playing computer games during the preschool period will probably impact the rate and type of children's cognitive developments in the future.

QSEN Checkpoint Question 28.6

Safety

John is a school-age child but still has difficulty learning Piaget's concept of conservation. What would this imply?

a. He doesn't understand why his mother insists he recycle plastic or metal soda cans.
b. He doesn't understand that, when crossing a two-way street, he must look both right and left.
c. He feels angry because his sister's piece of pie is long and thin where his is short and fat.
d. He tries to climb up onto the roof when playing with his imaginary friend.

Look in Appendix A for the best answer and rationale.

Kohlberg's Theory of Moral Development

One more developmental theory that has relevance to maternal and child health nursing is Kohlberg's (1927–1987) theory of moral development. A German psychologist, Kohlberg studied the reasoning ability of boys and, based on Piaget's development stages, developed a theory on the way children gain knowledge of right and wrong or moral reasoning. These stages, as described by Kohlberg (1984), are summarized in Table 28.7.

TABLE 28.7 Kohlberg's Stages of Moral Development

Age (in Years)	Stage	Description	Nursing Implications
Preconventional (Level I)			
2–3	1	Punishment/obedience orientation ("heteronymous morality"). Child does right because a parent tells him or her to and to avoid punishment.	Child needs help to determine what are right actions. Give clear instructions to avoid confusion.
4–7	2	Individualism. Instrumental purpose and exchange. Carries out actions to satisfy own needs rather than society's. Will do something for another if that person does something for him or her.	Child is unable to recognize that like situations require like actions. Unable to take responsibility for self-care, because meeting own needs interferes with this.
Conventional (Level II)			
7–10	3	Orientation to interpersonal relations of mutuality. Child follows rules because of a need to be a "good" person in own eyes and eyes of others.	Child enjoys helping others because this is "nice" behavior. Allow child to help with bed making and other such activities. Praise for desired behavior such as sharing.
10–12	4	Maintenance of social order, fixed rules, and authority. Child finds following rules satisfying. Follows rules of authority figures as well as parents in an effort to keep the "system" working.	Child often asks what are the rules and if something is "right." May have difficulty modifying a procedure because one method may not be "right." Follows self-care measures only if someone is there to enforce them.
Postconventional (Level III)			
Older than 12	5	Social contract, utilitarian law-making perspectives. Follows standards of society for the good of all people.	Adolescents can be responsible for self-care because they view this as a standard of adult behavior.
Older than 12	6	Universal ethical principle orientation. Follows internalized standards of conduct.	Many adults do not reach this level of moral development.

From Kohlberg, L. (1984). *The psychology of moral development.* New York, NY: Harper & Row, with permission.

Recognizing where a child is developmentally according to these stages can help identify how children may feel about an illness such as whether they think it is fair that they are ill. Recognizing moral reasoning also helps determine whether children can be depended on to carry out self-care activities such as administering their own medicine or whether children have internalized standards of conduct so they do not "cheat" when away from external control. Moral stages closely approximate cognitive stages of development because children must be able to think abstractly (be able to conceptualize an idea without a concrete picture) before being able to understand how rules apply even when no one is there to enforce them (Juujärvi, Pesso, & Myyry, 2011).

A Criticism of Kohlberg's Theory

Kohlberg's theory is frequently challenged as being male-oriented because his original research was conducted entirely with boys. Carol Gilligan (1993), a sociologist, argues that there are two modes of moral reasoning: the ethic of justice that focuses on individual rights, and the ethic of care that focuses on responsibilities in relationships. She suggests that girls may not score well on Kohlberg's scale because, being more concerned with relationships than are boys, they make moral decisions based on individual circumstances or the effect of their actions on others at a much younger age than boys, which skews their results on a standard male-influenced scale.

USING GROWTH AND DEVELOPMENT IN PRACTICE

An assessment of children's growth and development should be included in all children's nursing care plans because whether they are growing and developing within usual parameters is a significant mark of wellness. Because nurses do not work alone but as members of a health care team, Box 28.6 shows an interprofessional care map illustrating both nursing and team planning for supporting a child's growth and development.

BOX 28.6 Nursing Care Planning

AN INTERPROFESSIONAL CARE MAP FOR A CHILD WITH A DEVELOPMENTAL CONCERN

John Olson is a 6-year-old, mildly overweight boy brought into an emergency department because his leg is broken from a bicycle accident. His parents tell you that, although John has lived with them for 3 years, they find him cold and unloving. They ask you what they can do to change this.

Family Assessment Family lives in a three-bedroom house in suburbs. Father works as a plumber; mother has a part-time job as a substitute grade-school teacher.

Client Assessment At 4 months of age, John was taken away from his mother because she was not caring for him adequately. He was then moved back and forth among 12 different foster homes until he was finally adopted at age 3.5 years. His adoptive parents have 3-year-old twins of their own.

Nursing Diagnosis Interrupted family processes related to inability of child to meet parents' developmental expectations

Outcome Criteria Child demonstrates greater participation in family activities and improved response to parents' attempts to bond with him by 3 months' time.

Team Member Responsible	Assessment	Intervention	Rationale	Expected Outcome
Activities of Daily Living, Including Safety				
Nurse	Assess if family has thought through impact of bicycle accident on child's daily activities.	Suggest some obvious accommodations needed for cast care (e.g., no tub bathing, difficulty with stairs, no bike riding).	If a family is already under stress, an accident can compound family concerns.	Family members state they realize accidents are not anyone's "fault"; and are prepared to make adjustments needed.
Teamwork and Collaboration				
Nurse/Primary care provider	Assess if parents feel psychological counseling would be appropriate for child.	Assist parents with gaining a consultation if they feel they would welcome this.	Consultation with a skilled professional can offer parents information on specific actions to take.	Parents state whether they feel situation merits more skilled help at this time.

(continued on page 808)

BOX 28.6 Nursing Care Planning (continued)

Procedures/Medications				
Nurse/Primary care provider	Assess what emergency actions are necessary for a child with a fractured tibia.	Apply cast; give instructions for cast care. Keep pain or discomfort to a minimum.	Definite measures to prevent pain are important in promoting a sense of trust.	Client states he understands cast care; and states emergency department experience was at best an adventure, and at worst, not an ordeal.
Nutrition				
Nurse	Obtain a 24-hour recall dietary history to assess for usual calcium and vitamin D intake.	Suggest additional sources of calcium or vitamin D if needed.	Calcium is important for good bone healing and is absorbed best in the presence of vitamin D.	Client states he understands calcium will help healing and is willing to ingest more if needed.
Patient-Centered Care				
Nurse	Assess what parents understand about the development of trust in early life.	Suggest ways to initiate a sense of trust by demonstrating dependability and a warm, loving relationship.	Even if a sense of trust is not achieved as an infant, it can be achieved at a later developmental stage.	Parents state they are willing to identify and begin more active steps toward improving relationship with son.
Psychosocial/Spiritual/Emotional Needs				
Nurse	Assess what type of ideal child parents thought they were adopting.	Suggest measures that could bring parents and child closer together such as a "game night," always eating meals together, or quiet "talk times" before bed.	Identifying differences between expectations and reality can help people understand dissatisfactions.	Client and parents state they are willing to begin an active program of shared activities.
Informatics for Seamless Health Care Planning				
Nurse	Assess if client or parents have "walked through a day" to identify their child's needs after returning home.	Discuss with client and parents adjustments they recognize client will have to make to attend school with a cast in place.	Small needs not met can grow into major needs before a return appointment and can interfere further with a sense of trust.	Client and parents state they understand adjustments that need to be made and will work them out together with child.

What if... 28.4 You are interested in exploring one of the 2020 National Health Goals related to growth and development (see Box 28.1). Most government-sponsored money for nursing research is allotted based on these goals. What would be a possible research topic to explore pertinent to these goals that would be applicable to the Olson family and that would also advance evidence-based practice?

KEY POINTS FOR REVIEW

- Knowledge of growth and development is important in health promotion and illness prevention because it lays the basis for assessments and anticipatory guidance.
- Including growth and development guidelines in nursing care helps to achieve care that not only meets QSEN competencies but that also best meets a family's total needs.
- Genetic factors that influence growth and development are gender, ethnicity, intelligence, and health.
- Environmental influences include quality of nutrition, socioeconomic level, the parent–child relationship, ordinal position in the family, and environmental health.
- To meet growth and development milestones, children (like adults) need to follow basic guidelines for a healthy diet, such as eating a variety of foods, maintaining an ideal weight, avoiding extreme levels of saturated fat, eating foods with adequate starch and fiber, and avoiding too much sugar.
- Temperament is a child's characteristic manner of thinking, behaving, or reacting. Helping parents understand the effect of temperament is a nursing role.

- Common theories of development are Freud's psychoanalytic theory and Erikson's theory of psychosocial development. Both of these theories describe specific tasks children must complete at each stage of development to become a well-adapted adult.
- Piaget's theory of cognitive development describes ways children learn.
- Kohlberg advanced a theory of moral development, or how children use moral reasoning to solve problems.
- Although growth and development occur in known patterns, the rate that a child develops and grows varies from child to child. Caution parents not to be concerned that two siblings are very different as long as they both fit within usual parameters.

Critical Thinking Care Study

Andrew is a preschooler who "hates" his first days at preschool. He lives with his mother Berkley, a calculus teacher; his father Edgar, a physicist; and Molly, his 5-day-old baby sister. His mother is disappointed at his reaction to school. She tells you, "We worked so hard to prepare him for school. Taught him his whole alphabet and how to count to 100. He's so excited about learning he wanted to practice writing his name rather than go to a friend's birthday party." She asks you what could be wrong. How can she make his first school experience better?

1. What additional information would you like to know before you advise his mother? What are some reasons you can think of as to why he might not be enjoying preschool?
2. Could temperament be playing a role in why Andrew is not fitting in well at preschool? Are there other indications he doesn't approach new situations well?
3. As a preschooler, should Andrew be interested in exploring new things and going new places? Is there a reason he doesn't want to leave his house to go to school just now?

Patient Scenario
The McGray Family

Read about the McGray family, a family experiencing a growth and development concern, then answer the questions to further sharpen your skills and grow more familiar with NCLEX-type questions related to growth and development. Confirm your answers are correct by reading the rationales.

Visit http://thePoint.lww.com

Answers and Rationales

Looking for answers to the What If… and Critical Thinking Care Study questions?

Visit http://thePoint.lww.com

References

Barton, A. L., & Kirtley, M. S. (2012). Gender differences in the relationships among parenting styles and college student mental health. *Journal of American College Health, 60*(1), 21–26.

Black, M. M., Quigg, A. M., Hurley, K. M., et al. (2011). Iron deficiency and iron-deficiency anemia in the first two years of life: Strategies to prevent loss of developmental potential. *Nutrition Review, 69* (Suppl. 1), S64–S70.

Brandt, M. J. (2011). Sexism and gender inequality across 57 societies. *Psychological Science, 22*(11), 1413–1418.

Brownawell, A. M., Caers, W., Gibson, G. R., et al. (2012). Prebiotics and the health benefits of fiber: Current regulatory status, future research, and goals. *Journal of Nutrition, 142*(5), 962–974.

Burgess, J. N., & Broome, M. E. (2012). Perceptions of weight and body image among preschool children: A pilot study. *Pediatric Nursing, 38*(3), 147–152.

Butterworth, B., & Kovas, Y. (2013). Understanding neurocognitive developmental disorders can improve education for all. *Science, 340*(6130), 300–305.

Centers for Disease Control and Prevention. (2012). *Obesity rates among children in the U.S.* Atlanta, GA: Author.

Chess, S., & Thomas, A. (1985). Temperamental differences: A critical concept in child health care. *Pediatric Nursing, 11*(3), 167–171.

Danyliw, A. D., Vatanparast, H., Nikpartow, N., et al. (2012). Beverage patterns among Canadian children and relationship to overweight and obesity. *Applied Physiology, Nutrition & Metabolism, 37*(5), 900–906.

Dea, T. L. (2011). Pediatric obesity & type 2 diabetes. *MCN: American Journal of Maternal Child Nursing, 36*(1), 42–48.

Erikson, E. H. (1993). *Childhood & society.* New York, NY: W. W. Norton.

Feigelman, S. (2012). Overview and assessment of variability. In R. M. Kliegman, B. F. Stanton, J. W. Geme, et al. (Eds.), *Nelson textbook of pediatrics: Extra consult edition* (19th ed., pp. 192–212). Philadelphia, PA: Elsevier/Saunders.

Freud, S. (1962). *Three essays on the theory of sexuality.* New York, NY: Hearst Corporation.

Freud, S., & Brill, A. A. (1995). *The basic writings of Sigmund Freud.* New York, NY: Random House.

Gilligan, C. (1993). *In a different voice: Psychological theory and women's development.* Cambridge, MA: Harvard University Press.

Green, M., & Solnit, A. (1964). Reactions to the threatened loss of a child: A vulnerable child syndrome. *Pediatrics, 34*(8), 58–62.

Halfon, N., Stevens, G. D., Larson, K., et al. (2011). Duration of a well-child visit: Association with content, family-centeredness, and satisfaction. *Pediatrics, 128*(4), 657–664.

Hudson, J. L., Dodd, H. F., Lyneham, H. J., et al. (2011). Temperament and family environment in the development of anxiety disorder: Two-year follow-up. *Journal of the American Academy of Child & Adolescent Psychiatry, 50*(12), 1255–1264.

Johnston, M., Landers, S., Noble, L., et al. (2012). Breastfeeding and the use of human milk. *Pediatrics, 129*(3), e827–e841.

Jones, G. (2011). Early life nutrition and bone development in children. *Nestle Nutrition Workshop Series: Pediatric Programme, 2011*(68), 227–233.

Juujärvi, S., Pesso, K., & Myyry, L. (2011). Care-based ethical reasoning among first-year nursing and social services students. *Journal of Advanced Nursing, 67*(2), 418–427.

Kmietowicz, Z. (2012). Study identifies behaviours in young children that might prevent obesity. *BMJ: British Medical Journal, 344*(4), e2608.

Kohlberg, L. (1984). *The psychology of moral development.* New York, NY: Harper & Row.

Krebs, N. F., & Primak, L. E. (2011). Pediatric nutrition and nutritional disorders. In K. J. Marcdante, R. M. Kliegman, H. B. Jenson, et al. (Eds.), *Nelson essentials of pediatrics* (6th ed., pp. 103–122). Philadelphia, PA: Saunders/Elsevier.

Levine, D. A. (2011). Growth & development. In K. J. Marcdante, R. M. Kliegman, H. B. Jenson, et al. (Eds.), *Nelson essentials of pediatrics* (6th ed., pp. 13–44). Philadelphia, PA: Saunders/Elsevier.

Matook, S. A., Sullivan, M. C., Salisbury, A., et al. (2010). Variations of NICU sound by location and time of day. *Neonatal Network, 29*(2), 87–95.

Morgan, A. R. (2012). Determining genetic risk factors for pediatric type 2 diabetes. *Current Diabetes Reports, 12*(1), 88–92.

Mulholland, E. K., Griffiths, U. K., & Biellik, R. (2012). Measles in the 21st century. *New England Journal of Medicine, 366*(19), 1755–1757.

Naidoo, N., Pawitan, Y., Soong, R., et al. (2011). Human genetics and genomics a decade after the release of the draft sequence of the human genome. *Human Genomics, 5*(6), 577–622.

Newman, B. M., & Newman, P. R. (2011). Development through life: A psychosocial approach. In B. M. Newman & P. R. Newman, *Later adulthood* (pp. 526–559). Belmont, CA: Wadsworth Cengage.

Pastor, P. N., & Reuben, C. A. (2011). Emotional/behavioral difficulties and adolescent obesity: Effect of sex and Hispanic origin/race. *International Journal of Pediatric Obesity, 6*(5–6), 462–466.

Piaget, J. (1961). *The growth of logical thinking from childhood to adolescence.* New York, NY: Basic Books.

Pike, K., Jane-Pillow, J., & Lucas, J. S. (2012). Long term respiratory consequences of intrauterine growth restriction. *Seminars in Fetal & Neonatal Medicine, 17*(2):92–98.

Rossow, I., & Moan, I. S. (2012). Parental intoxication and adolescent suicidal behavior. *Archives of Suicide Research, 16*(1), 73–84.

Russell, S. T., Sinclair, K. O., Poteat, V. P., et al. (2012). Adolescent health and harassment based on discriminatory bias. *American Journal of Public Health, 102*(3), 493–495.

Rutherford-Hemming, T. (2012). Learning in simulated environments: Effect on learning transfer and clinical skill acquisition in nurse practitioner students. *Journal of Nursing Education, 51*(7), 403–406.

Sizer, F., & Whitney, E. (2011). The vitamins. In F. Sizer & E. Whitney (Eds.), *Nutrition: Concepts & controversies* (pp. 228–277). Belmont, CA: Wadsworth Cengage Learning.

Ting, W. H., Huang, C. Y., Tu, Y. K., et al. (2012). Association between weight status and depressive symptoms in adolescents: Role of weight perception, weight concern, and dietary restraint. *European Journal of Pediatrics, 171*(8), 1247–1255.

U.S. Department of Agriculture. (2012). *Choose MyPlate: A guide to daily food choices.* Washington, DC: Author.

U.S. Department of Health and Human Services. (2010). *Healthy people 2020.* Washington, DC: Author.

Vicedo, M. (2011). The social nature of the mother's tie to her child: John Bowlby's theory of attachment in post-war America. *British Journal for the History of Science, 44*(162, Pt. 3), 401–426.

Viner, R. M., Ozer, E. M., Denny, S., et al. (2012). Adolescence and the social determinants of health. *Lancet, 379*(9826), 1641–1652.

Wadsworth, B. J. (2003). *Piaget's theory of cognitive and affective development: Foundations of constructivism* (5th ed.). New York, NY: Longman.

Whitney, E. N., & Rolfes, S. R. (2012). Life cycle nutrition: Pregnancy & lactation. In *Understanding nutrition* (pp. 492–527). Belmont, CA: Wadsworth Publishing.

Chapter 29

Nursing Care of a Family With an Infant

KEY TERMS

- baby-bottle syndrome
- binocular vision
- deciduous teeth
- eighth-month anxiety
- extrusion reflex
- hand regard
- natal teeth
- neck-righting reflex
- neonatal teeth
- object permanence
- pincer grasp
- seborrhea
- social smile
- thumb opposition

OBJECTIVES

After mastering the contents of this chapter, you should be able to:

1. Describe normal infant growth and development and associated parental concerns.
2. Identify 2020 National Health Goals related to infant growth and development that nurses can help the nation achieve.
3. Assess an infant for normal growth and development milestones.
4. Formulate nursing diagnoses related to infant growth and development and associated parental concerns.
5. Identify expected outcomes to promote optimal infant growth and developmental needs as well as manage seamless transitions across differing health care settings.
6. Using the nursing process, plan nursing care that includes the six competencies of Quality & Safety Education for Nurses (QSEN): Patient-Centered Care, Teamwork & Collaboration, Evidence-Based Practice (EBP), Quality Improvement (QI), Safety, and Informatics.
7. Implement nursing care related to normal growth and development of an infant, such as encouraging eye–hand coordination.
8. Evaluate expected outcomes for achievement and effectiveness of care.
9. Integrate knowledge of infant growth and development with the interplay of nursing process, the six competencies of QSEN, and Family Nursing to promote quality maternal and child health nursing care.

You meet Ms. Simpson, 19 years old, at a pediatric clinic when she brings in her 2-month-old son, Bryan. She looks tired and tells you she is exhausted because her baby is "awake all night, crying constantly." She stopped breastfeeding and changed to formula to see if that would help. It didn't. She also began giving him cereal. That didn't help either. She tells you his bowel movements are normal. When you weigh Bryan, you find he has gained weight well. When you talk to him, he demonstrates a social smile.

Previous chapters described the newborn and the capabilities with which children are born. This chapter adds information about the dramatic changes, both physical and psychosocial, that occur during the first year. Such information can build a base for care and health teaching for the age group.

What condition common to early infancy might Ms. Simpson be describing? What factors might be playing a role? What suggestions could you make to help her enjoy caring for Bryan more?

BOX 29.1 Nursing Care Planning Based on 2020 National Health Goals

A number of 2020 National Health Goals focus on the promotion of health during the infant year. These include:

- Increase the proportion of mothers who exclusively breastfeed until 6 months of age from a baseline of 14.1% to 25.5%.
- Reduce the rate of infant deaths from a baseline of 6.9 out of 1,000 live births to 6.7 out of 1,000 live births.
- Increase immunization levels for universally recommended vaccines among young children for such diseases as diphtheria, tetanus, poliomyelitis, pertussis, measles, mumps, rubella, and varicella (chickenpox) from varying actual levels to the target level of 90%.
- Increase age-appropriate vehicle restraint system use in children aged 0 to 12 months from 86% to 95%.
- Decrease the number of infants who die from sudden infant death syndrome (SIDS) from 0.55 out of 1,000 live births to 0.50 out of 1,000 live births (U.S. Department of Health and Human Services [DHHS], 2010; see www.healthypeople.gov).

Nurses can help the nation achieve these goals by educating parents about the importance of using infant car seats, continuing exclusive breastfeeding for 6 months, and instigating measures to prevent SIDS such as placing infants to sleep on their backs.

Traditionally, infancy is designated as the period of time from 1 month to 1 year of age. In these important months, an infant undergoes such rapid development that parents sometimes believe their baby looks different and demonstrates new abilities every day. During this time, an infant typically triples birth weight and increases length by 50%. Babies' senses sharpen and, with the process of attachment to a primary caregiver, they form a first social relationship. Because of the growth and learning potential that occurs, this first year is a crucial one.

Without proper nutrition, a baby will not grow and physically thrive; without proper stimulation and nurturing care by a consistent caregiver, an infant may not develop a healthy interest in life or a feeling of security essential for future development (Olusanya & Renner, 2013). Box 29.1 highlights 2020 National Health Goals addressing this important developmental stage.

Nursing Process Overview

For Healthy Development of an Infant

Assessment

Nursing assessment of an infant begins with an interview with the primary caregiver. Important areas to discuss include nutrition, growth patterns, and development. An infant's height, weight, and head circumference are important indicators of growth, so they should be measured and plotted on standard growth charts, either the Centers for Disease Control and Prevention (CDC) or the World Health Organization (WHO) charts (Parsons, George, & Innis, 2011).

These charts represent average growth and can determine if the baby's growth remains within the same relative percentile at each checkup. Typical infant appearance is shown in Box 29.2.

The physical assessment of an infant must be done quickly yet thoroughly because a baby can tire or become hungry, making it difficult to judge overall behavior and temperament. It's best if a parent is present to make the infant feel comfortable. Using a calm, unhurried approach helps an infant feel safe enough to accept your interventions.

Nursing Diagnosis

Much of your assessment of an infant and family will focus on basic needs such as sleep, nutrition, and activity and the parents' adjustment to their new role. Examples of nursing diagnoses include:

- Ineffective breastfeeding related to maternal fatigue
- Disturbed sleep pattern (maternal) related to baby's need to nurse every 2 hours
- Deficient knowledge related to normal infant growth and development
- Imbalanced nutrition, less than body requirements, related to infant's difficulty sucking
- Health-seeking behaviors related to adjusting to parenthood
- Delayed growth and development related to lack of stimulating environment
- Risk for impaired parenting related to long hospitalization of infant
- Readiness for enhanced family coping related to increased financial support
- Social isolation (maternal) related to lack of adequate social support
- Ineffective role performance related to new responsibilities within the family

Outcome Identification and Planning

Outcomes established for infant care need to be realistic based on the family's new circumstances. Parents of infants, especially first-time parents, must do a lot of adjusting, and this takes time. Try to suggest activities that can be easily incorporated into the family's lifestyle. If your assessment data indicate that a child needs more exposure to language and you know both parents work during the day, for example, you might suggest the parents ask their child's caretaker to talk to their infant more. Encourage parents to spend additional time each evening reading or reciting nursery rhymes to their baby. Working together, these combined actions should increase the baby's language skills. Helpful Web sites about growth and development to recommend are the BabyCenter (www.BabyCenter.com) and the March of Dimes (www.MarchofDimes.com/baby). For questions about car seats, parents can consult the CDC (www.cdc.gov/motorvehiclesafety/child_passenger_safety/cps-factsheet.html). Other helpful Web sites to alert parents about safety are the American Association of Poison Control Centers (www.aapcc.org) and the American Academy of Pediatrics (AAP, www.aap.org). A site parents can check to see if a baby product has been recalled is the U.S. Consumer Product Safety Commission (www.CPSC.gov).

BOX 29.2 Nursing Care Planning Using Assessment

Appearance of the Average Infant

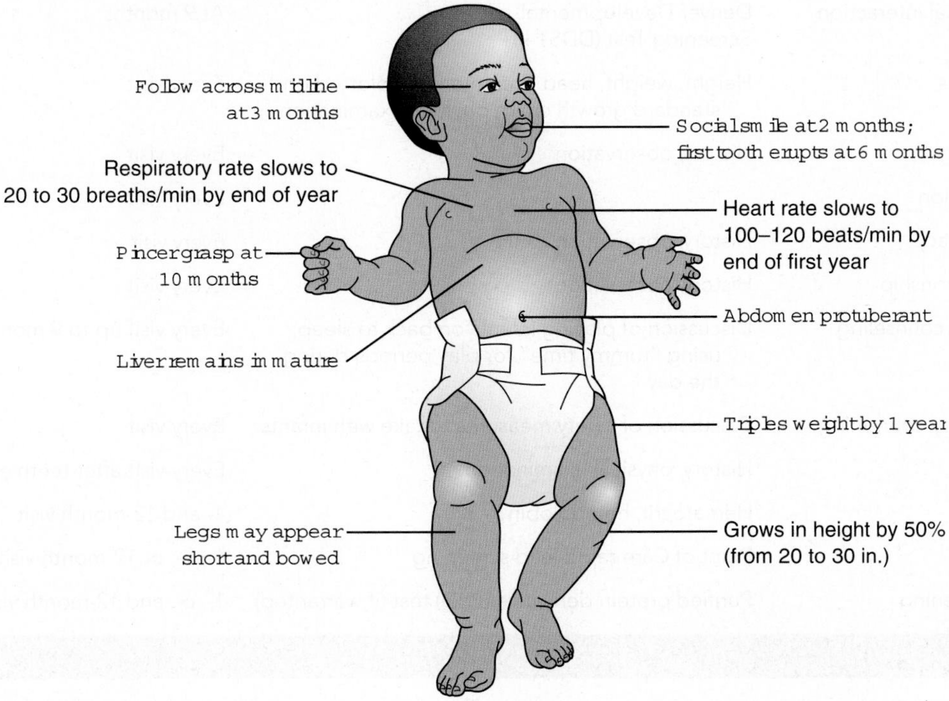
Follow across midline at 3 months
Social smile at 2 months; first tooth erupts at 6 months
Respiratory rate slows to 20 to 30 breaths/min by end of year
Heart rate slows to 100–120 beats/min by end of first year
Pincer grasp at 10 months
Abdomen protuberant
Liver remains immature
Triples weight by 1 year
Legs may appear short and bowed
Grows in height by 50% (from 20 to 30 in.)

Implementation

One of the most important interventions of the infant period is teaching new parents about normal growth and development milestones, such as the age range for rolling over or reaching for objects. Whenever possible, this information should be anticipatory so parents are not surprised by a new skill, and instead, are prepared for changes and developments before they occur.

Outcome Evaluation

Evaluate expected outcomes at each visit to detect that changes in growth and development are occurring. Helping parents understand the total developmental profile, not just a single element, provides the most important description of their child. Variation is so much the rule rather than the exception that a 2-month variation from the average during the infant year is considered normal. Many 4-month-old infants, for example, have mastered most of the 4-month skills and some of the 5-month skills, yet they may still be at a 3-month level on one or two other criteria.

Examples of expected outcomes include:

- Mother states she feels fatigued but able to cope with sleep disturbance from night waking.
- Parents state five actions they are taking daily to encourage bonding.
- Father states both he and spouse are adjusting to new role as parents.
- Parents verbalize appropriate techniques they use to stimulate infant.
- Infant demonstrates age-appropriate growth and development.
- Infant exhibits weight, height, and head and chest circumference within usual norms.

GROWTH AND DEVELOPMENT OF AN INFANT

Infants grow rapidly both in size and in their ability to perform tasks during their first year. A standard schedule for health care visits is for 2-week, 2-month, 4-month, 6-month, 9-month, and 12-month visits (AAP, 2012a). These visits are important for the infant because they provide time for immunizations and health assessments; they are also important for parents because they provide an opportunity for parents to ask questions about their child's growth pattern and developmental progress. They also provide opportunities for health care providers to assess for potential problems as they first appear.

Anticipatory guidance offered at these visits can help parents prepare for the rapid changes that mark the first year of life. When appropriate, encouraging parents to join clubs or networking groups is another way to help to increase their knowledge base and confidence level to care for their rapidly growing infant. Table 29.1 details the usual procedures done

TABLE 29.1 Health Maintenance Schedule, Infant Period

Physical Health	Physical Examination	Frequency
Developmental milestones including psychosocial interaction	History, observation Denver Developmental Screening Test (DDST II)	Every visit At 9 months
Growth milestones	Height, weight, head circumference plotted on standard growth chart; physical examination	Every visit
Vision and hearing	History, observation	Every visit
Physical examination		Every visit
Nutritional adequacy	History, observation	Every visit
Parent–child relationship	History, observation	Every visit
Sleep positioning counseling	Discussion of placing infants on back to sleep; using "tummy time" for play periods during the day	Every visit up to 9 months
Unintentional injury counseling	Discussion of safety measures to take with infants	Every visit
Dental health	History, physical examination	Every visit after teeth erupt
Anemia	Hematocrit, hemoglobin	4- and 12-month visit
Lead screening	Point of Care rapid lead screening	6-, 9-, or 12-month visit in high-risk areas
Tuberculosis screening	Purified protein derivative (PPD) test (if warranted)	1-, 6-, and 12-month visit
Immunizations		
Review of history and health record; teaching parent about any risks and side effects; administering immunization in accordance with health care agency policies		
Haemophilus influenzae type B	HIb	2-, 4-, 6-, and 12-month visits
Varicella	VAR	12-month visit
Inactivated poliomyelitis	IPV	2-, 4-, and 6-month visits
Pneumococcal disease	PCV	2-, 4-, 6-, and 12-month visits
Diphtheria, tetanus and pertussis (whooping cough)	DTaP	2-, 4-, 6-, and 12-15 months
Hepatitis B	HepB	Birth, 2-month, and 6- or 12-month visits
Rotavirus	RV	2-, 4-, and 6-month visit
Influenza	IIV	Yearly at 6-month or later visit
Mumps, measles, and rubella	MMR	12- or 15-month visit
Hepatitis A	HepA	12- or 15-month visit
Anticipatory Guidance		
Infant care	Active listening and health teaching	Every visit
Expected growth and developmental milestones before next visit	Health teaching	Every visit
Poison and unintentional injury prevention	Educate parents about infant safety, such as using car seats and locking up poisons; provide telephone number of national poison control center (800-122-1222)	Every visit
Problem Solving		
Any problems expressed by parent during course of the visit	Active listening and health teaching regarding nutrition, exercise, language development	Every visit

Centers for Disease Control and Prevention. (2013). *Recommended immunizations for children (birth through 6 years) United States, 2013.* Washington, DC: DHHS.

at infant health maintenance visits. The vaccines administered during the first year are discussed in Chapter 34 (also available at http://thePoint.lww.com/Pillitteri7e).

Physical Growth

The physiologic changes that occur in the infant year reflect both the increasing maturity and growth of body organs.

Weight

As a rule, most infants double their birth weight by 4 to 6 months and triple it by 1 year. During the first 6 months, infants typically average a weight gain of 2 lb per month. During the second 6 months, weight gain is approximately 1 lb per month. The average 1-year-old boy weighs 10 kg (22 lb); the average girl weighs 9.5 kg (21 lb). An infant's weight, however, is relevant only when plotted on a standard growth chart and compared to that child's own growth curve (available at http://thePoint.lww.com/Pillitteri7e).

Height

An infant increases in height during the first year by 50%, or grows from the average birth length of 20 in. to about 30 in. (50.8 to 76.2 cm). Height, like weight, is best assessed if it is plotted on a standard growth chart. Infant growth is most apparent in the trunk during the early months. During the second half of the first year, it becomes more apparent as lengthening of the legs occurs. At the end of the first year, the child's legs may still appear disproportionately short, however, and perhaps bowed. For accuracy, measure infants lying supine on a measuring board even if they are beginning to be able to stand (see Chapter 34, Box 34.9).

Head Circumference

By the end of the first year, the brain already reaches two thirds of its adult size. Head circumference increases rapidly during the infant period to reflect this rapid brain growth.

Some infants' heads appear asymmetric until the second half of the first year, especially if they are always placed on their back to sleep (which they should be), causing the skull bones to flatten in the back. Suggest to parents they continue to place the infant on the back to sleep but to spend "tummy time" daily with the infant placed in a prone position to prevent this flattening. This early head distortion will gradually correct itself as the child sleeps less and spends more time with the head in an erect position. Persistence of asymmetry suggests an infant is not receiving enough stimulation or is spending the majority of time lying in bed.

Body Proportion

Body proportion changes during the first year from that of a newborn to a more typical infant appearance. By the end of the infant period, the lower jaw is definitely prominent and remains that way throughout life.

The circumference of the chest is generally less than that of the head at birth by about 2 cm. It is even with the head circumference in some infants as early as 6 months and in most by 12 months. The abdomen remains protuberant until the child has been walking well for some time, generally well into the toddler period. Cervical, thoracic, and lumbar vertebral curves develop as infants hold up their head, sit, and walk. Lengthening of the lower extremities during the last 6 months of infancy readies the child for walking and often is the final growth that changes the appearance from "babylike" to "toddlerlike."

Body Systems

In the cardiovascular system, heart rate slows from 110 to 160 beats/min to 100 to 120 beats/min by the end of the first year. The heart continues to occupy a little over half the width of the chest. Pulse rate may slow with inhalation (sinus arrhythmia), but this does not become marked until preschool age. That the heart is becoming more efficient is shown by a decreasing pulse rate and a slightly elevated blood pressure (from an average of 80/40 to 100/60 mmHg).

Infants are prone to develop a physiologic anemia at 2 to 3 months of age. This occurs because the life of a typical red cell is 4 months, so the cells the child had at birth begin to disintegrate at that time, yet new cells are not yet being produced in adequate replacement numbers. Hemoglobin in an infant becomes totally converted from fetal to adult hemoglobin at 5 to 6 months of age. Infants may experience a decrease in serum iron levels at 6 to 9 months as the last of iron stores established in utero are used.

The respiratory rate of an infant slows from 30 to 60 breaths/min to 20 to 30 breaths/min by the end of the first year. Because the lumens of the respiratory tract remain small and mucus production by the tract to clear invading microorganisms is still inefficient, upper respiratory infections occur readily and tend to be more severe than in adults.

At birth, the gastrointestinal tract is immature in its ability to digest food and mechanically move it along. These functions mature gradually during the infant year. Although the ability to digest protein is present and effective at birth, the amount of amylase, which is necessary for the digestion of complex carbohydrates, is deficient until approximately the third month. Lipase, necessary for the digestion of saturated fat, is decreased in amount during the entire first year.

The liver of an infant remains immature, possibly causing an inadequate conjugation of drugs (if a drug should be necessary for treatment of illness) and the inefficient formation of carbohydrate, protein, and vitamins for storage. Until age 3 or 4 months, an **extrusion reflex** (food placed on an infant's tongue is thrust forward and out of the mouth) prevents some infants from eating effectively if they are offered solid food this early (not recommended). Newborns can drink from a cup as long as a parent controls the fluid flow. An infant can independently drink from a cup by age 8 or 10 months.

The kidneys remain immature and not as efficient at eliminating body wastes as in an adult. The endocrine system remains particularly immature in response to pituitary stimulation, such as adrenocorticotropic hormone, or insulin production from the pancreas. Without these hormones functioning effectively, an infant may not be able to respond to stress as effectively as an adult.

An infant's immune system becomes functional by at least 2 months of age; an infant can actively produce both immune globulin (Ig)G and IgM antibodies by 1 year. The levels of other immunoglobulins (IgA, IgE, and IgD) are not plentiful until preschool age, which is the reason why infants continue to need protection from infection (Goldson & Reynolds, 2011).

The ability to adjust to cold is mature by age 6 months. By this age, an infant can shiver in response to cold (which increases muscle activity and provides warmth) and has developed additional adipose tissue to serve as insulation. The amount of brown fat, which protected the newborn from cold, decreases during the first year as subcutaneous fat increases.

Although the fluid in body compartments shifts to some extent, extracellular fluid accounts for approximately 35% of an infant's body weight, with intracellular fluid accounting for approximately 40% by the end of the first year, in contrast to adult proportions of 20% and 40%, respectively. This proportional difference increases an infant's susceptibility to dehydration from illnesses, such as diarrhea, because loss of extracellular fluid could result in loss of over a third of an infant's body fluid.

Teeth

The first baby tooth (typically a central incisor) usually erupts at age 6 months, followed by a new one monthly. However, teething patterns can vary greatly among children. Figure 29.1 illustrates the usual ages of deciduous (baby teeth) eruption by tooth type.

Some newborns (about 1 in 2,000) may be born with teeth (**natal teeth**) or have teeth erupt in the first 4 weeks of life (**neonatal teeth**). The lower central incisors (see Fig. 29.1) are the teeth most frequently involved in this early growth. These very early teeth may be membranous and so may be reabsorbed (supernumerary or extra teeth). If they are loosely attached, they are usually removed before they loosen spontaneously and are aspirated by the infant. In most infants, however, natal or neonatal teeth are deciduous or are fixed firmly. These should not be removed because no other teeth will grow to replace them until the permanent teeth erupt at age 6 or 7. **Deciduous teeth** are essential for allowing proper

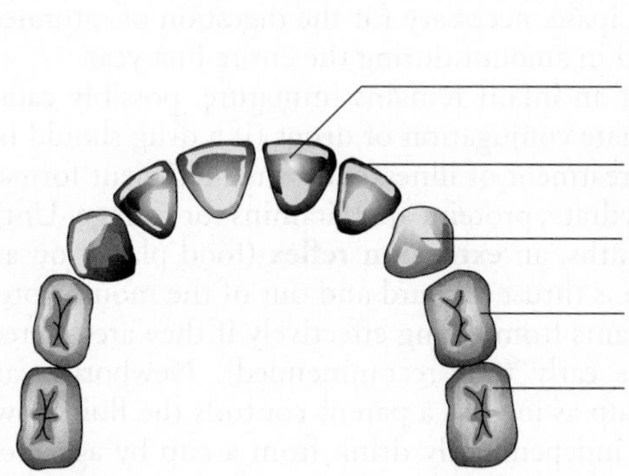

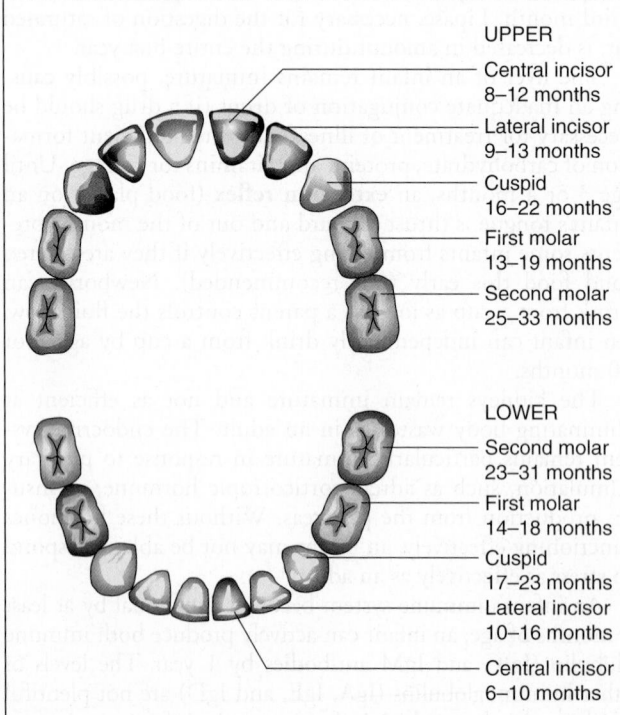

FIGURE 29.1 A typical eruption pattern of deciduous teeth.

growth of the dental arch. If they are injured, children need conscientious follow-up to be certain there is space for permanent teeth to erupt effectively or that permanent teeth are not discolored (de Amorim Lde, Estrela, & da Costa, 2011).

Motor Development

An average infant progresses through systematic motor growth during the first year, strongly reflecting the principles of cephalocaudal (head to toe) and gross to fine motor development. Control proceeds from head to trunk to lower extremities in a progressive, predictable sequence. As different infants show individual variations in accomplishing different tasks, the ages given here are only averages.

To assess motor development, both *gross motor development* (ability to accomplish large body movements) and *fine motor development*, measured by observing or testing *prehensile ability* (ability to coordinate hand movements), are evaluated.

Gross Motor Development

Four positions—ventral suspension, prone, sitting, and standing—are used to assess gross motor development.

Ventral Suspension Position. *Ventral suspension* refers to an infant's appearance when held in midair on a horizontal plane and supported by a hand under the abdomen (Fig. 29.2A). In this position, the newborn allows the head to hang down with little effort at control. One-month-old infants lift their head momentarily, then drop it again. Two-month-old infants hold their head in the same plane as the rest of their body, a major advance in muscle control. By 3 months, infants lift and maintain their head well above the plane of the rest of the body in ventral suspension.

A *Landau reflex* is a new reflex that develops at 3 months. When held in ventral suspension, the infant's head, legs, and spine extend. When the head is depressed, the hips, knees, and elbows flex. This reflex continues to be present in most infants during the second 6 months of life, but then it becomes increasingly difficult to demonstrate. It is an important reflex to assess because a child with motor weakness, cerebral palsy, or other neuromuscular defects will not be able to demonstrate the reflex.

At 6 to 9 months, an infant also demonstrates a *parachute reaction* from a ventral suspension position. This means that when infants are suddenly lowered toward an examining table, the arms extend as if to protect themselves from falling. Children with cerebral palsy do not demonstrate this response because they flex their extremities too tightly.

Prone Position. When lying on their stomach, newborns can turn their head to move it out of a position where breathing is impaired, but they cannot hold their head raised for an extended time (see Fig. 29.2B). By 1 month of age, they lift their head and turn it easily to the side. They still tend to keep their knees tucked under their abdomen, however, as they did as a newborn. Two-month-old infants can raise their head and maintain the position, but they cannot raise their chest high enough to look around yet. Their head is still held facing downward.

A 3-month-old child lifts the head and shoulders well off the table and looks around when prone. The pelvis is flat on the table, no longer elevated. Some children can turn from a prone to a side-lying position at this age.

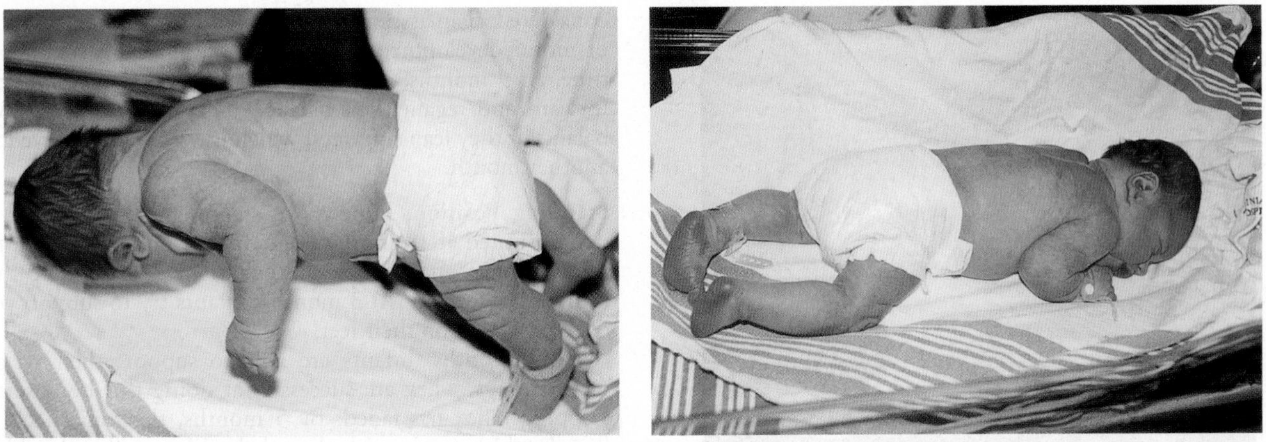

A B

FIGURE 29.2 **(A)** The ventral suspension position. **(B)** The prone position.

Four-month-old infants lift their chests off the bed and look around actively, turning their head from side to side. They are able to turn from front to back. The first time, this tends to occur as an extension of lifting the chest combined with a **neck-righting reflex**, which begins at this age. This reflex causes babies to lose their balance and roll sideways when lifting the head up. The baby is frightened by the sudden feeling of rolling free and probably cries. After this happens a few more times, however, a baby begins to delight in this new accomplishment.

Most babies turn front to back first and then, 1 month later, back to front. When taking a health history, ask which way a child turned first. Those with spasticity may turn first back to front. This is not necessarily an indication of spasticity, however, because some healthy babies turn back to front first also.

Five-month-old infants are able to rest weight on their forearms when prone. They can turn completely over, front to back and back to front. By 6 months, infants can raise their chests and the upper part of their abdomens off the table.

By 9 months, a child can creep from the prone position. Creeping means the child has the abdomen off the floor and moves one hand and one leg and then the other hand and leg, using the knees on the floor to locomote (Fig. 29.3).

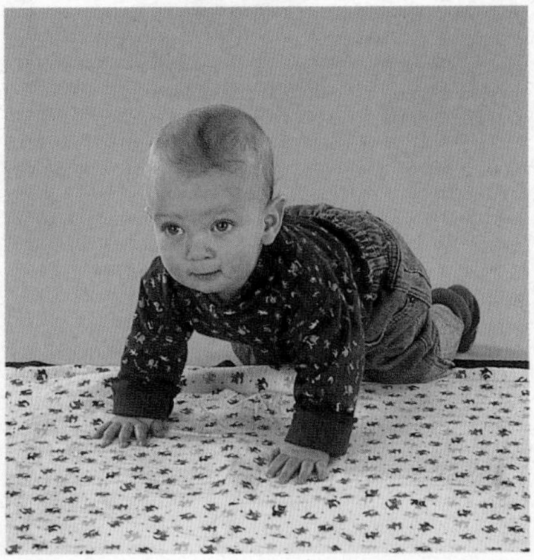

FIGURE 29.3 Creeping. When infants creep, they move forward with one arm and leg, then the other arm and leg, carrying the torso above and parallel to the floor.

Sitting Position. When placed on his or her back and then pulled to a sitting position, a newborn has extreme head lag; this lag is present until about 1 month (Fig. 29.4). In a sitting position, the back appears rounded and an infant demonstrates only momentary head control.

By 2 months, infants can hold their head fairly steady when sitting up, although their head does tend to bob forward and will still show head lag when pulled to a sitting position. A 4-month-old child reaches an important milestone by no longer demonstrating head lag when pulled to a sitting position.

A 5-month-old infant can be seen to straighten his or her back when held or propped in a sitting position. By 6 months, infants can sit momentarily without support. They anticipate being picked up and reach up with their hands from this position. Some parents expect a child this age to be able to sit securely and may be worried because their sitting posture is still extremely shaky when it is normal (Fig. 29.5). Infants are capable of movement by hitching or sliding backward from this position. Alert parents that an infant this young is capable of moving from one spot to

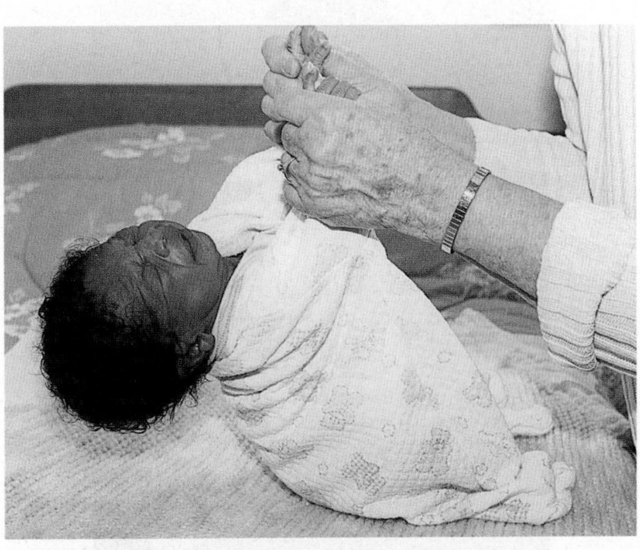

FIGURE 29.4 An infant is pulled to a sitting position to demonstrate head lag. Notice how evident this is in the very young infant.

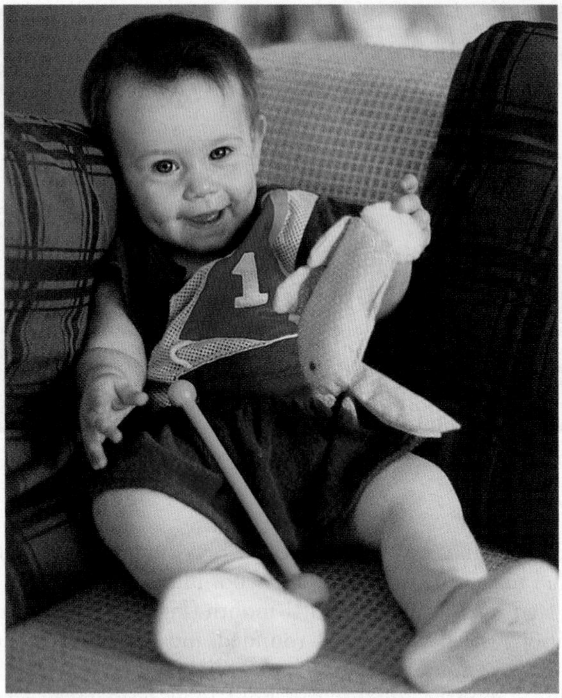

FIGURE 29.5 A 6-month-old infant not quite ready to sit on her own. Notice how she is propped with pillows to maintain the position.

another in this way so they are prepared for this and can prevent unintentional injuries.

A 7-month-old child can sit alone, but only when the hands are held forward for balance. An 8-month-old child can sit securely without any additional support (Fig. 29.6). This is a major milestone in development that should always be considered in an assessment. Children with delayed cognitive or motor development may not accomplish this step at this time. At 9 months, infants sit so steadily that they can lean forward and regain their balance. They may still lose their balance if they lean sideways, which is a skill not achieved for another month.

Standing Position. A newborn stepping reflex can still be demonstrated at 1 month of age. In a standing position, the infant's knees and hips flex rather than support more than momentary weight. At 3 months, infants try to support part of their weight on their feet.

At 4 months, infants are able to support their weight on their legs. They are successful at doing this because the stepping reflex has faded. By 5 months, the tonic neck reflex should be extinguished, and the Moro reflex should be fading.

By 6 months, infants nearly support their full weight when in a standing position. A 7-month-old child bounces with enjoyment in a standing position. Nine-month-olds can stand holding onto a coffee table if they are placed in that position. Ten-month-olds can pull themselves to a standing position by holding onto the side of a playpen or a low table, but they cannot let themselves down again as yet.

At around 11 months, an infant learns to "cruise" or move about the crib or room by holding onto objects such as the crib rails, chairs, walls, and low tables (Fig. 29.7). At 12 months, the child can stand alone at least momentarily. Some parents expect children to walk at this time and may be disappointed to see their child is merely standing still. A child has until about 22 months of age to walk and still be within the normal limit, however (Fig. 29.8).

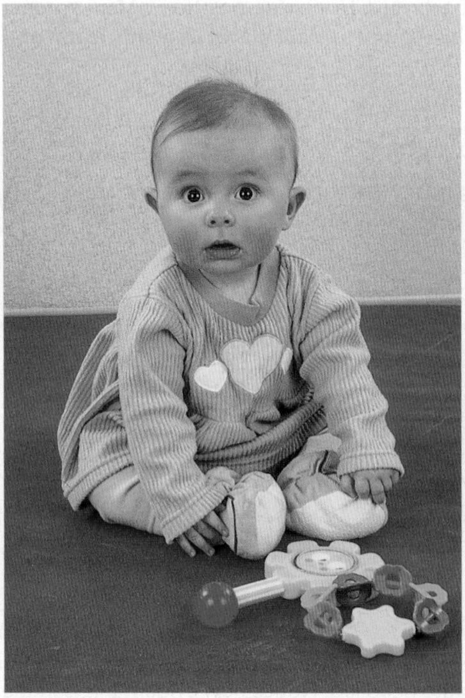

FIGURE 29.6 At 8 months of age, an infant sits independently.

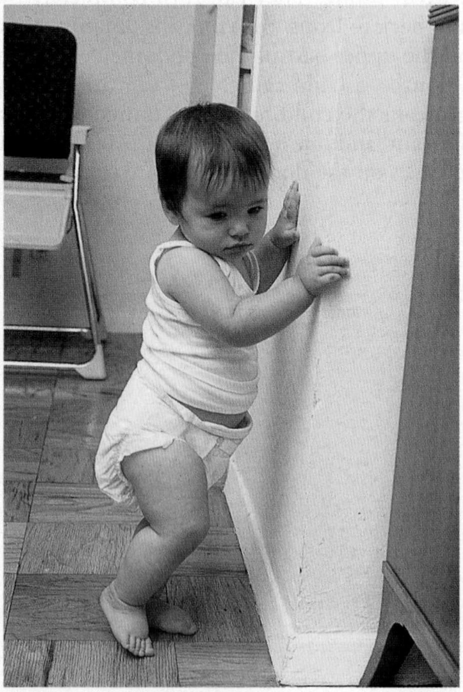

FIGURE 29.7 An 11-month-old child cruising along the walls. Further childproofing of the house will be necessary to keep the child safe. (Photo Researchers, Inc.)

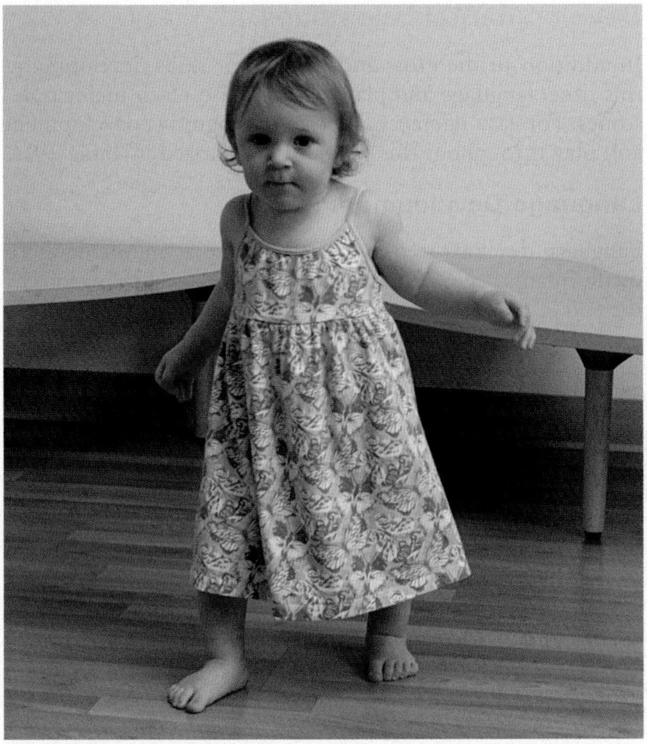

FIGURE 29.8 There is a wide variation in the age at which children take a first step, typically ranging from 8 to 15 months. Here, a child has mastered walking.

QSEN Checkpoint Question 29.1

Teamwork & Collaboration

Bryan is 2 months old and you are collaborating with the occupational therapist in his care. You and your colleague should plan care based on the knowledge that he should sit securely at what age?

a. 2.5 months
b. 6 months
c. 8 months
d. 12 months

Look in Appendix A for the best answer and rationale.

Fine Motor Development

One-month-old infants still have a strong grasp reflex so they hold their hands in fists so tightly that it is difficult to extend their fingers. As the grasp reflex fades, a 2-month-old infant will hold an object for a few minutes before dropping it. The hands are held open, not closed in fists.

By 3 months, infants reach for attractive objects in front of them. Their grasp is unpracticed, however, so they usually miss them. You can assure parents this is part of normal development so they do not think their child is nearsighted or farsighted or has poor coordination.

When they reach 4 months, infants bring their hands together and pull at their clothes. They will shake a rattle placed in their hand. **Thumb opposition** (ability to bring the thumb and fingers together) begins, but the motion is a scooping or raking one, not a picking-up one, and is not very accurate.

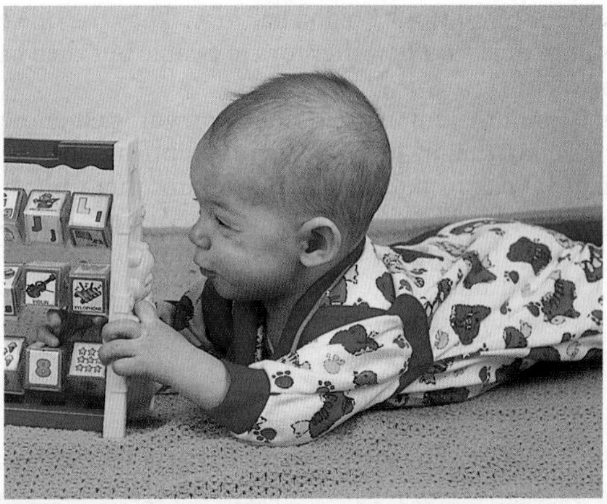

FIGURE 29.9 By age 4 months, an infant is able to manipulate large objects.

This limits the infant to handling large objects (Fig. 29.9). Palmar and plantar grasp reflexes have disappeared.

Five-month-old children can accept objects that are handed to them by grasping with the whole hand. They can reach and pick up objects without the object being offered and often play with their toes as objects. Fisting that persists beyond 5 months suggests a delay in motor development. Unilateral fisting suggests hemiparesis or paralysis on that side.

By 6 months, grasping has advanced to a point where a child can hold objects in both hands. Infants at this age will drop one toy when a second one is offered, however. They can hold a spoon and start to feed themselves (with much spilling). The Moro, the palmar grasp, and the tonic neck reflexes have completely faded. A Moro reflex that persists beyond this point should arouse suspicion of neurologic disease.

Seven-month-old infants can transfer toys from one hand to the other. They hold a first object when a second one is offered. By 8 months, random reaching and ineffective grasping disappear as a result of advanced eye–hand coordination.

A major milestone at 10 months is the ability to bring the thumb and first finger together in a **pincer grasp** (Fig. 29.10). This enables children to pick up small objects such as crumbs

FIGURE 29.10 An infant almost ready to demonstrate a pincer grasp.

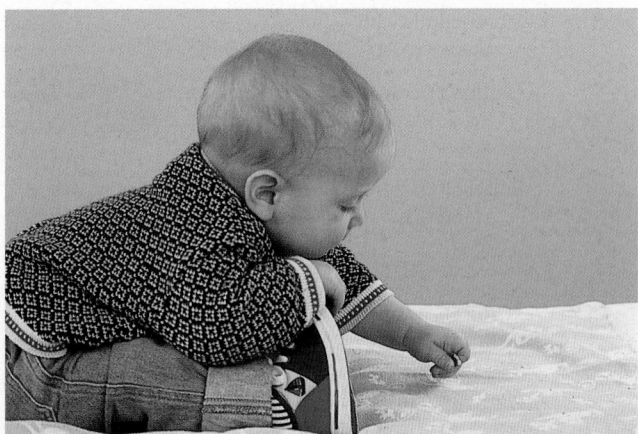

or pieces of cereal from a high chair tray. They use one finger to point to objects. They offer toys to people but then cannot release them.

At 12 months, infants can hold a crayon well enough to draw a semi-straight line. They enjoy putting objects such as small blocks in containers and taking them out again. They can hold a cup and spoon to feed themselves fairly well (if they have been allowed to practice) and can take off socks and push their hands into sleeves (again, if they have been allowed to practice). They can offer toys and release them.

Developmental Milestones

In addition to the gross and fine motor skills developing at this time, language and play behavior also reach major milestones. For easy reference, motor and cognitive development and play throughout this year are summarized in Table 29.2.

Language Development

Language develops step by step the same as motor development. Infants begin to make small, cooing (dovelike) sounds by the end of the first month. By 2 months, they can differentiate

TABLE 29.2 Summary of Infant Growth and Developmental Milestones

Month	Motor Development	Fine Motor Development	Socialization and Language	Time Reflexes Fade	Play
0–1	Largely reflex actions	Keeps hands fisted; able to follow object to midline with eyes			Enjoys watching face of primary caregiver; needs play time in prone position
2	Holds head up when prone	Demonstrates social smile	Makes cooing sounds; differentiates cry	Grasp reflex fading	Enjoys bright-colored mobiles
3	Holds head and chest up when prone	Follows object past midline with eyes	Laughs out loud	Landau reflex is strong	Spends time looking at hands (hand regard); "tummy time" important during the day
4	Turns back to front; no longer has head lag; bears partial weight on feet			Stepping, tonic neck, extrusion reflexes are fading	Needs space to practice turning
5	Should turn readily front to back and back to front			Tonic neck reflex fading	Handles rattles well
6	Beginning to show ability to sit	Uses palmar grasp	May say vowel sounds (*oh-oh*)	Moro & tonic neck reflex have faded	Enjoys bathtub toys, rubber ring for teething
7	Reaches out to be picked up; first tooth (central incisor) erupts	Transfers objects hand to hand	Shows beginning fear of strangers		Likes objects that are good size for transferring
8	Sits securely without support		Fear of strangers peaks		Enjoys manipulation, rattles, and toys of different textures
9	Creeps or crawls (abdomen off floor)		Says first word (*da-da*)		Needs safe space for creeping
10	Pulls self to standing	Uses pincer grasp (thumb and finger) to pick up small objects			Plays games like patty-cake and peek-a-boo
11	"Cruises" (walks with support)				"Cruising" can be main activity
12	Stands alone; some infants take first step	Holds cup and spoon well; helps to dress (pushes arm into sleeve)	Says two words plus *ma-ma* and *da-da*	Landau reflex fades	Likes toys that fit inside each other (pots and pans); nursery rhymes; will like pull toys as soon as walking

their cry. For example, parents can begin to distinguish a cry that means "hungry" from one that means "wet" or from one that means "lonely." This is an important milestone in development for an infant; asking if a parent can tell the difference in crying is a good way to assess how far a parent has progressed in the task of parenting (Mesman, Oster, & Camras, 2012). A first-time parent usually has more difficulty making the distinction in crying than one who has experienced this before.

In response to a nodding, smiling face, or a friendly tone of voice, a 3-month-old infant will squeal with pleasure or laugh out loud. The same as with differentiating a cry, this is an important step in development because it makes a baby even more fun to be with. Parents spend increased time with infants at this age, not just to care for them but because they enjoy watching them smile at attention.

By 4 months, infants are very "talkative," cooing, babbling, and gurgling when spoken to. They definitely laugh out loud. By 5 months, an infant says some simple vowel sounds (e.g., "goo-goo," "gah-gah").

At 6 months, infants learn the art of imitating. They may imitate a parent's cough, for example, or say "Oh!" as a way of attracting attention. The amount of talking infants do increases still more at 7 months. They can imitate vowel sounds well (e.g., "oh-oh," "ah-ah," "oo-oo"). By 9 months, an infant usually speaks a first word: "da-da" or "ba-ba." Occasionally, a mother may need reassurance that "da-da" for daddy is an easier syllable to pronounce than "ma-ma" for mommy. German mothers report the first word their babies say is "here," which is "da" in German. By 10 months, an infant masters another word such as "bye-bye" or "no." By 12 months, infants can generally say two words in addition to "ma-ma" and "da-da," and they use those two words with meaning.

QSEN Checkpoint Question 29.2

Informatics

Beginning verbal communication is one of the most important tasks that infants need to achieve. You should teach Bryan's mother that by 12 months of age he should display which of the following characteristics?

a. "Children this age can usually say around two words, plus 'ma-ma' and 'da-da.'"
b. "One-year-olds can usually say more words than they are able to understand."
c. "A 12-month-old child can express his or her basic needs verbally."
d. "An infant who is this age usually can't understand spoken words."

Look in Appendix A for the best answer and rationale.

Play

Parents often ask what toys their infant would enjoy. Because 1-month-olds can fix their eyes on an object, they are interested in watching a mobile over their crib or playpen. Mobiles are best if they are black and white or brightly colored and light enough in weight so they move when someone walks by. Be sure they face down toward the infant, not toward the adult standing beside the crib. Musical mobiles provide extra stimulation. One-month-old children also spend a great deal of time watching their parents' faces, appearing to enjoy this activity so much a face may become their favorite "toy." Help parents understand they are not spoiling infants by sitting and holding them for long periods of time, just studying each other, in these early months. Parents will enjoy recalling such calm moments later, when they are stacking blocks, winding up toys, or playing table games with their growing child.

Hearing is a second sense that is a source of pleasure for children in early infancy. Even newborns "listen" to the sound of a music box or a musical rattle. They stir and seem apprehensive at the sound of a raucous rattle. Two-month-old infants will hold light, small rattles for a short period of time but then drop them. They are very attuned to mobiles or cradle gyms strung across their crib. They continue to spend a great deal of time just watching the people around them.

Three-month-old infants can handle small blocks or small rattles. Four-month-olds need a playpen or a sheet spread on the floor so they have an opportunity to exercise their new skill of rolling over. Rolling over may be so intriguing that it can serve as a "toy" for the entire month.

Five-month-old infants are ready for a variety of objects to handle, such as plastic rings, blocks, squeeze toys, clothespins, rattles, and plastic keys. Check that all of these are small enough that an infant can lift them with one hand, yet big enough that he or she cannot possibly swallow them.

A 6-month-old child can sit steadily enough to be ready for bathtub toys such as rubber ducks or plastic boats if carefully supervised. Because they are starting to teethe, most at this age enjoy a teething ring to chew on.

Because 7-month-old infants can transfer toys, they are interested in items such as blocks, rattles, or plastic keys that are small enough to be transferred easily. As their mobility increases, they begin to be more interested in brightly colored balls or toys that previously rolled out of reach.

Eight-month-old infants are sensitive to differences in texture. They enjoy having toys with different feels to them, such as velvet, fur, and fuzzy, smooth, or rough items.

The 9-month-old infant needs the experience of creeping. This means time out of a crib or playpen so there is room to maneuver. Many 9-month-olds begin to enjoy toys that go inside one another, such as a nest of blocks or rings of assorted sizes that fit on a center post. Some are more interested in pots and pans that stack rather than toys.

By 10 months, infants are ready for peek-a-boo and will spend a long time playing the game with their hands or with a cloth over their head that they can easily reach and remove. They can clap, so they are also ready to play patty-cake. These games have a positive value, just as laughing out loud did for the 3-month-old. They make the baby feel like an active part of the household. A family feeling begins to grow as the baby begins to actively participate in this type of game.

By 11 months, children have learned to cruise or walk by holding on to low tables. They often find this so absorbing that they spend little time doing anything else during the month. Twelve-month-old infants enjoy putting things in and taking things out of containers. They like little boxes that fit inside one another or dropping small blocks into a larger box. As soon as they can walk, they will be interested in pull toys. A lot of time may be spent listening to someone saying nursery rhymes or listening to music.

Although watching television has an advantage to children during the preschool age because it can help them learn language, the AAP recommends infants not be exposed to television (AAP, 2012c). They don't need exposure to the amount of violence seen on TV (remember children's cartoons may be the worst offenders of this), and interaction with real people (their parents or siblings) is less confusing and a better experience for them.

What if... 29.1 Bryan's mother asks you what would be a good toy for him at 2 months of age. As a nurse, what would you recommend?

Development of Senses

Like other facets of development, maturation of the senses proceeds progressively during the infant year.

Vision

One-month-old infants are able to regard an object in the midline of their vision (something directly in front of themselves) as soon as it is brought in as close as about 18 in. (46 cm). They follow the object a short distance if it moves but not across the midline as yet. They study or regard a human face with a fixed stare. Two-month-old infants focus well (from about age 6 weeks) and so are able to follow moving objects with the eyes (although still not past the midline). The ability to follow and focus in this way is a major milestone in development, indicating that an infant has achieved **binocular vision**, or the ability to fuse two images into one (Fig. 29.11). Teach parents to make a point of initiating eye-to-eye contact with newborns right from birth as a method of stimulating vision as well as a way of promoting socialization.

Three-month-old infants can follow an object across their midline. They typically hold their hands in front of their face and study their fingers for long periods of time (**hand regard**). Blind children also demonstrate this phenomenon, however, so it may not be so much a test of vision as of cognitive or exploratory development. Up until 6 months of age, it is not unusual for infants to experience some difficulty with establishing eye coordination. After 3 months, however, an infant whose eyes still "cross" the majority of the time should be examined by a primary care provider to be certain the muscles that control side-to-side vision are not impaired.

Four-month-old infants are able to recognize familiar objects, such as a frequently seen bottle, rattle, or toy animal. They eagerly follow their parents' movements with their eyes. By 6 months, infants are capable of organized depth perception. This increases the accuracy of their reach for objects as they begin to perceive distances accurately.

Seven-month-olds pat their own image in a mirror. Their depth perception has matured to the extent that they can perform such tasks as transferring toys from hand to hand. By 10 months, an infant looks under a towel or around a corner for a concealed object (the beginning of **object permanence**, or an awareness that an object out of sight still exists).

Most parents are aware that infants enjoy mobiles and also a crib mirror. Occasionally, parents supply so many of these that they can overwhelm the infant with too many patterns and objects dangling above the crib. Ask parents to consider how all these trappings must appear from an infant's viewpoint.

In a hospital environment, because hospital walls tend to be bland, assess that infants receive adequate visual stimulation (Fig. 29.12). If a child's movement is restricted in any way, such as by a cast, move the position of a mobile or mirror from time to time to provide a new view. Photos of family members or pictures drawn by older brothers or sisters can be posted near the crib. Ask parents if there are any items from home that the infant would normally see during the course of the day while being fed, changed, or bathed. Bringing those items into the hospital, if possible, could help visual stimulation.

Hearing

That an infant can hear can be demonstrated at birth by the way a newborn quiets momentarily at a distinctive sound such as a bell or a squeaky rubber toy. By 1 month, this reaction is even more marked. Hearing awareness becomes so

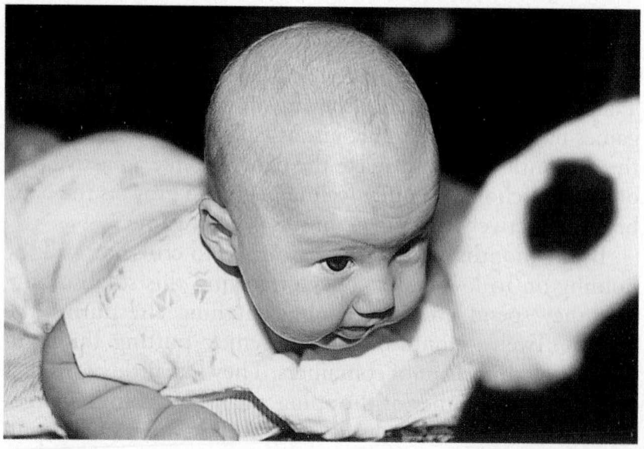

FIGURE 29.11 A 2-month-old infant focuses steadily and lifts her head up while prone. Note her interest in the stuffed bear.

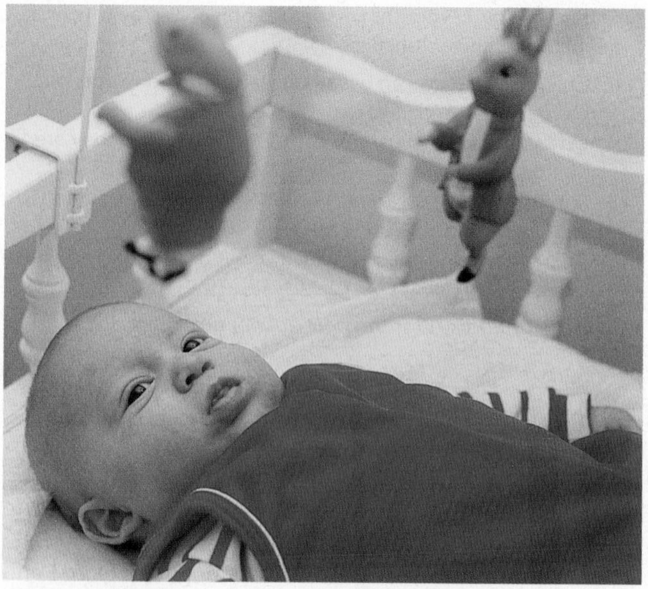

FIGURE 29.12 A 2-month-old infant enjoys watching a simple mobile.

BOX 29.3 Nursing Care Planning Based on Effective Communication

A health care visit for Bryan is over and you dress him while his mother talks to her health care provider.

Less Effective Communication	More Effective Communication
Nurse: Don't move, Bryan. And don't suck your thumb so I can put on your sweater. All done. Let's find your mother.	**Nurse:** Are you ready to go home? Your mother said you're going to pick up Daddy and then go shopping. Do you know about shopping? That's when you ride in a buggy while your mother buys things. Look what a cute yellow sweater you have. It matches the yellow duck on your shirt. Ducks say quack, quack, quack when they talk. Okay. You look ready. Let's find your mother.

Infants appreciate someone talking to them even if they don't understand the words. The first exchange includes only a minimum of words. The second example not only involves the infant but also helps develop vocabulary and the name of colors. Role modeling effective communication this way is important to help parents learn to incorporate language development as they give care.

acute by 2 months of age that infants will stop an activity at the sound of spoken words. Many 3-month-old infants turn their head to attempt to locate a sound. At 4 months of age, when infants hear a distinctive sound, they turn and look in that direction.

By 5 months of age, infants demonstrate they can localize sounds downward and to the side, by turning their head and looking down. Six-month-olds have progressed to being able to locate sounds made above them. By 10 months, infants can recognize their name and listen acutely when spoken to. By 12 months, infants can easily locate sounds in any direction and turn toward them. A vocabulary of two words plus "ma-ma" and "da-da" also demonstrates that an infant can hear.

All during the first year, infants appear to enjoy soft, musical sounds or soft, cooing voices (Box 29.3); they are startled by harsh, raucous rattles or loud bangs. Urge parents to choose for an infant's first toys ones that make these types of welcoming sounds. Recordings of maternal heart sounds can be soothing to very young infants. For the hospitalized infant, a recording of family voices might be a soothing reminder of their presence. Encourage parents to read to their child daily from the beginning of life through the early school-age years, not only because the sound of the parent's voice is comforting but also because this increases language development dramatically.

Touch

Infants need to be touched so they can experience skin-to-skin contact. Clothes should feel comfortable and soft rather than rough; diapers should be dry rather than wet. Teach parents to handle infants with assurance yet gentleness. Remind parents that right now their child is a baby; he or she will have time enough to become a strong man or woman later.

Taste

Infants demonstrate they have an acute sense of taste by turning away from or spitting out a taste they do not enjoy. When infants are introduced to solid food at about 6 months, urge parents to make mealtime a time for fostering trust as well as supplying nutrition by being certain feedings are done at an infant's pace and the amount offered fits the child's needs and not the parent's idea of how much should be eaten.

Smell

Infants can smell accurately within 1 or 2 hours after birth. They respond to an irritating smell by turning their head away from it. They appear to enjoy pleasant odors and learn early in life to identify the familiar smell of breast milk. Teach parents to be alert to substances that cause sneezing when sprayed into the air, such as room deodorizers or cleaning compounds, and to keep irritating odors of this nature out of their child's environment.

Emotional Development

Socialization, or learning how to interact with others, is an extensive phenomenon. One-month-old infants show they can differentiate between faces and other objects by studying a face or the picture of a face longer than other objects. They quiet and eat best for the person who has been their primary caregiver.

When an interested person nods and smiles at a 6-week-old infant, the infant smiles in return. This is a **social smile** and is a definite response to the interaction, not the faint, quick "smile" that younger infants, even newborns, demonstrate. It is a major milestone because it reflects growing maturity in a number of areas, most notably vision, motor control, and intelligence. Cognitively challenged children or children with spasticity may not demonstrate a social smile until much later in the infant year.

By 3 months, infants demonstrate increased social awareness by readily smiling at the sight of a parent's face (Fig. 29.13). Three-month-old infants laugh out loud at the sight of a funny face. By 4 months, when a person who has been playing with and entertaining an infant leaves, the infant is likely to cry or show that the interaction was enjoyable. Infants at this age recognize their primary caregiver

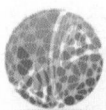

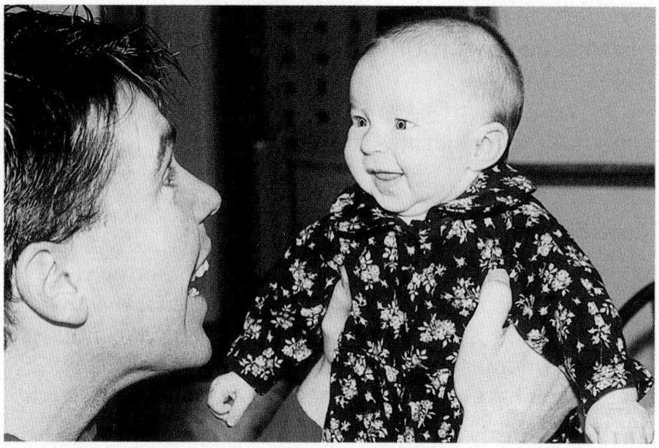

FIGURE 29.13 A 3-month-old smiles delightedly at her father's happy face. This indicates increased social awareness.

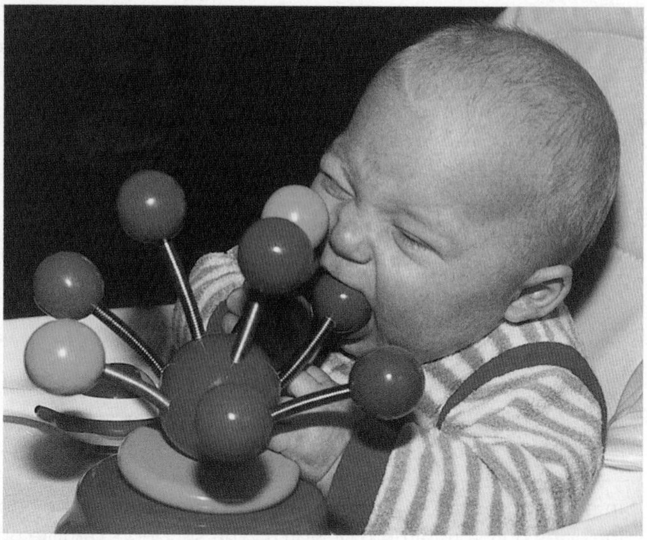

FIGURE 29.14 Infants explore the world by mouthing objects or fingering them. This also helps them separate self from environment.

and prefer that person's presence to others. By 5 months, infants may show displeasure when an object is taken away from them. This is a step beyond showing displeasure when a person leaves.

By 6 months, infants are increasingly aware of the difference between people who regularly care for them and strangers. They may begin to draw back from unfamiliar people. Seven-month-old infants begin to show obvious fear of strangers. They may cry when taken from their parent, attempt to cling to the parent, and reach out to be taken back. Parents may view this as a bad trait or a regression in socialization. Help them appreciate that it is actually a big step forward because it shows that their infant can differentiate between people and also can recognize the difference between persons to trust and others.

Fear of strangers reaches its height during the eighth month, so much so that this phenomenon is often termed **eighth-month anxiety**, or stranger anxiety (Levine, 2011). Remember that an infant at the height of this phase will not go willingly from a parent's arms to a nurse's arms. Taking a few minutes to talk to the child and parent first so you are perceived as a friend, not a stranger, is time well spent.

Nine-month-old infants are very aware of changes in tone of voice. They cry when scolded, not because they understand what is being said but because they sense their parent's displeasure. By 12 months, most children have overcome their fear of strangers and are alert and responsive again when approached. They like to play interactive nursery rhymes and rhythm games and "dance" with others. They also like being at the table for meals and joining in family activities.

Cognitive Development

In the first month of life, an infant mainly uses simple reflex activity. There is little evidence infants at this early age see themselves as separate from their environment. However, this does not mean they cannot respond actively or interact with people. They demonstrate they are very people oriented moments after birth by cuddling against an adult's chest.

Primary and Secondary Circular Reaction

By the third month of life, a child enters a cognitive stage identified by Piaget (1952) as *primary circular reaction*. During this time, the infant explores objects by grasping them with the hands or by mouthing them (Fig. 29.14). Infants appear to be unaware of what actions they can cause or what actions occur independently, however. For example, if an infant's hand should accidentally strike a mobile across the crib, the infant appears to enjoy watching the brightly colored birds move in front of him, but makes no attempt to hit the mobile again because he does not realize his hand caused the movement.

At about 6 months of age infants pass into a stage Piaget (1952) called *secondary circular reaction*. Now when infants reach for a mobile above the crib, hit it, and watch it move, they realize it was their hand that initiated the motion, and so they hit it again.

By 10 months, infants discover object permanence. Infants are ready for peek-a-boo once they have gained this concept. They know their parent still exists even when hiding behind a hand or blanket and wait excitedly for the parent to reappear.

As infants reach 1 year of age, they are capable of reproducing new events (they deliberately hit a mobile once, it moves, and they hit it again). They drop objects from a high chair or playpen and watch where they fall or roll. This is a frustrating activity for parents because it involves a great deal of reaching and picking up. It is an important activity for infants, however, because it confirms their awareness of the permanence of objects and how they are able to control events in their world.

QSEN Checkpoint Question 29.3

Quality Improvement

You are discussing object permanence with Bryan's mother. Which action by her infant would best illustrate that he understands object permanence?

a. The child looks for you after you walk away.
b. The child cries when either hungry or lonely.
c. The child prefers a large yellow ball to a small red one.
d. The child smiles when the mobile on his or her crib jingles.

Look in Appendix A for the best answer and rationale.

THE NURSING ROLE IN HEALTH PROMOTION OF AN INFANT AND FAMILY

The nursing role with infants is wide ranging because infants are so dependent on their caregivers for safety, learning, and emotional development.

Promoting Achievement of the Developmental Task: Trust Versus Mistrust

Erikson (1993) proposed that the developmental task of the infant period is to form a sense of trust. When an infant is hungry, a parent feeds and makes the infant comfortable again. When an infant is wet, a parent changes his or her diaper and the infant is dry again. When an infant is cold, a parent holds the baby closely. By these simple processes, infants learn to trust that when they have a need or are in distress, a parent will come and meet that need.

A synonym for trust in this connotation is love. By the way infants are handled, fed, talked to, and held, they learn to love and recognize they are loved. Infants who have numerous caregivers, who may be fed one day on a rigid schedule and the next only when they are hungry, who sometimes are treated roughly and sometimes gently, or who don't always have their needs met can have difficulty learning to trust (Box 29.4). If infants cannot trust, they cannot enjoy deeply satisfying interactions with others and may have difficulty trusting themselves, experiencing high self-esteem, and establishing close relationships as adults.

It is important for infants to establish the ability to love, or trust, early in life in this way because development is sequential. If a first developmental step is inadequate, this inadequacy can pervade all future steps. In reference to trust, the end result could be an adult unable to instill a sense of trust in his or her own child, perpetuating the inadequacy from generation to generation.

How do parents (or a nurse) encourage a sense of trust in an infant? Trust arises primarily from a sense of confidence that one can predict what is coming next. This does not mean parents should set up a rigid schedule of care for their infant. However, it does imply that parents should study their infant's reaction to activities and then establish a workable schedule based on that (e.g., breakfast, bath, playtime, nap, lunch, walk outside, quiet playtime, dinner, story, and bedtime). This gentle rhythm of care gives infants a sense of being able to predict what is going to happen and gives life consistency.

All little children thrive on routine such as the same story read over and over again, the same bedtime rituals, or the same spoon every day for lunch. Infancy is not too early for children to learn family traditions such as decorating for a holiday because this type of repetition can help them feel secure in their world. Some parents have difficulty accepting routine as important to a child. They may be so tired of their own work schedules that they want to raise their children as free spirits. Do not discourage this philosophy; however, you might suggest a few modifications to instill some order into infants' lives.

Just as it is important that there is a rhythm to the care, it is also important that the care is mainly given by one person (Fig. 29.15). This person can be the mother, father, grandparent, a conscientious babysitter, a foster parent, or anyone who can give consistent care. For infants ill at birth who are hospitalized for months, this person is often a primary nurse or case manager. You may have to encourage parents who are reluctant at first to interact with their infant not to feel self-conscious about talking to a baby who does not talk back. Pointing out the importance of such interactions and role modeling them while caring for children help parents use this type of stimulation as they care for their baby's physical needs.

Women who work outside their home during the first year of a baby's life (at least 90% of women) should try to arrange for one person to care for their child while they are away from home or choose a day care center that will provide

BOX 29.4 Nursing Care Planning to Respect Cultural Diversity

Although development follows set patterns during the infant year, the care of them is more dependent on cultural factors. One difference is in the way mothers carry their infants. Western mothers tend to carry infants in their arms and so have to put them down to work or into a stroller to shop. South American women carry their infants in shoulder slings or on their hips, positions that allow a woman to continue to work or walk while holding an infant close. Infants who are held with their legs outspread that way tend to develop deeper hip sockets and have less hip dysplasia (see Chapter 27).

The amount of infant bathing that is done is also inconsistent across cultures. In the United States, most infants are bathed daily. In colder climates or countries where warm, clean water is not readily available, infant bathing is more limited. The use of diapers varies also. In hot climates, infants are often not diapered. Being aware of these cultural differences leads to better understanding of the reasons for an individual woman's particular method of childrearing.

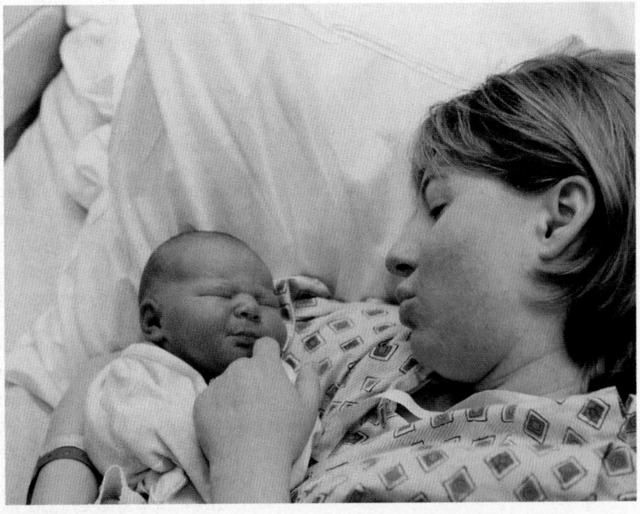

FIGURE 29.15 An infant's sense of trust develops through warm interpersonal relationships. Here, a mother and infant share a "together" moment.

a consistent caregiver. Urge them to discuss their methods of child care with alternative caregivers to prevent disrupting an infant's routine. When a child is admitted to a hospital, document and list this information on an infant's electronic record.

Urge parents to make certain that not only will the number of caretakers for their child be limited but also that caretakers will be actively interacting with their child. Passively caring for infants—not talking to them or touching or stroking them while feeding or changing them—amounts to little more than not being with them at all. An increasing number of parents are installing video cameras to make sure a caretaker is actively interacting with their baby to instill a sense of trust in their child. Nursing actions designed to help an ill infant develop a sense of trust in addition to individual caretaking are detailed in Table 29.3.

Promoting Infant Safety

Unintentional injuries are a leading cause of death in children from 1 month through 24 years of age. These are second only to acute infections as a cause of acute morbidity and primary care provider visits (CDC, 2011).

Most unintentional injuries in infancy occur because parents either underestimate or overestimate a child's ability. Nursing interventions that help parents become sensitive to their infant's developmental progress, therefore, not only help establish sound parent–child relationships but also guard infant safety (Box 29.5).

TABLE 29.3 Ways for Nurses to Help an Ill Infant Develop a Sense of Trust

Area of Care	Nursing Actions
Nutrition	Encourage mothers to continue to breastfeed if possible while their infant is hospitalized; provide privacy and support as necessary. If a parent is not present to do so, hold the infant no matter what feeding method is used (e.g., gavage, total parenteral, oral, enteral). If this is not possible, hold infants for a time after or between feedings so they receive holding equal to what they would ordinarily receive with being fed. If infant feeding is not oral, provide a pacifier (medical condition and parent preference considered) five or six times daily for sucking pleasure.
Dressing change	Use nonallergenic tape to avoid irritation while it is applied and reduce pain when removed. Use stockinette, rolled gauze, or Kling gauze to hold a bandage in place rather than tape if possible. To prevent chilling, be certain irrigation solutions are warm; keep exposure during dressing changes to a minimum. Restrain only those body parts necessary for safety. Describe what you are doing in a nonthreatening tone of voice as you give care to give comfort.
Medicine administration	Flavor oral medicine to disguise disagreeable taste. Never add medicine to formula to prevent changing the formula's taste. Comfort the infant after injections or intravenous insertion by holding and rocking, or immediately give the infant to a parent. Check intravenous sites frequently for infiltration and pain. Role model for parents how to hold the infant despite tubing and restraints.
Rest	Encourage parents to rock infants to sleep. Do this yourself if no parent is present. Always wake infants gently because it is frightening (for anyone) to be awakened by a stranger. If bed rest is necessary, check for irritated elbows, heels, and knees from rubbing against sheets; protect with long sleeves or pants or a Kling bandage.
Hygiene	Check the temperature of bath water for comfort and to prevent chilling or burning. Change diapers frequently to reduce discomfort from irritation. To avoid caries, begin toothbrushing with first tooth.
Pain	Hold and comfort an infant in pain. Do not ask parents to restrain a child for a painful procedure. Allow parents to comfort the child afterward because that is a better parent role. Reduce painful procedures to a minimum (e.g., combine blood drawing so only one puncture is necessary for many tests).
Stimulation	Remember that infants focus longest on a human face. Face them directly to talk to them. Provide a crib mirror or a mobile, because visual stimulation seems satisfying to an infant. If no mobile is available, create one from string or strips of adhesive tape, colored paper, cotton balls, or colored tongue blades. For safety, hang the mobile high enough for the infant to see but not reach. During the second half of the first year, infants need to try to crawl. Put a pad or sheet on the floor and encourage them to come to you while you stand by to offer reassurance. If contagion or immunosuppression is not a problem, bring the infant's crib to the nursing desk where the infant can still interact with you while you do necessary paperwork.

BOX 29.5 Nursing Care Planning Based on Family Teaching

UNINTENTIONAL INJURY PREVENTION MEASURES FOR INFANTS

Q. Bryan's mother is worried about keeping him safe. She asks, "How can I prevent accidents at this age?"
A. Here are some tips to help prevent specific types of unintentional injuries:

Potential Unintended Injury	Prevention Measures
General	Be aware that the frequency of injury is increased when parents are under stress. Take special precautions at these times. Choose babysitters carefully and explain and enforce all precautions when sitters are in charge.
Aspiration	Be certain any object an infant can grasp and bring to the mouth is either safe to eat or too big to fit in the mouth. Do not offer foods such as popcorn or peanuts, because these are easily aspirated. Store baby powder out of reach; inspect toys and pacifiers for small parts that could be aspirated if broken off.
Falls	Never leave an infant on an unprotected surface, such as a bed or couch, even if the infant is in an infant seat. Place a gate at the top and bottom of stairways; do not allow your infant to walk with a sharp object in the hands or mouth. Raise crib rails and make sure they are locked before walking away from the crib. Do not leave a child unattended in a high chair; avoid using an infant walker near a stairway.
Motor vehicle	Never transport an infant in an automobile unless the infant is buckled into an age-appropriate seat in the back seat of the car. Be aware of the proper technique for tethering the car seat to the car. Do not be distracted by an infant while driving. Do not leave an infant unattended in a parked car (the infant can become dehydrated from excess heat, can move the gear shift, or be abducted).
Suffocation	Allow no plastic bags within infant's reach; don't use pillows in cribs. Store unused appliances such as refrigerators or stoves with the doors removed. Buy a crib that is approved for safety (spacing of rails is not over 2 3/8 in. [6 cm] apart). Remove constricting clothing such as a bib or pacifier string from neck at bedtime.
Drowning	Do not leave infants alone in a bathtub or unsupervised near water (even buckets of cleaning water).
Animal bites	Do not allow an infant to approach a strange dog; supervise play with family pets.
Poisoning	Never present medication as a candy; buy medications in containers with safety caps; put away in a high cabinet immediately after use; and never leave medication in a pocket or handbag. Never take medication in front of infants. Place all medication and poisons in locked cabinets or overhead shelves. Do not use lead-based paint in any area of the home. Hang plants or set on high surfaces. Post telephone number of the national poison control center by the telephone (1-222-1222).
Burns	Test warmth of formula and food before feeding (use extra precaution with microwave warming). Do not smoke or drink hot liquids while holding or caring for an infant. Buy flame-retardant clothing for infants; turn handles of pans toward back of stove. Use a sunscreen on a child over 6 months when out in direct or indirect sunlight, and limit the child's sun exposure to less than 30 minutes at a time. If a vaporizer is used, use a cool-mist, not a hot-mist type; remain in room to monitor so child cannot reach vaporizer. Monitor infants carefully near candles. Do not leave infants unsupervised near hot-water faucets. Keep a screen in front of a fireplace or heater. Do not allow infants to blow out matches or candles (don't teach infants that fire is fun). Keep electric wires and cords out of reach; cover electrical outlets with safety plugs.
General	Be aware some infants are more active, curious, and impulsive and therefore more vulnerable to unintentional injury than others.

Aspiration Prevention

Aspiration is a chief injury threat to infants throughout the first year. Round, cylindrical objects are more dangerous than square or flexible objects in this regard. A 1-in. (3.2-cm) cylinder, such as a carrot or hot dog, is particularly dangerous because it can totally obstruct an infant's airway. A deflated balloon can be sucked into the mouth, obstructing the airway in the same way. Educate parents who feed their infant formula not to prop bottles. By doing this, they are overestimating their infant's ability to push the bottle away, sit up, turn the head to the side, cough, and clear the airway if milk should flow too rapidly into the mouth, allowing an infant to aspirate.

Other instances of aspiration occur because parents underestimate their infant's ability to grasp and place objects in their mouth. Even a newborn can wiggle to a new position to reach an attractive object such as a teddy bear with small button eyes. Newborns' grasp and sucking reflexes automatically cause them to grasp and pull the object into their mouth. Caution parents to be certain nothing comes within an infant's reach that would not be safe to put into the mouth. Using clothing without decorative buttons and checking toys and rattles to ensure they have no small parts that could snap off or fall out are good steps for parents to follow.

A test of whether a toy could be dangerous if an infant puts it inside the mouth is whether it fits inside a toilet paper roll. If it does, it is small enough to be aspirated. When solid foods are introduced, encourage parents to offer small pieces of hot dogs or grapes, not large chunks for this reason. Children under about 5 years of age should not be offered popcorn or peanuts because of the danger of aspiration.

As infants become more adept at handling toys, parents need to reassess toys for loose pieces or parts. If parents are going to offer an infant a pacifier, they should use one that has a one-piece construction with a flange large enough to keep it from completely entering the child's mouth (Fig. 29.16).

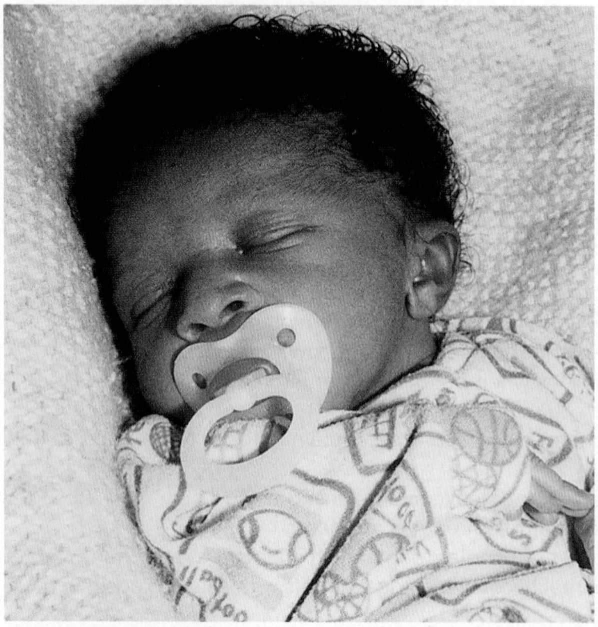

FIGURE 29.16 Many infants enjoy sucking on a pacifier to help them fall asleep. This may also help prevent sudden infant death syndrome.

QSEN Checkpoint Question 29.4

Evidence-Based Practice

Scalding injuries occur in infants when caretakers spill hot beverages while holding them in their lap or, toward the end of the first year, the infant is able to pull a pan of hot liquid off the stove. To confirm the incidence of this type of injury, researchers studied the admission records of an urban pediatric emergency department in Ireland. Of 280 children seen for burns, 161 (57%) were scalds. Of these, 79% occurred in children under 5 years of age, 65% were caused by hot beverages, 16% were caused by hot water, and 16% by hot food. The areas of children most affected were upper limbs and upper trunks. The researchers concluded that more parent education as to the danger of scalding is needed to reduce the number of these very painful injuries in young children (Yates, McKay, & Nicholson, 2011).

Based on the study, which remark by Bryan's mother would worry you most?

a. "I never drive without a cup of coffee in my cup holder."
b. "I'm going to switch to drinking tea to reduce my caffeine intake."
c. "I drank coffee during Bryan's pregnancy; it's why he's so high strung."
d. "I'm a coffee addict; I always have a fresh cup in my hand."

Look in Appendix A for the best answer and rationale.

Fall Prevention

Falls are a second major cause of infant injuries. As a preventive measure, no infant, beginning with a newborn, should be left unattended on a raised surface. Normal wiggling can bring even a newborn to the edge of a bed, couch, or table top, resulting in a fall.

Teach parents to be prepared for their infant to turn over by 2 months of age. From that time on, they must be especially vigilant not to leave the baby unattended on a changing table or counter. If the child sleeps in a crib, the mattress should be lowered to its bottom position so the height of the side rails increases; rails should be no more than 2⅜ in. apart, narrow enough so children cannot put their head between them. Two months is about the maximum length of time infants can safely sleep in a bassinet; they need the protection of a crib and high side rails before they turn over.

All of these safety precautions apply to the hospital environment as well as to the home. Be sure crib sides are raised and secure before you walk away from a crib, even for just a moment. Also ensure the space between the mattress and headboard is small enough that an infant's head could not become trapped. Make sure cords from nursing call bells or other equipment are out of an infant's reach.

Car Safety

Teaching car safety for infants (as well as for the whole family) is an important protective health measure. The use of car seats for newborns is discussed in Chapter 18. Infants should be placed in backward facing seats in the back seat because an inflating front seat airbag could suffocate an infant (AAP, 2012b). Backward-facing car seats should continue to be used without interruption until age 2 years, or until the child reaches the highest weight or height allowed by the car safety seat's manufacturer. If parents are firm about keeping infants in car seats even when they are fussy or impatient, children will eventually become more comfortable and accepting of car seats.

QSEN Checkpoint Question 29.5

Safety

You review infant safety with Bryan's mother. In light of your knowledge about the most common injuries among infants, it would be most important to teach her about preventing which of the following?

a. Drowning and hypersensitivities
b. Poisoning and suffocation
c. Auto accidents and burns
d. Aspiration and falls

Look in Appendix A for the best answer and rationale.

Safety With Siblings

As infants become more fun to play with at about 3 months of age, older brothers and sisters grow more interested in interacting with them. You may need to remind parents that children under about 5 years of age, as a group, are not responsible enough or knowledgeable enough about infants to be left unattended with them. They might introduce an unsafe toy or engage in play that is too rough for an infant. Some preschoolers may be so jealous of a new baby they will physically harm an infant if left alone.

Bathing and Swimming Safety

As babies begin to develop good back support, many parents begin to bathe them in an adult tub. Caution parents to never leave an infant unattended in a tub, even when propped up out of the water or sitting in a bath ring or bath seat. Normal wiggling can easily cause a baby to slip down under the water. This applies to a hospital setting as well.

Many communities offer infant swim programs for babies as young as 6 months. If an infant is enrolled in one of these programs, parents may become overconfident about their infant's ability to operate safely in water. Urge them to think carefully before enrolling their infant in such a program, because, although infants can dog paddle momentarily in a swimming pool, this action does not mean they can sustain that position for any length of time in a bathtub or pool by themselves. As a second danger, being able to swim momentarily may cause children to lose their instinctive fear of water and so be in more danger when around water than children who are still naturally more cautious. Such programs can also cause hypothermia and spread microorganisms because infants this age are not yet toilet trained. Exposure to chlorinated water might damage lung epithelium, which then has the possibility to become a precursor to childhood asthma (Klootwijk & Krul, 2011).

Childproofing

Toward the end of pregnancy, parents need to begin preparing for their infant's arrival by childproofing their home. As soon as infants begin teething at 5 to 6 months, they chew on any object within reach to lessen gumline pain. Remind parents to thoroughly check for possible sources of lead paint, such as painted cribs, playpen rails, or windowsills before this time to avoid lead poisoning (CDC, 2011). Paints safe for baby furniture should be marked "Safe for use on surfaces that might be chewed by children." If an infant is going to play on the floor, urge parents to move furniture in front of electrical fixtures or buy protective caps for outlets. Infants are especially fascinated by the holes in electric outlets and will probe them with (often wet) fingers. Parents may need to install safety gates at the top and bottom of stairways as additional safety measures before the infant crawls.

Urge parents to move all potentially poisonous substances from bottom cupboards and store them well out of their infant's reach. Infants of any age should not be left unattended in carriages, high chairs, grocery shopping carts, or strollers. Baby walkers are extremely dangerous because infants can maneuver them near stairways and fall the length of the stairs.

When infants begin creeping, remind parents to recheck bottom cupboards and stairways for safety. When the child begins to walk, higher areas, such as coffee tables, need to be cleared of dangerous items. In a hospital setting, assess low counter areas for dangerous objects. Do not leave possibly dangerous supplies in an infant's room.

By 10 months, achievement of a pincer grasp makes infants able to pick up very small objects. Remind parents to check play areas or areas such as tabletops for pins or other sharp objects that could be swallowed. At this point, some of an infant's toys may now be 10 months old and need to be checked to be certain they are still intact and safe.

Although infants can seem very independent and able to take care of themselves toward the end of the infant year, their judgment about what situations could be dangerous is immature. As soon as they can walk they're able to venture into the street or a swimming pool if not carefully supervised (Fig. 29.17). In a hospital setting, a 12-month-old child can

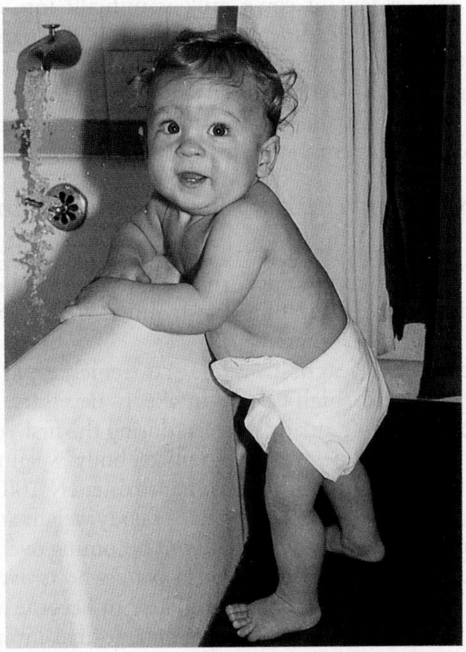

FIGURE 29.17 Once walking begins, the extended range of activities brings an infant in contact with potentially dangerous places or objects unless the house is childproofed. The bathroom is an important room in which to begin childproofing.

wander onto an elevator, out of the hospital, into a laboratory area, or fall down a flight of stairs if not supervised (Ibrahim, Wood, Margulies, et al., 2011).

What if...29.2 Bryan's mother is interested in "childproofing" her house? What questions would you want to ask to determine whether her house is safe for a 2 month old?

Promoting Nutritional Health of an Infant

The best food for an infant during the first 12 months of life (and the only food necessary for the first 4 to 6 months) is breast milk (see Chapter 19 for tips on breastfeeding). With breastfeeding, as long as the infant's mother is ingesting an adequate diet, no additional supplements such as iron or vitamins are necessary, except for fluoride if it is not included in the water supply (after 6 months of age) and possibly vitamin D. How long mothers continue to breastfeed is an individual choice, although it is recommended that infants be exclusively breastfed for 4 months. It is optimal if breastfeeding is then continued through the entire first year (Whitney & Rolfes, 2012). There is a suggestion that early weaning from breastfeeding can lead to an increased incidence of obesity (Townsend & Pitchford, 2012). There is a possibility that prolonged breastfeeding into the preschool period can limit nutrients and impair a child's growth.

For infants whose mothers choose not to or are unable to breastfeed, a commercial iron-fortified formula will supply adequate nutrition for the infant year (Krebs & Primak, 2011) (for types of commercial formulas, see http://thePoint.lww.com/Pillitteri7e). Supplementation is unnecessary with iron-fortified commercial formula although after 6 months, if the water supply does not contain fluoride, this may need to be supplemented. Infants who are changed to cow's milk before 1 year of age—a practice that is not recommended because the protein in cow's milk is difficult for an infant to digest, possibly leading to such intestinal irritation that slight but continuous gastrointestinal bleeding occurs, which results in anemia—should receive a supplementary form of vitamin C and iron and possibly fluoride to make up for the deficiency of these components in cow's milk.

Recommended Dietary Allowances for Infants

Because children's nutritional needs vary so much from infancy through adolescence, the recommended allowances of calories, protein, vitamins, and minerals also vary with each period of development.

The entire first year of life is one of extremely rapid growth, so a high-protein, high-calorie intake is necessary. Calorie allowances can be gradually reduced during the first year from a level of 120 calories per kilogram of body weight (50 to 55 calories per pound) at birth to approximately 100 calories per kilogram (45 calories per pound) of body weight at the end of the first year to prevent babies from becoming overweight.

Although heredity plays a role, a baby who is overweight during the first year of life is more likely to become an obese adult than one whose weight is within normal limits. Such long-term effects occur because overfeeding in early life may produce large numbers of excess fat cells (adipocytes) used to store fat. Because these cells are permanent and remain filled with fat, once they are present, weight regulation can become difficult throughout life. Breastfed infants gain less weight than those who are formula fed and so usually tend to be somewhat lighter in weight and have less risk of becoming overweight (Thilo & Rosenberg, 2011).

Introduction of Solid Food

From a nutritional standpoint, a normal full-term infant can thrive on breast milk or a commercial iron-fortified formula without the addition of any solid food until 4 to 6 months (Conti, Patel, & Bhat, 2011). Delaying solid food until this time also helps prevent overwhelming an infant's kidneys with a heavy solute load. Although difficult to document, it also may delay the development of food allergies in susceptible infants and be yet another way to help prevent future obesity (Gaffney, Kitsantas, & Cheema, 2012).

Most parents are eager to begin feeding their infant solid food, hoping this will help their child sleep through the night. So eager, in fact, some parents do begin food before the recommended time without apparent ill effects, possibly because much of the food is not processed by the gastrointestinal tract, but rather passes through undigested because of the immaturity of the digestive system, and decreased amounts of amylase and lipase (digestive enzymes).

Generally speaking, parents can tell infants are physiologically ready for solid food when they are nursing vigorously every 3 to 4 hours and do not seem satisfied or when they are taking more than 32 oz (960 ml) of formula a day and do not seem satisfied.

Introducing Solid Food. Infants are not ready to digest complex starches until amylase is present in saliva at approximately 2 to 3 months. Biting movements begin at approximately 3 months. Chewing movements do not begin until 7 to 9 months. Therefore, foods that require chewing should not be given until this age.

In addition to these cautions, the extrusion reflex needs to fade before infants accept food readily. With the extrusion reflex intact, when anything is placed on the anterior third of an infant's tongue, it is automatically extruded or thrust out of the mouth by the tongue (Fig. 29.18). This is a lifesaving

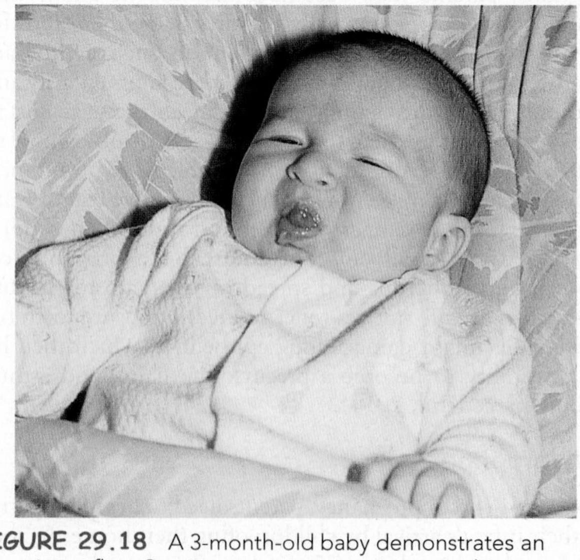

FIGURE 29.18 A 3-month-old baby demonstrates an extrusion reflex. Caution parents not to interpret this action as a food dislike but recognize it as the reflex action that it is.

reflex in early infancy because it prevents infants from swallowing or aspirating foreign objects that touch the mouth. The reflex fades at 3 to 4 months at about the same time the gastrointestinal tract has matured to be ready to digest solid food.

Techniques for Feeding Solid Food. The introduction of solid food begins a new type of interaction between parents and their infant and can require a period of adjustment (van Dijk, Hunnius, & van Geert, 2012). A typical pattern for the introduction of solid food beginning at 4 to 6 months includes:

- Iron-fortified infant cereal mixed with breast milk, orange juice, or formula; aids in preventing iron-deficiency anemia as well as is the least allergenic type of food and the most easily digested so is usually the first food offered.
- Vegetables (if using commercial types, begin with level 1 which contain a single ingredient and are pureed, then switch to level 2 at about 6 months, which are strained). These are a good source of vitamin A and add new texture and flavors to diet.
- Fruit (use level 1 foods, then change to level 2 at about 6 months, which are strained). These are the best sources of vitamin C and a good source of vitamin A.
- Meat is a good source of protein, iron, and B vitamins (level 3 foods, which have more texture, encourage chewing).
- At the end of the first year, egg yolk, a good source of iron, can be added.

Caution parents to omit wheat, tomatoes, oranges, fish, and egg whites if there are allergies in the family because these foods are those most likely to cause allergies. Also, parents should never use honey as a sweetener because it may contain botulism spores and never use cow's milk because it can cause microscopic intestinal bleeding.

Teach parents to offer new foods one at a time and to allow their child to eat that item for about 3 to 7 days before introducing another new food. This system helps parents to detect a possible food allergy in addition to allowing the infant to get used to the new experience.

A newborn's stomach can hold approximately 2 tablespoons (30 ml). By 1 year, a stomach can hold no more than about 1 cup (240 ml). For this reason, when they begin eating solid food, infants rarely take more than 2 tablespoons (30 ml) at a time.

It is best for the first solid food feeding if an infant is held in the parent's arms as if for breastfeeding or bottle feeding. This reduces the newness of the experience and minimizes the amount of stress associated with it. Some infants accept new experiences of this type readily, whereas other infants resist heartily. If an infant does not take readily to solid food, advise parents to wait a few days and then try again. Remind them this is not a contest to see whose child takes cereal, vegetables, or fruit first.

Babies have distinct taste preferences even at young ages and may spit out a food because they do not like the taste. Even after the extrusion reflex has faded, some infants continue to spit out food. This is because, when infants drink from a bottle or breast, they press their tongue and the nipple against their hard palate. When an infant tries to eat solid food using the same technique, it appears the child is spitting out the food. A parent who knows an infant's cues will be able to distinguish taste preferences from inadequate management of solid food. Box 29.6 lists pointers to help make the introduction of solid foods a positive experience.

If a parent is going to prepare baby food, the parent needs to avoid preparing spinach, carrots, beets, green beans, and squash because these can contain excessive amounts of nitrates that are not processed well by infants. Commercial baby food has the nitrates removed and so does not present this problem.

Cereal. Infant cereal is fortified with B vitamins and iron. It is supplied as a precooked, fine dry powder to which expressed breast milk, infant formula, or juice is added. Adding sugar to cereal is unnecessary. Extra sugar in the diet can lead to diarrhea in young infants and beginning caries in older infants.

Fortified cereal costs no more than unfortified cereal, so remind parents to buy the fortified product. The first cereal introduced is usually rice cereal, because fewer children are allergic to rice products than to wheat and corn products. Usually, this is offered twice a day, in the morning and

BOX 29.6 Nursing Care Planning to Empower a Family

TIPS TO HELP INTRODUCE SOLID FOODS TO INFANTS

Q. Bryan's mother has already started feeding him solid food. She asks, "When and how should I have begun food?"
A. It's best if infants are exclusively breastfed for 4 months so infants typically are ready for solid food at 4 to 6 months of age. Usual guidelines to help introduce solid foods include:

- Introduce one food at a time, waiting 3 to 7 days between new items.
- Introduce the food before formula or breastfeeding when the infant is hungry.
- Introduce small amounts of a new food (1 or 2 teaspoons) at a time.
- Respect infant food preferences; a child cannot be expected to like all new tastes equally well.
- Use only minimal to no salt and sugar on solid food to minimize the number of additives.
- Remember that the extrusion reflex is present for the first 4 to 6 months of life, so any food placed on an infant's tongue will be pushed forward and extruded.
- To prevent aspiration, *do not* place food in bottles to drink with formula.
- Even though you don't like a particular food, introduce it with a positive, "You'll like this" attitude. It could be your child's favorite.

evening. Once the child has taken rice cereal for 1 week, if they wish, parents can try another kind.

Caution parents not to mix cereal into the infant's bottle because, as it is necessary to cut a larger hole in the bottle nipple for the cereal and milk mixture to flow freely, there is a danger an infant may aspirate if the hole cut is too big or if the parent then uses that nipple for formula without cereal added. This practice also denies the child the opportunity of learning to eat from a spoon and experiencing different food tastes and textures.

Infant cereal is so rich in iron that parents should continue feeding it at least through the first year. Ideally, children should eat infant cereal until age 3 or 4 years, because few popularly advertised products can match the nutrients of fortified infant cereal.

Vegetables and Fruit. Because the iron content in vegetables is generally higher than that of fruits, vegetables are usually the second food added to the diet (at 5 to 7 months of age). To prepare their own, a parent simply cooks a vegetable and then blends or processes it so it does not have to be chewed. Caution parents not to add butter, sugar, or salt to the preparation because infants have difficulty digesting fats until almost the end of the first year and the added salt or sugar is unnecessary. By filling ice-cube trays with the blended vegetables, parents can make a 1-week supply and defrost a cube at a time. An ice cube is approximately 1 oz, or one fourth the size of a jar of baby food.

If parents use commercial baby food, they should begin with level 1 types (single ingredient and pureed) and feed from a dish rather than directly from the jar. This is because, if the spoon carries salivary enzymes from an infant's mouth back to the food jar, the enzymes will quickly liquefy what remains in the jar. Also, there is a danger of transferring bacteria (principally streptococci) from an infant's mouth to the jar. Then, if the parent keeps the jar for another feeding in the next 24 hours, bacteria will multiply rapidly because the contents serve as a culture medium. Baby food jars should be refrigerated once they are opened, and manufacturers recommend they be used no longer than 48 hours after they were first opened.

When vegetables are added to the diet, they are usually offered at lunch. Remind parents to offer both green and yellow vegetables. Help them to remember that their own dislike of a particular vegetable does not mean their child will feel the same way about it. If they do convey distaste for a food, their child will pick up on the feeling and may not like the vegetable either.

Fruit is usually offered 1 week after beginning vegetables (at 5 to 7 months of age). It can be given in addition to cereal for breakfast and dinner. Raw mashed banana is easy to prepare with just a fork; peaches are easily prepared in a blender. As with vegetables, parents should offer a selection so an infant is exposed to different tastes and textures.

Meat and Eggs. Meat is usually introduced at 6 months of age because this is the time an infant's iron stores are beginning to be depleted. Parents can grind a portion of the meat they have prepared for their own meal so it is tender, or they can use commercially prepared baby food. If they use commercial baby meat, remind them to use the plain meat preparations, not vegetable and meat dinners because these contain mostly vegetables. Chicken has the advantage of being low in cholesterol, but this is not a priority with infants. Beef and pork have more iron than chicken, so encourage parents to offer a variety. When meat is added to an infant's diet, it is usually added as part of the evening meal in place of cereal.

Egg yolks are offered at the end of the first year (8 to 10 months of age). Egg yolks contain the bulk of the iron content of eggs; the white contains the bulk of protein. Egg yolk alone should be given at first, because the protein of the egg white can lead to allergy or can be difficult for an infant to digest. Eggs may be hard-boiled (then a little formula or breast milk can be added to the mashed yolk to make it more liquid) or purchased as commercial baby food. Soft boiling or poaching is not usually recommended, because salmonella, the chief offending microorganism that may be in eggs, may not be killed by these methods. Also, thorough cooking makes protein easier to digest.

Table Food. With the introduction of solid food, encourage parents to establish a three-meal-a-day pattern, if that is the family's lifestyle, and to have the infant join the family at the table. If an individual infant is too distracted by the activity at a family table to eat well, parents may find the infant eats more if fed first and then given a cracker to chew on while just sitting at the table and being with the family.

Commercial junior foods are now prepared without excessive additives and are convenient for parents who have little time to prepare food. Generally, however, encourage parents to use homemade foods rather than relying on commercially prepared junior or toddler foods (often labeled as level 4 foods) as much as possible so the infant will have less difficulty switching to a parent's cooking when older.

Mashed potatoes or peas and cut-up meatloaf are examples of table foods that infants older than 6 months of age like to eat and busy parents can prepare quickly. If hot dogs are offered, caution parents to cut them into small bite-size portions; otherwise, their shape is dangerous if aspirated. As infants begin teething, they may enjoy dried bread or teething biscuits.

Remind parents that high chairs are one of the most dangerous pieces of baby equipment they own. Urge them to always fasten the restraint and never leave an infant unattended in a high chair, because even a 6 month old can squirm out of a chair with little effort. This is important to keep in mind as well when feeding infants in a hospital setting.

Establishment of Healthy Eating Patterns

Some parents may need to be reminded that there are no hard-and-fast rules for infant feeding. The "rules" are only guidelines based on what seems to work well with most infants. Encourage them to individualize their approach according to the cues their child is giving them for readiness and to understand that refusing a teaspoonful of carrots is refusing a teaspoonful of carrots and nothing more.

Most infants, however, eat hungrily, so feeding problems tend to be reported more frequently as a second-year or toddler problem than as an infant concern. If an infant does refuse to eat, ask the parents what foods they are offering. Have them list exactly the types and amounts of foods the child ate the day before (a 24-hour dietary recall history). It may be apparent from this that enough is being eaten in a day's time and the parents' expectations are unrealistic for the child's size and age.

If intake is inadequate and the child is, indeed, a fussy eater, ask about the parents' methods of feeding. For example, infants generally accept the new experience of eating from a spoon better when they are hungry, not when their stomach is full. Some babies, however, particularly those with an intense temperament, may be so hungry at mealtime that they cannot tolerate the frustration of spoon feeding until some of their hunger is relieved. They may need to drink 2 or 3 oz of formula or nurse at the breast for a few minutes before they will eat a spoonful of food.

If infants are fatigued or overstimulated, they also may not eat well. Providing a quiet environment away from older brothers or sisters or other distractions before mealtime might be a solution to this problem.

Encourage parents not to force infants to eat if they do not seem hungry. Healthy, happy infants will be hungry at mealtime and will eat. Those who refuse a meal may be tired, distracted, or perhaps ill. Forcing only leads to regurgitation or, if they are ill, vomiting. Infants who are eating and not thriving or not eating and therefore are not thriving should be examined by their primary care provider to determine if a cause such as a metabolic disorder or failure to thrive exists (see Chapters 48 and 55).

Weaning

Mothers are advised to continue breastfeeding for at least 6 months and, if possible, to continue breastfeeding for the full first year. Infants are capable of approximating their lips to a cup and they can drink effectively from one at about 9 months of age. The sucking reflex begins to diminish in intensity between 6 and 9 months, which makes this the time to consider weaning from a bottle.

To wean from either formula or breast milk, the parent needs to choose one feeding a day and begin offering fluid by the new method at that feeding. Choosing a time of day that is not an infant's fussy period is helpful; other than that, the time is unimportant. After 3 days to 1 week, when an infant has become acclimated to the one change, the parent then changes a second feeding and so on. Should an illness such as an upper respiratory infection occur or should the child have teething discomfort, there will be setbacks, so no set number of weeks should be prescribed to complete weaning. Infants usually need more fluid during hot weather than cold weather because of increased perspiration. This may make it more difficult to interest them in weaning to a cup during the summer.

Self-Feeding

At approximately 6 months of age, infants become interested in handling a spoon and beginning to feed themselves. Their coordination, unfortunately, has not developed enough for them to use a spoon without a great deal of spilling, so they are much more adept at feeding themselves with their fingers (Fig. 29.19). Parents concerned with neatness can spread newspapers, a plastic tablecloth, or a towel on the floor around a high chair to catch most of the dropped food, and then let the child practice. When an infant becomes fatigued or frustrated at attempts of self-feeding, a parent can then quietly help without making an issue of it.

When infants play with their food by squeezing it through their fingers or dabbing it in their hair, it is time to end the meal. Infants who are hungry eat; those who are full, play.

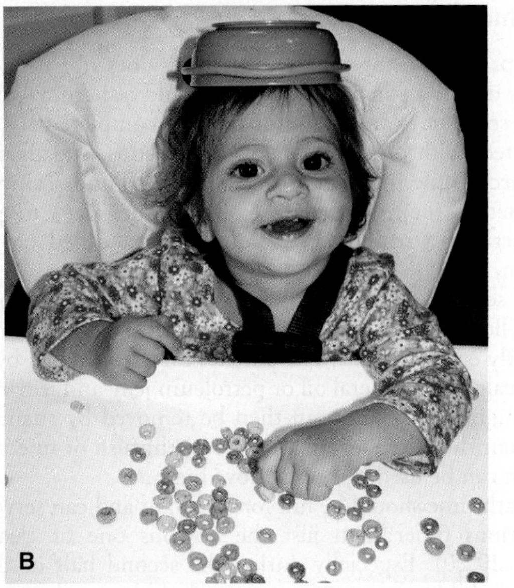
B

FIGURE 29.19 Self-feeding is not always a neat process for young children.

A Vegetarian Diet

An infant eating a vegetarian diet should continue to be breastfed or ingest an iron-fortified commercial formula for the entire first year. If a milk allergy is present, a soy-based formula can be substituted. As soon as they are introduced to solid food, they can begin vegetarian foods (Amit, 2010). As with all infants, an assortment of foods should be provided, including vegetables such as peas, potatoes, and carrots; fruits such as apples, prunes (which are high in iron), and bananas; infant cereal; tofu; wheat germ; legumes; brewer's yeast; and synthetic vitamin D. Feeding fortified cereal throughout the first year will ensure that iron stores are built. If the diet is to include dairy products, these can be added toward the end of the first year as usual.

Because vegetarian diets are high in fiber, infants who eat them may have more frequent and looser than usual bowel movements. Teach parents to change diapers frequently to avoid skin irritation. Using less fibrous, more concentrated forms of protein, such as tofu and powdered nuts rather than green vegetables, can minimize this problem.

A sound vegetarian diet can be easily designed for the older infant who prefers finger foods, because many vegetables, fruits, and grains such as pieces of oranges, peaches, tomatoes, and crackers are easily eaten this way.

Promoting Infant Development in Daily Activities

In the first year, caring for an infant—feeding, bathing, dressing, and so forth—occupies what may seem like nearly all of the parents' waking hours. All of these basic care-related activities provide important opportunities for parents and infants to get to know one another and to become used to each other's unique personalities and patterns. Nurses can play a key role in teaching parents about these activities and stressing their importance.

Bathing

Except in very hot weather, an infant does not need a bath every day. If a parent is tired and would not enjoy bath time or if some days are just too rushed, a complete bath can be omitted, with only the infant's face, hands, and diaper area washed. Some infants do need their head and scalp washed frequently (i.e., every day or every other day) to prevent **seborrhea**, a scaly scalp condition often called cradle cap (Lyon, 2011).

If seborrhea lesions do develop, they adhere to the scalp in yellow, crusty patches. The skin beneath them may be slightly erythematous. The patches can be softened by oiling the scalp with mineral oil or petroleum jelly and leaving it on overnight. The crusts can then be removed by shampooing the hair the next morning. A soft toothbrush or fine-toothed comb can be used to help remove them.

Bath time should be fun for an infant and can serve many functions other than just the obvious one of cleanliness (Fig. 29.20). Especially during the second half of the first year, a child enjoys poking at soap bubbles on the surface of the water or playing with bath toys. Bath time also helps an infant learn different textures and sensations and provides an opportunity to exercise and kick, as well as a good opportunity for a parent to touch and communicate with the child. Teach parents never to leave infants alone in a tub even if they are supported by an infant seat because they could easily slip under the water and drown.

Diaper-Area Care

The most effective means of promoting good diaper-area hygiene is to change diapers frequently, about every 2 to 4 hours. However, it is rarely good practice to interrupt the child's sleep to change diapers. If an infant develops a rash from sleeping in wet diapers, air drying or sleeping without a diaper may be a solution.

At each diaper change, parents should wash the skin with clear water or a commercial alcohol-free (and perfume-free if an infant has sensitive skin) diaper wipe, then pat or allow the skin to air dry. Routinely using an ointment such as Desitin or A&D ointment to keep urine and feces away from an infant's skin is good prophylaxis. Parents do not need to use baby powder. If they choose to use this, advise them to sprinkle the powder on their hands first, and then apply it to an infant's skin. Caution them not to shake the powder onto an infant to reduce the possibility of the infant breathing in or aspirating the powder. They should place the container out of the infant's reach afterward, or an infant could easily spill it into his mouth and aspirate it. Following a diaper change, remind parents to wash their hands to reduce the possibility of spreading infection.

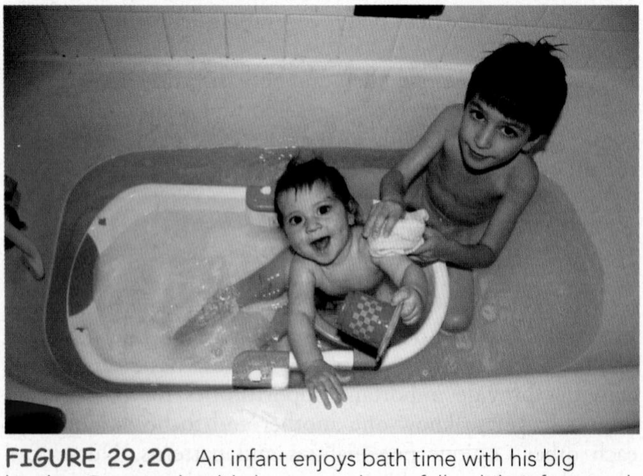

FIGURE 29.20 An infant enjoys bath time with his big brother. Parents should always watch carefully while infants and toddlers are in the tub.

Dental Care

It is well accepted that exposing developing teeth to fluoride is one of the most effective ways to promote healthy tooth formation and prevent tooth decay. A water level of 0.3 ppm fluoride in water is recommended because this is the level that protects tooth enamel best yet does not lead to staining of teeth. In communities where the water supply does not provide enough fluoride or where parents prefer to drink unfluoridated bottled water or use unfluoridated well water, the use of an oral fluoride supplement (fluoride drops) beginning at 6 months of age or the use of fluoride toothpaste or rinses after tooth eruption is recommended (AAP, 2011a). Urge parents to ask about the presence of fluoride in the drinking water in their community and help them to determine what, if any, supplementation is necessary.

Toothbrushing can begin even before teeth erupt by rubbing a soft washcloth over the gum pads. This eliminates plaque and reduces the presence of bacteria, creating a clean environment for the arrival of first teeth. Once teeth erupt, all surfaces should be brushed with a soft brush or washcloth once or twice a day. Children lack the coordination to brush effectively until they are school age, so parents must be responsible for this activity well past infancy (Milgrom & Chi, 2011). Toothpaste is not necessary for an infant, because it is the scrubbing that removes the plaque. An initial dental checkup should be made by 2 or 2.5 years of age, and checkups should continue at 6-month intervals until adulthood.

Dressing

Clothing for infants should be easy to launder and simply constructed, so neither dressing nor undressing are a struggle. When they begin to creep, infants need long pants to protect their knees. Until they begin to walk, they need only soft-soled shoes or merely socks or booties to keep their feet warm. Even when they begin walking, the soles of their shoes need only be firm enough to protect their feet against rough surfaces. Extremely hard soles and high ankle sides are unnecessary.

Sleep

Sleep needs and habits vary greatly among infants, but most require 10 to 12 hours of sleep at night and one or several naps during the day. Parents are advised to let a baby sleep in a separate space close by rather than in their bed so the parents do not awaken at every toss and squeak and possibly avoid infant suffocation. Doing so also allows infants to learn to quiet themselves and go back to sleep should they awaken briefly. Caution parents not to place pillows in an infant's crib. Always place an infant on his or her back to sleep because this position markedly reduces the incidence of sudden infant death syndrome (SIDS) (AAP, 2011b). In addition to supine positioning, use of a firm sleep surface, breastfeeding, room sharing without bed sharing, routine immunizations as shown in Table 29.1, considering the use of a pacifier, and avoidance of overheating, closed spaces, and exposure to tobacco smoke are other suggestions for helping to prevent the syndrome (Scollan-Koliopoulos & Koliopoulos, 2010) (see Chapter 26 for a further discussion of SIDS).

Exercise

Infants benefit from outings in a carriage or stroller because sunlight provides a natural source of vitamin D. In hot weather, caution parents to protect an infant from sunburn by exposing the child to the sun for only very short periods, beginning with 3 to 5 minutes the first day, a little more the next day, and so on up to 15 to 20 minutes at a time. The sun is most intense between 10 AM and 3 PM, so early mornings and late afternoons are the best times for infants to be outside. These short time spans are necessary because the use of sunscreen is not recommended in children until they are at least 6 months old.

Toward the end of the first year, infants need space to crawl and then to walk, such as in an enclosed outdoor play space. In addition to providing fresh air, going for leisurely walks while pointing out the sights of the world—trees, birds, dogs, houses, neighbors—helps children develop language and allows for quality time with a parent. Parents can judge how much outdoor clothing to put on an infant by how much they need themselves.

Caution parents to supervise infants using walkers because they can be seriously injured if they maneuver the walker too near a stairway and fall the length of the steps.

Promoting Healthy Family Functioning

A primary task of parents during the infant year is to learn to interpret infants' cues so they can better decipher their needs. This becomes an easier task by 2 months of age, when infants can indicate by their particular cry whether they are feeling cold, hungry, wet, or lonely.

Parental Concerns and Problems Related to Normal Infant Development

Some of the difficulties parents are apt to have in evaluating the health of infants are shown in Table 29.4. Both new and experienced parents may need reassurance and answers to questions about child care procedures or health during the infant period because they have not yet learned to interpret infant cues. The unique characteristics of each child require at least some adjustment from parents.

Teething

Most infants have little difficulty with teething, but some appear very distressed by the process. Generally, gums are sore and tender before a new tooth breaks the surface. As soon as the tooth is through, the tenderness passes (Kiran, Swati, Kamala, et al., 2011).

Because of this pain, infants can be resistant to chewing for a day or two and be slightly cranky, possibly because they are a little hungry from not eating as much as usual. High fever, seizures, vomiting or diarrhea, as well as earache are never normal signs of teething. An infant with any of these symptoms has an underlying infection or disease process that requires further evaluation.

Rubbing the gumline with a finger or a soft cloth can help a new tooth erupt and so can be effective (Plutzer, Spencer, & Keirse, 2011). Teething rings that can be placed in the refrigerator or freezer provide soothing coolness against tender gums. Remind parents that an infant who is teething will place almost any object in the mouth to chew on, so parents must screen articles within the baby's reach to be certain they are edible or safe to chew on.

Many over-the-counter medicines are sold for teething pain. As a rule, these should be discouraged, especially if they contain benzocaine, a topical anesthetic. If applied too far back in the throat, this could interfere with a gag reflex. Infant's or children's liquid acetaminophen (Tylenol) may be given for teething discomfort after parents check with their primary care provider for the correct dose. As a rule, they always need to check with their infant's health care provider before giving any over-the-counter drug this way to be certain that pain enough to warrant an analgesic is simple teething discomfort.

Thumb-Sucking

Sucking is a surprisingly strong need in early infancy: sonograms demonstrate thumb-sucking as early as in utero. Many infants begin to suck a thumb or finger at about 3 months of

TABLE 29.4 Common Difficulties Parents Experience in Evaluating the Health of Infants

Difficulty	Suggestions for Improving Assessment
Evaluating pain	Infants manifest pain by fussiness or crying if it is sharp pain. They reveal arm and leg pain by immobility of the body part; ear pain by brushing or tugging at the ear; and stomach pain by pulling up the legs against the abdomen.
Evaluating degree of reduced activity	Infant has lack of interest in smiling or interaction. May lie supine with legs nonflexed (frog-legged) as if exhausted.
Evaluating infant temperature	All parents should learn how to take an axillary or tympanic temperature so they can report a specific degree of fever rather than a subjective finding, such as "feels hot."
Evaluating amount of vomiting or diarrhea	Count the number of times vomiting and/or diarrhea has occurred. Estimating amount in comparison with what the child ate is helpful as well as estimating an amount (e.g., a cupful). Knowing whether diapers are "soaked" or "stained" with stool helps to estimate severity of diarrhea. Caution parents that vomiting and diarrhea are always serious in infants; if these occur, they should alert their primary health care provider and ask for advice.

age and continue the habit through the first few years of life. The sucking reflex peaks at 6 to 8 months, whereas thumb-sucking peaks at about 18 months.

Parents can be assured that thumb-sucking is normal and does not deform the jaw in infancy. It does not cause "baby talk" or any of the other speech concerns commonly attributed to it. Children who continue the habit into school age, however, can have changes in their dental arch that leads to asymmetric concerns such as crossbite (Montaldo, Montaldo, Cuccaro, et al., 2011). The best approach for parents is to be certain an infant has adequate sucking pleasure and then to ignore thumb-sucking. Making an issue of it rarely causes a child to stop; if anything, it may intensify and prolong it.

Use of Pacifiers

Whether to use pacifiers is a question that parents must settle for themselves depending on how they feel about them and their infant's needs. Benefits of pacifiers include: they appear to be comforting to an infant, they may aid in pain relief, and there is a decreased risk of SIDS. Risks associated with them are an increased incidence of acute otitis media (ear infection), possibly a negative impact on breastfeeding, and dental malocclusion, particularly if usage is greater than 2 to 3 years (Nelson, 2012).

An infant who completes a feeding and still seems restless and discontent, who actively searches for something to put into the mouth, or who sucks on hands and clothes may need a pacifier. Babies who have colic crave sucking and enjoy pacifiers because their abdomen hurts, and they interpret this as a hunger sensation. If a child is formula fed, parents should check nipples to be certain the holes are small and the rubber is sturdy so their infant can suck hard enough to derive pleasure. If the nipples are satisfactory, parents could offer a pacifier after feeding for more sucking. Theoretically, a child whose sucking needs are met in infancy will not crave as much oral stimulation later in life and is less likely to become a pencil chewer, cigarette smoker, nail biter, or the like.

A major drawback of pacifiers is the problem of cleanliness. They tend to fall on the floor or sidewalk and are then put back into an infant's mouth. If not well constructed, they may come apart and the nipple part may be aspirated. Hanging a pacifier on a string around an infant's neck could cause strangulation.

Parents should attempt to wean a child from a pacifier any time after 3 months of age and certainly during the time the sucking reflex is fading at 6 to 9 months. Weaning after this age is difficult because a pacifier becomes a comfort mechanism, like a warm blanket or fuzzy toy to which a child may continue to cling.

Head Banging

Some infants rhythmically bang their head against the bars of a crib for a period of time before they fall asleep, an action that can be a distressing behavior for parents. Besides fearing their children will hurt themselves, they may have heard blind children or those with mental illness or an autism spectrum disorder do this and worry their child is ill in some way.

Head banging in this limited fashion—beginning during the second half of the first year of life and continuing through to the preschool period, associated with naptime or bedtime, and lasting under 15 minutes—can be considered normal. Children use this measure to relax and fall asleep. Investigating stress factors operating in the house may be helpful. If some of the stress can be relieved (such as the parents' overestimation of the child's development, marital discord, illness in another family member), the head banging may decrease or it may have already become such an engrained habit that it will persist for months or even years.

Advise parents to pad the rails of cribs so infants cannot hurt themselves, and reassure them this is a normal mechanism for the relief of tension in children of this age. No therapy should be necessary. Excessive head banging done to the exclusion of normal development or activity, head banging past the preschool period, or if associated with other symptoms suggests a pathologic basis; such children need a referral for further evaluation (Singer, 2011).

Sleep Concerns

Sleep concerns develop in early infancy because of colic or because an otherwise healthy infant takes longer than usual to adjust to sleeping through the night. Breastfed babies tend to wake more often than those who are formula fed because breast milk is more easily digested, and so infants become hungry sooner. In late infancy, the problem of waking at night and remaining awake for an hour or more can become common. Although an infant may be content and not cry during this time, parents are reluctant to sleep while a child is awake, so they may become extremely fatigued. Suggestions for eliminating or at least coping with night waking include delaying bedtime by 1 hour, shortening afternoon naps, not responding immediately to infants at night so infants can have time to fall back to sleep on their own, and providing soft toys or music to allow infants to play quietly alone during this wakeful time.

Reassuring parents that infants take varying lengths of time to adjust to night sleeping is helpful in assuring them their child is not ill. Suggesting parents use the time they are awake at night to do things such as solve a problem at work, watch a late show, or plan a shopping list may help them view the situation as a constructive time rather than a concern. If infants have difficulty falling or staying asleep, this is not correlated with long-term sleep disorders (Price, Wake, Ukoumunne, et al., 2012).

Constipation

Breastfed infants are rarely constipated because their stools tend to be naturally loose. Constipation may occur in formula-fed infants from something as simple as if their diet is deficient in fluid. This can be corrected simply by offering more fluid.

Some parents misinterpret the normal pushing with bowel movements of a newborn and report that their infant is constipated. When infants defecate, their faces do turn red, and they grimace and grunt. As long as stools are not hard and contain no evidence of fresh blood (as might occur with a rectal fissure), this is not constipation but normal infant behavior.

If hard bowel movements are present beyond 5 or 6 months of age, encourage parents to check with the infant's primary health care provider about measures to relieve this. Adding foods with bulk, such as fruits or vegetables, and increasing fluid intake generally relieves the problem. Apple juice (3 or 4 oz) or prune juice (0.5 to 1 oz daily) may be given as a temporary measure.

All infants with a history of true constipation (exceedingly hard or no bowel movements) should be examined for an anal fissure or tight anal sphincter. Softening stools and thereby relieving the pain of defecation often solves the problem and helps the fissure to heal. If an unusually tight anal sphincter exists, parents will be given instructions to manually dilate the sphincter two or three times daily until it dilates sufficiently.

Hirschsprung disease (aganglionic megacolon, or lack of nerve innervation to a portion of the colon) may be manifested early in life as constipation. If no stool is present in the rectum of a constipated infant on rectal examination, this disease is suggested (Sundaram, Hoffenberg, Kramer, et al., 2011). A careful history must then be taken to assess for other symptoms of Hirschsprung disease: ribbonlike stools, bouts of diarrhea, and a distended abdomen (see Chapter 45).

Chronic constipation also may occur in children with congenital hypothyroidism (decreased functioning of the thyroid gland). Therefore, an infant with constipation also should be carefully observed for characteristic signs of hypothyroidism, such as lethargy, protruding tongue, and failure to meet developmental milestones (see Chapter 48). Infants with either of these disorders need therapy to correct the disorder.

Loose Stools

Many new parents are unfamiliar with the consistency or color of normal newborn stools, so they mistakenly report normal stooling as diarrhea. Stools of breastfed infants are generally softer than those of formula-fed infants. If a mother takes a laxative while breastfeeding, an infant's stools may be very loose. An infant who is formula fed can have loose stools if the formula is not diluted properly. Occasionally, loose stools may begin with the introduction of vegetables or fruit.

A serious reason for loose stools is celiac disease or the inability to process gluten (sometimes termed malabsorption syndrome) (see Chapter 45). The inability to digest fat and fat-soluble vitamins, accompanied by a distended abdomen, are other common symptoms of celiac disease; an infant needs a referral to a primary care provider for this.

When talking to a parent about loose stools, ask them how long the infant has been having them, the number of stools per day, their color and consistency, and whether there is any mucus or blood in them. Also, is there associated fever, cramping, or vomiting? Does an infant continue to eat well? Appear well? Seem to be thriving? Is an infant wetting at least six diapers daily?

Infants with associated signs and symptoms such as fever, cramping, vomiting, loss of appetite, a decrease in voiding, and weight loss should be examined by their health care provider because this suggests an infectious process. If in doubt as to whether their child is ill, teach parents to err on the side of phoning their care provider. Dehydration occurs rapidly in a small infant who is not eating and is losing body fluid through loose stools (Mehal, Esposito, Holman, et al., 2012).

Colic

Colic is paroxysmal abdominal pain that generally occurs in infants under 3 months of age and is marked by loud, intense crying (Shergill-Bonner, 2010). Infants pull their legs up against their abdomen, their faces become red and flushed, their fists clench, and their abdomens become tense. If offered a bottle, an infant with colic will suck vigorously for a few minutes as if starved, then stop as another wave of intestinal pain occurs.

The cause of colic is unclear and probably results for several reasons. It may occur in susceptible infants from overfeeding or from swallowing too much air while feeding. Formula-fed babies tend to have more symptoms than breastfed babies, possibly because they swallow more air while drinking or because formula is harder to digest.

Although infants continue to thrive despite colic, the condition should not be dismissed as unimportant. It is a distressing and frightening problem for parents because their infant is not only in acute pain but also the distress persists for hours, usually into the middle of the night, allowing no one in the family to get adequate rest. This creates a difficult beginning to a parent–child relationship, which needs to be strong and binding for parents to enjoy parenting and for an infant to thrive in their care.

Take a thorough history of an infant with signs of colic because an intestinal obstruction or infection can mimic an attack of colic and be misinterpreted by the casual interviewer. With colic, symptoms of abdominal pain typically last up to 3 hours a day and occur at least 3 days every week; bowel movements are normal. Constipation; narrow, ribbonlike stools; and the presence of blood or mucus suggest other problems.

If the infant is bottle fed, ask about the type of formula used, how it is prepared, and if parents hold the baby upright and burp the infant adequately after feeding. For a breastfed baby, ask about the mother's diet (is she avoiding "gassy" food such as cabbage?).

A number of interventions can be helpful to recommend to relieve colic symptoms. For example, both breastfed and formula-fed infants may feel more comfortable with small, frequent feedings to prevent distention and discomfort. Offering a pacifier can be comforting. Reducing stimuli, taking infants for car rides, or playing a music box that simulates the sound of a heartbeat are often reported as being helpful (Gahagan, 2011). Dietary changes have little effect, although there is some evidence using hydrolysed protein, probiotics or prebiotics, or a soy-based formula for bottle-fed babies may be helpful (Iacovou, Ralston, Muir, et al., 2011; Thomas & Greer, 2010).

Some parents try placing a hot water bottle on their infant's stomach for comfort, but this should be discouraged. A basic rule for any abdominal discomfort is to avoid heat in case appendicitis is developing. This is highly unlikely in so young an infant, but parents will remember they once used heat and may use it again when the child is older. Hot water bottles and heating pads also might burn the delicate skin of infants.

Caution parents to check with their primary care provider before using herbs or home remedies such as star anise to be certain what they have heard to be effective is safe for infants (Madden, Schmitz, & Fullerton, 2012). They should use the same precaution for chiropractic or acupressure therapy.

As a final measure, it is important to think of colic as a family problem or else a vicious circle may gradually begin. An infant cries and the parents may become tense and unsure of themselves. An infant then senses the tension and develops more colic. Some parents benefit from planning relief time from infant care to relieve their stress level and prevent this cycle. Box 29.7 shows an interprofessional care map illustrating both nursing and team planning to address such a problem as infant colic.

BOX 29.7 Nursing Care Planning

AN INTERPROFESSIONAL CARE MAP FOR AN INFANT WITH COLIC

You meet Ms. Simpson, 19 years old, at a pediatric clinic when she brings in her 2-month-old son, Bryan. She looks tired and she tells you she is exhausted because her baby is "awake all night, crying constantly." When you weigh Bryan, you find he has gained weight well. When you talk to him, he demonstrates a social smile.

Family Assessment Infant lives with single parent and her family (baby's grandfather, grandmother, 26-year-old uncle, and 22-year-old aunt). Mother works as an exotic dancer from 12 noon to 6 PM daily; grandmother cares for infant during this time.

Client Assessment Well-proportioned, 2-month-old male. Height and weight at 50th percentile on growth chart. Currently bottle-fed with intake of approximately 4 oz of commercial formula every 4 hours. Has two or three soft yellow stools daily. The mother reports, "His face gets red and he pulls his legs up against his belly and cries every night from 6 PM 'til 2 AM. Why is he so good for my mother in the afternoon but cries at night for me? Why does he hate me so much?"

The physical examination on Bryan was within normal limits. His nurse practitioner diagnosed colic as the cause of his crying.

Nursing Diagnosis Compromised family coping related to difficulty managing infant crying episodes

Outcome Criteria Parent voices increased confidence in caring for infant and increased feeling of control over situation within 1 week; infant sleeps for at least 1 hour during 6 PM to 2 AM period.

Team Member Responsible	Assessment	Intervention	Rationale	Expected Outcome
Activities of Daily Living, Including Safety				
Nurse	Assess what infant's total day is like to try to identify why crying seems confined to evenings.	Make suggestions as needed to see if different caregivers use consistency in care.	Infants with different caretakers can have difficulty adjusting to changing feeding techniques.	Parent details a day history for infant.
Teamwork and Collaboration				
Nurse/Nurse practitioner	Determine which nurse practitioner is available for care team.	Contact nurse practitioner to do a physical exam to ensure infant is healthy.	A physical exam will differentiate symptoms of colic from other, more serious problems.	Nurse practitioner completes the physical exam and makes recommendations.
Procedures/Medications for Quality Improvement				
Nurse/Primary care provider	Assess what steps parent has taken to try to relieve symptoms.	Suggest the use of a pacifier, sitting the infant upright, feeding in quiet environment, riding in car, etc.	Both sucking on a pacifier and an upright position may promote passage of gas.	Parent states she is willing to try new measures such as a pacifier.
Nutrition				
Nurse	Assess how parent prepares formula and technique used for feeding and burping infant.	Review methods for formula preparation, bottle holding, and burping as needed.	Proper techniques can minimize the amount of air swallowed.	Parent describes correct formula preparation and infant feeding methods. Confirms other family members are consistent.
Patient-Centered Care				
Nurse	Assess what parent knows about colic, including its incidence, usual timing, symptoms, etc.	Educate parent about common characteristics of colic, including duration, timing, and intensity of crying.	Education promotes better understanding of the problem, hopefully alleviating stress.	Parent states she understands how common colic is and that the crying is from pain, not related to her personally.

Psychosocial/Spiritual/Emotional Needs				
Nurse/Nurse practitioner	Assess why parent is taking the fact the infant cries only during her care time personally.	Reassure parent it's a coincidence colic occurs at the time she is giving care.	Reassurance that the problem is not the mother's fault can aid in objective problem solving.	Parent states she understands the problem is not a personal one.
Nurse	Assess parent's level of stress about constant crying.	Caution parent that crying in infants produces frustration in adults. Help plan respite time if necessary.	Acknowledging frustration helps to validate feelings. Time away can help relieve tension.	Parent states she is frustrated but also ready to work on solving the problem.
Informatics for Seamless Health Care Planning				
Nurse	Urge the parent to call for further suggestions if needed. Stress that colic usually resolves by 3 months of age.	Advise parent to contact clinic if measures are ineffective by 1 week.	Assurance that continuing support will be available can help relieve stress.	Parent agrees to call in 1 week if crying has not improved.

In about 85% of infants, colic disappears almost magically at 3 months of age, probably because it becomes easier to digest food and an infant maintains a more upright position by this time, which allows less gas to form.

What if... 29.3 Bryan's mother asks you if changing her work shift so her mother cares for Bryan during his "awake" time would help solve her problem. Would you agree with her?

Spitting Up

Almost all infants spit up, although formula-fed babies appear to do this more than breastfed babies. Parents who did not handle their infant much in the health care facility where their child was born may discover spitting up only after they take the baby home. They may interpret this as vomiting or think an infant is developing an infection. Ask them to carefully describe what they mean by "spitting up." How long has the baby been doing it? How frequently? What is the appearance of the spit-up milk? Almost all milk that is spit up smells at least faintly sour, but it should not contain blood or bile.

The baby who spits up a mouthful of milk (rolling down the chin) two or three times a day (or sometimes after every meal) is experiencing normal, early-infancy spitting up. Associated signs such as diarrhea, abdominal cramps, fever, cough, cold, or loss of activity suggest illness. If an infant is spitting up so forcefully that milk is projected 3 or 4 ft away, it may be the beginning of pyloric stenosis (an abnormally tight valve between the stomach and duodenum), which requires surgical intervention. If the spitting up is a large amount with each feeding, parents may be describing gastroesophageal reflux, in which a lax cardiac sphincter and esophagus allow for the regurgitation of gastric contents into the esophagus. This also requires medical attention (see Chapter 45).

Burping the baby thoroughly after a feeding often limits spitting up. Parents may try sitting an infant in an infant chair for half an hour after feeding. Changing formulas generally is of little value. Reassure parents spitting up decreases in amount as the baby becomes better at coordinating swallowing and digestive processes (the cardiac sphincter matures). In the meantime, a bib can protect the baby's clothing and the parent. After a few months, the child will naturally stay in an upright position longer, and gravity will help to correct the problem.

Diaper Dermatitis

Some infants have such sensitive skin that diaper dermatitis (diaper rash) is a problem from the first few days of life. It occurs for a number of reasons.

When parents do not change a child's diapers frequently, feces is left in contact with skin, and irritation may result in the perianal area. Urine that is left in diapers too long breaks down into ammonia, a chemical extremely irritating to infant skin. Ammonia dermatitis of this type is generally a problem in the second half of the first year of life, when an infant is producing a larger quantity of urine than before. For some infants, however, it is a problem from the first week.

Frequent diaper changing, applying an ointment, and exposing the diaper area to air may relieve the problem. Some infants may have to sleep without diapers at night to solve the problem. If a diaper area is covered with lesions that are bright red, with or without oozing, that last longer than 3 days, and appear as red pinpoint lesions, suspect a fungal (monilial or candidiasis) infection that will also need therapy (an antifungal medicine such as Nystatin). Fungal infections of this type are discussed in Chapter 43.

Whenever the entire diaper area is erythematous and irritated so the outline of the diaper on the skin can be identified, an allergy to the material in the diaper or to laundry products if a commercially washed or home-washed diaper is being used is suggested. Changing the brand or type of diaper or washing solution usually alleviates this problem.

Miliaria

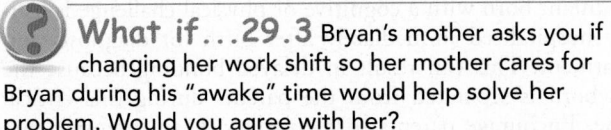

Miliaria, or prickly heat rash, occurs most often in warm weather or when babies are overdressed or sleep in overheated rooms. Clusters of pinpoint, reddened papules with occasional vesicles and pustules surrounded by erythema usually appear on the neck first and may spread upward to around the ears and onto the face or down onto the trunk.

Bathing an infant twice a day during hot weather, particularly if a small amount of baking soda is added to the bath water, may improve the rash. Eliminating sweating by reducing the amount of clothing on an infant or lowering the room temperature should bring almost immediate improvement and prevent further eruptions.

Baby-Bottle Tooth Decay Syndrome

Putting an infant to bed with a bottle can result in decay of all the upper teeth and the lower posterior teeth (Bishop, 2011) (Fig. 29.21). Decay occurs because, while an infant sleeps, liquid from the propped bottle continuously soaks the upper front teeth and lower back teeth (the lower front teeth are protected by the tongue). The problem, called **baby-bottle syndrome**, is most serious when the bottle is filled with sugar water, formula, milk, or fruit juice. The carbohydrate in these solutions ferments to organic acids that demineralize the tooth enamel until it decays.

To prevent this problem, advise parents never to put their baby to bed with a bottle. If parents insist a bottle is necessary to allow a baby to fall asleep, encourage them to fill it with water and use a nipple with a small hole to prevent the baby from receiving a large amount of fluid. If the baby refuses to drink anything but milk, the parents might dilute the milk with water more and more each night until the bottle contains water only.

Obesity in Infants

Obesity in infants is defined as a weight greater than the 90th to 95th percentile on a standardized height/weight chart. Obesity occurs when there is an abnormal increase in the number of fat cells because of excessive calorie intake. Preventing obesity in infants is important because the extra fat cells formed at this time are likely to remain throughout childhood and even into adulthood. If a child becomes obese because of overingesting milk, iron-deficiency anemia may also be present because of the low iron content of both breast and commercial milk. Once infant obesity begins, it is difficult to reverse, so prevention is the key (Taylor, Heath, Galland, et al., 2011).

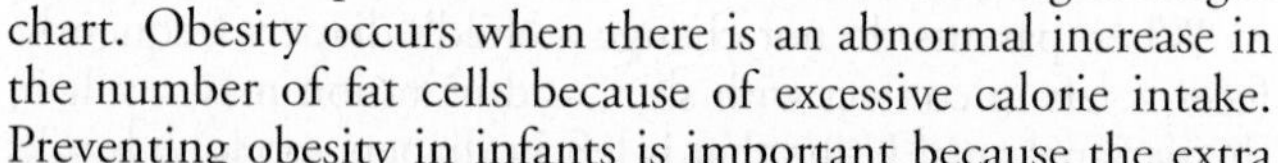

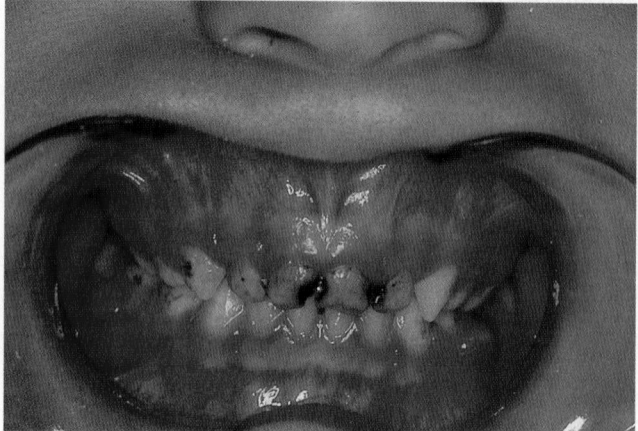

FIGURE 29.21 Baby-bottle syndrome. Notice the extensive decay in the upper teeth. (From K. L. Boyd, DDS/Custom Medical Stock Photograph.)

Overfeeding in infancy often occurs because parents were taught to eat everything on their plate, and they continue to instill this concept in their children. This appears to be the case most often with formula-fed infants whose parents urge them to empty their bottle or finish a cereal serving. It can occur any time parents automatically feed an infant when the child cries, rather than investigating what the cry might really mean. As a general rule, an infant should take no more than 32 oz of formula daily and shouldn't be breastfeeding more often than every 2 hours. When solid food is introduced, a bottle of water can be substituted for formula at one feeding to reduce calories. Nonfat milk should not be given because it contains so little fat that essential fatty acid requirements may not be sufficient to ensure cell growth.

Another way to help prevent obesity is to add a source of fiber, such as whole-grain cereal and raw fruit, to an infant's diet. These prolong the stomach-emptying time, so they can help reduce food intake. Caution parents about giving obese infants foods with high amounts of refined sugars, such as pudding, cake, cookies, and candy. Encourage parents to learn more about balanced nutrition and to provide this for their entire family.

Concerns of the Family With an Infant With Unique Needs

An infant born with a cognitive or physical challenge is usually hospitalized immediately after birth for diagnosis and treatment. This can result in delayed bonding because the newborn is separated from the parents during this critical time. Encourage parents to regularly visit an intensive care nursery to help form a strong parent–child attachment. If parents cannot visit, urge them to telephone the hospital as frequently as they can to ask about their child. E-mailing them photographs or posting them by the infant's crib for parents to take home are other ways to encourage bonding.

Many of the developmental events of the infant year (e.g., social smile, laughing out loud, reaching for an object, uttering the first word, sitting, talking) are activities that encourage parent–child interaction because they make an infant fun to be with and naturally make a parent want to spend more time with the child. Children who are cognitively challenged may not reach these milestones. Children who are physically challenged may be unable to achieve them as well if they cannot reach up and pat their mother's face or hold out arms to be picked up by the father. If infants leave the hospital with a cast or other equipment such as a ventilator for care, parents may be so concerned with these items that they cannot initiate normal singing and playing activities with their children.

To encourage a good parent–child relationship, point out the positive things the infant can do. Perhaps the child's facial expression says, "Pick me up," even though he doesn't reach up with his hands, or perhaps his eyes follow his mother's actions even though he can't yet call to her.

Helping parents to interact more fully with their infants this way helps to build a sense of trust in the infant. Keeping painful procedures to a minimum when infants are ill is also important in helping infants achieve a positive outlook on the world (Stevens, Abbott, Yamada, et al., 2011).

Without this sense of trust, children have difficulty expressing themselves to others, and they may not believe they are lovable or that people would want to interact with them. Physically challenged individuals, no matter what their ages, need people around them to give them help at whatever point they cannot meet their own needs. It is unfortunate when physically challenged children cannot reach out for help because they never developed a sense of trust.

Infants who are cognitively or physically challenged or chronically ill experience the same health and growth problems as other infants such as colic or diaper rash. Parents may be reluctant to mention these concerns at health care visits because they believe such problems pale in comparison to the child's primary illness or condition. When taking the health histories of children with chronic or long-standing medical problems, ask parents about these secondary concerns. "What about everyday things? Any problems there?" Treat these concerns seriously, so parents can feel confident about bringing them to your attention at future health care visits. Also mention they are part of normal infant development so parents can begin to view their child apart from his or her illness.

Discomfort from diaper rash and colic may actually occur more frequently in babies with other illnesses than those who are well because a parent may not want to "bother" an ill infant with physical care or burp the infant as long or as often as they would a well child. The bowel movements of physically disabled or chronically ill children may be looser than normal because of a liquid diet or medicine. Their urine may be more concentrated because of reduced intake. These conditions make diaper rash more apt to occur. Offering anticipatory guidance to parents can go a long way toward helping them avoid these special concerns of infancy.

QSEN Checkpoint Question 29.6

Patient-Centered Care

When planning care for an infant who has unique needs, you can best promote the parents' psychosocial well-being by which of the following means?

a. Lowering the family's expectations around their infant's skills
b. Clearly describing the etiology of the infant's development deficits
c. Encouraging the family to have more children
d. Emphasizing what the infant can do more than what he or she cannot do

Look in Appendix A for the best answer and rationale.

Nutrition for the Infant With Unique Needs

Ill infants may tire too easily to suck long enough to take in adequate feedings. If any degree of neurologic involvement exists, sucking and swallowing reflexes may not be coordinated. If an infant has some gastrointestinal disorders, feeding may be impossible.

To ensure adequate calorie and protein intake, infants may need to be maintained on nasogastric tube or gastrostomy feedings, or total parenteral nutrition. Because these methods limit the amount of sucking that is possible and sucking provides pleasure as well as satisfying thirst, this is a major loss. Provide an infant with nonnutritive sucking experiences such as a pacifier if possible (which is acceptable with the parent's and the infant's condition) to fill this need. Help parents find time each day to hold the infant equal to the time they would have held the child if fed by breast or bottle to make parenting more satisfying and more like the role they planned (Wilken, 2012).

Infants who are ill for a long time may not eat solid foods eagerly once they are introduced because they are not hungry enough to be interested in a new eating method. Help parents to experiment with different foods to find a taste that does appeal to ill children, or teach them to limit foods to only those that the child appears to like most from all five food groups.

What if...29.4 You are particularly interested in exploring one of the 2020 National Health Goals with respect to infant care (see Box 29.1). What would be a possible research topic to explore pertinent to this goal that would be applicable to Bryan and his family and that would also advance evidence-based practice?

Key Points for Review

- The infant period is from 1 month to 12 months of age. Children typically double their birth weight at 4 to 6 months and triple it at 1 year.
- Infants develop their first tooth at about 6 months; by 12 months, they have six to eight teeth.
- Important gross motor milestones during the infant year are lifting the chest off a bed at 2 months, sitting at 6 to 8 months, creeping at 9 months, "cruising" at 10 to 11 months, and walking at 12 months.
- Important fine motor accomplishments are the ability to pass an object from one hand to the other (7 months of age) and a pincer grasp (10 months of age).
- Important milestones of language development during the first year are differentiating a cry (2 months of age), making simple vowel sounds (5 to 6 months of age), and saying two words besides "ma-ma" and "da-da" (12 months of age). The more infants are spoken to, the easier it is for them to acquire language.
- Providing infants with proper toys for play helps development. All infant toys need to be checked to be certain they are too large to be aspirated (wider than a toilet paper roll).
- Important milestones of vision development are the ability to follow a moving object past the midline (3 months of age) and ability to focus securely without eyes crossing (6 months of age).
- According to Erikson (1993), the developmental task of the infant year is the development of a sense of trust versus mistrust. Helping parents spend quality time with their infant helps a sense of trust to develop and helps in planning nursing care that not only meets QSEN competencies but that also best meets the family's total needs.
- Safety is important. Infants must be protected from falls and the aspiration of small objects. Skills an infant cannot accomplish one day, such as crawling (which can lead to danger), may be accomplished the next.
- Solid food is generally introduced into an infant's diet at 5 to 6 months of age. Before infants can eat solid food, they must lose their extrusion reflex.

- Common concerns related to infant development include teething, thumb-sucking, use of pacifiers, sleep problems, constipation, colic, diaper dermatitis, baby-bottle syndrome (decayed teeth from sucking on a bottle of formula while they sleep), and obesity. Nurses play a key role in teaching parents about these problems and suggestions to deal with them.
- Remember that parent–infant attachment is critical to mental health. Urge parents to continue to give as much care as possible to ill infants to maintain this important relationship.

Critical Thinking Care Study

Alicia Scinta is a 3-month-old you meet in an emergency room because she has mild diarrhea. Her mother tells you Alicia is a "picky eater," and "no wonder she's sick."

Her mother works weekends as a drugstore clerk so Alicia is cared for at a child care center on the weekends. Her father, a university professor, tells you he'll watch her weekends "later on, when she's more fun."

1. Alicia's mother said she was a "picky eater." What questions would you want to ask to discover why she says that?
2. Alicia is cared for at a child care center every weekend. What questions would you want to ask about the center to evaluate if they are encouraging Alicia's infancy developmental task?
3. Mr. Scinta says he'll watch Alicia later "when she's more fun." What features of a 3-month-old could you point out to him to help convince him she is fun to care for now?

Patient Scenario

The Burrows Family

Read about the Burrows family, a family with an infant with a feeding problem, then answer the questions to further sharpen your skills and grow more familiar with NCLEX-type questions related to nursing care of a family with an infant. Confirm your answers are correct by reading the rationales.

Visit http://thePoint.lww.com

Answers and Rationales

Looking for answers to the What If. . . and Critical Thinking Care Study questions?

Visit http://thePoint.lww.com

References

American Academy of Pediatrics. (2011a). *Fluoride supplements.* Washington, DC: Author.

American Academy of Pediatrics. (2011b). SIDS and other sleep-related infant deaths. *Pediatrics, 128*(5), e1341–e1367.

American Academy of Pediatrics. (2012a). *Recommendations for preventive pediatric health care.* Washington, DC: Author.

American Academy of Pediatrics. (2012b). *Where we stand: Car seats for children.* Washington, DC: Author.

American Academy of Pediatrics. (2012c). *Where we stand: TV viewing time.* Washington, DC: Author.

Amit, M. (2010). Vegetarian diets in children and adolescents. *Paediatric Child Health, 5*(5), 303–314.

Bishop, W. P. (2011). Oral cavity. In K. J. Marcdante, R. M. Kliegman, H. B. Jenson, et al. (Eds.), *Nelson essentials of pediatrics* (6th ed., pp. 475–476). Philadelphia, PA: Saunders/Elsevier.

Centers for Disease Control and Prevention. (2011). Ten great public health achievements—United States, 2001–2010. *MMWR: Morbidity & Mortality Weekly Report, 60*(19), 619–623.

Conti, T. D., Patel, M., & Bhat, S. (2011). Breast-feeding & infant nutrition. In J. E. South-Paul, S. C. Matheny, & E. L. Lewis (Eds.), *Current diagnosis & treatment in family medicine* (3rd ed., pp. 28–35). Columbus, OH: McGraw-Hill.

de Amorim Lde, F., Estrela, C., & da Costa, L. R. (2011). Effects of traumatic dental injuries to primary teeth on permanent teeth. *Dental Traumatology, 27*(2), 117–121.

Erikson, E. (1993). *Childhood and society* (3rd ed.). New York, NY: W. W. Norton.

Gaffney, K. F., Kitsantas, P., & Cheema, J. (2012). Clinical practice guidelines for feeding behaviors and weight-for-age at 12 months. *Worldviews on Evidence Based Nursing, 9*(4), 234–242.

Gahagan, S. (2011). Crying and colic. In K. J. Marcdante, R. M. Kliegman, H. B. Jenson, et al. (Eds.), *Nelson essentials of pediatrics* (6th ed., pp. 45–47). Philadelphia, PA: Saunders/Elsevier.

Goldson, E., & Reynolds, A. (2011). Child development & behavior. In W. W. Hay, M. J. Levine, J. M. Sondheimer, et al. (Eds.), *Current pediatric diagnosis & treatment* (20th ed., pp. 64–103). Columbus, OH: McGraw-Hill.

Iacovou, M., Ralston, R. A., Muir, J., et al. (2011). Dietary management of infantile colic: A systematic review. *Maternal Child Health Journal, 16*(6), 1319–1331.

Ibrahim, N. G., Wood, J., Margulies, S. S., et al. (2011). Influence of age and fall type on head injuries in infants and toddlers. *International Journal of Development & Neuroscience, 30*(3), 201–206.

Kiran, K., Swati, T., Kamala, B. K., et al. (2011). Prevalence of systemic and local disturbances in infants during primary teeth eruption. *European Journal of Paediatric Dentistry, 12*(4), 249–252.

Klootwijk, T., & Krul, M. (2011). Some concerns remain about the proposed association between swimming and asthma. *American Journal of Respiratory Critical Care Medicine, 184*(12), 1419–1420.

Krebs, N. F., & Primak, L. E. (2011). Pediatric nutrition & nutritional disorders. In K. J. Marcdante, R. M. Kliegman, H. B. Jenson, et al. (Eds.), *Nelson essentials of pediatrics* (6th ed., pp. 103–107). Philadelphia, PA: Saunders/Elsevier.

Levine, D. A. (2011). Normal development. In K. J. Marcdante, R. M. Kliegman, H. B. Jenson, et al. (Eds.), *Nelson essentials of pediatrics* (6th ed., pp. 16–18). Philadelphia, PA: Saunders/Elsevier.

Lyon, V. B. (2011). Dermatology. In K. J. Marcdante, R. M. Kliegman, H. B. Jenson, et al. (Eds.), *Nelson essentials of pediatrics* (6th ed., pp. 713–734). Philadelphia, PA: Saunders/Elsevier.

Madden, G. R., Schmitz, K. H., & Fullerton, K. (2012). A case of infantile star anise toxicity. *Pediatric Emergency Care, 28*(3), 284–285.

Mehal, J. M., Esposito, D. H., Holman, R. C., et al. (2012). Risk factors for diarrhea-associated infant mortality in the United States, 2005–2007. *Pediatric Infectious Disease Journal, 31*(7), 717–721.

Mesman, J., Oster, H., & Camras, L. (2012). Parental sensitivity to infant distress: What do discrete negative emotions have to do with it? *Attachment & Human Development, 14*(4), 337–348.

Milgrom, P., & Chi, D. L. (2011). Prevention-centered caries management strategies during critical periods in early childhood. *Journal of the California Dental Association, 39*(10), 735–741.

Montaldo, L., Montaldo, P., Cuccaro, P., et al. (2011). Effects of feeding on non-nutritive sucking habits and implications on occlusion in mixed dentition. *International Journal of Paediatric Dentistry, 21*(1), 68–73.

Nelson, A. M. (2012). A comprehensive review of evidence and current recommendations related to pacifier usage. *Journal of Pediatric Nursing, 27*(6), 690–699.

Olusanya, B. O., & Renner, J. K. (2013). Pattern and characteristics of growth faltering in early infancy in an urban Sub-Saharan African setting. *Pediatrics & Neonatology, 54*(2),119–127.

Parsons, H. G., George, M. A., & Innis, S. M. (2011). Growth assessment in clinical practice: Whose growth curve? *Current Gastroenterology Reports, 13*(3), 286–292.

Piaget, J. (1952). *The origins of intelligence in children.* New York, NY: International University Press.

Plutzer, K., Spencer, A. J., & Keirse, M. J. (2011). How first-time mothers perceive and deal with teething symptoms: A randomized controlled trial. *Child: Care, Health and Development, 38*(2), 292–299.

Price, A. M., Wake, M., Ukoumunne, O. C., et al. (2012). Outcomes at six years of age for children with infant sleep problems: Longitudinal community-based study. *Sleep Medicine, 13*(8), 991–998.

Scollan-Koliopoulos, M., & Koliopoulos, J. S. (2010). Evaluation and management of apparent life-threatening events in infants. *Pediatric Nursing, 36*(2), 77–79.

Shergill-Bonner, R. (2010). Infantile colic: Practicalities of management, including dietary aspects. *Journal of Family Health Care, 20*(6), 206–209.

Singer, H. S. (2011). Stereotypic movement disorders. *Handbook of Clinical Neurology, 100*(1), 631–639.

Stevens, B. J., Abbott, L. K., Yamada, J., et al. (2011). Epidemiology and management of painful procedures in children in Canadian hospitals. *Canadian Medical Association Journal, 183*(7), E403–E410.

Sundaram, S., Hoffenberg, E., Kramer, R., et al. (2011). Gastrointestinal tract. In W. W. Hay, M. J. Levine, J. M. Sondheimer, et al. (Eds.), *Current Pediatric Diagnosis &Treatment* (20th ed., pp. 595–630). Columbus, OH: McGraw-Hill.

Taylor, B. J., Heath, A. L., Galland, B. C., et al. (2011). Prevention of overweight in infancy. *BioMedical Central (BMC) Public Health, 11*(1), 942.

Thilo, E. H., & Rosenberg, A. A. (2011). The newborn infant. In W. W. Hay, M. J. Levine, J. M. Sondheimer, et al. (Eds.), *Current pediatric diagnosis & treatment* (20th ed., pp. 1–63). Columbus, OH: McGraw-Hill.

Thomas, D. W., & Greer, F. R. (2010). Probiotics and prebiotics in pediatrics. *Pediatrics, 126*(6), 1217–1231.

Townsend, E., & Pitchford, N. J. (2012). Baby knows best? The impact of weaning style on food preferences and body mass index in early childhood in a case-controlled sample. *British Medical Journal, 2*(1), e000298.

U.S. Department of Health and Human Services. (2010). *Healthy people 2020.* Washington, DC: Author.

van Dijk, M., Hunnius, S., & van Geert, P. (2012). The dynamics of feeding during the introduction to solid food. *Infant Behavior & Development, 35*(2), 226–239.

Whitney, E. N., & Rolfes, S. R. (2012). Life cycle nutrition: Infant, childhood & adolescence. In E. N. Whitney & S. R. Rolfes, *Understanding nutrition* (pp. 528–573). Belmont, CA: Wadsworth Publishing.

Wilken, M. (2012). The impact of child tube feeding on maternal emotional state and identity: A qualitative meta-analysis. *Journal of Pediatric Nursing, 27*(3), 248–255.

Yates, J., McKay, M., & Nicholson, A. J. (2011). Patterns of scald injuries in children—Has anything changed? *Irish Medical Journal, 104*(9), 263–265.

Chapter 30

Nursing Care of a Family With a Toddler

KEY TERMS

- assimilation
- autonomy
- deferred imitation
- discipline
- lordosis
- parallel play
- preoperational thought
- punishment

OBJECTIVES

After mastering the contents of this chapter, you should be able to:

1. Describe normal growth and development of a toddler as well as common parental concerns.
2. Identify 2020 National Health Goals related to the toddler age group that nurses can help the nation achieve.
3. Assess a toddler for normal growth and development milestones.
4. Formulate nursing diagnoses related to toddler growth and development or parental concerns regarding growth and development.
5. Identify expected outcomes for nursing care of a toddler as well as help parents manage seamless transitions across differing health care settings.
6. Using the nursing process, plan nursing care that includes the six competencies of Quality & Safety Education for Nurses (QSEN): Patient-Centered Care, Teamwork & Collaboration, Evidence-Based Practice (EBP), Quality Improvement (QI), Safety, and Informatics.
7. Implement nursing care to promote normal growth and development of a toddler, such as discussing toddler developmental milestones with parents.
8. Evaluate expected outcomes for achievement and effectiveness of care.
9. Integrate knowledge of toddler growth and development with the interplay of nursing process, the six competencies of QSEN, and Family Nursing to promote quality maternal and child health nursing care.

Jason is a 2.5-year-old boy you see at a pediatric clinic. His mother tells you he has changed completely in the past 6 months from an easy-to-care-for baby into a "monster" who refuses to do anything she asks. The only word he says anymore is "no." He has a temper tantrum every night at dinner over some type of food. She tells you this has changed parenting from "fun" to "a real chore."

The previous chapter discussed the growth and development of infants and the abilities that infants develop in the first year. This chapter adds information about the dramatic changes, both physical and psychosocial, that occur during the toddler years and that form the basis for care and health teaching for this age group.

What advice could you give Jason's mother to help her regain a positive view of parenting?

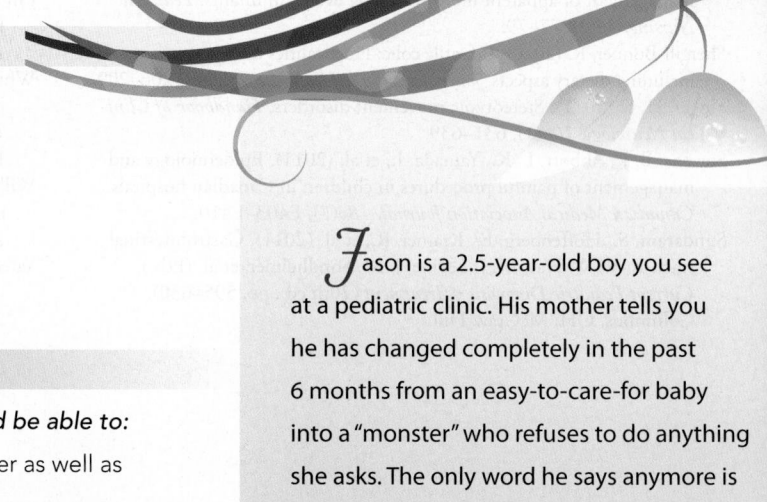

During the toddler period, the age span from 1 to 3 years, enormous changes take place in a child and, consequently, in a family. During this period, children accomplish a wide array of developmental tasks and change from largely immobile and preverbal infants who are dependent on caregivers for the fulfillment of most needs to walking, talking young children with a growing sense of **autonomy** (independence). To match this growth, parents must also change during this period.

If parents enjoyed caring for an infant because time could be spent rocking or singing to the child, they may not enjoy being the parents of a toddler because now their task is to support their child's growing independence by letting the child experiment with toys or other activities. In contrast, some parents thrive during this time as they enjoy playing with this more active child. Because healthy children and families are constantly being challenged by the process of normal development this way, parents often have questions about how to guide their child in different situations and how to cope with special needs and concerns relevant to this age (Nelson, 2013). Box 30.1 shows 2020 National Health Goals that speak to the toddler age group.

BOX 30.1 Nursing Care Planning Based on 2020 National Health Goals

A number of 2020 National Health Goals relate specifically to safety during the toddler years. These include:

- Increase the use of child automotive restraints in children 3 years of age and under from a baseline of 72% to 79%.
- Eliminate or improve elevated blood lead levels in children from a target level of 0.9% of children to a target level of 0%.
- Increase the percentage of persons 2 years of age and older who have had a dental visit in the past 12 months from a baseline of 44.5% to 49%.
- Maintain the rate of deaths caused by poisonings from a baseline at 13.1 out of 100,000 (U.S. Department of Health and Human Services [DHHS], 2010; see www.healthypeople.gov).

Nurses can help the nation achieve these goals by continuing to educate parents about the importance of using car seats and childproofing their homes against household and lead poisoning.

Nursing Process Overview

For Healthy Development of a Toddler

Assessment

Whether a child is seen for a routine checkup or has come to a health care center because of a specific health concern, assessment begins with a careful health history. Asking parents about a toddler's ability to carry out activities of daily living offers assessment information not only on the child's developmental progress but also offers important clues about the child–parent relationship. Because parents see their children daily, they are the best source of information and opinion on when a child seems to be acting "out of sorts" or "different" (a typical sign a child may not be feeling well).

Careful observation is another crucial element of the nursing assessment of a toddler, although toddlers may not show typical behavior at a health care visit (e.g., may not talk, may cling to a parent instead of demonstrating walking).

Nursing Diagnosis

Nursing diagnoses related to growth and development of toddlers usually focus on the parents' eagerness to learn more about the parameters of normal growth and development or issues of safety or care. Examples include:

- Health-seeking behaviors related to normal toddler development
- Deficient knowledge related to best method of toilet training
- Risk for injury related to impulsiveness of toddler
- Interrupted family process related to need for close supervision of 2-year-old
- Readiness for enhanced family coping related to parents' ability to adjust to new needs of child
- Risk for imbalanced nutrition, more than body requirements, related to fast food choices
- Disturbed sleep pattern related to lack of bedtime routine

Outcome Identification and Planning

To help parents resolve a concern during the toddler period, focus largely on family education and anticipatory guidance. Urge them to establish realistic goals and outcomes so they can meet the rapidly changing needs of their toddler and learn to cope with typical toddler behaviors. Otherwise, parents can expect too much of a toddler and grow frustrated instead of enjoying being a parent of a child this age. Helpful Web sites to recommend are the Healthy & Active Preschoolers (www.healthypreschoolers.com) and the March of Dimes (www.MarchofDimes.com). For questions about car seats, parents can consult the Centers for Disease Control and Prevention (CDC, www.cdc.gov/motorvehiclesafety/child_passenger_safety/cps-factsheet.html). Other helpful Web sites to alert parents about safety are the American Association of Poison Control Centers (www.aapcc.org) and the American Academy of Pediatrics (AAP, www.aap.org). The national toll-free telephone number for a poison control center is 800-222-1222. A site parents can check to see if a toddler product has been recalled is the U.S. Consumer Product Safety Commission (www.CPSC.gov).

Implementation

When teaching about typical toddler behavior, teach parents that a good rule is to think of a toddler as a visitor from a foreign land who wants to participate in everything the family is doing, but doesn't know the customs or the language. They need to help their toddler learn these the same as they would for a stranger.

Also teach parents not only how to approach a current problem but also how to learn adequate methods for resolving similar situations that are sure to arise in the future. If parents do not learn methods that can be applied throughout their child's growing years, they may win battles but lose wars. For instance, parents may find that if they promise a child a treat when the child is in the middle of a temper tantrum, that will stop the tantrum, but it will not prevent other tantrums from occurring in the future (and, in fact, may encourage them). Health visits provide opportunities to help parents learn healthier coping techniques as well as a time to demonstrate effective communication skills so parents can improve their interactions with their child.

Outcome Evaluation

Expected outcomes must be evaluated frequently during the toddler period because children change so much and learn so many new skills during this time that their abilities and associated parental concerns can change from day to day. Examples of expected outcomes include:

- Parents state child maintains a consistent bedtime routine within the next 2 weeks.
- Parents state they have childproofed their home by putting a lock on kitchen cupboards by next clinic visit.
- Grandmother states she has modified usual activities to conserve strength to care for toddler granddaughter by 1 week's time.

BOX 30.2 Nursing Care Planning Using Assessment

Appearance of the Average Toddler

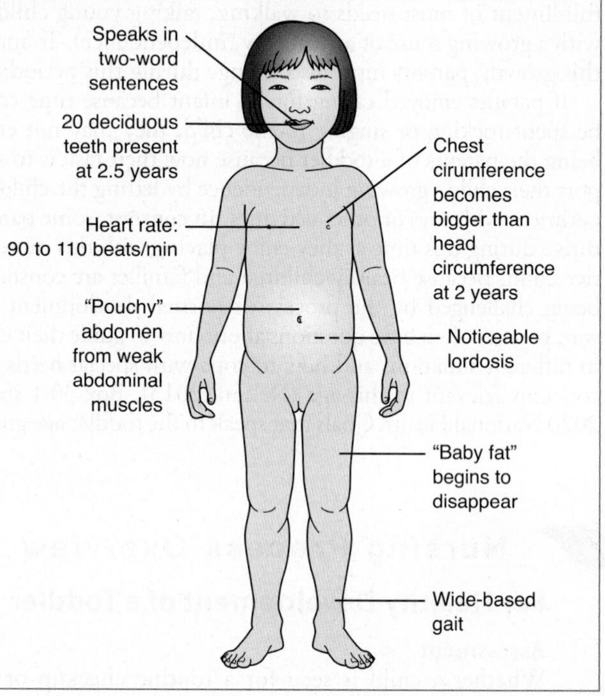

NURSING ASSESSMENT OF A TODDLER'S GROWTH AND DEVELOPMENT

An assessment of a toddler begins with the child's physical growth and skill development. Box 30.2 describes a typical toddler appearance. Table 30.1 provides some guidelines to help parents evaluate illness at this age.

Physical Growth

While toddlers are making great strides developmentally, their physical growth begins to slow.

Weight, Height, Head Circumference, and Body Mass Index

Plot weight and height on a standard growth chart for toddlers (available at http://thePoint.lww.com/Pillitteri7e) at each health care visit to determine if progress is normal for that particular child. If a child is not yet walking, continue to measure height with the child lying down. A child gains only about 5 to 6 lb (2.5 kg) and 5 in. (12 cm) a year during the toddler period, much less than the rate of growth during the infant year. As subcutaneous tissue, or baby fat, begins to disappear toward the end of the second year, the child changes from a plump baby into a leaner, more muscular little girl or boy. A toddler's appetite decreases accordingly, yet adequate intake of all nutrients is still essential to meet energy needs (Whitney & Rolfes, 2013).

Head circumference increases only about 2 cm during the second year compared to about 12 cm during the first year. Head circumference equals chest circumference at 6 months to 1 year of age. By 2 years, chest circumference should have grown greater than that of the head.

Body mass index (BMI) is usually calculated beginning with the toddler age to identify toddlers who are overweight or underweight. A good Web site to use to calculate a child's BMI is the CDC (http://apps.nccd.cdc.gov/dnpabmi/).

Body Contour

Toddlers tend to have a prominent abdomen because, although they are walking well, their abdominal muscles are not yet strong enough to support abdominal contents as well as they will be able to do later (Fig. 30.1A). They also have a forward curve of the spine at the sacral area **(lordosis)**. As they become more experienced at walking, this will correct itself naturally. In addition, many toddlers waddle or walk with a wide stance (see Fig. 30.1B). This stance seems to increase the lordotic curve, but it keeps them on their feet.

Body Systems

Body systems continue to mature during this time.

- Respirations slow slightly but continue to be mainly abdominal.
- Heart rate slows from 110 to 90 beats/min.
- Blood pressure increases to about 99/64 mmHg.
- The brain develops to about 90% of its adult size.
- In the respiratory system, the lumens of vessels enlarge progressively so the threat of lower respiratory infection lessens.
- Stomach secretions become more acid; therefore, gastrointestinal infections also become less common.

TABLE 30.1 Parental Difficulties in Evaluating Illness in Toddlers

Problem	Guidelines for Parents
Evaluating seriousness of illness	Toddlers typically answer "no" to almost all questions; therefore, a question such as "Does your arm hurt?" may bring a "no" response even if an arm does hurt. Observing children for indications of illness (e.g., holding an arm stiffly, rubbing abdomen, crying when they void) is more helpful. Many toddlers do not know the words to describe a feeling of nausea or a sore throat. They reveal these symptoms by not eating. If the child is normally a light eater, as many are, it is difficult for a parent to appreciate these signs.
Differentiating tiredness from illness	Toddlers tend to whine or sleep when they are either tired or ill. Reviewing the child's day and activities often helps to evaluate what is happening. If the child is not tired (it is not nap or bedtime) or if there is not a break in usual routine, crying and whining or temper tantrums suggest illness.
Evaluating nutritional intake	Toddlers are normally fussy eaters compared to infants. Evaluating children as to whether they are active and growing is better than assessing any one day's food intake.
Age-specific diseases to be aware of	The toddler period is an important age to assess speech development; children should be further evaluated if they cannot use simple sentences composed of a noun or pronoun and verb ("me go") by 2 years of age. As children begin to walk, they should be observed for an abnormal gait. Osteomyelitis (bone infection) occurs with a high frequency in toddlers; symptoms of limping, swollen joints, or arm or leg pain should be regarded as serious until ruled otherwise. Toddlers contract 10–12 mild upper respiratory infections a year. Otitis media (middle ear infection) may occur as a complication of these. The child with an upper respiratory infection who suddenly develops a high fever and pulls or manipulates his or her ears should be seen by a primary care provider. Children who attend day care programs have a high incidence of hepatitis A, *Giardia*, and *Shigella* infections. Teach parents to report jaundice or diarrhea promptly to a health care provider to detect these infections.

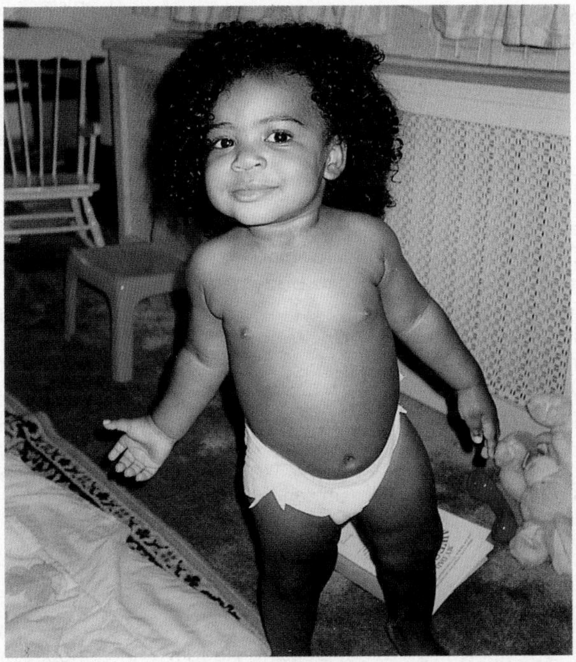
A

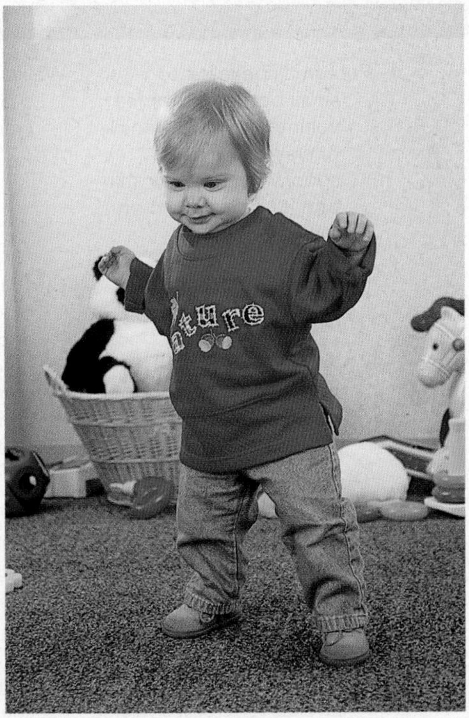
B

FIGURE 30.1 The physical characteristics of toddlers. **(A)** Toddlers typically have a prominent abdomen. **(B)** Toddlers typically walk with an unsteady gait for better stability.

- Stomach capacity increases to the point a child can eat three meals a day.
- Control of the urinary and anal sphincters becomes possible with complete myelination of the spinal cord so toilet training is possible.
- Immune globulin (Ig)G and IgM antibody production becomes mature at 2 years of age. The passive immunity obtained during intrauterine life is no longer operative.

QSEN Checkpoint Question 30.1

Quality Improvement

The father of Jason, the 2-year-old, has asked if it is normal for his son to spread his feet wide apart when he walks. After providing health education to Jason's father, which of his statements suggests that he received accurate teaching?

a. "Jason may be all right, but toddlers with dislocated hips also walk that way."
b. "A wide spaced gait is a common characteristic of toddlers."
c. "Most toddlers walk with feet close together to better stabilize themselves."
d. "His shoes may not have a good arch and this could be causing him to walk unsteadily."

Look in Appendix A for the best answer and rationale.

Teeth

Eight new teeth (the canines and the first molars) erupt during the second year. All 20 deciduous teeth are generally present by 2.5 to 3 years of age (Bishop, 2011).

Developmental Milestones

The developmental milestones of the toddler years are less numerous but no less dramatic than those of the infant year, because this is a period of slow and steady, not sudden, growth. Toddler development is influenced to some extent by the amount of social contact and the number of opportunities children have to explore and experience new degrees of independence. It is strongly influenced by individual readiness for a new skill. Table 30.2 highlights growth and development milestones of gross and fine motor skills, language, and play during the toddler years.

Language Development

Toddlerhood is a critical time for language development, although even this varies among children because to master language, children need practice time. A child who is 2 years old and does not talk in two-word, noun–verb simple sentences needs a careful assessment to determine the cause because this implies underdevelopment. Parents are often worried a lack of language means their child has an autism spectrum disorder (ASD) (Barbaro & Dissanayake, 2012).

TABLE 30.2 Milestones of Toddler Growth and Development

Age (in Months)	Fine Motor	Gross Motor	Language	Play
15	Puts small pellets into small bottles; scribbles voluntarily with a pencil or crayon; holds a spoon well but may still turn it upside down on the way to mouth	Walks alone well; can seat self in chair; can creep up stairs	4–6 words	Can stack two blocks; enjoys being read to; drops toys for adult to recover (exploring sense of permanence)
18	No longer rotates a spoon to bring it to mouth	Can run and jump in place; can walk up and down stairs holding onto a person's hand or railing; typically places both feet on one step before advancing	7–20 words; uses jargoning; names one body part	Imitates household chores such as dusting; begins parallel play (playing beside, not with, another child)
24	Can open doors by turning doorknobs; unscrew lids	Walks up stairs alone, still using both feet on same step at same time	50 words; two-word sentences (noun or pronoun and verb), such as "Daddy go," "Dog talks"	Parallel play evident
30	Makes simple lines or strokes for crosses with a pencil	Can jump down from chairs	Verbal language increasing steadily; knows full name; can name one color and holds up fingers to show age	Spends time playing house, imitating parents' actions; play is "rough-housing" or active

It is true that a delay in language can represent the first symptom of autism, but it also may only be a temporary phenomenon until the child fully grasps the essence of speech.

A word that is used frequently by toddlers and that is a manifestation of their developing autonomy is "no." Toddlers may use the word to mean they are refusing a task, that they do not understand it, or they may only be practicing a sound they have noticed has potent effects on those around them.

To learn other words, children need exposure to conversation and need to be read to often. Language develops quickest if parents respect what toddlers have to say so children grasp the use and purpose of language. Watching television promotes little learning because the activity is passive and it is difficult to discern how language causes action. The AAP (2012) recommends television viewing should be severely limited until at least 2 years of age.

Urge parents to encourage language development by naming objects (e.g., ball, block, music box, doll) as they play with their child or when they give the toddler something ("Here is your drink of water," "Let's put on these pajamas," and so on). This helps children grasp the fact that words are not meaningless sounds, but that they apply to people and objects and have uses. Always answering a child's questions is another good way to do this. Be certain answers for toddlers are simple and brief because they have such a short attention span.

Still other toddlers do not develop language readily because they are not called on to use it. When they point at an object, someone hands it to them; when they climb into their high chair, someone places a meal in front of them. To assess whether parents are encouraging language development, ask them what happens when the child wants something. Do they provide opportunities for the child to ask for things? Children should not be made to name an object before they can have it because their vocabulary is so limited, but parents can reinforce language by voicing the request (e.g., "You want the ball?"). Reading aloud is another effective way to strengthen vocabulary. Reading the exact words in a book is not as important at this age as is pointing to the pictures and describing what the picture shows, such as "See Jane throwing the ball?" "Look, that dog took that ball!" Reading this way can also have the additional benefit of strengthening parent–child bonds and offering respite for parents who are tired of more active games (Landry, Smith, Swank, et al., 2011).

Children who are very active may use fewer words than children who are less active because active children are too busy doing things to describe what it is they are doing. Such children probably have a large unexpressed vocabulary, however, or understand more words (comprehensive vocabulary) than can be expressed (expressive vocabulary).

Because children learn language from imitating what they hear, if they are spoken to in baby talk, their enunciation of words can be poor; if they hear examples of bad grammar, they will not use good grammar. Remind parents that pronouns are difficult for children to use correctly; many children are 3.5 or 4 years of age before they can separate the different uses of "I," "me," "him," and "her." Bilingual children often interchange words from both languages.

QSEN Checkpoint Question 30.2

Informatics

Toddlers learn a great deal about oral communication in the course of their development. Which of the following statements should you expect Jason, a 2-year-old, to have mastered?

a. "Red tomatoes."
b. "Daddy come."
c. "Old MacDonald."
d. "Please, please."

Look in Appendix A for the best answer and rationale.

Emotional Development

Children change a great deal in their ability to understand the world and how they relate to people during the toddler years.

Autonomy. The developmental task of the toddler years according to Erikson (1993) is the development of a *sense of autonomy versus shame or doubt*. Children who have learned to trust themselves and others during the infant year are better prepared to do this than those who have not learned to trust themselves or others.

To develop a sense of autonomy is to develop a sense of independence. A healthy level of autonomy is achieved when parents are able to balance independence with consistently sound rules for safety. Children who are constantly told not to try things because they will hurt themselves may be left with a stronger sense of doubt than confidence at the end of the toddler period. Children who are made to feel it is wrong to be independent may leave the toddler period with a stronger sense of shame than autonomy.

Infants appear to have difficulty differentiating between their bodies and those of others; they think of their bodies as extensions of their parents or their primary caregivers. When infants approach toddlerhood, they begin to make the differentiation. As they recognize they are separate individuals, toddlers also realize they do not always have to do what others want them to do. From this realization comes the reputation toddlers have for being negativistic, obstinate, and difficult to manage.

This reputation probably exists because parents misinterpret children's cues. For example, children's refusal to accept help putting on shoes may be seen by a parent as disobedience, whereas children may view this as insisting on performing a task they can do independently—a positive expression of autonomy.

Socialization. Once toddlers are walking well, they become resistant to sitting in laps and being cuddled. This is not lack of a desire for socialization but a function of being independent. At 15 months, children are still enthusiastic about interacting with people, providing those people are willing to follow them where they want to go. By 18 months, toddlers imitate the things they see a parent doing, such as "study" or "sweep," so they seek out parents to observe and imitate. By 2 or more years of age, children become aware of gender differences and may point to other children and identify them as "boy" or "girl."

FIGURE 30.2 Toddlers play beside, but not with, other children (parallel play).

Play Behavior. All during the toddler period, children play beside other children, not with them. This side-by-side play **(parallel play)** is not unfriendly but is a normal developmental sequence that occurs during the toddler period (Fig. 30.2). Caution parents that if two toddlers are going to play together, they must provide similar toys because an argument over one toy is likely to occur (Levine, 2011).

The toys toddlers enjoy most are those they can play with by themselves and that require action. Trucks they can make go, squeaky frogs they can squeeze, rocking horses they can ride, pegs they can pound, and a toy telephone they can talk into are all favorites. These are all toys children can control, giving them a sense of power in manipulation, which is an expression of autonomy (Fig. 30.3).

Some parents are not prepared for this change in play habits in their child. They wonder why a child who used to play quietly in his crib is now more interested in banging trucks together. However, they need only watch a toddler tug a pull toy, stop to see if it is following, walk again, and stop and look to see if it is still following to understand the feeling of accomplishment involved in manipulating toys.

At 15 months of age, children are still in a put-in, take-out stage, so they continue to enjoy stacks of boxes that fit inside each other. They enjoy throwing toys out of a playpen or from a high chair tray as long as someone will pick them up and return them again and again.

The 18-month-old child walks securely enough to enjoy pull toys. Toys should be strong enough to take a great deal of abuse because children this age may use toys in ways other than those for which they were designed. For example, an infant will sit and softly stroke a stuffed cat; however, a toddler will pick it up by the tail and swing it, pound it, or pull at it. There is no need for parents to correct children about the way they are using a toy as long as it is safe and appears to give satisfaction. If toddlers find a toy frustrating because they are holding or using it incorrectly, showing them the right way will ease frustration.

By age 2 years, when toddlers begin to spend time imitating adult actions in their play such as wrapping a doll and putting it to bed or "driving the car," they begin to use fewer toys than before. The act of imitating has become their play. By the end of the toddler period, both boys and girls begin to like roughhousing and spend at least part of every day in this very active, stimulating type of play (Fig. 30.4). Encouraging parents to schedule this type of play outdoors, where vases or other prized possessions cannot be broken, makes it more acceptable.

A child who feels a need for active play is notably not easy to get to sit down and eat, fall asleep, or play quiet games and so may be described as "trouble." It is good to explore with parents the amount of outside or roughhousing time they allow a child each day. Stroller walks are good because they provide fresh air and sunshine, but toddlers also need opportunities to engage in strenuous activity such as running and jumping (Hodges, Smith, Tidwell, et al., 2012). Because of this rough activity, most toddlers have at least one black-and-blue mark on their legs at all times from tripping over their feet while trying to run too fast or from jumping or bumping into a chair or doorway. Examine these and document their presence, but don't mistake them for child maltreatment (Hooker, Ward, & Verrinder, 2012).

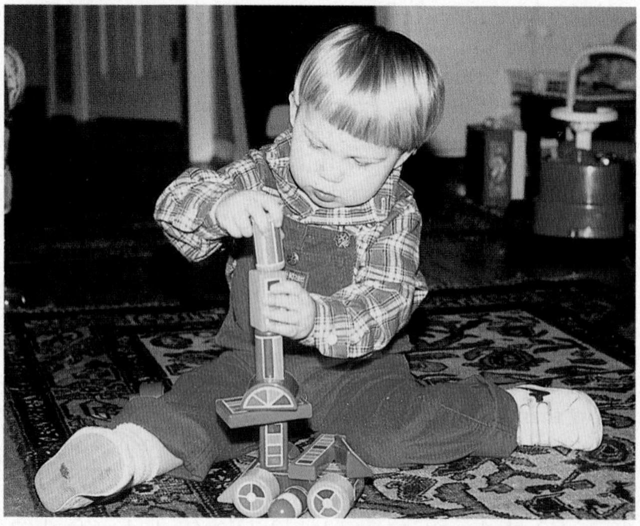

FIGURE 30.3 Toddlers enjoy toys they can manipulate.

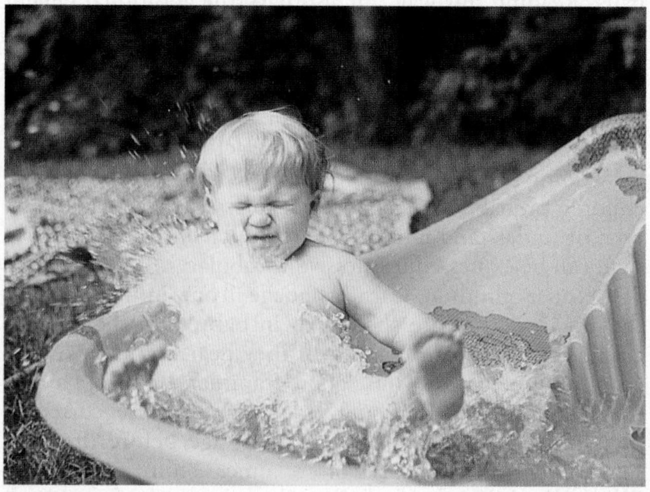

FIGURE 30.4 Toddlers usually enjoy rough and tumble play.

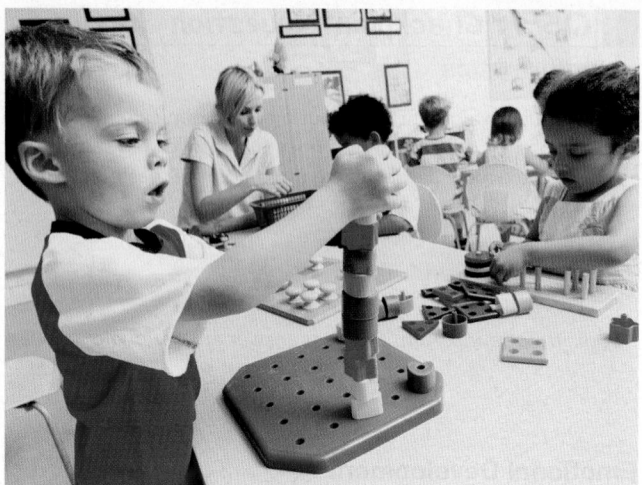

What if...30.1 Jason's mother tells you, "I arrange play dates for Jason but he never shares his toys. How can I make him do that?" How would you answer her?

Cognitive Development

As a toddler, a child enters the fifth and sixth stages of Piaget's sensorimotor thought (Piaget 1952). In these stages, toddlers are described as "little scientists" because of their interest in trying to discover new ways to handle objects or new results that different actions can achieve. For instance, by trial and error, toddlers discover that cats do not like baths and cookies on the center of a table can be reached by pulling them down using the tablecloth. Obviously, toddlers need supervision for these types of scientific investigations because they can lead to errors or injury.

Infants, when they want to retrieve a ball that rolled under a chair, crawl under the chair or along the same path the ball took. Many children at 15 months of age are able to follow a different path (walk in back of the chair) to obtain the object because they can project where it will stop rolling. This results from increased awareness that the ball is permanent and, even if it follows a different direction from the one the child must take, it will be there to retrieve.

By stage 6 of cognitive development (between 18 and 24 months of age), toddlers are able to try out various actions mentally rather than having to actually perform them—the beginning of problem solving or symbolic thought. Children at this stage are also able to remember an action and imitate it later **(deferred imitation)**; they can do such things as pretend to drive a car or put a baby to sleep because they have seen this previously and not just in the recent past. Object permanence becomes complete.

At the end of the toddler period, children enter a second major period of cognitive development termed **preoperational thought** and begin to use a process termed **assimilation**. Because they are not able to change their thoughts to fit a situation, they learn to change the situation (or how they perceive it). This ability is what causes toddlers to use toys in the "wrong" way. For example, if a child is given a toy hammer, instead of pounding with it, she may shake it to see if it rattles (i.e., the child has changed the toy's use to fit her thoughts, or used assimilation).

PLANNING AND IMPLEMENTATION FOR HEALTH PROMOTION OF A TODDLER AND FAMILY

Toddlers tend to develop many upper respiratory and ear infections but otherwise come to health care facilities most often for health maintenance visits (recommended at 15, 18, and 24 months of age) and for important immunizations. These visits allow you to focus on health promotion and provide the opportunity for early detection of any growth and development delays. Table 30.3 lists specific areas to assess during these visits.

Routine health maintenance visits also provide opportunities to support parents through the normal crises of the toddler period. Ways to encourage parents to promote healthy development of independence in their toddler include listening carefully to their concerns, asking questions to help separate the objective circumstances surrounding a problem from the parents' possible emotional biases, and providing guidelines on how to handle specific problems.

Promoting Toddler Safety

Accidents (unintentional injuries) are the major cause of death in infants through young adults in the United States (CDC, 2012a). Unintentional ingestions (poisoning) and auto accidents are the types of unintentional injuries that occur most frequently in toddlers (Beirens, van Beeck, Brug, et al., 2010).

Although poisoning can involve medicine such as acetaminophen (and there is a growing concern of illegal or prescription drug ingestions even in toddlers), it most often occurs from ingestion of cleaning products. Aspiration or ingestion of small objects such as watch or hearing aid batteries, pencil erasers, or parts of crayons is also a major danger for children of this age (Litovitz, Whitaker, & Clark, 2010). Urge parents to childproof their home by putting all poisonous products, drugs, and small objects out of reach by the time their infant is crawling, and certainly by the time their infant is walking, to avoid these problems (Lee & Marcdante, 2011).

Other unintentional injuries that occur frequently in toddlers include motor vehicle accidents, burns, falls, drowning, and playground injuries. These occur because toddlers' motor ability jumps ahead of their judgment. To prevent serious injury, teach parents to be alert as to what their toddler is doing at all times.

By the end of the toddler period, children can walk surely; if they are left outside to play, they can very quickly travel a block away. Because they have no judgment concerning moving cars, they walk across streets with no regard for oncoming cars. Because they cannot swim well, parents need to check whether backyard pools—another area prone to unintended injury—are securely fenced (Bowman, Aitken, Robbins, et al., 2012).

For safety in automobiles, parents should keep their toddlers in rear-facing seats until age 2 years, or until the child reaches the maximum height and weight for their particular seat. Following that, children need to ride in a car seat with a five-point restraint (Fig. 30.5). Car seats should be placed in the back seat so the child is not struck by the passenger seat airbag (AAP, 2013). Remind parents that it is unsafe to leave a toddler alone in a car. One way for a parent to be reminded that the child is in the back seat is to always place a purse or briefcase in the back seat alongside the child's car seat.

Toddlers need to wear a helmet as soon as they begin riding a tricycle. Although parents are becoming conscientious about using car seats, they are not as conscientious about using toddler or booster car seats or helmets for bicycle riding, so these are areas where health teaching is necessary (Macy, Clark, Freed, et al., 2012).

Some 15-month-old children are able to climb over the side rails of their cribs and enjoy exploring the house early in the morning before anyone else is awake. Parents might have to move their child to a regular bed with a side rail as early as

TABLE 30.3 Health Maintenance Schedule, Toddler Period

Well-Child Visits (Typically Scheduled at 15, 18, 24, and 30 Months)		
Area of Focus	**Methods**	**Frequency**
Health history	Health interview	Every visit
Physical health	Physical examination	Every visit
Developmental milestones	History and observation Formal Denver Developmental Screening Test (DDST-II)	Every visit 18- and 24-month visits
Autism spectrum disorder screening	Observation and language assessment	18- and 30-month visits
Growth milestones	Height and weight plotted on standard growth chart Head circumference Body mass index	Every visit 15-, 18-, and 24-month visits Beginning at 24-month visit
Nutrition	History, observation; height and weight information	Every visit
Parent–child relationship	History and observation	Every visit
Social/Behavior assessment	History and observation	Every visit
Vision and hearing	History and observation	Every visit
Dental health	History and physical examination; first dental appointment	18- or 34-month visit
Anemia	Hematocrit/hemoglobin	18-, 24-, and 30-month visits
Lead screening	Point of care rapid lead screening	Depending on risk level; 18- or 24-month visit
Tuberculosis	Purified protein derivative (PPD) test	18- or 24-month visit depending on prevalence in community
Urinalysis	Clean-catch urine	24-month visit
Dyslipidemia	Cholesterol level	24-month visit
Immunizations		
(Administer immunization in accordance with health care agency policies. Check history and past records, and inform caregiver about any risks and side effects before administration [www.cdc.gov/vaccines/schedules].)		
Diphtheria, tetanus, and pertussis	DTaP	15-month visit (4th)
Haemophilus influenzae type B	HiB	15-month visit (4th)
Pneumococcal vaccine	PVC	15-month visit if not previously immunized
Hepatitis A	HepA	12- or 18-month visit (1st & 2nd)
Hepatitis B	HepB	15- or 18-month visit (3rd)
Influenza	IIV	Yearly
Measles, mumps, and rubella	MMR	12- or 15-month visit (1st)
Inactivated poliomyelitis	IPV	12- or 15-month visit (3rd)
Varicella vaccine	VAR	12- or 15-month visit (1st)

Area of Focus	Methods	Frequency
Anticipatory Guidance		
Toddler care	Active listening and health teaching	Every visit
Expected growth and developmental milestones before next visit	Health teaching	Every visit
Poison and unintentional injury prevention	Educate parents about toddler safety, such as using car seats and bicycle helmets, locking up poisons, and such precautions as removing drawstrings from hooded clothing to prevent strangulation; provide telephone number of national poison control center (1-800-222-1222).	Every visit
Problem Solving		
Any problems expressed by caregiver during course of the visit	Active listening and health teaching regarding temper tantrums, toilet training, negativity	Every visit

From American Academy of Pediatrics, Committee on Practice and Ambulatory Medicine. (2012). *Recommendations for preventive pediatric health care*. Washington, DC: Author; Centers for Disease Control and Prevention. (2013). *Birth–18 years & "catch up" immunization schedules*. Washington, DC: Author.

this time to keep the child from falling when climbing out of a crib. A safety gate on the door of his or her room is another way to keep a toddler contained and safe.

As the child reaches 2 years of age and begins to imitate housework or repairing a car, parents must be sure the child does not use real cleaning compounds or sharp tools. Box 30.3 summarizes unintentional injury prevention measures to encourage parents to take with their toddler.

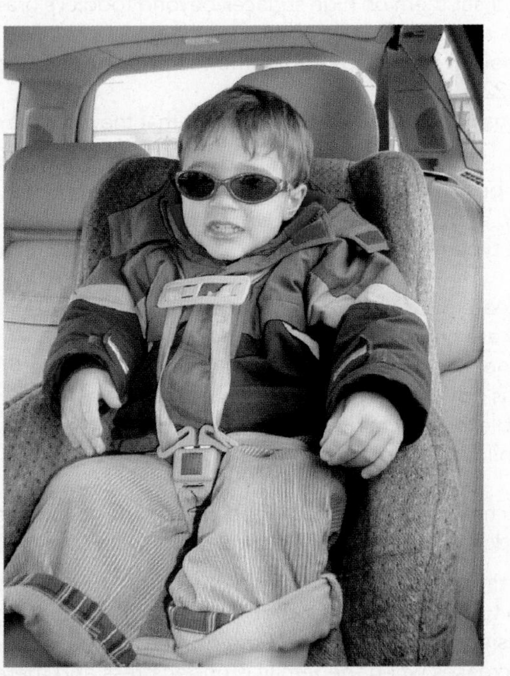

FIGURE 30.5 Toddlers should use a car seat with a five-point restraint while riding in an automobile until they are 2 years of age.

QSEN Checkpoint Question 30.3

Evidence-Based Practice

As television sets become larger and thinner, viewing becomes easier. To investigate if television sets can also be a threat to young children, researchers reviewed a Canadian trauma database over a 15-year period as to how many emergency room visits were caused by a television set falling onto a young child. They identified a total of 179 injuries (20 to 24 per year). Toddlers were the most frequently injured age group, and head and neck injuries were the most common consequences of a television pulled down onto a young child (Mills, Grushka, & Butterworth, 2012).

Based on the study and the AAP recommendations on television viewing, how would you advise Jason's parents?

a. Encourage Jason to watch television in his room where the television set is smaller.
b. Teach Jason to always watch television from a distance of no less than 12 feet.
c. Teach Jason to use the remote control so he can watch television safely by himself.
d. Allow Jason to watch television only when a parent is free to supervise his actions.

Look in Appendix A for the best answer and rationale.

Lead Screening

The CDC has set as a goal the elimination of elevated blood lead levels in children (CDC, 2012b). All children between the ages of 6 months and 6 years who live in communities with buildings built before 1950 and immigrant children who might have been exposed to sources of lead in another country should be tested for the presence of lead in their

BOX 30.3 Nursing Care Planning Based on Family Teaching

UNINTENTIONAL INJURY PREVENTION MEASURES FOR TODDLERS

Q. Jason's mother tells you, "My toddler is constantly on the go. How can I keep him safe?"
A. Injury prevention has to be constant while your child is a toddler. Try the following precautions:

Potential Unintended Injury	Prevention Measure
Motor vehicles	Maintain your child in a car seat; do not be distracted by the child from safe driving. Do not allow the child to play outside unsupervised. Do not allow the child to operate electronic garage doors or play near lawn mowers or snow blowers. Supervise toddlers with pedaling toys (e.g., look before crossing driveways, do not cross streets), but do not expect toddler will obey these rules at all times (i.e., stay close by).
Falls	Keep house windows closed or keep secure screens in place. Place gates at top and bottom of stairs. Supervise at playgrounds. Do not allow child to walk with sharp object in hand or mouth. Raise crib rails and check to make sure they are locked before walking away from crib.
Aspiration	Examine toys for small parts that could be aspirated; remove toys that appear dangerous. Do not feed toddler popcorn or nuts; caution child not to eat while running. Do not leave toddler alone with a balloon.
Drowning	Do not leave toddler alone in a bathtub or near water (including buckets of cleaning water). Fence pools; insist toddlers wear safety "floats" or life vests; supervise at all times when near water.
Animal bites	Do not allow toddler to approach strange dogs. Supervise child's play with family pets.
Poisoning	Never present medication as candy. Buy medications with childproof caps; put away immediately after use. Never take medication in front of child. Place all medication and poisons in locked cabinets or overhead shelves where child cannot reach them. Never leave medication in parents' purse or pocket where child can reach it. Always store food or substances in their original containers. Know the names of houseplants and find out if they are poisonous. (Call national poison control center for information: 800-222-1222.) If unsure if plants are safe, hang them or set them on high surfaces beyond toddler's grasp. Be certain small batteries or magnets are out of reach. Post telephone number of national poison control center by the telephone or add as a contact on a cell phone: (800-222-1222). Inspect toys to be certain if they were manufactured in another country that they are free of lead-based paint.
Burns	Cook on the back burners of stove if possible; turn handles of pots toward back of stove to prevent toddler from reaching up and pulling them down. If a vaporizer is used, use a cool-mist type rather than a steam vaporizer so child cannot be scalded. Keep screen in front of fireplace or heater. Monitor toddlers carefully when they are near lit candles. Do not leave toddlers unsupervised near hot-water faucets; check temperature setting for hot-water heater so thermostat is not over 125°F. Do not leave coffee/tea pots on a table where child can reach them. Never drink hot beverages when a child is sitting on your lap or playing within reach. Buy flame-retardant clothing. Do not allow toddlers to blow out matches (teach fire is not fun); store matches out of reach. Keep electric wires and cords out of toddlers' reach; cover electrical outlets with safety plugs.
General	Know whereabouts of toddlers at all times. Toddlers can climb onto chairs or high stools they could not manage before, can turn door knobs and go places they could not go before, and are able to pull a television set over on top of themselves. Be aware the frequency of injuries increases when the family is under stress and therefore less attentive to children. Special precautions must be taken at these times. Be aware some children are more active, curious, and impulsive and therefore more vulnerable to unintentional injury than others.

body (lead poisoning). Elevated lead levels are caused by eating, chewing, or sucking on objects (e.g., windowsills, paint chips, furniture) that are covered with lead-based paint. Although federal law has prohibited the use of lead in the manufacture of both interior and exterior paints since the mid-1970s, many older houses are still coated with lead-based paint. Additional sources of lead poisoning can include:

- Toys manufactured in countries where restrictions on lead are not enforced or cribs that were painted with lead-based paint
- Soil around the exterior of the house and contaminated food grown there
- Dust or fumes created by home renovation
- Pottery made with lead glazes or jewelry made from lead or lead alloys
- Colored print in newspapers or older lead-based water pipes
- Lead dust brought home on the clothing of parents who work with lead products such as batteries

Lead-based gasoline used to be a concern but is no longer available in the United States. Because lead is toxic to body tissue, ingestion of it leads to serious damage to the brain and nervous system, kidneys, and red blood cells. Levels as low as 5 μg/dl can cause learning and behavioral problems (CDC, 2012b). High levels may result in seizures, cognitive challenges, coma, and even death. Although 10 μg/dl was the standard to define lead toxicity for the past decade, the new lower level of 5 μg is proposed as the best way to help prevent minimal damage (Kuehn, 2012).

Beginning symptoms of lead poisoning include irritability, headache, fatigue, and abdominal pain. Often, however, there are no symptoms before damage occurs, which is why blood screening is essential. The CDC (2012b) recommends screening for all children between the ages of 9 and 12 months at least once and again at 18 or 24 months of age. A small amount of blood taken by a finger prick is analyzed. A positive result (over 5 μg/dl) must be confirmed by further testing. The long-term effects of lead poisoning and therapy are discussed in Chapter 52.

QSEN Checkpoint Question 30.4

Safety

Jason's grandmother often visits the family. When she does, she brings a number of medications with her. What precautions about unintentional poisoning would you like to see the family following?

a. Advise the grandmother to keep her medicine in her purse and stress that no one should open her purse but her.

b. Show Jason his grandmother's pills and emphasize that he is not permitted to touch them.

c. Assure the grandmother that as long as her vials of medicine have childproof caps, there is no danger.

d. Buy the grandmother a medicine case that locks and place it on a high shelf when she visits.

Look in Appendix A for the best answer and rationale.

Promoting Nutritional Health in Toddlers

Because growth slows abruptly after the first year of life, a toddler's appetite is usually less than an infant's. Children who ate hungrily 2 months earlier now may sit and play with their food. It is important to educate parents that, while the child is still an infant, this decline in food intake will occur, so they will not be concerned when it happens. Because the actual amount of food eaten daily varies from one child to another, teach parents to place a small amount of food on a plate and allow their child to eat it and ask for more rather than serve a large portion that the child cannot finish. One tablespoonful of each food served is a good start. Also, cleaning a plate gives a child a feeling of independent functioning, whereas leaving food uneaten suggests that parents expected something more.

Because mothers are urged to breastfeed for the entire first year, many mothers begin weaning from breastfeeding or bottle feeding during the toddler years. Recommend that mothers do this gradually in order to avoid confrontation. Additional tips for weaning are discussed in Chapter 29.

Allowing self-feeding is a major way to both strengthen independence in a toddler and improve the amount of food consumed. Offering finger foods such as pieces of chicken, slices of banana, pieces of cheese, and crackers, and allowing a choice between two types of food helps promote independence while exposing children to varied foods (Whitney & Rolfes, 2013). Toddlers usually prefer to eat the same type of food over and over because of the sense of security this offers. Most toddlers insist on feeding themselves and generally will resist eating if a parent insists on feeding them. An independent child may react to repeated attempts at being fed by refusing to eat at all.

Toddler Nutrition Requirements

Parents may become frustrated when trying to provide adequate nutrition for their toddler because of a toddler's varying and unpredictable appetite and food preferences. Although a toddler's daily food consumption may vary greatly, energy needs are generally met when sufficient food is supplied in a positive environment.

- Sedentary children ages 1 to 3 years should consume 1,000 kcal daily; active children in this age group may need up to 1,400 kcal daily (U.S. Department of Agriculture, 2012).
- Calories are best supplied by a variety of foods spaced into three meals a day.
- Protein and carbohydrate needs are often those most easily met during the toddler period; diets high in sugar should be avoided to help prevent toddler obesity.
- Fats should generally not be restricted for children under 2 years old; however, children over 2 years old should have a total fat intake between 30% and 35% of calories, with most fat coming from sources of polyunsaturated and monounsaturated fatty acids, such as fish, nuts, and vegetable oils, the same as adults.
- Trans fats should be kept to a minimum.
- Adequate calcium and phosphorus intake is important for bone mineralization. Milk should be whole milk until age 2 years, after which 2% milk can be introduced (Whitney & Rolfes, 2013).

A Vegetarian Diet

Vegetarian diets are adequate for toddlers if parents are well informed about needed vitamins and minerals (Chisholm, 2011). A vegetarian diet can be easily designed for a toddler who prefers finger foods because many vegetables, fruits, and grains such as pieces of oranges, peaches, raisins, chickpeas, and crackers are easily eaten this way. The use of fortified soy milk prevents fluid, protein, vitamin B_{12}, and calcium deficiencies. Tofu should be served often to supply protein.

Promoting Toddler Development in Daily Activities

A toddler's new independence and developing abilities in self-care, such as dressing, eating, and to a limited extent hygiene, present special challenges for parents. Learning how to promote autonomy yet maintain a safe, healthful environment should be a major goal for the family.

Dressing

By the end of the toddler period, most children can put on their own socks and underpants (Fig. 30.6). Some may also be able to pull on slacks, pullover shirts (the sleeves of a shirt often confuse a toddler), or simple dresses. Parents may be reluctant to encourage toddlers to dress themselves because it is easier and quicker for a parent to do so. Also, a toddler who is dressed by parents will (usually) be wearing clothes in the correct way. When toddlers dress themselves, they invariably put shoes on the wrong feet and shirt and pants on backwards. Encourage parents to give up perfection for the benefit of the child's developing sense of autonomy. If they feel they must change the child's clothes, urge them to begin with a positive statement, such as "You did a good job," before making the switch.

Don't judge whether the parents encourage self-dressing by what they do at a health care–setting visit. In this setting, parents may dress a child quickly to show the child that the examination is over, or they may simply be in a hurry to get home.

As soon as children are up on their feet and walking, they need shoe soles that are firm enough to provide protection from rough surfaces. However, toddlers do not need extremely firm or ankle-high shoes. Because a toddler's arches are still developing, it is better for their arches to provide foot support rather than having it provided by shoes. Sneakers are an ideal toddler shoe because the soles are hard enough for rough surfaces and arch support is limited.

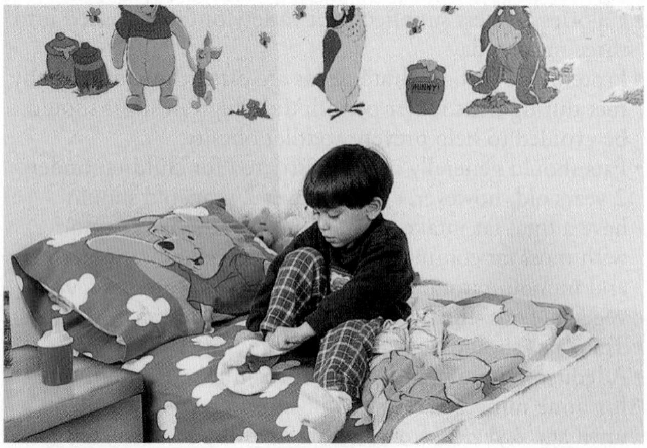

FIGURE 30.6 Getting dressed by himself is a fun morning activity for this older toddler.

Sleep

The amount of sleep children need gradually decreases as they grow older (Gahagan, 2011). They may begin the toddler period napping twice a day and sleeping 12 hours each night, and end it with one nap a day and only 8 hours of sleep at night. Parents who are not aware that the need for sleep declines at this time may view a child's disinterest in sleeping as a problem (about 10% of parents report toddler-age sleep problems (Byars, Yolton, Rausch, et al., 2012). If a child has difficulty falling asleep at night, it may be time to omit or shorten an afternoon nap. If a child is so short tempered at dinnertime that eating is impossible, perhaps the child needs two naps a day. Some toddlers begin having night terrors or awake crying from a bad dream and so may receive little sleep because they are reluctant to fall back asleep (Bhargava, 2011). Night terrors are further discussed in Chapter 31.

When toddlers are tired, they naturally fall asleep. They may begin to resist naps, however, as well as nighttime sleep as they become aware for the first time that activities go on while they sleep. Caution parents when they say, "We'll do this after naptime," that they wait until then to do it. Otherwise, a child may be reluctant to nap the next day for fear of missing another activity. Also, parents must be sure older siblings do not point out to a toddler all the exciting things a toddler missed while napping.

Other toddlers resist naptime as part of their developing negativism. Parents might minimize this by including a nap as part of lunchtime routine, not as a separate activity (i.e., the child always goes from the table directly to bed as if the two things are connected). The parent can state simply, "It's naptime now," and then give a secondary choice: "Do you want to sleep with your teddy bear or your rag doll?" Toward the end of the toddler period, when children are ready to omit their afternoon naps, they may still be agreeable to a "shoes off" or "quiet play" period until they begin to attend school full time.

As with any other activity of this period, a toddler loves a bedtime routine: bath, pajamas, a story, toothbrushing, being tucked into bed, having a drink of water, choosing a toy to sleep with, and turning out the lights. Parents must be careful, however, not to let a child maneuver them into such a long procedure that sleep is delayed considerably past the time initially set. Although toddlers need to be independent, they also need a feeling of security. Just as adults like to know there are guardrails along steep mountain roads, toddlers like to see parents as firm, consistent people who can be counted on to be reliable over and over, especially when they're tired.

Many toddlers are ready to be moved out of a crib into a youth bed or regular bed with protective side rails or a chair strategically placed beside it by the end of the toddler period. Remind parents to stress that sleeping in a regular bed does not give children the right to get in and out of bed as they choose. Some toddlers do well if they are allowed to sleep in a regular bed and a folding gate is placed across the door to their room. This arrangement gives them a feeling of independence but still keeps them safe. When first moved to a bed without side rails, many children are found sleeping on the floor of the room in the morning. There is no harm in this unless it is cold or drafty. Dressing the child in warm pajamas or putting a blanket on the floor might be solutions to help parents accept this.

Bathing

The time for a toddler's bath should depend on the parents' and the child's wishes and schedule. Some parents prefer to bathe a toddler before the evening meal because it has a quieting effect and prepares the child for eating; others prefer to give it at bedtime because it has a relaxing effect and helps a child sleep. However, the time is not as important as the attempt to establish a sense of routine and a sense that life has order. Learning to be independent is sometimes frightening, and there is security in knowing that certain events are predictable.

Toddlers usually enjoy bath time, and parents should make an effort to make it fun by providing a toy, such as a rubber duck or plastic fish. Bath time is usually so enjoyable for toddlers that parents can use it as a recreational activity or something to do on a rainy day when they can find nothing else to interest their child. Remind parents that although toddlers can sit well in a bathtub, it is still not safe to leave them unsupervised. They might slip and get their head under water or reach and turn on the hot-water faucet and scald themselves (Hutchings, Barnes, Maddocks, et al., 2010). Parents shouldn't add bubble bath to the water because its use is associated with vulvovaginitis and possibly urinary tract infections, especially in girls (Smith, 2011).

Dental Care

Toddlers often need between-meal snacks. To help prevent dental caries from frequent snacking, encourage parents to offer fruit (e.g., bananas, pieces of apple, orange slices) or protein foods (e.g., cheese, pieces of chicken) for snacks rather than high-carbohydrate items such as cookies to limit exposure of the child's teeth to carbohydrate (Smith & Riedford, 2012). Calcium (found in large amounts in milk, cheese, and yogurt) is especially important for the development of strong teeth and so are other good snack foods. In addition, children should continue to drink fluoridated water or, if not available, receive fluoride supplements so all new teeth form with cavity-resistant enamel (Tubert-Jeannin, Auclair, Amsallem, et al., 2011).

Remind parents not to put a child to bed with a bottle of milk or juice to help prevent the development of caries. Toddlers need a toothbrush they recognize as their own. Toward the end of the toddler period, they can begin to do the brushing themselves under supervision (almost all children need some supervision until about age 8 years). Remind parents that it is better for a child to brush thoroughly once a day, probably at bedtime, than to do it poorly many times a day. After brushing, parents can use dental floss to clean between their child's teeth and remove plaque.

Urge parents to schedule a first visit to a dentist skilled in pediatric dental care at about 12 months of age (and certainly no later than 24 months of age) for an assessment of dentition (Hoeft, Barker, & Masterson, 2011).

Parents can prepare their child for this first visit and subsequent visits by reading a story about a dentist visit, maintaining a positive attitude about the visit, avoiding the use of frightening words such as "drill" or "shot," and answering their child's questions honestly without going into too much detail. Because children rarely have cavities this early, the visit is usually painless and sets a positive stage for future dental supervision visits.

Promoting Healthy Family Functioning

Because learning self-reliance is the primary goal of a child during the toddler period, some parents who enjoyed caring for their child as an infant may find it difficult to have their authority challenged by a toddler. Help parents to understand their responses to these attempts at independence are crucial to the healthy development of their child. Although the child still needs firm limits to feel secure, a child must be given room to make independent decisions in areas the parents feel they do not need to control. Someone outside of the family, such as a nurse, can provide an important perspective on this issue.

At bedtime, naptime, or anytime they are tired, toddlers may become much more like their old selves, wanting to sit on a parent's lap and be rocked or picked up and carried. This does not signal babyish behavior or regression in a toddler; it is a natural state between infant and preschool ages.

Parental Concerns Associated With the Toddler Period

Parental concerns of the toddler period usually arise because of a conflict over autonomy.

Toilet Training

Toilet training is one of the biggest tasks a toddler tries to achieve. There are so many theories concerning toilet training that understanding the procedure can become one of the biggest tasks of this period for parents. Most first-time parents ask when to start, when training should be completed, and how to go about it (Box 30.4). You can explain to parents that toilet training is an individualized task for each child. It should begin and be completed according to a child's ability to accomplish it, not according to a set schedule (Kiddoo, 2012).

BOX 30.4 Nursing Care Planning to Respect Cultural Diversity

In the United States, toilet training is usually introduced during the toddler period. Like so many other aspects of childrearing, however, the time when parents begin these activities is culturally determined. In other countries, toilet training may be started as soon as a child can sit—at about 6 months. Although praise is used in the United States as a common means of encouraging toddlers to learn new tasks, other cultures believe praise could bring a child harm by attracting evil spirits; instead, strategies of shame or strict discipline are used. Being aware that childrearing practices are not consistent across the world is a help in understanding why parents approach childrearing problems differently and why childrearing advice must be individualized.

Before children can begin toilet training, they must have reached three important developmental levels, one physiologic and the other two cognitive:

- They must have control of rectal and urethral sphincters, usually achieved by the time they walk well.
- They must have a cognitive understanding of what it means to hold urine and stools until they can release them at a certain place and time.
- They must have a desire to delay immediate gratification for a more socially accepted action.

Because physiologic development is cephalocaudal, the rectal and urethral sphincters are not mature enough for control in most children until at least the end of the first year, when tracts of the spinal cord are myelinated to the anal level. A good way for a parent to know a child's development has reached this point is to wait until the child can walk well independently.

Toilet training need not start this early, however, because cognitively and socially, many children do not understand what is being asked of them until they are 2 or even 3 years old. The markers of readiness are subtle, but as a rule, children are ready for toilet training when they begin to be uncomfortable in wet diapers. They demonstrate this by pulling or tugging at soiled diapers, or they may bring a parent a clean diaper after they have soiled so they can be changed (Fig. 30.7).

Teach parents not to underestimate the difficulty of the task they are expecting their child to achieve. Toddlers live by a pleasure principle: they want what they want when they want it. Before they can complete toilet training, they must be able to give up an immediate pleasure—relieving themselves whenever they have the urge—to gain other pleasure later on—improved physical comfort and another step in growing up. Guidelines for how to toilet train a toddler are shown in Box 30.5.

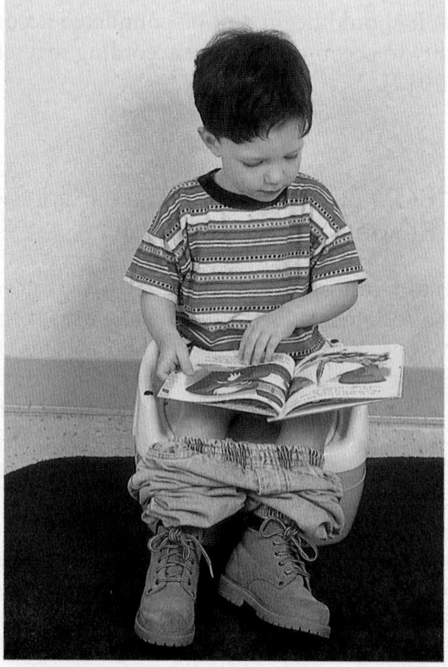

FIGURE 30.7 Toddlers are interested in toilet training as an expression of autonomy.

Some toddlers smear or play with feces, often at about the same time that toilet training is started. This occurs because they have become fully aware of body excretions but have no adult values toward them; stools seem little different from the modeling clay they play with. This activity can be minimized by providing toddlers with play substances of similar texture and by changing diapers immediately after defecation. Teach parents to accept this behavior for what it is: enjoyment of the body and of the self, and the discovery of a new substance. After a child is fully toilet trained, this activity rarely persists.

Ritualistic Behavior

Although toddlers spend a great deal of time every day investigating new ways to do things and trying activities they have never done before, they also enjoy ritualistic patterns. They will use only "their" spoon at mealtime or only "their" blanket at bedtime. They will not go outside unless a mother or father locates their favorite cap.

The child who seems to need an excessive number of objects to cling to or an excessive number of routines, however, may be trying to say, "I need more guidelines, more rules. Don't let me be quite so independent."

What if . . . 30.2 Jason's mother tells you he is toilet trained, but when he's admitted to the hospital for minor surgery he refuses to use the toilet. What would you do?

Negativism

As part of establishing their identities as separate individuals, toddlers typically go through a period of extreme negativism. They do not want to do anything a parent wants them to do. Their reply to every request is a very definite "no."

It is easy for parents to believe their authority is being questioned when this happens and to worry children are becoming so disrespectful they will have difficulty getting along in the world. They can be baffled by the extreme change from happy, cooperative infants who lived to please them to irritating, uncooperative toddlers. They may need some help to realize that this is not only a normal phenomenon of toddlerhood but also a positive stage in development. This change indicates toddlers have learned that they are separate individuals with separate needs. It is important toddlers do this if they are to grow up to be persons who are independent and able to take care of their own needs and desires.

Parents who went away from home for the first time for college or camp might remember they behaved similarly. They may recall they rarely slept or ate sensibly; they tried, in effect, to break every rule their parents used to enforce on them. Most regained their equilibrium in time to find a midpoint between irresponsible independence and common sense. If parents can recall such circumstances, it helps them to understand that this behavior in their toddler is not specific to the age but to the first feeling of independence. They can also remember they meant no vindictiveness by their behavior, so they can realize their child means none either. This understanding can help to put the child's "no" into a better light.

Once it runs its course, extreme negativism will pass. In the meantime, the more parents try to make children obey

BOX 30.5 Nursing Care Planning to Empower a Family

COMMON GUIDELINES FOR TOILET TRAINING

Q. Jason's mother asks you, "How can I tell if my 2-year-old is ready for potty training? And if he is, how do I start?"
A. Try the following suggestions:

1. Children are physically ready for toilet training when they can walk securely. Plan 1 or 2 weeks of psychological "readiness" activities such as showing your child "grown up" pants and how other family members use the toilet, activities that will help him realize the task of toilet training is a step toward growing up, not something only toddlers do.
2. Check that training pants pull down readily and slacks are free of complicated buttons or grippers; otherwise, your child will have accidents because he cannot undress quickly enough.
3. Purchase either a potty chair that sits on the floor or an infant seat that is placed on the regular toilet. If you choose a toilet seat, place a footstool in front of the toilet so your child has some support for his feet.
4. Begin with defecation training because this is so much easier to grasp than urination. Sit your child on the potty chair or toilet at the time he usually defecates, such as when he wakes up in the morning.
5. Praise your child if he does defecate. Remind him to wash his hands afterward.
6. Be careful not to flush the toilet while your child is sitting on it because 2-year-old children are unable to realize they will not be flushed away. Encourage your child to flush the toilet independently after you have helped him get redressed.
7. Do not allow a child to remain on a potty chair for much longer than 10 minutes (less than that if he is resistant). Also, do not allow your child to use the chair to eat or as a play table, so he doesn't become confused as to its purpose.
8. If your child does not seem ready on a day-to-day basis, return him to diapers for a short period. Be careful not to make this feel like failure or equate "good" with being dry and "bad" with being wet. Continue with readiness activities. Reintroduce training pants and attempt toilet training again when your child seems more ready.
9. When children have mastered defecation, it's time to include urination. Boys enjoy standing to urinate and aiming at objects in a toilet bowl, such as pieces of breakfast cereal.
10. Some toddlers have difficulty remaining dry at night until they are 3 to 4 years old. Do not pressure your child to accomplish nighttime dryness, but assume he is doing the best he can. Change him to training pants for the night by explaining (not punitively) that it is hard to keep dry while he sleeps. After your child has been dry during the night for about 1 month, he has probably mastered nighttime dryness.
11. Do not wake your child during the night and carry him to the bathroom to void. This system may keep him dry during the night, but it does not help him stay dry for long periods. It may even prolong nighttime wetness because it conditions him to void every 4 hours instead of retaining urine for 8 hours while he sleeps.

them, the more children are likely to resist. Some long-term parent–child interaction problems begin during this period because parents insist on being obeyed totally or are inconsistent in their approach.

A toddler's "no" can best be eliminated by limiting the number of questions asked of the child. A father does not really mean, for example, "Are you ready for dinner?" He means, "Come to the table. It's dinnertime." A mother asks, "Will you come take a bath now?" She means, "It's time for your bath." Making a statement instead of asking a question in this way can avoid a great many negative responses.

A toddler needs experience in making choices, however. To provide the opportunity to do this, a parent could give a secondary choice. "No" is not allowed for the major task, so the parent states, "It's bath time now" but then says, "Do you want to take your duck or your toy boat into the tub with you?" Other examples are, "It's lunchtime. Do you want to use a big or little plate?" or "It's time to go shopping. Do you want to wear your jacket or your sweater?" Although this solution is simple, it is one parents may not arrive at by themselves because finding a solution to a problem is always more difficult for the person in the middle of the problem than it is for an objective observer. Once they are helped to practice this approach, however, parents usually find it helpful in smoothing out the friction caused by the negativism of the toddler period (Box 30.6).

Discipline

Some parents ask during the last part of the infant year or the early toddler period when they should start to discipline their child, or when toddlers are old enough for punishment to be acceptable. Remind parents that discipline and punishment are not interchangeable terms. **Discipline** means setting rules or road signs so children know what is expected of them. **Punishment** is a consequence that results from a breakdown in discipline or the child's disregard of the rules that were learned.

Parents should begin to instill some sense of discipline early in life because part of it involves setting safety limits and protecting others or property (e.g., a child must stay away from the fireplace or heater, she must not go into the street, she must not hit other children). Enforcing most limits of this type arises out of the day-to-day interactions with the child and out of the rhythm of child care, not out of a set

BOX 30.6 Nursing Care Planning Based on Effective Communication

Jason's mother has brought 2-year-old Jason to the clinic for a health maintenance visit. Jason is rambunctious and uncooperative. His mother is obviously frustrated.

Less Effective Communication

Nurse: Come on, Jason, sit quietly so I can hear your heartbeat.
Jason: No!
Ms. Matthis: Jason, listen to the nurse.
Jason: No!
Nurse: If you promise to sit still, I'll let you play with the stethoscope.
Jason: Okay.

Jason plays with the stethoscope.

Ms. Matthis: Jason, now it's time to give the stethoscope back to the nurse.
Jason: No.
Nurse: I have work to do, Jason. I really must listen to your heart.

Ms. Matthis takes the stethoscope from Jason. Jason starts crying.

Ms. Matthis: If you stop crying and sit still, I'll take you for ice cream on our way home.
Jason: (whimpering a bit) Okay.
Nurse: Oh, those terrible twos!

More Effective Communication

Nurse: Jason, I need to listen to your heart so you must be very quiet. Would you rather sit quietly on the chair or the table?
Jason: Table.
Nurse: All right, Jason, jump up.

Jason climbs onto the table and starts to fidget.

Ms. Matthis: Jason, sit still for the nurse.
Jason: No!
Nurse: If you'd like, you can use the stethoscope for a few seconds. Do you want to listen to your mom's heart or my heart?
Jason: Mom's.
Nurse: Great, now we will both be very quiet so you can hear.

Jason listens to his mother's heart.

Nurse: Good, now it's my turn.
Jason: Okay. (Jason hands back the stethoscope.)

The nurse listens to Jason's heart.

Notice that, in the first scenario, the nurse and mother both bribe Jason. Jason finally does what they want, but the situation is still frustrating and his behavior change will not likely be long lasting. In the second scenario, the nurse demonstrates how to communicate better by offering choices. The situation is much more enjoyable for everyone.

procedure such as, "Today, I'm going to teach discipline." Two general rules to follow include:

1. Parents need to be consistent.
2. Rules are learned best if correct behavior is praised rather than wrong behavior punished.

A "time-out" is a technique to help children learn that actions have consequences. To use a time-out effectively, parents first need to be certain their child understands the rule they are trying to enforce (e.g., "You can't hit people. If you hit your brother, you'll have time-out."). Parents should give one warning. If the child repeats the behavior, parents select an area that is nonstimulating, such as a corner of a room or a hallway. The child is directed to go immediately to the time-out space. The child then sits there for a specified period of time. If the child cries or shows any other disruptive behavior, the time-out period doesn't begin until there is quiet. When the specified time has passed, the child can return to the family. A guide as to how long children should remain in their time-out chair is 1 minute per year of age (e.g., a 2-year-old would stay in the corner for 2 minutes). Using a timer that rings when time is up is an effective way to let children know when they can return to the family.

✔ QSEN Checkpoint Question 30.5

Teamwork & Collaboration

Jason's mother would prefer to use a time-out for punishment. What should you teach Jason's mother or his day care setting caregivers about the use of this technique?

a. The child should sit still for as many minutes as his age.
b. The child should sit still for as many minutes as he misbehaved.
c. Time-out activities can include quiet play or reading books.
d. Children are not ready for time-outs until school age.

Look in Appendix A for the best answer and rationale.

Separation Anxiety

As discussed in Chapter 29, fear of being separated from parents begins at about 6 months of age and persists throughout the preschool period. This universal fear in this age group is known as separation anxiety. Toddlers who have separation anxiety have difficulty accepting being separated from their primary caregiver to spend the day at a day care center or if they or their primary caregiver is hospitalized. Chapter 36 discusses nursing responsibility for care of toddlers in the hospital as well as the reactions of toddlers to the separation caused by hospitalization and the methods used to minimize these reactions.

Parents may ask what they can do about this problem. They believe they have a right to leave their child in a babysitter's or center's care, but how can they tolerate the crying at the door? Most toddlers react best to separation if a regular babysitter is employed or if the day care center has consistent caregivers. It helps if toddlers have fair warning they will have a babysitter. For example, they could be told, "Mommy is fixing dinner early because Mommy and Daddy are going to visit some friends tonight. Marsha is going to come and babysit for you. She'll put you to bed. When you wake up in the morning, Mommy and Daddy will be here again."

No matter how well prepared toddlers are, they may cry when the babysitter actually appears or may greet the babysitter warmly only to cry when the parents reach for their coats. It helps if parents say good-bye firmly, repeat the explanation they will be there when the child wakes in the morning, and then leave. Prolonged good-byes only lead to more crying. Sneaking out prevents crying and may ease the parents' guilt, but it can strengthen a child's fear of abandonment and so should be discouraged. This applies to leaving after hospital visits as well.

QSEN Checkpoint Question 30.6

Patient-Centered Care

Jason answers every request of his mother by saying, "No!" His mother admits that she is exasperated and embarrassed by this and she states that she is desperate to change this behavior. How can you best meet her expressed learning needs?

a. Have her tell Jason she doesn't want him to say no anymore.
b. Instruct her to answer all Jason's questions by saying, "No!"
c. Encourage her to reduce the number of questions she asks Jason.
d. Tell her to explain he is not using good communication skills.

Look in Appendix A for the best answer and rationale.

Temper Tantrums

Almost every toddler has a temper tantrum at one time or another. The child may kick; scream; stomp feet; shout, "No, no, no"; flail arms and legs; bite; or bang his or her head against the floor.

Temper tantrums occur as a natural consequence of toddlers' development. They occur because toddlers are independent enough to know what they want, but they do not have the vocabulary or the wisdom to express their feelings in a more socially acceptable way (Green, Whitney, & Potegal, 2011). For example, temper tantrums occur most often when children are tired, just before naptime or bedtime, or during a long shopping trip or visit. They may be a response to an unrealistic request by a parent, such as asking a child to comb her hair before she is coordinated enough to do so, asking her to pick up toys before she has a feeling of family responsibility, or asking her to share before she can understand what that means. Tantrums may also occur if parents are saying "no" too frequently with regard to such things as touching the coffee table, using a spoon, or running and jumping, thus making children feel constantly thwarted. A tantrum may also be a response to difficulty making choices or decisions or to pressure from activities such as toilet training. Such children need to express feelings in some way and do so with temper tantrums. These episodes are not only taxing for the parents but are also energy consuming for children.

Some children hold their breath as part of a temper tantrum until they become cyanotic. This occurs when a child is provoked; the child develops a distended chest (a halt after inspiration), often has air-filled cheeks, and shows increasing distress as the body registers oxygen want. Ignoring the child will make it an ineffective technique for expressing frustration or getting what is wanted. True breath holding is an unprovoked neurologic problem in which children, under stress, appear to "forget" to breathe in or halt breathing after expiration, usually at the peak of anger. They become so short of breath they slump to the floor. True breath holding needs follow-up to separate it from temper tantrums (see Chapter 49).

Box 30.7 offers suggestions for managing temper tantrums. Probably the best approach is for parents to simply tell a child that they disapprove of the tantrum and then ignore it. They might say, "I'll be in the bedroom. When you're done kicking, you come into the bedroom, too." Children who are left alone in a kitchen this way will usually not continue a tantrum but will stop after 1 or 2 minutes and rejoin their parents. Parents should then accept the child warmly and proceed as if the tantrum had not occurred. This same approach works well for nurses caring for hospitalized toddlers.

Nursing Diagnoses and Related Interventions

Nursing Diagnosis: Risk for compromised family coping related to toddler behavior

Outcome Evaluation: Family states temper tantrums now occur less than two times daily.

Helping parents correct problems early may limit the number of tantrums they must deal with; however, it will not prevent them because parents cannot anticipate all the circumstances that will cause this reaction. In fact, parents should not feel they must prevent all of them; after all, they are parents, not mind readers. As the child matures, increases his or her vocabulary, and is capable of better responses to stress situations, tantrums begin to fade by themselves. Box 30.8 shows an interprofessional care map illustrating both nursing and team planning to address such a problem as temper tantrums.

BOX 30.7 Nursing Care Planning Based on Family Teaching

MANAGING TODDLER'S TEMPER TANTRUMS

Q. Jason's mother tells you, "I've had it with temper tantrums. I can't stand to watch another one."
A. Here are suggestions to prevent them:

Try to determine the reason for the behavior:
- Do tantrums always occur just before bedtime? If so, you might schedule an earlier bedtime or an afternoon nap.
- Do tantrums occur every time you go shopping? If so, perhaps it would help to schedule two shorter trips each week rather than one long one.
- Do tantrums occur whenever you ask the child to do something? If so, is the child being asked to perform tasks that are not age appropriate?
- Do tantrums occur in response to not being able to make a decision? If so, you may have to limit the number of choices you are asking of the child.

Next, be certain it seems like a tantrum, not something more:
- Is there a possibility you are mistaking seizure activity for temper tantrums?
- Could you be confusing neurologic breath holding with a temper tantrum?

Lastly, think through what you do when the child has a tantrum:
- Do you give either material or emotional bribes (e.g., "Come and get a cookie")? This method is rarely effective because, by acceding to the child's wishes, you are encouraging your child to have more tantrums because they are so rewarding.
- Do you punish the child? Toddlers have a right to express opinions; they just need to be guided to learn a more controlled and mature way of doing that.
- Do you role model adult behavior in managing anger or frustration? For example, if your child shouts or kicks, do you respond, "I can shout as loud as you"? Instead of showing the child a better way to express feelings, this reinforces the way the child is responding.

BOX 30.8 Nursing Care Planning

AN INTERPROFESSIONAL CARE MAP FOR A TODDLER WITH TEMPER TANTRUMS

Jason is a 2.5-year-old boy you see at a pediatric clinic. His mother tells you he has changed completely in the past 6 months from an easy-to-care-for baby into a "monster" who refuses to do anything she asks. The only word he says anymore is "no." He has a temper tantrum every night at dinner over some type of food. She tells you this has changed parenting from "fun" to "a real chore."

Family Assessment Child lives with two parents in three-bedroom home. Father is a ferry boat captain; works 6 days a week. Mother works as a secretary at local university. Finances are "good. We've worked hard to get where we are."

Client Assessment Well-nourished 2-year-old boy. Physical findings within normal limits. Mother reports the child is having temper tantrums "at least 20 times a day. He throws himself on the floor and pounds his head and fists." Mother unable to describe any precipitating factors for the tantrums. She states, "He seems to have them just when I start to do something. I could be playing with him one minute, and then I get up to do something, like answer the phone or start dinner, and he starts." Mother reports picking up the child immediately because she fears he will hurt himself. "I just don't know what to do anymore."

Nursing Diagnosis Health-seeking behaviors related to measures for dealing with and reducing the number of temper tantrums.

Outcome Criteria Mother describes measures to manage tantrums and reports tantrums have decreased to fewer than four a day by end of 1 week.

Team Member Responsible	Assessment	Intervention	Rationale	Expected Outcome
Activities of Daily Living, Including Safety				
Nurse	Ask mother to describe a typical day; document when tantrums occur and situations that seem to provoke them.	Make suggestions to eliminate cause of distress as revealed by assessment.	Temper tantrums can increase with stress and inability of child to feel independent.	Mother reviews a typical day and identifies times when tantrums are most apt to occur.
Teamwork and Collaboration				
Nurse/Primary health care provider	Assess if child has possible neurologic symptoms.	Refer child for full neurologic workup if physical exam suggests the need.	Temper tantrums can be confused with seizures if a careful history is not taken.	Mother agrees to further neurologic testing if suggested.
Procedures/Medications for Quality Improvement				
Nurse/Nurse practitioner	Assess what measures mother thinks would prevent temper tantrums best.	Work with the mother to develop actions such as ignoring the tantrum and encouraging the mother not to pick up child unless there is actual danger of injury.	Temper tantrums are a method to express emotion. Rewarding the behavior prevents the child from learning more mature methods of coping with frustration.	Mother voices agreement to try suggested solutions and to telephone clinic in 3 days if there is no improvement.
Nutrition				
Nurse practitioner	Assess if child appears well nourished, and assess usual dietary pattern.	Because eating is a time when tantrums occur, review with mother if her actions are different at this time than others.	Eating is an area in which children want to express independence.	Mother lists foods that allow child independent eating, which she will try to serve, to keep meals tantrum free.
Patient-Centered Care				
Nurse	Assess mother's knowledge of toddler behavior and temper tantrums.	Review normal toddler growth and development, explaining that some temper tantrums during this period are natural occurrences.	Information about normal toddler growth and development provides a foundation for further teaching and instruction.	Mother states she understands tantrums occur because of toddler's limited capabilities to express desires.
Nurse	Assess why mother is so fearful her child will hurt himself during a tantrum.	Inform the mother that children rarely hurt themselves during tantrums.	Increased knowledge about the minimal risk of injury during tantrums should help to alleviate the mother's anxiety.	Mother states she has increased understanding about the danger of tantrums.
Psychosocial/Spiritual/Emotional Needs				
Nurse/Nurse practitioner	Assess what mother feels would be most helpful to relieve her degree of stress and frustration.	Suggest she arrange for "time out" breaks for herself by having husband or friend relieve her.	Short periods away from the child can allow her to regroup her thinking.	Mother describes a plan by which she can receive more help with child care from friend, because husband is home only 1 day per week.

BOX 30.8 Nursing Care Planning (continued)

Informatics for Seamless Health Care Planning				
Nurse/Nurse practitioner	Review with mother the plan for added support and interventions.	Instruct the mother to keep a diary of the child's behavior and measures used during the next week. Set up an appointment for a telephone conference next week to review the diary and discuss the child's behavior.	Keeping a diary and reviewing it aids in evaluating the child's behavior and the effectiveness of the methods used. A follow-up telephone call also provides an additional opportunity for feedback, teaching, and support.	Mother states she will follow suggestions for managing tantrums and will keep telephone and clinic appointments for follow-up care.

What if...30.3 Jason, when you are caring for him in the hospital, has a temper tantrum in the middle of a busy hallway. Would you ignore it or move him to a quieter place?

Concerns of the Family With a Toddler Who Has Unique Needs

It may be difficult for children with handicaps or disabilities to achieve a sense of autonomy or independence because they may never be totally independent. However, it is important for these children to develop as strong a sense of autonomy as possible so they see themselves as independent and can work to become increasingly self-sufficient as they grow older.

Nursing actions designed to help the challenged or chronically ill child develop a sense of autonomy are outlined in Table 30.4. Most important are such actions that allow toddlers to do as much for themselves as possible. If toddlers have physical limitations, for example, they may be unable to explore freely or may not have the physical ability to pound and manipulate toys as the average toddler does. They do, however, have the ability to work at a project while they sit in a chair at a table.

A toddler with a long-term illness or who is physically challenged can be expected to exhibit normal toddler behaviors, such as temper tantrums, and to have normal outlooks, such as negativism. Parents whose child is uncoordinated or has a neurologic disease may mistake temper tantrums for seizure activity. Investigate such activity carefully and explain to parents the difference between the two. Parents may also mistake particular toddlers' insistence on having their own way as a manifestation of illness. Remind these parents the behavior is more often an indication of age and development rather than of illness so that they can respond appropriately.

Toilet training is difficult for a child who is hospitalized at periodic intervals because success usually requires a consistent caregiver; in addition, hospitalization can result in regressive behaviors. If a chronically ill child has difficulty with ambulation, soiling accidents may occur beyond the usual age because of an inability to reach a bathroom easily.

Children who survive a long-term illness are sometimes referred to as medically fragile or vulnerable children (Green & Solnit, 1964). Some parents tend to protect and shelter such a child, and you may have to remind them that, even though the toddler is chronically ill, he or she will demand independence and has the right to explore. A child who uses a lower extremity prosthesis, for example, might prefer to crawl somewhere rather than wait for help to put the prosthesis in place. Although this degree of independence is good, parents may have to limit how it is expressed so the child will learn how to use the prosthesis (e.g., they could make a rule the child must use the prosthesis to walk but can choose whether to use a spoon when eating).

Autism Spectrum Disorder

Classical ASD is a complex range of neurodevelopment disorders characterized by communication difficulties, poor social interaction, and frequent repetitive and stereotyped movements (Fountain, Winter, & Bearman, 2012). It occurs in all ethnic and socioeconomic groups, as frequently as 1 in 88 children, and more frequently in boys than in girls. Milder forms of the disorder are termed Asperger syndrome, Rett syndrome, childhood disintegrative disorder, or pervasive developmental disorder not otherwise specified (usually referred to as PDD-NOS).

Symptoms begin to appear slightly in infancy but are usually obvious enough during the toddler years for parents to become concerned because their child tends not to speak any words, does not make eye contact with others, and has difficulty interacting with playmates, preferring instead to watch a spinning toy, water swirling down the toilet, or repeating sing-song repetitive phrases.

Children need to be screened for autism symptoms by 12 months of age and again at 18 and 24 months of age by observation and parent report. Additional symptoms and therapy for autism are discussed in Chapter 54.

Nutrition and the Physically Challenged or Chronically Ill Toddler

All toddlers need experience feeding themselves if at all possible, but allowing a child with neurologic deficits do this can be difficult for parents. Help them accept the accidents that occur, and suggest finger foods if possible.

TABLE 30.4 Nursing Interventions to Help a Physically Challenged or Chronically Ill Child Develop a Sense of Autonomy

Area	Nursing Action
Nutrition	A special diet may limit typical finger foods. Use imagination to offer other foods not usually eaten this way as finger foods. Allow child to help pour liquid diet for a tube feeding. Toddlers are frightened by vomiting because they have no control over it. Comfort afterward. Check for possibility that child is nauseated. Toddlers have no way to express this other than by not eating.
Dressing changes	A child can hold pieces of tape or put tape in place to maintain sense of control. The child can remove an old bandage if it is not contaminated. Allow the child to view his or her incision and watch dressing changes, explaining each step of a procedure as you perform it helps the child maintain control. Restrain only those body parts necessary during a procedure to allow a child a sense of control. Remove all supplies after a procedure or the child may "redo" the dressing.
Medication	Allow children no choice as to whether a medicine will be taken. Do allow a child to choose a "chaser," such as milk or juice, after oral medicine. Do not ask a toddler to indicate a choice of site for an injection or intravenous insertion. This is too advanced a decision for a toddler to handle.
Rest	Locate or create a ritual for bedtime (e.g., put child into bed, tuck him in, say, "Goodnight, Bobby." Tuck in bear. Say, "Goodnight, Bear"). Allow a choice of toy or cover but not a choice of bedtime or naptime hour.
Hygiene	Allow a child a choice of bathtub toy or clothing. Allow a child to wash face and hands to gain control of the situation. Allow the child to put toothpaste on a brush, but you should brush or "touch up" teeth afterward to ensure all plaque has been removed.
Pain	Encourage a child to express pain (e.g., "Say 'ouch' when I pull off the tape"). Help channel a child's self-expression to what is acceptable (the child may shout, for example, but may not kick).
Stimulation	Provide a toddler with a toy that can be manipulated, such as boxes that fit inside one another and can be taken out again, trucks that can be pushed, and pegs that can be pounded. In a health care setting, items can usually be found that fit together (e.g., boxes from central supply, plastic vials from the pharmacy). Another action toy: buy a nonlatex balloon and tie it to the crib side to be used as a punching bag; another one tied to the foot of the crib can serve as a leg exerciser.
Elimination	A child who is toilet trained needs to be encouraged to continue to use a potty chair or toilet during an illness. Help children with ureter or bowel stomas to help with changing bags so they are as independent in bowel function as possible.

If children are on a special diet, it may be difficult to prepare finger foods. If they are tube fed, they receive no experience at all with finger foods. For these children, parents should try to provide other, comparable experiences in independence, such as letting them choose what toy to take to bed or what clothing to wear.

What if . . . 30.4 You are particularly interested in exploring one of the 2020 National Health Goals with respect to toddler growth and development (see Box 30.1). What would be a possible research topic to explore pertinent to this goal that would be applicable to Jason's family and that would also advance evidence-based practice?

KEY POINTS FOR REVIEW

- Erikson's developmental task for the toddler period is to form a sense of autonomy or independence versus shame or doubt.
- Toddlers make great strides forward in development, but their physical growth slows.
- A critical milestone of toddler development is being able to form two-word sentences (a noun and a verb) by 2 years of age.
- Toddlers are capable of preoperational thought, or are able to deal much more constructively with symbols than they could while infants.
- Important aspects of toddler care are promoting safety, toddler development, and healthy family functioning because all three of these facets help in planning nursing care that not only meets QSEN competencies but that also best meets a family's total needs.
- Toddler appetites decrease from those of the infant, so children eat proportionally less than they did as infants.
- Common concerns of parents during the toddler period are toilet training, ritualistic behavior, negativism, temper tantrums, discipline, and separation anxiety.
- Promoting autonomy in the child who is physically challenged or chronically ill calls for creative planning because there may be many tasks that must be done for the child to be certain they are done safely.

Critical Thinking Care Study

Bobby is a 2.5-year-old boy you meet at a pediatric clinic because he has a "tummy ache." He lives with his single mother in a one-bedroom apartment on the third floor of a controlled rent building. His mother tells you he doesn't get outside much because she's afraid to walk to the local park because it is "owned" by a street gang. Bobby sleeps with her in a double bed. Yesterday, he got up before her; she found him sitting on a kitchen counter near the stove. She adds, "His father wants him to be a baseball player. I just want him to learn enough words so he can say when he needs to use a bathroom."

1. What are some safety precautions you would want to discuss with Bobby's mother?
2. The walls of this family's apartment are painted with automobile paint his father secured from his job as a car painter. Would you be concerned with the use of such paint?
3. Bobby does not speak in sentences as yet. What questions would you want to ask his mother to help determine if his development is delayed?

Patient Scenario:

The Wallace Family

Read about the Wallace family, a family with a toddler, then answer the questions to further sharpen your skills and grow more familiar with NCLEX-type questions related to toddler growth and development. Confirm your answers are correct by reading the rationales.

Visit http://thePoint.lww.com

Answers and Rationales

Looking for answers to the What if. . . and Critical Thinking Care Study questions?

Visit http://thePoint.lww.com

References

American Academy of Pediatrics. (2012). *Where we stand: TV viewing time.* Washington, DC: Author.

American Academy of Pediatrics. (2013). *Where we stand: Car seats for children.* Washington, DC: Author.

Barbaro, J., & Dissanayake, C. (2012). Developmental profiles of infants and toddlers with autism spectrum disorders identified prospectively in a community-based setting. *Journal of Autism & Developmental Disorders, 42*(9), 1939–1948.

Beirens, T. M., van Beeck, E. F., Brug, J., et al. (2010). Do parents with toddlers store poisonous products safely? *International Journal of Pediatrics, 2010*(7), 702827.

Bhargava, S. (2011). Diagnosis and management of common sleep problems in children. *Pediatric Review, 32*(3), 91–98.

Bishop, W. P. (2011). The oral cavity. In K. J. Marcdante, R. M. Kliegman, H. B. Jenson, et al. (Eds.), *Nelson essentials of pediatrics* (6th ed., pp. 475–476). Philadelphia, PA: Saunders/Elsevier.

Bowman, S. M., Aitken, M. E., Robbins, J. M., et al. (2012). Trends in U.S. pediatric drowning hospitalizations, 1993–2008. *Pediatrics, 129*(2), 275–281.

Byars, K. C., Yolton, K., Rausch, J., et al. (2012). Prevalence, patterns, and persistence of sleep problems in the first 3 years of life. *Pediatrics, 129*(2), 276–284.

Centers for Disease Control and Prevention. (2012a). *10 leading causes of death by age group, United States.* Atlanta, GA: Author.

Centers for Disease Control and Prevention. (2012b). *Childhood lead poisoning prevention program.* Atlanta, GA: Author.

Chisholm, K. (2011). Vegetarian diets in children. *Advance for NPs & PAs, 2*(1), 39–41.

Erikson, E. H. (1993). *Childhood and society.* New York, NY: W. W. Norton.

Fountain, C., Winter, A. S., & Bearman, P. S. (2012). Six developmental trajectories characterize children with autism. *Pediatrics, 129*(5), e1112–e1120.

Gahagan, S. (2011). Normal sleep and pediatric sleep disorders. In K. J. Marcdante, R. M. Kliegman, H. B. Jenson, et al. (Eds.), *Nelson essentials of pediatrics* (6th ed., pp. 57–62). Philadelphia, PA: Saunders/Elsevier.

Green, J. A., Whitney, P. G., & Potegal, M. (2011). Screaming, yelling, whining, and crying: Categorical and intensity differences in vocal expressions of anger and sadness in children's tantrums. *Emotion, 11*(5), 1124–1133.

Green, M., & Solnit, A. A. (1964). Reactions to the threatened loss of a child: A vulnerable child syndrome. *Pediatrics, 34*(2), 56–66.

Hodges, E. A., Smith, C., Tidwell, S., et al. (2012). Promoting physical activity in preschoolers to prevent obesity: A review of the literature. *Journal of Pediatric Nursing, 28*(1), 3–19.

Hoeft, K. S., Barker, J. C., & Masterson, E. E. (2011). Maternal beliefs and motivations for first dental visit by low-income Mexican American children in California. *Pediatric Dentistry, 33*(5), 392–398.

Hooker, L., Ward, B., & Verrinder, G. (2012). Domestic violence screening in maternal & child health nursing practice. *Contemporary Nurse, 42*(2), 198–215.

Hutchings, H., Barnes, P. M., Maddocks, A., et al. (2010). Burns in young children: A retrospective matched cohort study of health and developmental outcomes. *Child Care Health & Development, 36*(6), 787–794.

Kiddoo, D. A. (2012). Toilet training children: When to start and how to train. *Canadian Medical Association Journal, 184*(5), 511–512.

Kuehn, B. M. (2012). Panel advises tougher limits on lead exposure. *Journal of the American Medical Association, 307*(5), 445.

Landry, S. H., Smith, K. E., Swank, P. R., et al. (2011). The effects of a responsive parenting intervention on parent–child interactions during shared book reading. *Developmental Psychology, 48*(4), 969–986.

Lee, K. J., & Marcdante, K. J. (2011). Poisoning. In W. W. Hay, M. J. Levine, J. M. Sondheimer, et al. (Eds.), *Current pediatric diagnosis & treatment* (20th ed., pp. 158–163). Columbus, OH: McGraw-Hill.

Levine, D. A. (2011). Normal development. In K. J. Marcdante, R. M. Kliegman, H. B. Jenson, et al. (Eds.), *Nelson essentials of pediatrics* (6th ed., pp. 16–18). Philadelphia, PA: Saunders/Elsevier.

Litovitz, T., Whitaker, N., & Clark, L. (2010). Preventing battery ingestions: An analysis of 8648 cases. *Pediatrics, 125*(6), 1178–1183.

Macy, M. L., Clark, S. J., Freed, G. L., et al. (2012). Carpooling and booster seats: A national survey of parents. *Pediatrics, 129*(2), 290–298.

Mills, J., Grushka, J., & Butterworth, S. (2012). Television-related injuries in children—The British Columbia experience. *Journal of Pediatric Surgery, 47*(5), 991–995.

Nelson, T. (2013). The continuum of behavior guidance. *Dental Clinics of North America, 57*(1), 129–143.

Piaget, J. (1952). *The origins of intelligence in children.* New York, NY: International University Press.

Smith, G. A., & Riedford, K. (2012). Epidemiology of early childhood caries: Clinical application. *Journal of Pediatric Nursing.* Advance online publication.

Smith, S. (2011). Vulvovaginitis. In K. J. Marcdante, R. M. Kliegman, H. B. Jenson, et al. (Eds.), *Nelson essentials of pediatrics* (6th ed., pp. 415–46). Philadelphia, PA: Saunders/Elsevier.

Tubert-Jeannin, S., Auclair, C., Amsallem, E., et al. (2011). Fluoride supplements (tablets, drops, lozenges or chewing gums) for preventing dental caries in children. *Cochrane Database of Systematic Reviews,* (12), CD007592.

U.S. Department of Agriculture. (2005). *Choose my plate: A guide to daily food choices*. Washington, DC: USDA.

U.S. Department of Health and Human Services. (2010). *Healthy people 2020*. Washington, DC: Author.

Whitney, E. N., & Rolfes, S. R. (2013). Life cycle nutrition: Infancy, childhood and adolescence. In E. N. Whitey & S. R. Rolfes, *Understanding nutrition* (13th ed., pp. 504–550). New York, NY: Wadsworth/Cengage Learning.

Chapter 31

Nursing Care of a Family With a Preschool Child

KEY TERMS

- broken fluency
- bruxism
- conservation
- ectomorphic body build
- Electra complex
- endomorphic body build
- genu valgus
- intuitional thought
- Oedipus complex
- secondary stuttering

OBJECTIVES

After mastering the contents of this chapter, you should be able to:

1. Describe normal growth and development as well as common parental concerns of the preschool period.
2. Identify 2020 National Health Goals related to the preschool period that nurses can help the nation achieve.
3. Assess a preschooler for normal growth and developmental milestones.
4. Formulate nursing diagnoses related to preschool growth and development or common parental concerns.
5. Identify expected outcomes for nursing care of a preschooler as well as help parents manage seamless transitions across differing health care settings.
6. Using the nursing process, plan nursing care that includes the six competencies of Quality & Safety Education for Nurses (QSEN): Patient-Centered Care, Teamwork & Collaboration, Evidence-Based Practice (EBP), Quality Improvement (QI), Safety, and Informatics.
7. Implement nursing care related to normal growth and development of a preschooler, such as preparing a preschooler for an invasive procedure.
8. Evaluate expected outcomes for achievement and effectiveness of care.
9. Integrate knowledge of preschool growth and development with the interplay of nursing process, the six competencies of QSEN, and Family Nursing to promote quality maternal and child health nursing care.

Cathy Edwards is a 3-year-old you meet at a health maintenance visit. Her father cares for her at present because her mother is hospitalized with preterm labor for a second pregnancy. Her father tells you he is concerned because Cathy talks constantly with an imaginary friend named Emma. She makes up stories about events that can't possibly be true. When corrected, Cathy stutters so badly no one can understand her. Her father is also concerned because his daughter cries when he leaves her at daycare.

The previous chapter described toddler growth and development and the abilities children develop during that period. This chapter adds information about the changes, both physical and psychosocial, that occur during the preschool years. Such information builds a base for care and health teaching for this age group.

Is Cathy's father describing typical preschool behavior, or does Cathy need a referral to a child care specialist?

The preschool period traditionally includes the years 3, 4, and 5. Although physical growth slows considerably during this period, personality and cognitive growth continue at a rapid rate. Therefore, this is also an important period of growth for parents because they may be unsure how much independence and responsibility for self-care they should allow their rapidly maturing child. Most children of this age want to do things for themselves—choose their own clothing and dress themselves, feed themselves completely, wash their own hair, and so forth. As a result, parents of a preschooler may find their child dressed in one red and one green sock, going to preschool with unwashed ears, or trying to eat soup with a fork. They need reassurance that this behavior is typical because it is the way children explore and learn about new experiences (Fergusson, Boden, & Horwood, 2013).

Parents may also need some guidance in separating those tasks that a preschooler can accomplish independently from those that still require some adult supervision so they can set sensible limits. Setting limits this way protects children from harming themselves or others while participating in all the interesting experiences available to them. Box 31.1 lists 2020 National Health Goals related to this in-between toddler and school-age period.

BOX 31.1 Nursing Care Planning Based on 2020 National Health Goals

A number of 2020 National Health Goals are designed to target the preschool population. They include:

- Increase the number of states and the District of Columbia with laws requiring helmets for bicycle riders under 15 years of age, from 19 states to 27 states.
- Decrease acute middle ear infections (otitis media) among children from 246 out of 1,000 to 221 out of 1,000.
- Increase the proportion of children aged 19 to 35 months who receive the recommended doses of diphtheria, tetanus, and pertussis (DTaP); polio; MMR; Hib; hepatitis B; varicella; and PCV vaccines from 44.3% to 90%.
- Increase the rate of use of forward-facing child car seats among children age 1 to 3 years from a baseline of 72% to 79%.
- Reduce the proportion of children 3 to 11 years exposed to secondhand smoke from 52.2% to 47% (U.S. Department of Health and Human Services [DHHS], 2010; see www.healthypeople.gov).

Nurses can help the nation achieve these goals by alerting parents to these concerns as well as by serving as consultants at child care and preschool settings to be certain that preschoolers are protected against secondhand smoke, that recommended automobile restraints are used, and that children are fitted with helmets before beginning bicycle riding.

Nursing Process Overview

For Healthy Development of a Preschooler

Assessment

Regular assessment of a preschooler includes obtaining a health history and performing both a physical and developmental evaluation at health care visits. Preschoolers may speak very little during a health assessment; they may even revert to baby talk or babyish actions such as thumb-sucking if they find a health visit stressful. A history that details their usual performance level is therefore very important for accurate evaluation.

Assess a child's weight and height and body mass index (BMI) according to standard growth charts (available at http://thePoint.lww.com/Pillitteri7e). Keep in mind that these charts are based on average weights and heights of white American children, so children from other ethnic or cultural backgrounds may not completely conform with these norms (i.e., they may fall into the lower or upper percentiles). Also assess a child for general appearance. Does the child appear alert? Happy? Active? Preschoolers typically have 6 to 12 respiratory infections per year; therefore, many of them will have one at the time of a health assessment.

Nursing Diagnosis

Nursing diagnoses for preschoolers typically center on health promotion or unintentional injury prevention. Examples include:

- Health-seeking behaviors related to developmental expectations
- Risk for injury related to increased independence outside the home
- Delayed growth and development related to frequent illness
- Risk for imbalanced nutrition, more than body requirements, related to fast food choices
- Risk for poisoning related to maturational age of child
- Parental anxiety related to lack of understanding of childhood development

Outcome Identification and Planning

For many parents, preschool is a difficult time because a child is at an in-between stage—no longer an infant, although not yet ready for formal school. Planning and establishing expected outcomes for care of children at this age often begin with establishing a schedule for discussing normal preschool development with the parents. Planning for unintentional injury prevention such as how to cross streets safely becomes increasingly important as children begin to enjoy experiences away from home. It is also important to plan opportunities for adventurous activities and interaction with other children. Helpful Web sites for parents are the Healthy & Active Preschoolers (www.healthypreschoolers.com) and the March of Dimes (www.MarchofDimes.com/baby). For questions about car seats, parents can consult the Centers for Disease Control and Prevention (http://www.cdc.gov/features/passengersafety/). Other helpful Web sites to alert parents about safety are the American Association of Poison Control Centers (www.aapcc.org) and the American Academy of Pediatrics (www.aap.org). The national toll-free telephone number for a poison control center is 1-800-222-1222. A site parents can check to see if a preschool product has been recalled is the U.S. Consumer Product Safety Commission (www.CPSC.gov).

Implementation
Preschool children imitate moods as well as actions. An important nursing intervention, therefore, is role-playing a mood or attitude you would like a child to learn. To project an attitude that a health assessment is an enjoyable activity, you might suggest preschoolers participate by listening to their heart or coloring the table paper. Unintentional injury prevention is also best taught by role modeling (e.g., a parent always crosses streets at the corner, a parent doesn't start the car until seatbelts are in place).

Outcome Evaluation
An evaluation of expected outcomes needs to be continuous and frequent. Because growth during this period is more cognitive and emotional than physical, parents may report little growth. Evaluating specific areas can help them appreciate that progress has occurred. Examples of expected outcomes might include:

- Child states importance of holding parent's hand while crossing streets.
- Parent states realistic expectations of 3-year-old child's motor ability by next visit.
- Mother reports she has prepared her 4-year-old for new baby by next visit.

NURSING ASSESSMENT OF A PRESCHOOLER'S GROWTH AND DEVELOPMENT

An assessment of preschoolers needs to include physical, cognitive, and developmental growth (Box 31.2).

Physical Growth

A definite change in body contour occurs during the preschool years. The wide-legged gait, prominent lordosis, and protuberant abdomen of the toddler change to slimmer, taller, and much more childlike proportions. Contour changes are so definite that future body type—**ectomorphic body build** (slim body build) or **endomorphic body build** (large body build)—becomes apparent. Handedness also begins to be obvious. A major step forward is a child's ability to learn extended language, which is achieved not only by motor development but also by cognitive development. Children of this age who are exposed to more than one language or who live in a bilingual family have a unique opportunity to master two languages with relative ease because of this increased cognitive ability.

Lymphatic tissue begins to increase in size, particularly the tonsils; levels of immune globulin (Ig)G and IgA antibodies increase. These changes tend to make preschool illnesses more localized (e.g., an upper respiratory infection remains localized to the nose with little systemic fever).

Physiologic splitting of heart sounds may be present for the first time on auscultation; innocent heart murmurs may also be heard for the first time. This type of murmur occurs because of the changing size of the heart in reference to the thorax because the anteroposterior and transverse diameters of the chest have not yet reached adult proportions. Pulse rate decreases to about 85 beats/min, and blood pressure holds at about 100/60 mmHg.

The bladder is easily palpable above the symphysis pubis; voiding is frequent enough (9 or 10 times a day) that play must be interrupted, and voiding accidents may occur if a child becomes absorbed in an activity.

A child who earlier in life had an indeterminate longitudinal arch in the foot generally demonstrates a well-formed arch now. Muscles are noticeably stronger, so activities such as gymnastics become possible. Many children at the beginning of the period exhibit **genu valgus** (knock-knees); this disappears with increased skeletal growth at the end of the preschool period.

Weight, Height, Body Mass Index, and Head Circumference

Weight gain is slight during the preschool years; the average child gains only about 4.5 lb (2 kg) a year. During these years, appetite remains the same as it was during the toddler years, a level perhaps considerably less than some parents would like or expect.

Height gain is also minimal during this period: only 2 to 3.5 in. (6 to 8 cm) a year on average. Head circumference is not routinely measured at physical assessments on children over 2 years of age because it changes little after this time.

BOX 31.2 Nursing Care Planning Using Assessment

Appearance of the Average Preschooler

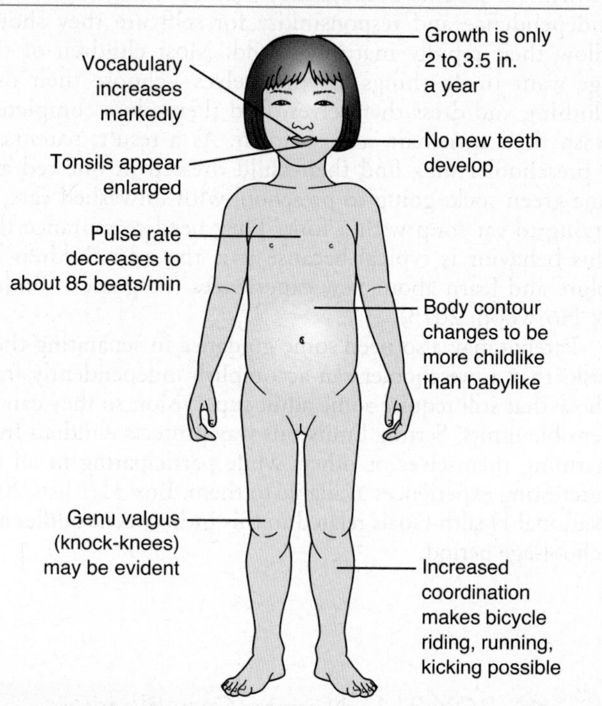
Growth is only 2 to 3.5 in. a year
Vocabulary increases markedly
No new teeth develop
Tonsils appear enlarged
Pulse rate decreases to about 85 beats/min
Body contour changes to be more childlike than babylike
Genu valgus (knock-knees) may be evident
Increased coordination makes bicycle riding, running, kicking possible

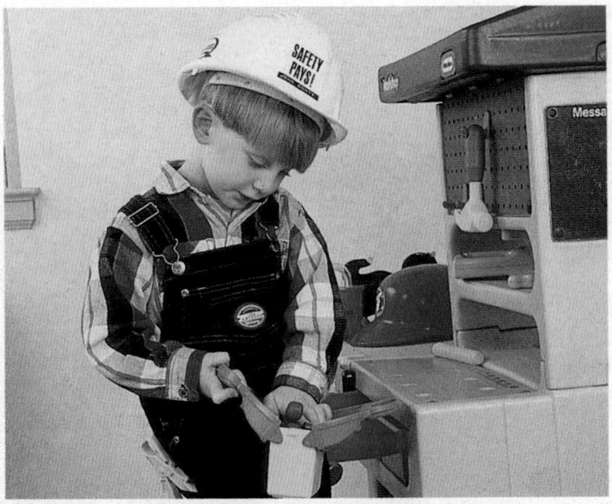

FIGURE 31.1 Preschoolers like to imitate the roles of adults as they learn about the world around them.

Teeth

Children generally have all 20 of their deciduous teeth by 3 years of age; permanent teeth don't replace these until school age. Preserving these teeth is important because they hold the position for the permanent teeth as the child's jaw grows larger. If a deciduous tooth has to be removed, children need conscientious follow up to be certain a space for a permanent tooth remains (de Amorim Lde, Estrela, & da Costa, 2011).

Developmental Milestones

Each year during the preschool period marks a major step forward in gross motor, fine motor, and language development. Play activities change focus dramatically as the preschooler learns new skills and understands more about the world (Fig. 31.1). Table 31.1 summarizes major milestones of the period.

Language Development

The extent of a 3-year-old child's vocabulary varies depending on how much the child has been encouraged to ask questions or participate in conversations (Box 31.3). A child typically, however, has a vocabulary of about 900 words and uses it to ask questions constantly, up to 400 a day, such as "Why is snow cold?", "How do worms hear?", and "What does your tongue do?" A child needs simple answers to such questions to encourage curiosity, vocabulary building, and questioning.

BOX 31.3 Nursing Care Planning to Respect Cultural Diversity

Whether children are allowed to ask questions is culturally determined and can make a difference in how much vocabulary a child uses. In a society in which children are expected to be seen and not heard, a preschool child may not have the same expressive vocabulary as a child who has been encouraged to ask questions. Recognition that differences among cultures can affect levels of development means assessments must be individualized and meaningful in terms of the cultural milieu.

Words that sound alike but mean different things such as "whether" and "weather" can be confounding to children of this age. If a parent tells a child her shoes should go on with the buckles on the outside, she may seem to understand but return in a few minutes to ask, "Why do I have to go outside to put on my shoes?"

Four- and 5-year-old children enjoy participating in mealtime conversation and can describe an incident from their day in great detail. Remember that preschoolers tend to imitate language exactly, so if they hear less-than-perfect language, this is the language pattern they adopt. They may imitate and use "bathroom language" because of the attention from adults this generates.

Preschoolers are egocentric, so they define objects in relation to themselves (e.g., a key is not a metal object but "what I use to open a door", a car is not a means of transportation but "what Mom uses to take me to school").

Play

Preschoolers do not need many toys because, with an imagination keener than it will be at any other time in life, they enjoy games that use imitation or pretending such as pretending they are a teacher, cowboy, firefighter, or store clerk. Many preschoolers have imaginary friends at this stage as a part of having such an active imagination (Nielsen, 2012). These are normal and often exist until children formally begin school.

Four- and 5-year-olds divide their time between roughhousing and imitative play. Five-year-olds become interested in group games or reciting songs they have learned in kindergarten or preschool.

TABLE 31.1 Summary of Preschool Growth and Development

Age (in Years)	Fine Motor Skills	Gross Motor Skills	Language	Play
3	Undresses self; stacks tower of blocks; draws a cross	Runs; alternates feet on stairs; rides tricycle; stands on one foot	Vocabulary of 900 words	Able to take turns; very imaginative
4	Can do simple buttons	Constantly in motion; jumps; skips	Vocabulary of 1,500 words	Pretending is major activity
5	Can draw a six-part figure; can lace shoes	Throws overhand	Vocabulary of 2,100 words	Likes games with numbers or letters

QSEN Checkpoint Question 31.1
Informatics

Cathy, 3 years old, constantly asks questions. When teaching her father about communication skills in children of this age, you should state that a child of Cathy's age typically asks how many questions in a day?

a. Around 50
b. 100 to 200
c. 300 to 400
d. 600 or more

Look in Appendix A for the best answer and rationale.

Emotional Development

Children change a great deal in their ability to understand their world and how they relate to other people during the preschool years.

Initiative

The developmental task for the preschool-age child is to achieve a sense of initiative versus guilt (Erikson, 1993). Children with a well-developed sense of initiative like to explore because they have discovered that learning new things is fun.

If children are criticized or punished for attempts at initiative, they can develop a sense of guilt for wanting to try new activities or to have new experiences. Those who leave the preschool period with a sense of guilt can carry it with them into school situations. They may even have difficulty later in life making decisions about everything from changing jobs to choosing an apartment because they cannot envision that they are capable of solving the associated problems that will come with change.

To gain a sense of initiative, preschoolers need exposure to a wide variety of experiences and play materials so they can learn as much about how things work as possible. They are ready to explore outside their homes such as enjoying a trip to the zoo or an amusement park (Fig. 31.2). They enjoy going with their family on vacation. These types of experiences lead to increased vocabulary (e.g., at the zoo, words such as giraffe, elephant, and bear come alive because they are transferred from abstract concepts to the actual animals).

Urge parents to provide play materials that encourage creative play, such as finger paints, soapy water to splash or blow into bubbles, sand to build castles, and modeling clay or homemade dough to mold into figures or make into pretend cookies. These are messy activities, so some parents prefer not to allow a child to indulge in them more than once a week, but any experience with free-form play is helpful.

Preschoolers tend to have such active imaginations that they need little guidance in this type of play. They smear both hands into clay or finger paint and create instinctively. What they make may not be recognizable; it is the enjoyment of feeling the material and how it manipulates that is the experience.

Imitation

Imitating the actions of the people around them peaks during preschool age. Role modeling this way should be fun and does not have to be accurate. If a boy is pretending to be a police officer who is busy putting out fires or a firefighter who is stopping playmates from speeding, the fact that he is freely imitating a role is more important than getting the role absolutely correct. If a parent is concerned that a child should recognize these roles more accurately, it is usually best not to stop the play, but rather, the next time they drive past the fire station, to explain that is where firefighters work and that their job is to put out fires.

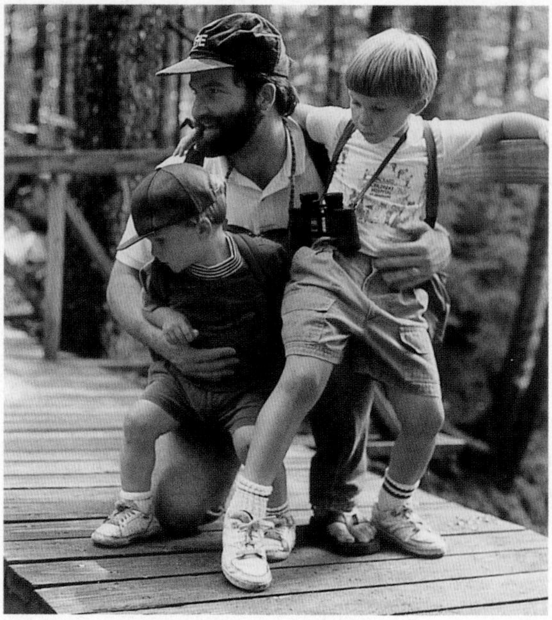

FIGURE 31.2 Preschoolers like exposure to new events and places. Here, a 3-year-old child is eager to explore the woods during a hike with the family.

Children generally imitate those activities best that they see their parents performing at home. A young girl will set the table for breakfast, eat with her "husband," help clean off the table, and leave for work. A young boy might work on his computer, pretend to feed a doll, and put the doll to bed as he has seen his father do with a younger sibling. In addition to learning what activities adults carry out at home, preschoolers should also be introduced to their parents' work environments. Such visits not only provide a visual context for the parent's job but also let a child learn such words as photocopier, assembly line, legal brief, or fax machine.

Fantasy

Toddlers cannot differentiate between fantasy and reality; they believe cartoon characters they see on television are real. Preschoolers, however, begin to make this differentiation. They may become so engrossed in a fantasy role, however, that they become afraid they seem to have lost their own identity or become "stuck" in the fantasy. Such intense involvement in play is part of "magical thinking," which is active at this age (i.e., believing thoughts and wishes can come true).

Parents sometimes strengthen this feeling without realizing it so they (and you) need to be careful in this regard. A preschooler, like Cathy for example, whom you care for in the hospital might be pretending she is a white rabbit. When you walk into her room, you are aware of the game, so say, "That's strange, I don't see Cathy anywhere. All I see is a white rabbit." Cathy may be frightened that she has actually become a white rabbit; how will she ever get home again? A better response from you would be to support the imitation—this is age-appropriate behavior and a good way of exploring roles—by saying instead, "What a nice white rabbit you're pretending to be." This both supports the fantasy and yet reassures the child she is still herself.

Oedipus and Electra Complexes

Although the development of Oedipus and Electra complexes may have been overstated by Freud—possibly because of gender bias—many children do appear to manifest such behavior (Erreich, 2011). An **Oedipus complex** refers to the strong emotional attachment a preschool boy demonstrates toward his mother; an **Electra complex** is the attachment of a preschool girl to her father. A daughter demonstrating this complex might prefer to always sit beside her father at the table, or she may ask for her father to tuck her in at night. She makes a point that she is "Daddy's girl." A mother who is not prepared for this behavior may feel hurt and cut off from family interaction. A father may feel the same way when his son wants to sit beside his mother and prefers her to be the one to tuck him in for the night.

Parents can be assured this phenomenon of competition and romance in preschoolers is a normal part of maturing. Some parents may need help in handling feelings of jealousy and anger, however, particularly if a child is vocal in expressing feelings toward a parent.

Gender Roles

Preschoolers begin to be aware of the difference between sexes and so need to be introduced to both gender roles. Encourage single parents to plan opportunities for their children to spend some time with adults other than themselves, such as a grandparent, a friend, or a relative of the opposite sex, for this experience. If a child is hospitalized during the preschool period, a nurse could readily fill this role.

Many parents do not want their child to grow up as they did, with a fixed gender role as a result of stereotyping. Help them understand that parents reinforce such attitudes by their actions as well as by their words. For example, a father may tell his son it is important for both boys and girls to do housework, but if the father never does dishes, he is teaching his son that managing a household is not a man's job.

Socialization

Because 3-year-olds are capable of sharing, they play with other children their age much more agreeably than do toddlers, which makes the preschool period become a sensitive and critical time for socialization. Preschoolers who are exposed to other playmates have an easier time learning to relate to people than those raised in an environment where they rarely see other children of the same age (Paulus & Moore, 2012) (Fig. 31.3).

Although 4-year-olds continue to enjoy play groups, they may become involved in arguments more than they did at age 3 years, especially as they become more certain of their role in the group. This development, like so many others, may make parents worry that a child is regressing. However, it is really forward movement that involves some testing and identification of their group role.

Five-year-olds begin to develop "best" friendships, perhaps on the basis of who they walk to school with or who lives closest to them. The elementary rule that an odd number of children will have difficulty playing well together generally pertains to children at this age: two or four will play, but three or five will quarrel.

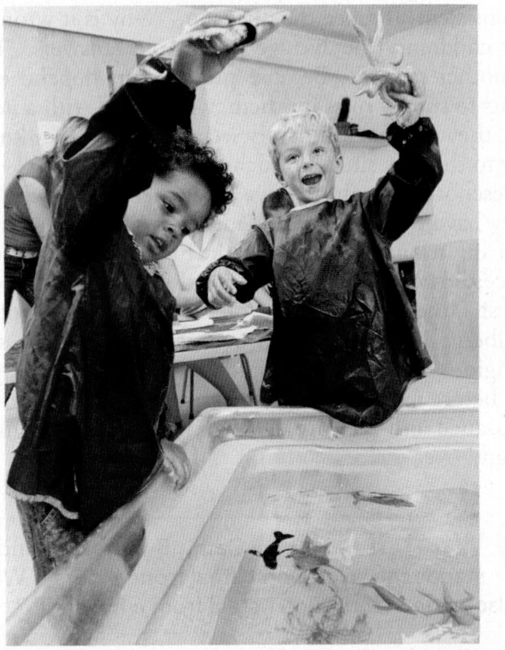

FIGURE 31.3 The preschool child moves past parallel play to make new friendships.

Cognitive Development

According to Piaget (1969), at 3 years of age, cognitive development is still preoperational. Although children during this period do enter a second phase called **intuitional thought**, they lack the insight to view themselves as others see them or to put themselves in another's place (this is termed *centering*). Because preschoolers cannot make this kind of mental substitution, they feel they are always right. It's important to remember this when explaining procedures to preschoolers. They cannot see your side of the situation, they cannot hurry because you must have something done by 10 o'clock, and they cannot hold still just because you want them to.

Also, preschoolers are not yet aware of the property of **conservation**. This means that if they have two balls of clay of equal size, but one is squashed flatter and wider than the other, they will insist the flatter one is bigger (because it is wider) or the intact one is bigger (because it is taller). They cannot see that only the form, not the amount, has changed. This inability to appreciate conservation has implications for nursing care because it means preschoolers are not able to comprehend that a procedure done two separate ways is the same procedure. If the nurse before you, for example, told a child to turn on his right side and then his left side while his bed was made, you may have to allow him to turn those same ways or he will insist you are making his bed wrong.

Moral and Spiritual Development

Children of preschool age determine right from wrong based on their parents' rules because they have little understanding of the rationale for these rules or even whether the rules are consistent. If asked the question, "Why is it wrong to hit other children?" the average preschooler answers, "Because my mother says so." Because preschoolers depend on their parents to supply rules for them, when faced with a new situation, they may have difficulty seeing the rules they know also apply to the new situation such as a hospital.

Preschoolers begin to have an elemental concept of God if they have been provided some form of religious training. Belief in an outside force aids in the development of conscience; however, preschoolers tend to do good out of self-interest rather than because of strong spiritual motivation (Kohlberg, 1984). Children at this age enjoy the security of religious holidays and religious rituals such as prayer and grace before meals because these rituals offer them the same reassurance and security as a familiar nursery rhyme read over and over.

What if...31.1 Cathy, 3 years old, understands the rule "Don't steal from a store". Would she also understand "Don't steal from a hospital"?

PLANNING AND IMPLEMENTATION FOR THE HEALTH PROMOTION OF A PRESCHOOLER AND FAMILY

Preschoolers are old enough to begin to take responsibility for their own actions. Children's safety, nutritional health, daily activities, and family functioning are all affected by this increased responsibility.

Promoting Preschooler Safety

As preschoolers broaden their horizons, safety issues must also widen. By age 4 years, children may project an attitude of independence and the ability to take care of their own needs. However, they still need supervision to be certain they do not injure themselves or other children while roughhousing and to ensure they do not stray too far from home. Their interest in learning adult roles may lead them to exploring the blades of a lawn mower or an electric saw or a neighbor's pool (Bowman, Aitken, Robbins, et al., 2012). Because they imitate adult roles so well, they may imitate taking medicine if they see family members doing so. It's also not too early to think about gun safety or being certain any gun in their home is locked away separate from its ammunition (Senger, Keijzer, Smith, et al., 2011).

A final area to consider is automobile safety. Preschoolers must be reminded repeatedly to buckle their booster seat and not to walk in back of or in front of automobiles. Otherwise, a preschooler's thought "I want to play with Mary across the street" can be so quick and so intense that the child will run into the middle of the street before remembering street safety rules. Additional safety points for the preschool period are summarized in Box 31.4.

Keeping Children Safe, Strong, and Free

The preschool years are not too early a time to educate children about the potential threat of harm from strangers or how to address bullying behavior from people (children or adults) they meet at preschool or at play (Jonson-Reid, Kohl, & Drake, 2012) through such measures as:

- Cautioning a child never to talk with or accept a ride from a stranger
- Teaching a child how to call for help in an emergency (yelling or running to a designated neighbor's house if outside, or dialing 911 if near a phone)
- Describing what police officers look like and explaining that police can help in an emergency situation
- Explaining that if children or adults ask them to keep secrets about anything that has made them uncomfortable, they should tell their parents or another trusted adult, even if they have promised to keep the secret
- Explaining that bullying behavior from other children is not to be tolerated and should be reported so they can receive help managing it

It is often difficult for parents to impart this type of information to preschoolers because they don't want to terrify their child about the world. They also can't imagine their child will ever be in a situation in which the information will be needed. If the information is presented in a calm and everyday manner, however, children can use it to begin to build safe habits that will help them later when they are old enough to walk home from school alone or play with their friends unsupervised.

Motor Vehicle and Bicycle Safety

Because of front seat airbags, preschoolers need to be buckled into car seats or booster seats in the back seat (American Academy of Pediatrics [AAP], 2012). Urge parents to stress the important role of seat belts in preventing injury and to make a rule that the car does not move until seat belts are fastened. Many preschoolers outgrow their car seats during this period (when they reach about 40 lb) and need to graduate to a booster-type seat. Remind parents to check the position of the shoulder harness in both types of seat so the belt doesn't cross a child's face or throat.

Preschool is also the right age to promote bicycle safety because falls off bicycles are a major cause of severe head injuries in this age group (Agarwal & Pruthi, 2010). To prevent such injuries, preschoolers need a safety helmet approved for children their age and size. Encourage parents who ride bicycles to demonstrate safe riding habits by wearing helmets as well. Seeing a parent routinely wearing a helmet may well be the most compelling reason for a preschooler to wear one.

What if...31.2 Cathy tells you she knows to not leave preschool with anyone who is strange. Is that the same as knowing not to leave with a stranger?

Promoting the Nutritional Health of a Preschooler

Like the toddler period, the preschool years are not a time of fast growth, so preschool children are not likely to have ravenous appetites (Raman, 2011). Being certain they get enough daily exercise helps to improve this. A sense of initiative, or learning how to do things, can be strengthened by allowing a child to prepare simple foods, such as making a sandwich or spreading jelly on toast.

Most children are hungry after preschool and enjoy a snack when they arrive home. Because sugary foods can dull

BOX 31.4 Nursing Care Planning to Empower a Family

COMMON SAFETY MEASURES TO PREVENT UNINTENTIONAL INJURIES TO PRESCHOOLERS

Q. Cathy's father says to you, "My preschooler is so active! How can I keep her safe?"
A. All of the safety measures that apply to toddlers also apply to preschoolers. In addition, try these tips:

Possible Unintentional Injury	Prevention Measure
Motor vehicles	Teach safety with tricycles (e.g., look before crossing driveways, do not cross streets).
	Teach the child to always hold hands with an adult before crossing a street.
	Teach parking lot safety (e.g., hold hands with an adult, do not run behind cars that could be backing up).
	Teach children to consistently wear helmets when beginning bicycle riding.
Falls	Always supervise a preschooler at a playground.
	Remove drawstrings from hooded clothing.
	Help the child to judge safe distances for jumping or safe heights for climbing.
Drowning	Teach beginning swimming.
Animal bites	Do not allow the child to approach strange dogs.
	Supervise the child's play with family pets.
Poisoning	Never present medication as a candy.
	Never take medication in front of a child.
	Never store food or substances in containers other than their own.
	Post the telephone number of the poison control center by the telephone or as a cell phone contact number (1-800-222-1222).
	Teach the child that medications are a serious substance and not for play.
Burns	Store matches in closed containers.
	Do not allow the preschooler to help light birthday candles, or fireplaces; fire is not fun or a "treat".
Community safety	Teach the preschooler that not all people are friends (e.g., "Do not talk to strangers or take candy from strangers").
	Define a stranger as someone the child does not know, not someone odd looking.
	Teach the child to say "no" to people whose touching he or she does not enjoy, including family members. (When a child is sexually maltreated, the offender is usually a family member or close family friend.)
General	Know the whereabouts of the preschooler at all times.
	Be aware the frequency of unintentional injuries increases when parents are under stress. Special precautions must be taken at these times.
	Some children are more active, curious, and impulsive and therefore more vulnerable to unintentional injuries than others.

a child's appetite for dinner and it is not too soon to begin measures to prevent childhood obesity, urge parents to offer snacks such as fruit, cheese, or milk rather than cookies and a soft drink or juice (Bevan & Reilly, 2011).

Preschool Nutrition Requirements

As with all age groups, foods selected for preschoolers should be based on MyPlate (www.choosemyplate.gov) recommendations, making certain to offer a variety of food (U.S. Department of Agriculture [USDA], 2012). Preschoolers may not eat a great deal of meat because it can be hard to chew. Many parents ask whether their preschooler needs to take supplementary vitamins to make up for this. As long as a child is eating foods from all five food groups and meets the criteria for a healthy child such as being alert and active with height and weight within normal averages, additional vitamins are probably unnecessary.

If parents do give vitamins, remind them that a child will undoubtedly view a vitamin as candy rather than medicine because of the attractive shapes and colors of preschool vitamins, so they must be stored out of reach. Caution parents not to give more vitamins than the recommended daily amount as well, or poisoning from high doses of fat-soluble vitamins or iron can result.

A Vegetarian Diet

A vegetarian diet is usually colorful and therefore appeals to preschoolers. Vegetables, fruits, and grains are also healthy snack foods.

If vegetarian diets are deficient in any aspects, it is usually in calcium, vitamin B_{12}, and vitamin D. Check to be sure a child is ingesting a variety of calcium sources (e.g., green leafy vegetables, milk products) because calcium is very important for bone growth. Vitamin D is found in fortified cereals and milk. Vitamin B_{12} is found almost exclusively in animal products, so a child on a vegetarian intake may need a supplemental source of this (Whitney & Rolfes, 2013).

Promoting the Development of the Preschooler in Daily Activities

The preschooler has often mastered the basic skills needed for most self-care activities, including feeding, dressing, washing (with supervision), and toothbrushing (again, with supervision).

Dressing

Many 3-year-olds and most 4-year-olds can dress themselves except for difficult buttons, although there may be a conflict over what the child will wear. Preschoolers prefer bright colors or prints and so may select items that are appealing in color rather than matching. As with other preschool activities, however, children need the experience of choosing their own clothes. One way for parents to solve the problem of mismatching is to fold together matching shirts and slacks so a child sees them as a set rather than individual pieces. If children insist on wearing mismatched clothing, urge parents to make no apologies for their appearance. A simple statement, "Mark chose his own clothes today" explains the situation. Anyone who understands preschoolers appreciates that the experience children gain in being able to select their own clothing is worth more than a perfect appearance by adult standards.

Sleep

Many toddlers, who go through a typical negative phase, resist taking naps no matter how tired they are. Preschoolers, however, are more aware of their needs; when they are tired, they often curl up on a couch or soft chair and fall asleep. Many, particularly those who attend afternoon child care or preschool, give up afternoon naps. If they nap at preschool, they may have some difficulty going to sleep at the usual bedtime established at home.

On some occasions, even though they may be tired, children in this age group may refuse to go to sleep because of fear of the dark and may wake at night terrified by a bad dream (Byars, Yolton, Rausch, et al., 2012). This means that preschoolers may need a night-light turned on, although they did not need one before. A helpful suggestion for parents is to screen out frightening stories or TV watching just prior to bedtime and to be certain when the light in their bedroom is dimmed, it has a soothing atmosphere (no staring teddy bears or evil smiling dolls). Box 31.5 is an interprofessional care map for a child with preschool fears.

✔ QSEN Checkpoint Question 31.2

Evidence-Based Practice

Many preschoolers have difficulty falling asleep or wake during the night with nightmares. To see if changes in the type of television watched could improve preschooler's sleep, researchers encouraged half of a group of families studied to replace television watching with quality educational and prosocial video content through use of an initial home visit and follow-up telephone calls over 6 months. Among the 565 children studied, the most common sleep problem was delayed sleep onset (38%). Results at the end of 18 months showed that children in the intervention group had significantly lower odds of any sleep problems (Garrison & Christakis, 2012).

Based on the study, which of the following would be the best advice you could give the Edwards family?

a. Don't allow Cathy to watch television until she is 5 years of age.
b. Encourage Cathy to watch specific DVDs that her parents choose for her.
c. Discuss with Cathy that TV does not necessarily reflect reality.
d. Allow her to only watch cartoons so she won't be seeing violence.

Look in Appendix A for the best answer and rationale.

Exercise

The preschool period is an active phase, so preschool play tends to be vigorous. Roughhousing helps relieve tension and should be allowed as long as it does not become destructive. In addition, preschoolers love time-honored games such as ring-around-the-rosy, London Bridge, or other more structured games they were not ready for as toddlers. Promoting these types of active games and reducing television watching can be steps toward helping children develop motor skills as well as prevent childhood obesity (Hodges, Smith, Tidwell, et al., 2012; Mitka, 2012).

Hygiene

Preschoolers can wash and dry their hands adequately if the faucet is regulated for them (so they do not scald themselves with hot water). When possible, parents should turn down the temperature of the water heater in their home to under 120°F to help prevent scalds.

Although preschoolers certainly sit well in bathtubs, they should still not be left unsupervised at bath time in case they decide to add more hot water or to practice swimming and then be unable to get their head out of the water again. Some girls develop vulvar irritation (and perhaps bladder infections) from exposure to bubble bath so parents shouldn't add such products to the water (Smith, 2011). Although not well studied, cranberry juice may help prevent these infections the same as in adult women (Goldman, 2012).

Children this age are not paragons of neatness and may not clean their hands thoroughly. Preschoolers do not clean

BOX 31.5 Nursing Care Planning

AN INTERPROFESSIONAL CARE MAP FOR A PRESCHOOLER WITH FEARS

Cathy Edwards is a 3-year-old whom you meet at a health maintenance visit. Her father tells you he is concerned because Cathy talks constantly with an imaginary friend named Emma. She makes up stories about events that can't possibly be true. When corrected, Cathy stutters so badly that no one can understand her. Her father is also concerned because his daughter cries when he leaves her at child care.

Family Assessment Family lives in rented apartment in inner city. Mother, a stay-at-home mom, is hospitalized with complications of a second pregnancy. Father works as city police detective.

Client Assessment A 3-year-old girl within normal limits for height, weight, and development. Child currently enrolled in all-day preschool program while mother is hospitalized. Father picks child up after his work. Father arrived late to pick child up from preschool last week. She states, "He forgot me." Child refuses to return to preschool. Cries, sticks finger in mouth to make herself vomit, and complains her stomach hurts when he tries to drop her off now.

Nursing Diagnosis Fear related to separation and abandonment during preschool period

Outcome Criteria Child verbalizes fear. Father demonstrates measures to minimize child's fears; reports by 2 weeks that crying episodes at school have decreased.

Team Member Responsible	Assessment	Intervention	Rationale	Expected Outcome
Activities of Daily Living, Including Safety				
Nurse	Ask father to detail a 24-hour day for the family to gain clear picture of child's role and capabilities.	Father describes differences in family life since wife has been hospitalized and strain it causes on Cathy.	People are unable to solve a problem until the extent of the problem is clear.	Father details a typical day as well as expresses his wish to continue or not continue the preschool experience for Cathy.
Teamwork and Collaboration				
Nurse/Nurse Practitioner	Assess if father feels referral to child guidance service is necessary to help reduce fear.	Encourage the father to talk with the preschool staff about the problem and common methods to decrease a child's fear.	Discussion with care providers can help reinforce the measures used by the father to provide consistency and thereby help to minimize a child's fears.	Father states he will consult with preschool staff to help solve problem.
Procedures/Medications for Quality Improvement				
Nurse	Assess what father knows about measures to reduce fear in preschoolers.	Instruct the father in measures to help reduce child's fear, such as reinforcing the time he will return. Will call if he's running late; post memo to self to pick her up.	Reassurance helps to reduce a child's fear of abandonment.	Father describes steps he will take to be certain he will not be late again at preschool for pickup.
Nutrition				
Nurse	Assess if child uses threat of vomiting at any other time.	Stress that effect of eating disorders potentially dangerous.	Frequent vomiting in young children can lead to fluid and electrolyte imbalances.	Father states whether he has ever seen pseudovomiting before.

(continued on page 878)

BOX 31.5 Nursing Care Planning (continued)

Patient-Centered Care				
Nurse/Nurse practitioner	Assess father's knowledge of typical preschool fears such as abandonment and fear of the dark.	Review with the father the typical fears experienced by the preschooler, including those of separation and abandonment.	Knowledge of normal growth and development helps to reduce the father's anxiety about the behavior and possible causes.	Father acknowledges he deals mainly with adults in his business; expresses desire to learn more about preschool period.
Psychosocial/Spiritual/Emotional Needs				
Nurse	Explore with child why she is so fearful her father will not return for her.	Encourage the father to set up a special time for himself and his daughter in the evening or on weekends so they have a consistent close time.	Special time for a father and daughter enhances the parent–child relationship. Consistently adhering to this time helps to foster a sense of trust and security and show he is dependable.	Father states he will plan for a special time each week, even if it is difficult to arrange because of wife's hospitalization and his irregular work schedule.
Informatics for Seamless Health Care Planning				
Nurse	Assess if father would find a follow-up telephone call helpful.	Arrange for a follow-up telephone call (if desired) in 1 week.	Follow-up provides additional support and means for evaluating the effectiveness of the methods used.	Father states he is receptive to follow-up care.

their fingernails or ears well, either, so these areas often need "touching up" by a parent or older sibling. Using a nonirritating shampoo and hanging a mobile over the tub so they have a reason to look up while their hair is rinsed helps make hair washing a fun procedure.

Care of Teeth

If independent toothbrushing was not started as a daily practice during the toddler years, it should be started during preschool (Smith & Riedford, 2012). One good toothbrushing period a day is often more effective than more frequent half-hearted attempts. Electric or battery-operated toothbrushes are favorites of preschoolers and can be used safely if the child is taught not to use it or any other electrical appliance near a basin of water. Although many preschoolers do well brushing their own teeth, parents must check that all tooth surfaces have been cleaned. Parents should also floss the child's teeth, because this is a skill beyond a preschooler's motor ability.

Preschoolers should continue to drink fluoridated water or receive a prescribed oral fluoride supplement if fluoride is not provided in the water supply (Tubert-Jeannin, Auclair, Amsallem, et al., 2011). Encouraging children to eat apples, carrots, chicken, or cheese for snacks rather than candy or sweets is yet another way to prevent tooth decay. If a child is allowed to chew gum, it should be the sugar-free variety.

A first visit to a dentist should be arranged no later than 3 years of age for an evaluation of tooth formation because deciduous (baby) teeth must be preserved to protect the dental arch. If a tooth has to be pulled for any reason, this can cause the permanent teeth to drift out of position or the jaw not to grow enough to accommodate them (Merlino & Gigli, 2012). Because this visit usually reveals no cavities, this should be a pain-free experience and should help implant the idea that dentists like to help rather than hurt.

Teeth grinding **(bruxism)** may begin at this age as a way of "letting go," similar to body rocking, which children do for a short time each night before falling asleep. Children who grind their teeth extensively may have greater than average anxiety. Children who have cerebral palsy may do this because of the spasticity of jaw muscles. If grinding is extensive, the crowns of the teeth can actually become abraded. The condition can advance to such an extent that tooth nerves become exposed and painful. If damage is evident, refer the family to a pediatric dentist so the teeth can be evaluated, repaired (capped), and conserved.

What if...31.3 **Cathy's father tells you she hates to take a bath and brush her teeth. What suggestions could you make to help her enjoy these bedtime activities more?**

Promoting Healthy Family Functioning

An important role of preschooler parents is to respect creativity. Some who enjoyed maintaining a gentle rhythm of care for an infant can have difficulty being the parents of a preschooler because more flexibility and creativity are required. Other parents come into their own as their child reaches 3 years; they delight in encouraging imaginative games and play.

Part of encouraging creativity is encouraging vocabulary building. One way for parents to do this is to read aloud to their child; another is to answer questions so the child sees language as an organized system of communication. Answering a preschooler's questions can be difficult, however, because the

BOX 31.6 Nursing Care Planning Based on Effective Communication

Cathy is being seen for a health maintenance visit. You overhear her father talking to his daughter in the waiting room.

Less Effective Communication

Cathy: Why do we have to wait so long?
Mr. Edwards: It's how things work here.
Cathy: Why?
Mr. Edwards: I have no idea.
Cathy: Why is that girl here? Is she sick?
Mr. Edwards: I have no idea.
Cathy: When are we going home?
Mr. Edwards: I have no idea.
Cathy: What's that girl's name?
Mr. Edwards: I have no idea.

More Effective Communication

Cathy: Why do we have to wait so long?
Mr. Edwards: It's how things work here.
Cathy: Why?
Mr. Edwards: People have to take turns. We're waiting for our turn.
Cathy: Why is that girl here? Is she sick?
Mr. Edwards: She might be. Some children are here because they're sick and some are just here for a checkup like you.
Cathy: When are we going home?
Mr. Edwards: As soon as the nurse practitioner checks you over.
Cathy: What's that girl's name?
Mr. Edwards: I don't know. Do you want to ask her?

Preschoolers ask 300 to 400 questions a day as they explore their world. In the first scenario, the father tries to discourage questions by offering almost no answers. In the second scenario, when he tries to answer the child's questions, he is not only supplying information but also is helping the child build vocabulary. Because preschoolers ask so many questions, you may have to encourage parents to continue to answer questions this way. Otherwise, discouraging questions can become the method of interaction.

questions are frequently philosophical, not fact finding such as, "Why is grass green?" A child may listen to an explanation of chlorophyll but then repeat the question, regardless of the clarity of the explanation, because the parent underestimated the depth of the question. The child did not want to know what makes grass green, but why, philosophically, it is not red, blue, or yellow. The obvious answer to that is, "I don't know." Parents who are confident can give this answer without feeling threatened. Parents who are less sure of themselves may feel extremely uncomfortable when they realize they do not know the answer to what a 4-year-old is asking (Box 31.6).

Discipline

Preschoolers have definite opinions on things such as what they want to eat, where they want to go, and what they want to wear and these opinions may bring them into opposition with parents. A major parental responsibility when this happens is to guide a child through these struggles without discouraging the child's right to have an opinion. A "time-out" is a useful technique for parents to correct behavior throughout the preschool years (see Chapter 30). Although the technique has some critics, it allows parents to discipline without using physical punishment and allows a child to learn a new way of behavior without extreme stress. Time-out periods should be as many minutes long as the child is old, so 3 to 5 minutes is appropriate for preschoolers.

Parental Concerns Associated With the Preschool Period

A number of common health problems and fears usually arise during the preschool years.

Common Health Problems of the Preschooler

The mortality of children during the preschool years is low and becoming lower every year as more infectious diseases are preventable. This results in the major cause of death being automobile accidents, followed by poisoning and falls (Centers for Disease Control and Prevention [CDC], 2012).

Even though the number of major illnesses is few in this age group, the number of minor illnesses, such as common colds and ear infections, are high. Children who live in homes in which parents smoke have a higher incidence of ear (otitis media) and respiratory infections than others (Yilmaz, Caylan, & Karacan, 2012). Children who attend child care or preschool programs also have an increased incidence of gastrointestinal disturbances (vomiting and diarrhea) and upper respiratory infections from the exposure to other children unless frequent hand washing is stressed at the setting (Sun & Sundell, 2011).

Children may demonstrate frequent whining or clinging behavior because of this parade of constant minor infections. Assess to be certain such constant illness is not causing parents to perceive a child as sickly or not able to cope with everyday life so they don't begin to discourage independence in favor of overprotection. As parents become more experienced in handling these conditions, their perception of whether an illness is serious or not and their ability to cope with them will change.

Table 31.2 shows the recommended health maintenance schedule for preschoolers. Table 31.3 lists common problems parents may have in evaluating a preschooler's illness.

TABLE 31.2 Health Maintenance Schedule, Preschool Period

Area of Focus	Methods	Frequency
Assessment		
Health history	Health interview	Every visit
Physical health	Physical examination	Every visit
Developmental milestones	History, observation Formal Denver Developmental Screening Test (DDST-II)	Every visit Before start of school
Growth milestones	Height and weight plotted on standard growth chart; body mass index (BMI) and physical examination	Every visit
Hypertension	Blood pressure	Every visit
Nutrition	History, observation; height and weight information	Every visit
Parent–child relationship	History and observation	Every visit
Social behavior	History and observation	Every visit
Vision and hearing defects	History and observation Preschool E stereo and audiometer testing	Every visit Before start of school
Autism spectrum disorder screening	History and observation	At 18 and 24 months
Dental health	History, physical examination	Every visit
Dyslipidemia	Cholesterol, triglycerides	24 months and 4 years
Lead	Blood analysis (depending on risk in area)	18 months and 3–4 years
Tuberculosis	Purified protein derivative (PPD) test (if there are high-risk factors)	Before start of school
Immunizations		
(Administer immunization in accordance with health care agency policies. Check history and past records, and inform caregiver about any risks and side effects before administration [www.cdc.gov/vaccines/schedules].)		
Diphtheria, pertussis, and tetanus	DTaP 5	Before start of school
Measles, mumps, and rubella (MMR)	MMR #2	Before start of school
Poliomyelitis (inactivated)	IPV #4	Before start of school
Varicella	VAR #2	Before start of school
Influenza	IIV	Yearly
Pneumococcal	Pneumococcal conjugate vaccine (PCV)	May be indicated before school in susceptible children
Anticipatory Guidance		
Preschool care	Active listening and health teaching	Every visit
Expected growth and developmental milestones before next visit	Active listening and health teaching	Every visit
Unintentional injury prevention	Counseling about street and personal safety	Every visit
Problem Solving		
Any problems expressed by caregiver during course of the visit	Active listening and health teaching regarding preschool illnesses and imaginative play	Every visit

From American Academy of Pediatrics, Committee on Practice and Ambulatory Medicine. (2012). *Recommendations for preventive pediatric health care.* Washington, DC: Author; Centers for Disease Control and Prevention. (2013). *Birth–18 years and "catch up" immunization schedules.* Washington, DC: Author

TABLE 31.3 Parental Difficulties Evaluating Health Problems in the Preschool Child

Difficulty	Helpful Suggestions for Parents
Evaluating seriousness of illness or condition	Preschoolers are eager to please and tend to answer all questions such as, "Does your stomach hurt?" with a yes. Observing the child for signs of illness (e.g., refusing to eat, holding an arm stiffly, having to go to the bathroom frequently) is often more productive as an evaluation technique.
Evaluating bowel and bladder problems	Preschoolers are independent in toilet habits for the first time, so parents do not have diaper contents to evaluate. Frequent trips to the bathroom, rubbing the abdomen, and holding genitals are the usual signs of bowel or bladder dysfunction.
Evaluating nutritional intake	Preschoolers begin to eat away from home at friends' houses or at child care, or stay overnight with grandparents for the first time, so parents have less opportunities to observe daily food intake as accurately as before. Observing whether a child is growing and is active is better than monitoring any one day's intake.
Evaluating bed-wetting	Many preschoolers continue to have occasional enuresis at night until school age. If other signs are present (e.g., pain, low-grade fever, listlessness), a child should have a urine culture because persistent bed-wetting can indicate a low-grade urinary tract infection.
Evaluating activity versus hyperactivity	Many lay magazines have articles on hyperactivity in children. Parents wonder whether their active child could be hyperactive. As a rule of thumb, if a child can sit through a meal (when he is hungry), watch a half-hour television show (that is his favorite), or sit still while his favorite story is read to him, he is not hyperactive.
Age-specific diseases to be aware of	Preschool age is a time for vision and hearing assessment because, for the first time, a child is able to be tested by a standard chart or by audiometry tests. Urinary tract infections tend to occur with a high frequency in preschool-age girls. A language assessment should be done if a child is not able to make wants known by complete, articulated sentences by age 3 years (exceptions are transposing *w* for *r* and broken fluency: "I want-want-want to go").

Common Fears of the Preschooler

Because preschoolers' imaginations are so active, this leads to a number of fears such as fear of the dark, mutilation, and separation or abandonment. These can rise in incidence when combined with the stress of an illness, hospitalization, or unsafe conditions in the child's community (Kushnir & Sadeh, 2011). Although most of these fears can be handled by comforting from parents, in some children, fears are so intense that they need therapy such as desensitization in order for the fear to be conquered.

Fear of the Dark. The tendency to fear the dark is an example of a fear heightened by a child's vivid imagination: a stuffed toy by daylight becomes a threatening monster at night. Children awaken screaming because of nightmares. They may be reluctant to go to bed or go back to sleep by themselves unless a light is left turned on or a parent sits nearby.

If parents are prepared for this fear and understand it is a phase of growth, they are better able to cope with it. It is generally helpful if they monitor the stimuli their children are exposed to, especially around bedtime. This includes television, adult discussions, and frightening stories. Parents are sometimes reluctant to leave a child's light on at night because they do not want to cater to the fear. Leaving on a dim night-light, however, can solve the problem and costs only pennies. Children who awake terrified and screaming need reassurance that they are safe and that whatever was chasing them was a dream and is not in their room (Fig. 31.4). Most preschoolers do not remember in the morning that they had such a dream; however, they remember for a lifetime that they received comfort when they needed it.

If parents take sensible precautions against fear of the dark or nightmares and a child continues to have this kind of disturbance every night, it may be a reaction to undue stress, which needs to be investigated and eliminated. Giving sleep medication to counteract the sleep disturbance does not solve the basic problem, so this is rarely recommended. Fear of the dark and sleep disturbances both can become intensified in a hospital setting and require careful planning to relieve (Linder & Christian, 2011).

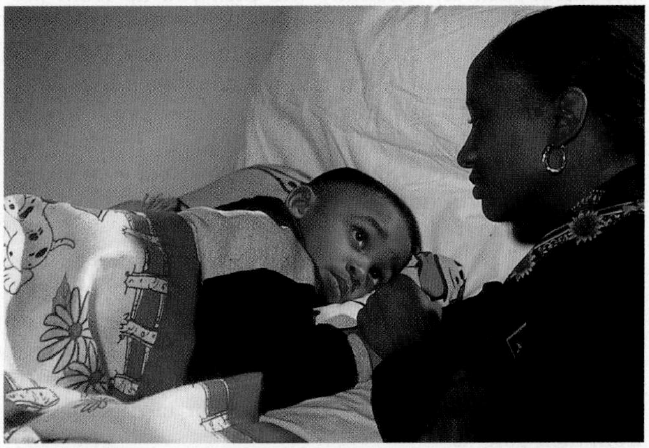

FIGURE 31.4 Having mom close by after a bad dream is a comfort to a preschooler.

Fear of Mutilation. Fear of mutilation is also significant during the preschool age, as revealed by the intense reaction of a preschooler to even a simple injury such as falling and scraping a knee or having a needle inserted for an immunization. A child cries afterward not only from the pain but also from the intrusiveness of the injury or procedure. Part of this fear arises because preschoolers do not know which body parts are essential and which ones—like an inch of scraped skin—can be easily replaced. Boys develop a fear of castration because, developmentally, they are more in tune with their body parts and are starting to identify with the same-sex parent as they go through the Oedipal phase.

Preschoolers can be worried that if some blood is taken out of their bodies, all of their blood will leak out. They often lift a bandage to peek at an incision or cut to see if their body is still intact underneath. They dislike procedures such as needlesticks, rectal temperature assessments, otoscopic examinations, or having a nasogastric tube passed into their stomach. They need good explanations of the limits of health care procedures, such as a tympanic thermometer does not hurt or a finger prick heals quickly, as well as distraction techniques in order to feel safe.

QSEN Checkpoint Question 31.3

Patient-Centered Care

Cathy's parent tells you she keeps the entire family awake at night because she is so afraid of the dark. What would be the best suggestion for helping her overcome this fear?

a. Assure her the room's window is locked so no one can kidnap her.
b. Suggest she temporarily sleep in the living room in front of the television set for safety.
c. Buy a night-light for her room and inspect the room to be certain it appears safe.
d. Teach her that her fear is not grounded in reality.

Look in Appendix A for the best answer and rationale.

Fear of Separation or Abandonment. Fear of separation is yet another major concern for preschoolers. Their sense of time is still so distorted that they cannot be comforted by assurances such as, "Mommy will pick you up from preschool at noon." Their sense of distance is also limited, so making a statement such as "I work only a block away" is not reassuring. Relating time and space to something a child knows better, such as meals, television shows, or a friend's house, is most effective. For example, stating, "Mommy will pick you up from preschool after you have had your snack" is apt to be more comforting than "Mommy will pick you up at 3 PM."

Caution parents to be sensitive to such fears when they talk about missing children or if they have their preschooler's photo or fingerprints taken for identification. Children whose chief fear is that they will be abandoned or kidnapped might not understand that fingerprints are being taken to keep them safe, only that someone might take them away from their parents.

A hospital admission or going to a new school often brings a child's fear of separation to the forefront. Help parents thoroughly prepare preschoolers for these experiences so they can survive them in sound mental health (see Chapter 35). Help them give clear instructions on when they will visit the child in the hospital.

Behavior Variations

A combination of a keen imagination and immature reasoning results in a number of other common behavior variations in preschoolers.

Telling Tall Tales. Stretching stories to make them seem more interesting is a phenomenon frequently encountered in preschoolers. For example, after a trip to the zoo, if you ask a preschooler, "What happened today?" a child perceives you want something exciting to have happened, and so might answer, "A bear jumped out of his cage and ate the boy next to me." This is not lying, but merely supplying an expected answer. Parents may be concerned that tall tales of this nature can lead to chronic lying if supported. Caution them, therefore, not to encourage this kind of storytelling, but instead help the child separate fact from fiction by saying, "That's a good story, but now tell me what really happened." This conveys the idea that the child has not told the truth, yet does not squash imagination or initiative (Talwar & Crossman, 2011). On the other hand, parents must be alert to respect that children may be telling the truth when they are reporting a happening such as an adult molesting them so they do not dismiss information as nothing important.

QSEN Checkpoint Question 31.4

Safety

Cathy's father, a police detective, tells you that he and his wife wish to take measures to prevent Cathy being kidnapped. What action should you recommend to this family?

a. Limit playdates to Cathy's own home.
b. Withdraw Cathy from daycare to limit her exposure to other adults.
c. Describe common kidnapping culprits the father knows.
d. Be certain Cathy understands not to leave daycare with anyone but her parents.

Look in Appendix A for the best answer and rationale.

Imaginary Friends. Many preschoolers have an imaginary friend who plays with them (Nielsen, 2012). They tell a parent to "wait for Eric" or to "set a place at the table for Lucy." Although imaginary friends are a normal, creative part of the preschool years and can be invented by children who are surrounded by real playmates as well as by those who have few friends, parents may find them disconcerting. If so, let parents know that as long as their child has exposure to real playmates and imaginary playmates do not take center stage in children's lives or prevent them from socializing with other children, they should not pose a problem and often leave as quickly as they come. In the meantime, pretend friends can encourage language development, may provide an outlet for a child to express innermost feelings, or serve as a handy scapegoat for behavior about which a child has some conflict.

Parents can help their preschooler separate fact from fantasy about their imaginary friend by saying, "I know Eric isn't real, but if you want to pretend, I'll set a place for him." This response helps a child understand what is real and what is fantasy without restricting imagination or creativity.

Difficulty Sharing. Sharing is a concept that first comes to be understood around the age of 3 years. Before this, children engage in parallel play (two children need two toys and two spaces to play because they cannot pass one toy back and forth or play together). Around 3 years of age, children begin to understand some things are theirs, some belong to others, and some can belong to both. For the first time, they can stand in line to wait for a drink, take turns using a shovel at a sandbox, and share a box of crayons. Sharing does not come easily, however; children who are ill or under stress have greater difficulty with it than usual.

Assure parents that sharing is a difficult concept to grasp, and, as with most skills, preschoolers need practice to understand and learn it (Sutherland & Friedman, 2012). Parents may need to help a child learn property rights as part of learning to share, such as, "This is my private drawer and no one touches what is in it but me." "That is your private box, and no one touches the things in it but you." "A shovel is ours and can be used by everyone playing in the sand pile." Defining limits and exposing children to these three categories (i.e., mine, yours, ours) helps them determine which objects belong to which category.

Regression. Some preschoolers, generally in relation to stress, revert to behavior they previously outgrew, such as thumb-sucking, negativism, loss of bladder control, and inability to separate from their parents. Although the stress that causes this may take many forms, it is usually the result of such things as a new baby in the family, a new school experience, seeing frightening and graphic television news or programming, stress in the home from financial or marital difficulties, or separation caused by hospitalization.

Help parents understand that regression in these circumstances is normal, and a child's thumb-sucking is little different from the parents' reaction to stress (e.g., smoking many cigarettes, nail biting, overeating), so it's easier for them to accept and understand. Obviously, removing the stress is the best way to help a child discontinue this behavior. The stresses mentioned, however, are not ones that are easily controlled. New babies cannot be returned, irreparable marriages cannot be patched together, frightening news happens every day, and hospitalizations do occur.

Techniques for minimizing the stress of hospitalization for preschoolers are discussed in Chapter 35. Children's reactions to severe and prolonged stress are discussed in Chapter 54. Children undergoing less severe stress can be assured that although situations are changing, the important aspect of their life—that someone still loves them and will continue to take care of them—is not. The manifestations of stress, such as thumb-sucking, are best ignored; calling them to a child's attention merely causes more stress because, in addition to experiencing the primary stress, it makes children aware they are not pleasing their parents.

Sibling Rivalry. Jealousy of a brother or sister may first become evident during the preschool period because this is the first time children have enough vocabulary to express how they feel (i.e., know a name to call) and partly because preschoolers are more aware of family roles and how responsibilities at home are divided (Snowling, 2011). For many children, this is also the time when a new brother or sister is born.

A firstborn child is rarely allowed the privileges of a second child. The parents are untried, unsure of how far they should let a first child venture or what level of responsibility a child could accept, allowing the firstborn to serve as the "trial run" for all children who come after. Children as young as preschool, however, can tell when a younger sibling is being allowed behavior that is not tolerated in them. They are little appeased by the explanation, "Your brother is just a baby."

To help preschoolers feel secure and to promote self-esteem during this time, reminding them that there are things they can do that a younger sibling is not allowed to do and supplying them with a private drawer or box for their things that parents or other children do not touch can be helpful. A private box serves as a defense against younger children who do not yet appreciate property rights.

Preparing for a New Sibling

Introduction of a new sibling is such a major happening that parents need to take special steps to be certain their preschooler will be prepared (Volling, 2012). There is no rule as to when this preparation should begin, but it should be before the time the child begins to feel the difference the new baby will make. This is perhaps when the mother first begins to look pregnant. It is certainly before parents begin to make physical preparations for the new child. It is always less frightening to understand why things are happening, no matter how distasteful they may be, rather than hear people whispering or having people obviously evading the issue. The unknown is always more fearful than a definite event because those can be faced and conquered.

Help parents not to underestimate the significance of a bed to a preschool child because it is security, consistency, and "home." If their preschooler is sleeping in the crib that will be used for the new baby, it's usually best if the preschooler can be moved to a bed about 3 months in advance of the birth. Parents might explain, "It's time to sleep in a new bed now because you're a big girl." The fact that the child is growing is a better reason for such a move than because a new brother or sister needs their bed. The latter may be a direct route to sibling rivalry and jealousy.

If children are to start preschool or child care, it's also best if they can do so either before the new baby is born or 2 or 3 months afterward. That way, children can perceive starting school as a result of maturity and not of being pushed out of the house by the new child.

If the mother will be hospitalized for the birth, parents should be certain their child is prepared for this separation. Because the mother is likely to go to the hospital during the night, it is unrealistic to expect a child to be happy to learn in the morning about the arrival of a new sibling when he realizes the new baby has taken away his mother. Some communities offer preparation for birth classes for preschoolers, the same as for parents, or include children in adult preparation courses to help them master this new experience.

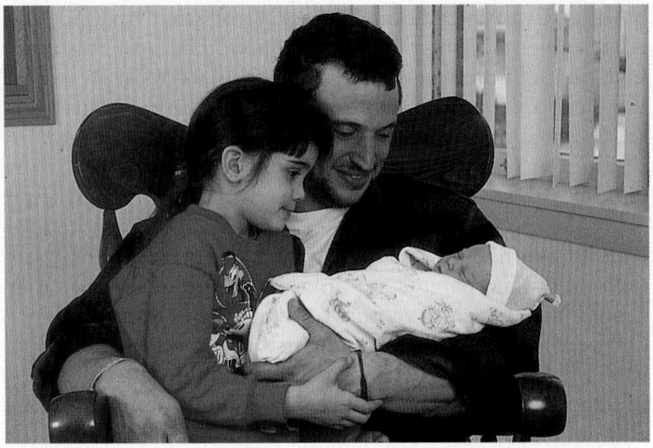

FIGURE 31.5 A preschooler greets a new baby sister. She feels special as dad explains how important it is to be a big sister.

Encourage women to maintain contact with their preschooler during the short time they are hospitalized for the new birth. Some preschoolers may react very coldly to their mothers, turning their head away and refusing to come to them after even a few days of separation when they return home. This is a reaction not to the new baby but to the separation, the same phenomenon that may occur when a child returns home after being hospitalized (see Chapter 35). Allowing the child to visit in the hospital can help relieve this type of separation anxiety.

Ask pregnant women or couples what kind of preparation they are making for older children and ask the mother of a new baby how everything is working out. Most parents find the problem of jealousy is bigger than they anticipated and welcome a few suggestions about how to provide more time for their preschooler during the day or which activities a preschooler would especially enjoy (Fig. 31.5 and Box 31.7).

QSEN Checkpoint Question 31.5

Teamwork & Collaboration

Cathy's family is expecting a new baby. When liaising with the birthing center nurse, you should promote which of the following as a means of fostering family bonding during this time of transition?

a. Take action to help Cathy spend as much time with her mother and the infant as possible.
b. Teach Cathy about the ways that her life might change after the birth of the baby.
c. Remind Cathy that her parents love her very much.
d. Explain to Cathy that she's very lucky because sisters grow up to become best friends.

Look in Appendix A for the best answer and rationale.

Sex Education

During the preschool age, children become acutely aware of the difference between boys and girls, possibly because it is a normal progression in development and possibly because this may be the first time they are exposed to the genitalia of the opposite sex as they watch while a new brother or sister has a diaper changed, they see other children using the bathroom at a preschool, or they see a parent nude.

Preschoolers' questions about genital organs are simple and fact finding; for example, "Why does James look like that?" or "How does Jasmine pee?" Explanations should be just as simple: "Boys look different from girls. The different part is called a penis." It is important that parents do not convey that these body parts are never to be talked about so they leave an open line of communication for sexual questions. Occasionally, girls attempt to void standing up as they have seen boys doing, and boys may try sitting down to void as they try to use this new body knowledge.

It is common for preschoolers to engage in masturbation while watching TV or before they fall asleep at night. The

BOX 31.7 Nursing Care Planning Based on Family Teaching

ANTICIPATORY GUIDANCE TO HELP MINIMIZE SIBLING RIVALRY

Q. Cathy's father says to you, "Cathy's acting jealous of her new sister and she's not even born yet. What can we do to reduce sibling jealousy?"

A. This isn't a simple problem, but the following suggestions might be helpful:

- After returning home from the hospital with the baby, devote attention to your preschooler and spend some special time together after the baby has gone to bed.
- When friends and family visit, encourage them to spend time with the preschooler as well as the baby. If they bring gifts for the baby, it is often wise for them to bring a small present for the preschooler as well.
- So your preschooler doesn't come to expect gifts (promoting sibling rivalry), teach her to help open the baby's gifts. Explain it is the baby's birthday and on her birthday she will receive gifts, too.
- Don't ask your preschooler a question such as, "Do you like your new sister?" It is better to express feelings of empathy such as, "New babies cry a lot. It's hard to get used to that, isn't it?"
- Provide special time for your preschooler during each day, so when you say, "Mother and Daddy love you just the same," it seems real. This might be a quiet time for talking or reading.
- While feeding the baby, read or tell a story to your preschooler. Some children enjoy feeding a doll while a parent feeds the baby or giving a doll a bath while the baby has one.

frequency of this may increase under stress, as does thumb-sucking. If observing a child doing this bothers parents, suggest they explain certain things are done in some places but not in others. Children can relate to this kind of direction without feeling inhibited, just as they can accept the fact they use a bathroom in private or eat only at the table. Calling unnecessary attention to the act can increase anxiety and cause increased, not decreased, activity.

Because this may be the time a new brother or sister comes into the family, it is also the most likely time for questions such as, "Where do babies come from?" Because a child is asking a simple fact-finding question, parents usually find a simple, factual answer to this type of question is best, such as, "Babies grow in a special place in a mother's body called a uterus." Saying "uterus" rather than "tummy" prevents children from envisioning babies and food all mixed together in their mother's stomach (Fig. 31.6).

It is so natural for preschoolers to ask about where babies come from that those who do not ask are exceptions and may not be asking because they sense from a preliminary exploratory question that the subject is closed. A parent could introduce the subject by visiting a new baby in the neighborhood with the child or pointing out a neighbor who is pregnant. Visiting new kittens or puppies can also offer the chance to introduce the subject. If a new brother or sister will be born at a birthing center or at home, many parents may want their preschooler to be present at the birth. Encourage parents to prepare children thoroughly for this experience, or else the sight of their mother in pain and the wonder of birth can become an overwhelming and negative experience rather than a positive one for them (see Chapter 14).

Preschool children generally do not ask how babies get inside mothers to start growing or how babies get out at the end of the process. Should they ask, an explanation might be, "When a woman and a man love each other and decide they want a baby, the man plants a seed inside the woman. The man's seed and the woman's seed grow together in the special place inside the mother into a new baby." Some parents prefer to say, "God plants a seed." This answer may leave preschool boys feeling cheated because men appear to have such a little role in this wondrous process. Perhaps a compromise statement is, "God helps the man plant a seed." If preschoolers ask how the baby gets out, an answer might be, "When the baby is ready, a doctor or nurse helps the baby out from the special place in her body by a passageway called a vagina."

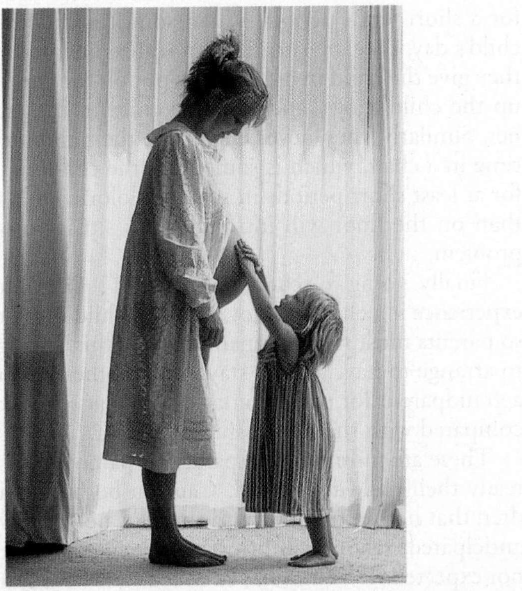

FIGURE 31.6 Preschool children have the beginnings of sexual awareness and are interested in learning where babies grow. (Taeke Henstra/Science Source/Photo Researchers, Inc.)

Many books for children explain where babies come from, including descriptions of sexual relations. These are helpful for parents to read to a child to increase understanding if they feel the child is ready for longer explanations.

QSEN Checkpoint Question 31.6

Quality Improvement

You are drafting an educational handout for parents of preschoolers that addresses the topic of sex education. What guideline should be included in this educational material?

a. Tell your child that you will explain these matters when they are old enough to start kindergarten.
b. Emphasize the fact that sexual intercourse between adults must always be consensual.
c. Describe some of the differences between boys and girls in clear and accurate terms.
d. Distract your child from questions about sexuality for as long as possible.

Look in Appendix A for the best answer and rationale.

Another important part of sex education for preschoolers is teaching them to avoid sexual maltreatment, such as not allowing anyone to touch their body unless they and their parents agree that it is all right (Pérez-Fuentes, Olfson, Villegas, et al., 2012). Because children have been taught this, remember to ask permission before giving nursing care that involves touching, especially before procedures such as catheterization or clean catch urines (see Chapter 32, Box 32.4).

Choosing a Preschool or Child Care Center

A school or child care experience is helpful for preschoolers because peer exposure appears to have a positive effect on social development (Gubbels, Van Kann, & Jansen, 2013). Children who have learned to be comfortable in a preschool group, for example, approach school comfortably and ready to learn; children who have played only infrequently in groups during the preschool age can be so busy adjusting to this new concept that they are left behind in learning new skills in kindergarten or first grade. Most parents enroll their child in a child care program because both parents work outside their home. A parent who is at home full time has to weigh whether it would be best for a child to have socialization experiences or to not diminish the family time this can create.

The terms "child care center," and "preschool" are often used interchangeably, so parents cannot depend on the name of a school to define its structure. Traditionally, the main purpose of a child care center is to provide child care while parents work or are otherwise occupied. A preschool is dedicated to stimulating children's sense of creativity and initiative and introducing them to new experiences and social contacts that they would not ordinarily receive at home. Head Start programs and many modern child care centers fulfill both functions (Wrobel, 2012).

If there are other 3- or 4-year-old children in a neighborhood with whom a child has almost daily contact and if a parent can supervise organized play dates and projects (providing peer interaction, in which working together is the key), a preschool program may not be necessary. However, if all the neighborhood children are either older or younger or there is only one other child available to play with during the day, a preschool experience will probably be beneficial. Parents with large families point out that their child gets ample exposure to groups because every meal is a "group session." This is not a peer group, however, so this situation does not offer the same experience as does preschool.

Be sure parents investigate preschools or child care centers carefully before they enroll their child to be certain their child will not only be safe there but also that the child will have an enjoyable experience. Guidelines to aid parents in this assessment are shown in Table 31.4.

To continue to evaluate their child's school experience, urge parents to make a habit of asking children what happened at school, what they learned, and the names of any new friends. For the remainder of the growing years, school will have important influences on their child's development. By taking an active role in education, parents influence what and how their child learns.

Child care centers may be responsible for the spread of infectious disease among those age 5 years and under because bringing together children from so many different homes to one setting each day increases the risk of spreading contagious disease. Preschoolers in child care settings may develop frequent upper respiratory infections or gastrointestinal illnesses. Outbreaks of cytomegalovirus and human parvovirus (fifth disease) make working in such centers a particular hazard to pregnant women because such illnesses are potentially teratogenic. To prevent the spread of infection, children need to wash their hands frequently and cover their mouths with their sleeve when coughing. Child care centers where infants are enrolled need to take special precautions against hepatitis A or parasitic infections because these can be spread by caregivers not washing their hands or not washing tables after changing diapers. Hepatitis may be subclinical in the preschooler, but other members of the preschooler's family can develop overt symptoms as the illness spreads through the family, making vaccinations against this important (CDC, 2011).

Preparing a Child for School

At the end of the preschool period, children begin a formal school experience as they enter kindergarten. Parents may wonder whether their child is old enough for this, especially if a child's birthday is in the late summer or early fall. If this is a concern, urge parents to discuss their concern with school officials to determine whether their child should be registered for kindergarten or delayed for a year. Because school involves a great deal of children's time and influences their future greatly, it's important for parents to take time to prepare preschoolers not only physically, by being certain their immunizations are up to date (see Table 31.2), but also emotionally.

Essential to this preparation is the parents' attitude. If school is discussed as something to look forward to, as an adventure that will be satisfying and rewarding, a child comes to look forward to it as a positive experience. If school is presented as a punishment ("Wait until you get into first grade—your teacher will make you behave"), there can be little delight in anticipating it.

If a child was not attending preschool, some parents may have to change their child's daily routine a few months in advance of beginning school to accustom the child to waking earlier or going to bed earlier. School has so many new components that it's wise for parents to try to eliminate as many distractions such as this as possible.

If a child is to ride a bus to school, a parent might take a child on a municipal bus as an introduction to this form of transportation. If a child is to walk to school, a trial walk is in order. In either instance, safety should be stressed such as, "Don't walk behind the bus because the driver can't see you" and "Wait for the crossing guard to help you cross the street."

If a child will be required to take a lunch to school, a parent can introduce this new experience by preparing a bagged lunch at home. If a child is to purchase lunch at school, the parent can play "cafeteria" at home by serving a buffet-style meal and letting the child practice walking from one dish to another to select food.

Some kindergartens suggest that children should know how to tie their shoes, can name basic colors, and can print their name before they begin. Parents should familiarize themselves with any such suggestions from the school, but the wisdom of requiring these skills can be questioned. Identifying colors should be established by this age, but some children are not coordinated enough at 4 to 5 years of age to tie their shoes or to print. A better contribution for parents to make toward their children's achievement in school is to instill in their children the concept that learning is fun, and that their child may not always be able to do all the things other children can do, but trying to do one's best is what is important. Trying to make children complete fine motor tasks for which they are not developmentally prepared does not instill that concept.

For children to do well in a formal school setting, they must be able to follow instructions and sit at a table and chair for a short work period. When some parents examine their child's day, they are surprised to realize how few instructions they give the child in a day. They put on the child's coat, pick up the child's toys, and lead the child to the table for dinner. Similarly, they never encourage their child to spend any time in a chair, which is something the child will have to do for at least short periods in school. Coloring at a table rather than on the floor will introduce this situation without any problem.

Finally, going to school is a form of separation and a new experience if a child has not attended child care or preschool, so parents must make preparations for this. It might be good to arrange to have a child stay with another caregiver such as a grandparent for part of a day. Staying at school can then be compared with that successful event.

These are minimum preparations parents can complete to ready their child for school. Caution both parents and children that no matter how hard they try, not everything can be anticipated; school will bring some new happenings that are not expected. If a child has been led to believe learning is fun and new experiences are enjoyable (creating a strong sense of initiative), solving these unpredictable problems is good preparation for the thousands of surprise experiences ahead.

TABLE 31.4 Questions to Use in Evaluating Child Care Centers

Question	Finding
Management	
How long has the center been in operation?	Length of operation does not necessarily indicate quality, but it allows you to locate other parents who have used the center to ask about their experience there.
Is the center licensed, registered, approved, or inspected by the appropriate agency?	Ask in your local community what agency has the responsibility for licensing child care centers. If not licensed, its quality is suspect.
What are the qualifications of staff members?	If staff members are teachers, more learning activities will be provided; staff should be qualified to perform cardiopulmonary resuscitation.
Is there a fast turnover rate of staff?	A fast turnover rate means little continuity of care will be provided (and probably suggests dissatisfaction with center administration).
What is the child–staff ratio?	A ratio of three or four children to one staff member provides time for quality interaction.
What is the center's policy on parental visits?	Parents should be able to drop in at any time. Be wary of facilities that restrict parental visiting in any way.
Physical Environment	
Is there adequate space in the center?	There should be opportunities for rough-and-tumble and imaginative play in addition to naptime areas and table activities.
Does the space appear safe?	Stairways should be fenced. No paint should be peeling.
Can children get in and out of the building easily?	A first-floor plan is safest. Fire exits should be well marked. An evacuation plan should be practiced.
Is there a safe play area for children outside?	Find out how often children are taken outside: once or twice a day, or only occasionally for "outings"?
Is there a quiet place for naps?	Ask if a child can nap if tired or has to wait until a set naptime.
Can the bathroom be reached easily?	Both potty chairs and small toilet seats should be available.
If food is provided, does it meet preschool recommendations?	Food should be "preschool friendly" and healthy, not just high-fat snacks.
Is there adequate refrigeration?	Food poisoning is a concern without refrigeration.
Staff Philosophy	
Are the caregivers warm and affectionate toward children?	Watch how they greet children. They should ask questions and listen to answers.
Do caregivers spend most of their time performing janitorial tasks (cleaning) or devoting their time to children?	It is best if the cleaning staff are separate from the care staff.
Is each child assigned to a particular caregiver on a continuing basis?	Ask caregivers to describe their care pattern; if this is not planned, little continuity of care results.
Are the children provided stimulating toys and equipment?	Imaginative items, such as a puppet theater, finger paint, and water play, should be included.
How do caregivers discipline children? Do they yell or treat the children roughly?	The method should reflect the parents' philosophy. Staff should be able to talk to children calmly without raising their voices in anger.
Is there a planned curriculum?	There should be specific goals the caregivers hope to accomplish.
Can the child pursue an individual interest?	Play or learning activities should be individualized.

(continued on page 888)

TABLE 31.4 Questions to Use in Evaluating Child Care Centers (continued)

Question	Finding
Health Care Protocols	
How does the center care for an ill child?	There should be access to a nurse. Staff should be able to evaluate for illness. They should know actions to take in an emergency.
What precautions do caregivers take to prevent the spread of infection?	The counter where diapers are changed should be wiped with a disinfectant; tissues and hand-washing facilities should be present.
Does the center follow good sanitary practices?	Be sure the center requires waterproof disposable diapers to minimize contamination of the environment and other children, and separates diaper-changing areas from other activities, especially anything related to food handling. Observe caregivers changing diapers. Do they wash hands after each change? Are children encouraged to wash their hands before eating?
Under what conditions are children not allowed to attend the center?	A center should have a very specific policy on what illness symptoms require a child to be kept home, and they should enforce this policy strictly. For instance, a runny nose may be acceptable, but a fever is not, and children with chickenpox should be kept at home until the lesions are covered with scabs. Children with special needs should be integrated into usual activities.
Children's Behavior	
Do the children appear happy and relaxed?	Observe for at least one morning.
Do children rush to greet any new visitors?	This could be a sign of boredom with their center's activities and a strong need for adult attention.

Broken Fluency

Developing language is such a complicated process that children from 2 to 6 years of age typically have some speech difficulty. A child may begin to repeat words or syllables, saying, "I-I-I want a n-n-new spoon-spoon-spoon." This is called **broken fluency** (repetition and prolongation of sounds, syllables, and words). It is often referred to as **secondary stuttering** because the child began to speak without this problem and then, during the preschool years, develops it. Unlike the adult who stutters, children are unaware that they are not being fluent unless it is called to their attention. You may need to remind parents that this is a part of normal development and, if accepted as such, will pass (Nippold & Packman, 2012). It is resolved most quickly if parents follow a few simple rules, including:

- Do not discuss in the child's presence that he or she is having difficulty with speech because this can make the child conscious of speech patterns and compound the problem.
- Listen with patience rather than interrupt or ask the child to speak more slowly or to start over. These actions make the child aware speech is repetitious, and broken fluency increases.
- Always talk to the child in a calm, simple way to role model slow speech. If adults talk quickly, the child imitates this pattern and has difficulty speaking clearly.
- Protect space for the child to talk if there are other children in the family. Rushing to say something before a second child interrupts is the same as rushing to conform to adult speech.
- Do not force a child to speak if he or she does not want to. Do not ask preschoolers to recite or sing for strangers.
- Do not reward a child for fluent speech or punish for nonfluent speech. Broken fluency is a developmental stage in language formation, not an indication of regression or a chronic speech pattern.

"Bathroom Language"

Many preschoolers imitate the vocabularies of their parents or older children in the family so well during this time that they incorporate swear words into their vocabularies if they hear these used. Parents may have to be reminded that children do not necessarily understand what the word they are using means; they have simply heard it, just as they have heard hundreds of other words and have decided to use it. Correction should be unemotional such as, "That's not a word I like to hear you say. When you're angry, why don't you say 'fudge' [or whatever]?" The correcting is no different from that involved when a child uses poor grammar. If parents become emotional, a child realizes the value of such a word and may continue using it for the attention it creates.

Concerns of the Family With a Preschooler With Unique Needs

Learning how to do things when you have physical or cognitive limitations can be very frustrating. A preschooler with a disability, however, has a greater need for problem-solving skills than the average child, because even simple procedures such as eating or getting dressed can be difficult if their physical challenge limits the options.

Physically challenged or chronically ill preschoolers should attend a preschool program if at all possible because of the

TABLE 31.5 Nursing Interventions to Encourage a Sense of Initiative in the Preschooler With Special Needs

Consideration	Nursing Actions
Nutrition	Serving toast or sandwiches cut into animal shapes with cookie cutters, cereal in the form of alphabet characters, or food arranged on a plate to make a face appeals to the imagination and may make a preschooler with a limited appetite more interested in eating. Respect the child's food preferences because trying to eat a nonfavorite food is difficult for everyone.
Dressing changes	Allow preschoolers to measure and cut tape or draw a face on it. Allow child to see the incision site. Explain the steps of dressing change as you work to reduce unknowns and areas of fear. Provide extra bandages to put on a doll so the child can see that bandages are not to be feared.
Medicine	Allow the child to choose a "chaser" such as juice or milk after oral medicine. Choosing a site for injection or intravenous line is too advanced for the preschooler; do not suggest such choices.
Rest	Provide a light in the room or bring the child's bed into the hallway so fear of the dark is reduced and the child can deal solely with problems based in the real world. Identify sounds the preschooler might hear in the hospital, such as an air conditioner turning on, and explain what these are.
Hygiene	Allow the child to choose bathtub toys and clothing to wear after a bath. Allow the child to wash his or her own hands and face. Allow the child to splash in water as a play activity as well as for cleanliness.
Pain	Encourage the preschooler to express pain. Allow the child to handle a syringe or suction catheter, and give "shots" or suction to a doll to alleviate anger or fear. Encourage the child to ask for analgesic if necessary.
Stimulation	Guessing games encourage a sense of initiative. Draw a dog or a house and ask the child to close his or her eyes while you add one more detail to the drawing, such as an ear or a chimney, then ask the child to identify the new item. Reverse the game and ask the child what you erased from the drawing, or allow the child to do his or her own drawing. Provide manipulative toys, such as finger paint, soapy water, clay, or dry cereal to use as sand. Allow the preschooler to accompany you to other departments is a way of teaching more about the hospital. Use "Simon Says" games not only for socialization but also to urge treatments, such as deep-breathing exercises. Encourage use of the playroom for socialization. Encourage the child to interact with his or her family by drawing pictures for siblings or telephoning home.

socialization benefits. If a child must remain in bed, parents may be reluctant to offer potentially messy experiences like finger paint. A large tray of dry oatmeal or other breakfast cereal with sand shovels or cars and trucks is a neater substitute activity for such a child. Although not necessarily tidy, these substances (which are available even in a hospital setting) can be vacuumed away easily at the finish of play. Table 31.5 lists nursing actions that can aid a chronically challenged child to solve problems and develop a sense of initiative.

Nutrition and the Preschooler With Special Needs

Experiences with eating help to reinforce a sense of initiative in preschoolers. Chronically ill preschoolers who are limited in the foods they can eat (e.g., perhaps they can eat only soft foods) or in their ability to help with food preparation may miss this reinforcement. If their appetite is diminished because of illness to the point where they take little or nothing orally, it is still important that they continue to join the family at meals if at all possible. In most households, this is a time for socialization, and preschoolers are ripe for the learning that goes with this type of daily interaction.

What if . . . 31.4 You are particularly interested in exploring one of the 2020 National Health Goals with respect to preschool growth and development (see Box 31.1). What would be a possible research topic to explore pertinent to this goal that would be applicable to Cathy's family and that would also advance evidence-based practice?

KEY POINTS FOR REVIEW

- Although preschoolers grow only slightly and gain just a little weight, they seem much taller than when they were toddlers because their contour changes to more childlike proportions.
- Erikson's developmental task for the preschool period is to gain a sense of initiative versus guilt, or to learn how to

do things. Play materials ideal for this age group are those that stimulate creativity, such as modeling clay or colored markers.

- Promoting childhood safety is a major role because preschoolers' active imaginations can lead them into dangerous situations; stressing this helps in planning nursing care that not only meets QSEN competencies but that also best meets a family's total needs.
- Common parental concerns during the preschool period are broken fluency, imaginary friends, difficulty sharing, and sibling rivalry. Preschoolers may develop a number of universal fears, such as fear of the dark, mutilation, and abandonment.
- The preschool age is often the time when a new sibling is born. Helping parents offer good preparation for this is necessary to prevent intense sibling rivalry.
- Preschoolers are still operating at a cognitive level that prevents them from understanding conservation (objects have not changed substance even if they have changed appearance).
- Preschoolers are self-centered (egocentric) so it is difficult for them to share and view someone else's side of a problem. They need good explanations of how a procedure will benefit them before they can agree to it.
- Many preschoolers begin preschool programs or child care. Late in the preschool period, they may be enrolled in kindergarten. Parents often appreciate guidance on how to prepare their children for these new experiences.
- Preschoolers who have special needs may have difficulty achieving a sense of initiative because they may be limited in their ability to participate in activities that stimulate initiative. They may need special playtimes set aside for stimulation and learning.

CRITICAL THINKING CARE STUDY

Calvin Saunders is a 4-year-old who lives with his single mom and 6-year-old brother, David. Calvin stays with his grandmother 2 days a week and with his father 3 days a week because his mother works full time in a local grocery store. His BMI is 27 (overweight).

1. At preschool, Calvin pushes and shoves other children rather than plays well with them. What suggestions could you make to his mother to improve his social relationships?
2. Calvin speaks with broken fluency. His mother jokes, "If he yelled 'fire,' we'd all burn to death before we understood him." She saw a movie where a king learned not to stutter by singing so, although it's expensive, she has enrolled Calvin in a boy's chorus. Is this her best approach to helping Calvin speak clearly?
3. Calvin's mother doesn't supervise Calvin or his older brother while they warm up snacks in the microwave. Is Calvin mature enough to do this independently?

Patient Scenario
The Tiffany Family

Read about the Tiffany family, a family with a preschooler, then answer the questions to further sharpen your skills and grow more familiar with NCLEX-type questions related to growth and development in the preschool-age child. Confirm your answers are correct by reading the rationales.

Visit http://thePoint.lww.com

Answers and Rationales

Looking for answers to the What if . . . and Critical Thinking Care Study questions?

Visit http://thePoint.lww.com

References

Agarwal, A., & Pruthi, M. (2010). Bicycle-spoke injuries of the foot in children. *Journal of Orthopedic Surgery, 18*(3), 338–341.

American Academy of Pediatrics. (2012). *Where we stand: Car seats for children.* Washington, DC: Author.

Bevan, A. L., & Reilly, S. M. (2011). Mothers' efforts to promote healthy nutrition and physical activity for their preschool children. *Nursing, 26*(5), 395–403.

Bowman, S. M., Aitken, M. E., Robbins, J. M., et al. (2012). Trends in US pediatric drowning hospitalizations, 1993–2008. *Pediatrics, 129*(2), 275–281.

Byars, K. C., Yolton, K., Rausch, J., et al. (2012). Prevalence, patterns, and persistence of sleep problems in the first 3 years of life. *Pediatrics, 129*(2), 276–284.

Centers for Disease Control and Prevention. (2011). National and state vaccination coverage among children aged 19–35 months—United States, 2010. *MMWR: Morbidity & Mortality Weekly Report, 60*(34), 1157–1163.

Centers for Disease Control and Prevention. (2012). *Injuries among children and adolescents.* Atlanta, GA: Author.

de Amorim Lde, F., Estrela, C., & da Costa, L. R. (2011). Effects of traumatic dental injuries to primary teeth on permanent teeth. *Dental Traumatology, 27*(2), 117–121.

Erikson, E. H. (1993). *Childhood & society.* New York, NY: W. W. Norton.

Erreich, A. (2011). More than enough guilt to go around: Oedipal guilt, survival guilt, separation guilt. *Journal of the American Psychoanalytical Association, 59*(1), 131–151.

Fergusson, D. M., Boden, J. M., & Horwood, L. J. (2013). Nine-year follow-up of a home-visitation program: A randomized trial. *Pediatrics, 131*(2), 297–303.

Garrison, M. M., & Christakis, D. A. (2012). The impact of a healthy media use intervention on sleep in preschool children. *Pediatrics, 130*(3), 492–499.

Goldman, R. D. (2012). Cranberry juice for urinary tract infection in children. *Canadian Family Physician, 58*(4), 398–401.

Gubbels, J. S., Van Kann, D. H., & Jansen, M. W. (2013). Play equipment, physical activity opportunities, and children's activity levels at childcare. *Journal of Environmental & Public Health,* 2012, 326520.

Hodges, E. A., Smith, C., Tidwell, S., et al. (2012). Promoting physical activity in preschoolers to prevent obesity. *Journal of Pediatric Nursing, 28*(1), 3–19.

Jonson-Reid, M., Kohl, P. L., & Drake, B. (2012). Child and adult outcomes of chronic child maltreatment. *Pediatrics, 129*(5), 839–845.

Kohlberg, L. (1984). *The psychology of moral development.* New York, NY: Harper & Row.

Kushnir, J., & Sadeh, A. (2011). Sleep of preschool children with nighttime fears. *Sleep Medicine, 12*(9), 870–874.

Linder, L. A., & Christian, B. J. (2011). Characteristics of the nighttime hospital bedside care environment (sound, light, and temperature) for children with cancer. *Cancer Nursing, 34*(3), 176–184.

Merlino, G., & Gigli, G. I. (2012). Sleep related movement disorders. *Neurological Sciences, 33*(3), 491–513.

Mitka, M. (2012). Programs to reduce childhood obesity seem to work, say Cochrane reviewers. *Journal of the American Medical Association, 307*(5), 444–445.

Nielsen, M. (2012). Imitation, pretend play, and childhood: Essential elements in the evolution of human culture? *Journal of Comparative Psychology, 126*(2), 170–181.

Nippold, M. A., & Packman, A. (2012). Managing stuttering beyond the preschool years. *Language, Speech & Hearing Services in Schools, 43*(3), 338–343.

Paulus, M., & Moore, C. (2012). Producing and understanding prosocial actions in early childhood. *Advances in Child Development & Behavior, 42*(8), 271–305.

Pérez-Fuentes, G., Olfson, M., Villegas, L., et al. (2012). Prevalence and correlates of child sexual abuse: A national study. *Comprehensive Psychiatry, 54*(1), 16–27.

Piaget, J. (1969). *The theory of stages in cognitive development.* New York, NY: McGraw-Hill.

Raman, L. (2011). Why do we eat? Children's and adults' understanding of why we eat different meals. *Journal of Genetic Psychology, 172*(4), 401–413.

Senger, C., Keijzer, R., Smith, G., et al. (2011). Pediatric firearm injuries: A 10-year single-center experience of 194 patients. *Journal of Pediatric Surgery, 46*(5), 927–932.

Smith, S. (2011). Vulvovaginitis. In K. J. Marcdante, R. M. Kliegman, H. B. Jenson, et al. (Eds.), *Nelson essentials of pediatrics* (6th ed., pp. 415–416). Philadelphia, PA: Saunders/Elsevier.

Smith, G. A., & Riedford, K. (2012). Epidemiology of early childhood caries: Clinical application. *Journal of Pediatric Nursing.* Advance online publication.

Snowling, M. J. (2011). Editorial: What's behind sibling rivalry: Checks and balances in the sibling relationship. *Journal of Child Psychology & Psychiatry & Allied Disciplines, 52*(6), 629–630.

Sun, Y., & Sundell, J. (2011). Early daycare attendance increases the risk for respiratory infections and asthma of children. *Journal of Asthma, 48*(8), 790–796.

Sutherland, S. L., & Friedman, O. (2012). Preschoolers acquire general knowledge by sharing in pretense. *Child Development, 83*(3), 1064–1071.

Talwar, V., & Crossman, A. (2011). From little white lies to filthy liars: The evolution of honesty and deception in young children. *Advances in Child Development & Behavior, 40*(4), 139–179.

Tubert-Jeannin, S., Auclair, C., Amsallem, E., et al. (2011). Fluoride supplements (tablets, drops, lozenges or chewing gums) for preventing dental caries in children. *Cochrane Database of Systematic Reviews, 2011*(12), CD007592.

U.S. Department of Agriculture. (2012). *Choose my plate: A guide to daily food choices*. Washington, DC: Author.

U.S. Department of Health and Human Services. (2010). *Healthy people 2020.* Washington, DC: Author.

Volling, B. L. (2012). Family transitions following the birth of a sibling: An empirical review of changes in the firstborn's adjustment. *Psychology Bulletin, 138*(3), 497–528.

Whitney, E. N., & Rolfes, S. R. (2013). Life cycle nutrition: Infancy, childhood and adolescence. In E. N. Whitney & S. R. Rolfes, *Understanding nutrition* (13th ed., pp. 504–550). New York, NY: Wadsworth/Cengage Learning.

Wrobel, S. (2012). From threat to opportunity: A Head Start program's response to state-funded pre-K. *Journal of Health &Human Services Administration, 35*(1), 74–105.

Yilmaz, G., Caylan, N. D., & Karacan, C. D. (2012). Effects of active and passive smoking on ear infections. *Current Infectious Disease Reports.* Advance online publication.

Chapter 32

Nursing Care of a Family With a School-Age Child

KEY TERMS

- accommodation
- caries
- class inclusion
- conservation
- decentering
- malocclusion
- nocturnal emissions

OBJECTIVES

After mastering the contents of this chapter, you should be able to:

1. Describe the normal growth and development pattern and common parental concerns of the school-age period.
2. Identify 2020 National Health Goals related to school-age children that nurses can help the nation achieve.
3. Assess a school-age child for normal growth and development milestones.
4. Formulate nursing diagnoses related to both school-age children and their families.
5. Establish expected outcomes for nursing care of school-age children to help children and parents manage seamless transitions across differing health care settings.
6. Using the nursing process, plan nursing care that includes the six competencies of Quality & Safety Education for Nurses (QSEN): Patient-Centered Care, Teamwork & Collaboration, Evidence-Based Practice (EBP), Quality Improvement (QI), Safety, and Informatics.
7. Implement nursing care to help achieve normal growth and development of a school-age child, such as counseling parents about helping their child adjust to a new school.
8. Evaluate expected outcomes for achievement and effectiveness of care.
9. Integrate knowledge of growth and development in school-age children with the interplay of nursing process, the six competencies of QSEN, and Family Nursing to promote quality maternal and child health nursing care.

Shelly Lewis is an 11-year-old girl who recently started middle school. Her mother tells you that Shelly, who is overweight, says she likes school and wants to try out for cheerleading, but she has developed a lot of nervous habits such as nail biting since she started attending her new school. Her mother asks you if this is "normal."

The previous chapter discussed the preschooler and the abilities children develop in those years. This chapter adds information about the changes, both physical and psychosocial, that occur during the school-age years. Such information builds a base for care and health teaching for this age group.

How would you advise Shelly's mother?

The term "school age" commonly refers to children between the ages of 6 and 12 years. Although these years represent a time of slow physical growth, cognitive growth and development continue to proceed at rapid rates. Because of this, there are many differences among children at each year of this age group. For example, 7- and 10-year-old children have very different needs and outlooks than do 11- and 12-year-old children. Because of these big differences, always assess children as individuals to understand the particular developmental needs of each child based on what developmental status has been achieved, not on what stage you think the child should have reached (Lowe, Godoy, Rhodes, et al., 2013).

Unlike the infant or toddler periods, when progress is marked by obvious new abilities and skills such as the ability to sit up or roll over or the ability to speak a full sentence, the development of a school-age child is much more subtle and may be marked by irregular mood swings; what the child enjoys on one occasion may not be acceptable on the next. For instance, a child may ask his parents for a guitar and lessons, but then after the family invests in these, he may quickly lose interest in music and prefer soccer. School-age children are also more influenced by the attitudes of their friends than previously. They may choose not to do something that was previously enjoyable because no friends are interested in the activity.

Parents who make too much of these likes and dislikes may find themselves engaged in unnecessary conflicts with their child. The school-age period is usually the first time children begin to make truly independent judgments. Because parents may not be prepared for this, additional conflicts with parents may develop. Box 32.1 lists 2020 National Health Goals related to the school-age period.

BOX 32.1 Nursing Care Planning Based on 2020 National Health Goals

A number of 2020 National Health Goals address the health of the school-age population:

- Increase the proportion of public and private schools that require daily physical education for elementary school students, from a baseline of 3.8% to a target of 4.2%; for middle school students, from 7.9% to 8.6%.
- Increase the proportion of public and private schools that require students to wear appropriate protective gear when engaged in school-sponsored physical activities from 76.8% to 84.5%.
- Reduce the proportion of children who have dental caries (in permanent or primary teeth) to no more than 49% from a baseline of 54.4%.
- Increase age-appropriate vehicle restraint system use in children from 78% to 86%.
- Increase the number of states that require helmet use by bicyclists from 19 to 27 states (U.S. Department of Health and Human Services [DHHS], 2010; see www.healthypeople.gov).

Nurses can help the nation achieve these goals by urging children to begin and maintain a consistent exercise program, to brush teeth and go for dental checkups regularly, and to follow safety rules for bicycles and automobiles.

Nursing Process Overview
For Healthy Development of a School-Age Child

Assessment

Use both history and physical examination to assess growth and development of school-age children. Include questions about school activities and progress. School-age children are interested and able to contribute to their own health history; to allow for this, it is useful to interview children 10 years or older, at least in part, without their parents present. During a physical examination, show your respect for children's adult-level modesty by furnishing a cover gown.

Parents of school-age children often mention behavioral issues or conflicts during yearly health visits. They may feel they are losing contact with their child during these years or are surprised by a particular behavior as their child begins to express more opinions and values.

In some instances, it may be necessary to obtain the opinion of school personnel (with the parents' permission) regarding a problem or even to just determine whether school personnel feel a problem exists. In some instances, a counselor's opinion may be necessary. If the problem is related to a medical condition, its effect on the family should also be assessed, because the illness of a child affects the functioning of the entire family.

Nursing Diagnosis

Common nursing diagnoses pertinent to growth and development during the school-age period include:

- Health-seeking behaviors related to normal school-age growth and development
- Readiness for enhanced parenting related to improved family living conditions
- Anxiety related to slow growth pattern of child
- Risk for injury related to deficient parental knowledge about safety precautions for a school-age child

Outcome Identification and Planning

When identifying expected outcomes and planning care, keep in mind that school-age children tend to enjoy small or short-term projects rather than long, involved ones. In her early school years, a child with diabetes, for example, may gain a feeling of achievement by learning to assess her own serum glucose level, but she may have difficulty continuing glucose assessments on a regular basis.

Behavior problems need to be well defined before outcomes are identified and interventions planned. Often, it is enough for parents to accept the problem as one consistent with normal growth and development. Helpful Web sites to recommend to parents to learn more about school-age growth and development are the American Academy of Pediatrics (AAP, www.aap.org) and the Centers for Disease Control and Prevention (CDC, www.CDC.gov). For questions about car restraints, parents can consult the CDC (http://www.cdc.gov/MotorVehicleSafety/Child_Passenger_Safety/CPS-Factsheet.html). For a discussion of cyberbullying, a good site to access is www.cyberbullying.us.

Implementation
School-age children are interested in learning about adult roles, so this means they will watch you to note your attitude as well as your actions in a given situation. When giving care, keep in mind that children this age feel more comfortable if they know the "hows" and "whys" of actions. This means that they may not cooperate with a procedure until they are given a satisfactory explanation of why it must be done.

Outcome Evaluation
Yearly health visits covering both physical and psychosocial development are important at this age. It may be useful for parents to look back on problems identified at the last visit and discuss if and how they were resolved. Often, some problems and conflicts fade away without anyone really noticing. As some problems recede, however, others may emerge. Make sure no underlying problem exists that prevents resolution. Examples of expected outcomes include:

- Parent states that he allows the child to make his own decisions (within acceptable limits) about how to spend an allowance.
- Child lists books she and her parents have read together in the past 2 weeks.
- Child states he understands his growth is within the usual guidelines, even though he is the shortest boy in his eighth-grade class.
- Child does not sustain injuries from sports activities during the summer recess.

GROWTH AND DEVELOPMENT OF A SCHOOL-AGE CHILD

The school-age period is a relatively long time span, and even though growth is slow, children grow and develop extensively during this time period.

Physical Growth

The average annual weight gain for a school-age child is approximately 3 to 5 lb (1.3 to 2.2 kg); the increase in height is 1 to 2 in. (2.5 to 5 cm). Children who did not lose a lordosis and knock-kneed appearance during the preschool period lose this now.

By 10 years of age, brain growth is complete, so fine motor coordination becomes refined. As the eye globe reaches its final shape at about this same time, an adult vision level is achieved. If the eruption of permanent teeth and growth of the jaw do not correlate with final head growth, malocclusion with teeth malalignment may be present (El-Dawlatly, Fayed, & Mostafa, 2012).

The immune globulins IgG and IgA each reach adult levels, and lymphatic tissue continues to grow in size until about age 9 years. The resulting abundance of tonsillar and adenoid tissue in early school children is often mistaken for disease because the tonsils seem to fill the entire back of the throat. This may also result in temporary conduction deafness from eustachian tube obstruction until the tissue recedes normally. The appendix is also lined with lymphatic tissue, so swelling of this tissue in the narrow tube can lead to trapped fecal material and inflammation (appendicitis) in the early school-age child (Bishop, 2011). Frontal sinuses develop at about 6 years, so sinus headaches become a possibility (before then, a headache in children is rarely caused by a sinus infection) (Smith, 2011).

The left ventricle of the heart enlarges to be strong enough to pump blood to the growing body. Innocent heart murmurs may become apparent due to this extra blood crossing heart valves. The pulse rate decreases to 70 to 80 beats/min; blood pressure rises to about 112/60 mmHg. Maturation of the respiratory system leads to increased oxygen–carbon dioxide exchange, which increases exertion ability and stamina. Scoliosis may become apparent for the first time in late childhood (Fletcher & Bruce, 2012). All school-age children over 8 years should be screened for this at all health appraisals (see Chapter 51).

Sexual Maturation

At a set point in brain maturity, the hypothalamus transmits an enzyme to the anterior pituitary gland to begin production of gonadotropic hormones, which then activate changes in the testes and ovaries to cause puberty. Hormone changes that occur with puberty are discussed in detail in Chapter 5. Table 32.1 describes the usual order in which secondary sex characteristics develop.

Timing of the onset of puberty varies widely, between 8 and 14 years of age (Edmonds, 2012), partly due to genetic and cultural differences, and is rated according to Tanner stages (shown in Chapter 33). The length of time it takes to pass through puberty until sexual maturity is complete also varies. Sexual maturation in girls usually occurs between the years of 12 and 18; in boys, between 14 and 20 years. Puberty is occurring increasingly earlier, however, and, in a class of 11-year-old sixth graders, it is not unusual to discover more than half of the girls are already menstruating. This change in the onset of puberty is important because it means, for sex education to be effective, parents or schools must introduce this material as early as when their children are in grade school. Precocious puberty is an abnormal onset of puberty and is discussed in Chapter 47.

Sexual and Physical Concerns. The changes in physical appearance that come with puberty can lead to concerns for both children and their parents. The school-age period is a time for parents to discuss with children the physical changes that will occur and the sexual responsibility these changes dictate. This is also a time to reinforce previous teaching with children that their body is their own, to be used only in the way they choose. Specific measures for children to help prevent sexual maltreatment are discussed later in this chapter. Nurses can play a major role in this type of education (Daley, 2011).

In both sexes, puberty brings changes in the sebaceous glands. Under the influence of androgen, glands become more active, setting the stage for acne (see Chapter 33). Vasomotor instability commonly leads to blushing; perspiration also increases.

Concerns of Girls. Prepubertal girls are usually taller by about 2 in. (5 cm) or more than preadolescent boys because their typical growth spurt begins earlier. In a culture in which boys are expected to be taller than girls, this can cause concern. Sometimes a girl notices the change in her pelvic contour

TABLE 32.1 Chronologic Development of Secondary Sex Characteristics

Age (in Years)	Boys	Girls
9–11	Prepubertal weight gain occurs.	Breasts: Elevation of papilla with breast bud formation; areolar diameter enlarges.
11–12	Sparse growth of straight, downy, slightly pigmented hair at base of penis. Scrotum becomes textured; growth of penis and testes begins. Sebaceous gland secretion increases. Perspiration increases.	Straight hair along the labia. Vaginal epithelium becomes cornified. pH of vaginal secretions becomes acidic; slight mucous vaginal discharge is present. Sebaceous gland secretion increases. Perspiration increases. Dramatic growth spurt.
12–13	Pubic hair present across pubis. Penis lengthens. Dramatic linear growth spurt. Breast enlargement may occur.	Pubic hair grows darker; spreads over entire pubis. Breasts enlarge, still no protrusion of nipples. Axillary hair present. Menarche occurs.

when she tries on a skirt or dress from the year before and realizes her hips are becoming broader. She may misinterpret this finding as a gain in weight and attempt a crash diet. You can assure her that broad bone structure of the hips is part of an adult female profile.

Girls are usually conscious of breast development. A girl who develops ahead of her peers may tend to slouch or wear loose clothing to hide the size of her breasts. Another girl studies herself in a mirror and wonders whether her breasts are going to develop enough. Breast development is not always symmetrical, so it is not unusual for a girl to have breasts of slightly different sizes. After the condition has been checked during a physical examination to assure her that no tumors are present to make one breast larger or that the other is diseased in some way to make it smaller, she can be reassured this development is normal. Supernumerary (additional) nipples may darken or increase in size at puberty. Be sure girls understand that a supernumerary nipple is affected by the hormones in her body in the same way as other breast tissue, so she isn't frightened by the accessory nipple enlarging with puberty or in a future pregnancy.

Early preparation for menstruation is an important preparation for future childbearing and for a girl's concept of herself as a woman (Marván & Molina-Abolnik, 2012) (Box 32.2). A girl who is told menstruation is a normal function that occurs every month in all healthy women has a different attitude toward her body than a girl who wakes up one morning to find blood on her pajamas and is told bluntly, "You'd better get used to that. You'll have to put up with it for the rest of your life." In the first instance, the girl can trust her body: it is doing what every woman's body does. In the second instance, the girl may feel her body is out of control. How can she accept and enjoy growing up if it involves something so unpredictable?

In addition to an explanation of the reason for menstrual flow, girls need an explanation of good hygiene and reassurance they can bathe, shower, and swim during their periods. They can use either sanitary napkins or tampons; if they choose tampons, they must take precautions to avoid toxic shock syndrome (see Chapter 47).

Girls also need to know that vaginal secretions will begin to be present. If this is not explained, a girl may fear needlessly she has contracted an infection. Explain that any secretions that cause vulvar irritation should be evaluated by a health care provider, because this does suggest infection.

Most girls have some menstrual irregularity during the first year or two after menarche (the start of menstruation). This occurs primarily because a girl's cycles are at first anovulatory. With added maturity and the onset of ovulation, cycles become more regular.

Irregular periods can cause concern because girls need to know when their periods will occur so they can get used to this new phenomenon and learn to trust their bodies (Horne & Critchley, 2012). A girl in college can explain matter-of-factly that she prefers not to go to the beach because she is having her period, but for a preadolescent, this topic may be too sophisticated and too emotionally charged to discuss openly. Preteenagers want to be able to plan activities to avoid having to make such explanations.

This means that menstrual irregularity can be a significant concern for preadolescents. A girl may fear that irregular periods indicate a hormone imbalance. She may worry about her future ability to conceive, or she may be ill informed about how conception occurs and may fear irregularity of her periods means that she is pregnant. Both malnourishment and obesity possibly influence menstrual regularity. Emotions can also affect consistent cycles. If irregularity continues beyond the first year, a careful history of the girl's nutrition; overall health; and school, social, and home adjustment should be taken. Dysmenorrhea, or painful menstruation, is discussed in Chapter 47.

For a nominal charge, manufacturers of sanitary napkins or tampons will mail an introductory kit of their products, together with well-illustrated, factual booklets, to introduce girls to menstruation. Such kits are useful if they supplement a parent's or a nurse's discussion, but they should not take the place of individual attention.

Concerns of Boys. Boys who are not prepared for the physical changes of puberty worry about them in the same way as girls. Just as girls become keenly aware of breast development, boys

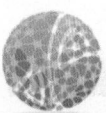

BOX 32.2 Nursing Care Planning Based on Effective Communication

Shelly, 11 years old, comes into the nurse's office at her school.

Less Effective Communication

Nurse: Hello, Shelly. What can I do for you?
Shelly: I'm having cramps.
Nurse: Are you having your period?
Shelly: No. I haven't started them yet.
Nurse: Can you describe your cramps to me?
Shelly: Both my sisters started their periods when they were 10.
Nurse: Are you sick to your stomach?
Shelly: I'm the only girl in my gym class who doesn't have her period yet.
Nurse: Let's talk about the cramps. What do you think is causing those?
Shelly: They're not really bad. I'll go back to class.

More Effective Communication

Nurse: Hello, Shelly. What can I do for you?
Shelly: I'm having cramps.
Nurse: Are you having your period?
Shelly: No. I haven't started them yet.
Nurse: Can you describe your cramps to me?
Shelly: Both my sisters started their periods when they were 10.
Nurse: Are you sick to your stomach?
Shelly: I'm the only girl in my gym class who doesn't have her period yet.
Nurse: You sound as if you're more worried about that than what you came in for.
Shelly: I need to know why I'm so different. Will I be able to have children?
Nurse: Let's talk about that.

In the past, when topics such as menstruation were discussed only in whispers and neither television nor magazines advertised tampons or medicine for menstrual discomfort, most 11-year-old children had little idea about what to expect at puberty. Today, with this information readily available, it is easy to forget that preadolescents still may not know much about what to expect at puberty. Through effective communication and listening, you can help them talk about their problems and concerns.

become aware of increasing genital size. If they do not know testicular development precedes penis growth, they can worry that their growth will be inadequate.

Hypertrophy of breast tissue (gynecomastia) can occur in prepubescent boys, most often in those who are stocky or obese. A youth with this condition may be concerned a breast tumor is present or may feel embarrassed about his growing breasts. He can be assured that this is a transitory phenomenon and, although it makes him self-conscious, will fade as soon as his male hormones become more mature and active.

Some boys can also become concerned because, although they have pubic hair, they cannot yet grow a beard or do not have chest hair, which are outward, easily recognized signs of maturity. You can assure them that pubic hair normally appears first, and that chest and facial hair may not grow until several years later.

As increased seminal fluid begins to be produced, boys begin to notice ejaculation during sleep, termed **nocturnal emissions** (Widaman & Helm, 2012). Preadolescent boys may believe the old myth that loss of seminal fluid is debilitating; also, boys may have heard the term "premature ejaculation" and worry this is a forewarning of a problem in years to come. Both are fallacies.

Teeth

Deciduous teeth are lost and permanent teeth erupt during the school-age period (Fig. 32.1). Because of this, the average child gains 28 teeth between 6 and 12 years of age: the central and lateral incisors; first, second, and third cuspids; and first and second molars (Fig. 32.2).

Developmental Milestones

As with all ages, you can measure school-age children's progress by whether they meet typical developmental milestones.

Gross Motor Development

School-age development is summarized in Table 32.2. At the beginning of the school-age period (age 6 years), children

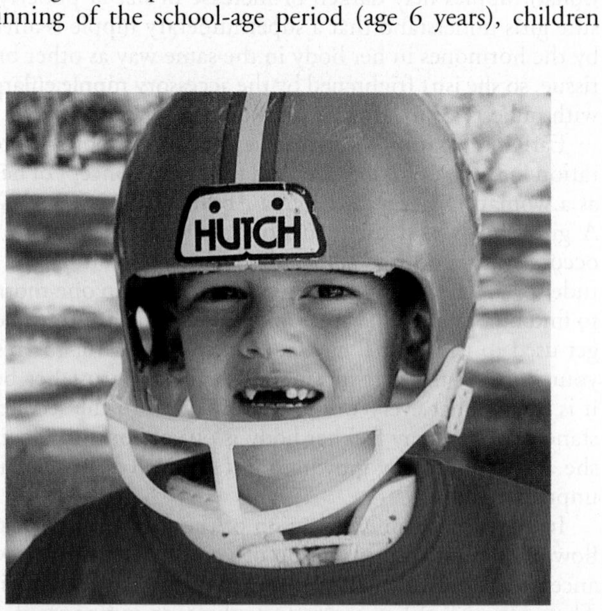

FIGURE 32.1 Early school-age children typically have a missing upper incisor as deciduous teeth are replaced by permanent teeth.

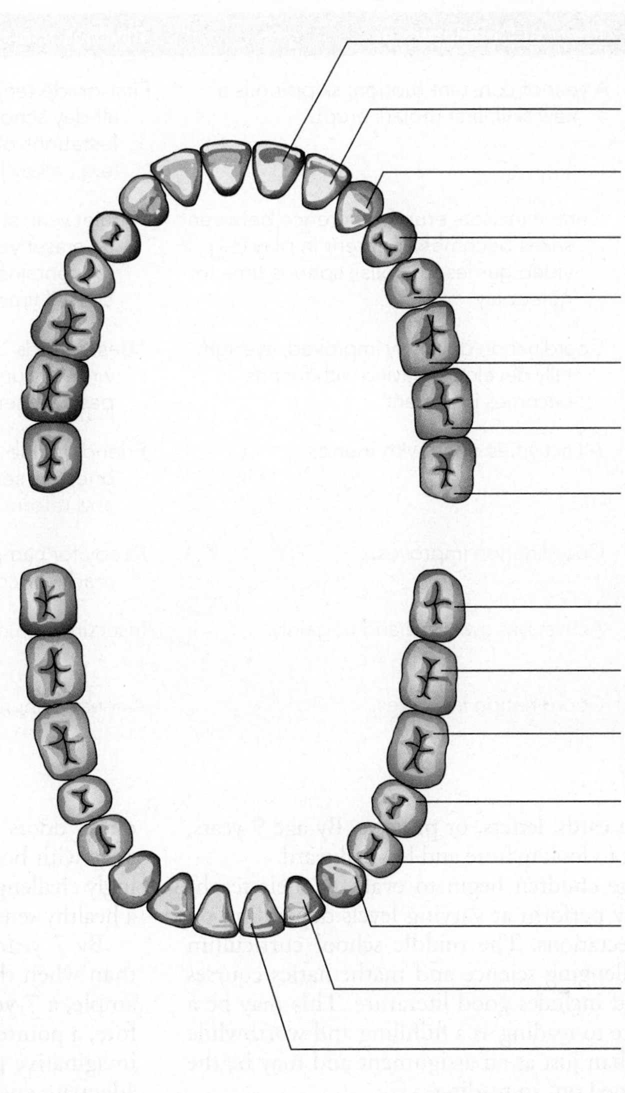

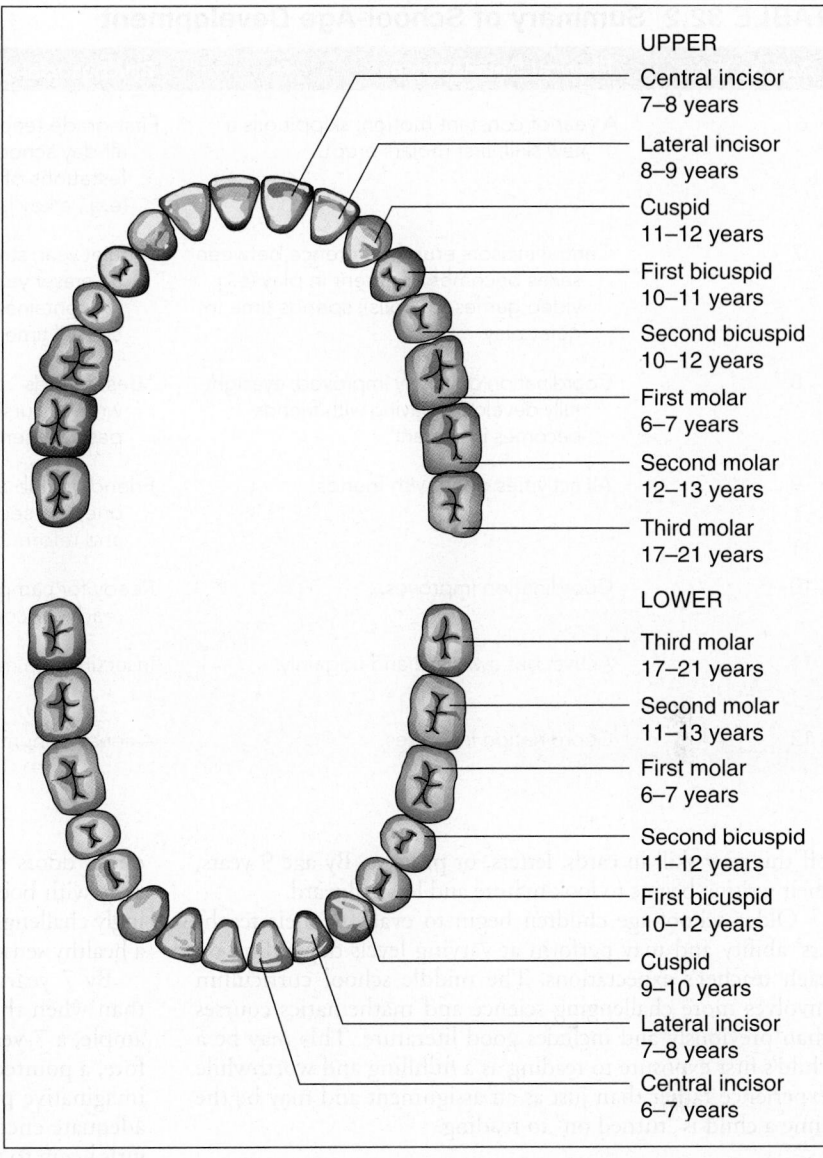

FIGURE 32.2 The eruption pattern of permanent teeth.

endlessly jump, tumble, skip, and hop. They have enough coordination to walk a straight line, many can ride a bicycle, and they learn to skip rope with practice.

A 7-year-old child appears quiet compared with a rough-and-tumble 6-year-old. Gender differences usually begin to manifest themselves in play: "girl games," such as dressing dolls, and "boy games," such as pretending to be pirates, develop.

The movements of 8-year-olds are more graceful than those of younger children, although, as their arms and legs grow, they may stumble on furniture or spill milk and food. They ride a bicycle well and enjoy sports such as gymnastics, soccer, and hockey.

Nine-year-olds are on the go constantly, as if they always have a deadline to meet. They have enough eye–hand coordination to enjoy baseball, basketball, and volleyball. By 10 years of age, children are more interested in perfecting their athletic skills than they were previously.

At 11 years of age, many children feel awkward because of their growth spurt and drop out of sports activities rather than look ungainly attempting them. They may channel their energy into constant motion instead: drumming fingers and tapping pencils or feet. This fall in sports participation may bother parents who see sports as the key to popularity, self-esteem, fitness, and teamwork.

Twelve-year-olds plunge into activities with intensity and concentration. They often enjoy participating in sports events for charities such as walkathons. They may be refreshingly cooperative around the house, able to handle a great deal of responsibility and complete given tasks.

Fine Motor Development

Six-year-olds can easily tie their shoelaces. They can cut and paste well and draw a person with good detail. They can print, although they may routinely reverse letters. Seven-year-olds concentrate on fine motor skills even more than they did the year before. This has been called the "eraser year" because children are never quite content with what they have done. They set too high a standard for themselves and then have difficulty performing at that level.

By 8 years of age, children's eyes are developed enough so they can read regular-size type. This can make reading a greater pleasure and school more enjoyable (Fig. 32.3). Eight-year-olds are able to write script in addition to print. They enjoy showing

TABLE 32.2 Summary of School-Age Development

Age (in Years)	Physical Development	Psychosocial and Cognitive Development
6	A year of constant motion; skipping is a new skill; first molars erupt.	First-grade teacher becomes authority figure; adjustment to all-day school may be difficult and may lead to nervous manifestations of fingernail biting, etc. Defines words by their use (e.g., a key is to unlock a door, not a metal object).
7	Central incisors erupt; difference between sexes becomes apparent in play (e.g., video games vs. dolls); spends time in quiet play.	A quiet year; striving for perfection leads to this year being called an eraser year. Learns conservation (e.g., water poured from tall container to a wide, flat one is the same amount of water); can tell time; can make simple change.
8	Coordination definitely improved; eyesight fully develops; playing with friends becomes important.	"Best friends" develop; whispering and giggling begin; can write in cursive as well as print; understands concepts of past, present, and future.
9	All activities done with friends.	Friend or club age; a 9-year-old club is formed to spite someone, has secret codes, is all boy or all girl; clubs disband and reform quickly.
10	Coordination improves.	Ready for camp away from home; collecting age; likes rules; ready for competitive games.
11	Active, but awkward and ungainly.	Insecure with members of opposite sex; repeats off-color jokes.
12	Coordination improves.	A sense of humor is present; is social and cooperative.

off this new skill in cards, letters, or projects. By age 9 years, their writing begins to look mature and less awkward.

Older school-age children begin to evaluate their teachers' ability and may perform at varying levels depending on each teacher's expectations. The middle school curriculum involves more challenging science and mathematics courses than previously and includes good literature. This may be a child's first exposure to reading as a fulfilling and worthwhile experience rather than just as an assignment and may be the time a child is "turned on" to reading.

Play

Play continues to be rough and tumble at age 6 years; however, when children discover reading as an enjoyable activity that opens doors to other worlds, they can begin to spend quiet time with books. Many children spend hours playing increasingly challenging video games, an activity that can either foster a healthy sense of competition or create isolation from others.

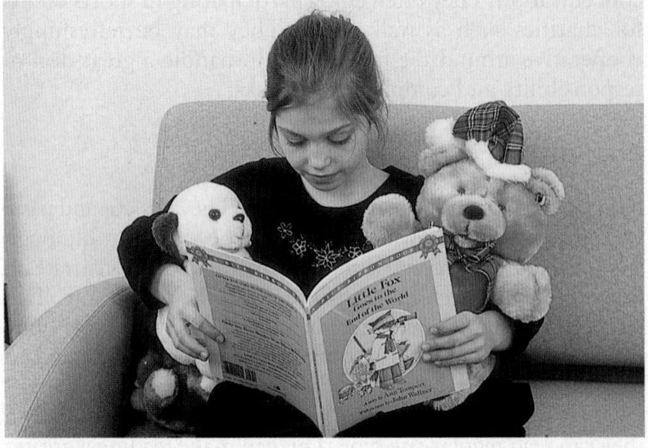

FIGURE 32.3 One of the biggest discoveries of childhood is that reading and writing are fun. These are activities that can help a child pass the hours during an illness.

By 7 years of age, children require more props for play than when they were younger. To be a police officer, for example, a 7-year-old may need a badge and gun, whereas before, a pointed finger sufficed. This is the start of a decline in imaginative play, which will continue unless a child receives adequate encouragement to use imagination. At age 7 years, girls begin to prefer teenage dolls if they didn't previously, and their coordination is good enough that they can button the miniature dresses and pull on the tiny boots.

Around 7 years of age, children also develop an interest in collecting items such as baseball cards, dolls, rocks, or marbles. The type of item is not as important as the quantity. These collections become structured as a child reaches 8 years of age; time is spent sorting and cataloging. Most girls and boys of this age also enjoy helping in the kitchen with jobs such as making cookies and salads or frosting cakes. They start to be more involved in simple science projects and experiments. Eight-year-olds also like table games but hate to lose, so they tend to avoid competitive games. They may change the rules in the middle of a game to keep from losing.

Nine-year-olds play hard. They wake in the morning, squeeze in some activity before school, and plan something the moment they arrive home again. They may have difficulty going to bed at night because they want to play just one more game. Play is rough; children are not as interested in perfecting their skills as they will be in another year. Some parents or coaches expect children of this age to be more interested in perfecting their skills, so conflicts can arise.

Many schools begin music lessons for children at about 9 years of age. Children do well if others in their group are

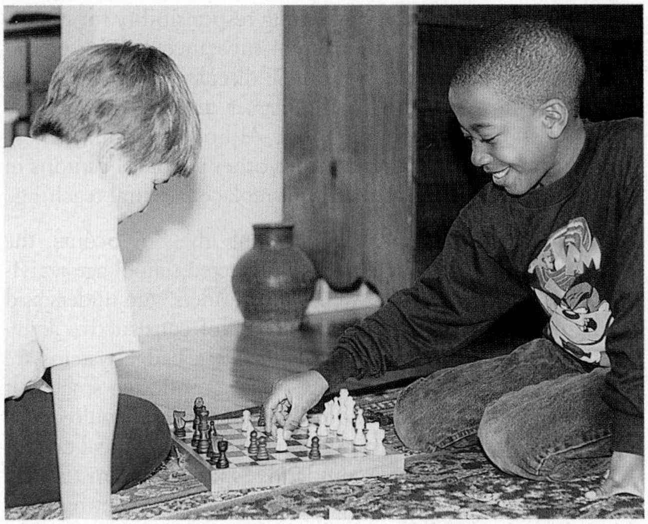

FIGURE 32.4 By 10 years of age, children are ready for competition. These two children enjoy a game of chess.

taking similar lessons. Talent for music or art becomes evident, and children respond with new interest in school or wherever they are exposed to these arts. Nine years of age is also a time when children discover that there are other children on the Internet who are waiting to talk to them in chat rooms or other social media. Because they are not yet wise enough to recognize the dangers that talking to strangers can create, this is an activity parents need to supervise (Briggs, Simon, & Simonsen, 2011).

Many 10-year-olds spend most of their time playing handheld or console games. Boys and girls play separately at age 10 years, although interest in the opposite sex is apparent. Boys show off as girls pass their group; girls talk loudly or giggle at the sight of a familiar boy. Girls become more interested in the way they look and dress. Slumber parties and campouts become increasingly popular. Children talk, giggle, and roughhouse into the middle of the night.

During their 10th year, children become very interested in rules and fairness. Before this time, they gave younger children breaks in games, allowing extra turns or hints. Now they strictly enforce rules (Fig. 32.4). Club activities become structured, with a president, a secretary, and rules of order.

Children age 11 and 12 years enjoy dancing to popular music and playing table games; they are accommodating enough again to be able to play with younger siblings who need the rules modified to their advantage. Time with friends is often spent just talking. If older school-age children use their bedroom as a place to meet with friends, they become more interested in seeing it is tidy. Twelve-year-olds typically like to do jobs such as raking leaves or babysitting for money. Both boys and girls seem to feel they are on the verge of something great and anxiously wait to turn 13 years old and become teenagers.

Language Development

Six-year-olds talk in full sentences, using language easily and with meaning. They no longer sound as though talking is an experiment but appear to have incorporated language permanently. They still define objects by their use (e.g., a key is to unlock a door, a fork is to eat with).

Most 7-year-olds can tell the time in hours, but they may have trouble with concepts such as "half past" and "quarter to," especially with the prevalence of digital clocks. They know the months of the year and can name the months in which holidays fall. They can add and subtract and make simple change (if they have had experience), so they can go with a parent to a store and make simple purchases. Much of children's talk is concerned with these concepts as they practice them and show them off for family or friends.

Because children discover "dirty" jokes at about age 9 years, they like to tell them to friends or try to understand those told by adults. They use swear words to express anger or just to show other children that they are growing up. They may have a short period of intense fascination with "bathroom language," as they did during the preschool years. As before, if parents want to discourage this, it should be made clear that they find such language unacceptable and they refrain from using it themselves in their child's presence.

By 12 years of age, children can carry on an adult conversation, although stories are limited because of a lack of experience.

Emotional Development

Ideally, children enter the school-age period with the ability to trust others and with a sense of respect for their own worth. They can accomplish small tasks independently because they have gained a sense of autonomy. They should have practiced or mimicked adult roles, learned to share, discovered that learning is an adventure, and grasped the idea that doing things is more important and more rewarding than watching things being done (a sense of initiative).

Developmental Task: Industry Versus Inferiority

During the early school years, children attempt to master their new developmental step: learning a sense of industry or accomplishment (Erikson, 1993). If gaining a sense of initiative can be defined as learning how to do things, then gaining a sense of industry is learning how to do things well.

If children are prevented from achieving a sense of industry or do not receive rewards for accomplishment, they can develop a feeling of inferiority or become convinced they cannot do things they actually can do. These children can have difficulty tackling new situations later in life (e.g., new job, new school, new responsibility) because they cannot envision how they will be successful in handling them. This can result in frustration in school or work activities.

The questions a preschool child asks reflect curiosity, such as "how," "why," and "what." During the early school years, children concentrate their questions on the "how" of tasks: "Is this the right way to do this?" "Am I making this right?" and "Is this good?" Often, school-age children will comment, "I can't do anything right" because their craft project falls short of expectations. School-age children need reassurance that they are doing things correctly and this reassurance is best if it comes immediately after a task is completed.

The books preferred by school-age children have many short chapters; children experience a sense of accomplishment as they finish each chapter. Small chores that can be completed quickly also give this type of reward. Children can survey their finished work and see they have done a good job. A child may dislike vacuuming, for instance, because the rug may not look very different when the task is complete. Picking up the scattered contents of a toy box, however, is a task that clearly makes a difference in the appearance of the room and so offers a reward.

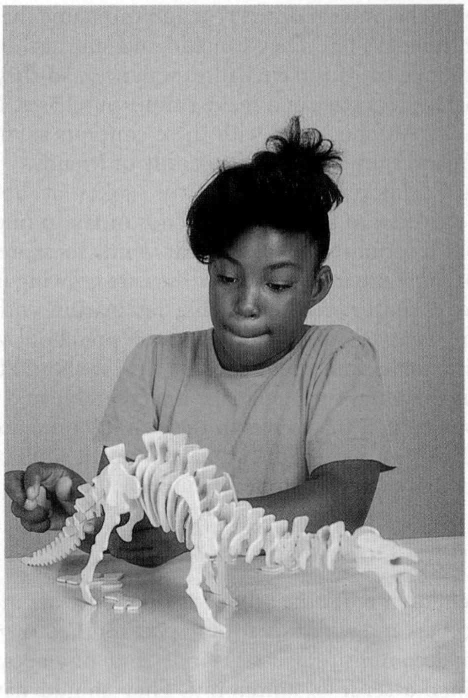

FIGURE 32.5 Assembling this simple model in a short time helps a school-age child gain a sense of industry. (© Stephen Frisch/Stock Boston.)

Hobbies and projects also are enjoyed best if they are small and can be finished within a short time. Most school-age children, for example, prefer putting together two or three fairly simple model-car kits to assembling one extremely complicated kit. The three kits offer three rewards, whereas the involved one delays the reward so long that the child may become bored and never complete it. With adolescence will come more respect for quality. Teenagers realize that if they want the better model, they will have to spend the extra energy and attention and that quality products involve quality work (Fig. 32.5).

Home as a Setting to Learn Industry. Parents of a school-age child may need to take a step forward in development along with their child. For the first time, they realize their child has begun to look to other role models than themselves. Parents who enjoyed fostering imagination in a preschooler may feel frustrated when a school-age child chooses to conform to rules and insists on the "right way" to do things. They may feel they have failed to encourage the child's creativity, but conformity is vital to children at this age. It is how they learn more about their world's rules.

Children 8 or 9 years of age begin to spend more and more time with their peers and less time with their family. They forget to do household chores they once enjoyed, such as setting the table or mowing the lawn, or they may do the work sloppily so they have more time to spend with their friends. Although this may seem like a regression in behavior, it is actually a step of independence away from the parents and into the larger world, a developmental step toward helping them become emotionally mature. This is an example of a new role the child is trying out, one of many that will be tried in the process of reaching maturity, when an eventual "right fit" is found.

School as a Setting to Learn Industry. Adjusting to and achieving in school are two of the major tasks for this age group. Ideally, a child's teacher will think of learning as fun and will encourage a child to plunge into new experiences.

Schools are increasingly assuming responsibility for education about sex, safety, avoidance of substances of abuse, and preparation for family living. These discussions are generally superficial, however, and if the classes are large, may raise more questions than they answer. Although learning these skills with peers helps children learn other people's opinions in these areas, such classes should not replace parental teaching.

Structured Activities. The Girl Scouts, the Boy Scouts, the Campfire Girls, and 4-H clubs are respected school-age activities. If the local chapters are well run by leaders who understand children's needs, they can provide hours of constructive activity and strengthen a sense of industry. Merit badge systems are geared to the needs of school-age children, offering small but frequent rewards. As with school activities, parents should determine the worth of each organization for their individual child.

Urge parents to evaluate competitive sports programs as well. Before children can compete successfully in these, they must be able to lose a game without feeling devastated—in other words, be able to say, "I lost because I played badly," not "I lost because I am a bad person." Children do not usually develop sufficient ego strength to do this until they are about 10 years old.

Another problem to consider with organized contact sports is the possibility of athletic injuries. Encourage parents to consider their child's maturity and the risk of injury (see Chapter 52) before they decide whether team competition is right for their child (Theisen, Frisch, Malisoux, et al., 2012).

Problem Solving. An important part of developing a sense of industry is learning how to solve problems. Parents and teachers can help children develop this skill by encouraging practice. When a child asks, "Is this the right way to do this?" a parent can encourage problem solving by saying, "Let's talk about possible ways of doing it" rather than offering a quick solution.

The world depends on machinery, so mishaps and breakdowns (and therefore sudden changes) do occur. A child who can create an indoor playhouse with a card table and blanket when it is too wet or cold to use an outdoor one will be able, as an adult, to problem solve another solution to a data distribution problem when a computer malfunctions. This attitude of optimism rather than pessimism toward problem solving produces adults who rarely say, "It can't be done." Just as important, it leaves these adults with confidence, a sense of pride, and feeling good about themselves because they have control of their environment and abilities.

✔ QSEN Checkpoint Question 32.1

Quality Improvement

According to Erikson, a sense of industry or accomplishment is the developmental task of the school-age period. When planning care, what would be the best activity to introduce to Shelly to help her achieve this?

a. Encourage her to establish a new club.
b. Suggest she begin a diary in which she records her secret thoughts.
c. Help her with spelling so over a year's time she becomes an expert at this.
d. Locate small projects she could complete in 1 day and feel rewarded.

Look in Appendix A for the best answer and rationale.

Learning to Live With Others. School-age children are sometimes so interested in tasks and in accomplishing physical projects that they forget they must work with people to achieve these goals. A good time to urge children to learn compassion and thoughtfulness toward others is during the early school years, when children are first exposed to large groups of other youngsters. Writing thank-you letters or shoveling an older neighbor's sidewalk are examples of activities that can help children develop empathy toward others.

Learning to give a present without receiving one in return or doing a favor without expecting a reward is also a part of this process, and this can be taught by example. Children should see their parents doing such things with an attitude not of "What will I get out of this?" but "What can I contribute?"

Children may show empathy toward others as early as 20 months, but cognitively they cannot relate others' experiences to their own until about 6 years of age. Therefore, it is usually ineffective to lecture a child by saying, "That was cruel to call Mary names." The child may feel she had every right to do so. A better technique is to ask children to put themselves in Mary's place for a minute and imagine how they would feel if they were Mary. A school-age child will generally be able to do this and understand why name-calling hurts. Following this, a simple statement such as, "It doesn't feel good to be called names, does it?" may suffice.

Socialization

Six-year-old children play in groups, but when they are tired or under stress, they usually prefer one-to-one contact. In a first-grade classroom, for example, students compete actively for a few minutes of special time with their teacher. At the end of a day, they enjoy spending individual time with parents. You may have to remind parents that this is not babyish behavior but that of a typical 6-year-old.

Seven-year-olds are increasingly aware of family roles and responsibility. Promises must be kept, because 7-year-olds view them as definite, firm commitments. Children this age tattle because they have such a strong sense of justice (Loke, Heyman, & Forgie, 2011). This tattling has the side effect of dissolving play groups quickly.

Eight-year-olds actively seek the company of other children. Most 8-year-old girls have a close girlfriend; boys have a close boyfriend. Girls begin to whisper among themselves as they share secrets with close friends, annoying both parents and teachers.

Nine-year-olds take the values of their peer group very seriously. They are much more interested in how other children dress than in what their parents want them to wear. This is typically the friend or club age because children form groups, usually "spite clubs." This means if there are four girls on the block, three form a club and exclude the fourth. The reason for exclusion is often unclear; it might be that the fourth child has a chronic disease, she has more or less money than the others, she was at the dentist's the day the club was formed, or simply that the club cannot exist unless there is someone to exclude. Such clubs typically have a secret password and secret meeting place. Membership is generally all girls or all boys.

If an excluded child does not react badly to being shut out, the club will probably disband after a few days because its purpose is lost. The next day, the excluded member may meet with two others and snub a different child. Parents need to use caution deciding whether to intervene with this type of play because loyalties shift quickly: the child who is club president today may be the excluded one tomorrow.

Because they are so ready for social interaction, 9-year-olds are ready for activities away from home, such as a week at camp. They can take care of their own needs and are mature enough to be separated from their parents for this length of time. Going to camp before this age usually results in homesickness and can be a negative introduction to being away from home.

Although 10-year-olds enjoy groups, they also enjoy privacy. They like having their own bedroom or at least their own dresser, where they can store a collection and know it is free from parents' or siblings' eyes. One of the best gifts for a 10-year-old is a box that locks.

Girls become increasingly interested in boys and vice versa by 11 years of age. Favorite activities are mixed-sex rather than single-sex ones. Children of this age are particularly insecure, however, and girls tend to dance with girls while boys talk together in corners. Better socialization patterns need not be rushed. Just as infants crawl before they walk, so 11-year-olds must attempt many awkward and uncomfortable social experiences before they become comfortable forming relationships with the opposite sex.

Twelve-year-olds feel more comfortable in social situations than they did the year before. Boys experience erections on small provocation and so may feel uncomfortable being pushed into boy–girl situations until they learn how to better control their bodies. Because some children develop faster than others, every group has some members who are almost adolescent and some who are still children, making social interactions sometimes difficult.

✔ QSEN Checkpoint Question 32.2

Informatics

Shelly belonged to a series of clubs when she was 9 years old. When you talk to her school nurse, what would you expect to hear the nurse cite as a typical characteristic of a 9-year-old's club?

a. Clubs have formal rules and regulations.
b. Clubs are designed to help shy children get outside of their "comfort zone."
c. Clubs invariably exclude one or more children.
d. Clubs always include both boys and girls.

Look in Appendix A for the best answer and rationale.

Cognitive Development

The age period from 5 to 11 years is a transitional stage where children undergo a shift from the preoperational thought they used as preschoolers to concrete operational thought or the ability to reason through any problem they can actually visualize (Piaget, 1969) (Fig. 32.6).

Children can use concrete operational thought because they learn several new concepts during school age, such as:

- **Decentering**, the ability to project one's self into other people's situations and see the world from their viewpoint rather than focusing only on their own view.
- **Accommodation**, the ability to adapt thought processes to fit what is perceived such as understanding that there can be more than one reason for other people's actions. A preschooler might expect to see the same nurse in the

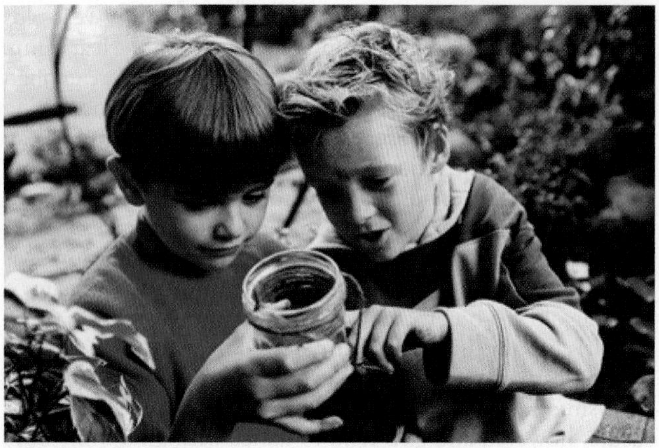

FIGURE 32.6 School-age children learn concrete operational thought or concentrate on phenomena they can actually see occurring. For example, children may have closely catalogued collections of action figures, science specimens, sports materials, or books and spend much time attending to and enhancing such collections.

morning who was there the evening before, whereas a school-age child will understand that different nurses work different shifts.

- **Conservation**, the ability to appreciate that a change in shape does not necessarily mean a change in size. If you pour 30 ml of cough medicine from a thin glass to a wide one, the preschooler will say that one glass holds more than the other; a school-age child will know that both glasses hold an equal amount.
- **Class inclusion**, the ability to understand that objects can belong to more than one classification. A preschooler is able to categorize items in only one way, for example, stones and shells are found at the beach; a school-age child can categorize them in many ways such as by different materials or by a difference in sizes and shapes, not just that they are found at the beach.

These cognitive developments lead to some of the typical changes and characteristics of the school-age period. Decentering enables a school-age child to feel compassion for others, which was not possible in younger years. Because understanding the principle of conservation is possible, a school-age child is not fooled by perceptions as often as before. The ability to classify objects leads to the collecting activities of the school-age period. Class inclusion is also necessary for learning mathematics and reading, systems that categorize numbers and words.

What if...32.1 You make Shelly's hospital bed one day and then give her an injection. What if the next day she begins to cry while you're making her bed because she "doesn't want a shot"? The lack of what cognitive process led her to believe your actions would be exactly the same the second day?

Moral and Spiritual Development

School-age children begin to mature in terms of moral development as they enter a stage of *preconventional reasoning*, sometimes as early as 5 years of age (Kohlberg, 1984). During this stage, if asked, "Why is it wrong to steal from your neighbor?" school-age children will answer, "The police say it's wrong," or "Because if you do, you'll go to jail." They concentrate on "niceness" or "fairness" and cannot see yet that stealing hurts their neighbor, the highest level of moral reasoning. Because they are still limited in their ability to understand others' views, they may interpret something as being right because it is good for them, not because it is right for humanity as a whole.

Remember that school-age children are rule oriented; when they ask for something, because they were good, they expect to receive what they are asking.

What if...32.2 When you tell Shelly it would be good if she lost some weight, she says you're not being fair. Is this a typical school age response?

HEALTH PROMOTION FOR A SCHOOL-AGE CHILD AND FAMILY

Because of still limited judgment, school-age children need guidelines in reference to safety, nutrition, and daily care. These are always excellent topics for discussion at health care visits.

Promoting School-Age Safety

School-age children are ready for time on their own without direct adult supervision. This means that they need good education on safety practices (Box 32.3). As with adults, unintentional injuries tend to occur when children are under stress or when their mind is not solely on their surroundings.

School age is not too early for parents to look at the effect of carrying heavy backpacks on children's posture. A backpack that weighs more than 10% of the child's body weight is enough to cause a child to have to lean forward chronically to bear the weight. This can lead to chronic back pain (Kistner, Fiebert, & Roach, 2012).

Sexual maltreatment is an unfortunate and all-too-common hazard for children. Teaching points to help children avoid sexual maltreatment are summarized in Box 32.4 (see also Chapter 55).

QSEN Checkpoint Question 32.3

Safety

Teaching safety is an important area to consider for school-age children. Which of the following would be the best advice?

a. "Keep your backpack filled to capacity to avoid falling on frequent trips back to your locker."
b. "As soon as you no longer need an automobile booster seat, you'll no longer need a seatbelt either."
c. "Gaining weight isn't serious in the school-age years; it only becomes a real problem after age 18 years."
d. "You're old enough to tell if you are sick or not; your mother's opinion isn't as important as when you were younger."

Look in Appendix A for the best answer and rationale.

BOX 32.3 Nursing Care Planning Based on Family Teaching

COMMON SAFETY MEASURES TO PREVENT UNINTENTIONAL INJURIES DURING THE SCHOOL YEARS

Q. Shelly's mother tells you, "She's constantly on the go. How can I keep her free from accidents when I'm not always with her?"

A. Putting preventive steps in place, such the ones that follow, is the key.

Source of Unintentional Injury	Preventive Measure
Motor vehicle	Encourage children to use seat belts and a booster seat if needed; role model seatbelt use. Teach street-crossing safety; stress that streets are no place for roughhousing, pushing, or shoving. Teach parking lot and school bus safety (e.g., do not walk in back of parked cars, wait for crossing guard).
Bicycle	Teach bicycle safety, including wearing a helmet and not giving "passengers" rides.
Community	Teach to avoid unsafe areas, such as train yards, grain silos, and back alleys. Stress to not go with strangers (parents can establish a code word with child; child does not leave school with anyone who does not know the word). Teach children to say "no" to anyone who touches them if they do not wish it, including family members (most sexual maltreatment is by a family member, not a stranger). Teach children not to arrange a meeting with people they meet on the Internet. For older school-age children, teach rules of safer sex so they know these rules before they need to use them a first time (see Chapter 5, Box 5.7).
Burns	Teach safety with candles, matches, and campfires and that fire is not fun. Also teach safety with beginning cooking skills (e.g., be certain to include microwave oven safety, such as closing firmly before turning on oven; not using metal containers). Teach safety with sun exposure; use sun block. Teach to not climb electric poles.
Falls	Educate that roughhousing on fences or climbing on roofs is hazardous. Teach skateboard, scooter, and skating safety.
Sports injuries	Teach that wearing appropriate equipment for sports (e.g., face masks for hockey; mouthpiece and cup for football; helmet for bicycle riding, skateboarding, or in-line skating; batting helmets for baseball) is not babyish, but smart management. Stress not to play to a point of exhaustion or in a sport beyond physical capability (no pitching baseballs or toe ballet for an early grade-school child). Use trampolines only with adult supervision to avoid serious neck injury.
Drowning	Teach how to swim; dares and roughhousing when diving or swimming are not appropriate. Stress not to swim beyond limits of capabilities.
Drugs	Help your child avoid all recreational drugs; prescription medicine should only be taken as directed. Teach to avoid tobacco and alcohol.
Firearms	Teach firearm safety. Keep firearms in locked cabinets with bullets separate from gun.
General	School-age children should keep adults informed as to where they are and what they are doing; cell phones can help with this. Be aware the frequency of unintentional injures increases when parents are under stress and therefore less attentive. Special precautions must be taken at these times. Caution that some children are more active, curious, and impulsive and therefore more vulnerable to unintentional injuries than others.

BOX 32.4 Nursing Care Planning Based on Family Teaching

TEACHING POINTS TO HELP CHILDREN AVOID SEXUAL MALTREATMENT

Q. Shelly's mother wants to protect her daughter from being abused sexually. She asks you, "What are good rules to teach children without scaring them?"

A. A number of suggestions include:

1. Your body is your property and you can decide who looks at it or touches it.
2. Secrets are fun things to keep. If a person asks you not to tell about something that was done to you that you didn't like, however, it's not a secret. It's all right to tell someone about it.
3. Don't go anywhere with a stranger (a stranger is someone you do not know, not someone "strange"). Don't be fooled by people asking you to give them directions or to go with them because your mother is sick or hurt or because they have lost a pet.
4. Being touched by someone you like is a good feeling. You don't have to allow anyone to touch you in a way you don't like. Don't allow yourself to be left alone with a person you are uncomfortable with because that person touches you in a way you don't like.
5. Avoid meeting with people you talk with on Internet chat sites because they may not be the age or the person whom they say they are.
6. A "private part" is the part of you a bathing suit touches. If anyone asks you to show them a private part or touches a private part, tell them to stop, and tell someone what happened.
7. If the person you tell doesn't believe you, keep telling people until someone does believe you.

Promoting Nutritional Health of a School-Age Child

Most school-age children have good appetites, although any meal is influenced by the day's activity. If children have had a full day of active play, they may come to the dinner table ready to eat anything. If a day was filled with frustration—a child received a poor mark in school, had an argument with a friend, or has a big game to think about—the child may pick and poke at food. This is no different from the way adults feel at times, and so should be respected.

Establishing Healthy Eating Patterns

School-age children need breakfast to provide enough energy to get them through active mornings at school. They eat best if parents get up in the morning and eat some themselves because children react badly to the instruction, "Do as I say, not as I do."

If children take a packed lunch to school, urge parents to allow them some say in the meal, because packed lunches become tedious for everyone after a while. Whether they take lunch or buy it at school, school-age children should know some elementary facts of nutrition so they do not trade a sandwich for cake or choose only desserts from the cafeteria. Ideally, children should receive guidance from school personnel, but this often is impossible in a busy lunchroom. Health care personnel, therefore, should play an active role in nutrition education at health maintenance visits.

Many children qualify for a free or reduced-price school lunch and breakfast (Hirschman & Chriqui, 2012). A government-regulated school lunch (type A) provides milk (8 oz), protein (2 oz), one starch serving, a vegetable (3/4 cup), and fruit (3/4 cup). Serving sizes vary according to age to provide one third of a child's nutrition requirements for a day (Fig. 32.7). Check that children are actually eating school lunches, not trading items they do not want, so they receive the full benefit of the program. Alert children with food allergies for such things as eggs or peanuts that they need to ask how food is prepared (Robinson & Ficca, 2012).

Most children are hungry after school and enjoy a snack when they arrive home. Because sugary foods may dull a child's appetite for dinner, urge parents to make the snack nutritious, such as fruit, cheese, or milk rather than cookies and a soft drink.

Early school age is not too young to put in place preventive measures against illnesses later in life. Eating salty foods, for example, can lead to hypertension. Excessive saturated fat can lead to the formation of artery plaques and cardiovascular disease (Harika, Cosgrove, Osendarp, et al., 2011). Enjoying too many soft drinks (soda) leads to childhood obesity (Caprio, 2012).

Teach parents to make every attempt to make mealtime a happy and enjoyable part of the day for everyone because some school-age children learn to eat as quickly as possible (and therefore incompletely) to escape from the table before something unpleasant happens, such as an argument they can sense is brewing.

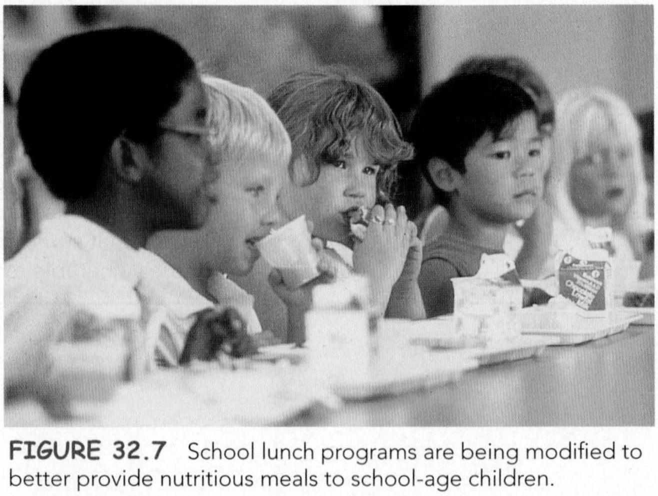

FIGURE 32.7 School lunch programs are being modified to better provide nutritious meals to school-age children.

Fostering Industry and Nutrition

As a part of fostering industry, school-age children usually enjoy helping to plan meals. They can prepare foods such as instant pudding, Jell-O, salads, scrambled eggs, and sandwiches. They may eat meals they have planned or prepared more willingly than ones that are just set in front of them.

Most parents would like children to develop better table manners. Because they are in a hurry to finish eating, school-age children tend to gulp their food. Many meals are interrupted by spilled milk. As children become teenagers and are more aware of the impression they make on others, manners often improve dramatically. It is usually comforting for parents to know children typically display better table manners in other people's homes than in their own.

Recommended Dietary Intakes

Although parents may have less to say about what a school-age child eats, it is important that the increasing energy requirements that come with this age (often in spurts) are met daily with foods of high nutritional value.

During the late school years, the recommended dietary intakes for children begin to be separated into different categories for girls then for boys because boys require more calories and other nutrients at this time. Both girls and boys require more iron in prepuberty than they did between the ages of 7 and 10 years. Adequate calcium and fluoride intake remains important to ensure good teeth and bone growth. A major deficit may be fiber because school-age children typically dislike vegetables.

A Vegetarian Diet

School-age children who are vegetarians need to learn aspects of vegetarian nutrition if they are going to eat in a school cafeteria or at other people's houses. Unfortunately, many school lunch programs offer mainly milk and meat or cheese foods, such as sloppy Joe sandwiches, macaroni and cheese, or pizza. These foods force children who are vegetarians to carry packed lunches. Vegetarian packed lunches can be varied day by day with foods such as cucumber, tomato, or peanut butter sandwiches on whole-grain bread; hot soups; salads; vegetable sticks; and fruit.

A potential problem to assess with vegetarian school-age children is whether they are obtaining enough protein and calcium so their body is prepared for the rapid growth spurt of puberty (Van Winckel, Vande Velde, De Bruyne, et al., 2011). Foods highest in calcium are green leafy vegetables such as spinach and turnip greens, enriched bread, and cereals. Soybeans, legumes, grains, and immature seeds such as green beans, lima beans, and corn are relatively high in protein. As with any individual on a vegetarian diet, children may need a vitamin B_{12} supplement because natural B_{12} is only supplied by animal sources. Encourage outside activities for sun exposure to increase vitamin D. Iron may need to be supplemented as well, especially in girls with heavy menstrual flows (Whitney & Rolfes, 2012).

Promoting Development of a School-Age Child in Daily Activities

With life centered on school activities and friends, a school-age child still needs parental guidance for most daily activities because the habits and lifestyle patterns gained during this period will form the basis for the patterns of living later in life. Figure 32.8 shows a day in the life of a family with school-age children. Along with nutritional needs, areas of concern for a school-age child and family include dressing, sleep needs, exercise, hygiene, and dental care.

Dress

Although school-age children can fully dress themselves, they are not skilled at taking care of their clothes until late in the school-age years. This is the right age, however (if not started already), to teach children the importance of caring for their own belongings. School-age children have definite opinions about clothing styles, often based on the likes of their friends, a popular sport, or a popular musician rather than the preferences of their parents. Help parents be aware that a child who wears different clothing than others may become the object of exclusion from a school club or group. In schools with a gang or bullying culture, children may not be able to wear a certain color or style lest they be mistaken for a gang member or become a bully's victim (White & Mason, 2011). For this reason, many schools have begun requiring school uniforms to avoid this problem.

Sleep

Sleep needs vary among individual children. Younger school-age children typically require 10 to 12 hours of sleep each night; older ones require about 8 to 10 hours. Most 6-year-olds are too old for naps but do require a quiet time after school to get them through the remainder of the day. Nighttime terrors may continue during the early school years and may actually increase during the first-grade year as a child reacts to the stress of beginning school.

During early school years, many children enjoy a quiet talk or a reading time at bedtime. At about age 9 years, when friends become important, children generally are ready to give up bedtime talks with parents in preference to phoning or text messaging a friend. Some parents may need some help to take at face value their child's statement, "I'm tired. I'd rather go to sleep," rather than feel rejected.

Children with television sets, electronic games, or smartphones in their bedrooms not only have shorter sleep times at night but also are more likely to be obese (Chahal, Fung, Kuhle, et al., 2012).

Exercise

School-age children need daily exercise. Although they go to school all day, they do not automatically receive much exercise because school is basically a sit-down activity. Children who are bussed or driven by a parent to school may therefore return home without having spent much time in active exercise.

Increasing time spent in exercise need not involve organized sports. It can come from neighborhood games, walking with parents or a dog, or bicycle riding. As children enter preadolescence, those with poor coordination may become reluctant to exercise. Urge them to participate in some form of daily exercise, however, or obesity or osteoporosis can result later in life (Eagle, Sheetz, Gurm, et al., 2012; Gunter, Almstedt, & Janz, 2012).

Hygiene

Children 6 or 7 years of age still need help in regulating bath water temperature and in cleaning their ears and fingernails. By age 8 years, children are generally capable of bathing

(text continues on page 908)

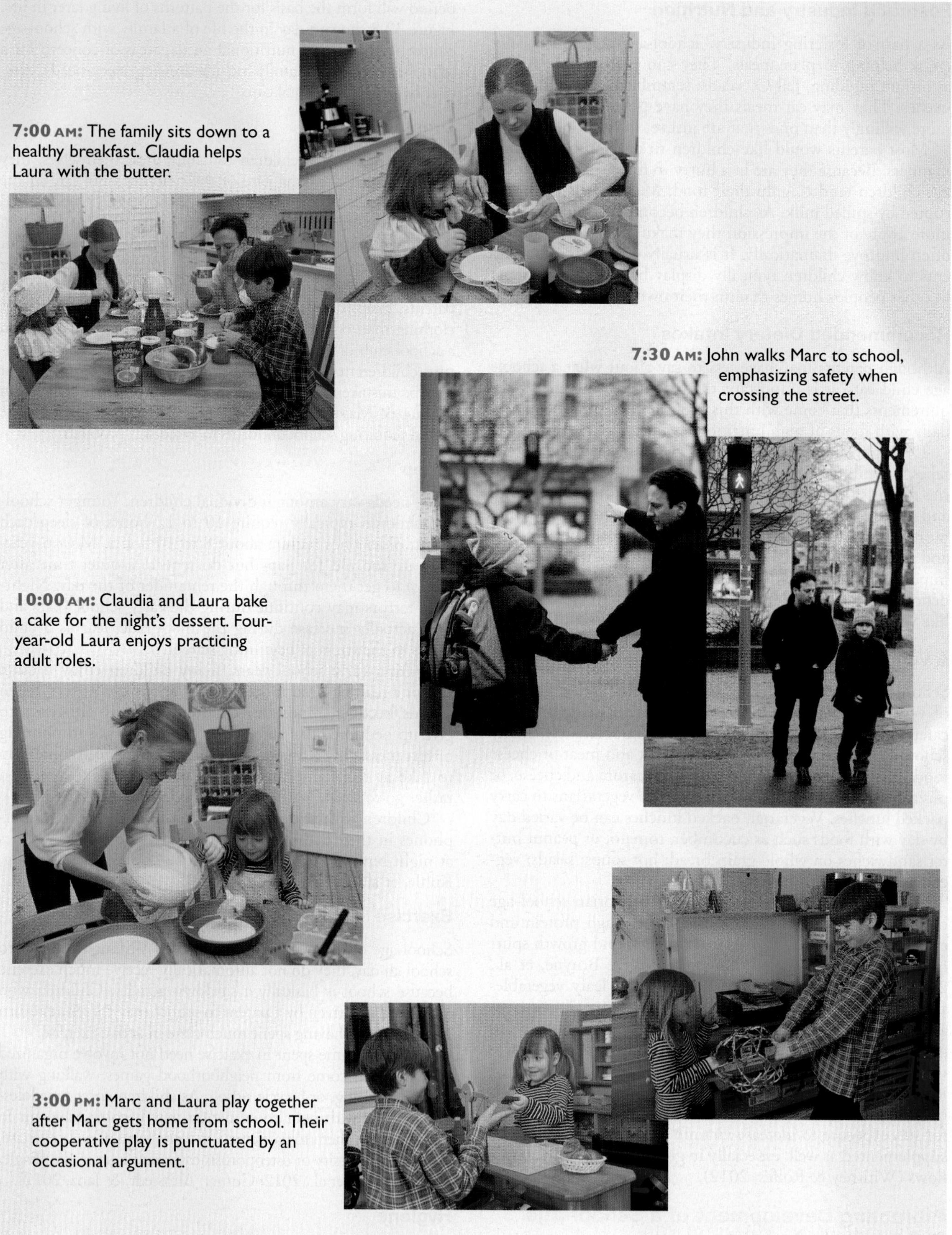

7:00 AM: The family sits down to a healthy breakfast. Claudia helps Laura with the butter.
7:30 AM: John walks Marc to school, emphasizing safety when crossing the street.
10:00 AM: Claudia and Laura bake a cake for the night's dessert. Four-year-old Laura enjoys practicing adult roles.
3:00 PM: Marc and Laura play together after Marc gets home from school. Their cooperative play is punctuated by an occasional argument.

FIGURE 32.8 A day in the life of a family with young children.

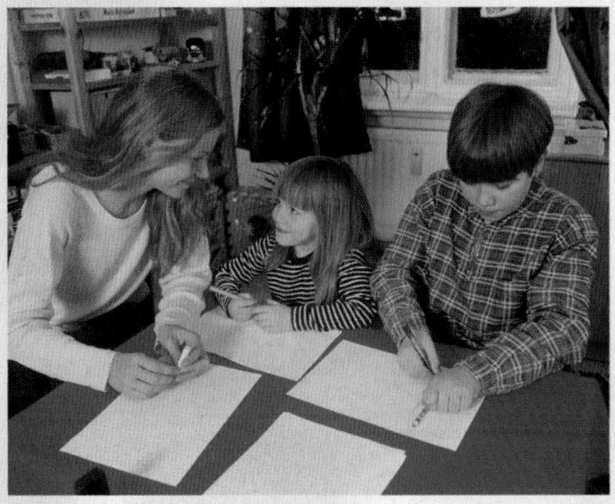

4:00 PM: Claudia helps Marc with his homework. Laura likes to draw alongside her big brother.

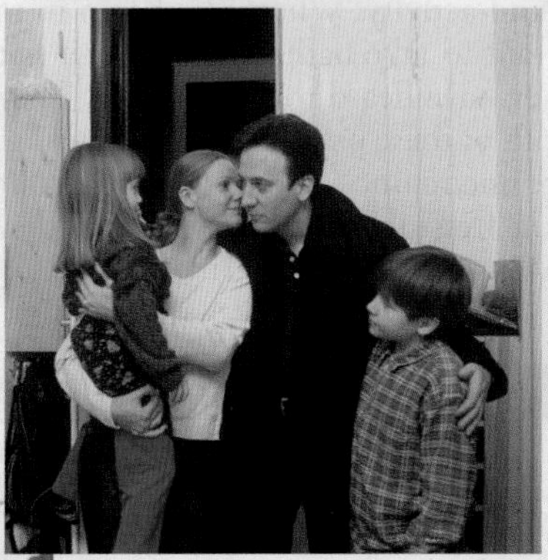

5:00 PM: The family greets John as he comes home from work.

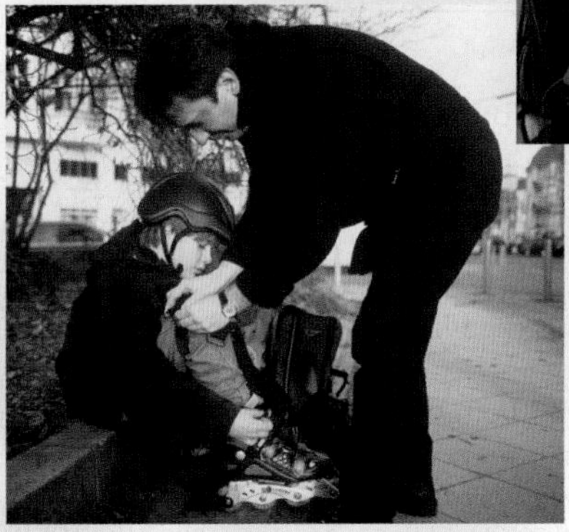

5:30 PM: John and Marc go rollerblading before dinner. John makes sure Marc's protective gear is in place.

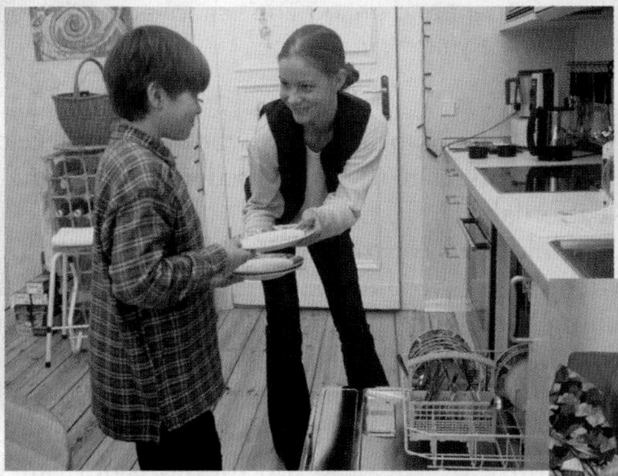

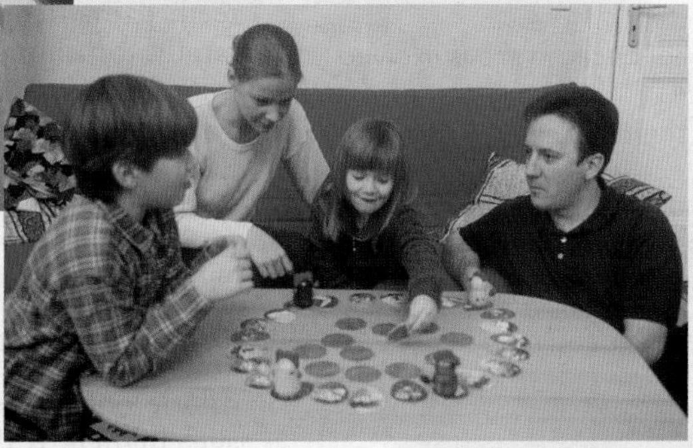

7:00 PM: After dinner, Marc helps with the dishes, then the family spends time together playing a game.

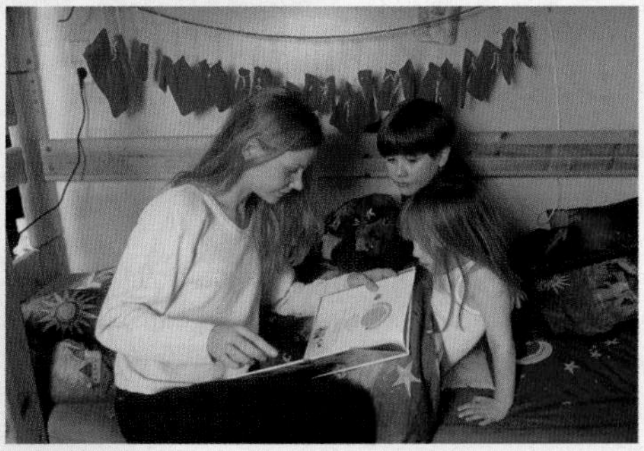

8:30 PM: Time to get ready for bed! Claudia helps the kids clean up and brush their teeth. And there's always time to read them a story.

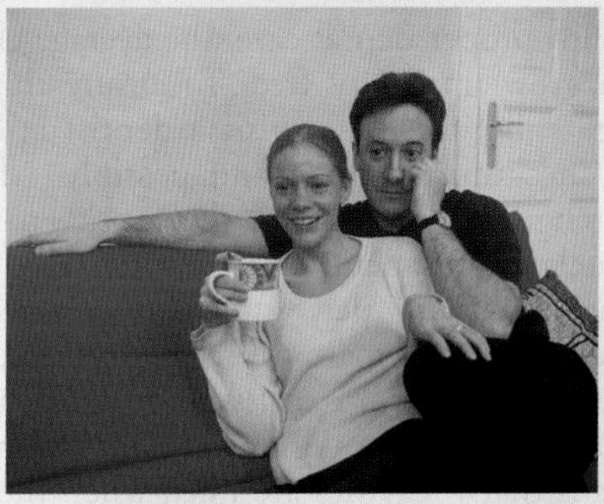

9:00 PM: John and Claudia relax together at the end of the day.

FIGURE 32.8 *(continued)*

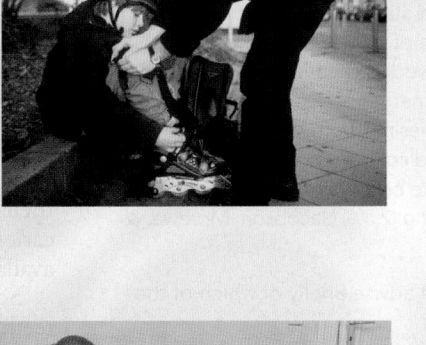

themselves but may not do it well because they are too busy to take the time or because they do not find bathing as important as do their parents.

Both boys and girls become interested in showering as they approach their teens. This can be encouraged because perspiration increases with puberty, along with sebaceous gland activity. When girls begin to menstruate, they may be afraid to take baths or wash their hair during their period if they have heard this is not safe. They need information that both of these practices are safe during their menses. Boys who are uncircumcised may develop inflammation under the foreskin from increased secretions if they do not wash regularly (Meng & Tanagho, 2013).

QSEN Checkpoint Question 32.4

Evidence-Based Practice

Shelly has told you she wants to try out for cheerleading. This is a sport appealing to school-age children and adolescents because of its combinations of dance and gymnastics, the friendships that can develop, and the school status it almost automatically creates. To investigate what type of injuries typically occur with cheerleading, researchers reviewed all cheerleading injuries (over 4,000) presented to U.S. emergency departments during a 5-year period. The types of injuries most often seen were sprains/strains (44%), fractures (16%), and contusions (16%). The activities resulting in the most injuries were body collisions (29%), stunting (19%), tumbling (11%), and tossing (2.5%) (Jacobson, Morawa, & Bir, 2012).

Based on the study, you would advise Shelly of which of the following?

a. Cheerleading will be good for her because she is likely to lose weight from the exercise.
b. She will need to drink an extra source of calcium every day to avoid broken bones.
c. She should pursue a sport or activity that is safer.
d. She should be aware that cheerleading may be beneficial to her but does carry some risks.

Look in Appendix A for the best answer and rationale.

Care of Teeth

With proper dental care, the average child today can expect to grow up cavity free. To ensure this happening, school-age children should visit a dentist at least twice yearly for a checkup, cleaning, and possibly a fluoride treatment to strengthen and harden the tooth enamel (Tubert-Jeannin, Auclair, Amsallem, et al., 2011) (Fig. 32.9). Remind them that not all bottled water is fluoridated so they don't want this to be their main source of drinking water. Some children develop a fear of dentists and, if a dentist visit was painful, want to avoid going at all. The advantage of frequent visits is that if cavities are filled when they are small, the drilling required is minimal and little pain is involved. If cavities are not treated promptly in this way but are allowed to grow large, the drilling can hurt, causing these children to refuse to go back to a dentist. More large cavities then grow, and a vicious cycle develops. Pedodontists specialize in caring for children's teeth and understand the developmental level of their patients. The parents of children who tend to develop caries might be encouraged to visit a pedodontist if one is available and affordable.

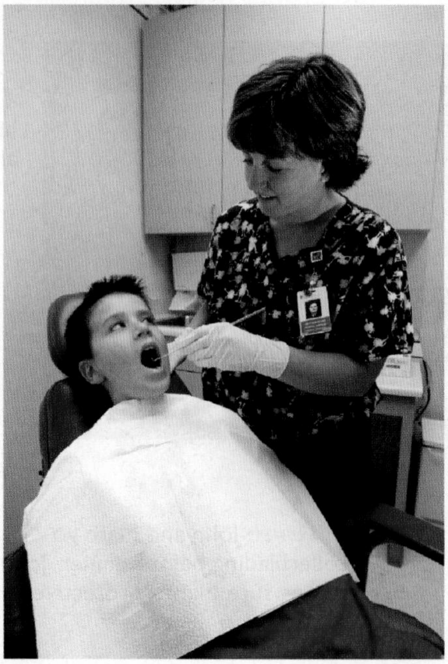

FIGURE 32.9 Dental caries are the number one health problem in school-age children. Stress to parents that good dental health is important and encourage school-age children to visit a dentist twice a year.

School-age children have to be reminded to brush their teeth daily. If brushing becomes an area of conflict for the family, brushing well once a day may be more effective than brushing more often but doing an inadequate job. For effective brushing, a child should use a soft toothbrush, fluoride-based toothpaste, and dental floss to clean between teeth to help remove plaque. Electric toothbrushes can be used safely by school-age children.

Snacks are best limited to high-protein foods such as chicken and cheese rather than candy. Fruits, vegetables, and cereals fortified with minerals and vitamins (not empty calorie ones) can all be fun after-school snacks for school-age children. If the child does eat candy, a type that is eaten quickly and dissolves quickly is better than slowly dissolving or sticky candy because these types stay in contact with the teeth longer.

QSEN Checkpoint Question 32.5

Teamwork & Collaboration

Shelly tells you she collected "a bushel" of candy on Halloween. Because of how common this phenomenon is, in consultation with a dental hygienist, you would teach children that what type of candy is less likely to cause dental caries?

a. Salt water taffy
b. A chocolate bar
c. Chewy caramels
d. Hard candy

Look in Appendix A for the best answer and rationale.

Promoting Healthy Family Functioning

At 6 years of age, most children have passed through a preschool phase of attraction for the parent of the opposite sex and identify again with the parent of the same sex (Freud, 1962). Children from single-parent homes or those with a parent who has difficulty being a good role model may need help in finding a suitable adult to serve as this important person in their life.

To their parents' annoyance, many 6-year-olds often quote their teacher as the final authority on all subjects. This may be the first time the parents see someone surpassing them in their child's eyes, and accepting the situation can be painful. Children also cite their friends as guides for behavior; for example, "Mary Jane doesn't have to go to bed until 10 o'clock," or "Carlos' mother lets him go to the movies every Saturday." Parents may require help to realize these remarks are a normal consequence of being exposed to other adults and children. A simple statement such as, "There are all kinds of ways to do things, but in our house, the rule is this" shows no criticism of Carlos' or Mary Jane's family, yet conveys a special and secure "our house" feeling.

Parents may also need to be reminded that even the simplest tasks of everyday life require repeated practice before they can be accomplished well. The way parents correct children as they learn these tasks influences children's opinions of themselves and their ability to continue learning. "Putting all the silverware in a pile is one way of putting it away; another way would be to divide spoons, forks, and knives separately" is always preferable to "What a silly way to put away silverware!" Comments such as, "Can't you do anything right?" or "Why don't you ever do what I say?" should always be avoided because children will rise only to the level expected of them.

If parents have difficulty telling what a child's completed project is supposed to be, the time-honored "Tell me about it" is preferable to "What is it?" It is good for parents to find a redeeming characteristic in a project, no matter how shakily it is put together: "I like the bright color you painted it" or "That must have been fun to make." Displaying and using children's gifts are part of having school-age children in a family. A finger painting hung on the refrigerator door enhances, not detracts from, the most elegant home. The best-dressed woman looks even more radiant wearing her child's necklace made of macaroni on a string. Both examples are gestures of love, which goes well with everything.

In talking to parents of school-age children, good questions to ask to estimate the degree of interaction that occurs in the home and whether parents are strengthening a child's sense of accomplishment include:

- How do they correct the child when he or she does something wrong?
- Do they display school projects?
- Does the child have chores that are his or hers to accomplish?
- Do they ask the child to participate in family decision making?

Common Health Problems of the School-Age Period

Children in their early school years may have many small health concerns such as head lice or ringworm (see Chapter 43). At the same time, they have one of the lowest rates of death and serious illness of any age group. The two causes of death seen most frequently are from unintentional injury and cancer. Minor illnesses are largely due to dental caries, gastrointestinal disturbances, and upper respiratory infections (Heron, 2012).

Because learning difficulties such as attention deficit hyperactivity disorder (ADHD) and autism spectrum disorders (ASDs) become marked at school age, they are also important parental concerns (see Chapter 54). Table 32.3 shows the usual health maintenance pattern for a school-age child (AAP, Committee on Practice and Ambulatory Medicine, 2012). Table 32.4 lists problems that parents may have in evaluating illnesses in school-age children.

Dental Caries

Caries (cavities) are progressive, destructive lesions or decalcification of the tooth enamel and dentin. When the pH of the tooth surface drops to 5.6 or below (which happens after children eat readily fermented carbohydrates, such as table sugar), acid microorganisms (acidogenic lactobacilli and aciduric streptococci) found in dental plaque attack the cementing medium of teeth and destroy it. Plaque tends to accumulate in deep grooves of the teeth and contact areas between teeth, making these areas most susceptible to dental decay. The enamel on primary teeth is thinner than on permanent teeth, so these are even more susceptible to destruction than permanent teeth. The distance from the enamel to the pulp is shorter also, so invasion of the tooth nerve can occur quickly. Neglected caries result in poor chewing and therefore poor digestion, abscesses and pain, and sometimes osteomyelitis (bone infection) if the jaw bone is involved.

As stated earlier, dental caries are largely preventable with proper brushing and use of fluoridated water or fluoride application. When caries do occur, it's important they be treated quickly and the child's dental hygiene practices be evaluated and improved if necessary. Most importantly, children must believe that they have a stake in the health of their teeth, so even though they are cavity free, they willingly undertake the self-care measures necessary to ensure healthy teeth with parental support rather than parental command (Wen, Goldberg, Marrs, et al., 2012).

Malocclusion

The upper jaw in children matures during early childhood along with skull growth; the lower jaw reaches maturity more slowly, forcing teeth to make a prolonged series of changes until they reach their final adult alignment and position. Good tooth occlusion, in which the upper teeth overlap the lower teeth by a small amount and teeth are evenly spaced and in good alignment, is necessary for optimal formation of teeth, health of the supporting tissue, optimal speech development, and what most people view as a pleasant physical appearance. **Malocclusion** (a deviation of tooth position from the normal) may be congenital due to conditions such as cleft palate, a small lower jaw, or familial traits tending toward malocclusion. The condition can result later on from constant mouth breathing or abnormal tongue position (tongue thrusting). Thumb-sucking is still another possibility if it persists past the time of eruption of the permanent front teeth (6 to 7 years) (Sandler, Madahar, & Murray, 2011). The loss of teeth due to extraction or an unintentional injury may lead to malocclusion if not properly treated so that alignment is maintained.

TABLE 32.3 Health Maintenance Schedule, School-Age Period

Area of Focus	Methods	Frequency
Assessment		
Health history	Health interview	Every visit
Physical health	Physical examination	Every visit
Developmental milestones	History and observation	Every visit
Growth milestones	Height and weight plotted on standard growth chart; body mass index (BMI) and physical examination	Every visit
Hypertension	Blood pressure	Every visit
Nutrition	History and observation; height and weight information	Every visit
Parent–child relationship	History and observation	Every visit
Behavior or school problems	History and observation	Every visit
Vision and hearing disorders	History and observation Formal Snellen or Titmus testing Audiometer testing	Every visit At 7–9 years and 10–12 years At 7–9 years and 10–12 years
Dental health	History and physical examination	Every visit
Scoliosis	Physical examination	Yearly after age 8 years
Thyroid	Physical examination and history	Every visit after age 10 years
Dyslipidemia	Cholesterol and triglycerides	6–8 years and 10–12 years
Tuberculosis	Purified protein derivative (PPD) skin test	Depending on prevalence of tuberculosis in community
Bacteriuria	Clean-catch urine	At 6–7 years
Anemia	Hematocrit and hemoglobin	At 7–8 years and 11–12 years
Immunizations		
Check history and past records, inform caregiver about any risks and side effects, and administer immunization in accordance with health care agency policies.		
Diphtheria, tetanus, and pertussis vaccine	(DTaP)	11–12 years
Hepatitis A vaccine	(HepA)	If not previously administered
Hepatitis B vaccine	(HepB)	If not administered in infancy or three injections were not completed
Human papillomavirus vaccine	(HPV or HPV4)	11 or 12 years; second injection 2 months later; third injection 6 months after first dose
Inactivated poliomyelitis vaccine	(IPV)	If four doses not previously administered
Influenza vaccine	(IIV)	Yearly
Meningococcal conjugate vaccine	(MCV4)	11–12 years
Pneumococcal vaccine	(PPSV)	To children at high risk
Measles, mumps, rubella vaccine	(MMR)	If two doses not previously administered
Varicella vaccine	(VAR)	At any age after 1 year if not previously immunized, or at 11–12 years if lacking reliable history of chickenpox

Area of Focus	Methods	Frequency
Anticipatory Guidance		
School-age care	Active listening and health teaching	Every visit
Expected growth and developmental milestones before next visit	Active listening and health teaching	Every visit
Unintentional injury prevention	Counseling about street and personal safety	Every visit
Problem Solving		
Any problems expressed by caregiver during course of the visit	Active listening and health teaching regarding cigarette smoking, substance abuse, sex education, school adjustment, etc.	Every visit

American Academy of Pediatrics, Committee on Practice and Ambulatory Medicine. (2012). *Recommendations for preventive pediatric health care*. Washington, DC: Author; Centers for Disease Control & Prevention. *Birth–18 years & "catch up" immunization schedules*. Washington, DC: Author.

Malocclusion may be either crossbite (sideways) or anterior or posterior. Children with a malocclusion should be evaluated by an orthodontist to see if orthodontic braces or other therapy is necessary. The time to begin correction varies with the extent of the malocclusion and jaw size. Braces are painful when they are first applied and at periodic visits when they are tightened to maintain pressure for further straightening. Some children develop mild, shallow ulcerations (canker sores) on the buccal membrane from friction of metal wires. Rubbing the offending wire with dental wax dulls the surface and gives relief. Oral acetaminophen or an agent such as Orajel (an over-the-counter drug) rubbed on the ulceration may also offer relief.

All children who wear braces need to brush their teeth well and be assessed periodically to see that they are brushing properly around the braces (a Waterpik is often recommended for thorough cleaning). They should use dental floss to remove plaque from around wires.

After the removal of braces, many children usually wear retainers to maintain the correction the braces achieved.

TABLE 32.4 Parental Difficulties Evaluating Health Problems in the School-Age Child

Difficulty	Helpful Suggestions for Parents
Evaluating seriousness of illness	For the first time, a school-age child may view illness as a way to avoid unpleasant activities (e.g., school, a coach who asks too much, household chores). Evaluating whether the child has symptoms when asked to do a favorite thing often reveals the difference between exaggeration and an ill child (e.g., too sick to eat spinach, not too sick to eat ice cream; too sick to go to school, not too sick to go ice skating). If the child uses symptoms of illness as a means of avoiding situations, parents must evaluate what it is about the situation they could improve or see if some change should be made in their expectations.
Evaluating nutritional intake	Many school-age children eat lunch at school, and they may spend weekends away from home and weeks away at camp. As with all ages, noting whether they are growing and active is better than monitoring any one day's food intake.
Evaluating puberty changes	There is a wide variation in the time secondary sex characteristics occur (8–17 years for girls; 10–20 years for boys). Children should be examined if and when they or their parents are concerned pubertal changes are delayed or appearing too early.
Age-specific diseases to be aware of	School age is a time to evaluate vision because vision changes occur with increased maturity of the eye globe. Squinting, rubbing the eyes, or poor marks in school may be signs of poor vision. Streptococcal sore throats occur frequently in early-school-age children. Those with sore throats should be examined by a health care provider to prevent complications, such as glomerulonephritis or rheumatic fever, from developing. Girls, in particular, must be evaluated for scoliosis (curvature of the spine). Parents may detect this by noticing that a girl's skirt hangs unevenly or bra straps are uneven. Parents may need to be cautioned that vomiting or a headache in the morning that passes fairly quickly (at about the same time the school bus leaves) may be a symptom of school phobia, but a physical examination is in order because these are also symptoms of other conditions. Absence seizures, a neurologic condition that typically arises in the school-age years, can be confused with behavior problems if observation is not thorough (see Chapter 49). Attention deficit hyperactivity disorder (ADHD) (see Chapter 54) can also lead to behavior or inattention disorders.

Although braces are wired into place, retainers are not. Loss of a retainer can be a problem if it must be removed when eating; check bedside food trays of school-age children before removing them to be certain a child has not placed a retainer on the tray.

Show appropriate sympathy and help children problem solve if they are bothered by the appearance of braces or wearing a retainer. Once thought of as implements to be made fun of, teeth braces have become such a common feature of life for schoolchildren that most children who wear them find comfort in not being the only one to suffer this indignity and, once used to their own appliances, experience little reluctance in letting their classmates see them. Some even view them as a mark of pride or a status symbol (Hamdan, Singh, & Rock, 2012).

Concerns and Problems of the School-Age Period

Two of the most important disorders of the school-age period are ADHD and ASDs because these interfere so dramatically with school progress (see Chapter 54). Other problems concern language, fears, and responsibility.

Nursing Diagnoses and Related Interventions

Nursing Diagnosis: Parental anxiety related to less-than-expected behavior of a school-age child

Outcome Evaluation: Parent states undesired behavior has decreased in frequency; parent feels less stress about the child's health or future.

Problems Associated With Language Development

The common speech problem of the preschool years is broken fluency; the most common problem of a school-age child is articulation. The child has difficulty pronouncing *s, z, th, l, r,* and *w* or substitutes *w* for *r* ("westroom" instead of "restroom") or *r* for *l* ("radies' room" instead of "ladies' room"). This is most noticeable during the first and second grades; it usually disappears by the third grade. Unless it persists, speech therapy for this normal developmental stage is not necessary.

Common Fears and Anxieties of a School-Age Child

School-age children are old enough to experience adult reactions to problems at home or school.

Anxiety Related to Beginning School. Adjusting to grade school is a big task for 6-year-olds. Even if they attended preschool, grade school is different: the rules are firmer, and the elective feeling (e.g., "If I don't like it, I can quit") no longer applies. School is for keeps until age 16 years or longer, a time span too long for a young child to even imagine. Also, where preschool learning was carried out through fun activities, part of every day in grade school involves obvious work (Box 32.5 shows an interprofessional care map for a child with school concerns). Some instances of anxiety may be a reflection of a parent's anxiety (Pass, Arteche, Cooper, et al., 2012).

Because school requires an adjustment, a health assessment of all school-age children should include an inquiry about progress in school by a question such as, "How is Shelly doing in school?" followed by a second question, "How does her teacher say she is doing?" If there is a discrepancy between those two answers, the situation bears study. Some parents may have to alter their expectations of how much their child should be achieving to conform to their child's actual ability. This can obviously be difficult.

One of the biggest tasks of the first year of school is learning to read. It is best if parents have prepared children for this by reading to them since infancy, pointing to the words and pictures as they read. This helps children realize that sentences flow from left to right and that the words, not the pictures, tell the story. Box 32.6 offers some useful hints to help parents encourage reading in their young school-age child.

Many first graders are capable of mature action at school but appear less mature when they return home. They may bite their fingernails, suck their thumb, or talk baby talk. Some develop tics (irregular movements of isolated muscle groups), such as wrinkling the forehead, shrugging the shoulders, clearing the throat, or frequently blinking. Such movements may occasionally be confused with seizure activity. Tics, however, disappear during sleep and occur mainly when the child is subjected to stress or anxiety. Scolding, nagging, threatening, or punishing does not stop either tics or nail biting, and invariably makes these problems worse. Methods such as using bad-flavored nail polish and restraining the child's hands to prevent nail biting are also ineffective.

These behaviors stop when the underlying stress is discovered and alleviated. Urge parents to spend some time with the child after school or in the evening so the child continues to feel secure in the family and does not feel pushed out by being sent to school. If such behavior manifestations persist despite attempts to eliminate their cause, the family might benefit from formal counseling, including temporary pharmacology support for the child (Pringsheim, Doja, Gorman, et al., 2012).

School Refusal or Phobia. School refusal is a fear of attending school. It is a type of "social phobia" similar to agoraphobia (fear of going outside the home) or separation anxiety disorder (SAD). Children who resist attending school this way develop physical signs of illness, such as vomiting, diarrhea, headache, or abdominal pain on school days. This lasts until after the school bus has left or the child is given permission to stay home for the day.

A particular child may be reacting to a situation such as a harsh teacher, having to shower in gym class, or facing a class bully every day. In these instances, counseling may help the child manage the situation better. School refusal may also occur if the child is overly dependent on the parents or may be reluctant to leave home because of worry that younger siblings will usurp the parents' affection. The anxiety of separation may also result because the parent is overprotective of the child or is the one having the most difficulty separating.

Because the problem of school refusal is usually only partly the child's, the entire family generally requires counseling to resolve the issue. As a rule, once it has been established that the child is free of any illness and the resistance

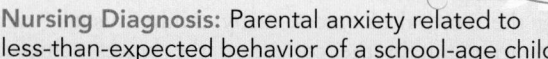

BOX 32.5 Nursing Care Planning

AN INTERPROFESSIONAL CARE MAP FOR A SCHOOL-AGED CHILD BEGINNING MIDDLE SCHOOL

Shelly Lewis is an 11-year-old girl who recently started middle school. Her mother tells you that, although Shelly, who is overweight, says she likes school and wants to try out for cheerleading, she has developed a lot of nervous habits such as nail biting since school started.

Family Assessment Child lives with mother, stepfather, and three younger stepsisters in a four-bedroom home. Family owns a boarding kennel for dogs; both parents work full time at business. Mother describes finances as "Okay. It's hard with a big family."

Client Assessment Child has been "chubby" since preschool. States she likes to read rather than play sports. Is in seventh grade (age appropriate). Observed to be restless in chair during conversation with mother about the new school. Mother states, "Her sisters have no trouble with change; she always does. Don't you think if she lost weight she'd fit in better?"

Nursing Diagnosis Anxiety related to beginning a new school.

Outcome Criteria Child states she feels more comfortable with new school setting; nail biting has decreased in intensity; child agrees to begin weight-reduction program.

Team Member Responsible	Assessment	Intervention	Rationale	Expected Outcome
Activities of Daily Living, Including Safety				
Nurse	Assess what activities client enjoys.	Review with client the advantages of participating in activities that involve more exercise than reading. Support cheerleading; suggest walking with a friend.	Effective weight reduction calls for increased exercise. Books on tape can supply reading enjoyment while walking.	Child states she will try some active activity for at least 20 minutes each day.
Teamwork and Collaboration				
Nurse/Nurse practitioner	Assess if child would be interested in a weight-reduction class at the health center.	Suggest different options available such as a weight-loss group or a commercial weight-reduction program.	Children respond well to group activities. Other group members supply friendship as well as increase motivation.	Child states whether she would like to join a weight-reduction group.
Procedures/Medications for Quality Improvement				
Nurse	Ask child to try to identify if she feels something is upsetting about the new school; if so, ask what it is.	Help child "walk through" a day at school and discuss how small changes could affect her fitting in to school.	Talking with the child allows her to share feelings and concerns openly and safely, possibly increasing her awareness of them and their impact on her.	Child describes a typical day and points she would like to see changed.
Nutrition				
Nurse/Nutritionist	Assess child's intake by 24-hour recall history.	Review with child changes that would reduce calories yet maintain her lifestyle.	Eleven-year-old children are old enough to take responsibility for what and when they eat.	Client reviews her dietary intake and makes at least three suggestions on things she will attempt to change.
Patient-Centered Care				
Nurse	Assess if family members appreciate the stress a new school setting can create.	Review with mother and child ways to reduce stress when encountering new situations, such as equating them with something already known.	It is easy for parents to view 11-year-olds as able to handle new situations better than they can because of pseudomaturity.	Mother states she may have been taking the change in school too lightly and agrees to offer more support.

(continued on page 914)

BOX 32.5 Nursing Care Planning (continued)

Psychosocial/Spiritual/Emotional Needs				
Nurse/Nurse practitioner	Assess family functioning with child's mother.	Stress that all children are individuals and what works for her stepsisters may not work for client.	Being constantly compared to siblings can create feelings of low self-esteem, which can lead to difficulty solving problems.	Mother states she will try to reduce comparisons to stepsisters to help reduce stress at home.
Informatics for Seamless Health Care Planning				
Nurse	Assess if child or mother thinks an early follow-up appointment would be helpful.	Arrange for a follow-up clinic appointment within 1 month with the mother and daughter if desired.	It is difficult for a family to make internal changes if they are too emotionally involved to be objective.	Mother and child express their preferences based on their future plans.

stems from separation anxiety or phobia, the child should be made to attend school. Reinforcement by parents to go to school this way helps to prevent problems such as school failure, peer ridicule, or a pattern of avoiding difficulties. Some children may benefit from a gradual program of school involvement, such as walking to school but not going in for one day, then going to school but staying for only 1 hour the next day, then staying for half a day, and so on until the child can stay all day every day. Give support to parents so they can matter-of-factly treat the child's illness symptoms (a great deal of reassurance that these symptoms are not major will be necessary) so they can take the child firmly to the bus or to the classroom.

Managing school refusal requires coordination among the school, the school nurse, and the health care provider who identifies the problem. A nurse is the ideal person to coordinate such efforts and to help parents allow the child some independence not only in going to school but also in other activities. A few children have such difficulty that they require formal counseling and pharmacologic therapy to overcome school refusal (Scheffer, 2011).

BOX 32.6 Nursing Care Planning to Respect Cultural Diversity

With the activities of children in modern cultures turning more toward electronic games than opening books, reading for pleasure is threatened with becoming a lost art. A number of tips for making reading more enjoyable and increase cultural understanding for children include:

- Read books yourself to set an example so your child thinks of reading as an adult activity. If you spend most of your free time watching television, your child will think reading is mainly for children and assume that it is not important.
- Make reading more fun by encouraging your child to make practical use of what he or she reads. Ask the child to read culturally different recipes while you cook or to read road signs during a car trip.
- Play a treasure hunt game where you hide a small object, such as a favorite toy, then write simple clues on slips of paper: "Look under a lamp," "Look in a book," and so on until your child has been led to the hidden object. Your child can develop writing skills by playing the same game for you to follow.
- Suggest to relatives that a gift certificate from a bookstore would be a good present. Let your child browse the store to select the book.
- Talk about books the child has read—what was good, what was bad, or what the child learned while reading.
- Read a book together as a bedtime family activity.

What if...32.3 Shelly's mother tells you the many nervous habits she began since starting middle school are increasing. What suggestions would you make to her mother regarding this?

Homeschooling

Because of religious or personal preference or because of disillusionment with the school system, a growing number of children are homeschooled today (Anthony & Burroughs, 2010). Because their main contact has been with well educated parents at home, the vocabulary of homeschooled children may be advanced or may suggest they are older than their actual age. When discussing homeschooling with parents, assess if children have peer experiences, perhaps through participation in community sports teams or clubs. Ask if they receive exposure to other cultures or families so they can better adjust to people different from themselves later on at college or at a job.

Children Who Spend Time Independently

Children whose parents both work outside the home may spend time alone without adult supervision for a part of each weekday. Such children have become a prominent concern because, in as many as 90% of families today in the United States, both parents work at least part time outside of the home. Few parents have work hours so flexible that they can always be at home when a child leaves for or returns from school. Extended family members who once watched children after school are often working as well or may no longer be close at hand; many communities are no longer close-knit enough to have neighbors who can be depended on to help out with informal child care.

A major concern of children staying home alone is that they will experience an increased number of unintentional injuries, delinquent behavior, alcohol or substance abuse, or decreased school performance from a lack of adult supervision. For children who are responsible and feel safe in their community, however, a short period of independence every day may actually be beneficial because it encourages problem solving in self-care (Mack, Dellinger, & West, 2012).

Suggestions for parents whose children must spend time alone before or after school are shown in Box 32.7. Many communities and schools offer special after-school programs so children do not have to be home alone. Nurses are in a position to educate parents about such services so their children can feel both safe and stimulated creatively during this time. Both Boy and Girl Scouts, the Boys & Girls Clubs of America, and Camp Fire USA are examples of organizations that offer programs in many neighborhoods to help children adjust to being home alone. Many communities also organize hotline numbers that a child who is alone can call if a problem arises. At health visits, assess whether parents and a child appear to have a concern with or are uncomfortable about after-school arrangements. For a child who is extremely fearful or impulsive or who finds problem solving difficult, time alone after school may not be appropriate. Determine the individual circumstances and recommend changes as appropriate.

Sex Education

It is important that school-age children be educated about pubertal changes and responsible sexual practices. Also, preteens should have adults they can turn to for answers to questions about sex. Ideally, these should be their parents, but because sex is an emotionally charged topic, some parents may be extremely uncomfortable discussing it with their children. As a result, health care personnel often become resource persons.

It's best if sex education is incorporated into health education classes throughout the school years in a manner that is appropriate to age and development. Topics to teach and discuss in a sex education course for both preadolescent boys and girls include:

- Reproductive organ function and physiology of reproduction, so children understand what menstruation is and why it occurs
- Secondary sexual characteristics, so children will understand what is happening in their bodies
- Male sexual functioning, including why the production of increased amounts of seminal fluid leads to nocturnal emissions
- The physiology of pregnancy and the possibility for unintended pregnancies, which will come with sexual maturity
- Responsibilities of sexual maturity
- Reproductive life planning measures and the principles of safer sex if appropriate to the cultural setting (see Chapters 5 and 6)

A sex education course that includes films and discussions is helpful but never answers all of a preteen's questions (most youngsters would rather avoid asking a question than risk appearing ignorant in front of their peers in such a setting). Handing children booklets or showing films with the words, "If you have any questions after you've read (or watched) this, come and ask me" is equally ineffective because it implies they should have no questions. Urge parents or other health educators to watch films or read booklets with children to show they are truly available to answer questions.

Stealing

During early school age, most children go through a period during which they steal loose change from their mother's purse or father's dresser. This usually happens at around 7 years of age, when children first learn how to make change and also discover the importance of money. Stealing occurs because, although a child is gaining an appreciation for money, this appreciation is not yet balanced by strong moral principles or an understanding of ownership.

Parents should explore the reason for the stealing, including:

- Do other children on the block receive an allowance and so have money for small items?
- Did their child make a bet that must be paid?
- Is a child buying a bully's friendship by purchasing gum or candy for that child?
- Does a child need more security and view money as security?

As a rule, early childhood stealing is best handled without a great deal of emotion. A parent should tell the child the money is missing. The importance of property rights should be reviewed: mother's and father's money is theirs, the child's money is the child's, and they are not interchangeable. Youngsters who continue to steal past 8 years of age may require counseling because they should have progressed beyond this normal developmental step by this age (Sourander, Fossum, Rønning, et al., 2012).

Some shoplifting occurs with early school-age children, but the major problem with this arises during preadolescence. Some of this happens for the same reason that past generations tipped over outhouses or untied the preacher's horse and buggy: it is a public act of rebellion against authority, a "coming of age" ritual. It usually occurs because of peer pressure such as when children believe they must have a certain type of clothing to belong to the "in" crowd. It can also be an initiation ritual for gang membership.

Shoplifting must be taken seriously by parents because it is a punishable crime, not a prank. Just as money missing from a purse should not be ignored, shoplifting should be confronted immediately to prevent children who succeed once from taking something even bigger the second time. Children should be asked how they came to possess the article and they should not be allowed to use it. Children should then be denied access to stores until they demonstrate more responsibility. A child who shoplifts more than once may need counseling because it reflects more than simple confusion about property rights.

BOX 32.7 Nursing Care Planning to Empower a Family

TIPS FOR CHILDREN WHO SPEND TIME INDEPENDENTLY AND THEIR PARENTS

Q. Shelly stays by herself after school for a half hour each week day. Her mother asks you, "What are good tips for being sure it's safe to let her do that?"

A. Think in a number of areas:

Safety Points for Children

Always lock doors and never show keys to others or indicate you stay home alone.

When answering the telephone, say a parent is busy, not absent from home.

Have a plan in the event you lose your key (e.g., stay with a neighbor).

Don't go into the house if the door is open or a window is broken.

Learn fire safety (practice a fire drill from all rooms of the house).

Check in with parents by telephone or laptop when you first arrive home.

Identify a caller before opening the door. Agree on a secret code word; you should not open the door or go with a person unless the person knows the word.

Learn how to change light bulbs safely if it will be dark before parents return home. If appropriate, learn how to change fuses or reset circuit-breaker switches.

Learn how to report a fire and telephone police (practice this with your parents).

Safety Responsibilities for Parents

Prepare a safety kit with bandages and such; include a flashlight in case of a power failure so children do not need to light candles.

Plan after-school snacks that do not require cooking to prevent burns.

Keep firearms locked, with the key in a place unknown to child.

Keep a list of emergency telephone numbers (including parents' work numbers) by the telephone.

Arrange with a neighbor who is usually home during the late afternoon for the child to stay there in an emergency.

If an older child will be watching a younger one, be certain both children understand the rules laid down and the degree of responsibility expected.

Be certain the child understands the rules that apply during other times also apply during independent time (e.g., never swim alone, do not play by the railroad tracks).

Parental Actions to Prevent Loneliness

Leave messages on the refrigerator or in the bathroom that just say "hi."

Leave a tape- or video-recorded message for the child to play when he or she first arrives home (make sure it is not full of tasks to do, but is a welcoming message).

Be certain to make parent–child time available after work to allow for quality relationship time.

Each morning, help the child plan an activity for that day so he or she has something purposeful to look forward to during the time alone.

Allow special privileges such as listening to music other members of the family do not like; consider allowing extra television hours during this time.

Consider getting a pet. Even a caged animal, such as a hamster or a bird, offers companionship in a quiet house.

Call the child if there will be a delay in arriving home; unexpected time alone is very frightening.

Encourage the child to read; fictional characters can serve as friends as well as help to pass time.

Urge the child to network with other children who spend time alone as to how they use time effectively; talking on the telephone or e-mailing another child reduces loneliness for both.

Parental Actions to Increase Socialization

Help the child plan after school activities such as joining a science club for one afternoon a week.

Explore sports programs at school or in the community because these often are held after school.

Explore after school programs at the school the child attends, or at a public library, a church, or a temple.

Network with other parents or ask for flex time so child supervision can be alternated after school.

Be certain the child has opportunities to socialize with friends on weekends or on days when either parent is home.

Parental Actions to Increase Self-Esteem

Praise the child for the ability to take care of himself or herself for short time intervals (e.g., rather than scold him or her that there are cracker crumbs on the carpet).

Walk with the child through the empty house and together identify sounds (e.g., the click of the furnace turning on, the refrigerator starting to defrost), so they can determine the cause of sounds when home alone and not be frightened.

Help the child to view the quiet as a beneficial time in which they can do some things more efficiently, such as homework, than at noisy times.

Do not allow the child to use their time alone role to provoke parental guilt. Allow children to have some say in family spending so they can see how their time alone (which allows both parents to work) contributes to family unity and progress.

As an overall principle, parents should set good examples if they expect their child to be honest. If one parent takes money from the other without permission, neither should be surprised to find their child attempting to do the same. If a parent unwraps items and eats them without paying for them in the supermarket, a parent cannot expect a child to do otherwise.

Violence or Terrorism

Children basically view their world as safe, so it is a shock when violence such as a school shooting or reports of terrorists enter their lives (Dowdell, 2012). Common recommendations for parents to help children feel safe when they hear of these instances include:

- Assure children they are safe; even if the violence is in their community, their parents are actively involved in being certain they are not in danger.
- Observe for signs of stress such as sleep disturbances, fatigue, lack of pleasure in activities, or signs of beginning substance abuse.
- Do not allow children or adolescents to view footage of traumatic events over and over, because this decreases their ability to feel safe.
- Watch news programs with children so it can be explained that the situation portrayed is not near them and that their child is safe.
- Explain that there are bad people in the world, and bad people do bad things, but not all people in a particular group or who look a particular way are bad. Lashing out at people who resemble them only causes more harm.
- Prepare a family disaster plan, including such things as bottled water, blankets, toiletries, pet supplies, appropriate clothing, flashlights, and information such as what immunizations their children have had (particularly tetanus) and, if a child is ill, a history of medical needs or care so that such items are ready in an emergency.
- Designate a "rally point" where the family will meet if ever separated by a disaster or evacuation (AAP, 2012b).

Some parents may be reluctant to talk to their children about a disaster plan for the family, believing that these preparations will frighten children unnecessarily, but such preparations should have the major effect of increasing a feeling of safety, not decreasing it. Fear of the unknown is always more intense than a fear of something tangible.

Bullying

A frequent reason school-age children cite for feeling so unhappy that they turn guns on classmates or commit suicide is because they were ridiculed or bullied to the point they could no longer take such abuse (Cooper, Clements, & Holt, 2012). Alert parents that Internet or texting bullying are both also possible, and that a bully doesn't have to be in fact-to-face contact with their child to be harmful.

Traits commonly associated with school-age bullies include:

- Advanced physical size and strength for their age
- Aggressive temperament (both male and female)
- Parents who are indifferent to the problem or are permissive with an aggressive child
- Parents who typically resort to physical punishment
- There is the presence of a child who is a "natural victim" (e.g., small, insecure, with low self-esteem)

Suggestions for school personnel to deal with bullies include:

- Supervise recreation periods closely.
- Intervene immediately to stop bullying.
- Insist if such behavior does not stop, both the school and parents will become involved.
- Advise parents to discuss bullying with their school-age child and help them understand that it should be reported to allow adults to intervene.

If bullying behavior is ingrained, therapy may be needed to correct the behavior. Stopping bullying helps not only the victim but also the bully because statistics show that children with this type of aggressive behavior in grade school are more apt to be incarcerated as adults than others (AAP, 2012a).

Recreational Drug Use

Once considered a college or high school problem, illegal drugs such as marijuana, cocaine, and amphetamines are now available to children as early as elementary school and certainly by the time they reach the seventh and eighth grades. Because they are available in so many homes, alcohol, inhalants, and prescription drugs have also become commonly abused by this age group (Blake & Davis, 2011; Young, Glover, & Havens, 2012). Parents should be particularly aware of children who may be taking adult antidepressant drugs from home medicine cabinets because this is associated with suicide in young children (Adegbite-Adeniyi, Gron, Rowles, et al., 2012).

The use of hard drugs and alcohol and ways to encourage children to avoid their use are discussed in Chapter 33. Inhalants, which are easily available to school-age children for abuse, include airplane glue (toluene) and aerosolized cooking oil. Children do not become physically addicted to glue but do become psychologically dependent on it. To achieve the desired effect, they drop quantities of the glue into a paper bag, then sniff the fumes to experience a feeling of exhilaration or giddiness. This may seem like a harmless procedure, but, in high concentrations, glue fumes can cause extensive liver damage or enough pulmonary edema to be fatal. Cooking spray or computer keyboard cleaner give this same effect. Because these products contain Freon, they can cause severe respiratory and cardiac irregularity (Baydala, 2010).

Children who report being happy and are able to communicate with their family are less likely to be regular users than others (Farmer & Hanratty, 2012). Parents should suspect recreational drug use if their child regularly appears irritable, inattentive, or drowsy.

Abuse of androgenic steroids or human growth hormone to enhance sports performance are yet other drugs that can be found in preteen children. Counsel children against this because abuse of steroids can lead to cardiovascular irregularities, uncontrollable aggressiveness, and possible cancer in later life (Oberlander & Henderson, 2012).

Cigarette smoking also begins in school-age children. With the sure knowledge that cigarette smoking plays a large part in the development of lung cancer and other serious respiratory illnesses, many parents assume their children will know better than to begin smoking. Smoking is viewed as an adult activity, however, so adopting the habit can be considered a giant step on the road to adulthood. Although the amount of cigarette advertising targeting young people as consumers has decreased, school-age children should still be taught to recognize advertising manipulation aimed at them. Caution children against experimenting with smokeless tobacco as well because this can lead to mouth and throat cancer, the same as smoking (Zhou, Michaud, Langevin, et al., 2012).

To discourage use of tobacco by school-age children, health care professionals and parents need to be role models of excellent nonsmoking health behavior in hope that children will follow their good examples.

QSEN Checkpoint Question 32.6

Patient-Centered Care

The school-age period is the time when many young people begin smoking. In order to design interventions that are effective and patient centered, you should begin by acknowledging which of the following?

a. Most children who try smoking do not like it.
b. The media have occasionally exaggerated the risks of smoking.
c. Many people view smoking as being an "adult" activity.
d. Children under puberty cannot become addicted to smoking.

Look in Appendix A for the best answer and rationale.

Concerns of the School-Age Child and Family With Unique Needs

A number of situations cause school-age children to have additional needs or concerns.

The Child of Alcoholic Parents

Children who live with an alcoholic parent are at greater risk for having emotional problems than others because of the frequent disruption in their lives (Serec, Svab, Kolšek, et al., 2012). In addition, because alcoholism may have a genetic base, children of alcoholics may be more likely to become alcoholics as adults. This makes it imperative for such children to learn effective coping behaviors. Immediate problems that can occur with children of alcoholic parents include:

- A feeling of guilt that they are the cause of the parent's drinking
- Constant worry that the alcoholic parent will become sick or die, leaving the child alone; at the same time, the child may fear the alcoholic parent and wish the parent would leave
- A feeling of shame that prevents the child from inviting friends home or asking for help
- Decreased ability to trust adults because the parent has been unreliable so many times
- Poor nutrition and decreasing grades in school because the alcoholic parent's behavior is so erratic that no regular schedule of bedtime or meals exists
- Anger at the alcoholic parent for drinking and at the nonalcoholic parent for not doing more to correct things
- Helplessness to change the situation

Such fears may be revealed by not only failing marks in school but also withdrawal from friends or social activities and delinquent behavior such as stealing. With adolescence may come depression, suicidal thoughts, or abuse of drugs or alcohol. School nurses are in an excellent position to identify such children, monitor their school progress, and refer them to organizations such as Al-Anon or Alateen (www.al-anon.alateen.org) for support.

The Child With a Long-Term Illness or Physical Cognitive Challenge

One of the biggest problems facing school-age children with a long-term illness or physical challenges is time lost from school. This threatens not only their academic achievement but also their relationships with peers because it may make the child the "odd person out" with respect to making friends or joining clubs. Whether children are on home care or hospitalized, helping them to keep in contact with friends by texting, e-mail, or letters can help foster the socialization that is so important for continued development. Keeping up with schooling, whether it is homeschool or a distant learning option, is also important and an area where school nurses can play an important role (Singer, 2012).

If at all possible, children with physical or cognitive challenges should attend regular schools and classes **(inclusion)** based on federal law (Public Law 99-457), which stipulates that all children have the right to equal education in the least restrictive environment possible (Sass-Lehrer & Bodner-Johnson, 1989). The decision as to which classroom would be best for an individual child is determined by a committee in each school system. You may need to advocate for a child with such a committee to demonstrate, for example, that although a child uses a wheelchair or needs continuous oxygen, the child will be able to contribute to regular classroom activities. It may be necessary to meet with a school nurse, teacher, or the child's classmates (with the parents' permission) to increase their understanding and acceptance of a child's illness or to help arrange a period each day with a special resource teacher.

Urge parents of children with physical or cognitive challenges to assign them household chores just like other children and to allow them to participate in peer activities, such as Girl or Boy Scouts, in which accomplishment is encouraged. It is important for such children to develop a sense of industry or accomplishment so they can persevere in measures that will help them to be as independent as possible in the future (Fig. 32.10).

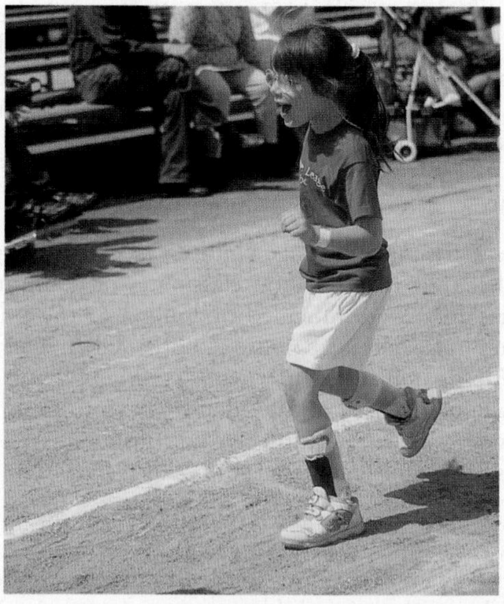

FIGURE 32.10 A school-age child who is physically challenged is elated at a finish line. This accomplishment can go far toward her developing a sense of industry. (© Jose Carillo/Stock Boston.)

TABLE 32.5 Nursing Actions That Encourage a Sense of Industry in the Physically Challenged or Chronically Ill School-Age Child

Category	Actions
Nutrition	Allow choices of food when possible and respect food preferences. Provide small food servings that child can finish, which encourages a sense of accomplishment.
Dressing	Ask for suggestions as to how bulky the child wants the dressing and where to apply tape.
Medicine	Teach the child the name and action of medicine. Encourage the child to keep track of medication times by clock or record. The child may feel more in control of injections or intravenous insertions if allowed to choose the site from among options offered. Allow the child to choose oral medicine form (capsules or liquid) if possible.
Rest	Establish clear rules for rest periods (e.g., reading or watching television is all right; playing a game is not).
Hygiene	Respect the modesty of a school-age child at an adult level. Allow as much choice as possible such as own clothing and timing of self-care.
Pain	Encourage the child to express and rate pain. Encourage the child to use distraction techniques, such as counting backward from 100 or imagery, during episodes of pain. Explain the source and cause of pain to give the child sense of mastery.
Stimulation	Encourage school work. Encourage activities that end in a product (e.g., putting together a picture puzzle rather than listening to a CD). Encourage paper-and-pencil games, such as connect the dots or tic-tac-toe. Card games provide social interaction and also encourage simple addition skills (make a deck from paper if one is not available). Don't suggest competitive games for children younger than age 10 years. Encourage using the playroom for socialization. Encourage the child to keep in contact with school friends by texting or e-mailing them.

When you are caring for a school-age child who is chronically ill or physically challenged, choose short-term activities that can be completed independently, as with all school-age children. Conversely, be careful not to insult a child with tasks that are obviously not age appropriate. Table 32.5 describes some nursing actions to help foster a sense of industry in children who are physically challenged or chronically ill.

Nutrition and the School-Age Child With a Challenge

Food preparation and washing the dishes are times for socializing in most households. A school-age child who cannot be involved in these activities because of a physical challenge may need extra time during the day to make up for these lost socializing experiences, such as a specific hour set aside for talking or sharing a project that can be accomplished in one sitting.

When eating in cafeterias or at a friend's home, children who must eat special diets are usually tempted to select the same food as everyone else rather than limit what they choose. They may decline invitations rather than admit to requiring a special diet or needing help with eating. Ask at health care visits if any of these problems are present. Help children with special diets to plan ways they could be comfortable in social food-based settings such as bringing a party snack that is appropriate and can be easily eaten, or how to politely decline particular foods. Help children who are hospitalized to select a diet that is enjoyable as well as nutritious.

The Overweight or Obese Child

In some communities, as many as 50% of school-age children are obese by body mass index guidelines. Some of these children have been overweight since infancy, and the natural prepubertal weight gain makes them become obese. Children with an endomorphic build (a natural tendency to accumulate body fat) are more likely to be obese at any time in life than those with a mesomorphic (normal) or ectomorphic (slender) build. Many families rely on fast-food meals several times a week, and such foods tend to be high in calories and fat and can lead to obesity. Soft drink machines in grade schools add to the problem (Krebs & Primak, 2011). Children of obese parents are also more apt to become obese, probably related to both genetic and environmental influences.

By preteen years, obese children begin to develop many of the same health problems as obese adults, such as hypertension, type 2 diabetes, and an elevated total cholesterol level, with possible atherosclerosis. They also may be ridiculed or bullied for their size and may be unable to participate on sports teams. This is strong evidence of the need for active measures to help preteens regulate their weight (Schantz, 2012).

Those who become so obese that friends leave them out of activities or they cannot play sports because they tire so quickly may develop such a poor self-image they have little motivation for self-improvement. The type of weight-reduction program that will probably work best is one that emphasizes long-term lifestyle changes and contains features such as:

- An intake of about 1,200 calories a day (no more than 30% as fat), with lifestyle changes such as a structured family meal, eliminating eating or snacking in front of the television, decreasing portion sizes, and eliminating sugar-rich drinks.
- An active exercise program, including monitoring and limiting time spent in physical inactivity (e.g., watching television, playing computer and video games, surfing the Internet, texting).
- A counseling program to discuss aspects such as self-image and motivation to reduce weight.

Total caloric intake should not be reduced too drastically in children because they need calories to form new body tissue for continued growth. Caution children not to try faddish high-protein diets (as most adults should not), because such diets do not supply enough carbohydrates and may produce a heavy renal solute load (the breakdown product of proteins) to the kidneys. It helps if children aim to lose 5 lb over a short time rather than 50 lb over a year. This short-term goal coincides better with the task of developing industry.

Surgical techniques such as an intestinal bypass or lap band surgery are obviously extreme measures and inappropriate for children. Obese children might request one, however, in an attempt to avoid the not insignificant difficulty of long-term weight loss.

Nursing Diagnoses and Related Interventions

Nursing Diagnosis: Altered family dynamics related to lack of motivation to reduce weight

Outcome Evaluation: Child states reasonable weight loss and exercise goals; discusses feelings about being overweight and reactions from schoolmates; expresses positive feelings about self-worth.

Motivating preteens to lose weight can be very difficult because they are not concerned when told that obese people do not live as long as slimmer persons or that they have more heart attacks because this will happen so far in the future. They do, however, have a great respect for adults who are sympathetic to their problems. They are also aware that slim children are usually the most popular, and they wish they could look that way. They follow better dietary regimens, therefore, if they are asked to do so by a respected adult, such as a nurse, or if they fear being left out of social interactions.

Overweight school-age children often do well if a dieters' club is formed; they are not too young to participate in formal weight-control organizations. Having tangible support from other group members helps them follow tedious and monotonous nutrition patterns. As a way of increasing daily activity, preadolescents do well with formal exercise classes because, again, they enjoy the support from other children. In addition, encourage them to increase informal exercise, such as walking to and from school or walking a dog. Encourage coaches of childhood sports to accept obese children as part of a team, not because the child will necessarily benefit the team, but because the exercise will benefit the child. Not only does exercise burn up calories, but if children's daylight hours are filled with activities and friends, they have less time to eat and spend less time in sedentary activities.

Lifestyle change is the ultimate goal for the entire family because obesity is usually a family problem. Rather than preparing special meals for just the obese child, the entire family probably needs to eat in a healthier manner. Because preadolescents do not generally prepare their own food, the person in the home who prepares meals requires as much information on the planned weight loss as the child. The old concepts that used to hold ("A clean plate is good" and "How can you leave food when people in other countries are starving?") may have to be changed so children and other family members reduce their intake appropriately. The importance of exercise should also be reflected in the home. Family members should not only encourage the obese child to exercise, but they should also partake in some form of daily activity with them.

There is some danger in pointing out to preadolescents that they are overweight because some children can become so obsessed with losing weight that they develop eating disorders (see Chapter 54). Stressing that children should "become healthier" or "improve stamina" may be better advice than talking about losing weight (Field, Sonneville, Micali, et al., 2012).

What if...32.4 You are particularly interested in exploring one of the 2020 National Health Goals with respect to school-age growth and development (see Box 32.1). What would be a possible research topic to explore pertinent to this goal that would be applicable to Shelly's family and that would also advance evidence-based practice?

Key Points for Review

- School-age children mature slowly but steadily. Their average annual weight gain is 3 to 5 lb; their increase in height is 1 to 2 in.
- At about age 10 years, children begin to develop secondary sex characteristics. Preparation for this helps them accept these changes positively.
- Deciduous teeth are lost and permanent teeth erupt during the school-age period.
- Erikson's developmental task for the school-age period is to gain a sense of industry, or how to do things well.
- Common health problems during the school-age period include minor respiratory and gastrointestinal infections as well as dental caries and malocclusion.
- Common parental concerns during this period are language development, fears and anxieties, and behavior problems such as stealing and exposure to recreational drugs. Treating preventive strategies regarding these helps in planning nursing care that not only meets QSEN competencies but that also best meets a family's total needs.
- As many as 90% of parents of school-age children are dual-earner families. This means that many school-age

children return home before their parents. Counseling families on ways to turn this independent time into a positive experience is helpful.

- Children in a concrete stage of operational thought are limited to understanding concepts that they can actually see. When health teaching, use concrete examples (actually let them hold a syringe, don't just talk about it) to increase their understanding.
- School-age children thrive on rules. It is confusing for them when rules are changed (e.g., medicine will now be taken four rather than three times a day) unless they have a clear explanation of why the change is occurring.
- School-age children look for good adult role models; it is hard for them to feel confidence in an adult who isn't honest with them or who fails to live up to their expectations by not following through on promises.
- School-age children with a family tendency toward obesity may become overweight. Helping the family learn a healthier lifestyle is important.

Critical Thinking Care Study

Georgia is a 6-year-old girl in the first grade whom you meet when working as a school nurse. She lives with her 10-year-old sister and her parents in a three-bedroom home. Her father works long shifts as a coal miner, and her mother cleans houses for a commercial housecleaning firm.

1. Georgia's mother tells you she received a note from her teacher asking her to help Georgia "speak more clearly." Is this a common concern with early school-age children? What further information do you need to know to evaluate whether this is a concern?
2. Georgia's teacher is also concerned because Georgia does not share well. Is this a developmental step that Georgia should have already mastered?
3. Georgia's mother wants her to be popular and so has enrolled her in dance classes two times per week, a school soccer club four times per week, violin lessons once per week, and a gymnastics class twice per week. Despite all the effort she puts in driving her daughter to all these sessions, the mother tells you Georgia doesn't act grateful. She asks you why Georgia isn't interested in making friends.

Patient Scenario

The Ralston Family

Read about the Ralston family, a family with a school-age child, then answer the questions to further sharpen your skills and grow more familiar with NCLEX-type questions related to growth and development in the school-age child. Confirm your answers are correct by reading the rationales.

Visit http://thePoint.lww.com

Answers and Rationales

Looking for answers to the What if . . . and Critical Thinking Care Study questions?

Visit http://thePoint.lww.com

References

Adegbite-Adeniyi, C., Gron, B., Rowles, B. M., et al. (2012). An update on antidepressant use and suicidality in pediatric depression. *Expert Opinion on Pharmacotherapy, 13*(15), 2119–2130.

American Academy of Pediatrics. (2012a). *Bullying: It's not okay.* Evanston, IL: Author.

American Academy of Pediatrics. (2012b). *Terrorism disaster fact sheet.* Evanston, IL: Author.

American Academy of Pediatrics, Committee on Practice and Ambulatory Medicine. (2012). *Recommendations for preventive pediatric health care.* Evanston, IL, Author.

Anthony, K. V., & Burroughs, S. (2010). Making the transition from traditional to home schooling: Home school family motivations. *Current Issues in Education, 13*(4), 1–30

Baydala, L. (2010). Inhalant abuse. *Paediatrics & Child Health, 5*(7), 443–454.

Bishop, W. P. (2011). The digestive system. In K. J. Marcdante, R. M. Kliegman, H. B. Jenson, et al. (Eds), *Nelson essentials of pediatrics* (6th ed., pp. 463–498). Philadelphia, PA: Saunders/Elsevier.

Blake, K., & Davis, V. (2011). Substance abuse. In K. J. Marcdante, R. M. Kliegman, H. B. Jenson, et al. (Eds.), *Nelson essentials of pediatrics* (6th ed., pp. 281–284). Philadelphia, PA: Saunders/Elsevier.

Briggs, P., Simon, W. T., & Simonsen, S. (2011). An exploratory study of Internet-initiated sexual offenses and the chat room sex offender. *Sexual Abuse, 23*(1), 72–91.

Caprio, S. (2012). Calories from soft drinks—Do they matter? *New England Journal of Medicine, 367*(15), 1462–1463.

Chahal, H., Fung, C., Kuhle, S., et al. (2012). Availability and night-time use of electronic entertainment and communication devices are associated with short sleep duration and obesity among Canadian children. *Pediatric Obesity, 8*(1), 42–51

Cooper, G. D., Clements, P. T., & Holt, K. E. (2012). Examining childhood bullying and adolescent suicide: Implications for school nurses. *Journal of School Nursing, 28*(8), 275–283.

Daley, A. M. (2011). Providing adolescent-friendly HPV education. *Nurse Practitioner, 36*(11), 35–40.

Dowdell, E. B. (2012). Urban seventh grade students: A report of health risk behaviors and exposure to violence. *Journal of School Nursing, 28*(2), 130–137.

Eagle, T. F., Sheetz, A., Gurm, R., et al. (2012). Understanding childhood obesity in America: Linkages between household income, community resources, and children's behaviors. *American Heart Journal, 163*(5), 836–843.

Edmonds, D. K. (2012). Puberty and its disorders. In D. K. Edmonds (Ed.), *Dewhurst's textbook of obstetrics & gynaecology* (8th ed., pp. 471–489). Oxford, UK: John Wiley & Son.

El-Dawlatly, M. M., Fayed, M. M., & Mostafa, Y. A. (2012). Deep overbite malocclusion: Analysis of the underlying components. *American Journal of Orthodontics & Dentofacial Orthopedics, 142*(4), 473–480.

Erikson, E. H. (1993). *Childhood and society.* New York, NY: W. W. Norton.

Farmer, S., & Hanratty, B. (2012). The relationship between subjective wellbeing, low income and substance use among schoolchildren in the north west of England: A cross-sectional study. *Journal of Public Health (Oxford), 34*(4), 512–522.

Field, A. E., Sonneville, K. R., Micali, N., et al. (2012). Prospective association of common eating disorders and adverse outcomes. *Pediatrics, 130*(2), e289–e295.

Fletcher, N. D., & Bruce, R. W. (2012). Early onset scoliosis: Current concepts and controversies. *Current Reviews in Musculoskeletal Medicine, 5*(2), 102–110.

Freud, S. (1962). *Three essays on the theory of sexuality.* New York, NY: Hearst Corporation.

Gunter, K. B., Almstedt, H. C., & Janz, K. F. (2012). Physical activity in childhood may be the key to optimizing lifespan skeletal health. *Exercise & Sport Science Reviews, 40*(1), 13–21.

Hamdan, A. M., Singh, V., & Rock., W. P. (2012). Assessment of the relationship between perceptions of dental aesthetics and demand for orthodontic treatment in 10–11 year old school children in Birmingham, UK. *Community Dental Health, 29*(1), 124–128.

Harika, R. K., Cosgrove, M. C., Osendarp, S. J., et al. (2011). Fatty acid intakes of children and adolescents are not in line with the dietary intake recommendations for future cardiovascular health. *British Journal of Nutrition, 106*(3), 307–316.

Heron, M. (2012). Deaths: Leading causes. *National Vital Statistics Reports, 60*(6), 1–90.

Hirschman, J., & Chriqui, J. F. (2012). School food and nutrition policy, monitoring and evaluation in the USA. *Public Health Nutrition, 25*(9), 1–7.

Horne, A. W., & Critchley, H. O. D. (2012). Menstrual problems: Heavy menstrual bleeding and primary dysmenorrhoea. In D. K. Edmonds (Ed.), *Dewhurst's textbook of obstetrics & gynaecology* (8th ed., pp. 534–543). Oxford, UK: John Wiley & Son.

Jacobson, N. A., Morawa, L. G., & Bir, C. A. (2012). Epidemiology of cheerleading injuries presenting to NEISS hospitals from 2002 to 2007. *Journal of Trauma & Acute Care Surgery, 72*(2), 521–526.

Kistner, F., Fiebert, I., & Roach, K. (2012). Effect of backpack load carriage on cervical posture in primary schoolchildren. *Work, 41*(1), 99–108.

Kohlberg, L. (1984). *The psychology of moral development.* New York, NY: Harper & Row.

Krebs, N. F., & Primak, L. E. (2011). Pediatric nutrition and nutritional disorders. In K. J. Marcdante, R. M. Kliegman, H. B. Jenson, et al. (Eds.), *Nelson essentials of pediatrics* (6th ed., pp. 103–122). Philadelphia, PA: Saunders/Elsevier.

Loke, I. C., Heyman, G. D., Forgie, J., et al. (2011). Children's moral evaluations of reporting the transgressions of peers: Age differences in evaluations of tattling. *Developmental Psychology, 47*(6), 1757–1762.

Lowe, S. R., Godoy, L., Rhodes, J. E., et al. (2013). Predicting mothers' reports of children's mental health three years after hurricane Katrina. *Journal of Applied Developmental Psychology, 34*(1), 17–27.

Mack, K. A., Dellinger, A., & West, B. A. (2012). Adult opinions about the age at which children can be left home alone, bathe alone, or bike alone: Second Injury Control and Risk Survey (ICARIS-2). *Journal of Safety Research, 43*(3), 223–226.

Marván, M. L., & Molina-Abolnik, M. (2012). Mexican adolescents' experience of menarche and attitudes toward menstruation: Role of communication between mothers and daughters. *Journal of Pediatric & Adolescent Gynecology, 25*(6), 358–363.

Meng, M. V., & Tanagho, E. A. (2013). Physical examination of the urinary tract. In J. McAninch & T. F. Lue (Eds.), *Smith & Tanagho's general urology* (18th ed., pp. 41–47). New York, NY: McGraw-Hill Publishing Company.

Oberlander, J. G., & Henderson, L. P. (2012). The Sturm und Drang of anabolic steroid use: Angst, anxiety, and aggression. *Trends in Neurosciences, 35*(6), 382–392.

Pass, L., Arteche, A., Cooper, P., et al. (2012). Doll play narratives about starting school in children of socially anxious mothers, and their relation to subsequent child school-based anxiety. *Journal of Abnormal Child Psychology, 40*(8), 1375–1384.

Piaget, J. (1969). *The theory of stages in cognitive development.* New York, NY: McGraw-Hill.

Pringsheim, T., Doja, A., Gorman, D., et al. (2012). Canadian guidelines for the evidence-based treatment of tic disorders: Pharmacotherapy. *Canadian Journal of Psychiatry, 57*(3), 133–143.

Robinson, J. M., & Ficca, M. (2012). Managing the student with severe food allergies. *The Journal of School Nursing, 28*(6), 187–194.

Sandler, P. J., Madahar, A. K., & Murray, A. (2011). Anterior open bite: Aetiology and management. *Dental Update, 38*(8), 522–524.

Sass-Lehrer, M., & Bodner-Johnson, B. (1989). Public Law 99–457: A new challenge to early intervention. *American Annals of the Dead, 134*(2), 71–77.

Schantz, S. (2012). Overweight and obesity in youth. *Journal of School Nursing, 28*(6), 167–168.

Scheffer, R. (2011). Anxiety and phobias. In K. J. Marcdante, R. M. Kliegman, H. B. Jenson, et al. (Eds.), *Nelson essentials of pediatrics* (6th ed., pp. 67–71). Philadelphia, PA: Saunders/Elsevier.

Serec, M., Svab, I., Kolšek, M., et al. (2012). Health-related lifestyle, physical and mental health in children of alcoholic parents. *Drug & Alcohol Review, 31*(7):861–870.

Singer, B. (2012). Perceptions of school nurses in the care of students with disabilities. *Journal of School Nursing.* Advance online publication.

Smith, S. (2011). Sinusitis. In K. J. Marcdante, R. M. Kliegman, H. B. Jenson, et al. (Eds.), *Nelson essentials of pediatrics* (6th ed., pp. 389–390). Philadelphia, PA: Saunders/Elsevier.

Sourander, A., Fossum, S., Rønning, J. A., et al. (2012). What is the long-term outcome of boys who steal at age eight? *Social Psychiatry & Psychiatric Epidemiology, 47*(9), 1391–1400.

Theisen, D., Frisch, A, Malisoux, L., et al. (2012). Injury risk is different in team and individual youth sport. *Journal of Science & Medicine in Sport, 16*(3), 200–204.

Tubert-Jeannin, S., Auclair, C., Amsallem, E., et al. (2011). Fluoride supplements (tablets, drops, lozenges or chewing gums) for preventing dental caries in children. *Cochrane Database of Systematic Reviews,* (12), CD007592.

U.S. Department of Health and Human Services. (2010). *Healthy people 2020.* Washington, DC: Author.

Van Winckel, M., Vande Velde, S., De Bruyne, R., et al. (2011). Clinical practice: Vegetarian infant and child nutrition. *European Journal of Pediatrics, 170*(12), 1489–1494.

Wen, A., Goldberg, D., Marrs, C. F., et al. (2012). Caries resistance as a function of age in an initially caries-free population. *Journal of Dental Research, 91*(7), 671–675.

White, R., & Mason, R. (2011). Bullying and gangs. *International Journal of Adolescent Medicine & Health, 24*(1), 57–62.

Whitney, E. N., & Rolfes, S. R. (2012). Life cycle nutrition: Infancy, childhood & adolescence. In *Understanding nutrition* (pp. 528–573). Belmont, CA: Wadsworth Publishing.

Widaman, K. F., & Helm, J. L. (2012). Nocturnal emissions: A failure to replicate. *American Journal of Psychology, 125*(1), 39–50.

Young, A. M., Glover, N., & Havens, J. R. (2012). Nonmedical use of prescription medications among adolescents in the United States: A systematic review. *Journal of Adolescent Health, 51*(1), 6–17.

Zhou, J., Michaud, D. S., Langevin, S. M., et al. (2012). Smokeless tobacco and risk of head and neck cancer: Evidence from a case-control study in New England. *International Journal of Cancer, 132*(8), 1911–1917.

Chapter 33

Nursing Care of a Family With an Adolescent

KEY TERMS

- adolescence
- comedones
- formal operational thought
- glycogen loading
- identity
- puberty
- role confusion
- stalking
- substance abuse

OBJECTIVES

After mastering the contents of this chapter, you should be able to:

1. Describe normal growth and development and common parental concerns of the adolescent period.
2. Identify 2020 National Health Goals related to adolescents that nurses could help the nation achieve.
3. Assess an adolescent for normal growth and development milestones.
4. Formulate nursing diagnoses related to adolescent growth and development or common parental concerns.
5. Identify expected outcomes for nursing care of an adolescent as well as help parents manage seamless transitions across differing health care settings.
6. Using the nursing process, plan nursing care that includes the six competencies of Quality & Safety Education for Nurses (QSEN): Patient-Centered Care, Teamwork & Collaboration, Evidence-Based Practice (EBP), Quality Improvement (QI), Safety, and Informatics.
7. Implement nursing care related to growth and development or special needs of an adolescent, such as organizing a discussion group on ways to prevent substance abuse.
8. Evaluate expected outcomes for achievement and effectiveness of care.
9. Integrate knowledge of adolescent growth and development with the interplay of nursing process, the six competencies of QSEN, and Family Nursing to promote quality maternal and child health nursing care.

Raul is a 15-year-old teenager you meet at an adolescent clinic. His chief concern is a head cold. He has numerous acne lesions on his forehead and cheeks. His parents tell you Raul seemed depressed for a long time after his girlfriend broke up with him but now seems happy again. They are pleased to see him maturing so much that he recently gave away his collection of baseball cards to a young neighbor. You mention to Raul a decongestant would probably make him feel better. He asks you how many pills it would take to kill someone, then jokes he was kidding. His health care provider prescribes a decongestant and suggests Raul return in 6 months.

The previous chapter discussed school-age children and the capabilities children develop during that time period. This chapter adds information about the changes, both physical and psychosocial, which occur during adolescence. Such information builds a base for care and health teaching for this age group.

Did Raul have some needs that were not met by his clinic visit?

Adolescence is generally defined as the period between ages 13 and 18 or 20 years, a time that serves as a transition between childhood and becoming a young adult. It can be divided into an early period (13 to 14 years), a middle period (15 to 16 years), and a late period (17 to 20 years). During all periods, adolescence is defined not so much by chronologic age as by physiologic, psychological, and sociologic changes. The drastic change in physical appearance and the change in expectations of others (especially parents) that occur during the period can lead to both emotional and physical health concerns (Sass & Kaplan, 2013).

Adolescents invariably feel a sense of pressure throughout this period because they are mature in some respects but still young in others. For example, an adolescent's sexual interests are awakening, yet personal or parental pressures discourage sexual exploration. An adolescent may not feel mature enough to live away from home, yet parents and teachers may urge the adolescent to apply for an out-of-town college. This duality causes a major dilemma or conflict for an adolescent, leading to many of the growth and developmental concerns of the age (Ahern & Norris, 2011). The 2020 National Health Goals related to adolescence are shown in Box 33.1.

BOX 33.1 Nursing Care Planning Based on 2020 National Health Goals

Health teaching in the adolescent years is important because healthy habits begun at this time can influence health over a lifetime. For this reason, a number of 2020 National Health Goals relate to adolescent health, including:

- Reduce the number of adolescents who are obese from a prevalence of 17.9% to 16.1%.
- Reduce the proportion of high school students engaging in binge drinking from 25.2% to 22.7%.
- Reduce cigarette use by adolescents from 19.5% to 16%.
- Reduce the rate of smokeless tobacco use by adolescents from 8.9% to 6.9%.
- Reduce the proportion of adolescents who are offered, sold, or given an illegal drug on school property from 22.7% to 20.4%.
- Reduce the proportion of adolescents who report they rode, during the previous 30 days, with a driver who was drinking alcohol from 28.3% to 25.5%.
- Reduce the rate of suicide attempts by adolescents from 1.9% to 1.7%.
- Increase the proportion of adolescents who meet current federal physical activity guidelines for aerobic physical activity from 18.4% to 20.2% (U.S. Department of Health and Human Services [DHHS], 2010; see www.healthypeople.gov).

Nurses can help the nation achieve these goals by educating adolescents about the use of cigarettes, smokeless tobacco, alcohol, and substance abuse, and by acting as support people for adolescents during times of crisis to help prevent self-injury or suicide.

Nursing Process Overview

For Healthy Development of an Adolescent

Assessment

Parents rarely bring adolescents for routine health maintenance visits the way they did when they were younger, and adolescents generally don't come to health care facilities on their own unless they are ill. Until adolescents need a physical examination for athletic or some other clearance, therefore, they are often not seen for health assessments. When adolescents are accompanied by their parents at health visits, it is best to obtain a health history separately from the adolescent to promote independence and responsibility for self-care. When performing physical examinations on adolescents, be aware they may be very self-conscious of their body. They need health assurance and appreciate comments such as "Your blood pressure is 120/70, which is healthy," so they can learn more about their rapidly changing bodies.

Nursing Diagnosis

Nursing diagnoses for adolescents can cover a wide range of topics. Frequently used diagnoses related to adolescents and their families include:

- Health-seeking behaviors related to normal growth and development
- Low self-esteem related to facial acne
- Anxiety related to concerns about normal growth and development
- Risk for injury related to peer pressure to use alcohol and drugs
- Readiness for enhanced parenting related to increased knowledge of teenage years

Outcome Identification and Planning

When planning care with adolescents, respect the fact that they have a strong desire to exert independence or do things their own way. This means they are not likely to adhere to a plan of care that disrupts their lifestyle or makes them appear different from others their age. Because of this, including them in planning is essential so the plan will be agreeable and accepted. Establishing a contract, such as asking an adolescent to agree to take medication daily, may be the most effective means to reach a mutual understanding.

Remember that adolescents are very oriented to the present, so a program that provides immediate results, such as increased respiratory function, will usually be carried out well. In contrast, a regimen oriented toward the future, with long-term goals such as preventing hypertension at middle age, may not be as successful. This does not mean it is not important to teach adolescents about the necessity of reducing future health risks—by eating well, not smoking, and generally taking care of their bodies—but that information will be best accepted if geared as much as possible to specific, short-term benefits to their health. Helpful Web sites for teenage referrals include:

- Mothers Against School Hazing (www.mashinc.org)
- Students Against Destructive Decisions (www.sadd.org)
- National Eating Disorder Foundation (www.nationaleatingdisorders.org)

- American Association of Suicidology (www.suicidology.org)
- Partnership for a Drug-Free America (www.drugfreeamerica.org)
- Al-Anon/Alateen (www.alateen.com)
- Planned Parenthood Federation of America, Inc. (www.plannedparenthood.org)
- Sexual Information and Education Council of the United States (SIECUS) (www.siecus.org)
- GLBT National Help Center (www.GLBTnationalhelpcenter.org) or 1-888-843-4564.

Implementation

Adolescents tend to do poorly with tasks someone tells them they *must* do. If they help to plan tasks, however, they typically carry them out successfully. Adolescents have little patience with adults who do not demonstrate the behavior they are being asked to achieve; a parent or nurse who smokes and asks an adolescent not to smoke, for example, will probably not be successful. For best results, evaluate how an intervention appears from an adolescent's standpoint before beginning teaching.

Outcome Evaluation

An evaluation of expected outcomes should include not only whether desired outcomes have been achieved but also whether adolescents are pleased with the outcome. Individuals will have difficulty accomplishing desired goals as adults unless they have high self-esteem that includes feeling secure in their new body image.

Examples of outcome criteria that might be established include:

- Client states she feels good about herself even though she is the shortest girl in her class.
- Client states he has not consumed alcohol in 2 weeks.
- Parents state they feel more confident about their ability to parent an adolescent.
- Client states she feels high self-esteem despite persistent facial acne.

GROWTH AND DEVELOPMENT OF AN ADOLESCENT

Adolescents both grow rapidly and mature dramatically during the period from age 13 to 18 to 20 years.

Physical Growth

The major milestones of physical development in the adolescent period are the onset of puberty at 8 to 12 years of age, and the cessation of body growth around 16 to 20 years (Sass & Kaplan, 2013). Between these milestones, physiologic growth and development of adult coordination occur. At first, the gain in physical growth is mostly in weight, leading to the stocky, slightly obese appearance of prepubescence; later comes the thin, gangly appearance of late adolescence.

Most girls are 1 to 2 in. (2.4 to 5 cm) taller than boys coming into adolescence but generally stop growing within 3 years from menarche and so are shorter than boys by the end of adolescence. Boys typically grow about 4 to 12 in. (10 to 30 cm) in height and gain about 15 to 65 lb (7 to 30 kg) during their teenage years. Girls grow 2 to 8 in. (5 to 20 cm) in height and gain 15 to 55 lb (7 to 25 kg). Growth stops with closure of the epiphyseal lines of the long bones, which occurs at about 16 or 17 years of age in females and about 18 to 20 years of age in males.

Because the heart and lungs increase in size more slowly than the rest of the body, adolescents may have insufficient energy and become fatigued trying to finish the various activities that interest them. Pulse rate and respiratory rate decrease slightly (to 70 beats/min and 20 breaths/min, respectively), and blood pressure increases slightly (to 120/70 mmHg) by late adolescence. With adulthood, blood pressure becomes slightly higher in males than in females because more force is necessary to distribute blood to the larger male body mass.

All during adolescence, androgen stimulates sebaceous glands to extreme activity, sometimes resulting in acne, a common adolescent skin problem. Apocrine sweat glands (i.e., glands present in the axillae and genital area, which produce a strong odor in response to emotional stimulation) form shortly after puberty. Adolescents begin to notice they must shower or bathe more frequently than when they were younger in order to be free of body odor because of this change.

Teeth

Adolescents gain their second molars at about 13 years of age and their third molars (wisdom teeth) between 18 and 21 years of age. Third molars may erupt as early as 14 to 15 years of age. The jaw reaches adult size only toward the end of adolescence, however. As a result, adolescents whose third molars erupt before the lengthening of the jaw is complete may experience pain and may need these molars extracted because they do not fit their jawline (Marciani, 2012).

What if . . . 33.1 Raul asks you if you think he's going to grow some more; being the shortest boy in his gym class makes him feel "left out." Also, he asks if his teeth are white enough. Are these common concerns of adolescents?

Puberty

Puberty is the time at which an individual first becomes capable of sexual reproduction. A girl has entered puberty when she begins to menstruate; a boy enters puberty when he begins to produce spermatozoa. These events usually occur between ages 11 and 14 years. The age of first menstruation in girls is gradually decreasing from a mean of 13 years to 12.4 years, which is probably related to more weight gain in girls (Ledger, 2012). Puberty creates many questions for early teenagers about what is normal and what is not (Marván & Molina-Abolnik, 2012).

Secondary Sex Changes

Secondary sex characteristics, such as body hair configuration and breast growth, are those characteristics that distinguish the sexes from each other but that play no direct part in reproduction. The secondary sex characteristics that began in the late school-age period (see Chapter 32) continue to develop during adolescence. Typical stages of sexual maturation are shown in Table 33.1.

Encourage parents to give adolescents more freedom in areas such as choosing their own clothes or after-school activities; at the same time, help parents continue to place some restrictions on adolescent behavior ("You must drive the car safely," "We must know where you go after school"). These are not unreasonable rules and actually help adolescents accept the responsibility that comes with independence.

Both parents and adolescents may need help to understand that emancipation does not mean severance of a relationship, but rather a change in a relationship as people who are independent of one another can have even better relationships than those who are dependent on one another. It can be helpful to remind parents this step is actually no different from the one children accomplished when they grew from infants to toddlers, when they changed from wanting to be held and rocked to wanting to run. If parents can think of it in this light, they will gain a better perspective and may realize they will not lose the children because they become adults. There are ex-wives and ex-husbands. There are no ex-children.

Late Adolescent Developmental Task: Intimacy Versus Isolation

Developing a sense of intimacy means a young adult is able to form long-term, meaningful relationships with persons of the opposite as well as their same sex (Erickson, 1993). Those who do not develop a sense of intimacy are left feeling isolated; in a crisis situation, they have no one to whom they feel they can turn to for help or support. A sense of intimacy is closely related to the sense of trust learned in the first year of life because, without the feeling that one can trust others, building a sense of intimacy is difficult.

Some adolescents require help from parents or other adults to differentiate between sound relationships and those that are based only on sexual attraction. Never do adolescents need an adult to listen to them more than when they are struggling with the heart-rending feelings of young love or wondering whether a particular love relationship is temporary or lasting.

Some parents may not be able to listen to their adolescent without interjecting their own opinions, because they worry that relationships based on infatuation will lead to a sexual relationship. Parents should feel an obligation to inform their children of their feelings about early sexual relationships. At the same time, they have to be realistic that some adolescents will not follow their advice as shown by the rising rates of teenage pregnancy and sexually transmitted diseases, including HIV (Centers for Disease Control and Prevention [CDC], 2012c). If parents suspect their adolescent is sexually active, counsel them to be certain their child is knowledgeable about safer sex practices (see Chapter 5, Box 5.7 and Chapter 22 for a discussion of adolescent pregnancy).

Some adolescents may believe intense sexual yearnings or peer pressure can be alleviated only by a sexual act. They can be reassured that they are pleasant people to be with because of the many fine qualities they possess and that sexual intercourse can be delayed until two persons have come to know these qualities in each other and have made a mutual commitment based on a deeper level than simply physical passion.

In our busy modern society in which adolescents engage in such a variety of activities, they may need help learning how to project themselves into another person's situation and to ask themselves how the world looks from that position. This concept, *empathy*, is the ability to understand the feelings of another, or, in other words, a developed sense of intimacy in its finest form.

Socialization

Early teenagers may feel more self-doubt than self-confidence when they meet another adolescent with whom they would like to begin a lasting relationship. The voices of most boys have not yet dependably deepened; this makes them unable to trust their voices to carry the serious tone they wish to convey. Most girls' bodies have not yet fully developed; they may look at themselves in a mirror and compare their profiles with those of models in popular magazines and feel inadequate.

Both male and female early adolescents tend to be loud and boisterous, particularly when someone whose attention they would like to attract is nearby. They are impulsive and very much like 2-year-old children in that they want what they want immediately, not when it is convenient for others.

Many 13-year-olds begin to experience "crushes," or infatuations with school mates. At this age, however, they may spend more time longing for someone than they do instituting an in-depth and rewarding relationship. They have too little experience with life and too limited a frame of reference yet to know how to offer a deep commitment to another or accept one from that person.

By age 14 years, teenagers have become quieter and more introspective. They are becoming used to their changing bodies, have more confidence in themselves, and feel more self-esteem.

Adolescents watch adults carefully during this period, searching for good role models with whom they can identify. They usually have a hero—a film star, writer, scientist, or athlete—whom they want to grow up to be like. They may form a friendship with an older adolescent, trying to imitate that person in everything from thoughts to clothing. If the older adolescent has dropped out of school or plays a particular sport, the younger person may express a wish to drop out or train for that sport too.

Idolization of famous people or older adolescents of this nature fades as adolescents become more interested in forming reciprocal friendships. Attachments to older adolescents are often severed abruptly and painfully as older teenagers make it clear they are more interested in being with people their own age. Rejection by an older member of a pair forces the younger member to turn to his or her own-age friends and ends the intense hero worship so typical of early adolescence.

Most 15-year-olds fall "in love" five or six times a year. However, many of these relationships are based on attraction because of physical appearance, not because of inner qualities or characteristics that are compatible with their own. Because infatuation is fleeting, it can lead to extremely intense but brief attachments that fade once the two young people discover they have little in common. Beginning romantic attachments this often, however, does not mean their feelings are any less strong or that they feel any less pain when the relationship ends (Fig. 33.4).

By age 16 years, boys are becoming sexually mature (although they continue to grow taller until about 18 years of age). Both sexes are better able to trust their bodies than they were the year before. By age 17, they tend to have adult values and responses to events. They have left behind the childish behaviors they used in early adolescence—shoving and punching—to get the attention of others.

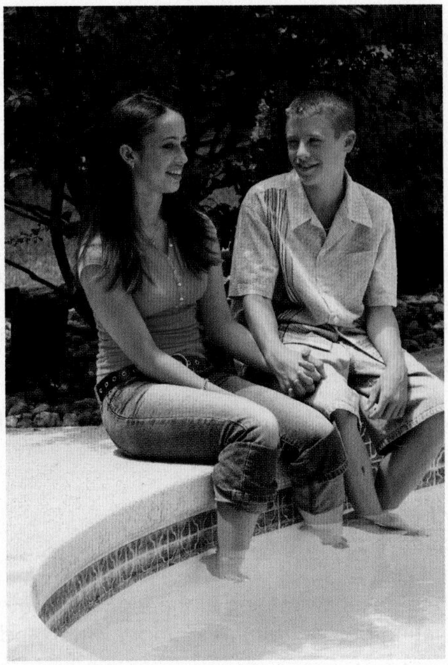

FIGURE 33.4 Although infatuation or love can be fleeting, adolescents may feel intensely for another.

Cognitive Development

The final stage of cognitive development, the stage of **formal operational thought**, begins at age 12 or 13 years and grows in depth over the adolescent years, although it may not be complete until about age 25 years (Piaget, 1969). This step involves the ability to think in abstract terms and use the scientific method (i.e., deductive reasoning) to arrive at conclusions. The problems that adolescents are asked to solve in school depend on this type of thought. Problem solving in any situation depends on the ability to think abstractly and logically.

With the ability to use scientific reasoning, adolescents can plan their future. They can create a hypothesis (What if I go to college? What if I don't?) and think through the probable consequences (In the long run, I'll earn more money, or I could begin earning money immediately).

Moral and Spiritual Development

Because adolescents enlarge their thought processes to include formal reasoning, they are able to respond to the question, "Why is it wrong to steal from your neighbor's house?" with "It would hurt my neighbor by requiring him to spend money to replace what I stole," rather than with the immature response of the school-age child, "The police will punish me." Some adolescents, however, may have difficulty envisioning a department store or a large corporation as capable of suffering economic loss from stealing, a concept that can contribute to the frequent practice of petty shoplifting at this age.

Almost all adolescents question the existence of God and any religious practices they have been taught (Kohlberg, 1984). This questioning is a natural part of forming a sense of identity and establishing a value system at a time in life when they draw away from their families.

✔ QSEN Checkpoint Question 33.2

Quality Improvement

You are evaluating some of the anticipatory guidance that you provided to Raul with the goal of fostering his sense of identity. Which of his following statements would suggest that he is successfully working toward this goal? *Select all that apply.*

a. I'm debating whether I'd like to be a pilot or a race car driver."
b. "I ask my parents at least once a week to let me do more things."
c. "I handle money at my part time job and it's sometimes tempting to take some of it."
d. "I'm getting used to being so much taller than my younger sister."

Look in Appendix A for the best answer and rationale.

HEALTH PROMOTION FOR AN ADOLESCENT AND FAMILY

Because their judgments are still limited, adolescents still need guidelines in reference to safety, nutrition, and daily care. These are always excellent topics for discussion at health care visits.

Promoting Adolescent Safety

Unintentional injuries, most commonly those involving motor vehicles, are the leading cause of death among adolescents. Although teenagers are at the peak of physical and sensorimotor functioning, their need to rebel against authority or to gain attention through risk-taking leads them to take careless actions, such as speeding or driving while intoxicated.

In the interest of an adolescent's safety and that of others, parents need to have the courage to insist on emotional maturity rather than age as the qualification for obtaining a driver's license. Adolescents needs to take seriously the graduated licensing requirements for their state so they not only learn the techniques of safe driving but also learn a sense of responsibility toward others (Elliott, Jacobsohn, Winston, et al., 2012).

Some adolescents dismiss seat belts as childish and so need extra instruction that it is wise to use every safety precaution available when in a motor vehicle (Chen, Cao, & Logan, 2012). Equally dangerous for adolescents are motorcycles, motorbikes, and motor scooters, which are appealing because of their low cost and convenience in parking. Both drivers and riders should wear safety helmets to prevent head injury, long pants to prevent leg burns from exhaust pipes, and a full body covering to prevent abrasions in case of an accident. Advise adolescents who choose these forms of transportation to be as familiar with safety rules as automobile drivers and to wait until they are emotionally mature enough to use sound driving judgment.

Although drowning tends to occur in younger children, it does occur in adolescents when good swimmers go beyond their capabilities on dares or in hopes of impressing friends. Teaching water safety, such as not swimming alone or when tired, is as important as teaching the mechanics of swimming (CDC, 2012b).

BOX 33.3 Nursing Care Planning to Empower a Family

MEASURES TO PREVENT UNINTENTIONAL INJURIES IN ADOLESCENTS

Q. Raul's mother tells you, "My son doesn't always use mature judgment. How can I keep him safe from accidents?"
A. Teaching the following points can be helpful to him:

Unintentional Injury	Health Teaching Measure
Motor vehicle	Always use a seat belt whether a driver or a passenger. Never use a cell phone or text while driving. Do not drink alcohol while driving and always refuse to ride with anyone who has been drinking (name a designated driver or arrange with your parents to be picked up or provide money for a taxi). Wear a helmet and long trousers as driver or passenger on a motorcycle. Accepting dares has no place in safe driving. Take graduated driver programs seriously so you learn safe driving habits for both two-wheel and four-wheel vehicles.
Firearms	Always consider all guns loaded and potentially lethal. Learn safe gun handling before attempting to clean a gun or hunt.
Drowning	Learn how to swim. Follow safe water rules, such as never swimming alone, no diving into the shallow end of swimming pools, no hyperventilating before swimming under water, and no swimming beyond one's own limit. Taking dares has no place in water safety.
Sports	Use protective equipment, such as face masks for hockey and pads and a helmet for football. Do not attempt to participate beyond physical limits. Keep well hydrated by drinking fluid before and after play. Careful preparation for sports through training is essential to safety. Recognize and set one's own limit for sports participation.

Other common causes of death in adolescents are homicide and self-harm (i.e., suicide) (Swahn, Ali, Bossarte, et al., 2012). These are related to the easy accessibility of guns when added to depression, binge drinking, and impulsivity. Gang violence and the desire to protect themselves are additional factors. Unintentional gunshot injuries increase in early adolescence, often for the same reason that drowning increases: youngsters want to impress friends by showing they can handle guns. Be certain that firearm safety is taught creatively through problem solving rather than lecturing, because teenagers tend to rebel against such lectures or claim that they have heard it all before.

Athletic injuries, especially overuse injuries from poor conditioning, tend to increase in number during adolescence because of the vigorous level of competition that occurs in organized sports (Khan, Thompson, Blair, et al., 2012). Types of athletic injuries are discussed in Chapter 52. Health teaching measures to prevent unintentional injuries, especially while participating in athletics, are summarized in Box 33.3.

Promoting Nutritional Health for an Adolescent

Adolescents experience such rapid growth that they may always feel hungry (Fig. 33.5). If their eating habits are unsupervised, because of peer pressure and when in a hurry to get to other activities, they tend to eat faddish or quick snack foods rather than more nutritionally sound ones. Some adolescents turn away from the basic MyPlate food groups to eat sweets, soft drinks, or empty-calorie snacks and so are left poorly nourished. This type of eating pattern, combined with a lack of exercise, also leads to obesity (Wengle, Hamilton, Manlhiot, et al., 2012).

One form of adolescent rebellion is to refuse to eat foods that parents stress as important. Parents who stock their kitchens with healthy snacks such as fruit and vegetables and who are willing to meet their adolescents half way in terms of food preferences can be more certain their child is eating nutritious foods than if such food aren't available. Giving an adolescent some responsibility for food planning or meals,

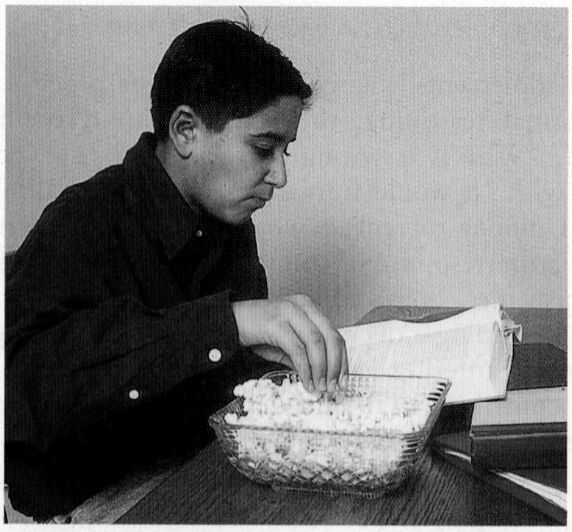

FIGURE 33.5 Adolescents experience rapid physical growth, so typically, they eat frequently. (© Billy Barnes/Stock Boston.)

such as making dinner every Wednesday night, can teach some important lessons about nutrition without conflict.

Adolescents who are slightly obese because of prepubertal changes may begin low-calorie or starvation diets during adolescence to lose weight. Some diet so excessively they develop eating disorders such as bulimia or anorexia nervosa (see Chapter 54). A weight-loss diet is appropriate during adolescence, but it must be supervised to ensure the adolescent is consuming sufficient calories and nutrients for growth. For example, many adolescents entirely omit breads and cereals to lose weight rather than just reducing the amounts they eat. Diets such as these can be deficient in vitamins B1 (thiamine) and B2 (riboflavin), which are necessary for growth.

Recommended Dietary Reference Intakes

An adolescent needs an increased number of calories over that needed previously to support the rapid body growth that occurs. Foods must come from a variety of sources to supply necessary amounts of carbohydrates, vitamins, protein, and minerals.

The nutrients that are most apt to be deficient in both male and female adolescent diets are iron, calcium, and zinc. Iron is necessary to meet expanding blood volume requirements. Females require a high iron intake not only because of this increasing blood volume but also because iron begins to be lost with menstruation. Girls with a heavy menstrual flow (i.e., menorrhagia) and especially those who participate in strenuous athletics may need to take an additional iron supplement to prevent iron-deficiency anemia (Fernández-Gaxiola & De-Regil, 2011; McClung, 2012) (see Chapter 44).

Increased calcium and vitamin D plus physical exercise are necessary for rapid skeletal growth as well as to "stockpile" calcium to prevent osteoporosis later in life (Chouinard, Randall Simpson, & Buchholz, 2012). Zinc is necessary for sexual maturation and final body growth. Good sources of iron are meat and green vegetables; calcium is abundant in milk and milk products; and meat and milk are also high in zinc.

Promoting Nutritional Health With a Varied Diet

Vegetarian Diets. Because vegetables generally contain fewer calories than meat, adolescents need to consume large amounts of them to achieve an adequate caloric intake from a vegetarian diet. Textured vegetable protein or tofu can be added to meals to increase the amount of protein supplied and help meet adolescent growth needs (Whitney & Rolfes, 2012). Some adolescents may find it difficult to follow a vegetarian diet because it makes them different from their peers and limits the foods they can eat at parties or at school, such as pizza, meat tortillas, or hot dogs. Whether to continue to follow this type of diet is a decision an adolescent must make as part of achieving a sense of identity. Be certain that adolescents who have become semi-vegetarians in order to lose weight add enough protein to their food intake to sustain their rapid body growth (Timko, Hormes, & Chubski, 2012).

Glycogen Loading. Athletes need more carbohydrate or energy than those who do not engage in strenuous activity; the source of carbohydrate that best sustains athletes comes from the breakdown of glycogen because this supplies a slow and steady release of glucose. **Glycogen loading** is a procedure used to ensure there is adequate glycogen to sustain energy through an athletic event. Several days before a sports event, athletes lower their carbohydrate intake and exercise heavily to deplete muscle glycogen stores. They then switch to a diet high in carbohydrate. With the renewed carbohydrate intake, muscle glycogen is stored at two to three times the usual level, which supplies them with up to twice the glucose needed for sustained energy (Bagnulo, 2012).

Although used by many high school athletes, the effects of frequent glycogen loading in this age group are not well studied and so should be done cautiously. As a rule, the goals of nutrition that are best for everyone, such as eating a well-balanced diet rather than a diet that interferes with carbohydrate, fluid, or fat intake, are also the best rules for athletes.

Promoting Development of an Adolescent in Daily Activities

Adequate sleep, hygiene, and exercise are important health education topics for adolescents as these become an adolescent's responsibility rather than the responsibility of the parents.

Dress and Hygiene

Adolescents are capable of total self-care and, because of their body awareness, may even be overly conscientious about personal hygiene and appearance. Both sexes try many types of shampoo, deodorant, breath fresheners, and toothpaste. They may take seriously (without admitting it) the content of ads showing that toothpastes or deodorants can help win an attractive person or gain instant success. Remember that, when caring for hospitalized adolescents, providing time for self-care, such as shampooing hair, is important to include in an adolescent's nursing care plan.

Adolescents can be acutely aware of how their peers dress. When hospitalized, most teenagers seem to improve markedly when allowed to wear their own clothing rather than a hospital gown. Needing to look like everyone else is undoubtedly a factor in adolescent shoplifting. Only during late adolescence do teenagers discover that who they really are shows through their clothing.

Care of Teeth

Adolescents are generally very conscientious about tooth brushing because of a fear of developing bad breath. They should continue to use a fluoride paste rather than a brand advertised as providing white teeth. They should also continue to drink fluoridated water to ensure firm enamel growth (Armfield, 2010), but they should also be careful to not use so much fluoride through the use of mouth rinses or toothpaste that they develop fluorosis (i.e., a blue discoloration of teeth). Teens with braces must be extremely conscientious about tooth brushing to prevent plaque buildup on hidden tooth surfaces. If they snack a great deal, and so their teeth are always exposed to bacterial erosion, some may develop a cavity for the first time during this period.

Sleep

Although it is widely believed everyone needs 8 hours of sleep a night, some need more and others can adjust to considerably less. Because protein synthesis occurs most readily during sleep and adolescents are building so many new cells, this age group may need proportionately more sleep than any other age group (Short, Gradisar, Lack, et al., 2012). In addition, because this is a busy time with extracurricular activities and also a stressful period similar to first grade, adolescents may sleep restlessly as their mind reworks the day's tensions. Even long periods of sleep, therefore, may not leave them feeling refreshed. This is why adolescents, admitted to a hospital for even a minor illness, for example, may sleep as if exhausted. Even though frequent lack of sleep can lead to chronic fatigue or depression, medication is not usually recommended for adolescents; instead, they are urged to reduce activity to get more sleep (Frost & Burns, 2012).

Exercise

Just as with younger children, adolescents need exercise every day both to maintain muscle tone and to provide an outlet for tension. Unlike younger children, however, and although they are constantly on the go, adolescents often receive very little real exercise. They may ride a bus to school, sit for classes, and sit at a mall after school and talk to friends. They have put in a full day, yet most of their time was spent sitting. Because of this, adolescents who have had an injury and must learn an activity such as crutch walking usually need to do muscle-strengthening exercises at first, just as adults must.

Adolescents who are involved in structured athletic activities do receive daily exercise. If they have not participated in competitive sports before, however, they may need advice on increasing exercise gradually so they do not overdo it and consequently develop muscle sprains or other overuse injuries (Hoang, Coel, Vidal, et al., 2012).

Sun Exposure

Because some adolescents spend a great deal of time outdoors participating in athletics, it is a critical time for them to avoid excessive sun exposure so they don't develop skin cancer (i.e., melanoma) from ultraviolet rays. Encourage teenagers to use sunscreen, avoid tanning beds, and report to their primary health care provider any skin mole that changes in shape or color. Do this as creatively as possible because teenagers have difficulty looking to the future and imagining how drastically the development of melanoma could affect their lives (Cohen, Brown, Haukness, et al., 2013).

Promoting Healthy Family Functioning

Early adolescents may have many disagreements with parents that stem partly from wanting more independence and partly from being so disappointed in their bodies. It may be helpful to counsel parents to appreciate that, although it is not easy to live with a teenager, it is equally difficult to be the teenager.

When a child reaches about age 15 years, parent–child friction tends to peak. By this age, adolescents have discovered from careful observation that most adults are far from perfect. Teachers they previously thought were all knowing are revealed to have very human shortcomings. School marks may slump as a reflection of this "fallen angel" syndrome.

Adolescents discover even more faults in their parents and wonder, for instance, how they can exist with such outdated ideas. Adolescents may follow health advice poorly because they view health care personnel in the same light.

By the time they are 16 years old, adolescents generally become more willing to listen and talk about problems. As a result, they may learn adults are not as inadequate as they previously thought. This changed perception does not mean an adolescent of 16 years is calm and quiet and free of parent–child discord. Adolescents may comprehend how hard it was for parents to get where they are, but they may not understand, for example, why they themselves are not allowed to stay out later than midnight on weekends.

Most 17-year-old adolescents, who have stayed in school, are usually high school seniors; for most of them, this year is likely to be stormy. Looking ahead to leaving a school system with which they may have been involved since they were very young may give them a feeling of losing security. Even if going away to college or beginning a full-time job seems exciting, it can also be an unwelcome change from the people and routines they feel so comfortable with to new contacts and new regulations that appear strange and even hostile.

The ambivalence that such feelings create makes some 17-year-olds enjoy having parents perpetuating family traditions such as the house decorated for a holiday in the same way as usual or being served a traditional birthday meal. This clinging to security is not a step backward but a preliminary working through to a time of separation that will be a major milestone in reaching maturity.

Unfortunately, as another way to prove they are old enough to leave high school and enter into a more mature college or work world, older adolescents may begin to experiment with drugs or alcohol, interpreting the use of these as the mark of being an adult (Lewis & Hession, 2012).

Common Health Problems of an Adolescent

A health maintenance schedule for the adolescent period and the assessments to be included at visits are shown in Table 33.2.

Hypertension

Hypertension is present if blood pressure is above the 95th percentile, or 127/81 mmHg for 16-year-old girls and 131/81 for 16-year-old boys for two consecutive readings in different settings. (Pulse, respiration, and blood pressure value charts are available at http://thePoint.lww.com/Pillitteri7e.) Adolescents who are obese, who are African American, who eat a diet high in salt, or who have a family history of hypertension are most susceptible to developing the condition. All children over 3 years of age should have their blood pressure routinely taken at all health assessments to detect this (American Academy of Pediatrics [AAP], 2012a). This is particularly important for adolescents because new medications plus education can help to greatly reduce the incidence of cardiovascular disease as they reach adulthood (Blake & Davis, 2011). Prevention and management of hypertension in children and adolescents are discussed in Chapter 41.

Poor Posture

Many adolescents, particularly those who reach adult height before their peers, demonstrate poor posture, a tendency to round shoulders and a shambling, slouchy walk to not be

TABLE 33.2 Health Maintenance Schedule, Adolescent Period

Area of Focus	Methods	Frequency
Assessment		
Developmental milestones	History, observation	Every visit
Growth milestones	Height, weight plotted on standard growth chart; body mass index (BMI), physical examination	Every visit
Hypertension	Blood pressure	Every visit
Nutrition	History, observation; height/weight, BMI information	Every visit
Dyslipidemia	Total cholesterol and triglycerides	At 18 years of age; earlier screening for children who have family members with the disorder
Parent–child relationship	History, observation	Every visit
Behavior or school problems	History, observation	Every visit
Substance abuse	History, observation	Every visit
Vision and hearing disorders	History, observation	Every visit
	Formal Snellen or Titmus testing	At 15 and 18 years of age
	Audiometer testing	If concern or high risk is present
Dental health	History, physical examination	Every visit; recommend a yearly checkup with dental health provider
Cervical dysplasia (Scoliosis)	Physical examination	Every visit at least to 16 years of age
Thyroid disease	Physical examination, history	Every visit
Tuberculosis	Purified protein derivative (PPD) test	Depending on prevalence of tuberculosis in community
Bacteriuria	Dipstick	Annually if sexually active
Anemia	Hematocrit or hemoglobin	Annually for menstruating females
Cervical or vaginal cancer	Pap test, pelvic examination	Every 1 to 3 years for sexually active females
Sexually transmitted diseases	History, observation	Every visit if sexually active
Immunizations		
	Check history and past records; inform caregiver about any risks and side effects; administer vaccine in accordance with health care agency policies.	
Hepatitis A vaccine	HepA	If not previously immunized
Hepatitis B vaccine	HepB	If not previously immunized
Human papillomavirus vaccine	HPV	If not previously vaccinated
Influenza vaccine	TIV (trivalent influenza vaccine) or LAIV	Yearly
Measles, mumps, rubella vaccine	MMR	If not previously vaccinated; do not give to pregnant adolescents

continues on page 936

TABLE 33.2 Health Maintenance Schedule, Adolescent Period (continued)

Area of Focus	Methods	Frequency
Meningococcal vaccine	MPV4	Booster at 16 years
Pneumococcal vaccine	PCV (pneumococcal conjugate vaccine)	To high-risk groups if not previously vaccinated
Tetanus and diphtheria vaccine	Tdap	If not previously immunized
Varicella vaccine	VAR	If not previously vaccinated
Anticipatory Guidance		
Adolescent care including violence and nutrition counseling	Active listening and health teaching	Every visit
Expected growth and developmental milestones before next visit	Active listening and health teaching	Every visit
Unintentional injury prevention	Counseling about street and personal safety	Every visit
Any problems expressed by caregiver or adolescent during visit	Active listening and health teaching	Every visit

From American Academy of Pediatrics. (2012b). *Recommendations for preventive pediatric health care*. Evanston, IL: Author.

taller than those around them. This is also due to the imbalance of growth that arises from the skeletal system growing a little more rapidly than the muscles attached to it. Girls, especially, may slouch so as not to appear taller than boys or to diminish the appearance of their breast size if they are developing more rapidly than their friends. Yet another reason may be related to carrying backpacks that are too heavy (Kistner, Fiebert, & Roach, 2012).

Urge children of both sexes to use good posture during these rapid-growth years. Assess posture at all adolescent health appraisals to detect the difference between simple poor posture and the beginning of spinal dysplasia or scoliosis (i.e., lateral curvature of the spine) (see Chapters 34 and 51).

Body Piercing and Tattoos

Body piercing and tattoos are a strong mark of adolescence (Stein & Jordan, 2012). Both sexes my have ears, lips, chins, navels, and breasts pierced and filled with studs, or tattoos applied to arms, legs, or their central body. Body piercings and tattoos have become a way for adolescents to make a statement of who they are and that they are different from their parents. Be certain they know the symptoms of infection at a piercing or tattoo site (e.g., redness, warmness, drainage, swelling, mild pain) and to report these to their health care provider if they occur because serious staphylococcal or streptococcal infections can occur at piercing sites. Caution adolescents that sharing needles for piercing or tattooing carries the same risk for contacting a blood-borne disease as sharing needles for intravenous drug use.

Fatigue

Because so many adolescents comment that they feel fatigued to some degree, it can be considered normal for the age group. However, fatigue may also be a beginning symptom of disease, so it is important that it is not underestimated as a concern. Always assess the diet, sleep patterns, and activity schedules of fatigued adolescents. Be aware that if the fatigue began as a short period of extreme tiredness, it suggests disease more so than a long, ill-defined report of always feeling tired.

If an adolescent's sleep and diet appear to be adequate, his or her activity schedule is reasonable, and a physical assessment suggests no illness, then the fatigue may be of emotional origin. It can be a means of avoiding school, conflict with parents (e.g., when children appear ill, parents are more sympathetic), or social situations (e.g., too tired to go to the mall). Those who are understimulated by school may develop fatigue as a sign of boredom.

Blood tests may be indicated to rule out anemia and common infections in adolescents, such as infectious mononucleosis (see Chapter 43). Chronic fatigue syndrome, although not seen as often in this age group as in adults, may also need to be ruled out (Lloyd, Chalder, & Rimes, 2012). If tests for these categories of conditions are normal, teenagers can be assured they are healthy and should be offered guidance to solve the problem with better diet, more sleep, fewer activities, and better problem-solving techniques to relieve tension.

Menstrual Irregularities

Menstrual irregularities can be a major health concern of adolescent girls as they learn to adjust to their individual body cycles. Chapter 47 discusses these problems in detail.

Acne

Acne is a self-limiting inflammatory disease that involves the sebaceous glands, which empty into hair shafts (the pilosebaceous unit). It is the most common skin disorder of adolescence, occurring in as many as 80% to 95% of adolescents (Morelli & Prok, 2012). It occurs slightly more frequently in boys than in girls. The peak age for the lesions occurring in girls is 14 to 17 years of age; for boys, 16 to 19 years of age. Although not proven, genetic factors may play a part in their development.

Changes associated with puberty that cause acne to develop include:

- As androgen levels rise in both sexes, sebaceous glands become active.
- The output of sebum, which is largely composed of lipids, mainly triglycerides, increases.
- Trapped sebum causes whiteheads, or closed **comedones**.
- As trapped sebum darkens from accumulation of melanin and oxidation of the fatty acid component on exposure to air, blackheads, or open comedones, form. Leakage of fatty acids cause a dermal inflammatory reaction.
- Bacteria (generally, *Propionibacterium acnes*) lodge and thrive in the retained secretions and ducts.

Acne is categorized as mild (i.e., comedones are present), moderate (i.e., papules and pustules are also present), or severe (i.e., cysts are present). The most common locations of acne lesions are the face, neck, back, upper arms, and chest (Fig. 33.6). Flare-ups are associated with emotional stress, menstrual periods, or the use of greasy hair creams or makeup that can further plug gland ducts. Lesions are less noticeable in summer months, probably because of increased exposure to the sun, which increases epidermal peeling, or because of a reduction in stress as a result of being out of school.

Assessment. Always ask adolescents at health assessments if they are troubled with acne and to what extent it interferes with their self-image because this can be a major cause of stress in adolescents. Inspect for facial, chest, and back lesions on physical examination.

Therapeutic Management. The goal of therapy for acne is threefold: (a) decrease sebum formation, (b) prevent comedones, and (c) control bacterial proliferation.

External Medication. Medications that are applied externally peel away the superficial skin layer to prevent sebum plugs from forming and are sufficient if only comedones are present. A common prescription medication is tretinoin (Retin-A cream). This reduces keratin formation and plugging of ducts. Caution adolescents using a vitamin A cream to avoid prolonged sun exposure and to use a sunblock of SPF 15 or higher because the preparation makes their skin more susceptible to ultraviolet rays (Karch, 2013). Additional creams frequently prescribed contain benzoyl peroxide or azelaic acid. Caution adolescents that, for the first week or two of therapy, peeling or oxidizing agents may make the complexion appear worse. If the adolescent has inflammatory lesions, topical antibiotic creams such as dapsone, tetracycline, or doxycycline may be prescribed to reduce the bacterial level on the skin. Tetracycline is not prescribed for children under age 12 years because it can cause permanent staining of teeth and may possibly interfere with growth of long bones. It is contraindicated for adolescents who are or may become pregnant as it is teratogenic (Simonart, 2012).

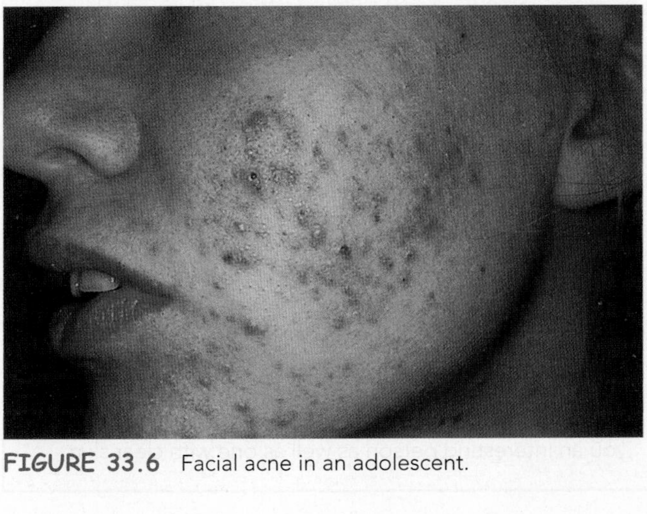

FIGURE 33.6 Facial acne in an adolescent.

Systemic Medication. In pustular and cystic acne, systemic (i.e., oral) antibiotics can be helpful. Tetracycline (500 mg twice daily the first week, then tapered to 250 mg daily for maintenance) is effective against the anaerobic bacteria that break down sebum to form irritating acids. Improvement is not generally seen for 2 weeks, so you may need to support adolescents to continue to take the medication during the waiting period. Without noticeable improvement, adolescents have a tendency to continue taking the higher dose or even increase the dose, hoping to initiate a faster effect.

Food impairs the absorption of oral tetracycline so the drug should be taken on an empty stomach (2 hours before or after eating). Adolescents must be certain of the date of expiration of the drug; outdated tetracycline breaks down into an extremely toxic composition. Females taking systemic antibiotics for long periods of time become susceptible to developing candidal vaginitis and need to be instructed about the symptoms of this: a white, pruritic vaginal discharge. As yet another precaution, because tetracycline may interfere with oral contraceptives, adolescent girls who are sexually active should use another method of birth control while taking the antibiotic. Alternative antibiotics prescribed are erythromycin or clindamycin. Although these drugs avoid the complications of tetracycline, they may not produce the same effective results.

Other Treatment Methods. Estrogen, alone or in combination with progesterone, suppresses sebaceous gland activity and, therefore, oral contraceptives are useful therapy in some girls with acne (Arrington, Patel, Gerancher, et al., 2012). Oral contraceptives taken for this reason carry the same precautions as when they are prescribed as a reproductive planning method: estrogen tends to close epiphyseal centers of long bones, causing bone growth to halt, and long-term therapy does have potential side effects, including embolism and thrombophlebitis. A last resort is administration of isotretinoin (a retinoid or vitamin A compound) for a short time (Lyon, 2011). Isotretinoin must be taken with caution, however, because it is extremely teratogenic and also has been linked to inflammatory bowel disease. It should not be taken at the same time as tetracycline or it can lead to brain edema. Many adolescents are left with some degree of scarring following teenage acne lesions. Laser therapy is a follow-up possibility to reduce the effect of scarring.

Nursing Diagnoses and Related Interventions

Nursing Diagnosis: Risk for low self-esteem related to the development of acne during adolescence and lack of knowledge regarding treatment possibilities

Outcome Evaluation: Adolescent verbalizes positive aspects of self; states acne does not affect self-image, or if client admits to feelings of negative self-esteem, is able to discuss feelings and concerns about condition; describes ways to prevent or reduce acne outbreaks and states realistic short- and long-term goals of treatment.

It is necessary to respect how devastating acne can be to some adolescents. The actual extent of the condition often is not as important as an adolescent's feelings about it. With a face constantly covered by red marks, it may be extremely difficult for adolescents to feel good about themselves.

When carrying out interventions, remember that acne is a potentially destructive disease; if left untreated, it can cause irreparable physical and emotional scarring. Therefore, advise parents and adolescents to seek medical treatment rather than self-medicate if the condition is severe. At the same time, being overly concerned may lead to becoming unduly self-conscious, which may affect performance in school and the establishment of social relationships. Common health teaching measures for the prevention and treatment of acne are summarized in Box 33.4.

QSEN Checkpoint Question 33.3

Patient-Centered Care

Raul is prescribed both a topical cream and oral tetracycline to treat his acne. What statements would let you know he needs additional health information (list all that apply)?

a. "I know acne is not contagious even though all my friends seem to have it."
b. "My girlfriend wants to borrow my tetracycline; I don't mind sharing it."
c. "I know not to take hot showers as hot water can create new lesions."
d. "I know not to eat chocolate because that always makes lesions worse."

Look in Appendix A for the best answer and rationale.

Obesity

Most overweight adolescents have obese parents, suggesting that both inheritance and environment play a part in the development of adolescent obesity. Obesity can interfere with developing a sense of identity if it is difficult for adolescents to like their reflection in a mirror or if they are always excluded from groups because of their weight. Because of stress related to weight, the attempted suicide rate for obese female adolescents is higher than for nonobese adolescents (Zhang, Yan, Li, et al., 2012).

Some adolescents may be unaware that their food intake is excessive because they have been told they need excess nutrients for healthy adolescent growth and everyone in their family eats large portions. Health teaching with these

BOX 33.4 Nursing Care Planning Based on Family Teaching

GUIDELINES FOR THE PREVENTION AND TREATMENT OF ACNE

Q. Raul says to you, "I've had acne for the last 3 months. How can I make this go away?"

A. Most adolescents have some acne lesions. Try the following suggestions:

- Do not pick or squeeze acne lesions, which ruptures glands and spreads sebum into the skin, thus increasing inflammation. The times you are most likely to do this are during periods of stress, such as when you are taking a test. When you find your hand on your face, distract yourself with some other motion, such as interlocking your fingers.
- Greasy hair preparations or tight sweatbands can both plug ducts of glands and increase comedone formation, so avoid these, if possible. For girls, makeup can plug ducts; using medicated makeup both covers and helps lesions heal.
- Topical acne preparations work by unplugging glands, so you must use them consistently for them to be effective. Plan enough time in the morning before school and a time in the evening to apply these. Post a chart by your bathroom mirror to remind yourself.
- Washing daily to remove irritating fatty acids is helpful. Excessive washing is not necessary and, in fact, can actually harm healing by rupturing glands.
- Oral medications work by reducing sebum secretions or preventing bacterial invasion. Again, these work only if you take them conscientiously. Make a chart to post in your bathroom or kitchen to remind yourself to take these. Remember, tetracycline must be taken on an empty stomach or it is not effective.
- Both topical and oral vitamin A make your skin very sensitive to sunlight. Avoid long exposures to sunlight, or you will sunburn readily.
- Although diet does not influence the development of acne lesions, you should eat a healthy, well-balanced diet for good general health.
- No acne medication works immediately. While you are waiting for lesions to heal, keep yourself occupied with a new activity (e.g., join a school club, try dancing lessons). When your skin is clear, these experiences will help make you an interesting person as well as one with clear skin.

adolescents may need to begin with a discussion of "normal" weight and standard food portions because, if they do not begin to own this problem as adolescents, they run a high risk of becoming obese adults.

If adolescents eat a diet too low in protein for any length of time, they can develop a faulty nitrogen balance, which can lead to seriously impaired growth. A diet of fewer than 1,400 to 1,600 calories per day, therefore, can rarely be tolerated by adolescents. They generally do better and will stick with a diet closer to 1,800 calories per day.

Nursing Diagnoses and Related Interventions

Nursing Diagnosis: Ineffective individual coping by overeating related to stresses of the adolescent period, which has led to obesity

Outcome Evaluation: Adolescent identifies stressful situations that lead to overeating; describes ways to avoid those situations or methods that would help coping with them.

Adolescents who are overweight because of stress need support until their pleasure in eating diminishes and their satisfaction with themselves as a "new" person or until their friends' satisfaction with them can sustain them. They may need to visit a health care facility once or twice a week for encouragement and praise for their efforts. National weight-control organizations are good to use if other adolescents also attend the meetings. They tend to be less effective if all the other members are adults because adolescents generally cannot relate to adult concerns. It's important an adolescent's self-esteem is maintained while losing weight or an adolescent may switch to binge eating or such severe dieting that the opposite—extreme weight loss—can occur (Sánchez-Carracedo, Neumark-Sztainer, & López-Guimerà, 2012).

In addition to reducing calories consumed, encourage activities that burn calories, such as swimming, gym classes, or walking their dog (Loprinzi, Cardinal, Loprinzi, et al., 2012). These activities are generally preferable to formal exercises, such as sit-ups and push-ups, which may be viewed as punishment.

Adolescents who use overeating as their main reaction to stress may require psychological counseling rather than diet counseling if they are to develop a more mature emotional response to stress. Behavior modification is sometimes successful with adolescents as a means of helping them lose weight, but it is rarely recommended for obesity alone (see Chapter 35).

General measures to help adolescents decrease overeating include:

- Making a detailed log of the amount they eat, the time, and the circumstances (including how they felt while they were eating), and then changing those circumstances
- Always eating in one place (the kitchen table) instead of while walking home from school or watching television
- Slowing the process of eating by counting mouthfuls and putting the fork down between bites, or being served food on small plates so helpings look larger

These measures may be of little use, however, unless they are combined with a suitable diet and adequate exercise. Despite all these interventions, weight reduction may not always be effective with adolescents. For some, a more realistic goal might be to prevent additional weight gain until they reach adulthood.

Concerns Regarding Sexuality and Sexual Activity

Due to increasing exposure to and acceptance of premarital sexual relations in society, more adolescents than ever before engage in high-risk sexual behaviors, exposing them to sexually transmitted infections or conception (Taylor & Joshi, 2012). Because of this, as part of routine health assessments of adolescents and preadolescents, ask if they are sexually active or are concerned about sexual risk behaviors.

Adolescents are usually interested in discussing sexuality concerns with a health care provider because they realize that without adequate protection, they are exposing themselves to HIV infection or other sexually transmitted diseases and to pregnancy. At the same time, it is an awkward topic for many to discuss. Some adolescents may feel trapped into engaging in sex even though they are unwilling because they perceive it as a way of keeping friends. For adolescents who want to have intercourse, the primary reasons given are sexual curiosity and affection for their partner. For adolescents who agree to have intercourse but do not really want to, the primary reasons given are peer pressure, curiosity, and affection for their partner (Katsufrakis & Nusbaum, 2011).

Counseling can help adolescents improve their perspective and also learn how to say no. In contrast, some adolescents would like to be sexually active but are not because they believe myths such as early sexual relations or masturbation will drain their strength or change their body so sexual relations later on will not be enjoyable. Unless these falsehoods are explored through discussion, adolescents who believe them may never be comfortable with sexual relationships.

Adolescence is also the time when teenagers deal with the realization that they are gay or lesbian. Although this orientation is something they have been aware of for years, actually facing it and accepting it is another step, and one that is difficult for many families (Bregman, Malik, Page, et al., 2013). Offer support to adolescents who are having difficulty telling their parents about their perceived sexual orientation. To their surprise, after telling their parents, they often discover their parents already knew before the concern was voiced.

Sometimes adolescents use a mild cold or a mild acne condition as a reason to come to a health care facility, where they hope someone will stumble onto their real concern about sexual activity. After asking adolescents at health maintenance

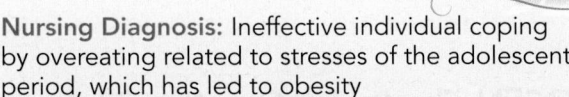

BOX 33.5 Nursing Care Planning Based on Family Teaching

HEALTH TEACHING GUIDELINES FOR ADOLESCENTS REGARDING SEXUALITY

Q. Raul asks you, "How will I know when I'm ready for sex?"
A. Here are a few common guidelines:

- It is your choice whether to participate in sexual relations. Do not be influenced by friends who may be exaggerating stories to impress you or who ask you to do something you do not want to do. When you say no, be firm and clear about your wishes.
- There is no 100% method to prevent pregnancy or a sexually transmitted infection (STI) except abstinence. Be direct with a sexual partner in discussing abstinence or reproductive and infection prevention measures.
- Sexual relations neither add to nor detract from your physical strength or general wellness.
- The mark of an adult sexual relationship is that the activity is pleasurable to both partners. If sexual partners are not interested in your enjoyment as well as their own, you should reconsider the relationship.
- There is no "normal" mode of sexual expression. Any activity that is pleasurable to both partners is "normal."
- Learn about safer sex techniques, and practice them (see Chapter 5, Box 5.7).

visits if they are sexually active, ask if they have any questions or problems they want to discuss with you, such as questions about contraception. Be certain they know about and are practicing safer sex measures (see Chapter 5, Box 5.7). General guidelines on counseling an adolescent with respect to sexual activity are summarized in Box 33.5.

Be certain to provide information on date rape and rape prevention in a discussion of sexual behaviors because adolescents are in a high-risk age group for date rape (Makin-Byrd & Bierman, 2013) (see Chapter 55). One form of date rape occurs when flunitrazepam (Rohypnol) (i.e., the "date-rape drug"), a colorless, odorless, and flavorless benzodiazepine drug, is dropped into a drink, causing drowsiness, impaired motor skills, and amnesia for a time (Karch, 2013). Adolescents who are seen for sexual assault who appear intoxicated or have amnesia for the event should be suspected of unknowingly ingesting flunitrazepam or another drug such as ketamine. In these instances, a urine specimen analysis will reveal the drug's metabolites or that the drug was ingested (D'Aloise & Chen, 2012).

Stalking

Stalking refers to repetitive, intrusive, and unwanted actions such as constant and threatening pursuit directed at an individual to gain the individual's attention or to evoke fear. Stalking may mainly take place as Internet correspondence (i.e., cyberstalking), such as sending unwanted e-mails or text messages (Briggs, Simon, & Simonsen, 2011). In some instances, the stalker goes so far as to attack a victim and even murder the victim.

Stalking behavior begins as early as adolescence. Although the usual stalker is a male who stalks a female who has rejected him, both males and females can become stalkers or victims (McNamara & Marsil, 2012). It is difficult to prevent stalking because no one can evaluate when they begin a relationship that it will end so badly. To avoid stalking, adolescents should be aware of and avoid situations where they will be vulnerable to being alone with a stalker and to report stalking to law enforcement officers so they can obtain a restraining order to prevent the stalker from coming near them again.

QSEN Checkpoint Question 33.4
Safety

Raul is depressed because his girlfriend broke up with him. Which of his statements could be interpreted as stalking?

a. "I keep her photo on my bedside stand so I can kiss her goodnight."
b. "We take the same route to school every day so I often still see her."
c. "I e-mail her every night to tell her what a huge mistake she's made."
d. "I took down her photo from Facebook but wish I could put it back."

Look in Appendix A for the best answer and rationale.

Concerns Regarding Hazing or Bullying

Bullying, which began during school age (see Chapter 32), can easily continue into adolescence and actually becomes more serious because this can be the time the bullied child has the ability to retaliate through self-destructive behavior or school violence.

Hazing, a form of organized bullying, refers to demeaning or humiliating rituals that prospective members have to undergo to join sororities, fraternities, adolescent gangs, or sports teams (Allan & Madden, 2011). Most rituals are secret and in the past were accepted as "rites of passage." In recent years, hazing has become so extreme the practice has moved out of the "just fun" category into activities that can cause physical and certainly psychological harm, such as being forced to wear demeaning clothing or engaging in crude or lewd skits. They can be extended to such an extreme that adolescents may be punched or kicked, sodomized, left out in the cold so long that frostbite develops, or forced to drink alcohol until they vomit, pass out, or even die from alcohol intoxication. Initiation for street gangs can require prospective members to steal or destroy property or even kill another person.

To help prevent this from happening to their child, urge parents to be aware of what clubs or organizations their adolescent joins and what the requirements for membership are. Help adolescents make sound decisions about what type of hazing their organization advocates by asking them about the subject at health assessments.

Concerns Regarding Substance Abuse

Substance abuse refers to the use of chemicals to improve a mental state or induce euphoria. This is so common among adolescents that as many as 50% of high school seniors report having experimented with some form of drug (CDC, 2012a). Use of drugs occurs in adolescence from a desire to expand consciousness, peer pressure, or a desire to feel more confident and mature; it also can be a form of adolescent rebellion related to childhood adversity or violence. Stages of drug use range from experimentation where teenagers try drugs to enhance social acceptance to regular use, where they actively seek the effect of drugs to relieve everyday stress (Benjet, Borges, Medina-Mora, et al., 2012).

Types of Abused Substances

Because adolescents may not have a large source of money, the drugs they most frequently abuse are those they can obtain on a limited budget and through limited contacts.

Prescription and Over-the-Counter Drugs. Adolescents may first begin drug experimentation by taking drugs prescribed for another family member or a pet such as sedatives, pain medication, ketamine (an anesthetic used in veterinary medicine), or cough syrup containing codeine or dextromethorphan (DXM). Called "pharming," adolescents who use drugs this way can easily overdose because they are unaware of usual dosages (Young, Glover, & Havens, 2012).

Methylphenidate (Ritalin) is a drug frequently prescribed for attention deficit hyperactivity disorder. Because Ritalin is a stimulant, when oral tablets are crushed and injected intravenously, they produce a feeling of giddiness and extreme well-being. Unfortunately, because they do not completely dissolve, the resultant small particles remaining in the bloodstream can result in complications such as pulmonary embolus or emphysema, so this is a very dangerous practice. Every house has a number of inhalants, such as oil-based cooking spray, gas, butane, or lighter fluid, that may be abused by adolescents. Inhalants can lead to cardiac failure from suffocation. Mephedrone, commonly called "bath salts," is a stimulant that creates an enjoyable "high" and is available for purchase online and so is easily obtained by adolescents (Hadlock, Webb, McFadden, et al., 2011). The effect of using it is seen more regularly in emergency departments as the cause of reckless driving or unconsciousness (Baumann, Partilla, & Lehner, 2013). Listed as a schedule 1 drug, it is now illegal to obtain.

Alcohol. As many as 90% of high school seniors report having consumed alcohol. As many as 25% of high school students report having engaged in episodic heavy or binge drinking. At least 10% of high school students report driving a car or other vehicle when they had been drinking alcohol. Nearly 30% of students report having ridden in a car or other vehicle driven by someone who had been drinking alcohol (CDC, 2012a).

Although alcohol use is correlated with motor vehicle accidents, homicide, and suicide in adolescents, it has never carried the social stigma of other drugs. Some parents are actually relieved when they learn their child's strange behavior on returning home from a party was caused by drunkenness and not illegal drugs. Alcohol use cannot be taken lightly, however, because it can cause diseases such as cirrhosis and is linked to destructive behaviors such as addiction, depression, and vulnerability to date rape.

Heredity has a definite role in the use of alcohol, but environment plays an equal part in whether an adolescent becomes a frequent user (Maimon & Browning, 2012). Remind parents they have a responsibility to set good examples for adolescents in the use of alcohol by not drinking indiscriminately.

Most adolescents will admit they use alcohol if asked two specific questions: "Do you drink alcohol?" and "When was your last drink?" Adolescents who answer yes to the first and "within the last 24 hours" to the second are candidates for further assessment.

Once adolescents admit they have come to rely on alcohol as a way to feel popular or reduce stress, an organization such as Alcoholics Anonymous can be invaluable in helping them stop drinking; innovative online programs geared especially for adolescents are also available. Encourage the remainder of their family to join Al-Anon, the organization for families of alcoholics, so both children and their families can restructure their lives to find satisfaction without the use of this drug.

Many adolescents are not the primary alcohol abuser in a family but are the children of alcoholic parents. Make an effort to identify this group of children as well, not only to prevent them from becoming users of alcohol but also to help them build self-esteem and coping abilities for the difficulties they face living in a possibly disorganized household.

✔ QSEN Checkpoint Question 33.5

Evidence-Based Practice

It has long been theorized there may be a "gateway" drug or one that, when used first, leads to further and more dangerous substance abuse. To determine whether alcohol, tobacco, or marijuana was the gateway drug, researchers obtained information on the drug use of a nationally representative sample of high school seniors. Results of the study showed alcohol was the gateway drug, leading to tobacco, marijuana, and then other illicit substances (Kirby & Barry, 2012).

Based on the previous study, which statement by Raul would give you the most concern?

a. "Some of my friends got hammered last weekend but I decided not to stick around."
b. "Some of my friends use weed; they tell me it really helps them relax."
c. "My parents said I could celebrate my next birthday by drinking my first beer."
d. "My mother eats some kind of chocolate almost every day. Is that hereditary?"

Look in Appendix A for the best answer and rationale.

Tobacco. Although it is well documented that cigarette smoking leads to increased cardiovascular and respiratory illnesses by middle age, every day, approximately 4,000 American youth aged 12 to 17 years of age try their first cigarette. As many as 20% of high school students report current cigarette use; about 14% report current cigar use. Eight percent of high school students report current smokeless tobacco use (CDC, 2012d).

Adolescents usually begin smoking because the habit conveys a stamp of maturity; smoking may be viewed as especially desirable by those who are having difficulty demonstrating maturity in other areas. Although at one time, proportionately more males than females smoked, adolescent girls now are the population most likely to begin smoking. One of the strongest determinants of whether adolescents will smoke a first cigarette is whether their friends smoke.

As cigar smoking is becoming more popular with adults, it also is becoming more popular with adolescents. "Smokeless tobacco" or chewing tobacco is also becoming more popular (Rath, Villanti, Abrams, et al., 2012). Although chewing tobacco does not have the potential dangers of smoking tobacco in relation to lung disease, it can cause gingival recession and lip and mouth cancer, and it can be just as habit-forming as cigarettes.

It has been well documented that adolescents are influenced to begin smoking by advertising (Widome, Brock, Noble, et al., 2013). Most school systems have extensive programs as early as grade school to caution children not to listen to cigarette advertising. Unfortunately, the ultimate danger of illness or death in middle age is not a strong threat to young persons who are interested only in the present.

More effective campaigns, therefore, might be those that point out that cigarette smoking causes foul-smelling hair, clothes, and breath, which detracts from physical appearance (i.e., "now" concerns). Helping adolescents find other methods to demonstrate their maturity, such as allowing them opportunities for increased decision making and emphasizing that being able to *not* smoke is a sign of true maturity, needs to be investigated. Urge adolescents who want to quit cigarette smoking to enroll in a group cigarette or online withdrawal program. Nicotine gum and nicotine patches have both been successfully used with adolescents (Larzelere & Williams, 2012).

Remember that adolescents are very reluctant to follow instructions that are given from a "do as I say, not as I do" standpoint. Nurses who smoke, therefore, can have extreme difficulty launching an effective campaign against the habit with adolescents. Stopping smoking can be especially difficult during periods of stress or inactivity. Trying to introduce such an action during exam week, for example, is not good planning. During an illness is also a bad time, unless not feeling well has reduced the urge to smoke. A return visit for follow-up and health maintenance care might be a better time to introduce the topic.

What if...33.2 Raul tells you during a history assessment that he does not smoke, but you smell cigarette smoke on his clothing. Although he says he doesn't use drugs, a number of blue-and-white capsules fall out of his shirt pocket when he unbuttons his shirt. What questions would you want to ask him to determine if he is smoking cigarettes or using drugs? What would be your next action if he does admit he is not only heavily into drugs but also does not intend to stop using them?

Performance-Enhancing Substance Abuse. Anabolic steroids are derivatives of the natural hormone testosterone. Common names are stanozolol, an oral compound, and testosterone propionate, an injectable form. Adolescents take steroids (obtained illegally) to enhance lean body mass and muscular development and so improve their athletic ability or appearance. These substances have side effects of euphoria and lessened fatigue, which make them doubly appealing.

Unfortunately, steroid use can lead to early closure of the epiphyseal line of long bones, acne, elevated triglyceride levels, hypertension, aggressiveness, possibly psychosis, abnormal liver function, and perhaps liver cancer. In addition, athletes using them and paying vigorous sports can die from ventricular hypertrophy (Montisci, El Mazloum, Cecchetto, et al., 2012).

Students using anabolic steroids need to be identified so they can be cautioned that the use of such drugs is illegal in sports competitions as well as being detrimental to their health. If needles are shared for administration, they additionally run the risk of acquiring hepatitis B or HIV infections.

Human growth hormone is a second drug used to enhance athletic performance. This increases muscle strength and stamina and is more difficult to detect than steroid use and so is also becoming a commonly abused substance in athletes (Baumann, 2012). It's dangerous in adolescents because side effects are joint pain and swelling and the development of diabetes.

Marijuana. Marijuana (widely known as "pot," "grass," or "weed"), derived from the leaves and stems of the Indian hemp plant *Cannabis sativa*, is the most frequently abused illicit substance, next to alcohol, used by adolescents (Kaul, 2013). It is generally rolled into cigarettes ("joints" or "reefers") and smoked, although it can also be mixed with food or sniffed. Scraping the resin from the flowering leaves produces a much stronger substance called hashish. Sinsemilla is a seedless form that is even more potent.

Breakdown products of marijuana are not readily eliminated from the body and remain in the fatty cells of the brain. This residue can create synaptic gaps that interfere with electrical brain waves and memory storage, especially for short-term memory. Physical and psychological effects of all forms of marijuana are euphoria and a sense of well-being, temporary impairment of coordination, rapid mood swings, decreased attention span, and loss of memory for recent events (up to 1 hour's time). Withdrawal symptoms include irritability, drowsiness, and cravings for high-carbohydrate snacks.

Long-term side effects can include pulmonary disorders such as sinusitis, bronchitis, emphysema, and perhaps lung cancer (which can develop after only 1 year of continual use compared with 20 years of cigarette use), as well as lack of sperm formation or subfertility in males (Fronczak, Kim, & Barqawi, 2012).

Because the drug is prescribed to relieve nausea and vomiting, adolescents may view it as harmless. Help them to realize marijuana is more than an amusing leisure activity or a way to relieve stress so they can put its long-term effects into perspective.

Amphetamines. Amphetamines are a group of drugs used in the treatment of hyperactivity and narcolepsy, among other central nervous system disorders. They are easily manufactured in "meth labs" in people's homes and so may be readily available to adolescents. Amphetamines are called "uppers" or "speed" because they give the user a false sense of well-being, alertness, or self-esteem. A newer, stronger form that produces intense symptoms is known as "ice." Some of the side effects of either form are aggressive or demanding behavior, paranoia, and extreme restlessness. Chronic methamphetamine abuse results in destruction of teeth enamel or blackened, crumbling teeth (Auten, Matteucci, Gaspary, et al., 2012). Amphetamines can be especially appealing to obese adolescents as they suppress the appetite and result in weight loss.

Cocaine. Cocaine is one of the most popular drugs of abuse for young adults; its use can begin in adolescents. The drug may be sniffed into the nose (snorted), smoked, or injected intravenously. Occasionally, it is combined with heroin (termed a "speedball") and injected. Common street names for cocaine are "snow" and "white lady" because of its fine, white powder. A stronger form, called "crack," is manufactured by heating cocaine powder with baking soda and water. This preparation process is dangerous in itself because it involves using volatile solvents that can ignite or explode. The resulting drug, often called "freebase" or "rock," is so strong it can cause immediate cardiac and respiratory arrhythmias (Paczynski & Gold, 2011).

It is difficult to document how many adolescents use cocaine, but estimates range from 3% to 9%. After absorption, blood levels rise rapidly for the first 20 minutes, peak at 60 minutes, and then decline over the next 3 hours. Although a toxic dose of cocaine is usually considered to be 600 to 700 mg, toxicity has been reported in as low as a 20 mg dose (a single line).

Cocaine produces the physical effects of increased pulse and respiration rates, increased temperature, increased blood pressure, and decreased appetite. Psychological effects produced are euphoria, excitement and restlessness, increased sociability, and possible hallucinations.

Toxic symptoms include seizures, tachyarrhythmias, tachypnea, hypertension, nausea and vomiting, abdominal pain, headaches, chills, and fever. It can be a major cause of cardiovascular arrest in young adults (Eisendrath & Lichtmacher, 2013). It may be a cause of adolescent automobile accidents because it creates such a sense of well-being and safety (Stoduto, Mann, Ialomiteanu, et al., 2012).

Cocaine is rarely ingested orally, but occasionally, adolescents swallow it when trying to hide a supply from parents or school personnel. Gastric acid destroys the action of cocaine, so unless the amount is extremely large, it is potentially harmless when swallowed in this way.

Teach adolescents that although cocaine sniffing may be fascinating and offer temporary pleasure and relief from stress, it also causes psychological dependency and is potentially extremely dangerous because of its cardiac and respiratory effects. Chronic inhalation of cocaine can cause ulceration in the mucous membrane of the nose, and injection of the substance exposes an adolescent to the risk of HIV and AIDS or hepatitis B. During pregnancy, it can cause separation of the placenta with potential fetal and maternal death (Mbah, Alio, Fombo, et al., 2012).

Hallucinogens. Examples of hallucinogenic drugs used by adolescents are lysergic acid diethylamide (LSD), dimethyltryptamine (DMT), 2,5-dimethoxy-4-methamphetamine (STP), phencyclidine hydrochloride (PCP), *Salvia divinorum*, mephedrone ("bath salts"), and methaqualone (Quaalude). The use of LSD has substantially increased in popularity since the 1960s when it first became available, because it is a drug that can be manufactured by an informed adolescent in a "kitchen lab." Methylenedioxymethamphetamine (MDMA, also known as "ecstasy") was previously used by some psychotherapists to make patients more receptive to therapy. It is now illegal as chronic use destroys the serotonin system of the brain, causing progressive decline of immediate and delayed memory and alterations in mood (Hittner & Schachne, 2012).

All of these drugs cause bizarre mind reactions such as distortion in vision, smell, or hearing. Adolescents report seeing colors more vividly than they have ever seen them before, hearing sounds so clear they cause physical pain, or perceiving themselves as being totally impervious to harm leading to "good trips" or "bad trips."

Recurrences or flashbacks of drug-induced experiences may, unfortunately, recur at unpredictable times and in unexpected places. Such flashbacks are not only disconcerting but can also be dangerous, especially if they occur while a person is driving a motor vehicle. They can be so frightening that some users believe they are becoming mentally deranged.

QSEN Checkpoint Question 33.6

Teamwork & Collaboration

At the conclusion of a long conversation, Raul admits he has experimented with cocaine. Which assessment finding would most strongly warrant a referral to addiction services?

a. Raul has frown lines in his forehead.
b. Raul has thin, fissured lips.
c. Raul's eyebrows appear thin.
d. Raul lacks nasal hair.

Look in Appendix A for the best answer and rationale.

Opiates. Opiates include drugs such as heroin, meperidine (Demerol), and morphine. At one time, these were not typically used by adolescents because they are expensive, but they are now gaining popularity among teens.

Opiates can be extremely dangerous because of their tendency to decrease one's respiratory rate. Addiction to them can cause such physiologic cravings in adolescents, like adults, that they may steal, defraud, and turn to prostitution to secure enough money to buy a day's supply. In addition to the direct danger of opiates, adolescents who use them risk the danger of contracting HIV and AIDS and hepatitis B infection if they share contaminated needles. "Snorting" heroin can lead to an acute cerebrovascular accident and death.

Methadone or levomethadyl acetate (LAAM) programs can be prescribed to help adolescents wean themselves from opiates (Eisendrath & Lichtmacher, 2013). Users report to a center every day and receive an oral dose of methadone, which fulfills the same physiologic need as heroin. Although methadone is a narcotic and its use can be associated with automobile accidents, because adolescents do not have to pay for it, they no longer have to steal or prostitute themselves to obtain it. It allows them to stay in school or hold a job and become productive citizens (Bramness, Skurtveit, Mørland, et al., 2012). Caution adolescents that they can feel "light-headed" from methadone, and that a methadone overdose can occur the same as with any narcotic. After a time, LAAM is gradually substituted for methadone. The advantage of LAAM over methadone is that its effect lasts longer—72 rather than 24 hours—so less frequent administration is necessary. If a methadone program is not available, pregnant adolescents may be treated with buprenorphine so their baby is not born opiate dependent (Heberlein, Leggio, Stichtenoth, et al., 2012).

Assessment of Substance Abuse

If adolescents trust health care personnel, they will generally admit if they have engaged in drug experimentation (Box 33.6). Clues they are using drugs are poor school attendance and general flawed reasoning, being diagnosed with hepatitis B, are HIV positive, or appearing to receive no benefit from usual analgesic agents. Physical symptoms that indicate specific substance abuse are summarized in Table 33.3.

Nursing Diagnoses and Related Interventions

Nursing Diagnosis: Risk for injury related to the use of alcohol or addictive chemical substances

Outcome Evaluation: Adolescent states he is not experimenting with drugs; can describe a way to respond to peers who encourage such use; shows no evidence of drug use such as lethargy, confusion, positive urine drug screen, or parental suspicion.

One of the greatest dangers of early drug experimentation is that it affects an adolescent's ability to solve problems, which creates a delay in maturity. Because adolescents may avoid adults who might detect their drug use, they remove themselves from exposure to adult role models.

Important teaching points for avoiding drug use include:

- Whether a drug is inhaled, swallowed, or injected, it still is absorbed, enters your body, and is therefore potentially harmful.
- Relying on drugs to give you courage to solve problems (or to help you forget you have problems) prevents you from learning to handle life situations and maturing.
- The bottom line of substance abuse is that you have the final say: you are the only one who can stop chemical dependency from happening.
- Despite their social acceptability, alcohol and nicotine are drugs. A short span of daily use of either can make you addicted.

Therapeutic communities or 24-hour facilities in which adolescents can live while they recover from chemical dependency may be necessary for some adolescents. The aim of all these programs is to increase adolescents' sense of self-esteem, improve problem-solving ability, realign them with society's values, and increase their self-awareness so they can function effectively without the aid of substances of abuse. Unfortunately, campaigns against substance abuse for adolescents have not been very successful, so the problem continues.

Adolescents who are no longer chemically dependent should be evaluated by a history and physical examination at all health care visits because, if the circumstances that initially caused them to become chemically dependent recur, they may return to a dependency pattern. A continuing relationship with health care personnel not only allows time for this evaluation but also provides concrete role models of nonchemical, productive behavior.

BOX 33.6 Nursing Care Planning Based on Effective Communication

You talk to Raul, age 15 years, in an adolescent clinic.

Less Effective Communication

Nurse: Here's a pamphlet about adolescents and drug use. I hope you haven't been using any.
Raul: No problem.
Nurse: Drugs can be really harmful. It takes an absolutely stupid person to use them.
Raul: No problem.
Nurse: Have you been doing any?
Raul: No problem.

More Effective Communication

Nurse: Here's a pamphlet about adolescents and drug use. I hope you haven't been using any.
Raul: No problem.
Nurse: Sometimes it's difficult to talk to parents or other adults about such things.
Raul: No problem.
Nurse: Have you been doing any?
Raul: No problem.

Raul answered with the same response in both conversations. Do you think he meant the same thing in both conversations? Was the nurse wise to announce that only stupid people use drugs and then ask if Raul was using any?

TABLE 33.3 Symptoms to Help Identify Substance Abusers

Drugs Used	Symptoms of Use	Dangers
Glue	Violence, drunken appearance, dreamy or blank expression; glue smears on clothing or fingers; tubes of glue, paper bags in possession	Lung, brain, or liver damage; death through suffocation or choking; anemia
Heroin, morphine, codeine	Stupor, drowsiness, needle marks on body, watery eyes, loss of appetite, bloodstains on shirt sleeve, runny nose; possession of needles or hypodermic syringes, cotton, tourniquet strings, burnt bottle caps or spoons, glassine envelopes	Death from overdose; addiction; liver and other infections due to unsterile needles
Cough medicines containing codeine	Drunken appearance, lack of coordination, confusion, excessive itching; possession of empty bottles of cough medicine	Addiction
Marijuana	Sleepiness, wandering mind, enlarged pupils, lack of coordination; discolored fingers, strong odor of burnt leaves; possession of small seeds in pocket lining, cigarette papers	Psychological dependence
Hallucinogens (LSD, DMT, PCP)	Severe hallucinations, feelings of detachment, incoherent speech, cold hands and feet, laughing and crying, vomiting, strong body odor; possession of cube sugar with discoloration in center	Suicidal tendencies, unpredictable behavior; chronic exposure may have neurologic effects
Stimulants (methamphetamine, cocaine)	Aggressive behavior, giggling, silliness, rapid speech, confused thinking, no appetite, extreme fatigue, black caries, dry mouth, shakiness, insomnia, absence of nasal hair; possession of pills or capsules of varying colors, possession of a glass pipe	Death from overdose; hallucinations; psychosis
Depressants (barbiturates, alcohol)	Drowsiness, stupor, dullness, slurred speech, drunken appearance, vomiting, odor of alcohol on breath; possession of pills or capsules of varying colors	Death or unconsciousness from overdose; addiction; seizures from withdrawal
Steroids	Aggressive behavior, increase in muscle strength and mass	Violent actions; possibly tumor growth

Concerns Regarding Depression and Self-Injury

Self-injury includes a range of self-destructive actions from cutting to suicide, the planned intent to end one's life. Cutting is found more frequently in girls than boys and can begin as early as grade school (Barrocas, Hankin, Young, et al., 2012).

Successful suicide occurs more frequently in males than in females, although more females apparently attempt suicide than males (a ratio of about 8:1). Adolescent suicides tend to be attempted most often in the spring or the fall, reflecting school stress at these times of year, and between 3 PM and midnight, reflecting depression that increases with the dark. Suicide is so common in adolescents it ranks third as a cause of death in the 15- to 19-year-old age group (Eaton, Kann, Kinchen, et al., 2012). This statistic may actually be underestimated because some well-meaning coroners may report these deaths as unintentional injuries to spare the family additional pain. Some automobile or hiking injuries, for example, may be attempts at self-destruction; in addition, some homicides may be caused by deliberately provoking another person in the hope of being killed.

Some degree of depression is present in most adolescents because they are not only losing their parents while they grow apart from them but also their carefree childhood (Fried, Williams, Cabral, et al., 2013). If school failure, loss of a girlfriend or boyfriend, loss of a competition with loss of self-esteem, or rejection by a peer group is superimposed on existing depression, the pressure may be great enough to cause some adolescents to attempt suicide. This makes the reasons for adolescent suicide varied: incest, maltreatment, increased chemical dependency, marital instability in the family, and poor problem-solving ability are all reasons that may lead an adolescent to decide death may be easier than coping with overwhelming problems.

Yet other reasons may involve anger with others, trying to get even, and manipulation (e.g., psychological blackmail) as a way of having one's needs met. Because some adolescents may be unable to believe a parent was at fault in the case of divorce, they may instead believe they somehow caused the parent to leave.

Assessment

Adolescents need to have thorough physical examinations at health maintenance visits to assure them they are in good physical health. Assess at these visits signs of depression such as anorexia, insomnia, excessive fatigue, or weight loss (Gampetro, Wojciechowski, & Siarkowski Amer, 2012). In younger adolescents, depression may be manifested not so much by appearing sad, but by behavior problems such as disobedience, temper tantrums, truancy, and running away. Self-destructive behavior or injury proneness; difficulties in school; acting out with chemicals, alcohol, or sexual promiscuity; or trouble with legal authorities may be further clues.

Occasionally, depressed adolescents find it so hard to be alone that they seek constant activity as a means of escape. Others may withdraw from contact with other people and become completely isolated. Either behavior needs to be detected through assessing activity and interaction levels.

Adolescents who attempt suicide do not fall into any one category, although many tend to be loners or have difficulty expressing their feelings to others and, therefore, do not receive emotional support from friends or family. Others appear to be "perfect" students, so friends or family do not see a need to counsel them. The stress of trying to continually achieve at a high level, however, is the trigger that provokes suicide. Gay and lesbian youths appear to have higher levels of suicide than others, reflecting the level of stress they may be experiencing. Assess for these lifestyles as well (Shields, Whitaker, Glassman, et al., 2012).

If another member of a family or a close friend commits suicide, the chance an adolescent will also do so is greater than usual. The anniversary of a family member's suicide is an especially vulnerable time because wishing to join the dead family member may appear attractive. Adolescent suicide rates may actually reach epidemic proportions after a popular student's suicide. Students who have Internet contacts may arrange a group suicide as a method of making a statement or gaining support.

Because suicide usually reflects a problem in family interaction, a family assessment is helpful. A thorough family history may reveal conflict with one or both parents or reveal how little support the adolescent receives at home. School friends may often be the ones who are first aware that an adolescent is contemplating suicide. Caution parents not to discount reports from their child's friends who tell them they are concerned.

Close to the chosen time of suicide, some adolescents demonstrate characteristic behaviors that show they are making preparations to end their life. Teach family and friends these typical danger signs (Box 33.7).

When caring for a child after a suicide attempt, ask enough questions on a health history so you can help to analyze whether an adolescent made a detailed suicide plan. For example, a young person who took four aspirins and left the empty aspirin container conspicuously on the kitchen counter just before his mother was due to arrive home from work is more likely to be only making a cry for help; one who took 100 aspirins and hid the container under the bed just after his mother left for 8 hours of work is much more apt to be making a serious attempt.

As you care for an adolescent in a health care facility, you may be the first to realize the boy or girl is not "just talking" about suicide (it is a fallacy that people who talk about suicide do not attempt it) but is someone with a definite, well-thought-out plan to accomplish it. An adolescent who has been admitted to a hospital unit after a serious suicide attempt may formulate a new plan that will be successful the next time unless some action is taken and the adolescent's life can be changed in some way (see Box 33.8 for an interprofessional care map for an adolescent with possible suicide intent).

BOX 33.7 Nursing Care Planning Based on Family Teaching

SUICIDE WARNING SIGNS

Q. Raul's father says to you, "Our neighbor's son recently committed suicide. What are warning signs of this to look for in our son?"

A. The following are commonly seen clues:

- Giving away prized possessions
- Organ donation questions, such as "How do you leave your body to a medical school?"
- Sudden, unexplained elevation of mood, which may indicate the individual has reached a decision about the suicide and feels relief
- Injury proneness, carelessness, and death wishes
- Decrease in verbal communication or a statement such as, "This is the last time you will see me"
- Withdrawal from peer activities or previously enjoyed events
- Previous attempt (80% of all completed suicides have been preceded by a failed attempt)
- Preference for art, music, and literature with themes of death
- Recent increase in interpersonal conflict with significant others
- Running away from home
- Recent experience of a friend or famous person committing suicide
- Inquiring about the hereafter
- Asking for information (supposedly for a friend) about suicide prevention and intervention
- Almost any sustained deviation from the normal pattern of behavior

BOX 33.8 Nursing Care Planning

AN INTERPROFESSIONAL CARE MAP FOR AN ADOLESCENT WITH POSSIBLE SUICIDE INTENT

Raul is a 15-year-old boy you meet at an adolescent clinic. His chief concern is a head cold. He has numerous acne lesions on his forehead and cheeks. His parents tell you Raul seemed depressed for a long time after his girlfriend broke up with him but now seems happy again. They are pleased to see him maturing so much; for example, he recently gave away his collection of baseball cards to a young neighbor. You mention to Raul a decongestant would probably make him feel better. He asks you how many pills it would take to kill someone, then jokes he was kidding.

Family Assessment Client lives with both parents and two younger siblings. Father manages a funeral parlor; mother works as a beautician for funeral parlor. Client describes finances as "all right, if you think burying people is a good way to earn money."

Client Assessment Fifteen-year-old male with history of acne for the last 6 months. Reports washing his face approximately five or six times a day with abrasive soap and covering lesions with cocoa butter cream twice a day. He states, "Look at me. I look terrible." Physical examination reveals scattered pustules and comedones on forehead and face. Two lesions on right cheek with large erythematous base and tender to touch. Remainder of physical examination unremarkable.

Nursing Diagnosis Risk for self-injury related to disappointing appearance because of acne lesions and lack of friendships

Outcome Criteria Adolescent states causes of acne; identifies measures for prevention and treatment; agrees to counseling to reestablish self-esteem

Team Member Responsible	Assessment	Intervention	Rationale	Expected Outcome
Activities of Daily Living, Including Safety				
Nurse/Nurse practitioner	Assess adolescent's understanding of acne and its causes.	Instruct adolescent in measures to prevent and control acne.	Gentle washing removes irritating fatty acids. Omit greasy creams.	Client states intent to follow recommendations to decrease acne symptoms.
Teamwork and Collaboration				
Nurse/Primary health care provider/Mental health counselor	Evaluate if client was joking or was serious about a self-injury attempt.	Schedule consultation if client may be contemplating self-injury.	Client shows typical signs of self-injury behavior.	Mental health counselor meets with client to make recommendations on client safety.
Procedures/Medications for Quality Improvement				
Nurse/Nurse practitioner	Assess what measures client has been using to self-treat acne.	Discuss treatment options available.	Discussion provides the adolescent with correct information on acne therapy.	Client describes full range of therapies available and what new measures he would be willing to try.
Nutrition				
Nurse/Nutritionist	Assess client's understanding of the effect of nutrition on acne.	Counsel client to follow a well-balanced diet.	No particular food is associated with development of acne, despite old beliefs.	Client states he understands food intake is not the major cause of acne.

(continued on page 948)

BOX 33.8 Nursing Care Planning (continued)

Patient-Centered Care				
Nurse	Assess family's communication level, overall coping techniques, and abilities.	Discuss how better communication can aid in helping adolescent cope with life changes.	Better communication among family members provides support for all family members.	Parents discuss family communication pattern and make suggestions for better patterns.
Psychosocial/Spiritual/Emotional Needs				
Nurse	Assess how acne affects client's self esteem.	Review and reinforce with adolescent positive attributes about self.	Positive attributes provide a foundation for rebuilding self-esteem.	Client states he knows that others value his friendship above his appearance.
Informatics for Seamless Health Care Planning				
Nurse/Nurse practitioner/ Mental health counselor	Assess with mental health counselor if it will be safe for client to return home.	Give client hotline telephone number and instruct to use as needed.	Knowing a support source is available can be as valuable as actually contacting the source.	Client assures staff he has the hotline number available and will call if needed.

Nursing Diagnoses and Related Interventions

Nursing Diagnosis: Risk for violence, self-directed, related to symptoms of depression or expressed desire to hurt oneself

Outcome Evaluation: Client expresses feelings of depression to health care providers or other adults; states he will contact support person should the desire to commit suicide become overwhelming.

Crisis intervention for adolescents who are contemplating suicide includes trying to alleviate their pain and depression and counseling them in an effort to help them change their perspective on the value of life. Be aware that establishing expected outcomes with adolescents who are contemplating suicide or who have made an attempt will be difficult because they are often too depressed to come up with alternative solutions to their problems (their goal was to kill themselves, not solve problems).

It is important not to underestimate adolescents' determination and capability to end their own life. In most instances, adolescents at this point need referral to a consultant who is well versed in suicide prevention to improve self-image and offer alternative solutions to problems.

As another measure, try to find out the things in the child's life that are still viewed as important; build a plan that will help view life as worth living enough to work through difficulties. Show them how no one can change everything, but everyone can make one or two changes that can make a difference. After these small changes are made, a domino effect can be created to change more and more of one's circumstances.

Because adolescents resort to suicide as a method of solving problems, helping all adolescents learn better problem-solving skills is a prime intervention strategy. Ask "what would happen if" questions such as "Suppose you did fail a course; what would be the worst that could happen?" Your help in this area is important because, generally, persons who are depressed do not have strong support people around them or do not believe anyone cares enough about them to help.

For an adolescent's safety, a period of observation on an adolescent or a psychiatric service is desirable after a suicide attempt to prevent the adolescent from inflicting personal injury again and to allow an assessment in a neutral setting, away from the stress that precipitated the attempt. Evidence for the effectiveness of selective serotonin reuptake inhibitors, as are used with adults, is limited with children; these medications have a black box warning to use with caution in persons under 25 years of age as some have been associated with elevating the mood of depressed children enough that they then are able to formulate a plan and commit suicide after taking them (Gibbons, Brown, Hur, et al., 2012).

The continuing evaluation by both history taking and physical examination should be ongoing because the young person who has attempted suicide once may attempt it again if support people and better problem-solving abilities are not available.

What if . . . 33.3 Raul seems unusually happy at a clinic visit when usually he is sad because of loss of his girlfriend. You know he recently gave away his collection of baseball cards to a neighborhood boy because "I won't need them where I'm going." Would you be concerned about him? If you learned he is about to leave to be an exchange student in England, would this affect your assessment?

Concerns of the Adolescent and Family With Unique Needs

Homeless youth (i.e., runaways) and adolescents who are disabled have specific concerns that need special attention.

Homeless or Runaway Youth

A *runaway* is commonly defined as an adolescent between the ages of 10 and 17 years who has been absent from home at least overnight without permission of a parent or guardian. Fortunately, most teenagers who run away do not go far or stay away long (under 1 week); about 1 in 20 adolescent runaways stays away as long as 1 year, and some never return home and become homeless youth. Runaway adolescents are most likely to be from either low- or high-income families. Stress factors such as family unemployment, alcoholism, sexual maltreatment, incest, attempted suicide, and poverty are frequent characteristics in their families (Moskowitz, Stein, & Lightfoot, 2012). They are slightly more likely to be male than female.

Assessment. Running away is usually preceded by an argument with parents that is often the last straw after a number of long-term disagreements. Other reasons may be personal concerns such as loneliness; pregnancy; and problems with friends, school, or the police. A school history often reveals frequent truancy, failing grades, possible drug use, and runaway behavior by friends. It is a sad fact that some adolescents are "throwaways" or cannot remain at home because they have been rejected by their families.

Common health reasons for which runaway adolescents are seen at health care facilities are sexually transmitted diseases, including HIV and AIDS, rape, pregnancy, substance abuse, hepatitis, and vaginitis. They also have a high incidence of suicide attempts (Palepu, Hubley, Russell, et al., 2012).

When caring for adolescents with these concerns, be certain to secure a thorough history so the fact that they are no longer living at home will not be overlooked. Do not reveal you are shocked by a report such as an adolescent has been sleeping on a park bench for 2 months, has been robbed, or steals to obtain money because this could prevent you from learning even greater concerns, such as having a sexually transmitted disease, being pregnant, or using drugs.

As they lack references for jobs and do not necessarily qualify for public assistance programs, homeless adolescents generally have no secure source of income. This can cause both males and females to resort to stealing or prostitution to support themselves. Legally, they are considered to be juvenile delinquents, so police are required to return them to their homes if discovered.

Because many adolescents who run away are not good problem solvers, setting goals with them may be difficult. A short-term goal to stay home through a holiday rather than a long-term one of finishing high school may be all you can achieve. Try to imagine yourself in the adolescent's circumstances to determine whether your health instructions or goals will be sensible for their lifestyle. As they have no money for food, giving them an instruction to eat iron-rich foods to prevent anemia, for example, may be ludicrous. If they do not have a source of running water, telling them to soak a lesion or change a dressing may be impossible. If they don't have a means of transportation, they may be unable to return to the health care facility for frequent follow-up visits so try to meet as many of the runaway's needs as possible at one visit. Remember that many runaways have associated school failure and so have poor health literacy; discuss the information with them as well as give them a pamphlet or written instructions.

Be certain, also, to ask if an adolescent wants to return home. Even though being homeless is high stress, and many adolescent runaways want to take the first step back toward their parents, they may not know how to begin the process or be certain they will be welcomed back at home. Check if they are familiar with the National Youth Crisis Hotline, which they can telephone day or night when they want to return home (1-800-448-4663 [1-800-HIT HOME]). Remember also they are runaways because, for some reason, their home was intolerable. Although they agree to return home, they may not remain there unless circumstances have been or can be changed.

A Physically Challenged or Chronically Ill Adolescent

Achieving a sense of identity may be difficult for adolescents who have a chronic illness or other challenges. It is vital, however, for such individuals to learn to look past their particular condition to their real selves. For example, a 16-year-old girl in a wheelchair must learn to perceive herself as a teenager who is intelligent, is a good conversationalist, has a good sense of humor, enjoys watching football, and only incidentally uses a wheelchair to ambulate.

Some of the biggest problems of chronically ill adolescents are likely to be difficulties in being as independent as they would like to be, achieving in school, and establishing intimate relationships. Those who cannot learn to drive when their friends are learning to do so, who are not invited to dances and parties because of a unique concern, or who are too hesitant to ask someone to go with them may feel acute loneliness and loss of self-esteem. Moreover, the loss of many hours of school due to illness or frequent hospitalization may result in the inability to pursue a desired career, at least a delay in doing so. Adolescence may be the first time these individuals realize certain occupations or opportunities, such as a military career, may be closed to them. As they prepare to leave the security of a familiar school system, it may be the first time they examine just how they will be able to function on their own. Some may come to realize they will never be able to do so with complete independence.

Chronic hospitalization or the realization they will never be free of symptoms can cause depression in such adolescents, placing them at high risk for substance abuse or self-injury. Helping these adolescents realize that even completely well people must compromise life decisions for other reasons such as lack of money, lack of qualifications, or other personal responsibilities helps them feel they are not so different

TABLE 33.4 Nursing Actions That Encourage a Sense of Identity in the Physically Challenged or Chronically Ill Adolescent

Category	Actions
Nutrition	If adolescent is on special diet, discuss role of food preferences with dietitian (e.g., hot dogs, pizza). Respect food preferences in all ways possible.
Dressing change	Allow adolescent to order supplies. Ask for suggestions as to final appearance of dressing. If soaks are included, have adolescent time the treatment. Allow adolescent to choose time for dressing change.
Medicine	Offer the adolescent a choice of site for injection or intravenous insertion to encourage a sense of control. Teach name, action, and possible side effects of medicine.
Rest	Contract with adolescent for time and length of rest periods.
Hygiene	Respect modesty as you would with an adult. Contract with adolescent for extent of self-care (e.g., will give own bath and make bed, not medicate self).
Pain	Encourage adolescent to express pain, and teach distraction technique for sharp pain, such as deep breathing and counting backward from 100. Encourage adolescent to ask for analgesics as needed.
Stimulation	Provide favorite music with earphones. Provide a radio to listen to talk shows to foster active involvement. Encourage school work (you may need to help adolescents divide up school assignments so they do not become overly fatigued and frustrated). Provide crossword puzzles or card games to increase socialization (make or have the adolescent make a card deck from pieces of paper if one is not available). Encourage adolescents to network with one another. Encourage adolescents to keep in contact with friends through texting, e-mail, or writing notes.

from others. The fact an adult is willing to make a time commitment to discuss their future with them can be enough to give these adolescents the self-esteem they need to alter aspirations and plans and find a future role consistent with their capabilities. Nursing actions to encourage a sense of identity in an adolescent with a long-term illness or who is physically challenged are summarized in Table 33.4.

Nutrition and the Chronically Ill Adolescent

Adolescents who are not fully mobile must be cautious of their total calorie intake because, as growth needs decline at the end of adolescence, they may become obese. They should also be knowledgeable about good nutrition, so they can participate in meal planning, an action that can help them feel a sense of control over this area of their life. Assess how often they have a chance to eat at fast-food restaurants; although this is not a source of excellent nutrition, eating there occasionally can provide an important social experience and a chance to be like their peers.

What if . . . 33.4 You are particularly interested in exploring one of the 2020 National Health Goals with respect to adolescent growth and development (see Box 33.1). What would be a possible research topic to explore that is pertinent to this goal that would be applicable to Raul's family and that would also advance evidence-based practice?

Key Points for Review

- The major milestones of development in the adolescent period are the onset of puberty and the cessation of body growth. Between these milestones, physical growth is rapid, although the development of adult coordination and thought processes is slow.
- The development of secondary sex characteristics is completed during adolescence. These are rated according to Tanner stages.
- The developmental task of an adolescent according to Erikson is to establish independence from parents by gaining a sense of identity versus role confusion. Therefore, adolescents usually respond best to health care personnel who respect their attempts at independence and who allow them as many choices as possible in care.
- Adolescents reach a point of cognitive development termed *formal operational thought*. With this gained, they are able to think in abstract terms and use rational thinking to arrive at conclusions.
- Adolescents need to consume adequate calories and especially protein, iron, calcium, and zinc to meet their increased growth needs, but at the same time, be certain they don't become overweight.
- Being an adolescent is difficult in today's world. Be aware that, to reduce stress, some adolescents may begin to abuse substances. Asking about an adolescent's drug experiences during a health assessment is not intruding on privacy.

Rather, it is a method of safe health interviewing and helps in planning nursing care that not only meets QSEN competencies but also best meets a family's total needs.

- Promoting adolescent safety is an important nursing role. Motor vehicle accidents, homicide, and suicide are leading causes of death in this age group.
- Common health problems in an adolescent are sometimes minor and include poor posture, fatigue, or acne; they can also be serious, such as beginning hypertension, substance abuse, and scoliosis. Identifying these problems and referring an adolescent for help are important nursing actions.

Critical Thinking Care Study

Genève is a 14-year-old who lives with her parents and an 8-year-old brother. They take a vacation for 2 weeks every summer at the beach.

1. Genève has asked her parents if she can bring her best friend, a 24-year-old neighbor, with her on vacation. Her parents ask you whether that would be a good idea. How would you respond?
2. Genève was stopped by security at a department store for shoplifting a red sweater she said she needed to wear to a party that evening. Her father paid for the sweater so she was not charged with shoplifting. Would you suggest her parents let her wear the sweater to the party?
3. Genève has her own television in her bedroom. Her parents tell you she often stays awake until 2 in the morning watching programs. Her parents ask you if they should monitor what she watches or if she is old enough to do this for herself.

Patient Scenario

The Pulvino Family

Read about the Pulvino family, a family with an adolescent, then answer the questions to further sharpen your skills and grow more familiar with NCLEX-type questions related to adolescent growth and development. Confirm your answers are correct by reading the rationales.

Visit http://thePoint.lww.com

Answers and Rationales

Looking for answers to the What If. . . and Critical Thinking Care Study questions?

Visit http://thePoint.lww.com

References

Ahern, N. R., & Norris, A. E. (2011). Examining factors that increase and decrease stress in adolescent community college students. *Journal of Pediatric Nursing, 28*(6), 530–540.

Allan, E. J., & Madden, M. (2011). The nature and extent of college student hazing. *International Journal of Adolescent Medicine & Health, 24*(1), 83–90.

American Academy of Pediatrics. (2012a). *High blood pressure in children.* Evanston, IL: Author.

Armfield, J. M. (2010). Community effectiveness of public water fluoridation in reducing children's dental disease. *Public Health Reports, 125*(5), 655–664.

Arrington, E. A., Patel, N. S., Gerancher, K., et al. (2012). Combined oral contraceptives for the treatment of acne: A practical guide. *Cutis, 90*(2), 83–90.

Auten, J. D., Matteucci, M. J., Gaspary, M. J., et al. (2012). Psychiatric implications of adolescent methamphetamine exposures. *Pediatric Emergency Care, 28*(1), 26–29.

Bagnulo, J. D. (2012). Carbohydrate. In I. Kohlstadt (Ed.), *Scientific evidence for musculskeletal, bariatric & sports nutrition.* Boca Raton, FL: Taylor & Francis.

Barrocas, A. L., Hankin, B. L., Young, J. F., et al. (2012). Rates of nonsuicidal self-injury in youth: Age, sex, and behavioral methods in a community sample. *Pediatrics, 130*(1), 39–45.

Baumann, G. P. (2012). Growth hormone doping in sports: A critical review of use and detection strategies. *Endocrine Reviews, 33*(2), 155–186.

Baumann, M. H., Partilla, J. S., & Lehner, K. R. (2013). Psychoactive "bath salts": Not so soothing. *European Journal of Pharmacology, 698*(1–3), 1–5.

Benjet, C., Borges, G., Medina-Mora, M. E., et al. (2012). Chronic childhood adversity and stages of substance use involvement in adolescents. *Drug & Alcohol Dependence.* Advance online publication.

Blake, K., & Davis, V. (2011) Adolescent medicine. In K. J. Marcdante, R. M. Kliegman, H. B. Jenson, et al. (Eds.), *Nelson essentials of pediatrics* (6th ed., pp. 265–284). Philadelphia, PA: Saunders/Elsevier.

Bramness, J. G., Skurtveit, S., Mørland, J., et al. (2012). An increased risk of motor vehicle accidents after prescription of methadone. *Addiction, 107*(5), 967–972.

Bregman, H. R., Malik, N. M., Page, M. J., et al. (2013). Identity profiles in lesbian, gay, and bisexual youth: The role of family influences. *Journal of Youth & Adolescence, 42*(3), 417–430.

Briggs, P., Simon, W. T., & Simonsen, S. (2011). An exploratory study of Internet-initiated sexual offenses and the chat room sex offender: Has the Internet enabled a new typology of sex offender? *Sexual Abuse, 23*(1), 72–91.

Centers for Disease Control and Prevention. (2012a). *Alcohol & drug use.* Atlanta, GA: Author.

Centers for Disease Control and Prevention. (2012b). Drowning—United States, 2005–2009. *MMWR: Morbidity & Mortality Weekly Report, 61*(19), 344–347.

Centers for Disease Control and Prevention. (2012c). *Sexually transmitted disease surveillance.* Atlanta, GA: Author.

Centers for Disease Control and Prevention. (2012d). *Youth & tobacco use: Fact sheet.* Atlanta, GA: Author.

Chen, H., Cao, L., & Logan, D. B. (2012). Analysis of risk factors affecting the severity of intersection crashes by logistic regression. *Traffic Injury Prevention, 13*(3), 300–307.

Chouinard, L. E., Randall Simpson, J., & Buchholz, A. C. (2012). Predictors of bone mineral density in a convenience sample of young Caucasian adults living in southern Ontario. *Applied Physiology, Nutrition & Metabolism, 37*(4), 706–714.

Cohen, L., Brown, J., Haukness, H., et al. (2013). Sun protection counseling by pediatricians has little effect on parent and child sun protection behavior. *Journal of Pediatrics, 162*(2), 381–386.

D'Aloise, P., & Chen, H. (2012). Rapid determination of flunitrazepam in alcoholic beverages by desorption electrospray ionization-mass spectrometry. *Science & Justice, 52*(1), 2–8.

Eaton, D. K., Kann, L., Kinchen, S., et al. (2012). Youth risk behavior surveillance—United States, 2011. *Morbidity & Mortality Weekly Report, 61*(4), 1–162.

Eisendrath, S. J., & Lichtmacher, J. E. (2013). Substance use disorders. In M. Papadakis & S. J. McPhee (Eds.), *Current medical diagnosis & treatment, 2013* (52nd ed., pp. 1079–1087). New York, NY: McGraw-Hill/Lange.

Elliott, M. R., Jacobsohn, L., Winston, F. K., et al. (2012). Determining subgroups of teens for targeted driving injury prevention strategies: A latent class analysis approach. *Traffic Injury Prevention, 13*(3), 258–264.

Erikson, E. H. (1993). *Childhood and society.* New York, NY: W. W. Norton.

Fernández-Gaxiola, A. C., & De-Regil, L. M. (2011). Intermittent iron supplementation for reducing anaemia and its associated impairments in menstruating women. *Cochrane Database of Systematic Reviews,* (12), CD009218.

Fried, L. E., Williams, S., Cabral, H., et al. (2013). Differences in risk factors for suicide attempts among 9th and 11th grade youth: A longitudinal perspective. *Journal of School Nursing, 29*(2), 113–122.

Fronczak, C. M., Kim, E. D., & Barqawi, A. B. (2012). The insults of illicit drug use on male fertility. *Journal of Andrology, 33*(4), 515–528.

Frost, L. A., & Burns, C. E. (2012). Sleep and rest. In C. E. Burns, A. M. Dunn, M. A. Brady, et al. (Eds.), *Pediatric primary care* (5th ed., pp. 256–273). Philadelphia, PA: Elsevier/Saunders.

Gampetro, P., Wojciechowski, E. A., & Siarkowski Amer, E. (2012). Life concerns and perceptions of care in adolescents with mental health care needs: A qualitative study in a school-based health clinic. *Pediatric Nursing, 38*(1), 23–30.

Garzon, D. L., & Dunn, A. M. (2013). Developmental management of adolescents. In C. E. Burns, A. M. Dunn, M. A. Brady, et al. (Eds.), *Pediatric primary care* (5th ed., pp. 110–131). Philadelphia, PA: Elsevier/Saunders.

Gibbons, R. D., Brown, C. H., Hur, K., et al. (2012). Suicidal thoughts and behavior with antidepressant treatment: Reanalysis of the randomized placebo-controlled studies of fluoxetine and venlafaxine. *Archives of General Psychiatry, 69*(6), 580–587.

Gilligan, C. (1982). *In a different voice: Psychological theory and women's development.* Cambridge, MA: Harvard University Press.

Hadlock, G. C., Webb, K. M., McFadden, L. M., et al. (2011). 4-Methylmethcathinone (mephedrone): Neuropharmacological effects of a designer stimulant of abuse. *Journal of Pharmacology & Experimental Therapeutics, 339*(2), 530–536.

Heberlein, A., Leggio, L., Stichtenoth, D., et al. (2012). The treatment of alcohol and opioid dependence in pregnant women. *Current Opinion in Psychiatry, 25*(6), 559–564.

Hittner, J. B., & Schachne, E. R. (2012). Meta-analysis of the association between ecstasy use and risky sexual behavior. *Addictive Behavior, 37*(7), 790–796.

Hoang, Q. B., Coel, R. A., Vidal, A., et al. (2012). Sports medicine. In W. Hay, M. Levin, R. Deterding, et al. (Eds.), *Current diagnosis & treatment pediatrics* (21st ed., pp. 849–880). New York, NY: McGraw-Hill/Lange.

Karch, A. M. (2013). *2013 Lippincott's nursing drug guide.* Philadelphia, PA: Lippincott Williams & Wilkins.

Katsufrakis, P. J., & Nusbaum, M. R. H. (2011). Adolescent sexuality. In J. E. South-Paul, S. C. Matheny, & E. L. Lewis (Eds.), *Current diagnosis & treatment in family medicine* (3rd ed., pp. 122–130). Columbus, OH: McGraw-Hill/Lange.

Kaul, K. (2013). Adolescent substance abuse. In W. Hay, M. Levin, R. Deterding, et al. (Eds.), *Current diagnosis & treatment pediatrics* (21st ed., pp. 153–166). New York, NY: McGraw-Hill/Lange.

Khan, K. M., Thompson, A. M., Blair, S. N., et al. (2012). Sport and exercise as contributors to the health of nations. *Lancet, 380*(9836), 59–64.

Kirby, T., & Barry, A. E. (2012). Alcohol as a gateway drug: A study of U.S. 12th graders. *Journal of School Health, 82*(8), 371–379.

Kistner, F., Fiebert, I., & Roach, K. (2012). Effect of backpack load carriage on cervical posture in primary schoolchildren. *Work, 41*(1), 99–108.

Kohlberg, L. (1984). *The psychology of moral development.* New York, NY: Harper & Row.

Larzelere, M. M., & Williams, D. E. (2012). Promoting smoking cessation. *American Family Physician, 85*(6), 591–598.

Ledger, W. L. (2012). The menstrual cycle. In D. K. Edmonds. (Ed.) *Dewhurst's textbook of obstetrics & gynaecology* (8th ed, pp. 487–494). Oxford: John Wiley & Son.

Lewis, T. P., & Hession, C. (2012). Alcohol use: From childhood through adolescence. *Journal of Pediatric Nursing, 27*(5), e50–e58.

Lloyd, S., Chalder, T., & Rimes, K. A. (2012). Family-focused cognitive behaviour therapy versus psycho-education for adolescents with chronic fatigue syndrome. *Behavior Research & Therapy, 50*(11), 719–725.

Loprinzi, P. D., Cardinal, B. J., Loprinzi, K. L., et al. (2012). Benefits and environmental determinants of physical activity in children and adolescents. *Obesity Facts, 5*(4), 597–610.

Lyon, V. B. (2011). Dermatology. In K. J. Marcdante, R. M. Kliegman, H. B. Jenson, et al. (Eds.), *Nelson essentials of pediatrics* (6th ed., pp. 713–734). Philadelphia, PA: Saunders/Elsevier.

Maimon, D., & Browning, C. R. (2012). Underage drinking, alcohol sales and collective efficacy: Informal control and opportunity in the study of alcohol use. *Social Science Research, 41*(4), 977–990.

Makin-Byrd, K., & Bierman, K. L. (2013). Individual and family predictors of the perpetration of dating violence and victimization in late adolescence. *Journal of Youth & Adolescence, 42*(4), 536–550.

Marciani, R. D. (2012). Complications of third molar surgery and their management. *Atlas of the Oral & Maxillofacial Surgery Clinics of North America, 20*(2), 233–251.

Marván, M. L., & Molina-Abolnik, M. (2012). Mexican adolescents' experience of menarche and attitudes toward menstruation. *Journal of Pediatric & Adolescent Gynecology, 25*(6), 358–363.

Mbah, A. K., Alio, A. P., Fombo, D. W., et al. (2012). Association between cocaine abuse in pregnancy and placenta-associated syndromes using propensity score matching approach. *Early Human Development, 88*(6), 333–337.

McClung, J. P. (2012). Iron status and the female athlete. *Journal of Trace Elements in Medicine & Biology, 26*(2–3), 124–126.

McNamara, C. L., & Marsil, D. F. (2012). The prevalence of stalking among college students: The disparity between researcher- and self-identified victimization. *Journal of American College Health, 60*(2), 168–174.

Montisci, M., El Mazloum, R., Cecchetto, G., et al. (2012). Anabolic androgenic steroids abuse and cardiac death in athletes: Morphological and toxicological findings in four fatal cases. *Forensic Science International, 217*(1–3), e13–e18.

Morelli, J. G., & Prok, L. D. (2012). Acne. In W. Hay, M. Levin, R. Deterding, et al. (Eds.), *Current diagnosis & treatment pediatrics* (21st ed., pp. 411–412). New York, NY: McGraw-Hill/Lange.

Moskowitz, A., Stein, J. A., & Lightfoot, M. (2012). The mediating roles of stress and maladaptive behaviors on self-harm and suicide attempts among runaway and homeless youth. *Journal of Youth & Adolescence.* Advance online publication.

Paczynski, R. P., & Gold, M. S. (2011). Cocaine and crack. In P. Ruiz & E. Strain (Eds.), *Lowinson and Ruiz's substance abuse: A comprehensive textbook* (5th ed., pp. 191–213). Philadelphia, PA: Wolters Kluwer/Lippincott Williams & Wilkins.

Palepu, A., Hubley, A. M., Russell, L. B., et al. (2012). Quality of life themes in Canadian adults and street youth who are homeless or hard-to-house: A multi-site focus group study. *Health & Quality of Life Outcomes, 10*(8), 93.

Piaget, J. (1969). *The theory of stages in cognitive development.* New York, NY: McGraw-Hill.

Rath, J. M., Villanti, A. C., Abrams, D. B., et al. (2012). Patterns of tobacco use and dual use in U.S. young adults: The missing link between youth prevention and adult cessation. *Journal of Environmental & Public Health.* Advance online publication. doi: 10.1155/2012/679134

Sánchez-Carracedo, D., Neumark-Sztainer, D., & López-Guimerà, G. (2012). Integrated prevention of obesity and eating disorders: Barriers, developments and opportunities. *Public Health Nutrition, 2012*(3), 1–15.

Sass, A. E., & Kaplan, D. W. (2013). Adolescence. In W. Hay, M. Levin, R. Deterding, et al. (Eds.), *Current diagnosis & treatment pediatrics* (21st ed., pp. 113–152). New York, NY: McGraw-Hill/Lange.

Shields, J. P., Whitaker, K., Glassman, J., et al. (2012). Impact of victimization on risk of suicide among lesbian, gay, and bisexual high school students in San Francisco. *Journal of Adolescent Health, 50*(4), 418–420.

Short, M. A., Gradisar, M., Lack, L. C., et al. (2012). A cross-cultural comparison of sleep duration between U.S. and Australian adolescents. *Health Education & Behavior.* Advance online publication.

Simonart, T. (2012). Newer approaches to the treatment of acne vulgaris. *American Journal of Clinical Dermatology, 13*(6), 357–364.

Stein, T., & Jordan, J. D. (2012). Health considerations for oral piercing and the policies that influence them. *Texas Dental Journal, 129*(7), 687–693.

Stoduto, G., Mann, R. E., Ialomiteanu, A., et al. (2012). Examining the link between collision involvement and cocaine use. *Drug & Alcohol Dependence, 123*(1–3), 260–263.

Swahn, M. H., Ali, B., Bossarte, R. M., et al. (2012). Self-harm and suicide attempts among high-risk, urban youth in the U.S.: Shared and unique risk and protective factors. *International Journal of Environmental Research & Public Health, 9*(1), 178–191.

Tanner, J. M. (1962). *Growth at adolescence* (2nd ed.). Oxford, UK: Blackwell.

Taylor, M., & Joshi, A. (2012). Surveys assessing STI related health information needs of adolescent population. *Technology &Health Care, 20*(4), 247–261.

Timko, C. A., Hormes, J. M., & Chubski, J. (2012). Will the real vegetarian please stand up? An investigation of dietary restraint and eating disorder symptoms in vegetarians versus non-vegetarians. *Appetite, 58*(3), 982–990.

U.S. Department of Health and Human Services. (2010). *Healthy people 2020*. Washington, DC: Author.

Wengle, J. G., Hamilton, J. K., Manlhiot, C., et al. (2012). The 'Golden Keys' to health—A healthy lifestyle intervention with randomized individual mentorship for overweight and obesity in adolescents. *Paediatric & Child Health, 6*(8), 473–478.

Whitney, E. N., & Rolfes, S. R. (2012). Life cycle nutrition: Infancy, childhood & adolescence. In E. N. Whitney & S. R. Rolfes (Eds.), *Understanding nutrition* (pp. 528–573). Belmont, CA: Wadsworth Publishing.

Widome, R., Brock, B., Noble, P., et al. (2013). The relationship of neighborhood demographic characteristics to point-of-scale tobacco advertising and marketing. *Ethnicity & Health, 18*(2), 136–151.

Young, A. M., Glover, N., & Havens, J. R. (2012). Nonmedical use of prescription medications among adolescents in the United States: A systematic review. *Journal of Adolescent Health, 51*(1), 6–17.

Zhang, J., Yan, F., Li, Y., et al. (2012). Body mass index and suicidal behaviors: A critical review of epidemiological evidence. *Journal of Affective Disorders*. Advance online publication.

Chapter 34

Child Health Assessment

KEY TERMS

- antitoxins
- audiogram
- auscultation
- bruit
- chief concern
- conjunctivitis
- deep tendon reflexes
- diaphragmatic excursion
- epispadias
- esotropia
- exotropia
- gamma globulin
- geographic tongue
- hordeolum
- hydrocele
- hypospadias
- inspection
- intelligence
- intercostal spaces
- kwashiorkor
- palpation
- percussion
- physiologic splitting
- point of maximum impulse
- ptosis
- retractions
- review of systems
- sinus arrhythmia
- strabismus
- temperament
- toxoid
- turgor
- varicocele

OBJECTIVES

After mastering the contents of this chapter, you should be able to:

1. Describe the purposes and techniques of health assessment in children of all ages.
2. Identify 2020 National Health Goals related to health assessment of children that nurses can help the nation achieve.
3. Assess a child and family by health interview, physical examination, and developmental screening.
4. Formulate nursing diagnoses based on health assessment findings.
5. Identify expected outcomes based on health assessment findings as well as help parents manage seamless transitions across differing health care settings.
6. Using the nursing process, plan nursing care that includes the six competencies of Quality & Safety Education for Nurses (QSEN): Patient-Centered Care, Teamwork & Collaboration, Evidence-Based Practice (EBP), Quality Improvement (QI), Safety, and Informatics.
7. Implement nursing care, such as conducting an age-appropriate health interview or physical examination by modifying techniques based on the child's age.
8. Evaluate expected outcomes for achievement and effectiveness of care.
9. Integrate knowledge of health assessment with the interplay of nursing process, the six competencies of QSEN, and Family Nursing to promote quality maternal and child health nursing care.

Keoto Wiser is a 13-year-old you meet in an ambulatory clinic. Her father has brought both her and her 2-year-old sister, Candy, for health assessment before Keoto begins seventh grade. He knows they both need an immunization update. Her father is worried Keoto doesn't see well because she always sits close to the television set. He's concerned that if glasses are prescribed, his daughter won't be able to play on her school's soccer team.

Previous chapters described the normal growth and development of children. This chapter adds information about techniques for assessing the health of children, including history taking; physical examination, related screening procedures for hearing, vision, and development; and recommended immunizations. This information builds a base for care and health teaching for differing age groups throughout childhood.

What questions would you want to ask Keoto? What screening tests for vision would be best for this 13-year-old? What could you do to help her adjust to wearing glasses if they are prescribed?

A nursing assessment is not only the first step in the nursing process but also the fundamental means by which health care personnel establish and maintain contact with children and their families throughout childhood. Child health assessment is especially important as an opportunity to provide families with information about health promotion, signs of health and illness, and expected developmental progress in children. This anticipatory guidance can have a long lasting and positive impact on the health of children and their families (Cameron, Rice, Sparkman, et al., 2013).

An effective assessment for the maternal–child population first requires you to be familiar with health maintenance standards and usual findings, because this knowledge is essential to the ability to recognize illness. Most health screening procedures are performed in ambulatory settings such as pediatric clinics, health care offices, community clinics, and schools, but they can be used to evaluate children in all settings, including during hospitalizations.

Sometimes it is necessary to complete just a partial history or a partial physical examination, such as when a child is referred for a vision examination. This chapter, however, covers all aspects of physical examination so that, when necessary, a complete examination can be performed. Assessment procedures specific to particular illnesses are discussed in later chapters with the illness they detect. Box 34.1 lists 2020 National Health Goals related to health assessment in children.

BOX 34.1 Nursing Care Planning Based on 2020 National Health Goals

A number of 2020 National Health Goals directly relate to health assessment of children:

- Developmental: Increase the proportion of children with a diagnosed condition identified through newborn screening who have an annual assessment of services needed and received.
- Increase the proportion of children and youth, 17 years of age and younger, who have a specific source of ongoing care from a baseline of 94.3% to a target of 100%.
- Increase the proportion of adolescents aged 12 to 19 years who have had a hearing examination in the past 5 years from a baseline of 79.3% to 87.2%.
- Increase the proportion of preschool children aged 5 years and under who receive vision screening from a baseline of 40.1% to a target of 44.1%.
- Achieve and maintain effective vaccination coverage levels for universally recommended vaccines among young children from baselines of 85% (DTaP), 94% (hepatitis B), 57% (*Haemophilus influenzae* type b), 94% (poliomyelitis), 91% (varicella), and 92% (MMR) to a target level of 90% (U.S. Department of Health and Human Services [DHHS], 2010; see www.healthypeople.gov).

Nurses can help the nation achieve these goals by actively participating in health assessment, including vision and hearing, and conscientiously screening for and administering vaccines.

Nursing Process Overview
For Health Assessment of the Child and Family

Assessment

Health assessment can be a positive, educational experience for the child and family if time is taken to listen carefully to the family's concerns and responses to questions. Never rush either an interview or a physical examination. Be sure children have time to familiarize themselves with the environment and the equipment that will be used. The recommendations for standard preventive child health care for the United States are available at http://thePoint.lww.com/Pillitteri7e.

Nursing Diagnosis

Nursing diagnoses related to health assessment most commonly speak to a health concern identified at the time of the assessment. When establishing nursing diagnoses, however, be certain not to overlook diagnoses that accentuate the healthy functioning of a child and family in addition to addressing any specific problems that have been identified. These wellness diagnoses are crucial components of the entire assessment picture. For instance, the nursing diagnosis of "Impaired social interaction related to lack of self-esteem secondary to disability" would be appropriate for a 4-year-old child who ambulates by wheelchair who, according to the parents, feels uncomfortable around other children. If the parents have difficulty adapting to their child's disability but are eager to accept advice from health care experts on how to provide the most stimulating environment for their child, the diagnosis "Readiness for enhanced family coping" would also be appropriate. Using both these diagnoses allows the development of a plan of care that takes advantage in the best way of this family's strengths.

Outcome Identification and Planning

Health promotion and illness prevention are vital parts of outcome identification following a health assessment. Helping parents plan for their child's next developmental stage or keeping them aware of important safety measures is also important. Remind parents about future immunizations that will be needed and be certain they know when to schedule the next health care visit. A current immunization schedule is always available at the Centers for Disease Control and Prevention (CDC) Web site (www.CDC.gov). Growth charts for children are available at both the CDC Web site (www.CDC.gov/growthcharts) and the World Health Organization (WHO) Web site (www.WHO.int/childgrowth).

Implementation

Health interviewing and physical examination both require a great deal of skill, skills that can only be perfected through practice. To perfect skills and judgment with children of different ages, take advantage of every opportunity by practicing interviewing and physical examination techniques with them.

Outcome Evaluation

Health assessment of children is an ongoing process that does not end when the first database is created. Because children change so much, data must be added at all future interactions so the database remains current and meaningful. Examples suggesting expected outcomes have been achieved include:

- After a health examination, parents state that they are satisfied with their child's motor development.
- After Snellen test, the child states that she is aware that her vision needs correction.
- The parents state they will continue to assess their child's growth by weighing the child weekly.

HEALTH HISTORY: ESTABLISHING A DATABASE

The assessment of a young child begins with an interview of the child's parents. An adolescent or preadolescent may choose to be interviewed without the parents present, although many preadolescents and adolescents still prefer to have a parent with them for support.

The purpose of a health interview is to gather information that will direct physical or laboratory examinations to complete a thorough health evaluation. An extensive interview not only elicits facts such as parental problems in childrearing or detection of future health problems, but also lays a foundation for health education and health promotion. Important principles of child health interviewing include establishing a conducive interview setting, formulating the right types of questions to ask, and organizing the information collected.

Interview Setting

An interview is best conducted in a private room with all parties seated comfortably (Fig. 34.1); if not seated, a health care provider can appear rushed and is also unable to interact at eye level. During the interview, be certain to call the parents by their names. This lets them know that their input and opinions about how their child is developing are valued. A question such as, "Does Candy speak in sentences yet, Mr. Wiser?" is far more personal and a better form than, "Does baby sit up yet?" As children grow, they are able to answer questions themselves.

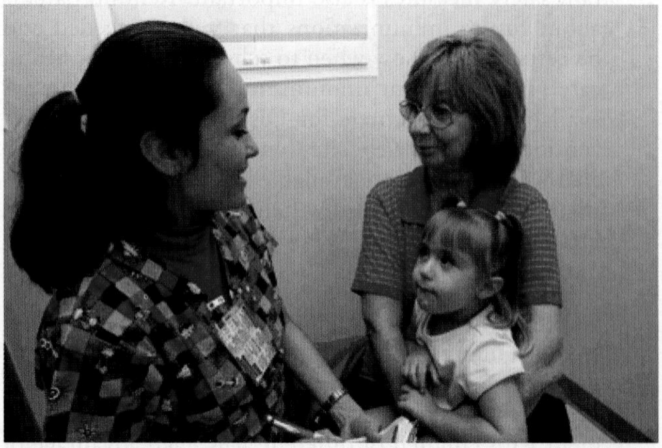

FIGURE 34.1 Maintaining good eye contact and allowing children to play as active a part as possible in the assessment process are important for good health interviewing.

Types of Questions Asked

The phrasing of questions varies depending on the type of answer desired. Closed-ended and open-ended questions are two types of effective questions; compound, expansive, and leading questions, in contrast, are three types of questions to avoid.

Closed-Ended Questions

This simplest form of question directly asks for a fact, such as, "Did you take Candy's temperature?" This is an effective type of question if a particular point is being sought. It is limited in scope, however, because the response usually will be a "yes" or a "no," with no further elaboration.

Open-Ended Questions

An open-ended question allows for elaboration. In contrast to the closed-ended question, "What did you do for Candy?" is open ended. The parent will answer with a list of all the things he did, such as, he took Candy's temperature, had her lie on the couch, gave her extra fluid, and so on. It is important to ask open-ended questions with school-age children and adolescents so they are encouraged to fully describe a problem (Box 34.2).

Compound Questions

Compound questions should be avoided if all possible because the information they elicit is often inaccurate and must be followed by a clarifying question. An example is, "Did Candy have nausea and vomiting?" The parent answers "yes," but it remains unknown whether Candy had vomiting and nausea, just vomiting, or just nausea because the question included multiple possibilities.

Expansive Questions

Expansive questions are open-ended questions gone wrong because the question being asked is too vague to answer. "What can you tell me about Candy?" leaves a parent wondering where to start. "How has Candy been since her last visit?" limits the question and makes it answerable.

Leading Questions

Leading questions supply their own answers and so they should also be avoided. "Candy has had all her immunizations, hasn't she?" implies that Candy should have had them and perhaps implies that the parent is a poor caregiver if he responds with anything other than "yes." The result of such an exchange could be a child left vulnerable to disease.

BOX 34.2 Nursing Care Planning Based on Effective Communication

A second reason Keoto's father has brought her to your ambulatory clinic is because she has noticed frequency and burning on urination.

Less Effective Communication

Nurse: Hello, Keoto. What's the reason you've come into clinic today?
Mr. Wiser: It hurts when she urinates.
Nurse: When did she first notice that?
Mr. Wiser: She started complaining about it this morning.
Nurse: Has she had any blood in her urine?
Mr. Wiser: She hasn't said anything about that. The important thing is the pain.
Nurse: Okay. I'm sure we'll need a urine specimen for culture. Let's get that started.

More Effective Communication

Nurse: Hello, Keoto. What's the reason you've come into clinic today?
Mr. Wiser: It hurts when she urinates.
Nurse: Let's let Keoto answer for herself, Mr. Wiser. Tell me what you think is the problem, Keoto.
Keoto: It hurts when I go to the bathroom.
Nurse: When did you first notice that?
Mr. Wiser: She started complaining about it yesterday.
Nurse: Keoto, when do *you* think it started?
Keoto: About an hour after I came in from my date last night.
Nurse: Have you had any blood in your urine?
Mr. Wiser: She hasn't said anything about that.
Nurse: Keoto, have you noticed your urine is red or dark brown?
Keoto: I had bright blood last night.
Nurse: Let me take you down to the lavatory and explain about a urine specimen. While we're there, I'd like to ask you some more questions about last night.

At about 10 years of age, children are able to supply much of a health history by themselves. As children become teenagers, it is increasingly important for them to do this because they may not have shared a total history with a parent. In this scenario, for example, when the child is asked directly for information, she supplied more than when her history was given by the father. Some urinary tract infections occur in girls after their first sexual relations. It would be important to ask Keoto if she is sexually active (what her "date" last night included), not only to document the probable cause of the urinary tract infection but also to be certain she is knowledgeable about pregnancy prevention and safer sex practices.

Contents of a Health Interview

Data gathering for an initial health assessment can be divided into nine sections:

1. Introduction and explanation
2. Demographic data
3. Chief concern
4. History of chief concern
5. Health and family profile
6. Day history
7. Past health history, including pregnancy history
8. Family health history
9. Review of systems

At return visits, the categories used generally include only introduction and explanation, chief concern, health and family profile, interval history, and day history.

Using Transition Statements

While conducting a health interview, be certain to make a transition statement before shifting from one section of an interview to another because, without a transition, a parent can possibly misinterpret a question's significance. For instance, if a parent has been providing information on the family's hospital insurance policy and, without a transition, is asked whether the child has been vomiting, a parent may think the interviewer believes the child needs hospitalization when that is not the intent at all. A statement such as, "Before we talk about Keoto's current symptoms, let me ask you some general questions about your family so I can get to know you better," is an example of a good transition statement.

Introductions and Explanations

As a matter of courtesy, you should introduce yourself to parents and children and introduce what topics you will be discussing. "Hello, Mr. Wiser, I'm Janet Dickson, a nurse here in the One-Day Surgery Department. I'd like to ask you some questions about Candy" is an example of a suitable introduction. Because some families have never had the benefit of in-depth health care, it is also helpful to include a statement about the subjects that will be discussed during the interview. For example, "So that I can get a picture of Candy's overall health, I'd like to ask you questions about not just why you've brought her here today, but her birth history, and any past concerns you've had," would be appropriate. Hearing that, parents begin to concentrate on those areas because they realize health care providers in this setting are interested not just in Candy's health on this particular day, but in her total health.

Demographic Data

Demographic data refers to data such as a child's name, address, gender, social security number, and the name of the person who will be providing information. To provide culturally competent care and make provisions for special needs, a child's culture, ethnicity, place of birth, religious or spiritual practices, and primary and secondary language should also be identified (Box 34.3).

Be certain to identify the child's primary caregiver. If the parents are divorced or deceased, it is especially important to identify who has custody of the child or who has the right to sign a consent for health care treatment.

Chief Concerns

The first topic parents want to talk about is the reason they have brought their child to the health care agency on this day, or the **chief concern**. An effective way to elicit this information is to ask directly, "Why did you bring Candy to the clinic today, Mr. Wiser?" Such an opening allows the parent freedom to answer in a number of areas of concern: physical, emotional, nutritional, or developmental. If asked, "How is Candy feeling today?" or "Is Candy ill?" a parent is left to think about only physical aspects and may not voice the biggest concern: Candy's teething difficulty or frequent temper tantrums. Record the chief concern in the child's electronic record exactly as it is stated ("She has constant headaches," not, "Headache") because the parent's description often not only reveals information about a disease condition but the depth of the parent's concern about the symptom (Levine, 2011).

BOX 34.3 Nursing Care Planning to Respect Cultural Diversity

Health assessment findings in children differ depending on racial and ethnic characteristics. Whether people establish eye contact with an interviewer, for example, is a characteristic that is culturally determined. Assessing for cyanosis, as another example, is more difficult in dark-skinned than in fair-skinned children (the mucous membrane is the best place to detect this). Because height and weight charts are standardized on middle-class Caucasian children, measurements of children who do not fit this description may not plot well on these charts. In Vietnam, touching the head of a child during a physical assessment is thought to be harmful because the head is considered to be the seat of the soul.

Recognizing that people hold differing cultural expectations and characteristics such as these can help in establishing rapport with children and their families and can help make health assessment more thorough and meaningful.

Some cultures are much more aware of the danger of communicable diseases in childhood than others and so advocate for all children to be immunized against these disorders. Even if awareness about the danger of disease spreading exists, however, it does not mean all people in a community are conscientious about having their children immunized. Other factors, such as cost and convenience, religious beliefs, and safety concerns, are also important.

The Amish are an example of a group who do not encourage immunization. Being aware immunization rates are not consistent from place to place aids in understanding the importance of planning health education and health surveillance based on findings gained from health assessment.

History of Chief Concerns

Once a parent has voiced a chief concern, ask him or her to describe at least six aspects of the problem, including:

1. Duration
2. Intensity
3. Frequency
4. Description
5. Associated symptoms
6. Actions taken

Duration refers to the length of time a specific symptom such as vomiting or the parent's concern about the child's symptom has been present. The intensity, in this example, refers to the kind of vomiting the child is having (e.g., drooling, spitting up, actual vomiting). The description is the amount (e.g., a cupful, a mouthful) and color (e.g., whether it contains blood, bile, mucus). Associated symptoms might include fever, abdominal pain, difficulty eating, or signs of respiratory illness. A good question to use to obtain associated symptoms is, "Is Candy ill in any other way?"

Knowing the parent's actions helps to establish ineffective actions or whether anything a parent has been doing, such as offering a great deal of fluid to replace that which was vomited, has actually made the illness worse. This information also reveals the parent's response to caring for an ill child. The parent who says, "I tucked her into bed and gave her a little tea to drink" is different from one who replies, "Nothing. I fall apart when my child is ill." If the child is going to return home under the parents' care, the parents in the second example need more instructions and support before they leave the health care setting than the first parents.

During this phase of the interview, it is also important to gather information to see if a parent has other related or additional health concerns. "Is there anything else that worries you about Candy?" is a good way to elicit this information. Unless asked about a second concern this way (e.g., the parent is also concerned about frequent temper tantrums; as soon as he arrives home and he knows Candy will begin stomping her feet in the car, unwilling to go into the house), the parent will feel that the health care Candy received was less than adequate because he did not receive help with this concern.

Do not assume parents will always reveal their most important concern in the initial minute of an interview; discussing certain symptoms such as constipation can be embarrassing for parents. It also can be frightening to put a fear that their child has a serious illness into words. As long as a concern hangs as a nebulous thought in the mind, it is easy to tell oneself it may not be true. Only when a parent voices the thought ("Do you think Candy is mentally handicapped?" "Do you think this is leukemia?" "Could this be inherited?") does the fear become real. Before parents dare to speak openly this way, they must trust health care providers not to treat their statement lightly. For this reason, it is helpful to repeat the question about a second concern once more at the very end of the interview to be certain other concerns were not missed.

Health and Family Profiles

A family profile includes documentation of the circumstances in which the child lives. A good introduction to a health and family profile is a sentence such as, "Before we talk about any past illnesses or happenings with Candy, let me ask you some questions about your family as a whole."

Important information concerning the family includes:

- Is the parent married, single, or divorced?
- What is the family type (e.g., nuclear, extended, blended)?
- How many children are in the family?
- What are the family's living arrangements?
- What are the parents' occupations? (This helps establish the family's socioeconomic level and time available for child care.)
- If both parents work outside the home, how do they manage child care?

Obtaining a family profile is sometimes delayed by medical interviewers until the end of the interview, when, theoretically, a parent or child is more comfortable and will answer these personal questions more readily. However, by following a nursing model and obtaining the information earlier in the interview, you can better assess the child and evaluate data.

Day Histories

The child's current skills, sleep patterns, hygiene practices, eating habits, and interactions with the family can all be elicited by asking a parent to describe a typical day. Day histories are fun to obtain because most parents are eager to describe their day with their child and information gained this way is surprisingly rich and pertinent, much more so than if parents are just asked how their child sleeps, eats, or plays.

Begin by asking, "Was yesterday a fairly typical day?" (The parent says yes, it was.) "Describe for me everything Candy did yesterday, beginning with when she first woke up." Some parents offer this information in great detail; with others, it is necessary to backtrack for particular details, such as, "What did she eat for breakfast? Does she use a fork and spoon? Does she sit in a high chair or on your lap?"

Play. Play is the work of children and so reveals a great deal about a child's development and overall well-being. Important questions to ask about play include:

- Is the child kept in a playpen or given room to run?
- What is the child's favorite toy?
- Does she play active, chasing games or engage in quiet, pretending types of activities?
- Do you (the parent) read to the child?
- Do you (the parent) play with the child or let the child play alone? (This allows for an estimation of the quality of interaction during the day.)

Sleep. Every child needs adequate rest for healthy growth and development. Poor sleep patterns can often reveal a psychosocial or physical health problem. Important questions regarding sleep include:

- How long does the child sleep at night?
- How long does she nap (if appropriate for age)?
- Is falling asleep a problem?
- Where does she sleep? Does she have night terrors?
- Does she sleepwalk?
- Does she wet her bed (if the child is toilet trained)?

Hygiene. Good hygiene practices promote healthy teeth, gums, and skin; prevent infections; and improve self-esteem. Poor hygiene may reflect neglect, depression, substance abuse, or inability of the household to have hot water. Important questions regarding hygiene include:

- How much self-care does the child do?
- Can the child shower or bathe independently?
- Does the child brush her teeth? How often? Does she floss regularly? (Responses depend on the age of the child.)
- Does the child wash her hands before snacks and meals?
- Has there been a recent change in hygiene practices?

Nutrition. Nutritional assessment is an important portion of a health assessment because it strongly influences health (Whitney & Rolfes, 2012). Characteristics of a nutritionally healthy child that can be revealed by assessment are summarized in Table 34.1. Food and nutrient intake risk factors are summarized in Box 34.4.

Taking a history of a child's food intake can help determine whether there are any foods missing in a typical meal plan or if any quantities seem inadequate or excessive. Be certain to assess not only the quantity of food taken but also the quality; for example, for an infant, cereal should be iron fortified.

Food intake is best obtained by including this as part of a typical day (24-hour recall) history, listing what the child ate for

TABLE 34.1 Physical Signs of Adequate Nutrition

Assessment	Finding
Overall impression	Alert, with good energy level; positive mood
Hair	Shiny, strong, with good body
Eyes	Good eyesight, particularly at night; conjunctiva moist and not pale
Mouth	No cavities in teeth; no swollen or inflamed gingivae; no cracks or fissures at corners of mouth; mucous membrane moist and pink; tongue smooth and nontender
Neck	Normal contour of thyroid gland
Skin	Smooth; normal color and turgor; no ecchymotic or petechial areas present
Extremities	Normal muscle mass and circumference; normal strength and mobility; normal reflexes; legs not bowed; no tender joints or edema present
Gastrointestinal	No diarrhea or constipation present
Finger and toenails	Smooth, pink; not cracked or broken
Height and weight	Within normal limits on growth chart and body mass index (BMI)
Blood pressure	Normal for age

BOX 34.4 Food and Nutrient Intake Risk Factors

History or evidence of any of the following may pose a potential nutritional risk:

- Intake less or greater than standard for age, for calories, protein, vitamins, or minerals
- Unusual food habits, such as pica, faddism, and meal skipping
- Inappropriate use of supplements (excessive vitamins, minerals, fortified food products)
- A health care provider's prescription for nothing by mouth (NPO) or a clear liquid diet for more than 3 days without enteral or parenteral nutrition
- Minimal or no intake from a major food group
- Fluid intake less than output
- Eating disorders such as bulimia
- Food allergies
- Restricted diet, such as a restricted potassium diet for kidney disease

each meal and between meals as well. With an older child, the 24-hour recall can be a joint parent–child venture. Providing this history can be difficult for parents if the child consumes some meals at home and others at day care or school. It may be necessary to ask for a weekend history to get a complete picture.

When assessing an adolescent, take a 24-hour recall nutritional history without a parent present, if possible. In front of a parent, adolescents may add nutritional foods to a food intake history or leave out foods they have eaten such as milkshakes, potato chips, or pizza to avoid a lecture later; however, they may also leave out healthy items or add less desirable ones because they may enjoy the obvious parental disapproval, indicative of their rebellion against adult authority.

After taking a history of a child's food intake, determine whether the child is receiving foods that comply with the MyPlate recommendations (U.S. Department of Agriculture [USDA], 2012; www.ChooseMyPlate.gov). If whole food groups are absent or grossly inadequate, a follow-up evaluation should include a food frequency record as a verification to see if the 24-hour recall was truly representative of a usual day. Remember, children do not have to eat food from all groups at every meal as long as they eat from them every day. If parents think in terms of days rather than meals, it allows them to exert less pressure regarding what the child eats at each meal.

Be certain to consider the role of food preferences and cultural, lifestyle, religious, and financial variations when assessing food intake as well as the number of meals eaten at home versus outside the home, how traditional meals are cooked, and the pattern of meals. Do not appear critical of a child's diet as you record a history. If you convey dismay at erratic eating habits, parents or older children (especially adolescents) may begin to fabricate a food history to make it seem more acceptable to you.

Past Health Histories

For a past health history, ask whether a child has ever had any serious illnesses. Parents do not generally think of childhood diseases such as measles, chickenpox, and mumps as serious illnesses; inquire about these separately. Also inquire about the child's immunization history and whether immunizations are up to date for the child's age (see the discussion of immunizations later in this chapter.) Has a child had any accidents (unintentional injuries)? Any surgery? Parents may not think of a tonsillectomy as surgery because there were no stitches; ask about that separately. Did a child ever ingest anything that was inedible or harmful? Has a child been hospitalized for any reason? How many times has a child been seen in an emergency room? These last questions provide information about the degree of adult supervision, and possibly clues to maltreatment (Wood, Pecker, Russo, et al., 2012).

Information about the outcomes of past illnesses is as important to obtain as information about the illnesses themselves. If the child had otitis media (i.e., middle ear infection) at age 2 years and recovered without complications, the parent has every reason to be confident the child will also get better from a present illness because there is confidence in health care personnel. If the child was left with a hearing difficulty from the previous illness, parents may not be as trustful of the care being given to their child now; they may need extra support to follow instructions. This is important information to gain before planning care.

QSEN Checkpoint Question 34.1

Evidence-Based Practice

To investigate what poisons young children typically ingest, researchers studied the records of children under 6 years of age who were seen at a major children's hospital. Among 928 poisonings, 41% were found to be from household products; 20% from over-the-counter drugs; 7% from prescription narcotics/sedatives; 29% from other prescription drugs; and about 1% each from alcohol, illicit drugs, or other substances (Wood et al., 2012).

Based on the previous study, which would be the most important question to ask Candy's father?

a. "Has Candy tried to drink something that you're drinking?"
b. "Do you keep all your prescription drugs securely locked?"
c. "What do you keep in the cupboards below your sinks?"
d. "Where do you store the alcoholic beverages in your house?"

Look in Appendix A for the best answer and rationale.

Pregnancy Histories

The health of children is affected by their mother's health during pregnancy. For children under 5 years of age, therefore, a pregnancy history is usually obtained. Document which pregnancy this was for the mother. Were there complications in any of her pregnancies? Induced abortions or miscarriages? Stillbirths? Children born prematurely?

A history of the pregnancy of the child being assessed can begin with a question such as, "How was your pregnancy with Candy?" This allows the mother to answer in both physical and emotional areas. After exploring details mentioned by the mother, ask about specific events that are known to occur with pregnancy that may have had an effect on a fetus, such as:

- Did the mother have any complications such as bleeding, falls, swelling of hands and feet, high blood pressure, or unusual weight gain?

- Did she take any medication?
- Were any X-ray films or sonograms taken other than a routine one to date the pregnancy?
- Did she smoke cigarettes, drink alcohol, or use recreational drugs while she was pregnant?
- Did the pregnancy end early or late?

Because life contingencies such as loss of finances or illness in the family during a pregnancy may affect a parent's ability to form a bond with a child, the emotional experiences of a woman during pregnancy are also important to obtain. Ask if the pregnancy was intentional. A question such as, "A lot of pregnancies come as a sort of surprise. Is that how it was with Candy?" or "Some women want to have children and some don't. How was it with you?" lets parents know you will nonjudgmentally accept any answer they give.

Next, review the labor and birth by including such questions as:

- How long was labor? Was it what you expected it to be?
- Were there any complications? Was the birth vaginal or cesarean?
- Was anesthesia used for birth?
- Was the baby born vertex (i.e., head first) or breech?

Then ask about the health of the child immediately after birth, including:

- Did the baby cry right away?
- Did the infant room in or need care in a special nursery?
- Did the infant need special procedures or equipment?
- Was there cyanosis or jaundice?
- Was the infant discharged from the birth setting with the mother?
- How did the parents feel about having a boy or a girl?
- How did it feel for them to be new parents?

Family Health Histories

Because some diseases are inherited or familial, it is important to know which ones tend to occur in a family. Ask if any family member has a condition, such as cardiac disease (childhood or adult type), kidney disease, congenital anomalies, seizures, diabetes (type 1 or 2), tuberculosis, a sexually transmitted infection, allergies, or is cognitively challenged.

Review of Systems

The last step in a health interview is a summary of body symptoms or a **review of systems**. Once more, make certain to introduce this part of the history with a transition statement. Otherwise, parents may think the local problem they were describing (e.g., vomiting) has spread to other body systems. A statement, such as, "I'd like to ask about different parts of Candy's body, from her head down to her toes, just to be certain I didn't miss anything" provides such a transition.

Although the important items to be covered in a review of systems differ according to the age of the child, a basic list is shown in Box 34.5.

A review of systems covers a lot of ground, but it generally takes no more than 5 minutes. However, do not rush through the questions so quickly that a parent does not have time to answer or begins to believe this part of the interview is only an unimportant exercise ("Has Candy ever had nausea/vomiting/diarrhea/painful joints/broken bones?") Each question is important. If a child has any of the symptoms described, an entirely new area of the child's health needs to be explored.

BOX 34.5 Review of Systems

The following questions provide a guide when completing a review of systems:

Overall health: What is the general state of health? Is the child taking any prescription medications? Over-the-counter medications? Home or folk remedies, such as herbal remedies?

Neuropsychiatric symptoms: Has the child ever had a head injury? Seizures? Attention problems? Depression? Aggressive behavior? Has the parent ever had such difficulty rousing the child that the parent believed the child was unconscious? Is there any concern about suspected substance abuse?

Eyes: Has the child ever had difficulty with eyes not focusing? Eye infection? Does the parent have any reason to believe the child does not see well? Does the child wear eyeglasses or contact lenses?

Ears: Ear infections? Drainage from the ears? Ear aches? Tubes in ears? Any infection from piercing? Reason to believe the child does not hear well?

Nose: Frequent drainage or cold symptoms? Difficulty breathing? Nosebleeds?

Mouth: Difficulty with teeth or teething? Mouth infections? Has the child seen a dentist (if older than 2 years of age)? Does the child chew tobacco?

Throat: Throat infections? Difficulty swallowing?

Neck: Masses or swelling? Stiffness? Does the child hold the head and neck straight? (Torticollis or wry neck will make a child hold the head crookedly; children with poor vision also may cock their heads to the side to try to see better.)

Chest: Is breast development in girls appropriate for age? Any pain in breasts?

Lungs: Breathing problems? Infections? Pneumonia? Asthma? Does the child smoke any substance?

Heart: Has a health care provider ever said there was difficulty? What exactly was said?

Gastrointestinal system: Has there been an eating problem? Frequent nausea? Vomiting? Diarrhea? Constipation? Is the child toilet trained? Any difficulty with this?

Genitourinary system: Pain or burning on urination? Blood in urine? Does the child have a good urine stream? If a girl is age 10 years or older, has she started menstruation? Any concerns with menstruation? If an adolescent male, has he begun testicular self-examination? If an adolescent, is the child sexually active? Knows safer sex practices? Uses contraception? Wants more information on contraception? Ever had a sexually transmitted infection (STI)? (To protect privacy, it is essential to ask the adolescent, not the parents, questions regarding sexuality.)

Extremities: Painful or swollen joints? Broken bones? Muscle sprains? Is the parent pleased with the child's coordination?

Skin: Rashes? Lesions such as warts?

Immunizations: What immunizations has the child received to date? Are they up to date?

Conclusion

A health history should close with one last open-ended question: "Is there anything more about Candy we should know?" or "Is there anything I didn't mention you want to ask about?" A parent may have been reluctant to bring up something earlier. Asking this final question gives a parent a final opportunity to reveal a concern.

QSEN Checkpoint Question 34.2

Quality Improvement

With the participation of her father, you obtain a health history from Keoto. What question should you ask at the end of this and every interview?

a. "Where do you think we should go from here?"
b. "Is there anything else you'd like to discuss?"
c. "Are you still feeling okay?"
d. "Am I a good interviewer? I'm trying hard."

Look in Appendix A for the best answer and rationale.

PHYSICAL ASSESSMENT

Mastery of physical examination technique is essential to incorporating physical assessment data into the assessment step of the nursing process, so a physical assessment, along with health interviewing, is one of the most frequently practiced skills of a nurse. The scope and extent of a pediatric physical assessment will vary, like health interviewing, depending on the circumstances of each health contact. At a first health care encounter, for example, children usually receive a complete physical examination. Later on, only a single focus may be required to obtain the information needed. If a child has a gastrointestinal disorder, for example, an assessment might be only a brief, multisystem examination followed by concentration on the gastrointestinal system (i.e., mouth, abdomen, rectum, fluid status).

Purpose and Techniques

The actual process of a physical examination involves four separate techniques:

1. **Inspection**
2. **Palpation**
3. **Percussion**
4. **Auscultation**

These techniques are usually carried out in the listed order in each area of the body except the abdomen (auscultation should follow inspection and precede palpation of the abdomen because handling the abdomen may obliterate bowel sounds). The findings from these techniques strengthen or validate history findings and help determine whether a concern requires immediate action (Box 34.6).

Effective use of physical assessment skills takes practice. Palpating an abdomen, for example, is a simple procedure; recognizing abdominal pathology through palpation is a more complicated skill. It is difficult to distinguish between normal liver tissue and a distended liver, for example, until both these conditions have been felt many times.

BOX 34.6 Techniques of Physical Examination

Inspection: Examining a child or adolescent initially with your eyes or nose, and being alert to visual indications or odors that may point to a health problem.

Palpation: Examining by touch, either light or deep. Use light palpation before deep palpation so the child or adolescent does not tense muscles and make light palpation difficult. The tips of your fingers are most sensitive to texture, vibration, consistency, and contour; the back of your hand is most sensitive to warmth. *If a child has a sensitive or painful body part, palpate that area last.* Otherwise, the child may be unwilling to allow you to touch other parts for fear of additional pain.

Percussion: The assessment of a body structure by determining the sound you hear in response to striking the part with an examining finger and then interpreting the sound. Dense body areas such as bone have a dull, flat sound; those filled with air, such as lungs, are resonant. If an organ is stretched (e.g., a distended bladder), it has a hyperresonant or low and hollow sound. An organ stretched to an even greater point of distention has a tympanic or extremely hollow, ringing sound.

Auscultation: Listening to sounds that are either discernible to the ear (e.g., wheezing or heavy breathing) or, as in most instances, made louder by means of a stethoscope. Always listen for four qualities of sound: duration, frequency, intensity (i.e., loudness), and pitch (i.e., high or low).

Equipment, Setting, and Approach

When performing a complete physical assessment, you'll need the following equipment: a thermometer, a stethoscope, a tongue depressor, an ophthalmoscope, an otoscope, a sphygmomanometer, a tape measure, a tuning fork, a reflex (percussion) hammer, examination gloves, and perhaps a client drape or gown. Nurses who work in community settings or clients' homes must be sure to carry with them any equipment that may be needed.

Be certain to provide privacy and that the temperature in an examining room is comfortable. Change paper table covers between children to avoid possible spread of illness.

During a complete physical examination, every part of the child's body should be exposed for inspection. To protect against chilling and to provide for modesty, expose body parts individually and only for the amount of time necessary for the examination. Because examining body parts such as the mouth or an open lesion exposes your hands to body fluids, as part of infection control precautions, wear gloves as appropriate during an examination.

People have the right not to have another person touch their body unless they permit them to do so. It is essential, therefore, to inform children that it is necessary to touch them for a physical examination, and tell them what is happening at each step during the examination so they know when they will be touched. For instance, say, "Next I want to look at your throat" to prevent surprises. If some action will cause discomfort, such as deep palpation of the abdomen, offer fair warning, such as, "You'll feel pressure for a minute."

Assume that adolescents will cooperate in placing themselves in whatever position is required to inspect body parts unless they are short of breath or in some other way unable to cooperate. Small children may not cooperate readily and so may need to be restrained during an examination of such body parts as the nose, throat, and ears. Proper restraint enables an examiner to see well and also to ensure an instrument such as an otoscope will not accidentally cause injury. As a rule, do not ask parents to restrain during any procedure in which the child will feel threatened or feel pain; parents are best used as protectors and comforters after the procedure. If a parent does volunteer to restrain a child, urge them to do this with a positive approach such as, "I'll help you keep your head still."

Variations for Age and Developmental Stage

Techniques of physical examination need to be tailored to the age and developmental stage of the individual child being assessed. Expected findings also depend on the child's age and developmental stage.

The Newborn

All newborns receive a physical examination immediately after birth and again after the first 24 hours of life. When examining newborns, cover body areas that are not being directly examined or perform the exam under a radiant heat warmer because maintaining body temperature is difficult for the newborn (Sargant, Sen, & Marden, 2012). Take axillary or tympanic temperatures to prevent rupture of rectal mucosa. Assess the heart rate apically because peripheral pulses may be too faint to be counted accurately. Be certain to obtain femoral pulses in newborns to rule out coarctation of the aorta. Include newborn reflexes, head circumference, and an assessment of gestational age (see Chapter 18) as routine parts of the examination. Taking blood pressure is not necessary because this value is unreliable in newborns. If possible, examine newborns with the parents present and use this assessment time to teach them about normal appearance and development.

The Infant

Infants are usually examined most effectively if a parent holds them during most of the examination. Use an "isn't this fun?" or "this is a game" approach with the infant. As a rule, assess heart and lung function first; do intrusive procedures such as ear and throat assessment last so an infant does not cry and complicate the remainder of the examination. Blood pressure is still not taken routinely. Include assessment of newborn reflexes until 6 months of age; continue to take the heart rate apically and the temperature in the axilla or by tympanic membrane. Measure head circumference for a full year.

Toward the end of the first year, children become fearful of strangers. Taking an extra minute to become well acquainted with an infant at the beginning of an examination can help to counteract this problem. Remember, infants calm to the tone of your voice as much as they do to what you actually say. They can be distracted by brightly colored toys while you listen to their heart or lungs. Offering a bottle of water or pacifier may be necessary during a heart assessment.

The Toddler and Preschooler

Ask parents to remove clothing or allow a toddler or preschooler to do this independently so it is less threatening. Children this age may be very afraid of examining equipment. To alleviate their fears, let them handle items such as stethoscopes, otoscopes, and blood pressure cuffs before the examination (Fig. 34.2). Leave intrusive procedures such as assessment of the genitalia, ears, and throat until last. Give generous praise for cooperation (anything short of hysterical screaming or kicking is good cooperation for intrusive procedures in this age group). Box 34.7 describes ways parents can prepare children of this age for assessment.

Begin to include blood pressure as part of routine assessment at 3 years of age; taking an oral temperature by an electronic thermometer, rather than a tympanic temperature, can also begin at this age. Children up to school age often need to be restrained for ear and throat examinations because they grow fearful about procedures performed on a part of the body they cannot see (e.g., ears) or about a throat examination that may be uncomfortable. Before beginning an examination, establish a good rapport with the child's parents, because children this age sense parental trust or suspicion.

The School-Age Child and Adolescent

Some children of this age may still be unaware of what a physical examination includes and whether it will cause discomfort. Offer good explanations so they are not frightened by the unknown. Provide older children with a choice about having a parent with them during the examination. Comment on body parts as you examine them to teach about good health such as, "Your heart sounds good. And your ears look fine." Sometimes adolescents are so concerned with a part of their body (e.g., a supernumerary nipple) that they are unable to voice this concern. A comment such as, "This is a supernumerary (extra) nipple. Does it ever worry you that you have that?" may help an adolescent or young adult talk about what has indeed been a concern for years. Use a head-to-toe procedure; leave genitalia for last. Be certain to assess height and weight because more children in this age group are obese than ever before.

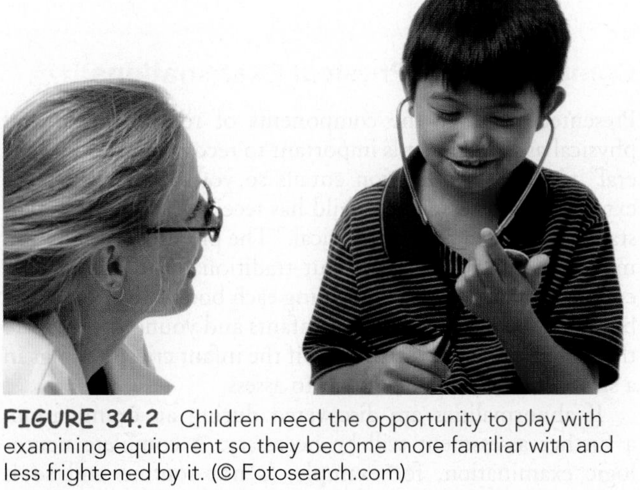

FIGURE 34.2 Children need the opportunity to play with examining equipment so they become more familiar with and less frightened by it. (© Fotosearch.com)

BOX 34.7 Nursing Care Planning to Empower a Family

SUGGESTIONS FOR PREPARING A CHILD FOR A HEALTH ASSESSMENT

Q. Candy's father asks you, "How can I best prepare my 2-year-old for a preschool health exam?"
A. Here are some suggestions to help prepare a child for a health assessment:

- Promote the attitude that a health visit will be a positive experience.
- Bring a comfort item from home (e.g., a favorite doll or toy).
- Never threaten the child that if she is not good, a health care provider will punish her.
- Review with your daughter what she can expect during an assessment, such as a health care provider will ask questions of her parent; she or he will then look at the child's head, hands, etc.
- If she has been taught not to let strangers touch her body (as she should have been taught), reassure her it is all right for the health care provider to examine her.
- Dress your daughter in clothing that is easy to remove and replace so you can dress her quickly after an examination to rapidly assure her that the examination is over.

It is increasingly important to take blood pressure beginning in early school age also because, as more children are overweight, more have elevated blood pressure (Riley & Bluhm, 2012). Because obesity in school-age children and adolescents is also associated with the development of type 2 diabetes mellitus and future cardiovascular disorders (Rendall, Weden, Fernandes, et al., 2012), as well as an association between overweight and self-harm (Heneghan, Heinberg, Windover, et al., 2012), signs of these need to be assessed as well. School-age children and adolescents are particularly modest. Respect this by careful use of gowns or drapes. Include a breast exam for adolescent girls and teach testicular self-examination for boys beginning at about age 13 years.

QSEN Checkpoint Question 34.3

Patient-Centered Care

Keoto's sister is 2 years old and appears fearful of medical equipment. To preserve her comfort, you can exclude blood pressure measurement from your assessment until what age?

a. 2.5 years
b. 3 years
c. 5 years
d. 7 years

Look in Appendix A for the best answer and rationale.

Components of Physical Examinations

Presented here are the components of routine or general physical assessment. It is important to recognize what a "general" physical examination entails so you can interpret the extent of the assessment a child has received when the parent states, "He had a routine physical." The physical examination may be done in any order, but traditionally the order proceeds from head to toe, examining each body part thoroughly before moving on to the next. Infants and young children are the exception, however, because if the infant cries, findings in a specific area become difficult to assess.

If abnormalities are discovered during an examination, a further assessment will be necessary. A complete neurologic examination, for example, is not routine and so is not included here (see Chapter 49 for details of a complete neurologic examination).

Vital Signs Assessment

Vital signs refer to temperature, pulse, respiration, blood pressure, and whether the child has pain (i.e., the state of vital bodily functions including heart and lung function, metabolic rate, and comfort level). Temperature is an important assessment in children because it can reveal a subtle infection that has not as yet become obvious by other signs. Because of the important information these provide, measurements of vital signs are recorded not only with complete physical examinations but in many other instances of care. Techniques of these measurements and the nursing responsibilities that accompany them are discussed in Chapter 37. Remember, blood pressure in children can be elevated if they are anxious in a medical setting, the same as happens to adults and so needs to be evaluated in light of that (Flynn, Zhang, Solar-Yohay, et al., 2012).

General Appearance

General appearance establishes an overall impression of a child's health as well as reveals specific body areas that will need a detailed assessment (Fig. 34.3 and Box 34.8). Be certain to include such areas as:

- Does the child appear well or ill overall?
- Is the child's height and weight proportional?
- Does the child appear well nourished? Appear underweight or overweight?
- What is the child's color? Pale? Yellow (jaundiced)? Cyanotic (blue)?
- Is posture normal? (Children who are in pain often assume an abnormal posture for relief.)
- What is the child's hygiene level? (Fatigue or illness can cause poor hygiene.)
- Are lesions or symptoms of a specific illness present?
- Are there any significant body odors (Table 34.2)?
- Does the child appear relaxed or distressed? Lethargic or active?
- Is breathing easy or distressed?

If the child appears to have pain, ask the child to rate it on a child-appropriate pain scale, such as the Faces scale, to better determine the degree of pain (Ely, Chen-Lim, Zarnowsky, et al., 2012).

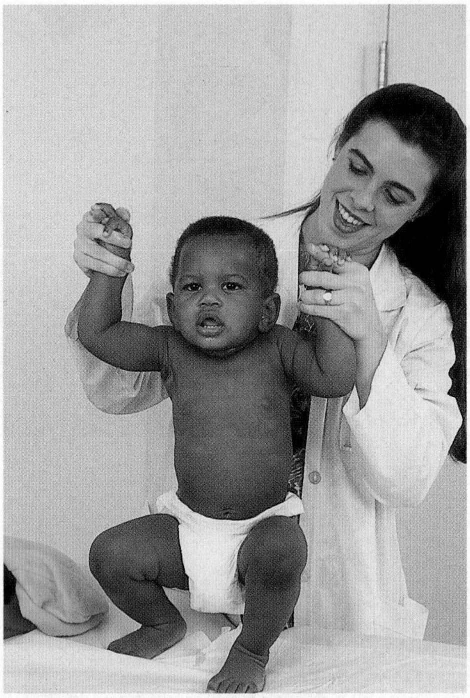

FIGURE 34.3 A general appearance assessment reveals that this child is well proportioned and active.

Mental Status Assessment

A mental status assessment is also made early in an examination as a complement to general appearance. As with general appearance, additional information is gained on mental status throughout the entire examination.

Begin by assessing a child's level of consciousness: Is the child alert? Next, assess orientation, or if the child is aware of person, place, and time (i.e., awareness of who they are, where they are, and the date) if the child is over preschool age. If an infant, does the child "attune" or look aware of surroundings? Assess the appropriateness of behavior and mood (e.g., Is a child hostile, frightened, relaxed?). At some point in the examination of children older than preschool age, ask questions that test recent memory (e.g., what they ate for breakfast) and distant memory (e.g., the name of their first-grade teacher).

Body Measurements

Body measurements are important determinants of health in children because, with chronic illness, the body expends so many nutrients combating the destructive process of the disease that normal height and weight cannot be maintained. Conversely, being overweight (i.e., obesity) needs to be documented because this can lead to illnesses such as heart and lung disease later in life.

Weight. Until they can stand well, infants are weighed nude laying or sitting on an infant scale (diapers can be heavy in proportion to total body weight). Always keep a protective hand over an infant on an infant scale (hovering but not touching) because infants squirm readily and there is danger of them falling (Fig. 34.4A,B). Cover both infant scales and adult scales with scale paper before weighing to prevent the spread of infection from one child to another.

BOX 34.8 Nursing Care Planning Using Assessment

Assessing the Child for General Well Health

History
- → Demographic data
- → Chief concern
- → History of chief concern
- → Health and family profile
- → Past health history
- → Family health history
- → Review of systems

Physical examination
- → General appearance
- → Vital signs

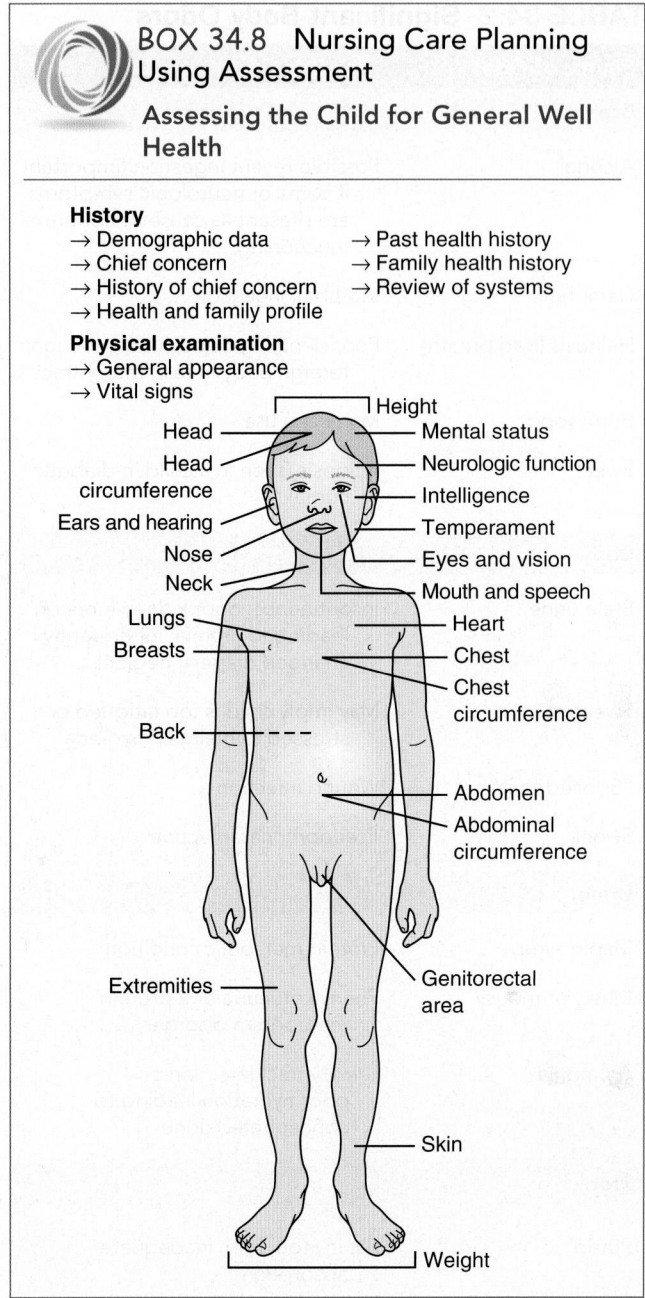

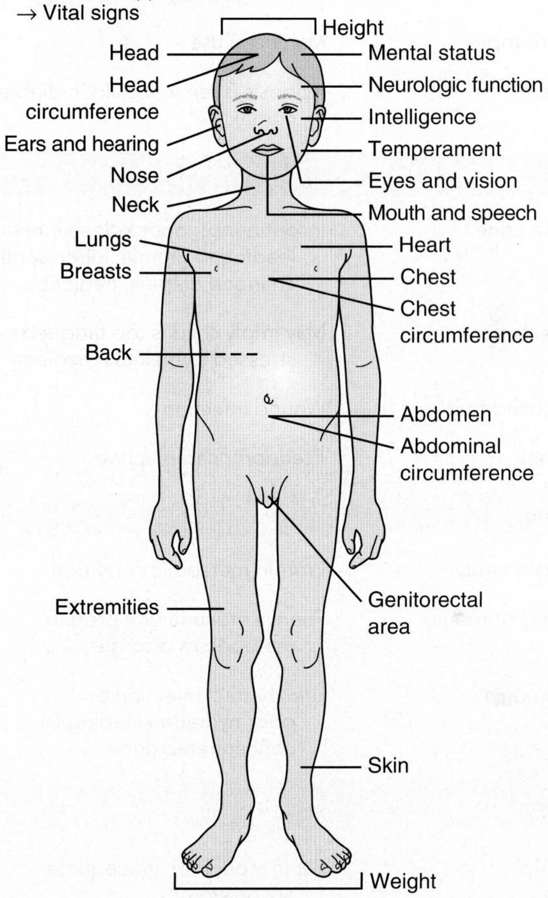

Children older than 2 years of age are weighed on standing scales, in street clothes (no shoes), or if in a hospital, in a gown or pajamas (Fig. 34.4C). If children are going to have serial weights (i.e., weighed every day), be sure they wear the same clothing every time they are weighed so any discrepancy in weight is truly a difference in body weight and not due to more or less clothing. Also take serial weights at the same time each day (preferably before breakfast) on the same scale for greatest accuracy.

Most children and their parents want to know their weight. To convert from kilograms to pounds, multiply the kilogram amount by 2.2 (50 kg × 2.2 = 110 lb). To assess whether weight is average for height, compare the child's weight with a standardized height/weight graph (available at http://thePoint.lww.com/Pillitteri7e). On these standardized graphs, all weights between the 10th and 90th percentiles

TABLE 34.2 Significant Body Odors

Source of Odor	Possible Cause
Breath	
Alcohol	Possible recent ingestion (important if coma or neurologic symptoms are present as cause of abnormal functioning)
Camphor	Mothball ingestion
Halitosis (bad breath)	Poor dental hygiene, lung infection; foreign body in respiratory tract
Burnt rope	Marijuana use
Sweet	Acidosis (seen in a child in diabetic coma)
Body	
Stale urine	Incontinence; poor kidney function leading to uremia; infrequently changed diapers; neglect
Sweat	May imply child is too fatigued or stressed to maintain hygiene
"Spoiled fruit"	Wound infection
Sweet	*Pseudomonas* infection
Urine	
Maple syrup	Protein metabolic condition
Musty or mousy	Phenylketonuria or a protein metabolism disorder
Ammonia	Urinary tract infection or poor hydration leading to concentrated urine
Stool	
Putrid	Fat in stool from inadequate absorption

are considered normal (statistically, a range of weights that includes two standard deviations from the mean or the 50th percentile). All children with weight below the 25th or above the 75th percentiles need close examination because they are moving close to the end points of the usual weight continuum.

As important as it is for children's weight to fall between the 10th and 90th percentile on growth charts, it is also important that, over time, the weight follows one of the percentile curves; in other words, children should not be at the 70th percentile the first time they are weighed, and a month later, at the 80th or 40th percentile. Although both readings are within the normal range, they reflect a weight change that would need investigation. A child is defined as "failing to thrive" if height or weight drops below the third percentile on a standardized growth chart (Jaffe, 2011). Any height or weight in this category definitely needs to be reported so its cause can be investigated. Identifying

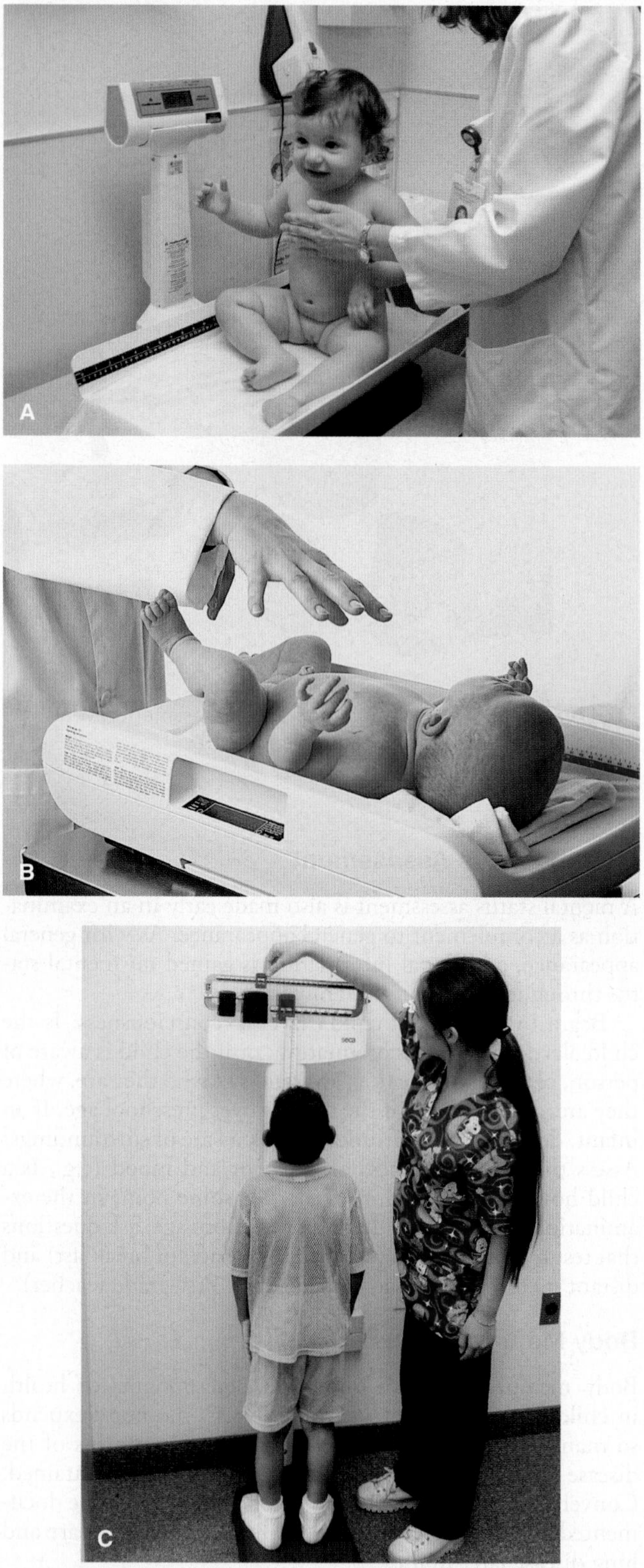

FIGURE 34.4 **(A,B)** Weighing an infant. Note the protective hand to ensure the infant's safety. **(C)** Weighing an older child.

that one is overweight is equally important because this can lead to so many illnesses later on in life (Water, 2011).

U.S. growth charts were compiled by the CDC in the 1960s when almost all infants were formula fed, not breastfed, so breastfed infants tend to score lower on these charts than might be expected (often at the 25th percentile). The WHO has published growth charts that better reflect the weight of breastfed infants. It can be helpful to plot infant weight on these alternative growth charts to reassure parents that their breastfed infant is thriving (de Onis, Onyango, Borghi, et al., 2012).

Another method to determine whether a child's weight is consistent with height is to compute his or her body mass index (BMI) by using a Web site such as www.cdc.gov.

Height. In children, height is as good a determinant of health and normal nutrition as is weight. For tips on accurately measuring the height of infants and older children, see Box 34.9.

Following a measurement, plot the height of children on a standard graph, the same as for weight. Height and weight should follow the same percentiles. Remember that height/weight charts have been standardized for middle-class Caucasian American children, so there will be variations among children from different cultural backgrounds. The important thing to look for is consistency in measurements over time (i.e., always at the same percentile).

What if...34.1 Keoto, 13 years old, weighs 93 lb. Would you be concerned? What if 6 months earlier she weighed 110 lb and a year earlier she weighed 105 lb?

Head Circumference. Head circumference is measured at birth and routinely on physical assessment until 1 or 2 years of age. Head growth occurs because the brain is growing, so head circumference reflects brain growth and potential neurologic function. The measurement is made by placing a tape measure around the infant's head just above the eyebrows and around the most prominent portion of the back of the head (i.e., the occipital prominence) (Fig. 34.5). Babies generally push any object away from their head, so it may be more difficult than it seems to carry out this simple procedure. Plot measurements on a standardized graph (see Growth Charts available at http://thePoint.lww.com/Pillitteri7e). Head circumference should correlate with the child's length; that is, if length is in the 40th percentile, head circumference also should be. If measurements of head circumference plot at different percentiles over time, this should be reported because it implies brain or skull growth is in some way abnormal and needs to be investigated.

Chest and Abdominal Circumference. Measurements of chest and abdominal circumference are not done routinely, but rather, only when specific pathology warrants. Chest circumference is measured at the nipple line, and the abdominal circumference is measured at the level of the umbilicus.

Skin

Skin is assessed in conjunction with the examination of each body region. Always assess temperature, color, dryness, texture, **turgor** (i.e., amount of fluid in body tissue), and the presence of any lesions such as a rash that might reveal a communicable illness.

Table 34.3 summarizes various findings that may be detected on skin examination. Be certain there is adequate lighting, especially when assessing dark-skinned children. Also be certain to examine a child's total skin surface at some point during an examination. If necessary, remove and replace adhesive bandages or other dressings that could hide important findings (e.g., possible maltreatment).

The Newborn and Infant. Newborns may appear ruddy because, as their layer of subcutaneous fat is thin, the intense redness of their blood circulation is visible. Erythema toxicum (i.e., newborn rash) or birthmarks (e.g., hemangiomas, Mongolian spots, nevi) may be present (see Chapter 18). After the first few days of life, a diaper rash may be present.

The Toddler, Preschooler, and School-Age Child. Many children this age have minor lesions from mosquito bites or from flea bites if they own a pet. They also typically have a number of ecchymotic spots on their lower extremities from bumping into objects during active play. Ecchymotic spots on upper extremities are less common and may suggest a blood coagulation problem or maltreatment (Troiano, 2011). Lesions, scratch marks, or excessive dryness can reveal atopic dermatitis, a common childhood disorder (Spiewak, 2012).

The Adolescent or Young Adult. At least a few acne lesions on the face or back are usually present in an adolescent. Lesions or rashes caused by allergies to cosmetics also may be seen. If a child has a tattoo or a body piercing, assess the site for inflammation to be certain an infection is not present. Look carefully for moles that are very dark, have uneven borders, or have recently changed shape because these are signs of melanoma or skin cancer (de Maleissye, Beauchet, Saiag, et al., 2012).

The Head

To examine a child's head, slide a hand over the skull, assessing for irregular configurations or tenderness. Most children have a prominent occipital outgrowth; do not mistake this natural head contour for an abnormality. Assess the texture and cleanliness of hair. Children who are well nourished usually have hair of good texture; poorly nourished children tend to have dry, brittle, or limp hair. If hair is exceptionally oily, it may suggest a lack of adequate hygiene, possibly from fatigue due to an unidentified illness. If a serious protein deficiency such as **kwashiorkor** is present, the hair becomes striped with dark and light color, because dark hair forms during periods of good protein intake and the light color forms during periods of protein deficiency. Patches of hair loss (i.e., alopecia) suggest a fungal infection (e.g., tinea capitis), child maltreatment, or a possible drug reaction (chemotherapy will cause total hair loss, not patches).

The Newborn and Infant. In a newborn, the head usually shows molding (i.e., an elongated shape due to pressure against the cervix before birth). A caput succedaneum or cephalohematoma from the pressure of birth may be present (see Chapter 18). Skull suture lines are palpable. In both newborns and infants, sit the child upright and palpate the skull for the presence of fontanelles (i.e., the places where the skull bones fuse). The anterior fontanelle is diamond shaped and measures 2 to 3 cm (0.8 to 1.2 in.) in width and 3 to 4 cm (1.2 to 1.6 in.) in length. The posterior fontanelle is triangular and measures approximately 1 cm (0.5 in.) in length (see Chapter 15, Fig. 15.2).

With the infant sitting, fontanelles should be felt as soft spots, but should not appear indented (a sign of dehydration)

BOX 34.9 Nursing Care Planning Using Procedures

MEASURING A CHILD'S HEIGHT

Purpose: To assess for optimal growth.

PROCEDURE	PRINCIPLE
Infant	
1. Until they can stand securely (at approximately age 2 years), measure infants lying down on a measuring frame or an examining table.	1. Promotes accuracy.
2. Align the infant's head snugly against the top bar of the measuring frame and ask an assistant to secure it there. Parents can help you restrain infants for height measurements because it is a painless procedure.	2. Provides a starting point for measurement.
3. Straighten the infant's body (Fig. A).	3. Knees are difficult to straighten in infants because they usually keep them flexed.

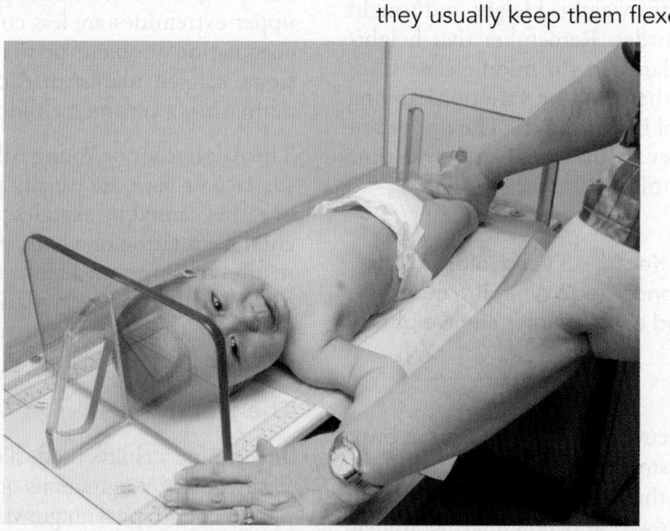

A

PROCEDURE	PRINCIPLE
4. Hold the infant's feet in a vertical position. Bring the foot board up snugly against the bottom of the foot.	4. Completes measurement.
5. If an examining table is used instead of a measuring frame, mark the spots at the top of the child's head and bottom of the feet on the table paper, then measure between the marks with a tape measure.	5. Provides for an alternative approach.
6. Plot height measurements on a standard graph.	6. Allows for interpretation of findings.
Older Child	
1. Have the child remove shoes and step onto the scale.	1. Promotes accuracy.
2. Ask the child to stand straight with head held level.	2. Puts the child in the proper position for accurate measurement.
3. Align the measuring bar of a standing scale with the top of the child's head.	3. Determines the measurement.
4. If a scale with a measuring bar is not available, place a flat object such as a clipboard on the child's head in a horizontal position and read the height at the point at which the object touches a measuring tape on the back of the scale or a flat wall surface (Fig. B).	4. Provides for an alternative approach.
5. Plot height measurement on a standard graph.	5. Allows for interpretation of findings.

MEASURING A CHILD'S HEIGHT

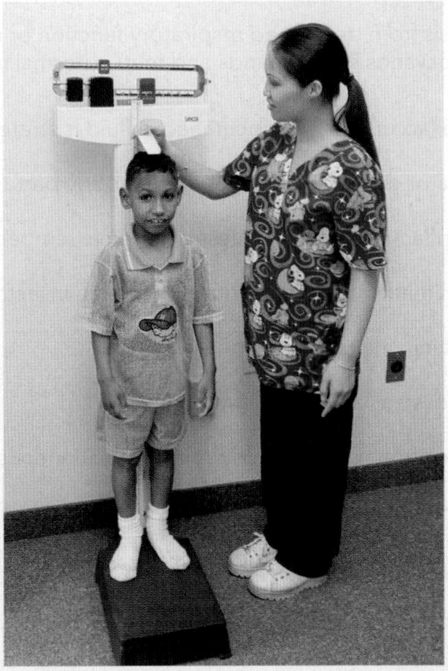

or bulging (a sign of increased intracranial pressure). When an infant cries, cerebral pressure increases, so with crying, the fontanelles may feel tense, and sometimes the fluctuation of a pulse can even be observed. The anterior fontanelle normally closes at 12 to 18 months and the posterior fontanelle by the end of 2 months and so should not be palpable after these times. The closing of fontanelles too early or too late can indicate decreased or increased brain or ventricle growth and is, therefore, a serious finding.

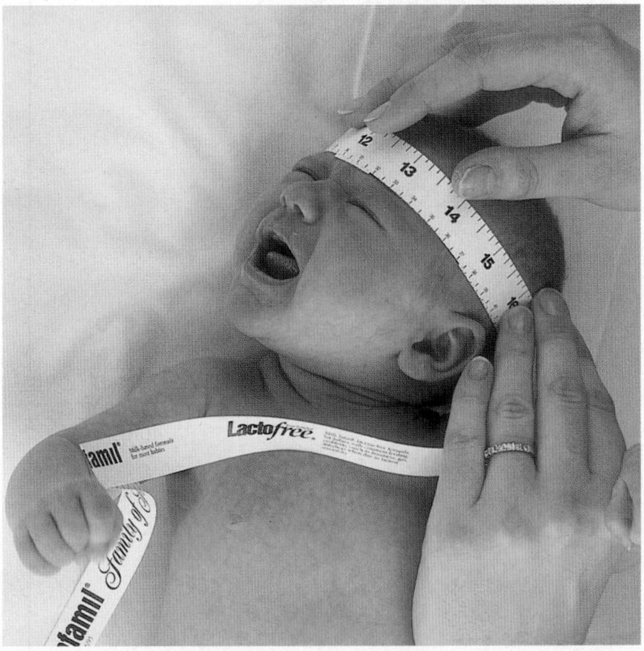

FIGURE 34.5 Measuring head circumference. The measuring tape passes just above the eyebrows and around the prominent posterior aspect of the head.

A scalp problem commonly encountered in infants is seborrhea (i.e., scaling, greasy-appearing, salmon-colored patches), or "cradle cap." You can advise parents that increasing the frequency of hair washing to once a day and applying baby oil to the scalp typically reduces this problem.

The Toddler, Preschooler, and School-Age Child. Examine the hair of children who attend school or day care carefully for small white-yellow, sand-sized particles attached to hair strands, which are the eggs (i.e., nits) of pediculi (i.e., head lice). Pediculi can spread easily in school-age children due to sharing of combs and towels in school. Nits cling and cannot be readily removed from the hair by running fingers the length of the hair (Shmidt & Levitt, 2012). The child may have recent scratch marks on the scalp or state that the scalp feels itchy.

Also examine the scalp carefully for round circular areas (perhaps weeping in the center, crusting and scaling on the edges) that would suggest tinea capitis (i.e., ringworm, which is a fungal infection). Like pediculi, fungal infections can easily spread among school-age children; a prescription medication is necessary to best cure both conditions (see Chapter 43).

The Adolescent and Young Adult. Both adolescents and young adults may streak their hair with dye or arrange it in a way that requires gel, hair extensions, or use of a curling iron. Inspect to see that their scalp and hair are healthy underneath the styling.

The Eyes

Observe eyes for symmetry and signs of redness (i.e., erythema), frequent blinking, crusting, squinting, or rubbing as these are signs of **conjunctivitis**, an infection of the thin conjunctiva that covers the eye globe (Braverman, 2012).

TABLE 34.3 Skin Findings in Children That Suggest Illness

Finding	Indication
Central bluish color	Cyanosis from decreased respiratory function or cyanotic heart disease; acrocyanosis (blue hands and feet) is normal in newborns for first 48 hours.
White color	Edema (accumulated subcutaneous fluid is stretching the skin).
Pale color	Anemia or decreased circulation to a body part.
Reddened area	Local inflammation or increased systemic temperature.
Linear abrasion	Scratch marks from local irritation from an insect bite or allergic reaction.
Ecchymoses (black and blue marks)	Recent injury to skin.
Petechiae (pinpoint blood marks)	Blood dyscrasia (poor clotting ability).
Yellow color	Jaundice from increased bilirubin in subcutaneous tissue; carotenemia (excess carotene in skin).
Moistness	Excess perspiration from elevated temperature.
Localized cold temperature	Decreased circulation to particular body part.
Warm temperature	Local irritation or elevated systemic temperature.
Poor turgor	Dehydration.
Rash	Infectious childhood illness, excessive heat, or allergy.

Also observe lids and lashes for redness or abnormalities to detect a **hordeolum** or stye (i.e., an infection of the gland that lubricates an eyelash). Both conditions require an antibiotic for therapy (see Chapter 50).

Assess the location of eyes in relation to the nose (i.e., not unusually wide or narrow spaced) and the relationship of the globe to the socket (i.e., neither sunken nor protruding from the socket [exophthalmos]). Abnormalities in these areas occur in chromosomal or metabolic illnesses such as hyperthyroidism. Inspect the sclera of the eye for spots of hemorrhage (i.e., subconjunctival hemorrhage) or yellowing. African American children often have a slight yellowing of the sclera and small black spots on the sclera; do not mistake these for abnormal findings. Assess that no sclera shows above the pupil (if it does, this is termed a sunset sign, a possible indication of increased intracranial pressure).

Palpate each eye globe with the eyelid closed to assess for tenseness, a finding suggesting glaucoma (although this is rare in children). Determine whether the eyelids completely close; edema or neurologic illnesses may shorten eyelids so they cannot close. Lastly, determine whether the lids retract far enough so they do not obscure vision when the child opens his or her eyes. When a lid obscures vision (**ptosis**), it generally denotes neurologic involvement. The difference in Western and Eastern eye creases is shown in Figure 34.6.

Examine the inner lining of the lower eyelid (i.e., the conjunctiva) by pulling the lid down slightly with your fingertip. Here, the mucous membrane should appear moist and not pale. In children with anemia, it often appears pale; for a child with an allergy or infection, it may appear unusually red and irritated. Do not initiate a blink reflex by touching the cornea with a wisp of cotton, as is done in adults, as this is momentarily painful and frightening for children.

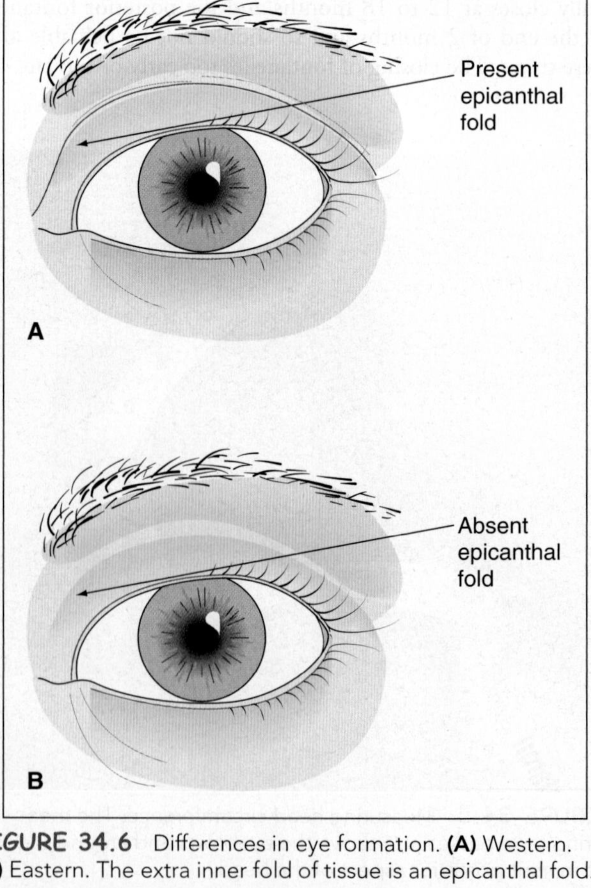

FIGURE 34.6 Differences in eye formation. **(A)** Western. **(B)** Eastern. The extra inner fold of tissue is an epicanthal fold.

In addition, observe whether the eyes appear to be in good alignment. **Strabismus** refers to eyes that are not evenly aligned. If an eye is always turning in, the condition is termed **esotropia**; if it always turns out, this is termed **exotropia**. Two screening procedures for straight eye alignment include the Hirschberg test and the cover test. During a Hirschberg test, the light of an otoscope should reflect evenly off both pupils if they are in equal alignment (Fig. 34.7).

To perform a cover test (Fig. 34.8), perform the following steps:

- Have children look at an attractive object approximately 4 ft in front of them.
- Hold a 3″ × 5″ card over the left eye for a count of five. If any degree of strabismus is present, the eye will wander to its misaligned position while covered.
- Remove the card and observe the eye for movement.
- As the child again fixes vision on the specified object, the eye will move back into line, revealing the misalignment.
- Repeat the process with the right eye.

Some children, particularly preschoolers with wide epicanthic folds, may appear at a quick glance, to show misalignment. A cover test is helpful in these children because there will be no eye movement after removal of the card, demonstrating that they have no actual misalignment, only the temporary appearance of that. Reasons for true misalignment are discussed in Chapter 50.

To test the eyes for their ability to focus in all fields of vision:

- Ask the child to follow a moving light (or catch the attention of an infant with a moving light) while holding the child's chin stationary.
- Move the light out to the side, then up, and then down.
- Cross to the opposite side and move it up and down.
- Bring the light back to the midline and observe whether the child's eyes converge (follow the light in to the nose). Infants under 3 months of age cannot follow past the midline; the eyes of children under school age do not converge well.

If the pupil constricts (i.e., reduces in size) in response to the light, it is confirmation that the third cranial nerve is intact. For this test, it is best to approach the child's eye

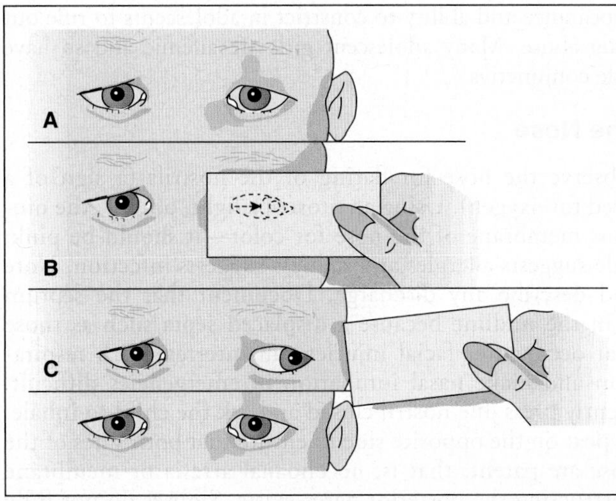

FIGURE 34.8 The cover test. **(A)** The child's eyes appear to be in good alignment. **(B)** The left eye is covered for 5 seconds. **(C)** When the card is removed, the left eye is seen to move perceptibly back to good alignment. This movement indicates it "drifted" into a deviant position while covered; that is, an exophoria (misalignment) is present.

from the forehead so the light suddenly appears on the pupil rather than advancing it toward the child slowly because this makes the pupil constrict more dramatically. When one pupil constricts in response to a bright light, this is termed *direct constriction*; constriction should also occur in the opposite eye (i.e., *consensual constriction*). Record that pupils are equal in size and react to light as PERL (pupils equal, react to light). If the pupil converges (i.e., moves to follow a light in toward the nose), this is charted as PEARL or PERLA (pupils equal, react to light, accommodate).

For a final step, shine a flashlight or ophthalmoscope light into the pupil. A red reflex or the red pupil that occurs with a flash photo should appear. This is evidence that the retina is intact and the lens and cornea are clear (i.e., no tumor, cataract, scarring, or infection is present).

The Newborn and Infant. Newborns often have a small, bright-red spot on the sclera (i.e., a subconjunctival hemorrhage) because the pressure of birth ruptured a small conjunctival blood vessel. This is normal and will fade in 7 to 10 days as the blood is absorbed.

Newborns and infants can easily be tested for a red reflex, but until they are about 3 months, they cannot follow an object or light across the midline or follow a light into all six positions of gaze. Assessing for a red reflex is especially important in newborns because a congenital cataract can lead to a loss of central vision if not discovered early.

The Toddler and Preschooler. Most young children are reluctant to let someone look into their eyes. Explaining what will happen during an eye examination is important to reduce the child's anxiety about this part of the assessment.

The School-Age Child and Adolescent. Many older children wear contact lenses (a red reflex is visible with a contact lens in place), and others may be nervous about having their eyes examined because they know they should be wearing prescribed eyeglasses but are not wearing them because they do not like their appearance. Observe carefully for pupillary

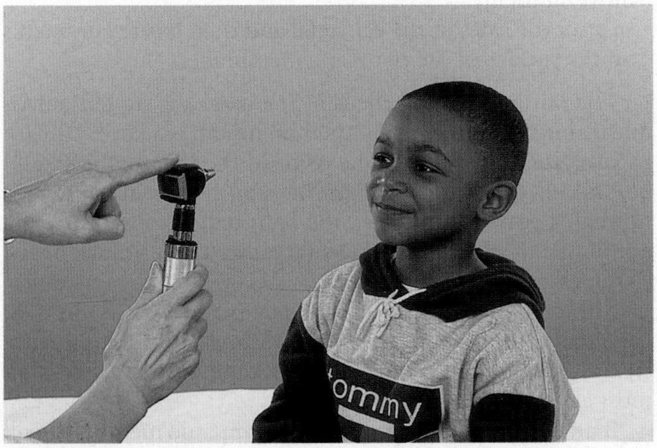

FIGURE 34.7 Testing good eye alignment by the Hirschberg's test. The child is asked to look directly at the light of the otoscope. The light reflex on the pupils of both eyes will be equal if the eyes are in straight alignment.

appearance and ability to constrict in adolescents to rule out drug abuse. Many adolescent girls are anemic and so have pale conjunctiva.

The Nose

Observe the nose for flaring of the nostrils (a sign of a need for oxygen). Using an otoscope light, observe the mucous membrane of the nose for color—it should be pink; pale suggests allergies and redness suggests infection. Note and describe any discharge. Document that the septum is in the midline because a displaced septa such as those that occur after facial injuries can interfere with respiration and make nasal intubation in emergencies difficult. Gently press one nostril closed and ask the child to inhale. Repeat on the opposite side to ensure that both sides of the nose are patent; that is, no choanal atresia or membrane obstructing the posterior nares exists. Sinuses do not fully develop until about 6 years. For children 6 years or older, palpate the areas over the frontal and maxillary sinuses for tenderness, which is a symptom of sinus infection. Assess the sense of smell in school-age children and adolescents by asking them to identify a familiar odor such as chocolate or an orange.

The Newborn and Infant. Infants are obligate nose breathers. They cannot coordinate mouth breathing, so they become disturbed when the nose is temporarily blocked to check for patency; do this only momentarily to avoid discomfort. Most newborns have milia (i.e., small white papules) on the surface of the nose, which are of no consequence.

The Older Child. Many children preschool age and older have upper respiratory infections that cause reddened nasal mucous membranes and a purulent discharge. In contrast, allergies cause a clear discharge and pale mucous membranes. Children who have dry mucosa due to dry air, which leads to cracking and nosebleeds, may be reluctant to allow inspection of their nose. Adolescents who sniff cocaine lose nasal hair and may have excoriations or abscesses in the mucous membrane. If the child has a nose piercing, inspect the site for redness or drainage.

Ears

Observe ears for proper alignment. In the average child, a line drawn from the inner canthus of the eye to the outer canthus and then to the ear will touch the top of the pinna of the ear (Fig. 34.9). Ears set lower than this are associated with chromosomal disorders such as trisomy 13. Observe the opening to the ear canal for any discharge. Touch the pinna and watch for evidence of pain, which is a sign of external canal infections. Observe the area immediately in front of the ear for a dermal sinus or skin tag, findings that are usually innocent but may be associated with kidney abnormalities. Observe the ear lobes for redness or drainage from infected piercing sites, if applicable.

To examine the ear canal:

- Select the smallest size otoscope tip possible that will still give adequate visibility.
- Straighten the ear canal by pulling the pinna gently down and back in the child under 2 years of age and up and back in the older child.
- Insert an otoscope tip into the external canal.

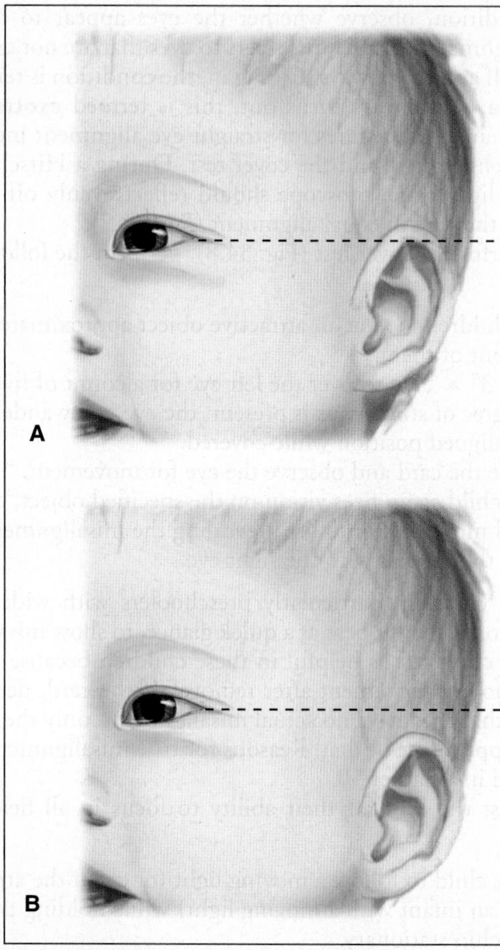

FIGURE 34.9 Normal ear alignment. When a line is drawn from the inner canthus through the outer canthus of the eye to the ear, the top of the ear pinna should meet the line **(A)**. Abnormal ear alignment **(B)** is associated with certain chromosomal abnormalities.

- Be certain to rest the instrument on your hand, not on the child's head (Fig. 34.10). In this position, the otoscope will move with the child, avoiding the danger the plastic tip will scratch the canal if the child should move suddenly.
- Inspect the sides of the ear canal and then locate landmarks on the surface of the tympanic membrane.

The outline of the malleus of the inner ear should be visible through the translucent membrane and is a key landmark to visualize (Fig. 34.11). The color of the membrane should be pinkish gray; usually, if the tension of the membrane is normal, a cone of light (i.e., the light reflex) should be present in one of the lower corners (at either the 5 o'clock or the 7 o'clock position).

Although many children have wax (i.e., cerumen) in their ear canals, which appears as a dark-brown, glistening substance, viewing the tympanic membrane past the wax is almost always possible.

If an ear infection is present, the tympanic membrane will appear reddened and will often bulge forward so the malleus is no longer discernible and the cone of light is absent (Yoon, Kelley, & Friedman, 2012).

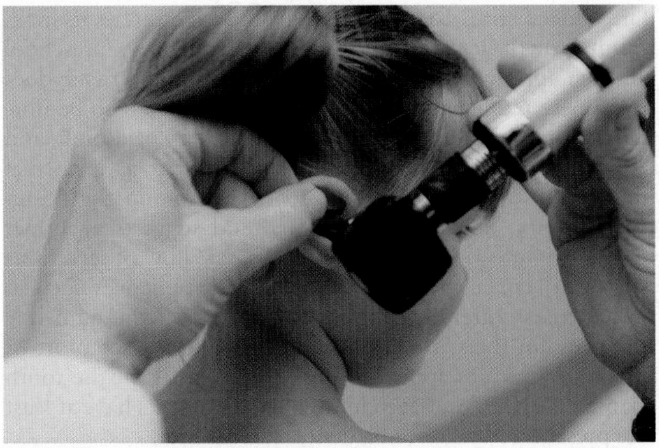

FIGURE 34.10 An otoscopic examination. Note how the nurse's hand rests between the otoscope and the child's head. Should the child move, no injury to the tympanic membrane will be sustained with this technique because the otoscope will move with the child's head.

If there is fluid in the middle ear, it may be possible to see bubbles of air through the membrane. With chronic middle ear disease (i.e., serous otitis media), the tympanic membrane may be retracted, the malleus will then be extremely prominent, and the cone of light will be missing. If the membrane has been torn from trauma or rupture, the jagged edge and opening to the middle ear are discernible. Inspect also for any ulcerated areas that could be a cholesteatoma or an ingrowing tumor, most often seen on the upper part of the membrane (see Chapter 50).

Although not a routine procedure, the mobility of the eardrum can be tested by injecting a column of air into the ear canal against the drum by a pneumatic attachment on an otoscope, which looks like the bulb of a blood pressure cuff (Fig. 34.12). A normal drum is freely mobile and can be seen to move with pressure on the bulb; one with fluid behind it has decreased mobility. Before introducing air, warn the child that air against the membrane will tickle.

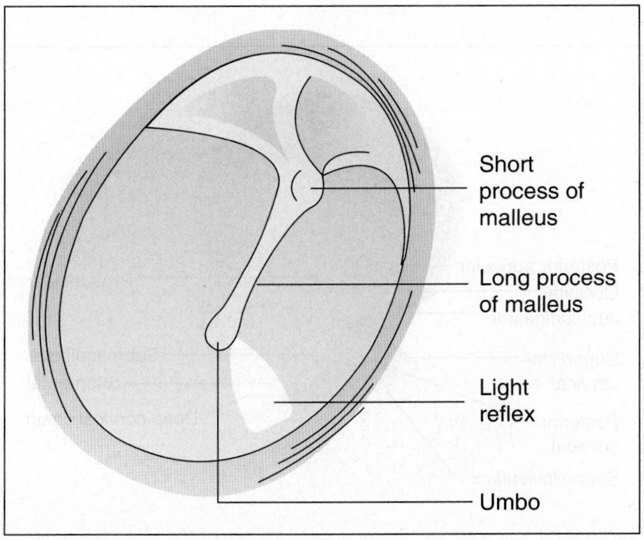

FIGURE 34.11 A tympanic membrane as viewed with an otoscope.

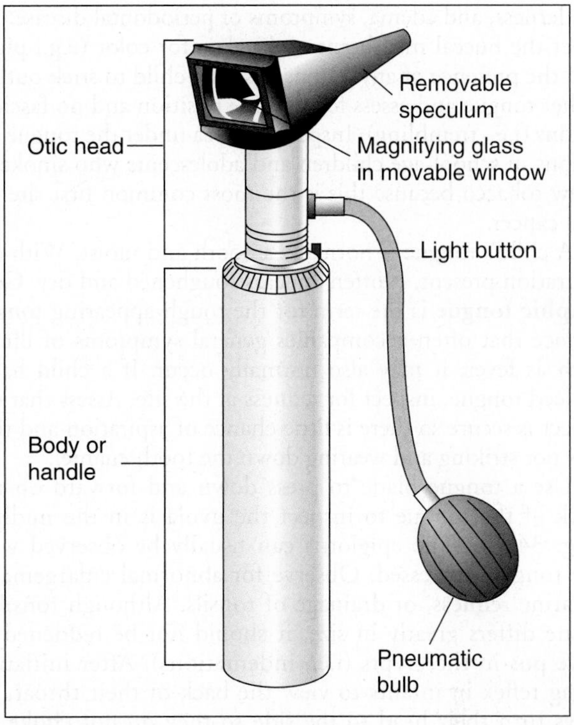

FIGURE 34.12 An otoscope with pneumatic attachment.

Finally, appraise hearing. Appraisal for this can be done grossly in older children by assessing their response to your questions. Distract an infant with a toy; then make a sound behind the infant's back, out of peripheral vision, and watch if there is a response. Hearing infants will show some noticeable reaction, although they have difficulty looking directly toward or locating the sound until about 4 months of age.

The Newborn and Infant. Many newborns still have amniotic fluid or vernix caseosa in their ear canal, so inspecting the ear canal is ineffective. Be certain to assess for ear level and normal pinna contour. Assess gross hearing ability, for example, by watching the infant startle to a sudden sound or quiet to the calming effect of quiet talking.

The Older Child. Middle ear infection (i.e., otitis media) is a common childhood illness. This causes the ear to be painful when examined. An external ear infection (often called swimmer's ear) causes any movement of the pinna to be painful. Explaining what is happening during the examination helps to allay a child's fear of having an instrument pressed into the ear. Beginning with preschool age, children may have myringotomy tubes (i.e., small circular plastic tubes placed into the tympanic membrane) to relieve chronic fluid collected in the middle ear. Inspect that the area surrounding the tube is not inflamed and the tube is not merely lying in the external canal and no longer inserted into the membrane (see Chapter 50).

The Mouth

Assess the external appearance of the lips for symmetry and color. Ask the child to smile and frown to evaluate the mobility of facial muscles. Count the number of teeth present and assess their condition (e.g., number missing or cavities present). Inspect the gum line (i.e., gingivae) for redness, tenderness, and edema, symptoms of periodontal disease. Inspect the buccal membrane and palate for color (e.g., pink) and the presence of any lesions. Ask the child to stick out his or her tongue and assess for midline position and no fasciculations (i.e., trembling). Inspect the area under the tongue for lesions in school-age children and adolescents who smoke or chew tobacco because this is the most common first site for oral cancer.

A child's tongue is normally smooth and moist. With dehydration present, it often appears roughened and dry. **Geographic tongue** is the term for the rough-appearing tongue surface that often accompanies general symptoms of illness such as fever; it may also normally occur. If a child has a pierced tongue, inspect for redness at the site. Assess that the object is secure so there is little chance of aspiration and that it is not striking and wearing down the tooth enamel.

Use a tongue blade to press down and forward on the back of the tongue to inspect the uvula is in the midline (Fig. 34.13). The epiglottis can usually be observed with the tongue depressed. Observe for abnormal enlargement, palatine redness, or drainage of tonsils. Although tonsillar tissue differs greatly in size, it should not be reddened or have pus in the crypts (i.e., indentations). After initiating a gag reflex in infants to view the back of their throat, always turn their head to the side so they do not choke on any saliva that accumulated in the mouth during the throat examination because infants are less able to manage this than are adults.

Do not depress the tongue of any child who is suspected to have epiglottitis or whose glottis is inflamed. Symptoms of this condition are a sore throat, drooling, high fever, difficulty with respiration, dysphagia, and a barking cough. If a swollen, inflamed epiglottis rises with the pressure of a tongue blade, it can obstruct the respiratory tract so completely that the child is immediately unable to breathe.

The Newborn and Infant. Many newborns have considerable mucus in their mouths because they are less able to handle swallowing due to immature muscle coordination. If a newborn has teeth, evaluate them for stability; if teeth are loose, they may need to be removed to prevent aspiration. Assess for white patches that do not scrape away from the buccal membrane or tongue (i.e., thrush), a common but abnormal finding in infants that requires antifungal therapy (see Chapter 43).

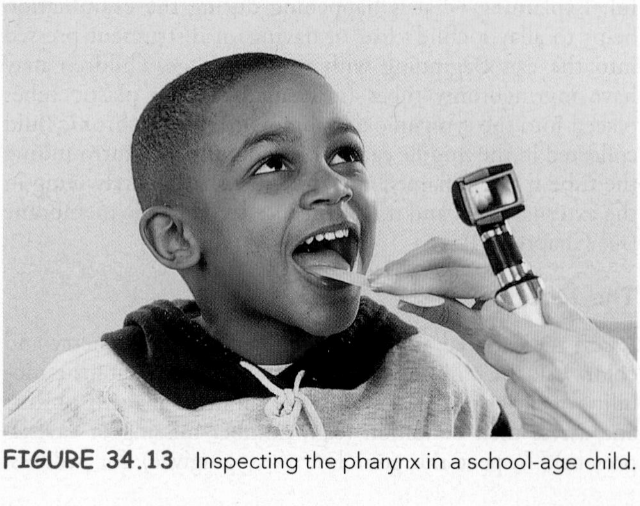

FIGURE 34.13 Inspecting the pharynx in a school-age child.

The Older Child. Tonsillar tissue in children reaches its maximum growth at early school age, making many preschool children appear to be "all tonsils." As long as the tissue does not appear reddened or tender, you can assume it to be normal for the age. Many children have irregular, pale-pink, and elevated projections on the posterior pharynx as a normal finding. A stream of mucopurulent discharge in the posterior pharynx, however, is not usual and suggests an upper respiratory infection and that a "postnasal" flow of secretions is present. For a child with orthodontic appliances such as braces, assess carefully for pinpoint ulcers on the gum line to be certain the wires are not causing undue discomfort or infection. Cavities appear as dark-brown areas on the tooth enamel. Many school-age children or adolescents have at least one present and will need a dental care referral.

QSEN Checkpoint Question 34.4

Teamwork & Collaboration

Pressing a tongue blade against the back of the throat causes a gag reflex. When would you want your team members to know it is important *not* to elicit a gag reflex?

a. When a child is under 5 years of age
b. When a child has symptoms of epiglottitis
c. When a boy has a possible inguinal hernia
d. When a girl has a geographic tongue

Look in Appendix A for the best answer and rationale.

The Neck

Assess the neck for symmetry (the trachea should be in the midline; any deviation suggests lung or thyroid pathology). Observe the outline of the thyroid gland (barely noticeable before puberty) because it is obscured by the sternocleidomastoid muscle, on the anterior neck, to be certain it is not swollen or tender. Palpate the area in front of the ear, which is the location of the parotid gland, and smooth a hand over the location of lymph nodes at the sides of the neck and under the chin to palpate for swelling. Figure 34.14 shows

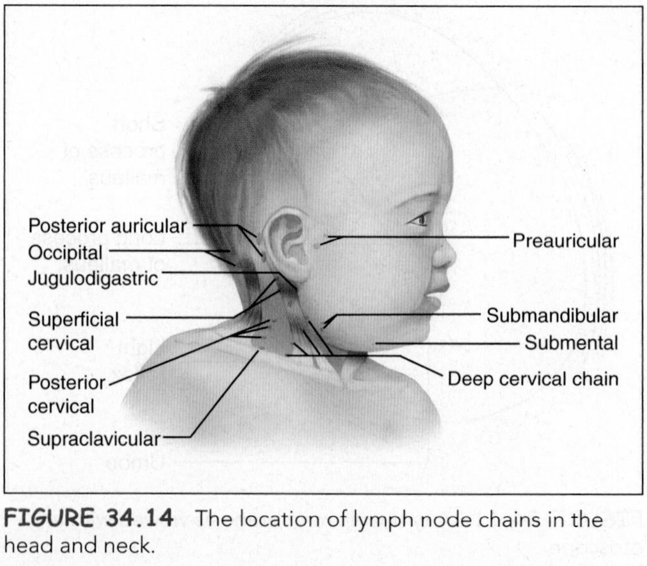

FIGURE 34.14 The location of lymph node chains in the head and neck.

the location of lymph node chains of the head and neck. Because children have so many upper respiratory infections, a few nodes that are freely movable, about the size of peas, termed "shotty" nodes because they simulate the feel of buckshot under the skin, are often present. Commonly, preauricular and postauricular nodes are palpable after ear infections, and postoccipital nodes are palpable after a scalp infection. Submental nodes generally denote a tooth abscess. Palpable submaxillary, anterior, and posterior cervical nodes follow throat infections.

Ask the child to move the head (or move it for the child) through flexion (i.e., touch chin to chest) and extension (i.e., raise chin as high as possible), and turn it right and left (i.e., rotation) to see that a child does all of these movements easily. Pain on forward flexion is an important sign because it can be caused by neurologic (i.e., meningeal) irritation or is a sign of meningitis.

The Newborn and Infant. With infants, always assess the ability to control the head by laying the infant supine and pulling the child to a sitting position. Babies younger than 4 months of age will let their heads lag backward as they are pulled up this way, and they will right their heads only as they reach a sitting position. After 4 months, infants should bring their head up with no head lag if their neuromuscular coordination is adequate for their age. This simple but important test yields information about overall neuromuscular control as well as neck strength.

The Adolescent. In adolescents, be certain to palpate the thyroid gland for both symmetry and possible nodes. To do this, press on the right side of the gland, which will cause it to be more prominent on the left side. Palpate the left half to discern any irregularities (areas of hardness). Repeat on the right side. A finding of a thyroid node needs to be investigated as it may be only an innocent transient cyst, or it may be the first indication of thyroid malignancy. Many adolescents have a normal increase in the size of the thyroid at puberty; this hypertrophy should not be accompanied by any nodes.

The Chest

For ease in specifying the location of chest pathology, the chest is divided into sections by imaginary lines drawn through the midclavicle, midmammary, and midsternum points on the front; the midaxilla on the side; and the midscapula on the back. Pathology is described in terms of these lines such as "abnormal lung sound heard at left midaxillary line." Other helpful means of locating pathology is by the suprasternal notch, the ribs, and the spaces between them **(intercostal spaces)**. Intercostal spaces are numbered according to the ribs immediately above them (Fig. 34.15). Inspect both front and back surfaces of the chest for symmetry of appearance and motion. Inspect for **retractions** or indentation of intercostal spaces or the suprasternal and substernal areas that reflect difficult respirations. Assess the proportion of the anteroposterior to the lateral diameter (normally 1:2). Children with chronic lung disease develop a broad (i.e., barrel) chest or a chest that is more rounded than usual. This and other chest abnormalities are shown in Figure 34.16. An infant with a diaphragmatic hernia (i.e., intestine herniated into the chest cavity) may have a chest enlarged on that side. An infant with atelectasis (i.e., collapsed lung) may have a chest that is smaller on the affected side. If a child has an enlarged heart, the left side of the chest may appear larger.

The Breasts

The degree of breast assessment depends on the child's age and development. As part of a usual breast assessment, inspect and palpate the breasts of all children to detect any abnormalities.

The Newborn. Both male and female newborns may have breast edema from the influence of maternal hormones. A few drops of clear fluid may be present from the nipples. This is normal and will fade in a few days time. Document if a supernumerary nipple is present for baseline data.

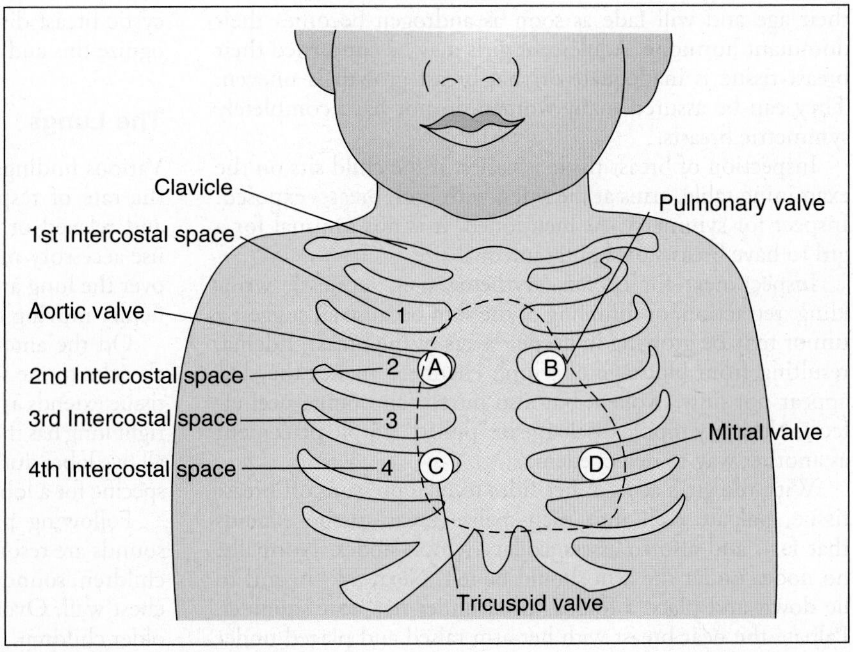

FIGURE 34.15 Intercostal (between rib) spaces are numbered according to the ribs immediately above them. The points *(A, B, C, D)* are the locations where the sounds of the heart valves radiate or where they can be heard best.

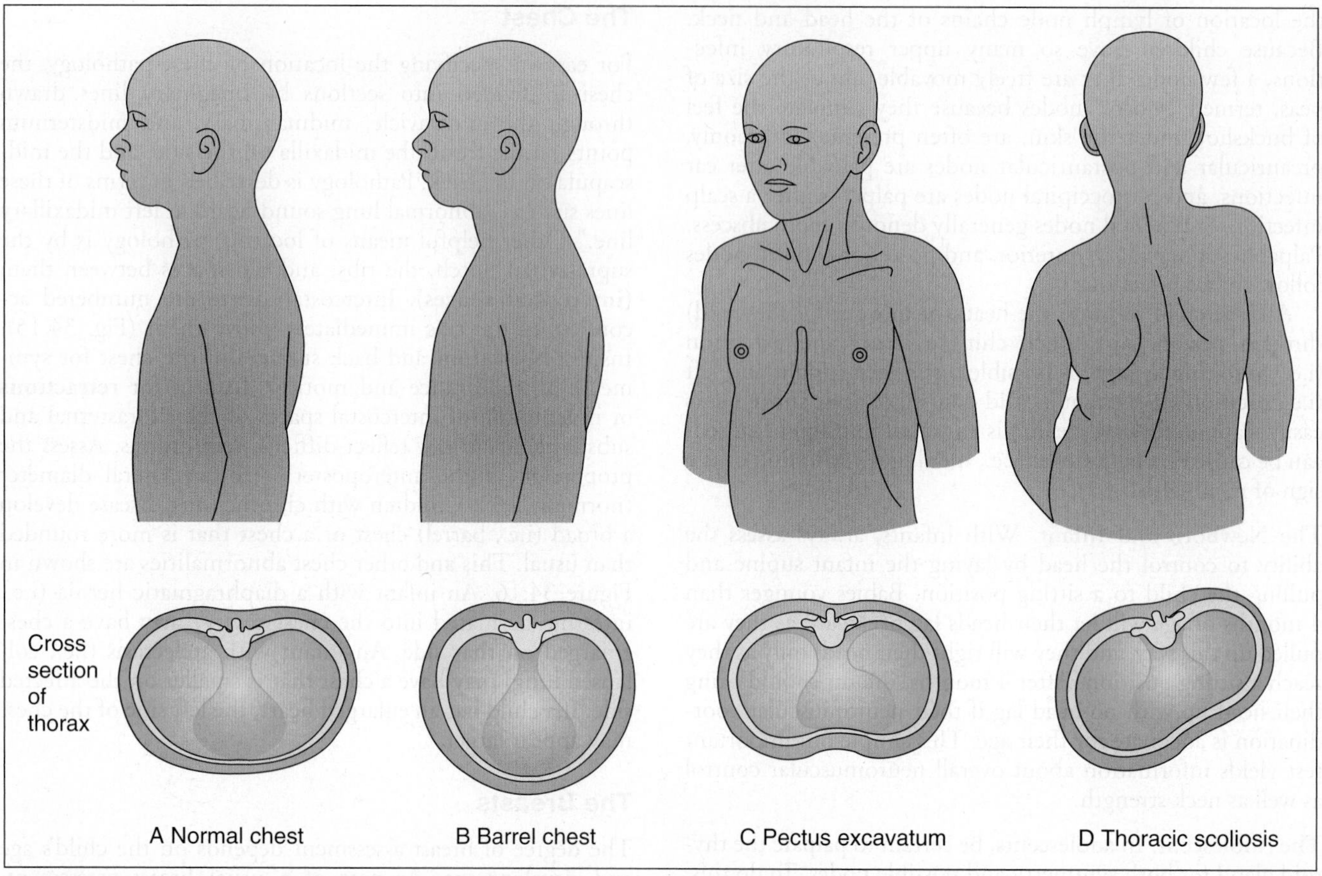

FIGURE 34.16 Chest contours that can be assessed by inspection. **(A)** Normal chest. **(B)** Barrel chest. **(C)** Funnel chest (pectus excavatum). **(D)** Thoracic kyphoscoliosis.

The School-Age Child and Adolescent. Do a breast examination on all girls past puberty. If a girl younger than 8 years is beginning breast development, precocious puberty (see Chapter 48) should be suspected. Many preadolescent boys develop hypertrophy of breast tissue due to increased hormonal influences (i.e., gynecomastia); such boys may be concerned and will need reassurance that this is normal for their age and will fade as soon as androgen becomes their dominant hormone. Adolescent girls may be concerned their breast tissue is inadequate or that breast growth is uneven. They can be assured many women do not have completely symmetric breasts.

Inspection of breast tissue is easiest if the child sits on the examining table, arms at the sides, with both breasts exposed. Inspect for symmetry. As mentioned, it is not unusual for a girl to have breasts of slightly unequal size.

Inspect next for edema, erythema (i.e., redness), wrinkling, retraction, or dimpling of the skin because all suggest a tumor may be growing in deeper layers of the breast. Edema, resulting from blockage of lymph channels, makes the skin appear not only swollen, but also pitted (an orange-peel effect). Note any nipple discharge or "pulled" nipple placement as another way to detect edema.

With the girl's arms at her sides to take pressure off breast tissue, palpate well into each axilla (breast tissue extends that far), and also to assess axillary lymph nodes. Normally, no nodes under the arm should be felt. Next, ask the girl to lie down and place a folded towel under her near shoulder. Palpate the near breast with her arm raised and placed under her head because this spreads out breast tissue; begin at the nipple and palpate outward in a circular motion. The lower edge of each breast feels hard; do not mistake this or rib prominences underneath for a tumor. Repeat on the other side. Although self-breast exams are no longer recommended, it's good to teach adolescents breast awareness or to know what their breasts normally feel like so if a condition such as fibrocystic breast disease should develop, they will be able to recognize this and report it to their primary health care provider.

The Lungs

Various findings reveal respiratory distress in children. Assess the rate of respirations and whether respirations seem easy and relaxed or stressed; note if it's necessary for a child to use accessory muscles to achieve effective ventilation. Palpate over the lung area for vibrations that suggest air is having difficulty moving through small air passages.

On the anterior chest, lung tissue extends from above the clavicles to the sixth or eighth rib. On the posterior chest, lung tissue extends as low as the 10th to 12th thoracic vertebrae. The right lung has three lobes; the left, only two. Attempt to evaluate all five lobes during lung assessment because lung disease can be specific for a lobe rather than involve the entire lung.

Following palpation, percuss lung tissue. Normal lung sounds are resonant in older children; in infants and younger children, sounds are hyperresonant due to the thinness of the chest wall. Overexpanded lungs will sound hyperresonant in older children, and lungs filled with fluid sound dull in older

TABLE 34.4 Breath Sounds Heard on Auscultation

Sound	Characteristics
Vesicular	Soft, low-pitched sound, heard over periphery of lungs; inspiration longer than expiration. Normal.
Bronchovesicular	Soft, medium-pitched sound, heard over major bronchi; inspiration equals expiration. Normal.
Bronchial	Loud, high-pitched sound, heard over trachea; expiration longer than inspiration. Normal.
Rhonchi	A snoring sound made by air moving through mucus in bronchi. Normal.
Rales (also called crackles)	Crackling or crinkling sounds (like cellophane) are created by air moving through fluid in alveoli. Abnormal.
Wheezing	Whistling on expiration made by air being pushed through narrowed bronchi. Abnormal; seen in children with asthma or foreign body obstruction.
Stridor	Crowing or rooster-like sound made by air being pulled through a constricted larynx. Abnormal; seen in children with upper respiratory obstruction.

children and less resonant in younger children. The lower anterior lobe of the right lung will sound dull because the liver covers it on the anterior surface below the fourth or fifth intercostal space. The space over the heart will also percuss as dull.

Diaphragmatic excursion (i.e., the distance the diaphragm descends with inhalation) is an estimation of lung volume. To establish this, perform the following steps:

- Ask the child to take a deep breath and hold it.
- Percuss downward to locate the bottom of the lungs (the percussion note changes from resonant to flat at that point).
- Ask the child to expire fully and momentarily hold that position.
- Percuss upward to locate the expired or empty lung position (the percussion note changes from flat to resonant).

The difference between these two points is the diaphragmatic excursion. Children who have overexpanded lungs from obstructive disease have little diaphragmatic excursion in relation to others.

Auscultate breath sounds by listening with the diaphragm of a stethoscope over each lung lobe while a child inhales and exhales (preferably with the mouth open). Listen both anteriorly and posteriorly; compare the left side with the right side for equal findings. Usual breath sounds are slightly longer on inspiration than expiration. Consider whether there are any abnormal sounds. Table 34.4 describes usual breath sounds and transmitted airway sounds as well as adventitious sounds that, if heard, might reflect illness.

The Newborn and Infant. Infants cannot breathe in and out on request. Try to listen to breath sounds early in an examination, because breath sounds are difficult to hear clearly over the sound of crying.

The Heart

Heart assessment begins with asking children if they have ever noticed any cardiac symptoms such as pain. Visual inspection to see if there is a point on the chest where the heartbeat can be observed follows this. This point represents the location of the left ventricle or the point where the apical heartbeat can be heard best. In children younger than 7 years of age, this point is generally lateral to the nipple line and at the fourth intercostal space. In children older than 4 years, it is at the nipple line or just medial to it and at the fifth intercostal space. This point is termed the **point of maximum impulse** (PMI) and is observable in approximately 50% of children.

Percuss the left side of the chest to discern the left side of the heart. Percussing in from the axilla, the sound will become dull as the heart is identified. Normally, the percussion note changes from resonant (i.e., percussing over lung) to flat (i.e., percussing over heart) midway between the midaxillary and midmammary line. A heart located further to the left than this suggests enlargement.

Heart Sounds

To assess heart function, first listen over the heart and record the rate (Fig. 34.17). Compare this to the child's age to determine if it is normal. To hear differences in first and second heart sounds, auscultate at the four main points in the following

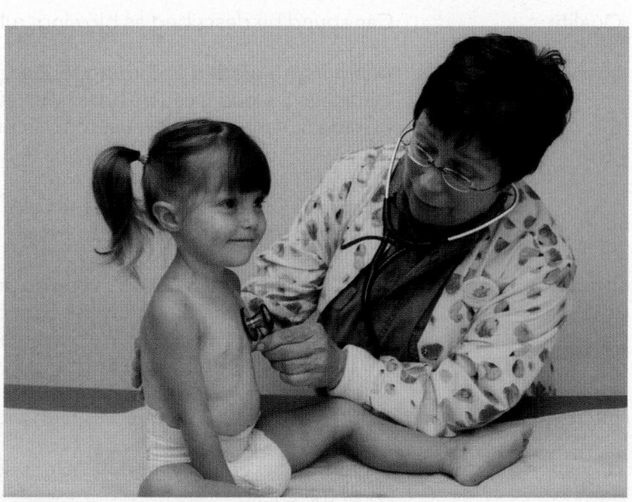

FIGURE 34.17 Auscultating heart sounds.

TABLE 34.5 Heart Sounds Heard on Auscultation

Sound	Cause
S_1 (first heart sound)	Closure of tricuspid and mitral valves with beginning of ventricular contraction (systole)
S_2 (second heart sound)	Closure of pulmonary and aortic valves with beginning of atrial contraction (diastole)
S_3 (third heart sound)	Rapid ventricular filling
S_4 (fourth heart sound)	Abnormal filling of ventricles

bullets. Although these are not the anatomic locations of heart valves, they are the sites to which the sounds of the valves radiate and can be heard best in children (see Fig. 34.15).

- The mitral valve is heard best at the fourth or fifth left intercostal space at the nipple line.
- The tricuspid valve is heard best near the base of the sternum (fourth or fifth right intercostal space).
- The pulmonary valve is heard best at the second left intercostal space.
- The aortic valve is heard best at the second right intercostal space.

Table 34.5 describes normal and abnormal heart sounds, which may be heard on auscultation. Abnormal sounds are heard best if you listen first through the diaphragm of the stethoscope, followed by the bell.

To understand heart sounds, recall heart physiology. The first sound heard (S_1) is that of the mitral and tricuspid valves closing and the ventricles contracting (described as a "lub" sound). The second sound (S_2; described as a "dub" sound) is made by the closure of the aortic and pulmonary valves and atrial contraction. The first sound is generally longer and lower pitched than the second. Over the heart ventricles it is louder, but at other sites tends to be slightly quieter.

The rhythm of the heart sounds should be regular. **Sinus arrhythmia** is a normal but marked heart rate increase that occurs as a child inspires and a marked decrease in heart rate as the child expires, and is frequently noted in school-age children and adolescents. Ask a child to take and hold a breath, and the rhythm of the heart should remain steady.

Another variation in heart sounds occurs because with inspiration and the resulting increase of pressure in the lungs, the pulmonary valve closes slightly later than the aortic valve. This is termed **physiologic splitting** and is heard as a "lub d-dub" sound. As long as this is associated with inspiration, it is a normal finding. Splitting that is always present implies there is difficulty with the pulmonary valve closing and suggests pathology.

At times, a distinct third heart sound (S_3) may be heard due to rapid filling of the ventricles. Although this is not necessarily a serious finding, further investigation is warranted. The presence of a fourth heart sound (S_4) generally signifies heart pathology because this sound (a gallop rhythm) is caused by an abnormal filling of the ventricles, which causes increased pressure on values.

Lastly, listen for heart murmurs. These are caused by the sound of blood flowing with difficulty or in an abnormal pathway within the heart (sounds like a swishing sound) and can be either innocent (i.e., functional) or pathogenic (i.e., organic). If a heart is pumping with abnormal force, there may be a palpable vibration, termed a *thrill*, on the chest wall. Palpate the precordium (i.e., area over the heart) for evidence of this (feels like a cat purring) or a heave (a definite outward chest movement), which also denotes a struggling heart. On hearing or palpating any accessory heart sounds or movements, describe them with reference to Table 34.6.

TABLE 34.6 Description of Accessory Heart Sounds

Assessment	Information to be Gathered
Location	At which listening post is the sound most distinct?
Quality	Can sound be described as blowing, rubbing, rasping, or musical?
Intensity	*Murmurs* are graded according to the following criteria: - Grade 6: So loud it can be heard with stethoscope not touching the chest wall; has a thrill (palpable vibration). - Grade 5: Very loud but must touch stethoscope to chest to hear; has a thrill. - Grade 4: Loud; may or may not have a thrill. - Grade 3: Moderately loud; no thrill. - Grade 2: Quiet, but easily discernible. - Grade 1: Very quiet; difficult to hear.
Timing	When in relation to S_1 and S_2, did you hear the murmur? A sound superimposed between S_1 and S_2 is a *systolic murmur*, one between S_2 and the next S_1 is a *diastolic murmur*. Innocent murmurs (functional, denoting no pathology) are usually systolic, although there are exceptions to this. Pathologic murmurs are more likely to be diastolic.
Pitch	Can the sound be described as high pitched or low pitched?
Radiation and thrills	Is there an accompanying thrill? Does sound radiate so it can be heard at another location, such as the back of the chest?

All unusual heart sounds need further identification and investigation as to their cause. The skills of listening to and identifying normal and abnormal heart sounds require considerable practice. Determining the cause of an abnormal heart sound requires a cardiac specialist. However, determining that an abnormal sound exists and securing proper referral is an important nursing role.

The Newborn, Infant, and Toddler. Listen to heart sounds in young children early in an examination, before a child begins to cry, because it is almost impossible to evaluate heart sounds over the sound of crying. Allowing a parent to hold a child while listening to the heart helps reduce fear.

The School-Age Child and Adolescent. Listen carefully for sounds of murmurs in children of school age and older. Be particularly conscientious with student athletes; it seems paradoxical that they could have heart disease, but if present, this could be fatal to them during athletic events (Patel & Elliott, 2012). Refer them to their primary health care provider for further evaluation if any abnormalities are detected. Parents are always frightened by an unusual heart sound, but unless the child has other symptoms, they can be assured that although you are referring them, most murmurs are innocent (i.e., functional) and caused only by the normal flow of blood across valves.

✔ QSEN Checkpoint Question 34.5

Informatics

You are using your stethoscope to auscultate the sound of Keoto's mitral heart value closing. The best location to listen would be which of the following?

a. Over the anterior sternum
b. The right 9th or 10th intercostal space
c. The left interior rim of the left clavicle
d. The fourth or fifth left intercostal space at the nipple line

Look in Appendix A for the best answer and rationale.

The Abdomen

The abdomen is anatomically divided into four quadrants. The quadrants and the organs that lie within them are shown in Figure 34.18. To assess an abdomen, first inspect the surface for symmetry and contour. It will be slightly protuberant in infants and scaphoid in older children. Note any skin lesions or scars.

Auscultate the abdomen for bowel sounds before palpating, because palpating may alter bowel action (i.e., peristalsis) and therefore disturb bowel sounds. Bowel sounds can normally be heard in all quadrants of the abdomen. They are high "pinging" sounds that occur normally at intervals of approximately 5 to 10 seconds, and because they are high-pitched sounds, are heard best with the bell of a stethoscope. If the bowel is distended, the sounds occur more frequently; if the bowel is blocked, so there is no movement of contents, sounds will be absent below the obstruction. Listen for 3 to 5 minutes before concluding that no bowel sounds are present to be certain they are not just widely spaced.

Next, listen along the middle of the abdomen over the aorta for irregular sounds. A **bruit** is a swishing or blowing sound that occurs if there is an outpouching of the aorta (i.e., an aneurysm), a condition that can be congenital, although it usually occurs with aging.

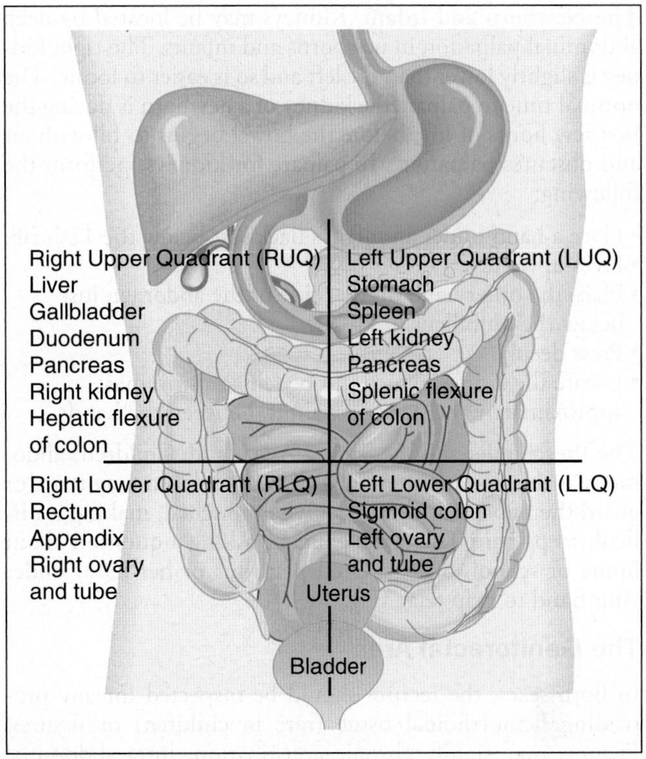

FIGURE 34.18 The quadrants of the abdomen and underlying structures.

Palpate the abdomen in a systematic manner (e.g., the lower left quadrant, upper left quadrant, upper right quadrant, lower left quadrant) to include all four quadrants. First palpate lightly, then deeply. Ascertain whether any area is tender by watching the child's face while palpating; observe for guarding or the child tensing the abdominal muscles to keep you from pressing deeply at that point. If a child indicates that any portion of the abdomen is tender, begin assessment at the farthest point and work toward the tender area. If no tenderness is present, the order of palpation is unimportant as long as it is thorough. Note any hard areas or masses. If a tender area is detected, attempt to elicit rebound tenderness to determine its cause. To do this, press on the abdomen, then lift your hand suddenly. This causes internal organs to vibrate. Although all children do not show this sign, the occurrence of more pain with the vibration than with the original pressure is one of the standard diagnostic criteria for appendicitis (Santillanes, Simms, Gausche-Hill, et al., 2012).

When palpating from the right lower quadrant to the right upper quadrant, the hand will bump against the lower edge of the liver 1 to 2 cm below the right ribs. On the left side, the lower edge of the spleen may be discernible in the same way. A liver or spleen larger than this is suggestive of disease. Lastly, palpate the umbilicus to try to identify the presence of an umbilical hernia. A fascial ring at the umbilicus of more than 2 cm in diameter in an infant denotes a ring of fascia larger than will normally close spontaneously; when this is present, the child will generally need surgery to prevent an umbilical hernia. Liver, spleen, and bladder size can all be documented further by percussion.

The Newborn and Infant. Kidneys may be located by deep abdominal palpation in newborns and infants. The right kidney is slightly lower than the left and so is easier to locate. The optimal time to palpate the kidney of a newborn is during the first few hours of life, before the bowel begins to fill with air and obscures palpation. To palpate for kidneys, perform the following:

- Place a hand under an infant's back just below the 12th rib.
- Press upward.
- Place the other hand on that side of the abdomen just below the umbilicus.
- Press deeply.
- Locate the kidney, which can be felt as a firm mass approximately the size of a walnut, between the hands.

The Preschooler and the School-Age Child. Children's abdomens at this age are often ticklish, and children may tense or guard their abdominal muscles when touched, making it difficult to palpate. Distract a child by asking a question about home or school, or let a child place his or her hand under your hand to help relax (Fig. 34.19).

The Genitorectal Area

In both sexes, the rectum should be inspected for any protruding hemorrhoidal tissue (rare in children) or fissures. Fissures may signify chronic constipation, intra-abdominal pressure, or sexual maltreatment.

The Female Genitalia. Inspection of the external genitalia and an assessment of femoral nodes are included in every complete health assessment in girls (Braverman & Breech, 2010). An external examination consists of inspecting for the Tanner stage of pubic hair growth and configuration (i.e., an inverted triangle) and inspection of external genitalia (i.e., clitoris, labia majora, and labia minora) for normal contours. Look for signs of discharge or irritation. A vaginal discharge that suggests infection or a fourchette tear in a young child may be an indication of sexual maltreatment, and in an adolescent, this can be an indication of rape (Berkowitz, 2011).

A pelvic examination is usually scheduled at the time the girl becomes sexually active, at 21 years of age, or at the first sign of a gynecologic disorder (American Academy of Pediatrics [AAP], 2012). The technique for internal pelvic examinations is discussed in Chapter 11.

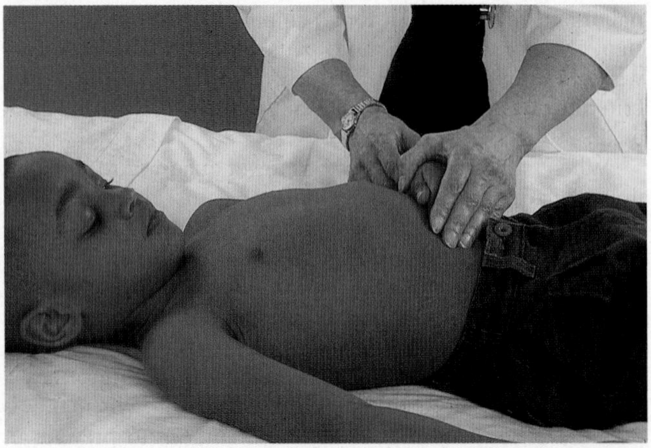

FIGURE 34.19 Decrease ticklishness during abdominal palpation by placing the child's hand under yours.

The Male Genitalia. Inspection of male genitalia consists of observing:

- The distribution and the Tanner stage of pubic hair, which has a diamond shape.
- The penis, for lesions that might suggest a sexually transmitted infection.
- Appearance and placement of the urethral opening, which should be slit-like and centered at the penis tip. Note whether the boy is circumcised because boys who are uncircumcised have more urinary tract infections than those who are circumcised (Dubrovsky, Foster, Jednak, et al., 2012); repeated urinary tract infections can cause scarring of the meatal opening, making it small and round.
- The ability to retract the foreskin, if a boy is uncircumcised. *Phimosis* exists when the foreskin of a child older than 6 to 12 months is too tight to retract.

Hypospadias means the urethral opening is located on the inferior or ventral (i.e., under) surface of the penis; **epispadias** denotes a urethral opening on the superior or dorsal (i.e., upper) surface. Both these conditions need to be identified. If more than a slight deviation is present, repair is usually initiated before school age because such a urethral placement may interfere with self-image if not corrected. During adulthood, it can interfere with fertility.

Inspect the scrotum for size and the presence of testes. In most boys, the left testicle is slightly lower than the right, so the scrotum does not appear truly symmetric. Palpate to check that both testes are present by placing one hand at the top of the scrotum over the inguinal ring and then palpating the testis on that side (see Chapter 18, Fig. 18.21). This hand position prevents the testis from slipping up into the inguinal ring and appearing to be absent on palpation. Any swelling or mass in the scrotum needs to be identified. The most likely cause of such a condition is a **hydrocele** (i.e., a fluid-filled sac), but it could represent a serious finding such as testicular cancer in adolescents. Hydroceles can be transilluminated; when a flashlight is held in back of the scrotum, the fluid-filled cyst glows. A **varicocele** (i.e., enlarged veins of the epididymis) may be palpated. These are not important findings in young boys, but they could possibly interfere with fertility later in life.

Assess the urethral meatus for any discharge that could reveal a sexually transmitted infection, such as gonorrhea, or any lesions that would suggest herpes simplex type 2 infection or syphilis (see Chapter 47). Palpate femoral nodes (located in the groin and on the inner surface of the upper thigh) for any swelling, which suggests infection. Beginning at puberty, teach boys to do testicular palpations every month. The technique for this is described in Box 34.10.

To assess for the presence of an inguinal hernia in an infant, simply observe the groin area for any bulging, especially while the infant is crying. In the school-age child or adolescent, with the child standing, place a fingertip against the inguinal ring in the groin area and ask the child to cough. If the tendency for a hernia is present, coughing tightens the abdominal muscles and forces the abdominal contents to bulge against the finger.

The Extremities

Observe the upper extremities for good color and warmth. Because changes in fingernails can be a sign of overall ill health, inspect them for color, contour, and shape (Shah

BOX 34.10 Nursing Care Planning Based on Family Teaching

TESTICULAR SELF-EXAMINATION

Q. Keoto's father asks you, "What is the best technique for testicular self-examination?"

A. Starting in their adolescent years, all males need to perform testicular self-examination once a month. Follow these guidelines:

- Select a certain day each month (e.g., first day, last day) to perform the examination.
- Perform the examination in or immediately after a shower, because warmth makes scrotal skin relaxed.
- Gently roll each testicle between your thumb and fingers, feeling for any hard lumps or nodules, a change in consistency, or a difference in size.
- Also feel for the epididymis, found at the rear of the testes. It should feel like a strong cord.
- Remember that for most males, one testicle is slightly larger than the other and hangs a little lower in the scrotal sac.
- If you notice any changes in size, tenderness, or unusual mass, call or visit your health care provider.

& Rubin, 2012). Normally, nails are pink (or deeply pigmented in darker skinned children), smooth, and convex. They should feel hard to the touch but not so brittle that they break readily. Signs of bitten fingernails in the school-age child may reflect a high level of stress. A blue or purple tinge denotes cyanosis; a yellow tinge denotes jaundice. Children who have decreased respiratory function or heart disease develop clubbed fingers (Fig. 34.20); children with endocarditis often have characteristic linear hemorrhages under the nails.

Iron-deficiency anemia may cause extremely concave surfaces of fingernails (spoon shaped). Press against a fingernail, release the pressure, and time the refilling interval (should be under 5 seconds). Count the fingers and check for webbing between fingers. Examine that fingerprints are present. Distinctive dermatoglyphics are present on fingertips from the third month of intrauterine life; these are unique to every person and show patterns of circular grooves. Abnormal fingerprints may occur with chromosomal anomalies. Check also for normal palmar creases. Children with chromosomal abnormalities may have only one central palm crease (i.e., a simian line) on each hand rather than the normal three (see Chapter 7). Check the wrist, elbow, and shoulder joints for movement and for normal range of motion; palpate joints for swelling or warmth. Palpate to be certain no lymph nodes are present in the antecubital space; palpate to check that a radial pulse is present.

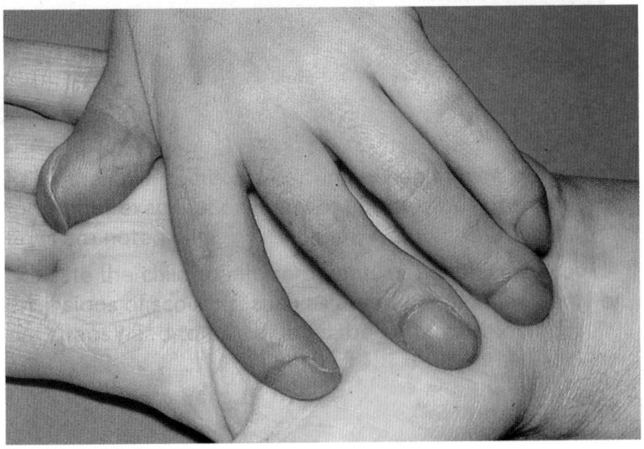

FIGURE 34.20 Clubbed fingers are a sign of cyanosis from heart or respiratory disease. (NMSB/Custom Medical Stock Photo.)

Inspect the lower extremities for color and warmth. Count the toes and check for webbing between toes. Check the ankle, knee, and hip joints for normal range of motion. Check for developmental hip dysplasia in infants by attempting to abduct the hips fully (see Chapter 18, Fig. 18.22). Palpate to ensure no enlarged lymph nodes are present in the groin or popliteal areas and that femoral pulses are present and equal bilaterally. Ask the older child to walk, and observe for ease of gait, limping, or any foot displacement such as toeing in or out. Toddlers typically walk with a wide-based gait; they walk best if allowed to walk toward their parent (a safe action) rather than away. Remember many adolescents are self-conscious and slouch or amble rather than present their true, natural gait. Children who limp need a further evaluation. A limp can be due to something as simple as a blister on the foot from wearing new shoes, or can be a sign of a serious hip or bone condition (Perry, Green, Bruce, et al., 2012).

The Back

Inspect the back for symmetry and the spinal column for any deviation. Inspect the base of the spine for a dermal sinus (i.e., a pinpoint opening) or a tuft of hair or a hemangioma that might reveal spina bifida occulta (i.e., a defect of the bony structure of the canal). Also inspect for any dimpling that might denote a dermal cyst (i.e., pilonidal cyst). This is an innocent finding unless it becomes infected or connects to deeper tissue layers. Assess for tenderness along the spinal column by palpating each vertebra because chronic lower back pain can be present as early as school age (King, Chambers, Huguet, et al., 2011).

A routine assessment of the school-age child beginning at 12 years of age and through adolescence should include screening for scoliosis (i.e., sideways curvature of the spine) (Walter, 2011). Box 34.11 details the steps to follow for a scoliosis screening exam (see Chapter 51 for more details on scoliosis).

Neurologic Function

A full neurologic examination takes at least 20 minutes to complete, so this is not included in a routine physical examination. It is important, however, to assess for **deep tendon reflexes** (such as triceps, biceps, patellar, and Achilles

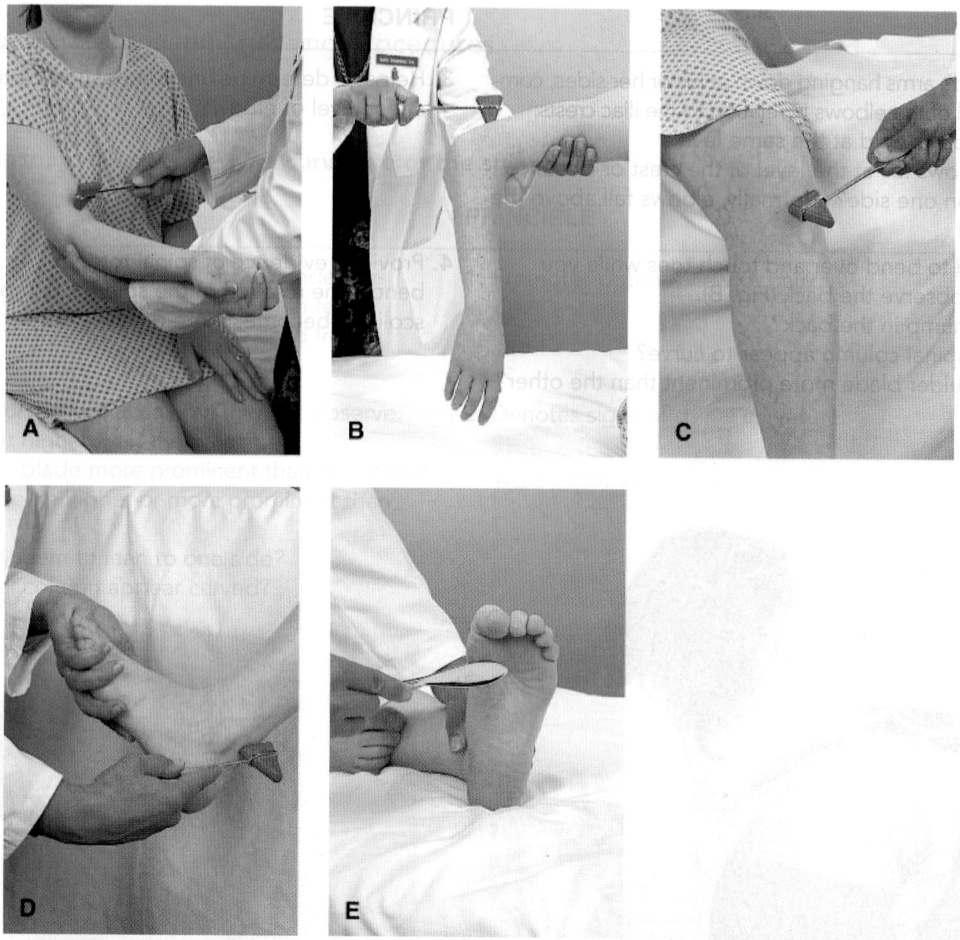

FIGURE 34.21 Techniques for eliciting major reflexes. **(A)** The biceps reflex. **(B)** The triceps reflex. **(C)** The patellar reflex. **(D)** The ankle or Achilles reflex. **(E)** The Babinski response. (From Weber, J., & Kelley, J. [2003]. Health assessment in nursing [2nd ed.]. Philadelphia, PA: Lippincott Williams & Wilkins. Images © B. Proud.)

reflexes) to test for motor and sensory function and balance and coordination. Techniques for eliciting deep tendon reflexes are shown in Figure 34.21. Grade reflexes according to the scale is shown in Table 34.7. The biceps reflex tests the fifth and sixth cervical nerves; the triceps reflex tests the seventh and eighth cervical; the patellar reflex tests the second, third, and fourth lumbar; and the Achilles reflex tests the first and second sacral. Test the sole of the foot for a Babinski reflex (see Chapter 18, Fig. 18.9). Fanning of the toes will occur in an infant younger than 3 months of age; a downward reflex of the toes will occur beyond 3 months of age. (Some normal infants demonstrate a flaring Babinski response until they are 2 years of age and, in the absence of other neurologic findings, this is not significant.)

Test for superficial reflexes: abdominal reflexes in both sexes, and a cremasteric reflex in boys. An abdominal reflex is elicited by lightly stroking each quadrant of the abdomen. Normally, the umbilicus moves perceptibly toward the stroke. Presence of the reflex indicates integrity of the 10th thoracic nerve and the first lumbar nerve of the spinal cord. A cremasteric reflex is elicited by stroking the medial aspect of the thigh in boys. With this, the testes move perceptibly upward. The presence of this reflex indicates integrity of the first and second lumbar nerves.

TABLE 34.7 Grading of Deep Tendon Reflexes

Grade	Interpretation
4+	Hyperactive; extremely marked reaction; abnormal
3+	Stronger than average, but within normal range
2+	Average response
1+	Less than average response, but within normal range
0	No response; abnormal

Motor and Sensory Function

Test general facial nerve function by asking a child to make a face. The child's ability to grasp with the hands and push against a surface with the feet establishes general motor ability. Recall whether the child's gait was adequate when observed walking to assess for balance and coordination.

To test sensory function, ask children to close their eyes and identify the location where you touch them at (at least) six points on different body parts.

What if...34.2 Although you know children should be completely undressed for physical examinations so all body surfaces can be inspected, Candy's father says he doesn't want Candy undressed because the exam room is too cold. What if he did not want to remove a Band-Aid from Candy's back?

VISION ASSESSMENT

Assessing vision is an important part of a physical assessment because good vision is so important to childhood development. The extent and type of testing depends on the age of the child.

Any child with congenital anomalies, low birth weight, or fetal alcohol syndrome is at risk for eye abnormalities, as is a child who received oxygen at birth. During an assessment, if you notice an unreported eye injury or infection or signs of neglected vision, make a special note. Because the average parent is careful of a child's eyes, these findings may be indicative of child neglect.

Vision Screening

Routine vision screening is usually begun at 3 years of age. Parents can provide important clues to possible problems; therefore, listen carefully any time a parent expresses concern about or questions a child's ability to see well. Common vision screening, indicators, and techniques for children of different ages are summarized in Table 34.8.

TABLE 34.8 Common Vision Screening Indicators and Procedures

Age	Common Test
Newborn	General appearance* Ability to follow moving object to midline; focus steadily on an object at 10–12 in.
Infant and toddler	General appearance* Ability to follow light past midline
Age 3 years to school age	General appearance* Random dot E for stereopsis (depth perception) Allen cards or preschool E chart for visual acuity Ishihara's plates for color awareness
School age to adult	General appearance* Snellen test for visual acuity

*Note redness, blinking, squinting, crusting of eyes, or tilting of head.

The Newborn and Infant. Newborns should be able to focus on a moving object such as a finger and follow it to the midline. Infants see black and white objects better than they do colored objects. They seem to see objects that are at a distance of about 19 cm [8 to 10 in.]) best. Ask parents if an infant's eyes follow them as they move around the room. Does an infant who is older than 6 weeks return their smile? Do the parents have any reason to think their child has difficulty seeing?

The Toddler and Preschooler. Ask parents if their children do any of the following, which may be signs of vision problems:

- Rub their eyes, blink frequently, squint, or frown
- Cover one eye to look at objects
- Tilt the head to see things better
- Stumble over objects in their path
- Hold books and toys extremely close or extremely far away to look at them

Asking whether children sit close to a television set is meaningless because almost all children sit closer than necessary if allowed.

The School-Age Child and Adolescent. Ask the parents if their child:

- Reports difficulty seeing
- Reports frequent headaches
- Does poorly with class work
- Avoids sports that require long-distance vision, such as baseball or softball
- Avoids watching movies
- Skips over words when reading aloud
- Reports blurriness or double vision
- Has reddened conjunctivae or drainage from the eyes
- Blinks at bright light

Techniques of Vision Testing

Vision is tested by asking a child to read a standardized eye chart. All children need good orientation to such testing so they can appreciate that this is not a test in the usual sense of the word; otherwise, they may be unusually anxious or try to "pass" it by cheating. Vision testing needs to be started in the preschool period, so children with amblyopia (i.e., lazy eye; see Chapter 50), a potentially serious vision disorder, can be identified while the condition is still correctable (Archer, 2012). In addition to usual testing, a digital photo of the child's face can be used to help identify strabismus (i.e., uneven gaze or eyes not symmetrically aligned).

The Snellen Chart. As soon as children can identify letters of the alphabet (i.e., early school age), their vision can be tested by use of a Snellen eye chart. Because this chart is standardized, set procedures must be followed when using it to test vision (Box 34.12).

The Preschool E Chart. Between 3 years of age and the age when children can read the alphabet, they can be tested by use of a preschool E chart (Fig. 34.22). This chart is also helpful to test children who are cognitively challenged or those who do not speak fluent English. The procedure is similar to that of the standard Snellen chart:

1. The child stands 20 ft from the chart and reads first with the right eye, then with the left, then with both eyes.

BOX 34.12 Nursing Care Planning Using Procedures

SNELLEN EYE CHART ASSESSMENT

Purpose: To assess vision.

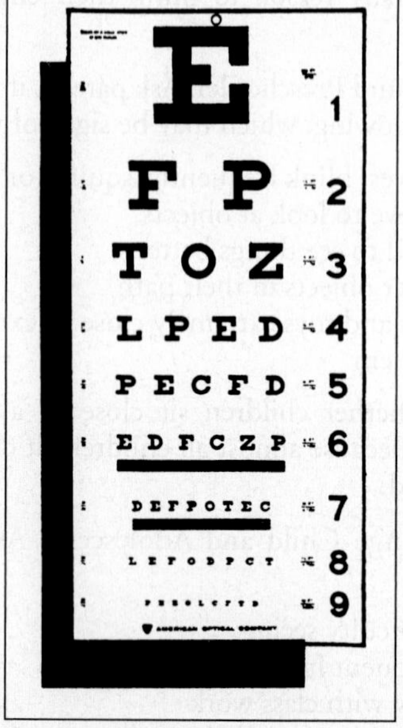

PROCEDURE	PRINCIPLE
1. Hang the chart so the 20-ft line is at the child's eye level.	1. The child who has to look up or down must look farther than the child who is looking straight across at the chart. A possible solution to avoid moving the chart is to have smaller children stand and taller children sit. To accommodate children in wheelchairs, the chart needs to be lowered (or have all children sit for the test).
2. Provide a good light for the chart and place it so there is no glare. A light intensity of 20-ft candles is recommended.	2. Appropriate lighting provides for optimal test conditions.
3. Measure a distance of 20 ft from the chart. Mark the floor at this point with a piece of masking tape or other similar mark. For younger children, it is helpful to cut out paper footprints and paste them to the floor with the heels of the footprints touching the 20-ft line. If the child sits in a chair, the back legs of the chair should touch the 20-ft line.	3. Twenty feet is the optimal distance from the chart for testing.
4. Provide the child being examined with a 3″ × 5″ card to cover the eye not being tested.	4. Covering the other eye allows for one eye to be tested at a time.
5. If the child wears glasses, screen first with the glasses in place. Do not screen the child first without glasses and then with them, because this forces the child to strain to read the chart.	5. Testing with corrective lenses screens for corrected eyesight. After squinting, a child may have difficulty readjusting to reading with glasses, and this makes the prescription appear too weak or too strong.
6. To begin testing, tell the child to stand with shoes on the footprints (heels against the line), keep both eyes open, and cover the left eye with the occluding card. Be certain the child does not press the card against the eye (instead, the edge of the card should rest across the child's nose).	6. Covering the eye not being tested provides one eye to be tested at a time. Pressure will cause blurred vision when the child removes the card to test that eye.

PROCEDURE	PRINCIPLE
7. Begin at the 40-ft line of the chart and, using a pointer or pencil, point to each symbol on the line from left to right (the order in which children are taught to read). If the child reads the majority of symbols in a line, the line is passed satisfactorily.	7. Starting at the 40-ft line is the standardized testing procedure.
8. If the child "passes" the 40-ft line, have the child read the 30- and 20-ft lines or the last line the child can read. Record the last line read. If the child fails to read the 40-ft line satisfactorily, then begin at the top of the chart and move downward to identify the last line the child can read. Record this reading. Because the 200-ft, 100-ft, and 70-ft lines have so few symbols, the child must read all the symbols on them to have read them satisfactorily.	8. Moving to the 30-ft line or less reflects use of the standardized testing procedure.
9. Visual acuity is always stated as a fraction. The top number is the distance in feet the child stands from the chart (always 20). The bottom of the fraction represents the last line the child read correctly. The adult with good (average) vision can read the 20-ft line from 20 ft away and thus is said to have 20/20 vision.	9. Using a fraction for visual acuity is the standardized reporting procedure.
10. It is important to test the eyes separately, then together. For example, suppose Keoto reads all the symbols on the 40-ft line with her right eye, but she misses three out of four on the 30-ft line. Her visual acuity for her right eye is 20/40 (the distance from the chart/the last line she read correctly). With her left eye, she reads the 40-ft, 30-ft, and 20-ft lines correctly. Her vision in that eye is 20/20. With both eyes, Keoto reads the 40-ft, 30-ft, and 20-ft lines correctly. Her visual acuity for both eyes is therefore 20/20.	10. If only this last reading were taken, the right eye weakness (a symptom of amblyopia or "lazy eye") would be missed.
11. Observe children for straining or squinting as they read the chart.	11. By squinting and changing the shape of the eyeball, children can improve vision and will score higher; therefore, children will appear to see better than they actually do in everyday situations.

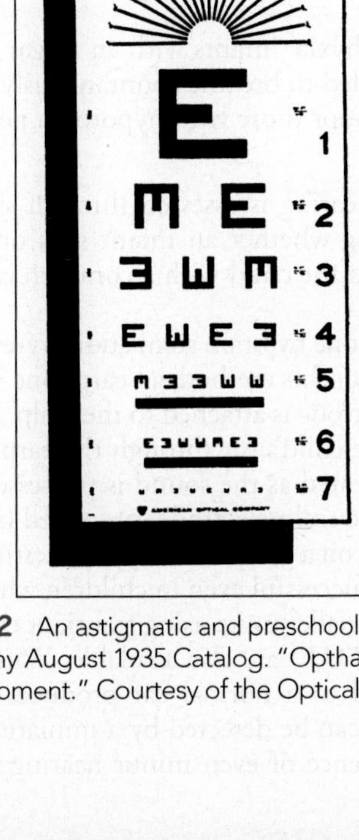

FIGURE 34.22 An astigmatic and preschool E chart. American Optical Company August 1935 Catalog. "Opthamalogical Instruments and Equipment." Courtesy of the Optical Heritage Museum.

Young children do not understand the importance of not pressing the card against their eye and of not peeking, so a second person is often needed to hold the occluder card for children of this age.

2. Compare the E on the chart with a table with three legs and ask the child which way the legs of the table point. By 3 years of age, children are familiar with tables, but the letter E may still be a strange symbol. Tell the child to point with the entire arm and hand in the direction the legs point so you do not confuse the hand motion.
3. Ask the child to begin by looking at the 40-ft line, as with a standard Snellen chart, and work downward until the child passes all lines or cannot read the majority of symbols on a line. Record the distance from the chart and the last line read correctly (20 over the last correct line).

The National Association for the Prevention of Blindness Home Test. A home eye test is available from the National Association for the Prevention of Blindness for parents to test children ages 3 to 6 years at home. It is similar to the preschool E chart except it is smaller and the child stands only 10 ft away. The test can help alert parents that a child needs a professional eye examination. Home tests can be given or suggested to parents whose child is tired or who, for some other reason, does not test well in a health care facility (Prevent Blindness America [PBA], 2012).

Allen Cards. Allen cards consist of pictures of common objects such as a horse and rider, a car, a house, and a birthday cake. The cards are shown to the child at a 15-ft distance and the child is asked to identify the pictures (proof the child sees them). Be certain children have time to examine the cards before the test so you're sure they know the names of the objects.

STYCAR Cards. For this test, a child is given cards with nine letters: H, C, O, L, U, T, X, V, and A. The child holds up the card that matches the one you point to on a STYCAR chart.

Titmus Vision Tester. Another useful method for testing the vision of children is the Titmus Vision Tester, the same instrument used by many motor vehicle licensing offices. As the child looks into the eyepieces of the machine, alphabet letters, or preschool Es are projected onto a screen for the child to identify. Closed vision testers such as the Titmus have an advantage over wall charts in that a child is less easily distracted during testing. Also, because children cannot see the vision chart beforehand, they cannot memorize the letters while waiting to be tested.

Vision Color Awareness Testing. The inability to discern colors is a sex-linked recessive characteristic that occurs in males rather than in females, although females carry the recessive gene for the disorder. All male children should be screened once for the disorder during their early school years.

To test a child for color awareness, ask the child to identify the colored stripes at the top of a Snellen eye chart or show the child a series of colored diagrams (i.e., Ishihara plates). With the latter, a person with color vision is able to see hidden figures such as butterflies, but people with red-green or yellow-blue color vision deficits cannot. Detecting a color vision deficit in children is important because many educational materials and some occupations depend on the ability to identify color. Even such a simple childhood pleasure as riding a bicycle safely on city streets depends on being able to distinguish colors, such as deciphering red from green on a traffic light.

Vision Referrals

Always screen children twice before referring them to their primary care provider. Some children do not perform well on eye tests because they are too easily distracted or do not know their alphabet as well as they pretend (e.g., they may say they do not see a letter when they really mean they do not know or remember its name). Testing twice helps eliminate or identify this type of misleading result.

After a second screening, the following children generally require a vision referral:

- Preschool children (3 to 5 years of age) who have 20/50 vision or less in one or both eyes
- Children 6 years of age or older who have 20/40 vision or less in one or both eyes
- Any child with a two-line difference between the eyes, as this might be a beginning of amblyopia
- Any child who states or shows other symptoms of visual difficulty (PBA, 2012)

What if... 34.3 Keoto's father expresses concern she may have a vision problem because she always sits very close to a television set. Keoto doesn't want to be tested because, she "will never wear glasses." What questions on history would be important to ask her? What type of eye chart would you use with Keoto to assess her vision?

HEARING ASSESSMENT

A thorough health assessment should also include an evaluation of hearing, including both history and observation, because good hearing is so important for the development of age-appropriate skills. Parents and grandparents are usually attuned to hearing difficulty in children and may be suspicious of it in advance of its official detection. When taking an auditory history, therefore, be certain to ask the accompanying adult or parent an overall question such as, "Do you have any reason to believe your child doesn't hear as well as other children?"

Auditory Screening

Routine screening for adequate hearing levels is usually begun at 3 years of age. Testing requires knowledge of the technique, use of an audiometer, and a quiet, undistracted setting.

The Newborn and Infant. All infants should be screened at birth. Those most apt to be born with a hearing difficulty are those with:

- A history of childhood hearing impairment in the family
- Perinatal infection, such as cytomegalovirus, rubella, herpes, toxoplasmosis, or syphilis
- Anatomic malformations involving the head or neck
- Birth weight less than 1,500 g
- Hyperbilirubinemia at a level exceeding indication for exchange transfusion
- Bacterial meningitis, especially when caused by *Haemophilus influenzae*
- Severe birth asphyxia: infants with an Apgar score of 0 to 3, those who failed to breathe spontaneously within 10 minutes of birth, or those with hypotonia persisting to 2 hours of age

A newborn's hearing is assessed through simple response testing—observing whether an infant stirs or responds to a sound delivered to the child with a commercial sound device (CDC, 2012a).

It can also be done by brain stem auditory-evoked response (BAER) testing. For this method, an earphone is placed on the infant and an electrode is attached to the scalp. When sound is transmitted to the child's ear through the earphone, the electrical potential created as the sound is processed by the brain stem is read by the scalp electrode, processed by a microcomputer, and plotted on a graph. This type of testing may be used at any age and is successful even in children who are comatose or anesthetized. Smaller units using transient evoked *otoacoustic* emissions (TEOAE) are also available. With these, a click stimulus delivered to a normal ear produces an echo from the cochlea. This can be detected by a miniature microphone to reveal the presence of even minor hearing loss. Although

TABLE 34.9 Levels of Hearing Loss

Hearing Loss (dB Level)	Hearing Level Present
Slight (less than 30 dB)	Inability to hear whispered words or faint speech No speech challenge present Possible lack of awareness of hearing difficulty Achievement in school and home is attained by leaning forward, speaking loudly
Mild (30–50 dB)	Beginning speech challenge may be present Difficulty hearing if not facing speaker; some difficulty with hearing normal conversation
Moderate (55–70 dB)	Speech challenge present, possibly requiring speech therapy Difficulty hearing normal conversation
Severe (70–90 dB)	Difficulty hearing any but nearby loud voice Vowels easier to hear than consonants Speech therapy required for clear speech Possible ability to still hear loud sounds such as jets or whistle of train
Profound (more than 90 dB)	Almost no sound heard

newborn hearing screening can lead to false-positive results because many infants of this age are still sleepy from birth analgesia and may have fluid- or vernix-filled ear canals, a repeat test usually decreases the incidence of false-positive results.

The Older Child. Older children who are at risk for hearing loss are those who have been exposed to loud noises such as an explosion or loud music, were of low birth weight, have congenital anomalies, have a repaired cleft palate, or have had repeated ear infections. During history taking, ask children if they ever worry if they have difficulty hearing. Be certain not to confuse difficulty hearing with shyness or recalcitrance in answering. Also ask them how they are doing in school. Some children with a minimal hearing impairment are considered to have behavioral problems in school because they do not follow directions well, when in fact they may be unable to hear the instruction. Children with an ear infection (i.e., otitis media) or allergies should be tested after the fluid in their ears clears because their hearing may be temporarily affected by these conditions. Almost all children have some cerumen (i.e., ear wax) in their ear canals; only when this becomes impacted is it a cause of hearing loss (Jones & Kacmarynski, 2012).

Principles of Audiometric Assessment

With proper instruction in technique, nurses conduct audiometric testing in schools and other ambulatory settings.

Frequency. Sound is the result of vibration; the frequency of sound is the number of vibrations a sound creates per second. When frequency is increased, the pitch of the sound increases. For audiometric testing, frequency is measured in hertz units. Normal speech sounds fall into a narrow range of 500 to 2,000 Hz; so, to function adequately and speak effectively, a child must be able to hear in this range. Children are tested for a wider frequency range than this, however, from 500 to 6,000 Hz, on a routine screening assessment.

Loudness. Decibels are an expression of the intensity or loudness of a sound (or vigor of the vibrations). A decibel level of 0 dB is the softest sound that can be heard. Normal conversation is held at approximately 50 to 60 dB. The sound level at which inner ear damage can occur is about 90 dB. Sound levels of 140 dB are so intense they actually cause pain. Screening audiometry is done at 25 dB.

Hearing Loss. Table 34.9 lists levels of hearing loss and the effect of hearing loss on conversation and speech. If children can hear all frequencies at the 25-dB level, they have passed an audiometric screening check. If a child fails to hear two or more frequencies at 25 dB, in either or both ears, the child has failed and should be referred to the primary care provider or an otologist. An **audiogram** is a record of audiometric testing. Figure 34.23 shows an audiogram of a child with normal hearing in the right ear (the child heard all frequencies at the 20-dB level), but with an inability to hear sounds softer than 45 dB in the left ear at frequencies of 1,000, 2,000, and 4,000 Hz.

Acoustic Impedance Testing

Acoustic impedance testing is based on the principle that sound entering the ear canal meets resistance at the tympanic membrane. If the middle ear is functioning normally, there will be a symmetric pattern of resistance on a tympanogram printout. If the middle ear is not functioning normally, the level of resistance will be greater or less, and so the pattern will be abnormal.

Acoustic impedance testing is performed by audiologists. For the assessment, the ear to be tested is plugged with a rubber disc. Sound is then administered to the ear through the center of the disk. The resistance met at the eardrum is registered and recorded as a graph. Tympanograms are inaccurate in children younger than 7 months of age because the tympanic membrane is too compliant under that age to register normal impedance.

Conduction Loss Testing

Both the Rinne and the Weber tests are used to perform assessments that can be used to identify conduction loss in older children (Box 34.13).

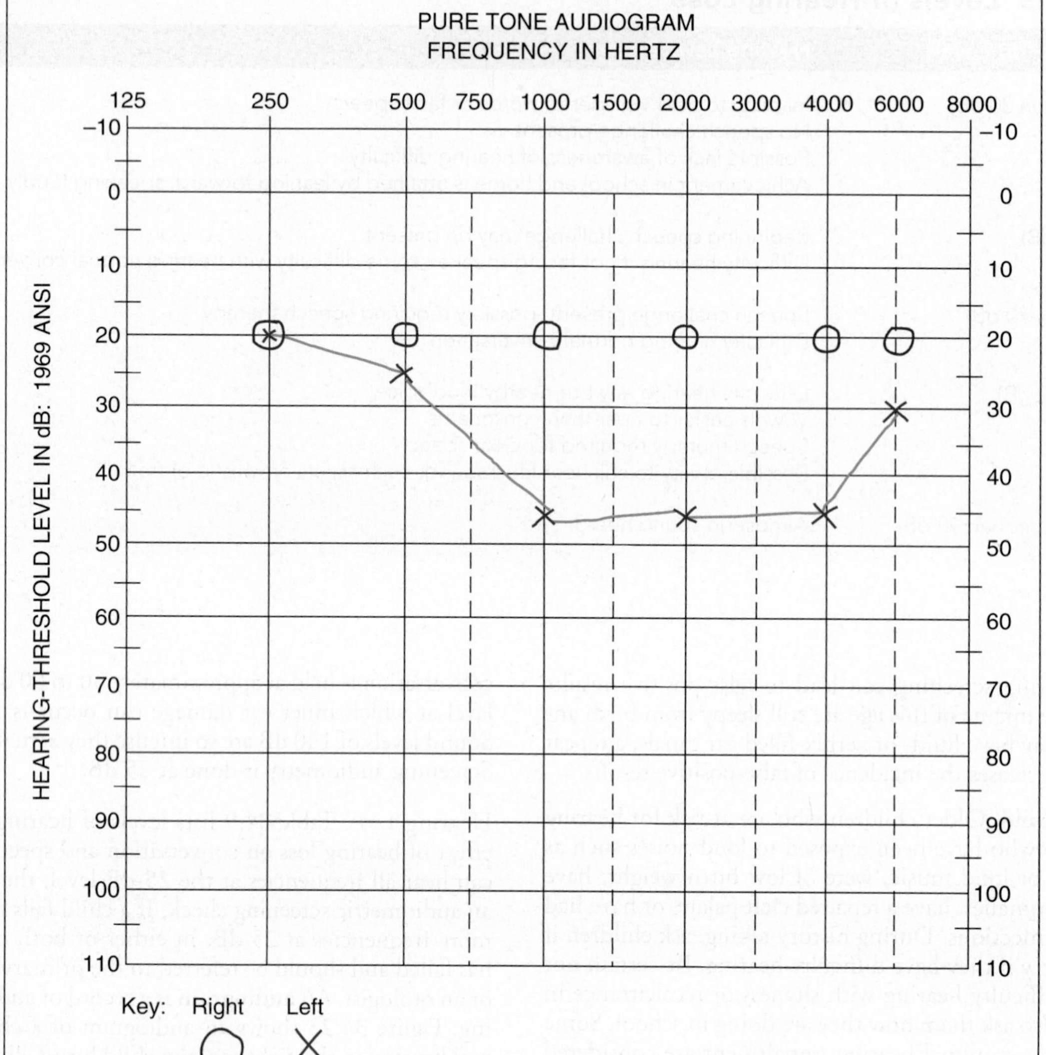

FIGURE 34.23 An audiogram done as a screening procedure. Notice that hearing is normal in the right ear (all frequencies are heard at the 20-dB level). In the left ear, there is hearing loss (the frequencies 1,000, 2,000, and 4,000 Hz are heard only at the 45-dB level). (Courtesy of Dr. H. Schill, Speech Pathology and Audiology Department, Boston University.)

SPEECH ASSESSMENT

Speech problems are directly related to hearing problems: infants who do not hear will make preliminary babbling sounds but then will not develop intelligible speech because they cannot hear speech sounds to repeat. Speech difficulties may also be related to:

- Motor development, such as when a child does not have enough control of tongue and facial muscles to be able to form words properly
- Cognitive development, such as when a cognitively challenged child cannot grasp the concept of speech or word use until later than usual, or possibly not at all
- Cultural influences, such as when parents speak two languages, making it difficult for a child to accurately learn and articulate either language or if parents spoke "baby talk" for so long that the child mimicked that instead of pronouncing words clearly

Speech screening begins by asking children a few simple questions to determine their language pattern. Also ask parents if they have noticed any difficulties with their child's pronunciation or comprehension. Standardized tests, such as the Denver Articulation Screening Examination (DASE), may also be administered.

Denver Articulation Screening Examination

The DASE is designed to detect significant developmental delays as well as normal variations in the acquisition of speech sounds. Because it is a standardized test, its directions must be followed precisely. The test is only standardized for use with English-speaking children.

Administration. Before the test, explain that the child will need to repeat the words she hears you speak. Give enough examples that you are certain she understands what she is to do: "When I say 'boat,' then you say 'boat.'" When you are certain

BOX 34.13 Rinne and Weber Tests

Rinne and Weber tests are assessments for air and bone conduction.

Rinne Test

Strike a 500-Hz tuning fork and hold the stem of it against the child's mastoid bone. Ask the child to say when the tuning fork's ringing sound can no longer be heard. When the child says it is no longer audible, move the fork forward so it is at the auditory meatus (Fig. A). Because air conduction is normally better than bone conduction, the child should hear it when it is held in front of the meatus, although it can no longer be heard when it was held against the bone. If the child does not hear it when it is brought forward, then the child's air conduction is probably reduced.

Weber Test

Strike a 500-Hz tuning fork and hold the stem of it against the top of the child's head (Fig. B). The child with normal hearing in both ears will hear the sound equally well with both ears. If the child has an air conduction loss in one ear, the child will hear the sound better in that ear than in the good ear. The test must be used in conjunction with other evaluation tools because if the sound is intensified in one ear, it may mean that there is no hearing perception (i.e., there is nerve loss) in the opposite ear.

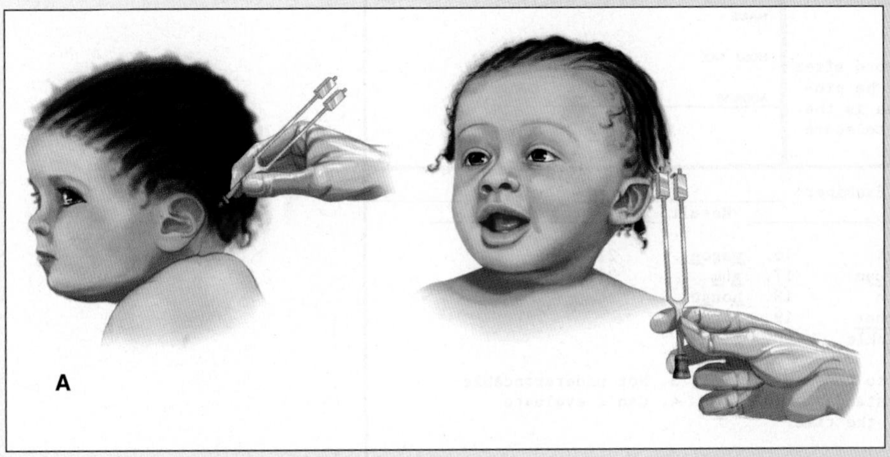

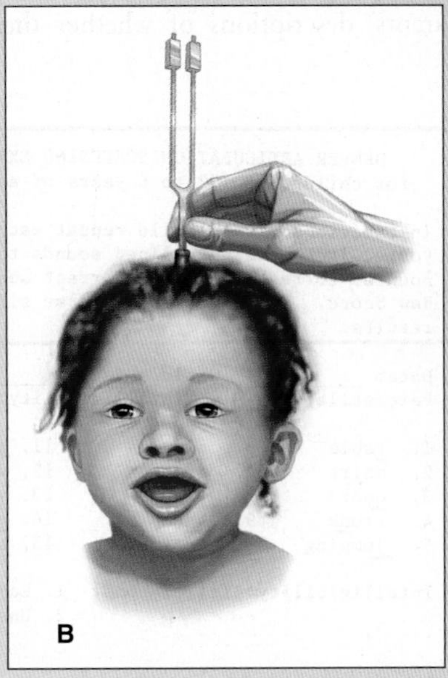

the child understands the directions, say each of the 22 words shown on the DASE form (Fig. 34.24A). Convey the impression that there are no right or wrong answers. Give the child approval for responding and following directions correctly, no matter how inaccurately the child repeats the word.

Scoring. The DASE is designed for use with children between the ages of 2.5 and 6 years. In scoring, consider the child's age to be the closest previous age shown on the percentile rank chart (Fig. 34.24B). Score the child's pronunciation of the underlined sounds or blends in each word on the test form. A perfect raw score is 30 correctly articulated sounds. Match this raw score on the percentile rank chart with the column representing the child's age. The number at which the raw score line and the age column meet is the percentile rank of the child (how the child compares with other children of that age). Percentiles shown above the heavy line are abnormal; those below the line are normal. For example, a 3-year-old who says only 12 sounds correctly ranks in the ninth percentile (abnormal ranking); a 3-year-old who scores 20 sounds correctly ranks in the 58th percentile (normal ranking).

In addition to determining the percentile ranking, rate the child's spontaneous speech in terms of intelligibility as 1, easy to understand; 2, understandable half the time; 3, not understandable; or 4, cannot evaluate (e.g., maybe the child did not speak in sentences or phrases during your contact time). Score intelligibility according to the chart in Figure 34.24B. For a final score, rate the child's total test result (e.g., normal or abnormal on the DASE or intelligibility).

Children who score abnormally on this screening test should be retested in about 2 weeks. If they still score abnormally, they should be referred for a complete speech evaluation.

DEVELOPMENTAL APPRAISAL

It would be ideal if children demonstrated all the developmental skills they are capable of every time they are asked to demonstrate them. Rarely, however, do they accomplish this. Infants become hungry, sleepy, or upset during testing. Older children may become shy. Therefore, a portion of developmental information, especially developmental milestones, on almost all health assessment must be elicited by history taking.

Developmental Histories

Many parents keep careful records of their first child's development, a less careful record of their second, a scanty record of the third, and so on. Information, therefore, generally depends on parents' memories.

If parents cannot recall the month during which a skill was first demonstrated, ask them to try to remember in terms of holidays or seasons when they first saw the child performing the skill. They may not recall, for example, at which month their infant first used a pincer grasp (grasped cleanly with index finger and thumb), but do recall the child pinched the ear of the family dog at a summer picnic.

If parents seem to have no recall at all of developmental milestones and these are important to the child's present evaluation, suggest they ask other family members or look through family photographs to jog their memories and to call back with as much information as they can gather.

The CDC has developmental norms listed on their Web site (www.CDC.gov) that parents can use to compare their child's progress (CDC, 2012b). In addition to getting the parents' descriptions of whether their child has mastered these skills, it is helpful to watch a child perform skills and rate them according to standard criteria.

Denver II Developmental Screening Test

The Denver II Developmental Screening Test (available at http://thePoint.lww.com/Pillitteri7e) is the most widely used tool to assess early childhood development (Frankenburg, 1994). Four categories are rated:

1. Personal–social
2. Fine motor–adaptive
3. Language
4. Gross motor skills

Administration. The Denver II should ideally be administered when a child is approximately 3 or 4 months of age,

DENVER ARTICULATION SCREENING EXAM
for children 2 1/2 to 6 years of age

Instructions: Have child repeat each word after you. Circle the underlined sounds that he pronounces correctly. Total correct sounds is the Raw Score. Use charts on reverse side to score results.

NAME
HOSP. NO.
ADDRESS

Date: ______ Child's Age: ______ Examiner: ______ Raw Score: ______
Percentile: ______ Intelligibility: ______ Result: ______

1. table	6. zipper	11. sock	16. wagon	21. leaf
2. shirt	7. grapes	12. vacuum	17. gum	22. carrot
3. door	8. flag	13. yarn	18. house	
4. trunk	9. thumb	14. mother	19. pencil	
5. jumping	10. toothbrush	15. twinkle	20. fish	

Intelligibility: (circle one) 1. Easy to understand 2. Understandable 1/2 the time. 3. Not understandable 4. Can't evaluate

Comments:

Date: ______ Child's Age: ______ Examiner: ______ Raw Score ______
Percentile: ______ Intelligibility: ______ Result: ______

1. table	6. zipper	11. sock	16. wagon	21. leaf
2. shirt	7. grapes	12. vacuum	17. gum	22. carrot
3. door	8. flag	13. yarn	18. house	
4. trunk	9. thumb	14. mother	19. pencil	
5. jumping	10. toothbrush	15. twinkle	20. fish	

Intelligibility: (circle one) 1. Easy to understand 2. Understandable 1/2 the time. 3. Not understandable 4. Can't evaluate

Comments:

Date: ______ Child's Age: ______ Examiner: ______ Raw Score ______
Percentile: ______ Intelligibility: ______ Result: ______

1. table	6. zipper	11. sock	16. wagon	21. leaf
2. shirt	7. grapes	12. vacuum	17. gum	22. carrot
3. door	8. flag	13. yarn	18. house	
4. trunk	9. thumb	14. mother	19. pencil	
5. jumping	10. toothbrush	15. twinkle	20. fish	

Intelligibility: (circle one) 1. Easy to understand 2. Understandable 1/2 the time. 3. Not understandable 4. Can't evaluate

Comments:

A

FIGURE 34.24 The Denver Articulation Screening Exam (DASE). **(A)** The test form. *(continued)*

To score DASE words: Note Raw Score for child's performance. Match raw score line (extreme left of chart) with column representing child's age (to the closest previous age group). Where raw score line and age column meet number in that square denotes percentile rank of child's performance when compared to other children that age. Percentiles above heavy line are ABNORMAL percentiles, below heavy line are NORMAL.

PERCENTILE RANK

Raw Score	2.5 yr.	3.0	3.5	4.0	4.5	5.0	5.5	6 years
2	1							
3	2							
4	5							
5	9							
6	16							
7	23							
8	31	2						
9	37	4	1					
10	42	6	2					
11	48	7	4					
12	54	9	6	1	1			
13	58	12	9	2	3	1	1	
14	62	17	11	5	4	2	2	
15	68	23	15	9	5	3	2	
16	75	31	19	12	5	4	3	
17	79	38	25	15	6	6	4	
18	83	46	31	19	8	7	4	
19	86	51	38	24	10	9	5	1
20	89	58	45	30	12	11	7	3
21	92	65	52	36	15	15	9	4
22	94	72	58	43	18	19	12	5
23	96	77	63	50	22	24	15	7
24	97	82	70	58	29	29	20	15
25	99	87	78	66	36	34	26	17
26	99	91	84	75	46	43	34	24
27		94	89	82	57	54	44	34
28		96	94	88	70	68	59	47
29		98	98	94	84	84	77	68
30		100	100	100	100	100	100	100

To Score intelligibility:

	NORMAL	ABNORMAL
2 1/2 years	Understandable 1/2 the time, or, "easy"	Not Understandable
3 years and older	Easy to understand	Understandable 1/2 time Not understandable

Test Result: 1. NORMAL on Dase and Intelligibility = NORMAL
2. ABNORMAL on Dase and/or Intelligibility = ABNORMAL

* If abnormal on initial screening rescreen within 2 weeks. If abnormal again child should be referred for complete speech evaluation.

B

FIGURE 34.24 *(continued)*
(B) The percentile rank form. (Reprinted by permission. Denver Developmental Materials, Inc.

again at about 10 months, and again at 3 years. It is a supplement to the developmental evaluation by history that should be a part of every well-child assessment.

The materials to administer the test must be purchased as a kit. They include a skein of red wool, a box of raisins, a small bottle, a bell, a rattle with a narrow handle, a tennis ball, 10 1-in. brightly colored blocks, a small plastic doll, a toy baby bottle, a plastic cup, and a pencil.

Although administration of the Denver II is not difficult, it should not be attempted except by health care providers trained specifically in its procedures and interpretation. This precaution is necessary to ensure the validity of its developmental norms. Periodic retraining and proficiency testing are recommended, so administrators sustain a high degree of accuracy in administration.

Caution a parent before administration that this is not a test of intelligence but of the child's level of development or ability to perform age-appropriate tasks.

The child's inability to perform a task that most children of the same age can accomplish indicates a delay in that area. Further evaluation is then needed to determine the reason for this delay.

Scoring. The child is scored P (passed), F (failed), R (refused), or N.O. (no opportunity) on each item according to guidelines in the instruction manual. Each item is represented on the Denver II test form by a bar showing the ages by which 25%, 50%, 75%, and 90% of children normally have mastered that item. For example, on the form, 25% of children are expected to demonstrate the task "plays pat-a-cake" at 7 months, 50% perform this between 9 and 10 months, 75% between 10 and 11 months, and 90% by ages 11 to 12 months. A description of each task and an interpretation of performance are detailed in the manual.

Prescreening Test. A Denver Prescreening Developmental Questionnaire (R-PDQII) is available in addition to the

Denver II. The PDQII is a questionnaire completed by the parents addressing 10 developmental items. A child who scores 8 out of 10 or fewer should be retested in approximately 2 weeks. If the initial score is under 6 or the retest score is 8 or below, the child should be referred for Denver II testing. Encouraging parents to complete a questionnaire this way is helpful because it can detect developmental delays that otherwise might be missed in a busy office or clinic.

INTELLIGENCE

Children must learn many important concepts or ideas such as near and far, number sequences, how to judge time intervals, how to reason and solve problems, and how to judge weight before they can function effectively in the world.

This type of learning—gaining concepts—is cognitive learning and is measured by intelligence tests. **Intelligence** can be defined as the ability to think abstractly, to adjust to new situations, and to profit from experience. Almost everyone has their intelligence quotient (IQ) rated at some point in a school career. Although intelligence tests are not part of routine health appraisals, it is helpful to be familiar with those that are used for childhood measurements because these findings can help predict a child's school success.

The IQ is the ratio of mental age as measured by an intelligence test to chronologic age. To determine IQ, the formula is

(mental age ÷ chronologic age) × 100.

A child aged 9 years old (i.e., chronologic age) who passes all the items on an intelligence test that an average 9-year-old child is expected to pass would be

(9 [mental age] ÷ 9 [chronologic age]) × 100 = 100 (child's IQ).

If a child passes no more items than the average 5-year-old child would pass, the IQ would be

(5 [mental age] ÷ 9 [chronologic age]) × 100 = 55.

If a child passed all the items that a 12-year-old child normally passes, the IQ would be

(12 [mental age] ÷ 9 [chronologic age]) × 100 = 133.

Intelligence scores are not always accurate; for instance, children may score poorly because of test anxiety. Cultural bias and past experience can also affect scores. Labeling children by IQ and classifying them into divisions based on IQ is no longer used as extensively as in the past. It must be done with considerable thought and study.

It is difficult to test very young children with any degree of accuracy because they lack the ability to complete tasks in the areas used for scoring intelligence tests, including comprehension, imagination, reasoning, memory, and vocabulary. The most common tests used with infants include the Cattell Infant Intelligence Scale, the Bayley Mental Scale, and the Gesell Developmental Schedule. These tests rely heavily on perceptual and motor skills as rating devices.

The two most frequently used tests for older children are the Wechsler Intelligence Scale for Children and the Stanford–Binet test. The results of these can be made available, with parental permission, to child health care teams if they can demonstrate to school officials that such information is necessary for total health care or planning. If the information is unavailable, the child can be referred to a psychologist or a psychological testing clinic for assessment at the time of a disease diagnosis.

Goodenough-Harris Drawing Test

A Goodenough-Harris Drawing Test is a quick intelligence measurement that can be administered without special training to children between 3 and 10 years of age (Goodenough, 1926). To administer this, give a child a pencil and paper and tell the child to draw a person. Urge the child to draw carefully and take enough time to do it well.

The child receives one point for each of the items listed in Box 34.14 that are demonstrated in the drawing. For each four points scored, 1 year is added to a base age of 3 years to calculate the child's mental age. The picture shown in Figure 34.25, for example, was drawn by a 4.5-year-old: it received eight points. The child's IQ level is therefore

(5.0 [mental age] ÷ 4.5[chronologic age]) × 100 = 111.

Scores on the test are reasonably reliable, correlating well with a Stanford–Binet test, although results may not be as reliable with children who are mentally ill. A child who scores significantly lower than chronologic age (after allowing for fatigue, illness, strange surroundings, nervousness, physical ability to use a pencil, and previous practice using a pencil and paper) should be referred for more refined testing.

TEMPERAMENT

Temperament refers to a child's innate behavioral characteristics, such as activity level, rhythmicity, tendency to approach or withdraw, and adaptability to situations (see Chapter 28). A child with an "easy" temperament is generally adaptable and easy to care for; in contrast, a child with a "difficult" temperament will almost invariably create childrearing concerns. Helping parents assess their child's temperament helps them, in turn, recognize their child's uniqueness and so anticipate and ideally prevent personality conflicts as a child grows older and expresses identified reactions to situations. If a behavior or parent–child interaction problem is already present, a nursing assessment can be useful to determine whether temperament is a factor in the problem and to assist parents with constructive solutions (Thomas & Chess, 1977).

IMMUNIZATIONS

One of the most important health assessment and promotion measures for children is to verify their immunization status is up to date (see Recommended Childhood and Adolescent Immunization Schedule, available at http://thePoint.lww.com/Pillitteri7e).

Teach parents about the importance of having their children immunized and the need to be able to describe the number and type of immunizations a child has received. If gaps are present in a child's number of immunizations, remind the child's primary care provider about this lack in protection and prepare to administer the necessary vaccines.

Help parents understand that although diseases such as measles and mumps are referred to as common childhood illnesses,

BOX 34.14 Goodenough-Harris Drawing Test

Score one point for each characteristic listed as follows that is present on the drawing. For every four points scored, add 1 year to a base mental age of 3 years.

1. Head present
2. Legs present
3. Arms present
4a. Trunk present
4b. Length of trunk greater than breadth
4c. Shoulders indicated
5a. Both arms and legs attached to trunk
5b. Legs attached to trunk; arms attached to trunk at correct point
6a. Neck present
6b. Neck outline continuous with head, trunk, or both
7a. Eyes present
7b. Nose present
7c. Mouth present
7d. Nose and mouth in two dimensions; two lips shown
7e. Nostrils indicated
8a. Hair shown
8b. Hair nontransparent, over more than circumference
9a. Clothing present
9b. Two articles of clothing nontransparent
9c. No transparencies, both sleeves and trousers shown
9d. Four or more articles of clothing definitely indicated
9e. Costume complete, without incongruities
10a. Fingers shown
10b. Correct number of fingers shown
10c. Fingers in two dimensions; length greater than breadth, angle less than 180°
10d. Opposition of thumb shown
10e. Hand shown distinct from fingers or arms
11a. Arm joint shown, either elbow, shoulder, or both
11b. Leg joint shown, either knee, hip, or both
12a. Head in proportion
12b. Arms in proportion
12c. Legs in proportion
12d. Feet in proportion
12e. Both arms and legs in two dimensions
13. Heel shown
14a. Firm lines without overlapping at junctions
14b. Firm lines with correct joining
14c. Head outline more than circle
14d. Trunk outline more than circle
14e. Outline of arms and legs without narrowing at point of junction with body
14f. Features symmetric, correct position
15a. Ears present
15b. Ears in correct position and proportion
16a. Eye detail: brow and lashes shown
16b. Eye detail: pupil shown
16c. Eye detail: proportion correct
16d. Eye detail: glance directed to front in profile drawing
17a. Both chin and forehead present
17b. Projection of chin shown

From Goodenough, F. L. (1926). *Measurement of intelligence by drawings.* New York, NY: World Book Company. Revised Harris, D. B. (1963), *Children's drawings as measures of intellectual maturity.* New York, NY: Harcourt, Brace & World, Inc. Reprinted with permission from Estate of Dale B. Harris.

they are potentially serious and possibly lead to complications such as pneumonia and encephalitis (see Chapter 43).

Types of Immunizations

Vaccines are the solutions used to immunize children in order to provide artificially acquired active or passive immunity (see Box 34.15 for the definition of active and passive immunity).

Vaccines are prepared in a number of forms. Attenuated vaccines are made from live organisms that have been reduced in virulence to a point where they will not cause active disease but will ensure a good antibody response. Because they are

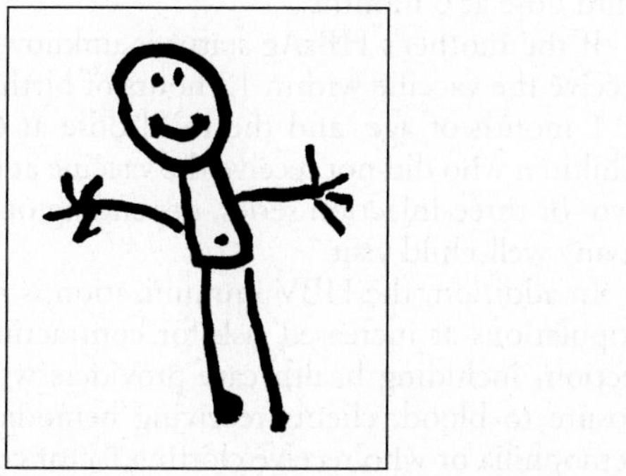

FIGURE 34.25 An eight-point drawing, as scored on the Goodenough-Harris Drawing Test.

strong solutions, a single dose usually provides a good degree of active immunity.

Because some bacteria, such as diphtheria, cause disease by producing a toxin, the vaccine against such a disease, a **toxoid**, is actually an extract of the toxin with reduced virulence. The antibodies produced against toxin-producing bacteria are called **antitoxins**.

Gamma globulin is serum obtained from the pooled blood of many people. Because it combines the serum of many people, it probably has antibody protection against measles, rubella, poliomyelitis, varicella, and hepatitis B, among many other infectious diseases. When administered, it offers artificially acquired passive immunity.

Immune serums are serums available against specific diseases such as diphtheria, tetanus, the pit viper snake, the black widow spider, and respiratory syncytial virus. Like general immune globulin, these provide passive immunity.

Childhood Immunizations

The American Academy of Pediatrics and the CDC both issue specific recommendations for childhood immunization (available at http://thePoint.lww.com/Pillitteri7e).

The Diphtheria, Tetanus, Pertussis Vaccine

Diphtheria, tetanus toxoid, and acellular pertussis (i.e., whooping cough) (DTaP) vaccines are supplied in a single vial as

BOX 34.15 Active Versus Passive Immunity

Immunity, the ability to combat a particular antigen, may be either active or passive.

Active Immunity. When a child produces antibodies after the natural invasion of a pathogen (e.g., the child has measles), the child develops *naturally acquired active immunity*. Active antibodies (or the child's ability to produce antibodies rapidly should the specific antigen [measles] invade again) last a lifetime. When pathogens are artificially injected into the child by immunization, the child receives *artificially acquired active immunity*. If the specific antigen should enter again, antibodies will be produced against the pathogen that are just as lasting as those produced in naturally acquired active immunity.

Passive Immunity. IgG antibodies a woman possesses either through immunization or through having had a disease are transferred across the placenta to a fetus in utero. Because the fetus does not make these antibodies but merely receives them, this is termed *naturally acquired passive immunity*. Passive immunity usually lasts only a few months, although some antibodies transferred across the placenta, such as those for measles, have been isolated up to age 1 year (which is why measles immunization must be delayed until 15 months of age).

When children are exposed to a disease against which they have no antibodies, antibodies made synthetically or obtained from animal serum may be injected into the child to give rapid immunity (*artificially acquired passive immunity*). Like naturally acquired passive antibodies, these last only approximately 6 weeks. A child who is susceptible to tetanus, for example, would receive tetanus antibodies after a stab wound to ensure she has protection against the tetanus virus.

DTaP and given in one intramuscular injection. It is recommended that children receive a primary series of four immunizations with the vaccine (at 2, 4, 6, and 15 to 18 months of age). A booster is then given between 4 and 6 years of age, or before entry into school. Because whooping cough outbreaks have occurred in the teenage and young adult population, a combined injection of the DTaP vaccine is recommended at 11 to 12 years of age. Teenagers who did not receive the booster at 11 to 12 years of age or who received only a diphtheria/tetanus (Td) injection at that time are encouraged to receive one dose of DTaP 5 years after the last Td/DTaP dose. It is recommended that young adults continue with tetanus prophylaxis every 10 years throughout life to keep their tetanus immunizations current.

Side effects to these vaccines include drowsiness, fretfulness, low-grade fever, and redness and pain at the injection site. A pertussis vaccination may not be recommended for children who have a progressive or unstable neurologic disorder. A Td vaccine can be substituted for these children.

The Polio Vaccine

Inactivated polio vaccine (IPV) contains all three strains of poliovirus and is the preferred type for routine immunization. It is administered in a primary series of three doses and given along with DTaP at 2, 4, and 6 to 18 months of age with a fourth booster dose given between the ages of 4 and 6 years, or before school entry (CDC, 2012c).

The Measles, Mumps, Rubella Vaccine

The measles, mumps, and rubella (MMR) vaccine is furnished in one injection and routinely administered between 12 and 15 months of age. A second dose of MMR is generally given between the ages of 4 to 6 years, or if the child did not receive this dose at 4 to 6 years of age, it is given at 11 to 12 years of age. The first dose is delayed until the end of the first year because children receive a great deal of passive immunity to measles from their mothers while they are in utero. Until this passive immunity has faded, the injected vaccine would be neutralized by passive antibodies and no immunity would result. For the same reason, children who have recently received immune globulin or other blood products that contain antibodies should not receive an MMR vaccination for about 3 months because the passively acquired antibodies could interfere with the child's immune response to the vaccine.

Side effects to the vaccine include transient rash and a fever, which may begin 5 to 12 days after vaccination and last several days. Adverse reactions include joint pain, low-grade fever, rash, and lymphadenopathy 5 to 12 days after vaccination.

Before the vaccine is administered, children should be skin tested for tuberculosis because the measles virus can cause tuberculosis to become systemic. Tuberculosis skin tests also may show false-negative reactions if given shortly after a measles immunization (i.e., a child who has active tuberculosis would be wrongly identified as not having the illness).

Formerly, there was a concern the administration of the MMR vaccine was associated with the development of autism in children, as symptoms of autism often begin to be apparent during the second year or close to the time of MMR vaccine administration. Further research has shown there to be no causal relationship between the vaccine and autism (Uno, Uchiyama, Kurosawa, et al., 2012). Parents may ask about this association, however, or may refuse to have their child immunized against MMR for this reason (Luthy, Beckstrand, Callister, et al., 2012).

The Hepatitis B Vaccine

The vaccine for hepatitis B virus (HBV) is recommended for all infants in the United States because hepatitis B is associated with liver cancer later in life. Three doses are required. Those infants born to hepatitis B surface antigen (HBsAg)-negative mothers should receive the first dose in the newborn period before hospital discharge, a second dose at 1 or 2 months and a third dose at 6 or 18 months. Those born to HBsAg-positive mothers should receive hepatitis B immune globulin within 12 hours of birth plus HBV. A second dose of HBV is then recommended at 1 to 2 months of age and a third dose at 6 months.

If the mother's HBsAg status is unknown, infants should receive the vaccine within 12 hours of birth, the second dose at 1 month of age, and the third dose at 6 months of age. Children who did not receive the vaccine at birth may begin a two- or three-injection series, depending on the vaccine used at any well-child visit.

In addition, the HBV immunization is recommended for populations at increased risk for contracting hepatitis B infection, including health care providers with significant exposure to blood, clients receiving hemodialysis, those with hemophilia or who receive clotting factor concentrates, those who take illicit injectable drugs, and sexually active individuals with multiple sexual partners.

The Hepatitis A Vaccine

Two doses of hepatitis A vaccine, administered 6 months apart, are recommended for all children between 1 and 2 years of age. Children who did not receive this as toddlers can be vaccinated against hepatitis A at any time.

The Rotavirus Vaccine

Rotaviruses are responsible for the majority of severe gastrointestinal disease in infants, so immunization against these viruses is important for preventing outbreaks of diarrhea in infants, particularly those who attend a day care setting. The vaccine is given at 2, 4, and 6 months of age. No doses should be given after children reach 32 weeks of age.

Haemophilus influenzae Type B Vaccine

Haemophilus influenzae type B conjugate vaccine (Hib) protects against *H. influenzae* bacteria, a major cause of meningitis in children. You may need to explain the difference between *H. influenzae* (a bacteria) and the influenza virus so that parents do not think a "flu shot" protects against this. Several formulations of this vaccine are available; depending on the individual vaccine, they are administered in a two-dose (at age 2 and 4 months of age) or a three-dose regimen (at 2, 4, and 6 months of age, with an additional booster at 12 months of age). Local reactions include tenderness at the injection site. Reactions such as crying and fever may occur (CDC, 2012c).

The Varicella Vaccine

The varicella (i.e., chickenpox) vaccine was a difficult vaccine to develop because of the complex structure of the herpes zoster virus. It's an important vaccine because once a generation of children has been successfully immunized, it should mark the end of an epidemic childhood illness. Infants may receive varicella vaccine at any visit after their first birthday (usually scheduled at 12 to 18 months of age) and again at 4 to 6 years of age. Those who did not receive the vaccine as infants and who lack a reliable history of chickenpox should be immunized during adolescence with two doses of vaccine, administered at least 1 month apart.

The Pneumococcal Pneumonia Vaccine

The pneumococcal vaccine is recommended for all children between 2 and 23 months of age. The vaccine is administered at 2, 4, 6, and 12 months of age and provides protection for 6 to 10 years (AAP, 2013). It is especially recommended for children (and adults) who would be prone to a pneumococcal infection (e.g., those with pulmonary or cardiac disease, those without a spleen, those who are immunosuppressed).

The Human Papillomavirus Vaccine

The human papillomavirus (HPV) is associated with the development of cervical cancer in women. It is recommended that all preteens (male and female) receive three injections of this vaccine beginning at 11 to 12 years of age. The second dose should be administered 2 months after the first dose and the third dose should be given 6 months after the first dose. Those who did not receive the vaccine in early adolescence can receive it at any time, with the proper monthly intervals for administration. Some teenagers who have taken abstinence pledges not to have sexual relations until they are married may state they do not need the vaccine. Counseling them about the safety of being immunized in case they change their mind about abstinence or to be protected when they become sexually active may be necessary.

The Meningococcal Vaccine

Children who have immunologic deficiencies or have had their spleen removed due to trauma or those receiving therapy for a blood dyscrasia are prone to develop meningitis caused by meningococcal bacteria. Children in these high-risk groups are, therefore, advised to receive a meningococcal vaccine between 2 and 10 years of age. Because meningitis occurs frequently on college campuses, previously unvaccinated college freshmen living in dormitories should also receive the vaccine.

The Lyme Disease Vaccine

Lyme disease is a serious and debilitating infection caused by *Borrelia burgdorferi* and transmitted by the bite of a deer tick. A vaccine to guard against it is no longer available. Children who contract the disease can be successfully treated with antibiotics to minimize the disease. Tips for preventing Lyme disease are shown in Chapter 43.

The Influenza Vaccine

Influenza is caused by A, B, or C retroviruses, which mutate so easily that it has been impossible to design a vaccine that is effective for more than 1 year. All children—infants through adolescents—and particularly those who have chronic pulmonary or cardiovascular disorders or are immunosuppressed should receive a yearly injection of the vaccine (CDC, 2012c).

The Anthrax and Smallpox Vaccines

Anthrax is a potentially fatal disease caused by a gram-positive, spore-forming *Bacillus anthracis* and spread by farm animal feces. It is extremely rare, but parents may ask about a vaccine for it because of the threat of biologic warfare associated with terrorism. A vaccine is available for people in high-risk occupations, such as hunters, taxidermists, or veterinarians, but it is not recommended for children.

Smallpox is an extremely infectious disease caused by the smallpox virus and transmitted by direct or indirect contact. Smallpox vaccination has not been required in the United States for over 30 years because the disease is theoretically extinct across the world. As with anthrax, parents may ask about a smallpox vaccination because it is a disease associated with biologic warfare and terrorism. Both a vaccine (active artificial immunity) and passive artificial immunity are available should a child be exposed to the virus. In some high-risk communities, health care providers are asked to be immunized to be certain they will not contract the virus if a terrorist attack should occur (Sato, Tomio, Tanaka, et al., 2011).

Administration of Immunizations

Current immunization recommendations are available at http://thePoint.lww.com/Pillitteri7e. Assess both well children at health maintenance visits and ill children at clinic or hospital admission to identify those who need their immunizations updated according to this schedule. Children who are seriously ill should not receive immunizations, but a slight upper respiratory tract infection (e.g., a stuffy nose with no fever) is not a contraindication. So many infants and preschoolers have common cold symptoms (the average toddler has 10 to 12 colds a year), if children were not immunized at health maintenance visits when they have slight cold symptoms, many would never receive basic immunizations. Catch-up schedules for children who did not receive primary immunizations or who are behind in an immunization schedule are also available at http://thePoint.lww.com/Pillitteri7e. Because these schedules change yearly based on the introduction of new vaccines or new potential health threats, consult the American Academy of Pediatrics Web site (www.aap.org) or the CDC Web site (www.CDC.gov) for up-to-date information before immunizing a specific child.

When preparing to administer an immunization, be certain to follow the manufacturer's recommendations for storage and handling of vaccines, such as whether the vaccine should not be exposed to light or whether it needs refrigeration. Failure to follow these precautions may significantly reduce the potency and effectiveness of vaccines.

Children With Unique Needs

Children with chronic illnesses may be hospitalized at the time an immunization is due and so fall behind schedule. Children who miss the scheduled time for an immunization do not need to have the series started over, but rather, should simply continue at the point they left off.

Primary care providers may choose to alter the sequence of immunization schedules if specific infections are prevalent at the time. For example, the measles vaccine might be given on a first health maintenance visit (providing a child is older than 12 months of age) if an epidemic was underway in the community at the time.

Children who are immunosuppressed, receiving corticosteroids, or receiving chemotherapy or radiation therapy should not receive live virus vaccines. The live attenuated viruses such as measles, rubella, oral polio (OPV) and mumps must not be given to girls who are pregnant because these vaccines could cross the placenta, thus causing disease in the fetus. Before traveling internationally, parents should consult their local public health service to see what additional vaccines are required for children for overseas travel.

Although MMR vaccines are prepared from chick embryo cultures, egg sensitivities are not likely to occur because egg albumin and yolk components of the egg are absent from the culture. However, children with egg allergy should have their allergist's permission for immunization to rule out the possibility of a hypersensitivity reaction.

Parental Education

A major reason parents do not bring children for routine immunizations is that they do not know what is required or have misconceptions about immunity. Fully inform parents and, when old enough, children about what immunizations are recommended. When vaccines are given, be certain parents know what is being given and what side effects may be expected. Because children may develop a low-grade fever after any immunization, counsel parents they may need to give acetaminophen (Tylenol) or children's ibuprofen for a fever higher than 101°F (38.4°C).

Unfavorable reactions are most likely to occur within a few hours or days of administration. With live attenuated virus vaccines, viruses can multiply, so reactions may occur up to 30 days later. With the rubella vaccine, a reaction (serum sickness) may occur up to 60 days later. Ask parents to report any untoward symptoms of immunization.

When giving a vaccine, record the date, type of vaccine, vaccine manufacturer, lot number, and name and address of the vaccine provider so that, if a vaccine reaction should occur, the instance can be investigated. Make a copy of the child's immunization record for the parents and urge them to keep good track of such a record. They will need this information to admit their child to school and to feel safe in the event an epidemic of a particular disease occurs. They will need to know their child's record of tetanus immunizations if the child should receive a puncture wound so that the correct therapy can be given for this.

QSEN Checkpoint Question 34.6

Safety

Keoto's father wants to be sure Keoto's immunizations are up to date. When is the immunization for human papillomavirus (HPV) recommended?

a. At 12 to 18 months of age
b. Before kindergarten entrance
c. At 16 years of age
d. At 11 to 12 years of age

Look in Appendix A for the best answer and rationale.

CONCLUDING A HEALTH ASSESSMENT

At every health maintenance visit, inform parents and the child (or ask the child's primary care provider to inform them, depending on agency policy) of any available results of screening procedures performed. After learning the results, some parents may require counseling to assist them with health or behavior concerns. Box 34.16 shows an interprofessional care map illustrating both nursing and team planning for a child in need of a pre-sports health assessment.

Ask parents if they have any other remaining questions. If the health assessment revealed some health concerns and follow-up procedures are planned, be certain parents understand the reason for the upcoming tests. Suggest to parents that follow-up phone calls are welcome after they return home from a health assessment so additional questions can be answered. Provide parents with the best hours to call so someone will be available to answer questions for them.

What if...34.4 You are particularly interested in exploring one of the 2020 National Health Goals with respect to health assessment (see Box 34.1). What would be a possible research topic to explore that is pertinent to this goal, applicable to Keoto's family, and that would also advance evidence-based practice?

BOX 34.16 Nursing Care Planning

AN INTERPROFESSIONAL CARE MAP FOR A CHILD IN NEED OF A PRE-SPORTS HEALTH ASSESSMENT

Keoto Wiser is a 13-year-old you meet in an ambulatory clinic. Her father has brought her for health assessment before Keoto begins seventh grade.

Family Assessment Child lives with two parents and 2-year-old sister, Candy. Father works as a paramedic for the fire department; mother is a notary public employed by a bank. Father rates finances as "good."

Child Assessment Keoto was born with a lung cyst that required removal not only of the cyst but also a portion of her left upper lung lobe at 6 months of age. Her father is concerned her lessened lung size may make her ineligible for competitive sports participation. He asks if carbohydrate loading would give her enough energy to make up for any decreased lung function. He's also concerned she may need eyeglasses because she always sits close to the television set. He asks you if wearing glasses could decrease her chance of being chosen for a sports team.

Nursing Diagnosis Anxiety related to ability to participate in school sports program

Outcome Criteria Client participates in school sports program to the degree dictated by physical findings.

Team Member Responsible	Assessment	Intervention	Rationale	Expected Outcome
Activities of Daily Living, Including Safety				
Nurse	Assess child's development by taking a 24-hour day history.	Discuss with parent and child any areas that cause concern.	Parents can "get behind" in expectations of child, as preteenage children grow and develop rapidly.	Parent or child gives day history and discusses any areas seen as problematic.
Teamwork and Collaboration				
Nurse/Primary health care provider	Determine name of health care provider who determines eligibility for sports teams at child's school.	Consult with identified health care provider to determine eligibility rules for sports.	Schools may have restrictions on children who do not have both pairs of duplicate organs such as lungs.	Qualifications for sports participation are obtained and outlined for parents and child.
Procedures/Medications for Quality Improvement				
Nurse/Primary health care provider	Obtain health assessment, particularly with regard to stamina and past ability to participate in sports activities.	Perform complete physical examination focusing on heart, lung, and muscle status.	Physical examination can reveal additional findings regarding lung capacity and stamina.	A physical examination yields information on child's overall health.
Nurse	Assess whether child is familiar with Snellen vision testing.	Assess child's eyesight using a Snellen eye chart.	A Snellen eye chart is a standardized test for vision appraisal.	Child completes eye exam and is told results.
Nutrition				
Nurse/Nutritionist	Assess what parents and child know about carbohydrate loading.	Counsel regarding disadvantages of carbohydrate loading for children.	Children and parents who are well informed can make better choices for nutrition practices.	Parent and child state they understand carbohydrate loading is not recommended for children.
Patient-Centered Care				
Nurse	Assess past health history and recommended immunizations.	Review with parents and child the child's current immunization status and any immunizations needed.	Parents are often unfamiliar with required immunizations and so need to be reminded of recommended schedules.	Parents and child agree to any immunization necessary before child returns to school.

(continued on page 1000)

BOX 34.16 Nursing Care Planning (continued)

Psychosocial/Spiritual/Emotional Needs				
Nurse	Assess what will be child's likely reaction if she cannot participate in her school's sports program or needs to wear eyeglasses.	If child is unable to participate in school sports, review with child other options: joining a club, petition school sports committee, etc. Discuss advantage of clear vision.	Planning ahead can help child adjust to less-than-desired results if these occur.	Child lists alternate ways to participate with other children at school, if sports are not an option, or describes a sensible plan for petitioning for an exception to rules.
Informatics for Seamless Health Care Planning				
Nurse	Assess if parents or child have had questions answered during the health assessment.	Answer remaining questions, if any; schedule a return visit as needed.	If questions remain unanswered at the health assessment, needs haven't been fully met.	Parents and child state they have no further questions; describe plans for next action.

KEY POINTS FOR REVIEW

- Health assessment always causes some degree of apprehension for both parents and children because of the worry that an illness will be detected. Giving reassurance of wellness during examinations helps to alleviate this worry.
- A health history is an important part of an assessment. The purpose is to gather information that will supplement physical or laboratory examinations to provide a more thorough health evaluation.
- A health history includes an introduction, chief concern, family profile, history of past illnesses, day history, family health history, and review of systems.
- A physical examination involves four techniques: inspection, palpation, percussion, and auscultation. Techniques and approaches must be varied according to the child's age.
- Be certain to use examining instruments safely, such as supporting an otoscope base so that, if a child moves, the otoscope moves with the child. Be certain young children are not left unsupervised on an examining table as this could cause a fall.
- The components of a physical examination include vital sign assessment, general appearance, mental status assessment, body measurements, and an assessment from head to toes.
- Adolescent boys can be taught testicular self-examination at the time of a health appraisal. Self-breast examinations for females should be done by the examiner but is no longer thought to reveal enough information to be practical as a preventive measure.
- A vision assessment consists of asking children to read a standardized chart such as a Snellen or Preschool E Chart, cover testing, or color discrimination assessment.
- A hearing assessment consists of such assessments as audiometric testing and Rinne and Weber tests.
- Determining a child's development is an important part of total assessment. The Denver II Developmental Screening Test and the DASE are specific development tests used.
- The Goodenough-Harris Drawing Test correlates well with IQ and is an easy test to administer to children between the ages of 3 and 10 years to assess intelligence.
- An assessment of immunization status is included as part of a health assessment. Childhood immunizations are a major safeguard for children against common childhood illnesses; being certain they receive what is needed at each health care visit not only helps in planning nursing care that meets QSEN guidelines but also helps to keep a child safe.

CRITICAL THINKING CARE STUDY

Suzanne is a 6-year-old you meet at a school-based clinic. You notice from her attendance record that she misses about 4 days of school every month for "constipation." As she walks down the hallway, you notice she walks on her tiptoes.

1. Suzanne's mother tells you Suzanne walks on her tiptoes because she learned to do that so her father, who works nights, won't be awakened during the day. Would you want to examine Suzanne's gait any further?
2. Suzanne's mother confirms Suzanne has almost "constant constipation." Her mother explains that it is because Suzanne never eats vegetables. On examination, you locate a hard mass in her upper right quadrant. Would you want to ask more questions about Suzanne's constipation?
3. Suzanne tells you she often doesn't eat lunch at school because she forgets her lunch money. Would you want to assess Suzanne's short-term or long-term memory?

Patient Scenario
The Diller Family

Read about the Diller family, a family with a 15-month-old, then answer the questions to further sharpen your skills and grow more familiar with NCLEX-type questions related to child health assessment. Confirm your answers are correct by reading the rationales.

Visit http://thePoint.lww.com

Answers and Rationales

Looking for answers to the What If… and Critical Thinking Care Study questions?

Visit http://thePoint.lww.com

References

American Academy of Pediatrics. (2012). *Recommendations for preventive pediatric health care.* Evanston, IL: Author.

American Academy of Pediatrics. (2013). *Your teen's yearly checkup.* Evanston, IL: Author.

Archer, S. M. (2012). Are amblyopia treatments really all equal? Is that even the right question? *American Orthoptic Journal, 62*(1), 1–3.

Berkowitz, C. D. (2011). Healing of genital injuries. *Journal of Child Sexual Abuse, 20*(5), 537–547.

Braverman, P. K., & Breech L. (2010). American Academy of Pediatrics. Clinical report—Gynecologic examination for adolescents in the pediatric office setting. *Pediatrics, 126*(3), 583–590.

Braverman, R. S. (2012). The eye. In W. W. Hay, M. J. Levin, R. R. Deterding, et al. (Eds.), *Current diagnosis & treatment pediatrics* (21st ed., pp. 424–464). Columbus, OH: McGraw-Hill/Lange.

Cameron, J. R., Rice, D. C., Sparkman, G., et al. (2013). Childhood temperament-based anticipatory guidance in an HMO setting: A longitudinal study. *Journal of Community Psychology, 41*(2), 236–248.

Centers for Disease Control and Prevention. (2012a). CDC grand rounds: Newborn screening and improved outcomes. *MMWR: Morbidity & Mortality Weekly Report, 61*(21), 390–393.

Centers for Disease Control and Prevention. (2012b). *Developmental milestones.* Washington, DC: Author.

Centers for Disease Control and Prevention. (2012c). *Immunization schedules.* Washington, DC: Author.

de Maleissye, M. F., Beauchet, A., Saiag, P., et al. (2012). Sunscreen use and melanocytic nevi in children: A systematic review. *Pediatric Dermatology, 30*(1), 51–59.

de Onis, M., Onyango, A., Borghi, E., et al. (2012). Worldwide implementation of the WHO Child Growth Standards. *Public Health Nutrition, 15*(9), 1603–1610.

Dubrovsky, A. S., Foster, B. J., Jednak, R., et al. (2012). Visibility of the urethral meatus and risk of urinary tract infections in uncircumcised boys. *CMAJ: Canadian Medical Association Journal, 184*(15), E796–E803.

Ely, E., Chen-Lim, M. L., Zarnowsky, C., et al. (2012). Finding the evidence to change practice for assessing pain in children who are cognitively impaired. *Journal of Pediatric Nursing, 27*(4), 402–410.

Flynn, J., Zhang, Y., Solar-Yohay, S., et al. (2012). Clinical and demographic characteristics of children with hypertension. *Hypertension, 60*(4), 1047–1054.

Frankenburg, W. K. (1994). Preventing developmental delays: Is developmental screening sufficient? *Pediatrics, 93*(4), 586–589.

Goodenough, F. L. (1926). *Measurement of intelligence by drawings.* New York, NY: World Book Company.

Heneghan, H. M., Heinberg, L., Windover, A., et al. (2012). Weighing the evidence for an association between obesity and suicide risk. *Surgery for Obesity & Related Diseases, 8*(1), 98–107.

Jaffe, A. C. (2011). Failure to thrive: Current clinical concepts. *Pediatrics in Review, 32*(3), 100–108.

Jones, J. L. P., & Kacmarynski, D. S. F. (2012). Hearing loss and balance disorders. In N. L. Shapero (Ed.), *Handbook of pediatric otolaryngology.* Hackensack, NJ: World Scientific Publishing.

King, S., Chambers, C. T., Huguet, A., et al. (2011). The epidemiology of chronic pain in children and adolescents revisited: A systematic review. *Pain, 152*(12), 2729–2738.

Levine, D. A. (2011). Evaluation of the well child. In K. J. Marcdante, R. M. Kliegman, H. B. Jenson, et al. (Eds.), *Nelson essentials of pediatrics* (6th ed., pp. 24–30). Philadelphia, PA: Saunders/Elsevier.

Luthy, K. E., Beckstrand, R. L., Callister, L. C., et al. (2012). Reasons parents exempt children from receiving immunizations. *Journal of School Nursing, 28*(2), 153–160.

Patel, V., & Elliott, P. (2012). Sudden death in athletes. *Clinical Medicine, 12*(3), 253–256.

Perry, D. C., Green, D. J., Bruce, C. E., et al. (2012). Abnormalities of vascular structure and function in children with perthes disease. *Pediatrics, 130*(1), e126–131.

Prevent Blindness America. (2012). *Distant vision test for younger children.* Chicago, IL: Author.

Rendall, M. S., Weden, M. M., Fernandes, M., et al. (2012). Hispanic and black U.S. children's paths to high adolescent obesity prevalence. *Pediatric Obesity, 7*(6), 423–435.

Riley, M., & Bluhm, B. (2012). High blood pressure in children and adolescents. *American Family Physician, 85*(7), 693–700.

Santillanes, G., Simms, S., Gausche-Hill, M., et al. (2012). Prospective evaluation of a clinical practice guideline for diagnosis of appendicitis in children. *Academy of Emergency Medicine, 19*(8), 886–893.

Sargant, N., Sen, E. S., & Marden, B. (2012). Too cold for comfort: A neonate with severe hypothermia. *Emergency Medicine Journal, 29*(5), 420–421.

Sato, H., Tomio, J., Tanaka, Y., et al. (2011). The public acceptance of smallpox vaccination to fight bioterrorism in Japan: Results of a large-scale opinion survey in Japan. *Environmental Health & Preventive Medicine, 16*(5), 290–298.

Shah, K. N., & Rubin, A. I. (2012). Nail disorders as signs of pediatric systemic disease. *Current Problem in Pediatric & Adolescent Health Care, 42*(8), 204–211.

Shmidt, E. & Levitt, J. (2012). Dermatologic infestations. *International Journal of Dermatology, 51*(2), 131–141.

Spiewak, R. (2012). Contact dermatitis in atopic individuals. *Current Opinion in Allergy & Clinical Immunology, 12*(5), 491–497.

Thomas, A., & Chess, S. (1977). *Temperament and development.* New York, NY: Brunner/Mazel.

Troiano, M. (2011). Child abuse. *Nursing Clinics of North America, 46*(4), 413–422.

Uno, Y., Uchiyama, T., Kurosawa, M., et al. (2012). The combined measles, mumps, and rubella vaccines and the total number of vaccines are not associated with development of autism spectrum disorder: The first case-control study in Asia. *Vaccine, 30*(28), 4292–4298.

U.S. Department of Agriculture. (2012). *Choose my plate: A guide to daily food choices.* Washington, DC: Author.

U.S. Department of Health and Human Services. (2010). *Healthy people 2020.* Washington, DC: Author.

Walter, K. D. (2011). Orthopedic assessment. In K. J. Marcdante, R. M. Kliegman, H. B. Jenson, et al. (Eds.), *Nelson essentials of pediatrics* (6th ed., pp. 735–762). Philadelphia, PA: Saunders/Elsevier.

Water, T. (2011). Critical moments in preschool obesity: The call for nurses and communities to assess and intervene. *Contemporary Nurse, 40*(1), 60–70.

Whitney, E. N., & Rolfes, S. R. (2012). Life cycle nutrition: Infancy, childhood & adolescence. In E. N. Whitney & S. R. Rolfes, *Understanding nutrition* (pp. 528–573). Belmont, CA: Wadsworth Publishing.

Wood, J. N., Pecker, L. H., Russo, M. E., et al. (2012). Evaluation and referral for child maltreatment in pediatric poisoning victims. *Child Abuse & Neglect, 36*(4), 362–369.

Yoon, P. J., Kelley, P. E., & Friedman, N. R. (2012). Ear, nose & throat. In W. W. Hay, M. J. Levine, J. M. Sondheimer, et al. (Eds.), *Current pediatric diagnosis & treatment* (20th ed., pp. 477–509). Columbus, OH: McGraw-Hill.

Chapter 35

Communication and Teaching With Children and Families

KEY TERMS

- affective learning
- behavioral therapy
- clarifying
- cognitive learning
- communication
- demonstration
- empathy
- feedback
- focusing
- health literacy
- nontherapeutic communication
- paraphrasing
- perception checking
- positive reinforcement
- psychomotor learning
- redemonstration
- reflecting
- therapeutic communication

OBJECTIVES

After mastering the contents of this chapter, you should be able to:

1. Describe principles of effective communication as well as teaching and learning as they relate to health teaching with children.
2. Identify 2020 National Health Goals related to communication and teaching with children that nurses can help the nation achieve.
3. Assess children for their ability to communicate and their readiness to learn.
4. Formulate nursing diagnoses related to communication and health teaching with children.
5. Identify expected outcomes for a specific child based on the child's age, developmental maturity, emotional needs, and communication or learning style to better enable parents to manage seamless transitions across differing health care settings.
6. Using the nursing process, plan nursing care that includes the six competencies of Quality & Safety Education for Nurses (QSEN): Patient-Centered Care, Teamwork & Collaboration, Evidence-Based Practice (EBP), Quality Improvement (QI), Safety, and Informatics.
7. Implement health teaching, such as creating a puppet show using principles of effective communication and teaching and learning.
8. Evaluate expected outcomes for achievement and effectiveness of care.
9. Integrate knowledge of communication and teaching with the interplay of nursing process, the six competencies of QSEN, and Family Nursing to promote quality maternal and child health nursing care.

You meet two patients of very different ages in an outpatient clinic. Wolf Whitefeather is a 3-year-old boy who is scheduled for repair of syndactyly (webbed fingers) next week. His mother tells you his favorite activity is coloring. She is concerned he will be hard to entertain after surgery because the large pressure bandage he will have afterward will prevent him from using that hand. "I don't even want to begin to talk to him about surgery," she tells you.

Barry Sandoz is a 16-year-old with a recurring peptic ulcer. His mother tells you health teaching with Barry will be ineffective because he never listens to a thing adults say.

Previous chapters discussed normal growth and development and how children's understanding increases with age. This chapter adds information about techniques for effective communication and health teaching with children and adolescents. This type of information is what builds a successful base for disease prevention and health promotion as well as increases health literacy.

(Continued on next page)

(Continued from previous page)

What would be a good strategy for teaching 3-year-old Wolf about his surgery? Would you try to teach Barry more about his condition, or not? How would your communication with these children vary because of their age difference?

Health literacy is an individual's ability to read, understand, and use health care information to make decisions and follow instructions (Taylor, Nicolle, & Maguire, 2013). Both communication and health teaching are independent nursing actions that are important for increasing health literacy, helping children learn more about their illness, and providing better measures to use to stay well. Increasing health literacy is especially important when preparing a child for surgery or some other health care procedure.

Communication is fundamental to social interaction and is one of the first and most important skills children learn (Cruz, Quittner, Marker, et al., 2013). It can be either a formal or informal exchange. Health teaching can also be both formal, such as teaching a group of preschoolers about hospitalization, or informal, such as assuring a parent a child is getting enough nutrition even though the child snacks rather than sits down to regular meals. It may be offered to an individual child or to a group of children with similar learning needs. Health teaching is so important, that a number of 2020 National Health Goals speak to it (Box 35.1).

BOX 35.1 Nursing Care Planning Based on 2020 National Health Goals

A number of 2020 National Health Goals address good communication and health teaching because it is such an important mechanism of preventive health care.

- Increase the proportion of schools that provide school health education from a baseline of 35.2% to 38.7% for elementary school; from 56.9% to 62.2% for middle school; and from 76.8% to 84.5% for high school.
- Increase the health literacy of the population by increasing the proportion of persons who report their health care provider always gave them easy-to-understand instructions about what to do to take care of their illness or health condition (developmental).
- Increase the proportion of persons who report their health care providers have satisfactory communication skills by increasing the proportion of persons who report their health care provider always explained things so they could understand them from 60% to 66%.
- Increase the proportion of local health departments that have established culturally appropriate and linguistically competent community health-promotion and disease-prevention programs (developmental) (U.S. Department of Health and Human Services [DHHS], 2010; see www.healthypeople.gov).

Nurses can help the nation achieve these goals by consulting with schools and health care organizations to develop what health teaching programs are needed and then teaching in such programs.

Nursing Process Overview
For Health Teaching With Children

Assessment
Communication and health teaching are best accomplished when they are placed within the context of the nursing process. Learner needs and characteristics, teacher characteristics, available support people, and the level of content are all factors that affect learning and whether communication will be received. Assessing these allows for nursing diagnoses that clearly state the specific health needs to be formulated.

Nursing Diagnosis
Common examples of nursing diagnoses related to communication or health teaching include:

- Risk for impaired verbal communication related to use of Russian as primary language
- Deficient knowledge related to importance of taking medicine daily
- Health-seeking behaviors related to ways to improve the child's nutritional intake
- Impaired verbal communication related to placement of endotracheal tube
- Anxiety related to perceived amount of material needed to be learned for home care of child

Outcome Identification and Planning
After formulating a nursing diagnosis, an individualized plan for communication or teaching should be constructed. The plan should detail not only what is to be communicated or learned but also methods to accomplish this and how it can be evaluated. The most effective way to ensure expected outcomes are achieved is to ask a child or family to join in the planning. Be certain outcomes are concrete and measurable (not "Child will discuss general aspects of his disease," but "Child will list three steps to help prevent disease reoccurrence"). Helpful tips for health education can be found at the American Association for Health Education Web site (http://www.aahperd.org/aahe) as well as that of the American Academy of Pediatrics (AAP; www.AAP.org).

Implementation
The step of implementation involves the actual carrying out of the communication or teaching. Teaching children is not always easy and requires practice and knowledge of each child's particular developmental level and needs.

Outcome Evaluation
As a final step of communication or teaching, what was communicated or learned must be evaluated to be certain learning occurred. A new plan may need to be developed and teaching continued if communication or learning proves to be less than optimal. Examples of outcome criteria include:

- Child demonstrates good technique for self-injection of insulin.

- Child demonstrates anger using language rather than punching wall.
- Child lists five foods to include in a high-protein diet.
- Family demonstrates improved family communication techniques by next clinic visit.
- Parents demonstrate effective cardiopulmonary resuscitation technique at home visit.

COMMUNICATION

Communication is the exchange of ideas between two or more persons. It can be verbal (i.e., using words) or nonverbal (i.e., using actions such as touch or eye contact, or a remote system such as mail or e-mail). Communication is important in the care of children because it can make or break an effective relationship. As a process, communication is divided into two major categories: *nontherapeutic* (i.e., casual, everyday conversation) and *therapeutic* (i.e., helpful, constructive interchanges).

Nontherapeutic Communication

Nontherapeutic communication is identified by its lack of structure or planning; that is, it lacks deliberate purpose other than socializing. Dinner conversation is an example of nontherapeutic communication.

Therapeutic Communication

Therapeutic communication is an interaction between two people that is planned (e.g., you deliberately intend to determine how a child truly feels), has structure (e.g., you use specific wording techniques that will encourage a truthful response), and is helpful and constructive (e.g., at the end of the exchange you will know more about the child than you did at the beginning, and ideally, the child will know more about a particular problem or concern) (Forchuk, 2010).

In some instances, there is no cure for a child you care for—no surgery, no medication, and no pain relief. If you practice therapeutic communication, however, you still have something to offer this child: support by your words or nonverbal communication such as touch. In perspective, this is often the most valued, most appreciated, and most helpful aspect of care (Svavarsdottir, Tryggvadottir, & Sigurdardottir, 2012).

Components of Good Communication

Communication can be broken down and diagrammed according to its essential components: the encoder, the code, the decoder, and response or feedback (Arnold, 2011) (Fig. 35.1).

The Encoder

The encoder is a person who desires to share a thought or feeling with someone else and so originates a message. This person molds this thought into a form suitable for transferring to another person (i.e., a code). Communication can be ineffective if a person omits cognitive processing or speaks without thinking; chooses the wrong words for the message; or accompanies the spoken words with a facial expression, tone of voice, or gesture that is inappropriate for the message.

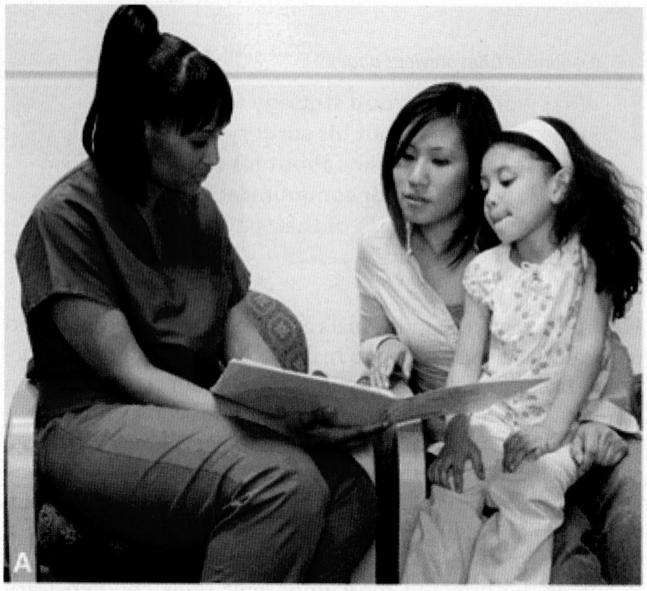

FIGURE 35.1 Health teaching is an interactive process, in which both a teacher and a learner share in the learning experience.

The Code

The code is the message that is conveyed and includes the medium or system used to convey it. Although this usually involves a simple spoken system, messages can also be conveyed by such methods as a painting, writing a poem or novel, Morse code, Braille, by electronic devices such as through text messaging, a movie projector, or over the telephone. Communication can be ineffective when a person chooses the wrong medium for a message; for instance, delivering a lecture with many technical words when a drawing would have made the message much clearer, or e-mailing when confronting a person directly would have had more impact.

The Decoder

The receiver (decoder) is the person who not only receives the message (i.e., hears it, reads it, views it) but also interprets or decodes its meaning (i.e., cognitive processing). Messages are interpreted in light of the receiver's previous knowledge. They may be misinterpreted if a receiver's store of knowledge is too different from that of the sender or if the receiver misses part of the transmission, such as a wink accompanying the spoken words that would have let the receiver know the sender was joking. Under stress, children tend to narrow their ability to receive information to a small area of concern (i.e., they center). Children who are extremely anxious, therefore, may not receive or be unable to interpret a message because of anxiety, even though both the sender and the message components of the communication were adequate.

Feedback or Response

Feedback is the reply the decoder returns to the sender to acknowledge the message has been received and interpreted. This could be a spoken statement, a nod of the head, a facial grimace, a return e-mail, or the sudden slamming of a telephone receiver. With feedback, the roles of sender and receiver become reversed and another communication cycle is begun. Communication can be ineffective if children do not offer feedback (i.e., the message was neither received nor understood) or if they offer feedback before the message is fully interpreted (i.e., acting before thinking). When you are caring for children with sensory challenges such as vision or hearing, you may need to change your usual feedback mechanisms in order to be understood because a nod of the head or quiet response may not be received. When a child is from a culture different than yours, it may require sensitive adaptation to be fully heard or to hear and understand.

The Development of Language

The development of language involves not only physically being able to form and voice words but also the comprehension of what they mean and how they are used (Box 35.2). One of the first responses an infant makes at birth is to cry. This first cry is important because it both signals that the infant is breathing well and also announces to the parents the birth is real, therefore stimulating the beginning of parent–child interactions.

By 2 years of age, children have mastered language well enough to be able to put two-word sentences (a noun and a verb) together. By preschool age, they not only have a vocabulary of about 900 words but also can code them into simple jokes or stories (Levine, 2011). Even children with cognitive challenges, although they may interpret jokes differently, still appreciate them (Degabriele & Walsh, 2010).

BOX 35.2 Nursing Care Planning Using Assessment

Assessing the Child's Learning and Communication Capabilities

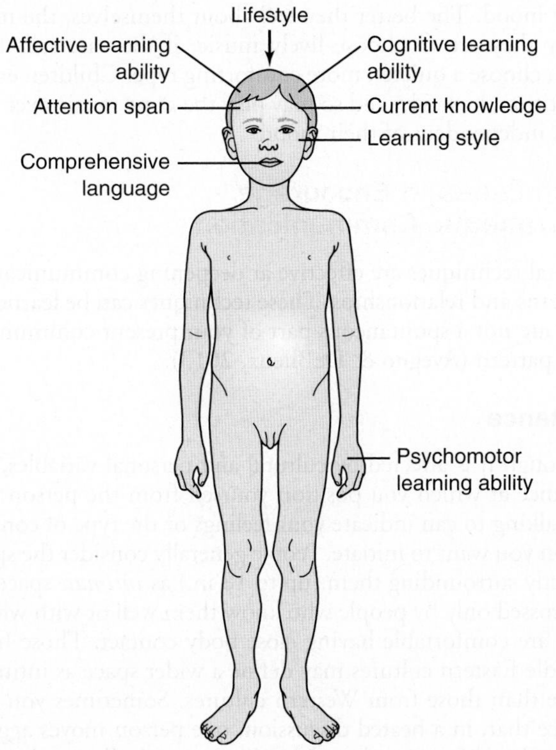

School-age children enlarge their ability to communicate from oral exchanges to use of the telephone and various electronic devices. They can write poetry and, by the end of the period, show an adult sense of humor by the jokes they create. Adolescents progress to a new phase in which they originate new words for objects or feelings ("cool" and "whatever" as responses). This form of communication helps them separate their world from adults and keep their adolescent culture separate.

Levels of Communication

Not every conversation you engage in has the same depth level, nor should it. Throughout the day, a person may use as many as five levels, from clichés to peak communication.

The First-Level: Cliché Conversation

Cliché conversation is pleasant chatting or comments such as, "Have a nice day" between people who do not intend for their relationship to extend beyond a superficial level. It is important when meeting a child for the first time that you introduce yourself not only with your name but also with your position and function (e.g., "I'm a student nurse who is going to take care of you"; "I'm a nurse who will be visiting you in your home"). This information leads the family to move the conversation from the cliché level to a more meaningful one.

The Second Level: Fact Reporting

Fact reporting is simply stating facts about oneself (a child says, "I'm 12; I'm in sixth grade"). Fact reporting is necessary for you to understand children, but it does not tell you anything about their feelings or needs. Children can move from this level to a higher level of communication only when they feel they can trust you with more information.

The Third Level: Shared Personal Ideas and Judgments

When children know you well, they are able to share ideas such as, "I always wanted to be an astronaut," and judgments such as, "This is too hard for me." This level of communication exposes them to a loss of self-esteem if their views are not respected. It is the level that is the beginning of therapeutic interactions.

The Fourth Level: Shared Feelings

It is difficult to share feelings until you truly trust another person because feelings are fragile concepts, easily destroyed and crushed by inept or uncaring comments. Listen carefully for an expression of feeling from children such as, "I hate always being sick." These admissions are telling you much more than how a child feels today; they represent trust in you and the depth of the relationship the child has established with you.

The Fifth Level: Peak Communication

The fifth level of communication is a sense of oneness, or being able to know what the other person is experiencing without any words being voiced. It sometimes occurs spontaneously in high-intensity situations but generally arises out of long-term relationships.

Nonverbal Communication

Nonverbal communication, such as wrinkling the nose, can be especially important in areas such as intensive care units when a child may be unable to speak because of endotracheal tubes and ventilators. Nonverbal communication can be expressed in a number of ways.

General Appearance

Children who have high self-esteem tend to maintain good body hygiene and care about their appearance. Those who are depressed may not feel the effort involved in grooming is worthwhile. Personal hygiene varies, however, and it is difficult to assess on your first contact with a child. What you see as ill-kempt may be neat and trim for that particular child; what you think of as well groomed may be comparatively sloppy for the child on that day.

Be aware that your impression of how children look or dress registers very strongly in your subconscious. Do not let an unconscious dislike for something such as body piercings or tattoos cause you to draw back. Preparing to give nursing care is not the same kind of activity as evaluating whether you wish to invite that person to dinner.

Body Posture and Gait

Children who feel good about themselves usually assume an upright body posture and walk rapidly and surely; those who are depressed or insecure tend to slouch and move more timidly; and those who are threatened tend to either draw back or act aggressively. Children who are in agreement with you usually maintain eye contact with you as you speak to them. Very depressed or insecure children do not do that (they feel too inferior), nor do children who are very angry. Remember that children from some cultures may not meet your gaze because it is not culturally appropriate (Box 35.3).

Humor

Some people have a natural knack for finding humor in any situation; others do not instinctively have this quality and so must cultivate it. Those who can laugh at their own mistakes are usually enjoyable people to have around because their laughter at themselves suggests that, when you make a mistake, they will be able to accept it the same way (or at least not be angry about it).

Be careful of the use of humor with children, however, because they are usually school age before they appreciate most adult jokes. If they are fatigued or ill, they may be looking for a support person to be with them more than one who is amusing. You can often measure the fall in a child's anxiety after a procedure by noting the first time the child responds to you with a humorous statement. Remember, though, laughter and joking can also be signs of increasing anxiety. Ascertain whether a child really finds a situation amusing or would rather have a serious caregiver.

BOX 35.3 Nursing Care Planning to Respect Cultural Diversity

Cultural differences between a teacher and a learner can complicate techniques of health teaching and the evaluation of its effectiveness. Even when language is not a barrier, the way children show they are listening or comprehending may vary from culture to culture. Looking directly at a speaker, for example, is considered disrespectful in some Asian countries. The "OK" sign traditional in the United States can be interpreted as vulgar, not positive, in Spain. In South Africa and some Middle Eastern countries, a "thumbs up" sign is insulting. In India, the way people move their head to express yes and no can be opposite to those used in the United States. A hand raised in a "stop" position may not be interpreted as halt by a child from a Middle Eastern culture but as a "go ahead" direction.

Being aware of these cultural differences is important when planning health teaching for diverse cultural groups so neither teaching nor reactions to teaching are misinterpreted.

Drawings

A useful nonverbal technique to learn how children feel about a frightening experience is to ask them to draw a picture of what happened or a picture of themselves. A child hospitalized for heart surgery, for example, might draw her heart prominently. She's revealing that she realizes she cannot survive if something happens to such an important body part.

A child's use of color may be a clue as to mood (happy children tend to use bright colors; depressed children use black or dark colors). A child with high self-esteem usually fills the full page with a drawing; one with less self-esteem crowds a drawing into a corner. These observations are quite variable, however, as a child may have had only a black crayon with which to color or may be saving the rest of the paper for a second drawing.

Music

The type of music to which children listen often also conveys their mood. The better they feel about themselves, the more likely they are to choose lively music; if they are sad, they often choose a quieter, more comforting type. Children enjoy repetition, however, and so may play the same music over and over, independent of their mood.

Techniques to Encourage Therapeutic Communication

Several techniques are effective at deepening communication patterns and relationships. These techniques can be learned if they are not a spontaneous part of your present communication pattern (Avegno & DeBlieux, 2013).

Distance

Although it is affected by cultural and personal variables, the distance at which you position yourself from the person you are talking to can indicate your feelings or the type of conversation you want to initiate. People generally consider the space directly surrounding them (up to 18 in.) as *intimate* space, to be crossed only by people who know them well or with whom they are comfortable having close body contact. Those from Middle Eastern cultures may define a wider space as intimate space than those from Western cultures. Sometimes you will notice that, in a heated discussion, one person moves aggressively into this space; the other will automatically step back to protect it. People in elevators usually separate themselves from others by this much space if the car is not full.

Whenever you touch a child, you violate intimate space, so always tell them when you are about to touch them ("I'm going change your bandage now"). If a child agrees to let you enter this space, it means they see you as safe, protective, and helpful.

The space between 18 in. to 4 ft is sensed by most people as *personal* space. This is the distance people usually stand apart from each other for casual conversation or hand shaking. When you stand by the side of a crib or bed or sit next to a person at home, you are within this space. It is a concerned, I-care-about-you distance but does not invade intimate space.

The distance between 4 ft and 12 ft is *social* space, the usual distance used to conduct business or to teach a class. Conversation spoken at this distance is readily heard by others. Do not use social space to ask a personal question. If you ask a child, "How are you feeling?" as you pass by in a hallway, for example, the child will probably answer, "Fine, thank you," a programmed reply almost everyone is taught in early childhood. In contrast, if you ask that same question from a personal or intimate distance, in a more private setting, the answer might be, "I'm scared I'm never going home again."

Although it is carried out miles apart, most people perceive texting, speaking on the telephone, or using mail or e-mail as either social or personal space. The tone of voice or the words used help to differentiate which area it appears to be. A message such as, "Have I got news for you!" suggests social space. "Can you keep a secret?" brings it into personal space.

The distance beyond 12 ft is *public* space. To communicate from this distance, you need to shout and privacy is not respected. Waving to a friend in a hallway or across a parking lot is an example of public space communication.

✔ QSEN Checkpoint Question 35.1

Patient-Centered Care

You want to review some health educational materials with Barry, age 16 years. In order to maximize his learning and his comfort level, this activity should take place in which type of physical space?

a. Intimate space
b. Social space
c. Public space
d. Personal space

Look in Appendix A for the best answer and rationale.

Genuineness and Truthfulness

Genuineness is a quality of projecting sincerity or being yourself. Children can have difficulty trusting you and therefore may be unable to move to a deep relationship with you if you change your behavior from one day to the next, such as from maximum patience one day to short-tempered the next, because this causes them to have to spend energy testing to see who you are on that particular day. The way to achieve a feeling of genuineness is being true to yourself, not trying to be what you are not, as the insecurity that comes from pretending can manifest itself as negative feelings such as aggressiveness or a bored attitude.

Warmth

Warmth is an innate quality some people manifest more spontaneously than others. Basic ways in which warmth is demonstrated are direct eye contact, use of a gentle tone of voice, listening attentively, approaching a child within a comfortable space of 1 to 4 ft, and using touch appropriately. Warmth is a quality you display best when you know another person well. Therefore, any action that helps you to know a person better (e.g., taking a health history, talking about school or family or how a child feels about the present situation) not only lets you plan care but also allows you to become increasingly comfortable with the child and creates opportunities to deepen the warmth of your relationship.

Empathy

Empathy is the ability to put yourself in another person's place and understand and be sensitive to the feelings of another (McMillan & Shannon, 2011). People who are capable of empathy are the best support people because they can anticipate a child's reactions or fears. Feeling empathy is emotionally draining because, when you assume another person's emotions, you experience them at the same depth as that person. Nurses who are capable of empathy need to surround themselves with good support people so they have refueling resources when they need them.

Gestures

Children vary a great deal in the gestures they use to accompany their spoken words. Although gestures are culturally influenced, it is also an individual trait. Be careful not to assess emotion only by a child's gestures. Some children wave their arms wildly describing an everyday occurrence; others would use that degree of expression only when in extreme distress. Be aware also that your own gestures are not always read well by children. A verbal statement that you approve of something is contradicted by placing your arms across your chest in a disapproving, stern manner.

Facial Expressions

Facial expressions are an important accompanying gesture to words. Clenched teeth, frowns, and smiles are easily interpreted by most people. The degree of pain a child is experiencing may be more evident by distressed facial expressions than words. Your approval or disapproval of an action may be more evident in your face than in your words.

Touch

Touch is the most intimate and meaningful of nonverbal techniques. When words are inadequate, touch rarely is. Learn to use touch such as clapping a child's shoulder or squeezing a hand to accompany reassuring words or in place of words as a strong support signal (e.g., I'm here; I understand; it's all right to be afraid). Be aware, however, that some children enjoy being touched more than others. Due to individual preferences or cultural variations, some children are not used to being touched or hugged. Assess individually for the appropriateness of using touch.

Attentive Listening

No one likes to talk to someone who does not appear to be listening or responding. Good listening, therefore, like speaking, is not passive but active. Be aware that your posture reveals to a great extent whether you are listening (e.g., sitting, not standing, to convey you are not on the run; leaning forward, not backward; stooping to meet a child's level). Nodding, maintaining eye contact, and stopping all other activities are strong indicators that you are attuned to what is being said. Making it clear you are attentively listening indicates you value what the other person is saying. Children who feel valued are much more likely to confide feelings and concerns than those who sense you do not consider them important.

In some instances, it is necessary to repeat a part of what a child said, interject an appropriate "uh-huh" or "m-m-m," or make a direct statement ("I'm listening. Go on") to indicate you are listening. Be certain, when you are listening to the 20th child on any given day, you do not exhibit "end-of-the-day" behavior. To be therapeutic, you have to give everyone's concerns the same alert attention (Box 35.4).

Reflecting

Reflecting is a technique, like attentive listening, that is so simple that its importance is easy to discount. **Reflecting** is restating the last word or phrase a child has said when there is a pause in the communication. A child says, "I'm worried," and then stops. You repeat the last word. "Worried?" The child, assured you are listening and interested, will generally enlarge on the first statement: "I'm worried I'll be too short of breath to make the football team this year." In contrast, adolescents may not respond well to reflection; they may interpret it as imitating them, not seeking information.

Clarifying

Clarifying consists of repeating statements others have made so you can be certain you understood them. This is particularly helpful if a child has been describing a set of symptoms or series of actions. A statement such as, "Let me see if I understand this. You said you always get the pain first in your stomach. Then it spreads to your chest," clarifies or makes clear what you have heard. If you are not quoting correctly, the child will interrupt and restate the problem: "No, the chest pain comes first."

Paraphrasing

Paraphrasing is restating what the child has said not only to assure the child you have heard correctly (as in clarifying) but also to help the child explain a thought. In clarifying, you repeat a child's exact words; in paraphrasing, you retain the meaning of the words but repeat them in a clearer or more condensed form. The child says, for example, "I don't talk about my problems with my parents." A paraphrasing statement might be, "You're telling me you and your parents haven't discussed home care. Is that right?" When paraphrasing, ask for confirmation that your interpretation is correct; otherwise, you may find yourself putting words in children's mouths.

When the topic is embarrassing or emotionally charged (e.g., an adolescent discussing sexual orientation), the child might use such vague terms that the explanation becomes difficult to follow. Paraphrasing using basic terms would let him know not only that you understand him but also that, if he can describe the problem better with such words than with medical terminology, it is all right to do that.

Perception Checking

Perception checking documents a feeling or emotion reported to you. This makes it a step deeper than paraphrasing. In paraphrasing, you document a statement or fact; in perception checking, you document a feeling or emotion. The child says for the second time, "I'm not at all worried about surgery. I mean, what could happen?" You say, "You're telling me you're not worried, but the number of times you've said it makes me wonder if you really are worried. Are you?"

Always ask for validation that your perception is correct so you do not make false assumptions. Perception checking is helpful because, as a rule, children are not ready to deal with emotions until they can admit they are experiencing them. When you bring an emotion out in this way, it allows them to confront it and deal with it for the first time. They may also lose their reluctance to admit other worries because you have implied that worrying is acceptable.

BOX 35.4 Nursing Care Planning Based on Family Teaching

LISTENING TO CHILDREN

Q. Barry's mother says to you, "My son always tells me I don't listen to him. How can I be a better listener?"

A. Try the following tips:

1. Stop talking. You cannot listen if you are talking.
2. Look and act interested. Don't read or write while he talks. Listen to understand rather than to reply.
3. Remove distractions. Do not doodle, tap, or shuffle papers. Turn off the television or put down your cell phone.
4. Empathize. Try to put yourself in your child's place so you can appreciate his point of view.
5. Be patient. Allow plenty of time. Do not interrupt. Do not edge toward the door as if you're about to walk away.
6. Hold your temper, argument, or criticism. An angry person can easily misinterpret the meaning of words.
7. Ask questions. This is proof that you have been listening.
8. Stop talking. This is the first and last suggestion, because all others depend on it.

What if...35.1 Because Barry Sandoz's family has hypercholesterolemia, Barry, 16 years old, needs to begin a low-cholesterol diet. He needs to learn more about foods so he can eat safely in the school cafeteria. Who would be the most important person to teach about Barry's diet? Barry? His mother who prepares his food? Or his father who does the grocery shopping?

Focusing

Focusing helps children to center on a subject you suspect is causing them anxiety because they comment about it indirectly or else completely avoid it. It is done by repeating something they said ("You mentioned you feel tired all the time") or by mentioning the avoided topic ("You haven't said a word about how you feel about this surgery"). Once a subject is brought up for discussion, most children respond to it. As long as it can be avoided, however, they do not have to face the problem and won't begin to solve it.

Supportive Statements

Supportive statements let children know you accept their behavior or at least appreciate they have dealt well with unfortunate circumstances. For example, an adolescent says, "My girlfriend dumped me while I've been here in the hospital." Such a statement deserves a supportive reply such as, "That must not feel good." The adolescent will take this response to mean you want to discuss the topic and, encouraged by your support, may elaborate on it because it still affects him.

Silence

If you ask a question and a child does not respond immediately, it is natural to ask another question or perhaps change the subject, assuming the child is not interested in the topic. This is a social custom that prevents you from putting someone into the awkward position of having to discuss a sensitive topic. Silence, however, can be an effective therapeutic technique. If you ask an emotion-laden question (e.g., "Are you worried?") and the child does not answer immediately, allow a period of silence to pass. Because you do not hurry to fill in the silence, the child is likely to respond (by hurrying an answer). When this happens, the answer is usually spontaneous and often open and uninhibited. In other instances, a child may answer the question deliberately and cautiously and, because you have provided a period of time to answer, may offer additional information.

Do not overdo silence, however, either by the number of times you use it or the length of time you allow it to extend. In this era of constant noise, many individuals are extremely uncomfortable with silence. Too much silence can also indicate to a child that you are not interested enough to maintain the conversation.

Process Recording

Process recording is a method to examine how effective you are at therapeutic communication. After your next interaction with a child, draw three columns on a sheet of paper. Take a few minutes to write down in the left column a statement the child made to you. In the middle column, write what you thought on hearing the statement. In a third column, write your response. Try to record both statements and responses verbatim or as close to the actual words used as possible. The average person can accurately recall about 3 minutes of communication this way.

Next, examine your responses to each statement by asking: Did I encourage the child to tell me more by my response, or did I block communication? Were my responses supportive, critical, or trite? Did I check perceptions or did I just assume I understood correctly what was told to me? See Box 35.5 for an example of a process recording with an adolescent.

QSEN Checkpoint Question 35.2

Informatics

You have heard from a colleague that Barry, 16 years old, hates school. When considering the use of informatics to respond to this statement, which principle should guide your actions?

a. Communication is most effective when it is enhanced by cutting-edge technology.
b. Referral to an appropriate, evidence-based Web site can likely resolve this issue.
c. Technology cannot usually substitute for skilled interpersonal communication.
d. Communication skills are being replaced by technologic innovation in nursing.

Look in Appendix A for the best answer and rationale.

Factors That Can Interfere With Effective Communication

Because so much of nursing care is influenced by verbal communication, it is important to avoid miscalculations in communication and to recognize common situations in which meanings can easily be distorted.

Age and Developmental Level

Age and developmental levels are important to communication abilities because they influence vocabulary and reading ability so greatly. Newborns and infants are amazingly perceptive regarding nonverbal communication. They quiet readily at a gentle tone of voice, and they show discomfort if an adult shouts or handles them roughly. Toddlers and preschoolers remain just as adept at reading nonverbal communication signals. They much prefer a happy approach (e.g., "Isn't this fun?") rather than a stern one. Because of their short attention span, their concentration wanders after about 5 minutes of time spent on an explanation. Older children are ready to listen to spoken words, although they are still attentive to nonverbal actions. They like role models and so are very opposed to "do as I say, not as I do" advice. They are ready to ask questions and use techniques, such as reflection, to be certain they understand what you have just said.

Intellectual or Behavioral Level

Intellectual level, like age, affects vocabulary and ability both to encode and decode messages. It influences the number of languages a child speaks, reading ability, and the depth of explanation a child is capable of understanding. Children

TABLE 35.3 Ways to Incorporate Informal Teaching Into Nursing Care

Activity	Type of Teaching
Medication administration	Children as young as early school age should know the type, action, and any expected side effects of all medication they are taking. Present medicine not by saying, "Here is your pill" but rather, "Here is your [name of medication]. It should help your temperature come back to normal. After you take this, you might feel yourself start to sweat. That means it's working."
Vital sign measurement	When taking vital signs such as blood pressure, temperature, and pulse, tell children what normal levels are, such as, "Your blood pressure is 100/70 mmHg. That's normal." If the child is in a high-risk category for hypertension, add some prevention measures to teaching.
Any procedure	Always tell children the purpose and principle of procedures. For instance, do not say, "You need to drink a lot of fluid" but rather, "You need to drink a lot of fluid because . . ."
Dressing changes	Dressing changes provide an opportunity to teach the danger of introducing infection into an open wound. The parents or child may not change this dressing, but they will apply bandages to small cuts in the future and so will benefit from teaching.
Mealtime	Provide information about nutrition, such as, "I know you're not hungry enough to eat the entire sandwich, but could you try the meat? Meat is high in protein and that's important for healing."
Hygiene	Emphasize the necessity for covering the mouth with a shirt sleeve to prevent the spread of upper respiratory infections or good perineal hygiene (i.e., wiping front to back in girls) to decrease the possibility of urinary tract infections.
Physical assessment	Assure children that their body parts are healthy as you examine them (e.g., "Your hair feels squeaky clean and strong") as both education and reassurance. Explain the importance and technique of self-testicular examination.
Positioning	Don't just reposition children in bed. Teach the hazards of immobility and how a change of position and ambulation increases circulation and respiratory function.
Sleep	Teach that sleep is a healing therapy and so should not be considered a waste of time.
Bowel elimination	Teach children elimination patterns vary, and that occasional variations in their elimination patterns are normal but stools should not be loose or black or painful.

Alternative Settings Versus Institutional Teaching. Health teaching in a health care agency usually focuses on immediate, acute care concerns. Teaching in a school may focus on topics such as basic health promotion and hygiene, reproductive and sex education, and drug abuse prevention. Teaching in the home may focus on medication regimens, dressing changes, or measures to prevent complications of a particular illness. It may also involve helping a child and parents adapt a procedure to the home setting, such as accommodating a wheelchair or oxygen therapy. Be certain parents know how to obtain the supplies they will need to learn and perform the procedure in the home.

Teaching in the home offers the advantage of being able to assess a child's environment, interactions with other family members, and overall family functioning. This may yield data that prove useful to further planning and implementation of care. It may also provide an opportunity to include other family members—siblings, grandparents, and so forth—in the teaching plan; this can strengthen the impact of teaching and ensure all family members understand the procedures in the same way. Always include evaluation as a step of teaching in all settings so you can feel confident that learning has occurred.

What if . . . 35.2 You organize a discussion group of adolescents on special diets so they can learn more about healthy nutrition in general. Barry, who needs to follow a low-cholesterol diet, says he won't participate in the group because nutrition is a "childish" subject. Would you insist he come to the meetings, or take the extra time to teach good nutrition to Barry at his bedside?

Determining Teaching Strategies

Because children's knowledge base, capabilities, learning styles, and attention spans vary so much, teaching strategies are most effective when they are both intermixed and selected in response to the individual child to be taught. The more interactive the method, the more appealing it is apt to be.

Lecture. Lecture (or directly explaining information) is the most efficient and time-saving method of offering information to both individual children and to groups. A lecture, however, does not allow for much participation, and it is effective only in short, well-structured periods. It is rarely effective for children who are not yet school age.

Demonstration. **Demonstration** is actually performing a procedure, such as a dressing change or instillation of eye drops, so the child can clearly see how the procedure should be done. Do not demonstrate a procedure unless you have all the necessary equipment to do it. If you have to stop in the middle of a demonstration to say, "Be sure to use a sterile syringe, not what I'm using," the poor technique demonstrated may be the lesson learned, not the good technique. The purpose of demonstration is to show how the procedure is actually done; having to imagine steps is little different than reading about it. School-age children, because of their stage of cognitive development (i.e., concrete operations), learn best by demonstration.

Redemonstration. To determine whether a child has truly grasped a demonstration, ask the child to perform a **redemonstration**, or an exact imitation of the procedure (Fig. 35.3). This is best if it immediately follows demonstration. Praise the effort to redemonstrate even if the redemonstration was not of the quality desired. No one likes to be put on the spot, and children may be unwilling to expose themselves again by a second redemonstration if criticized. Children do not have to follow your motions exactly because there are many different ways to do almost everything, as long as their technique accomplishes the same goal. An effective way to correct a wrong action is to say, "That's one way of doing that; you might find it easier, though, to. . . ." This type of criticism is nonthreatening because it acknowledges the child's effort in a positive way before offering a correction.

Discussion. Discussion is a shared learning experience in which children ask questions about particular concerns and you answer based on the child's individual circumstances. At the end of the discussion, hopefully all questions are answered and the problems are solved. The first time children are introduced to a subject, they tend to ask few questions because they do not know enough about the illness or health issue as yet to anticipate concerns. As their knowledge increases, so does their ability to project and modify information to fit their own lifestyle. Remember, children tend to think in the present: a problem that will arise once tomorrow is usually viewed as more important than one that can be predicted will arise repeatedly in years to come. Because this technique recognizes and respects their opinions, school-age children and adolescents enjoy discussion.

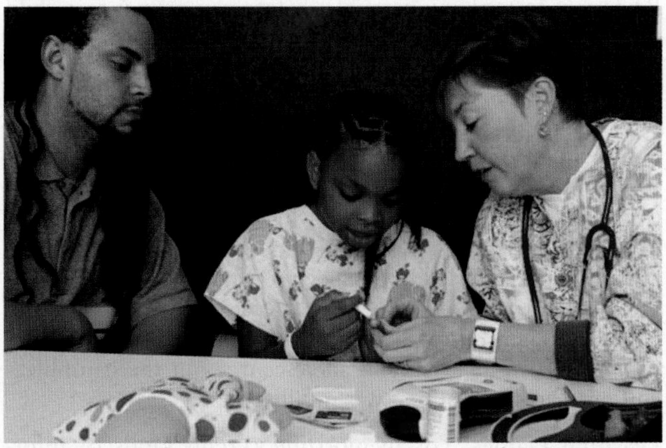

FIGURE 35.3 A school-age child redemonstrates blood glucose monitoring.

Role Modeling. Role modeling is demonstrating a certain attitude or behavior that you want a child to learn. Be certain when health teaching not only to present facts but also to radiate a positive role-modeling attitude because children pick up on role modeling cues as readily as a spoken message. Showing annoyance at getting a bubble out of a syringe demonstrates, for example, that giving injections is frustrating; showing a bored attitude toward nutrition implies eating well is boring.

Role modeling is an important technique used to teach new parents newborn care; as they watch a nurse hold, comfort, and talk to their newborn, they quickly learn to model these behaviors.

Behavioral Therapy. Typically, learning occurs best with **positive reinforcement** (e.g., a child tries to understand a new procedure, is praised for the effort, and tries even harder). **Behavioral therapy**, also called *behavior modification*, is a term used for a system aimed at *erasing* some form of behavior that interferes with healthy functioning. It was originally designed to help people who are cognitively challenged erase socially unacceptable behavior. Currently, it has many uses, including as a way to control disruptive classroom behavior. The basic premise of behavior modification is that a child is rewarded for healthful behavior, whereas unhealthful behavior is ignored or unrewarded. For example, a cognitively challenged child may have a socially unacceptable habit of constantly rocking back and forth. The child is not scolded or criticized for rocking, but the action is ignored. The preferred behavior (e.g., sitting for 5 minutes without rocking), however, is praised. Children respond best to behavior modification if, in addition to praise, they receive a tangible reward such as a star on a chart or an extra privilege for good behavior.

A behavior modification program must be discussed with the child before it is begun, because no behavior can be modified—just as no new behavior can be learned—until a child truly wants a change to occur. It might be necessary to ask older children to sign a learning contract to be certain both teacher and learner agree on the method to be used. Many older children are able to use self-rewards to reinforce a behavior modification program such as rewarding themselves by playing a video game or going to a movie after an afternoon of efficient studying or an hour of doing breathing exercises.

Behavior modification must be used with common sense and concern so children are not being manipulated more than they are being helped to achieve a more healthful lifestyle. It is a legitimate device to use to encourage children to do as much self-care as possible or to reduce anxiety disorders (May, Rudy, Davis, et al., 2012).

Trying to modify beliefs or values, not actions, by behavior modification is considered unethical and is one reason why behavior modification is often criticized as a learning technique for children. However, some behavior changes also require a change in values to be effective and long term. For example, a child's behavior of talking back to parents can be extinguished by ignoring or not responding to the behavior and by praising polite communication. This method teaches the child to value improved communication and parental approval in order to meet his or her needs.

Selecting Teaching Tools

Teaching tools are the mechanical devices used to present content. They vary based on content, teacher/learner characteristics, and environment.

Visual Aids. "A picture is worth a thousand words" is not an idle quotation but a realistic one. Because small children know little about their bodies or where body organs are located, using visual aids such as drawings or photographs of anatomy can be very helpful to explain disease. Figure 35.4 shows abdominal contents as an example of such a drawing. You could use such an illustration to show a preschooler how food moves through the body. Figure 35.5 is an example of a good tool to use while naming body parts. Pointing to a figure drawing and saying, "This is the part of your tummy you're going to have fixed," is less threatening than actually pointing to the child's abdomen. Clarifying body parts this way is important because young children may have no clear understanding of where a body part such as a hand ends and an arm begins.

Do not be afraid to draw a picture of a heart, a kidney, a bladder, or any other organ to make a point about anatomic structure. Children are more interested in understanding procedures or the reason for a health maintenance measure than criticizing your artwork because they likely do not know anatomy well enough to be able to tell if a drawing is distorted.

Pamphlets. Pamphlets or information sheets are helpful teaching aids with school-age children, adolescents, and parents (Pile, 2013). These usually contain brief, easy to read, and easily understood information and are often cleverly illustrated with cartoon characters to make them enjoyable for a wide age range. Be certain to read any pamphlet before you offer it to a child to be certain the information included in it is accurate. Medical advances occur so quickly that a 1-year-old pamphlet may contain a gross inaccuracy in the light of subsequent knowledge.

If a pamphlet contains some statements that are inaccurate or that do not apply to a child, do not simply cross out the information that would be contradictory before offering it (most children deliberately read what they have been told not to read). Instead, take the time to explain why it doesn't apply. Also, do not be misled into believing that because children are given clever pamphlets, they will necessarily read them and learn from them. Sit with a school-age child and read the pamphlet together. Talk with an adolescent about the pamphlet's contents later to ensure it was not just tossed aside.

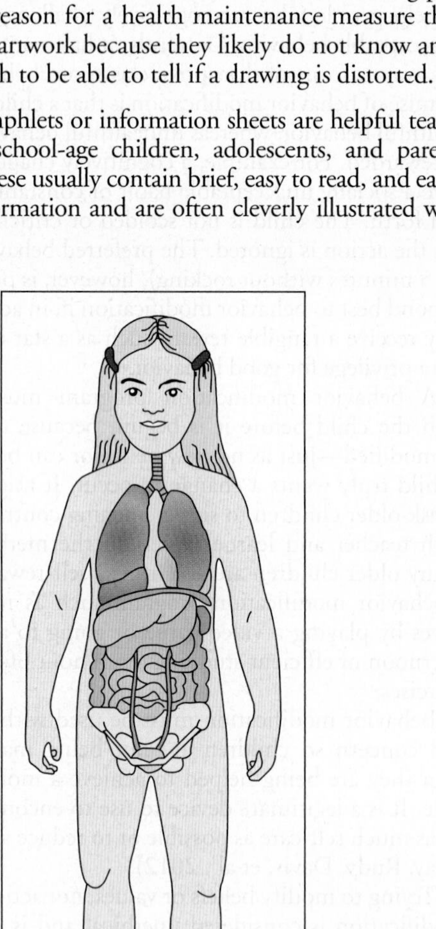

FIGURE 35.4 Anatomic drawings are helpful to illustrate basic health education topics and health care procedures.

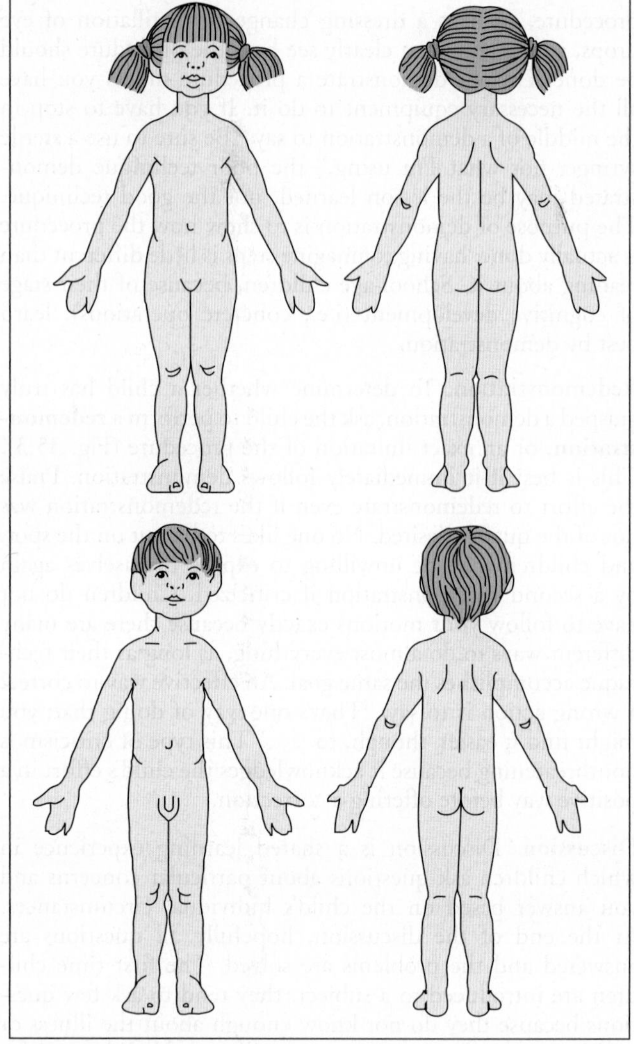

FIGURE 35.5 Simple line drawings such as these can be used to explain to a child exactly what part of his or her body will be "fixed" in surgery. For many children, having this pointed out on a drawing seems much less intrusive than having it pointed to on their own bodies.

Learning Games. For memorizing certain kinds of information, such as what foods are high or low in potassium or sodium, flash cards can be a helpful learning tool. Many children over 10 years of age (the age the average child is ready for competition) enjoy playing trivia-type board games. For health teaching, instead of using the game's categories of information, make up new cards with questions such as, "Where is insulin produced in your body?" Children learn information quickly this way because the reward for learning is immediate (e.g., they get to move their token on the board). Having parents play the game with their child can effectively educate parents at the same time.

Word scrambles are easy games to develop. Crossword puzzles are fairly easy to design; one might be developed to address the important activities for a child to do after surgery such as deep breathing, exercising legs, and not eating immediately.

Videos. Many health care agencies, homes, schools, and community centers have video playback equipment, such as a DVD player, that can be used to show a short video or PowerPoint presentation as part of a health education program. Most households have CD or DVD players, so discs can be sent home for families to view. Viewing such programs can offer children a sense of power in that the program seems to be talking directly to them. Such a program can also be used over and over to refresh children's knowledge of the steps they need to take to remain well (Crawford, Texter, Hurt, et al., 2012). As with pamphlets, view the material first before showing it to a child and be certain the vocabulary used will be appropriate for an individual child or family.

Playing video or electronic games can be used to urge children to exercise, although the worth of these must be carefully compared to more traditional forms of exercise such as walking or joining a sports team (Primack, Carroll, McNamara, et al., 2012).

QSEN Checkpoint Question 35.4

Safety

You want to teach Barry more about his hypercholesterolemia and he has expressed a preference for video resources. In order to ensure that such videos are safe, age-appropriate, and accurate, you should do which of the following?

a. Preview any potential video resources before referring them to Barry.
b. Encourage Barry to search YouTube and then report back to you.
c. Emphasize the fact that written materials are usually preferable to video materials.
d. Refer Barry to his local public library and have him liaise with a librarian.

Look in Appendix A for the best answer and rationale.

Puppets and Dolls. Many children are shy about talking to strangers. This shyness, in addition to their concern about what will happen to them, may make it difficult for them to discuss or explain what they know about their health, illness, or intended surgery. However, they may be able to open up to an uncritical puppet or doll because they see this as a usual part of play (Meghan, 2012). Box 35.7 shows an interprofessional care map illustrating both nursing and team planning for a preschooler having surgery. Preschool children are particularly receptive to puppets and dolls because, with their imagination at its peak, they believe the puppet or doll is actually talking to them.

Teaching preschool children about what to expect from a hospital experience is often taught by using a series of puppets or dolls to represent different hospital personnel such as a surgeon, a nurse, and a nurse's assistant. Children can practice giving the doll "shots" or submitting it to the procedures they will experience (see Chapter 36 for a discussion of therapeutic play).

Mass Media. Television and radio are examples of effective mass media that are used to teach many children about self-help or self-care. Consulting on the topics to present or helping develop the material used in these types of health messages can be an important role for nurses. Messages originated for these media must be attention getting and brief to compete with the programs and commercial messages that precede or follow them.

Computers and Internet. Many children learn to solve problems using computers as early as preschool age. Using an Internet application to answer questions about an illness or prepare children for surgery is effective because this type of activity can be both entertaining and informative (Whittemore, Jaser, Jeon, et al., 2012). Caution children not all information posted on the Web is reliable, and participating in chat rooms can lead not only to the information they were seeking but also to exposure to Internet predators (Briggs, Simon, & Simonsen, 2011).

Preparing Teaching Supplies

To avoid having to reorganize equipment or instructions each time a procedure is taught, put together a basket or box containing all the information and equipment needed to teach a particular task. This helps ensure that teaching will not only be organized but also economical in that everyone on a hospital unit is not opening new equipment for demonstrations. It also helps to ensure everyone is teaching the same information. Nothing is more confusing to someone learning a new skill than to be taught two different principles or techniques for doing something.

Implementing the Plan

Health teaching can begin immediately after contact with a child and should flow easily if goals have been well developed and strategies for teaching have been carefully designed.

Using Designated Teachers

Many health care agencies, including home care agencies, have specific people who are available for health teaching about specific subjects such as diabetes, stomal care, respiratory exercises, or drug abuse prevention. Using such people is helpful because they know all the "tricks of the trade" for teaching that particular subject.

Some children do not learn as well from such designated teachers, however, because they see them only infrequently, unlike a primary nurse, whom they may see daily. Some parents react badly to the thought that, if it takes an expert to tell them about the care needed, how can they possibly learn it? They may also find it inconvenient to be told their questions

BOX 35.7 Nursing Care Planning

AN INTERPROFESSIONAL CARE MAP FOR A PRESCHOOLER HAVING SURGERY

Wolf Whitefeather is a 3-year-old boy who is scheduled for repair of syndactyly (webbed fingers) next week.

Family Assessment Client lives with mother in two-bedroom mobile home. Parents separated. Mother works at local hospital in Medical Billing. Grandmother does child care 4 hours a day; child attends Head Start program in afternoon. Mother describes finances as "I'm making it." Father will visit after surgery; mother has custodial authority.

Client Assessment Favorite activity: coloring. His mother is concerned Wolf will be hard to entertain after surgery because the large pressure bandage he will have in place will prevent him from using that hand. "I don't even want to begin to talk to him about surgery," she added. When nervous or frightened, child has a habit of biting his hand; he has done this constantly since admission.

Nursing Diagnosis Deficient knowledge related to what to expect in surgery

Outcome Criteria Child describes expected outcomes of surgery. Demonstrates a minimum of nervous behaviors such as biting hand, can play "Simon Says" for hand exercises postsurgery, and describes how pain will be relieved by a "special button" (patient-controlled analgesia).

Teaching Points Child is shy with strangers; mother states he learns best by "hands-on" experiences; "cocks head" when puzzled. Also learns better from his mother than from his father (father tends to be authoritarian).

Cognitive Learning to Be Taught Why surgery is necessary

Psychomotor Skills to Be Taught To keep hand in elevated position after surgery

Affective Aspects to Be Taught Accepts surgery as a growth experience

Team Member Responsible	Assessment	Intervention	Rationale	Expected Outcome
Activities of Daily Living, Including Safety				
Nurse	Assess what child and parent understand about care necessary postoperatively.	Introduce postoperative hand exercises child will need to do by playing "Simon Says."	Games are an appealing way to keep the preschooler interested and motivated in doing exercises.	Child demonstrates opening and closing hand to help prevent contractions postprocedure.
Teamwork and Collaboration				
Nurse/Surgical health care provider	Assess which anesthesia team member will be available for operating room and postoperative pain management.	Request anesthesia/ analgesia consult.	Child is too young to be cooperative during surgery; needs pain relief afterward.	Anesthesia service meets with child and parent; determines best form of pain management and anesthesia.
Procedures/Medications for Quality Improvement				
Nurse/Surgical health care provider	Assess health history.	Complete the physical exam.	Health assessment helps ensure readiness for surgery.	Child cooperates with the history and exam.
Nurse	Assess Wolf's and parent's knowledge of surgery and postoperative procedures.	Introduce dressing and show how child's hand will be suspended postoperatively by letting Wolf dress and suspend puppet's hand.	Therapeutic play provides an excellent medium for teaching and learning with toddlers and preschoolers.	Child demonstrates he understands how hand will be positioned by showing position with puppet.

Nutrition				
Nurse	Assess if child and parent know child will be nothing by mouth (NPO) for general anesthesia for surgery.	Teach parent importance of NPO preoperatively and immediately postoperatively.	Maintaining NPO status helps prevent aspiration with anesthesia.	Child and parent state they understand need for NPO status and will adhere to requirement.
Patient-Centered Care				
Nurse	Assess child's cognitive level and ability to learn and who is child's main support person.	Using puppets, teach that the child's hand will be washed with antiseptic solution before surgery.	Reducing skin bacteria prior to surgery can help prevent osteomyelitis.	Child cooperates with preprocedure washes. Names mother as person he wants with him.
Psychosocial/Spiritual/Emotional Needs				
Nurse/Pain management team member	Assess what past experiences, if any, the child has had with pain.	Teach child he will have pain after surgery but it can be relieved by a "special button" on his intravenous pump.	Explaining how pain will be relieved before surgery can help reduce amount of stress after surgery.	Child and parent state they know there will be pain and understand method to be used for control.
Informatics for Seamless Health Care Planning				
Nurse	Assess if child and parent feel equipped to change bandages, carry out hand exercises at home, and have return appointment.	Review with parent a schedule of care based on Head Start and grandmother involvement.	Helping a parent walk through how post-procedure activities can be managed helps ensure adherence.	Mother states she has a plan for how to consistently arrange care given by three caregivers, and will keep return appointment.

QSEN Checkpoint Question 35.5

Evidence-Based Practice

Preparing children for surgery can be time consuming if done as a face-to-face instruction. To determine if a Web-based instructional program could be as effective at reducing children's anxiety about surgery as one-on-one instruction, researchers studied the differences between 75 children who watched an Internet "virtual surgery tour" program and 75 children who received face-to-face instruction. Although the results of the study showed no measurable change in children's emotional distress between those who watched the virtual tour and those who received one-on-one instruction, the knowledge level of children in the Web-based group was significantly higher. Interestingly, parents' anxiety increased by watching the virtual tour program (Tourigny, Clendinneng, Chartrand, et al., 2011).

Based on the previous study, which of the following would you recommend for Wolf, 3 years old, if he seemed exceptionally anxious before surgery?

a. Face-to-face instruction is preferable because it is most effective.
b. He has no reason to feel anxious because 1-day surgery is finished so quickly.
c. He should be given the choice between a Web-based program or face-to-face instruction.
d. He, like most preschoolers, is too young to understand an explanation of his surgery.

Look in Appendix A for the best answer and rationale.

cannot be answered until the following day when the designated teacher is available to answer them. Be certain that if a designated teacher does teach a subject, you coordinate your teaching with that person. Make a point of introducing the person to the child so the child does not view the person as a suspicious stranger.

Parent Education

With very young children, parents as well as children need teaching. It's good practice with all children to be certain that at least one adult in the household has the necessary information or can perform the required skill as well as the child. If at all possible, allowing for cultural beliefs that may dictate child care responsibilities in the family, let the child choose this person because the individual who everyone assumes is a child's chief support person may not be the person the child perceives as the most reliable choice for a health care backup. This person, when identified, needs as much information as the child about why the health measure is important.

What if...35.3 Wolf, 3 years old, refuses to tell you whether he has pain because you are a "stranger" and he doesn't talk to strangers. What would you do?

Evaluating the Effectiveness of Teaching

Evaluation, or assessing whether teaching has been effective, is the final step in teaching. It is optimum if evaluation occurs not only after the teaching plan has been implemented but also throughout the entire learning process. This ongoing evaluation helps both teacher and learner modify the teaching plan to better meet changing needs.

There is some advantage in asking children questions before and after teaching to prove that teaching was effective and that the child has safely learned a new health care measure. Demonstration of a change of behavior or attitude, however, is the real proof that learning has occurred.

QSEN Checkpoint Question 35.6

Teamwork & Collaboration

You want Wolf, 3 years of age, to know how to do the hand exercises he will need to do after surgery. When collaborating with the physiotherapist, which technique below would probably be most effective with Wolf?

a. A pamphlet you read together
b. A lecture from a sports hero
c. Playing a game of Simon Says
d. A group discussion on hand pain

Look in Appendix A for the best answer and rationale.

HEALTH TEACHING FOR A SURGICAL EXPERIENCE

Teaching to prepare a child for surgery is an example of teaching that requires planning for several stages of learning. The child and the child's parents often feel anxious about surgery because this is always a potentially frightening experience. Therefore, teaching must first address this anxiety. Such preparation differs according to the type of surgery being performed, but certain activities apply to all surgery and all children.

A psychological preparation of both the child and parents is aimed at reducing a child's fears about the procedure and consists primarily of providing health teaching and opportunities for therapeutic play. A physical preparation includes providing for restrictions on food and fluid intake before surgery, preparing the incision site on the child's skin, and arranging for transportation of the child to surgery. Because many children's surgical procedures are done on an ambulatory basis, parents often perform a part of physical preparation in preparation for the surgery as well as postoperative care and so must have clear instructions as to their responsibility. Do not downplay a family's fears, but allow the child and family opportunities to express their concerns as part of the teaching/learning process.

Assessing Current Level of Knowledge

On admission to the health care setting, whether the surgery will include a 1-day or longer hospitalization experience, elicit from parents what preparation they have made for this experience and what specifically they have told their child about what will happen. It's good to also ask whether a child's concerns about the experience seem more or less than the parents had anticipated. To see if the child is emotionally prepared, ask if there has been an unpleasant surgery or hospitalization in the family recently that the child might have heard discussed, or if the child has seen anything recently on a medical show on TV that might have been upsetting?

Emotional Preparation

Preparing a child emotionally for surgery requires minimizing fears common to all children such as fear of separation, fear of mutilation, or fear of death. Give careful explanations of what the procedure will entail and describe any specific equipment or techniques that will be used, such as anesthesia, eye bandages, nasogastric tubes, sutures, or special aftercare. Be certain all preparation is appropriate to the child's age. Most children who need surgery receive a general anesthetic rather than a local or regional anesthetic, as might be used with adults, because this minimizes their fears of intrusive or mutilating procedures, and because children who are not yet adolescent are not mature enough to cooperate adequately during surgery if they are not fully anesthetized.

It is best to prepare a child for a major experience like this in stages rather than all at once because it is difficult to absorb so much information in a short time span. However, contact before surgery may be limited to only one office or clinic visit, or the morning of surgery, so time constraints can force information to be more compacted.

Be certain to discuss presurgery preparations such as necessary blood work and not eating the morning of surgery. If the child will have general anesthesia, it is important to emphasize that anesthetized sleep is "special" sleep. Otherwise, toddlers or preschoolers may be reluctant to fall asleep after surgery for fear people will come and do strange things to them. Do not say a child will be "put to sleep" (dogs and cats who are "put to sleep" are never seen again). To help prepare a young child for surgery, a doll's abdomen could be washed, a hospital gown put on, and an injection given to make the doll sleepy. It could be carried to a cart made from a cardboard box. After saying goodbye to its parents, the doll could be wheeled to surgery by a puppet nurse.

The surgery procedure should be discussed but minimized. "After you're asleep, the doctor will fix your tummy. You won't feel anything because of the special sleep. When you wake up, you'll be in a room called a recovery room where you'll stay until you're wide awake." Be honest concerning pain, "Your tummy will feel sore afterward, but I'll give you something to make it feel better" is a fair statement.

It is important to alert children that personnel in surgery wear surgical masks. Assure toddlers and preschoolers the persons behind the masks are doctors and nurses, some of whom the child has probably already met, not superheroes or bandits.

It is also good to mention recovery rooms in preparation, because this is often an area parents neglect to mention. In fact, parents may not be aware that, in some institutions, they will

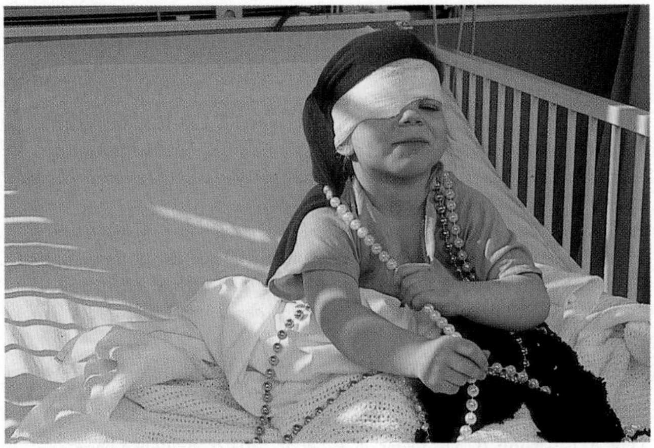

FIGURE 35.6 Pretending to be a pirate helps this young child prepare for having to wear an eye patch after surgery.

not be allowed in the recovery room and may have promised the child, "As soon as you wake up, I'll be there." Clarify the parents' misconceptions about recovery rooms, and reiterate the child will get to see his parents back in his own room once he is fully awake. This both makes the parents' preparation correct and saves the child from feeling deceived.

Explain postsurgery items, such as the use of oxygen, monitors, bedpans, bandages, or intravenous equipment. Furnishing a doll with such equipment is especially helpful in preparing younger children (Fig. 35.6). This play level is less stressful for preschoolers, rather than being taken to an intensive care unit where they can feel overwhelmed by the sight of actual monitors and ventilators. After surgery, be certain to evaluate whether a child's preparation was adequate, both to document the experience was as trauma free as it could have been and to evaluate your expertise in teaching children.

What if...35.4 You are particularly interested in exploring one of the 2020 National Health Goals with respect to communication and teaching with children (see Box 35.1)? What would be a possible research topic to explore pertinent to this goal that would be applicable to Barry's or Wolf's family and that would also advance evidence-based practice?

Key Points for Review

- Communication is the exchange of ideas between two or more persons. It can be verbal or nonverbal.
- Therapeutic communication is a planned interaction, has structure, and is constructive. Nontherapeutic communication lacks deliberate purpose other than socializing.
- Successful communication requires an encoder, a code, a decoder, and feedback or a response.
- Levels of communication include: (1) cliché, (2) fact reporting, (3) shared ideas, (4) shared feelings, and (5) peak communication.
- Typical methods of nonverbal communication are using distance, gestures, body posture, touch, use of drawings, and empathy.
- Techniques that encourage therapeutic communication are attentive listening, open-ended questions, reflecting, clarifying, paraphrasing, perception checking, focusing, supportive statements, and silence.
- Some situations require special communication techniques such as interacting with demanding or shy children, children who are visually or hearing challenged, or children who are not proficient in English.
- Establishing a teacher/learner relationship based on mutual input and setting expected outcomes are effective ways to meet the unique needs and goals of a child and family as well as to help in planning nursing care that meets QSEN competencies.
- There are three types of learning: cognitive, psychomotor, and affective. For something to be learned well, all of these areas may need to be involved.
- To individualize a teaching program for a child, assess the child's attention span, cognitive or intellectual capability, lifestyle, and learning style and your own teaching strengths and limitations.
- In many instances, there is a great deal of material a child must learn about an illness. If possible, divide material into lessons that can be taught immediately and lessons that can be taught at return health visits.
- The format and strategies of teaching used with children vary depending on a child's age and developmental level. Various types to consider are formal versus informal, single or group teaching, lecture, discussion, and role-playing.
- Behavior modification is a special technique aimed at erasing some form of behavior that interferes with good health.
- Children learn many other things besides health information every day. This may make the retention of information not as great as you would like. You may need to schedule frequent reviews and updates to keep information current.

Critical Thinking Care Study

Lucy is a 7-year-old who is scheduled to have her tonsils removed. She lives with her mother and father in a central city apartment. Her father works as a taxi driver. Her mother is a stay-at-home mom. Lucy is home schooled because she is cognitively challenged due to a birth injury and because she doesn't want other children to "laugh at her because she's in a special class." Her mother does not know her exact developmental age but says, "She can't begin to comprehend" second grade work. Because Lucy is becoming overweight, you'd like to teach her more about the importance of exercise so hopefully she can include some every day into her home schooling schedule.

1. You schedule a hospital tour every week for children who will have a tonsillectomy the following week. Lucy's mother replies she doesn't want to take advantage of this learning opportunity. Are you surprised by this? Is declining the tour in Lucy's best interest?
2. Following Lucy's tonsillectomy, you bring your teaching basket about exercise to her bedside. Lucy refuses to look at anything you show her; instead, she just concentrates on putting shoes on her doll. Would you continue teaching?

3. Lucy's mother has told you she doesn't know Lucy's developmental age. Would it be important for her to have a psychology consult prior to surgery so you could be certain your preparation for surgery will be effective?

Patient Scenario

The Henrietta Family

Read about the Henrietta family, a family with a child who needs added health teaching, then answer the questions to further sharpen your skills and grow more familiar with NCLEX-type questions related to communication and teaching children and families. Confirm your answers are correct by reading the rationales.

Visit http://thePoint.lww.com

Answers and Rationales

Looking for answers to the What If. . . and Critical Thinking Care Study questions?

Visit http:thePoint.lww.com

References

Arnold, E. C. (2011). Theoretical perspectives and contemporary dynamics. In E. C. Arnold & K. U. Boggs (Eds.), *Interpersonal relationships: Professional communication skills for nurses* (6th ed., pp. 1–21). Philadelphia, PA: Elsevier/Saunders.

Avegno, J., & DeBlieux, P. M. C. (2013). Characteristics of great teachers. In R. L. Rogers, A. Mattu, M. Winters, et al. (Eds.), *Practical teaching in emergency medicine* (pp. 159–167). Hoboken, NJ: Wiley-Blackwell.

Başkale, H., & Bahar, Z. (2011). Outcomes of nutrition knowledge and healthy food choices in 5- to 6-year-old children who received a nutrition intervention based on Piaget's theory. *Journal for Specialists in Pediatric Nursing, 16*(4), 263–279.

Briggs, P., Simon, W. T., & Simonsen, S. (2011). An exploratory study of Internet-initiated sexual offenses and the chat room sex offender. *Sexual Abuse, 23*(1), 72–91.

Coplan, R. J., Rose-Krasnor, L., Weeks, M., et al. (2013). Alone is a crowd: Social motivations, social withdrawal, and socioemotional functioning in later childhood. *Developmental Psychology, 49*(5), 861–875.

Crawford, D., Texter, T., Hurt, K., et al. (2012). Traditional nurse instruction versus 2 session nurse instruction plus DVD for teaching ostomy care. *Journal of Wound, Ostomy & Continence Nursing, 39*(5), 529–537.

Cruz, I., Quittner, A. L., Marker, C., et al. (2013). Identification of effective strategies to promote language in deaf children with cochlear implants. *Child Development, 84*(2):543–559.

Decarlo, D. K., McGwin, G. Jr., Bixler, M. L., et al. (2012). Impact of pediatric vision impairment on daily life: Results of focus groups. *Optometry & Vision Science, 89*(9), 1409–1416.

Degabriele, J., & Walsh, I. P. (2010). Humour appreciation and comprehension in children with intellectual disability. *Journal of Intellectual Disabilities Research, 54*(6), 525–537.

Deibel, M. D., & Wagner, M. J. (2013). Small group discussion skills. In R. L. Rogers, A. Mattu, M. Winters, et al. (Eds.), *Practical teaching in emergency medicine* (pp. 180–191). Hoboken, NJ: Wiley-Blackwell.

Erikson, E. H. (1993). *Childhood and society.* New York, NY: W. W. Norton.

Espelage, D. L., Basile, K. C., & Hamburger, M. E. (2012). Bullying perpetration and subsequent sexual violence perpetration among middle school students. *Journal of Adolescent Health, 50*(1), 60–65.

Forchuk, C. (2010). Communication & the therapeutic relationship. In W. Austin & M. A. Boyd (Eds.), *Psychiatric mental health nursing for Canadian practice* (2nd ed.). Philadelphia, PA: Lippincott Williams & Wilkins.

Hee, H. I., Lim, E. H., Tan, Q. C., et al. (2012). Effect of preoperative education on behaviour of children during induction of anaesthesia: A randomised clinical trial of efficacy. *Anaesthesia & Intensive Care, 40*(5), 795–802.

Johnson, N. L., Lashley, J., Stonek, A. V., et al. (2012). Children with developmental disabilities at a pediatric hospital: Staff education to prevent and manage challenging behaviors. *Journal of Pediatric Nursing, 27*(6), 742–749.

Kirk, K. I., Prusick, L., French, B., et al. (2012). Assessing spoken word recognition in children who are deaf or hard of hearing: A translational approach. *Journal of the American Academy of Audiology, 23*(6), 464–475.

Kohlberg, L. (1984). *The psychology of moral development.* New York, NY: Harper & Row.

Levine, D. A. (2011). Growth & development. In K. J. Marcdante, R. M. Kliegman, H. B. Jenson, et al. (Eds.), *Nelson essentials of pediatrics* (6th ed., pp. 13–44). Philadelphia, PA: Saunders/Elsevier.

May, A. C., Rudy, B. M., Davis, T. E., et al. (2012). Evidence-based behavioral treatment of dog phobia with young children: Two case examples. *Behavior Modification, 37*(1), 143–160.

McMillan, L. R., & Shannon, D. (2011). Program evaluation of nursing school instruction in measuring students' perceived competence to empathetically communicate with patients. *Nursing Education Perspectives, 32*(3), 150–154.

Meghan, L. (2012). Children at play: An innovative method for studying and teaching nutritional behaviors. *Pediatric Nursing, 38*(3), 139–143.

Metsiou, K., Papadopoulos, K., & Agaliotis, I. (2011). Adaptive behavior of primary school students with visual impairments: The impact of educational settings. *Research in Developmental Disabilities, 32*(6), 2340–2345.

Munjal, S. K., Panda, N. K., & Pathak, A. (2010). Dynamics of hearing status in closed head injury. *Journal of Neurotrauma, 27*(2), 309–316.

Olino, T. M., Durbin, C. E., Klein, D. N., et al. (2013). Gender differences in young children's temperament traits: Comparisons across observational and parent-report methods. *Journal of Personality, 81*(2), 119–129.

Piaget, J. (1969). *The origins of intelligence in children.* New York, NY: International Universities Press.

Pile, D. (2013). Does using an asthma prompting form improve asthma care in a pediatric office? *Journal of Pediatric Nursing, 28*(3), 275–281.

Primack, B. A., Carroll, M. V., McNamara, M., et al. (2012). Role of video games in improving health-related outcomes: A systematic review. *American Journal of Preventive Medicine, 42*(6), 630–638.

Singer, B. (2012). Perceptions of school nurses in the care of students with disabilities. *Journal of School Nursing.* Advance online publication.

Smith, M., Hubbard, J. A., & Laurenceau, J. P. (2011). Profiles of anger control in second-grade children: Examination of self-report, observational, and physiological components. *Journal of Experimental Child Psychology, 110*(2), 213–226.

Svavarsdottir, E. K., Tryggvadottir, G. B., & Sigurdardottir, A. O. (2012). Knowledge translation in family nursing: Does a short-term therapeutic conversation intervention benefit families of children and adolescents in a hospital setting? *Journal of Family Nursing, 18*(3), 303–327.

Taylor, S. P., Nicolle, C., & Maguire, M. (2013). Cross-cultural communication barriers in health care. *Nursing Standard, 27*(31), 35–43.

Tourigny, J., Clendinneng, D., Chartrand, J., et al. (2011). Evaluation of a virtual tour for children undergoing same-day surgery and their parents. *Pediatric Nursing, 37*(4), 177–183.

U.S. Department of Health and Human Services. (2010). *Healthy people 2020.* Washington, DC: Author.

Whittemore, R., Jaser, S. S., Jeon, S., et al. (2012). An Internet coping skills training program for youth with type 1 diabetes: Six-month outcomes. *Nursing Research, 61*(6), 395–404.

Williams, C. (2012). Promoting vocabulary learning in young children who are deaf and hard of hearing: Translating research into practice. *American Annals of the Deaf, 156*(5), 501–508.

Yang, C., & Chen, C. M. (2012). Effects of post-discharge telephone calls on the rate of emergency department visits in paediatric patients. *Journal of Paediatric & Child Health, 48*(10), 931–935.

Unit 6

The Nursing Role in Supporting the Health of Ill Children and Their Families

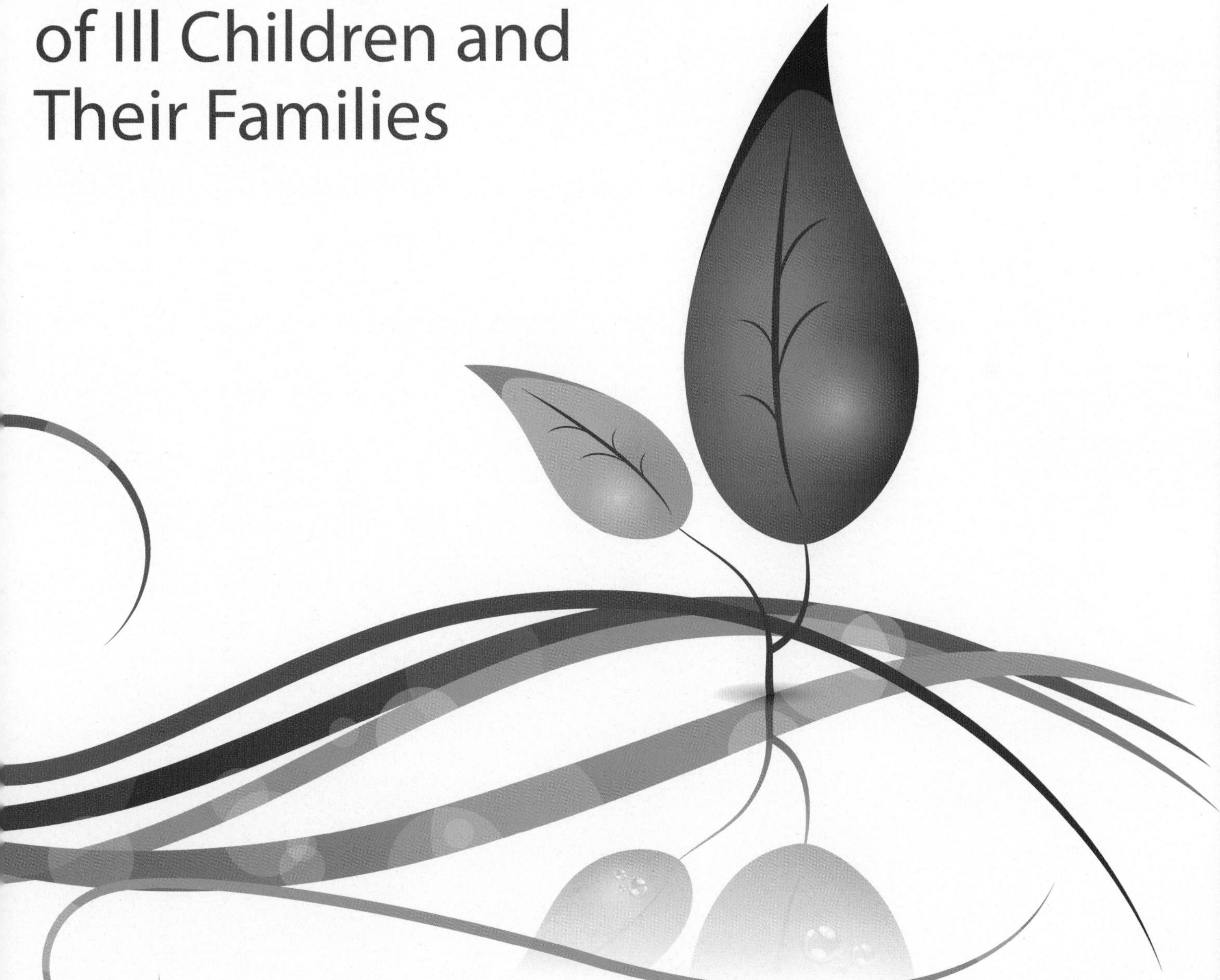

Chapter 36

Nursing Care of a Family With an Ill Child

KEY TERMS

- calorie counting
- case management nursing
- non–rapid eye movement (NREM) sleep
- play therapy
- primary nursing
- rapid eye movement (REM) sleep
- sensory deprivation
- sensory overload
- sleep deprivation
- therapeutic play

OBJECTIVES

After mastering the contents of this chapter, you should be able to:

1. Describe illness and illness experiences as they must appear to children.
2. Identify 2020 National Health Goals related to the care of ill children that nurses can help the nation achieve.
3. Assess the impact of an illness, especially one requiring a hospital stay, on a child.
4. Formulate nursing diagnoses related to the stress of illness in children.
5. Establish expected outcomes for an ill child to help manage a childhood illness as well as manage seamless transitions across differing health care settings.
6. Plan nursing care to reduce the stress of illness, such as helping parents plan for ambulatory care or therapeutic play.
7. Using the nursing process, plan nursing care that includes the six competencies of Quality & Safety Education for Nurses (QSEN): Patient-Centered Care, Teamwork & Collaboration, Evidence-Based Practice (EBP), Quality Improvement (QI), Safety, and Informatics.
8. Evaluate expected outcomes for achievement and effectiveness of care.
9. Integrate knowledge of a child's response to illness with the interplay of nursing process, the six competencies of QSEN, and Family Nursing to promote quality maternal and child health nursing care.

Becky is a 7-year-old whose foot was unintentionally burned by a campfire. She is going to be admitted to the hospital for a 1-day surgery to have the wound debrided. Becky's parents tell you that Becky "hasn't been herself" since the injury. She has reverted to temper tantrums and sulking, more like a 3-year-old than one of school age. Even though she has been told eating meat is important because it provides protein for healing, she refuses to eat anything but Jell-O or soup. In the admission suite of the hospital, she picked up a doll and twisted its leg off. "How can we get our old daughter back again?" her mother asks you.

Previous chapters described the normal growth and development of children and their special needs at each stage of development. This chapter adds information about the additional needs of children when they become ill. Such information builds a basis for nursing care and health teaching.

Becky is obviously showing some effects of her unintentional injury. What type of additional explanation might be helpful to her? What advice would you give her mother to help her better prepare Becky for the upcoming debridement procedure?

BOX 36.1 Nursing Care Planning Based on 2020 National Health Goals

Illness and hospitalization can be major stressors for children; therefore, three 2020 National Health Goals speak directly to this:

- Increase the proportion of children with special health care needs who have access to a medical home from 47.1% to 51.8%.
- Increase the proportion of children aged 0 to 11 years with special health care needs who receive their care in family-centered, comprehensive, and coordinated systems from 20.4% to 22.4%.
- Increase the proportion of children aged 0 to 11 years with special health care needs who receive their care in family-centered, comprehensive, and coordinated systems from 20.4% to 22.4% (U.S. Department of Health and Human Services [DHHS], 2010; see www.healthypeople.gov).

Nurses can help the nation achieve these goals by helping reduce the stress of hospitalization or health care so families use preventive services to help children stay well rather than totally use emergent or ill child care services.

Illnesses that require the attention of health care professionals are outside the usual occurrences of childhood, so most children typically have little knowledge about them. Helping a child and family prepare for or adjust to such an experience is a fundamental nursing role. This role goes well beyond just providing information on what to expect throughout an illness. It involves providing emotional support as well.

Research has repeatedly shown that unrestricted visitation in health care settings increases family satisfaction, improves children's morale, and can improve communication among the staff, the client, and the family (Whitton & Pittiglio, 2011). In response to this, nurses need to provide orientation programs before hospital admissions, advocate for the use of therapeutic play, and be more open to parental visiting and overnight stay policies even in intensive care areas if these are not already in effect (Zempsky, Palermo, Corsi, et al., 2013). In addition, nurses can help families establish a therapeutic environment for the care of an ill child in the home after a hospitalization. Box 36.1 shows 2020 National Health Goals concerned with children and illness.

Nursing Process Overview

For an Ill Child

Assessment

An assessment for an ill child begins with an interview of the child and parents to identify ways they think the illness will change their lives. This could include a wide range of situations such as increased expenses, changes in schedules to visit or stay with a hospitalized child, the need for one parent to take a leave from work to care for an ill child at home, the need to schedule frequent ambulatory visits, consultation to handle body image changes, and the need to arrange for child care for other children. Because these needs change as the course of an illness changes, the assessment must be ongoing.

Nursing Diagnosis

Nursing diagnoses vary greatly depending on the extent of a child's illness, the care needed, and the age of the child. Those often used with families of children seen in ambulatory and in-hospital settings include:

- Health-seeking behaviors related to lack of knowledge regarding illness
- Anxiety related to pending hospital admission
- Risk for social isolation related to hospitalization
- Fear related to being away from home for the first time
- Activity intolerance related to fatigue from illness
- Potential for unintentional injury related to high-tech therapy equipment

Outcome Identification and Planning

Planning for the care of an ill child requires consideration of all aspects of the child's and the family's life: financial, social, and personal. When children become ill, many of their needs, such as those for nutrition, play, and family support, change. If a child will need long-term care or hospitalization, the entire family may find their priorities changing. Unless these changing needs are examined, recognized, and met, a child may achieve physical wellness again but not mental or emotional health, leaving a family severely disadvantaged. Identifying additional needs in this way and putting in place necessary services or interventions is an important nursing role. An organization that offers helpful information on the hospitalization of children for both parents and health care providers is the Association for Early Learning Leaders (www.earlylearningleaders.org).

Implementation

Five hazards that may occur with children with all illnesses are (1) experiencing harm or injury, such as physical discomfort, pain, mutilation, and death; (2) being separated from routines, parents, peers, and respected adults; (3) facing the unknown (new and strange sights and sounds and happenings); (4) facing uncertain limits (unclear definition of acceptable and expected behavior); and (5) experiencing a loss of control (loss of competence or loss of the ability to make decisions).

Being aware of these potential problems is important to guard against those that are preventable and to reduce a child's concern associated with those that cannot be prevented (such as facing new sights and sounds). Discussing these hazards with older children is important so that implementations to reduce their impact can be tailored to each child. Reading to a child, role-playing, and puppetry are all useful techniques for reducing the number of new experiences and easing the impact on the child.

Outcome Evaluation

An evaluation of expected outcomes for ill children should include specific measures such as whether discomfort was kept to a minimum during the experience. Indicators to evaluate outcomes that are long term should include whether children were able to return to usual behaviors after the experience. The following are examples that suggest achievement of outcomes regarding a hospital experience:

- Parents state their level of anxiety regarding hospitalization of their infant is now at a tolerable level.
- Parents have effectively changed work schedules to be able to stay with their child in the hospital.
- Social isolation of a toddler is minimized through a case manager nursing assignment.

THE MEANING OF ILLNESS TO CHILDREN

The response of children to illness depends on their cognitive ability, past experiences, and level of knowledge. It parallels cognitive development (see Chapter 28). From early school age, children generally know quite a bit about the workings of their major body parts. As general guidelines, early grade-school children are usually able to name the function of the heart, lungs, and stomach. They may not be able to do that for the bowel, kidneys, or bladder, however, because of the difficulty some parents have in discussing these body parts with their children.

Younger children may think the cause of illness is magical (no one knows where it comes from) or that it occurs as a consequence of breaking a rule such as walking in the rain or eating candy after school. With this perspective, they may also think getting well again is possible only if they follow another set of rules, such as staying in bed and taking medicine. By fourth grade, children are generally aware of the role germs play in illness but may be fooled by thinking that all illnesses are caused by germs. Because of this, they may see a passive role for themselves in getting well, because illness comes from outside influences. At about eighth grade, children are able to voice an understanding that illnesses can occur from several causes, such as being susceptible to chickenpox because they did not get a vaccine or if they carelessly caused an unintentional injury. Once children understand this, they can take an active role in getting better.

An illness in a child is a stress, especially if it includes hospitalization (Litke, Pikulska, & Wegner, 2012). Knowing how children of each age view illnesses affects the planning of nursing care and influences how explanations should be worded. For example, saying you are going to "stick" a child for blood work could be interpreted by young children as meaning you are actually going to put a stick in their arm. Saying a child will receive dye for a test could be interpreted as meaning the child will "die" during the procedure. Explanations of procedures can sound confusing if words sound alike or have double meanings (e.g., "drawing" as in making a picture versus "drawing" blood). Because of these distorted perceptions, explanations of procedures do not always relieve children's stress.

Differences in Responses of Children and Adults to Illness

Keeping in mind that children are not just small adults is important when evaluating how children react to illness, perceive an illness, or react to health care (Fig. 36.1). Their body images, for example, as evidenced in their drawings, are different from those of adults. They may have difficulty telling which body parts are indispensable and which are not (this is why it is wise to talk to preschool and early school-age children about "fixing" body parts, such as tonsils, rather than "taking them out").

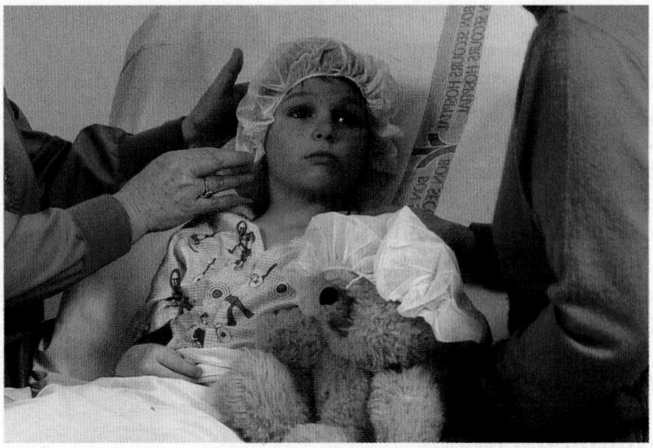

FIGURE 36.1 Illness is potentially traumatic because of the unknown and because of the pain and discomfort that may be involved. Children need extra attention and reassurance to calm their fears.

Inability to Communicate

Very young children do not have the vocabulary to describe symptoms. Children younger than 5 years of age have a great deal of difficulty describing a headache, for example. Dizziness and nausea can be equally bewildering because young children do not know the words to express these phenomena.

By the time children reach school age, most can describe symptoms with accuracy. They may intensify their concerns, however, if they believe someone expects symptoms to be more serious. They may minimize symptoms if they are afraid that an illness will interfere with an activity they want to do.

Because of this, evaluate a child's symptoms as much by observation as by a child's report. A crying, whining preschooler who is "just not herself" probably has a symptom she cannot describe. A school-age child who guards her abdomen (i.e., keeps abdominal muscles rigid) is in pain just as clearly as a child who verbalizes a source of discomfort.

Inability to Monitor Own Care and Manage Fear

Adults who are ill often ask questions about medications prescribed for them or procedures they are scheduled to undergo. If a hospitalized adult knows he is to receive a diuretic three times a day and by 10 AM has not been offered it as yet, he usually reminds someone of the oversight. School-age and younger children cannot monitor their own care this way because they may not know which medicine or procedures they are scheduled to receive. If they do know, they may be confused about the time. In addition, children have fears that adults do not experience. The infant, for example, probably fears separation above all else; the toddler and preschooler enlarge their fears to include separation, the dark, intrusive procedures, and mutilation of body parts. The school-age child and adolescent may be concerned about the loss of body parts, loss of life, and loss of friends. Adults have fears also, but most have learned to cope with them. Children in a strange environment (such as a hospital) have not learned coping skills as yet and so require proportionally more support and active intervention to manage their stress and fears. Otherwise, hospitalization, particularly if it follows trauma from unintentional injury, can result in posttraumatic stress disorder (PTSD) or the development of characteristic symptoms, such as difficulty falling asleep, outbursts of anger, difficulty concentrating, difficulty completing tasks, or experiencing symptoms such as stomachaches or headaches (Duzinski, Lawson, Maxson, et al., 2012). They may also re-experience the traumatic event through dreams or flashbacks (Landolt, Ystrom, Sennhauser, et al., 2012).

Nutritional Needs

In addition to psychological differences, there are major physiologic differences in the way illnesses affect children compared with adults related to different physiologic needs and how they respond to imbalances that occur (Citty, 2011).

For example, children need more nutrients (calories, protein, minerals, and vitamins) per pound of body weight than adults because their basic metabolic rate is faster, and they must take in not only enough to maintain body tissues but also enough to allow for growth. The infant, for example, requires 120 kcal/kg of body weight per day; the adult requires only 30 to 35 kcal/kg of body weight per day. An ill child who must limit food intake because of nausea or vomiting, therefore, may require hospitalization for intravenous therapy, even though this might not be necessary for an adult under the same circumstances.

Fluid and Electrolyte Balance

In the adult, extracellular water (the water held in plasma and outside body cells) represents approximately 23% of total body water; in a newborn, extracellular water is closer to 40%. This means that an infant does not have as much water stored in the cells as an adult and so is more likely to lose a devastating amount of body water with diarrhea or vomiting. Because of this, there is no such thing as "only diarrhea" in a child younger than 1 year. The full implications of both vomiting and diarrhea are discussed in Chapter 45.

Systemic Response to Illness

Because their bodies are immature, young children tend to respond to disease systemically rather than locally. The child with pneumonia, for example, may be brought to an emergency department not because of a cough (although the child has one) but because of accompanying systemic symptoms such as fever, vomiting, and diarrhea. In fact, nausea and vomiting occur so frequently in children with any type of illness that these symptoms do not have the diagnostic value that they have in adults. Systemic reactions of these kinds can delay diagnosis and therapy and can cause increased fluid and nutrient loss, circumstances that compound the initial illness.

Age-Specific Diseases

Because of their growth requirements and their immaturity, children tend to be susceptible to some diseases that do not affect adults. For example, because infants are growing, a lack of vitamin D will cause rickets or abnormal bone growth, but this same lack does not cause these conditions in adults. Most adults have achieved immunity to common infectious diseases; children, however, are very susceptible to illnesses such as measles, mumps, and chickenpox. Children younger than 5 years of age who have a high temperature may respond with generalized seizures (febrile seizures), a phenomenon that rarely occurs after this age (Scanlon & Cook, 2010).

CARE OF THE ILL CHILD AND FAMILY IN THE HOSPITAL

The mother, father, family, and caregivers of children admitted to intensive care units (ICUs) or neonatal intensive care units (NICUs) can be predicted to experience a high degree of stress during their child's hospitalization both because of the severity of their child's illness and the high-tech pediatric ICU (PICU) or NICU setting. They can experience a second round of stress when their child is transferred from a NICU or PICU to a regular hospital unit.

Based on the theory that hospitalization creates a high degree of stress for children, only after careful agreement that a child cannot be managed successfully on an ambulatory basis is a child admitted to the hospital for inpatient care. This can be a shock for parents because, in the past, most children with head injuries, for example, were automatically hospitalized overnight for observation. Today, unless a child is unconscious or shows other signs of neurologic injury, the child will be sent home to be observed by parents for signs of increasing intracranial pressure.

This change in care requires nurses to spend the time that used to be spent giving care to children to now teaching parents skills such as how to take a pulse or evaluate consciousness. Teaching parents who are under stress requires patience because people under stress, as a general rule, can have difficulty comprehending instructions. However, because psychological trauma and excessive health care costs are prevented by allowing a child to return home, it is important teaching.

Children who are seen in the emergency departments for acute gastritis and vomiting were also once automatically admitted to the hospital so they could receive intravenous fluid. Today, they are given an oral hydrating solution or probiotics so they possibly may not need to be admitted (Blush & Matzo, 2012).

As yet another example, many pediatric surgery procedures such as a tonsillectomy or herniorrhaphy are now done on an ambulatory basis in order to prevent the major problem of separation anxiety. Unfortunately, this does not necessarily reduce parents' apprehension about the procedure. Some parents may actually feel less confident and more anxious with ambulatory procedures than they would have with in-hospital admissions because they sense that their responsibility for preparation and follow-up care will be significantly greater (Frisch, Johnson, Timmons, et al., 2010). They often comment that modern care is not as good as when children were admitted, and that this change is a result of cost containment by insurance companies. Although it is true that short hospital stays reduce cost, it is helpful to inform parents that ambulatory or outpatient procedures are as safe as those performed with hospital admissions, and that ambulatory procedures can be helpful in preventing the detrimental effects of separation related to hospitalization.

The Effect of Hospital Separation and Children: Decreasing Separation Anxiety

The importance of a primary caregiver to the emotional life of a child is difficult to explain, but the intensity of the relationship can be demonstrated. As early as 4 months of age, an infant registers disapproval if a primary caregiver walks away. At 5 months of age, an infant registers anxiety when strangers are present or when a person other than the usual caregiver gives care. Infants fix their eyes on the stranger, become restless, perhaps thrash arms or legs, and begin to cry. This activity peaks at approximately 8 months of age, so it is commonly called "8-month anxiety." It is a developmental milestone that shows that an infant is able to distinguish a primary caregiver from other persons. It also means the child has reached a vulnerable stage in emotional development and will react poorly to separation or the threat of it (Brumariu & Kerns, 2010).

In many instances, toddlers and preschoolers can be as affected by separation as infants and even express their feelings better, louder, and longer. Although many toddlers and preschoolers attend day care and have had prior experiences with separation, others may have had only limited experiences being away from their parents. Being hospitalized may be the first time they are away from parents in a strange setting or away from home overnight. The effect of separation can become especially intense in young children before they are able to understand time because statements such as "Mom will visit again tomorrow" or "Dad will be here by 6 o'clock" are meaningless unless they know what "tomorrow" or "6 o'clock" means.

School-age children and adolescents react better than younger children to the separation imposed by hospitalization because they have experiences they can use for comparison. They have been to school for whole days, perhaps they have stayed with a grandparent or a friend overnight, and they may have been to a summer camp. This can make hospitalization a time for developing self-esteem and confidence in their ability to be independent. Even in light of this, ill school-age children and adolescents appreciate their parents being near them and reassurance that their parents will be there to support them through this crisis.

Remember that being separated may create an equally difficult time for parents. You may need to spend time with them assuring them that their child will receive good care at all times, even if they have to leave for a work commitment or to care for other children at home.

To appreciate why preventing separation is so important, it is helpful to review the research that provided the foundation for this method of care. Spitz (1945) was one of the first researchers who documented the effects of separation on children. He observed children in a penal nursery and in a foundling home who had been separated from their mothers for both short and long periods of time. From this observation, he was able to document that infant's growth and development slowed the longer they were away from their parent. Bowlby (1951) conducted additional studies with children separated from their parents during World War II. Building on Spitz's and Bowlby's work, Robertson (1958) applied these effects to the hospitalization of children and supplied labels for separation effects. Although defined over 50 years ago, these findings are still applicable to children today.

Reducing the ill effects of separation and hospitalization to the extent possible should be a high priority for all health care providers (Abraham & Moretz, 2012a; Abraham & Moretz, 2012b). Nurses play a major role in this on both direct care and management levels. Unfortunately, even despite the best preparation by parents or nurses, not all of these effects of hospitalization can be prevented.

QSEN Checkpoint Question 36.1

Teamwork & Collaboration

You are collaborating with your interprofessional team in the care of Becky, age 7 years. The social worker believes that she is showing the first signs of separation anxiety. What evidence would prompt the social worker to draw this conclusion?

a. Loud, demanding crying
b. Silent, sullen protesting
c. Quiet introspective thought
d. Inability to respond verbally

Look in Appendix A for the best answer and rationale.

Preparing the Ill Child and Family for Hospitalization

Many childhood illnesses such as febrile seizures, appendicitis, poisonings, and asthma attacks strike suddenly, making advance preparation for hospital admission impossible. However, when hospitalizations such as orthopedic or second-stage surgeries are scheduled, advance preparation is very possible. The preparations parents make for a child obviously vary depending on the child's age and individual experiences. No matter what the child's age, it is a good rule for parents to always convey a positive attitude toward the coming hospitalization or surgery. Statements such as, "They'll make you behave in the hospital" or "Wait until you have to stay in bed all day" are the kind of statements you can guide parents to avoid.

Children may worry unnecessarily if they are told about their approaching hospitalization too far in advance. Conversely, few things are more frightening for children than to hear a conversation halt as they enter a room or to hear adults spelling out unknown words. As a rule, therefore, children between 2 and 7 years of age should be told about a scheduled ambulatory or inpatient hospitalization as many days before the procedure as the child's age in years. For example, a 2-year-old should be informed 2 days before hospitalization; a 4-year-old, 4 days before; and so forth. Children older than 7 years of age can be told as soon as the parents are aware of it.

On the day of hospital admission, it is important for you to ask the parents what preparation they have done to ensure the child and family accurately understand the child's condition and upcoming procedures. Based on that, you can provide further health teaching and clear up any misunderstandings as necessary (Box 36.2).

BOX 36.2 Nursing Care Planning Based on Effective Communication

Becky, 7 years old, is admitted to your ambulatory surgery unit for burn debridement. Becky and her mother arrive together on the unit.

Less Effective Communication

Nurse: Hello, Becky. How are you?
Becky: Good.
Nurse: Do you know why you're coming into the hospital?
Mrs. Miller: We've talked about surgery. She knows that's why she's here.
Nurse: Did you bring a favorite toy, Becky?
Becky: I brought a book to color.
Nurse: You sound ready. Let's get you admitted.

More Effective Communication

Nurse: Hello, Becky. How are you?
Becky: Good.
Nurse: Do you know why you're coming into the hospital?
Mrs. Miller: We've talked about surgery. She knows that's why she's here.
Nurse: Tell me why you're here yourself, Becky.
Becky: To read a book. I brought a book.
Nurse: Let's talk about everything you told her, Mrs. Miller.
Mrs. Miller: Well, I didn't want to introduce anything scary.
Nurse: Let's take some time and talk about the whole procedure.

The poor communication in the above example happened because the nurse assumed that when the parent said she had prepared her daughter, she had prepared her in the same way the nurse would have prepared her. The communication improved when the nurse stopped assuming the level of preparation and asked direct questions of the mother and child about what they knew.

Nursing Diagnoses and Related Interventions

Nursing Diagnosis: Deficient knowledge related to preparation for hospitalization

Outcome Evaluation: Parents and child both state they feel prepared for hospitalization; child has brought some personal item important to self. Child describes with accuracy and detail appropriate to age the reason for hospital stay; asks questions and expresses feelings appropriate to age about hospitalization.

Preparing Family Caregivers: Planning for hospitalization should begin as soon as parents know hospitalization will be necessary. Some parents, however, may be so concerned about the reason for hospitalization that they cannot begin to prepare their child until they are better prepared themselves. Easing parental concerns regarding illness and hospitalization is particularly important because children can keenly sense a parent's stress. Even though a parent says, "Don't worry, everything will be all right," a child can sense if parents really do not believe everything will be all right.

As part of preparation, urge parents to ask questions about things such as what diagnostic procedures will be necessary, how long the hospital stay will be, and what kind of dressings or other equipment will be used so they can be as familiar as possible with what will happen. Being well informed in this way should (at least theoretically) reduce their worry as much as possible.

If you are practicing in a medical office or clinic when surgery or a hospital admission is first proposed, become familiar with what parents can expect so you can serve as the parents' backup informant. Many parents ask a nurse to repeat their primary care provider's explanation for a procedure or to have instructions clarified to be certain they have understood everything correctly. If parents arrive at a hospital unit with questions still unanswered fill in gaps immediately and continue to educate as new questions or concerns arise.

Preparing an Infant: Because an infant cannot understand explanations of surgery or treatments, oral preparation is minimal. Remind parents to pack special items such as a favorite toy, blanket, or pacifier, because these objects provide a special kind of security for which there is no substitute.

The infant's primary caregiver should plan to spend a great deal of time in the hospital with the infant. Be certain that a parent who will be rooming-in has made plans for older children or a spouse or other obligations ahead of time. If a parent cannot arrange to room-in, make plans to have a consistent nurse assigned to the infant because this can both help decrease concern in the parents and help minimize separation anxiety in the infant.

Preparing a Toddler or Preschooler: Three chief fears of toddlers or preschoolers are fear of the unknown, fear of abandonment or separation, and fear of mutilation. Preparation for children of this age, therefore, should clearly aim at alleviating these three fears. Bringing a favorite toy or personal item such as a blanket can help. Referred to as "transitional objects," these items are symbols of the longed-for return home. Some parents buy a new toy to replace a child's favorite one because they are ashamed of a teddy bear with one ear or one eye missing. A new bear may mean nothing to the child, however, and clinging to it does not offer the same comfort as their favorite toy.

When making hospital beds or changing paper on examining tables, be alert for ragged blankets and threadbare stuffed animals because it's easy for these to cling to sheets and be easily discarded. Throw nothing away in a child's room without first asking a child or parent if it is important. What looks like a useless alphabet block to you may mean security and home to a 2-year-old.

When young children are admitted to a hospital in an emergency, parents rarely have time to bring toys. In these instances, suggest that a parent give a child a familiar object of theirs, such as the parent's wallet (money and papers removed) or a sweater. Notice how a child will hold these in the same way as a favorite toy. The child's outside shoes can serve this same purpose because the child interprets their presence as meaning, that because shoes walk home, they will also be returning home at the end of hospitalization.

Several helpful books about hospitalization are available for parents to read with children and to also learn more about children's health care (Box 36.3). These can be obtained from local bookstores, libraries, or Internet book sites, or by writing directly to the publishers. For preschool preparation, parents could read one of these books to a child, adapting the story to include information specific to their child. Some books fail to orient children well to hospitalization because they are too sweet (as if the child were going to a picnic rather than a hospital). Others may omit pertinent facts, such as surgery will involve some pain (and that the child will be given medicine so the pain will go away) or that when bed rest is required, the child will have to use a bedpan. Young children need to be oriented to this because it is difficult for toddlers and preschoolers to go anywhere but in a toilet because they have just been toilet trained and told repeatedly they must use the bathroom.

Because the imagination of preschoolers is at a peak, role-playing can be an effective means of preparing a child of this age for a new experience. To do this, a parent could encourage a child to act out a hospitalization experience with puppets or dolls. Or, the child could change into pajamas and get into bed. The parent could then act out a physical examination, a meal in bed, a bedpan (a round cake pan simulates this), or anesthesia administration (a strainer can be used for an induction mask). At the end of the session, the parent should stress that when the child's tummy or throat is better, the child will be able to change back to street clothes and come home. Remind parents that it is always better to use the word "fix" rather than "cut" when talking about surgery with young children, because "cut" automatically suggests pain and mutilation.

BOX 36.3 Books on Hospitalization for Children

Bourgeois, P., & Clark, B. (2000). *Franklin goes to the hospital.* New York, NY: Scholastic Publishers. (Grades pre-K to 3)

Bridwell, N. (2011). *Clifford visits the hospital.* New York, NY: Scholastic Publishers. (Grades pre-K to 3)

Civardi, A. (2005). *Going to the hospital.* Tulsa, OK: Usborne Publishers. (Infant to preschool)

Mills, J. C., & Sebern, B. (2003). *Little tree: A story for children with serious medical illness.* Washington, DC: Magination Press. (Early school age)

Rey, H. A. (1999). *Curious George goes to the hospital.* Boston, MA: Houghton Mifflin Co. (Grades 2 to 3)

Ross, T. (2013). *I don't want to go to the hospital!* London, United Kingdom: Andersen Press Picture Books. (Early school age)

Slanina, A. M. (2011). *The adventures of Annie Mouse: Baby brother goes to the hospital.* Harrisville, PA: Anna Mouse Books Publishing. (School age)

Preparing a School-Age Child or Adolescent: School-age children enjoy reading, so books about surgery and hospitalization can be helpful for preparation. Be sure both school-age children and adolescents receive factual explanations of what will happen during surgery. This should also include what will *not* happen; for example, surgery will require a small abdominal incision, but it will *not* create a scar that will show when wearing a bathing suit.

If parents do not have enough information to be able to answer a school-age child's questions, remind them that few people know everything, and caution them that their best response may be, "I don't know" rather than a guess. This prevents a child from feeling betrayed when the real answer is different from the one the parent supplied.

Many community hospitals sponsor hospital orientation programs for children's groups or school groups during which hospitalization is discussed. These programs are beneficial because they lay a foundation for all children about what to expect in a hospitalization; then, if they must be admitted on an emergency basis, they may not be so frightened. Programs are offered by nurses at the hospital or on visits to children's groups or schools (Fig. 36.2). Box 36.4 provides guidelines for setting up hospital tours or discussions for early school-age children.

At approximately 9 years of age, when children first begin to understand the full meaning of death, parents need to be especially careful to explain that an anesthetic causes a "special sleep," not that a child is "put to sleep." Animals that are put to sleep are not seen again. Talking to another child who has undergone the same experience and come through it intact is yet another helpful way to introduce children and adolescents to hospitalization. Although parents cannot usually supply such a person in advance, on admission to the hospital, a visit to a recovering patient is often possible and is a constructive way to give reassurance.

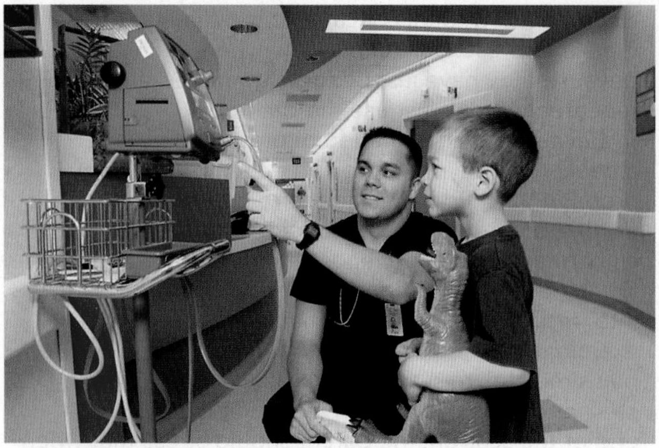

FIGURE 36.2 Children learn what to expect from hospitalization by becoming familiar with some of the equipment that might be used.

If hospitalization is to be more than 1 week long, parents need to think about how their child will continue schooling. Advise them to ask their care provider at what point the child will be able to do homework. Many school systems provide tutors, and children's hospitals often have their own teachers from the local school system to carry out this service so children don't fall behind due to hospitalization (Eaton, 2012).

What if . . . 36.1 You notice the mother of Becky's roommate, a 2-year-old, brought pots and pans to the hospital as her child's favorite play items. Would you suggest that she bring an actual toy?

BOX 36.4 Guidelines for Conducting Hospital Tours With Early School-Age Children

1. Keep groups small (about 10 children per group) so individual reactions to the presentation can be assessed.
2. Allow or encourage parents to join the tour so their concerns about the hospital can also be relieved.
3. Conduct the tour for only 20 to 30 minutes to meet the short attention span of children.
4. Use an indirect method to present various aspects of a hospital that would be exceptionally anxiety producing such as the intensive care unit (ICU) or an operating room, by using puppets, films, or a PowerPoint slide show. Include nonthreatening features such as a hospital playroom.
5. Present explanations about hospitalization in concrete terms and at the child's level of understanding. Include only what the child will see, hear, and feel.
6. Avoid dwelling on unpleasant and threatening events or intrusive procedures, such as blood drawing or anesthesia, that may create apprehension.
7. Allow children opportunities to ask questions.
8. Allow children opportunities to play with dolls and hospital equipment to decrease anxiety and satisfy curiosity.

QSEN Checkpoint Question 36.2

Evidence-Based Practice

Preparing children and their families for surgery is crucial and also challenging. After observing and gathering feedback from children and their families, the author and the perioperative nurses at a surgical center developed a program focusing on the learning needs of such clients. Specifically, customizable educational interventions were created that included both education initiatives and a hands-on experience. The program was shown to successfully educate pediatric patients and their parents about the entire perioperative process. A major outcome of the intervention was reduced anxiety about surgery on the part of both patients and their families (Adams, 2011).

Based on the study, what would be the best outcome to establish after teaching Becky and her family about surgical process and her anticipated course of recovery?

a. Becky and her family will adhere to preoperative and postoperative instructions.
b. Becky will be able to describe the reasons why a surgical intervention is necessary.
c. Becky will state that she understands the basic principles of asepsis better than before the teaching.
d. Becky will state that she feels less anxious about the prospect of having her foot debrided.

Look in Appendix A for the best answer and rationale.

Preparing a Child With a Different Cultural Background: Perhaps the most important aspect to consider when preparing a child from a different culture for hospitalization is to identify if there are traditions or practices that will be in opposition to usual health care facility practices. Ask enough questions and practice good listening skills to gain information about the particular needs of a child and his or her family. When cultural differences do exist, be prepared to act as a liaison between the family and the health care team. If a different language is interfering with communication, a medical translator may be necessary in this preparation phase. Provide the opportunity for parents to voice their fears and ask questions, and allow time and opportunity for discussion and effective communication.

Preparing a Child With Unique Concerns or Who Is Chronically Ill: Children with unique physical concerns or those who are chronically ill frequently come to ambulatory health care settings for care; they also are often admitted to the hospital for care, and possibly remain in the hospital for an extended time followed by continuing care at home. Think through ways in which a new hospitalization or visit will be like past ones and other ways in which it will be different to determine how best to prepare each child. Help children to maintain contact with their families and school friends during a long hospitalization by encouraging telephone calls, e-mails, text messaging, letters, and visits.

Admitting the Ill Child and Family

Whether an ambulatory or inpatient hospital unit admission, children and parents need to be admitted as a single entity to encourage parents to feel that they are true partners in care (Fig. 36.3). A child coming to a hospital for an elective admission generally arrives at a reception area where significant facts are obtained, such as name, age, address, and hospital insurance coverage. The child and parents are then brought to the hospital unit. Remember that first impressions count. If parents are left standing at a counter while nurses chat, they can easily feel that no one appreciates their concern and that possibly their child will not receive optimal care. Some days are busier than others and it is true that at certain times on a children's unit all nurses are busy finishing treatments for other children. Even so, one nurse should take the time to meet and greet the parents and child and find a comfortable place for the family to wait until someone is available to orient them to the unit. When introducing yourself to children, stoop down so that your face is level with the child's face. Call the child by his or her name or ask for a nickname. Calling all children "honey" or "pumpkin" can cause children to worry they will be confused with another child.

All children should have an armband attached which lists their name and hospital chart number. Because their hands are not much larger than their wrists and their feet are not much larger than their ankles, small infants often need two bands in place as an extra safeguard. If a band should fall off, secure it back onto the child; never tape it to the crib or bedside stand because this will not provide adequate protection. Any time the infant is away from the crib, the child no longer has identification and, for example, could be given a lethal medicine unintentionally before the mistake is realized.

BOX 36.5 Nursing Care Planning Using Assessment

Assessing a Child for the Effects of an Illness

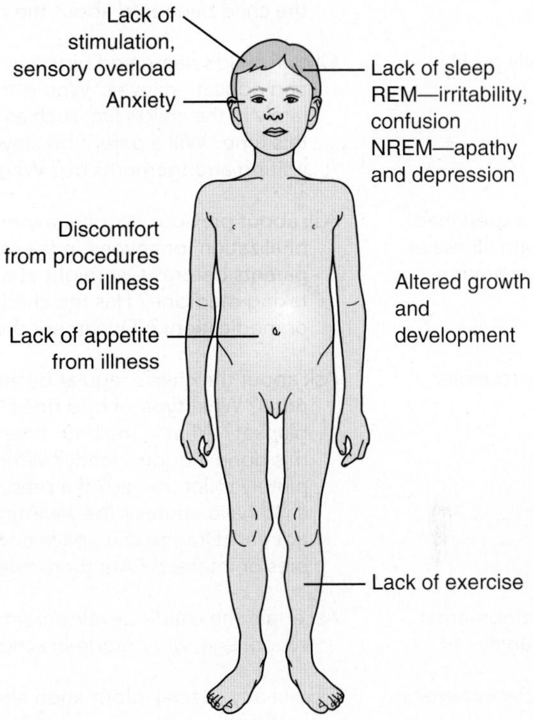

Assessment on Admission

Assess each child's level of preparation for a hospitalization on admission (Box 36.5). Be aware of not only what the child describes orally but also what any facial expressions or nervous manifestations may be indicating.

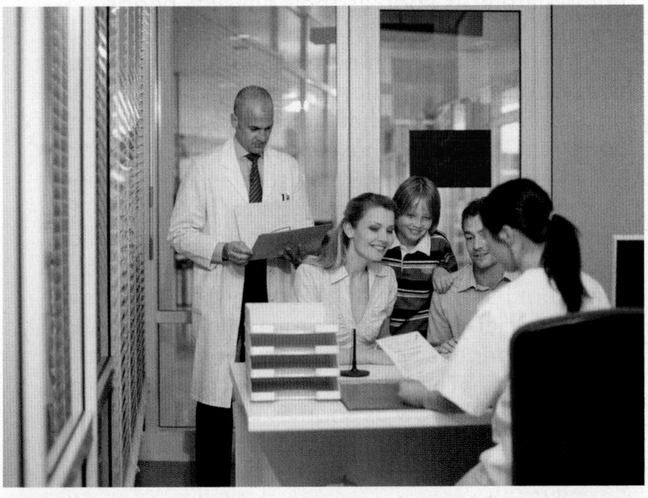

FIGURE 36.3 A child is admitted to a hospital unit. Notice how the nurse engages all the family's members (© F1online digitale Bildagentur GmbH/Alamy).

Interview parents on hospital admission for a nursing history to obtain the information needed to plan nursing care (see Chapter 34 for a description of a full child database interview history). Many hospitals have information checklists for parents to bring with them. Obtaining information in this way is highly efficient, but it may not be as satisfying to worried parents as hearing a nurse taking a few minutes to ask questions personally or to specifically review the completed form. Typical information that is necessary to obtain about a child and that should be included in a plan of care is shown in Table 36.1. Box 36.6 shows an interprofessional care map illustrating both nursing and team planning for a child admitted for 1-day surgery.

Make a note of any medication or food allergy on the child's plan of care and, if pertinent, post this information by the child's bed because, unlike an adult, a child cannot call these things to the attention of health care personnel when food or medication is offered.

Take and record the child's temperature, pulse, and respirations. Measure height and weight to determine overall growth and to allow for the determination of safe medication dosages. Whether blood pressure needs to be taken depends on the child's age (usually obtained in children over 3 years of age) and condition. Obtain a specimen for urinalysis as another routine procedure. Be sure to explain all equipment used and allow the child to touch and handle the equipment as much as possible to help reduce fear.

TABLE 36.1 Information Necessary for the Child's Plan of Care on Admission

Area of Information	Specific Knowledge
Chief concern	Determine what the parents' understanding is of why the child is being admitted. (This view may differ widely from the family care provider's view regarding the reason the child is being admitted.) What has the child been told about the reason for hospitalization?
Family profile	Obtain child's name and birthday. Who lives at home (including pets)? Ask about the parents' occupation and education levels. Who is the child's primary caregiver? Have there been any disruptive happenings lately in the child's life, such as a move or a divorce, that would make the child particularly insecure at this time? Will a parent be staying with the child? If parents are separated or divorced, what will the visiting arrangements be? Who has legal authority to sign medical permission?
Past experience with illness or separation	Ask about previous hospital experiences and how the child feels about them. Has there been a recent hospitalization for anyone in the family that resulted in a bad outcome? Has the child been away from the parents before? Overnight at a grandparent's? Summer camp? What is the child's past experience with taking medicine? Has the child swallowed pills before? Does the child have any known allergies to food or medications? (Document these by asking for exact symptoms and happenings.)
Daily routines	Ask about the child's regular bedtime and sleep times. Does the child nap? Is there an important bedtime ritual? What type of bed does the child sleep in at home? Does the child sleep with a favorite toy or blanket? What is the bath time routine? Does the child need help brushing teeth or combing hair or is this done independently? What words does the child use for voiding and defecating? Is the child completely toilet trained? If a preschooler, is the child accustomed to using a potty chair or toilet? Does the child have enuresis (bed-wetting)? What is the child's usual meal plan? Are there foods the child does not eat? Did the child pack a favorite toy for the hospital? What are the child's favorite games and hobbies or interests? Are there television programs the parents especially like the child to see or not see?
Developmental survey	Ascertain the child's developmental level. Does child feed self? Use a spoon, cup, bottle? Dress self? If school age, what grade in school?
Special information	Obtain any special information about the child the parents think would make him or her more comfortable in the hospital.

Inspect for gross motor ability when weighing a child and measuring height. Listen for language ability (although children in strange situations may say nothing). Perform a physical examination (see Chapter 34) to gain the information necessary for nursing diagnosis and planning.

The way children deal with hospitalization is based on the same factors that determine how they deal with any crisis: perception of the event, whether support people are available, and effectiveness of past coping experiences or skills. After an assessment, analyze whether a child's coping ability seems to be enough to balance the hazards of inpatient or ambulatory care hospitalization.

Nursing Diagnoses and Related Interventions

Nursing Diagnosis: Parental and child anxiety related to the need for the child's hospitalization

Outcome Evaluation: Parents and child accurately state the reason for the child's hospital admission and therapy the child will receive; state that although worried, they feel confident they can manage their apprehension.

To help reduce family anxiety regarding hospitalization, be certain a family is oriented to a hospital stay by discussing the need for hospitalization and what they can expect when the hospitalization is first suggested to them in an ambulatory care setting. When children are admitted for emergency care, this type of orientation must be completed immediately, as soon as their physical needs are met.

On admission, both parents and the child need at least basic information. If the child's diagnosis is uncertain, tell them what steps are being taken to confirm it. It helps if these steps are named specifically (e.g., blood work, X-ray studies, observation, recording of vital signs, calling in a consultant). Be certain they know the tentative plan for the child (e.g., complete bed rest, infection control procedures until the results of blood work or cultures are back, special diet, special procedures). If the primary care provider has written no directions as yet, be honest (e.g., "The specific plan of care isn't written yet. I'll let you know as soon as I'm sure what it will be."). Although this answer does not provide a family with information, it does tell them you appreciate how difficult and worrisome a child's hospitalization experience can be.

BOX 36.6 Nursing Care Planning

AN INTERPROFESSIONAL CARE MAP FOR A CHILD HAVING 1-DAY SURGERY

Becky is a 7-year-old who burned her foot in a campfire accident. She is going to be admitted to the hospital for 1-day surgery to have the wound debrided.

Family Assessment Child lives with parents and two older brothers (10 and 14 years of age) in a three-bedroom suburban home. Father works as sound technician at a recording studio; mother was a grade-school teacher, now is stay-at-home mom; home schools all three children. Father rates finances as, "All right. We have everything we need."

Client Assessment Client burned left foot on a campfire while on a family weekend camping trip. Was playing hide and seek with brothers and ran into the fire. Treated at local hospital for third-degree burn; transferred to burn center for follow-up care. Becky's parents tell you that Becky "hasn't been herself" since the injury. She has reverted to temper tantrums and sulking, more like a 3-year-old than one of early school age. Even though she has been told eating meat is important because it provides protein for healing, she refuses to eat anything but Jell-O or soup. In the admission suite of the hospital, she picked up a doll and twisted its leg off. "What can I do with her?" her mother asks you. "How can we get our old daughter back again?"

Nursing Diagnosis Anxiety related to hospital admission and burn debridement

Outcome Criteria Child accurately describes what debridement will entail; cooperates with procedures with age-appropriate responses. Describes measures she will need to take after returning home to aid burn healing.

Team Member Responsible	Assessment	Intervention	Rationale	Expected Outcome
Activities of Daily Living, Including Safety				
Nurse	Assess the degree of self-care child usually carries out.	Allow child maximum inclusion in procedures.	Ability to carry out self-care helps "normalize" hospital procedures.	Child participates in self-care to extent possible with post-procedure bandage.
Teamwork and Consultation				
Nurse/Child life specialist	Consult with Child Life service on what type of therapeutic play would be most beneficial.	Conduct therapeutic play with child before and after debridement procedure.	Therapeutic play can be helpful to children to relieve their anxiety about a painful procedure.	Child participates in therapeutic play and demonstrates less anxious behaviors following debridement.
Procedures/Medications for Quality Improvement				
Nurse	Assess what is the child's greatest concern about the debridement procedure.	Prepare child for surgery, stressing anesthesia will be used to relieve pain during procedure and analgesia will be available after procedure.	A clear understanding of what is to happen helps relieve concern, and knowing pain relief is available is invaluable to well-being.	Child and parent state they understand what procedure will entail, and child cooperates in age-appropriate ways.
Nutrition				
Nurse/Nutritionist	Assess what are child's favorite foods.	Suggest ways mother could incorporate protein into soup (meat or beans) to increase protein in child's diet.	Jell-O is a protein source, and adding meat to what child eats will provide protein yet respect the child's choice of food.	Mother details ways she can increase child's protein intake without opposing child's food preferences.

(continued on page 1040)

BOX 36.6 Nursing Care Planning (continued)

Patient-Centered Care				
Nurse/Nurse practitioner	Assess what child and parent understand about debridement procedure.	Educate family about procedure and pre- and postoperative care.	Well-prepared child and the family can better cooperate with care to make the experience a positive one for child.	Child and parents ask questions about the procedure; state they understand what it will entail.
Psychosocial/Spiritual/Emotional Needs				
Nurse/Nurse practitioner	Take history about unintentional injury resulting in severe burn.	Review with mother what she believes has caused the change in child's attitude. Does she think the child or parents feel guilty about the child's injury?	Children can believe they are being punished by procedures if they believe an injury was their fault; guilt can also influence parent's relationship with child.	Child and parent state they both should have been more diligent to avoid the unintentional injury, but these do happen even in the best circumstances.
Informatics for Seamless Health Care Planning				
Nurse	Assess what will be a typical day for the child after returning home.	Plan with parent what measures child will need to carry out to keep the bandage clean, to exercise the foot, and to return to home schooling.	Prospective planning can help avoid problems in home care.	Child and parent review a typical day and decide on actions that will promote healing.
Nurse/Primary health care provider	Assess when follow-up visit will be necessary.	Schedule follow-up visit as determined by primary health care provider.	A follow-up visit will help ensure the burn is healing without further complications.	Child and parent state they understand importance of follow-up visit and will keep appointment.

If a child is admitted from the emergency room, parents may have little understanding of their child's condition or the treatment plan. Conversely, someone might have taken a great deal of time to explain what was happening while the child was being cared for in the emergency department. Ask them what they have been told and if they have any further questions about their child's condition or the course of treatment they want to discuss with the inpatient facility's health care team.

Ideally, a parent should be prepared to stay with the child, but if the admission was an emergency one, a parent may have to leave rather than remain because of other obligations. If this happens, be certain the parent sees the child's room before leaving because it is important for children to feel confident that their parents know where they can be found when the parents return. If there are other children in the room, introduce the new child to them. Let children wear their own clothes if possible rather than change into hospital gowns for a greater sense of control.

Promoting a Positive Hospital Stay

Several nursing actions lay an important foundation for creating a successful, rather than an unsuccessful, hospital experience.

Minimizing Length of Hospital Stay

Hospitalizations for children should be limited to the shortest time possible. To help reduce the days of hospitalization, be certain that diagnostic procedures are scheduled at the child's, not the hospital's, convenience so no child has to stay in a hospital longer than is necessary. Pressure from a concerned nurse can make a big difference in a department's willingness to cooperate with scheduling.

Providing Continuity of Care

To ensure that children are exposed to as few caregivers as possible and to maintain the consistency and quality of care, nursing assignments are best if one nurse gives as much care to the same child as possible (either **primary nursing** or **case management nursing**) (Fig. 36.4). These staffing patterns

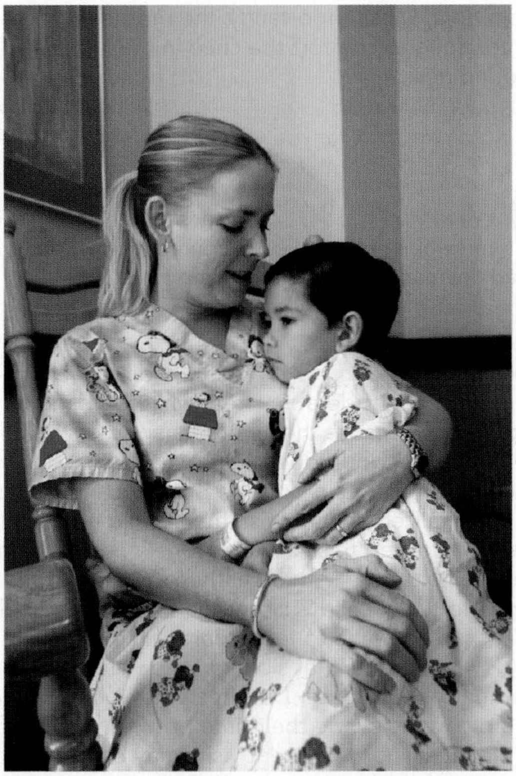

FIGURE 36.4 Hospitalized children should have one nurse who is "theirs" to minimize the effect of separation from parents (primary care nursing).

allow the same nurse to admit the child, take the nursing history, establish nursing diagnoses, set goals for care in cooperation with the parents and the child, and evaluate progress toward achieving goals. It allows children to have one main nurse to call their own. It's also helpful to parents because it allows them to establish a meaningful contact with the hospital staff and maintains continuity of care, planning, and implementation.

Nursing Diagnoses and Related Interventions

Nursing Diagnosis: Anxiety of child related to separation during hospitalization

Outcome Evaluation: Child actively relates to hospital personnel and hospital routine in ways appropriate to child's age and stage of development; manifests a minimum of nervous symptoms.

Promoting Open Parent Visiting: When possible, young children should have a parent room-in with them when they are in the hospital (Fig. 36.5). Even children 10 to 12 years of age enjoy short time spans alone but also continue to enjoy the feeling of security rooming-in provides. Because a parent will be sleeping alongside the child, check the room has

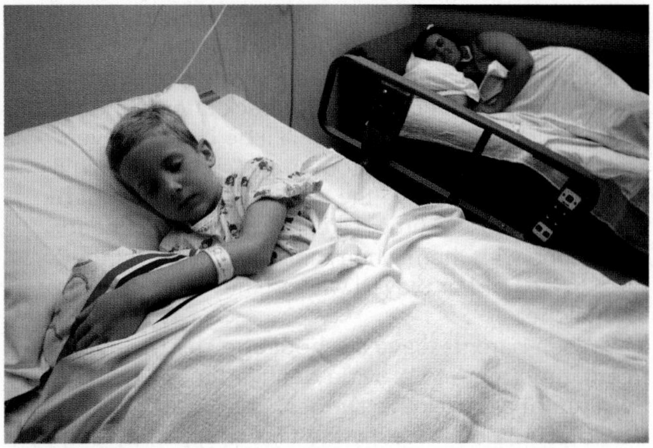

FIGURE 36.5 Rooming-in helps alleviate separation anxiety for both the child and the parent.

a parent as well as a child bed. When parents were first allowed to sleep over in children's units, it was thought their presence would reduce the need for nursing care. In many instances, because so much parental education is needed, requirements for health care personnel actually increase.

If parents cannot stay continuously, they may ask for help in smoothing the transition of coming or going. You may need to remind them that when a toddler first sees parents after being separated, a common reaction might be to ignore them (a sign of despair). This is a defense mechanism: "I won't show you I love you until you show me you love me; that way I won't be hurt again." If a parent's reaction to being treated this way causes the parent to play with a child in the next bed—a "well, be that way then" reaction—the toddler's worst fears are fulfilled: a parent has forgotten about him. To avoid this type of interaction, urge parents to speak to the child for a few minutes or try to interest the child in a toy despite the child's "cold shoulder"; after a short time, a child will generally reach out to be comforted and will act relieved the parents are there.

Parents often need help in saying goodbye when it is time to leave a child so they can eat a meal or go home for the night (if the parent is not sleeping in). Assure parents that although someone will not be in their child's room every minute while they are gone, the child will be well cared for. When the parents of an infant are leaving, go into the room a few minutes before they leave and hold or play with the infant. Help a parent to say once, "I have to go now," and then leave. Prolonged departures only delay the process and do not reduce the amount of crying that may occur. After parents leave, hold and rock infants to let them know that they are safe even though their preferred caregiver is no longer present.

If the parents of a toddler or preschooler have to leave, urge them first to give a warning they will soon have to go: "I have to leave in a minute to fix dinner for Daddy." When the time to go has come, the parent should say firmly that it is time to go and then explain the time he or she will return. Time for a preschooler is best measured in terms of events rather than clock hours. "I'll be back after you've eaten supper," is better than "I'll be back at seven"; and "after you wake up tomorrow," is better than 8 AM as these times give the child a concrete event by which to measure time. Like infants, toddlers need someone with them when their parents leave; they like to be held or played with so they know they are not alone.

When parents leave a school-age child or adolescent, urge them to provide definite times when they will return and to leave suggestions for activities a child could do to occupy the time (e.g., "Why don't you finish your book? Get a start on your homework and I'll check it when I come back"). Remind them it is more comforting to name a specific time, "I'll be back around 9 tomorrow morning" rather than a vague time period such as, "I'll be back sometime tomorrow."

When a child has to leave the patient unit for surgery, it may be especially difficult for parents to separate. Reminding them that the surgery is important and helping them manage this is an important part of preoperative nursing care.

Providing Opportunities for Parents to Participate in Child's Care: One of the most stressful parts of a child's hospitalization is the parents feeling that their parental role is diminished (Agazio & Buckley, 2012). Participating in their child's care can make parents feel more in control, thereby reducing their unease, which then hopefully transmits to reducing anxiety in their child. Encourage parents, therefore, to give as much care as possible during a hospital stay, such as bathing or feeding their child, giving oral medicine, helping with procedures such as warm soaks, or assessing that their child is awake from anesthesia. Most parents are eager to help and do these things spontaneously. Be certain they have proper instruction on the tasks they will be able to do. Be sure parents who change diapers or feed children know whether the number of diaper changes or the amount of food intake needs to be recorded; ask them to report when they do these things or write them down on a flow sheet attached to the child's door or crib. Do not ask them to restrain children for a procedure that will be painful because their main job should be to comfort. Occasionally, parents may be reluctant to give care for fear of being judged inadequate. You can assure them they are the persons from whom their child would most like to receive care.

Because children may be especially apprehensive about undergoing a procedure without a parent present, there is rarely any reason a parent cannot accompany a child into a treatment room to help with undressing, measuring weight and height, and taking a temperature or accompanying a child to another department for a procedure such as a sonogram or blood work. Most importantly, the mother or father can continue to comfort the child in these strange surroundings.

What if...36.2 Becky's father does not call you when her intravenous pump alarms that it is finished. Instead, he resets the pump himself.

Supporting Sibling Visitations: Children in a family are under considerable stress while a sibling is hospitalized because their world changes as much as the parents' world does (Lehna, 2010). Sibling visitation refers to allowing the brothers and sisters of a hospitalized child to visit the ill child along with parents. Allowing this alleviates loneliness on both sides, helps prevent other children at home from imagining the ill child is sicker than is true, and helps the ill child continue to feel a part of the family. Check with parents that siblings who visit are free of communicable disease. During a visit, you may need to help parents divide their time between the ill child and siblings (short, frequent visits may be better for young children than long ones). Before a visit, ensure that the ill child's room is safe for younger children's visits by removing poisonous substances or electric wires within reach.

Minimizing Negative Effects of Procedures: Ill children often undergo numerous diagnostic and therapeutic procedures that have the potential to cause pain, fear, and anxiety. Details related to specific procedures are discussed in Chapter 37. General guidelines designed to make any procedure less painful or frightening are discussed in the following sections.

Nursing Diagnosis: Fear related to diagnostic or therapeutic procedures

Outcome Evaluation: Child voices satisfaction with comfort measures; describes self-participation in a procedure; rates experience as no less than "tolerable" after the procedure.

Reducing or Eliminating Pain: Some pain and discomfort are unavoidable in association with health care. Limit this whenever possible, however, by such measures as advocating for the use of intermittent infusion devices such as heparin locks (see Chapter 38) to eliminate multiple punctures for intravenous medication or blood sampling, providing traditional comforts such as a change of clothing or position, or talking about a favorite subject. Children respond well to alternative therapy techniques, such as distraction or imagery, to reduce pain. Listening to music can also be effective (Barry, O'Callaghan, Wheeler, et al., 2010). Children do not always express discomfort as freely as adults so closer assessments before and

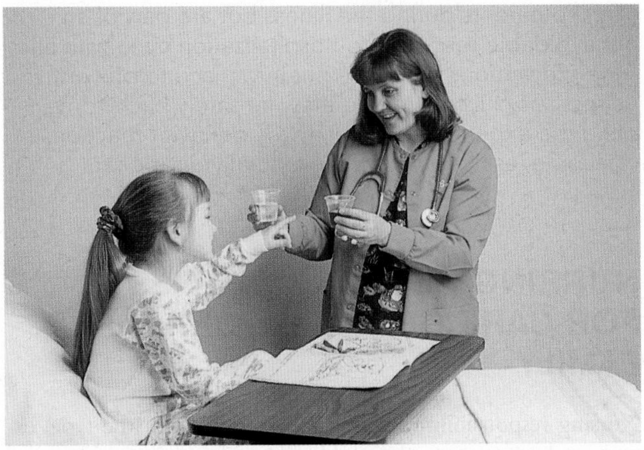

FIGURE 36.6 Include children in procedures whenever possible to offer them a feeling of control. Here, a nurse gives a child a choice of fluids to drink with her medication.

after a procedure may be necessary to reveal how they truly feel about a procedure.

Maintaining the Child's Bed as a Safe Area: To assure children that their bed is an area that is safe, all painful procedures should be done in a treatment room or another department, away from the child's bed. Be certain this rule is not broken by "just one time" venipunctures or intravenous insertions because only one painful experience at the bedside can be enough to significantly decrease a child's feeling of safety. Remember that finger punctures for blood work, although done quickly, can cause as much pain and stress as a venipuncture. In addition, dressing changes, although not necessarily painful, can cause worry and so should be done in a treatment room, not at a child's bedside.

Helping Children Maintain Control: Events are always more frightening if they appear to be beyond our control. Explaining to children what will happen, including what they will feel or what they will see and helping them to make choices whenever possible, limits this type of fear because these actions offer a sense of control (Fig. 36.6). In almost any procedure, there is some choice a child can make (e.g., whether or not to use a straw to drink, deciding what size of tape to use on a bandage, or deciding which direction to walk down the hallway). Letting a child sit in on the signing of a consent form by parents can be an additional way to help a child feel a sense of control.

Providing Adequate Play Facilities

Play is often described as the work of children because it is the medium through which they learn. To continue usual growth and development during hospitalization, they need to be able to play as normally as possible. The best children's hospital units are equipped with a playroom or play space that is maintained as a "pain-free" zone. No medical procedures, not even painless ones, should be performed in this area because, even if a procedure is not painful, it can be frightening. Children who are on bed rest need toys or crafts supplied for them.

Therapeutic play is play designed to help children express their feelings about painful or frightening procedures (DeCourcey, Russell, & Keister, 2010). The uses of therapeutic play and guidelines for providing this are discussed later in this chapter.

Setting Limits on Behavior

Setting limits on behavior can help promote a positive hospital stay because it can help to provide a sense of security and safety. Average children are motivated to follow instructions and demonstrate good behavior during a hospital stay because they want to get well again and return home as soon as possible. Occasional children who misbehave in a hospital setting usually do so because they lack a clear understanding of what is expected of them or are making a strong statement that their personal needs have not been recognized and met.

A child who needs frequent reminders to stop running in the hallway, for example, is probably bored with staying in a room. Providing more activities (playing a board game) or allowing more structured exercise (letting the child accompany a nursing aide to take a blood specimen to a laboratory) can prevent further unsafe activity.

Children who refuse to cooperate for procedures generally do so out of fear of the unknown rather than deliberate misbehavior. The better prepared a child is for such a procedure, therefore, the better a child is apt to accept it (Anson, Edmundson, & Teasley, 2010). For potentially painful procedures such as a bone marrow aspiration, lumbar puncture, blood sampling, or cast removal, any behavior short of hysterical screaming can be considered "good" behavior. If limit setting is necessary, such as with a child who hits or bites other children, confer with the child's parents about the need for limit setting and what measures they would suggest. Gain their cooperation and approval so that what you do is consistent with their usual care. Using "time-out" periods or removing the child to a nonstimulating area for a short time could be an effective measure. Be certain a child understands time-out rules (e.g., if the child bites or hits again, sitting alone for a designated period will be necessary). The next time the child does misbehave, give one warning that the behavior is against the rules; if the behavior continues, take the child to the time-out spot. If the child is disruptive, begin timing the period from when the child quiets down. When the child has been quiet for the specified duration (usually 1 minute per year of age), the child can leave the time-out place and rejoin activities.

Discharge Planning

Discharge planning is not only an important link between the hospital and the home but it is also a final way to create a satisfying hospital experience.

Nursing Diagnoses and Related Interventions

Nursing Diagnosis: Parental health-seeking behaviors related to care for child at home after hospital discharge

Outcome Evaluation: Parents state accurately the care their child will need at home; describe and demonstrate any procedures they will need to perform with child.

Many children, particularly those who are having surgery, are hospitalized for only a few hours, and, as soon as they are able to take and retain fluid and have voided once, they are discharged. It is vitally important that nurses anticipate what will be a child's discharge needs so the discharge process is one of continuity with hospital care (Williams, Eilers, Heermann, et al., 2012).

If a child has been admitted to an ambulatory care unit, preparation for discharge should begin at almost the same time as admission. If some procedures will need to be continued at home, allow parents to perform them in the hospital at least once so they can become comfortable with the necessary technique and discover any problems while help is still available. Suppose parents will be doing warm sterile soaks for an open lesion at home. Urge them to think through the steps they will need to follow. How will they sterilize the water? Where can they buy dressings? Will they be able to afford them? What can they use to keep the soaks warm for 20 minutes? What suggestions can they think of for keeping the child quiet and content for 20 minutes, so the child doesn't move a great deal and knock off the dressing? These are small problems, one by one, but can become big ones if they're not worked out before a parent returns home with them unanswered. Urge them not to leave this kind of question unanswered until the last minute, because then there will not be time left to solve such problems.

Discharge planners can be indispensable in helping ready parents for home care. Some parents will require follow-up help in their homes provided by a community or home health care nurse. Be certain not to leave the full responsibility for teaching procedures or medicine administration to these home care nurses, knowing they will soon be on board, because parents need to know what they must do on the first day before this further help arrives. Double check that parents have the phone number of a person to contact if plans do not work out as anticipated and that they have a return appointment for follow-up care.

Many preschool children manifest behavior problems such as thumb-sucking, bed-wetting, temper tantrums, and nightmares after returning home from a hospital stay; school-age children may manifest these behaviors to a lesser extent. You can assure parents that these behaviors do not happen because the child has been "spoiled" by the hospital staff or by the parents during the illness but are part of an unavoidable response to hospitalization even with all the precautions that were put into place to prevent stress. As children realize they are safely back home and the experience is over, these behavior reactions become less frequent and eventually disappear.

NURSING RESPONSIBILITIES FOR CARE OF THE ILL CHILD AND FAMILY

Nursing responsibilities will vary, naturally, with the type, extent, and seriousness of a child's illness, age, care setting, and individual circumstances. Chapter 37 discusses specific responsibilities related to diagnostic tests or interventions. Chapter 39 discusses the important role of promoting comfort in an ill child. A number of responsibilities such as promotion of normal growth and development, sleep, stimulation, and play are more global, cross all ages and phases of care, and are discussed here.

Promoting Growth and Development of the Ill Child

It is easy for children to fall behind in growth and development because of an illness unless health care providers monitor for and strengthen this.

Nursing Diagnoses and Related Interventions

Nursing Diagnosis: Risk for delayed growth and development related to the effects of illness

Outcome Evaluation: Child demonstrates only limited signs of regression to previous stage; is able to continue doing the activities most recently accomplished.

Illness represents a crisis event and, in a crisis state, children, like adults, can grow from the experience or, in contrast, can be overwhelmed and regress.

The Ill Infant: To promote optimal growth and development in infants, try to change their usual routine as little as possible. Sameness provides security to a child this young and encourages the development of trust. An infant who is used to sleeping in a bassinet, for example, may feel loose and insecure in a large crib. Swaddling such a child in a receiving blanket in a large crib would help to offer the same close, bound feeling of a smaller sleeping area. Providing a singular room in a NICU has been shown to improve parent satisfaction with care because it removes the parents from the noise and tension of the larger, unstructured room (Stevens, Helseth, Khan, et al., 2011).

Also, change the infant's diet as little as possible. Unless a child is diagnosed with failure to thrive or is obviously underweight, illness is not an ideal period in which to introduce new foods or formula. Breastfeeding should be continued if at all possible. If a mother cannot be at the hospital constantly, urge her to pump milk, freeze it, and bring it in so her child can continue to receive the immunologic protection of breast milk. Overall, because infants cannot begin to understand the strange feelings accompanying illness, they need increased swaddling and comforting. As their condition improves, be certain they are provided with stimulation and play opportunities suitable for their age.

The Ill Toddler and Preschooler: Because illness can limit autonomy and prevent children from learning how to do new things, try to find opportunities to promote both autonomy in toddlers and initiative in preschoolers. One way to accomplish this is to encourage children to make choices about their care whenever possible. Choosing the color to use to cross off a dose of medication in a medication schedule, for example, is the kind of task that can help encourage initiative in a preschooler.

Toddlers and preschoolers who are not used to sleeping in cribs at home may resent being placed in a crib in a hospital unless you explain to them, "All our beds here have side rails." Watch energetic toddlers closely to be certain they do not attempt to climb over crib rails to get out of bed. A child who does try might be safer sleeping in a bed than a crib or may need a safety crib cover when a parent is not in the room.

As with infants, illness is a poor time to change the eating habits of toddlers and preschoolers. Because children of this age insist on self-feeding, they often eat better at a small table than using a tray in bed. Many child care units organize "toddler tables" so children this age can eat together. Supervise children carefully if they are eating with others to be certain they eat only their own food, not food belonging to someone else. Also be certain they're not so distracted by other children that they don't eat. All children may eat better when a parent joins them for a meal.

Illness is also a poor time to introduce toilet training, even if this is an appropriate activity for the child's age. However, if parents have already begun toilet training, continue this if possible, so you don't disturb a usual routine.

The Ill School-Age Child: Ill school-age children need to continue to work on a sense of industry or learning more about how and why things are done. Explaining specific procedures and involving them as much as possible in planning their care is an effective way to do this.

Remember, few children who are ill are at their best and so they may not act as mature as usual. A 7-year-old, for example, whose parents describe him as very mature may begin to function (and whine) at the level of a 3-year-old. School-age children who do well with competition when they are healthy may do poorly with competition when they are ill, reverting to playing types of games they would normally dismiss as too young for them. Make a point of not holding children of any age to their chronologic age while ill to avoid asking more of them than they are able to accomplish.

School-age children usually enjoy sharing a room with another child close in age so they can play games together. They need to continue schooling, provided their condition will allow it. Because it is age appropriate, ill children generally do well working with a parent or tutor on school activities. It is such a normal, everyday activity that it provides security to an otherwise insecure day. It is also a reassuring sign that they are expected to get better and to return to school when hospitalization is over.

Working on projects such as needlecraft, writing for brochures about the place the family plans to visit on vacation next year, or viewing videos on science or nature are activities that not only help pass the time but that also encourage learning. Remember, school-age children also are developing moral responsibility and so may find comfort in spiritual practices. Ways to assist with spiritual needs during a hospitalization are shown in Table 36.2.

TABLE 36.2 Nursing Interventions to Meet Children's Spiritual Needs

Action	Implementation
Prayers	Ask on hospital admission whether a child follows religious practices such as saying grace with meals or a prayer at bedtime. Write it on the plan of care so all nurses know to provide time for this. Remember, saying grace may also apply to unconventional meals, such as a tube feeding. Bedtime prayers may be especially important to young children because they lend security in a strange environment.
Religious services	Many children of school age and older enjoy attending a religious service in a hospital chapel. Include time for this in the plan of care and be certain transportation by wheelchair or cart is available.
Visits from clergy	Many school-age children and adolescents enjoy an active recreation or social program at a religious facility when well; therefore, they enjoy a visit from their clergy when they are ill, not only for its religious importance but also as for support from a respected adult. Free the child's time as necessary for such visits.
Religious articles	A child's parent may wish to attach a religious article to the child's clothing or pillow or to post it over the bed. Be careful when changing linen or gowns that you do not throw away such articles. Mark their presence and importance on the child's plan of care.

Encourage school-age children to carry out as much self-care as usual, and, if being cared for at home, to continue to contribute to household routines, such as helping with dishes or picking up after themselves as much as they are able. This not only takes some burden off caregivers but also sends a signal that people expect this illness to pass and the child to become a full family member again.

The Ill Adolescent: An adolescent who is struggling to develop a sense of identity may find it difficult to be ill because the limitations imposed by an illness make the development of a sense of identity so difficult. If possible, help adolescents to continue to participate in activities they did before becoming ill to help them feel that their world is not totally changing. Encourage them to maintain self-care activities and good hygiene practices to help preserve self-esteem.

Illness can be especially difficult for adolescents also because peer relationships are so important to them and a hospitalization automatically interferes with those. They may miss acting in a school play, being chosen for a sports team, or competing for a scholarship. A girlfriend or boyfriend may break off a relationship. To help avoid feelings of exclusion and hurt, urge them to welcome visitors from their peer group. Suggest texting or e-mailing as easy ways to keep in contact with friends and maintain relationships with individuals who are important to them while separated from them.

Adolescents usually appreciate being hospitalized in a special adolescent unit or at least in a room free of childish decor. Be certain to welcome parents with the same considerations as on other children's units; fear of procedures and pain of separation are not limited to the younger than 13 years of age set. Although many adolescents enjoy having parents stay overnight because it is reassuring to know that they are concerned, they may also enjoy being separated (assuming everything is going well) and so may not want their parents present all day and night.

Often, adolescents convey a blasé attitude toward procedures (e.g., having an X-ray taken is nothing, surgery is a cinch, a cast change is a snap). Listen carefully to make certain adolescents really feel this way and are not trying to convince themselves that a procedure is harmless. Remember that adolescents are extremely worried about their body parts. Make certain they know what is going to happen in surgery or in other departments because it is easy to assume from their attitude they know more than they do.

Promoting Nutritional Health of the Ill Child

Nursing responsibilities related to nutrition for ill children include maintaining optimal nutritional status in the face of an illness or therapy that interferes with adequate intake, correcting nutritional deficiencies or otherwise aiding children and families to follow the nutritional care plan devised by the health care team, and educating a child and family regarding specific nutritional needs as well as overall sound nutritional health. Specific procedures for promoting nutrition such as measuring fluid intake and output and providing enteral feedings, gastrostomy tube feedings, and total parenteral nutrition are described in Chapter 37.

Nursing Diagnoses and Related Interventions

Nursing Diagnosis: Risk for imbalanced nutrition, less than body requirements, related to lack of appetite

Outcome Evaluation: Child maintains skin turgor and age- and size-determined weight pattern; ingests 80% of prescribed diet daily.

An acute illness in a child, such as pneumonia, is often accompanied by a loss of appetite; gastrointestinal illnesses frequently cause nausea and vomiting. Because most acute illnesses last only a few days, there is no need for children to eat more than a small amount during this time as long as they can drink fluid. Trying to force them to eat only increases nausea and vomiting, which increases the possibility of creating an electrolyte imbalance. When an illness lasts for more than a few days, however, providing adequate nutrition becomes increasingly important because children need nutrients not only to repair ill or diseased tissue but also to maintain normal childhood growth.

Important points to address when planning nutrition for ill children are summarized in Table 36.3. Children who are hospitalized often tolerate hospital-prepared food, which can be repetitious and bland, better than adults. Provided that it is the kind of food they like, such as hot dogs and hamburgers, these may appeal to children more than the elaborate dishes with spices and sauces preferred by adults. Children who are receiving care at home need as much nursing supervision of their nutrition as those in health care agencies (possibly more) because they may not have a dietitian planning meals to ensure adequate nutrition. Assess not only the quantity but also the quality of food to ensure that intake is optimal. If prescribed, ask whether nutrition supplements are being offered to increase intake (Cota & Allen, 2010).

Encouraging Fluid Intake: Increasing oral fluid intake has traditionally been termed "forcing fluid." It is better to avoid this term with children, however, because they can interpret the instruction to mean that someone is going to physically force them to swallow fluid. A physician's prescription should state in detail the amount of fluid a child is to receive during 24 hours, because the amount differs so much for different ages. The following are some practical guidelines for encouraging fluid intake at any age:

- Offer small, full glasses frequently rather than larger, half-full glasses; children are mid–school

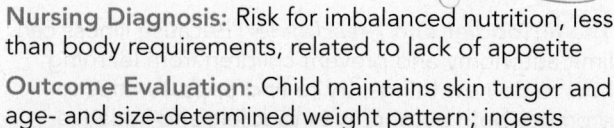

TABLE 36.3 Areas to Consider When Planning Nutrition for Ill Children

Area	Importance
Meaning of food	Early in life, infants learn to associate eating with being held and loved; if they cannot eat for some reason, such as while waiting for surgery, they may view the restriction as punishment or a restriction of love. Encourage a parent to sit and rock them or read to them to lessen this uncomfortable time.
Opportunity for socialization	Mealtime is an ideal time for family members to socialize and share their day; being separated from family for meals can create loneliness and, consequently, a poor appetite. Urge parents to visit at mealtime if possible, so "sharing a day" can continue.
Level of stress	Children under stress may either feel a loss of appetite or experience a need to snack frequently; this can make it necessary to be certain children maintain adequate intake if not hungry and that, when hungry, their snacks are nutritious.
Custom and culture	Food customs are important; for example, many children like foods served separately and resist eating them if they are mixed into a casserole. They like best the foods they typically eat at home. If possible, ask if a parent could bring in a favorite food treat to stimulate appetite.
Environment	Hunger is associated with the sight and smell of food; many children are normally in the kitchen and help prepare meals; they may not feel as hungry, therefore, when food is served to them without their having seen and smelled it being prepared. Allowing them to pick what foods they want for meals, if possible, gives them at least some sense of food preparation and selection.

age before they evaluate the amount of fluid in a container rather than the size of the container.

- Determine the child's favorite fluid, and then offer it, if appropriate.
- Try changes of temperature in fluid offered (e.g., hot cocoa, then cold juice, then hot soup) for variety. Broth can be a nice change of liquid (many commercial types are quick to prepare, but be aware of their high sodium content).
- Popsicles and Jell-O count as fluids.
- Children can drink more of a clear fluid (e.g., ginger ale, water) than a thicker fluid (e.g., milk shakes, cream soups) because thicker fluids are absorbed from the stomach much more slowly.
- Suggest soothing beverages such as Kool-Aid or milk for children with mouth lesions. They may be unable to drink fruit juices because the acid content stings their mouths; carbonated beverages may also cause discomfort.
- Because ice melts to one half its volume, count a glass of ice chips as only a half-full glass of fluid.
- Unless contraindicated, let children drink fluids with a straw; this is a novelty to many who do not normally use these and so encourages intake.
- Introduce a game, such as Simon Says (Simon says, "Drink") or a board game in which a child takes turns and with each turn has to take a drink. One can also use play as a method of teaching nutrition and sound dietary habits to children (Lynch, 2012).

Encouraging Food Intake: **Calorie counting**, as the name implies, involves counting the number of calories that children ingest each day. To do this, record all the foods that a child eats during each 24-hour period, being certain to include snacks, candy, or gum. A dietitian then will analyze the list and determine the caloric intake. Be certain when doing this that you describe the types of food and amounts (i.e., not "some toast," but "half a slice of whole wheat toast"). Be sure that everyone caring for the child (including parents) is aware that calories are being counted so that they also record this information accurately.

QSEN Checkpoint Question 36.3

Quality Improvement

You want to encourage Becky to drink a lot of water to promote hydration. Last time you made rounds, she drank an entire 10-oz glass at once and vomited several minutes later. Considering the failed attempt to encourage oral hydration, what would be your best next course of action?

a. Teach Becky about the consequences of failing to drink sufficient water.
b. Set up a plan with Becky and her parents to provide small glasses of water frequently.
c. Continue to offer her large glasses of water so she does not have to drink so often.
d. Alert her that if she does not increase her fluid intake she will likely have to receive IV fluids.

Look in Appendix A for the best answer and rationale.

PROMOTING SAFETY FOR THE ILL CHILD

A prime consideration of nursing interventions is to keep children safe during illness care.

Nursing Diagnoses and Related Interventions

Nursing Diagnosis: Risk for injury related to procedures or therapy necessary for care

Outcome Evaluation: Child remains free of injury, such as a fall from bed or injury from medical equipment.

Promoting safety for children is a responsibility for all health care providers. Care of a child who is ill and being cared for at home includes assessing the safety of the house and providing family teaching. It also includes making provisions for emergencies. For example, a family may need to install a counter-level telephone or purchase a cell phone so a child in a wheelchair can call for emergency help. Parents might also need to make a plan for how to evacuate an ill child from the home in an emergency such as a fire.

Safety on a children's unit or clinic is the responsibility of all health care providers, from the administrator of the institution to part-time health care personnel. Important steps to follow to make a child health care environment a safer place include:

- Always be sure of the location of all children in your care.
- Ensure that doors or gates are provided near stairways or elevators.
- Ensure that doors of health care facilities have working alarms to prevent children from going out and to prevent strangers from coming in.
- Be sure windows are covered by screens or guards so children cannot climb up on sills and fall out.
- Check that the side rails of beds and cribs are in good repair and raised appropriately.
- Always raise bedside rails after a child has received preoperative or sedative medication.
- Test a crib rail after it is raised to ensure the lock has caught so the rail will remain raised.
- Push bedside tables or stands away from cribs so a child cannot climb over the railing and use the stand as a step down.
- Be certain crib caps are available for small children to prevent them from climbing out of bed.
- Fasten the seat belt restraint for infants in high chairs. Never leave an infant in a high chair (at home or in a hospital) without someone close enough to reach the child because infants can easily squirm out of a high chair restraint.
- Ensure that electrical cords or appliances such as hair dryers are not used in bathrooms, where they could come in contact with water.
- Be careful of the placement of television/call cords or Venetian blind cords so they cannot lead to strangulation.
- Never leave children younger than 5 years of age alone in a bathtub; they could turn on the hot water and scald themselves or slip under the water and drown.
- Never leave equipment or items that would be harmful to eat within the reach of children.
- Adhere to all fire precaution measures.
- Closely follow standard infection precautions to prevent the spread of infections.

Promoting Fire Safety: Fire precautions both in the home and in the hospital are essential in preserving the safety of children. Adults can usually take responsibility for removing themselves from a burning structure, but children depend on care providers. Ensure that there is a plan of action in case of a fire and that everyone in the home, in the clinic, or on a hospital unit knows it. To be certain a home is safe, having a smoke detector on each floor is a wise precaution. A downstairs bedroom is not only safest in case of a fire but also allows a child more self-care ability. Fire departments supply free decals for the bedroom windows of children or those with a unique concern so they can be easily located in a fire. Parents can contact their local fire department for this safety measure.

Electrical equipment such as respiratory and cardiac monitors, radiant heat warmers, special-care equipment, and electrical heating pads are often used in the care of children. Do not use equipment with frayed cords or equipment that is not properly grounded. Plugs should be three pronged for extra safety; do not overload circuits with additional plugs. Electrical outlets should have safety caps to cover them when they are not in use so toddlers cannot poke objects into them and electrocute themselves.

Adhering to Standard Infection Precautions: In every health care setting, closely follow standard infection precautions to protect ill children, the family, and staff from infections (Waltman, Schenk, Martin, et al., 2011). Because of a compromised immune system, ill children may be more susceptible to repeat or secondary infections than usual, especially drug-resistant strains of bacteria such as methicillin-resistant *Staphylococcus aureus* (MRSA), which can spread easily if not everyone is conscientious about precautions. A proper hand-washing technique, disposal of tissues and waste materials, and efforts to minimize exposure of other ill children or adults are all effective methods to decrease the risk of infection. For more details on infection control, see Chapter 43.

PROMOTING ADEQUATE SLEEP FOR THE ILL CHILD

Ill children need adequate rest and sleep so their body tissues can effectively use nutrients for repair and normal growth can continue (Meltzer, Davis, & Mindell, 2012). Children may not sleep well when they are ill because of discomfort, pain, the administration of medications, or intensified symptoms of chronic sleep problems. They may not sleep well in a hospital because it is a strange setting; they may have to undergo so many procedures that they also do not nap or rest as much

TABLE 36.4 Stages of Sleep in Children

Stage	Description	Nursing Implications
Non–rapid eye movement (NREM) Stage I	A feeling of drifting or falling. Often described as twilight sleep. Temperature and heart rate decrease slightly; electroencephalogram (EEG) waves show peaked, frequent (alpha) waves.	A child can be roused easily from this early sleep by the slightest noise or silent presence of another person in the room. Reduce noise level in room to promote sleep.
NREM Stage II	Sleep deepens. Temperature and heart rate decrease slightly more.	It is more difficult to wake a child from sleep when this point is reached.
NREM Stage III	Sleep deepens still further. An EEG tracing reveals mixed spindle and slow (delta) waves. Temperature and heart rate decrease further. This period lasts about 10 min.	It is very difficult to wake a child from stage III sleep. Use patience to wake a child fully to offer medicine.
NREM Stage IV	Approximately 20–30 min after beginning to fall asleep, a child enters stage IV sleep. Respirations and heart rate slow even more, and blood pressure and temperature decrease; EEG shows slow, steady (delta) waves. Children remain at a stage IV sleep level for approximately 30 min, then progress back through stages III and II until they then pass into a phase of REM sleep.	Children may be confused and unable to orient themselves readily if awakened from stage IV sleep. Use patience until a child is fully awake, particularly if asking a question.
Rapid eye movement (REM)	Eyes move in rapid, involuntary motions. Respirations are irregular; body turnings, movements, and penile erections may occur. Lasts 10 to 30 min and then a new sleep cycle with NREM sleep begins.	Dreaming occurs during REM sleep. Although children appear to be close to waking because of the active eye movements, they are really very soundly asleep. Children may wake afraid and crying, disturbed by a frightening dream.

during the day as usual. Children who are recovering from trauma such as injuries from a car accident or burns may be unable to sleep because of nightmares about the accident. These nightmares can cause them to suffer sleep deprivation in the same way as a child who is frequently awakened for procedures during the night. Encourage parents to stay with these children for support and comfort. Remember, though, that parents who sleep in hospital rooms do not obtain adequate sleep either (Meltzer et al., 2012). Although their presence is healthy for children, it can lower the parent's ability to handle stress or interpret happenings.

Sleep Patterns

Sleep is influenced by apprehension level, state of health, habit, medication, and environment at the time of sleep. Stages of sleep are summarized in Table 36.4. Figure 36.7A shows a pattern of normal sleep. As a sleep cycle begins, children first enter **non–rapid eye movement (NREM) sleep**. This type of sleep occurs in up to 80% of total sleep time. As children fall deeper and deeper asleep, they pass from stage I to stages II, III, and IV of NREM sleep over a period of 20 to 30 minutes. **Rapid eye movement (REM) sleep** follows. In infants, most of sleep time is REM sleep, whereas young adults have the least amount of this type of sleep. The sleep pattern of a child who is awakened frequently during the night for procedures would resemble that shown in Figure 36.7B.

The purpose of NREM sleep, the first phase of sleep, is rest and restoration of the body; this stage keeps body cells functioning and healthy. During the periods of stages III and IV NREM sleep, the secretion of growth hormone (somatotropic hormone) from the pituitary is at its highest level. Growth hormone is necessary for protein synthesis, for the growth of new cells, and for the repair and maintenance of all cells. Corticosteroids and adrenaline from the adrenal gland, which are instrumental in the catabolism or breakdown of cells, are at their lowest levels. This balance of hormones produces the ideal combination for protein synthesis and cell growth and repair.

The purpose of REM sleep is less clear. The rapid eye movements may serve to coordinate binocular vision. Dreams that occur during this time apparently serve as a release of tension or help to integrate new knowledge and experiences with the old in the brain's memory system. Vital signs may fall during NREM sleep. During REM sleep, vital signs rise to near normal levels. These periods of REM sleep interspersed with NREM sleep, therefore, may be a fail-safe measure to prevent vital signs from falling too low during sleep.

Sleep Deprivation

Infants are dependent on sleep to promote brain development. Deprivation of sleep from 2 to 4 hours in healthy infants has been studied and thought to lead to short-term variations in cardiac function as well as an increase in apnic events (Allen, 2012). Children who do not receive enough sleep can suffer **sleep deprivation**, just as adults do. After approximately 4 days of poor sleep, this can cause them to experience difficulty in concentrating and episodes of disorientation and misperception.

If the sleep loss is mainly REM deprivation, children show symptoms of irritability and difficulty concentrating. Lack

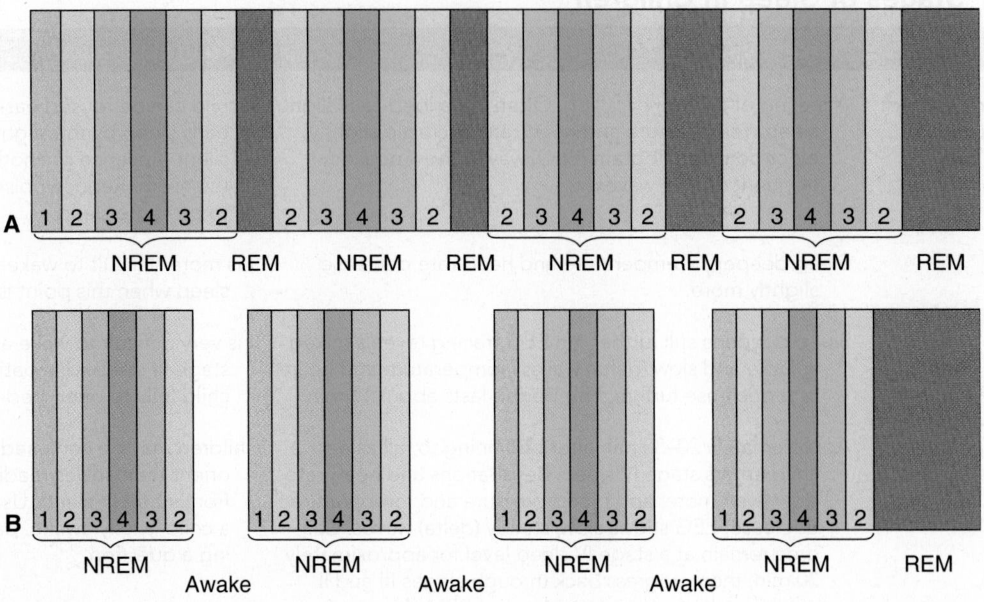

FIGURE 36.7 Sleep patterns. **(A)** A normal sleep pattern. Notice how the periods of rapid eye movement (REM) sleep increase in length during the last half of the night. **(B)** The sleep pattern of a child who has been awakened frequently during the night. Notice how little REM sleep is present.

of stage IV NREM sleep, in contrast, tends to cause apathy, physical fatigue, and depression and can slow recovery. This is the same phenomenon that can happen in adolescents if they are studying for exams. It easily occurs in younger children during illness if they are awakened frequently for treatments.

Nursing Diagnoses and Related Interventions

Nursing Diagnosis: Disturbed sleep pattern related to timing of medication, discomfort, or sleep disorder

Outcome Evaluation: Child sleeps through the night without interruption (when therapeutic regimen allows); is alert and active during the day; is able to take nap during the day if that is part of his or her usual sleep schedule.

Because sleep is so important for ill children, you need to take special steps to ensure that children are able to sleep during an illness. Be certain children are as free of pain and worry as possible. Try to let them maintain as normal a bedtime routine as possible (e.g., bath, change to nightclothes, nighttime story, prayers). Provide an atmosphere conducive to sleep (e.g., lights out, quiet surroundings, reassuring support people). Children who are bored with bed rest may catnap constantly during the day and then be wide awake at night. Providing more interesting activities for them during the day can help reduce their naps and increase nighttime sleep.

Managing Chronic Sleep Problems: Some children may have chronic sleep problems such as night terrors, nocturnal enuresis, somnambulism (sleepwalking), sleep talking, and sleep apnea. These sleep problems can intensify with illness and can increase sleep deprivation in ill children.

Somnambulism is a common sleep problem in children. It apparently occurs during NREM sleep, probably during the deepest part of stage IV. It is frightening for children to wake and realize they have been sleepwalking. Sleepwalking can be potentially dangerous when children are ill because, while getting out of bed, they could dislodge intravenous tubing or oxygen equipment. It is untrue that sleepwalkers should not be wakened; instead, wake them gently, help them get reoriented, and then return them to bed after reassuring them they are safe. Be certain that the side rails are raised on the bed of a child who tends to sleepwalk. In a hospital, it may be necessary to move a child's bed out into the hallway at night near the nurses' desk if a parent will not be sleeping over so the child can be observed for sleepwalking.

Sleeptalking seems to occur during REM sleep. Dreaming of some frightening or puzzling situation, a child calls out a name or instruction such as, "Stop!" Because illness is a stressful situation that increases anxiety, sleeptalking may also occur at an increased rate during this time. It is unnecessary to wake a child who is sleeptalking unless the child is thrashing about and would dislodge equipment such as intravenous tubing. However, because sleeptalking usually results from a frightening dream, waking the child gently can be comforting. Parents may need to be assured that sleeptalking is harmless and will probably subside when their child is well again.

Some children are prone to night terrors, or wake up screaming approximately 20 minutes after they fall asleep. The condition tends to be familial. Waking children and comforting them helps everyone in the house or hospital unit return to sleep. In the morning, children rarely remember the incident.

Sleep apnea is the cessation of respirations during sleep for 20 seconds or more. It tends to occur more frequently in obese children, possibly because of the increased weight of their chest. It may contribute to sudden infant death syndrome or failure to thrive (Scollan-Koliopoulos & Koliopoulos, 2010) (see Chapters 26 and 55). Infants who are diagnosed with sleep apnea may be prescribed respiratory monitors to evaluate their breathing pattern and warn against any cessation of respirations.

PROMOTING ADEQUATE STIMULATION FOR THE ILL CHILD

Children are in constant interaction with both their internal environment (body) and their external environment (surroundings) by means of their five senses and the central nervous system. This makes them capable of responding to changes in the environment and, by so doing, meet basic needs. Any illness that changes their ability to respond to their environment can cause either sensory deprivation or sensory overstimulation.

Sensory Deprivation

Sensory deprivation is the condition of being deprived of, or lacking, adequate sensory, social, physical, or cognitive stimulation. When this happens, children tend to lose the ability to make decisions and become easily confused and depressed. Some children are more prone to sensory deprivation than others.

Ill children may have sensory deprivation because they are confined to their homes or hospital rooms and their varied activities such as school, sports, and clubs are replaced with hours of watching television or playing video games. Hospital regulations for ICUs may limit parental visiting. When parental interaction is limited this way, children generally receive less-than-normal cognitive stimulation. Such children need cognitive stimulation from warm, reassuring health care personnel to replace this.

Children with hearing or visual deficits are more prone than others to sensory deprivation. Children with forms of sensory nerve loss or those receiving chemotherapy may lose their sense of touch, taste, or proprioception (the sense of where they are in space). After losing these forms of perception, children may draw back from interacting with other people because they are self-conscious about the loss, so they may be further deprived of social and cognitive stimulation. Techniques for interacting with sensory-deprived children are discussed in Chapter 50.

Some children receive medication to lessen awareness of the stimulating factors in their environment. To ensure they do not suffer sensory deprivation, give them definite orientation measures, such as always mentioning the time of day and the day of the week in conversations with them. At the same time, they often must have overly stimulating factors reduced, such as the number of visitors, so that perceptions can be interpreted clearly.

Nursing Diagnoses and Related Interventions

Nursing Diagnosis: Deficient diversional activity related to lack of appropriate toys and peers

Outcome Evaluation: Child demonstrates alert and interested attitude toward self-care and play activities.

Providing Stimulation for the Child on Bed Rest: Children on bed rest cannot secure materials for cognitive stimulation by themselves or participate in physical activities, except to a limited degree. A room where walls and windows offer no visual appeal and therapeutic equipment provides the only sound offers them little sensory stimulation. If no one comes into the room, they may suffer from social deprivation. When possible, encourage a child with restricted mobility to move out of bed into a wheelchair; this can provide some mobility and transportation to a place of interest, such as near a window or, in a hospital, near the nurses' desk. Watching television, a common activity for children on bed rest, actually can overstimulate the infant or child's brain and can create decreased socialization in all children (Arthur, 2010). In addition, children can be exposed to inappropriate programming if this is not carefully monitored.

Occasionally, a child must remain in bed to reduce stimulation for reasons such as to rest the heart or to increase kidney function, but generally, bed rest is prescribed mainly to inactivate one part of the body, such as a fractured bone. When possible, other stimulation, such as a favorite toy, games, books, or simply talking with someone, must be provided for these children to help them maintain physical bed rest; otherwise, they become bored and irritable and thrash and turn instead of lying still (Fig. 36.8).

If a child is home on bed rest and the bedroom is away from the main activities of the home, encourage family members to include the ill child in as many family activities as possible (e.g., bring the television set into the child's bedroom so the entire family gathers there, set up a card table in the room so everyone can eat there) or encourage the child to join the rest of the family for activities by resting on the couch in the living room, a lounge chair in the backyard, or a chair in the kitchen. This principle applies to hospitalized children as well. A toddler, for example, may rest in a parent's lap rather than in a bed.

Providing Stimulation for Children on Transmission-Based Precautions: Children who are placed on transmission-based precautions because of the

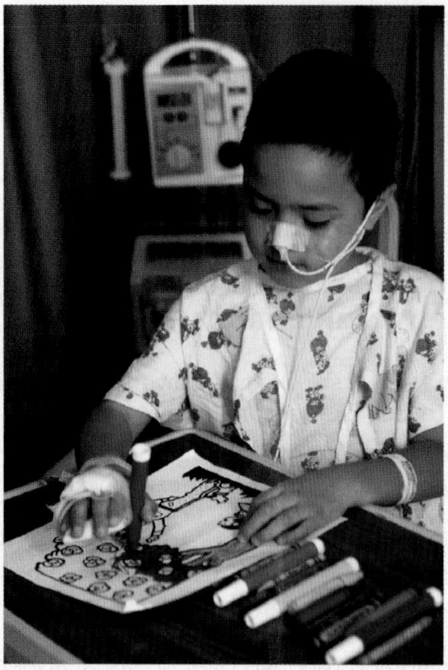

FIGURE 36.8 Children on bed rest need stimulation. Here, a young child enjoys coloring.

possibility of contagious illness may experience severe sensory deprivation if everyone who enters the room must wear a gown and mask or if the number of visitors must be kept to a minimum. If gloves are part of precautions, a child can experience a significant loss of skin-to-skin contact as well. Transmission-based precautions are discussed in Chapter 43. Careful planning must be done to ensure that a child who is isolated this way is not psychologically isolated and that every possible measure is carried out to maintain sensory, social, physical, and cognitive stimulation. For example, try to visit with a child at a time in addition to those times in which you must perform procedures so you can simply talk, place the bed so the child can see out of the room, encourage the child to text message or Facetime friends, make posters for the walls so they're no longer bare, or encourage interactive play such as with electronic games. For ideas on providing stimulation to children in specific age groups, refer to Chapters 29 to 33.

Providing valid, reliable Internet resources for immune-suppressed adolescents with chronic conditions wanting to socialize with other adolescents can be an alternative to direct socialization and also decrease the risk of contracting a communicable illness. However, Internet use should be strictly monitored for safety factors (Jacobs & Popick, 2012).

Sensory Overload

Sensory overload, in contrast to deprivation, occurs when children receive more stimulation than they can tolerate or process. Children with sensory overload react similarly to those with sensory deprivation or feel confused, unable to make decisions, and feel severely fatigued. Sometimes it is difficult to determine the cause of these symptoms (whether they are caused by sensory deprivation or overload) unless assessed carefully.

The lights in ICUs, for example, are never turned out. Although children may find this comforting, it can also result in excessive stimulation. In addition to constant light, there is excessive sound such as the whir of machines, the buzzing of ventilators, the ringing of alarms, or the mix of voices in consultation. Noise levels in the NICU have been studied as a factor influencing the function of a premature infant's brain through alterations in cerebral blood flow, which then possibly slows development and adjustment to the outside world (Elser, Holditch-Davis, Levy, et al., 2012). Using indirect lighting whenever possible, reducing unnecessary conversations, and covering incubators for "quiet times" are all measures used to reduce these types of stimulation.

Most ICUs have no windows because the wall space is used for monitoring equipment; therefore, night and day are not easily distinguished. It is easy for a child to become confused about time and place in such a setting. Orient children to the time of day by making frequent references to it or by providing calendars and clocks. For children who are cared for at home in a family room where people talk constantly, the television is always on, and activity never ceases, sensory overload may also occur. If necessary, provide eye covers or ear plugs to reduce stimulation.

✔ QSEN Checkpoint Question 36.4

Patient-Centered Care

Becky's mother is worried Becky will have a traumatic hospital experience. Which of the following would you advise her to do to help make Becky's hospitalization less traumatic?

a. Suggest she keep her visits short so Becky can spend time with her nurse.
b. After visiting, don't tell Becky she is leaving. Just try to slip quietly away.
c. Insist Becky have blood drawn by her bed because she fears the treatment room.
d. Take Becky to the playroom, a place where she can feel free from being hurt.

Look in Appendix A for the best answer and rationale.

PROMOTING PLAY FOR THE ILL CHILD

Play, often described as "the work of children," is an invaluable component of child health care. Providing a space and opportunity for play can help children feel more comfortable and allow for an important release of energy for children who are confined to a room or bed. Play also may be used to help assess children's level of knowledge and feelings about their condition so that more individualized nursing care can be planned. Depending on a child's age, play can also be a useful tool in health teaching (see Chapter 35).

BOX 36.7 Nursing Care Planning Based on Family Teaching

UNDERSTANDING DIFFERENT PLAY TYPES

Q. Becky's mother tells you, "When Becky was younger, she didn't like toys as much as the boxes they came in. What's normal for children and play?"

A. Children play differently at different ages. Examples of typical play patterns include:

Type of Play/Age	Description	Example
Observation/Infant	Child watches particular play intently, although not actively engaged in it.	Watching a mobile
Parallel/Toddler	Two children play side by side but seldom attempt to interact with each other.	Playing separately with a similar push toy
Associative/Preschooler	Children play together in a similar activity; there is little organization of responsibilities.	Engaging in typical backyard play
Cooperative/School Age	Children play with an organized structure or compete for desired goal or outcome.	Playing organized games with rules

Defining play is not a simple task because play activities vary greatly from child to child and among different age, cultural, and socioeconomic groups. A common definition is that play is any voluntary activity engaged in for the purpose of enjoyment. If a child views an activity as enjoyment, therefore, no matter what it is and whether it would be fun or not for an adult, it is play.

Play is clearly the means by which children develop increasing cognitive, psychomotor, and social capabilities. Touching a soft rabbit, passing colored blocks from one hand to the other, pounding with a plastic hammer, feeding a doll, and playing board games are all ways in which children are exposed to and learn about different textures and colors, experience the feeling of possessing and owning, and learn about competition, winning, and losing. A soft toy tells a child more clearly than can be described that this is what the word "soft" means. Colored blocks reveal how parts can join to make a whole, how things stacked too high will fall (there are limits one cannot go beyond), and practice makes perfect. As children talk with playmates during play, they develop both language and social skills. The repetitive acts involved in most games encourage the development of musculoskeletal skills. Therefore, play is not something children do when they have nothing else to do, but rather, it is something children *have* to do. During illness, it provides a feeling of security because it is an activity that has continuity with everyday life.

The manner in which children play differs as they mature. Types of play and the age groups in which these types are seen most frequently are shown in Box 36.7.

Assessing Child Health Through Play

Children who are acutely ill do not play or play very little because they do not have the strength, the attention span, or the interest in activities required for play. They continue, however, to enjoy being read to, and they find comfort in holding a favorite toy even if they do not actively manipulate it. Once children are over the acute phase of an illness, interest in play returns. Therefore, whether a child is spontaneously playing is a good index of health. The toys children use at play are a good indication of their growth and development level and emotional state.

The average parent knows a child's play preferences and current favorite game or toy. Asking for this information at a health interview helps to assess a child's developmental level and whether it is age appropriate. It also helps to assess the quality of parenting (if parents view play as important or are familiar with the child's activities).

Providing Play in Ambulatory Settings

Children in ambulatory departments are under a great deal of stress. They sit in a waiting room and glance fearfully at the door that leads to the examining room. They hear children crying beyond the door and wait in terror for what lies in store for them when it is their turn.

Parents may know that when their child is coming to a hospital to be admitted, they should pack the child's favorite toy. Often, they do not think of an ambulatory visit as a sufficiently threatening circumstance to warrant bringing a favorite toy, however, so the child has nothing to play with. In addition, having a parent sit beside them is so comforting they may ignore or hesitate moving 4 ft away to get the toys furnished by the health care facility unless they are urged to do so.

It is best if ambulatory departments are stocked with toys that can be played with quickly and by single children. There should be a low table and chairs so a parent can come to a table and play with a child. Examining rooms should have toys also, which may be used to distract a child while a procedure such as an ear examination is performed and because the wait in an examining room may be as long as the wait in a waiting room. Well siblings who accompany a parent and sick child to the facility can play with toys to distract them as well so that a parent can concentrate on the ailing child. Some hospitals furnish computer games for older children for this reason. Examples of ways that play can be used in an ambulatory care setting are shown in Table 36.5.

TABLE 36.5 Ways to Incorporate Play Into Nursing Care

Nursing Care	Play Activity
Aid with physical assessment	Distract child's attention with puppet during respiratory and cardiac assessment. Play Simon Says to encourage child to take deep breaths for respiratory assessment. Allow child to listen to own heart with a stethoscope. Play Follow the Leader to assess gait. Draw a face on the tongue blade used to assess the throat. Show child how to "blow out" the otoscope light. Draw child's outline on the table examining paper and give it to the child to take home to color.
Health teaching	Use puppets as a teacher. Create word scrambles or crossword puzzles.

Providing Play in the Hospital

Ideally, all hospital units in which children are cared for should have a play space big enough for most of the children on the unit to come to. There should be enough space to accommodate children who are not fully ambulatory, such as those with casts or who are in wheelchairs (Fig. 36.9). Tables for board games and play materials such as crayons and paints should be available. Children can release a great deal of anger or tension by splashing water, squeezing or pouring sand, or smearing finger paint.

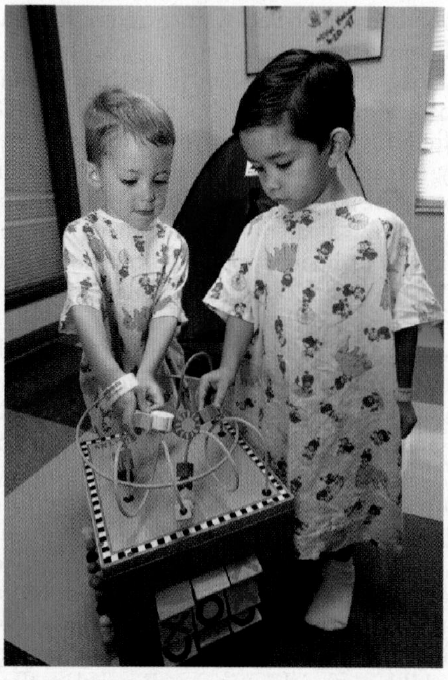

FIGURE 36.9 Children enjoying themselves in a hospital playroom, which is spacious and well equipped with age-appropriate toys and activities.

School-age children can play games such as shuffleboard or tossing sand bags for tension relief and competition. Adolescents enjoy table tennis and pool tables. A great deal of "play" in older school-age children and adolescents centers on conversation with peers they meet in the playroom.

Children who are hospitalized for 1 week or more may enjoy putting on a puppet show or playing school, store, or house. It is good if a corner of a playroom is devoted to this kind of imaginative play, with a structure that will serve as a store front, puppet stage, house, or school and where dolls, cribs, empty food boxes and cans, and puppets are provided. Large blocks (6 in. × 12 in.) are available for playrooms so that such structures can be built and rebuilt each day. For ill children, the blocks are best if made of cardboard covered with contact paper or foam (which can be easily cleaned for infection control), not wood, because ill children tire easily when lifting heavier wood blocks. Table 36.6 lists games that require no equipment other than that which is readily available on a nursing unit for children who have brought nothing of their own to play with or who have grown bored with existing games.

Providing play equipment and supervision for a recreational play program, in most instances, is economically feasible through donations and volunteers. Generally, toys for a playroom can be secured through donations from clubs in the community. For safety reasons, children need to be supervised while they play. Because they do not feel well in a hospital or are shy in these different surroundings, they usually enjoy having a concerned adult to watch over them and suggest new activities. Such adults may be volunteers. Supervision is an excellent after-school activity for members of a future nurses' club. Ideally, child support or play specialists supervise such play.

If play supervisors are unavailable through other sources, the nursing staff must free such personnel as necessary to lead play activities. This shows that play is important (e.g., supervising finger painting is as important a duty for assistive personnel as straightening beds, organizing a puppet show for long-term clients is as important as giving a bed bath). A clear sign that the nurses on a particular children's unit understand little about their young patients' needs is a locked playroom door and the explanation, "We have no one to staff it."

Providing Play for Children on Bed Rest

Children who are on bed rest, at home or in a hospital, need to have play periods built into their day. The length of time for play and the toys individual children can play with depend on their age and physical and emotional states. Suggestions for play activities for children on bed rest are shown in Table 36.7.

Infants need toys in their cribs, such as mobiles, blocks, soft toys, and rattles. They also need to be out of cribs, sitting on a parent's or a nurse's lap, or sitting in strollers or swings. As soon as they are able, they need some time on the floor (with a sheet under them) to practice crawling or walking. At about 3 months, when infants discover their hands, those become that month's "toys." For a child learning to crawl, "cruise," or walk, that activity is the toy or interest for the month.

Toddlers need put-in and take-out types of toys such as blocks that can be repeatedly dropped into a bottle or that can be stacked to play with in bed. They enjoy listening to songs and nursery rhymes. Toddlers are in constant motion. They

TABLE 36.6 Games and Activities Using Materials Available on a Nursing Unit

Age	Activity
Infant	Make a mobile from roller gauze and colored tongue blades to hang over a crib. Ask the pharmacy or central supply for different-size boxes to use for put-in, take-out toys. (Do not use round vials from pharmacy; if accidentally aspirated, these can completely occlude the airway.) Draw a smiling face on a piece of paper. Hang it so the child can see it. Play patty-cake, "so big," and peek-a-boo.
Toddler	Ask central supply for boxes to use as blocks for stacking. Tie roller gauze to a glove box for a pull toy. Sing or recite familiar nursery rhymes.
Preschool	Play Simon Says or Mother, May I. Draw a picture of a dog; ask child to close eyes; add an additional feature to the dog; ask child to guess the added part; repeat until a full picture is drawn. Make a puppet from a lunch bag or draw a face on your hand with a marker. Cut out a picture from a newspaper or a magazine (or draw a picture); cut it into large puzzle pieces. Pour breakfast cereal into a basin; furnish boxes to pour and spoons to dig. Furnish chart paper and a magic marker for coloring. Make modeling clay from 1 cup salt, 0.5 cup flour, 0.5 cup water from diet kitchen. Play ring-around-the-rosey or London Bridge.
School age	Play I Spy or charades. Make a deck of cards to play Go Fish or Old Maid; invent cards such as Nicholas Nurse, Doctor Dolittle, Irene Intern, Polly Patient Play Hangman. Furnish scale or table paper and a marker for a huge drawing or sign. Hide an object in the child's room and have the child look for it (have the child name places for you to look if the child cannot be out of bed).
Adolescent	Color squares on a chart form to make a checker board. Have adolescent make a deck of cards to use for Hearts or Rummy. Compete to see how many words an adolescent can make from the letters in his or her name. Compete to guess whether the next person to enter the room will be a man or woman, the next car to go by window will be red or black, and so forth. Compete to see who can name the most episodes of a favorite TV show.

TABLE 36.7 Play Activities for Children on Bed Rest

Care Measure	Play Activities
Bathing	Allow children to play in bath water with water toys.
Encouraging fluid	Hold a pretend "tea party" for a preschooler and drink "tea" with important but imaginary guests. Play a board game with a school-age child in which each turn starts with taking a drink. Draw a circle and let the child color in a section each time a drink is taken. Play Simon Says, in which Simon says, "Drink."
Deep breathing exercises	Have child blow soap bubbles in a glass of soapy water with a straw. Have child blow a cotton ball across the surface of a bedside table. Play Simon Says, in which Simon says, "Take a deep breath." Allow the child to score points for reaching a high number on an incentive spirometer.
Muscle-strengthening exercises	Have children throw bean bags or large wads of paper (computer waste) at a wastebasket. Play Simon Says, in which Simon says, "Raise your arms," and so forth. Have children throw and catch a ball. Have children squeeze and mold modeling clay. Help preschoolers pretend they are butterflies, airplanes, and so forth.
Procedures such as blood transfusion	Save a favorite game or activity only for these times.
Health teaching	Use puppets as teacher. Make up board games, word scrambles, and crossword puzzles.

need to be out of bed as much as their physical condition allows, playing with take-apart, put-together, or pull-and-push toys. Preschoolers need creative materials such as modeling clay or sand. School-age children need quiet games such as books or crayons or markers by their bedside. They also enjoy radios, compact disk players, or iPods. Most activities for hospitalized children must be short-term projects because children are called away for treatments or procedures, and because, when they are ill, their attention span is shorter than usual. Short-term projects always appeal to the school-age child because they help a child of this age achieve a sense of industry.

Watching television is a nonparticipant activity, so it is not the best activity for children. There is some value, however, in watching nature programs or specials on television that depict school-age children in real-life situations coping with problems common to the child's age group. Encouraging parents or friends to watch a game show with a school-age child and help the child guess the solution to a puzzle or watch "Sesame Street" with a preschooler can make the activity a participatory one. Watching a DVD with an adolescent and then discussing the people and their problems can also turn television watching into active participation.

Safety With Play

Be certain to screen all toys for safety. They should be washable to prevent spreading disease, with no sharp edges and no small parts that could be swallowed or aspirated. A cylinder 1 in. in diameter, such as a rubber hot dog, is the most dangerous size for a toy because it totally occludes the trachea if it is aspirated. A toy smaller than this would cause only partial obstruction; something larger could not be inhaled into the trachea. As a rule, if a toy can fit through the center of a toilet tissue tube, it is too small for safe play.

Be certain toys offered will not lead children into danger. Tossing a ball to a toddler on bed rest is generally a safe activity. One who has a large cast in place, however, might lean over to retrieve a dropped ball and fall out of bed. Chasing a ball could lead to collisions with door frames or oxygen equipment.

If children become bored with a toy because it is not stimulating enough or they have had it for too long a time, they may begin to use the toy in an unsafe way. After toddlers grow tired of stacking blocks, for example, they may begin to throw them. Children who normally play safely with modeling clay but who are on a restricted diet may eat it because they are hungry. Knowing where children are and what activity they are engaged in at all times is the best prevention against unsafe play.

For the child cared for at home, parents may need to purchase new toys. This is especially true if the bulk of the toys they furnished previously were for outside play such as balls, in-line skates, or skateboards. Because of an illness, they may now need to provide more "sit-down" toys such as markers, puzzles, or board games.

Child Support Programs

Child support programs are incorporated into major children's hospitals and are an integral feature of child health care (Hart & Walton, 2010). As part of a child support program, a specialist offers children the opportunity to reenact and thereby master the unease associated with illness. Through therapeutic play, child specialists provide programs that prepare children for hospitalization and, once hospitalized, prepare children for surgery or for procedures that could be painful. They consult with parents about good toys to choose for home care. These specialists also help children air their frustration about painful or intrusive procedures, prevent social isolation of children by means of an active recreation program, and ensure that the total health care environment is conducive to children's well-being.

Such a program not only aids in promoting children's mental health but also leads to more cooperative responses of children to treatments or procedures. It is complementary to play programs initiated by nurses.

QSEN Checkpoint Question 36.5

Safety

You are worried Becky's 2-year-old roommate might aspirate a toy the family friend brought in for her. Which of the following items is most likely to be aspirated, and therefore poses the greatest risk to safety?

a. Puzzle pieces
b. Clothing for a baby doll
c. Crayons
d. Blocks that are 1-in. square

Look in Appendix A for the best answer and rationale.

Therapeutic Play

Anything almost automatically becomes less threatening when a person can talk about it. Many children cannot talk about what is happening to them during illness, however, because of fear or because their vocabulary is so limited they cannot describe their feelings.

Because play is the language of children, children who have difficulty voicing their thoughts in words can often speak clearly through play. **Play therapy** is a psychoanalytic technique used by psychiatrists to help children understand their feelings, thoughts, and motivations better. In play therapy, the therapist attempts to interpret the child's verbal and nonverbal cues. Interpreting nonverbal cues and helping the child understand them this way requires the skill of a psychiatric nurse–clinician or others with specialized training. **Therapeutic play** is a play technique that can be used by all nurses to better understand children's feelings and thoughts (Cochran, Cochran, Fuss, et al., 2010). For therapeutic play, only the child's verbal cues are used as responses.

Therapeutic play can be divided into three types:

1. Energy release
2. Dramatic play
3. Creative play

Energy Release

Children release energy by pounding, hitting, running, punching, or shouting. Furnishing children with materials that allow them to do these things helps them release anxiety as well. Toddlers enjoy pounding pegs with a plastic hammer or pretending to cut wood with a toy saw. Other examples include giving modeling clay to a preschooler (an anxious child often pounds it flat; a relaxed child, however, will build it into shapes) or tying a Mylar balloon to an overbed trapeze for a school-age child or adolescent to punch.

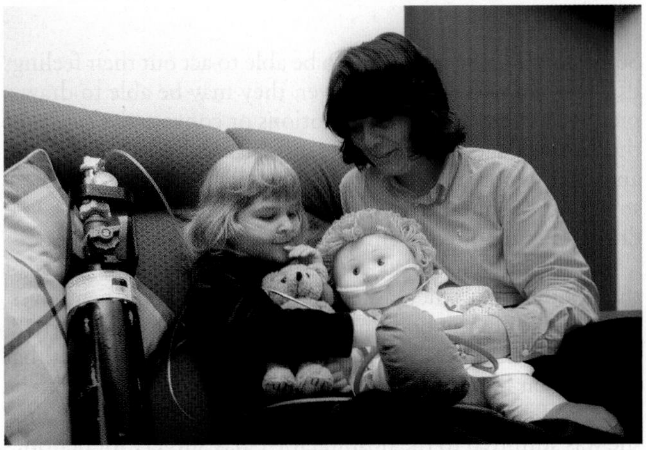

FIGURE 36.10 Therapeutic play allows children the opportunity to voice their fears of illness and procedures (© Janine Wiedel Photolibrary/Alamy).

Dramatic Play

Dramatic play is acting out an anxiety-producing situation. It is most effective with preschool children because they are at the peak of imagination. During illness, the situations about which children need to express feelings are illness related, and therefore the equipment needed for therapeutic play is common health care equipment, such as dolls, doll beds, play stethoscopes, IV equipment, syringes, masks, and gowns. Puppets of doctors, nurses, mothers, fathers, and children help young children express their feelings. Anatomically correct dolls are used to help children describe their feelings about sexual maltreatment.

It is good to have a play session with a child near the beginning of an illness to see whether the child communicates any fears about this experience through play. This initial session also serves as a way of preparing the child for events that will occur during the illness (Fig. 36.10). Repeat a play session after any painful or traumatic procedure such as surgery so that the child can express new feelings. A list of procedures that fall into this category is shown in Table 36.8. If such play sessions reveal fears, a child should be scheduled for other play sessions, perhaps once daily.

Furnish children with a wide range of equipment and then let them choose those items with which they wish to play. Children invariably choose a piece of equipment that has been used with them. They poke at a doll with a syringe without a needle or with a small rubber tube attached to simulate a needle or enjoy giving it a "shot." They wrap the doll in bandages or put tubes into its mouth or stomach, acting out things that were done to them or that they saw done to other children on a nursing unit or at a clinic visit they fear will be done to

TABLE 36.8 Therapeutic Play Techniques for Children After Procedures

Procedure	Play Activity (Provide a doll and . . .)
X-ray	A table and box labeled "X-ray machine"; children sometimes worry X-rays will injure them, just as laser rays in science fiction shows do. Handling a "machine" can reduce anxiety.
Blood drawing	Syringe, alcohol wipes, tourniquet, or finger lancets; remember that finger sticks are as frightening for children as needles.
Clean-catch urine	Alcohol wipes and a collection cup; children are often more embarrassed by urine collection than adults realize.
Intravenous therapy	Intravenous tubing, as well as tape and an armboard; some children are as angry about being restrained as having the needle inserted.
Endoscopy such as bronchoscopy, cystoscopy	Catheters or a penlight to simulate an endoscope.
Scans	Intravenous fluid and tubing, because scans usually require the intravenous injection of isotopes.
Bone marrow	Alcohol wipes, syringe.
Electroencephalogram (EEG), electrocardiogram (ECG)	Electrode leads that attach to a box; children might be afraid of these procedures because of their fear of electricity.
Surgery	An anesthesia mask and a blunt kitchen knife; watch and listen for where the child cuts and how the experience is described.
Dental examination	Suction catheter, a penlight to simulate a drill, and a 4 in. × 4 in. piece of plastic to simulate a dental dam; some children are angered by the use of plastic in their mouth.
Dressing changes	Gauze and adhesive tape.
Cast application or removal	Provide plaster to soak and apply; simulate a cast cutter with an electric razor or hair dryer.
Nasogastric tube insertion, enema, catheterization	Appropriate tubes.
Temperature assessment	Thermometer.

them. Allow play to be nondirective (let children proceed at their own pace, choosing freely what equipment to play with and what they want to do with equipment). As a child works through an experience this way, the experience becomes less fearful and the child gains increased control over it.

Observe for children who may be using equipment in an unusual way, such as hitting dolls with stethoscopes or poking them in the eye with a thermometer (suggesting they are confused about the purpose of such equipment or are acting out for another reason). Such behavior can alert you to the importance of explaining the purpose of equipment to children. Listen to what children say as they play. A comment such as, "I'm giving shots to all the bad dolls" suggests the child thinks injections are punishment. It would be important to stress the next time the child needs an injection that medicine is to make the child feel well again. A comment such as, "This doll is going to surgery, so you won't have her anymore" could suggest the child thinks she will not return from surgery (she may have heard a family member describe someone who died after surgery and is asking for reassurance that such a thing is not going to happen to her). Do not be surprised about the force with which children insert nasogastric tubes into dolls. In part, this reflects how they perceive these procedures, but it also represents energy or nervous release, in the way that pounding or hitting releases anger.

To better understand how a child feels, repeat what the child says verbally: "You're giving the bad dolls shots?" or ask the child to tell you more about the activity: "Do you think that's the only kind of children who get shots—bad children?" Do not rush to reassure ("Don't worry, that isn't going to happen to you"). Quick reassurance tells children they should not ask any more questions or that the topic is not open for discussion.

Sometimes, even children who seem well prepared may be taken by surprise during a procedure. For example, 7-year-old Tanya, seen in an ambulatory setting for a diagnostic workup after a urinary tract infection, showed little interest in dolls and syringes and tubing in the playroom. She had been prepared by her mother for the experience and seemed to understand what would happen during her X-ray procedure. After returning from the X-ray room, where she had a voiding cystourethrogram, however, she was obviously upset. Her nurse brought her a rag doll, a doctor and a nurse figure, a play X-ray machine, and some tubing that could simulate a urinary catheter and encouraged Tanya to play with them. Tanya picked up the girl doll and put her under the X-ray machine. She imitated the doctor doll shouting, "Pee in front of everybody!" Tanya's mother had not realized that she would have to void during a cystourethrogram and so had not prepared her for that. Tanya felt betrayed by not being really prepared for this embarrassing situation. Her play brought her emotion out in the open, where it could be talked about and handled. When Tanya was scheduled the next day for ureteral reflux surgery, her nurse was alerted to make the preparation absolutely thorough.

Children older than 9 or 10 years of age find playing with dolls too childish to be of benefit. They enjoy handling syringes, however, and being able to see and handle such equipment as nasogastric tubes in advance of their being placed. Active handling helps to eliminate fear because it identifies exactly what the child has to face, and it meets their concrete-level learning needs.

Creative Play

Some children are too angry to be able to act out their feelings through dramatic play. However, they may be able to draw a picture that expresses their emotions or conveys the extent of their knowledge. To encourage this, give a child a blank paper and crayons or markers. If a child seems reluctant to draw something spontaneously, suggest a topic: "Why don't you draw a picture of yourself?"

Some children are so concerned with particular parts of their bodies that when asked to draw pictures of themselves, they draw only the body part about which they are worried. Such children generally are saying they need to talk about that part of their body, to be given reassurance that it is going to be all right. Figure 36.11A shows a picture drawn by Becky when she was admitted to the hospital for 1-day surgery for debridement of a campfire burn on her left foot. She stated on admission that she was being admitted to have the burn on her foot "cleaned out." This sounds like a child who understands what debridement involves. Note, however, that the figure she drew has no left leg. One has to wonder whether she was concerned that she was going to surgery to have more than debridement. After the word "debridement" was explained to her, she drew the picture in Figure 36.11B. The child in the drawing now has a left and a right leg, with the left leg covered by a bandage. Through a drawing, this child was able to say something she could not express without this help.

Many ill children draw pictures that reflect punitive images: a boy or girl tied to a bed or shut behind bars, or doctors and nurses frowning at them, obviously unhappy with them (Fig. 36.12). Such children may need assurance that they are not being punished, but rather, that they need to stay in bed or are being cared for by doctors and nurses to be made well. Other children draw pictures that are symbolic of death: airplanes crashing, boats sinking, buildings on fire, or children in graveyards. They need assurance that they will not die.

Other concerns such as fear of abandonment and loss of independence may also be manifested in drawings. For example, preschoolers may draw a child in one corner of a picture and an adult in a far corner. They may comment that the parent cannot find the child because she's gone to the hospital. They need to be reassured that their parents know where they are and, although they're not there constantly, they will visit them each day after work.

Older school-age children and adolescents may not be interested in drawing but can be interested in making a list of procedures or experiences they like and dislike. Examine the dislike list for procedures such as "shots" or "chemo." Mark the nursing care plan for nurses to take special time to explain these procedures and to offer special support when they must be done.

What if... 36.3 While you're playing with her, Becky draws a purple person with only three body parts. Would this worry you? Why or why not?

Guidelines for Conducting Therapeutic Play

Use common sense when conducting therapeutic play. Be certain, for example, not to interpret a child's black and gloomy drawing as meaning the child is depressed when a

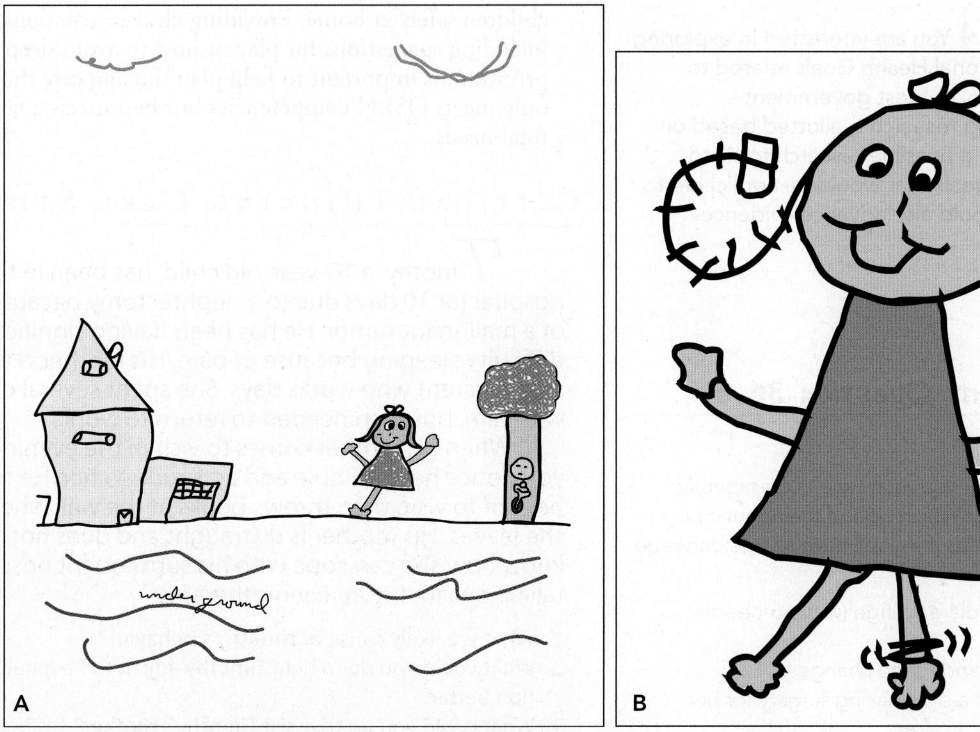

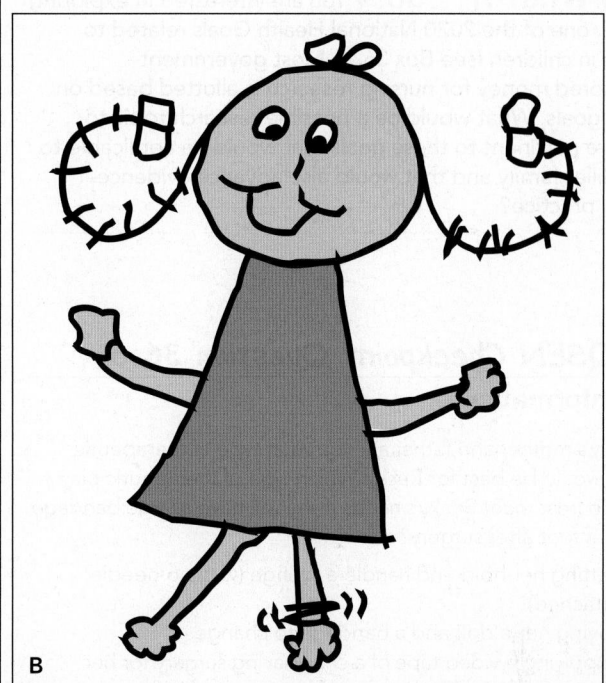

FIGURE 36.11 **(A)** Children who are concerned about body parts may draw pictures with that part missing or exaggerated. Note the missing left leg here. **(B)** After reassurance that her leg will be all right, the girl who did the drawing in **A** now draws a girl with two legs.

black marker was the only one available. Many children 4 to 5 years of age draw a person lacking many body parts because that is the best human form they can draw.

Remember, too, that all children occasionally treat dolls badly. A 2-year-old who pounds and bangs a rag doll may not be expressing anger toward the doll image at all, but may be intent on discovering the feel of a new texture and is unaware for the moment that the object is a doll.

A conference with health care team members, including a psychologist or a psychiatric nurse specialist, may be needed if a child continues to express mutilating behavior after normal reassurance. Guidelines for conducting therapeutic play are summarized in Box 36.8.

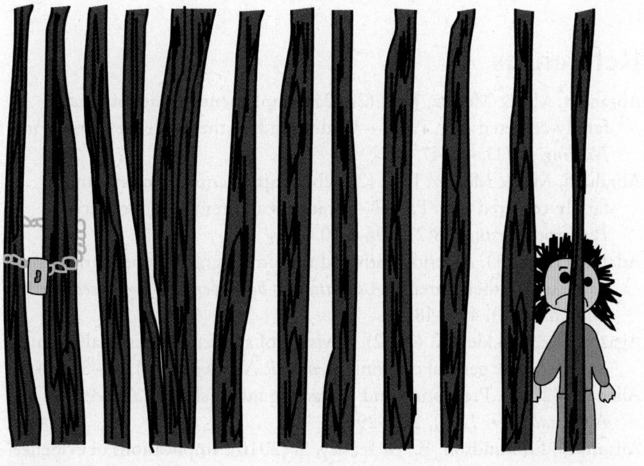

FIGURE 36.12 A picture drawn by a hospitalized child. Note the prisonlike appearance of the crib. (Courtesy of Rita Crever.)

BOX 36.8 Guidelines for Therapeutic Play

1. Allow children to choose the articles with which they want to play (something may be too frightening for a child to play with immediately, or more time may be needed to work up to the activity).
2. Provide the materials specific to the child's experiences of which you are aware, such as a nasogastric tube, syringe, or bandages, but do not supply only those things; a child may have misunderstandings and fears of situations you cannot know about.
3. Allow play to be unstructured; let children use the materials however they wish. If a child seems uninterested in materials, initiate play such as giving a doll an injection to see if this reduces the child's fear enough to be able to handle items.
4. If a child cannot manipulate materials for some reason such as a large cast or traction, ask the child what would be good for you to do with an item.
5. Reflect only what the child expresses (verbal expression).
6. Do not criticize play; this inhibits further expression.
7. Use a therapeutic response; not "Don't worry, that won't happen," but "Are you worried that could happen?"
8. Ask children to describe paintings; not "That's a good picture of yourself," but "Tell me about your picture."
9. Do not be reluctant to use real equipment such as real catheters and blood lancets. Handling real equipment best helps to reduce stress.
10. Supervise therapeutic play, because some equipment could cause an injury (and therapeutically responding to the child's comments is necessary).

What if...36.4 You are interested in exploring one of the 2020 National Health Goals related to illness in children (see Box 36.1). Most government-sponsored money for nursing research is allotted based on these goals. What would be a possible research topic to explore pertinent to these goals that would be applicable to the Miller family and that would also advance evidence-based practice?

QSEN Checkpoint Question 36.6
Informatics

Becky's mother and father ask you what type of therapeutic play would be best for Becky. Which type of therapeutic play would best meet Becky's needs if she will have a large bandage on her foot after surgery?

a. Letting her hold and handle a syringe (with no needle attached)
b. Giving her a doll and a bandage to change
c. Supplying a video tape of a child having surgery for her to watch
d. Giving her a book to read about a child's hospitalization experience

Look in Appendix A for the best answer and rationale.

Key Points for Review

- Illnesses may be more traumatic for children than for adults because of children's inability to communicate and monitor their own care and because they have different nutrition, fluid, and electrolyte needs. The stress of hospitalization can be so acute that it can result in PTSD.
- Separation from parents because of hospitalization can have permanent psychological effects on children. Methods to reduce this include keeping hospital stays as brief as possible, promoting open parent and sibling visiting, and providing primary or case management nursing.
- Currently, many medical procedures can be done on an ambulatory basis. Advocating for care to be done in such settings is a nursing responsibility.
- The presence of parents during health care can help reduce trauma to children. Making parents as welcome as possible in health care facilities makes it possible for them to room-in. Include parents in both the planning and the implementation of care. Parents reinfect children with fear if their own fear is not reduced.
- Preschoolers may have the most difficult time during hospitalization because they have so many fears. Preparation and promotion of therapeutic play may be essential to reduce trauma to a tolerable level.
- Because hospitalizations currently are so brief, parents need good discharge instructions to continue to care for children safely at home. Providing clear instructions, including suggestions for play or how to avoid sleep deprivation, is important to help plan nursing care that not only meets QSEN competencies but best meets a family's total needs.

Critical Thinking Care Study

Timothy, a 10-year-old child, has been in the hospital for 10 days due to a nephrectomy because of a malignant tumor. He has been having significant difficulty sleeping because of pain. His mother is a single parent who works days. She spent several days with him, but then needed to return to work.

When his mother comes to visit in the evenings, you notice he is irritable and acts rude to her. He tells her not to visit, then throws books at the wall when she leaves. His mother is distraught and does not know how she can cope with his subsequent hospitalizations for future chemotherapy.

1. What is a likely cause of Timothy's behavior?
2. What could you do to help Timothy adjust to hospitalization better?
3. What could you do to assist Timothy's mother?

Patient Scenario
The Century Family

Read about the Century family, a family with a school-age child with cerebral palsy, then answer the questions to further sharpen your skills and grow more familiar with NCLEX-type questions related to supporting the health of ill children and their families. Confirm your answers are correct by reading the rationales.

Visit http://thePoint.lww.com

Answers and Rationales

Looking for answers to the What if . . . and Critical Thinking Care Study questions?

Visit http://thePoint.lww.com

References

Abraham, M., & Moretz, J. G. (2012a). Implementing patient- and family-centered care. Part I—Understanding the challenges. *Pediatric Nursing, 38*(1), 44–47.

Abraham, M., & Moretz, J. G. (2012b). Implementing patient- and family-centered care. Part II—Strategies and resources for success. *Pediatric Nursing, 38*(2), 106–110.

Adams, H. (2011). A perioperative education program for pediatric patients and their parents. *Association of periOperative Registered Nurses Journal, 93*(4), 472–481.

Agazio, J., & Buckley, K. (2012). Revision of a parental stress scale for use on a pediatric general care unit. *Pediatric Nursing, 38*(2), 82–87.

Allen, K. (2012). Promoting and protecting infant sleep. *Advances in Neonatal Care, 12*(5), 288–291.

Anson, L., Edmundson, E., & Teasley, S. (2010). Implications of evidence based venipuncture practice in a pediatric health care magnet facility. *Journal of Continuing Education in Nursing, 41*(4), 179–185.

Arthur, N. (2010). Technology and television for babies and toddlers. *Children and Libraries, 8*(2), 58–59.

Barry, P., O'Callaghan, C., Wheeler, G., et al. (2010). Music therapy CD creation for initial pediatric radiation therapy, A mixed methods analysis. *Journal of Music Therapy, 47*(3), 233–263.

Blush, R., & Matzo, M. (2012). Acute infectious diarrhea. *American Journal of Nursing, 112*(8), 65–68.

Bowlby, J. (1951). *Maternal care and mental health. Bulletin of the World Health Organization.* Geneva, Switzerland: World Health Organization.

Brumariu, L. E., & Kerns, K. A. (2010). Mother–child attachment patterns and different types of anxiety symptoms: Is there specificity of relations? *Child Psychiatry & Human Development, 41*(6), 663–674.

Citty, S. W. (2011). Empowering nurses to improve patient nutrition. *Nursing, 41*(11), 51–53.

Cochran, J. L. Cochran, N. H., Fuss A., et al. (2010). Outcomes and stages of child-centered play therapy for a child with highly disruptive behavior driven by self–concept issues. *Journal of Humanistic Counseling, Education and Development, 49*(2), 231–246.

Cota, B. M., & Allen, P. J. (2010). The developmental origins of health and disease hypothesis. *Pediatric Nursing, 36*(3), 157–167.

DeCourcey, M., Russell, A. C., & Keister, K. (2010). Animal-assisted therapy: Evaluation and implementation of a complementary therapy to improve the psychological and physiological health of critically ill patients. *Dimensions of Critical Care Nursing, 29*(5), 211–214.

Duzinski, S. V., Lawson, K. A., Maxson, R. T., et al. (2012). The association between positive screen for future persistent posttraumatic stress symptoms and injury incident variables in the pediatric trauma care setting. *Journal of Trauma & Acute Care Surgery, 72*(6), 1640–1646.

Eaton, S. (2012). Addressing the effects of missing school for children with medical needs. *Pediatric Nursing, 38*(5), 271–277.

Elser, H., Holditch-Davis, D., Levy, J., et al. (2012). The effects of environmental noise and infant position on cerebral oxygenation. *Advances in Neonatal Care, 12*(55), 518–527.

Frisch, A. M., Johnson, A., Timmons, S., et al. (2010). Nurse practitioner role in preparing families for pediatric outpatient surgery. *Pediatric Nursing, 36*(1), 41–47.

Hart, R., & Walton, M. (2010). Magic as a therapeutic intervention to promote coping in hospitalized pediatric patients. *Pediatric Nursing, 36*(1), 11–17.

Jacobs, H., & Popick, R. (2012). Utilization of internet resources for adolescents coping with chronic conditions. *Pediatric Nursing, 38*(4), 228–231.

Landolt, M. A., Ystrom, E., Sennhauser, F. H., et al. (2012). The mutual prospective influence of child and parental post-traumatic stress symptoms in pediatric patients. *Journal of Child Psychology & Psychiatry & Allied Disciplines, 53*(7), 767–774.

Lehna, C. (2010). Sibling experiences after a major childhood burn injury. *Pediatric Nursing, 36*(5), 245–251.

Litke, J., Pikulska, A., & Wegner, T. (2012). Management of perioperative stress in children and parents: The preoperative period. *Anaesthesiology Intensive Therapy, 44*(3), 165–169.

Lynch, M. (2012) Children at play: An innovative method for studying and teaching nutritional behaviors. *Pediatric Nursing, 38*(3), 139–143.

Meltzer, L., Davis, K. F., & Mindell, J. (2012). Patient and parent sleep in a children's hospital. *Pediatric Nursing, 38*(2), 64–71.

Robertson, J. (1958). *Young children in hospitals.* London, United Kingdom: Tavistock.

Scanlon, A., & Cook, S. S. (2010). Febrile seizures, genetic (generalized) epilepsy with febrile seizures plus, and Dravet's syndrome. *Journal of Specialists in Pediatric Nursing, 15*(2), 154–159.

Scollan-Koliopoulos, M., & Koliopoulos, J. (2010). Evaluation and management of apparent life threatening events in infants. *Pediatric Nursing, 36*(2), 77–83.

Spitz, R. A. (1945). Hospitalism: An inquiry into the genesis of psychiatric conditions in early childhood. *Psychoanalytic Study of the Child, 1*(3), 53–59.

Stevens, D. C., Helseth, C. C., Khan, M. A., et al. (2011). A comparison of parent satisfaction in an open-bay and single-family room neonatal intensive care unit. *HERD: Health Environments Research & Design Journal, 4*(3), 110–123.

U.S. Department of Health and Human Services. (2010). *Healthy people 2020.* Washington, DC: Author.

Waltman, P. A., Schenk, L. K., Martin, T. M., et al. (2011). Effects of student participation in hand hygiene monitoring on knowledge and perception of infection control practices. *Journal of Nursing Education, 50*(4), 216–221.

Whitton, S., & Pittiglio, L. (2011). Critical care open visiting hours. *Critical Care Nursing Quarterly, 34*(4), 361–366.

Williams, L., Eilers, J., Heermann, J., et al. (2012). The lived experience of parents and guardians providing care for child transplant recipients. *Progress in Transplantation, 22*(4), 393–402.

Zempsky, W. T., Palermo, T. M., Corsi, J. M., et al. (2013). Daily changes in pain, mood and physical function in children hospitalized for sickle cell disease pain. *Pain Research & Management, 18*(1):33–38.

Chapter 37

Nursing Care of a Family When a Child Needs Diagnostic or Therapeutic Modalities

KEY TERMS

- aspiration studies
- bronchoscopy
- clean-catch urine specimen
- colonoscopy
- computed tomography (CT)
- electrical impulse studies
- endoscopy
- magnetic resonance imaging (MRI)
- positron emission tomography (PET)
- radiopharmaceuticals
- single-photon emission computed tomography (SPECT)
- total parenteral nutrition (TPN)
- ultrasound

OBJECTIVES

After mastering the contents of this chapter, you should be able to:

1. Describe common nursing interventions used in the health care of children to aid diagnosis and therapy.
2. Identify 2020 National Health Goals related to diagnostic and therapeutic procedures for children that nurses can help the nation achieve.
3. Assess children regarding their developmental stage and knowledge level before beginning diagnostic or therapeutic procedures.
4. Formulate nursing diagnoses related to common diagnostic or therapeutic procedures used with children.
5. Identify expected outcomes for a child who needs a diagnostic or therapeutic procedure as well as help families manage seamless transitions across differing health care settings.
6. Using the nursing process, plan nursing care that includes the six competencies of Quality & Safety Education for Nurses (QSEN): Patient-Centered Care, Teamwork & Collaboration, Evidence-Based Practice (EBP), Quality Improvement (QI), Safety, and Informatics.
7. Implement nursing care relevant to diagnostic or therapeutic procedures, such as preparing a child for magnetic resonance imaging.
8. Evaluate expected outcomes for achievement and effectiveness of care.
9. Integrate knowledge of common diagnostic and therapeutic procedures with the interplay of nursing process, the six competencies of QSEN, and Family Nursing to promote quality maternal and child health nursing care.

Felipe Ramos is a preschooler who is scheduled to have a magnetic resonance imaging (MRI) study because he was shoved off a 6-ft high slide at a playground and hit his head. "How can I agree to this?" his mother asks you through an interpreter. "He's already upset because of the bullying. When he's afraid of the dark, how can I allow him to be wheeled into a long dark machine that way?"

Previous chapters described the growth and development of well children. This chapter adds information about how to care for children who are having diagnostic or therapeutic procedures. This is important information because it builds a base for both care and health teaching.

How would you explain the MRI procedure to Felipe to make the procedure more acceptable to him?

BOX 37.1 Nursing Care Planning Based on 2020 National Health Goals

2020 National Health Goals speak to efforts to keep children well so they need a minimal number of diagnostic or therapy procedures.

- Reduce hospitalizations for asthma among children under age 5 years from a baseline of 41.4% to a target level of 18.1%.
- Increase age-appropriate vehicle restraint systems in children aged 4 to 7 years from a baseline of 43% to a target level of 47%.
- Increase the number of adolescents who have had a wellness checkup in the past 12 months from 68.7% to 75.6%. (U.S. Department of Health and Human Services [DHHS], 2010; see www.healthypeople.gov).

Nurses can help the nation achieve these goals by providing health counseling to parents and children to help prevent children from becoming ill and subsequently requiring hospitalization, such as teaching sound nutrition and common practices on avoiding unintentional injury.

Illness can be particularly stressful if many diagnostic and therapeutic procedures are necessary for diagnosis or care. In today's health care climate, there is less time for teaching and preparation than was once available, so good planning and follow-through are essential when procedures are scheduled (Jackson & Thalange, 2013). Chapter 36 described measures to make an illness experience more positive. Health teaching, discussed in Chapter 35, is also a cornerstone in this process.

Many nursing actions offer an opportunity to accomplish several goals. Supporting a child and family during a diagnostic procedure, for instance, cannot only aid in an efficient diagnosis but may also help establish a trusting relationship between the family and health care providers that will make all future interactions more successful. This chapter describes the most common diagnostic and therapeutic techniques used in the care of ill children, including modifications needed to make these procedures safe and to reduce associated stress, depending on the child's age and condition. Box 37.1 shows 2020 National Health Goals that address this area of child health practice.

Nursing Process Overview

For a Child Who Needs Diagnostic or Therapeutic Procedures

Assessment

Before performing procedures such as assisting with a diagnostic test or collecting laboratory specimens, first carefully evaluate a child's age and developmental stage, as well as any special needs a child may have. Even the most common and painless procedures create a certain amount of stress for children and parents. During complex diagnostic procedures, this stress level is almost certain to increase even further due to fear of the unknown. Unfamiliar people (e.g., doctors, nurses, other health team members), high-tech supplies and equipment, and strange surroundings all add up to a frightening experience for most adults; imagine how frightening they are to children.

It is important to acknowledge that many procedures that involve highly technologic equipment may be painful or uncomfortable for a child, especially if the child has a chronic disease. Assess a child's level of anxiety associated with a procedure as well as the child's knowledge concerning a technique before initiating the procedure or beginning health teaching. Pointing out a child's past experience with similar procedures can lay a foundation for increased cooperation.

Nursing Diagnosis

Common nursing diagnoses related to diagnostic and therapeutic procedures are as varied as the procedures themselves. Some examples include:

- Fear related to new and strange surroundings of the procedure room
- Pain related to a lumbar puncture procedure
- Deficient knowledge related to the technique for 24-hour urine collection
- Deficient diversionary activity related to hospitalization and lengthy procedures
- Imbalanced nutrition, less than body requirements, related to need for food restriction preprocedure and postprocedure
- Risk of injury related to need for intrusive procedures

Outcome Identification and Planning

Procedures can produce stress in addition to the anxiety caused by a primary illness. An important nursing goal, therefore, is to perform procedures and complete interventions with the least amount of anxiety possible. To achieve this goal, plan specific ways to prepare children in advance and apply the best communication techniques possible to explain a procedure at the level of understanding and developmental stage appropriate for each child. Consideration should be given to the number of diagnostic or therapeutic procedures and the time frame in which they are performed. Some children may have less anxiety if diagnostic tests are scheduled over several days to preserve the child's coping ability. Conversely, some older children (and parents) do better if they can complete all necessary tests in 1 day to reduce the anxiety produced by the anticipation of more testing still to come.

Helpful Web sites to assist parents in preparing their children for procedures are KidsHealth (www.kidshealth.org) and the Mayo Clinic Web site (www.mayoclinic.com).

Implementation

Whether assisting with a procedure or performing a therapeutic intervention, it is necessary to function in several roles simultaneously: organizing supplies, performing (or assisting with) the procedure, providing active support to the child and parents, and observing and then documenting the child's reactions. As a final follow-through step, plan for introducing therapeutic play techniques that would be helpful in relieving stress caused by the procedure.

Outcome Evaluation

Evaluating expected outcomes related to diagnostic and therapeutic procedures is not only helpful in determining the effect of the procedure on a child but also aids in future planning should other procedures be required. Recording that a particular child who did not appear nervous during a procedure later admitted to being "more scared than I've ever been before," for example, can help another nurse provide reassurance to this child, even if the child is successful at masking emotions the next time the procedure is performed. Examples suggesting achievement of expected outcomes include:

- The child reports the ability to cope with a second bone marrow aspiration.
- The child lists steps for successful 24-hour urine collection at home.
- The child participates in 1 hour of active exercise daily.
- The child eats a minimum of 1,000 calories per day.
- The child experiences minimal loss of blood, less than 10 ml, during a diagnostic procedure.
- The parent outlines plan to use alternative therapies to reduce the child's anxiety.

NURSING RESPONSIBILITIES WITH DIAGNOSTIC AND THERAPEUTIC TECHNIQUES

The most efficient way to reduce children's stress from hospitalization is to reduce the number of hospitalizations necessary. If that cannot be accomplished, then the next step is reducing the number of diagnostic or therapeutic procedures children have to undergo. Despite these attempts, some children, such as those who are chronically ill or are dependent on technology such as a ventilator, require 24-hour care in either a health care setting or their home. Children who show initial symptoms of an illness need diagnostic procedures in order for their condition to be confirmed and therapy can begin.

When hospitalization is indicated in these ways, the stress of the experience can be reduced for both the child and parents if procedures are carried out in the least stressful way possible (Litke, Pikulska, & Wegner, 2012). When performing or assisting with procedures on children, remember to maintain safety and legal responsibilities for care such as:

- Verify that an informed consent is obtained, as needed.
- Utilize the electronic health record to verify the prescription for the procedure.
- Explain the procedure to the child and parents to be certain both are well informed.
- Schedule the procedure.
- Prepare the child physically and psychologically.
- Obtain necessary equipment for the procedure.
- Accompany a child to a treatment room or hospital department where the procedure will be performed.
- Coordinate and collaborate with other health care providers to ensure the safety and efficacy of all procedures.
- Provide support during the procedure, using the least amount of restraint possible.
- Ensure adherence to standard infection precautions.
- Assess a child's response to the procedure.
- Provide care to a child and specimens obtained once the procedure is completed.
- Document the outcome of the procedure and the child's reaction to the procedure.

Obtaining Informed Consent

Informed consent is legally required and must be obtained before any procedure or treatment that has the risk of causing injury to the child is performed. The benefits and risks of the treatment or procedure must be discussed along with the risks if the treatment or procedure was not performed. Although obtaining consent is the physician's responsibility, assuring that it is obtained is a nursing responsibility. Acting as an advocate for a family if they do not understand the consent form, the procedure, or the risks of the procedure is an important nursing role. Be certain the rights of emancipated minors are respected and that, in single-parent families, the custodial parent is the one who is asked to give the permission (Lane & Kohlenberg, 2012).

Explaining Procedures

To be able to explain procedures clearly and answer questions about them appropriately, try to observe as many procedures as you can. After any procedure, asking children to describe what sensations they experienced can help them work through possibly frightening situations (often called "debriefing") and can also increase your knowledge of common procedures.

As a general guide, before a procedure, a child needs a detailed description of what to expect, such as, "I'll clean your finger. You will feel a small pinprick," as well as an explanation of:

- Why the procedure is being performed (e.g., "Your doctor needs to look at your blood to see why you're so sick")
- Where the procedure will be done (e.g., the X-ray department, a treatment room)
- Any unusual sensations to be expected during the procedure (e.g., "The alcohol I use to clean your skin will feel cold")
- Any pain involved (e.g., "The needle will sting, although I'll put some cream on first to dull the feeling")
- Any equipment that will be unfamiliar such as a magnetic resonance imaging (MRI) machine
- The approximate length of time the procedure will take
- Any special care after the procedure (e.g., "You will need to lie quietly for 15 minutes afterward")

Be certain to use age-appropriate language when explaining procedures. Also be careful not to use words that might be confusing during an explanation, such as "transducer" or "electrode," without defining them. Try to associate the procedure with something you know the child is already familiar and comfortable with, such as describing an X-ray machine as "a big camera." Try not to use the word "test" in explanations because school-age children associate the word "test" with a pass/fail situation. Wondering if they "passed" a procedure can make them unduly worried afterward.

If you are unfamiliar with what a procedure entails, do not guess the answers to a child's questions because nothing is more confusing than being told two different versions of an answer to the same question. Most technical personnel will take the time to describe important information a child should know about a study or procedure so you can relay this information to the child or parent; having a well-informed child makes the technician's job easier. Remember, a child is apt to have difficulty relaxing if a parent is still anxious. Be certain, therefore, that parents as well as the child receive an explanation of the procedure. Encourage them to stay with their child during the procedure, if possible, because they can be extremely helpful in reducing the threatening aspects of a procedure (Forsey, Salmon, Eden, et al., 2011).

Scheduling

If a child is having more than one diagnostic procedure in a day, try to arrange for the child to have time for meals and some free play time between the procedures. If food or fluid must be restricted, monitor the child's degree of discomfort and physiologic needs related to the restriction. Advocate as necessary for sufficient periods of time between examinations so a child can eat, or for decreased time between procedures so the time spent without food or fluid is limited. Ask if, even with a fluid limitation, whether small sips of water or ice chips would be acceptable to decrease a child's thirst (Haemer, Primark, & Krebs, 2011).

Preparing a Child and Family Physically and Psychologically

Physical preparation varies with each procedure to be performed. In many instances, preparing a child for an examination, such as a barium enema, involves another procedure such as a saline enema, so that physical preparation also becomes education for the actual examination. In all instances, explain both the preparative and actual procedures, and allow the child to ask questions since appropriate explanations aid in reducing anxiety and fear (Box 37.2).

About 60 minutes before a procedure, children may be given oral chloral hydrate to relieve both apprehension and make them feel sleepy. For painful procedures or those that demand extreme cooperation, such as a bronchoscopy (see section on Direct Visualization Procedures), children may be administered conscious sedation (Havidich & Cravero, 2012). Used in both ambulatory and inpatient settings, conscious sedation results in a depressed level of consciousness

BOX 37.2 Nursing Care Planning to Respect Cultural Diversity

Professional nursing practice must continually adapt to the changing values and beliefs of the population it serves. The diversity of the population is reflected in pediatric patients and their families, many of whom are from various cultural backgrounds, have a language other than English as their primary language, have difficulty reading English so have questionable health or reading literacy, and may be overwhelmed by the information and expectations of adaptation to a new health care system. Translators should be available to comply with the Joint Commission (TJC) standards in health care to ensure effective communication. Be certain when health teaching concerning procedures or handing out written instructions that you first assess a child and parent to be sure they understand or can read English.

induced by the intravenous administration of a sedative such as midazolam in combination with a narcotic such as morphine sulfate and perhaps a short-acting hypnotic. It is administered by an anesthesiologist or a nurse specially prepared in the technique (Adler, Kawa, Hilden, et al., 2011).

While under conscious sedation, children are able to maintain their ability to breathe independently and also respond appropriately to verbal commands such as, "Lift your head." They feel minimal pain, however, because of the analgesic administered. Before the technique is started, emergency equipment, including respiratory and pharmacologic measures, must be on hand. The child's level of consciousness and ability to respond, heart rate, respiratory rate, blood pressure, and oxygen saturation must be monitored throughout the procedure. Using conscious sedation is an excellent technique to allow children to accept a potentially painful procedure both emotionally and physically. If it will be used, be certain a child is prepared not only for the diagnostic procedure but for the use of conscious sedation as well.

Accompanying the Child

If a procedure will be done at a different site from the primary care clinic or hospital unit with which a child is comfortable, ideally, a nurse whom the child knows should accompany the child to the other department and remain with the child for the procedure, or at least until the child has met a primary person who will be responsible for the procedure. If a parent is available, having a parent accompany a child is also of invaluable help. Although arranging the time to be present may prove difficult for a working family, most parents are eager to do this. Older children do well with being accompanied by only a nursing assistant, as long as they have been introduced in advance to the new person who will give them care.

Before leaving the child's patient care unit or clinic, ask the child to void for comfort unless this is contraindicated by the procedure. Check for any medication or specific baseline assessment procedures such as a blood pressure recording that should be given or done before leaving the unit for another department, in case the child will be away from the primary unit for an extended time. If a child is an inpatient, also check that the identification band is securely in place and readily visible despite any intravenous equipment. In most health care settings, variations of the SBAR (Situation, Background, Assessment, Recommendation) or ISBAR (Introduction, Situation, Background, Assessment, Recommendation) format is implemented for interdisciplinary/interdepartmental communication to be certain preparation procedures follow the Joint Commission standards on communication (The Joint Commission, 2010). If there will be a considerable wait in another department, ask children if they would like to bring along an activity such as a game or book. In addition, hallways can be cool. Provide adequate blankets for comfort, especially for infants, because their temperature-control mechanisms are underdeveloped their temperature can fall quickly. Always use cart straps and side rails for safety as safety is a priority during all procedures performed on children (Jain, Petrillo-Albarano, & Parks, 2013).

Providing Support

Children do well with diagnostic and evaluative procedures as long as they have adequate support from a concerned provider or parent with them. Try to provide support both verbally (i.e., explain what is going to happen, assure the child everything is going well) and nonverbally (e.g., a hand on the arm or a nearby presence). After a procedure, be certain the child has a favorite toy with which to play to help reduce the effect of the experience.

Modifying Procedures According to a Child's Age and Developmental Stage

It is important to consider a child's age and potential understanding of procedures when planning the number and order of tests and the way they will be performed.

The Infant

The number of painful or uncomfortable procedures done on infants should be kept to an absolute minimum to avoid interfering with an infant's developing sense of trust. Be particularly responsible about obtaining blood specimens (which can deplete an infant's small blood stores) and X-ray procedures (which are possibly harmful to immature bone marrow). You should advocate for limitation of these procedures, and can help parents understand why these procedures are being limited and that their infant's care is not compromised by performing fewer diagnostic procedures.

At the time of a procedure, advocate for parents to be able to accompany their infant to hospital departments and remain during procedures to offer support. Some parents may ask to hold their child during a procedure that causes pain, but do not ask parents to restrain the child during such a procedure. Their role should be supportive and comforting, not one that causes pain.

Infants become dehydrated quickly, so the time they can remain nothing by mouth (NPO) for procedures must not exceed 6 hours. You may need to advocate time for breastfeeding before and after a procedure for the comfort of both the infant and mother. If a procedure continues for longer than 3 to 4 hours, provide the mother a room in which to use a breast pump, if needed. Assess the infant's temperature to guard against extremes. Have a blanket available to prevent chilling.

After procedures, pick up infants and actively comfort them (e.g., children of any age like a hug or honest compliment for their cooperation).

The Toddler and Preschooler

Toddlers and preschoolers resist any diagnostic testing that involves any degree of discomfort or pain or any procedure that is unfamiliar to them. Give children of this age short explanations of what to expect close to the time of the procedure so that little time can be spent worrying. Try to associate any new equipment with things that they are already familiar, such as comparing an MRI to a giant cell phone camera. If possible, introduce any equipment that will be used in procedures such as a nasogastric tube in a play session with a doll so the child can handle the new object and see that the doll is not injured or minds having the tube inserted.

The School-Age Child and Adolescent

School-age children are concrete thinkers and so are interested in the theory and reason for procedures. They can often be persuaded to cooperate for a procedure by being promised a look at their X-ray or a point-of-care meter readout afterward. Be careful, however, to ensure that viewing the results is actually possible before promising this to children; otherwise, it can be difficult to obtain any further cooperation. Adolescents may project an air of maturity or sophistication beyond their years to remain in control of themselves in the face of frightening procedures. Do not be misled into thinking an adolescent would not appreciate an explanation or a comforting hand on a shoulder during a procedure.

What if...37.1 Felipe who is scheduled for a cranial MRI puts his hands over his ears and refuses to listen to your explanation of what will happen during the MRI. How could you give an explanation to him? Why do you think he is acting this way?

Promoting Safety During Procedures

Whether a procedure will be safe depends a great deal on the nursing planning and support that accompanies the procedure. Children are unable to guard their own safety because they are unable to form mature judgments, a situation that leaves them vulnerable to harm unless their caregivers give special consideration to promoting safety during procedures.

Nursing Diagnoses and Related Interventions

Nursing Diagnosis: Risk for injury related to diagnostic procedure

Outcome Evaluation: Child remains free of injury from diagnostic equipment; voices afterward that procedure was not as frightening as anticipated.

As the first safety measure, before performing any procedure, and even before offering food or a medication, read the name on a child's identification armband. If an armband must be removed because it interferes with an intravenous infusion site, cut it away but immediately anchor it to another extremity with adhesive tape. Ask the admissions department to provide a new armband as soon as possible. Do not leave the old one off while waiting for a replacement band because this leaves the child susceptible to the danger of mistaken identity during the waiting period.

Because of their natural curiosity, children tend to fuss with equipment to see what will happen if they turn a knob or spin a dial. This means they need close monitoring while procedures are performed to ensure they do not touch any buttons or in other way unintentionally harm themselves. After a procedure, be certain to remove all equipment from a room. Otherwise, for example, children may pick up scissors or forceps left at bedsides and injure an eye, or they may drink antiseptics such as alcohol or povidone-iodine left at their bedside and poison themselves. Syringes and needles can cause puncture wounds. Infants and young children can choke on small objects such as needle covers.

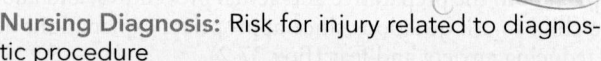

Use of Restraints

The purpose of a restraint during a procedure is to keep a child safe from injury. Always use the least amount of restraint necessary and apply with care because, if improperly applied, restraints can cause extreme stress and may not make a difference in outcome (Michelotti, Long, & Leber, 2012). Children can have difficulty distinguishing between restraint and punishment, so restraint should never be used more often or for a longer time frame than necessary. Be certain there is a primary care provider's prescription for a restraint, and that parents receive an explanation for the need to restrain their child (e.g., "Because of a particular danger of this procedure, it is safer if your child has a reminder to not bend his arm").

If a restraint is in place, check it every 15 minutes to be certain it is not occluding circulation; remove it temporarily every hour so the body part can be exercised provided the exercise does not dislodge a device or interfere with a treatment. No part of a child's body other than that which is necessary should be restrained. When infants have scalp vein infusions in place, such as for injection of a radioactive isotope for a nuclear medicine scan, for example, their arms may need to be immobilized so they do not touch the infusion site. Their trunk may need to be immobilized so they do not turn. Their lower extremities, however, do not need to be restrained so they can still actively kick and exercise. When a nurse or a parent is with a child, in most instances, all restraints can be removed. Various types of restraints commonly used are described in Table 37.1 and shown in Figure 37.1.

Providing Care After Procedures

After a procedure, assess how well a child reacted to the procedure by both observation and history. Allowing children to explain what happened helps them retrace the procedure in

TABLE 37.1 Safety With Restraints

Type of Restraint	Purpose	Method
Wheelchairs and carts	Promote safety while transporting children to and from a health care facility procedure department.	For a wheelchair, use a vest restraint. Attach straps to the frame of the wheelchair with enough slack so the child has some mobility. For a cart, fasten a restraining belt and raise the side rails. Even with restraints in place, never leave a child unattended in hallways outside departments in a wheelchair or on a cart. Not only is this unsafe because the child may attempt to get down from the cart or wheelchair but also the anxiety of waiting in a strange department for a procedure without a support person with them may be too acute for young children to handle.
Clove-hitch restraints	Secure one arm or leg for a procedure, such as an intravenous infusion.	Use disposable restraints, gauze, or soft muslin tape. Soft muslin tape "gives" a little if the child exerts pressure against it so it will not pull too tight and reduce circulation or cause pain. Tie the restraint as shown in Figure 37.1A. If a child struggles against restraints, fold several layers of soft gauze around the wrist or ankle under the restraint. Secure the restraint to the underpart of the bed. Never tie restraints to side rails; when a side rail is lowered, it will jerk the child's arm or leg and possibly cause an injury. Release arm and leg restraints whenever someone can be with the child to keep the limb in the desired position.
Jacket restraints	Restrain children younger than 6 months in a supine position.	Fasten the ties at the back of the jacket. Tie strips attached to the sides of the jacket under the mattress to keep the child in one position (see Fig. 37.1B). Assess that the restraint is not pressing against the neck or could be causing interference with a child's airway.
Elbow restraints	Prevent children from touching the head or face (e.g., following facial surgery).	Dress the baby in a long-sleeved shirt to prevent irritation from the restraint. Slip a commercial restraint such a NoNoSleeve up over the infant's arm and secure it by the Velcro strips (see Fig. 37.1C). Assess the infant's fingers to be certain the sleeve is not too tight that it interferes with circulation.
Mummy restraints	Temporarily immobilize young children for a procedure involving the head, neck, or throat (e.g., during insertion of a nasogastric tube or blood drawing).	Use this only for the duration of the procedure because it is a total body restraint. Follow the steps shown in Figure 37.1D. If the child is exceptionally strong, a few safety pins can be used to hold the restraint even more firmly in place. For the infant who needs continuous observation for respiratory function, fold the mummy restraint so the chest is exposed. For newborns or infants, use a Papoose Board, a commercial restraint used in the same way as a full or mummy restraint (see Fig. 37.1E).

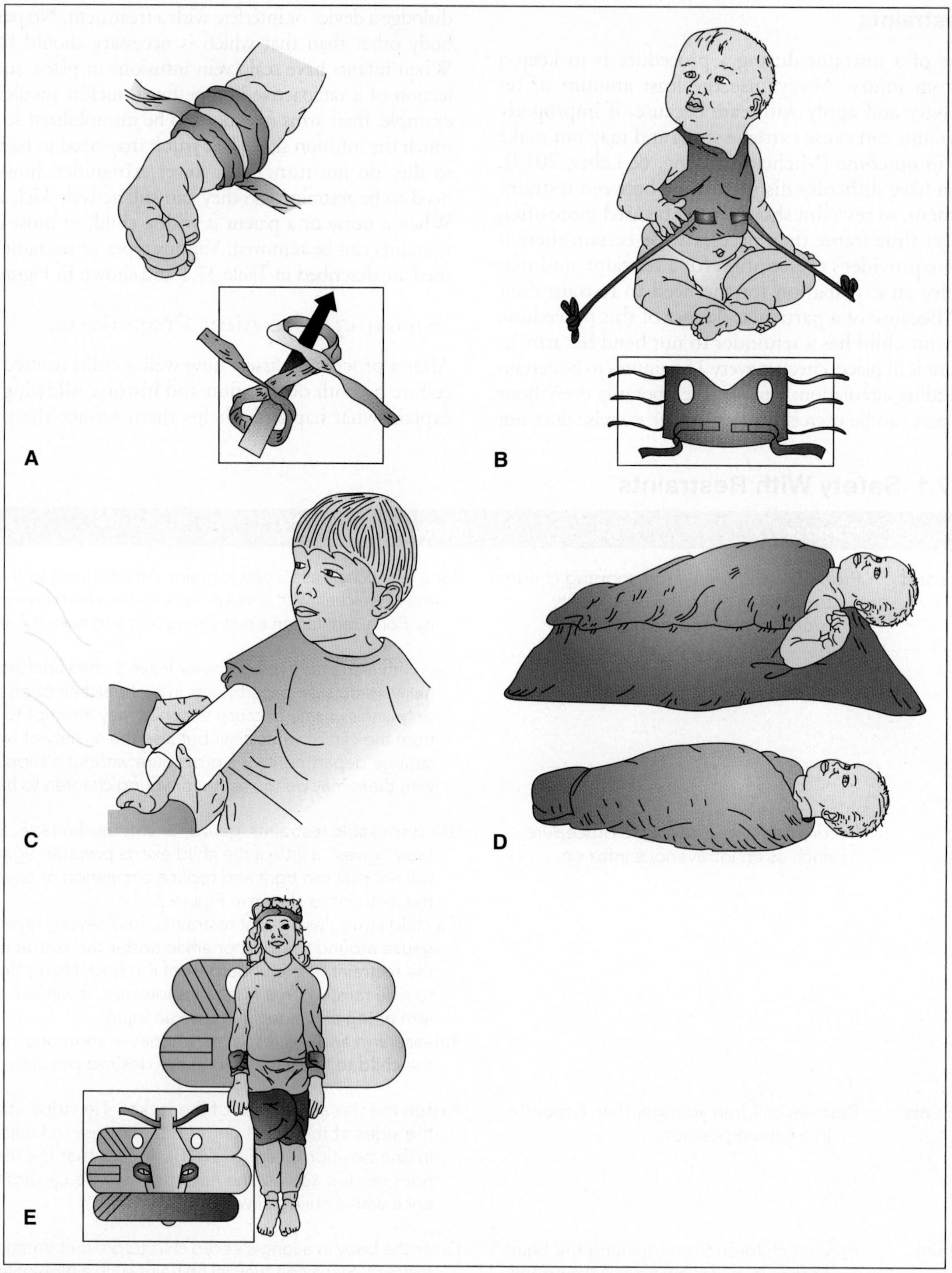

FIGURE 37.1 Types of restraints. **(A)** A clove-hitch restraint. **(B)** A jacket restraint. **(C)** A NoNo-Sleeve or commercial elbow restraint. **(D)** A mummy restraint. **(E)** A Papoose Board.

their mind so they can conquer their fear of it. Fill in gaps in information as necessary to improve a child's perception of the procedure. Provide therapeutic play, as necessary, to help reduce anxiety (see Chapter 36).

Be certain tissue samples obtained after a procedure, such as bone marrow aspiration, are sent to the proper laboratory for analysis as soon as possible. Guard against specimens being dropped or improperly labeled; children do not have extra body fluids, such as blood, to sacrifice for additional specimen collection.

If conscious sedation was used, children may be discharged home or to an inpatient hospital unit as early as 30 minutes after the procedure if they are awake and oriented; have a patent airway; respiratory status is without retraction, stridor, or wheezing; and oxygen saturation is 95% or greater on room air. Blood pressure, heart rate, and respiratory rates should be age-appropriate, and the child should be reasonably free of pain. Using a postanesthesia score sheet (Fig. 37.2) is an effective method to rate recovery from anesthesia and to be certain all these criteria are met.

Postanesthesia Assessment

Activity:	Description:	Score:
Activity	Able to move four extremities	2
	Able to move two extremities	1
	Able to move no extremities	0
Respiration	Regular, able to deep breathe/cough	2
	Dyspnea, limited and obstructed breathing	1
	Apneic	0
Circulation	BP within 20 mmHg of preprocedure	2
	BP within 20–25 mmHg of preprocedure	1
	BP 25 mmHg above or below preprocedure level	0
Level of consciousness	Awake, alert	5
	Drowsy, but easily aroused	4
	Stupor, aroused by vigorous stimuli	2
	Responds to pain only	1
	No response to pain	0
Skin color	Preprocedure color, warm, dry	2
	Pale, dusky, blotchy, clammy	1
	Cyanotic, diaphoretic, cold	0
Ambulation	Ambulates with minimum help	5
	Ambulates with minimum support	4
	Unable to ambulate	2

FIGURE 37.2 A postanesthesia recovery score. A passing score is at least 10 with a level of consciousness score no lower than 4. (From Tolia, V., Peters, J. M., & Gilger, M. A. [2000]. Sedation for pediatric endoscopic procedures. *Journal of Pediatric Gastroenterology and Nutrition, 30*[5], 477–485.)

Parents often have questions about what care their child will need after they return home after having conscious sedation. Tips for parents about this are highlighted in Box 37.3.

✔ QSEN Checkpoint Question 37.1

Safety

You are going to restrain Felipe to obtain a blood sample from his hand. What type of restraint would be best to use?

a. Ask his mother to hold him tightly on her lap.
b. Apply a jacket restraint to confine his body.
c. Ask a fellow nurse to hold his hand firmly.
d. Use a mummy restraint so he can't be hurt.

Look in Appendix A for the best answer and rationale.

MEASURING VITAL SIGNS

Vital signs for children consist of temperature, pulse, respiratory rate, blood pressure, and pain assessment. All vital signs need to be recorded conscientiously and with knowledge of the child's underlying condition so they can be meaningfully analyzed. Be especially alert that assessing any of these measures is not enough; if they are abnormal or if a child has pain, a measure to relieve the problem needs to be initiated. Average pulse rates, respiration rates, and blood pressures for children of different ages, because these differ according to the size and age of the child, can be viewed at http://thePoint.lww.com/Pillitteri7e. Pain assessment and management is discussed in Chapter 39.

Temperature

Normal temperature values in children are the same as in adults: axillary, 97.6°F (36.5°C); oral or tympanic, 98.6°F (37.0°C); and rectal, 99.6°F (37.6°C). Thermometers that assess the tympanic membrane temperature are ideal for assessment in children because they register within 2 seconds and therefore cause less fear because a child only has to be restrained for a few seconds (Fig. 37.3A) (Pappas, 2012). Tympanic membrane temperatures, however, may not be effective in newborns because the vernix is still present in their ears.

In newborns, take the temperature using the axilla instead. Never take it rectally because of the danger of damaging their fragile rectal mucosa with a thermometer (Fig. 37.3B). Children receiving chemotherapy have fragile rectal mucosa as well and so should not have their temperature routinely assessed using the rectum.

For a tympanic temperature recording, straighten the ear canal by pulling down on the earlobe in a child younger than age 2 years and pulling up on the pinna of the child older than age 2 years. Insert the tip of the tympanic thermometer gently into the child's ear canal directing the sensor beam toward the center of the tympanic membrane. Even if the child has earwax, tympanic membrane temperature is not affected, so the reading is consistently accurate within seconds. By 4 years of age, children are usually old enough to close their mouth sufficiently for oral temperature recording by use of an electronic thermometer.

For an axillary recording, place the tip of an electronic thermometer in the axilla and hold the child's arm down to the side to keep the thermometer firmly in place until it registers. For the rare occasions when a rectal temperature must be taken, insert the electronic thermometer only to the length of the tip (0.5 in.) in infants, and not over 1 in. in older children, and hold it in place for 5 minutes.

BOX 37.3 Nursing Care Planning Based on Family Teaching

CARE AFTER CONSCIOUS SEDATION

Q. Felipe's mother says to you, "If my son receives conscious sedation for his MRI, what special care will he need when he comes home?"

A. Here are some tips to help you:

- Most children sleep for at least an hour after leaving the health care facility. Some feel sleepy for the remainder of the day.
- Do not allow the child to walk alone for at least 4 hours. The child may suddenly feel dizzy and fall without warning.
- Wait until getting home to give the child something to eat or drink to avoid car sickness because conscious sedation may cause children to feel nauseated more easily than usual.
- For the first 12 hours, do not ask him to do any activity that requires alertness, coordination, or balance, such as riding a bicycle, swimming, or doing homework because the sedative can affect coordination and balance.
- Remember that the child may forget things readily for the rest of the day. This forgetfulness should go away, however, after a night's sleep.
- Conscious sedation may cause children to behave in unexpected ways, such as losing self-control or becoming very emotional. By the next day, the child's usual behavior should return.
- Give infants clear liquids (e.g., water, apple juice, tea) after getting home. Wait approximately 30 minutes to make sure the child does not choke or vomit. Then breast milk, formula, or other foods may be given.
- Do not allow older children to drink until their hands are steady enough to hold a cup without help to be certain they are awake enough to keep from choking. Wait approximately 30 minutes after first drinking fluid. If there is no vomiting or choking, the child can be given food.
- Call your primary care provider if the child has pain or recurrent vomiting, or if any of the effects above last for more than 12 hours.

Pulse Rate

As children grow older, the heart rate slows and the range of normal values narrows. If possible, measure a child's pulse rate while the child is at rest. An apical pulse (i.e., listening at the heart apex through a stethoscope) is taken in children younger than 1 year of age because their radial (i.e., wrist) pulse is too faint to be palpated accurately. In an infant, the point of maximum intensity, or the point on the chest wall where the heartbeat can be heard most distinctly, is just above and outside the left nipple (i.e., just lateral to the midclavicular line at the third or fourth intercostal space). This point gradually becomes more medial and slightly lower up to 7 years of age. By 7 years of age, it is at the fourth or fifth interspace at the midclavicular line as in adults. For greatest accuracy, count the pulse rate for 1 full minute.

Respiratory Rate

Respirations also should be measured before an infant is disturbed because the respiratory rate increases with crying. Take this, if possible, while a child is sitting in a parent's lap or lying quietly in a crib before lowering the side rail. Infants tend to breathe with their abdominal muscles so it is just as accurate to take respirations by counting movements of the abdomen as it is to count chest movements. Again, for greatest accuracy, count respirations for 1 full minute.

Blood Pressure

Blood pressure is included in the routine physical assessment of all children older than 3 years of age. As the incidence of obesity in children increases, recording this becomes

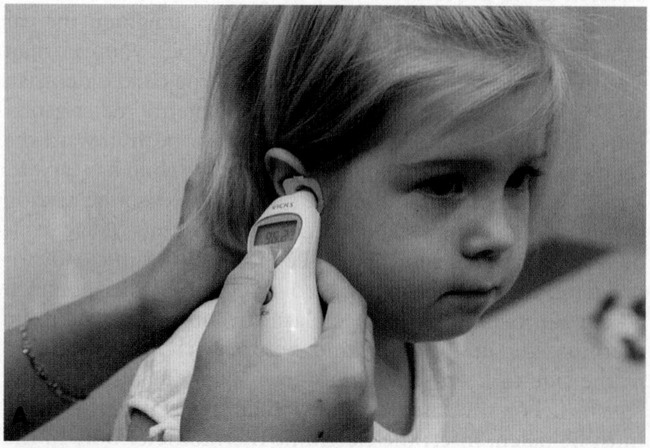

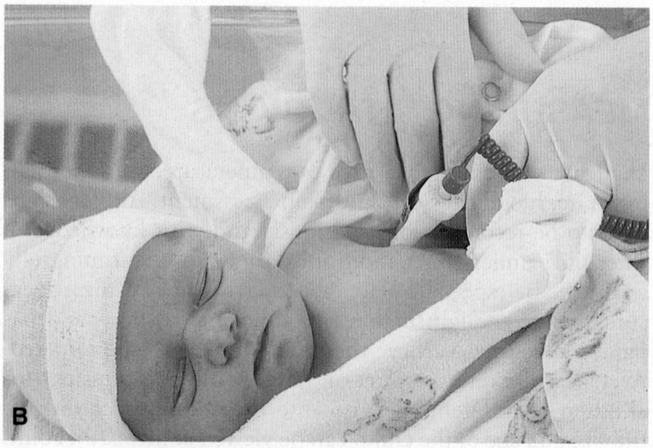

FIGURE 37.3 Temperature taking. **(A)** Tympanic membrane temperature. **(B)** Axillary temperature.

increasingly more important to detect children with accompanying hypertension (Ho, Garnett, Baur, et al., 2012). Offer a good explanation of the procedure, especially to young children, because wrapping their arm and feeling the pressure applied can be frightening if they are not prepared for it.

Systolic pressure in children is read as the manometer pressure is dropping and at the point where the first sound is heard. The point at which the sound disappears is considered the diastolic pressure. Blood pressure can be difficult to measure in infants because the cuff used must be no more than two-thirds and not less than one-half the length of their upper arm; a wider cuff gives a lower reading and a narrower cuff gives a higher reading (Fig. 37.4). Doppler ultrasound blood pressure, which bounces high-frequency sound waves off blood moving through a vein, is especially effective when continuous monitoring is necessary for infants because it can be set to record at specified times and the result is obtained so much faster. If a Doppler lead is placed over an artery, either the movement of the blood (i.e., pulse wave) or its tension (i.e., blood pressure) can be registered on a digital readout or monitor print or the sound of the pulse waves can be broadcast for auscultatory assessment.

Preschoolers and school-age children enjoy watching the digital readout numbers, so digital recording also works well with these age groups. Direct measurement (i.e., intra-arterial monitoring by an indwelling catheter into the radial or femoral artery) is used with children who are critically ill and is described in Chapter 41.

If a child's arms are not free for blood pressure recording, blood pressure may be recorded by wrapping a cuff over the thigh and palpating or auscultating the popliteal pulse behind the knee. In infants younger than 1 year of age, the thigh and arm blood pressure should be equal. In children older than 1 year of age, the systolic pressure in the thigh tends to be 10 to 40 mmHg higher, whereas diastolic pressure remains the same. If the thigh blood pressure reading is lower than that in the arm, coarctation of the aorta or an interference with circulation to the lower extremities may be the cause.

When assessing blood pressure, be certain to pay attention to the pulse pressure—the difference between systolic and diastolic readings—in addition to the actual numbers because both an unusually wide (more than 50 mmHg) or narrow (less than 10 mmHg) range may suggest congenital heart disease. An abnormally narrow pulse pressure, for instance, is a sign of aortic stenosis. An abnormally low diastolic pressure (causing a wide pulse pressure) occurs with patent ductus arteriosus.

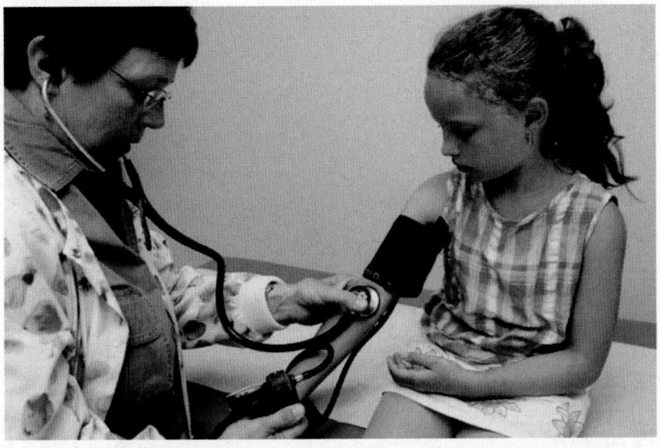

FIGURE 37.4 Blood pressure measurements are essential during routine health assessments and before diagnostic or therapeutic procedures. Here, a nurse assesses a child's blood pressure during a routine examination.

REDUCING ELEVATED TEMPERATURE IN CHILDREN

Fever is such a common symptom in children that reducing temperature, or giving a parent instructions on how to reduce a child's temperature at home, is a common intervention with children.

Nursing Diagnoses and Related Interventions

Nursing Diagnosis: Risk for hyperthermia related to illness or interference with temperature regulation from medication or surgery

Outcome Evaluation: Child's tympanic temperature returns to 98.6°F (37°C) within 2 hours.

Because the temperature-regulating mechanism in children is immature, fever tends to be more marked than in adults, and may even be out of proportion to the seriousness or extent of their disease. A high temperature occurs because a child's temperature-regulating point (set point) has been elevated. The child's temperature, therefore, cannot be reduced until the set point returns (or is returned) to normal.

Acetaminophen (Tylenol) and ibuprofen (Motrin or Advil) are excellent antipyretics, and so, are the drugs most often prescribed if a child has an oral or tympanic temperature of more than 101°F (38.3°C) or an axilla temperature of more than 100.5°F (38.0°C) (Box 37.4).

Typically, one or the other of these is prescribed every 4 hours, although with severe fever, they can be rotated every 4 hours (Smith & Goldman, 2012). Parents often do not give the full dose of antipyretics because they are afraid their child will have an adverse reaction to them, and therefore their child's fever is not sufficiently reduced. Encourage them to give a full dose of the antipyretic every 4 hours, up to the prescribed number of doses a day, until their child's temperature is reduced. Also, teach parents that fever is actually a body protection measure and, unless it is exceptionally high (more than 106°F [41.1°C]), it does no specific harm. In fact, there is some evidence that fever may be of value in helping to combat infection, because it aids in destroying microorganisms. Caution parents not to leave the antipyretic within the child's reach after administration or children can help themselves to more of the "good tasting" medicine, possibly resulting in liver or kidney toxicity (Karch, 2013). Caution parents also to never give acetylsalicylic acid (aspirin) to children with fever because aspirin is associated with Reye syndrome, a

BOX 37.4 Nursing Care Planning Based on Responsibility for Pharmacology

IBUPROFEN (ADVIL, PEDIAPROFEN)

Action: Used to reduce inflammation, fever, and mild-to-moderate pain
Pregnancy Risk Category: B; D if used in last trimester
Dosage: (For fever or pain) Individually based on child's weight, not over 4 doses in 24 hours.
Possible Adverse Effects: Gastric upset, headache, dizziness, nausea, occult blood loss, prolonged bleeding, peptic ulceration (Karch, 2013)

Nursing Implications

- Use with caution in children who have gastrointestinal irritation because ibuprofen causes gastric irritation.
- Encourage fluid intake; ibuprofen may cause renal failure if child becomes dehydrated.
- Administer this medication with food or drink to minimize gastrointestinal irritation.
- Do not give to infants under 6 months of age without health care provider's approval.
- Always use the measuring device supplied by the manufacturer, not a kitchen spoon, for dosage accuracy.

severe neurologic disorder (Morris & Jackson, 2013) (see Chapter 49).

Many parents dress febrile children warmly in flannel pajamas to keep them from "getting a chill." This actually increases the child's temperature and does not prevent the shaking, trembling reaction that comes with a high fever. In addition to antipyretic administration, therefore, suggest parents dress children with a fever in lightweight clothing, such as summer pajamas. They can remove all clothing but the diaper from an infant. Placing a cool cloth (not ice) on a child's forehead often feels comforting and can help prevent a headache. Sponging children with ice water used to be prescribed on a routine basis to reduce fever, but the practice may lead to extreme chilling and shock to an immature nervous system, and has little advantage over the use of oral antipyretics.

COMMON DIAGNOSTIC PROCEDURES

Diagnostic and therapeutic procedures used with children vary depending on a child's condition and age but are similar to those used with adults. Blood, urine, and stool studies are commonly prescribed. Respiratory illnesses require special procedures and are discussed in Chapter 40. Biopsies (i.e., surgical procedures to remove tissue for examination) are done to detect malignancy and are discussed in Chapter 53. Stress or exercise testing for cardiovascular pathology is discussed in Chapter 41.

Electrical Impulse Studies

As their name implies, **electrical impulse studies** are those that include electrical conduction. Children need special preparation for studies such as electrocardiograms (ECGs) (Fig. 37.5) or electroencephalograms (EEGs) because they have been warned not to play with electric wires and so may worry about being burned or electrocuted. You can assure a child the electricity passes from their body to the machine, not the other way around. Except for electromyelograms (i.e., study of the conduction paths of the spinal cord), you can also assure them these tests are painless. The electrodes are attached to the body by paste or sticky tape, which is easily removed afterward. If possible, give the child a portion of the test strip afterward to keep as a souvenir.

X-Ray Studies

A variety of X-ray studies are used to inspect internal body tissues. These range from simple flat-plate views to the more complicated computed tomography (CT) scan or studies using contrast dye.

Flat-Plate X-Rays

X-rays are used to diagnose and evaluate the progress of illnesses as well as assess the placement of apparatuses such as gastrointestinal feeding tubes. As a rule, children accept X-rays without protest because the X-ray machine can be compared with a camera, an instrument with which they are familiar (Fig. 37.6). Caution children that, although you or

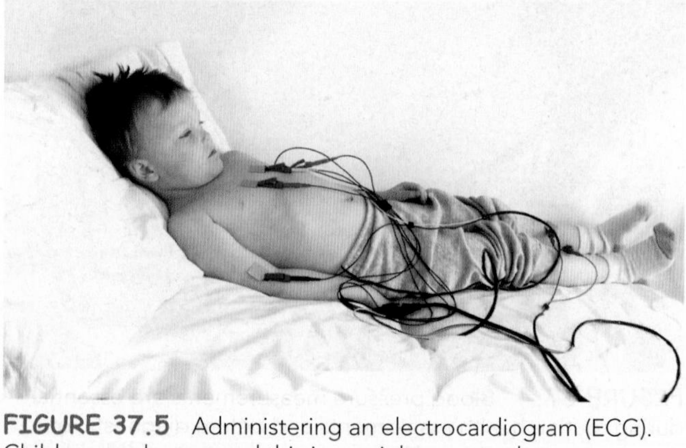

FIGURE 37.5 Administering an electrocardiogram (ECG). Children can be assured this is a painless procedure (© Fotosearch.com).

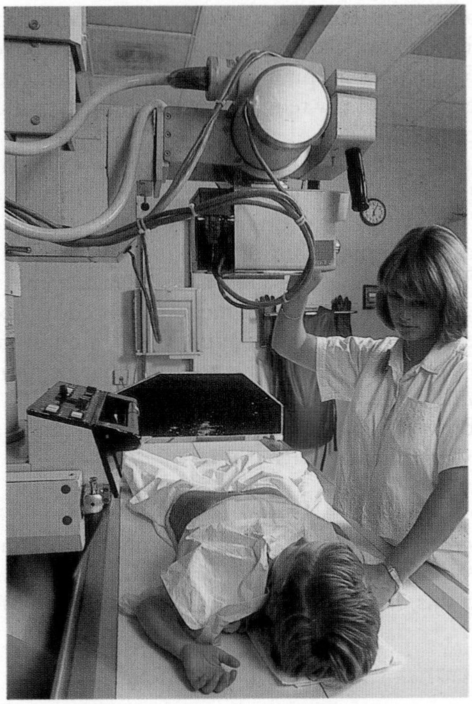

FIGURE 37.6 Positioning of a child for an X-ray. (© Bachmann/Stock Boston.)

a parent will be able to accompany them to the X-ray department, you will not be allowed to stay in the room while the picture is actually taken. If it is necessary for you to remain in the room to help restrain a child, a lead apron and lead glove protection must be provided for you. Such protection is also necessary if a portable X-ray will be taken at a child's or infant's bedside.

Dye Contrast Studies

To visualize a body cavity, radiopaque dye may be swallowed, instilled by enema, or administered intravenously and then revealed by X-ray. Caution the child who is asked to drink barium for a gastrointestinal study that, even if flavored, it does not taste terribly good (more like warm thick milk). If a child is going to receive a contrast medium intravenously, be certain to check whether the child is allergic to iodine before the procedure because most intravenous solutions contain this. As the contrast dye is injected, the child may feel a hot flush, a sensation that can be frightening if the child is unprepared for this. Try not to use the word "dye" when describing a contrast medium to prevent young children from worrying they will be dyed like an Easter egg or will "die." Use the phrase "special medicine" instead.

Children easily grow bored during this type of procedure because of the time involved waiting for the contrast medium to reach and outline the specific organ to be studied. Have the child take along an activity to the exam room to make the time pass faster. If children are not allowed to eat for the duration of a long procedure, be certain they receive supervision, or else, not realizing the importance of this, they may decide to snack. Ensure that parents understand children do not "radiate" X-rays or radioactivity after the procedure, so they will not be afraid to hold a child closely for comfort.

Computed Tomography

Computed tomography (CT) is an X-ray procedure in which many views of an organ or body part are obtained to represent what the organ would look like if it were cut into thin slices. As with any X-ray, dense structures appear white and less dense structures appear gray to black on the films.

The procedure may include injection of an iodine-based radioisotope contrast medium. If this is necessary, the study may be referred to as **positron emission tomography (PET)** or **single-photon emission computed tomography (SPECT)**.

Because a CT scan involves so many films, it can become a lengthy procedure. Also, the machinery is complex, large, and potentially frightening (Fig. 37.7A). It's important for children to lie still during the long procedure to avoid creating shadows on the film. To help them do this for such an extended period, they may be given a sedative, such as chloral hydrate or conscious sedation, before the procedure to make them sleepy. You can assure parents that although the radiation exposure from CT scans occurs over a long period of time, such low doses are used that the actual exposure is comparable to a regular X-ray. However, like regular X-rays, repeated CT scans can carry a threat of excessive radiation exposure and so need to be limited in number (Natale, Joseph, Rogers, et al., 2012).

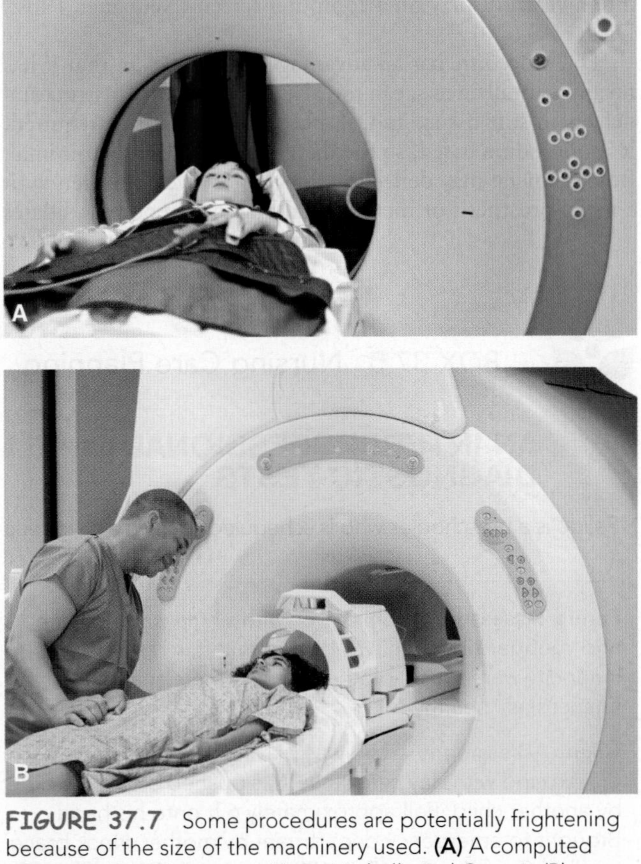

FIGURE 37.7 Some procedures are potentially frightening because of the size of the machinery used. **(A)** A computed tomography (CT) scanner. (From Michelle Del Guercio/Photo Researchers, Inc.) **(B)** A magnetic resonance imaging (MRI) scanner (© Fotosearch.com).

QSEN Checkpoint Question 37.2

Informatics

Felipe's mother is relieved that he does not need a CT scan because she tells you she "would not have not allowed that." What would be your best response to her?

a. "X-rays are almost never used for children under 4 years so you don't have to worry."
b. "Aren't you prepared to take some risks to ensure Felipe's well-being?"
c. "If, at any point, Felipe does need an X-ray, be prepared to change your mind."
d. "What is the reason you wouldn't have allowed a CT scan for your son?"

Look in Appendix A for the best answer and rationale.

Magnetic Resonance Imaging

Magnetic resonance imaging (MRI) combines a magnetic field, radiofrequency, and computer technology to produce diagnostic images that aid in the diagnosis of disorders such as the cause of renal or brain pathology. The child lies on a moving pallet that is pushed into the core of the machine, the magnet (Fig. 37.7B). When the magnetic field surrounding the child is turned on, it causes tissue atoms to line up in a parallel fashion. As radio waves are turned on and off, the atoms change position. This change is sensed and converted into a visual display on a computer screen (Neubauer, Pabst, Dick, et al., 2012).

The procedure has an advantage over X-rays in that it has no apparent ill effects, can reveal astonishingly clear structural defects in soft tissue, and, if a contrast medium is required, it is not iodine based, so the danger of a reaction is minimal. Because metal may deflect the magnetic waves, children with a metal prosthesis or metal dental braces are poor candidates for the procedure. Hairpins and eye makeup (which often has a metallic base), watches, or other jewelry should be removed. Be certain a child's hospital gown does not have a metal snap at the neckline and any religious medals pinned to their gown are removed.

When the radio waves are turned on and off during the procedure, a booming noise can be heard. Prepare children for this sound (which is often compared with the sound of drums) as well as the feeling of claustrophobia they may experience. Except for cranial exams, headphones can be provided to decrease the noise. Because the total procedure (excluding cranial examinations) may take up to 45 minutes, for some children a sedative or conscious sedation may be indicated so they can lie quietly for this length of time (Slynn & Hulkes, 2012). Box 37.5 shows an interprofessional care map for a child having a cranial MRI exam.

What if... 37.2 Felipe's mother repeats to you that he is very frightened of dark places. Knowing this, how would you prepare him for an MRI?

Ultrasound

Ultrasound is a painless procedure in which images of internal tissue and organs, such as the appendix, are produced by the use of sound waves (Dingemann & Ure, 2012). Because it is noninvasive, children accept ultrasound easily and may even enjoy watching the oscilloscope screen during the procedure. Alert a child that the clear gel, which is applied to the skin over the body part to be studied, may feel cool and sticky. Compare the transducer that is used on the body surface to pick up internal images to a television camera so it is not viewed as something strange (Fig. 37.8). Be certain that parents understand ultrasound is not an X-ray, so they can remain in the room to comfort their child during the procedure. Because ultrasound appears to have no long-term effects, it can be repeated over and over for serial determinations.

BOX 37.5 Nursing Care Planning

AN INTERPROFESSIONAL CARE MAP FOR A CHILD IN NEED OF DIAGNOSTIC TESTS

Felipe is a preschooler who is scheduled to have a magnetic resonance imaging (MRI) study for a possible head injury.

Family Assessment Child lives with single-parent mother and younger sibling in two-bedroom loft in refurbished inner-city warehouse. Mother is a commercial artist. Rates finances as "healthy."

Client Assessment Child was playing at community playground with day care staff. Was pushed off top of slide by another child. Fell approximately 6 ft onto his head. Brought to emergency department by mother. Neck brace applied. Temperature (T) = 100.6 tympanic; Pulse (P) = 90; Blood pressure (BP) = 100/65 mmHg. Crying from pain in neck and upper back. "How can I agree to an MRI?" his mother asks you. "Because he's afraid of the dark, how can I allow him to be wheeled into a long dark machine?"

Nursing Diagnosis Anxiety (child and parent) related to necessary diagnostic procedure

Outcome Criteria Mother listens to explanation of advantages of MRI for diagnosis of head, neck, or spine injury. Voices agreement to allow procedure. Helps prepare child for anxiety-filled experience.

Team Member Responsible	Assessment	Intervention	Rationale	Expected Outcome
Activities of Daily Living, Including Safety				
Nurse	Take history to assess if child has change of behavior from usual.	Review with parent that traumatic events can affect all body systems.	Head injury, if severe, can affect vital signs and cognitive processing.	Parent states she feels child is reacting as usual except for neck pain.
Teamwork and Collaboration				
Nurse/Primary care provider	Assess if further neurologic consultation will be necessary following physical and neurologic exam.	Consult as necessary with neurologist about child's condition and continued care based on MRI findings.	A 6-ft fall could cause considerable intracranial swelling depending on whether child broke fall.	Neurologist on call completes necessary consult and any needed additional procedures.
Procedures/Medications for Quality Improvement				
Nurse/Pain management team	Ask child to rate pain using poker chip technique.	Explain MRI procedure to parent and child. Assist with conscience sedation.	Conscious sedation will allow child to sleep during an otherwise frightening procedure.	Consent for conscious sedation is obtained. Sedation is used during procedure without complications.
Nutrition				
Nurse	Assess last time child ate or drank.	Keep child nothing by mouth (NPO) prior to procedure.	Conscious sedation can cause aspiration in children with full stomachs.	Child remains NPO until postprocedure.
Patient-Centered Care				
Nurse/Nurse practitioner	Assess parent's understanding of the need and technique of MRI.	Fill in gaps of knowledge for parent about procedure.	A well-informed parent is able to make well-informed decisions about care.	Mother states she understands why procedure is needed.
Psychosocial/Spiritual/Emotional Needs				
Nurse	Assess if child is still frightened from bullying episode at playground.	Review with child that bad things can happen to good people.	Discussion of an injury can help to relieve guilt and increase self-esteem.	Child discusses what happened; states he knows incident was not his fault.
Informatics for Seamless Health Care Planning				
Nurse/Primary care provider	Assess if parent understands importance of assessing child's respirations and pulse every 4 hours after return home.	Review with parent technique for respiration and pulse assessment.	A decreasing pulse or respiratory rate can indicate increased intracranial pressure.	Parent confirms she will be able to take vital signs accurately; will notify emergency department if vital signs vary from norms given to her.

Nuclear Medicine Studies

Radiopharmaceuticals are radioactive-combined substances that, when given orally or by injection, flow to designated body organs. When a scintillation machine (a form of Geiger counter) is passed over the organ where the radiopharmaceutical has collected, the pattern of the collected material outlines the organ. The pattern can then be reproduced as a screen image or a photograph.

Parents may worry that a child will be harmed by exposure to a radioactive substance (Alexander, 2012). You can assure them that the dose of radiation in these studies is no greater than that used for a diagnostic X-ray, so this is not a danger. Tagged iodine (iodine-131) frequently is the medium used for such studies, so be certain to ask if the child is allergic to iodine. A second danger of iodine is that it will go immediately to the thyroid gland rather than the organ to be studied if injected intravenously, with the result that enough concentrated radioactivity could accumulate in the thyroid gland to destroy it. For this reason, a blocking agent such as potassium perchlorate, which prevents accumulation in the thyroid gland, may be required prior to the test. Always check

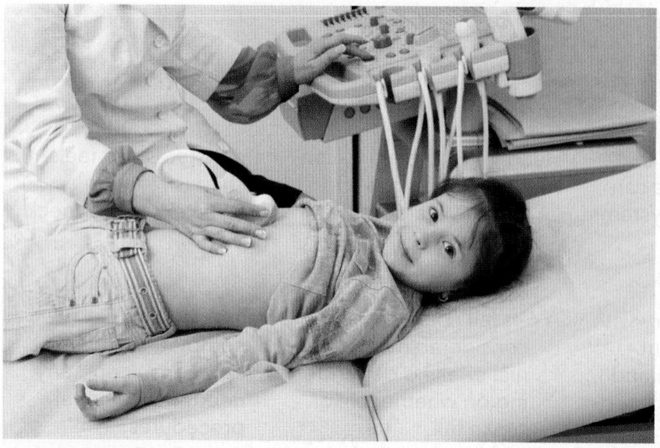

FIGURE 37.8 Ultrasound can be potentially frightening for children unless they receive good preparation because they don't understand the concept of sound waves (© iStockphoto/Thinkstock).

whether a blocking agent is required before transporting a child to the nuclear medicine department to be certain administration of this is not overlooked.

Direct Visualization Procedures

Direct visualization procedures involve the observation of an internal body cavity by way of a thin tube inserted through a body surface opening. Types of direct visualization include endoscopy, bronchoscopy, and colonoscopy.

Endoscopy

Endoscopy involves the use of an endoscope, which is passed through the mouth, to examine the gastrointestinal tract and has become a common method of diagnosis for gastrointestinal disorders in children. The procedure is also used as an emergency measure to remove objects such as quarters or safety pins swallowed by children (Bishop, 2011).When first developed, endoscopes were straight and stiff metal instruments, so their use was limited. Currently, they are fiberscopes, which are extremely flexible and easily maneuvered, so these examinations are not nearly as uncomfortable as before.

The thought of having a tube passed down your throat, however, can be very frightening. Even after children understand what the procedure will consist of, they can still be very uncomfortable at the thought of a tube being passed into them. Before the procedure, children must remain on an NPO status for between 4 and 6 hours. They will need a sedative or conscious sedation so they can lie quietly for the time required. Good support during both the anxious time waiting for the procedure and during the procedure is crucial. Ask whether the child can have a digital photograph taken during the procedure to keep as a scrapbook souvenir.

Because the endoscope is passed through the throat, edema of the throat may occur from the pressure on the esophagus and pharynx. This means that the child requires close observation afterward for at least an hour to be certain edema is not interfering with respirations or causing discomfort. Observe closely the first time the child drinks after the procedure to ensure that the gag reflex is intact despite throat edema or the effect of a local pharyngeal anesthetic that may have been sprayed into the throat before the procedure.

Bronchoscopy

Bronchoscopy is the direct visualization of the larynx, trachea, and bronchi through a lit, flexible, fiberoptic tube (i.e., a bronchofiberscope). The procedure is used with children who have aspirated a foreign object, such as a peanut, or to take culture and biopsy specimens (Goyal, Nayar, Gogia, et al., 2012).

Before the procedure, the child may be given atropine by injection to reduce bronchial secretions and to encourage bronchial relaxation. Typically, the throat is sprayed with a local pharyngeal anesthetic to numb the area. Conscious sedation is then administered. Any manipulation of the airway has the potential to cause increased bronchial secretions and edema, leading to narrowing of the airway following the procedure. An ice bag applied postprocedure to the neck often helps reduce the possibility of edema and can relieve throat discomfort. Closely observe the child's respiratory function and airway patency for at least the next 4 hours. Observe children carefully the first time they drink after the procedure to be certain their gag reflex is intact and they do not choke.

Colonoscopy

Colonoscopy is an endoscopic examination of the large intestine with a flexible fiberscope that is inserted through the anus and advanced as far as the ileocecal valve. Air is then infused to expand the bowel walls for good visualization. The technique allows the colon walls to be visualized; if abnormalities are found, photographs can be taken for analysis. It is used to diagnose inflammatory bowel disease or to obtain biopsies if a malignancy is suspected (Thakkar, Alsarraj, Fong, et al., 2012).

Before the procedure, children are given a clear liquid diet for about 24 hours. Then, they are asked to drink an isotonic saline laxative that causes fluid diarrhea so their bowel is clean for the procedure. It can be difficult for younger children to drink as much of the laxative solution as is needed so their bowel is cleared completely of stool. Playing games such as Simon Says can be helpful to gain their cooperation. If a child cannot swallow all the laxative, a saline enema may be necessary. Conscious sedation is used during the procedure to reduce discomfort.

Children may pass a great deal of flatus in the first 12 hours because of the air introduced during the procedure. If the procedure was done on an ambulatory basis, children are discharged about 2 hours after the procedure (but they are kept NPO during that time to allow the bowel to have a brief rest). Be certain parents have instructions on what observations they should make and report if they occur after they return home, such as abdominal pain, blood in stool, weakness, or paleness (signs of bowel bleeding) especially if a polyp was removed or a biopsy specimen was obtained. Even with conscious sedation, colonoscopies are difficult procedures for children to accept. Give generous praise afterward for their cooperation with both the preparation for the procedure and the actual procedure.

Aspiration Studies

Aspiration studies, which are the removal of body fluids by such techniques as lumbar puncture or bone marrow aspiration, are always anxiety-causing procedures. The size of the needle that will be used can be frightening to parents and children alike. Children may need a sedative or conscious sedation so that they lie quietly during the procedure. Support and restrain children by talking and using touch as appropriate. Assess for bleeding at the puncture site after the procedure and apply pressure as needed to halt bleeding completely. After a lumbar puncture, remind children to remain quiet and with their head flat to help prevent a postprocedure headache (see Chapter 49 for specific procedural details).

COLLECTING SPECIMENS FOR ANALYSIS

The collection of body fluids, secretions, and excretions is a collaborative nursing function essential to the complete assessment of a child. Elements of these fluids are measured by a variety of means; findings can be used to help diagnose an illness, evaluate the progress of a condition, or evaluate a child's response to therapy. As with all procedures, use standard infection precautions regardless of the source from which the sample is taken. Be certain precautions are maintained through the entire process, from obtaining, transporting, discarding, or storing specimens.

Obtaining Blood Specimens

Never underestimate how frightening having a blood specimen taken can be to a child. For many children, their past experience with losing blood has involved a nosebleed or a cut knee and the discomfort or pain they felt. They have had injections for immunizations also, so they know that injections sting. Putting the two experiences together makes collecting a blood specimen an extremely terrifying process. For these reasons, make certain children receive good preparation both before and during the procedure. Blood specimens should always be obtained away from a child's bedside, if possible, to keep the room and bed as "safe" areas. Applying a Band-Aid afterward to cover the needle site provides physical as well as psychological support.

Venipuncture

For very small infants, the usual sites for venipuncture (entrance into a vein) are the same as for adults: the superficial veins of the dorsal surface of the hand or the antecubital fossa. In a few instances, the jugular or femoral vein can also be used (Fig. 37.9). Apply an anesthetic cream such as EMLA (Eutectic Mixture of Local Anesthesia) before venipuncture if possible to reduce pain (Schreiber, Ronfani, Chiaffoni, et al., 2012) (see Chapter 39), and liberally use distraction techniques such as "I spy" or blowing bubbles for preschoolers, and videos or computer programs for school-age children and adolescents (Hanrahan, McCarthy, Kleiber, et al., 2012).

Offer children a simple explanation of the procedure: "I need to take some blood from your hand. First, I'll put some cream on your skin so when I come back to take the blood in a little while, you'll feel only a pinprick because of the cream." Let the child know you understand how difficult it is to agree to the procedure. Using a statement such as, "No one likes to have blood taken; I'm going to do this as quickly as possible" is always a better approach than, "Be a big girl" or "Come on, show me how much of a big boy you can be" as the second approach shames a child who is unable to hold still. Try not to say "drawing blood," as this sounds as if you're proposing an activity with crayons, not a procedure that will cause discomfort (Box 37.6).

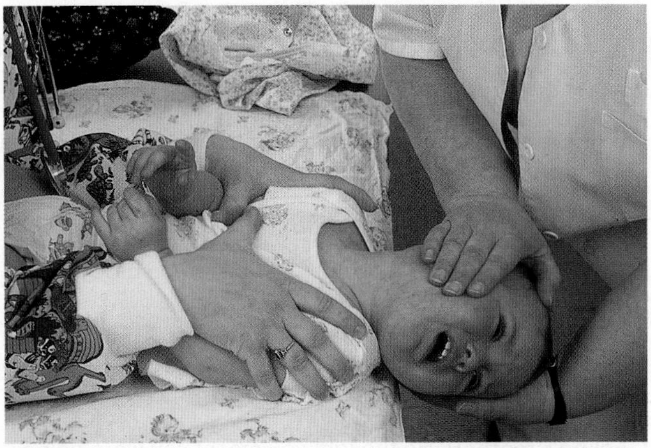

FIGURE 37.9 Positioning for jugular venipuncture. The infant's head is held sideways over the edge of the table by one nurse, while the body is restrained by a second nurse.

Preschoolers may worry that they will lose all their blood during the procedure because they have no concept of how much blood their body contains. Assure them they have lots to spare. Many children younger than school age may have to be restrained for blood sampling, because no matter how cooperative or brave they might be initially, the minute they see the needle, they can be too overwhelmed with fear to hold still.

✔ QSEN Checkpoint Question 37.3

Evidence-Based Practice

One of the biggest problems with trying to reduce pain from a procedure such as a venipuncture or an injection is that anesthetic creams don't take effect until 30 minutes to an hour. To test whether a commercial device called a "Buzzy" (made of plastic and shaped like a large bee, which turns cold and gently vibrates when strapped to a child's upper arm) could serve as an effective distraction technique to immediately reduce pain, researchers randomly selected 120 children aged 6 to 12 years who were going to have a venipuncture. Half of them served as a control group with no intervention for pain; the other group had the Buzzy device applied before and during the procedure. Results showed children who had the Buzzy device applied rated their pain and anxiety as significantly lower than the group who did not receive any intervention. Use of the apparatus did not cause a significant difference in the success of the blood specimen collection procedure (Inal & Kelleci, 2012).

Based on the previous study, the next time Felipe needs to have blood drawn, your best action would be which of the following?

a. Assess Felipe's pain and anxiety levels before and after venipuncture.
b. Explain that venipuncture feels much the same as a mild bee sting.
c. Plan a distraction technique for him that his mother thinks would be effective.
d. Explain to Felipe that you will try to distract him before performing the procedure.

Look in Appendix A for the best answer and rationale.

BOX 37.6 Nursing Care Planning Based on Effective Communication

Felipe is a 4-year-old who is going to have several diagnostic studies. He's coloring a picture when you approach him to obtain a blood specimen for electrolyte levels.

Less Effective Communication

Nurse: Hi, Felipe! Is it all right if I draw some blood?
Felipe: Okay.
Nurse: Hold out your arm for me.
Felipe: Are you drawing on me?
Nurse: I'm going to wipe off your arm, then prick your skin. (Felipe begins crying.)
Felipe's mother: He thought you meant you were going to color with him.

More Effective Communication

Nurse: Hi, Felipe. Remember I put some cream on your hand earlier? Now I need to take some blood from your arm. I'll wipe off your arm, then prick your skin. It'll only hurt like a small pinprick.

The nurse in the first scenario makes two mistakes in introducing a procedure: making the activity seem like a game and also asking for permission to carry it out. In the second scenario, the nurse both explains what she needs to do and why it is important. It is easy to forget that what a word means to you may not be interpreted the same way by a young child.

Capillary Puncture

Capillary blood heel or fingertip punctures are often obtained for glucose and hematocrit determinations. Apply an anesthetic cream before the procedure to reduce discomfort if needed; however, be careful when applying this to a finger that the child doesn't lick this off and anesthetize their tongue or throat. Be certain to use the side of the finger, not the center, for the puncture to reduce discomfort afterward; for heel punctures, use the lateral aspect of the heel to avoid striking the medial plantar artery or the periosteum of the bone (Fig. 37.10). Comfort the child afterward because fingertip punctures seem minor but can be more painful than a venipuncture afterward.

In many settings, laboratory analysis such as glucose level can then be completed immediately using a commercial meter (a point-of-care or POST test) (Whitmore, 2012). Be certain when completing POST tests that you document completely and accurately because your documentation, rather than a technician's, will serve as the only basis for continuation of care or a change in care.

QSEN Checkpoint Question 37.4

Patient-Centered Care

Felipe will be having a fingertip puncture for serum glucose. What would be the best instruction to empower him before the procedure?

a. "It won't hurt a bit; it's only a small finger prick."
b. "Why don't you choose which finger you'd like me to use."
c. "Most other boys your age don't mind this at all."
d. "Make sure you hold still, otherwise you won't get a special treat."

Look in Appendix A for the best answer and rationale.

Obtaining Urine Specimens

Depending on the type of test required, urine may be collected with a usual voiding, after the external meatus has been cleaned (i.e., a clean-catch specimen), by catheterization, or by suprapubic aspiration. A specimen may require a single specimen or collection of all the urine voided in a 24-hour period.

Routine Urinalysis

Routine urinalysis requires only a single voided specimen. The specimen will then be analyzed for appearance, glucose, specific gravity, and microscopic analysis. Specimens must always be collected in clean containers to prevent contamination.

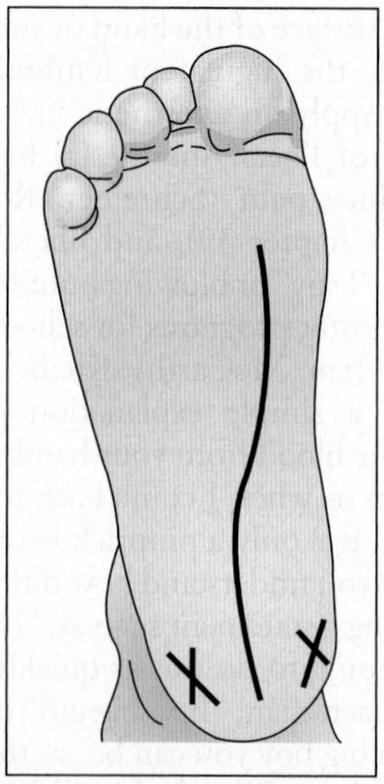

FIGURE 37.10 Sites for a capillary blood heel puncture. Choose a site to the right or left on the heel to avoid the medial artery.

The Infant and Toddler. An infant or a child who has not been toilet trained cannot be expected to urinate on command, so a collecting device must be attached to the genitalia to collect their next voiding.

For girls, wash the perineum to remove any fecal matter, then rinse with water and be certain to dry the site where the collecting device will be attached to ensure good adherence. For boys, wash the penis, and rinse and thoroughly dry the same way. Be certain skin is dry and free from powder, lotions, and oils (Fig. 37.11A). Apply the adhesive side of the collection device firmly and smoothly to the skin (any folds or wrinkling will cause leakage) to cover the urethral opening.

If an infant attempts to loosen the collector, cover the device with a diaper to keep it out of reach. Otherwise, leave the device visible so that it can be observed for urine output. Offer the child something to drink to encourage voiding. Most infants void shortly after a feeding, so if the collector is applied just before a regular feeding, voiding will probably result soon afterward. Remove the collector as soon as the infant voids and transfer the specimen to a specimen cup by cutting a bottom corner of the bag.

Urine may be aspirated from diapers for tests such as specific gravity, dipstick protein, pH, or glucose (Fig. 37.11B). Current disposable diapers, however, are designed to trap urine in the material so effectively, they can make it impossible to squeeze out a specimen. Placing cotton balls inside the diaper can be a help because these can be squeezed for additional urine.

The Preschooler and School-Age Child. It may be difficult to obtain routine urine specimens from preschoolers or toilet-trained toddlers because they can void only when they feel a definite urge to do so, not on command. Another problem is language. It is not unprofessional to use words such as "pee-pee" if this is what the child will understand. Provide a potty chair if one is available; if not, put a urine collection cap device on a toilet. A generally successful approach with a child this age is to act as if voiding is not a difficult procedure. Offer the child a glass of water or other fluid, and ask a parent to reinforce the request to void so that the child knows a parent approves. Do not encourage children to drink more than one glass of fluid to induce voiding, or else their urine production may be so diluted the specific gravity, protein, and glucose levels can be inaccurate. A school-age child is usually able to void when asked, although the child may find it more difficult than the adult.

The Adolescent. Adolescents are usually knowledgeable and cooperative about providing urine specimens. As with adults, give them a clean specimen container and tell them what is needed. Unless they have voided recently, they usually are able to void on command. Remember, however, that adolescents are concerned and self-conscious about body functions and therefore are often reluctant to carry a urine specimen

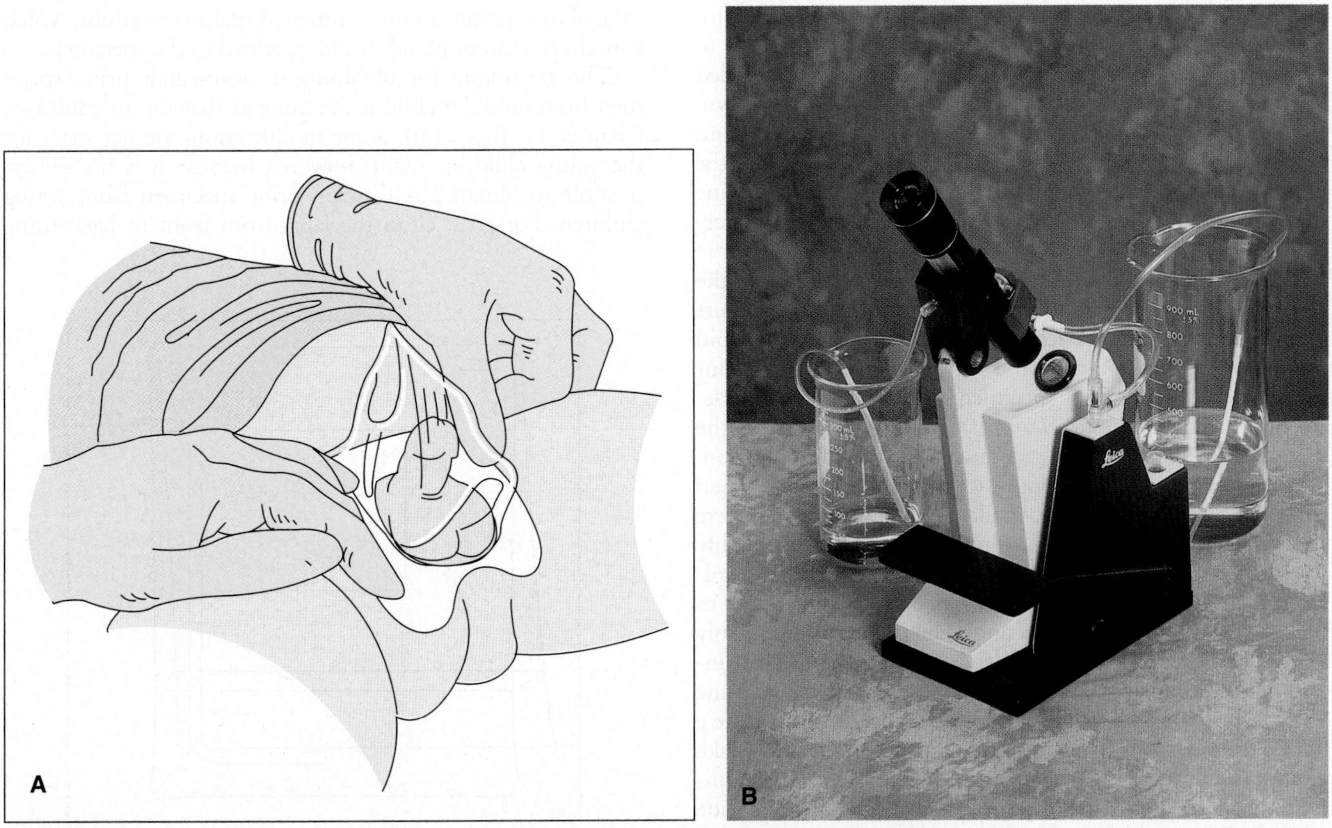

FIGURE 37.11 **(A)** A urine collector for infants. The trick to making the collector adhere is to be certain the child's skin is dry. **(B)** Testing specific gravity of urine with a refractometer. The advantage of this is that only one drop of urine is required.

through a crowded waiting room to the desk area. They may be too self-conscious to void if they know someone is nearby, for example, just outside a curtain waiting for them. Send them to a nearby bathroom with a closed door, or leave the area to give them privacy. Collect the specimen from them immediately so they do not have to carry it themselves.

Some adolescents are suspicious that a urine specimen is being requested for drug testing. Providing a good explanation of its actual purpose relieves this fear. If you are in doubt regarding whether the fluid returned to you is urine, not water, assess its specific gravity. Water has a specific gravity of 1.000; urine will have a specific gravity more than this (1.003 to 1.030).

Adolescent girls may be embarrassed to mention they are menstruating so be sure to ask an adolescent girl about this before she voids. To prevent having a urine specimen contaminated by menstrual blood, which changes the specific gravity, protein, and red blood cell analysis, ask the girl who is menstruating to wash her perineum well with soap and water and rinse and dry it to remove menstrual blood. Next, supply a tampon or a cotton ball for her to insert gently into her vagina just before voiding (and to remove it following voiding). Mark the specimen "possibly contaminated by menstrual blood" even though it does not appear discolored, because microscopic red blood cells may be present.

Twenty-Four–Hour Urine Specimens

Although a urinalysis of a single urine specimen will indicate the presence of substances such as protein or glucose, a 24-hour urine specimen may be necessary to determine how much of a substance is excreted during a full day (quantitative analysis). To begin a 24-hour urine collection, ask a child to void (with an infant, attach a collecting bag and wait for the child to void). This specimen (i.e., the discard specimen) is discarded so that a specific time for the ensuing collection is known. If the urine collection was started early in the morning and this first specimen was counted as part of the collection, the urine collected during the next 24 hours would include urine that had been forming all night, resulting in an approximately 32-hour collection period that would distort the analysis.

Record the start of the collection period as the time of the discarded urine. Save all urine voided for the next 24 hours and place it in one collection bottle. Have the child void (or watch for an infant to void) at the end of the 24-hour period and add the final specimen to the collection bottle. Record the time of the collection as being from the time of the discarded urine to the final specimen added to the collection.

For an infant, use a 24-hour rather than a single specimen urine collector. These types of collectors, however, will adhere for this length of time only if a child's perineum is thoroughly dry at the time of application. Also, before applying the collector, apply tincture of benzoin or a commercial product to make the skin somewhat tacky and to help the collector firmly adhere to the skin. After the collector is applied, place the infant in a semi-Fowler's position, if possible, to encourage urine to flow freely into the collector. It may be necessary to place a diaper on the infant to keep the apparatus out of sight. Make certain the tubing from the collector is pinned out of the infant's reach or the infant may pull the collector free. Provide activities for the child, and make sure the parents understand they can pick up infants and hold them during this time as long as they take care not to kink or pull the tubing.

To keep the bacterial count to a minimum, 24-hour collection containers are generally kept on ice; after each voiding, pour the new specimen into the larger container, which is kept refrigerated for the 24-hour period and until it can be transported to the laboratory for analysis. Because a preservative (considered a hazardous chemical) is added to the large container for some types of collections, be certain older children know to void into a smaller container and then add this to the large container, or never void directly into the chemical-added container. Appropriate warning labels should be visible on the container to alert anyone handling the container. The Material Safety Data Sheet (MSDS) should be included with the handling instructions.

With active infants, fitting them with a colostomy bag applied to cover the urinary meatus may be more effective than using a collector with tubing because this allows them more mobility (Fig. 37.12). For this, puncture a small hole in the corner of the top of the colostomy bag. Insert a small feeding tube through this into the bottom of the bag and then apply the bag to the child's perineum. When the child voids, attach a syringe to the feeding tube and aspirate the urine. Transfer the specimen to the collection bottle. For the active toddler, this collector may be the only type that is acceptable to obtain a day-long specimen.

Clean-Catch Specimens

A **clean-catch urine specimen** is prescribed when a urine culture for bacteria is needed. The objective is to obtain urine that is uncontaminated by external organisms, which would increase the organism count of the urine. Specimens used for protein or blood analysis may be ordered as clean-catch specimens because this careful cleaning also reduces the possibility that vaginal or foreskin (in uncircumcised males) secretions, which contain protein or blood, could be added to the specimen.

The technique for obtaining a clean-catch urine specimen from an older child is the same as that for an adult (see Chapter 11, Box 11.6). Some modifications are necessary for the young child or infant, however, because it is not always possible to obtain a midstream urine specimen from young children. For girls, clean the labia from front to back using

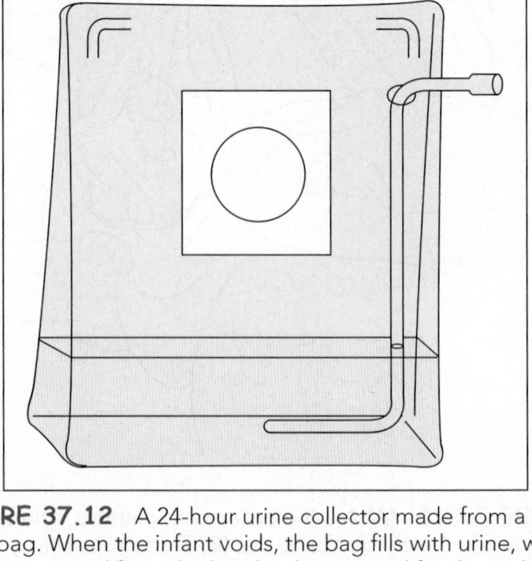

FIGURE 37.12 A 24-hour urine collector made from a colostomy bag. When the infant voids, the bag fills with urine, which can be aspirated from the bag by the inserted feeding tube.

a cleansing pad or cotton balls saturated with the agency's designated cleaning solution for each wipe. Rinse with cotton balls saturated with sterile water. Repeat the procedure to clean the labia minora. For boys, clean the tip of the penis and scrotum to remove any fecal matter. Clean the tip of the penis with cotton balls and the designated cleaning solution, then rinse with cotton balls saturated in sterile water.

To collect a specimen from a young child, ask the child to void into a sterile emesis basin or sterile container attached to a toilet or potty seat after you have washed the perineum or penis. Then use a sterile container to interrupt the urine stream to obtain the specimen. If the child voids only a small amount, send that in the sterile container marked "not midstream." To collect a specimen from an infant, wash the genitalia and apply a sterile urine collector. If the infant does not void within 2 hours, remove the collecting bag and recleanse the perineum or penis because some microorganisms will have collected after this period of time. After the area is cleansed again, reapply a new sterile bag. Again, mark specimens collected with this method as "not midstream" or "obtained by a collector" for laboratory purposes.

Clean-catch urine specimens have a major advantage over bladder catheterized specimens: they are not invasive, so they carry no risk of introducing a bladder infection, and if clean-catch specimens are obtained with care, they practically eliminate the need for catheterization. A clean-catch specimen with a bacterial colony count of more than 100,000 per milliliter is considered a positive specimen, or evidence that a urinary tract infection exists.

It is almost impossible for young girls to wash their perineum thoroughly because they cannot see it well, so they usually need assistance. Young boys also must be assisted to wash until they have enough coordination to do it themselves. Be aware that this can be embarrassing for children. Ask a parent to confirm for a child that the procedure is all right, because they have been told not to let adults touch this part of their body.

To be certain school-age children and adolescents understand the procedure, have them repeat the instructions you gave to them, then send them to a nearby bathroom to carry out the procedure by themselves.

Suprapubic Aspiration

Suprapubic aspiration is the withdrawal of urine from the bladder of a child who is not old enough or in some other way cannot cooperate enough so that a clean-catch or catheterized specimen can be obtained. The procedure is done by inserting a sterile needle into the bladder through the anterior wall of the abdomen. Suprapubic aspiration is usually done by primary care providers, although nurses in specialty units may also perform this procedure. A successful suprapubic aspiration depends on the following steps:

1. Apply EMLA cream to lessen the discomfort 30 minutes to 1 hour before the procedure.
2. Secure a sterile syringe and needle and designated antiseptic solution.
3. Clean the anterior abdominal wall with the antiseptic.
4. Block the urinary meatus by pressure from a gloved finger to confine urine in the bladder.
5. Insert the needle on the syringe just above the pubis into the bladder.

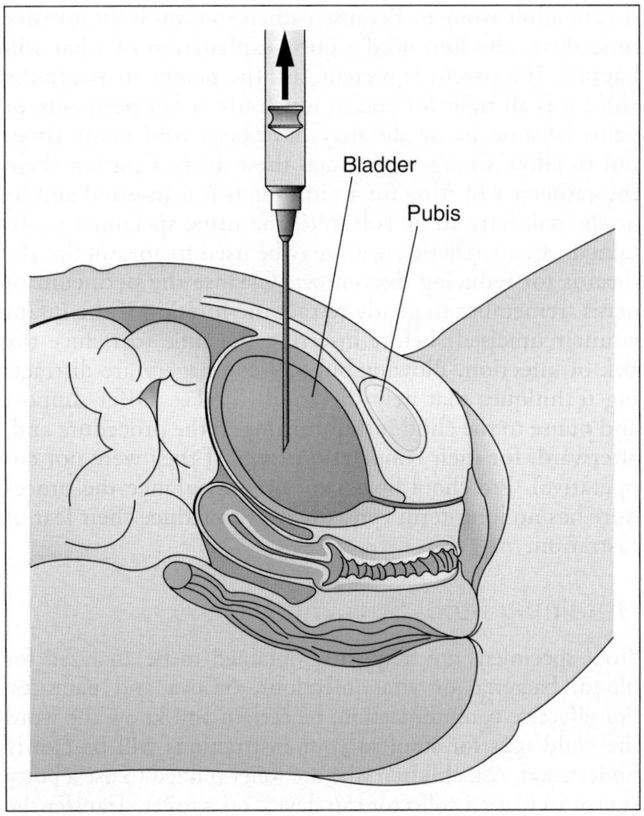

FIGURE 37.13 A suprapubic bladder aspiration. The full bladder is easily accessible by an abdominal puncture.

6. Aspirate urine through the needle into the syringe, then withdraw the syringe and needle.
7. Comfort the infant or child afterward because the sight of the needle is frightening, it may cause some pain, and some restraint is necessary.

Withdrawal of urine by suprapubic aspiration is effective because the bladder is the most anterior of abdominal organs and, when distended with urine, is easily accessible just under the abdominal wall (Fig. 37.13). However, the needle can cause a bladder spasm, and can produce a moment of sharp discomfort as the needle is inserted. Be certain parents understand why the urine specimen is needed and the reason for the method being used, as they may not be familiar with this procedure. Theoretically, the risk of bladder infection from needle insertion is less than that from catheter insertion so, in addition to being a method to obtain a urine specimen for culture, it can also help prevent a urinary tract infection (Tosif, Baker, Oakley, et al., 2012).

Catheterization

Bladder catheterization is accomplished most easily in children up to school age if a small (#5 or #8) feeding tube is used instead of a urinary catheter because such a thin tube passes readily through the meatus of even an infant. Before beginning catheterization, be certain to observe the perineum of girls to locate the urinary meatus because it is not as readily observable in infants and young children as it is in adult women. Because catheterization is an invasive procedure, children need a good explanation of what will happen. If a parent is present, ask the parent to assure the child it is all right for you to touch his or her perineum or penis because he or she may have been told many times not to allow strangers to touch these areas. Caution them the catheter will sting for an instant as it is inserted and he or she will have to lie still until the urine specimen is obtained. An anesthetic cream may be used to anesthetize the meatus for reducing discomfort. Cleanse the perineum or penis (remember to gently retract the foreskin if the infant is uncircumcised) before inserting the tube to reduce the risk of infection. Blowing bubbles or imagery are distracting techniques that help the child to relax. Offer support and praise to the child for submitting to the procedure and, afterward, for their cooperation (even if they were not cooperative). Preschool boys may need assurance the procedure has no long-term consequences to reduce their fear of castration.

Obtaining Stool Specimens

Stool specimens are frequently obtained to be analyzed for blood, bacterial or viral infections, or ova and parasites. For effective communication, be certain you know the word the child uses for stool so your instructions will be clearly understood. Ask children who are toilet trained to use a potty seat or to place a collector cap device on a toilet. Transfer the specimen to a laboratory collection cup using tongue blades. To obtain a specimen from a child who is not toilet trained, scrape stool from a diaper using tongue blades and place it in a stool collection cup. Some stool specimens need a preservative added to the container. If it is important to keep urine from contaminating the stool specimen, place a separate urine collector bag on the infant. Ask an older child to void first into the toilet, then defecate into the potty seat or collection device.

Be certain that stool specimens are sent to the laboratory promptly so they do not dry and have to be collected a second time, because most children need at least 24 more hours to produce a stool specimen. If the stool specimen is for ova and parasites, do not refrigerate it because refrigeration destroys the organisms to be analyzed; instead, see that it arrives in the laboratory in less than 1 hour after collection, so parasites can be readily detected.

QSEN Checkpoint Question 37.5

Teamwork & Collaboration

Felipe needs to have a 24-hour urine specimen collected and this will require you to coordinate your care with nurses on subsequent shifts. To ensure you have an accurately timed collection, when would you identify the collection's start point?

a. The time you discard the first void
b. The first time he voids in the morning
c. A set time, which is most often 0700
d. At the time of his first void after the discarded urine

Look in Appendix A for the best answer and rationale.

ASSISTANCE WITH ELIMINATION

Two aspects of intestinal elimination that require special care are administration of enemas and ostomy care.

Administering Enemas

Enemas are rarely used with children unless they are used as therapy for fecal impaction, Hirschsprung disease, a part of preparation for surgery, or an X-ray study. If an enema is necessary, offer a careful explanation of what the child can expect.

Commercial enemas, such as Fleet enemas, are not routinely administered to children younger than 2 years of age because of the harsh action of the sodium biphosphate and sodium phosphate they contain. Tap water is not used either because, as it is not isotonic, it causes rapid shifts of fluid in body compartments, possibly leading to water intoxication. Although a solution of milk and molasses may be used in an emergency department to relieve a fecal impaction, normal saline (0.9% sodium chloride) is the usual solution used. It can be made by parents at home by adding 1 teaspoonful of salt to 1 pint (500 ml) of water.

As the sizes of children's bowels vary greatly, the usual amounts of enema solutions used are:

- Infant: Less than 250 ml (exact amount should be stipulated by primary care provider's prescription)
- Preschooler: 250–350 ml
- School-age child: 300–500 ml
- Adolescent: 500 ml

For an infant, use a small, soft catheter (#10 to #12 French) in place of an enema tip to prevent rectal trauma. Lubricate the catheter generously with a water-soluble lubricant and insert it only 2 to 3 in. (5 to 7 cm) in children and only 1 in. (2.5 cm) in infants. Be certain to hold the solution container no more than 1 ft above the level of the sigmoid colon (12 to 15 in. above the bed surface) so the solution flows at a controlled rate. If a child experiences intestinal cramping, clamp the tubing to halt the flow temporarily and wait until the cramping passes before instilling any more fluid. An older child can be instructed to open the mouth and take deep breaths to reduce guarding of abdominal muscles and to help the cramping sensation pass. The amount of solution used in infants is so small that this is not usually a problem.

Until late school age, children cannot retain an enema as adults can (rarely more than 5 to 10 minutes). For this reason, be certain the bathroom the child will use is available before administering the enema.

Infants and children up to ages 3 or 4 years cannot retain enema solutions at all, so hold the buttocks together for a short time to prevent immediate expulsion of the solution, or pad the edge of a bedpan so it is not cold or sharp, and rest their pelvis on it following the procedure. Elevate the child's upper body by placing a pillow under the upper body for better positioning and comfort. If the enema solution is to be retained, such as an oil solution, hold the child's buttocks together for a count of 10 after administration.

After any type of enema administration, praise a child for cooperating. Allow a preschooler an opportunity for therapeutic play, because this is a frightening, intrusive procedure.

Providing Ostomy Care

An ostomy is a surgically formed opening from an internal structure to the surface of the body. Ostomies in newborns are created in the gastrointestinal (GI) system to relieve bowel obstruction caused by conditions such as ileal atresia, necrotizing enterocolitis, and imperforate anus. In older children, GI ostomies are constructed for conditions such as inflammatory bowel syndrome and Hirschsprung disorder (Sharma & Gupta, 2012). If an ostomy is created in the ileum (i.e., an ileostomy), the stoma is located on the right side of the abdomen and drains liquid stool, which is extremely irritating to the skin because of the digestive enzymes it contains. If an ostomy is created in the sigmoid portion of the bowel (i.e., a colostomy), the stoma is on the left lower abdomen and passes normally formed stool (Fig. 37.14).

An ileostomy requires the use of a collecting ostomy appliance to contain acid stool and to prevent excoriation of the abdominal skin. Older children also may use an appliance with a colostomy. For an infant with a colostomy, parents may choose (with support and advice) to use an appliance or just apply a diaper.

Two basic problems commonly arise when using an ostomy appliance with an infant: It may be difficult to locate one small enough to contain liquid drainage without leaking, and the skin under the appliance may become extremely irritated. Consulting with a wound ostomy continence nurse (WOCN) can be helpful to resolve these problems. As a rule, clear plastic, ringless colostomy bags are more easily cut to fit the size of the stoma, and the contour and size of an infant's abdomen than bags with a ring attached. Be certain when using a commercial skin sealant to harden the skin surrounding the stoma that you apply it according to the brand directions and fan to dry. If a spray is used, protect the infant's face so that the child does not inhale the solution. Tuck the chosen stoma collection appliance inside the diaper to help keep the infant from pulling it loose.

Check the appliance or bag for collecting stool at least every 4 hours. To protect the underlying skin, do not remove a self-adhering bag if it is full, but drain collected stool from the bottom of the appliance into a basin or paper cup for disposal. To reduce odor, flush the appliance bag with a warm water and soap solution, using a bulb-type syringe (an Asepto syringe), and rinse with clear water. The collection bag may stay in place for as long as 1 week if properly secured. To remove a bag that was placed with a sealant, be certain to use the designated solvent to prevent pulling or harming the underlying skin. After removal, wash the skin with soap and water or the solvent can become an irritant. Because most infants enjoy tub bathing, a long, soaking bath is an excellent way to loosen an adherent appliance.

If a parent chooses not to use an appliance, stool will be discharged onto the abdomen three or four times a day, similarly to the usual newborn or infant stool pattern. Wash and dry the stoma and surrounding skin area well after defecation. Follow your agency's protocol for skin care, such as applying karaya powder or a skin protection cream. Apply ample absorbent gauze (fluffed) and an absorbent pad over the stoma. Secure in place with nonadhesive tape or a binder. Without an appliance in place, stool is kept from touching the skin only by the protection of the ointment and frequent changing of the dressing, so assess for stool about every 4 hours. Turning an infant from side to side after every feeding can be helpful in keeping stool from flowing continuously to one side. Leaving the abdominal skin exposed to air for at least 1 hour per day also helps protect skin integrity.

Stress to parents caring for an infant with an ostomy that little is different from usual because all parents must change their infant's diapers frequently and clean the diaper area. Stress that the stoma has no nerves, so a parent can feel free to wash it without hurting the child and that compression against the stoma will not cause a child pain so the parent can feel comfortable placing an infant on the abdomen or holding the infant closely against his or her body for comfort.

Colostomies are rarely irrigated in children. On occasion, to prepare a child for second-stage abdominal surgery, irrigation of the "blind-end" bowel (i.e., the bowel between the rectum and colostomy) of a double-barreled colostomy may be prescribed daily to keep it lubricated and to maintain bowel tone. The exact amount of fluid to be used should be specified

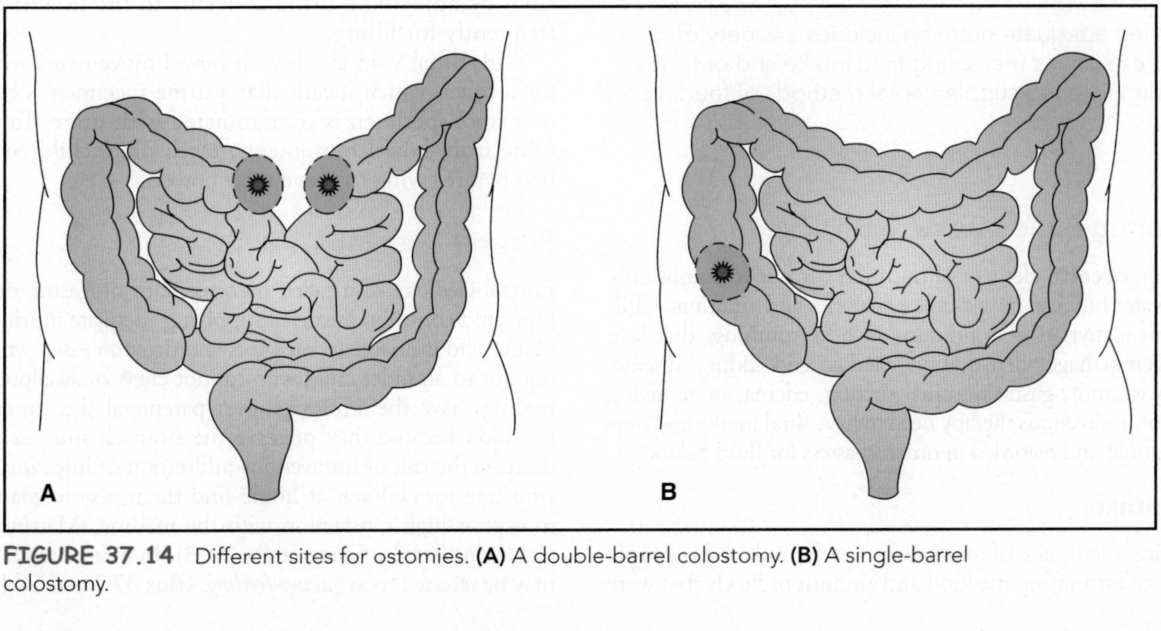

FIGURE 37.14 Different sites for ostomies. **(A)** A double-barrel colostomy. **(B)** A single-barrel colostomy.

by the primary care provider; typically, the amount is small in infants, only 40 to 100 ml. Normal saline (0.9% sodium chloride) should be used in place of tap water, which could lead to water intoxication because tap water is not isotonic.

Children who have had a colostomy since infancy adapt well to having it because they have never known another method of defecation. Suggest that parents begin toilet training for urine control at the usual time (2 to 3 years of age). In contrast, school-age children often have a great deal of difficulty adjusting to a new colostomy. Encourage children to perform complete self-care as soon as possible to develop early independence. Preschool children usually benefit from therapeutic play that helps them work through their feelings about a colostomy. Provide some time for older children to discuss concerns about being accepted by others and how to answer questions from other children about a colostomy. Adolescents with a colostomy may have questions regarding sexuality and need reassurance that this should not interfere with intimate relationships.

NUTRITIONAL CARE

Almost all illnesses affect the nutritional and fluid balance status of children; therefore, assessment of these areas sheds a great deal of light on their general health. If a child is not able to take in oral food, it can be supplemented by enteral feeding, gastrostomy, or total parenteral nutrition (TPN) depending on the child's need for nutrients.

Nursing Diagnoses and Related Interventions

Nursing Diagnosis: Risk for imbalanced nutrition, less than body requirements, related to chronic illness

Outcome Evaluation: Skin turgor remains good; no signs of dehydration are present; child gains a minimum of 1 lb weekly as evidence that nutritional need is being met.

Supplying adequate nutrition includes a variety of measures such as measuring fluid intake and output and administering supplemental methods of feeding.

Measuring Fluid Intake and Output

Fluid is an essential element of nutrition because it cannot only supply water but also be a source of calories and vitamins. Children with a myriad of conditions such as vomiting, diarrhea, burns, hemorrhage, dehydration, cardiac and kidney disease, draining wounds, gastrointestinal suction, edema, or receiving diuretic or intravenous therapy need to have fluid intake and output measured and recorded in order to assess for fluid balance.

Fluid Intake

Estimating the intake of infants who are formula fed is simply a matter of estimating the kind and amount of fluids that were swallowed. Intake in breastfed infants is merely recorded as "breastfed for however minutes." If it is necessary to estimate the amount more closely than this, an infant can be weighed before and after a feeding. The difference in weight (measured in grams) is calculated to establish the number of milliliters of breast milk ingested (1 g = 1 ml).

With preschool children, be certain to record fluids ingested during snacks as well as meals, because children this age may drink more with snacks than with meals. At approximately 10 years of age, children can be depended on to record their own intake as long as they have a list of how many milliliters are contained in each glass or cup they swallow (an average cup is 150 ml; a glass, 180 ml). Remind them that soup, flavored frozen ice such as Popsicles, gelatin, sherbet, and ice cream are liquids (they liquefy at room temperature so should be counted as fluid).

Fluid Output

A single episode of vomiting is common in childhood and, because it is self-limiting, usually requires no special treatment. Extensive vomiting, however, can lead to dehydration and/or electrolyte imbalance. Measuring the amount a child vomits (i.e., emesis) can be challenging if it spills onto clothing or bed linen. When this happens, estimate the amount in relation to the amount of food or fluid the child recently ate; include the number of episodes, a description of the color of the vomitus (e.g., red or black may contain blood; green may contain bile), and whether it was composed of clear fluid or undigested food. Remind the child's parents or the child of the importance of noting the amount if more vomiting occurs; supply a graduated measuring container at the child's bedside.

Diapers can be readily used as a method of measuring urine output. Weigh a diaper before it is placed on an infant and record this weight conspicuously (e.g., mark it on the front of the plastic covering with a ballpoint pen). Reweigh the diaper after it is wet and subtract the difference to determine the amount of urine present. This difference will be in grams but because 1 g = 1 ml, the amount can be recorded in milliliters. In infants who have liquid stools, it is difficult to separate stool from urine because these blend together in a diaper. Separate urine from stool by applying a urine collector to the infant; check it frequently for filling.

Girls often void along with bowel movements when they use a toilet, which means that a urine specimen is easily lost or a stool specimen is contaminated with urine. To separate urine from bowel movements, teach older children to void first before trying to move their bowels.

Enteral Feedings

Enteral feedings, also called nasogastric or orogastric tube feedings, are a common means of supplying adequate nutrition to an infant who is unable to suck (or who tires too easily when sucking), or to an older child who cannot chew or swallow. Enteral feedings have the advantage over parenteral (i.e., intravenous) nutrition because they preserve the stomach mucosa and also decrease the risk of intravenous infiltration or infection. Parents who care for children at home find them easy to manage and so express high satisfaction with the method (Martínez-Costa, Calderón, Pedrón-Giner, et al., 2013). In infants, such feedings may be referred to as *gavage feedings* (Box 37.7 and Table 37.2).

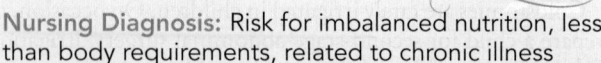

BOX 37.7 Nursing Care Planning Using Procedures

INITIATING AN ENTERAL FEEDING FOR AN INFANT

Purpose: To supply nutrition by an enteral tube.

PROCEDURE	PRINCIPLE
1. Loosely swaddle the infant using a mummy restraint.	1. Mummy restraints effectively contain arms and legs without causing any unwarranted pressure on the infant.
2. Measure the space from the bridge of the infant's nose to the earlobe then to a point halfway between the xiphoid process and the umbilicus using a #8 or #10 feeding tube. If the child is older than 1 year of age, measure from the bridge of the nose to the earlobe to the xiphoid process (Fig. A).	2. Measuring the tube ensures it will be long enough to enter the stomach. If a tube is passed too far, it will curl and end up in the esophagus; if not passed far enough, it will also be in the esophagus. Both situations could lead to aspiration of the feeding.

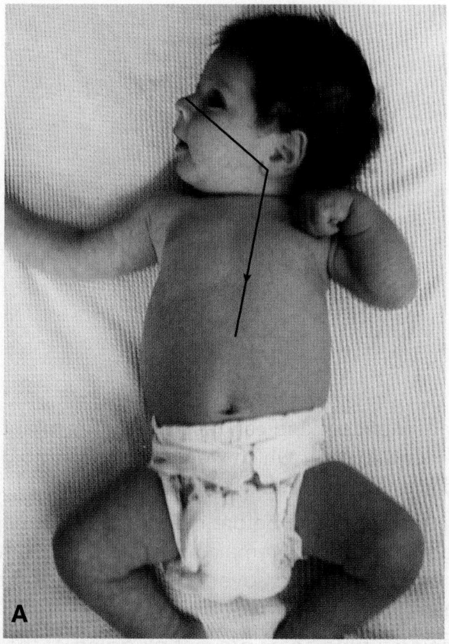

A

PROCEDURE	PRINCIPLE
3. Mark the tube at the measured point with a small clamp or piece of tape. Lubricate the tip of the catheter with water.	3. Water lubrication helps the tube pass through the esophagus without trauma. Don't use an oil lubricant because, although the tube is going to be passed into the stomach, occasionally it can unintentionally pass into the trachea. Oil left in the trachea could lead to lipoid pneumonia, a complication an infant already burdened with a disease may not be able to tolerate.
4. Pass the catheter with gentle pressure to the point of the clamp or tape. If the catheter is inadvertently passed into the trachea rather than the esophagus, the infant usually will cough and become dyspneic. If this happens, withdraw and replace the catheter.	4. Using gentle pressure helps to ensure comfort and safety.
5. Assess the catheter for position (confirm that it is not in the trachea) before administering a feeding (see Table 37.2).	5. Assessing for proper placement helps to ensure the feeding will enter the stomach, not the infant's respiratory tract.
6. Aspirate stomach contents to assess amount. If the amount aspirated is small (a few milliliters), merely replace it at the beginning of the feeding. If large (large is determined by comparing it to the care provider's nutrition prescription), replace it through the tubing, and reduce the amount of the feeding by that amount.	6. Assessing stomach content amount aids in determining if the previous feeding was absorbed. Replacing stomach secretions rather than discarding them helps prevent electrolyte loss.

(continued on page 1086)

BOX 37.7 Nursing Care Planning Using Procedures (continued)

INITIATING AN ENTERAL FEEDING FOR AN INFANT

PROCEDURE	PRINCIPLE
7. After being certain the catheter is in the stomach, attach a syringe or special feeding funnel to the tube. Elevate the infant's head and chest slightly to encourage fluid to flow downward into the stomach.	7. Elevating the infant's upper body allows the feeding to flow by gravity.
8. Add the specific kind and amount of feeding prescribed to the syringe or funnel and allow it to flow by gravity into the infant's stomach. Don't elevate the syringe end of the tube more than 12 in. above the infant's abdomen (Fig. B).	8. Excessive elevation can cause the feeding to flow too quickly, filling the esophagus and increasing the risk for aspiration. Hurrying feedings by using the plunger of the syringe or a bulb attachment for more pressure also can lead to aspiration.

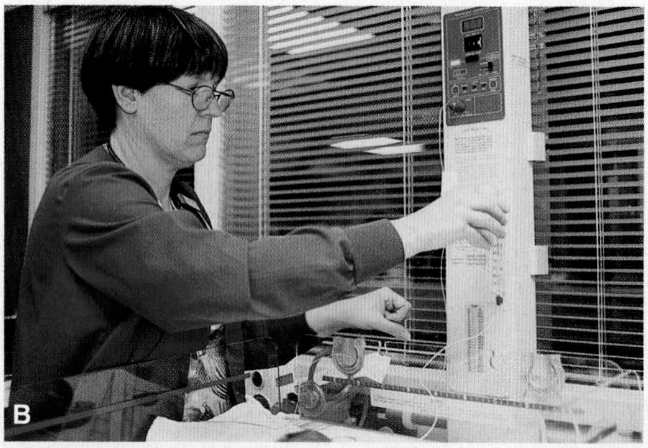
B

PROCEDURE	PRINCIPLE
9. Offer a pacifier (nonnutrient sucking) during the feeding if the infant appears to enjoy this.	9. Nonnutrient sucking can help satisfy the infant's normal need to suck, which would otherwise go unsatisfied with enteral feedings.
10. When the feeding has passed through the tube, reclamp the tube securely and gently and rapidly withdraw it.	10. Clamping the tube before it is withdrawn is important to prevent any milk remaining in the tube from flowing out as the tube is removed, thereby reducing the risk of aspiration.
11. If the tube is to remain in place, flush it with 1 to 5 ml of clear water and cap it.	11. Flushing a tube helps prevent plugging of the tube with the feeding solution. Capping a tube helps to prevent air and bacteria from entering.
12. If the tube is to be left in place, tape it below the nose and to the cheek. Do not tape it to the forehead.	12. Taping a tube to the forehead can put pressure on the anterior naris, leading to ulceration.
13. Burp the baby after an enteral feeding the same as you would after bottle or breastfeeding. If a parent is present, encourage him or her to do this.	13. Burping helps to prevent air accumulation and regurgitation of the feeding. Encouraging parental participation aids in promoting close contact, which is essential to the baby's development.
14. Unswaddle and place the infant on the right side with the head slightly elevated or hold and rock the infant in this position.	14. Placing on the right side helps the feeding solution enter the pyloric valve, thus promoting stomach emptying.
15. Assess that the infant appears comfortable. If a parent observed the procedure, answer any questions or concerns.	15. Assessing the infant after the feeding aids in outcome evaluation. Helping parents feel comfortable with alternative feeding methods can promote bonding with the infant.

Whether enteral catheters should be passed through the nares or the mouth is controversial. Because newborns are obligate nasal breathers and passing a catheter through the nose may obstruct their breathing space, most tubes are inserted orally in small infants (Bohnhorst, Cech, Peter, et al., 2010).

Orogastric insertion can also decrease the possibility of striking the vagal nerve in the back of the throat and causing bradycardia. For older children, insertion through a nostril is often more comfortable. To prevent irritation or ulcer formation from the tube rubbing against the tip of the nose, always tape nasogastric tubes to the child's cheek rather than the forehead to secure it in place.

TABLE 37.2 Methods to Determine Feeding Tube Placement

Method	Considerations
1. If an X-ray is obtained to document correct tube placement, measure the length of the tube evident at that time. Remeasure the length of tube before a feeding to document that the tube has not pulled out or advanced further.	This system has inherent problems because it requires an X-ray and does not verify that the tube is actually in the stomach, but it can be used if it is health care policy.
2. Attach a syringe to the end of the tube and aspirate stomach contents. Test for pH (below 7 is acidic), which reveals the tube is in the stomach.	In most instances, stomach contents aspirated this way are returned to the stomach before the feeding; in small infants, the amount of stomach contents is subtracted from the prescribed amount of feeding. Because stomach contents are highly acid, discarding them at each feeding could lead to alkalosis.
3. Inject 5 ml air into the feeding tube and listen over the stomach with a stethoscope to the sound of injected air.	The injected air is heard as a whistling or growling sound. Do not use an adult-size stethoscope on small infants to listen for it; the diaphragm of the stethoscope will be partially over lung, and where one is hearing the air injection is unknown.

Because tubes are radiopaque, their placement or that they extend into the stomach can be confirmed by X-ray. Table 37.2 describes other methods to use to be certain before a feeding the tube is not in the trachea or has pulled out so is actually just resting in the back of the throat.

Although children with long-term neurologic disabilities may have enteral tubes left in place for continuous feedings administered by an enteric feeding pump, most children are generally offered bolus or intermittent feedings at what would be a usual meal time, rather than continuous infusions, to more closely mimic a normal feeding pattern. The nutrition formula infused should be at room temperature to prevent chilling the child. Before a feeding, be certain to elevate the child's upper trunk 30 to 40 degrees (i.e., a semi-Fowler's position) so the fluid will flow downward into the stomach and not upward into the esophagus, possibly causing aspiration into the trachea. For infants, you can do this by holding the infant in your lap or placing the infant in an infant seat. For an older child, use pillows or elevate the head of the bed. For small infants, it is often necessary to aspirate stomach contents before a feeding as this reveals whether an infant is absorbing the quantity of fluid given as well as confirms the tube's placement is in the stomach. After noting the amount and type of fluid aspirated, unless prescribed otherwise, replace this fluid so the child does not lose the electrolytes or stomach enzymes it contains.

Following this, to administer a feeding, attach a syringe to the tube and allow the specified amount of nutrition formula to flow by gravity into the tube. Don't use the barrel of the syringe to force the feeding forward in order to prevent reflux and possible aspiration. Most infants enjoy having a pacifier for nonnutritive sucking during a feeding. This action helps to maintain or strengthen the sucking reflex for later when the child returns to oral feedings.

At the end of the feeding, flush the tube with 1 to 5 ml of water to clear it of the feeding solution, prevent blockage, and maintain patency. Keep the child's head elevated for at least 1 hour after a feeding to help prevent esophageal reflux. Provide mouth care at least twice a day to encourage salivation in children who are receiving nasogastric tube feedings; otherwise, their mouths can become dry and prone to the formation of mucosal ulcers.

Gastrostomy Tube Feedings

A gastrostomy tube is one inserted under regional anesthesia through an abdominal puncture site into the stomach and used for nutritional formula feedings (Fig. 37.15). The method may be necessary for children who cannot swallow, have an esophageal stricture, or who need long-term enteral feedings (Bishay, Lakshminarayanan, Arnaud, et al., 2012). The tube used in children is usually an indwelling urinary catheter (i.e., a Foley catheter) rather than a true gastrostomy tube because these are smaller in size, can be removed easily, and changed should they become plugged. In addition, the balloon used to secure the tube is small enough so it does not obscure and fill the small stomach space. As with nasogastric feedings, gastrostomy feedings should be at room temperature to prevent chilling and given at spaced times to simulate meal times. Be certain to aspirate for stomach secretions to assess absorption and placement before the feeding, then allow the formula to flow by gravity only, not forced. If a child has had esophageal surgery, suspend the unclamped tube in an elevated position after the feeding because leaving the tube unclamped and elevated this way ensures that if the child should vomit, vomitus will be evacuated from the stomach by the tube rather than past new sutures in the esophagus. Cover the open end of the tube with a clean piece of porous gauze to reduce bacterial colonization.

Because infants who are fed by gastrostomy tube miss the pleasure of sucking the same as those fed by nasogastric tubes, offer a pacifier to suck on during the procedure unless contraindicated. Talk or sing to the child as if the feeding were being given orally.

The biggest problem with managing gastrostomy tubes is they may not fit snugly, so formula or irritating gastric secretions can leak around the tube onto the abdominal skin. Clean the skin around the tube daily with a product such as half-strength hydrogen peroxide, and protect the skin with a commercial protection cream as directed by the manufacturer's instructions. If a gastrostomy tube remains in place for a long period of time, the tube can move into the duodenum through the pyloric sphincter and cause obstruction. Observe and report any vomiting, abdominal distention, or brown or

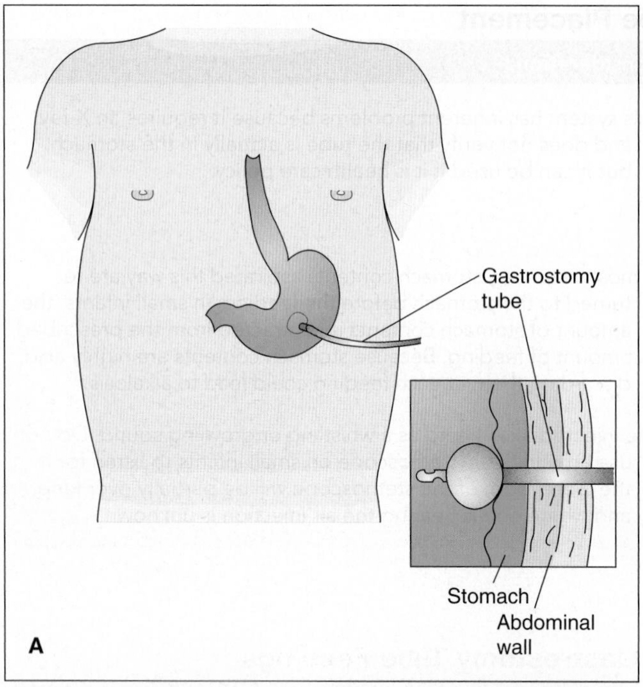

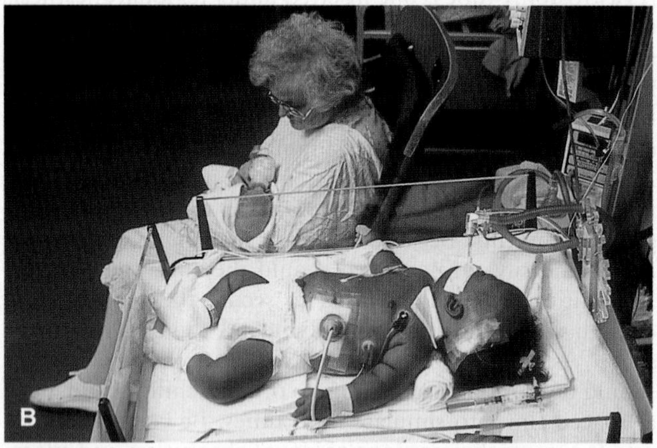

FIGURE 37.15 Children who are ill often need supplemental feedings by nasogastric or gastrostomy tube feedings. **(A)** Internal placement of a gastrostomy tube. **(B)** An infant with a gastrostomy tube in place. (From W. McIntyre/Photo Researchers, Inc.)

green tube drainage, which could be duodenal secretions that would suggest the tube has moved. Stomach secretions are acid, and duodenal secretions are alkaline. Therefore, testing residual aspiration fluid before a feeding to see that it is acid is a guarantee the tube is in the stomach. Also, putting a mark on the tube with an indelible pen lets you check that the tube has not migrated further into the gastrointestinal tract but is remaining securely in place.

Tubes are replaced approximately every 6 weeks. To replace a tube, deflate the catheter balloon by withdrawing the water in it, and then gently pull the tube free. Insert a clean catheter into the stomach opening approximately 1 in. beyond the balloon, then inflate the balloon with 2 to 4 ml water. Apply skin protection and tape the tube into place.

Help parents to view gastrostomy feeding as merely an alternative way of feeding rather than a totally different one. Provide opportunities for parents and caregivers to participate and learn the feeding procedure. Be certain they

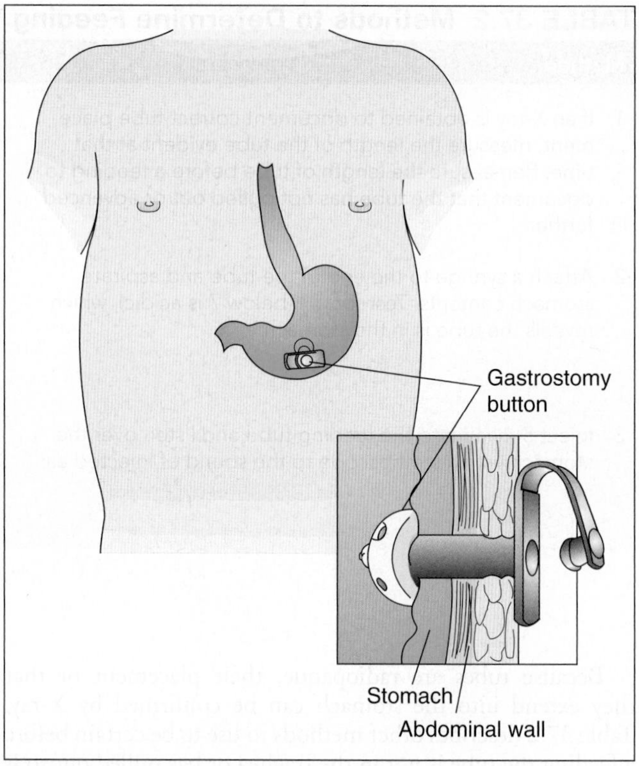

FIGURE 37.16 Placement of a gastrostomy button.

are comfortable with the procedure before the child is discharged from the hospital. Reinforce with them the understanding that it does not hurt their child to have pressure put against the tube so they do not worry about holding their child snugly.

If a child is going to need gastrostomy feedings for an extended time, a gastrostomy button will usually be implanted for easier stomach access, to prevent skin irritation, and to prevent ulceration of the stomach mucosa from the internal balloon (Fig. 37.16). For feeding with a button in place, a catheter is inserted through the device for a feeding and removed following the feeding. Advantages of gastrostomy buttons are the cosmetic benefit because only a small access device is visible instead of a bulky tube, and there is a lessened incidence of skin irritation.

What if . . . 37.3 The child in the hospital room next to Felipe has a gastrostomy button in place, with which she will be discharged. Her mother tells you she's going to take her daughter to a restaurant as soon as they're discharged as she thinks "eating out" is an excellent way to teach table manners. Would you agree with her that this is a good idea?

Total Parenteral Nutrition

Total parenteral nutrition (TPN), or nutrition administered intravenously, has become one of the most important therapies for children who have gastrointestinal illnesses that prevent proper absorption of basic caloric or fluid requirements or respiratory illnesses that make infants too exhausted to suck.

Nursing Diagnoses and Related Interventions

Nursing Diagnosis: Imbalanced nutrition, less than body requirements, related to malabsorption of nutrients

Outcome Evaluation: Skin turgor is good; no signs of dehydration are present; child loses no weight during therapy; intestinal cramps and distention lessen.

Traditional intravenous therapy contains fluid, electrolytes, and sugars but not protein and fat, ingredients which are essential for the maintenance and growth of body tissues. With TPN, all of a child's nutritional needs can be met by a concentrated hypertonic solution containing glucose, vitamins, electrolytes, trace minerals, and protein. An intralipid solution (emulsified fat able to be administered intravenously) given once or twice per week, supplies needed fatty acids. Children with chronic diarrhea or vomiting, inflammatory bowel disease, bowel obstruction, anorexia, or extreme immaturity are examples of children who benefit greatly from TPN.

TPN solutions may be administered via a central intravenous access site or via a peripherally inserted central venous catheter (PICC line) (Pittiruti, Brutti, Celentano, et al., 2012). If a central access site is chosen, a catheter is inserted through the right external jugular vein into the superior vena cava, or directly into the subclavian vein under strict aseptic conditions (see Chapter 38). The catheter is secured at the site of insertion with sutures and covered with a sterile dressing to help reduce bacterial invasion. A major vein of this type is chosen to avoid inflammation reactions and resulting venous thrombosis from the high-caloric and high-osmotic fluid that will be infused.

The TPN solution is prepared in a pharmacy under sterile conditions according to prescription. A Millipore filter, which removes small particles in the solution that might cause an embolus to form, is inserted into the tubing. Because the solution is concentrated, it is administered by means of a constant infusion pump so the rate can be governed. As a general rule, if the rate should fall behind, do not increase it the next hour to make up the amount of fluid, as serious cardiovascular overload could result because the fluid is so concentrated.

Infection is a major danger of TPN because the solution is a perfect medium for the growth of bacteria or *Candida* organisms. The dressing over the insertion site and the intravenous tubing need to be changed every 48 hours or as needed according to the Centers for Disease Control and Prevention (CDC) Guidelines for Prevention of Intravascular Catheter-Related Infections (O'Grady, Alexander, Burns, et al., 2011). Don't use the tubing for obtaining blood or for adding medications (unless a double-barreled tube is used), because such processes have the potential to introduce infection. Use sterile technique to change both the bags of solution and the dressing so infection is not introduced. Inspect the insertion site at the time of a dressing change for indications of local infection, such as redness, tenderness, or discharge because infection at the insertion site can lead to a serious sepsis or thrombosis (Niedner, Huskins, Colantuoni, et al., 2011).

A second major problem that can occur with TPN is dehydration. This occurs because a TPN solution contains approximately twice the amount of glucose normally administered in an intravenous solution to ensure that the amino acids in the solution will be used for protein synthesis, not for energy. Dehydration can occur when the kidneys recognize the amount of glucose in the bloodstream as excessive and begin to reduce it by excreting it (the same phenomenon that leads to high urine output in persons with diabetes mellitus). Before TPN is started and during the administration, test urine for glucose and specific gravity with each voiding. If two or more consecutive samples indicate a 3+ or 4+ glucose level, either the rate of the infusion or the amount of glucose in the solution may need to be decreased, or insulin may need to be added to the solution to counteract the excess glucose. Generally, decreasing the concentration of glucose and then gradually increasing it again allows the child's body to adjust to the glucose overload without problems.

After the first few days of TPN, a rebound effect (i.e., the child's body produces increased insulin) may cause hypoglycemia. A urine sample that suddenly is negative for glucose after several serial specimens have been highly positive, therefore, is not necessarily an encouraging sign; rather, it may be a warning the child's glucose level has become dangerously low. The TPN solution should never be discontinued abruptly, but rather, should be gradually tapered, or hypoglycemia could also occur. If a TPN catheter should be accidentally pulled out by a child, notify the child's primary health care provider immediately and apply pressure to the insertion site to halt bleeding. The child must be immediately assessed for the effect of loss of blood and closely observed for signs of hypoglycemia (e.g., lethargy, lack of motor coordination, fidgeting, seizures). Parents need to be alerted to these steps if managing a child with parenteral nutrition on home care.

Remember that, to a child, eating is more than a means of receiving nourishment; it is also a means of receiving comfort and love. Even though children are able to voice the reason they must have TPN and appear to understand they are receiving all the needed nutrients by infusion, they still may miss eating food and the natural social interaction that comes with it. While in a hospital, they may be upset by the smell of food from a hospital unit kitchen or by the fact playmates have to leave to eat a meal. Finding an activity for a child receiving TPN while other children eat, such as helping to check unit supplies or stamping laboratory slips, can be helpful to supply the interaction a child misses. Make certain parents arrange for special times each day with the child to make up for the time normally spent interacting at meals.

Some children tolerate TPN better if they can be allowed chewing gum or occasional hard candy; advocate for these as necessary. Remind the child to continue tooth brushing twice a day to keep oral mucous membrane healthy because he or she is not chewing. An infant may enjoy the sucking pleasure from a pacifier.

QSEN Checkpoint Question 37.6

Quality Improvement

Felipe's primary health care provider asks you to keep as accurate a record as possible of Felipe's intake and output while he is undergoing diagnostic testing. Felipe vomits without warning on his gown and the floor. How should you document this form of output to ensure an accurate assessment?

a. Estimate the amount of emesis and describe the character in his health record.
b. Describe the event in Felipe's health record and note that it was not possible to gauge the quantity.
c. Weigh his soiled gown and compare the weight to a clean gown of the same size.
d. Ask his mother to tell you the approximate amount that he vomited.

Look in Appendix A for the best answer and rationale.

HOT AND COLD THERAPY

Children who sustain muscle sprains or undergo procedures such as bronchoscopy or tonsillectomy may have cold applications prescribed to prevent swelling or edema, help control hemorrhage, or provide an analgesic effect. Ice packs are left in place for about 20 minutes. To prevent frostbite, never place an ice pack directly on the skin; instead, insert a towel between the pack and the skin. Document the type of application, duration of the therapy, and the condition of the skin before and after the treatment.

Local application of heat may be prescribed to relieve congestion and pain by increasing circulation through vasodilation and muscle relaxation (Box 37.8). Heat may also be prescribed to help resolve superficial inflammation and hasten the formation and drainage of abscesses or absorption from subcutaneous tissue if IV fluid infiltrated. It is important to not leave either hot or cold compresses in place continuously or a rebound effect that blocks their effectiveness may occur. Always assess the skin before and after the treatment to be certain tissue damage (e.g., a burn) did not occur from treatment. If you are using a heating pad to maintain warmth in a young child, set the temperature dial, then tape it in place so the child cannot spin the dial and increase the temperature beyond a safe level.

WOUND CARE

Children frequently have a dressing or bandage put in place to cover a surgical incision or sutured laceration. Such dressings are the same as those used with adults except in size, material, and methods used to secure them. Keeping a dressing dry to avoid introducing infection to the wound in infants and toddlers who are not toilet trained can be a major problem if the dressing is near the diaper area. In many instances after surgery, collodion (i.e., a clear substance similar to nail polish) or other commercially available "wound glues" are used to cover the incision because these solutions not only replace stitches but also keep the incision line from coming in contact with urine or feces. These materials allow good visualization of the healing surface as well because they are clear. Assure parents that such a covering is adequate and actually preferable if the incision is in the groin such as from a hernia repair. They are also preferable if an incision or laceration is on the face because they tend to heal with less scarring than if sutures were used.

BOX 37.8 Nursing Care Planning to Empower a Family

GUIDELINES FOR HOT AND COLD APPLICATIONS WITH CHILDREN

Q. Felipe's mother tells you, "I need to apply cold compresses to my child's head to reduce swelling. How do I do this?"
A. When applying any type of hot or cold therapy such as cold or warm compresses, use the following guidelines:

- Apply neither heat nor cold for longer than 20 minutes unless prescribed because, after that time, the vasoconstriction caused by cold and the vasodilatation caused by heat begins to reverse.
- When using electrical sources of heat with toddlers and preschoolers, never make a game of plugging in and pulling out the apparatus that makes the light come on or a dial glow. Otherwise, the child may play with it after you leave.
- Supply a special activity for a child to enjoy while a hot or cold application is in place (e.g., playing a board game, reading a story to the child), so that the procedure is not viewed as a chore but as a pleasant time to look forward to.
- Put tape on the gauge of an electric appliance at the point where you want it, so that you will be able to tell if the child changes the setting.
- To be certain solutions or heat sources are not too hot, always test them with your inner wrist or the dorsal surface of your hand before applying them to the child.
- Do not apply ice packs or ice directly to the skin. Cover the pack or ice with a towel or other cover such as dish towel to prevent frostbite and cell damage from cold.
- Be cautious using heat or cold applications with a child who is receiving an analgesic because the child's perception of heat or cold may be reduced and the site could easily be burned.

If a gauze dressing is used near the diaper area, it can be covered with plastic and held in place with nonadhesive, waterproof tape to protect it from becoming soiled. Be certain when cutting plastic to cover a dressing not to leave an extra piece behind in the crib as a child could pull this over the head and suffocate.

Occlusive dressings (e.g., hydrogel sheets, hydrocolloids, polyurethane films) are dressings especially designed to keep a healing surface clean and dry. Be certain to apply and remove these according to each product's directions or agency policy to protect irritating the skin underneath.

Apply Band-Aids generously after venipuncture or finger punctures because young children find bandages comforting and accept them as a "badge of courage."

Use nonadhesive tape (e.g., silk, paper) or secure a dressing with a nonadhering bandage (Kling) or roller gauze instead of adhesive tape to protect sensitive skin. Don't be surprised to see a young child pull a dressing loose and inspect what is underneath. Do not discourage children from looking at their incision during dressing changes. Even if the area looks raw and unhealed, it may look better than what the child envisioned was under the dressing.

What if . . . 37.4 You are particularly interested in exploring one of the 2020 National Health Goals with respect to diagnostic or therapeutic procedures in children (see Box 37.1). Most government-sponsored money for nursing research is allotted based on these goals. What would be a possible research topic to explore pertinent to these goals that would be applicable to Felipe's family and that would advance evidence-based practice?

Key Points for Review

- Preparing children for procedures reduces anxiety. Prepare a child and parents by trying to relate a procedure to something a child is already familiar with, such as comparing an X-ray machine to a camera.
- Include parents in both the planning and implementation of care because parents can reinfect children with fear if their own fear is uncontrolled. Try to give explanations on two levels: "I'm going to change the dressing on her suture line" for a parent; "I'm going to put a clean bandage on your tummy" for the child.
- Minimize the number of painful procedures; for instance, combine blood sampling procedures, if possible.
- Perform any procedures that will cause pain in a treatment room or away from the child's bedside so the bed remains a "safe" place.
- Perform treatments without chilling or exposure. Respect modesty even in very young children.
- Allow a child to voice anger or fear of a procedure. Provide therapeutic play after a procedure to help reduce these reactions.
- Children feel more secure with adults who are confident in their actions. Practice as necessary the steps of a procedure before you begin so you can demonstrate confidence and skill.
- Once you have announced that a procedure needs to be done, proceed to do it; waiting for something to happen is often as stressful as actually having it done.
- Involve children in procedures to implement care that not only meets QSEN competencies but also best meets a family's total needs. Allow a child to examine electrodes or apply gel for electrode contact before a procedure, for example. Give children a portion of an ECG strip as a badge of courage after the procedure, or let children apply their own adhesive bandage.
- Praise children for cooperation even if none was visibly obvious. For painful procedures, any behavior short of hysterical screaming counts as cooperation.
- Following the use of conscious sedation, observe children carefully until they are fully awake. Check for the return of the child's gag reflex before offering any fluids to minimize the risk of aspiration.
- Help make feeding by a route such as a gastrostomy tube as close to normal as possible by talking to the child to simulate mealtime conversation and socialization.

Critical Thinking Care Study

Donald Kohl is an 8-year-old whose father has brought him to the emergency room because he has been vomiting all morning and, over the past hour, has developed sharp pain in his right lower abdomen. You need to schedule him for an ultrasound to rule out appendicitis. Because Donald's parents are divorced and the father is not the custodial parent, he phones Donald's mother. She screams at him for being completely incompetent at child care and tells him, "Don't you dare sign anything until I can get there."

1. Because it will take a minimum of 45 minutes for Donald's mother to arrive, you are concerned that long a delay in having the ultrasound could be a significant threat to Donald's health because, if he has appendicitis, his appendix could rupture during that time. Would you ask the father to sign the permission despite his wife's opinion or wait for the mother to arrive?
2. Donald has had three X-rays over the past year because he broke his right tibia in an auto accident due to a combination of him not having his seatbelt fastened and his father's unsafe driving. His father asks you, in light of the radiation Donald has already received over the past year, if an ultrasound will be safe for him. Would you explain this is an emergency so diagnosing whether his son has appendicitis is more important than evaluating the degree of radiation?
3. You talk to Mrs. Kohl on her cell phone while she is in her car and she says it will be all right if you draw blood for a white blood count on Donald. As he's already anxious, would it be more important to apply anesthetic cream to his venipuncture site to help reduce pain or obtain the blood sample immediately?

Patient Scenario

The Gordon Family

Read about the Gordon family, a family with a child who needs gastrostomy feedings, then answer the questions to further sharpen your skills and grow more familiar with NCLEX-type questions related to when a child needs diagnostic and therapeutic modalities. Confirm your answers are correct by reading the rationales.

Visit http://thePoint.lww.com

Answers and Rationales

Looking for answers to the What If… and Critical Thinking Care Study questions?

Visit http://thePoint.lww.com

References

Adler, D. G., Kawa, C., Hilden, K., et al. (2011). Nurse-administered propofol sedation is safe for patients with obstructive sleep apnea undergoing routine endoscopy: A pilot study. *Digestive Diseases & Sciences, 56*(9), 2666–2671.

Alexander, M. (2012). Managing patient stress in pediatric radiology. *Radiologic Technology, 83*(6),549–660.

Bishay, M., Lakshminarayanan, B., Arnaud, A., et al. (2012). The role of parenteral nutrition following surgery for duodenal atresia or stenosis. *Pediatric Surgery International, 29*(2), 191–195.

Bishop, W. F. (2011). The digestive system. In K. J. Marcdante, R. M. Kliegman, H. B. Jenson, et al. (Eds.), *Nelson essentials of pediatrics* (6th ed., pp. 463–498). Philadelphia, PA: Saunders/Elsevier.

Bohnhorst, B., Cech, K., Peter, C., et al. (2010). Oral versus nasal route for placing feeding tubes: No effect on hypoxemia and bradycardia in infants with apnea of prematurity. *Neonatology, 98*(2), 143–149.

Dingemann, J., & Ure, B. 2012). Imaging and the use of scores for the diagnosis of appendicitis in children. *European Journal of Pediatric Surgery, 22*(3), 195–200.

Forsey, M., Salmon, P., Eden, T., et al. (2011). Comparing doctors' and nurses' accounts of how they provide emotional care for parents of children with acute lymphoblastic leukaemia. *Psychooncology, 22*(2), 260–267.

Goyal, R., Nayar, S., Gogia, P., et al. (2012). Extraction of tracheobronchial foreign bodies in children and adults with rigid and flexible bronchoscopy. *Journal of Bronchology & Interventional Pulmonology, 19*(1), 35–43.

Haemer, M, Primark, L. E. & Krebs, N. R. (2011). Normal childhood nutrition & its disorders. In W. W. Hay, M. J. Levin, J. M. Sondheimer, et al. (Eds.), *Current pediatric diagnosis and treatment* (20th ed, pp. 288–315.). New York, NY: McGraw-Hill.

Hanrahan, K., McCarthy, A. M., Kleiber, C., et al. (2012). Building a computer program to support children, parents, and distraction during healthcare procedures. *Computers, Informatics, Nursing, 30*(10), 554–561.

Havidich, J. E., & Cravero, J. P. (2012).The current status of procedural sedation for pediatric patients in out-of-operating room locations. *Current Opinion in Anaesthesiology, 25*(4), 453–460.

Ho, M., Garnett, S. P., Baur, L., et al. (2012). Effectiveness of lifestyle interventions in child obesity: Systematic review with meta-analysis. *Pediatrics, 130*(6), e1647–e1671.

Inal, S., & Kelleci, M. (2012). Relief of pain during blood specimen collection in pediatric patients. *MCN: American Journal of Maternal Child Nursing, 37*(5), 339–345.

Jackson, L., & Thalange, N. (2013). Assessing childhood illness. In N. Thalange, R. Beach, D. Booth, et al. (Eds.), *Essentials of paediatrics* (2nd ed., pp. 1–6). Philadelphia, PA: Elsevier/Saunders.

Jain, R., Petrillo-Albarano, T., Parks, W. J., et al. (2013). Efficacy and safety of deep sedation by non-anesthesiologists for cardiac MRI in children. *Pediatric Radiology, 43*(5), 605–611.

Karch, A. M. (2013). *2013 Lippincott's nursing drug guide.* Philadelphia, PA: Lippincott Williams & Wilkins.

Lane, S., & Kohlenberg, E. (2012). Emancipated minors: Health policy and implications for nursing. *Journal of Pediatric Nursing, 27*(5), 533–548.

Litke, J., Pikulska, A., & Wegner, T. (2012). Management of perioperative stress in children and parents: The preoperative period. *Anaesthesiology Intensive Therapy, 44*(3), 165–169.

Martínez-Costa, C., Calderón, C., Pedrón-Giner, C., et al. (2013). Psychometric properties of the structured Satisfaction Questionnaire with Gastrostomy Feeding (SAGA-8) for caregivers of children with gastrostomy tube nutritional support. *Journal of Human Nutrition & Dietetics, 26*(2), 191–197.

Michelotti, B., Long, R. E., Leber, D., et al. (2012). Should surgeons use arm restraints after cleft surgery? *Annals of Plastic Surgery, 69*(4), 387–388.

Morris, M. A., & Jackson, L. (2013). Digestion & nutrition. In N. Thalange, R. Beach, D. Booth, et al. (Eds.), *Essentials of paediatrics* (2nd ed., pp. 159–182). Philadelphia, PA: Elsevier/Saunders.

Natale, J. E., Joseph, J. G., Rogers, A. J., et al. (2012). Cranial computed tomography use among children with minor blunt head trauma: Association with race/ethnicity. *Archives of Pediatric & Adolescent Medicine, 166*(8), 732–737.

Neubauer, H., Pabst, T., Dick, A., et al. (2012). Small-bowel MRI in children and young adults with Crohn disease: Retrospective head-to-head comparison of contrast-enhanced and diffusion-weighted MRI. *Pediatric Radiology, 43*(1), 103–114.

Niedner, M. F., Huskins, W. C., Colantuoni, E., et al. (2011). Epidemiology of central line-associated bloodstream infections in the pediatric intensive care unit. *Infection Control & Hospital Epidemiology, 32*(12), 1200–1208.

O'Grady, N. P., Alexander, M., Burns, L. A., et al. (2011). *2011 Guidelines for the prevention of intravascular catheter-related infections.* Atlanta, GA: Centers for Disease Control and Prevention.

Pappas, M. (2012). Understanding the different methods for taking a temperature. *NASN School Nurse, 27*(5), 254–255.

Pittiruti, M., Brutti, A., Celentano, D., et al. (2012). Clinical experience with power-injectable PICCs in intensive care patients. *Critical Care, 16*(1), R21.

Schreiber, S., Ronfani, L., Chiaffoni, G. P., et al. (2012). Does EMLA cream application interfere with the success of venipuncture or venous cannulation? *European Journal of Pediatrics, 172*(2), 265–268.

Sharma, S., & Gupta, D. K. (2012). Hirschsprung's disease presenting beyond infancy: Surgical options and postoperative outcome. *Pediatric Surgery International, 28*(1), 5–8.

Slynn, C., & Hulkes, C. (2012). Developing a nurse-led child sedation service. *Nursing Children & Young People, 24*(6), 20–22.

Smith, C., & Goldman, R. D. (2012). Alternating acetaminophen and ibuprofen for pain in children. *Canadian Family Physician, 58*(6), 645–647.

Thakkar, K., Alsarraj, A., Fong, E., et al. (2012). Prevalence of colorectal polyps in pediatric colonoscopy. *Digestive Diseases & Sciences, 57*(4), 1050–1055.

The Joint Commission. (2010). *Advancing effective communication, cultural competence, and patient- and family-centered care: A roadmap for hospitals.* Oakbrook Terrace, IL: Author.

Tosif, S., Baker, A., Oakley, E., et al. (2012). Contamination rates of different urine collection methods for the diagnosis of urinary tract infections in young children: An observational cohort study. *Journal of Paediatrics & Child Health, 48*(8), 659–664.

U.S. Department of Health and Human Services. (2010). *Healthy people 2020.* Washington, DC: Author.

Whitmore, C. (2012). Blood glucose monitoring: An overview. *British Journal of Nursing, 21*(10), 583–587.

Chapter 38

Nursing Care of a Family When a Child Needs Medication Administration or Intravenous Therapy

KEY TERMS

- absorption
- distribution
- excretion
- intermittent infusion devices
- intracath
- metabolism
- pharmacokinetics
- vascular access ports (VAPs)
- weight-based dosage

OBJECTIVES

After mastering the contents of this chapter, you should be able to:

1. Describe common methods of medication and intravenous (IV) therapy used in the health care of children.
2. Identify 2020 National Health Goals related to medication or IV therapy that nurses can help the nation achieve.
3. Assess the developmental stage and knowledge level of children and adolescents before beginning medication or IV therapy.
4. Formulate nursing diagnoses related to medication or IV therapy with children.
5. Identify expected outcomes to meet the needs of children receiving medication or IV therapy as well as manage seamless transitions across differing health care settings.
6. Using the nursing process, plan nursing care that includes the six competencies of Quality & Safety Education for Nurses (QSEN): Patient-Centered Care, Teamwork & Collaboration, Evidence-Based Practice (EBP), Quality Improvement (QI), Safety, and Informatics.
7. Implement nursing interventions concerned with medication and IV therapy and children, such as introducing patient-controlled analgesia or calculating weight-based dosing of medications with a milligram per kilogram system.
8. Evaluate expected outcomes for achievement and effectiveness of care.
9. Integrate knowledge of medication and IV therapy with the interplay of nursing process, the six competencies of QSEN, and Family Nursing to promote quality maternal and child health nursing care.

Terry, an 8-year-old with Down syndrome, is brought to the emergency department by her parents because she has pain in her ankle. She is diagnosed with osteomyelitis, a bone infection. When you give her a tablet of acetaminophen (Tylenol) for pain, she spits it out. She does the same when you repeat with a second tablet. Her mother tells you Terry can't swallow pills. Her father tells you, "You'll have to give her an IV."

Previous chapters described the difficulty children may have adjusting to illness and also diagnostic and therapeutic procedures that are frequently used with children. This chapter adds information about techniques for administering medication and intravenous (IV) therapy to children. Because therapy for almost all illnesses today involves some form of medicine or IV administration, and safe medication administration is one of the most important parts of a child health nurse's role, this information is pertinent to the care of almost all children.

What would be an effective technique to help Terry learn to swallow pills? How would you gain her cooperation?

Most adults immediately grasp that taking a medicine you offer them will be important to relieve whatever symptoms they are experiencing from an illness. Because children do not necessarily have this same level of understanding, they may resist taking medicine unless its importance is thoroughly explained to them and the medication is given to them by a method that best meets their preference. Many children do not have enough coordination to swallow tablets or pills until they are 6 or 7 years of age, and many adolescents still "don't like pills." This might mean getting a child to agree to try an oral medication only if it is furnished in a liquid or meltaway form. Almost all children fear intrusive procedures. This can make them forcibly resist accepting medication given by a rectal, nasal, intramuscular (IM), or IV route. Because children range in size from as small as 1 lb (0.5 kg) if preterm to more than 200 lb (90.9 kg) by late adolescence, there is no "standard" dose of medicine for children. This can make it difficult to determine the correct dose unless a **weight-based dosage** system is used; or a child weighing 100 lb receives 10 times the amount of most medicines than does the child who weighs 10 lb (Ghaleb, Barber, Franklin, et al., 2010). The recent rise in childhood obesity has complicated correct dosing further because overweight can result in a child receiving too little of a drug or a drug dose exceeding maximum dosing recommendations. In addition, children have difficulty reporting adverse effects of medicine as accurately as adults. This can make it difficult to determine if side effects or adverse effects are occurring. All these things make medicine administration for children one of the most challenging interventions in nursing (Walsh, Mazor, Roblin, et al., 2013). The 2020 National Health Goals that address this area of child health practice are shown in Box 38.1.

BOX 38.1 Nursing Care Planning Based on 2020 National Health Goals

When administering medicine to children or teaching children and parents how to take or give medicine, remember that medicines can be as dangerous in overdoses as they are helpful in the correct doses. They can be ineffective if a dose is inadequate or missed. Drugs also must be stored safely to avoid poisoning. National Health Goals that speak to medicine administration include:

- Reduce emergency department (ED) visits for medication overdoses among children less than 5 years of age from 32.8% to a target level of 29.5%.
- Increase the proportion of at-risk adolescents aged 12 to 17 years who, in the past year, refrained from using alcohol for the first time from 85.8% to a target level of 94.4%.
- Reduce the proportion of adolescents reporting the use of alcohol or any illicit drugs during the past 30 days from 18.4% to 16.6%.
- Reduce the past year nonmedical use of any psychotherapeutic drug (including pain relievers, tranquilizers, stimulants, and sedatives) from 6.1% of persons aged 12 years and older to 5.5% (U.S. Department of Health and Human Services [DHHS], 2010; see www.healthypeople.gov).

Nurses can help the nation achieve these goals by educating parents about safe drug storage (locked in elevated cabinets) and teaching children and parents about effective nonpharmacologic ways to relieve stress or anxiety to help reduce drug dependence.

Nursing Process Overview

For a Child Needing Medication/Intravenous Therapy

Assessment

Because children vary so greatly in size and individual need, administering medication to children begins by assessing the child's weight in kilograms so that weight-based dosing can occur. For some medications, such as chemotherapy, height and weight are both used to calculate dosage (body surface area dosage). Also crucial to the assessment is the child's developmental age. This is important because it reveals if a child can swallow oral medicine or will be able to use such self-medication methods as patient-controlled analgesia; in addition, it will help you determine which site would be best for an IM or IV injection. Also assess the child's chronologic age and cognitive level to aid in planning the level of explanation that will be needed. Including an assessment of the child's past experience with taking medicine and if the family has access and the financial means to buy the medicine can help predict whether the child will actually receive the medicine and what the child's response to medicine administration might be.

Following the administration of the medicine, careful observation must continue to determine if the medication is having its desired effect or if any unwanted or adverse effects are occurring (Dickinson, Wagner, Shaw, et al., 2012).

Nursing Diagnosis

Common nursing diagnoses related to medicine administration vary widely. Some examples include:

- Disturbed sleep pattern related to q4h (every 4 hours) timing of medication administration
- Deficient knowledge related to action and side effects of medicine
- Fear related to IV administration of medicine
- Discomfort related to side effect of medicine
- Health-seeking behaviors by parent related to desire to learn more about different types of medicine available for the child's illness

Outcome Identification and Planning

Planning the administration of medicine for children involves the same safe rules of administration as those for adults. Extra consideration is necessary at each step, however, because determining the right form and route of medicine such as liquid or capsule and oral or IM, varies so widely. Establishing a dose that is accurate for the size of the child can involve recalculating the dose using a milligram per kilogram formula, or a nomogram that shows body surface area. The schedule for administration must be not only one that is effective for the drug's action but also one that will not interfere with school activities, eating, or sleep.

Explain to children the effects that can be expected from any medicine. Be certain to give this explanation at an age-appropriate level, and be sure it is consistent with any prior explanation that a parent or other health care provider has supplied. The American Academy of Pediatrics (AAP) Web site (www.aap.org) offers information on general medicine administration and tips on how to read medicine labels, so is a useful site to recommend to parents.

Implementation

Medicine and IV interventions with children include both administering medicine to ill children as well as teaching parents and children how to continue to take the medicine when at home or at school. As long as the child is uncomfortable or has definite disease symptoms, parents tend to give medicine conscientiously. However, when symptoms fade, a child returns to school, or the family returns to its busy everyday schedule, it is easy for parents to forget to give medicine. This can leave children open to a recurrence of the condition or symptoms, such as pain or recurrent infection, because the organisms causing the illness were only suppressed, not killed. The classic example is strep throat—the child feels better, the medicine is stopped before completed, and, in the worst case scenario, rheumatic fever results, possibly causing damage to the heart valves (see Chapter 41). Helping parents fill out administration schedules to post in a readily visible location, such as on the refrigerator or a bathroom mirror, or leaving reminder messages on their smartphones can be as important as explaining the drug's action to help ensure all doses of medicine will be given.

Outcome Evaluation

Expected outcomes associated with medication administration should ensure that a child receives the medicine as prescribed and that the medicine has the desired effect. Specific examples suggesting outcome achievement include:

- Child states she understands she must continue to take thyroid hormone for a lifetime.
- Parents list the adverse effects of prescribed drug and state the telephone number they will call if adverse symptoms occur.
- Parents demonstrate the correct dose using the medication delivery device (oral syringe) that they will use at home.
- Adolescent describes an administration program that includes four doses daily but allows time for sports activities after school.
- Child agrees to allow IV therapy if it is inserted into his nondominant hand.
- Adolescent states he realizes his prescribed medicine is for his illness alone so it or other medicines in the family medicine cabinet are not to be shared with friends.

MEDICATION ADMINISTRATION

Medications in children are given by a variety of routes: orally, intranasally, transdermally, topically, rectally, and via injection (subcutaneous, intradermal, IM, IV, intraosseous, or epidural) or by inhalation. Epidural administration is described in Chapter 16 because this route is also frequently used with women in labor. Inhalation techniques are discussed in Chapter 40 with respiratory illnesses.

To administer drugs safely, it is important to have a good understanding of **pharmacokinetics**, or the way drugs are absorbed, distributed throughout the body, metabolized, inactivated, and excreted.

Pharmacokinetics in Children

The four basic processes of absorption, distribution, metabolism, and excretion determine the intensity and duration of a drug's action. The immaturity of body systems in children (and especially in newborns) plays a major role in drug action throughout each of these processes (Johnson & Rostami-Hodjegan, 2010).

Absorption

Drug **absorption** (the transfer of the drug from its point of entry in the body into the bloodstream) is influenced by the route of administration as well as by the concentration and acidity of the drug. Some routes of administration in children are limited and so are rarely used. For example, children younger than school age usually cannot hold tablets under their tongue for sublingual administration; they tend to swallow them instead. The small muscle size of young children limits sites for IM injection. Infants pull off transdermal patches because they do not understand they are important. The gastrointestinal system may be so immature at birth that gastrointestinal absorption can be ineffective. Vomiting and diarrhea, frequent symptoms of childhood illnesses, also interfere with absorption because a drug does not remain in the gastrointestinal tract long enough to be absorbed.

Distribution

Distribution refers to the movement of the drug through the bloodstream to a specific site of action. Children tend to have more fluid held in interstitial spaces and less in intracellular spaces than adults so drugs may not be distributed as quickly as in adults. Many drugs are distributed bound to serum albumin (which is manufactured by the liver), so adequate albumen must be present for the drug to reach its site of action. This binding action limits the amount of free drug in the circulation, thereby providing protection against toxic levels of a drug. As free drug is used, the bound drug is released to maintain a therapeutic level. Newborns with immature liver function may not have enough serum albumin to transport drugs readily. This is particularly true if elevated bilirubin levels are present, because bilirubin is also carried by serum albumin. Bound to serum albumin this way, bilirubin is harmless. In free form, however, it can leave the bloodstream and enter other body tissues. If it enters the brain cells, it destroys their ability to function (acute bilirubin encephalopathy). If a newborn who has a high level of bilirubin from destruction of fetal hemoglobin receives a drug such as a sulfonamide that competes for albumin binding sites, a large quantity of bilirubin may be left unbound and the infant may develop acute bilirubin encephalopathy or may not receive benefit from the sulfonamide because it cannot be carried to the infection site. In addition, newborns have sluggish peripheral circulation, so distribution to arms or legs in children this young may not be effective. Any child with cardiovascular disease also may have limited distribution of drugs because of general poor circulation.

Metabolism

Metabolism involves conversion of the drug into an active form (biotransformation) or into an inactive form (inactivation). Because a child's basic metabolic rate is faster than that of an adult, certain drugs are metabolized more rapidly in children. This means that the drug must be administered more frequently to a child to maintain effective drug levels than it would be in adults. Whether drugs are coadministered can also make a difference because this could cause the drugs to metabolize more quickly or more slowly than usual. Some drugs, such as the salicylates and chloramphenicol, are metabolized directly by liver enzymes. Because liver enzymes are not fully developed in newborns, these drugs cannot be metabolized and so can reach toxic levels rapidly. Older children with liver disease who have impaired liver enzymes also have a decreased ability to inactivate or transform drugs.

Excretion

Excretion (the elimination of raw drug or drug metabolites, a process that largely prevents properly administered drugs from becoming toxic) is potentially limited until about 12 months of age, when kidney function becomes mature. If a child has kidney disease, excretion potential is limited at any age. A few drugs, such as digitoxin, are excreted in bile. Most newborns have sluggish bile formation, so excretion of these drugs is questionable. Monitoring intake and output is important in children receiving drugs to be certain urine excretion or an outlet for drug metabolites is adequate.

QSEN Checkpoint Question 38.1

Informatics

After Terry receives an antibiotic, her body must distribute it to the site where it will act. Which assessment parameter addresses her body's ability to distribute a drug?

a. Terry's renal function
b. Terry's arterial blood gases
c. Terry's plasma protein levels
d. Terry's gallbladder function

Look in Appendix A for the best answer and rationale.

Adverse Drug Effects in Children

Children respond to drugs in much the same way as adults, but they may experience unique or exaggerated side effects because of immature liver function or rapid metabolism during periods of rapid growth. The newborn may suffer adverse effects from drugs taken by the mother prenatally or from drugs transferred in breast milk.

Safe Storage of Drugs

Because young children do not appreciate that overdoses of medicine can be serious and even fatal, they may help themselves to additional doses of medicine and poison themselves. This can occur with prescription medications, over-the-counter medication, and even alternative/complementary medications (Zuzak, Rauber-Luthy, & Simoes-West, 2010).

Adolescents can deliberately take extra doses of drugs such as steroids or pain medicine, hoping for an added effect. Oxycodone (OxyContin), for example, is an analgesic that may be prescribed for adolescents and also is frequently abused by them. Methylphenidate (Ritalin), administered to children with attention deficit hyperactivity disorder, is a second prescription drug that may also be frequently abused (Roux, Carrieri, Keijzer, et al., 2011).

Adults always need to be certain to store medicine in a safe place. Because poisoning from medicine is a frequent type of poisoning in preschool children, children's medicine—whether prescription, over-the-counter, or alternative/complimentary—should be secured in a *locked* and safe place.

In most homes, this is in a locked medicine cabinet or a locked drawer above the height their child can reach; a motivated toddler can climb so well that just placing medicines "out of reach" is not sufficient. Remind parents that most childhood poisonings occur when a family is under stress because, during these times, the family may forget usual procedures and leave medications unlocked or within reach. Be certain to teach parents that they should never take medicine in front of children; children may imitate this action with the parent's medication when the parents are out of sight. Another caution is not to pour or prepare medicine in the dark. Because almost all medicine bottles dispensed from local pharmacies look and feel the same, it is easy to pour the wrong liquid, extract the wrong pills, or read the bottle instructions incorrectly without adequate light.

Remember that these same rules apply in a health care setting. A toddler walking past a medicine cart at a hospital, for example, could easily remove a handful of pills and swallow them, thinking they are candy. For the same reason, never leave medicine on a bedside table for children to take later if they are playing a game or taking a shower because a nearby preschooler could take the medicine first.

The Safe Administration of Drugs

Administering drugs safely to children requires about 10 "rights"; in other words, that you first determine that you are giving the right drug (and right drug form) to the right child, in the right dosage and by the right route, at the right time for the right action. Afterward, you observe for the right response, and use the right documentation. You also need to ensure that the parents or child have the right information about the medicine.

Right Medicine/Right Drug Form

Most medication errors are made in situations where the number of medications being given is high and speed in administration is crucial. Intensive care units and emergency departments, therefore, are the highest areas at risk for medication errors, often because of interruptions during the medication administration process (Kalisch & Aebersold, 2010; Pham, Story, Hicks, et al., 2011). Errors can occur because prescribers may write a prescription using either generic or trade names. As the number of medicines available increases yearly, so does the possibility that two drugs will have similar names. These factors make the step in medicine administration of identifying that you have the correct drug in the correct form even more important than ever.

What if...38.1 Terry's father tells you Terry is such a "picky eater" that she rarely eats a full meal. When should he give Terry a medicine that should be taken with a meal?

Right Child

When asked what is their name, children cannot be depended on to reply with their correct name. Anxious to please, a preschooler will answer the question, "Are you Johnny Jones?" with "yes." He may also, however, agree with any other name you propose. School-age children who want to avoid taking a medicine may deny they are the person whose name you called. To prevent these types of errors, never ask children their names for identification. Instead, read their identification arm bands and compare them with the medication sheet or electronic record. In ambulatory care settings or homes, ask a parent to confirm the child's identity; to include the child, ask for their date of birth (or their age for younger children).

Right Dosage

The correct dosage of most drugs for children is based on weight-based dosing. However, for drugs such as chemotherapy, the dosage is based on a body surface area using a nomogram (Fig. 38.1). To calculate surface area using such a chart, find the child's height in the left column (e.g., 40 cm); next, find the child's weight in the right column (e.g., 20 kg). Hold a ruler or straightedge to connect the two points. The mark at which the ruler crosses the center column is the child's body surface area (e.g., 0.38 m^2). Before administering any medication to a child, confirm that the dose prescribed is correct for the child's weight or the child's body surface area. Take and record height and weight measurements conscientiously at health visits or on hospital admission (or daily, if

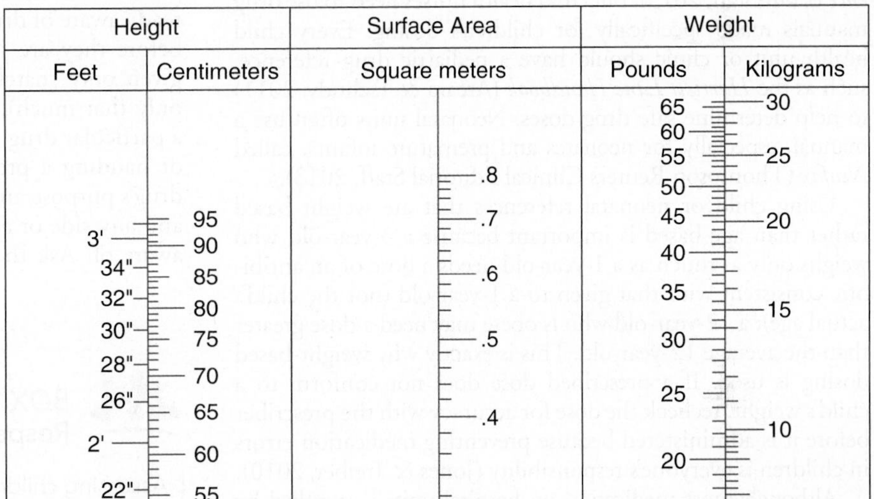

FIGURE 38.1 A nomogram to estimate body surface area. To use such a chart, draw a line from the child's height to the child's weight. The point at which it crosses the middle line is the child's surface area.

BOX 38.2 Nursing Care Planning Based on Responsibility for Pharmacology

To calculate a fractional drug dose use the formula:

$$\frac{\text{Strength Desired (D)}}{\text{Strength You Have (H)}} \times \frac{\text{Quantity Desired (QD)}}{\text{Quantity You Have (QH)}} = \text{Answer}$$

For example, you have a prescription for 90 mg acetaminophen. Acetaminophen is supplied as 125 mg drug in 5 ml liquid. Using the formula:

$$\frac{\text{90 mg (D)}}{\text{125 mg (H)}} \times \frac{\text{QD (what you are asking)}}{\text{5 ml (QH)}} = ?$$

Cross multiply: $125\ QD = 450(5 \times 90)$

Divide the number on the left by the number on the right: $450 \div 125 = 3.6$ ml (the amount you will need to administer).

important, during an admission) to obtain this information for dose calculation.

Adult patient providers often use the *Physicians' Desk Reference* (PDR Staff, 2013), but child health nurses need to use drug manuals made specifically for children's dosing. Every child health unit or clinic should have a pediatric drug reference, such as the *Harriett Lane Handbook* (Arcara & Tschudy, 2011) to help determine safe drug doses. Neonatal units often use a manual, especially for neonates and premature infants, called *Neofax* (Thompson Reuters Clinical Editorial Staff, 2013).

Using child or neonatal references that are weight based rather than age based is important because a 3-year-old who weighs only as much as a 1-year-old needs a dose of an antibiotic consistent with that given to a 1-year-old (not the child's actual age); a 12-year-old who is obese may need a dose greater than the average 12-year-old. This is exactly why weight-based dosing is used. If a prescribed dose does not conform to a child's weight, recheck the dose for accuracy with the prescriber before it is administered because preventing medication errors in children is everyone's responsibility (Jones & Treiber, 2010).

Although most medication on hospital units is supplied by the pharmacy in unit doses, nurses may still need to occasionally calculate fractional dosages (Box 38.2). When talking to parents about giving medicine, stress that if a medicine comes supplied with a dosing cap, it is best to use that to measure the correct dose (Pham et al., 2011). If there is no dosing cap, then an oral medicine syringe or dropper are the next best methods to measure liquid medicine because the "teaspoons" in their kitchen drawer are rarely exactly 5 ml. If they do not have any of these measuring devices, encourage them to use cooking measuring spoons for more accurate dosing (Yin, Mendelsohn, Wolf, et al., 2010).

Right Route and Time

Possible routes of administration for medicine in children are discussed in the following sections. Each of these methods requires special techniques, because most children do not enjoy taking medicine and need strong support during administration. Proper spacing of time between doses is also necessary for accurate medication uptake, but choosing the right time of day for parents to give medicine (e.g., planning doses for 11 PM and 7 AM instead of 8 PM and 4 AM) can positively impact the ability of a family to successfully complete the medication as prescribed.

Right Information and Documentation

Because so many medications are advertised directly today on television or in magazines, many parents and children are already aware of drug names and the action of individual drugs before they are prescribed. However, since they have been given only snatches of information (or listened to or read only that much), they also may have misconceptions about a particular drug. Be certain when giving medicine to a child or handing a prescription to a parent that you review the drug's purpose and action, when and how it should be taken, and any side or adverse effects the parent or child should be aware of. Ask them if they have any questions (Box 38.3).

BOX 38.3 Nursing Care Planning to Respect Cultural Diversity

Assessing children's attitudes about the worth or wisdom of medicine is important because attitudes are not consistent across cultures. Some families, for example, would rather depend on an herb or home remedy rather than a prescribed medicine. Because of this, a family may accept a prescription but then not fill it or administer the medicine. A herbal remedy they use may duplicate or counteract a prescribed medicine's effect. Socioeconomic factors effect medicine administration as well because medicine is expensive and difficult to afford for many families who do not have health insurance.

As part of health histories, always ask if a child commonly takes any type of herbal or home remedy or if the child has been given anything specific for the present illness. Because medicine is expensive, when discussing a prescription with parents, ask them if they think they will have any difficulty with obtaining or giving it, as well as assessing for the medicine's effect, or returning for a follow-up appointment to evaluate the medicine's effect. Such inquiries allow parents to say they have questions about the medicine or are uncertain whether they should give it because of a cultural belief.

Remember that people under stress do not "hear" well, so although the prescriber may have reviewed this same information with parents when the prescription was written, this may be the first time they actually hear it. Children as young as 5 or 6 years of age are able to identify adverse or side effects, so be certain your explanation of drug action includes them as well (de Maria, Lussier, & Bajcar, 2011). Correct documentation assures other health care providers that a drug was administered and allows for continuity of care (Elliott & Liu, 2010).

QSEN Checkpoint Question 38.2

Safety

Suppose you are going to give acetaminophen (Tylenol) to Terry in the emergency department and she has no ID band currently in place. What would be the best way to identify her?

a. Ask her to tell you what her name is.
b. Tell her you need to know her name.
c. Ask a parent to identify her for you.
d. Ask to see her school student card.

Look in Appendix A for the best answer and rationale.

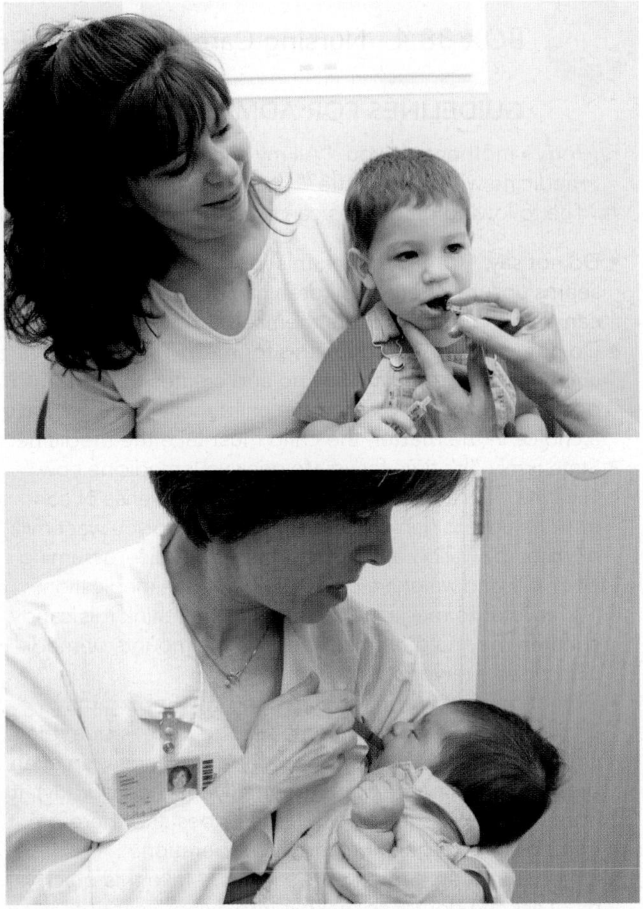

FIGURE 38.2 To administer oral medicine with a syringe, place the medicine at the side of the child's mouth. Note that infants should be positioned at least at a 45-degree angle.

Oral Administration

Children younger than 9 years of age often have difficulty swallowing tablets. For children younger than 3 years of age, it is virtually impossible. Most oral medication for young children, therefore, is furnished in liquid, chewable, or melt-away forms (El-Alfy, Sari, Lee, et al., 2010).

In infants, oral medication can be given with a medicine dropper or a unit dose syringe (without a needle). Never give medicine with the child lying completely flat; otherwise, a child could choke and aspirate. Instead, gently restrain the child's arms and head by holding the child against your body with the head raised. A crying child is already opening his or her mouth for you; otherwise, gently open the mouth by pressing on the child's chin. Be certain the end of the syringe or dropper rests at the side of the infant's mouth to help prevent aspiration (Fig. 38.2). Press the bulb of the medicine dropper or use the plunger of the syringe so that the fluid flows slowly into the side of the child's mouth. An infant also may be given fluid from a small glass or spoon. Allow the fluid to flow a little at a time so that the child has time to swallow between small sips. Because oral solutions are pleasantly flavored, most infants resist the first drop but then suck the remainder of the medicine into their mouth.

Even though the medicine tastes good, the firm pressure used in giving medicine to infants may cause them to be frightened afterward. Take the time to sit and comfort (or let a parent do this) after giving medication. These actions are as important as checking the correct dosage of the drug because protecting a child's mental health is as important as protecting the child's physical health.

Preschoolers and early school-age children respond well to rewards such as stickers that they can paste into a book each time they take their medicine. For older children, hand them the glass of medicine or a tablet alongside a glass of fluid as if you expect them to take it (Box 38.4). If a child has difficulty swallowing tablets, they can possibly be crushed and added to a teaspoonful of applesauce or a flavored syrup. If pills are not to be chewed (e.g., capsules, enteric-coated tablets), be certain to tell the child not to chew them.

Some children may be old enough to swallow tablets but have never done it before. To let them practice learning how to do this, give them small bits of ice to use for practice; these melt rapidly and so do not stick in the back of the throat or esophagus. Tell the child to put the ice on the back of the tongue, tip the head slightly to the side, take a sip of water, and swallow the water. Give generous praise for learning this new skill. Some people suggest using easily dissolved chocolate candy for practice but you don't want to suggest medicine is the same as candy so ice or small sections of tofu (which also dissolves easily) are better to use.

Another useful technique to help a child swallow pills is to push them into a teaspoonful of ice cream or pudding. Children tend not to chew this type of food; rather, as they swallow the pudding, they also swallow the pill. If using this technique, push the pill into the ice cream or pudding in front of the child so it's obvious what you're doing. The intent is not to hide the pill or fool the child, but to help the child learn to swallow the medicine (Box 38.5).

BOX 38.4 Nursing Care Planning to Empower a Family

GUIDELINES FOR ADMINISTERING ORAL MEDICATION

Q. Terry's mother tells you, "All my children fight me anytime they need to take medicine. How can I get them to take medicine without a battle?"

A. The following guidelines can often help make the task a bit easier:

- Do not say, "*Can* you drink this for me?" If an adult seems unsure whether children can do a task, children can develop grave doubts themselves.
- Do not say, "*Will* you drink this for me?" This leaves a child the opportunity to say no and creates the awkward position of having to admit the child really does not have a choice in the matter; the child must take the medicine.
- State firmly, "It's time for you to drink your medicine now." Give the child a secondary choice to allow a sense of control: "It's time to drink your medicine now; do you want milk or water to swallow after it?" is a suitable choice, assuming both milk and water are compatible with the medication.
- Never refer to medicine as candy. If they think it is candy, children may help themselves to fatal amounts of medicine when everyone's back is turned.
- Do not bribe children to take medicine. Bribing may work for one dose, but when a second dose is due, the child will ask for a bigger bribe; for a third dose, an even bigger one. At some point (generally reached quickly), it is impossible to supply such large bribes and therefore it is impossible to gain the child's cooperation.
- Do not threaten. Statements such as, "Take this quickly or I'll ask the doctor to make it into a shot" cannot be followed through. The child calls the bluff (many medicines do not come in a form that can be injected intramuscularly), and once more the child is in control. A statement such as, "Take this or I'll call your doctor" is also unfair (the physician has been made the villain) and ultimately undermines your authority (you must not have much power, or you would not need help).
- Children expect honesty from adults; therefore, do not lie about the taste of medicine. If in doubt about the taste, taste it (with the obvious exception of drugs such as digoxin). Most children's medicines are artificially flavored with raspberry, orange, or cherry syrup, so they do not taste bad.
- If a medicine tastes bitter, mix it with a spoonful of strained applesauce or a teaspoonful of flavored syrup. Do not mix medicine with a full jar of baby food, because the child will then have to eat the entire jar of food to get all of the medicine. As a rule, encourage children to take liquid medicine straight, then follow it with a pleasant-tasting drink to take away any bitter taste.
- If a medicine is supplied in tablet form, you could crush or dissolve it in with syrup or applesauce for a better taste if appropriate. Be certain before removing the particles from a capsule that the medicine will work properly when not in capsule form: some are encapsulated to keep them from dissolving in the stomach and to bring them into the intestine, where they have a therapeutic effect. The same precaution must be followed when giving enteric-coated tablets.
- Never leave medicine by a child's bed or chair for the child to take "in a minute" or "after your shower." The child may become involved with another activity "in a minute" and will not take it, or a smaller child could find the medicine appealing and swallow it.

BOX 38.5 Nursing Care Planning Based on Effective Communication

You want to give acetaminophen (Tylenol) to Terry, 8 years old, to help relieve her pain.

Less Effective Communication

Nurse: I have your medicine, Terry. Swallow these for me?
Terry: No. My ankle is too sore.
Nurse: If you don't swallow them, I'll have to give you medicine that tastes even worse.
Terry: That's okay. If it helps my ankle.
Nurse: Well, I can't do that. This is the medicine you have to take.
Terry: Then I'm not going to take it.

More Effective Communication

Nurse: I have your medicine, Terry. Swallow these for me.
Terry: No. My ankle is too sore.
Nurse: That's why I want you to swallow the pills. It'll take away the hurt.
Terry: I'd rather get a shot, my ankle is so sore.
Nurse: This type of medicine has to be swallowed. Do you want orange juice or soda pop to drink with them?
Terry: Soda pop.
Nurse: Good. Take a big swallow and they'll be gone.

The nurse in the first scenario makes some important medication administration errors: first, he *asks* the child if she will swallow the tablets rather than *telling* her to swallow them; second, he threatens the child; even worse, he threatens with a measure he cannot enforce (acetaminophen is the only medicine prescribed). When the child refuses the request and contradicts his threat, he is left powerless. A better approach is shown in the second scenario. Here, the nurse explains the advantage of taking the medicine and conveys that he expects cooperation. Allowing a secondary choice, such as a choice of beverage, offers the child a sense of control, but does not allow her to say no to the primary request.

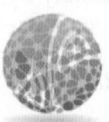

QSEN Checkpoint Question 38.3

Teamwork & Collaboration

Although Terry is 8 years old, she doesn't know how to swallow pills. If you needed to delegate the administration of an oral medication to a licensed practical nurse, what instruction would you provide to your colleague?

a. "Draw a picture of a child swallowing medicine and talk about it."
b. "Tell the child that all medicine tastes sweet so she'll take it readily."
c. Give the child a small ice chip to use to practice swallowing."
d. "Tip the child's head forward to avoid the possibility of choking."

Look in Appendix A for the best answer and rationale.

Intranasal Administration

Because nasal drops and sprays are easy to administer, more medications are supplied in these forms every year (Wolfe & Braude, 2010). Having someone drop medicine into the nose can feel very uncomfortable for a child, however, so from a child's perspective, these can be very frightening. Tell the child that you understand the medicine may feel odd, but it is important to help the child get better. Explain what you are going to do by a statement such as: "I'm going to place two drops of medicine into your nose. Then I want you to sniff for me [demonstrate]. Then I'll put two drops into the other side of your nose and I want you to sniff again. And then we're done."

Turn the child or ask the child to turn onto his or her back. A school-age child can extend the head over the side of the bed so that it is lower than the trunk. Preschoolers generally are too frightened by this strange position and do better with a pillow under their shoulders so that their head extends over the pillow and rests downward. Infant may need to be restrained in a mummy restraint for nose drop administration if they struggle to keep the syringe or dropper away from their nose (see Chapter 37 for a discussion of appropriate restraints).

Instill the appropriate number of drops into one nostril. Turn the child's head to the side—to the left after the left nostril, to the right after the right nostril—so that the medicine stays in the nose longer. If the child is a preschooler or older, ask him or her to further "sniff" the medicine so that it goes far back into their nose. If a child gets up immediately, the medicine will flow out and will be less effective. Therefore, have the child remain in the head-flat position for at least 1 minute to be certain the medicine remains in contact with the mucous membrane of the nose. Give children high praise even if they did not cooperate well because it lets children know that you understand how hard it was for them to stay still while the medicine was instilled.

Children over about age 6 years can use nasal sprays competently after they have been introduced to the technique. Acknowledge that spraying a liquid into the nose is uncomfortable because it tickles or causes a sneezing sensation. Have the child sit or stand upright, hold the spray bottle upright with the tip just inside one side of the nose, and gently squeeze the spray bottle. In most instances, a child should then tip the head to the side (the right side for the right nostril, the left side for the left nostril) or sniff, depending on the bottle instructions, for best absorption. The administration is then repeated for the second nostril. Stress that although this form of medication administration seems simple and "fun," drugs are well absorbed across the nasal mucosa so this route is an effective means of drug administration and can be a route for important and even life-sustaining drugs. Spray bottles should be individually prescribed for children and should not be used by any other child to prevent the spread of disease organisms. Because influenza vaccine is now supplied in this form, in the near future, children will be more familiar with this route of medicine administration and, hopefully, less resistant to the method (Flood, Ryan, Rousculp, et al., 2011).

Ophthalmic Administration

Eye medications, in particular, antibiotics to treat eye infections, are administered by being dropped into the conjunctival sac of the eye (Wong & Nischal, 2010). This type of administration, like nose drops, is frightening for children because they have been warned many times never to put anything into their eyes. Also, children know that getting something such as dust in their eye can be very painful. As a result, infants and preschoolers generally must be restrained in a mummy restraint for eye drop administration. Always explain what you are going to do and that the medicine will not hurt (assuming that is true). Place the child on his or her back. Open the eyes of infants and preschoolers by gently but firmly pressing on the lower lid with the thumb and on the upper lid with the index finger. A school-age child or adolescent will open their eyes cooperatively, but you may need to rest a hand on the eyelid to keep the eye open long enough for the drug to be administered (Fig. 38.3). Be certain your fingernails are cut short to avoid scratching the child's cornea.

Instill the correct number of drops into the conjunctiva of the lower lid. Allow the eyelid to close. Avoid placing the drops directly on the cornea, because that can be painful. To prevent the conjunctiva from drying, do not hold the eyelids apart any longer than necessary. After the child has blinked two or three times, allow the child to get up. Give praise for their cooperation even if cooperation was not evident; the child accomplished a major feat by allowing you to touch and invade their eyes in this way.

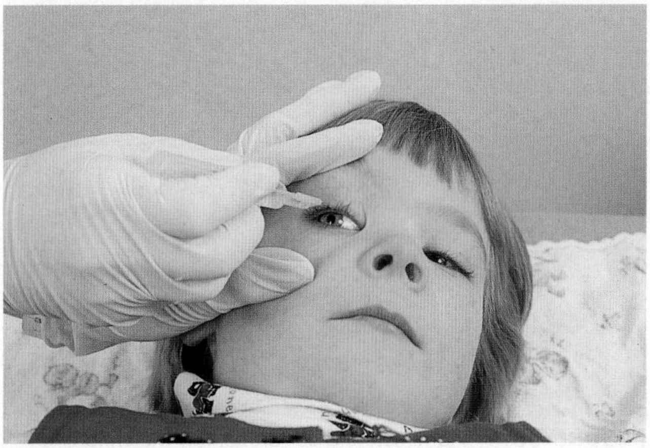

FIGURE 38.3 Administering eye drops.

To instill an ophthalmic ointment, apply a fine line of the ointment along the inside rim of the conjunctival sac, working from the inner to the outer eye canthus. Always work from the inner to the outer canthus because if the eye is pus filled, applying medication under pressure toward the midline could force pus across to the other eye or down into the lacrimal duct. Eye medicine should be individually prescribed and not used by other children because if even the tip of the dropper or tube touches the conjunctival sac, it is contaminated with body fluid and any germs that were there.

Otic Administration

Otic administration refers to administering medicine, primarily drops, into the ear canal. Like other forms of medicine, this is difficult for children to accept because they have been told many times not to put anything into their ears. Also, because ear drops are generally administered for an earache, which is sharp, excruciating pain, a child may worry having medicine put into the ear will make the pain even worse. In addition, a child cannot watch what is happening (which is always frightening). Assuming that you have been honest with the child up to this point, remind the child, "Remember how I told you the injection would hurt a little? Well, if this would hurt, I'd tell you now, too. But this doesn't hurt." Remind the child that ear drops can feel odd, however, as if someone were tickling their ear.

Ear drops must always be used at room temperature or warmed slightly because cold fluid, such as medication taken from a refrigerator, does cause pain and may also cause severe vertigo as it touches the tympanic membrane.

Turn the child or ask the child to turn onto his or her back, or use a mummy restraint as necessary for an infant. Turn the child's head to one side (Fig. 38.4). The slant of the ear canal in children is shown in Chapter 50. If the child is younger than 2 years of age, straighten the external ear canal by pulling the pinna down and back. If the child is older than 2 years of age, pull the pinna of the ear up and back. Instill the specified number of drops into the ear canal. Hold the child's head in the sideways position while you count to 60 to ensure the medication fills the entire ear canal. Praise the child for cooperating during such a difficult procedure.

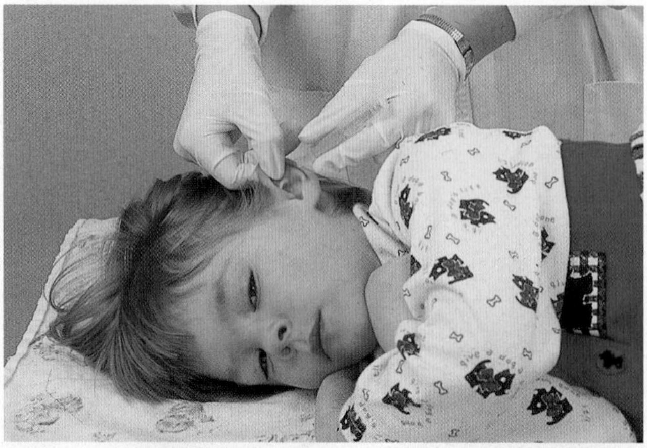

FIGURE 38.4 Administering ear drops. For the child over 2 years old of age, the pinna of the ear is pulled up and back.

Rectal Administration

A good route for administering medication to children who are having a seizure or who are unconscious is by rectal insertion, because this not only allows a drug to be absorbed across the mucous membrane of the intestine but also avoids the danger of aspiration (de Haan, van der Geest, Doelman, et al., 2010). Rectal administration may also be used to give a drug such as Tylenol to young children who refuse to swallow oral medicine or to those who are vomiting. Most children, however, rate this as the least desirable method for receiving medication because of privacy issues, so it is not a major route of administration. Absorption rates also vary widely, so dosing is inconsistent and this is not a route preferred by most health care providers.

Some medications given by this route are administered by rectal suppository; a few are given by retention enema. Because the child cannot see what is happening with rectal administration, a child can be easily frightened by this procedure. Show the child the medication so the child can be certain that it is not an injection. Having been honest with the child up to this point is helpful again: "If it were anything else, I would tell you so."

Many suppositories are supplied already lubricated. If not, add a drop of water-based lubricant such as K-Y Jelly to the tip. Use a glove and insert the suppository gently but quickly beyond the rectal sphincters (approximately 0.5 in. or as far as the first knuckle of your little finger for infants, and approximately 1 in. or as far as the first knuckle of your index finger for older children). Withdraw your finger and press the child's buttocks together firmly for a count of approximately 10, or until the child's urge to evacuate the suppository passes.

If the medication is to be administered by a retention enema to a young child, use usual enema technique, but with as small an amount of fluid as possible so the child can retain it. Press the child's buttocks firmly together for approximately 15 seconds after administering the enema or a child will expel the solution almost immediately and the medicine will be lost. Using a distraction technique, such as asking the child to count backward or to say the alphabet backward, are ways to help a defecation reflex to pass. Remember, any invasive procedure is particularly threatening to a preschooler. Give lavish praise for cooperation.

What if . . . 38.2 Terry's mother tells you her child's school has a "no drug" policy, so Terry will not be able to take her oral antibiotic at school. What would you advise her to do?

Transdermal/Topical Administration

Children who have a skin irritation or who need medicine to relieve itching or dryness may have topical creams or lotions prescribed. Most children accept this type of application well because the medicine seems easy to apply and brings about almost immediate relief. Children as young as toddlers can help apply this type of medicine with your supervision. Be certain they wash their hands afterward so they do not lick any extra off their fingers and inadvertently take it orally.

Several children's medicines are available by transdermal patch, because absorption of drugs through the skin can be yet another effective and pain-free route for administration. Be certain the child's skin is dry and intact at the site where the patch will be applied. Apply a patch over the trunk or a

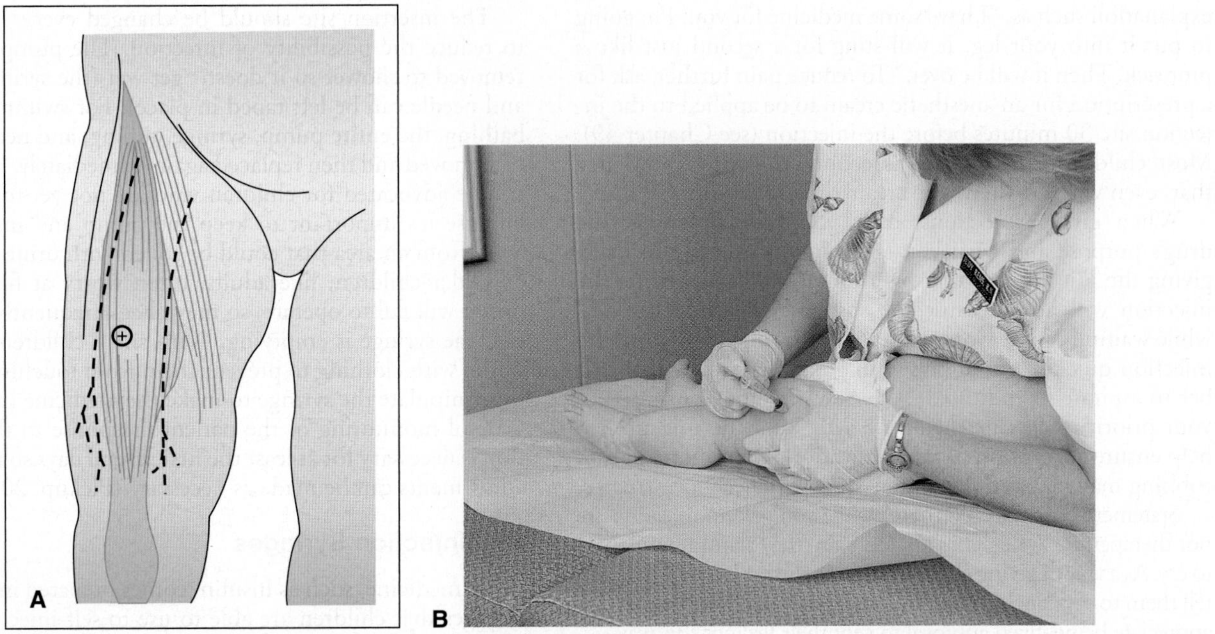

FIGURE 38.5 **(A)** For infants under walking age, use the vastus lateralis muscle for intramuscular injections. **(B)** The technique for administering an intramuscular injection to an infant. Note the way the nurse uses her body to restrain and stabilize the infant.

major muscle, not on distal extremities, for best absorption. Assess the skin under the patch every time a patch is changed to be certain the site is not becoming irritated because an irritated site might cause more than usual absorption. If possible, change the site every time a new patch is applied to decrease the possibility of irritation to the skin from the patch.

Young children tend to remove transdermal patches the same as they do Band-Aids because of normal curiosity about what is underneath. Putting clothes on the young child immediately so the patch is out of sight is helpful. Assess infants carefully to be certain they have not pulled off the patch and are chewing on it as this can lead to drug toxicity. Be certain as well that patches applied to children wearing diapers are not placed where a leaking diaper could wet the patch and irritate the skin or dilute the medicine.

Intramuscular and Subcutaneous Administration

IM injections are rarely prescribed for children admitted to the hospital because many children do not have sufficient muscle mass for easy deposition of medication, and they are also painful. However, IM injections may be used in an emergency department and are commonly used for immunization. For IM injections in infants, the mandatory site for administration is the vastus lateralis muscle of the anterior thigh (Fig. 38.5). Use the lateral aspect rather than the medial portion because this site is not as tender and should cause less pain. Using the gluteal muscle in children younger than 1 year of age is extremely hazardous because this muscle does not develop until a child walks. This means the sciatic nerve occupies a larger portion of the area than later on and could be permanently damaged by gluteal injections. Figure 38.5 shows an effective restraining technique for giving injections to infants. In older children, as in adults, the deltoid muscle (Fig. 38.6A) or a ventrogluteal site (see Fig. 38.6B) should be used.

Never give injections to children who are sleeping, even if they are infants, in the hope they will not wake up and notice what is happening because they will wake up and will be terrified at being attacked. Instead, always give a short explanation of what you are about to do to a child or play with the baby until they are awake and aware. Be honest about the pain involved; try to describe it accurately so that the child knows it has limits (a small amount of pain for a short time) with an

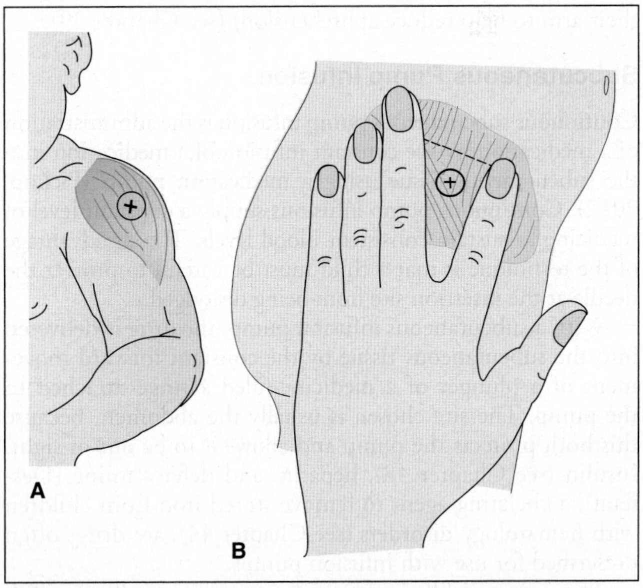

FIGURE 38.6 Sites for intramuscular injection. **(A)** In older children, the deltoid muscle is an acceptable site. **(B)** A ventrogluteal site may also be used in older children. Place the heel of the hand on the greater trochanter and the index finger angled toward the child's anterosuperior iliac crest, spreading the middle finger along the crest posteriorly. The triangle formed by the space between the index and middle fingers is the correct site.

explanation such as, "I have some medicine for you. I'm going to put it into your leg. It will sting for a second just like a pinprick. Then it will be over." To reduce pain further, ask for a prescription for an anesthetic cream to be applied to the injection site 30 minutes before the injection (see Chapter 39). Most children react well to injections if you acknowledge that, even with an anesthetic cream, injections can still hurt.

When giving injections, once you have described the drug's purpose and what you are going to do, do not delay giving the injection further by elaborating on how little the injection will hurt because the suspense the child can feel while waiting can be worse than the actual injection. Give the injection quickly, but always with good technique. Remember to aspirate (if indicated). Quickness counts, but safety is your priority. Massage the area briefly after the injection to help ensure absorption of the medication, but remember that rubbing may be painful and may be experienced as intrusive.

Statements such as "Don't cry" while you give an injection are not therapeutic. When children feel pain, they should be allowed to cry. As a way of giving children a better sense of control, you can tell them to say "ouch" when the needle is inserted. Most children appreciate being given approval to vent their feelings this way.

If necessary, ask for help in restraining a child when giving an injection to ensure safe administration. Evaluate children individually, however, because school-age children may be proud they are able to lie still and being restrained would shame them. Always hold and comfort a young child after all painful procedures or let a parent do it after an injection.

Record the site of any injection as well as the medication injected, so that sites can be rotated for better absorption. For subcutaneous immunizations, use the same injection sites, the lateral aspect of the thigh or upper arm, and inject the vaccine at a 45-degree angle.

If children are going to receive a series of injections, you can teach them distraction techniques such as imagery (e.g., thinking of the needle as a long thin rocket ship landing on their arm to help reduce apprehension) (see Chapter 39).

Subcutaneous Pump Infusion

Continuous subcutaneous pump infusion is the administration of a medication by the constant infusion of a medication into the subcutaneous tissue using a medication pump (Pickup, 2012). Continuous pump infusions supply a constant level of medicine to sustain consistent blood levels. The disadvantage of the technique is that a child must be careful to protect the needle at the insertion site from being dislodged.

With a subcutaneous infusion pump, the drug is delivered into the subcutaneous tissue by the constant forward movement of a plunger of a medicine-filled syringe attached to the pump. The site chosen is usually the abdomen, because this both protects the pump and allows it to be out of sight. Insulin (see Chapter 48), heparin, and deferoxamine (Desferal), a chelating agent to remove stored iron from children with hematology disorders (see Chapter 44), are drugs often prescribed for use with infusion pumps.

The syringe is filled with medicine, and a small tube with the needle attached at the distal end is attached to the hub of the syringe. The syringe is then clamped to the pump, the skin site is cleaned with alcohol, and the needle is inserted at a 45-degree angle (the usual subcutaneous insertion technique). As soon as the needle is taped in place, the pump is turned on (see Chapter 20, Fig. 20.5).

The insertion site should be changed every 1 to 2 days to reduce the possibility of infection. The pump should be removed to shower so it doesn't get wet (the syringe, tubing, and needle can be left taped in place). For swimming or tub bathing, the entire pump, syringe, tubing, and needle should be removed and then replaced again immediately. Pumps may not be advocated for children who are not yet toilet trained because it's important to keep the pump and insertion site away from an area that could be soiled with urine or stool.

Older children, like adults, often worry at first that the pump will fail to operate, so they check frequently to be certain the syringe is emptying. With small children, cover the pump with clothing to prevent them from touching or trying to manipulate the syringe to make the medicine infuse faster. Careful monitoring of the patient's response to the medication is necessary for at least the first several days so that dosage adjustments can be made as necessary (Pickup, 2012).

Autoinjection Syringes

Some medicine, such as insulin, comes prepared in autoinject syringes that children are able to use to self-inject as soon as they are about 5 or 6 years old. Such injectable syringes have advantages in that they are prefilled with the correct amount of medicine, and the needle is small and the spring that causes the needle to inject the medication acts so quickly that the injection is almost painless. You may need to remind preschool children not to play with the syringe or school-age children not to use it as a weapon against their friends or they could unintentionally inject their thumb with the medicine. The use of EpiPens, which are filled with epinephrine (used to counteract anaphylactic reactions to allergens), is described in Chapter 42.

QSEN Checkpoint Question 38.4
Quality Improvement

Suppose Terry, 8 years old, needs to have ear drops administered. If you consult the unit's policies and procedures, you should expect what directive?

a. Have the child self-administer the drops to give the child a sense of control.
b. Refrigerate the drug for at least 30 minutes so it numbs the ear canal.
c. Pull the pinna of the child's ear down to straighten the canal.
d. Keep the child's head turned to the side to help retain the drops.

Look in Appendix A for the best answer and rationale.

INTRAVENOUS THERAPY

In the past, IV therapy was used extensively as a rapid means of hydrating children who had become dehydrated because of diarrhea. Today, oral rehydration therapy is most often used in this way (Passariello, Terrin, de Marco, et al., 2011). IV therapy is a fast and effective means of maintaining a fluid and electrolyte balance, producing therapeutic levels of drugs in the body quickly, to provide nutritional support and offer blood or blood product replacement, however, so it still has a common place in children's care. The amount, type, and rate of IV fluids for children are prescribed carefully to prevent fluid overload. IV fluid may be infused into a peripheral vein, a central venous access device, or a peripherally inserted central venous catheter.

Despite its common use, IV therapy with children is not without problems. Because children move about a great deal and tend to remove bandages, all IV access sites must be assessed at least hourly for signs of infiltration. With movement, peripheral IV catheters can poke through fragile veins, central access devices can become dislodged, and ports can disconnect from the internal tubing, especially with the activity level of some of the most playful children. When carefully inspecting sites, assume things are not all right or "go looking for trouble," because it is better to err on the side of caution in order to notice any swelling or disconnected port quickly.

Infection is another problem associated with IV access. If a line becomes infected, it usually must be removed, which may involve surgery for a centrally placed device. To avoid infection, insertion sites must be changed using a sterile technique as well as be carefully monitored. Keeping an IV site wrapped with something such as Kling gauze may help protect a curious toddler from removing the dressing and disrupting the site.

Determining Fluid and Caloric Needs of the Child

IV fluid administered to children and infants must be isotonic (exerts the same osmotic pressure as their bloodstream) to prevent the destruction of red blood cells or the development of water intoxication. The use of isotonic fluid prevents fluid shifting from the bloodstream into interstitial tissue (as would happen if the IV fluid were hypotonic) or fluid shifting from interstitial tissue into the bloodstream (as would happen if the IV fluid were hypertonic). A 0.9% normal saline is the IV fluid most commonly used in children because it is isotonic (Neville, Sandemann, Rubenstein, et al., 2010). Dextrose 10% in 0.9% sodium chloride is an example of a hypertonic solution that might be used to cause fluid to shift into the bloodstream to relieve cerebral edema for a child with a head injury.

It is important to understand the principles of IV therapy, including the fluid and caloric needs of children (which differ significantly from those of the adult) so you can act as a second level of protection against overhydration, underhydration, or electrolyte imbalances such as hyponatremia (Hanna & Saberi, 2010).

Table 38.1 shows a typical method of calculating fluid requirements for children. Fluids administered using this table should ideally contain at least 5% dextrose, 0.9% saline, and 20 mEq potassium per liter so nutrients for energy and electrolytes are also replaced. For example, according to Table 38.1, a child weighing 45 kg would need 2,000 ml of a maintenance solution. A flow rate would be calculated for this amount (2,000 ml fluid in 24 hours = 83 ml/hr).

TABLE 38.1 Calculating Fluid Requirements for Children

Body Weight	Fluid Requirement per 24 Hours
Up to 10 kg	100 ml/kg
11–20 kg	1,000 ml + 50 ml/kg for each additional kilogram over 10 kg
More than 20 kg	1,500 ml + 20 ml/kg for each additional kilogram over 20 kg

Obtaining Venous Access

The needle size for IV therapy varies depending on the solution and the rate at which it will be administered. Commonly used needle sizes include 22 gauge, 24 gauge, 25 gauge, or 27 gauge in newborns. "Butterfly" needles (also termed "scalp vein needles" because they were originally designed for use in infant scalp veins) are metal needles with a flange of plastic added on both sides of the needle hub to give the person starting the infusion a wider surface to grasp, thereby making it easier to guide needle placement. A length of narrow tubing leads from the needle to the fluid administration tubing, which must be flushed with IV solution before the needle is inserted to avoid an air embolus.

Sites frequently used for IV insertion in young children or infants include the veins on the dorsal surface of the hand or on the flexor surface of the wrist. Leg and foot veins also may be used. In infants, another site is a scalp vein over the temporal area. Seeing IV fluid infusing into a scalp vein can be frightening for parents because it looks like a much more serious procedure than an infusion administered into a hand. You can explain to parents that scalp vein infusion is just another site to use to administer fluid or medicine to infants and ultimately might cause the least discomfort for their child because needles there do not infiltrate readily (Box 38.6). If any hair will be shaved away to place such a needle, be certain to save the hair for the parents, because this may be baby's first "haircut."

Preschoolers and older children often express a preference regarding where they want an infusion inserted. Offer a choice, if possible, or suggest the nondominant hand. Act as the child's advocate and see that wishes are respected.

Children who have IV infusions for long periods may require the placement of an **intracath** (a slim, pliable catheter threaded into a vein). The advantage of this type of device is that it cannot be dislodged as easily as a normally inserted IV needle, allowing a child the ability to move about more freely.

For all children (including adolescents), IV infusions are usually secured in place with at least a small arm board. Although children may say they will be careful not to move their arms, without an arm board, it is easy to move unintentionally to turn off the television set or reach for something that fell off the bed and accidentally dislodge the needle. Tape a board to the arm of an older child with the words, "This is just to remind you to keep your arm still", an explanation that is more acceptable than if children think you doubt their ability to hold their hands still.

Determining the Rate and Amount of Fluid Administration

Because children's hearts and circulatory systems are smaller than those of adults, IV fluid must be infused at a slower rate to keep the child's cardiovascular system from becoming quickly overloaded. Therefore, just as in medication administration, supervising the amount of solution infused is

BOX 38.6 Nursing Care Planning Using Procedures

INITIATING A SCALP VEIN INFUSION IN AN INFANT

Purpose: To provide a route for intravenous therapy

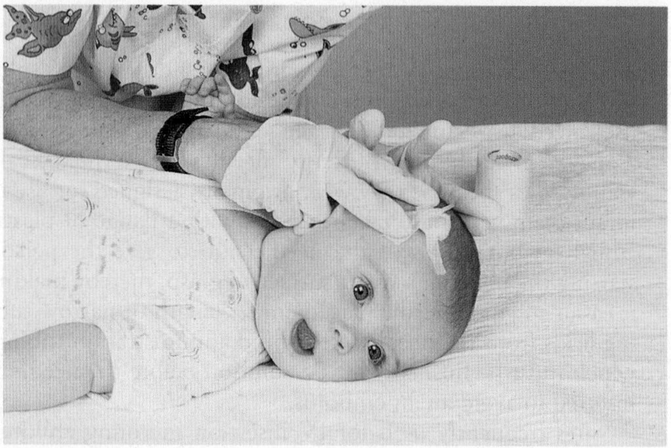

PROCEDURE	PRINCIPLE
1. Apply an anesthetic cream to the chosen site.	1. An anesthetic cream decreases discomfort.
2. In about 30 minutes (the time for the anesthetic cream to take effect), adequately restrain the infant using a mummy restraint.	2. Restraining the infant promotes safety. Trying to hold the infant's arms and legs still without a restraint can be exhausting.
3. Press the child's head to the side and hold it firmly in that position, with one hand on the occiput and the other securing the front of the head. Be certain the hand resting over the child's face does not obstruct the child's breathing.	3. This positions the child without interfering with respirations.
4. Lather the site over the temporal bone with a cleaning solution and carefully shave the hair. Ask parents if they want to save the clippings of hair if it is their child's first haircut. Assure them the hair will grow back in quickly.	4. The cleaning solution potentially reduces the possibility of nicks to the scalp. Hair removal allows a clear view of the insertion site and possibly reduces the risk of infection.
5. Place a rubber band around the infant's head at the level of the forehead.	5. A tourniquet is needed to dilate scalp veins.
6. Wash the shaved area with an antiseptic solution.	6. Washing the scalp further reduces the possibility of infection.
7. Insert a special small scalp vein needle or polytetrafluoroethylene (Teflon) catheter into a vein on her temple.	7. Use of an appropriate insertion device establishes a fluid route.
8. Continue to hold the infant firmly until the needle is securely taped in place and until satisfied the infusion is running well.	8. Securing the infant and device ensures an effective insertion site.
9. Cover the infusion needle with a piece of gauze (a plastic protector taped onto the site provides additional protection).	9. Covering the site keeps the infant from brushing the needle out of place when the infant turns her head.
10. If necessary, pin the shirt sleeves of the baby to the sides of the diaper or use a trunk or jacket restraint to prevent the infant from touching the insertion site.	10. Pinning the shirt keeps the infant from brushing at the site. Using restraints also prevents the infant from turning over.
11. Spend some time comforting the child, talking and smiling or lightly touching and stroking. Many infants enjoy sucking a pacifier or a bottle of glucose water during or after painful procedures; being held and rocked is the best comfort.	11. The infant may be frightened by the pinprick of the needle insertion, as well as by having been held so firmly for a length of time.

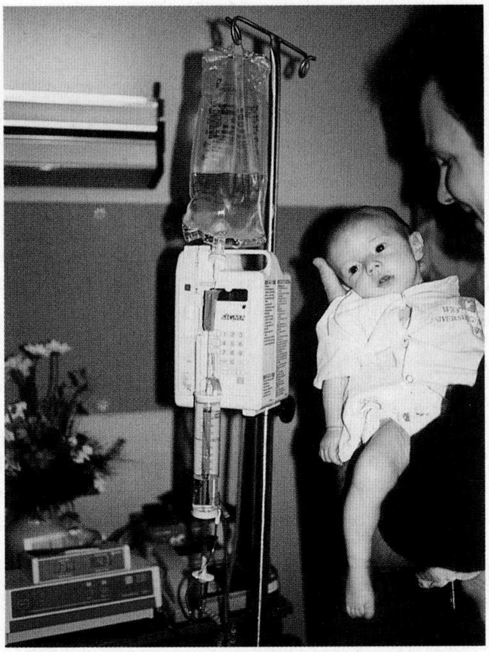

FIGURE 38.7 An infusion pump and calibrated infusion chamber are safety features used with children's intravenous infusions.

critical. Automatic rate-flow infusion pumps are mandatory when giving potent medications and always for small children because they regulate the flow accurately to a few drops per minute (Fig. 38.7). Overloading of IV fluid in infants and children can also be prevented by use of fluid chambers, devices that allow only 50 to 100 ml of fluid into the drip chamber at a time. With these in place, even if the pump fails, only the amount of fluid in the drip chamber will be allowed to enter the child's circulation, not the entire contents of the bag suspended above the child's head.

A third fluid safety measure is the use of a minidropper, a device that reduces the size of the drop in the control chamber to 60 drops per ml (in adult administration sets, there are 10 to 15 drops per ml). With an adult dropper in place, an infusion regulated to administer 30 ml/hr drops at a rate of 7 or 8 drops per minute, thus making it difficult to regulate. With a minidropper in place, the drops are smaller, so the same infusion (still providing the same amount of fluid per hour) drops at 30 drops per minute. This flow is easier to regulate and provides more accurate IV administration.

Keep a careful record of both the rate and amount of IV fluid administered to guard against fluid overload. At least once an hour, record the type and amount of fluid; the rate of flow (including the number of drops per minute); and, for a cross-check, the amount of fluid remaining in the pediatric IV fluid chamber. Signs of fluid overload are those of congestive heart failure and include increased pulse rate and blood pressure. As the heart becomes overwhelmed by excessive fluid, blood pressure falls and signs of edema develop. In addition to observing for changes in vital signs such as these, assess the specific gravity of urine at least every 4 hours to detect extremely dilute urine (specific gravity under 1.003), which suggests that the child is excreting a large quantity of fluid in an effort to reduce overloaded circulating volume.

It is difficult for children to lie still and wait for an IV infusion to finish (see Box 38.7, an interprofessional care map for a child receiving intravenous medication). Try to provide children with quiet activities that will not interfere with the infusion. If a child will have medicine administration daily, help the child plan a special activity such as play a board game, listen to special music, or watch a favorite TV program, an activity reserved for only that time so IV infusion time is changed from a dreaded activity to a "can't wait for"

BOX 38.7 Nursing Care Planning

AN INTERPROFESSIONAL CARE MAP FOR A CHILD RECEIVING MEDICATION

Terry is an 8-year-old with Down syndrome whom you meet in the emergency room. She has been diagnosed with osteomyelitis, a bone infection at her ankle. When you gave her a tablet of acetaminophen (Tylenol) for pain, she spit it out. Her mother tells you Terry cannot swallow pills. Her father tells you, "You'll have to give her an IV."

Family Assessment: Child is the youngest of four siblings. Lives with parents and other siblings in five-bedroom home on dairy farm. Parents rate finances as, "Fine, as long as people keep drinking milk."

Client Assessment: Child diagnosed with Down syndrome at birth; IQ approximately 60. Lacerated right foot on farm equipment in fall from hay loft 2 weeks ago. Laceration cleaned and bandaged by mother; not seen by health care provider. Today, wound has not healed, is open and erythematous; foot swollen; pain radiates up leg from foot. X-ray reveals abscess in bone. Child is so frightened by injections; she screams at the sight of any kind of needle. Placed on bed rest and prescribed an intravenous (IV) antibiotic and Demerol for pain.

Nursing Diagnosis: Pain related to disease process (infection) in foot

Outcome Evaluation: Child rates pain on pain scale as 2 or below; cooperates with IV medication therapy to supply antibiotic and pain relief.

(continued on page 1108)

BOX 38.7 Nursing Care Planning (continued)

Team Member Responsible	Assessment	Intervention	Rationale	Expected Outcome
Activities of Daily Living, Including Safety				
Nurse	Assess what self-care measures child will be able to complete by herself while on bed rest.	Explain resting foot and maintaining IV therapy are crucial measures.	Non–weight-bearing and antibiotic therapy will best cure the condition and relieve pain.	Child, nurse, and parent agree on plan of care for activities of daily living.
Teamwork and Collaboration				
Nurse/Primary care provider	Assess if pain management team advice will be necessary.	Meet with pain consultant to discuss problem: child is in pain but needs to remain still for IV therapy.	Sustained antibiotic therapy is necessary to treat bone infection; consultation can help avoid infiltration.	Pain management consultant meets with child and parent as appropriate; agrees on pain management plan.
Procedures/Medications for Quality Improvement				
Nurse	Assess if child has a preference for IV therapy site.	Begin IV therapy in nondominant hand if possible.	Allowing a child as much choice as possible helps to prevent a feeling of entrapment.	Child helps to identify insertion site; cooperates to the best of her ability with IV insertion.
Nutrition				
Nurse	Assess if child has had past experience with eating in bed.	Discuss with child and parent the importance of continuing nutrition while on bed rest. Suggest taking pain medication before meals.	Hospitalization can be a major stress to children. Pain can interfere with nutrition.	Child helps to choose foods from hospital menu that she would like to eat.
Patient-Centered Care				
Nurse	Assess if child has had experience with IV therapy in the past.	Review importance and plan for IV therapy with child and parents.	Knowledgeable patients and parents can aid in the success of therapy.	Child and parents state they understand why antibiotic and analgesia is needed and why administration method is required.
Psychosocial/Spiritual/Emotional Needs				
Nurse	Explore (if known) why child is so afraid of needles. Ask child to rate pain by FACES Pain Scale hourly.	Discuss advantages of IV therapy, which will minimize injections yet supply antibiotic.	Fear of needles is common in children; advocating for IV therapy rather than IM injection can help relieve this fear.	Child states she understands IV therapy will involve a needle but needle will be inserted only once. Rates pain hourly.
Informatics for Seamless Health Care Planning				
Nurse	Assess if parents have questions about child's care at home.	Explain the importance of continuing IV, then oral antibiotic. Practice swallowing pills with ice chips to ready child for oral administration.	Continuing antibiotic administration will be necessary to combat deep-seated infection.	Parents state they understand importance of continuing medicine administration. Keep follow-up visit for evaluation.

activity. Be sure parents understand the importance of the IV therapy and help guard the infusion site while they are with their child. Infants who receive total fluids by IV infusion may enjoy sucking on a pacifier to fulfill their oral needs, although if the infant will return to breastfeeding soon, the mother may not want a pacifier offered. Wrapping an infant's or preschooler's infusion site with gauze so that it is no longer interesting to them prevents them from playing with the needle and accidentally dislodging it.

QSEN Checkpoint Question 38.5

Evidence-Based Practice

To investigate whether the viewing of cartoons can reduce the perception of pain in pediatric patients, younger children who presented to a major emergency department were randomized to watch a Barney cartoon in Spanish or English, and older children were randomized to view a Tarzan cartoon in either of the same two languages during painful procedures. Younger children were assessed 5 minutes before the procedure, during the procedure, and 5 minutes after the procedure using either a Poker Chip Tool or FACES Pain Scale. Older children were assessed at the same time interval using self-reporting and a visual analog scale. Results revealed children who watched the cartoons rated their pain as significantly lower than those who did not watch the cartoons (Downey & Zun, 2012).

Based on the previous study, if Terry were watching television as you approached her to insert an IV cannula, what would be your best action?

a. Temporarily turn off the TV so she can clearly hear your instructions.
b. Ask Terry's mother to turn the TV set to the cartoon channel.
c. Put on a *Barney* DVD for Terry to watch.
d. Allow Terry to continue to watch the current channel.

Look in Appendix A for the best answer and rationale.

Intravenous Medication Administration

Medications may be added to an IV line as a small, one-time administration (bolus), a fluid chamber infusion, or by piggyback for larger children. As with any medication administration, identify the child before adding medicine to an IV line. Also ensure that the drug to be injected is compatible with the IV fluid being infused.

To administer medicine by a bolus technique, clamp the IV tubing above the medicine port in the IV line, clean the port with alcohol, insert the needleless syringe filled with the prescribed medicine into the port, and inject the medicine slowly and gently based on the manufacturer's instructions. Once the medication has been given, remove the syringe and reopen the IV line immediately to allow the IV solution to flush the medicine into the child.

For small children and infants, fluid chamber administration is used. A small amount of maintenance fluid (usually 10 to 20 ml) is placed in the fluid chamber, and the medication is inserted through the chamber port using a needleless syringe. When the fluid has infused and the chamber is empty, a small amount of maintenance fluid is placed in the chamber as a flush. When complete, the chamber is used again for maintenance fluid at the maintenance rate.

For a piggyback infusion of medicine, medication is provided by the pharmacy prepared and diluted in small fluid-filled plastic bags. To begin a piggyback infusion, hang the piggyback bag, clean the medicine port on the IV line, and insert the piggyback system into the port. Lower the level of the main infusion bag and adjust the flow rate to that desired to allow the piggyback system to operate. As soon as the piggyback bag has emptied, elevate the maintenance bag of fluid again and make certain the IV line is flowing well and at the proper rate.

Children accept piggyback administrations of fluid well because it seems no different from receiving maintenance IV fluid. Older children can take an active role in alerting health care providers that the total medication amount has infused and it is time to return to maintenance fluid.

Analgesics are commonly administered to older children by patient-controlled analgesia machines (Franson, 2010). Because these machines are set with lockout time intervals, they are safe to use with children as young as early school age (see Chapter 39). Although, when programmed, such pumps help protect against medication errors, they are not foolproof and so need to be monitored when in use with children.

What if... 38.3 Terry's mother tells you she does not believe in introducing any "foreign" substance into her child's body, so she does not want her to have IV medicine. How would you counsel her?

Using Intermittent Infusion Devices

Intermittent infusion devices, sometimes called heparin locks, are devices that maintain open venous access for medicine administration while allowing children to be free of IV tubing so that they can be out of bed and more active (Fig. 38.8). A vein on the back of the hand is generally chosen as the IV site. Scalp vein tubing is used and capped at the end with a specially designed rubber stopper or a commercial trap. The tubing is filled with a dilute solution of heparin or normal saline through the rubber stopper and flushed again with solution every 2 to 8 hours (depending on hospital policy) to keep it patent. Be certain the tubing and stopper

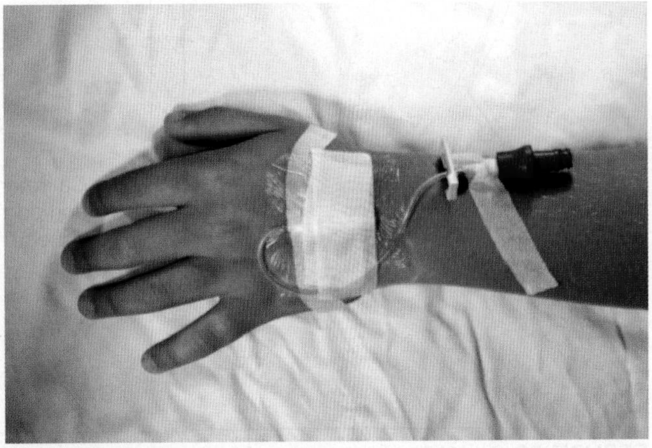

FIGURE 38.8 An intermittent infusion device in place. Advocating for this type of apparatus minimizes pain.

are both firmly secured to the wrist and, if necessary, an arm board is taped in place to remind the child to protect the site from trauma.

Children who are hospitalized or receiving home care for a long time and who need only IV medication, not additional fluid, are good candidates for such devices because IV medicine can be added to the site as needed without further venipunctures. Intermittent infusion devices also can be used if frequent venous blood samples are required because this also protects against additional venipunctures. Similar devices may be inserted into arteries when arterial blood is required, for example, for the child who is having blood gases monitored frequently.

Using Central Venous Access Catheters and Devices

Venous access for long-term IV therapy can be obtained using a tunneled catheter inserted into the vena cava just outside the right atrium; the catheter then exits the chest just under the clavicle for easy access (Fig. 38.9). Typical catheters used

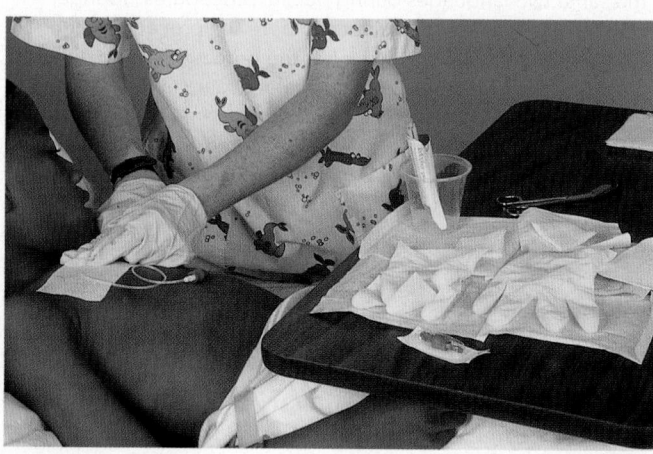

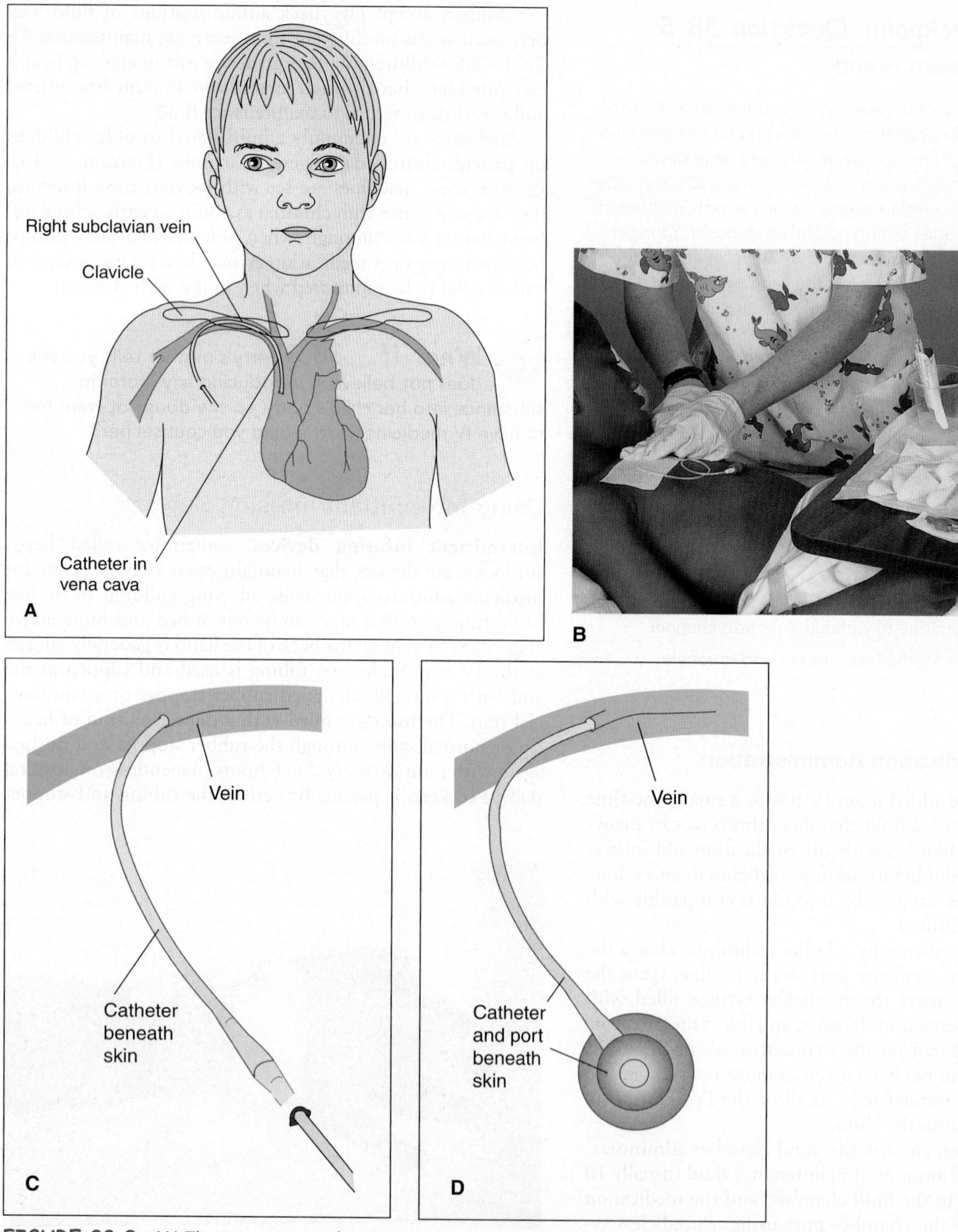

FIGURE 38.9 **(A)** The insertion site for placement of a central venous catheter for intravenous infusion. **(B)** Changing a dressing for a central venous catheter. **(C)** The central venous catheter beneath the skin. **(D)** A vascular access port (VAP) device beneath the skin.

in this way include Broviac, Hickman, and Groshong types. Such catheters have a wrinkle-resistant fabric (Dacron) cuff that adheres to the subcutaneous tissue and helps to seal the catheter in place and keep out infection. These catheters are usually inserted in the operating room, because tunneling under the skin is required and general anesthesia is preferred. These semipermanent catheters are used to administer bolus or continuous infusions of medications and fluid (Handrup, Moller, Frydenberg, et al., 2010). Care of the catheter (depending on agency policy) consists of daily or weekly changes of dressings over the exit site and periodic irrigation with heparin or saline to ensure patency.

Such catheters are advantageous because discomfort from further skin punctures is avoided. One disadvantage is that the catheter could become snagged on something and accidentally be pulled out. If this happens, it is an emergency situation because the child could lose an appreciable amount of blood from the point of entrance into a vein as major as the vena cava. Unless there is a waterproof dressing covering the insertion site, children with central venous catheters in place are usually not allowed to swim or take showers to avoid infection. Another disadvantage is the potential for profuse bleeding or air embolus if the IV tubing becomes disconnected from the catheter. A filter should be used at all times to prevent air embolus, and connections should be carefully secured and monitored. Infections must be prevented or the catheter will likely need to be removed.

Vascular access ports (VAPs) are small plastic infusion devices that are implanted under the skin, usually on the anterior chest just under the clavicle, for long-term fluid or medication administration via bolus or continuous administration (see Fig. 38.9D). A small catheter threads from the port internally into a central vein. After skin cleansing, blood samples can be removed or medication can be injected by a puncture through the chest skin into the port. Although this device requires a skin puncture (which causes pain), it may be well accepted by children because it is not as visible as a central venous catheter, no dressing is required, and it allows a full range of activities, such as showering and swimming. Be certain when accessing these ports to use only the needle supplied by the manufacturer, because a regular needle tends to "core" or remove a small circle of the membrane over the port and destroy the integrity of the device. Use an anesthetic cream to decrease discomfort as necessary before the skin puncture. As with central lines, air emboli, bleeding from a disconnected line, and infection are major concerns with VAPs also.

Yet another route of IV access are peripherally inserted central catheters (PICC lines) for therapy (Levy, Bendet, Samra, et al., 2010). These are advantageous particularly for home care because they can remain in place for up to 4 months without being changed. For this, a catheter is inserted into an arm vein (usually at the antecubital space into the median, cephalic, or basilic vein) and advanced until the tip rests in the superior vena cava. If a shorter catheter is used, the tip will rest closer to the head of the clavicle (a midline insertion).

Drugs commonly administered by PICC lines are antibiotics and analgesics. After medication is administered, the line is flushed with a small amount of a solution such as normal saline. The dressing over the insertion site is changed periodically according to agency policy.

Many parents seem more comfortable with this type of insertion than with a central venous catheter because it appears so much more like a routine IV. Newborns can have a catheter inserted into an umbilical vessel, with fluid and medications being administered by that route (see Chapter 26).

Remember that when caring for children with central venous access systems in place, all these types have the potential to result in hemorrhage, infection, air embolism, and thrombosis. Be certain to use strict aseptic techniques when changing the dressings over them to prevent infections because this is a major area of emphasis (O'Grady, Alexander, Burns, et al., 2011).

QSEN Checkpoint Question 38.4

Patient-Centered Care

Terry has her IV site changed to her dominant hand. She has stated that she is "bored and kind of sad." What would be the best activity for her while her medication infuses?

a. Listening to a story you read
b. Playing kick ball in the hallway
c. Playing Simon Says with her parents
d. Building a tower in the play area with another child

Look in Appendix A for the best answer and rationale.

Administering an Intraosseous Infusion

Intraosseous infusion is the infusion of fluid into the bone marrow cavity of a long bone, usually the distal or proximal tibia, the distal femur, or the iliac crest (Nagler & Krauss, 2011). Because the bone marrow communicates directly with the circulatory system, fluid reaches the bloodstream as quickly by this route as if it were administered intravenously. All fluids that can be administered intravenously, including whole blood or medication, can also be administered by this route.

Intraosseous infusion is used in an emergency when it is difficult to establish usual IV access or in a child with such extensive burns that the usual sites for IV infusion are not available. It is a temporary measure until a usual route of administration can be obtained because of the danger of osteomyelitis, a devastating infection with long-term effects to bone marrow. It must be initiated with a sterile technique and, if continued for an extended time, the infusion point is rotated about every 2 to 3 days to minimize the risk of infection.

Intraosseous infusion is painful as the needle enters the bone marrow cavity. Prepare the child for this and offer support.

Steps to initiate an intraosseous infusion include:

1. The skin over the chosen site is cleaned as per protocol and anesthetized with a local anesthetic.
2. A small incision is made into the skin with a scalpel blade.
3 A large hypodermic or bone marrow needle is inserted through the incision into the cavity of the bone.
4. To ensure the needle tip has reached the bone marrow cavity, a syringe is attached to the needle and bone marrow is aspirated.
5. When bone marrow is obtained, the syringe is removed and IV tubing, including a filter and the fluid to be administered, is attached to the needle and opened to a gravity flow.
6. A dressing with additional antiseptic is then applied over the needle site.

7. A restraint is applied to the leg to help the child hold the leg still.

Tubing and dressings must be changed as per protocol (approximately every 48 hours for the tubing and approximately every 24 hours for the dressing), again, to reduce the possibility of infection. Assess for a distal pulse and adequate temperature and color of the leg every hour throughout the infusion to ensure there is adequate circulation to the extremity. To optimize assessment, place a pulse oximeter on a toe distal to the infusion and monitor waveform. If the needle should become dislodged, symptoms of circulatory impairment or pain and taut skin over the site occur.

Occasionally during fluid administration, a bone chip or thick marrow will occlude an intraosseous needle and slow the infusion. If this occurs, a stylet passed through the needle clears it and allows for continued fluid administration.

What if...38.4 You are interested in exploring one of the 2020 National Health Goals with respect to the administration of medicine in children (see Box 38.1). Most government-sponsored money for nursing research is allotted based on these goals. What would be a possible research topic to explore pertinent to these goals that would be applicable to Terry and her family and that would also advance evidence-based practice?

KEY POINTS FOR REVIEW

- The effectiveness of medicines varies depending on the pharmacokinetics (absorption, distribution, metabolism, and excretion) of the drug.
- The principles of safe medicine administration for adults also apply to children: right medicine, right child, right dose, right route, right time, and right patient instructions.
- The correct drug dose in children is usually calculated according to the child's body weight. Body surface area, determined by using a nomogram, may also be used.
- Use adequate restraints as needed when giving medicine to be certain children will not inadvertently be harmed in the process.
- In children, the majority of medications are given orally or intravenously to avoid the discomfort of other routes. Subcutaneous pumps infuse medicine such as insulin.
- IV therapy may be administered peripherally or via a central venous access site. A scalp vein is a common IV site used for infants.
- An intraosseous infusion is used in an emergency when it is difficult to establish usual IV access or in a child with such extensive burns that the usual sites for IV infusion are not available.
- Teach parents safe actions for giving medicine at home so children can continue to receive accurate doses after hospital discharge and ensure they understand the importance of storing medications in a locked area; such thoroughness helps in planning care that not only meets QSEN competencies but also best meets a family's total needs.

CRITICAL THINKING CARE STUDY

Casey is a previously healthy 4-year-old boy brought to the pediatric emergency room by his parents because he has diarrhea and has been refusing to eat today. He says his throat hurts too much for him to swallow and wants something to "stop the pain." Upon examination, Casey is found to be mildly to moderately dehydrated. Pain medication (acetaminophen) and an oral rehydration solution (Pedialyte) are prescribed. His throat swab reveals he has a "strep throat," so he is also started on a course of oral antibiotics.

1. Casey has been prescribed two oral medications plus an oral rehydration solution, yet one of his chief concerns is that his throat hurts too much for him to swallow. How would you approach this problem?
2. Suppose Casey vomits the rehydration solution so his primary care provider asks you to begin an IV infusion with him. How would you approach him to do this?
3. Casey has 2-year-old twin sisters and a new baby brother, 6 months old, at home. What would be important safety precautions to remind his parents about before he is discharged from the emergency room?

Patient Scenario

The Lewis Family

Read about the Lewis family, a family with concerns about long-term medicine administration, then answer the questions to further sharpen your skills and grow more familiar with NCLEX-type questions related to medication administration. Confirm your answers are correct by reading the rationales.

Visit http://thePoint.lww.com

Answers and Rationales

Looking for answers to the What If… and Critical Thinking Care Study questions?

Visit http://thePoint.lww.com

References

Arcara, A., & Tschudy, M. (2011). *The Harriett Lane handbook* (19th ed.) Maryland Heights, MO: Mosby.

de Haan, G., van der Geest, P., Doelman, G., et al. (2010). A comparison of midazolam nasal spray and diazepam rectal solution for the residential treatment of seizure exacerbations. *Epilepsia, 51*(3), 478–482.

de Maria, C., Lussier, M., & Bajcar, J. (2011). What do children know about medications? A review of the literature to guide clinical practice *Canadian Family Physician, 57*(3), 291–295.

Dickinson, C. J., Wagner, D. S., Shaw, B. E., et al. (2012). A systematic approach to improving medication safety in a pediatric intensive care unit. *Critical Care Nursing Quarterly, 35*(1), 15–26.

Downey, L. V., & Zun, L. S. (2012). The impact of watching cartoons for distraction during painful procedures in the emergency department. *Pediatric Emergency Care, 28*(10), 1033–1035.

El-Alfy, M., Sari, T. T., Lee, C. L., et al. (2010). The safety, tolerability, and efficacy of a liquid formulation of deferiprone in young children with transfusion iron overload. *Journal of Pediatric Hematology/Oncology, 32*(8), 601–605.

Elliott, M., & Liu, Y. (2010). The nine rights of medication administration: An overview. *British Journal of Nursing, 19*(5), 300–305.

Flood, E. M., Ryan, K. J., Rousculp, M. D., et al. (2011). A survey of children's preferences for influenza vaccine attributes. *Vaccine, 29*(26), 4334–4340.

Franson, H. E. (2010). Postoperative patient-controlled analgesia in the pediatric population: A literature review. *AANA: Journal of the American Association of Nurse Anesthetists, 78*(5), 374–378.

Ghaleb, M. A., Barber, N., Franklin, B. D., et al. (2010). The incidence and nature of prescribing and medication administration errors in paediatric inpatients. *Archives of Disease in Childhood, 95*(2), 113–118.

Handrup, M. M., Moller, J. K., Frydenberg, M., et al. (2010). Placing of tunneled central venous catheters prior to induction chemotherapy in children with acute lymphoblastic leukemia. *Pediatric Blood & Cancer, 55*(2), 309–313.

Hanna, M., & Saberi, M. S. (2010). Incidence of hyponatremia in children with gastroenteritis treated with hypotonic intravenous fluids. *Pediatric Nephrology, 25*(8), 1471–1475.

Johnson, T. N., & Rostami-Hodjegan, A. R. (2010). Resurgence in the use of physiologically based pharmakinetic models in pediatric clinical pharmacology. *Pediatric Anesthesia, 21*(3), 291–301.

Jones, J. H., & Treiber, L. (2010). When the 5 rights go wrong: Medication errors from the nursing perspective. *Journal of Nursing Care Quality, 25*(3), 240–247.

Kalisch, B. J., & Aebersold, M. (2010). Interruptions and multitasking in nursing care. *Joint Commission Journal on Quality and Patient Safety, 36*(3), 126–132.

Levy, I., Bendet, M., Samra, Z., et al. (2010). Infectious complications of peripherally inserted central venous catheters in children. *Pediatric Infectious Disease Journal, 29*(5), 426–429.

Nagler, J., & Krauss, B. (2011). Intraosseous catheter placement in children. *New England Journal of Medicine, 364*(8), e14.

Neville, K. A., Sandemann, D. J., Rubenstein, A., et al. (2010). Prevention of hyponatremia during maintenance intravenous fluid administration: A prospective randomized study of fluid type versus fluid rate. *The Journal of Pediatrics, 156*(2), 313–319.

O'Grady, N. P., Alexander, M., Burns, L., et al. (2011). Guidelines for the prevention of intravascular catheter-related infections. *Clinical Infectious Diseases, 52*(9), e162–e193.

Passariello, A., Terrin, G., de Marco, G., et al. (2011). Efficacy of a new hypotonic oral rehydration solution containing zinc and prebiotics in the treatment of childhood acute diarrhea: A randomized controlled trial. *Journal of Pediatrics, 158*(2), 288–292.

PDR Staff. (2013). *Physicians' desk reference* (67th ed.). Montvale, NJ: PDR Network.

Pham, J. C., Story, J. L., Hicks, R. W., et al. (2011). National study on the frequency, types, causes, and consequences of voluntarily reported emergency department medication errors. *The Journal of Emergency Medicine, 40*(5), 485–492.

Pickup, J. C. (2012). Insulin-pump therapy for type I diabetes mellitus. *New England Journal of Medicine, 366*(17), 1616–1624.

Roux, P., Carrieri, M. P., Keijzer, L., et al. (2011). Reducing harm from injecting pharmaceutical tablet or capsule material by injecting drug users. *Drug & Alcohol Review, 30*(3), 287–290.

Thompson Reuters Clinical Editorial Staff. (2013). *Neofax* (26th ed.). Montvale, NJ: PDR Network.

U.S. Department of Health and Human Services. (2010). *Healthy people 2020.* Washington, DC: Author.

Walsh, K. E., Mazor, K. M., Roblin, D., et al. (2013). Multisite parent-centered risk assessment to reduce pediatric oral chemotherapy errors. *Journal of Oncology Practice, 9*(1), e1–e7.

Wolfe, T. R., & Braude, D. A. (2010). Intranasal medication delivery for children: A brief update. *Pediatrics, 126*(3), 532–537.

Wong, I. B. Y., & Nischal, K. K. (2010). Managing a child with an external ocular disease. *Journal of American Association for Pediatric Ophthalmology and Strabismus, 14*(1), 68–77.

Yin, H. S., Mendelsohn, A. L., Wolf, M. S., et al. (2010). Parent's medication administration errors: Role of dosing instruments and health literacy. *Archives of Pediatric and Adolescent Medicine, 164*(2), 181–186.

Zuzak, T. J., Rauber-Luthy, C., & Simoes-West, A. P. (2010). Accidental intakes of remedies from complementary and alternative medicine in children. *European Journal of Pediatrics, 169*(6), 681–688.

Chapter 39

Pain Management in Children

KEY TERMS

- acute pain
- chronic pain
- conscious sedation
- cutaneous pain
- distraction
- epidural analgesia
- gate control theory
- nociceptors
- pain
- pain threshold
- pain tolerance
- patient-controlled analgesia (PCA)
- referred pain
- somatic pain
- substitution of meaning
- thought stopping
- transcutaneous electrical nerve stimulation (TENS)
- visceral pain

OBJECTIVES

After mastering the contents of this chapter, you should be able to:

1. Describe the major methods and techniques of pain management for children.
2. Identify 2020 National Health Goals related to pain management in children that nurses can help the nation achieve.
3. Assess a child regarding whether pain management is needed or adequate.
4. Formulate nursing diagnoses for a child in pain.
5. Identify expected outcomes associated with management of pain in children as well as help families manage seamless transitions across differing health care settings.
6. Using the nursing process, plan nursing care that includes the six competencies of Quality & Safety Education for Nurses (QSEN): Patient-Centered Care, Teamwork & Collaboration, Evidence-Based Practice (EBP), Quality Improvement (QI), Safety, and Informatics.
7. Implement nursing care related to a child in pain, such as suggesting an alternative therapy.
8. Evaluate outcomes for achievement and effectiveness of care for a child in pain.
9. Integrate knowledge of pain management in children with the interplay of nursing process, the six competencies of QSEN, and Family Nursing to promote quality maternal and child health nursing care.

Robin Harvey is a 3-year-old girl who was admitted to your hospital unit and has just returned from a bone marrow aspiration to rule out the possibility of leukemia. Robin received intravenous (IV) morphine sulfate during the procedure. Her mother asks you if Robin could have some more. "I know she's not having pain yet," her mother tells you, "but I want her to have something before the pain comes back."

Previous chapters described the growth and development of children and general care of ill children. This chapter adds information about the care of children when they need pain management. Such information builds a base for care and health teaching in a crucial area.

Is this mother's assessment or Robin's pain apt to be accurate or should you ask Robin herself about pain? Would anticipating pain in this way be the best intervention for Robin?

Pain is a difficult concept to define because it is a subjective symptom (experienced by the person), not an objective one (able to be determined by observation), and is unique to each person. Because it respects children's opinion of where and how much pain they feel, McCaffery's (1979) classic description of pain is the one most useful to use with children: "The sensation of pain is whatever the person experiencing it says it is, and it exists whenever the person says it does."

For children, because pain is such a different sensation than usual, pain is not only a hurting sensation but it can also be a very confusing one—the child did not anticipate the pain, does not have words to explain how it feels, and cannot always understand its cause. In addition, preschoolers and younger children lack an understanding of time, which makes it difficult to explain to them when the pain will go away. This can leave them feeling frustrated or angry while they wait for someone to give them relief.

Children's perception of the situation influences their response to how much pain they feel. This means that children experiencing procedures that are less intrusive but who feel maximum anxiety from them may describe the degree of pain felt as more intense than they otherwise might have because of the accompanying anxiety (Vervoort, Eccleston, Goubert, et al., 2010).

Both helping children describe the type and extent of pain they are feeling and performing active interventions to relieve pain are some of the most important nursing roles in children's care. Assessing for pain is so important that pain can be considered the "fifth vital sign" (Harrison, Elia, Royle, et al., 2013).

The 2020 National Health Goals that speak to pain management are shown in Box 39.1.

BOX 39.1 Nursing Care Planning Based on 2020 National Health Goals

Several 2020 National Health Goals speak directly to alleviating pain in several different areas:

- Reduce the proportion of patients suffering from untreated pain due to a lack of access to pain treatment.
- Reduce serious injuries from the use of pain medicines.
- Reduce the number of non–U.S. Food and Drug Administration (FDA)-approved pain medications on the market.
- Reduce deaths from the use of pain medicines (U.S. Department of Health and Human Services [DHHS], 2010; see www.healthypeople.gov).

Nurses can help the nation reduce pain among children by active management of pain as well as by teaching children about the importance of avoiding painful unintentional injuries by the use of safety belts and bicycle helmets.

Nursing Process Overview

For a Child in Pain

Assessment

Children, like adults, experience pain individually depending on the type and cause of the pain, their temperament, their previous experience with pain, and their expectation of relief. Infants and young children cannot verbalize what they are feeling and so have the most trouble communicating how they feel.

Beginning as young as 3 years of age, children can indicate by pointing to a body part where they feel pain. They can also learn to express the degree of pain through a system such as comparing its intensity to a number of poker chips or drawings of faces. Older school-age children and adolescents can rate their pain on a scale of 1 to 10. Be aware that some children may be reluctant to admit pain because they are trying to be brave. Some may be reluctant to say they have pain because they are afraid they will receive a "shot" to relieve it, which will cause more pain. As a rule, including an assessment of pain level along with a vital sign measurement is an efficient way to ensure pain is assessed.

Nursing Diagnosis

Nursing diagnoses for children with pain focus not only on the pain but also on the stress, fear, or anxiety that pain produces. Examples of nursing diagnoses include:

- Pain related to an invasive procedure
- Fear related to anticipation of painful procedure
- Disturbed sleep pattern related to chronic pain
- Anxiety related to planned dressing changes that cause pain

Outcome Identification and Planning

The mark of efficient pain control is to anticipate when pain will occur and plan interventions to prevent it rather than let it occur and then relieve it. Three common reasons why nurses and other pediatric providers may not provide adequate pain relief to children include a belief that infants and young children do not experience pain, a fear children will become addicted to pain relief medications, and a fear of causing respiratory depression from analgesics. Infants and young children do experience pain, and there is little chance that children receiving narcotics during a short hospital stay will become narcotic dependent or that opiates cause greater respiratory depression in children than in adults (Fanning, Stucke, Christensen, et al., 2012). A good referral for parents is the American Academy of Pediatrics (AAP) Web site (www.aap.org) where pain management suggestions are available.

Implementation

Implementation for pain relief includes choosing the specific method of pain relief that is best for each child. Everyone involved in a child's care needs to be aware of the signs and symptoms that an individual child uses to express pain and specific ways that will help the child manage pain. If children are reluctant to admit they have pain because of the fear of receiving an injection, advocate for an oral form of analgesia or an intermittent IV infusion device or patient-controlled analgesia as appropriate options. Many parents are unsure about the safety of using strong analgesics for pain relief and so may give less than the prescribed dose. Therefore, educating parents about the need for pain relief, proper doses, and taking actions to involve them in the assessment and evaluation process are essential. Planning and assisting with complementary therapies is yet another area to consider.

Outcome Evaluation

An evaluation of expected outcomes is a key aspect of managing pain because no one pain relief measure is effective for everyone. After a child is given an analgesic, look for nonverbal clues, assess vital signs, and listen to the child's statements about pain to determine whether a drug was effective. Based on these findings, it may become clear that the technique of pain management being used may need to be modified or increased. A new technique may need to be added to the regimen so a child receives maximum pain relief.

Possible examples indicating achievement of expected outcomes include:

- Child states pain is now at a tolerable level that will not interfere with activity or sleep.
- Adolescent says she has managed her fear through imagery.
- Child rates pain as no greater than 2 on a 1-to-10 scale.
- Child describes ways he will help reduce pain when it returns.
- Child resumes age-appropriate behaviors following analgesia administration.

THE PHYSIOLOGY OF PAIN

As in adults, acute pain in children usually occurs for one of four reasons: reduced pH alterations, which cause depletion of oxygen in tissues, pressure on tissue, external injury, or overstretching of body cavities with fluid or air. Chronic pain often involves irritation of tissue, which occurs from the pain of shingles, fibromyalgia, or long-term back pain. The stimulus causing pain is not always visible or measurable. In addition, anxiety can lead to increased pain regardless of the physical stimuli.

Pain conduction consists of four major steps: transduction (sensing the pain sensation), transmission (routing the pain sensation to the spinal cord), perception (the brain interprets the sensation as pain), and modulation (steps the body takes to relive pain).

Transduction begins in the peripheral nerves when a mechanical, thermal, or chemical stimulus activates **nociceptors**, a specialized group of sensory receptors. Several neurotransmitters (e.g., substance P) are also stimulated and involved in conducting pain. Sharp pain impulses are conducted by both A-α and A-β fibers (large fibers that are myelinated and conduct the response at a rapid rate). In contrast, light pressure and vibration are conducted by A-δ and C fibers, fibers that are smaller and that conduct at a slower rate.

Pain impulses join central nervous system (CNS) fibers in the dorsal horn of the spinal cord. Here, the impulses are projected upward to the brain, where they will be perceived as pain.

- **Acute pain** means sharp pain. It generally occurs abruptly after an injury. The pain of a pin prink is an example.
- **Chronic pain** is pain that lasts for a prolonged period or beyond the time span anticipated for healing. Acute pain usually causes extreme distress and anxiety; chronic pain can lead to depression and less ability to achieve as the threshold to sense pain apparently lowers and creates a "feedback loop" (Palermo, Eccleston, Lewandowski, et al., 2010).
- **Cutaneous pain** is pain that arises from superficial structures such as the skin and mucous membrane. A paper cut is an example.
- **Somatic pain** is pain that originates from deep body structures such as muscles or bones. The pain of a sprained ankle is somatic pain.
- **Visceral pain** involves sensations that arise from internal organs such as the intestines. The pain of appendicitis is visceral pain.
- **Referred pain** is pain that is perceived at a site distant from its point of origin. The pain of right lower lobe pneumonia, for example, is often first thought to be abdominal pain because the pain is referred, or felt in the abdomen.

A child's **pain threshold** refers to the point at which the child first senses pain. This varies greatly from person to person and is probably most influenced by heredity. All people also have a point above which they are not willing to bear any additional pain. This is a person's **pain tolerance**. Pain tolerance levels are probably most affected by cultural influences.

When pain is felt, the pituitary and hypothalamus glands both respond reflexively by releasing *endorphins* or polypeptide compounds that simulate opiates in their ability to produce analgesia and a sense of well-being. Children also consciously try to modify pain by physical actions such as shifting position or rubbing the body part.

Several theories have been proposed to explain the transmission of pain and how pain can best be managed. Of these, the gate control theory is the best known.

QSEN Checkpoint Question 39.1

Informatics

Robin, 3 years of age, has just returned from having a bone marrow biopsy. Your documentation in her electronic health record would note the presence of what type of pain?

a. Cutaneous pain
b. Somatic pain
c. Visceral pain
d. Neuropathic pain

Look in Appendix A for the best answer and rationale.

Gate Control Theory of Pain

The **gate control theory** of pain (Melzack & Wall, 1965) attempts to explain how pain impulses travel from a site of injury to the brain, where the impulse is registered. This theory envisions gating mechanisms in the substantia gelatinosa of the dorsal horn of the spinal cord that, when activated, can halt an impulse at that level of the cord. This prevents the pain impulse from being received at the brain level and interpreted as pain. Gating mechanisms can be stimulated by three techniques: cutaneous stimulation, distraction, and anxiety reduction.

Cutaneous stimulation (skin stimulation) has an effect because, when the peripheral nerves next to an injury site are stimulated, the ability of the A-δ or C fiber nerves at the injury site responsible for transmitting pain impulses appears to decrease. Rubbing an injured part such as a stubbed toe and applying heat or cold to the site are types of maneuvers that suppress pain because these actions activate the nearby peripheral fibers. This technique is especially effective with children because the rubbing is not only comforting from a physical standpoint but also conveys psychological warmth.

Distraction allows the cells of the brainstem that register an impulse as pain to be preoccupied with other stimuli so a pain impulse cannot register. Having a child focus intently on an action or a thought or telling a child to say "ouch" while an injection is administered are common uses of this technique. For a child in pain after a procedure, a gift of a Mylar balloon or their favorite toy to hug can be wonderful distractions.

Pain impulses are perceived more quickly by the brain if anxiety is present. Therefore, any attempt to reduce a child's anxiety as much as possible, such as teaching a school-age child what to expect with a procedure so there are no surprises, can help reduce the intensity of pain. In addition to teaching when something is going to happen, be certain you also teach when nothing is going to happen. Being told a clinic visit is just for a checkup and so will not involve painful procedures allows a child to relax and feel less anxiety.

The effectiveness of gate control theory techniques varies with a child's age, ability to cooperate, degree of pain, and time allowed for learning and applying pain management techniques. Because memory may influence the sensation of pain (expecting to have pain produces anxiety, which increases pain), these techniques are best taught to children before they begin to have pain. In all instances, children should know to use them just before or at the moment they first feel the pain. If they wait until pain is intense, the pain may be so distracting that they cannot concentrate on using a technique. Children who were able to use a distraction technique in the past but can no longer do so need to be evaluated for what has changed. Is it their ability to cope with the pain, or is the pain increasing in intensity?

ASSESSING THE TYPE AND DEGREE OF PAIN

Pain assessment can be difficult with children, not only because children have difficulty describing pain but also because some children will suffer with pain rather than report it, unaware that someone could make it go away. Other children may distract themselves by methods such as concentrating on play. Others may sleep, not from comfort but from the exhaustion caused by the pain. Cultural differences also influence how pain is expressed (Box 39.2). All of these factors can make using only subjective measures to assess pain, such as observation, misleading.

BOX 39.2 Nursing Care Planning to Respect Cultural Diversity

Because children may have difficulty describing pain in a manner that adults can understand, it is difficult to assess the extent of their discomfort. Also, because pain is an individualized sensation, it may be experienced and expressed differently by different children. In some families, for example, pain may be expressed very openly and freely. In others, children are expected to be stoic about pain. The expression of pain is culturally determined in this way; therefore, two children who have the same degree of pain may express it very differently (Palermo et al., 2010).

Parents may be unclear and don't intervene with pain assessment or control because they assume health care providers are experts on pain control. Health care providers, on the other hand, may depend on parents to speak up if their child is in pain. Discussing how pain will be assessed, everyone's role, and what is available for pain relief clearly and openly early in a treatment program help ensures that these misunderstandings do not occur. Be certain that you also frequently reassess pain to be certain interventions such as the administration of an analgesic, distraction, or improved positioning are effective.

Keeping in mind each child's developmental level as well as chronologic age are important when assessing pain because assessment varies widely from that of a nonverbal infant to a very verbal adolescent (Box 39.3).

The Infant

In the past, it was believed that infants do not feel pain because of incomplete myelination of peripheral nerves. Evidence-based practice has shown this not to be true because myelination is not necessary for pain perception.

A second argument in the past against needing to provide pain relief for infants was that they have no memory. It can be shown, however, that physiologic changes occur with pain even in preterm infants, so even with a lack of memory, it is clear that pain is experienced. Even newborns instinctively guard a body part by holding an extremity still or tensing the abdomen. Other clues are diffuse body movements; tears; a high-pitched, harsh cry; a stiff posture; alterations in facial expression such as

BOX 39.3 Nursing Care Planning Using Assessment

Assessing a Child With Pain

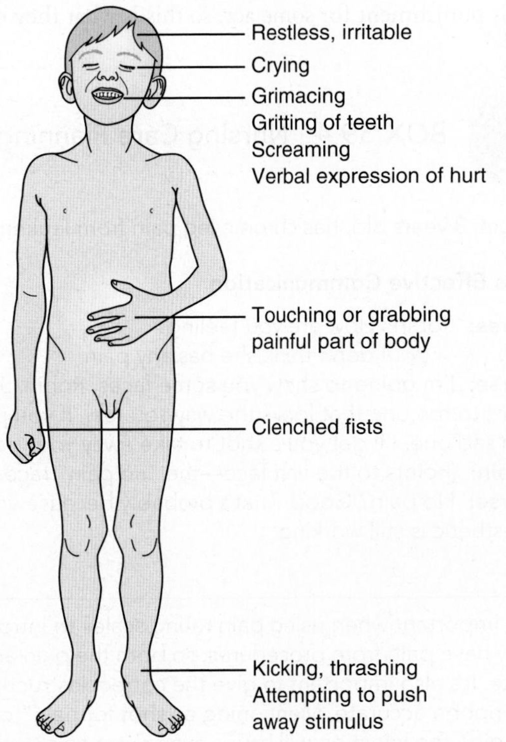

eyes squeezed shut; a quivering chin; lack of play; and fisting (Schiavenato, Butler-O'Hare, & Scovanner, 2011). Perhaps the chief mark in infants, however, is that when pain is present, they cannot be comforted completely. Preterm neonates particularly may have a difficult time organizing a distress response to cue a health care provider to the presence of pain. When working with any infant, be sensitive to situations that could cause pain and try to reduce them to the maximum extent possible.

The Toddler and the Preschooler

Determining when and how much pain is present continues to be difficult with toddlers and preschoolers because they may not have a word in their limited vocabularies to describe the sensation they feel because words such as "sharp," "nagging," or "aching" have little meaning until a child has experienced each type (Box 39.4). Parents often encourage children of this age to refer to pain as "my boo-boo" or some other like word, so children often are not sure if what you mean by the word "pain" (to be most accurate in assessment, use the child's term for pain or teach the child that "pain" is the same as "boo-boo"). Children also can have difficulty comparing the pain they feel now to past pain (e.g., is it better or worse?) because they have had so little experience with pain. For some toddlers, pain is such a strange sensation that, aside from crying in response to it, they may react aggressively (e.g., pounding, rocking) as if to fight it off. They also may avoid being touched or held.

Preschool children can describe that they have pain but continue to have difficulty describing its intensity. They begin to use comforting mechanisms, such as gritting teeth, pressing a hand against a forehead, pulling on their ear, holding their throat, rubbing an arm, or grimacing, to control or express pain. Some preschoolers do not think to mention they have pain because they believe it is something to be expected or, because of their egocentric thinking, they assume adults are already aware of their pain. They also may think pain is punishment for some act, so this is what they deserve. It is sometimes difficult to comfort children of this age during painful procedures by a statement such as "It's only for a minute" because they do not yet have a perception of time.

Still other behavior changes you may see in preschoolers are regression or withdrawal. To help evaluate if they have pain, ask yourself, "What would this child normally be doing?" (e.g., playing, eating, sleeping). Input from parents on how their child usually behaves can be valuable in an evaluation. If a trial dose of analgesia is used, you can then evaluate behavior changes after the dose is given. Children who resume their usual behavior after analgesia were probably in pain before the analgesia took effect.

The School-Age Child and the Adolescent

Children who think concretely (preadolescents) can have difficulty envisioning that a word like "sharp" applies both to knives and to the feeling in their abdomen. Because of this, they continue to have difficulty describing pain. They may also assume, like preschoolers, that you, as an authority figure, already know they have pain.

Some children of school age will regress with pain such as returning to baby talk or lying in a fetal position. If pain will last only an instant, such as with an injection, children this age are old enough to control the pain through nonpharmacologic activities such as distraction techniques.

Children may be in middle school before they can understand how to use a numerical pain rating scale or that the scale intensifies from left to right. Doing some preassessment work with them, such as giving them 10 different-sized triangles and asking them to arrange them from smallest to largest, is a good way to evaluate if they understand incremental measurements or "least to most" and are primed to describe pain intensity in a measurable way. A scale of 1 to 5 can be used in younger children if 1 to 10 seems overwhelming. If it seems clearer, you can turn a pain rating scale vertically so it measures bottom (little pain) to top (a lot of pain) to help a child learn incremental measurement.

BOX 39.4 Nursing Care Planning Based on Effective Communication

Robin, 3 years old, has chronic leg pain from leukemia. You want to assess her level of pain.

Less Effective Communication

Nurse: Robin? How are you feeling?
Mrs. Harvey: I don't think she has any pain.
Nurse: I'm going to show you some faces, Robin. Just point to the one that looks the way you feel. If you point to a sad one, I'll get you a shot to take away your pain.
Robin: (Points to the first face—the "no pain" face.)
Nurse: No pain? Good. That's probably because your anesthetic is still working.

More Effective Communication

Nurse: Robin? How are you feeling?
Mrs. Harvey: I don't think she has any pain.
Nurse: Robin? Remember the faces we looked at this morning before surgery? I want you to use them to tell me how you feel. This one means "no hurt." This one means "the most hurt you could have." Point to the one that shows how much hurt you have.
Robin: (Points to the middle face—the "hurts even more" face.)

It is important when using pain rating scales to introduce them to children before surgery or before they have pain from procedures, so both the pain and the rating tool are not new to the child all at once. It's also important to give the correct instructions for standardized assessment tools, or the results will not be accurate. Mentioning a "shot for pain" can cause children not to report pain because they imagine the injection will cause even more pain, rather than relieve it.

TABLE 39.1 Common Fallacies About Pain in Children

Fallacy	Fact
Nurses can accurately estimate children's pain from their actions and so do not need to rely on children's self-reports.	Nurses commonly underestimate children's pain from physical appearance or activity.
Young children, particularly newborns, do not feel pain.	Newborns and children do feel pain.
A child who resumes usual activity or who sleeps cannot be in pain.	Some children distract themselves with play or music while in pain. They may sleep from exhaustion from the pain.
Because of the possible adverse effects, narcotic analgesics are too dangerous for young children.	In the proper dose, narcotics can be used safely with children, including low–birth-weight infants.
Experiencing pain will not harm an infant or young child.	Newborns with pain can become cyanotic and bradycardic; no one knows the psychological stress of pain at this age.
If children deny they are feeling pain, you should believe them.	Children may deny pain to avoid a procedure, such as an injection, which they view as more painful. They may be afraid, fearing that they are being punished, or believe others know how they feel.

Adolescents are able to use adult pain scales for assessment and also commonly use adult mechanisms for controlling pain such as grimacing or verbal outbursts. Some try to be stoic or not show pain in order to avoid stereotypes of "crybaby" or "chicken." This tendency makes an assessment for body motions that could indicate pain, such as clenched hands, clenched teeth, rapid breathing, and guarding (tensing) of body parts, doubly important to observe.

PAIN ASSESSMENT

Common fallacies about pain in children are shown in Table 39.1. Although monitoring for physiologic findings such as a change in pulse or blood pressure may give some indication that a child is under stress, these are not the most dependable indicators of pain because pain is a subjective symptom. Once children can speak, asking them to tell you about their pain (self-reporting or using a pain rating scale) becomes the most accurate method for assessment (Downey & Zun, 2012).

A variety of pain rating scales have been devised to use with children. None have been proven to be consistently better than the others, mainly because both children and the type of pain they can be experiencing vary so much. As a rule, pick a well-documented effective scale and urge your care team to use that consistently for each child rather than asking a child to adapt to different assessment techniques. Be sure to follow the specific instructions for that scale.

The Pain Experience Inventory

The Pain Experience Inventory is a tool consisting of eight questions for children and eight questions for the child's parents. It is designed to elicit the terms a child uses to denote pain and what actions a child thinks will best alleviate pain. Such a form can be used when a child is admitted to an acute care facility or on an initial home care visit (Box 39.5). If possible, it should be used before the child has pain.

The CRIES Neonatal Postoperative Pain Measurement Scale

The CRIES Neonatal Postoperative Pain Measurement Scale is a 10-point scale named for five physiologic and behavioral variables commonly associated with neonatal pain: C = crying; R = requires increased oxygen administration; I = increased vital signs; E = expression; S = sleeplessness (Krechel & Bildner, 1995) (Table 39.2).

Each area of concern is scored from 0 to 2. Infants with a total score of 4 or more are most likely to be in pain and need

BOX 39.5 Pain Experience Inventory

Questions for the Child

Tell me what pain is.
Tell me about any hurt you have had before.
What do you do when you hurt?
Do you tell others when you hurt?
What do you want others to do for you when you hurt?
What do you *not* want others to do for you when you hurt?
What helps the most to take away your hurt?
Is there anything special you would like me to know about you when you hurt? (If yes, have the child describe.)

Questions for Parents

Describe any pain your child has had before.
How does your child usually react to pain?
Does your child tell you or others when pain is experienced?
How do you know when your child is in pain?
What do you do for your child when your child is hurting?
What does your child do to help relieve pain?
Which of these actions work best to decrease or take away your child's pain?
Is there anything special that you would like me to know about your child and pain? (If yes, have the parents describe.) (Hester & Barcus, 1986)

TABLE 39.2 The CRIES Neonatal Postoperative Pain Measurement Scale

	Infant's Score		
Assessment	0	1	2
Crying	No cry or cry is not high pitched.	Cry is high pitched but baby is easily consolable.	Cry is high pitched and baby is inconsolable.
Oxygen required for SpO_2 <95%	No oxygen required.	≤30% oxygen required.	>30% oxygen required.
Increased vital signs	Heart rate and blood pressure unchanged or less than baseline.	Baseline heart rate or blood pressure increased <20% of baseline.	Baseline heart rate or blood pressure increased ≥20% of baseline.
Expression	No grimace present.	Grimace alone is present.	Grimace and noncry vocalization grunt is present.
Sleepless	Infant has been continually asleep for past hour.	Infant has wakened at frequent intervals for past hour.	Infant has been awake constantly.
Total infant score			

From Krechel, S. W., & Bildner, J. (1995). CRIES: A new neonatal postoperative pain management score. *Pediatric Anesthesia, 5*(1), 53.

interventions to reduce discomfort. The scale cannot be used with infants who are intubated or paralyzed for ventilatory assistance because they would have no score for crying, and because, if their faces are obscured, it is difficult to rate them for facial expression.

The COMFORT Behavior Scale

The COMFORT Behavior Scale is a pain rating scale devised by nurses to rate pain in very young infants (Boerlage, Ista, de Jong, et al., 2012; van Dijk, Peters, van Deventer, et al., 2005). On the first part of the scale, six different categories (alertness, calmness/agitation, crying, physical movement, muscle tone, and facial expression) are rated from 1 to 5. The lowest score is 6 (no pain), and 30 is the highest (a great deal of pain). In addition to rating physical parameters, the infant is then observed for 2 minutes and the evaluation of the baby's pain is documented on an analog (1-to-10) visual scale.

The FLACC Pain Assessment Tool

The FLACC Pain Assessment Tool is a scale by which health care providers can rate a young child's pain when a child cannot give input, such as during circumcision (Merkel, Voepel-Lewis, & Malviya, 2002). It incorporates five types of behaviors that can be used to rate pain: facial expression, leg movement, activity, cry, and consolability. Because a child does not provide active input, older children may prefer a pain rating system in which they actively participate.

The Poker Chip Tool

The Poker Chip Tool (Hester & Barcus, 1986) uses four red poker chips placed in a horizontal line in front of the child. The technique can be used with children as young as 4 years of age, provided the child has some concept of "more" or "less." To use the tool, tell the child, "These are pieces of hurt." Beginning at the chip nearest the child's left hand and ending at the one nearest the child's right hand, point to the chips and say, "This is a little bit of hurt, this is a little more hurt, this is more hurt, and this [the fourth chip] is the most hurt you could ever have." Then ask the child, "How many pieces of hurt do you have right now?" Children without pain will reply they don't hurt; others will point to one of the poker chips. To gain more understanding of how much pain the child is feeling, clarify the child's answer by a follow-up question such as, "Oh, you have a little hurt? Tell me about that." This is an effective tool for young children because the poker chips are concrete items and children are concrete thinkers (Fig. 39.1).

Wong-Baker FACES Pain Rating Scale

This scale consists of six cartoonlike faces ranging from smiling to tearful (Fig. 39.2). Explain to the child that each face from left to right corresponds to a person who has no hurt up to a lot of hurt (Wong & Baker, 1996). Use the words under each face to describe the amount of pain the face represents. Next, ask the child to choose the face that best describes the child's pain, and record the number under the face the child chooses. The scale is popular with young children and can be used for those as young as 3 years of age (Pagé, Katz, Stinson, et al., 2012). The scale appeals to health care providers as well because it is

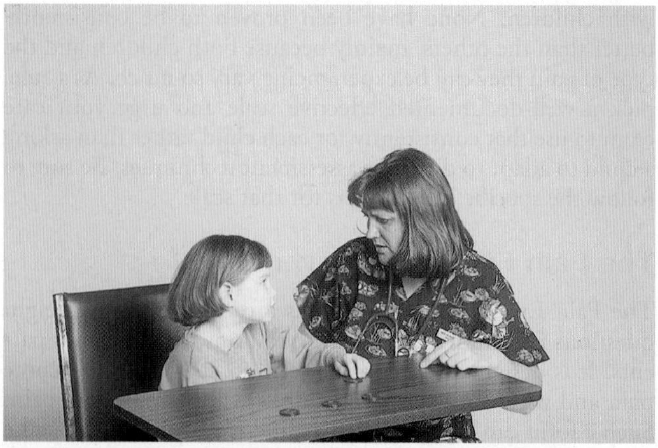

FIGURE 39.1 Use a pain rating tool to assess children's pain. Here, a child points to the poker chip indicating the degree of pain she is experiencing.

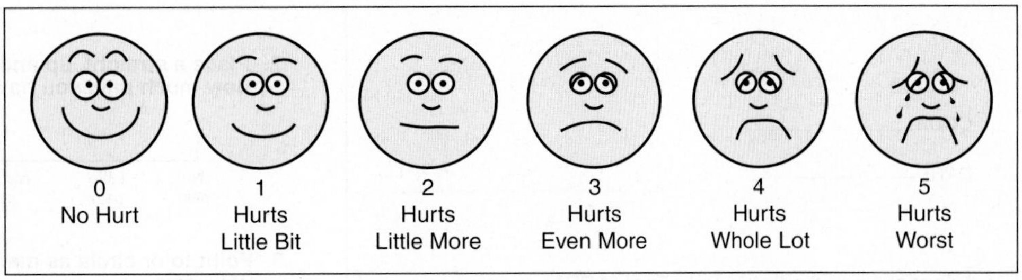

FIGURE 39.2 Wong-Baker FACES Pain Rating Scale. (Copyright 1983, Wong Baker FACES Foundation, www.WongBakerFACES.org Used with permission. Originally published in Whaley & Wong's Nursing Care of Infants and Children. © Elsevier Inc.)

cute; however, because it is not as concrete a measure as the Poker Chip Tool, it may not be as effective with all children.

The Oucher Pain Rating Scale

The Oucher Pain Rating Scale (Beyer, Denyes, & Villarruel, 1992) consists of six photographs of children's faces representing "no hurt" to "biggest hurt you could ever have." Also included is a vertical scale with numbers from 0 to 100. To use the photograph portion, point to each photograph and explain what each photo represents. Ask the child to point to the photo that best represents the child's degree of hurt.

To use the numbered scale portion, point to each section of the scale and explain that 0 means "no hurt"; 1 to 29 means "a little hurt"; 30 to 69 means "middle hurt"; 70 to 99 means "big hurt"; and 100 means "the biggest hurt you could ever have." Ask the child to point to the section of the scale that represents the present level of hurt. Children as young as 3 years of age can use the tool by pointing to the photograph that best describes their level of pain. If the child can count to 100 by ones and understands the concept of increasing value, the numbered scale can be used. The Oucher scale has Caucasian, African American, and Hispanic American photograph versions. If children are most comfortable with the tool, allow them to select the version they want to use or present the version that most closely matches the cultural characteristics of the child.

The Numerical or Visual Analog Scale

The numerical or visual analog scale (Fig. 39.3) uses a line with end points marked "0 = no pain" on the left and "10 = worst pain" on the right. Divisions along the line are marked in units from 1 to 9. Explain to children that the left end of the line (0) means that a person feels no pain. At the other end is a 10, which means that a person feels the worst pain possible. The numbers 1 to 9 in the middle are for "a little pain" to "a lot of pain." Ask children to choose a number that best describes their pain. As soon as they can count and have a concept of "less to more," children are ready to use a numerical scale. Be certain to show school-age children the scale; do not just say score your pain from 0 to 10. Until children reach late adolescence, they use concrete thought processes and so need the help of seeing the line to rate their pain best.

The Adolescent Pediatric Pain Tool

The Adolescent Pediatric Pain Tool (APPT) combines a visual activity and a numerical scale (Savedra, Tesler, Holzemer, et al., 1992). On one half of the form (Fig. 39.4) is an outline figure showing the anterior and posterior view of a child. To use the tool, tell a child to color in the figure drawing at the point where pain is felt. In addition, on the right side of the form, tell the child to rate the present pain in reference to "no pain," "little pain," "medium pain," "large pain," and "worst possible pain." For a third activity, tell children to point to or circle as many words as possible on the form that describe their pain (words such as horrible, pounding, cutting, and stinging). The scale is suggested for use in children 8 through 17 years of age. Because many children below this age group need so much help reading and interpreting the multitude of words that describe pain, it makes the form impractical for them. This is a useful tool for involving parents to talk with their child about pain. Reading the words together helps children examine the type, location, and level of pain they are experiencing. It also helps parents to better understand what their child is experiencing.

Logs and Diaries

Having children keep logs or diaries in which they note when pain occurs and the intensity of the pain each time it occurs can be useful for assessing children with chronic but intermittent pain. Examining such a diary not only reveals when pain occurs but also provides direction for pain management. For example, if the diary shows the child always awakens with pain in the morning, the child may need a longer acting analgesic to take at bedtime; if pain is worse during weekends spent at a grandparent's house, investigate whether something

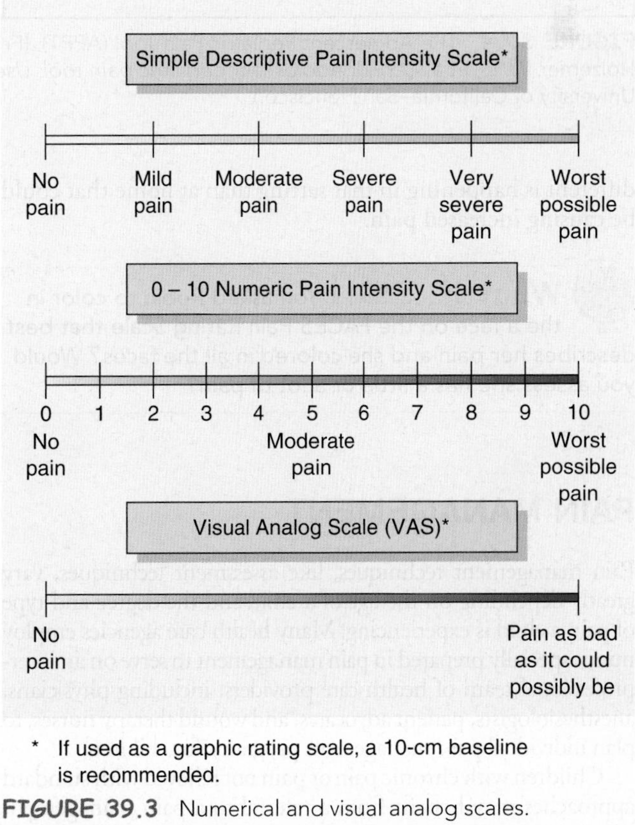

FIGURE 39.3 Numerical and visual analog scales.

CODE________________

DATE________________

Adolescent and Pediatric Pain Tool (APPT)

1. INSTRUCTIONS

Color in the areas on these drawings to show where you have pain. Make the marks as big or as small as the place where the pain is.

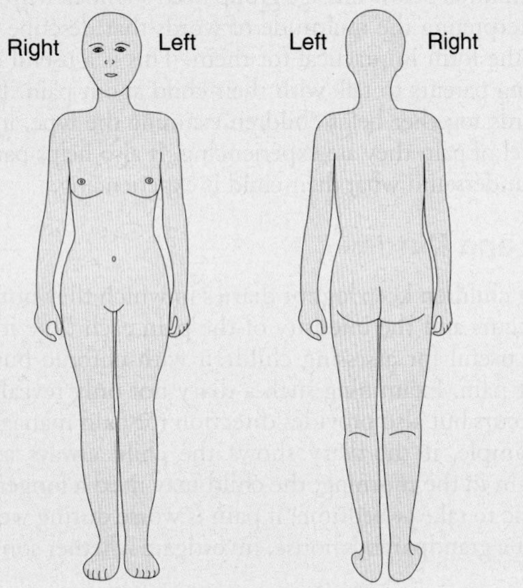

2. Place a straight, up and down mark on this line to show how much pain you have.

No pain | Little pain | Medium pain | Large pain | Worst possible pain

3. Point to or circle as many of these words that describe your pain

1	5	10	15
annoying	blistering	awful	off and on
bad	burning	deadly	once in a while
horrible	hot	dying	sneaks up
miserable	6	killing	sometimes
terrible	cramping	11	steady
uncomfortable	crushing	crying	
2	like a pinch	frightening	If you like you may add other words:
aching	pinching	screaming	
hurting	pressure	terrifying	
like an ache	7	12	
like a hurt	itching	dizzy	
sore	like a scratch	sickening	________
3	like a sting	suffocating	________
beating	scratching	13	________
hitting	stinging	never goes away	
pounding	8	uncontrollable	
punching	shocking	14	
throbbing	shooting	always	For office use only
4	splitting	comes and goes	
biting	9	comes on all of a sudden	
cutting	numb	constant	
like a pin	stiff	continuous	
like a sharp knife	swollen	forever	
pin like	tight		
sharp			
stabbing			

For office use only

BSA:			
IS:			
#S (2-9)	____/37=	____	%
#A (10-12)	____/11=	____	%
#E (1,13)	____/8=	____	%
#T (14,15)	____/11=	____	%
Total	____/67=	____	%

FIGURE 39.4 The Adolescent Pediatric Pain Tool (APPT). (From Savedra, M. C., Tesler, M. D., Holzemer, W. L., et al. [1992]. *Adolescent pediatric pain tool: User's manual.* San Francisco, CA: University of California–San Francisco.)

different is happening in that setting than at home that could be causing increased pain.

What if...39.1 You asked Robin to color in the a face on the FACES Pain Rating Scale that best describes her pain and she colored in all the faces? Would you assess she has a little or a lot of pain?

PAIN MANAGEMENT

Pain management techniques, like assessment techniques, vary greatly depending on the age of a child and the degree and type of pain a child is experiencing. Many health care agencies employ nurses specially prepared in pain management to serve on an interprofessional team of health care providers, including physicians, anesthesiologists, patient advocates, and wound therapy nurses, to plan individual pain management programs for children.

Children with chronic pain or pain not relieved with standard approaches may benefit from a referral to a pain management specialist or team because relief of frequent pain episodes or prolonged pain may require intense, consistent assessments and interventions, which are difficult to achieve in an acute care setting or during infrequent office visits. Whatever assessment tools or methods of pain relief are used, the staff should all become familiar and comfortable with their use so interventions do not vary based on the health care provider.

A good rule for determining whether children need pain relief for a procedure is to remember that if the procedure would cause pain in an adult, it will also cause pain in a child. Many health care professionals such as physicians or X-ray or endoscopic assistants perform procedures with a child that could cause pain. Assist these team members in scheduling procedures at times when a child can be administered optimal pain relief. Help them institute nonpharmacologic measures of pain management such as distraction because often a combination of nonpharmacologic and pharmacologic methods work best (Riddell, Racine, Turcotte, et al., 2012).

General measures to alleviate pain based primarily on the gate control theory of pain management are summarized in Box 39.6. Box 39.7 shows an interprofessional care map for a child requiring pain management based on these guidelines.

BOX 39.6 Nursing Care Planning Based on Family Teaching

PAIN MANAGEMENT WITH CHILDREN

Q. Mrs. Harvey asks you, "How can I be sure I can keep my daughter pain free after we return home?"
A. Here are some tips on ways to offer pain relief in addition to just giving medicine:

- Let the child know you want very much to try to take away the pain and so are happy to work with her to relieve it. Use a positive approach: "This medicine will take away your pain," not "Take this and let's hope it works."
- Administer pain medication before pain becomes intense to help *prevent* pain rather than just relieve it. If a child is in the hospital, inform the staff if a particular approach works or does not work.
- Never just give an analgesic. Make the child comfortable in ways such as straightening the sheets or offering a back rub.
- Ask your child about measures she thinks will be helpful, such as an additional pillow, the television turned on, or a favorite toy nearby.
- Help your child talk about and describe the pain she is experiencing. This can help make it more concrete and not as psychologically frightening.
- Relieve anxiety about other phases of life, if possible. Relaxation reduces muscle strain and tension that can add to pain.
- Offer emotional support. Pain never seems as bad when a support person is present. Reassuring your child that she is loved and that you will be there for her can be very comforting.
- Try not to use such statements as, "Be a big girl" or "Stop crying" when a child is in pain from a procedure such as an injection. Say instead, "It's all right to cry. I know it hurts," to avoid shaming a child who cannot stop crying.

BOX 39.7 Nursing Care Planning

AN INTERPROFESSIONAL CARE MAP FOR A CHILD REQUIRING PAIN MANAGEMENT

Robin Harvey, a 3-year-old girl admitted to your hospital unit, has just returned from a bone marrow aspiration to rule out the possibility of leukemia. Robin received intravenous (IV) morphine sulfate during the procedure. Unfortunately, the bone marrow obtained for analysis is not adequate, so a repeat procedure is scheduled for 3 hours from now.

Family Assessment Child is only daughter of two parents. Father works as a welder in a local steel mill; mother works part time at a local convenience store. Family rates finances as, "Doing good."

Client Assessment A 3-year-old girl with a history of frequent nosebleeds, petechiae, and bruising admitted for diagnostic testing. First experience with hospitalization. Screams at the sight of a syringe and needle. Both parents at bedside talking with child. Child upset and crying, "Don't let them hurt me!"

Nursing Diagnoses Anxiety related to fear of the unknown and anticipation of painful procedure.

Outcome Criteria Child identifies pain as no higher than 1 with Oucher Pain Rating Scale; exhibits few to no nonverbal indicators of pain; exhibits age-appropriate coping behaviors, including the use of one nonpharmacologic pain relief technique.

Team Member Responsible	Assessment	Intervention	Rationale	Expected Outcome
Activities of Daily Living, Including Safety				
Nurse	Assess if IV morphine provided adequate pain relief for last procedure.	Review with parents the necessity for the repeat procedure and possible methods to help child with pain.	Being prepared for coming procedure can reduce anxiety in both parents and child.	Parents state they understand why repeat procedure must be done; are satisfied with repeat pain relief measures to be used.

(continued on page 1124)

BOX 39.7 Nursing Care Planning (continued)

Nurse	Assess vital signs and the child's present pain rating.	Engage the child in quiet activities for the first hour postprocedure.	The child is at risk for bleeding from the puncture site. Quiet activities reduce the risk for bleeding and also provide distraction.	Vital signs remain stable; pain rating is not over 1 on child rating scale. Child colors quietly.
Teamwork and Collaboration				
Nurse/Primary health care provider	Assess if pain management team member is available for consultation.	Consult with pain management team member for best pain relief for frightened preschool child.	Well-planned pain relief can best meet the needs of an anxious child.	Pain management team member meets with parents and child; determines best method of pain relief.
Procedures/Medications for Quality Improvement				
Nurse	Assess if repeat bone aspiration site is free of inflammation.	Apply anesthetic cream to aspiration site and cover with an occlusive dressing 1 hour before scheduled procedure.	Anesthetic cream helps reduce pain. An occlusive dressing enhances absorption and tissue penetration.	The child cooperates with application procedure. Occlusive dressing remains in place preprocedure.
Nutrition				
Nurse	Assess when the child last ate.	Keep the child nothing by mouth (NPO) for 30 minutes preprocedure.	Nausea from heavy analgesia can lead to aspiration if stomach is full.	Parents state they understand temporary restriction for fluid.
Patient-Centered Care				
Nurse	Assess what the child and parents believe was most traumatic aspect of previous bone marrow aspiration.	Review with the child that a feeling of pressure with needle insertion will occur.	Anticipatory knowledge of events and feelings helps to prepare the child and aids in coping.	Parents state they feel prepared for new procedure; will support child through the procedure.
Nurse	Assess if pain assessment tool was used with child during previous procedure.	Introduce the child to Oucher Pain Rating Scale.	Introducing the child to the tool prior to the onset of pain minimizes anxiety and so can increase the tool's usefulness and accuracy in determining the level of pain.	Child rates her pain preprocedure to demonstrate she understands how to use the scale. Number sets a baseline for comparison postprocedure.
Psychosocial/Spiritual/Emotional Needs				
Nurse	Assess if the child has had experience with therapeutic play.	Provide opportunities for therapeutic play with a doll and syringe before and after the procedure.	Therapeutic play helps the child express her feelings about painful procedures and possibly reduces anxiety.	The child plays with doll and syringe under nurse supervision; does not demonstrate behavior suggestive of extreme anxiety or fright.
Informatics for Seamless Health Care Planning				
Nurse	Assess if the child is free of pain postprocedure and if parents received adequate information on the outcome of the procedure.	Ask the child to rate pain on the Oucher Scale; ask parents if they have received a procedure report and understand the results.	A postprocedure evaluation helps to meet further needs of the child and parents and improves skills of health care providers.	Child rates pain as 1 or below on a pain rating scale. Parents state they have results of the procedure and they understand the next step needed for diagnosis and treatment.

What if...39.2 A nurse who works with you tells you she doesn't want to use a self-report tool with Robin because she feels that such tools replace her nursing judgment. You'd like her to use one. How would you justify your view to her? What are the pros and cons of pain assessment tools?

NONPHARMACOLOGIC PAIN MANAGEMENT FOR CHILDREN

Nonpharmacologic pain relief measures (often called alternative or complementary therapies) can be used either independently or as complements to pharmacologic pain relief.

Distraction

Distraction techniques aim at shifting a child's focus from pain to another activity or interest (Fig. 39.5). Blowing soap bubbles, for example, could be used during an injection to accomplish this. If oral glucose is offered to infants during painful procedures, the pain they experience appears to be significantly less (Kassab, Sheehy, King, et al., 2011). It is hypothesized that drinking glucose not only serves as a distraction technique but also activates endorphins and produces a central analgesic effect (Harrison, Beggs, & Stevens, 2012). Breastfeeding may also be used in this way but is not advised to avoid the infant making an association between breastfeeding and pain. When helping parents choose a distraction technique such as blowing soap bubbles with their child, be certain they do not interpret "distraction" as just talking to the child or suggesting a video game to divert attention. Although these are distractions, a distraction activity must require concentration; simple distractions can allow pain to break through.

Substitution of Meaning or Imagery

Substitution of meaning or guided imagery is a distraction technique to help a child place another meaning (a nonpainful one) on a painful procedure (Kline, Turnbull, & LaBruna, 2010). Children are often more adept at imagery than adults because their imagination is less inhibited. This technique works well with both quick, simple procedures such as venipunctures and chronic pain. Success with this technique requires practice, however, so it may have limited application in an acute care setting. As an example, a child could imagine a venipuncture needle as a silver rocket ship probing the moon or a submarine diving under the water to escape a torpedo just in time. Be certain a child thinks of a specific image. Help the child elaborate on the image to make it more concrete each time it is used by asking questions such as: "What color is the rocket ship?" "Are there stripes on the sides?" and "What does the pilot look like?" This helps the child's mind stay on the image and not the venipuncture pain.

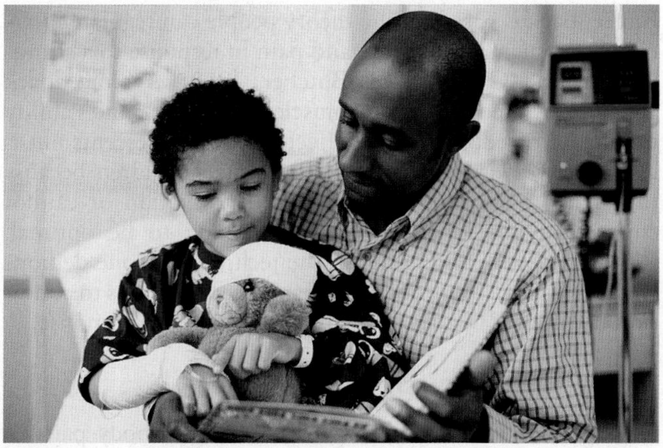

FIGURE 39.5 A parent using distraction (reading a book) as a pain management technique.

QSEN Checkpoint Question 39.2

Evidence-Based Practice

Parents, as a rule, are anxious to stay with their children while they have painful procedures. To investigate whether parents' reassurance during a painful procedure reduced or intensified children's fear, researchers observed 100 children (40 boys, 60 girls) 5 to 10 years old and their parents (86 mothers, 14 fathers) while the child had a venipuncture. Spontaneous parent–child interactions during the procedure were captured and used for a video-mediated recall task in which the children viewed instances of parental reassurance and then distraction and rated their parents' fear and happiness. Second, the children were asked to rate the intensity of parental fear and happiness for 12 video vignettes showing an actor posing as a parent during venipuncture. For both tasks, the children provided higher ratings of fear during reassurance than during distraction as if they realized their parent might be saying "Don't worry" but facial expression or tone of voice radiated worry (McMurtry, Chambers, McGrath, et al., 2010).

Based on the previous study, when Robin has her next bone marrow biopsy, which of the following would you do?

a. Ask her mother if she and her husband would step outside the room.
b. Suggest her mother just nod her head but not talk during the procedure.
c. Ask her mother how best to draw Robin's attention elsewhere.
d. Suggest that Robin's parents avoid the words, "Don't worry" when talking.

Look in Appendix A for the best answer and rationale.

Thought Stopping

Thought stopping is a technique in which children learn to stop anxious thoughts by substituting a positive or relaxing thought in its place. As with imagery, this technique requires practice before it can be used in a painful situation. It may be most helpful in relieving anticipatory anxiety, a negative force that not only increases a pain experience during a procedure but also makes the time before it full of anxiety as well. For this technique, help children think of a set of positive things about the approaching feared procedure. For a bone marrow aspiration, for example, this might include, "It doesn't take long; my father will be with me; it's important to help me get better." Whenever children start to think about the impending procedure, they should stop whatever they are doing and recite the list of positive thoughts to themselves if others are present or out loud if they are alone or only important support people are present. Children can then return to a usual activity. Every time the anxious thoughts appear, however, a child should stop and recite the list again (Curtis, Wingert, & Ali, 2012).

Thought stopping is different from merely saying, "Don't think about it," because the technique does not suppress thoughts; rather, it changes them into positive ones. It also gives children a feeling of control. The secret for success is for the child to use the technique every time the disturbing, anxious thoughts appear even if, at first, such thoughts crowd in as frequently as every few minutes.

Hypnosis

Hypnosis is not a common pain management technique with children but can be effective if a child is properly trained in the technique (Kuttner, 2012). For best results, a child needs to train with a therapist before anticipated pain, so at the time of the pain, the child can produce a trancelike state to effectively avoid sensing pain.

Aromatherapy and Essential Oils

Aromatherapy is based on the principle that the sense of smell plays a significant role in overall health. When an essential oil is inhaled, its molecules are transported via the olfactory system to the limbic system in the brain. The brain then responds to particular aromas with emotional responses. When applied externally, the oils are absorbed by the skin and then carried throughout the body. Essential oils may be able to penetrate cell walls and transport nutrients or oxygen to the inside of cells. Jasmine and lavender are oils thought to be responsible for relieving pain (Miller, Jacob, & Hockenberry, 2011).

Magnet Therapy

Magnet therapy is based on the belief that magnets can control or shift body energy lines to restore health or relieve pain. Magnets can be applied as jewelry or sewn into clothing or shoes. Although many people find relief from magnet therapy, the relief may be more of a placebo effect than an actual change in pain level (Lee & Raja, 2011). Copper also is believed to have pain-relieving ability and is often incorporated into rings and bracelets for this reason.

Music Therapy

The use of music for calming or improving well-being can be effective for all ages of children or adolescents, even as young as preterm infants. It works to relieve pain because it can be relaxing and also serves as a distraction (Nguyen, Nilsson, Hellstrom, et al., 2010). A child who is "blasting" music from a phone or iPad may not actually enjoy hearing the music that loud but needs that level of distraction to feel free of pain.

Yoga and Meditation

Yoga, a term derived from the Sanskrit word for "union," involves a series of exercises that were originally designed to bring people who practice it closer to God. It offers a significant variety of proven health benefits, such as increasing the efficiency of the heart, slowing the respiratory rate, lowering blood pressure, promoting relaxation, reducing stress, and allaying anxiety. Exercises consist of deep-breathing exercises, body postures to stretch and strengthen muscles, and meditation to focus the mind and relax the body. Yoga may be helpful at reducing pain through its ability to create total relaxation and possibly through distraction or the release of endorphins (Evans, Moieni, Sternlieb, et al., 2012).

Acupuncture and Acupressure

Acupuncture involves the insertion of needles into critical positions (meridian lines) in the body to achieve pain relief (Chiou & Nurko, 2010). Acupressure involves applying deep pressure at the same points. Although acupuncture is almost painless, children can be very afraid of it at first because of the sight of the needles. This level of stress can make it not as attractive an option for pain management with children as acupressure. Children who consent to either technique, however, particularly those with chronic pain, report that the overall process is pleasant and the method offers relief from stress (Das, Nayak, & Margaret, 2011).

Crystal or Gemstone Therapy

Some people believe gemstones or crystals have healing powers when they are arranged in certain positions around the body. If these are being used, be careful when changing bedding or rearranging equipment in a child's room that you do not tip them over or move them. A child may feel they may lose their pain-relieving powers if placed in a different position (Zuzak, Bonková, Careddu, et al., 2013).

Herbal Therapies

Specific herbs are frequently used for relieving pain or for generally improving children's health. Some examples include chamomile tea (inflammation reduction), garlic (anti-inflammatory reduction, anticancer prevention), ginger (nausea or vomiting reduction), goldenrod (urinary tract inflammation reduction), or peppermint (abdominal pain relief) (Hunt & Ernst, 2011). Always ask when taking health histories if a child is being given any herbs to be informed about common herbs and to be certain what the child is receiving will complement, not interfere with, the effects of prescribed pain medication.

Biofeedback

Biofeedback is based on the theory people can regulate internal events such as heart rate and pain in response to a stimulus (Myrvik, Campbell, & Butcher, 2012). A biofeedback apparatus is used to measure muscle tone or the child's ability to relax. Biofeedback can be effective with adolescents but is less effective with school-age and younger children because they tend to resist the biofeedback information or cannot concentrate for long enough for training to be optimal. Although some children grasp the technique in one demonstration session, most need to attend several sessions to condition themselves to adequately regulate their pain response.

Therapeutic Touch and Massage

Massage is the use of rubbing or kneading of body parts to aid circulation and relax muscles. Therapeutic touch is the use of touch to provide comfort and relieve pain (Hall, 2012).

Therapeutic touch is based on the principal that the body contains energy fields. When these are plentiful and arranged correctly, they lead to health; when they are in lesser supply, ill health results. Although therapeutic touch may serve as a form of distraction, proponents believe it is possible to redirect energy fields to increase the supply and the release of endorphins.

Transcutaneous Electrical Nerve Stimulation

Transcutaneous electrical nerve stimulation (TENS) involves applying small electrodes to the dermatomes that supply the body portion where pain is experienced (Ali, Drendel, Kircher, et al., 2010). When children sense pain, they push a button on a control box, which then delivers a small electrical current to the skin. The principle underlying this technique is the same as rubbing an injured part or acupressure—the current interferes with the transmission of the pain impulse across small nerve fibers.

TENS can be used to manage either acute or chronic pain. Some children (and parents) dislike TENS therapy because they are nervous about the electric current. Assure them that the current is a very mild one and will not harm their child. TENS is not recommended if the child is incontinent or has a wound that is likely to cause the electrodes to get wet. Skin should also be monitored for irritation from the TENS pads.

Heat or Cold Application

Cold reduces pain by constricting capillaries and therefore reducing vessel permeability and edema and pressure at an injured site. After the first 24 hours of an injury, applying heat may be more helpful because this dilates capillaries, increases blood flow to the area, and again helps reduce edema.

QSEN Checkpoint Question 39.3

Quality Improvement

The algorithm on the pediatric unit for addressing pain in children includes teaching Robin guided imagery to help reduce pain. What is the rationale for using this technique to manage children's pain?

a. Children's pain is generally not as acute as that of adults.
b. IV pain relief is poorly distributed in children.
c. Children's imaginations are at their peak in life.
d. Children are typically more relaxed than adults.

Look in Appendix A for the best answer and rationale.

PHARMACOLOGIC PAIN RELIEF

Pharmacologic pain relief refers to the administration of a wide variety of analgesic medications. Many children need analgesic agents in addition to nonpharmacologic techniques for pain relief, especially for acute pain. Medications can be applied topically or given orally, intramuscularly, intravenously, or by epidural injection. As a rule, intramuscularly administered analgesia should be avoided in children because children dislike injections and have a limited number of adequate injection sites. Be certain children understand that it is acceptable to ask for medication for pain because they may not know they can do so unless this is stressed by health care providers. Be very careful when administering pain medications to children that, even if you are hurrying to provide pain relief, you use all the usual medication safeguards because mistakes can have a very serious outcome. Always check medication doses in a pharmacology reference designed specifically for children or neonates (see Chapter 38).

Topical Anesthetic Cream

To reduce the pain of procedures such as venipuncture, lumbar puncture, and bone marrow aspiration, a local anesthetic cream that contains 4% lidocaine can be used (Jorge, Feres, & Teles, 2011; Poonai, Alawi, Rieder, et al., 2012).

The cream is applied to the skin, and the site is then covered with an occlusive dressing or plastic wrap to keep young children from wiping away or tasting the cream. The time needed for effect between different brands varies from 30 minutes to 1 hour and so must be applied within that time frame before an expected procedure (Box 39.8). Parents can apply anesthetic cream at home before bringing a child to a clinic visit for a procedure such as bone marrow aspiration to avoid a long waiting time (Fig. 39.6). Caution them not to allow their child to remove the dressing because the cream could anesthetize the gag reflex if eaten or cause eye damage if rubbed into the eyes. They are effective with procedures such as venipuncture, intramuscular (IM), or subcutaneous injections. They also can be used effectively for pain relief with circumcision (Rosen, 2010). EMLA cream, a combination of local anesthetics, is a popular cream used, but has to be applied at least 1 hour before the procedure; however, it can be applied up to 3 hours before a procedure and still be effective. A newer compound, ELA-MAX (LMX), containing only lidocaine, takes effect in 30 minutes or less (Crowley, Storer, Heaton, et al., 2011). It can be purchased without a prescription, but, as an over-the-counter medication, is often not reimbursed by insurance companies.

What if...39.3 Robin is scheduled to have blood drawn at 10 AM and, to prepare her for this, you apply an anesthetic cream, which takes an hour to be effective, at 9 AM. However, the technician who will take the blood arrives early. Would you ask the technician to wait, or explain to Robin that the cream is not going to work?

Oral Analgesia

Oral analgesia is advantageous because it is cost-effective and relatively easy to administer. Many analgesics are supplied in liquid form and flavored with cherry or grape syrup to disguise unpleasant tastes. Caution parents that even though such drugs taste sweet, they should never refer to them as "candy." Reinforce with parents the need for proper storage (locked in a cabinet or out of the child's reach) because, otherwise, children may help themselves to more of the pleasantly flavored "candy" when the parent leaves the room. Toxicity from too frequent or overly large doses of acetaminophen is the number one reason for poisoning in small children and can lead to severe liver damage in children (Karch, 2013).

BOX 39.8 Nursing Care Planning Based on Responsibility for Pharmacology

EMLA CREAM

Classification: EMLA (eutectic mixture of local anesthetics) is a topical anesthetic cream containing lidocaine and prilocaine.

Action: Acts to anesthetize skin before potentially painful procedures (Karch, 2013).

Pregnancy Risk Category: B

Dosage: Dollop of cream to intended skin site for at least 1 hour before procedure (2 to 3 hours before deeper procedures such as lumbar puncture or bone marrow aspiration)

Possible Adverse Effects: Hypersensitivity and itching

Nursing Implications

- Explain to the child that the cream will help prevent pain during a procedure.
- Wash the site with soap and water; don't use alcohol because this removes body oil, which is necessary for the effective action of the anesthetic.
- Apply a dollop of cream to the intended site and cover with a transparent occlusive dressing at least 1 hour before the procedure. Do not rub cream into the skin.
- If the cream is to be applied at home, instruct the parents how to apply the cream and the occlusive dressing. Suggest the parents use plastic wrap for the occlusive dressing.
- Instruct the child not to touch the dressing while it is in place. If necessary, cover the occlusive dressing with an opaque material to prevent the child from touching or playing with it.
- Just before the procedure, remove the dressing and then wipe the skin to remove the cream.
- Observe the skin. Look for reddened or blanched skin, which indicates that the drug has penetrated the skin.
- Do not use the drug for a child with a known history of sensitivity or allergy to local anesthetics such as lidocaine.
- The drug is not approved for use in infants younger than 1 month, although it is frequently used for circumcisions after research showed it was tolerated well by neonates for that procedure (Rosen, 2010).

Nonsteroidal anti-inflammatory drugs (NSAIDs) such as ibuprofen or naproxen are excellent for reducing pain because, as their name implies, they reduce inflammation as well as pain in conditions such as sprained ankles or rheumatic conditions. Long-term administration of any NSAID can lead to severe gastric irritation, so this category of analgesics should not be used longer than prescribed. Help parents giving any analgesia around the clock for several days to make out a medication sheet to hang on their refrigerator door or some other method to remind them when the next dose will be due and alert them not to give drug doses too close together.

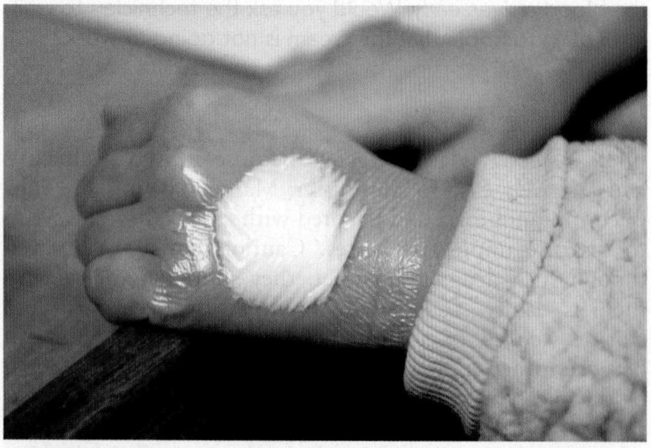

FIGURE 39.6 The local anesthetic cream can be applied to a child's hand and held in place with a transparent dressing at home prior to surgery (© Sheldon Levis/Alamy).

Children should not receive acetylsalicylic acid (aspirin) for pain relief, especially in the presence of flulike symptoms, because there is an association between aspirin administration and the development of Reye syndrome, a severe neurologic disorder (see Chapter 49).

For managing severe or acute pain, such as postoperative pain or the pain of a sickle-cell crisis, opioids, such as morphine, oxycodone, and hydromorphone (Dilaudid), are frequently prescribed. Because this class of drugs is also referred to as narcotics, parents may be reluctant to give their children these medications out of concern that their child will become addicted. Acknowledge their concern, but reassure them the risk for addiction during short-term use is remote. Reinforce that the main concern is supplying adequate pain relief for their child.

QSEN Checkpoint Question 39.4

Safety

Robin's primary health care provider has prescribed both an oral analgesic and an IV antibiotic for her. What is the most important thing you need to know before you can safely administer these medications?

a. Which medicine Robin's mother prefers you give
b. Robin's weight and the recommended doses based on her weight
c. Robin's precise age, because some medications are not prescribed for infants
d. Robin's ability to participate in nonpharmacologic interventions

Look in Appendix A for the best answer and rationale.

Intramuscular Injection

Although opiates are available as IM injections, analgesia for children is rarely given by this route because the number of suitable injection sites in children is limited, injections are associated with pain on administration, and such an injection can produce great fear in children. An IM injection also can lead to several risks, including uneven absorption, unpredictable onset of action, and nerve and tissue damage. As a rule, other routes are used whenever possible.

Intravenous Administration

IV administration of analgesia, the most rapid-acting route, is the method of choice in emergency situations, in the child with acute pain, and in a child requiring frequent doses of analgesia but in whom the gastrointestinal tract cannot be used. Common opioids given by this route include morphine, fentanyl, and hydromorphone (Dilaudid). Hydromorphone is 8 to 10 times stronger than morphine but very similar in action. Fentanyl has a shorter duration of action than morphine but works quickly and produces less side effects such as pruritus and vasodilatation. These features make it an ideal drug to use for short, painful procedures, such as debriding a burn or inserting a chest tube to relieve a pneumothorax.

Opiate analgesics can be given by bolus injection or by continuous infusion. If doses will be given periodically by an IV line, advocate for the use of an intermittent infusion device to avoid repeated venipunctures with each dose or the need for a confining IV line to be in place. If a child's pain is frequent or constant so a continuous IV line is necessary, advocate for a patient-controlled pump to offer the child a sense of control and rapid analgesia. As the child becomes able to take medications by mouth, oral forms of analgesics will then be administered. When switching from IV to oral medications, be certain the oral medication is supplied in an equianalgesic dose.

All opioids have the potential to decrease respiratory rate, although this is not a worry with accurate dosing. Other side effects include nausea, pruritus, vasodilatation, cough suppression, and constipation. If toxicity with opioids should occur, naloxone (Narcan), an opiate antagonist, can be administered to counteract the effects.

Patient-Controlled Analgesia

Patient-controlled analgesia (PCA) allows a child or a parent to self-administer boluses of medication, usually opioids, with an IV medication pump (see also Chapter 16). Children as young as 5 or 6 years of age are able to assess when they need a bolus of medicine and press the button on the pump to deliver the new dose through an established IV line. Parents or a nurse are able to administer a new dose to children younger than this. Morphine is a common analgesic used for PCA administration (Anghelescu, Faughnan, Oakes, et al., 2012). The pump is set with a lock-out time so that after each dose, the pump will not release further medication even if the button is pushed again; because of this, children cannot overmedicate themselves. If pain is constant, a continuous infusion should be used so that pain relief continues even while the child sleeps. The pump can still be programmed for bolus dosing to cover episodes of increased pain.

QSEN Checkpoint Question 39.5

Patient-Centered Care

Robin, 3 years old, received analgesia intravenously. Her mother has asked the care team if she would possibly be a candidate for PCA. What advantage of PCA would you discuss with this mother?

a. The child can gain a sense of control over his or her pain.
b. The child can have his or her pain relieved without the risk of adverse effects.
c. The child requires less nursing care in order to have his or her pain relieved.
d. The child's pain will change from acute pain to chronic pain.

Look in Appendix A for the best answer and rationale.

Conscious Sedation

Conscious sedation refers to a state of depressed consciousness usually obtained through IV analgesia therapy (Havidich & Cravero, 2012). The technique allows a child to be both pain free and sedated for a procedure. Unlike the use of general anesthesia, protective reflexes are left intact and a child can respond to instructions during the procedure. The technique is used for painful procedures such as dental extractions, wound care, and bone marrow aspiration, as well as for magnetic resonance imaging and endoscopy, both of which require a child to lie still for a long period of time and can be potentially frightening. Drugs used for conscious sedation can be something as common as chloral hydrate or as involved as a sedative-hypnotic-analgesic combination, which relieves both anxiety and pain and depresses the child's memory of the event. In many health care settings, conscious sedation is administered and monitored by nurses specially prepared in the technique (Fig. 39.7).

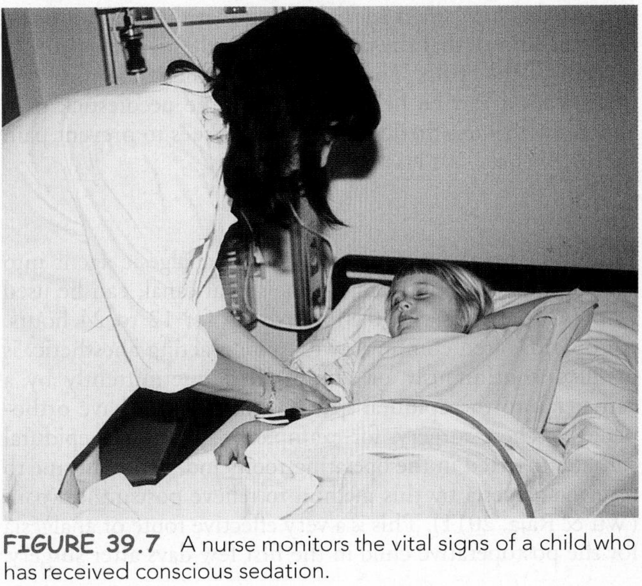

FIGURE 39.7 A nurse monitors the vital signs of a child who has received conscious sedation.

QSEN Checkpoint Question 39.6

Teamwork & Collaboration

Robin is scheduled for conscious sedation to have a repeat bone marrow aspiration. Your colleague will accompany Robin and her mother to the procedure and you will subsequently join them and the other members of the care team. How should you instruct your colleague to explain conscious sedation to Robin?

a. "You'll be given a special medicine to knock you out."
b. "I'll give you some medicine, but you will still be awake and feel everything."
c. "Conscious sedation is an analgesic, not an anesthetic, method of pain relief."
d. "I'll give you medicine so you'll be very sleepy but can still talk to me."

Look in Appendix A for the best answer and rationale.

Intranasal Administration

Intranasal administration is becoming an attractive way to dispense medicine for children because it's easy for parents to administer and the medicine absorbs well from the nasal mucous membrane. Influenza vaccine, for example, is now available in an intranasal form (Flood, Ryan, Rousculp, et al., 2011; Wolfe & Braude, 2010). Midazolam (Versed) is a short-acting adjuvant sedative that can be administered intranasally by nasal drops or nasal spray before surgery or procedures such as nuclear medicine scanning (Karch, 2013). Because it has a very short duration of action, it may require repeat administration. Because it has no analgesic action, an analgesic should be administered concurrently if the procedure will be painful.

Local Anesthesia Injection

Local anesthetics stop pain transmission by blocking nerve conduction of the impulse at the site of pain. Children receive local anesthetic injections, such as lidocaine, before procedures such as bone marrow aspiration, peritoneal dialysis, or suturing of lacerations. For many children, the sight of the anesthetic needle is so frightening that they cannot listen to the assurance that the momentary needlestick will actually prevent further pain. The use of an anesthetic cream before the injection can be helpful to relieve the needlestick pain and allow the anesthetic to numb the tissues to prevent pain (Crowley et al., 2011).

Epidural Analgesia

Epidural analgesia, an injection of an analgesic agent into the epidural space just outside the spinal canal, can be used to provide analgesia to the lower body for 12 to 24 hours. An opioid, often combined with a long-acting anesthetic, is instilled continuously or administered intermittently by a catheter into the epidural space. Children who have orthopedic or chest surgery, for example, may have an epidural catheter inserted in the operating room and then continue to receive analgesia by this method to relieve postsurgical pain (Wu & Raja, 2011). This is a very effective route of analgesia for the postoperative child in the first few days after surgery. Because it is commonly used for childbirth, it is discussed further in Chapter 16.

Some parents may be reluctant to allow this type of analgesia because they equate it with spinal anesthesia, which they know can cause severe headaches. You can assure them that an epidural needle does not enter the cerebrospinal fluid, so spinal headaches are extremely rare.

ONGOING PAIN RELIEF

Because of early discharge and the increased use of ambulatory surgery, many children return home on a pain management routine. Be certain children (and parents) are provided with support and follow-up to the extent necessary to continue adequate pain management in the home. Otherwise, the lack of pain relief at home can be overwhelming.

Either oral or IV analgesia can be administered by parents in a home setting. Be certain that parents have instructions on dosing, administration, frequency, expected outcomes, and expected level of relief. Provide them with the name and telephone number of a health care professional whom they can call if they have questions about pain management (Johnston, Barrington, Taddio, et al., 2011).

What if . . . 39.4 You are interested in exploring one of the 2020 National Health Goals related to pain management and children (see Box 39.1). Most government-sponsored money for nursing research is allotted based on these goals. What would be a possible research topic to explore pertinent to these goals that would be applicable to the Harvey family and that would also advance evidence-based practice?

KEY POINTS FOR REVIEW

- Many children and infants are undermedicated for pain relief because of common misperceptions by health care personnel, such as infants do not feel or remember pain. Infants do experience pain and so need pain management the same as all other groups.
- Inviting parents and the child, if preschool age or older, to participate in assessment and pain management is an important aspect of pain therapy. It not only helps in planning nursing care that meets QSEN competencies, but it also best meets the family's total needs.
- Pain in children is best assessed by means of a standardized self-report tool such as the Poker Chip or Wong-Baker FACES Pain Rating Scale tools. Without self-report forms, both nurses and parents may underestimate children's pain.
- Many nonpharmacologic pain relief measures such as imagery, distraction, and TENS are available for children based on the gate control theory of pain management.
- Many children benefit from a combination of nonpharmacologic and pharmacologic methods of pain management such as an oral analgesic followed by a distraction technique.
- Anesthetic cream to help dull the pain of injections or other brief procedures can be helpful to allow for suturing or venipunctures. Think ahead to use these because a child has to wait 30 to 60 minutes to feel the anesthetic effect.

- Few analgesics are administered intramuscularly to children. For acute pain, IV administration has become the method of choice. PCA, a technique that gives a child a sense of control, can be used effectively with children.
- Conscious sedation is useful with potentially frightening procedures. With this, protective reflexes are left intact, and the child can respond to instructions during the procedure.

Critical Thinking Care Study

Robert is a full-term male newborn. His parents are considering circumcision, but are unsure of the procedure and the level of pain it will cause. Robert is a healthy newborn with no health issues that would contraindicate the procedure.

1. Suppose the doctor who comes to circumcise Robert doesn't like to use an anesthetic for the procedure because it requires additional time. "I've done over a thousand of these," she tells you. "Not one complained to me afterward about how much it hurt." Because she supervises the births of only a few babies a year at your health care facility, would you try to change her opinion?
2. Suppose your health care setting policy requires an anesthetic cream to be used. What could you do for comfort for Robert over and above that?
3. Nurses often sit on institutional review boards (IRBs) to approve research protocols to be certain research respects patient safety and well-being. If you were a member of a hospital IRB, would you approve a study to investigate whether a new anesthetic cream or a placebo caused less pain in newborns having circumcisions?

Patient Scenario

The Merriman Family

Read about the Merriman family, a family whose child needs pain management, then answer the questions to further sharpen your skills and grow more familiar with NCLEX-type questions related to pain management in children. Confirm your answers are correct by reading the rationales.

Visit http://thePoint.lww.com

Answers and Rationales

Looking for answers to the What If . . . and Critical Thinking Care Study questions?

Visit http://thePoint.lww.com

REFERENCES

Ali, S., Drendel, A. L., Kircher, J., et al. (2010). Pain management of musculoskeletal injuries in children: Current state and future directions. *Pediatric Emergency Care, 26*(7), 518–524.

Anghelescu, D. L., Faughnan, L. G., Oakes, L. L., et al. (2012). Parent-controlled PCA for pain management in pediatric oncology: Is it safe? *Journal of Pediatric Hematology/Oncology, 34*(6), 416–420.

Beyer, J. E., Denyes, M. J., & Villarruel, A. M. (1992). The creation, validation, and continuing development of the Oucher: A measure of pain intensity in children. *Journal of Pediatric Nursing, 7*(5), 335–346.

Boerlage, A. A., Ista, E., de Jong, M., et al. (2012). The COMFORT behavior scale: Is a shorter observation period feasible? *Pediatric Critical Care Medicine, 13*(2), e124–e125.

Chiou, E., & Nurko, S. (2010). Management of functional abdominal pain and irritable bowel syndrome in children and adolescents. *Expert Review of Gastroenterology & Hepatology, 4*(3), 293–304.

Crowley, M. A., Storer, A., Heaton, K., et al. (2011). Emergency nursing resource: Needle-related procedural pain in pediatric patients in the emergency department. *Journal of Emergency Nursing, 37*(3), 246–251.

Curtis, S., Wingert, A., & Ali, S. (2012). The *Cochrane Library* and procedural pain in children: An overview of reviews. *Evidence-Based Child Health: A Cochrane Review Journal, 7*(5), 1363–1399.

Das, R., Nayak, B. S., & Margaret, B. (2011). Acupressure and physical stress among high school students. *Holistic Nursing Practice, 25*(2), 97–104.

Downey, L. V., & Zun, L. S. (2012). The impact of watching cartoons for distraction during painful procedures in the emergency department. *Pediatric Emergency Care, 28*(10), 1033–1035.

Evans, S., Moieni, M., Sternlieb, B., et al. (2012). Yoga for youth in pain: The UCLA pediatric pain program model. *Holistic Nursing Practice, 26*(5), 262–271.

Fanning, J. J., Stucke, A. G., Christensen, M. A., et al. (2012). Perioperative opiate requirements in children with previous opiate infusion. *Paediatric Anaesthesia, 22*(3), 203–208.

Flood, E. M., Ryan, K. J., Rousculp, M. D., et al. (2011). A survey of children's preferences for influenza vaccine attributes. *Vaccine, 29*(26), 4334–4340.

Hall, R. W. (2012). Anesthesia and analgesia in the NICU. *Clinical Perinatology, 39*(1), 239–254.

Harrison, D., Beggs, S., & Stevens, B. (2012). Sucrose for procedural pain management in infants. *Pediatrics, 130*(5), 918–925.

Harrison, D., Elia, S., Royle, J., et al. (2013). Pain management strategies used during early childhood immunisation in Victoria. *Journal of Paediatric Child Health, 49*(4), 313–318.

Havidich, J. E., & Cravero, J. P. (2012). The current status of procedural sedation for pediatric patients in out-of-operating room locations. *Current Opinion in Anaesthesiology, 25*(4), 453–460.

Hester, N. O., & Barcus, C. S. (1986). Assessment and management of pain in children. *Pediatrics: Nursing Update, 1*(14), 2–6.

Hunt, K., & Ernst, E. (2011). The evidence-base for complementary medicine in children: A critical overview of systematic reviews. *Archives of Disease in Childhood, 96*(8), 769–776.

Johnston, C., Barrington, K. J., Taddio, A., et al. (2011). Pain in Canadian NICUs: Have we improved over the past 12 years? *Clinical Journal of Pain, 27*(3), 225–232.

Jorge, L. L., Feres, C. C., & Teles, V. E. P. (2011). Topical preparations for pain relief: Efficacy and patient adherence. *Journal of Pain Research, 20*(4), 11–24.

Karch, A. M. (2013). *2013 Lippincott's nursing drug guide.* Philadelphia, PA: Lippincott Williams & Wilkins.

Kassab, M., Sheehy, A., King, M., et al. (2011). A double-blind randomized controlled trial of 25% oral glucose for pain relief in 2-month old infants undergoing immunization. *International Journal of Nursing Studies, 49*(3), 249–256.

Kline, W. H., Turnbull, A., LaBruna, V. E., et al. (2010). Enhancing pain management in the PICU by teaching guided mental imagery: A quality-improvement project. *Journal of Pediatric Psychology, 35*(1), 25–31.

Krechel, S. W., & Bildner, J. (1995). CRIES: A new neonatal postoperative pain measurement score. *Paediatric Anesthesia, 5*(1), 53–57.

Kuttner, L. (2012). Pediatric hypnosis: Pre-, peri-, and post-anesthesia. *Paediatric Anaesthesia, 22*(6), 573–577.

Lee, F. H., & Raja, S. N. (2011). Complementary and alternative medicine in chronic pain. *Pain, 152*(1), 28–30.

McCaffery, M. (1979). *Nursing management of the patient with pain* (2nd ed.). New York, NY: J. B. Lippincott.

McMurtry, C. M., Chambers, C. T., McGrath, P. J., et al. (2010). When "don't worry" communicates fear: Children's perceptions of parental reassurance and distraction during a painful medical procedure. *Pain, 150*(1), 52–58.

Melzack, R., & Wall, P. (1965). Pain mechanisms: A new theory. *Science, 150*(4), 971–976.

Merkel, S., Voepel-Lewis, T., & Malviya, S. (2002). Pain assessment in infants and young children: The FLACC scale. *American Journal of Nursing, 102*(10), 55–58.

Miller, E., Jacob, E., & Hockenberry, M. J. (2011). Nausea, pain, fatigue, and multiple symptoms in hospitalized children with cancer. *Oncology Nursing Forum, 38*(5), e382–e393.

Myrvik, M. P., Campbell, A. D., & Butcher, J. L. (2012). Single-session biofeedback-assisted relaxation training in children with sickle cell disease. *Journal of Pediatric Hematology/ Oncology, 34*(5), 340–343.

Nguyen, T. N., Nilsson, S., Hellstrom, A., et al. (2010). Music therapy to reduce pain and anxiety in children with cancer undergoing lumbar puncture: A randomized clinical trial. *Journal of Pediatric Oncology Nursing, 27*(3), 146–155.

Pagé, M. G., Katz, J., Stinson, J., et al. (2012). Validation of the numerical rating scale for pain intensity and unpleasantness in pediatric acute postoperative pain: Sensitivity to change over time. *Journal of Pain, 13*(4), 359–369.

Palermo, T. N., Eccleston, C., Lewandowski, A. S., et al. (2010). Randomized controlled trials of psychological therapies for management of chronic pain in children and adolescents: An updated meta-analytic review. *Pain, 148*(3), 387–397.

Poonai, N., Alawi, K., Rieder, M., et al. (2012). A comparison of amethocaine and liposomal lidocaine cream as a pain reliever before venipuncture in children: A randomized control trial. *Pediatric Emergency Care, 28*(2), 104–108.

Riddell, P., Racine, N. M., Turcotte, K., et al. (2012). Non-pharmacological management of infant and young child procedural pain. *Evidence-Based Child Health: A Cochrane Review Journal, 7*(6), 1905–2121.

Rosen, M. (2010). Anesthesia for ritual circumcision in neonates. *Pediatric Anesthesia, 20*(12), 1124–1127.

Savedra, M. C., Tesler, M. D., Holzemer, W. L., et al. (1992). *Adolescent pediatric pain tool: User's manual.* San Francisco, CA: University of California/San Francisco.

Schiavenato, M., Butler-O'Hare, M., & Scovanner, P. (2011). Exploring the association between pain intensity and facial display in term newborns. *Pain Research and Management, 16*(1), 10–12.

Shockley, R. A., & Rickett, K. (2011). What's the best way to control circumcision pain in newborns? *The Journal of Family Practice, 60*(4), 233a–233b.

U.S. Department of Health and Human Services. (2010). *Healthy people 2020.* Washington, DC: Author.

van Dijk, M., Peters, J. W., van Deventer, P., et al. (2005). The COMFORT Behavior Scale: A tool for assessing pain and sedation in infants. *American Journal of Nursing, 105*(1), 33–36.

Vervoort, T., Eccleston, C., Goubert, L., et al. (2010). Children's catastrophic thinking about their pain predicts pain and disability 6 months later. *European Journal of Pain, 14*(1), 90–96.

Wolfe, T. R., & Braude, D. A. (2010). Intranasal medication delivery for children: A brief update. *Pediatrics, 126*(3), 532–537.

Wong, D., & Baker, C. (1996). *Reference manual for the Wong-Baker FACES pain rating scale.* Duarte, CA: CHNMC.

Wu, C. L., & Raja, S. N. (2011). Treatment of acute postoperative pain. *Lancet, 377*(9784), 2215–2225.

Zuzak, T. J., Bonková, J., Careddu, D. A., et al. (2013). Use of complementary and alternative medicine by children in Europe. *Complementary Therapies in Medicine, 21*(1), S32–S47.

Unit 7

The Nursing Role in Restoring and Maintaining the Health of Children and Families With Physiologic Disorders

Chapter 40

Nursing Care of a Family When a Child Has a Respiratory Disorder

KEY TERMS

- adventitious sounds
- anoxia
- arterial blood gases (ABGs)
- aspiration
- atelectasis
- clubbing
- cyanosis
- expiration
- hypoxemia
- hypoxia
- inspiration
- paroxysmal coughing
- percussion
- pneumothorax
- rales
- retraction
- steatorrhea
- stridor
- tachypnea
- tracheostomy
- tracheotomy
- vibration
- wheezing

OBJECTIVES

After mastering the contents of this chapter, you should be able to:

1. Describe common respiratory disorders in children.
2. Identify 2020 National Health Goals related to children with respiratory disorders that nurses can help the nation achieve.
3. Assess a child with a respiratory disorder.
4. Formulate nursing diagnoses related to respiratory disorders in children.
5. Identify expected outcomes that address the priority needs of a child with a respiratory disorder to help him or her manage seamless transitions across differing health care settings.
6. Using the nursing process, plan nursing care that includes the six competencies of Quality & Safety Education for Nurses (QSEN): Patient-Centered Care, Teamwork & Collaboration, Evidence-Based Practice (EBP), Quality Improvement (QI), Safety, and Informatics.
7. Implement nursing care for a child with a respiratory disorder, such as administering oxygen.
8. Evaluate expected outcomes for achievement and effectiveness of care.
9. Integrate knowledge of respiratory disorders in children with the interplay of nursing process, the six competencies of QSEN, and Family Nursing to achieve quality maternal and child health nursing care.

Michael is a 6-year-old who is brought to the emergency department by paramedics who responded to an emergency call by his grandmother at his home. Michael has a sharp, barking cough, is crying loudly, and is obviously short of breath. "He can't breathe!" his grandmother shouts at you. "I gave him some chocolate. Is he allergic to that?" Michael is diagnosed as having laryngotracheobronchitis (croup) and admitted to an ambulatory care unit.

Previous chapters described the growth and development of well children. This chapter adds information about the dramatic changes, both physical and psychosocial, that occur when children develop respiratory disorders.

What emergency care does Michael need? Given Michael's description, what would lead you to believe his airway is not yet completely obstructed?

Respiratory disorders are among the most common causes of illness and hospitalization in children (Kirk, 2013). Overall, respiratory dysfunction in children tends to be more serious than in adults because the lumens of a child's respiratory tract are smaller and therefore more likely to become obstructed. Because respiratory disorders range from minor illnesses, such as a simple upper respiratory tract infection, to life-threatening lower respiratory tract diseases, such as pneumonia, and because the level of acuity can change quickly, respiratory disorders are often difficult for parents to evaluate. Both a child and parents need a great deal of nursing support when disease interferes with breathing, because even very young children may panic when breathing becomes labored. Early diagnosis and treatment are essential for preventing a minor problem from turning into a more serious one (Hafeez, Ronca, & Maldonado, 2011).

Because respiratory disorders are such a common cause of childhood illness and hospitalization, 2020 National Health Goals have been established for children with respiratory illnesses (Box 40.1).

BOX 40.1 Nursing Care Planning Based on 2020 National Health Goals

Because reducing the incidence of respiration illness in children could greatly reduce the number of emergency room visits and school days missed, a number of 2020 National Health Goals focus on respiratory illness:

- Reduce hospitalizations for asthma in children under 5 years of age from a baseline of 41.4 out of 10,000 children to a target level of 18.1 out of 10,000 children.
- Reduce invasive pneumococcal infections in children under 5 years from 20.3 out of 100,000 children to 12.0 out of 100,000 children.
- Reduce the number of courses of antibiotic prescribed solely for the common cold from 1,728 out of 100,000 children to 864 out of 100,000 children.
- Increase the proportion of children 6 months to 2 years of age who are immunized yearly against seasonal influenza from 25% to 80%.
- Increase the proportion of children 2 to 4 years of age who are immunized yearly against seasonal influenza from 23% to 80% (U.S. Department of Health and Human Services [DHHS], 2010; see www.healthypeople.gov).

Nurses can help the nation achieve these goals by teaching children ways to help avoid respiratory infections such as good hand washing, and reminding parents to come for child health maintenance visits so that children can receive pneumococcal immunization and yearly influenza immunization.

Nursing Process Overview

For a Child With a Respiratory Disorder

Assessment

Respiratory illness can begin as early as moments after birth if a neonate has difficulty initiating a first breath or establishing regular respirations. Rating a neonate using an Apgar score can help to quickly identify a newborn who may be experiencing respiratory difficulty at this early stage.

It is important to establish both the onset and duration of the problem so that its seriousness can be rapidly determined. An episode of sudden coughing is suggestive of an acute respiratory disorder. Infants who cannot finish a bottle feeding because of exhaustion or rapid breathing or children who cannot run with other children because they cannot catch their breath should be suspected of having a chronic respiratory disorder.

A child admitted to the hospital with a respiratory disorder is usually in an acute stage of illness. A child's condition may worsen rapidly in the first few hours until a prescribed medication, such as an antibiotic or steroid bronchodilator, begins to take effect. Nursing assessment findings that show a child is developing tachypnea or retractions may be the first indication of a child's worsening condition.

Nursing Diagnosis

Nursing diagnoses established for children with respiratory disorders focus both on the alteration in mechanisms of breathing and on the emotional distress such problems can create. "Ineffective airway clearance" is a common diagnostic category used in this area. The problem may be related to any one of a variety of factors, such as ineffective cough, fatigue, weakness, viscous secretions, pain, aspiration (inhalation of a foreign object into the airway), or lack of knowledge about the importance of coughing.

Examples of nursing diagnoses include:

- Activity intolerance related to insufficient oxygenation
- Fatigue related to impaired gas exchange
- Fear related to inability to breathe without effort
- Impaired gas exchange related to excessive mucous production
- Impaired social interaction related to difficulty in keeping up with physical activities of peers
- Ineffective breathing pattern related to decreased energy and fatigue
- Deficient knowledge related to the need for continued treatment

Outcome Identification and Planning

If a child is experiencing an acute respiratory problem, the expected outcomes and plan of care will focus on supporting the child and family through prescribed therapy and keeping parents informed about their child's health status and response to treatment. Often, the treatment period for respiratory illness is prolonged, so parents of children with chronic conditions need to learn how to continue therapy at home. Helping parents to plan programs of exercise and teaching chest physiotherapy and the actions of prescribed medications are important nursing activities. Parents also need to understand that their approach to these programs must change as their child grows older. For example, with an infant, parents simply need to perform the prescribed procedures. A game might be a good way to get a toddler or preschooler to breathe deeply (e.g., "Simon says, cough. Simon says, take five deep breaths"). Parents need to plan exercise programs for school-age children and adolescents around their school day; otherwise, children may have difficulty carrying out the program or do so only sporadically. If parents include other family members, such as older siblings or grandparents, in a respiratory therapy program, this may help to diffuse the burden of care and also to unite the family in working toward a common goal. Helpful Web sites for parents to consult about respiratory illnesses are www.kidshealth.org and www.everydayhealth.com. Some organizations to recommend as support to parents of the child with a respiratory disorder include the American Lung Association (www.lung.org), the National Asthma Education and Prevention Program (www.nhlbi.nih.gov/about/naepp), the Easter Seals Foundation (www.easterseals.com), and the Cystic Fibrosis Foundation (www.cff.org).

Implementation

Collaborative nursing interventions in the care of a child with respiratory dysfunction include suctioning to remove respiratory secretions, administering oxygen, and providing humidification and expectorant therapy to help maintain clear airways. Some of the most important nursing interventions in this area are independent nursing functions, such as placing a child in an upright position to help the child cough more effectively, providing an interesting game to teach a child the importance of strengthening chest muscles, supporting a child and family through the anxiety created when a child is not breathing normally, and teaching parents of a child with chronic respiratory dysfunction the basics of percussion or chest physiotherapy techniques. All of these interventions require sound nursing judgment and skill to carry out or teach effectively.

Outcome Evaluation

An acute respiratory illness such as pneumonia is extremely frightening for parents as well as the child. After the child has recovered, talk with the parents to determine whether they have come to terms with their fear and can treat the child as a well child again. Otherwise, overprotection of a child by the parents may result in a well but overly dependent child. Nursing evaluation can help to prevent this.

Expected outcomes for a child with chronic respiratory disease will change as a child grows and develops. No matter what the specific concerns are, however, evaluation should always include examination of how well an individual child and his or her family as a whole have adapted to managing the limitations imposed by the disorder while maintaining a lifestyle that fosters growth and development for all family members.

Examples of expected outcomes that would indicate achievement of goals include:

- Infant, at 3 months of age, maintains respiratory rate of at least 30 breaths/min.
- Child describes a simplified program of school activities he will maintain to reduce fatigue.
- Child's Po_2 is maintained at 80 to 100 mmHg in room air.
- Child lists steps she will take if breathing becomes impaired while at school.
- Parents demonstrate correct techniques for performing respiratory therapy at home.

ANATOMY AND PHYSIOLOGY OF THE RESPIRATORY SYSTEM

The respiratory system can be separated into two divisions: the upper respiratory tract, composed of the nose, paranasal sinuses, pharynx, larynx, and epiglottis; and the lower tract, composed of the bronchi, bronchioles, and alveoli. Through **inspiration** (breathing in), the respiratory system delivers warmed and moistened air to the alveoli, transports oxygen across the alveolar membrane to hemoglobin-laden red blood cells, and allows carbon dioxide to diffuse from red blood cells back into the alveoli. Through **expiration** (breathing out), carbon dioxide–filled air is discharged to the outside. Levels of oxygen and carbon dioxide in the lungs, blood, and body cells are shown in Figure 40.1.

Respiratory Tract Differences in Children

Because the respiratory tract continues to mature during childhood, children have several important differences in respiratory

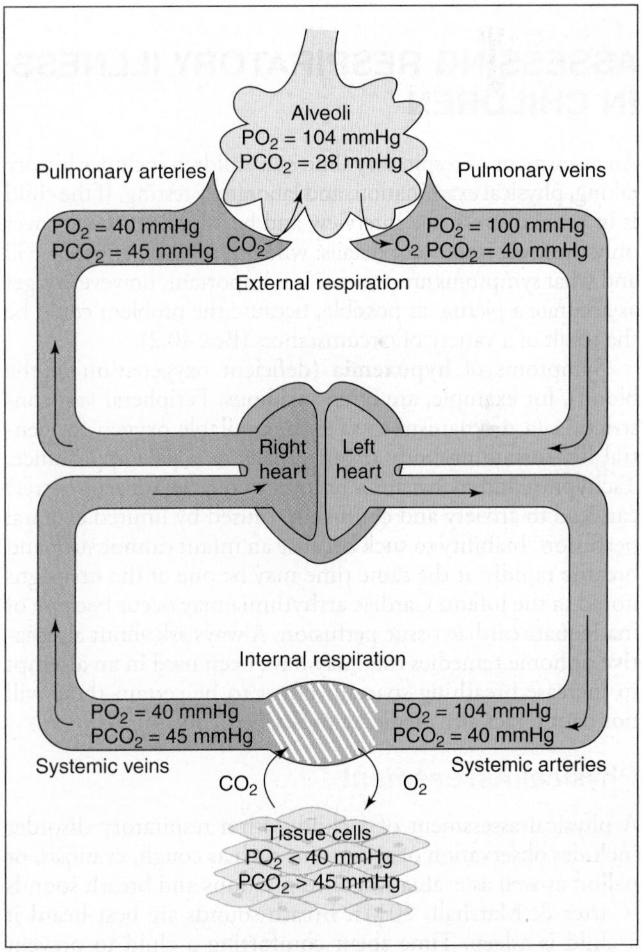

FIGURE 40.1 Partial pressure of gas (millimeter of mercury [mmHg]) as measured in peripheral and systemic circulation. Because of the differences in partial pressure of the gases in the different areas, O_2 moves from alveoli to pulmonary capillaries (i.e., the gas moves from the area of greater concentration to one of a lesser concentration). When it reaches the tissue capillaries, O_2 partial pressure in cells is less, so O_2 goes into the tissues and CO_2 moves out.

anatomy and physiology from adults. The ethmoidal and maxillary sinuses are present at birth, but the frontal sinuses (the sinuses most frequently involved in sinus infection) and the sphenoidal sinuses do not develop until 6 to 8 years of age. Because there is such rapid growth of lymphoid tissue, tonsillar tissue becomes normally enlarged in early school-age children.

Respiratory mucus functions as a cleaning agent by moving invading organisms or other particles out of the lungs. However, newborns produce little respiratory mucus, which makes them more susceptible to respiratory infections than older children. Excessive production of mucus in children up to 2 years of age can actually lead to obstruction because the bronchial lumens are so small in children of this age.

In infants, the walls of the airways have less cartilage than in older children and adults and so are not as strong and more likely to collapse after expiration. An advantage of immature development is that a lessened amount of smooth muscle in the airway means an infant does not develop bronchospasm as readily as an older child or adult. Therefore, **wheezing** (the sound of air being pushed through constricted bronchioles) may not be a prominent finding in infants even when the lumen of the airway is severely compromised.

ASSESSING RESPIRATORY ILLNESS IN CHILDREN

An assessment of respiratory illness in children includes history taking, physical examination, and laboratory testing. If the child is in acute distress, the interview and health history may cover only the most important details: when the child first became ill and what symptoms are present. It is important, however, to get as accurate a picture as possible, because the problem could be the result of a variety of circumstances (Box 40.2).

Symptoms of **hypoxemia** (deficient oxygenation of the blood), for example, are often insidious. Peripheral vasoconstriction (a mechanism to save the available oxygen for central life-sustaining body organs) leads to a pale appearance. Tachypnea and tachycardia (efforts to oxygenate cells better) can lead to anxiety and confusion, caused by limited cerebral perfusion. Inability to suck because an infant cannot suck and breathe rapidly at the same time may be one of the first signs noted in the infant. Cardiac arrhythmia may occur because of inadequate cardiac tissue perfusion. Always ask about alternative or home remedies that may have been used in an attempt to increase breathing space or effort to be certain these will not counteract any medicine prescribed (Box 40.3).

Physical Assessment

A physical assessment of a child with a respiratory disorder includes observation of symptoms such as cough, cyanosis, or pallor, as well as evaluation of respirations and breath sounds (Carter & Marshall, 2011). Breath sounds are best heard if a child is asleep. Time spent comforting a child to prevent crying is time well spent.

Cough

A cough reflex is initiated by stimulation of the nerves of the respiratory tract mucosa by the presence of dust, chemicals, mucus, or inflammation. The sound of coughing is caused by rapid expiratory air movement past the glottis. Coughing is a useful procedure to clear excess mucus or foreign bodies from the respiratory tract. It only becomes harmful and needs suppression when there is no mucus or debris to be expelled and the amount of coughing becomes exhausting. This might occur with respiratory tract inflammation. **Paroxysmal**

> **BOX 40.2 Nursing Care Planning Using Assessment**
>
> **Assessing a Child for Signs and Symptoms of Respiratory Dysfunction**
>
> **History**
>
> *Chief concern:* Cough, rapid respirations, noisy breathing, rhinitis, reddened sore throat, lethargy, cyanosis, difficulty sucking, fever.
>
> *Past medical history:* Poor weight gain, difficulty with respirations at birth, prematurity.
>
> *Family history:* History of family member with asthma; other family members with respiratory infection.
>
> **Physical examination**

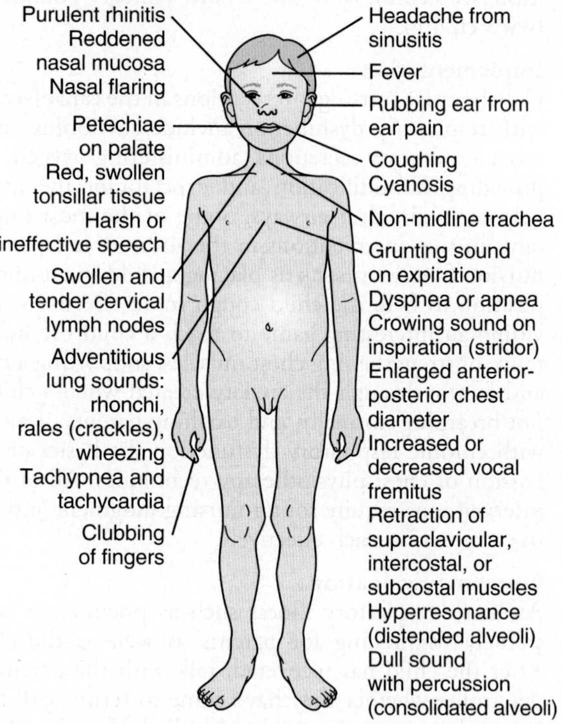

> **BOX 40.3 Nursing Care Planning to Respect Cultural Diversity**
>
> Upper respiratory illnesses occur universally, making them a concern of parents the world over. Home remedies for such illnesses vary greatly, however. Hanging garlic around a child's neck is a frequent therapy in Mediterranean countries. "Cupping" or applying pressure to the back to "draw out" an infection (which leaves red circular ecchymotic marks on the child's back) may be used in Asian cultures. Although the therapeutic value of these remedies may not be proved, it is important to the nurse–patient and nurse–family relationships to respect family traditions.

coughing refers to a series of expiratory coughs after a deep inspiration. Commonly, this occurs in children with pertussis (whooping cough) or in those who have aspirated a foreign body or a liquid they attempted to drink.

Although helpful in removing mucus, coughing does increase chest pressure and so may decrease venous return to the heart. This lowers cardiac output and can lead to fainting (syncope). Paroxysmal coughing may increase the pressure in the central venous circulation to such an extent that bleeding into the central nervous system (CNS) can result. Because young children often vomit after a series of coughs, they may be initially suspected of having a gastric disturbance even though their main illness is respiratory.

Rate and Depth of Respirations

Tachypnea (an increased respiratory rate) often is the first indicator of airway obstruction in young children. Assess not only the rate but also the depth and quality of respirations to assess **anoxia** (lack of oxygen in body cells).

Retractions

When children must inspire more forcefully than normal to inflate their lungs because of an airway obstruction or stiff, noncompliant lungs (as in newborns with pulmonary dysplasia), intrapleural pressure is decreased to the point that the nonrigid parts of the chest (the intercostal spaces) draw inward, creating **retractions** (Fig. 40.2). Retractions occur more commonly in newborns and infants than in older children because the intercostal muscles are weaker and less developed in younger children. Retraction of upper chest muscles (supraclavicular or suprasternal) suggests upper airway obstruction; retraction of intercostal or subcostal muscles suggests lower airway obstruction.

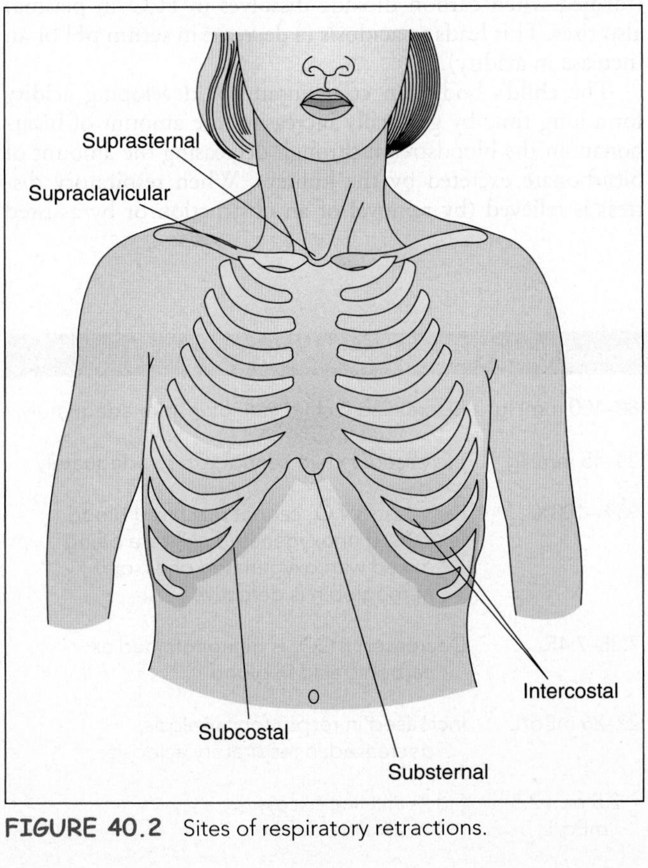

FIGURE 40.2 Sites of respiratory retractions.

Restlessness

When children or infants have decreased oxygen in body cells (**hypoxia**), they become anxious and restless. Be careful not to interpret the excessive movements of infants with respiratory distress as a sign that they are improving. Anxious or restless stirring may be a signal that respiratory obstruction is becoming acute or it may be one of the first signs of airway obstruction.

Cyanosis

Cyanosis (a blue tinge to the skin) indicates hypoxia. It becomes apparent when the Po_2 is under 40 mmHg or the level of unoxygenated hemoglobin increases to over 3 g per 100 ml because oxygenated red blood cells in the circulation are what give blood its red color. If children have a low unoxygenated red blood cell count (below 5g/100 ml), cyanosis may not be apparent because there are not enough unoxygenated red blood cells to give the arterial blood its blue tinge. The degree of cyanosis present, therefore, is not always an accurate indication of the degree of airway difficulty. When children have accompanying peripheral vasoconstriction caused by shock, cyanosis of the extremities also may or may not be apparent.

As the Po_2 drops and cyanosis results, children increase respiratory effort in an attempt to supply more oxygen to tissues. When they do this, the difference in pressure between the intralumen of a not yet fully developed trachea and the surrounding tissue becomes so great that the trachea may collapse, thus compounding the obstruction problem.

Clubbing of Fingers

Children with chronic respiratory illnesses often develop **clubbing** of the fingers, a change in the angle between the fingernail and nail bed because of increased capillary growth in the fingertips (Fig. 40.3). The increased capillary growth occurs as the body attempts to supply more oxygen routes (more capillaries) to distal body cells.

Adventitious Sounds

Normal breath sounds are reviewed in Chapter 34. Pathologic conditions cause **adventitious sounds** (extra or abnormal breathing sounds), which can be heard on lung assessment in children with respiratory disorders.

The vibrations produced as air is forced past an obstruction, such as mucus in the nose or pharynx, cause a snoring sound (*rhonchi*). If the obstruction is at the base of the tongue or in the larynx, a harsher, strident sound on inspiration (*stridor)* occurs. If an obstruction is in the lower trachea or bronchioles, an expiratory whistle sound (*wheezing*) occurs. If alveoli become fluid filled, fine crackling sounds (**rales**) are heard. Diminished or absent breath sounds occur when the alveoli are so fluid filled that little or no air can enter them.

Chest Diameters

With chronic obstructive lung disease, children may be unable to exhale completely, thus allowing air to be chronically trapped in lung alveoli (hyperinflation). This produces an elongated anteroposterior diameter of the chest, sometimes

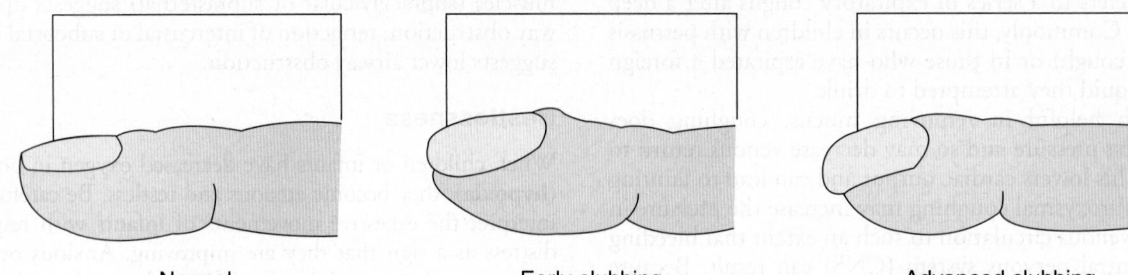

FIGURE 40.3 Clubbing of the fingers. (*Left*) The angle between the nail and digit is normally about 20 degrees in a child. (*Center*) Flattened angle represents early stage of clubbing. (*Right*) In advanced clubbing, the nail is rounded over the end of the finger. Note also that the distal phalanx is bulbous and of greater depth than the proximal portion of the finger (interphalangeal depth).

termed a "pigeon breast." There is an accompanying tympanic or hyperresonant (loud and hollow) sound heard on percussion (see later discussion on chest physiotherapy) over lung spaces.

Laboratory Tests

Several laboratory tests can be used to confirm or rule out the presence of a respiratory disorder and to help identify the cause and severity of the problem. These include an analysis of arterial blood gases, nasopharyngeal culture, and sputum analysis.

Blood Gas Analysis

Blood gas analysis is an invasive method for determining the effectiveness of ventilation and acid–base status. Table 40.1 shows the normal values of **arterial blood gases (ABGs)**—the amount of oxygen and carbon dioxide in the blood.

Blood gas analysis provides important information about oxygenation of the blood because values may indicate not only whether the arterial partial pressure of oxygen (Po_2) is adequate, but also whether the oxygen saturation of hemoglobin is adequate. The oxygen saturation level will fall if adequate oxygen cannot reach the bloodstream because of respiratory distress or if the hemoglobin is defective and cannot carry a full complement of oxygen (as with sickle-cell anemia or thalassemia major). If a child has a severe anemia, the saturation level may be adequate (95% to 100%), but body cells may still not be receiving enough oxygen because of the limited number of red blood cells carrying oxygen. With increased or decreased Pco_2, a low pH, or decreased temperature, the ability of hemoglobin to accept oxygen diminishes so, again, cells may become hypoxic.

Pco_2 measures the efficiency of ventilation. In children who are hypoventilating (breathing very shallowly), Pco_2 will be increased because they cannot blow off CO_2; in children who are hyperventilating (breathing deeply), Pco_2 will be decreased because children are blowing off too much. When children cannot evacuate accumulated CO_2 because of an obstruction or hypoventilation, the partial pressure of CO_2 in the arterial blood rises and the concentration of carbonic acid (formed when carbon dioxide dissolves in H_2O in plasma) also rises. This leads to acidosis (a decrease in serum pH or an increase in acidity).

The child's body can compensate for developing acidity for a long time by gradually increasing the amount of bicarbonate in the bloodstream through decreasing the amount of bicarbonate excreted by the kidneys. When respiratory distress is relieved (by removal of an obstruction or by assisted

TABLE 40.1 Arterial Blood Gas Values

Measure	Definition	Normal Value	Clinical Significance
Po_2	Partial pressure of oxygen in arterial blood	80–100 mmHg	Decreased if child cannot inspire adequately
Pco_2	Partial pressure of carbon dioxide in arterial blood	35–45 mmHg	Increased if child cannot expire adequately
O_2 saturation	The percentage of hemoglobin carrying oxygen	95%–100%	Decreased if O_2 cannot reach red blood cells, if unoxygenated cells are being mixed with oxygenated ones, or if hemoglobin is defective
pH	The hydrogen ion concentration of blood	7.35–7.45	Decreased if CO_2 is being retained as carbonic acid in blood
HCO_3	The bicarbonate concentration in blood	22–26 mEq/L	Increased in respiratory alkalosis; decreased in respiratory acidosis
Base excess	Bicarbonate available for buffering	−2.5 or +2.5 mEq/L	(+) = alkaline excess (−) = alkaline deficit

TABLE 40.2 Comparison of Respiratory Alkalosis and Respiratory Acidosis

Acid–Base Condition	Cause	Findings
Respiratory alkalosis	Hyperventilation	Rapid, deep breathing Confusion, unconsciousness Elevated plasma pH (above 7.45) Elevated urine pH (above 7.0) Decreased Pco_2 (below 40 mmHg) Plasma bicarbonate — Initially normal — Compensated: below 20 mEq/L Base excess: 0 or a negative reading such as −4
Respiratory acidosis	Hypoventilation trapping carbon dioxide in alveoli	Shallow breathing; inability to expire freely Confusion, disorientation Decreased plasma pH (below 7.35) Decreased urine pH (below 6.00) Elevated Pco_2 (over 40 mmHg) Plasma bicarbonate — Initially normal or elevated — Compensated: above 25 mEq/L Base excess: 0 or a positive reading such as +4

ventilation), the amount of bicarbonate present in the bloodstream may exceed the amount of acid produced at that point, and the child's condition may change from acidosis to alkalosis. With alkalosis, the respiratory rate decreases as the child tries to conserve CO_2. As a result, periods of apnea may occur. Children require close observation during this time, including frequent blood gas and electrolyte determinations, to ensure prompt treatment so these changes can be detected and reversed. Table 40.2 compares respiratory alkalosis and respiratory acidosis. Box 40.4 shows steps for evaluating ABGs.

To analyze blood gases, arterial blood rather than venous blood must be used (arterial blood will reflect how well the

BOX 40.4 A Quick Assessment of Arterial Blood Gases

Use a systematic format to assess arterial blood gases (ABGs) quickly:

1. Evaluate the pH: Normally, pH falls between 7.35 and 7.45. A pH below 7.35 denotes acidemia; one above 7.45 reflects alkalemia. If the patient has more than one acid–base imbalance at work, the pH identifies the process in control.
2. Evaluate Pco_2: The partial pressure of arterial CO_2 (Pco_2) normally ranges between 35 and 45 mmHg. A Pco_2 greater than 45 mmHg indicates ventilatory failure and respiratory acidosis from CO_2 accumulation. A Pco_2 less than 35 mmHg indicates alveolar hyperventilation and respiratory alkalosis.
3. Evaluate HCO_3: A bicarbonate (HCO_3^-) less than 22 mEq/L or a base excess (BE) less than −2 mEq/L denotes metabolic acidosis. A bicarbonate level greater than 26 mEq/L or a BE greater than 2 mEq/L reflects metabolic alkalosis. If the two measurements conflict, the BE is the better indicator of metabolic status.
4. Determine which is the primary and which is the compensating disorder: Often, two acid–base imbalances coincide; one is primary, the other is the body's attempt to return the pH to normal. When both the Pco_2 and the HCO_3^- are abnormal, one denotes the primary acid–base disorder and the other denotes the compensating disorder.
   a. To decide which is which, check the pH. *Only a process of acidosis can make the pH acidic; only a process of alkalosis can make the pH alkaline.* For example, if steps 2 and 3 indicate that the patient has respiratory acidosis and metabolic alkalosis and the pH is 7.25, the primary disorder must be respiratory acidosis. The remaining disorder is compensating for the primary problem.
   b. When pH rises (becomes alkalotic), Pco_2 decreases in amount (will be below 35 mmHg). When pH decreases (becomes acidotic), Pco_2 increases (will be above 45 mmHg). When an opposite problem exists this way (pH increased; Pco_2 decreased), the problem is respiratory in origin.
   c. pH and HCO_3^- normally move in the same direction (when pH is elevated, HCO_3^- is elevated). When these two measurements correspond this way (pH decreased, HCO_3^- decreased), then the cause of the problem is metabolic in origin.
   d. Three states of compensation are possible: *noncompensation,* reflected in an alteration of only Pco_2 or HCO_3^-; *partial compensation,* in which both Pco_2 and HCO_3^- are abnormal and, because compensation is incomplete, the pH is also abnormal; and *complete compensation,* in which both Pco_2 and HCO_3^- are abnormal but, because compensation is complete, the pH is normal. To identify the primary disorder when compensation is complete, consider a pH between 7.35 and 7.40 indicative of primary acidosis and a pH between 7.40 and 7.45 indicative of primary alkalosis.
5. Evaluate oxygenation: Normally, Po_2 remains between 80 and 100 mmHg. A Po_2 between 60 and 80 mmHg reflects mild hypoxemia; between 40 and 60 mmHg, moderate hypoxemia; and below 40 mmHg, severe hypoxemia.
6. Interpret the findings: Your final analysis should include the degree of compensation, the primary disorder, and the oxygenation status (e.g., "partially compensated respiratory acidosis with moderate hypoxemia").

BOX 40.5 The Allen Test

Before obtaining an arterial blood gas (ABG) from the radial artery, it is important to establish that a child has collateral circulation to the hand. Otherwise, the needle puncture may block the artery and block blood flow to the hand.

To prove that there is collateral circulation, compress both the radial and ulnar arteries on the inner side of the wrist and elevate the hand until color disappears. Release the pressure over the ulnar artery and observe for a color change in the hand. If the hand does not turn pink (proof the blood has flowed into the hand), the radial artery on that wrist should not be used for catheter insertion.

lungs are oxygenating the blood, whereas venous blood will reflect only the oxygenation of the particular extremity from which the blood was drawn). In the young infant, the temporal artery may be used as a site for blood gases; in newborns, an umbilical artery catheter can be used. In older children, the radial artery is the site of choice because of the collateral circulation present at the wrist. (If clotting should occur in the radial artery, the hand would still be well nourished by collateral circulation; see the Allen test in Box 40.5.)

For an ABG assessment, a specimen is withdrawn into a heparinized syringe (to prevent clotting). After any arterial puncture, always firmly compress the site. Otherwise, blood from the punctured vessel can seep into subcutaneous tissue, possibly causing a large hematoma and obscuring the site for further assessment. If frequent specimen collections are required, an arterial catheter, inserted either peripherally or centrally, may be used. Doing so allows frequent specimen collections without the trauma of additional punctures. Be sure to apply dressings over the area where an arterial catheter exits the skin to help prevent a young child from fussing or playing with the site. Soft restraints, such as an elbow or hand restraint, may be needed to keep a child from dislodging the catheter.

In small infants, when it is impossible to obtain arterial blood directly, heel or finger punctures may be used. Warm the heel or finger for about 20 minutes with a warm compress before the procedure because this will increase local blood flow so much that the blood gas levels of the capillaries approach those of arteries.

Be certain to note the use of oxygen, if any, and its liter flow on laboratory slips for ABG assessments. Also note the site where the specimen was obtained. While being transported to the laboratory, keep ABG specimens on ice to ensure accurate results (CO_2 levels decline in room air). It is important to deliver the ABG specimen to the laboratory immediately following the blood draw, as delaying delivery can result in the specimen being unusable.

The oxygen saturation of hemoglobin can also be obtained noninvasively using pulse oximetry.

Pulse Oximetry. Pulse oximetry is a noninvasive technique for measuring oxygen saturation. For the measurement, a sensor and a photodetector are placed around a vascular bed, most often a finger for a child or a foot for an infant (Fig. 40.4). Infrared light is directed through the finger from the sensor to the photodetector. Because hemoglobin absorbs light waves differently when it is bound to oxygen than when it is not, the oximeter can detect the degree of oxygen saturation (Sao_2) in the hemoglobin.

Oxygen saturation is closely aligned with Po_2 (Fig. 40.5). When Sao_2 is 95%, the Po_2 is within the normal range of 80 to 100 mmHg. When Sao_2 has fallen to 90%, the Po_2 is 60 mmHg. An easy rule to remember with regard to the relationship between Sao_2 and Po_2 is the 60 to 30 and 90 to 60 rule: when Sao_2 is 60, Po_2 is 30; when Sao_2 is 90, Po_2 is 60. Any Sao_2 reading under 90, therefore, is a cause for concern.

One advantage of pulse oximetry is that it is noninvasive. A second advantage is that the continuous monitoring provided by a pulse oximeter allows you to modify your care appropriately. If an oxygen level should begin to fall while you are handling an infant, for example, you could immediately stop care until the infant's Po_2 again returns to

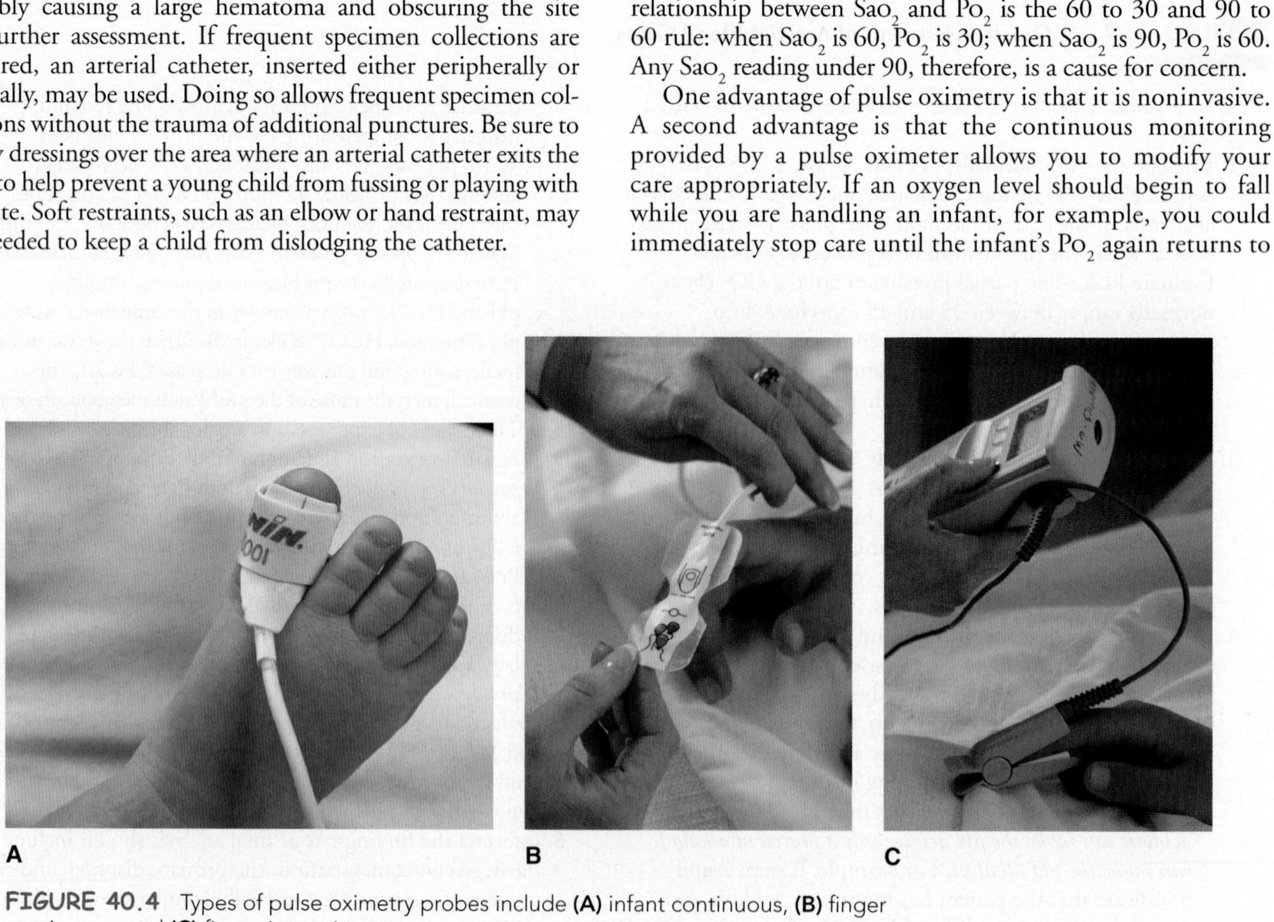

A B C

FIGURE 40.4 Types of pulse oximetry probes include **(A)** infant continuous, **(B)** finger continuous, and **(C)** finger intermittent.

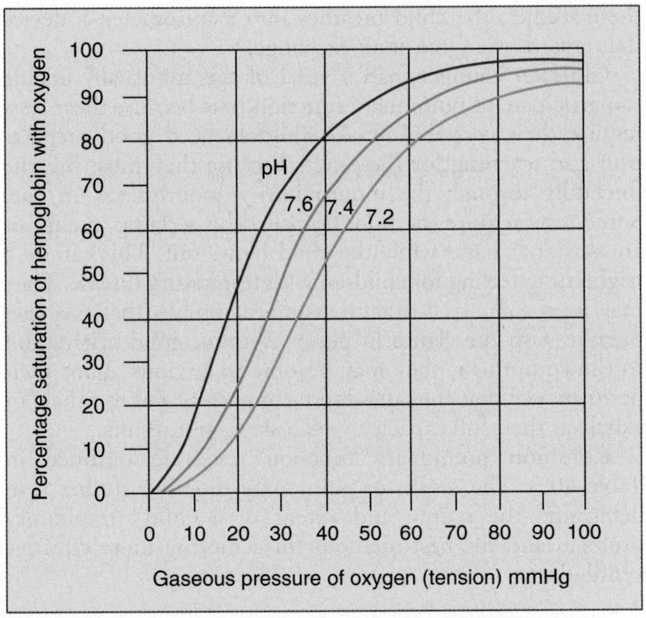

FIGURE 40.5 The oxyhemoglobin dissociation curve.

normal. A disadvantage is that the sensor is small and must be checked frequently to see that it remains in place. Excess light in a room can distort the reading. Therefore, the sensor may need to be covered with a blanket in a neonatal intensive care unit or a brightly lit nursery for readings to be accurate. Young children also tend to remove the sensors just as they frequently remove adhesive bandages from their fingers.

QSEN Checkpoint Question 40.1

Evidence-Based Practice

Pediatric patients often receive oxygen therapy as part of their care when they are diagnosed with a respiratory condition. In order to monitor whether they are receiving enough oxygen, continuous pulse oximetry monitoring is often prescribed. A pulse oximetry alarm is set to ring when the oximetry results are either lower or higher than the preset limits so quick interventions can be taken. To assess if nurses consistently set prescribed alert levels on oximeters with preterm infants, nurse researchers in a neonatal intensive care nursery reviewed prescribed alarm settings. Results of the study showed correct limits were set only 68% to 79% of the time (Armbruster, Schmidt, Poets, et al., 2010).

Based on the previous study, what would be your best action in reference to the oximeter of Michael, age 6 years?

a. Turn off the alarm as long as Michael's mother will be sleeping in the room with him.
b. Confirm the alarm limit settings as part of your safety checks during Michael's nursing care.
c. Set the alarm limits 10% lower or 10% higher to ensure they sound within safe limits.
d. Remove the oximeter periodically so you remain familiar with the sound of the alarm.

Look in Appendix A for the best answer and rationale.

Nasopharyngeal Culture

When done efficiently, nasopharyngeal cultures cause little discomfort and reveal a great deal of information about the microorganisms causing a disease. However, most children are terribly frightened by having something placed in their noses or throats and so may resist accordingly. Firm, calm support during the procedure while you touch a moistened swab to the mucus membrane of the nose or throat is essential. Nose and throat cultures can reveal only the organisms present in the upper respiratory tract. As a result, they may not show organisms causing a lower respiratory tract infection. A throat culture will miss pathogenic organisms if the culture tip is not touched to the infected aspect of the pharynx.

Respiratory Syncytial Virus Nasal Washings

Nasal washings are obtained to diagnose an infection by the respiratory syncytial virus (RSV). For this, a child is placed in the supine position, and 1 to 2 ml of sterile normal saline is dropped with a sterile needleless syringe into one nostril. The nose is then aspirated using a small, sterile bulb syringe. The secretions removed are placed in a sterile container to be sent to the laboratory for analysis. Nasal washings are even more uncomfortable for children than nasal swabbings because of the saline that is instilled. Provide comfort to a child afterward and assure the child the specimen collection is over.

Sputum Analysis

Because they cannot raise sputum with a cough, sputum collection is rarely feasible in children younger than school age. Older children, however, are able to cough and expectorate sputum. Teach them exactly what you want (a specimen of what they are coughing up, not just clearing from the back of their throat). Then ask them to breathe in and out several times, cough deeply, and spit mucus they have raised into a sterile specimen container.

Diagnostic Procedures

In addition to cultures, several other diagnostic procedures are used to identify respiratory disorders in children. Many of these procedures are also used with adults, with modifications to account for the physical and developmental differences of children. Bronchoscopy (visualization of the bronchi through a bronchoscope) is discussed in Chapter 37.

Chest Radiography

Chest X-ray films will show areas of infiltration or consolidation in the lungs; if a foreign body is opaque, an X-ray study will show its location. Chest X-ray films are more difficult to obtain in infants than in older children because infants cannot take a breath and hold it when instructed. It is therefore difficult to picture the lungs at their most expanded position. Computed tomography (CT) scans may be ordered for children with chronic lung disease because this technique can best mark disease progress.

Bronchography

On a chest X-ray, the air-filled larynx, trachea, and major bronchi are revealed as dark spaces. Any obstruction or distortion in the organs is apparent. For further definition of structures, a radiopaque solution may be introduced into the respiratory tract by an ultrasonic nebulizer or by a catheter inserted into the trachea before the X-ray study is performed. Children may require conscious sedation for this because nebulization or having a catheter passed into the airway can be frightening. Afterward, children may have increased mucus production from bronchial irritation by the procedure. Observe them carefully after such a procedure for possible respiratory obstruction from accumulating mucus.

Pulmonary Function Studies

The process of ventilation, or the work of breathing, involves three main forces: (1) an inertial force that must be overcome to change the speed and direction of air when the lungs change from exhalation to inhalation; (2) an elastic force to help the lungs expand with inhalation; and (3) the flow resistance force or resistance to the movement of air through the bronchial tree that must be overcome. Flow resistance must be at a minimum for best ventilation. It becomes increased when the bronchioles are narrowed or plugged with mucus. Pulmonary function tests measure the forces of inertia, elasticity, and flow resistance. Peak flow, a commonly used measure, is the amount of air that can be moved out of the lungs with a forceful breath.

The alveoli of the lungs are never completely empty at the end of expiration because as the bronchioles collapse, they trap a residual amount of air in the alveoli. In contrast, alveoli are never completely filled on inspiration because their potential for expansion exceeds that necessary for good respiratory function. Children with obstructive lung diseases such as asthma or bronchiolitis have some difficulty moving air into the lungs, but they have even more difficulty moving air out of the lungs so greatly expand the size of the alveoli. Even if they do expire the same amount of air as the average child, they expire it over a longer period. Children with restrictive ventilatory disorders, such as neuromuscular disorders, have equal difficulty with inspiration and expiration.

Several lung capacity studies can be done to determine the degree of obstruction or restricted ventilation ability. For these studies, the child breathes into a spirometer, a device that records the force of air exchange.

Children younger than 4 years of age are usually unable to participate in pulmonary function tests because these tests require their cooperation. All children need good preparation and teaching for these tests because they must breathe forcefully through the mouth into a mouthpiece on cue. Some tests require the nose be closed by a clamp, a clip, or an assistant's hand while the child blows out. This can be a frightening feeling for children with respiratory disease. They may need some trial runs to assure themselves that they can breathe with the clamp in place. Without good orientation to the equipment, they may become so anxious about their performance that they develop tachypnea or fail to inhale or exhale at their full capacity, which skews test results.

Common pulmonary function tests are outlined in Table 40.3. The results of pulmonary function studies help determine the nature and extent of a child's respiratory problem and the best methods for achieving more effective ventilation.

HEALTH PROMOTION AND RISK MANAGEMENT

Several ways to promote respiratory health are available for parents and children. The common cold is the most frequent respiratory disorder seen in children and is spread through families easily. Teach children as young as toddlers to help avoid spreading colds by washing their hands, properly disposing of tissues, and blocking a cough by their shirt or blouse sleeve. The incidence of *Haemophilus influenzae* type B (HIB), the cause of bronchiolitis, as well as influenza can be reduced by ensuring that children receive their routine immunizations against these (HIB and influenza vaccine). Be certain that children with chronic respiratory illnesses receive the pneumococcal vaccine as well. Reducing respiratory irritation by reducing secondary smoke can help prevent upper respiratory infections and can reduce the incidence of asthma attacks as well as otitis media (middle ear infections).

TABLE 40.3 Pulmonary Function Tests

Test	Measurement	Clinical Implications
Vital capacity (VC)	The maximum amount of air expelled after a maximum inspiration	Decreased if bronchial lumens are narrowed or obstructed
Tidal volume (TV)	The amount of air inhaled and exhaled in a normal respiratory movement	Decreased if bronchial lumens are constricted
Residual volume	The amount of air remaining in the lungs after a maximum expiration	Increased if there is air trapping in alveoli, as in obstructive lung disease
Functional residual capacity (FRC)	The volume of air remaining in the lungs after a normal expiration	Increased if ability to breathe out is impaired
Forced expiratory volume (FEV)	The amount of air expired in 1 second	Decreased in obstructive disease that prevents free expiration
Peak flow	The strength of air expired in a forceful expiration	Decreased in obstructive disease that prevents free expiration

THERAPEUTIC TECHNIQUES USED IN THE TREATMENT OF RESPIRATORY ILLNESS IN CHILDREN

The primary goal of nursing interventions in the care of children with respiratory disorders is to maintain or reestablish the airway to help ensure that adequate oxygen reaches the blood. Often, this includes interventions aimed at liquefying and removing mucus secretions so they do not clog the bronchial pathways. Such clogging prevents adequate oxygenation and contributes to the development of bronchial and alveolar infections.

Expectorant Therapy

Any irritation of the respiratory tract causes the production of large amounts of mucus. The amount produced can become so great that the natural mechanisms for clearing it (coughing and upward cilia action) are no longer adequate. If a child is breathing rapidly because of respiratory distress, the frequent passage of air over the mucus tends to dry it and make it more viscous, thus compounding the removal problem. Instilling saline nose drops or using saline nasal sprays can be effective at moistening and loosening dried mucus in the nose (Sylvester, Carr, & Nix, 2013).

Vaporizers

Humidification is the provision of moisture to the airway. Vaporizers do this by emitting a stream of air moistened by fine droplets of water into the air, providing either a cool or a warm mist to the entire room. Caution parents when using warm mist that a serious scald burn can result if children accidentally pull a vaporizer onto themselves. To avoid this type of accident, they should be certain the vaporizer is placed up and out of reach of the child. Although cool mist can create a clammy atmosphere in a room, this can be advantageous for a child who also has a fever by helping to cool and moisten the whole environment. Caution parents to clean vaporizers thoroughly after use to prevent the growth of *Pseudomonas* or other pathogenic organisms.

Nebulizers

Nebulizers are mechanical devices that provide a stream of moistened air directly into the respiratory tract. Most are hand-held masks that fit over the nose and mouth and are attached to an electrical pump as a power source (Fig. 40.6). Ultrasonic nebulization delivers such minuscule droplets into the respiratory tract that even the smallest bronchioles can be moistened. Nebulizers also serve as an important means for the delivery of respiratory tract medications because such as antibiotics or bronchodilators can be combined with the nebulized mist and sprayed into the lungs (Dolovich & Dhand, 2011).

Many children find nebulizer treatments uncomfortable because the feel of the mist in their upper respiratory tract can be frightening or irritating. Assure them that aerosol administration is the most effective route for moisture and medication to reach and cause an effect in their respiratory tract. During aerosol medication administration, watch carefully for signs

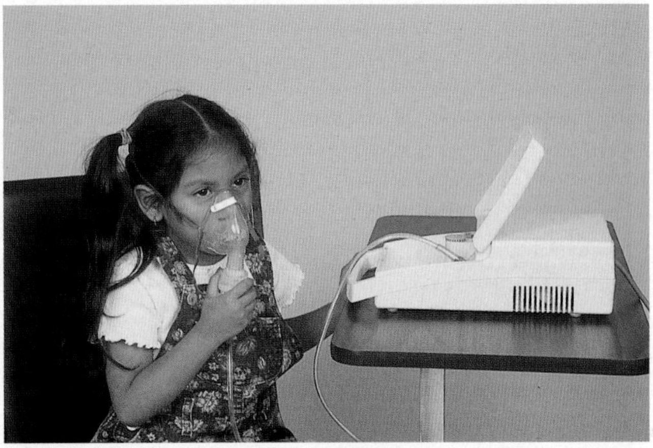

FIGURE 40.6 A child using a nebulizer.

of both local tracheal or bronchial effect (e.g., spasm, edema) that might result from airway irritation as well as systemic symptoms that might result from absorption of a medication by the membrane.

Coughing

As a rule, encourage coughing rather than suppress it in children because it is an effective method of raising mucus. Changing a child's position and suggesting mild exercise or deep breathing are helpful techniques to initiate coughing. Caution parents not to give cough syrup routinely to children as many produce little effect and the risk of overdose, incorrect dosing, and adverse events is greater than the benefit of the syrup (Chang, 2010).

Mucus-Clearing Devices

A mucus-clearing device (a Flutter device) can be used to aid in the removal of mucus. This device looks like a small plastic pipe. A stainless-steel ball inside the device moves when the child breathes out, causing vibrations in the lungs (Fig. 40.7). This vibration helps loosen mucus so that it can be moved up the airway and expectorated. This device is used most frequently with children who have cystic fibrosis or pneumonia to help remove mucus from the lungs.

Chest Physiotherapy

Simply changing a child's position helps mucus to move, initiate a cough reflex, and be expelled. When a child is positioned so the chest is lower than the abdomen, gravity aids in the removal of mucus from the lower lobes and bronchi. When a child sits upright, gravity aids drainage from the upper lobes into the bronchi. When lying supine, anterior alveoli drain; when prone, posterior alveoli drain. Frequent changes of position are important, therefore, to prevent mucus from pooling in certain lung areas. If a child has a localized mucus problem, lying predominantly in one position can encourage drainage of that lung segment. When the child is repositioned and the mucus drains into new bronchi, this will often result in a cough from irritation caused by this new drainage.

Three techniques are involved with chest physiotherapy (CPT) to further loosen mucus for expectoration: postural drainage, percussion, and vibration. Each technique can be

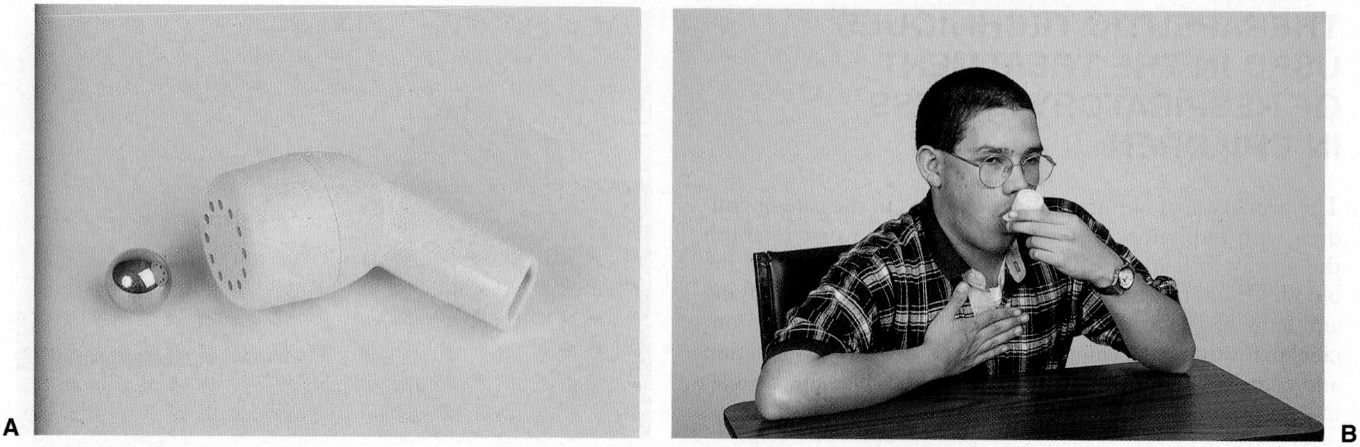

FIGURE 40.7 **(A)** Flutter device. The metal ball (shown) is enclosed in the chamber and causes the vibration. **(B)** An adolescent using a flutter device.

used alone, but they are usually more effective at moving mucus toward the main stem bronchus when performed together.

Although chest physiotherapy is done by respiratory therapists, you will need to integrate the activity into care because CPT is best scheduled before meals or at least an hour after a meal so the subsequent coughing does not cause vomiting. Although CPT takes approximately 30 minutes each time, because these techniques are tiring, you may need to remain with the child to be certain the child can tolerate the different position changes and the techniques. Provide mouthwash to the child after the procedure if age appropriate as coughed sputum may taste unpleasant. Use standard infection precautions to throw away soiled tissues.

Common postural drainage positions for the infant are shown in Figure 40.8. An infant may be positioned on your lap, whereas a slant board or other surface is needed for postural drainage with an older child. **Percussion** involves striking a cupped or curved palm against the chest to determine the consistency of tissue beneath the surface area. This technique causes a loud, thumping noise that sounds as if it hurts, but you can assure a child or parents it does not. In infants and some small children, a specialized device, a nipple, or a small oxygen mask may be used if the palm of the hand is too big (Fig. 40.9). These devices concentrate the motion and may increase the amount of mucus removed.

Vibration is done by pressing a vibrating hand against a child's chest during exhalation. Like percussion, it mechanically loosens and helps move tenacious secretions upward. Vibration also may be accomplished by a mechanical vibrator or a vibrating vest.

If a child is going to need continued CPT at home, one or both parents will need to learn the technique before their child is discharged so that it can be continued conscientiously. The technique is used most frequently with children with bronchiolitis or cystic fibrosis (Dmello, Nayak, & Matuschak, 2010).

What if...40.1 Michael needs to cough to expectorate bronchial mucus but he refuses to try to cough. How would you convince him to do that?

Therapy to Improve Oxygenation

Improving oxygenation almost automatically relieves breathing distress.

Oxygen Administration

Oxygen administration elevates the arterial oxygen saturation level by supplying more oxygen to red blood cells through the respiratory tract. Oxygen may be delivered to infants by flooding an incubator, and for all ages, by a mask or cannula.

Nasal catheters provide a concentration of approximately 50% with an oxygen flow of 4 l/min. Most children do not like nasal prongs or catheters because they are intrusive. Assess their nostrils carefully when using these as the pressure of prongs can cause areas of necrosis, particularly on the nasal septum.

A snug-fitting oxygen mask is a method for supplying nearly 100% oxygen and is the method frequently used in emergencies (Fig. 40.10). Masks, like prongs or catheters, are often not well tolerated by children because they tend to slip and obstruct their view. If necessary, let them hold a mask rather than strapping it in place to allow the child more control.

Regardless of the delivery method used, oxygen must be administered warmed and moistened. Without proper humidification, oxygen dries mucous membranes and thickens secretions, compounding breathing difficulty. Oxygen, like any other drug, requires careful administration and a follow-up assessment. If concentrations are too low, oxygen is not therapeutic; in concentrations greater than those desired, it can be toxic. If newborns are subjected to oxygen concentrations over 100 mmHg for an extended time, retinopathy of prematurity can occur (see Chapter 26). In any child, administering oxygen concentrations of 70% to 80% for an extended period may lead to a thickening of the lung alveoli and a loss of lung pliancy (i.e., oxygen toxicity or bronchopulmonary dysplasia). For these reasons, oxygen should not be given in high concentrations for long periods unless adequate facilities for blood gas analysis or oximetry are available (Bassham, Kane, Mackeil-White, et al., 2012).

When caring for a child with any form of oxygen equipment, follow safety rules. Because oxygen supports combustion, keep open flames away from oxygen and minimize the

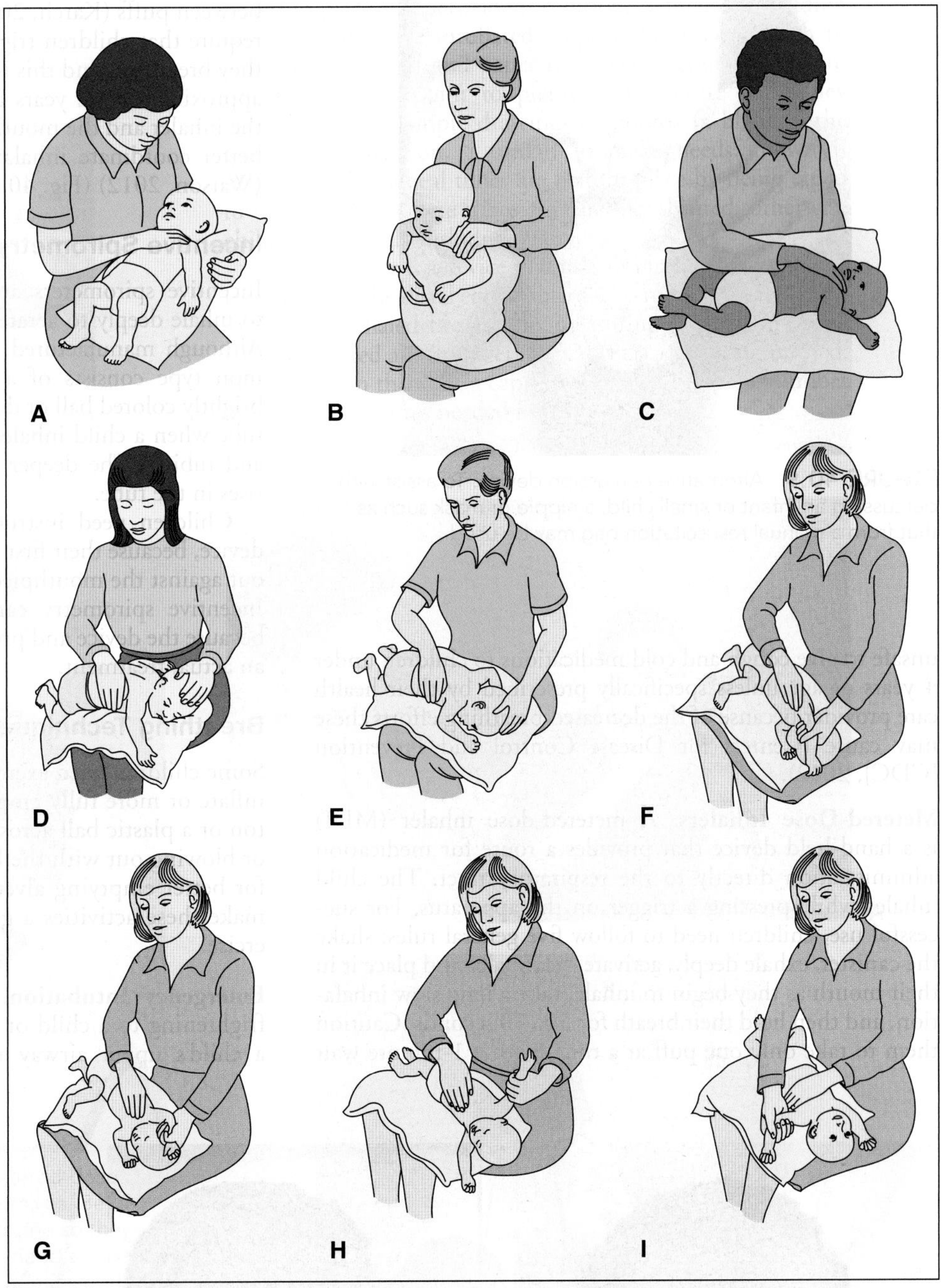

FIGURE 40.8 Positions for bronchial drainage for major segments of all lobes in infants. This procedure is most readily performed with the infant in your lap, with your hand on the chest over the area to be cupped or vibrated. **(A)** The apical segment of left upper lobe. **(B)** The posterior segment of left upper lobe. **(C)** The anterior segment of left upper lobe. **(D)** The superior segment of right lower lobe. **(E)** The posterior basal segment of right lower lobe. **(F)** The lateral basal segment of right lower lobe. **(G)** The anterior basal segment of right lower lobe. **(H)** The medial and lateral segments of right middle lobe. **(I)** The lingular segments (superior and inferior) of left upper lobe.

risks of sparks. Because oxygen is humidified, the equipment is a good source of microbial contaminants and so should be changed according to your agency's policy or at least once a week to keep bacterial counts within safe limits.

Pharmacologic Therapy

Children experience difficulty with exchange of air when their airways become obstructed because of unusual mucus production, bronchoconstriction, or inflammation. Several drugs may be used in children to reverse these processes. Nasal sprays such as normal saline can be administered to moisten and loosen nasal secretions. Antihistamines given by this route can reduce mucus production and thereby enlarge the airway. Corticosteroids taken either orally or by inhalation reduce inflammation and so also enlarge the airway. Decongestants cause vasoconstriction, leading to shrinkage of the mucous membranes, as yet another way to enlarge breathing space. Expectorants such as guaifenesin (Robitussin) can help an older child expectorate mucus. Most of these agents also cause drowsiness, however, so doses must be regulated, especially in adolescents who will be driving. Bronchodilators such as albuterol (Ventolin), terbutaline (Brethine), and levalbuterol (Xopenex) are examples of drugs used to open the lower airway. Antibiotics may be given intravenously, intramuscularly, orally, or inhaled through nebulization to reduce infection and limit purulent mucus and inflammation. Because there are so many different approaches available to aid breathing, parents can be confused about the action of each medicine their child is prescribed. Caution them it is

Tracheostomy

A **tracheostomy** is an opening into the trachea to create an artificial airway to relieve respiratory obstruction that has occurred above that point (Mitchell, Hussey, Setzen, et al., 2013). The procedure to create the airway is called a **tracheotomy**, and the resultant airway is called the tracheostomy. Tracheostomies also may be used as a route for suctioning mucus when accumulating mucus causes lower airway obstruction. Long-term respiratory assistance is the most frequent use of a tracheostomy today (Serra, Cocuzza, Longo, et al., 2012).

A danger of tracheostomies is that they eliminate the warming and filtering action of the nose and pharynx, making children more susceptible to infection. However, if an obstruction is in the pharynx, so noninvasive oxygen administration by a mask or prongs as well as endotracheal intubation is impossible, tracheotomies can be lifesaving.

Tracheotomies are done more easily on the flat surface of a treatment room table than on a bed or crib, so it is generally best to carry a child immediately to a treatment room for the procedure. For a tracheotomy, the cricoid cartilage of the trachea is swabbed with an antiseptic; if readily available, a local anesthetic may be injected into the cartilage ring. (This is not necessary in the unconscious child.) An incision is made just under the ring of cartilage, and a tracheostomy tube with its obturator in place is inserted into the opening (Fig. 40.13A). When the obturator is removed, the child can breathe through the hollow tracheostomy tube (Fig. 40.13B). Have suction equipment available for immediate use to clear any blood caused by the incision, which is minimal, and any obstructing mucus from the trachea.

A few sutures may be necessary at the tube insertion site to halt bleeding or to reduce the size of the incision so the tube fits snugly. As children begin to breathe normally and, if unconscious, regain consciousness, they often thrash and push at people around them, both from oxygen deficit and from fright. They call for a parent but can make no sound, adding to their fright. Assure children everything is all right even though they cannot speak. A school-age child can understand a simple explanation such as, "You can't speak right now because of the tube in your throat, but that's all right." As soon as children's respirations are even and they are no longer experiencing acute respiratory distress, show them how, by placing a finger over the tracheostomy tube opening, air will again flow past their larynx and they can speak. If this causes a child to become short of breath, supply a paper and pencil or chalkboard for communication.

Be certain parents understand why the tube is in place and how important it is that it remain patent. Assure them it is a temporary measure to provide oxygen, provided this is true. Children have difficulty relaxing enough to accept this strange new way of breathing until their parents can relax and accept it also; therefore, if they were not present in the room for the procedure, encourage them to visit the child as soon as possible to assure themselves their child is again all right. Some children hyperventilate, not because of respiratory difficulty, but because of this fear.

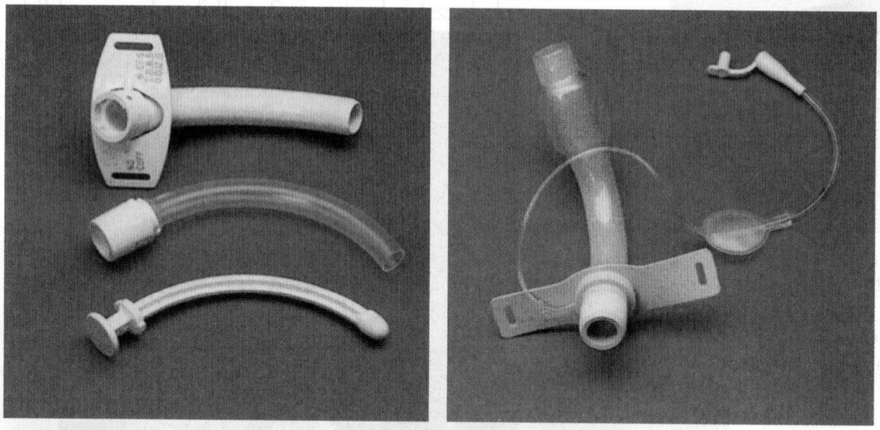

A

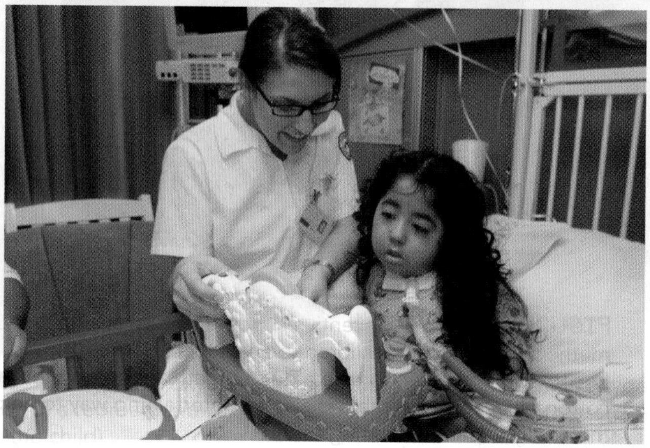

B

FIGURE 40.13 **(A)** Tracheostomy tubes: (*left*) a plastic tube, inner cannula, and obturator; (*right*) a plastic, cuffed tube. **(B)** The tracheostomy collar allows for humidification of inspired air or supplemental oxygen.

Suctioning Technique. Most tracheostomy tubes used with children today are plastic. They do not include an inner cannula, which would require removal and regular cleaning. Most children, however, do require frequent suctioning (perhaps as often as every 15 minutes) to keep their airway free of mucus. Use sterile technique to prevent introducing microorganisms, and suction gently yet thoroughly. Ineffective suctioning does not remove obstructive mucus and, because of irritation, can actually cause more mucus to form. Be certain you know how deeply to suction. Some children need only the length of the tracheostomy tube suctioned so that the catheter does not touch and irritate the tracheal mucosa. Others need to be deeply suctioned to reduce the possibility mucus will become so copious or so thick that it obstructs the trachea below the tube.

Because suctioning removes air as well as secretions from the trachea, children may become oxygen deprived during the procedure. Although not evidence based, preoxygenating them by "bagging" or administering oxygen for approximately 5 minutes before the procedure may help reduce this problem (Cardone & Lepe, 2010). Young children may need to wear elbow restraints while being suctioned to keep their hands away from the sterile catheter. In addition, restraints may be necessary at all times when they are alone to prevent them from fussing with the tracheostomy tube and accidentally removing it.

Tracheostomy tubes are held in place by cloth ties that fasten at the back of the child's neck. Change ties when they become soiled or loose, and check them frequently to be certain they remain tied. Children may fuss with and untie such things, whereas adults will not. Assess that the ties fit snugly but also allow for one finger to be inserted underneath them so they do not rub and cause pain. For preschoolers or younger children, it is a good idea to cover the tracheostomy opening with a gauze square tied to the child's neck like a bib while they eat to prevent crumbs or spilled liquids from entering the tracheostomy opening.

Caution parents:

- Not to give their child small toys that could fit into the lumen of the tube and cause obstruction.
- To keep the use of sprays such as room fresheners to a minimum so they won't be irritating to the exposed trachea.
- To keep cold air from blowing against the tracheostomy opening because this can cause tracheal spasm (e.g., cover the child's throat with a loose fleece scarf when outside in cold weather).
- To inspect stuffed toys to be certain they are intact and do not shed (e.g., fur or stuffing could enter the tube).
- To supervise play with other children so they don't place anything in the tube. Stay with the child in the bathtub to be certain water does not splash into the tube.

When caring for children with tracheostomies, check on them frequently to assess for possible respiratory difficulty. Spend time playing with them or just sitting and rocking them so they can think of you in ways other than as the person who comes to suction them. If parents cannot stay with the child, assure them that you check on their child more frequently than what is necessary for suctioning alone, so they can feel confident if the child should have another episode of acute obstruction, someone will be nearby. If the tracheostomy tube is to be left in place after discharge from the hospital, be certain parents have enough experience with changing tubes if that will be necessary or suctioning so they can safely care for their child at home (Peacock & Stanik-Hutt, 2013).

Each child is considered individually with regard to when it is time to remove a tracheostomy tube. Tubes are generally sealed off partially by adhesive tape or a commercial occlusion device for a day or two before removal; then they are completely occluded (but not removed) for another day to provide a weaning period where suctioning is still possible if it is needed.

Occasionally, children cough so forcefully that they dislodge a tracheostomy tube. Because the incision site usually does not close completely to occlude the tracheal opening when a tube is dislodged, the child still has a patent airway so as long as the child is not in distress, this is not an emergency. Always keep a new tube and inserter (obturator) at the bedside so these are available if replacement is necessary. Slide the obturator into the tube and gently replace it in the tracheal opening. Remove the obturator and secure the new tube in place. If you do this quickly yet calmly, the average child is not alarmed and so will not protest. If, however, a child senses your excitement or if you indicate that something is terribly wrong, a child may begin to cry and turn away, making it difficult to replace the tube without assistance.

Assisted Ventilation

When children cannot breathe effectively enough to improve oxygen saturation to a sufficient level, assisted ventilation may be necessary (Abadesso, Nunes, Silvestre, et al., 2012). Positive-pressure machines deliver moistened or nebulized air or oxygen to the lungs under enough pressure and with appropriate timing to produce artificial, periodic inflation of alveoli, and they rely on the elastic recoil of the lungs to empty the alveoli.

Some commonly used terms associated with ventilator therapy are shown in Table 40.4. Children who need respiratory assistance are frightened. A great many fight ventilators or refuse to lie quietly and let the ventilator breathe for them. Pancuronium (Pavulon) in conjunction with sedation and pain medication such as Ativan and fentanyl, may be administered intravenously to a point of abolishing spontaneous respiratory action in order to overcome resistance and allow mechanical ventilation to be accomplished at lower pressures. Clearly, children who receive pancuronium have no spontaneous respiratory function and need critical observation and frequent oximetry because they depend totally on caregivers at that point.

Noninvasive ventilation is the preferred method of ventilation with children, although if ventilation will be used for a prolonged period, children will usually require either a tracheotomy or endotracheal intubation (Fig. 40.14). Infants need a nasogastric tube inserted to prevent stomach distention from air entering the esophagus with a ventilator in place. Providing adequate nutrition may be a challenge, but enteric (nasogastric) feedings or total parenteral nutrition solves this concern. Providing a balance of rest, stimulation, and assurance for the child is a challenge for nursing personnel and parents.

Even as resistant as children may be at the beginning of ventilator assistance, once children become accustomed to assisted ventilation, it can be difficult to discontinue a

TABLE 40.4 Terms Commonly Used With Ventilator Therapy

Term	Definition	Clinical Application
IMV	Intermittent mandatory ventilation	Number of mandatory breaths the ventilator will deliver each hour. A child may breathe most of the time without assistance, but a set (mandatory) number of breaths per minute is delivered to ensure adequate lung expansion and oxygenation.
PEEP	Positive end-expiratory pressure	Pressure delivered to lungs at the end of each expiration to keep alveoli from collapsing on expiration and to ensure adequate oxygenation.
Sigh	A deep inhalation delivered by the ventilator	Method used to fully inflate the lungs several times each minute.
CPAP	Continuous positive airway pressure	A constant pressure exerted on the alveoli to keep them from collapsing on expiration.
FIO_2	Concentration of oxygen the child is receiving (inspiring)	A child on oxygen therapy will have an FIO_2 from 22% to 100%.

device (Gizzi, Moretti, & Agostino, 2011). This is most pronounced in adolescents, who are very aware of the role of oxygen and proper ventilation for life function. You may need to provide several trial periods free of the ventilator with you remaining close by so children can be assured that if they do have difficulty breathing, someone is standing by to help. Many children are too afraid to fall asleep on the first night off a ventilator unless someone is with them and has assured them they will be there through the night.

Lung Transplantation

Lung transplantation is a possibility for children with a chronic respiratory illness such as cystic fibrosis (Vandemheen, Aaron, Poirer, et al., 2010). The transplant may involve a single lung or both lungs, or it can be done in conjunction with heart transplantation if chronic respiratory disease has caused ventricular hypertrophy of the heart. The donor lung can be from a live donor or a cadaver.

As with any organ transplantation, children need continued immunosuppression therapy with drugs such as cyclosporine or azathioprine (Imuran) following a lung transplant to decrease cell-mediated immunity. Although this level of immunosuppression is the key to successful transplantation, it also makes posttransplant children susceptible to fungal, bacterial, and viral lung infections. In addition, families

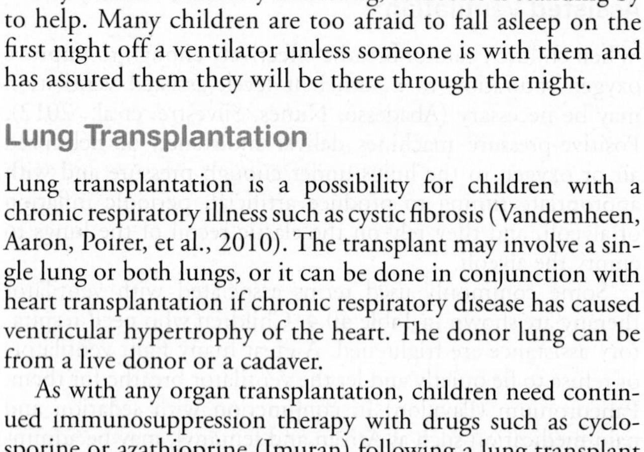

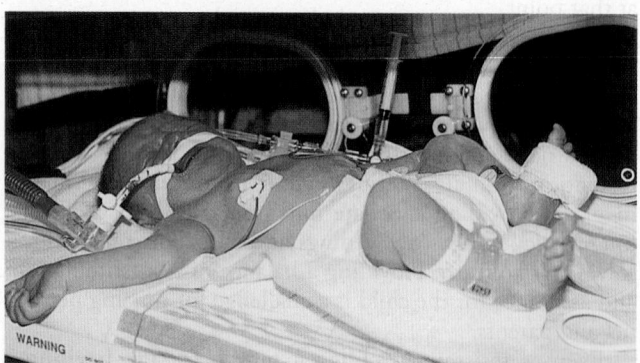

FIGURE 40.14 An infant with an endotracheal tube receiving assisted ventilation.

experience a tremendous psychosocial toll as they wait to see whether the new transplant will be rejected. With the transplanted lung in place, children may need to have chest physiotherapy or use a portable spirometry device daily to help mobilize secretions resulting from loss of nerve innervation or a reaction to accumulating mucus in the transplant.

DISORDERS OF THE UPPER RESPIRATORY TRACT

The upper respiratory tract warms, humidifies, and filters the air that enters the body (Fig. 40.15). Because the structures of the upper respiratory tract constantly come into contact with a barrage of foreign organisms, including pathogens, this can lead to airway irritation and infection. Congenital malformations of respiratory structures also cause some upper respiratory tract disorders.

Choanal Atresia

Choanal atresia is congenital obstruction of the posterior nares by an obstructing membrane or bony growth, which prevents a newborn from drawing air through the nose and down into the nasopharynx (Eladl, 2010). It may occur either unilaterally or bilaterally.

Newborns up to approximately 3 months of age are naturally nose breathers, so infants born with choanal atresia almost immediately develop signs of respiratory distress after birth as they attempt to breathe through their nose for the first time. Passing a soft #8 or #10 French catheter through the posterior nares to the stomach is a part of birthing room procedure in many health care facilities and confirms immediately that no atresia is present.

Choanal atresia can also be assessed by holding the newborn's mouth closed, then gently compressing first one nostril, then the other. If atresia is present, infants will struggle as they experience air hunger when their mouth is closed. Their color improves when they open their mouth to cry. Atresia is also suggested if infants struggle and become cyanotic at feedings because they cannot suck and breathe through the mouth simultaneously.

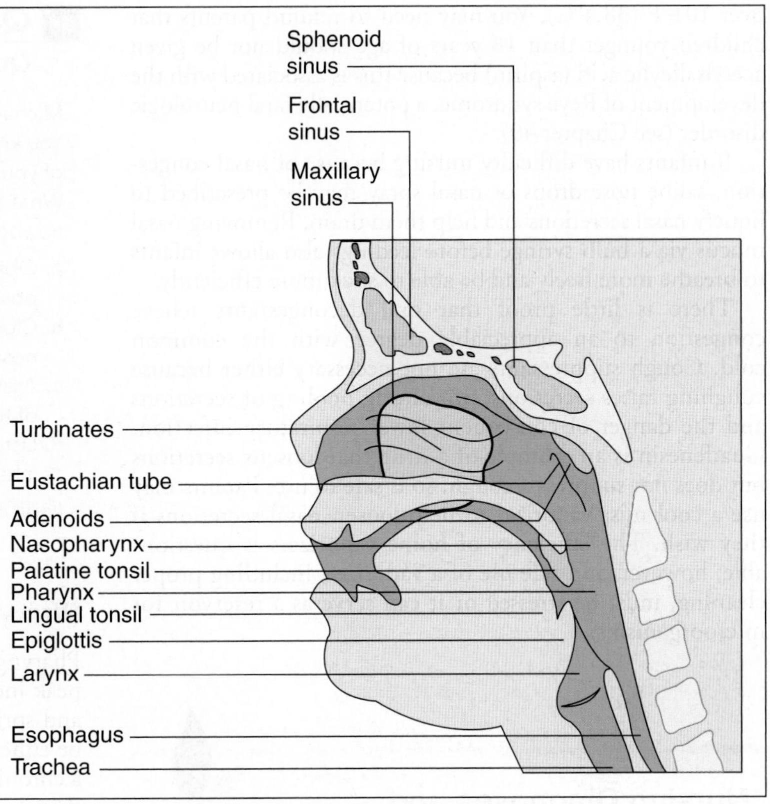

FIGURE 40.15 Structures of the upper respiratory tract.

The treatment for choanal atresia is either local piercing of the obstructing membrane or surgical removal of the bony growth. Because infants with choanal atresia have such difficulty with feeding, they may receive intravenous fluid to maintain their glucose and fluid level until surgery can be performed. Some infants may need an oral airway inserted to ensure they continue to breathe through their mouths. Following surgery, children should have no further difficulty or symptoms.

Acute Nasopharyngitis (Common Cold)

The common cold is the most frequent infectious disease in children; in fact, toddlers can have as many as 10 to 12 colds a year. School-age children and adolescents have as many as 8 to 10 yearly because infection is spread so readily in classrooms. The incubation period for the common cold is typically 2 to 3 days. Most occur in the fall and winter (Science, Johnstone, Roth, et al., 2012).

Upper respiratory infections are caused by one of several viruses, most predominantly by rhinovirus, coxsackievirus, RSV, adenovirus, and parainfluenza and influenza viruses. Children who are in ill health from some other cause, or if their immune system is compromised, are more susceptible than others to the cold viruses. Although difficult to prove, stress factors also appear to play a role in the development of the common cold.

Assessment

Symptoms begin with nasal congestion, a watery rhinitis, and a low-grade fever. The mucous membrane of the nose becomes edematous and inflamed, constricting airway space and causing difficulty breathing. Posterior rhinitis, plus local irritation, leads to pharyngitis (sore throat). As upper airway secretions drain into the trachea, this leads to a cough. Cervical lymph nodes may be swollen and palpable. The process lasts about a week and then symptoms fade. In some children, a thick, purulent nasal discharge occurs because bacteria such as streptococci invade the irritated nasal mucous membrane and cause a secondary purulent infection.

Infants can be critically ill yet not develop a fever because their temperature-regulating system is still immature. With the common cold, they often develop a fever elevated out of proportion to the symptoms, possibly as high as 102° to 104°F (38.8° to 40°C). Infants also may develop secondary symptoms, such as vomiting and diarrhea, as a general response. Because they cannot suck and breathe through their mouth at the same time, they refuse feedings, which can lead to dehydration. Older children rarely develop as high a fever, rarely above 102°F (38.8°C). Because older children can breathe through their mouth, nasal congestion does not seem as acute.

Therapeutic Management

There is no specific treatment for a common cold. Although many parents ask to have antibiotics prescribed, because colds are caused by a virus, antibiotics are not effective unless a secondary bacterial invasion has occurred. If a child has a fever, it can be controlled by an antipyretic such as acetaminophen (Tylenol) or children's ibuprofen (Motrin). Help parents understand these drugs are effective only in controlling fever symptoms; they do not reduce congestion or "cure" the cold. Therefore, they should not be given unless the child has a fever, which is generally defined as an oral temperature over 101°F (38.4°C). You may need to remind parents that children younger than 18 years of age should not be given acetylsalicylic acid (aspirin) because this is associated with the development of Reye syndrome, a potentially fatal neurologic disorder (see Chapter 49).

If infants have difficulty nursing because of nasal congestion, saline nose drops or nasal spray may be prescribed to liquefy nasal secretions and help them drain. Removing nasal mucus via a bulb syringe before feedings also allows infants to breathe more freely and be able to suck more efficiently.

There is little proof that oral decongestants relieve congestion to an appreciable degree with the common cold. Cough suppressants are not necessary either because coughing raises secretions, preventing pooling of secretions and the danger of consequent lower respiratory infection. Guaifenesin is an example of a drug that loosens secretions but does not suppress a cough, so is safe to use. Parents may use a cool mist vaporizer to help loosen nasal secretions if they wish. The efficiency of home vaporizers is questionable, however, and safe use of a vaporizer, including proper cleaning, must be stressed or it can serve as a reservoir for microorganisms.

Nursing Diagnoses and Related Interventions

Nursing Diagnosis: Parental health-seeking behaviors related to management of child's upper respiratory symptoms

Outcome Evaluation: Parents state intention to use cool mist vaporizer to loosen secretions, to encourage oral fluid, to administer an antipyretic to reduce fever, and to avoid cough medicine.

Care of the child with a cold is primarily supportive until the infection runs its course. Because they may have a loss of appetite, children may prefer simple liquids to solid food for the first few days of the illness. Parents generally ask whether children should remain on bed rest. Children characteristically restrict their activity when ill, so with acute cold symptoms, children often naturally curl up on the couch and sleep. One of the best ways parents can judge when children are improving is to note they have begun to increase their activity or are "acting like themselves" again.

Because the symptoms in infants are so out of proportion to the seriousness of the disorder, parents may need assurance that a cold in an infant is only a cold and nothing more. A possible complication of a cold is otitis media (middle ear infection) because the common precursor for otitis media is a viral upper respiratory tract infection. Instruct parents about this possibility and the need to report symptoms suggestive of this infection, such as sudden elevated temperature and ear pain (Hoberman, Paradise, Rockette, et al., 2011).

QSEN Checkpoint Question 40.2

Quality Improvement

Michael's history reveals he was born with choanal atresia. You know that screening protocols on the birthing unit of your hospital specify assessments for this condition. What assessment at birth may be performed to determine if newborns have this condition?

a. Observe if the infant can breathe well while lying in a prone position.
b. Close his mouth and observe if he can breathe through his nose.
c. Assess if the infant's palatine tonsils are blocking the back of the throat.
d. Listen for the sound of either stridor or wheezing on inhalation.

Look in Appendix A for the best answer and rationale.

Pharyngitis

Pharyngitis is infection and inflammation of the throat. The peak incidence occurs between 5 to 15 years of age in winter and spring, with an incubation period of 2 to 5 days. It may be either bacterial or viral in origin. It may occur as a result of a chronic allergy in which there is constant postnasal discharge that results in a secondary irritation. At least a slight pharyngitis usually accompanies all common upper respiratory infections.

Viral Pharyngitis

The causative agent of pharyngitis is usually an adenovirus (Martin, 2010). The symptoms are generally mild: a sore throat, fever, rhinorrhea, cough, and general malaise. On a physical assessment, regional lymph nodes may be enlarged. Erythema will be present in the back of the pharynx and the palatine arch. Laboratory studies will usually indicate an increased white blood cell count.

If the inflammation is mild, children rarely need more than an oral analgesic such as acetaminophen or ibuprofen for comfort. Warm heat applied to the external neck area using a warm towel or heating pad also can feel soothing. By school age, children are capable of gargling with a solution such as warm water to help reduce the pain. Before this age, children tend to swallow the solution unless the procedure is well explained and demonstrated to them.

Because children's throats feel so sore, they often prefer liquids to solid food. Infants, especially, must be observed closely until the inflammation and tenderness diminish to be certain they are taking in sufficient fluid to prevent dehydration.

Streptococcal Pharyngitis

Group A β-hemolytic streptococcus is the organism most frequently involved in bacterial pharyngitis in children. All streptococcal infections must be taken seriously because they can lead to cardiac and kidney damage from an accompanying autoimmune process (Altamimi, Khalil, Khalaiwi, et al., 2012).

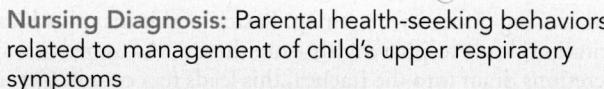

Assessment. Streptococcal infections are generally more severe than viral infections. The back of the throat and palatine tonsils are usually markedly erythematous (bright red); the tonsils are enlarged and there may be a white exudate in the tonsillar crypts. Petechiae may be present on the palate. A child typically appears ill with a high fever, an extremely sore throat, difficulty swallowing, and overall lethargy. Temperature is usually elevated to as high as 104°F (40°C) and the child frequently has a headache. Swollen abdominal lymph nodes may cause abdominal pain. A throat culture, often completed as a quick office procedure, confirms the presence of the *Streptococcus* bacteria.

Therapeutic Management. Treatment consists of a full 10-day course of an oral antibiotic such as penicillin G or clindamycin. Cephalosporins or broad-spectrum macrolides such as erythromycin may be prescribed if resistant organisms are known to be in the community. Help parents understand the importance of completing the full prescribed days of therapy in order to ensure all the streptococci are eradicated. If they are not, the child may develop a hypersensitivity or autoimmune reaction to group A streptococci that can result in glomerulonephritis or rheumatic fever (although the chance of these occurring is probably as low as 1%) (Chiappini, Regoli, Bonsignori, et al., 2011).

Because symptoms of acute glomerulonephritis (blood and protein in urine) appear 1 to 2 weeks after the pharyngitis, children may be asked to return to the health care facility with a urine specimen to be examined for protein so that developing acute glomerulonephritis can be detected.

Instruct parents about the importance of rest, relief of throat pain, and maintaining hydration, the same actions as for a common cold. To ensure a child receives the full antibiotic course, help parents make a reminder sheet to place on a cabinet or refrigerator door or leave memos to themselves by smartphones. Because it is impossible for parents to discriminate between a pharyngitis caused by a virus (and needing no therapy other than comfort measures) and a streptococcal pharyngitis (needing definite therapy to prevent life-threatening illnesses), a child with pharyngitis should always be brought to a health care facility for diagnosis.

QSEN Checkpoint Question 40.3

Teamwork & Collaboration

Michael has had two streptococcal pharyngitis infections in the past. You would want your team members to know to remind parents of children with streptococcal pharyngitis to give the full course of prescribed antibiotic because, without this, a few children develop a complication such as:

a. Lymphedema or epiglottitis
b. Dental abscesses
c. Heart or kidney disease
d. Lung abscesses or emphysema

Look in Appendix A for the best answer and rationale.

Retropharyngeal Abscess

In infants, the lymph nodes, which drain the nasopharynx, are located just behind the posterior pharynx wall; therefore, following an acute nasopharyngitis or pharyngitis, these nodes may become infected. Because these nodes disappear by preschool age, the problem is usually limited to young infants (Lin & Lee, 2011).

Assessment. Typically, infants have an upper respiratory tract infection or sore throat for a few days. Suddenly, they develop a high fever, refuse to eat, and may drool because they cannot swallow saliva past the obstruction in the back of their throat. They begin to "snore" with respirations as the pharynx becomes further occluded. To allow themselves more breathing space, they may hyperextend the head, which is a very unusual position for infants.

A physical assessment reveals enlargement of the regional lymph nodes, although the mass in the posterior pharynx may not be visible if it is below the point of vision. An ultrasound will reveal the bulging tissue in the pharynx. Laboratory studies will reveal leukocytosis.

Therapeutic Management. Because the most common cause of retropharyngeal abscess is group A β-hemolytic streptococcus, either benzathine penicillin G or penicillin V is effective. As a result of their poor swallowing, infants' mouths may need to be suctioned to remove secretions. While doing this, be careful not to touch the suction catheter to the posterior pharynx because this might rupture the abscess, possibly leading to aspiration of the abscess contents (producing respiratory obstruction or a pneumonia caused by the aspirated purulent material). Blood vessels invade some retropharyngeal abscesses, so rupture of the structure also could lead to profuse bleeding, which is dangerous to the child both because of the loss of blood from a major artery such as the carotid artery and because the blood could be aspirated.

Place infants in a side-lying position to allow difficult-to-swallow mouth secretions to drain forward. Limit oral intake to fluids as irritation from a hard food such as a toast crust (a food often recommended for teething) is another way the abscess could rupture.

Although some postpharyngeal abscesses resolve on their own, some need to be incised by a surgeon to promote drainage. This is done with the child in a Trendelenburg position so that drainage from the abscess can be suctioned away to prevent aspiration. After surgery, maintain the child in a Trendelenburg or a side position as prescribed to encourage further drainage and continue to prevent aspiration. Monitor vital signs closely and observe any drainage from infants' mouths to detect fresh bleeding. Bleeding may also be revealed by frequent swallowing. Increased respiratory rate suggests airway obstruction.

Oral fluid is introduced as soon as an infant's swallowing and gag reflexes are intact after surgery. Although the throat is undoubtedly still sore, most infants suck eagerly and need supplemental intravenous fluid administration following surgery for only a short time.

On admission to the hospital, parents may have been thoroughly frightened by the extent of their child's symptoms (e.g., gurgling or snoring sound, high temperature, dyspnea). Encourage parents to give care while in the hospital to help them allay their fears and regain confidence in their ability to both trust their judgment and to care for the child again.

Tonsillitis

Tonsillar tissue is lymphoid tissue that filters pathogenic organisms from the head and neck area. Tonsillitis refers to infection and inflammation of the palatine tonsils, which are located on both sides of the pharynx. Adenitis refers to infection and inflammation of the adenoid (pharyngeal) tonsils, which are located in the pharynx. Additional tonsils are located at the entrance to the eustachian tubes (the tubal tonsils) and at the base of the tongue (lingual tonsils). All four types of tonsils, referred to collectively as Waldeyer ring, are easily infected because of the bacteria that pass through or are screened through them with lymph.

Assessment

Infection of the palatine tonsils presents with all of the symptoms of a severe pharyngitis. Children drool because their throat is too sore to effectively swallow saliva (dysphagia). They may describe swallowing as so painful it feels as if they are swallowing bits of metal or glass. In addition, they usually have a high fever and are lethargic. Tonsillar tissue appears bright red and may be so enlarged that the two areas of palatine tonsillar tissue meet in the midline. Pus can be detected on or expelled from the tonsillar crypts (Lin & Lee, 2011).

In addition to fever, lethargy, pharyngeal pain, and edema, if adenoidal tissue is infected, the child also develops a nasal quality of speech, mouth breathing, difficulty hearing, and perhaps halitosis or sleep apnea from pressure of the swollen tonsil tissue against the posterior throat or eustachian tubes. Long-term obstruction from blocked eustachian tubes can lead to serous and acute otitis media.

Tonsillitis most commonly occurs in school-age children. In children younger than 3 years of age, the cause is often viral. In school-age children, the organism is generally a group A β-hemolytic streptococcus (Martin, 2010). Both types can be identified by a throat culture.

Therapeutic Management

Therapy for bacterial tonsillitis includes an antipyretic for fever, an analgesic for pain, and a full 7- to 10-day course of an antibiotic such as penicillin or amoxicillin. If the cause is viral, no therapy other than comfort or fever reduction strategies is necessary. Although the pain of the infection will subside a day or two after the antibiotic administration is begun, remind parents that children need the full course of antibiotic to eradicate streptococci completely from the back of the throat. Following a tonsillar infection, tonsillar tissue may remain hypertrophied, or it may atrophy and actually appear smaller than it did previously.

Tonsillectomy. Tonsillectomy is removal of the palatine tonsils. *Adenoidectomy* is removal of the pharyngeal tonsils. In the past, tonsillectomy was recommended for children after one episode of tonsillitis. This is no longer recommended because tonsillar tissue is an important component of the immune system. Chronic tonsillitis is about the only reason for removal of palatine tonsils. Adenoids may be removed if they are so hypertrophied they cause obstruction or sleep apnea.

During a tonsillectomy, tonsillar tissue is removed by ligation or by laser surgery. Because sutures are not usually placed, the chance for hemorrhage after this type of surgery is higher than after surgery involving a closed incision. The danger of aspiration of blood at the time of surgery and the danger of a general anesthetic also compound the risk.

Tonsillectomy or adenoidectomy is never done while the organs are infected, because an operation at such a time might spread pathogenic organisms into the bloodstream, causing septicemia. Help parents understand although the child's tonsils are very painful, it is beneficial to schedule surgery for a later date. Most parents report an improvement in their child's general health and performance after tonsillectomy surgery because this ends the chronic infections.

Nursing Diagnoses and Related Interventions

Nursing Diagnosis: Risk for fluid volume deficit related to blood loss from surgery

Outcome Evaluation: Child's pulse and blood pressure remain normal for age; there is an absence of extensive bleeding; intake and output are within acceptable parameters.

Tonsillectomies are done as ambulatory or 1-day surgery following completion of a history and physical examination and laboratory tests, including bleeding and clotting times, complete blood count, and urinalysis. Teach parents to use common sense in their child's care during the week before hospital admission so the child does not develop a cold or recurrent tonsillitis at the time planned for surgery. An important aspect of the presurgery assessment is to observe for loose teeth because, if present, these could be dislodged during surgery and aspirated. Make certain the presence of loose teeth is noted in the child's electronic record so the anesthesiologist can be aware of this.

Following surgery, observe vital signs carefully to make certain the child is not bleeding from the denuded surgical area. Place the child on his or her side or abdomen with a pillow under the chest so that the head is lower than the chest to allow blood and unswallowed saliva to drain from the child's mouth rather than back to the pharynx, where it might be aspirated (Fig. 40.16).

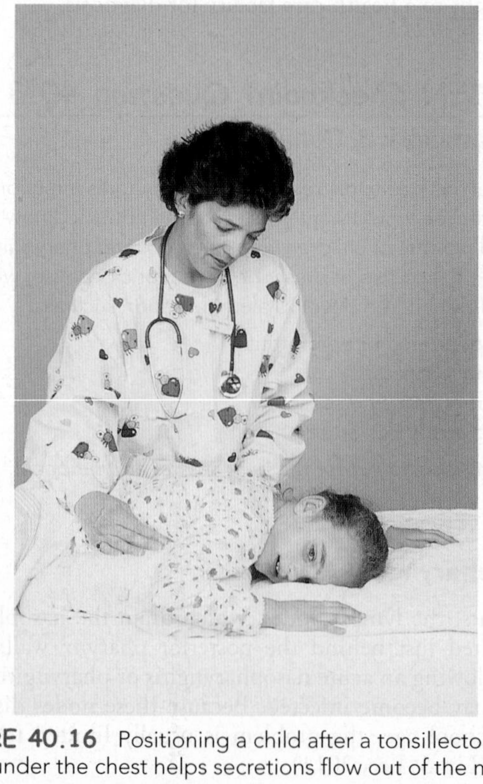

FIGURE 40.16 Positioning a child after a tonsillectomy. The pillow under the chest helps secretions flow out of the mouth.

If hemorrhage should occur after tonsillectomy, it can be acute and intense. Because children swallow any blood that is oozing from the surgical site, a child can be bleeding heavily, however, and yet little blood will be apparent. To detect if the child is bleeding, assess for subtle signs of hemorrhage, such as an increasing pulse or respiratory rate, frequent swallowing, throat clearing, or a feeling of anxiety. A child's first line of defense against hemorrhage is a nurse who recognizes these subtle signs of bleeding before the bleeding becomes so intense that signs of hypovolemic shock occur.

If you find that the surgical site is bleeding, elevate the child's head to reduce vascular pressure on the operative site and notify the child's primary care provider. If bleeding is heavy, the child may need to be returned to surgery for a suture or two to halt bleeding.

The most dangerous periods for a child after a tonsillectomy are the first 24 hours, when the clots covering the denuded surgical area are forming, and days 5 to 7, when the clots begin to lyse or dissolve. If new granulation tissue has not yet formed when the clots dissolve, hemorrhage from the denuded surface can occur at this time (Isaacson, 2012).

If children have no complications from surgery, are able to swallow fluids, and have voided, they are discharged later the same day of surgery. Be certain parents have received careful instructions concerning the danger signs to watch for during the first day home (e.g., frequent swallowing, clearing the throat, increasing restlessness). They are usually also advised to restrict their child's activity (e.g., no gymnastics, no competitive sports) until after the seventh day, when firm healing should have taken place. Be certain the parents have a return appointment to a health care facility approximately 2 weeks after surgery for follow-up assessment to make certain the surgical area has healed without complication.

Nursing Diagnosis: Pain related to surgical procedure

Outcome Evaluation: Child states level of pain is tolerable.

A tonsillectomy is an uncomfortable and painful procedure. Be certain children receive good preparation for both the procedure and for the sensations they will experience afterward. Some children develop a mild earache after surgery for the first week in addition to a painful throat, probably caused by shifting pressure on the eustachian tube. Although tonsils are removed, it is better to talk about tonsils being "fixed" rather than taken out as children may be extremely frightened to know a body part will be removed, however small it is.

Liquid analgesics are better tolerated than pills or tablets following surgery because they are easier to swallow. Rectal administration is a possibility for very young children. Most children are thirsty immediately after surgery, and drinking is helpful because swallowing fluid causes active pharyngeal movement, thus increasing the blood supply to the area and reducing edema and pain. Children may have been promised by well-meaning relatives they can have all the ice cream they want after a tonsillectomy. Because milk products form tenacious secretions that are difficult to swallow, ice cream is not a food of choice. Offer instead frequent sips of clear liquid, Popsicles, or ice chips. Avoid acidic and citric juices because these sting the denuded tissue. Carbonated beverages also can irritate unless they stand for a time to become "flat." Avoid red fluid such as Kool-Aid, which, if vomited, could be mistaken for swallowed blood.

Children are then gradually advanced after 24 to 48 hours to a diet of soft foods such as gelatin, mashed potatoes, soups, and cooked fruits. Alert parents they should continue to eat only soft foods for the first week (e.g., no toast crusts or other foods that could cause pharyngeal irritation if not chewed well). Be certain parents know whom they should call (clinic, hospital, or primary care provider) if they have a question or concern about their child's condition or care.

Epistaxis

Epistaxis (nosebleed) is extremely common in children and usually occurs from trauma, such as picking at the nose, from falling, or from being hit on the nose by another child (Robertson, King, & Tomkinson, 2010). In homes that lack humidification, a hot, dry environment causes mucous membranes to dry and be susceptible to cracking and bleeding. Nosebleeds may also occur after strenuous exercise, with hemolytic disorders such as sickle-cell anemia, or may be associated with nasal polyps, sinusitis, or allergic rhinitis. Some families appear to show a familial predisposition to them.

Nosebleeds are always frightening because of the sudden visible bleeding and the choking sensation of blood running down the back of the nasopharynx. The fear, however, and the amount of blood that can be seen is generally out of proportion to the seriousness of the bleeding.

Keep children with nosebleeds in an upright position with their head tilted slightly forward to minimize the amount of blood pressure in nasal vessels and to keep blood moving forward, not back into the nasopharynx. Apply pressure to the cartilage on the sides of the nose with your fingers for about 10 minutes (Fig. 40.17). Make every effort to quiet the child and to help stop crying, because crying increases pressure in the blood vessels of the head and prolongs bleeding. If these simple measures do not control the bleeding, epinephrine (1:1,000) may be applied to the bleeding site to constrict blood vessels. A cotton or gauze nasal pack may be necessary to provide continued pressure. Every child has an occasional nosebleed. Chronic nasal bleeding, however, should be investigated to rule out a systemic disease or blood disorder.

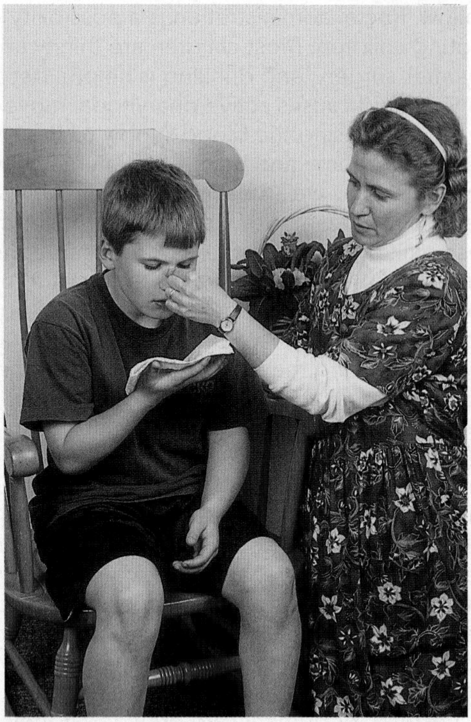

FIGURE 40.17 Emergency therapy for a nosebleed is to sit the child up and apply pressure to the sides of the nose.

QSEN Checkpoint Question 40.4

Patient-Centered Care

Michael's 4-year-old roommate in the care unit is scheduled for a tonsillectomy later today. In order to ensure that your nursing care is empathic and patient centered, what food would be best to offer the roommate following his surgery?

a. Grilled cheese sandwich
b. Tomato juice and crackers
c. Potato chips and dip
d. A cold green ice pop

Look in Appendix A for the best answer and rationale.

Sinusitis

Sinusitis is infection and inflammation of the sinus cavities. It rarely occurs in children younger than 6 years of age because the frontal sinuses do not develop fully until that age. It can occur either as a primary infection or a secondary one in older children when streptococcal, staphylococcal, or *H. influenzae* organisms spread from the nasal cavity to the sinuses (DeMuri & Wald, 2012). Children develop a fever, a purulent nasal discharge, headache, and tenderness over the affected sinus. A nose and throat culture will identify the infectious organism.

Treatment for acute sinusitis consists of an antipyretic for fever, an analgesic for pain, and an antibiotic for the specific organism involved. Oxymetazoline hydrochloride (Afrin), supplied as nose drops or a nasal spray, shrinks the edematous mucous membranes and allows infected material to drain from the sinuses and relieve pain. To avoid a rebound effect, caution parents that this type of nasal spray should be used for only 3 days at a time; otherwise, it actually causes more nasal congestion than was present originally. Warm compresses to the sinus area may also encourage drainage and relieve pain.

Sinusitis is often considered to be a minor illness. It needs to be treated, however, because it can have serious complications if the infection spreads from the sinuses to invade the facial bone (osteomyelitis) or the middle ear (otitis media). Chronic sinusitis can also interfere with school and social interactions because of the constant pain.

Laryngitis

Laryngitis is inflammation of the larynx, which results in brassy, hoarse voice sounds or the inability to make audible voice sounds. It may occur as a complication of pharyngitis or from excessive use of the voice, as in shouting or loud cheering. Laryngitis is as annoying for children as it is for adults. Sips of fluid (either warm or cold, whichever feels best) offer relief from the annoying tickling sensation often present. The most effective measure, however, is for the child to rest the voice for at least 24 hours until inflammation subsides. For infants with laryngitis, attempt to meet their needs before they have to cry for things. Simply caution older children not to speak. Provide them with a paper and pencil or chalkboard for communication.

Congenital Laryngomalacia/Tracheomalacia

Congenital laryngomalacia means that an infant's laryngeal structure is weaker than normal and collapses more than usual on inspiration (Adil, Rager, & Carr, 2011). This produces laryngeal **stridor** (a high-pitched crowing sound on inspiration) present from birth and possibly intensified when the infant is in a supine position or when sucking.

Assessment

The infant's sternum and intercostal spaces may retract on inspiration because of the increased effort needed to pull air into the trachea past the collapsed cartilage rings. Many infants with this condition must stop sucking frequently during a feeding to maintain adequate ventilation and to rest from their exhausting respiratory effort.

Therapeutic Management

Most children with congenital laryngomalacia need no routine therapy other than to have parents feed them slowly and provide rest periods as needed. The condition improves as infants mature and cartilage in the larynx becomes stronger at about 1 year of age. When parents wake at night and listen in a quiet house to the sound of stridor, it seems unbearably loud and can make it difficult for them to believe it is safe for them to care for the infant at home.

Many parents sleep at night with the child's crib next to their bed or with one hand resting on the infant's chest so they can be assured during the night the child is continuing to breathe. Because of this, assess at health care visits whether the parents are receiving enough sleep and are not becoming too exhausted to be able to continue their daily activities. Showing them a weight chart that demonstrates their child is growing and thriving despite this problem can be reassuring.

Be certain that parents know the importance of bringing the child for early care if signs of an upper respiratory tract infection should develop because, with this, laryngeal collapse will be even more intense and a complete obstruction of the trachea could occur. At any point, if stridor becomes more intense, advise parents to have the infant seen by their primary care provider because this generally indicates a beginning obstruction and probably the beginning of an upper respiratory tract infection. As parents become more accustomed to the sound their infant makes while breathing, they become astute reporters of change in their infant's condition. Listen to them carefully when they report a change to prevent overlooking this important information.

Croup (Laryngotracheobronchitis)

Croup (inflammation of the larynx, trachea, and major bronchi) is one of the most frightening diseases of early childhood for both parents and children. In children between 6 months and 3 years of age, the cause of croup is usually a viral infection such as parainfluenza virus (Schomacker, Schaap-Nutt, Collins, et al., 2012).

Assessment

With croup, children typically have only minimal signs at bedtime. Temperature is normal or only mildly elevated. During the night, however, they develop a barking cough (croupy cough), inspiratory stridor, and marked retractions from inflammation of the larynx, trachea, and major bronchi. They wake in extreme respiratory distress. These severe symptoms typically last several hours and then, except for a rattling cough, subside by morning. Cyanosis is rarely present, but the danger of glottal obstruction from the laryngeal inflammation and hypoxemia is very real (Kilic, Ünüvar, Sütçü, et al., 2012).

Therapeutic Management

One emergency method of relieving croup symptoms is for a parent to run the shower or hot water tap in a bathroom until the room fills with steam, then keep the child in this warm, moist environment because this relaxes the airway and widens the bronchi lumens. If this does not relieve symptoms, parents should bring the child to an emergency department for further evaluation and care. At the health care facility, pulse oximetry is helpful to document whether hypoxemia is present. Cool moist air combined with a corticosteroid, such as dexamethasone, or racemic epinephrine, given by nebulizer, usually reduces inflammation and produces effective bronchodilation to open the airway. Intravenous therapy may be prescribed to keep the child well hydrated because it is difficult to swallow past the inflamed throat. Maintain accurate intake and output records and test urine specific gravity to ensure hydration remains adequate.

Nursing Diagnoses and Related Interventions

Nursing Diagnosis: Ineffective airway clearance related to edema and constriction of airway

Outcome Evaluation: Respiratory rate is not above 22 breaths/min; no cyanosis is present; Po_2 is 80 to 100 mmHg; and Sao_2 is over 95%.

Attach a sensor for pulse oximetry monitoring and remain constantly with a child with croup, not only to observe closely for increasing respiratory distress but also to reduce the child's anxiety. Take vital signs as often as every 15 minutes, because extreme restlessness and thrashing, increased stridor, increased heart and respiratory rates, and cyanosis are all symptoms of oxygen deprivation. In some children, it is difficult to distinguish their fright from the newness of the experience (and their sense of their parents' fright) from the anxiety that comes from oxygen deprivation, so try to keep the child calm and occupied with a favorite activity.

Laryngospasm with total occlusion of the airway can occur if a child's gag reflex is elicited or when the child is crying. Therefore, *do not elicit a gag reflex in any child with a croupy, barking cough*, and provide comfort to prevent crying. If symptoms worsen so oxygen saturations falls, a tracheostomy or endotracheal intubation along with oxygen therapy may be necessary.

Croup is a frightening disease for parents because their child is both suddenly and severely ill. When the symptoms disappear by morning, however, parents may feel foolish they rushed to a hospital with the child in the middle of the night. Assure them that their initial judgment was correct. When they brought the child in, the child was seriously ill. Parents may be reluctant to see their child discharged in the morning until they can be convinced their child is now well enough to go home. Box 40.6 shows an interprofessional care map illustrating both nursing and team planning for a child with laryngotracheobronchitis.

What if...40.2 Michael, who had loud stridor when he was admitted, suddenly has no stridor present. Would you be relieved (i.e., his condition must be improving) or worried (i.e., his airway may be so blocked not enough air is entering to make the sound of stridor)? How should you respond?

Epiglottitis

Epiglottitis is inflammation of the epiglottis, which is the flap of cartilage that covers the opening to the larynx to keep out food and fluid during swallowing. Although it is rare, inflammation of the epiglottis is an emergency because the swollen epiglottis

BOX 40.6 Nursing Care Planning

AN INTERPROFESSIONAL CARE MAP FOR A CHILD WITH LARYNGOTRACHEOBRONCHITIS (CROUP)

Michael is a 4-year-old who is brought to the emergency department by paramedics who responded to an emergency call by his grandmother at his home. He has a sharp, barking cough, is crying loudly, and is obviously short of breath. His grandmother shouts at you, "I gave him some chocolate. Is he allergic to that?" Michael is diagnosed as having laryngotracheobronchitis (croup) and admitted to an ambulatory care unit.

Family Assessment Child lives with two parents in four-bedroom suburban home. Father works as a bartender at local restaurant; mother works part time as a beautician. Parents are out of town on vacation. Were notified of child's condition and gave oral permission for therapy by telephone to W. Burton, MD (witnessed by C. Finacca, RN); will fax consent and signatures from vacation hotel.

Client Assessment Child was born with choanal atresia. Is allergic to seafood, especially shrimp (develops hives and shortness of breath). Age-acceptable parameters for height and weight. Has had a "slight head cold" for last 2 days; woke from nap this afternoon gasping for breath. Has audible stridor. Tympanic temperature 102.2°F (39.0°C); pulse 146 beats/min; respirations 40 breaths/min. Nasal flaring and intercostal retractions noted. Sharp, frequent, nonproductive cough.

Nursing Diagnosis Fear related to inability to breathe without effort, heightened by absence of parents.

Outcome Criteria Respiratory rate, oxygen saturation, and arterial blood gas levels are within age-acceptable parameters without the use of supplemental oxygen. No stridor is present on auscultation. Child states he can breathe more easily; is aware parents are concerned although absent.

Team Member Responsible	Assessment	Intervention	Rationale	Expected Outcome
Activities of Daily Living, Including Safety				
Nurse	Assess if child is able to complete any self-care despite fatigue and shortness of breath.	Place the child in a semi-Fowler's to high Fowler's position. Reposition the child frequently.	An upright position facilitates breathing and promotes optimal lung expansion by lowering diaphragm. Frequent repositioning prevents pooling and stasis of secretions.	Child cooperates with procedures to extent possible, given degree of fatigue and fear.
Teamwork and Collaboration				
Nurse/Nurse practitioner/ Anesthesiologist	Assess if anesthesiologist is available.	Consult with anesthesiologist about the possibility that intubation or tracheostomy may be necessary.	If tracheolaryngeal edema occludes airway, intubation or tracheostomy can be lifesaving.	Anesthesiology team examines child; prepares equipment for emergency intubation if necessary.
Procedures/Medications for Quality Improvement				
Nurse	Assess temperature by tympanic thermometer.	Administer acetaminophen liquid orally as prescribed.	Oral temperature would be inaccurate because of rapid respirations.	Child's temperature decreases one degree per hour until it reaches 98.6°F.
Nurse	Assess if child has experience with vital sign procedures or breath sound assessment.	Assess pulse, respirations, and lung sounds every 15 minutes. Attach pulse oximeter to finger.	An increasing pulse or respiratory rate or increased stridor can signal decreasing oxygenation.	Child agrees to allow chest leads to be applied to monitor heart rate. Pulse and respiratory rate do not increase any further.

Nurse	Assess if child has ever received medicine by nebulizer or humidifier.	Administer racemic epinephrine by nebulizer every 3 hours as prescribed. Keep room infused with cold humidification.	Epinephrine causes bronchodilation, widening the lumens of the airway. Cold moisture helps reduce inflammation and moisten mucus.	Child cooperates with nebulizer therapy to extent possible, given fear. Respiratory rate and stridor decrease following treatment.
Nurse	Assess which method of oxygen administration (face mask or nasal prongs) would be most acceptable to child.	Administer humidified oxygen at prescribed rate. Obtain arterial blood gases (ABGs) as ordered and monitor oxygen saturation levels via pulse oximetry.	Humidified oxygen improves ventilation without drying the mucous membranes to reduce hypoxemia. ABGs and pulse oximetry provide objective evidence of the child's oxygenation.	Child chooses method for oxygen administration; cooperates with oxygen administration; Po_2 and Sao_2 improve to adequate levels.
Nutrition				
Nurse	Assess what is child's favorite fluid to drink.	Offer the child sips of fluid frequently. Maintain prescribed intravenous (IV) fluid.	Dehydration can occur from rapid respirations. Adequate hydration helps moisten mucus.	Child drinks 80% of fluid offered; IV is maintained at prescribed rate.
Patient-Centered Care				
Nurse	Assess grandparent's knowledge of child's condition.	Review that croup is a viral infection, not an allergic disorder.	Understanding why a disease occurs can help grandparent to not feel guilty about the chocolate	Grandparent states she understands the cause of croup, its usual course, and its prognosis.
Psychosocial/Spiritual/Emotional Needs				
Nurse/Nurse practitioner/ Child life specialist	Assess if child has had prior experiences with hospitalization.	Use play to encourage the child to cough, deeply breathe, and drink fluid.	Games and play are effective methods for encouraging fluid intake in a child.	Child states he understands procedures are to help him breathe, not punishment for eating candy.
Informatics for Seamless Health Care Planning				
Nurse/ Respiratory therapist	Assess if grandparent knows action to take if child should develop croup again.	Review child's condition and the careful watching grandparent will need to continue.	Croup is a frightening illness. Good preparation will help grandparent respond to condition.	Grandparent states she is better prepared to care for child, and will telephone primary care provider or 911 if child's symptoms return.

cannot rise and allow the airway to open. It occurs most frequently in children from 2 to about 8 years of age (Smith, 2011).

Epiglottitis can be either bacterial or viral in origin. *H. influenzae* type B has been replaced as the most common bacterial cause of the disorder followed by pneumococci, streptococci, or staphylococci. Echovirus and RSV also can cause the disorder.

Assessment

Symptoms begin as those of a mild upper respiratory tract infection. After 1 or 2 days, as inflammation spreads to the epiglottis, the child suddenly develops severe inspiratory stridor, a high fever, hoarseness, and a very sore throat. Children may have such difficulty swallowing that they drool saliva. They may protrude their tongue to increase free movement in the pharynx.

If a child's gag reflex is stimulated with a tongue blade, the swollen and inflamed epiglottis can be seen to rise in the back of the throat as a cherry-red structure. It can be so edematous, however, that the gagging procedure causes complete obstruction of the glottis and shuts off the ability of the child to inhale. Therefore, in children with symptoms of epiglottitis (e.g., dysphagia, inspiratory stridor, cough, fever, and hoarseness), *never attempt to visualize the epiglottis directly with a tongue blade or obtain a throat culture* unless a means of providing an artificial airway, such as tracheostomy or endotracheal intubation, is immediately available. This is especially important for the nurse who functions in an expanded role and performs physical assessments and routinely elicits gag reflexes.

When epiglottitis is present, laboratory studies will show leukocytosis (20,000 to 30,000 mm^3), with the proportion of neutrophils increased. A blood culture will reveal if septicemia is present; pulse oximetry is necessary to evaluate respiratory sufficiency. A lateral neck X-ray film or ultrasound will reveal the enlarged epiglottis. Do not allow a child with possible epiglottitis to go to these departments for assessment accompanied only by parents or a nursing aide in case obstruction occurs away from immediate emergency measures.

Therapeutic Management

Children need moist air to reduce the epiglottal inflammation. If cyanosis is present, they need oxygen. An antibiotic, such as a third-generation cephalosporin like cefotaxime, may be prescribed until a throat culture indicates the need for a specific antibiotic drug. Because they cannot swallow, children need intravenous fluid therapy to maintain hydration. They may need a prophylactic tracheostomy or endotracheal intubation to prevent total airway obstruction, although it is often difficult to intubate children with epiglottitis because the tube cannot be passed beyond the edematous epiglottis. After antibiotic therapy begins, the epiglottal inflammation recedes rapidly. By 12 to 24 hours, it has reduced enough that the intubation may be removed. Alert parents to continue antibiotic administration for the full 7 to 10 days prescribed. Siblings of the ill child may be prescribed prophylactic antibiotic therapy to prevent them from developing the same symptoms.

Initially, the symptoms of epiglottitis are not unlike those of croup. As a result, parents may not realize the extent of the occlusion in their child, especially if the child has had croup on other occasions. They may question why a prophylactic tracheostomy or intubation was necessary this time when it was not used when the child had croup. Explain to them the difference between the two diseases (Table 40.5).

Some infants with epiglottitis die because obstruction occurs before a tracheotomy or intubation can be accomplished. If this should happen, parents can be assured they could not have realized the seriousness of their child's symptoms. Support them as they regain confidence in themselves as parents and in their ability to judge their other children's health.

✔ QSEN Checkpoint Question 40.5
Safety

Michael has a barking cough, sore throat, and fever. You want to see if his throat looks sore and swollen. What is the safest and most accurate way of performing this assessment?

a. Gag him with a tongue blade so you can inspect his tonsils.
b. Ask him to press down on his tongue with one of his fingers.
c. Elicit a gag reflex using only one of your gloved fingers.
d. Ask him to open his mouth and inspect his throat visually.

Look in Appendix A for the best answer and rationale.

Aspiration

Aspiration (inhalation of a foreign object into the airway) occurs most frequently in infants and toddlers. When a child aspirates a foreign object such as a coin or a peanut, the immediate reaction is choking and hard, forceful coughing. Usually, this dislodges the object. However, if the airway becomes so obstructed no coughing or speech is possible, intervention is essential. A series of back blows or subdiaphragmatic abdominal thrusts may be used with children, the same as

TABLE 40.5 Comparison of Laryngotracheobronchitis (Croup) and Epiglottitis

Assessment	Laryngotracheobronchitis	Epiglottitis
Causative organism	Usually viral	Usually pneumococci or streptococci
Usual age of child	6 months–3 years	3–6 years
Seasonal occurrence	Late fall and winter	None
Onset pattern	Preceded by upper respiratory infection; cough becomes worse at night	Preceded by upper respiratory infection; suddenly very ill
Presence of fever	Low grade	Elevated to about 103°F
Appearance	Retractions and stridor; prolonged inspiratory phase of respirations; not very ill appearing	Drooling; very ill appearing; neck hyperextended to breathe (do not attempt to view enlarged epiglottis, or immediate airway obstruction can occur)
Cough	Sharp, barking	Muffled cough
X-ray findings	Lateral neck X-ray showing subglottal narrowing	Lateral neck X-ray showing enlarged epiglottis
Possible complications	Asphyxia because of subglottic obstruction	Asphyxia because of supraglottic obstruction

for adults. This recommendation does not extend to infants, however, because of the great risk of rupturing the liver (American Heart Association [AHA], 2010).

For subdiaphragmatic abdominal thrusts, stand behind the child and place a fist just under the child's diaphragm, a point immediately below the anterior rib cage. Embrace the child, grip your fist with your other hand, and pull back and up with a rapid thrust. The pressure created by this action of pushing up on the diaphragm forces the aspirated material out of the trachea (Fig. 40.18).

If a child is lying on his or her back at the time of the aspiration, stand at the head of the bed or table, place your hands in the same position as described previously, and exert the same inward and upward thrust. A subdiaphragmatic abdominal maneuver may cause a child to vomit as well as expel an aspirated object so turn the child's head to the side to prevent aspiration of vomitus.

For infants, use back thrusts to dislodge an aspirated object. Turn the infant prone over your arm and administer up to five quick back blows forcefully between the infant's shoulder blades, using the heel of the hand (Fig. 40.19A). If the object is not expelled, turn the infant while carefully supporting the head and neck and hold the infant in a supine position draped over your thigh. Be sure to keep the infant's head lower than his or her chest. Provide up to five quick downward thrusts in the lower third of the sternum (Fig. 40.19B). This is generally enough to dislodge the foreign object. If it is not effective, alert the emergency response system and begin cardiac massage (see Chapter 41).

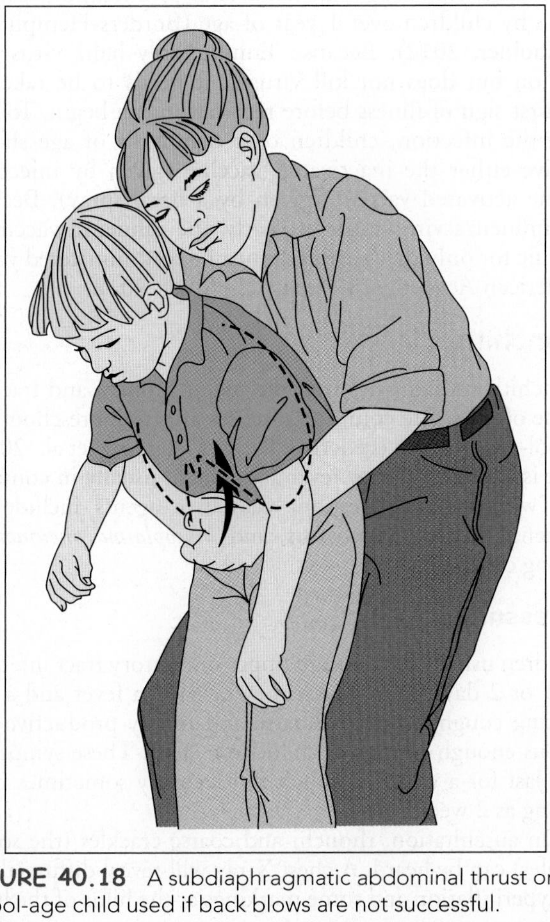

FIGURE 40.18 A subdiaphragmatic abdominal thrust on a school-age child used if back blows are not successful.

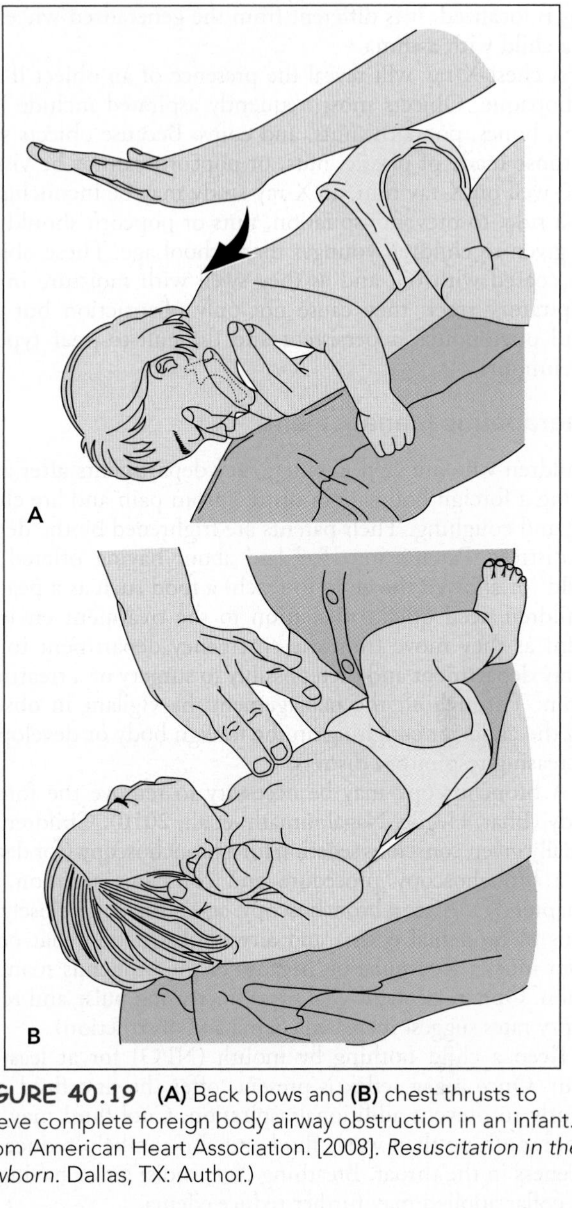

FIGURE 40.19 **(A)** Back blows and **(B)** chest thrusts to relieve complete foreign body airway obstruction in an infant. (From American Heart Association. [2008]. *Resuscitation in the newborn*. Dallas, TX: Author.)

Bronchial Obstruction

The right main bronchus is straighter and has a larger lumen than the left bronchus in children older than 2 years of age. For this reason, an aspirated foreign object that is not large enough to obstruct the trachea may lodge in the right bronchus, obstructing a portion or all of the right lung. The alveoli distal to the obstruction will collapse as the air remaining in them becomes absorbed (atelectasis), or hyperinflation and pneumothorax may occur if the foreign body serves as a ball valve, allowing air to enter but not leave the alveoli (see later discussion on disorders of the lower respiratory tract).

Assessment

After aspirating a small foreign body, the child generally coughs violently and may become dyspneic. If the article is not expelled, hemoptysis, fever, purulent sputum, and leukocytosis will generally result as infection develops. Localized wheezing (a high whistling sound on expiration made by air passing through the narrowed lumen) may occur. Because this is localized, it is different from the generalized wheezing of a child with asthma.

A chest X-ray will reveal the presence of an object if it is radiopaque. Objects most frequently aspirated include buttons, bones, popcorn, nuts, and coins. Because objects such as those made of plastic, nuts, or popcorn cannot be visualized well on X-ray film, an X-ray study may be inconclusive. As a rule, to prevent aspiration, nuts or popcorn should not be given to children younger than school age. These objects are coated with oil, and as they swell with moisture in the respiratory tract, they cause not only obstruction but also lipid pneumonia, a persistent and difficult-to-treat type of pneumonia.

Therapeutic Management

Children who are seen in emergency departments after aspirating a foreign body are in distress from pain and are choking and coughing. Their parents are frightened by the degree of distress. Parents may feel bad about having offered the child (or allowed the child to reach) a food such as a peanut. Children need quick orientation to the treatment environment as they move from the emergency department to the X-ray department and then possibly to surgery or a treatment room. Throughout the management, be vigilant in observing the child for coughing up the foreign body or developing increasing respiratory distress.

A bronchoscopy may be necessary to remove the foreign body (Bhat, Hegde, Nagalotimath, et al., 2010). Children are usually given conscious sedation for a bronchoscopy (for details of a bronchoscopy procedure and conscious sedation, see Chapter 37). After a bronchoscopy, assess the child closely for signs of bronchial edema and airway obstruction that occur from mucus accumulation because of the bronchus manipulation. Obtain frequent vital signs (increasing pulse and respiratory rates suggest increased edema and obstruction).

Keep a child nothing by mouth (NPO) for at least an hour. Once a gag reflex is present, offer the first fluid cautiously to prevent additional aspiration. Cool fluid may feel more soothing than warm fluid and also can help reduce the soreness in the throat. Breathing cool, moist air or having an ice collar applied may further reduce edema.

Obviously, parents need to be cautioned about the dangers of aspiration to keep this from happening again. Do not lecture, however. Parents whose child has just been through this experience already recognize the danger of aspiration and realize they need to be more careful in the future.

DISORDERS OF THE LOWER RESPIRATORY TRACT

The structures of the lower respiratory tract are subject to infection by the same pathogens that attack the upper respiratory tract. Although these illnesses, such as bronchiectasis, can begin as a simple infection, a danger is they will lead to secondary pneumonia and chronic illness.

Bronchiectasis

Bronchiectasis is chronic dilatation and plugging of the bronchi, which can follow pneumonia, but often occurs as the aftermath of aspiration of a foreign body that was not removed (Brashers, 2012). Children will develop a chronic cough with mucopurulent sputum (Kirk, 2013). Young infants may have accompanying wheezing or stridor. If a large area of lung is involved, children may have cyanosis. As the disease becomes chronic, children develop symptoms of chronic lung disease, such as clubbing of the fingers and easy fatigability. Their physical growth may become restricted. Their chest may become enlarged from overinflation of alveoli caused by air trapped behind inflamed bronchi.

Inhaled mucolytic agents or bronchodilators and chest physiotherapy may be necessary to raise the tenacious sputum. An antibiotic will be necessary if infection is present. If the cause of the bronchiectasis is an aspirated seed or nut, this must be identified and removed before the chronic process can be relieved. In rare instances, surgery to remove the affected lung portion may be necessary.

Influenza

Influenza involves inflammation and infection of the major airways. It is caused by the orthomyxovirus influenza type A, B, or C. It is marked by a cough, fever, fatigue, aching pains, a sore throat, and often accompanying gastrointestinal symptoms such as vomiting or diarrhea. The disease spreads readily through a home or a classroom because children are contagious on the day before symptoms appear and for about the next 5 days. Although most children recover from influenza without incident, it is a potentially serious illness because it can lead to bronchitis or pneumonia.

Children usually need an antipyretic such as acetaminophen (Tylenol) to control fever. Oseltamivir (Tamiflu), a new antiviral drug that halts viral proliferation, can be taken by children over 1 year of age (Borders-Hemphill & Mosholder, 2012). Because Tamiflu only halts virus replication but does not kill viruses, it needs to be taken at the first sign of illness before replication can begin. To prevent the infection, children over 6 months of age should receive either the inactivated vaccine (given by injection) or the activated vaccine (given by a nasal spray). Because the influenza virus mutates yearly, the influenza vaccine is specific for only that year and must be readministered yearly (American Academy of Pediatrics [AAP], 2012).

Bronchitis

Bronchitis (inflammation of the major bronchi and trachea) is one of the more common illnesses affecting preschool and school-age children (Federico, Kirby, Deterding, et al., 2011).

It is characterized by fever and cough, usually in conjunction with nasal congestion. Causative agents include the influenza viruses, adenovirus, and *Mycoplasma pneumoniae*, among others.

Assessment

Children usually have a mild upper respiratory tract infection for 1 or 2 days, after which they develop a fever and a dry, hacking cough, which is hoarse and mildly productive and serious enough to wake a child from sleep. These symptoms may last for a week, although full recovery sometimes takes as long as 2 weeks.

On auscultation, rhonchi and coarse crackles (the sound of rales) can be heard. A chest X-ray will reveal diffuse alveolar hyperinflation and some markings at the hilus of the lung.

Therapeutic Management

Therapy is aimed at relieving respiratory symptoms, reducing fever, and maintaining adequate hydration. An antibiotic will be prescribed for bacterial infections. If mucus is viscous, an expectorant may be necessary to help the child raise sputum. It is important children with bronchitis cough to expectorate accumulating sputum, so cough syrups to suppress coughing should not be used.

Bronchiolitis

Bronchiolitis is inflammation of the fine bronchioles and small bronchi. The infection occurs most often in the winter and spring and is the most common lower respiratory illness in children younger than 2 years of age, peaking in incidence at 6 months of age (Kelsall-Knight, 2012). Many children who develop asthma later in life have numerous instances of bronchiolitis during their first year of life. Viruses, such as adenovirus, parainfluenza virus, and RSV, in particular, appear to be the pathogens most responsible for the infection (Black & Brennan, 2011).

Assessment

Typically, infants have 1 or 2 days of an upper respiratory tract infection, then suddenly begin to demonstrate an increased respiratory rate, nasal flaring, and intercostal and subcostal retractions on inspiration. They may have a mild fever, leukocytosis, and an increased erythrocyte sedimentation rate, indicating the amount of bronchial inflammation present. Both accumulating mucus and inflammation block the small bronchioles, so air can no longer enter or leave alveoli freely; therefore, alveolar hyperinflation occurs from air being able to enter more easily than leaving inflamed, narrowed bronchioles. This increases the expiratory phase of respiration and can create wheezing. After initial hyperinflation, areas of atelectasis in alveoli may occur as the air that cannot be expired is absorbed. Tachycardia and cyanosis develop from hypoxia. Infants soon become exhausted from rapid respirations. A chest X-ray reveals pulmonary infiltrates caused by a secondary infection or collapse of alveoli (atelectasis). Pulse oximetry shows low oxygen saturation. A throat culture will identify the offending organism.

Therapeutic Management

For children with less severe symptoms, antipyretics, adequate hydration, and maintaining a watchful eye for progression to more serious illness is all that is necessary. Hospitalization is warranted for children in severe distress such as when an infant is tachypneic, has marked retractions, seems listless, or has a history of poor fluid intake. Children with chronic pulmonary disease may receive anti-RSV immunoglobulin if RSV is identified as the causative agent.

If symptoms are severe, children need humidified oxygen to counteract hypoxemia and adequate hydration to keep respiratory membranes moist. Nebulized bronchodilators, epinephrine, and anti-inflammatory medications such as nebulized budesonide (a glucocorticoid steroid) may be used, although there is little evidence they make a major difference in reducing symptoms. Feeding is often a problem because infants tire easily and therefore cannot finish a feeding. Intravenous fluids may be given for the first 1 or 2 days of illness to eliminate the need for oral feeding.

Some children's symptoms are so severe that they need ventilatory assistance or extracorporeal membrane oxygenation (the same as that used for heart surgery) to maintain adequate oxygenation. All infants with bronchiolitis need to be carefully observed because if RSV is the cause, apnea may occur (Smith, 2011). Because RSV infection spreads readily from one child to the next, infants should be isolated for care. Nursing care should be organized so nurses do not care for other infants than those infected with RSV.

The disease peaks in severity between 48 to 72 hours. Recurrent apneic episodes are rare, so home monitoring for apneic episodes is usually not necessary. Two products are available for the prevention of RSV infection: RSV immune globulin intravenous (RSV-IGIV), made from RSV antibody–positive donor serum, and palivizumab, a humanized monoclonal antibody produced by recombinant DNA technology. These may be given prophylactically to premature infants during the winter months (Kirk, 2013).

The acute phase of bronchiolitis lasts 2 or 3 days. After this time, the child's condition improves rapidly. Although mortality from bronchiolitis is less than 1%, it is a serious disorder of infancy; without treatment, a larger number of infants certainly would die. Some children develop an increased incidence of airway hyperreactivity that may persist for years and be manifested later as asthma (Carter & Marshall, 2011).

Nursing Diagnoses and Related Interventions

Nursing Diagnosis: Parental anxiety related to respiratory distress in child

Outcome Evaluation: Parents state their anxiety level is tolerable as signs and symptoms of disease decrease.

Be certain the parents of a child with bronchiolitis receive a good explanation of their child's condition. Most parents are aware of bronchi but are unfamiliar with the word *bronchiole*. This leaves them unsure how a simple cold has become so severe and if they should have sought medical attention sooner. Assure them bronchiolitis begins as only a cold and that it was impossible to know that this cold would take a more serious turn to help them regain confidence in themselves as parents.

Asthma

Asthma, an immediate hypersensitivity (type I) response, is the most common chronic illness in children, accounting for a large number of days of absenteeism from school and many hospital admissions each year. It tends to occur initially before 5 years of age, although in these early years, it may be diagnosed as frequent occurrences of bronchiolitis rather than asthma (Table 40.6). The condition may be intermittent, with symptom-free periods, or chronic, with continuous symptoms (Upton & Thalange, 2013).

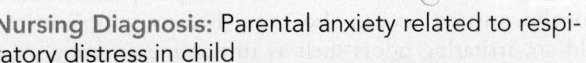

TABLE 40.6 Comparison of Bronchiolitis, Pneumonia, and Asthma

Assessment	Bronchiolitis	Pneumonia	Asthma
Cause	Usually respiratory syncytial virus	Possibly bacterial (pneumococcal, or *Haemophilus influenzae*), viral, or mycoplasmal; possibly secondary to aspiration	Hypersensitivity type I immune response
Age of child	Under 2 years	All through childhood	Onset: 1–5 years
Onset pattern	Follows an upper respiratory infection	Follows an upper respiratory infection	Follows initiation by an allergen
Appearance	Fatigued, anxious, shallow respirations, increasing anteroposterior diameter of chest	Fatigued, anxious, shallow respirations	Wheezing, exhausted, frightened
Cough	Paroxysmal, dry	Productive, harsh cough	Paroxysmal, with thick mucus production
Fever	Low grade	Elevated	None
Auscultatory sounds	Barely audible breath sounds, rales, expiratory wheezing	Decreased breath sounds, rales	Wheezing

Asthma tends to occur in children with atopy or those who tend to be hypersensitive to allergens. When an allergen invades, mast cells release histamine and leukotrienes that result in diffuse obstructive and restrictive changes in the airway because of a triad of inflammation, bronchoconstriction, and increased mucus production. Most children with asthma can be shown to have sensitization to inhalant antigens such as pollens, molds, house dust, or peanuts. Severe bronchoconstriction can also occur because of exposure to cold air, irritating odors such as turpentine or smog, or air pollutants such as cigarette smoke. Although there may be a seasonal factor responsible for a particular child's symptoms, most children have multiple sensitivities so are affected all year long. Aspirin can be a trigger, so caution adolescents with asthma that if they begin to take aspirin as an adult, it may initiate an attack.

Mechanism of Disease

Asthma primarily affects the small airways. The processes of bronchospasm, inflammation of bronchial mucosa, and increased bronchial secretions (mucus) act together to reduce the size of the airway lumen, leading to the major symptom of acute respiratory distress. Bronchial constriction occurs because of stimulation of the parasympathetic nervous system (the cholinergic-mediated system), which initiates smooth muscle constriction. Inflammation and mucus production occur because of mast cell activation to release leukotrienes, histamine, and prostaglandins. Once viewed as a long-term, poorly controlled disorder, newer therapy makes asthma a reversible or manageable disorder (McColley & Morty, 2012).

Assessment

The word *asthma* is derived from the Greek word for "panting," a description of the child's distress. Typically, an episode begins with a dry cough. Children then develop increasing difficulty exhaling as it becomes more and more difficult for them to force air through the narrowed lumen of the bronchioles that are not only inflamed and swollen but also filled with mucus. Typical dyspnea and wheezing (the sound caused by air being pushed forcibly past obstructed bronchioles) associated with the disorder begin. Wheezing is heard primarily on expiration because the lumen of bronchioles are narrower during exhalation than inhalation; although, if the reaction is severe, wheezing may be heard on inspiration as well. If a child coughs up mucus, it is generally copious and may contain white casts bearing the shape of the bronchi from which it was dislodged.

History. An assessment should include a thorough history of the development of a child's symptoms; for example, what the child was doing at the time of the attack, and what actions were taken by the parents or child to decrease or arrest the symptoms. After the acute attack has passed, take time to ask a parent or the child to describe the home environment, including any pets, the child's bedroom, outdoor play space, classroom environment, and type of heating in the house, to see whether more environmental control could reduce allergen triggers and future occurrences.

Physical Assessment. In some children, the initial wheezing is evident only by stethoscope auscultation; in others, it is so loud it can be heard by simply listening. Because asthma affects all lobes of the lungs and although the wheezing may be more prominent in one lobe than in another, it is generally audible in all lung fields (audible wheezing in only one lobe suggests only one bronchus is plugged or a foreign body such as a peanut is more likely responsible than asthma for wheezing). The child may have central cyanosis. The eosinophil count will be elevated.

A bronchospasm leads to CO_2 trapping and retention; therefore, arterial oxygen saturation monitored by a pulse oximeter will begin to decrease because of the child's inability to fully aerate the lungs. The child becomes frightened because of an acute feeling of suffocation. A peak flow meter can be used to assess the child's ability to exhale (Fig. 40.20).

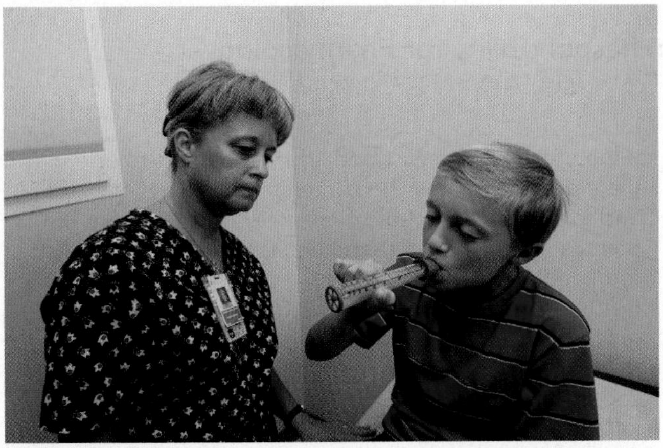

FIGURE 40.20 Here a child with asthma practices using a peak flow meter to track his peak expiratory flow readings on a daily basis.

Air-filled lungs are hyperresonant to percussion or they make a louder, more hollow noise on percussion than usual. With normal respiration, the inspiration phase of breathing is longer than the expiration phase. During an asthma attack, however, a child must work so hard to exhale that the expiration phase becomes longer than the inspiration phase. Time the two phases to demonstrate this. Also observe for retractions (the chest wall is drawn inward with breaths) because children have to use intercostal accessory muscles to achieve full breaths.

As constriction becomes acute, the sound of wheezing may decrease because so little air can leave the alveoli. Hypoxemia and possibly cyanosis will become severe. When blood gases show an increased PCO_2 level and the sound of wheezing suddenly stops, respiratory failure is imminent.

During attacks, children with asthma are generally more comfortable in a sitting or standing position rather than lying down. If seated in a chair, they lean forward and raise their shoulders to give themselves more breathing space. Because of this, do not urge children to "lie down and relax," because this can cause not only severe anxiety but also increased difficulty in breathing. Children who do agree to lie down are either at the end of an attack and beginning to feel less threatened by the dyspnea or are so exhausted by the paroxysms of coughing that they no longer have the strength to sit upright.

Over time, as children have many bouts of asthma, systemic symptoms develop such as a shield-like or barrel-shaped chest from constant overinflation of air in alveoli. Clubbing of the fingers (from the growth of excess capillaries initiated when oxygen deprivation is sensed in distal parts) may be noticeable. If children have been treated for a long period with high doses of steroids, they may fall behind in growth and so may be shorter than usual.

Pulmonary Function Studies

Good pulmonary function depends on good ventilation (both drawing adequate air into the lungs and expelling it again), adequate transfer of gases across the alveolar capillary membranes, and adequate volume and distribution of pulmonary capillary blood flow to transport oxygen to body cells. In children with asthma, the vital capacity (i.e., the air that they are able to exhale) may be low or the capacity may be normal, but because of narrowed bronchioles as a result of bronchospasm, the expiratory rate will be abnormally long (more than 10 seconds, rather than the normal 2 or 3 seconds). If a child has bronchial plugging, the vital capacity will be low because of air absorption behind blocked bronchi. A gross measure of vital capacity is to ask a child to pretend your finger is a candle and try to blow it out. A child with an average vital capacity should be able to blow forcefully. Children with asthma may not have enough expiratory pressure to do this.

Peak Expiratory Flow Rate Monitoring. Children with asthma often use a home peak flow meter daily to measure gross changes in peak expiratory flow and to help in planning an appropriate therapeutic regimen. Children with asthma should be able to tell you their usual reading and personal best score.

To use a peak flow meter, a child places the indicator on the apparatus at the bottom of the numbered scale and takes a deep breath. The child then places the meter in his or her mouth and blows out as hard and fast as possible. The child then repeats this two more times and records the highest number achieved as the peak flow meter result. During a 2-week period when a child feels well, this should be done daily. The highest number achieved during this time is recorded as the child's personal best.

Children are assigned "zones" to rate their expiratory compliance:

- The green zone (80% to 100% of their personal best) means no asthma symptoms are present, and they should take their routine medications.
- The yellow zone (50% to 80% of personal best) signals caution. An episode of asthma may be beginning.
- The red zone (below 50% of personal best) indicates an asthma episode is beginning. Children should immediately take their prescribed medication such as an inhaled Beta-2 agonist, then repeat the peak flow assessment. If the second reading is not in the green zone, their parents should alert their primary care provider of the impending asthma attack.

Therapeutic Management

Therapy for children with asthma involves planning for the three goals of all allergic disorders: (1) avoidance of the allergen by environmental control; (2) skin testing and hyposensitization to identified allergens; and (3) relief of symptoms by pharmacologic agents (see Chapter 42). Parents need good instructions to be able to continue to address all three concerns over an extended period of time (Kovesi, Schuh, Spier, et al., 2010).

Cough suppressants are contraindicated with asthma because, as a rule, as long as children can continue to cough up mucus, they are not in serious danger. When they stop coughing up mucus, thick plugs form that can then lead to pneumonia, atelectasis, and further acidosis.

A child with mild but persistent asthma usually is prescribed an inhaled anti-inflammatory corticosteroid such as fluticasone (Flovent) either daily or every other day (not taking the steroid everyday may allow for more growth) (Chauhan, Chartrand, & Ducharme, 2012). Children who have moderate persistent symptoms usually are prescribed

BOX 40.7 Nursing Care Planning Based on Responsibility for Pharmacology

Classification: Cromolyn sodium is a mast cell inhibitor.
Action: Inhibits the release of histamine, slow-releasing substance of anaphylaxis, and leukotriene, thereby decreasing the overall allergic response. In asthma, it is used prophylactically to prevent severe bronchospasms (Karch, 2013).
Pregnancy Risk Category: B
Dosage: Initially, 20 mg inhaled (via spinhaler or as nebulized solution) four times daily at regular intervals; one ampule orally four times daily one-half hour before meals and at bedtime (ampule is not recommended for use in children under the age of 5 years)
Possible Adverse Effects: Dizziness, headache, nausea, dry and irritated throat, cough, nasal congestion, epistaxis, sneezing

Nursing Implications

- Instruct parents and child that this drug is not effective in an acute attack.
- Caution child and parents to take the drug exactly as prescribed and to continue other agents, such as bronchodilators.
- Instruct child and parents in the use of metered-dose inhaler or nebulizer for administration of cromolyn sodium.
- If the oral form is prescribed, instruct parents to open the ampule and pour the contents into a glass of water and to wait for the medication to dissolve. Caution parents not to substitute the oral form for the inhalant form and vice versa.
- Instruct parents and child to watch for a possible recurrence of asthma symptoms if dosage is decreased.
- Know that this drug is only given once the acute episode is over and the child's airway is clear, to prevent a further episode.
- Caution child and parents not to exceed the number of ordered puffs via inhaler, to prevent possible tolerance to drug.
- If more than one inhalation is ordered, advise child to wait 1 to 2 minutes before taking the second puff.
- If the child is also receiving an inhaled bronchodilator, advise the child and parents to have the child use the bronchodilator first to open the airway and then wait approximately 5 minutes before using the cromolyn sodium, to maximize its effectiveness.

a long-acting bronchodilator at bedtime in addition to the inhaled anti-inflammatory corticosteroid. Children who have severe persistent asthma symptoms may take a high dose of both an oral corticosteroid and an inhaled corticosteroid daily as well as a long-acting bronchodilator at bedtime.

In addition, children may be prescribed a long-acting Beta-2 agonist bronchodilator, such as terbutaline, albuterol, or budesonide, to use if an attack should begin. Cromolyn sodium is a mast cell stabilizer and may be given by a nebulizer or metered-dose inhaler (see Fig. 40.6 and Fig. 40.11A,B) to prevent bronchoconstriction and thereby prevent the symptoms of asthma (Box 40.7). Cromolyn sodium is not effective once symptoms have begun, so children need to take it before they find themselves in a "trigger" situation such as visiting at a friend's house where there will be cigarette smoke (Kovesi et al., 2010).

Another group of drugs used in the chronic treatment of asthma for children over 6 years of age are leukotriene receptor antagonists such as montelukast (Singulair) (Blakey & Wardlaw, 2012).

If children are to receive medication by nebulizer or inhaler, be certain they know how to use these properly. It is easy for children to take this type of medication lightly because of the belief that it is "not really medicine" because it is not swallowed. As a result, an overdose from constant use of nebulizers or MDIs can occur.

Dehydration occurs rapidly in children during an asthma attack because they have decreased oral intake (e.g., children stop drinking because they are coughing, or coughing makes them vomit and parents stop offering fluid) as well as increased insensible loss that occurs from tachypnea. Dehydration is destructive because it may contribute to increased mucus plugging and further airway obstruction. Encourage children to continue to drink fluids (ask about favorite beverages and offer small sips of them); although milk or milk products should be avoided because they cause thick mucus and difficulty swallowing. In an emergency setting, an intravenous line may be established to supply continuous fluid therapy and to also provide a route for emergency drug administration.

Nursing Diagnoses and Related Interventions

Nursing Diagnosis: Fear related to sudden onset of asthma attack

Outcome Evaluation: Parents and child express confidence in their ability to prevent attacks and effectively manage any that occur.

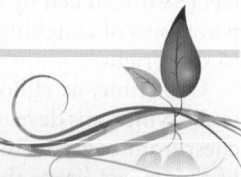

Asthma is a frightening disease. At the time it is diagnosed, parents may have already gone through a long period of wondering why their child was always tired and had episodes of difficulty with breathing. After

diagnosis, parents may be afraid to allow a child to sleep overnight away from them or to leave the child alone with a babysitter. Help parents find a middle ground, allowing the child enough freedom for growth and development while still being certain the child is safe. Taking steps to slow breathing, better emptying alveoli through pursed-lip breathing, and administering medications to prevent symptoms are key measures for children to learn. Many children have long periods without attacks. When a new one occurs after a long absence, it is almost as frightening as the original attack because everything seems so new again.

Nursing Diagnosis: Health-seeking behaviors related to prevention of and treatment for asthma attacks

Outcome Evaluation: Parents and child accurately state triggers that cause an attack; and child correctly demonstrates breathing exercises, use of inhaler, and peak expiratory flow meter.

Children need to learn how to avoid possible triggers through environmental control. If foods are a trigger, children need to learn to be responsible for their own diets so they can avoid these foods. Children as young as 6 years of age can learn what foods they cannot eat and can take responsibility for telling a friend's parent or a schoolteacher that they must not eat certain foods. They must learn to use a metered-dose inhaler or nebulizer if prescribed. At the same time, they must not become inhaler dependent, use the inhaler constantly, or be afraid to go anywhere without it because this will invariably result in their using the inhaler much more often than is necessary.

To prevent children with asthma from losing chest mobility and to decrease their tendency to develop a barrel chest, they can be taught several breathing or mobility exercises to do daily at home. Such exercises are aimed at increasing expiratory function (diaphragmatic or side expansion breathing). Recommended activities include bending side to side, bending forward and touching the left foot with the right hand, and swinging the arms rhythmically in front of the body like a windmill (jumping jacks). These exercises can be incorporated into a family participation time; parents (and nurses) who do mobility exercises with children find the exercises are helpful to them as well because they help tighten the abdominal muscles. Using an incentive spirometer daily is another method for children to exercise the lungs and keep chest muscles supple.

The prognosis in children who develop asthma is good if they adhere to their treatment regimen. Although children do not "outgrow" asthma, most of them do become free of symptoms as adults, probably because the lumens of major airways enlarge with adulthood.

In light of this, be careful not to convey to parents the impression that asthma is a disease that will be simply outgrown so parents maintain careful environmental control, conscientious administration of medication, and hyposensitization, if indicated, to keep the child free of symptoms during childhood.

QSEN Checkpoint Question 40.6

Informatics

You want to teach Michael's 3-year-old roommate about peak flow testing. During this diagnostic test, what instruction should you provide?

a. "Hold your breath until I say, and then cough forcefully."
b. "When I put the meter in your mouth, take a big, deep breath."
c. "I need you to blow out through the meter as hard and fast as you can."
d. "Breathe like you usually do when I put the meter against your mouth."

Look in Appendix A for the best answer and rationale.

Status Asthmaticus

Under ordinary circumstances, an asthma attack responds readily to the aerosol administration of a bronchodilator such as albuterol, terbutaline, levalbuterol (Xopenex), or salmeterol (Serevent). When children fail to respond and an attack continues, they are in *status asthmaticus*. This is an extreme emergency because, if the attack cannot be relieved, the child may die of heart failure caused by the combination of exhaustion, atelectasis, and respiratory acidosis from bronchial plugging (Bhogal, McGillivray, Bourbeau, et al., 2012).

Assessment

A child with status asthmaticus is in acute respiratory distress. Both heart rate and respiratory rate are elevated. Both oxygen saturation and Po_2 are low; Pco_2 is elevated because the bronchi are so constricted the child cannot exhale, resulting in CO_2 accumulation. The rising Pco_2 rapidly leads to acidosis. In contrast to the loud wheezing initially heard in an asthma attack, children with status asthmaticus may have so little air passing in or out of their lungs that breath sounds may be limited. Pulse oximetry will reveal the low oxygen saturation level.

Status asthmaticus is often initiated by a respiratory infection, which acts as the triggering mechanism for the prolonged attack. If this occurs, obtain cultures from coughed sputum and be prepared to administer a broad-spectrum antibiotic until the culture results are available. Be certain the sputum obtained for culture was coughed from deep in the respiratory tract and not just from the back of the child's throat.

Therapeutic Management

By definition, a child in status asthmaticus has failed to respond to first-line therapy (Dehò, Lutman, Montgomery, et al., 2010). Continuous nebulization with an inhaled Beta-2 agonist and intravenous corticosteroids may be necessary to reduce symptoms. Oxygen is given by face mask or nasal prongs to maintain the Po_2 at more than 90 mmHg. These methods supply good oxygen concentrations and yet leave the child's face unobscured for easy observation. It is best administered at a concentration of 30% to 40%, not 100%; if concentrations greater than 40% are needed, a Venturi mask that allows for rebreathing may be used. Some children in severe status asthmaticus

from inhalation as vapors from the stomach rise and are inhaled. As bronchial edema occurs from irritation and inflammation, respirations become shallow, increased in rate, and dyspneic.

A physical assessment shows an increased percussion sound caused by the presence of air trapped in the alveoli beyond the point of inflammation. Rales may be heard as air passes through collecting mucus. Because air cannot reach and inflate the alveoli fully, breath sounds may be diminished. The inflammation reaction from hydrocarbon aspiration may lead to such occlusion that emphysema (pocketing of air in alveoli) occurs, causing rupture of the alveoli into the pleural space, with consequent pneumothorax and atelectasis.

Therapeutic Management. Irritation from fumes of hydrocarbon ingestion may occur when children initially swallow the fluid. If they are given an emetic to induce vomiting, it can cause them to aspirate vomitus or cause additional irritation. After any poisoning, parents should telephone the national poison control center (1-800-122-2222) and ask for advice rather than induce vomiting to prevent this secondary complication. In the emergency room, nasogastric lavage must be done by health care personnel with great care to remove the substance from the stomach while preventing inhalation.

The child is usually admitted to a hospital observation unit for a short time to be certain respirations are stabilizing. Obtain vital signs and carefully observe the child's general appearance for evidence of increased respiratory tract obstruction or increasing drowsiness or other symptoms of CNS involvement from CNS intoxication. Cool, moist air administered by a nebulizer with supplemental oxygen may be prescribed to decrease lung inflammation. If febrile, a child needs an antipyretic. Frequent changes of position will prevent pooling of secretions, which could lead to a secondary infection. Chest physiotherapy will help to move secretions and reduce areas of stasis. Often, children who swallow a household cleaner or other substance are aware they should not have been handling substances kept under the sink. As a result, they cannot help but interpret the hospitalization, blood drawing, and other uncomfortable procedures as punishments for their action. They may benefit from therapeutic play with puppets or dolls that will help alleviate their guilt and anger at being "punished" so severely.

Hydrocarbon pneumonia is slow to resolve, so the child will be ill for some time. After the illness, reinforce with parents the need to keep poisons in a safe place. Offer a listening ear so they can explain they were unaware of the extreme danger of these everyday household products.

Atelectasis

Atelectasis is the collapse of lung alveoli. It may occur in children as a primary or secondary condition. It must be considered as a possibility in all children with respiratory distress.

Primary Atelectasis

Primary atelectasis occurs in newborns who are preterm and so do not breathe with enough respiratory strength at birth to inflate lung tissue or in those who are so lacking in surfactant, the lipoprotein that helps alveoli expand at birth, that alveoli cannot expand. It also may occur if infants have mucus or meconium plugs in the trachea (Dargaville, 2012).

When primary atelectasis occurs, the newborn's respirations become irregular, with nasal flaring and apnea. After a few minutes, a respiratory grunt and cyanosis may occur. The sound of a respiratory grunt is caused by the newborn's glottis closing on expiration. At first, this is a helpful action because it increases pressure in the respiratory tract, keeps alveoli from collapsing, and allows for better alveoli exchange surfaces. This action is also tiring, however. As the infant tires, hypoxemia will increase, and the infant will become hypotonic and flaccid. The Apgar score will invariably be low.

As infants cry or are administered oxygen, more alveoli become aerated and cyanosis may decrease. The cause of the atelectasis must be established, however, so that therapy directed to the specific cause can be initiated.

Secondary Atelectasis

Secondary atelectasis occurs in children when they have a respiratory tract obstruction that prevents air from entering a portion of the alveoli (Federico et al., 2011). As the residual air in the alveoli is absorbed, the alveoli collapse. The causes of obstruction in children include mucus plugs that may occur with chronic respiratory disease or aspiration of foreign objects. In some children, atelectasis occurs because of pressure on lung tissue from outside forces, such as compression from a diaphragmatic hernia, scoliosis, or enlarged thoracic lymph nodes (Fig. 40.21).

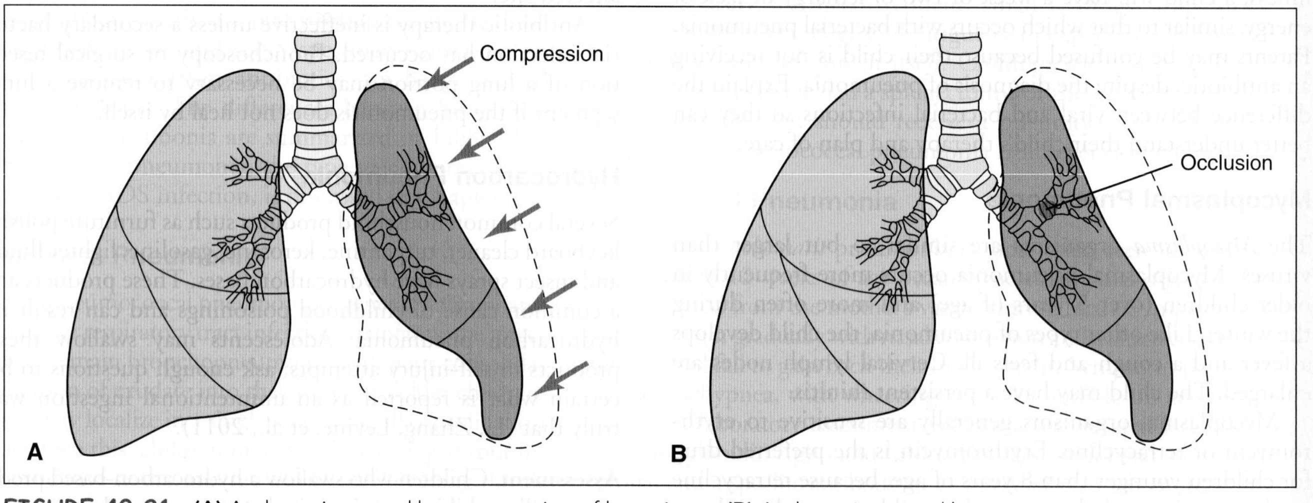

FIGURE 40.21 **(A)** Atelectasis caused by compression of lung tissue. **(B)** Atelectasis caused by obstruction.

The signs of secondary atelectasis depend on the degree of collapse. Asymmetry of the chest may be noticed. Breath sounds on the affected side are decreased. If the process is extensive, tachypnea and cyanosis will be present. A chest X-ray will show the collapsed alveoli (a "whiteout"). Children with atelectasis are prone to secondary infection because mucus, which provides a good medium for bacteria, becomes stagnant without air exchange.

Therapeutic Management. Atelectasis caused by inspiration of a foreign object will not be relieved until the object is removed by bronchoscopy. Atelectasis caused by a mucus plug will resolve when the plug resolves or is moved or expectorated. Children may need oxygen and assisted ventilation to maintain adequate respiratory function until this time (Carter & Marshall, 2011).

Make certain the chest of a child with atelectasis is kept free from pressure so that the lungs can expand as fully as possible to allow as much breathing space as possible. If restraints are being used to keep an infant positioned, make certain that body restraints do not cross the chest area or interfere with chest expansion. Check clothing to be certain it is loose and nonbinding. Make certain the child's arms are not positioned across the chest, where their weight could interfere with deep inspiration.

A semi-Fowler's position generally allows for the best lung expansion because it lowers abdominal contents and increases chest space. Increase the humidity of the child's environment to prevent further bronchial plugging; suction and chest physiotherapy may be necessary to keep the respiratory tract clear and free of mucus. Observe closely for increased respirations or cyanosis, as these indicate failing oxygenation.

Pneumothorax

Pneumothorax is the presence of atmospheric air in the pleural space; its presence causes the alveoli to collapse (atelectasis) (Fig. 40.22). Pneumothorax in children usually occurs when air seeps from ruptured alveoli and collects in the pleural cavity. It also can occur when external puncture wounds allow air to enter the chest (Janssen & Cardillo, 2011).

Pneumothorax occurs in approximately 1% of newborns, probably because of rupture of the alveoli from the extreme intrathoracic pressure needed to initiate a first inspiration. The infant develops tachypnea, grunting respirations, flaring of the nares, and cyanosis. Auscultation reveals absent or decreased breath sounds on the affected side. Percussion may not be revealing, despite the hollow air space; because so much air is present, the chest may be hyperresonant. A more revealing sign may be the shift of the apical pulse (mediastinal shift) away from the site of the pneumothorax and the resulting atelectasis. A chest film will show the darkened area of the air-filled pleural space.

A child with a pneumothorax needs oxygen therapy to relieve respiratory distress. A thoracotomy catheter or needle may be placed through the chest wall into the pleural space and atmospheric air aspirated or low-pressure suction with water-seal drainage applied to remove accumulated air. In most children with pneumothorax, symptoms are relieved within 24 hours after suction is begun. The use of water-seal drainage with children is discussed in Chapter 41.

If the air in the pleural space is from a puncture wound such as a stab wound, cover the chest wound immediately with an impervious material, such as petrolatum gauze, to prevent further air from entering and to help decrease the possibility of atelectasis. In an emergency, an impervious object can be your gloved hand.

Pneumothorax is always a potentially serious respiratory concern. The extent of the symptoms and the outcome will depend on the cause of entry of air into the pleural space and whether it can be removed.

Bronchopulmonary Dysplasia

Bronchopulmonary dysplasia (BPD) is chronic pulmonary involvement that can occur in infants who are treated for acute respiratory distress in the first days of life (Hayes, Feola, Murphy, et al., 2010). The condition frequently presents in infants who were born preterm and received mechanical ventilation for respiratory distress syndrome at birth. The condition is thought to occur from a combination of surfactant deficiency (which is decreased from lung trauma),

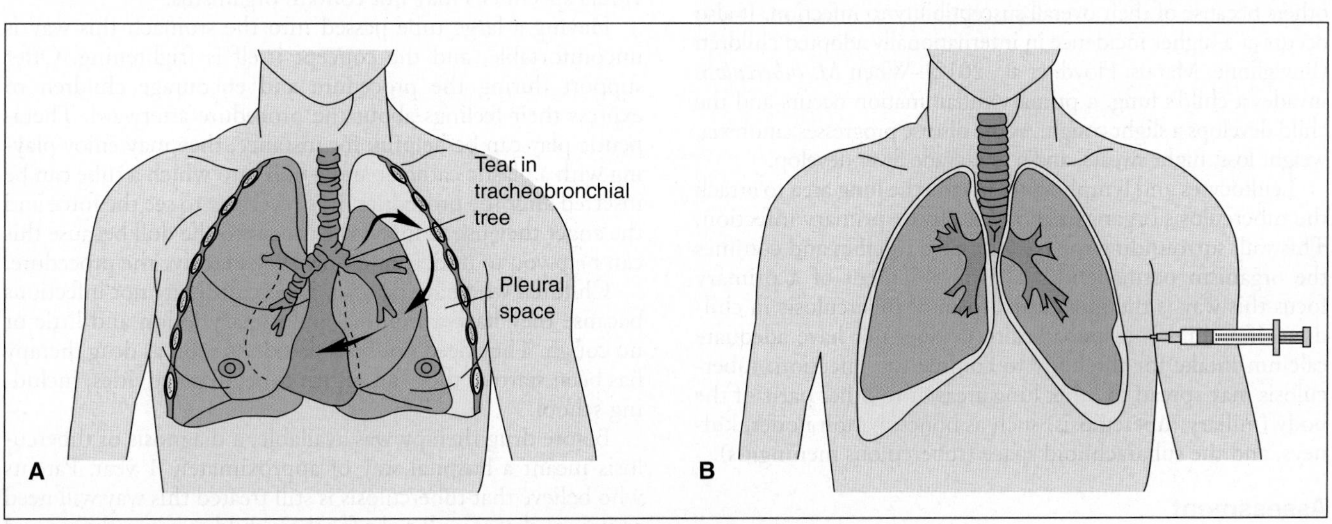

FIGURE 40.22 **(A)** A pneumothorax. A tear in the tracheobronchial tree has caused air to move into the pleural space; the lung collapses and the mediastinum shifts to the unaffected side. **(B)** Aspiration of air from the pleural space allows lung to reexpand after a pneumothorax.

barotrauma (lung damage from ventilator pressure), oxygen toxicity (from high levels needed to counteract the original respiratory distress), and continuing inflammation.

Infants with BPD develop tachypnea, retractions, nasal flaring, tachycardia, oxygen dependence, and abnormal X-ray findings that show areas of overinflation, inflammation, and atelectasis. As the inflamed surfaces heal, the infant is left with fibrotic scarring. On auscultation, decreased air movement can be detected.

The clinical course ranges from a mild need for increased oxygen requirements that will gradually resolve over a few months to a severe disease requiring chronic tracheostomy and mechanical ventilation for as long as the first 2 years of life. A respiratory infection at any time greatly compromises the infant's ability to breathe.

Administration of caffeine and careful monitoring to keep oxygen administration at the lowest level possible help prevent the disorder (Greenough & Ahmed, 2013). Administration of a corticosteroid to reduce inflammation and a bronchodilator by nebulizer can improve respiratory function.

Infants need to be monitored carefully for nutrition and fluid intake, especially if they are ventilator-dependent. Because of the long hospitalization involved, parents need support to continue to visit and care for the child as what seemed to be a miracle at birth (their very small newborn survived) becomes years of specialized and expensive health care.

Tuberculosis

Tuberculosis is a highly contagious pulmonary disease that affects children worldwide (Winston & Menzies, 2012). The causative agent is *Mycobacterium tuberculosis* (tubercle bacillus). The mode of transmission is inhalation of infected droplets. The incubation period is 2 to 10 weeks.

Children generally contract this disease from someone in the immediate family. When any member of a family contracts tuberculosis, all family members must be tested via a Mantoux skin test to screen for the disease. In some children, known exposure to an infected person is not determined, and the disease is first detected when symptoms appear. Children who are homeless or severely impoverished, have HIV, or who have a chronic illness or malnutrition tend to be more susceptible than others because of their overall susceptibility to infection. It also occurs at a higher incidence in internationally adopted children (Raviglione, Marais, Floyd, et al., 2012). When *M. tuberculosis* invades a child's lung, a primary inflammation occurs and the child develops a slight cough. As the disease progresses, anorexia, weight loss, night sweats, and a low-grade fever develop.

Leukocytes and lymphocytes invade the lung area to attack the tuberculosis organism and wall off the primary infection. This wall surrounding the bacteria then calcifies and confines the organism permanently. The development of a primary focus this way is the most usual form of tuberculosis in children. If a child is in poor health or does not have adequate calcium intake for the body to confine the infection, tuberculosis may spread to other lung areas or to other parts of the body (miliary tuberculosis) such as bones, lymph nodes, kidneys, and the subarachnoid space (tuberculous meningitis).

Assessment

All children should have a tuberculin test as part of basic preventive health care at 9 to 12 months of age, and yearly thereafter if they live in a high-risk area for tuberculosis. The test should not be done immediately after measles immunization or the test can read falsely negative (i.e., a child with tuberculosis will be considered free of the disease). Also, the measles vaccine (MMR) can cause primary tuberculosis to become miliary; it is important, therefore, to have a negative tuberculin result before administering this vaccine.

For a Mantoux test, also called a purified protein derivative (PPD) test, 5 units of protein derivative vaccine is injected intradermally, usually on the left lower arm. A health care professional inspects the area in 72 hours and notes the reaction. A positive reaction (the formation of a 5- to 15-mm reddened induration) indicates the child has been exposed to tuberculosis or has developed antibodies to the foreign products of the tuberculosis organism. Children with positive reactions need follow-up with a chest X-ray to ascertain whether a current infection exists. Skin testing should not be done on children who are known to have had tuberculosis because such a child will have such an intense reaction that the skin at the site of the test may slough and necrose.

In the early course of tuberculosis, because the initial focus of the tuberculosis is so small, it may not be evident on a chest X-ray. As local inflammation occurs, however, cloudiness in the inflamed area will be noticeable on the film, as will calcification as it occurs.

To confirm a diagnosis of active disease, sputum is analyzed. Make certain children understand that you want them to expectorate mucus raised from the lungs, not just from the back of the throat for a sputum specimen. Have a child demonstrate a deep cough to you so you can be sure he or she understands what is expected. Infants and children younger than 5 years of age do not expectorate sputum but swallow it. In young children, therefore, a gastric lavage may be necessary to obtain the sputum specimen. (Because tuberculosis bacteria are acid fast, they are not destroyed by gastric secretions and so can be obtained if a nasogastric tube is passed into the stomach.) Schedule this test early in the morning before the child eats in order to prevent vomiting and to allow for the collection of large numbers of organisms that the child coughed up and swallowed during the night. Analyses of sputum are generally done for 3 consecutive days because individual specimens may not contain organisms.

Having a large tube passed into the stomach this way is uncomfortable, and the concept itself is frightening. Offer support during the procedure and encourage children to express their feelings about the procedure afterward. Therapeutic play can be helpful; for instance, they may enjoy playing with a plastic catheter and a doll into which a tube can be inserted after the procedure. It is revealing to see the force and the anger they use to insert the tube into the doll because this can help you to understand how they perceive the procedure.

Children who have primary tuberculosis are not infectious because they have a minimal pulmonary lesion and little or no cough. They need not be isolated. As soon as drug therapy has been started, they can return to regular activities, including school.

Before drug therapy was available, a diagnosis of tuberculosis meant a hospital stay of approximately 1 year. Parents who believe that tuberculosis is still treated this way will need assurance that it is all right for their child to return home and attend school regularly as soon as their child begins taking medication.

Therapeutic Management

Several medications are effective against tuberculosis. Isoniazid (INH) is the drug of choice. INH may produce peripheral neurologic symptoms if pyridoxine (vitamin B_6) is not administered concurrently. Rifampin is a secondary drug often used in combination with INH. Para-aminosalicylic acid (PAS) is bacteriostatic to *M. tuberculosis* and for a long time served as the mainstay of therapy. However, PAS administration may lead to gastrointestinal disturbances in children, and so is not currently used as often today. If it is prescribed, it should be administered after meals, never on an empty stomach.

Ethambutol is used with older children. It must be used with caution with infants because one side effect is optic neuritis. The inability to do adequate eye examinations in children under school age to discover this side effect can make ethambutol unsafe for long-term use.

In addition to drug therapy, children should ingest a diet high in protein, calcium, and pyridoxine, especially if INH is being used because these nutrients are necessary to wall off organisms in lung tissue.

Because tuberculosis therapy can last up to 18 months, major concerns during treatment are that the tuberculosis organism will become resistant to commonly used drugs and that parents may not continue to administer the drugs for this long of a period. Children should have periodic chest X-rays for the rest of their life to make certain the disease does not reactivate later in life. A woman who had tuberculosis as a child should tell her primary care provider about this when she becomes pregnant because lung changes that occur in pregnancy as a result of the pressure of the growing uterus against the lungs can break down calcifications and reactivate tuberculosis. Children who develop another chronic disease that interferes with appetite, and therefore with calcium intake, can also have a high risk of reactivation of calcium-contained tuberculosis.

Assess at health care visits that children who have had tuberculosis receive regular childhood immunizations, especially the pertussis (whooping cough) vaccine because the paroxysmal cough caused by this illness could easily reactivate tuberculosis lesions.

What if...40.3 Michael has a PPD test and it is positive. Would you allow him to continue to play with other children on the hospital unit or isolate him until he's been on an antibiotic for 24 hours?

Cystic Fibrosis

Children with cystic fibrosis (CF) have a generalized dysfunction of the exocrine glands (Brashers, 2012). Mucus secretions of the body, particularly in the pancreas and the lungs, are so tenacious that they have difficulty flowing through gland ducts. There is also a marked electrolyte change in the secretions of the sweat glands; chloride concentration of sweat can be two to five times above normal. The cause of the disorder is an abnormality of the long arm of chromosome 7. This results in the inability to transport small molecules across cell membranes, which leads to dehydration of epithelial cells in the airway and pancreas and to dry secretions.

The disorder is inherited as an autosomal recessive trait and occurs in approximately 1 in 2,500 live births. It occurs most commonly in Caucasian children and rarely in Black or Asian children. Although the disease can be fatal in early life, the current life expectancy for a cystic fibrosis patient who is born today is approximately 60 years (Cohen-Cymberknoh, Shoseyov, & Kerem, 2011). The availability of lung transplantation makes this full life expectancy possible. Because the gene that causes the disorder can be isolated, chorionic villi sampling or amniocentesis can be done early in pregnancy to detect fetuses who have the disease. All newborns can be screened at birth by a simple heel puncture blood sample for the disorder (Laguna, Lin, Wang, et al., 2012). In the future, it is expected that gene therapy will be available to reverse the effect of the involved gene.

Boys with CF may not be able to reproduce because they have persistent plugging and blocking of the vas deferens from tenacious seminal fluid. Girls may have such thick cervical secretions that sperm motility is limited. Alternative insemination or in vitro fertilization are options for those who desire to become pregnant.

Pancreas Involvement

The acinar cells of the pancreas normally produce lipase, trypsin, and amylase, enzymes that flow into the duodenum to digest fat, protein, and carbohydrate. With CF, these enzyme secretions become so thickened that they plug the ducts; eventually, there is such back pressure on the acinar cells that they atrophy and then are no longer capable of producing the enzymes. The islets of Langerhans and insulin production are little influenced by this process until late in the disease because they have endocrine (ductless) activity.

Without pancreatic enzymes in the duodenum, children are unable to digest fat, protein, and some sugars. The child's stools become large, bulky, and greasy (**steatorrhea**). The intestinal flora increases because of the undigested food; this, when combined with the fat in the stool, gives the stool an extremely foul odor, often compared to that of a cat's stool. The bulk of feces in the intestine leads to a protuberant abdomen. Without therapy, because children are benefiting from only about 50% of the food they ingest, they show signs of malnutrition—emaciated extremities and loose, flabby folds of skin on their buttocks. The fat-soluble vitamins, particularly vitamins A, D, and E, cannot be absorbed because fat is not absorbed, so children develop symptoms of low levels of these vitamins. These four symptoms—malnutrition, protuberant abdomen, steatorrhea, and fat-soluble vitamin deficiencies—are the same four symptoms that occur with celiac disease (malabsorption syndrome), so they are referred to as a celiac syndrome (see Chapter 45).

Meconium in a newborn is normally thick and tenacious. In approximately 10% of children with CF, it may be so thick because pancreatic enzymes are lacking that it obstructs the intestine (meconium ileus). The newborn develops abdominal distention with no passage of stool. This is suspected in any infant who does not pass a stool by 24 hours of life (Wainwright, 2011). Rectal prolapse from straining to evacuate hard stool is another common finding in infants with CF.

Lung Involvement

Thickened mucus pools in bronchioles. Pockets of infection then begin in these secretions. The organisms most frequently cultured are *Staphylococcus aureus, Pseudomonas aeruginosa*, and *H. influenzae*. Secondary emphysema (overinflated alveoli) occurs because air cannot be pushed past the thick mucus on expiration, when all bronchi are narrower than they are on inspiration. The anteroposterior diameter of the chest becomes enlarged. Bronchiectasis and pneumonia can occur. Respiratory acidosis may develop because obstruction interferes with the ability to exhale carbon dioxide. Atelectasis occurs as a result of absorption of air from alveoli behind blocked bronchioles. The child's fingers become clubbed because of the inadequate peripheral tissue perfusion.

Sweat Gland Involvement

Although the sweat glands themselves do not appear to be changed in structure, the level of chloride to sodium in perspiration is increased two to five times above normal. Some parents report that they knew their newborn had the disease before they had laboratory tests done because when they kissed their child, they could taste such strong salt in the perspiration.

Assessment. If CF is not diagnosed by a screening blood sample at birth, it can be diagnosed by documenting the chromosomal abnormality or by the history and the combination of the abnormal concentration of chloride in sweat, the absence of pancreatic enzymes in the duodenum, the presence of immunoreactive trypsinogen in the blood, and pulmonary involvement.

CF may be suspected in a newborn when a newborn loses the normal amount of weight at birth (5% to 10% of birth weight), but then, because the infant cannot make use of the fat in milk, does not gain it back at the usual time of 7 to 10 days and perhaps not until 4 to 6 weeks of age. Nurses often weigh newborn babies and infants at well-child health visits, and therefore, may be the first to detect this lack of weight gain. Nurses may also be the first health care provider to suspect CF because meconium is so tenacious that an infant is unable to pass stool (meconium ileus). Immunoreactive trypsin (IRT) will be present in blood serum because obstruction in the pancreas occurs as early as during fetal life.

Children who are not diagnosed at birth may be seen in a health care setting at about 1 month of age because of a feeding problem. Using only about 50% of their intake because of their poor digestive function, they are always hungry. This causes them to eat so ravenously they tend to swallow air, which leads to colic or abdominal distention and vomiting. The appearance of typical CF stools (large and greasy) is an important finding because children with simple colic do not show these changes in stool consistency.

Respiratory infections develop at 4 to 6 months of age. Even at this early stage of the disease, wheezing and rhonchi may be heard on chest auscultation. By the time a child with CF is a preschooler, a cough is a prominent finding. On percussion, the chest is hyperresonant, reflecting the emphysema present. Rales and rhonchi are heard. Clubbing of the fingers may already be apparent. It is rare for a child to go undiagnosed beyond this time because the symptoms of the illness have become so persistent and evident.

Sweat Testing. Sweat testing is a time-honored method for detecting the abnormal salt concentrations in sweat in children with CF. Sweat is collected by placing a filter paper on the skin for a length of time; it is then analyzed for sodium chloride content. With chromosomal determination is available, sweat tests are no longer necessary, but parents may ask about the procedure if they hear about it from friends. A normal concentration of sodium chloride in sweat is 20 mEq/l; a level of more than 60 mEq/l of sodium chloride in children is diagnostic of CF.

Duodenal Analysis. An analysis of duodenal secretions for detection of pancreatic enzymes reveals the extent of the pancreatic involvement. This is done by passing a nasogastric tube into the duodenum and then aspirating secretions for analysis. This test may take a considerable amount of time because the tube is allowed to pass through the pylorus and into the duodenum by natural peristaltic action. You can tell a tube has passed from the stomach into the duodenum by aspirating secretions from the tube and testing them for their pH levels. Stomach secretions are acid (pH less than 7.0), and duodenal secretions are alkaline (pH more than 7.0). The initial insertion of the tube typically is frightening to children because they may choke and gag as it passes the pharynx. Children, however, are generally surprised that once the initial insertion is done, the tube is not uncomfortable. They need a great deal of support during the procedure, however, because it is so unusual and initially so uncomfortable. A duodenal analysis may also be done by endoscopy; for this, the child usually receives conscious sedation (Havidich & Cravero, 2012). The secretions removed from the duodenum are sent to the laboratory for analysis of trypsin content, the easiest pancreatic enzyme to assay. Keep the secretions cold during transport. They should be analyzed immediately for accurate results.

Stool Analysis. Stool may be collected and analyzed for fat content and lack of trypsin, although a description of the large greasy appearance may be all that is necessary.

Pulmonary Testing. A chest X-ray generally confirms the extent of the pulmonary involvement; pockets of emphysema and perhaps beginning pneumonia infiltration are present. Pulmonary function tests may be done to determine the extent of atelectasis and emphysema.

Therapeutic Management. Therapy for children with CF consists of measures to reduce the involvement of the pancreas, lungs, and sweat glands. Because so many organs are involved, care works best if it is a collaborative process (Cohen-Cymberknoh et al., 2011).

Nursing Diagnoses and Related Interventions

Nursing Diagnosis: Imbalanced nutrition, less than body requirements, related to inability to digest fat

Outcome Evaluation: Child's height and weight follow percentile growth curves; quantity of stool decreases; signs and symptoms of vitamin deficiency are absent.

Children with CF are placed on a high-calorie, high-protein, and moderate-fat diet. Water-miscible forms of vitamins A, D, and E are supplemented. Medium-chain triglycerides are used with the diet because these are more readily digested than other oils. During the hot months of the year, extra salt may be added to food to replace that lost though perspiration.

Generally, infants with CF cannot be totally breastfed because there is not enough protein in breast milk for them and such infants need large amounts because they cannot make use of all the protein they ingest. Breastfeeding with supplementary formula is required. Some of these children, unfortunately, are initially diagnosed as having a milk allergy and are treated by being placed on a soybean formula. This does not contain enough protein either, and their malnutrition greatly increases while they are taking this formula. A high-protein formula, such as Probana, is generally recommended as a supplement.

Because children with CF have a ravenous appetite, they eat well. Before each meal or snack, they need to take a synthetic pancreatic enzyme, pancreatic lipase (Cotazym or Pancrease), to replace the enzyme they cannot produce (Box 40.9). These synthetic enzymes are supplied in large capsules that must be opened for young children because they cannot swallow such a big capsule; infants, in particular, may not have enough gastric acids to dissolve the capsule. The powder from the capsule is then added to a small amount (no more than a teaspoonful) of food. It should not be added to hot food because a large portion of enzyme activity can be destroyed. Also, it must not be added to the infant's bottle of formula, because the infant may not drink the entire bottle and therefore will not receive the total benefit of the enzyme. When children are taking a synthetic source of pancreatic enzyme this way, the size of stools and the accompanying foul odor decreases. Children also begin to gain weight.

In adolescence, children may have a great deal of difficulty eating enough to maintain weight, even with enzyme therapy, because their growth spurt requires so many additional calories.

If children with CF become overheated, they begin to lose excessive sodium and chloride through perspiration and become dehydrated. Caution parents to keep their house temperature at 72°F or below and to offer water frequently. They also need to supervise outside play to guard against overexertion or heat exposure.

Nursing Diagnosis: Ineffective airway clearance related to inability to clear mucus from the respiratory tract

Outcome Evaluation: Child's temperature is below 100.4°F (38.0°C); Po_2 is 80 to 90 mmHg; Pco_2 is less than 40 mmHg; oxygen saturation is 92% to 100%.

Unfortunately, the pulmonary effects of CF progress despite supplementation with the pancreatic enzyme; infection from plugged airways is always a possibility. Therefore, it is important to try to keep bronchial secretions as moist and freely flowing as possible so they can drain from the bronchial tree. This is done by frequent nebulization or aerosol therapy followed by chest physiotherapy.

Be certain to observe children with CF frequently because their condition can change rapidly. If a portion of a lung becomes obstructed from a plug of mucus, a child can quickly experience respiratory difficulty. The right side of the heart tends to enlarge in children with chronic respiratory disease because the congestion in the lungs increases pressure in the pulmonary artery and the right ventricle. After a period of stress or exercise, children may begin to show signs of cardiac failure because their already enlarged heart cannot compensate any further.

BOX 40.9 Nursing Care Planning Based on Responsibility for Pharmacology

PANCRELIPASE (COTAZYM)

Classification: Pancrelipase is an enzyme replacement.
Action: Used to aid digestion in children with cystic fibrosis (Karch, 2013).
Pregnancy Risk Category: C
Dosage:

- Children 6 months to 1 year of age: 2,000 units orally per meal
- Children 1 to 6 years of age: 4,000 to 8,000 units orally with each meal and 4,000 units with snacks
- Children 7 to 12 years of age: 4,000 to 12,000 units orally with each meal and with snacks

Possible Adverse Effects: Nausea, abdominal cramps, diarrhea, hypersensitivity

Nursing Implications

- Administer the drug before or with meals and snacks. Instruct parents and child to do the same.
- Caution child and parents to avoid inhaling powder or spilling it on the hands because it may irritate the skin or mucous membranes.
- Do not crush or let the child chew the enteric form of the drug. Break open the capsule and mix with 1 teaspoon of food.
- Instruct the child and parents about possible adverse effects and encourage them to contact their health care provider should any become severe.

Humidified Oxygen. Oxygen is supplied to children by mask, prongs, ventilators, or nebulizers. Mist can be supplied by an ultrasonic compressor and delivered through a nebulizer mask, which makes the droplet size so small that the mist reaches the smallest bronchial spaces.

Aerosol Therapy. Three or four times a day, children may be given aerosol therapy by means of a nebulizer to provide antibiotics or bronchodilators. Antibiotics are specifically determined by culture. A mucolytic, such as acetylcysteine (Mucomyst), can be added to the mist to aid in diluting and liquefying secretions. Children's coughs will become loose and productive after using aerosol therapy. Provide a box of tissues so a child can cough up these loose secretions. Observe children to ensure that they can cough and keep the airway clear. Never give cough syrups to suppress a cough because getting secretions out is essential for air exchange and to prevent infection. Likewise, question a prescription for codeine as an analgesic because codeine suppresses the cough reflex.

Chest Physiotherapy. Because the bronchial secretions with CF are so tenacious, even with liquefaction by mist or aerosol therapy, children may be unable to expectorate them. To aid drainage of secretions, children need chest physiotherapy frequently, as many as three or four times a day.

Activity. Children with CF should maintain normal activities as much as possible. When confined to bed, they need frequent position changes so that, at various times of the day, all lobes of their lungs will be encouraged to drain by being in a superior position. Be certain they sit up part of each day to drain the upper lobes. This change in position also helps to prevent skin breakdown over bony prominences.

Respiratory Hygiene. The sputum that a child coughs up may have a disagreeable taste or odor. Offer frequent mouth care, tooth brushing, and a good-tasting mouthwash to make the child's mouth feel fresh.

Nursing Diagnosis: Risk for impaired skin integrity related to acid stools

Outcome Evaluation: Child's skin does not exhibit areas of erythema or ulceration; rectal prolapse is not present.

Until children are regulated on pancreatic enzymes, their stool is particularly irritating because of its high fat content. Children who are not toilet trained need to have their diapers changed immediately after they wet the diaper or pass stool so that they do not develop skin irritation and breakdown in the diaper area.

After a bowel movement, check the rectum for rectal prolapse. Because of weak musculature of the rectal area, this is a common complication. A prolapse of rectal mucosa appears as a bright-red mass protruding from the anal sphincter. This mucosa must be replaced promptly before its blood supply is compromised. Place the child on the slant board used for chest physiotherapy with the head lower than the buttocks; then, with a lubricated, gloved hand, gently replace the prolapsed rectal mass. Afterward, compress the buttocks together to maintain gentle pressure on the anus for a few minutes. This occurs much less frequently in children who are receiving pancreatic enzymes than in those who are not, because the incidence of rectal prolapse decreases with better nutrition.

Nursing Diagnosis: Risk for compromised family coping related to chronic illness in a child

Outcome Evaluation: Family members state they have adequate resources to cope with current circumstances.

The parents of children with CF are asked to assume a great deal of responsibility for care of their child. Begin discharge planning when a child is first admitted to a hospital in terms of what changes need to be made to accommodate the child at home and familiarizing parents with the necessary care measures. For example, many children with this disorder sleep with oxygen by cannula at night when they are at home. Parents need to be taught the functions of oxygen and how to regulate the flow. This type of learning is most effective if a little is taught every day (e.g., "Could you turn the oxygen on for me, Mrs. Smith? I'm ready to tuck Brian in to sleep" rather than a sit-down, let-me-tell-you-how-oxygen-works lecture given close to the day of discharge). Teach parents how to do chest physiotherapy the same way.

Because they will be spending a great deal of time caring for their child, the family will have to think through how such care needs will affect their home life. They will need to balance work, care of the child, and care of the rest of the family. Many parents become fatigued after the first week of having the child at home, believing that if they fall soundly asleep at night, they may not hear their child call to them if in distress. As they grow more confident in their ability to evaluate their child's condition before bedtime, their apprehension will lessen. Real confidence, however, may not come for months, even years. This may always be a problem for some parents.

Be sure that parents have the telephone number of the health care provider they should call if they feel overwhelmed. Encourage parents to join a support group, so that there are other people available who understand and to whom they can voice their concerns. At these times, one of the most important needs they have is to verbalize to someone what it feels like to be the parent of a child with CF, including feelings of guilt they may be experiencing because the disease is inherited.

Adequate Rest and Comfort. Any child who has compromised lung function has a degree of dyspnea that leads to exhaustion. To counteract this, provide periods of rest during the day, but do not group too many activities or procedures together all at once because this could exhaust a child. Plan a rest period before meals so that a child is not too tired to eat. Also plan for a long rest period before chest physiotherapy so that the child will be able to tolerate it better. Achieving a balance between allowing periods of rest and yet not doing all procedures at once is not an easy task.

Growth and Development. Children need to be exposed to as many normal life experiences as possible. This may be difficult because it is important not to tire the child out or expose the child to crowds of people (possibly increasing the risk for infection). Assist parents with planning age-appropriate activities with the child.

Children should attend regular school if possible so they are provided with socialization experiences with other children. If this is not possible, a home tutor can be arranged for them. Urge children to participate to the extent they can in physical fitness activities in school or with friends. Use a reminder sheet as needed so they can remember to take pancreatic enzymes with them if they are going to be eating lunch in the school cafeteria or outside the home.

Continuing Care. Ensure that children with CF receive periodic health assessments and routine childhood immunizations. It is not unusual for children with a chronic disease to fall behind in routine checkups and immunizations if they are hospitalized at the times these are routinely done. It is particularly important that children with CF receive the pertussis and measles vaccines because these two infections cause severe respiratory complications. Children also should receive influenza, meningococcal, and pneumococcal vaccines.

As children with CF reach adolescence, they are candidates for lung transplants. Some of these are done as lower lobe transplants from a living donor. People who donate a single lobe in this manner report that they feel little loss of lung capacity afterward. A lung transplant is advantageous for children with CF because the new lung does not possess the defective gene that caused mucus to be so thick. Life expectancy can also greatly improve.

What if...40.4 You are particularly interested in exploring one of the 2020 National Health Goals with respect to respiratory disorders and children (see Box 40.1). Most government-sponsored money for nursing research is allotted based on these goals. What would be a possible research topic to explore pertinent to these goals that would be applicable to Michael and his family and that would also advance evidence-based practice?

KEY POINTS FOR REVIEW

- Respiratory tract disorders tend to occur more frequently in children than adults because the lumens of children's bronchi are narrow and obstruction and infection are more likely to occur. Families are frightened at the sight of their child not breathing and need assurance. Planning nursing care that includes assurance not only meets QSEN competencies but also best meets the family's total needs.
- Infants with respiratory illness need extremely close observation because they cannot describe oxygen deprivation.
- Young children do not comprehend the fact that oxygen supports combustion. Observe children receiving oxygen therapy more frequently than adults to be certain that no flames, such as birthday candles, are brought within 10 ft of an oxygen source.
- Acute nasopharyngitis (the common cold) is the most common infectious disease in children. There is no specific therapy for a common cold other than comfort measures.
- Tonsillitis is infection and inflammation of the palatine tonsils. Adenitis is infection and inflammation of the adenoid tonsils. Children with recurring infections may have their tonsils surgically removed.
- Laryngotracheobronchitis (croup) is inflammation of the larynx, trachea, and major bronchi. Epiglottitis is inflammation of the epiglottis. Both of these conditions can cause severe impairment of the airway. Children with epiglottitis should never be assessed for a gag reflex with a tongue blade because the elevated epiglottis can completely occlude the airway.
- Bronchitis is inflammation of the major bronchi and trachea. Bronchiolitis is inflammation of the fine bronchioles. Both conditions are caused by a bacterial or viral invasion.
- Respiratory syncytial virus infection is an infection that accounts for the majority of lower respiratory infections in young children. Infants with RSV infections must be observed closely because they are prone to apnea.
- Pneumonia may occur from a variety of organisms (viral, pneumococcal, chlamydial, mycoplasmal, lipidic, and hydrocarbonic). Except for viral pneumonia, children need specific antibiotics depending on the organism present.
- Asthma, a type I hypersensitivity reaction, is a diffuse and obstructive airway disease with wheezing as the most common symptom. Newer drugs such as leukotriene receptor antagonists and careful environmental control have aided in the management of asthma.
- Tuberculosis is a lung infection that is growing in incidence, with some strains becoming very resistant to the usual therapy. The entire family needs drug therapy if one member develops a primary lesion.
- Cystic fibrosis is a disease in which there is generalized dysfunction of the exocrine glands. This results in malabsorption and tenacious pulmonary secretions, leading to infection and pneumonia. Lung transplantation can be used to replace the diseased lung tissue and to increase the child's life span.

Critical Thinking Care Study

Amanda is a 14-year-old with chronic asthma whom you meet in the emergency room. She is allergic to cats, goldenrod, and tomatoes. She lives with her mother; her parents have been divorced for the past 6 months. This afternoon, she attended a birthday party for a school friend. As soon as she returned home her respiratory rate increased, she gasped for breath, and began wheezing. Her father, a fireman, whom she's been staying with for the weekend, came home from work still in his rubber coat and boots to bring her to the hospital. While you talk to him to obtain a history, he keeps glancing at his watch.

1. Amanda's father keeps looking at his watch while he waits for you to take vital signs on Amanda. When you ask her if anything happened at the party she could identify as an asthma "trigger," she shakes her head rapidly. Would you want to ask her any more questions?
2. Amanda admits she doesn't take her medications regularly because it isn't "cool." What suggestions could you give her to make her feel better about taking medicine?
3. Amanda was suspended from school last month because she rang the fire alarm, and she is banned from entering her local convenience store because she was caught stealing candy from there. When you ask her why these things happened, she answers, "because I have asthma." What questions would you want to ask her to see if she's using her illness as an excuse for bad behavior?

Patient Scenario
The Denman Family

Read about the Denman family, a family with an adolescent with CF, then answer the questions to further sharpen your skills and grow more familiar with NCLEX-type questions related to respiratory illness in children. Confirm your answers are correct by reading the rationales.

Visit http://thePoint.lww.com

Answers and Rationales

Looking for answers to the What If. . . and Critical Thinking Care Study questions?

Visit http://thePoint.lww.com

References

Abadesso, C., Nunes, P., Silvestre, C., et al. (2012). Non-invasive ventilation in acute respiratory failure in children. *Pediatric Reports, 4*(2), e16.

Adil, E., Rager, T., & Carr, M. (2012). Location of airway obstruction in term and preterm infants with laryngomalacia. *American Journal of Otolaryngology, 33*(4), 437–440.

Altamimi, S., Khalil, A., Khalaiwi, K. A., et al. (2012). Short-term late-generation antibiotics versus longer term penicillin for acute streptococcal pharyngitis in children. *Cochrane Database of Systematic Reviews, 2012*(8), CD004872.

American Academy of Pediatrics. (2012). *Inactivated influenza vaccine 2012-13: What you need to know.* Elk Grove, IL: Author.

American Heart Association. (2010). *Pediatric advanced life support provider manual.* Dallas, TX: Author.

Armbruster, J., Schmidt, B., Poets, C. F., et al. (2010). Nurses' compliance with alarm limits for pulse oximetry: Qualitative study. *Journal of Perinatology, 30*(8), 531–534.

Bassham, B. S., Kane, I., Mackeil-White, K., et al. (2012). Difficult airways, difficult physiology and difficult technology: Respiratory treatment of the special needs child. *Pediatric Emergency Medicine, 13*(2), 81–90.

Bhat, K. V., Hegde, J. S., Nagalotimath, U. S., et al. (2010). Evaluation of computed tomography virtual bronchoscopy in paediatric tracheobronchial foreign body aspiration. *Journal of Laryngology and Otology, 124*(8), 875–879.

Bhogal, S. K., McGillivray, D., Bourbeau, J., et al. (2012). Early administration of systemic corticosteroids reduces hospital admission rates for children with moderate and severe asthma exacerbation. *Annals of Emergency Medicine, 60*(1), 84–91.

Black, A., & Brennan, R. A. (2011). Breathing easy: Implementing a bronchiolitis protocol. *Pediatric Nursing, 37*(3), 129–135.

Blakey, J. D., & Wardlaw, A. J. (2012). What is severe asthma? *Clinical & Experimental Allergy, 42*(5), 617–624.

Borders-Hemphill, V., & Mosholder, A. (2012). U.S. utilization patterns of influenza antiviral medications during the 2009 H1N1 influenza pandemic. *Influenza & Other Respiratory Viruses, 6*(6), e129–e133.

Brashers, V. L. (2012). Alterations in pulmonary function. In S. E. Huether & K. L. McCance, (Eds.), *Understanding pathophysiology* (pp. 678–706). St. Louis, MO: Elsevier/Mosby.

Cardone, G., & Lepe, M. (2010). Tracheostomy: Complications in fresh postoperative and late postoperative settings. *Clinical Pediatric Emergency Medicine, 11*(2), 122–129.

Carter, E. R. & Marshall, S. G. (2011). The respiratory system. In K. J. Marcdante, R. M. Kliegman, H. B. Jenson, et al. *Nelson essentials of pediatrics* (6th ed., pp. 499–524). Philadelphia: Saunders/Elsevier.

Centers for Disease Control & Prevention. (2012). *Cold and cough medicines.* Atlanta, GA: Author.

Chang, A. B. (2010). Pediatric cough: Children are not miniature adults. *Lung, 188*(Suppl. 1), S33–S40.

Chauhan, B. F., Chartrand, C., & Ducharme, F. M. (2012). Intermittent versus daily inhaled corticosteroids for persistent asthma in children and adults. *Cochrane Database of Systematic Reviews,* (12), CD009611.

Chiappini, E., Regoli, M., Bonsignori, F., et al. (2011). Analysis of different recommendations from international guidelines for the management of acute pharyngitis in adults and children. *Clinical Therapeutics, 33*(1), 48–58.

Cohen-Cymberknoh, M., Shoseyov, D., & Kerem, E. (2011). Managing cystic fibrosis: Strategies that increase life expectancy and improve quality of life. *American Journal of Respiratory and Critical Care Medicine, 183*(11), 1463–1471.

Dargaville, P. A. (2012). Respiratory support in meconium aspiration syndrome: A practical guide. *International Journal of Pediatrics,* 2012: 965159.

Dehò, A., Lutman, D., Montgomery, M., et al. (2010). Emergency management of children with acute severe asthma requiring transfer to intensive care. *Emergency Medical Journal, 27*(11), 834–837.

DeMuri, G. P., & Wald, E. R. (2012). Clinical practice. Acute bacterial sinusitis in children. *New England Journal of Medicine, 367*(12), 1128–1134.

Dmello, D., Nayak, R. P., & Matuschak, G. M. (2010). High-frequency percussive ventilation for airway clearance in cystic fibrosis: A brief report. *Lung, 188*(6), 511–513.

Dolovich, M. B., & Dhand, R. (2011). Aerosol drug delivery: Developments in device design and clinical use. *The Lancet, 377*(9770), 1032–1044.

Eladl, H. M. (2010). Transnasal endoscopic repair of bilateral congenital choanal atresia: Controversies. *Journal of Laryngology and Otology, 124*(4), 387–392.

Faksh, A., Wax, J. R., Lucas, F. L., et al. (2011). Preterm premature rupture of membranes ≥32 weeks' gestation: Impact of revised practice guidelines. *American Journal of Obstetrics & Gynecology, 205*(4), 340.e1–e5.

Federico, M. J., Kirby, G. S., Deterding, R. R., et al. (2011). Respiratory tract & mediastinum. In W. Hay, M. Levin, R. Deterding, et al. (Eds.), *Current diagnosis & treatment pediatrics* (21st ed., pp. 487–584). New York, NY: McGraw-Hill/Lange.

Gizzi, C., Moretti, C., & Agostino, R. (2011). Weaning from mechanical ventilation. *Journal of Maternal-Fetal & Neonatal Medicine, 24*(Suppl. 1), 61–63.

Greenough, A., & Ahmed, N. (2013). Perinatal prevention of bronchopulmonary dysplasia. *Journal of Perinatal Medicine, 41*(1), 119–126.

Hafeez, W., Ronca, L. T., & Maldonado, T. E. (2011). Pediatric advanced life support update for the emergency physician. *Clinical Pediatric Emergency Medicine, 12*(4), 255–265.

Havidich, J. E., & Cravero, J. P. (2012). The current status of procedural sedation for pediatric patients in out-of-operating room locations. *Current Opinion in Anaesthesiology, 25*(4), 453–460.

Hayes, D., Feola, D. J., Murphy, B. S., et al. (2010). Pathogenesis of bronchopulmonary dysplasia. *Respiration, 79*(5), 425–436.

Hoberman, A. H., Paradise, J. L., Rockette, H. E., et al. (2011). Treatment of acute otitis media in children under 2 years of age. *New England Journal of Medicine, 364*(2), 105–115.

Isaacson, G. (2012). Tonsillectomy healing. *Annals of Otology, Rhinology & Laryngology, 121*(10), 645–649.

Janssen, J., & Cardillo, G. (2011). Primary spontaneous pneumothorax: Towards outpatient treatment and abandoning chest tube drainage. *Respiration, 82*(2), 201–203.

Karch, A. M. (2013). *2013 Lippincott's nursing drug guide*. Philadelphia, PA: Lippincott Williams & Wilkins.

Kelsall-Knight, L. (2012). Clinical assessment and management of a child with bronchiolitis. *Nursing Children & Young People, 24*(8), 29–34.

Kilic, A., Ünüvar, E., Sütçü, M., et al. (2012). Acute obstructive respiratory tract diseases in a pediatric emergency unit: Evidence-based evaluation. *Pediatric Emergency Care, 28*(12), 1321–1327.

Kirk, A. (2013). Pulmonary disease. In M. M. Tschudy & K. M. Arcara (Eds.), *The Harriet Lane handbook* (19th ed., pp. 584–605). Philadelphia, PA: Elsevier/Mosby.

Kovesi, T., Schuh, S., Spier, S., et al. (2010). Achieving control of asthma in preschoolers. *Canadian Medical Association Journal, 182*(4), E172–E183.

Kugel, G., Gerlach, R. W., Aboushala, A., et al. (2011). Long-term use of 6.5% hydrogen peroxide bleaching strips on tetracycline stain: A clinical study. *Compendium of Continuing Education in Dentistry, 32*(8), 50–56.

Laguna, T. A., Lin, N., Wang, Q., et al. (2012). Comparison of quantitative sweat chloride methods after positive newborn screen for cystic fibrosis. *Pediatric Pulmonology, 47*(8), 736–742.

Li, L., Zhang, X., Levine, B., et al. (2011). Trends and pattern of drug abuse deaths in Maryland teenagers. *Journal of Forensic Sciences, 56*(4), 1029–1033.

Lim, W. J., Mohammed-Akram, R., Carson, K. V., et al. (2012). Non-invasive positive pressure ventilation for treatment of respiratory failure due to severe acute exacerbations of asthma. *Cochrane Database of Systematic Reviews,* (12), CD004360.

Lin, Y., & Lee, J. (2011). Bilateral peritonsillar abscesses complicating acute tonsillitis. *Canadian Medical Association, 183*(11), 1276–1279.

Marchiori, E., Zanetti, G., Fontes, F. B., et al. (2012). Optimizing the utility of high-resolution computed tomography in diagnosing exogenous lipoid pneumonia. *Heart Lung, 41*(2), 207–208.

Martin, J. M. (2010). Pharyngitis and streptococcal throat infections. *Pediatric Annals, 39*(1), 22–27.

McColley, S. A., & Morty, R. E. (2012). Update in pediatric lung disease 2011. *American Journal of Respiratory and Critical Care Medicine, 186*(1), 30–34.

Mishra, K. N., Bhardwaj, P., Mishra, A., et al. (2011). Acute *Chlamydia trachomatis* respiratory infection in infants. *Journal of Global Infectious Diseases, 3*(3), 216–220.

Mitchell, R. B., Hussey, H. M., Setzen, G., et al. (2013). Clinical consensus statement: Tracheostomy care. *Otolaryngology: Head & Neck Surgery, 148*(1), 6–20.

Peacock, J., & Stanik-Hutt, J. (2013). Translating best care practices to improve nursing documentation regarding pediatric patients dependent on home mechanical ventilation and tracheostomy tube support: A quality improvement initiative. *Home Healthcare Nurse, 31*(1), 10–17.

Raviglione, M., Marais, B., Floyd, K., et al. (2012). Scaling up interventions to achieve global tuberculosis control: Progress and new developments. *The Lancet, 379*(9829), 1902–1913.

Robertson, A., King, R., & Tomkinson, A. (2010). Frequency and management of epistaxis in schools. *Journal of Laryngology and Otolaryngology, 124*(3), 302–305.

Schomacker, H., Schaap-Nutt, A., Collins, P. L., et al. (2012). Pathogenesis of acute respiratory illness caused by human parainfluenza viruses. *Current Opinion in Virology, 2*(3), 294–299.

Science, M., Johnstone, J., Roth, D. E., et al. (2012). Zinc for the treatment of the common cold: A systematic review and meta-analysis of randomized control trials. *Canadian Medical Journal, 184*(10), E551–E561.

Serra, A., Cocuzza, S., Longo, M. R., et al. (2012). Tracheostomy in childhood: New causes for an old strategy. *European Review for Medical & Pharmacological Sciences, 16*(12), 1719–1722.

Smith, S. (2011). Infectious diseases. In K. J. Marcdante, R. M. Kliegman, H. B. Jenson, et al. (Eds.), *Nelson essentials of pediatrics* (6th ed., pp. 355–462). Philadelphia, PA: Saunders/Elsevier.

Sylvester, D. C., Carr, S., & Nix, P. (2013). Maximal medical therapy for chronic rhinosinusitis: A survey of otolaryngology consultants in the United Kingdom. *International Forum of Allergy & Rhinology, 3*(2), 129–132.

Upton, C., & Thalange, N. (2013). Respiration. In N. Thalange, R. Beach, D. Booth, et al. (Eds.), *Essentials of paediatrics* (2nd ed., pp. 99–118). Philadelphia, PA: Elsevier/Saunders.

U.S. Department of Health and Human Services. (2010). *Healthy people 2020*. Washington, DC: Author.

Vandemheen, K. L., Aaron, S. D., Poirer, C., et al. (2010). Development of a decision aid for adult cystic fibrosis patients considering referral for lung transplantation. *Progress in Transplantation, 20*(1), 81–87.

Wainwright, C. E. (2011). Treatment of cystic fibrosis following infant screening. *Therapy, 8*(6), 613–622.

Watson, P. (2012). Inhaler spacer devices to treat asthma in children. *Nursing Times, 108*(46), 18–20.

Winston, C. A., & Menzies, H. J. (2012). Pediatric and adolescent tuberculosis in the United States, 2008-2010. *Pediatrics, 130*(6), e1425–e1432.

Chapter 41

Nursing Care of a Family When a Child Has a Cardiovascular Disorder

KEY TERMS

- acyanotic heart disease
- afterload
- balloon angioplasty
- cardiac catheterization
- congestive heart failure
- contractility
- cyanosis
- cyanotic heart disease
- diastole
- innocent heart murmur
- organic heart murmur
- polycythemia
- postcardiac surgery syndrome
- postperfusion syndrome
- preload
- systole
- vasculitis

OBJECTIVES

After mastering the contents of this chapter, you should be able to:

1. Describe the common cardiovascular disorders of childhood.
2. Identify 2020 National Health Goals related to children with cardiovascular disorders that nurses can help the nation achieve.
3. Assess a child with a cardiovascular dysfunction.
4. Formulate nursing diagnoses for a child with a cardiovascular disorder.
5. Establish outcomes based on the priority needs of a child with a cardiovascular disorder that can help the family manage seamless transitions across different health care settings.
6. Using the nursing process, plan nursing care that includes the six competencies of Quality & Safety Education for Nurses (QSEN): Patient-Centered Care, Teamwork & Collaboration, Evidence-Based Practice (EBP), Quality Improvement (QI), Safety, and Informatics.
7. Implement nursing care for a child with a cardiovascular disorder, such as teaching about the importance of taking prescribed medication.
8. Evaluate expected outcomes for achievement and effectiveness of care.
9. Integrate knowledge of cardiovascular disorders with the interplay of nursing process, the six competencies of QSEN, and Family Nursing to promote quality maternal and child health nursing care.

Megan is a newborn who was born with tetralogy of Fallot. By 1 hour of age, she developed rapid respirations, tachycardia, and cyanosis. An echocardiogram revealed the typical four structural disorders of the syndrome. Megan's parents will be taking her home this afternoon for 2 months to await cardiac surgery. They tell you their primary care provider instructed them to "watch her carefully" during that time. "What does that mean?" they ask you. "Exactly what should we watch for?"

Previous chapters described the growth and development of well infants and children and care of children when ill. This chapter adds information about the child who is ill with a cardiovascular disorder and the stress that such a serious diagnosis places on families. Such information builds a base for care and health teaching for children with these disorders.

What advice would you offer Megan's parents?

The cardiovascular system, the body system on which all other systems depend, consists of the heart, which acts as a pump; the blood, which provides the fluid and cells for transport of oxygen, nutrients, regulatory substances such as hormones, enzymes, and antibodies, and the evacuation of waste products; and the blood vessels, which provide the means and routes for transport throughout the body. The system has a great capacity to adapt to changing body needs by adjusting the rate and force of heart pumping, modifying the size of the blood vessels, and altering the volume and composition of the blood (Lange & Hillis, 2013).

Most cardiovascular disorders in children occur as a result of a congenital anomaly; either the heart develops inadequately in utero, or the heart cannot adapt to extrauterine life for some reason. Open-heart surgery often is the only therapy that will correct the primary congenital concern. Children also may experience acquired cardiovascular disorders, such as rheumatic fever or Kawasaki syndrome, disorders that can also lead to inadequate heart function.

Cardiovascular disorders are frightening for both children and parents, as even small children realize the importance of their heart to sustain life. For the families of children with a cardiovascular disorder, understanding the functioning of the heart and circulation is an important first step toward coping with the illness. Box 41.1 shows 2020 National Health Goals that address achieving cardiovascular health through health promotion and disease prevention, measures that can begin in childhood and adolescence.

BOX 41.1 Nursing Care Planning Based on 2020 National Health Goals

Cardiovascular illness is a major health problem in adults. Because the illness and its effects can be prevented or at least minimized by instituting measures early in childhood, a number of 2020 National Health Goals address ways parents and children can modify nutrition or exercise to achieve better cardiovascular health:

- Increase the proportion of adolescents who meet current federal physical activity guidelines for aerobic physical activity and for muscle-strengthening activity from a baseline of 18.4% to a target of 20.2%.
- Reduce the proportion of children age 2 to 5 years who are considered obese from 10.7% to 9.6%.
- Reduce consumption of calories from solid fats in the population age 2 years and older from a baseline of 18.9 to 16.7.
- Reduce the proportion of children and adolescents with hypertension from 3.5% to 3.2% (U.S. Department of Health and Human Services [DHHS], 2010; see www.healthypeople.gov).

Nurses can help the nation achieve these goals by educating parents and children about the importance of reducing obesity and planning exercise and nutrition programs for sound cardiovascular health. It is equally important for nurses to caution parents not to start their children on reduced-fat diets until they are 2 years old, to allow for myelination of nerve cells.

Nursing Process Overview

For Care of a Child With a Cardiovascular Disorder

Assessment

Assessment of a child with a cardiovascular disorder includes both careful history taking and physical examination, because many of the signs and symptoms of heart disease in children are subtle. A variety of diagnostic studies such as echocardiography, electrocardiography, or cardiac catheterization may be used to confirm the diagnosis and prepare a child for surgery. Teaching about these tests and providing psychological support to children and their families are two major responsibilities of nurses throughout the assessment process.

Remember that hypertension, hypercholesterolemia, and congenital heart disorders occur at higher incidences in some families than others because these disorders tend to be familial. Hypertension, for example, occurs at a higher rate in African Americans than in other groups. Nurses have a responsibility to educate adolescents about the importance of maintaining a sensible weight and sodium intake and reducing saturated fat and cholesterol intake in an attempt to minimize these familial disorders.

Nursing Diagnosis

Nursing diagnoses associated with heart disease in children usually address the effect of poor circulation to body tissues or the effect a serious disorder can create for the child or parents. Examples include:

- Decreased cardiac output related to congenital structural disorder
- Ineffective tissue perfusion related to inadequate cardiac output
- Deficient knowledge related to care of the child pre- and postoperatively
- Fear related to lack of knowledge about child's illness
- Interrupted family processes related to stresses of diagnosis and care responsibilities
- Ineffective coping related to lack of adequate support people
- Impaired parenting related to inability to bond with critically ill newborn

If the concerns in the latter three diagnoses are not identified when a child is ill, they may continue long after a child is treated and returns home.

If a child will be undergoing surgery or cardiac catheterization, nursing diagnoses will focus on the psychological needs of the child and family for preparation and postprocedure care in addition to physical concerns after the procedure such as hypothermia related to cooling during surgery and powerlessness related to conscious sedation during cardiac catheterization.

Outcome Identification and Planning

Nursing planning is essential to help parents and children understand heart anatomy because a sound knowledge base can help them understand the need for diagnostic testing. Additional teaching is necessary to prepare parents and children for procedures or surgery and recovery at home. Teaching parents to conscientiously administer cardiac medications is another area where planning plays an important role. Organizations that are helpful for referral are the American Heart Association (AHA) (www.heart.org), the Cardiovascular Disease Foundation (www.cvdf.org), the Congenital Heart Information Network (www.tchin.org), and the U.S. Department of Health and Human Services Organ Procurement and Transplantation Network (http://optn.transplant.hrsa.gov).

Implementation

Nursing interventions in the care of children with a cardiovascular disorder include teaching, providing an opportunity for children and their families to express fears about a child's illness and treatment plan, providing physiologic and psychological support such as comfort measures after surgery, and caring for a child in cardiac failure. An equally important role is teaching prevention of heart disease such as promoting nonsmoking and exercise, maintaining appropriate weight, and eating a low-fat diet.

Outcome Evaluation

Outcome evaluation should include both immediate and future outcomes for the child and family because cardiac disorders may be long term. Important short-term outcomes involve receiving adequate support during procedures and treatment. If long-term care becomes necessary, evaluating the family's ability to think of their child not in terms of illness, but in terms of wellness and providing opportunities for parents to express their concerns about their child's status are important.

Examples suggesting achievement of outcomes are:

- The child's heart rate remains within accepted parameters for age.
- The child demonstrates age-appropriate coping skills related to diagnosis and possible surgery.
- The parents demonstrate competence with procedures required for care of their child.
- The parents exhibit positive coping skills related to their child's diagnosis and required care to foster optimal growth and development in their child.
- The parents verbalize positive aspects about their child.

THE CARDIOVASCULAR SYSTEM

Embryologic development of the heart is described in Chapter 9; cardiac adaptations at birth are described in Chapter 18. After these birth adaptations, the heart can be thought of as consisting of two pumps: one on the right side that pumps blood to the lungs, where it is oxygenated before returning to the left side of the heart, and one on the left side that moves the oxygenated blood to peripheral tissues through systemic arteries. After supplying nutrients and collecting wastes, the blood returns through the veins to the right side of the heart, where the cycle begins again (Fig. 41.1). Contraction of the heart chambers is termed **systole**; relaxation is termed **diastole**.

Most heart disease in children occurs because the heart formed inappropriately in utero or the embryonic structures necessary for fetal life such as the ductus arteriosus did not close at birth. Because pressure and volume on the left side of the heart are greater than on the right side, when there is connection between the left and right heart chambers, unoxygenated blood will flow through the connecting opening (from the left side to the right side) and mix with oxygenated blood, or flow from the area of stronger heart action to the area of weaker heart action.

Cardiac output is the volume of blood pumped by the ventricles each minute. It is affected by three main factors: **preload** (the volume of blood in the ventricles at the end of

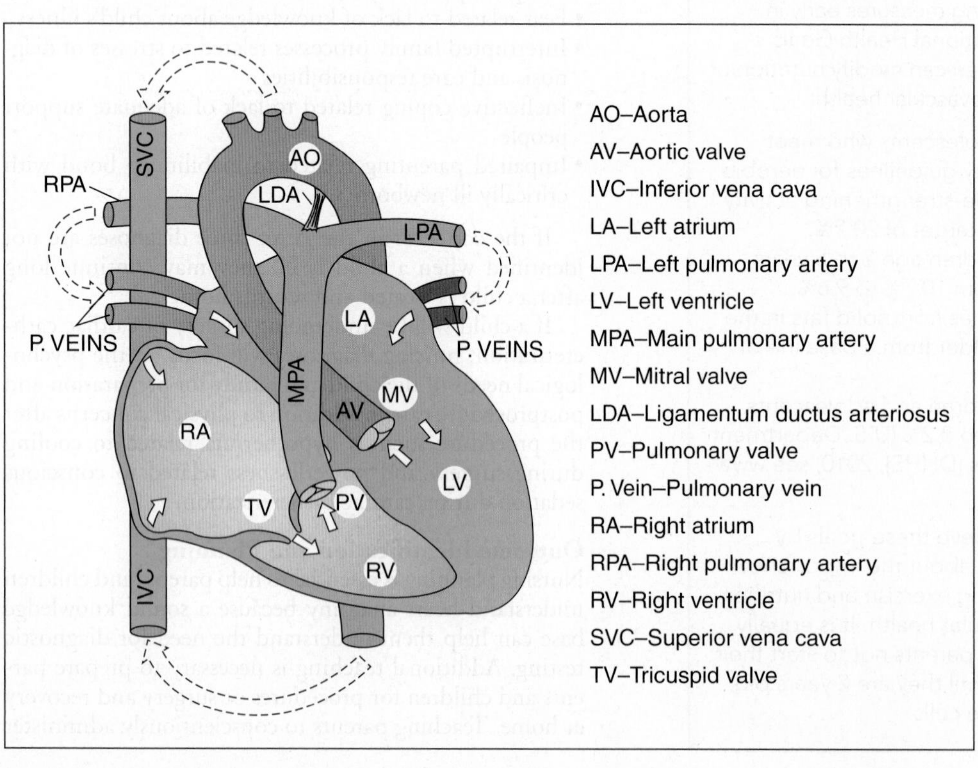

FIGURE 41.1 Anatomy of the normal heart.

diastole or the point just before contraction), **contractility** (or the ability of the ventricles to stretch), and **afterload** (the resistance against which the ventricles must pump). Much of the therapy of heart disease is aimed at reducing preload and afterload and increasing contractility to promote better cardiac output.

ASSESSMENT OF HEART DISORDERS IN CHILDREN

Because all children with heart disorders have an increased risk of poor tissue perfusion, which may affect growth and development, developmental and physical testing is incorporated into assessment.

History

A family history is important for assessment because some congenital heart disorders, such as atrial septal defects (ASDs), may have a polygenic inheritance pattern. Because the heart arises from the same embryonic origin as the kidney, heart disorders often occur in conjunction with renal disease. Heart disorders also occur as an anomaly in chromosomal disorders such as Down syndrome.

As a result of technologic advances in prenatal care, such as prenatal ultrasound, which can show poor heart action or an enlarged heart, heart disease may be recognized as early as fetal life. In the newborn period, because the newborn heart rate is so rapid, the extra sounds of abnormal circulation can be difficult to hear, so heart disease may not be detected until about 2 weeks after birth. Heart disease may first be detected when the infant who is breathing rapidly because of tachycardia and tachypnea has to stop sucking on a bottle or breast frequently to breathe or to rest.

Be certain a history includes a pregnancy history to try to determine whether an intrauterine insult such as toxoplasmosis, cytomegalovirus, or rubella infection could have led to poor fetal formation. Ask also whether the mother took any medication during pregnancy, whether nutrition was adequate, or whether she was exposed to any radiation, because these may also contribute to congenital heart disorders.

A mark of older children with heart disease is that they notice easy fatigue. Ask how much activity it takes before a child feels tired: an hour of strenuous play or a short walk? Be sure parents are not confusing sedentary activities (the child who prefers to sit and read) with activities that are the result of fatigue such as coming home from school and falling asleep day after day.

Infants who have difficulty oxygenating blood tend to assume a knee–chest position, whereas older children often voluntarily squat; these positions trap blood in the lower extremities because of the sharp bend at the knee and hip, allowing the child to oxygenate the blood remaining in the upper body more fully and easily. Also ask about frequency of infections, because children with heart disease have a higher incidence of lower respiratory tract infections than do other children, most likely due to less than usual pulmonary circulation. Ask about perspiration because children with left-to-right cardiac shunts may perspire excessively as a result of sympathetic nerve stimulation. They are able to effectively produce urine only when cardiac function is adequate to perfuse kidneys. To assess kidney output, evaluate how often an infant wets diapers or an older child voids. Edema from retained fluid that cannot be voided is a late sign of heart disease in children. If it does occur, periorbital edema (swelling around the eyes) generally occurs first.

Cyanosis (a blue tinge to the skin) will occur if a shunt is allowing deoxygenated blood to enter the arterial system. Such infants also generally fail to thrive or look light in weight. Children with coarctation of the aorta, discussed later in the chapter, will have nosebleeds and headaches from high blood pressure in the head and upper extremities. Because of corresponding low blood pressure in the lower extremities, the child may report pain in the legs on running (often described by parents as "growing pains").

Physical Assessment

Physical assessment of a child with a suspected heart disorder begins with measuring height and weight and plotting these findings on a standard growth chart. A thorough physical examination should then be done, with particular emphasis on certain body parts or systems (Box 41.2).

Because a major part of the physical assessment will include inspection, palpation, and auscultation of the chest for heart function, it is best if a child is relaxed and not

BOX 41.2 Nursing Care Planning Using Assessment

Assessing a Child With a Cardiovascular Disorder

History

Chief concern: Fatigue, cyanosis, frequent upper respiratory infections, feeding difficulty, poor weight gain, growth failure.

Past medical history: Infection during pregnancy, difficulty with resuscitation at birth.

Family history: Other members with heart disorders.

Physical examination

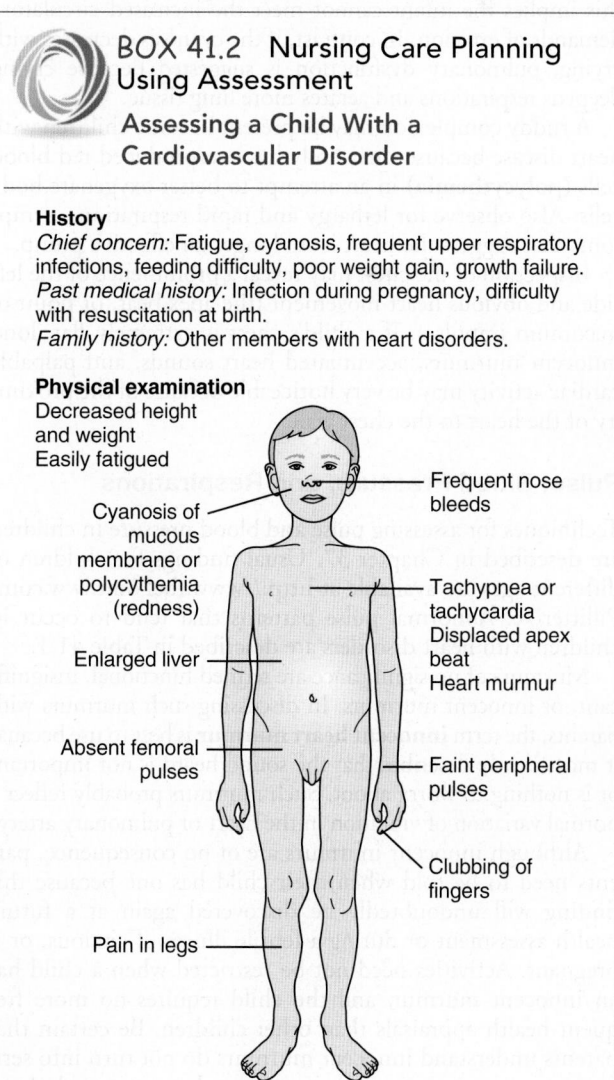

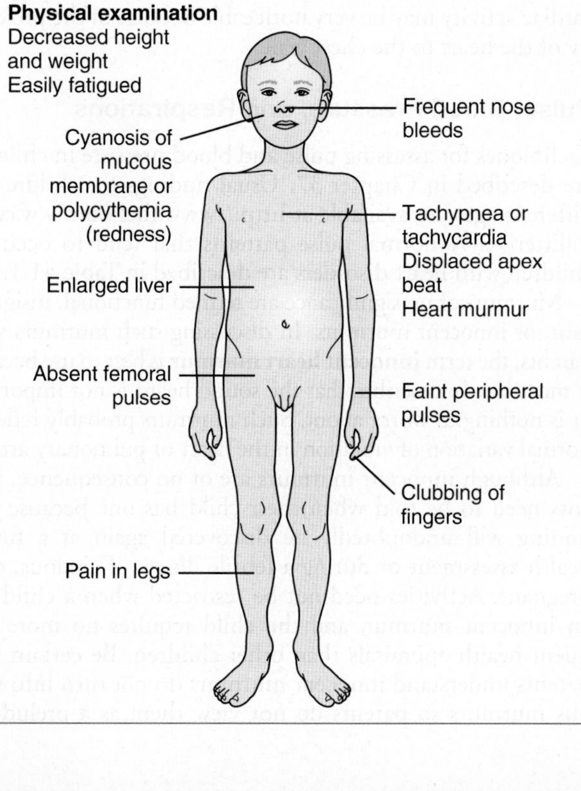

crying. Play with both children and infants if possible before an examination so they are acquainted and not afraid of you. Provide age-appropriate toys to distract a child as necessary. Often, a bottle of formula or breast milk (or ask the mother to breastfeed) can help comfort an infant enough that you can effectively listen to his or her heart.

General Appearance

Be certain to inspect toes and fingers (particularly the thumbs) for clubbing and color and measure capillary refill time by applying slight pressure on a fingernail and then quickly releasing, because these are indications of poor blood perfusion. When pressure is applied to a fingernail or toenail, it will blanch white and then quickly return to pink in a child with good circulation and oxygenation. In a child with poor tissue perfusion, the pink color returns slowly (more than 5 seconds).

The mucous membranes of the mouth are the most likely place for cyanosis to be visible, so always assess the buccal membrane and lips for a blue color, although any time hemoglobin is reduced below 4 to 6 g/100 ml, cyanosis may not be evident because the severe anemia masks it. At birth, if cyanosis persists over 20 minutes (except for acrocyanosis), this suggests serious cardiopulmonary dysfunction. As a general rule, if cyanosis increases with crying, cardiac dysfunction is suggested, because this implies the infant cannot meet the increased circulatory demands of exertion. In contrast, if the cyanosis decreases with crying, pulmonary dysfunction is suggested because crying deepens respirations and aerates more lung tissue.

A ruddy complexion may be present in some children with heart disease because their body has overproduced red blood cells **(polycythemia)** in an attempt to better oxygenate body cells. Also observe for lethargy and rapid respirations, symptoms that suggest the heart is no longer an effective pump.

Inspection of the chest may reveal a prominence of the left side and obvious heart movement (the apex beat, or point of maximum impulse). If a child's chest is extremely flat, loud innocent murmurs, accentuated heart sounds, and palpable cardiac activity may be very noticeable because of the proximity of the heart to the chest wall.

Pulse, Blood Pressure, and Respirations

Techniques for assessing pulse and blood pressure in children are described in Chapter 37. Usual findings for children of different ages are available at http://www.thePoint.lww.com/Pillitteri7e. Abnormal pulse patterns that tend to occur in children with heart disorders are described in Table 41.1.

Murmurs of no significance are termed functional, insignificant, or innocent murmurs. In discussing such murmurs with parents, the term **innocent heart murmur** is best to use because it most clearly describes that the sound heard is not important or is nothing to worry about. Such murmurs probably reflect a normal variation of vibration in the heart or pulmonary artery.

Although innocent murmurs are of no consequence, parents need to be told when their child has one because this finding will undoubtedly be discovered again at a future health assessment or during a febrile illness, if anxious, or if pregnant. Activities need not be restricted when a child has an innocent murmur, and the child requires no more frequent health appraisals than other children. Be certain that parents understand innocent murmurs do not turn into serious murmurs so parents do not view them as a prelude to heart disease. At future health assessments, parents may need to be reassured again that a murmur is innocent.

If a murmur is present as the result of heart disease or a congenital disorder, it is an **organic heart murmur**. The characteristics of innocent and organic murmurs are compared in Table 41.2.

To help differentiate innocent from organic murmurs, describe any murmur that you hear on physical assessment according to:

- Its position in the cardiac cycle, that is, early systolic, midsystolic, late diastolic, etc.
- Duration (how long the sound lasts in seconds)
- Quality (blowing, rasping, rumbling)
- Pitch (high- or low-sounding noise)
- Intensity (loudness)
- Location (where it is heard best or the point of maximum intensity)
- Presence of a thrill (a palpable purring sensation)
- The response of the murmur to exercise or change of position

TABLE 41.1 Abnormal Pulse Patterns

Pulse Pattern	Description
Tachycardia	Tachycardia in children is typically defined as a pulse rate of more than 160 beats/min in an infant and more than 100 beats/min at 3 years of age or older. Tachycardia is particularly significant if it persists during sleep, when the possibility of excitement and activity is removed.
Water hammer pulse	Very forceful and bounding pulse (Corrigan's pulse); capillary pulsations possibly apparent even in the fingernails; suggestive of cardiac insufficiency, as in patent ductus arteriosus
Pulsus alternans	A pulse of one strong beat and one weak beat; suggestive of myocardial weakness
Dicrotic pulse	A double radial pulse for every apical beat; symptomatic of aortic stenosis
Thready pulse	Weak and usually rapid pulse; suggestive of ineffective heart action

TABLE 41.2 Comparison of Innocent and Organic Murmurs

Characteristic	Innocent	Organic
Timing	Systolic	Systolic or diastolic
Duration	Short	Longer
Quality	Soft, musical	Harsh, blowing
Intensity	Soft	Loud
Position in which heard	Usually supine position	Heard in all positions

The intensity, or loudness, of the murmur is graded according to standard criteria shown in Table 34.6, Chapter 34.

What if... 41.1 You notice that Megan, who has tetralogy of Fallot, at 2 months old always draws her knees up tightly against her chest. Would you allow her to do this or urge her to leave her legs straight to prevent stasis of blood flow and help prevent thrombophlebitis?

Diagnostic Tests

The diagnostic studies performed on a child with suspected heart disease vary with the specific anomaly suspected.

Electrocardiogram

An *electrocardiogram* (ECG) is a written record of the electrical voltages generated by the contracting heart and provides information about heart rate, rhythm, state of the myocardium, presence or absence of hypertrophy (thickening of the heart walls), ischemia or necrosis due to inadequate cardiac circulation, abnormalities of conduction, or the effect of various drugs and electrolyte imbalances on the heart.

A heartbeat is initiated by the sinoatrial (SA) node in the right atrial wall near the entrance of the superior vena cava. From the SA node, the electrical impulse spreads over the atria, reaching the atrioventricular (AV) node in the lower right atrium. From there, it spreads through the AV bundle (bundle of His) and the Purkinje fibers to the walls and septum of the ventricles. At the point that the ventricles have filled, the electrical flow reaches a peak and ventricles contract.

A usual ECG wave form consists of an atrial wave (the P wave, denoting atrial contraction), a brief hesitation before the AV node is activated, then a prominent peak as the ventricles contract (the QRS spike), another brief hesitation, and then a large slow wave caused by ventricular recovery (the T wave). Some children may have an incompletely understood additional slow wave (the U wave; Fig. 41.2). On the tracing, a longer than usual P wave suggests the atria are hypertrophied, making it take longer than usual for the electrical conduction to spread over the atria. A lengthened P-R interval suggests there is a difficulty with coordination between the SA and AV nodes (first-degree heart block). A heightened R wave indicates ventricular hypertrophy is present. An R wave that is decreased in height suggests the ventricles are not contracting fully, as happens if they are surrounded by fluid (pericarditis). Elongation of the T wave occurs in hyperkalemia; depression of the T wave is associated with anoxia; depression of the ST segment is associated with abnormal calcium levels.

QSEN Checkpoint Question 41.1

Informatics

Megan has been diagnosed as having tetralogy of Fallot, a congenital heart disorder. With this disorder, the right ventricle tends to become distended because extra blood flows into it across a septal wall defect. Which pattern on an ECG would let you know ventricular hypertrophy has occurred?

a. A long, slow P wave
b. An elongated T wave
c. A high and wide R wave
d. A flat but wide P-R interval

Look in Appendix A for the best answer and rationale.

X-Ray Studies

X-ray examination can furnish an accurate picture of the heart size and suggest the contour and size of the heart chambers as well as whether fluid is collecting in the lungs or pulmonary artery from poor heart function. X-ray is also frequently used to confirm the placement of pacemaker leads.

Fluoroscopy is a form of X-ray that provides a motion-picture record of the size and configuration of the heart, great vessels, lungs, thoracic cage, and diaphragm. Because prolonged observation is necessary to record this information, special precautions must be taken to protect a child and health care personnel from radiation during the assessment.

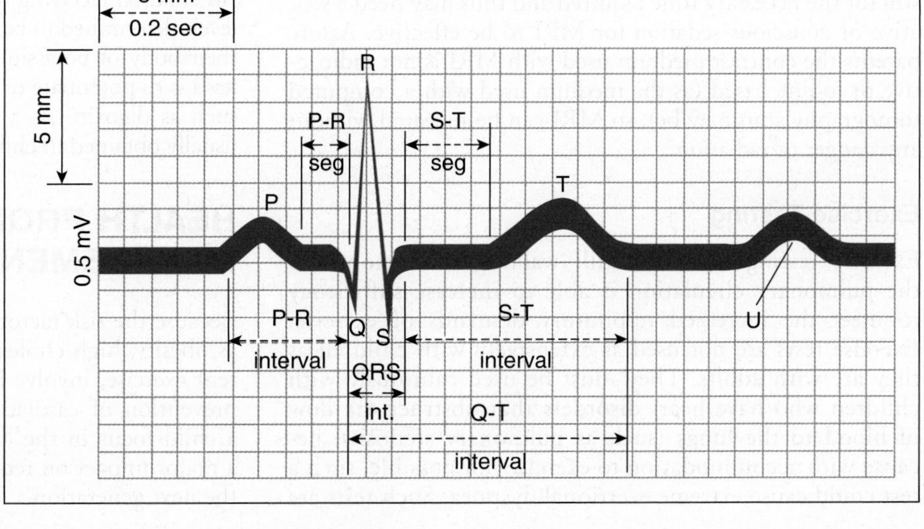

FIGURE 41.2 A normal ECG configuration.

In radioangiocardiography, a radioactive substance such as technetium is injected intravenously into the bloodstream. As the substance circulates through the heart, it can be traced and recorded on video to demonstrate, in particular, septal shunts.

Echocardiography

Echocardiography, or ultrasound cardiography, has become the primary diagnostic test for congenital heart disease (Bharucha & Mertens, 2013). For this, high-frequency sound waves, directed toward the heart, are used to locate and study the movement and dimensions of cardiac structures, such as the size of chambers; thickness of walls; relationship of major vessels to chambers; and the thickness, motion, and pressure gradients of valves. The technique is referred to as M-mode when a single beam is used to reveal chamber contractility; two-dimensional if it is used to reveal chamber and vessel size; and Doppler technique, which reveals the velocity of blood flow. You can remind parents that echocardiography does not use X-rays, so it can be repeated at frequent intervals without exposing their child to the possible risk of radiation. In some children, it may be done using a transesophageal probe to better reveal fetal heart chambers. Used during pregnancy, it can reveal heart anomalies as early as 18 weeks into a pregnancy, allowing health care personnel to be prepared with immediate resuscitation or other procedures at the baby's birth (Donofrio, Levy, Schuette, et al., 2013).

Phonocardiography and Magnetic Resonance Imaging

A *phonocardiogram* is a diagram of heart sounds translated into electrical energy by a microphone placed on the child's chest and then recorded as a diagrammatic representation of heart sounds. The technique can measure the timing of heart sounds that occur too quickly or at too high or too low a sound frequency for the human ear to detect by direct auscultation. Magnetic resonance imaging (MRI), using large magnets and radio-frequency waves, may be used in conjunction with a phonocardiogram to evaluate heart structure or blood flow to account for the recorded sounds (Meziani, Debbal, & Atbi, 2012). Small children may be frightened by the size of an MRI machine and not able to lie still for the necessary time required and thus may need a sedative or conscious sedation for MRI to be effective. Assure parents the contrast medium used with MRI is not radioactive or iodine based (as the medium used with a computed tomography scan may be), so MRI can be repeated without any danger of radiation.

Exercise Testing

Exercise testing uses treadmill walking to demonstrate the pulmonary circulation is able to increase sufficiency to meet the increased respiratory demands of exercise. Exercise tests are not used as extensively with children as they are with adults. They must be used cautiously with children who have heart disorders that obstruct the flow of blood to the lungs (such as pulmonary stenosis), because with accommodation to exercise not possible, such a test could cause extreme exertional dyspnea. Such tests are difficult to perform successfully with young children because they require the child's cooperation (Kyle, Macicek, Lindle, et al., 2012).

Laboratory Tests

Children with heart disease usually undergo a number of blood serum tests to support the diagnosis of heart disease or to rule out anemia or clotting disorders. Hematocrit or hemoglobin studies are usually obtained to assess the rate of erythrocyte production, which may increase in an attempt to produce more oxygen-carrying red blood cells. If the increase in the number of red blood cells is extreme (polycythemia), there will be a corresponding increase in blood volume and possibly an increase in blood viscosity. Newborns are normally slightly polycythemic, so in newborns, polycythemia is typically defined as a hemoglobin level over 25 g/100 ml or a hematocrit level over 70%. In an older child, polycythemia is defined as a hemoglobin level over 16 g/100 ml or a hematocrit level over 55%. An erythrocyte sedimentation rate (ESR) is an additional test that may be prescribed because an elevated ESR level denotes inflammation or documents that an inflammatory process, such as occurs with rheumatic fever, Kawasaki syndrome, or myocarditis, is present (Xiu-Yu, Jia-Yu, Qiang, et al., 2010).

Blood gas levels also are determined. To test for this, a child is given 100% oxygen for about 15 minutes. If the child still has a partial pressure of oxygen (Po_2) less than 150 mmHg after this time, a shunt directing deoxygenated blood into oxygenated blood can be suspected. Oxygen saturation levels also are assessed using pulse oximetry; children with a deoxygenated to oxygenated shunt will have a lower than normal oxygen saturation level (below 92% compared to a usual level of 95% to 98%).

Before cardiac catheterization or cardiac surgery, blood clotting must be assessed so prothrombin time, partial thromboplastin time, and platelet count will be completed before the procedure. Some children with polycythemia from heart disease have an associated reduced platelet count (thrombocytopenia). Because platelet formation is necessary for blood coagulation after surgery, such children may have this corrected before cardiac surgery with a platelet infusion.

In children with congestive heart failure (CHF) who have obvious edema, a serum sodium level may be obtained to ensure an increased sodium level is not adding to the edema formation. All children receiving diuretics typically have serum potassium levels determined to be certain diuretic therapy is not depleting their body of potassium. An effect of a low serum potassium level is to potentiate or increase the effect of cardiac glycosides, such as digoxin. As a result, serum potassium levels are also usually obtained in children receiving these medications.

HEALTH PROMOTION AND RISK MANAGEMENT

Because the risk factors that lead to adult heart disease, such as obesity, high cholesterol serum levels, and lack of consistent exercise, involve health habits that begin in childhood, prevention of cardiac disease has shifted from an adult to a child focus in the hope that early interventions will have a major impact on reducing the incidence of heart disease in the next generation.

Risk Management for Congenital Heart Disease

The cause of congenital heart disease often cannot be documented, although it is associated with familial patterns of inheritance and possibly triggers such as rubella (German measles) and varicella (chickenpox) infection during pregnancy. Women need to enter pregnancy fully immunized to help prevent infection during pregnancy. Parents who have a family member born with a heart disorder need to be aware that other children born to them need to be carefully screened prenatally and at birth for a similar disorder.

Risk Management for Acquired Heart Disease

Acquired heart diseases in children that have identified risk factors include rheumatic fever, hypertension, and hyperlipidemia. Rheumatic fever is an autoimmune response that follows a group A beta-hemolytic streptococcal infection. Ensuring that all children who have a streptococcal infection such as streptococcal pharyngitis or impetigo receive adequate antibiotic therapy is essential in preventing the complication of rheumatic fever (Altamimi, Khalil, Khalaiwi, et al., 2012).

Although hypertension (elevated blood pressure) is associated with a genetic predisposition, a high intake of sodium (such as table salt), lack of exercise, and obesity increase the chances a susceptible child will develop the disorder by late childhood (Underwood, Averhart, Dean, et al., 2012). If infants are never introduced to high-sodium foods, perhaps by the time they are selecting their own meals, they will continue to eat a low-sodium diet, helping to prevent the development of hypertension in later life. For this reason, baby food manufacturers have stopped adding salt and monosodium glutamate to infant food. Urging school-age children and adolescents to reduce their intake of canned soups, cheese, lunch meats, and hot dogs, all foods with high sodium contents, can reduce salt intake in these age groups. School nurses can play an important role in this effort by monitoring the foods served daily in school cafeterias and advocating for more nutritious menus. Beginning when a child is 3 years of age, blood pressure should be included as part of routine assessment to detect as early as possible whether hypertension is developing (American Academy of Pediatrics [AAP], 2012).

Although the tendency toward hyperlipidemia is also inherited, a diet high in saturated fat has been implicated in the development of the syndrome. It is important that fat intake not be restricted in infants because they need fat and the calories it provides for neuro growth. School-age children and adolescents, however, should reduce their fat intake to 30% of total calories (the same recommendation as for adults). Children from high-risk families (a family member has had an early myocardial infarction or hyperlipidemia prior to the age of 50 years) should be regularly screened for elevated cholesterol and triglyceride levels beginning at about 3 years of age at health care visits. Children with low-density lipoprotein (LDL) levels greater than 130 mg/dl on two successive tests should receive nutritional counseling and instruction about a regular exercise program to enhance their health (AAP, 2012).

NURSING CARE OF THE CHILD WITH A CARDIAC DISORDER

Most parents have many questions about how to care for a child born with heart disease. Encourage them to learn as much as possible about their child's disorder and give care to their newborn in the hospital so they can feel more secure in caring for the infant at home. Be certain parents are aware that not all children with heart disease have the same disease or need the same degree of activity or intake restriction so parents do not unnecessarily limit their infant's activities or types of food. Caring for an older child who develops a heart disease is equally intimidating. Offer support at health care visits to help parents feel confident they know the child's medication regimen and any signs or symptoms they should report immediately to the child's primary health care provider.

Nursing Diagnoses and Related Interventions

Nursing diagnoses for children with cardiac disease need to address both physical and psychosocial care.

Nursing Diagnosis: Parental health-seeking behaviors related to desire to be informed about child's cardiac disorder

Outcome Evaluation: Parents accurately state the nature of their child's illness and unique needs of their child; parents state they will telephone or e-mail the child's primary health care provider if they have any questions or concerns.

Provide or Review Information About Care. Parents generally ask questions such as, "Is it safe to let a baby with heart disease cry?" The answer, of course, depends on the individual child's condition. If the infant has a cardiac disorder such as tetralogy of Fallot in which hypercyanotic episodes tend to develop, the baby should not be allowed to cry for long periods of time (no baby should). However, crying for a few minutes while a parent warms formula or fully awakens at night to breastfeed will, as a rule, not harm the baby.

Another common question is, "Does our child need special nutrition?" As with all newborns, breastfeeding is the preferred method of feeding, and the average infant with heart disease can be successful at this. Because anemia stresses the heart, infants may be prescribed an iron or iron and vitamin supplement to prevent iron deficiency anemia during the first year. Because some infants with congenital heart disease tire readily, frequent small feedings during the day are usually taken better than three large meals. If a child is an extremely poor eater, a high-calorie formula (24 calories per ounce) or enteral or gastrostomy feedings may be necessary to supply enough calories for growth.

"How much activity can we allow the baby?" is a third question that is often asked. Again, the answer to this depends on the type and extent of the heart disorder, but, as a rule, infants or young children naturally limit their own activity or stop exercising when they are fatigued. Parents may need some guidance, however, in knowing when to set sensible limits. Playing a game such as chasing a ball or roughhousing with siblings, for example, may not be advisable. Encourage parents to observe their infant carefully, especially when new activities are introduced, so they can recognize the first signs of respiratory distress or the point at which the child is beginning to exceed exercise tolerance.

Although children with congenital heart disorders are usually followed by a cardiologist for health supervision, it's important they are also followed by health care personnel for routine care so they receive usual childhood immunizations and health guidance. As a rule, parents need to bring infants with heart disorders for prompt treatment for minor illnesses, especially upper respiratory infections as the fever that can accompany a common cold can increase the metabolic rate of a child who has a severe congenital heart disorder to beyond the point at which the child's heart can compensate. Hydration must be monitored so dehydration does not occur in children with polycythemia so the polycythemia does not become so severe that clotting or thrombophlebitis results.

Remind parents that children with many types of congenital heart disorders or rheumatic fever need prophylactic low-dose aspirin therapy to avoid blood clotting; although becoming a controversial practice, they may be prescribed antibiotic therapy such as oral amoxicillin before oral surgery (tooth extractions or tonsils removed) to prevent streptococcal organisms, generally present in the mouth, from leading to infectious endocarditis if the organisms enter the bloodstream during surgery (Dinsbach, 2012).

Children with congenital heart disorders should receive routine immunizations and influenza vaccines and should be considered as candidates for the pneumonia vaccine.

Review Steps for Follow-Up Care and Emergencies. Before parents leave the hospital with a newborn who has a congenital heart disorder, be certain they have the name and number of the health care professional to call if they have a question about their infant's health. Review with them the steps to take if their child should become cyanotic, such as placing the child in a knee–chest position. Be certain they also have an appointment for a first health assessment so they can feel assured that the responsibility of caring for this child will not be theirs alone but will be shared by concerned health care personnel (Marino, Lipkin, Newburger, et al., 2012). If they become unsure of whether their child is in distress or ill, urge them to err on the side of caution by telephoning or bringing the child to their primary care setting, because everyone who cares for infants or children with heart disease appreciates the responsibility parents feel and the difficulty they can have in making health judgments about their child.

Teach parents cardiopulmonary resuscitation (CPR) (discussed later in the chapter) before they leave the hospital so they appreciate that "hands on" CPR is not recommended for children as it is for adults (American Heart Association [AHA], 2010).

The Child Having a Cardiac Catheterization

Cardiac catheterization, a procedure in which a small radiopaque catheter is passed through a major vein in the arm, leg, or neck into the heart to secure blood samples or inject dye, is a major method used to evaluate cardiac function (Schneider, 2011). *Diagnostic* cardiac catheterization is used to diagnose specific heart disorders in anticipation of surgery. *Interventional* cardiac catheterization is used to correct an abnormality, such as dilating a narrowed valve by the use of a balloon catheter or other device. With both types, the pressure of blood flow in all heart chambers and total cardiac output can be evaluated. Blood specimens can be obtained to determine oxygen saturation levels, or a contrast medium can be injected for angiography or magnetic resonance scanning. Electrodes can be introduced to record electrical activity and diagnose arrhythmias.

This procedure is usually completed as ambulatory or 1-day surgery using conscious sedation. Children have a chest X-ray, ECG, serum electrolyte analysis, and blood typed and crossmatched before the procedure. Be certain to measure and record height and weight because this information is used to determine catheter size and the amount of sedation to be administered. Also record pedal pulses are present because this measurement will be repeated afterward to ensure the blood vessel chosen for catheterization is functioning well. Because the vessel site chosen for catheterization must not be infected at the time of catheterization (or obscured by a hematoma), never draw blood specimens from the projected catheterization entry site before the procedure (generally a femoral vein). Children scheduled for the procedure are usually kept nothing by mouth (NPO) for 2 to 4 hours beforehand to reduce the danger of vomiting and aspiration during the procedure.

In the cardiac catheterization room, after the child is sedated, ECG and pulse oximetry leads are attached. The site for catheter insertion is locally anesthetized with a eutectic mixture of local anesthetics (EMLA) cream or intradermal lidocaine, and a catheter is threaded through a large-bore needle into a blood vessel. The specific vessel used differs according to the technique being planned. In neonates, an umbilical artery may be catheterized. For right-side heart catheterization, a right femoral vein or a vein in the antecubital fossa usually is used. Left-side heart catheterization can be performed using either a venous or an arterial approach. If done by the arterial route, a catheter is inserted into either the femoral or brachial artery. If a venous route is used, the catheter is inserted into the right femoral vein. Under fluoroscopy, the catheter is advanced to the right atrium and then

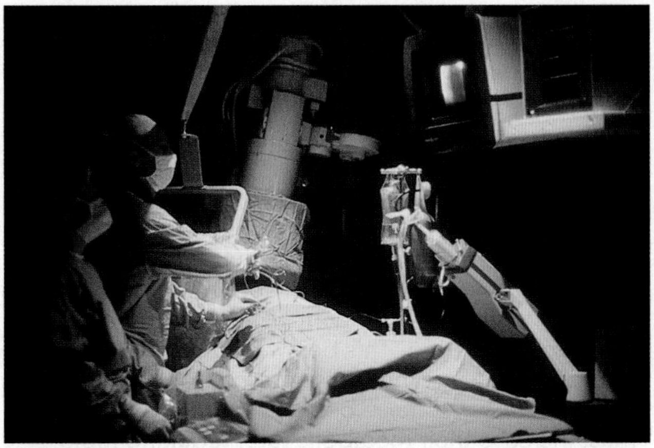

FIGURE 41.3 A child undergoing a cardiac catheterization. (© Hough/Custom Medical Stock Photograph.)

through the foramen ovale. Once the catheter is in a selected heart chamber, a contrast medium can be injected to outline the heart configuration on X-ray or MRI (Fig. 41.3).

Cardiac catheterization has a low mortality rate, less than 0.1% when done as an elective procedure and approximately 2% to 5% when performed in a severely distressed child (Kern & King, 2013). Arrhythmias may occur while the catheter is being passed through the heart chambers or when the contrast medium is introduced. Such arrhythmias generally are transitory or stop abruptly with withdrawal of the catheter. Other complications that may occur are inadvertent perforation of the heart, bleeding from the insertion site (secondary to heparin introduced into the catheter to reduce the possibility of clot formation), and thrombophlebitis (from platelet aggregation due to irritation by the catheter). However, because cardiac catheterization may be necessary so a surgeon can visualize and plan a cardiac repair, it's generally agreed that the benefits of the procedure outweigh these risks.

Nursing Diagnoses and Related Interventions: Preprocedure Phase

Cardiac catheterization is a stress-filled procedure for parents because its outcome will dictate whether their child's heart can be successfully repaired.

Nursing Diagnosis: Anxiety related to possible outcome of cardiac catheterization procedure.

Outcome Evaluation: Parents state goal of procedure and reasons for preparation and aftercare measures; parents state they are able to manage anxiety while waiting for results.

Because most cardiac catheterizations are done with children under conscious sedation, children may need more information about what is going to happen during this procedure than they will need for cardiac surgery, when they will be fully anesthetized. Both parents and children may need a review of heart anatomy before they can appreciate the path of the catheter.

Try and provide an explanation of the procedure to the child with the parents present, if possible, so parents can reinforce the information as needed. After this explanation, provide parents with a more detailed explanation if they want one, allowing time for questions they do not want to ask in the child's presence.

Be aware that consenting to a cardiac catheterization brings with it the realization that cardiac surgery may be necessary. As a result, parents may be so concerned with what the procedure may reveal that they have difficulty listening well to preprocedure explanations. To reduce the child's anxiety, allow parents to accompany their child to the catheterization room and, if possible and appropriate, remain there for support until the child is sedated.

Older children enjoy a tour of the cardiac catheterization area and the opportunity to meet the personnel. For small children, because they can become overwhelmed by seeing the actual room, try building a facsimile room out of small cardboard boxes (representing the X-ray machine, the fluoroscopy screen, the ECG machine, and so forth) with a puppet or small doll as the patient. Dress other puppets in surgery suits and masks and have them act out what the child can expect to happen.

If children have never seen ECG leads or restraints before, let them touch and feel them. Caution them that the total procedure may be as long as 3 to 4 hours and that they will need to lie still during this time. Help them master imagery or another stress-reduction technique to help reduce apprehension while waiting for the procedure.

Do not underestimate what children know about their heart's purpose and function; even preschoolers know their heart is vital to their body. Reassure them, therefore, that people are only taking a look at their heart during this procedure, not cutting it or removing any part of it, assuming that is true.

Caution children that the lights will be turned off in the room so people can see the fluoroscopy (TV) screen better. Assure them that when the catheter is inserted, it won't hurt. They may, however, feel a momentary uncomfortable rapid beating of their heart. When the contrast medium is injected, they may feel a stinging sensation. Do not say that "dye" will be injected because young children can misinterpret that as "die." Instead, say "medicine" or "medium." Let children know that after the procedure, a pressure dressing will be placed over the catheter insertion site to reduce the risk of bleeding. They will need to keep that extremity flat and unbent to prevent the dressing from loosening.

Nursing Diagnoses and Related Interventions: Postprocedure Phase

Nursing Diagnosis: Risk for ineffective cardiopulmonary and peripheral tissue perfusion related to cardiac catheterization

Outcome Evaluation: Child's vital signs remain within established parameters; there is absence of arrhythmia; absence of bleeding or hematoma formation at catheter insertion site; pulse present distal to catheter insertion site.

When a child returns from the procedure, assess the pressure dressing over the catheter insertion site to be certain the dressing is snug and intact and no bleeding is present. Assess the site every 5 minutes for the first 15 minutes, every 15 minutes for 1 hour, then hourly to verify that there is no bleeding. Instruct the child not to bend the hip (if the femoral site was used) or the elbow (if the brachial site was used) to keep the pressure dressing secure and to prevent hematoma formation. This is particularly important when an artery was used for catheterization because a loose dressing on an artery can cause a large blood loss in a very short time. If there is bleeding at the insertion site, apply firm, continuous pressure and notify the care provider who performed the procedure immediately.

Because cardiac arrhythmias and bradycardia may occur from the mechanical action of the catheter having touched the conduction nodes of the heart, assess pulse, color, and circulation (blanch the toe- or fingernail on the leg or arm that was used for catheter insertion and watch to see that it turns pink again readily) at frequent intervals (about every 15 minutes) for the first several hours to help detect whether arrhythmias or obstruction is occurring. In the immediate postcatheterization period, a child's blood pressure may be 10% to 15% lower than the precatheterization level because of the hypotensive effect of the contrast medium. Keep the child flat in bed for 4 to 6 hours until the child is completely awake from conscious sedation to help both oozing at the insertion site and postural hypotension, which can occur when a child rises suddenly after lying flat while under sedation.

Be alert for other signs of arrhythmias, such as older children describing their heart as "fluttering" or "skipping beats." Small children cannot describe the odd feeling that accompanies an arrhythmia. Be alert, therefore, for signs of increasing anxiety in children because this may be the child's only way of reporting these feelings. Counting the pulse for a full minute also helps detect irregular beats.

Infants need intravenous (IV) fluid during the procedure and for several hours afterward to prevent dehydration, which could result from being NPO for a long period of time. If an infant is polycythemic, IV fluid also helps minimize the risk of vessel thrombi. Regulate IV fluid carefully to prevent CHF that could occur from fluid overload.

As a final assessment, take a temperature immediately after the procedure to determine a baseline. Some children will have a transient elevation in temperature due to physiologic dehydration as a result of having been NPO or as a reaction to the contrast medium. Others have slightly subnormal temperature because they were resting in a cool procedure room for a lengthy period. This below-normal body temperature quickly compromises respiratory and heart action because, to raise body temperature, infants must increase their metabolic rate, requiring rapid breathing and increased heart action, which can lead to exhaustion. Infants may need to be placed under radiant heat warmers to help regain and maintain normal body temperature.

Children often appreciate being asked to describe their experience afterward (debriefing). Saying out loud how frightened they were—by the X-ray machine being pushed in over them or by the thought of a tube going all the way into their heart—helps alleviate their fear and allows better acceptance of the procedure. Offer praise for their cooperation during a very stressful experience. Introduce therapeutic play if needed.

If oxygen was administered during the catheterization procedure, it may be continued for a period of time after the procedure to reduce the stress of respirations and help prevent apnea, sternal retractions, or dyspnea. Like arrhythmias, dyspnea, bradycardia, and blood pressure anomalies will be transient, but all should be reported so they can be evaluated.

Nursing Diagnosis: Risk for infection related to presence of cardiac catheterization incision site

Outcome Evaluation: The child's temperature remains less than 100.4°F (38.0°C) tympanic; the catheter insertion site appears free of erythema or drainage.

If the dressing for a cardiac catheterization is over the femoral artery or vein in a non–toilet-trained child, be certain to keep it clean of stool and urine. If necessary, waterproof the dressing with plastic to keep it dry. Alert parents to observe the catheter insertion site daily for redness and to monitor their child's temperature daily for about 3 days. They should omit tub baths and strenuous exercise for their child for 2 to 3 days to aid healing.

What if...41.2 Megan is scheduled for a cardiac catheterization. Why is it important to assess for cardiac arrhythmias and a pedal pulse on the leg where the catheter was inserted after this procedure?

The Child Scheduled for Cardiac Surgery

Open-heart or intracardiac catheterization surgery remains the chief cure for congenital heart disease. Because there are many different types of congenital heart disorders, there are many different procedures available to correct them. Open-heart surgery is made possible by the use of cardiopulmonary bypass or extracorporeal membrane oxygenation (ECMO). With this, the venous return to the heart is diverted from the right atrium or inferior and superior vena cava to a heart–lung machine, where it is artificially oxygenated. It is returned to the child's body's arterial system by way of the aorta, bypassing the heart. Because the heart is kept practically bloodless by the blood shunting, it then can be opened and repaired (Bernstein, 2012). Very ill infants may be maintained on ECMO before surgery or afterward using the same technique.

During surgery, hypothermia is used to reduce the child's body temperature to 68° to 79°F (20° to 26°C) in order to reduce the child's metabolic needs and slow the heart rate. If extreme hypothermia is used (59° to 68°F [15° to 20°C]), usually in an infant, the body temperature drops so low that the heart stops beating and the surgeon can then repair the heart in a quiet and bloodless field. Measuring temperature to be certain the infant is rewarmed is a major responsibility after surgery.

Preoperative Care

Before surgery, obtain vital signs (blood pressure, temperature, pulse, and respirations) to establish baselines; count pulse and respiratory rates for a full minute for accuracy. Some children may need baseline pulse determinations done at several pulse points or blood pressures taken in both upper and lower extremities. Before obtaining a blood pressure, have a child rest for about 15 minutes and take the recording with the child lying down so it closely mimics what the child's position will be following surgery. Also record height and weight because these parameters are necessary for the estimation of blood volume for the heart–lung machine as well as for medication dosages. Weight also is helpful to estimate blood loss or edema after surgery. In children receiving digoxin, it is usually withheld 24 hours before surgery because cardiac surgery may cause arrhythmias in the presence of cardiac glycosides.

An enema may be given to keep children from straining to pass stool and placing additional strain on the newly operated heart in the immediate postoperative period. Most children and parents are startled to learn that cardiac surgery may be performed through the sternal bone or the back, not over the left side of the chest, so they may question why one of those areas is being prepped for the incision.

Nursing Diagnoses and Related Interventions: Preoperative Phase

Nursing Diagnosis: Deficient knowledge related to cardiac surgery and its outcome

Outcome Evaluation: Parents and child accurately state the reason for surgery and expected outcome.

Bringing a child to the hospital and agreeing to cardiac surgery is a large responsibility for parents because although they want their child to be cured, they are also aware there is a definite risk from this surgery. As parents, they may have been protecting and guarding their child for months or years; they feel no less protective the morning of surgery. For this reason, parents of children being readied for cardiac surgery may watch preoperative procedures more carefully than usual. Parents usually appreciate a visit to the intensive care unit (ICU) before surgery. Be certain they have an opportunity to meet the ICU staff, especially if those nurses are not the same ones who are caring for the child preoperatively. Be certain to prepare them for the amount of equipment that will surround their child after surgery, such as a cardiac monitor, oxygen and IV equipment, chest tubes, and a ventilator (Fig. 41.4).

Prepare Child for Surgery and Postoperative Care. A good rule is to try and prepare the child for surgery with the parents present to allow parents the opportunity to reinforce your teaching. This also demonstrates to children that their parents approve and feel secure with these surgery plans. Because many children scheduled for cardiac surgery have already had a cardiac catheterization, talking to them about their previous hospitalization experience can be helpful to reveal things they are worrying about. Any misconceptions they have can then be discussed and clarified. Be certain to explain that anesthesia is a "special sleep" from which they will have no difficulty waking.

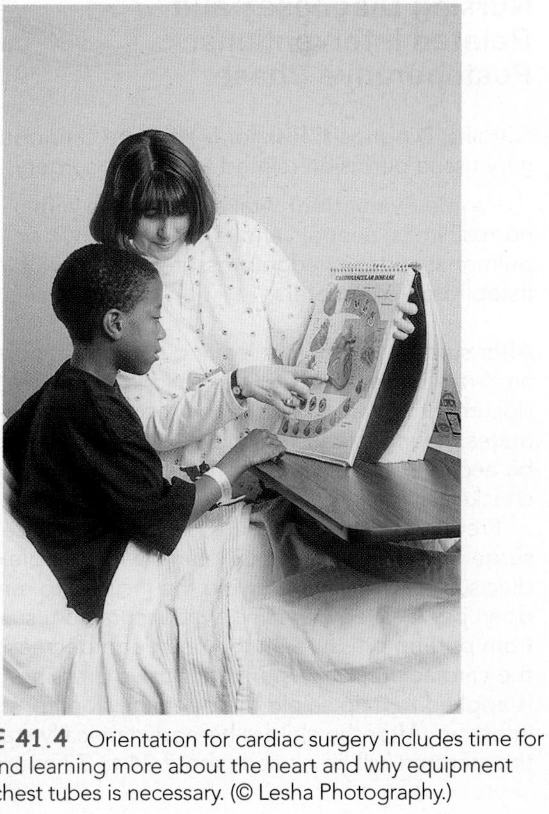

FIGURE 41.4 Orientation for cardiac surgery includes time for talking and learning more about the heart and why equipment such as chest tubes is necessary. (© Lesha Photography.)

Meeting the anesthesiologist and receiving reassurance directly from the person who will be watching over them while they are asleep is often helpful. After the child is fully prepared, ask parents if they need additional time to discuss the surgical procedure and ask questions they might not have wished to ask in front of their child.

When discussing postoperative care, parents and older children can be taken to the ICU where they will return after surgery and be shown the equipment that will surround them. For younger children, it may be helpful to make models of the equipment so it's not so overwhelming.

Because the child will need to cough and deep-breathe and use incentive spirometry to help the lungs expand after surgery, introduce these exercises and the idea of chest tubes and oxygen preoperatively so a child can learn that these will be expected. Caution both the child and parents that chest tubes must stay in place until it is time for them to be removed so if children want to turn over with tubes in place, they will need to ask for help to prevent the tubes from being dislodged. Caution parents also that the chest-tube drainage reservoir must remain below the level of the child's chest so collected fluid doesn't infuse back into the child. Comparing ECG leads to being "hooked up" like an astronaut is often appealing to children. Orienting children to oxygen equipment is discussed in Chapter 40.

Nursing Diagnoses and Related Interventions: Postoperative Phase

Nursing Diagnosis: Risk for ineffective cardiopulmonary tissue perfusion related to cardiac surgery

Outcome Evaluation: Vital signs remain within normal limits; central venous pressure (CVP) or pulmonary artery wedge pressure remains within established parameters.

After surgery and before leaving the operating room, an X-ray film is taken and the child is weighed to document the amount of blood loss. Future estimates of lung expansion and whether edema could be accumulating from poor heart function will be checked against these two measurements.

Frequently, sternal closure is delayed after cardiac surgery, especially on small infants with complex cardiac surgical repairs. Allowing the incision to remain open prevents any swelling that occurs from surgery from putting pressure on the heart and decreasing the cardiac output. A sterile occlusive dressing is applied to help shield the open incision from infection. After the child is hemodynamically stable, the sternum will be closed (about 24 to 72 hours) either in the ICU or the operating suite. The nursing care for the child with an open sternotomy includes the same diligent care as for all children who have had cardiac surgery plus extreme prevention of and monitoring for infection (Pye & McDonnell, 2010).

Taking accurate vital signs, as often as every 15 minutes, is essential in the immediate postoperative period. Continuous cardiac monitoring and assisted ventilation with endotracheal intubation also are usually necessary. Blood pressure will be monitored directly by means of an intra-arterial catheter or indirectly with an automated blood pressure recording device. Hemodynamic monitoring by way of a pulmonary artery or central venous catheter will reveal information on chamber pressures and oxygen saturation (Fig. 41.5).

Carefully monitor and record all IV fluid administered to the child because fluid overload can pose a severe threat to a recently repaired heart. If a child is voiding adequately after surgery, it indicates the kidneys are receiving an adequate blood flow or the heart is working effectively. An indwelling urinary (Foley) catheter, therefore, is inserted at the time of surgery so urine output can be carefully measured and recorded postoperatively (should be 1 ml/kg/hr). Be certain to mark the amount of urine drainage present when the child first returns from surgery so that lack of or diminished urinary output will not be missed or misinterpreted. Individual samples can then be removed and tested for specific gravity and pH as an additional assessment (a specific gravity below 1.010 implies the kidneys are not concentrating urine well, perhaps because of the overall stress of surgery). The pH should remain slightly acid; however, extreme acidity suggests respiratory acidosis from poor pulmonary perfusion.

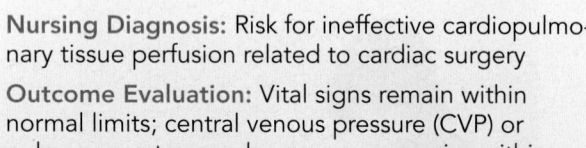

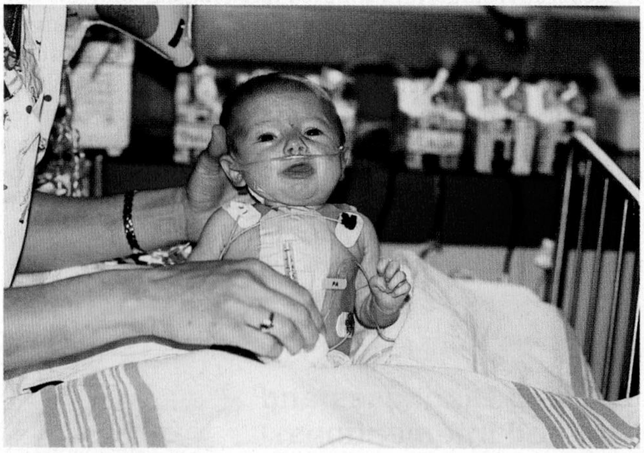

FIGURE 41.5 Because children after cardiac surgery typically have a myriad of wires and tubes attached to monitors, pumps, and equipment, parents need to be prepared for how their child will look. As the child's condition improves, use of the equipment is discontinued. Here, an infant is 2 days post-cardiac surgery. Note his level of alertness and the use of only a few monitoring devices and equipment. (© Caroline Brown, RNC, MS, DEd.)

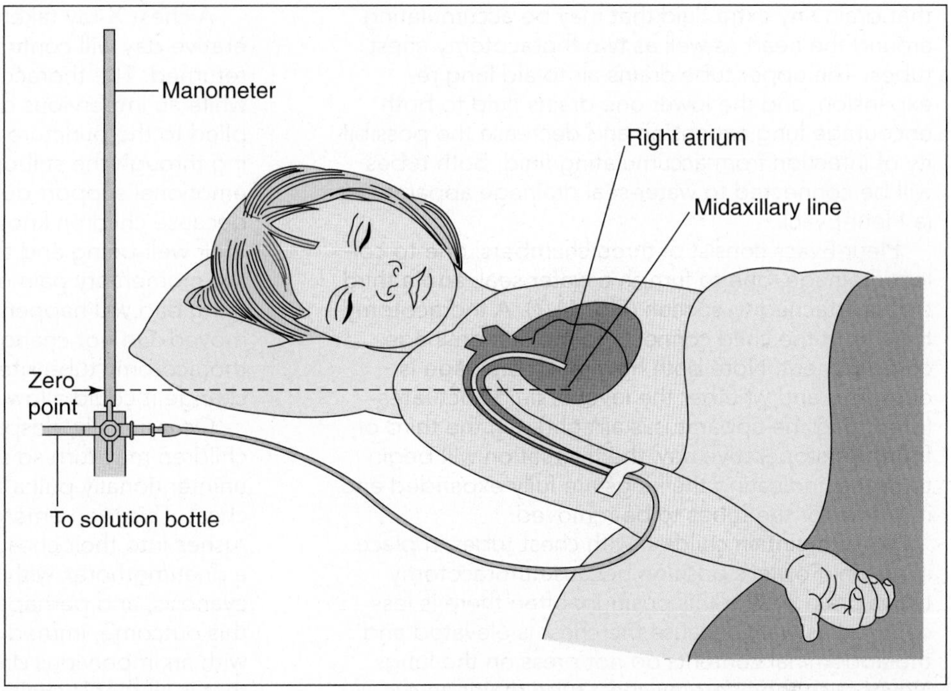

FIGURE 41.6 A central venous pressure catheter may be inserted after cardiac surgery to monitor fluid volume. The zero point on the scale is at the level of the right atrium.

Oxygen saturation level is monitored by pulse oximetry. Laboratory tests such as arterial blood gases (Po_2 and partial pressure of carbon dioxide [Pco_2]), hemoglobin, hematocrit, clotting time, and electrolytes (particularly sodium and potassium) will also be monitored closely to assess postoperative cardiac and pulmonary function. A drug such as dopamine may be administered to improve cardiac output.

Central Venous Pressure Monitoring. CVP is recorded by means of a catheter inserted into a brachial, jugular, or subclavian vein and threaded into the vena cava just outside the right atrium (Fig. 41.6). CVP reflects the child's fluid volume status. A usual level is 2 to 6 mmHg. This level will rise with CHF because the heart cannot manage all of the blood arriving at the atria.

Pulmonary Artery Pressure Monitoring. To assess pressure in the left side of the heart parallel to CVP measurement, a multilumen pulmonary artery catheter, such as a Swan-Ganz, can be threaded through the venous circulation, then through the right side of the heart and the pulmonary valve, into the pulmonary artery. The pressure in the artery (usually at 9 to 18 mmHg) registers as a waveform on a cardiac monitor to reflect both the resistance of the lungs to the passage of blood (pulmonary artery resistance) and the ability of the left side of the heart to handle the circulating fluid volume returning from the lungs.

Nursing Diagnosis: Impaired gas exchange related to unexpanded lung space and collection of lung excretions

Outcome Evaluation: Child's respiratory rate remains within age-appropriate parameters; there is no sound of rales (crackles) or other adventitious breath sounds; chest tubes function effectively.

Measures to Prevent Pooling of Secretions in Lungs. Suction as necessary while a child is receiving ventilatory assistance to prevent pooling of secretions in the respiratory tract. Assist with chest physiotherapy (percussion and vibration) as needed to help keep lung secretions mobile. As soon as the endotracheal tube and ventilator are removed, encourage the child to cough and deep-breathe or use an incentive spirometer at hourly intervals as other ways to mobilize secretions. Although children may have practiced such procedures preoperatively, they have difficulty carrying them out postoperatively because, unless continuous epidural anesthesia is used for pain relief, coughing or deep breathing is very painful. To minimize pain, administer prescribed analgesia or alert the child to use the patient-controlled analgesia (PCA) pump 10 to 15 minutes before it is time to deep-breathe. For optimal effectiveness, demonstrating coughing again, or deep breathing with the child, may be necessary. Be certain parents understand that games such as blowing cotton balls or using an incentive spirometer are not really games but important exercises to help achieve lung expansion. Otherwise, they can interpret these exercises as too tiring for the child and discourage them.

Some children will have pacing wires attached to their heart that exit both sides of their sternum and are attached to a pacemaker if heart stimulation is needed. In addition, most children have one or two mediastinal tubes inserted just below their sternum that drain any extra fluid that may be accumulating around the heart as well as two thoracotomy chest tubes. The upper tube drains air to aid lung re-expansion, and the lower one drains fluid to both encourage lung expansion and decrease the possibility of infection from accumulating fluid. Both tubes will be connected to water-seal drainage apparatuses (a Pleur-Evac).

Pleur-Evacs consist of three chambers: one to collect drainage, one to furnish a water seal, and a third that is attached to suction (Fig. 41.7). A thoracotomy tube from the child connects to the first drainage compartment. Note both how much drainage is occurring and whether the level of fluid fluctuates (proof that the apparatus is airtight). On the third or fourth postoperative day, the fluctuation will begin to cease, indicating the lungs are fully expanded and it is time for the tubes to be removed.

Try to maintain children with chest tubes in place in a semi-Fowler's position because thoracotomy tubes drain best in this position; often there is less dyspnea as well, because the chest is elevated and the abdominal contents do not press on the lungs. Never raise thoracotomy chest tube drainage systems above the level of the child's chest so fluid does not flow back from the tube into the pleural space. Assess daily that tube connections are secure and that the Pleur-Evac is not cracked or broken. If broken, air could enter the chest cavity and collapse the child's lungs (pneumothorax).

Mark the amount of fluid level in the collecting chamber immediately after surgery, then continue to mark the level of fluid in the drainage chamber every hour so the hourly amount of drainage can be evaluated (approximately 5 ml/kg/hr is typical). Inspect the color of the drainage fluid as this may be blood-tinged but should not contain fresh blood or clots. If it does, it suggests active bleeding, which should not be present.

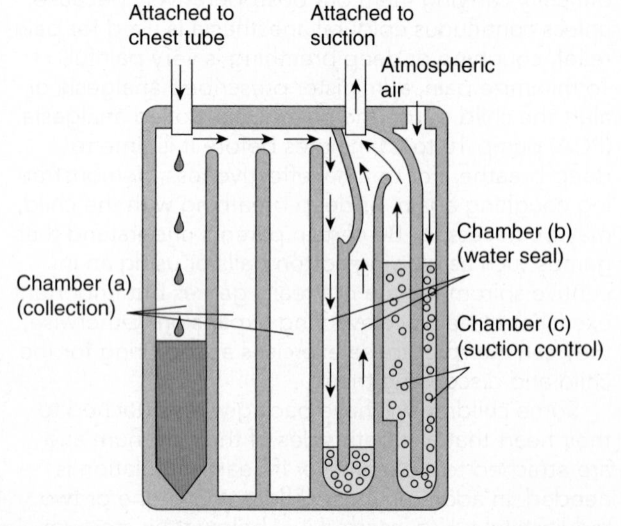

FIGURE 41.7 Pleur-Evac system for chest tube drainage.

A chest X-ray taken on the third or fourth postoperative day will confirm that full lung expansion has returned. The thoracotomy tubes are then removed while an impervious dressing is simultaneously applied to the puncture site to prevent air from entering through the still-open puncture wounds. Provide emotional support during thoracotomy tube removal, because children know the tubes were important for their well-being and they may worry not only about the momentary pain of removal but also that something bad will happen to them with the tubes removed. Do not change the dressing over the former thoracotomy tube site, because lifting the dressing to change it could allow air to enter.

Occasionally, despite being cautioned not to, children may turn so suddenly after surgery that they unintentionally pull a thoracotomy tube out of their chest. This is an emergency situation because, if air rushes into their chest from the tube site, it can cause a pneumothorax with sudden dyspnea, tachycardia, cyanosis, and perhaps sharp chest pain. To prevent this outcome, immediately cover the puncture site with an impervious dressing (or your gloved hand if that is all that is available) until help arrives.

If a tube connection comes loose, creating a slow air leak, less dramatic symptoms such as restlessness and apprehension accompanying gradually increasing dyspnea are more apt to occur. If this happens, clamp the tube close to the child's chest to prevent further air from entering the chest. In both instance, the child may need emergency oxygen administered to counteract the decreased amount of air exchange space created as a result of partial lung collapse. Remaining calm while righting the situation is a major way to help the child remain calm, avoiding increasing respiratory rate and oxygen demand.

Nursing Diagnosis: Risk for infection related to surgical incision and tube sites

Outcome Evaluation: Child's temperature remains at or below 100.4°F (38.0°C) tympanic; incision site is clean, dry, and without evidence of erythema or foul drainage.

Some children are begun on a prophylactic course of a broad-spectrum antibiotic before surgery. If so, this will be continued for 24 to 48 hours postoperatively. To detect whether infection could be beginning, frequently monitor temperature postoperatively. Frequently assess the dressing over the surgical incision and the points of insertion of the thoracotomy tubes for drainage and erythema. Use strict aseptic technique when changing the incisional dressing to avoid introducing pathogens.

Nursing Diagnosis: Hypothermia related to cooling during surgery

Outcome Evaluation: Child's temperature is above 96.8°F (36.0°C) tympanic. Capillary refill is less than 5 seconds.

If hypothermia was induced for surgery, the child's temperature will be so low postoperatively that a hyperthermia blanket, warm blankets, or radiant heat may be necessary to elevate the temperature to normal. Alternatively, in some children, temperature may rise above normal because of an inflammatory response that occurs because of the hypothermia. Unless infection is developing, these temperature readings will gradually return to normal in a few days.

Nursing Diagnosis: Risk for excess or deficient fluid volume related to fluid shifts accompanying cardiac surgery

Outcome Evaluation: Child maintains weight; skin turgor is good; CVP or pulmonary artery pressure remains within established parameters.

Children tend to develop hypervolemia after cardiac surgery because of increased production of aldosterone by the adrenal glands and an increase in antidiuretic hormone secretion by the pituitary gland in response to stress. Also, if cardiopulmonary bypass was used, some fluid may have been shifted from the intravascular system to the interstitial spaces during surgery. After surgery, as this fluid returns by osmosis to the vessels, it creates additional hypervolemia. An individual child, however, may have experienced excessive bleeding because of the heparin used during surgery and subsequently develop hypovolemia.

Monitor central venous or pulmonary artery pressures carefully to evaluate which hemodynamic status is occurring. Monitor IV fluid administration carefully to be certain hypovolemia is corrected or to prevent fluid overload. Typically, oral fluid intake is withheld for at least the first 24 hours after surgery. Once bowel sounds have returned, oral fluids can be introduced gradually.

Nursing Diagnosis: Parental anxiety related to lack of knowledge of postoperative routine and exercises

Outcome Evaluation: Family members accurately state plans for child's postoperative recovery; family members relate less anxiety after teaching and support.

Most children recover amazingly quickly from heart surgery. Passive range-of-motion exercises are usually prescribed for the day of surgery. By 24 hours, children are out of bed and ambulating. Encourage parents to do as much as they want to do for their child's care during this period because it can be difficult for them to accept that the surgery is over and their child is now a well child (or will be at the end of the surgery recovery period).

Offering the child sips of water or playing a game with the child helps parents see their child is returning to usual activities. Be certain, however, in the midst of the postoperative excitement, the child receives adequate rest the first postoperative days. To manage this, you may need to monitor and regulate visits by staff or outside visitors to be certain a child is undisturbed for sustained rest periods. Urge parents to read to children or listen to music with them as a way to provide quiet rest periods. Caution parents not to pick up an infant under the arms to hold the child, because this pulls on the chest incision. Show them how to lift an infant by placing their hands under the shoulders and buttocks instead.

Once the immediate postoperative period has passed, the child will be moved from the ICU to a routine patient unit. This is a major step toward recovery but also may be a difficult move for both the child and the parents because they have developed confidence in the ICU staff and are reluctant to entrust their child to new personnel (even if the patient unit is the one to which the child was initially admitted before surgery). It helps the transition if the regular nursing staff visits the child daily in the ICU. As a general rule, place children returning from the ICU in a room near the nursing station, and place the bed so it can be easily seen from the hallway to assure parents that although you are not providing the constant attendance the child received in the ICU, you are continuing to be very observant and aware of the child's needs. Stopping to look in every time you pass the room is another way to reassure the family you are always close by. Allow parents the opportunity to voice their concern over the change in personnel and surroundings. Accepting this change can help prepare them for the day of hospital discharge, when they will be observing and caring for their child on their own.

At hospital discharge, parents need a clear explanation of any restriction in activity they need to enforce. Be sure they have an appointment for a return visit for the child and the telephone number they should call if they have any questions regarding their child's care. Remember that the protectiveness they felt for the child before surgery does not diminish instantly. They may find themselves saying, "Don't run" for months after the child has been allowed full activity. Provide a listening ear for their concerns, which may include expressing a feeling that they are not as important to their child as they were before surgery when the child was ill. Emphasize to them that well children also need continued parental supervision and guidance to help them adjust to this dramatic change in their life (Box 41.3).

Complications of Cardiac Surgery

Morbidity and mortality have been significantly decreased due to advances in surgical techniques and postoperative nursing care; however, complications of heart surgery still occur because of the use of cardiopulmonary bypass and the extent of the surgery. Hemorrhage may occur because heparin is necessary to prevent blood coagulation during the cardiopulmonary bypass. Although protamine sulfate (the antidote for heparin) is administered IV immediately after surgery, some heparin can remain in the child's system. To detect early signs

BOX 41.3 Nursing Care Planning Based on Effective Communication

Megan is a 2-month-old infant who is being discharged after cardiac surgery. You stop at her hospital room to give discharge instructions to her mother.

Less Effective Communication

Nurse: Good morning, Mrs. Carver. Let me review a few instructions with you.
Mrs. Carver: The most important thing you can tell me is how to keep a baby on bed rest.
Nurse: Most infants are exhausted from surgery, but just let her assume her usual activities as she likes.
Mrs. Carver: She likes to kick a mobile. It'll be hard to keep her from doing that.
Nurse: Her appetite should be back to normal in a few days. Be sure to check back with the clinic if it doesn't improve.
Mrs. Carver: I don't understand how she'll eat well if she has to be in bed all the time.
Nurse: Megan will need to continue to take digoxin until she returns for her checkup in 1 week. Do you have any questions about the dose?
Mrs. Carver: No. It'll be hard to get her to cooperate, though, when she's unhappy about having to stay in bed all the time.
Nurse: You'll also need to check the incision daily and report any redness or increasing pain.
Mrs. Carver: I can do that. It's the bed rest I'm worried about.
Nurse: Good. Wait here, until I call transportation to take you downstairs. I hope you brought a car seat. You know that's important.

More Effective Communication

Nurse: Good morning, Mrs. Carver. Let me review a few instructions with you.
Mrs. Carver: The most important thing you can tell me is how to keep a baby on bed rest.
Nurse: Most infants are exhausted from surgery, but just let her assume her usual activities as she likes.
Mrs. Carver: She likes to kick a mobile in bed. It'll be hard to keep her from doing that.
Nurse: Her appetite should be back to normal in a few days. Be sure to check back with the clinic if it doesn't improve.
Mrs. Carver: I don't understand how she'll eat well if she has to be in bed all the time.
Nurse: You've mentioned bed rest several times. Let's talk about what that means with an infant.

Because cardiac surgery is such serious surgery, most parents assume it will take their child a very long time to recover from it. In the above scenarios, the mother has overestimated the time it will take her child to return to normal activities. Only when really listening to what the mother is saying, rather than just continuing to review discharge instructions, does the nurse recognize the mother has not heard the first instruction—let the child return to activities at as near normal a level as possible.

of bleeding, monitor the coagulation time and vital signs and observe thoracotomy tube or incision site drainage.

Shock, another possible complication, is revealed by hypotension, oliguria, acidosis, and cyanosis. Shock may result from hypovolemia or cardiac tamponade (bleeding into the heart muscle or pericardium, interfering with the heart's ability to contract forcibly), or it may be a reaction to prolonged extracorporeal perfusion. It is treated according to individual needs, including plasma volume expanders, continued mechanical ventilation, and perhaps a return to surgery to stop the bleeding. Heart block or arrhythmias may occur as the result of edema or trauma compromising the effectiveness of the bundle of His (Bernstein, 2012). An artificial pacemaker may be inserted to correct these problems.

Neurologic symptoms, also a possible complication, may occur if the child experienced hypoxia during surgery. If the child had congestive heart disease before surgery, this may persist for a week or more after surgery. If it occurs as a new entity, it suggests the surgery caused a stricture to circulation at some point, causing either the right or left side of the heart to become overwhelmed. Measures for treating postoperative CHF are the same as those in children who have this syndrome from any cause.

A **postcardiac surgery syndrome** may develop at the end of the first postoperative week. This is a febrile illness with pericarditis and pleurisy (fluid collecting in the pleural space) that appears to be a benign inflammatory response to the surgical procedure. Anti-inflammatory therapy and bed rest reduce the symptoms, although the symptoms may recur again months after surgery.

Postperfusion syndrome may occur 3 to 12 weeks after surgery in response to the use of cardiopulmonary bypass during surgery. The child develops a fever, an enlarged spleen, general malaise, and a maculopapular rash. Increased liver size also may be present. The white blood cell count reveals a leukocytosis, with lymphocytes as the predominant cell type. Such a reaction may be caused by a cytomegalovirus infection contracted from the donor blood used in the cardiopulmonary bypass machine. The illness runs a short course, with no permanent effect.

QSEN Checkpoint Question 41.2

Evidence-Based Practice

Infections after pediatric cardiac surgery are a common complication, occurring in as many as 30% of children. To discover whether a bedside prediction rule could be used to estimate the risk of postoperative infection, researchers analyzed the outcomes of 412 surgeries done at a major medical center over a 3-year period. Results showed that children most likely to develop an infection were those age less than 6 months, those who remained in a postoperative pediatric ICU (PICU) longer than 48 hours, or those who had an open sternum for longer than 48 hours (Algra, Driessen, Schadenberg, et al., 2012).

Based on the previous study, which finding in Megan after cardiac surgery would be most predictive that she might develop a postoperative infection?

a. Her sternum was closed after the first 24 hours.
b. She was transferred from the PICU as soon as possible.
c. She was operated on when she was 2 months old.
d. Her birth weight was 7 lb, 7 oz.

Look in Appendix A for the best answer and rationale.

The Child With an Artificial Valve Replacement

A number of congenital heart anomalies, such as aortic stenosis, and diseases, such as rheumatic fever or Kawasaki syndrome, can require artificial heart valve replacement (Myers, Cikirikcioglu, Tissot, et al., 2012). Valve replacement is technically more complicated in children than adults because children's hearts are smaller. Because children will have a valve in place for the length of their life, they may need the valve replaced again later in life. The administration of the long-term anticoagulation therapy necessary to prevent clots from forming at the valve site must be weighed against the problem of extensive bleeding from normal childhood unintentional injuries.

Artificial valves are made of synthetic material (prosthetic) or obtained from human donors (homografts). After surgery to place the artificial valve, a child will be given an anticoagulant such as heparin or warfarin sodium (Coumadin) to prevent thrombi from forming at the valve implantation site. Antiplatelet therapy (administration of acetylsalicylic acid [aspirin] and dipyridamole [Persantine]) also may be prescribed. Aspirin works by decreasing platelet aggregation; dipyridamole decreases platelet adhesiveness. The dosage for all these drugs must be periodically monitored by blood analysis to ensure they remain adequate as the child grows.

If a child should develop a bacterial infection with an artificial valve in place, organisms tend to cluster and colonize at the valve site. For this reason, children with artificial valves are rated as high risk for developing infectious endocarditis and thus may be prescribed prophylactic antibiotic therapy to prevent endocarditis. Additional therapy with amoxicillin may be prescribed if a child is scheduled for dental work or any other invasive procedure (Dinsbach, 2012).

Adolescent girls need counseling about avoiding pregnancy until they become adults because the artificial valve may be unable to accommodate both the increased blood volume associated with pregnancy and an adolescent growth spurt. In addition, because warfarin is teratogenic, an adolescent contemplating pregnancy needs to have her medication changed to a heparin regimen before conception. Question whether girls with artificial valves in place should be prescribed an estrogen-based birth control pill, because an increased estrogen level can increase blood coagulation and possibly lead to thrombi.

Hemolytic anemia is yet another complication that may occur from artificial valve replacement. This occurs because the extreme turbulence of blood through the prosthetic valve apparently results in breakage and destruction of red blood cells. Periodic blood replacement may be necessary if the hemolytic process persists.

The Child Undergoing Cardiac Transplantation

Children who have a hypoplastic left ventricle or extensive cardiomyopathy from any cause can be candidates for heart transplantation (Paris, Moore, & Schreiber, 2012). While waiting for a donor heart to be available, children may be maintained on ECMO or a ventricular assist device (Almond, Singh, Gauvreau, et al., 2011).

Ventricular Assist Devices

A ventricular assist device is a small pump, implanted in the child's chest, that pumps blood either from an incision in the left ventricle into an incision in the aorta or from the right ventricle into the pulmonary artery when ventricles are too weakened to achieve this without additional help (Brancaccio, Filippelli, Michielon, et al., 2012). A cord from the pump exits from a small puncture site in the child's upper abdomen and is connected to a battery pack. When the child is discharged from the hospital, be certain parents know how often the power pack must be recharged (usually every 24 hours); if the child remains in the hospital, be certain charging times are conscientiously followed.

A totally artificial heart (the SynCardia) has been approved by the U.S. Food and Drug Administration as a second means of establishing a bridge to transplantation (Slepian, Alemu, Soares, et al., 2013). Children who have ventricular assist devices or the artificial heart in place may have altered pulse rates as the pump may move blood continuously, not in ventricular bursts. Observe small children carefully when such devices are in place because they can move blood too rapidly for the child's small circulatory volume or the child's lung space may be compromised because of the small chest size.

Cardiac Transplant

Children who will be having heart transplants may be at home or in the hospital when their family is notified a donor heart is available. At the site where the donor heart is available, the donor heart is perfused with a balanced electrolyte solution and chilled immediately to maintain its function during transport. If there will be a delay in transplant, function can be maintained by using cardiopulmonary bypass technique. For the transplant procedure, the damaged recipient heart is removed except for the upper portion of the right atrium, which contains the SA node. The major cardiac vessels are reattached, and intrathoracic hemodynamic monitoring lines and ventricle pacing wires are implanted. Transplanted hearts beat normally except, because they do not have autonomic nervous system control, the heart varies its rate in response to the amount of blood arriving, or response is one to catecholamines rather than by nervous system control. An ECG will show two P waves (one from the residual original heart and one from the donor heart) because both SA nodes are still intact.

Postoperative care is similar to that for any child undergoing cardiac surgery. The child has the same potential problems of decreased cardiac output, impaired gas exchange, risk for infection, imbalanced nutrition, and ineffective family coping. If the SA node is not functioning regularly, children will demonstrate arrhythmias, which may need a pacemaker assist.

Although a long-term consequence of cardiac transplantation is severe atherosclerosis, apparently as a result of inflammation, rejection of the transplant is the number one cause of death in cardiac transplant patients (Ameduri, Zheng, Schechtman, et al., 2012).

To avoid rejection, an antithymocyte antibody preparation and drugs such as cyclosporine, prednisone, methotrexate, tacrolimus, and azathioprine are commonly prescribed to achieve immunosuppression. If rejection does occur, it is seen in three separate forms: hyperacute, acute, or chronic. Hyperacute rejection occurs immediately and is marked by coronary thrombosis. Acute rejection occurs in about 7 days; the child develops a low-grade fever, tachycardia, edema, and ECG changes. Cardiac catheterization is usually performed a week after transplant to obtain a biopsy sample from the heart muscle to evaluate for signs of acute rejection (tissue necrosis will have started to occur). Long-term or chronic rejection may not begin until about 6 months. Regardless of when rejection begins, additional antithymocyte globulin (ATG) or other immunosuppressants will be infused to help stop the process.

Once past the rejection period, most children adjust well to cardiac transplant as they begin to participate in usual growth and development activities. Depending on the specific protocol, they may be scheduled to return to the transplant center yearly for a repeat cardiac catheterization and evaluation of progress.

The Child With a Pacemaker

A child whose heart has ineffective SA node function or has difficulty in transmitting impulses from the SA node to the ventricles may have an artificial pacemaker inserted to stimulate the ventricles electronically. A usual pacing system consists of two components: a pulse generator that contains the battery and wire leads that connect to the heart. Most leads placed in children are attached to the epicardium (the outside wall of the heart) by sutures. The generator is placed under the skin in the subxyphoid or mid or lower abdomen. Heart disorders that will need pacing can be detected as early as during intrauterine life by fetal monitoring; in these infants, pacemakers can be implanted as soon as they are born (Gil-Jaurena, Castillo, & Rubio, 2012).

The functions of the most common type of pacemaker are denoted by either a three- or five-letter code. With the three-letter system, the first letter identifies the chamber paced, the second the chamber sensed, and the third the pacemaker's response to the intrinsic activity of the heart. If a fourth letter is used, it denotes whether rate modulation is possible; a fifth letter denotes whether antitachyarrhythmia function, such as the ability to produce a shock to defibrillate, is possible (Vijayaraman & Ellenbogen, 2013). For example, a pacemaker that is set to pace the ***v***entricle, sense the ***v***entricle, and be ***i***nhibited (cannot modify the rate and does not respond as long as the heart initiates a normal beat) is a VVI pacemaker.

Teach the parents of the child with a pacemaker how to take the child's pulse, because they will need to do this daily at home, and to report any alterations in the pulse rate to their primary care provider until it is certain the paced rate is appropriate for their child. They also may need to telephone the health care center periodically and transmit a recording of the child's heart action to the center by means of a telephone attachment to ensure the paced rate remains accurate.

Some parents stay awake at night worrying batteries in their child's pacemaker will suddenly stop operating and their child will die during the night. As a result, they may be reluctant to take a vacation separate from the child or allow the child to go away to a summer camp. How long a pacemaker battery lasts depends on the percentage of time pacing is needed (continuous or intermittent), the battery energy output in amplitude (the amount of battery voltage needed to create each pacing impulse), and the pulse width (the length of time the impulse is being delivered). With usual pacemaker parameters, however, a battery can last as long as 12 to 15 years. In all instances, parents can be reassured that pacemaker batteries lose power slowly, not abruptly. They will have ample time to recognize weakening batteries through signs in their child such as dizziness, fatigue, fainting, or a slow pulse rate and arrange to have the pacemaker replaced before the child's heart would fail.

Occasionally, pacemaker leads in the right ventricle of infants lie in such close proximity to the diaphragm that they stimulate the diaphragm to contract with each ventricular contraction causing constant hiccupping. If this occurs, the leads may need a position adjustment. A small problem occurs when, in some infants, there is not room in their chest to implant the generator deeply so it triggers airport security systems.

Help parents learn to inspect toys for safety because, as a rule, toys with magnets or those that emit an electrical current can interfere with a pacemaker's operation. Question the prescription for an MRI (which involves the use of magnets) or electrocautery (which involves the use of electricity) with children with pacemakers in place. Caution parents that children should avoid contact sports such as football that could damage the pacemaker. Sports that involve a high degree of shoulder action that could dislodge pacemaker leads, such as gymnastics and basketball, should be limited (Beery, Smith, Kudel, et al., 2011).

CONGENITAL HEART DISORDERS

About 8% of term newborns and 9% to 10% of preterm infants are born with a congenital cardiovascular abnormality (Darst, Collins, & Miyamoto, 2012). These disorders affect equal numbers of male and female infants, but specific disorders show a tendency toward sex differentiation. Patent ductus arteriosus (PDA) and ASD, for example, are found more commonly in girls. Valvular aortic stenosis, coarctation of the aorta, tetralogy of Fallot, and transposition of the great vessels occur more often in boys.

The usual cause of congenital heart disorders is failure of the heart structure to progress beyond an early stage of embryonic development. Maternal rubella is an example of an infection known to lead to disorders such as PDA or pulmonary or aortic stenosis. ASD and ventricular septal defect (VSD) may have genetic causes because they tend to be familial (Wang, Wang, Zhao, et al., 2012).

Classification

Formerly, congenital heart disorders were classified based on the physical sign of cyanosis, or these disorders were classified as either cyanotic or acyanotic disorders.

Acyanotic heart disease involves heart or circulatory anomalies that involve either a stricture to the flow of blood or a shunt that moves blood from the arterial to the venous system (oxygenated to unoxygenated blood, or *left-to-right shunts*). These disorders cause the heart to function as an ineffective pump and make the child prone to CHF. **Cyanotic heart disease** occurs when blood is shunted from the venous to the arterial system as a result of abnormal communication between the two systems (deoxygenated blood to oxygenated blood, or *right-to-left shunts*). Although helpful, this classification system has inherent difficulties because children with acyanotic heart disease can develop cyanosis, and children with cyanotic disease may not exhibit cyanosis until they are seriously ill.

Although the terms cyanotic and noncyanotic heart disease are still commonly used, congenital heart disorders are formally classified according to the hemodynamic and blood flow patterns that they create rather than the presence of cyanosis, allowing a more uniform and predictable set of signs and symptoms to be described.

Disorders With Increased Pulmonary Blood Flow

Congenital heart disorders associated with increased pulmonary blood flow involve blood flow from the left side of the heart, which is under greater pressure, to the right side of the heart, which is under less pressure, through some abnormal opening or connection between the two systems or the great arteries.

Ventricular Septal Defect

VSD, the most common type of congenital cardiac disorder seen, occurs in about 4 to 5 of every 1,000 live births (van der Linde, Konings, Slager, et al., 2011). With this disorder, an opening is present in the septum between the two ventricles. Blood shunts from left to right across the septum (an acyanotic disorder) impairing the efficiency of the heart because blood that should be forced into the aorta and out to the body from contraction of the left ventricle shunts back into the pulmonary circulation, resulting in right ventricular hypertrophy and increased pressure in the pulmonary artery (Fig. 41.8).

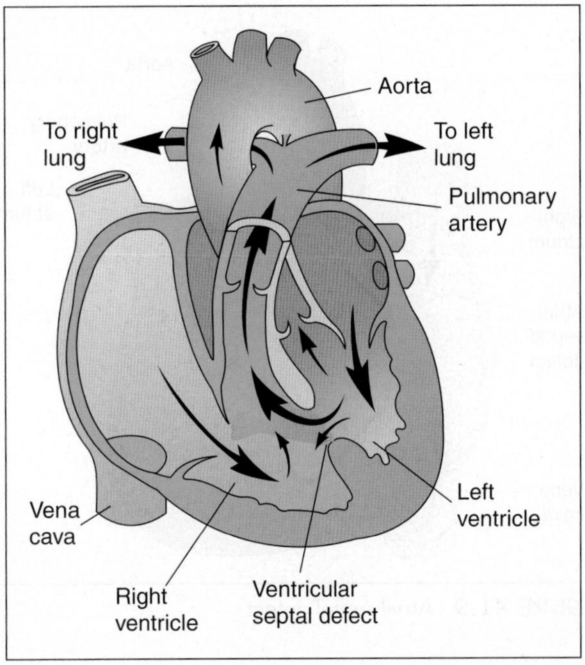

FIGURE 41.8 A ventricular septal defect.

Assessment. The typical murmur of a VSD may not be heard at birth because, with incomplete opening of the lung alveoli, there is such high pulmonary artery resistance that little blood is shunted through the defect. At about 4 to 8 weeks of age, as shunting begins, the infant begins to demonstrate easy fatigue; a loud, harsh systolic murmur becomes evident along the left sternal border at the third or fourth interspace; and a thrill (vibration) also may be palpable. The diagnosis of VSD is based on examination by chest X-ray, ECG, and echocardiography with color flow Doppler or an MRI, which reveals the right ventricular hypertrophy and possibly pulmonary artery dilatation from the increased blood flow.

Therapeutic Management. Because up to 85% of VSDs are so small they close spontaneously, many children are managed by only close observation during the first years of life, perhaps with administration of a diuretic or digoxin to help prevent fluid from accumulating in the lungs (Bernstein, 2012). Those that do not close spontaneously can be closed by placement of a septal occluder device during cardiac catheterization to prevent chronic pulmonary artery hypertension from developing or the heart from becoming infected (endocarditis) because of the recirculating and stagnant blood flow. Over time, septal tissue then grows across the synthetic device and knits it firmly into place.

Postoperatively, listen carefully for arrhythmias because edema in the septum can interfere with conduction from the AV node to the ventricles. If there are no complications, children can expect to participate in usual activities or have no restrictions after the repair.

Atrial Septal Defect

An ASD is an abnormal communication between the two atria, allowing blood to shift from the left to the right atrium (an acyanotic disorder) resulting in an increase in blood volume in the right side of the heart, right ventricular hypertrophy, and an increased pulmonary artery blood flow, the same as with a VSD (Fig. 41.9). The disorder is more common in girls than boys. Approximately 80% are so small they close spontaneously (Lange & Hillis, 2013).

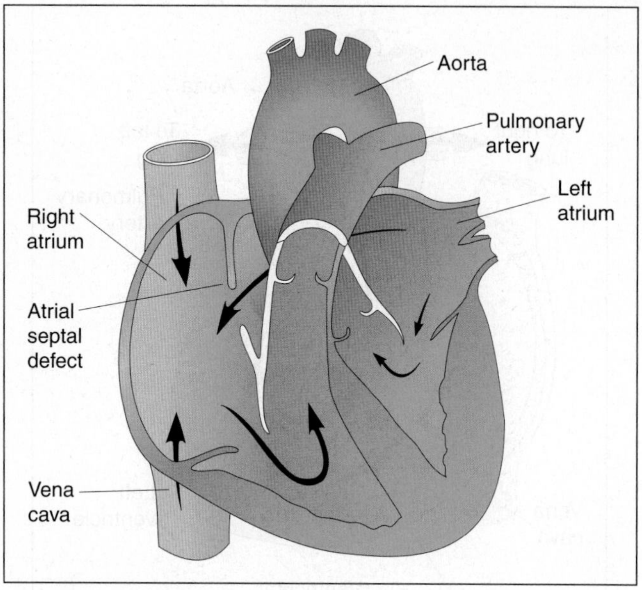

FIGURE 41.9 Atrial septal defect.

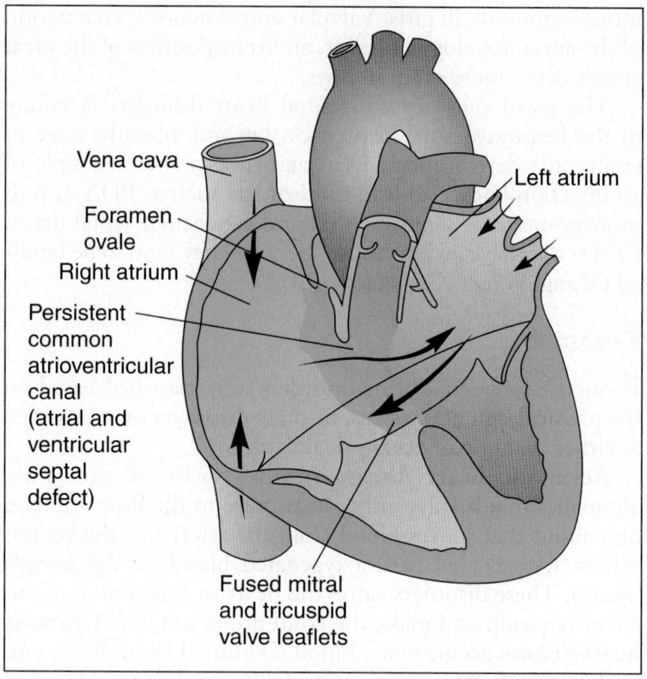

FIGURE 41.10 Atrioventricular canal defect.

Assessment. A sign of ASD is a harsh systolic murmur heard over the second or third interspace (the pulmonic area) because of the extra amount of shunted blood crossing the pulmonic valve. As the volume of this blood crossing the pulmonic valve causes the valve to close 1 or 2 seconds later than the aortic valve, the second heart sound will be auscultated as split (a lub-dub-dub sound), a finding almost always diagnostic of ASD.

Echocardiography with color flow Doppler will generally reveal the enlarged right side of the heart and the increased pulmonary circulation. Cardiac catheterization reveals the separation in the atrial septum and the increased oxygen saturation in the right atrium.

Therapeutic Management. Surgery to close the disorder is usually done electively by cardiac catheterization between 1 and 3 years of age. That the disorder be closed is particularly important in girls, because the abnormal blood flow can cause emboli during pregnancy (Li, Margraf, Kluck, et al., 2012). In the cardiac catheterization laboratory, the edges of the opening in the septum are approximated and filled in with a septal occluder device. Postoperatively, carefully observe the child for arrhythmias because edema of the right atrium could interfere with SA node function. Assuming the surgery is uncomplicated, children can expect a normal quality and length of life with no activity restrictions afterward.

Atrioventricular Canal Defect

Atrioventricular canal defect (AVCD), also called an endocardial cushion defect, results from incomplete fusion of the endocardial cushion or the septum of the heart at the junction of the atria and the ventricles possibly involving both the mitral and tricuspid valves (Fig. 41.10). Although blood flow is generally left to right, if the defect is extensive, blood may be mixed between all four heart chambers. Although rare in the general population, as many as 20% of children with trisomy 21 (Down syndrome) who have heart disease have this type of congenital cardiac disorder (Kucik, Shin, Siffel, et al., 2013).

The disorder leads to the same symptoms as ASDs (right ventricular hypertrophy, increased pulmonary blood flow, and fixed S2 splitting). An ECG often will reveal first-degree heart block as impulse conduction is halted before the AV node. Echocardiography will confirm the diagnosis. To reduce the amount of pressure in the pulmonary artery, a band may be placed on the pulmonary artery, preventing so much blood from entering it in selected infants. Surgery, however, is always necessary for a final repair because these disorders tend to be too large to close spontaneously. Because surgery may involve a valve repair as well as a septal repair, mitral and tricuspid insufficiency from poor valve function may occur at a later date.

Postoperatively, closely observe children for jaundice resulting from red blood cell destruction if red cells are destroyed by the newly constructed valves. Both prophylactic anticoagulation and antibiotic therapy will be prescribed postoperatively if artificial valve replacement was necessary. With the artificial valves in place, children should be able to lead an active life afterward.

Patent Ductus Arteriosus

The ductus arteriosus is an accessory fetal structure that connects the pulmonary artery to the aorta. If it fails to close at birth (closure begins with the first breath and is usually complete between 7 and 14 days of age, although full closure may not occur until 3 months of age), blood will shunt from the aorta (oxygenated blood) to the pulmonary artery (deoxygenated blood) because of the higher pressure in the aorta. The shunted blood returns to the left atrium of the heart, passes to the left ventricle, out to the aorta, and shunts back to the pulmonary artery, causing increased pressure in the pulmonary circulation from the extra shunted blood; this leads to right ventricle hypertrophy and ineffective heart action (Fig. 41.11). It occurs most often in infants who are preterm or have difficulty establishing respirations at birth.

Assessment. PDAs are twice as common in girls as in boys and occur at a higher incidence at higher altitudes. In preterm

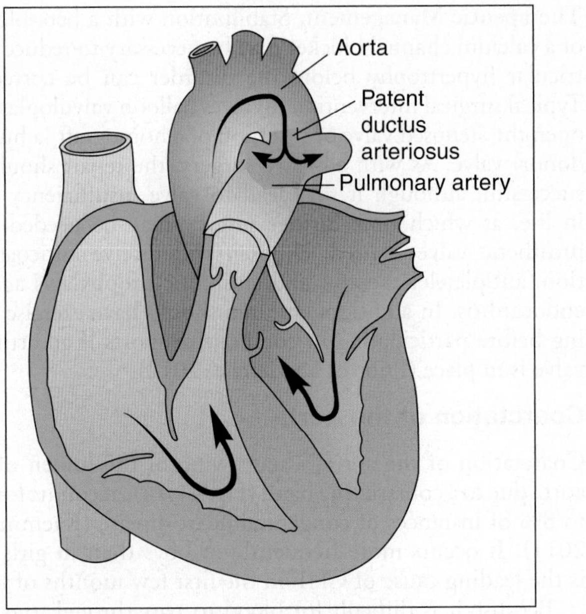

FIGURE 41.11 Patent ductus arteriosus.

infants, the incidence may be as high as 20% to 60%. On physical examination, the child usually has a wide pulse pressure (the difference between systolic and diastolic blood pressures). The diastolic pressure, a measure of peripheral resistance, is low because of the shunt or runoff of blood, which reduces resistance. A typical continuous (systolic and diastolic) "machinery" murmur can be heard at the upper left sternal border or under the left clavicle in older children. In newborns, the murmur may not be quite so characteristic, perhaps a short grade II or III harsh systolic sound. An ECG will usually not reveal the shunting, although it may show ventricle enlargement if the shunt is large. Echocardiography provides good visualization of the patent ductus. Cardiac catheterization is generally not necessary for diagnosis but may be performed to rule out associated disorders.

Therapeutic Management. One reason that the ductus arteriosus remains open in fetal life is a combination of stimulation by prostaglandins, particularly prostaglandin E_1 (PGE_1), released from the placenta and the low oxygen level of fetal blood. At birth, when the placenta is no longer present and the infant takes a first breath, the PGE_1 level falls, the blood oxygen saturation increases, and the ductus arteriosus is stimulated to close.

Closure of the ductus is necessary or the child will remain at risk for CHF from the increased amount of blood pouring back into the pulmonary artery and infectious endocarditis developing from the recirculating blood and potential stasis in the pulmonary artery (Evans, 2012). Infants in whom spontaneous closure does not occur may be prescribed IV indomethacin or ibuprofen, prostaglandin inhibitors, to effect closure. If indomethacin is given, assess for possible side effects, including reduced glomerular filtration, impaired platelet aggregation, and diminished gastrointestinal and cerebral blood flow. Because it has much fewer side effects, ibuprofen rather than indomethacin is becoming the drug of choice; it can even be used as prophylaxis in preterm infants.

If medical management fails to bring about closure of the ductus arteriosus, the disorder can be closed by insertion of Dacron-coated stainless-steel coils by interventional cardiac catheterization when the child is 6 months to 1 year of age. Exceptionally large disorders can be closed surgically by ductal ligation or by surgery performed using only three small thoracotomy incisions on the chest and not requiring extracorporeal circulation.

Disorders With Obstruction to Blood Flow

A number of congenital anomalies cause the blood flow leaving the heart to be obstructed because a vessel or a valve is narrower than usual. Pressure from blood flow increases prior to the narrowing and decreases after the narrowing. These are problematic disorders in that they prohibit enough blood from reaching its intended site, the lungs or the rest of the body; they threaten to overwhelm the heart because of backpressure.

Pulmonary Stenosis

Pulmonary stenosis, a narrowing of the pulmonary valve or the pulmonary artery just distal to the valve, accounts for about 10% of congenital heart anomalies (Fig. 41.12) (Bernstein, 2012). Inability of the right ventricle to evacuate blood by way of the pulmonary artery because of the obstruction leads to right ventricular hypertrophy.

Assessment. Infants with pulmonary artery stenosis may be asymptomatic or have signs of mild right-sided CHF. If the narrowing is severe, cyanosis may be present from inability of adequate blood to reach the lungs for oxygenation or right-to-left shunting across the foramen ovale because of the increased right-sided heart pressure. A typical systolic ejection murmur, grade IV or V crescendo–decrescendo in quality, can be heard, usually loudest at the upper left sternal border, possibly radiating to the suprasternal notch. The second heart sound is usually widely split because of late closure of the pulmonary valve. An ECG or echocardiography will reveal right ventricular hypertrophy. Cardiac catheterization is rarely nec-

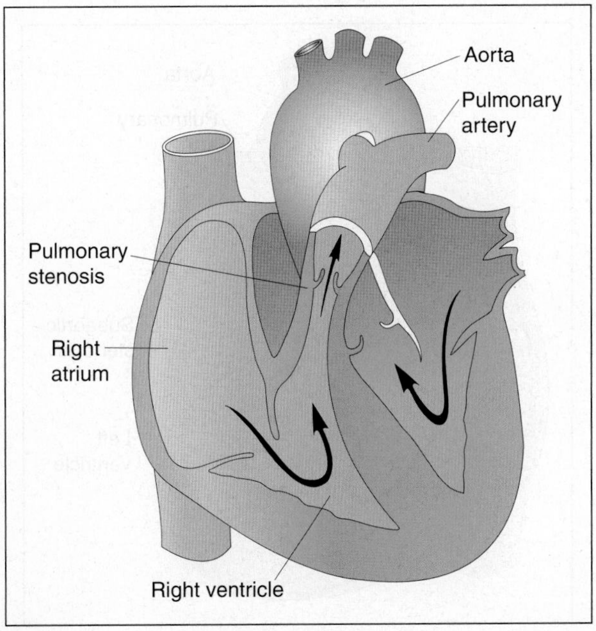

FIGURE 41.12 Pulmonary stenosis.

essary for diagnosis but is used for interventional enlargement of the stenosed valve.

Therapeutic Management. Management of the disorder depends on the severity of the stenosis and the child's age. **Balloon angioplasty** by way of cardiac catheterization is the procedure of choice. With this procedure, a catheter with an uninflated balloon at its tip is inserted and passed through the heart into the stenosed valve. As the balloon is inflated, it breaks valve adhesions and relieves the stenosis. Following the procedure, although children may always have a residual heart murmur, they can expect to have a normal life span.

Aortic Stenosis

Stenosis, or stricture, of the aortic valve prevents blood from passing freely from the left ventricle of the heart into the aorta. Because the heart cannot force blood through the strictured valve, increased pressure and hypertrophy occur in the left ventricle (Fig. 41.13). If this pressure becomes acute, pressure in the left atrium will increase as well, resulting in back-pressure in pulmonary veins and possibly pulmonary edema. Aortic stenosis accounts for about 10% of congenital cardiac abnormalities (Darst et al., 2012).

Assessment. Most infants with aortic stenosis are asymptomatic, but physical assessment will reveal a typical murmur, a rough systolic sound heard loudest in the second right interspace (the aortic space). If the valve stenosis is severe, decreased cardiac output evidenced by faint pulses, hypotension, tachycardia, and inability to suck for long periods may be present. As the child grows and is more active, chest pain similar to angina occurs, because the coronary arteries cannot receive adequate blood with strenuous exercise. Sudden death can occur when the amount of oxygen needed by the heart muscle on exertion far exceeds what is available (Asif, Rao, & Drezner, 2013).

ECG or echocardiography will reveal left ventricular hypertrophy. Cardiac catheterization is rarely necessary unless interventional therapy by this route is planned.

Therapeutic Management. Stabilization with a beta-blocker or a calcium channel blocker may be necessary to reduce ventricular hypertrophy before the disorder can be corrected. Typical surgical intervention involves balloon valvuloplasty to open the stenosed valve or insertion of a homograft (a human donor) valve. As with all valve surgery, the repair should be successful, although it may lead to valve insufficiency later in life, at which time further surgery may be needed. If a prosthetic valve is used, children will receive anticoagulation, antiplatelet therapy, and antibiotic prophylaxis against endocarditis. In addition, children should have exercise testing before participating in competitive sports if an artificial valve is in place (Prior & La Gerche, 2012).

Coarctation of the Aorta

Coarctation of the aorta, a narrowing of the lumen of the aorta due to a constricting band (Fig. 41.14), accounts for 5% to 8% of instances of congenital heart disease (Kaemmerer, 2011). It occurs more frequently in boys than in girls and is the leading cause of CHF in the first few months of life.

Because it is difficult for blood to pass through the narrowed lumen of the aorta, blood pressure increases proximal to the coarctation and decreases distal to it, resulting in increased blood pressure in the heart and upper portions of the body. By preschool age, the elevated upper body blood pressure begins to produce headaches and vertigo. Because a child under 3 years of age has difficulty describing these sensations, exceptional irritability may be the main clue that such symptoms are present. By school age, epistaxis (nosebleed) and cerebrovascular accident, an event not generally associated with children, can occur from this dangerously elevated blood pressure. Children begin to experience leg pain on exertion because of the diminished blood supply to their lower extremities.

Assessment. If the coarctation is slight, absence of palpable femoral pulses from the decreased blood pressure in the lower body may be the only symptom seen. To help detect this, always include evaluation of femoral pulses in all

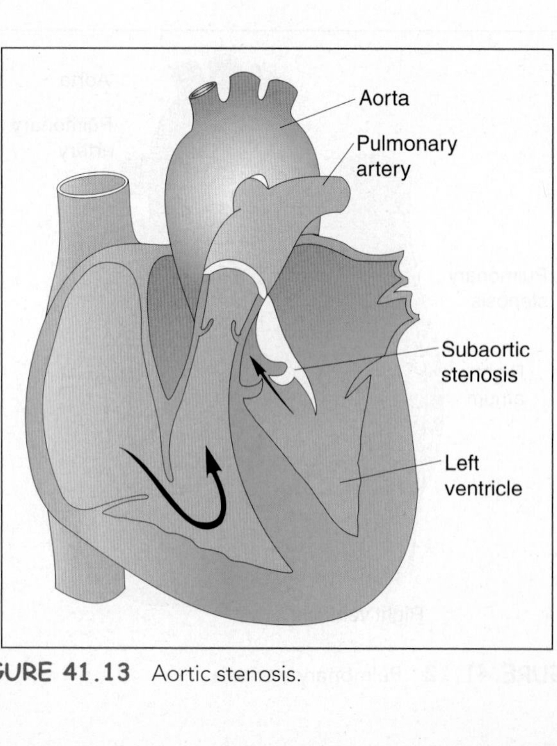

FIGURE 41.13 Aortic stenosis.

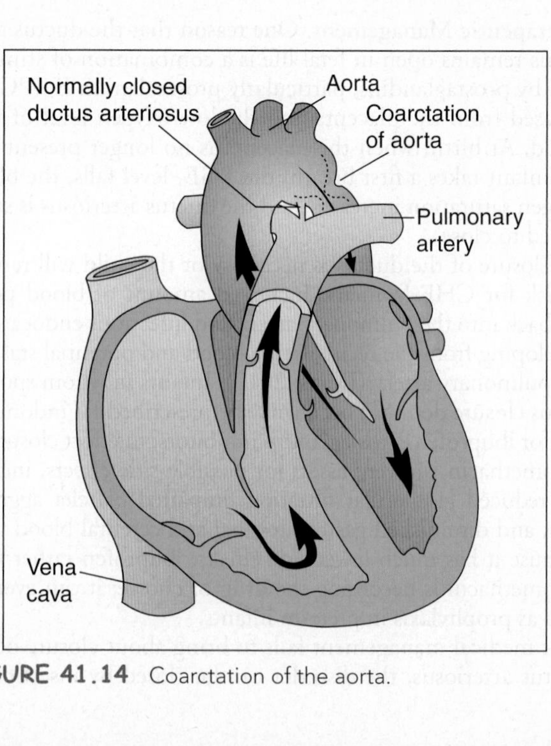

FIGURE 41.14 Coarctation of the aorta.

initial newborn assessments and admission inspections to newborn nurseries. A child who has an obstruction proximal to the left subclavian artery may have absent brachial pulses as well. Because collateral circulation is necessary to allow blood to flow around the constricted aorta, collateral arteries enlarge and may be seen on the ribs as obvious nodules.

The diagnosis of coarctation of the aorta may be made based on the history and physical assessment. On examination, the blood pressure in the arms will be at least 20 mmHg higher than in the legs, a reversal of the normal pattern. Echocardiography, ECG, MRI, or X-ray examination will reveal left-sided heart enlargement from back-pressure and also notching of the ribs from the enlarged collateral vessels. Occasionally, a soft or moderately loud systolic murmur, especially prominent at the base of the heart, will be present, but the sound is variable in position, intensity, and character, and the absence of a murmur does not rule out a stricture of the aorta.

Therapeutic Management. Management of coarctation of the aorta is by interventional angiography (a balloon catheter) or surgery. With surgery, the narrowed portion of the aorta is removed and the new ends of the aorta are anastomosed. A graft of transplanted subclavian artery or a prosthetic stent may be necessary if the narrowed section is so extensive an anastomosis cannot be accomplished readily.

Before surgery can be performed, a number of infants may require therapy with digoxin and diuretics in order to reduce the severity of hypertension and CHF.

It is ideal if children can achieve the greater part of their adult height before surgical correction, as this can prevent a strain on the incision line as they grow. At the same time, in terms of self-image, correction is best done before children begin to think of themselves as chronically ill or before they develop a complication, such as chronic hypertension. Girls must have the disorder repaired before childbearing age, or the extra blood volume that occurs during pregnancy can cause CHF. Surgical repair is usually scheduled, therefore, by 2 years of age. Following surgery, because abdominal vessels are receiving more blood than they did previously, this can result in temporary but generalized abdominal discomfort. Some children continue to have elevated upper body hypertension after the repair because there is still some aortic narrowing. If so, they may need continued treatment with antihypertensive agents. Some children require repeat balloon angioplasty at adolescence to re-enlarge the aortic lumen and help reduce this upper body hypertension.

Disorders With Mixed Blood Flow

Mixed disorders are cardiac anomalies that involve mixing of blood from the pulmonary and systemic circulation in the heart chambers. This mixing results in a relative deoxygenation of systemic blood flow, although cyanosis is not always visible.

Transposition of the Great Arteries

In transposition of the great arteries, the aorta arises from the right ventricle instead of the left, and the pulmonary artery arises from the left ventricle instead of the right. Blood enters the heart from the vena cava to the right atrium, then flows to the right ventricle, and goes out into

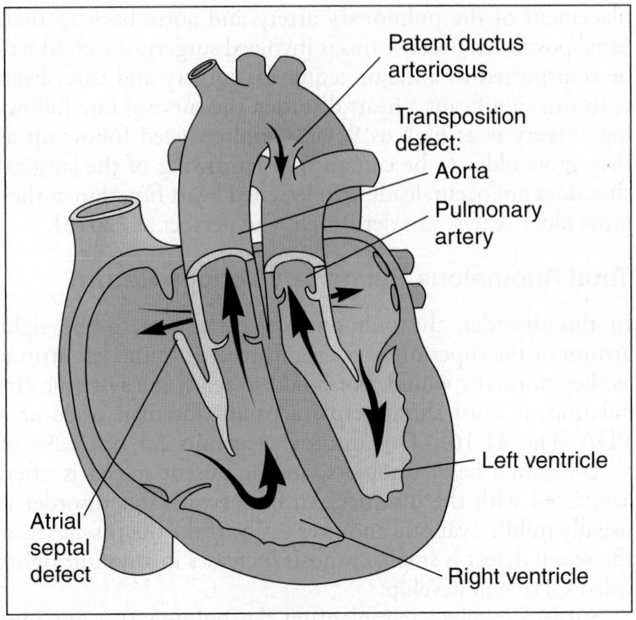

FIGURE 41.15 Transposition of the great arteries.

the aorta to the body completely deoxygenated; it returns again by the vena cava. A secondary source of blood enters the heart from the pulmonary veins, goes to the left atrium, left ventricle, and out the pulmonary artery to the lungs to be oxygenated, and returns to the left atrium, a second closed circulatory system (Fig. 41.15). This severe disorder is incompatible with life because the oxygenated blood never reaches the aorta. Fortunately, in most instances, ASD and VSD are also present, turning the entire heart into a mixed circulatory system that does supply some oxygen to body cells. Transposition tends to occur in large newborns (9 to 10 lb) and occurs more often in boys than in girls. The disorder accounts for about 5% of congenital heart anomalies (Lange & Hillis, 2013).

Assessment. Infants with this disorder are usually cyanotic from the moment of birth. There may not be a heart murmur present, or there may be various murmurs, depending on the shunting of blood through atrial or ventricular defects or through the ductus arteriosus, which usually remains open. Echocardiography generally reveals the enlarged heart. Cardiac catheterization will reveal the low oxygen saturation resulting from the mixing of blood in the heart chambers.

Therapeutic Management. If no septal defect exists or if the defect is too small to allow enough mixing of blood to sustain life, PGE_1, a prostaglandin, will be administered to keep the ductus arteriosus patent and allow for a route of blood between the aorta and pulmonary artery. A balloon atrial septal pull-through operation may be done by cardiac catheterization to enlarge the septal openings. With this procedure, a deflated balloon catheter is passed from the right atrium through the foramen ovale into the left atrium. The balloon is then inflated, and the catheter is drawn back into the right atrium, enlarging the opening of the foramen ovale and creating an artificial ASD.

Surgical correction of transposition of the great arteries (an arterial switch procedure) is done at 1 week to 3 months of age and consists of, as the name implies, switching the placement of the pulmonary artery and aorta back to their usual positions. Because this is involved surgery, the child will be transported to a major center for surgery and care. Even with this significant a heart disorder, the survival rate following surgery is as high as 95%. Children need follow-up as they grow older to be certain that narrowing of the surgical sites does not occur, leading to lessened heart function as they grow older (Ruys, van der Bosch, Cuypers, et al., 2013).

Total Anomalous Pulmonary Venous Return

In this disorder, the pulmonary veins return to the right atrium or the superior vena cava instead of to the left atrium as they normally would. For blood to reach the systemic circulation, it must shunt across a patent foramen ovale or a PDA (Fig. 41.16). This disorder accounts for only 2% of all congenital heart disorders, and an absent spleen is often associated with the disorder. An infant with this disorder is usually mildly cyanotic and tires easily. If the ductus closes or the septal defect is small, cyanosis increases in amount; right-sided CHF will develop.

Surgery involves reimplanting the pulmonary veins into the left atrium. Until this can be scheduled, the child may be maintained on a continuous IV infusion containing PGE_1 to help keep the ductus arteriosus open; a balloon atrial septal pull-through procedure may be done to enlarge a small foramen ovale and allow better mixing of blood (Koneti, Kandraju, Kanchi, et al., 2012).

Truncus Arteriosus

Truncus arteriosus is a rare disorder (approximately 1% of initial cardiac lesions) in which one major artery or "trunk" arises from the left and right ventricles in place of separate aorta and pulmonary artery vessels (Fig. 41.17). There is a VSD accompanying this; the child is cyanotic and may have a typical VSD murmur. Repair involves restructuring the common trunk to create separate vessels. Some children will need a second surgical procedure by school age as their heart outgrows the graft inserted to separate the aorta and pulmonary artery (Panwar, Bradleym, & Kavarana, 2012).

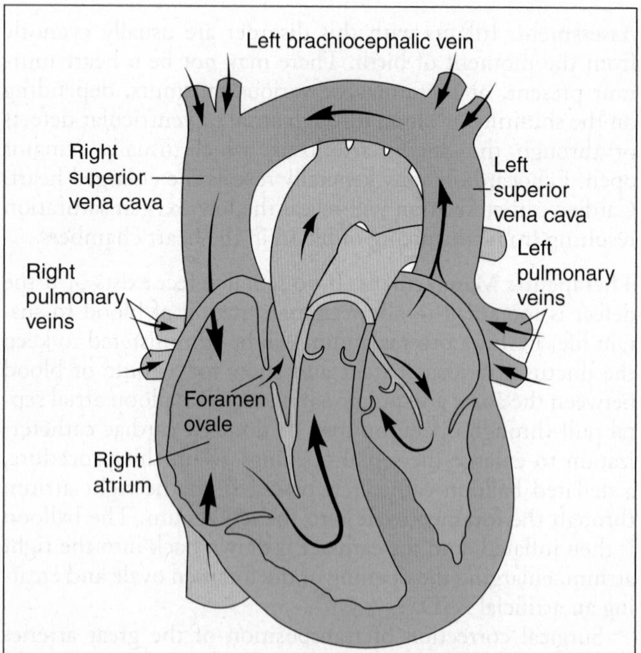

FIGURE 41.16 Total anomalous pulmonary venous return.

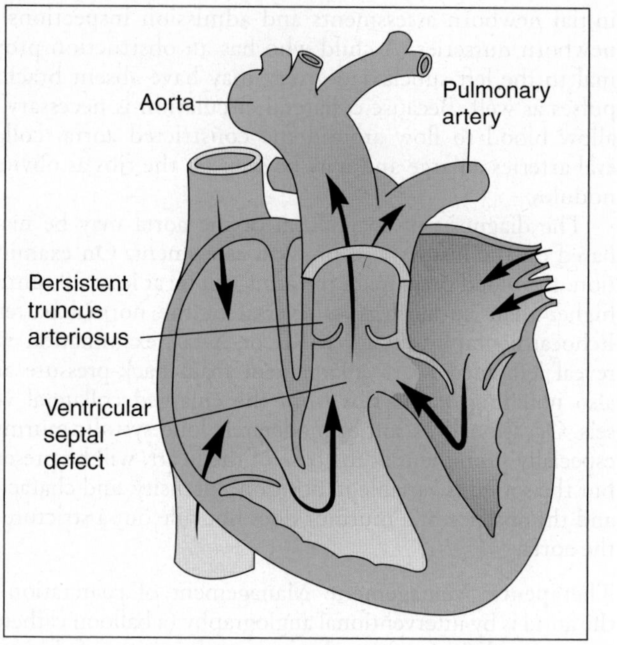

FIGURE 41.17 Truncus arteriosus.

Hypoplastic Left Heart Syndrome

In hypoplastic left heart syndrome, a rare disorder accounting for only 1% to 3% of congenital heart disease, the left ventricle is nonfunctional or lacks adequate strength to pump blood into the systemic circulation. In addition, there may be accompanying mitral or aortic valve atresia. As the right ventricle struggles to maintain the entire heart action, it greatly hypertrophies (Naguib, Dewhirst, Winch, et al., 2013).

The disorder may be detected by ultrasound prenatally. At birth, mild to moderate cyanosis develops within a few hours after birth as deoxygenated blood is shunted across the foramen ovale into the left atria because of the greater pressure on the right side of the heart. Echocardiography effectively diagnoses this condition. Prostaglandin therapy to maintain a PDA will be initiated to increase blood supply to the aorta. Inhaled nitrogen combined with oxygen may be prescribed to decrease Po_2 as this can increase pulmonary resistance and allow the right side of the heart to shift more blood into the left heart and aorta. Surgery has had significant success in this syndrome, using a three-stage procedure in restructuring the heart for adequate circulation.

Surgery begins with a Norwood procedure including a right ventricle–pulmonary artery shunt performed in the first week of life, followed by a Glenn procedure completed between 3 and 8 months. Finally, a Fontan procedure is performed between 18 months and 3 years of age for a final repair. Where once only heart transplant could correct this anomaly, with the improvements in survival rates with the three-stage reconstruction, heart transplantation is now reserved for children with unsuccessful surgical outcomes (Bondy, 2010).

Disorders With Decreased Pulmonary Blood Flow

As the category implies, disorders with decreased pulmonary blood flow involve some type of obstruction to blood flow in the pulmonary artery. Because of the obstruction, pressure increases in the right side of the heart. If an ASD or VSD also is present, deoxygenated blood may shunt into oxygenated blood.

Tricuspid Atresia

Tricuspid atresia is an extremely serious disorder because with this, the tricuspid valve is completely closed, allowing no blood to flow from the right atrium to the right ventricle or reach the lungs. In most infants, blood crosses through the patent foramen ovale into the left atrium, bypassing the lungs and the step of oxygenation. It reaches the lungs for oxygenation by being shunted back through a PDA (Fig. 41.18). As long as the foramen ovale and ductus arteriosus remain open, the child can obtain adequate oxygenation. At the point these close, however, the infant will develop extreme cyanosis, tachycardia, and dyspnea. An IV infusion of PGE_1 is begun to ensure the ductus remains open. Surgery consists of the construction of a vena cava–to–pulmonary artery shunt, which deflects more blood to the lungs, or a Fontan procedure (sometimes termed a Glenn shunt baffle), which restructures the right side of the heart.

Tetralogy of Fallot

Tetralogy of Fallot, one of the first types of congenital heart disease ever described, occurs in about 5% to 10% of children with congenital cardiac disease (Bacha, 2012). It is called a tetralogy because four anomalies are present: pulmonary stenosis, VSD (usually large), dextroposition (overriding) of the aorta, and hypertrophy of the right ventricle. Because of the pulmonary stenosis, pressure increases in the right side of the heart, causing blood to shunt from the right ventricle into the left ventricle and the overriding aorta. The extra effort involved to force blood through the stenosed pulmonary artery causes the fourth deformity, hypertrophy of the right ventricle (Fig. 41.19).

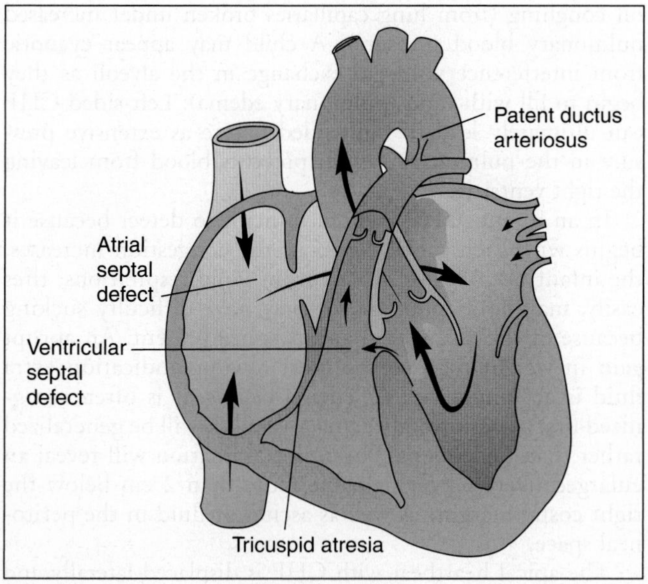

FIGURE 41.18 Tricuspid atresia.

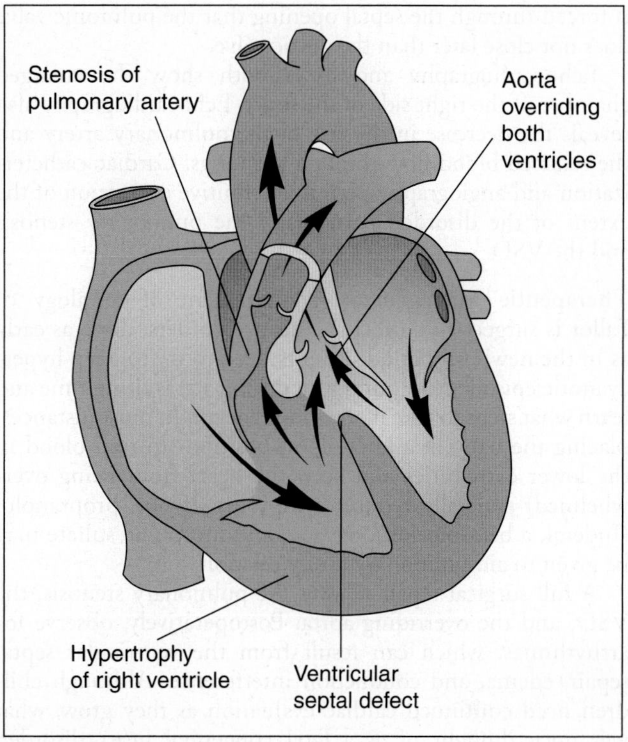

FIGURE 41.19 Tetralogy of Fallot.

Assessment. Although this is an extremely serious form of heart disease, newborns may not exhibit a high degree of cyanosis immediately after birth. As they become more active, however, their skin acquires a bluish tint. Polycythemia (an increase in the number of red blood cells) occurs as the body attempts to provide enough red blood cells to supply oxygen to all body parts. This creates an additional potential danger because the increased concentration of red blood cells causes the blood to become thick (increased viscosity), and clots in blood vessels may occur, resulting in complications such as thrombophlebitis, embolism, or cerebrovascular accident.

If the heart disorder is not corrected, a child will generally develop severe dyspnea, growth restriction, and clubbing of the fingers. The child tends to assume a squatting or a knee–chest position when resting because this offers physiologic relief to the overstressed heart by trapping blood in the lower extremities (Sharkey & Sharma, 2012). Children may develop syncope (fainting) and hypercyanotic episodes (sometimes called tet spells) caused by a temporary decreased blood and oxygen supply to the brain usually following prolonged crying or exertion. This can be so extreme, if long term, that children develop a cognitive challenge.

Tetralogy of Fallot is suspected based on the history and physical symptoms, including a loud, harsh, widely transmitted murmur or a soft, scratchy, localized systolic murmur in the left second, third, or fourth parasternal interspace. Although there is pulmonary artery narrowing, splitting of the second heart sound rarely occurs because so much blood is forced through the septal opening that the pulmonic valve does not close later than the aortic valve.

Echocardiography and ECG both show the enlarged chamber of the right side of the heart. Echocardiography also reveals the decrease in the size of the pulmonary artery and the reduced blood flow through the lungs. Cardiac catheterization and angiography permit a definitive evaluation of the extent of the disorder, particularly the pulmonary stenosis and the VSD.

Therapeutic Management. Management of tetralogy of Fallot is surgery to correct the heart disorders, done as early as in the newborn period. Parents need to try to keep hypercyanotic episodes to a minimum during any waiting time and learn what steps to take if one should occur. In most instances, placing the baby in a knee–chest position (to trap blood in the lower extremities and keep the heart from being overwhelmed) generally reduces symptoms. If not, propranolol (Inderal, a beta-blocker), oxygen, and morphine sulfate may be given to aid pulmonary artery dilation.

A full surgical repair relieves the pulmonary stenosis, the VSD, and the overriding aorta. Postoperatively, observe for arrhythmias, which can result from the ventricular septal repair, edema, and conduction interference. Although children need continued cardiac evaluation as they grow, what was once thought of as a fatal congenital heart disorder, tetralogy of Fallot is now a treatable disorder with a full life expectancy.

✔ QSEN Checkpoint Question 41.3

Safety

A danger for children with tetralogy of Fallot is that they develop "tet spells," or sudden periods of extreme cyanosis, often following exertion. When teaching Megan's parents to respond to such events, what should you encourage them to do first?

a. Take Megan's pulse and respiratory rate.
b. Place Megan in a knee–chest position.
c. Set Megan upright in her infant car seat or a high chair.
d. Begin chest compressions.

Look in Appendix A for the best answer and rationale.

ACQUIRED HEART DISEASE

Acquired heart disease in children results from a number of different conditions, any of which can lead to CHF.

Congestive Heart Failure

Congestive heart failure occurs when the myocardium of the heart is overwhelmed and unable to pump and circulate enough blood to supply oxygen and nutrients to body cells. It usually occurs as a result of a congenital heart disorder during the first year of life, following cardiac surgery, or later on from a disease such as rheumatic fever, Kawasaki syndrome, or infectious endocarditis, conditions that weaken the heart muscle. The presence of severe anemia, hypocalcemia, and myocarditis can contribute to the heart's inability to function effectively (Dinardo, 2013).

Because blood cannot be pumped forward, it pools in the heart (excessive preload) or in the pulmonary or venous systems. The heart has two main compensatory methods to increase cardiac output and move blood forward. The first is to increase the number of ventricle beats per minute. The second is to lengthen muscle fibers so the ventricles are able to manage more blood with each heart stroke (ventricular hypertrophy). As long as these adaptations are able to maintain adequate cardiac output, the signs of CHF are not delectable. The heart's capacity for compensation is limited, however, particularly in infants, so, eventually, signs and symptoms of ventricular failure will surface.

Sympathetic nervous system stimulation causes the frequently seen symptoms of excessive sweating and pallor. As blood flow to the kidneys decreases, the glomerular filtration rate slows, resulting in stimulation of the renin–angiotensin system. This causes fluid and sodium to be retained in order to supply more blood flow to the kidneys. Both increased aldosterone secretion by the adrenal glands and increased antidiuretic hormone secretion by the pituitary gland join in to promote additional sodium retention. The additional fluid retained results in dependent edema.

Assessment

One of the first signs of CHF is tachycardia as the heart attempts to beat faster to move blood forward more effectively; this is quickly followed by tachypnea or rapid breathing to supply enough oxygen for blood transport. When a child has primary right-sided CHF, increased venous pressure and hepatomegaly (enlarged liver) occur from backpressure in the portal circulation. The child may feel irritable and restless from abdominal pain caused by the liver distention. Lower extremity edema, usually a primary sign in adults, tends to occur as a late sign of CHF in children (Box 41.4).

With left-sided CHF, back-pressure causes blood to accumulate in the pulmonary system causing orthopnea (difficulty breathing except in an upright position because of increased pulmonary congestion). The sound of rales (crackles) can be heard on auscultation; the child may produce bloody sputum on coughing (from lung capillaries broken under increased pulmonary blood pressure). A child may appear cyanotic from interference with gas exchange in the alveoli as they begin to fill with fluid (pulmonary edema). Left-sided CHF can ultimately lead to right-sided failure as extensive pressure in the pulmonary system prevents blood from leaving the right ventricle.

In an infant, CHF is often difficult to detect because it begins with such subtle signs. As the congestion increases, the infant becomes breathless from rapid respirations, tires easily, may be diaphoretic, or may have difficulty sucking because of the exhaustion and dyspnea present. An abrupt gain in weight may be the most obvious indication extra fluid is accumulating. As edema begins, it is often recognized first as periorbital edema; overall, it will be generalized rather than dependent. Physical examination will reveal an enlarged liver (a liver palpable more than 2 cm below the right costal margin) as well as ascites or fluid in the peritoneal space.

The apical heartbeat with CHF is displaced laterally and downward. As a rule, if the width of the heart can be per-

BOX 41.4 Nursing Care Planning Using Assessment

Assessing a Child With Congestive Heart Failure

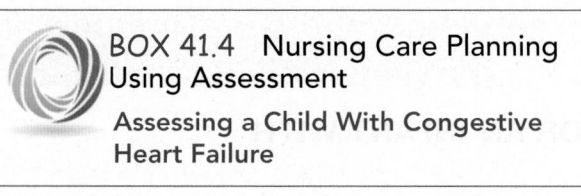

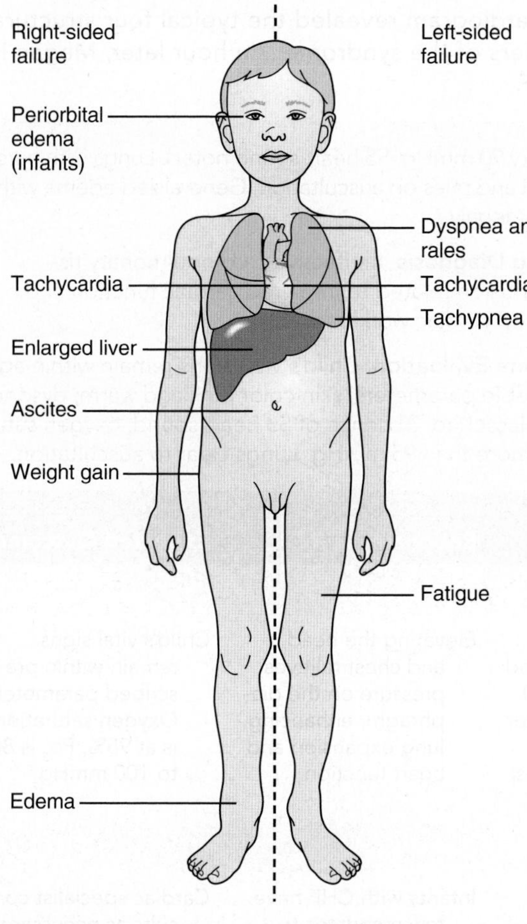

cussed as more than half the width of the chest (in a child over 1 year of age), it means the heart is enlarged. In addition, a galloping heart rhythm or an accentuated third heart sound may be heard because of the sudden distention of the ventricle during the rapid filling phase. CHF is confirmed by an echocardiograph. Ventricular hypertrophy can also be confirmed by ECG.

Therapeutic Management

Therapy for CHF consists of reducing the workload of the heart by measures such as evacuating the accumulated fluid with diuretics (reduces preload), slowing the heart rate and strengthening cardiac function by administering an inotropic (heart-strengthening) drug (increases contractility), and reducing afterload with a vasodilator.

A commonly used diuretic is furosemide (Lasix). The most common drug used to increase contractility and slow tachycardia is digoxin. Typical drugs used to decrease afterload are propranolol, a beta-blocker, or captopril, an angiotensin-converting enzyme (ACE) inhibitor (Karch, 2013).

Nursing Diagnoses and Related Interventions

Be certain outcomes established for the care of a child with congestive heart disease are realistic in light of the child's overall condition as well as individualized for each child. Interventions focus on helping support heart function and helping parents deal with this crisis until the child's heart is strong enough to maintain strong heart action. Box 41.5 shows an interprofessional care map illustrating both nursing and team planning for an infant with CHF.

Nursing Diagnosis: Ineffective cardiopulmonary and peripheral tissue perfusion related to inadequate heart function

Outcome Evaluation: Child's pulse, blood pressure, and respiratory rate are within acceptable parameters for age group; abnormal heart sounds, edema, and ascites are absent.

Provide for Rest Periods. Rest, a major aspect of care for a child with CHF, reduces the metabolic rate and, thus, also decreases myocardial and body oxygen demand. Most children with CHF feel more comfortable in a semi-Fowler's position than in a supine position because the chest-elevated position lowers the abdominal contents, enlarging the thoracic cavity and allowing easier, more comfortable lung expansion. Babies are most comfortable in an infant seat, which supports them in a semi-Fowler's position. Sedation with morphine may be necessary to encourage bed rest in some children. Most children with CHF, however, automatically limit their activity, so the need for sedation must be considered on an individual basis.

Organize nursing care to allow periods of sustained rest. At the same time, do not attempt to perform too many procedures at once or you will exhaust the child. Be certain the child's parents understand exactly how much rest the child is to have each day. Does it mean a child may eat by herself, or must she be fed? Does it mean bathroom privileges or not? Playtime or not? Unless children are exceptionally exhausted, most children need to be entertained or played with to remain on bed rest. Activities such as watching television, being read to, or listening to music are the type of activities that can promote better rest than if the child is expected to rest quietly without any diversion.

Provide Oxygen as Necessary. If a child has dyspnea, hypoxemia, or cyanosis, supplemental oxygen by way of mask or nasal prongs is usually necessary.

Remember oxygen is actually a drug and must be prescribed according to amount or oxygen parameters except when associated with resuscitation. Oxygen saturation should be monitored with pulse oximetry. If a child is receiving oxygen by nasal prongs, assess the nostrils about every 4 hours to detect

BOX 41.5 Nursing Care Planning

AN INTERPROFESSIONAL CARE MAP FOR AN INFANT WITH CONGESTIVE HEART FAILURE

Megan is a newborn who was born with tetralogy of Fallot. At 1 hour of age, she developed rapid respirations, tachycardia, and cyanosis. An echocardiogram revealed the typical four structural disorders of the syndrome. An hour later, Megan is in CHF.

Family Assessment Child's parents were divorced 1 month ago; dual custody of infant granted. Child will spend weekdays with mother, weekends with father. Father is a city bus driver; mother is a paralegal. Father to pay child support; with child support, mother rates finances as "workable."

Client Criteria One-hour-old infant girl who appears pale to cyanotic, tachycardic, and dyspneic. Child born by vaginal birth; Apgars 9 and 6. Afebrile; pulse, 150 beats/min; respirations, 36 breaths/min. Oxygen saturation via pulse oximetry 90 mmHg. S3 heart sound noted. Lungs with harsh rhonchi and rales on auscultation. Generalized edema with hepatomegaly.

Nursing Diagnosis Ineffective cardiopulmonary tissue perfusion related to impaired cardiac function and increased cardiac workload

Outcome Evaluation Child's vital signs remain within age-acceptable parameters; skin color pink and warm; dyspnea seems lessened. Absence of S3 heart sound; oxygen saturation more than 95 mmHg. Lungs clear to auscultation.

Team Member Responsible	Assessment	Intervention	Rationale	Expected Outcome
Activities of Daily Living, Including Safety				
Nurse	Assess vital signs and heart and lung sounds, as prescribed. Monitor oxygen saturation level via pulse oximetry.	Place infant in infant seat to elevate head and chest 30 to 60 degrees. Administer oxygen as prescribed. Protect rest time.	Elevating the head and chest relieves pressure on the diaphragm, enhancing lung expansion and heart function.	Child's vital signs remain within prescribed parameters. Oxygen saturation is at 95%. Po_2 is 80 to 100 mmHg.
Teamwork and Collaboration				
Nurse/Primary health care provider	Determine whether additional consultation will be necessary.	Consult with cardiac specialist team on call as necessary.	Infants with CHF have few resources to use to compensate for failing heart action.	Cardiac specialist consults as necessary to better stabilize infant's condition.
Procedures/Medications for Quality Improvement				
Nurse	Assess apical pulse before administering digoxin. Obtain serum digoxin levels as necessary.	Administer digoxin as prescribed.	Digoxin improves myocardial contractility.	Infant receives digoxin based on adequate heart rate and serum level.
Nurse	Obtain baseline weight. Assess electrolytes for hypokalemia before administering diuretics.	Monitor weight daily at same time. Administer diuretics, such as furosemide, as prescribed	Weight is an indicator of fluid balance. Diuretics reduce edema and diminish afterload. Potassium can be removed with urine.	Infant receives diuretics as prescribed, based on weight and potassium status.
Nurse/Respiratory therapist	Assess oxygen saturation with continuous pulse oximetry.	Administer oxygen by nasal cannula.	Oxygen enhances tissue perfusion; nasal cannula provides oxygen without obscuring infant's face.	Infant's oxygen saturation remains at 95% or above.

Nutrition				
Nurse	Assess child's intake and output for adequacy.	Assist mother to feed 24 calories per ounce of commercial formula every 4 hours as prescribed. Allow to rest halfway through feeding.	Eating requires energy expenditure, which could compromise heart function and interfere with nutrition.	Infant takes in prescribed formula without evidence of undue fatigue. Mother states she is comfortable feeding ill infant.
Patient-Centered Care				
Nurse	Assess parents' understanding of child's condition.	Educate parents as needed about congenital heart disease and CHF.	Parents need an understanding of child's illness to respect need for rest and medications.	Parents both state that they understand child's condition; necessary because both will be caregivers.
Psychosocial/Spiritual/Emotional Needs				
Nurse/Nurse practitioner	Assess whether parents feel they have enough emotional support to care for an ill infant at home while waiting for cardiac surgery at 2 months.	Discuss necessity for vigilance and keeping infant free of infection.	Respiratory infection could quickly worsen child's condition.	Parents state they understand the strain caring for an ill infant can cause. Have made arrangements for continuous care.
Informatics for Seamless Health Care Planning				
Nurse	Assess whether parents are familiar with cardiopulmonary resuscitation (CPR) technique for infants.	Teach parents infant CPR technique using CPR mannequin. Schedule appointment for 1-week follow-up visit.	Well-prepared parents can be the child's first line of defense. Weekly evaluation will help ascertain whether child's condition remains stable until corrective surgery.	Parents correctly demonstrate infant CPR technique on CPR mannequin. State they understand importance of follow-up visit and will keep appointment.

irritation and breakdown of the interior nostrils. Be certain to orient a child to oxygen equipment before you bring it to the bedside so you don't increase apprehension at the site of strange equipment. Once oxygen is started, however, children generally experience such relief from dyspnea that any remaining apprehension quickly disappears.

Administer Drugs as Prescribed to Improve Heart Action. Digoxin, a cardiac glycoside made from digitalis, acts directly on the heart to increase the contractility of the myocardium (and the force of contraction) and thus slows the heart rate. When it is first prescribed, an ECG and serum digoxin level are generally obtained before a second or third dose to assess that the dose is adequate and daily maintenance doses can begin.

Before administering a dose of digoxin, to be certain the child's heart rate is not already abnormally slow, always obtain a child's apical pulse. As a safety rule, the pulse rate should be above 100 beats/min in infants and above 70 beats/min in older children. As soon as digoxin begins to improve the strength of the heart's contraction, diuresis begins to relieve any edema present. Changes in the ECG (a lengthening of the P-R interval or a depression of the S-T segment) confirm digitalization has taken place.

The "window" between effective digitalization and digoxin toxicity is very narrow. Monitor serum digoxin levels closely, therefore, as prescribed. Observe for symptoms of toxicity such as anorexia, nausea and vomiting, dizziness, diarrhea, headache, arrhythmia, and bradycardia.

BOX 41.6 Nursing Care Planning to Empower a Family

GIVING DIGOXIN SAFELY AT HOME

Q. Megan's mother says to you, "The doctor has prescribed our daughter digoxin to take at home. Are there any special things we should do?"

A. Use the guidelines below to ensure safe digoxin administration at home:

- Always assess an apical pulse before administration; do not administer the drug if your child's heart rate is below 100 beats/min (or as specifically instructed as she grows older).
- Always use only a clearly marked syringe so the dose given is accurate and consistent.
- Do not change the amount or timing of the dose without specific instructions from your primary care provider.
- If you omit a single dose, give the next dose on time as prescribed. If you omit more than one dose, telephone your primary care provider for further instructions.
- Give digoxin 1 hour before or 2 hours after feeding, to avoid a dose being lost if the child spits up.
- If a dose is vomited, do not repeat the dose. Give the next dose at the scheduled time. If the child vomits the next dose, call your primary care provider as this could be a sign of toxicity.

Many children are discharged to home care on long-term administration of digoxin. Be certain parents understand the drug's correct dose and frequency of administration. Help them choose a specific time for administration to which they can adhere faithfully. Urge them to make out a reminder sheet or leave a reminder on their smartphone to help them remember to give the drug. Additional instructions for home administration of digoxin are shown in Box 41.6.

Diuretics such as furosemide (Lasix) may be administered as well to decrease pulmonary edema (which will reduce afterload). Taking a daily weight (at the same time, with the same scale, and the child in the same clothing or nude) is a good way to gauge the diuretic's effectiveness. Because large quantities of fluid can be lost through diuretics, remember that large amounts of potassium can be lost also, leading to hypokalemia (low serum potassium levels). To detect this, monitor urine output (typical urine output is 1 to 2 ml/kg/hr) and serum electrolyte levels, including the potassium level. Preventing hypokalemia is doubly important if a child is receiving digoxin because hypokalemia increases the risk of digoxin toxicity.

Hydrochlorothiazide is a typical diuretic used for long-term therapy in children. Because this is a thiazide diuretic, it can lead to extensive potassium excretion so a diet high in potassium and perhaps oral potassium supplementation may be prescribed to maintain potassium levels. Remember, if liquid potassium is prescribed, this is irritating to the gastrointestinal tract and should be given mixed with fruit juice.

QSEN Checkpoint Question 41.4

Quality Improvement

Children with CHF are often prescribed digoxin. Knowing that this drug possesses a high risk for adverse effects, you have provided educational materials to Megan's parents. Which statement by Megan's mother would alert you that she has not received all the education that she needs?

a. "I know the drug will slow down Megan's heart rate."
b. "It's important I give the exact dose every time."
c. "If I happen to miss a dose, I'll make sure not to 'double-dose' afterward."
d. "Nausea and vomiting are expected side effects for the first few weeks of treatment."

Look in Appendix A for the best answer and rationale.

Nursing Diagnosis: Risk for imbalanced nutrition, less than body requirements, related to fatigue

Outcome Evaluation: Child maintains percentile curve on growth chart; skin turgor remains good.

Maintaining proper nutrition may be a problem for children with CHF because they tire so easily. Eating six to eight small meals daily is often less tiring than eating three large meals. Smaller meals also prevent the child's stomach from pressing upward on the diaphragm and compromising an enlarged heart. Sucking is hard work, so infants may need to drink smaller amounts frequently to maintain adequate fluid intake or receive a higher calorie formula or fortified breast milk to allow for adequate calories without added fluid volume.

Nursing Diagnosis: Fear related to child's ill appearance and possible disease outcome

Outcome Evaluation: Parents and child openly discuss fears and concerns, actively question, and express confidence in treatment plan and health care team.

By school age, children with CHF are old enough to appreciate the seriousness of their condition. To help their heart work more efficiently, they may lie stiffly in bed, afraid to move or burden their already overtaxed heart with even simple activities such as turning pages in a book. Offer reassurance that, although their heart is a little behind in its action, the oxygen and medication they are receiving is making it stronger. If hospitalized, assure them people are checking on them frequently, both during and in between procedures. Offer time to talk or use therapeutic play so they can express their fears.

Parents of a child with CHF need the same assurance (provided the statements are true) because they are as frightened as the child by their child's obviously ill appearance. It is often helpful to point out subtle signs of improvement to parents that they may not notice on their own, such as a slower heart rate or slower, less distressed respirations.

If the child will be cared for at home, review CPR technique to be certain parents know how to use this in an emergency. Be certain they have a follow-up appointment scheduled and a telephone number they can call if they have any concerns about their child's condition.

✔ QSEN Checkpoint Question 41.5

Patient-Centered Care

Suppose Megan develops long-term CHF subsequent to tetralogy of Fallot. At school age, how could you best reconcile her physical limitations with her need for stimulation and activity?

a. Plan activities that are achievable and engaging, yet not overly physical.
b. Offer Megan rewards for challenging her physical stamina.
c. Lower Megan's expectations for activity and engagement until her condition resolves.
d. Teach her to focus solely on reading, writing, and other indoor pursuits.

Look in Appendix A for the best answer and rationale.

Persistent Pulmonary Hypertension

Persistent pulmonary hypertension (PPH) results when the high pulmonary vascular resistance present at birth, because of unopened alveoli, fails to resolve. The disorder occurs most often in full-term infants who have experienced perinatal asphyxia from conditions such as postterm birth (Lange & Hillis, 2013). The disorder occurs because hypoxia and acidosis from respiratory difficulty cause vasoconstriction of the pulmonary artery. The infant develops tachypnea, and pulse oximetry reveals a low Po_2 from inability of blood to perfuse the lungs. The resulting hypoxia and acidosis cause even greater vasoconstriction of the pulmonary artery. An echocardiogram shows right-to-left shunting across the patent ductus or foramen ovale.

Treatment consists of supportive therapy such as oxygen, ventilation, IV glucose to provide calories, antibiotics to combat infection, medications to reduce pulmonary resistance, and other drugs, such as low-dose dopamine, to elevate systemic blood pressure. Surfactant administration also has promising effects for vasodilation and reduced resistance (Karch, 2013). Inhaled nitric oxide is still another technique to promote pulmonary vasodilatation (Oishi, Datar, & Fineman, 2011). Infants who do not respond to these usual measures may require ECMO to allow the lungs to rest until adequate pulmonary vasodilatation and the return of alveoli perfusion can be achieved.

PPH is a severe threat to newborns, because of both the original insult from respiratory distress that produced the syndrome and the prolonged therapy course. As a result, a newborn may be left with a neurologic challenge from severe hypoxia and inadequate brain cell oxygen perfusion even after the hypertension improves.

Rheumatic Fever

Rheumatic fever is an autoimmune disease that occurs as a reaction to a group A beta-hemolytic streptococcal infection (Tandon, 2012). Inflammation from the immune response leads to fibrin deposits on the endocardium and valves, in particular the mitral valve, as well as in the major body joints. The source of the streptococcal infection is often an incident of pharyngitis, tonsillitis, scarlet fever, "strep throat," or impetigo. Although the development of rheumatic fever has declined greatly in recent years, the disease has not been eradicated, and in some inner cities and developing countries, the incidence is rising (Smith, Lester-Smith, Zurynski, et al., 2011). It occurs most often in children 6 to 15 years of age, with a peak incidence at 8 years. It is seen most often in poor, crowded urban areas. Because children do not develop immunity to streptococcal infections, streptococcal infections can recur; rheumatic fever can also recur.

The symptoms of the original streptococcal infection subside in a few days with or without antimicrobial therapy. Children appear well again. After 1 to 3 weeks, however, if the child was not treated with an appropriate antibiotic for the original infection, the onset of rheumatic fever symptoms can begin. Because nurses are the primary people who advise parents when to seek health care and how to adhere to medicine administration, nurses have contributed greatly to the decline of this disorder.

Assessment

The signs and symptoms of rheumatic fever are divided into major and minor symptoms according to the Jones criteria (Box 41.7). Of these, the heart involvement is the most serious. The child usually has a systolic murmur from mitral insufficiency and prolonged P-R and Q-T intervals on an ECG that reflect inflammation and slowing of impulse conduction. Sydenham chorea (sudden involuntary movement of the limbs) is a striking symptom that occurs in some children (Cardoso, 2011). This loss of voluntary muscle control, which results in dysfunctional speech and poor hand control, is due to inflammation of basal ganglia and occurs more often in girls than boys and most often in children between 7 and 14 years of age (rarely after age 20 years). The presence of dysfunctional speech can be demonstrated by asking the child to count rapidly. Children with chorea begin with clear speech, but then suddenly the sounds become garbled or they cannot speak for several seconds. If asked to protrude the tongue, children cannot keep from making undulating, jerky movements. If asked to extend their arms in front of them, they soon hyperextend their wrists and fingers. Hand grasp

BOX 41.7 Nursing Care Planning Using Assessment

Assessing a Child With Rheumatic Fever

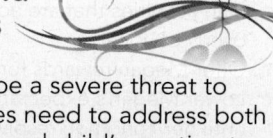

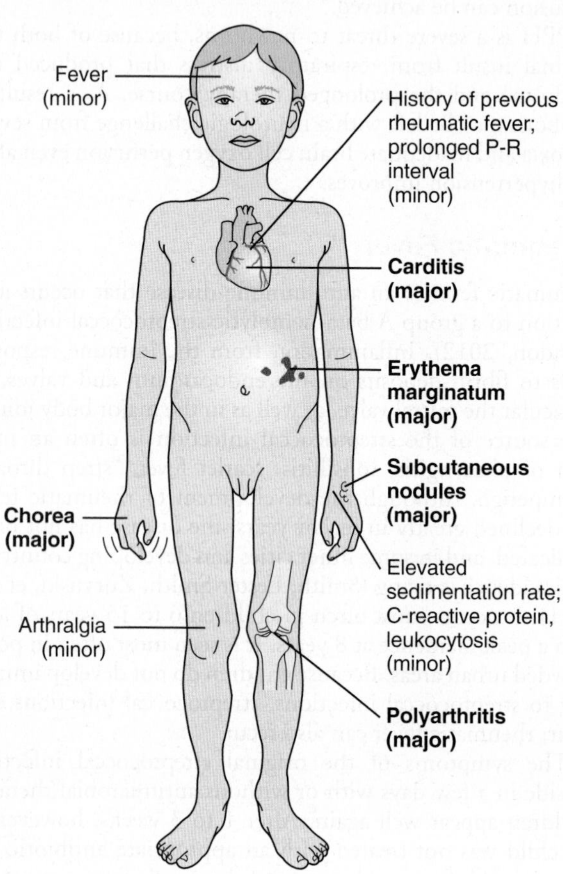

may be weak or may consist of spasmodic contractions and relaxation. If asked to smile, the facial expression may change rapidly from a "Cheshire cat" grin to a flat, expressionless affect or grimace.

Erythema marginatum, a macular rash found predominantly on the trunk; subcutaneous nodules (painless lumps) on tendon sheaths by the joints; and tender swollen large joints (polyarthritis) are additional frequent symptoms. Important laboratory findings include the presence of an antibody antistreptococcal titer (ASO) and increased ESR and C-reactive protein levels, proof the child had a resent streptococcal infection (Ralph & Carapetis, 2013).

Therapeutic Management

The course of rheumatic fever is about 6 to 8 weeks. Children are maintained on bed rest only during the acute phase of illness or until congestive heart disease is not present, the ESR decreases, and the C-reactive protein level and pulse rate return to normal. Because pulse rate is a valuable sign of improvement, monitoring vital signs is essential during and after the acute phase. Obtain an apical pulse for a full minute for best results. Taking it while the child is asleep as well as when the child is awake helps to measure the effect of activity on the pulse rate, another way to judge that inflammation is decreasing and the child's heart action is improving.

A course of penicillin therapy or a single intramuscular injection of benzathine penicillin will be prescribed to eliminate any group A beta-hemolytic streptococci remaining in the child's body. Oral ibuprofen or a corticosteroid may be prescribed to reduce inflammation and joint pain. Remember that possible side effects of corticosteroid therapy include hirsutism, a round moon face (Cushing syndrome), and an increased susceptibility to infection. Help children understand that these are a response to the drug and will fade when the medicine is halted.

Phenobarbital and diazepam are both effective in reducing the purposeless movements of chorea. If CHF is present, measures to reduce symptoms such as use of digoxin and diuretics will be prescribed.

The prognosis for the child with rheumatic fever depends on the extent of myocardial involvement. If Aschoff bodies (fibrin deposits) form on heart valves, permanent valve dysfunction, especially of the mitral valve, may occur. This is especially hazardous for girls, because either mitral insufficiency or stenosis may lead to CHF during pregnancy. As a result, some children need mitral valve replacement to restore heart function. Usually, there are no residual effects from joint or chorea involvement.

Nursing Diagnoses and Related Interventions

Because rheumatic fever can be a severe threat to heart health, nursing diagnoses need to address both physical care and the parents' and child's reaction to the serious diagnosis.

Nursing Diagnosis: Risk for nonadherence to drug therapy related to knowledge deficit about importance of long-term therapy

Outcome Evaluation: Child takes oral penicillin daily; absence of symptoms of throat infection; vital signs are within age-acceptable parameters.

Children who have had rheumatic fever must be prevented from contracting the disease again to prevent valve damage (or further valve damage) from occurring. To prevent further streptococcal infections, they are prescribed prophylactic antibiotic therapy either as a monthly injection of benzathine penicillin G or daily oral doses of aqueous penicillin (penicillin V) for at least 5 years after the initial attack, or until they are 18 years of age. If some valve involvement is present, taking oral penicillin indefinitely may be recommended.

Although it's becoming controversial, additional prophylactic measures may be recommended when dental or tonsillar surgery is planned, because, with an open incision in the mouth, there is risk for streptococcal invasion of the bloodstream (Dinsbach, 2012).

Nursing Diagnosis: Situational low self-esteem related to chorea movements secondary to rheumatic fever

Outcome Evaluation: Child expresses frustration with inability to control movements; child continues to feed and dress self with help as needed.

Children with chorea may be emotionally unstable and cry easily as well as have difficulty feeding themselves or working with small objects. Try to emphasize the transitory nature of this symptom; stress that you appreciate it is frustrating to have to be fed and to be unable to use your hands meaningfully, but this lack of coordination will pass without permanent effects. Provide toys and games that do not require fine coordination. Pad bedrails if necessary so a child on bed rest doesn't injure legs or arms by unintentionally striking them against the rails.

Kawasaki Syndrome

Kawasaki syndrome (mucocutaneous lymph node syndrome) is a febrile, multisystem disorder that occurs almost exclusively in children before the age of puberty; its incidence is so high that it has replaced rheumatic fever as the most likely cause of acquired heart disease in children. It tends to occur in late winter and spring and more in boys than girls. **Vasculitis** (inflammation of blood vessels) is a principal (and life-threatening) symptom because it can lead to formation of aneurysms or myocardial infarction.

The cause is unknown, but it appears to develop in genetically predisposed individuals after exposure to an as-yet-unidentified infectious agent. After the infection (perhaps an upper respiratory one), altered immune function leads to an increase in antibody production. Circulating immune (antibody–antigen) complexes begin to bind to the vascular endothelium, causing inflammation. This leads to aneurysms, platelet accumulation, and the formation of thrombi or obstruction in the heart and blood vessels.

Assessment

Kawasaki syndrome begins with an acute phase (stage I) of high fever (102° to 104°F [39.0° to 40.0°C]) that does not respond well to antipyretics (Box 41.8). The child acts lethargic or irritable and may have reddened and swollen hands and feet. Soon the mucous membrane of the eyes becomes inflamed (conjunctivitis) and the child develops a "strawberry" tongue plus red, cracked lips. A variety of rashes, often confined to the trunk or diaper area, may occur. Cervical lymph nodes appear swollen. As internal lymph nodes enlarge, children may develop abdominal pain, anorexia, and either diarrhea or bowel obstruction that occurs from swollen abdominal lymph nodes. Joints may be so swollen and reddened they simulate an arthritic process. White blood cell count and the ESR will both be elevated.

About 10 days after the onset, a subacute phase begins. The skin desquamates, particularly on the palms and soles. The platelet count rises, increasing the possibility of clotting, particularly in the fingertips, and if extreme, can result in necrosis of the fingertips or toes as blood circulation is decreased beyond a clot. If an aneurysm forms in a coronary artery, accumulating thrombi or rupture of the aneurysm can lead to decreased blood circulation and a myocardial infarction.

A convalescent phase (stage II) begins at about the 25th day and lasts until about 40 days. The last stage (stage III) is the time period after 40 days until the ESR returns to normal.

BOX 41.8 Nursing Care Planning Using Assessment

Assessing a Child With Kawasaki Syndrome

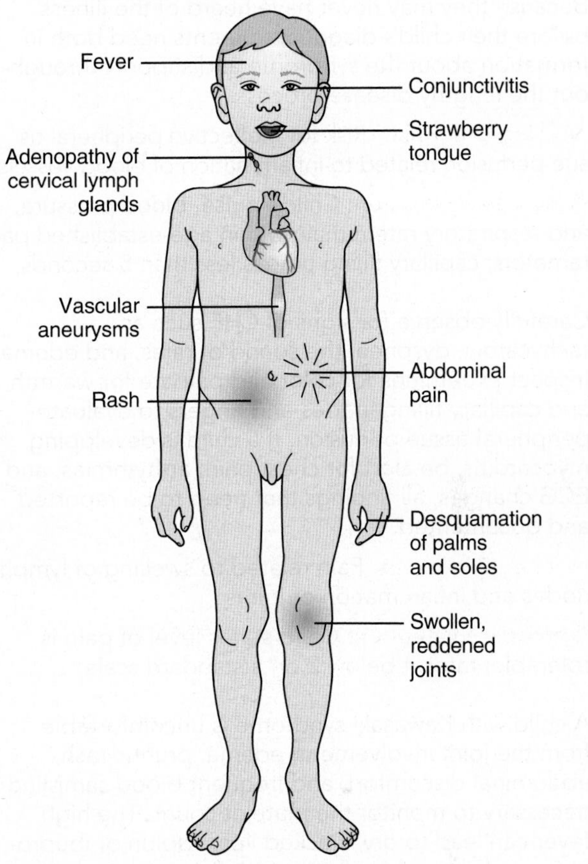

Therapeutic Management

The administration of acetylsalicylic acid (aspirin), ibuprofen, or other platelet receptor inhibitors is prescribed to decrease inflammation and block further platelet aggregation (Karch, 2013). Administration of IV immune globulin (IVIG) is a possibility to reduce the immune response (Dominguez & Anderson, 2013). Caution parents that children should not receive routine immunizations while taking IVIG or the immunization will be ineffective. Steroids are also contraindicated because these may increase aneurysm formation. If the child is left with coronary artery disease from stenosis or aneurysms of the coronary arteries, coronary artery bypass surgery may be necessary in the future.

Nursing Diagnoses and Related Interventions

Kawasaki syndrome is a frightening illness because of the danger of a coronary artery aneurysm forming. Because they may never have heard of the illness before their child's diagnosis, parents need both information about the syndrome and support throughout the lengthy disease process.

Nursing Diagnosis: Risk for ineffective peripheral tissue perfusion related to inflammation of blood vessels

Outcome Evaluation: Child's pulse, blood pressure, and respiratory rate remain within age-established parameters; capillary filling time is less than 5 seconds.

Carefully observe for signs of CHF such as tachycardia, dyspnea, the sound of rales, and edema. Inspect extremities for color and palpate for warmth and capillary filling in toes and fingers to evaluate peripheral tissue perfusion. If a child is developing myocarditis, be alert for chest pain, arrhythmias, and ECG changes, all findings that need to be reported and documented.

Nursing Diagnosis: Pain related to swelling of lymph nodes and inflammation of joints

Outcome Evaluation: Child states level of pain is tolerable; rates it below 2 on a standard scale.

A child with Kawasaki syndrome is uncomfortable from the joint involvement, edema, pruritic rash, abdominal discomfort, and frequent blood sampling necessary to monitor the platelet count. The high fever can lead to dry, cracked lips. Aspirin or ibuprofen, administered for their anti-inflammatory action, helps reduce both the pain and itchiness (which is a low level of pain). Provide additional comfort measures such as rocking and holding or distraction. Try to protect edematous areas from pressure; make certain clothing is not constricting and irritating areas of rash. Applying lip balm helps protect lips from drying and cracking.

Because the child's fever remains high, offer extra fluid to help maintain hydration and reduce mouth tenderness. Keep the child free of heavy blankets or clothing, and prevent overexertion. Monitor IV fluid to prevent fluid overload.

Children with Kawasaki syndrome lose their appetite and generally eat poorly because of the systemic illness, mouth soreness from cracks and fissures, and abdominal pressure from swollen lymph nodes. Carefully monitor and record the child's intake and output to be certain intake is adequate. Observe for signs of gastrointestinal obstruction, such as vomiting. Encourage the child to continue brushing his or her teeth (use a soft toothbrush or a commercial swab), even though the oral mucous membrane is tender, to prevent tooth decay or ulcer formation. Soft, nonirritating foods such as gelatin (Jell-O) may be better tolerated than foods that require chewing or acidic fluids, such as orange juice, which might sting.

Most children with Kawasaki syndrome recover fully, although if they experienced coronary artery involvement, they will need conscientious follow-up; a few may need cardiac bypass surgery to improve coronary artery circulation.

What if...41.3 Megan's hospital roommate, who has Kawasaki syndrome, has ibuprofen prescribed every 4 hours but tells you she no longer has pain or fever. Should you continue to give the ibuprofen?

Infectious Endocarditis

Infectious endocarditis is inflammation and infection of the endocardium or valves of the heart. It may occur in a child without heart disease but more commonly occurs as a complication of congenital heart disease such as tetralogy of Fallot, VSD, or coarctation of the aorta. The infection is generally caused by streptococci of the viridans type, although staphylococcal or fungal organisms may be at fault. The streptococcal infection tends to invade the body during oral surgery, such as with dental extractions. It also can enter from a urinary tract infection or a skin infection, such as impetigo. As the disease progresses, vegetation composed of bacteria, fibrin, and blood appears on the endocardium of the valves and heart chambers. The invasion tends to occur more commonly on the left side of the heart, although if a heart disorder is present, erosion begins at the site of the disorder. Over a period of time, the invading process destroys the endocardial lining of the heart, underlying muscle, and valves (Johnson, Boyce, Cetta, et al., 2012).

Assessment

The onset of the illness is insidious. Children often appear pale, with anorexia and weight loss, arthralgia (pain in joints), malaise, chills, or periods of sweating, especially at night. As the vegetative process begins to erode the heart's valves, significant murmurs become audible and signs of CHF appear. Petechiae of the conjunctiva or oral mucosa or hemorrhages of the fingernails or toenails (that simulate a splinter inserted under the nail) are still other signs. On physical assessment, the spleen may be enlarged; the child may notice left upper quadrant abdominal pain from infarction of the spleen. Laboratory studies will reveal proteinuria or hematuria; a normochromic, normocytic anemia from red blood cells being destroyed by the uneven heart valves; leukocytosis; and an increased ESR. An echocardiogram will show the growths on the heart valves. A blood culture will reveal and confirm the presence of the invading organism.

Therapeutic Management

Children with unrepaired congenital heart disease, those who have a prosthetic patch, or those who have had rheumatic fever are typically prescribed prophylactic administration of an antibiotic before ear, nose, throat, tonsil, or mouth surgery (and before childbirth) to help prevent infectious endocarditis. If endocarditis occurs despite these preventive measures, therapy is directed toward the underlying infection and supportive measures to reduce CHF. Because the invading organism is generally *Streptococcus*, a penicillinase-resistant penicillin such as nafcillin or a combination of vancomycin, gentamicin, and rifampin is prescribed and given IV through a central venous access device. Children need long-term follow-up care to be certain the invading organism is fully eliminated and the disease process has halted. Once the organism is eliminated, the prognosis is good unless an embolus from the vegetation on the valves causes a complication such as renal occlusion or cerebrovascular accident (Wei, Wu, Sy, et al., 2010).

Arrhythmias

Children have fewer cardiac arrhythmias than adults, but the number of these is increasing as more and more children survive congenital heart disease because of cardiac surgery but are left with a cardiac arrhythmia due to septal trauma. Better means of monitoring cardiac rhythm patterns through the use of Holter monitors has also made detection of cardiac arrhythmias easier. Remember not to confuse normal sinus arrhythmia (the heart slows during inspiration but increases again on expiration), which tends to occur in school-age children, with a cardiac arrhythmia.

Ventricular tachycardia and atrial fibrillation are syndromes that occur because of multiple or abnormal initiation of the heartbeat and can occur following surgery for congenital heart disease. These can cause episodes of syncope, palpitations, and exercise intolerance. If bradycardia occurs, it can be treated with a drug such as atropine to counteract vagal stimulation and increase heart rate; digoxin is commonly used for decreasing and strengthening the heart rate if needed. A few children may require pacemakers implanted to maintain a steady heart rhythm (Beery et al., 2011). Cryoablation and radioablation are nonsurgical transvenous catheter techniques that can permanently disrupt an abnormal arrhythmia focus.

Hypertension

Primary hypertension occurs in only about 1% of children, and most hypertension seen in children is usually associated with a secondary disorder such as kidney disease, coarctation of the aorta, Cushing syndrome, primary hyperaldosteronism, adrenogenital syndrome, pheochromocytoma (a tumor of the adrenal gland), metabolic syndrome, or brain tumor. It has a higher incidence among black children than other ethnic groups and in children who are obese.

It is difficult to define hypertension in children because normal blood pressure varies with the age of the child. A systolic pressure reading above the 95th percentile for a given age may be used as a practical criterion (AAP, 2012).

Assessment

Beginning at 3 years of age, blood pressure should be included as part of routine health assessment. To ensure accuracy, be sure a child is relaxed, after at least 1 or 2 minutes of rest, before taking a blood pressure. When children are discovered on routine physical assessment to have hypertension, the reading should be repeated at a successive visit to confirm that the abnormal reading was not a reaction to the stress of the examination or some other emotional event of that day.

When a child is discovered to be hypertensive, a number of additional studies are prescribed to discover whether an underlying disease condition exists. For example, blood pressure recording of both lower and upper extremities helps to rule out coarctation of the aorta, and a urine specimen for analysis of blood or microalbuminuria may be taken to detect kidney disease. Further studies to rule out adrenal disease or increased intracranial pressure may be prescribed if these preliminary assessment procedures do not reveal a cause for the hypertension (AAP, 2012).

Therapeutic Management

Therapy to reduce hypertension caused by a secondary illness is therapy for the secondary disease. If essential hypertension (elevated blood pressure for no identifiable reason) is present and a child is obese, a weight-reducing diet with an increased level of exercise is recommended. Salt intake is rarely limited in children, although it may be recommended if salt intake has been excessive; adolescent girls are advised to use another reproductive life planning choice than estrogen-based oral contraceptives because these can elevate blood pressure. In adolescents, increasing the amount of sleep may also be helpful in reducing stress and development of hypertension (Narang, Manlhiot, Davies-Shaw, et al., 2012). Unfortunately, because mild hypertension produces few symptoms, often children do not adhere to nutritional suggestions or suggested exercise programs so their hypertension doesn't decrease. For these children, a single medication such as an ACE inhibitor (e.g., captopril [Capoten]) may be prescribed. A diuretic such as hydrochlorothiazide may also be added.

Children with hypertension need continued counseling at health care visits so they're aware of the long-term detrimental effects of hypertension (increased risk of heart and blood vessel disease) and, hopefully, can see the benefits of taking medication (Herouvi, Karanasios, Karayianni, et al., 2013).

Dyslipidemia

Dyslipidemia (increased lipids in blood serum) can involve both cholesterol and triglycerides. Risk factors include familial hypercholesterolemia, a dominantly inherited disease occurring in 5% to 25% of children; obesity; a sedentary lifestyle; and a high-fat diet (AAP, 2012). For this reason, all children of parents with premature coronary artery disease (disease before the age of 55 years) or a family history of hypercholesterolemia (parents with blood cholesterol levels above 200 mg/dl or LDL levels above 130 mg/dl) should be screened for total serum cholesterol, because of the association between high total cholesterol and LDL and the incidence of coronary artery disease. This is particularly important if the child smokes, is obese, or has a sedentary lifestyle.

Acceptable levels of total cholesterol and LDL in children are less than those in adults: 170 mg/dl and less than 110 mg/dl, respectively. Total cholesterol and LDL levels are considered borderline if they are 170 to 199 mg/dl and 110 to 129 mg/dl, respectively; they are high if over 200 mg/dl and 130 mg/dl, respectively (National Heart, Lung, and Blood Institute, 2012).

If the total triglyceride, cholesterol, or LDL levels are found to be elevated, the child's diet should be regulated and an exercise program begun in an attempt to lower these levels. Adolescents may be placed on the AHA's Step 1 Diet (look for foods with less than 6.5 g total fat, 1 g or less of saturated fat, less than 0.5 g of trans fats, and cholesterol of 20 g or less) to attempt to bring them into adulthood with sound nutritional habits (AHA, 2013). Younger children rarely are placed on low-fat diets because they need calories for growth. Use of low-fat diets in infants under 2 years of age is even less common because fat is needed for myelinization of nerve fibers.

If the child becomes an adolescent and the diet has not been effective, one of the many cholesterol-reducing agents such as cholestyramine (Questran) may be prescribed. These agents reduce the cholesterol level by binding bile acids and decreasing their reabsorption. Side effects of these drugs include large, bulky stools and possible gastrointestinal discomfort. If this therapy is ineffective, an HMG-CoA inhibitor such as atorvastatin (Lipitor) may be prescribed.

Because hypercholesterolemia has no symptoms, it is difficult to motivate children to continue a special diet and take medication unless the entire family changes to a lower fat diet and exercises more. Children need continued counseling at health care visits so they understand the damage that excess lipids can cause to coronary arteries (Lipshultz, Schaechter, Carrillo, et al., 2012).

Cardiomyopathy

The term "cardiomyopathy" refers to a structural or functional abnormality of the ventricular myocardium that occurs following an infection such as adenovirus, cytomegalovirus, or HIV/AIDS infection and results in severe dilation of the left ventricle or both ventricles (Mares & Bar-Cohen, 2012). This impairs systolic function and leads to CHF. Idiopathic dilated cardiomyopathy is a rare form that presents before 2 years of age, usually after a viral respiratory or gastrointestinal illness. Hypertrophic cardiomyopathy is a relatively common autosomal dominant disease that tends to show symptoms in young adults.

In an older child, symptoms appear gradually. Physical examination will reveal an ill-appearing child in severe respiratory distress. Peripheral pulses are weak, and blood pressure is decreased. Pulsus alternans (beat-to-beat variation) and an enlarged liver from back-pressure are both common findings. A chest X-ray, echocardiogram, and ECG all reveal the enlarged heart.

Therapy is directed at controlling the CHF by bed rest, fluid restriction, and pharmacologic agents to decrease the cardiac load, improve myocardial contractility, and decrease afterload. Immune globulin may be helpful in reversing the process. If a child fails to respond to medical therapy, cardiac transplantation is a final solution.

CARDIOPULMONARY ARREST

Children with heart disease are at high risk for cardiopulmonary arrest, although this may occur in any child for reasons such as airway obstruction, trauma, an anaphylactic reaction, central nervous system depression, drowning, or electrocution. Exact management of cardiopulmonary arrest may vary according to the cause of the arrest and the age of the patient, but the basic considerations are the same.

Many health care facilities and public buildings provide automated external defibrillators (AEDs) for use in cardiac resuscitation. Nurses who respond to emergencies need to familiarize themselves with this equipment as well as CPR technique (AHA, 2010).

Assessment

Respiratory failure is the most frequent cause of cardiac arrest because anoxia in the heart muscle quickly leads to cardiac arrest. When cardiac arrest occurs, no audible heart sounds or pulses can be obtained. No blood pressure can be recorded (do not waste time trying to obtain one). If a cardiac monitor was attached before the arrest, it will show no ECG complex. This is a helpful assessment if available, but again, do not waste time attaching monitor leads if they are not already in place. The outcome for the child in arrest will depend to a great extent on the speed with which resuscitation is begun, so it is better to err on the side of unnecessary resuscitation rather than delayed resuscitation. The steps for resuscitation can be remembered as "CAB" (***c***hest compressions, ***a***irway, and ***b***reathing); this may be followed by defibrillation. The health care professional should spend no more than 10 seconds checking for responsiveness or pulse before beginning effective chest compressions.

Chest Compressions

The depth of chest compressions on a child should be one third the anterior–posterior diameter depth of the child's chest (about 1½ in. in an infant and 2 in. in an older child); be certain to allow full recoil of the chest between compressions, and compressions should be at a rate of 100 per minute (Figs. 41.20 and 41.21). If the resuscitation attempt is successful, the child's color will improve (especially the oral mucous membrane, which is readily visible) and the carotid pulse will become palpable.

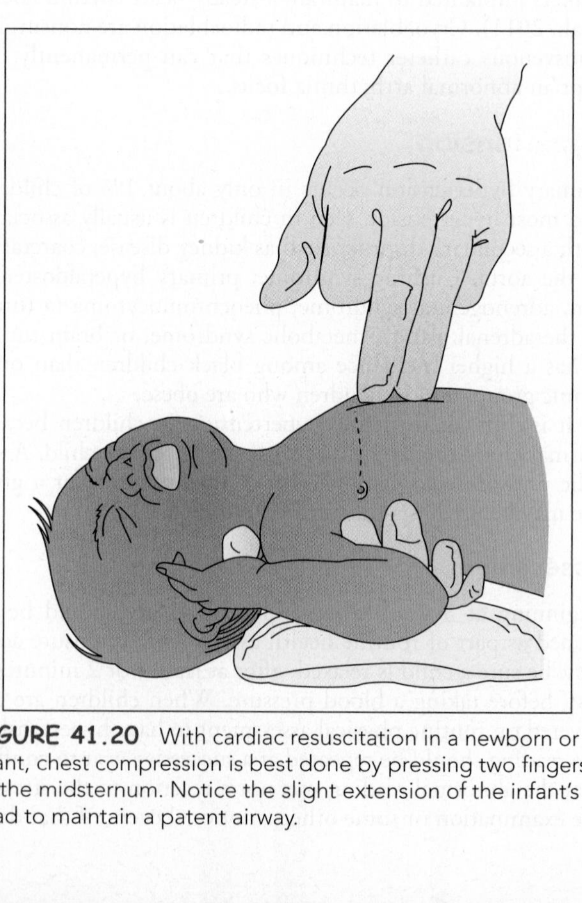

FIGURE 41.20 With cardiac resuscitation in a newborn or infant, chest compression is best done by pressing two fingers on the midsternum. Notice the slight extension of the infant's head to maintain a patent airway.

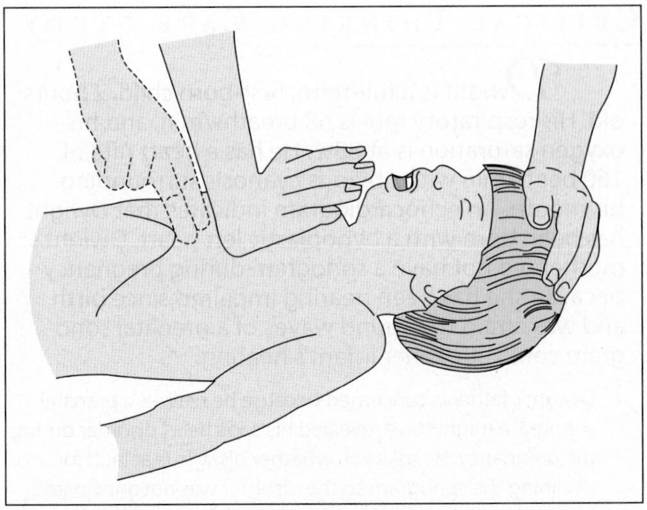

FIGURE 41.21 Locating hand position for cardiac compression in an older child.

Airway

Emergency equipment such as an Ambu-bag should be readily available in all health care settings so that mouth-to-mouth resuscitation is not necessary. If no breathing bag is available, use a protective one-way valve mask for mouth-to-mouth resuscitation to protect yourself from body secretions.

For small infants, place the bag mask over the infant's mouth and nose, creating a seal. For larger infants and children, make a bag-to-mouth seal, pinching the child's nose tightly with the thumb and forefingers. Provide two slow breaths (1 to 1.5 seconds per breath). It may be necessary to adjust the head-tilt chin position to obtain optimal airway patency, although this should not be done if neck or spine trauma is suspected (AHA, 2010).

Breathing

For a single rescuer, the ratio of compression to airway is 30:2, and for two rescuers, the ratio is 15:2. Minimize any interruptions for less than 10 seconds. Do not lift your fingers or hands off the chest during breaths because doing so requires time spent to properly reposition them. Also make sure to maintain a patent airway by using the head-tilt chin lift using the hand not performing the compressions.

If oxygen is available, attach it to the resuscitation bag at a rate of about 4 L/min. However, do not wait for oxygen if it is not available. Room air's oxygen content is about 21%, so additional oxygen is helpful but not necessary for resuscitation. Observe the child's chest with each breath you administer to see if it rises. When the AED arrives, attach it and follow directions as to whether further shock or continued CPR is needed.

These three techniques (chest compressions, airway, and breathing) will provide adequate oxygenation to major body organs for several minutes until additional personnel arrive who can then initiate further resuscitation measures. The outcome of these secondary measures depends on how well and promptly the initial measures were performed.

QSEN Checkpoint Question 41.6

Teamwork & Collaboration

It is important that all members of the care team be certified to perform CPR. What action should you perform first if you have to administer CPR?

a. Ready a defibrillator and place it on standby.
b. Take and record her carotid or apical pulse.
c. Blow two strong breaths of air into her mouth.
d. Begin chest compressions at a rate of 100 per minute.

Look in Appendix A for the best answer and rationale.

Secondary Measures

IV access for drug administration is a fourth step of resuscitation. If it is not possible after several attempts to locate an accessible vein, such as could happen in a severely burned child, an intraosseous catheter can be inserted (see Chapter 38). Drugs administered through an intraosseous route reach the circulation as rapidly as IV administration because of the rich blood supply in bone. Drugs such as epinephrine, lidocaine, and atropine also may be given by an endotracheal tube, again, if IV administration is not available. The dose of drugs given by an endotracheal route is larger than that used for IV administration. The drug is first diluted with normal saline, administered by a catheter inserted deeply into the endotracheal tube, and followed by an additional 1 or 2 ml of normal saline and several positive-pressure breaths to move the drug into the lungs.

Psychological Support

A cardiopulmonary arrest is an acute emergency, and everyone who arrives at the scene should know the next step needed and what course of action to take (Pye, Kane, & Jones, 2010). As soon as children begin to respond to resuscitation, be aware that they begin to hear. They may be frightened by the number of people and all the equipment surrounding them as well as vivid memories of frightening body sensations they experienced just before going into cardiac arrest. A child may regain consciousness, therefore, struggling and fighting. Assure the child as quickly as possible that everyone is there to help. It is extremely frightening for parents to see their child suddenly stop breathing. Although it was comforting to see emergency personnel arrive promptly and efficiently, parents are as frightened as the child to realize their child is ill enough to need such skilled personnel. Provide specific information to them on the child's condition as soon as it is available, therefore, and keep them updated (Litak, 2012). If they were not in the room during the resuscitation, allow them to see their child as soon as possible afterward so they can assure themselves their child is breathing and has heart function again. Be certain they know that any follow-up procedures such as ECG monitoring or blood-gas measurements are being scheduled to prevent another emergency, not because anything new is happening. In contrast, offer support to help them begin grieving if the child does not survive the resuscitation attempt (Litak, 2012).

What if . . . 41.4 You are particularly interested in exploring one of the 2020 National Health Goals related to achieving cardiovascular health in childhood (see Box 41.1). What would be a possible research topic to explore pertinent to this goal that would be applicable to Megan's family and also advance evidence-based practice?

Key Points for Review

- Cardiovascular disorders in children may be either structural, such as congenital heart disease, or acquired, such as Kawasaki syndrome, rheumatic fever, or cardiomyopathy. Assessment of children with heart disease includes history and physical examination. Echocardiogram, MRI, and cardiac catheterization are procedures used frequently for diagnosis.
- Congenital heart disorders are classified as those associated with increased pulmonary blood flow, decreased pulmonary blood flow, obstruction to blood flow, and mixed blood flow.
- Common signs of CHF seen in children include tachycardia, tachypnea, enlarged liver, dyspnea, and cyanosis. Signs tend to be subtle in infants and may be manifested chiefly by difficulty in feeding from exhaustion and dyspnea.
- Hypertension in children usually occurs as a result of a secondary disorder. Helping families limit saturated fat intake and follow a consistent exercise program to help children avoid obesity and heart disease in later life is a strategy that not only meets QSEN competencies but also best meets the family's total needs.
- Surgical repair, heart transplant, and pacemaker insertion are all possible therapies for children born with congenital heart disease.
- The families of children undergoing cardiac surgery need a great deal of support from health care personnel so they can cope with this major event in order to be able to provide effective support to their child.
- Postcardiac surgery syndrome and postperfusion syndrome are two complications that may occur after cardiac surgery related to the extracorporeal circulation used during the procedure.
- Rheumatic fever is an autoimmune disease that occurs after a group A beta-hemolytic streptococcal infection. Taking prophylactic penicillin after the illness until age 18 years helps prevent further recurrence and cardiac involvement. Some children with congenital heart disease may also need this same protective routine.
- Kawasaki syndrome results from altered immune function. An inflammation of blood vessels leads to platelet aggregation and formation of thrombi and aneurysms. Infectious endocarditis is an infection of the endocardium of the heart. It may be a complication of congenital heart disease.
- Children with heart disease are at high risk for cardiopulmonary arrest. Nurses and parents need to know how to perform CPR to be prepared for this emergency.

Critical Thinking Care Study

Dwight is a full-term, first-born child, 2 hours old. His respiratory rate is 68 breaths/min, and his oxygen saturation is at 88%. He has a heart rate of 160 beats/min with obvious cyanosis surrounding his mouth. An echocardiogram indicates that Dwight has been born with a hypoplastic left heart. Dwight's mother did not have a sonogram during pregnancy because she has been hearing impaired since birth and was afraid the sound waves of a prenatal sonogram could affect her infant's hearing.

1. Dwight's father is concerned because he realizes a prenatal sonogram might have revealed his son's heart disorder during the pregnancy. He asks you whether his wife is at fault for declining the sonogram so the disorder was not anticipated or whether he is at fault for not realizing the sonogram might have been important. How should you respond?
2. You are preparing a prostaglandin infusion for Dwight. How would you explain to the father the purpose of this infusion?
3. Dwight's father tells you he is worried his health insurance will not cover the three separate surgeries described by the cardiac surgeon. "Is he trying to make money off of us?" he asks you. "Or are the three procedures really necessary?" How should you respond?

Patient Scenario

The Tamel Family

Read about the Tamel family, a family with a child with rheumatic fever, then answer the questions to further sharpen your skills and grow more familiar with NCLEX-type questions related to cardiac disorders in children. Confirm your answers are correct by reading the rationales.

Visit http://thePoint.lww.com

Answers and Rationales

Looking for answers to the What if . . . and Critical Thinking Care Study questions?

Visit http://thePoint.lww.com

References

Algra, S. O., Driessen, M. M., Schadenberg, A. W., et al. (2012). Bedside prediction rule for infections after pediatric cardiac surgery. *Intensive Care Medicine, 38*(3), 474–481.

Almond, C. S., Singh, T. P., Gauvreau, K., et al. (2011). Extracorporeal membrane oxygenation for bridge to heart transplantation among children in the United States. *Circulation, 123*(25), 2975–2984.

Altamimi, S., Khalil, A., Khalaiwi, K. A., et al. (2012). Short-term late-generation antibiotics versus longer term penicillin for acute streptococcal pharyngitis in children. *Cochrane Database of Systematic Reviews,* (8), CD004872.

Ameduri, R. K., Zheng, J., Schechtman, K. B., et al. (2012). Has late rejection decreased in pediatric heart transplantation in the current era? A multi-institutional study. *Journal of Heart & Lung Transplantation, 31*(9), 980–986.

American Academy of Pediatrics. (2012). *Recommendations for preventive pediatric health care.* Evanston, IL: Author.

American Heart Association. (2010). *Pediatric advanced life support.* Dallas, TX: Author.

American Heart Association. (2013). *Heart-check mark nutrition guidelines.* Dallas, TX: Author.

Asif, I. M., Rao, A. L., & Drezner, J. A. (2013). Sudden cardiac death in young athletes: What is the role of screening? *Current Opinion in Cardiology, 28*(1), 55–62.

Bacha, E. (2012). Valve-sparing options in tetralogy of Fallot surgery. *Seminars in Thoracic & Cardiovascular Surgery: Pediatric Cardiac Surgery Annual, 15*(1), 24–26.

Beery, T. A., Smith, C. R., Kudel, I., et al. (2011). Measuring sports participation decisional conflict in youth with cardiac pacemakers and/or ICDs. *Journal of Advanced Nursing, 67*(4), 821–828.

Bernstein, D. (2012). Congenital heart disease. In R. M. Kliegman, B. F. Stanton, J. W. St. Geme III, et al. (Eds.), *Nelson textbook of pediatrics* (19th ed., pp. 1549–1600). Philadelphia, PA: Saunders/Elsevier.

Bharucha, T., & Mertens, L. (2013). Recent advances in pediatric echocardiography. *Expert Review of Cardiovascular Therapy, 11*(1), 31–47.

Bondy, C. A. (2010). Hypoplastic left heart syndrome. *The New England Journal of Medicine, 362*(21), 1533–1544.

Brancaccio, G., Filippelli, S., Michielon, G., et al. (2012). Ventricular assist devices as a bridge to heart transplantation or as destination therapy in pediatric patients. *Transplant Proceedings, 44*(7), 2007–2012.

Cardoso, F. (2011). Sydenham chorea. *Handbook of Clinical Neurology, 100*(1), 221–229.

Darst, J. R., Collins, K. K., & Miyamoto, S. D. (2012). Cardiovascular diseases. In W. Hay, M. Levin, R. Deterding, et al. *Current diagnosis & treatment pediatrics* (21st ed., pp. 561-622). New York, NY: McGraw-Hill/Lange.

Dinardo, J. A. (2013). Heart failure associated with adult congenital heart disease. *Seminars in Cardiothoracic & Vascular Anesthesia, 17*(1), 44–54.

Dinsbach, N. A. (2012). Antibiotics in dentistry: Bacteremia, antibiotic prophylaxis, and antibiotic misuse. *General Dentistry, 60*(3), 200–207.

Dominguez, S. R., & Anderson, M. S. (2013). Advances in the treatment of Kawasaki disease. *Current Opinion in Pediatrics, 25*(1), 103–109.

Donofrio, M. T., Levy, R. J., Schuette, J. J., et al. (2013). Specialized delivery room planning for fetuses with critical congenital heart disease. *American Journal of Cardiology, 111*(5), 737–747.

Evans, N. (2012). Preterm patent ductus arteriosus: Should we treat it? *Journal of Paediatrics & Child Health, 48*(9), 753–758.

Gil-Jaurena, J. M., Castillo, R., & Rubio, L. (2012). Intrapericardial pacemaker in a 2-kilogram newborn. *Cardiology in the Young, 22*(4), 459–460.

Herouvi, D., Karanasios, E., Karayianni, C., et al. (2013). Cardiovascular disease in childhood: The role of obesity. *European Journal of Pediatrics, 172*(6), 721–732.

Johnson, J. A., Boyce, T. G., Cetta, F., et al. (2012). Infective endocarditis in the pediatric patient: Review. *Mayo Clinic Proceeding, 87*(7), 629–635.

Kaemmerer, H. (2011). Aortic coarctation and interrupted aortic arch. In M. A. Gatzoulis, G. D. Webb, & P. E. F. Daubeney (Eds.), *Diagnosis and management of adult congenital heart disease* (2nd ed., pp. 261–270). Philadelphia, PA: Elsevier.

Karch, A. M. (2013). *2013 Lippincott's nursing drug guide.* Philadelphia, PA: Lippincott Williams & Wilkins.

Kern, M. J., & King, S. B., III. (2013). Cardiac catheterization and coronary angiography. In R. Walsh, J. Fang, & V. Fuster (Eds.), *Hurst's the heart manual of cardiology* (13th ed., pp. 79–91). New York, NY: McGraw-Hill.

Koneti, N. R., Kandraju, H., Kanchi, V., et al. (2012). Endovascular stenting of the obstructed vertical vein in a neonate with supracardiac total anomalous pulmonary venous return. *Annals of Pediatric Cardiology, 5*(1), 75–77.

Kucik, J. E., Shin, M., Siffel, C., et al. (2013). Trends in survival among children with Down syndrome in 10 regions of the United States. *Pediatrics, 131*(1), e27–e36.

Kyle, W. B., Macicek, S. L., Lindle, K. A., et al. (2012). Limited utility of exercise stress tests in the evaluation of children with chest pain. *Congenital Heart Disease, 7*(5), 455–459.

Lange, R. A., & Hillis, L. D. (2013). Congenital heart disease. In E. T. Bope & R. D. Kellerman, *Conn's current therapy* (pp. 425–429). Philadelphia, PA: Elsevier/Saunders.

Li, Y., Margraf, J., Kluck, B., et al. (2012). Thrombolytic therapy for ischemic stroke secondary to paradoxical embolism in pregnancy: A case report and literature review. *Neurologist, 18*(1), 44–48.

Lipshultz, S. E., Schaechter, J., Carrillo, A., et al. (2012). Can the consequences of universal cholesterol screening during childhood prevent cardiovascular disease and thus reduce long-term health care costs? *Pediatric Endocrinology Review, 9*(4), 698–705.

Litak, D. (2012). Parental presence during child resuscitation: A critical review of a research article. *Journal of Perioperative Practice, 22*(2), 63–66.

Mares, J. C., & Bar-Cohen, Y. (2012). Tachycardia-induced cardiomyopathy in a 1-month-old infant. *Case Reports in Pediatrics, 2012*, 513690.

Marino, B. S., Lipkin, P. H., Newburger, J. W., et al. (2012). Neurodevelopmental outcomes in children with congenital heart disease. *Circulation, 126*(9), 1143–1172.

Meziani, F., Debbal, S. M., & Atbi, A. (2012). Analysis of phonocardiogram signals using wavelet transform. *Journal of Medical Engineering & Technology, 36*(6), 283–302.

Myers, P. O., Cikirikcioglu, M., Tissot, C., et al. (2012). Triple valve repair in children with rheumatic heart disease: Long-term experience. *Journal of Heart Valve Disease, 21*(5), 650–654.

Naguib, A. N., Dewhirst, E., Winch, P. D., et al. (2013). Pain management after comprehensive stage 2 repair for hypoplastic left heart syndrome. *Pediatric Cardiology, 34*(1), 52–58.

Narang, I., Manlhiot, C., Davies-Shaw, J., et al. (2012). Sleep disturbance and cardiovascular risk in adolescents. *CMAJ: Canadian Medical Association Journal, 184*(17), E913–E920.

National Heart, Lung, and Blood Institute. (2012). *Third report of the Expert Panel on Detection, Evaluation, and Treatment of the High Blood Cholesterol in Adults (Adult Treatment Panel III): Executive summary.* Bethesda, MD: Author.

Oishi, P., Datar, S. A., & Fineman, J. R. (2011) Advances in the management of pediatric pulmonary hypertension. *Respiratory Care, 56*(9), 1314–1340.

Panwar, S., Bradleym, S. M., & Kavarana, M. N. (2012). Truncus arteriosus and unbalanced complete atrioventricular septal defect: Pulmonary protection in the neonate. *Annals of Thoracic Surgery, 94*(6), e151–e153.

Paris, J. J., Moore, M. P., & Schreiber, M. D. (2012). Physician counseling, informed consent and parental decision making for infants with hypoplastic left-heart syndrome. *Journal of Perinatology, 32*(10), 748–751.

Prior, D. L., & La Gerche, A. (2012). The athlete's heart. *Heart, 98*(12), 947–955.

Pye, S., Kane, J., & Jones, A. (2010). Parental presence during pediatric resuscitation: The use of simulation training for cardiac intensive care nurses. *Journal for Specialists in Pediatric Nursing, 15*(2), 172–175.

Pye, S., & McDonnell, M. (2010). Nursing considerations for children undergoing delayed sternal closure after surgery for congenital heart disease. *Critical Care Nurse, 30*(3), 50–61.

Ralph, A. P., & Carapetis, J. R. (2013). Group A streptococcal diseases and their global burden. *Current Topics in Microbiology & Immunology, 368*, 1–27.

Ruys, T. P., van der Bosch, A. E., Cuypers, J. A., et al. (2013). Long-term outcome and quality of life after arterial switch operation: A prospective study with a historical comparison. *Congenital Heart Disease.* Advance online publication.

Schneider, D. S. (2011). The cardiovascular system. In K. J. Marcdante, R. M. Kliegman, H. B. Jenson, et al. (Eds), *Nelson essentials of pediatrics* (6th ed., pp. 525–554). Philadelphia, PA: Saunders/Elsevier.

Sharkey, A. M., & Sharma, A. (2012). Tetralogy of Fallot: Anatomic variants and their impact on surgical management. *Seminars in Cardiothoracic & Vascular Anesthesia, 16*(2), 88–96.

Slepian, M. J., Alemu, Y., Soares, J. S., et al. (2013). The Syncardia(TM) total artificial heart: In vivo, in vitro, and computational modeling studies. *Journal of Biomechanics, 46*(2), 266–275.

Smith, M. T., Lester-Smith, D., Zurynski, Y., et al. (2011). Persistence of acute rheumatic fever in a tertiary children's hospital. *Journal of Paediatrics and Child Health, 47*(4), 198–203.

Tandon, R. (2012). Rheumatic fever pathogenesis: Approach as research needs change. *Annals of Pediatric Cardiology, 5*(2), 169–178.

Underwood, S. M., Averhart, L., Dean, A., et al. (2012). Clinical evaluation and follow-up of body mass and blood pressure in pre-elementary school children: Program review. *Journal of the National Black Nurses Association, 23*(1), 8–15.

U.S. Department of Health and Human Services. (2010). *Healthy people 2020*. Washington, DC: Author.

van der Linde, D., Konings, E. E., Slager, M. A., et al. (2011). Birth prevalence of congenital heart disease worldwide: A systematic review and meta-analysis. *Journal of the American College of Cardiology, 58*(21), 2241–2247.

Vijayaraman, P., & Ellenbogen, K. A. (2013). Bradyarrhythmias & pacing. In R. Walsh, J. Fang, & V. Fuster (Eds.), *Hurst's the heart manual of cardiology* (13th ed., pp. 133–143). New York, NY: McGraw-Hill.

Wang, X., Wang, J., Zhao, P., et al. (2012). Familial congenital heart disease: Data collection and preliminary analysis. *Cardiology in the Young, 22*(10), 1–6.

Wei, H. H., Wu, K. G., Sy, L. B., et al. (2010). Infectious endocarditis in pediatric patients: Analysis of 19 cases presenting at a medical center. *Journal of Microbiology, Immunology & Infection, 43*(5), 430–437.

Xiu-Yu, S., Jia-Yu, H., Qiang, H., et al. (2010). Platelet count and erythrocyte sedimentation rate are good predictors of Kawasaki syndrome: ROC analysis. *Journal of Clinical Laboratory Analysis, 24*(6), 385–388.

Chapter 42

Nursing Care of a Family When a Child Has an Immune Disorder

KEY TERMS

- allergen
- anaphylaxis
- antigen
- atopic dermatitis
- autoimmunity
- cell-mediated immunity
- chemotaxis
- complement
- cytotoxic response
- delayed hypersensitivity
- environmental control
- humoral immunity
- hypersensitivity response
- hyposensitization
- immune response
- immunity
- immunogen
- immunoglobulins
- lymphokines
- lysis
- macrophages
- phagocytosis
- tolerance

OBJECTIVES

After mastering the contents of this chapter, you should be able to:

1. Describe the immune process as it relates to childhood illnesses.
2. Identify 2020 National Health Goals related to immune disorders in children that nurses can help the nation achieve.
3. Assess a child with a disorder of the immune system.
4. Formulate nursing diagnoses for a child with a disorder of the immune system.
5. Establish outcomes for a child with a disorder of the immune system that can help the family manage seamless transitions across different health care settings.
6. Using the nursing process, plan nursing care that includes the six competencies of Quality & Safety Education for Nurses (QSEN): Patient-Centered Care, Teamwork & Collaboration, Evidence-Based Practice (EBP), Quality Improvement (QI), Safety, and Informatics.
7. Implement nursing care for a child with an immune disorder, such as teaching about environmental control.
8. Evaluate expected outcomes for achievement and effectiveness of care.
9. Integrate knowledge of immune disorders with the interplay of nursing process, the six competencies of QSEN, and Family Nursing to promote quality maternal and child health nursing care.

Dexter Goodenough is a 6-year-old boy you meet in an ambulatory clinic. He had atopic dermatitis (infantile eczema) as an infant. Today, his eyes look reddened and are watering; his nose is draining a clear discharge. His mother tells you he is constantly listless and other children have started to bully him because of his appearance and the fact he has a peanut allergy. His grades are "terrible" because his rhinitis symptoms begin the minute he gets to school. Dexter is diagnosed as having atopic rhinitis (hay fever). "Thank heavens," his mother exclaims. "I thought when I heard he had an immune system disease, he had AIDS. What a relief to know it's only another allergy."

Previous chapters described normal growth and development of children. This chapter adds information about the dramatic changes, both physical and psychosocial, that can occur when a child is born with or develops a disorder of the immune system.

In light of the effect this condition is having on Dexter's life, is this "only" an allergy? What additional information would you want his mother to know about his condition? Knowing his problem is worse at school, what environmental control measures would you want to suggest for Dexter?

The immune system consists of a complex network of cells interacting to protect the body against invasion by foreign substances. The study of the immune system is a growing field as more diseases are being attributed, at least in part, to malfunctioning of the immune system, making it important to have an understanding of how the immune system works in health and disease in order to provide safe nursing care (Hellmann & Imboden, 2013).

Disorders of the immune system include deficiencies of immune substances and function that affect the body's ability to ward off infection (immunodeficiency disorders), abnormal and excessive immune response to foreign substances (hypersensitivity disorders, or allergies), and abnormal and excessive immune response to one's self (autoimmune disorders). The immune system holds the key to understanding a major illness such as HIV/AIDS and possibly why cancers occur. Immunodeficiencies and examples of allergic disorders are described in this chapter. Autoimmune disorders, which include a wide range of illnesses, often affect a particular body system and so are described in the chapter that discusses the affected system (e.g., juvenile arthritis, which affects the joints, is discussed in Chapter 51). The 2020 National Health Goals related to immune disorders and children are shown in Box 42.1.

BOX 42.1 Nursing Care Planning Based on 2020 National Health Goals

Allergies affect at least 25% of the population, therefore, efforts to reduce them are reflected in several 2020 National Health Goals:

- Reduce indoor allergen levels such as cockroach allergens in settled dust from a baseline of 0.51 units to 0.46 units.
- Increase the proportion of the nation's elementary, middle, and high schools that have an indoor air quality management program to promote a healthy and safe physical school environment from a baseline of 51.4% to a target level of 56.5%.
- Reduce new cases of perinatally acquired AIDS from a baseline of 28 cases yearly to 25 new cases yearly.
- Reduce new AIDS cases among adolescents and adults from a baseline of 14.4 new cases per 100,000 to a target level of 13.0 new cases per 100,000.
- Increase the proportion of sexually active unmarried females aged 15 to 44 years who use condoms from a baseline of 34.5% to a target level of 38% (U.S. Department of Health and Human Services [DHHS], 2012; see www.healthypeople.com).

Nurses can help the nation achieve these goals by advocating for improved air quality in schools, initiating educational programs for children and adolescents that includes teaching about the way HIV is transmitted (sexual relations and unclean intravenous needles) and protective measures they can take to avoid contracting the disease (using safer sex practices and not using intravenous drugs).

Nursing Process Overview

For a Child With an Immune Disorder

Assessment

The purpose of the immune system is to provide protection to the body from invading organisms or antigens. A deficiency of *immunocompetent* cells (cells capable of resisting these types of foreign invaders) or alteration in their function can limit this protection. An assessment focuses on an analysis of blood components, particularly, the white blood cells, to determine exactly what components are altered, missing, or not functioning properly. When the immune system reacts excessively or inappropriately to the invasion of certain antigens, a thorough history and analysis of presenting symptoms becomes the best way to identify the problem and to develop appropriate interventions.

Nursing Diagnosis

Examples of nursing diagnoses associated with immune dysfunction include:

- Risk for infection related to altered immune response
- Impaired skin integrity related to inadequate lymphocyte protection
- Activity intolerance related to chronic illness
- Risk for delayed growth and development related to chronicity of HIV/AIDS
- Risk for infection due to altered skin integrity

Nursing diagnoses for children experiencing allergic responses because of an altered response focus on the particular allergic symptoms. Examples of these include:

- Situational low self-esteem related to symptoms of contact dermatitis
- Ineffective breathing pattern related to bronchospasm of anaphylaxis
- Anxiety related to continuing allergic response
- Powerlessness related to difficulty determining cause of allergy

Outcome Identification and Planning

Outcome identification and planning for a child with an immune disorder should focus both on present and future concerns. Relief of immediate symptoms is the first priority followed by planning for long-term care and prevention of future attacks. Examples of organizations helpful for supplying information to parents or children are the National Eczema Association (www.nationaleczema.org) and the Asthma and Allergy Foundation of America (www.aafa.org).

Implementation

A major nursing intervention in the care of children with immune disorders is client and family teaching. The family of a child with an immunodeficiency may need help in identifying ways to keep the child from contracting life-threatening infections while at the same time providing enough stimulation and social contact to promote normal growth and development. The family of a child with a chronic allergic disorder needs to learn ways to help their child avoid triggers or situations that provoke the allergy response, but at the same time, not keep the child so isolated or fearful that the child misses out on important experiences.

Outcome Evaluation

Outcome evaluation with immune disorders must be ongoing because new triggers for allergies can arise at any time. New therapies for disease processes such as HIV/AIDS are constantly being investigated. Because the field of immunology is continually evolving, theories about immune diseases and associated treatments change year to year. This means that health care providers need to keep abreast of the latest developments. Emphasize to parents that they need to know the latest technologic information as well, especially as it relates to providing a safe environment for their child. Examples of outcomes suggesting the achievement of goals include:

- The child voices high self-esteem even if contact dermatitis rash has not completely faded.
- The child's pulse oximetry is maintained at 95% or above with minimal wheezing.
- The child and parents are able to adhere to the plan of care.
- The child lists three actions he takes daily to help feel a greater sense of control and well-being.
- The child demonstrates achievement of developmental milestones within age-acceptable parameters despite chronic illness.

THE IMMUNE SYSTEM

The immune system functions to protect the body from invasion by foreign substances by several mechanisms. First, body surfaces such as the skin, cilia, and mucous membrane act as physical protective barriers. If an invading pathogen does get through this first barrier, **phagocytosis**, or the destruction of the invaders, begins. **Macrophages** (mature white blood cells) engulf, ingest, and neutralize the pathogen. At the same time, an inflammatory response creates vascular and cellular changes that help to rid the body of dead tissue and the inactivated antigens. The immune system maintains cells ready to attack this way whenever necessary, directing the efforts of macrophages and supplementing the inflammatory response as necessary. It also singles out specific antigens for interactions (*antibody–antigen reactions*). This immune response not only furnishes immediate protection but also creates a template for how to destroy that particular antigen again in the future.

Immune Response

The **immune response** is the body's action plan devised to combat invading organisms or substances by leukocyte and antibody activity. An **antigen** is any foreign substance (molecule) capable of stimulating an immune response. Most antigens are proteins, but other large molecules such as polysaccharides may also function the same way. Penicillin, although not antigenic by itself, can become antigenic when it combines with a higher weight molecule, usually a protein (a process called *hapten formation*). If an antigen is one that can be readily destroyed by an immune response, and **immunity** (the ability to destroy like antigens) results, the antigen may be referred to as a simple **immunogen**.

If, during the immune response, mediating substances are released that cause tissue injury and allergic symptoms, the antigen is termed an **allergen**. Allergens can enter the body through a variety of routes. They may be ingested (foods such as eggs or wheat), inhaled (pollen, dust, or mold spores), injected (drugs), or absorbed across the skin or mucous membranes (poison ivy).

Immune System Organs and Cells

The organs of the immune system consist of the lymph nodes, bone marrow, thymus, spleen, and tonsils. Bone marrow produces two types of lymphocytes, *B lymphocytes* and *T lymphocytes*. After being produced, lymphocytes travel throughout the lymphoid system and are stored in the lymph nodes and spleen. Both T and B lymphocytes are able to recognize invading organisms and attack specific antigens (Fig. 42.1).

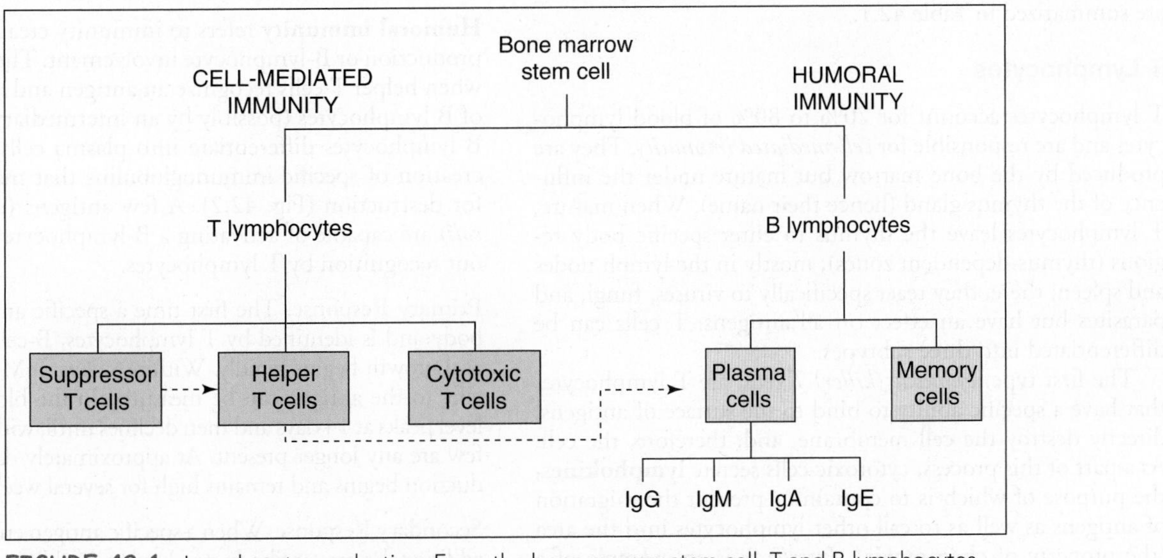

FIGURE 42.1 Lymphocyte production. From the bone marrow stem cell, T and B lymphocytes are formed. T-lymphocyte action leads to cell-mediated immunity. B-lymphocyte action results in humoral immunity. Ig, immunoglobulin.

TABLE 42.1 Locations and Functions of Immunoglobulins

Immunoglobulin	Description
IgM	Effective in agglutinating antigens as well as lysing cell walls; discovered early in the course of an infection in the bloodstream.
IgG	Most frequently occurring antibody in plasma; during secondary response, it is the major immunoglobulin to be synthesized. It freely diffuses into extravascular spaces to contact antigens. In prenatal life, it diffuses across the placenta to supply passive immune protection to the fetus until the infant can effectively produce immunoglobulins. It has the major responsibility for neutralizing bacterial toxins and in activating phagocytosis (destruction of bacteria).
IgA	Found in external body secretions such as saliva, sweat, tears, mucus, bile, and colostrum. It provides defense against pathogens on exposed surfaces, especially those of the gastrointestinal tract and respiratory tract, and works, apparently, by preventing adherence of pathogens to mucosal cells.
IgD	Found in plasma. It may be the receptor that binds antigens to lymphocyte surfaces.
IgE	Involved in immediate hypersensitivity reactions. It exists bound to mast cells on tissue surfaces. When contacted by an antigen, cellular granules are released. It is associated with allergy and parasitic infections.

B Lymphocytes

Originating in the bone marrow (the reason for their name), B lymphocytes develop into *plasma cells* and *memory cells* when exposed to antigens. Plasma cells secrete large quantities of **immunoglobulins** (Ig) or antibodies, which bind to and destroy specific antigens (termed *humoral immunity*). When an antibody is formed in response to a particular antigen this way, it is specific to that antigen. An antibody against the pertussis antigen, for instance, will not have any effect on the tetanus antigen. *Memory cells* are responsible for retaining the formula or ability to produce specific immunoglobulins. Immunoglobulins are classified as IgG, IgA, IgM, IgD, and IgE. Those involved in immunity include IgG, IgA, and IgM. IgM reaches adult levels at approximately 1 year of age, IgG at 4 years, and IgA at adolescence (Fuleihan, 2011).

IgE is primarily responsible for allergic or hypersensitivity responses and is present at proportions capable of extreme response early in infancy. The functions of immunoglobulins are summarized in Table 42.1.

T Lymphocytes

T lymphocytes account for 70% to 80% of blood lymphocytes and are responsible for *cell-mediated immunity*. They are produced by the bone marrow but mature under the influence of the thymus gland (hence their name). When mature, T lymphocytes leave the thymus to enter specific body regions (thymus-dependent zones), mostly in the lymph nodes and spleen; there, they react specifically to viruses, fungi, and parasites but have an effect on all antigens. T cells can be differentiated into three subtypes.

The first type, *cytotoxic (killer) T cells*, are T lymphocytes that have a specific ability to bind to the surface of antigens, directly destroy the cell membrane, and, therefore, the cell. As a part of this process, cytotoxic cells secrete **lymphokines**, the purpose of which is to contain or prevent the migration of antigens as well as to call other lymphocytes into the area (the property of **chemotaxis**). *Interferon* is an example of a lymphokine widely discussed because it is important to prevent viral spread.

A second type, *helper T cells* (CD4 cells), serve the purpose of stimulating B lymphocytes to divide and mature into plasma cells so they can begin secreting immunoglobulins. The IgA antibody response, especially, depends on stimulation by helper T cells. Helper T cells can be identified in blood because of specific markers on their surface. Analysis of these (CD4 counts) is an important assessment criteria used to determine if antiretroviral therapy is beginning to be successful in the treatment of AIDS (Boyd, 2011).

The third type, *suppressor T cells*, are specific cells that reduce the production of immunoglobulins against a specific antigen and prevent their overproduction.

Types of Immunity

The action of B and T lymphocytes leads to two different types of immunity: humoral and cell mediated.

Humoral Immunity

Humoral immunity refers to immunity created by antibody production or B-lymphocyte involvement. The process begins when helper T cells recognize an antigen and cause activation of B lymphocytes (possibly by an intermediary macrophage). B lymphocytes differentiate into plasma cells and begin the creation of specific immunoglobulins that mark the antigen for destruction (Fig. 42.2). A few antigens (e.g., *Escherichia coli*) are capable of activating a B-lymphocyte response without recognition by T lymphocytes.

Primary Response. The first time a specific antigen enters the body and is identified by T lymphocytes, B-cell differentiation and growth begins rapidly. Within 6 days, IgM antibodies specific to the antigen can be measured in the bloodstream. This level peaks at 14 days and then declines until, within a few weeks, few are any longer present. At approximately day 10, IgG production begins and remains high for several weeks (Fig. 42.3).

Secondary Response. When a specific antigen enters the body an additional time, antibody production is able to begin immediately again because of memory cells. The main type of immunoglobulin produced in a secondary response is IgG (see Fig. 42.3).

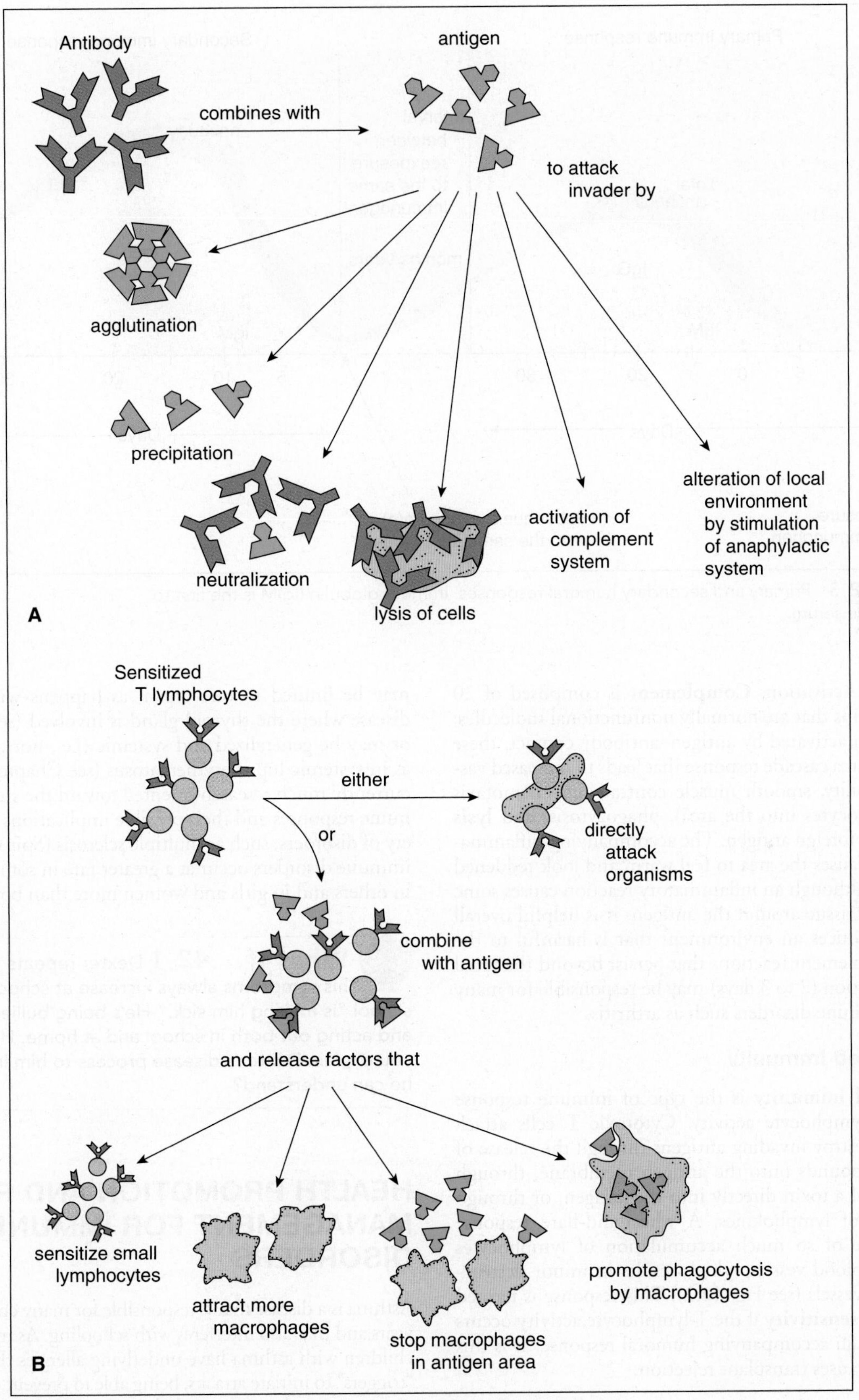

FIGURE 42.2 Mechanism of immunity response. **(A)** Humoral immunity. **(B)** Cell-mediated immunity.

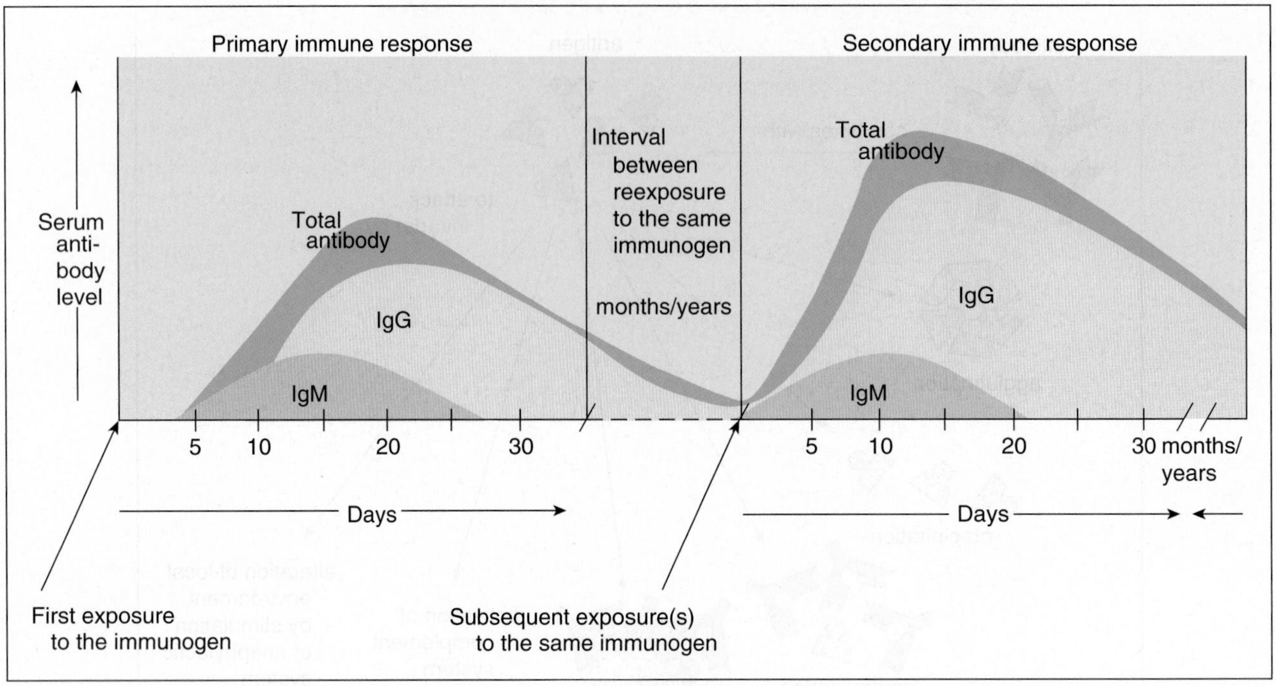

FIGURE 42.3 Primary and secondary humoral responses. Immunoglobulin (Ig)M is the first to appear in the serum.

Complement Activation. **Complement** is composed of 20 different proteins that are normally nonfunctional molecules; however, when activated by antigen–antibody contact, these molecules begin a cascade response that leads to increased vascular permeability, smooth muscle contraction, chemotaxis ("calling" leukocytes into the area), phagocytosis, and **lysis** (killing) of the foreign antigen. The accompanying inflammatory reaction causes the area to feel warm and look reddened and swollen. Although an inflammatory reaction causes some local injury to tissue around the antigen, it is helpful overall because it produces an environment that is harmful to the antigen. Complement reactions that persist beyond the usual time for resolution (2 to 3 days) may be responsible for many of the autoimmune disorders such as arthritis.

Cell-Mediated Immunity

Cell-mediated immunity is the type of immune response caused by T-lymphocyte activity. Cytotoxic T cells attack and directly destroy invading antigens through the release of chemical compounds onto the antigen membrane, through the injection of a toxin directly into the antigen, or through the secretion of lymphokines. A wheal-and-flare response occurs because of so much accumulation of lymphocytes around small blood vessels, which results in minor destruction of blood vessels (see Fig. 42.2). This response is termed **delayed hypersensitivity** if the T-lymphocyte activity occurs solely without an accompanying humoral response. It is this response that causes transplant rejection.

Autoimmunity

Autoimmunity is the result of the immune system being unable to distinguish self from nonself, causing the immune system to carry out immune responses against normal cells and tissue rather than invading antigens. Autoimmune responses may be limited to one organ, as happens with Hashimoto disease where the thyroid gland is involved (see Chapter 48) or may be generalized and systemic (i.e., not organ specific), as in systemic lupus erythematosus (see Chapter 20). There is currently much research oriented toward the study of autoimmune responses and their possible implications in a wide variety of disorders, such as multiple sclerosis (Spiro, 2012). Autoimmune disorders occur at a greater rate in some families than in others and in girls and women more than boys and men.

What if...42.1 Dexter repeats for you that his symptoms always increase at school or that school "is making him sick." He's being bullied at school and acting out both in school and at home. How would you explain Dexter's disease process to him in language he can understand?

HEALTH PROMOTION AND RISK MANAGEMENT FOR IMMUNE DISORDERS

Asthma is a disease that is responsible for many emergency room visits and that also interferes with schooling. As many as 90% of children with asthma have underlying allergies that serve as the "triggers" to initiate attacks; being able to prevent or reduce allergic responses, therefore, could have a major impact on the health of children (Covar, Fleischer, & Boguniewicz, 2012). It is hard to document that exclusive breastfeeding and the late introduction of solid food, methods once recommended as ways to prevent allergies, truly have an effect (Lack, 2012). Parents should still be encouraged to breastfeed and delay the introduction of solid

BOX 42.2 Nursing Care Planning to Empower a Family

AVOIDING SECONDARY SMOKE

Q. Dexter's mother says to you, "Neither my husband nor I smoke, but some of our relatives and friends do. How can we keep our child from being exposed to secondary smoke?"

A. The following guidelines should be helpful:

- Declare your home and car smoke-free zones.
- If family members smoke, ask them to smoke outside. Because smoke adheres to people's clothing, suggest a person change clothing after smoking before holding a young baby.
- If at a restaurant, ask to sit in a no-smoking area, or visit only smoke-free restaurants.
- If staying at a hotel, ask for a nonsmoking room.
- Do not be reluctant to ask people around your child at a social gathering to stop smoking.
- Encourage your friends or family members who smoke to begin quit-smoking courses (for their own benefit as well as yours).

foods until 6 months because of other reasons, including the impact of other milks on an infant's immature gastrointestinal tract. Environmental control to reduce the number of allergens in a home is well documented and can have long-term effects in reducing allergy symptoms (Scott, Roberts, Kurukulaaratchy, et al., 2012). This should begin when parents choose furnishings for a child's room, such as eliminating wool blankets, choosing toys carefully, and keeping the room free of dust. Keeping the house free of secondary smoke and using a minimum of washing compounds or spray products such as room deodorants so children are exposed to as few chemical products as possible are other steps to take (Box 42.2). Urge parents to follow these rules from the time the child is born, rather than wait for the child to develop allergic rhinitis or atopic dermatitis and then have to put these measures into effect. Latex is a common substance that causes an allergy in children, so it's important that the amount of latex used in health care settings is kept to a minimum especially when children at high risk (those with a history of multiple surgical procedures, a history of hay fever, rhinitis, asthma, eczema, or an allergy to tropical fruits) are cared for (Mercurio, 2011). Yet another category of environmental pollutants, such as exhaust from automobiles or ash from forest fires, adds to the number of allergic responses in children.

Because some families are more prone to allergies than others, there are communities that have a higher incidence of children with allergies than others. As a result, these communities may have more services and specialists to treat these children, a situation that develops a "community culture" of allergy acceptance and treatment. Children typically may leave school early for immunotherapy. School cafeterias commonly offer allergy-free foods. In other communities where fewer children have allergies, a child with an allergy is viewed as unique or not typical, and so may need additional support from health care providers (Stewart, Letourneau, Masuda, et al., 2012).

Allergies are a type of disorder that typically causes chronic rather than acute symptoms. For this reason, children who develop allergies often need to be encouraged to be vigilant in taking their medicine. For the same reason, once parents begin a child on an immunotherapy program, they may need to be encouraged to continue it. It helps if children and their parents understand how allergic reactions lead to symptoms and how important it is for them to play a role in their own therapy.

Although it is probably impossible to keep children with atopic allergies completely free of reactions and manifestations of allergies, parents who know of familial allergy patterns can take some preventive steps in this direction. If parents are going to prepare allergy-free foods, be certain they consider the child's likes and dislikes and think through the child's weekly intake to ensure that the child will receive all essential nutrients. If a child eats at school or has a meal prepared every day at a child care center, remind parents to make sure the center, babysitter, or school dietitian is aware of the child's allergies. If a child is allergic to wheat products and cannot eat bread for sandwiches, preparing a bag lunch for school may be a difficult daily problem that only good planning can eliminate. Fortunately, many nonwheat alternatives are available for those needing gluten-free or wheat-free diets (Susanna & Prabhasankar, 2012). Remind parents to read food labels so they can clearly identify these.

The parents of children with immune deficiencies may need to be reminded periodically to take measures to keep their children free of disease, such as keeping immunizations updated and seeking help immediately for infections. If a child's allergies involve pollen sensitivities, planning vacations at a time when the pollen count is lowest may make the vacation more pleasant for the family. If desensitization against a specific pollen is necessary, assist parents in planning to start desensitization early enough that it will be effective by the time the pollen count of the offending allergen rises.

Health promotion is also important to prevent HIV/AIDS. Teaching children safer sex practices is an important part of this. All health care providers can help prevent the spread of HIV/AIDS by using standard infection precautions.

✔ QSEN Checkpoint Question 42.1

Safety

Dexter is at his primary care provider's office and you've been asked to assist with his physical examination. What safety intervention should you use with Dexter because he's known to have many allergies?

a. Assess his blood pressure using a new blood pressure cuff.
b. Distract him by showing him a tropical fish tank.
c. Spot check his oxygen saturation using pulse oximetry.
d. Use nonlatex gloves to conduct the examination.

Look in Appendix A for the best answer and rationale.

IMMUNODEFICIENCY DISORDERS

When any one portion of the immune system is not functioning adequately, an immunodeficiency results. The immunodeficiency disorder may be primary (congenital) or acquired (secondary to viral invasion or exposure to a toxic substance). Only a part or the entire system may fail in its goal of protecting the body from invading organisms. It cannot be overemphasized that live vaccines and nonirradiated blood should be avoided if an immune deficiency is suspected (Woo & Bahna, 2011).

Primary (Congenital) Immunodeficiency

Children with primary congenital immunodeficiencies are born without or with inadequate amounts of immune substances. Usually these deficiencies become apparent relatively early in life. However, it may take a few months for B-lymphocyte deficiencies to produce symptoms, because a newborn is born with enough maternal IgG (which crossed the placenta during pregnancy) to supply protection for approximately the first 6 months of life.

B-Lymphocyte Deficiencies

There are varying degrees of B-lymphocyte deficiencies called hypogammaglobulinemia. Agammaglobulinemia is characterized by an almost complete absence of B cells and humoral immunity (Ochs & Hitzig, 2012).

Hypogammaglobulinemia. Hypogammaglobulinemia can occur as a result of an assault on the immune system such as from chemotherapy or a critical illness. However, most often it results from an inherited X-linked recessive gene (Hauk, Johnston, & Liu, 2011). At approximately 6 months of age, when passively transferred maternal antibodies fade, male infants begin to develop frequent bacterial respiratory, digestive, or throat infections. Autoimmune diseases such as juvenile arthritis and systemic lupus erythematosus may occur in later life. The cellular or T-lymphocyte response remains adequate, allowing the child to resist viral, fungal, and parasitic infections.

This deficiency is treated with intravenous or subcutaneous immune globulin (IG) injections to supply immunoglobulins. Bone marrow transplantation is a long-term solution to restore immune competency. Help parents set up a schedule for IG injections so these are not forgotten. Both parents and children need to be taught the importance of recognizing symptoms of infection early so the child receives treatment as early as possible and possibly additional IG.

Common Variable Immunoglobulin Deficiencies. The most common disorder in this group is deficiency of IgA in surface secretions (Resnick & Cunningham-Rundles, 2012). The overall level of B lymphocytes is normal, but IgA production is reduced or absent, perhaps because of an increase of IgA suppressor cells or a defect in helper T cells that are important for IgA synthesis. Without IgA, infections of body surfaces exposed to the external environment and normally protected by mucus secretions such as sinusitis, upper respiratory tract illness, and inflammatory bowel disease begin to occur. There are also associated atopic diseases (allergies) because without IgA on the surface mucosa, many more antigens than usual can enter the body, thus permitting more antigens to interact with IgE and produce allergic symptoms.

A danger of this chronic irritation is that these large numbers of antigens can predispose exposed tissue to malignant transformation, causing malignancy of the respiratory, gastrointestinal, and lymphoid systems to occur at a greater incidence than usual. As yet another concern, there is an increased risk that an antibody will cross-react with a self-antigen to cause an autoimmune illness such as systemic lupus erythematosus. IgA deficiency can occur as a secondary type because of treatment with phenytoin (an anticonvulsant) and penicillamine (a copper chelating agent). IG contains little IgA, so therapy with IG does not greatly reduce IgA deficiency symptoms.

T-Lymphocyte Deficiencies

T-lymphocyte immunodeficiencies involve inadequate numbers or inadequate functioning of one or more types of T lymphocytes; this affects cell-mediated immunity and also, because of helper T-lymphocyte function, possibly humoral immunity as well. Di George syndrome is a chromosomal disorder in which there is deletion of a small piece of chromosome 22. This leads to not only a T-cell defect but also misshaped or low-set ears, a smaller than usual mandible, an absent thymus, neonatal tetany, and congenital heart disease (Woo & Bahna, 2010).

Combined T- and B-Lymphocyte Deficiency

Severe combined immunodeficiencies (SCID) are a group of inherited rare disorders associated with large defects in T- and B-cell immunity (Hellmann & Imboden, 2013). SCID is caused by a developmental abnormality (sometimes but not always related to the absence of a particular enzyme), which prevents the formation of T lymphocytes (a stem cell abnormality). This, in turn, prevents the maturation of both T and B lymphocytes. Children cannot respond directly to antigen invasion and no antibodies are produced. The definitive treatment for children with SCID is correction of the immunologic defect by hematopoietic stem cell transplantation, possibly from cord blood (Accetta Pedersen, Verbsky, & Routes, 2011).

Secondary (Acquired) Immunodeficiency

Secondary immunodeficiency, or loss of immune system response, can occur from factors such as severe systemic infection, cancer, renal disease, radiation therapy, severe stress, malnutrition, immunosuppressive therapy, and aging. There can be complete or partial loss of both B- and T-lymphocyte response.

Stress appears to alter the immune response by stimulating the release of corticosteroids from the adrenal gland. This suppresses the inflammatory response by inhibiting macrophage action. Immunosuppressive drugs, such as prednisone, also act to suppress the inflammatory response. The action of radiation or chemotherapy limits the function of or destroys rapidly growing cells and so destroys both T and B lymphocytes because these are rapidly growing and dividing cells. Extreme infection is yet another cause for a decreased immune response because the body's continued ability to combat infection becomes exhausted.

Malnutrition depletes the body of protein necessary for immune system function; renal disease with protein loss will also deplete the amount of protein available for new lymphocyte production.

HIV Infection and AIDS

The HIV virus is a slowly replicating rotovirus and has at least two main divisions, HIV-1 and HIV-2, followed by a variety of further subtypes. The virus acts by attacking the lymphoreticular system, in particular CD4-bearing helper

T lymphocytes. The virus enters the cell, substitutes its own RNA and DNA for the cell's DNA, and begins to replicate, destroying the lymphocytes in the process and the ability to initiate an effective B-lymphocyte response.

There is no effective way to destroy the virus, so it remains in the body for life and can activate if the immune system becomes even more depressed. Because B-lymphocyte or humoral immune function, which initiates the production of antibodies, is affected, antibody formation will be decreased (hypogammaglobulinemia). When monocytes and macrophages become affected as well, the person with HIV infection cannot resist usual infections such as the common cold. When the CD4 count falls below 500 cells/mm^3 or the viral load rises above 5,000 copies/ml, it is difficult for infected individuals to resist opportunistic infections such as fungal infections. The final result is that both the immune response and the ability to screen and remove malignant cells from the body are lost (Smith, 2011).

Transmission. HIV infection is spread by exposure to blood and other body secretions through sexual contact, the sharing of contaminated needles for injection, the transfusion of contaminated blood or blood products, perinatally from mother to fetus or newborn, and possibly through breastfeeding. Children could also acquire the infection because of sexual maltreatment. Health care providers must maintain vigilance to guard against needle punctures, as these injuries can be a direct source of blood transfer.

Although it is decreasing in incidence, the transmission of HIV from mother to child by placental spread is still the most common reason for childhood HIV infection in the United States. Children with hemophilia no longer have a high incidence of the disease because blood products are now screened for the virus. Transmission of HIV through sexual activity is a growing concern for adolescents and an important area where health education is needed (Sawyer, Afifi, Bearinger, et al., 2012). HIV is not transmitted by animals or through usual, casual contact, such as shaking hands or kissing, or in households, day care centers, or schools.

Assessment. HIV has a long incubation period of about 10 years in adults. The disorder appears to progress more rapidly in children and infants, however, who receive the virus through placental transmission (if they do not receive treatment). These individuals are usually HIV positive by 6 months and develop clinical signs by 1 to 3 years of age. Children who receive the virus from another source usually convert to HIV positivity by 2 to 6 weeks, or at least by 6 months after exposure. During this preconversion time, a child may display preliminary symptoms such as poor resistance to infection, fever, swollen lymph nodes, respiratory tract infections, and oral candidiasis.

All infants born to infected mothers test positive for antibodies to the virus at birth because of passive antibody transmission (which persists for about 18 months). The disease is diagnosed, therefore, by recovery of the HIV antigen in children under this age and antibodies to the virus in children over this age. Tests to detect the antigen are termed PCR (polymerase chain reaction) tests; those for the antibody are termed ELISA (enzyme-linked immunosorbent assay) or Western blot confirmation. CD4 counts are used to document the disease status and predict disease progression. Normal counts vary somewhat according to age because the lymphocyte count normally varies by age, but a count of 500 ml to 1,500 ml is a healthy count.

The Centers for Disease Control and Prevention (CDC, 1994) classification of HIV infection in children has three categories:

- Category A, *Mildly Symptomatic*: Two or more symptoms such as enlarged lymph nodes, liver, or spleen, or recurrent or persistent upper respiratory infections, sinusitis, or otitis media are present.
- Category B, *Moderately Symptomatic*: More serious illnesses such as oropharyngeal candidiasis, bacterial meningitis, pneumonia, sepsis, cardiomyopathy, cytomegalovirus infection, hepatitis, herpes simplex virus (HSV), bronchitis, pneumonitis, or esophagitis, herpes zoster (shingles), lymphoid interstitial pneumonia (LIP), pulmonary lymphoid hyperplasia complex, or toxoplasmosis are present.
- Category C, *Severely Symptomatic (AIDS)*: Serious bacterial infections such as septicemia, mycobacterial pneumonia, meningitis, bone or joint infection, abscess of an internal organ or body cavity; candidiasis (esophageal or pulmonary), encephalopathy, herpes simplex lasting over 1 month, histoplasmosis, lymphoma, tuberculosis, *Pneumocystis carinii* pneumonia (PCP; a form of pneumonia caused by a yeastlike fungus), and Kaposi sarcoma (a malignancy that causes large purple/blue tumors to grow from the lining of capillaries) have occurred.

Therapeutic Management. Because of advances in general health care, increased birth control education focused on the needs of HIV-positive women, as well as the availability of antiretroviral medications, the number of infants born with HIV infection is decreasing (Gay, Hardee, & Croce-Galis, 2011). Those infants who are born with HIV, once thought to have a short life expectancy, now have an opportunity for long-term survival.

Nursing Diagnoses and Related Interventions

Nursing Diagnosis: Risk for infection related to decreased immune function

Outcome Evaluation: Child's temperature is within normal parameters; no cough or skin lesions are present.

Combating HIV infection and maintaining an effective CD4 count requires continuous specific antiretroviral medications to prevent progressive deterioration of the immune system and to provide prophylactic measures against opportunistic infections. The introduction of Highly Active Antiretroviral Therapy (HAART) in pediatric HIV/AIDS treatment has made the difference between an acute disease where 60% of children died by age 6 years to a life expectancy of 40 to 50 years (Shulman, 2011). Four classes of drugs are the mainstay of therapy: nucleoside reverse transcriptase inhibitors (NRTIs), nonnucleoside reverse transcriptase inhibitors (NNRTIs), protease inhibitors, and integrase strand transfer inhibitors. NRTIs are designed to block the production of viral DNA, limiting the ability of the virus to infect cells; zidovudine is an example (Box 42.3). NNRTIs also inhibit the DNA synthesis of viruses but act at different sites on the

the child keep a chart of when symptoms are worse and better often helps identify a specific allergen. Children with allergic rhinitis (hay fever), for example, have more symptoms on a windy day and fewer after a rainstorm (the rain washes pollen out of the air). A record that details when symptoms start—on arising, or only after the child reaches school, as another example—also can help identify an allergen.

Laboratory Testing

Few laboratory tests are helpful in establishing a diagnosis of allergy. A radioallergosorbent test (RAST) may be prescribed. A determination of IgE serum antibodies can also be helpful. Because allergies tend to raise an eosinophil count, most children with allergies have 5% or more of eosinophils on a differential count and a total eosinophil count of 250 or more cells/mm^3. Another main cause of an increased eosinophil count, however, is invasion by ova or parasites, which is why a stool specimen for ova and parasites is generally collected to rule out these problems as the cause of the increased eosinophil count.

Skin Testing

Skin testing is done to detect the presence of IgE in the skin, or to isolate an antigen (allergen) to which the IgE is responding or to which a child is sensitive. When an allergen is introduced into the child's skin and the child is sensitive to that allergen, a wheal or flare response will appear at the site of the test from the release of histamine, which leads to local vasodilation. Because this reaction appears quickly, the test should be read in 20 minutes. Systemic or aerosol administration of an antihistamine will inhibit the flare response, so be certain the child has not received these drugs for 8 hours before skin testing. Corticosteroid therapy does not affect immediate skin reactivity and so may be continued during skin testing.

Skin testing may be done by applying a patch or using a scratch or an intracutaneous injection technique. Patch testing has become the method of choice because it is painless and also more efficient. For the child with rare allergies not typically provided by commercial patches, scratch or intracutaneous testing still may be necessary. Scratch testing is done by placing a drop of allergen solution on the skin, then scratching through the drop of liquid with a sterile needle. A relatively concentrated extract of allergen must be used for scratch testing because little allergen actually enters the child's skin.

Intracutaneous injections are done by injecting a small amount of a solution of allergen below the epidermis of the skin. This is usually done on the forearm so that if a sensitivity reaction does occur, a tourniquet could be applied proximal to the test site to prevent further absorption of the antigen. If the categories to be tested are extensive, the back can be used as well for testing. Solutions used for intracutaneous injections are more dilute than those used for scratch testing (1:500 dilution compared with 1:5 for scratch testing). If helping with allergen testing, the extracts are not interchangeable from a group prepared for scratch testing to a group prepared for intracutaneous injections (or vice versa).

Because intracutaneous injections are given just below the epidermal layer of skin, they are almost painless. This is the same phenomenon as passing a needle or pin under the top layer of skin of a fingertip, a trick every school-age child does at least once to the horror of friends. The child needs a great deal of support for this type of skin testing, however, because it looks as if it will be painful and the sight of a needle may be frightening.

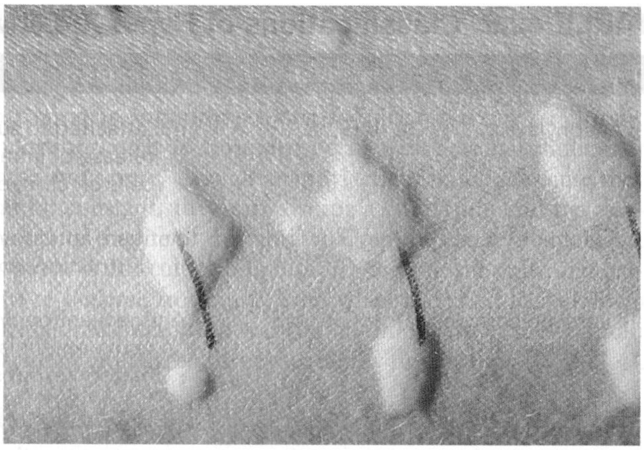

FIGURE 42.4 Allergy skin testing. Note the positive reactions. (© SPL/Custom Medical Stock Photograph.)

The allergens chosen for skin testing depend on the child's symptoms. Few children need more than 30 test media tried. This is because most allergies are worse at certain times of the year, and only the allergens prevalent at that time of year need to be evaluated. With all forms of skin testing, if the child is allergic to the test solution, a wheal and erythema (redness) will occur at the test site (Fig. 42.4). The size of the reaction is then measured and graded as 1+ to 4+, or as slight, moderate, or marked.

Always have a syringe filled with 1 ml epinephrine (Adrenalin) 1:1,000 on hand to counteract an unexpected anaphylactic reaction from skin testing (Box 42.5). Epinephrine is given intramuscularly in doses of 0.01 mg/kg, up to 0.3 mg. Children should stay in the health care setting for at least 30 minutes after skin testing so they will be there at the time such a reaction is most apt to occur.

Skin testing with food extracts is largely ineffective, although this may be used to identify foods associated with irritable bowel syndrome (Stierstorfer, Sha, & Sasson, 2013). In most instances, food allergies are best identified by eliminating a suspected food from the diet and observing whether there is an improvement in symptoms. After a time of improvement, the food is reintroduced. If it is one to which the child is allergic, symptoms will return with its reintroduction (termed "rechallenging") (Calvani, Berti, Fiocchi, et al., 2012).

Therapeutic Management

No matter what the symptoms of a child's allergy, there are three goals for therapy: reduce the child's exposure to the allergen, hyposensitize the child to produce a state of increased clinical **tolerance** (i.e., a state of not responding) to the allergen, or modify the child's response to the allergen with a pharmacologic agent.

Reducing the child's exposure to the allergen is possible when the offending allergen is a drug, food, or irritant. Reducing exposure is much more difficult when the child is found to be allergic to molds, dust, feathers, or other substances found almost everywhere.

Environmental Control

Environmental control means removal of as many common allergens as possible from a child's environment. Common measures of environmental control are shown in Table 42.3

BOX 42.5 Nursing Care Planning Based on Responsibility for Pharmacology

EPINEPHRINE HYDROCHLORIDE (ADRENALIN)

Classification: Epinephrine is a sympathomimetic drug.

Action: Acts on both α- and β-receptor sites of sympathetic receptor cells to cause increased blood pressure and heart rate. It also relaxes the smooth muscles of the bronchi. It is used to counteract the symptoms of anaphylaxis (Karch, 2013).

Pregnancy Risk Category: C

Dosage: 0.01 mg/kg, up to 0.3 mg of a 1:1,000 solution intramuscularly into the vastus lateralis of the thigh every 20 min for up to 4 doses. This may be followed by an individualized intravenous bolus if symptoms still persist.

Possible Adverse Effects: Anxiety, restlessness, headache, nausea, arrhythmias, hypertension, palpitations, pallor

Nursing Implications

- Be sure to calculate the drug dosage and check the solution strength carefully; solution is available in different concentrations, and epinephrine is a very potent drug.
- Obtain blood pressure, pulse, and respirations and auscultate breath sounds before and immediately after administration. Assess the child for signs indicating the resolution of anaphylaxis.
- Rotate injection sites to prevent necrosis at the site.
- Have a rapidly acting α-adrenergic blocking agent or vasodilator readily available in case of a hypertensive reaction, or have a β-adrenergic blocking agent readily available in case of arrhythmias.
- Protect the drug from light and heat. Use only solutions that are clear and colorless.

TABLE 42.3 Common Measures for Environmental Control of Allergens

Area of Concern	Measures	Rationale
Child's bedroom	Encase mattress and pillow in sturdy plastic, which is impervious to house mites.	Reduces dust and dust mites.
	Cover the zipper of plastic pillow and mattress case with adhesive tape.	Keeps dust confined.
	Use blankets or quilts made of or stuffed with smooth, synthetic material; avoid wool.	Minimizes dust; wool is a good dust collector or may be an allergen itself.
	Take down any ornamental items, such as a bed canopy.	Prevents dust collection.
	Remove stuffed chairs and replace with wooden ones.	Removes dust collectors.
	Remove venetian blinds and curtains that need to be dry cleaned; replace with easily laundered types.	Removes dust collectors.
	Remove stuffed toys unless filled with synthetic material.	Removes dust collectors and possible sources of allergens.
	Remove aquariums and plants.	Removes mold spores.
	Clean closet so it contains only currently used items.	Eliminates dust collectors.
	Remove any fur or woolen items from the child's wardrobe.	Removes possible allergens.
Living or television room	Remove all carpets. If a rug is necessary, vacuum at least weekly; replace an animal hair pad with a foam rubber one.	Avoids containers for dust collection.
	Provide a wooden chair, not a stuffed one, for sitting.	Provides space free from allergens
	Vacuum floor surfaces frequently.	Minimizes dust collection.
	Use a piece of linoleum or plastic laminate surface on top of carpet if the child sits on the floor.	Provides space free from allergens.
Bathroom	Use nonscented toilet paper, soaps, and cleaners.	Minimizes exposure to potential irritants.
School room	Have child sit away from blackboard, caged animals, or fish tanks.	Minimizes exposure to chalk, mold spores, and animal dander, which are allergens.
	Keep locker free of collectibles.	Reduces dust collection.
General	Purchase a dehumidifier; add compounds to paint to decrease mold spores.	Reduces mold spores.
	Use high-efficiency particulate air (HEPA) filters on furnaces and vacuums.	Filters air of possible allergens.
	Keep a favorite pet but do not purchase a new pet.	Reduces exposure to animal dander.
	Dust daily with a moist cloth.	Controls dust better than dry dusting.

BOX 42.6 Nursing Care Planning Based on Effective Communication

The Goodenough family has been instructed on environmental control measures because Dexter has severe allergic rhinitis. Despite this, Dexter's symptoms have not improved. You meet with his parents to confirm they are carrying out recommended measures.

Less Effective Communication

Nurse: Have you made the changes around your house we discussed to reduce dust?
Mrs. Goodenough: As many as we can.
Nurse: What about Dexter's bedroom? Do you have the mattress covered? Any frilly curtains taken down? His stuffed animals taken out?
Mrs. Goodenough: I've done everything I can.
Nurse: It's important he has a protected floor space in the living room and that he doesn't sit in overstuffed chairs.
Mrs. Goodenough: I've done everything I can.
Nurse: Well, you sound in good shape. It's puzzling, though, why Dexter's symptoms haven't improved.

More Effective Communication

Nurse: Have you made the changes around your house we discussed to reduce dust?
Mrs. Goodenough: As many as we can.
Nurse: What about Dexter's bedroom? Do you have the mattress covered? Any frilly curtains taken down? His stuffed animals taken out?
Mrs. Goodenough: I've done everything I can.
Nurse: Describe for me exactly what you've done.
Mrs. Goodenough: I covered the mattress. I had to leave the curtains up, though, because they match the rug. I took out a lot of the toys, but had to leave the stuffed bears because they were gifts from his grandmother.
Nurse: Let's review again what environmental control means and the effect it can have on reducing Dexter's symptoms.

By taking the parent's statement she has done "everything possible" to mean she has done everything that needs to be done, the nurse makes an incorrect assumption. Following up by asking the parent to be more specific reveals better information.

and Box 42.6. Some parents carry out instructions to reduce potential allergens in their house without difficulty, but for others, the process can seem too involved to undertake. Help parents understand that environmental control can make a great deal of difference in their child's symptoms and, if environmental control is effective with their child, this is preferable to long-term medication use or hyposensitization, which involves many health care visits and the injection or oral administration of allergens (Reisacher, 2011).

Pharmacologic Therapy

A number of pharmacologic preparations can be used to reduce the symptoms of childhood allergies. Intranasal cromolyn sodium can be used prophylactically to prevent symptoms. Second- and third-generation antihistamines, such as cetirizine (Zyrtec) and loratadine (Claritin), cause little drowsiness yet effectively block histamine release and, as a result, control itching, sneezing, and rhinorrhea. If the child's mouth feels dry while taking an antihistamine, sucking on a sugarless lozenge can help. Parents should notify the child's primary health care provider if the child develops a lower respiratory infection because antihistamines should not be continued when secretions need to be kept moist to encourage expectoration. Decongestants, such as pseudoephedrine (Sudafed), decrease nasal edema and can help enlarge breathing space, and so may also be prescribed. Intranasal corticosteroids reduce inflammation, producing an effect similar to decongestants and may be the drug of choice (Greiner, Hellings, Rotiroti, et al., 2011). Question the use of an antihistamine if a child has glucose-6-phosphate dehydrogenase deficiency because the action of an antihistamine can cause severe hemolysis in these children.

Hyposensitization

Hyposensitization, or immunotherapy, is done when the child's allergy symptoms cannot be controlled by avoidance of an allergen or conventional drug therapy. It can be accomplished by subcutaneous injections or drops given sublingually.

Hyposensitization works by increasing the plasma concentration of IgG antibodies, which then act to prevent or block IgE antibodies from coming in contact with an allergen. For the injection method, after specific allergens have been recognized with skin testing, small amounts of allergy extracts, which are dilute enough to be clinically subreactive, are injected into the child subcutaneously at 3- to 5-day intervals. The dose of antigen is increased in strength each time until the peak concentration that does not give clinical symptoms is reached. Following hyposensitization, the child's allergy symptoms should be greatly reduced or absent. Unfortunately, the child then needs periodic injections every 3 to 4 weeks to maintain hyposensitization to the allergen.

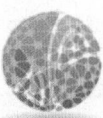

Sublingual immunotherapy (SLIT) administration of chosen allergen solutions is growing in use because it has the advantage of being painless, can be self or parent administered, and produces results equal to that of other therapies (Frati, Incorvaia, Lombardi, et al., 2012). If children are going to have an anaphylactic reaction to an injected or sublingual allergen, it generally occurs within 30 minutes after the injection. Therefore, always have children wait in the health care setting for 30 minutes after an injection before leaving. Caution parents to observe their child for this after sublingual administration.

Immunotherapy is generally continued for 2 to 3 years because the longer it is used, the longer the period of relief from symptoms after it is stopped. Be certain parents know from the beginning of treatment that this therapy will not "cure" their child. However, it can make their child symptom free or decrease symptoms for a length of time. It may also prevent a mild atopic disorder such as hay fever (allergic rhinitis) from turning into a severe atopic disorder such as asthma (see Chapter 40). Be certain children have adequate education and preparation if injection procedures are used. Help them understand the importance of returning for additional injections.

QSEN Checkpoint Question 42.3

Patient-Centered Care

Dexter's mother asks you about the potential risks and benefits of hyposensitization, stating that some Web sites she has consulted convey dire warnings against the practice. What potential benefit would you describe to Dexter's mother to alleviate her anxiety?

a. Dexter will recover more quickly from infections.
b. Dexter will be protected against secondary infections.
c. Dexter's level of helpful immunoglobulins will be increased.
d. The overall health of Dexter's immune system will be increased.

Look in Appendix A for the best answer and rationale.

COMMON IMMUNE REACTIONS

Anaphylactic Shock

Anaphylactic shock is an immediate, life-threatening, type I hypersensitivity reaction that occurs after exposure to an allergen in a previously sensitized child. Anaphylactic shock must be treated immediately because it can be fatal.

Assessment

Initially, a child may become nauseated, with vomiting and diarrhea, because of the sudden increase in gastrointestinal secretions produced by the stimulation of histamine. This is followed by urticaria (itching) and angioedema (swelling). Next, bronchospasm can become so severe that the child becomes dyspneic, hypoxemic, and then hypoxic. As blood vessels dilate, blood pressure and pulse rate fall. Seizures and death can follow as soon as 10 minutes after the allergen was introduced into the child's body.

It is sometimes difficult to distinguish anaphylactic shock from fainting (syncope). Children, however, as a rule, do not faint after an injection or a bee sting, which are common causes of anaphylactic shock. Syncope also rarely occurs if a person is lying down, so if the reaction occurred while the child was lying on a treatment table, it is most likely that the reaction is anaphylactic. Another way to differentiate the two types is with syncope, although the child may appear pale, fall to the ground, and be momentarily unconscious, pulse and blood pressure remain normal. The child can be readily aroused by gentle shaking or after breathing amyl nitrite (smelling salts). In contrast, the child with an anaphylactic reaction cannot be roused this way.

Therapeutic Management

Preventing and recognizing anaphylaxis are as important as knowing how to respond when it occurs. Before giving drugs that are known to have a high incidence of anaphylactic reactions such as penicillin, cephalosporins, aspirin, or antitoxin serums, check the child's electronic record to be certain no prior reactions have been noted; be certain as well to ask parents if their child has ever had a previous reaction to the drug. If in doubt, withhold the drug until its safety for the child can be confirmed. Urge children (and adults) who have a known hypersensitivity reaction to any injectable substance to wear a bracelet or necklace identifying the substance to which they are allergic. Some children object to this safety measure because they do not want to look conspicuous, but stress to them this could be a lifesaving measure. Generally, children who have hypersensitivity reactions to insect stings are advised to undergo hyposensitization therapy because they cannot totally avoid insects.

Epinephrine, injected intramuscularly, is the drug of choice for the treatment of anaphylaxis (Phillips, Lockey, Fox, et al., 2011). For maximum effectiveness, if anaphylaxis follows an injection or an insect sting, inject the epinephrine into the vastus lateralis muscle of the thigh or the opposite arm. Additional emergency interventions to take in a health care setting are summarized in Box 42.7.

If a sensitized child receives an injection or is stung by an insect while at home, parents must know the proper procedure to follow for anaphylactic shock so they can give their child immediate help. They need to notify the emergency response system (911) that their child is having a severe reaction. In place of a tourniquet, they can apply ice to the injection or sting site to slow absorption. If a child has been prescribed an antihistamine, they should administer that; caution them, however, not to attempt to give any oral medications if the child is comatose. Parents should have an emergency kit (Ana-Kit), an insect sting treatment kit that contains measured doses of epinephrine (often in a device called an EpiPen, which injects the epinephrine; Box 42.8), and an antihistamine on hand. Parents and children need practice to inject an EpiPen correctly or they can accidentally puncture their thumb, thus creating circulation problems in their own hand (Sheikh, Simons, Barbour, et al., 2012).

An evaluation of the child after an anaphylactic reaction involves not only a physical examination but also an evaluation to help the child avoid such a serious reaction again. This involves health teaching about the substance that caused the reaction and related substances that could have the same effect.

BOX 42.7 Emergency Measures for Anaphylactic Shock

Anaphylaxis is a true emergency, so fast interventions are necessary.

- Position the child with the head level with the body to counteract hypotension.
- Administer aqueous epinephrine (Adrenalin) 1:1,000 intramuscularly at a dosage of 0.01 mg/kg of body weight up to 0.3 mg. This relieves laryngeal edema and severe bronchospasm by widening the airway.
- Notify the cardiac arrest team because both respiratory and cardiac arrest may occur.
- If hypoxia is present, administer oxygen by mask or nasal cannula.
- Anticipate the need for an intravenous (IV) fluid line as a route for a vasopressor such as dopamine and fluid to help restore blood pressure.
- If an insect sting was the cause of the condition, a tourniquet, applied above the site of the bite, may be prescribed to limit absorption of the insect venom into the bloodstream.
- Anticipate use of a nebulized bronchodilator such as albuterol to halt wheezing or diphenhydramine (Benadryl) intramuscularly or IV if urticaria (itching and swelling) is present.
- If the child is experiencing seizures, turn the child onto his or her side and prepare to administer an antiseizure medication such as phenobarbital or diazepam.
- A corticosteroid may be administered as a second-line drug. This does not act immediately but does reduce inflammation. IV methylprednisolone is a typical drug given.
- Keep the child and family members calm; anxiety adds to bronchospasm and decreases breathing ability.

QSEN Checkpoint Question 42.4

Teamwork & Collaboration

Any child can have an anaphylactic reaction to a food, drug, or vaccine and Dexter is at risk because of his allergy history. If you were a school nurse, and Dexter, who weighs 48 kg, had an anaphylactic reaction after you gave him a vaccine, the correct dose of epinephrine for you or a staff member to give him would be:

a. 0.048 mg
b. 0.48 mg
c. 4.8 mg
d. 8.4 mg

Look in Appendix A for the best answer and rationale.

Urticaria and Angioedema

Urticaria, or hives, refers to flat wheals surrounded by erythema arising from the chorion layer of skin; they are intensely pruritic (often described as a burning sensation). Elevations may occur so closely together that they tend to coalesce (blend together); dilatation of capillaries and venules with increased permeability occurs around the lesions. The cause of urticaria is a type I or immediate hypersensitivity reaction created by the release of histamine from an antibody–antigen reaction, similar to but of lesser intensity than anaphylaxis. In chronic urticaria, no causative allergen may be found.

Angioedema is edema of the skin and subcutaneous tissue. This occurs most frequently on the eyelids, hands, feet, genitalia, and lips—areas where skin is loosely bound by subcutaneous tissue. Angioedema can be distinguished from other edemas because it is not dependent, is generally asymmetrically distributed, and usually occurs in conjunction with urticaria.

BOX 42.8 Nursing Care Planning Based on Family Teaching

GUIDELINES FOR USING AN EpiPen

Q. Dexter's father says to you, "If my child is stung by a bee, I'm supposed to inject epinephrine. How do I do that?"

A. It is important you think about this in advance, because, from the moment your child is stung, it will be an emergency situation.

- Purchase an EpiPen, a commercial syringe with a designated dose of epinephrine for use in emergencies.
- If necessary, purchase additional EpiPens so you have one at home, provide one for your child's school, and maybe keep one in your car to avoid having to remember to carry one with you.
- Store EpiPens at room temperature; don't refrigerate.
- Inspect the color of the solution in the EpiPen once a month; replace it if it is cloudy or discolored.
- If your child is stung, remove the gray safety cap from the device and wipe the outer fleshy portion of your child's thigh with an alcohol wipe.
- Place the EpiPen against the thigh until the device activates and inject the solution into your child's thigh. If necessary, you can place the device on top of your child's clothing. The needle is long enough to pass through the clothing and into your child's skin.
- Be careful before injecting that you are holding the EpiPen with the needle toward your child. If not, you will accidentally inject your own thumb (a serious circumstance, because the dose of epinephrine could seriously injure your thumb).
- Keep in mind that the EpiPen is designed so that not all the solution in the pen will be ejected. Do not try to give the remainder of the solution.
- Remember that epinephrine will control symptoms for about 20 minutes. Therefore, after administering the dose, call 911 for transportation assistance or transport your child to an emergency facility for further care.

With severe angioedema, the larynx may be involved. This is a serious type because laryngeal edema could be so extreme that it leads to airway obstruction and, subsequently, asphyxiation and death.

The allergens that most frequently cause urticaria and angioedema include drugs, foods, and insect stings. In some children, exposure to hot or cold can also cause these reactions. All children need their causative agent identified so it can be avoided. Although a rare event, children who have a reaction to hot or cold must especially be identified because, if they swim in cold water, the sudden release of histamine could cause dizziness so severe that they could drown. Immediate therapy for urticaria or angioedema is a intramuscular epinephrine injection or the administration of an oral antihistamine. For long-term therapy, corticosteroids may be prescribed; cyclosporine (an immunosuppressant) and omalizumab (Xolair), a monoclonal antibody, are usually reserved for older adolescents or adults (Kaplan, 2012).

Serum Sickness

Serum sickness is an inflammatory reaction that occurs in the blood vessel walls and surrounding tissue, causing tissue damage, fever, malaise, lymphadenopathy, arthralgia, urticaria, and arthritis as common symptoms. It is usually caused by drugs, infectious agents, vaccines, or blood products (Fuleihan, 2011). Examples of foreign sera given to children include tetanus antitoxin, diphtheria antitoxin, and rabies antiserum, all obtained from horse serum. Although penicillin is usually thought of the antibiotic most apt to cause a reaction, one of the most common antibiotics causing serum sickness in children is the cephalosporin drug cefaclor (Ceclor) (Cruz & Bahna, 2011).

Assessment

Symptoms of serum sickness begin 7 to 12 days after the serum injection. If a child has previously received the same type of foreign serum, symptoms may occur as early as 1 to 5 days. Children notice itching, edema, and erythema at the injection site. There is generalized urticaria (hives) with or without angioedema (generalized edema). Erythematous maculopapular rashes, erythema multiforme (a generalized macular eruption with dark red papules), or purpura (hemorrhage into the skin), fever, arthralgia (joint pain), and swollen regional lymph nodes near the site of the injection may all follow. Some children experience nausea, vomiting, and abdominal pain. In the most extreme instances, the child's nervous system can be involved and optic neuritis, stupor, and coma may occur. If edema is severe, laryngeal edema will become the paramount symptom that needs attention and treatment.

Therapeutic Management

Serum sickness lasts days or weeks. In its usual form (symptoms limited to urticaria, edema, arthralgia, or pruritus), the treatment is only symptomatic by the administration of an antihistamine or epinephrine to relieve the urticaria followed by a nonsteroidal anti-inflammatory drug (NSAID) such as ibuprofen (Motrin) or a corticosteroid to relieve the fever and joint pain because the condition will improve by itself with time.

Like anaphylactic reactions, serum sickness reactions are frightening to children and parents. Be certain that parents understand why the reaction occurred (their child has a low threshold of sensitization to this particular substance), that it was not anyone's fault, and that it did not occur from the administration of the wrong compound (assuming that proper precautions to ascertain sensitivity to the solution were taken before the incident). Because serum sickness mimics so many other disorders, parents need reassurance that their child does not have arthritis (the arthralgia may make them think their child has this) and that their child will not have long-term effects.

Be certain that they understand the child should not receive the foreign serum or drug that was responsible for this primary occurrence again. Otherwise, if administered again, the manifestation of the reaction could be anaphylaxis. Urge children to wear a bracelet or necklace stating the substance to which they are hypersensitive. Parents need to be certain the child's immunizations (and records) are kept current so there is never a need to give sera such as tetanus or diphtheria antitoxins because they were underimmunized.

ATOPIC DISORDERS

Individuals with atopic disease are prone to all types of allergic responses. Three disorders occur most frequently: hay fever (allergic rhinitis), eczema (atopic dermatitis), and asthma (discussed with other respiratory diseases in Chapter 40). The gene responsible for an immune response is located near the human leukocyte antigen that is responsible for graft rejections. In certain children, a tendency for sensitivity to antigens or abnormality of this gene is apparently inherited. These children have a higher than normal production of IgE antibodies, which makes them more responsive to allergens than other people.

Because such diseases show a familial tendency, different family members may have different symptoms. In one family, for example, the father may have allergic rhinitis, one child may have asthma, and another may have atopic dermatitis.

Allergic Rhinitis

Allergic rhinitis is associated with an IgE-mediated inflammatory response to allergen exposure. It is closely associated with and may be a precursor to asthma (Ciprandi, Signori, Tosca, et al., 2011). It is also one of the most common chronic conditions affecting people in the United States with estimates of 35 to 50 million people affected; incidences are increasing, especially among the pediatric population (Blaiss, 2010).

Assessment

Common symptoms of allergic rhinitis include sneezing, nasal engorgement, and a profuse watery nasal discharge. The mucous membrane of the nose is generally paler than normal. It may be edematous, adding to nasal congestion. The eyes tend to water. The conjunctivae may be pruritic, often with a distinctive pebbly appearance. Children constantly rub their noses in an upward motion, termed an "allergic salute." Over a long period, rubbing the nose this way leads to a horizontal crease across the tip of the nose, called an allergic crease or Dienne line. Because of congestion in the nose, there tends to be back-pressure to the blood circulation around the eye orbit, which leads to blackened areas under the eyes, termed allergic shiners (Fig. 42.5).

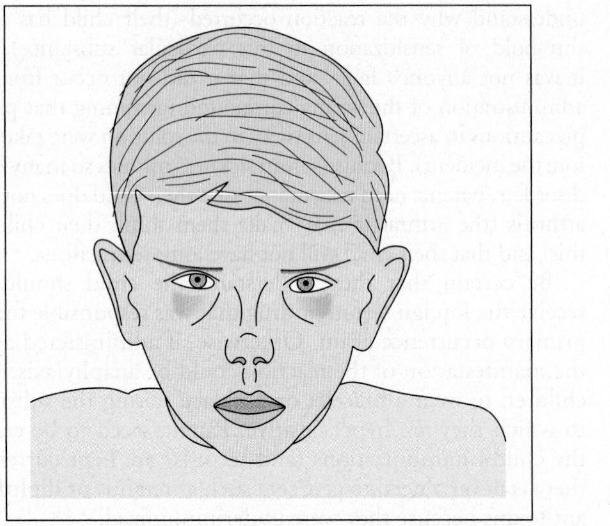

FIGURE 42.5 Back-pressure to the blood circulation around the eye orbit from allergic rhinitis may lead to dark areas under the eyes (allergic shiners). The frequent rubbing of the nose in an upward direction can lead to a peculiar horizontal crease (Dennie line).

Children older than 6 years of age (when frontal sinuses develop) may report full frontal headaches that become even more marked with adolescence. Some children have many symptoms—they feel exhausted and lethargic and do not function well in school. Recurrent otitis media may occur because of swollen pharyngeal tissue (eustachian tubes are blocked to the middle ear). A smear of the nasal discharge will reveal an increased eosinophil count (more than 10% of the white cell count). A RAST analysis may reveal the offending allergens.

The allergens that usually cause allergic rhinitis are pollens or molds rather than foods or drugs. Many children are brought to a health care setting during peak pollen months because parents think they have a constant "summer cold." However, with an upper respiratory infection, the mucous membrane of the nose is more apt to be reddened than pale, and the secretions draining from the nose are apt to be thick white or yellow rather than the thin, watery secretions of allergic rhinitis. Children with an upper respiratory infection often also have a fever, whereas children with allergic rhinitis do not. Yet another differentiation is, with an upper respiratory infection, a sore throat and cervical adenopathy may be present, whereas these rarely accompany allergic rhinitis.

Therapeutic Management

Allergic rhinitis is managed by a three-prong program: avoidance of offending allergens, use of pharmacologic agents (antihistamines, leukotriene inhibitors, or corticosteroids), or immunotherapy. It may be impossible for some children to avoid all the allergens that cause symptoms because the child has sensitivity to so many pollens or grasses. If children always show symptoms at one particular time of the year, parents may be able to carry out environmental control for that period of the year to limit symptoms.

Parents usually ask how sick children should be before they need to see an allergist about skin testing and definitive treatment. As a rule, if the child's symptoms are increasing in intensity, if there is associated lower respiratory tract involvement, or if the condition interferes with activities in which the child wants to participate, the child needs testing and treatment. Those with minor symptoms can be managed by environmental control and medications such as intranasal antihistamines or corticosteroids to reduce symptoms.

Help parents, as necessary, to make out reminder sheets for the administration of medications so symptoms can be prevented, not treated after they appear. It's helpful if children and parents choose an antihistamine that causes the least amount of drowsiness so this doesn't interfere with schoolwork or, if an adolescent, with safe driving. Review with parents that if nasal antihistamine sprays are given for more than 3 days, a rebound effect can occur (the nasal mucosa becomes more edematous rather than less edematous) and symptoms will appear to worsen rather than improve.

Allergic rhinitis is often considered a minor illness by parents, something children will outgrow. However, while the condition exists, it may not be a minor illness for the child if it keeps the child from interacting with peers because going outside intensifies symptoms. Box 42.9 shows an interprofessional care map illustrating both nursing and team planning for a child with allergic rhinitis.

QSEN Checkpoint Question 42.5

Quality Improvement

Dexter is atopic, or prone to allergies. When planning his care, what desired outcome should you prioritize?

a. Dexter states that his symptoms do not interfere with being able to play with his friends.
b. Dexter is able to describe the cause of his allergic response.
c. Dexter states that he no longer has allergies.
d. Dexter states he enjoys taking medicine to prevent his allergy symptoms.

Look in Appendix A for the best answer and rationale.

Perennial Allergic Rhinitis

Allergic rhinitis becomes perennial (year round) when the allergen is one that is present in the environment year round, such as house dust mites or pet hair. Although the child's symptoms may not result in the obvious distress associated with seasonal allergic rhinitis, the child needs treatment just as much because the symptoms otherwise never go away. In addition, serous otitis media can accompany the disorder as a long-term consequence (see Chapter 50). Because the agent that causes perennial allergic rhinitis is often something in the house, environmental control as well as sublingual immunotherapy can play a big role in the control of the allergic symptoms (Wise & Schlosser, 2012).

Atopic Dermatitis (Infantile Eczema)

Atopic dermatitis is primarily a disease of infants, beginning as early as the second month of life and possibly lasting until the child is 2 to 3 years old. It may be related to food allergy because it tends to occur more often in formula-fed infants than in breastfed infants and is more common if infants are fed solid food before 6 months. Sweating, heat, tight clothing, and contact irritants such as soap tend to increase the pruritus. Symptoms may be more annoying in the winter, when additional irritating clothing is present, with marked improvement in the summer.

Assessment

With infantile atopic dermatitis, capillary permeability increases, causing a loss of serous fluid out into the tissues.

BOX 42.9 Nursing Care Planning

AN INTERPROFESSIONAL CARE MAP FOR A CHILD WITH ALLERGIC RHINITIS

Dexter Goodenough is a 6-year-old boy you meet in an ambulatory setting. His mother has just been told he has allergic rhinitis (hay fever). "Thank heavens," his mother exclaims. "I thought when I heard he had an immune system disease he had AIDS. What a relief it's only an allergy."

Family Assessment Child lives with his mother and stepfather in a beachfront cottage. Also in the family is a brother, 8 years old; a stepbrother, 16 years old; and a paternal grandmother. His stepfather owns a jewelry store. His mother is a stay-at-home mom. Finances are rated as "not a problem."

Client Assessment Child has documented peanut allergy. Child's eyes are reddened and watery; nose drains a clear discharge. His mother tells you he frequently has a headache and is constantly listless. Other children at school have started to bully him because of his appearance. His grades are "terrible" because the minute he gets to school, his symptoms begin. Dexter is prescribed an antihistamine and environmental control.

Nursing Diagnosis Situational low self-esteem related to feelings of inadequacy and embarrassment

Outcome Criteria Client states he is able to function in school despite allergy symptoms and discomfort; is taking active measures to avoid allergens; will report bullying to school official.

Team Member Responsible	Assessment	Intervention	Rationale	Expected Outcome
Activities of Daily Living, Including Safety				
Nurse	Assess what Dexter's classroom is like to identify potential allergens, because child's symptoms are most intense when he is at school.	Discuss potential source of allergens with mother; ask her to meet with teacher to see if modifications could be made.	Environmental control can reduce the number of allergens that cause symptoms.	Mother visits classroom as necessary to suggest changes such as moving Dexter's seat further away from the hamster cage.
Teamwork and Collaboration				
Nurse/Primary health care provider	Assess if child's symptoms could be reduced with hyposensitization.	Arrange a consultation with allergist about the possibility of hyposensitization.	Hyposensitization can greatly reduce allergy symptoms if specific allergens can be identified.	Parent and child meet with allergist to discuss the possibility of sublingual hyposensitization if antihistamine is not effective.
Procedures/Medications for Quality Improvement				
Nurse	Assess if child has had experience with taking medicine.	Help mother set up a medicine chart that will help with antihistamine adherence.	Allergy medicine is most effective when it is taken conscientiously.	Parent states she will be conscientious about antihistamine administration.
Nutrition				
Nurse/Nutritionist	Assess if there are any foods the child or mother feel contribute to allergy symptoms. Ask how he manages the peanut allergy.	If foods other than peanuts are identified, review with mother the list of foods to avoid.	Respiratory allergens are more likely involved in allergic rhinitis, but foods should be ruled out.	Mother and child describe any foods that cause discomfort for child and measures to avoid them.

(continued on page 1244)

BOX 42.9 Nursing Care Planning (continued)

Patient-Centered Care				
Nurse	Assess environmental aspects at home that could be causing the child's symptoms.	Discuss environmental control with parents.	Reducing allergens in the home can also aid in reducing the child's symptoms.	Parents agree to any modifications necessary in their home.
Nurse	Assess if the child is exposed to secondary smoke in the home.	Educate family on the damage that secondary smoke can cause.	Secondary smoke is a potent allergen that also contributes to lung and heart disease.	Parents agree to make their home smoke free.
Psychosocial/Spiritual/Emotional Needs				
Nurse/Social work counselor	Assess the extent of ridicule the child undergoes at school.	Discuss coping measures with child; urge mother to report bullying to school authorities.	Psychological health is as important as physical health.	Child describes experiences at school are improving; states he is no longer bullied about allergy symptoms.
Informatics for Seamless Health Care Planning				
Nurse	Assess if parent has other questions about child's allergies.	Schedule a follow-up visit for reevaluation of new medication.	A range of medicine types are available for allergy control; therefore, if one isn't effective, another can be selected and prescribed.	Mother states she understands the importance of a follow-up visit and will keep appointment.

Children develop papular and vesicular skin eruptions with surrounding erythema. The vesicles rupture and exude yellow, sticky secretions that form crusts on the skin as they dry. An increased eosinophil count reveals that the condition is allergy based. Because the lesions are extremely pruritic, the child scratches and further irritates the lesions, causing linear excoriations. Secondary infections of open lesions may then occur. As the infected lesions heal, the skin becomes depigmented and lichenified (shiny), and dry, flaky scales form. If a secondary infection occurs, the infant may have a low-grade fever and puss-filled lesions, and local lymph nodes may be swollen.

The common sites for lesions include the scalp and forehead, the cheeks, neck, behind the ears, and the extensor surfaces of the extremities (Fig. 42.6). In contrast, the palms of the hands and the soles of the feet are usually uninvolved. Because the lesions feel so uncomfortable, children with infantile atopic dermatitis become fussy and irritable. They may not eat well because of this generalized discomfort.

Although infantile atopic dermatitis is generally diagnosed based on a family history (by considering other allergic individuals in the family) and noticing the characteristic lesions and their patterns, it is sometimes difficult to distinguish from seborrheic dermatitis (cradle cap; see Chapter 29). The findings in seborrheic dermatitis and infantile atopic dermatitis are contrasted in Table 42.4. A child with seborrheic dermatitis needs little therapy than soaking the scales in mineral oil, then lifting them away; infants with infantile atopic dermatitis must be referred for long-term therapy. Because untreated phenylketonuria (PKU) can lead to atopic dermatitis, children with infantile atopic dermatitis need to have a repeat test for PKU to be certain this is ruled out (Seashore, 2011).

Skin testing is usually ineffective because, although the allergen causing infantile atopic dermatitis may be a pollen, dust or mold spore, it is often a food allergen.

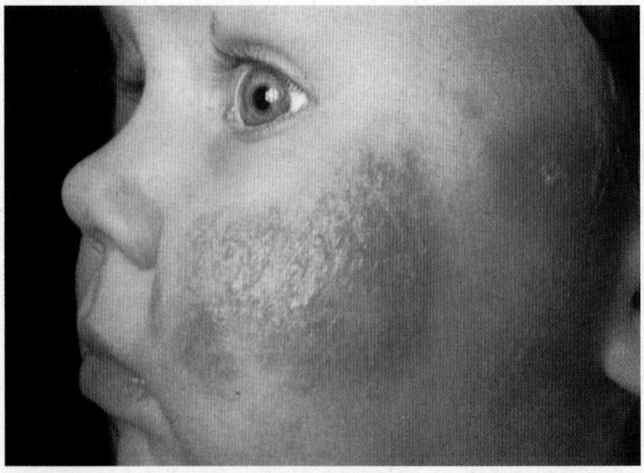

FIGURE 42.6 An infant with atopic dermatitis. (From Sauer, G. C., & Hall, J. C. [1996]. *Manual of skin diseases* [7th ed.]. Philadelphia, PA: Lippincott-Raven Publishers.)

TABLE 42.4 Comparison of Seborrheic Dermatitis and Atopic Dermatitis

Finding	Seborrheic Dermatitis	Atopic Dermatitis
Age at onset	0–6 months	2–6 months
Length of disease	Rarely 1 year	2–3 years
Mood of child	Happy; parents happy	Irritable; parents tired
Location of lesions	Scalp, behind ears, near umbilicus	Cheeks, extensor surfaces, some flexor surfaces
Types of lesions	Salmon-colored erythematous lesions with greasy scales	Papulovesicular erythematous lesions with weeping and crusting
Itching	No	Severe
Depigmentation	No	Yes
Lichenification	No	Yes
White dermographism	No	Yes
Eosinophilia	No nasal mucus or blood eosinophilia	Nasal mucus or blood eosinophilia
IgE serum levels	Low	High

Therapeutic Management

The treatment of atopic dermatitis is aimed at reducing the amount of allergen exposure, if such allergens can be identified. The most likely foods to which infants are allergic are milk, eggs, wheat, chocolate, fish, tomatoes, and peanuts. The use of elimination diets to identify food allergens is discussed later in this chapter. A second major consideration in treatment is aimed at reducing pruritus so children do not irritate lesions and cause secondary infections by scratching. Hydrating the skin by bathing or applying wet dressings (wet with tap water or Burow's solution) for 15 to 20 minutes, followed by the application of a moisturizer such as Eucerin is helpful. While infants are having wet dressings applied, be conscientious that they don't become chilled, especially if a large portion of the body is to be covered with the dressings. Use a stockinette dressing with holes cut out for the eyes, nose, and mouth pulled over the head to hold wet dressings in place so you don't have to use any form of tape. To prevent corneal irritation, be careful that dressings don't come in contact with the eyes.

Some infants will be prescribed an antihistamine to reduce itching. Topical steroids such as 1% hydrocortisone cream also effectively relieve the discomfort and appearance of lesions by reducing the inflammation and pruritus. If the lesions are dry, a corticosteroid ointment is most effective; if moist, a lotion may be most effective. Applying the cream or lotion and then covering the area with an occlusive dressing such as plastic wrap overnight may speed the healing process and keep the infant's hands away from the dressing. If the lesions are secondarily infected, hydrocortisone mixed with an antibiotic base (generally, neomycin) may be prescribed. Caution parents not to discontinue the application of cortisone cream abruptly. Although absorption with topical application is limited, some does occur and suppresses adrenal gland functioning. Phasing out the use of the cream slowly allows the infant's adrenal response (ability to produce epinephrine) to gradually return to a usual level and be available for an emergency. Also caution parents not to overuse cortisone cream. More is not better and may increase the risk of systemic absorption. Because of these precautions with steroid creams, children over 2 years old may be prescribed the immunomodulator tacrolimus (Protopic) or pimecrolimus (Elidel). These drugs have been associated with serious side effects and, as a result, have been U.S. Food and Drug Administration (FDA) approved only with a black box warning that these drugs need to be prescribed at the minimal possible dose (Nicol, 2011).

Nursing Diagnoses and Related Interventions

Nursing Diagnosis: Risk for impaired parenting related to feelings of inadequacy secondary to infant's chronic atopic dermatitis

Outcome Evaluation: Parents express confidence in their ability to follow recommended therapy; express positive aspects of infant; hold and interact with infant warmly.

Parents of children with infantile atopic dermatitis need a great deal of support through the course of the disease because infants can become extremely irritable from the constant pruritus. No matter how hard parents try, they do not seem to be able to make their child happy. Parents need a listening ear so they can vent these concerns and maintain their self-esteem as parents. Attending support groups with other parents also can help meet this need.

Nursing Diagnosis: Impaired skin integrity related to infantile atopic dermatitis

Outcome Evaluation: Infant does not scratch lesions; parents state infant is less irritable and easier to care for; lesions show signs of healing.

When lesions begin to heal, a skin emollient and moisturizer, such as Eucerin, or baths with a substance to lubricate the skin, such as Alpha Keri, are prescribed to prevent excessive skin dryness. Be certain that parents know that the infant should soak in the bath with the lubricant for approximately 15 minutes, then be patted dry, not rubbed, so lesions are not aggravated. Caution them not to use soap for bathing, because it can be drying.

Suggest that parents trim the infant's fingernails short or cover the hands with cotton socks to prevent scratching. Let them know that exposure to the herpes virus can cause a generalized reaction. This means that they should screen babysitters or alert child care personnel with active herpes lesions not to care for their infant while atopic dermatitis is active.

In most infants, the lesions of infantile atopic dermatitis clear by the time they are 3 years old. Unless secondary infection with scarring has occurred, the skin surface will not be marked. Many of these children go on to develop other allergies, however. In the preschool years, parents may report that the child has "one cold after another" (allergic rhinitis). By early school years, the child may show signs of asthma.

Atopic Dermatitis in the Older Child

Atopic dermatitis that occurs at later ages is prominent on the flexor surface of the extremities and on the dorsal surfaces of the wrists and ankles. It often occurs in the eyebrows; if the child scratches the lesions, hair loss and scant eyebrows can result. Depigmentation or hyperpigmentation is usually noticed as lesions fade; lichenification can be marked. Often, the child's fingernails have a glossy sheen caused by the buffing action of constant rubbing and scratching. In some children, an "itch–scratch cycle" occurs as a response to stress and leads to an exacerbation of symptoms. For example, children who feel pressured in school to achieve or who are upset because their parents are about to be divorced, rub their skin, a nervous, comforting mannerism; the rubbing or scratching leads to irritation of lesions. The lesions itch intensely and the child scratches even more vigorously because of the increased discomfort. The accelerated scratching leads to an increased number of lesions, the increased number or lesions leads to more scratching, and so on.

Therapeutic Management

Atopic dermatitis is a difficult disease for older children because they realize the scratching leads to depigmentation or lichenification, but they're unable to stop scratching because the itching is so intense. Adolescents, especially, are acutely aware of their appearance, so this can be an especially difficult illness for them. Suggest they use only a prescription soap (or none at all) to prevent skin drying. Avoiding swimming in chlorinated pools may also help. If children are required to swim in school, encourage them to shower well afterward to remove chlorine from the skin as well as apply a skin emollient and moisturizer such as Eucerin after coming out of the water. After a period of activity in which sweating occurs, such as gymnastics, suggest the child take a shower to remove perspiration so this doesn't irritate the skin. Avoiding tight clothing at the flexor portions of the extremities is also important. As a final precaution, urge children not to use medication intended for acne cover-up because these medications are designed to dry the skin and will increase itching with atopic dermatitis.

Medical treatment is basically the same as for the infant with atopic dermatitis: keeping the skin hydrated and identifying allergens and any psychological problems that are initiating an itch–scratch cycle. The application of hydrocortisone cream or phototherapy with ultraviolet light both can make a big difference in helping lesions improve.

An evaluation for the older child with atopic dermatitis should include evaluating not only how well the lesions are healing but also how well the child is adjusting to school and family in light of having this irritating disorder.

What if... 42.2 **When Dexter had atopic dermatitis (infantile eczema) as an infant, almost his entire face was covered with weeping, crusting lesions and his forehead was lined with scratch marks. His mother was exhausted because Dexter never slept because of the constant itching. What suggestions could you have made to his mother to make him more comfortable? What could you suggest she do for herself?**

DRUG AND FOOD ALLERGIES

Drug Allergies

One of the hazards of giving any medication is the risk that a child may experience a reaction to it or exhibit allergic symptoms (Caubet & Eigenmann, 2012). Because reactions to drugs differ, it is important to be familiar with the differences between an allergic reaction, a toxic reaction, or a known side effect to a drug because a child might be exhibiting a toxic or side reaction rather than an allergic one.

A *toxic reaction* is one that occurs when a child has received too much of a drug. *Side effects* of drugs are those that are known to occur in addition to a therapeutic effect. When an *allergic effect* occurs, a range of unpredictable symptoms occur. With the exception of acetylsalicylic acid (aspirin) and NSAIDs, allergies rarely occur to orally administered drugs. Children with atopic diseases appear to be most prone to allergic drug reactions, although anyone can have such a reaction.

A drug itself may not be an allergen, but when the drug combines with body protein, it becomes an allergen, which is why allergic responses occur not with the initial administration of a drug, but only after the protein interaction (hapten formation or sensitivity) has occurred. When drugs are applied to the skin or mucous membrane, the chance of a drug allergy is highest.

Skin manifestations seen frequently include urticaria, angioedema, allergic contact dermatitis, pruritus, and purpura. Respiratory symptoms include wheezing or rhinitis. Thrombocytopenia and hemolytic anemia may develop. Anaphylactic shock and serum sickness may occur. As mentioned previously, children with a known drug allergy should wear a medical identification bracelet stating the drug to which they are sensitive.

Injectable drugs that are frequently involved in allergic reactions are cephalosporins, penicillin, and vaccines. In most instances, discontinuing the drug or never again administering the drug or vaccine is the only therapy needed. If urticaria or serum sickness occurs, an antihistamine (such as diphenhydramine hydrochloride [Benadryl]) may be needed to relieve the symptoms. If anaphylaxis results, the treatment would be the same as for any anaphylaxis.

Food Allergies

Food allergies are an abnormal immune response caused by exposure to a particular food protein. They can be IgE-mediated, cell-mediated, or mixed reactions, although IgE-mediated (type 1 hypersensitivity) reactions account for most food reactions (Robison & Pongracic, 2012). Symptoms of food allergies vary greatly among children, but urticaria, angioedema, pruritus, abdominal pain, colic, cramps, diarrhea, respiratory symptoms, and atopic dermatitis are common (Wallengren, 2011). They occur more often in boys than in girls and in infants born of women over 35 years of age (Karpa, Paul, Leckie, et al., 2012).

A symptom such as urticaria begins to manifest itself only minutes after an offending food is eaten. Additional symptoms may be delayed, often making the offending food difficult to recognize. Whole protein is probably the cause of immediate reactions; delayed reactions are probably the result of sensitivity to some protein breakdown product.

Skin testing is unreliable with food allergies as a whole and delayed reactions in particular, because it is done with whole protein extracts and allergies to partial breakdown proteins will not be detected. The most common foods that cause immediate allergy symptoms include egg whites, fish and other seafood, berries, and nuts. Delayed food reactions are commonly caused by cereals (wheat and corn), milk, chocolate, pork, legumes, white potatoes, beef, food additives and colorings, and oranges. If children are allergic to milk, caution them that they are probably allergic to milk products as well. Children who are allergic to eggs often cannot eat any foods that contain eggs, such as pudding or baked goods. Whether children who are allergic to eggs should receive vaccines that contain egg protein has to be evaluated in light of the importance of the vaccine in preventing a serious childhood illness (Hui & Macdonald, 2011).

Assessment

Young children cannot describe why they do not enjoy eating a particular food because they do not know the word for "headache," "stomachache," or "itchiness," but they do tend to avoid foods that affect them, which often earns them a reputation of being "fussy eaters." This is not diagnostic of food allergies, however, because children may refuse to eat foods as a form of toddler rebellion or may be reported as fussy eaters because parents are expecting them to eat more than their small size requires.

Encouraging a child or the parents to keep a food diary or a record of everything a child eats each day and then documenting if any symptoms occurred is often the best way to spot offending foods. A food that is found on lists when symptoms were few, but not on days when the child is in distress, is not an offending food. A food that appears only on "bad days," however, can be strongly suspected as being an allergen.

An elimination diet is a traditional method to detect food allergens. For this, parents feed the child only foods that rarely cause allergy, such as rice, lamb, carrots, peas, and sweet potatoes, for about 7 days. Then they add, one by one, at 2- to 3-day intervals, foods that are suspected of causing the allergy. When a food is introduced in this way, the child must be encouraged to eat a lot of it that day. If symptoms occur, the food is then eliminated from the child's meals on a permanent basis. If no symptoms occur, the child can continue to eat the food.

Therapeutic Management

The easiest treatment for a food allergy is to permanently eliminate offending foods from the child's diet. This is relatively easy to do if there are only a few offending foods, but it becomes difficult when the foods are great in number or, like milk, wheat, or eggs, are found in many products. If many foods are involved, the child's nutrition status (whether the child is growing adequately and increasing in weight) needs to be assessed at health care visits. For some children, sublingual immunotherapy will be prescribed so they can eat a more varied diet (Traister, Green, Mitchell, et al., 2012).

Urge parents to become careful shoppers and read labels carefully to be certain the foods they are buying do not contain products to which their child is sensitive. Help school-age children learn to choose foods they can safely eat at the school cafeteria or at summer camp to avoid reactions.

Milk Hypersensitivity

The true incidence of milk hypersensitivity is probably not as high as the number of diagnoses made. Allergy to milk occurs in infancy and is typified by failure to gain weight, diarrhea, perhaps vomiting, and abdominal pain. Because these symptoms also occur in gastrointestinal disorders, infants with colic (characterized by abdominal pain, no change in stools, and no failure to gain weight), those with lactase deficiency (they cannot ingest the lactose in milk) or those with a gastroenteritis infection (have nausea and vomiting) may be incorrectly diagnosed as having a milk allergy. The existence of milk allergy is yet another reason to promote breastfeeding because milk allergy is almost nonexistent with this. Changing a formula-fed infant to a hydrolyzed protein-based or soybean formula usually decreases symptoms dramatically.

Caution parents to read food labels carefully to be certain frozen foods or hot dogs, for example, do not contain milk because milk can be used as filler in these products. Because milk is a major source of vitamin D and calcium, children who are forced to avoid all milk, and milk products may need a vitamin and calcium supplement. Milk allergy usually lasts until 3 to 5 years of age (Koletzko, Niggemann, Arato, et al., 2012). To establish whether the problem is truly a milk allergy, milk can be reintroduced every 6 to 12 months. If the problem is a true milk allergy, signs will recur. Oral immunotherapy can be used for preschool and school-age children in whom an allergy persists.

Peanut Hypersensitivity

Peanut and tree nut ingestions are the cause of more than 85% of fatalities caused by food anaphylaxis in the United States (Robison & Pongracic, 2012). School nurses need to be very aware of this danger and may need to advocate for "peanut-free" lunch rooms (Pistiner & Lee, 2012). Desensitization to peanuts may be required to minimize children's responses as it's difficult for a child to always avoid peanuts, especially at social events.

QSEN Checkpoint Question 42.6

Evidence-Based Practice

Food allergies are an important concern for nurses working in child care or preschool settings because such sites may be where a child eats an allergenic food and experiences a possibly fatal reaction. To examine the circumstances of why allergic reactions in young children occur, researchers collected data on 512 infants aged 3 to 15 months who had documented allergies to milk or egg.

The incidence of reactions in the study group was less than one reaction per child per year. Reactions occurred mostly because of unintentional exposure to milk or egg through label-reading errors and cross-contact. In 50% of reactions, the offending food was provided by a person other than a parent. Of the reactions, 29% were severe enough that the child was treated with epinephrine. Factors resulting in undertreatment included a lack of recognition of the severity of symptoms, epinephrine being unavailable, and fears about epinephrine administration (Fleischer, Perry, Atkins, et al., 2012).

Based on the previous study and the fact that Dexter is allergic to peanuts, which statement by Dexter's mother would give you the most concern?

a. "I pack his lunch every day so I'll know what he eats."
b. "Dexter is a good kid and always willing to share."
c. "If he goes to a party, I ask if peanuts will be served."
d. "I try to limit Dexter's food to things I know are safe."

Look in Appendix A for the best answer and rationale.

STINGING INSECT HYPERSENSITIVITY

Children may have severe hypersensitivity reactions to stings from bees, wasps, hornets, or yellow jackets (Yavuz, Sahiner, Buyuktiryaki, et al., 2012). Although a serum sickness reaction may occur, the usual reaction to these stings is an immediate type I hypersensitivity reaction (anaphylaxis).

Assessment

The first time a child is stung, the total reaction is probably only local edema at the site. The second time, generalized urticaria, pruritus, and edema may develop. The third time, symptoms may progress to wheezing and dyspnea. The next time, the reaction could be so severe that shock and death result. The progression of symptoms may be slower than this (involving 10 to 12 stings) if the stings occur far apart; if the stings are received close together (1 or 2 days apart, or even 3 weeks apart), the progression to fatal symptoms may occur as early as the second or third exposure.

Once a child is sensitized, the time interval between the fatal sting and death becomes extremely short, approximately 10 minutes. For this reason, these children must be identified so they can be given medication to combat shock immediately (there is no time to transport them for emergency care).

Therapeutic Management

The best way to protect children with allergies to stinging insects is to begin hyposensitization by immunotherapy against insect stings after the first reaction. An extract of wasp, yellow jacket, hornet, and honeybee venom accomplishes this.

The child who has not been hyposensitized must be treated immediately after the sting by an injection of epinephrine (EpiPens are available for self-injection; see Box 42.8). If children are going on a hiking or camping expedition away from parents, caution parents that their child needs to learn to self-administer this or be certain that a responsible adult accompanying them will be able to do it. Someone at school should be given the responsibility of administering this if a child is stung during recess or an outside gym period. If a school nurse is in attendance, this certainly is the nurse's responsibility. In schools where there is no full-time nurse, however, another person must be designated and taught how to give the injection. If the child has an antihistamine medication in addition to epinephrine, this should be taken also. Ice applied to the site minimizes the amount of venom absorbed. The child should then be transported to a health care setting in case additional epinephrine is needed (the initial injection will be effective for only approximately 20 minutes).

Teach children who are allergic to stinging insects ways to avoid them such as not using scented preparations such as hair spray, deodorants, lotions, or perfume because these attract insects. They also should not go outside barefoot because bees are often found in ground clover. They should not be assigned household chores such as mowing the lawn or weeding the garden, actions that might stir up bees. Because insects tend to cluster around garbage containers, taking out the trash is also an inappropriate chore for these children. Whenever they are out of doors, they should have a fast-acting insecticide handy to use on flying insects. Encourage them to refrain from drinking out of open soda cans at outside activities because bees and wasps are drawn to the sugar in the soda, but the child may be unaware that an insect has entered the open can.

What if...42.3 Dexter's school does not have a plan for managing students with immune disorders. After obtaining a parent's permission to discuss his care with the school nurse, how could you involve the nurse more in Dexter's plan of care?

CONTACT DERMATITIS

Contact dermatitis is an example of a delayed or type IV hypersensitivity response; it is a reaction to skin contact with an allergen (a substance irritating to the child only

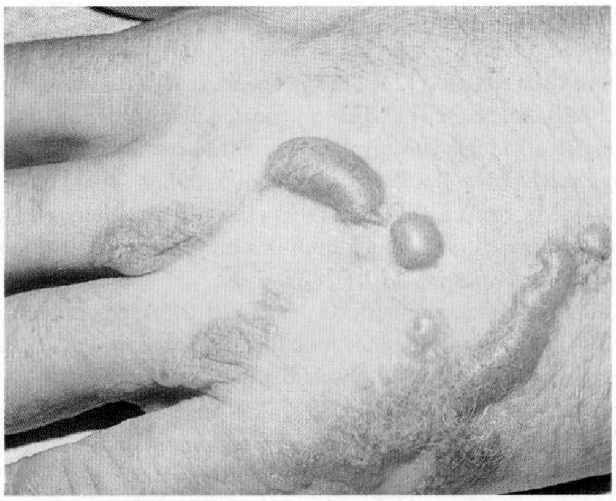

FIGURE 42.7 Poison ivy on a child's hand. (© Beckman/Custom Medical Stock Photograph.)

with prior sensitization). The first reaction is generally erythema, followed by intensely pruritic papules and then vesicles. The allergen causing the irritation is often suggested by the part of the child's body that is affected. For example, dermatitis from a diaper-washing compound appears in the diaper area. Allergy to cosmetics appears on the face. Oozing at the site of pierced ears suggests an allergy to the nickel used in earring posts. Poison ivy appears on the hands and arms where the child brushed against the plant (Fig. 42.7). Children who have had repeated surgeries such as those with spina bifida, are at high risk of developing allergies to latex and will have lesions where the latex touches them (Bernardini, Catania, Caffarelli, et al., 2011). Footwear, because of the chemicals used to tan leather, is also a frequent offender.

Assessment

Patch testing may be used to identify contact dermatitis allergens. A child should not be taking a corticosteroid at the time of patch testing because these drugs reduce delayed hypersensitivity reactions. However, a child may continue to take antihistamines or sympathomimetic drugs because these do not interfere. After 48 hours, the patches used for testing are removed and the reactions are graded 1+ to 4+, the same as in regular skin testing.

Therapeutic Management

Treatment for contact dermatitis consists of removing the identified allergen from the child's environment. In children, this is generally not difficult to do. In adults, because allergens may be work related, this is much more difficult.

Dressings moistened with water, saline, or Burow's solution relieves itching. Calamine and Caladryl lotion are also generally effective. Hydrocortisone lotions or creams reduce itching and also promote healing. Baths with baking soda or oatmeal in the water may be helpful if a large area of the body is involved. Some children may need a sedative to relieve their discomfort during the period of intense pruritus. As with all allergies, nurses need to document contact allergies on electronic health records so all health care providers can be aware of them and guard against a reaction.

What if... 42.4 You are particularly interested in exploring one of the 2020 National Health Goals with respect to immune disorders and children (see Box 42.1). What would be a possible research topic to explore pertinent to this goal that would be applicable to Dexter and his family and that would also advance evidence-based practice?

KEY POINTS FOR REVIEW

- An antigen is a foreign substance capable of stimulating an immune response. The immune system protects the body from invasion by such substances.
- Humoral immunity refers to immunity created by antibody production originated by B lymphocytes. Cell-mediated immunity refers to T-lymphocyte involvement.
- Autoimmunity results from an inability to distinguish self from nonself, causing the immune system to carry out immune responses against normal cells.
- Immunodeficiency disorders can be primary (which occur at birth), such as B-lymphocyte and T-lymphocyte deficiencies, or secondary (which occur later in childhood), such as AIDS.
- HIV/AIDS is spread by the retrovirus HIV through blood and body secretions. Conscientious use of standard infection precautions is essential to prevent transmission.
- Allergic disorders occur as a result of an abnormal antigen–antibody response.
- Immune disorders, as a category, are long-term disorders, and children must participate in their own care to remain well, such as avoiding allergens or conscientiously taking a medication to suppress reactions. Involving children from the start both helps them play an active role in their own care and helps to plan nursing care that not only meets QSEN competencies but that also best meets a family's total needs.
- Anaphylactic shock is an acute type I hypersensitivity reaction characterized by extreme vasodilation and bronchoconstriction. If action is not taken immediately, the reaction can be fatal. Epinephrine is the drug of choice to reduce symptoms.
- Atopic disorders include allergic rhinitis (hay fever), atopic dermatitis, and asthma.
- Environmental control refers to ways to reduce the number of allergens to which children are exposed.
- Hyposensitization by subcutaneous or sublingual immunotherapy is a method to increase the plasma concentration of IgG antibodies to prevent or block IgE antibody formation and allergic symptoms.

CRITICAL THINKING CARE STUDY

Kayla is a 14-year-old girl with a diagnosis of multiple allergies, among them strawberries, eggs, shellfish, and cats. Although she admits she doesn't take her prescribed antihistamine on a regular basis (it wouldn't be "cool" for her friends to see it in her purse), she's concerned because her running nose and frequent cough have been growing worse over the last 6 months. Because she finds her family "old fashioned," she spends a lot of time at her new best friend's house. The community where she lives is a coastal one where shellfish is a popular food (her best friend's mother is a waitress at a seafood restaurant). Kayla had an episode last month when she was taken to the local emergency room with sudden shortness of breath because she was at the restaurant with a group of friends and "forgot" about her allergy.

1. What may be a reason that Kayla's allergy symptoms are worsening?
2. How can you work with Kayla to create a plan of care that minimizes the impact of her allergies on her social life and development and that creates a safe environment for her as well?
3. Kayla has been advised to carry an EpiPen with her at all times. She usually "forgets," however, and leaves it at home. How would you approach Kayla to teach her the importance of having the EpiPen with her at all times? What facts or safety concerns would you want to discuss with Kayla?

Patient Scenario

The Tustin Family

Read about the Tustin family, a family with an adolescent with atopic dermatitis, then answer the questions to further sharpen your skills and grow more familiar with NCLEX-type questions related immune disorders. Confirm your answers are correct by reading the rationales.

Visit http://thePoint.lww.com

Answers and Rationales

Looking for answers to the What if . . . and Critical Thinking Care Study questions?

Visit http://thePoint.lww.com

References

Accetta Pedersen, D., Verbsky, J., & Routes, J. (2011). Screening newborns for primary T-cell immunodeficiency: Consensus and controversy. *Expert Review of Clinical Immunology, 7*(6), 761–768.

Bernardini, R., Catania, P., Caffarelli, C., et al. (2011). Perioperative latex allergy. *International Journal of Immunopathology & Pharmacology, 24* (3, Suppl.), S55–S60.

Blaiss, M. (2010). Allergic rhinitis. Direct and indirect costs. *Allergy and Asthma Proceedings, 31*(5), 375–380.

Boyd, S. (2011). Management of HIV infection in treatment-naive patients: A review of the most current recommendations. *American Journal of Health System Pharmacy, 68*(11), 991–1001.

Calvani, M., Berti, I., Fiocchi, A., et al. (2012). Oral food challenge: Safety, adherence to guidelines and predictive value of skin prick testing. *Pediatric Allergy & Immunology, 23*(8), 755–761

Caubet, J. C., & Eigenmann, P. A. (2012). Diagnostic issues in pediatric drug allergy. *Current Opinion in Allergy & Clinical Immunology, 12*(4), 341–347.

Centers for Disease Control and Prevention. (1994). 1994 Revised classification system of human immunodeficiency virus infection in children less than 13 years of age. *Morbidity & Mortality Weekly Report, 43*(RR-12), 1–10.

Ciprandi, G., Signori, A., Tosca, M. A., et al. (2011). Spirometric abnormalities in patients with allergic rhinitis: Indicator of an "asthma march"? *American Journal of Rhinology & Allergy, 25*(5), e181–e185.

Covar, R. A., Fleischer, D. M., & Boguniewicz, M. (2012). Allergic disorders. In W. Hay, M. Levin, R. Deterding, et al. (Eds.), *Current diagnosis & treatment pediatrics* (21st ed., pp. 1123–1157). New York, NY: McGraw-Hill/Lange.

Cruz, N., & Bahna, S. (2011). Fever, urticarial, lymphadenopathy, and protracted arthralgia and myalgia resistant to corticosteroid therapy. *Allergy and Asthma Proceedings, 32*(5), 395–398.

Fleischer, D. M., Perry, T. T., Atkins, D., et al. (2012). Allergic reactions to foods in preschool-aged children in a prospective observational food allergy study. *Pediatrics, 130*(1), e25–e32.

Frati, F., Incorvaia, C., Lombardi, C., et al. (2012). Allergen immunotherapy: 100 years, but it does not look like. *European Annals of Allergy & Clinical Immunology, 44*(3), 99–106.

Fuleihan, R. (2011). Immunology. In K. J. Marcdante, R. M. Kliegman, H. B. Jenson, et al. (Eds.), *Nelson essentials of pediatrics* (6th ed., pp. 285–306). Philadelphia, PA: Saunders/Elsevier.

Gay, J., Hardee, K., Croce-Galis, M., et al. (2011). What works to meet the sexual and reproductive health needs of women living with HIV/AIDS. *Journal of the International AIDS Society, 14*(1), 56.

Getahun, H., Raviglione, M., Varma, J., et al. (2012). CDC Grand Rounds: The TB/HIV syndemic. *Morbidity and Mortality Weekly Report, 61*(26), 484–489.

Greiner, A. N., Hellings, P. W., Rotiroti, G., et al. (2011). Allergic rhinitis. *Lancet, 378*(9809), 2112–2122.

Hauk, P. J., Johnston, R. B., & Liu, A. H. (2011). Immunodeficiency. In K. J. Marcdante, R. M. Kliegman, H. B. Jenson, et al. (Eds.), *Nelson essentials of pediatrics* (6th ed., pp. 990–1010). Philadelphia, PA: Saunders/Elsevier.

Haywood, P. (2012). Highlights from the 19th AIDS Conference. *Lancet Infectious Diseases, 12*(9), 666–667.

Hellmann, D. B., & Imboden, J. B. (2013). Musculoskeletal and immunological disorders. In M. Papadakis & S. J. McPhee (Eds.), *Current medical diagnosis & treatment* (52nd ed., pp. 809–869). New York, NY: McGraw-Hill/Lange.

Hoyt, M. J., Storm, D. S., Aaron, E., et al. (2012). Preconception and contraceptive care for women living with HIV. *Infectious Diseases in Obstetrics & Gynecology, 2012*, 604183.

Hui, C. P., & Macdonald, N. E. (2011). Use of influenza vaccines in children with an egg allergy. *Paediatrics & Child Health, 16*(8), 491–492.

Johnston, R., & Barré-Sinoussi, F. (2012). Controversies in HIV cure research. *Journal of the International AIDS Society, 15*(1), 16.

Kaplan, A. P. (2012). Treatment of chronic spontaneous urticaria. *Allergy, Asthma & Immunology Research, 4*(6), 326–331.

Karch, A. M. (2013). *2013 Lippincott's nursing drug guide.* Philadelphia, PA: Lippincott Williams & Wilkins.

Karpa, K. D., Paul, I. M., Leckie, J. A., et al. (2012). A retrospective chart review to identify perinatal factors associated with food allergies. *Nutrition Journal, 11*(1), 87–88.

Koletzko, S., Niggemann, B., Arato, A., et al. (2012). Diagnostic approach and management of cow's-milk protein allergy in infants and children. *Journal of Pediatric Gastroenterology Nutrition, 55*(2), 221–229.

Lack, G. (2012). Update on risk factors for food allergy. *Journal of Allergy & Clinical Immunology, 129*(5), 1187–1197.

Levison, J., Williams, L., Moore, A., et al. (2011). Increasing use of rapid HIV testing in labor and delivery among women with no prenatal care: A local initiative. *Maternal and Child Health Journal, 15*(6), 822–826.

McLean, S., Chandler, D., Nurmatov, U., et al. (2011). Telehealthcare for asthma: A Cochrane review. *Canadian Medical Association Journal, 183*(11), E733–E742.

Mercurio, J. (2011). Creating a latex-safe perioperative environment. *OR Nurse, 5*(6), 18–25.

Natchu, U. C., Liu, E., Duggan, C., et al. (2012). Exclusive breastfeeding reduces risk of mortality in infants up to 6 mo of age born to HIV-positive Tanzanian women. *American Journal of Clinical Nutrition, 96*(5), 1071–1078.

Nicol, N. (2011). Efficacy and safety considerations in topical treatments for atopic dermatitis. *Pediatric Nursing, 37*(6), 295–301.

Ochs, H. D., & Hitzig, W. H. (2012). History of primary immunodeficiency diseases. *Current Opinion in Allergy & Clinical Immunology, 12*(6), 577–587.

Phillips, J., Lockey, R., Fox, R., et al. (2011). Systemic reactions to subcutaneous allergen immunotherapy and the response to epinephrine. *Allergy and Asthma Proceedings, 32*(4), 288–294.

Pistiner, M., & Lee, J. J. (2012). Creating a new community of support for students with food allergies. *NASN School Nurse, 27*(5), 260–266.

Reisacher, W. R. (2011). Allergy treatment: Environmental control strategies. *Otolaryngologic Clinics of North America, 44*(3), 711–725.

Resnick, E. S., & Cunningham-Rundles, C. (2012). The many faces of the clinical picture of common variable immune deficiency. *Current Opinion in Allergy & Clinical Immunology, 12*(6), 595–601.

Robison, R., & Pongracic, J. (2012). Food allergy. *Allergy and Asthma Proceedings, 33*(Suppl. 1), S77–S79.

Sawyer, S., Afifi, R., Bearinger, L., et al. (2012). Adolescence: A foundation for future health. *The Lancet, 379*(9826), 1630–1640.

Scott, M., Roberts, G., Kurukulaaratchy, R. J., et al. (2012). Multifaceted allergen avoidance during infancy reduces asthma during childhood with the effect persisting until age 18 years. *Thorax, 67*(12), 1046–1051.

Seashore, M. R. (2011). Metabolic disorders. In K. J. Marcdante, R. M. Kliegman, H. B. Jenson, et al. (Eds.), *Nelson essentials of pediatrics* (6th ed., pp. 187–210). Philadelphia, PA: Saunders/Elsevier.

Sheikh, A., Simons, F. E., Barbour, V., et al. (2012). Adrenaline auto-injectors for the treatment of anaphylaxis with and without cardiovascular collapse in the community. *Cochrane Database of Systematic Reviews,*(8), CD008935.

Shulman, S. (2011). Thirty years of pediatric HIV/AIDS treatment: A time of breakthroughs, innovation. *Pediatrics Annals, 40*(7), 340–341.

Smith, S. (2011). Infectious diseases. In K. J. Marcdante, R. M. Kliegman, H. B. Jenson, et al. (Eds.), *Nelson essentials of pediatrics* (6th ed., pp. 355–462). Philadelphia, PA: Saunders/Elsevier.

Spiro, D. B. (2012). Early onset multiple sclerosis: A review for nurse practitioners. *Journal of Pediatric Health Care, 26*(6), 399–408.

Stewart, M., Letourneau, N., Masuda, J. R., et al. (2012). Support needs and preferences of young adolescents with asthma and allergies. *Journal of Pediatric Nursing, 27*(5), 479–490.

Stierstorfer, M. B., Sha, C. T., & Sasson, M. (2013). Food patch testing for irritable bowel syndrome. *Journal of the American Academy of Dermatology, 68*(3), 377–384.

Susanna, S., & Prabhasankar, P. (2012). Quality, microstructure, biochemical and immunochemical characteristics of hypoallergenic pasta. *Food Science &Technology International, 18*(4), 403–411.

Traister, R. S., Green, T. D., Mitchell, L., et al. (2012). Community opinions regarding oral immunotherapy for food allergies. *Annals of Allergy, Asthma & Immunology, 109*(5), 319–323.

U.S. Department of Health and Human Services. (2010). *Healthy people 2020.* Washington, DC.

Wallengren, J. (2011). Identification of core competencies for primary care of allergy patients using a modified Delphi technique. *BMC Medical Education, 11*(12), 1–18.

Wise, S. K., & Schlosser, R. J. (2012). Evidence-based practice: Sublingual immunotherapy for allergic rhinitis. *Otolaryngologic Clinics of North America, 45*(5), 1045–1054.

Woo, C., & Bahna, S. (2011). Evaluation of the child with immune deficiency disorder. *Pediatric Annals, 40*(4), 205–211.

Yavuz, S. T., Sahiner, U. M., Buyuktiryaki, B., et al. (2012). Clinical features of children with venom allergy and risk factors for severe systemic reactions. *International Archives of Allergy & Immunology, 160*(3), 313–321.

Chapter 43

Nursing Care of a Family When a Child Has an Infectious Disorder

KEY TERMS

- catarrhal stage
- chain of infection
- convalescent period
- enanthem
- exanthem
- exotoxin
- fomites
- incubation period
- interferon
- Koplik spots
- mode of transmission
- portal of entry
- portal of exit
- prodromal period
- reservoir
- septicemia
- susceptible host

OBJECTIVES

After mastering the contents of this chapter, you should be able to:

1. Describe the causes and course of common infectious disorders of childhood.
2. Identify 2020 National Health Goals related to infectious disorders in children that nurses could help the nation achieve.
3. Assess a child with an infectious disorder.
4. Formulate nursing diagnoses for a child with an infectious disorder.
5. Establish outcomes to help a family manage an infectious disorder as well as manage seamless transitions across differing health care settings.
6. Using the nursing process, plan nursing care that includes the six competencies of Quality & Safety Education for Nurses (QSEN): Patient-Centered Care, Teamwork & Collaboration, Evidence-Based Practice (EBP), Quality Improvement (QI), Safety, and Informatics.
7. Plan nursing care for a child with an infectious disorder, such as helping them understand infectious precautions.
8. Evaluate expected outcomes for the achievement and effectiveness of care.
9. Integrate knowledge of infectious diseases with the interplay of nursing process, the six competencies of QSEN, and Family Nursing to achieve quality maternal and child health nursing care.

Marty Ireland, a 10-year-old boy, was admitted to the hospital yesterday for appendicitis. This morning after surgery, his throat is painful and his arms are covered by a very itchy, red, macular (flat) rash. He was diagnosed as having scarlet fever. His family works as migrant farm workers. "His sister is home with mono," his mother tells you. "How could our family get two infections plus appendicitis all in 1 week?"

Previous chapters described the growth and development of well children. This chapter adds information about the dramatic changes, both physical and psychosocial, that can occur when children contract an infectious disorder. It's important to know about the spread and care of these diseases because many of them spread easily to other children.

How would you respond to Marty's mother? Is it most likely that Marty contracted this new disease while he was in the hospital, or before he was admitted? What is a measure you would recommend to help reduce the itching?

BOX 43.1 Nursing Care Planning Based on 2020 National Health Goals

Several 2020 National Health Goals address ways to prevent and reduce the incidence of infectious disease in children.

- Reduce, eliminate, or maintain elimination of vaccine-preventable diseases such as measles from 115 infected children per year to a target of 30 children per year.
- Achieve and maintain effective vaccination coverage levels for universally recommended vaccines such as the diphtheria, tetanus, and acellular pertussis (DTaP) vaccine among young children from 84% to 90%.
- Increase the number of states that use electronic data from rabies surveillance to inform public health prevention programs from 8 states to 29 states.
- Reduce central-line–associated bloodstream infections (developmental).
- Reduce invasive health care–associated methicillin-resistant *Staphylococcus aureus* (HA-MRSA) infections from 26 per 100,000 people to 6.5 per 100,000 people (U.S. Department of Health and Human Services [DHHS], 2010; see www.healthypeople.gov).

Nurses can help the nation achieve these goals by educating parents about the importance of immunizations and ways to avoid infections. They can also help prevent the spread of infection in hospital units by scrupulously adhering to infection control precautions.

Despite the number of preventive measures available, infectious diseases remain a leading cause of morbidity in children (Beach & Thalange, 2013). Nurses can play a key role in reducing the incidence of these disorders by educating parents about how they are spread and appropriate preventive steps. It's important to be able to recognize their signs and symptoms because nurses are often the first health care provider to see evidence of infection as they triage children in emergency rooms or at school. Several 2020 National Health Goals, shown in Box 43.1, relate to the prevention of infectious disorders in children.

Nursing Process Overview

For a Child With an Infectious Disorder

Assessment

Many infectious diseases begin subtly. Parents report symptoms such as, "he doesn't act like himself" or "she's so listless." A day or so later, a rash develops. With many disorders, children are infectious just before and just after the rash appears. Rashes can be difficult to identify, so it is important to obtain as full a description and history of the rash as possible.

Nursing Diagnosis

Common nursing diagnoses used with children directly related to the infectious process include:

- Pain related to pruritus from skin lesions
- Impaired skin integrity related to rash, pruritus, and scratching
- Risk for infection related to presence of infective organism in sibling or family member
- Altered body temperature (fever) related to systemic infection
- Fluid volume deficit related to insensible fluid loss from increased body temperature
- Knowledge deficit (learning) related to disease prognosis, prevention, and treatment

Additional diagnoses when children must be separated from others to prevent infection transmission might include:

- Social isolation related to precautions required to prevent infection transmission
- Deficient diversional activity related to activity restriction and precautions to prevent disease transmission

Outcome Identification and Planning

When establishing outcomes for care of children with infectious disorders, include those that help parents deal with the current infection and also prevent another infection such as teaching about necessary infection control precautions and immunizations. Parents often ask about communicability to their other children and to the infected child's playmates or schoolmates, so these issues need to be addressed. Planning care for a child who requires restrictions to prevent disease transmission requires a thoughtful consideration to prevent boredom. Two organizations helpful for referral are the National Foundation for Infectious Diseases (www.nfid.org) and the Centers for Disease Control and Prevention (www.cdc.gov).

Implementation

Nursing responsibilities when caring for a child with an infectious disorder depend on the setting in which the child is seen. Often, a child will not be brought into a clinic if the disease can be easily identified over the telephone. Counseling parents about techniques to relieve the irritation of rashes or other symptoms can then be relayed to parents over the telephone or by e-mail as well. Administering antibiotics and being alert for potential adverse effects are other major nursing responsibilities.

Outcome Evaluation

An evaluation of outcomes for a child with an infectious disease should determine not only whether the child is returning to wellness but also whether the child and family have learned more about ways to prevent infectious diseases. If one member of the family has a decreased immune response due to steroid or chemotherapy, prevention of transmission takes on even greater importance.

Examples of expected outcomes that would indicate achievement of goals include:

- Child states pain from pruritus and skin lesions is at a tolerable level.
- Siblings and family members remain free of signs and symptoms of the infectious disorder.
- Parent names diversional activities she has planned to keep the child occupied.
- Parent verbalizes how to prevent transmission of infectious disease to other family members.

THE INFECTIOUS PROCESS

Pathogens are any organism that causes disease and can be classified into five types of microorganisms: viruses, bacteria, rickettsiae, helminths, and fungi. The properties of these organisms are discussed in conjunction with the common diseases that they cause.

Stages of Infectious Disease

Infectious diseases follow certain stages, during which the communicability (i.e., ability to be spread to others) or severity of the illness can be predicted (Fig. 43.1).

- The **incubation period** is the time between the invasion of an organism and the onset of symptoms of infection. During this time, microorganisms grow and multiply. Although incubation periods vary depending on the pathogen, a common interval is 7 to 10 days (although it can be longer). The incubation period for tetanus, for example, is 2 to 21 days.
- A **prodromal period** is the time between the beginning of nonspecific symptoms such as lethargy, low-grade fever, fatigue, and malaise and the onset of disease-specific symptoms such as a rash. Children are infectious (capable of spreading the microorganisms to others) during the prodromal period, but because their symptoms are so vague at this point, they do not yet realize that they need to take precautions against spreading disease. During the prodromal period, therefore, infectious diseases spread readily through communities from a person with the disease to any susceptible individual. Fortunately, prodromal stages are generally short, ranging from hours to a few days.
- *Illness* is the stage during which specific symptoms either related to the body organ affected or to the entire body (systemic symptoms) occur, such as fever, increased white blood cell count, or headache. Many childhood infections have an accompanying specific rash on the skin **(exanthem)** or mucous membrane **(enanthem)** (Box 43.2).
- The **convalescent period** is the interval between when symptoms first begin to fade and when the child returns to a healthy baseline. Because fatigue is often an accompanying symptom of infection, the convalescent period (or the time until full energy is restored) may often take longer than anticipated.

Chain of Infection

The **chain of infection** is the method by which organisms are spread and enter a new individual to cause disease.

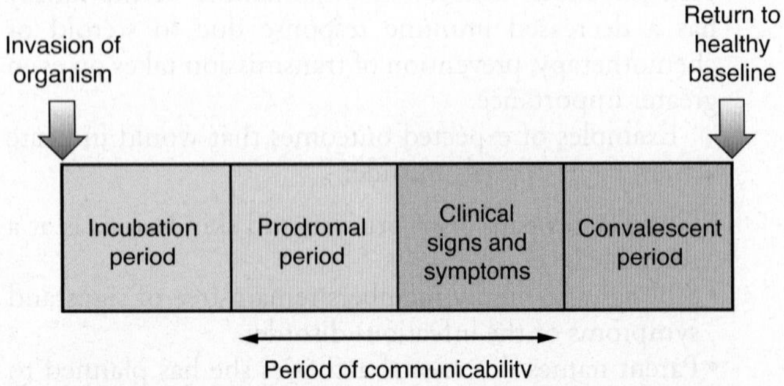

FIGURE 43.1 The time frame for infectious diseases. Period of communicability is the time during which the disease can be transmitted to other people.

BOX 43.2 Nursing Care Planning Using Assessment

Assessing a Child For Common Signs and Symptoms of Infectious Disorders

History

Chief concern: Does child have a fever, general malaise, vomiting, or diarrhea? Was child recently exposed to someone with an infection?

Past medical history: Are child's immunizations current?

Physical examination

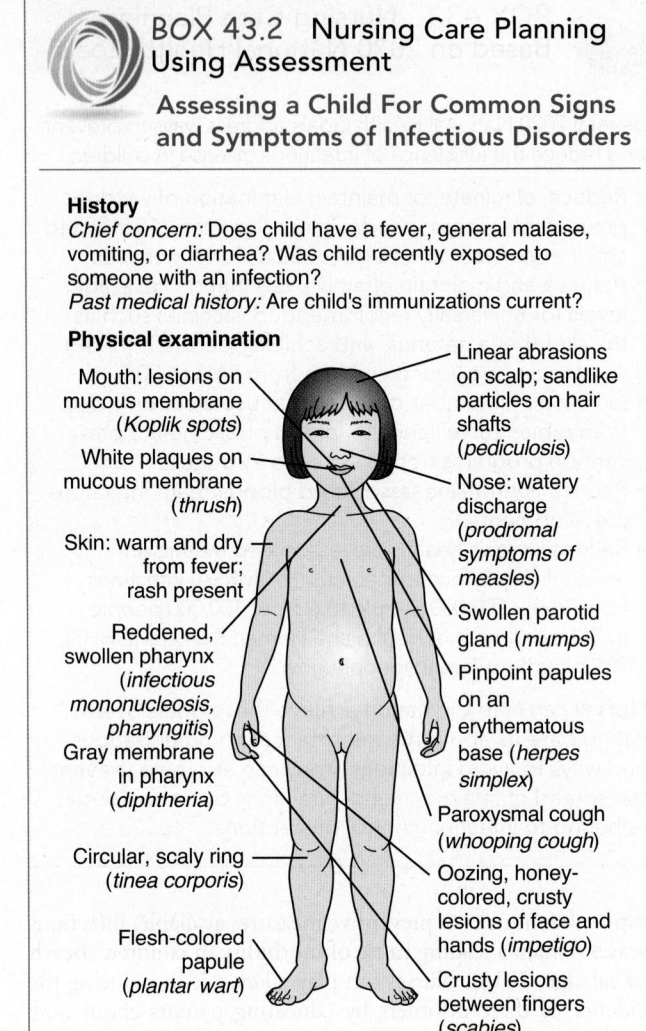

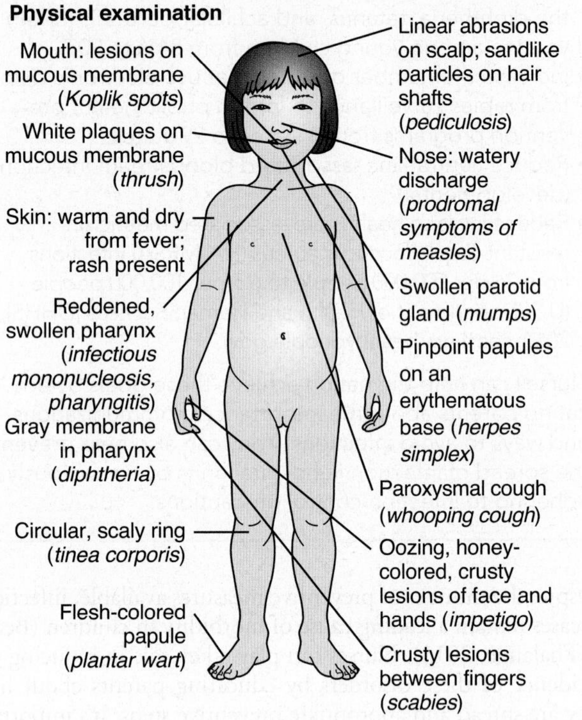

Breaking the chain at one of its susceptible points is the most efficient way to prevent infection from spreading (Smith, 2011). Nurses are instrumental in doing this by teaching parents activities such as good hand washing; they serve as first-line defenders against infections in health care facilities.

Reservoir

The **reservoir** is the container or place in which an organism grows and reproduces. The reservoir would be another person with the disease, a contaminated object such as a kitchen counter, or an animal or insect. A major role of immunizations is to help limit organisms' use of children as reservoirs for growth.

Portal of Exit

The **portal of exit** is the route by which an organism leaves an infected child's body to be spread to others. Organisms can be carried out of the body by upper respiratory excretions, feces, vomitus, saliva, urine, vaginal secretions, blood, or lesion secretions (Table 43.1). To break a chain of infection

TABLE 43.1 Methods by Which Infections Spread

Portal of Exit	Means of Transmission	Portal of Entry	Prevention Measures
Blood	Arthropod vectors Blood sampling Transfusion	Injection into the bloodstream	Decreasing exposure to vectors Careful handling of blood sampling equipment Prescreening of blood for organisms such as HIV or hepatitis B
Respiratory secretions	Airborne droplets Fomites	Respiratory tract	Wearing a mask Droplet and airborne precautions Hand washing
Feces	Water, food Fomites Vectors such as flies	Gastrointestinal tract	Hand washing before eating, after using bathroom, or after handling diapers
Exudate from lesions	Direct contact Contact with soiled dressings	Skin, mucous membranes	Contact precautions Self-screening for sexual contacts Gloves

at this point, follow a good aseptic technique and prescribed transmission-based precautions such as wearing a gown, gloves, or mask and/or face shield as appropriate. Be certain to wash after contact with any body secretions as well as after coming into contact with any of the previous portal of exits. Also be certain to supply an adequate number of disposable tissues to any child coughing or sneezing so droplet or airborne spread from these sources can be limited. Stress that hand washing is the most effective way to prevent the spread of infection.

QSEN Checkpoint Question 43.1

Evidence-Based Practice

Because effective and frequent hand washing is so important in preventing the spread of infection, researchers studied what factors most influence effective hand washing practices in children by investigating the practices of 2,323 sixth-grade students plus 2,089 of their parents. Results of the study showed that health literacy, parents' hand washing practices, parent and child bonding, and a greater amount of shared time together all had significant correlations with children's hand hygiene practices (Song, Kim, & Park, 2012).

Based on the previous study, what would be the most effective way to ensure Marty, the 10-year-old, consistently washes his hands before meals?

a. Continue to remind him to wash his hands as often as possible.
b. Talk to Marty's mother about the importance of modeling good hand hygiene practices.
c. Explain to Marty the role that bacteria play in the transmission of illness.
d. Stress that washing his hands makes him look grown-up and responsible.

Look in Appendix A for the best answer and rationale.

Means of Transmission

The **mode of transmission** refers to whether the infection is spread by *direct* or *indirect* contact. Sexually transmitted infections, for example, are spread by skin-to-skin or direct contact. Other infections are spread indirectly by **fomites**—inanimate objects such as soil, food, water, bedding, towels, combs, nonrefrigerated food, or drinking glasses. Insects, rats, or other vermin (vectors) also cause indirect spread.

The most common means of indirect contact, however, is the spread of mouth and nose secretions (droplet infection) through talking, sneezing, coughing, breathing, kissing, and sharing drinking glasses or straws. Some droplets containing pathogenic organisms are spread immediately to another individual in this way. Some droplets fall to the ground, where the organisms dry and then are spread by dust. If small, the organisms become suspended in the air (airborne transmission) and can move with the wind to infect people at a distance. A common respiratory tract infection is an example of an illness spread by indirect contact.

To break a chain of infection at this point, use transmission-based precautions as appropriate and wash hands before, between, and after client care. Teach parents and children good hand washing techniques and other measures as necessary.

Portal of Entry

The **portal of entry** refers to the opening through which a pathogen can enter a child's body such as by inhalation, ingestion, or breaks in the skin from bites, abrasions, or burns. To break a chain of infection at this point, teach children to wash their hands after sneezing or coughing, before eating, and after using the bathroom. Teach girls to wipe their perineum from front to back after defecating or voiding to prevent organisms from spreading from the rectum to the urethra. Teach parents to wash cuts and abrasions before bandaging them.

TABLE 43.2 Types and Functions of White Blood Cells (Leukocytes)

Type	Percentage of Total Count	Origin	Function
Granular Forms			
Neutrophils	60% at birth; 33% at 2 years of age; 60% thereafter	Bone marrow	Active in acute bacterial infections
Eosinophils	1%–4%	Bone marrow	Increased in parasitic infection
Basophils	0.0%–0.5%	Bone marrow	Increased with inflammation
Nongranular Forms			
Lymphocytes	30% at birth; 50% at 2 years of age; 30% thereafter	Bone marrow	T lymphocytes (stored in the thymus gland) directly react with invading antigens; B lymphocytes from bone marrow produce antibodies that inactivate antigens
Monocytes	5%–10%	Bone marrow	Serve as a backup for neutrophils in acute infection; macrophages are mature form

Susceptible Host

For infection to occur, one more step must be present: the child must be susceptible to the infection **(susceptible host)**. Certain characteristics make some individuals more prone to infection than others, including:

- Age: Infection occurs most readily in the very young and the very old.
- Gender: Girls, for example, have more urinary tract infections than boys.
- Virulence: Some organisms are stronger than others or cause disease more readily.
- Body defenses: Physical, chemical, and immune responses all protect against foreign invaders. Children with immunosuppression are more susceptible than others. Infants who are breastfed are less susceptible than formula-fed infants.

The Body's Immune Response to Organisms

When a foreign organism (antigen) enters the body, it can be destroyed by the phagocytic (cell-engulfing) action of white blood cells, which seek it out or by activation of the body's immune system. Phagocytes are unique white blood cells (neutrophils) that are capable of cell destruction. Monocytes serve as backup cells for phagocytosis. The different actions of all the white blood cells are summarized in Table 43.2.

The action of phagocytes on organisms produces pus (remnants of the organisms, phagocytes, and destroyed tissue). Children and parents alike may need a review of the purpose of pus because they may think its presence indicates that an infection is becoming worse. More likely, it indicates phagocytosis is occurring and the infection is resolving.

If bacteria escape the action of the phagocytes, they enter the blood and lymph systems and are then transported to other body locations, activating the immune system. Pathogenic organisms in the bloodstream create **septicemia** (blood infection), which is always a serious development because it means the organism is being spread systemically.

With activation of the immune system, B lymphocytes (humoral immunity) and T lymphocytes (cell-mediated immunity) begin to be produced. B lymphocytes form antibodies specific to offending antigens that either actively destroy them or activate *complement*, a special body protein that is capable of lysing (dissolving) cells (see Chapter 42).

T lymphocytes (thymus dependent) are often called killer cells because they can destroy antigens by either direct contact or by the release of lymphokines. An example of a lymphokine is **interferon**, which is a substance that appears to prevent cells from being host to more than one virus at a time. This is why it is rare to see a child with two viral diseases at the same time, although it is not impossible to see a child with both a viral and a bacterial disease (e.g., perhaps scarlet fever and a common cold) at the same time. This is also why two virus vaccines are not given to a child at the same time unless they are specially designed to be given together (e.g., measles, mumps, and rubella). (See Chapter 42 for a more detailed discussion of the immune response and Chapter 34 for a discussion of immunizations.)

HEALTH PROMOTION AND RISK MANAGEMENT

Preventing infectious diseases is important because these disorders are responsible not only for a high percentage of illnesses but also of hospital admissions in children. Prevention begins with being certain all children are in general good health. Adequate nutrition is important to provide protein and vitamins to supply adequate white blood cells so that both phagocytic and antibody-producing B lymphocytes are available to destroy invading organisms.

A second important step is to be certain all parents are aware of the need for their children to be immunized. Nurses need to ensure immunizations are offered to children at health care visits so their immunizations can be kept up to date (Daley, O'Leary, & Nyquist, 2012).

It is important that parents also understand that although diseases such as scarlet fever, chickenpox (varicella), and mumps (infectious parotitis) are referred to as "common" childhood illnesses, they have the potential to be extremely serious and can lead to complications such as pneumonia and encephalitis. This is why, when children develop typical childhood communicable diseases, they need to be seen by a primary health care provider so the risk of these complications can be minimized.

The responsibility expected of parents and children to help prevent the spread of communicable diseases differs from country to country and varies among cultures. In the United States, both federal and state governments have taken an active role in preventing the spread of such diseases by requiring children to have immunizations against the most common illnesses. Parents are expected to obtain such immunizations for children by school age. Schools and school nurses, as well as the school system's frontline health officers, take an active role in enforcing these regulations. Community health nurses serve an important role in administering immunizations and counseling families on how to prevent the spread of disease in their homes. Nurses also have an obligation to be certain parents are aware of the latest studies available on the safety of vaccines. Unfortunately, some vaccines were associated with the development of autism spectrum disorder in the past, causing some parents to be reluctant to have their child immunized against any illnesses. Up-to-date evidence has shown there is no association between autism spectrum disorder and vaccines, so the number of children being vaccinated is again increasing (Lewis, Bernal, Shay, et al., 2010).

Developing countries have a great deal of difficulty maintaining this same level of disease prevention. Remember, when caring for children newly arrived from another country, that the child may not have the same level of immunization as usually seen. This opens an important area of health teaching, because the parents may not be aware of the importance of immunizations, which ones are required, or what community services are available to supply them.

Preventing the Spread of Infections

Nosocomial or health care–associated infections (HAI) are infections that are contracted while in a hospital or other health care setting. They represent a major threat to hospitalized children because the overall rate of hospital-acquired infections in children range from 0% in low-risk settings to 23% in high-risk settings such as intensive care units. Children younger than 2 years of age, children with a nutritional deficit, those who are immunosuppressed, those who have indwelling vascular lines or catheters, are receiving multiple antibiotic therapy, or who remain in the hospital for longer than 72 hours are at highest risk for contracting such an infection (Duval, 2010). Nurses provide a line of defense against such infections by adhering to a strict aseptic technique, such as frequent and thorough hand washing, and by following protective transmission-based precautions when indicated (Askarian, Yadollahi, Kuochak, et al., 2011). Summaries of standard infection precautions and transmission-based infection control precautions are available at http://thePoint.lww.com/Pillitteri7e and in Box 43.3.

What if...43.1 You realize Marty, who was diagnosed as having scarlet fever a day after surgery for appendicitis, must have been infectious while he was in surgery because that was his prodromal period. Will everyone, including yourself, who has been exposed to him need to be administered an antibiotic to keep from contracting the infection?

CARING FOR THE CHILD WITH AN INFECTIOUS DISEASE

As almost all childhood infectious diseases include a fever or rash, nursing care must address identification and relief of these symptoms.

Nursing Diagnoses and Related Interventions

Nursing Diagnosis: Pain related to pruritus from skin lesions

Outcome Evaluation: Child states he is more comfortable; reports less itching; is not seen scratching rash; no signs of excessive scratching or bleeding are present.

Providing comfort for the pruritus of skin lesions is important for many childhood infections. No matter what agent is causing the disease, a rash tends to be extremely itchy and uncomfortable. Fortunately, several simple remedies are available for reducing discomfort (Box 43.4).

Some parents wrongly bundle up children who have rashes, believing that the extra clothing prevents a rash from turning inward and affecting the heart. In reality, bundling only serves to make a rash more uncomfortable and probably increases any accompanying fever. Although none of the previous measures are apt to be 100% effective, a second advantage is that they give a parent a constructive and comforting activity to carry out.

Most infectious diseases also involve fever. Measures to combat fever in children are discussed in Chapter 37.

Nursing Diagnosis: Social isolation related to required activity restriction associated with precautions to prevent disease transmission

Outcome Evaluation: Child states reasons for restrictions; expresses interest in activities proposed by nurses or parents.

A child who is restricted from others because of infection control precautions can begin to feel lonely and depressed unless stimulation and social needs are met.

BOX 43.3 Standard and Transmission-Based Precautions for Infection Control

To reduce the risk of disease transmission in the health care setting:

1. Wash hands immediately with a non-antimicrobial soap and water before and after examining patients and after any contact with blood, body fluids, and contaminated items whether or not you wear gloves.
2. Wear clean, nonsterile gloves anytime contact with blood, body fluids, mucous membranes, or broken skin is likely. Change gloves between tasks or procedures on the same patient. Before going to another patient, remove gloves, wash hands, and then put on new gloves.
3. Wear a mask, protective eyewear, and gown during any patient care activity when splashes or sprays of body fluids are likely. Remove the soiled gown and wash hands as soon as possible.
4. Make sure contaminated nondisposable equipment is not reused with another patient until it has been cleaned, disinfected, and sterilized properly. Do not recap needles. Dispose of nonreusable needles, syringes, and other sharp patient care instruments in puncture-resistant containers.
5. Routinely clean and disinfect frequently touched surfaces including beds, bed rails, examination tables, and bedside tables.
6. Do not touch linens soiled with blood or body fluids with bare hands. Use plastic bags to transport soiled linen.
7. Place a patient whose blood or body fluids are likely to contaminate surfaces or other patients in an isolation room or area.
8. Minimize the use of invasive procedures to avoid the potential for injury and accidental exposure. Use oral rather than injectable medications whenever possible.
9. When a specific diagnosis is made, find out how the disease is transmitted. Use precautions according to the transmission risk.

Airborne Precautions

Airborne precautions reduce the risk of small-particle organisms being transmitted through the air as microorganisms carried by this route can be carried widely. If airborne transmission is possible:

1. Place the patient in a single-patient isolation room that is not air-conditioned or where air is not circulated to the rest of the health care facility. Make sure the room has a door that can be closed.
2. Wear a high-efficiency particulate air (HEPA) or other biosafety mask when in the patient's room.
3. Limit movement of the patient from the room to other areas. Place a surgical mask on a patient who must be moved.

Droplet Precautions

Droplet precautions reduce the risk of pathogens being spread through large-particle droplet contact by acts such as coughing, sneezing, and talking or through procedures such as suctioning or bronchoscopy. Large droplets do not remain suspended in the air for long periods and generally travel only short distances, so close proximity is required for the spread of disease. If droplet transmission is possible:

1. Place the patient in a single-patient isolation room.
2. Wear a HEPA or other biosafety mask when caring for the patient.
3. Limit movement of the patient from the room to other areas. If the patient must be moved, place a surgical mask on the patient.

Contact Precautions

Contact precautions reduce the risk of transmission of pathogens by direct contact such as skin-to-skin contact (shaking hands) or indirect contact through an intermediate object such as a comb or soiled dressing. If contact transmission is possible:

1. Place the patient in an isolation room and limit access.
2. Wear gloves during contact with the patient and with infectious body fluids or contaminated items.
3. Wear a disposable gown when in the patient's room.
4. Limit movement of the patient from the isolation room to other areas.
5. Avoid sharing equipment between patients. Designate equipment for each patient if supplies allow. If sharing equipment is unavoidable, clean and disinfect it before use with the next patient.

From Siegel, J. D., Rhinehart, E., Jackson, M., et al., (2007). *Guidelines for isolation precautions: Preventing transmission of infectious agents in healthcare settings*. Atlanta, GA: Centers for Disease Control and Prevention.

In a hospital setting, make as few trips as possible in and out of the room to limit the possibility of pathogen spread; however, do not make care visits seem hurried. If there is a procedure scheduled at 9:00 AM and another at 9:30 AM, for example, stay in the room rather than leave to return again, if possible. Use the time to read a story to the child, play a card game, or explore ways for the child to connect with friends and family through texting or via the Internet.

You may need to remind parents that they must follow these precautions, like all hospital personnel, when they visit. Some parents feel so self-conscious about having to wash and gown that they may stay away rather than visit. Helping them feel comfortable with these procedures so they continue to visit is a nursing responsibility. Remember that when children are admitted to a hospital, parents may not hear everything said to them during admission because of their anxiety. If the gowning technique was explained at the time of admission, therefore, do not assume parents will remember the next day what was said. Explain and reinforce the technique as many times as necessary to prevent them from exposing themselves to an infectious organism.

Parents may be reluctant to give children who require transmission-based precautions their favorite toy, thinking it will have to be destroyed after contagious precautions are discontinued. There are few toys, however, that cannot be scrubbed with soap and water so there is no reason to restrict such

BOX 43.4 Nursing Care Planning Based on Family Teaching

RELIEVING THE ITCHINESS OF A RASH

Q. Marty's mother says to you, "Our son is miserable because his rash is so itchy. What can we do to help him?"

A. Itching is a very uncomfortable sensation. Use the following to help relieve the itch of a rash:

- Dress your child in light cotton clothing so overheating and perspiration do not occur. Perspiration can make itching worse.
- Avoid wool clothing, because it can irritate the skin and increase itching.
- Offer adequate fluid to maintain good hydration because dry skin increases discomfort.
- Keep your child's fingernails short to avoid injury to the skin from scratching.
- Teach your child to press on an itchy area rather than scratching to relieve discomfort; cold cloths or compresses applied to an area can also be helpful.
- Administer an analgesic, such as acetaminophen, as needed for comfort.
- Adding a few teaspoonfuls of baking soda to bath water can be soothing. Use lukewarm rather than hot water.
- Keep in mind that some children need an antihistamine such as diphenhydramine (Benadryl) to reduce itching. Ask your primary care provider about using this medication.

items. Never leave children in a room before checking that they have a toy to play with or an activity that will keep them busy for the length of time they will be alone. See Chapter 36 for a discussion of interventions that can be used to promote adequate stimulation for a child requiring transmission-based precautions as well as the role of a child life specialist to help locate and provide stimulating activities for children.

VIRAL INFECTIONS

Viruses are the smallest infectious agents known, and are so small that they cannot be seen through an ordinary microscope. They actually are not true cells because they contain either RNA or DNA, but not both. Because they are incomplete in this way, viruses cannot replicate on their own but only by invading bacteria, plant, animal, or human cells and using the biochemical products of those cells to function. Although body cells may not look to be outwardly altered by a viral invasion, they can fail to function or die because of lysis of internal components or rupture. Symptoms usually do not become apparent until many cells have been invaded in this way, creating a long incubation period. Some viruses are capable of invading only specific cells. The Epstein–Barr virus, for example, invades only B lymphocytes, HIV viruses invade CD4 T lymphocytes, and influenza viruses affect specific receptor sites in tracheal cells. Other viruses are not so selective.

Viral Exanthems

The majority of childhood exanthems (rashes) are caused by viruses; each of these diseases has specific symptoms, characteristic lesions, and a specific distribution or pattern to the rash that allows it to be identified (Figs. 43.2 and 43.3).

Exanthem Subitum (Roseola Infantum)

- Causative agent: Human herpesvirus 6 (HHV-6)
- Incubation period: Approximately 10 days
- Period of communicability: During febrile period
- Mode of transmission: Unknown
- Immunity: Contracting the disease offers lasting natural immunity; no artificial immunity is available

Assessment. Roseola is a disease with severe symptoms, although the illness itself is mild. It generally occurs in children between 6 months to 3 years of age, and mainly in the spring and fall, although it can occur at any time of the year. The first symptom is a high fever (104° to 105°F [40.0° to 40.6°C]). Infants become irritable and anorexic, although even with this high a fever, usually remain playful and alert. Their pharynx may appear slightly inflamed; the occipital, cervical, and postauricular lymph nodes may be enlarged. If blood composition is studied, the total white blood count is usually decreased, with the proportion of lymphocytes increased.

After 3 or 4 days, the fever falls abruptly and a distinctive rash of discrete, rose-pink macules approximately 2 to 3 mm in size and flat with the skin surface appears (see Fig. 43.3). The lesions occur most prominently on the trunk, fade on pressure, and last 1 to 2 days. The rash is darker than that of rubella or measles and, aside from the slightly reddened throat, children have no accompanying coryza (upper respiratory symptoms), conjunctivitis, or cough. The condition is diagnosed based on the physical signs and symptoms with the hallmark appearance of a rash appearing immediately after the sharp decline in fever (Porth, 2011).

Therapeutic Management. Treatment focuses on measures to reduce the discomfort of the rash and fever such as acetaminophen (Tylenol) or ibuprofen (Motrin). The most frequent complication of roseola is a febrile seizure with the onset of the disease because the temperature rises so rapidly. Management of this type of seizure is discussed in Chapter 49.

There are no long-term effects of roseola. If an infant should develop this exanthem in the hospital, follow standard infection precautions.

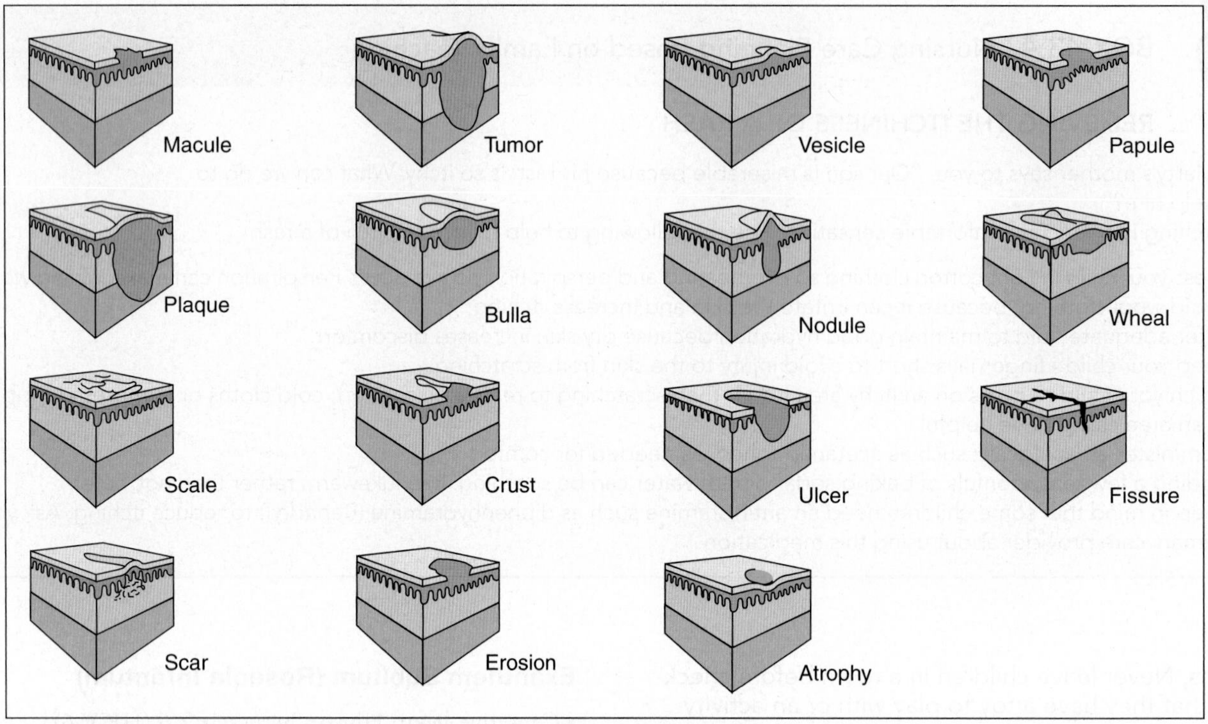

FIGURE 43.2 Primary and secondary skin lesions and their characteristics.

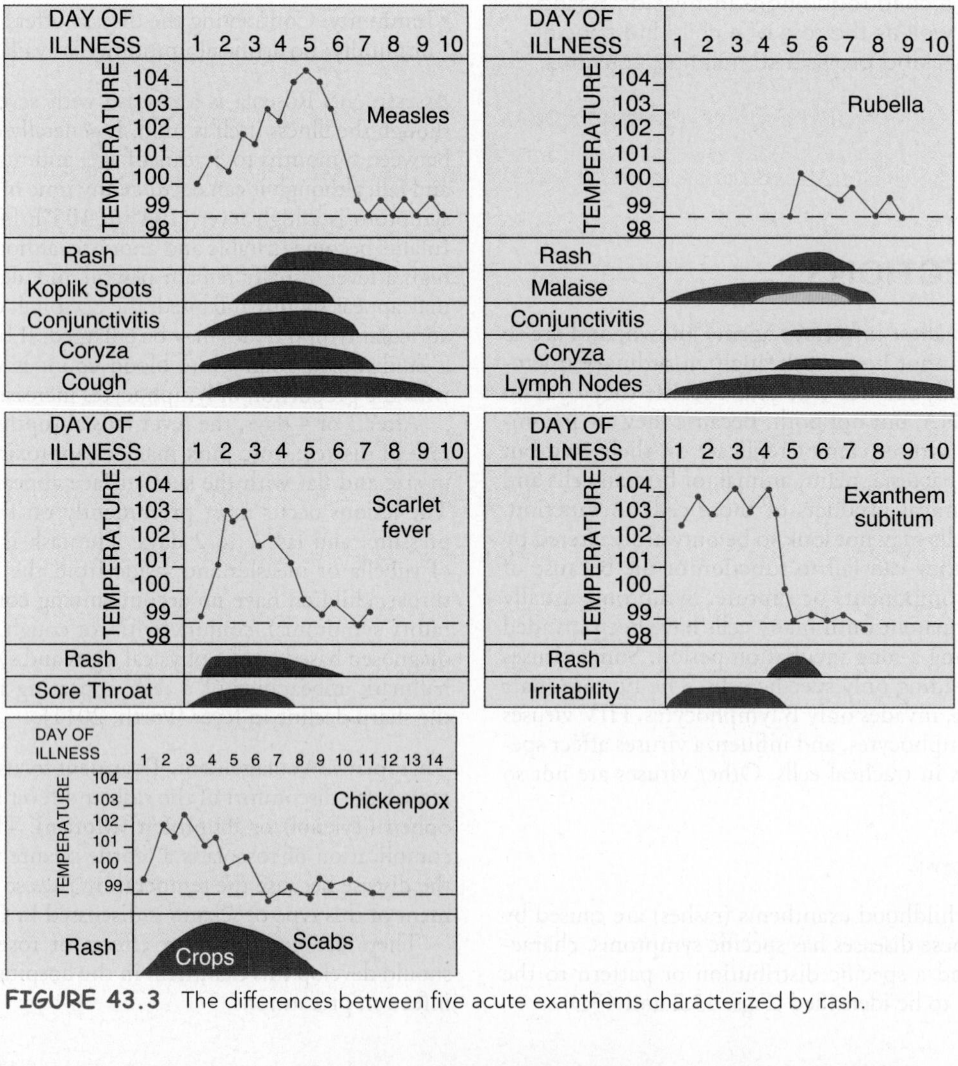

FIGURE 43.3 The differences between five acute exanthems characterized by rash.

Rubella (German Measles)

- Causative agent: Rubella virus
- Incubation period: 14 to 21 days
- Period of communicability: 7 days before to approximately 5 days after the rash appears
- Mode of transmission: Direct and indirect contact with droplets
- Immunity: Contracting the disease offers lasting natural immunity; a high rubella antibody titer reveals infection has occurred
- Active artificial immunity: Attenuated live virus vaccine (e.g., measles, mumps, and rubella vaccine)
- Passive artificial immunity: Immune serum globulin is considered for pregnant women

Assessment. Rubella (often called German or 3-day measles) is rarely seen today, but when it does occur, it is seen most commonly during the spring and mostly affects older school-age and adolescent children. The symptoms begin with a 1- to 5-day prodromal period, during which children have a low-grade fever, headache, malaise, anorexia, mild conjunctivitis, possibly a sore throat, a mild cough, congestion, coryza, and swollen lymph nodes such as those in the suboccipital, postauricular, and cervical chains (Levin & Weinberg, 2012).

After the 1 to 5 days of prodromal signs, a discrete pink-red maculopapular rash (see Fig. 43.3) begins on the face, then spreads downward to the trunk and extremities. On the third day, the rash disappears. There is generally no desquamation (peeling); if present, it is primarily fine flaking of the skin. Fever with rubella is not marked, although arthritis (joint pain) with effusion into the joints occurs in some children on the second or third day and lasting as long as 5 to 10 days.

Therapeutic Management. Children need comfort measures for the rash and an antipyretic such as acetaminophen (Tylenol) or ibuprofen (Motrin) for fever or joint pain. If a child develops rubella while in the hospital, follow droplet precautions for 7 days after the onset of the rash in addition to standard infection precautions.

If a woman contracts rubella while pregnant, it can cause extensive congenital malformation in the fetus (see Chapter 12). Because of this, it can never be considered a simple disease. It is so important that girls are immunized against it before they reach childbearing age, that the vaccine is included in the MMR vaccine. Because the vaccine contains a live virus, it is not recommended to obtain this immunization while pregnant (Centers for Disease Control and Prevention [CDC], 2012).

✔ QSEN Checkpoint Question 43.2

Safety

Suppose you are preparing to enter Marty's room. Because his infection involves potential airborne transmission, what isolation precautions should you use?

a. Goggles and nonsterile gloves
b. Gown and nonsterile gloves
c. Mask, gown, and nonsterile gloves
d. No precautions provided Marty wears a mask

Look in Appendix A for the best answer and rationale.

Measles (Rubeola)

- Causative agent: Measles virus
- Incubation period: 10 to 12 days
- Period of communicability: Fifth day of incubation period through the first few days of rash
- Mode of transmission: Direct or indirect contact with droplets
- Immunity: Contracting the disease offers lasting natural immunity
- Active artificial immunity: Attenuated live measles vaccine (e.g., MMR)
- Passive artificial immunity: Immune serum globulin

Assessment. Measles is sometimes called brown or black, regular, or 7-day measles to differentiate it from rubella (German, or 3-day, measles). Like rubella, because of high vaccination rates, it is rarely seen today except for periodic outbreaks that occur, usually in the winter or early spring, in underimmunized immigrant populations or underimmunized college-age populations (Moss & Griffin, 2012). When it does occur, it can be a devastating illness because of the serious complications that can occur.

The disease has a 10- to 11-day prodromal period during which postauricular, cervical, and occipital lymph nodes become enlarged and the child develops a high fever (103° to 104°F [39.5° to 40.0°C]) along with malaise. By the second day of the prodromal period, coryza (rhinitis and a sore throat), conjunctivitis with photophobia (sensitivity to light), and a cough develop. **Koplik spots** (small, irregular, bright-red spots with a blue-white center point) appear on the buccal membrane. Unfortunately, the coryza of measles is indistinguishable from that of a common cold (nasal congestion; a mucopurulent discharge; and a deep brassy, bronchial cough) when it begins. As a result, many children with measles are diagnosed as having a simple upper respiratory infection at this point and so, are encouraged to attend school, which easily spreads the disease.

Koplik spots are hallmark symptoms because they do not appear with any other exanthem. They usually appear first on the buccal membrane opposite the molars and then extend to cover the entire buccal surface (Fig. 43.4). The raised base of the spots may coalesce so much that the blue-white centers stand out like grains of salt on a wide erythematous base.

By the fourth day of fever, a deep-red maculopapular rash begins at the hairline of the forehead, behind the ears, and at the back of the neck and then spreads to the face, the neck, upper extremities, trunk, and finally, the lower extremities

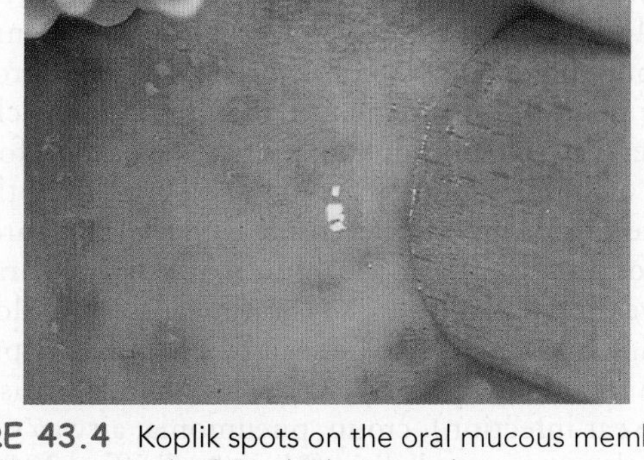

FIGURE 43.4 Koplik spots on the oral mucous membrane. (© SPL/Custom Medical Stock Photograph.)

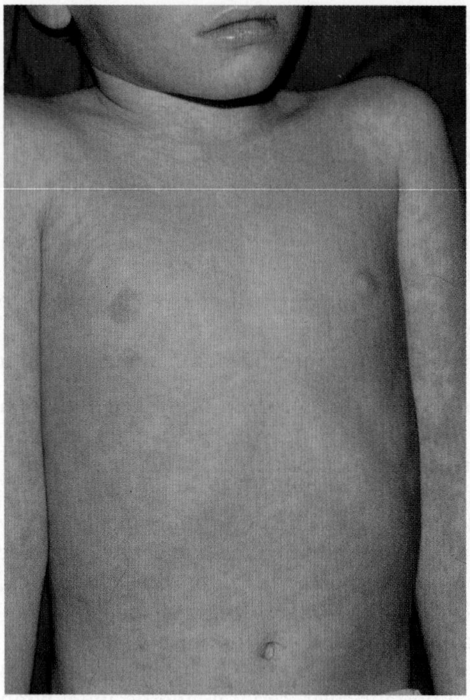

FIGURE 43.5 The typical rash of measles on a child's upper body. (© NMSB/Custom Medical Stock Photograph.)

(Fig. 43.5). After several days, the rash typically turns from red to brown. While the rash is red, it fades on pressure; when it is brown, it does not fade. This differentiates it from the rash of scarlet fever, which always fades on pressure. After 5 to 6 days, the rash fades, leaving a fine desquamation of skin cells behind. It is important to note the skin of the hands and feet does not desquamate, a feature again differentiating it from scarlet fever.

Children with measles appear very ill because their cough is loud and frequent, the coryza is acute, the fever is high, and the rash is pruritic. Fortunately, on the third or fourth day, when their temperature begins to fall, the other symptoms clear quickly and children begin to feel better. Fever that lasts beyond the third or fourth day of a rash or coughing that continues generally suggests one of the complications of measles, such as pneumonia, has occurred.

Therapeutic Management. Children with measles need comfort measures for the rash and an antipyretic for the fever. Nasal drainage does not respond to decongestants, so the skin below a child's nose may become excoriated from the constant nasal discharge. Applying a lubricating jelly or an emollient (e.g., A&D ointment) to the area may help prevent excoriation. A cough suppressant to reduce coughing can be helpful; otherwise, the throat can become painful from frequent irritation. Because children with measles have photophobia, it can be painful for them to look at bright lights, so it may be painful for them to watch television or use electronic devices. They are often more comfortable with the blinds or curtains drawn or when wearing dark glasses, so these measures should be instituted. Children need to be seen by a health care provider because the complications of measles include otitis media (middle ear infection), croup, pneumonia, airway obstruction, and acute encephalitis (Moss & Griffin, 2012). If a child is hospitalized, follow airborne precautions for the duration of the illness in addition to standard infection precautions.

Chickenpox (Varicella)

- Causative agent: Varicella-zoster virus
- Incubation period: 10 to 21 days
- Period of communicability: 1 day before the rash to 5 to 6 days after its appearance when all the vesicles have crusted
- Mode of transmission: Highly contagious; spread by direct or indirect contact of saliva or open vesicles
- Immunity: Contracting the disease offers lasting natural immunity to chickenpox; however, because the same virus causes herpes zoster, the virus may be reactivated at a later time as herpes zoster (shingles).
- Active artificial immunity: Attenuated live virus vaccine
- Passive artificial immunity: There is little passive placental immunity to chickenpox. Children who are immunosuppressed, such as those with leukemia or HIV/AIDS, or those who are being treated with corticosteroids are offered varicella-zoster immune globulin (VZIG) within 72 hours of exposure to help prevent or modify disease symptoms.

Assessment. Chickenpox is another common childhood infection that is decreasing in incidence because of required immunization. The people most prone to it are those who have not been immunized, such as immigrant children and college students. The disease is marked by a low-grade fever, malaise, and, in 24 hours, the appearance of a distinctive rash (see Fig. 43.3). Varicella lesions first begin as a macula, then progress rapidly within 6 to 8 hours to a papule, and then a vesicle that becomes umbilicated and then forms a crust. Each lesion is approximately 2 to 3 mm in diameter and is surrounded by an erythematous area. When the first crop of lesions appears, the child's temperature usually rises markedly to 104° or 105°F (40.0° or 40.6°C).

Most of chickenpox lesions are found on the trunk, although the face, scalp, palate, and neck also may be involved. They appear in approximately three separate series or crops, with each new lesion moving through progressive stages (Fig. 43.6). At some point, all four stages of lesions (macule, papule, vesicle, and crust) may be present.

Therapeutic Management. If the scabs from crusting are allowed to fall off naturally and lesions do not become secondarily infected, no scarring results. Scabs that are removed prematurely, however, may leave a white, round, slightly indented scar at the site. For this reason, it is important that children do not scratch and remove scabs. However, because the chickenpox rash is extremely pruritic, preventing scratching becomes a difficult problem for parents. A prescribed antihistamine usually helps to reduce the itchiness to a bearable level, and an antipyretic will counteract the high fever. Acyclovir, an antiviral, may be prescribed to reduce the number of lesions and shorten the course of the illness (Karch, 2013). The development of Reye syndrome (see Chapter 49) has been associated with aspirin use during varicella and influenza virus illnesses, so caution parents to avoid aspirin and instead use acetaminophen or ibuprofen to control fever.

If the child is hospitalized, in addition to standard infection precautions, follow airborne and contact precautions until all lesions are crusted. Children may return to school

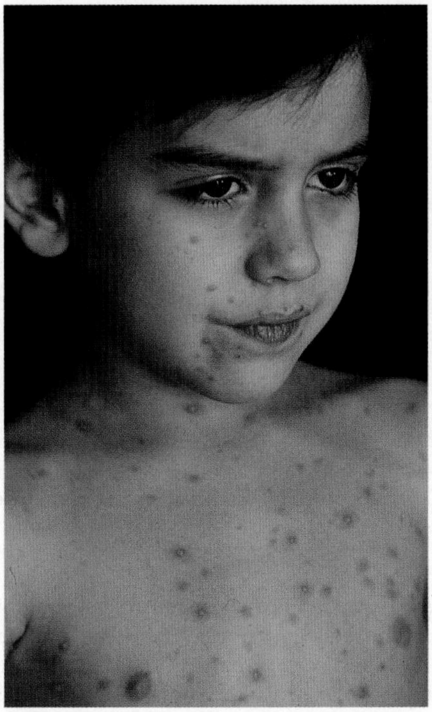

FIGURE 43.6 An older school-age boy with varicella. (© Martin/Custom Medical Stock Photograph.)

as soon as all the lesions are crusted (i.e., the crusts are not infectious). Complications include secondary infections of the lesions, pneumonia, and encephalitis.

Herpes Zoster

Herpes zoster is caused by the varicella-zoster virus, the same virus that causes chickenpox (Donohue, Kieke, Garguillo, et al., 2010). Apparently, the first time the virus invades, children demonstrate the symptoms of chickenpox. With a second invasion, herpes zoster symptoms appear due to reactivation of a latent virus. Herpes zoster, therefore, tends to occur in older children or young adults, although it can occur at any age.

The first manifestations are pruritus and cutaneous vesicular lesions on erythematous bases that follow the distributions of the lumbar and thoracic nerves (usually on the trunk, face, or upper back) and cause deep, nagging pain (Fig. 43.7).

Treatment for herpes zoster includes analgesia for pain and measures to reduce pruritus. Acyclovir, which inhibits viral DNA synthesis, may be effective at limiting the disease. Administration of VZIG may minimize symptoms.

Smallpox (Variola)

Smallpox is a disease that has been extinct in the world since 1995. Health care providers need to be able to recognize symptoms of it, however, because viruses, colonies of which are stored in various laboratories throughout the world, could be used as an agent of biologic terrorism (Anderson & Bokor, 2012).

The causative agent is the smallpox virus. The incubation period is 7 to 17 days, with a period of communicability from the onset of the rash until all crusts have been shed.

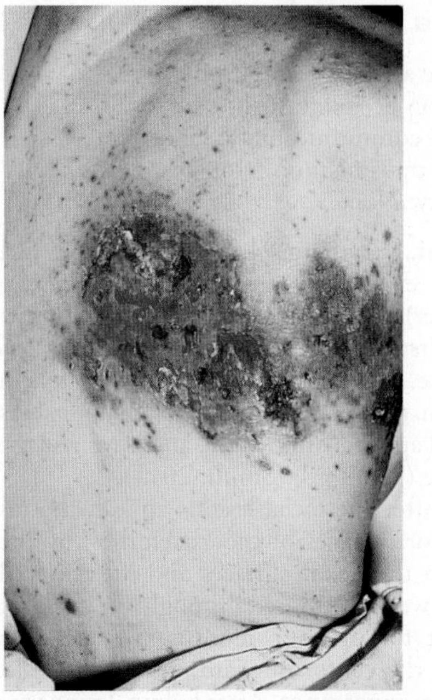

FIGURE 43.7 Herpes zoster on a child's back. (© Dr. P. Marazzi/SPL/Science Source/Photo Researchers.)

Vaccination is no longer recommended; if exposed, vaccinia immune globulin (VIG) might reduce the disease process. The disease begins with a 3- to 4-day prodromal period of chills, fever, headache, and vomiting. A rash and high fever appear on about the third day. The lesions, most prominent on the distal extremities and face, begin as macules, then progress to papules, vesicles, and pustules, eventually crusting over a 10- to 14-day period.

Although the lesions of smallpox resemble those of chickenpox, they can be differentiated by the appearance of the pustular stage (not seen with chickenpox) and the fact that they arise as one crop of lesions, all progress at the same rate, and the crusts are contagious.

Smallpox is a serious illness; its mortality rate is as high as 50% and it can be spread readily by direct or indirect contact from one infected person to another. Disease symptoms can be modified by administration of VIG and an antibiotic to prevent secondary infection of lesions. Oxygen or other measures to support respiratory and cardiac function should be provided as necessary, or these systems can fail.

QSEN Checkpoint Question 43.3

Patient-Centered Care

Marty's rash is causing him to scratch his skin. In order to maintain skin integrity and promote comfort, which of the following actions should you prioritize in his plan of care?

a. Ask Marty to rate his pain level on a pain scale.
b. Administer an antihistamine as prescribed.
c. Instruct Marty not to ever scratch the lesions.
d. Cover his hands and fingernails with mittens.

Look in Appendix A for the best answer and rationale.

Erythema Infectiosum ("Fifth Disease")

- Causative agent: Parvovirus B19
- Incubation period: 6 to 14 days
- Period of communicability: Uncertain
- Mode of transmission: Droplet
- Immunity: None

Assessment. Erythema infectiosum (the fifth important childhood exanthem after measles, rubella, varicella, and scarlet fever) occurs most often in children 2 to 12 years of age. The first phase of the infection includes fever, headache, and malaise. A week later, a rash, which erupts in three stages, appears. In the first stage, a maculopapular rash that is intensely red appears on the face, and is termed a "slapped face" appearance (Fig. 43.8) (Smith, 2011).

A day after the facial lesions appear, the rash spreads to the extensor surfaces of the extremities; by the next day, it appears on the flexor surfaces and the trunk. These lesions last for 1 week or more, although the facial rash may still be present for up to 3 months. When lesions fade, they fade from the center outward, giving the lesions a distinctive lacelike appearance. After fading, lesions may reappear if precipitated by skin irritation such as trauma, sunlight, heat, or cold. Some children develop joint pain and inflammation as well.

Therapeutic Management. Treatment is typically supportive, with antipyretics and analgesics and comfort measures for the rash (see Box 43.4). There are no known complications of fifth disease for a child; it is teratogenic in a fetus, however, so children with this disorder should avoid contact with pregnant women. Use droplet precautions in a hospital. Children can return to school as soon as the rash appears because they are no longer infectious after this point.

Pityriasis Rosea

- Causative agent: Unknown; associated with HHV-6
- Incubation period: Unknown
- Period of communicability: Unknown
- Mode of transmission: Unknown
- Immunity: Apparently none

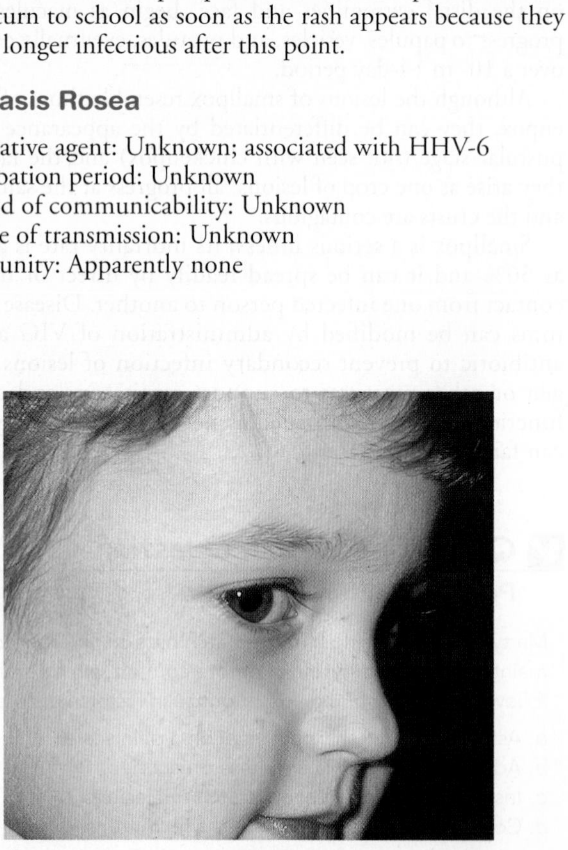

FIGURE 43.8 The "slapped face" appearance of fifth disease. (© Dr. P. Marazzi/SPL/Science Source/Photo Researchers.)

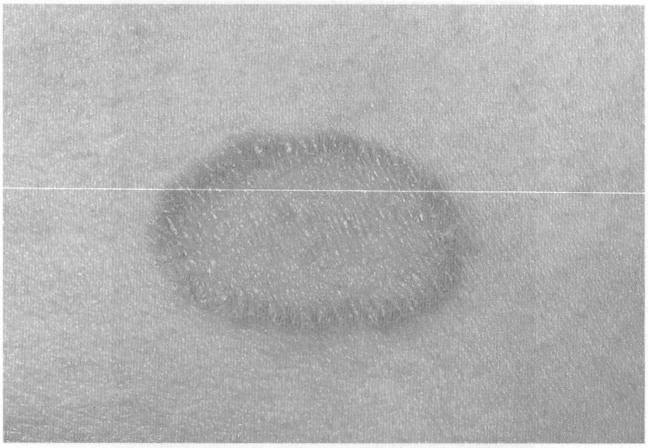

FIGURE 43.9 The "herald patch" of pityriasis rosea. (© Dr. H. C. Robinson/SPL/Science Source/Photo Researchers.)

Pityriasis rosea tends to occur in school-age and older children. Children may notice a short, mild prodromal period of fever and sore throat. A herald patch, an erythematous round lesion with a scaly border usually appearing on the trunk, is the first obvious lesion (Fig. 43.9). Approximately 1 week after the appearance of the herald patch, a generalized rash of papules, vesicles, or urticaria appears, usually also confined to the trunk. The rash follows skin lines, giving it the unique configuration of a Christmas tree (Zawar & Chuh, 2012).

The rash lasts 6 to 8 weeks. It is pruritic and, because it lasts so long, is particularly worrisome to children and parents. Because the lesions, particularly the herald patch, are scaly at the edges, they are often confused with tinea corporis (ringworm). Treatment is limited to oral antihistamines and other comfort measures for rash.

Pityriasis rosea appears to have no sequelae or complications; in fact, it is difficult to demonstrate in what manner it is infectious. It is a baffling rash of childhood, but children with it need to be seen by a health care provider so it can be differentiated from severe exanthems.

Enteroviruses

There are three main types of enteroviruses: echoviruses (33 subdivisions), coxsackievirus A (24 subdivisions) and coxsackievirus B (6 types), and polioviruses (3 subdivisions). All three types cause illness in children.

Echovirus Infections

The echoviruses are responsible for a number of childhood diseases, including aseptic meningitis, diarrhea, acute respiratory illness, and maculopapular rashes. Although potentially serious, such infections are usually benign and self-limiting. Treatment involves supportive measures such as an antipyretic for fever and comfort measures for the rash. If a child is hospitalized, follow contact precautions for the duration of the illness in addition to standard infection precautions.

Coxsackievirus Infections

The coxsackievirus groups are responsible, like the echovirus groups, for a variety of diseases. One of the most frequently seen diseases caused by coxsackievirus A is herpangina. With this, children develop an abrupt elevation of temperature, up to 104° or 105°F (40.0° or 40.6°C), which lasts 1 to 4 days. Anorexia, difficulty swallowing, sore throat, headache, abdominal pain, and vomiting may also be present. Small lesions, generally discrete grayish vesicles and pinpoint in size, appear on the tonsillar fauces, soft palate, and uvula (Lam, 2010). These gradually change to shallow ulcers surrounded by a red areola by the following day. After a few more days, they disappear and the temperature returns to normal. There are generally no complications.

Children need a soft or liquid diet while their mouth and throat are sore. If a child is hospitalized, follow contact precautions for the duration of the illness in addition to standard infection precautions.

Poliovirus Infections: Poliomyelitis (Infantile Paralysis)

- Causative agent: Poliovirus
- Incubation period: 7 to 14 days
- Period of communicability: Greatest shortly before and after onset of symptoms, when virus is present in the throat and feces (1 to 6 weeks)
- Mode of transmission: Direct and indirect contact
- Immunity: Contracting the disease causes active immunity against the one strain of virus causing the illness
- Active artificial immunity: Inactivated polio virus (IPV) vaccine
- Passive artificial immunity: None

Polio is Greek for "gray," the color of the spinal cord after it atrophies from the effect of the poliomyelitis virus. No longer seen in the United States thanks to effective vaccination programs, poliomyelitis is still seen around the world, particularly in India and parts of Africa, so immigrant children may be susceptible. The illness may be caused by any of the three strains of poliovirus, which is why children are immunized with the trivalent (three-strain) vaccine.

Assessment. The poliovirus enters the child's gastrointestinal tract, where it multiplies and produces symptoms such as fever, headache, nausea, vomiting, abdominal pain, and mild stiffness of the neck, back, and legs.

As the virus invades the central nervous system, these initial symptoms change to intense pain and tremors of the extremities and then paralysis. Swallowing becomes difficult if laryngeal paralysis occurs; respiratory paralysis can halt respirations (CDC, 2011a).

Therapeutic Management. Treatment for poliomyelitis is bed rest with analgesia and moist hot packs to relieve pain. If the respiratory muscles are involved, long-term ventilation may be necessary. Survivors tend to develop progressive muscle atrophy (postpoliomyelitis muscular atrophy syndrome) or severe arthritis in late adulthood, which further reduces their ability to be self-sufficient (Gonzalez, Olsson, & Borg, 2010).

Viral Infections of the Integumentary System

Viral infections of the skin include herpes infections and warts (verrucae).

Herpesvirus Infections

Herpesviruses are responsible for both facial and genital lesions in children.

- Causative agent: Herpes simplex or herpes type 1 or type 2 virus
- Incubation period: 2 to 12 days
- Period of communicability: Greatest early in the course of the infection
- Mode of transmission: Direct contact
- Immunity: Immunity to a primary herpes response is gained after one incident. There is no immunity to recurrent herpes infections, however, because the virus lies dormant in the neurons of local ganglia until it is activated by stress, sun exposure, fever, other illness, or menstruation.

Acute Herpetic Gingivostomatitis. Acute herpetic gingivostomatitis is the most common form of herpes simplex invasion in young children (Usatine & Tinitigan, 2010). An example of the primary (not the recurrent) response, it occurs most often in children aged 1 to 4 years. Children develop a high fever (104° to 105°F [40.0° to 40.6°C]), are restless, and have anorexia with an edematous and erythematous pharynx. Their gum line is also swollen, reddened, and bleeds easily. White plaques or shallow ulcers with red areolae appear on the buccal mucosa, tongue, and palate and perhaps on the tonsillar fauces. The anterior cervical lymph nodes are usually enlarged and tender. The disease runs its course in 5 to 14 days.

Children may need an antipyretic to reduce fever. They also need soft, acid-free foods they can eat with minimal irritation or abrasion. Popsicles and Jell-O are soothing against inflamed mucous membranes. Oral acyclovir helps with healing. Use contact precautions with hospitalized children to avoid contact with lesions. Although usually mild, the disease can become serious, especially in infants, if the mouth becomes so sore that an infant cannot swallow, which then leads to dehydration.

Herpes Simplex (Herpes Labialis). Herpes simplex infection, popularly known as a cold sore or fever blister, represents the recurrent form of a type 1 herpesvirus invasion that remains dormant in the ganglia of the trigeminal or fifth cranial nerve. Herpes simplex typically appears as a cluster of painful, grouped vesicles surrounded by an erythematous base on the lips or skin surrounding the mouth. After 2 or 3 days, vesicles crust and then gradually dry. Topical or oral acyclovir reduces pain and increases healing. Because children can feel conspicuous about the appearance of the lesion, they may need counseling to assure them the lesion is not as obvious to others as it seems to them.

Acute Herpetic Vulvovaginitis (Genital Herpes). Genital herpes is caused by the human herpesvirus type 2, which remains dormant in the ganglia of the sacral nerves. Because this form is spread primarily by sexual contact, it is discussed in Chapter 47 with other sexually transmitted infections. Normally, children rarely contract this form, so the occurrence in a young child suggests child sexual maltreatment (Reading, Hughes, Hill, et al., 2011).

Warts (Verrucae)

Warts, one of the most common dermatologic diseases in children, are caused by the papillomavirus. The virus has an incubation period of 1 to 6 months. The mode of transmission is unknown, but it is probably by direct contact (Swanson & Canty, 2013).

Warts appear as flesh-colored, dirty-appearing papules that generally occur on the dorsal surface of the hands. Plantar warts appear on the soles of the feet and are painful when children walk. These can be differentiated from calluses in that they obliterate skin lines as they grow, whereas calluses do not.

Warts on the hands or the face generally are removed if they are cosmetically unattractive to children. Plantar warts may have to be removed because of the discomfort they cause. Parents can use over-the-counter wart-removing preparations, such as Compound W (a salicylic acid solution), to dissolve them. Application of a stronger prescription salicylic acid solution may be prescribed to remove plantar warts. Carbon dioxide snow, liquid nitrogen, electrodessication, and cryotherapy are other methods also available for removal, but these methods are painful and rarely necessary.

Children need reassurance that people do not catch warts from frogs or toads and that, even if left without any treatment, warts will eventually fade by themselves after about 24 months. Anogenital warts need special consideration because, like herpes type 2 lesions, they can be a mark of sexual maltreatment. They can be prevented by the human papillomavirus (HPV) vaccination, which is recommended for all children at 12 to 14 years of age (Thornsberry & English, 2012).

Viruses Causing Central Nervous System Diseases

Viruses are the causative agent for central nervous system disorders such as rabies, encephalitis, and meningitis. Encephalitis and meningitis are discussed in Chapter 49.

Rabies

- Causative agent: Rabies virus
- Incubation period: 2 to 6 weeks, possibly as long as 12 months
- Period of communicability: 3 to 5 days before the onset of symptoms through the course of the disease
- Mode of transmission: The bite of rabid animals; rarely through saliva from infected animals being transferred to an open lesion on a child's skin
- Immunity: Contracting the disease apparently offers active immunity, but few people have ever survived the illness to verify this
- Active artificial immunity: Human diploid cell rabies vaccine
- Passive artificial immunity: Rabies immune globulin (RIG)

Any warm-blooded animal can contract rabies. Although most people assume dogs are the most common source of infection, wild animals, such as skunks, squirrels, raccoons, and bats, constitute the primary sources of rabies infection in the United States. Children are bitten more often by dogs, however, and therefore, more children are treated for dog or cat bites. Rodents are seldom found to be rabid. Bites from other children do not cause rabies, although therapy is required because such bites usually contain streptococci.

When a child is bitten by an infected animal, the virus migrates from the bite area to the child's central nervous system over several days time, damaging cranial nerve and spinal cord nuclei. Negri bodies (cytoplasmic inclusion bodies) can be isolated from nerve cells to confirm the diagnosis (Jackson, 2011).

Assessment. After the long incubation period of the virus, children begin to show prodromal signs of malaise, fever, anorexia, nausea, sore throat, drowsiness, irritability, and restlessness. They may notice numbness or hyperesthesia at the area of the bite and along the course of the involved nerves. The white blood cell count begins to reveal a slight leukocytosis. If tested, the cerebrospinal fluid shows only a slight elevation in protein and cells. Symptoms such as high fever, anxiety, and hyperexcitability increase; involuntary twitching and generalized seizures may occur. When children try to drink, they experience violent contractions of the muscles of the mouth leading to drooling of saliva. This phenomena gives the disease its former name: hydrophobia ("water fear") (Jackson, 2011).

As symptoms progress, children will become comatose, with possible total body paralysis. Peripheral vascular collapse and death can follow as quickly as 5 or 6 days later. Postmortem examination will reveal the diagnostic Negri bodies in brain cells.

Therapeutic Management. Once the disease process begins, rabies is almost invariably fatal, so the key is prevention of the active process. All children who receive an animal bite should be seen by a health care provider to evaluate the circumstances surrounding the bite and to decide whether rabies prevention measures should begin, a decision which must be made immediately if treatment is to be effective.

Take a history of the incident to determine the type of animal that caused the bite. Most children can be certain they know the type of animal if it was a dog or cat, but they may be unsure if it was a wild animal. Be careful not to lead children into naming an animal just to please, such as, "Was it a skunk? A raccoon? A squirrel?" When names are suggested in this way, children may choose an animal name as if they are answering a multiple choice question, not because they are certain of the type of animal. Instead, ask children to describe the animal; from that description, establish what kind of animal must have bitten the child. It helps in rural health care facilities to have a picture book of animals handy so preschoolers, in particular, can identify the animal from a photo. Ask also how the animal acted because a rabid animal usually runs blindly, often staggering; it may dribble saliva rather than swallow it. It is easy for parents to assess whether a household pet is acting unusual in this way. It can be more difficult to assess the actions of a wild animal because the fear it experiences at being trapped or cornered may make it run about frantically.

An unprovoked attack is much more suggestive that the animal is rabid, rather than if the bite happened during a provoked attack. Let children know that they will not be punished if they were found to be provoking an animal so they feel free to say so. Listen for statements such as "I was only hugging him" or "I was just feeding him" because such actions sound innocent, but may have constituted a provoked attack to the animal.

The kind of wound a child receives and the immunity status of the animal are also instrumental in deciding whether treatment will be necessary. A bite mark is much more serious than a scratch from an animal's claws, for example. If the animal was properly immunized against rabies, it will rarely transmit the virus. Whether rabies exists in the community at the time of the attack is yet another factor that influences the decision. If there have been no other reported instances in domestic animals, the chance that this dog bite is serious in terms of rabies is lower than if dogs with rabies have been reported in the area.

Inspect the wound carefully to see whether it shows teeth marks or scratch marks. Wash the wound well with an antiseptic solution. If puncture wounds are present, the wound must not be sutured and closed because tetanus (organisms that are anaerobic and grow in deep, closed wounds where oxygen does not reach) can develop in the wound in addition to rabies. The animal that caused the bite should be located, if possible, and confined for 5 to 10 days. If it develops any signs of rabies during this period, it will be destroyed and the brain will be examined for evidence of rabies. You can assure people that domestic animals are not destroyed unless they show signs of rabies or otherwise they may resist surrendering an animal for observation.

If the animal is found to be rabid, children receive both the rabies vaccine and an antirabies serum (RIG). This applies also if the animal escapes and its condition is unknown (i.e., it is assumed to be rabid). A portion of the RIG dose is injected into the wound site and the remainder is given intramuscularly. Antirabies vaccine is given immediately (day 0) and then again on days 3, 7, and 14 (Karch, 2013).

It may seem contradictory to give an active immunization serum (i.e., administering antigen to children) when they have received an animal bite, which administers antigen to them. This is done, however, because the rabies virus has a long incubation period before antibody production is stimulated; administering RIG provides antibodies against the rabies virus immediately. Administering the rabies vaccine allows the child to begin additional antibody formation so that by the time the rabies virus from the bite begins to have an effect (2 to 6 weeks after the bite), the child has developed sufficient antibodies to combat it and prevent the illness.

West Nile Virus Disease

Although the West Nile virus may be transmitted by contaminated blood products, it is usually spread by the bite of a mosquito after the mosquito has bitten and acquired the infection from a natural host such as an infected bird, horse, squirrel, or reptile (Murray, Walker, & Gould, 2011).

Fortunately, most children who contract the disease remain asymptomatic. A small number develop flulike symptoms such as fever, fatigue, and malaise. The infection is serious, however, because some develop encephalitis, with symptoms such as mental confusion, lethargy, photophobia, headache, muscle weakness, and coma, leading to death. West Nile virus disease is diagnosed when antibodies to the virus are recovered from blood serum. There is no evidence-based therapy for the disorder, except for supportive measures to maintain function; however, ribavirin and intravenous immunoglobulin (IVIG) have been used to reduce symptoms. There is also currently no vaccine for this condition.

Parents can help prevent the spread of West Nile virus disease by adhering to the "5D's" (Murray et al., 2011):

- Instruct children to stay inside between **D**usk and **D**awn when mosquitoes are most prevalent.
- **D**rain standing water so there are few opportunities for mosquitoes to breed.
- **D**ress should include long pants and long sleeves when outside.
- Apply mosquito repellant that contains **D**EET (use a concentration not over 30% and apply only once a day. Don't place it on children's hands so they don't ingest it or use with infants younger than 2 months of age).

Other Viral Infections

Mumps (Epidemic Parotitis)

- Causative agent: Mumps virus
- Incubation period: 14 to 21 days
- Period of communicability: Shortly before and after onset of parotitis
- Mode of transmission: Direct or indirect contact
- Immunity: Contracting the disease gives lasting natural immunity
- Active artificial immunity: Attenuated live mumps vaccine (MMR)
- Passive artificial immunity: Mumps immune globulin

Assessment. Mumps is now a rare disease in the United States due to successful immunization programs. If it does occur, it is most likely to be in adolescents who have not been immunized. If the disease occurs, it begins with fever, headache, anorexia, and malaise. Within 24 hours, pain on chewing and an "earache" occurs. When the child points to the site of the earache, however, the child does not point to the ear, but rather, the jawline just in front of the earlobe, which is the site of the parotid gland. By the next day, the gland appears swollen and feels tender, and the ear becomes displaced upward and backward. Boys may also develop testicular pain and swelling (orchitis).

It is often difficult to differentiate mumps from submaxillary adenitis (swelling of lymph nodes). The best method of differentiation is to place a hand along the child's jawline. If the major amount of swelling is above the hand, it is probably mumps. If the largest amount of swelling is below the handline, it is probably adenitis (Fig. 43.10).

Therapeutic Management. Because chewing movements are so painful, children may need soft, bland, or liquid foods until the major portion of the swelling recedes (about 6 days). They may need an analgesic for pain and an antipyretic for fever. Children are infectious prior to and for a few days after parotid swelling appears and should be excluded from school until after this time. If a child is hospitalized, follow droplet precautions in addition to standard infection precautions.

Some parents worry that because their child had swelling only on one side, their child will develop mumps on the opposite side in the future. One attack of mumps gives lasting immunity, however, so the child will not contract the disease again. If a child does appear to have contracted mumps twice, the diagnosis was probably confused with cervical adenitis either time.

Mumps is a potentially serious illness because several serious complications, such as meningoencephalitis or severe permanent hearing impairment from neuritis of the auditory nerve, can develop. If mumps orchitis develops, only a single testis is usually involved, which swells rapidly and is painful and tender. As soon as the fever declines, testicular swelling also decreases, although the tenderness may exist for weeks. Although atrophy of the testis may result, leading to a low sperm count, the chance mumps orchitis will lead to complete subfertility is rare (Rundell, 2013).

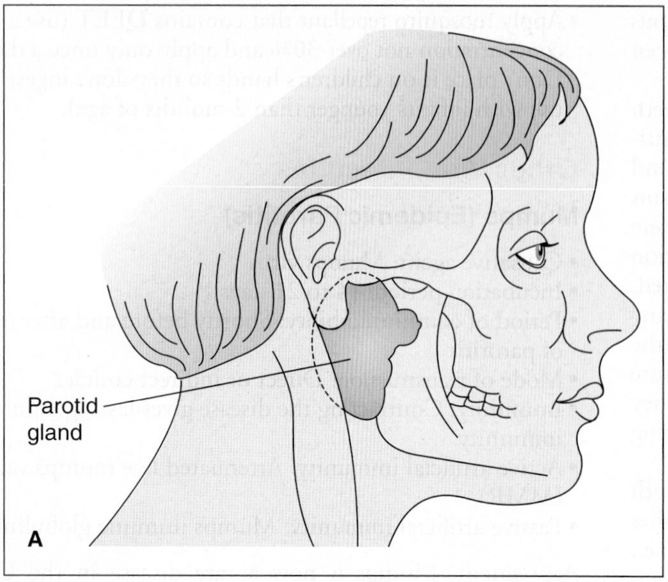

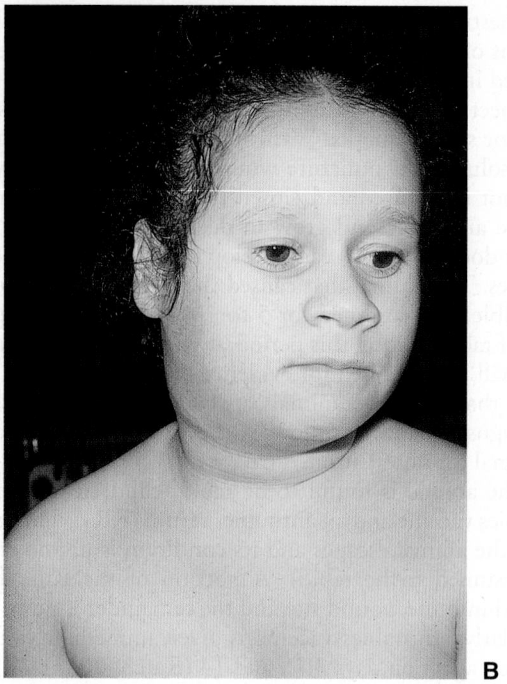

FIGURE 43.10 Epidemic parotitis. **(A)** The parotid gland is located just in front of the ear. **(B)** A boy with parotitis (mumps). (© Morris Huberland/Science Source/Photo Researchers.)

QSEN Checkpoint Question 43.4

Teamwork & Collaboration

A nurse on your care team calls into work ill because she's worried she has contracted mumps (infectious parotitis). Which of the following symptoms is most associated with mumps?

a. A productive cough and a severe runny nose
b. Pronounced swelling behind both of her ears
c. Swelling above the jaw line in front of one ear
d. Adenoid tonsils are reddened and swollen and hurt

Look in Appendix A for the best answer and rationale.

Infectious Mononucleosis

- Causative agent: Epstein–Barr virus
- Incubation period: Unknown; probably 2 to 8 weeks
- Period of communicability: Unknown; probably only during acute illness
- Mode of transmission: Direct and indirect contact
- Immunity: One episode apparently gives lasting immunity. No vaccination is available.

Infectious mononucleosis is also known as glandular fever or, because it was first discovered as a disease that is transferred readily from one person to another by kissing, the *kissing disease*. It occurs most commonly in adolescents and young adults, although it may occur at any age of the child (Katz, 2013). Complications that can occur include meningitis or encephalitis.

Assessment. Following an incubation period of 4 to 8 weeks, the beginning symptoms include chills, fever, headache, anorexia, and malaise. Children develop enlarged lymph nodes and a severe sore throat accompanied by a high fever (103°F [39.5°C]).

The cervical lymph nodes are the ones most markedly affected and feel firm and tender to touch; swallowing is painful. The tonsils are enlarged, reddened, and often covered by a thick, white membrane; petechiae appear on the palate (Fig. 43.11). If the mesenteric lymph nodes enlarge, children may experience abdominal pain so sharp that it simulates appendicitis. If the spleen enlarges, it places the child at risk for spontaneous rupture. Other symptoms that may occur are hepatitis, a maculopapular eruption similar to the rash of rubella, pneumonitis, and central nervous system involvement such as encephalitis, meningitis, or polyneuritis.

On a blood smear, lymphocytosis (lymphocytes representing more than 50% of the total white blood cell count) will be present. A positive Monospot test, which can be reported in minutes, or a heterophile antibody test, which must be analyzed in a laboratory, along with the increased number of atypical lymphocytes apparent on a blood slide, confirms the diagnosis. Antibodies against the Epstein–Barr virus can be assessed in blood serum for a final confirmation.

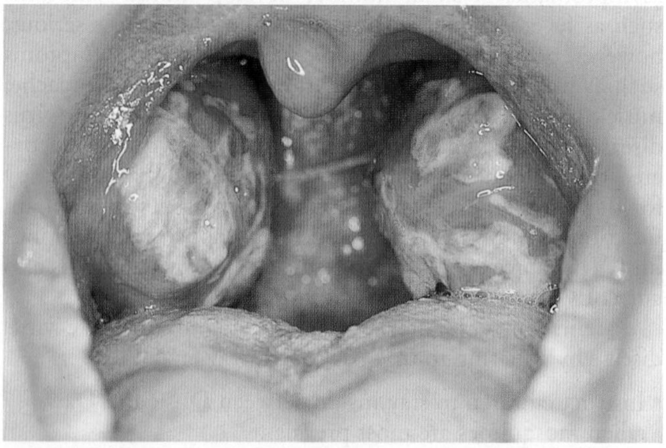

FIGURE 43.11 The appearance of the tonsils in a child with infectious mononucleosis. Note the degree of erythema, enlargement, and purulent covering. (© Dr. P. Marazzi/SPL/Science Source/Photo Researchers.)

Therapeutic Management. Children with infectious mononucleosis need bed rest during the acute stage of the illness (i.e., 2 to 3 weeks) because, with the splenomegaly, there is a danger of spleen rupture with any trauma to that area. If a child is hospitalized, follow standard infection precautions. Be careful in helping children with this disease turn in bed so no pressure is placed over the splenic area. If palpating the spleen, do so gently to avoid inadvertent rupture.

Teach children and parents the importance of maintaining a good fluid intake despite the sore throat; cool, nonacidic fluids are often tolerated best. Caution children they may notice weakness and general fatigue for up to 2 to 3 months after the illness and to avoid contact sports as long as their spleen is enlarged. Because infectious mononucleosis occurs primarily in adolescents or young adults, it may interrupt school or career plans. Help these young adults to voice their frustration with this illness. Offer support to help them through this unexpected interruption in their life (Porth, 2011).

Hantavirus Pulmonary Syndrome Infection

The hantavirus is a member of the arbovirus group. The virus infects small rodents and perhaps cats who have eaten mice. Outbreaks occur sporadically, usually in families who have camped in an area with infected rodents. Symptoms such as fever, muscle aches, thrombocytopenia, gastrointestinal upset, and hypotension occur 1 to 5 weeks after exposure. Death can occur from rapidly progressive pulmonary edema or kidney failure (Heyman, Thoma, Marié, et al., 2012). Supportive care is necessary, as antiviral medications do not seem to be effective and there is no cure or vaccine available. Caution families not to touch dead mice and to have mice exterminated from their homes to avoid the possibility of contracting this disease.

QSEN Checkpoint Question 43.5

Quality Improvement

Marty's sister is home with "mono," or infectious mononucleosis. In the event that she requires hospital care, assessment protocols should emphasize what action?

a. Lymph nodes should be palpated before being percussed.
b. The spleen should be palpated gently to prevent rupture.
c. Lymph nodes should be assessed by Doppler.
d. Petechiae should be lightly massaged.

Look in Appendix A for the best answer and rationale.

BACTERIAL INFECTIONS

Bacteria are independent, living organisms with a nucleus that contains both DNA and RNA. They reproduce by fission, in which one cell enlarges and duplicates itself, then divides into two equal parts. They occur in three main shapes: spheres (cocci), rods (bacilli), and spirals (spirochetes).

Types of bacteria can be distinguished after they are fixed onto a laboratory slide and then stained. Bacteria that stain violet are said to be gram-positive organisms and those that stain red are gram-negative organisms. Those that cannot be decolorized with acid after being stained are acid-fast. As some bacteria grow, they produce **exotoxins**, or poisons. When this happens, disease symptoms arise not from the bacteria itself but from the effect of the toxins on the body. Tetanus, botulism, scarlet fever, and diphtheria are examples of diseases caused by the systemic spread of toxins produced by bacteria.

Streptococcal Diseases

Streptococci, which are gram-positive organisms, are found normally in the respiratory, alimentary, and female genital tracts and produce a myriad of types of infection. Most severe diseases in children result from infection with *Streptococcus pyogenes* (β-hemolytic streptococci, group A). A β-hemolytic, group B streptococcal infection can be contracted from vaginal secretions at birth (see Chapter 26) and so tends to occur in newborns. Streptococcal pharyngeal infections are discussed in Chapter 40 with other throat infections. Rheumatic fever and glomerulonephritis, conditions that may result as an autoimmune response to streptococci, are discussed in Chapters 41 and 46, respectively.

Scarlet Fever

- Causative agent: β-hemolytic streptococci, group A
- Incubation period: 2 to 5 days
- Period of communicability: Greatest during acute phase of respiratory illness; 1 to 7 days
- Mode of transmission: Direct contact and large droplets
- Immunity: One episode of disease gives lasting immunity to scarlet fever toxin. No vaccination is available.

Assessment. Scarlet fever occurs most commonly in the 6- to 12-year-old age group, although it may be seen in preschoolers. The incidence is highest in temperate climates, and the disease occurs usually in late winter or early spring.

Symptoms begin abruptly and are those of streptococcal pharyngitis: fever, sore throat, perhaps headache, chills, a rapid pulse, and malaise. As the β-hemolytic, group A streptococcus grows in the child's body, it produces several toxins; erythrogenic toxin is the one responsible for a rash that appears 12 to 48 hours after the onset of the pharyngeal symptoms (see Fig. 43.3). The fever is high (103° to 104°F [39.5° to 40.0°C]) on the first day of throat symptoms and again on the day the rash appears, but then gradually returns to normal.

The rash is unique in that it is both enanthematous and exanthematous (i.e., on both the mucous membrane and the skin). The skin rash typically is red with pinpoint lesions that blanch on pressure and feel as rough as sandpaper. They tend to be densest on the trunk and very prominent in skin folds (Pastia's sign). The rash persists for approximately 1 week. It desquamates, with large areas of skin peeling off in fine flakes (Patel, Lambert, Gagna, et al., 2011).

In addition to the rash, the tonsils appear inflamed and enlarged and are usually covered with white exudate. The palate may be covered with reddened punctiform (pinpoint) lesions and perhaps scattered petechiae. The tongue, during the first 2 days of the illness, is white and appears furry. By day 3, papillae enlarge and protrude through the white coat, giving the tongue a "white strawberry" appearance. By day 4 or 5, the white coat disappears and the prominent papillae of the tongue give it a "red strawberry" appearance. A "strawberry tongue" is a hallmark symptom of scarlet fever and helps to differentiate the disease from other rashes or pharyngeal infections. A throat culture, which reveals streptococci along with the rash, is diagnostic.

Therapeutic Management. Children with scarlet fever usually appear ill. They may need an analgesic and antipyretic, such as acetaminophen (Tylenol) or children's ibuprofen (Motrin) for pain and fever. They need a soft or liquid diet for a few days until their throat soreness has diminished enough that their throat is not too sore to eat. Comfort measures are important for the rash. Because the underlying cause of the illness is a streptococcal infection, a course of antibiotics is prescribed (Beach & Thalange, 2013). Caution parents to give the full amount prescribed for the full course prescribed to prevent the complications of β-hemolytic, group A streptococcal infections (acute glomerulonephritis or rheumatic fever). If a child is hospitalized, follow droplet precautions until 24 hours after therapy is started, in addition to standard infection precautions, because the child is infectious until this time (see Box 43.3). Box 43.5 shows an interprofessional care map illustrating both nursing and team planning for a hospitalized child with scarlet fever.

QSEN Checkpoint Question 43.6

Informatics

Marty, who has scarlet fever, is missing his school friends so is eager to return to school. Because he received an antibiotic, when should you inform the school nurse that it would be safe for him to return to school?

a. Whenever he feels that he is strong enough
b. Forty-eight hours after his spleen has returned to usual size
c. As soon as his fever is within normal range
d. Twenty-four hours after he began the antibiotic

Look in Appendix A for the best answer and rationale.

Impetigo

- Causative agent: β-Hemolytic streptococcus, group A (nonbullous); *Staphylococcus aureus* (bullous) or methicillin-resistant *Staphylococcus aureus* (MRSA)
- Incubation period: 2 to 5 days
- Period of communicability: From outbreak of lesions until lesions are healed
- Mode of transmission: Direct contact with lesions
- Immunity: None

Parents may be upset at being told their child has impetigo because the lesions (which are dirty and crusty appearing) have been associated in the past with poverty and poor hygiene. It is common to see several children in a family with identical impetigo lesions because it is spread by direct contact.

Assessment. Impetigo begins as a single papulovesicular lesion surrounded by localized erythema. Soon, more vesicles appear and become purulent, ooze, and form honey-colored crusts (Fig. 43.12). They are found most commonly on the face and extremities. They are often seen as secondary infections of insect bites or in children who have body piercings. If there are several lesions, children may have local swollen lymph nodes.

Therapeutic Management. Treatment is oral administration of penicillin or erythromycin or the application of mupirocin (Bactroban) ointment for 7 to 10 days (Box 43.6). The lesions heal most quickly if a parent or the child also washes the crusts daily with soap and water.

Although rare, complications of rheumatic fever or acute glomerulonephritis may occur after impetigo, as with other streptococcal infections. If a child develops impetigo while in the hospital, follow contact precautions until 24 hours after initiation of the antibiotic. If the infection does not heal or seems to be growing worse, parents need to notify their health care provider because impetigo can be caused by MRSA, which will need a systemic antibiotic for therapy rather than a topical cream (Odell, 2010).

Cat-Scratch Disease

- Causative agent: *Bartonella henselae* bacteria
- Incubation period: 3 to 10 days
- Period of communicability: Unknown
- Mode of transmission: Bite or scratch from a cat or kitten
- Immunity: One episode of disease gives lasting immunity; no passive artificial immunity

Cat-scratch disease occurs most commonly in preschool children because children at that age play roughly with cats or pick them up and so receive scratches. At the time the child contracts the disease, the cat does not appear ill.

The first symptom for the child is a single skin papule or pustule that lasts 1 to 3 weeks. Approximately 1 to 2 weeks after the scratch, a single lymph node of the head, neck, or axilla becomes severely swollen. The swelling generally lasts several months.

Some children also have a low-grade fever and malaise. Occasionally, central nervous system involvement, such as encephalitis or meningitis, occurs. A positive reaction to a skin test of cat-scratch disease antigen will be present. This, along with the history of a cat scratch and the aspiration of sterile pus from the enlarged lymph node, is diagnostic. Treatment is symptomatic, although an antibiotic may be prescribed to help shorten the course of the disease. Children may need an analgesic to relieve pain from the swollen lymph node. Aspiration of the involved node may be necessary to relieve pain and make swallowing easier (Klotz, Ianas, & Elliott, 2011).

Parents may ask if the cat should be destroyed. Because an attack of cat-scratch disease gives lifetime immunity and fewer than 10% of children scratched by the same cat contract cat-scratch disease, there is no need to destroy the cat for an act it may have seen as defending its safety.

Staphylococcal Infections

Staphylococcal organisms are gram positive. Colonies of them are normally found on the skin surface; therefore, they are commonly the organisms involved in skin infections (pyodermas). Because the organisms grow rapidly in cream foods that are not well refrigerated, such as potato salad or cream pies, they are also often the organisms involved in summer food poisoning episodes. Because food poisoning produces gastrointestinal symptoms, these infections are discussed in Chapter 45.

Furunculosis (Boils)

A furuncle is a staphylococcal infection of a hair follicle. A yellow pustule forms at the site. There is localized redness, pain, and edema of the surrounding skin. Moist heat for

BOX 43.5 Nursing Care Planning

AN INTERPROFESSIONAL CARE MAP FOR A HOSPITALIZED CHILD WITH SCARLET FEVER

Marty, a 10-year-old boy, was admitted to the hospital yesterday for appendicitis. This morning after surgery, his throat is painful and his arms are covered by a very itchy, red, macular rash. He was diagnosed as having scarlet fever. "His sister is home with mono," his mother tells you. "How could our family get two infections plus appendicitis all in 1 week?"

Family Assessment Child has three siblings: a 16-year-old sister and two brothers, 6 years and 10 days old. Parents are migrant crop workers. Family moves yearly from Florida to Connecticut to follow crops. Mother rates finances as: "We have no money."

Client Assessment Macular, pinpoint erythematous rash on abdomen, groin folds, and chest. Lesions blanch with pressure. Groin and elbow areas hyperpigmented. Child scratching constantly. Uvula and pharynx beefy red. Tonsils inflamed and enlarged with white exudate. Temperature: 103°F (39.5°C). Pinpoint lesions with two or three scattered petechiae noted on palate. Tongue white and furry. Throat culture positive for streptococcus. Other physical examination findings within normal limits for postoperative course. Child upset and crying, saying, "I wish my Mom was here to stay with me. I can't even go to the playroom." Mother usually visits once a day in the late afternoon.

Nursing Diagnosis Social isolation related to required restrictions associated with infection-control precautions

Outcome Evaluation Child states reason for restrictions, identifies time when restrictions will be lifted, and expresses interest in activities proposed.

Team Member Responsible	Assessment	Intervention	Rationale	Expected Outcome
Activities of Daily Living, Including Safety				
Nurse	Assess what child understands about how communicable diseases are spread.	Review the reason for restrictions and infection control precautions. Institute droplet precautions.	Child may associate precautions and restrictions with feelings of being punished. Droplet precautions help reduce the spread of the disease.	Child states he understands reason for isolation. Cooperates to maintain infection precautions.
Nurse	Assess what play activity would provide stimulation.	Visit the child frequently, and provide him with opportunities for therapeutic play.	Frequent visits help to decrease feelings of being alone. Therapeutic play helps the child deal with resentment about condition.	Child states that although he wants to go to playroom, he has found an enjoyable activity to occupy his time in his hospital room.
Teamwork & Collaboration				
Nurse/Primary health care provider	Determine whether hospital infection control committee is aware of contagious illness in a postoperative patient.	Consult with infection control members on the possibility that surgical personnel may have been exposed to scarlet fever.	Scarlet fever is contagious for 1 to 7 days prior to the outbreak of a rash.	Infection control officer states she is aware of possible spread of illness and the need for penicillin for exposed health care personnel.
Procedures/Medications for Quality Improvement				
Nurse	Determine whether child has ever had a reaction to penicillin.	Begin antibiotic therapy as prescribed.	Penicillin is effective for group A β-hemolytic streptococcus, the causative organism of scarlet fever.	Child's parents are contacted and report child has not had a previous reaction to penicillin. Child takes oral penicillin as prescribed.

(continued on page 1272)

BOX 43.5 Nursing Care Planning (continued)

Nurse	Ask child to rate pain of sore throat and itchiness of rash on scale of 1 to 10.	Administer analgesia and antihistamine prescribed. Caution child that antihistamine may make him feel sleepy.	An antihistamine such as Benadryl can greatly reduce the pruritus of a rash.	Child states the itchiness of rash and pain of sore throat have decreased to tolerable levels.
Nutrition				
Nurse/ Nutritionist	Assess what fluid child would find most appealing to drink.	Provide frequent oral fluids. When soft diet is begun (child is post-op appendicitis), provide soft foods.	Adequate fluid intake is important to prevent skin dryness, which increases discomfort. A soft or liquid diet is less irritating to the child's sore throat.	Child identifies favorite fluid to drink. States he is able to eat soft foods even with painful throat.
Patient-Centered Care				
Nurse/ Primary care provider	Determine whether other members of family will need a prophylactic antibiotic.	Explain the purpose of prophylactic penicillin for susceptible family members.	Because family members were near the child during the prodromal period, they are susceptible to also contracting the disease.	Parent identifies susceptible family members; states she will be able to fill prescription and supervise to be sure they take prescribed antibiotic.
Psychosocial/Spiritual/Emotional Needs				
Nurse	Assess whether child and parent understand the cause of scarlet fever.	Discuss that the spread of infectious diseases is not related to "good or bad" values.	Mother voiced she was concerned because two diseases happened to her child at the same time.	Mother and child state they understand diseases are caused by infectious organisms, not moral status.
Informatics for Seamless Health Care Planning				
Nurse	Assess if parent is aware the child's rash will be itchy for about 1 week.	Discuss possible measures the parent can take to reduce pruritus (e.g., loose clothing, cool compresses) and measures to reduce pain of sore throat (e.g., analgesic).	If children scratch pruritic lesions, they can cause a secondary infection. Sore throats interfere with comfort and an ability to eat well.	Parent states she understands common measures to reduce pruritus and will begin them.

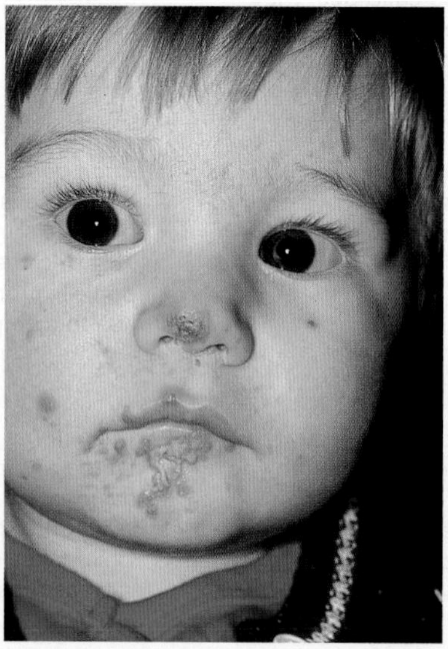

FIGURE 43.12 Impetigo in a toddler. Note the honey-colored crust appearance of some of the lesions. (© Dr. P. Marazzi/SPL/Science Source/Photo Researchers.)

20 minutes applied to the lesion can help relieve pain. Urge children not to rupture these lesions but rather to allow them to run their self-limiting course so the infection is not spread to surrounding tissue and does not become a cellulitis.

Cellulitis

Cellulitis is staphylococcal inflammation of the deeper layers of skin. It occurs generally on the extremities or face, or surrounding wounds. The skin feels warm to the touch and is edematous and reddened. Warm soaks help relieve pain and inflammation. Therapy is a systemic antibiotic.

Methicillin-Resistant *Staphylococcus aureus*

MRSA is a strain of staphylococcus that causes skin infections and has become resistant to common broad-spectrum antibiotics. When an infection occurs in a health care setting, it is referred to as health care–associated MRSA or HA-MRSA. If it occurs in a community setting, it is termed community-associated methicillin-resistant *Staphylococcus aureus* (CA-MRSA). Children with weakened immune systems are at the greatest risk for contracting the infection.

BOX 43.6 Nursing Care Planning Based on Responsibility for Pharmacology

MUPIROCIN (BACTROBAN)

Classification: Mupirocin is a topical antibiotic.
Action: Mupirocin is used to treat impetigo caused by *Staphylococcus aureus* and *Streptococcus pyogenes*.
Pregnancy Risk Category: B
Dosage: Small amount applied three times a day to the affected areas for 10 days duration
Possible Adverse Effects: Erythema, dry skin, pruritus, burning, stinging (Karch, 2013)

Nursing Implications

- Advise parents to wash the lesions with soap and water and pat dry before applying ointment to soften crusts for better absorption.
- Caution parents that causative organisms are infectious by direct contact. Instruct them to wash their own hands before and after applying the ointment.
- Although the lesions may begin to improve before 10 days have elapsed, urge parents to continue to use the ointment to ensure eradication of the causative bacteria.
- Instruct parents to use caution if applying the ointment around the eyes because the ointment is irritating to the eyes.

An infection usually begins as a boil. It can spread to become a painful abscess or invade deeper body structures such as joints and heart valves. Children who are identified as having MRSA are isolated to help prevent the spread of the bacteria to others. Vancomycin is the drug of choice for treatment of hospital-based lesions because the bacteria are still susceptible to its design. Trimethoprim-sulfamethoxazole is commonly used with community infections. Use strict standard infection precaution measures when caring for a child with an MRSA infection. Teach children the best way to prevent staphylococcal infections of the skin is good hand washing and reporting skin wounds to a health care provider before an open wound can become infected (Upshaw-Owens & Bailey, 2012).

Scalded Skin Disease

Scalded skin disease (Ritter disease) is a staphylococcal infection seen primarily in neonates. Newborns develop rough-textured skin and general erythema, especially on areas that encounter friction. Large bullae (vesicles) filled with clear fluid form. The epidermis separates in large sheets and desquamates, leaving a raw, red, glistening, and scalded-looking surface. Children need intensive intravenous antibiotic therapy to survive this extreme infection (Neylon, O'Connell, Sleven, et al., 2010).

Other Bacterial Infections

Diphtheria

- Causative agent: *Corynebacterium diphtheriae* (Klebs–Löffler bacillus)
- Incubation period: 2 to 6 days
- Period of communicability: Rarely more than 2 weeks to 4 weeks in untreated persons; 1 to 2 days in children treated with antibiotics
- Mode of transmission: Direct or indirect contact with respiratory secretions
- Immunity: Contracting the disease gives lasting natural immunity
- Active artificial immunity: Diphtheria toxin given as part of diphtheria, tetanus, and pertussis (DTaP) vaccine
- Passive artificial immunity: Diphtheria antitoxin

Assessment. Diphtheria is an illness that should be extinct because of available immunizations; however, it still occurs in isolated outbreaks. Diphtheria bacilli invade and grow in the nasopharynx of children, and produce an exotoxin (a potent protein poison) that causes massive cell necrosis and inflammation. The necrosing material lends itself well to the growth of the bacilli, so the bacilli reproduce rapidly. The inflammation and necrosing cells form a characteristic gray membrane on the nasopharynx. This may extend up into the nose and down into the major bronchi, causing a purulent nasal discharge and a brassy cough. The toxin is absorbed from the membrane surface and spreads systemically by the bloodstream to affect major organs, such as the heart and nervous system. If untreated, myocarditis with heart failure and conduction disturbances may occur. Central nervous system involvement can include severe neuritis with paralysis of the diaphragm and pharyngeal and laryngeal muscles. The diagnosis of diphtheria is made based on clinical appearance and on a throat culture, which reveals the presence of the diphtheria bacilli (Ogle & Anderson, 2012).

Therapeutic Management. Treatment involves intravenous administration of antitoxin in large doses. In addition, children are given penicillin or erythromycin intravenously. Complete bed rest is crucial during the acute stage of the illness. Droplet precautions must be followed until cultures are negative. Children need careful observation at all times to prevent airway obstruction. If obstruction occurs, endotracheal intubation may be necessary.

Because the diphtheria vaccine is included in routine immunizations for infants, diphtheria is almost extinct in the United States. However, isolated instances do occur, and when they do, prompt recognition and treatment are necessary.

Whooping Cough (Pertussis)

- Causative agent: *Bordetella pertussis*
- Incubation period: 5 to 21 days
- Mode of transmission: Direct or indirect contact
- Period of communicability: Greatest in catarrhal (respiratory illness) stage
- Immunity: Contracting the disease offers lasting natural immunity

- Active artificial immunity: Pertussis vaccine given as part of DTaP vaccine
- Passive artificial immunity: Pertussis immune serum globulin

Pertussis is a serious disease of childhood but, like diphtheria, has become quite rare in the United States because of required immunizations. It still occurs sporadically and is actually making a comeback in some locales, particularly with underimmunized adolescents (Spratling & Carmon, 2010).

Assessment. Pertussis manifests itself in three steps: the catarrhal stage, the paroxysmal stage, and the convalescent stage. The **catarrhal stage** begins with upper respiratory symptoms such as coryza, sneezing, lacrimation, cough, and a low-grade fever, symptoms subtle enough they may at first be mistaken for those of a common cold. This first period lasts 1 to 2 weeks.

The paroxysmal stage lasts 4 to 6 weeks. During this time, the cough changes from a mild one to paroxysmal, involving 5 to 10 short, rapid coughs, followed by a rapid inspiration, which causes the "whoop" or high-pitched crowing sound of whooping cough. Children are in obvious distress while coughing. They may become cyanotic or red faced, and their nose may drain thick, tenacious mucus. They often vomit after a paroxysm of coughing, and they feel exhausted afterward from the effort.

During the convalescent stage, there is a gradual cessation of the coughing and vomiting. During the next year, however, if children develop an upper respiratory infection, they may again have a return of the paroxysmal coughing with vomiting.

Pertussis is diagnosed by its striking symptoms, although in children younger than 6 months of age, the "whoop" of the cough may be absent, making it more difficult to diagnose. The *B. pertussis* bacillus may be cultured from nasopharyngeal secretions during the catarrhal and paroxysmal stages. The white blood cell count, particularly the lymphocyte count, is markedly increased to as high as 20,000 to 30,000/mm^3 (normal levels are 5,000 to 10,000/mm^3).

Therapeutic Management. Children with pertussis are maintained on bed rest until the paroxysms of coughing subside. Urge parents to keep them secluded from environmental factors, such as cigarette smoke and dust, and to avoid strenuous activities because these initiate coughing episodes. Nutrition may become a problem if the child is constantly coughing and vomiting. As a rule, frequent small meals are vomited less than larger meals and so should be encouraged.

A full 10-day course of erythromycin or azithromycin may be prescribed because these drugs have the potential to shorten the period of communicability and may shorten the duration of symptoms. Droplet precautions are used until 5 days after a child starts antibiotic therapy. Complications of pertussis include alkalosis and dehydration caused by vomiting and pneumonia, atelectasis, or emphysema from plugged bronchioles. Epistaxis, subconjunctival and subarachnoid bleeding, or seizures from asphyxia as a result of severe paroxysms of coughing may also occur. Infants with pertussis may be admitted to a health care facility for observation because they become dehydrated or may have such tenacious secretions that they need airway suction. For safety, place an intercom in the infant's room so you can identify severe coughing even when not in the room.

Prevention. Little passive immunity is transferred across the placenta, so children in their early months are particularly susceptible to the disease. It is the reason that, at 2 months, the pertussis vaccine (in the form of the DTaP vaccine) is one of the first immunizations scheduled (Atkinson, Wolfe, & Hamborsky, 2011).

What if... 43.2 An adolescent who has pertussis vomits after an episode of coughing. Should you urge him to try to eat again immediately, or do you think he would be too nauseated to do so?

Anthrax

- Causative agent: *Bacillus anthracis*, a bacteria
- Incubation period: 1 to 7 days (inhalational), 1 to 12 days (cutaneous), 1 to 7 days (gastrointestinal)
- Mode of transmission: Originally contracted from contact with the feces of infected cows or sheep; not transmissible from person to person
- Immunity: Unstudied
- Active artificial immunity: A vaccine is available for people in high-risk occupations, such as veterinarians, but it is not recommended for children
- Passive artificial immunity: Not available

Anthrax is an acute infectious disease that is contracted from exposure to the anthrax bacteria or its spores. As the organism grows inside the human body, a toxin is produced that causes the bulk of the symptoms. Children, like adults, may be affected by all three clinical forms: cutaneous, inhalational, or gastrointestinal.

Inhalational anthrax has a mortality rate of over 90%. It begins with a brief prodromal period of flulike symptoms, followed shortly by dyspnea, severe systemic shock, and marked evidence of mediastinal widening and pleural effusion on X-ray. Because it can be fatal and spreads through coughing, anthrax has been proposed as bacteria that could be used in bioterrorism (Woodward, 2012).

Cutaneous anthrax is characterized by a skin lesion that begins as a papule, then passes through a vesicle stage, to a painless depressed black eschar. Fever, malaise, headache, and regional swollen lymph nodes may accompany the skin lesion. The mortality of cutaneous anthrax is as low as 1% with antibiotic therapy.

Gastrointestinal anthrax is contracted by eating undercooked meat infected with the organism. The child develops severe abdominal pain, fever, bloody diarrhea, and septicemia. The mortality rate for this form is about 25%.

If exposed to anthrax, prophylaxis with ciprofloxacin (Cipro) for those older than 18 years of age and doxycycline for younger patients are the drugs of choice. Drug therapy is continued for 60 days because of the potential persistence of and difficulty in killing spores.

Tetanus (Lockjaw)

- Causative agent: *Clostridium tetani*
- Incubation period: 3 days to 3 weeks
- Period of communicability: None
- Mode of transmission: Direct or indirect contamination of a closed wound

- Immunity: Development of the disease gives lasting natural immunity
- Active artificial immunity: Tetanus toxoid contained in DTaP vaccine
- Passive artificial immunity: Tetanus immune globulin

Tetanus, a highly fatal disease if untreated, is caused by an anaerobic, spore-forming bacillus found in soil and the excretions of animals. It enters the body through an open wound. If the wound is deep, such as a stab wound, where the distal end of the wound is shut off from an oxygen source, tetanus bacilli begin to reproduce. The organism may also enter through a burn site, which crusts, thus creating an anaerobic environment. As the bacilli grow, they produce exotoxins that cause the disease symptoms by affecting the motor nuclei of the central nervous system (Afshar, Raju, Ansell, et al., 2011).

The entrance site of the bacillus does not appear infected (no pus or reddened area is present unless a secondary infection also exists). After the incubation period, the exotoxins have developed to such an extent, however, that they are capable of disrupting the nervous system. In the United States, most children are vaccinated against tetanus. In developing countries, it continues to have a high incidence, caused by infection of an entry point such as the umbilical cord at birth (Bairwa, Rajput, Khanna, et al., 2012).

Assessment. The first symptoms that are noticeable are stiffness of the neck and jaw (lockjaw). Within 24 to 48 hours, muscular rigidity of the trunk and extremities develops. The back becomes arched (opisthotonos), the abdominal muscles are stiff and boardlike, and the face assumes an unusual appearance, with wrinkling of the forehead and distortion of the corners of the mouth (a "sardonic grin" sign). Any stimulation, such as a sudden noise, a bright light, or a touch, causes painful, paroxysmal spasms. The sensorium is clear throughout the course of the disease, so the child is aware of the pain associated with the muscle spasms. As these spasms begin to include the larynx, respiratory obstruction and death by asphyxiation can occur.

Therapeutic Management. A child needs to be cared for in a quiet, stimulation-free room with total parenteral nutrition, sedation, and a muscle relaxant to prevent aspiration from muscle spasms. If the wound is filled with necrotic tissue, it may be debrided to ensure no secondary infections arise. Tetanus immune globulin (human) is administered to supply passive antitoxins; parenteral penicillin G or erythromycin will be administered to reduce the number of growing forms of the bacillus. A child may need to be intubated and mechanical ventilation begun to maintain respiratory function.

Prevention. Tetanus is a serious disease, but it can be prevented through active immunization and suitable booster immunizations. Children routinely receive tetanus immunization as part of routine DTaP immunization with a booster dose at school age; thereafter, they should receive a booster dose every 10 years. At the time of a wound, the wound site should be cleaned well with soap and water and a suitable antiseptic. It should not be sutured but should be left open to heal by secondary intention to reduce the possibility of an anaerobic pocket forming in the wound. If the child received basic immunization against tetanus and it has been fewer than 10 years since the last injection, no booster or antitoxin management is needed at the time of the wound.

If a child's immunization record cannot be obtained, or if it has been more than 10 years since the child received a booster injection or an initial injection for tetanus, a child will be treated with a booster injection and tetanus immune globulin. The booster injection provides tetanus antigen to the child. The booster injection will cause the body to "remember" how to make tetanus antibodies so, by the time the invading tetanus organisms from the wound have passed their long incubation period (3 days to 3 weeks), the child will have antibodies in the system prepared to eradicate the organisms. If the initial immunizations were incomplete or are unknown, in addition to tetanus antigen, the child will also receive the passive antibodies included in tetanus immune globulin (Lee & McCallin, 2011).

Lyme Disease

- Causative agent: *Borrelia burgdorferi*, a spirochete
- Incubation period: 3 to 30 days
- Period of communicability: Not communicable from one person to another
- Mode of transmission: Deer tick
- Active artificial immunity: Lyme disease vaccine
- Passive artificial immunity: Immune globulin

Lyme disease is caused by a spirochete, *B. burgdorferi*, which is transmitted by a tick frequently carried on deer (Esposito, Bosis, Sabatini, et al., 2013). The disease is the most frequently reported vector-borne infection in the United States, occurring most often in the summer and early fall and on the east coast (it is named after the city in Connecticut where it was first identified). A vaccine for the disease is not currently available, because the manufacturer ceased production in 2002, due to low demand (CDC, 2011b).

Almost immediately after a tick bite, an erythematous papule is noticeable at the site, which spreads over the next 3 to 30 days (the incubation period) to become a large, round ring with a raised swollen border (erythema chronicum migrans) (Fig. 43.13). This is followed by systemic involvement that can lead to cardiac, musculoskeletal, and neurologic symptoms. Cardiac involvement may be so severe that it includes heart block from atrioventricular conduction abnormalities. Neurologic symptoms commonly include stiff neck, headache,

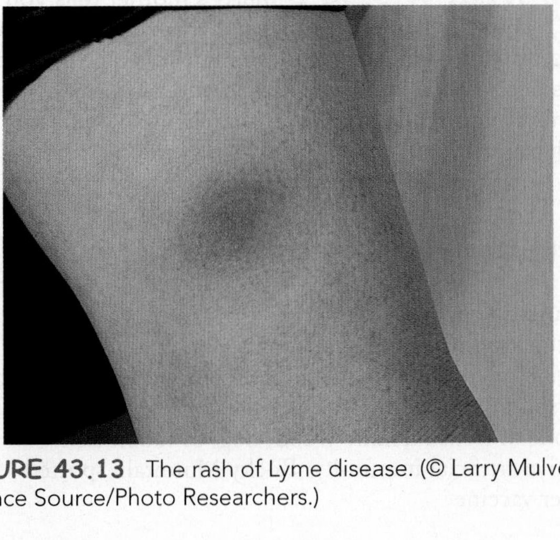

FIGURE 43.13 The rash of Lyme disease. (© Larry Mulvehill/ Science Source/Photo Researchers.)

BOX 43.7 Nursing Care Planning to Empower a Family

TIPS FOR AVOIDING EXPOSURE TO LYME DISEASE

Q. Marty's father tells you, "My children love to play in the woods, but I'm so afraid they'll get Lyme disease. What can I do to protect them?"

A. Here are some suggestions to help reduce the risk of exposure:

- Wear protective clothing when hiking or playing in wooded areas, such as long sleeves, high necklines, and long slacks. Tuck bottom of slacks into socks or boots.
- Wear light-colored clothing so any tick present on clothing can be readily observed.
- Inspect skin for ticks thoroughly after hiking or playing in wooded areas. Remove any ticks found with tweezers.
- Report any area of inflammation that might be a tick bite to a health care provider for early diagnosis.

and cranial nerve palsy. Musculoskeletal symptoms include painful swollen arthritic joints, particularly in the knee.

Amoxicillin is administered at the time of the bite to young children, whereas doxycycline is given to those older than 8 years of age. Encourage parents to inspect the skin of children who have been playing in wooded areas for tick bites to help identify the disorder before debilitating symptoms occur (CDC, 2011b). Other suggestions for avoiding Lyme disease are shown in Box 43.7.

OTHER INFECTIOUS PATHOGENS

Rickettsial Diseases

Rickettsiae are organisms that resemble viruses both in size and in their inability to reproduce except inside the cells of a host organism. They reproduce by fission, however, as bacteria do; like bacteria, they are complete organisms containing both RNA and DNA. They multiply inside ticks, lice, mites, or fleas (arthropods) without causing disease. They are transmitted to humans through the bite or feces of the infected arthropod. An exception is Q fever, which is spread by droplet infection. All rickettsial diseases include fever, trigger an immune response, and almost all include a rash caused by rickettsial multiplication in the endothelial cells of small blood vessels.

What if...43.3 Marty's mother tells you she's always been afraid her children would contact Lyme disease because, in the winter, the family picks both limes and lemons in Florida. Could you assure her Marty will never contract Lyme disease while in an orchard picking fruit?

Rocky Mountain Spotted Fever

- Causative agent: *Rickettsia rickettsii*
- Incubation period: 3 to 12 days
- Period of communicability: Not communicable from one person to another
- Mode of transmission: Wood, dog, or rabbit tick
- Active artificial immunity: Rocky Mountain spotted fever vaccine

Rocky Mountain spotted fever is the second most common rickettsial disease seen in the United States. It is most prevalent in the western United States and is transmitted by tick bites (Graham, Stockley, & Goldman, 2011).

It occurs most often during the spring and early summer, when ticks are most plentiful. A reddened area develops at the site of the tick bite. In 2 to 8 days, a typical rash, persistent headache, fever (as high as 104°F [40°C]), and mental confusion begin. The rash is distinctive, beginning with reddened macules, which then changes to petechiae. It begins on the wrists and ankles, then spreads up the arms and legs onto the trunk. Unlike most rashes, it can cover the palms and soles (Fig. 43.14).

In untreated children, symptoms worsen to include central nervous system involvement (stiff neck and seizures) and cardiac and pulmonary symptoms such as heart failure and pneumonia.

Rocky Mountain spotted fever was a serious childhood illness before antibiotic therapy was available, and it still has the potential to be serious if the symptoms are not reported when they first occur. First-line therapy is with doxycycline for 7 to 10 days, and should be initiated within the first 5 days of the appearance of symptoms. Caution parents to administer the drug for the full course of therapy to ensure disease eradication and to prevent the risk of complications.

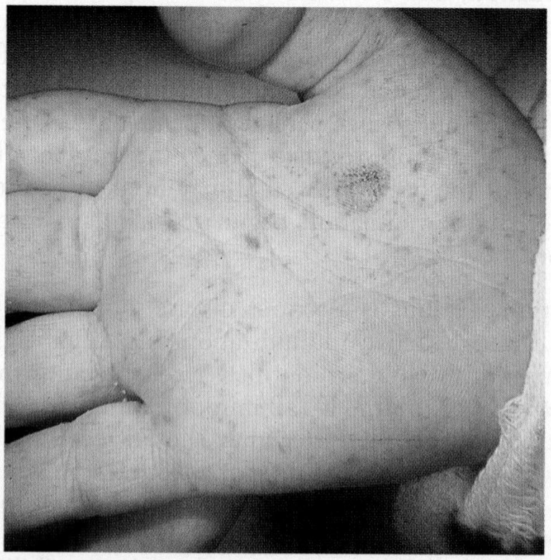

FIGURE 43.14 The typical rash of Rocky Mountain spotted fever. (Courtesy of Stuart Starr, MD, The Children's Hospital of Philadelphia.)

TABLE 43.3 Common Parasitic Infections

Infection	Organism	Symptoms	Treatment
Pediculosis capitis	Head lice	Small, white flecks on hair shaft (nits or eggs of lice); extreme pruritus	Wash hair with shampoo such as lindane (Kwell) and comb nits from hair with fine-toothed comb. Wash bed sheets and recently worn clothes; vacuum pillows, mattresses, or other items unable to be washed. Teach children not to exchange combs, hair barrettes, or other personal items.
Pediculosis	Pubic lice	Same as for head lice except on pubic hair	Same as head lice.
Scabies	Female mite (*Acarus scabiei*)	Black burrow filled with mite feces 1–2 in. long, usually between fingers and toes, on palms, or in axilla or groin	Caution that adolescent groin infestations might be spread by physical intimacy. Wash area with lindane (Kwell) lotion or permethrin (Elimite).

Psittacosis

Psittacosis, caused by *Chlamydia psittaci*, is a disease transmitted to children through the inhalation of dried secretions of birds, such as parakeets, macaws, parrots, cockatiels, turkeys, and ducks. Although the bird does not appear ill, children develop symptoms of an upper respiratory infection, such as pneumonia, possibly a low-grade fever, a dry cough, weakness, an enlarged spleen, and anorexia out of proportion to the fever. The course of the disease is as long as 3 to 4 weeks. Treatment is with an antibiotic such as doxycycline (Stewardson & Grayson, 2010).

Parasitic Infections

Parasites are organisms that live on and obtain their food supply from other organisms. Although many of these can cause illness, ones frequently associated with children include head lice and scabies (Table 43.3). Parents are often embarrassed when they learn their child has one of these illnesses. You can reassure them that these infestations could happen to any child (Box 43.8).

Helminthic Infections

Helminths are pathogenic or parasitic worms. They include roundworms (nematodes), flukes (trematodes), or tapeworms (cestodes). Most helminths begin life when the eggs or larvae are eliminated in the feces or urine of humans. They are then transmitted to the oral cavity by contaminated foods or hands. Because children tend to be careless about washing their hands before eating or tend to suck their thumbs, it makes them prone to these infections (Rote, 2012).

Roundworms (Ascariasis)

The roundworm parasite lives in the intestinal tract. Larvae, which hatch from the ingested eggs, penetrate the intestinal

BOX 43.8 Nursing Care Planning Based on Effective Communication

When Marty's 6-year-old brother Joshua visits him, you notice Joshua has scratch marks on his neck and forehead. His hair shafts are covered by sandlike particles. You suspect he has pediculosis capitis or head lice.

Less Effective Communication

Nurse: Mrs. Ireland, I'm wondering if you've noticed these sandlike particles in your son's hair.
Mrs. Ireland: Well, you know boys. They don't always wash well.
Nurse: I'm concerned they may be the eggs of head lice.
Mrs. Ireland: We're not that poor. Don't insult us.
Nurse: Like you said, it's probably something else.

More Effective Communication

Nurse: Mrs. Ireland, I'm wondering if you've noticed these sandlike particles in your son's hair.
Mrs. Ireland: Well, you know boys. They don't always wash well.
Nurse: I'm concerned they may be the eggs of head lice.
Mrs. Ireland: We're not that poor. Don't insult us.
Nurse: Let's talk about head lice, and how easy it is for anyone to get them.

The previous scenario is an example of what can happen if people believe the myth that communicable diseases are always associated with poor hygiene or poverty. Head lice can be spread easily in locker rooms or classrooms, so any child can contract them.

wall and enter the circulation. From there, they may migrate to any body tissue. Children develop a loss of appetite and perhaps nausea and vomiting. Intestinal obstruction may occur from a mass of roundworms in the intestine. Ascariasis can be prevented by the sanitary disposal of feces to prevent contamination of the soil. A single dose of an anthelmintic such as pyrantel pamoate (Antiminth) controls the infection.

Hookworms

Hookworm eggs, like roundworm eggs, are found in human feces. They enter children's bodies through the skin and then migrate to the intestinal tract, where they attach themselves onto the intestinal villi and suck blood from the intestinal wall to sustain themselves. If a great number of hookworms are present, severe anemia may result. Treatment is with anthelmintics. Children may also need therapy for the anemia.

Pinworms

Pinworms are small, white, threadlike worms that live in the cecum. At night, the female pinworm migrates down the intestinal tract and out of the anus to deposit eggs on the skin in the anal and perianal region. The movement of the worms causes the anal area to itch, and the child will awaken at night crying and scratching. Some of the eggs are then carried from the child's fingernails to the mouth. After being ingested, they hatch in the child's intestinal tract, and the cycle is repeated (Wang, Hwang, & Chen, 2010).

The worms are large enough that they can be seen if the child's buttocks are separated. Pressing a piece of cellophane tape against the anus, then inspecting it under a microscope will generally reveal pinworm eggs.

Treatment is with a single dose of mebendazole (Vermox) or pyrantel pamoate (Antiminth) (Lee & McCallin, 2011). Underclothing, bedding, towels, and nightclothes should be washed before reuse. In addition, all family members need to be treated for pinworm infestation because the worms are easily transmitted from person to person. Teach children to avoid nail biting and to wash their hands before food preparation or eating to avoid transfer of pinworm eggs and to prevent this type of infection.

Protozoan Infections

Protozoa are unicellular organisms. They absorb fluid through their cell membrane and can move from place to place by pseudopod, flagella, or cilia action. They are most pathogenic in the gastrointestinal, genitourinary, and circulatory systems. Some protozoa reproduce by simple binary fission, whereas other forms have complex life cycles. They have the ability to form cysts or surround themselves with a membrane, which makes them resistant to destruction.

Giardiasis

Giardia lamblia is a protozoan infection responsible for epidemic outbreaks of diarrhea, particularly in travelers to Europe and in day care centers in the United States (Karon, Hanni, Mohle-Boetani, et al., 2010).

Transmission occurs when the child ingests the cysts of the organism from unclean hands. The cysts then develop in the intestine into the mature form of the organism, causing symptoms such as diarrhea, weight loss, abdominal cramps, and nausea after an incubation time of 3 to 25 days. Diagnosis is made by history and recognition of the mature form of the organism in the stool or on duodenal aspiration. Therapy is with metronidazole (Flagyl) for 7 days (Wright, 2012).

Fungal Infections

Fungi are larger than bacteria; some are unicellular (yeasts), but generally they are multicellular (molds). Deep mycoses invade internal organs. Transmission is by the inhalation of spores. Subcutaneous mycoses invade the skin, subcutaneous tissue, and bone. Infections usually occur from introduction of the fungi into a wound. Superficial mycoses invade only the hair, skin, or nails.

Superficial Fungal Infections

Four superficial fungal infections seen frequently in children are tinea cruris, pedis, capitis, and corporis.

Tinea Cruris. Tinea cruris (jock itch) occurs on the inner thighs and scrotum. The area appears reddened and is very pruritic. Local application of clotrimazole (Lotrimin) or econazole (Spectazole) liquid or powder destroys the infection (Karch, 2013).

Tinea Pedis. Tinea pedis (athlete's foot) produces pruritic, pinpoint vesicles with fissuring between the toes and on the plantar surface of the foot. It is treated with liquid preparations of an antifungal agent such as clotrimazole (Lotrimin).

Tinea Capitis. Tinea capitis (ringworm of the scalp) begins as the infection of a single hair follicle but then spreads rapidly in a circular pattern to produce a lesion approximately 1 in. in diameter. The hairs involved in the lesion generally break off and the circle becomes filled with dirty-appearing scales.

Treatment is with an antifungal such as griseofulvin, which is given orally. Adolescents should be cautioned not to consume alcohol while taking this drug because this may cause tachycardia. Safety of the drug during pregnancy is not established. Caution children to avoid strong sunlight during therapy because photosensitivity may occur (Gupta & Drummond-Main, 2013).

Tinea capitis is not as contagious as was once assumed. Children do not need to have their head shaved or be kept home from school, although they should be cautioned not to exchange towels, combs, or other potential fomites. The course of the disease can be lengthy, perhaps as long as 3 months, before all lesions have faded (Petros, 2010).

Tinea Corporis. Tinea corporis (ringworm of the body) is an infection of the epidermal layer of the skin. It presents as a scaly ring of inflammation with a clear area in the center, which can occur anywhere on the body (Fig. 43.15). Treatment is with a topical antifungal agent such as clotrimazole (Lotrimin).

Candidiasis

Candida albicans is the fungus responsible for candidal (monilial) infections. Candidal organisms grow in the vagina of many adult women and adolescents (candidal vaginitis) (see Chapter 47). Newborns born vaginally may develop an infection of the mucous membrane of the mouth (thrush

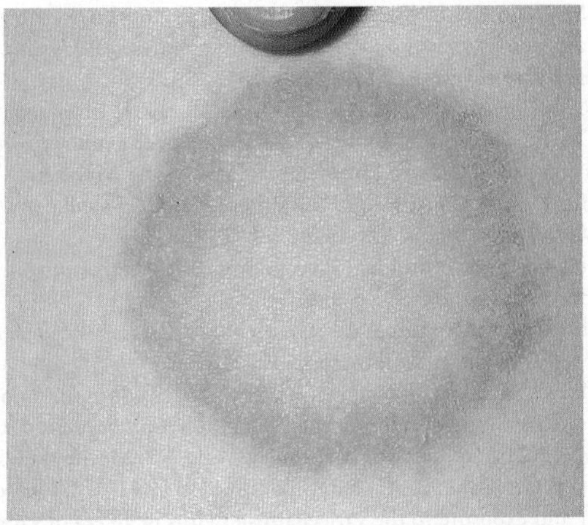

FIGURE 43.15 Ringworm (tinea corporis). The fungus spreads rapidly, producing a circular, ringlike lesion. (© SPL/ Science Source/Photo Researchers.)

or oral candidal infection) from exposure at birth. Thrush is characterized by white plaques on an erythematous base on the buccal membrane and the surface of the tongue. It resembles a milk curd left from a recent milk feeding. Thrush plaques do not scrape away, however, whereas milk curds do. The infant's mouth is painful and he or she may not suck well due to the inflammation and local pain.

C. albicans can also cause a severe, bright red, sharply circumscribed diaper-area rash (Fig. 43.16). The rash is marked by its intense color, satellite lesions are usually present, and it does not improve with usual diaper rash measures, such as application of a protective ointment, frequent changing of diapers, or exposure to air.

Nystatin is an example of an effective antifungal drug (Karch, 2013). For oral candidiasis, it is generally administered by mouth approximately four times a day. Teach parents to drop the liquid into the mouth after feedings so it will remain in contact with the lesions rather than being washed away immediately by a feeding. For diaper rash, a nystatin ointment is prescribed.

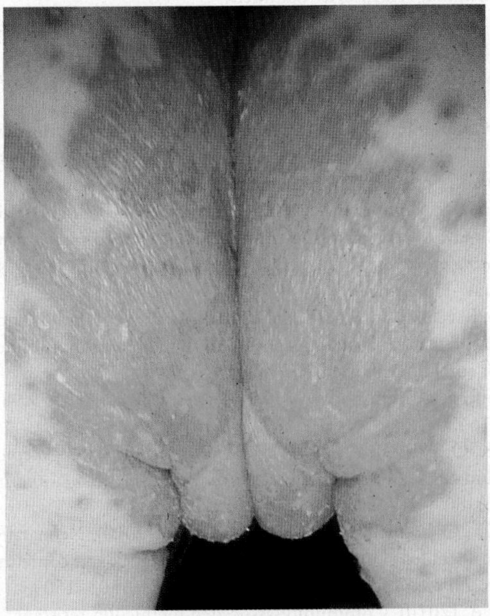

FIGURE 43.16 Monilial (candidiasis) diaper rash. Note the intense red color of the rash and the satellite lesions. (© Custom Medical Stock Photograph.)

There is a tendency to think of thrush as a common, almost expected disease of infants. Candidiasis can become a systemic infection, however, and it can spread easily through a newborn population such as a nursery or child care facility (Antaya, 2010).

What if... 43.4 You are particularly interested in exploring one of the 2020 National Health Goals related to infectious diseases in children (see Box 43.1). What would be a possible research topic to explore pertinent to this goal that would be applicable to Marty and his family and that would also advance evidence-based practice?

KEY POINTS FOR REVIEW

- The incubation period of an infectious disease is the time between the invasion of an organism and the onset of symptoms. The prodromal period is the time between the beginning of nonspecific symptoms and specific ones and the time when children are most infectious. Illness is the stage during which specific symptoms are evident. The convalescent period is the interval between the time symptoms begin to fade and the time the child returns to baseline health.
- The chain of infection depends on the presence of a reservoir, a portal of exit, a mode of transmission, a portal of entry, and a susceptible host. To reduce the spread of infection, use standard infection precautions to break the chain of infection. Transmission-based precautions—airborne, droplet, and contact—also may be necessary.
- Common viral infections of childhood include exanthem subitum (roseola), rubella (German measles), measles (rubeola), chickenpox (varicella), herpes zoster, erythema infectiosum (fifth disease), pityriasis rosea, mumps (epidemic parotitis), infectious mononucleosis, and cat-scratch disease. Other important viral infections include poliomyelitis (now almost extinct), herpesvirus infections, verrucae (warts), rabies, and West Nile virus disease.
- Common streptococcal diseases include scarlet fever and impetigo. Staphylococcal infections include furunculosis (boils), cellulitis, and scalded skin disease. Outbreaks of diphtheria, whooping cough (pertussis), and tetanus (lockjaw) still occur.
- Common tick-borne diseases are Rocky Mountain spotted fever and Lyme disease. Parasitic infections are pediculosis capitis (head lice), pediculosis pubis, and scabies. Helminthic infections include roundworms, hookworms, and pinworms. Fungal infections are tinea capitis and tinea corporis, both of which are forms of ringworm.
- Teaching parents and children about infection control measures and the need for keeping immunizations up to date is essential not only for reducing the risk of infectious disorders in children but also for meeting QSEN competencies and best meeting the family's total needs.

Critical Thinking Care Study

Barbie is a 10-year-old you meet while working as a nurse at a resident summer camp. Both her forearms and lower legs have several papular lesions that feel very itchy and are surrounded by erythema; a number have honey-colored drainage and some crusting. Four days ago was "sleep out," day so she spent the night in a tent with three friends but didn't sleep well because "mosquitoes bit me all night." Barbie's parents return from their vacation to be certain their daughter is all right, but they seem angry and frustrated. The mother tells you, "We thought camp would be a good experience for Barbie to separate her from a boyfriend she likes a lot but we have qualms about that now. Look at her; she'll probably end up with scars from this."

1. What do you suspect is the cause of the scattered lesions?
2. Given how impetigo is transmitted to others, what implications does its presence have for infection control practices in the camp setting?
3. What if you learn Barbie has never had more immunizations than those she received as an infant because her mother believes the danger of vaccines is higher than contracting "simple childhood infections"? Would immunization have prevented Barbie from contracting impetigo? Would you recommend she receive routine immunizations now or, at 10 years of age, is she no longer in much danger from common contagious illnesses?

Patient Scenario

The Sukioto Family

Read about the Sukioto family, a family whose adolescent has an infectious disease, then answer the questions to further sharpen your skills and grow more familiar with NCLEX-type questions related to infectious disorders. Confirm your answers are correct by reading the rationales.

Visit http://thePoint.lww.com

Answers and Rationales

Looking for answers to the What If. . . and Critical Thinking Care Study questions?

Visit http://thePoint.lww.com

References

Afshar, M., Raju, M., Ansell, D., et al. (2011). Narrative review: Tetanus—A health threat after natural disasters in developing countries. *Annals of Internal Medicine, 154*(5), 329–335.

Anderson, P. D., & Bokor, G. (2012). Bioterrorism: Pathogens as weapons. *Journal of Pharmacy Practice, 25*(5), 521–529.

Antaya, R. J. (2010). Blisters and pustules in the newborn. *Pediatric Annals, 39*(10), 635–645.

Askarian, M., Yadollahi, M., Kuochak, F., et al. (2011). Precautions for health care workers to avoid hepatitis B and C virus infection. *International Journal of Occupational & Environmental Medicine, 2*(4), 191–198.

Atkinson, W., Wolfe, C., & Hamborsky, J. (Eds.). (2011). *The pink book: Epidemiology & prevention of vaccine-preventable diseases* (12th ed.). Waldorf, MD: Public Health Foundation.

Bairwa, M., Rajput, M., Khanna, P., et al. (2012). India is on the way forward to maternal and neonatal tetanus elimination! *Human Vaccines & Immunotherapeutics, 8*(8), 1129–1131.

Beach, R., & Thalange, N. (2013). Infectious disease & immunity. In N. Thalange, R. Beach, D. Booth, et al. (Eds.), *Essentials of paediatrics* (2nd ed., pp. 231–246). Philadelphia, PA: Elsevier/Saunders.

Centers for Disease Control and Prevention (2011a). *A polio-free U.S. thanks to vaccine efforts*. Washington, DC: Author.

Centers for Disease Control and Prevention (2011b). *Preventing tick bites*. Atlanta, GA: Author.

Centers for Disease Control and Prevention. (2012). *Rubella: Be sure your child gets vaccinated*. Washington, DC: Author.

Daley, M. F., O'Leary, S. T., & Nyquist, A. C. (2012). Immunization. In W. Hay, M. Levin, R. Deterding, et al. (Eds.), *Current diagnosis & treatment pediatrics* (21st ed., pp. 254–288). New York, NY: McGraw-Hill/Lange.

Donohue, J. G., Kieke, B. A., Gargiullo, P. M., et al. (2010). Herpes zoster and exposure to the varicella zoster virus in an era of varicella vaccination. *American Journal of Public Health, 100*(6), 1116–1122.

Duval, L. (2010). Infection control 101. *Nephrology Nursing Journal, 37*(5), 485–489.

Esposito, S., Bosis, S., Sabatini, C., et al. (2013). *Borrelia burgdorferi* infection and Lyme disease in children. *International Journal of Infectious Disease, 17*(3), e153–e158.

Gonzalez, H., Olsson, T., & Borg, K. (2010). Management of post-polio syndrome. *Lancet Neurology, 9*(6): 634–642.

Graham, J., Stockley, K., & Goldman, R. D. (2011). Tick-borne illnesses: A CME update. *Pediatric Emergency Care, 27*(2), 141–117.

Gupta, A. K., & Drummond-Main, C. (2013). Meta-analysis of randomized, controlled trials comparing particular doses of griseofulvin and terbinafine for the treatment of tinea capitis. *Pediatric Dermatology, 30*(1), 1–6.

Heyman, P., Thoma, B. R., Marié, J. L., et al. (2012). In search for factors that drive hantavirus epidemics. *Frontiers in Physiology, 2*(3), 237.

Jackson, A. (2011). Rabies in the critical care unit: Diagnostic and therapeutic approaches. *The Canadian Journal of Neurological Sciences, 38*(5), 689–695.

Karch, A. M. (2013). *2013 Lippincott's nursing drug guide*. Philadelphia, PA: Lippincott Williams & Wilkins.

Karon, A. E., Hanni, K. D., Mohle-Boetani, J. C., et al. (2010). Giardiasis outbreak at a camp after installation of a slow-sand filtration water-treatment system. *Epidemiology and Infections, 139*(5), 713–717.

Katz, B. Z. (2013). Infectious mononucleosis & other Epstein-Barr Virus associated lymphoproliferative disorders. In E. T. Bope & R. D. Kellerman (Eds.), *Conn's current therapy 2013* (pp. 104–105). Philadelphia, PA: Elsevier/Saunders.

Klotz, S. A., Ianas, V., & Elliott, S. P. (2011). Cat-scratch disease. *American Family Physician, 83*(2), 152–155.

Lam, J. M. (2010). Characterizing viral exanthems. *Pediatric Health, 4*(6), 623–635.

Lee, B., & McCallin, T. (2011). Microbiology & infectious disease. In M. M. Tschudy & K. M. Arcara (Eds.), *The Harriet Lane handbook* (19th ed., pp. 405–455). Philadelphia, PA: Elsevier Mosby.

Levin, M. J., & Weinberg, A. (2012). Infections, viral & rickettsial. In W. Hay, M. Levin, R. Deterding, et al. (Eds.), *Current diagnosis & treatment pediatrics* (21st ed., pp. 1177–1219). New York, NY: McGraw-Hill/Lange.

Lewis, E., Bernal, P., Shay, D., et al. (2010). Immunoglobulins and risk of autism prenatal and infant exposure to thimerosal from vaccines and risk of autism. *Pediatrics, 126*(4), 656–664.

Moss, W. J., & Griffin, D. E. (2012). Measles. *The Lancet, 379*(9811), 153–164.

Murray, K. O., Walker, C., & Gould, E. (2011). The virology, epidemiology, and clinical impact of West Nile virus. *Epidemiology and Infection, 139*(6), 807–817.

Neylon, O., O'Connell, N. H., Slevin, B., et al. (2010). Neonatal staphylococcal scalded skin syndrome: Clinical outbreak and containment review. *European Journal of Pediatrics, 169*(12), 1503–1509.

Odell, C. A. (2010). Community-associated methicillin-resistant *Staphylococcus aureus* (CA-MRSA) skin infections. *Current Opinion in Pediatrics, 22*(3), 273–277.

Ogle, J. W., & Anderson, M. S. (2012). Bacterial infections. In W. Hay, M. Levin, R. Deterding, et al. (Eds.), *Current diagnosis & treatment pediatrics* (21st ed., pp. 1230–1293). New York, NY: McGraw-Hill/Lange.

Patel, L. M., Lambert, P. J., Gagna, C. E., et al. (2011). Cutaneous signs of systemic disease. *Clinics in Dermatology, 29*(5), 511–522.

Petros, H. M. (2010). What's your assessment? *Dermatology Nursing, 22*(1), 1–4.

Porth, C. M. (2011). *Essentials of pathophysiology* (3rd ed.). Philadelphia, PA: Lippincott Williams & Wilkins.

Reading, R., Hughes, G., Hill, J., et al. (2011). Genital herpes in children under 11 years and investigations for sexual abuse. *Archives of Disease in Childhood, 96*(8), 752–757.

Rote, N. S. (2012). Infections & defects in mechanisms of defense. In S. E. Huether & K. L. McCance (Eds.), *Understanding pathophysiology* (5th ed., pp. 165–203). St. Louis, MO: Elsevier Mosby.

Rundell, K. (2013). Mumps. In E. T. Bope & R. D. Kellerman (Eds.), *Conn's current therapy 2013.* Philadelphia, PA: Elsevier/Saunders.

Siegel, J. D., Rhinehart, E., Jackson, M., et al. (2007). *Guidelines for isolation precautions: Preventing transmission of infectious agents in healthcare settings.* Atlanta, GA: Centers for Disease Control and Prevention.

Smith, S. (2011). Infectious diseases. In K. J. Marcdante, R. M. Kliegman, H. B. Jenson, et al. (Eds.), *Nelson essentials of pediatrics* (6th ed., pp. 355–462). Philadelphia, PA: Saunders/Elsevier.

Song, I. H., Kim, S. A., & Park, W. S. (2012). Family factors associated with children's handwashing hygiene behavior. *Journal of Child Health Care.* Advance online publication.

Spratling, R., & Carmon, M. (2010). Pertussis: An overview of the disease, immunization, and trends for nurses. *Pediatric Nursing, 36*(5), 239–244.

Stewardson, A. J., & Grayson, M. L. (2010). Psittacosis. *Infectious Disease Clinics of North America, 24*(1), 7–25.

Swanson, A., & Canty, K. (2013). Common pediatric skin conditions with protracted courses: A therapeutic update. *Dermatology Clinics, 31*(2), 239–249.

Thornsberry, L., & English, J. C. III. (2012). Evidence-based treatment and prevention of external genital warts in female pediatric and adolescent patients. *Journal of Pediatric & Adolescent Gynecology, 25*(2), 150–154.

Upshaw-Owens, M., & Bailey, C. A. (2012). Preventing hospital-associated infection: MRSA. *Medsurg Nursing, 21*(2), 77–81.

Usatine, R. P., & Tinitigan, R. (2010). Nongenital herpes simplex virus. *American Family Physician, 82*(9), 1075–1082.

U.S. Department of Health and Human Services. (2010). *Healthy people 2020.* Washington, DC: Author.

Wang, L. C., Hwang, K. P., & Chen, E. R. (2010). *Enteriobius vermicularis* infection in schoolchildren. *Epidemiology and Infections, 138*(1), 28–36.

Woodward, C. (2012). Vaccinating children against anthrax. *CMAJ: Canadian Medical Association Journal, 184*(11), E577–E578.

Wright, S. G. (2012). Protozoan infections of the gastrointestinal tract. *Infectious Disease Clinics of North America, 26*(2), 323–339.

Zawar, V., & Chuh, A. (2012). Follicular pityriasis rosea. A case report and a new classification of clinical variants of the disease. *Journal of Dermatology Case Reports, 6*(2), 36–39.

Chapter 44

Nursing Care of a Family When a Child Has a Hematologic Disorder

KEY TERMS

- allogeneic transplantation
- autologous transplantation
- blood dyscrasias
- erythroblasts
- erythrocytes
- erythropoietin
- granulocytes
- hemochromatosis
- hemolysis
- hemosiderosis
- leukocytes
- megakaryocytes
- pancytopenia
- petechiae
- plethora
- poikilocytic
- priapism
- purpura
- reticulocyte
- syngeneic transplantation
- thrombocytes
- thrombocytopenia

OBJECTIVES

After mastering the contents of this chapter, you should be able to:

1. Describe the major hematologic disorders of childhood.
2. Identify 2020 National Health Goals related to children with hematologic disorders that nurses could help the nation achieve.
3. Assess a child with a hematologic disorder such as sickle-cell anemia.
4. Formulate nursing diagnoses related to a child with a hematologic disorder.
5. Identify expected outcomes for a child with a hematologic disorder to help parents manage seamless transitions across differing health care settings.
6. Using the nursing process, plan nursing care that includes the six competencies of Quality & Safety Education for Nurses (QSEN): Patient-Centered Care, Teamwork & Collaboration, Evidence-Based Practice (EBP), Quality Improvement (QI), Safety, and Informatics.
7. Implement nursing care related to a child with a hematologic disorder, such as reducing the possibility of infection.
8. Evaluate expected outcomes for achievement and effectiveness of care.
9. Integrate knowledge of childhood disorders of the blood with the interplay of nursing process, the six competencies of QSEN, and Family Nursing to promote quality maternal and child health nursing care.

Lana is a 4-year-old girl diagnosed with thalassemia major whom you meet at a pediatric clinic. She has a prominent mandible and wide-spaced upper front teeth from overgrowth of bone marrow centers. Joey is a 7-year-old with sickle-cell anemia who attends the same clinic. His growth is only in the fifth percentile, and he's had two vaso-occlusive crises in the past year. "Why did this happen to our families?" Lana's mother asks you. "What can we do to help our children have better lives?"

Previous chapters described the growth and development of well children. This chapter adds information about the dramatic changes, both physical and psychosocial, that occur when children have a hematologic disorder.

What additional health teaching does Lana's mother need so she can better understand hematologic diseases?

The blood and blood-forming tissues that make up the hematologic system play a vital role in body metabolism because they transport oxygen and nutrients to body cells, remove carbon dioxide from cells, and initiate blood coagulation when vessels are injured. As a result of all of these functions, any alteration in the substance or function of blood can have immediate and life-threatening effects on the functioning of all body systems (Zempsky, Palermo, Corsi, et al., 2013).

Hematologic disorders, often called **blood dyscrasias**, occur when components of the blood are formed incorrectly or either increase or decrease in amount beyond normal ranges. Most blood dyscrasias in children originate in the bone marrow, where blood cells are formed. They do not occur at equal rates in all countries, because many of these disorders are inherited. Sickle-cell anemia, for example, occurs mainly in African Americans; thalassemia occurs in children of Mediterranean heritage. Being aware of the differences in the incidence of blood dyscrasias this way can be helpful in planning care and providing health care services for children and communities. Treatment for blood disorders vary as well based on cultural influences. Families who are Jehovah's Witnesses, for example may refuse blood transfusions, a common therapy for blood disorders, on religious grounds (Kitney, Kanani, & De Souza, 2012). Box 44.1 shows 2020 National Health Goals related to blood disorders.

BOX 44.1 Nursing Care Planning Based on 2020 National Health Goals

2020 National Health Goals speak to ways to improve children's health. Because both iron-deficiency and sickle-cell anemia are seen worldwide, improving care in these areas could have a dramatic effect on both national and world health.

- Reduce the incidence of iron deficiency among children aged 1 to 2 years from a baseline of 15.9% to a target level of 14.3%; in children aged 3 to 4 years, from 5.3% to 4.3%.
- Reduce the incidence of iron deficiency among adolescents 12 to 18 years of age from 10.4% to 9.4%.
- Reduce the proportion of persons with hemophilia who develop reduced joint mobility due to bleeding into joints from 82.9% to 74.6%.
- (Developmental) Reduce hospitalization due to preventable complications of sickle-cell disease yearly among children aged 9 years and under.
- Increase the proportion of children with special health care needs who have access to a medical home from 47.1% to 51.8% (U.S. Department of Health and Human Services [DHHS], 2010; see www.healthypeople.gov).

Nurses can help the nation achieve these goals by educating parents about the importance of women taking an iron supplement during pregnancy, encouraging iron-rich food sources for young children, and educating adolescents about healthy diets. Being certain that parents are well informed about preventive measures for children with all types of hematologic disorders could help reduce hospital admissions.

Nursing Process Overview

For a Child With a Hematologic Disorder

Assessment

Many of the symptoms of hematologic disorders begin insidiously, with symptoms such as pallor, lethargy, and bruising. These are such minor symptoms that parents may not bring their child to a health care facility for some time. When they do, they are surprised to learn such subtle symptoms signify the presence of a serious illness.

Children with iron deficiency, for example, aside from appearing pale and irritable, look plump and "healthy." It takes careful history taking to reveal the possibility of an iron deficiency.

Nursing Diagnosis

When a child is diagnosed with an inherited disorder, parents may feel guilty or blame themselves or their partner for their child's disease. This can make it difficult for a family to act together to support a child during an illness when members need intensive support themselves. Examples of nursing diagnoses that address the entire family include:

- Deficient knowledge related to the cause of the child's illness
- Imbalanced nutrition, less than body requirements, related to family pattern of not eating iron-rich foods
- Anxiety related to frequent blood-sampling procedures
- Pain related to tissue ischemia
- Compromised family coping related to long-term care needs of child with a chronic hematologic disorder

Outcome Identification and Planning

When helping parents plan outcomes, be certain that the outcomes planned are realistic for both the child and family. It may not be possible to reduce the number of blood-sampling procedures, for example, but a child can be helped, with distraction techniques, to deal with the pain and anxiety that the procedures produce.

Children with hematologic disorders often are prescribed a long-term medication such as a corticosteroid. When a child appears very ill, parents are usually very conscientious about giving such medicine. When a child has a disorder with few symptoms, however, like a blood dyscrasia, it is easy for parents to forget to give the medication. In addition, a child may refuse to take the medication for a long time because it tastes bad or upsets the stomach. Planning, therefore, includes helping parents devise ways to disguise the taste or remember to give medication over the long term. If a child will be restricted in activity for long periods because the immune system is compromised as a part of the illness, planning must include ways to keep the child engaged with friends to promote development. Parents may need help investigating possible resources for education and support to do this.

Some organizations helpful for referral are the Aplastic Anemia & MDS International Foundation (www.aplastic.org), the Sickle-cell Disease Association of America (www.sicklecelldisease.org), the American Society of Pediatric Hematology and Oncology (www.aspho.org), and the National Hemophilia Foundation (www.hemophilia.org).

Implementation

Nursing interventions for children with hematologic disorders range from helping to obtain blood specimens for testing to assisting with blood or hematopoietic stem cell transfusions. Remember that a finger puncture for blood is often as painful as a venipuncture (and more painful afterward because the fingertip hurts when the child attempts to use it). Suggesting that blood be drawn by means of an intermittent device and applying an anesthetic cream (mixtures of lidocaine and prilocaine) before finger punctures or venipunctures are effective measures to help reduce pain and improve cooperation with these procedures and so are important to initiate. Even so, children may need some therapeutic playtime with a syringe and a doll to express their anger about constant invasion by needles.

Outcome Evaluation

An evaluation focuses on whether short-term outcomes such as moderation of pain or elimination of anxiety in a child undergoing diagnosis or treatment were achieved and that progress is being made toward the achievement of long-term outcomes such as improving the ability of the family to manage the stress of raising a child with a chronic illness or dealing with frequently occurring health crises.

Examples of expected outcomes that suggest goals were achieved include:

- Parents correctly state the most frequent causes of iron-deficiency anemia.
- Child states she feels better able to cope with blood-sampling procedures through the use of imagery.
- Parents describe realistic plans to ensure adherence to long-term medication administration.
- Parents voice that they understand the importance of preventing dehydration in their school-age child with sickle-cell anemia.

ANATOMY AND PHYSIOLOGY OF THE HEMATOPOIETIC SYSTEM

Blood components originate in the bone marrow, circulate through blood vessels, and ultimately are destroyed by the spleen.

Blood Formation and Components

The total volume of blood in the human body is roughly proportional to body weight: 85 ml/kg at birth, 75 ml/kg at 6 months of age, and 70 ml/kg after the first year. Although the *blood plasma* is important in diseases that cause vomiting and diarrhea (when this fluid may become depleted, leading to dehydration), plasma is not a major site of hematologic disease. The formed elements—the erythrocytes (red blood cells [RBCs]), leukocytes (white blood cells [WBCs]), and thrombocytes (platelets)—are the portions most affected by hematologic disorders in children.

Erythrocytes (Red Blood Cells)

Erythrocytes (RBCs) function chiefly to transport oxygen to and carry carbon dioxide away from body cells. They are formed in the bone marrow under the stimulation of **erythropoietin**, a hormone formed by the kidneys that is produced whenever a child has tissue hypoxia. Children with kidney disease often have a low number of RBCs because erythropoietin secretion is inadequate in diseased kidneys. *Polycythemia*, or an overproduction of RBCs, can occur in children who experience prolonged systemic hypoxia because of erythropoietin overproduction (Rote & McCance, 2012).

At birth, an infant has approximately 5 million RBCs per cubic millimeter of blood. This concentration diminishes rapidly in the first months, reaching a low of approximately 4.1 million/mm^3 at 3 to 4 months of age. The number then slowly increases until adolescence, when the adult value of approximately 4.9 million/mm^3 is reached.

RBCs form first as **erythroblasts** (large, nucleated cells), then mature through normoblast and **reticulocyte** stages, to mature, nonnucleated erythrocytes. An elevated reticulocyte count (more than 1% of the total count) indicates that rapid production of new RBCs is occurring. At the end of their life span (about 120 days), erythrocytes are destroyed through phagocytosis by reticuloendothelial cells, found in the highest proportion in the spleen.

Hemoglobin. The component of RBCs that allows them to carry out the transport of oxygen is *hemoglobin*, composed of globin, a protein, and heme, an iron-containing pigment. It is the heme portion that combines with oxygen and carbon dioxide for transport.

The hemoglobin in erythrocytes during fetal life differs from that formed after birth. Fetal hemoglobin is composed of two α and two γ polypeptide chains. At birth, 40% to 70% of the infant's hemoglobin is this type (hemoglobin F). During the first 6 months of life, this is gradually replaced by adult hemoglobin (hemoglobin A), which is composed of two α and two β chains. For this reason, diseases such as sickle-cell anemia or the thalassemias, which are disorders of the β chains, do not become apparent clinically until this hemoglobin change has occurred (at approximately 6 months of age). Because some hemoglobin A is present, however, even in early intrauterine life, they can be diagnosed prenatally by hemoglobin analysis or electrophoresis in fetal or newborn life (Kline, 2012).

Hemoglobin levels are highest at birth (13.7 to 20.1 g/100 ml); they reach a low at approximately 3 months of age (9.5 to 14.5 g/100 ml), and then gradually rise again until adult values are reached at puberty (11 to 16 g/100 ml).

Bilirubin. After an RBC reaches its life span of approximately 120 days, it disintegrates and its protein component is preserved by the reticuloendothelial cells of the liver and spleen for further use. Iron is reused by the bone marrow to construct new RBCs. As the heme portion is degraded, it is converted into protoporphyrin; protoporphyrin is then further broken down into indirect bilirubin. Indirect bilirubin is fat soluble and so cannot be excreted by the kidneys. It is therefore converted by the liver enzyme glucuronyl transferase into *direct bilirubin*, which is water soluble and excreted in bile.

In the newborn, generally liver function is so immature that the conversion from indirect to direct bilirubin is difficult, allowing a portion of bilirubin to remain in the indirect form. When the level of indirect bilirubin in the blood rises to more than 7 mg/100 ml, it permeates outside the circulatory system, and the infant begins to show signs of yellowing or jaundice from the color of bilirubin. At any point in life, if excessive **hemolysis** (destruction) of RBCs occurs from other than usual causes, a child will also show signs of jaundice.

Leukocytes (White Blood Cells)

Leukocytes (WBCs) are nucleated cells and few in number compared with RBCs (there is approximately only 1 WBC to every 500 RBCs). Their primary function is defense against antigen invasion; their life span varies from approximately 6 hours to unknown intervals. With the exception of neutropenia (a reduced number of WBCs), leukocytes are not major hematologic concerns; because they are important in immune disorders and malignancies, they are further discussed in Chapters 42 and 53.

Thrombocytes (Platelets)

Thrombocytes are round, nonnucleated bodies formed by the bone marrow; their function is capillary hemostasis and primary coagulation. The usual number is 150,000 to 300,000/mm^3 after the first year. Immature thrombocytes are termed **megakaryocytes**. If large numbers of these are present in serum, it indicates that a rapid production of platelets is occurring.

Blood Coagulation

Effective blood coagulation depends on a complex series of four events, including a combination of blood and tissue factors released from the plasma (the intrinsic pathway) and from injured tissue (the extrinsic pathway) (Schwartz, Rote, & McCance, 2012). The numbers of coagulation factors refer to the order in which factors were discovered, not to the order of action in coagulation. The plasma-released factors include factors VIII, IX, and XII. Factors released from injured tissues are a tissue factor (an incomplete thromboplastin or factor III), plus factors VII and X. Together, these pathways unite to form factor V.

When a vessel is injured, vasoconstriction occurs in the area proximal to the injury, thus narrowing the vessel lumen and reducing the amount of blood that can flow to the injured area. Platelets begin to adhere to the damaged vessel site and to one another, forming a platelet plug and initiating the first stage of clotting (Fig. 44.1).

In the second stage, factors from either the intrinsic or the extrinsic system combine with platelet phospholipids to form complete thromboplastin. In the third stage, thromboplastin converts prothrombin (factor II) to thrombin if ionized calcium is present. The production of prothrombin and factors VII, IX, and X all depend on the presence of vitamin K. This stage will be incomplete, therefore, if levels of any of factors VIII through XII, vitamin K, or calcium are deficient.

In the fourth stage, thrombin converts fibrinogen (factor I) to fibrin. Fibrin strands form a mesh incorporating RBCs, WBCs, and platelets to form a permanent protective seal at the site of injury. Factor XIII (fibrin stabilizing factor) then acts to make the fibrin clot insoluble and permanent.

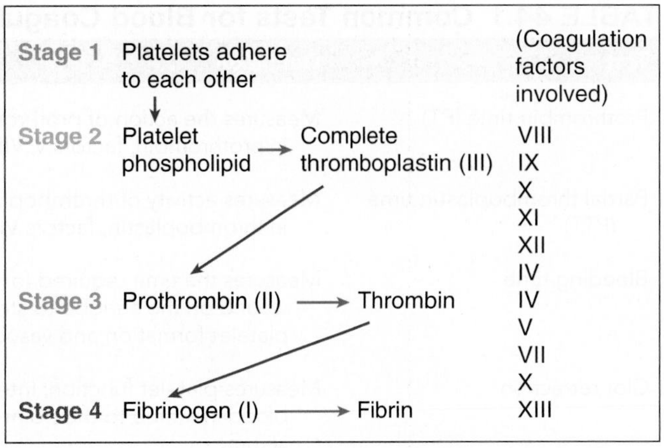

FIGURE 44.1 The steps in blood coagulation.

To prevent too much coagulation after the seal is complete, plasminogen is then converted to plasmin (a fibrinolysin) near the injury to halt the clotting sequence. Common tests for blood coagulation are described in Table 44.1.

ASSESSMENT OF AND THERAPEUTIC TECHNIQUES FOR HEMATOLOGIC DISORDERS

An assessment of children with hematologic disorders begins with a history to identify inherited disorders. For a specific diagnosis, children generally require several diagnostic procedures such as blood cell or bone marrow analysis.

Bone Marrow Aspiration and Biopsy

Bone marrow aspiration provides samples of bone marrow so the type and quantity of cells being produced can be determined (Panepinto & Scott, 2011). In children, the aspiration sites used are the iliac crests or spines (rather than the sternum, which is commonly used in adults) (Fig. 44.2) because performing the test at these sites is usually less frightening for children. These sites also have the largest marrow compartments during childhood. In neonates, the anterior tibia can be used as an additional site.

For a bone marrow aspiration, following conscious sedation, a child lies prone on a hard surface such as a treatment table because pressure is needed to insert the needle through the surface of the bone into the marrow compartment. Topical anesthesia may be applied to help reduce pain (Hjortholm, Jaddini, Hałaburda, et al., 2013).

The area of the aspiration is cleaned with an antiseptic solution and draped. The overlying skin is infiltrated with a local anesthetic and then a large-bore needle and stylus is introduced through the overlying tissue into the bone. When the marrow cavity is reached, the stylus is removed, a syringe is attached to the needle, and bone marrow is aspirated (which appears as thick blood in the syringe). The syringe is then removed, and the marrow obtained is expelled onto a slide, sprayed with a preservative, and taken to a laboratory for analysis. Pressure must be applied to the puncture site immediately afterward to prevent bleeding. A pressure dressing is then applied to maintain pressure and to continue to halt bleeding.

TABLE 44.1 Common Tests for Blood Coagulation

Test	Definition	Normal Value
Prothrombin time (PT)	Measures the action of prothrombin; reveals deficiencies in prothrombin, factors V, VII, and X.	11–13 s (PT) or 2.0–3.0 International Normalized Ratio (INR)
Partial thromboplastin time (PTT)	Measures activity of thromboplastin; reveals deficiencies in thromboplastin, factors VIII–XII.	30–45 s
Bleeding time	Measures the time required for bleeding at a stab wound on the earlobe to stop; reveals deficiencies in platelet formation and vasoconstrictive ability.	3–10 min
Clot retraction	Measures platelet function; interval from placement of blood in a tube to the point clot shrinks and expels serum.	Retraction at side of test tube should be present by 1 hr; complete in 24 hr
Tourniquet	Measures capillary fragility and platelet function; response of tissue to application of tourniquet to forearm for 5–10 min.	0–2 petechiae per 2-cm area
Prothrombin consumption time	Evaluates thromboplastin function; if clot formation used a great deal of prothrombin (as it should), serum prothrombin time will be brief; prolongation denotes defects in thromboplastin function.	Approximately 20 s
Thromboplastin generation time	Tests basic ability to form thromboplastin; distinguishes factor VIII from factor IX disorders.	12 s or less
Plasma fibrinogen	Measures stage 4 clotting process or level of fibrinogen in blood.	200–400 mg/100 ml plasma
Venous clotting time (Lee-White clotting time)	Measures factor deficits in stages 2 and 4.	9–12 min

A child will feel pain from the local anesthetic injection and hard pressure while the needle is inserted. Some report a sharp pain when the marrow is actually aspirated. If conscious sedation is used, monitor vital signs until the child is fully awake. Monitor pulse and blood pressure and observe the dressing every 15 minutes for the first hour after the procedure to be certain no bleeding is occurring. Keep the child fairly quiet for the first hour by playing a quiet game or other activity. Because bone marrow aspiration is a painful and invasive procedure, allow young children an opportunity for therapeutic play with a doll and syringe to help them express their feelings about the procedure. If the procedure was done as an ambulatory one, instruct parents to take the child's temperature 12 and 24 hours after the procedure to detect infection.

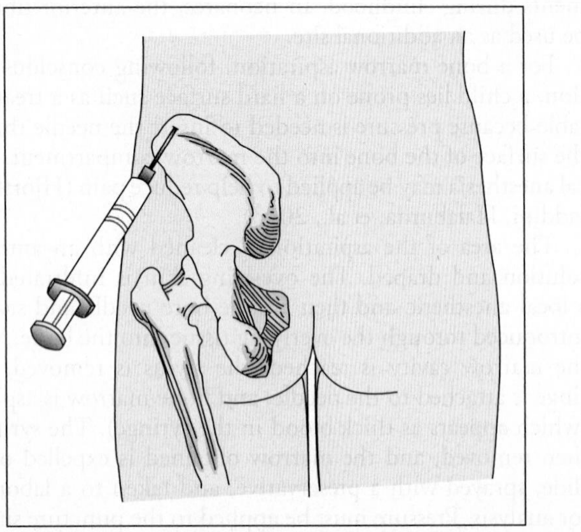

FIGURE 44.2 A common site used for bone marrow aspiration in children is the iliac crest. In neonates, the anterior tibia may be used.

Blood Transfusion

Transfusions of blood or its products are commonly used in the treatment of blood disorders, and may include whole blood, packed RBCs, washed RBCs (as much "foreign" matter is removed as possible to reduce the possibility of an antagonistic reaction), plasma, plasma factors, platelets, WBCs, and albumin. No matter what the blood product, it's important that it has been carefully matched with the child's blood type and is infused with a solution as nearly isotonic as possible (normal saline). If blood should be given with a hypertonic solution, this will cause fluid to be drawn out of the transfused RBCs, causing them to shrink and be useless; if blood is infused with a hypotonic solution, fluid will be drawn into the cells, causing them to burst, and again, be destroyed.

Packed RBCs are the most common form of transfusion used with children because they help minimize the risk of fluid overload. The usual amount of blood transfused is typically 15 ml/kg of body weight. The commonly accepted rate for transfusions in a child is 10 ml/kg/hr unless the child has hypovolemic shock and volume equilibrium needs to be established quickly. An infusion of packed RBCs at a proportion of 15 ml/kg will raise the hematocrit level 5 points. A transfusion of platelets will elevate the platelet count by approximately 10,000 cells. Platelets last only approximately 10 days, however, so transfusions must be repeated every 10 days to maintain a functioning platelet level (Panepinto & Scott, 2011).

Even if given slowly, a blood transfusion is always a strain on a child's circulation beyond that of a regular intravenous infusion because the circulatory system must accommodate such a thick, difficult-to-mobilize fluid.

Before any transfusion, ensure a signed consent form is obtained that respects sociocultural or religious beliefs. Obtain vital signs to establish a baseline and monitor these about every 15 minutes during the first hour and about every half hour for the remainder of the transfusion. Keep the infusion rate slow for the first 15 minutes; then, if no reaction occurs, increase the rate to about 10 ml/kg/hr or as otherwise prescribed. Common symptoms of blood transfusion reactions that may occur are shown in Table 44.2.

To prevent children from becoming bored or attempting to increase the infusion rate to speed up the process, think of and provide an enjoyable activity for children during transfusions.

Hematopoietic Stem Cell Transplantation

Stem cell transplantation is the intravenous infusion of hematopoietic stem cells from bone marrow obtained by marrow aspiration or from peripheral or umbilical cord blood drawn from a compatible donor to reestablish marrow function in a child with deficient or nonfunctioning bone marrow.

Stem cell transplantation has become a relatively common procedure for children with blood disorders such as acquired aplastic anemia, sickle-cell disease, thalassemia, leukemia, and some forms of immune dysfunction diseases.

TABLE 44.2 Common Symptoms of Blood Transfusion Reactions

Symptoms	Cause	Time of Occurrence	Nursing Interventions
Headache, chills, back pain, dyspnea, hypotension, hemoglobinuria (blood in urine)	Anaphylactic reaction to incompatible blood; agglutination of red blood cells occurs; kidney tubules may become blocked, resulting in kidney failure	Immediately after start of transfusion.	Discontinue transfusion. Maintain normal saline infusion for accessible intravenous (IV) line. Administer oxygen as necessary. Anticipate administration of a diuretic to increase renal tubule flow and reduce tubule plugging and/or heparin to reduce IV coagulation.
Pruritus, urticaria (hives), wheezing	Allergy to protein components of transfusion	Within first hour after start of transfusion	Discontinue transfusion temporarily. Give oxygen as needed. Anticipate administration for antihistamine to reduce symptoms.
Increased temperature	Possible contaminant in transfused blood	Approximately 1 hr after start of transfusion	Discontinue transfusion. Obtain blood culture to rule out or identify bacterial invasion.
Increased pulse, dyspnea	Circulatory overload	During course of transfusion	Discontinue transfusion; give oxygen as needed. Provide supportive care for pulmonary edema or congestive heart failure, which may develop. Anticipate administration of diuretic to increase excretion of excess fluid.
Muscle cramping, twitching of extremities, seizure	Acid-citrate-dextrose anticoagulant in transfusion combines with serum calcium and causes hypocalcemia	During course of transfusion	Discontinue transfusion. Anticipate administration of calcium gluconate intravenously to restore calcium level.
Fever, jaundice, lethargy, tenderness over liver	Hepatitis from contaminated transfusion	Weeks or months after transfusion	Obtain transfusion history of any child with hepatitis symptoms. Refer for care of hepatitis.
Bronze-colored skin	Hemosiderosis or deposition of iron in skin from transfusion	After repeated transfusions	Support self-esteem with altered body image. Administer iron-chelating agent (deferoxamine) as prescribed to help reduce level of accumulating iron.

Although a stressful procedure to undertake, it offers children the opportunity for a complete reversal of symptoms. However, there is no guarantee that the grafted cells will be accepted by the recipient or that improvement will occur, but with good tissue compatibility in the absence of infection, it can be effective in most children (Thompson, Ceja, & Yang, 2012).

Stem cell transplantation can be allogeneic, syngeneic, or autologous. **Allogeneic transplantation** is the transfer of stem cells from an immune-compatible (histocompatible) donor, usually a sibling, or from a national cord blood bank or national volunteer donor registry (Petrini, 2013). **Syngeneic transplantation** (which is rare) involves a donor and recipient who are genetically identical (i.e., identical twins). **Autologous transplantation** involves use of the child's own stem cells removed from cord blood banked at the time of the child's birth. If this is not available, in some instances, stem cells can be aspirated from the child's bone marrow or obtained from circulating blood, treated to remove abnormal cells, and then reinfused.

Hematopoietic stem cells are recovered from a donor's circulating peripheral blood after the stimulation of stem cell production by a cytokine or stem cell colony-stimulating factor. Success is most likely if the recipient has not already received multiple blood transfusions that have sensitized the child to blood products and the donated stem cells are a close human leukocyte antigen (HLA) match to the child's blood. Siblings have about a 25% chance of being HLA compatible with the ill child.

To prevent a child's T lymphocytes from rejecting the newly transplanted donor stem cells, total body irradiation to destroy the child's marrow or an immunosuppressive drug such as cyclophosphamide (Cytoxan) is administered intravenously to the child before the procedure. This is a difficult time for the child because, even with antiemetic therapy, both total body irradiation and the immunosuppressive drug cause extreme nausea, vomiting, and diarrhea.

If the marrow will be taken directly from a donor rather than from peripheral blood, on the day of the procedure, the donor is admitted to the hospital for a 1-day stay and receives epidural anesthesia or conscious sedation because multiple bone marrow aspirations from the posterior iliac crests are necessary for retrieval. The marrow is strained to remove fat and bone particles and any other unwanted cells. An anticoagulant is added to prevent clotting and it is then infused intravenously into the recipient's bloodstream.

Because an infused hematopoietic stem cell solution is fairly thick, the infusion takes 60 to 90 minutes. Do not use the filter that is normally used for the infusion of blood products, because this would filter out marrow tissue. Monitor the child's cardiac rate and rhythm during the infusion to detect circulatory overload or pulmonary emboli from unfiltered particles.

Fever and chills are common reactions to a hematopoietic stem cell transplant infusion. Acetaminophen (Tylenol) or diphenhydramine hydrochloride (Benadryl) may be prescribed to reduce this reaction. After the infusion, take the child's temperature at 1 hour and then about every 4 hours to detect an infection that could occur because the child's WBCs are nonfunctional from radiation or immunosuppression. Reinforce strict hand washing and limit the child's diet to cooked foods to reduce exposure to bacteria.

Almost immediately after the infusion, stem cells begin to migrate from the child's bloodstream into the marrow. If *engraftment* occurs (the transplant is accepted), new RBCs can be detected in the peripheral blood in approximately 3 weeks. The WBC count will be measured daily to be certain WBCs are regenerating, although WBCs and platelet cells may not return to normal for up to 1 year after the transplant. Bone marrow aspirations or venous blood samples are then scheduled at regular intervals over the next year to assess the growth of the new marrow.

What if...44.1 Lana's 12-year-old sister donates hematopoietic stem cells to Lana, but the transplant is not successful. The sister tells you she knew it wouldn't be successful because she and Lana are more rivals than compatible sisters. Could sibling rivalry this way have made a difference in the success of the procedure?

Nursing Diagnoses and Related Interventions

Because it takes a long time for the success or failure of stem cell transplantation to be documented, the procedure almost always produces anxiety not just in the child but also in the donor and the entire family.

Nursing Diagnosis: Anxiety related to long period of waiting to receive results of hematopoietic stem cell transplant and necessary extended restrictions and infection control precautions in hospital or at home.

Outcome Evaluation: Parents state they are managing their level of anxiety, are carrying out infection restrictions as prescribed, and are expressing satisfaction with child's ongoing development.

Be certain when discussing the risks of a stem cell transplant that both the child who received the transplant and the donor understand they are not responsible for the outcome of the procedure because its success does not depend on their behavior or what kind of person they are but on immunologic factors over which they have no control.

Because not all hematopoietic stem cell transplants are successful, some children will die of the original disease that necessitated the transplant. And, even if the transplant was successful, another risk is that a child will develop an infection despite all precautions and die of sepsis in the weeks immediately after the transplant.

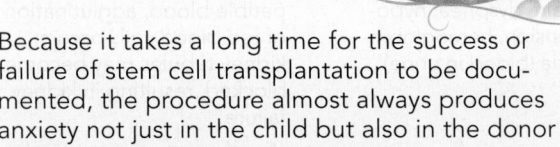

To prevent the child from contracting an infection until the WBC count returns to a safe range, children are restricted from interacting with other children either by remaining in the hospital or by employing visiting restrictions at home. Be certain to visit the room of an isolated child frequently and provide sterilized play materials the child can enjoy as appropriate. Because raw vegetables and fruits have the potential to carry germs, thick-skinned fruits such as bananas and oranges can be given soon after the procedure, but unwashed foods are typically avoided because these are foods most likely to carry bacteria.

Be certain children are well prepared for all procedures. Allow them to make as many choices as they can about their care to help them preserve a sense of control over their lives. Encourage periods of therapeutic play into their care so they can begin to express their anger and frustration at the number of intravenous therapies or follow-up bone marrow aspirations they require. Frequent visits by their parents and measures to help the child cope with pain, such as imagery, can help them accept one more painful procedure.

Ask the parents if they have made provisions for schoolwork as soon as the child has a return of RBCs in the peripheral blood (about 3 weeks). Help them locate a support group in their community if they feel this will be helpful. Be certain they feel free to call the transplant center after discharge to discuss any problems (Cooke, Grant, & Gemmill, 2012). Once the danger of infection has passed and the restrictions can be discontinued, some parents may still be reluctant to allow their child outside or to interact with other children. This makes frequent follow-ups by e-mail or texting for the next year necessary to not only ensure that the child is free of infection but also to assess whether the parents allow their child to pursue age-appropriate activities to encourage growth and development.

Graft-Versus-Host Disease

Graft-versus-host disease (GVHD) is a potentially lethal immunologic response of donor T cells to the tissue of the bone marrow recipient (Alousi, Bolaños-Meade, & Lee, 2013). The symptoms range from mild to severe and generally include a rash and general malaise beginning 7 to 14 days after the transplant. Severe symptoms include high fever and diarrhea and liver and spleen enlargement.

Because there is no known cure for GVHD, prevention is essential. Careful tissue typing, intravenous administration of a corticosteroid and an immunosuppressant before transplant, and irradiation of blood products (which helps to inactivate mature T lymphocytes) before the infusion all can help reduce the incidence of this complication. Immunosuppressant drugs such as methotrexate or cyclosporine work by killing all rapidly growing cells, including WBCs and T lymphocytes, so administration of these drugs after transplantation cannot be continued or they would also interfere with the growth of the host's new stem cells. Administration of corticosteroids or antithymocyte globulin (ATG), an immune serum, can be continued and may decrease the severity of GVHD; be certain parents understand the importance of this so, if prescribed, they give them conscientiously (Theurich, Fischmann, Shimabukuro-Vornhagen, et al., 2012).

QSEN Checkpoint Question 44.1

Patient-Centered Care

Lana, who has thalassemia major, is scheduled for a bone marrow transplant, and her mother is highly anxious about this upcoming procedure. Which of the following statements is most accurate and best exemplifies patient-centered care?

a. "If you can hold her still during the procedure, the pain will pass more quickly for her."
b. "We will go to great lengths to make sure Lana doesn't develop an infection."
c. "Lana will need to lie still while the new bone marrow infuses into her bones."
d. "She will not need any further bone marrow aspirations after this."

Look in Appendix A for the best answer and rationale.

Splenectomy

One of the purposes of the spleen is to remove damaged or aged blood cells. This poses a problem with diseases such as sickle-cell anemia and the thalassemias because the spleen interprets the typical cells of these diseases as damaged and destroys them. This causes children with these disorders to have a continuous anemia, with hemoglobin levels as low as 5 to 9 g/ml. In some children, therefore, removal of the spleen (splenectomy) will not cure the basic defect of the blood cells but will limit the degree of anemia. Splenectomy formerly required a large abdominal incision but today it can be performed by laparoscopy so, although still a procedure with risks, it does not require as long a recovery period (Deng, Maharjan, Tang, et al., 2012).

A second function of the spleen is to strain blood particles that might lead to blood clots as well as invading microorganisms from the blood plasma so phagocytes and lymphocytes can destroy them. This causes children who have had their spleen removed to be very susceptible to both thrombophlebitis and pneumococcal infections because these substances are no longer removed systematically from the body (Rodeghiero & Ruggeri, 2012). After surgery, oral penicillin is typically given as a prophylactic antibiotic for a year or two to guard against infection. Assess to be certain the child also receives *Haemophilus influenzae* type b (Hib) and pneumococcal and meningococcal vaccines for further protection. Review with parents the signs of infection (e.g., cough, fever, general malaise), and encourage them to report any such signs immediately to their primary care provider.

HEALTH PROMOTION AND RISK MANAGEMENT

Hematologic disorders cover a wide range of diseases, both inherited and as an immunosuppressive response to infection, so they produce multiple symptoms in children (Box 44.2). Health promotion and disease prevention, therefore, begins with ensuring families have access to genetic counseling so they can be aware of the incidence of a disorder in their family and the potential for the disease to develop in their child.

BOX 44.2 Nursing Care Planning Using Assessment

Assessing a Child With a Hematologic Disorder

History

Chief concern: Fatigue, easy bruising, epistaxis.
Past medical history: Low birthweight; blood loss at birth; lack of vitamin K administration at birth.
Nutrition: "Picky eater" or presence of pica. Increasd milk intake.
Past illnesses: History of recent illness; history of recent medicine ingestion.
Family history: Inherited blood disorder; parents known to have sickle-cell trait, thalassemia minor, or hemophilia in family.

Physical examination

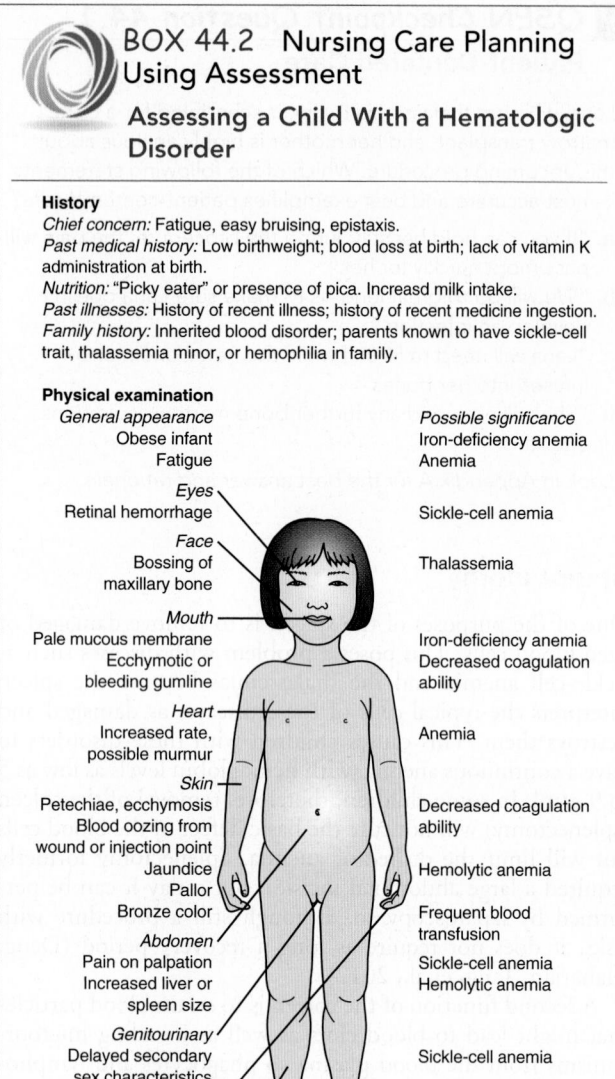

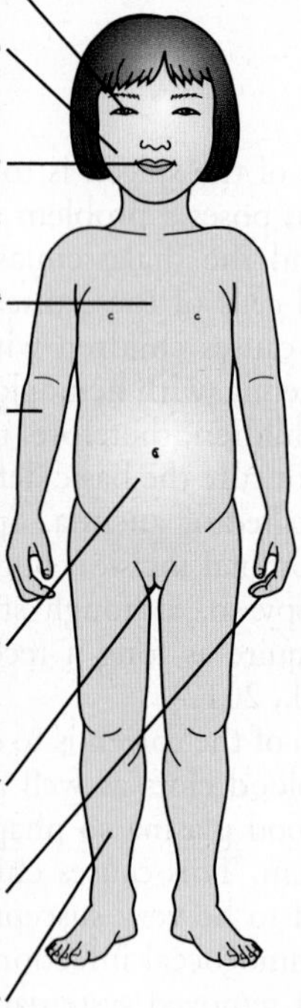

	Possible significance
General appearance	
Obese infant	Iron-deficiency anemia
Fatigue	Anemia
Eyes	
Retinal hemorrhage	Sickle-cell anemia
Face	
Bossing of maxillary bone	Thalassemia
Mouth	
Pale mucous membrane	Iron-deficiency anemia
Ecchymotic or bleeding gumline	Decreased coagulation ability
Heart	
Increased rate, possible murmur	Anemia
Skin	
Petechiae, ecchymosis	Decreased coagulation ability
Blood oozing from wound or injection point	
Jaundice	Hemolytic anemia
Pallor	
Bronze color	Frequent blood transfusion
Abdomen	
Pain on palpation	Sickle-cell anemia
Increased liver or spleen size	Hemolytic anemia
Genitourinary	
Delayed secondary sex characteristics	Sickle-cell anemia
Extremities	
Spoon-shaped nails	Iron-deficiency anemia
Joint swelling, pain	Hemophilia, sickle-cell crisis
Neurologic	
Weak muscle tone	Iron-deficiency anemia

The most frequently occurring anemia in children, iron-deficiency anemia, could be virtually eliminated if all infants were breastfed and those infants who are formula fed were fed iron-fortified formula for the full first year. The disorder occurs again with a high incidence in adolescents because adolescent diets tend to be low in meat and green vegetables, the chief dietary sources of iron. Adolescents who begin pseudo-vegetarian diets are another group especially prone to developing the disorder. Counseling parents of young children to maintain well-child health care visits and urging adolescents to ingest iron-rich foods could have a major impact on decreasing the incidence of the disorder.

Aplastic anemia, or the inability to form blood elements, can be acquired if a child is exposed to a toxic drug or chemical. Educating parents about the importance of keeping poisons out of the reach of children and being aware of toxic substances in their community could help decrease the incidence of this disorder. Because children with hematologic disorders may have a changed physical appearance and also need to avoid contact sports to prevent bleeding episodes, they may be the victims of bullying or stigmas; be certain parents talk with their children about this so children know to report bullying rather than continue to be a victim (Jenerette, Brewer, Crandell, et al., 2012).

DISORDERS OF THE RED BLOOD CELLS

Most RBC disorders fall into the category of the anemias, or a reduction in the number or function of erythrocytes. Polycythemia, or an increase in the number of RBCs, can also occur and, because it can lead to blood clots, may be as dangerous to a child as a reduction in RBC production.

Anemia occurs when the rate of RBC production falls below that of cell destruction, or when there is a loss of RBCs, causing their number and the hemoglobin level to fall below that of production. Anemias are classified according to the changes seen in RBC numbers or configuration, or according to the source of the problem. Although any reduction in the amount of circulating hemoglobin lessens the oxygen-carrying capacity, clinical symptoms are not usually apparent until the hemoglobin level reaches 7 to 8 g/100 ml. Average values for hemoglobin and RBC number are available at http://thePoint.lww.com/Pillitteri7e.

Normochromic, Normocytic Anemias

Normochromic (normal color), normocytic (normal cell size) anemias occur because of impaired production of erythrocytes by the bone marrow or by abnormal or uncompensated loss of circulating RBCs, as with acute hemorrhage. The RBCs appear normal in both color and size; however, there simply are too few of them for effective oxygen transport.

Acute Blood-Loss Anemia

Blood loss that is sufficient to cause anemia can occur from trauma such as an automobile accident with internal bleeding; from acute nephritis in which blood is lost in the urine; or in the newborn from disorders such as placenta previa, premature separation of the placenta, maternal–fetal or twin-to-twin transfusion, or trauma to the cord or placenta. In childhood, it can occur from the action of long-term intestinal parasites such as a tapeworm or hookworm or, in small infants, bedbug bites (Studdiford, Conniff, Trayes, et al., 2012).

With sudden blood loss, children immediately appear pale. Because their heart must push the reduced amount of blood through their body more rapidly than usual, tachycardia will occur. Children will also begin to breathe rapidly because body cells are still not able to receive adequate oxygen. Newborns may have gasping respirations, intercostal retractions, and cyanosis. Children with rapid heart and respiratory rates due to this do not respond well to oxygen therapy because they lack RBCs to transport and use the oxygen. They become listless and inactive, dizzy, and possibly, comatose.

This type of acute blood-loss anemia generally is transitory because the sudden reduction in available oxygen stimulates the release of erythropoietin from the kidney and a regeneration response in the bone marrow. The reticulocyte count rises, which is evidence that the bone marrow is trying to increase production of erythrocytes to meet the sudden shortage.

Treatment involves control of bleeding by addressing its underlying cause and transfusing additional RBCs. Lie the child flat to provide as much circulation as possible to brain cells. Keep the child warm with blankets; place the infant in an incubator or under a radiant heat warmer. Until blood is available for transfusion, a blood expander such as plasma or intravenous fluid such as normal saline or Ringer's lactate may be given to expand blood volume and improve blood pressure. With such emergency steps, the situation should be transitory with no long-term consequences.

Anemia of Acute Infection

Acute infection or inflammation, especially in infants, can cause increased destruction or decreased production of erythrocytes. Common conditions that do this include osteomyelitis and ulcerative colitis. Management involves treatment of the underlying condition. When the condition is reversed, blood values will return to normal.

Anemia of Renal Disease

Either acute or chronic renal disease can cause loss of function in kidney cells, which causes an accompanying decrease in erythropoietin production, resulting in a normocytic, normochromic anemia. Administration of recombinant human erythropoietin can increase RBC production and correct the anemia, but not the renal disease (Lum, 2012).

Anemia of Neoplastic Disease

Malignant growths such as leukemia or lymphoma (common neoplasms of childhood) result in normochromic, normocytic anemias because the invasion of bone marrow by proliferating neoplastic cells impairs RBC production. There may be accompanying blood loss if platelet formation also is decreased. The treatment of such an anemia involves measures designed to achieve remission of the neoplastic process and transfusion to increase the erythrocyte count.

Hypersplenism

Under usual conditions, blood filters rapidly through the spleen. If the spleen becomes enlarged, however, blood cells pass through more slowly, with more cells being destroyed in the process. This increased destruction of RBCs can cause anemia and may lead to pancytopenia (deficiency of all cell elements of blood). Virtually any underlying splenic condition can cause this syndrome.

Therapeutic management consists of treating the underlying splenic disorder, and includes a possible splenectomy.

Aplastic Anemias

Aplastic anemias result from depression of hematopoietic activity in the bone marrow. The formation and development of WBCs, platelets, and RBCs can all be affected (Rovó, Tichelli, & Dufour, 2013).

Congenital aplastic anemia (Fanconi syndrome) is inherited as an autosomal recessive trait. A child is born with several congenital anomalies, such as skeletal and renal abnormalities, hypogenitalism, and short stature. Between 4 and 12 years of age, the child begins to manifest symptoms of **pancytopenia**, or a reduction of all blood cell components (Linker & Damon, 2012).

Acquired aplastic anemia is a decrease in bone marrow production, which occurs if a child is excessively exposed to radiation, drugs, or chemicals known to cause bone marrow damage. Exposure to insecticides and chemotherapeutic drugs temporarily causes this. Other examples of drugs that cause acquired aplastic anemia include chloramphenicol, sulfonamides, arsenic (contained in rat poison, sometimes eaten by children), hydantoin, benzene, or quinine. A serious infection such as meningococcal pneumonia might cause autoimmunologic suppression of the bone marrow, which then also results in this condition.

Assessment. When symptoms begin, a child appears pale, fatigues easily, and has anorexia from the lowered RBC count and tissue hypoxia. Because of reduced platelet formation **(thrombocytopenia),** the child bruises easily or develops **petechiae** (pinpoint, macular, purplish-red spots caused by an intradermal or submucous hemorrhage). A child may have excessive nosebleeds or gastrointestinal bleeding. As a result of a decrease in WBCs (neutropenia), a child may contract an increased number of infections and respond poorly to antibiotic therapy. Observe closely for signs of cardiac decompensation such as tachycardia, tachypnea, shortness of breath, or cyanosis from the long-term increased workload of all these effects on the heart. Bone marrow samples will show a reduced number of blood elements, and blood-forming spaces will be infiltrated by fatty tissue (Kline, 2012).

The child is apt to be irritable because of the fatigue and recurring symptoms. Parents may feel distressed if the illness originated from exposure to a chemical they should have kept away from their child, such as an insecticide. This can cause parents to have less confidence in health care personnel if the illness followed treatment with a drug such as chloramphenicol. They may wonder how they can trust in a drug to cure the illness if they believe a prescribed drug caused the illness.

Therapeutic Management. The first step in therapy is to immediately discontinue any drug or chemical suspected of causing the bone marrow dysfunction and removing the substance from the child's environment to avoid exposure. The ultimate therapy for both congenital and acquired aplastic anemia is hematopoietic stem cell transplantation (Korthof, Békássy, & Hussein, 2013). If a donor cannot be located, the disease is managed by a variety of procedures to supplement blood or to suppress T-lymphocyte–dependent autoimmune responses while waiting for a histocompatible donor. Packed RBCs, platelet transfusions, cyclosporine, ATG, and an RBC-stimulating factor such as erythropoietin are generally necessary to maintain adequate blood elements. Some children show improvement with a course of an oral corticosteroid (prednisone) to further decrease the immune response or a course of testosterone to stimulate RBC growth. Be certain to observe a child well when administering ATG intravenously because of the high risk for anaphylaxis.

For children who receive a hematopoietic stem cell transplant, chances of complete recovery are good. For others, the course will be uncertain. A decreased WBC count leaves the child open to infection. The decreased platelet count may persist for years after other blood elements have returned to normal, producing long-term problems of bleeding, especially petechiae or purpura (Box 44.3).

BOX 44.3 Nursing Care Planning to Empower a Family

TECHNIQUES FOR REDUCING BLEEDING WITH THROMBOCYTOPENIA

Q. Lana's mother asks you, "What precautions do you take to limit black and blue spots on Lana when her platelet count is low?"

A. "We try, as a team, to do the following."

- Limit the number of blood-drawing procedures; combine samples whenever possible.
- Use a blood pressure cuff instead of a tourniquet to reduce the number of petechiae.
- Apply pressure to any puncture site for a full 5 minutes before applying a bandage.
- Minimize the use of adhesive tape to the skin (pulling for removal may tear the skin and cause petechiae).
- Pad side and crib rails to prevent bruising. Assess the need for routine blood pressure determinations because tight cuffs can lead to petechiae.
- Protect intravenous sites to avoid numerous reinsertions.
- Administer medication orally or by intravenous infusion when appropriate to minimize the number of subcutaneous or intramuscular injection sites.
- Assess that the child is using a soft toothbrush and is offered foods that can be chewed without irritation (e.g., avoid toast crusts).
- Check toys for sharp corners, which may cause scratches. Urge the child to be careful with paper, because paper cuts can bleed out of proportion to their size.
- Distract the child from rough play; suggest stimulating but quiet activities to minimize risk of injury.

Nursing Diagnoses and Related Interventions

Nursing diagnoses need to speak to not only the physical symptoms of aplastic anemia but also the continual stress the parents feel if laboratory reports do not reveal a dramatic change in their child's blood cell production. It may be helpful to urge them to deal with this problem by facing only one day or one blood test at a time rather than trying to dwell on the outcomes of all the blood tests to come.

Nursing Diagnosis: Risk for disturbed body image related to changed appearance occurring as medication side effects

Outcome Evaluation: Child views self as a worthwhile person; does not appear to be excessively shy or reluctant to interact with peers.

Children who receive corticosteroids such as prednisone to suppress the immune response almost always experience some of the drug's side effects, such as a cushingoid appearance, hirsutism, hypertension, and marked weight gain. Long-term therapy with testosterone can result in masculinizing effects, such as growth of facial and body hair, the development of acne, and deepening of the voice. Be certain both children and their parents know these effects are related to the medication and will fade when the medication is withdrawn.

Adolescents may have an especially difficult time accepting weight gain and increased acne and so need a chance to express their feelings about their changed appearance. Reinforce and emphasize things they are doing well such as how well they are managing this unexpected turn in their life.

Hypoplastic Anemias

Hypoplastic anemias also result from depression of hematopoietic activity in bone marrow and can also be either congenital or acquired. Unlike aplastic anemias, however, in which WBCs, RBCs, and platelets are all affected, with hypoplastic anemias, only RBCs are affected.

Congenital hypoplastic anemia (Blackfan–Diamond syndrome) is a rare disorder apparently caused by an inherent defect in RBC formation that affects both sexes and shows symptoms as early as the first 6 to 8 months of life (Sakaguchi, Nakanishi, & Kojima, 2013). An acquired form of this can be caused by infection with parvovirus 19, the infectious agent that causes fifth disease (Morinet, Leruez-Ville, Pillet, et al., 2011).

The onset of a hypoplastic anemia is insidious, and at first it may be difficult to differentiate from iron-deficiency anemia. With iron-deficiency anemia, blood cells appear hypochromic and microcytic and are few in number; however, in hypoplastic anemia, they are not only few in number but also their structure is normochromic and normocytic.

With the acquired type, the reduction of RBCs is transient, so no therapy other than monitoring is necessary. Children with the congenital form receive corticosteroid therapy along with transfusions of packed RBCs to raise erythrocyte levels. As a result of the necessary number of transfusions, **hemosiderosis** (a deposition of iron in body tissue) can occur. An iron chelation program such as subcutaneous infusion of deferoxamine (Desferal) may be started concurrently with transfusions to bind with iron and aid its excretion from the body in urine. Although an oral form is available for children over 10 years of age, this is usually given by a subcutaneous infusion pump over an 8-hour period for 5 or 6 nights a week. Remind the parent to assess that the child is voiding as usual and that his or her specific gravity is normal (1.003 to 1.030) before beginning an infusion so iron removed from tissues can be excreted (Karch, 2013).

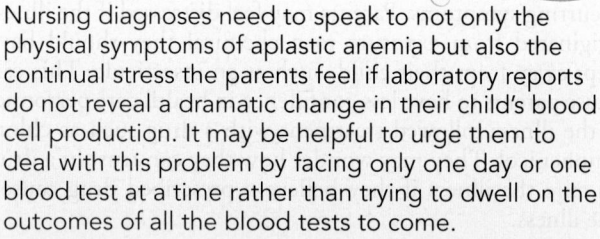

To begin such an infusion, an area beside the scapula or on the thigh is cleaned with alcohol and a short 25-gauge needle is inserted at a low angle into the subcutaneous tissue and

attached to an infusion pump by intravenous tubing. In addition to the assessments of voiding and specific gravity, periodic slit-lamp eye examinations should be scheduled to check for cataract formation, a possible adverse effect of deferoxamine.

Although congenital hypoplastic anemia has to be thought of as a chronic condition, about one fourth of affected children will undergo spontaneous permanent remission before the age of 13 years. If not, they are candidates for hematopoietic stem cell transplantation. As with aplastic anemia, both the child and the parents need support from health care personnel to help them accept the many procedures and tests required before full remission is finally achieved.

QSEN Checkpoint Question 44.2

Informatics

Lana has received iron chelation therapy by deferoxamine in the past. Which statement by her mother would best assure you she understands the use and action of iron chelation therapy?

a. "I know the drug acts to remove excess iron from my child."
b. "I have to check Lana's pulse before I turn on the pump."
c. "The drug is used to increase the level of iron in bone cells."
d. "The drug has minimal side effects, so I can't really give it wrong."

Look in Appendix A for the best answer and rationale.

Hypochromic Anemias

When hemoglobin production is inadequate, erythrocytes appear pale (hypochromia) and are also usually reduced in diameter (microcytic).

Iron-Deficiency Anemia

Although the incidence of iron-deficiency anemia is decreasing in the United States due to improved infant nutrition, it is still the most common anemia of infancy and childhood, occurring whenever the intake of dietary iron is inadequate. Without adequate iron, hemoglobin cannot be incorporated into RBCs.

Children are at a higher risk for iron-deficiency anemia than adults because they need more daily iron in proportion to their body weight to maintain an adequate iron level than do adults—a daily intake of 11 to 15 mg of iron. This type of anemia occurs most often between the ages of 9 months and 3 years from infants drinking more milk than they are eating iron-rich foods (Ziegler, 2011). Its frequency rises again in adolescence, when iron requirements increase, especially for girls who are menstruating. It is also found at a high incidence in overweight teenagers if they ingest most of their calories from high-carbohydrate, not iron-rich, foods (Moschonis, Chrousos, Lionis, et al., 2012).

The Infant. A newborn usually has enough iron in reserve to last for the first 6 months of life. After that, the infant needs iron incorporated into the diet. Because iron stores are laid down near the end of gestation, infants born preterm will have fewer iron stores than those born at term and so tend to develop iron-deficiency anemia before 5 to 6 months. Women with iron deficiency during pregnancy tend to give birth to iron-deficient babies because the babies do not receive iron stores. As a preventive measure, preterm infants and those whose mother was iron deficient during pregnancy may be given an iron supplement beginning at about 2 months of age.

Infants born with structural defects of the gastrointestinal system, such as gastroesophageal reflux or chalasia (where an immature valve exists between the esophagus and stomach resulting in regurgitation) or pyloric stenosis (narrowing between the stomach and duodenum, resulting in vomiting), are particularly prone to iron-deficiency anemia because iron is not adequately digested. Infants with chronic diarrhea may not be able to make use of iron due to inadequate absorption. If infants are fed cow's milk rather than breast milk, so much minimal gastrointestinal bleeding may occur that iron deficiency anemia may develop.

Urging parents to breastfeed or use iron-fortified formula as well as introduce iron-fortified cereal as a "first food" are important health teaching measures to prevent this form of anemia. Occasionally, infants can become constipated while ingesting iron-rich formula, but this is the exception rather than the rule.

Older Children. In children older than 2 years of age, chronic blood loss is the most frequent cause of iron-deficiency anemia caused by gastrointestinal tract lesions such as polyps, ulcerative colitis, Crohn disease, protein-induced enteropathies, parasitic infestation, or frequent epistaxis. Adolescent girls with heavy menstrual periods can become iron deficient when this is combined with frequent attempts to diet or with overconsumption of snack foods that are low in iron.

Assessment. Common symptoms of iron-deficiency anemia are shown in Box 44.4. The mark of iron-deficiency anemia

BOX 44.4 Nursing Care Planning Using Assessment

Assessing a Child With Iron-Deficiency Anemia

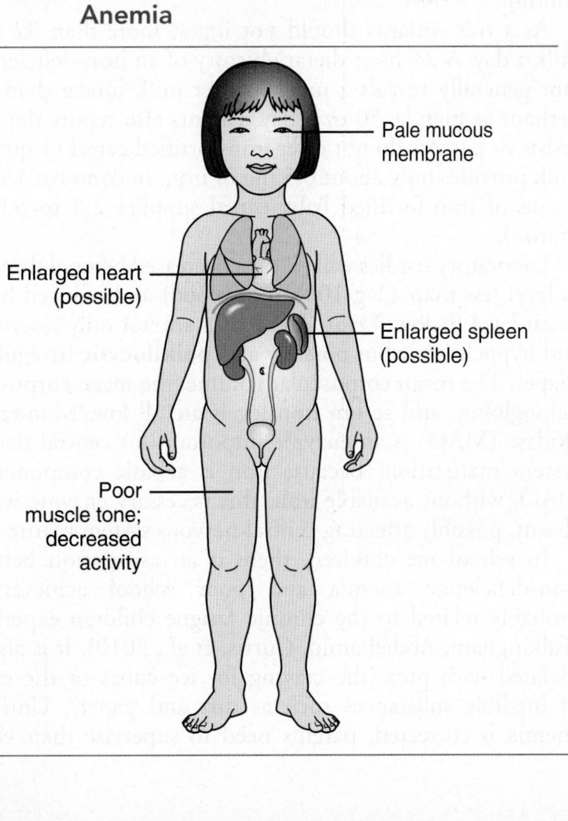

BOX 44.5 Nursing Care Planning Based on Responsibility for Pharmacology

FERROUS SULFATE (FEOSOL)

Classification: Ferrous sulfate is an iron salt.

Action: Supplies iron for red cell production. It elevates the serum iron concentration and then is converted to hemoglobin or trapped in the reticuloendothelial cells for storage and eventual conversion to a usable form of iron (Karch, 2013).

Pregnancy Risk Category: A

Dosage: For severe iron-deficiency anemia: 4 to 6 mg/kg/d, in three divided doses. For mild iron-deficiency anemia: 3 mg/kg/d in two divided doses.

Possible Adverse Effects: Gastrointestinal upset, anorexia, nausea, vomiting, constipation, dark stools, stained teeth (liquid preparations)

Nursing Implications

- Instruct parents to administer the drug on an empty stomach with water to enhance absorption. If this causes gastrointestinal irritation, administer it after meals. Avoid giving it with milk or tea because these interfere with absorption.
- If the liquid preparation is ordered, advise parents to mix it with water or juice to mask the taste. Have the child drink the medication through a straw to avoid staining the teeth.
- Remember that iron is absorbed best in the presence of an acid. Suggest parents give the iron with a citrus juice such as orange juice to help absorption. Some children may be prescribed vitamin C to take concurrently to increase absorption.
- Inform the child and parents that iron may turn stools black.
- Encourage parents to include high-fiber foods in the child's diet to minimize the risk of constipation.
- Reinforce the need for thorough brushing of teeth to prevent staining.
- Remind parents about the need for follow-up blood studies to evaluate the effectiveness of the drug.

is pale conjunctiva. Because this pallor develops slowly, however, parents may describe their child as "fair skinned" especially when their face develops the same pale appearance.

With extended iron deficiency, infants develop poor muscle tone and reduced activity. Their heart may enlarge and, on auscultation, demonstrate a soft systolic precordial murmur as the heart beats faster in an attempt to supply body cells with more oxygen. The spleen may be slightly enlarged. Fingernails typically become spoon shaped or depressed in contour.

As a rule, infants should not ingest more than 32 oz of milk a day. A 24-hour dietary history of an iron-deficient infant generally reveals a much higher milk intake than this, perhaps as high as 50 oz a day. Parents also report the child resists or parents do not offer iron-fortified cereal (1 quart of milk provides only about 0.5 mg of iron; in contrast, 1 tablespoon of iron-fortified baby cereal supplies 2.5 to 5.0 mg of iron).

Laboratory studies will reveal a decreased hemoglobin level (a level less than 11 g/100 ml of blood) and reduced hematocrit level (below 33%). The RBCs are not only microcytic and hypochromic but possibly also **poikilocytic** (irregular in shape). The mean corpuscular volume, the mean corpuscular hemoglobin, and serum iron levels are all low. Monoamine oxidase (MAO) is an enzyme important for central nervous system maturation. Because iron is a basic component of MAO, without available iron, this necessary enzyme will be absent, possibly affecting central nervous system maturation.

In school-age children, there is an association between iron-deficiency anemia and poor school achievement, probably related to the chronic fatigue children experience (Falkingham, Abdelhamid, Curtis, et al., 2010). It is also associated with pica (the craving for ice cubes or the eating of inedible substances such as dirt and paper). Until the anemia is corrected, parents need to supervise their child's environment to keep inedible materials out of his or her reach (Khan & Tisman, 2010).

Therapeutic Management. Therapy for iron-deficiency anemia focuses on treatment of the underlying cause: the lack of iron. An iron compound such as ferrous sulfate for 4 to 6 weeks is the drug of choice to improve RBC formation and replace iron stores (Box 44.5) (Costa, Bracco, Gomes, et al., 2011). In addition, the diet of the child must be changed to one rich in iron and vitamin C, which enhances iron absorption.

Nursing Diagnoses and Related Interventions

Nursing Diagnosis: Imbalanced nutrition, less than body requirements, related to inadequate ingestion of iron

Outcome Evaluation: Parents report child's dietary intake includes iron-rich foods; parents administer ferrous sulfate as prescribed; serum iron levels increase to normal by 6 months.

When planning care for an infant with iron-deficiency anemia, it is helpful to minimize the child's activities to prevent fatigue, particularly at mealtime, because a fatigued child is more reluctant to eat any food, let alone iron-rich foods.

Counsel parents on measures to improve their infant's nutrition, such as adding iron-rich foods while decreasing formula or breast milk intake. If the child is not fond of meat, suggest parents substitute cheese, eggs, green vegetables, or fortified cereal. Because iron-rich foods are often expensive, remind parents that these items are important and they should not substitute less expensive, high-carbohydrate foods for them. Help them also devise a reminder system so they can manage to give the iron supplement over a long period of time. Alert parents to possible side effects, such as stomach irritation, constipation, and that liquid iron preparations can stain teeth if not taken through a straw. Iron is absorbed best with an accompanying acid medium, so ascorbic acid may also be prescribed (or the parent should be advised to give the iron medication with orange juice) to increase absorption. To avoid constipation, the child may need additional fiber like that supplied by green leafy vegetables. If oral iron is not tolerated or if there is a doubt the child will take it, an iron–dextran injection (Imferon) can be given intramuscularly, although this is extremely irritating and stains the skin unless it is given by deep Z-track intramuscular injection.

Of all age groups, adolescents tend to do the least well with taking medicine consistently. Help them plan a daily time for taking their iron supplement with a medication reminder chart. At first, they may reject this as childish, but assure them that everyone needs some sort of aid to remember such things. Review with them the iron-rich foods they will need to eat daily and that an iron supplement is only a supplement if taken with iron-rich foods.

After 7 days of iron therapy, a reticulocyte count is usually obtained. If elevated, this means the child is now receiving enough iron that erythrocytes are now proliferating and correcting the anemia. Iron medication is taken for at least 4 to 6 weeks after the RBC count has returned to normal so iron stores are rebuilt as well. In some children, maintenance therapy may continue for as long as a year.

Chronic Infection Anemia

Acute infection interferes with RBC production, producing a normochromic, normocytic anemia. When infections are chronic, however, anemia of a hypochromic, microcytic type occurs, which is probably caused by impaired iron metabolism. The degree of anemia is rarely as severe as that occurring with iron deficiency; administration of iron will have little effect until the infection is controlled (Aguilar, Moraleda, Quintó, et al., 2012).

Macrocytic (Megaloblastic) Anemias

A macrocytic anemia is one in which the RBCs appear abnormally large (Lum, 2012). Such cells are actually immature erythrocytes or megaloblasts (nucleated immature red cells) so these anemias are often also referred to as megaloblastic anemias. Because these anemias are caused by nutritional deficiencies, they occur most often in developing countries.

Anemia of Folic Acid Deficiency

A deficiency of folic acid combined with vitamin C deficiency produces an anemia in which the erythrocytes grow abnormally large. There is often accompanying neutropenia and thrombocytopenia. Although the mean corpuscular hemoglobin concentration will be normal, the mean corpuscular volume and mean corpuscular hemoglobin will both be increased. Bone marrow contains megaloblasts, indicating inhibition of the production of erythrocytes at an early stage. Megaloblastic arrest, or inability of RBCs to mature past this early stage, may occur in the first year of life from the continued use of infant food containing too little folic acid or from an infant drinking goat's milk, which tends to be deficient in folic acid. Treatment is daily oral administration of folic acid. With this treatment, the response is dramatic.

Pernicious Anemia (Vitamin B_{12} Deficiency)

Vitamin B_{12} is necessary for the maturation of RBCs. Pernicious anemia results from a deficiency in or an inability of the body to use the vitamin (Scott & Molloy, 2012). In children, the cause is more often a lack of ingestion of vitamin B_{12} rather than poor absorption. Adolescents may be deficient in vitamin B_{12} if they are ingesting a long-term, poorly formulated vegetarian diet because the vitamin is found primarily in foods of animal origin (Andres, 2012).

For vitamin B_{12} to be absorbed from the intestine, an intrinsic factor must be present in the gastric mucosa. If a child is born with an intrinsic factor deficiency, symptoms occur as early as the first 2 years of life. The child appears pale, anorexic, and irritable, with chronic diarrhea. The tongue appears smooth and beefy red due to papillary atrophy. If not identified and treated at that point, neuropathologic findings such as ataxia, hyporeflexia, paresthesia, and a positive Babinski reflex will develop.

The rate and efficiency of absorption of vitamin B_{12} can be tested by the ingestion of the radioactively tagged vitamin when a dose of intrinsic factor is also measured. If the anemia is identified as being caused by a B_{12}-deficient diet, temporary injections of B_{12} will reverse the symptoms. If the anemia is caused by lack of the intrinsic factor, lifelong monthly intramuscular injections of B_{12} may be necessary.

Hemolytic Anemias

Hemolytic anemias are those in which the number of erythrocytes is low because there is increased erythrocyte destruction. The destruction may be caused by fundamental abnormalities in erythrocyte structure or by extracellular destruction forces.

Congenital Spherocytosis

Congenital spherocytosis is a hemolytic anemia that occurs most frequently in the white Northern European population and is inherited as an autosomal dominant trait. RBCs are small and have a short life span apparently due to abnormalities of the protein of the cell membrane that make them unusually permeable to sodium (Casale & Perrotta, 2011).

The anemia can be noticeable shortly after birth, although symptoms may not be recognized until later in the first year as the abnormal cells swell, rupture, and then are destroyed by the spleen creating a severe anemia. Chronic jaundice and splenomegaly also develop. Because the cells are so small, the mean corpuscular hemoglobin concentration will be increased. Gallstones may be present in older school-age children and adolescents because of the continuous hemolysis, bilirubin release, and incorporation of bilirubin into gallstones.

Infections can precipitate a crisis or cause bone marrow failure. During such a period, the anemia increases rapidly as the hemolysis continues. Blood transfusion will be necessary to maintain a sufficient number of circulating erythrocytes until the crisis passes.

The diagnosis of the disease is based on family history, the obvious hemolysis, and the presence of the abnormal spherocytes. The treatment generally is a splenectomy at approximately 5 to 6 years. This measure will increase the number of RBCs present but will not alter their abnormal structure.

Glucose-6-Phosphate Dehydrogenase Deficiency

The enzyme glucose-6-phosphate dehydrogenase (G6PD) is necessary for maintenance of RBC life; lack of the enzyme results in premature destruction of RBCs. The disease is transmitted as a sex-linked recessive trait and occurs most frequently in children of African American, Asian, Sephardic Jewish, and Mediterranean descent (approximately 10% of African American males have the disorder) (Panepinto & Scott, 2011).

G6PD disease occurs in two identifiable forms. Children with a congenital nonspherocytic type develop hemolysis, jaundice, and splenomegaly and may have aplastic crises. Other children have a drug-induced form in which the blood pattern is normal until the child is exposed to fava beans or drugs such as antipyretics, sulfonamides, antimalarials, and naphthoquinones (the most common drug in these groups is acetylsalicylic acid [aspirin]). Approximately 2 days after ingestion of such an oxidant drug, the child begins to show evidence of hemolysis, a low-grade fever, and perhaps back pain. A blood smear will show *Heinz bodies* (oddly shaped particles in RBCs).

The degree of RBC destruction depends on the drug and the extent of exposure to it. Occasionally, a newborn is seen with marked hemolysis because the mother ingested an initiating drug during pregnancy.

G6PD deficiency may be diagnosed by a rapid enzyme screening test or electrophoretic analysis of RBCs. The drug-induced type usually is self-limiting, and if a child is not exposed to substances that cause hemolysis, blood transfusions are rarely necessary. Be certain that both parents and children know about the abnormality in the child's metabolism so they can avoid common drugs such as acetylsalicylic acid.

Sickle-Cell Anemia

Sickle-cell anemia is an autosomal recessive inherited disorder carried on the β chain of hemoglobin; the amino acid valine takes the place of the normally appearing glutamic acid. With this, the erythrocytes become characteristically elongated and crescent shaped (sickled) when they are submitted to low oxygen tension (less than 60% to 70%), a low blood pH (acidosis), or increased blood viscosity, such as occurs with dehydration or hypoxia. When RBCs sickle or change to an elongated shape, they cannot move freely through vessels. Stasis and further sickling occurs (a *sickle-cell crisis*). Blood flow halts and tissue distal to the blockage becomes ischemic, resulting in acute pain and cell destruction (Linker & Damon, 2012).

Because fetal hemoglobin contains a γ, not a β, chain, the disease usually will not result in clinical symptoms until a child's hemoglobin changes from the fetal to the adult form at approximately 6 months. However, the disease can be diagnosed prenatally by chorionic villi sampling or from cord blood during amniocentesis. If these were not done, it will be identified at birth by neonatal screening (Forman, Coye, Levy-Fisch, et al., 2013).

Sickle-cell disease occurs in about 1 out of every 400 African American infants in the United States. The sickle-cell trait (a child carries a gene for the disease but does not have active symptoms) occurs in approximately 8% of African Americans (Hastings, Torkildson, & Agwaral, 2012).

The form of hemoglobin in this disorder is designated hemoglobin S. A child with sickle-cell disease is said to have hemoglobin SS (homozygous involvement). Both parents of the child with the disease will have a combination of usual adult and hemoglobin S types or be carriers (heterozygous) of the *sickle-cell trait* (hemoglobin AS). People with the trait produce enough normal hemoglobin to compensate for any hemoglobin that is sickled and therefore show no symptoms. A child with the disease (homozygous) produces no normal hemoglobin and so will demonstrate characteristic symptoms of sickle-cell anemia. A very few children have combinations of hemoglobin S and hemoglobin C or E, which leads to chronic mild anemia.

QSEN Checkpoint Question 44.3

Evidence-Based Practice

The sickle-cell trait (hemoglobin AS) occurs in about 8% of African Americans and, although typically benign, there is some concern that intense physical exercise in such individuals could lead to cardiac deaths from occlusive crises. To investigate if this occurs, researchers examined the U.S. Sudden Death in Athletes Registry. Of 271 African American football deaths in the registry, 7% (1 in 14) were known to have the sickle-cell trait. Each athlete experienced collapse with gradual deterioration over several minutes during vigorous or exhaustive physical exertion, usually during conditioning drills, typically early in the training season, and when the outdoor temperature was at or above 80°F (Harris, Haas, Eichner, et al., 2012).

Based on the previous study, which would be the best exercise for Joey, who has sickle-cell disease, and his father who has the sickle-cell trait?

a. Playing video games with each other
b. Joining a swimming program at their local YMCA
c. Watching sports together on TV each evening
d. Organizing a touch (no contact) football game each weekend

Look in Appendix A for the best answer and rationale.

Sickle-Cell Crisis. *Sickle-cell crisis* is the term used to denote a sudden, severe onset of sickling. There is pooling of many new sickled cells in blood vessels causing consequent tissue hypoxia beyond the blockage (a *vaso-occlusive crisis*). Such a crisis is most apt to occur when a child has a gastrointestinal illness causing dehydration, a respiratory infection that results in lowered oxygen exchange and a lowered arterial oxygen level, or after extremely strenuous exercise (enough to lead to tissue hypoxia); however, sometimes, no obvious cause of a crisis can be found (Boxes 44.6 and 44.7). Symptoms

BOX 44.6 Nursing Care Planning Using Assessment

Assessing a Child With Sickle-Cell Crisis

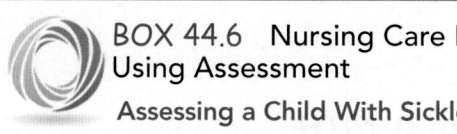

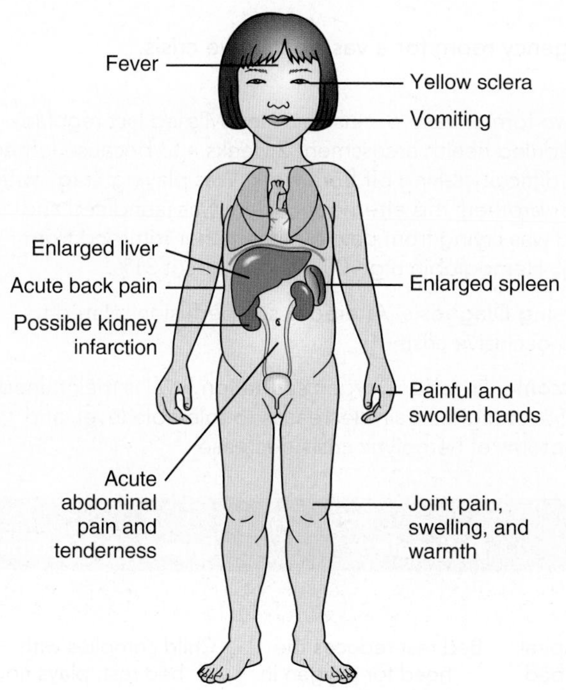

are sudden, severe, and painful (Box 44.8 Nursing Care Planning, an interprofessional care map for the child with sickle-cell anemia). A laboratory report will reveal a hemoglobin level of only 6 to 8 g/100 ml. A peripheral blood smear will demonstrate sickled cells. Bilirubin and reticulocyte levels will be increased and the WBC count is often elevated to 12,000 to 20,000/mm^3.

Further complications that may occur are aseptic necrosis of the head of the femur or humerus causing sharp joint pain or a cerebrovascular accident that occurs from a blocked artery, resulting in loss of motor function, coma, seizures, or even death. If there is renal involvement, hematuria or flank pain may be present.

Other types of crisis that may occur include:

- A *sequestration crisis* occurs when there is splenic sequestration of RBCs or severe anemia occurs due to pooling and increased destruction of sickled cells in the liver and spleen. Shock symptoms occur from hypovolemia. The spleen is enlarged and tender.
- A *hyperhemolytic crisis* occurs when there is increased destruction of RBCs.
- A *megaloblastic crisis* occurs if the child has folic acid or vitamin B deficiency (new RBCs cannot be fully formed due to lack of these ingredients).
- An *aplastic crisis* occurs when there is a sudden decrease in RBC production. This form usually occurs with infection. It creates a severe anemia.

Assessment for Sickle-Cell Anemia. Sickle-cell anemia is diagnosed at birth because of required blood-spot screening. At approximately 6 months of age, children begin to show initial signs of fever and anemia. Stasis of blood and infarction may occur in a body part, leading to local pain. Some infants

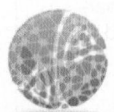

BOX 44.7 Nursing Care Planning Based on Effective Communication

Joey, who has sickle-cell disease, is seen in the emergency department with a new vaso-occlusive crisis. His right knee is discolored by a large brush burn. He's crying from pain.

Less Effective Communication

Nurse: Hello, Mr. Harrow. I need to ask some questions to see if anything triggered this new crisis.
Mr. Harrow: He better not have been doing something he's not allowed to do.
Nurse: His knee looks like he may have fallen. Were you running, Joey? So you got dehydrated?
Mr. Harrow: He better not say he was doing that.
Nurse: Joey, how did you hurt your knee?
Joey: I don't know.
Nurse: Okay. Let's get you better and not worry about what started this.

More Effective Communication

Nurse: Hello, Mr. Harrow. I need to ask some questions to see if anything triggered this new crisis.
Mr. Harrow: He better not have been doing something he's not allowed to do.
Nurse: His knee looks like he may have fallen. Were you running, Joey? So you got dehydrated?
Mr. Harrow: He better not say he was doing that.
Nurse: Mr. Harrow, why don't we let Joey tell us how he thinks the accident happened? Then later on, we can talk about what are good rules for him to be following.

Children with sickle-cell anemia have to follow what seems like a great many rules to avoid clotting or bleeding episodes, such as not playing contact sports or playing too hard in the sun. In an emergency room, it's important that both children and parents recognize the priority at the moment is obtaining an accurate history rather than assigning blame. Here, the nurse takes an active step to help the parent move past a broken rule so therapy can be started.

BOX 44.8 Nursing Care Planning

AN INTERPROFESSIONAL CARE MAP FOR A CHILD WITH SICKLE-CELL ANEMIA

Joey is a 7-year-old with sickle-cell anemia you see in the emergency room for a vaso-occlusive crisis.

Family Assessment Child lives with two older brothers (10 and 12 years of age) and both parents in a three-bedroom home. Father works as a distributor for a local water bottling company. Mother, an X-ray technician, is temporarily on duty with the National Guard in the Middle East. Father rates finances as, "Not good. Medical bills are killing us."

Client Assessment Thin, early school-age child with weight at fifth percentile for age. Was screened and diagnosed with sickle-cell anemia at birth. Described as "picky eater"; has eaten little since mother was deployed because he doesn't like father's cooking. Has a history of two former vaso-occlusive crises. Missed last regularly scheduled health assessment 2 weeks ago because father had difficulty taking off from work. Was playing "tag" with older brothers this afternoon. Sclera was jaundiced and child was crying from pain by time father returned from work. Hemoglobin 6 g/100 ml; hematocrit 31%.

Nursing Diagnosis Altered tissue perfusion related to vaso-occlusive crisis

Outcome Criteria Oxygen saturation level is maintained at 95% or higher, pain decreases to tolerable level, and symptoms of hemolytic crisis decrease.

Team Member Responsible	Assessment	Intervention	Rationale	Expected Outcome
Activities of Daily Living, Including Safety				
Nurse	Assess if child understands he will need to remain in bed.	Admit child to hospital unit; restrict to bed rest.	Bed rest reduces the need for oxygen in body cells.	Child complies with bed rest; plays non-action games with parent or health care personnel.
Teamwork and Collaboration				
Nurse/Primary care provider	Assess if hematology service is needed for consult.	Meet with hematology service as needed for emergency and long-range planning	Repeated vaso-occlusive crises suggest family needs better management strategies.	Hematology service meets with parent and child as indicated.
Procedures/Medications for Quality Improvement				
Nurse/Nurse practitioner	Assess degree of child's pain by use of FACES pain scale.	Administer prescribed analgesic as needed.	Vaso-occlusive crises can cause sharp pain that requires strong analgesia.	Child rates pain as no higher than 2 following analgesia administration.
Nurse	Assess oxygen saturation level by continuous pulse oximetry.	Administer oxygen by nasal prongs to keep oxygen saturation above 95% or as prescribed.	Oxygen saturation decreases because sickled cells are unable to carry a full complement of oxygen.	Child cooperates with pulse oximetry and oxygen administration. Oxygen saturation remains above 95%.
Nurse	Determine whether child has been taking folic acid and hydroxyurea at home.	Administer medications to initiate red blood cell (RBC) production as prescribed.	Folic acid and hydroxyurea help to build new RBCs to replace those that have been hemolyzed.	Child takes medication cooperatively.

Nutrition				
Nurse	Assess child's intake and output.	Begin oral rehydration or intravenous (IV) therapy as prescribed.	Restoring hydration reduces sickle-cell clotting.	Child names best hand to start IV infusion; drinks prescribed fluid.
Nurse/Nutritionist	Assess child's usual nutrition intake by 24-hour dietary recall history.	Demonstrate child's reduced weight to parent. Plan ways to increase calorie intake.	Even "picky eaters" need to take in enough food daily to meet growth and maintenance needs.	Parent states he will try harder to serve foods the child likes; child voices intent to eat at least one meat helping daily.
Patient-Centered Care				
Nurse	Assess family members' understanding of the causes of sickle-cell vaso-occlusive crises.	Review with family members the importance of child avoiding dehydration and oxygen deficiency.	Dehydration leads to clumping of sickled cells, cutting off circulation in distant body parts.	Family members state they are aware they must be as responsible as the child for avoiding sickling circumstances.
Psychosocial/Spiritual/Emotional Needs				
Nurse	Assess the stress level of family in light of absent mother and child with chronic illness.	Review with family ways to maintain a tight knit family unit (e.g., game night, common activities) to maintain family unity until mother returns.	When families miss a support person, they need to rally together to devise other support methods.	Father states he will try harder to meet children's needs, although worrying about keeping his job and his wife's safety are major concerns.
Informatics for Seamless Health Care Planning				
Nurse	Determine whether parent has any questions about care of his or her child.	Schedule a follow-up visit in 3 days following hospital discharge for evaluation as prescribed.	Care of a chronically ill child can be a major strain on a family. Follow-up visits help share responsibility for care.	Father states he understands importance of follow-up visit and will keep appointment with child.

have swelling of the hands and feet (a hand–foot syndrome) probably caused by aseptic infarction of the bones of the hands and feet. As they grow, children tend to have a slight build and characteristically long arms and legs. They may have a protruding abdomen because of an enlarged spleen and liver. In adolescence, the spleen size may decrease in size from repeated infarction and atrophy, leaving the teenager more susceptible to infection than usual because the spleen can no longer filter bacteria. Pneumococcal meningitis and salmonella-induced osteomyelitis become frequent illnesses; the child needs prophylactic antibiotics and pneumococcal and *Hib* vaccines to prevent these infections (Ngwube, Jackson, Dixon, et al., 2012).

During late childhood or adolescence, an acute chest syndrome with symptoms of fever, tachypnea, wheezing, or cough that leads to pneumonia may begin to occur (Livesay & Ruppert, 2012). The syndrome develops because, when areas of the lung become inflamed and hypoxic, sickle cells adhere to the irritated endothelium and then fail to be reoxygenated. Blood transfusion is used to increase the oxygen-carrying capacity of the blood, and broad-spectrum antibiotics are given to resolve the pneumonia.

Another change that may occur is stasis of blood flow because of cirrhosis of the liver (fibrotic degeneration), which will eventually occur from infarcts and tissue scarring. The kidneys may have subsequent scarring also, so kidney function may be decreased. Eye sclera become icteric (yellowed) from release of bilirubin from destruction of the sickled cells; small retinal occlusions may lead to decreased vision. Cell clusters in the blood vessels of the penis may cause **priapism**, or a persistent, painful erection (Linker & Damon, 2012).

Therapeutic Management. The child in a sickle-cell crisis has three primary needs: pain relief, adequate hydration, and oxygenation to prevent further sickling and halt the crisis.

Acetaminophen (Tylenol) may be adequate pain relief for some children; for others, a narcotic analgesic such as intravenous morphine may be necessary. Once children are pain free and able to relax, the metabolic demand for oxygen is reduced and sickling begins to end. Hydration is generally accomplished with intensive intravenous fluid replacement therapy. The acidosis that develops from tissue hypoxia must be corrected by electrolyte replacement. As a rule, because some kidney infarction may have occurred, do not administer potassium intravenously until kidney function has been determined (e.g., the child voids). Otherwise, excessive potassium levels can lead to cardiac arrhythmias. If infection appears to be the precipitator for a sickling crisis, blood and urine cultures, a chest X-ray, and a complete blood count will be taken and the infection will be treated by antibiotics. Blood transfusion (usually packed RBCs) may be necessary to maintain the hemoglobin above 12 g/100 ml (termed hypertransfusion) (Marouf, 2011).

Hydroxyurea, an antineoplastic agent that has the potential to increase the strength and oxygenation capacity of sickled cells (Ponnampalam & Thalange, 2013). Given orally, a side effect of the drug is anorexia, so children need their nutrition intake monitored while taking the drug to be certain it is adequate.

If none of the previous measures appears to be effective, children may be given an exchange transfusion to remove most of the sickled cells and replace them with normal cells. Hematopoietic stem cell transplantation is a permanent solution to the disorder and is advocated for the child who does not respond to usual therapies (Thompson et al., 2012).

QSEN Checkpoint Question 44.4

Quality Improvement

Joey, who has sickle-cell anemia, is being treated for sickle-cell crisis. Which statement by his father would best assure you that Joey is receiving adequate nursing care?

a. "He never used to understand why he had these crises, but now he can describe the reason."
b. "He says that his pain is actually quite manageable now."
c. "He says that the nurses he's met so far are such nice people."
d. "He's looking forward to getting home, but he really doesn't mind it here."

Look in Appendix A for the best answer and rationale.

Nursing Diagnoses and Related Interventions

Because, like most anemias, sickle-cell disease is a chronic process, nursing diagnoses need to consider both short- and long-term goals.

Nursing Diagnosis: Ineffective tissue perfusion related to generalized infarcts due to sickling

Outcome Evaluation: Child's respiratory rate is 16 to 20 breaths/min; cyanosis is absent; arterial blood gases within acceptable parameters, including Pco_2 = 40 mmHg, Po_2 = 80 to 90 mmHg, oxygen saturation of 95%; urine output greater than 1 ml/kg/hr.

Oxygen may be administered by either nasal cannula or mask if arterial blood gases reveal a low Po_2 level. High concentrations of oxygen are used with caution because hypoxia is a stimulant to erythrocyte production, which is badly needed to replace damaged cells. Monitor the flow rate carefully, therefore, and use pulse oximetry to evaluate oxygen saturation levels for changes. Encourage bed rest to reduce oxygen expenditure.

Nursing Diagnosis: Ineffective health maintenance related to lack of knowledge regarding long-term needs of child with sickle-cell anemia

Outcome Evaluation: Parents accurately describe disease process and identify special precautions necessary to prevent a sickle-cell crisis.

In many children, episodes of sickling grow less severe as the child reaches adolescence. Other children experience such devastating episodes in early childhood that, without a stem cell transplant, the disease becomes fatal at an early age.

Between crises, parents need to focus care on preventing recurring crises. Although the hemoglobin level of children may remain as low as 6 to 9 g/100 ml, children adjust well to this chronic state. Caution parents that children who receive frequent blood transfusions should not be given supplementary iron or iron-fortified formula or vitamins because they may receive too much iron; high levels of excess iron are deposited in body tissues (**hemochromatosis**) to a point of staining body tissue or being incorporated into body tissue with fibrotic scarring (hemosiderosis). Oral folic acid may be prescribed to help rebuild hemolyzed RBCs. They need to monitor urine output and may be asked to test urine for specific gravity and hematuria to detect the extent or presence of kidney damage occurring from minor infarcts. Some children who have had kidney infarcts and a lessened ability to concentrate urine have chronic nocturnal enuresis (bed-wetting).

Be certain that children receive childhood immunizations so they are not vulnerable to common childhood infections such as measles or pertussis and receive meningococcal, pneumococcal, and haemophilus influenzae type B vaccines to prevent those specific infections. If children are prescribed oral penicillin as prophylaxis against infection, help the parents determine a method to remember or remind conscientious administration of this.

Caution parents to bring their child to a health care facility at the first indication of infection. Some parents are reluctant to do this, afraid that they will be labeled overprotective. Assure them that health care personnel are knowledgeable about sickle-cell anemia and that they know that a child with even a minor infection could become very ill.

Children should attend regular school and should be allowed to participate in all school activities except contact sports (such as football), which could result in rupture of an enlarged spleen or liver. Long-distance running is also inadvisable because it can lead to dehydration. During the summer, parents need to offer the child frequent drinks to prevent dehydration, especially on long hikes and at the beach. Caution parents against taking the child on board an unpressurized aircraft in which the oxygen concentration may fall during flight.

Children with sickle-cell disease are at high risk if they need surgery because the hours of being held on nothing-by-mouth status, as well as being unable to eat afterward, may lead to dehydration; anesthesia may cause a transient hypoxia leading to sickling. Caution parents that even for a simple operation such as tooth extraction, they must alert health care personnel about their child's condition.

Because puberty is delayed in some children, both parents and children may need counseling to accept this; although they can be assured once puberty changes do occur, they are adequate and just appear later than usual. Children may need support and positive reinforcement during their growth years to enhance their self-esteem as they learn how to deal with the results of a chronic hematologic disorder (Box 44.9).

What if...44.2 Joey's parent tells you he restricts Joey, who has sickle-cell anemia, from drinking any fluid after 4 PM to prevent bed-wetting. Is this a good solution to bed-wetting for a child with sickle-cell disease? How would you counsel this parent?

Thalassemias

The thalassemias are autosomal recessive anemias associated with abnormalities of the β chain of adult hemoglobin (HgbA). Although these anemias occur most frequently in the Mediterranean population, they also occur in children of African and Asian heritage (Ponnampalam & Thalange, 2013).

Thalassemia Minor (Heterozygous β-Thalassemia)

Children with thalassemia minor, a mild form of this anemia, produce a combination of both defective β hemoglobin and normal hemoglobin. The condition represents the heterozygous form of the disorder and can be compared with children having the sickle-cell trait. Because there is some normal production, the RBC count is usually normal, but the hemoglobin concentration will be decreased by 2 to 3 g/100 ml below usual levels. The blood cells are moderately hypochromic and microcytic because of the poor hemoglobin formation.

Children may have no symptoms other than pallor. They require no treatment, and life expectancy is normal. They should not receive a routine iron supplement because their inability to incorporate it well into hemoglobin may cause them to accumulate too much iron.

Thalassemia Major (Homozygous β-Thalassemia)

Thalassemia major is also called Cooley anemia or Mediterranean anemia. It is diagnosed at birth by a blood spot test. Because this is a β-chain hemoglobin defect, symptoms do not become apparent until a child's fetal hemoglobin has largely been replaced by adult hemoglobin during the second half of the first year of life. Effects of thalassemia major on body systems are summarized in Table 44.3. Unable to produce normal β hemoglobin, the child shows symptoms of anemia, including pallor, irritability, and anorexia (Holstein & Hohl, 2012).

BOX 44.9 Nursing Care Planning Based on Family Teaching

SCHOOL SAFETY PRECAUTIONS FOR CHILDREN WITH SICKLE-CELL DISEASE

Q. Joey's father says to you, "What precautions should I discuss with my son's teacher so I know he's safe at school?"

A. Some common suggestions include:

- Be certain your child either takes fluid with him or buys adequate fluid for lunch because he needs to maintain a high fluid intake to prevent blood from becoming thick.
- Provide additional fluid in the summer, when dehydration is more apt to happen. Anticipate ways to provide fluid during long hikes or school trips; time spent on a hot beach may need to be limited.
- Learn about sources high in folic acid, such as vegetables and fruit, and be certain these foods are included in your son's packed lunch or selected from a cafeteria every day.
- With the exception of contact sports (to avoid damage to an enlarged spleen) and long-distance running (to prevent dehydration), encourage your son to participate in normal school activities.
- Know that bed-wetting may occur as part of the illness. Encourage your son to take baths in the morning if this occurs so his clothes don't smell of urine.
- Maintain routine health care such as immunizations to prevent common childhood illnesses such as measles and mumps, which cause fever and dehydration.
- Have the school nurse call you for any sign of illness, such as an upper respiratory infection, so therapy can be started immediately.

TABLE 44.3 Effects of Thalassemia Major

Body Organ or System	Effect of Abnormal Cell Production
Bone marrow	Overstimulation of bone marrow leads to increased facial-mandibular growth
Skin	Bronze-colored from hemosiderosis and jaundice
Spleen	Splenomegaly
Liver and gallbladder	Cirrhosis and cholelithiasis
Pancreas	Destruction of islet cells and diabetes mellitus
Heart	Failure from circulatory overload

RBCs are both hypochromic and microcytic. Fragmented poikilocytes and basophilic stippling (unevenness of hemoglobin concentration) are also usually present. The hemoglobin level is less than 5 g/100 ml. The serum iron level is high because iron is not being incorporated into hemoglobin; iron saturation will be 100%.

Assessment. To maintain a functional level of hemoglobin, the bone marrow hypertrophies in an attempt to produce more RBCs, causing bone pain and the formation of target cells or large macrocytes that are short lived and nonfunctional. The hyperactivity of the bone marrow results in characteristic changes in the shape of the skull (parietal and frontal bossing) and protrusion of the upper teeth, with marked malocclusion. The base of the nose may be broad and flattened; the eyes may be slanted with an epicanthal fold, as in Down syndrome. An X-ray of the bone shows marked osteoporotic (of lessened density) tissue, which can lead to fractures. The child may have both an enlarged spleen and liver due to excessive iron deposits and fibrotic scarring in the liver and the spleen from increased attempts to destroy defective RBCs. Abdominal pressure from the enlarged spleen may cause anorexia and vomiting. Epistaxis is common; diabetes mellitus may result from pancreatic hemosiderosis (deposition of iron); and cardiac dilatation with arrhythmias and heart failure may result in myocardial fibrosis caused by invasion of iron.

Therapeutic Management. Stem cell transplantation is the ultimate cure for the disorder. While waiting for a matched donor, digitalis, diuretics, and a low-sodium diet may be prescribed to prevent heart failure. Transfusion of packed RBCs every 2 to 4 weeks (hypertransfusion therapy) can be used to maintain hemoglobin between 10 and 12 g/100 ml because, with this level of hemoglobin, erythropoiesis is suppressed and cosmetic facial alterations, osteoporosis, and cardiac dilatation are minimized. Hypertransfusion therapy also reduces the possibility that a splenectomy will be necessary. Frequent blood transfusions, unfortunately, increase the risk of blood-borne diseases, such as hepatitis B, and hemosiderosis, so children need an oral iron-chelating agent to remove this excessive store of iron, such as deferasirox or deferoxamine (Berdoukas, Farmaki, Carson, et al., 2012).

A splenectomy may become necessary to reduce discomfort and also to reduce the rate of RBC hemolysis and the number of transfusions needed. Bone marrow stem cell transplantation can offer a cure. Even without stem cell transplantation, the overall prognosis of thalassemia is improving, although it is still grave. Most children with the disease die of cardiac failure during adolescence or as young adults if they do not receive a hematopoietic stem cell transplant.

Nursing Diagnoses and Related Interventions

Nursing Diagnosis: Risk for situational low self-esteem related to changed physical appearance

Outcome Evaluation: Child states she can accept altered appearance and interacts with peers.

Children with thalassemia major may have delayed growth and sexual maturation. They may develop a marked change in facial appearance because of the overgrowth of marrow-producing centers of the facial bones, which will be permanent. In addition, the child who receives frequent blood transfusions may develop such hemosiderosis that skin color appears bronze.

Children should be allowed as much activity as possible and should attend regular school to maintain a nearly normal childhood. Discussions about other children's reactions to their changing facial appearance and how people are evaluated by who they are and not what they look like can be helpful.

What if...44.3 The last time you saw Lana she was fair skinned, but at a clinic visit today you notice her skin looks a lot darker. She tells you she and her mother both spent time at a tanning salon to get ready for a vacation in the sun. Would you admire her new tan or worry if her darkened skin is caused by something else?

Autoimmune Acquired Hemolytic Anemia

Occasionally, autoimmune antibodies (abnormal antibodies of the immunoglobulin [Ig]G class) attach themselves to RBCs, destroying them or causing hemolysis. This can occur at any age, and its origin is generally unknown, although the disorder is associated with malignancy, viral infections, or collagen diseases such as rheumatoid arthritis or systemic lupus erythematosus. A child may recently have had an upper respiratory infection, measles, or varicella virus infection (chickenpox). The disorder may occur after the administration of drugs such as quinine, phenacetin, sulfonamides, or penicillin (Garratty, 2012).

Assessment. The onset of symptoms is insidious. Children usually develop a low-grade fever, anorexia, lethargy, pallor, and icterus from release of indirect bilirubin from the hemolyzed cells. Both urine and stools appear dark as the excess bilirubin is excreted. In a few children, the illness begins abruptly with high fever, hemoglobinuria, marked jaundice, and enlarged liver and spleen.

Laboratory findings reveal RBCs have become extremely small and round (spherocytosis). The reticulocyte count will be increased as the body attempts to form replacement RBCs. A direct Coombs test result is positive, indicating the presence of antibodies attached to red cells. Hemoglobin levels may fall as low as 6 g/100 ml.

Therapeutic Management. In some children, the disease process runs a limited course and no treatment is necessary. In others, a single blood transfusion may correct the disturbance. It is difficult to cross-match blood for transfusion for these children, however, because the red cell antibody tends to clump or agglutinate all blood tested. If cross-matching is impossible, the child may be given type O, Rh-negative blood, which doesn't need to match. Carefully observe the child especially during any transfusion for signs of transfusion reaction.

If anemia is persistent, corticosteroid therapy (oral prednisone) to reduce the immune response is generally effective, increasing the RBC count and hemoglobin concentration in a short period. If this is not effective, splenectomy or stronger immunosuppressive agents such as cyclophosphamide (Cytoxan) or azathioprine (Imuran) are necessary to reduce antibody formation.

Often, it is difficult for parents to understand the process causing their child's condition. How could their child's body turn on itself this way? How long will this last? What will stop it from happening again? Because there are no certain answers to these questions, provide parents and children with support as they wait for this unexplainable process to run its course and for their child to be well again.

QSEN Checkpoint Question 44.5

Teamwork & Collaboration

Autoimmune acquired hemolytic anemia can occur in any child. You would want your team members to know the usual cause of this disorder is:

a. Allergy to the protein found in fish or shrimp
b. A mutant gene similar to sickle-cell anemia
c. An elevated (increased) eosinophil cell count
d. Antibody production against red blood cells

Look in Appendix A for the best answer and rationale.

Polycythemia

Polycythemia is an increase in the number of RBCs (Giona, Teofili, Moleti, et al., 2012). The condition results from increased erythropoiesis, which occurs as a compensatory response to insufficient oxygenation of the blood in order to help supply more oxygen to body cells. Although this may occur as a hereditary form, chronic pulmonary disease and congenital heart disease are the usual causes of polycythemia in childhood. Also, it may occur from the lower oxygen level maintained during intrauterine life in newborns or with twin transfusion at birth (one twin receives excess blood while a second twin is anemic).

Plethora (marked reddened appearance of the skin) occurs because of the increase in total RBC volume. Erythrocytes are usually macrocytic (large) and the hemoglobin content is high. This means the mean corpuscular hemoglobin will be elevated; the mean corpuscular hemoglobin concentration, however, will be normal, indicating that, although many in number, each erythrocyte is normally saturated with hemoglobin. The RBC count may be as high as 7 million/mm^3. Hemoglobin levels may be as high as 23 g/100 ml.

Treatment of polycythemia involves treatment of the underlying cause. Because of the high blood viscosity from so many crowded blood cells, cerebrovascular accident or emboli may occur. The risk increases particularly if the child becomes dehydrated, such as with fever or during surgery. A program of low-dose aspirin to help prevent clotting, or exchange transfusion or phlebotomy to reduce the RBC count may be necessary.

DISORDERS OF BLOOD COAGULATION

Platelets are necessary for blood coagulation, so disorders that limit the number of platelets limit the effectiveness of this process. A normal platelet level is 150,000/mm^3. Thrombocytopenia (decreased platelet count) is defined as a platelet count of less than 40,000/mm^3. Thrombocytopenia often leads to purpura, or blood seeping from vessels into the skin. In one rare disorder, children are born with thrombocytopenia and are also missing the radius bone in the forearm (thrombocytopenia-absent radius [TAR] syndrome).

Purpuras

Purpura refers to a hemorrhagic rash or small hemorrhages in the superficial layer of skin. Two main types of purpura occur in children: idiopathic thrombocytopenia purpura and Henoch–Schönlein syndrome.

Idiopathic Thrombocytopenic Purpura

Idiopathic thrombocytopenic purpura (ITP) is the result of a decrease in the number of circulating platelets in the presence of adequate megakaryocytes (precursors to platelets). The cause is unknown, but it is thought to result from an increased rate of platelet destruction due to an antiplatelet antibody that destroys platelets, making this an autoimmune illness (Arnold, 2012).

In most instances, ITP occurs approximately 2 weeks after a viral infection such as rubella, rubeola, varicella, or an upper respiratory tract infection. Congenital ITP may occur in the newborn of a woman who has had ITP during pregnancy. An antiplatelet factor apparently crosses the placenta and causes platelet destruction in the newborn in the same way that Rh incompatibility or hemolytic disease of the newborn develops (see Chapter 26). However, in ITP, the platelets, not the RBCs, are sensitized.

Assessment. Manifestations often begin abruptly, first evidenced as miniature petechiae or as large areas of asymmetric ecchymosis most prominent over the legs, although they may occur anywhere on the body (Fig. 44.3). Epistaxis or bleeding into joints may be present.

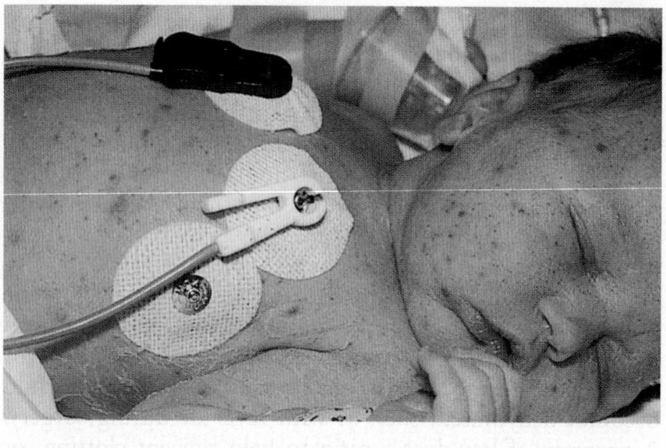

FIGURE 44.3 An infant with idiopathic thrombocytopenia purpura (ITP). Notice the tiny petechiae and larger ecchymotic areas. (From Zitelli, B. J., & Davis, H. W. [1997]. *Atlas of pediatric physical diagnosis* [3rd ed.]. St. Louis, MO: Mosby–Year Book, Inc.)

Laboratory studies reveal marked thrombocytopenia. The platelet count may be as low as 20,000/mm^3. Bone marrow examination reveals a normal number of megakaryocytes.

Therapeutic Management. Oral prednisone to reduce the immune response and intravenous immunoglobulin (IVIG) or, in Rh-positive children, anti-D immunoglobulin to supply anti-ITP antibodies are used to treat ITP. Platelet transfusion will temporarily increase the platelet count, but because the life span of platelets is relatively short, a platelet transfusion has only limited effect. Children with central nervous system bleeding may require a splenectomy, although this is rarely necessary.

If the child experiences joint pain from bleeding, acetaminophen (Tylenol) rather than salicylates or ibuprofen is prescribed for pain because both salicylates and ibuprofen increase the chance for bleeding as they prevent the aggregation of platelets at wound sites.

In most children, ITP runs a limited, 1- to 3-month course. A few children develop chronic ITP. A course of immunosuppressive drugs may be attempted if the chronic state persists. All children need to be vaccinated against the viral diseases of childhood so that diseases such as rubella, rubeola, and varicella are eradicated and can no longer lead to this defective coagulation process.

Nursing Diagnoses and Related Interventions

Nursing Diagnosis: Health-seeking behaviors related to injury-prevention measures

Outcome Evaluation: Parents state precautions they will take to reduce possibility of bleeding, repeat correct dose and timing of medication therapy, child's skin is free of ecchymotic areas, and platelet count rises to normal values.

The techniques for reducing bleeding described earlier in the chapter, such as padding surfaces where the child plays (see Box 44.3), can be used to reduce the possibility of bleeding for the child with ITP. Parents cannot eliminate the possibility of a serious bleeding injury, however, until the platelet count returns to normal. The chief danger to the child from ITP, aside from the psychological stress of a perplexing illness, is intracranial hemorrhage. Although this is rare, be alert for signs such as persistent headache, nuchal rigidity, and lethargy.

Nursing Diagnosis: Risk for compromised family coping related to diagnosis of child's illness

Outcome Evaluation: Parents state that they understand the nature of their child's illness and have identified ways to carry out daily activities despite the illness.

Because symptoms such as the easy bruising of ITP mimics the beginning signs of leukemia, parents may be extremely frightened when symptoms first occur. You can assure them after the diagnosis is made that this bruising is not and will not lead to leukemia. A child may have so many bruises that the parents are initially suspected of child maltreatment. This can cause them to become very defensive and angry at health care personnel. Allow them time to express their anger and regain confidence in their health care team.

It is always bewildering for parents to be told that no one knows exactly what is causing their child's illness. To feel comfortable that health care personnel can manage their child's care without knowing the exact cause, parents need careful explanations of all procedures.

Henoch–Schönlein Syndrome

Henoch–Schönlein purpura (also called anaphylactoid purpura) is caused by increased vessel permeability. Although no definite allergic correlation can be identified, it is generally considered to be a hypersensitivity reaction to an invading allergen. It occurs most frequently in children between 2 and 8 years of age, and more frequently in boys than girls (Liu & Zhang, 2012). Usually, there is a history of a mild infection before the outbreak of symptoms. The syndrome presents (because of the purpura) as a possible platelet disorder until a differential diagnosis is made.

Assessment. The purpural rash occurs typically on the buttocks, posterior thighs, and extensor surface of the arms and legs (Fig. 44.4). The tips of the ears may be involved. The rash begins as a crop of urticarial lesions that change to pink maculopapules. These become hemorrhagic (bright red) and then fade, leaving brown macular spots that remain for several weeks. The child's joints are tender and swollen. The child may have gastrointestinal symptoms such as abdominal pain, vomiting, or blood in stools. Gross or microscopic hematuria may be present from kidney involvement. A biopsy shows **granulocytes** (white blood cells) in the walls of small arterioles.

Laboratory studies show a normal platelet count. The child's sedimentation rate, WBC count, and eosinophil count are elevated.

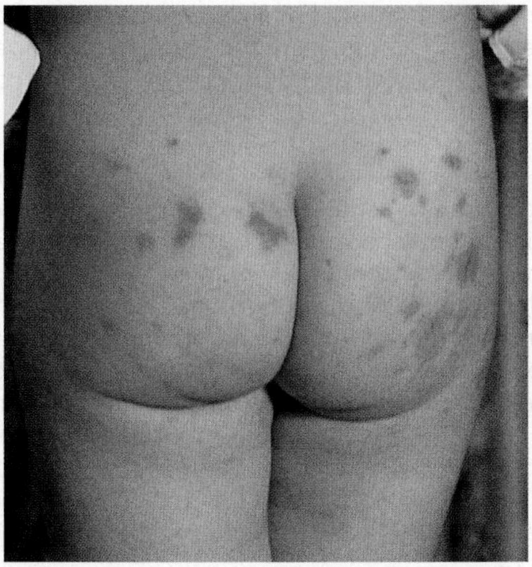

FIGURE 44.4 The distinctive purpural rash of Henoch–Schönlein syndrome appearing on the buttocks of a young child. (From Zitelli, B. J., & Davis, H. W. [1997]. *Atlas of pediatric physical diagnosis* [3rd ed.]. St. Louis, MO: Mosby–Year Book, Inc.)

Therapeutic Management. Treatment involves oral corticosteroid therapy (prednisone) and mild analgesics for a short period. Nose and throat cultures rule out continuing bacterial involvement. Urine should be assessed for protein and glucose to detect kidney involvement. Typically, the disease runs a course of 4 to 6 weeks. A few children develop chronic nephritis as a complication (Jauhola, Ronkainen, & Koskimies, 2012).

QSEN Checkpoint Question 44.6

Safety

Suppose Lana develops idiopathic thrombocytopenia purpura (ITP) after a viral infection. Which of the following would be an important nursing action?

a. Caution Lana and her mother that she will bruise easily.
b. Show Lana how to do a finger-stick test for glucose.
c. Tell Lana to report if she develops a sharp headache.
d. Show her mother how to test Lana's urine for protein.

Look in Appendix A for the best answer and rationale.

Hemophilias

Hemophilias are inherited disorders of blood coagulation. There are numerous types, each involving a deficiency of a different blood coagulation factor.

Hemophilia A (Factor VIII Deficiency)

The classic form of hemophilia is caused by deficiency of the coagulation component factor VIII, the antihemophilic factor, and transmitted as a sex-linked recessive trait. In the United States, the incidence is approximately 1 in 10,000 white males. A female carrier may have slightly lowered but sufficient levels of the factor VIII component so that she does not manifest a bleeding disorder. Males with the disease also have varying levels of factor VIII; their bleeding tendency varies accordingly, from mild to severe (Chitlur & Kulkarni, 2013).

Factor VIII is an intrinsic factor of coagulation; its absence causes the intrinsic system for manufacturing thromboplastin to be incomplete. The child's coagulation ability is not totally absent because the extrinsic or tissue system remains intact. Because of this system, the child's blood will eventually coagulate after an injury.

Assessment. Hemophilia often is recognized first in the infant who bleeds excessively after circumcision. If the disease has not shown itself for several generations in a family, the parents may be unaware of its existence. For this reason, all infants need careful and thoughtful observation after circumcision. Because infants do not receive many injuries, children's bleeding tendencies may not become apparent until they become active (e.g., crawling, climbing, or walking).

Suddenly, the lower extremities (where the child bumps things) become heavily bruised. There is soft tissue bleeding and painful hemorrhage into joints, which become swollen and warm. Repeated bleeding into a joint this way causes damage to the synovial membrane (hemarthrosis), possibly resulting in severe loss of joint mobility (Solimeno, Luck, Fondanesche, et al., 2012).

Severe bleeding may also occur into the gastrointestinal tract, peritoneal cavity, or central nervous system. Although nosebleeds are common, they are not as severe as with the platelet deficiency syndromes. The platelet count and prothrombin time are both normal; the whole blood clotting time is either markedly prolonged or normal, depending on the level of factor VIII present. A thromboplastin generation test will be abnormal. Partial thromboplastin time (PTT) is the test that best reveals the low levels of factor VIII. It's important that children with hemophilia be identified by such tests before surgery; otherwise, fatal bleeding could occur.

Therapeutic Management. With even minor abrasions, bleeding can be controlled by the administration of factor VIII supplied by fresh whole blood, fresh or frozen plasma, or a concentrate of factor VIII. The concentrate is supplied as a powdered form that can be stored at home and reconstituted as needed. For most bleeding episodes, one bag of concentrate per 5 kg of body weight is usually sufficient to provide protection for approximately 12 hours; another transfusion may be necessary after that time. In some children, the administration of desmopressin (DDAVP), which stimulates the release of factor VIII, may also help prevent bleeding.

In a few children, antibodies (termed inhibitors) to factor VIII develop, rendering the factor ineffective. If this happens, ε-aminocaproic acid, a fibrinolytic enzyme that helps to stabilize clot formation and promote wound healing, can be self-administered every 6 hours if needed. Children with inhibitors to factor VIII can also be given a factor IX concentrate (Proplex or Konyne). This concentrate enters the coagulation cascade after factor VIII and halts bleeding at that point.

Nursing Diagnoses and Related Interventions

Nursing Diagnosis: Parental health-seeking behaviors related to strategies for protecting child from injury

Outcome Evaluation: Child's skin is free of ecchymotic areas, frequent epistaxis is absent, blood pressure is within age-appropriate parameters, and swelling or warmth at joints is absent.

Parents need information both about how to prevent bleeding episodes and how to respond when one does occur. To help prevent injuries, help parents set appropriate limits for activity. An active infant, for example, may need to have crib sides padded and all toys should be inspected for sharp edges or parts. Older children need to self-monitor activities such as roughhousing and sports participation needs to be evaluated as to whether it will be safe. On the other hand, parents need to be certain their child is not so inactive that obesity occurs (Wong, Majumdar, Adams, et al., 2011).

Parents (and the child at about age 10 years) can be taught to reconstruct and administer a replacement factor intravenously to prevent bleeding immediately after an injury. Although the child needs to be assessed by a health care provider, this action, combined with pressure applied to the bleeding site, immobilization of the injured extremity, and an ice pack applied locally, almost always eliminates the need for hospital admission. "Butterfly bandages" are used in place of suturing for lacerations whenever possible, because sutures create additional puncture sites that could bleed.

Nursing Diagnosis: Pain related to joint infiltration by blood

Outcome Evaluation: Child states pain is at a tolerable level.

The child with hemophiliac bleeding experiences discomfort because of the bleeding into joints and may be frightened because his parents are so frightened. Acetaminophen (Tylenol) rather than ibuprofen is ordered as an analgesic because ibuprofen may prolong bleeding. As soon as effective levels of factor VIII have been provided, the pain in the bleeding joint is generally relieved, despite the continued heat or swelling. Be certain that when joints are immobilized, they are in good alignment. As soon as the acute bleeding episode has halted (approximately 48 hours), help the child perform passive range of motion as prescribed to maintain function.

Nursing Diagnosis: Risk for interrupted family processes related to fears regarding child's prognosis and long-term nature of illness

Outcome Evaluation: Family members voice their fear regarding illness, state they are able to cope despite stress level, and demonstrate positive coping responses.

Parents of children with hemophilia are frightened during a time of acute bleeding, not just because of what is currently happening but also because they may have seen other family members or even a previous child die of the disease. Be certain to give them a chance to talk about how the bleeding began (e.g., "I should have noticed that toy had a sharp edge," "He fell from his bike. I should have watched him more closely"). It is extremely important for parents to allow the child to lead a normal life, so remind them when they do this that it is impossible to prevent all injuries (Neufeld, Recht, Sabio, et al., 2012).

von Willebrand Disease

von Willebrand disease, an inherited autosomal dominant disorder, affects both sexes and is often referred to as angiohemophilia (Blombäck, Eikenboom, Lane, et al., 2012). Along with a factor VIII defect, there is also an inability of the platelets to aggregate and the blood vessels to constrict to aid in coagulation. Bleeding time is prolonged, with most hemorrhages occurring from mucous membrane sites.

Epistaxis is a major problem, because all children tend to rub or pick at their nose as a nervous mechanism. In girls, menstrual flow is unusually heavy and may cause embarrassment from stained clothing. Childbirth is obviously a risk for women with von Willebrand disease, so women must be monitored closely for 9 months and again during the postpartal period (Weiss, 2012). Bleeding is controlled with factor VIII replenishment as with hemophilia, or by administration of DDAVP, which stimulates factor VIII release.

Christmas Disease (Hemophilia B, Factor IX Deficiency)

Christmas disease, caused by factor IX deficiency, is transmitted as a sex-linked recessive trait. Only approximately 15% of people with hemophilia have this form. Treatment is with a concentrate of factor IX, which is available for home administration (Linker & Damon, 2012).

Hemophilia C (Factor XI Deficiency)

Hemophilia C, or plasma thromboplastin antecedent deficiency, is caused by factor XI deficiency, is transmitted as an autosomal recessive trait, and occurs in both sexes. The symptoms are generally mild compared with those in children with factor VIII or factor IX deficiencies. Bleeding episodes are treated with administration of DDAVP or transfusion of fresh blood or plasma.

Disseminated Intravascular Coagulation

Disseminated intravascular coagulation (DIC) is an acquired disorder of blood clotting that results from excessive trauma or some similar underlying stimulus, such as an acute infection or trauma (Rote & McCance, 2012).

A child begins to develop petechiae or have uncontrolled bleeding from puncture sites from injections or intravenous therapy. Ecchymoses and petechiae form on the skin. Observe all children with a serious illness carefully for signs such as these of increased bleeding to help identify that this is happening. DIC is also discussed in Chapter 21 as a frequent complication of bleeding disorders in pregnancy.

What if... 44.4 You are particularly interested in exploring one of the 2020 National Health Goals with respect to hematologic disorders and children (see Box 44.1). What would be a possible research topic to explore pertinent to this goal that would be applicable to Lana's or Joey's family and that would also advance evidence-based practice?

Key Points for Review

- Hematopoietic stem cell transplantation is the main therapy for numerous blood dyscrasias. Transplantation can be allogeneic (from a histocompatible donor), autologous (using the child's own marrow or umbilical cord blood), or syngeneic (the donor and recipient are identical twins).
- Splenectomy, another possible treatment, may increase a child's susceptibility to pneumococcal infections. Assess whether a child has received pneumococcal vaccine after a splenectomy.
- Disorders of the RBCs that commonly occur in children include acute blood loss anemia and anemia of acute infection. Aplastic and hypoplastic anemias occur from depression of hematopoietic activity in bone marrow. These anemias can be congenital or acquired.
- A major hypochromic anemia that develops in children is iron-deficiency anemia. Children invariably fatigue easily because they cannot oxygenate body cells well. Their care must include measures to keep them from tiring; oxygen administration may be necessary.
- Macrocytic anemias occur from folic acid deficiency and pernicious anemia (vitamin B_{12} deficiency).
- Hemolytic anemias include congenital spherocytosis, glucose-6-dehydrogenase deficiency, sickle-cell anemia, thalassemia, and autoimmune acquired hemolytic anemia. Sickle-cell anemia occurs most often in African American children.
- Disorders of blood coagulation include the purpuras (ITP and Henoch–Schönlein syndrome), DIC, and the hemophilias.
- Children with blood coagulation disorders must carefully guard against injury. This includes monitoring types of toys and activities. It may also include padding a crib or side rail.
- Disorders of the blood tend to be long-term illnesses. Education of the parents and child is important to promote adaptation to the condition and enhance long-term medication therapy that not only meets QSEN competencies but also best meets a family's total needs.

Critical Thinking Care Study

Tooley James is a 12-year-old you meet at an emergent care clinic. Tooley has sickle-cell anemia and is awaiting a stem cell transplant. He had a splenectomy 2 years ago. He lives with his older sister Michele (18 years of age), his mother (32 years of age), and his grandmother (76 years of age). Tooley's mother works two jobs to support the family (as an assembly line worker making paper products during the day and as a waitress at a local restaurant in the evening). Tooley is responsible for taking his folic acid and his hydroxyurea daily as well as "staying clear of infections" independently.

1. He's at the clinic today because "a kid shoved him" on his way home from school. His sister offered to bring him to the hospital, but because she has a cold Tooley refused to ride in the car with her. By the time his mother returned home from her second job his right knee was visibly swollen, he had pain "all over," and was gasping for breath. Tooley knows it's important to avoid infections, but did he make a good decision about his care?
2. Tooley needs some emergency measures in your clinic. What are the three main measures you anticipate he will need? Should you explore further how his injury happened?
3. Tooley's mother tells you Tooley's school grades have fallen from Bs to Cs and Ds over the past year. When you ask him why this is happening, he tells you, "If I don't get a transplant, how will it matter what my grades are?" Is that a typical preadolescent attitude or would you worry Tooley is becoming depressed about his situation?

Patient Scenario

The Winston Family

Read about the Winston family, a family with a child with a hematologic disorder, then answer the questions to further sharpen your skills and grow more familiar with NCLEX-type questions related to hematologic disorders. Confirm your answers are correct by reading the rationales.

Visit http://thePoint.lww.com

Answers and Rationales

Looking for answers to the What If. . . and Critical Thinking Care Study questions?

Visit http://thePoint.lww.com

References

Aguilar, R., Moraleda, C., Quintó, L., et al. (2012). Challenges in the diagnosis of iron deficiency in children exposed to high prevalence of infections. *PloS One, 7*(11), e50584.

Alousi, A. M., Bolaños-Meade, J., & Lee, S. J. (2013). Graft-versus-host disease: State of the science. *Biology of Blood & Marrow Transplantation, 19*(1, Suppl.), S102–S108.

Andres, E. (2012). Pernicious anemia & other megaloblastic anemias. In E. T. Bope & R. D. Kellerman (Eds.), *Conn's current therapy* (pp. 842–844). Philadelphia, PA: Elsevier/Saunders.

Arnold, D. M. (2012). Immune thrombocytopenia: Getting back to basics. *American Journal of Hematology, 87*(9), 841–842.

Berdoukas, V., Farmaki, K., Carson, S., et al. (2012). Treating thalassemia major-related iron overload: The role of deferiprone. *Journal of Blood Medicine, 2112*(3), 119–129.

Blombäck, M., Eikenboom, J., Lane, D., et al. (2012). von Willebrand disease biology. *Haemophilia, 18*(Suppl. 4), 141–147.

Casale, M., & Perrotta, S. (2011). Splenectomy for hereditary spherocytosis: Complete, partial or not at all? *Expert Review of Hematology, 4*(6), 627–635.

Chitlur, M., & Kulkarni, R. (2013). Hemophilia & related conditions. In E. T. Bope & R. D. Kellerman (Eds.), *Conn's current therapy* (pp. 803–809). Philadelphia, PA: Elsevier/Saunders.

Cooke, L., Grant, M., & Gemmill, R. (2012). Discharge needs of allogeneic transplantation recipients. *Clinical Journal of Oncology Nursing, 16*(4), E142–E149.

Costa, J. T., Bracco, M. M., Gomes, P. A., et al. (2011). Prevalence of anemia among preschoolers and response to iron supplementation. *Journal of Pediatrics, 87*(1), 76–79.

Deng, X. G., Maharjan, A., Tang, J., et al. (2012). A modified laparoscopic splenectomy for massive splenomegaly in children with hematological disorder: A single institute retrospective clinical research. *Pediatric Surgery International, 28*(12), 1201–1209.

Falkingham, M., Abdelhamid, A., Curtis, P., et al. (2010). The effects of oral iron supplementation on cognition in older children and adults: A systematic review and meta-analysis. *Nutrition Journal, 25*(9), 4–5.

Forman, J., Coyle, F., Levy-Fisch, J., et al. (2013). Screening criteria: The need to deal with new developments and ethical issues in newborn metabolic screening. *Journal of Community Genetics, 4*(1), 59–67.

Garratty, G. (2012). Immune hemolytic anemia caused by drugs. *Expert Opinion on Drug Safety, 11*(4), 635–642.

Giona, F., Teofili, L., Moleti, M. L., et al. (2012). Thrombocythemia and polycythemia in patients younger than 20 years at diagnosis: Clinical and biologic features, treatment, and long-term outcome. *Blood, 119*(10), 2219–2227.

Harris, K. M., Haas, T. S., Eichner, E. R., et al. (2012). Sickle cell trait associated with sudden death in competitive athletes. *American Journal of Cardiology, 110*(8), 1185–1188.

Hastings, C. A., Torkildson, J. C., & Agwaral, A. K. (2012). Sickle cell disease. In C. A. Hastings, J. C. Torkildson, & A. K. Agwaral (Eds.), *Handbook of pediatric hematology & oncology* (2nd ed., pp. 18–35). Hobokin, NJ: John Wiley & Son.

Hjortholm, N., Jaddini, E., Hałaburda, K., et al. (2013). Strategies of pain reduction during the bone marrow biopsy. *Annals of Hematology, 92*(2), 145–149.

Holstein, S. A., & Hohl, R. J. (2012). Thalassemia. In E. T. Bope & R. D. Kellerman (Eds.), *Conn's current therapy* (pp. 865–869). Philadelphia, PA: Elsevier/Saunders.

Jauhola, O., Ronkainen, J., & Koskimies, O., et al. (2012). Outcome of Henoch-Schönlein purpura 8 years after treatment with a placebo or prednisone at disease onset. *Pediatric Nephrology, 27*(6), 933–939.

Jenerette, C., Brewer, C. A., Crandell, J., et al. (2012). Preliminary validity and reliability of the sickle cell disease health-related stigma scale. *Issues in Mental Health Nursing, 33*(6), 363–369.

Karch, A. M. (2013). *2013 Lippincott's nursing drug guide*. Philadelphia, PA: Lippincott Williams & Wilkins.

Khan, Y., & Tisman, G. (2010). Pica in iron deficiency: A case series. *Journal of Medical Case Reports, 12*(4), 86.

Kitney, L., Kanani, R., & De Souza, C. (2012). A Jehovah's Witness adolescent with pancytopenia. *Canadian Medical Association Journal, 184*(9), 1055–1059.

Kline, N. E. (2012). Alterations of hematologic function in children. In S. E. Huether & K. L. McCance (Eds.), *Understanding pathophysiology* (5th ed., pp. 535–550). New York, NY: Elsevier Publishing.

Korthof, E. T., Békássy, A. N., & Hussein, A. A. (2013). Management of acquired aplastic anemia in children. *Bone Marrow Transplantation, 48*(2), 191–195.

Linker, C. A., & Damon, L. E. (2012). Blood disorders. In J. E. McPhee & M. A. Papadakis (Eds.), *Current medical diagnosis and treatment* (51st ed., pp. 475–519). Columbus, OH: McGraw-Hill/Lange.

Liu, A., & Zhang, H. (2012). Detection of antiphospholipid antibody in children with Henoch-Schönlein purpura and central nervous system involvement. *Pediatric Neurology, 47*(3), 167–170.

Livesay, S., & Ruppert, S. D. (2012). Acute chest syndrome of sickle cell disease. *Critical Care Nursing Quarterly, 35*(2), 183–195.

Lum, G. M. (2012). Kidney and urinary tract. In W. W. Hay, M. J. Levine, J. M. Sondheimer, et al. (Eds.), *Current pediatric diagnosis & treatment* (20th ed., pp. 717–739). Columbus, OH: McGraw-Hill.

Marouf, R. (2011). Blood transfusion in sickle cell disease. *Hemoglobin, 35*(5–6), 495–502.

Morinet, F., Leruez-Ville, M., Pillet, S., et al. (2011). Concise review: Anemia caused by viruses. *Stem Cells, 29*(11), 1656–1660.

Moschonis, G., Chrousos, G. P., Lionis, C., et al. (2012). Association of total body and visceral fat mass with iron deficiency in preadolescents. *British Journal of Nutrition, 108*(4), 710–719.

Neufeld, E. J., Recht, M., Sabio, H., et al. (2012). Effect of acute bleeding on daily quality of life assessments in patients with congenital hemophilia with inhibitors and their families. *Value in Health, 15*(6), 916–925.

Ngwube, A., Jackson, S., Dixon, T., et al. (2012). Disseminated Salmonella osteomyelitis in a 2-year-old with sickle cell disease. *Clinical Pediatrics, 51*(6), 594–601.

Panepinto, J. A., & Scott, J. P. (2011). Hematology. In. K. J. Marcdante, R. M. Kliegman, H. B. Jenson, et al. *Nelson essentials of pediatrics* (6th ed., pp. 555-584.). Philadelphia, PA: Saunders/Elsevier.

Petrini, C. (2013). Ethical issues in umbilical cord blood banking: A comparative analysis of documents from national and international institutions. *Transfusion, 53*(4), 902–910.

Ponnampalam, J., & Thalange, N. (2013). Blood & cancer. In N. Thalange, R. Beach, D. Booth, et al. (Eds.), *Essentials of paediatrics* (2nd ed., pp. 59–78). Philadelphia, PA: Elsevier/Saunders.

Rodeghiero, F., & Ruggeri, M. (2012). Short- and long-term risks of splenectomy for benign haematological disorders: Should we revisit the indications? *British Journal of Haematology, 158*(1), 16–29.

Rote, N. S., & McCance, K. L. (2012). Structure & function of the hematologic system. In S. E. Huether & K. L. McCance (Eds.), *Understanding pathophysiology* (5th ed., pp. 477–495). New York, NY: Elsevier Publishing.

Rovó, A., Tichelli, A., & Dufour, C. (2012). Diagnosis of acquired aplastic anemia. *Bone Marrow Transplantation, 48*(2), 162–167.

Sakaguchi, H., Nakanishi, K., & Kojima, S. (2013). Inherited bone marrow failure syndromes in 2012. *International Journal of Hematology, 97*(1), 20–29.

Schwartz, A., Rote, N. S., & McCance, K. L. (2012). Alterations of hematologic function. In S. E. Huether & K. L. McCance (Eds.), *Understanding pathophysiology* (5th ed., pp. 500–534). New York, NY: Elsevier Publishing.

Scott, J. M., & Molloy, A. M. (2012). The discovery of vitamin b(12). *Annals of Nutrition & Metabolism, 61*(3), 239–245.

Solimeno, L., Luck, J., Fondanesche, C., et al. (2012). Knee arthropathy: When things go wrong. *Haemophilia, 18*(Suppl. 4), 105–111.

Studdiford, J. S., Conniff, K. M., Trayes, K. P., et al. (2012). Bedbug infestation. *American Family Physician, 86*(7), 653–658.

Theurich, S., Fischmann, H., Shimabukuro-Vornhagen, A., et al. (2012). Polyclonal anti-thymocyte globulins for the prophylaxis of graft-versus-host disease after allogeneic stem cell or bone marrow transplantation in adults. *Cochrane Database of Systematic Reviews,* (9), CD009159.

Thompson, L. M., Ceja, M. E., & Yang, S. P. (2012). Stem cell transplantation for treatment of sickle cell disease: Bone marrow versus cord blood transplants. *American Journal of Health-System Pharmacy. 69*(15), 1295–1302.

U.S. Department of Health and Human Services. (2010). *Healthy people 2020*. Washington, DC: Author.

Weiss, J. A. (2012). Just heavy menses or something more? Raising awareness of von Willebrand disease. *American Journal of Nursing, 112*(6), 38–44.

Wong, T. E., Majumdar, S., Adams, E., et al. (2011). Overweight and obesity in hemophilia: A systematic review of the literature. *American Journal of Preventive Medicine, 41*(6, Suppl. 4), S369–S375.

Zempsky, W. T., Palermo, T. M., Corsi, J. M., et al. (2013). Daily changes in pain, mood and physical function in children hospitalized for sickle cell disease pain. *Pain Research & Management, 18*(1):33–38.

Ziegler, E. E. (2011). Consumption of cow's milk as a cause of iron deficiency in infants and toddlers. *Nutrition Reviews, 69*(Suppl. 1), S37–S42.

Chapter 45

Nursing Care of a Family When a Child Has a Gastrointestinal Disorder

KEY TERMS

- beriberi
- dehydration
- gastroesophageal reflux
- inguinal hernia
- insensible loss
- intussusception
- keratomalacia
- kwashiorkor
- liver transplantation
- McBurney's point
- Meckel's diverticulum
- necrotizing enterocolitis
- nutritional marasmus
- overhydration
- pellagra
- rickets
- scurvy
- steatorrhea
- volvulus
- xerophthalmia

OBJECTIVES

After mastering the contents of this chapter, you should be able to:

1. Describe common gastrointestinal disorders seen in children.
2. Identify 2020 National Health Goals related to gastrointestinal disorders in children that nurses can help the nation achieve.
3. Assess a child with a gastrointestinal disorder.
4. Formulate nursing diagnoses for a child with a gastrointestinal disorder.
5. Identify expected outcomes for a child with a gastrointestinal disorder as well as how to manage seamless transitions across differing health care settings.
6. Using the nursing process, plan nursing care that includes the six competencies of Quality & Safety Education for Nurses (QSEN): Patient-Centered Care, Teamwork & Collaboration, Evidence-Based Practice (EBP), Quality Improvement (QI), Safety, and Informatics.
7. Implement nursing care for a child with a gastrointestinal disorder, such as preparing the child for surgery.
8. Evaluate expected outcomes for achievement and effectiveness of care.
9. Integrate knowledge of gastrointestinal disorders in children with the interplay of nursing process, the six competencies of QSEN, and Family Nursing to promote quality maternal and child health nursing care.

Barry Abraham is a 2-year-old boy diagnosed with celiac disease who you see at a birthday party. His abdomen is protuberant, yet his arms and legs seem thin and wasted. He refuses to eat a piece of birthday cake even though his mother sits beside him insisting he eat it. "See the problem I have with him?" she asks you. "He eats nothing. When he does, he gets diarrhea."

Previous chapters described the growth and development of well children and the nursing care for children with disorders of other systems. This chapter adds information about the dramatic changes, both physical and psychosocial, that can occur when children develop gastrointestinal disorders. Such information builds a base for care and health teaching for children with these disorders.

Does Barry's mother understand her son's disease? Is she choosing wise food selections for him?

Because the gastrointestinal (GI) system is so long and so diverse, a multitude of possible disorders can occur along the tract, including both congenital disorders and acquired illnesses. Also, because the GI system is responsible for taking in and processing nutrients for all parts of the body, any problem with the system can quickly affect other body systems and, if not adequately treated, can affect overall health, growth, and development (Sachar & Walfish, 2013).

Because it can be difficult to appreciate the seriousness of a GI illness, parents often are surprised to learn that what they thought was a simple "stomach flu" has caused a serious electrolyte imbalance and possibly a life-threatening state for their child. Some GI disorders require both parents and the child to learn new nutritional patterns. As children grow older, counseling to help them maintain self-esteem and learn nutritional requirements so they can become independent is vital. Food poisoning and hepatitis are examples of GI illnesses that are so pervasive that 2020 National Health Goals have been set to limit their incidence (Box 45.1).

BOX 45.1 Nursing Care Planning Based on 2020 National Health Goals

Nutrition deficiencies, unsafe food preparation, and hepatitis are three areas that could be reduced in incidence if people knew more about them and took active interventions to reduce their occurrence or spread. 2020 National Health Goals addressing these include:

- Increase the contribution of fruits and vegetables to the diets of the population aged 2 years from 0.5 cup of fruits per 1,000 calories to 0.9 cup per 1,000 calories.
- Achieve and maintain effective vaccination coverage levels for universally recommended vaccines among young children and older (three doses of hepatitis B vaccine and two doses of hepatitis A vaccine by 19 to 35 months of age).
- Reduce infections caused by key pathogens transmitted commonly through food (including *Escherichia coli* (from 200 to 180 cases per year), *Listeria* (from 0.3 to 0.2 cases per 100,000 population per year), and *Salmonella* (from 15.2 to 11.4 cases per 100,000 population per year).
- Increase the proportion of consumers who follow key food safety practices of "Chill: refrigerate promptly" from 88.1% to 91.1% (U.S. Department of Health and Human Services [DHHS], 2010; see www.healthypeople.gov).

Nurses can help the nation achieve these goals by counseling parents about safe food preparation and the need for children to ingest adequate fiber from fruit and vegetables for sound bowel function, by serving as consultants to day care providers to reduce the spread of stool contamination and by actively administering hepatitis A and B vaccines to infants and adolescents to eradicate these forms of the illness in another generation.

Nursing Process Overview

For a Child With a Gastrointestinal Disorder

Assessment

Children with GI disorders quickly need to be assessed for signs of fluid loss, such as poor skin turgor, dry mucous membranes, or lack of tearing. When talking to parents about a child's symptoms, ask exactly what they mean when they say "spitting up" or "a little vomiting" to be certain you're talking about the same amount. Also ask how many times a child has voided or how many diapers have been wet in the past 24 hours, and whether this is less than usual. Compare the child's current weight with past weight measurements, if available. Unless the child is an adolescent who has been actively dieting, there is never a normal reason for weight loss in children.

As a rule, all children with diarrhea, especially small children, need to be seen by a health care provider because fluid and electrolyte changes occur rapidly in children because of the greater percentage of fluid held extracellularly rather than intracellularly.

For many children, a GI tract disorder is largely diagnosed by presenting symptoms such as those just described. In other instances, X-ray studies with a contrast medium (barium) or an endoscopic examination may be needed to confirm the presence of an anomaly. Ultrasound or magnetic resonance imaging (MRI) also may be helpful. Another important assessment area is laboratory testing for electrolyte balance through serum analysis or fluid concentration through urinalysis.

Nursing Diagnosis

Nursing diagnoses relevant to children with GI disorders invariably center on imbalanced nutrition because most GI diseases alter the kind and amount of nutrients ingested or absorbed into the body in some way. In addition, because feeding is one of the primary ways mothers bond with their newborns and the process of eating and the types of food eaten are integral components of family life and culture, any disruption caused by an illness can place a strain on the entire family. Examples of nursing diagnoses include:

- Impaired parenting related to interference with establishing the parent–infant bond
- Interrupted family processes related to a chronic illness in child
- Risk for deficient fluid volume related to chronic diarrhea
- Imbalanced nutrition, less than body requirements, related to malabsorption of necessary nutrients
- Situational low self-esteem related to feelings of being different resulting from special dietary restrictions

Outcome Identification and Planning

Be certain when helping plan a new nutritional pattern for a child that you include the person who actually prepares or supervises the child's nutrition. In many instances, some of the foods that a child eats are prepared by a babysitter, day care center staff, the child's other parent, or a grandparent. Many children eat breakfast and lunch at school cafeterias. That means it may be necessary to contact school staff to ask them to make meal exceptions for a child or to supervise a choice of foods (or to see that a child eats only the packaged lunch brought to school, not extra items the child trades for with friends).

Some parents are unfamiliar with basic food categories and the importance of providing food from the MyPlate nutrition guidelines (www.ChooseMyPlate.gov). When a special diet is requested, parents may have little understanding of which foods have high or low fiber content, or which foods are "bland" or "clear." Many parents have difficulty keeping children restricted to nothing by mouth (NPO) for tests or to rest the GI tract because they know dehydration happens quickly in infants (which is true). They need support to follow the necessary restrictions when this action is so opposed to basic parenting, such as giving food.

If feedings will be given by nasogastric or gastrostomy tube, parents need enough practice to be proficient with the equipment and the technique before they are given the responsibility of doing it alone at home. If a child is going to gag or become distressed when a new oral or nasal tube is passed, parents need to have this happen where there are calm, supportive people nearby, not when they are by themselves at home.

Agencies that might be helpful for referral to parents are the Celiac Disease Foundation (www.celiac.org), the Crohn's & Colitis Foundation of America (www.ccfa.org), the International Foundation for Functional Gastrointestinal Disorders (www.iffgd.org), and the North American Society for Pediatric Gastroenterology and Nutrition (www.naspgn.org).

Implementation

Never underestimate the difficulty family members may experience adapting to alternative nutrition methods such as total parenteral nutrition, enteric or gastrostomy feedings, or caring for a child with a colostomy. Parents need a great deal of support to adapt their busy life to these alternative methods of feeding or care.

GI disorders that occur at birth are discussed in Chapter 27. Insertion of a nasogastric tube, enteral and parenteral nutrition, and administration of an enema are discussed in Chapter 37. Be certain to give clear, simple explanations, and praise both parents and child after they demonstrate these procedures. Children can easily interpret enemas as punishment because of the extreme intrusiveness. Provide therapeutic play before and after these procedures to reduce children's anxiety.

Outcome Evaluation

Recording children's height and weight is a primary method to evaluate nutritional outcomes. Even if a diet is limited in a special way, if it is adequate, children should gain weight and maintain growth.

Because children will ultimately be responsible for their own nutrition, expected outcomes should include making certain children gradually learn more about their specific nutritional measures so they can become increasingly responsible for their own intake. Often, only when they are at this stage can their parents feel secure enough to let them stay overnight with a friend, visit a relative in a distant city, or go to summer camp—activities that become important to children as they reach school age.

Children who require special nutritional plans need to be evaluated for self-esteem at periodic health visits. Do children think of themselves as inferior to or different from others because of food restrictions? What kind of positive experiences can be offered to such children, or what can parents do to provide children with experiences that would improve self-esteem?

Some examples of expected outcomes include:

- Child lists examples of gluten-free foods to select for lunch from the school cafeteria menu.
- Parent states steps she will take to seek medical care if her child has a second episode of severe diarrhea.
- Family members state they have adjusted to care of their child with liver disease.

ANATOMY AND PHYSIOLOGY OF THE GASTROINTESTINAL SYSTEM

Digestion occurs the same in children and infants as it does in adults beginning with the mouth, where food is broken down into small particles and mixed with saliva. Digestion continues in the stomach and small intestine.

The esophagus pierces the diaphragm to serve as a passageway to the stomach (Fig. 45.1). At the junction of the esophagus and the stomach is the gastroesophageal (cardiac) sphincter. In some newborns, this sphincter is so lax that fluid regurgitates into the esophagus (gastroesophageal reflux). At the distal end of the stomach is the pyloric sphincter. In some infants, this valve is narrowed (stenosed), preventing food from flowing out of the stomach freely (pyloric stenosis). Originally, it was believed that the stomach was sterile because the action of hydrochloric acid could easily kill invading organisms and limit infections. However, since the discovery that a bacterium, *Helicobacter pylori*, is the cause of peptic ulcer disease, it is now obvious that organisms can and do survive in the stomach. The small intestine is divided into three sections: the duodenum, the jejunum, and the ileum. The large intestine is divided into the cecum, the ascending colon, the transverse colon, the descending colon, the sigmoid colon, and the rectum. The appendix, which frequently becomes diseased in children, is attached to the cecum.

DIAGNOSTIC AND THERAPEUTIC TECHNIQUES

Several typical procedures, such as a fiber optic endoscopy, small intestine wireless enteroscopy, colonoscopy, and a barium enema, are used in the diagnosis and therapy of GI disorders (Barth, 2011). Children need good preparation for all of these procedures because they are all potentially frightening (Hardee, 2012). If children receive conscious sedation for a procedure, they need preparation for this as well as for the actual procedure.

Therapy may include alternative methods of feeding such as enteral (nasogastric or gastrostomy tube feedings) or nutrition sources such as total parenteral nutrition and intravenous (IV) therapy to rest the GI tract. A colostomy or ileostomy may be created to further rest the GI tract. Because

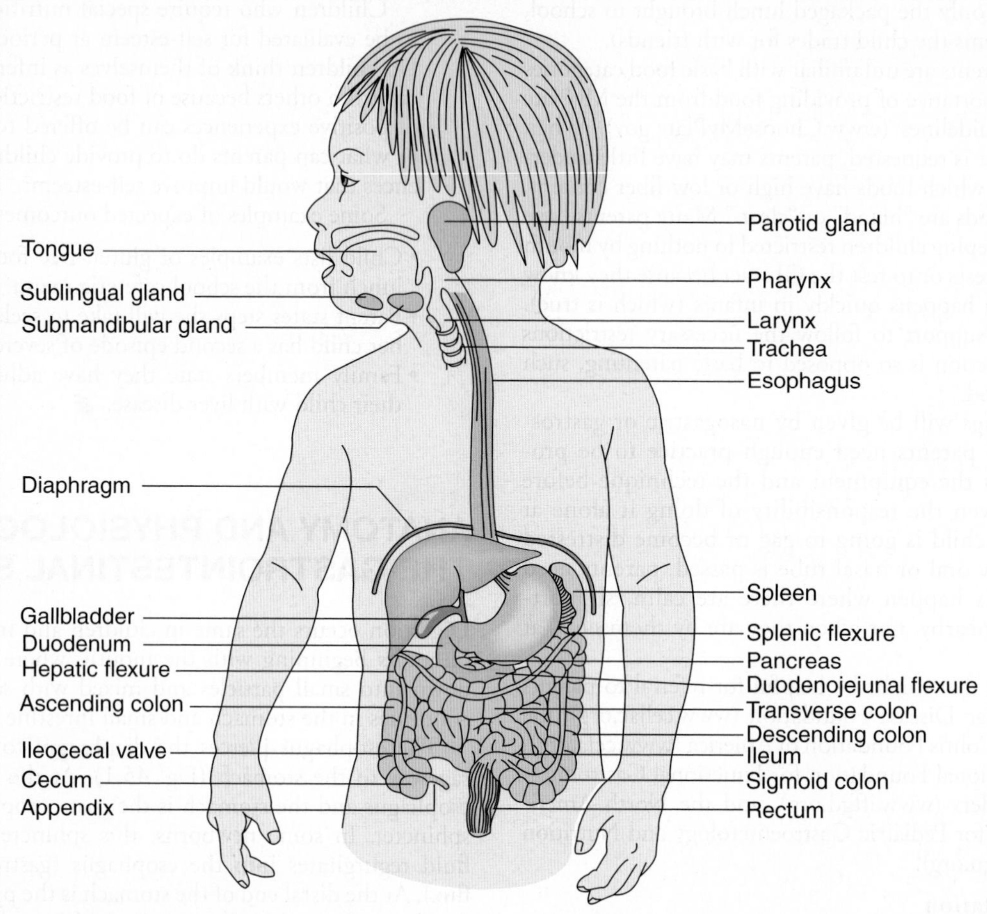

FIGURE 45.1 The gastrointestinal tract.

these are used for other disorders as well, these procedures, their meaning, their impact on children, and nursing responsibilities are discussed in Chapters 37 and 38.

HEALTH PROMOTION AND RISK MANAGEMENT

Health promotion related to GI disorders focuses on a wide area because the causes of these disorders cover a wide range. Some disorders, such as appendicitis, cannot be prevented because they occur from unpredictable causes. Other disorders, such as celiac disease (sensitivity or abnormal immunologic response to protein), involve genetic aspects that cannot be changed. Still others, such as Crohn disease and ulcerative colitis, are associated with an autoimmune response. Other conditions, such as vomiting and diarrhea, are often caused by foods that were refrigerated improperly or are spread through improper hand washing and so can be prevented. Hepatitis can be prevented through good hand washing (for hepatitis A) and immunization (for both hepatitis A and B). Vitamin and protein deficiency disorders can be prevented by educating parents about the importance of a consistently healthy diet. A vaccine to prevent rotavirus infections (taken by mouth so it is painless) is recommended for infants (Centers for Disease Control and Prevention [CDC], 2011).

Because any interference in nutrition pervades many aspects of children's lives, families often need help with planning care. Help families plan the necessary adaptations to their lifestyle to prevent the disease from interfering with family functioning (e.g., Will day care center personnel do gastrostomy feedings? Will a nursery school accept a child with a colostomy? Can a child select a gluten-free diet at the school cafeteria?). All families should be encouraged to eat at least one meal a day together so they can have time to share experiences and "touch base" with each other. For the family with a child who has a feeding problem such as a gastrostomy feeding or total parenteral nutrition, this can be difficult. Urge such families to bring the child to the table for a social time even if the child cannot eat with the family. If watching family members eat while the child cannot eat is too difficult, urge the family to provide a "together" time in some other way so the child does not miss out on this valuable family activity.

Some GI disorders in children, such as aganglionic megacolon, are diagnosed late because parents think the child's refusal to eat is just the sign of being a "picky eater" or a manifestation of 2-year-old autonomy. Educating parents about normal nutrition and how to distinguish things such as vomiting from illness from normal "spitting up," or severe diarrhea from a simple GI upset helps parents bring their children for care at the earliest possible time. Early intervention prevents the child from becoming dehydrated and seriously ill.

FLUID, ELECTROLYTE, AND ACID–BASE IMBALANCES

Because the GI system is the main route by which substances are taken into the body, it can be a major source of fluid and electrolyte loss if vomiting or diarrhea occurs (Smith, 2011). Retaining fluid is of greater importance in the body chemistry of infants than that of adults because fluid constitutes a greater fraction of the infant's total weight. In adults, body water accounts for approximately 60% of total weight. In infants, it accounts for as much as 75% to 80% of total weight; in children, it averages approximately 65% to 70%.

Fluid is distributed in three body compartments: (a) intracellular (within cells), 35% to 40% of body weight; (b) interstitial (surrounding cells), 20% of body weight; and (c) intravascular (blood plasma), 5% of body weight. Together, the interstitial and the intravascular fluid are often referred to as *extracellular fluid* (ECF), totaling 25% of body weight. In infants, the extracellular fluid portion is much greater, totaling up to 45% of total body weight (Fig. 45.2). In young children, this amount is 30%; in adolescents, it is 25%.

Fluid is normally obtained by the body through oral ingestion of fluid and by the water formed in the metabolic breakdown of food. Primarily, fluid is lost from the body in urine and feces. Minor losses **(insensible losses)** occur from evaporation from skin and lungs and from saliva, which is of little importance except in children with tracheostomies or those requiring nasopharyngeal suction. Infants do not concentrate urine as well as adults because their kidneys are immature. As a result, they have a proportionally greater loss of fluid in their urine. In infants, the relatively greater surface area to body mass also causes a greater insensible loss. When diarrhea occurs, or when a child becomes diaphoretic because of fever, the fluid output can be markedly increased, quickly leading to **dehydration** (excessive loss of fluid) (Porth, 2011). To avoid dehydration, fluid requirements for infants and children are shown in Table 45.1.

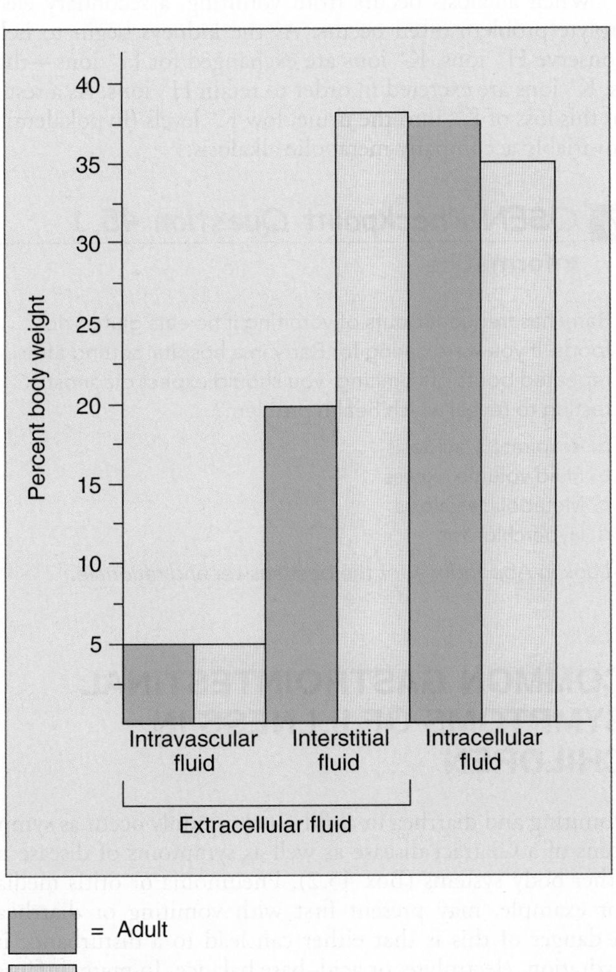

FIGURE 45.2 The distribution of fluid in body compartments.

TABLE 45.1 A Method to Calculate Fluid Requirement

Body Weight	Fluid Requirement per 24 Hours
Up to 10 kg	100 ml/kg
11–20 kg	1,000 ml + 50 ml/kg for each additional kilogram over 10 kg
More than 20 kg	1,500 ml + 20 ml/kg for each additional kilogram over 20 kg

Fluid Imbalances

Under most circumstances, water and salt are lost in proportion to each other, termed *isotonic dehydration*. Occasionally, water is lost out of proportion to salt, and water depletion or *hypertonic dehydration* occurs. If electrolytes are lost out of proportion to water, this is termed *hypotonic dehydration*. Each of these abnormal states produces specific symptoms.

Isotonic Dehydration

Isotonic dehydration occurs when a child's body loses more water than it absorbs (as with diarrhea) or absorbs less fluid than it excretes (as with nausea and vomiting). The main result of isotonic dehydration is a decrease in the volume of blood serum. Typical signs and symptoms of isotonic dehydration are summarized in Table 45.2.

TABLE 45.2 Signs and Symptoms of Dehydration

	Isotonic	Hypotonic	Hypertonic
Thirst	Mild	Moderate	Extreme
Skin turgor	Poor	Very poor	Moderate
Skin consistency	Dry	Clammy	Moderate
Skin temperature	Cool	Cool	Warm
Urine output	Decreased	Decreased	Decreased
Activity	Irritable	Lethargic	Very lethargic
Serum sodium level	Normal	Reduced	Increased

What if... 45.1 Barry's mother tells you her primary care provider has told her to "force fluids" for Barry whenever he has diarrhea. She asks how much she should force the child to drink. How would you answer her?

Hypertonic Dehydration

When water is lost in a greater proportion than electrolytes, hypertonic dehydration occurs. This might occur in a child with nausea (thus preventing fluid intake) and fever (which increases fluid loss through perspiration); profuse diarrhea, where there is a greater loss of fluid than salt; or renal disease associated with polyuria such as nephrosis with diuresis. Electrolytes such as sodium, chloride, and bicarbonate concentrate in the blood. The red blood cell count and hematocrit will be elevated because the blood is more concentrated than usual. Additional signs and symptoms are summarized in Table 45.2.

Hypotonic Dehydration

With hypotonic dehydration, there is a disproportionately high loss of electrolytes in proportion to fluid loss. The plasma concentration of sodium and chloride are low. This could result from excessive loss of electrolytes by vomiting, from an increased loss of salt from diuresis, or from diseases such as adrenocortical insufficiency or diabetic acidosis. In order to achieve an electrolyte balance, the kidneys begin to excrete more fluid to bring the proportion of electrolytes and fluid back in balance, leading to a secondary extracellular dehydration (see Table 45.2).

Overhydration

Overhydration, or excessive body fluid intake, can be as serious as dehydration. It generally occurs in children who are receiving IV fluid and can lead to cardiovascular and cardiac failure.

When large quantities of salt-poor fluid (hypotonic solutions) such as tap water are ingested or are given by enema, the body transfers water from the extracellular space into the intracellular space to restore normal osmotic relationships. This transfer results in intracellular edema manifested by a headache, nausea, vomiting, dimness and blurring of vision, cramps, muscle twitching, and seizures. A situation in which intracellular edema may occur is when tap water enemas are given to a child with aganglionic disease of the intestine.

Acid–Base Imbalance

When vomiting or diarrhea occurs, the GI system often is involved with two severe acid–base imbalances: metabolic acidosis and metabolic alkalosis. Whether body serum is becoming acidotic is determined by analyzing a sample of arterial blood for blood gases. The pH of blood is normally slightly alkaline, ranging from 7.35 to 7.45. The amount of dissolved carbon dioxide in arterial blood (Pco_2) is normally 35 to 45 mmHg. The level of bicarbonate (HCO_3) in arterial blood is normally 22 to 26 mEq/L.

Metabolic Acidosis

Metabolic acidosis results from diarrhea because a great deal of sodium is lost with stool. This excessive loss of Na^+ causes the body to conserve H^+ ions in an attempt to keep the total number of positive and negative ions in serum balanced. With metabolic acidosis, an arterial blood gas analysis will reveal a decreased pH (under 7.35) and a low HCO_3 value (near or below 22 mEq/L). The lower the HCO_3 value is, the more Na^+ ions that have presumably been lost or the more extensive the diarrhea has been. The child breathes rapidly (hyperpnea) to "blow off" CO_2 to prevent it from combining with H_2O and reforming HCO_3. Urine becomes more acidic as ammonia formation in the urine is increased.

Metabolic Alkalosis

With vomiting, a great deal of hydrochloric acid is lost. When Cl^- ions are lost this way, the body has to decrease the number of H^+ ions present so the number of positive and negative charges remains balanced. This causes the child to become alkalotic because the number of H^+ ions becomes proportionately lower than the number of OH^- ions present. The lungs attempt to conserve CO_2 and water by slowing respirations (hypopnea). The excessive CO_2 retained by this maneuver dissolves in the blood as carbonic acid and then is converted into excessive H^+ and HCO_3^-. With metabolic alkalosis, therefore, the serum HCO_3 will invariably be high. The higher the value, presumably the more Cl^- ions have been lost or the more extensive the vomiting has been. The child will breathe slowly and shallowly; pH will be elevated (near or above 7.45), and HCO_3 level will be near or above 28 mEq/L.

When alkalosis occurs from vomiting, a secondary electrolyte problem often occurs. As the kidneys begin to help conserve H^+ ions, K^+ ions are exchanged for H^+ ions—that is, K^+ ions are excreted in order to retain H^+ ions. As a result of this loss of K^+ into the urine, low K^+ levels (hypokalemia) invariably accompany metabolic alkalosis.

QSEN Checkpoint Question 45.1

Informatics

Barry has frequent bouts of vomiting if he eats gluten-rich foods. If you were caring for Barry in a hospital setting after repeated bouts of vomiting, you should expect diagnostic testing to reveal which health problem?

a. Respiratory acidosis
b. Fluid volume excess
c. Metabolic alkalosis
d. Hyperchlorosis

Look in Appendix A for the best answer and rationale.

COMMON GASTROINTESTINAL SYMPTOMS OF ILLNESS IN CHILDREN

Vomiting and diarrhea in children commonly occur as symptoms of a GI tract disease as well as symptoms of disease in other body systems (Box 45.2). Pneumonia or otitis media, for example, may present first with vomiting or diarrhea. A danger of this is that either can lead to a disturbance in hydration, electrolyte, or acid–base balance. In many infants, vomiting and diarrhea can be more threatening to the child than the primary disease.

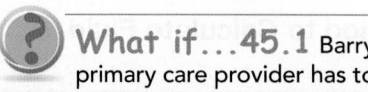

BOX 45.2 Nursing Care Planning Using Assessment

Assessing a Child With Altered Gastrointestinal Function

History

Chief concern: Vomiting, diarrhea, constipation, abdominal pain, abdominal distention, weight below normal standard, lethargy, paleness.
Past medical history: History of past vomiting or diarrhea or abdominal pain; hydramnios in pregnancy.
Family history: Relatives have a similar disorder; high stress level because of home or school environment.

Physical examination

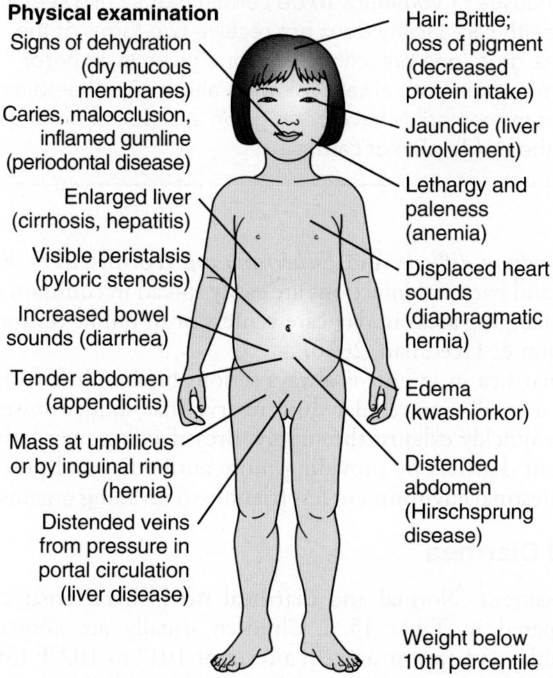

Vomiting

Many children with vomiting are suffering from a mild gastroenteritis (infection) caused by a viral or bacterial organism. The adolescent who is pregnant may mistake the normal nausea and vomiting of pregnancy for an illness. Some children develop persistent or cyclic vomiting (Lee, Abbott, Mahlangu, et al., 2012).

Assessment

In describing symptoms of vomiting, be certain to differentiate between the various terms that are used (Table 45.3). It is important that vomiting be thoroughly described this way because different conditions are marked by different forms of vomiting, and a correct description of the child's actions can aid greatly in a diagnosis.

Therapeutic Management

The treatment for vomiting is to withhold food from the stomach for a time because, if there is nothing in the stomach, vomiting cannot occur. Many parents treat vomiting in the opposite way. Every time a child vomits, they attempt to feed the child again. The child vomits again and they feed again, and so on. This prolongs the vomiting and intensifies the potential for electrolyte imbalance.

Nursing Diagnoses and Related Interventions

Nursing Diagnosis: Risk for deficient fluid volume related to vomiting

Outcome Evaluation: Skin turgor remains good; specific gravity of urine is 1.003 to 1.030, urine output is more than 1 ml/kg/hr; episodes of vomiting decrease in frequency and amount.

TABLE 45.3 Differentiation Between Regurgitation and Vomiting

Characteristic	Regurgitation	Vomiting
Timing	Occurs with feeding	Timing unrelated to feeding
Forcefulness	Runs out of mouth with *little force*	Forceful: often projected 1 ft away from the infant; *projectile vomiting*: projected as much as 4 ft (most often associated with pyloric stenosis)
Description	Smells barely sour; only slightly curdled	Extremely sour smelling and curdled, yellow, green, clear or watery, or black or blood tinged
Distress	Nonpainful; no appearance of distress; may even smile as if sensation is enjoyable	Possible crying just before vomiting as if abdominal pain is present, and after vomiting as if the force of action is frightening
Duration	Occurs once per feeding	Continuing until stomach is empty; followed by dry retching
Amount	1–2 tsp	Full stomach contents

On average, a period of 3 to 6 hours' time is usually sufficient to withhold all food or fluid for the older child. After this period of fasting, offer a few ice chips, then water in small amounts—approximately 1 tbsp every 15 minutes, four times; then 2 tbsp every half hour, four times. Popsicles can be substituted for water. If this is retained, children can be given small sips of clear liquids, such as tea, ginger ale, or a rehydration fluid such as Pedialyte. The World Health Organization provides a home recipe for fluid rehydration of 2 tbsp of sugar with 1/4 tsp of table salt and 1/4 teaspoon of baking soda dissolved in 1L (1 qt) of water (Victoria, Bryce, Fontaine, et al., 2000).

Children may become hungry and want whole glasses of fluid, but keeping the quantity to small sips prevents vomiting. Once the child is able to retain sips of clear liquids, the child can be offered portions of broth, clear soup, and skim milk in addition to clear liquids. Dry crackers or toast will help assuage hunger. By the second day, children can take a soft diet; by the third day, they should be back to their regular diet.

For the infant, introduce fluid after a fasting period of approximately 3 hours in the same slow manner: 1 tbsp every 15 minutes for 2 hours, then 1 oz every 2 hours for the next 12 to 18 hours. Glucose water or a commercial hydration solution such as Pedialyte may be given as fluid during this time to help the infant maintain electrolyte balance. Infants progress gradually, as do older children, to clear liquids or breast milk, then a soft diet, then a regular diet. If vomiting is prolonged, infants may need IV therapy to restore hydration (Moritz & Ayus, 2011). Assure parents that if children receive a small amount of fluid and do not vomit it, they will ultimately receive more fluid than if they take a large amount, but because of gastroenteritis, they vomit that amount. Stress that stomach secretions are lost along with vomitus each time, and the preservation of these stomach secretions is equally important. Antiemetic medicine is rarely necessary for children because acute gastroenteritis is a self-limiting condition and vomiting may actually be helpful if it rids the child's body of toxic substances. If vomiting is severe, however, an antiemetic such as promethazine (Phenergan) or ondansetron (Zofran) may be prescribed. Always ask parents if they have used an herbal remedy to stop vomiting to be certain that any medication prescribed will be safe with the alternative treatment (Box 45.3).

Diarrhea

Diarrhea that is acute is usually associated with infection; chronic diarrhea is more likely related to a malabsorption or inflammatory cause. *Giardia lamblia* is a frequent protozoan infection that causes diarrhea. The most common viral pathogens that invade the GI tract include rotaviruses and adenoviruses (Rabin, 2011). The most common bacterial pathogens include *Campylobacter jejuni*, *Salmonella*, *Clostridium difficile*, and *Escherichia coli* (Porth, 2011). Both viral and bacterial infections are easily spread in common diaper changing areas in day care centers or in public restrooms (Rimon & Freedman, 2010).

Diarrhea in infants is always serious because infants have such a small extracellular fluid reserve that sudden losses of water quickly exhaust the supply. Breastfeeding may actively prevent diarrhea by providing more antibodies and possibly an intestinal environment less friendly to invading organisms.

BOX 45.3 Nursing Care Planning to Respect Cultural Diversity

The incidence of GI illnesses varies among communities. Vomiting and diarrhea, for example, tend to occur because of food poisoning in communities where refrigeration is less than optimal and from eating raw meat or unprocessed cheese. Celiac disease occurs most frequently in children of Northern European ancestry. Because constipation, vomiting, and diarrhea are so common, every culture has home remedies for these symptoms: cascara for constipation; psyllium for diarrhea; and ginger, peppermint, licorice, or chamomile tea for nausea or vomiting. To be certain that a child seen in a health care facility does not receive two forms of the same drug (one prescribed and one given in an herb form by a parent), always ask what alternative therapies or home remedies have been given and document these on the child's plan of care.

Mild Diarrhea

Assessment. Normal and diarrheal stool characteristics are compared in Table 45.4. Children usually are anorectic, irritable, and appear unwell; a fever of 101° to 102°F (38.4° to 39.0°C) may be present. The episodes of diarrhea consist of 2 to 10 loose, watery bowel movements per day.

TABLE 45.4 Differentiation Between Normal Stool and Diarrheal Stool in an Infant

Characteristic	Infant Normal Stool	Diarrheal Stool
Frequency	1–3 daily	Unlimited number
Color	Yellow	Green
Effort of expulsion	Some pushing effort	Effortless; may be explosive
pH	More than 7.0 (alkaline)	Less than 7.0 (acidic)
Odor	Odorless	Sweet or foul smelling
Occult blood	Negative	Positive; blood may be overt
Reducing substances	Negative	Positive

The mucous membrane of the mouth appears dry and the skin feels warm, although skin turgor will not yet be decreased. The pulse may be rapid and out of proportion to the low-grade fever. Urine output is usually normal.

Therapeutic Management. At this stage, diarrhea is not yet serious, and children can be cared for at home. As with vomiting, treatment for diarrhea involves resting the GI tract, but this is necessary for only a short time. At the end of approximately 1 hour, parents can begin to offer an oral rehydration solution such as Pedialyte in small amounts on a regimen similar to that for vomiting (Smith, 2011). For breastfed infants, breastfeeding should continue. Probiotics (dietary supplements containing potentially beneficial bacteria or yeasts) to change the bacterial flora of the intestine may be administered (McFarland, 2010). Children also may need measures to reduce their elevated temperature.

Caution parents to contact their health care provider prior to initiating over-the-counter drugs such as loperamide (Imodium) or bismuth subsalicylate (Kaopectate) to halt diarrhea because, as a rule, toxic levels of these can occur quickly (Karch, 2013). Caution parents to wash their hands after changing diapers to prevent the spread of infection to themselves and to notify their health care provider if fever, pain, or diarrhea worsens.

Infants may develop a temporary lactase deficiency after diarrhea that leads to lactose intolerance. With this, a child cannot take formula or breast milk without new diarrhea beginning. Parents should alert their health care provider if they feel this is happening because the infant will initially need to be introduced to a lactose-free formula before being returned to the usual formula or breast milk.

Severe Diarrhea

Severe diarrhea may result from progressive mild diarrhea, or it may begin in a severe form.

Assessment. Infants with severe diarrhea appear obviously ill. Rectal temperature is often as high as 103° to 104°F (39.5° to 40.0°C). Both pulse and respirations are weak and rapid, and the skin is pale and cool. Infants may be apprehensive, listless, and lethargic. Obvious signs of dehydration such as a depressed fontanelle, sunken eyes, and poor skin turgor are usually present. The episodes of diarrhea usually consist of a movement of liquid green stool perhaps mixed with mucus and blood, passed with explosive force every few minutes. Urine output will be scanty and concentrated. Laboratory findings will show elevated hematocrit, hemoglobin, and serum protein levels because of the dehydration. Electrolyte determinations will indicate a metabolic acidosis (Huether, 2012).

It is difficult to measure the amount of fluid a child has lost with diarrhea, but an estimate can be derived from the loss in body weight, if known. For example, if a child weighed 10.4 kg yesterday at a health maintenance visit and today weighs 8.9 kg, the child has lost more than 10% of body weight. A loss of 2.5% to 5% of body weight suggests mild dehydration. Severe diarrhea quickly causes a 5% to 15% loss of body weight, which suggests severe dehydration. Any infant who has lost 10% or more of body weight requires immediate treatment.

Therapeutic Management. Treatment focuses on regulating electrolyte and fluid balance by initiating a temporary rest for the GI tract, oral or IV rehydration therapy, and discovering the organism responsible for the diarrhea.

All children with severe diarrhea or diarrhea that persists longer than 24 hours should have a stool culture taken to determine if infection is causing the diarrhea, and if so, a definite antibiotic therapy can be prescribed. Because a side effect of many antibiotics is diarrhea, antibiotics should not routinely be used to treat diarrhea without an identifiable bacterial cause. Stool cultures may be taken from the rectum or from stool in a diaper or a bedpan.

Blood serum specimens need to be drawn for a hemoglobin level (an estimation of hydration as well as anemia); white blood cell and differential counts (to attempt to establish whether infection is present); and determinations of P_{CO_2}, Cl^-, Na^+, K^+, and pH (to establish electrolyte needs). If a child can drink, the most effective way to replace fluid is by offering oral rehydration therapy. For a child who will not drink, an IV solution such as normal saline or 5% glucose in normal saline is begun to provide replacement of fluid, sodium, and calories.

Although infants usually have a potassium depletion, potassium is not given until it is established that the child is not in renal failure because giving a potassium IV when the body has no outlet for excessive potassium can lead to excessively high potassium levels and heart block. *Before this initial IV fluid is changed to a potassium solution, therefore, be certain the infant or child has voided—proof that the kidneys are functioning.*

Enough fluid must be given not only to replace the deficit that has occurred but also to replace the continuing loss until the diarrhea improves. If an infant has lost less than 5% of total body weight, his or her fluid deficit is approximately 50 ml/kg of body weight. If an infant has lost 10% of body weight, he or she needs approximately 100 ml/kg of body weight to replace the fluid deficit. If the weight loss suggests a 12% to 15% loss of body fluid, the infant requires 125 ml/kg of body weight to replace the fluid lost. This fluid will be given rapidly in the first 3 to 6 hours, and then it will be slowed to a maintenance rate. Once infants void, a potassium additive can be prescribed to restore serum potassium.

Nursing Diagnoses and Related Interventions

Nursing Diagnosis: Deficient fluid volume related to loss of fluid through diarrhea

Outcome Evaluation: Skin turgor remains good; specific gravity of urine is 1.003 to 1.030, urine output is more than 1 ml/kg/hr; and bowel movements are formed and fewer than four per day. Stool tests negative for reducing substances and blood pH is 7.41.

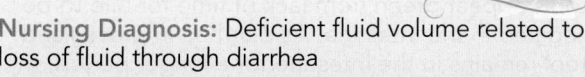

Promote Hydration and Comfort. During the time an infant is NPO, wet the infant's lips with a moisturizing cream or jelly such as Vaseline if they appear

to be dry. Offer a pacifier to suck if this seems to comfort him or her. (Infants want to suck because they are very thirsty and, if they have intestinal cramping with the diarrhea, they interpret this as hunger.) As the infant's condition improves, oral intake can be increased, changing to a soft then a regular diet.

If the child with severe diarrhea also has a fever, measures to reduce the fever will be necessary (see Chapter 37). Do not obtain rectal temperatures to assess fever because stimulating the anal sphincter could initiate more diarrhea. Change diapers frequently, assess perianal skin for irritation from liquid stools, and keep the skin clean and dry.

Record Fluid Intake and Output

Much of the nursing care of children with diarrhea focuses on careful recording of fluid intake and output. For children with severe dehydration, oral rehydration or IV therapy serves as their lifeline. Be certain to maintain proper functioning of an IV infusion and site if this is used by use of an arm board or soft restraints to prevent catheter dislodgment or interference with the infusion. If soft restraints are used, remember to release them every hour and passively exercise the child's extremities. Be certain parents understand why the IV infusion is important so they will understand the need for the soft restraints.

In children who are not toilet trained, it is important to separate urine from stool so the appearance of the stool can be accurately described and measured. Because current diapers contain a gel that quickly absorbs urine, apply a disposable urine collection bag to the infant so you can be assured the infant is voiding, thus confirming kidney function.

For each stool passed, record its color, consistency, odor, size, and the presence of any blood or mucus. Weigh soiled diapers to reveal the number of grams of stool in the diaper (1 g = 1 ml fluid). Testing the stool for acidity and for reducing substances (e.g., sugars) indicates how quickly the stool has passed through the irritated tract. A stool that is both positive for sugar and with a pH below 7.0 (acid) indicates diarrhea is acute because so little absorption of sugar has occurred (sugar is normally absorbed rapidly from ingested food). Diarrheal stools appear green from lack of time for bile to be modified in the intestine. As diarrhea improves and stool remains in the intestine for a longer period, the stool deepens in color and the acid and sugar contents fade. Testing stools for occult blood shows the extent of bowel irritation that is occurring from the acid stool. As the diarrhea improves and the irritation to the bowel lessens, the finding of occult blood also disappears.

Nursing Diagnosis: Risk for impaired skin integrity related to presence of diarrheal stool on skin

Outcome Evaluation: Skin in diaper area is not erythematous or ulcerated.

Because diarrheal stool is extremely irritating to the skin, change diapers immediately after infants pass any stool. Wash the skin of the diaper area well after each stool, and, if agency policy advises, cover it with an ointment such as Vaseline or A&D Ointment to protect it from further irritation. If the child is older, caution the child to wipe away stool thoroughly.

If infants already have skin excoriation from the number of stools they have had at home, an ointment such as Desitin may help soothe the irritated skin. Exposing infants' buttocks to air also is generally helpful in healing irritations. Assure older children that a stool "accident" because of diarrhea is not "shameful" or "babyish" but to be expected because they are so ill.

Nursing Diagnosis: Anxiety related to traumatic experience

Outcome Evaluation: Child interacts with parents in age-appropriate way; can be comforted after painful procedures.

All children with diarrhea are assumed to have an infectious form of gastroenteritis and therefore need contact and standard infection precautions until their condition is ruled otherwise. To counteract the discomfort of diarrhea, children need the security of someone to stay with them. Be sure to take time during initial procedures to touch and soothe children and talk to them; once the initial admission procedures are done, sit by the bed and hold the child or gently stroke the child's head. Encourage parents to give as much care as possible. Children need this support to counteract the strange world into which they have suddenly been plunged.

Bacterial Infectious Diseases That Cause Diarrhea and Vomiting

A number of common microorganisms are responsible for the majority of diarrheal infections in children. Common methods to prevent contracting an infection from these organisms are shown in Box 45.4.

Salmonellosis

- Causative agent: One of the *Salmonella* bacteria
- Incubation period: 6 to 72 hours for intraluminal type; 7 to 14 days for extraluminal type
- Period of communicability: As long as organisms are being excreted (may be as long as 3 months)
- Mode of transmission: Ingestion of contaminated food, especially chicken and raw eggs

Listeriosis

- Causative agent: *Listeria monocytogenes*
- Incubation period: Variable, ranging from 1 day to more than 3 weeks
- Mode of transmission: Ingestion of unpasteurized milk or cheeses or vegetables grown in contaminated soil. The infection is particularly important to avoid during pregnancy because infections during pregnancy can lead to miscarriage or stillbirth, prematurity, or infection of the newborn.

BOX 45.4 Nursing Care Planning to Empower a Family

PREVENTING *SALMONELLA*- OR *LISTERIA*-CAUSED GASTROENTERITIS

Q. Barry's mother says to you, "I hear so much about food poisoning. How can I protect my family against that?"

A. Anyone can get food poisoning. However, it can be prevented by using the following measures:

- Wash your hands well before preparing any foods, especially chicken and eggs.
- Remember that chicken may have been contaminated with *Salmonella* at the factory where it was prepared. Wash your hands well after handling raw chicken to prevent the spread of infection to other foods being prepared.
- Clean cutting boards or food preparation surfaces with hot, soapy water and dry thoroughly after use to prevent them from becoming reservoirs of infection. Use plastic cutting boards and avoid wooden cutting boards because they may be more difficult to clean.
- Make a habit of preparing chicken last, after other foods are prepared.
- Cook eggs well (do not use raw eggs in milkshakes; cook soft-boiled or poached eggs for at least 3 minutes).
- Refrigerate chicken and eggs after preparation.
- Wash hands well after playing with or feeding a pet turtle or changing the turtle's water because turtles can also transmit *Salmonella*.
- Wash raw vegetables thoroughly before eating.
- Avoid soft cheeses such as feta, Brie, Camembert, blue-veined, and Mexican queso fresco cheese. Hard cheeses; processed cheeses, including sliced cheese, cream cheese, cheese spreads, and cottage cheese; and yogurt need not be avoided.
- Cook leftover foods or ready-to-eat foods such as hot dogs until steaming hot before eating.
- Avoid foods from delicatessen counters such as prepared salads, meats, and cheeses, or heat/reheat these foods until steaming before eating.
- Avoid refrigerated pâtés and other meat spreads or heat and/or reheat these foods before eating; canned or shelf-stable pâté and meat spreads need not be avoided.
- Avoid raw or unpasteurized milk, including goat's milk, or milk products or foods that contain unpasteurized milk or milk products.

Shigellosis (Dysentery)

- Causative agent: Organisms of the genus *Shigella*
- Incubation period: 1 to 7 days
- Period of communicability: Approximately 1 to 4 weeks
- Mode of transmission: Contaminated food, water, or milk products

Staphylococcal Food Poisoning

- Causative agent: Staphylococcal enterotoxin produced by some strains of *Staphylococcus aureus*
- Incubation period: 1 to 7 hours
- Period of communicability: Carriers may contaminate food as long as they harbor the organism
- Mode of transmission: Ingestion of contaminated food such as creamed foods (e.g., potato salad)

QSEN Checkpoint Question 45.2

Patient-Centered Care

What if Barry's mother tells you that she is anxious about the possibility of "food poisoning" and that she particularly wants to prevent *Salmonella* poisoning in her family? Which of the following actions would you suggest?

a. Urge family members to keep their immunizations up to date.
b. Avoid excessive intake of dairy products.
c. Don't cut vegetables on a cutting board used to cut raw chicken.
d. Wash fruits such as strawberries and grapes with soap and water before eating.

Look in Appendix A for the best answer and rationale.

Protozoan or Viral Diarrhea

Most protozoan- or viral-caused diarrhea results in loose, watery stools. The chief therapy for these is oral rehydration solutions. Children who are cultured with *Giardia lamblia* may be prescribed metronidazole (Flagyl).

COMMON DISORDERS OF THE STOMACH AND DUODENUM

Disorders of the upper GI tract in children tend to involve inadequate function of the gastroesophageal valve or infection.

Gastroesophageal Reflux

Gastroesophageal reflux or the regurgitation of stomach secretions into the esophagus through the gastroesophageal (cardiac) valve occurs mainly in infants and adolescents.

Gastroesophageal Reflux in Infants

Gastroesophageal reflux in infants occurs when the gastroesophageal (cardiac) sphincter and the lower portion of the esophagus spasm, which then allows easy regurgitation of gastric contents into the esophagus. It usually starts within 1 week after birth and may be associated with a hiatal hernia. Children with cerebral palsy or other neurologic involvement are at particular risk. The regurgitation occurs almost immediately after feeding or when the infant is laid down after a feeding. If the amount of the reflux is large or constant, an infant does not retain sufficient calories and will fail to thrive. In addition, aspiration pneumonia or esophageal stricture from the constant reflux of hydrochloric acid into the esophagus can occur (Sundaram, Hoffenberg, Kramer, et al., 2011).

Assessment. History suggests the diagnosis. If vomiting occurs, it is effortless and small in amount. The child may be irritable and may experience periods of apnea. Inserting a probe or catheter through the nose into the distal esophagus and determining the pH from secretions can show whether gastric secretions are entering the esophagus (if the pH is less than 7.0, then acid is present). Esophageal manometry is used to measure the strength of the esophageal sphincter. A fiber optic endoscopy or esophagography (barium swallow) will further show the involved sphincter and the reflux of stomach contents into the esophagus, especially if the infant is tilted downward on a slant board.

Therapeutic Management. The traditional treatment of GI reflux is to feed infants a formula thickened with rice cereal (1 tbsp of cereal per 1 oz of formula or breast milk) while holding them in an upright position and then keeping them upright in an infant chair for 1 hour after feeding so gravity can help prevent reflux (Srivastava, Jackson, & Barnhart, 2010). An H_2 receptor antagonist such as ranitidine (Zantac) or a proton pump inhibitor such as omeprazole (Prilosec) may be prescribed daily to reduce the possibility of the stomach acid contents irritating the esophagus.

In infants, gastroesophageal reflux is usually a self-limiting condition. As the esophageal sphincter matures and the child begins to eat solid food or is maintained in a more upright position, the problem disappears. If not, botulinum toxin may be injected into the lower esophageal sphincter to temporarily relieve symptoms of obstruction. If such medical therapy is ineffective, a laparoscopic or surgical myotomy procedure (narrowing of the esophageal sphincter) may be performed. After this procedure, the child will temporarily have a nasogastric tube attached to intermittent low suction. Assess nasogastric tube drainage and any vomitus for coffee-colored drainage after the first 24 hours (it is a normal finding in the first 24 hours), which would indicate bleeding from the surgical site. When infants are first fed after surgery, they may display signs of abdominal discomfort and distention because food can no longer reflux into the esophagus as readily as it could before. As their stomach adjusts to this, however, symptoms will fade. Before this happens, however, the distention may be so extreme that it leads to bradycardia and dyspnea. Be alert for the development of these important signs and symptoms.

Gastrointestinal Reflux in Adolescents

Gastroesophageal reflux disease (GERD) affects about 20% of adults, and gastric irritation symptoms frequently begin in adolescence. Reflux at this age occurs when the adolescent lies supine or when intra-abdominal pressure is increased by a full stomach, lifting or bending, or tight clothing. It is potentially dangerous because it can lead to erosion of the esophagus with perforation or stricture and is associated with the development of esophageal cancer in later life (Wang & Souza, 2011).

The typical symptom is heartburn that occurs 30 to 60 minutes after a meal. Diagnosis is based on history (typical symptoms of heartburn) and, if symptoms are severe, an endoscopy to reveal the irritated esophagus (esophagitis). The goal of treatment is to provide symptomatic relief and to heal any esophagitis identified.

To prevent reflux, adolescents should avoid lying down until 3 hours after a meal and should sleep at night with their upper body elevated on a foam wedge or extra pillow. They should avoid acidic foods such as tomato products, citrus fruits, or spicy foods. Avoiding foods that delay gastric emptying such as fatty foods, chocolate, or alcohol and eating smaller portions may also be helpful. Generally, losing some weight if overweight, avoiding bending over after meals, and removing tight belts are also recommended steps.

Taking an over-the-counter antacid relieves pain immediately by decreasing the concentration of the stomach acid. H_2 receptor antagonists such as cimetidine (Pepcid) or ranitidine (Zantac) are also available over the counter and can be taken before meals to prevent heartburn. Proton pump inhibitors such as omeprazole (Prilosec) (both over-the-counter and prescription) or rabeprazole (AcipHex) (prescription), drugs that halt the release of stomach acids, offer the best long-term relief. Adolescents generally take these for 6 to 8 months until esophageal healing is complete.

As with adults, esophageal reflux in adolescents may return. Some adults require surgery in later life to relieve esophageal strictures or recurring ulcers from returning.

Nursing Diagnoses and Related Interventions

Nursing Diagnosis: Risk for imbalanced nutrition, less than body requirements, related to regurgitation of food with infant esophageal reflux

Outcome Evaluation: Skin fold returns to place quickly when turgor is assessed, specific gravity of urine is 1.003 to 1.030; intake is appropriate for age and weight.

Teach parents the importance of monitoring intake, output (urination), and weight. Also reinforce the need to keep the infant upright, such as in an infant seat, after a feeding. Be certain parents understand how much cereal to mix with formula or breast milk. Encourage parents to feed the infant during the short time that the infant remains in the hospital after surgery so that they can regain their confidence as parents.

Pyloric Stenosis

The pyloric sphincter is the opening between the lower portion of the stomach and the beginning portion of the intestine (the duodenum). If hypertrophy or hyperplasia of the muscle surrounding the sphincter occurs, it is difficult for the stomach to empty, a condition called *pyloric stenosis* (Fig. 45.3). The incidence is high, approximately 1:150 in males and 1:750 in females. It tends to occur most frequently in first-born white male infants. The exact cause is unknown, but multifactorial inheritance is the likely cause.

Assessment

With this condition, at 4 to 6 weeks of age, infants typically begin to vomit almost immediately after each feeding. The vomiting

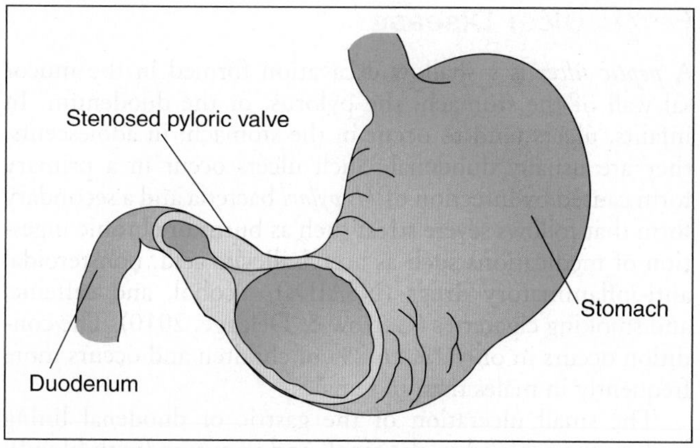

FIGURE 45.3 Pyloric stenosis. Fluid is unable to pass easily through the stenosed and hypertrophied pyloric valve.

grows increasingly forceful until it is projectile, possibly projecting as much as 3 to 4 ft (Pandya & Heiss, 2012).

Pyloric stenosis occurs less frequently in breastfed infants than in formula-fed infants. Breastfed infants begin having symptoms at 6 weeks, whereas formula-fed infants typically begin having symptoms at closer to 4 weeks of age because the curd of breast milk is smaller than that of cow's milk and it passes through a hypertrophied muscle more easily.

Vomitus usually smells sour because it has reached the stomach and has been in contact with digestive enzymes. There will never be bile in the vomitus because the feeding does not reach the duodenum to become mixed with bile. Infants are usually hungry immediately after vomiting because they are not nauseated. Although it is difficult to assess whether nausea is present in infants, signs such as a disinterest in eating, excessive drooling, or chewing on the tongue may suggest this.

Many infants have signs of dehydration such as dry mucous membrane of the mouth, sunken fontanelles, fever, decreased urine output, poor skin turgor, and weight loss from the vomiting when they are first seen. Alkalosis may be present because of the excessive loss of chloride from the loss of stomach fluid, along with accompanying hypochloremia, hypokalemia, and starvation. Hypopnea (slowed respirations) occurs as the body attempts to compensate for the alkalosis. This will cause the HCO_3 content of plasma generally to be above 30 mEq/L (normal levels are 22 to 28 mEq/L). Tetany may occur with alkalosis because the increased HCO_3^- ions may combine with Ca^{2+} ions in trying to affect homeostasis and thereby lowering the level of ionized calcium.

A definitive diagnosis can be made by watching the infant drink. If a pyloric stenosis is present, the sphincter feels round and firm, approximately the size of an olive in the right abdomen. As the infant drinks, gastric peristaltic waves pass from left to right across the abdomen. The olive-size lump becomes more prominent and the infant vomits with projectile emesis. If the diagnosis is still in doubt, an ultrasound will show a hypertrophied sphincter (Iqbal, Rivard, Mortellaro, et al., 2012). An endoscopy also may be used for diagnosis by directly visualizing the hypertrophied sphincter.

Therapeutic Management

Treatment is surgical or laparoscopic correction (a pyloromyotomy), which is performed before electrolyte imbalance occurs from the vomiting or before hypoglycemia occurs from the lack of food. Before surgery, if electrolyte imbalance, dehydration, and starvation have already occurred, these must be corrected by administration of IV fluid, usually isotonic saline or 5% glucose in saline. Oral feedings are withheld to prevent further electrolyte depletion. An infant who is receiving only IV fluid generally needs a pacifier to meet nonnutritive sucking needs and be comfortable. If tetany is present, verified by a low calcium level on blood analysis, IV calcium also must be administered. The infant usually needs additional potassium, but as a rule this cannot be administered until it is determined the child's kidneys are functioning (e.g., the child is voiding). Otherwise, the potassium buildup could cause cardiac arrhythmias.

For surgical correction, the muscle of the pylorus is split down to the mucosa, allowing for a larger lumen. Although the procedure sounds simple, it is technically difficult to perform, and there is a high risk for infection following surgery because the abdominal incision is near the diaper area.

The overall prognosis for infants with pyloric stenosis is excellent if the condition is discovered before an electrolyte imbalance occurs.

Nursing Diagnoses and Related Interventions

Nursing Diagnosis: Risk for deficient fluid volume related to inability to retain food

Outcome Evaluation: Skin turgor remains good; specific gravity of urine is 1.003 to 1.030; vomiting episodes have ceased; weight is within acceptable, age-appropriate parameters.

Preoperative Care Preoperative management for pyloric stenosis consists of fluid and electrolyte replacement based on laboratory determinations. Carefully note the frequency of urination, the specific gravity of the urine, and the number of stools passed to help assess dehydration and starvation. Parents may be impatient with preoperative management because it may take 24 hours or more to restore a severe fluid imbalance. They ask why their child can't have immediate surgery. Explaining that infants cannot go to surgery with an electrolyte imbalance is helpful so parents know the hours before surgery are as important to the welfare of their child as the operation itself.

Postoperative Care Infants will return from surgery or laparoscopy with an IV line in place. The postoperative feeding regimen differs from one surgeon to another but usually involves frequent feedings of small amounts of fluid that are gradually increased over time as tolerated. Approximately 4 to 6 hours after surgery, infants are started on a small amount of an oral rehydrating solution by bottle. If no vomiting occurs, the amount is increased or half-strength formula or breastfeeding is begun. Finally, by 24 to 48 hours, infants can take their full formula diet or can be fully breastfed. They are usually discharged from the hospital at the end of 48 hours.

Postoperatively, it is important that infants ingest a small amount of fluid because fluid passing through the sphincter helps to keep adhesions of the sphincter from forming. At the same time, it is important that infants not be given any more than the amount of fluid prescribed at any given time so the surgical repair site is not stretched from an overdistended stomach. As the amount taken orally increases, the IV fluid will be decreased and then discontinued. Infants should be burped well after a feeding so there is no pressure from air in the stomach. Lay them on their right side after feeding so that if vomiting does occur, there is little chance of aspiration and the flow of fluid through the pyloric valve is aided by gravity. Continue to monitor daily weights to confirm the child is receiving adequate intake. Although postoperative vomiting is commonly experienced, it should be reported immediately because the physiologic cause of the vomiting may be related to delayed gastric emptying, advancing feedings too rapidly, or edema at the operative site, all of which need to be corrected. A few infants develop short-term diarrhea (dumping syndrome) after surgery because of rapid functioning of the pyloric sphincter, but this tends to resolve without additional therapy.

Nursing Diagnosis: Risk for infection at site of surgical incision related to danger of contamination from feces because of proximity of incision to diaper area

Outcome Evaluation: Infant's temperature is not above 98.6°F (37.0°C) tympanic; incision is clean, dry, and intact without erythema or drainage.

The surgical incision for pyloric stenosis may be covered with collodion, a solution similar to clear nail polish, or a similar commercial compound to help keep urine and feces from touching it. Keep diapers folded low to prevent the incision line from being contaminated, and change diapers frequently. If the incision is exposed to feces, wash the collodion thoroughly with soap and water.

Nursing Diagnosis: Risk for impaired parenting related to infant's feeding difficulty and illness

Outcome Evaluation: Parents hold and feed infant; express positive characteristics about infant.

Encourage the parents to "room-in" with their child so they can grow comfortable and confident in caring for the child again. When the child first began vomiting so forcefully, parents may have felt they were doing something wrong and so may have lost confidence in themselves as parents. Explain to them that the vomiting was caused by a physical problem and not by anything they did.

Hospitalization often occurs near the infant's second month, when the child would normally receive diphtheria-tetanus-pertussis, rotavirus, pneumococcal, oral poliomyelitis, and *Haemophilus influenzae* immunizations. If the child is otherwise healthy, ask if they could be administered before discharge so the child's immunization status remains current. This also might serve to remind parents that getting back to normal means regular health care visits for vaccines and checkups.

Peptic Ulcer Disease

A *peptic ulcer* is a shallow excavation formed in the mucosal wall of the stomach, the pylorus, or the duodenum. In infants, ulcers tend to occur in the stomach; in adolescents, they are usually duodenal. Such ulcers occur in a primary form caused by infection of *H. pylori* bacteria and a secondary form that follows severe stress such as burns or chronic ingestion of medications such as acetylsalicylic acid, nonsteroidal anti-inflammatory drugs (NSAIDs), alcohol, and caffeine, and smoking cigarettes (Garrow & Delegge, 2010). The condition occurs in only 1% to 2% of children and occurs more frequently in males than in females.

The small ulceration of the gastric or duodenal lining leads to pain, blood in the stool, and vomiting (with blood). If left uncorrected, peptic ulcer disease can lead to bowel or stomach perforation with acute hemorrhage or pyloric obstruction. A chronic ulcer condition may lead to anemia from the constant, gradual blood loss.

Assessment

An ulcer occurring in a neonate usually presents with hematemesis (blood in vomitus) or melena (blood in the stool). Such ulcers are usually superficial and heal rapidly, although they can lead to rupture, with symptoms of respiratory distress, abdominal distention, vomiting, and, if extensive, cardiovascular collapse. If an ulcer occurs in a toddler, the first symptoms are usually anorexia or vomiting. Bleeding follows in several weeks. If an ulcer begins when children are of preschool or early school age, pain may be the presenting symptom. The child may report pain as mild, severe, colicky, or continuous. It is often poorly localized, although it may be in the epigastric area as in adults. If the pain occurs in the right lower quadrant, it may be confused with appendicitis.

In school-age children and adolescents, symptoms are generally those of the adult—a gnawing or aching pain in the epigastric area before meals that is relieved by eating. Vomiting (because of spasm and edema of the pylorus) occurs in a small number of children. On abdominal palpation, epigastric tenderness is present.

A fiber optic endoscopy is the most reliable diagnostic test to confirm the diagnosis of peptic ulcer disease; it allows for visual inspection and cultures for *H. pylori*. In many children, little increase in gastric activity can be demonstrated by gastric analysis. Children with this condition must have blood tests done periodically to be monitored for blood loss anemia.

Therapeutic Management

Children with peptic ulcer disease are treated with a combination of medications to reduce the bacteria count and suppress gastric acidity. Adolescents are prescribed an antibiotic such as amoxicillin or clarithromycin (Biaxin) and a proton pump inhibitor such as omeprazole (Prilosec). Bismuth subsalicylate (Pepto-Bismol) is soothing and mildly antibiotic and so may be prescribed concurrently. Younger children are prescribed cimetidine (Tagamet) because safe levels of omeprazole have yet to be established for this age group. With current therapy, only a few children experience the potential complications of perforation, blood loss anemia, and intestinal obstruction, although some school-age children and adolescents will have recurring symptoms when they grow older. Most important to prevent an ulcer reoccurring seems to be the evacuation of *H. pylori* from the child's stomach or intestine (Bashinskaya, Nahed, Redjal, et al., 2011).

Nursing Diagnoses and Related Interventions

Having peptic ulcer disease can be difficult for children because it is painful, and remembering to take medicine daily can be a problem.

Nursing Diagnosis: Pain related to ulceration in intestinal tract

Outcome Evaluation: Child exhibits verbal and nonverbal signs of decreased pain; appears comfortable and without excessive crying.

Children with peptic ulcer disease should be able to eat a usual diet while avoiding heavily spiced food such as pizza or sausage if such food causes discomfort. Work with them to devise a schedule so they can remember to take their medications.

Be certain the outcomes planned are realistic because it may not be possible to relieve symptoms of peptic ulcers immediately. However, children can be helped immediately to understand why the pain occurs and what they can do to help relieve it.

✔ QSEN Checkpoint Question 45.3

Quality Improvement

Barry's mother is concerned that her new baby will develop pyloric stenosis. To detect vomiting from this, you would assess the infant at what time?

a. Immediately after feeding
b. An hour after feeding
c. On arising in the morning
d. When the infant cries

Look in Appendix A for the best answer and rationale.

HEPATIC DISORDERS

Hepatic disorders include both congenital disorders, such as obstruction or atresia of the biliary duct, and acquired disorders, such as hepatitis or cirrhosis.

Liver Function

In infants, 1 or 2 cm of liver is readily and normally palpable under the diaphragm on the right side of their abdomen. An organ essential for the normal metabolism of carbohydrates, proteins, and fats, the liver plays a major role in the maintenance of normal blood sugar levels by changing glucose to glycogen and storing it until needed by body cells. It then reverses the process and changes glycogen back to glucose and releases it into the blood when cells need it (Huether, 2012). It assists in the catabolism of fatty acids and protein and serves as a temporary storage space for both fat and protein.

By the means of the enzyme glucuronosyltransferase, the liver is responsible for converting indirect (or unconjugated) bilirubin into direct (or conjugated) bilirubin so it can be excreted in bile and eliminated from the body. This is an important function in the newborn, and jaundice can result if the level of glucuronosyltransferase is low because of immaturity.

Lastly, the liver manufactures bile, a secretion necessary for the digestion of fat; fibrinogen and prothrombin, substances essential for blood clotting; heparin, a substance necessary to keep blood from clotting in intact vessels; and blood proteins, which are necessary for cell growth and repair. It destroys red blood cells and detoxifies many harmful absorbed substances, such as drugs. The liver is a life-sustaining organ because of all these functions; therefore, any disorder involving the liver is always serious.

Hepatitis

Hepatitis (inflammation and infection of the liver) is caused by invasion of the hepatitis A, B, C, D, or E virus (CDC, 2012).

Hepatitis A

- Causative agent: A picornavirus, hepatitis A virus (HAV)
- Incubation period: 25 days on average
- Period of communicability: Highest during 2 weeks preceding onset of symptoms
- Mode of transmission: In children, ingestion of fecally contaminated water or shellfish; day care center spread from contaminated changing tables
- Immunity: Natural; one episode induces immunity for the specific type of virus
- Active artificial immunity: HAV vaccine (recommended for all children 12 to 23 months of age, workers in day care centers, and certain international travelers)
- Passive artificial immunity: Immune globulin

Hepatitis B

- Causative agent: A hepadnavirus; hepatitis B virus (HBV)
- Incubation period: 120 days on average
- Period of communicability: Later part of incubation period and during the acute stage
- Mode of transmission: Transfusion of contaminated blood and plasma or semen; inoculation by a contaminated syringe or needle through IV drug use; may be spread to fetus if mother has infection in third trimester of pregnancy
- Immunity: Natural; one episode induces immunity for the specific type of virus
- Active artificial immunity: HBV vaccine (recommended for routine immunization beginning at birth and also to all health care providers) (CDC, 2012)
- Passive artificial immunity: Specific hepatitis B immune serum globulin

Hepatitis C, D, and E

Although hepatitis A and B are the viruses that most frequently cause hepatitis, hepatitis C, D, and E viruses may also be involved. Hepatitis C (HCV) is a single-strand RNA virus. Transmission, as with HBV, is primarily by blood or blood products, IV drug use, or sexual contact. The virus produces mild symptoms of disease, but there is a high incidence of chronic infection with the virus.

Hepatitis D (HDV), or the delta form, is similar to HBV in transmission, although it apparently requires a coexisting HBV infection to be activated. Disease symptoms are mild, but there is a high incidence of fulminant hepatitis after the initial infection.

The E form of hepatitis is enterically transmitted similarly to hepatitis A (e.g., fecally contaminated water). Disease symptoms from the E virus can range from asymptomatic to mild to chronic liver disease (Faramawi, Johnson, Chen, et al., 2011).

Assessment. No matter which virus is involved, hepatitis is a generalized body infection with specific and intense liver effects. Type A occurs in children of all ages and accounts for approximately 30% of instances. Hepatitis B tends to occur in newborns from placental–fetal transfer and in adolescents after intimate contact or the use of contaminated syringes for drug injection.

Clinically, it is impossible to differentiate the type of hepatitis from the signs that are present. All hepatitis viruses cause liver cell destruction, leading to increased serum aspartate aminotransferase (AST), alanine aminotransferase (ALT), and alkaline phosphatase levels. Albumin synthesis decreases, and bile formation and excretion are impaired. The type of virus causing the disease can be determined by the recognition of a specific antibody against the virus such as anti-HAV immunoglobulin (Ig)M or anti-HBV IgM.

With hepatitis A, children notice a headache, fever, and anorexia. Jaundice occurs as liver function slows. This lasts for approximately 1 week, and then symptoms fade with a full recovery. Symptoms of hepatitis B are more marked. Children report generalized aching, right upper quadrant pain, and a headache. They may have a low-grade fever. They feel ill and become fretful from pruritus (itching). After 3 to 7 days of such symptoms, the color of the urine becomes darker (brown) because of the excretion of bilirubin. In another 2 days, the sclerae of the eyes become jaundiced; soon, the child has generalized jaundice. With generalized jaundice, there is little excretion of bilirubin into the stool, so the stools become white or gray. This icteric (jaundiced) phase lasts for a few days to 2 weeks. Some children have an anicteric form of infection, in which they develop the beginning symptoms but then never develop the jaundice. However, they are as infectious as children with overt jaundice.

Laboratory studies will show elevations of the liver enzymes AST (SGOT) and ALT (SGPT). Levels of bilirubin are increased in the urine. Bile pigments in the stool are decreased. Serum bilirubin levels are increased.

QSEN Checkpoint Question 45.4

Safety

Barry's family likes to celebrate family events by eating crab, lobster, and shrimp. What form of hepatitis is most apt to be contracted by eating contaminated shellfish?

a. Hepatitis B
b. Hepatitis A
c. Hepatitis E
d. Hepatitis C

Look in Appendix A for the best answer and rationale.

Therapeutic Management. All health care providers should receive prophylaxis against hepatitis with the hepatitis B vaccine. Newborns should also receive routine immunization against HBV. All women should be screened during pregnancy for hepatitis B surface antigen (HBsAg). Infants born to hepatitis-positive mothers should receive both hepatitis B immune globulin (HBIG) and active immunization at birth to prevent them from contracting the disease (Roznovsky, Orsagova, Kloudova, et al., 2010). Hepatitis A vaccine is available for health care providers and included in routine immunization programs for infants beginning at 1 year of age (CDC, 2012).

Strict hand washing and infection control precautions are mandatory when caring for children with hepatitis. Feces must be disposed of carefully because the type A virus can be cultured from feces. Syringes and needles must be disposed of with caution because the type B virus can be transmitted by blood. Contacts should receive immune globulin (hepatitis A) or HBIG as appropriate.

The treatment for hepatitis A is increased rest and maintenance of a good caloric intake. A low-fat diet, once recommended, is not required and, in any event, is difficult to enforce. Children are generally hungrier at breakfast than later in the day, so encourage them to eat a healthy breakfast. They should not return to school or a day care center until 2 weeks after the onset of symptoms to guard against spreading the infection.

Lamivudine (Epivir) is an antiviral agent that may be effective at reducing viral replication with hepatitis B. Interferon also may be prescribed. Of those with type B, 90% will recover completely, but 10% will develop chronic hepatitis and become hepatitis carriers. Hepatitis B is always potentially serious because newborns who contract the disease at birth have an increased risk for liver carcinoma later in life (Bailey, Shiau, Zola, et al., 2011). Because hepatitis B is a sexually transmitted disease, preadolescent children with the infection need to be screened for the possibility of sexual maltreatment (Leder, 2012).

Nursing Diagnoses and Related Interventions

Nursing Diagnosis: Pain related to pruritus of jaundice and liver inflammation

Outcome Evaluation: Child states level of itching is tolerable, no scratch marks on skin; reports right upper quadrant pain is minimal.

Pruritus from jaundice results in extreme discomfort for some children A cool bath and being certain a child is not overheated and not perspiring usually reduces the itching. Skin moisturizers such as Eucerin or an antihistamine may also be helpful. Cholestyramine (Questran) is a bile acid sequestrant, which binds bile in the GI tract to prevent its reabsorption and so may be prescribed. Teaching a child distraction techniques such as putting pressure on a pruritic area or trying imagery to lessen the urge to scratch are also helpful measures.

Chronic Hepatitis

Hepatitis is considered chronic when it persists for longer than 6 months. This is most often the result of a hepatitis B, D, or C infection. Abnormal liver enzyme levels and a liver biopsy establish the diagnosis and can also predict the severity. With chronic hepatitis, fatty infiltration and bile duct damage can occur. The disease may progress to cirrhosis and eventually liver failure. Therapy is supportive to compensate for decreased liver function (Sundaram et al., 2011).

Fulminant Hepatic Failure

Fulminant hepatic failure is present when acute, massive necrosis or sudden, severe impairment of liver function occurs, leading to liver failure and hepatic encephalopathy. Acetaminophen (Tylenol) toxicity is the most likely etiology. Hepatic encephalopathy, or invasion of brain cells by ammonia, occurs because of the inability of the liver to detoxify the ammonia being constantly produced by the intestine in the process of digestion (Garcovich, Zocco, Roccarina, et al., 2012).

Children may show mental aberrations such as confusion, drowsiness, or disorientation. Treatment involves reducing protein intake and administering lactulose to prevent absorption of ammonia in the colon or administering nonabsorbable antibiotics such as neomycin to decrease the production of ammonia by the intestinal bacteria. Liver transplantation (surgical replacement of a malfunctioning liver by a donor liver) may be necessary. If a full donor liver is not available, a lobe can be removed from a living donor such as a parent and transplanted into a child. The donor is then able to regenerate the lost lobe of the liver without long-term effects.

Obstruction of the Bile Ducts

Obstruction of the bile ducts in children generally occurs from congenital biliary atresia, stenosis, or absence of the duct. It also can occur from the plugging of biliary secretions, although this is rare. When the bile duct is obstructed, bile, unable to enter the intestinal tract, accumulates in the liver. Bile pigments (direct bilirubin) enter the bloodstream and jaundice occurs, which increases in intensity daily.

Assessment

Although bile duct obstruction is a congenital disorder, the chief sign (jaundice) does not develop until approximately 2 weeks of age. This delay differentiates it clinically from physiologic jaundice, which occurs in almost all newborns on the third day of life, or the jaundice of Rh or ABO isoimmunization, which typically occurs during the first 24 hours of life. Laboratory findings will also distinguish this type of jaundice from other types because, with physiologic and isoimmunization jaundice, there is a rise in indirect bilirubin; in the jaundice of bile duct obstruction, there is a rise in direct bilirubin. Alkaline phosphatase levels will also be elevated. The AST (SGOT) level is normal in the early phase but later becomes abnormal, when prolonged obstruction and back-pressure cause liver cell damage. In addition, because bile salts, which are necessary for fat and fat-soluble vitamin absorption, are not reaching the intestine, absorption of fat and fat-soluble vitamins (vitamins A, D, E, and K) becomes poor. Calcium absorption, which depends on vitamin D absorption, will fail as well. The infant's stools appear light in color from a lack of bile pigments. The pressure on the liver from the obstruction becomes so acute with time that cell destruction or cirrhosis occurs. Ultimately, without liver transplantation, death from liver failure will result (Kaido, Mori, Ogura, et al., 2012).

Therapeutic Management

Before treatment is begun, appropriate blood work and a liver biopsy under local anesthesia may be obtained to rule out hepatitis. Duodenal secretions may be collected by endoscopy to assess for bile. Radionuclide imaging to show that bile ducts are not patent may confirm the diagnosis. If the problem appears to only be a mucus plug in the duct, children may be given magnesium sulfate (installed into the duodenum to relax the bile duct) or a dehydrocholic acid (Decholin) IV to stimulate the flow of bile. If atresia of the bile duct is the problem, surgical correction is the treatment (a Kasai procedure). With this surgery, a loop of bowel is sutured next to the liver to create a fistula for bile flow between the liver and intestine. A double-barreled colostomy is then created (an enterostomy). Bile flows out of the proximal loop into a collecting bag. It is periodically returned to the distal loop of intestine by injection. After 6 to 12 weeks, the colostomy is closed when a normal bile flow has been established. Surgical correction may not be possible in all infants because the atresia may occur too far back in the liver to be in an operable area. Liver transplantation is then needed for children with extensive involvement or in whom a Kasai procedure is not successful.

Nursing Diagnoses and Related Interventions

Nursing Diagnosis: Risk for imbalanced nutrition, less than body requirements, related to inability to digest fat

Outcome Evaluation: Infant's weight remains in same percentile on standardized growth curve, absence of signs of vitamin deficiency such as cracked lips or altered bone growth; dietary record reflects intake of adequate nutrients.

Preoperative Care Infants who are admitted for surgery for bile duct obstruction are placed on a low-fat, high-carbohydrate diet preoperatively. They are given water-soluble forms of vitamins A, D, and K to improve vitamin levels. If the vitamin K level is too low, coagulation may be affected, so vitamin K may be administered parenterally until prothrombin levels rise to normal limits. Infants will also be well hydrated with parenteral fluids.

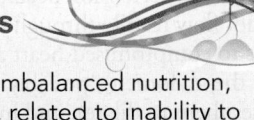

Postoperative Care Following surgery, infants return with a nasogastric tube in place attached to low intermittent suction. Observe carefully for abdominal distention because paralytic ileus, or bowel dysfunction, is a frequent complication of this type of surgery. The nasogastric tube will be left in place until peristalsis has returned. Gradually, children will be introduced to oral fluids and, eventually, to a normal diet. If the repair is successful, the child's stools change to a yellow and then brown (normal stool) color after surgery. Therefore, a description of stools is an important postoperative observation.

If bile flow is inadequate after surgery, infants will remain on a medium-fat, high-carbohydrate diet or receive total parenteral nutrition while they await transplantation surgery.

Nonalcoholic Fatty Liver Syndrome and Cirrhosis

Nonalcoholic fatty liver syndrome is the accumulation of fatty deposits in the liver and is usually associated with obesity. As obesity is increasing in school-age children and adolescents, this condition is also increasing in incidence (Vajro, Lenta, Socha, et al., 2012). *Cirrhosis* is fibrotic scarring of the liver. Cirrhosis means "yellow," or the typical color of hepatic scar tissue. It rarely occurs in children, although it may be seen as a result of congenital biliary atresia or as a complication of chronic illnesses such as protracted hepatitis, sickle-cell anemia, or cystic fibrosis.

When fibrotic infiltrates replace normal liver cells, total liver function becomes impaired, resulting in a decreased ability to detoxify toxic substances, decreased protein synthesis, inability to produce prothrombin, decreased ability to produce bile, and, possibly, hypoglycemia. Children will have large, fatty stools resulting from the decrease in bile production; avitaminosis of fat-soluble vitamins; symptoms of hemorrhage from decreased clotting ability; and anemia.

Portal hypertension occurs from back-pressure of blood that cannot flow readily through the scarred organ (Fig. 45.4). This leads to compromised heart action, *ascites* (an exudate of fluid into the abdomen), possibly esophageal varices (back-pressure causes them to dilate), and hypersplenism (D'Antiga, 2012).

Cholestyramine (Questran) may be prescribed to stimulate bile flow and reduce reabsorption of bile into the circulation to minimize jaundice. Once fatty or fibrotic infiltration begins, however, there is no way to reverse the changes. Nursing care focuses on promoting comfort, providing adequate nutrition by a high-carbohydrate, medium-chain–triglyceride diet, and preventing further involvement until liver transplantation can be scheduled.

Esophageal Varices

Esophageal varices (distended veins in the esophagus) are a frequent complication of liver disorders such as cirrhosis (Hussey, Kelleher, & Ling, 2010). They generally form at the distal end of the esophagus near the stomach because of back-pressure on the veins resulting from increased portal circulation blood pressure. Varices may bleed if children cough vigorously or strain to pass stool. Gastric reflux into the distal esophagus may irritate and erode the fine covering of the distended vessels, causing rupture.

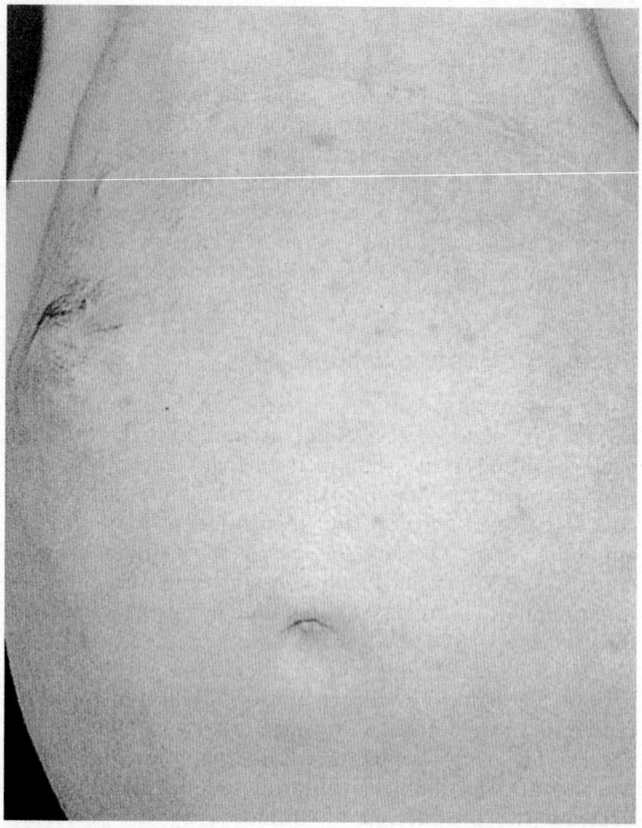

FIGURE 45.4 A child with cirrhosis of the liver. Note the abdominal distention and development of prominent, tortuous veins secondary to portal hypertension. (From Zitelli, B. J., & Davis, H. W. [1997]. *Atlas of pediatric physical diagnosis* [3rd ed.]. St. Louis: Mosby–Year Book, Inc.)

A rupture of esophageal varices is an emergency because children can lose a large quantity of blood quickly from the engorged vessels. Vasopressin or nitroglycerin may be given by IV to lessen hypertension and reduce the hemorrhage. An injection of a sclerosing agent into the varicosed veins may be attempted to decrease their size. An iced saline nasogastric lavage may be instituted to promote vasoconstriction. A Sengstaken–Blakemore tube or Linton-Nachlas catheter may be passed into the stomach. After insertion, balloons on the sides of these catheters are inflated to apply pressure against the bleeding vessels. As with an external tourniquet, the compression must be reduced for 5 to 10 minutes every 6 to 8 hours, or tissue necrosis can result.

Following one episode of bleeding, children must be monitored for future bleeding episodes. Frequent vital sign measurements and testing of stool and any vomitus for the presence of blood will indicate if new bleeding is occurring.

Liver Transplantation

Liver transplantation is the surgical replacement of a malfunctioning liver by a donor liver. Child-size donor livers are not readily available, so the waiting time for surgery may be months. Adult livers can be reduced in size for transplantation or a lobe of a liver from a living donor can be used. Often, the child is extremely ill with ascites, GI bleeding, extreme pruritus, hepatic encephalopathy, or renal dysfunction before the surgery. This makes nursing care after liver transplantation in a child complex because it involves taking care of a child who has had major surgery and who normally would be categorized as too ill to undergo surgery.

Despite the severity of illness and the length of surgery, however, children tend to recover quickly after liver transplantation (Mouzaki & Ng, 2010). Both children and parents must have thorough preoperative preparation so they understand the seriousness of the surgery and the possibility that the graft will be rejected. It helps to introduce the parents to others whose children have successfully undergone the procedure so they have support people available for this critical time.

Preoperative Management

Preoperative management consists of keeping the child in the best physiologic condition possible so that, when a liver is available, the transplantation can be performed. For many children, this includes dialysis and severe nutritional restrictions.

Surgical Procedure

Liver transplantation is a time-consuming procedure and requires a wide subcostal incision. The vena cava is temporarily clamped during the removal of the natural liver to prevent bleeding, which means that all IV lines must be placed in the upper extremities.

Postoperative Management

Rejection of a liver transplant is most often because of the function of T lymphocytes. Careful tissue matching (human leukocyte antigen [HLA] matching) is necessary to reduce the possibility of stimulating T-cell rejection. To further reduce the action of T lymphocytes, children are given an immunosuppressive drug such as mycophenolate mofetil (CellCept), cyclosporine (Sandimmune), or tacrolimus (Prograf) before the transplantation.

Children may need assisted ventilation for approximately 24 hours postoperatively to prevent pulmonary complications such as atelectasis and pneumonia because the large abdominal incision makes coughing and deep breathing difficult. In addition, ascites places pressure against the diaphragm, interfering with lung expansion, and preoperative pulmonary edema may be present. After discontinuation of mechanical ventilation and extubation, chest physiotherapy may be started to mobilize lung secretions.

Advocate for adequate pain control. Frequently assess blood pressure, capillary refill, peripheral pulses, and skin color to ensure adequate cardiovascular function, which is important for good tissue perfusion of the transplanted liver. The child may have a central venous pressure line or an arterial line such as a Swan-Ganz catheter inserted to assess hemodynamic status. Assess neurologic status hourly using a modified Glasgow Coma Scale (see Chapter 52).

Usually, a child is positioned flat for the first 24 hours to prevent cerebral air emboli, which may result from any air remaining in the transplanted liver. Typically, children have a nasogastric tube inserted during surgery that is attached to low intermittent suction postoperatively. Irrigate the tube according to agency policy to maintain patency. Assess the gastric pH by aspirating stomach contents every 4 hours; based on this assessment, administer antacids or H_2 receptor antagonists such as cimetidine or mucosal protectants as prescribed to help prevent a stress ulcer. If preoperative esophageal varices are present, assess nasogastric drainage carefully for frank or occult blood.

A T-tube inserted into the bile duct for drainage allows the amount of bile being produced by the new liver to be evaluated. Once bowel sounds become active, nasogastric suction and the T-tube are usually discontinued and liquids and then solid foods are introduced gradually. If vomiting occurs and is persistent, total parenteral nutrition may be used for 3 or 4 days to rest the intestinal tract before fluid is reintroduced.

Hypoglycemia is a major danger postoperatively because glucose levels are regulated by the liver, and the transplanted organ may not function efficiently at first. Assess serum glucose levels hourly by finger-stick puncture. A 10% solution of dextrose IV may be necessary to prevent hypoglycemia.

Sodium, potassium, chloride, and calcium levels are evaluated approximately every 6 to 8 hours to be certain electrolyte balance is maintained. Even if a low potassium level is detected, potassium is rarely added to IV solutions because of the risk that renal failure has occurred because of the stress of surgery. Plus, if the graft begins to necrose, the breakdown of cells will release potassium, elevating the level even more. Continuous cardiac monitoring is usually necessary to detect hyperkalemia (hyperkalemia causes elevation of T waves or ventricular fibrillation), hypokalemia (causes small T waves and a U wave), or other arrhythmias.

Many children develop hypertension within 72 hours after surgery. This occurs because of alterations in the renin–angiotensin system because of the not yet fully functioning transplanted liver or as a side effect of cyclosporine, tacrolimus, and steroid therapy, which is continued postoperatively to guard against transplant rejection. IV therapy with hypotensive agents such as hydralazine (Apresoline) and nitroprusside may be needed to reduce hypertension. In contrast, hypotension will occur if the transplanted liver becomes dysfunctional or if there is bleeding caused by poor blood coagulation. To help detect bleeding, observe and record abdominal girth, the incision line, and drainage from any catheters or tubes placed in the incision to allow peritoneal secretions to drain.

A warming blanket may be required postoperatively to maintain normal body temperature after the long exposure of surgery. Take axillary or tympanic, not rectal, temperatures, because many children with liver damage have hemorrhoids that could rupture from the trauma of a thermometer insertion. Prevent the child from unnecessary exposure during procedures and care to help restore and maintain normal body temperature.

Nursing Diagnoses and Related Interventions

Nursing Diagnosis: Risk for infection related to administration of immunosuppressive medication

Outcome Evaluation: Temperature remains within normal range; no exudate or inflammation around abdominal incision is present.

BOX 46.1 Nursing Care Planning Based on 2020 National Health Goals

Renal disease can lead to long-term illness, so preventing it is important to improving the health of the nation. 2020 National Health Goals that address this concern are:

- Reduce the rate of new cases of end-stage renal disease from a baseline of 300 per 1 million population to a target rate of 221 per 1 million population.
- Increase the proportion of patients with treated chronic kidney failure who receive a transplant within 3 years of end-stage renal disease from a baseline of 17.1% to 18.8% (U.S. Department of Health and Human Services [DHHS], 2010; see www.healthypeople.gov).

Nurses can help the nation achieve these goals by educating parents to give antibiotics conscientiously for streptococcal throat infections and being active advocates for organ transplant procedures.

Normally, the urinary system maintains the proper balance of fluid and electrolytes in the blood. When disease occurs, such as with structural abnormalities or kidney malfunction, children may be left with excessive amounts of fluid in the body or with an imbalance of electrolytes essential to body functioning that becomes long term (Ring & Huether, 2013).

Unfortunately, because symptoms may be vague or because children or parents do not realize the seriousness of urinary tract disease (or are embarrassed to discuss it), children may not be evaluated at the first sign of illness, making health education to increase the awareness of the symptoms of urinary tract and kidney disorders an important area of family health teaching. Box 46.1 shows 2020 National Health Goals related to renal disorders and children.

Nursing Process Overview

For Care of a Child With a Renal or Urinary Tract Disorder

Assessment

Because the symptoms of many urinary tract and renal disorders, such as mild abdominal pain, slowly increasing edema, or low-grade fever, are subtle, school nurses play an important role in recognizing the seriousness of such minor symptoms and making referrals for care.

A hallmark symptom of kidney or bladder infection is pain. Be sure to assess the degree of any pain, including its location and intensity, before administering an analgesic or antispasmodic to aid with diagnosis or prognosis. Obtaining urine specimens is another important means of helping with assessment.

Nursing Diagnosis

Nursing diagnoses used with children with urinary tract or renal disorders are related to the symptoms these disorders cause plus the effect chronic disease can have on a family. Some examples include:

- Pain related to bladder irritation from urinary tract infection
- Excess fluid volume related to decreased kidney function and fluid accumulation
- Fear related to as yet unknown outcome of kidney transplantation
- Imbalanced nutrition, less than body requirements, related to effects of dietary restrictions
- Social isolation related to immunosuppressant therapy
- Interrupted family processes related to the effects and stresses of child's chronic illness
- Compromised family coping related to the chronic nature of child's illness

Outcome Identification and Planning

Be certain that outcomes established for care are relevant to a child's age and condition. If renal disease becomes chronic, expected outcomes may need to be modified frequently to meet changing needs.

Planning for a child with a urinary tract or renal disorder often involves helping parents remember to give medicine. A child with nephrotic syndrome or a renal transplant, for example, may need to take three or four different types of medicine every day. Be certain parents understand the types of medicine prescribed and the expected action and side effects of each. If the school a child attends has a zero tolerance policy for taking medication at school, children need a schedule that allows them to take medicine before they leave home in the morning or after they return in the afternoon.

Help parents schedule times for hemodialysis or peritoneal dialysis as well as for care of their other children and their work schedules. This should help them achieve balance among all tasks that need to be done. If a child develops severe renal impairment, parents may be asked to make a decision regarding kidney removal and transplantation. Provide them with ample time for discussion about this because offering to be a living kidney donor is a major life step. Examples of organizations that are helpful for referral include the National Kidney Foundation (www.kidney.org), the Polycystic Kidney Disease Foundation (www.pkdcure.org), the Urology Care Foundation (www.urologyhealth.org), and the Kidney Dialysis Foundation (www.kdf.org.sg).

Implementation

Both parents and children may not fully understand the function of the urinary system because it is not a system that receives much discussion. For example, they may confuse the words "ureter" and "urethra." Nurses can play major roles as resource persons, explaining anatomy, tests and procedures, and why such tests are being done.

Many children with kidney disease take a corticosteroid for immunosuppression and so develop a typical cushingoid appearance with edema or ascites, making them appear obese. This can lead to teasing or bullying by classmates because of their "different" appearance. Contacting the school nurse or making the reason for the child's appearance known to the child's teacher may be necessary (with the child's and parents' permission) to help minimize this. Frequent contact and discussion with the child's siblings are also important to help them understand the reason for so many tests and health care visits as well as why their sibling is receiving so much attention.

If kidney damage becomes extensive and the child's kidneys fail or a transplant is rejected, nursing care needs to be refocused on helping the family to face the possibility of the child's death. Caring for children with a near fatal or fatal diagnosis is discussed in Chapter 56.

Outcome Evaluation

Children with urinary or renal disease often need follow-up care after their acute illness to be certain their kidneys and bladder have returned to functioning adequately. Even though their child is being followed by a specialty renal group or clinic, remind parents that routine health maintenance such as routine childhood immunizations (although children taking steroids or other immunosuppressive therapy should not receive live virus vaccines) is still important

Examples suggesting achievement of outcomes are:

- Child reports that pain is at a tolerable level and decreasing in intensity after treatment.
- Family members state they are able to cope with long-term illness in their child.
- Child states the purpose of a low-sodium diet and lists the ingredients of a low-sodium meal.
- Child states she can accept the need for kidney transplantation.
- Child states the precautions he must follow to reduce possibility of infection while on immunosuppressive therapy.

ANATOMY AND PHYSIOLOGY OF THE KIDNEYS

Embryonic development of the urinary tract is discussed in Chapter 9. Figure 46.1 identifies the structures of the tract. Kidneys in children are located slightly lower in relation to the ribs than in adults. They also do not have as much perinephric fat to pad them, making them more susceptible to trauma.

Kidney Filtration

The glomeruli in the kidney filter water and solutes from the blood. The process is only effective, however, if the blood pressure is higher in the arteries going into the kidneys than in the internal tubular arteries. Urine production is also dependent on the blood pressure being lower in the arteries leaving the kidneys than in the internal tubular arteries. For this reason, renal function must be assessed carefully in children who have either decreased or increased blood pressure for any reason.

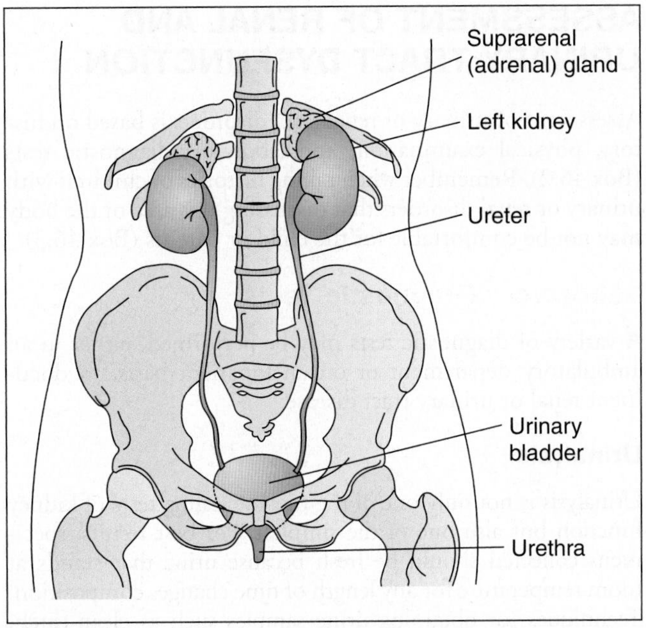

FIGURE 46.1 The urinary system.

Urine

Approximate urine output from different age groups is shown in Table 46.1. A significant decrease in urine production is *oliguria*; absence of urine production is *anuria*.

When renal disease occurs and glomerular or tubular function becomes impaired, nonprotein nitrogenous substances such as creatinine, urea, ammonia, and purine bodies are retained in the blood rather than being excreted. The amount of urea in urine is an indirect indication of kidney and liver function.

Creatinine is a product released during muscle cell metabolism. The amount excreted in urine normally remains constant, regardless of the amount of protein in the diet or body processes. When it is less in amount, therefore, it means kidneys are not functioning as well as usual. *Casts* are formed when there is an abnormal condition that causes the kidney tubule to become lined with protein formed from red and white blood cells, epithelial cells, or fatty cells that harden into the shape of the tubule. After urine washes the casts out, they can be detected by microscopic examination of urine. Because protein deposits in this way only when fluid is slow-moving, their presence suggests slow filtration.

TABLE 46.1 Child's Average Urine Output in 24 Hours

Age	Amount of Urine (ml)
6 months–2 years	540–600
2–5 years	500–780
5–8 years	600–1,200
8–14 years	1,000–1,500
Over 14 years	1,500

ASSESSMENT OF RENAL AND URINARY TRACT DYSFUNCTION

Assessment of urinary or renal tract disorders is based on history, physical examination, and laboratory/diagnostic tests (Box 46.2). Remember when taking histories of children with urinary or renal disorders that discussing this area of the body may not be comfortable for the child or parents (Box 46.3).

Laboratory/Diagnostic Tests

A variety of diagnostic tests may be performed, either in an ambulatory department or on an inpatient basis, to document renal or urinary tract disease.

Urinalysis

Urinalysis is not only one of the most revealing tests of kidney function but also one of the simplest. For best results, specimens collected should be fresh because urine that stands at room temperature for any length of time changes composition. Techniques for obtaining urine samples such as clean-catch, catheterization, 24-hour collections, suprapubic aspiration, and urinalysis are described in Chapter 37. A chemical reagent strip can be used to detect glucose, protein, and occult blood and to measure pH. Specific gravity is best determined by use of a refractometer (requires only a single drop; see Chapter 37).

> **BOX 46.2 Nursing Care Planning Using Assessment**
>
> **Assessing a Child for Renal and Urinary Tract Dysfunction**
>
> **History**
> *Chief concern:* Child reports burning or cries on urination; bloody or "dark" urine, frequency of urination; abdominal pain, flank pain, enuresis. Parents report increase in size of abdomen, periorbital edema, poor appetite, frequent thirst, weight gain, strong odor to urine; diaper rash in infants. A school-age child may be described as a behavior problem because he or she frequently asks to use the bathroom.
> *Family history:* History of renal disease, such as polycystic kidney, enuresis; hypertension.
> *Pregnancy history:* Exposure to nephrotoxic drugs (antibiotics) during pregnancy. Oligohydramnios at birth.
> *Past illness history:* Child recently had a throat or skin infection.
>
> **Physical assessment**
> *General appearance*
> Fatigue, paleness
> Growth restriction
> Low-grade temperature

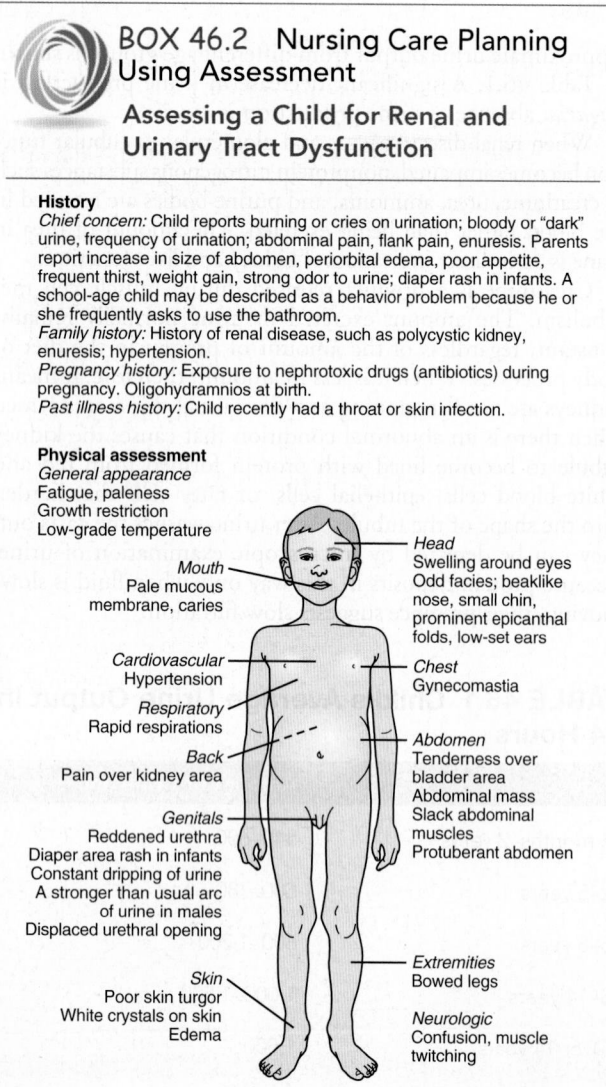

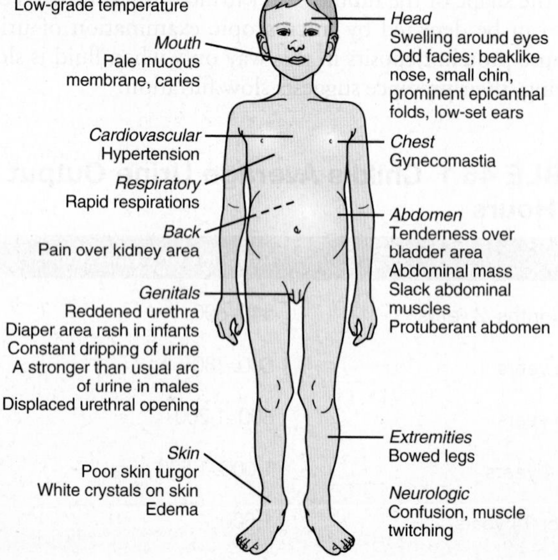

> **BOX 46.3 Nursing Care Planning to Respect Cultural Diversity**
>
> As a general rule, because elimination functions are typically regarded as private, this is not a body system that all people discuss as comfortably as they do illnesses of other body systems. The more modesty is stressed in a culture, the more difficult it may be for people to ask questions about this system's disorders. By being aware that this is a difficult area for parents to discuss, health care personnel can better observe whether added health education is needed when caring for a child with one of these disorders.

Urine Culture

A urinary tract infection (UTI), or the presence of bacteria in urine, is diagnosed by urine culture. Because bladder catheterization can introduce bacteria into the bladder and is also painful and intrusive, most urine specimens in children are obtained by a clean-catch procedure or sterile suprapubic aspiration (see Chapter 37). Several instant-read commercial kits for culturing urine are available and accurate.

Radioisotope Scanning

The administration of radioisotopes (a technetium scan) is another way to assess glomeruli filtration ability. For this, radioactively tagged substances are given intravenously; the rate at which these substances flow through the kidney and are excreted in urine is then determined. The level of radioisotopes used in these studies is small, and urinating removes the substance from the body immediately afterward. You can assure parents that children do not remain radioactive after the procedure, so that parents are not afraid to stay near their children or to hold them.

Blood Studies

A blood urea nitrogen (BUN) test measures the level of urea in blood or how well the kidneys can clear urea from the bloodstream. A normal value is 5 to 20 mg/100 ml.

Glomerular filtration rate is the rate at which substances are filtered from the blood to the urine. It is measured by the amount of creatinine (the breakdown product of creatine from muscle contraction) in blood serum or excreted in 24 hours as determined by a 24-hour urine sample. A normal creatinine clearance rate is 100 ml/min. A normal urine creatinine level is 0.7 to 1.5 mg/100 ml; creatinine in blood serum rarely exceeds 1 mg/dl (Huether, 2013).

Ultrasonography and Magnetic Resonance Imaging

Either a *sonogram* or *magnetic resonance imaging* (MRI) can show differing sizes of kidneys or ureters and illustrate the difference between solid or cystic kidney masses. Because they do not involve X-rays, both ultrasound and MRI may be repeated at frequent intervals for follow-up without danger of radiation exposure (Nelson, Chow, Rosoklija, et al., 2012). When explaining ultrasound and MRI tests, compare the machines used to a camera so it's an object familiar to children and not as frightening.

X-Ray Studies

A flat-plate abdominal radiograph can provide information about the size and contour of the kidneys and may be referred to as a *KUB* (*k*idney, *u*reters, and *b*ladder). *Computed tomography* (CT) scans of the kidneys reveal both the size and density of kidney structures and adequacy of urine flow. Conscious sedation may be given before a CT scan because the size of a CT scanner can be frightening and a child must lie still for an extended time during the procedure. If a contrast medium will be injected to better outline urine flow, be certain to ask about allergy to iodine before the study (the injected medium is iodine based). As with magnet resonance screening, comparing the machine used to a camera can help reduce fear. When preparing children for a test with an injected medium, say "medicine," not "dye" (or compare coloring kidneys to coloring with crayons), so the child doesn't mistake the word "dye" for "die." Caution children that they may experience flushing of the face, warmth, and a salty taste in their mouth after the injection of the "medicine." Because a support person is not allowed to remain in the room during the procedure, thoroughly prepare children so they can comfortably remain still for the procedure.

Intravenous Pyelogram. An *intravenous pyelogram* (IVP) is an X-ray study of the upper urinary tract. It used to be a mainstay of diagnosis for kidney disorders but now is used less frequently as a result of the preferred use of ultrasounds, MRIs, or CT scans. For the procedure, a radiopaque dye is injected into a peripheral vein, circulates through the bloodstream, and is almost immediately identified as a foreign substance by the kidneys and filtered out into the urine by the glomeruli. X-ray films taken at frequent intervals show the outline of collecting systems in the kidney and of the ureters as the radiopaque dye passes through them.

Voiding Cystourethrogram. A *voiding cystourethrogram* (VCUG), a study of the lower urinary tract, reveals the structure of the urethra and bladder and the presence of reflux into the ureters (Lum, 2012). After bladder catheterization, a radiopaque dye is injected into the bladder, and the catheter is then removed. The child is asked to void into a bedpan while serial X-ray films are taken. Although the catheterization is unpleasant, being asked to void while they are being observed may be the most stressful part of the procedure for children because they have been taught that voiding is a private act. Be sure children are told in advance that they will be asked to do this and that it is all right if a stranger watches them (something they have been taught to avoid as well). A first voiding after catheterization may be painful, but you can assure children this is usually only a one-time occurrence. Pouring warm water over the perineal area while sitting on a toilet or sitting in a bathtub of warm water and voiding into the water may help relieve pain if they worry about having pain at the time of a second voiding. Most children, once they void this second time and realize that it is not painful, usually have no further difficulty.

A VCUG should not be done if a child has an active UTI because there is danger the radiopaque material injected into the bladder could spread bacteria from the infection into the ureters and kidneys. Therefore, report any symptoms of a UTI, such as frequency, pain on voiding, or low back pain, to the radiologic service before the procedure. A clean-catch urine specimen for culture may be prescribed before the VCUG to rule out infection if there is doubt whether one is present.

Cystoscopy

Cystoscopy, or examination of the bladder and ureter openings by direct examination with a cystoscope introduced into the bladder through the urethra, is done to evaluate for possible vesicoureteral reflux or urethral stenosis. Radiopaque dye may be introduced into the bladder at the time of cystoscopy so the bladder can be visualized on X-ray or by ultrasound. During the procedure, small catheters can be threaded into the ureters for the introduction of dye to outline them (retrograde pyelography). Because the procedure is painful and requires a child to lie still, it is usually done under conscious sedation. As with catheterization, the first voiding may be painful. Once allowed, urge children to drink fluid so they urinate frequently to flush out any pathogens introduced at the time of the procedure.

✔ QSEN Checkpoint Question 46.1

Teamwork & Collaboration

Carey had a VCUG last year to help diagnose whether she had vesicoureteral reflux. If you had collaborated with the radiology technician to ensure an accurate test that did not cause distress for Carey, what would you have emphasized in order to achieve these goals?

a. The technician will have to read the instructions for the test to Carey.
b. Lying in a large, metal tube is frightening for most children.
c. Children often feel uncomfortable voiding in public.
d. The dye capsules may be too large for Carey to swallow.

Look in Appendix A for the best answer and rationale.

Renal Biopsy

Renal biopsy involves passing a thin biopsy needle into the kidney through the skin over the kidney. The procedure is used to diagnose the extent of renal disease and thereby predict disease outcome or progress or reveal beginning rejection of a transplanted kidney (Tse, Yadav, Herrema, et al., 2013).

Renal biopsy may be done in an older child under only local anesthesia, but conscious sedation may be necessary for a younger child who cannot cooperate easily. The kidney is located first by ultrasound to accurately locate the best place for the biopsy. The child lies prone with a sandbag under the abdomen for firmness. If the procedure is done under a local anesthetic, prepare children for the feel of a pinprick as the local anesthetic is injected; after this, they should not feel any further pain. They will feel pressure, however, as the biopsy needle is inserted. Caution children they need to lie still while the biopsy specimen is taken (if the child moves suddenly, the needle might puncture a renal artery or vein or tear vital glomeruli). Be certain children have support people to remain with them for this procedure so they have someone to hold their hand or comfort them when they feel the pressure of the needle.

After the biopsy, press a sterile gauze square against the biopsy site for approximately 15 minutes to halt bleeding, and then apply a pressure dressing. Caution parents beforehand that a large dressing will be used so they don't think the size of the dressing reflects the size of the specimen taken (the amount of tissue removed is actually no more than the lumen of the needle used, or about the size of a pencil lead).

Measure vital signs and observe the biopsy site every 15 minutes for at least the first hour afterward. Do not lift the dressing to assess bleeding, because doing so destroys the protective function of the pressure dressing. If the procedure is done on an ambulatory basis, children can be discharged 2 to 4 hours after the procedure if vital signs are stable and they have voided. Encourage children to drink a considerable amount of fluid (a glass every hour while awake) during the first 24 hours to keep urine flowing freely and prevent blood from clotting in the kidney tubules and blocking urine flow. Play games with the child, if necessary, to encourage a high fluid intake (the child must take a drink each time before a turn at a game, or play "Simon Says" and have Simon frequently say, "Drink").

The first voiding after renal biopsy is invariably blood-tinged. Advise parents to keep children on restricted activity for 24 hours or until no more hematuria is present. Instruct parents how to keep serial urine samples, comparing each specimen with the previous one, to detect whether hematuria is becoming more or less marked. When urine no longer appears bloody, they can test it for occult blood a final time to confirm even minimum bleeding has stopped. A hematocrit level may be prescribed 24 hours after the procedure to ensure that bleeding is not continuing.

What if . . . 46.1 Carey's grandmother telephones you after a kidney biopsy and says Carey is voiding black urine. She asks you if there is a possibility she is voiding blood. What recommendations would you make to the grandmother?

THERAPEUTIC MEASURES FOR THE MANAGEMENT OF RENAL DISEASE

Because kidney function is necessary for life, if it deteriorates, therapies to replace renal function must be instituted.

Peritoneal Dialysis

Dialysis is the separation and removal of solutes from body fluid by diffusion through a semipermeable membrane. *Peritoneal dialysis* uses the membrane of the peritoneal cavity to do this. Hemodialysis circulates blood through an outside synthetic membrane to do this. Unlike hemodialysis, peritoneal dialysis does not require elaborate equipment or expense, but it does take more time. Peritoneal dialysis may be used as a temporary measure for children who experience sudden renal failure caused by trauma or shock. It is also used for fairly long periods with children with chronic renal disease to allow them to live until kidney transplantation can be arranged (Issa, Lankireddy, & Kukla, 2012).

It is usually begun when the serum creatinine level reaches 10 mg/100 ml. Other indications are congestive heart failure, BUN of more than 100 mg/100 ml, hyperkalemia (potassium level of more than 6 mEq/L), and uremic encephalopathy (confusion or coma). Continuous peritoneal dialysis allows the procedure to be done at home because less rigorous monitoring of the procedure is necessary.

Performing Peritoneal Dialysis

Before peritoneal dialysis begins, a child's weight and vital signs need to be obtained to provide baseline information. Ask the child to void to reduce bladder size so the bladder occupies as little anterior space as possible; if a child cannot void, catheterization may be necessary. Following this, the child's abdomen is cleaned just below the umbilicus with an antiseptic solution and covered with a sterile drape; a local anesthetic is injected into the abdominal wall, and a large-bore needle is inserted into the peritoneal cavity. If ascites fluid is present, a quantity of this fluid is removed, and then a warmed hypertonic glucose solution (approximately 50 to 100 ml/kg of body weight) or a commercial dialysis solution is infused by gravity flow into the peritoneal cavity. This distends the abdominal wall and allows safe insertion of a peritoneal catheter, which is sutured into place and covered with a sterile dressing (Fig. 46.2). This catheter will remain in place for the duration of dialysis.

As for any procedure, children need to be well prepared for peritoneal dialysis, but if the procedure is presented in a matter-of-fact way, children usually accept it with no more apprehension than IV therapy as both procedures involve a needle penetration. Caution children they will feel the initial prick of the needle that administers the local anesthetic but then will feel only pressure after that as the peritoneal needle or catheter is inserted. The procedure is intrusive, however, and frightening. Provide opportunities for therapeutic play such as letting the child handle a cloth doll, a dialysis tube, IV tubing, a doll's bed, or syringes and needles afterward.

With the dialysis tube in place, a prescribed amount of dialysis solution is then infused into the peritoneal cavity by gravity drainage. This takes approximately 10 minutes and is recorded as *inflow* time. Be certain the infusion fluid is warmed to room temperature to prevent the child from becoming chilled; warming the solution in a basin of warm water or with the use of commercial warm packs so it is near body temperature also appears to improve diffusion

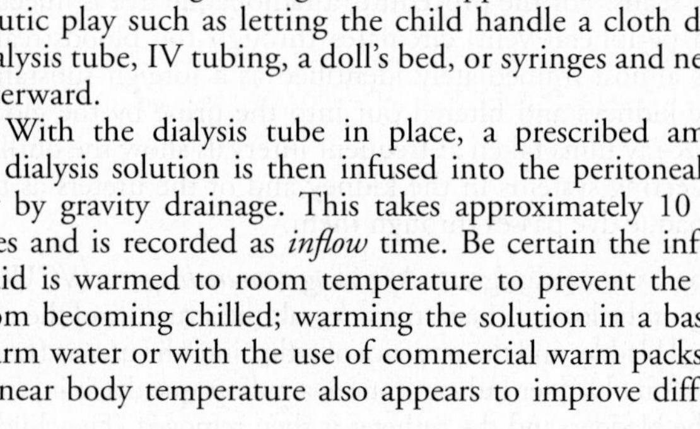

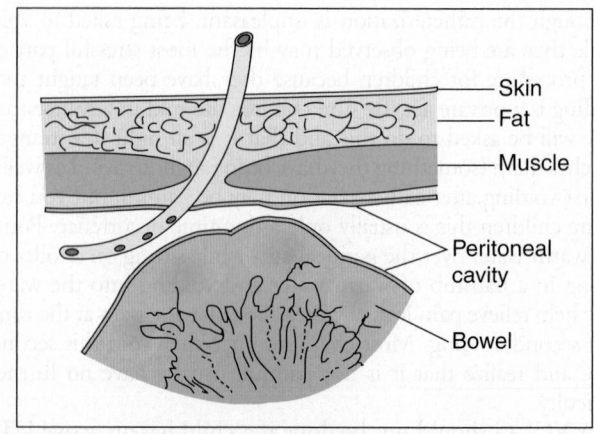

FIGURE 46.2 Insertion site for a peritoneal dialysis catheter.

efficiency. Heparin may be added to the first infusion to keep any initial bleeding from the abdominal puncture from plugging the tube.

The infused fluid is allowed to remain in the child's peritoneal cavity for 15 to 60 minutes (called the *equilibrium* or *dwell time*) while fluid, urea, and electrolytes move by osmosis from extracellular spaces into the hypertonic solution. After the designated equilibrium time has passed, drain the fluid from the peritoneal catheter into a collecting bottle (this takes approximately 10 minutes and is recorded as *outflow* time). More fluid generally drains from the peritoneal cavity than was infused, because excessive fluid has diffused across the peritoneum, reducing accumulated peritoneal or ascitic fluid.

Peritoneal dialysis may be conducted continuously for periods of 12 to 72 hours, depending on the effectiveness of the procedure in restoring serum creatinine and BUN levels to normal.

Monitor vital signs at least every hour while children are undergoing peritoneal dialysis. Frequent blood studies are necessary during periods of peritoneal dialysis to determine electrolyte concentrations. If electrolyte imbalances occur, electrolytes may be added to the infusion solution or administered IV. During each new infusion period and while the solution is in the abdomen, carefully observe for shortness of breath, because the fluid exerts upward pressure on the diaphragm. Elevating the head of the bed a little usually helps to increase breathing space and ease respirations. If either tachycardia or hypotension occurs, this suggests that hypovolemia is occurring or fluid is moving too rapidly into the peritoneal cavity. An increasing temperature (after 24 hours) suggests peritoneal infection (Sayed, Abu-Aisha, Ahmed, et al., 2012).

Follow the agency's policy for cleaning and covering the end of the peritoneal catheter if there are periods when dialysis is halted (Fig. 46.3). The longer the peritoneal catheter remains in place, the greater is the risk of infection. Always assess the tube insertion site daily for redness or drainage. Use palpation to assess the abdomen for guarding or tenderness (rigidity suggest peritonitis or infection). Ask children to report any abdominal pain or diarrhea.

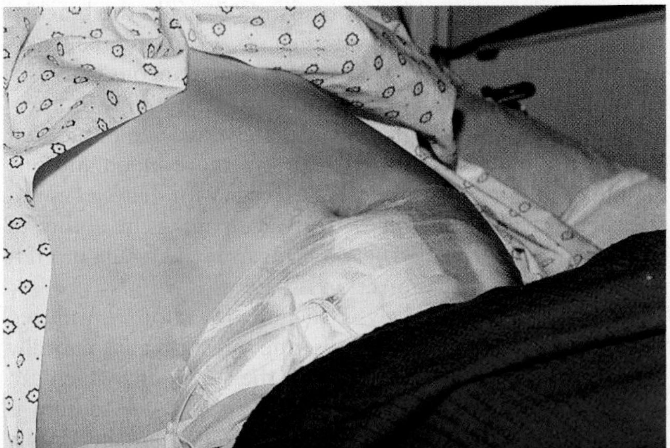

FIGURE 46.3 Peritoneal catheter inserted into a child's abdomen. A secure dressing surrounds the insertion site to prevent infection. (Courtesy of Karen M. Polise, MSN, RN, Division of Nephrology, The Children's Hospital of Philadelphia.)

Once cycles of dialysis begin, children often grow bored lying in bed waiting for this procedure to be finished. Plan interaction for these times—perhaps a toy or game that is allowed only during the procedure, so that the time remains special. Children generally do not feel hungry while having peritoneal dialysis, because the bulk of peritoneal fluid causes pressure on the stomach and makes them feel uncomfortably full, so they usually prefer a liquid diet or small frequent feedings during this time. So that children can feel they have a sense of control over what is happening, let them help with the procedure by doing such things as recording the amount of solution infused and drained and allowing them to select liquids they like for meals.

Peritoneal dialysis is a simple yet important procedure. Help parents understand its importance for their child so they can demonstrate a positive attitude toward it because their acceptance of the procedure helps the child accept it as well.

Continuous Cycling Peritoneal Dialysis

Continuous cycling peritoneal dialysis (CCPD) allows a child to go to school or participate in other activities while receiving dialysis (Davenport, 2012). With CCPD, a permanent dialysis catheter is inserted and sutured into place at the abdomen. Although commercial devices may be used, for the simplest method, the child or parent attaches a bag of dialysis fluid and tubing to this and infuses a prescribed dialysis solution by gravity drainage; the bag and tubing are then rolled into a compact square under the child's clothes. The infused solution remains in the child for 4 to 6 hours during the day (8 hours at night); the dialysate bag is then lowered, and the solution drains from the peritoneal cavity into it. The bag and fluid are then discarded and a new bag of dialysate solution is attached and raised, and new solution is infused.

CCPD requires careful monitoring and attention by the child or family so there is a record of the amount of fluid infused. Children on CCPD can participate in gym programs but should not participate in contact sports or swimming. Teach parents to think ahead for holidays or family trips so they do not run short of supplies.

Because CCPD is continuous, electrolytes in the bloodstream are maintained at more constant levels than when intermittent dialysis is used. A great deal of potassium is removed, however, so caution is needed or children may become hypokalemic (Lum, 2012). The main advantage is that CCPD allows greater freedom for children to attend school. There are disadvantages, however, such as infection resulting from the long-term placement of the catheter and dehydration or hypernatremia resulting from excess fluid removal. Because the tube remains in place at all times and the peritoneal solution constantly distends the abdomen, the child appears obese and clothing is difficult to fit, frequently reminding the child of the illness. Possible complications of CCPD are summarized in Table 46.2.

What if...46.2 Carey, who receives CCPD, wants to go to her church camp this summer. Her grandmother asks you whether this would be a good experience for her. What factors would you want to know about the camp? About Carey? About her dialysis regimen?

TABLE 46.2 Possible Complications of Continuous Cycling Peritoneal Dialysis

Assessment	Problem	Interventions
Redness, pain, or swelling at tube insertion site	Infection	Report findings; take culture of site; administer antibiotics or other site care as prescribed.
Abdominal pain, increased temperature, nausea and vomiting, cloudy return in drainage solution	Peritonitis	Report findings; administer antibiotics as prescribed; auscultate for bowel sounds with vital sign assessment.
Cramps as fluid is infused	Irritation of peritoneal cavity	Infuse solutions more slowly; warm temperature of solution to body temperature.
Difficulty with infusion or drainage of fluid	Kinked or clotted tubing; malpositioned catheter	Assess tubing for kinking; change position of child; ask child to cough to increase abdominal pressure; add prescribed amount of heparin to dialysate bag (prevents clotting).
Weight increase; moist cough, shortness of breath	Fluid overload	Assess blood pressure and weight; decrease sodium and fluid oral intake as prescribed; possibly decrease strength of dialysis fluid as prescribed.
Weight loss, hypotension, poor skin turgor, tachycardia	Fluid loss	Assess blood pressure and weight; increase fluid and sodium intake as prescribed.
Blood-tinged dialysis return	Ruptured capillary vessel	Report findings; assess pulse and blood pressure; observe for further bleeding in drainage; flush catheter with prescribed amount of heparin to keep clots from forming.

Hemodialysis

Hemodialysis removes body wastes by using an external membrane as the diffusion surface. For hemodialysis, a catheter is inserted into an artery and blood is removed from the child and circulated through a dialysis coil. Urea and electrolytes in the blood diffuse into the surrounding fluid bath as the blood passes through the coil (Hothi, Stronach, & Harvey, 2013). After diffusion is complete, the blood is returned to the child's venous circulation (Fig. 46.4).

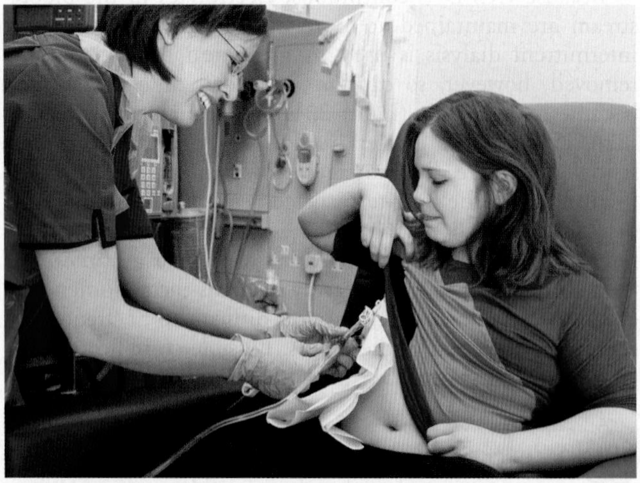

FIGURE 46.4 A nurse preparing a 10-year-old girl for a hemodialysis session. A subclavian catheter from the child is connected to the hemodialysis equipment (in the background). Blood flows from the child through the catheter to the hemodialysis equipment and is then returned to the child's venous circulation (© Life in View/Science Source).

Hemodialysis can be done as a continuous process, but it is so effective that 3 hours of hemodialysis accomplish as much as 12 hours of peritoneal dialysis. Children who have renal failure or whose kidneys have been removed while they await a kidney transplant can be maintained almost indefinitely by hemodialysis sessions two or three times a week or by continuous ultrafiltration or continuous arteriovenous hemofiltration. It can be used in infants as well as older children (Quinlan, Bates, Sheils, et al., 2013).

To establish a site for initial blood removal, children may have a double-lumen central catheter inserted into a central vein, such as the subclavian or internal jugular vein. A permanent technique is subcutaneous anastomosis of a vein and artery, creating an arteriovenous fistula (usually the brachial artery and brachiocephalic vein; Fig. 46.5A) or internal anastomosis of the artery and vein using a subcutaneous graft (see Fig. 46.5B). The possibility of infection is reduced with internal anastomosis, although, unfortunately, two venipunctures, one from a low point in the shunt to remove blood and one high in the shunt to return it, are necessary for dialysis (use an anesthetic cream beforehand to reduce pain). The ability to feel a thrill (vibration) or hear a bruit over the fistula or graft site is proof that the connection is patent.

The risks of hemodialysis include infection introduced with venipuncture (severe because the infection automatically becomes septicemia) and clotting of the access site, which can lead to emboli. During hemodialysis, if too much sodium is removed, muscle cramping may occur. A "first use" syndrome or symptoms such as dizziness or muscle cramping can occur from a reaction to the fibers in the dialysis machine coil. If urea is moved from the blood at too rapid a rate—faster than urea can be shifted from the brain into the blood—children may begin to show signs of confusion, vomiting, dizziness, visual blurring, or hallucinations from a *dialysis disequilibrium syndrome.*

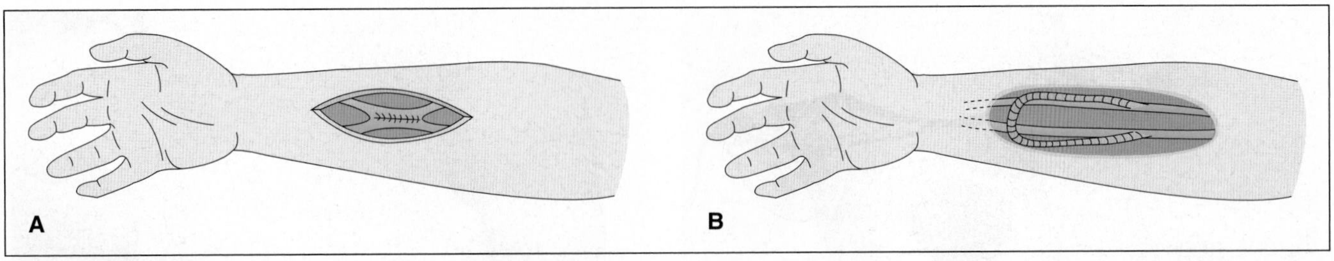

FIGURE 46.5 (A) An internal arteriovenous fistula. (B) An internal arteriovenous graft.

This occurs because, as osmotic pressure is greater in the brain than the blood, fluid shifts into the brain, resulting in cerebral edema. Hemodialysis must be temporarily halted if these symptoms occur to allow equalization.

Children grow as bored during hemodialysis as they do during peritoneal dialysis. Help parents provide stimulating activities such as a playing a board game or reading a favorite story, which are only used during that time period. When children's kidneys are removed prior to transplantation, they must remain on a continuous program of hemodialysis. These children may come to resent a machine as "owning" or "controlling" them as they become aware they cannot exist apart from it (Bayhakki & Hatthakit, 2012). Allowing them to plan special activities to do during hemodialysis time can help not only to pass the time but also to give them a feeling of control.

HEALTH PROMOTION AND RISK MANAGEMENT

Several important interventions can help prevent urinary and renal disease in children. The first intervention is to educate parents and caregivers about wiping from front to back when changing diapers of female infants. The second intervention is to prevent UTI in girls by beginning education about perineal hygiene measures from the time they are first toilet trained. Remind parents of simple ways to prevent UTI, such as not allowing children to bathe with bubble bath. Teach parents to recognize that abnormally colored urine (red, black, or cloudy) should not be dismissed because this could be the beginning of a UTI or kidney disease.

Educating parents about the importance of giving the full course of antibiotics prescribed for UTIs can help prevent return reinfection; giving the full course of antibiotics after a streptococcal infection can help prevent acute glomerulonephritis.

STRUCTURAL ABNORMALITIES OF THE URINARY TRACT

Because the urinary tract is a system of hollow tubes, congenital disorders can rise from faulty recanalization in intrauterine life.

Patent Urachus

When the bladder first forms in utero, it is joined to the umbilicus by a narrow tube, the *urachus*. If this fails to close during embryologic development, a fistula is left between the bladder and umbilicus (**patent urachus**). This occurs more commonly in males than in females. Nurses are frequently the ones to discover this condition as they notice clear fluid draining from the base of the umbilical cord while changing a newborn's diaper. If you test the fluid with nitrazine paper for pH, its acid content will identify it as urine. An ultrasound will confirm the patent connection.

A few patent urachus abnormalities heal spontaneously, but most require surgical correction to prevent pathogens from entering the fistula site and causing persistent bladder infection. This is done in the immediate neonatal period using only a small subumbilical incision (Tsai & Yeh, 2011).

Exstrophy of the Bladder

Exstrophy of the bladder is a midline closure defect that occurs during the embryonic period of gestation (first 8 weeks). As a result, the bladder lies open and exposed on the abdomen. It occurs more frequently in males than females by a ratio of 2:1 (Mahan, 2011).

Assessment

Exstrophy is often detected by fetal ultrasound as the lack of an anterior wall of the bladder and a lack of anterior skin covering the lower anterior abdomen are revealed (Fig. 46.6A). At birth, the bladder appears bright red and continually drains urine from the open surface. In both sexes, pelvic bone defects, particularly nonclosure of the pubic arch, may be present. In males, the penis may be unformed or malformed. In females, the urethra may be abnormally formed. Urethral defects in males such as epispadias—the opening of the urinary meatus on the dorsal or superior surface of the penis—are also common. The skin around the bladder quickly becomes excoriated because of constant exposure to acid urine. Kidney infection can occur from ascending organisms from the open bladder. When children with this disorder begin to walk, they may demonstrate a "waddling" gait from the effect of the nonfused pubic arch.

Therapeutic Management

The treatment of bladder exstrophy begins with surgical closure of the bladder and, if necessary, the anterior abdominal wall and construction of a urethra (see Fig. 46.6B).

Preoperative Interventions. To minimize the possibility of infection in the bladder while the infant waits for initial surgery, keep the exposed bladder covered by a sterile plastic bowel bag to prevent the bladder surface from adhering to bedclothes or diapers and being injured. To prevent the skin of the abdomen from excoriation, consult a wound, ostomy, and continence nurse for the best approach, which usually involves a protective substance such as A&D Ointment,

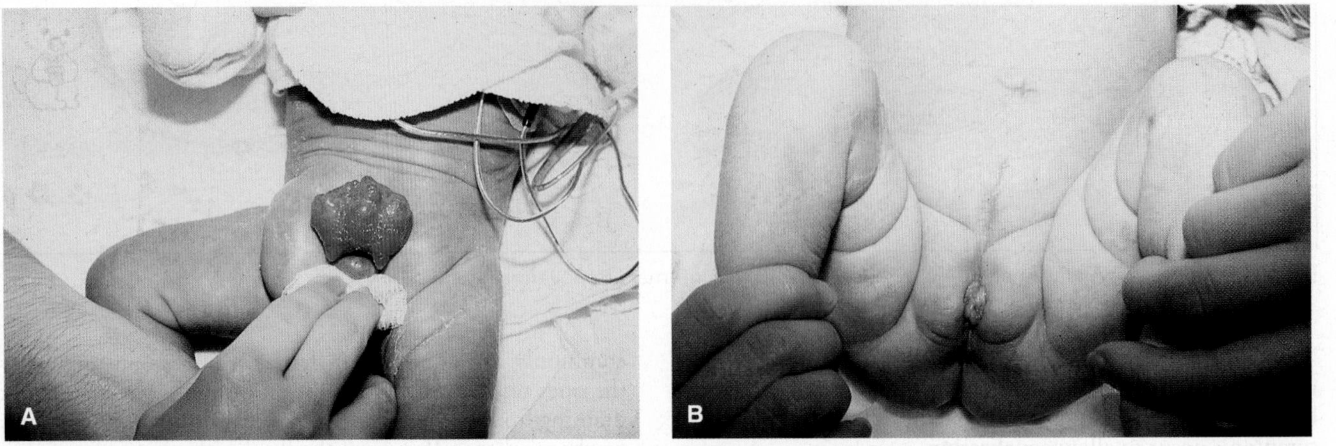

FIGURE 46.6 Bladder exstrophy. **(A)** Prior to surgical reconstruction. Note the bright-red color of the bladder. **(B)** Following surgical reconstruction. (Courtesy of Karen M. Polise, MSN, RN, Division of Nephrology, The Children's Hospital of Philadelphia.)

Karaya Gum, or Maalox. To prevent further separation of the symphysis, the infant's legs may be flexed, brought together, and wrapped in Ace bandages to hold them in that position. If this is done, do not separate the infant's legs to apply diapers; just place them under the child instead. Be certain to change diapers promptly after defecation so feces is not brought forward to the open bladder. Position the infant on the back so urine drains freely. Sponge bathe rather than tub bathe the infant to prevent water from entering the ureters and becoming a source of infection.

Help parents to view their child as perfect in all other ways but the unusual bladder formation. In some instances, the bladder repair will not be done immediately, so parents will need instructions on how to care for the child at home while waiting for surgery.

Postoperative Interventions. Surgery is completed as either a one-step or two-step procedure. In the first step, the bladder tissue is reconstructed; in the second, a urethra is created. After bladder construction, a suprapubic or indwelling urethral catheter for urine drainage will be in place to allow the newly constructed bladder to rest. Keep the infant positioned on the back or in an infant chair to prevent feces from coming forward and contaminating the incision line. Immediately after surgery, urine draining from the catheter may be blood stained, but this should clear after the first few hours. Children may experience sharp painful bladder contractions for the first few days after surgery. Provide enough analgesia or an antispasmodic to keep the child comfortable. To prevent the nonfused pubic bone from separating and putting stress on the suture line, at the time of surgery, the child may be fitted with an external fixation device to hold the pubic bones in approximation until they fuse (4 to 6 weeks).

After the second-stage urethra repair, children can be expected to experience some stress incontinence (loss of urine on physical exertion) from the constructed urethra. When they are older, Kegel exercises can help strengthen the perineal muscles and reduce this concern.

For some children, so little bladder tissue is present that surgical reconstruction isn't possible, so the bladder remnants are surgically removed and a ureterocecal implantation (ureters directed into the small intestine) or a *continent urinary reservoir* (an artificial bladder) is constructed (Fig. 46.7) (Elshal, Abdelhalim, Hafez, et al., 2012).

For continent urinary diversion, a small segment of the intestine is separated from the intestinal tract. The intestinal tract is then anastomosed so the gastrointestinal tract is maintained. The separated segment is attached to the internal abdominal wall using the appendix to create an artificial urethra. The ureters are anastomosed to this segment.

Urine drains from the kidneys into the ureters and then into the collecting bowel segment. The parent or child catheterizes the abdominal urethra three or four times daily to empty urine. The procedure is theoretically simple, but it is

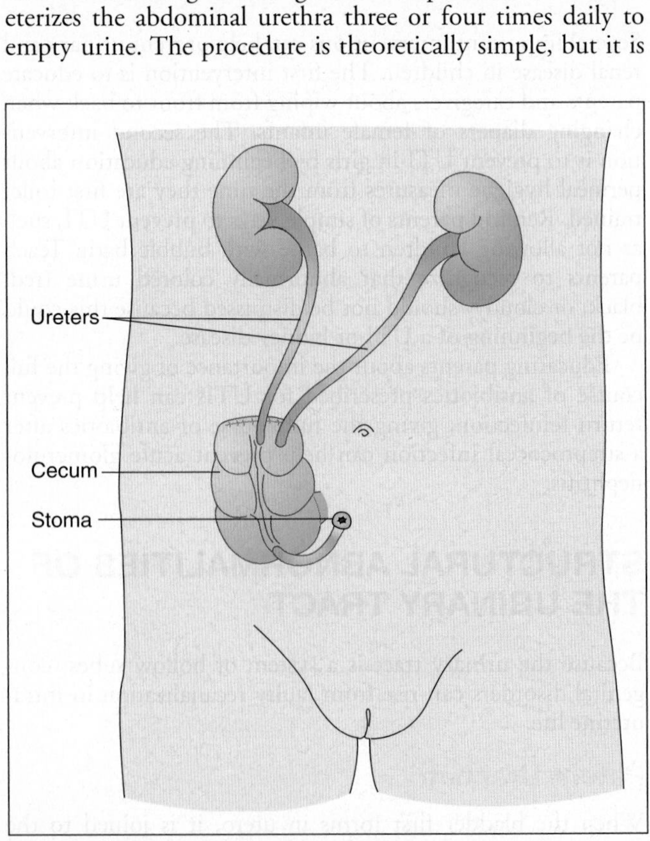

FIGURE 46.7 A continent urine reservoir. A portion of intestine is isolated; the attached ureters drain into it. The appendix creates an abdominal stoma for catheterization.

technically difficult to accomplish. Parents need a good review of anatomy to aid their understanding of the procedure. As the child reaches school age and begins school activities, such as showering, that expose the condition to others, adjusting to a continent urinary reservoir can be difficult. Ensure that the child has a plan for follow-up care during the school years and in adolescence so the function of the reservoir and also the child's adjustment can continue to be assessed.

Hypospadias

Hypospadias is a urethral defect in which the urethral opening is not at the end of the penis but on the ventral (lower) aspect of the penis (Fig. 46.8A) (Spinoit, Poelaert, Groen, et al., 2013). It is a fairly common anomaly, occurring in approximately 1 in 300 male newborns. It tends to be familial or may occur from a multifactorial genetic focus. **Epispadias** is a similar defect in which the opening is on the dorsal surface of the penis (see Fig. 46.8B).

Assessment

Be certain to inspect all male newborns at birth for hypospadias or epispadias as part of a routine physical examination. The degree of hypospadias may be minimal (on the glans but inferior in site) or maximal (at the midshaft or at the penal-scrotal junction). Many newborns with hypospadias have an accompanying short *chordee*—a fibrous band that causes the penis to curve downward (often called a cobra-head appearance; see Fig. 46.8C). Also inspect carefully for *cryptorchidism* (undescended testes), which is often found in conjunction with hypospadias.

If the penis defect is so extensive that sex determination is unclear, sex cell karyotyping or DNA analysis (see Chapter 7) will be done. Parents may have difficulty discussing this condition with relatives or health care personnel because it is a sensitive area for them. Help parents work through these feelings by allowing them to talk about the disorder and by answering their questions honestly and openly about what the condition includes.

Therapeutic Management

Children with hypospadias should not be circumcised because, at the time of the repair, the surgeon may wish to use a portion of the foreskin for the repair. In the newborn, the surgical procedure may be a *meatotomy*—a procedure in which the urethra is extended to a usual position—to establish better urinary function. When the child is older (age 12 to 18 months), adherent chordee can be released. If the repair will be extensive, all surgery may be delayed until the child is 3 to 4 years of age. To encourage penis growth and make the procedure easier, the child may have testosterone cream applied to the penis or receive injections of human growth hormone until surgery. It's important that hypospadias be corrected before school age if at all possible so the child looks and feels like other males. If left uncorrected, in later years, a meatal opening at an inferior penile site may interfere with fertility, because it does not allow sperm to be deposited close to the female cervix during coitus (Vidal, Gorduza, Haraux, et al., 2010).

After surgical repair, a urethral urinary drainage catheter will be inserted to allow urine output without putting tension against the urethral sutures. The child may notice painful bladder spasms as long as the catheter is in place (3 to 7 days), so an analgesic such as acetaminophen (Tylenol) and an anticholinergic medication such as oxybutynin (Ditropan) may be prescribed for pain relief. After hypospadias repair, children can be expected to have usual urinary and reproductive function unless accompanying anomalies of the penis were present.

INFECTIONS OF THE URINARY SYSTEM AND RELATED DISORDERS

As the urinary system drains to the outside of the body, infection can easily spread to the bladder or kidneys.

Urinary Tract Infection

UTI occurs more often in females than in males at a ratio of about 8% in girls to 2% in boys (Lum, 2012). Urinary pathogens appear to enter the urinary tract most often as an ascending infection from the perineum and are gram-negative rods such as *Escherichia coli*. UTIs also occur as a health care–acquired infection in children who have urinary catheters.

UTIs occur more often in girls than boys because the urethra is shorter in girls and, because it is located close to the vagina and anus, vulvovaginitis or rectal bacteria can easily spread to the urethra. Changing diapers frequently can help reduce the risk for infection in infants. Girls should be taught early (when they are toilet-trained) to wipe themselves

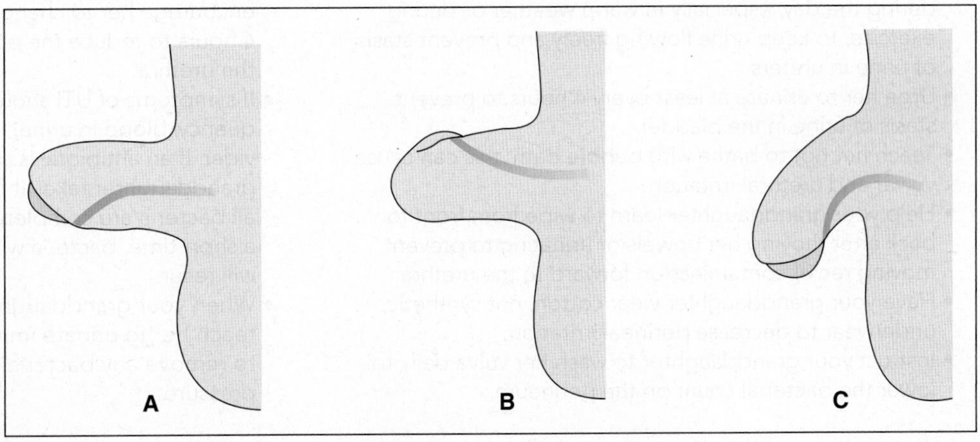

FIGURE 46.8 Urethral defects. **(A)** Hypospadias. **(B)** Epispadias. **(C)** Hypospadias with chordee.

from front to back after voiding and defecating to avoid contaminating the urethra. There is a suggested correlation between the use of products such as bubble bath, feminine hygiene sprays, and hot tubs and UTI in girls, so use of these should be discouraged or minimized (Gaylord & Peterson-Smith, 2012). Additional measures to prevent UTIs are summarized in Box 46.4.

It's important that UTIs are treated so they do not spread to involve the kidneys (pyelonephritis) and cause permanent damage. Girls who have more than two UTIs or boys with their first UTI should be referred to a urologist to determine whether they have a congenital anomaly such as an urethral stenosis or bladder–ureter reflux that causes recurrent urinary stasis.

Assessment

Although it may be possible to locate a UTI precisely as urethritis, cystitis, ureteritis, or pyelonephritis, the signs and symptoms in young children often are not clear-cut, so all types are referred to as a UTI. The typical symptoms that occur in older children or in adults—pain on urination, frequency, burning, and hematuria—may not be present in young children, so UTI is suspected when a child has a fever with no demonstrable cause on physical examination. If the infection is confined to the bladder (cystitis), the child may have a low-grade fever, mild abdominal pain, and enuresis (bed-wetting). If the infection is a pyelonephritis, the symptoms generally are more acute, with high fever, abdominal or flank pain, vomiting, and malaise.

Urine for culture can be collected by a clean-catch technique, suprapubic aspiration, or catheterization, so bacteria from the vulva or foreskin do not contaminate the sample and give a false reading. Suprapubic aspiration is generally limited to infants because the sight of the syringe is so frightening to older children; plus, the procedure can introduce infection. Catheterization, also frightening and a potential source of infection, is limited in children of all ages.

Urine obtained from suprapubic aspiration is generally sterile, so any growth from this source is significant. A clean-catch urine specimen is said to be positive for bacteriuria if the bacterial colony count is more than 100,000 per ml. A count of less than 10,000 per ml is considered a negative culture. If the count is between 10,000 and 100,000 per ml or if the urine is positive for proteinuria (which could happen because of the presence of bacteria), the count is usually repeated. In addition to identifying the responsible organism, microscopic examination of the urine specimen may indicate the presence of red blood cells (hematuria) caused by bacterial irritation of the bladder mucosa. The presence of either red or white blood cells or bacteria tends to make urine more alkaline, so the pH of the sample will be elevated (greater than 7).

Therapeutic Management

The medical treatment for UTI is the oral administration of a broad-spectrum antibiotic such as sulfamethoxazole-trimethoprim (Bactrim) or amoxicillin, or an antibiotic specific to the causative organism that is cultured (Paintsil, 2013). In addition to the antibiotic, a child needs to drink a large quantity of fluid to "flush" the infection out of the urinary tract, particularly if a sulfa drug is prescribed because these can cause urinary crystals in concentrated urine. Cranberry juice is often recommended as being highly effective in acidifying urine and making it more resistant to bacterial growth. In actual practice, there is little evidence of its effectiveness, so offer any fluid the child will drink readily. If the child experiences moderate to severe pain on urination that interferes with the ability to void, suggest the child sit in a bathtub of warm water and void into the water. A mild analgesic, such as acetaminophen (Tylenol), may help reduce pain enough to allow voiding.

BOX 46.4 Nursing Care Planning to Empower a Family

PREVENTING URINARY TRACT INFECTION IN FEMALES

Q. Carey's grandmother tells you, "Carey had two urinary tract infections last year. How can we prevent that from happening again?"

A. Here are some important tips to help prevent urinary tract infection (UTI):

- Encourage your granddaughter to drink fluid periodically during the day, especially in warm weather or during exercise, to keep urine flowing freely and prevent stasis of urine in ureters.
- Urge her to urinate at least every 4 hours to prevent stasis of urine in the bladder.
- Teach her not to bathe with bubble bath; this can cause vulvar and urethral irritation.
- Help your granddaughter learn to wipe from front to back after moving her bowels or urinating to prevent moving rectal contamination forward to the urethra.
- Have your granddaughter wear cotton, not synthetic, underwear to decrease perineal irritation.
- Instruct your granddaughter to wash her vulva daily to lower the bacterial count on the perineum.
- When your granddaughter begins menstruating, encourage her to change sanitary pads at least every 4 hours to reduce the possible growth of bacteria near the urethra.
- If symptoms of UTI should occur (pain on urination, frequency, blood in urine), call your primary health care provider. If an antibiotic is prescribed, make sure that your granddaughter takes it for the full prescribed course, so all bacteria are completely eradicated. Otherwise, after a short time, bacteria will proliferate, and the infection will recur.
- When your granddaughter becomes sexually active, teach her to urinate immediately after intercourse to remove any bacteria forced into the urethra by pressure.

Remind parents that with a UTI, treatment with antibiotics must be continued for the full prescription or the infection will return. Help parents create a reminder system, such as a sheet of paper for the refrigerator door or a reminder on their smartphone, to help ensure adherence. A repeat clean-catch urine sample is usually obtained at 72 hours to assess the effectiveness of the antibiotic treatment and to be certain the bacterial count is being reduced.

After recurrent UTIs, children may be prescribed a prophylactic antibiotic for 6 months. At periodic health checkups for the next few years, the child should void a clean-catch specimen for culture or microscopic analysis so it is certain that a low-grade infection does not still exist.

"Honeymoon" Cystitis

Honeymoon cystitis refers to UTI seen in young women shortly after they initiate a first sexual relationship caused by the local irritation and inflammation that results from coitus.

Like most UTIs, these respond quickly to antibiotic therapy. Voiding as soon as possible after coitus may help to flush pathogenic organisms from the urethra and prevent such infections. When cystitis is seen in an adolescent girl, it is an alert that a girl may be sexually active. In addition to the need for counseling about personal hygiene measures to prevent UTI, the girl may need information about safer sex (see Box 5.7 in Chapter 5), reproductive planning, and symptoms of sexually transmitted infections. Recurrent UTIs in a school-age or preschool girl may suggest sexual maltreatment (Beck, Bekker, & Van Driel, 2010).

✔ QSEN Checkpoint Question 46.2

Quality Improvement

Carey's grandmother is concerned because Carey had two UTIs last year. Which of her following statements best shows that Carey's grandmother received adequate teaching on the prevention of UTIs?

a. "I won't allow Carey to drink too much milk or eat foods like yogurt."
b. "I'll try to have Carey bathe with bath salts to discourage bacteria in her groin area."
c. "I'll be certain to administer all of the antibiotic pills that the doctor prescribes."
d. "I'll make sure that Carey doesn't overexert herself when she's playing with her friends."

Look in Appendix A for the best answer and rationale.

Vesicoureteral Reflux

Normally, urine flows from the ureters into the bladder, with almost no flow reentering the ureters from the bladder because the ureters enter the bladder obliquely and a bladder skin flap or "valve" obscures the end of the ureter, preventing backflow. **Vesicoureteral reflux** refers to retrograde flow of urine from the bladder into the ureters (Batinic, Miloševic, Topalovic-Grkovic, et al., 2012). This reflux of urine occurs with micturition (voiding) when the bladder contracts (Fig. 46.9) because the valve that guards the entrance from the bladder to the ureter is defective, either from birth or because of scarring from repeated UTIs; bladder pressure is stronger than usual; or ureters are implanted at unusual angles.

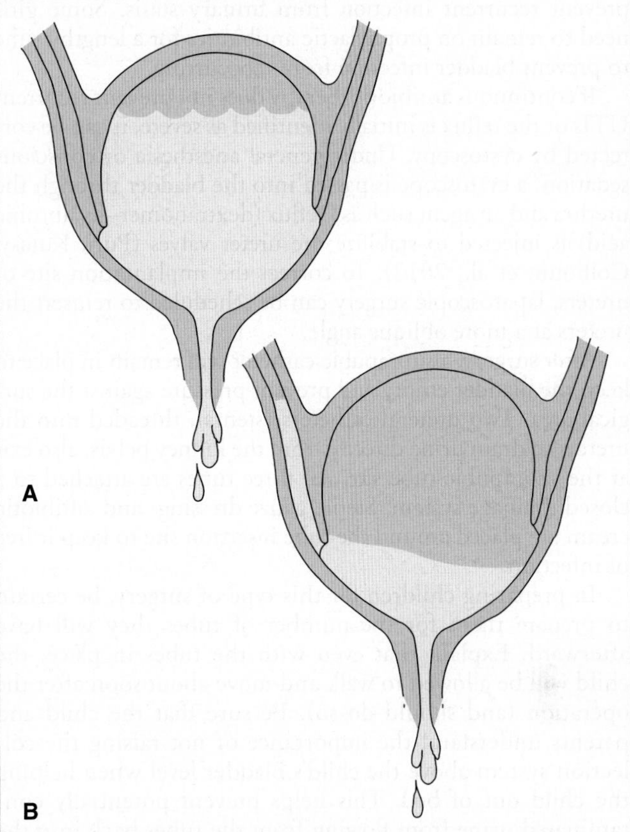

FIGURE 46.9 Vesicoureteral reflux. **(A)** Normal voiding pattern. **(B)** Reflux into ureters with voiding.

Reflux has the potential to lead to bladder infection because urine is retained in the ureters after voiding, and stasis of any fluid is subject to infection. The capacity for normal bladder tissue to lyse bacteria also becomes reduced because of the large residual urine volume that is always present. If the reflex is enough that it leads to back-pressure on the kidneys, it has the potential to lead to nephron destruction and, subsequently, hydronephrosis or dilatation of the renal pelvis. As the condition tends to appear in families, it is most likely caused by a heterogeneous gene disorder (Hunziker & Puri, 2012).

Assessment

A child with reflux is usually first seen by health care personnel because of a history of repeated UTIs. A VCUG, CT scan, MRI, cystoscopy, or cystography with contrast material will show the ureteral reflux. Based on diagnostic studies, reflux is graded from I to V by degree of reflux, with grade V being the most serious.

Therapeutic Management

The majority of instances of vesicoureteral reflux resolve with maturity without a need for surgery. Until this normal growth occurs, however, the condition must be treated to decrease the possibility of glomerular scarring from infection or back-pressure (Passamaneck, 2011). Teaching double voiding (having the child void and then in a few minutes attempt to void again) may help to empty the bladder more fully and prevent recurrent infection from urinary stasis. Some girls need to remain on prophylactic antibiotics for a lengthy time to prevent bladder infection from reoccurring.

If continuous antibiotic therapy does not prevent recurrent UTIs or the reflux is initially identified as severe, it can be corrected by cystoscopy. Under general anesthesia or conscious sedation, a cystoscope is passed into the bladder through the urethra and an agent such as Deflux (dextranomer–hyaluronic acid) is injected to stabilize the ureter valves (Puri, Kutasy, Colhoun, et al., 2012). To correct the implantation site of ureters, laparoscopic surgery can be scheduled to reinsert the ureters at a more oblique angle.

After surgery, a suprapubic catheter will remain in place to keep the bladder empty and prevent pressure against the surgical area. Two ureteral catheters (stents), threaded into the ureters to drain urine directly from the kidney pelvis, also exit at the suprapubic tube site. All three tubes are attached to a closed drainage system. Sterile gauze dressings and antibiotic cream are placed around the tube insertion site to keep it free of infection.

In preparing children for this type of surgery, be certain to prepare them for the number of tubes they will have afterward. Explain that even with the tubes in place, the child will be allowed to walk and move about soon after the operation (and should do so). Be sure that the child and parents understand the importance of not raising the collection system above the child's bladder level when helping the child out of bed. This helps prevent potentially contaminated urine from flowing from the tubes back into the bladder or ureters.

Urine will drain primarily from the stents for approximately the first 3 days after surgery; thereafter, drainage will flow around the stents and will be mainly from the suprapubic tube. As long as they are in place, it's important to assess that both stents are draining to ensure kidney production is equal on both sides. Observe the suprapubic tube and stent drainage closely for color or clots (should not be over pinpoint in size), and measure the amount and record it every hour for the first 24 hours and then about every 4 hours following that. Initially, drainage from the bladder catheter will be bloody, but this should clear in 1 or 2 days. To show that urine is clearing of blood, obtain serial urine specimens each time collecting bags are emptied and label them with the time of removal. Comparing the color of these samples will show that urine is clearing of blood. School-age children can help label the containers, which can help add to their sense of accomplishment and control over the situation.

To help keep the ends of stents or the suprapubic tube from becoming contaminated, an antiseptic solution may be prescribed to be placed in the drainage bags to limit the growth of bacteria in the collecting urine. Be certain any amount of additional fluid added is subtracted from the output amount so the urine output is accurately recorded. As soon as urine drainage from the stent catheters has decreased and blood has cleared, the stent catheters will be removed. Many children are frightened because they worry this will be painful. You can assure them this is a simple procedure and can be done before hospital discharge or at an ambulatory visit without anesthesia.

Incisional pain and painful bladder spasms may be present for the first 3 days after surgery, so antispasmodics are usually prescribed to reduce bladder spasm. Not touching or moving the suprapubic tube also helps to reduce spasms because this limits bladder irritation. The suprapubic tube is removed between 4 and 7 days after surgery (again, a nearly painless procedure). There may be slight urine leakage from the puncture site of the tube for 1 or 2 days after removal of the tube. Keep a sterile dressing in place to absorb the leaking urine. Remind the child and parents to avoid tub baths until the suprapubic tube site has closed completely.

A few children continue to have bladder reflux after ureter reimplantation. All children need follow-up care such as repeated urine cultures or perhaps an IVP or ultrasound at a later date to establish that surgery was effective in halting the reflux.

Hydronephrosis

Hydronephrosis is enlargement of the pelvis of the kidney with urine as a result of back-pressure in the ureter. The back-pressure is generally caused by obstruction, either of the ureter or of the point where the ureter joins the bladder, as with vesicoureteral reflux. Although this may occur at any age, it occurs most often in the first 6 months of life and is often diagnosed by ultrasound during intrauterine life (Yamaçake & Nguyen, 2013).

The condition is usually asymptomatic. The infant may have repeated UTIs caused by urinary stasis (difficult to detect in a young child except as general irritability or crying on voiding). Elevated blood pressure caused by increasing tubular pressure (which activates the renin–angiotensin system) may be detected on a routine health assessment, although blood pressure is not taken routinely in infants. With severe back-pressure, the infant will eventually experience flank or abdominal pain. Abdominal palpation may reveal an abdominal mass (the dilated kidney pelvis). An IVP or ultrasound will reveal the enlarged pelvis and the point of obstruction.

Hydronephrosis is a serious disorder because, if the pressure in the pelvis becomes too acute, back-pressure on the kidney can interfere with tubular function or destroy the nephrons. The treatment is surgical correction of the obstruction before glomerular or tubular destruction occurs.

DISORDERS AFFECTING NORMAL URINARY ELIMINATION

Interferences with urine elimination can arise from innocent conditions such as enuresis or extremely serious disorders such as kidney agenesis.

Enuresis

Enuresis is involuntary passage of urine past the age when a child should be expected to have attained bladder control (Fleming, 2012). Because this is expected at 2 to 3 years of age for daytime and age 4 years for nighttime, enuresis is said to occur at approximately 5 to 7 years. Enuresis may be nocturnal (occurs only at night), diurnal (occurs during the day), or both. It is primary if bladder training was never achieved and is considered acquired or secondary if control was established but has now been lost.

Most enuresis is nocturnal. It is found more frequently in boys than in girls. It also tends to be familial (if it is present in a child, one of the parents probably experienced it, too).

Assessment

Children with enuresis who are older than 5 years of age need an evaluation to determine whether there is an organic cause for the disorder. During history taking, ask how parents have tried to correct the problem; identify whether it is primarily a problem for the child or the parents (treatment will be most effective if the child wants the situation corrected). Assess whether there are stresses in the family, such as parents who expect more mature behavior of a child than the child can manage, the introduction of a new brother or sister, an uncomfortable school situation such as bullying, or marital discord.

If children wet only on nights when they are exceptionally tired or troubled, a functional rather than an organic cause is suggested. If children wet only when they are engrossed in an interesting activity, they may simply need more reminders to empty their bladder. If children have symptoms other than bed-wetting, such as abdominal pain, burning, or frequency, UTI is suggested. It is a common practice for many parents to lift children out of bed every night and take them to the bathroom so they don't bed wet. At any point parents stop this practice, children may begin bed-wetting because they have been conditioned to empty their bladder at that time of night.

Some children with enuresis have abnormal electroencephalographic patterns. Other children with the same abnormal patterns do not have enuresis, however, so this by itself is not a sufficiently specific finding to be helpful. In others, bed-wetting seems to occur as children pass from a period of rapid eye movement sleep pattern to a type IV level, or it is primarily a sleep disorder. It may be associated with small bladder capacity (which would explain why the condition is familial).

Although usually not necessary to aid diagnosis, an IVP, VCUG, or ultrasound may be prescribed to rule out organic disease, and a clean-catch urine specimen may be prescribed to rule out bacteriuria. Assess specific gravity, protein, and glucose of urine to rule out a defect in urine concentration or reveal evidence of nephron disease.

Therapeutic Management

The treatment of enuresis can be complex because the cause is generally unknown. If stress factors have been identified, not all of these can be eliminated because certain circumstances, such as the birth of a new sibling, cannot be changed, but frank discussion with children regarding what causes the stress and attempts to help them cope better with their daytime activities may lessen incidents.

In many children, it helps to limit fluids after dinner. Remind parents, however, that not all children are able to go without a drink from dinner until breakfast without growing exceedingly thirsty. Caution parents of children with sickle-cell anemia not to restrict fluid this way because increased sickling of cells occurs with dehydration.

Alarm bells that ring when children wet at night can be effective in some children. This type of system does not actually stop bed-wetting, but a sensor registers wetness and wakes the child, and then the child stops voiding and gets up and uses the bathroom. Over time, this type of conditioning may be effective, but once the urine alarm is removed, children may relapse. Bladder-stretching exercises—drinking a large quantity of water and then refraining from voiding as long as possible—to increase the functional size of the bladder may also be helpful in some children. A bladder that can hold 300 to 350 ml of fluid will generally be large enough to contain urine during a night's sleep.

If these measures are not effective, synthetic antidiuretic hormone (ADH; desmopressin [DDAVP]) administered intranasally or orally is the drug of choice to reduce urinary output and enuresis (Deshpande, Caldwell, & Sureshkumar, 2012) (Box 46.5).

Although enuresis is not a major problem in relation to other urinary or renal disorders, it can become a major problem for a family. As a general measure, children who wet their beds need to take baths in the morning rather than at bedtime to minimize urine odor and avoid bullying. Parents may find planning a vacation with hotel stays difficult. They may

BOX 46.5 Nursing Care Planning Based on Responsibility for Pharmacology

DESMOPRESSIN ACETATE (DDAVP)

Classification: A synthetic form of human antidiuretic hormone

Action: Promotes resorption of water in the renal tubule or decreases bladder filling; drug of choice for enuresis (Karch, 2013)

Pregnancy Risk Category: B

Dosage: In children 6 years of age and older, 20 μg (0.2 ml) intranasally at bedtime, possibly increasing the dose up to 40 μg if necessary; or 0.2 mg orally at bedtime, titrated up to 0.6 mg to obtain the desired response

Possible Adverse Effects: Transient headache, nausea, flushing, mild abdominal cramps, fluid retention

Nursing Implications

- Instruct parents and child that child should restrict fluid after dinnertime in addition to taking medication.
- Teach parents and child the proper method for intranasal administration; refrigerate the solution after use.
- Caution child and parents that nasal administration is less effective if the child develops a cold with draining rhinitis.

resent the daily linen washing. Children may exclude themselves from activities such as slumber parties or camping trips with friends to avoid embarrassment.

Enuresis may occur in hospitalized children because of the stress of their new surroundings. Preschool children may experience it because they are uncomfortable using strange bathrooms or do not understand which bathroom is theirs to use. As a rule, place as little stress or importance on enuresis as possible during an illness, and encourage parents to do the same.

Postural (Orthostatic) Proteinuria

A few children will spill albumin into the urine when they stand upright for an extended period (**postural proteinuria**, also called postural albuminuria). The amount of spilling decreases when they rest in a supine position. To identify a possible cause for the condition, an MRI of kidneys and ureters may be prescribed. To document that the proteinuria is related to posture, collect urine after the child has been recumbent during the night (a first-voided specimen) and then again after the child has been up and active for several hours. Make certain when collecting these urine specimens to record the child's activity accurately. If the child stood by the crib rail crying for a parent or was held in a nurse's lap for most of the night, the urine may show protein in the morning specimen because it is not truly a "resting specimen." Likewise, the "active" specimen should be collected after the child was truly active, not lying in a supine position reading a book for most of the time. Play a game if necessary, such as follow the leader, so the child is active.

Unless the MRI reveals an obstructive cause, postural proteinuria apparently results from the effect of gravity and thus needs no therapy. However, be certain to document the condition because some of these children do have obstructive disorders that need further identification (Milani, Mazzoni, Burdick, et al., 2010).

Kidney Agenesis

Agenesis means lack of growth (literally, lack of a beginning) or that no organ formed in utero. Absence of kidneys in a newborn is suggested when the volume of amniotic fluid on ultrasound or at birth is severely less than usual (oligohydramnios), indicating that fetal urine was not added to the volume of amniotic fluid. The infant often has *Potter syndrome* or accompanying misshapen, low-set ears and hypoplastic (stiff, inflexible) lungs from compression caused by the lack of amniotic fluid in utero (Tsai, Manchester, & Elias, 2012). Bilateral absence of kidneys is obviously incompatible with life unless a renal transplantation can be accomplished; the associated condition of nonfunctioning lungs, however, lessens the infant's eligibility for a successful transplantation.

Polycystic Kidney

Polycystic kidney implies that large, fluid-filled cysts have formed in place of normal kidney tissue. The most frequent type of polycystic kidney seen in children is inherited as an autosomal recessive trait. A more rare form is inherited as an autosomal dominant trait (Mahan, 2011). With either type, there is abnormal development of the collecting tubules. The kidneys grow large and feel soft and spongy. If the disorder is bilateral, an infant will not be able to pass urine so the mother will develop oligohydramnios during pregnancy. The newborn can have a flattened nose or *micrognathia* (small jaw), findings of Potter syndrome. A sonogram during pregnancy or at birth will reveal the fluid-filled cysts.

If the condition is unilateral, urine production will be decreased (oliguria), not absent. For this reason and because kidneys are difficult to locate in newborns, a unilateral polycystic kidney may be missed until later in life, when, with increased kidney growth, an abdominal mass can be palpated. The cystic growth offers such resistance to blood circulation that systemic hypertension often results by school age.

In many children, the condition is associated with a cerebral aneurysm, and the liver is filled with identical cysts. This is most evident later in life when increased difficulty with portal circulation occurs (blood cannot perfuse the cystic liver structures either).

The treatment for polycystic formation is surgical removal of the diseased kidney if only one is cystic. If both kidneys are cystic, treatment is renal transplantation (difficult in the young child, because few infant kidneys are available for transplantation and because of the technical challenge presented by such small blood vessels). Because this kidney disease is inherited, parents, and children at adolescence, need genetic counseling to inform them that future children may have this problem.

Renal Hypoplasia

Hypoplasia means reduced growth, so hypoplastic kidneys are small and underdeveloped and contain fewer lobes than usual. In addition to having poor kidney function, hypertension from stenosis of the renal arteries may develop. If hypoplasia is bilateral, the child may need a kidney transplant in later life to maintain kidney function and prevent extreme hypertension.

Prune Belly Syndrome

Prune belly syndrome is severe urinary tract dilation that develops as early as intrauterine life. Occurring mainly in boys, the severe dilation of ureters and the bladder causes back-pressure and destruction of kidneys. The infant is born with oligohydramnios and pulmonary dysplasia because of the lack of amniotic fluid in utero (Hassett, Smith, & Holland, 2012).

The condition is marked by the presence of three symptoms: deficiency of usual abdominal muscle tone, bilateral undescended testes, and the dilated faulty development of the bladder and upper urinary tract. The infant's abdomen appears wrinkled (like a prune) because of the poorly developed abdominal muscles (Fig. 46.10). Without surgical remodeling, the infant will develop repeated UTIs, leading eventually to end-stage renal disease. Teach parents to protect their child's abdomen from trauma, such as can happen from lap belts or baby walkers because their child lacks abdominal support, while waiting for muscle transplant procedures to create more abdominal support (Fearon & Varkarakis, 2012). Some children need kidney transplants as they reach school age because of destruction of glomeruli from continual back-pressure of urine on nephrons.

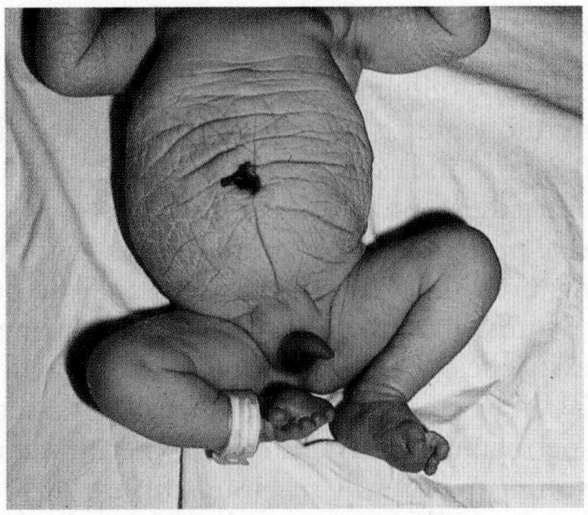

FIGURE 46.10 Prune belly syndrome. (Courtesy of Karen M. Polise, MSN, RN, Division of Nephrology, The Children's Hospital of Philadelphia.)

Acute Poststreptococcal Glomerulonephritis

Glomerulonephritis, inflammation of the glomeruli of the kidney, may occur as a separate entity but usually occurs in children as an immune complex disease after infection with nephritogenic streptococci (most commonly subtypes of group A beta-hemolytic streptococci) where complement, a cascade of proteins activated by antigen–antibody reactions, plugs or obstructs glomeruli. Immunoglobulin G (IgG) antibodies against streptococci can be detected in the bloodstream of children with acute glomerulonephritis, proof the illness follows a streptococcal infection (Kambham, 2012).

Intravascular coagulation occurs in the minute renal vessels; ischemic damage from this leads to scarring and decreased glomerular function. The glomerular filtration rate decreases, leading to an accumulation of sodium and water in the bloodstream. The inflammation of the glomeruli allows protein molecules to escape into the urine.

Assessment

Acute glomerulonephritis is most common in children between the ages of 5 and 10 years, the age group most susceptible to streptococcal infections. Boys appear to develop the disease more often than girls; it occurs more often during the winter and spring, as do pharyngeal streptococcal infections. The child typically has a history of a recent respiratory infection (within 7 to 14 days) or impetigo (within 3 weeks). All children who have had a "strep" throat, tonsillitis, otitis media, or impetigo caused by a streptococcal infection, ideally, should have a urinalysis 2 weeks after the infection to evaluate that glomerulonephritis is not occurring. Many children do not receive this follow-up step, however, because of lack of health insurance coverage or compliance.

The disorder is announced by a sudden onset of hematuria and proteinuria. Urinary sediment will contain white blood cells, epithelial cells, and hyaline, granular, and red blood cell casts. Testing a single specimen of urine will show 1+ to 4+ protein; a 24-hour urine specimen may contain as much as 1 g of protein (normally, urine contains none).

The hematuria is usually so extreme that the child's urine appears tea-colored, reddish-brown, or smoky. After these initial urine changes, the child develops oliguria. Specific gravity of urine becomes elevated. Hypertension from hypervolemia occurs. The child may have abdominal pain, a low-grade fever, edema, anorexia, vomiting, or headache. There may be cardiac involvement such as orthopnea, cardiac enlargement, enlarged liver, pulmonary edema, a galloping heart rhythm, or heart failure because of the difficulty in managing the excessive plasma fluid.

Blood analysis will indicate a lowered blood protein level (hypoalbuminemia) caused by the massive proteinuria. As the child's blood volume expands, a mild anemia will also develop. As in all inflammatory diseases, the erythrocyte sedimentation rate will increase. Because the glomeruli cannot filter properly, concentrations of urea, nonprotein nitrogen (BUN), and creatinine in blood will increase.

If blood pressure reaches 160/100 mmHg as part of the expanding circulatory volume, encephalopathy may occur, with symptoms of headache, irritability, seizures, vomiting, coma or lethargy, and perhaps transitory paralysis, symptoms all caused by *cerebral ischemia* (vasoconstriction of cerebral vessels that occurs to reduce cranial pressure).

Therapeutic Management

In most children, acute glomerulonephritis runs a limited, short-term, 1- to 2-week, benign course, and during this time, there is little specific therapy other than to alleviate symptoms of the disorder. A course of antibiotics may be prescribed to be certain all streptococci are removed from the child's system. Diuretics are of little value because obstructed glomeruli cannot be made to function, although a course of ethacrynic acid or furosemide (Lasix) may be tried. If heart failure occurs, keeping the child in a semi-Fowler's position, digitalization, and oxygen administration are helpful. If diastolic blood pressure rises to more than 90 mmHg, antihypertensive therapy with an antihypertensive such as labetalol will be prescribed. Phosphate binders, such as aluminum hydroxide to reduce phosphate absorption in the gastrointestinal tract, or a potassium-removing resin agent, such as sodium polystyrene sulfonate (Kayexalate), may be necessary in children who have rising phosphate and potassium levels because the kidneys are unable to clear these from the circulation.

Diet is controversial. Although restricting salt may limit edema and limiting protein intake may reduce the amount of protein lost in urine, most children who are losing large quantities of protein actually need more protein to supplement this loss. Most children do well, therefore, on a usual diet for their age. Weighing the child every day and calculating intake and output are important assessments to follow the course and extent of the disease.

Bed rest is unnecessary, although it's good to encourage children to participate in quiet play activities rather than active exercise. After 1 or 2 weeks, they can attend school and engage in their usual activities, although competitive activity is limited until kidney function has returned to normal (about 2 months). Caution parents that the results of a urine protein test may remain abnormal for up to a year, so if their child has this test done as a routine screening procedure at a health checkup, they don't worry that the finding means reinfection or the beginning of further disease.

A few children will not completely recover from acute glomerulonephritis but will develop chronic nephritis. These children apparently suffer destruction from the initial inflammation that destroys renal function (Praga & Morales, 2013).

Nursing Diagnoses and Related Interventions

Nursing care for the child with glomerulonephritis centers on helping alleviate symptoms and allowing the child to adjust to his or her sudden change in appearance.

Nursing Diagnosis: Situational low self-esteem, related to feelings of responsibility for onset of serious illness

Outcome Evaluation: Child (parent) admits feeling guilty about inadequate treatment of initial infection; discusses plans and ways to maintain health at this point; participates in care.

Glomerulonephritis is a frightening disease for both children and their parents because it begins so abruptly. Children may be frightened by the initial hematuria and upset at the appearance of periorbital edema, which makes their reflection in the mirror seem so strange to them. Children as young as early school age are aware that kidneys are necessary for life and thus appreciate the seriousness of kidney disease.

If children were prescribed penicillin for pharyngitis 2 weeks before the development of the condition but refused to take it, they and their parents often need to talk about their feelings. To help them understand that the outcome of the original neglected therapy does not have to result in a bad outcome, provide frequent reports of subtle positive changes in the child's condition, such as "Her blood pressure is not as high as before; she doesn't need medicine for that anymore." or "She weighs 2 pounds less today than 4 days ago; that generally means her kidneys are beginning to function more efficiently."

Be certain that parents know the date and place of a return visit for follow-up care. Because this is a perplexing disease, be certain they have a telephone number to call if they have questions about their child's care or condition. Acute glomerulonephritis tends not to recur with subsequent streptococcal infections, so prophylactic penicillin to prevent further streptococcal infections is not necessary.

QSEN Checkpoint Question 46.3

Patient-Centered Care

Carey's grandmother tells you that Carey had symptoms of acute glomerulonephritis last week that were greatly distressing to her. Which symptom Carey reported is a typical first symptom of glomerulonephritis?

a. Carey said her left knee hurt, although she didn't remember bumping it.
b. Carey asked her grandmother why there was blood in the toilet bowl.
c. Carey cried because she was starting to experience cramps.
d. Carey told her grandmother her stomach hurt after using the bathroom.

Look in Appendix A for the best answer and rationale.

Chronic Glomerulonephritis

Although chronic glomerulonephritis occasionally follows acute glomerulonephritis or nephrotic syndrome, it also occurs as a primary disease (or after acute glomerulonephritis that was clinically so mild it was undiagnosed). The child is found to have proteinuria at a routine health assessment. Further investigation indicates hypertension and the presence of red cell or white cell casts and occult blood in urine with low specific gravity (below 1.003). Blood studies may indicate an increased BUN or creatinine level. An MRI or a renal biopsy will reveal permanent destruction of glomeruli membranes.

The disorder may result in either diffuse or local nephron damage. In both instances, the undamaged nephrons increase their glomerular filtration rate to compensate for the damaged nephrons. At some point in this chronic disease destruction process, however, compensatory mechanisms begin to fail, and renal insufficiency or failure results. **Alport syndrome**, which also includes hearing loss and ocular changes, is progressive chronic glomerulonephritis inherited as an X-linked or autosomal recessive disorder (Kruegel, Rubel, & Gross, 2013).

With chronic glomerulonephritis, if the child has acute symptoms of edema, hematuria, hypertension, or oliguria, bed rest may be necessary. If children have only a chronic manifestation, such as proteinuria, and if they feel well, they can maintain normal activity, including attending school. Children should not engage in competitive activities such as contact sports, however, because of the risk of kidney injury.

Therapy is nonspecific and directed at symptom relief rather than the disease process or its cause, which is unknown. Therapy with antihypertensive drugs such as hydralazine (Apresoline) or with diuretics to increase urine output such as ethacrynic acid (Edecrin) can be helpful. Corticosteroid therapy may reduce or halt the progress of the disorder by reducing inflammation. Children have difficulty accepting long-term corticosteroid therapy because of the side effects, in particular the typical "moon face" and extra body hair (Cushing syndrome) that develop. Talk with them about these body changes and assure them that these changes will reverse when the drug is discontinued.

Children receiving corticosteroids are at an increased risk for developing infections because of the immunosuppressive activity of these drugs. Be certain parents know how to take their child's temperature and to report the earliest signs of infection as well as shield their child from other children (and health care personnel) with infections.

Generally, the prognosis for children with chronic glomerulonephritis is not encouraging because, although the illness runs a long-term course, eventually it leads to renal insufficiency and renal failure (Kraut, 2013). Kidney transplantation is a possibility to replace a diseased kidney. Children can be maintained for long periods by peritoneal dialysis or hemodialysis while waiting for a transplant.

Although most children are adolescents or young adults before the disease runs its ultimate course, because children as young as early school age are aware of the importance of kidney function, most are aware of the likely outcome of their disease at an early age. They indicate that they appreciate having health care personnel face this outcome with them honestly while they wait for kidney transplantation to prolong their life.

Nephrotic Syndrome (Nephrosis)

Nephrosis is altered glomerular permeability apparently due to an autoimmune process or a T-lymphocyte dysfunction that results in fusion of the glomeruli membrane surfaces, which, in turn, leads to abnormal loss of protein in urine. The highest incidence is at 3 years of age, and it occurs more often in boys than in girls (Mahan, 2011).

Nephrotic syndrome occurs in three forms: (a) congenital, as an autosomal recessive disorder; (b) secondary, as a progression of glomerulonephritis or in connection with systemic diseases such as sickle-cell anemia or systemic lupus erythematosus (SLE); and (c) idiopathic (primary). The congenital form is rare; the idiopathic form is most common (Praga & Morales, 2013).

Nephrosis can be further classified according to the amount of membrane destruction: minimal change nephrotic syndrome (MCNS), focal glomerulosclerosis (FGS), and membranoproliferative glomerulonephritis (MPGN). MCNS is the type most often seen in children (80%). As the name implies, with this type, little scarring of glomeruli occurs. Both of the other types involve scarring of glomeruli, and these children will have a poorer response to therapy (Hodson & Craig, 2013).

The four characteristic symptoms of nephrotic syndrome are proteinuria, edema, hypoalbuminemia (low serum albumin level), and hyperlipidemia (increased blood lipid level) (Richardson, 2012). Proteinuria occurs because increased glomerular permeability leads to protein loss in the urine and, subsequently, hypoalbuminemia. With a low level of protein in the bloodstream, osmotic pressure causes fluid to shift from the bloodstream into interstitial tissue, causing the edema. As the blood volume decreases, the kidneys begin to conserve sodium and water, adding to the potential for edema. The hyperlipidemia occurs because the liver increases production of lipoproteins to try to compensate for protein loss. Lipids are too large to be lost in urine, so they rise to high levels in the blood serum. Some children have such high lipid levels that, when blood is drawn and placed into a test tube, a circle of white fat forms across the top. Figure 46.11 illustrates the process that leads to these usual symptoms.

Assessment

Symptoms invariably begin insidiously. Edema tends to be dependent, or occur in the lower parts of the body. Children develop swelling around the eyes (periorbital edema) when they wake in the morning if they slept with their head flat on the bed. Parents may notice that clothing no longer fits a child around the waist, because edematous fluid is beginning to collect in the abdominal cavity (ascites). It is easy for parents to dismiss these first symptoms as those of an upper respiratory tract infection and the normal "paunchy" belly of a toddler or preschooler. As edema progresses, however, the child's skin becomes pale, stretched, and taut. In boys, scrotal edema becomes extremely marked. Ascites may become so extensive that the resultant pressure on the stomach and intestine leads to anorexia, vomiting, or diarrhea. Because of poor nutrition, the child's growth may decline and the child may become malnourished, yet the child will appear deceptively obese because of the extensive abdominal edema. When the abdominal ascites presses against the diaphragm, children may develop difficulty breathing. Parents report that children are irritable and fussy, probably from the feeling of abdominal fullness and generalized edema (Fig. 46.12). In addition, an increased risk for clotting can occur from the decreased intravascular fluid volume.

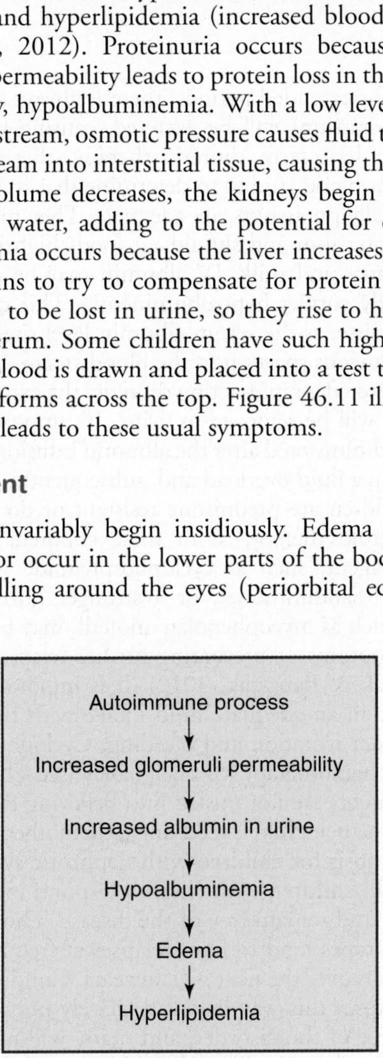

FIGURE 46.11 The process that results in the signs and symptoms of nephrotic syndrome.

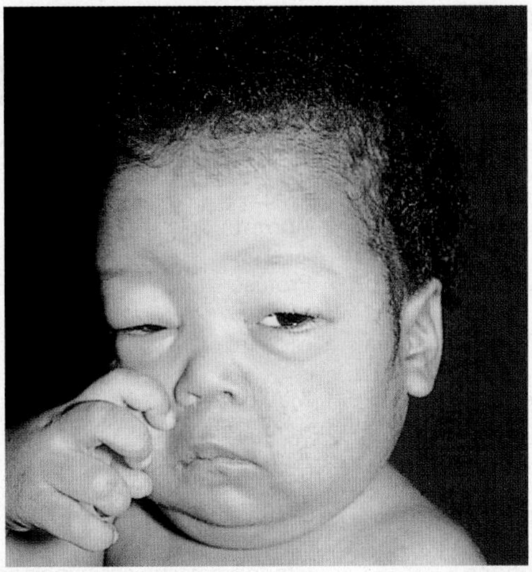

FIGURE 46.12 A 2-year-old child with nephrotic syndrome. Note the extensive edema of the face and hand. (From Zitelli, B. J., & Davis, H. W. [1997]. *Atlas of pediatric physical diagnosis* [3rd ed.]. St. Louis, MO: Mosby–Year Book, Inc.)

Laboratory studies will reveal marked proteinuria. A single test will show a 1+ to 4+ protein; a 24-hour total urine test will show up to 15 g of protein (normally, urine contains no protein). The protein loss with nephrotic syndrome is almost entirely albumin, differentiating it from the proteinuria of glomerulonephritis, in which protein loss tends to be nonspecific. Some children with nephrotic syndrome exhibit hematuria at the onset, but it is minimal in contrast to that seen with acute glomerulonephritis. The erythrocyte sedimentation rate (demonstrating the inflammation of the glomeruli membrane) is elevated. Features of acute glomerulonephritis and nephrotic syndrome are compared in Table 46.3. An MRI or renal biopsy may be done to determine whether there is scarring of the glomerular membrane and to document the type of nephrotic syndrome present.

Therapeutic Management

Therapy for nephrotic syndrome is directed toward reducing the proteinuria and subsequently the edema with a course of corticosteroids, such as IV methylprednisolone or oral

TABLE 46.3 Comparison of Features of Acute Glomerulonephritis and Nephrotic Syndrome

Factor	Acute Glomerulonephritis	Nephrotic Syndrome
Cause	Immune reaction to group A beta-hemolytic streptococcal infection	Idiopathic or an autoimmune process or a congenital inherited type
Onset	Abrupt	Insidious
Hematuria	Profuse	Rare
Edema	Mild	Extreme
Hypertension	Marked	Mild
Hyperlipidemia	Rare or mild	Marked
Peak age frequency	5–10 years	2–3 years
Interventions	Limited activity; antihypertensives as needed; symptomatic therapy for congestive heart failure	Corticosteroid and cyclophosphamide administration; possibly diuretic and potassium supplements
Diet	Normal for age	Normal for age with some salt restriction
Prevention	Prevention or thorough treatment of group A beta-hemolytic streptococcal infections	None known

prednisone, and keeping the child free of infection while the immune system is suppressed by these drugs. An initial dose of prednisone is given until diuresis without protein loss is accomplished; the dosage is then reduced for maintenance and continued for as long as 1 to 2 months.

Instruct parents to test the first urine specimen of the day for protein with a chemical reagent strip and keep an accurate chart showing the pattern of protein loss. Approximately once a week, parents are usually asked to collect a 24-hour urine specimen so total protein loss can be measured.

After an initial 4 weeks of therapy, prednisone is generally given every other day rather than every day. This is because prednisone has the potential to halt growth and to suppress adrenal gland secretion, side effects which can be reduced if the drug is given on alternate days, resulting in less alteration of adrenal steroid production (Karch, 2013). Parents may need to be assured that alternate-day therapy is best to keep them from changing the schedule to every day or giving twice the calculated dose by adding extra tablets on alternate days as an attempt to make their child well sooner. Prednisone tastes bitter, so parents may welcome suggestions regarding how to disguise the taste, such as by mixing it with applesauce or flavored syrup.

Be certain that both the parents and the child are aware long-term administration of prednisone will cause a cushingoid appearance or a "moon face," extra fat at the base of the neck, and increased body hair. Be certain also that parents know to plan ahead for pharmacy refills so prednisone therapy is not stopped abruptly because an abrupt stop can lead to adrenal insufficiency.

Diuretics are not commonly used to reduce the edema of nephrosis because they tend to decrease blood volume, which is already decreased, possibly leading to acute renal failure. Children who respond poorly to prednisone alone, however, may need diuretic therapy with a drug such as furosemide (Lasix) to initiate more kidney function. When children are taking furosemide for extended periods, there is always a danger that too much potassium will be excreted, causing hypokalemia. Children on long-term diuretic therapy, therefore, usually need frequent blood studies to determine that their electrolyte levels, especially potassium, are adequate. They may need supplemental potassium and should eat foods high in potassium such as bananas and milk. IV albumin may be administered to temporarily correct hypoalbuminemia. This causes edema to lessen because, as the serum albumin level rises, fluid shifts from subcutaneous spaces into the bloodstream. If the child is then administered a rapid-acting diuretic, the extra fluid in the bloodstream will be removed as urine. It's important that the diuretic be administered after the albumin infusion or the child could develop a fluid overload and, subsequently, heart failure.

Some children are prednisone resistant or do not respond to corticosteroid therapy. With these children, a course of a cytotoxic agent, such as cyclophosphamide (Cytoxan) or cyclosporine (Sandimmune), or a stronger immunosuppressant agent, such as mycophenolate mofetil, may be effective in reducing symptoms or preventing further relapses of the disease (Banaszak & Banaszak, 2012). It is important to ensure children take in an adequate fluid intake with these drugs to prevent bladder irritation and bleeding. Cyclophosphamide is also used in chemotherapy for malignancy (see Chapter 53), so be certain parents are not misled into believing their child has cancer because their child is receiving a chemotherapeutic drug.

The prognosis for children with nephrotic syndrome varies. Almost all children with MCNS respond initially to steroid therapy and remain free of the disease. Those with FGS and MPGN types tend to have relapses at frequent or infrequent intervals over the next several years. Children who have frequent relapses this way have a relatively poorer chance of ever being free of the disorder, and many will need a kidney transplantation later in life. All children and families need emotional support while the disease runs a long-term course.

QSEN Checkpoint Question 46.4

Safety

Suppose Carey is subsequently diagnosed with nephrotic syndrome. What action would be best to teach the grandmother?

a. Caution her grandmother to not feed her foods high in salt because salt irritates glomeruli.
b. Encourage her to walk to school daily for exercise.
c. Teach her grandmother to test Carey's urine for protein using a dipstick.
d. Teach her grandmother how to take Carey's tympanic temperature daily.

Look in Appendix A for the best answer and rationale.

Nursing Diagnoses and Related Interventions

Nursing interventions with nephrotic syndrome center on diminishing symptoms such as edema and proteinuria.

Nursing Diagnosis: Imbalanced nutrition, less than body requirements, related to poor appetite, restricted diet, and protein loss

Outcome Evaluation: Child follows normal growth curve on standard growth chart.

With nephrosis, a good protein intake is necessary to offset protein loss. A good potassium intake through consumption of fruits and fruit juices, particularly bananas, is necessary to maintain sufficient serum potassium levels, if the child is receiving a potassium-losing diuretic (Table 46.4). Although important, eating sufficient protein may be difficult because abdominal ascites can lead to a poor appetite. During acute phases of the disease, fluid or sodium may be temporarily restricted. If this is so, most children are happiest with many small glasses of fluid spaced throughout the day, rather than several large drinks. It may help to make a chart showing the amount of fluid a child can drink each day. As fluid is given, color in a portion of the chart corresponding to the amount given to allow the child to tell from the uncolored portion how much more fluid is allowed that day, a much easier method for toddlers and preschoolers (the age group usually affected by this disease) to understand rather than hearing fluid measured in milliliters or even glassfuls.

Children need to be weighed daily to detect if fluid accumulation is continuing (caution parents to use the same scale with the child in the same clothing and measure at the same time of day for best accuracy). Review with them how to measure intake and output as well. If the child is hospitalized, taking pulse rate and blood pressure every 4 hours will help detect hypovolemia from excessive fluid shifts to interstitial tissue.

TABLE 46.4 Foods High in Potassium

Food Group	Examples
Fruits	Bananas, peaches, prunes, raisins, oranges, orange juice
Vegetables	Carrots, celery, lima beans, potatoes, collards, dandelion greens, spinach
Protein	Nuts, peanuts, red meat
Dairy products	Milk, whole or skim; low-sodium milk
Miscellaneous	Salt substitutes, chocolate and cocoa, bran

Nursing Diagnosis: Risk for impaired skin integrity related to edema

Outcome Evaluation: Child's skin is intact without erythema.

Edematous skin tends to break down easily, so children with nephrotic syndrome need frequent position changes while in bed. Check clothing to make certain an elastic band at the waist of pajamas or other constricting parts is not too tight. Place soft gauze between skin surfaces, especially around the scrotum, to help prevent skin irritation. Remember edematous tissue does not heal well, so breaks in the skin can easily become secondarily infected. Change frequently the diapers of children who are not toilet-trained and thoroughly clean their skin with each change to prevent skin breakdown and infection in the diaper area. Because medications are poorly absorbed from edematous skin areas, keep intramuscular or subcutaneous injections to a minimum. Advocate for oral medication if at all possible (see Box 46.6, an interprofessional care map illustrating both nursing and team planning for a child with nephrotic syndrome).

Children are generally more comfortable if they sleep with their head elevated in a semi-Fowler's position rather than a supine or prone position because this reduces periorbital edema. If children do sleep in a head-flat position, edema can be so severe in the morning their eyes are swollen completely shut or their tongues are so swollen, they cannot speak. Suggest ways parents can provide a semi-Fowler's position at home, such as by placing extra pillows on the child's bed or slipping a cardboard box under the head of the mattress to raise that end of the mattress.

What if . . . 46.3 You need to give an intramuscular injection to Carey, who has extensive dependent edema from nephrotic syndrome. Would it be best to inject into a thigh or deltoid muscle, and why?

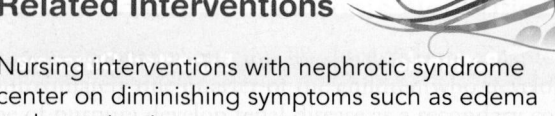

KIDNEY TRANSPLANTATION

The ultimate possibility for prolonging the life of children with renal failure is kidney transplantation. With complete renal failure, children who have extensive hypertension may have their damaged kidneys removed and be placed on hemodialysis or CCPD to await kidney transplantation. Kidney removal this way is an important step for both the parents and the child because although parents realize their child's kidneys are no longer functioning, this step removes all hope that a miracle might make them function once more. Parents may ask whether it is possible to leave one of the child's kidneys, because only one kidney will be transplanted (not recommended, because the hypertension would continue). Be certain that parents have a thorough explanation of why hypertension is destructive and that it could lead to a cerebrovascular accident or coronary artery disease. Help them understand that their child's renal biopsy shows that, short of a miracle, their child's kidneys will not function again, and so their removal is not a loss but only recognition of a loss.

Preoperative Care

Kidney transplantation is most effective (the kidney is less likely to be rejected) if the kidney is taken from a living twin, parent, or sibling (Butani, Troppmann, & Perez, 2012). Rejection occurs at a higher incidence if a kidney comes from a cadaver or recently deceased child. Most people consider that children should be of legal age to give consent to supply a kidney for transplantation, so few children have a sibling who is eligible to donate a kidney. Transplanted kidneys are placed in the abdomen, not the usual kidney space. Transplanting one from an adult into a child who weighs less than 10 kg can be difficult because of the difference in the size of the arteries and veins, which must be matched, and because of the possibility of hypertension, excessive diuresis, and abdominal complications (from the lack of space).

Many children anticipate that the characteristics of the donor will be transmitted to them by the kidney, so they are reluctant to accept the kidney of a family member with a character trait they do not like (perhaps a bad temper). You can assure them that transplanted organs do not carry this type of concern with them.

People who are ineligible to donate a kidney include those with multiple bilateral small renal arteries, bilateral renal disease, renal infection, advanced medical illness, severe obesity, or hypertension. Although kidney removal can be done by laparoscopy, donors must understand that removal of a kidney involves major surgery. Tests kidney donors can expect to have preoperatively include human leukocyte antigen (HLA) typing, electrolyte blood analysis, complete blood count, bleeding time, urinalysis and urine culture, 24-hour urine sample for protein, a renal arteriogram, and IV pyelography. Donors will have urine samples collected after surgery to assess that their remaining kidney is capable of maintaining full function and that they are still in good health.

Before surgery, children who are to receive a transplant may be dialyzed to clear their body of excessive potassium and fluid. If the donated kidney will be from a relative, there is adequate time for thorough preoperative preparation of this type. If the donor kidney is from a cadaver, the announcement of surgery will be sudden, and time for preoperative instruction and procedures may be limited.

✔ QSEN Checkpoint Question 46.6

Evidence-Based Practice

When kidney disease becomes chronic, it places a great burden on parents' energy and finances. To investigate how parents feel about caring for a child with chronic kidney disease, researchers interviewed parents of 20 children with chronic kidney disease recruited from two pediatric hospitals. Results of the study revealed four major themes: parents had to struggle to accept the diagnosis and permanence of their child's disorder; parents found continuous caregiving stressful, exhausting, and overwhelming; spousal tension and sibling neglect occurred; and parents felt they needed support from their health care providers (Tong, Lowe, Sainsbury, et al., 2010).

Based on the previous study, if Carey developed chronic kidney disease, which action by you would be most helpful?

a. Assure the grandmother she can call the clinic at any time if she has a concern.
b. Ask the grandmother to keep a daily record of conversations she has with Carey.
c. Review with the grandmother ways that Carey will require even more care in the future.
d. Help the grandmother learn to say "no" when other family members ask her to help them.

Look in Appendix A for the best answer and rationale.

Human Leukocyte Antigen Typing

HLAs are a group of antigens found on the surfaces of all cells with a nucleus, including blood components such as leukocytes and platelets. The name is derived from the fact they were first identified on white blood cells. Such antigens are inherited from both parents and are specific for each individual. They are carried on the short arm of chromosome 6 in each cell and denote tissue type or determine which tissue the immune system will identify as foreign tissue. They also serve as the basis for paternity typing and may cause reactions to blood product transfusions and bone marrow and organ transplants.

When two people have the same, or mostly the same, HLA antigens, they are said to be *histocompatible*. Identical twins have complete histocompatibility; family members have partial histocompatibility; any two people can have histocompatibility on at least one antigen site.

Children who are awaiting kidney transplantation are HLA typed, and this information is circulated to major medical centers. When a kidney is available for transplantation, the child's tissue type is compared with the donor kidney, and factors such as "best match," general condition, size of the child, and length of time the child has been on the waiting list are considered. The chance of receiving a kidney is increased today because, with new immunosuppressive drugs, even donor kidneys that are not fully matched have a chance to successfully graft.

Postoperative Care

After renal transplantation, children are cared for in an environment that is as sterile as possible as they are placed on immunosuppressive therapy such as cyclosporine,

BOX 46.7 Nursing Care Planning Based on Effective Communication

Carey's grandmother tells you Carey has "changed completely" since she became ill with acute glomerulonephritis.

Less Effective Communication

Nurse: Mrs. Hendricks, in what way has Carey changed?
Mrs. Hendricks: She used to whine all the time, and constantly ask for things. Now she entertains herself. It's like heaven.
Nurse: That sounds wonderful. Let's review her medicine routine to be sure that's going well.
Mrs. Hendricks: That's another thing she does perfectly: never fusses a bit about anything she has to take.

More Effective Communication

Nurse: Mrs. Hendricks, in what way has Carey changed?
Mrs. Hendricks: She used to whine all the time, and constantly ask for things. Now she entertains herself. It's like heaven.
Nurse: Do you think she's acting a little too perfect?
Mrs. Hendricks: Well, it does seem a bit strange.
Nurse: Do you think she feels responsible for being sick? Could she be worrying that if she misbehaves, her medicine will stop working?
Mrs. Hendricks: I never thought of that. I would feel better if she started to act like her old self.

What the grandmother above is describing is a "honeymoon" period that children may pass through after being told their kidneys are injured because they know how important kidneys are for life. Parents often need help seeing this for what it is, so they can begin to reassure children that behaving perfectly will not influence the outcome of their illness and that, because they loved them as they were, they will continue to love them regardless.

azathioprine (Imuran), and methylprednisolone (Solu-Medrol), and possibly antilymphocyte globulin and antithymocyte globulin to reduce the possibility of kidney rejection. Although some transplanted kidneys begin to function immediately, hemodialysis may be continued until the implanted kidney can fully function after the insult of transplantation.

Children may pass through a "honeymoon" period after the transplantation or a period during which a child models perfect behavior on the belief the success of the transplant depends on good behavior rather than the condition of renal veins and arteries, the transplanted kidney, or antigen–antibody formation (Box 46.7).

Children with end-stage renal disease are usually behind in growth at the time of a transplant. Although the rate of growth will be improved after kidney transplantation, they may never reach full height, related to the already lost growth plus need for corticosteroid maintenance therapy to continue immunosuppression.

Transplant Rejection

Acute transplant rejection, if it occurs, usually develops within the first 3 months after transplantation. Children begin to develop fever, proteinuria, oliguria, weight gain, hypertension, and tenderness over the kidney. Serum creatinine and BUN levels will rise. Increasing the dose of immunosuppressants may be effective in stopping this type of rejection.

Rejection may also be *chronic*, in which the transplanted kidney gradually loses function after the first 6 months. Hypertension and anemia result. An MRI or a biopsy will show vascular changes such as narrowing of arterial lumens and interstitial changes such as fibrosis and tubular atrophy. This type of rejection is difficult to halt, although it may be such a slow, steady process that it will be 2 or 3 years before the kidney actually fails. If a kidney is rejected, it is removed, and a child is returned to a program of hemodialysis. Because one kidney was rejected does not mean a second transplant will also be rejected. Unfortunately, because the number of kidneys available for transplantation is limited, kidney rejection of this type becomes an ominous sign for the child's long-term survival.

Malignant disease is more common in transplantation recipients than in the normal population, probably because of the long-term immunosuppression (Ponticelli & Graziani, 2012). The original disease for which the child underwent transplantation, such as glomerulonephritis, may also recur in the transplanted kidney. During adolescence, typically an age of poor adherence to medication regimens, monitor kidney recipients closely to be certain they are taking their immunosuppressive therapy. Parents cannot help but overprotect the child after a kidney transplant; they worry a roughhousing session with a sibling or playing a game such as baseball may injure the transplanted kidney. The child may be afraid to engage in any activity for the same reason. Ask at health care visits if the family needs help to return to a healthy lifestyle after this major life change.

What if . . . 46.4 You are particularly interested in exploring one of the 2020 National Health Goals regarding renal disorders of children (see Box 46.1). What would be a possible research topic to explore pertinent to this goal that would be applicable to Carey's family and also advance evidence-based practice?

Key Points for Review

- Many urinary tract disorders, such as polycystic kidneys, urethral obstruction, and bladder exstrophy, are evident on a fetal ultrasound. Early identification on fetal ultrasound allows therapy to begin in utero or immediately at birth.
- Many urinary tract disorders, such as polycystic kidneys or chronic renal failure, are long-term conditions requiring years of therapy. Be certain parents are well informed about their child's condition so they can continue to participate in planning their child's care that not only meets QSEN competencies but also best meets the family's total needs.
- Congenital structural abnormalities of the urinary tract include patent urachus, exstrophy of the bladder, hypospadias, and epispadias. Surgical correction is required for all of these, but the outcome should be favorable.
- UTI tends to occur more often in girls than boys. "Honeymoon cystitis" refers to a UTI occurring with first-time sexual intercourse. Preventing recurring infections is important to prevent spread of the infection to the kidneys.
- Vesicoureteral reflux is the backflow of urine into ureters with voiding because the valve that guards the entrance to the ureters is lax or the ureters are misplaced. Surgical correction may be necessary to prevent repeated UTI.
- Kidney dysfunction can occur for structural reasons such as kidney agenesis, polycystic kidney, and renal hypoplasia, all conditions that limit kidney function.
- Acute poststreptococcal glomerulonephritis is inflammation of the glomeruli after a streptococcal infection. It is characterized by an acute episode of hematuria and proteinuria but typically runs a short-term course.
- Nephrotic syndrome is an immunologic process that results in altered glomerular permeability and can lead to a self-limiting or long-term course.
- Diminished kidney function leads to both fluid and electrolyte imbalances. Creative techniques are necessary to encourage children to continue to ingest a restricted-protein diet.
- When renal failure is either acute or chronic, peritoneal dialysis or hemodialysis may be used to remove body wastes until kidney function can be restored.
- Kidney transplantation is the ultimate option for children with kidney failure. It requires extensive surgery and requires the child to remain on immunosuppressive therapy to counteract transplant rejection.

Critical Thinking Care Study

Jamie is a 16-year-old teenager with chronic kidney disease. He lives with his mother and a younger sister, 10 years old. He's homeschooled because he has to miss 3 days of school each week for hemodialysis.

1. You notice that, although Jamie is supposed to limit the amount of potassium he ingests, when offered a choice between popcorn with orange juice or raisins and milk for an afternoon snack he chose the raisins and milk. Was that his best choice?
2. Jamie appears obese because of the long-term use of immunosuppressants. You hear him brag to his girlfriend that he has lost more weight than her as part of a New Year's resolution pact. You also notice, according to Jamie's medicine reminder sheet, that he has missed taking two doses of prednisone. Would omitting taking prednisone cause him to lose weight? What could be the effect of omitting his prescribed prednisone?
3. Jamie's mother wants him to learn to drive so he can travel to the dialysis center by himself. Jamie says he can't do that because dialysis makes him feel dizzy and nauseated. Are those common symptoms of dialysis? As his dialysis nurse, what could you do to reduce his symptoms?

Patient Scenario

The Maggio Family

Read about the Maggio family, a family whose school-age child has a urinary tract infection, then answer the questions to further sharpen your skills and grow more familiar with NCLEX-type questions related to urinary and renal disorders in children. Confirm your answers are correct by reading the rationales.

Visit http://thePoint.lww.com

Answers and Rationales

Looking for answers to the What if . . . and Critical Thinking Care Study questions?

Visit http://thePoint.lww.com

References

Banaszak, B., & Banaszak, P. (2012). The increasing incidence of initial steroid resistance in childhood nephrotic syndrome. *Pediatric Nephrology, 27*(6), 927–932.

Bayhakki, A., & Hatthakit, U. (2012). Lived experiences of patients on hemodialysis: A meta-synthesis. *Nephrology Nursing Journal, 39*(4), 295–304.

Batinic, D., Miloševic, D., Topalovic-Grkovic, M., et al. (2012). Vesicoureteral reflux and urodynamic dysfunction. *Urology International.* Advance online publication.

Beck, J., Bekker, M., Van Driel, M., et al. (2010). Female sexual abuse evaluation in the urological practice: Results of a Dutch survey. *Journal of Sexual Medicine, 7*(4, Pt. 1), 1464–1468.

Braun, L., Sood, V., Hogue, S., et al. (2012). High burden and unmet patient needs in chronic kidney disease. *International Journal of Nephrology Renovascular Disease,* (5), 151–163.

Butani, L., Troppmann, C., & Perez, R. V. (2012). Outcomes of children receiving en bloc renal transplants from small pediatric donors. *Pediatric Transplantation, 17*(1), 55–58.

Davenport, A. (2012). Portable or wearable peritoneal devices—The next step forward for peritoneal dialysis? *Advances in Peritoneal Dialysis, 28*(3), 97–101.

Deshpande, A. V., Caldwell, P. H., & Sureshkumar, P. (2012). Drugs for nocturnal enuresis in children (other than desmopressin and tricyclics). *Cochrane Database of Systematic Reviews,* (12), CD002238.

Elshal, A. M., Abdelhalim, A., Hafez, A. T., et al. (2012). Ileal urinary reservoir in pediatric population: Objective assessment of long-term sequelae with time-to-event analysis. *Urology, 79*(5), 1126–1131.

Fearon, J. A., & Varkarakis, G. (2012). Dynamic abdominoplasty for the treatment of prune belly syndrome. *Plastic Reconstructive Surgery, 130*(3), 648–657.

Fleming, E. (2012). Supporting children with nocturnal enuresis. *Nursing Times, 108*(41), 22–25.

Gaylord, N. M., & Peterson-Smith, A. M. (2012). Genitourinary disorders. In C. E. Burns, A. M. Dunn, M. A. Brady, et al. (Eds.), *Pediatric primary care* (5th ed., pp. 809–843). Philadelphia, PA: Elsevier/Saunders.

Geerdes-Fenge, H. F., Löbermann, M., Nürnberg, M., et al. (2013). Ciprofloxacin reduces the risk of hemolytic uremic syndrome in patients with *Escherichia coli* O104:H4-associated diarrhea. *Infection*. Advance online publication.

Hassett, S., Smith, G. H., & Holland, A. J. (2012). Prune belly syndrome. *Pediatric Surgery International, 28*(3), 219–228.

Hodson, E. M., & Craig, J. C. (2013). Corticosteroid therapy for steroid-sensitive nephrotic syndrome in children: Dose or duration? *Journal of the American Society of Nephrology, 24*(1), 7–9.

Hothi, D. K., Stronach, L., & Harvey, E. (2013). Home haemodialysis. *Pediatric Nephrology, 28*(5), 721–730.

Huether, S. E. (2013). Structure and function of the renal and urologic systems. In S. E. Huether & K. L. McCance (Eds.), *Understanding pathophysiology* (5th ed., pp. 724–764). New York, NY: Elsevier Publishing.

Hunziker, M., & Puri, P. (2012). Familial vesicoureteral reflux and reflux related morbidity in relatives of index patients with high grade vesicoureteral reflux. *Journal of Urology, 188*(4, Suppl.), 1463–1466.

Issa, N., Lankireddy, S., & Kukla, A. (2012). Should peritoneal dialysis be the preferred therapy pre-kidney transplantation? *Advances in Peritoneal Dialysis, 28*(1), 89–93.

Jauhola, O., Ronkainen, J., Koskimies, O., et al. (2012). Outcome of Henoch-Schönlein purpura 8 years after treatment with a placebo or prednisone at disease onset. *Pediatric Nephrology, 27*(6), 933–939.

Kambham, N. (2012). Postinfectious glomerulonephritis. *Advances in Anatomic Pathology, 19*(5), 338–347.

Karch, A. M. (2013). *2013 Lippincott's nursing drug guide*. Philadelphia, PA: Lippincott Williams & Wilkins.

Kraut, J. A. (2013). Chronic kidney failure. In E. T. Bope & R. D. Kellerman (Eds.), *Conn's current therapy* (pp. 877–881). Philadelphia, PA: Elsevier/Saunders.

Kruegel, J., Rubel, D., & Gross, O. (2013). Alport syndrome—Insights from basic and clinical research. *Nature Reviews: Nephrology, 9*(3), 170–178.

Lateef, A., & Petri, M. (2012). Unmet medical needs in systemic lupus erythematosus. *Arthritis Research Therapy, 14*(Suppl. 4), S4.

Lum, G. M. (2012). Kidney and urinary tract. In W. Hay, M. Levin, R. Deterding, et al. (Eds.), *Current diagnosis & treatment pediatrics* (21st ed., pp. 717–739). New York, NY: McGraw-Hill/Lange.

Mahan, J. D. (2011). Nephrology and urology. In K. J. Marcdante, R. M. Kliegman, H. B. Jenson, et al. (Eds.), *Nelson essentials of pediatrics* (6th ed., pp. 607–624). Philadelphia, PA: Saunders/Elsevier.

Milani, G. P., Mazzoni, M. B., Burdick, L., et al. (2010). Postural proteinuria associated with left renal vein entrapment: A follow-up evaluation. *American Journal of Kidney Disease, 55*(6), e29–e31.

Nelson, C. P., Chow, J. S., Rosoklija, I., et al. (2012). Patient and family impact of pediatric genitourinary diagnostic imaging tests. *Journal of Urology, 188*(4, Suppl.), 1601–1607.

Paintsil, E. (2013). Update on recent guidelines for the management of urinary tract infections in children: The shifting paradigm. *Current Opinion in Pediatrics, 25*(1), 88–94.

Passamaneck, M. (2011). The changing paradigm for the management of pediatric vesicoureteral reflux. *Urology Nursing, 31*(6), 363–366.

Ponticelli, C., & Graziani, G. (2012). Education and counseling of renal transplant recipients. *Journal of Nephrology*, 25(6), 879–889.

Praga, M., & Morales, E. (2013). Primary glomerular disease. In E. T. Bope & R. D. Kellerman (Eds.), *Conn's current therapy* (pp. 891–894). Philadelphia, PA: Elsevier/Saunders.

Puri, P., Kutasy, B., Colhoun, E., et al. (2012). Single center experience with endoscopic subureteral dextranomer/hyaluronic acid injection as first line treatment in 1,551 children with intermediate and high grade vesicoureteral reflux. *Journal of Urology, 188*(4, Suppl.), 1485–1489.

Quinlan, C., Bates, M., Sheils, A., et al. (2013). Chronic hemodialysis in children weighing less than 10 kg. *Pediatric Nephrology, 28*(5), 803–809.

Richardson, M. A. (2012). The many faces of minimal change nephrotic syndrome: An overview and case study. *Nephrology Nursing Journal, 39*(5), 365–374.

Ring, P., & Huether, S. E. (2013). Alternations of renal and urinary tract function in children. In S. E. Huether & K. L. McCance (Eds.), *Understanding pathophysiology* (5th ed., pp. 764–773). New York, NY: Elsevier Publishing.

Sayed, S. A., Abu-Aisha, H., Ahmed, M. E., et al. (2012). Effect of the patient's knowledge on peritonitis rates in peritoneal dialysis. *Peritoneal Dialysis International*. Advance online publication.

Spinoit, A. F., Poelaert, F., Groen, L. A., et al. (2013). Hypospadias repair in a single reference centre: Long term follow-up is mandatory to detect the real complication rate. *Journal of Urology, 189*(6), 2276–2281.

Steele, M. R., Belostotsky, V., & Lau, K. K. (2012). The dangers of substance abuse in adolescents with chronic kidney disease: A review of the literature. *CANNT Journal: Official Publication of the Canadian Association of Nephrology Nurses and Technologists, 22*(1), 15–22.

Tong, A., Henning, P., Wong, G., et al. (2013). Experiences and perspectives of adolescents and young adults with advanced CKD. *American Journal of Kidney Disease, 61*(3), 375–384.

Tong, A., Lowe, A., Sainsbury, P., et al. (2010). Parental perspectives on caring for a child with chronic kidney disease: An in-depth interview study. *Child Care Health & Development, 36*(4), 549–557.

Tsai, A. C., Manchester, D. K., & Elias, E. R. (2012). Genetics and dysmorphology. In W. Hay, M. Levin, R. Deterding, et al. (Eds.), *Current diagnosis & treatment pediatrics* (21st ed., pp. 1088–1122). New York, NY: McGraw-Hill/Lange.

Tsai, M. S., & Yeh, M. L. (2011). Images in clinical medicine. Patent urachus. *New England Journal of Medicine, 365*(14), 1328.

Tse, Y., Yadav, P., Herrema, I., et al. (2013). Performing renal biopsies in children under general anesthesia in the lateral position. *Pediatric Nephrology, 28*(4), 671–673.

U.S. Department of Health and Human Services. (2010). *Healthy people 2020*. Washington, DC: Author.

Vidal, I., Gorduza, D. B., Haraux, E., et al. (2010). Surgical options in disorders of sex development (DSD) with ambiguous genitalia. *Best Practice & Research: Clinical Endocrinology & Metabolism, 24*(2), 311–324.

Wesseling-Perry, K. (2013). Bone disease in pediatric chronic kidney disease. *Pediatric Nephrology, 28*(4), 569–576.

Yamaçake, K. G., & Nguyen, H. T. (2013). Current management of antenatal hydronephrosis. *Pediatric Nephrology, 28*(2), 237–243.

Chapter 47

Nursing Care of a Family When a Child Has a Reproductive Disorder

KEY TERMS

- amenorrhea
- anovulatory
- cryptorchidism
- dysmenorrhea
- endometriosis
- fibrocystic breast disease
- gynecomastia
- hermaphrodite
- hydrocele
- menorrhagia
- metrorrhagia
- mittelschmerz
- orchiectomy
- orchiopexy
- pelvic inflammatory disease (PID)
- premenstrual dysphoric disorder (PDD)
- sexually transmitted infection (STI)
- toxic shock syndrome (TSS)
- varicocele
- vulvovaginitis

OBJECTIVES

After mastering the contents of this chapter, you should be able to:

1. Describe common reproductive disorders in children.
2. Identify 2020 National Health Goals related to reproductive disorders that nurses can help the nation achieve.
3. Assess a child with a reproductive disorder.
4. Formulate nursing diagnoses for a child with a reproductive disorder.
5. Establish expected outcomes for a child with a reproductive disorder that help children and parents manage seamless transitions across differing health care settings.
6. Using the nursing process, plan nursing care that includes the six competencies of Quality & Safety Education for Nurses (QSEN): Patient-Centered Care, Teamwork & Collaboration, Evidence-Based Practice (EBP), Quality Improvement (QI), Safety, and Informatics.
7. Implement nursing care for a child with a reproductive disorder, such as teaching about normal menstruation.
8. Evaluate expected outcomes for achievement and effectiveness of care.
9. Integrate knowledge of children's reproductive disorders with the interplay of nursing process, the six competencies of QSEN, and Family Nursing to promote quality maternal and child health nursing care.

Navi is a 15-year-old girl you meet in a pediatric clinic. She has a purulent vaginal discharge and burning on urination; she is diagnosed with gonorrhea. When you ask her if she is sexually active, she says no; she thinks she contracted the infection from sharing a towel in a locker room. As she leaves the clinic, you hear her tell the receptionist, "I'm glad I got this early in life. Now I won't have to worry about getting it again."

Previous chapters described the growth and development of well children and health concerns that occur in other body systems. This chapter adds information about the dramatic changes, both physical and psychosocial, that occur when children develop reproductive disorders. Such information forms the basis for care and health teaching in this area.

What kind of health education does Navi need?

BOX 47.1 Nursing Care Planning Based on 2020 National Health Goals

Because sexually transmitted infections (STIs) not only cause short-term distress as a result of painful lesions but also can have long-term implications for fertility and future childbearing, several 2020 National Health Goals specifically address these and include:

- Reduce the proportion of adolescents with *Chlamydia trachomatis* infections seen in family planning clinics from a baseline of 7.4% to a target of 6.7%.
- Reduce the annual incidence of new cases of gonorrhea in adolescent females from a baseline of 285/100,000 cases to no more than 257/100,000 cases and, in adolescent males, from 220/100,000 cases to 198/100,000 cases.
- Reduce the incidence of primary syphilis in adolescent females from a baseline of 1.5/100,000 cases to no more than 1.4/100,000 cases and, in adolescent males, from 7.6/100,000 cases to 6.8/100,000 cases.
- Reduce the incidence of congenital syphilis from a baseline of 10.1/100,000 live births to 9.1/100,000 live births.
- Reduce the incidence of genital herpes from a baseline of 10.5% to no more than 9.5%.
- Reduce the proportion of females with human papillomavirus (HPV) infection (Developmental).
- Reduce the incidence of pelvic inflammatory disease among women aged 15 through 44 years from a baseline of 3.9% to no more than 3.5% (U.S. Department of Health and Human Services [DHHS], 2010; see www.healthypeople.gov).

Nurses can help the nation achieve these goals by educating adolescents about effective ways to prevent STIs and how to recognize the signs and symptoms of these illnesses.

Reproductive disorders in children range from mild infections to serious anatomic malformations. All of these disorders require prompt and careful treatment so children can reach adulthood in good reproductive health, with unaltered fertility, and with a positive sense of sexuality. Reproductive infections may suggest child maltreatment, so children with these also need careful assessment to rule out this possibility (Dubowitz, 2013) (see Chapter 55). The 2020 National Health Goals related to reproductive disorders in children are highlighted in Box 47.1.

Nursing Process Overview

For Care of a Child With a Reproductive Disorder

Assessment

Assessment of reproductive health begins with the first physical examination at birth and continues at health assessments throughout childhood and adolescence. Because this is a sensitive area for many people to discuss, parents may not be as comfortable inquiring about or describing disorders of the reproductive tract as they are about discussing other areas. Unless they have clear, thorough explanations of the condition and prescribed therapy, their reluctance to pursue the subject may leave them confused or misinformed. Even young children can sense that a health problem affecting genitalia is viewed by some adults as different from other disorders and so may not ask as many questions as they do about other concerns.

Nursing Diagnosis

Nursing diagnoses formulated for reproductive illnesses in children focus not only on the result of the disease symptoms but also on the anxiety this type of disorder can cause. Examples of nursing diagnoses include:

- Risk for infection transmission related to lack of knowledge of safer sex practices
- Pain related to symptoms of vaginal infection
- Disturbed body image related to fibrocystic breast disease
- Anxiety related to absence or irregularity of menstrual periods in adolescent
- Fear related to surgery on genital organs

Outcome Identification and Planning

An assessment of a child's knowledge about the reproductive system and ways illness can affect reproductive and sexual functioning forms the foundation for developing appropriate outcomes. Educating the child about reproductive health may be one of the first areas to plan. When establishing expected outcomes with adolescents, work with them to establish a plan that will involve them in the decision-making process.

Organizations helpful for referral to parents or adolescents include the National Women's Health Network (www.nwhn.org), the National Adolescent and Young Adult Health Information Center (nahic.ucsf.edu), and the Centers for Disease Control and Prevention (www.cdc.gov).

Implementation

Interventions for children with reproductive disorders should always include education about reproductive functioning and measures for maintaining reproductive and sexual health. Health education regarding the importance of testicular self-examination for adolescent males should be stressed at health care visits (see Chapter 34). Guidelines for teaching about menstrual health and safer sex to protect against unintended pregnancy or sexually transmitted infections (STIs) (covered in Chapter 5) are also important.

Essential nursing interventions also include supporting parents and children through difficult decisions about procedures and providing close observation and empathic counseling after surgery. For example, surgery for undescended testes is a procedure that can be traumatic for a child, especially if it is performed during a developmental stage in which a boy views such surgery as castrating (a psychological reason in addition to a physical reason as to why it is done early in life). As all children with any reproductive disorder reach puberty, they need honest explanations about any effect such a condition will have on interpersonal relationships, sexual functioning, or childbearing.

Outcome Evaluation

The responses of children to reproductive dysfunction vary both with the severity of the condition and with the specific age and fears of the child. It is safe to assume, however, that children who have experienced such a health problem are at risk for a loss of self-esteem or confusion about their body image. Therefore, outcome evaluation should include a long-term evaluation of the child's coping abilities and self-image. If a child contracts an STI, the evaluation should also address the child's knowledge about avoiding STIs in the future and willingness to seek help should an infection recur.

The following are examples suggesting achievement of outcomes:

- Adolescent states discomfort from vaginal infection is tolerable after beginning medication.
- Adolescent states she is able to view self as competent despite fibrocystic breast disease.
- Child states that she is able to wait 6 months without worrying about not yet beginning her menstrual periods.
- Child states he feels less fearful about impending surgery after talking with his health care provider.

ASSESSING REPRODUCTIVE DISORDERS IN CHILDREN

Reproductive disorders in children may be congenital or acquired, so assessments for these must be ongoing throughout childhood (Box 47.2).

As with other parts of a health interview, questions regarding reproductive health are generally addressed to the parents until the child is able to answer history questions reliably and independently. Once a girl has reached adolescence, a gynecologic history (Box 47.3) should be included in the health assessment. To preserve their privacy, adolescents of both genders may prefer to not be accompanied by a parent during a physical examination for a reproductive disorder.

Adolescents who are worried that they may have contracted an STI or suspect they have become pregnant often visit health care facilities without parents. Before they can admit this chief concern, however, they may "test" a health care provider by eliciting a reaction to a minor problem. Be aware that an adolescent who consults a health care provider with a seemingly minor concern may be simply misinterpreting symptoms, and the adolescent actually may be seeking help for another problem. Asking the adolescent, "Is there anything else that worries you? Is there any other way we can help you today?" may help you elicit the adolescent's primary concern (Box 47.4).

A pelvic examination is unnecessary for girls who have not yet reached adolescence. However, if vaginal walls need to be inspected (because of an inflammation, infection, or the suspicion of sexual maltreatment), an otoscope and ear tip can be used in place of a speculum. Cotton-tipped applicators can be used to take culture specimens without causing discomfort.

BOX 47.2 Nursing Care Planning Using Assessment

Assessing a Child With a Reproductive Disorder

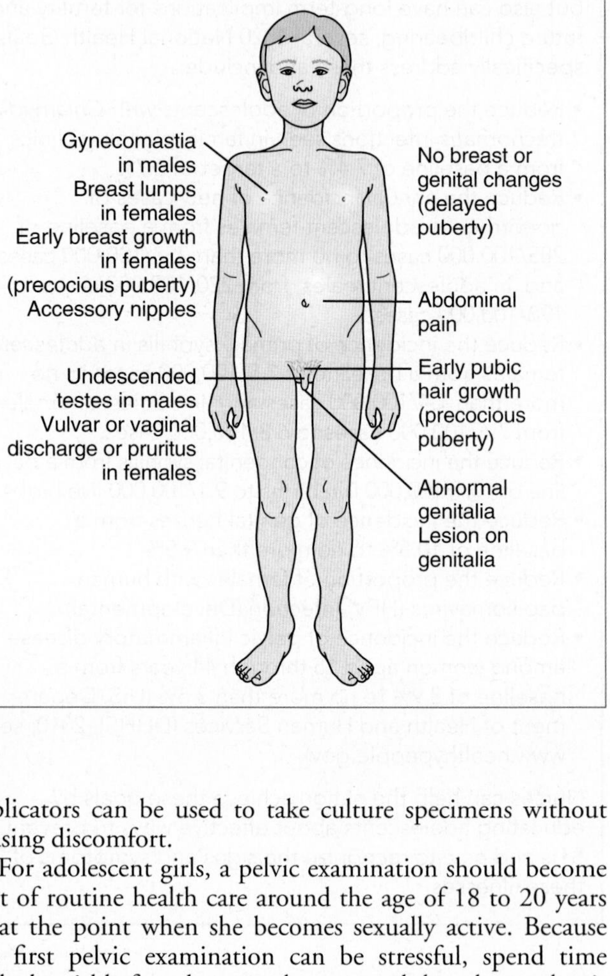

For adolescent girls, a pelvic examination should become part of routine health care around the age of 18 to 20 years or at the point when she becomes sexually active. Because the first pelvic examination can be stressful, spend time with the girl before the procedure to teach her about what is being assessed. A three-dimensional model of internal organs and some representative instruments may be more useful when describing the examination than a verbal description of anatomy.

Health care facilities should have a small speculum for examining young girls. For their comfort, warm the speculum first. Let the girl look at and handle a speculum before one is used. Remember that different cultures have different attitudes toward reproductive disorders. Adolescents from Middle Eastern countries, for example, are extremely modest, and so may be extremely uncomfortable having pelvic examinations. Girls from these countries may be more comfortable if the examiner is a woman. Remaining beside an adolescent as a support person also helps to reduce the stress the teen may be experiencing. To protect her self-esteem, be sure she meets the person who will examine her before she is placed in a lithotomy position.

If a young adolescent is uncomfortable in a lithotomy position, she can be examined in a dorsal recumbent position instead (see Chapter 11 for information on assisting with a pelvic examination). Allow an adolescent to choose whether she wants a parent to remain in the room with her.

BOX 47.3 Taking a Gynecologic History

When assessing an adolescent for a gynecologic health history, be especially conscious of an adolescent's sense of modesty and need for privacy.

Menstrual History

At what age did you begin menstruating? When was your last menstrual period?

How often do your menstrual periods occur? How long do they usually last?

What is the amount of menstrual flow? (Document by number of pads or tampons used.)

Do you experience discomfort? (Document if discomfort occurs on first day or all days, and action taken to relieve it.)

Do any sisters or your mother have discomfort or pain during their menstrual periods (endometriosis is familial)?

Do you experience any symptoms of irritability, moodiness, headache, or diarrhea (premenstrual dysphoric disorder) 1 or 2 days before menses?

Reproductive Tract History

Have you or do you have a vaginal discharge? (Document amount and whether pad is necessary; include duration, frequency, description, associated symptoms, and actions taken.)

Is there vaginal itching (pruritus)? Or vaginal odor?

Have you had reproductive tract surgery? Have you ever been pregnant? Have you ever had an abortion or miscarriage?

Sexual History

Are you currently sexually active? What is the gender of your partner?

Have you had a sexually transmitted infection such as herpes, gonorrhea, or syphilis?

Do you experience any discomfort during sexual activity (dyspareunia) or any spotting afterward (postcoital spotting)?

Do you have any concerns about frequency, position, or partner's satisfaction with coitus? Do you experience orgasm?

Contraception History

Do you use any type of birth control? If so, what contraceptive do you use? (Document length of time used, satisfaction, and any problems.)

Breast Health

Have you ever noticed any abnormality such as a lump, discharge, or pain in your breasts?

Have you ever had breast surgery?

Have you breastfed a child?

Do you have a yearly breast examination by a health care provider?

BOX 47.4 Nursing Care Planning Based on Effective Communication

Navi, age 15 years, is seen at your pediatric clinic. She has mild upper respiratory tract symptoms.

Less Effective Communication

Nurse: Navi? Doctor Jensen doesn't believe you need anything for your cold. Just drink a little extra fluid and take it easy for a couple days.
Navi: Don't I need a prescription? Some penicillin or something?
Nurse: No. Colds are caused by viruses. Penicillin isn't necessary.
Navi: I want to be sure I get over this. I'd really like an antibiotic of some kind.
Nurse: One really isn't necessary.
Navi: I have a bad cough. I don't think I mentioned that.
Nurse: Doctor Jensen listened to your chest. You don't have anything serious there.
Navi: My stomach doesn't feel very good either. Can't I have something?
Nurse: Sorry. Goodbye now.

More Effective Communication

Nurse: Navi? Doctor Jensen doesn't believe you need anything for your cold. Just drink a little extra fluid and take it easy for a couple days.
Navi: Don't I need a prescription? Some penicillin or something?
Nurse: No. Colds are caused by viruses. Penicillin isn't necessary.
Navi: I want to be sure I get over this. I'd really like an antibiotic of some kind.
Nurse: One really isn't necessary.
Navi: I have a bad cough. I don't think I mentioned that.
Nurse: Doctor Jensen listened to your chest. You don't have anything serious there.
Navi: My stomach doesn't feel very good either. Can't I have something?
Nurse: It seems you're having more symptoms than you originally mentioned. Are you worried about something other than cold symptoms?
Navi: Well, I have this rash and . . .
Nurse: And . . . ?
Navi: I'm scared I might have a sex disease.

Adolescents can have difficulty discussing reproductive tract symptoms. Here, an adolescent tries to obtain an antibiotic by describing respiratory or abdominal symptoms. Being alert to this possibility helps you to recognize a "growing" history of this type.

HEALTH PROMOTION AND RISK MANAGEMENT

Newborns need a thorough examination at birth to rule out congenital reproductive disorders so these can be diagnosed and management can begin. All children need education about how to make sexually healthy decisions and how to care for their bodies (Doswell, Braxter, Cha, et al., 2011). Adolescents may state they are not interested in this information because they are choosing abstinence. It is still important to provide the education with regard to making sexually healthy decisions and reward positive choices for staying healthy.

DISORDERS CAUSED BY ALTERED REPRODUCTIVE DEVELOPMENT

Genetic sex or *biologic gender* (sex chromosomes XX or XY) is determined at conception. However, development of the reproductive system, including external genitalia, occurs over two distinct periods. Reproductive organs and genitalia begin to differentiate in utero by the eighth week, with growth and refinement occurring over the next several months. A second phase occurs with specific endocrine changes triggered during puberty and is the period of maturation of primary and secondary sexual characteristics.

Ambiguous genitalia, a rare condition that occurs during fetal development, is an example of a first-stage disorder; precocious puberty or delayed puberty are examples of second-phase disorders.

Ambiguous Genitalia

Ambiguous genitalia refers to genitalia that are not clearly defined in a newborn (Malone, Hall-Craggs, Mouriquand, et al., 2012). Although external sexual structures generally follow from the presence of the XX or XY chromosomes, a diagnosis of ambiguous genitalia means external sexual organs in the child did not follow this normal course of development, so that, at birth, they are so incompletely or abnormally formed that it is impossible to clearly determine the child's gender by simple observation. For instance, a male infant with *hypospadias* (urethral opening on the underside of the penis) and cryptorchidism (undescended testes) may appear more female than male on first inspection (see Chapter 46 for a discussion of hypospadias).

A female fetus can become "masculinized" if exposed to androgen in utero. The most common cause of this is *congenital adrenocortical syndrome*. The adrenal gland produces androgen instead of adequate cortisone, causing the clitoris to become the size of a typical newborn male's penis (Mattila, Fagerholm, Santtila, et al., 2012) (see Chapter 48).

If testosterone was produced in utero but development of the müllerian duct (female) was not suppressed, a child may be intersexed (formerly termed **hermaphrodite**), with both ovaries and testes and either male or female external genitalia. Children with ambiguous genitalia are often termed pseudointersexed because, as infants, they have some external features of both sexes, although only either ovaries or testes (or neither) are present.

Assessment

If there is any question about a child's gender, karyotyping or a DNA analysis establishes whether the child is genetically male or female (see Chapter 7). *Laparoscopy* (introduction of a narrow laparoscope into the abdominal cavity through a half-inch incision under the umbilicus) or possibly exploratory surgery may be necessary to determine if ovaries or undescended testes are present. Intravenous pyelography or ultrasound can be used to establish whether a complete urinary tract is present.

Therapeutic Management

Once the child's true chromosomal gender has been documented by chromosome or DNA analysis, the extent of necessary reconstructive surgery is determined in consultation with the parents. This may involve correction of a hypospadias or cryptorchidism, removal of labial adhesions, or surgical removal of an enlarged clitoris. If removal of an enlarged clitoris seems necessary, parents must consider what the absence of this organ will mean to the girl in terms of later sexual enjoyment. Parents are well advised to delay this type of surgery until adolescence when the girl can decide for herself whether she wants this done. If a vagina will be constructed, surgery for this is usually delayed until adolescence as well when growth is complete (Jospe, 2011).

If an infant is chromosomally male but does not have an adequate penis, a decision to raise the child as a female might be made, although construction of an artificial penis is more likely. Nonfunctioning ovaries or testes are generally removed to prevent malignancy later in life.

Nursing Diagnoses and Related Interventions

The birth of a child with a perplexing disorder produces a particularly high level of stress, possibly hampering parents' ability to think calmly about their situation and make plans.

Nursing Diagnosis: Anxiety related to ambiguous gender of child at birth

Outcome Evaluation: Parents voice willingness to support treatment plan, including additional necessary tests; and state they are prepared to make decisions with guidance from health care team.

If the gender of a child is unclear, the parents should be told this immediately. If first told their child is a boy, only to be told 24 hours later that the child is chromosomally a girl, then parents may find this difficult to accept. During this period when the baby's gender is yet to be determined, avoid calling the baby "it." Rather, say "the baby" or "your child." Explain how sexual organs form in utero and that every child has the potential to be externally female or male.

To promote bonding, help parents understand that their child is otherwise perfect (assuming this is true). As the child grows, additional counseling may be needed for both the parents and the child to provide education about the full meaning of the congenital disorder.

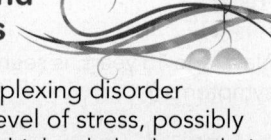

BOX 47.5 Nursing Care Planning Based on Responsibility for Pharmacology

LEUPROLIDE ACETATE (LUPRON DEPOT-PED)

Classification: Leuprolide is a hormonal agent, specifically a luteinizing hormone-releasing hormone (LH-RH) agonist.
Action: Occupies pituitary gonadotropin-releasing hormone (GnRH) receptors, preventing GnRH from functioning, thereby reducing the level of testosterone or estrogen in the body (Karch, 2013).
Pregnancy Risk Category: X
Dosage: Intramuscular (IM) injection every 3 months.
Possible Adverse Effects: Nausea, vomiting, anorexia, hot flashes, headache, pain at injection site

Nursing Implications

- Administer only with the syringe supplied with the drug.
- Vary injection sites to decrease local irritation.
- Monitor injection sites for bruising and rash.
- Because injections are given only every 3 months, assist parents with preparing a calendar so they know when the next injection will be due.

Precocious Puberty

Although precocious puberty (the development of breasts or pubic hair before 8 years of age) can occur in both sexes, the condition is most often seen in girls. Such early development may be only a reflection of early maturation, but is traditionally considered precocious sexual development (Faizah, Zuhanis, Rahmah, et al., 2012). Development may be limited to just breast tissue but can proceed to complete secondary sex characteristics, spermatogenesis, or menstrual function.

The condition is caused by the early production of gonadotropins by the pituitary gland; gonadotropins then stimulate the ovaries or testes to produce sex hormones. Such stimulation can occur because of a pituitary tumor, cyst, or traumatic injury to the third ventricle next to the pituitary gland. It also can occur because of estrogen-secreting cysts or tumors of the ovary or testosterone-secreting cysts of the testes. In rare instances, it occurs because of an estrogen- or testosterone-secreting adrenal tumor. In girls, ingestion of a mother's oral contraceptive pills can initiate menarche-like changes. Overstimulation by the enzyme aromatase, which converts androgens into estrogens by a process called aromatization, may be yet another cause (Pavone & Bulun, 2012).

In children with precocious puberty, a pituitary tumor must be ruled out. If no physical cause, such as a tumor, is detected, the phenomenon appears to occur only because the *gonadostat* of the hypothalamus (the trigger that begins the development of secondary sex characteristics) has turned on several years too early.

Assessment

With precocious puberty, children have accelerated skeletal maturation as well as increased breast and genital development. Girls have menstrual bleeding yet have little pubic or axillary hair because of still low androgen secretion. Boys have obvious genital growth. The diagnosis of early puberty is confirmed by serum analysis for estrogen or androgen, which will be at adult levels.

Therapeutic Management

Children need therapy, not only because of their outward appearance but also because if epiphyseal lines of long bones close early, they will be left unnecessarily short in stature. A synthetic analog to gonadotropin-releasing hormone (GnRH) is available as leuprolide acetate (Lupron) (Box 47.5). Administration of this analog desensitizes GnRH receptors, making stimulation by GnRH ineffective and halting sexual maturation at the point to which it has advanced (Karch, 2013). Therapy may also include use of aromatase inhibitors, which are able to block the enzyme aromatase and therefore decrease signs of estrogen effects (Pavone & Bulun, 2012).

Nursing Diagnoses and Related Interventions

Nursing Diagnosis: Disturbed body image related to precocious puberty

Outcome Evaluation: Child voices an understanding of what is happening and does not evidence excessive shyness or reluctance to interact with peers.

Children who develop precociously may have difficulty interacting with peers because they appear so different from other members of their age group. Parents may worry about a child becoming sexually active, and particularly about girls becoming pregnant. Both parents and children need reassurance that, after reaching the age of normal puberty, the child will maintain normal growth, development, and appearance.

Help parents to understand that their child is fully fertile and able to inseminate or conceive. Oral contraceptives, however, are not advisable for girls this young, because the estrogen in them also causes early closure of epiphyseal lines, possibly stunting the child's growth further.

Parents may need to be reminded also, that, although their child appears to be much older, the changes are only in sexual characteristics. Household tasks, responsibility, and expectations must be geared to the child's chronologic age, not to his or her outward appearance.

Delayed Puberty

Secondary sex characteristics are normally present by age 14 years in girls and 15 years in boys. Delayed puberty, as the name implies, is the failure of pubertal changes to occur at the usual age. The family history of many of these children reveals a family tendency for late maturation. If so, the child needs a thorough physical examination to disclose whether some secondary sex characteristics are present or endocrine stimulation is beginning.

Most girls worry considerably about delayed menstruation, but, once reassured that their development is merely delayed, they are usually willing to wait for menarche to occur on its own. If girls have not begun to menstruate by age 17 years and pathology has been ruled out, menstrual cycles can be initiated by administering estrogen. Similarly, boys who are distressed by their lack of development may receive testosterone supplements to stimulate pubic hair and genital growth, but again, patience may allow usual maturation to occur.

✔ QSEN Checkpoint Question 47.1

Informatics

Suppose Navi, 15 years of age, had undergone diagnostic testing and been diagnosed with precocious puberty. What advice would you give her parents?

a. Restrict the amount of physical and mental stimulation she receives daily to halt abnormal growth.
b. Although her sexual appearance is advanced, she is not able to conceive.
c. Treat her appropriately for her chronologic age, rather than her physical appearance.
d. Do not allow her to eat processed meats, which contain growth hormones.

Look in Appendix A for the best answer and rationale.

REPRODUCTIVE DISORDERS IN MALES

Common reproductive disorders in males include structural alterations in the penis or testes such as phimosis and cryptorchidism, inflammation such as balanoposthitis, and, in adolescents, testicular cancer.

Balanitis (Balanoposthitis)

Balanoposthitis is inflammation of the glans and prepuce of the penis. It tends to occur in uncircumcised boys, is usually caused by poor hygiene, or may accompany a urethritis or a regional dermatitis (Morris, Waskett, Banerjee, et al., 2012).

Assessment

The prepuce and glans appear red and swollen, and there may be a purulent discharge. The boy may have difficulty voiding because of crusting at the meatal opening and because acidic urine touching the denuded surface of the glans causes pain.

Therapeutic Management

Any discharge should be cultured to rule out an STI such as gonorrhea. Medical treatment involves local application of heat by warm wet soaks or warm baths. A local antibiotic ointment may be prescribed. If *phimosis* (a tight foreskin) appears to be contributing to the condition, circumcision may be advocated after the inflammation subsides to prevent the condition from recurring.

Although balanoposthitis is painful, a boy may tolerate the discomfort for several days because he may be worried it was caused by masturbation (which can contribute to the irritation) or by sexual activity and may be reluctant to seek help for fear of being criticized. He can be reassured that the problem is local and will have no long-range effect.

Phimosis and Paraphimosis

Phimosis is the inability to retract the foreskin from the glans of the penis. The foreskin is tight at birth and may even be held fast by adhesions and so, in newborns, cannot (and should not) be retracted. After a few months, the adhesions dissolve and the foreskin becomes retractable; if it does not, the infant has phimosis (Shahid, 2012). If a foreskin is extremely tight, it can interfere with voiding. Balanoposthitis may develop because the foreskin cannot be retracted for cleaning. Circumcision of newborns (discussed in Chapter 18) is no longer routinely advised but is used to relieve phimosis. Paraphimosis is the inability to replace the prepuce over the glans once it has been retracted. This is an emergency situation to address before circulation to the glans is impaired.

Cryptorchidism

Cryptorchidism is failure of one or both testes to descend from the abdominal cavity into the scrotum (Kollin, Stukenborg, Nurmio, et al., 2012). Normally, testes descend into the scrotal sac during months 7 to 9 of intrauterine life. They may descend any time up to 6 months after birth, but they rarely descend after that time (Mahan, 2011).

The cause of undescended testes is unclear. Testes apparently descend because of stimulation by testosterone; hence, a lower than usual level of testosterone production may prevent descent. Fibrous bands at the inguinal ring or inadequate length of spermatic vessels may prevent descent. The condition is found in about 3 out of every 1,000 male newborns; it occurs most often in premature or low-birth–weight babies (Gaylord & Petersen-Smith, 2013).

Assessment

Early detection of undescended testes is important because the warmth of the abdominal cavity may inhibit development of the testes, ultimately affecting spermatogenesis. After puberty, sperm production deteriorates rapidly in undescended testes, and the testes may even undergo a malignant change (Maule, Malavassi, & Richiardi, 2012). Anchoring the testes in the scrotal sac does not guarantee malignancy can be prevented, but it will allow the boy to perform preventive measures such as testicular self-examination.

Some boys may be diagnosed with undescended testes when, if an examining room is chilly, the testes have retracted to make palpation assessment difficult. Excessive palpation or stroking of the inner thigh may also stimulate the cremasteric reflex and cause retraction. In these instances, testes descend when the child is standing or after a warm bath.

Laparoscopy is effective at identifying whether an undescended testis is at the inguinal ring (true undescended testis) or ectopic (still in the abdomen). Because testes arise from the same germ tissue as the kidneys, the kidney function of a child with ectopic testes is usually evaluated as well. If undescended testes and other factors such as ambiguous genitals pose questions about the child's gender, a *karyotype* may be done to determine the child's true gender.

Therapeutic Management

Because the testes sometimes descend spontaneously during the first year of life, treatment is usually delayed for 1 year, possibly 2 years. Boys may be given a short course of chorionic gonadotropin hormone for about 5 days to see if testicular descent can be stimulated. If this is not successful, surgery **(orchiopexy)** by laparoscopy will then correct the condition (McIntosh, Scrimgeour, Youngson, et al., 2012).

Nursing Diagnoses and Related Interventions

If an orchiopexy is scheduled, the focus is on parent and child teaching, preoperative preparation, and postoperative care.

Nursing Diagnosis: Deficient knowledge related to parents' and child's inexperience with surgical procedure and postoperative treatment plan

Outcome Evaluation: Parents (and child, if old enough) accurately describe what will be accomplished by surgery.

Boys who are old enough to understand why they need surgery need good preparation for this. Use an anatomically correct picture to point out the exact site where surgery will be performed. Reassure the boy that the penis itself will not be cut. Although the child may not voice a fear of mutilation, you can assume it exists, especially in preschool children.

During surgery, internal sutures may be inserted to hold the testis in place. Although the child may be discharged from the hospital on the same day, his activity will be limited until approximately the second day after surgery to ensure the internal suture line remains intact.

Nursing Diagnosis: Disturbed body image related to change in physical appearance

Outcome Evaluation: Child (if verbal) states he views himself as a whole person and interacts with peers without excessive shyness or hesitancy.

The postoperative evaluation should reveal that the suture line is healing well and that both testes can be palpated in the scrotum. It should also address the boy's feelings about the surgery and the changes in his body. He may need an opportunity to express his fears about mutilation or castration by playing with puppets or dolls after surgery. In years to come, even after a repair, boys who had bilateral cryptorchidism may be less fertile. When boys reach puberty, teach testicular self-examination to assess any early symptoms of malignancy, such as nodules or abnormal growth (see Chapter 34).

Hydrocele

When a testis descends into the scrotum in utero, it is preceded by a fold of tissue, the *processus vaginalis*. Occasionally, fluid (termed a **hydrocele**) collects in this fold. In utero, the fluid can be revealed by ultrasound. At birth, the fluid causes the scrotum of the newborn to appear enlarged (Lao, Fitzgibbons, & Cusick, 2012). Its presence can be revealed by ultrasound or *transillumination* (the shining of a light through the scrotal sac causes the area to glow). If the hydrocele is uncomplicated, the fluid will gradually be reabsorbed, so no treatment is necessary. The child's parents can be assured that the hydrocele is only excess fluid and the scrotal enlargement is not caused by an abnormal testis, tumor, or hernia.

Hydroceles may form later in life due to *inguinal hernias* (abdominal contents extruding into the scrotum through the inguinal ring, with accompanying fluid). If this happens, when the hernia is repaired, the hydrocele will be reabsorbed (see Chapter 45). Injection of a drug to decrease fluid production (*sclerotherapy*) may also be effective for older youths.

Varicocele

A **varicocele** is abnormal dilation of the veins of the spermatic cord (Fig. 47.1). It is important to identify varicoceles in adolescents because, although it may not cause a difference, the increased heat and congestion in the testicles is a

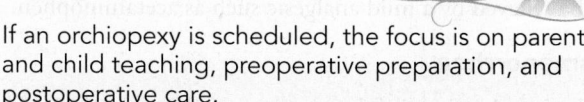

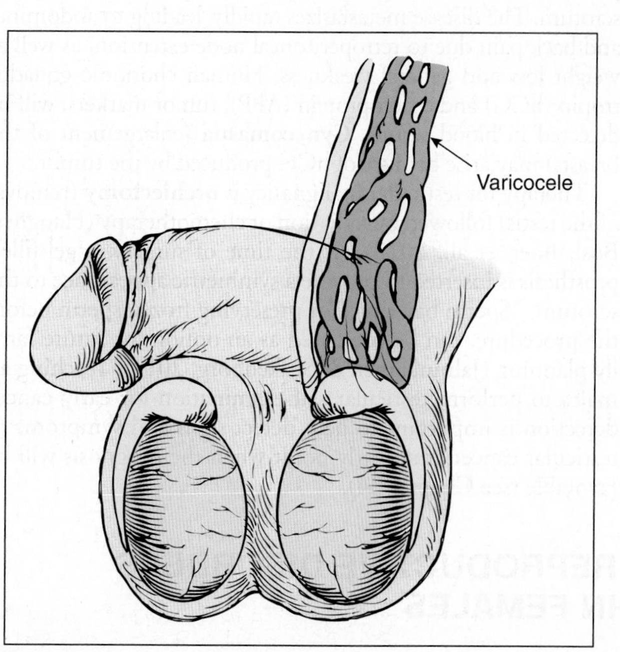

FIGURE 47.1 A varicocele. Identifying a varicocele in adolescent males is important because the condition may be associated with subfertility.

possible cause of subfertility (Fine & Poppas, 2012). If fertility becomes a concern, the varicocele can be surgically removed. The adolescent will experience some local tenderness and edema for a few days after surgery. This can be minimized by applying ice for the first few hours postoperatively.

What if...47.1 Ryan, Navi's boyfriend, was born with undescended testes. He had surgery for this when he was 2 years old. He's concerned now that he is at high risk for testicular cancer. How would you counsel him?

Testicular Torsion

Testicular torsion (twisting of the spermatic cord) is a surgical emergency. Although it can be present in newborns, it occurs most frequently during early adolescence in connection with a sports activity (Jospe, 2011). Less than normal testicular support apparently allows the spermatic cord to twist.

The boy experiences immediate severe scrotal pain and perhaps nausea and vomiting from the extent of the pain. The testis feels tender to palpation, and edema begins to develop. If the condition is not recognized promptly (within 4 hours), irreversible change in the testis can occur from lack of circulation to the organ. Boys need to be educated about the phenomenon so that they report symptoms promptly. Fortunately, the torsion can usually be reduced manually under ultrasound guidance (Sung, Setty, & Castro-Aragon, 2012). Laparoscopic surgery, however, may be necessary to reduce the torsion and to reestablish circulation.

Testicular Cancer

Testicular cancer is rare (only 1% of all malignancies) but can be an adolescent concern because it tends to occur between ages 15 and 35 years (Masterson & Beck, 2012). Symptoms include painless testicular enlargement and a feeling of heaviness in the scrotum. The disease metastasizes rapidly, leading to abdominal and back pain due to retroperitoneal node extension, as well as weight loss and general weakness. Human chorionic gonadotropin (hCG) and α-fetoprotein (AFP), tumor markers, will be detected in blood serum. **Gynecomastia** (enlargement of the breasts) may arise because of hCG produced by the tumor.

Therapy for testicular malignancy is **orchiectomy** (removal of the testis) followed by radiation or chemotherapy (Haugnes, Bosl, Boer, et al., 2012). At the time of surgery, a gel-filled prosthesis is inserted to provide a symmetric appearance to the scrotum. "Sperm banking," or preserving frozen sperm before the procedure, can be presented as an option for future family planning (Jahnukainen & Stukenborg, 2012). Teaching all males to perform testicular self-examination for early cancer detection is important to help detect signs and symptoms of testicular cancer at an early point when the prognosis will be favorable (see Chapter 34).

REPRODUCTIVE DISORDERS IN FEMALES

The most frequent reproductive disorders in females involve vaginal or menstrual irregularities. Other disorders are caused by physiologic or structural alterations of the reproductive organs such as imperforate hymen, pelvic inflammatory disease (PID), or infections caused by STIs.

Menstrual Disorders

Because menstruation is an ongoing process throughout half of a woman's life, an irregularity such as painful cycles can exert a major influence on her daily activities and life plans. Menstrual disorders in adolescents fall into two categories: (a) menstruation that is painful or uncomfortable and (b) infrequent or too frequent cycles (Gerlt & Smith, 2013).

Mittelschmerz

Some adolescents experience abdominal pain during ovulation from the release of accompanying prostaglandins. Pain at this time may also be caused by a drop or two of follicular fluid or blood spilling into the abdominal cavity. Called **mittelschmerz**, the pain can range from a few sharp cramps to several hours of discomfort. It is typically felt on one side of the abdomen (near an ovary) and may be accompanied by scant vaginal spotting.

An advantage of mittelschmerz is that it clearly marks ovulation. If pain is felt in the right lower quadrant, it should be differentiated from appendicitis; a lack of associated appendicitis symptoms such as nausea, vomiting, fever, abdominal guarding, and rebound tenderness does this. Mittelschmerz can be relieved by a mild analgesic such as acetaminophen.

Dysmenorrhea

Dysmenorrhea is painful menstruation (Munro, 2012). The pain is caused by the release of prostaglandins in response to tissue destruction during the ischemic phase of the menstrual cycle, which leads to smooth muscle contraction and uterine pain.

Although dysmenorrhea is exceedingly common, it needs to be investigated because it can also be a preliminary symptom of an underlying disorder such as PID, uterine myomas (tumors), or endometriosis (abnormal formation of endometrial tissue).

Assessment. During the first year or two of menstruation, dysmenorrhea rarely occurs because early menstrual cycles are usually **anovulatory** (without ovulation). As ovulation begins, typical menstrual discomfort also begins. As many as 80% of adolescents have some discomfort with menstruation; in as many as 10%, the discomfort seriously interferes with daily living (Harel, 2012).

It is categorized as *primary* if it occurs in the absence of organic disease; it is *secondary* if it occurs as a result of organic disease. Symptoms each month may begin with a "bloated" feeling and light cramping 24 hours before a menstrual flow. Colicky (sharp) pain is superimposed on a dull, nagging pain across the lower abdomen, and an "aching, pulling" sensation of the vulva and inner thighs when the flow begins. Some adolescents have mild diarrhea as well. Mild breast tenderness, abdominal distention, nausea, vomiting, and headache are other symptoms that may also be present.

Therapeutic Management. Dysmenorrhea can usually be controlled by a nonsteroidal anti-inflammatory drug (NSAID) such as ibuprofen (Advil, Motrin). Be certain girls know not to take these drugs on an empty stomach because they can be extremely irritating to gastric mucosa. If symptoms do not respond to NSAIDs, hormonal treatment, such as combined estrogen and progestin oral contraceptive pills (COCs) can be tried. These prevent pain by preventing ovulation, which was the cause of the pain. If preferred, adolescents can choose to be prescribed long-acting oral contraceptives so that they have menstrual periods only every 3 months. One disadvantage of COC therapy is the possible adverse effects of long-term estrogen administration such as thrombophlebitis or early closure of epiphyseal lines of long bones.

If dysmenorrhea does not improve within 6 months with the use of NSAIDs and COCs, a laparoscopy is indicated to look for endometriosis, the most common reason for secondary dysmenorrhea (Templeman, 2012).

Nursing Diagnoses and Related Interventions

Nursing Diagnosis: Pain related to menstrual period

Outcome Evaluation: Client states she feels some control over pain through nonpharmacologic or pharmacologic methods.

Several nonpharmacologic solutions such as yoga and exercise may help relieve dysmenorrhea (Chien, Chang, & Liu, 2013). Decreasing sodium intake for a few days before an expected menstrual flow by omitting salty foods such as potato chips and luncheon meats may help reduce "bloated" feelings. Abdominal breathing (breathing in and out slowly, allowing the abdominal wall to rise with each inhalation) may also be helpful. Applying heat to the abdomen with a heating pad or taking a hot shower or bath may relax muscle tension and relieve pain (Navvabi-Rigi, Kerman-Saravi, Navidian, et al., 2012). Abdominal massage (effleurage or light massage) or acupressure are still other options (Gharloghi, Torkzahrani, Akbarzadeh, et al., 2012). Adolescents who remain sexually active during their menses may discover an orgasm helps relieve pelvic engorgement and cramping.

If girls are going to apply heat to their abdomen, caution them not to do this until their menstrual flow actually begins because if the pain is actually from an inflamed appendix, heat could cause rupture of the appendix and life-threatening peritonitis.

QSEN Checkpoint Question 47.2

Evidence-Based Practice

Nonpharmacologic interventions are being used with increasing frequency to help reduce the pain of dysmenorrhea. To discover if yoga exercises could achieve this, a researcher recruited 92 female students, 18 to 22 years of age. Half of them were assigned to an experimental group where they were taught and asked to perform yoga poses during the second half of their next cycle. Results of the study showed a significant difference in both the pain intensity and duration between the experimental group and the control group during their next menstrual period (Rakhshaee, 2011).

Based on the previous study, what would you recommend to Navi?

a. Make a list of menstrual symptoms each month because listing them helps reduce discomfort.
b. Nonpharmacologic measures can help you cope psychologically with your pain.
c. Some exercise programs can genuinely help reduce menstrual pain.
d. The more vigorous the exercise you do, the less pain you're likely to have.

Look in Appendix A for the best answer and rationale.

Menorrhagia

Menorrhagia is an abnormally heavy menstrual flow, usually defined as greater than 80 ml per menses or a flow that soaks more than one pad or tampon an hour. It tends to occur in girls close to puberty because, without ovulation and subsequent progesterone secretion, estrogen secretion causes extreme proliferation of endometrium. There is often also an unusual amount of menstrual flow in girls using intrauterine devices (IUDs). With oral contraceptives, the flow is often light; for this reason, it may seem alarmingly heavy once pills are discontinued, when this is just a return of the adolescent's normal flow.

Heavy flows need to be investigated, however, as they also can indicate endometriosis (see later discussion), a systemic disease (anemia), a blood dyscrasia such as a clotting defect, or a uterine abnormality such as a myoma (fibroid) tumor. It can be a symptom of infection such as PID, an indication of early pregnancy loss that is coincidentally occurring at the time of an expected menstrual period, or can occur from breakthrough bleeding from an oral contraceptive.

Assessment and Therapy. It is difficult to determine when a menstrual flow is abnormally heavy, but because a sanitary pad or tampon holds approximately 25 ml of fluid, if a pad or tampon is saturated in less than 1 hour, the flow is heavier than usual.

The adolescent who is losing excessive blood because of anovulatory cycles may be prescribed progesterone during the luteal phase to prevent proliferative growth during this phase of the cycle; if the ability to conceive is unimportant, adolescents may be prescribed a low-dose oral contraceptive or GnRH inhibitor to decrease the flow. If anemia is occurring from the heavy blood loss, an iron supplementation may be necessary to restore sufficient hemoglobin formation (Fernández-Gaxiola & De-Regil, 2011).

Metrorrhagia

Metrorrhagia is bleeding between menstrual periods (Davidson, Dipiero, Govoni, et al., 2011). This is normal in some adolescents who have spotting at the time of ovulation ("mittelstaining"). It may also occur in teenagers taking oral contraceptives (breakthrough bleeding) during the first

3 or 4 months of use. It also can occur from vaginal irritation caused by infection or spotting from a temporarily low level of progesterone production, which leads to endometrial sloughing (dysfunctional uterine bleeding or a luteal phase defect), although this condition most often occurs near the end of the reproductive years, not the beginning.

If metrorrhagia occurs for more than one menstrual cycle in a teenager who is not taking oral contraceptives, she needs to be referred to her primary care provider for examination, because abnormal vaginal bleeding is an early sign of uterine or cervical carcinoma or an ovarian cyst (Stapley & Hamilton, 2011). Endometrium ablation, used with premenopausal women to halt metrorrhagia, is not recommended for adolescents (Fernández-Gaxiola & De-Regil, 2011). Prescription of a COC that will reduce the amount of a menstrual flow is recommended instead (Davidson et al., 2011).

Menstrual Migraine

A *menstrual migraine headache* refers to a sharp, disabling headache, often accompanied by nausea or vomiting or vision changes, which occurs at the same time as a menstrual flow (Karlı, Baykan, Ertas, et al., 2012). This is probably caused by the drop in estrogen, which occurs immediately prior to a menstrual flow. Therapy is NSAIDs, which decrease inflammation, or sumatriptan (triptan), which reduces swollen blood vessels. Menstrual migraines seem to be more intense in adolescents taking birth control pills so those who tend to have these should be counseled to use another form of reproductive planning (Hershey, 2012). Any form of migraine headache is frightening because of its sharp intensity; assure girls this is not an uncommon symptom to accompany menstrual flows. Although this doesn't relieve the pain, it can help adolescents not read more into the symptom than it warrants.

Endometriosis

Endometriosis is the abnormal growth of extrauterine endometrial cells, often in the cul-de-sac of the peritoneal cavity or on the uterine ligaments or ovaries, and is one of the main causes of dysmenorrhea in adolescents (Kennedy & Koninckx, 2012; Templeman, 2012). This abnormal tissue results from excessive endometrial production and a reflux of blood and tissue through the fallopian tubes during a menstrual flow. The condition tends to occur most often in white nulliparous women, but there is also a familial tendency in which daughters of women with endometriosis develop symptoms of dysmenorrhea early in life.

The excessive production of endometrial tissue can be related to a deficient immunologic response. In many women, it appears to be related to excess estrogen production or a failed luteal menstrual phase caused by not ovulating or ovulating irregularly. The resulting proliferation of tissue forces the menstrual flow into the fallopian tubes.

Dysmenorrhea occurs as the abnormal tissue begins to slough in the same manner as the uterine lining in response to estrogen and progesterone stimulation and withdrawal. This causes inflammation of surrounding tissue in the abdominal cavity and a release of prostaglandins. Abnormal tissue in the pelvic cul-de-sac can cause *dyspareunia* (painful coitus) because it puts pressure on the posterior vagina. Subfertility may result if the fallopian tubes become immobilized and blocked by tissue implants or adhesions, preventing peristaltic motion and transport of ova (see Chapter 9). Adolescents with endometritis may want to consider having children early in life before overgrowth of the endometrium becomes so extensive that it begins to interfere with conception.

Assessment. Pelvic examination may show the uterus is displaced by tender, fixed, palpable nodules. Nodules in the cul-de-sac or on an ovary may be palpable and painful.

Therapeutic Management. Treatment for endometriosis can be medical or surgical, depending on the extent of the condition. Estrogen/progesterone-based oral contraceptives may reduce the amount of extrusion into the peritoneal cavity because the tissue sloughs under the influence of the progesterone. Danazol (Danocrine), a synthetic androgen, can be prescribed to help shrink the abnormal tissue. Administration of a GnRH agonist, such as leuprolide acetate (Lupron), can reduce hormone stimulation and cause the same effect (see Box 47.5). Aromatase inhibitors, which reduce estrogen levels, are still another solution (Gunderson & Yates, 2011). A laparotomy with excision by laser surgery is the most effective measure, but, because this is a highly invasive procedure, a course of conservative medical treatment may be tried first.

Amenorrhea

Amenorrhea, or absence of a menstrual flow, strongly suggests pregnancy but is by no means definitive, because it can also result from tension, anxiety, fatigue, chronic illness, extreme dieting, or strenuous exercise. Amenorrhea as a sign of pregnancy is discussed in Chapter 10. Competitive swimmers, long-distance runners (50 to 75 miles weekly), and ballet dancers may notice their intensive training causes menstrual periods to become scant and irregular, a phenomenon related to their low ratio of body fat to body muscle; this leads to excessive secretion of prolactin. An elevation in prolactin then causes a decrease in GnRH from the hypothalamus, followed by declines in follicle-stimulating hormone (FSH), follicular development, and estrogen secretion. Menstrual cycles usually return to normal within a few months after discontinuation of strenuous training and conditioning, although this may take up to 1 year (Arends, Cheung, Barrack, et al., 2012).

Adolescents who wish to maintain a normal cycle while training for a sports event may take bromocriptine (Parlodel), which reduces high prolactin levels by its action on the hypothalamus. Many adolescents, however, view the absence of menstrual periods as a benefit of sports training. If a menstrual flow is delayed and pregnancy is suspected, bromocriptine should be discontinued because it is potentially teratogenic.

Amenorrhea also occurs among females who diet excessively, partially as a natural defense mechanism to limit ovulation and also probably as a means of conserving body fluid. Adolescents with *anorexia nervosa* or *bulimia* (eating disorders described in Chapter 54) often develop amenorrhea after approximately 3 months of excessive dieting or binging and dieting; as in athletes, this is caused by an increase in prolactin (Dominé, Dadoumont, & Bourguignon, 2012).

What if... 47.2 Navi returns to your clinic in 6 months and tells you she hasn't had a menstrual flow for 3 months. Would your first suspicion be that she is pregnant? What questions would you want to ask her?

Premenstrual Dysphoric Disorder

Premenstrual dysphoric disorder (PDD) is a condition that occurs in the luteal phase of the menstrual cycle and is relieved by the onset of menses. Because of the variety of possible symptoms, as many as 3% to 8% of women experience some degree of PDD, such as anxiety, fatigue, abdominal bloating, headache, irritability, or depression, and these may begin as early as adolescence. For a small subset of these women, these symptoms become so extreme that they are incapacitating (Dennerstein, Lehert, & Heinemann, 2012).

The cause of PDD is unproven, but, contrary to previous beliefs, it must be due to more than a drop in progesterone just before menses. A syndrome similar to PDD can occur in women after tubal ligation; with this, apparently a decrease in the blood supply to the ovary results in decreased luteal function. In some women, a vitamin B–complex deficiency may lead to estrogen excess, causing an abnormal ratio of estrogen to progesterone. Other related causes may be poor renal clearance leading to water retention, or hypoglycemia leading to a surge of epinephrine and low calcium levels and interference with serotonin synthesis.

Because symptoms of PDD vary from cycle to cycle and throughout life, therapy is aimed at correcting specific symptoms (Steinberg, Cardoso, Martinez, et al., 2012). Adolescents who think they have PDD should keep a diary of when symptoms occur. They should be certain their diet is high in vitamins and calcium and low in salt. Agents that suppress ovarian function, such as oral contraceptives or the GnRH agonist leuprolide, may be prescribed. If depression is a major symptom, an antidepressant may be prescribed, although antidepressants (especially serotonin-reuptake inhibitors) are prescribed with caution in adolescents because they may be responsible for an increase in suicidal behavior (Adegbite-Adeniyi, Gron, Rowles, et al., 2012).

Additional Reproductive Disorders in Females

Female Circumcision

Female circumcision is the incision and removal of the clitoris (Gele, Johansen, & Sundby, 2012). There is no medical reason or advantage of the procedure, but, performed just prior to puberty, it is regarded as a coming of age ritual or religious practice in some cultures. Both a painful and mutilating procedure, it is not legal in the United States. You may, however, see adolescents or women in gynecology and pregnancy care settings who have had this done in another country. A major complication of the procedure is that women may have difficulty with conception or childbirth because of vulvar scarring and perineal contraction.

Imperforate Hymen

The *hymen* is the membranous ring of tissue that partly obstructs the vaginal opening. An *imperforate hymen* totally occludes the vagina, preventing the escape of vaginal secretions and menstrual blood (Karasahin, Keskin, & Ercan, 2012).

Before menarche, a girl with an imperforate hymen usually has no symptoms. With the onset of menstruation, however, the menstrual flow builds up in the vagina, causing increased pressure in the vagina and uterus and, eventually, abdominal pain. Palpation of the abdomen reveals a lower abdominal mass. On vaginal examination, an intact, bulging hymen is evident. The treatment is surgical incision or removal of the hymenal tissue. The girl may have local pain after the incision, which can be relieved by a mild analgesic and warm baths.

Because most girls of early menstrual age have scant knowledge of anatomy, pictures of the reproductive tract can help to explain that this is a local and minor problem. Once relieved, it will not interfere with sexual relations or future childbearing.

Polycystic Ovary Syndrome (PCOS)

Polycystic ovary syndrome (PCOS) is the most frequent cause of ovulation failure seen today. It is found in about 10% of women of childbearing age (Connor, 2012). Adolescents with the syndrome begin to develop an increased androgen (male hormone) level, which then prevents follicular ovarian cysts from maturing, a situation that leads to typical symptoms of irregular or missed menstrual cycles, acne, excessive hair growth (hirsutism), being overweight, male pattern baldness, type 2 diabetes, and most important, an absence of ovulation. Insulin is a hormone that causes an increase in androgen, so excessive insulin appears to be the root of the disorder. The condition may have a genetic tendency because the condition is often seen in siblings or daughters (Balen, 2012).

Assessment for the disorder includes a thorough history and physical exam, a pelvic exam to determine the consistency and size of ovaries, and perhaps an ovarian ultrasound for the same purpose. Serum androgen and glucose levels will also be assessed.

Because the exact cause of polycystic ovaries is not known, treatment is aimed at relieving the symptoms. Many adolescents with the syndrome are obese, therefore, weight loss by increasing lean meat, fruits, and vegetables and decreasing the amount of concentrated carbohydrates in their diet is encouraged. This eating pattern also lowers blood glucose levels, improves the body's use of insulin, and helps to normalize testosterone secretion. If a woman is morbidly obese, bariatric surgery may be recommended because this will achieve the same result.

A COC may be prescribed because this changes the ratio of estrogen and testosterone produced, leading to better regulated menstrual cycles. To prevent type 2 diabetes from developing, metformin (Glucophage) may be prescribed, which is yet another method to reduce blood glucose levels. If the adolescent or woman wants to become pregnant, fertility medications such as a course of clomiphene (Clomid) to stimulate ovulation may be suggested. Two final therapies to help achieve pregnancy are in vitro fertilization (IVF) (see Chapter 8) and ovarian drilling, a surgery technique done by laparoscopy that reduces the size of the ovaries and limits the amount of testosterone the ovaries are able to produce. To decrease hair growth and reduce acne symptoms, antiandrogens such as spironolactone (Aldactone) or finasteride (Propecia) can be tried. Caution women that finasteride is teratogenic and so should not be used if they intend to become pregnant, and it should be discontinued during pregnancy (Stout & Stumpf, 2010).

PCOS is a perplexing disorder because it produces such a wide range of symptoms, and responses to therapy may not be immediate. Support from health care providers is important, especially if the woman wants to become pregnant and realizes her condition is not going to readily allow this to happen.

QSEN Checkpoint Question 47.3

Quality Improvement

The symptoms of polycystic ovary syndrome can begin with adolescence. If Navi had this, you would want her to describe which of the following facts following an educational session?

a. Polycystic ovary syndrome can be easily treated with an antibiotic.
b. This condition can cause both obesity and interfere with future fertility.
c. The condition usually fades with full maturity at the end of adolescence.
d. Polycystic ovaries are easy to identify because they are so painful.

Look in Appendix A for the best answer and rationale.

Toxic Shock Syndrome

Toxic shock syndrome (TSS) is an infection that is usually caused by toxin-producing strains of *Staphylococcus aureus*. Although organisms can enter the body by other means, they typically enter through vaginal walls that have been damaged by the insertion of tampons at the time of a menstrual period (Edmonds, 2012). Once occurring at epidemic proportions because of superabsorbent tampons, it now can be prevented by simple steps (Box 47.6).

Assessment. The symptoms of TSS are a high temperature (over 102°F [38.9°C]), vomiting and diarrhea, hypotension, severe muscle pain, decreased platelet count, and a macular (sunburn-like) rash that desquamates on palms and soles. As the infection progresses, septic shock develops; renal, liver, and central nervous system functions fail, leading to disorientation and confusion.

Some adolescents have mild diarrhea as a normal accompaniment to dysmenorrhea, but any female who develops fever with diarrhea and vomiting during a menstrual period should suspect TSS and telephone her primary care provider.

Therapeutic Management. Women or adolescents with suspected TSS need a careful vaginal examination and removal of any tampon particles, as well as cervical and vaginal cultures for *S. aureus*. Iodine douches may reduce the number of organisms present vaginally. A penicillinase-resistant antibiotic such as the cephalosporins, oxacillins, or clindamycins, is prescribed. Intravenous fluid therapy to restore circulating fluid volume or a vasopressor such as dopamine (Intropin) may be necessary to increase blood pressure. Osmotic therapy to shift fluid back into the intravascular circulation is important to prevent renal and cardiac failure. Recovery occurs in 7 to 10 days with adequate therapy; however, fatigue and weakness may last for months.

TSS recurrence can occur, probably because the organism was not completely eliminated from the body. That makes it important for girls to complete their entire antibiotic prescription and in the future to use the lowest absorbency tampon appropriate for their individual flow.

Vulvovaginitis

In **vulvovaginitis**, inflammation of the vulva or vagina is accompanied by pain, odor, pruritus, and a vaginal discharge (Rome, 2012). Vaginal bleeding may also be present. The condition may occur in a girl of any age, but it tends to be more frequent as girls reach puberty probably because the change to adult pH and the presence of vaginal secretions make the vagina more receptive to infections. Box 47.7 discusses common measures to relieve vulvovaginal discomfort.

Preschool and School-Age Children. Vaginal discharge may occur before menarche, but bleeding is rarely seen at this age. If vaginal bleeding does occur, it is usually caused by irritation caused by an inserted foreign object into the vagina, infestation of pinworms, or daily bubble baths (which can lead to urinary tract infections [UTIs] as well as vulvar irritation). It could also be due to urethral bleeding from cystitis (bladder infection) or rectal pruritus, which has led to scratching and rectal bleeding. Precocious puberty is yet another disorder that must be ruled out. Finally, whether sexual maltreatment

BOX 47.6 Nursing Care Planning to Empower a Family

MEASURES TO PREVENT TOXIC SHOCK SYNDROME (TSS)

Q. Navi says to you, "I use tampons. How can I make sure I don't get toxic shock syndrome?"

A. The following measures can help prevent the syndrome:

- Use the lowest absorbency tampon possible that is still adequate for your individual flow.
- Alternate use of tampons with use of sanitary pads. Change tampons at least every 4 hours.
- Avoid handling the portion of the tampon that will be inserted vaginally.
- Do not use tampons near the end of a menstrual flow, when excessive vaginal dryness can result from scant flow.
- Do not insert more than one tampon at a time to avoid abrasions and to keep the vaginal walls from becoming too dry.
- Avoid deodorant tampons, deodorant sanitary pads, and feminine hygiene sprays; these products can irritate the vulvar–vaginal lining.
- If fever, vomiting, or diarrhea occurs during a menstrual period, discontinue tampon use and immediately consult your health care provider, because these are symptoms of TSS.
- Anyone who has had one episode of TSS is well advised not to use tampons again until two vaginal cultures for *Staphylococcus aureus*, the bacteria usually responsible for TSS, are negative.

BOX 47.7 Nursing Care Planning Based on Family Teaching

TIPS FOR RELIEVING THE PAIN OF VULVOVAGINITIS

Q. Navi says to you, "My bottom is irritated from my vaginal discharge. What can I do to relieve that?"
A. Here are some tips that might help:

- Wash the area twice a day with mild, nonperfumed soap and water, and pat dry to remove secretions and decrease irritation. Always wash and dry from front to back to prevent spreading rectal contamination forward.
- Take a tub bath or apply warm, moist compresses three times a day to soothe the area and to keep it free of irritating drainage.
- After drying the cleansed area, apply cornstarch for comfort and to absorb residual moisture.
- Avoid bubble baths and feminine hygiene sprays because the ingredients in these may cause additional local irritation as well as may contribute to urinary tract infections.
- Take acetaminophen (Tylenol) or a nonsteroidal anti-inflammatory drug (NSAID) such as ibuprofen every 4 hours. These are both analgesics and so relieve pain and reduce itching, a mild pain sensation.
- Avoid scratching, which may increase abrasions and introduce a secondary infection. Instead, apply a cold compress to relieve the itching sensation.
- Wear cotton underwear, which allows air to circulate and moisture to evaporate, rather than nylon or silk, which prevents air circulation and retains moisture.
- Sleep without underwear.
- Use an anesthetic spray or hydrocortisone cream if prescribed.
- If an antibiotic has been prescribed for a vaginal infection, take it conscientiously because only after the infection subsides will the vaginal discharge and itching clear.

has occurred must be investigated because it could be a cause of any bleeding, tenderness, or infection (see Chapter 55).

Treatment for pinworm is discussed in Chapter 43. If there is a foreign body in the vagina, it obviously should be removed by a vaginal examination. This may be difficult for young girls to accept because, unless a small speculum is used, vaginal manipulation and stretching can be painful. Application of a local antibiotic ointment or warm baths afterward may be prescribed to prevent infection and inflammation after removal of the object.

A few preschool or school-age children develop a vaginitis due to *Streptococcus* or to *Escherichia coli* introduced from the anus by improper perineal care after voiding or bowel movements. A tight hymen then traps the microorganisms in the vagina and leads to infection. The girl may need an antibiotic prescribed for this and needs to be reminded to wipe from front to back after voiding or bowel movements to help prevent this from occurring again.

Adolescents. As a girl enters puberty, she may notice a slight vaginal discharge caused by increased vaginal secretions. As long as she has no other symptoms, you can reassure her this is normal. To keep from developing vulvar irritation, caution girls to wear cotton underpants rather than nylon (so that moisture is absorbed better) and to dry the vulva thoroughly after bathing or swimming. Daily washing of the perineum and frequent changing of tampons or sanitary pads during menstruation helps prevent chafing or stasis of menstrual blood and so helps prevent irritation and odor.

Pelvic Inflammatory Disease

PID is infection of the pelvic organs: the uterus, fallopian tubes, ovaries, and their supporting structures (Guile & Keller, 2011). The infection can extend so far it causes pelvic peritonitis. Although sexual transmission accounts for approximately 75% of all instances of PID (gonorrheal and chlamydial organisms are frequently responsible), infections from other causes such as *E. coli* or *Streptococcus* can occur and may be as severe. Adolescents and young adults, those with multiple sexual partners, and those who don't use condoms have a higher incidence of PID than other groups (Ross, 2012).

PID usually begins with a cervical infection that then spreads by surface invasion along the uterine endometrium and then out to the fallopian tubes and ovaries. It is most likely to occur at the end of a menstrual period, because menstrual blood provides an excellent growth medium for bacteria and there is loss of the normal barrier of cervical mucus during this time.

Assessment. With acute PID, a woman or adolescent notices severe pain in the lower abdomen. She may have an accompanying heavy, purulent discharge. As the infection progresses, she develops a fever, and leukocytosis and an elevated erythrocyte sedimentation rate will be present. During a pelvic examination, any manipulation of the cervix causes severe pain, making it difficult to palpate the ovaries because of tenderness and abdominal guarding. As peritoneal tissue becomes inflamed and edematous, a purulent exudate, forms in the tubes. If the process is untreated, it enters a chronic phase and fibrotic scarring with stricture of the fallopian tubes results. With this chronic phase, the abdominal pain lessens but dyspareunia and dysmenorrhea may be extreme. If the ovaries are affected, intermenstrual spotting may occur. A diagnosis can be aided by ultrasound or laparoscopy.

Therapeutic Management. Therapy involves administration of analgesia for comfort plus a broad-spectrum antibiotic such as doxycycline (Vibramycin) or clindamycin

(Cleocin). In some women, a pelvic abscess forms and must be drained through the cul-de-sac before healing can occur. Women who have IUDs in place do not need to have them removed because these do not interfere with therapy (Tepper, Steenland, Gaffield, et al., 2012).

Women who have had one episode of PID have an increased chance of a second occurrence, because the immune protection of the tubes and ovaries may have been damaged. They should avoid coitus during menstruation, when their protective mechanisms are lowest, and be certain their sexual partner is also not infected with the organism that caused the original infection. Early childbearing or in vitro fertilization may be necessary for some women because extensive tubal scarring impaired their fertility. It is important for adolescents to recognize the symptoms of PID and to seek early help to avoid these worst case outcomes.

BREAST DISORDERS

Although males have few breast disorders, they can occur in either males or females.

Gynecomastia (enlarged breast tissue) may occur temporarily in preadolescent boys in response to a rising estrogen level. Particularly noticeable in obese males, this enlargement fades with a normal increase in testosterone production with puberty (Dickson, 2012). It may also occur in teens who participate in body-building sports as a result of steroid use. If this is the cause, counseling regarding the danger of performance-enhancing drug use is crucial.

Accessory (Supernumerary) Nipples

As the name implies, *accessory nipples* are additional breast nipples (Gowen, 2011). They tend to occur along the mammary lines and can be present in either male or female (Fig. 47.2). They are present from birth but usually are not as protuberant as true nipples; they also lack areolar pigmentation. Parents should be told what they are so they can inform their child later about this, because some growth in accessory nipples may occur at puberty or during pregnancy in response to estrogen stimulation. If girls are unaware they have an accessory nipple and think it is a large mole, they may be worried they have skin cancer when these changes occur.

In a few instances, actual breast tissue is present beneath the accessory nipple. If so, it is subject to the same diseases as other breast tissue such as fibrocystic disease or breast cancer (Osswald, Osswald, & Elston, 2011). If the accessory nipple or accessory breast tissue is cosmetically distressing to an adolescent, it can be removed by simple surgical excision.

Breast Hypertrophy

Breast hypertrophy is abnormal enlargement of breast tissue. In the average girl, progesterone levels are low until menstruation cycles are fully established. Breast development halts after puberty, as soon as progesterone levels rise to mature strength. If the time span between puberty and maturation is a lengthy one, breast growth lasts for longer than usual, resulting in larger than usual breasts.

Breast hypertrophy can lead to both physical and emotional stress because a girl may feel pain and fatigue in her back or shoulders from the weight of heavy breast tissue. In addition, she may feel self-conscious and try to minimize her breast size by slouching, resulting in poor posture or rounded shoulders. Pregnancy and lactation may be particularly difficult times, because breasts that are already large become even heavier with milk formation. Hearing comments such as, "I wish I had your problem," rather than receiving support and understanding from parents, peers, and health care providers does not relieve her concerns.

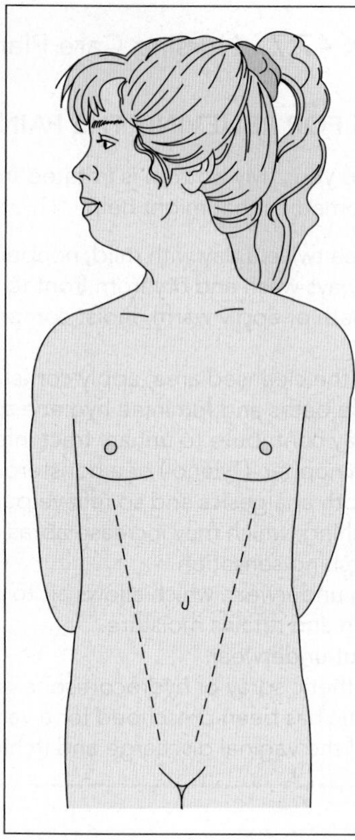

FIGURE 47.2 Nipple lines, along which accessory nipples occur.

Be certain adolescents with large breasts conscientiously schedule a yearly breast examination with their health care provider because it is easier for a cancerous lesion to escape detection in large amounts of breast tissue than in smaller breasts.

If breast hypertrophy is so extreme that it interferes with a girl's physical and emotional well-being, surgical breast reduction is a possibility (Hammond & Loffredo, 2012). Adolescents need to seriously consider the consequences of this procedure, however, before undertaking it at this early age. If a large amount of glandular tissue is removed, breastfeeding might no longer be an option. The adolescent also needs to be told realistically that changing her physical appearance will reduce physical discomfort, but changing her self-concept must come from within.

Breast Hypoplasia

Breast hypoplasia is less-than-average breast size. In most instances, this does not represent a decreased amount of glandular or functional breast tissue but a reduced amount of fatty tissue. If having small breasts interferes with self-esteem, a girl can have surgical augmentation by a silicon or a saline implant inserted under the breast tissue to increase breast size but, again, this needs careful consideration regarding whether it is necessary at this young age. Be certain the girl understands that her breast tissue is not replaced by the implant, and that she still needs breast examinations because she could still develop breast cancer in later years.

Breasts with implants in place may feel firmer than usual on palpation due to the formation of a fibrotic band or capsule around the implant. Decreased nipple sensation may be present for approximately 1 year after the procedure.

Breast implants do not interfere with breastfeeding because they are placed behind the milk glands. A traumatic blow to the breast, such as could occur from an automobile accident, requires examination by the augmentation surgeon to be certain the implant did not rupture, causing its contents to leak into the bloodstream or breast tissue.

Fat Necrosis

If breast tissue is struck during a fall or other traumatic injury such as injury from a seatbelt, it can become tender, painful, inflamed, or reddened (Hurt & Lipsett, 2011). A few days after the injury, necrosis or disintegration occurs in the fatty layer. As the area heals, fibrotic scar tissue forms leaving a firm, palpable lump in the breast. It is not freely movable; it can, however, cause skin or nipple retraction or dimpling on the skin surface. Unlike malignant breast growths that also show this "orange peel" sign, posttraumatic breast lumps tend to be well delineated because of the scar tissue.

It is generally recommended that such fibrotic areas be biopsied and then excised. The procedure is a minor one, usually leaves little scarring, and the adolescent no longer needs to worry about the lump in her breast afterward.

Fibrocystic Breast Disease

Fibrocystic breast disease is the most common benign breast condition in women of all ages (De Silva, 2012). It can occur as early as puberty, when estrogen rises to adult levels. More commonly, however, it is found in older adolescents. Round, fluid-filled, and freely movable cysts form in the connective breast tissue (Fig. 47.3). The consistency of these lesions varies with the menstrual cycle, changing from firm to soft, depending on the amount of serous fluid present. The lesions tend to shrink or disappear during pregnancy and lactation, and they tend to fade with menopause.

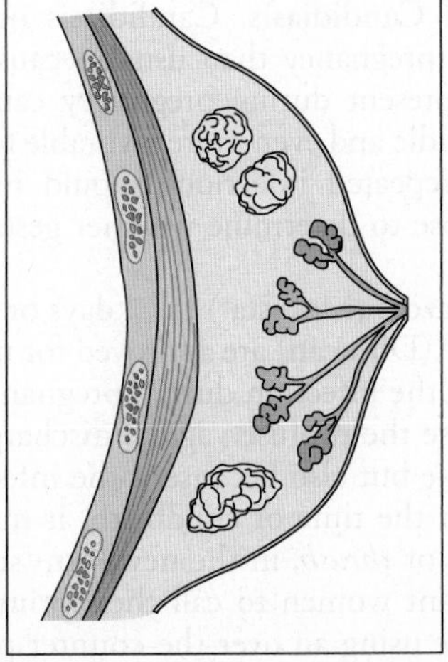

FIGURE 47.3 Round, fluid-filled cysts form in breast tissue in fibrocystic breast disease.

Decreased sodium intake or short-term use of a mild diuretic just before menses can reduce fluid retention and the size of the cysts. Discontinuing smoking can help as well. Because fibrocystic breasts feel tender and "stretched," this can interfere with active sports and other strenuous activity. This discomfort can usually be relieved with a simple analgesic, such as acetaminophen (Tylenol), an NSAID, or warm compresses, avoidance of trauma, and firm bra support. The formation of fibrocystic lesions may be increased in some women with the use of methylxanthines found in caffeine, theophylline, and theobromine, so avoiding foods such as coffee, cola drinks, tea, chocolate, some toffee candy, and medications that contain caffeine helps reduce pain.

If these measures do not decrease fibrocystic symptoms, cysts may be aspirated under a local anesthetic by injection of a thin sterile needle attached to a small syringe. This procedure not only reduces the size of the cyst but also provides fluid for biopsy (Hurt & Lipsett, 2011).

In addition to being physically distressed, women with fibrocystic breasts may worry that each lump could be malignant. Breast carcinoma does occur in women with fibrocystic breast disease, but fibrocystic lesions do not directly lead to this. Breast cancer, however, may not be discovered before a woman seeks a health consultation because a woman assumes all her breast lesions are benign. Therefore, in addition to a yearly breast examination, women with fibrocystic breast disease need an annual breast ultrasound or magnetic resonance imaging (MRI) to efficiently locate and identify that the cysts are benign.

Fibroadenoma

Fibroadenomas are tumors that consist of both fibrotic and glandular components that occur in response to estrogen stimulation (Ng, Mrad, & Brown, 2011). They may increase in size during adolescence, during pregnancy and lactation, or when a woman takes an estrogen source such as an oral contraceptive.

Unlike fibrocystic lesions, fibroadenomas feel round and well delineated, are painless and freely movable, and do not tend to cause skin retraction. Occasionally, they calcify and feel extremely hard. Like fibrocystic lesions, the presence of them can be distressing but they do not appear to become malignant.

Such tumors can be surgically excised so a woman no longer has to worry about them. Because the incision is small, it leaves little scarring at the site.

✔ QSEN Checkpoint Question 47.4

Safety

Navi, 15 years of age, asks if it would be safe for her to have breast augmentation. What advice would you give her?

a. She would not likely be able to breastfeed after undergoing augmentation.
b. Breast implants increase her risk of developing fibrocystic disease.
c. It is safe for girls her age to have this surgery, but careful consideration is needed.
d. Implants increase her risk of breast cancer in later life.

Look in Appendix A for the best answer and rationale.

Mastitis

Mastitis is inflammation or infection of the breast. Because this usually occurs as a complication of breastfeeding, it is discussed in Chapter 19.

SEXUALLY TRANSMITTED INFECTIONS

STIs are diseases that are spread through sexual contact with an infected partner. They range in severity from easily treated infections, such as trichomoniasis, to human immunodeficiency virus (HIV) infection, which, despite advances in therapy, is life threatening. If these diseases are discovered in young children, the possibility of sexual maltreatment has to be considered (Hammerschlag, 2011). They may be spread among heterosexual partners as well as women who have sex with women or men who have sex with men (Muzny, Sunesara, Martin, et al., 2012; Peate, 2012).

Abstinence or condom use provides the best protection against STIs. Additional measures include voiding immediately and washing genitals well with soap and water after coitus, as well as choosing sexual partners who are at low risk for infection (i.e., avoiding persons who are intravenous drug users or those with multiple sexual partners). Educating adolescents about safer sex practices, including the need for condom use (see Chapter 5) and the importance of health screening for these disorders, is an important nursing responsibility. Pay particular attention to adolescents who do not have a strong family support system because it may be particularly difficult for these youth to receive correct information about preventing STIs (Hudson, 2012).

STIs are becoming more difficult to treat because the causative organisms are becoming increasingly resistant to antibiotics. Always reinforce the fact that little immunity develops from STIs, so such diseases can be contracted repeatedly. In most instances, an infected partner should also be treated or the disease can recur from cross infection.

Several STIs, such as syphilis, are known to be teratogenic. All of them are suspected of being a causative factor of preterm birth. Chapter 12 discusses care for the newborn affected by such diseases.

Candidiasis

Candidiasis is a vaginal infection spread by the fungus *Candida*, an organism that thrives on glycogen (Rome, 2012). Candidiasis is so common that as many as 90% of women will have it sometime in their life. Because oral contraceptives produce a pseudopregnancy state, adolescents using oral contraceptives tend to have frequent vaginal candidal infections. If being treated with an antibiotic for another infection (which destroys normal vaginal flora and lets fungal organisms grow more readily), they are also particularly susceptible to this infection. Incidence is also strongly associated with immune suppression and diabetes mellitus, because hyperglycemia provides the perfect glucose-rich environment for candidal growth.

Assessment

Because of the scant mucus production in the period before menses, symptoms may be most acute at this time. The adolescent will notice vulvar and vaginal reddening, burning and itching, and even bleeding from hairline fissures. A thick, cream cheese–like discharge can usually be observed at the vaginal outlet. Internally, the vagina shows white "patches" that cannot be scraped away without bleeding on the walls. There may be accompanying pain on coitus or on tampon insertion. Candidal infections can also be present at other body sites, such as the oral cavity or a moist area such as the umbilicus. In immunosuppressed individuals, candidal infections can become systemic (Edmonds, 2012).

Candidal infections are diagnosed by removing a sample of the discharge from the vaginal wall and placing it on a glass slide. Three or four drops of a 20% potassium hydroxide (KOH) solution are then added, and the mixture is protected by a coverslip. Under a microscope, typical fungal hyphae indicate the presence of *Candida* organisms (Table 47.1). An at-home test kit (Vagasil Screening Kit) is available, which gives results instantly. A woman inserts a pH wand into her vagina and in a few seconds compares the color of the swab to a pH color chart. If the reading is above 5.0, it suggests she may have a bacterial infection and should see her health care provider. A pH level of 4.5 plus itching and/or burning, unusual discharge, or a yeasty odor suggests a yeast infection, and it would be all right for her to use an over-the-counter treatment.

Therapeutic Management

Therapy for candidal infections includes vaginal tablets or cream applications of antifungal preparations such as over-the-counter miconazole (Monistat) or clotrimazole (Lotrimin) once a day for 3 to 7 days. Oral fluconazole (Diflucan) can be administered as a one-time dose. Teach women to insert antifungal tablets or creams at bedtime so the drug does not drain from the vagina immediately afterward. Treatment should not be interrupted until it is complete, even during a menstrual period.

If a girl has frequent candidal infections, her urine should be tested for glucose to rule out diabetes mellitus. If she is using an oral contraceptive, she might be counseled to use another reproductive planning method. If an adolescent is sexually active, treatment of the male partner may be necessary to break a reinfection cycle (McGreal & Wood, 2012).

Pregnancy and Candidiasis. Candidiasis occurs more frequently during pregnancy than usual because the increased estrogen level present during pregnancy causes the vaginal pH to be less acidic and even more favorable for yeast growth. Women with repeated infections should have their urine tested for glucose to determine whether gestational diabetes is present.

Both miconazole (Monistat) for 7 days or a single dose of oral fluconazole (Diflucan) are approved for use during pregnancy. Treating the infection during pregnancy is important not only because the profuse vaginal discharge and pruritus is uncomfortable but also because if the infection is present in the vagina at the time of childbirth, it may cause a candidal infection, or *thrush*, in the newborn (see Chapter 43). Caution pregnant women to call their primary health care providers before using an over-the-counter product to double check that the product is safe to use during pregnancy and also so the primary care provider can know a vaginal

TABLE 47.1 Common Vulvovaginal Infections

Causative Agent	Symptoms	Common Therapy
Candida albicans	Vulvar reddening and pruritus; thick, white, cheese-like vaginal discharge	Clotrimazole (Lotrimin) or miconazole (Monistat) vaginal suppositories or fluconazole (Diflucan) orally; bathing with dilute sodium bicarbonate solution may relieve pruritus
Trichomonas	Thin, irritating, frothy, gray-green discharge; strong, putrid odor; itching	Metronidazole (Flagyl) or tinidazole (Tindamax) orally; douching with weak vinegar solution to reduce pruritus
Herpesvirus type II	Painful pinpoint vesicles on an erythematous base with a watery vaginal discharge possible; voiding may be irritating and painful	Bathing with dilute sodium bicarbonate solution, applying lubricating jelly to lesions, or an oral analgesic such as ibuprofen may be necessary for pain relief; topically applied acyclovir (Zovirax) helps heal lesions
Gardnerella	Edema and reddening of vulva; milky gray discharge; fishlike odor	Metronidazole (Flagyl) or clindamycin
Chlamydia trachomatis	Watery, gray-white vaginal discharge; vulvar itching	Tetracycline or doxycycline; erythromycin during pregnancy
Neisseria gonorrhoeae	Possibly symptomless; may have profuse yellow-green vaginal discharge	Ceftriaxone and doxycycline
Enterobius vermicularis (pinworm)	Rectal pruritus, especially on rising in the morning	Oral administration of an anthelmintic, such as mebendazole (Vermox)
Treponema pallidum (syphilis)	Painless ulcer on vulva or vagina	Benzathine penicillin, administered intramuscularly
Streptococcus	Vaginitis, vulvar itching; edema and reddening of vulva	Antibiotic such as amoxicillin
Foreign body	Vaginal discharge; odor	Removal of foreign body during pelvic examination

infection is occurring because a candidal infection may be associated with preterm birth (Roberts, Rickard, Kotsiou, et al., 2011).

What if...47.3 Navi tells you she feels protected from contracting an STI because she knows she is up to date with her immunizations. How would you counsel her?

Trichomoniasis

Trichomonas vaginalis is a single-cell protozoan that is spread by coitus and affects between 3% and 13% of adult men and women, in the United States (Sehgal, Goyal, & Sehgal, 2012).. The incubation period is 4 to 20 days. A serious consequence of trichomoniasis is that infection can cause such genital inflammation that it makes it easier for the person to be infected with the HIV virus or to pass the HIV virus on to a sex partner (Centers for Disease Control and Prevention [CDC], 2012a).

Assessment

With a trichomonal infection, females may notice only a slight vaginal discharge or else notice extreme vaginal itching and a frothy white or grayish-green vaginal discharge. The upper vagina looks reddened and may have pinpoint petechiae. In some women, these changes can be so extreme, a Pap test taken during this time may be misinterpreted as showing abnormal tissue. Males with the same infection tend not to report any symptoms.

The infection is diagnosed by microscopic examination of a sample of the vaginal discharge; trichomonads typically appear as rounded, mobile structures.

Therapeutic Management

Oral metronidazole (Flagyl) or tinidazole (Tindamax) eradicates trichomonal infections. Use of condoms by sexual partners help prevent recurrence of *Trichomonas* in both parties. Because metronidazole interacts with alcohol (to cause acute nausea and vomiting), caution older adolescents and women to not drink alcoholic beverages during the course of treatment with this drug.

Pregnancy and Trichomoniasis. Trichomoniasis infections are associated with preterm labor, premature rupture of membranes, and postcesarean infection. The drug of choice during pregnancy is single-dose oral metronidazole. Although classified as a Class B pregnancy drug, it may not be prescribed during the first semester of pregnancy to avoid detrimental fetal effects (Karch, 2013).

Bacterial Vaginosis

Bacterial vaginosis is the invasion of an organism such as *Gardnerella vaginalis*, which thrives in the vagina because of the reduced oxygen level (Singh, Zenilman, Brown, et al., 2013).

An intensely pruritic vaginal discharge appears milky-white to gray and has a fishlike odor. Microscopic examination of the discharge shows gram-negative rods adhering to vaginal epithelial cells (termed *clue cells*). Like trichomoniasis, bacterial vaginosis can increase a woman's susceptibility to other STIs, such as herpes simplex virus (HSV), chlamydia, and gonorrhea, as well as HIV (CDC, 2012b).

The treatment is oral or vaginal metronidazole for 7 days. The woman's sexual partner should also be treated to prevent recurrence of the infection. Therapy with probiotic lactobacilli to change vaginal organisms is a future possibility for prevention (Li, McCormick, Bocking, et al., 2012).

Pregnancy and Bacterial Vaginosis

The treatment during pregnancy is oral metronidazole or clindamycin for 7 days in order to prevent preterm labor as well as premature rupture of the membranes (Bennett, 2012).

QSEN Checkpoint Question 47.5

Teamwork & Collaboration

Candidal vaginal infections can occur as an opportunistic infection when adolescents are prescribed antibiotics. You would refer an adolescent for medical treatment of this problem if she reported which of the following?

a. Many yellow pinpoint vaginal lesions
b. Green-tinged pruritic vaginal walls
c. White, cheeselike vaginal discharge
d. Vaginal atrophy with final scarring

Look in Appendix A for the best answer and rationale.

Chlamydia trachomatis Infection

Chlamydia trachomatis infections have become the most common bacterial cause of STIs in the United States (Tharpe & Farley, 2012). The incubation period is 1 to 5 weeks; symptoms include a heavy, grayish-white discharge and vulvar itching. Diagnosis is made by identification of the organism, which can be done at the point of care. Therapy is oral doxycycline for 7 days or azithromycin as a single dose. Because the infection has become so common, most public health departments require that the infection be reported to the health department, the same as other STIs such as gonorrhea. Because there is a strong association between gonorrhea and *Chlamydia*, if a chlamydial infection is documented, women are usually tested for gonorrhea as well. Long-term effects of chlamydial infections are PID, possibly leading to subfertility.

Pregnancy and *Chlamydia*

Screening for *Chlamydia* via a vaginal culture is usually done during a woman's first prenatal visit. If a woman has multiple sexual partners, screening may be repeated again in the third trimester. Doxycycline (Vibramycin), the therapy for nonpregnant women, is contraindicated during pregnancy because of possible fetal long-bone deformities; azithromycin (Zithromax) or amoxicillin (Amoxil) are used instead. A woman's partner also should be treated to prevent her from becoming reinfected.

It's important that chlamydial infections be treated during pregnancy because they are associated with premature rupture of the membranes, preterm labor, and endometritis in the postpartum period. An infant who is born while a chlamydial infection is present can develop conjunctivitis or pneumonia after birth (see Chapters 50 and 40).

Human Papillomavirus

The human papillomavirus (HPV) causes fibrous tissue overgrowth (sometime called genital warts) on the external vulva, vagina, or cervix (condyloma acuminatum). At first, lesions appear as discrete papillary structures; they then spread, enlarge, and coalesce to form large, cauliflower-like lesions. The infection may be present in as many as 10% to 30% of women and is most common in women who have multiple sexual partners. Children (both male and female) who develop an HPV infection should be further investigated for sexual maltreatment (Hammerschlag, 2011). Therapy for such lesions is aimed at dissolving the lesions and also ending any secondary infection present. Small growths often fade by themselves, although they can be removed by applying podophyllin (Podofin), a wart removal medication. Large lesions are removed by laser therapy, cryocautery, laser, or knife excision. With cryocautery, edema at the site is evident immediately; lesions become gangrenous, and sloughing occurs in 7 days, with healing complete in 4 to 6 weeks with only slight depigmentation at the site. Warm baths and a lidocaine cream may be soothing during the healing period.

HPV infections are serious because they are associated with the development of penile and cervical cancer later in life (D'Hauwers, Depuydt, Bogers, et al., 2012). Related to this, women who have had one episode of infection should be conscientious about having yearly Pap tests for the rest of their lives, and men should conscientiously inspect their penis for any abnormal growths or ulcers. The vaccines, Gardasil or Cervarix, are recommended as part of routine administration to both early teenage girls and boys to prevent such infections. Approach the subject of immunization with parents and teenagers with sensitivity because some parents and children are not ready to admit they might be or will soon become sexually active and need this protection (Reynolds & O'Connell, 2012). Immunizing teenagers against an HPV infection should reduce not only the incidence of HPV infections in the future but also the rate of cervical and penile cancer as well (Markman, 2013).

Pregnancy and Human Papillomavirus Infection

HPV lesions tend to increase in size during pregnancy because of the high vascular flow in the pelvic area. They may become secondarily ulcerated and infected; when this occurs, a foul vulvar odor may develop.

Podophyllum is contraindicated during pregnancy because of possible toxic effects on the fetus. Trichloroacetic acid (TCA) or bichloroacetic acid (BCA) applied to the lesions weekly may be effective and can be used during pregnancy. Women who do not find the lesions bothersome may choose to leave them in place until the postpartum period and have them removed then. Remind them, in the meantime, that the lesions are infectious and can spread to a sexual partner.

The presence of vulvar lesions appears to have no effect on the fetus during pregnancy, but if they are so large they obstruct the birth canal for birth, a cesarean birth may be scheduled.

Herpes Genitalis (Herpes Simplex Type 2)

Genital herpes is caused by *herpesvirus hominis* type 2 (also called herpes simplex virus type 2 or HSV-2). This is one of four similar herpesviruses: cytomegalovirus, Epstein–Barr, varicella zoster, and herpes types 1 and 2. Genital herpes occurs in epidemic proportions in the United States, and its incidence appears to be growing yearly (Stohl & Satin, 2011). Although the virus can be contained, unlike most other STIs there is no known cure. The disease involves a lifelong process, therefore, and, although it may not be a direct precursor to cervical cancer, women with cervical cancer tend to have more antibodies against herpes genitalis than others or probably have been exposed to the virus more than others. The virus is spread by skin-to-skin contact, entering through a break in the skin or mucous membrane. In the newborn, acquired at birth, the virus can be systemic or even fatal (see Chapter 26).

Assessment

Herpes is diagnosed by culture of the lesion secretion from its location on the vulva, vagina, cervix, or penis or by isolation of HSV antibodies in blood serum. The incubation period is 3 to 14 days. On first contact, extensive primary lesions originate as a group of pinpoint vesicles on an erythematous base. Within a few days, the vesicles ulcerate and become moist, painful, draining, and open lesions. An adolescent may have accompanying flu-like symptoms with increased temperature; vaginal lesions may cause a profuse discharge. Pain is intense on contact with clothing or acidic urine. Diagnosis of the disorder is made by the appearance of the lesions and on the results of a Pap smear and an enzyme-linked immunosorbent assay (ELISA).

After this primary stage, which lasts approximately 1 week, lesions heal but the virus lingers in a latent form in the sensory nerve ganglia. The condition can flare up and become an active infection again during illness, just prior to menstruation, fever, overexposure to sunlight, or stress. This secondary response usually produces only local lesions rather than systemic symptoms.

Therapeutic Management

Both acyclovir (Zovirax) and valacyclovir (Valtrex) are examples of antivirals that can control the virus by interfering with DNA reproduction and decreasing symptoms (Stohl & Satin, 2011). Topical imiquimod (Aldara) or foscarnet (Foscavir) may be prescribed for resistant lesions. If applying a topical ointment or vaginal gel to a client, be certain to protect yourself with a finger cot or glove so you do not contract the virus or absorb the drug. Warm baths three times a day may be helpful to reduce discomfort for the client. An emollient (A&D Ointment) can also reduce discomfort, although its moisture tends to prolong the active period of the lesions. Infected people need to inform their partners when they have any active lesions and either avoid sexual contact or use a condom to decrease the danger of spreading the virus.

Because of the possible association with cervical cancer, any female with genital herpes should have yearly Pap tests for the rest of her life, and men need to self-inspect for recurrent lesions.

Pregnancy and Herpes Simplex Virus Type 2 Infection. If a woman contracts a herpes type 2 infection during pregnancy, herpes can be transmitted across the placenta to cause congenital infection in the newborn. If primary or secondary active lesions in the vagina or on the vulva are present at the time of birth, herpes infection can be transmitted to the newborn at birth. When this occurs, a severe systemic infection that is often fatal can result (see Chapter 26). To help avoid transmission, women with active lesions are usually scheduled for cesarean birth (Jaiyeoba, Amaya, Soper, et al., 2012).

The drug of choice for the treatment of herpes infection during pregnancy is the same as for nonpregnant women (acyclovir [Zovirax] or valacyclovir [Valtrex]) (Karch, 2013). Women can reduce the pain of the lesions by taking baths or applying warm, moist tea bags to the area.

Hepatitis B and Hepatitis C

Both hepatitis B and hepatitis C can be spread by semen as well as blood and therefore are considered STIs. These are discussed in Chapter 45, with other forms of hepatitis. Because hepatitis B can be spread by sexual intercourse, adolescents who did not receive immunization against this as an infant and who are sexually active need immunization.

Gonorrhea

Gonorrhea is transmitted by *Neisseria gonorrhoeae*, a gram-positive diplococcus, which thrives on the mucus membrane of the vagina or penis (O'Connor & Shubkin, 2012). In males, symptoms include *urethritis* (pain on urination and frequency of urination) and a urethral discharge, which appear after a 2- to 7-day incubation period. Untreated, the infection spreads easily among sexual partners and may spread to the testes, scarring the tubules and causing permanent sterility. It often occurs concurrently with a chlamydial infection.

Although symptoms of gonorrhea in females are not as visible, there may be a slight yellowish vaginal discharge. The Bartholin glands may become inflamed and painful. If left untreated, the infection can spread to pelvic organs, most notably the fallopian tubes, can cause PID, and, as in males, tubal scarring with permanent sterility. In both males and females, if systemic involvement occurs, arthritis or heart disease can develop.

Assessment

A urine culture for the gonococcal bacillus, in addition to vaginal, urethral, and perhaps anal and oral cultures, should be obtained on all children with vulvovaginitis or a urethral discharge to rule out gonorrhea because, if gonorrhea is detected, child maltreatment needs to be ruled out.

Therapeutic Management

One intramuscular injection of ceftriaxone (Rocephin) plus 7 days of oral doxycycline (Vibramycin) or azithromycin (Zithromax) is the current recommended therapy because this treatment regimen is effective for gonorrhea, chlamydia, and syphilis (Kirkcaldy, 2012). Sexual partners should receive the same treatment (Box 47.8, Nursing Care

BOX 47.8 Nursing Care Planning

AN INTERPROFESSIONAL CARE MAP FOR AN ADOLESCENT WITH GONORRHEA

Navi is a 15-year-old female high school student you meet at a pediatric clinic. She describes intense vulvar irritation from a yellowish-green vaginal discharge.

Family Assessment Navi lives with mother in a studio apartment in inner city. Mother works at home as a freelance journalist. Mother describes finances as "good."

Client Assessment Well-proportioned female; sexual maturity Tanner stage 3. Menarche at 12 years; periods every 30 days; duration 6 days. Sexually active for approximately 1 year with same partner. "He doesn't use a condom anymore because I'm the only one he's dating."

Vulva reddened and excoriated. Yellow-green discharge noted at vaginal introitus. Reddened areas noted on vaginal walls. One dose of intramuscular (IM) ceftriaxone (Rocephin), plus oral doxycycline (Vibramycin) prescribed for 7 days. She says, "I think I got this from a towel I borrowed in gym class. Does my boyfriend need treated too?"

Nursing Diagnosis Deficient knowledge related to cause and treatment of sexually transmitted infection (STI).

Outcome Evaluation Adolescent states she understands cause of STI; reports boyfriend has an appointment within 48 hours for evaluation.

Team Member Responsible	Assessment	Intervention	Rationale	Expected Outcome
Activities of Daily Living, Including Safety				
Nurse	Assess whether adolescent understands importance of washing hands after using bathroom and avoiding sexual intercourse during treatment.	Discuss how disease can be spread to boyfriend or to other body parts by unclean hands.	Gonorrhea is particularly hazardous because it can cause eye infections with corneal scarring.	Adolescent states she will take precautions to wash hands well; will avoid sexual intercourse until repeat culture.
Teamwork and Collaboration				
Nurse/STI counselor	Confer with STI counselor as to whether disease is a reportable one.	Meet with STI counselor regarding procedure for STI contacts.	Gonorrhea is a reportable disease.	STI counselor assumes responsibility for securing STI contacts.
Procedures/Medications for Quality Improvement				
Nurse	Assess whether adolescent has experience with taking medicine. Assess if a reminder sheet would be helpful.	Administer ceftriaxone (Rocephin) IM; give instructions for oral doxycycline (Vibramycin) for 7 days as prescribed.	The antibiotics chosen for gonorrhea treatment are also effective against chlamydia, which is frequently associated with gonorrhea.	Adolescent accepts IM injection; states she understands importance of taking oral antibiotic for full 7 days.
Nurse	Assess whether adolescent has access to a bathtub at home.	Recommend the use of warm bath before and after school.	Warm baths are soothing and help keep the vulva free of irritation.	Adolescent states she will use home bathtub for Sitz baths twice daily and will wash tub well after use.
Nutrition				
Not applicable (N/A)	N/A	N/A	N/A	N/A

Patient-Centered Care				
Nurse	Assess whether adolescent is aware STIs are spread through sexual intercourse not a towel exchange.	Teach adolescent about the cause, means of spread, and treatment for gonorrhea.	Adolescent must be aware of the spread of STIs to prevent them in the future.	Adolescent states she understands STIs are spread by sexual relations.
Psychosocial/Spiritual/Emotional Needs				
Nurse	Assess intensity of adolescent's pruritus or pain from vulvitis on a scale of 1 to 10.	Discuss the use of acetaminophen or ibuprofen for pain and pruritus as needed.	Acetaminophen and ibuprofen are effective analgesics for mild pain and itching.	Adolescent describes correct dosage of analgesics and states intention to use them.
Nurse/STI counselor	Assess whether adolescent has had sexual contacts other than current boyfriend.	Ask adolescent to name any additional sexual contacts.	Sexual contacts need to be notified so they can also receive treatment.	Adolescent names any other sexual contacts; possibility of rape or sexual maltreatment is ruled out.
Informatics for Seamless Health Care Planning				
Nurse	Assess whether adolescent understands, in the light of contracting this disease, that she must ask boyfriend to use a condom for sexual relations.	Discuss the possibility that, because he contracted an STI, his relationship with her may not be monogamous.	STI was spread to her by a sexual contact.	Adolescent states she will be more conscientious about insisting boyfriend use a condom.
Nurse	Assess whether adolescent or parent has any questions about disease or therapy.	Schedule adolescent for a return appointment in 1 week for repeat culture.	A repeat culture will reveal whether antibiotic therapy has been effective.	Child and parent state they understand the importance of a repeat culture and return appointment.

Planning, an interprofessional care map for an adolescent with an STI).

Approximately 24 hours after beginning treatment, gonorrhea is no longer infectious. Approximately 7 days after treatment, however, a client should return for a follow-up culture to verify the disease has been completely eradicated (few adolescents take this precaution without urging). Most states require gonorrhea be reported to the health department; adolescents are asked to name sexual contacts to help prevent the disease spread. Without being told who put them at risk, these people can then be notified by a health department investigator that they have been exposed to a particular STI and need treatment.

Pregnancy and Gonorrhea. Gonorrhea is associated with spontaneous miscarriage, preterm birth, and endometritis in the postpartum period. Pregnant women cannot be administered doxycycline because it has the potential to be teratogenic. Instead, they are prescribed azithromycin. It is important that gonorrhea be identified and treated during pregnancy because, if the infection is present at the time of birth, it can cause a severe eye infection, which can lead to blindness in the newborn (ophthalmia neonatorum; see Chapter 26).

✔ QSEN Checkpoint Question 47.6

Patient-Centered Care

Navi does not seem concerned about the possibility she could contract gonorrhea again. What additional health teaching does she need to better understand how this disease is spread?

a. The microorganism of gonorrhea is not likely to survive unless there is frequent intercourse.
b. It is possible for the gonorrhea organism to be spread by anal/penile contact.
c. The low pH of saliva prevents this from being spread by oral/penile contact.
d. Gonorrhea is a virus that can be treated effectively if diagnosed early.

Look in Appendix A for the best answer and rationale.

Syphilis

Syphilis is a systemic disease transmitted by the spirochete *Treponema pallidum* (O'Connor & Shubkin, 2012). Like gonorrhea and chlamydia, its occurrence must be reported to public health departments.

After an incubation period of 10 to 90 days, a deep ulcer (termed a *chancre*), which is usually painless despite its size, appears usually on the genitalia (penis or labia) or in the vagina, on the mouth, lips, or rectal area from oral–genital or genital–anal contact. Swollen lymph nodes may also be present but these are likely to be less noticed by the affected person. Without treatment, a chancre lasts approximately 6 weeks and then fades.

About 2 to 4 weeks after the chancre disappears, a generalized, macular, copper-colored rash appears. Rare among rashes, it covers the soles and the palms as well as extremities and the body. There may be secondary symptoms of generalized illness, such as a low-grade fever. A serologic test for syphilis taken at this time yields a positive result. With or without treatment, this stage of syphilis also fades.

The next stage is a latency period that may last from only a few years to several decades. The only indication of the disease at this point is a serologic test, which continues to yield a positive result.

The final stage of syphilis is a destructive neurologic disease that involves major body organs, such as the heart and the nervous system, with symptoms such as blindness, paralysis, mental confusion, slurred speech, and lack of coordination. If this third stage is not identified and treated, it can become fatal.

Assessment

Syphilis is diagnosed by recognition of the various symptoms of the three stages and by serologic serum tests, such as the Venereal Disease Research Laboratory test (VDRL), the automated reagin test (ART), the rapid plasma reagin test (RPR), or the fluorescent treponemal antibody–absorption test (FTA-ABS).

Therapeutic Management

Benzathine penicillin G, given intramuscularly in two sites, is effective therapy. For the adolescent who is sensitive to penicillin, either oral erythromycin or tetracycline can be given for 10 to 15 days. Sexual partners are treated in the same way as the person with an active infection. Therapy effectively arrests the disease at whatever stage it has reached. After therapy, adolescents may experience a sudden episode of hypotension, fever, tachycardia, and muscle aches (a Jarisch-Herxheimer reaction caused by the sudden destruction of spirochetes). The reaction lasts about 24 hours and then fades. Because syphilis can be treated so easily, one would think it would be easy to eradicate. In reality, however, because the primary chancre is painless, many people are either unaware of it or choose to ignore it, thereby transmitting the disease to unsuspecting sexual partners. Be certain adolescents are screened for disease symptoms by both history and physical exam at health care visits and receive accurate information about symptoms and safer sex practices to prevent the disease (White, Alter, Irvin, et al., 2012). They also need to be assured they can report the disease to health care personnel and name sexual contacts without fear of being criticized.

Pregnancy and Syphilis. Early in pregnancy (before week 18), the placenta appears to provide some protection against syphilis. After this time, however, the spirochete crosses the placenta freely and may be responsible for spontaneous miscarriage, preterm labor, stillbirth, or congenital anomalies in the newborn (see Chapter 12). All pregnant women are screened for syphilis at a first prenatal visit with a VDRL, ART, or FTA-ABS antibody reaction test. Those who have multiple sexual partners are typically tested again at about week 36 of pregnancy. In some institutions, women are screened again at the beginning of labor, and their newborns are screened for congenital syphilis by a cord blood sample. One injection of benzathine penicillin G is the drug of choice for the treatment of syphilis during pregnancy the same as for those who are not pregnant. If the woman has syphilis, her infant needs penicillin therapy at birth as well (Patel, Klinger, O'Toole, et al., 2012).

If a woman contracted syphilis during pregnancy but it was unrecognized and untreated, and so the newborn is untreated, a congenital form of the disease can occur in the newborn. Severely infected infants will be stillborn; others, less infected, are born with congenital anomalies. Wear gloves to handle such infants because moist lesions (the cord and nasal secretions) may be infectious.

Unlike adults, the infant does not develop a chancre but about a week after birth, will develop a typical copper-colored rash, most prominent over the face, soles of feet, and palms of hands. The infant's nose may show a severe rhinitis (stuffiness). An X-ray of the long bones reveals changes of epiphyseal lines at about 1 to 3 months of age. By 5 to 6 months, these bone changes may no longer be visible and so may be missed.

When the child's permanent teeth erupt at 5 or 6 years of age, the tops may be pegged or notched (Hutchinson's teeth), tend to be of poor quality and decay easily. If the disease remains untreated even with these symptoms, interstitial keratitis, an inflammatory reaction of the cornea that can result in scarring and blindness, may develop by school age. As the disease progresses further, it may become tertiary or lead to severe neurologic symptoms.

Group B Streptococcal Infection

Although streptococcus B infection is a less publicized disease than STIs such as herpes type 2 or gonorrhea, it may actually occur at a higher incidence than those diseases (Page-Ramsey, Johnstone, Kim, et al., 2012). If contracted during pregnancy, consequences can include UTIs, intra-amniotic infections, perhaps preterm birth, and postpartum endometritis.

Pregnant women are generally screened for streptococcus B at 35 to 38 weeks of pregnancy to prevent their newborn from becoming infected from placental transfer or from direct contact with vaginal secretions at birth. If they become infected, neonates can develop severe pneumonia, sepsis, respiratory distress syndrome, or meningitis (see Chapter 26).

A broad-spectrum penicillin such as ampicillin is the treatment of choice. Women who experience rupture of membranes at less than 37 weeks of pregnancy and so have not yet been screened may be treated with intravenous ampicillin during labor to reduce the risk of spreading the infection to the newborn.

Human Immunodeficiency Virus

HIV is carried by semen as well as other body fluids, so, although not officially listed as such, is an STI. Invasion of the virus is discussed with other immune system disorders in Chapter 42.

What if . . . 47.4 You are particularly interested in exploring one of the 2020 National Health Goals with respect to reproductive disorders in children (see Box 47.1). What would be a possible research topic to explore pertinent to this goal that would be applicable to Navi's family and that would also advance evidence-based practice?

KEY POINTS FOR REVIEW

- Children who are born with a reproductive tract disorder frequently adjust well when young. They may need counseling at puberty or when they become aware of the impact of their disorder on sexual functioning or their ability to reproduce.
- The cause of ambiguous genitalia is unknown but may be related to the level of testosterone produced in utero. The true gender of children is established by a karyotype of chromosomes.
- The development of breast or pubic hair before age 8 years is considered precocious sexual development. Children may be treated with a synthetic analog of GnRH to reduce development. Without effective support, such children are at high risk for disturbed body image.
- Delayed puberty is the failure to develop secondary sex characteristics by the age of 17 years. Girls may be administered estrogen to promote development; boys may be administered testosterone.
- Balanoposthitis (inflammation of the glans and prepuce of the penis) and phimosis (constricted foreskin) occur in boys. Phimosis can be treated with circumcision.
- Cryptorchidism is failure of one or both testes to descend during intrauterine life. The condition is surgically corrected to prevent subfertility and to make it possible to detect testicular cancer later in life.
- Testicular cancer is rare but tends to occur in young men. Boys need to be taught testicular self-examination for early detection.
- Dysmenorrhea, or painful menstruation, occurs frequently in adolescent girls. Therapy is the use of a prostaglandin inhibitor such as ibuprofen.
- Untreated endometriosis (the abnormal growth of extrauterine endometrial tissue) can lead to subfertility later in life. Therapy is the administration of a synthetic androgen or GnRH receptor inhibitor or surgery to reduce the size of the abnormal tissue.
- Vulvovaginitis (inflammation of the vulva and vagina) and PID are infections that can occur in adolescents. Therapy to prevent fallopian tube scarring and subfertility later in life is essential. In addition, girls need to be taught ways to avoid TSS from the use of menstrual tampons. Vulvovaginitis in young girls needs to be investigated for the possibility of sexual maltreatment.
- Conditions such as fibrocystic breast disease can occur in adolescents. Teaching to reduce the intake of caffeine and sodium can minimize symptoms and also help in planning nursing care that not only meets QSEN competencies but also best meets an adolescent's total needs.
- STIs such as candidiasis, trichomoniasis, *C. trachomatis* infection, genital warts, herpes genitalis, gonorrhea, and syphilis are increasing in incidence in the adolescent population. An important health-teaching area for adolescents is the need to follow safer sex practices.
- When teaching about STIs, it is important to stress that they do not confer immunity and therefore can be contracted more than once. If an STI occurs in a young child, the potential for child maltreatment should be investigated.

CRITICAL THINKING CARE STUDY

Melinda is a 16-year-old teenager you meet at an adolescent clinic. Her parents are divorced and she lives with her father.

1. Melinda is concerned because she has little breast development as of yet and only began having menstrual periods last week. She asks you if she is going to be underdeveloped.
2. Melinda's boyfriend wants to have sex with her. Because he has an unrepaired hypospadias, he has assured her she can't get pregnant. Should she believe him?
3. Melinda tells you she learned everything she knows about sexual relations and contraception from the Internet because her father has difficulty discussing such things with her. Is this a good source of information for her?

Patient Scenario

The Kalulopidus Family

Read about the Kalulopidus family, a family with a preschooler with a reproductive system concern, then answer the questions to further sharpen your skills and grow more familiar with NCLEX-type questions related to reproductive disorders. Confirm your answers are correct by reading the rationales.

Visit http://thePoint.lww.com.

Answers and Rationales

Looking for answers to the What If. . . and Critical Thinking Care Study questions?

Visit http://thePoint.lww.com.

References

Adegbite-Adeniyi, C., Gron, B., Rowles, B. M, et al. (2012). An update on antidepressant use and suicidality in pediatric depression. *Expert Opinion in Pharmacotherapy, 13*(15), 2119–2130.

Arends, J .C., Cheung, M. Y., Barrack, M. T., et al. (2012). Restoration of menses with nonpharmacologic therapy in college athletes with menstrual disturbances: A 5-year retrospective study. *International Journal of Sport, Nutrition & Exercise Metabolism, 22*(2), 98–108.

Balen, A. (2012). Polycystic ovary syndrome and secondary amenorrhea. In D. K. Edmonds (Ed.), *Dewhurst's textbook of obstetrics & gynaecology* (8th ed., pp. 513–533). Oxford, UK: John Wiley & Son.

Bennett, P. (2012). Preterm labour. In D. K. Edmonds (Ed.) *Dewhurst's textbook of obstetrics & gynaecology* (8th ed., pp. 338–355). Oxford, UK: John Wiley & Son.

Centers for Disease Control and Prevention. (2012a). *Bacterial vaginosis fact sheet.* Washington, DC: Author.

Centers for Disease Control and Prevention. (2012b). *Trichomoniasis fact sheet.* Washington, DC: Author.

Chien, L. W., Chang, H. C., & Liu, C. F. (2013). Effect of yoga on serum homocysteine and nitric oxide levels in adolescent women with and without dysmenorrhea. *Journal of Alternative & Complementary Medicine, 19*(1), 20–23.

Connor, E. L. (2012). Adolescent polycystic ovary syndrome. *Adolescent Medicine, 23*(1), 164–177.

Davidson, B. R., Dipiero, C. M., Govoni, K. D., et al. (2011). Abnormal uterine bleeding during the reproductive years. *Journal of Midwifery & Women's Health, 57*(3), 248–254.

Dennerstein, L., Lehert, P., & Heinemann, K. (2012). Epidemiology of premenstrual symptoms and disorders. *Menopause International, 18*(2), 48–51.

De Silva, N. K. (2012). Breast disorders in the female adolescent. *Adolescent Medicine, 23*(1), 34–52.

D'Hauwers, K. W., Depuydt, C. E., Bogers, J. J., et al. (2012). Human papillomavirus, lichen sclerosus and penile cancer. *Vaccine, 30*(46), 6573–6577.

Dickson, G. (2012). Gynecomastia. *American Family Physician, 85*(7), 716–722.

Dominé, F., Dadoumont, C., & Bourguignon, J. P. (2012). Eating disorders throughout female adolescence. *Endocrine Development, 22*(7), 271–286.

Doswell, W. M., Braxter, B. J., Cha, E., et al. (2011). Testing the theory of reasoned action in explaining sexual behavior among African American young teen girls. *Journal of Pediatric Nursing, 26*(6), e45–e54.

Dubowitz, H. (2013). Neglect in children. *Pediatric Annals, 2*(4), 73–77.

Edmonds, D. K. (2012). Benign diseases of the vagina, cervix & ovary. In D. K. Edmonds (Ed.), *Dewhurst's textbook of obstetrics & gynaecology* (6th ed., pp. 706–714). Oxford, UK: John Wiley & Son.

Faizah, M., Zuhanis, A., Rahmah, R., et al. (2012). Precocious puberty in children: A review of imaging findings. *Biomedical Imaging & Intervention Journal, 8*(1), e6.

Fernández-Gaxiola, A. C., & De-Regil, L. M. (2011). Intermittent iron supplementation for reducing anaemia and its associated impairments in menstruating women. *Cochrane Database of Systematic Reviews,* (12), CD009218.

Fine, R. G., & Poppas, D. P. (2012). Varicocele: Standard and alternative indications for repair. *Current Opinion in Urology, 22*(6), 513–516.

Gaylord, M. N., & Petersen-Smith, A. M. (2013). Genitourinary disorders. In E. E. Burns & A. M. Dunn (Eds.), *Pediatric primary care* (5th ed., pp. 809–843) Philadelphia, PA: Elsevier/Saunders.

Gele, A. A., Johansen, E. B., & Sundby, J. (2012). When female circumcision comes to the West: Attitudes toward the practice among Somali Immigrants in Oslo. *BMC Public Health, 12*(1), 697.

Gerlt, T., & Smith, N. B. (2013). Gynecologic disorders. In E. E. Burns & A. M. Dunn (Eds.), *Pediatric primary care* (5th ed., pp. 844–876) Philadelphia, PA: Elsevier/Saunders.

Gharloghi, S., Torkzahrani, S., Akbarzadeh, A. R., et al. (2012). The effects of acupressure on severity of primary dysmenorrhea. *Patient Preference & Adherence, 6*(2), 137–142.

Gowen, C. W. (2011). Assessment of the mother, fetus & newborn. In K. J. Marcdante, R. M. Kliegman, H. B. Jenson, et al. (Eds.), *Nelson essentials of pediatrics* (6th ed., pp. 213–231). Philadelphia, PA: Saunders/Elsevier.

Guile, M. W., & Keller, J. (2011). Infections of the genital tract. In K. J. Hurt, M. W. Guile, J. L. Bienstock, et al. (Eds.), *The Johns Hopkins manual of gynecology and obstetrics* (4th ed., pp. 322–339). Philadelphia, PA: Lippincott Williams & Wilkins.

Gunderson, C., & Yates, M. (2011). Menstrual disorders: Endometriosis, dysmenorrhea & premenstrual dysphoric syndrome. In K. J. Hurt, M. W. Guile, J. L. Bienstock, et al. (Eds.), *The Johns Hopkins manual of gynecology and obstetrics* (4th ed., pp. 454–463). Philadelphia, PA: Lippincott Williams & Wilkins.

Hammerschlag, M. R. (2011). Sexual assault and abuse of children. *Clinical Infectious Diseases, 53*(Suppl. 3), S103–S109.

Hammond, D. C., & Loffredo, M. (2012). Breast reduction. *Plastic Reconstructive Surgery, 129*(5), 829e–839e.

Harel, Z. (2012). Dysmenorrhea in adolescents and young adults: An update on pharmacological treatments and management strategies. *Expert Opinion in Pharmacotherapy, 13*(15), 2157–2170.

Haugnes, H. S., Bosl, G. J., Boer, H., et al. (2012). Long-term and late effects of germ cell testicular cancer treatment and implications for follow-up. *Journal of Clinical Oncology, 30*(30), 3752–3763.

Hershey, A. D. (2012). Perimenstrual headache in adolescence. *Current Pain & Headache Reports, 16*(5), 474–476.

Hudson, A. L. (2012). Where do youth in foster care receive information about preventing unplanned pregnancy and sexually transmitted infections? *Journal of Pediatric Nursing, 27*(5), 443–450.

Hurt, K. J., & Lipsett, P. A. (2011). Breast diseases. In K. J. Hurt, M. W. Guile, J. L. Bienstock, et al. (Eds.), *The Johns Hopkins manual of gynecology and obstetrics* (4th ed., pp. 15–32). Philadelphia, PA: Lippincott Williams & Wilkins.

Jahnukainen, K., & Stukenborg, J. B. (2012). Present and future prospects of male fertility preservation for children and adolescents. *Journal of Clinical & Endocrinology Metabolism, 97*(12), 4341–4351.

Jaiyeoba, O., Amaya, M. I., Soper, D. E., et al. (2012). Preventing neonatal transmission of herpes simplex virus. *Clinical Obstetrics & Gynecology, 55*(2), 510–520.

Jospe, N. (2011). Endrocrinology. In K. J. Marcdante, R. M. Kliegman, H. B. Jenson, et al. (Eds.), *Nelson essentials of pediatrics* (6th ed., pp. 625–670). Philadelphia, PA: Saunders/Elsevier.

Karasahin, K. E., Keskin, U., & Ercan, C. M. (2012). A uterovaginal septum and imperforate hymen with a double pyocolpos. *Human Reproduction, 27*(9), 2879–2880.

Karch, A. M. (2013). *2013 Lippincott's nursing drug guide.* Philadelphia, PA: Lippincott Williams & Wilkins.

Karlı, N., Baykan, B., Ertaş, M., et al. (2012). Impact of sex hormonal changes on tension-type headache and migraine: A cross-sectional population-based survey in 2,600 women. *Journal of Headache & Pain, 13*(7), 557–565.

Kennedy, S., & Koninckx, P. (2012). Endometriosis. In D. K. Edmonds (Ed.), *Dewhurst's textbook of obstetrics & gynaecology* (8th ed., pp. 615–616). Oxford, UK: John Wiley & Son.

Kirkcaldy, R. D. (2012). New treatment guidelines for gonorrhea: Antibiotic change. *CDC Expert Commentary*. Retrieved from http://www.medscape.com/viewarticle/768883.

Kollin, C., Stukenborg, J. B., Nurmio, M., et al. (2012). Boys with undescended testes. *Journal of Clinical Endocrinology & Metabolism, 97*(12), 4588–4595.

Lao, O. B., Fitzgibbons, R. J. Jr., & Cusick, R. A. (2012). Pediatric inguinal hernias, hydroceles, and undescended testicles. *Surgical Clinics of North America, 92*(3), 487–504.

Li, J., McCormick, J., Bocking, A., et al. (2012). Importance of vaginal microbes in reproductive health. *Reproductive Sciences, 19*(3), 235–242.

Mahan, J. D. (2011). Nephrology & urology. In K. J. Marcdante, R. M. Kliegman, H. B. Jenson, et al. (Eds.), *Nelson essentials of pediatrics* (6th ed., pp. 607–621). Philadelphia, PA: Saunders/Elsevier.

Malone, P. S., Hall-Craggs, M. A., Mouriquand, P. D., et al. (2012). The anatomical assessment of disorders of sex development (DSD). *Journal of Pediatric Urology, 8*(6), 585–591.

Markman, M. (2013). Risk of cervical cancer after HPV vaccination. *Current Pharmaceutical Design, 19*(8), 1488–1489.

Masterson, T. A., & Beck, S. D. W. (2013). Testicular cancer: Clinical signs & symptoms. In P. T. Scardino, W. N. Linehan, M. J. Zelefsky, et al. (Eds.), *Comprehensive textbook of genitourinary oncology.* Philadelphia, PA: Lippincott Williams & Wilkins.

Mattila, A. K., Fagerholm, R., Santtila, P., et al. (2012). Gender identity and gender role orientation in female assigned patients with disorders of sex development. *Journal of Urology, 188*(5), 1930–1934.

Maule, M., Malavassi, J. L., & Richiardi, L. (2012). Age at puberty and risk of testicular cancer: A meta-analysis. *International Journal of Andrology, 35*(6), 828–834.

McGreal, S., & Wood, P. (2012). Recurrent vaginal discharge in children. *Journal of Pediatric & Adolescent Gynecology*. Advance online publication.

McIntosh, L. A., Scrimgeour, D., Youngson, G. G., et al. (2012). The risk of failure after primary orchidopexy: An 18 year review. *Journal of Pediatric Urology.* Advance online publication. pii: S1477–5131(12)00225–2.

Morris, B. J., Waskett, J. H., Banerjee, J., et al. (2012). A 'snip' in time: What is the best age to circumcise? *BMC Pediatrics,* (12), 20–22.

Munro, M. G. (2012). Classification of menstrual bleeding disorders. *Reviews in Endocrine & Metabolic Disorders, 13*(4), 225–234.

Muzny, C. A., Sunesara, I. R., Martin, D. H., et al. (2012). Sexually transmitted infections and risk behaviors among African American women who have sex with women: Does sex with men make a difference? *Sexually Transmitted Diseases, 38*(12), 1118–1125.

Navvabi-Rigi, S. D., Kerman-Saravi, F., Navidian, A., et al. (2012). Comparing the analgesic effect of heat patch containing iron chip and ibuprofen for primary dysmenorrhea: A randomized controlled trial. *BMC Women's Health, 12*(1), 25.

Ng, W. K., Mrad, M. A., & Brown, M. H. (2011). Juvenile fibroadenoma of the breast: Treatment and literature review. *Canadian Journal of Plastic Surgery, 19*(3), 105–107.

O'Connor, C. A., & Shubkin, C. D. (2012). Adolescent STIs for primary care providers. *Current Opinion in Pediatrics, 24*(5), 647–655.

Osswald, S. S., Osswald, M. B., & Elston, D. M. (2011). Ectopic breasts: Familial functional axillary breasts and breast cancer arising in an axillary breast. *Cutis, 87*(6), 300–304.

Patel, S. J., Klinger, E. J., O'Toole, D., et al. (2012). Missed opportunities for preventing congenital syphilis infection in New York City. *Obstetrics & Gynecology, 120*(4), 882–888.

Page-Ramsey, S. M., Johnstone, S. K., Kim, D., et al. (2012). Prevalence of group B Streptococcus colonization in subsequent pregnancies of group B Streptococcus-colonized versus noncolonized women. *American Journal of Perinatology.* Advance online publication.

Pavone, M. E., & Bulun, S. E. (2012). Aromatase inhibitors for the treatment of endometriosis. *Fertility & Sterility, 98*(6), 1370–1379.

Peate, I. (2012). Sexually transmitted infections in men who have sex with men. *British Journal of Nursing, 21*(13), 811–815.

Rakhshaee, Z. (2011). Effect of three yoga poses (cobra, cat and fish poses) in women with primary dysmenorrhea: A randomized clinical trial. *Journal of Pediatric & Adolescent Gynecology, 24*(4), 192–196.

Reynolds, D., & O'Connell, K. A. (2012). Testing a model for parental acceptance of human papillomavirus vaccine in 9- to 18-year-old girls: A theory-guided study. *Journal of Pediatric Nursing, 27*(6), 614–625.

Roberts, C. L., Rickard, K., Kotsiou, G., et al. (2011). Treatment of asymptomatic vaginal candidiasis in pregnancy to prevent preterm birth: An open-label pilot randomized controlled trial. *BMC Pregnancy & Childbirth, 11*(3), 18–19.

Rome, E. S. (2012). Vulvovaginitis and other common vulvar disorders in children. *Endocrine Development, 22*(7), 72–83.

Ross, J. D. C. (2012). Pelvic infection. In D. K. Edmonds (Ed.), *Dewhurst's textbook of obstetrics & gynaecology* (8th ed., pp. 597–606). Oxford, UK: John Wiley & Son.

Sehgal, R., Goyal, K., & Sehgal, A. (2012). Trichomoniasis and lactoferrin: Future prospects. *Infectious Diseases in Obstetrics & Gynecology.* Advance online publication. doi: 10.1155/2012/536037.

Shahid, S. K. (2012). Phimosis in children. *ISRN Urology.* Advance online publication. doi: 10.5402/2012/707329.

Singh, R. H., Zenilman, J. M., Brown, K. M., et al. (2013). The role of physical examination in diagnosing common causes of vaginitis: A prospective study. *Sexually Transmitted Infections, 89*(3), 185–190.

Stapley, S., & Hamilton, W. (2011). Gynaecological symptoms reported by young women: Examining the potential for earlier diagnosis of cervical cancer. *Family Practice, 28*(6), 592–598.

Steinberg, E. M., Cardoso, G. M., Martinez, P. E., et al. (2012). Rapid response to fluoxetine in women with premenstrual dysphoric disorder. *Depression & Anxiety, 29*(6), 531–540.

Stohl, H., & Satin, J. J. (2011). Perinatal infection. In K. J. Hurt, M. W. Guile, J. L. Bienstock, et al (Eds.), *The Johns Hopkins manual of gynecology and obstetrics* (4th ed., pp. 137–153). Philadelphia, PA: Lippincott Williams & Wilkins.

Stout, S. M., & Stumpf, J. L. (2010). Finasteride treatment of hair loss in women. *Annals of Pharmacotherapy, 44*(6), 1090–1097.

Sung, E. K., Setty, B. N., & Castro-Aragon, I. (2012). Sonography of the pediatric scrotum: Emphasis on the Ts—Torsion, trauma, and tumors. *AJR: American Journal of Roentgenology, 198*(5), 996–1003.

Templeman, C. (2012). Adolescent endometriosis. *Current Opinion in Obstetrics & Gynecology, 24*(5), 288–292.

Tepper, N. K., Steenland, M. W., Gaffield, M. E., et al. (2012). Retention of intrauterine devices in women who acquire pelvic inflammatory disease: A systematic review. *Contraception.* Advance online publication.

Tharpe, N. L., & Farley, C. (2012). Clinical care of the woman with reproductive health problems. In N. L. Tharpe & C. Farley (Eds.), *Clinical practice guidelines for midwifery & woman's health* (pp. 327–420). Burlington, MA: Jones & Bartlett Learning.

U.S. Department of Health and Human Services. (2010). *Healthy people 2020.* Washington, DC: Author.

White, D. A., Alter, H. J., Irvin, N. A., et al. (2012). Low rate of syphilis screening among high-risk emergency department patients tested for gonorrhea and Chlamydia infections. *Sexually Transmitted Diseases, 39*(4), 286–290.

Chapter 48

Nursing Care of a Family When a Child Has an Endocrine or a Metabolic Disorder

KEY TERMS

- carpopedal spasm
- exophthalmos
- glycosuria
- hormones
- hyperglycemia
- hypoglycemia
- hypothalamus
- ketoacidosis
- latent tetany
- manifest tetany
- pedal spasm
- polydipsia
- polyuria
- sella turcica
- Somogyi phenomenon

OBJECTIVES

After mastering the contents of this chapter, you should be able to:

1. Describe the structure and function of the endocrine glands and why metabolic illnesses occur.
2. Identify 2020 National Health Goals related to childhood endocrine or metabolic disorders that nurses can help the nation achieve.
3. Assess a child with a disorder of endocrine or metabolic function.
4. Formulate nursing diagnoses for a child with altered endocrine or metabolic function.
5. Establish expected outcomes for a child with endocrine or metabolic dysfunction as well as help parents manage seamless transitions across differing health care settings.
6. Using the nursing process, plan nursing care that includes the six competencies of Quality & Safety Education for Nurses (QSEN): Patient-Centered Care, Teamwork & Collaboration, Evidence-Based Practice (EPB), Quality Improvement (QI), Safety, and Informatics.
7. Implement nursing care such as teaching long-term medicine administration to a child with an endocrine or metabolic disorder.
8. Evaluate expected outcomes for achievement and effectiveness of care.
9. Integrate knowledge of endocrine and metabolic disorders with the interplay of nursing process, the six competencies of QSEN, and Family Nursing to ensure quality maternal and child health nursing care.

Rob Tebecco is a 16-year-old boy with type 1 diabetes whom you meet in the emergency department, where he was taken after he became comatose while ice skating. His diabetes was diagnosed when he was 7 years old. His records indicate that his disease has generally been under good control over the past years, but in the last 6 months, he has "forgotten" to take his insulin at least once a week. When you ask him about this, he tells you that ice skating practice every morning and a new girlfriend have occupied his time and interrupted what used to be a strict schedule of home-cooked meals and a rigid routine.

Previous chapters described the growth and development of well children. This chapter adds information about the dramatic changes, both physical and psychosocial, that occur when children develop an endocrine or metabolic disorder. This is important information because it builds a base for care and health teaching.

Is Rob's history unusual for an adolescent? What health teaching do you think will most help him reestablish control?

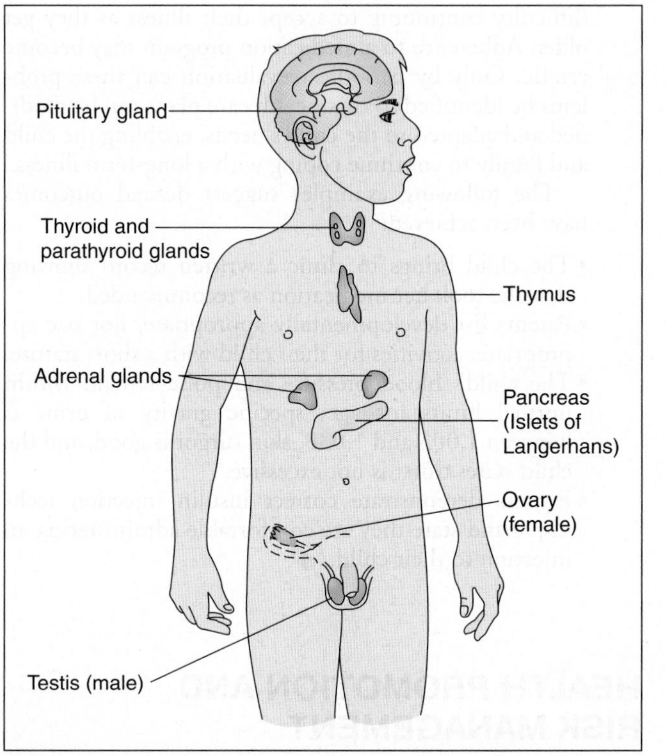

FIGURE 48.1 The location of the endocrine glands.

The endocrine system is composed of a small group of ductless glands that work together with the neurologic system to regulate and coordinate all body systems (Fig. 48.1). The glands produce **hormones**, which are secreted into surrounding tissue and picked up by the bloodstream, where they act individually and in concert to turn on or turn off various organ functions. (The word "hormone" is from the Greek *hormaein*, which means "to set in motion.") Each gland of the endocrine system acts on a specific target (or designated) organ or has specific duties that are necessary for regulating body processes (Thalange & Beach, 2013).

The inadequate secretion of hormones or dysfunction of the glands results in a variety of disorders, most of which have long-term implications. Parents—and children, as soon as they are old enough—need to understand the causes and symptoms of these diseases so they can participate in their long-term plan of care. Box 48.1 shows 2020 National Health Goals related to endocrine and metabolic disorders in children.

BOX 48.1 Nursing Care Planning Based on 2020 National Health Goals

Endocrine disorders tend to be long term and so cause lifetime consequences. Reducing the incidence of these or improving care has long-term implications. A sample of 2020 National Health Goals related to these include:

- Reduce the diabetes-related death rate from a baseline of 77 per 100,000 to no more than 46 per 100,000 people.
- Increase the proportion of persons with diabetes who receive formal diabetes education from a baseline of 56.8% to a target of 62.5%.
- Reduce the proportion of children aged 3 to 10 years diagnosed with a disorder through newborn blood spot screening who experience developmental delay requiring special education services from 15.1% to a target level of 13.5%.
- Increase the proportion of children with long-term illnesses who have access to a medical home from 57.5% of children under 18 years to 63.3% (U.S Department of Health and Human Services [DHHS], 2010; see www.healthypeople.gov).
- Nurses can help the nation achieve these goals by educating children with diabetes about their care and being certain newborns receive blood spot testing so children with these disorders not only can be identified as early in life as possible but receive continuing care in a "medical home." As the number of home births increases, it's important to evaluate at well child health care visits if a child did receive routine blood spot testing at birth or whether this should be obtained at a later date.

Nursing Process Overview

For Care of a Child With an Endocrine or Metabolic Disorder

Assessment

Endocrine and metabolic disorders, as a group, commonly cause changes in growth and a child's social, physical, and perhaps cognitive development. If not identified at birth, the disorder is usually detected when a child's height and weight are measured at a health care visit and found to be above or below a typical measurement for that age. An acute loss in weight is often the first symptom of type 1 diabetes mellitus in children. Thyroid deficiencies or type 2 diabetes mellitus (T2D) may be revealed by being overweight. Pituitary difficulties may be revealed by unusually short or tall stature.

To obtain information on activity in the child, take a day history by asking a parent or child to describe all of the child's actions on a typical day because this type of information yields clues that are helpful in distinguishing between a normally "quiet" child and one who is experiencing inactivity and chronic fatigue as a result of decreased endocrine function. For example, the quiet child lies down after school and reads, whereas the ill child lies down and sleeps. The healthy child appears to "go constantly" but can sit through a favorite television program or a meal. The child with increased thyroid hormone production may be unable to sit quietly at all.

Also assess dietary and elimination habits. Extreme thirst or appetite may occur with an endocrine disorder such as diabetes insipidus or type 1 diabetes mellitus. Frequent voiding in children most often reflects a urinary tract infection, but it may be evidence of excessive urine excretion (**polyuria**), possibly from pituitary dysfunction or diabetes mellitus. A child's general appearance may reveal early or late puberty changes, scaling or dry or darkening skin, drooping eyelids, protrusion of the eyeballs (**exophthalmos**), or poor muscle tone, all indications of endocrine disorders.

Nursing Diagnosis

Because endocrine glands control vital body functions, nursing diagnoses relevant to children with endocrine or metabolic disorders include both physiologic functions and the child's response to those changes. Some examples of such nursing diagnoses include:

- Deficient fluid volume related to constant excessive loss of fluid through urination
- Risk for imbalanced nutrition, less than body requirements, related to an inability to use glucose because of diabetes mellitus
- Disturbed body image related to abnormal height
- Health-seeking behaviors related to the self-administration of insulin
- Deficient knowledge related to long-term treatment needs
- Fear related to the potential illness outcome
- Anticipatory grieving related to presumed losses associated with diagnosis of long-term illness
- Interrupted family processes related to the child's chronic illness

Outcome Identification and Planning

Although most endocrine and metabolic disorders have long-term implications, parents and children may find it easier to work with outcomes that are initially short-term—particularly if they are having difficulty accepting the diagnosis and the long-term nature of the disorder. Because symptoms usually are not acute, children may easily forget to take (or parents may forget to give) necessary medications. Helping parents create reminder charts or set alerts on their smartphones are effective measures to increase compliance.

Evaluate both the school and home situation for any child with a chronic illness. You may need to help teachers better understand the child's health problem (with the parents' permission) so that they do not make excessive or inappropriate demands such as insisting that a child with hyperthyroidism submit neat handwriting assignments when the child cannot do so.

Selected organizations that are helpful for referral to parents include the American Diabetes Association (www.diabetes.org), the Congenital Adrenal Hyperplasia Support Group (www.cah.org.uk), Little People of America (www.lpaonline.org), and the National Tay–Sachs & Allied Diseases (www.ntsad.org).

Implementation

Interventions for children with endocrine or metabolic disorders must always be carried out with long-term aspects of care in mind. Bribing children to take medicine, for example, is never good practice with any child. It has no place with children who must continue to take a medication for the rest of their lives (bribery quickly becomes ineffective). As children reach maturity and can better understand their disorder, compliance increases as they begin to understand the way in which their daily medication is necessary to replace a missing endocrine component.

Outcome Evaluation

Children with disorders of endocrine or metabolic function need periodic evaluations throughout childhood because growth and changing activities necessitate changes in medication dosages or schedules. These checkups provide good opportunities for health teaching to equip children to meet new situations that arise as they mature. For example, body appearance such as being like, not unlike, their peers becomes increasingly important as children enter adolescence. Because of this, seemingly well-adjusted school-age children may develop extreme difficulty continuing to accept their illness as they get older. Adherence to a medication program may become erratic. Only by periodic reevaluation can these problems be identified so that health care plans can be modified and adapted to the child's needs, enabling the child and family to continue coping with a long-term illness.

The following examples suggest desired outcomes have been achieved:

- The child brings to clinic a written record showing that she took her medication as recommended.
- Parents list developmentally appropriate, not size appropriate, activities for their child with a short stature.
- The child's blood pressure and pulse remain within normal limits for age, specific gravity of urine is between 1.003 and 1.030, skin turgor is good, and the child states thirst is not excessive.
- Parents demonstrate correct insulin injection technique and state they are comfortable administering an injection to their child.

HEALTH PROMOTION AND RISK MANAGEMENT

Many endocrine and metabolic disorders are inherited; therefore, education and genetic counseling are important preventive measures (Box 48.2).

BOX 48.2 Nursing Care Planning Using Assessment

Assessing a Child With an Endocrine Disorder

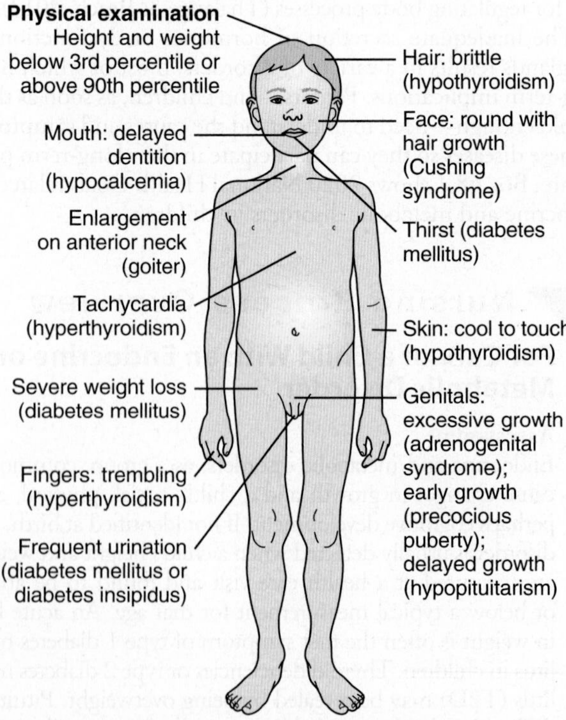

TABLE 48.1 Common Pituitary Hormones and Their Purposes

Pituitary Hormone	Source and Target Organs	Actions and Effects
Antidiuretic hormone (ADH)	Secreted by the neurohypophysis *Target organ:* Kidney	ADH helps regulate fluid volume by regulating urine output. By decreasing urine output, it increases the volume of extracellular fluid volume; when secretion of ADH is low, urinary output increases. Factors such as trauma, pain, anxiety, and exposure to high temperatures all increase ADH release.
Corticotropin (ACTH)	Secreted by the adenohypophysis *Target organ:* Adrenal glands	ACTH stimulates the adrenal gland to produce glucocorticoid and mineralocorticoid hormones. Increased production of adrenal gland secretions decreases ACTH production and vice versa.
Somatotropin (growth hormone [GH])	Secreted by the adenohypophysis *Target organ:* None; acts on all body cells	GH increases bone and cartilage growth by increasing the gastrointestinal absorption of calcium. If GH production is inhibited, undergrowth will occur; if GH production is excessive, overgrowth will occur.
Thyrotropin (TSH)	Secreted by the adenohypophysis *Target organ:* Thyroid gland	TSH stimulates the thyroid gland to produce thyroid hormones (thyroxine and triiodothyronine). Too little TSH leads to atrophy and inactivity of the thyroid gland; too much TSH causes hypertrophy (increase in size) and hyperplasia (increase in the number of cells) of the gland.

T2D is strongly associated with obesity so is at an epidemic incidence because obesity in school-age children is also at epidemic proportions (Dea, 2011). School nurses can be instrumental not only in counseling and helping students manage this disorder during school hours but also in helping prevent T2D by serving as an advisor to what foods and snacks ought to be available in school settings.

THE PITUITARY GLAND

The work of the pituitary gland is directed by the **hypothalamus**, an organ located in the center of the brain and which serves as the regulator of the autonomic nervous system. About 1 cm long, 1.0 to 1.5 cm wide, and 0.5 cm thick, the pituitary gland rests in the **sella turcica**, a depression of the sphenoid bone.

The gland is divided into several distinct regions: the anterior lobe, or *adenohypophysis*; the posterior lobe, or *neurohypophysis*; and the intermediate lobe, or *pars intermedia*, which lies between the anterior and posterior lobes. Altogether, these divisions store and release eight different hormones. Four of these—the antidiuretic hormone (ADH), thyrotropin, corticotropin, and somatotropin—are prominently involved in childhood illnesses (Table 48.1).

PITUITARY GLAND DISORDERS

Illnesses caused by pituitary dysfunction can result from a tumor growing in either the pituitary gland or the hypothalamus, interference with circulation to the gland, trauma, inflammation, structural abnormalities, erratic or nonfunctional feedback mechanisms, and, possibly, autoimmune responses. Interference due to these reasons can result in hypopituitarism (lack of growth hormone), hyperpituitarism (excess secretion of growth hormone), or diabetes insipidus (undersecretion of ADH).

Growth Hormone Deficiency

If production of human growth hormone (GH, or somatotropin) is deficient, children are not able to grow to full size (Dahlgren, 2011). As a result, children may appear well proportioned but measure well below the average on a standard growth chart. Deficient production of GH may result from a nonmalignant cystic tumor of embryonic origin that places pressure on the pituitary gland or from increased intracranial pressure as a result of trauma. In most children with hypopituitarism, however, the cause of the defect is unknown; it may have a genetic origin.

If hypopituitarism is not treated, predicting exactly what height a child will reach is difficult because height varies with each individual. Without treatment, however, most children will not reach more than 3 or 4 ft in height.

Assessment

The child with deficient production of GH is usually normal in size and weight at birth. Within the first few years of life, however, the child begins to fall below the third percentile of height and weight on growth charts. The face appears infantile because the mandible is recessed and immature and the nose is usually small. The child's teeth may be crowded in a small jaw (and may erupt late). The child's voice may be high pitched, and the onset of pubic, facial, and axillary hair and genital growth will be delayed. The history, physical findings, and a decreased level of circulating GH contribute to the diagnosis.

A pituitary tumor must be ruled out as the cause of decreased GH production. Sudden halted growth suggests a tumor; gradual failure suggests an idiopathic involvement. A history of vision loss, headache, an increase in head circumference, nausea, and vomiting (signs of increased intracranial pressure) also suggest a pituitary tumor. Growth failure may be so marked in some children that the parents may be suspected of child neglect.

BOX 48.3 Nursing Care Planning Based on Responsibility for Pharmacology

SOMATROPIN (NUTROPIN, HUMATROPE)

Classification: Somatropin is an example of a recombinant human growth hormone (rhGH).
Action: Used for the long-term treatment of children who have growth failure from inadequate production of pituitary hormone, renal failure, or Turner syndrome (Ross, Quigley, Cao, et al., 2011).
Pregnancy Risk Category: C
Dosage: Somatropin dosage is individualized. The drug is administered by injection either SC or intramuscularly.
Possible Adverse Effects: Injection site pain, glucose intolerance, hypothyroidism, bone problems (particularly the hip), blood abnormalities, rare intracranial hypertension in first 8 weeks of therapy

Nursing Implications

- Advise parents that X-rays of the wrist or hip will be performed before therapy begins. Thereafter, parents should be alert for limping or knee or hip pain, which should be reported to their primary health care provider because slipped capital epiphysis is associated with rhGH supplementation.
- Reinforce the need for periodic thyroid function tests and funduscopic examination to detect rare intracranial hypertension.
- Alert parents that rhGH may interact with glucocorticoid therapy such as prednisone, causing a decrease in the effectiveness of the rhGH. Urge parents to inform all health care providers that the child is receiving rhGH to avoid this type of interaction.

Ross, J. M. D., Quigley, C., Cao, D., et al. (2011). Growth hormone plus childhood low dose estrogen in Turner syndrome. *New England Journal of Medicine, 364*(13), 1230–1242.

As part of the history taking, evaluate the family history for traits of short stature or constitutional delay (familial late development). If at all possible, obtain estimates of the parents' height and siblings' height and weight during their periods of growth. Assess the child's prenatal and birth history for any suggestion of intrauterine growth restriction. Assess also for any severe head trauma that could have injured the pituitary gland, or chronic illness, such as a heart, kidney, or intestinal disorder, that could have contributed to the decreased level of growth. Take a 24-hour nutrition history to see if "picky eating habits" are extensive enough to halt growth. Be certain to assess not only the child's actual height but also his or her feelings about being short.

A physical assessment, including a funduscopic examination, neurologic testing, and blood analysis for hypothyroidism, hypoadrenalism, hypoaldosteronism, and growth factor–binding proteins are also helpful in ruling out a lesion or tumor. Bone age is established by a wrist X-ray (epiphyseal closure of long bones is delayed with GH deficiency but is proportional to the height delay). A skull series, computed tomography (CT) scanning, magnetic resonance imaging (MRI), or ultrasound will be prescribed to detect possible enlargement of the sella turcica, which would suggest a pituitary tumor.

Therapeutic Management

GH deficiency is treated by the administration of intramuscular (IM) recombinant human growth hormone (rhGH) usually given daily at bedtime, the time of day at which GH normally peaks (Graber & Rapaport, 2012) (Box 48.3). In addition, some children may need suppression of luteinizing hormone–releasing hormone (LHRH, or gonadotropin-releasing hormone [GnRH]) to delay epiphyseal closure. Other children may need supplements of gonadotropin or other pituitary hormones if these are determined to be deficient as well (Box 48.4 shows tips for the long-term administration of medicine to children).

BOX 48.4 Nursing Care Planning to Empower a Family

GUIDELINES FOR SUCCESSFUL LONG-TERM MEDICINE ADMINISTRATION

Q. Rob's father asks you, "What are good rules for long-term medicine administration?"
A. To be successful giving medicine over a long period of time, build the administration of it into your family's general routine through such measures as:

- Begin involving your child as early as possible in medicine administration by explaining what it is and why the child needs to take it.
- Plan times for medication administration that allow for a normal lifestyle, such as not having to wake up at 2 AM or having to interrupt a meal for an injection.
- Be aware of the life span of the medicine so that medication does not expire.
- Be certain to anticipate the need to obtain prescriptions before vacations, summer camp, or holidays so medicine is always available.
- If an intramuscular, subcutaneous, or intravenous medication is prescribed, not only the child but also at least one parent should learn the injection technique to ensure adherence.

GH has been used irresponsibly by athletes in the hope that it will improve muscle growth and overall stamina. Caution children that the use of the drug when there is no medical reason for it is potentially dangerous and so they should not share the drug with friends or take excessive doses themselves (Baumann, 2012). Because they have delayed epiphyseal closure, if treatment is begun early, children can expect to reach a height individually targeted for them. Once epiphyseal lines of long bones close (with adolescence), GH will be tapered and stopped.

Nursing Diagnoses and Related Interventions

Nursing Diagnosis: Situational low self-esteem related to short stature

Outcome Evaluation: Child speaks positively about self; identifies friends and activities enjoyed with peers.

If a child has been consistently behind in growth since early life, parents may simply assume in early childhood that the child is going to be short as an adult. The parents then may become concerned that something is wrong only after the child reaches puberty and fails to develop secondary sex characteristics. If an investigation at that time reveals the child's true problem is a lack of GH, parents may feel guilty that they did not become alarmed earlier. They may feel resentment toward health care personnel who did not alert them to the problem earlier. Encourage parents to discuss these feelings and provide support to help them accept their child in this new light as well as participate in making the new plan of care a success (Box 48.5). Children with short stature tend to report feelings of lower quality of life largely related to discrimination (Geisler, Lass, Reinsch, et al., 2012). You may need to remind parents to assign duties and responsibilities to children that match their chronologic age, not their physical size, in order to promote children's feelings of maturity and self-esteem. Because children different in any way from their peers may be the victims of bullying, alert parents to this possibility and assess for this at well-child visits to help protect the child's quality of life (Box 48.6).

Growth Hormone Excess

An overproduction of GH usually is caused by a benign tumor of the anterior pituitary (an adenoma). If the overproduction occurs before the epiphyseal lines of the long bones have closed, excessive or overgrowth will result. Weight will become excessive also, but it is proportional to height.

BOX 48.5 Nursing Care Planning Based on Effective Communication

Rob, a 16-year-old with diabetes, is short in stature. While observing him and his mother, you notice Rob is wearing clothes more suitable for a preteen than an adolescent.

Less Effective Communication

Nurse: Mrs. Tebecco, do you have any questions about Rob's care?
Mrs. Tebecco: No. I'm worried, though, that he'll be wanting a driver's license soon. I'm lucky he's so short he can't really drive yet.
Nurse: Is he happy being so short?
Mrs. Tebecco: It's made him better at gymnastics than the taller boys. Probably because he looks so much younger than he is.
Nurse: Well, that's good. Sometimes it's hard for children with a chronic disease to be happy.

More Effective Communication

Nurse: Mrs. Tebecco, do you have any questions about Rob's care?
Mrs. Tebecco: No. I'm worried, though, that he'll be wanting a driver's license soon. I'm lucky he's so short he can't really drive yet.
Nurse: Is he happy being so short?
Mrs. Tebecco: It's made him better at gymnastics than the taller boys. Probably because he looks so much younger than he is.
Nurse: But how does he feel about his size? How do you think he'll feel in the future?
Mrs. Tebecco: I don't even think about that. I don't want to lose my baby.
Nurse: Let's talk a bit about how his growing up makes both of you feel before we review his insulin injection technique.

Many children with endocrine or metabolic disorders are short in stature. This characteristic causes them to be viewed as cute and petite by parents, and some parents express that they enjoy their child's short stature; it makes it seem as if the child will remain a child longer and not grow up and be independent. Exploring how parents and the child feel about this misperception can help them see that all children grow older chronologically even if they appear still young and so need activities and interests related to their chronologic age, not their appearance age.

BOX 48.6 Nursing Care Planning to Respect Cultural Diversity

The way people view endocrine disorders can be culturally influenced. Because many of these disorders are inherited, they tend to cluster in various populations, so either the incidence of the condition in family or friends is high, or else people know nothing about the condition. In the past, because many endocrine disorders led to changes in body appearance, particularly overgrowth or undergrowth, and because the reason for these changes was poorly understood, children with these disorders found themselves poorly accepted by peers. Being aware of the way these diseases used to be viewed aids in understanding a parent's anxiety at diagnosis of these disorders and helps with nursing care planning to include reassurance and modern concepts of therapy.

The skull circumference typically exceeds usual, and the fontanelles may close late or not at all. After epiphyseal lines close, *acromegaly* (enlargement of the bones of the head and soft parts of the hands and feet) begin to be evident. The tongue can become so enlarged and thickened that it protrudes from the mouth, giving the child a dull, apathetic appearance and making it difficult to articulate words. If the condition remains untreated, a child may reach a height of more than 8 ft.

If X-rays or ultrasounds of the skull reveal that the sella turcica is enlarged or that a tumor is present, laser surgery to remove the tumor or cryosurgery (freezing of tissue) is the primary treatment. If no tumor is present, a GH antagonist such as bromocriptine (Parlodel) taken orally or octreotide (Sandostatin) taken by injection can slow the production of GH. When GH secretion is halted in this way, other hormones may also be affected; therefore, the child may need to receive supplemental thyroid extract, cortisol, and gonadotropin hormones in later life. A more permanent therapy is irradiation or radioactive implants of the pituitary gland, again to halt GH production. It is difficult for a child always to be bigger and taller than playmates, and problems such as buying clothes or fitting into airline seats continue to be very real and distressing in adulthood. Counseling them about maintaining self-esteem and making the adjustments necessary to accommodate their larger than usual size is a nursing responsibility.

QSEN Checkpoint Question 48.1

Quality Improvement

Sandy, Rob's 14-year-old girlfriend, often comes to your pediatric clinic with him. Rob and Sandy first met at the endocrine clinic because Sandy has hypopituitarism. Which of Sandy's statements would make you believe she needs more education about her disorder? Select all that apply.

a. "Taking growth hormone subcutaneously is a bother; I hope I'll be changed to pills soon."
b. "I know I have to take growth hormone for life but it's okay; I'll be all right."
c. "Growth hormone makes me pee a lot; I asked for a locker near the bathroom."
d. "Growth hormone turned my cheeks red, but I cover it with makeup so it's okay."
e. "I'm determined not to let this take away my quality of life."

Look in Appendix A for the best answer and rationale.

Diabetes Insipidus

Diabetes insipidus is a disease in which there is decreased release of ADH by the pituitary gland (Chamarthi, Morris, Kaiser, et al., 2010). This causes less reabsorption of fluid in the kidney tubules. Urine becomes extremely dilute, and a great deal of fluid is lost from the body. Diabetes insipidus may reflect an X-linked dominant trait, or it may be transmitted by an autosomal recessive gene. It may also result from a lesion, tumor, or injury to the posterior pituitary, or it may have an unknown cause. In a rare type of diabetes insipidus, pituitary function is adequate, but the kidneys' nephrons are not sensitive to ADH (a kidney-related etiology).

Assessment

The child with diabetes insipidus experiences excessive thirst (**polydipsia**) that is relieved only by drinking large amounts of water; there is accompanying polyuria. The specific gravity of the urine will be as low as 1.001 to 1.005 (normal values are more often 1.010 to 1.030). Urine output may reach 4 to 10 L in a 24-hour period (normal range, 1 to 2 L), depending on age.

Because so much fluid is lost, sodium becomes concentrated or hypernatremia occurs with symptoms of irritability, weakness, lethargy, fever, headache, and seizures. The signs and symptoms usually appear gradually. Parents may notice the polyuria first as bed-wetting in a toilet-trained child or weight loss because of the large loss of fluid. If the condition remains untreated, the child is in danger of losing such a large quantity of water that dehydration and death can result.

MRI, CT scanning, or an ultrasound study of the skull reveals whether a lesion or tumor is present. A further test is the administration of vasopressin (Pitressin) to rule out kidney disease. For this, after the child's urine output has been measured to establish a baseline, vasopressin is administered. The drug decreases the blood pressure, alerting the kidney to retain more fluid in order to maintain vascular pressure. If the fault that is causing the dilute urine is with the pituitary gland, not the kidneys, the child's urine output will decrease; if the fault is with the kidneys, urine will remain dilute and excessive in amount because the diseased kidneys cannot concentrate fluid.

Therapeutic Management

Surgery is the treatment of choice if a tumor is present. If the cause is idiopathic, the condition can be controlled by the administration of desmopressin (DDAVP), an arginine vasopressin. In an emergency, this drug can be given intravenously (IV). For long-term use, it is given intranasally or orally (Lemon & Crannage, 2011). If desmopressin is given as an intranasal spray, this may cause nasal irritation; the route will not be effective if the child develops an upper respiratory tract infection with swollen mucous membranes. Caution children that they will notice an increasing urine output just before the next dose is due so they can arrange their day according to where bathrooms are located.

Nursing Diagnoses and Related Interventions

Nursing Diagnosis: Risk for deficient fluid volume related to constant, excessive loss of fluid through urination

Outcome Evaluation: Child's blood pressure and pulse are within normal limits for age; specific gravity of urine is between 1.003 and 1.030; skin turgor is good; child states thirst is not excessive.

Teach About Long-Term Therapy: Be certain to explain the difference between diabetes insipidus and diabetes mellitus so the family is not confused about the differences in therapy. Help the family establish a routine to ensure the child receives adequate fluid to discourage a feeling of thirst and has access to bathroom facilities possibly more frequently than others. Review suggestions for long-term medicine administration with them (see Box 48.4).

Encourage Communication: Caution parents that, when seeking any type of health care, they should always notify health care providers that the child has diabetes insipidus. For example, surgery poses particular dangers because of the fluid restrictions that accompany most procedures. Encourage children to wear a medical alert tag identifying them as having diabetes insipidus. Urge parents to inform school personnel that the child may need to use the bathroom frequently and to plan on frequent bathroom stops and adequate fluid intake on long trips or activity-filled days.

Syndrome of Inappropriate Antidiuretic Hormone

The syndrome of inappropriate antidiuretic hormone (SIADH) is a rare condition in which there is overproduction of ADH by the posterior pituitary gland. This results in a decrease in urine production, which leads to water intoxication. As sodium levels fall in proportion to water, the child develops hyponatremia or a lowered sodium plasma level. SIADH can be caused by central nervous system infections such as bacterial meningitis (see Chapter 49), long-term positive pressure ventilation, or pituitary compression such as could occur from edema or a tumor.

Mild symptoms of hyponatremia are weight gain, concentrated urine (increased specific gravity), nausea, and vomiting. As the hyponatremia grows more severe, coma or seizures occur from brain edema.

Therapy consists of restriction of fluid and supplementation of sodium by IV fluid if needed. Demeclocycline (Declomycin), a tetracycline antibiotic that has the side effect of blocking the action of ADH in renal tubules and reducing resorption of water, may be prescribed (Wang, Shiang, Chen, et al., 2011).

THE THYROID GLAND

The thyroid gland, located at the front of the neck, is responsible for controlling the rate of metabolism in the body through the hormones thyroxine (T_4) and triiodothyronine (T_3), which are produced by its follicular cells.

Assessment of Thyroid Function

Radioimmunoassay of T_4 and T_3 is a specific blood study to determine how much protein-bound iodine (PBI) is present in serum. Ask if a child has recently taken large amounts of cough medicine containing iodide or underwent a study using an iodine-based contrast medium (e.g., urography, bronchography) recently before the study or PBI levels may be abnormally elevated. The small amount of iodine ingested from iodized salt does not affect PBI levels.

Children who have low circulating albumin levels can have abnormally low PBI levels because iodine is carried bound to protein. Phenytoin (Dilantin), a common anticonvulsant medication prescribed for children with recurrent seizures, may displace thyroxine from binding globulin and further contribute to low PBI levels.

Another test of thyroid function is a radioactive iodine uptake test. The child is given an oral dose of a solution containing radioactive iodine (^{123}I). The thyroid gland "traps" this iodine, and, 24 hours later, after the maximum amount has been trapped, the amount of radioactive iodine present can be determined. It is important in this type of test that the child swallows all the solution. In infants, the solution usually is given as a gavage feeding, so that accuracy of the dose can be ensured.

An uptake of less than 10% of the test dose suggests hypothyroidism. If the child vomits after ingesting the substance, this event should be recorded and called to the attention of the laboratory; it will obviously result in a lower uptake value because only a part of the actual dose will be available for uptake. Be certain that the child does not receive iodine or thyroid extract in any other form during the 24-hour test time because this would compete with uptake of the radioactive iodine and, again, produce a falsely low value.

THYROID GLAND DISORDERS

Congenital Hypothyroidism

Thyroid hypofunction causes reduced production of both T_4 and T_3. Congenital hypofunction (reduced or absent function) occurs as a result of an absent or nonfunctioning thyroid gland in a newborn. There has been a large increase in the incidence of congenital hypothyroidism in the United States in the last two decades (Allen & Fomenko, 2011). Researchers are attempting to determine if this increase reflects a true increase in the disorder possibly due to environmental factors, due to better screening methods, or results from an increase in transient hypothyroidism (lessened thyroid function caused by a low iodine level in the mother or autoimmune antibodies that crossed the placenta). The increased incidence is associated with Caucasians, is evident more in infant girls than boys, and in newborns of either low birth weight or a birth weight over 4,500 g (Hinton, Harris, Borgfeld, et al., 2010; Shapira, Lloyd-Puryear, & Boyle, 2010).

Congenital hypothyroidism or an indication that the infant's thyroid is not functioning well may not be noticeable at birth because the mother's thyroid hormones (unless she ingested less than usual amounts of iodine) maintain adequate levels in the fetus during pregnancy. The symptoms of the disorder become apparent during the first 3 months of life in a formula-fed infant and at about 6 months in a breastfed infant. Because congenital hypothyroidism leads to both severe, progressive physical and cognitive challenges, early diagnosis is crucial.

Assessment

A screening test for hypothyroidism is mandatory at birth in the United States in all 50 states (using the same few drops of blood obtained for a phenylketonuria [PKU] blood spot test) (Allen & Fomenko, 2011). If an infant should miss this screening procedure, an early sign that parents report is that their child sleeps excessively, but because the tongue is enlarged, they notice respiratory difficulty, noisy respirations, or obstruction. The child may also suck poorly because of sluggishness or choking from the enlarged tongue. The skin of the extremities usually feels cold, dry, and perhaps scaly and the child does not perspire. Pulse, respiratory rate, and body temperature all become subnormal. Prolonged jaundice may be present due to the immature liver's inability to conjugate bilirubin. Anemia may increase the child's lethargy and fatigue.

On a physical exam, the hair is brittle and dry and the child's neck appears short and thick. The facial expression is dull and open mouthed because of the infant's attempts to breathe around the enlarged tongue. The extremities appear short and fat; as muscles become hypotonic, deep tendon reflexes decrease and the infant develops a floppy, rag-doll appearance. Generalized obesity usually occurs. Dentition will be delayed, or teeth may be defective when they do erupt.

The hypotonia affects the intestinal tract as well, so the infant develops chronic constipation; the abdomen enlarges because of intestinal distention and poor muscle tone (Fig. 48.2). Many infants have an umbilical hernia. Infants have low radioactive iodine uptake levels, low serum T_4 and T_3 levels, and elevated thyroid-stimulating factor. Blood lipids are increased. An X-ray may reveal delayed bone growth. An ultrasound reveals a small or absent thyroid gland. Untreated, the condition will result in severe irreversible cognitive deterioration or delay (Olney, Grosse, & Vogt, 2010).

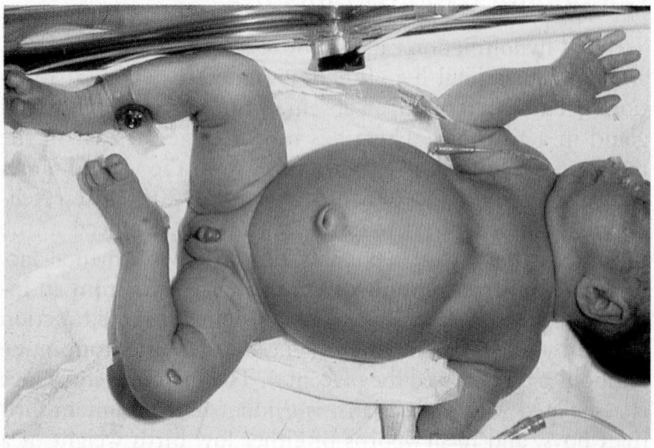

FIGURE 48.2 An infant with congenital hypothyroidism. Notice the short, thick neck and enlarged abdomen. (© David/NMSB/Custom Medical Stock Photograph.)

Therapeutic Management

Transient hypothyroidism usually fades by 3 months' time. The treatment for true hypothyroidism is the oral administration of synthetic thyroid hormone (sodium levothyroxine). A small dose is given at first, and then the dose is gradually increased to therapeutic levels. The child needs to continue taking the synthetic thyroid hormone indefinitely to supplement that which the thyroid does not make. Supplemental vitamin D may also be given to prevent the development of rickets when, with the administration of thyroid hormone, rapid bone growth begins (Plaut & McLellan, 2011).

Further cognitive challenges can be prevented as soon as therapy is started, but any degree of impairment that was already present cannot be reversed, making the disorder one of the most preventable causes of mental development delay known (LaFranchi, 2011).

Be certain the parents know the rules for long-term medication administration with children, particularly the rule about not putting medicine in a large amount of food (thyroxine tablets must be crushed and added to food or a small amount of formula or breast milk) and being certain they have medicine during holidays or vacations. Periodic monitoring of T_4 and T_3 helps to ensure an appropriate medication dosage. If the dose of thyroid hormone is not adequate, the T_4 level will remain low and there will be few signs of clinical improvement. If the dose is too high, the T_4 level will rise and the child will show signs of hyperthyroidism: irritability, fever, rapid pulse, and perhaps vomiting, diarrhea, and weight loss.

Acquired Hypothyroidism (Hashimoto Thyroiditis)

Hashimoto disease is the most common form of acquired hypothyroidism in childhood; the age at onset is most often 10 to 11 years. There may be a family history of thyroid disease and it occurs more often in girls than in boys. The decrease in thyroid secretion is caused by the development of an autoimmune phenomenon that interferes with thyroid production.

Assessment

The excretion of thyroid-stimulating hormone (TSH) from the pituitary increases when thyroid hormone production decreases in an attempt by the pituitary gland to increase thyroid function. In response to the increased level of TSH, hypertrophy of the thyroid gland (goiter) can occur, and body growth is impaired by a lack of thyroxine, with prominent symptoms of obesity, lethargy, and delayed sexual development.

Antithyroid antibodies will be present in serum if the illness was caused by an autoimmune process. If the thyroid enlarges, it may become nodular as well. Although in childhood, a nodular thyroid is usually benign, an investigation into the possibility this could be a thyroid malignancy must be considered. For diagnosis, children are administered radioactive iodine. If the nodes are benign, there is generally a rapid uptake of radioactive iodine ("hot nodes"). If there is no uptake ("cold nodes"), carcinoma is a much more likely diagnosis (which is rare at this age).

Therapeutic Management

Treatment for acquired hypothyroidism is the administration of synthetic thyroid hormone (sodium levothyroxine), the same as for congenital hypothyroidism. With adequate dosage, the obesity diminishes and growth begins again. It is important that the disease be recognized as early as possible so there is time to stimulate growth before the epiphyseal lines close at puberty.

If acquired hypothyroidism exists in a woman during pregnancy, her infant can be born cognitively challenged because there was not enough iodine present for fetal growth. It is important, therefore, that girls with this syndrome be identified before they reach childbearing age.

What if...48.1 Rob's mother tells you that her sister (his aunt) is 3 months pregnant and was prescribed Synthroid (synthetic thyroid hormone) but "forgets to take it most days and really cannot afford it." What would you do?

Hyperthyroidism (Graves Disease)

Hyperthyroidism is oversecretion of thyroid hormones by the thyroid gland. Neonatal Graves disease develops in the newborns of 1% to 2% of pregnant women who have the disease. Like transient hypothyroidism, this usually resolves between 3 to 12 weeks of age with no long-term results as the maternal antibodies are cleared (Snyder, Berch, Najjar, et al., 2011).

In older children, overactivity of the thyroid gland can occur from the glands being overstimulated by TSH from the pituitary gland due to a pituitary tumor. More frequently, however, hyperthyroidism in children is caused by an autoimmune reaction that results in overproduction of immunoglobulin G (IgG), which stimulates the thyroid gland to overproduce thyroxine. An exophthalmos-producing pituitary substance causes the prominent-appearing eyes that accompany hyperthyroidism in some children.

Assessment

Some children may have a genetic predisposition to development of the disorder, although Graves disease often follows a viral illness or a period of stress. With overproduction of T_3 and T_4, children gradually experience nervousness, tremors, loss of muscle strength, and easy fatigue. Their basal metabolic rate, blood pressure, and pulse all increase. Their skin feels moist and they perspire freely. They always feel hungry, and, although they eat constantly, do not gain weight and may even lose weight because of the increased basal metabolic rate. On X-ray, bone age will appear advanced beyond the chronologic age of the child. Unless the condition is treated, the child is not likely to reach usual adult height because epiphyseal lines of long bones will close before full height can be attained.

The thyroid gland, which usually is not prominent in children, appears as a swelling on the anterior neck as goiter develops. In a few children, the eye globes become prominent (exophthalmia), giving the child a wide-eyed, staring appearance. Laboratory tests show elevated T_4 and T_3 levels and increased radioactive iodine uptake. TSH is low or absent because the thyroid is being stimulated by antibodies, not by the pituitary gland. Ultrasound will reveal the enlarged thyroid.

Therapeutic Management

Therapy consists first of a course of a β-adrenergic blocking agent, such as propranolol, to decrease the antibody response. After this, the child is placed on an antithyroid drug, such as propylthiouracil (PTU) or methimazole (Tapazole), to suppress the formation of thyroxine. While the child is taking these drugs, the blood is monitored for leukopenia (decreased white blood cell count) and thrombocytopenia (decreased platelet count)—side effects of these drugs. If either of these results, the drug is discontinued until the white blood cell or platelet count returns to normal, so the child does not develop an infection or experience spontaneous bleeding.

Because the thyroid stores considerable thyroid hormone that must be used up first before thyroxine levels decline, it takes about 2 weeks for these drugs to have an effect. The child needs to continue to take the drug for 2 to 3 years before the condition "burns itself out." The exophthalmos may not recede, but it will not become worse once therapy is instituted.

If the child has a toxic reaction to medical management (severely lowered white blood cell count or platelet count) or is noncompliant about taking the medicine, radioiodine ablative therapy with ^{131}I or thyroid surgery to reduce the size of the thyroid gland can be accomplished. This has long-term effects, however, because after both radioiodine ablative therapy and thyroidectomy, supplemental thyroid hormone therapy may need to be taken indefinitely because the gland is no longer able to produce an adequate amount (Léger & Carel, 2013). It is important that adolescent girls be carefully regulated before they consider childbearing because hyperthyroidism during pregnancy can lead to neonatal hyperthyroidism in a fetus.

Nursing Diagnoses and Related Interventions

Nursing Diagnosis: Situational low self-esteem related to lack of coordination and presence of prominent goiter or exophthalmia

Outcome Evaluation: Child states positive traits about self and identifies friends and activities enjoyed; is not the victim of bullying because of unusual appearance.

Hyperthyroidism begins gradually and so may become fairly involved before it is detected. Suspect children at puberty of having hyperthyroidism if they are losing weight or have behavior problems in school, which occur because of the hand or tongue tremors that make it hard for them to write or speak and the nervousness that makes them unable to sit still during class.

Offer parents support to supervise medication administration so they can be certain the child takes the prescribed medicine every day. Caution children not to stop taking the medicine abruptly, or a thyroxine crisis (sudden onset of extreme symptoms of hyperthyroidism) can occur. Parents may ask if their child can have surgery as a cure so that long-term administration of medicine will not be required. Help them understand that surgery may not dispel the need for medication; if a large portion of the thyroid gland is removed, it may be necessary for their child to take medicine indefinitely to make up for the missing gland. In any event, it is preferable to try a course of medical management before resorting to surgery.

QSEN Checkpoint Question 48.2
Patient-Centered Care

Rob has a cousin who has developed hyperthyroidism with puberty. If you were a school nurse, you might need to support her in dealing with which of the following effects of this health problem?

a. Slow, lethargic movements
b. Swollen, protuberant abdomen
c. Jittery, nervous mannerisms
d. Reduced intellectual processing

Look in Appendix A for the best answer and rationale.

THE ADRENAL GLAND

The two adrenal glands are located retroperitoneally, just above the kidneys. They are made up of two distinct divisions; together, these divisions protect the body against acute and chronic forms of stress. Three hormones—cortisol (a glucocorticoid responsible for glucose and protein metabolism and preventing inflammation), androgen (a steroid hormone responsible for muscle development), and aldosterone (a mineralocorticoid hormone necessary for sodium and fluid balance) are important in childhood illnesses.

ADRENAL GLAND DISORDERS

Disorders of the adrenal glands cause either hypofunction, which can lead to acute or chronic production of necessary hormones, or hyperfunction (overactivity), which most often leads to overproduction of androgen or cortisol.

Acute Adrenocortical Insufficiency

Insufficiency (hypofunction) of the adrenal gland can occur in either an acute or chronic form. In either type, the function of the entire gland suddenly becomes nonproductive. Usually, this occurs following a severe overwhelming body infection such as meningococcemia. It also can occur when corticosteroid therapy such as prednisone, which has been maintained at high levels for a long period, is abruptly stopped and the gland does not return to usual function.

Assessment

With acute adrenocortical insufficiency, the child's blood pressure drops to extremely low levels, the child appears ashen gray, and the pulse will be weak. Temperature gradually becomes elevated; dehydration and **hypoglycemia** (an abnormally low concentration of blood glucose) become marked because cortisol is no longer present to regulate this. As sodium and chloride blood levels fall from a lack of aldosterone production, the potassium level becomes elevated due to the usual inverse relationship between sodium and potassium values. The child appears prostrate and seizures may occur. Without treatment, death can occur abruptly (Thalange & Beach, 2013).

Therapeutic Management

Acute adrenocortical insufficiency is a medical emergency. Treatment involves the immediate replacement of cortisol (with IV hydrocortisone sodium succinate [Solu-Cortef]); the administration of deoxycorticosterone acetate (DOCA), the synthetic equivalent of aldosterone; and IV 5% glucose in normal saline solution to restore blood pressure, sodium, and blood glucose levels. A vasoconstrictor may be necessary to elevate the blood pressure.

Although acute adrenal insufficiency is seen less often now than in the past because of the availability of antibiotics that quickly halt the course of infectious disease because more conditions are being treated with corticosteroids than ever before, the chance the syndrome will occur from sudden withdrawal of high-dose steroids is actually increasing.

Congenital Adrenal Hyperplasia

Congenital adrenal hyperplasia is a syndrome that is inherited as an autosomal recessive trait and which causes the adrenal glands to not be able to synthesize cortisol. Because the adrenal gland is unable to produce cortisol, the level of adrenocorticotropic hormone (ACTH) secreted by the pituitary increases in an attempt to stimulate the gland to increase function. Although the adrenals enlarge (hyperplasia) under the effect of ACTH, they still cannot produce cortisol; instead, they overproduce androgen.

Assessment

The excessive androgen production during intrauterine life causes the genital organs in a male fetus to "overgrow," or increase in size; it masculinizes a female fetus (i.e., the clitoris is so enlarged that it appears to be a penis; if the labia are fused, she appears to be a boy with undescended testes and hypospadias (Fig. 48.3) (Zeitler, Barker, Travers, et al., 2011). Other female organs appear normal, although a sinus between the urethra and vagina may be present (see the discussion of ambiguous genitalia in Chapter 47). If the condition is not recognized at birth and the child remains untreated, bone age will advance so the epiphyseal lines of the long bones close early, preventing the child from reaching a usual adult height; pubic and axillary hair, acne, and a deep masculine voice will appear precociously. At puberty, there will be no breast development or menstruation.

By 3 or 4 years of age, untreated boys develop acne and a deep, mature voice; pubic hair and still greater enlargement of the penis, scrotum, and prostate occur. In contrast, the testes do not enlarge and so appear small in relation to the size of the penis. Spermatogenesis does not occur with puberty, leaving the child infertile.

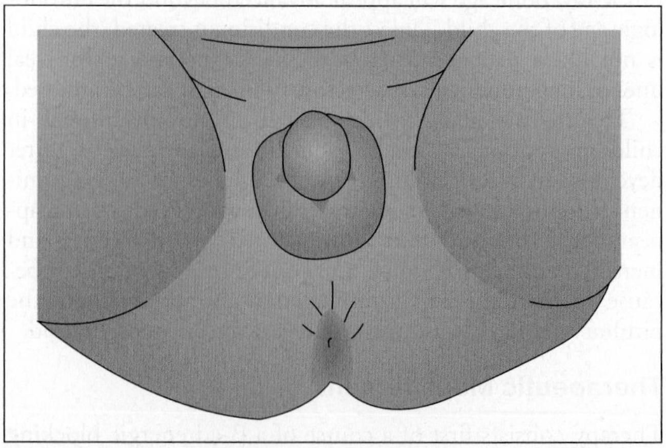

FIGURE 48.3 A female infant with congenital adrenogenital hyperplasia. Note the fused labia and abnormally enlarged clitoris.

It is possible to identify the fetus with congenital adrenogenital hyperplasia as early as 6 to 8 weeks of pregnancy by means of maternal serum analysis and at 15 weeks by amniocentesis (see Chapter 9). Although controversial, treatment of a mother with dexamethasone (a corticosteroid), which crosses the placenta to the fetus, can prevent masculinization in the fetus for the remainder of the pregnancy. The newborn will then need hydrocortisone administration after birth for continuing therapy.

The condition is usually diagnosed not during pregnancy, however, but in infancy by serum analysis, which shows the increased level of androgen. By determining the levels of other adrenal hormones, the exact degree of the metabolic defect in production of cortisol can be measured.

Therapeutic Management

The ultimate goal of therapy is to replace the cortisol that is missing, thereby suppressing ACTH concentrations and normalizing adrenal size and androgen production, a goal that seems quite simple but is actually very difficult to achieve (Dauber, Kellogg, & Majzoub, 2010). For therapy, both male and female infants are given a corticosteroid agent, such as oral hydrocortisone, to replace what they cannot produce naturally. When a corticosteroid is given to the child in this way, stimulation by ACTH decreases, the production of androgen returns to normal limits, and no further masculinization occurs. Because corticosteroid therapy needs to continue indefinitely, the child needs periodic analysis of serum cortisol levels and growth measurements to estimate the effectiveness of the therapy. Children may need to have a routine dose increased when they are undergoing periods of stress, such as during surgery or infection. They may need support throughout life if their body image is distorted because of body changes at birth.

Nursing Diagnoses and Related Interventions

Nursing Diagnosis: Situational low self-esteem related to genital formation at variance with true gender

Outcome Evaluation: Child identifies positive traits about self and describes activities enjoyed with peers; expresses satisfaction with gender identity; does not report bullying from peers.

All newborns need an extensive physical examination at birth so chromosomal girls with this syndrome are not wrongly identified as male. It is sometimes recommended to parents that a girl's enlarged clitoris be reduced by plastic surgery in infancy. This treatment is controversial, however, because even with finer surgical techniques, clitoral reduction can also result in reduced clitoral sensation. A girl should have the right to make this decision for herself, however, so, as a rule, surgery is delayed until the girl is old enough to understand what will be the implication of not having clitoral sensation on her sexual enjoyment (Jospe, 2011).

Parents of females with congenital adrenogenital hyperplasia may need a great deal of support during the first few days of their child's life because they may voice that their child is imperfect in an embarrassing, hard-to-explain way. When they are the results of the chromosome analysis, parents may react with grief for the loss of the son they first thought had been born to them. Parents need support from health care personnel who recognize that the child is simply lacking the ability to produce cortisol but is complete in every other way.

Salt-Losing Form of Congenital Adrenogenital Hyperplasia

If there is a complete blockage of cortisol formation, aldosterone production will also be deficient. Without adequate aldosterone, salt is not retained by the body, so fluid is not retained. Almost immediately after birth, affected infants begin to have vomiting, diarrhea, anorexia, loss of weight, and extreme dehydration (Dauber et al., 2010). If these symptoms remain untreated, the extreme loss of salt and fluid can lead to collapse and death as early as 48 to 72 hours after birth.

About one third of children with congenital adrenogenital hyperplasia are affected by this complete deficiency. Because boys with this syndrome appear normal at birth, the symptoms may be incorrectly diagnosed as infection or as failure to thrive. In girls, because of the ambiguous genitalia, the correct diagnosis can be made more easily.

Assessment

The salt-losing form must be detected before an infant reaches an irreversible point of salt depletion. (The reason newborns are weighed at birth and again at 24 hours is to detect this condition.) Weighing infants at each well-child health checkup is also important because, in boys, the inability to gain back their birth weight may be the first sign of the syndrome.

Therapeutic Management

Children with this form of congenital adrenogenital hyperplasia need to be supplemented with hydrocortisone, an increased salt intake, and DOCA, a synthetic aldosterone, in order to maintain a balance of fluid and electrolytes. A long-acting form of DOCA can be given once a month intramuscularly. Capsules of DOCA can also be implanted subcutaneously (SC) as another form of long-acting therapy. As the child grows older, fludrocortisone (Florinef), a mineralocorticoid, may be given orally to aid salt retention.

Nursing Diagnoses and Related Interventions

Nursing Diagnosis: Risk for deficient fluid volume related to loss of body fluid

Outcome Evaluation: Child's skin turgor remains good; specific gravity of urine is between 1.003 and 1.030.

Teach parents about the body's critical need to balance aldosterone, salt, and water, so they understand the drastic consequences if their child skips a dose of medication. Otherwise, they may underestimate that salt, although an "extra" in their own diet, is as vital to their child's intake as digitalis is in heart disease or insulin is in diabetes. Help them to set up a schedule as necessary for measuring their child's weight, giving medication, or measuring urine output.

Cushing Syndrome

Cushing syndrome is caused by overproduction of the adrenal hormone cortisol; this usually results from increased ACTH production due to either a pituitary or adrenal cortex tumor. The peak age of occurrence is 6 or 7 years, but the syndrome can occur as early as infancy. The inappropriate use of high-potency steroid creams for diaper dermatitis my be a possible cause (Fraser & Van Uum, 2010). The overproduction of cortisol results in increased glucose production; this causes fat to accumulate on the cheeks, chin, and trunk, causing a moon-faced, stocky appearance. Cortisol is catabolic, so protein wasting also occurs. This leads to muscle wasting, making the extremities appear thin in contrast to the trunk, and loss of calcium in bones (osteoporosis). Cortisol also suppresses the immune system, so humoral immunity is decreased, leaving children susceptible to infections. Additionally, it causes vasoconstriction, so extreme hypertension may occur.

Yet other effects are hyperpigmentation (the child's face appears unusually red, especially the cheeks), which occurs from the melanin-stimulating properties of ACTH; abnormal masculinization or feminization, which occurs from overproduction of androgen or estrogen; and poor wound healing, which results from reduced protein regulation. Purple striae resulting from collagen deficit appear on the child's hips, abdomen, and thighs, similar to those seen in pregnancy (Fig. 48.4).

Polyuria begins to develop as the body tries to excrete increased glucose levels. Growth ceases, and, if the condition is not reversed before the epiphyseal lines close, short stature will result.

Children who receive high doses of synthetic corticosteroids, such as prednisone, over a long period may develop the same symptoms as those observed in Cushing syndrome (termed a *cushingoid appearance*). Children who are obese may have elevated levels of plasma corticosteroids and so be wrongly diagnosed as having Cushing syndrome. However, with this, the child's growth is not impaired, so these elevated levels of corticosteroids are secondary to the obesity, not the cause.

Assessment

The serum of children with Cushing syndrome reveals an elevated plasma cortisol and increased urinary free-cortisol levels. A dexamethasone suppression test may be administered for diagnosis. For this test, a child is administered a dose of dexamethasone (a glucocorticoid); if the child has the syndrome, the plasma level of adrenal cortisol will fall. It will not fall in children with adrenocortical tumors because the tumor continues to stimulate the adrenal glands to oversecretion. If cosyntropin (Cortrosyn), a synthetic corticotropin, or ACTH is administered, plasma cortisol levels will normally rise. In children with an adrenal tumor, the gland is already functioning at full capacity, so no cortisol elevation occurs. A CT scan or ultrasound reveals the enlarged adrenal or pituitary gland, confirming the diagnosis.

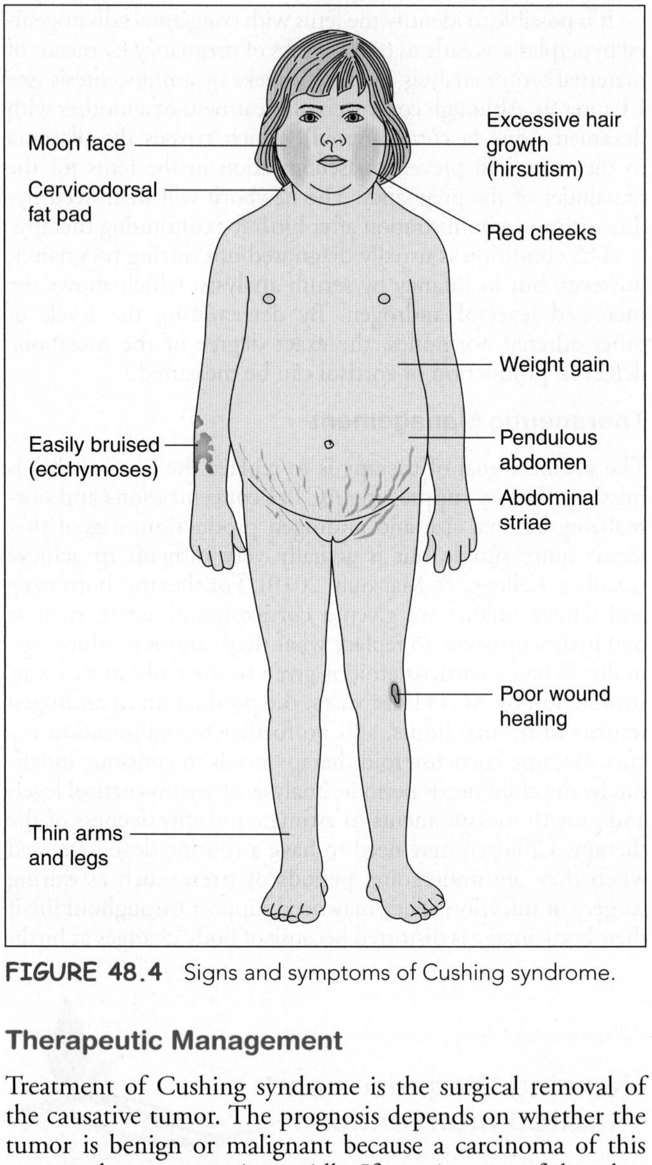

FIGURE 48.4 Signs and symptoms of Cushing syndrome.

Therapeutic Management

Treatment of Cushing syndrome is the surgical removal of the causative tumor. The prognosis depends on whether the tumor is benign or malignant because a carcinoma of this type tends to metastasize rapidly. If a major part of the adrenal glands are surgically removed, the child will need replacement cortisol therapy indefinitely.

If a major portion of the pituitary gland is removed because the problem was overproduction of ACTH, the replacement of all pituitary hormones may be necessary. After adrenal surgery, observe the child carefully for signs of shock: without epinephrine also produced by the gland, the body's ability to maintain blood pressure is severely compromised, and severe hypotension can result.

QSEN Checkpoint Question 48.3

Informatics

Rob has his adrenal gland function assessed through diagnostic testing. What is the effect on a child when sufficient aldosterone cannot be produced?

a. Substantially fewer red blood cells are produced.
b. There is an overall decreased urine output.
c. An excessive amount of sodium is lost in urine.
d. The child's growth rate increases abnormally.

Look in Appendix A for the best answer and rationale.

THE PANCREAS

The pancreas is a unique organ in that it has both endocrine (ductless) and exocrine (with duct) types of tissue. The *islets of Langerhans* form the endocrine portion, alpha islet cells have the responsibility to secrete glucagon, and beta islet cells secrete insulin.

Insulin is essential for carbohydrate metabolism and is also important in the metabolism of both fats and protein. It is formed from amino acids at a rate between 35 to 50 units per day in adults and proportionately less in children. When serum glucose that passes through the pancreas exceeds 100 mg/dl, beta cells immediately begin insulin production. When serum glucose levels are low, production decreases.

Insulin production is also stimulated by gastrin, a gastrointestinal hormone that rises when the stomach is full, as well as the levels of glucagon, cortisol, growth hormone, progesterone, and estrogen. Increasing levels of epinephrine or norepinephrine inhibit the secretion of insulin in order to preserve glucose for "flight or fight."

The principal childhood disorders associated with pancreatic dysfunction are type 1 and type 2 diabetes mellitus and cystic fibrosis. Because the nursing care for children with cystic fibrosis includes many respiratory care procedures, it is discussed in Chapter 40.

Type 1 Diabetes Mellitus

Type 1 diabetes mellitus is a disorder that involves an absolute or relative deficiency of insulin, which is in contrast to type 2, where insulin production is only reduced (Table 48.2). Type 1 diabetes is equal in incidence in boys and girls and affects approximately 1 of every 500 children and adolescents in the United States (Dashiff, Riley, Abdullatif, et al., 2011).

Etiology

The disease apparently results from immunologic damage to islet cells in susceptible individuals. Why autoimmune destruction of islet cells occurs is unknown, but children with the disorder have a high frequency of certain human leukocyte antigens (HLA), particularly HLA-DR3 and HLA-DR4, located on chromosome 6, that may lead to susceptibility. If one child in a family has diabetes, the chance that a sibling will also develop the illness is higher than in other families, because siblings also tend to have one of the specific HLA antigens that are associated with the disease.

Disease Process

Insulin can be thought of as a compound that opens the doors to body cells, allowing them to admit glucose, which is needed for functioning. It does not play a major role in glucose transport into the brain, erythrocytes, leukocytes, intestinal mucosa, or kidney epithelium. These cells, therefore, can survive insulin deficiency but not glucose deficiency.

If glucose is unable to enter body cells because of a lack of insulin, it builds up in the bloodstream (**hyperglycemia**). As soon as the kidneys detect hyperglycemia (greater than the renal threshold of about 160 mg/dl), the kidneys attempt to lower it to normal levels by excreting excess glucose into the urine, causing **glycosuria**, accompanied by a large loss of body fluid (polyuria). Excess fluid loss, in turn, triggers the thirst response (polydipsia), producing the three cardinal symptoms of diabetes: polyuria, polydipsia, and hyperglycemia.

Because body cells are unable to use glucose but still need a source of energy, the body begins to break down protein and fat. If large amounts of fat are metabolized this way, weight loss occurs and ketone bodies, the acid end product of fat

TABLE 48.2 Comparison of Type 1 and Type 2 Diabetes

Assessment	Type 1	Type 2
Age at onset	5–7 years or at puberty	40–65 years (may occur in adolescents as maturity-onset diabetes of youth [MODY])
Type of onset	Abrupt	Gradual
Weight changes	Marked weight loss often initial sign	Associated with obesity
Other symptoms	Polydipsia and polyphagia Polyuria (often begins as bed-wetting) Fatigue (marks fall in school) Blurred vision (marks fall in school) Mood changes (may cause behavior problems in school)	Polydipsia Polyuria Fatigue Blurred vision Mood changes
Therapy	Hypoglycemia agents never effective; insulin required No dietary foods used; should count carbohydrates plus evaluate blood glucose levels to help determine insulin dosage. Commonsense foot care for growing children	Diet, oral hypoglycemic agents, or insulin Nutrition concentrates on no excess weight gain and balanced intake of carbohydrates, protein, and fat Meticulous skin and foot care necessary
Period of remission	Period of remission for 1–12 months ("honeymoon period") generally after initial diagnosis	Not demonstrable

breakdown, begin to accumulate in the bloodstream (creating high serum cholesterol levels and ketoacidosis) and spill into the urine as ketones. Potassium and phosphate, attempting to serve as buffers, pass from body cells into the bloodstream. From there they are evacuated, causing a loss of these important electrolytes.

Untreated diabetic children, therefore, lose weight, are acidotic due to the buildup of ketone bodies in their blood, are dehydrated because of the loss of water, and experience an electrolyte imbalance because of the loss of potassium and phosphate in urine. Because large amounts of protein and fat are being used for energy instead of glucose, children lack the necessary components for growth; they therefore remain short in stature and underweight.

Assessment

Although children may be prediabetic for some time, the onset of symptoms in childhood is usually abrupt. Parents notice increased thirst and increased urination (which may be recognized first as bed-wetting [enuresis] in a previously toilet-trained child). The dehydration may cause constipation.

Laboratory Studies. In some children, diabetes is detected at a routine health screening. For others, although the disease has been progressing internally for some time, outward symptoms have such an abrupt onset that the child is in a coma from acidosis and hyperglycemia by the time it is detected. Laboratory studies usually show a random plasma glucose level greater than 200 mg/dl (normal range, 70 to 110 mg/dl fasting; 90 to 180 mg/dl not fasting) and significant glycosuria (Table 48.3).

Two diagnostic tests, the fasting blood glucose test and the random blood glucose test, are used to confirm diabetes. A diagnosis of diabetes is established if one of the following three criteria is present on two separate occasions:

- Symptoms of diabetes plus a random blood glucose level greater than 200 mg/dl
- A fasting blood glucose level greater than 126 mg/dl
- A 2-hour plasma glucose level greater than 200 mg/dl during a 75-g oral glucose tolerance test (GTT)

Typically, a GTT involves the oral ingestion of a concentrated glucose solution followed by blood glucose levels drawn at fasting (baseline), after 1 hour, and after 2 hours. The test is difficult for children to undergo because it requires them to fast for 8 hours, drink an overly sweet solution, and submit to painful, intrusive procedures (routine application of lidocaine/prilocaine [EMLA] cream to finger stick or venipuncture sites and use of intermittent infusion devices greatly reduces this problem). Do not take blood for glucose analysis from functioning IV tubing to try to help with pain because the glucose in the IV solution will cause the serum reading to be abnormally high.

TABLE 48.3 Acceptable Blood Glucose Ranges for Children With Type 1 Diabetes

Timing	Value (mg/dl)
Before a meal	70–110
1 hr after a meal	90–180
2 hr after a meal	80–150
Between 2 AM and 4 AM	70–120

Other Diagnostic Tests. If diabetes is detected, the diagnostic workup also usually includes an analysis of blood samples for pH, partial pressure of carbon dioxide (Pco_2), sodium, and potassium levels; a white blood cell count; and a glycosylated hemoglobin (HbA_{1c}) evaluation. Normally, the hemoglobin in red blood cells carry only a trace of glucose. If serum glucose is excessive, however, excess glucose attaches itself to hemoglobin molecules, creating glycosylated hemoglobin. In nondiabetic children, the usual HbA_{1c} value is 1.8 to 4.0. A value greater than 6.0 reflects an excessive level of serum glucose. Measuring glycosylated hemoglobin has advantages because it not only provides information on what is the child's present serum glucose level but what the serum glucose levels have been during the preceding 3 to 4 months (red blood cells have a life span of 120 days).

If the potassium level of the blood is low, a child may need an electrocardiogram to observe for T-wave abnormalities, the mark of potassium deficiency. The white blood cell count of a child with diabetes may be elevated even though no infection is present, apparently as a response to the ketoacidosis. The presence of infection must always be suspected, however, because it is often a precipitant to a diabetic crisis. For this reason, nose and throat cultures may be obtained as well.

Therapeutic Management

Therapy for children with type 1 diabetes involves five measures: insulin administration, regulation of nutrition and exercise, stress management, and blood glucose and urine ketone monitoring. The standard of care in the United States regarding a child with newly diagnosed diabetes involves a hospital admission of approximately 3 days, which includes extensive education involving caretakers and the child (Schmidt, Bernaix, Chiappetta, et al., 2012).

The Initial Regulation of Insulin. When children are first diagnosed with diabetes, they are usually hyperglycemic and perhaps ketoacidotic. To correct the metabolic imbalance, they are given insulin administered IV at a dose of 0.1 to 0.2 units per kilogram of body weight per hour. This initial IV infusion of insulin is then gradually reduced once the blood glucose level is lower than 200 mg/dl. Ideally, within 12 hours, the acidosis is considerably less than when a child was admitted to the hospital, and the serum glucose level is near the normal range. The insulin given for emergency replacement this way is regular (short-acting) insulin such as Humulin-R, because this is the form that takes effect most quickly.

It may seem that, in a child with diabetes in a state of acidosis, the administration of glucose would not be warranted. Because the child is being given insulin, however, body cells soon become ready to use glucose, so they require, incorporate, and use available glucose quickly. If more glucose is not provided, cells are forced to continue to break down fats and protein, and the acidosis can increase, not decrease. Glucose, therefore, may be added to the infusion.

TABLE 48.4 Common Types of Human Insulin

Preparation	Onset	Peak Effect	Duration of Effect (hr)
Lispro (Humalog)	Immediate	30 min–1 hr	3–4
Aspart	15 min	30–40 min	3–5
Regular (Humulin-R)	0.5–1.0 hr	2–4 hr	5–7
Lantus	1 hr	5 hr	24
Humulin-N	1–2 hr	4–12 hr	24+
Humulin-L	1–3 hr	6–14 hr	24+
Humulin-U	6 hr	16–18 hr	36+

From Karch, A. M. (2013). *2013 Lippincott's nursing drug guide.* Philadelphia, PA: Lippincott Williams & Wilkins.

After 24 hours, as the child's serum glucose returns to normal, oral feedings may replace the IV route. Further management in the days after this first crucial 24-hour period is based on serum glucose determinations. A child may remain on regular insulin given SC alone (given three or four times a day) for the first 1 or 2 days. Typically, intermediate-acting insulin is then added as soon as oral fluids are taken, usually on the second day of therapy.

Insulin Administration. Types of insulin vary as to their time of onset, peak action, and duration of action (Table 48.4). Children can be regulated on a variety of insulin programs, but typically receive a combined insulin dose of 0.4 to 0.7 units per kilogram of body weight daily in two divided doses (one before breakfast and one before dinner); adolescents may need as much as 1.2 units per kilogram daily divided into the two doses. The most common mixture of insulin used with children is a combination of an intermediate-acting insulin and a regular insulin, usually in a 2:1 ratio or 0.75 units of the intermediate-acting insulin to 0.33 units regular insulin, and given in the same syringe, although this prescription varies for individual children. The morning dose is two thirds of the total daily dose; the evening dose is the remaining one third.

The advantage of using two different types of insulin is that the peak effects occur at different times. Because the peak time of short-acting insulins is 3 to 4 hours, the child who takes insulin before breakfast will notice a maximum effect between 10 AM and 12 noon. The peak effect period of the intermediate-acting insulin is 8 to 14 hours, or late afternoon, just before dinner. These are important times to remember because these are the times when a child is most apt to experience symptoms of hypoglycemia.

Some children require a program of insulin therapy that includes three or even four injections daily in order to prevent hyperglycemia. Although these regimens are not popular with children, multiple injections allow for greater variation in activity and calorie consumption.

Part of the education of parents is to allow them to vary their child's insulin doses based on an insulin algorithm or protocol influenced by the child's level of activity and the size of meals consumed for that day (referred to as "thinking scales"). The time between the insulin injection and a meal is known as "lag time." If a child's premeal blood glucose level is above a target range, parents learn that increasing the lag time or delaying the meal will help prevent hyperglycemia. If the blood glucose is low at a premeal test, decreasing the lag time could help prevent hypoglycemia. If it is anticipated that the child will eat an unusually large meal such as at a special birthday dinner, parents can increase the size of the premeal regular insulin injection. If the child is to participate in a strenuous sport in the afternoon that will use glucose, the regular insulin injection can be decreased. Lantus is a new long-acting insulin that is supplied in an injectable pen and lasts 24 hours. A disadvantage of this insulin is its pH, which is so low it cannot be mixed in a syringe with other insulins. In some children, glucose levels can be regulated on Lantus plus three doses of regular insulin before meals.

Injection Technique. Teach parents that when insulins are mixed in one syringe, the regular or short-acting insulin should be drawn into the syringe first. Then, if mixing accidentally occurs in the bottle, the time of effectiveness of the short-acting insulin (which needs to be kept short-acting for emergency treatment) will not be lengthened by the addition of the intermediate-acting insulin.

Insulin is always injected SC except in emergencies, when half the required dose may be given IV. Subcutaneous tissue injection sites used most frequently in children include those of the upper outer arms and the outer aspects of the thighs (Fig. 48.5). The abdominal subcutaneous tissue injection sites commonly

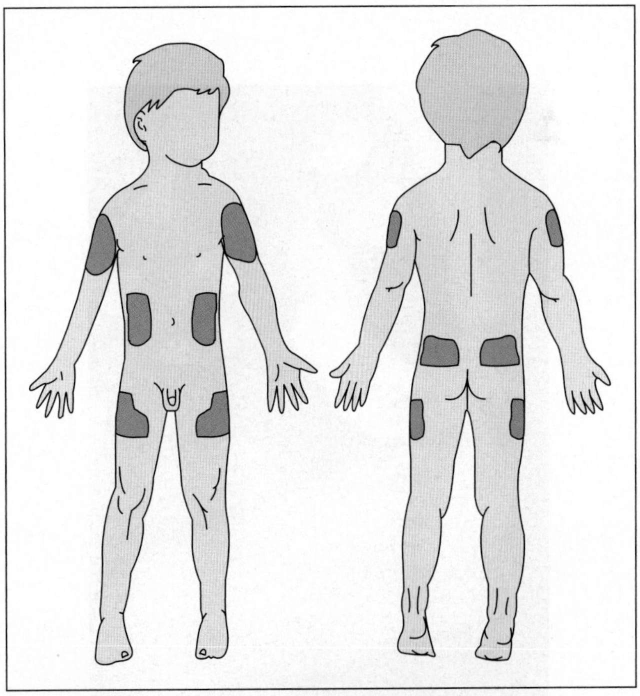

FIGURE 48.5 According to the American Diabetes Association, insulin injection sites in children and adults are the upper outer portions of the arms; the thighs, 4 in. below the hip and 4 in. above the knee (adjusted proportionally for children); and the abdominal area just above and just below the waist. The navel and a circular area just around it are excluded as injection sites. In some children, the abdominal area may not be an appropriate injection site.

used in adults can be adequate sites, but most children dislike this site because abdominal skin is tender. Encourage children or parents to rotate sites in a pattern based on their planned activity. Absorption, for example, is increased if the muscles under the injection site are exercised, so it is best to choose sites that will not be exercised soon after the injection. If a child will be jogging after an injection, for example, the thigh probably should not be used. Similarly, if the child will be playing tennis, the injection probably should not be given in the dominant arm.

Work out a plan of rotation with children so that everyone who will be giving injections knows what injection site should be used next. In the hospital, record the injection site in the child's record or nursing plan, so each nurse can check it before an injection and not repeat an injection site. This is less of a problem now that synthetic human insulin is used, but if the same injection site is used repeatedly, a great deal of subcutaneous atrophy (lipodystrophy) can occur, causing deep pockmarks.

Children quickly learn that, if they continuously give injections in the same site, scar tissue (lipohypertrophy) forms there, and no pain will be felt on injection (a situation sometimes called subcutaneous insulin resistance syndrome [SIRS]). This is a dangerous practice, however, because as lipohypertrophy occurs, insulin no longer absorbs well from the site. To be effective, the dose has to be increased beyond what the child actually needs for glucose metabolism because a portion of each dose is "locked" in the tissue. Should the child then inject this larger dose of insulin into a new site, there is a potential for overdose (which would cause hypoglycemia).

Although parents should keep additional bottles of insulin in the refrigerator to increase the insulin's shelf life, insulin should be administered at room temperature because this diminishes subcutaneous atrophy and ensures peak effectiveness.

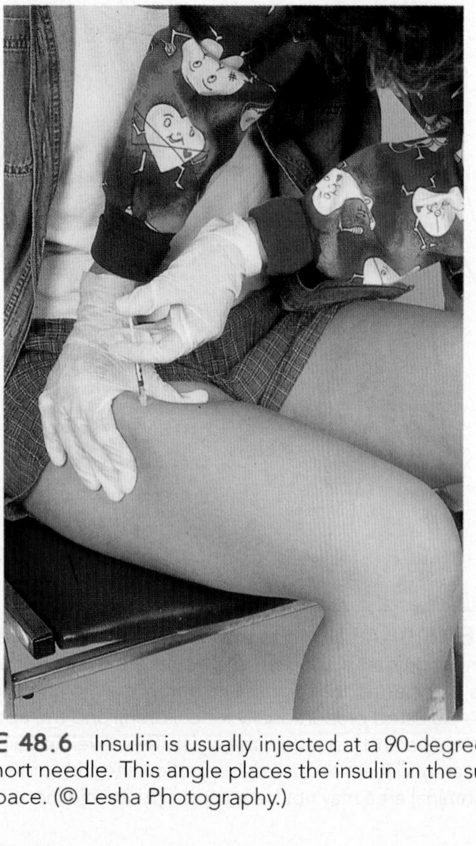

FIGURE 48.6 Insulin is usually injected at a 90-degree angle with a short needle. This angle places the insulin in the subcutaneous space. (© Lesha Photography.)

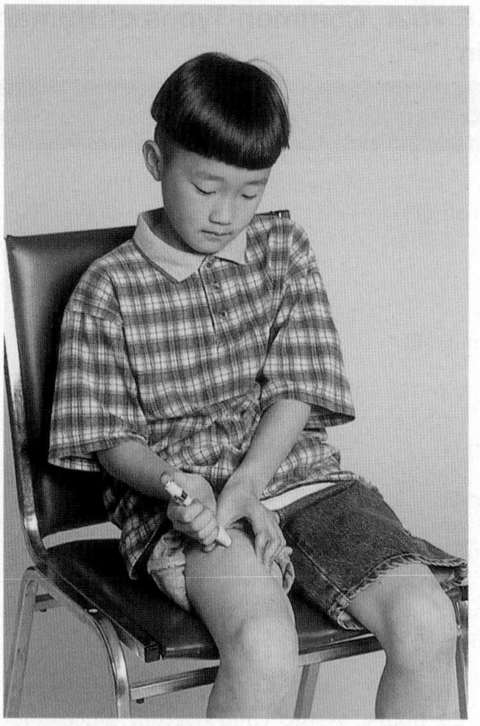

FIGURE 48.7 The injection of insulin by an automatic device. (© Lesha Photography.)

Because a short needle (less than 0.4 in.) is used, insulin can be injected at a 90-degree angle (Fig. 48.6). Although this is not a usual subcutaneous injection technique, because the needle is so short, the insulin will be deposited into the subcutaneous tissue. This technique is easier for children to learn, because it takes less coordination to administer an injection at a 90-degree angle than at a 45-degree subcutaneous angle. Automatic injection devices are available, such as pens and jet injectors, which are easy for children to use, come with prepared doses, promote early independence, and can be given with the 90-degree technique (Fig. 48.7).

Insulin Pumps. An insulin pump is an automatic device approximately the size of an iPhone. It delivers insulin at a constant rate, so it regulates serum glucose levels better than periodic injections (Buchko, Artz, Dayhoff, et al., 2012). To use a pump, a syringe of regular insulin is placed in the pump chamber; a length of thin polyethylene tubing leads to the child's abdomen, where it is implanted into the subcutaneous tissue of the abdomen by a small-gauge needle. Women who develop gestational diabetes also use insulin pumps; therefore, these are illustrated and the care is described in Chapter 20. Most children adjust well to pump therapy and prefer it to daily injections.

Inhalation Insulin. Inhalation insulin is not available as yet but may be in the future; production of it is in experimental trials. Difficulties with development are constructing an accurate delivery system and determining how the development of a cold or allergies that cause edema of the nasal membrane will affect drug absorption (Boss, Petrucci, & Lorber, 2012).

Nutrition. In order to know how much insulin to give before a meal, parents need to learn to count the total carbohydrate

BOX 48.7 Nursing Care Planning Based on Family Teaching

NUTRITIONAL GUIDELINES FOR CHILDREN WITH TYPE 1 DIABETES

Q. Rob's mother is concerned that Rob, as an adolescent, doesn't eat well. She asks you, "How can we make sure our child, who has diabetes, gets adequate nutrition?"

A. Here are some nutritional guidelines to help you:

- Be certain you understand your child's insulin-to-carbohydrate ratio and how to use this to plan meals. As a rule, foods high in carbohydrates are fruit and vegetables, "starchy foods" such as bread or pasta, milk and yogurt, and "sugary" foods such as candy bars or cake.
- Be aware of food portions. The total carbohydrate on a package of pasta refers to what one serving of pasta will contain, not the whole box of pasta.
- Provide three meals throughout the day, plus three snacks. A total daily caloric intake divided to provide 20% as breakfast, 20% as lunch, 30% as dinner, and 10% as morning, afternoon, and evening snacks help distribute carbohydrates throughout the day.
- Do not use dietetic food. This food is expensive and not necessary.
- Urge your child not to omit meals. Getting him to eat at every meal calls for creative planning so he likes the foods served and eats readily.
- Maintain a positive outlook by stressing the foods your child is allowed to eat, not those he should avoid.
- Steer clear of concentrated carbohydrate sources, such as candy bars, and be sure to include foods with adequate fiber, such as broccoli, because fiber helps prevent hyperglycemia.
- Keep complex carbohydrates available to be eaten before exercise, such as swimming or a softball game, to provide a sustained carbohydrate energy source to prevent hypoglycemia.
- Teach children about carbohydrate counting as early as possible so they can wisely select what to eat at school or at a friend's home and can begin independent self-care.

amount in food by carefully reading food labels. An insulin-to-carbohydrate ratio is then calculated individually for each child depending on age and activity to guide insulin administration. For example, if a child is prescribed an insulin-to-carbohydrate ratio of 1 unit of insulin to each 10 g of carbohydrates and the meal the child will be served contains 50 g carbohydrates, the parent would administer 5 units of regular insulin before the meal.

An overall meal pattern should include three spaced meals that are high in fiber plus a snack in the midmorning, midafternoon, and evening to keep carbohydrate amounts as level as possible during the day. Most parents need to meet with a nutritionist to discuss what a "meal high in fiber" means, how to become adept at carbohydrate counting, and what meals are best to serve to their age child. General rules are shown in Box 48.7.

Self-Blood Glucose Monitoring. Children as young as early school age can learn the techniques of finger puncture and reading a computerized monitor. Using a spring-loaded injection pen helps minimize pain; an automatic readout monitor simplifies the procedure (Fig. 48.8). Children are adolescents, however, before they can be counted on to independently monitor their serum glucose levels on a daily basis.

Urine Testing. Urine testing is not used routinely but is used to test for ketonuria if the child develops a gastrointestinal "flu" and is not able to eat. Acetone revealed by a test strip is a sign fat is being used for energy, or that the child is becoming acidotic.

The "Honeymoon" Period. After a child's diagnosis has been confirmed and the blood glucose level has been initially regulated by insulin, a honeymoon period may follow, during which only a minimal amount of insulin, or none at all, is needed for glucose regulation. This apparently occurs because the exogenous insulin stimulates the islet cells to produce a small amount of natural insulin, as if they are being reminded of their function. After a month or even up to a year, however, the islet cells will begin to fail once again, and diabetic symptoms will recur. This can be upsetting to parents if they began to believe their child was wrongly diagnosed or that a cure had taken place. Caution both the parents and the child that symptoms will inevitably recur.

Stress Adjustment. Whenever children with diabetes undergo a stressful situation, either emotionally or physically, they may need increased insulin to maintain glucose homeostasis.

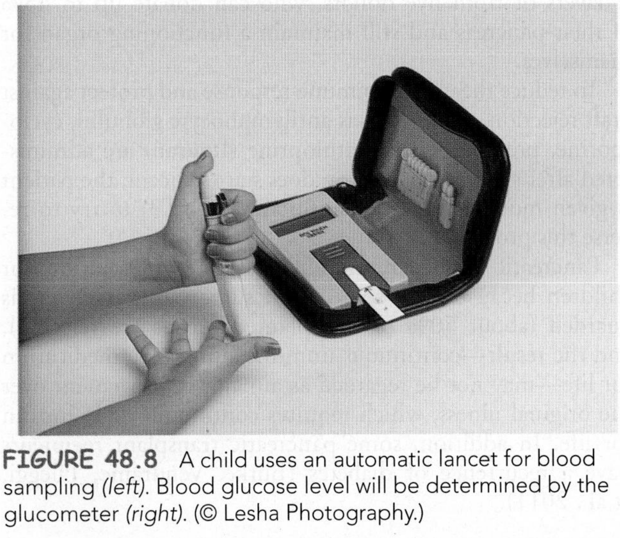

FIGURE 48.8 A child uses an automatic lancet for blood sampling *(left)*. Blood glucose level will be determined by the glucometer *(right)*. (© Lesha Photography.)

When children are seen at health care facilities for periodic checkups, ask them whether they are having any difficulty with blood testing or insulin injection and how things are at home and at school to detect their stress level.

Try to interview children separately from their parents, so they can feel free to talk about anything that may be happening or going wrong. If a child is experiencing stress because of school, parents may have to meet with school officials to help them view the child as well, not ill, so that they will allow participation in all activities, including sports. Sometimes, children are embarrassed to have to do blood glucose testing in school, especially in a public lavatory. It may be easier for them if they can go to the nurse's office for privacy when testing.

Complications. If an infection occurs and the child's temperature rises, insulin resistance increases, causing a need for additional insulin. Teach parents to notify their primary health care provider if their child appears to be ill (particularly if the child is nauseated or vomiting) for careful observation and a change in insulin dosage if necessary. If a child with diabetes is scheduled for surgery, careful regulation on the day of surgery and in the immediate postoperative period is essential, especially if oral fluids will be restricted.

Many long-term body changes such as arteriosclerosis (hardening of artery walls), which can lead to general poor circulation and kidney disease, and thickening of retinal capillaries and cataract formation, which ultimately can result in blindness, occurring because of chronic hyperglycemia, are not a major part of disease management in childhood because their onset does not begin until adulthood. It is not too early, however, when discussing hyperglycemia to mention that it does have long-term effects if not regulated beginning in childhood.

Pancreas Transplantation. For children who develop severe kidney disease or arteriosclerosis, pancreas transplantation may be considered to prevent further damage. In contrast to other organ transplantation procedures, the child's pancreas is not removed entirely prior to transplant. This is because the portion that supplies digestive enzymes is still functioning and so is left in place. The digestive enzymes of the new pancreas are diverted into the intestine or bladder, or the pancreatic ducts can be sclerosed so the digestive enzymes do not leave the transplanted organ. Grafts may be taken from cadavers or from live donors, who can donate up to 45% of their pancreas and still maintain a functioning organ for themselves.

To reduce the child's immune response and protect against graft rejection, drugs such as antilymphocyte globulin, cyclosporine, prednisone, or azathioprine (Imuran) are administered after surgery. If rejection does start to occur, the patient is given monoclonal T-cell antibodies (OKT3) to try to reverse this process.

Pancreatic transplantation is a last resort solution for children because it involves major surgery, the outcome is guarded (about 50% of transplanted organs are rejected), and the result—continuous immunosuppressive medication for life—may not be regarded as a major improvement over the original illness, which requires continuous daily insulin for life. In addition, some pancreatic transplant recipients have a recurrence of diabetes (Burke, Vendrame, Pileggi, et al., 2011).

Nursing Diagnoses and Related Interventions

Nursing Diagnosis: Health-seeking behaviors related to self-administration of insulin, balanced exercise, and nutrition

Outcome Evaluation: Child demonstrates insulin injection technique to nurse, describes steps correctly, and discusses plans for an exercise and nutrition program.

Self-Administration of Insulin: From about 8 years of age, children can be taught to administer their own insulin (Fig. 48.9). Many children younger than this do not have the dexterity to handle a syringe or an understanding of the importance of sterile technique and proper dosage. They may skip injections if they are tired or busy.

Do not underestimate how difficult it is for children to learn to give injections to themselves. Although it may seem like a two-step process (draw up the medication, and then inject it), in actuality, more than 25 steps are involved.

If the child has to mix insulins, the number of steps increases. Besides lacking dexterity and adult-level fine motor skills, children have to face injecting themselves. There is no such thing as getting used to injections. Children grow used to the *idea* of self-injection, not to the injections themselves.

Even if children are taught to give their own insulin from the beginning, at least one adult in the family should be taught to give it as well. There will be days when the child refuses to administer his or her own insulin or is not feeling well and needs to have or appreciates having someone administer it. Parents may have a hard time giving their child a painful injection; teaching them to view it as a helping action helps to alleviate their distress.

Exercise: Exercise is an important component of care because it uses up carbohydrates and helps reduce

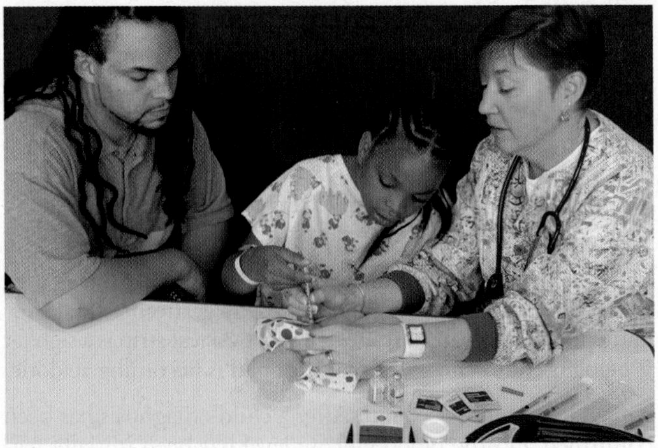

FIGURE 48.9 A school-age child practices insulin administration using a teaching doll for practice.

hyperglycemia. No type of exercise is restricted for children with diabetes. A problem that arises with vigorous exercise, however, is the development of hypoglycemia due to increased absorption of insulin from the injection site and use of glucose by active body cells. One way to minimize this effect is to choose the injection site that is least likely to be exercised. Another method is to eat additional carbohydrates or decrease the regular insulin injection according to an established protocol before exercise.

Teach children to design a consistent daily exercise program such as briskly walking the dog or 10 minutes of aerobics every day before school. Once a daily program is established, the child needs to continue this type of exercise every day (including weekends) to avoid becoming hyperglycemic on days of no exercise. If this process is not explained, parents may attempt to keep the child relatively quiet, unaware that exercise is actually healthful.

Hygiene: Skin care, particularly foot care, is extremely important for adults with diabetes, because arteriosclerosis causes loss of circulation to the feet, and decreased circulation leads to poor healing ability. This is not as important a concern with children, but they (and all children) should be taught to cut their toenails straight across, to prevent ingrown toenails, and to tend to cuts and scrapes promptly so that healing can begin right away. Properly fitted shoes are essential. Girls may need to be reminded of good perineal care to prevent vaginal infections.

Nursing Diagnosis: Parental anxiety related to newly diagnosed diabetes mellitus in their child

Outcome Evaluation: Parents accurately describe their child's illness and treatment and ways in which the disease will affect their lifestyle. They state a specific plan for daily routine child care and identify potential problems in the schedule and ways they can be managed.

Parents whose child is newly diagnosed with diabetes mellitus have a great deal of new responsibility. Be certain they have the telephone number of the health care facility, liaison, or home care person to call during the first days of home management so they have someone to consult before they give insulin the first several times.

Encourage the Expression of Feelings: Although parents may be aware that other family members have the disease, they may be surprised that diabetes has occurred in their child. Both the parents and the child need time to describe their perception of diabetes. If there are other family members with the illness, children may have heard many false stories about the disorder and may have been told how difficult it was in the past to achieve insulin control. These misconceptions need to be corrected so children can begin to accept their diagnosis and view themselves as basically well except for faulty insulin release.

What if...48.2 Rob wants to try out for soccer on his school team, but the soccer coach thinks children with diabetes should be excluded from sports. Because Rob doesn't always take his insulin reliably, would you agree with the coach?

Establish a Mode of Supervision and Support: Children with diabetes need frequent health supervision visits, approximately every 3 months. Those who appear to accept their diagnosis initially may have difficulty later, when their true feelings about their disorder surface. When they reach adolescence and are rebelling against a multitude of things, they may choose to rebel against blood glucose testing and insulin administration. Assess that children with diabetes have supportive friends to help them through "bad days." Make sure the parents can identify support people and others to contact if they have problems or questions. Sometimes what is needed most from health care personnel is understanding and appreciation of the difficulties encountered by children living with diabetes.

Teach Hypoglycemic Management: An episode of hypoglycemia is an extremely serious condition and must be prevented, if possible, because if it is not recognized and treated, it can lead to coma and seizures. Severe glucose depletion can lead to permanent brain damage with mental and motor impairment, because brain cells need glucose for metabolism.

Symptoms of hypoglycemia occur when the blood glucose level falls to about 60 mg/dl. At this point, there is no glycosuria. It results from the administration of too much insulin, excessive exercise (because exercise uses up glucose), or failure to eat enough food. Typically, beginning symptoms include nervousness, weakness, dizziness, sweating, or tremors. In many children, the first signs of hypoglycemia are behavior problems: temper tantrums, stubbornness, silliness, irritability, or simply "not acting like usual self." A few children become insensitive to the symptoms of hypoglycemia (termed *hypoglycemia unawareness*) and are then unable to recognize that it is occurring. Such children need more blood glucose determinations built into their routine.

When the signs of hypoglycemia are recognized, a child needs an immediate source of carbohydrates. Fifteen grams of a fast-acting carbohydrate such as that contained in a half glass of orange juice or regular soda is recommended. It is easy for children always to carry glucose tablets or hard candy such as Lifesavers with them to have them available for these times. If there is no improvement in symptoms and the blood glucose level has not risen by 15 mg/dl after 15 minutes, more carbohydrates (perhaps juice) should be given.

If the child is comatose when first discovered or is too upset or uncooperative to take oral sugar, parents can inject a specified dose of glucagon hydrochloride intramuscularly. This converts the glycogen that is stored in the liver into glucose. Usually, enough glycogen is converted after the drug injection to bring the child out of the coma, after which an oral form of glucose can be given. The drug will not be effective, however, if the child's supply of glycogen is depleted.

If parents cannot give their child an injection and oral sugar cannot be given, honey, corn syrup, cake icing gel, or glucose can be rubbed onto the gums or inside the cheek (of course, parents should be taught how to prevent aspiration) or corn syrup can be given as an enema. As soon as children are out of the coma or are cooperative, they should take a source of complex carbohydrates, such as crackers or whole wheat toast, to prevent further hypoglycemia. The primary health care provider needs to be notified of the incident so that its cause can be determined and steps can be taken to prevent hypoglycemia from occurring again.

Urge parents to anticipate occasions when hypoglycemia is likely to occur and to take preventive measures if possible. Hypoglycemia is most likely to occur, for example, at the peak effective time of the insulins being given, such as just before lunch or just before dinner. This means that many children who are attending school need to be scheduled for the first lunch period, not the second, or need a snack before lunch. Encourage the child and parents to discuss lunch times with the school nurse so appropriate meal planning is coordinated with the child's insulin schedule. Follow-ups at 6-month intervals are important so adjustments to account for changes in growth and school schedules can be made.

If children are going to engage in an active sport, such as swimming, tennis, or basketball, they should ingest a source of sugar before participation. This precaution is extremely important before swimming because a child who suddenly becomes weak in the middle of a pool may be unable to reach the side safely. Although eating before swimming is something that children typically are taught not to do, the child with diabetes must be taught to break this rule. This should be done sensibly, of course—before swimming, the child should eat a complex carbohydrate, such as crackers, not a full meal. Day and residential camps are available to help children learn more about diabetes and common measures other athletic children use to prevent hypoglycemia.

Occasionally, insulin overuse and persistent hypoglycemia cause a rebound hyperglycemic response; this is referred to as the **Somogyi phenomenon**. This phenomenon is suspected when children have nighttime (2 AM or 3 AM) hypoglycemia followed by high early-morning hyperglycemia. These children need to be referred to their health care provider because they actually need less insulin rather than more to correct the problem.

Teach Signs of Ketoacidosis: Because hyperglycemia leads to diabetic **ketoacidosis** (DKA), it is a metabolic emergency (Donahey & Folse, 2012). It may be difficult for parents to distinguish between hypoglycemia (occurring from too much insulin) and hyperglycemia (occurring from too little insulin for the level of glucose present in the bloodstream) because hyperglycemia presents with almost the same symptoms as hypoglycemia: irritability, vomiting and abdominal pain, and behavior changes such as temper tantrums.

If a parent does not know whether the problem is hypoglycemia or hyperglycemia, the child should be offered a carbohydrate, as if the problem were hypoglycemia. This is because the added carbohydrate will do no harm if the problem is already hyperglycemia, whereas giving insulin is harmful if the cause is hypoglycemia. An inability to void is a good clue that the problem is hypoglycemia because, with hyperglycemia, urine output is copious—one of the primary signs of diabetes. The real key to differentiating ketoacidosis from hypoglycemia, however, is the blood glucose level. Assessing the blood glucose concentration by finger stick solves the problem of whether symptoms relate to hypoglycemia or hyperglycemia. For quick reference, a comparison of hypoglycemia and hyperglycemia is shown in Table 48.5.

If ketoacidosis is not relieved when it first begins, it becomes severe with deep and rapid respirations (Kussmaul breathing) as the body attempts to "blow off" carbon dioxide and lessen the acidotic state. The child's breath smells sweet because of the presence of ketone bodies, and the pulse rate may be rapid. Signs of dehydration, including dry mucous membranes and skin, sunken eyeballs, and no tears, may be present. This is typically the picture when children are first diagnosed as having diabetes. It is also seen in children with diabetes who develop gastroenteritis and so eat poorly for several meals. Because the child is not eating well, parents may omit giving insulin. In actuality, because of an increased metabolic rate due to fever, parents need to consult with their primary care provider because the child may need more insulin and glucose than usual during these times. Box 48.8 shows an interprofessional care map for a child with diabetes type 1 to show how aspects of care need coordination.

QSEN Checkpoint Question 48.4

Teamwork & Collaboration

Rob tells you that when he was first diagnosed with diabetes mellitus, he experienced a "honeymoon" period. You would want all of your team members to recognize that this would be demonstrated by which of the following signs?

a. He developed an unnatural craving for sweets.
b. His metabolism increased because of glucose stimulation.
c. He became lightheaded or "giddy" every afternoon.
d. His need for injected insulin was drastically reduced.

Look in Appendix A for the best answer and rationale.

TABLE 48.5 Comparison of Hypoglycemia and Hyperglycemia

Comparison Factor	Hypoglycemia	Hyperglycemia
Cause	Excessive insulin injection Limited food intake Excessive exercise	Inadequate insulin injection Excessive food intake Stress from infection, surgery, etc.
Symptoms	Hunger Lethargy and sensorial changes Sweating Pallor Seizures Coma	Glycosuria and ketonuria Polyuria, polydipsia; vomiting Kussmaul respirations Flushing and dehydration Sweet (acetone) breath Lowered sodium, potassium, bicarbonate, chloride, and phosphate levels; decreased CO_2 combining power Coma
Danger	Brain cells need glucose for function and survival	Fatty acids used and ketoacidosis develops
Major nursing interventions	Administration of source of glucose by oral or intravenous route Education to prevent recurrences	Reestablishment of electrolyte balance and hydration Education to prevent recurrences

BOX 48.8 Nursing Care Planning

AN INTERPROFESSIONAL CARE MAP FOR AN ADOLESCENT WITH TYPE 1 DIABETES MELLITUS

Rob Tebecco is a 16-year-old boy with type 1 diabetes whom you meet in the emergency department, where he was taken after he became comatose while ice skating. He has had diabetes since he was 7 years of age; he was managing his insulin administration well up until 6 months ago when he began to "forget" to take his insulin at least once a week. When you ask him about this, he tells you ice skating practice every morning and a new girlfriend have occupied his time and interrupted what used to be a strict schedule of home-cooked meals and a rigid routine.

Family Assessment Adolescent lives with one younger sister and parents. Father works as Zamboni operator at a professional hockey arena. Mother works part time at the local post office. Family rates finances as, "We have everything we need."

Client Assessment Child was skating at local ice rink when he suddenly collapsed. Was brought to the emergency department by the emergency medical technician service, unconscious and breathing deeply. Breath smelled sweet. Blood glucose was 700 mg/dl. Received regular insulin intravenously (IV). As soon as blood glucose returned to normal, he regained consciousness. Arterial blood gases: pH, 7.20; Pco_2, 10 mmHg; HCO_3, 10 mEq/ml. Right heel has red and inflamed ulcer.

Currently takes short-acting and intermediate-acting insulin every morning before breakfast and again before dinner with self-injection device. Child performs finger-stick blood glucose levels four times a day. Blood glucose levels normally range between 105 and 115 mg/dl. Dietary history reveals three meals per day with midmorning, afternoon, and bedtime snack. Rob states, "Okay. I'm ready to do better. That was scary to black out."

Nursing Diagnosis Health-seeking behaviors related to need to follow a more conscientious diabetes regimen.

Outcome Evaluation Child and parents voice intention to be more conscientious about insulin administration and serum glucose testing. Child voices willingness to try insulin pump therapy.

Team Member Responsible	Assessment	Intervention	Rationale	Expected Outcome
Activities of Daily Living, Including Safety				
Nurse	Explore with child and parents their understanding of the interrelationship of nutrition, exercise, and diabetes.	Review and reinforce the importance of insulin administration, blood glucose monitoring, and exercise.	Explore and provide baseline information for identifying teaching needs and developing possible strategies.	Adolescent and parent state they understand new regimen; glucose levels do not fluctuate higher than 126 mg/dl.

(continued on page 1422)

BOX 48.8 Nursing Care Planning (continued)

Teamwork and Collaboration				
Nurse/Primary care provider	Assess whether adolescent would be a good candidate for insulin pump therapy to increase adherence.	Consult with diabetic service team to present the new method of insulin administration.	Use of an insulin pump offers a continuous supply of insulin; can be advantageous for busy adolescent.	Diabetic service team meets with adolescent and parent to present possibility of using insulin pump.
Procedures/Medications for Quality Improvement				
Nurse	Assess adolescent's level of understanding about the action of insulin with pump therapy.	Demonstrate and observe the adolescent draw up and refill the insulin syringe, and begin insulin pump infusion.	Adolescent's return demonstration best reveals whether he understands how to maintain the insulin pump.	Adolescent demonstrates proper preparation and administration of the insulin pump.
Nutrition				
Nurse/Nutritionist	Assess adolescent's usual meal pattern; determine who prepares food and whether adolescent counts carbohydrates.	Review importance of regular meals plus a bedtime snack to keep glucose within consistent levels with the insulin pump.	Irregular meal patterns can cause hypoglycemia with pump therapy.	Parents and adolescent state they will try to estimate carbohydrate count better; adolescent will test blood glucose according to set schedule.
Patient-Centered Care				
Nurse/Diabetic service team member	Assess whether adolescent and parents are aware of actions to take if hypoglycemic symptoms should occur with pump therapy.	Review signs and symptoms of hypoglycemia; review need to always carry a source of carbohydrate.	Having a readily available source of carbohydrate helps raise blood glucose levels quickly should hypoglycemia occur.	Adolescent and parents describe signs of hypoglycemia and action of carbohydrates to prevent this.
Nurse/Diabetic service team member	Assess whether adolescent and parents are aware of necessity to safeguard feet against trauma.	Review necessity to wear properly fitting shoes and skates and to clean any cuts or scrapes promptly.	Diabetes can result in decreased circulation to the feet and slowed healing, increasing the possibility for infection, which can ultimately affect glucose control.	Adolescent states he will be more conscientious about foot care; acknowledges foot infection may have contributed to his ketoacidosis episode.
Psychosocial/Spiritual/Emotional Needs				
Nurse/Nurse practitioner	Assess whether child's busy schedule allows for adequate diabetic control.	Encourage parents to discuss adolescent's needs with him and ways he could modify his schedule to better accommodate his diabetic routine.	Poor medicine adherence may be a way adolescents express their identity.	Parents and child plot out a weekly schedule that allows both freedom for new activities and for conscientious diabetic care.
Informatics for Seamless Health Care Planning				
Nurse	Assess whether child has experience with keeping a diabetic care journal.	Suggest the adolescent keeps a written diary of blood glucose levels, dietary intake (including snacks), and any symptoms of hypo- or hyperglycemia.	A written diary provides objective evidence for evaluating the new regimen and can indicate the need for possible changes or adjustments.	Adolescent agrees to keep a detailed journal until returning to clinic for a follow-up visit.
Nurse	Assess whether the adolescent or parents have any additional questions.	Arrange for a follow-up appointment in 1 week; encourage adolescent and parents to call with any questions or concerns.	Follow-up visit provides a means for evaluating the effectiveness of the new regimen and child's adaptation.	Adolescent and parents state they understand importance of follow-up visit for regulation of insulin pump therapy.

Type 2 Diabetes Mellitus

T2D, characterized by diminished insulin secretion, is a separate disease from type 1 diabetes because it is not caused by autoimmune factors (Sherr & Weinzimer, 2012). Usually, children with T2D do not need daily insulin because their disease can be managed with diet alone or with diet and an oral hypoglycemic agent. Once thought to occur only in older adults, T2D is now seen as early as in overweight school-aged children (Caprio, 2012). Other influencing factors are a strong family history of diabetes; children from African, Hispanic, Asian, or Native Indian descent; those who eat a diet high in fats and carbohydrates; and those who do not exercise regularly. Development of polycystic ovary syndrome (PCOS) (see Chapter 8) is also strongly associated with the disorder. At the time of diagnosis, it may not be possible for the classification to be correctly determined because symptoms and findings are so similar.

Symptoms often become apparent for the first time at puberty because increasing sex hormones naturally increase insulin resistance, creating a need for more insulin production. Children's urine will show glucose but few ketones. Children experience lessened amounts of thirst or increased urination. About 90% of children with T2D have dark shiny patches on the skin (*acanthosis nigricans*), which are most often found between the fingers and between the toes, on the back of the neck ("dirty neck"), and in axillary creases (Stephen, Gungor, & Douty, 2012). Children whose family has a history of T2D, are from susceptible genetic groups, or have symptoms such as acanthosis nigricans or high blood pressure should be screened by a fasting blood sugar test at puberty and again every 2 years.

With this type of diabetes, because the pancreatic islet cells are still able to minimally function, the pancreas continues to secrete at least small amounts of insulin. Therapy, therefore, consists of nutrition and exercise, the same as for type 1 diabetes, combined with an oral antiglycemic agent such as a biguanide (Metformin), which decreases the amount of glucose produced by the liver and increases insulin sensitivity in both the liver and muscle cells.

T2D is a chronic condition that will extend into adulthood and be present for life. Eventfully it leads to atherosclerosis with thickening of arteries and capillaries, kidney disease, poor healing ability, and blindness because of poor circulation to body organs. In order to prevent these complications, children who develop T2D need good instruction in how to manage their illness so, whether they are home with their parents supervising their care or away from home at camp or college, they can prevent hyperglycemia and the irritation to blood vessels which that causes.

QSEN Checkpoint Question 48.5

Safety

Rob needs to adjust his regular insulin dose to the amount of carbohydrates he eats in order to prevent dangerous complications of his disease. If his insulin-to-carbohydrate ratio is 1:10, how many units of insulin should he inject if his lunch will consist of a hotdog on a bun (24 g), 1 cup chicken noodle soup (7 g), an apple (19 g), and a glass of milk (25 g)?

a. 3 units
b. 7.5 units
c. 9 units
d. 12 units

Look in Appendix A for the best answer and rationale.

THE PARATHYROID GLANDS

The four parathyroid glands, located posterior and adjacent to the thyroid gland, regulate serum levels of calcium in the body by controlling the rate of bone metabolism through the secretion of parathyroid hormone. This hormone is unique in that it is not under the control of the pituitary gland, but rather is controlled by a negative feedback from the circulating serum levels of calcium and how much vitamin D is present to allow absorption of calcium from the gastrointestinal tract into the bloodstream.

Hypocalcemia

Hypocalcemia is a lowered blood calcium level that occurs to some extent in all newborns before they begin sucking well. It occurs because phosphorus and calcium levels are always maintained in an inverse proportion to each other in the bloodstream (if phosphorus levels rise, calcium levels decrease, and vice versa). Hypocalcemia may be caused, therefore, by a change in either calcium or phosphorus metabolism (Thomas, Smith, White, et al., 2012).

Assessment

Hypocalcemia tends to occur in infants who experienced birth anoxia (phosphorus is released with anoxia), in immature infants (the parathyroid glands are immature), and in infants of women with diabetes (it tends to accompany the hypoglycemia that occurs in these infants shortly after birth).

The chief sign of hypocalcemia is neuromuscular irritability, referred to as **latent tetany**. This occurs if the blood calcium level falls below 7.5 mg/dl. The newborn will demonstrate jitteriness when handled or if the infant has been crying for an extended period.

Four methods are used to produce the clinical manifestations of tetany for diagnosis, as shown in Table 48.6. Any of these tests are helpful in determining whether a newborn's jitteriness is a result of hypocalcemia or a central nervous system concern.

If the blood calcium level falls well below 7 mg/dl, **manifest tetany** may result, which is commonly observed as muscular twitching and a **carpopedal spasm** (abduction of the hand and flexion of the wrist with the thumb positioned across the palm). In **pedal spasm** (foot spasm), the foot is extended, the

TABLE 48.6 Tests for Detection of Hypocalcemia

Sign	Description
Chvostek	When skin anterior to external ear (just over sixth cranial nerve) is tapped, facial muscles surrounding eye, nose, and mouth contract unilaterally.
Trousseau	When upper arm is constricted by tourniquet for 2–3 min and area becomes blanched, carpal spasm is elicited (hand abducts, wrist flexes, thumb is positioned across cupped palm).
Peroneal	When fibular side of leg over peroneal nerve is tapped, foot abducts and dorsiflexes.

toes flex, and the sole of the foot cups. Without therapy at this point, generalized seizures or spasm of the larynx, with the infant emitting a high-pitched, crowing sound on inspiration, can occur. If the spasm is prolonged, respirations may cease.

Therapeutic Management

Treatment is aimed at increasing the calcium level in the blood above the point of latent tetany. This can be administered orally as 10% calcium chloride if the infant can and will suck. Otherwise, it will be given IV as a 10% solution of calcium gluconate. Newborns who are having generalized seizures may require anticonvulsant therapy in addition to the calcium gluconate to halt the seizures. Emergency equipment for intubation to relieve laryngospasm should be available.

After immediate therapy to increase the low blood calcium levels, infants are given oral calcium therapy until their calcium level stabilizes at greater than 7.5 mg/dl. Because vitamin D is necessary for the absorption of calcium from the gastrointestinal tract, the infant also may be given a vitamin D supplement such as calcitriol.

METABOLIC DISORDERS (INBORN ERRORS OF METABOLISM)

Many causes of hormonal deficiency or excess in children are not related to the endocrine glands and the highly complex system of feedback and communication between these glands and the pituitary, but rather are due to inherited biochemical disorders that disrupt the metabolism of amino acids, proteins, carbohydrates, or lipids. Many of these disorders are evident at or soon after birth and can cause irreversible cognitive challenge and early death, making early detection and treatment crucial. Gene therapy is expected to be available in the future to reverse symptoms of these disorders (van Karnebeek & Stockler, 2012).

Phenylketonuria

PKU is a disease of metabolism, which is inherited as an autosomal recessive trait. The infant lacks the liver enzyme phenylalanine hydroxylase, which is necessary to convert phenylalanine, an essential amino acid, into tyrosine (a precursor of epinephrine, thyroxine, and melanin). As a result, excessive phenylalanine levels build up in the bloodstream and tissues, causing permanent damage to brain tissue and leaving children severely cognitively challenged.

The metabolite phenylpyruvic acid (a breakdown product of phenylalanine) spills into the urine to give the disorder its name. It causes urine to have a typical musty or "mousy" odor that is so strong that it often pervades not only the urine but the entire child.

As the disease progresses, because tyrosine is necessary for building body pigment and thyroxine, the child becomes blue eyed with very fair skin and light blonde hair. Without adequate thyroxine, the child fails to meet average growth standards. Many children develop an accompanying seizure disorder. The skin is prone to eczema (atopic dermatitis). There is such a strong association between these two disorders that all infants with atopic dermatitis need to be rescreened for PKU at a well-child visit (Millington & Thalange, 2013).

PKU is found in 1 of every 10,000 births in the United States; it occurs rarely in people of African or Jewish ancestry. If the condition remains untreated, the child will be left with an IQ below 20, muscular hypertonicity and spasticity, and possible recurrent seizures. PKU cannot be detected by amniocentesis as a routine screening measure because the phenylalanine level does not rise in utero while the infant is still under the control of the mother's enzyme system. Recombinant DNA techniques can be used for carrier detection and prenatal diagnosis from maternal serum.

Assessment

Early identification of the disorder is essential to prevent the child from becoming severely cognitively challenged. Because of this, all infants in the United States are screened at birth by blood spot analysis after receiving 2 full days of breast or formula feedings. If an infant is born at home or is discharged from a hospital or birthing center before the second day of life, remind the parents to have the test performed on the second or third day after birth. If a newborn did not suck well, so there is a question as to whether the baby received adequate milk for the test to be effective, the test can be repeated at the second week of life during a health care visit.

Therapeutic Management

Dietary restriction has been the main treatment of PKU for over 50 years and still remains the main therapy. In addition to this, large neutral amino acids have been suggested as an alternative treatment to improve outcomes (van Spronsen, de Groot, Hoeksma, et al., 2010). The drug sapropterin (Kuvan), which works by increasing tolerance to phenylalanine, has been approved by the U.S. Food and Drug Administration (FDA) for treatment (Cunningham, Bausell, Brown, et al., 2012).

To begin dietary regulation, infants in whom this disease is detected during the first few days of life are placed on a formula that is extremely low in phenylalanine, such as Lofenalac. A dietitian may recommend a mother who wants to breastfeed do so on a limited basis so the child does receive some phenylalanine (this essential amino acid is necessary for growth and repair of body cells). Unfortunately, a low amino acid formula can cause stools to be loose and has a rather disagreeable taste; therefore, some infants may resist drinking the formula after tasting breast milk.

Providing nutrition for a child with PKU becomes a difficult task as the child grows older because there is no natural protein with both a low phenylalanine concentration and normal levels of other essential amino acids. This means dietary management of PKU must consist of a balancing act between the child consuming enough nutrition to support growth and development and not consuming enough protein to increase the blood phenylalanine level (MacDonald, Rocha, van Rijn, et al., 2011).

Foods highest in phenylalanine are those that are rich in protein, such as meats, eggs, and milk. Foods low in phenylalanine include orange juice, bananas, potatoes, lettuce, spinach, and peas. A formula such as Lofenalac can be used to prepare treat foods, such as ice cream, milk shakes, birthday cakes, and puddings (foods that would otherwise be forbidden because they are made with milk). Children need their blood and urine monitored frequently for phenylalanine levels (which should be below 8 mg/dl). Hemoglobin levels should also be closely monitored to ensure the child is not becoming anemic, because iron is found primarily in protein-rich foods, which the child must avoid. Because the diet tends to be high in carbohydrates to replace protein, children need to be screened for obesity at health care visits as well.

Be certain to offer parents the opportunity to express their feelings about the difficulty of maintaining a young child on such a restricted diet. Also assess the child's ability to cope with the illness because, by the time they reach adolescence, they tend to grow very tired of the constant testing and restrictive diet.

What if...48.3 You are helping at a preschool and notice a teacher's assistant urging Rob's cousin Mike, who has PKU, to drink his milk. When you suggest milk might not be good for him, the assistant says, "Of course it is. Milk is nature's perfect food." How would you respond, knowing it's only one time and one glass of milk?

At one time, it was thought children could discontinue the diet when they reached adolescence to solve the problem of compliance. The current advice is for children to follow the diet indefinitely, therefore, because discontinuing the diet may lead to some detrimental consequences, such as a lack of muscle strength. A woman who has PKU must anticipate when she wants to have children as an adult; if she has not been following her diet conscientiously, she needs to return to a strict low-phenylalanine diet for about 3 months before conception and must remain on the diet for the duration of pregnancy (see Chapter 13). Otherwise, her fetus will be exposed to high levels of phenylalanine during pregnancy and will be born cognitively challenged.

Maple Syrup Urine Disease

Maple syrup urine disease is a rare disorder, inherited as an autosomal recessive trait, in which there is a defect in metabolism of the amino acids leucine, isoleucine, and valine, which leads to cerebral degeneration similar to that observed in children with PKU.

Infants who have the disorder appear well at birth but quickly begin to show signs of feeding difficulty, loss of the Moro reflex, and irregular respirations. The symptoms progress rapidly to *opisthotonos*, generalized muscular rigidity, and seizures. If the condition remains untreated, an infant may die of the disease as early as 2 to 4 weeks of age. Fortunately, prenatal detection is possible by analyzing cells obtained by amniocentesis or from maternal serum (Drake & Gibson, 2010). Also, like PKU, all infants in the United States are screened at birth for the disorder (Chen, Mei, Kalman, et al., 2012).

Although the disorder is rare, it is mentioned here because nurses are the health care personnel who are often the first ones to detect the disorder because, on the first or second day of life, the urine of the child develops the characteristic odor of maple syrup (hence the name of the disease) due to the presence of ketoacids. Being aware of the disorder prevents discounting the pleasant urine odor not as an innocent finding but as the mark of a severe metabolic disorder.

Therapeutic Management

If maple syrup urine disease is diagnosed during the first day or two of life and the child is placed on a well-controlled diet that is high in thiamine and low in the amino acids leucine, isoleucine, and valine, cerebral degeneration can be prevented, just as it can be prevented in PKU. Such a diet is extremely difficult to maintain, however, because of its low protein content. Parents need intensive nutritional counseling. Hemodialysis or peritoneal dialysis may be necessary to temporarily reduce abnormal serum levels at birth or during a childhood infection, when catabolism of cells releases increased amino acids into the bloodstream.

Galactosemia

Galactosemia is a disorder of carbohydrate metabolism that is characterized by abnormal amounts of galactose in the blood (*galactosemia*) and in the urine (*galactosuria*). It occurs in about 1 in every 60,000 births, most often as an inborn error of metabolism, which is transmitted as an autosomal recessive trait. The child is deficient in the liver enzyme galactose-1-phosphate uridyltransferase (Listernick, 2012).

Lactose (the sugar found in milk) normally is broken down into galactose and glucose; galactose is then further broken down into additional glucose. Without the galactose 1-phosphate uridyltransferase enzyme, this second step, the conversion of galactose into glucose, cannot take place, and galactose builds up in the bloodstream and spills out into the urine. When it reaches toxic levels in the bloodstream, it destroys body cells.

Assessment

Symptoms appear as soon as the child begins formula or breastfeeding and include lethargy, hypotonia, and perhaps diarrhea and vomiting. The liver enlarges as cirrhosis develops. Jaundice is often present and persistent, and bilateral cataracts develop. If the condition remains untreated, symptoms can worsen so rapidly, a child may die by 3 days of age. Untreated children who survive beyond this time may be cognitively challenged and have bilateral cataracts.

Diagnosis is made by measuring the level of the affected enzyme in the red blood cells. A screening test (the Beutler test) can be used to analyze cord blood if a child is known to be at risk for the disorder.

Therapeutic Management

The treatment of galactosemia consists of placing the infant on a diet free of galactose or giving the child formula made with milk substitutes such as casein hydrolysates (Nutramigen). Once the child's condition is regulated on this diet, symptoms of the disease do not progress; however, any neurologic or cataract damage that is already present will persist. The duration of the restricted diet is controversial, but probably should be followed for life.

QSEN Checkpoint Question 48.6

Evidence-Based Practice

Because parents have so much influence on how children adjust to having a long-term illness, researchers administered a questionnaire to a total of 185 parents with children 1 to 19 years of age divided into three groups: one where the children had either PKU or galactosemia; one where the children were healthy; and a third group where the children had a chronic illness, which was likely to interfere with a long life span. Results of the study revealed that the parents of children with PKU or galactosemia rated their quality of life equal with that of parents of healthy children, and far above that of parents whose child could have a short life span. Factors that influenced their quality of life most were the presence of support people (a positive effect) and loss of friends (a negative effect) (Ten Hoedt, Maurice-Stam, Boelen, et al., 2011).

Based on the previous study, which comment by LaRoya, a 12-year-old girl who comes to your clinic because she has galactosemia, would make you believe her family's quality life is not ideal?

a. "My mother still loves to cook, although no one comes over anymore."
b. "We go to church every Sunday; my dad helps teach church school."
c. "We've lived in the same house for 10 years; the carpet is getting old."
d. "My grandmother is hard of hearing, so we have to shout so she hears us."

Look in Appendix A for the best answer and rationale.

Glycogen Storage Disease

Glycogen storage disease refers to a group of genetically transmitted disorders that involve altered production and use of glycogen in the body. Twelve of the 13 described types are inherited as autosomal recessive traits; the other is a sex-linked disorder.

Glycogen is normally stored in the liver to provide a reserve supply of glucose. When the body needs glucose for energy, this glycogen is transformed back to glucose. In children with glycogen storage disease, glycogen is deposited normally, but an enzyme deficiency prevents retransformation of the glycogen back to glucose.

In one form of this disorder (type II, or Pompe disease), children deposit large stores of glycogen not only in the liver but also in the muscle and heart (Rajan & Abdel-Hamid, 2012). The muscles begin to feel hard on palpation due to the deposits of glycogen. The heart becomes enlarged, and often an arrhythmia will be present. Without therapy, children with this form usually die of heart failure before they reach adulthood.

Assessment

Because the liver must store such a large supply of glycogen, it increases so much in size that the abdomen protrudes. Over a long period, the child's growth will be stunted because there is only glucose available for energy, not for growth. If hypoglycemic episodes have been severe, brain damage may result. Many children have a tendency toward epistaxis or hemorrhage and are at risk when having surgery performed because of an impaired clotting ability due to decreased platelet adhesiveness. They are susceptible to periods of hypoglycemia, because their only source of ready glucose is their oral intake. The development of gout from deposition of uric acid crystals in joints may also occur (Zychowicz, 2011).

Therapeutic Management

Children with glycogen storage disease need to eat a high-carbohydrate diet with snacks between meals to prevent hypoglycemia. In addition, a continuous glucose nasogastric or gastrostomy feeding during the night may be necessary to prevent hypoglycemia while sleeping. Therapy with diazoxide (Proglycem), an antihypoglycemic drug that inhibits insulin release, may help regulate the glucose level to provide additional growth. Liver transplantation may be a possibility, but it will not cure the basic enzyme deficiency.

Tay-Sachs Disease (Infantile GM2 Gangliosidosis)

Tay-Sachs disease is an autosomal recessively inherited disease in which the infant lacks hexosaminidase A, an enzyme necessary for lipid metabolism. Without this enzyme, lipid deposits accumulate on nerve cells, leading to severe cognitive challenge due to deposits on brain cells, and blindness due to deposits on optic nerve cells (Bley, Giannikopoulos, Hayden, et al., 2011).

Tay-Sachs disease is found primarily in the Ashkenazi Jewish population (Eastern European Jewish ancestry). Children generally appear well in the first few months of life except for an extreme Moro reflex and mild hypotonia. If left untreated, at about 6 months of age, they begin to lose head control and are unable to sit up or roll over without support. On an ophthalmoscopic examination, a characteristic cherry-red macula is noticeable (caused by lipid deposits). By 1 year of age, children will have developed symptoms of spasticity and are unable to perform even simple motor tasks. By 2 years of age, generalized seizures and blindness will have occurred. Most children die of cachexia (malnutrition) and pneumonia by 3 to 5 years of age.

There is no cure for Tay-Sachs disease. The disorder may be detected in utero by amniocentesis. Carriers for the disease trait may be identified by hexosaminidase A assay.

What if...48.4 You are particularly interested in exploring one of the 2020 National Health Goals with respect to endocrine or metabolic disorders (see Box 48.1). What would be a possible research topic to explore pertinent to this goal that would be applicable to Rob's family and that would also advance evidence-based practice?

Key Points for Review

- Endocrine disorders are almost all long-term disorders. Helping parents and children remember to take medicine on a long-term basis is an important nursing responsibility that not only meets QSEN competencies but that also best meets the family's total needs.
- Children with endocrine or metabolic disorders often develop height or weight discrepancies. Help children continue to maintain high self-esteem by concentrating on the things they are able to do despite a growth lag.
- GH deficiency, a pituitary disorder, results in extremely short stature if left untreated. Therapy for children consists of the injection of synthetic GH. Children can experience situational low self-esteem if they do not receive adequate emotional support from significant others.
- Other pituitary disorders include GH excess and diabetes insipidus. With GH excess, there is an overgrowth of body tissues. With diabetes insipidus, there is a decreased release of ADH, which leads to polyuria. Therapy is the administration of desmopressin, an arginine vasopressin.

- Congenital hypothyroidism occurs as a result of an absent or nonfunctioning thyroid gland. The condition is discovered by a blood spot test at birth. Therapy is the oral administration of synthetic thyroid hormone.
- Acquired hypothyroidism (Hashimoto disease) is an autoimmune phenomenon that interferes with thyroid gland function. Therapy is the administration of synthetic thyroid hormone.
- Hyperthyroidism is caused by overproduction of thyroid hormones. It leads to jitteriness and tachycardia. It is treated by medication to suppress thyroxine release.
- Acute adrenocortical insufficiency is an emergency situation in which there is abrupt nonfunction of the adrenal glands. Congenital adrenogenital hyperplasia is an inherited disorder in which girls are born masculinized. Both girls or boys may be unable to retain sodium, resulting in rapid fluid loss. Therapy is the administration of hydrocortisone and also aldosterone if sodium loss is present.
- Cushing syndrome is caused by the overproduction of cortisol by the adrenal gland, which is usually caused by a tumor in the gland. Children appear abnormally obese. Therapy is the surgical removal of the tumor.
- The most frequently occurring pancreatic disorder is type 1 diabetes mellitus, an autoimmune process that destroys insulin-producing islet cells. Therapy is a combination of insulin, diet, and exercise. Type 2 diabetes is now occurring in children, especially those who are obese. Therapy is diet, exercise, and an oral antiglycemic agent.
- Hypocalcemia, a parathyroid gland disorder, results in a lowered blood calcium level, causing tetany to develop. Therapy is the administration of calcium.
- Various disorders of metabolism that interfere with carbohydrate, amino acid, or fat metabolism occur in children. Representative of these are PKU, galactosemia, and Tay-Sachs disease.

CRITICAL THINKING CARE STUDY

Cassie is a 4-year-old child who has hypocalcemia because of inadequate parathyroid function caused by being struck in the neck by a baseball when she was 2 years of age. She takes a daily supplement of both vitamin D and calcium and she is urged to eat a diet high in calcium. She has begun to be increasingly uncooperative about taking her medication. Her mother worries that, as Cassie grows older, she will refuse her medication completely.

1. Cassie's mother is worried her daughter will gain weight drinking whole milk and so serves her nonfat milk. She adds chocolate syrup to it to change the taste. This morning she realized Cassie gave her 10-year-old brother her glass of milk to drink. Does serving nonfat milk or adding chocolate to it change the calcium content of milk? What actions could you take to help Cassie's mother increase Cassie's cooperation with drinking more milk?
2. Cassie's mother tells you she is at "the end of her rope" with trying to get Cassie to take her medicine. She's so frustrated that she's stopped trying to give her vitamin D because "it's only a vitamin." What suggestions could you make to help the mother increase Cassie's medicine compliance?
3. The teacher at the preschool Cassie attends has told her mother that Cassie refuses to hold a pencil when it's time to practice alphabet letters. She "acts out" by holding her hands together, "pretending they hurt" instead. She's asked the mother to reinforce with Cassie the importance of learning letters to be ready for kindergarten. How would you suggest the mother handle this?

Patient Scenario

The Adamine Family

Read about the Adamine family, a family with a child with diabetes insipidus, then answer the questions to further sharpen your skills and grow more familiar with NCLEX-type questions related to endocrine and metabolic disorders. Confirm your answers are correct by reading the rationales.

Visit http://thePoint.lww.com

Answers and Rationales

Looking for answers to the What if . . . and Critical Thinking Care Study questions?

Visit http://thePoint.lww.com

References

Allen, P. J., & Fomenko, S. D. (2011). Congenital hypothyroidism. *Pediatric Nursing, 37*(6), 324–326.

Baumann, G. P. (2012). Growth hormone doping in sports: A critical review of use and detection strategies. *Endocrine Reviews, 33*(2), 155–186.

Bley, A. E., Giannikopoulos, O. A., Hayden, D., et al. (2011). Natural history of infantile G(M2) gangliosidosis. *Pediatrics, 128*(5), e1233–e1241.

Boss, A. H., Petrucci, R., & Lorber, D. (2012). Coverage of prandial insulin requirements by means of an ultra-rapid-acting inhaled insulin. *Journal of Diabetes Science & Technology, 6*(4), 773–779.

Buchko, B., Artz, B., Dayhoff, S., et al. (2012). Improving care of patients with insulin pumps during hospitalization: Translating the evidence. *Journal of Nursing Care Quality, 27*(4), 333–340.

Burke, G. W. III, Vendrame, F., Pileggi, A., et al. (2011). Recurrence of autoimmunity following pancreas transplantation. *Current Diabetes Reports, 11*(5), 413–419.

Caprio, S. (2012). Development of type 2 diabetes mellitus in the obese adolescent: A growing challenge. *Endocrine Practice, 18*(5), 791–795.

Chamarthi, B., Morris, C. A., Kaiser, U. B., et al. (2010). Clinical problem-solving: Stalking the diagnosis. *The New England Journal of Medicine, 362*(9), 834–839.

Chen, B., Mei, J., Kalman, L., et al. (2012). Good laboratory practices for biochemical genetic testing and newborn screening for inherited metabolic diseases. *MMWR: Morbidity & Mortality Weekly Report, 61*(2), 1–44.

Cunningham, A., Bausell, H., Brown, M., et al. (2012). Recommendations for the use of sapropterin in phenylketonuria. *Molecular Genetics & Metabolism, 106*(3), 269–276.

Dahlgren, J. (2011). Metabolic benefits of growth hormone therapy in idiopathic short stature. *Hormone Research in Paediatrics, 76*(Suppl. 3), 56–58.

Dashiff, C., Riley, B. H., Abdullatif, H., et al. (2011). Parents' experiences supporting self-management of middle adolescents with type 1 diabetes mellitus. *Pediatric Nursing, 37*(6), 304–310.

Dauber, A., Kellogg, M., & Majzoub, J. (2010). Monitoring of therapy in congenital adrenal hyperplasia. *Clinical Chemistry, 56*(8), 1245–1251.

Dea, T. L. (2011). Pediatric obesity & type 2 diabetes. *MCN: American Journal of Maternal Child Nursing, 36*(1), 42–48.

Donahey, E., & Folse, S. (2012). Management of diabetic ketoacidosis. *Advanced Emergency Nursing Journal, 34*(3), 209–215.

Drake, E., & Gibson, M. (2010). Update on expanded newborn screening: Issues for consideration. *Nursing for Women's Health, 14*(3), 199–211.

Fraser, L. A., & Van Uum, S. (2010). Work-up for Cushing syndrome. *CMAJ: Canadian Medical Association Journal, 182*(6), 584–587.

Geisler, A., Lass, N., Reinsch, N., et al. (2012). Quality of life in children and adolescents with growth hormone deficiency: Association with growth hormone treatment. *Hormone Research in Paediatrics, 78*(2), 94–99.

Graber, E., & Rapaport, R. (2012). Growth and growth disorders in children and adolescents. *Pediatric Annals, 41*(4), e1–e9.

Hinton, C. F., Harris, K. B., Borgfeld, L., et al. (2010). Trends in incidence rates of congential hypothyroidism related to select demographic factors. *Pediatrics, 125*(Suppl. 2), S37–S47.

Jospe, N. (2011). Endocrinology. In K. J. Marcdante, R. M. Kliegman, H. B. Jenson, et al. (Eds.), *Nelson essentials of pediatrics* (6th ed., pp. 625–670). Philadelphia, PA: Saunders/Elsevier.

Karch, A. M. (2013). *2013 Lippincott's nursing drug guide.* Philadelphia, PA: Lippincott Williams & Wilkins.

LaFranchi, S. H. (2011). Approach to the diagnosis and treatment of neonatal hypothyroidism. *Journal of Clinical Endocrinology & Metabolism, 96*(10), 2959–2967.

Léger, J., & Carel, J. C. (2013). Hyperthyroidism in childhood: Causes, when and how to treat. *Journal of Clinical Research in Pediatric Endocrinology, 5*(Suppl. 1), 50–56.

Lemon, S. J., & Crannage, A. (2011). Pharmacologic anticoagulation reversal in the emergency department. *Advanced Emergency Nursing Journal, 33*(3), 212–223.

Listernick, R. (2012). A 2 month old with hyperbilirubinemia. *Pediatric Annals, 41*(3), 94–97.

MacDonald, A., Rocha, J. C., van Rijn, M., et al. (2011). Nutrition in phenylketonuria. *Molecular Genetics & Metabolism, 104*(Suppl. 1), S10–18.

Millington, G., & Thalange, N. (2013). Skin. In N. Thalange, R. Beach, D. Booth, et al. (Eds.), *Essentials of paediatrics* (2nd ed., pp. 79–88). Philadelphia, PA: Elsevier/Saunders.

Olney, R. S., Grosse, S. D., & Vogt, R. F. (2010). Prevalence of congenital hypothyroidism—Current trends and future directions: Workshop summary. *Pediatrics, 125*(Suppl. 2), S31–S36.

Plaut, D., & McLellan, W. (2011). Vitamin D. *Journal of Continuing Education Topics and Issues, 13*(1), 6–9.

Rajan, D. S., & Abdel-Hamid, H. (2012). Child neurology: Pompe disease: New horizons. *Neurology, 79*(23), e197–e200.

Ross, J. M. D., Quigley, C., Cao, D., et al. (2011). Growth hormone plus childhood low dose estrogen in Turner syndrome. *New England Journal of Medicine, 364*(13), 1230–1242.

Schmidt, C. A., Bernaix, L. W., Chiappetta, M., et al. (2012). In-hospital survival skills training for type 1 diabetes: Perceptions of children and parents. *Maternal Child Nursing, 37*(2), 88–94.

Shapira, S. K., Lloyd-Puryear, M. A., & Boyle, C. (2010). Future research directions to identify causes of the increasing incidence rate of congenital hypothyroidism in the United States. *Pediatrics, 125*(Suppl. 2), S64–S68.

Sherr, J., & Weinzimer, S. (2012). Diabetes types 1 and 2 in the pediatric population. *Pediatric Annals, 41*(2), 1–7.

Snyder, R., Berch, B., Najjar, J., et al. (2011). Neonatal Graves disease and recurrent goiter. *American Surgeon, 77*(3), 380–382.

Stephen, M. D., Gungor, N., & Douty, D. R. (2012). Type 2 diabetes mellitus in a young girl: Ominous presentation and atypical course. *Journal of Pediatric & Endocrinology Metabolism, 25*(5–6), 577–580.

Ten Hoedt, A. E., Maurice-Stam, H., Boelen, C. C., et al. (2011). Parenting a child with phenylketonuria or galactosemia: Implications for health-related quality of life. *Journal of Inherited Metabolic Disease, 34*(2), 391–398.

Thalange, N., & Beach, R. (2013). Endocrinology & metabolism. In N. Thalange, R. Beach, D. Booth, et al. (Eds.), *Essentials of paediatrics* (2nd ed., pp. 139–158). Philadelphia, PA: Elsevier/Saunders.

Thomas, T. C., Smith, J. M., White, P. C., et al. (2012). Transient neonatal hypocalcemia: Presentation and outcomes. *Pediatrics, 129*(6), e1461–e1467.

U.S. Department of Health and Human Services. (2010). *Healthy people 2020.* Washington, DC: Author.

van Karnebeek, C. D., & Stockler, S. (2012). Treatable inborn errors of metabolism causing intellectual disability: A systematic literature review. *Molecular Genetics & Metabolism, 105*(3), 368–381.

van Spronsen, F. J., de Groot, M. J., Hoeksma, M., et al. (2010). Large neutral amino acids in the treatment of PKU: From theory to practice. *Journal of Inherited Metabolic Disease, 33*(6), 671–676.

Wang, C. C., Shiang, J. C., Chen, J. T., et al. (2011). Syndrome of inappropriate secretion of antidiuretic hormone associated with localized herpes zoster ophthalmicus. *Journal of General Internal Medicine, 26*(2), 216–220.

Zeitler, P. S., Barker, J. M., Travers, S. H., et al. (2011). Endocrine disorders. In W. Hay, M. Levin, R. Deterding, et al. (Eds.), *Current diagnosis & treatment pediatrics* (21st ed., pp. 1011–1052). New York, NY: McGraw-Hill/Lange.

Zychowicz, M. (2011). Gout: No longer the disease of kings. *Orthopaedic Nursing, 30*(5), 322–330.

Chapter 49

Nursing Care of a Family When a Child Has a Neurologic Disorder

KEY TERMS

- astereognosis
- automatisms
- autonomic dysreflexia
- choreoathetosis
- choreoid
- decerebrate posturing
- decorticate posturing
- diplegia
- dyskinetic
- graphesthesia
- hemiplegia
- infantile spasms
- kinesthesia
- paraplegia
- pulse pressure
- quadriplegia
- status epilepticus
- stereognosis

OBJECTIVES

After mastering the contents of this chapter, you should be able to:

1. Describe common neurologic disorders in children.
2. Identify 2020 National Health Goals related to neurologic disorders in children that nurses can help the nation achieve.
3. Assess a child with a neurologic disorder.
4. Formulate nursing diagnoses for a child with a neurologic disorder.
5. Establish expected outcomes for a child with a neurologic disorder to help the family manage seamless transitions across differing health care settings.
6. Using the nursing process, plan nursing care that includes the six competencies of Quality & Safety Education for Nurses (QSEN): Patient-Centered Care, Teamwork & Collaboration, Evidence-Based Practice (EBP), Quality Improvement (QI), Safety, and Informatics.
7. Implement nursing care, such as monitoring medicine effectiveness, for a child with a neurologic disorder.
8. Evaluate expected outcomes for achievement and effectiveness of care.
9. Integrate knowledge of neurologic disorders and the interplay of nursing process, the six competencies of QSEN, and Family Nursing to promote quality maternal and child health nursing care.

Tasha is a 3-year-old girl you meet in an emergency department because she's had a seizure. Her mother grabs your arm, visibly upset. "Her sister has cerebral palsy and seizures. Does this mean Tasha has cerebral palsy too?" she asks you.

Previous chapters described normal growth and development in children and nursing care of children with disorders of other systems. This chapter adds information about the dramatic changes, both physical and psychosocial, that occur when a child is born with or develops a neurologic disorder. Such information builds a base for care and health teaching for children with these disorders.

What education does this parent need about cerebral palsy or recurrent seizures?

Neurologic disorders encompass a wide array of problems resulting from congenital disorders, infection, or trauma. Many of these disorders severely alter the child's life; some result in life-threatening complications. Whenever possible, prevention must be the highest priority for keeping the nervous system healthy because, in the future, stem cell research may offer a cure for neurologic disorders, but for now, because neural tissue does not regenerate like other body tissue, any nervous system degeneration is likely to be permanent. Therefore, nursing care focuses on prevention or measures to help the child and family develop strategies for dealing with the associated loss in mental or physical functioning, making the child comfortable, and providing an environment conducive to the child's development and self-esteem (Parachuri & Inglese, 2013). 2020 National Health Goals related to neurologic disorders in children are shown in Box 49.1.

BOX 49.1 Nursing Care Planning Based on 2020 National Health Goals

Neurologic disorders are major causes of long-term disability in children. 2020 National Health Goals that address these disorders are:

- Increase the proportion of children or youth with disabilities who spend at least 80% of their time in regular education programs from a baseline of 56.8% to a target level of 73.8%.
- Reduce the number of people 21 years of age and younger with disabilities who are in congregate care facilities from a baseline of 28,890 to 26,001.
- Increase the proportion of people with epilepsy or uncontrolled seizures who receive appropriate medical care.
- Reduce emergency department visits for nonfatal traumatic brain injuries from 407.2/100,000 population to 366.3/100,000 (U.S. Department of Health and Human Services [DHHS], 2010; see www.healthypeople.gov).

Nurses can help the nation achieve these goals through helping to prevent neurologic injury by educating children and parents about the use of helmets for bicycle and motorcycle safety, by administering and teaching paramedical personnel to administer safe care at accident scenes so children's heads and necks are protected, and by decreasing the possible spread of bacterial meningitis through good hand washing and infection control precautions in hospitals.

Nursing Process Overview

For Care of a Child With a Neurologic System Disorder

Assessment

Neurologic disorders often begin with vague symptoms. Parents may report that their child seems to be "walking strangely" or is "just not herself," making a thorough history and neurologic examination imperative for isolating the cause of the concern.

The neurologic examination covers six areas of neurologic functioning as well as motor and sensory functioning. If more information is needed following an exam, additional diagnostic tests will be prescribed. The parents and child need considerable support throughout the assessment process, because, although the neurologic examination can be made "fun" for a child, other procedures such as a computed tomography (CT) scan or lumbar puncture can be frightening. Additionally, the anxiety of not knowing what is wrong and fearing the worst can make the waiting period for test results especially difficult for the child's parents.

Nursing Diagnosis

Nursing diagnoses for children with neurologic disorders vary according to the child's needs and level of functioning. Initially, a child may need emergency care and constant observation; later on, maintenance care to retain function is the priority. If the child has surgery, nursing diagnoses need to address not only immediate preoperative and postoperative care but also long-term care such as rehabilitation and home care. Three common nursing diagnoses that apply to almost all neurologic disorders are:

- Risk for disuse syndrome related to neurologic deficit affecting one area of functioning
- Interrupted family processes related to stress associated with the long-term effects of neurologic involvement
- Health-seeking behaviors related to care of a child with neurologic involvement

Other nursing diagnoses are specific for disorders and thus are described along with specific disorders.

Outcome Identification and Planning

Be realistic when establishing expected outcomes because children who have permanent limitations will not be able to achieve progress in all areas. When neurologic disorders are first diagnosed, parents may be so stressed that they may be able to focus only on short-term aspects of care, such as whether the child will survive meningitis or whether the child has stopped convulsing. Later, they'll be able to concentrate on the long-term picture: What type of education setting will be best for their child? What type of exercise program will be required?

Before a diagnosis is confirmed, parents may attribute their child's functional deficits to immaturity (she is not walking yet because she is simply too young). This can make them unable to make plans because they have not fully acknowledged their child's neurologic deficits. Only when parents begin to adjust to the new reality are they ready to participate in planning and problem solving.

Numerous organizations are available for assistance and support, such as the Epilepsy Foundation of America (www.epilepsyfoundation.org), the National Information Center for Children and Youth With Disabilities (www.nichcy.org), the Children's Tumor Foundation (www.ctf.org), the National Spinal Cord Injury Association (www.spinalcord.org), and the United Cerebral Palsy Association (www.ucp.org).

Implementation

Nursing interventions for a child with a neurologic problem must address both short-term and long-term needs. A lot of nursing care involves modeling care, such

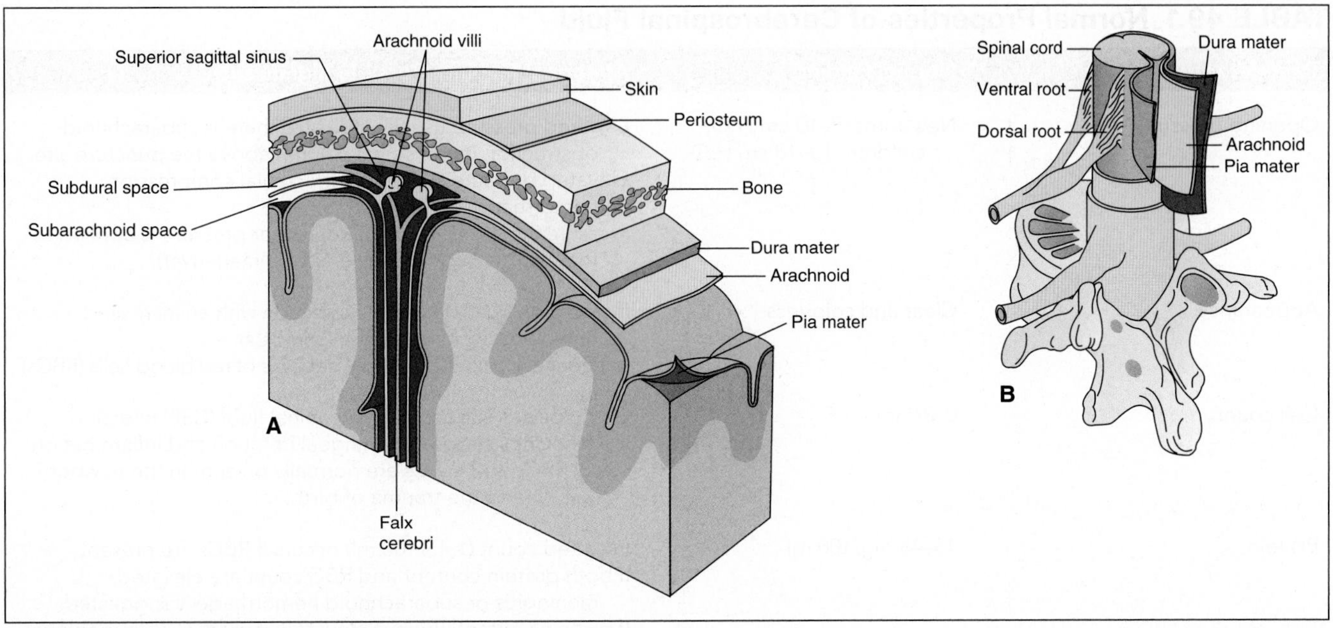

FIGURE 49.1 Meninges of the **(A)** brain and **(B)** spinal cord.

as how to gently handle an infant with increased intracranial pressure (ICP) and how to turn an infant on the side during a seizure to prevent choking, and reviewing needed medications with parents—actions that give parents confidence to be able to care for their child at home.

Outcome Evaluation

Evaluation of a child with a neurologic disorder should address not only the child's progress in regaining physical function but also the child's level of self-esteem. Some examples indicating achievement of possible outcomes are:

- The child states he is aware of potential for injury related to recurrent seizures.
- Family members state they are able to maintain family cohesiveness yet sustain contact with hospitalized child.
- The child practices exercises daily to reduce possibility of contracture from disuse syndrome.

ANATOMY AND PHYSIOLOGY OF THE NERVOUS SYSTEM

Nerve cells (*neurons*) are unique among body cells in that, instead of being compact, they consist of a cell nucleus and extensions: one axon and several dendrites. The *dendrite* transmits impulses to the cell nucleus; the *axon* transmits impulses away from the cell nucleus to body organs. These cells vary in size, ranging from a few inches to several feet long, reaching from distant body sites such as the feet, through the spinal cord, and to the brain. Although their great length is vital to motor and sensory function, it also makes nerve cells more susceptible than other body cells to injury.

The nervous system is not fully functioning at birth; it continues to mature through the first 12 years of life. Two separate systems are involved: the *peripheral nervous system (PNS)* and the *central nervous system (CNS)*. The PNS consists of the cranial nerves, the spinal nerves, and the somatic and visceral divisions. The CNS includes the brain and the spinal cord (Fig. 49.1) surrounded by the cerebrospinal fluid (CSF), the skull, and three membranes or meninges (the *dura mater*, a fibrous, connective tissue containing many blood vessels; the *arachnoid membrane*, a delicate serous membrane; and the *pia mater*, a vascular membrane) that protect the brain and spinal cord from trauma.

The properties of CSF are shown in Table 49.1. Basically, it is a colorless, alkaline fluid with a specific gravity of approximately 1.004 to 1.008, containing traces of protein, glucose, lymphocytes, and body salts.

ASSESSING THE CHILD WITH A NEUROLOGIC DISORDER

Because neurologic symptoms, such as headache, an unsteady gait, or lethargy, are often insidious, both a thorough history and a neurologic examination are needed to reveal the cause and extent of such symptoms (Box 49.2).

Health History

A child's history may first reveal symptoms of a neurologic disorder. Because many neurologic problems that are evidenced in infants and young children result from injury that occurred in utero, it is important to obtain the mother's pregnancy history as well.

At primary care visits, always ask parents about their child's developmental milestones and ability to perform age-appropriate tasks successfully. A Denver Developmental Screening Test can be used to indicate whether a parent's concern about a preschool child is well founded. The ability to perform well in school is important documentation for an older child.

TABLE 49.1 Normal Properties of Cerebrospinal Fluid

Parameter	Normal Finding	Abnormal Finding: Possible Significance
Opening pressure	Newborns: 8–10 cm H_2O; children: 10–18 cm H_2O	Lowered pressure usually indicates there is subarachnoid obstruction in the spinal column above the puncture site. Elevated pressure suggests intracranial compression, hemorrhage, or infection. Pressure increases if a child coughs or pressure is applied to the external jugular vein (Valsalva maneuver).
Appearance	Clear and colorless	If cloudy, indicates possible infection with an increased number of white blood cells (WBCs). If reddened, color is probably because of red blood cells (RBCs).
Cell count	0–8/mm^3	Granulocytes suggest cerebrospinal fluid (CSF) infection. Lymphocytes suggest meningeal irritation and inflammation. A few RBCs and WBCs are normally present in the newborn CSF due to the trauma of birth.
Protein	15–45 mg/100 ml	Elevated count (>45/100 ml) occurs if RBCs are present. If both protein content and RBC count are elevated, meningitis or subarachnoid hemorrhage is suggested. If protein content alone is elevated, it more likely suggests a degenerative process such as multiple sclerosis.
Glucose	60%–80% of serum glucose level	Bacterial meningitis causes a marked decrease in CSF glucose; invasion of fungi, yeast, tuberculosis, or protozoans into the CSF results in some decrease in glucose level. Viral infections do not cause a decrease in CSF glucose and may occasionally cause a slight increase.
Albumin/globulin (A/G) ratio	8:1	Increased level suggests infection or an A/G ratio neurologic disorder.

Neurologic Examination

A complete neurologic examination takes at least 20 minutes and requires both patience and skill to keep a child's attention while observing for possible indications of neurologic disease. For a full examination, six areas are assessed: cerebral, cranial nerve, cerebellar, motor, sensory, and reflex function.

Cerebral Function

Both general and specific cerebral functions need to be evaluated by assessing level of consciousness, orientation, intelligence, performance, mood, and general behavior (Rust, 2011). Children do best when these types of tests are presented as a game. Be certain to convey that there are no right or wrong answers because children who believe that they have failed these tests may not respond well to further testing.

The best way to evaluate a child's level of consciousness is through conversation. Note any drowsiness or lethargy. Allow the child to answer questions without prompting, and listen carefully to be certain the answer is appropriate to the question.

Orientation refers to whether children are aware of who they are, where they are, and what day it is (person, place, and time). Be certain to take into account a child's age and development because children younger than 4 years of age, for example, may not know both their first and last names. Children may be of school age before they know their address. Children younger than 7 or 8 years of age may have difficulty with the days of the week, confusing "yesterday" with "today" or "tomorrow." Intellectual performance (IQ) can be determined by the child's score on a standard intelligence test. Estimates of intellectual function can be made by asking the child questions on common topics.

Immediate recall is the ability to retain a concept for a short time, such as being able to remember a series of numbers and repeat them (a child of 4 years can usually repeat three digits; a child older than 6 years can repeat five digits). *Recent memory* covers a slightly longer period of time. To measure this, show the preschool child an object such as a key and ask him to remember it, because later you will ask him to tell you what it was. After about 5 minutes, ask whether he remembers what object you showed him. Ask older children what they ate for breakfast to test recent memory.

Remote memory is long-term recall. Ask preschoolers what they ate for breakfast that morning or for dinner the night before because, for them, that was a long time ago; ask older children what was the name of their first-grade teacher because most people remember this information their whole life.

Specific cerebral function can be measured by assessing language, sensory interpretation, and motor integration. When assessing language, listen to the child's ability to articulate. Remember, when listening to speech, many preschoolers substitute "w" for "r," saying "west time" instead of "rest time"; be aware that pronunciation is altered if English is not the child's primary language.

Stereognosis refers to the ability of a child to recognize an object by touch; it is a test of sensory interpretation. For this, ask

BOX 49.2 Nursing Care Planning Using Assessment

Assessing a Child for Signs and Symptoms of a Neurologic Disorder

History

Chief concern: Seizure, loss of consciousness, delay in developmental tasks, headache, clumsiness at motor tasks.
Past medical history: Infection during pregnancy; difficult birth; difficulty with initiating respirations at birth; head injury from fall or unintentional injury.
Family medical history: History of seizures or headaches in other family members.

Physical examination

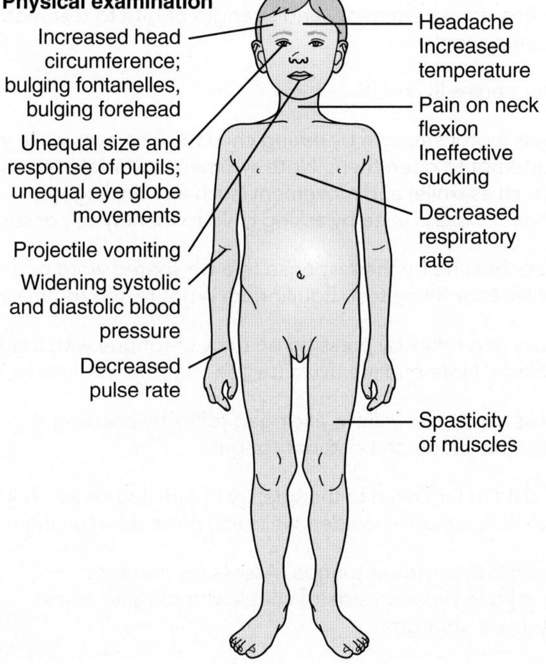

a child to close his or her eyes; then place a familiar object, such as a key, a penny, or a bottle cap, in her hand and ask her to identify it. This is a skill even preschoolers are able to do successfully.

Graphesthesia is the ability to recognize a shape that has been traced on the skin. Ask a child to close his or her eyes; trace first a circle and then a square on the back of his or her hand, and then ask him or her whether the shapes are the same or different. Be sure the child understands the concept of "different" by first showing him objects such as two keys and a bottle cap and documenting that he is able to identify the keys as being the same and the bottle cap as being different. For older children, trace numbers (8, 3, 0, and 1 work well) and ask the child to identify each one.

Kinesthesia is the ability to distinguish movement. Have a child close her eyes and extend her hands in front of her. Raise one of her fingers and ask her whether it is up or down. Hold the finger by its sides so that your other fingers do not brush against the child's palm or the back of her hand and reveal the finger position. Repeat the same movement with a toe on each foot. For preschoolers, be certain to first determine whether the child understands the concept of up and down.

To measure motor integration, ask a child to perform a complex motor skill, such as folding a piece of paper and putting it into an envelope. A child of 4 years or older should be able to do this neatly.

Children do best when these tests are presented as a game. Be certain to convey that there are no right or wrong answers. A child who believes that he has failed these tests may not respond well to further testing.

Cranial Nerve Function

Testing for cranial nerve function consists of assessing each pair of cranial nerves separately. Cranial nerves and methods of cranial nerve testing are described in Table 49.2. Methods to test pupil constriction and ability to follow into fields of gaze are described in Chapter 34.

Cerebellar Function

Tests for cerebellar function are tests for balance and coordination. To test these, observe the child walk to assess whether the walk is natural (most children walk at least a little self-consciously when they know they are being observed, so watch them also as they enter the exam room and move around for other activities). Ask the child to stand on one foot; a child as young as 4 years should be able to do this for as long as 5 seconds. Ask the child to attempt a tandem walk (walk a straight line, one foot directly in front of the other, heel touching toe) (Fig. 49.2A). A child older than 4 years of age should be able to do this for about four consecutive steps. Ask the child to touch his nose with his finger and then to reach and touch your finger with the same hand (held about 1½ feet in front of him) (see Fig. 49.2B). Tell him to repeat this action, and move your finger to a new position each time. The average child rarely reaches past your finger or stops before touching it.

Ask the child to pat one knee with the palm of the hand, then quickly turn the hand over and pat the knee with the back of the hand; repeat over and over, one hand at a time. The majority of children are able to do this rapid, coordinated motion without much difficulty. Preschoolers will "mirror" the movement of the actively moving hand by moving the inactive hand as well. Older children should not demonstrate this (or should show only a small amount of movement).

Other tests are to ask the child to touch each finger on one hand with the thumb of that hand in rapid succession or ask him to run the heel of one foot down the front of his other leg while he is lying supine (children should be able to do this without "running off" the leg). With the child lying on the examining table, ask him to close his eyes and draw a circle or figure 8 in the air with his foot (children should also be able to do this without difficulty).

Tests of cerebellar function such as these are fun for children to do, as long as they know that there are no passes or failures. Show approval for effort even if they are having difficulty with a task, so that they have confidence to try another one.

Motor Function

Motor function is measured by evaluating muscle size, strength, and tone. Begin by comparing the size and symmetry of extremities. If in doubt about either of these, measure the circumference of the calves and thighs or upper and lower arms with a tape measure. Palpate muscles for tone. Move the extremities through passive range of motion to evaluate symmetry, spasticity, and flaccidity bilaterally. To test for strength, ask the child to extend her arms in front of her and then resist

TABLE 49.2 Cranial Nerve Function

Cranial Nerve	Function	Assessment
I (olfactory)	Sense of smell	Assess child's ability to recognize common odors such as peanut butter or an orange while eyes are closed.
II (optic)	Vision	Assess vision fields and visual acuity; examine retinas.
III (oculomotor)	Motor control and sensation for eye muscles and upper eyelid	Assess pupillary size, equality, reaction to light and ability to follow an object in all directions. Note any nystagmus (an abnormal jerking motion).
IV (trochlear)	Movement of major eye globe muscles	As for nerve III.
V (trigeminal)	Mastication muscles and some facial sensations	Assess ability to discern light touch to test sensory component; assess symmetry and strength of bite to test motor component.
VI (abducens)	Movement and muscle sense of eye globe	As for nerves III and IV.
VII (facial)	Impulses for facial muscles, salivation, and taste	Assess motor strength by asking child to close eyes while you attempt to open them. Note symmetry of facial expression (such as smile) and movement (such as wrinkling forehead). Assess taste by asking child to identify salt or sugar.
VIII (acoustic)	Equilibrium and hearing	Assess hearing by the response to a whispered word or a Weber or Rinne test. Equilibrium is not tested routinely.
IX (glossopharyngeal)	Motor impulses to heart; sensation from pharynx, thorax, and abdominal organs	Assess gag reflex by pressing on back of tongue with tongue blade. Note midline uvula (tested together with nerve X).
X (vagus)	Swallowing and gag reflexes	Assess ability to swallow; elicit gag reflex by pressing a tongue blade on posterior tongue.
XI (accessory)	Impulses to striated muscles of pharynx and shoulders	Ask child to turn head to the side; try to turn it to center. Ask the child to elevate shoulders while you press down on them.
XII (hypoglossal)	Motor impulses to tongue and skeletal muscles; sensation from skin and viscera	Ask child to protrude tongue. Assess for tremors. Ask child to press on side of cheek with tongue; assess tongue strength.

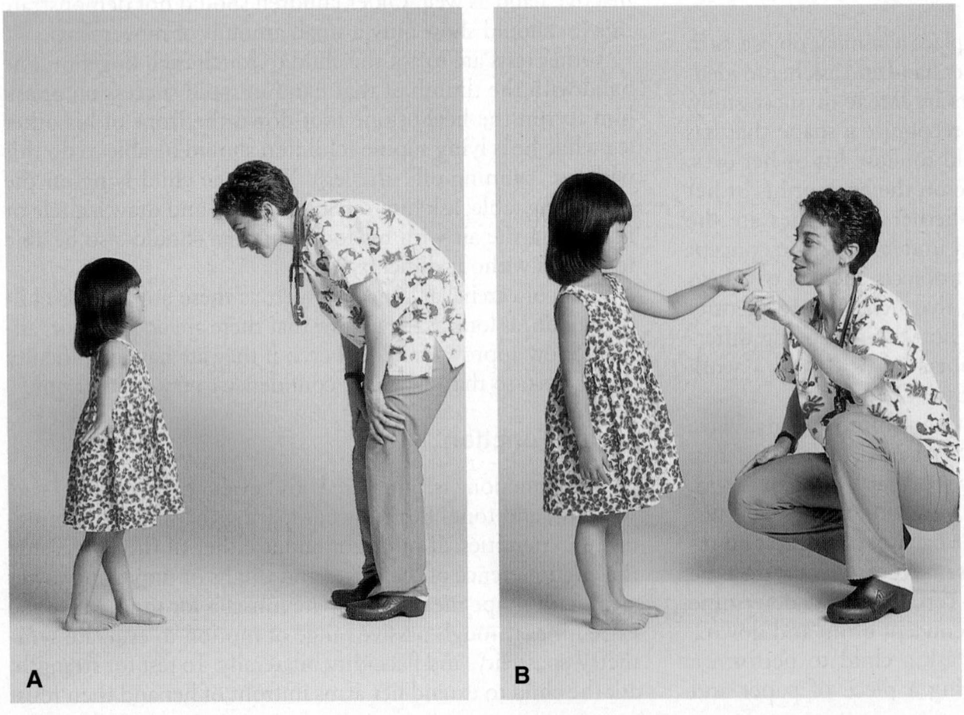

FIGURE 49.2 Cerebellar function tests. **(A)** A child attempting a tandem walk. **(B)** Nose-to-finger test. (© Lesha Photography.)

your action as you push down or up on her hands or push them out to the side. Do the same with the lower extremities.

Sensory Function

If children's sensory systems are intact, they should be able to distinguish light touch, pain, vibration, hot, and cold. Have a child close his eyes and then ask him to point to the spot where you touch him with an object. Light touch is tested by using a wisp of cotton, deep pressure by pressure of your finger, pain by a safety pin, and temperature by test tubes filled with hot or cold water. Vibration is tested by touching the child's bony prominences (iliac crest, elbows, knees) with a vibrating tuning fork. Warn the child that on pin testing, he will feel a momentary prick. Otherwise, he may be unwilling to close his eyes again for further testing.

Reflex Testing

Deep tendon reflex testing, which is part of a primary physical assessment (see Chapter 34), is also a basic part of a neurologic assessment. In newborns, reflex testing is especially important because the infant cannot perform tasks on command to demonstrate the full range of neurologic function (see Chapter 18).

QSEN Checkpoint Question 49.1

Patient-Centered Care

Tasha, 3 years old, is scheduled for a full neurologic examination. What would be the best explanation to prepare her for this?

a. "You'll need to answer questions carefully so you can pass this test."
b. "I'll be asking you to move in different ways, almost like a game."
c. "I need to find out how healthy or unhealthy your brain seems to be."
d. "Seizures can be caused by a brain tumor, so that needs to be ruled out."

Look in Appendix A for the best answer and rationale.

Diagnostic Testing

A variety of diagnostic tests may be prescribed to provide additional information should any abnormalities be detected in the health history, physical examination, or neurologic examination. Many of these tests are invasive, so if you are scheduling these, be certain both the child and family are well prepared for these procedures; try to schedule the least invasive procedures first to better elicit the child's cooperation. So explanations will be well understood, take into account not only the child's chronologic age but also the child's level of cognitive functioning. Provide an explanation that includes not only physically what will happen but also a description of any sensory experiences the child might undergo such as anything they might feel, hear, smell, or taste.

Lumbar Puncture

Lumbar puncture, the introduction of a needle into the subarachnoid space (under the arachnoid membrane) at the level of L4 or L5 to withdraw CSF for analysis, is used most frequently with children to diagnose hemorrhage or infection in the CNS or to diagnose an obstruction of CSF flow. The procedure is contraindicated if the skin over the needle insertion site is infected (to avoid introducing pathogens into the CSF) or if there is a suspected elevation of CSF pressure (if ICP is elevated, the higher pressure in the intracranial space could cause the brainstem to be drawn down into the spinal cord space, compressing the medulla and compromising the action of the cardiac and respiratory centers). To limit pain, EMLA or lidocaine cream should be applied to the puncture site 1 hour before the procedure. Alternatively, the child may be administered conscious sedation for the procedure (see Chapter 39).

For a lumbar puncture, a newborn is seated upright with the head bent forward (Fig. 49.3A). The older infant or child is placed on one side on the examining table. Help the child flex the head forward, flex the knees against the abdomen, and arch the back as much as possible; this position opens the space between the lumbar vertebrae, facilitating needle insertion (see Fig. 49.3B). You might describe the position as "rolling into a ball" or "folding up like an astronaut in a

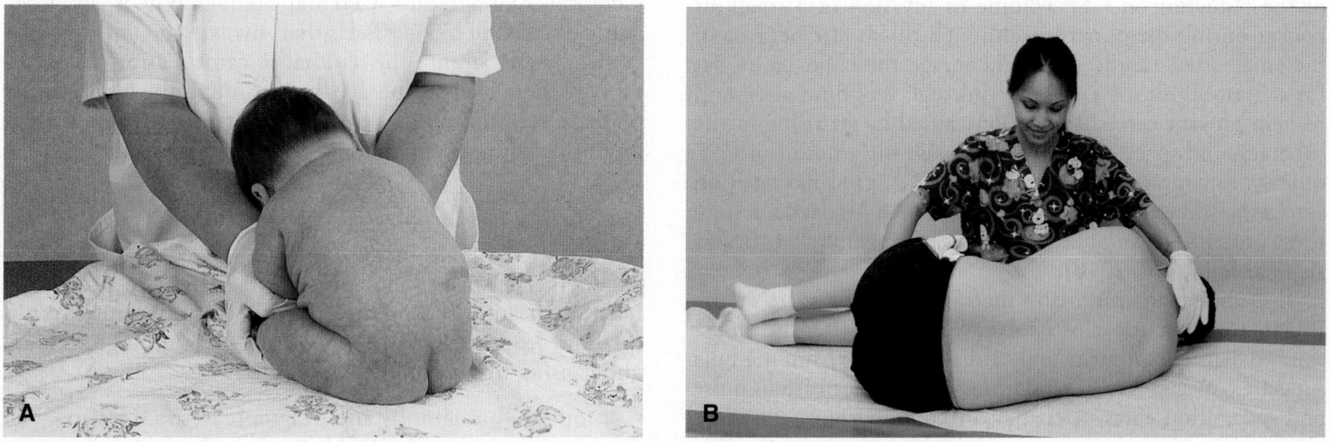

FIGURE 49.3 **(A)** Positioning an infant for a lumbar puncture. (© Barbara Proud.) **(B)** Positioning an older child for a lumbar puncture.

small spaceship" to associate it with something they know about. Children younger than school age need to be held in this position, because they may be so frightened by someone working on their back unseen that they are unable to hold this arched position (they try to turn over or turn their head to see what is happening). It helps a school-age child or adolescent if you stand by the table facing him and gently rest your hand on the back of the head, as a reminder to keep it bent forward. Talking quietly with the child not only assists in calming the child but also helps assess their respiratory status as they are "curled up." Closely observe an infant for any respiratory distress.

Children need good preparation for a lumbar puncture, because they cannot see what is happening. Be certain they know the health care provider performing the procedure will wash their back with a solution that feels cold and then inject a local anesthetic that might sting for a moment (if an analgesic cream was not applied before the procedure). Caution children they will feel pressure but not pain as the lumbar puncture needle is inserted. Occasionally, the needle will press against a dorsal nerve root and the child will experience a shooting pain down one leg. If this happens, reassure the child this feeling passes quickly and does not indicate an injury.

When the insertion stylette is removed and CSF drips from the end of the needle, the procedure has been successful. An initial pressure reading is made. To confirm the subarachnoid space in the cord is patent with that in the skull, the examiner may ask a child who is older than 3 years of age to cough; for an infant, the examiner may ask you to press on the child's external jugular vein. If either of these measures causes an increase of CSF pressure, it indicates that fluid is flowing freely through the subarachnoid space. Typically, three tubes of CSF, containing 2 to 3 ml each, are collected, a closing pressure reading is taken, and the needle is withdrawn. Samples are usually sent for culture, sensitivity, glucose level, and presence of red blood cells. The first sample obtained may contain blood or skin pathogens from the puncture, so it should not be the sample sent for determination of red blood cell content or culture. Additional evaluations requested might be albumin/globulin ratio or gamma-globulin level (an increased level of gamma-globulin is suggestive of multiple sclerosis or meningitis).

Lumbar puncture involves at least momentary pain, so children need to be comforted afterward. A few children may develop a headache after a lumbar puncture as a result of the reduction in CSF volume or invasion of a small air pocket during the puncture, although this is rare because of the small-sized needle used. Encourage the child to lie flat for at least 30 minutes and to drink a glass of fluid afterward to help prevent cerebral irritation caused by air rising in the subarachnoid space and to help increase the amount of CSF quickly. Encourage parents to hold an infant in a flat position across their knees. Some children develop a headache despite these precautions and need an analgesic for pain relief (Bezov, Ashina, & Lipton, 2010).

If a child had minimally increased CSF pressure at the time of the puncture, closely observe the child after the procedure to detect respiratory and cardiac difficulty from medulla pressure. An increase in blood pressure or a decrease in pulse and respiration rates, a change in consciousness, pupillary changes, or a decrease in motor ability are all important signs of increased intracranial compression.

✔ QSEN Checkpoint Question 49.2

Teamwork & Collaboration

Tasha's diagnostic workup will include a lumbar puncture. When collaborating with the physician to perform this procedure, what nursing action should you prioritize?

a. Explain to Tasha that her back will be washed with a cold liquid.

b. Apply EMLA cream to Tasha's lumbar region 5 to 10 minutes before the procedure.

c. Reassure Tasha that the procedure will not hurt.

d. Help Tasha into a prone position on the procedure table.

Look in Appendix A for the best answer and rationale.

Ventricular Tap

In infants, CSF may be obtained by a subdural tap into a ventricle through the anterior fontanelle. A small space on the scalp over the insertion site is shaved or clipped, and the area is prepared with an antiseptic. The infant's head must be held firmly in a supine position to prevent movement during the procedure so the needle does not strike and lacerate meningeal tissue.

Fluid must always be removed from this site slowly, rather than suddenly, to prevent a sudden shift in pressure that could cause intracranial hemorrhage. After the procedure, a pressure dressing is applied to the site, and the infant is placed in a semi-Fowler's position to prevent additional drainage from the puncture site. After the procedure, comfort the infant or allow the parents to do so to both reduce the stress of a painful procedure and prevent the infant from crying excessively, an action that could increase ICP and loss of additional CSF.

X-Ray Techniques

A flat-plate skull X-ray film may be used to obtain information about increased ICP or skull defects such as fracture or craniosynostosis (premature knitting of cranial sutures). Increased ICP is suggested if skull sutures appear separated on the X-ray. If the ICP is chronic, other subtle changes, such as a flattening of the sella turcica or an increase in the convolutions of the inner table of the skull, may be present.

Cerebral Angiography. Cerebral angiography is an X-ray study of cerebral blood vessels that involves the injection of a contrast material into the femoral or carotid artery. Serial X-rays are then taken as the dye flows through the blood vessels of the cerebrum, and any vessel defects or space-occupying lesions occluding cranial blood vessels are revealed.

Myelography. Myelography is the X-ray study of the spinal cord following the introduction of a contrast material into the CSF by lumbar puncture to reveal the presence of space-occupying lesions of the spinal cord. After the procedure, keep the head of the child's bed elevated to prevent contrast medium from reaching the meninges surrounding the brain and causing irritation.

Computed Tomography and Magnetic Resonance Imaging. Computed tomography (CT) involves the use of X-rays to reveal densities at multiple levels or layers of brain tissue and is helpful to confirm the presence of a brain tumor or other encroaching lesions. Single-photon emission computed tomography (SPECT) is a similar procedure used mainly for blood flow evaluation. Magnetic resonance imaging (MRI) uses magnetic fields to show differences in tissue composition, revealing normal versus abnormal brain tissue. Both CT and MRI are discussed in greater detail in Chapter 37.

Nuclear Medicine Studies (Brain Scan and Positron Emission Tomography)

Brain Scan. For a brain scan, a radioactive material is injected intravenously, and after a fixed time during which the injected material is deposited in cerebral tissue, radioactivity levels over the skull are measured. If the blood–brain barrier is not functioning, the radioactive material will accumulate in specific areas, suggesting possible tumor, subdural hematoma, abscess, or encephalitis.

Positron Emission Tomography. The diagnostic technique of positron emission tomography (PET) involves imaging after injection of positron-emitting radiopharmaceuticals into a vein. These radioactive substances accumulate at diseased areas of the brain or spinal cord. PET is extremely accurate in identifying seizure foci.

Echoencephalography (Ultrasound of Head or Spinal Cord)

Echoencephalography involves the projection of ultrasound (high-frequency sound waves above the audible range) toward the child's head or spinal cord (a type of ultrasound). The technique may be used to outline the ventricles of the brain. Because this technique of scanning is noninvasive, produces no discomfort, and has no known complications, it may be repeated frequently to monitor changes in the size of ventricles or an invading lesion and is particularly effective in infants with open fontanelles. This noninvasive technique is often used in neonatal intensive care units to monitor intraventricular hemorrhages and other problems frequently encountered by preterm infants.

Electroencephalography

The electroencephalogram (EEG) reflects the electrical patterns of the brain summarizing the physical and chemical interactions within the brain at the time of the test (Rapin, 2011). An EEG tracing typically indicates four types of waves: delta (1 to 3 waves per second), theta (4 to 7 waves per second), alpha (8 to 12 waves per second), and beta (13 to 20 waves per second).

To reduce extraneous movements of the eyes, head, or muscles that would affect the tracing, the child must be cooperative and quiet during the procedure. Traditionally, therefore, parents are asked to keep their child up later than usual the night before the exam so the child will fall asleep during the test. Caution children that the room will probably be darkened to help them rest. You can compare the electrode wires attached to their scalp with adhesive paste to those attached to astronauts in space. Reassure them that attaching the electrodes is not painful. Try to avoid using the word *electrical* because children as young as 3 years of age know electrical wires are dangerous and can hurt them. They cannot relax if they are worried they may be shocked or even electrocuted by the procedure.

Children who are unable to lie still and cooperate even after a careful explanation may need a sedative or conscious sedation, although sedation alters the electrical pattern of the cortex and thus is avoided if possible (Britton & Kosa, 2010). For example, chloral hydrate, a frequently used sedative for this procedure, may increase the fast activity of brain waves; chlorpromazine (Thorazine) is known to increase slow activity. Because some seizure medications also cause changes in brain waves, be certain to note on the child's electronic record what medications the child is currently receiving. Be certain that parents have specific instructions as to whether they should give or omit any antiseizure medication on the morning of testing.

Although EEGs can show important information about brain activity, they are not helpful in all circumstances because about 15% of children who have no cranial trauma or seizure activity demonstrate some abnormality on an EEG. They may not reveal a brain tumor because most of brain tumors in children are in the posterior fossa, which is not revealed on an EEG. On inspection of the symmetry of brain waves in different hemispheres, local lesions such as a hematoma may be suggested. An EEG is most beneficial in diagnosing absence seizures. The typical pattern with this disorder is discussed later in this chapter.

Visual stimulation, such as having a child look at a whirling disk, may be used in connection with an EEG, because various types of electrical discharges increase with rapid eye movements. In a child who is sensitive to this type of stimulation, the testing may produce a seizure. If this occurs, the child can be very disturbed and disoriented after the procedure. Describe what has happened, letting him know the seizure is over and he's okay.

Following an EEG, children will be sleepy if they have been sedated or had an EEG while sleep-deprived. Allow them to sleep as long as needed.

HEALTH PROMOTION AND RISK MANAGEMENT

Health promotion for nervous system health begins prenatally with measures to ensure optimal fetal growth and development and prevention of problems associated with anoxia. It continues throughout childhood with routine health maintenance visits, screening for possible neurologic or developmental problems, and timely immunizations to prevent sequelae of childhood infections such as measles or chickenpox. Nurses play a key role in providing education to parents about the importance of prenatal care, obtaining immunizations, and completing medication therapy to ensure complete resolution of an infection.

Parents may also need anticipatory guidance about safety measures to prevent injury, specifically, head and spinal cord injury by the use of seat belts or child restraints while riding in automobiles and protective gear when playing contact sports. Remind parents that children should wear helmets when riding or using anything that can move faster than the child can run such as scooters, roller skates/blades, ice skates, horses, skies, skateboards or snowboards, bicycles, or motorcycles (Riesch, Kedrowski, Brown, et al., 2012). For a child with seizures, parents need instructions to prevent injury during a seizure (see later discussion) and to administer antiseizure medications conscientiously.

For a child with a long-term neurologic disorder, rehabilitation and early intervention play a major role in reducing the risk of complications and in promoting the child's and family's optimal level of functioning.

INCREASED INTRACRANIAL PRESSURE

Increased ICP is not a single disorder but a group of signs and symptoms that occur with many neurologic disorders (Table 49.3). When caring for a child with a potential neurologic disorder, these are always important signs to assess or detect (Sigurtà, Zanaboni, Canavesi, et al., 2013). Increased ICP occurs because of an increase in the CSF volume, blood entering the CSF, cerebral edema, head trauma or infection, space-occupying lesions such as brain tumors, or the development of hydrocephalus or Guillain-Barré syndrome.

The rate at which symptoms develop depends on the cause and the ability of the child's skull to expand to accommodate the increased pressure. Children with open fontanelles, for example, can withstand more pressure without brain damage than can older children, whose suture lines and fontanelles have closed.

Assessment

Assessment of ICP may involve only a few quick procedures, such as obtaining vital signs, evaluating pupil response, and determining level of consciousness and motor and sensory function, or it may include more elaborate electronic monitoring.

Because symptoms are subtle at first, the initial signs children may show are headache, irritability, or restlessness. Growing pressure on the brainstem, which controls respiration and cardiac activity, soon causes pulse and respiration rates to slow. Compression of cranial vessels leads to a compensatory increase in blood pressure (or **pulse pressure**, the gap between the systolic and diastolic blood pressures). Pressure on the hypothalamus, the temperature-regulating center of the body, causes an increase in body temperature. An older child may be able to report symptoms such as diplopia (double vision). On funduscopic examination, papilledema may be detected. Always compare a new assessment of these against all recordings taken in the last 24 hours so a progressive change can be detected.

If ocular changes such as a dilated pupil occur, this indicates pressure is increasing posterior to the eye globe, causing compression of the second cranial nerve. Record any tendency toward strabismus, nystagmus (constant eye movement), or "sunset eyes" (white sclera showing over the top of the cornea), or inability to follow the light into any quadrant. Be sure to be specific about what you document. "Inability to follow light," for example, is not as informative as "Inability to follow light into left superior field; vertical nystagmus noted as child follows light into other fields."

An additional test for ICP is a "doll's eye" reflex. If a child lies supine and you turn his head gently but rapidly to the right, the eyes will normally turn toward the left, and vice versa. If a child has increased ICP, this phenomenon will be absent (a test useful in assessing a comatose child who is unable to cooperate by following a light).

Assess the child's level of consciousness, because if the child is alert but unable to comprehend surroundings, time, or place, this may be the first indication of increased ICP. As pressure continues to increase, a pseudo-awake state will occur, in which the child is awake but unable to follow light or locate a noise. Finally, the child becomes fully comatose, unable to be roused by any stimuli. Levels of coma are rated by the Glasgow Coma Scale, discussed in Chapter 52 in connection with assessment for head trauma.

Children, like adults, generally become disoriented about time first, then place, and then self. It's good to explain to a child that you will be periodically asking seemingly simple questions, such as asking the child for his name or to identify the day of the week. Otherwise, a child may quickly become annoyed with your questions, refuse to answer them, make up silly answers, or pretend to be asleep to avoid having to answer.

Be aware that many children, even when healthy, are groggy when they first awaken, especially if they have been

TABLE 49.3 Signs and Symptoms of Increased Intracranial Pressure

Sign or Symptom	Indication of Increased Intracranial Pressure
Increased head circumference	An increase >2 cm per month in first 3 months of life, >1 cm per month in the second 3 months, and >0.5 cm per month for the next 6 months
Fontanelle changes	Anterior fontanelle tense and bulging; closing late
Vomiting	Occurring in the absence of nausea, on awakening in morning or after nap; possibly projectile
Eye changes	Diplopia (double vision) from pressure on abducens nerves; white of sclera evident over pupil (setting sun sign); limited visual fields, papilledema
Vital sign changes	Elevated temperature and blood pressure; decreased pulse and respiration rates
Pain	Headache, often present on awakening and standing; increasing with straining at stool (Valsalva maneuver) or holding breath
Mentation	Irritability, altered consciousness such as sleepiness

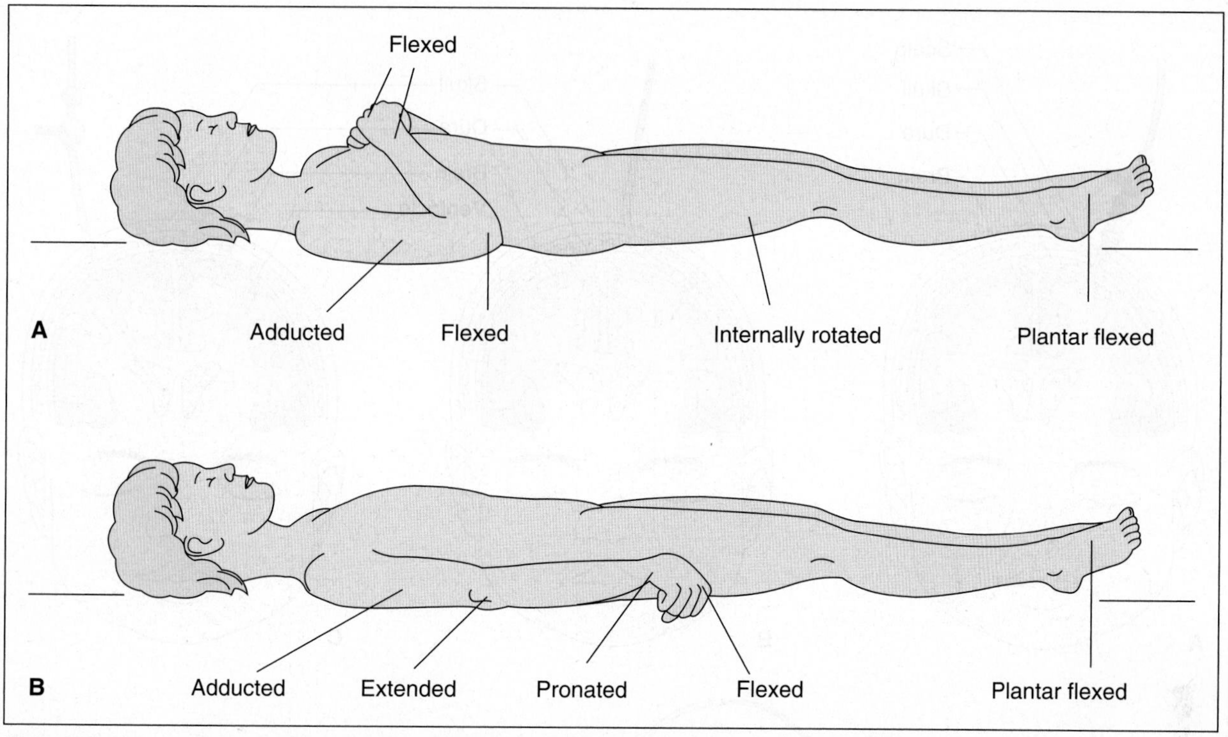

FIGURE 49.4 **(A)** Decorticate posturing. **(B)** Decerebrate posturing.

dreaming. Make sure children are fully awake, therefore, before attempting to determine level of consciousness. Be certain also you are asking questions appropriate to the child's age. Preschoolers, for example, do not usually know their whole name or the day of the week and may not know concepts such as *morning* or *night*. To assess consciousness in children this age, it is often more productive, every hour, to show them a colored block, a piece of fruit, or a cartoon character known to the child and ask them to name it. You may need to remind parents you are asking questions to assess their child's level of consciousness, not to quiz the child as to whether he knows colors so they don't answer for the child.

A good way to test an infant's level of consciousness is to determine whether the child responds (attunes) to sounds, such as a familiar music box or voices, or reaches for an attractive object you offer. Motor ability can be assessed by asking a child to perform some simple motor task, such as squeezing your hand, pushing against your hand with both feet, or performing rapid, alternating hand movements, such as turning a hand over and back several times. Evaluate cranial nerves grossly by having the child make a face, close the eyes tightly, or smile. Be certain to evaluate whether the facial responses are equal and symmetric bilaterally. Test deep tendon reflexes, because these decrease in intensity with decreased level of consciousness.

As a final assessment, carefully observe a child's resting posture because when motor control grows weaker because of loss of cell function, characteristic posturing (primitive reflexes) occurs. Cerebral loss is shown mainly by **decorticate posturing**: the child's arms are adducted and flexed on the chest with wrists flexed, hands fisted; the lower extremities are extended and internally rotated; the feet are plantar flexed (Fig. 49.4A). **Decerebrate posturing**, which occurs when the midbrain is not functional, is characterized by rigid extension and adduction of the arms and pronation of the wrists with the fingers flexed; the legs are held extended with the feet plantar flexed (see Fig. 49.4B).

Seizures are a sign of increased ICP, so if these occur, the child's ICP is becoming greatly compromised.

Intracranial Pressure Monitoring

ICP can be measured by several additional methods:

- An intraventricular catheter inserted through the anterior fontanelle
- A subdural screw or bolt inserted through a burr hole in the skull
- A fiberoptic sensor implanted into the epidural space (or the anterior fontanelle in an infant) (Fig. 49.5)

Intraventricular catheters (see Fig. 49.5C) are threaded into the lateral ventricle, filled with normal saline, and then connected to an external pressure monitor (Bailey, Liesemer, Statler, et al., 2012). As pressure in the ventricle fluctuates, it registers through the filled catheter onto an oscilloscope screen plus a written printout. This method is advantageous over simple scanning because it also enables CSF drainage and administration of medication through the catheter.

ICP in children normally ranges from 1 to 10 mmHg; a level greater than 15 mmHg needs further assessment. As blood pressure rises and falls with the influx of blood through vessels, so does ICP. On a monitor, this appears as A waves (plateau waves), B waves (short-duration waves), or C waves (small, rhythmic bursts). If brain ischemia is present, wave patterns change even before there is a deviation in blood pressure or pulse rate (Fig. 49.6). Because A waves appear to reflect brain ischemia, they can be used to signal when a child needs more oxygen.

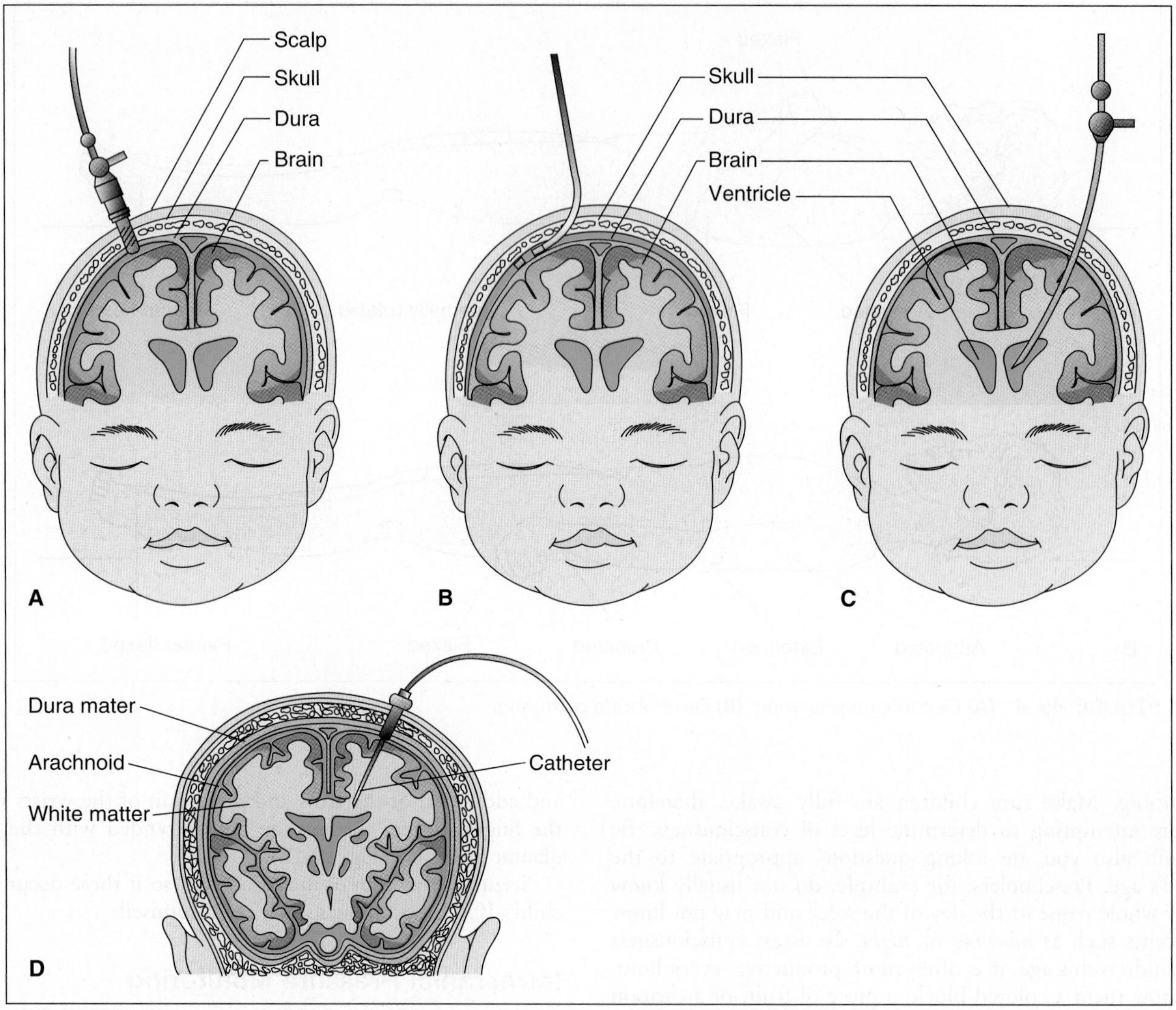

FIGURE 49.5 Devices used to monitor intracranial pressure. **(A)** Subarachnoid screw. **(B)** Epidural sensor. **(C)** Intraventricular catheter. **(D)** Intraparenchymal monitoring.

ICP monitoring also supplies information on cerebral perfusion pressure (CPP) or the amount of cerebral blood flow available to the brain (Box 49.3) because, if ICP ever exceeds arterial blood pressure (arises above about 50 mmHg), cerebral vessels can become obstructed (Budohoski, Zweifel, Kasprowicz, et al., 2012).

Parents can have difficulty accepting procedures such as the insertion of intraventricular catheters or screws. Explaining the brain's anatomy can help them understand that the catheter or screw is inserted into a hollow space and thus does not puncture or tear brain tissue. Be sure to explain that this type of monitoring is advantageous, not only because it enables early detection should problems arise but also because it helps to reduce the risk of further injury or complications.

Therapeutic Management

The cause of ICP must be identified and remedied as quickly as possible to prevent brain injury or compression to the brainstem, which can lead to both cardiac and respiratory failure. Actions such as coughing, vomiting, and sneezing and rapid administration of IV fluid increase ICP. When a parent is burping an infant after a feeding, caution them to be careful not to put pressure on the jugular veins, because this is another action that increases ICP. Placing a child in a semi-Fowler's position (use an infant seat for babies) or administering a corticosteroid such as dexamethasone (Decadron) can effectively reduce cerebral edema and its accompanying pressure. An osmotic diuretic, such as mannitol, given IV, causes a shift of fluid from extravascular compartments into the vascular stream (from brain tissue into blood vessels), so it also reduces pressure. Children usually have an indwelling urinary catheter inserted before beginning an osmotic diuretic to ensure that the child's kidneys are able to successfully excrete the intravessel fluid and prevent backpressure on the heart. If the ICP is caused by excessive fluid accumulating in the brain's ventricles, a ventricular tap may be necessary for immediate reduction of pressure.

Because increased ICP is a sign of an underlying disorder, after the pressure is reduced, the underlying cause must then be identified and rectified or the pressure will rise again from the original disorder.

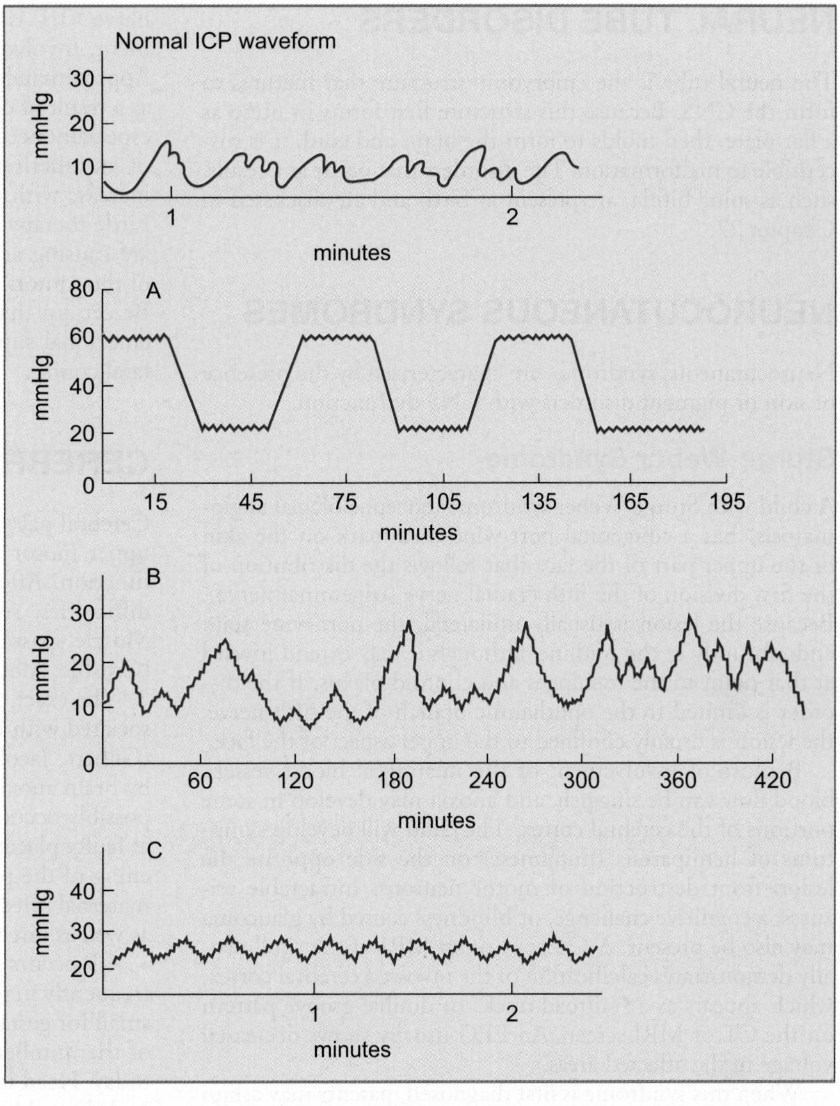

FIGURE 49.6 Normal intracranial pressure (ICP) waveform and generalized shapes of the three types of ICP waves: A waves or plateau waves, B waves, and C waves.

BOX 49.3 Calculating Cerebral Perfusion Pressure

Cerebral perfusion pressure (CPP) ranges from about 60 to 150 mmHg. If it is too low, it suggests blood is having difficulty circulating to brain cells; if it rises too high, it can also result in brain ischemia from the increased intracranial pressure (ICP). CPP is calculated by subtracting the mean ICP from the mean arterial pressure (MAP) or:

$$\text{MAP} - \text{ICP} = \text{CPP}$$

MAP is determined by subtracting the diastolic blood pressure (DBP) level from the systolic blood pressure (SBP) level, then dividing the result by 3, and adding that sum to 80 or:

$$\text{MAP} = \frac{(\text{SBP} - \text{DBP})}{3} + 80$$

To calculate CPP in a child with a blood pressure of 100/70 mmHg and an ICP of 10 mmHg, for example, first calculate the MAP:

$$\frac{(100 - 70)}{3} + 80 = 90 \text{ mmHg}$$

Next calculate the CPP:

$$90 - 10 = 80 \text{ mmHg (the child's CPP or a normal value)}$$

NEURAL TUBE DISORDERS

The neural tube is the embryonic structure that matures to form the CNS. Because this structure first forms in utero as a flat plate, then molds to form the brain and cord, it is susceptible to malformation. The disorders that occur as a result, such as spina bifida, are present at birth and are discussed in Chapter 27.

NEUROCUTANEOUS SYNDROMES

Neurocutaneous syndromes are characterized by the presence of skin or pigment disorders with CNS dysfunction.

Sturge-Weber Syndrome

A child with Sturge-Weber syndrome (encephalofacial angiomatosis) has a congenital port-wine birthmark on the skin of the upper part of the face that follows the distribution of the first division of the fifth cranial nerve (trigeminal nerve). Because the lesion is usually unilateral, the port-wine stain ends abruptly at the midline, although it may extend inward at that point to the meninges and choroid plexus. If the disorder is limited to the ophthalmic branch of the fifth nerve, the lesion is usually confined to the upper aspect of the face.

Because of involvement of the meningeal blood vessels, blood flow can be sluggish, and anoxia may develop in some portions of the cerebral cortex. The child will develop symptoms of hemiparesis (numbness) on the side opposite the lesion from destruction of motor neurons. Intractable seizures, a cognitive challenge, or blindness caused by glaucoma may also be present. A CT scan or an MRI of the skull usually demonstrates calcification of the involved cerebral cortex, which appears as a "railroad track" or double-groove pattern on the CT or MRI screen. An EEG usually shows decreased voltage in the affected areas.

When this syndrome is first diagnosed, parents may ask to have the skin lesion surgically removed in the belief that this will correct their child's condition. Unfortunately, because the lesion is not just a surface phenomenon, it's important that parents understand the need for long-term follow-up, particularly if the child has accompanying seizures that require long-term antiseizure therapy (Lo, Marchuk, Ball, et al., 2012).

Neurofibromatosis (von Recklinghausen Disease)

Neurofibromatosis is the unexplained development of subcutaneous tumors. The disorder can occur as a mutation, or it can be inherited as an autosomal dominant trait carried on the long arm of chromosome 17. It occurs in approximately 1 of every 4,000 live births and may be diagnosed prenatally (Ardern-Holmes & North, 2011). As an infant, the child typically shows irregular but excessive skin pigmentation. Later in childhood, pigmented nevi or café-au-lait ("coffee with cream") spots appear that tend to follow the paths of cutaneous nerves (six or more spots larger than 1 cm in diameter are diagnostic). By puberty, multiple soft cutaneous tumors begin to form in the child's skin along nerve pathways, and the child may develop seizures. Subcutaneous tumors develop by young adulthood. The acoustic nerve (cranial nerve VIII) is frequently involved, leading to hearing impairment. Involvement of the optic nerve can lead to vision loss. Approximately 8% of patients become cognitively challenged as a result of cerebral tumor formation or deterioration. Girls especially need to be aware of the disorder, not only because of its inheritance pattern but because tumor formation can increase with pregnancy (Chetty, Shaffer, & Norton, 2011). Little therapy is available to halt the tumor growth. If lesions are causing acoustic or optic degeneration, surgical removal of the tumors may be attempted to preserve hearing or sight. Be certain that both the parents and child have a source of emotional support through the disease's slow but invariably fatal course.

CEREBRAL PALSY

Cerebral palsy (CP) is a group of nonprogressive disorders of upper motor neuron impairment that result in motor dysfunction. Affected children also may have speech or ocular difficulties, seizures, cognitive challenges, or hyperactivity. Muscle spasticity can lead to orthopedic or gait difficulties (Crosbie, Alhusaini, Dean, et al., 2012).

The exact cause of CP is unknown, but the disorder is associated with low birth weight, preterm birth, or birth injury (Gilbert, Jacoby, Xing, et al., 2010). It apparently is caused by brain anoxia leading to cell destruction of the motor tracts possibly occurring during intrauterine life from a reason such as faulty placental implantation, placenta previa, or early loosening of the placenta. Nutritional deficiencies, drug use, and maternal infections such as cytomegalovirus or toxoplasmosis, as well as direct birth injury, may also contribute to the cause.

CP occurs in approximately 2 of every 1,000 births, most frequently in very-low-birth-weight infants and those who are small for gestational age; it is increasing in incidence because of the number of very-low-birth-weight infants who survive today. Head injury such as from child maltreatment or automobile accidents also may lead to CP symptoms. Infections such as meningitis or encephalitis can result in CP symptoms as well.

Types of Cerebral Palsy

CP has been classified in various ways, but traditionally, it is divided into two main categories based on the type of neuromuscular involvement: a pyramidal or spastic type (approximately 40% of affected children) and an extrapyramidal (dyskinetic) type, which is further subdivided into ataxic (approximately 10%), athetoid (approximately 30%), and mixed (approximately 10%) (Moster, Wilcox, Voilset, et al., 2010).

Spastic Type

Spasticity is excessive tone in the voluntary muscles that results from loss of upper motor neurons. A child with spastic CP has hypertonic muscles, abnormal clonus, exaggeration of deep tendon reflexes, abnormal reflexes such as a positive Babinski reflex, and continuation of neonatal reflexes, such as the tonic neck reflex, well past the age at which these usually disappear. If infants with CP are held in a ventral suspension position, they arch their backs and extend their arms and legs abnormally. They fail to demonstrate a parachute reflex if lowered suddenly and tend to assume a "scissors gait" because tight adductor thigh muscles cause their legs to cross when held upright. This involvement may be so severe that it leads to a subluxated hip. By school age, tightening of the heel cord can become so severe that children walk on their toes, unable to stretch their heel to touch the ground (Fig. 49.7).

Spastic involvement may affect both extremities on one side (**hemiplegia**), all four extremities (**quadriplegia**), or primarily the lower extremities (**diplegia** or **paraplegia**). Children with hemiplegia usually have greater involvement in the arm than the leg. The involved arm may be shorter and may have a smaller muscle circumference than the other arm. Most children with hemiplegia have difficulty identifying objects placed in their involved hand when their eyes are closed (**astereognosis**).

In older children, leg involvement may be detected most easily by examining the child's shoes as, because the child does not put the heel all the way down on the involved side, one shoe heel will be much more worn than the other. On physical examination, it may be difficult to abduct the involved hip fully, extend the knee, or dorsiflex the foot.

A child with quadriplegia invariably has impaired speech (pseudobulbar palsy) but may or may not be cognitively challenged. Swallowing saliva may be so difficult that the child drools and has difficulty swallowing food (Lewis, 2011).

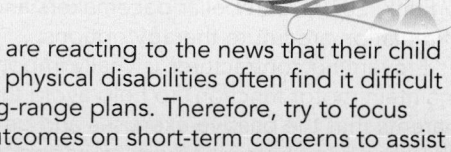

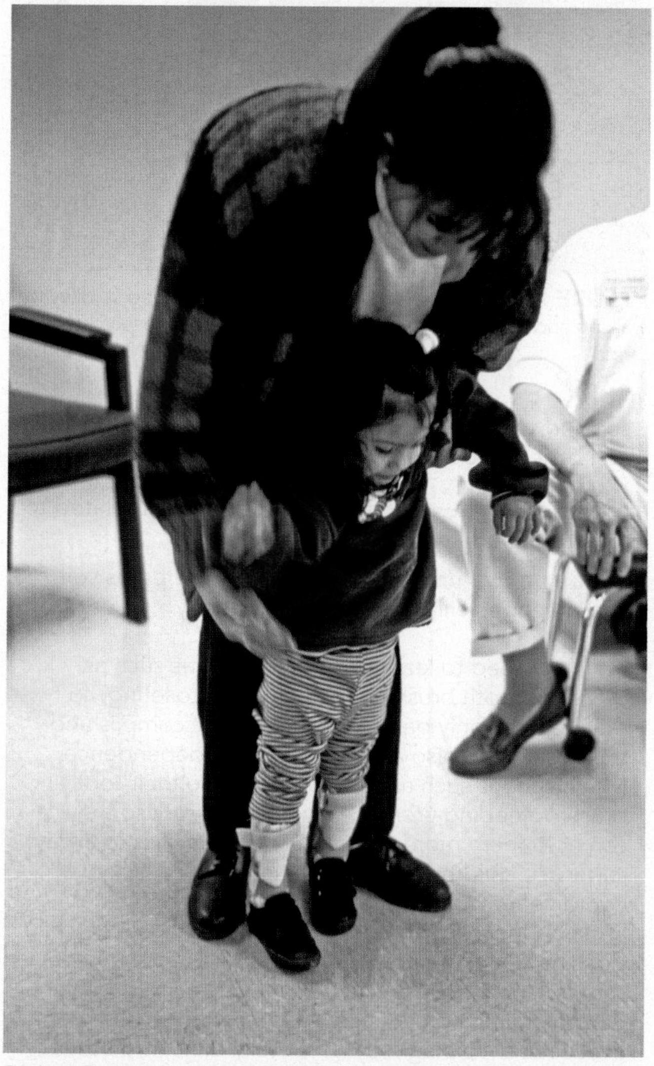

FIGURE 49.7 Physical therapy can help a child with cerebral palsy to lengthen the heel cords. (© Tina Manley/Alamy.)

Dyskinetic or Athetoid Type

The athetoid type of CP involves abnormal involuntary movement (*athetoid* means "wormlike"). Early in life, the child appears limp and flaccid. Later, in place of voluntary movement, children make slow, writhing motions. This can involve all four extremities, plus the face, neck, and tongue. Because of the poor tongue and swallowing movements, the child drools and speech is difficult to understand. Under emotional stress, the involuntary movements may become irregular and jerking (**choreoid**) with disordered muscle tone (**dyskinetic**).

Ataxic Type

Children with ataxic involvement have an awkward, wide-based gait. On neurologic examination, they are unable to perform fine coordinated motions, the finger-to-nose test, or rapid, repetitive movements (tests of cerebellar function).

Mixed Type

Some children show symptoms of both spasticity and athetoid or ataxic and athetoid movements. This combination obviously results in a severe degree of physical impairment.

Assessment

The diagnosis of CP is based on history and physical assessment. Any episode of possible anoxia during prenatal life or at birth should be documented. Determining the extent of involvement in an infant is difficult, so the full extent of the disorder may not be recognized until the child attempts complex motor skills, such as walking or coloring.

Children with all forms of CP may have sensory alterations such as strabismus, refractive disorders, visual perception problems, visual field defects, and speech disorders such as abnormal rhythm or articulation. They may show an attention deficit disorder or autism spectrum syndrome. Cognitive challenge and recurrent seizures also frequently accompany all types of the disorder. A skull X-ray or ultrasound may show cerebral asymmetry. An EEG may be abnormal, although the pattern is highly variable.

Nursing Diagnoses and Related Interventions

Parents who are reacting to the news that their child has multiple physical disabilities often find it difficult to make long-range plans. Therefore, try to focus expected outcomes on short-term concerns to assist with family functioning.

Nursing Diagnosis: Deficient knowledge related to understanding of complex disease condition

Outcome Evaluation: Parents state that they understand the cause of the disease is unknown but it is not progressive.

It's important for parents to understand that CP is nonprogressive and that the brain damage that occurred during pregnancy or at birth will not extend. The child's condition may seem to grow more apparent with age, however, as the child is expected to complete fine motor tasks. Without follow-up care, contractures from spasticity can result, further reducing existing motor function.

Caution parents also that CP is a single name for a wide variety of disorders of varying consequence. Although another child they know may have such severe CP that he has no useful function in his extremities, this does not mean their own child will be affected to the same extent. Conversely, although they know someone with CP who is able to hold a full-time job, their child may not be able to do so as well. Each child needs individual assessment so the child's maximum potential can be evaluated.

Nursing Diagnosis: Risk for disuse syndrome related to spasticity of muscle groups

Outcome Evaluation: Child walks with a minimum of support or equipment; skin and tissue remain intact.

Children with CP need promotion of any function that is not already impaired to prevent further loss of function and allow them to master the highest level of self-care, communication, ambulation, education, nutrition, and establishment of self-esteem they can achieve.

Learning to be ambulatory is an important part of self-care, because it plays a large role in determining how independent the child can become. Walking can be difficult for the child to master because of lack of muscle coordination. Following surgery to lengthen heel tendons, assisted ambulation devices such as wheeled walkers may be necessary (Fig. 49.8). There are no drugs that cure CP, but a number can help relieve spasticity. Dopaminergic drugs, such as carbidopa/levodopa (Sinemet), widely used in Parkinson disease, increase the level of dopamine and, therefore, reduce rigidity. Muscle relaxants such as baclofen (Lioresal), given either orally or administered continuously by an infusion pump, and benzodiazepines such as diazepam (Valium) can also help with smoother muscle movement (Gray, Morton, Brimlow, et al., 2012). Administration of botulism toxin (Botox) has been successful in some children to relieve spasticity and aid in walking (Placzek, Siebold, & Funk, 2010). Cerebellar pacemakers and vagal stimulation are future therapy options.

Preventing contractures is vitally important to maintain motor function. To help avoid these, teach parents that the passive exercises and games their child has been prescribed are an important part of their child's therapy and must be done consistently each day. To further prevent contractures, partial lightweight leg braces may be prescribed to encourage children to bring their heels down and to keep heel cords from tightening. If leg braces are prescribed, parents may need some encouragement and support to insist a child wears them because it is the constant stretching that offers best results.

FIGURE 49.8 Wheeled walkers give a child added stability for walking and keep heel cords from shortening. (© fotosearch.com.)

Nursing Diagnosis: Risk for self-care deficit related to impaired mobility

Outcome Evaluation: Child feeds and dresses self and manages elimination independently.

Children need to learn self-care measures such as dressing, tooth brushing, bathing, and toileting, so they can not only gain self-esteem by accomplishing these tasks but also achieve optimal independence. Modifications such as straps attached to their toothbrush or feeding utensils may be necessary so they can hold them more securely. Advise parents to always supervise children during bathing because lack of coordination could cause them to slip under water and drown. Toileting is often difficult because the child does not have the muscle group coordination necessary to achieve successful bowel evacuation. A high-fiber diet helps prevent constipation and aids bowel evacuation. Voiding may be equally difficult, because the child may lack sufficient voluntary muscle control.

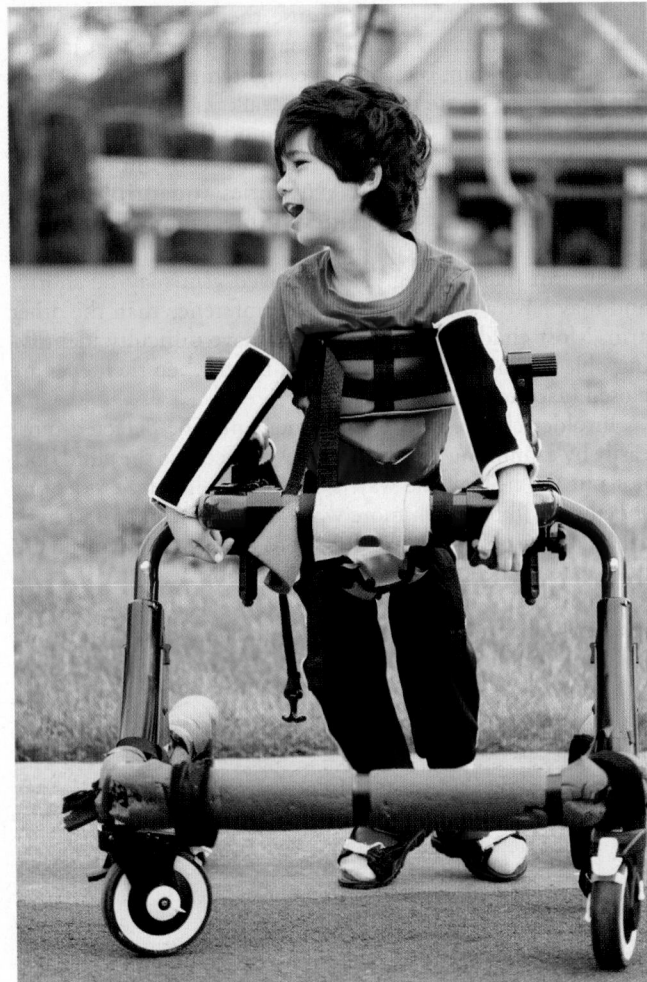

Parents may need considerable support and guidance to allow a child to complete self-care tasks independently, because doing so often requires extreme patience. Letting a child perform these activities, however, helps to instill confidence and self-esteem in the child and helps allow the child to reach his or her maximum potential.

Nursing Diagnosis: Risk for delayed growth and development related to activity restriction secondary to CP

Outcome Evaluation: Child receives environmental stimulation; expresses interest in people and activities around him; attends school setting that is as free of restrictions as possible.

Children with CP may be unable to pursue stimulating activities and surroundings because they are not fully mobile. Therefore, encourage parents to bring these things to them as well as be certain toys and activities are appropriate to the child's intellectual, developmental, and motor levels, not the child's chronologic age. Some children need more stimulating activities than others because they have difficulty concentrating on one activity for any length of time.

A preschool program is important to provide exposure to the outside world. If at all possible, school-age children with CP should be mainstreamed so that they can learn alongside other children. You may need to advocate that a child be placed in a school setting that is consistent with intellectual abilities.

Nursing Diagnosis: Risk for imbalanced nutrition, less than body requirements, related to difficulty sucking in infancy or difficulty feeding self in an older child

Outcome Evaluation: Child's weight remains within 5th to 95th percentile on height–weight chart; skin turgor remains good; specific gravity of urine is 1.003 to 1.030.

Providing adequate nutrition to children with CP can be difficult because they often have difficulty sucking because uncoordinated movements of the tongue, lips, and jaw and tongue thrusting make this difficult. They may tend to push food out of their mouth (a retained primitive reflex) rather than swallow smoothly. Older children may have difficulty holding and controlling a spoon to bring food to their mouths. Parents may need guidance in finding a feeding pattern that works for their child. Manually controlling the jaw may help control the head, correct neck and trunk hyperextension, and stabilize the jaw to assist with feeding. If a child cannot chew or swallow well, a liquid or soft diet may be necessary. A hyperactive gag reflex or symptoms of gastroesophageal reflux may cause children to vomit after feeding. Positioning infants upright after feeding helps to prevent aspiration if vomiting occurs.

Nursing Diagnosis: Impaired verbal communication related to neurologic impairment

Outcome Evaluation: Child can verbally make needs known to strangers and family members.

Most children with CP benefit from speech therapy, which helps them learn to speak slowly and to coordinate their lips and tongue to form speech sounds. Be patient when talking to them so they feel comfortable taking their time to form words deliberately. For the child who cannot speak clearly, provide an alternative form of communication, such as flash cards, a picture board, or a touch-screen computer to aid communication.

Long-Term Care

Because CP is not always diagnosed early in infancy, parents may not learn their child has a chronic disorder until 2 to 4 years later. Listen to parents during health care visits and encourage them to discuss the difficulties of daily living, such as feeding problems. Offer them support as needed if they grieve because their child is not able to accomplish all of the major things they had wished for during pregnancy or feel defeated by the day-to-day strain of caring for their child's multiple special needs. Care of a child with a chronic illness is discussed further in Chapter 56.

QSEN Checkpoint Question 49.3

Informatics

Tasha's sister Wanda was diagnosed with CP as an infant. What information would you want her parents to know about her prognosis?

a. Symptoms of CP typically begin to wane just after puberty.
b. The severity of cognitive deficits parallels the severity of physical deficits.
c. CP may occasionally be caused by a childhood vaccine reaction.
d. Symptoms may seem to grow worse as fine motor skill is needed.

Look in Appendix A for the best answer and rationale.

INFECTION

Infection of the nervous system is always potentially serious. It typically occurs from illnesses such as meningitis, encephalitis, Guillain-Barré syndrome, Reye syndrome, and botulism.

Bacterial Meningitis

Meningitis is, as the name implies, infection of the cerebral meninges. It tends to occur most frequently in children younger than 24 months of age and most often in winter. The organisms most frequently seen are *Streptococcus pneumoniae* or group B *Streptococcus*. In children younger than 2 months of age, *Escherichia coli* is a common cause. If children with myelomeningocele develop meningitis, *Pseudomonas* infection may be the causative agent. Children who have had a splenectomy are particularly susceptible to pneumococcal meningitis unless they have received a pneumococcal vaccine. *Haemophilus influenzae*, once a major cause of meningitis, is now rarely seen because of routine immunization against this organism (Greenberg-Kushnir, Haskin, Yarden-Bilavsky, et al., 2012).

Pathologic organisms usually spread to the meninges from upper respiratory tract infections, by lymphatic drainage possibly through the mastoid or frontal sinuses, or by direct introduction through a lumbar puncture or skull fracture. Once organisms enter the meningeal space, they multiply rapidly and then spread throughout the CSF to invade brain tissue through the meningeal folds, which extend down into the brain itself. Brain abscess or invasion of the infection into cranial nerves can result in blindness, hearing impairment, or facial paralysis. If a thick exudate accumulates in the narrow aqueduct of Sylvius, it can cause obstruction leading to hydrocephalus. Brain tissue edema can put pressure on the pituitary gland, causing increased production of antidiuretic hormone, resulting in the syndrome of inappropriate antidiuretic hormone secretion (SIADH), causing hyponatremia.

Assessment

Children usually have had 2 or 3 days of upper respiratory tract infection prior to the development of meningitis. They then grow increasingly irritable because of an intense headache. They experience sharp pain when they bend their head forward. In the newborn, symptoms such as poor sucking, weak cry, or lethargy develop. As the disease progresses, signs of meningeal irritability then occur, as evidenced by positive Brudzinski and Kernig signs.

Children may hold their back arched and their neck hyperextended (opisthotonos). If third and sixth cranial nerve paralysis occurs, a child will not be able to follow a light through full visual fields. If the fontanelles are open, they bulge upward and feel tense; if they are closed, papilledema may develop. If the meningitis is caused by *H. influenzae*, the child may develop septic arthritis. If it is caused by *Neisseria meningitidis*, a papular or purple petechial skin rash may occur (Pace & Pollard, 2012).

After this beginning of a myriad of general symptoms, sudden cardiovascular shock, seizures, nuchal rigidity, or apnea can occur. Because the infant has open fontanelles, nuchal rigidity appears late and is not as useful a sign for diagnosis as in the older child. As a rule, a child with a high temperature who then has a seizure is assumed to have meningitis until CSF findings prove otherwise.

CSF analysis obtained by lumbar puncture confirms the diagnosis. CSF results indicative of meningitis include increased white blood cell and protein levels, increased ICP, and a glucose level less than 60% of blood glucose (because bacteria have fed on the glucose). In addition to supplying blood for glucose level, blood is cultured and examined for increased WBC count. If the child has had close association with someone with tuberculosis, a tuberculin skin test to rule out tuberculosis meningitis will be done. A CT scan, MRI, or ultrasound study will be prescribed to examine for brain abscess.

Therapeutic Management

Antibiotic therapy as indicated by sensitivity studies is the primary therapy. Intrathecal injections (directly into the CSF) may also be necessary, especially because the blood–brain barrier may prevent the chosen antibiotic from passing freely into the CSF. In some children, it takes a month before the CSF cell count returns to normal. A corticosteroid such as dexamethasone or the osmotic diuretic mannitol may be administered to reduce ICP and help prevent hearing loss.

In addition to standard precautions, children with meningitis are placed on respiratory precautions for 24 hours after the start of antibiotic therapy to prevent transmission of the infection to other family members or health care providers. In addition, an antibiotic may be prescribed prophylactically for the child's immediate family members or for playmates who have been in close contact with the child.

Meningitis is always a serious disorder, because it can run a rapid, fulminating, and possibly fatal course. If symptoms are recognized early and treatment is effective, however, a child will recover with no sequelae. Neurologic sequelae, such as learning problems, seizures, hearing and cognitive challenges, and inability to concentrate urine from lessened antidiuretic hormone secretion, must be assessed in the weeks to come because these can be long-term consequences.

What if... 49.1 The cause of Tasha's seizure is found to be bacterial meningitis. Because she has severe neck pain whenever she is moved, her mother asks you not to be so concerned about measuring intake and output, so her daughter can rest. Would you follow that advice? Suppose you call Tasha's name and she does not answer you? Why is this a particular cause of concern in a child with meningitis?

Nursing Diagnoses and Related Interventions

If a child has meningitis, the parents may feel responsible for the illness because they knew the child had an upper respiratory infection. They may ask if they could have prevented meningitis if only they had taken the child to their primary care provider as soon as the respiratory symptoms began. You can assure them the symptoms of meningitis occur so insidiously that no one can appreciate what disease process is at work from the first generalized signs.

Be certain to orient parents to infection control techniques if the child is isolated so they can feel comfortable caring for their child.

Nursing Diagnosis: Pain related to meningeal irritation

Outcome Evaluation: Child states pain is tolerable and shows no facial grimacing or other signs of discomfort.

For a child with meningitis, dealing with the number of invasive procedures, such as lumbar puncture, venipuncture, and IV therapy, necessary can make a hospital stay difficult. Remember that children feel pain when their head is flexed forward, so they usually are more comfortable without a pillow. Be careful not to flex their neck forward when turning or positioning them.

Although children would probably benefit from puppet play or coloring, activities that could help them express how they feel about so many intrusive procedures, frequently they are too uncomfortable to play and thus are not able to be comforted by these measures. Be certain that children receive a good explanation of everything that is happening and extra attention from health care personnel, not just when they perform painful procedures but so children can feel secure. Help parents understand that their child's acute irritableness is caused by the disease process and not by anything they did or are doing so they can continue to interact with the child. You can assure them that, as their child recovers, irritability will lessen and the child will begin to show more interest in communicating feelings. Promote rest by keeping stimulation in the room to a minimum.

Nursing Diagnosis: Risk for ineffective tissue perfusion (cerebral), related to increased ICP

Outcome Evaluation: Child's vital signs return to normal; child is alert and oriented; motor, cognitive, and sensory functions are within acceptable parameters for the child's age; specific gravity of urine is 1.003 to 1.030.

Observe the child carefully for signs of increased ICP such as increased blood pressure or slowed pulse rate. Carefully monitor the rate of all IV infusions to prevent overhydration and increased ICP. Measure urine specific gravity to detect oversecretion or undersecretion of antidiuretic hormone because of pituitary pressure. Measure the child's head circumference, and weigh the child daily. Monitor hearing acuity (reduced if there is compression of the eighth cranial nerve) by asking an older child a question or observing whether an infant listens to a music box or to your voice.

Group B Streptococcal Infection

A major cause of meningitis in newborns is group B streptococci. The organism is contracted either in utero or from secretions in the birth canal. It can spread to other newborns in a hospital nursery if good hand washing technique is not used.

Colonization can result in either an early-onset or a late-onset illness. With the early-onset form, symptoms of pneumonia become apparent in the first few hours of life. The late-onset type leads to meningitis instead of pneumonia.

With meningitis, at approximately 2 weeks of age, the infant gradually becomes lethargic and develops a fever and upper respiratory tract symptoms. The fontanelles bulge from increased ICP. The disease is extremely serious as mortality from the infection is approximately 25%; surviving infants may develop neurologic consequences such as hydrocephalus or seizures (Libster, Edwards, Levent, et al., 2012). Treatment is with antibiotics that are effective against the group B *Streptococcus*, such as ampicillin and cephalosporins. Because it can be difficult for parents to understand how their infant suddenly became so ill, they may need considerable support in immediately caring for the infant or if the infant is left neurologically challenged.

QSEN Checkpoint Question 49.4

Quality Improvement

Tasha is diagnosed as having bacterial meningitis, and her plan of care is being amended in light of this diagnostic finding. How long should the care team maintain respiratory precautions for this condition after Tasha begins an antibiotic?

a. 4 hours
b. 24 hours
c. Until her core body temperature returns to normal
d. Until her arterial blood gases return to normal

Look in Appendix A for the best answer and rationale.

Encephalitis

Encephalitis is an inflammation of brain tissue and, possibly, the meninges as well (Kneen, Michael, Menson, et al., 2012). It can arise from protozoan, bacterial, fungal, or viral invasions. Enteroviruses are the most frequent cause, followed by arboviruses such as the togavirus. Several encephalitis viruses, such as those that cause St. Louis encephalitis, West Nile encephalitis, and Eastern equine encephalitis, are borne by mosquitoes and thus are seen most often during the summer months. Encephalitis also can result from direct invasion of the CSF during lumbar puncture. Yet another cause is as a complication of childhood diseases such as measles, mumps, or chickenpox. In order to prevent the disease, therefore, it is crucial children receive immunization against childhood diseases and use mosquito repellents when in mosquito-infested areas.

Assessment

Symptoms of encephalitis begin either gradually or suddenly and include symptoms such as headache, high temperature, ataxia (loss of usual muscle movements), muscle weakness or paralysis, diplopia, confusion, and irritability; if meninges are also involved, signs of meningeal irritation, such as nuchal rigidity and a positive Brudzinski or Kernig sign, may also be present. A child becomes increasingly lethargic and eventually comatose.

The diagnosis is made by the history and physical assessment. CSF evaluation will reveal an elevated leukocyte count and an elevated protein level. An EEG will demonstrate widespread cerebral involvement. A brain biopsy, usually taken from the temporal lobe or infected CSF, identifies the virus.

Therapeutic Management

Treatment for a child with encephalitis is primarily supportive. An antipyretic is prescribed to control fever. Mechanical ventilation may be required to maintain the child's respirations during the acute phase. A variety of medications, such as acyclovir (Zovirax), an antiviral agent, and carbamazepine (Tegretol), an anticonvulsant, may be prescribed. A steroid such as dexamethasone or an osmotic diuretic such as mannitol may be needed to decrease brain edema and ICP.

Encephalitis is always a serious diagnosis because, although a child may recover from the initial attack without further symptoms, there can be residual neurologic damage, such as seizures or learning disabilities. Parents may find it hard to believe their child is so seriously ill at first because in the beginning of the illness, their child only seemed tired and had a slight headache. They can find it even harder to accept that permanent impairment, such as a learning disability, could result. This makes follow-up care after hospitalization important both for the child's rehabilitation and to help parents deal with their grief, shock, and possible anger over this devastating turn of events in their life.

Reye Syndrome

Reye syndrome is acute encephalopathy with accompanying fatty infiltration of the liver, heart, lungs, pancreas, and skeletal muscle. It occurs in children from 1 to 18 years of age regardless of gender (Ninove, Daniel, Gallou, et al., 2011).

The cause is unknown, but symptoms such as lethargy, vomiting, confusion, and combativeness usually occur after a viral infection such as varicella (chickenpox) or influenza that was treated with acetylsalicylic acid (aspirin). Treatment is supportive. Untreated, the condition leads to coma and death. Anticipatory guidance to parents and children about avoiding the use of aspirin during viral infections has almost prevented the syndrome (Bennett, Starko, Thomsen, et al., 2012).

Guillain-Barré Syndrome

Guillain-Barré syndrome (inflammatory polyradiculoneuropathy) is a perplexing syndrome that occurs in about 1 in every 100,000 children. Both motor and sensory portions of peripheral nerves are affected. Boys develop it more often than girls (Yuki & Hartung, 2012). With successful widespread polio eradication efforts, Guillain-Barré syndrome is now the most common cause of acute and subacute flaccid paralysis in childhood (Rosen, 2012).

The cause of the condition is unknown, but it is suspected that the reaction is immune mediated, occurring after upper respiratory tract or gastrointestinal illnesses or, rarely, immunizations. Inflammation of the nerve fibers apparently causes temporary demyelinization of the nerve sheaths.

Assessment

Children experience peripheral neuritis several days after the primary infection. Tendon reflexes begin to decrease and then become absent. Muscle paralysis and paresthesia (loss of sensation) begin first in the legs and then spread to involve the arms, trunk, and head. The symmetric nature of the disorder helps to differentiate it from other types of paraplegia. Cranial nerve involvement leads to facial weakness and difficulty in swallowing. As the respiratory muscles become involved, spontaneous respirations are no longer possible, leading to respiratory involvement severe enough to warrant mechanical ventilation.

A significant laboratory finding is an elevated CSF protein level. An EEG may show denervation and decreased nerve conduction velocity.

Therapeutic Management

Treatment of Guillain-Barré syndrome is supportive until the paralysis peaks at 3 weeks and then is followed by gradual recovery. A course of prednisone to halt the autoimmune response may be tried, but its use is controversial. Plasmapheresis or transfusion of immune serum globulin may shorten the course of the illness. Cardiac and respiratory function must be closely monitored. All patients should be given subcutaneous fractionated or unfractionated heparin and support stockings until they are able to walk independently to prevent deep vein thrombosis.

Other necessary measures include prevention of the effects of extreme immobility while guarding respiratory function. An indwelling urinary catheter is usually inserted to monitor urine output. Enteral or total parenteral nutrition may be used to support protein and carbohydrate needs. If the child has discomfort from neuritis, adequate analgesia is necessary.

To prevent muscle contractures and effects of immobility, turning and repositioning every 2 hours is important in addition to passive range-of-motion exercises about every 4 hours. Be certain to provide adequate stimulation for the long weeks when the child is unable to perform any care independently. Fortunately, despite the long period of mandatory ventilation therapy, most children recover completely, without any residual effects of the syndrome, although some may continue to have minor problems such as residual weakness.

Botulism

Botulism occurs when spores of *Clostridium botulinum* colonize and produce toxins in the intestine. The disease cannot be transmitted from person to person and usually occurs in infants younger than 6 months of age (Chalk, Benstead, & Keezer, 2011). The source of the spores is often unknown, but honey may be frequently contaminated with the spores and thus should not be given to infants (Kumar, Lorenc, Robinson, et al., 2011).

Symptoms occur within a few hours after ingestion of the contaminated food. Almost immediately, there is generalized weakness, hypotonia, listlessness, a weak cry, and a diminished gag reflex, followed by a flaccid paralysis of the bulbar muscles that leads to diminished respiratory function. The organism can be cultured from stools or serum. Electromyography may be helpful to support the diagnosis. Treatment is supportive care. Human-derived botulinum immune globulin may stop the progress of the disease.

INFLAMMATORY DISORDERS

Two neurologic inflammatory disorders are found frequently in adolescents.

Carpal Tunnel Syndrome

Carpal tunnel syndrome is nerve compression of the median nerve that passes through the carpal tunnel at the wrist (Luckhaupt, Dalhamer, Ward, et al., 2013). Compression of the nerve causes numbness and sharp pain and burning in the thumb and the second, third, and fourth fingers of the hand. Word processing, texting, and video games have turned this previously adult disorder into a disorder that occurs in children as well. Pain usually occurs at night and is enough to keep a child awake. The usual therapy is application of a splint to the wrist, which holds the wrist in a neutral (not flexed and not extended) position. An oral anti-inflammatory medication and perhaps a corticosteroid injection into the inflamed wrist both help to relieve pain. If these therapies are not successful, the stricture at the carpal canal can be relieved surgically.

Facial Palsy (Bell Palsy)

Facial palsy is facial paralysis of the seventh (facial) cranial nerve, the nerve that innervates the muscles of facial expression. The syndrome occurs abruptly and may be associated with herpes or Lyme disease infection or occur as a result of cold air from skiing or from riding in a convertible. Therapy in adults consists of prednisone to reduce inflammation and acyclovir if the syndrome is herpes related. In children, prednisone use is variable. If the child is unable to close the eye on the affected side, eye drops three or four times daily will be needed. Although recovery is slow, usually takes about 4 months, most children recover without any permanent disability (McNamara, Doyle, McKay, et al., 2013).

PAROXYSMAL DISORDERS

A paroxysmal disorder is one that occurs suddenly and recurrently. Seizures, headaches, and breath-holding spells are the most frequent types seen in childhood.

Epilepsy (Recurrent Seizures)

A *seizure* is an involuntary contraction of muscle caused by abnormal electrical brain discharges. Approximately 5% of children will have at least one seizure by the time they reach adulthood (Baldin, Ludvigsson, Mixa, et al., 2012). These episodes are always frightening to parents and other children because of the intensity. Although about 50% of seizures are idiopathic (unknown cause), they also can be attributed to infection, trauma, or tumor growth. Familial or polygenic inheritance may be responsible. Because they are not so much a disease as a symptom of an underlying disorder, all seizures need to be investigated.

The term *epilepsy* comes from a Greek word meaning "to take hold of." Because the word has stigmas of cognitive challenge, behavioral disorders, institutionalization, or unexplainable strangeness attached to it, a preferred term is *recurrent seizures* because this term explains the disease process without the effect of discrimination (Box 49.4).

BOX 49.4 Nursing Care Planning to Respect Cultural Diversity

The degree of understanding about the cause of disorders such as recurrent seizures varies in different cultures. The often unknown cause of recurrent (idiopathic) seizures has lead to them being attributed to an invasion by evil spirits or the effect of curses. Many people today still fear that recurrent seizures will lead to cognitive impairment. Many parents worry that their child will be refused admission to a school or refused a job as an adult because they are viewed as so unpredictable. Being aware of these common misconceptions can help you appreciate parents' anxiety about the diagnosis of recurrent seizures, an anxiety that can accentuate the need for parent education and careful planning to maintain self-esteem in their child.

The types and causes of seizures vary with age and are classified into two major categories: partial and generalized seizures. As the name implies, with partial seizures, only one area of the brain is involved; with generalized seizures, the disturbance appears to involve the entire brain; loss of consciousness usually occurs. It's important that seizures be differentiated by their degree of severity and type, so that parents can know any special precautions they need to take for their child and appropriate management and drug therapy can be instituted.

Seizures in the Newborn Period

Seizure activity in the newborn period may be difficult to recognize because it may consist only of twitching of the head, arms, or eyes; smacking of the lips; slight cyanosis; and perhaps respiratory difficulty or apnea. Afterward, the infant may appear limp and flaccid. Whereas seizures in older children are often of unknown cause, 75% of seizures in neonates have a known cause such as trauma and anoxia from intrauterine life or birth; metabolic disorders, such as hypoglycemia, hypocalcemia or lack of pyridoxine (vitamin B_6); neonatal infection; or acute bilirubin encephalopathy caused by a blood incompatibility.

Because of the nervous system's immaturity, EEGs in the newborn may be normal despite extensive disease. A noticeably abnormal EEG in the newborn period, therefore, generally means a poor prognosis, indicating that involvement this early in life must be severe. Because almost 20% of all newborns have abnormal CSF values compared with adult standards (protein is increased, and there may be a few red blood cells from rupture of subarachnoid capillaries from the pressure of birth), lumbar puncture also is not conclusive.

High doses of antiseizure medication may be needed to control seizures in newborns because they metabolize drugs more rapidly than older children. In adults, for example, phenobarbital may be administered in the range of 1.5 mg/kg body weight per day. In newborns, the dose might be as high as 3 to 10 mg/kg/day.

Seizures in the Infant and Toddler Periods

Seizures commonly seen in this age group are **infantile spasms**, a form of generalized seizure often called "salaam" or "jackknife" seizures, or infantile myoclonic seizures. These are characterized by very rapid movements of the trunk with sudden strong contractions of most of the body, including flexion and adduction of the limbs, or the infant suddenly slumps forward from a sitting position or falls from a standing position. The episode may occur singly or in clusters as frequently as 100 times a day.

In approximately 50% of affected children, there is an identifiable cause such as trauma, a metabolic disease such as phenylketonuria, or a viral invasion such as herpes or cytomegalovirus. In other children, the spasms apparently result from a failure of normal organized electrical activity in the brain. Approximately 90% of infants with this type of involvement will be developmentally delayed as intellectual development appears to halt and even regress after the pattern of seizures begins. Most children with infantile spasms show high-amplitude slow waves and spikes, a chaotic discharge called *hypsarrhythmia* on an EEG tracing.

These seizures occur slightly more often in males than females, occur in 2 to 3 per 10,000 live births, have a family history in 3% to 6% of cases, and only spontaneously stop in 30% of children (Go, Mackay, Weiss, et al., 2012). Because the response to treatment with antiseizure therapy tends to be poor, parenteral adrenocorticotropic hormone (ACTH) therapy, prednisone, or high-dose vigabatrin, an amino acid, are used in its place. High-dose valproate or a newer antiseizure agent such as topiramate (Topamax) may be used in children who do not respond to usual therapy, as well as pyridoxine (vitamin B_6) or a ketogenic diet (see below), but research shows none to be as effective as ACTH, especially for preserving neurodevelopmental outcomes (Go et al., 2012). In most children, the seizure phenomenon seems to "burn itself out" by 2 years of age. Any associated cognitive or developmental delay remains, however, so children need good follow-up planning and care.

Seizures Caused by Poisoning or Drugs. The possibility of poisoning has to be considered in any child who has a first seizure. Although this is most likely to occur between 6 months and 3 years of age, it must be considered again in adolescence, when drugs may be intentionally self-administered. Seizures also can be a late symptom of encephalopathy caused by lead poisoning (see Chapter 52).

Seizures in Children Older Than 3 Years of Age

Febrile Seizures. Seizures associated with high fever (102° to 104°F [38.9° to 40.0°C]) are the most common type seen in preschool children, although these can occur as late as 7 years of age. They are most serious if they occur under 6 months of age. Such seizures may occur after immunization with live vaccines because these most commonly produce fevers. The seizure is usually a generalized tonic–clonic pattern, which lasts for 15 to 20 seconds. An EEG tracing afterward is usually normal. There also is usually a history of other family members having had similar seizures.

The seizure is apparently due to a sudden spike of temperature, not a gradual incline. The seizure only lasts 1 to 2 minutes or less. Although quickly over, such seizures must be taken seriously and investigated for a possible cause, because meningitis often manifests initially with high fever and a seizure this same way (American Academy of Pediatrics [AAP], 2011).

Prevention of Febrile Seizures. Because these seizures arise with high fever, they are largely preventable. If ibuprofen or acetaminophen is given to keep a developing fever below 101°F (38.4°C), the seizures rarely occur. They happen most often when a child develops a fever at night, when a parent is not aware of it, or when a parent is reluctant to give ibuprofen or acetaminophen in large enough doses to be therapeutic. Because the recommended doses of these medicines vary with the type (liquid or pills), caution parents to read the bottle label carefully before administration to be certain they are administering the correct dosage. At one time, febrile seizures were thought to be preventable by giving phenobarbital during an upper respiratory tract infection; this is no longer recommended because phenobarbital takes 2 or 3 days to reach a therapeutic blood level, and by this time, a seizure would already have occurred. If a second febrile seizure does occur, diazepam (Valium) may be prescribed for the parents to administer the next time the child has a high fever (AAP, 2011).

Teach parents that every child who has a febrile seizure must be seen by a health care provider to rule out meningitis and to be aware that it will be assumed by emergency room personnel that the child has meningitis until it is ruled out by a complete neurologic workup.

Therapeutic Management. After a febrile seizure subsides, parents should sponge the child with tepid water to reduce the fever quickly. Advise them not to put the child in a bathtub of water to do this because it would be easy for the child to slip under water should a second seizure occur. Caution parents not to apply alcohol or cold water because extreme cooling causes shock to an immature nervous system; in addition, alcohol can be absorbed by the skin or the fumes can be inhaled in toxic amounts, compounding the child's problems. Parents should not attempt to give oral medications such as acetaminophen, because the child will be in a drowsy, or *postictal*, state after the seizure and might aspirate the medicine. Suppositories may be given at the appropriate dose. If attempts to reduce the child's temperature by sponging are unsuccessful, advise parents to put cool washcloths on the child's forehead, axillary, and groin areas and transport the child, lightly clothed, to a health care facility for immediate evaluation.

At the health care facility, a lumbar puncture will be performed to rule out meningitis. If warranted, antipyretic drugs to reduce the fever below seizure levels will be administered. Appropriate antibiotic therapy will be prescribed if an infection is documented.

Many parents need to be reassured that febrile seizures do not lead to brain damage and that the child is almost always completely well afterward.

What if... 49.2 Tasha's mother refuses to allow her to play with other children because she's worried Tasha will contract an upper respiratory infection from one of them and then have a febrile seizure. Is the mother taking a safe precaution or overreacting to the possibility of a seizure?

Complex Partial (Psychomotor or Temporal Lobe) Seizures. More than half of children who develop recurrent seizures during school age have an idiopathic type or the cause of the seizures cannot be discovered. Despite this, medication can effectively control these seizures in almost all affected children. Some seizures in this age group occur because of organic causes such as laceration of brain tissue from an automobile accident or fall, an enlarging brain tumor, hemorrhage due to a blood dyscrasia, infection (meningitis or encephalitis), anoxia, or toxic conditions such as lead poisoning that have left residual damage. The possibility that brain trauma could have been caused by child maltreatment is always another possibility to consider.

Complex partial (psychomotor) seizures vary greatly in extent and symptoms and tend to be a difficult type to control. The child may notice a slight *aura*, or sensation a seizure is about to occur, but this is rarely as definite as that seen with tonic–clonic seizures. Results of a CT or MRI scan and EEG will invariably be normal.

This type of seizure often begins with a sudden change in posture, such as an arm dropping suddenly to the side. Other motor, sensory, and behavioral signs might include

automatisms (complex purposeless movements, such as lip smacking, fumbling hand movements, intense running, or screaming). A few children may then slump to the ground, unconscious. Circumoral pallor develops due to a halt in respirations. The child begins breathing again almost immediately and usually regains consciousness in less than 5 minutes. He or she may feel slightly drowsy afterward but does not have an actual postictal stage or a period of sustained unconsciousness as seen with tonic–clonic seizures.

Common drugs used to treat this type of seizure include carbamazepine (Tegretol) (Box 49.5) or valproate (Depakene). Carbamazepine can lead to neutropenia, so white blood cell counts need to be monitored during therapy. If these drugs are not effective, surgery to remove the epileptogenic focus or the implantation of a vagus nerve stimulator can be used to significantly reduce seizure frequency. If seizures cannot be controlled fully, parents need to anticipate potentially hazardous situations during their child's day, such as having to cross a busy street on the way to school or riding a bicycle. State regulations vary, but the majority of adolescents are not eligible to secure a permit to drive until they are cleared by their primary care provider (after about a year free of seizures) to protect their own safety and that of others.

Partial (Focal) Seizures. Partial seizures originate from a specific brain area. A typical partial seizure with motor signs begins in the fingers and spreads to the wrist, arm, and face in a clonic contraction. If the movement remains localized, there will be no loss of consciousness. If the spread is extensive, the seizure can cross the midline and become generalized and, at that point, is impossible to differentiate from a full generalized tonic–clonic seizure. This makes it important, therefore, to observe children carefully as a seizure begins to distinguish whether it began with local signs such as numbness, tingling, paresthesia, or pain all associated with one brain area. Documenting the spread can help localize the spot in the brain that first initiated the abnormal electrical discharge or be instrumental in detecting the location of a rapidly growing brain tumor.

Absence Seizures. Absence seizures, formerly known as petit mal seizures, are a type of generalized seizure (Tatum, Ho, & Benbadis, 2010). They occur more often in girls than boys, usually occur in school-age children between 4 and 12 years, and consist of a staring spell that lasts for a few seconds. A child might be reciting in class, for example, when he pauses and stares for 1 to 5 seconds and then continues the recitation as if he is unaware time has passed. Rhythmic blinking and twitching of the mouth or an extremity may accompany the staring. As many as 100 seizures can occur during a day. An EEG usually shows a typical 3-Hz wave and slow-wave discharge (Mariani, Rossi, & Vojani, 2011).

Children with absence episodes usually have normal intelligence but may have failing school marks, be accused of daydreaming in school, or be referred to the school nurse for behavior problems because they miss so many of a teacher's instructions.

On a neurologic exam, the presence of absence seizures can usually be demonstrated by asking a child to hyperventilate while they count out loud. If they are susceptible to such seizures, they typically breathe in and out deeply, possibly 10 times, stop and stare for 3 seconds, then continue to hyperventilate and count, unaware that they paused.

No first aid measures are necessary for absence seizures, and downplaying the importance of these episodes helps children maintain a positive self-image. They can be controlled by ethosuximide (Zarontin), valproate, or "off-label" lamotrigine (Robotham, 2011). If seizures are fully controlled by medication, children can participate in normal school activities and ride a bicycle or motorcycle. If seizures cannot be controlled

BOX 49.5 Nursing Care Planning Based on Responsibility for Pharmacology

CARBAMAZEPINE (TEGRETOL)

Classification: Carbamazepine is an antiseizure medication.

Action: Exact mechanism of action is unknown, but it is believed to inhibit polysynaptic responses and block posttetanic potentiation (Karch, 2013).

Pregnancy Risk Category: C

Dosage: Initially in children 6 to 12 years of age, 10 mg/kg/24 hr orally twice a day on the first day (maximum dose 100 mg), increased gradually in 100-mg increments at 1-week intervals until best response is achieved, or 10 to 30 mg/kg/day in divided doses three or four times a day. Not to exceed 1,000 mg/day.

Possible Adverse Effects: Dizziness, drowsiness, behavioral changes, nausea, vomiting, abnormal liver function tests, bone marrow depression, rash, photosensitivity

Nursing Implications

- Advise parents to administer the drug with food to minimize gastrointestinal upset.
- Remind parents to obtain serum drug levels as prescribed to monitor for effectiveness and to prevent possible toxicity; also obtain liver function studies and blood cell counts to detect marrow depression.
- Suggest that parents obtain a medical alert bracelet and have the child wear it in case of a seizure.
- Instruct parents to not give sleep-inducing or over-the-counter drugs because these can interact with antiseizure medication to cause dangerous synergistic effects. Caution adolescents to avoid alcohol.
- Caution parents not to discontinue the drug abruptly or change the dose unless ordered by the health care provider.
- Instruct parents to notify their health care provider if the child develops bruising, bleeding, or signs of infection because these could be signs of bone marrow depression.

fully, parents need to anticipate potentially hazardous situations during the child's day to prevent risky activities such as swimming alone.

Approximately one third to one half of all children with absence seizures "outgrow" them by adulthood. This does not mean that treatment is not necessary during childhood, however, in order to keep the child safe and maintain self-esteem. Follow-up health supervision is necessary during adolescence because some children's seizure pattern changes from absence involvement to tonic–clonic involvement as they approach adulthood.

Tonic–Clonic Seizures. Typical tonic–clonic seizures (formerly termed grand mal seizures) are generalized seizures usually consisting of three stages: a prodromal period of hours or days or an aura, or warning, immediately before the seizure that a seizure is about to occur; a tonic–clonic stage; and, finally, a postictal stage.

The prodromal period may consist of drowsiness, dizziness, malaise, lack of coordination, or tension. As a child reaches school age, the child may be able to predict from these vague preliminary feelings when a seizure is about to occur.

An aura reflects the portion of the brain in which the seizure originates. Smelling unpleasant odors (often reported as feces) denotes activity in the medial portion of the temporal lobe. Seeing flashing lights suggests the occipital area, repeated hallucinations arise from the temporal lobe, numbness of an extremity relates to the opposite parietal lobe, and a "Cheshire-cat grin" relates to the frontal lobe. Young children, unable to describe or understand an aura, may scream in fright or run to their parent at its onset. Noting exactly what symptoms the child experiences during this time helps to localize the involved brain portion.

The next phase is the tonic stage. All muscles of the body contract, extremities stiffen, the face distorts, air is pushed through the glottis from contraction of the chest muscles to produce a guttural cry, and the child falls to the ground. Although this phase lasts only about 20 seconds, because the respiratory muscles remain contracted during this time, the child may experience hypoxia and begin to appear cyanotic. Contraction of the throat prevents swallowing, so saliva collects in the mouth. A few children bite their tongue when the jaws contract and thus have bleeding from their mouth.

The seizure then enters a clonic stage, in which muscles of the body rapidly contract and relax, producing quick, jerky motions. The child may blow bubbles from foamy or bloody saliva and will be incontinent of stool and urine. This phase usually lasts 20 to 30 seconds.

Following this tonic–clonic period, the child falls into a sound sleep, the *postictal period.* He or she will sleep soundly for 1 to 4 hours rousing only to painful stimuli. When children awake, they often experience a severe headache. They have no memory of the seizure.

In some children, seizures occur only at night. The child wakes in the morning with a sore tongue, blood on the pillow, or a bed wet with urine. In a child with persistent bedwetting, the possibility this may be occurring from nocturnal seizures should be considered.

Children with this type of seizure may or may not have an abnormal EEG pattern. If an abnormal pattern is found, other family members may be found to have similarly abnormal EEG patterns, although they do not have symptoms.

Therapy includes the daily administration of an antiseizure medication such as valproate (Depakene) and carbamazepine (Tegretol). Phenobarbital may be administered to young children.

Medications are usually continued until the child has been seizure free for 2 to 3 years. No antiseizure medication should be stopped suddenly (it should be tapered) because rapid withdrawal may precipitate a seizure. In addition to medication, some children may be prescribed a ketogenic diet or a diet high in fat and low in protein and carbohydrate. This combination of nutrients creates a high level of ketones, which appears to decrease myoclonic or tonic–clonic seizure activity. Because the diet is monotonous for children and difficult for parents to prepare, however, it may be hard for children to eat this for a long time (Kossoff, Bosarge, Miranda, et al., 2010).

Status Epilepticus. **Status epilepticus** refers to a seizure that lasts continuously for longer than 30 minutes or a series of seizures from which the child does not return to the previous level of consciousness (Dobrin, 2013; Singh, Stephens, Berl, et al., 2010). This is an emergency situation requiring immediate treatment before exhaustion, respiratory failure, permanent brain injury, or death occurs. An IV benzodiazepine drug such as diazepam (Valium) or lorazepam (Ativan) halts seizures dramatically. Diazepam must be administered with extreme caution, however, based on the child's drug history because the drug is incompatible with many other medications, and any accidental infiltration into subcutaneous tissue causes extensive tissue sloughing. Parents can be instructed on how to administer diazepam by enema at home. Lorazepam (Ativan), a long-acting benzodiazepine used for children older than 2 years of age, provides a longer duration of action and also less respiratory depression (Karch, 2013). Both oxygen to relieve cyanosis and administering a medication to halt the seizure may be necessary; obtaining blood to monitor for glucose may reveal that hypoglycemia needs to be corrected.

QSEN Checkpoint Question 49.5

Evidence-Based Practice

Recurrent seizures can be depressing for children and parents if the seizures are difficult to eliminate with therapy. To investigate whether improved coping behaviors could minimize depressive symptoms, nurse researchers asked 76 children, age 9 to 17 years, who had recurrent seizures, to complete two questionnaires designed to reveal depression and coping ability. As expected, better coping ability was correlated with less depression. A surprising result of the study was that 27% of children expressed thoughts of self-injury or suicide (Wagner, Ferguson, & Smith, 2012).

Based on the previous study, if Tasha is found to have recurrent seizures, which statement by her at a health care visit, after she becomes a school-ager, would concern you the most?

a. "I forget to take my medicine twice last week; I have to try harder."
b. "I feel really sad when children call me names because I have seizures."
c. "I don't like having to miss school because of clinic visits."
d. "I think my medicine is giving me headaches; maybe I need glasses."

Look in Appendix A for the best answer and rationale.

Assessment of the Child With Seizures

It's important that a thorough pregnancy history be obtained on any child with seizures. Events that occurred immediately before the seizure and an accurate description of the seizure itself also should be recorded. Investigate the child's overall behavior in the last few weeks such as bed-wetting or failing marks in school because these might be signs of absence or nocturnal seizures that have occurred but gone unnoticed.

A complete physical and neurologic examination and blood studies are necessary to rule out metabolic or infectious processes. Prepare a child for a lumbar puncture to rule out meningitis or bleeding into the CSF. A CT scan, MRI, skull radiograph, or EEG may be obtained as indicated. Caution children during the EEG that they may be stimulated with rhythm patterns or flashing lights or asked to hyperventilate to see whether a seizure can be provoked.

Nursing Diagnoses and Related Interventions

Nursing Diagnosis: Risk for injury related to recurrent seizures

Outcome Evaluation: Child exhibits no signs of aspiration or traumatic injury.

Help a child having a partial seizure to a sitting position to protect against falling. Turn a child who has fallen to the floor onto the side so fluid will drain from the mouth and not be aspirated. Protecting a child from being hurt during a tonic–clonic seizure is crucial, but restraining the child's thrashing extremities is not advisable, because it is difficult for an adult to do so and could result in injury to the parent or child because of the amount of force needed to keep the child still (Box 49.6). Do not insert anything between the child's teeth to stop tongue biting because this is rarely necessary and can result in broken and aspirated teeth.

Remaining calm is an important responsibility because it is reassuring for parents to see someone calm and in control of a situation that seems to be very out of control. If the child passes rapidly from one seizure into another (status epilepticus), be prepared to provide supplemental oxygen and administer antiseizure therapy as needed.

Nursing Diagnosis: Interrupted family processes related to diagnosis of long-term illness in child

Outcome Evaluation: Child, parents, and other family members express fears and questions about disease to health care team; parents discuss ways to accommodate the illness in their daily life, such as medication schedules, school accommodations, sports activities, plans for vacation, and discipline.

As soon as the diagnosis of a seizure disorder is made, parents and children need to be told that it is likely to signify a long-term disorder because, although seizures can be controlled with medication, these do not change or cure the underlying cause of the seizures. Box 49.7 shows an interprofessional care map illustrating both nursing and team planning for a child with recurrent seizures. Most children are given tablets rather than liquid medication, because the latter tends to settle at the bottom of the bottle, resulting in overdiluted or overconcentrated doses that can allow seizures to break through at the end of the prescription period. To avoid this happening, caution parents to shake liquid medication thoroughly before every dose. Parents need to establish ways to remember to

BOX 49.6 Nursing Care Planning Based on Family Teaching

SAFETY DURING SEIZURES

Q. Tasha's mother asks you, "What can we do to be certain she doesn't get hurt during a seizure?"
A. Here are the usual actions to help keep her safe:

- Remain calm.
- Move away furniture or any sharp objects.
- Turn your child gently on her side, or on her abdomen with her head turned to the side, to prevent aspiration of unswallowed mouth secretions.
- Do not restrain her other than to keep her head turned to the side. Restraining a child could result in injury because of the amount of force necessary.
- Do not attempt to place an object between the child's teeth to prevent tongue biting. Trying to force an object into the mouth could break or loosen teeth.
- Be aware that a child having this type of seizure may have some slight cyanosis during the tonic and clonic stages, but these stages are so short that administering oxygen is not needed.
- After any seizure, telephone your primary care provider about the seizure so arrangements for any necessary follow-up care can be initiated.
- If your child should pass rapidly from one seizure into another (status epilepticus), she may need supplemental oxygen or medicine to stop the seizure. If this happens, telephone your emergency medical service number (911).

BOX 49.7 Nursing Care Planning

AN INTERPROFESSIONAL CARE MAP FOR A CHILD WITH RECURRENT SEIZURES

Tasha is a 3-year-old girl who was brought to the emergency department by her mother because she had a seizure. Her mother grabs your arm, visibly upset. "Her sister has cerebral palsy and seizures. Does this mean Tasha has cerebral palsy too?" she asks you.

Family Assessment Parents are divorced. Child lives in a two-bedroom apartment with mother and a 6-year-old sibling; attends child care daily from 9 AM to 3 PM. Neighbor watches her from 3 to 6 PM, when mother returns from work as a research librarian.

Client Assessment Well-proportioned preschooler sleeping soundly on left side since admission. Had first seizure 2 hours ago; a second one 30 minutes ago. Temperature at 103.4°F. Other vital signs within age-appropriate parameters. Reacts to painful stimuli only. Deep tendon reflexes depressed. Mother reports, "I kept her home from child care because she has a cold. Suddenly, she fell to the floor and started shaking. I called 911, and they brought her here." Apparent pain on forward flexion of the neck. Lumbar puncture performed; pressures within normal limits; specimens sent for cell count, glucose, and culture.

Nursing Diagnosis Risk for injury related to diminished level of consciousness resulting from seizure episode

Outcome Criteria Child is conscious within the hour. Exhibits no signs of aspiration or traumatic injury.

Team Member Responsible	Assessment	Intervention	Rationale	Expected Outcome
Activities of Daily Living, Including Safety				
Nurse	Assess whether mother was aware child's temperature was elevated. Assess whether child has continued pain on dorsiflexion of neck.	Keep child on side to help ensure an open airway until alert and responsive. Ask if mother has a thermometer to take any future fevers.	Side-lying position reduces risk for aspiration. Pain on dorsiflexion of neck and irritability are symptoms of meningitis.	Mother states she understands importance of taking temperature in the future; difficult to evaluate pain as child is unconscious.
Teamwork and Collaboration				
Nurse/Primary care provider	Assess in light of this second seizure and spinal tap results whether neurologic service should be consulted.	Consult with neurologic service, if indicated, about management of child.	A second seizure suggests this may be more than a simple response to elevated fever.	Neurologic service meets with mother and child as appropriate based on findings.
Procedures/Medications for Quality Improvement				
Nurse	Assess whether child has had a lumbar puncture or intravenous (IV) fluid administration before.	Assist with lumbar puncture and specimen collection. Begin IV fluid administration as prescribed.	Lumbar puncture is a frightening procedure for both child and parent. IV line supplies an emergency medicine route if needed for seizure control or infection therapy.	Mother states she understands reason for procedure and gives consent. IV line is established and safeguarded with board for unresponsive child.
Nurse	Assess whether mother understands why respiratory precautions are necessary.	Obtain equipment for respiratory precautions as needed.	Diagnosis could be meningitis, which is contagious by contact with nasal secretions.	Mother states she understands the importance of precautions. Respiratory precautions are readied.
Nutrition				
Nurse	Assess child's level of consciousness using a Glasgow Coma Scale.	Do not give anything by mouth until the child is fully awake, alert, and oriented and the gag reflex is intact.	Giving oral fluids too early increases risk for aspiration.	Child receives no oral fluid until she is awake and aware.

Patient-Centered Care				
Nurse/Nurse practitioner	Assess what mother knows about febrile seizures and meningitis.	Teach that a febrile seizure is more of a symptom of fever than a long-term condition. A meningeal infection could be very serious.	Understanding the basis for febrile seizures and meningitis can help the parent understand the basis for emergency care.	Mother states she understands child's current status and possible future implications.
Psychosocial/Spiritual/Emotional Needs				
Nurse	Assess whether mother needs to contact a support person if her child's diagnosis is found to be serious.	Help mother contact a support person if she feels this would be helpful.	A support person can be vital to help a parent withstand an ominous diagnosis.	Mother contacts support person as needed.
Informatics for Seamless Health Care Planning				
Nurse	Assess whether parent has any further questions about child's condition before transfer to pediatric intensive care unit.	Answer any remaining questions to make transfer as comfortable for parent and child as possible.	A parent gains confidence in emergency department staff and may find it difficult to change to new health care providers.	Mother states she understands that if meningitis or recurrent seizures are diagnosed, her child needs ongoing care.

buy medicine so they always have an adequate supply, especially if they are taking a trip away from home or need to provide enough for holidays.

Be certain the child receives health maintenance care during childhood to be certain that the medication dosage remains adequate with continued growth. To document that serum levels of drugs are adequate, children need periodic blood sampling.

Provide parents with as much information as possible about the cause of their child's seizures because it's almost always easier to deal with a known disease, not an unexplainable and unpredictable one. Although the cause of the seizures is unknown, you can assure them that treatment is known; new antiseizure medications are being introduced yearly into therapy.

General guidelines for safe administration of antiseizure medications to stress with parents include:

- Caution children to be careful around motor vehicles and electrical equipment, because many antiseizure medications cause drowsiness.
- Advise the child and parents to observe for easy bruising, because some antiseizure medicines may suppress bone marrow function.
- Caution the adolescent to avoid alcohol while taking antiseizure medications, because alcohol can potentiate the CNS effects of these medications.
- Use caution when administering antiseizure medications to children with liver disease. Because many of these drugs are metabolized by the liver, they may not be fully effective in such children.
- Caution the child and parents not to discontinue antiseizure therapy abruptly, because this may lead to uncontrolled seizures.
- Remind parents about the need for follow-up blood tests to evaluate the drug level. Maintaining a therapeutic blood level enhances the drug's effectiveness and minimizes the risk for toxicity.

Discuss with parents the need to treat children with seizures the same as other family members. Scolding children, asking them to do household chores, or insisting they do their homework will not cause seizures. A few children with absence seizures can initiate them by hyperventilating and may try to manipulate those around them by doing this to gain sympathy. The few children who use this extreme form of manipulation may need to be referred for counseling.

Assure parents also that occasional seizures in children are not harmful. Unless status epilepticus occurs and the child becomes anoxic, the chance their child will be injured during a seizure is remote. Knowing this helps parents not to worry about the child becoming cognitively challenged or about other misconceptions regarding seizures. Although some children who have seizures are cognitively challenged, this impairment and the seizures were caused by the same event; the seizures did not cause the impairment. At every health care visit, be certain parents have time to ask questions about their child's care and to express concerns. There are so many "scare stories" about seizures that every parent is likely to believe some of these stories unless counseled otherwise (Box 49.8).

As a rule, children with seizures should attend regular school and participate in physical education classes and active sports (with possible exceptions such as scuba or sky diving or rock climbing). Many teachers are concerned about the responsibility of having a child with seizures assigned to their class. Contact the school nurse (with the parents' permission) to help them learn about the success of modern seizure control.

In many children, seizures increase or intensify at puberty, probably as the result of glandular changes or the need for an increased medicine dosage because of preadolescent growth. All antiseizure medications are potentially teratogenic to a

BOX 49.8 Nursing Care Planning Based on Effective Communication

Tasha, 3 years old, had a febrile seizure and was diagnosed as having meningitis. You talk to her mother about the seizure.

Less Effective Communication

Nurse: Mrs. Jarman, can you describe what happened?
Mrs. Jarman: She started shaking all over. It was really frightening.
Nurse: Did she voice any symptoms before the seizure?
Mrs. Jarman: No, just started shaking.
Nurse: That must have been frightening.
Mrs. Jarman: Thinking about what it did to her is scarier.
Nurse: Well, lucky thing she's fine now.

More Effective Communication

Nurse: Mrs. Jarman, can you describe what happened?
Mrs. Jarman: She started shaking all over. It was really frightening.
Nurse: Did she voice any symptoms before the seizure?
Mrs. Jarman: No, just started shaking.
Nurse: That must have been frightening.
Mrs. Jarman: Thinking about what it did to her is scarier.
Nurse: Did to her?
Mrs. Jarman: I know seizures cause mental retardation. Our neighbor's son has them, and he's severely retarded.
Nurse: Let's talk about this a little more.

In the first scenario, although the nurse responds with a therapeutic statement ("That must have been frightening"), she fails to identify a misconception verbalized by the mother. In the second scenario, the nurse identifies the concern and attempts to clarify it, providing an opportunity for teaching.

fetus, so be certain adolescent girls are aware of this so they can choose to delay childbearing until later in life, when their medication can be reduced or even discontinued.

QSEN Checkpoint Question 49.6
Safety

Suppose Tasha has a tonic–clonic seizure while in the hospital. Which of the following items should you keep available at the bedside for a child known to have generalized seizures? (Select all that apply.)

a. Suction
b. Tracheostomy tube
c. Oxygen
d. Call bell
e. Padded tongue blade

Look in Appendix A for the best answer and rationale.

Breath Holding

Breath holding is a phenomenon that occurs in young children when they are stressed or angry. The child breathes in and, because of anger or stress, does not breathe out again or else breathes out and then does not inhale again. As brain cells become anoxic, the child appears cyanotic and slumps to the floor, momentarily unconscious. With loss of consciousness, the child begins breathing again, color returns, and the child awakens. Breath holding this way is frightening to parents but results from the immaturity of the child's neurologic control. This differs from a temper tantrum, in which a child deliberately attempts to hold his breath and then passes out (see Chapter 30). The child needs no immediate therapy except reassurance the episode is over. Breath holding may be associated with iron-deficiency anemia; if this is discovered, iron supplementation may be prescribed as medication to decrease the breath-holding episodes (Zehetner, Orr, Buckmaster, et al., 2010).

Headache

Headache in children younger than school age used to be considered rare, but young children can report "hair hurt" or have fussiness from allergies and viral inflammation of the upper respiratory tract that cause headaches. A toddler who has both vomiting and a headache should be evaluated because these are common signs of brain tumor, one of the most common tumors of childhood (Cleves & Rothner, 2011). Headache may also occur with a fever because of increased ICP caused by increased cerebral blood flow. As children reach school age, headaches may occur as a result of conditions as simple as eyestrain and sinusitis or, again, as serious as a brain tumor.

Headache pain results because of meningeal or vascular irritation, not from the brain itself because brain tissue is insensitive to pain. Because of this insensitivity, a cerebral tumor can be present for a lengthy time before meningeal irritation is enough that pain symptoms become apparent. With a brain tumor, pain becomes intense on changing body position, so a young child who reports a headache shortly after getting up in the morning should be carefully evaluated. Pain from a brain tumor is also usually occipital, so asking the child to indicate where it hurts helps determine whether a tumor could be the cause.

Tension or Stress Headache

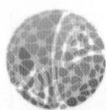

When children are studying intently or taking a test, contraction of their neck muscles from tension can cause temporary ischemia to the head. This type of headache is usually experienced as a dull, steady pain across the forehead, the temporal area, or the back of the neck. Children with these symptoms should have their vision tested, because poor eyesight may be the reason they hunch over their books. Stress headaches are relieved by simple analgesics, such as acetaminophen or ibuprofen, or by sleep or application of a cool compress. Advising children to take frequent "stretches" while studying can help avoid muscle tension and stress and reduce the number of headaches experienced.

Sinus Headache

Sinus headache usually accompanies sinusitis or is associated with inflammation and possible obstruction of the sinuses and is discussed in Chapter 40.

Migraine Headache

Migraine headache refers to a specific type of headache that may or may not begin with an aura or visual disturbance such as diplopia or a zigzag pattern across the visual field. The pain that follows is usually unilateral and extremely intense, with throbbing that is moderate to severe. The headache is aggravated by routine physical activity or menstrual periods; it may be compounded by nausea and vomiting and intolerance to bright lights and noise (Cleves & Rothner, 2011).

The cause of migraine headache is not well understood but probably results from abnormal constriction of intracranial arteries that temporarily reduces cerebral blood supply. The reduction in blood flow is then followed by compensating overdistention of cranial blood vessels. The aura accompanying such headaches results from the temporary ischemia that occurs in between those two processes. Some children who have migraine headaches have an abnormal EEG, but a normal EEG does not rule out the reality of the headaches.

Most children with migraine headache have a positive family history, or someone else in the family also has the same type of headache. A migraine syndrome may be inherited as a dominant trait.

Assessment. To help assess the cause of a headache, obtain a thorough history, including:

- When the headache usually occurs
- The events preceding it (to detect an aura)
- Its usual duration, frequency, intensity, description, and associated symptoms
- Any actions taken to treat the headache

The child needs a thorough physical examination, including funduscopic examination, to rule out papilledema. Blood pressure must be measured to rule out hypertension. If an aura is documented, an EEG will be prescribed to investigate a seizure as the basis of the headache.

Therapeutic Management. At the time of the headache, sleep or lying down may be necessary to relieve the pain and vomiting. Acetaminophen and nonsteroidal anti-inflammatory drugs are the first-line medical treatment for headaches in children, including migraines. Ergotamine tartrate (Cafergot), a vasoconstrictor, may be prescribed in addition for some children. Almotriptan, a member of the triptan family of drugs, is approved by the U.S. Food and Drug Administration for migraine in adolescents and may also be helpful. Verapamil and other calcium channel blockers that result in vasodilation and thus prevent hypertension may be prescribed prophylactically (Gelfand, Fullerton, & Goadsby, 2010). Frequent headaches interfere with a child's ability to achieve in school. Children may need to be reassured that even though their headaches are intense and even incapacitating, migraine headaches are benign and will not lead to any other condition so they can keep their headaches in perspective. Follow-up visits are necessary to confirm that they are not growing worse so treatment is remaining adequate (El-Chammas, Keyes, Thompson, et al., 2013).

If other family members have migraine headaches, counsel them that their reactions to their headaches influence their child's reaction to a headache. If the mother goes to bed for the day when she has a migraine headache, for example, she cannot expect her child to go to school when the child has a headache.

SPINAL CORD INJURY

Because of the resilience of their vertebrae, children have fewer spinal cord injuries than adults. However, the incidence among adolescents is increasing, especially among male adolescents, because more teenagers are involved in motor vehicle accidents, particularly motorcycle or off-road vehicle accidents, than previously (Martin-Herz, Zatzick, & McMahon, 2012). Another frequent cause of spinal cord injury is diving into too-shallow water at beaches or backyard pools. Spinal cord injury without radiologic abnormality (SCIWORA) syndrome may occur, so any child with a multiple traumatic injury needs to be assessed for spinal cord damage. Stabilizing the neck at the accident scene is the best protection against further injury in these children (Hazinski, 2012).

Recovery Phases

Spinal injuries result when the spinal cord becomes compressed or severed by the vertebrae; further cord damage can result from hemorrhage, edema, or inflammation at the injury site as the blood supply becomes impeded. Table 49.4 summarizes functional ability that will probably be present after spinal cord injury at different vertebral levels. Predictions such as these of useful body function cannot be made accurately at the time of the injury, however. Three phases of recovery must first take place.

First Recovery Phase

Immediately after the injury, the child experiences a *spinal shock syndrome* or loss of autonomic nervous system function (loss of nerve fibers traveling through the anterior horn of the spinal canal), leading to loss of motor function, sensation, reflex activity, and the presence of flaccid paralysis in body areas below the level of the injury. If a cervical or high thoracic injury is present, there will be loss of or decreased respiratory function because of flaccidity of the diaphragm or loss of the accessory muscles of the chest. At all levels, the child has no ability to sweat or shiver to change body temperature below the level of the lesion because of loss of autonomic nerve control; therefore, hypothermia or hyperthermia always becomes a threat. Blood vessels below the level of the injury are no longer able to constrict, so blood tends to pool in the lower body,

TABLE 49.4 Functional Ability After Spinal Cord Injury

Injury Site	Highest Key Functions Still Present	Effects and Possible Interventions
C1–3	Head and neck muscles intact	Respiratory paralysis from loss of phrenic nerve innervation; will need ventilatory assistance No voluntary motion below chin; possibly able to learn to use mouth to control pen for writing and mouth stick to reach objects
C4	Diaphragm intact	Loss of motor function of upper and lower extremities and trunk; able to learn to use abdominal muscles to breathe independently
C5	Shoulder control; biceps, deltoid function	Able to feed self and operate wheelchair if fitted with self-care aids
C6	Forearm pronation; wrist extension	Use of upper extremities for self-care; can transfer to wheelchair and so have increased independence
C7	Triceps function	Able to transfer to wheelchair readily; increasing independence
C8	Thumb and finger function	Able to do fine motor tasks; increases self-care ability
T1–7	Intercostal muscles (able to breathe with chest, not abdominal, muscles)	Full use of upper extremities but is still dependent on wheelchair Possibly able to drive car with hand controls Possibly able to have high leg braces fitted for standing
T10–12	Abdominal muscles	Use of long leg braces and four-point crutch to ambulate
L2–4	Hip flexion Leg extension	Use of long or short leg braces to ambulate
L5–S1	Gluteus maximus muscle function	Able to walk without aids
S4	Bladder and anal sphincter control	Able to control bladder and bowel function Penile erection and ejaculation possible

leading to yet another concern—upper body hypotension, especially if the upper body is elevated. Loss of bladder control occurs if the bladder is left flaccid (it overdistends and continually overflows). Loss of control in the bowel allows it to become equally distended; bowel sounds will be absent. This phase of spinal cord injury lasts from 1 to 6 weeks. As a rule, the shorter the phase of spinal shock, the better is the final outcome.

Administration of a corticosteroid can help reduce edema and possibly protect function of the spinal cord during this phase. A vasopressor agent such as dopamine may be prescribed to maintain blood pressure and perfusion to the cord.

Second Recovery Phase

During the second phase of recovery, the flaccid paralysis of the shock phase is replaced by spastic paralysis. Normally, motor impulses begin in the brain cortex and are transmitted to the medulla, where they cross to the opposite side of the cord; they then travel down the descending motor tracts of the spinal cord. They synapse in the anterior horn of the spinal cord and travel by way of the spinal and peripheral nerves to the designated muscle group, which they set in motion. The nerve pathways of the brain and the descending tracts are termed *upper motor neurons*. Those in the anterior horn cells and the spinal and peripheral nerves are termed *lower motor neurons*. Whether a motor neuron has upper or lower function, therefore, does not depend on its height in the spinal tract but rather on its position in relation to an anterior horn: between the brain and the anterior horn, it is an upper motor neuron; between the anterior horn and the point of innervation, it is a lower motor neuron (Fig. 49.9).

Spasticity in the second phase is caused by the loss of upper level control or transmission of meaningful innervation to the anterior horn. Lacking upper motor neuron function because of a severed cord, the lower motor neurons or reflex arcs cause the muscles to contract and remain that way. Parents and children are quick to interpret the sudden spastic movement of a lower extremity as meaningful activity. This is particularly easy to believe with infants, who cannot tell you they have no control or cannot stop their legs from contracting. Differences between upper and lower neuron damage are listed in Table 49.5. If the injury is very low in the spinal tract, affecting mostly lower motor neurons, the muscles will remain flaccid, because the lower motor neurons cannot send impulses for contraction.

During this phase, if the child's bladder is allowed to fill, the resultant sensory stimulation relayed to the damaged cord can initiate a powerful sympathetic reflex reaction (**autonomic dysreflexia**). The child will experience extreme hypertension, tachycardia, flushed face, and severe occipital headache. This is an emergency situation because if the severe hypertension is not relieved, cerebrovascular accident can result (Pellatt, 2010). Assess that the child's urinary catheter is not obstructed, so urine can flow freely and reduce the sensory stimulation. Also, frequently assess for signs of urinary tract infection such as elevated temperature or cloudy urine, because urinary complications remain the leading cause of morbidity and the most common infection for individuals with spinal cord injury (Eves & Rivera, 2010).

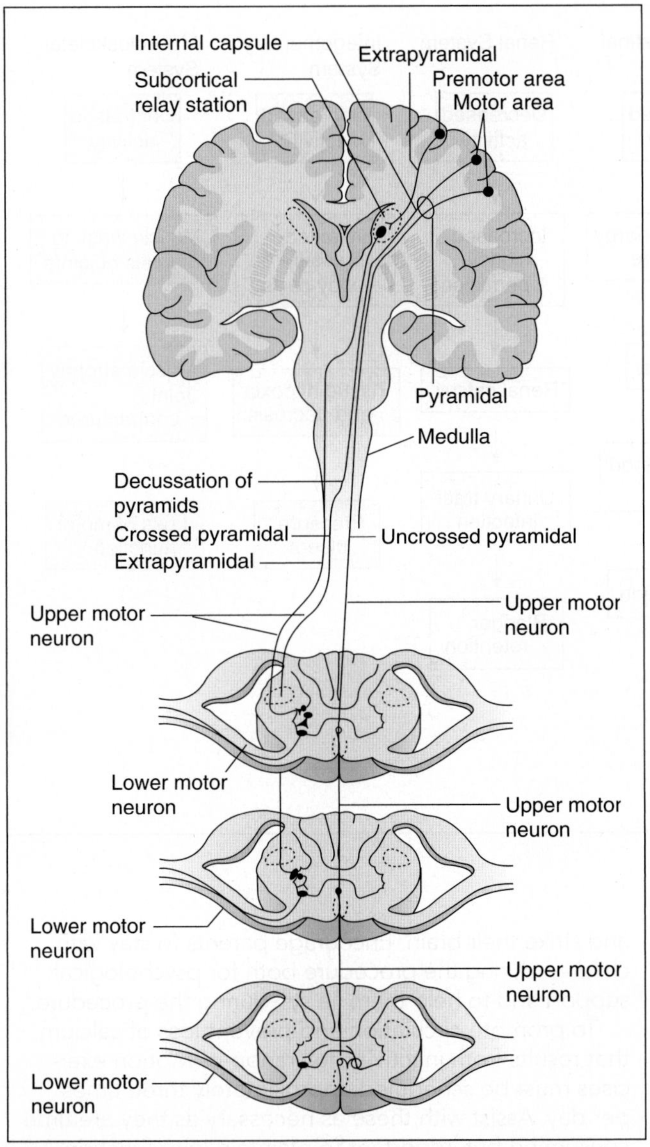

FIGURE 49.9 Diagram of motor pathways between the cerebral cortex, one of the subcortical relay stations, and lower motor neurons in the spinal cord. Decussation (crossing of fibers) means that each side of the brain controls skeletal muscles on the opposite side of the body.

Third Recovery Phase

The third phase of recovery from spinal cord injury is learning to live with the final outcome, or permanent limitation of motor and sensory function. If the compression of the spinal cord was only caused by edema that is then relieved, no permanent motor and sensory disability will occur.

Assessment of Spinal Cord Injury

Cervical and thoracolumbar areas of the spine are the ones most likely to sustain injury, but spinal cord injury should be suspected whenever a child has sustained a forceful trauma of any kind. Do not move a child with suspected spinal cord injury at the scene of the injury until the back and head can be supported in a straight line to prevent further injury to the spinal column from twisting or bending. In the emergency department, as a general rule, do not attempt to move the child from a stretcher to an examining table until spinal X-ray films have been obtained; if helping move the child onto the X-ray table, use a gentle log-rolling technique to avoid additional movement or injury. If resuscitation is necessary, be certain to maintain the child's head in a neutral position, not hyperextended. To keep the neck immobilized, if a child is wearing a football, bicycle, or motorcycle helmet or a neck brace, do not remove these (Nayduch, 2010). Help maintain spinal immobilization during such procedures as obtaining blood samples or a neurologic assessment.

Nursing Diagnoses and Related Interventions

During the first phase of recovery, a child's major problems are those that result from almost complete immobility: pressure ulcers on bony prominences, loss of appetite and subsequent poor nutrition from depression or being kept in a supine position, urinary calculi caused by excessive calcium loss from bones, atrophy of flaccid muscle groups, and urinary retention and bladder infection. These effects of immobility are presented in Figure 49.10.

TABLE 49.5 Characteristics of Upper and Lower Motor Nerve Injury After Spinal Shock Phase

Finding	Upper Motor Lesion	Lower Motor Lesion
Spasticity	Present	Absent (flaccidity present)
Clonus	Present, increased	Absent
Tendon reflexes	Increased	Absent
Babinski reflex	Present	Absent
Reflexes below level of lesion	Present	Absent
Reflex at level of lesion	Absent	Absent
Atrophy of muscles	Absent or present only to slight degree	Present (muscle fasciculations may be present)

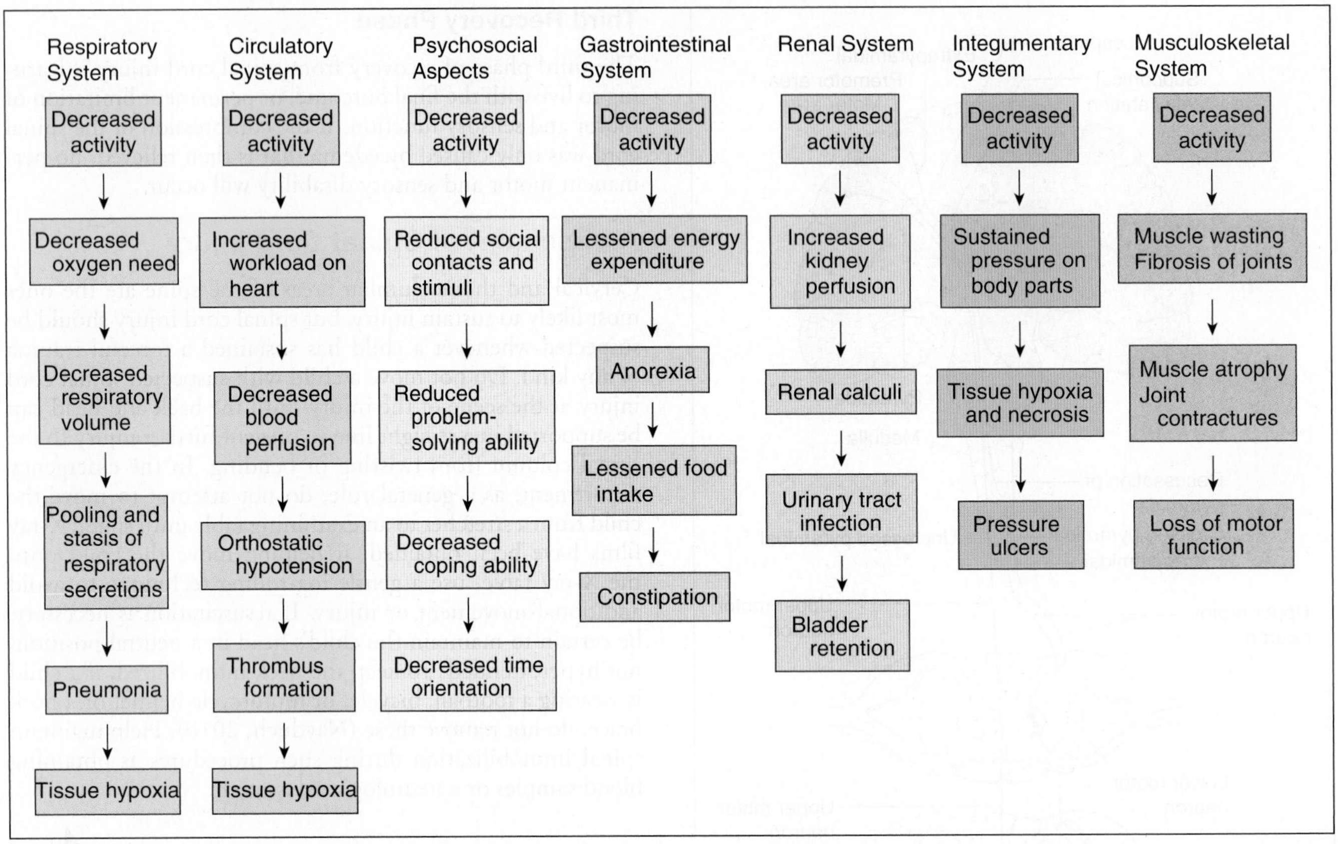

FIGURE 49.10 Effects of immobilization.

Nursing Diagnosis: Impaired physical mobility related to effects of spinal cord injury

Outcome Evaluation: Child ambulates with a minimum of artificial support and equipment; participates in exercise program within limitations.

To relieve edema at the injury site and prevent further injury, IV corticosteroids will be administered. Children may be placed in cervical traction with Crutchfield tongs and a traction belt (Fig. 49.11) or with halo traction (see Chapter 51). Having tongs inserted into the skull is a very frightening procedure for children because they worry the tongs will burrow into their skull and strike their brain. Encourage parents to stay with children during the procedure both for psychological support and to help them lie still during the procedure.

To promote circulation and prevent loss of calcium that results from inactivity, full range-of-motion exercises must be scheduled approximately three times per day. Assist with these as necessary as they are time consuming but important to maintain joint function.

During the second phase of recovery, when spasticity of muscle groups occurs, preventing contractures becomes the chief concern. Specialized splints, boots, or even hightop sneakers may be used to prevent foot drop (Fig. 49.12). If children have upper extremity mobility but will be left with lower extremity paralysis, exercises to strengthen the upper extremity muscle groups are needed so children will be strong enough to lift themselves from a bed to a wheelchair or raise themselves with a trapeze over the bed when changing positions. Holding legs and arms at the joints while moving is a good technique to help reduce muscle spasms.

One major problem of ambulation after spinal cord injury is helping a child's body readjust to a vertical position after being maintained in the supine position for so long. In the new upright position, blood tends to pool in dilated blood vessels below the level of the spinal injury, resulting in a pseudohypovolemia and hypotension. The first time a child sits up or stands, this may occur to such an extent that the child faints. Gradually increasing the angle of the bed helps the

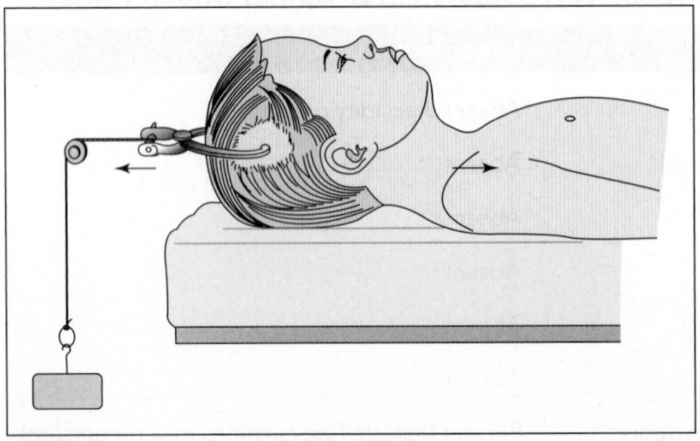

FIGURE 49.11 Crutchfield tongs used to create spinal traction.

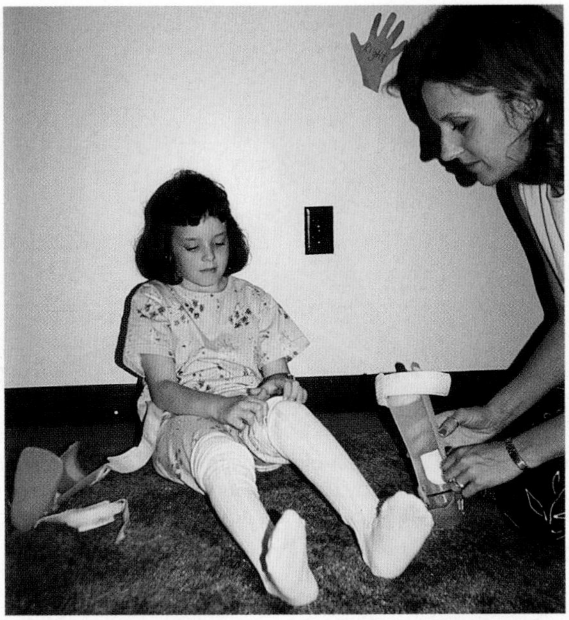

FIGURE 49.12 Specialized splints are used for a child with a low spinal cord injury to prevent contractures and foot drop. Here the physical therapist prepares to apply the splint to the child's leg. (Photograph courtesy of Sue Moses.)

child become acclimated to the upright position without experiencing so much vascular pooling.

Nursing Diagnosis: Self-care deficit related to spinal cord injury

Outcome Evaluation: Child states intention of taking over self-care; practices using equipment for eating, bathing, and toileting; participates in one new aspect of self-care each week.

As soon as possible, children should be introduced to self-help methods for activities of daily living. You may need to encourage parents to allow a child to become as self-sufficient as possible or not to take over complete care. The child may well outlive them and will someday need to be able to function as independently as possible without them.

Remember, without autonomic nervous system function, a child is unable to sweat and becomes hyperthermic if covered too warmly; if not covered warmly enough, the capillaries dilate, and the child loses considerable heat into the environment. If the room temperature cools at night, be careful to dress the child appropriately for sleeping.

Specific measures for bowel evacuation may be necessary, depending on the level of the injury. A bowel program incorporating the use of stool softeners, suppositories, and bowel retraining may be required. The child and parents need support and instructions in accomplishing this task and gaining independence as it may take weeks or months to accomplish.

For some children and parents, the first day of using a wheelchair is exciting (proof that the child can be partially ambulatory). For others, it is the day on which they are forced to face the reality that they cannot undo the results of the injury and that their child has a permanent lifelong disability. If parents have almost overcome their grief and accepted their child's disability, the introduction of a symbol of disability such as a wheelchair or long leg braces may bring new grieving and a sense of loss.

When the child reaches sexual maturity, limitations in this area may become a child's chief concern. If a male has had an upper motor neuron injury, he will not be able to achieve spontaneous erection or ejaculation. However, with manual stimulation of the penis (stimulation of lower motor neuron function), he may be able to achieve an erection and engage in coitus even though ejaculation and fertility remain limited. With most spinal cord injuries, a female is not able to experience orgasm but is able to conceive and bear children.

The limitations caused by a spinal cord injury become especially evident to the child (and the parents) when choosing a vocation and selecting an appropriate school program (remember children cannot be denied regular schooling by federal law in the United States, even with a severe physical disability). Counseling and rehabilitation are crucial aspects to achieve an optimal level of functioning and independence.

Nursing Diagnosis: Risk for impaired gas exchange related to spinal cord injury

Outcome Evaluation: Respiratory rate is within acceptable parameters; lungs are clear; airway is patent.

If the cervical level of the cord is involved, a child will need ventilatory assistance. The child may be intubated at first, but orotracheal or nasotracheal intubation is only a temporary measure to maintain a patent airway. At a later date, a tracheostomy will be done for long-term airway management and to prevent sloughing of pharyngeal tissue from the constant pressure of the intubation tube. If a tracheotomy tube is required, be certain parents receive thorough instructions on caring for the tracheostomy and, if necessary, working with a mechanical ventilator. A phrenic nerve pacemaker may be used to stimulate the diaphragm to contract and initiate respirations. If the child has a thoracic-level injury (which is rare because the rib cage gives extra strength to thoracic vertebrae), the child will be able to breathe independently but will have reduced vital capacity. Periodic positive-pressure breathing treatments may be necessary to encourage increased lung filling. Be careful when positioning a child not to compromise chest movement with equipment or other restricting objects. Other respiratory care measures, such as suctioning and chest physiotherapy, also help maintain chest function.

Nursing Diagnosis: Risk for impaired skin integrity related to immobility

Outcome Evaluation: Child's skin remains clean, dry, and intact without signs of erythema or ulceration.

To prevent skin breakdown, turn children about every 2 hours (always being certain to logroll or maintain immobilization with a striker frame or a continuously moving, automatically controlled bed). The use of an alternating-pressure mattress may also be helpful. With loss of sensation in body parts, the child is unable to report skin irritation from a wrinkled sheet or wet clothing. If the child is incontinent, change the linen immediately to prevent skin breakdown. Once children begin to be ambulatory, check their legs and buttocks regularly to prevent pressure ulcers caused by sitting in a wheelchair or using leg braces (McCaskey, Kirk, & Gerdes, 2011).

Nursing Diagnosis: Risk for impaired urinary elimination related to spinal cord injury

Outcome Evaluation: Child's urine output is adequate for intake; child identifies measures to assist with voiding; child demonstrates procedure for self-catheterization.

To prevent urinary retention during the first phase of recovery, a Foley catheter is usually inserted, or the bladder can be emptied by periodic suprapubic aspiration or intermittent catheterization. Second-stage spasticity causes periodic reflex emptying. The bladder rarely empties completely, however, so problems of stasis and infection continue. To live independently, the child needs to learn self-catheterization to empty the bladder (see Chapter 46).

Nursing Diagnosis: Anticipatory grieving related to loss of function secondary to spinal cord injury

Outcome Evaluation: Child and parents openly discuss their feelings about the injury and its effect on their lives.

The second recovery phase is the time for parents and children to begin thinking about what this degree of disability will mean to them as a family and to face what adjustments they will need to make. Children and parents typically react to the initial diagnosis with grief. They may still be in denial or shock when the second phase begins. With no sudden miracle cure in sight, they may begin to move through stages of anger, bargaining, depression, and then acceptance (the injury happened; we must go on from this point). They need assistance and support to work through all of these feeling, however. Both the parents and the child may need counseling to reach acceptance (Fig. 49.13).

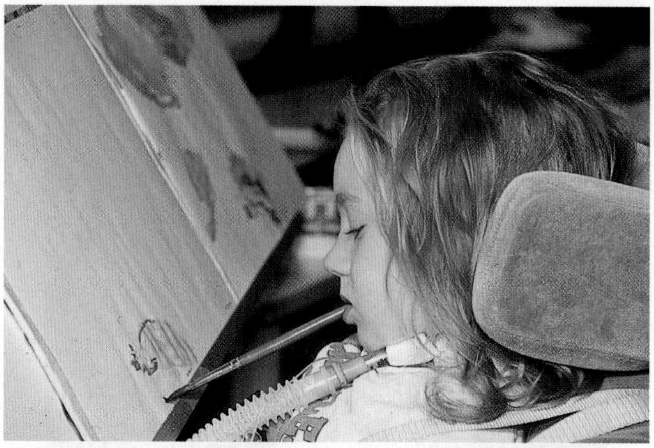

FIGURE 49.13 A 6-year-old girl with a cervical spine injury adapts to her disability by using her mouth to hold a paintbrush and participate in age-appropriate activities. (© Elisa Peterson/ Stock Boston.)

What if...49.3 Tasha's father, a high school science teacher, asks you to help him design a program to teach teenagers how to prevent spinal cord injury. What topics would be best to include?

ATAXIC DISORDERS

Ataxia is failure of muscular coordination or irregularity of muscle action. Ataxic disorders are often manifested by an awkward gait or lack of coordination. Causes of ataxia differ, but degeneration of cerebellar or vestibular function is always involved.

Ataxia-Telangiectasia

Ataxia-telangiectasia, transmitted as an autosomal recessive trait attributable to a defect of chromosome 11, is a primary immunodeficiency disorder that results in progressive cerebellar degeneration. This is a multisystem disease with neurologic and immunologic aspects. In addition, endocrine abnormalities may occur, and there is an increased risk of cancer, particularly brain tumor. Telangiectasias (red vascular markings) appear on the conjunctiva and skin at the flexor creases (McGrath-Morrow, Gower, Rothblum-Oviatt, et al., 2010).

Both immunologic and neurologic symptoms of this disorder vary in severity and onset. Serum immunoglobulin A (IgA) and IgE levels may be low, and there is often evidence of reduced T-cell function. Children develop frequent infections (primarily sinopulmonary) because of the immunologic deficits. Tonsillar tissue in the pharynx appears scant.

Neurologic symptoms caused by the degeneration process can usually be detected in early infancy when developmental milestones are not met. Children develop an awkward gait when they begin to walk. **Choreoathetosis** (rapid, purposeless movements), nystagmus, an intention tremor, or scoliosis may develop. Children may be unable to move their eyes or follow movement through visual fields. Eye changes (conjunctival telangiectasia) develop by 5 years of age. Unfortunately, there is no effective treatment. Children with this disorder often die in late adolescence of infection, respiratory failure, or a malignant brain tumor.

Friedreich Ataxia

Friedreich ataxia, which is carried on the short arm of chromosome 9 as an autosomal recessive trait, involves a variety of degenerative symptoms (Koeppen, 2011). Symptoms such as progressive cerebellar and spinal cord dysfunction occur in late adolescence. Teenagers develop a progressive gait disturbance, a lack of coordinated arm movements, a high-arched foot (pes cavus), hammer toes, and scoliosis. The combined symptoms of a positive Babinski reflex, absence of deep tendon reflexes in the ankle, and ataxia are strongly diagnostic. Neurologic examination shows difficulty in recognizing foot position (whether the foot is moved up or down). If the ataxia remains untreated, death occurs in young adulthood from myocardial failure. Antioxidant therapy such as high-dose idebenone may help to delay this outcome by reducing ventricular hypertrophy (Lynch, Regner, Schadt, et al., 2012).

What if... 49.4 You are interested in exploring one of the 2020 National Health Goals related to children with neurologic disorders (see Box 49.1). Most government-sponsored money for nursing research is allotted based on these goals. What would be a possible research topic to explore pertinent to these goals that would be applicable to Tasha's family and also advance evidence-based practice?

Key Points for Review

- Nerve cells are unique in that they do not regenerate if damaged, tending to make neurologic diseases long-term illnesses. Parents and children alike need support from health care providers to cope with problems that continue to occur over a long period. Planning nursing care to achieve this not only meets QSEN competencies but hopefully also meets the family's total needs.
- Increased ICP arises from an increase in the volume of CSF or from blood accumulation, cerebral edema, or space-occupying lesions. Vital sign changes such as increased temperature and blood pressure and decreased pulse and respirations begin as subtle changes. Always compare assessments with previous levels to detect that a consistent, although minor, change is occurring.
- CP is a nonprogressive disorder of upper motor neurons. The exact cause is usually unknown, but the condition is associated with anoxia occurring before, during, or shortly after birth. Four major types are identified: spastic (excessive tone in the voluntary muscles), dyskinetic or athetoid (abnormal involuntary movement), atonic (decreased muscle tone), and mixed (symptoms of both spasticity and athetoid movements).
- Meningitis is infection of the cerebral meninges, caused most frequently by bacterial invasion. Children need follow-up afterward to monitor for hearing acuity and impaired secretion of antidiuretic hormone.
- Encephalitis is inflammation of brain tissue. This is always a serious diagnosis, because the child may be left with residual neurologic damage, such as seizures or learning disabilities.
- Reye syndrome is acute encephalitis with accompanying fatty infiltration of the liver, heart, and lungs; it most frequently occurs if a child with a viral infection is administered acetylsalicylic acid (aspirin) and is the reason children should not be administered aspirin for fever.
- Guillain-Barré syndrome is inflammation of motor and sensory nerves. The reaction may be immune mediated, occurring after an upper respiratory tract illness. Temporary demyelinization of the nerve sheaths causes loss of function.
- Botulism occurs when spores of *C. botulinum* produce toxins in the intestine. Because honey can be a source of the organism, it should not be given to infants.
- Recurrent seizures are involuntary contractions of muscles caused by abnormal electrical brain discharges. Common types seen in children include febrile seizures, infantile spasms, partial (focal) seizures, absence seizures, and tonic–clonic seizures. Therapy is administration of antiseizure drugs.
- Spinal cord injury is occurring at increased rates in children involved in sports and motor vehicle accidents. Children pass through a first, second, and third recovery phase after the injury until they reach a final outcome.

Critical Thinking Care Study

Darien Fisher is a 12-year-old boy you see in the emergency room because he was brought to the hospital by ambulance after having a tonic–clonic seizure at basketball practice. His parents are divorced, so Darien lives with his mother and two younger brothers in a trailer park during weekdays. On the weekend, he lives with his father on a houseboat.

1. The emergency room physician asked Mrs. Fisher for permission to do a lumbar puncture on Darien but she refused because she remembered what a terrible headache she had after receiving spinal anesthesia for Darien's birth. Would you agree that lumbar punctures often lead to severe headaches? What are some things you could do to help prevent a headache in Darien?
2. Darien is prescribed Tegretol for recurrent seizures. His mother is concerned he won't take it on weekends because his father is "all fun—nothing serious." Would you agree with her that she's right in refusing to allow Darien to visit his father on weekends?
3. Darien is concerned that he won't be allowed to play on his school basketball team if he has another seizure. Are recurrent seizures aggravated by strenuous activity? Would preventing him from playing be good advice?

Patient Scenario

The Cardowski Family

Read about the Cardowski family, a family with an adolescent who has experienced a spinal cord injury, then answer the questions to further sharpen your skills and grow more familiar with NCLEX-type questions related to neurologic disorders in children. Confirm your answers are correct by reading the rationales.

Visit http://thePoint.lww.com

Answers and Rationales

Looking for answers to the What if . . . and Critical Thinking Care Study questions?

Visit http://thePoint.lww.com

References

American Academy of Pediatrics. (2011). Febrile seizures: Guidelines for the neurodiagnostic evaluation of the child with a simple febrile seizure. *Pediatrics, 127*(2), 389–394.

Ardern-Holmes, S. L., & North, K. N. (2011). Therapeutics for childhood neurofibromatosis type 1 and type 2. *Current Treatment Options in Neurology, 13*(6), 529–543.

Bailey, B. M., Liesemer, K., Statler, K. D., et al. (2012). Monitoring and prediction of intracranial hypertension in pediatric traumatic brain injury: Clinical factors and initial head computed tomography. *Journal of Trauma & Acute Care Surgery, 72*(1), 263–270.

Baldin, E., Ludvigsson, P., Mixa, O., et al. (2012). Prevalence of recurrent symptoms and their association with epilepsy and febrile seizures in school-aged children: A community-based survey in Iceland. *Epilepsy & Behavior, 23*(3), 315–319.

Bennett, C. L., Starko, K. M., Thomsen, H. S., et al. (2012). Linking drugs to obscure illnesses: Lessons from pure red cell aplasia, nephrogenic systemic fibrosis, and Reye's syndrome. *Journal of General Internal Medicine, 27*(2), 1697–1703.

Bezov, D., Ashina, S., & Lipton, R. (2010). Post-dural puncture headache: Part II—Prevention, management, and prognosis. *Headache: The Journal of Head and Face Pain, 50*(9), 1482–1498.

Britton, J. W., & Kosa, S. C. (2010). The clinical value of chloral hydrate in the routine electroencephalogram. *Epilepsy Research, 88*(2–3), 215–220.

Budohoski, K. P., Zweifel, C., Kasprowicz, M., et al. (2012). What comes first? The dynamics of cerebral oxygenation and blood flow in response to changes in arterial pressure and intracranial pressure after head injury. *British Journal of Anaesthesia, 108*(1), 89–99.

Chalk, C., Benstead, T. J., & Keezer, M. (2011). Medical treatment for botulism. *Cochrane Database of Systematic Reviews,* (3), CD008123.

Chetty, S. P., Shaffer, B. L., & Norton, M. E. (2011). Management of pregnancy in women with genetic disorders: Part 2: Inborn errors of metabolism, cystic fibrosis, neurofibromatosis type 1, and Turner syndrome in pregnancy. *Obstetrics & Gynecology Survey, 66*(12), 765–776.

Cleves, C., & Rothner, A. D. (2011). Headache in children and adolescents: Evaluation and diagnosis, including migraine and its subtypes. In S. J. Tepper & D. E. Tepper (Eds.), *The Cleveland Clinic manual of headache therapy* (pp. 81–92). New York, NY: Springer.

Crosbie, J., Alhusaini, A. A., Dean, C. M., et al. (2012). Plantarflexor muscle and spatiotemporal gait characteristics of children with hemiplegic cerebral palsy: An observational study. *Developmental Neurorehabilitation, 15*(2), 114–119.

Dobrin, S. (2013). Seizures & epilepsy in adolescents & adults. In E. T. Bope & R. D. Kellerman (Eds.), *Conn's current therapy* (pp. 646–654). Philadelphia, PA: Elsevier/Saunders.

El-Chammas, K., Keyes, J., Thompson, N., et al. (2013). Pharmacologic treatment of pediatric headaches: A meta-analysis. *JAMA: Journal of the American Medical Association Pediatrics, 167*(3), 250–258.

Eves, F. J., & Rivera, N. (2010). Prevention of urinary tract infection in persons with spinal cord injury in home health care. *Home Healthcare Nurse, 28*(4), 230–241.

Gelfand, A. A., Fullerton, H. J., & Goadsby, P. J. (2010). Child neurology: Migraine with aura in children. *Neurology, 75*(5), e16–e19.

Gilbert, W. M., Jacoby, B. N., Xing, G., et al. (2010). Adverse obstetrical events are associated with significant risk of cerebral palsy. *American Journal of Obstetrics and Gynecology, 203*(4), 328.e1–328.e5.

Go, C. Y., Mackay, M. T., Weiss, S. K., et al. (2012). Evidence-based guidelines update: Medical treatment of infantile spasms. *Neurology, 78*(24), 1974–1980.

Gray, N., Morton, R. E., Brimlow, K., et al. (2012). Goals and outcomes for non ambulant children receiving continuous infusion of intrathecal baclofen. *European Journal of Paediatric Neurology, 16*(5), 443–448.

Greenberg-Kushnir, N., Haskin, O., Yarden-Bilavsky, H., et al. (2012). *Haemophilus influenzae* type b meningitis in the short period after vaccination: A reminder of the phenomenon of apparent vaccine failure. *Case Reports in Infectious Diseases, 2012*, 950107.

Hazinski, M. F. (2012). Neurological disorders. In M. F. Hazinski (Ed.), *Nursing care of the critically ill child* (pp. 587–678). St. Louis, MO: Elsevier Health Sciences.

Karch, A. M. (2013). *2013 Lippincott's nursing drug guide.* Philadelphia, PA: Lippincott Williams & Wilkins.

Kneen, R., Michael, D. B., Menson, E., et al. (2012). The management of suspected viral encephalitis in children. *The Journal of Infection, 64*(5), 449–477.

Koeppen, A. H. (2011). Friedreich's ataxia: Pathology, pathogenesis, and molecular genetics. *Journal of the Neurological Sciences, 303*(1–2), 1–12.

Kossoff, E. H., Bosarge, J. L., Miranda, M. J., et al. (2010). Will seizure control improve by switching from the modified Atkins diet to the traditional ketogenic diet? *Epilepsia, 51*(12), 2496–2499.

Kumar, R., Lorenc, A., Robinson, N., et al. (2011). Parents' and primary healthcare practitioners' perspectives on the safety of honey and other traditional paediatric healthcare approaches. *Child: Care, Health & Development, 37*(5), 734–743.

Lewis, D. W. (2011). Neurology. In K. J. Marcdante, R. M. Kliegman, H. B. Jenson, et al. (Eds.), *Nelson essentials of pediatrics* (6th ed., pp. 671–700). Philadelphia, PA: Saunders/Elsevier.

Libster, R., Edwards, K. M., Levent, F., et al. (2012). Long-term outcomes of group B streptococcal meningitis. *Pediatrics, 130*(1), e8–e15.

Lo, W., Marchuk, D. A., Ball, K. L., et al. (2012). Updates and future horizons on the understanding, diagnosis and treatment of Sturge-Weber syndrome brain involvement. *Developmental Medicine & Child Neurology, 54*(3), 214–223.

Luckhaupt, S. E., Dalhamer, J. M., Ward, B. W., et al. (2013). Prevalence and work-relatedness of carpal tunnel syndrome in the working population. *American Journal of Industrial Medicine, 56*(6), 615–624.

Lynch, D. R., Regner, S. R., Schadt, K. A., et al. (2012). Management and therapy for cardiomyopathy in Friedeirch's ataxia. *Expert Reviews of Cardiovascular Therapy, 10*(6), 767–777.

Mariani, E., Rossi, L. N., & Vojani, S. (2011). Interictal paroxysmal EEG abnormalities in childhood absence seizures. *Seizures, 20*(4), 299–304.

Martin-Herz, S. P., Zatzick, D. F., & McMahon, R. J. (2012). Health-related quality of life in children and adolescents following traumatic injury: A review. *Clinical Child and Family Psychology Review, 15*(3), 192–214.

McCaskey, M. S., Kirk, L., & Gerdes, C. (2011). Preventing skin breakdown in the immobile child in the home care setting. *Home Healthcare Nurse, 29*(4), 248–255.

McGrath-Morrow, S. A., Gower, W. A., Rothblum-Oviatt, C., et al. (2010). Evaluation and management of pulmonary disease in ataxia-telangiectasia. *Pediatric Pulmonology, 45*(9), 847–859.

McNamara, R., Doyle, J., McKay, M., et al. (2013). Medium term outcome in Bell's palsy in children. *Emergency Medicine Journal, 30*(6), 444–446.

Moster, D., Wilcox, A. J., Voilset, S. E., et al. (2010). Cerebral palsy among term and postterm births. *JAMA: Journal of the American Medical Association, 304*(9), 976–982.

Nayduch, D. A. (2010). Back to basics: Identifying and managing acute spinal cord injury. *Nursing, 40*(9), 24–31.

Ninove, L., Daniel, L., Gallou, J., et al. (2011). Fatal case of Reye's syndrome associated with H3N2 influenza virus infection and salicylate intake in a 12-year-old patient. *Clinical Microbiology and Infection, 17*(1), 95–97.

Pace, D., & Pollard, A. J. (2012). Meningococcal disease: Clinical presentation and sequelae. *Vaccine, 30*(2), B3–B39.

Parachuri, V., & Inglese, C. (2013). Neurological problems in the adolescent population. *Adolescent Medicine State of the Art Reviews, 24*(1), 1–28.

Pellatt, G. C. (2010). Spinal surgery for acute traumatic spinal cord injury: Implications for nursing. *British Journal of Neuroscience Nursing, 6*(6), 271–275.

Placzek, R., Siebold, D., & Funk, J. F. (2010). Development of treatment concepts for the use of botulinum toxin A in children with cerebral palsy. *Toxins, 2*(9), 2258–2271.

Rapin, I. (2011). Child neurologists as evaluators of developmental disorders. *Seminars in Pediatric Neurology, 18*(2), 104–109.

Riesch, S. K., Kedrowski, K., Brown, R. L., et al. (2012). Health-risk behaviors among a sample of US pre-adolescents: Types, frequency, and predictive factors. *International Journal of Nursing Studies.* Advance online publication.

Robotham, D. (2011). Neurology. In K. Arcara & M. Tschudy (Eds.), *The Harriett Lane handbook: A manuel for pediatric house officers* (pp. 504–523). St. Louis, MO: Mosby.

Rosen, B. A. (2012). Guillain-Barré syndrome. *Pediatrics in Review, 33*(4), 164–171.

Rust, R. (2011). What the child neurologist should know at the conclusion of training: History taking, examination, and formulation (and a few other generalizations). *Seminars in Pediatric Neurology, 18*(2), 59–65.

Sigurtà, A., Zanaboni, C., Canavesi, K., et al. (2013). Intensive care for pediatric traumatic brain injury. *Intensive Care Medicine, 39*(1), 129–136.

Singh, R. K., Stephens, S., Berl, M. M., et al. (2010). Prospective study of new-onset seizures presenting as status epilepticus in childhood. *Neurology, 74*(8), 636–642.

Tatum, W. O., Ho, S., & Benbadis, S. R. (2010). Polyspike ictal onset absence seizures. *Journal of Clinical Neurophysiology, 27*(2), 93–99.

U.S. Department of Health and Human Services. (2010). Healthy people 2020. Washington, D.C.: Author.

Wagner, J. L., Ferguson, P. L., & Smith, G. (2012). The relationship of coping behaviors to depressive symptoms in youth with epilepsy: An examination of caregiver and youth proxy report. *Epilepsy & Behavior, 24*(1), 86–92.

Yuki, N., & Hartung, H. (2012). Guillain-Barré syndrome. *New England Journal of Medicine, 366*(24), 2294–2304.

Zehetner, A. A., Orr, N., Buckmaster, A., et al. (2010). Iron supplementation for breath-holding attacks in children. *Journal of Pediatrics & Child Health, 46*(6), 357–360.

Chapter 50

Nursing Care of a Family When a Child Has a Vision or Hearing Disorder

KEY TERMS

- accommodation
- amblyopia
- astigmatism
- diplopia
- enucleation
- fovea centralis
- goniotomy
- hyperopia
- light refraction
- myopia
- nystagmus
- orthoptics
- photophobia
- ptosis
- stereopsis
- strabismus
- tympanocentesis

OBJECTIVES

After mastering the contents of this chapter, you should be able to:

1. Describe the structure and function of the eyes and ears and disorders of these organs as they affect children.
2. Identify 2020 National Health Goals related to vision and hearing disorders of children that nurses could help the nation achieve.
3. Assess a child who has a disorder of vision or hearing.
4. Formulate nursing diagnoses related to a child with a disorder of vision or hearing.
5. Establish expected outcomes for a child with a disorder of vision or hearing to help parents manage seamless transitions across differing health care settings.
6. Using the nursing process, plan nursing care that includes the six competencies of Quality & Safety Education for Nurses (QSEN): Patient-Centered Care, Teamwork & Collaboration, Evidence-Based Practice (EBP), Quality Improvement (QI), Safety, and Informatics.
7. Implement nursing care to meet the specific needs of a child who has a disorder of the eyes or ears, such as educating parents about the symptoms of otitis media.
8. Evaluate expected outcomes for achievement and effectiveness of care.
9. Integrate knowledge of childhood disorders of the eyes or ears with the interplay of nursing process, the six competencies of QSEN, and Family Nursing to promote quality maternal and child health nursing care.

Carla Vander, a 6-year-old child, is brought to your pediatric clinic for evaluation. Her mother states, "She was born deaf and with a cataract. Today, she has pain in her ear and her left eye is red. How could a bad eye or an ear without a functioning nerve get infected?"

Previous chapters discussed the growth and development of well children. This chapter adds information about the changes, both physical and psychosocial, that occur when a child develops a disorder of the eyes (vision) or ears (hearing). This is important information because it builds a base for care and health teaching.

How would you answer Ms. Vander? What additional information does she need to know about eye and ear disorders?

Any interference with vision or hearing poses a threat to normal growth and development, because so much of what and how a child learns about the world is achieved through these sensory organs. Infants first learn how to interact with others by watching their parents' faces, for example. They learn to speak by listening to words spoken to them. They continue to depend on sensory input for stimulation and to protect their safety throughout life (LaRoche, 2013).

Eye and ear disorders may be transitory. However, they always have the potential for becoming long-term illnesses if they permanently affect vision and hearing. This is an area, therefore, in which health promotion, illness prevention, and health rehabilitation are all vital aspects of nursing care. Because of the importance of vision and hearing, 2020 National Health Goals have been established in relation to them (Box 50.1).

Nursing Process Overview

For Care of a Child With a Vision or Hearing Disorder

Assessment

All newborns should be assessed for their ability to focus on or see an examiner's face and to follow an object from the periphery to the midline. Observe the infant closely to ensure that this response is evoked by sight, not by the sound of your voice. If it's unclear whether a newborn can see, vision can be further tested by optokinetic nystagmus testing.

Assessing newborn infants for hearing loss is an equally important part of newborn care. This can be done by assessing if newborns quiet to the sound of a soothing voice. Most hospitals further routinely test newborn hearing with an audible sound before newborns are discharged from the facility.

Throughout childhood, children should be assessed by history for both vision and hearing disorders. In addition, children also should be assessed for their ability to speak clearly and appropriately for their age, because language development is influenced by hearing. Because hearing and vision assessment are part of routine physical exams, the techniques of these are discussed in Chapter 34.

Nursing Diagnosis

Teaching health promotion measures to safeguard vision and hearing is one of the most important roles in nursing. Examples of nursing diagnoses in this area include:

- Health-seeking behaviors related to the prevention of trauma to the eyes or ears
- Deficient knowledge related to the importance of early diagnosis and treatment of eye or ear infections
- Self-care deficit related to impaired visual acuity
- Risk for injury related to hearing loss
- Risk for situational low self-esteem related to long-term vision deficit
- Impaired verbal communication related to congenital hearing deficit
- Social isolation related to effects of hearing loss
- Risk for complicated grieving related to child's loss of sight

BOX 50.1 Nursing Care Planning Based on 2020 National Health Goals

Adequate vision and hearing ability are necessary for normal growth and development, therefore, several 2020 National Health Goals focus on prevention, early detection, treatment, and rehabilitation of eye and hearing health. These include:

- Increase the proportion of preschool children aged 5 years and younger who receive vision screening from a baseline of 40.1% to 44.1%.
- Reduce blindness and visual impairment in children and adolescents aged 17 years and younger from 28.2 per 1,000 children to 25.4 per 1,000.
- Reduce visual impairment in children aged 12 years and older from 136.1 per 1,000 population to 122.5 per 1,000.
- Increase the use of personal protective eyewear in recreational activities and hazardous situations around the home from 16.5% to 18.2% of children and adolescents aged 6 to 17 years.
- Reduce otitis media in children and adolescents from 246.1 persons per 1,000 persons under age 18 years to 221.5 per 1,000.
- Increase the proportion of persons with hearing impairments who have ever used a hearing aid or assistive listening devices or who have cochlear implants (developmental).
- Increase the proportion of persons who have had a hearing examination on schedule from 79.3% to 87.2% of adolescents aged 12 to 19 years (U.S. Department of Health and Human Services [DHHS], 2010: see www.healthypeople.gov).

Nurses can help the nation achieve these goals by screening for vision and hearing at all well-child assessments, paying particular attention to those children who had low birth weight, were cared for in neonatal intensive care units, or who were excessively exposed to loud noises such as loud music.

- Risk for parental role strain related to responsibilities of caring for a sensory impaired child
- Readiness for enhanced family coping related to child's traumatic injury and subsequent loss of vision in one eye

Outcome Identification and Planning

Be certain that expected outcomes established are realistic and address areas in which treatment can have some impact. By listening attentively to the concerns of parents and those of the child and by providing useful anticipatory guidance, you can help to increase a child's ability to function effectively. Because many eye and ear disorders cause pain, helping parents reduce pain in their child is a major nursing responsibility. Be certain that expected outcomes address preventive aspects of care in all areas of daily living.

When parents learn a child will have a vision or hearing disorder, they usually need help in planning for schooling and activities such as toilet training and self-care. Discuss with them the importance of talking to and touching their infant so the infant learns how to communicate and learn about the world through his or her functioning senses. Most children with sensory disorders benefit from very early preschool education programs because this exposes them to interesting and stimulating tasks while their initiative is strongest.

Many parents whose infant screens positive for hearing loss in the hospital do not follow up with additional hearing screening as recommended probably because of inadequate communication about the concern or a lack of health insurance (Shulman, Besculides, Saltzman, et al., 2010). Internet resources that can be helpful to parents are the Alexander Graham Bell Association for the Deaf and Hard of Hearing (www.agbell.org); the American Foundation for the Blind (www.afb.org); the American Speech-Language-Hearing Association (www.asha.org); Lighthouse International (www.lighthouse.org); the National Federation of the Blind (www.nfb.org); Learning Ally (www.learningally.org); and the National Association of the Deaf (www.nad.org).

Implementation

A disorder of the eyes or ears can range from an acute, onetime illness to a chronic and developmentally debilitating condition if steps are not taken to treat the initial problem quickly and completely. However, even the most rigorous preventive care and attention cannot avert the occurrence of some serious disorders affecting vision and hearing. Nursing care must then focus on helping the child and parents adjust to the condition, ensuring that the child receives the stimulation needed to grow and develop on a usual continuum.

Nursing interventions for a child with a disorder of the eyes or ears range from providing anticipatory guidance and teaching children and parents measures to promote eye and ear health to preparing a child for surgery. Nursing interventions also include helping a child and parents adjust to aids that are used to improve hearing, speech, or sight.

Outcome Evaluation

Continuing follow-ups with hearing and vision concerns is essential so self-esteem can be evaluated. Do children think of themselves as well or ill? As people able to do things or as disabled? Some parents may require help with their own feelings of worth (feeling inferior to other parents is common among parents of children with disabilities) before they can help their children. Be certain to evaluate if they're able to "let go" so their child can attend school.

Examples of expected outcomes include:

- Parent states she understands that antibiotics are no longer prescribed for simple otitis media.
- Parents state concrete plans for enrolling child in a hearing-impaired preschool program.
- The child wears corrective lenses for a major portion of each day.
- The child with a hearing disorder communicates effectively with health care providers by lip reading or writing out her needs.

HEALTH PROMOTION AND RISK MANAGEMENT

Vision can be assessed shortly after birth by eliciting a blink reflex and the ability to follow a moving object. All babies should be screened by a formal method for hearing loss before leaving the hospital or no later than 1 month of age (Centers for Disease Control and Prevention [CDC], 2012). Such tests give reassurance to worried parents that their child's vision and hearing is adequate or set the stage for early interventions if their child is visually or hearing challenged. School nurses play a vital role in the continuing assessment of vision or hearing as well as being instrumental in laying a foundation for steps that parents and children need to take to maintain vision and hearing health (Box 50.2).

A history and physical examination performed at each health maintenance visit can provide important clues to possible problems or the need for further evaluation. General guidelines for evaluation are listed in Table 50.1. During these visits, be certain to offer parents opportunities to ask questions and voice any concerns they may have regarding their child.

Children with vision or hearing disorders need to attend regular classrooms in school, if possible, so that they can have contact with seeing and hearing children to promote growth and development. If a child has a vision or hearing impairment, assist the parents with measures to adapt the child's environment to meet safety needs while promoting growth, development, and independence as much as possible. Help them to supplement verbal explanations with tactile and

BOX 50.2 Nursing Care Planning Using Assessment

Assessing a Child for Vision or Hearing Disorders

History

Chief concern: Are symptoms of vision or hearing difficulty present—blurriness of vision, squinting, turning head, leaning toward speaker, ignoring instructions?

Past health history: Has child had any exposure to loud noises? Eye trauma? Ear infection?

Family medical history: Do any family members have a hearing disorder? What is the vision level of parents?

Physical assessment

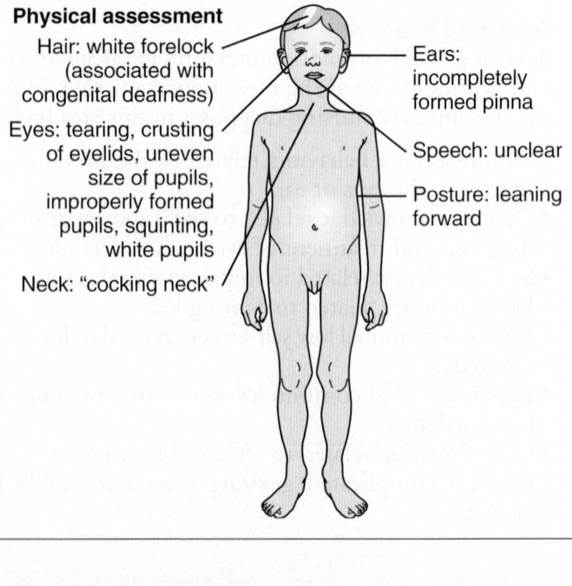

TABLE 50.1 Assessment Parameters for Vision and Hearing Screening

Age	Vision Assessment Parameters	Hearing Assessment Parameters
Infant	Ability to follow objects Corneal (blink) reflex Ability to turn to light stimuli	Startle reflex at hearing sound (at birth) Ability to track sounds (3–6 months) Ability to recognize sounds (6–8 months) Ability to locate sounds (8–12 months)
Toddler	Corneal light reflex Cover test Smooth ocular movements Hand–eye coordination	Ability to react to soft sounds (whispers) Ability to form a noun–verb sentence by 2 years Ability to follow simple directions Awareness of pitch and tone
Preschooler	Corneal light reflex Cover test Snellen E chart (or modification)	Pure tone audiometry (starting at age 4 years) Understandable language with increasing vocabulary
School age	Visual acuity testing every 1–2 years	Pure tone audiometry at ages 6, 8, and 11 years
Adolescent	Visual acuity testing every 1–2 years	Pure tone audiometry at ages 14 and 18 years

visual aids as appropriate as well as allow the child to use drawings, writing, gestures, a talking picture board, text messaging, and/or e-mail to respond and communicate. Assess whether parents are interested in investigating a cochlear implant for a hearing-challenged child. Be certain parents are familiar with measures to prevent eye and ear infections, so that these do not lead to long-term problems. Assess that children receive adequate vitamin A because, although not common in the United States, a deficiency of this may cause diminished night vision or even blindness (Dudek, 2010).

Caution children that exposure to high levels of sound over a period of time can permanently lower the level at which they hear. Music heard through earbuds, for example, is at about 110 dB (compared to 50 to 60 dB, the level of usual conversation). Rock concerts expose listeners to decibels as high as 120 to 140 dB. To lessen the danger of such exposure, urge students to invest in quality earplugs, don't listen through them for long time intervals, and listen to music at the lowest level possible. At music concerts, they should not sit near loud speakers and should wear foam earplugs to decrease the sound level (Box 50.3).

VISION

Vision occurs because light rays reflect from an object through the corneas, aqueous humors, lenses, and vitreous humors to the retinas (Fig. 50.1). If any of these structures have defects, light rays may not be able to reach the retinas or focus correctly there, resulting in a vision disorder. Both retinas are studded with *rods*, which are instrumental for night vision and for detecting movement in the visual field, and *cones*, which register daylight and color vision. The **fovea centralis** (the center of the macula) is an area of closely packed cones on the retinas where color is best perceived.

Each eye globe must not only develop good central and peripheral vision but also learn to work with the other eye to fuse or interpret a dual image as one (*single binocular vision*). Infants with poor eye alignment cannot establish single binocular vision but have **diplopia**, or double vision, instead.

Stereopsis

Stereopsis is depth perception, or the ability to see objects as three-dimensional. Children with vision loss in one eye do not develop stereopsis and, consequently, tend to reach farther or closer than the actual distance of an object when attempting to grasp it. They have difficulty learning to ride a bicycle and have great difficulty driving a car safely. Lack of stereopsis can be detected by a depth perception test such as the *Stereo-Fly* dot test, a test where the image of a fly is constructed from a series of colored dots. When asked to touch the fly's wings, a child with good depth perception touches them accurately. A child with poor depth perception touches a spot 2 or 3 in. above the pattern.

Accommodation

Accommodation is the adjustment the eye makes to focus on a close image. To do this, the eyes converge (look medially) and the pupils constrict. To test for accommodation, ask a child (over 6 months of age) to follow a penlight as you move it in toward the nose. Children who cannot accommodate are unable to fuse their vision to follow a penlight toward their nose this way; instead, they demonstrate double vision (diplopia). Poor accommodation is important to recognize because it can lead to headaches, poor reading ability, and difficulty achieving in school.

DISORDERS THAT INTERFERE WITH VISION

Eye disorders in children are always potentially serious because, if permanent vision impairment occurs, a child's functioning at many everyday tasks can be severely compromised.

Refractive Errors

Refractive errors that cause visual impairment are one of the most common visual deficits in school-age children (Pi, Chen, Liu, et al., 2010). **Light refraction** refers to the manner in

BOX 50.3 Nursing Care Planning Based on Family Teaching

PROTECTING VISION AND HEARING

Q. Carla's mother says to you, "What can we do to protect our children from having problems with their eyes and ears?"
A. Here are some helpful tips to protect children's vision and hearing:

To protect vision:

- Place infants and small children in a car seat (for older children, use a seat belt) when in a car to keep them from hitting the dashboard or front seat in the event of an accident.
- Do not allow infants to hold sharp objects because the object could strike the eye as the infant brings the hand to the mouth to suck his or her thumb.
- Do not allow children to carry sharp objects such as lollipop sticks in their hands while walking. If they fall, the object could puncture their eye.
- Caution older children to use eye-protection measures, such as goggles, when working with projects, such as soldering metal, in school or at home.
- Encourage the use of proper athletic facial protective gear when playing sports.
- Teach children not to place any medication in their eyes that is not prescribed by a health care provider; do not use outdated eye medication because it may become contaminated with bacteria or may change in composition with time.
- Wear a hat or ultraviolet (UV) coated lenses when outdoors, especially for children with light-colored eyes.
- Caution children that chemicals can cause burns to the eye; alert them to the emergency shower installations in science rooms that are used to wash away any spilled chemical from their eyes. Chemical burns may be worse in children who have contact lenses in place because chemicals can flow under the lens and remain in contact with the cornea longer.
- Teach children not to wear contact lenses for longer intervals than recommended by the manufacturer to prevent drying and a lack of oxygen supply to the cornea.

To prevent hearing loss:

- Keep children away from high noise levels, such as loud toys or electronic games. While in loud environments, protect ears with earplugs or earmuffs.
- Teach children to avoid chronic exposure to loud noises, such as can occur with radios and earbuds/earphones.
- Secure prompt treatment for pharyngitis (fever and sore throat) because this condition can lead to otitis media (middle ear infection).
- Caution children not to put anything in their ear canals because they could puncture their eardrums.
- Be certain children's immunizations are kept up to date because illnesses such as parotitis (mumps) or bacterial meningitis can lead to hearing loss.

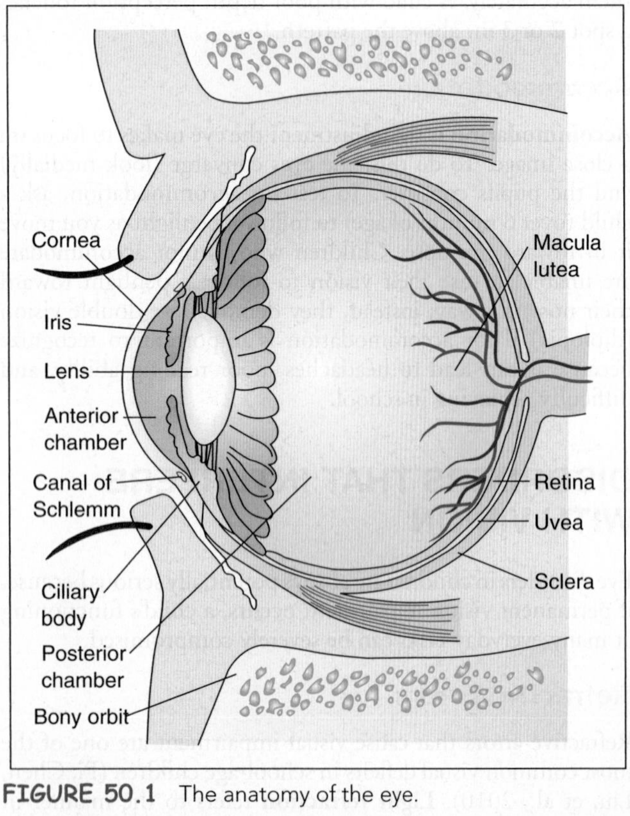

FIGURE 50.1 The anatomy of the eye.

which light is bent as it passes through the lens. Normally, this bending causes a ray of light to fall directly on the retina (Fig. 50.2A). Because the depth of the eye globe in infants and children increases with age, the light rays do not always focus onto the retina accurately as the child grows older, but at a point behind the retina. This results in **hyperopia** (farsightedness), in which vision is blurry at a close range and clear at a far range. It is important to remember that this normal hyperopia of preschoolers needs no correction when performing vision screening with children of this age because at about 5 years of age, as a result of developmental changes, hyperopia will begin to diminish. Some children, however, remain hyperopic. Focusing on close objects requires such strong accommodation that these children often develop headaches or dizziness while doing schoolwork. A finding of hyperopia in a school-age child is cause for referral so that the child can get a prescription for glasses with a convex lens (see Fig. 50.2B).

Myopia (nearsightedness) occurs when light rays focus anterior to the retina, causing objects that are far away to be unfocused. Typically, this develops around age 8 years and then progresses (Belden, DeFriez, & Huether, 2013). These children can read a book or a computer screen immediately in front of them but are unable to read the blackboard clearly from a distance. They have difficulty reading signs across the street or playing baseball. Myopia tends to plateau as the child reaches adolescence. Children with myopia need corrective (concave) lenses to enable them to see at a distance (see Fig. 50.2C).

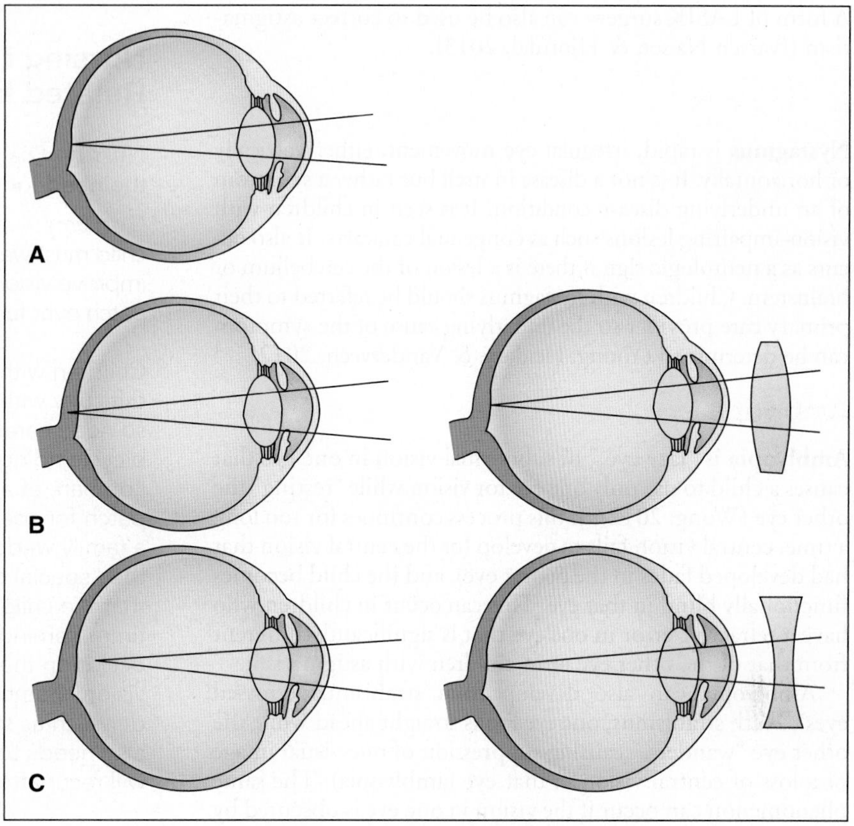

FIGURE 50.2 Corrective lenses for refractive errors of vision. **(A)** Normal vision. **(B)** Convex lens for hyperopia (farsightedness). **(C)** Concave lens for myopia (nearsightedness).

Myopia has a familial tendency, so if both parents are myopic, their children should be screened yearly during the early school years. Because children with myopia try to focus on objects by squinting or rubbing their eyes, any child who reports difficulty seeing or who shows mannerisms suggestive of refraction errors—rubbing the eyes, tearing, blinking, squinting, or pressing on the eyes—should be screened for visual difficulty.

It is possible for contact lenses to be fitted for even young infants. Children as young as 5 years of age are capable of putting them in and taking them out if taught properly. Contact lenses are a big responsibility, however; they require conscientious cleaning or changing to prevent eye irritation or infection. Children are usually about 12 years of age before they can be relied on to take appropriate care of contact lenses independently.

Young children may resist wearing glasses because they're worried they'll be bullied if they wear them. If glasses are needed, however, encourage children to give them a fair try. In most instances, glasses improve vision to such an extent that, after trying them, children will appreciate the difference they make and continue to wear them. Some children may need continued encouragement to keep wearing glasses, however, until they are old enough for contact lenses or surgical correction. Advise parents to choose frames fitted with safety glass (shatterproof) lenses so that, if the lenses accidentally break, the child's eyes will not be injured.

By late adolescence, children can have laser surgery (known as laser in situ keratomileusis [LASIK] or photorefractive keratectomy [PRK]) to permanently change the contour of the cornea and correct refractive vision errors.

Laser In Situ Keratomileusis and Photorefractive Keratectomy

LASIK and PRK are both laser surgery correction procedures for either myopia or hyperopia (Paysse, Tychsen, & Stahl, 2012). These involve an incision under the cornea to change the contour of the eye globe so that light rays fall more accurately on the retina. Postoperatively, children may have disturbed tear functioning for 1 or more months and so need to instill artificial tears or ointments to prevent surface damage. Because having the procedure carried out before the child's eye globe has reached its adult size would require the surgery to be repeated with maturity, the youngest age at which LASIK therapy is appropriate is controversial; most authorities recommend this not be done before 21 years of age to allow for natural eye contour changes to occur. The exception to this is children who have amblyopia or strabismus (see later in the chapter) (Alió, Wolter, Piñero, et al., 2011).

Astigmatism

Astigmatism is an irregular curvature of the cornea, causing light to focus incorrectly on the retina, resulting in an uneven quality of vision. When children with astigmatism look at the letter T, for example, they may see the crossbar but not the letter stem. If they focus on the stem, they cannot see the crossbar. On any given page of print, therefore, they may see only half the letters or can have great difficulty reading or following written instructions. They may report headache and vertigo after doing close work. Even though their vision appears deceptively normal on vision screening tests (they are able to see all of the numbers on a chart by tilting their head), these children need to be referred to an ophthalmologist on the basis of their other problems such as vertigo, headaches, and difficulty with reading. Corrective lenses for close work relieve the symptoms and restore functional vision. Contact lenses may be even more helpful, because they actually smooth out the curvature of the cornea.

A form of LASIK surgery can also be used to correct astigmatism (Ivarsen Næser, & Hjortdal, 2013).

Nystagmus

Nystagmus is rapid, irregular eye movement, either vertically or horizontally. It is not a disease in itself but rather a symptom of an underlying disease condition. It is seen in children with vision-impairing lesions such as congenital cataracts. It also occurs as a neurologic sign if there is a lesion of the cerebellum or brainstem. Children with nystagmus should be referred to their primary care provider so the underlying cause of the symptom can be determined (Young, Heidary, & Vanderveen, 2012).

Amblyopia

Amblyopia is "lazy eye," or subnormal vision in one eye that causes a child to use only one eye for vision while "resting" the other eye (Wong, 2012). If this process continues for too long a time, central vision fails to develop (or the central vision that had developed fades in the poorer eye), and the child becomes functionally blind in that eye. This can occur in children who have a refractive error in one eye that is significantly different from that of the other eye or in children with astigmatism.

Amblyopia can also develop from strabismus (crossed eyes). With strabismus, one eye looks straight ahead while the other eye "wanders," causing suppression of one visual image or a loss of central vision in that eye (amblyopia). The same phenomenon can occur if the vision in one eye is obscured by a lid that does not open fully (ptosis).

Assessment

The U.S. Preventive Services Task Force (USPSTF, 2011) for Vision Screening recommends vision screening for all children at least once between the ages of 3 and 5 years to detect amblyopia. If a child has amblyopia, a screening exam such as a preschool E chart (see Chapter 34) typically demonstrates 20/50 vision (which is normal for preschool age) in one eye, but the other eye shows lessened vision (perhaps as different as 20/100).

Therapeutic Management

Treatment for amblyopia is most successful among children under the age of 7 years, but there is evidence to show a response to treatment for children between 7 and 13 years of age (Holmes, Lazar, Melia, et al., 2011). Treatment can consist of wearing correcting lenses (glasses), covering the good eye with a patch, or a combination of the two (Taylor, Powell, Hatt, et al., 2012). Wearing a patch over the good eye forces the child to use the poor eye, thus developing vision in that eye. Usually, children have some difficulty initially adjusting to a patch because they are unable to see well from the unpatched eye. They may report headaches or dizziness and notice poor depth perception. Only constant attempts to see with the weaker eye, however, will improve binocular vision, so parents have to enforce patching if prescribed (Chou, Dana, & Bougatsos, 2011).

The patch should be removed for 1 hour each day to prevent amblyopia from developing in the nonamblyopic eye. If patching does not produce the anticipated result, LASIK surgery to improve the refractive error may be necessary (Paysse et al., 2012). Yet a further option is the administration of levodopa in addition to occlusion therapy because this almost immediately improves vision in both eyes (Yang, Luo, Liao, et al., 2012).

Nursing Diagnoses and Related Interventions

Nursing Diagnosis: Deficient knowledge related to the need for consistent wearing of eye patch

Outcome Evaluation: Parents state the reason their child must wear a patch over the functioning eye is to improve vision in the poorly functioning eye. Child wears patch over functioning eye for all but 1 hour per day.

Children with an eye patch in place may have more difficulty with motor coordination than others and so need careful supervision with activities such as bicycle riding or crossing a street safely (Roefs, Tjiam, Looman, et al., 2012). A child may beg to remove the patch for special occasions, such as a birthday party or a family wedding, or just for an hour. If this is allowed, the "special occasions" may soon become so frequent that the child is wearing the patch for only half the time. Remind parents how important it is to adhere to occlusion therapy so that their child will achieve good vision. If amblyopia occurs secondary to another disorder such as strabismus or ptosis, the primary problem also needs to be corrected. Otherwise, the amblyopia will recur after the patching is completed.

QSEN Checkpoint Question 50.1

Patient-Centered Care

What if Carla, who is 6 years old, develops amblyopia? Which statement by her mother would assure you that her learning needs are being met?

a. "I place the patch over her weak eye to enhance the vision in her stronger eye."
b. "I place the patch over her good eye to allow the weaker eye to strengthen."
c. "I alternate the patch between eyes every other day so both eyes strengthen."
d. "I can take off the patch while Carla eats to make it easier for her."

Look in Appendix A for the best answer and rationale.

Color Vision Deficit (Color Blindness)

Color deficit is, as the name implies, the inability to perceive color correctly. It occurs in 4% to 8% of boys because one of the sets of cones of the retina that perceive red, green, or blue is absent. It is inherited as a sex-linked disorder, although there is also a high incidence in children with hemophilia, congenital nystagmus, or glucose-6-phosphate dehydrogenase deficiency (Birch, 2012).

The vision problem may involve the inability to distinguish red from green or blue from yellow. A small proportion of children are unable to see any colors. It can be detected by the use of color plates or discs for children as young as preschool age. Children with normal vision see numbers or patterns on these plates, whereas children with a color vision deficit see only a jumble of dots or unclear images.

There is currently no therapy for color vision deficit because the condition is caused by a genetic mutation. The deficit is categorized based on severity. It's important that the loss of color perception is detected early so the child is not asked to complete color identification assignments in preschool and can learn to appreciate color changes in traffic signals or other color-dependent signs necessary for safety.

Some children associate color blindness with total "blindness" and fear they will eventually lose their eyesight. Reassure them that, although color blindness means they have a loss of color discrimination, their loss is limited to that one area.

STRUCTURAL PROBLEMS OF THE EYE

Structural problems of the eye tend to be congenital or already present at birth.

Coloboma

A *coloboma* is an example of an incomplete closure of the facial cleft. The incomplete closure may involve only the lower eyelid (there is a notch in the lid). It may involve the iris, giving it the shape of a keyhole, rather than a circle (Fig. 50.3). It may involve the ciliary body, the lens, the choroid, the retina, and the optic nerve. Children with any degree of coloboma should be referred to an ophthalmologist for further investigation to determine the extent of the condition. Children with only iris involvement have no decline in vision; those with retina and optic nerve coloboma will have some vision impairment in the affected eye (Braverman, 2012).

Hypertelorism

Hypertelorism is congenital, abnormally wide-spaced eyes. Children with wide epicanthal folds by the inner canthus may appear to have wide-spaced eyes, but, when the distance between the pupils is measured and compared with standards for the child's age, the true condition is revealed. Detecting true hypertelorism in children is important, because this condition is associated with chromosomal abnormalities, most notably Waardenburg syndrome, which also involves congenital hearing impairment. Children with this syndrome also have a white forelock of hair, different-colored irises, and eyebrows that tend to grow together in the center line, all signs not necessarily noticeable in newborns. Therefore, wide-spaced eyes, because of a broad-bridged nose, are the chief clue in a newborn that the child can hear no sound and will need close follow-up to determine whether cochlear implants or hearing aids can provide their ability to hear.

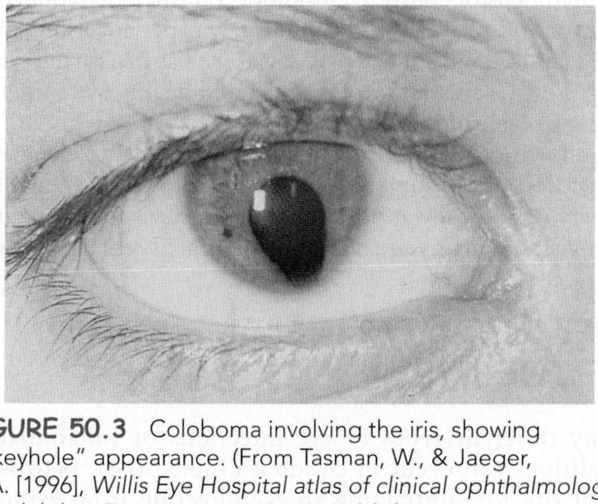

FIGURE 50.3 Coloboma involving the iris, showing a "keyhole" appearance. (From Tasman, W., & Jaeger, E. A. [1996], *Willis Eye Hospital atlas of clinical ophthalmology.* Philadelphia, PA: Lippincott-Raven Publishers.)

Ptosis

Ptosis is the inability to raise the upper eyelid the usual distance so the eyelid always remains slightly closed. With this, children tend to wrinkle their forehead and raise their eyebrows more than usual in an attempt to lift the eyelid further or cock their heads back to see under the lowered lid. The condition may be congenital (frequently hereditary and bilateral) or acquired (usually unilateral). It may be a result of injury to the lid or levator muscle, injury to the third cranial nerve, or from the development of myasthenia gravis (see Chapter 51) (Lewis, 2011). If the third cranial nerve has been injured, paralysis of one or more of the other muscles supplied by that nerve will also be affected and a child will exhibit:

- A dilated pupil
- An inability to rotate the eye globe upward, medially, or downward
- Weakness of accommodation (looking at near objects)

After a careful investigation of the cause has been completed, ptosis is corrected surgically. The correction is usually important to the child from a cosmetic standpoint, but if the ptosis is unilateral, and more importantly, if the lid obstructs vision, early surgery is necessary to prevent the development of amblyopia (from a lack of use of the closed eye). Be certain that parents understand it's important that ptosis be corrected during the preschool period because, if they wait until the child is older, although the ptosis can be corrected at that later date, the amblyopia cannot.

Strabismus

Strabismus is unequally aligned eyes (cross-eyes) caused by an imbalance of the extraocular muscles that control the movement of the eye globes, similar to the handling of reins of a horse (Fig. 50.4). Approximately 1% to 2% of children demonstrate some degree of strabismus. The condition does not favor either gender, social status, or geographic area; about 30% of children have a history of a similar strabismus in the family.

With strabismus, the resting position of one eye, instead of facing forward, will be *divergent* (turned out) or *convergent* (turned in). One pupil may appear higher than the other (vertical strabismus). The strabismus may be monocular, in which the same eye deviates constantly, or it may be an alternating strabismus, in which one eye and then the other deviates.

Assessment

Infants' eyes may cross occasionally until 6 weeks of age. If infants demonstrate a constant strabismus, refer them to their primary care provider at any time; if they still demonstrate occasional strabismus past 6 months, refer them at that point.

Definite deviations are obvious at a physical exam (Fig. 50.5). Note if the deviation is *exotropia* (an eye turns out), *esotropia* (an eye turns in), or *hypertropia* (an eye turns up). If the deviation is not so obvious or occurs only when the child is fatigued or ill and, therefore, less able to maintain fixation, the terms used are *exophoria*, *esophoria*, and *hyperphoria*. If the

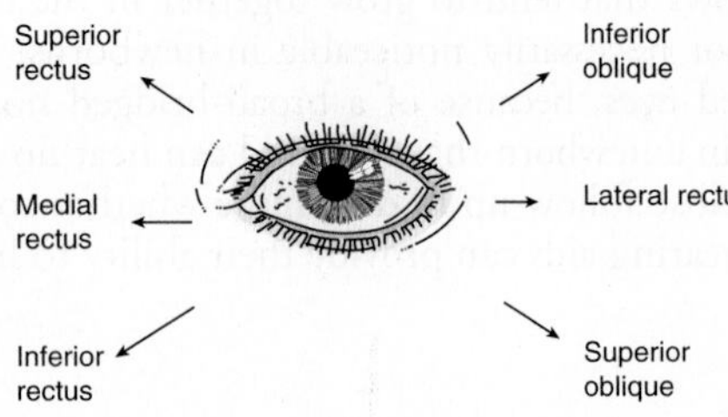

Eye muscle	Action	Innervation
Superior rectus	Turns eye up and medially	Oculomotor (third cranial) nerve
Medial rectus	Turns eye inward	Oculomotor (third cranial) nerve
Inferior rectus	Turns eye down and medially	Oculomotor (third cranial) nerve
Lateral rectus	Turns eye out	Abducens (sixth cranial) nerve
Superior oblique	Turns eye down and laterally	Trochlear (fourth cranial) nerve
Inferior oblique	Turns eye up and laterally	Oculomotor (third cranial) nerve

FIGURE 50.4 The extraocular eye muscles.

parents report that the deviation occurs only when the child is tired or sick, attempt to assess the strabismus at such a time, because then the deviation will be most striking.

Strabismus may be detected best when children are asked to examine a nearby object, because, to do this, they must turn both eyes medially, or *converge*, to focus at the short distance. If they are farsighted in one eye, they will have to turn the affected eye in more than the other, causing esotropia. If one eye is nearsighted, they will not need to turn that eye in as far as the other one; this results in divergence or exotropia.

Some children have a latent strabismus, or appear to have straight vision. Because they are only able to maintain fusion at the expense of eyestrain, however, they develop symptoms such as headache; tired, irritated eyes; and perhaps even nausea and vomiting.

Children who have flat, broad-bridged noses, a narrow interpupillary distance, and an epicanthal fold, or oval-shaped palpebral fissures may appear to have strabismus (pseudostrabismus) because less white sclera is visible in the inner margin of the eye than usual. A cover test reveals the true condition. If pseudostrabismus is present, the covered eye will not move after being uncovered because it only appears to be turned medially due to the obscured sclera at the inner canthus. The Hirschberg test is another method of detecting true strabismus (see Chapter 34).

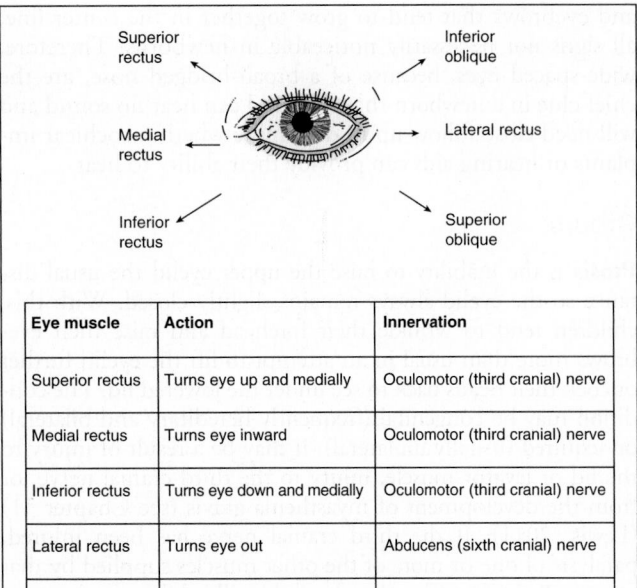

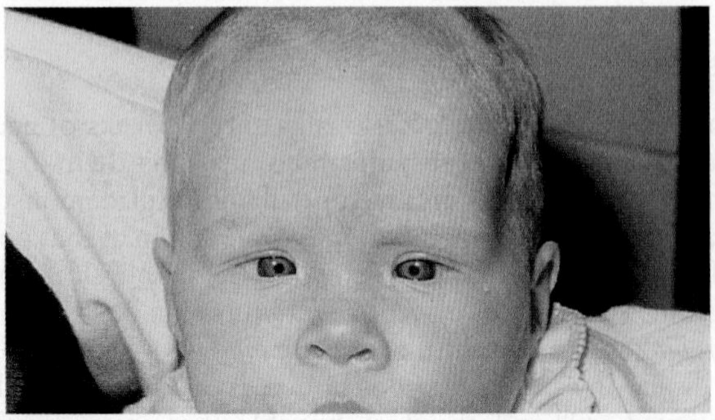

FIGURE 50.5 Strabismus (esotropia) in an infant.

Once strabismus is detected, it is important to attempt to discern whether it is concomitant (measures the same in all directions of gaze) or nonconcomitant (greater in one direction than in another, often called *paralytic strabismus*). Concomitant (nonparalytic) strabismus is the most usual type found in children. All the muscles of the eye are capable of functioning, but they do not function together. The deviation is equally apparent in all directions of gaze.

Paralytic strabismus is caused by paralysis of a muscle or nerve, perhaps from an injury (such as a birth injury), or an invading lesion. The eyes appear straight except when they are moved in the direction of the paralyzed muscle. Then double vision occurs, and the crossed eye is evident. Such children often close one eye or tilt their head to decrease the double vision. They may tilt their head so much that they appear to have a torticollis, or "wry neck"—an orthopedic rather than an eye problem. They may appear clumsy because of the diplopia. Because they are too young to describe double vision and how nauseated this makes them feel, they may express this by fussiness or whining.

Therapeutic Management

The therapy for strabismus depends on the cause of the problem. If the fusion mechanism is weak, eye exercises (**orthoptics**) can strengthen the weak muscle. If eyes are diverging because of farsightedness or nearsightedness, the child needs glasses or contact lenses to correct the basic visual defect. Surgical treatment can be used to permanently align the extraocular muscles if the cause is due to muscle strength. Another option is to use botulism toxin as a means of temporarily paralyzing the extraocular muscles. The use of botulism toxin is still considered investigative, however, and has no clear recommendations and varied effectiveness in children (Rowe & Noonan, 2012).

A side effect of strabismus can be amblyopia because, to avoid double vision, the child suppresses the vision in one eye. For this reason, eye correction for strabismus must be done early in life, before 7 years of age. Some children, because of an accommodation problem caused by hyperopia in one eye, outgrow the condition as the normal hyperopia of the preschooler lessens. This does not always occur, however. Even if the child's eyes appear to be straighter later, an amblyopia may be present that could have been prevented by earlier treatment.

After strabismus surgery, eye patches are not usually required. Postoperatively, antibiotic ointment is applied to the eye for 2 or 3 days. The child may experience some pain on eye movement for the first day as well as nausea and vomiting. Further nursing care for the child having eye surgery is discussed later in this chapter.

Follow-up visits after surgery are necessary to determine the success of the surgery. Retest children who have had this surgery periodically at health maintenance visits to be certain their vision remains equal and eye alignment remains straight.

INFECTION OR INFLAMMATION OF THE EYE

Many different types of eye infections or inflammatory conditions can occur in children (Table 50.2). Newborns are at risk for contracting an eye infection from exposure

TABLE 50.2 Infectious and Inflammatory Eye Disorders

Disorder	Description/Cause	Signs and Symptoms	Treatment
Stye	Infection of a ciliary gland (a modified sweat gland) that enters into the hair follicle at the lid margin; most commonly caused by *Staphylococcus*	Pain and redness at a localized point on the lid margin with possible edema of the lid out of proportion to the severity of the disease; preauricular lymph node swelling and tenderness.	Hot, moist compresses for 15–20 minutes four times daily; antibiotic ointment application after the compresses (possible); incision and drainage (when the stye points [develops a head]); nose and throat cultures for *Staphylococcus*. Follow-up evaluation for repeated episodes to rule out other debilitating diseases such as diabetes mellitus or anemia. Visual acuity assessment (although styes are not associated with refraction error, they occur when children rub their eyes excessively possibly because of problems with visual acuity).
Chalazion	Low-grade granulation tissue tumor of the *meibomian*, or tarsal, gland on the eyelid; cause unknown but may be a result of a low-grade infection produced by retained secretion in the gland	Small, slow-growing, hard, but painless nodule on the lid; skin freely movable over it; absence of inflammation or edema	Nodule may resolve spontaneously, evacuating itself onto the conjunctival surface of the lid; incision and drainage if no spontaneous remission, followed by antibiotic ointment application to prevent secondary gland infection. If ptosis is present in a child younger than 7–8 years of age, surgical removal is performed to prevent possible subsequent amblyopia.
Blepharitis marginalis	Inflammation of the eyelid margin; usually a local infection caused by *Staphylococcus*; possibly an extension of seborrheic dermatitis (cradle cap)	Eyelid margin reddened, possibly covered by hard, dirty-yellow crusts that stick tenaciously to the lid margin and lashes; styes possibly present secondary to the presence of *Staphylococcus*	Application of an antibiotic ointment six to eight times a day to the lower conjunctival rim; removal of crusts with a moistened cotton applicator after the lid margins have been covered by wet compresses for 10–15 minutes. If condition persists, systemic antibiotic therapy is used to reduce the presence of *Staphylococcus* on the skin surface.
Conjunctivitis	Inflammation of the conjunctiva; causes are numerous, including ophthalmia neonatorum (exposure to gonococcus bacillus; see Chapter 26) and bacterial, viral, and fungal organisms	Eyes watery with reddened conjunctiva and sensitivity to light; sticking of eyelids with pustular drainage	Application of an antibiotic ointment applied from inner to outer canthus to prevent spread of infection to other eye; follow-up visit is mandatory to be certain infection clears.
Inclusion blennorrhea	*Chlamydia* organism	Acute inflammation usually occurring on the 5th to 14th day after birth; conjunctiva reddened with tearing; eye discharge	Systemic antibiotic such as erythromycin.
Acute catarrhal conjunctivitis	Commonly called "pinkeye," usually caused by a virus or irritation from a foreign body; most frequently caused by *Haemophilus influenzae* and *Streptococcus pneumoniae*	Conjunctiva fiery red with tearing; mucopurulent or purulent discharge	Antibiotic ointment or drops three to four times daily for 7 days (redness usually disappears within 48 hours); avoid rubbing and transmitting infection to unaffected eye. Cool, moist compresses to affected eye.

(continues on page 1476)

TABLE 50.2 Infectious and Inflammatory Eye Disorders (continued)

Disorder	Description/Cause	Signs and Symptoms	Treatment
Herpetic conjunctivitis	Herpes simplex viral infection (may occur along with development of facial herpes lesion)	Series of pinpoint vesicles on the conjunctiva; on fluorescein stain, vesicles stain bright green and are readily evident	Referral to ophthalmologist (can spread easily and become a corneal infection with resultant opacity and permanent scarring). Antibiotics are ineffective; steroids avoided. Idoxuridine (Herplex), specific for herpesvirus, is possibly effective in limiting corneal involvement.
Allergic conjunctivitis	Hypersensitivity to specific allergen; usually seasonal	Eyelid edema; profuse tearing and severe itching	Treatment of underlying allergy; cool, moist compresses
Keratitis	Inflammation and infection of the superficial layers of the cornea; may accompany or be a complication of conjunctivitis; may result when a foreign body strikes the cornea	Acute pain, tearing, photophobia (intolerance to light), and redness	Referral to ophthalmologist for therapy (infection could lead to corneal scarring, resulting in vision impairment [light rays unable to enter the eye normally]).
Periorbital cellulitis	Cellulitis (infection of subcutaneous tissue) most often caused by extension of a superficial infection after an open break in the skin, such as a mosquito bite or scratch near the eye	Swelling around and in the eye with possible damage to eye globe or optic nerve	Intravenous antibiotic therapy.
Dacryostenosis	Blockage of the nasolacrimal duct; primarily in newborns because of a membrane obscuring distal end of duct or plugging by epithelial debris	Painless lump in the inner canthus; tearing; usually unilateral	Gentle pressure to inner aspect of each eye at each feeding in attempt to "milk" secretions down into duct; ophthalmologic probing of gland duct if condition not corrected spontaneously after age 6 months.
Dacryocystitis	Inflammation of nasolacrimal duct; possibly secondary to dacryostenosis (from fluid stasis) or from nasal mucosal swelling and infected mucus being forced back into duct	Acute pain in inner canthus (from presence of infected sac); complaints of pain in back of eye or possibly in the eye itself	Local and systemic antibiotics; possible probing of duct to free obstruction and allow for free drainage; antihistamines for children with chronic allergies or sinusitis to reduce nasal congestion.

to a variety of organisms while passing through the birth canal (see Chapter 26). Although it is a controversial practice, in most hospitals, antibiotic ointment is placed in each newborn's eye after birth to prevent serious eye infections (USPSTF, 2012). Small children contract infections by rubbing their eyes with unclean hands. School-age children are exposed to many infectious agents from other children in school classrooms or by participating in sports activities. Regardless of how the infection was contracted, be certain parents have specific instructions about instilling eye drops or applying ointment, preventing the transmission of infection, applying compresses, and completing systemic antibiotic therapy. Having eye medication applied can be frightening for children, because they worry a health care provider's or a parent's hand will slip and cut their eye. If they have pain, they may be especially reluctant to let anyone touch their eye.

QSEN Checkpoint Question 50.2

Quality Improvement

Carla is diagnosed as having a bacterial conjunctivitis of her right eye and your unit has a standardized care plan and educational materials that address this common diagnosis. What instruction would you want to check in these clinical resources?

a. Keep the infected eye tightly closed by covering it with clean gauze.
b. Do not apply the eye drops for more than 3 days in order to prevent a rebound.
c. Clean the eye discharge away from the inner to the outer canthus.
d. Caution Carla not to blow her nose for the next 24 hours.

Look in Appendix A for the best answer and rationale.

TRAUMATIC INJURY TO THE EYE

Children account for 20% to 50% of ocular injury admissions to emergency rooms (Acar, Tok, Acar, et al., 2011). These injuries may be caused by a variety of situations, such as improper use of fireworks, sports injuries, dirt, pieces off toys, fighting with others, and even fingernail scratches (Shope, Rieg, & Kathiria, 2010).

Assessment

Children who have eye injuries are usually in acute pain immediately after the injury. Their eyes tear and are sensitive to light, and they blink rapidly. Vision may be blurred or lost in the affected eye. Because of the pain and the fear of not being able to see clearly, most children are very reluctant to let anyone examine or touch their injured eye. A few drops of a topical anesthetic instilled into the eye may be necessary to relieve the pain and allow the eye to be opened for examination. Even after the anesthetic is applied, the child needs a thorough explanation that an examiner is "just looking" (provided this is true). Even after an anesthetic application, a child may not be able to open the eye readily for inspection because the acute pain of the injury can cause either the eyelid to close by reflex spasm or eyelid edema to form so quickly that these interfere with the eye's ability to open. Do not confuse these physical problems with an unwillingness to open the eye.

To visualize the inner surface of the lower lid and the bottom half of the eye globe, press firmly on the lower lid with your fingertip until it turns out. The inner surface of the upper lid and the upper portion of the eye globe can best be visualized if the upper eyelid is everted. Ask the child to look downward. Grasp the eyelashes and gently stretch the upper eyelid downward. Place the stick of a cotton-tipped applicator horizontally against the center of the upper lid. While still grasping the eyelashes, pull the eyelid upward and over the applicator until it is everted (Fig. 50.6). Gently press the everted eyelid against the eyebrow to maintain the everted position. Be careful not to exert pressure on the eye globe during the procedure in case a penetrating injury from a foreign body is present to prevent further embedding the object into the eye globe.

A foreign body, such as a speck of dirt or a fragment of glass, often clings to the inside of the upper lid and can be readily removed by touching it with a moistened, sterile, cotton-tipped applicator while the lid is everted. Keep an eyelid everted no longer than is necessary while you remove the object because the eye globe begins drying as soon as it is exposed. Magnetic resonance imaging (MRI) and ultrasound are excellent methods for documenting internal eye damage or corneal scarring from an injury (Mohammadi, Zandian, Fakhraie, et al., 2012).

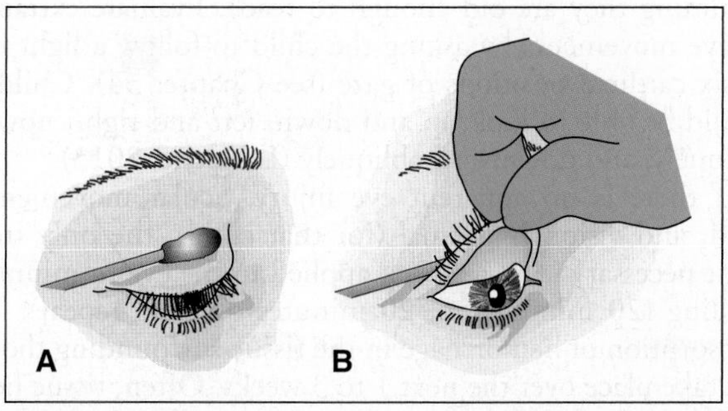

FIGURE 50.6 The technique for everting the upper eyelid for examination and foreign body removal. **(A)** Place a cotton applicator across the upper eyelid. **(B)** Pull the eyelid outward and upward over the applicator.

Nursing Diagnoses and Related Interventions

Nursing Diagnosis: Parental role conflict related to feelings of guilt about unintentional injury affecting child's vision

Outcome Evaluation: Parents accurately state child's treatment plan and expected outcome; child and parents talk openly about the injury and ways to prevent future injuries; parents participate actively in child's care and in decision making with health care providers regarding follow-up care.

Eye injuries are almost always serious in children because of the pain and the potential threat to vision. Both parents and children are apt to feel guilty that an injury occurred. Parents may have difficulty handling this emergency because they are angry at their child and even more angry at themselves for not supervising the child or teaching the child more about eye safety. Children may need help understanding that, although this injury might have been prevented, unintentional injuries do happen. Doing so can help them maintain a sense of self-esteem. Parents also may need counseling to reestablish their feelings of worth as parents (Box 50.4).

After eye trauma, the degree of vision in the child's affected eye as well as the status of the parent–child relationship needs to be evaluated because guilt about the injury, in either the parent or the child, can interfere with this relationship. After an eye injury, most children do not need future warnings about protecting their eyes, but it is still beneficial to reinforce eye safety measures with them.

Foreign Bodies

Foreign bodies such as sand or dirt that are loose on the conjunctiva can be removed by irrigation with a sterile normal saline solution or by gentle wiping with a well-moistened, sterile, cotton-tipped applicator after the eyelid is everted. After the removal, if the conjunctiva is touched with a strip of filter paper impregnated with fluorescein stain, any corneal ulceration or abrasion from the foreign body will stain green and be readily apparent. If the foreign body is easily removed and no corneal ulceration or injury is present, no further treatment is necessary. The child will blink a few times after the upper lid is returned to its place, but, in a matter of minutes, the child will report feeling "fine" again. If the

BOX 50.4 Nursing Care Planning Based on Effective Communication

Carla's older brother, Jon, a 7-year-old, is brought to the emergency department by his mother after his right eye was hit by a baseball.

Less Effective Communication

Nurse: Hello, Mrs. Vander. How did this injury happen?
Ms. Vander: He was playing catch with his cousin in the backyard.
Nurse: Is he hurt anywhere else?
Ms. Vander: No, but I didn't see exactly what happened. I should have been watching him more closely.
Nurse: Does he have pain?
Ms. Vander: Just a little. I shouldn't have left him out there with his cousin. What kind of a mother am I?
Nurse: Try and be calm. Your nurse practitioner will be in shortly to examine Jon.

More Effective Communication

Nurse: Hello, Mrs. Vander. How did this injury happen?
Ms. Vander: He was playing catch with his cousin in the backyard.
Nurse: Is he hurt anywhere else?
Ms. Vander: No. I should have been watching him more closely.
Nurse: Watching him more closely?
Ms. Vander: I should have been outside supervising them. What kind of a mother am I?
Nurse: Let's talk a little more about this.

In the first scenario, the nurse focuses on assessing the events surrounding the injury. Although this is important information, the nurse fails to identify the mother's feelings. In the second scenario, the nurse actively listens to the mother and so elicits information not just about the injury but also about her feelings.

fluorescein stain shows any corneal ulceration, refer the child to an ophthalmologist for follow-up care.

If a foreign body adheres to the cornea, it needs to be removed by an ophthalmologist, because, if the foreign body is metallic and has been in contact with the cornea for a period of hours, a rust ring can form around the particle. This rust ring must be removed as well as the object, or it will continue to act as a foreign body. After corneal injury, corneal tissue begins to regenerate. To aid this, the eye is washed with an antibiotic solution and then closed and patched. Assess that the patch is secure enough to keep the eyelid closed, yet does not put undue pressure on the eye. Caution the child that the patch must be left in place to prevent the delicate regenerating corneal epithelium from being rubbed off until it is well healed and secure once more.

If a foreign object is relatively large, such as a BB bullet, lollipop stick, or piece of broken glass, the fact that it has punctured the eye globe is usually apparent on first inspection. In these instances, the child also needs to be examined by an ophthalmologist. Surgery may be necessary to explore the depth of the puncture and to save the child's sight in that eye. Iron or copper fragments must be removed to prevent rust formation and continued irritation.

An extremely serious (although rare) complication called *sympathetic ophthalmia*, or inflammation of the opposite eye, may result if the uveal tract was involved in a penetrating injury. As a result, an autoimmune inflammatory response occurs in the noninjured eye, possibly leading to blindness in that eye. This complication can be prevented by the administration of a corticosteroid and antibiotics to reduce inflammation in the injured eye. If this is unsuccessful, removal (**enucleation**) of the injured eye may be necessary to prevent the other eye from being affected. If the vision in the injured eye appears to be destroyed, a decision for removal is not difficult for parents to make. If the vision is not totally destroyed, however, deciding to remove the injured eye is an extremely difficult decision for parents to be asked to make. Fortunately, immediate treatment with corticosteroids and antibiotics has significantly reduced the incidence of this complication; if these are prescribed, be certain parents understand the importance of giving the full course of these (Edelson, 2013).

Contusion Injuries

Many eye injuries happen not from a sharp object striking the eye but from blunt trauma such as being hit in the eye by a baseball, a fist, a soccer ball, or an automobile dashboard. With this type of injury, the eyelid and the surrounding tissue, including the intraorbital tissue, hemorrhages and becomes edematous (Scruggs, Scruggs, Stukenborg, et al., 2012).

The simplest form of contusion injury is a "black eye." When this occurs, inspect the eye globe (including a funduscopic examination) and assess vision in the eye. If a vision chart is not available, vision can be assessed by having children tell you how many fingers they can count at a distance of about 6 ft (assuming they are old enough to count accurately) or by having them read a printed page at reading distance (assuming they are old enough to read). Evaluate extraocular eye movements by asking the child to follow a light into all six cardinal positions of gaze (see Chapter 34). Children should be able to look up and down, left and right, upward obliquely, and downward obliquely (LaRoche, 2013).

If there is no apparent eye injury, ocular movement is good, and vision is normal (for that child), the only treatment necessary is an ice pack applied to the eye to minimize swelling (20 minutes on, 20 minutes off, and repeat). The reabsorption of hemorrhage in the tissue surrounding the eye will take place over the next 1 to 3 weeks. Often, tissue hemorrhage extends across the nose and surrounds the other eye the day after the injury. You can assure both the parents and the child that this is not a worsening of the condition, but rather mainly evidence of the severity of the initial blow.

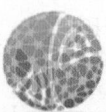

Limited eye movement or reports of diplopia (double vision) are strong evidence a "blowout" fracture of the floor of the orbit (the maxillary bone) has occurred, and the fracture line is trapping intraorbital tissue and preventing the eye globe from moving freely. Refer these children to an ophthalmologist because surgery is needed to free the entrapped tissue, prevent interference with vascular flow, and restore normal eye movements.

After a blunt contusion to the eye globe, if findings such as a dilated, fixed, or cloudy pupil; a cloudy lens or cornea; a loss of vision in the eye; or visible blood in the anterior chamber (hyphema) are present, these conditions indicate that dislocation of the lens or retinal detachment may have occurred. Again, immediate evaluation by an ophthalmologist is necessary.

Eyelid Injuries

Eyelid injuries may accompany eye globe injuries, or they may be the only finding present after a foreign body has struck the eye. Although such injuries appear to be trivial, don't dismiss them lightly. Refer the child to a primary care provider for care because a deep laceration of the eyelid can cause a permanent ptosis. A laceration to the inner canthal area can disrupt the lacrimal drainage system (dacryostenosis).

What if...50.1 You are asked to teach Carla Vander's first grade class on ways to prevent eye injuries. What suggestions would you include? How would your teaching plan be different if the class was for 16-year-old students?

INNER EYE CONDITIONS

Inner eye conditions are those that affect the lens, the retina, or the aqueous humor.

Cataracts

A *cataract* is marked opacity of the lens. This may be present at birth, or it may become apparent in early childhood. Some children have cataracts as a dominantly inherited condition, whereas in others, it may be as a result of another disease process such as galactosemia or scarring from an injury. A few children develop cataracts as a result of steroid use or radiation exposure. If the opacity occurs on the anterior surface of the lens, the cause is thought to be a birth injury or possibly contact between the lens and the cornea during intrauterine life. If the opacity is located at the edge of the lens, it may be a result of nutritional deficiency during intrauterine life, such as hypocalcemia. A quarter of infants born to women who were exposed to or contracted rubella may develop cataracts (Greener, 2011).

Assessment

When you inspect the pupil of a child with a cataract, the red reflex elicited by shining a light into the pupil appears white. Older children may report blurred vision because of cataract formation. In the infant, this can be detected by lack of response to a smile or an inability to reach and grasp a nearby object. The infant may also demonstrate nystagmus from being unable to focus the eye on objects. A few other conditions, such as retinoblastoma, retinopathy of prematurity, congenital glaucoma, or an abscess of the posterior chamber, simulate this appearance.

Therapeutic Management

Treatment of childhood cataract is the surgical removal of the cloudy lens, followed by insertion of an internal intraocular lens. If the total lens is involved, this may be done as early as 3 months of age. If this is not done before 6 years of age, amblyopia may result.

With modern surgical techniques, the incision is so small that eye patching is not necessary. Infants may be given a sedative to help them rest for 24 hours to keep them from rubbing their eyes. Introduce fluids cautiously after eye surgery so nausea and vomiting do not occur because vomiting increases intraocular pressure (IOP), which could injure the suture line. Encourage parents to stay with their infant and to help with care so the infant does not cry, because crying also increases IOP. Infants can be expected to have some discomfort but, in general, they should not have acute pain after surgery. If they are unusually restless, fussy, or cry as if in pain, report this. Although this could be unrelated to the surgery, it may be a sign of increased IOP from hemorrhage or from occlusion of the canal of Schlemm, causing a developing glaucoma.

As a rule, children will be given a mydriatic agent to dilate the pupil and steroids to prevent postoperative development of pupillary adhesions. If the eye that had the cataract is now amblyopic, patching the better eye (as with usual amblyopia correction) may be necessary to improve vision.

Parents of children with congenital cataracts need support to carry out the procedures necessary and to give the long-term medication and corrective measures needed. Outcome evaluations should include children's current vision status and also how they view themselves in light of this early vision problem (Lim, Rubab, Chan, et al., 2012).

QSEN Checkpoint Question 50.3

Safety

If Carla, the 6-year-old who has strabismus, has to have corrective eye surgery, why would the prevention of vomiting from anesthetic be a high priority?

a. Vomitus could be splashed into the eye.
b. Loss of sodium threatens the integrity of the new lens.
c. Vomiting increases IOP.
d. Loss of fluid causes the globe diameter to shrink.

Look in Appendix A for the best answer and rationale.

Congenital Glaucoma

Childhood glaucoma is a condition of the eye characterized by increased IOP, potential damage to the optic nerve, and possibility, vision loss (Yeung & Walton, 2012). Normally, aqueous humor, produced by the ciliary body, flows from the posterior chamber through the pupil to the anterior chamber; it is excreted through the canal of Schlemm at the lateral angle into the venous circulation (Fig. 50.7). In congenital glaucoma, a developmental anomaly in the angle of the

Blind children often want to be told what is on their food tray when it is first presented to them. Name the foods so they can identify tastes with names as well as the location of the foods on the plate. Do not hesitate to use food colors: "Those are green beans; this is an orange; those are red beets" as these words are names as well as colors. Visually challenged preschoolers enjoy the same finger foods as sighted children. Children with severe vision disorders have difficulty getting food from spoons or forks to their mouths neatly. However, they should not be spoon-fed just because it is neater and faster; eating is an important self-care skill a blind child must learn in order to be independent as an adult.

Be certain to offer frequent descriptions of what is happening or planned for children with visual impairments. They cannot see their surgical dressing, for example, so encourage them to feel it. They cannot see the intravenous infusion, but they can feel the tubing and the arm board that is holding their arm in place.

Parents of a severely visually challenged child usually plan to room-in with their child during a hospitalization experience. Review with the parents their routine at mealtime and bedtime, their child's favorite toy, what word is used for voiding, and so on, and post it conspicuously or pass this information on to the entire nursing staff. Only when parents have confidence in you and the other staff members will they be able to leave their child in your care to meet their own needs, such as going to a coffee shop for a meal.

STRUCTURE AND FUNCTION OF THE EARS

Ear anatomy is shown in Figure 50.8. Most diseases of the ear in children involve the external and middle portions.

The Physiology of Hearing Loss

Hearing loss is termed a *conduction loss* if there is interference with sound reaching the inner ear (difficulty with the external canal, the tympanic membrane, or the ossicles). It is termed *nerve* or *sensorineural loss* if the inner ear or the eighth cranial nerve is affected. Conduction loss occurs in children if the external canal is obstructed with cerumen (wax) or a foreign object, if the tympanic membrane is damaged or immobile, or if the middle ear is filled with fluid, as occurs in *serous otitis media*. Sensorineural loss results from diseases that affect the transmission of sound sensation to the cerebral cortex or because of a pathologic condition of the cochlea. In children, nerve damage is usually congenital, although it can occur after drug therapy, an infection such as meningitis or rubella, or exposure to loud sound (Hendry, Farley, & McLafferty, 2012).

Because diseases such as Treacher Collins syndrome, otosclerosis, osteogenesis imperfecta, and Waardenburg syndrome that lead to inherited hearing challenges tend to be autosomal dominant, there is a strong chance they will occur in future siblings of the hearing-challenged child. Genetic counseling can aid in increasing parental awareness of this possibility.

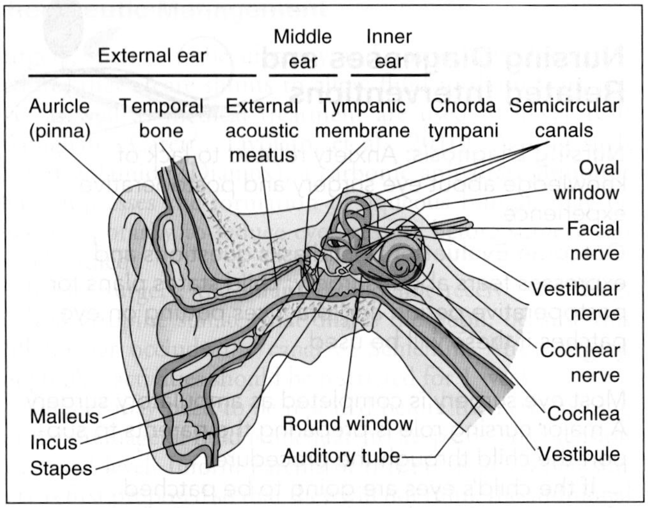

FIGURE 50.8 The structures of the ear.

Hearing Impairment

Approximately 12,000 infants, or 2 to 3 out of 1,000 children born in the United States are hard of hearing or deaf (National Institute on Deafness and Other Communication Disorders [NIDCD], 2012). Without newborn screening, these children may not be diagnosed with hearing loss until 2.5 to 3 years of age when development delays such as a lack of speech are identified (Shulman et al., 2010).

Hearing impairment occurs in many different degrees and is rated by level of severity (Table 50.3). Causes of slight

TABLE 50.3 Levels of Hearing Impairment

Decibel Level (dB)	Hearing Level Present
Slight (<30)	Unable to hear whispered words or faint speech No speech impairment present May not be aware of hearing difficulty Achieves well in school and home by compensating (such as leaning forward, speaking loudly)
Mild (30–50)	Beginning speech impairment may be present Difficulty hearing if not facing speaker; some difficulty with normal conversation
Moderate (55–70)	Speech impairment present; may require speech therapy Difficulty with normal conversation
Severe (70–90)	Difficulty with any sounds but nearby loud voice Hears vowels more easily than consonants Requires speech therapy for clear speech May still hear loud sounds, such as jets or train whistles
Profound (>90)	Hears almost no sound

hearing impairment include serous otitis media, trauma from such things as inflating automobile airbags, and untreated acute otitis media with rupture of the tympanic membrane.

The discovery that a child is hearing challenged is almost always a shock to parents because 9 out of 10 children born deaf are born to hearing parents (NIDCD, 2012). Children with hearing deficits should be exposed to language programs for hearing-impaired children as soon as possible so they have an optimum chance for language development and effective communication (Fig. 50.9).

For children who have conductive losses, an improvement in hearing usually can be achieved by use of a hearing aid (which intensifies the level of sound waves). Children who have inner ear or nerve deafness, however, cannot expect this kind of improvement. Parents of children with neural deafness need an explanation of the difference so they do not continue to search for a "cure" for their child or spend a great deal of money for hearing aids or alternative therapies, hoping a different brand, model, or technique will help their child.

Hearing Aids and Cochlear Implants

Hearing aids pick up sound through a microphone, convert the sound waves into electrical impulses, and amplify them across the tympanic membrane. They are powered by batteries that must be changed periodically.

Hearing aids are designed to be as inconspicuous as possible so children will not feel self-conscious wearing them. The receiver of the hearing aid may be incorporated into eyeglasses, molded into a plastic form that fits behind or into the ear, or housed in a small box (the size of a cell phone) that children wear on a cord around their neck or carry in a blouse or shirt pocket. Sound amplification systems are available to assist children in the classroom, such as personal frequency modulation systems in which the teacher wears a microphone that transmits directly to the child's hearing device (Wilson, Marinac, Pitty, et al., 2011). Teach children to remove hearing aids before washing their hair, showering, or swimming and to turn them off when removed to preserve the life of the batteries.

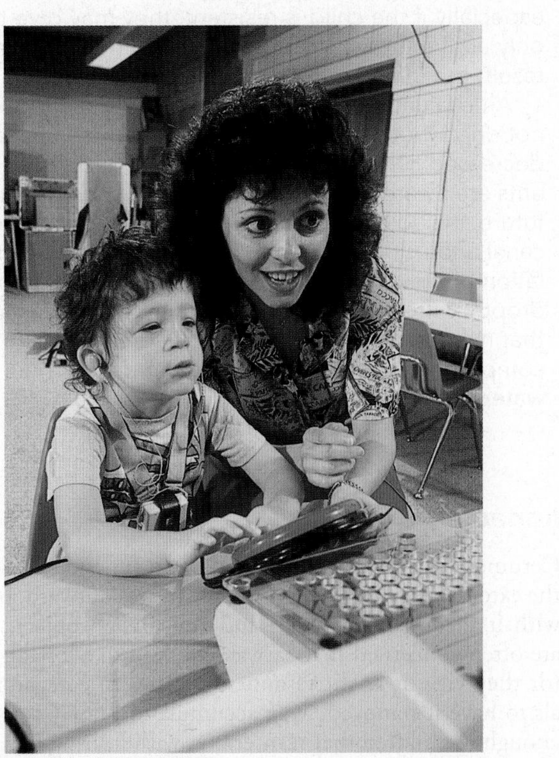

FIGURE 50.9 A hearing-challenged young girl learning to use the computer with the aid of a speech therapist. (© Bob Daemmrich/Stock Boston.)

Children with a hearing impairment may grow self-conscious about wearing a hearing aid at school and may be the victims of bullying. Encourage children to report bullying so it can be stopped. Be certain they value themselves as someone capable of overcoming great odds rather than as someone with a disability to hide.

Cochlear implants are mechanical devices consisting of a microphone, a speech processor, a transmitter/receiver, and an arrangement of electrodes that send impulses from the receiver directly to the auditory nerve. The auditory nerve then transmits the impulses to the brain where they are interpreted as words or common noises. The implant consists of an external portion that sits behind the ear and a second portion that is surgically implanted under the skin (Lenarz, Pau, & Paasche, 2012).

Approximately 28,400 children in the United States have received cochlear implants (NIDCD, 2012). These implants do not restore normal hearing, but do allow for sounds to be received. Many children report hearing as "muffled" or "under water" but adequate for communication. Months of training may be necessary to help a child interpret these distorted impulses correctly. Some hearing-challenged adults are reluctant to consent to a cochlear implant for their child because they believe the change from a hearing-challenged to a non–hearing-challenged status will remove their child from their deaf culture. Support parents with the choice they make regarding this; at the end of adolescence, children who have not received a cochlear implant can independently make the choice whether to have one. Children who spoke with an impediment before cochlear implantation usually need speech therapy afterward to improve their speech pattern because their pronunciation of words is so ingrained at that point.

Speech Therapy

If children who are hearing challenged are to interact as fully as possible with the world around them, they need an intensive program of speech therapy. Whether children should be introduced to sign language early is controversial; some therapists believe learning sign language early is helpful because it allows children to express their needs early, whereas others believe that, by learning sign language, children decrease their need to learn to articulate speech sounds or to lip read and, for those reasons, learning sign language should not be encouraged. It is true that, for real independence and to perform in regular school classes, children need to communicate by means other than sign language. For children with a profound impairment, however, learning speech sounds may be a long-term process, making sign language necessary for contact with the world around them until they can learn to speak.

What if... 50.3 You discover Carla, who is hearing challenged, refuses to wear her hearing aid because another child at her school made fun of it. What suggestions could you make to her parents to help her better accept wearing her hearing aid?

DISORDERS OF THE EAR

Ear disorders are always serious in children because hearing is such an important function for the growing child. Methods to assess hearing are discussed in Chapter 34.

External Otitis

External otitis (otitis externa) is inflammation of the external ear canal. Although external ear inflammation rarely threatens hearing or causes permanent damage, it does cause discomfort in the form of itching and sometimes extreme pain (CDC, 2011).

Assessment

The history of children with external otitis usually reveals that they have recently been swimming, which is why this condition is popularly called *swimmer's ear*. It also can occur if a young child pushes a foreign object, such as a peanut, into the ear canal. Unlike a middle ear infection (otitis media), there is no history of a recent respiratory infection. Children first notice itching of the canal, then pain. When the external ear is touched, the pain becomes acute. The moisture in the canal left from swimming or from decay of a food substance has caused inflammation, and a secondary infection then can occur in the closed space. *Pseudomonas* and *Candida* are agents frequently involved in these infections. On otoscopic examination, the pain may be found to be due to the sharply localized, tender swelling of a furuncle, or the entire canal may be swollen shut and tender to the touch. Fungal infections tend to turn the canal brown or black; although, if mold forms around a foreign body, such as the tip of a cotton applicator, it may appear white or gray. The skin under the object will be moist, red, and eroded.

If doing a first assessment on a child, be certain to visualize the tympanic membrane if possible to be certain it is intact and that it is not inflamed or to verify if the inflammation is about to extend into the middle ear. Before the tympanic membrane can be visualized clearly, it is often necessary to remove superficial debris from the canal. A Weber test (discussed in Chapter 34) should show that hearing is not decreased in the affected ear. If the sound of a tuning fork vibrates louder in the affected ear, it suggests otitis media is present.

Removing debris by an ear curette from an infected external canal requires both patience and skill. Children must lie still for the procedure to prevent them from suddenly turning their head and causing the curette to puncture the tympanic membrane and so they may need to be restrained. If the debris in the canal is hard and difficult to remove, it can be softened and loosened by touching it with a hydrogen peroxide–soaked cotton applicator or, alternatively, by dropping 2% acetic acid into the canal and allowing this to stand for a few minutes. Don't irrigate the external canal until it has been shown that the tympanic membrane is intact so that infected material is not washed through a rupture into the middle ear.

Therapeutic Management

The treatment of otitis externa differs according to the organism causing the infection. If the canal is so swollen that ear drops cannot flow back into the canal, a cotton wick moistened with Burow's solution may be threaded into the canal. The cotton extending out into the auricle is kept moistened by rewetting it periodically for the next 24 hours with Burow's solution. This usually reduces the swelling of the canal to a point where further cleaning can be accomplished.

Ear drops containing hydrocortisone, an antibiotic, or an antifungal mixture may be prescribed. Hydrocortisone reduces inflammation, and the antibiotic or antifungal preparation will reduce the infection. If ear pain is present, an analgesic, such as acetaminophen or ibuprofen, may be necessary to control discomfort. It is important that children keep the ear canal dry until the inflammation subsides, so they need to avoid swimming and washing their hair during this time. If they shower, they should first insert ear plugs into the external meatus or wear a shower cap to keep out moisture.

Nursing Diagnoses and Related Interventions

Nursing Diagnosis: Deficient knowledge related to technique for ear drop instillation or other care measures

Outcome Evaluation: Parents demonstrate proper instillation of ear drops; parents state the importance of continuing prescribed treatment to completion.

Administering ear drops can be a challenging task for parents because children invariably are reluctant to have any fluid dripped into their ear. Demonstrate to parents how this is done (see Chapter 38) before they leave the health care facility. Caution them to give the medication for the full period prescribed. Otherwise, especially if the child is resistant, they may give them only until the pain subsides (24 to 48 hours). As a result, the infection may recur in another week.

An evaluation after external otitis should include not only whether the inflammation and pain have decreased but also whether the child and the parents are aware of how to prevent the condition in the future, including not putting any object into the ear canal and using ear plugs during swimming. Instillation of a dilute alcohol or acetic acid solution by dropper after swimming is a prophylactic measure that may be recommended for children who swim competitively or who spend a great deal of time in water to help keep the ear canal dry.

Impacted Cerumen

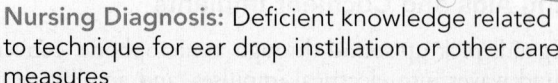

Cerumen (earwax) serves the important function of cleansing the external ear canal as it gradually moves outward, bringing with it shed epithelial cells and any foreign object. Parents are often concerned that earwax will lead to a loss of hearing (or they view it as dirty) and so ask health care professionals to have it removed. Wax accumulation rarely is extensive enough in children that it interferes with hearing and removing it can diminish its protective function, so it should not be removed routinely. Using cotton-tipped applicators to clean ears as a regular practice can also scratch an ear canal, causing an invasion site for a secondary infection. This practice may also push accumulated cerumen farther into the ear canal, causing a true plugging of wax.

Commercial softeners are available if cerumen accumulates to such an extent that hearing is affected. In some instances, a dilute solution of hydrogen peroxide may be necessary to dissolve cerumen. Again, this should not be done regularly because this will keep the ear canal constantly moist, an environment that leads to external otitis. For most children, the basic rule—never put anything smaller than an elbow in a child's ear—is the best rule.

QSEN Checkpoint Question 50.5

Evidence-Based Practice

A concern about the many mobile electronic devices available today is that increased noise exposure will cause neurologic hearing injury. To investigate if hearing loss was present in teenagers who typically listened to music through earplugs, researchers tested the hearing of 381 first-year university students and then asked them to self-report their history of music exposure. The results of the study showed those students with a high level of recreational noise exposure had lower hearing thresholds than those students with less recreational noise exposure (Tung & Chao, 2013).

Based on the previous study, which action by Carla's teenage brother would give you the most concern?

a. He listens to music on his computer while he does his homework.
b. He typically listens to sports news on the radio while he eats.
c. He plays varsity basketball in a noisy gymnasium once a week.
d. He listens to music with earbuds when he rides the bus and subway.

Look in Appendix A for the best answer and rationale.

Acute Otitis Media

Inflammation of the middle ear (otitis media) is one of the most prevalent diseases of childhood (Yoon, Kelley, & Friedman, 2012). It occurs most often in children 6 to 36 months of age and again at 4 to 6 years. Children most susceptible to it are males, Alaskan and Native American children, those with cleft palate, and infants who are formula-fed rather than breastfed. Formula-feeding leads to this because infants are held in a more slanted position while feeding, allowing milk to enter the eustachian tube. The incidence of otitis media is highest in the winter and spring because it frequently follows an upper respiratory infection and is higher in homes in which a parent smokes cigarettes (Jones, Hassanien, Cook, et al., 2012). Although it occurs frequently, otitis media is a potentially serious disease of childhood because permanent damage can occur to middle ear structures, leading to permanent hearing impairment.

Assessment

Acute otitis media usually occurs following a respiratory tract infection. Children have a "cold," rhinitis, and perhaps a low-grade fever for several days. Suddenly, their fever peaks to about 102°F (38°C) and sharp, constant pain begins in one or both ears. Older children can verbalize they have pain and point to where the pain is felt. Infants, unable to do this, become extremely irritable and frequently pull or tug at the affected ear in an attempt to gain relief from pain. On examination, the external canal is usually free of wax because the warmth of the inflammation and fever melts the wax and moves it more readily out of the canal. In contrast to an external ear canal infection, the discomfort they feel does not increase on manipulation of the auricle. Palpate the mastoid process behind the ear to be certain it doesn't feel tender to your touch. If it does, the infection probably has spread out of the middle ear into the mastoid cells, a very serious complication because it could spread from there to become meningitis.

The appearance of a normal eardrum shows the outline of the malleus (see Chapter 34). With an infection, the tympanic membrane appears inflamed or reddened. It may bulge forward into the external canal because of fluid and edema behind it. The landmarks of the tympanic membrane, the malleus and incus, can be visualized only poorly or not at all. The light reflex of the otoscope will not be as definite as usual because of the "pushed out" or convex shape of the eardrum. There is decreased mobility on a pneumatic examination. If a culture seems necessary, a **tympanocentesis** (withdrawal of fluid from the middle ear through the tympanic membrane) can be performed to obtain fluid for culture.

Therapeutic Management

Most middle ear infections are caused by *Streptococcus pneumoniae*, *Haemophilus influenzae* (especially in children younger than 5 years of age), or *Streptococcus pyrogenes*. Most otitis media infections resolve spontaneously, however, so antibiotic therapy is currently not recommended. Children who have a systemic infection or an individual difference in recovery time, however, may still have an antibiotic prescribed (Klein, 2011; Thornton, Parrish, & Swords, 2011).

Children need an analgesic and antipyretic such as acetaminophen (Tylenol). Decongestant nose drops to open the eustachian tubes and allow air to be admitted to the middle ear may also be helpful. These are given for only 2 to 3 days because, if they are given longer, a rebound effect can occur, causing edema and a subsequent increase in mucous membrane inflammation. Providing a smoke-free home environment can help prevent further episodes of otitis media (Herbert, Gagnon, Rennick, et al., 2011).

During the course of otitis media, most children experience a conductive hearing loss; this may last as long as 6 months after the acute infection. Caution parents about this so they will not think the infection is growing worse if they first notice the impairment after they arrive home from the health care facility. They also need to know about the possible hearing loss so that, if the child is routinely screened for hearing in school during the next 6 months, they can account for the hearing loss. If a child still has a conductive hearing loss after 6 months (or has other symptoms), the child should be examined again to see whether a new infection or serous otitis media has developed. Box 50.5 shows an interprofessional care map illustrating both nursing and team planning for a child with otitis media.

Otitis Media With Effusion

Otitis media with effusion occurs when otitis media becomes chronic. Normally, the middle ear is an air-filled cavity; air is supplied to it each time the eustachian tube opens with swallowing, yawning, or chewing. If this source of air to the

BOX 50.5 Nursing Care Planning

AN INTERPROFESSIONAL CARE MAP FOR A CHILD WITH OTITIS MEDIA

Carla Vander, a 6-year-old, is brought to your pediatric clinic for evaluation. Her mother states, "She was born with a hearing loss and a cataract. Today, her eye is red and she has pain in her ear. Can you see her quickly so I can get an antibiotic for the ear infection before the drugstore closes?"

Family Assessment Child lives with parents and two brothers, 7 and 14 years old, in three-bedroom suburban cottage. Father works as a travel agent; mother is a grade school librarian. Father describes finances as "middle class."

Client Assessment Child has had two previous ear infections in the past 8 months. Child had a clear, watery nasal discharge and slight cough for 2 days. Today has thick, purulent, nasal drainage. Temperature this morning was 102.2°F (39.0°C). Observed tugging vigorously on right ear.

On examination, right tympanic membrane is erythematous and bulging, with poor mobility on pneumoscopy. Left ear examination unremarkable. Child is diagnosed with otitis media of the right ear.

Nursing Diagnosis Pain related to inflammation and erythema secondary to ear infection

Outcome Evaluation Child no longer tugs at right ear; tympanic membrane no longer reddened or bulging; child rates pain as no higher than 2 on a FACES pain scale.

Team Member Responsible	Assessment	Intervention	Rationale	Expected Outcome
Activities of Daily Living, Including Safety				
Nurse	Assess whether child is able to sleep or wakes with pain.	Suggest mother give prescribed antihistamine at bedtime. Urge child to sleep with affected ear up.	Antihistamines can make children sleepy. Sleeping on affected ear can put pressure on eustachian tube, which can increase pain.	Mother reports child is able to sleep through the night.
Teamwork and Collaboration				
Nurse/Primary care provider	Assess whether child has susceptibility to ear infections or whether this could be reoccurrence of a former infection.	Meet with ear, nose, and throat service to consult on cause of frequent otitis media.	Otitis media is painful so can affect quality of life.	Consultant meets with mother to discuss cause of frequent ear infections.
Procedures/Medications for Quality Improvement				
Nurse	Assess whether child has experience with taking oral medicine; rate child's level of pain by FACES pain scale.	Instruct the mother to administer acetaminophen every 4 hours or ibuprofen every 8 hours, and how to instill saline nose drops.	Acetaminophen and ibuprofen are effective analgesics and antipyretics for this degree of pain; nose drops relieve nasal inflammation.	Child is able to take oral medicine cooperatively; rates pain level as not above 2 on FACES pain scale.
Nutrition				
Nurse	Assess what soft foods and fluids child likes to eat.	Encourage mother to offer liquids and soft foods.	Movement of the eustachian tube, such as with chewing, may increase pain.	Child names some foods and fluid she is willing to eat; eats less than usual, but adequate amount.

Patient-Centered Care				
Nurse	Assess how much mother and child understand about the cause of otitis media and the newer, no-antibiotic approach to treatment.	Educate the mother about the common characteristics of otitis media; reassure mother the infection will resolve without an antibiotic.	Education promotes better understanding of the problem, alleviating some of the stress and anxiety associated with it.	Mother states her prime goal is to get child well again; will follow primary care provider's recommendation for care.
Psychosocial/Spiritual/Emotional Needs				
Nurse	Assess how much experience mother has with care of an ill child.	Teach mother that otitis media usually resolves without the need for an antibiotic.	Correct information helps mother accept a lack of antibiotic prescription.	Mother states she feels capable of caring for child without antibiotic prescription.
Informatics for Seamless Health Care Planning				
Nurse	Assess whether child or parents have any questions about care that they still need answered.	Instruct the mother to contact the clinic or health care provider if there is no improvement within 24 to 48 hours or if the child exhibits increased pain.	Lack of improvement within 24 to 48 hours indicates the need for further evaluation; increased pain may indicate excessive fluid accumulation, which could lead to tympanic rupture.	Mother has clinic telephone number; will telephone if symptoms of complications occur.

middle ear is closed off due to inflammation or edema of the eustachian tube, the epithelial cells of the middle ear begin to secrete a thin, watery mucus. Over time, the compartment becomes so filled with this and the fluid becomes so thick and tenacious that it appears gluelike. Some children notice a feeling of fullness or the sound of popping or ringing in their ears. There may be a drop in hearing of 20 to 40 dB because of the inability of the ossicles to function effectively. Involvement is usually bilateral. The condition occurs most frequently in children 3 to 10 years of age (Murakami, Tutumi, & Watanabe, 2012).

Assessment

With otitis media with effusion, a child experiences muffled hearing and a feeling of pressure in the ear. Otoscopic examination may show a level of fluid behind the tympanic membrane. However, a fluid line will be visible only if there is also a quantity of air in the middle ear to contrast with it. As the collected fluid becomes thick, it tends to retract the eardrum. This makes the malleus more prominent and perhaps displaced to a horizontal angle as the membrane is retracted around it; the light reflex from the otoscope light becomes distorted. If a pneumatic otoscope is used, gentle introduction of air against the eardrum produces no movement of the tympanic membrane (as there would be normally).

Therapeutic Management

Therapy for otitis media with effusion may be long term. If the condition appears to be intensified by inflammation from an allergy, measures to control the allergy must be initiated. These may include avoidance of the allergen, hyposensitization, or pharmacologic alteration of the allergic response (see Chapter 42).

Definitive medical treatment is aimed at supplying air to the middle ear. For mild involvement, the daily administration of an antihistamine or a nasal decongestant to shrink the mucous membrane of the eustachian tube may be enough to achieve an air supply. In a few children, the eustachian tube is blocked by enlarged adenoids, and their removal is indicated. Fluid from the middle ear can be removed by tympanocentesis (a needle inserted through the tympanic membrane); however, the fluid usually returns unless some intervention to introduce air into the middle ear (tubal myringotomy) is undertaken.

Tubal Myringotomy. A source of air can be supplied to the middle ear by the insertion of small plastic (Teflon) tubes inserted through the tympanic membrane (tympanostomy). The insertion of such tubes is done by a myringotomy at a point in the tympanic membrane that is not instrumental for hearing, so the tube does not interfere with hearing (Fig. 50.10). Myringotomy tubes can be placed in one or both ears as an ambulatory procedure after the local injection of lidocaine (Xylocaine). Tubes tend to be extruded after 6 to 12 months. For most children, this period is long enough to halt the secretory process of the middle ear. In others, tubes must be reinserted to continue the aeration.

When myringotomy tubes are in place, the child has to be careful to not allow water to enter the ears. It's better if they bathe rather than shower, but showering is all right if ear plugs are used, especially while washing hair. Similarly, swimming is either contraindicated or allowed only with ear plugs in place.

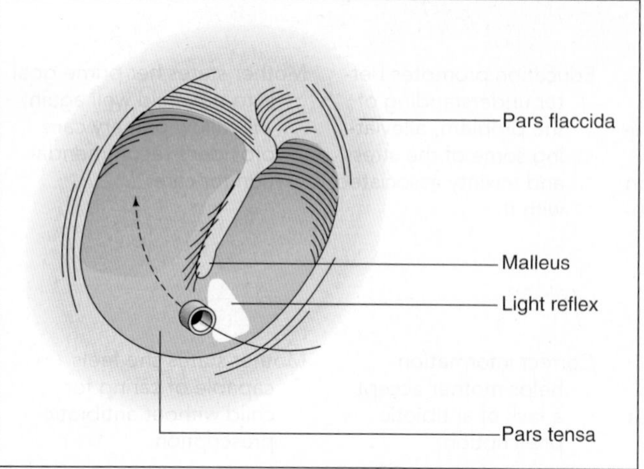

FIGURE 50.10 A myringotomy tube provides air to the middle ear to prevent otitis media with effusion.

Because the course of the process is long term, the hearing impairment associated with the condition may also be long term. Urge parents to notify the school nurse that their child has reduced hearing because of the middle ear fluid and has myringotomy tubes in place. Children may need to be changed to a front seat in a classroom so they do not miss important class content or discussion until the condition improves.

QSEN Checkpoint Question 50.6

Informatics

Carla is diagnosed as having otitis media. When interpreting the documentation in Carla's electronic health record, you should be cognizant that this diagnosis differs from otitis externa in what way?

a. Otitis media occurs from swimming; otitis externa typically follows a common cold.
b. Otitis media involves the middle ear; otitis externa involves the outer canal.
c. Otitis media involves the eardrum; otitis externa involves the cochlear nerve.
d. Otitis media does not cause pain; otitis externa produces throbbing pain.

Look in Appendix A for the best answer and rationale.

Cholesteatoma

Cholesteatoma is a lesion of the pars flaccida, or the upper portion of the tympanic membrane. A retraction cyst forms, and there is necrosis of the pars flaccida with foul-smelling drainage from the external canal. If the retraction cyst is not discovered and surgically removed at this point, it grows gradually deeper and deeper until it eventually invades the mastoid cells. It can progress to mastoiditis, meningitis, and possibly facial nerve paralysis if it is not surgically removed. Any child with foul-smelling drainage from the ear, therefore, should be referred to a primary care provider for further investigation to rule out this problem (Kuo, Shiao, Liao, et al., 2012).

THE HOSPITALIZED CHILD WITH A HEARING IMPAIRMENT

Conversation is usually held between 50 and 60 dB so a hearing loss greater than 49 dB is sufficient enough to interfere with hearing conversation and developing language. Like those who are visually challenged, children with hearing loss may be hospitalized as a direct consequence of their ear disorder or from other health problems. It can be difficult for parents to prepare children who cannot hear for hospitalization because words such as "surgery," "tonsils," "hurts," "operating room," and "recovery room" are new to them. Showing the child a book with pictures demonstrating what is going to happen is helpful. Allowing children time to play with dolls or puppets can help them understand hospital routine. Because children who are hearing challenged may not be as well prepared for hospitalization as those without a hearing impairment, make an extra effort on admission to ensure they receive such instruction.

Always allow hearing-challenged children to see you before you touch them because they will not find this nearly as intrusive as being touched without warning. If children are sleeping when you approach them, use a light touch to waken them gently. Some children turn off their hearing aid or remove it while they sleep. You may need to turn it on before you call them to wake them, or they may need to replace the hearing aid as soon as they awaken. Children as young as 2 years of age are effective lip readers as long as you are facing them. Position yourself at eye level, so the child can view your face. In a group, help the child follow conversation by directing the child to the person who is speaking. Assign consistent staff members to decrease the number of people with whom the child must attempt to communicate. Have a staff person accompany the child and stay with the child in all departments to help with communication.

Do not underestimate the intelligence level of hearing-challenged children. Because they do not speak clearly, others may assume hearing-challenged children are cognitively challenged. As a result, they may not be given information that the average hearing child receives, such as explanations of how things work. On a hospital unit, hearing-challenged children, locked in a silent world, are unable to express how they feel about procedures. They need help from health care personnel who understand this and take more than the usual amount of time to offer them explanations and support.

Ask parents of children who are hearing challenged to draw pictures or demonstrate the sign language symbols their children use for important words such as "pain," "drink," and "bathroom." Encourage children to use or draw pictures of what they want if they are still too young to write words and if you cannot understand what they are saying.

Hearing-challenged children have the right to be provided with a sign language interpreter during care. Advocate for this, especially if the parents will not be continually present.

What if . . . 50.4 You are particularly interested in exploring one of the 2020 National Health Goals with respect to vision and hearing disorders in children (see Box 50.1). What would be a possible research topic to explore pertinent to this goal that would be applicable to Carla's family and that would also advance evidence-based practice?

Key Points for Review

- Teaching preventive measures to avoid eye and hearing injuries (using proper eye protection during sports or play and wearing goggles or ear protection as appropriate) and screening children for sensory impairments are important nursing roles.
- Refractive errors of vision such as myopia and hyperopia are the most common eye disorders in children. Amblyopia is subnormal vision in one eye. Children with these disorders need correction at the time the disorder is recognized to prevent further vision distortion.
- Coloboma is congenital and involves the incomplete closure of the pupil or lower eyelid. Ptosis is the inability to open the upper eyelid normally. Ptosis needs correction to avoid the development of amblyopia. Strabismus is unequally aligned eyes. Like ptosis, it can lead to amblyopia if not corrected.
- Infections of the lids, such as styes or chalazia, can occur in children. Conjunctivitis (inflammation of the conjunctiva) often manifests with acute symptoms. An antibiotic is necessary for therapy.
- Eye injuries such as penetration by a foreign body need a follow-up after treatment to be certain vision remains adequate.
- Children who are either vision or hearing challenged need special preparation and orientation for a hospital or ambulatory health visit that not only meets QSEN competencies but that also best meets a family's total needs.
- Help children who are vision challenged to work through new experiences by letting them feel equipment as much as possible. Guide their hands through the steps of a new procedure you are teaching them.
- Otitis media (a middle ear infection) is a common childhood illness. Some children who have otitis media with effusion have myringotomy tubes inserted to relieve pressure and to supply air access to the middle ear.
- Use photographs, drawings, or demonstrations with hearing-challenged children to help them learn new skills. Contact a sign language interpreter as appropriate to be certain that children understand instructions.

Critical Thinking Care Study

Hannah, 11 years old, wears glasses because of a severe refractive difference in her eyes. She has had a severe hearing impairment since birth and so wears a hearing aid. She is admitted to your hospital unit for dehydration secondary to influenza. Her father tells you Hannah is proficient in American Sign Language and can also read lips fairly well.

1. What special precautions do you need to take to ensure Hannah is safe in the hospital environment?
2. Hannah's parents are separated; she spends 1 week a month with her mother and the other 3 weeks with her father. Her father worries she doesn't wear her glasses during the week she's with her mother. Her mother tells you she doesn't wear them when she's with her father. What suggestions could you make to remind her to wear the glasses?
3. You notice Hannah doesn't like the taste of the oral rehydrating solution, which she needs to drink to restore her fluid volume. When you check to see if she drank all of it, even though you know you faced her squarely and spoke loudly, she says she didn't hear you tell her to drink it. What would be a better way to communicate with Hannah?

Patient Scenario

The Coach Family

Read about he Coach family, a family with a child experiencing a vision disorder, then answer the questions to further sharpen your skills and grow more familiar with NCLEX-type questions related to vision or hearing disorders. Confirm your answers are correct by reading the rationales.

Visit http://thePoint.lww.com

Answers and Rationales

Looking for answers to the What if . . . and Critical Thinking Care Study questions?

Visit http://thePoint.lww.com

References

Acar, U., Tok, O., Acar, D., et al. (2011). A new ocular trauma score in pediatric penetrating eye injuries. *Eye, 25*(3), 370–374.

Alió, J. L., Wolter, N. V., Piñero, D. P., et al. (2010). Pediatric refractive surgery and its role in the treatment of amblyopia: Meta-analysis of the peer-reviewed literature. *Journal of Refractive Surgery,* 27(5), 364–374.

Babighain, S., Caretti, L., Tavolato, M., et al. (2010). Examiner laser trabeculotomy vs 180 degrees selective laser trabeculoplasty in primary open-angle glaucoma. *Eye, 24*(4), 632–638.

Belden, J., DeFriez, C., & Huether, S. E. (2013). The special senses. In S. E. Huether & K. L. McCance (Eds.), *Understanding pathophysiology* (5th ed., pp. 335–339). New York, NY: Elsevier Publishing.

Birch, J. (2012). Worldwide prevalence of red-green color deficiency. *Journal of the Optical Society of America, 29*(3), 313–320.

Braverman, R. S. (2012). The eye. In W. W. Hay, M. J. Levine, J. M. Sondheimer, et al. (Eds.), *Current pediatric diagnosis & treatment* (20th ed., pp. 401–441). Columbus, OH: McGraw-Hill.

Centers for Disease Control and Prevention. (2011). Estimated burden of acute otitis externa—United States. *MMWR: Morbidity & Mortality Weekly Report, 60*(19), 605–609.

Centers for Disease Control and Prevention. (2012). *Newborn screening.* Atlanta, GA: Author.

Chou, R., Dana, T., & Bougatsos, C. (2011). Screening for visual impairment in children ages 1–5 years. *Pediatrics, 127*(2), e442–e479.

Dudek, S. (2010). Nutrition for infants, children and adolescents. In S. Dudek (Ed.), *Nutrition essentials for nursing practice* (6th ed., pp. 272–296). Philadelphia, PA: Lippincott Williams & Wilkins.

Edelson, O. (2013). Uveitis. In C. S. Hoyt & D. Taylor (Eds.), *Pediatric ophthalmology & strabismus* (pp. 377–392). Philadelphia, PA: Elsevier/Saunders.

Greener, M. (2011). The tragedy of congenital abnormalities. *Nurse Prescribing, 9*(3), 117–121.

Hendry, C., Farley, A., & McLafferty, E. (2012). Anatomy and physiology of the senses. *Nursing Standard, 27*(5), 35–42.

Herbert, R. J., Gagnon, A. J., Rennick, J. E., et al. (2011). 'Do it for the kids': Barriers and facilitators to smoke-free homes and vehicles. *Pediatric Nursing, 37*(2), 33–37.

Holmes, J., Lazar, E., Melia, M., et al. (2011). Effect of age on response to amblyopia treatment in children. *Archives of Ophthalmology, 129*(11), 1451–1457.

Ivarsen, A., Næser, K., & Hjortdal, J. (2013). Laser in situ keratomileusis for high astigmatism in myopic and hyperopic eyes. *Journal of Cataract & Refractive Surgery, 39*(1), 74–80.

Jones, L. L., Hassanien, A., Cook, D. G., et al. (2012). Parental smoking and the risk of middle ear disease in children: A systematic review and meta-analysis. *Archives of Pediatric & Adolescence Medicine, 166*(1), 18–27.

Klein, J. (2011). Is acute otitis media a treatable disease? *The New England Journal of Medicine, 364*(2), 168–169.

Kuo, C. L., Shiao, A. S., Liao, W. H., et al. (2012). How long is long enough to follow up children after cholesteatoma surgery? A 29-year study. *Laryngoscope, 122*(11), 2568–2573.

LaRoche, G. R. (2013). Examination, history and special tests in pediatric ophthalmology. In C. S. Hoyt & D. Taylor (Eds.), *Pediatric ophthalmology & strabismus* (pp. 45–54). Philadelphia, PA: Elsevier/Saunders.

Lenarz, T., Pau, H. W., & Paasche, G. (2012). Cochlear implants. *Current Pharmacology & Biotechnology.* Advance online publication.

Lewis, D. W. (2011). Neurology. In K. J. Marcdante, R. M. Kliegman, H. B. Jenson, et al. (Eds.), *Nelson essentials of pediatrics* (6th ed., pp. 671–712). Philadelphia, PA: Saunders/Elsevier.

Lim, Z., Rubab, S., Chan, Y. H., et al. (2012). Management and outcomes of cataract in children: The Toronto experience. *JAAPOS: Journal of the American Association of Pediatric Ophthalmology & Strabismus, 16*(3), 249–254.

Mohammadi, S. F., Zandian, M., Fakhraie, G., et al. (2012). Ultrasound biomicroscopy findings in fireworks-related blunt eye injuries. *European Journal of Ophthalmology, 22*(3), 342–348.

Murakami, A., Tutumi, T., & Watanabe, K. (2012). Middle ear effusion and fungi. *Annals of Otology, Rhinology & Laryngology, 121*(9), 609–614.

National Dissemination Center for Children with Disabilities. (2012). *Categories of disabilities.* Washington, DC: Author.

National Institute on Deafness and Other Communication Disorders. (2012). *Statistics about hearing disorders, ear infections, and deafness.* Hyattsville, MD: National Center for Health Statistics.

Ou, Y., & Caprioli, J. (2012). Surgical management of pediatric glaucoma. *Developmental Ophthalmology, 50*(4), 157–172.

Papadopoulos, M., Brookes, J. L., & Khaw, P. T. (2013). Pediatric glaucoma. In C. S. Hoyt & D. Taylor (Eds.), *Pediatric ophthalmology & strabismus* (pp. 353–367). Philadelphia, PA: Elsevier/Saunders.

Paysse, E. A., Tychsen, L., & Stahl, E. (2012). Pediatric refractive surgery: Corneal and intraocular techniques and beyond. *Journal of the American Association of Pediatric Ophthalmology & Strabismus, 16*(3), 291–297.

Pi, L., Chen, L., Liu, Q., et al. (2010). Refractive status and prevalence of refractive errors in suburban school-aged children. *International Journal of Medical Sciences, 7*(6), 342–353.

Rahi, J. S., & Gilbert, C. E. (2012). Epidemiology and the world wide impact of visual impairment in children. In C. S. Hoyt & D. Taylor (Eds.), *Pediatric ophthalmology & strabismus* (pp. 1–9). Philadelphia, PA: Elsevier/Saunders.

Roefs, A. M., Tjiam, A. M., Looman, C. W., et al. (2012). Comfort of wear and material properties of eye patches for amblyopia treatment and the influence on compliance. *Strabismus, 20*(1), 3–10.

Rowe, F., & Noonan, C. (2012). Botulinum toxin for the treatment of strabismus. *Cochrane Database of Systematic Reviews,* (2), CD006499.

Scruggs, D., Scruggs, R., Stukenborg, G., et al. (2012). Ocular injuries in trauma patients. *Journal of Trauma & Acute Care Surgery, 73*(5), 1308–1312.

Shope, T. R., Rieg, T. S., & Kathiria, N. N. (2010). Corneal abrasions in young infants. *Pediatrics, 125*(3), e565–e569.

Shulman, S., Besculides, M., Saltzman, A., et al. (2010). Evaluation of the universal newborn hearing and screening and intervention program. *Pediatrics, 126*(1), S19–S27.

Taylor, K., Powell, C., Hatt, S., et al. (2012). Interventions for unilateral and bilateral refractive amblyopia. *Cochrane Database of Systematic Reviews,* (4), CD005137.

Thornton, K., Parrish, F., & Swords, C. (2011). Topical vs. systemic treatments for acute otitis media. *Pediatric Nursing, 37*(5), 263–267.

Tung, C. Y., & Chao, K. P. (2013). Effect of recreational noise exposure on hearing impairment among teenage students. *Research in Developmental Disabilities, 34*(1), 126–132.

U.S. Department of Health and Human Services. (2010). *Healthy people 2020.* Washington, DC: Author.

U.S. Preventive Services Task Force. (2011). Recommendation statement: Vision screening for children 1 to 5 years of age. *Pediatrics, 127*(2), 340–346.

U.S. Preventive Services Task Force. (2012). Ocular prophylaxis for gonococcal ophthalmia neonatorum: Reaffirmation recommendation statement. *American Family Physician, 85*(2), 195–196.

Wilson, W. J., Marinac, J., Pitty, K., et al. (2011). The use of sound-field amplification devices in different types of classrooms. *Language, Speech & Hearing Services in Schools, 42*(4), 395–407.

Wong, A. M. (2012). New concepts concerning the neural mechanisms of amblyopia and their clinical implications. *Canadian Journal of Ophthalmology, 47*(5), 399–409.

Yang, X., Luo, D., Liao, M., et al. (2012). Efficacy and tolerance of levodopa to treat amblyopia: A systematic review and meta-analysis. *European Journal of Ophthalmology.* Advance online publication.

Yeung, H., & Walton, D. (2012). Recognizing childhood glaucoma in the primary pediatric setting. *Contemporary Pediatrics, 29*(5), 32–40.

Yoon, P. J., Kelley, P. E., & Friedman, N. R. (2012). Ear, nose & throat. In W. Hay, M. Levin, R. Deterding, et al. (Eds.), *Current diagnosis & treatment pediatrics* (21st ed., pp. 452–486). New York, NY: McGraw-Hill/Lange.

Young, M. P., Heidary, G., & Vanderveen, D. K. (2012). Relationship between the timing of cataract surgery and development of nystagmus in patients with bilateral infantile cataracts. *JAAPOS: Journal of the American Association of Pediatric Ophthalmology & Strabismus, 16*(6), 554–557.

Chapter 51

Nursing Care of a Family When a Child Has a Musculoskeletal Disorder

KEY TERMS

- apposition
- arthroscopy
- cartilage
- compartment syndrome
- diaphysis
- distraction
- epiphyseal plate
- epiphysis
- fracture
- malleoli
- metaphysis
- myopathy
- periosteum
- remodeling
- resorption
- sequestrum
- traction

OBJECTIVES

After mastering the contents of this chapter, you should be able to:

1. Describe common musculoskeletal disorders in children.
2. Identify 2020 National Health Goals related to musculoskeletal disorders in children that nurses can help the nation achieve.
3. Assess a child with a musculoskeletal disorder.
4. Formulate nursing diagnoses related to a child with a musculoskeletal disorder.
5. Establish expected outcomes for a child with a musculoskeletal disorder that help children and parents manage seamless transitions across differing health care settings.
6. Using the nursing process, plan nursing care that includes the six competencies of Quality & Safety Education for Nurses (QSEN): Patient-Centered Care, Teamwork & Collaboration, Evidence-Based Practice (EBP), Quality Improvement (QI), Safety, and Informatics.
7. Implement nursing care, such as helping a child with a musculoskeletal disorder meet optimal ambulation capacity.
8. Evaluate expected outcomes for achievement and effectiveness of care.
9. Integrate knowledge of children's musculoskeletal disorders with the interplay of nursing process, the six competencies of QSEN, and Family Nursing to promote quality maternal and child health nursing care.

Jeffrey, a 13-year-old boy, accompanies his mother and 3-year-old sister into the hospital emergency room because his sister has pain in her arm after a fall. As you talk to Jeffrey, you notice his left lower leg is swollen, warm to the touch, and painful. When he takes off his shirt, you notice his spine is not straight. His mother tells you she noticed an infected mosquito bite on his leg 2 weeks ago. After further evaluation, Jeffrey's sister is diagnosed with a fracture of her ulna; Jeffrey is diagnosed with osteomyelitis. His mother asks you, "I know our family is prone to orthopedic problems, but how could a bone infection happen from such a simple thing as an insect bite? Are you sure he's not developing muscular dystrophy like his uncle? Or just having growing pains?"

Previous chapters described the growth and development of well children and the nursing care of children with a disorder of other body systems. This chapter adds information about the dramatic changes, both physical and psychosocial, which can

(Continued on next page)

(Continued from previous page)

occur when a child develops a musculoskeletal disorder.

What other information does Jeffrey's mother need to know about bone infections? How would you explain to her what has happened?

The skeletal system, composed of more than 200 bones connected by the joints and tendons, provides the structural casing or protective armor for the internal organs of the body and supplies the body with red and white blood cells grown in the central marrow. Skeletal muscles, which are attached to the bones by connective tissue, tendons, and ligaments, allow for voluntary movement, including gross motor activities, such as running, and fine motor activities, such as writing. Together, the skeletal and muscular systems both support the body and make coordinated movement possible.

Because their bones and muscles are still growing, children suffer from disorders of the musculoskeletal system more frequently than do adults. However, because bones are still growing, fractures (breaks in the continuity or structure of bone) heal much more quickly than in adults. If a growth plate is injured by trauma or infection, however, so that bone growth halts, an injury that might be simple in an adult becomes extremely serious in a child (Copley, Kinsler, Gheen, et al., 2013). Nurses play a key role in teaching parents ways to expose children who have muscular or skeletal disorders to the same sorts of stimuli that might be experienced if they were able to move around independently. Because the maintenance of musculoskeletal function and locomotion is so important, these are addressed by 2020 National Health Goals (Box 51.1).

BOX 51.1 Nursing Care Planning Based on 2020 National Health Goals

To maintain a healthy musculoskeletal system, proper exercise is necessary. Several 2020 National Health Goals address this, including:

- Increase the proportion of the nation's public and private schools that require daily physical education for elementary grade students from a baseline of 3.8% to 4.2%.
- Increase the proportion of the nation's public and private schools that require daily physical education for middle or junior high students from a baseline of 7.9% to 8.6% and for senior high students from 2.1% to 2.3%.
- Increase the proportion of adolescents who meet current federal physical activity guidelines for aerobic physical activity and for muscle-strengthening activity (developmental).
- Increase the proportion of children and adolescents aged 2 years through 12th grade who view television, videos, or play video games for no more than 2 hours a day from 78.9% to 86.8%.
- Increase the proportion of trips that children and adolescents make by walking (Developmental) (U.S. Department of Health and Human Services [DHHS], 2010; see www.healthypeople.gov).

Nurses can help the nation achieve these goals by educating children about the importance of physical activity, serving as consultants for school systems in designing physical education programs, and being certain to ask children about their usual activity level at health maintenance visits.

Nursing Process Overview

For Care of a Child With a Musculoskeletal Disorder

Assessment

Unlike many other diseases in children, disorders of the skeletal system usually manifest with specific, localized symptoms; therefore, parents usually bring children to health care facilities early in the course of such illnesses. Disorders of the muscles or joints, however, such as juvenile rheumatoid arthritis (JRA) may manifest insidiously; when the disorder is diagnosed, parents may feel guilty for not having sought health care earlier.

One condition whose seriousness parents may underestimate is a childhood limp. A limp is never normal, and it may be the first manifestation of a serious hip or knee problem. When weighing or measuring children at health care visits, take the opportunity to assess gait (whether a child walks naturally or stiffly, on tiptoes or on the whole foot; whether the feet are in good alignment; and whether the back is held straight). Such assessments may detect that a child brought to a health care center because of an upper respiratory condition, for example, has another, perhaps more important, musculoskeletal problem requiring an evaluation. Because scoliosis is a common spinal deformity requiring early detection, school nurses have direct responsibility for instituting scoliosis screening programs in their schools (Magee, Kenney, & Mullin, 2012). Because these screenings, however, do not detect all children who have the condition, and so this needs to be repeated at health care visits. Because skeletal injuries can be a sign of child maltreatment, careful history taking is necessary at all health visits to also rule out this possibility.

Nursing Diagnosis

The nursing diagnoses most frequently identified for children with musculoskeletal disorders include those that deal with pain, lack of mobility, and, because of immobilization, a need for diversional activities. Children, especially adolescents, who require a walker or other equipment to aid in skeletal support or locomotion may encounter problems with self-esteem. Examples of some typical nursing diagnoses include:

- Pain related to chronic inflammation of joints
- Impaired physical mobility related to a cast on the leg

- Deficient diversional activities related to a need for imposed activity restriction for 4 weeks
- Situational low self-esteem related to the continuous use of a body brace

Outcome Identification and Planning

Many musculoskeletal problems in children require long-term care. Despite current therapies, some disorders may leave a child with a permanent disability. Before a child is discharged from an ambulatory or inpatient setting, help parents plan how they will manage any necessary restrictions at home. For example, at first, a cast on an arm seems exciting: it is something for a school-age child to show off and an excuse not to write in school. After a few days, however, the cast may feel more frustrating than enjoyable. Take the time, therefore, to review what wearing the cast will mean to the child in everyday situations. Will the cast fit through required school uniform shirts with tight cuffs? Will a preschooler with a large cast fit into a car seat? If the child must stay home from school, do the parents know how to arrange for tutoring? If both parents work outside their home, will they need to arrange for child care?

Depending on the child's and family's circumstances, the answers to these problems can differ greatly. Taking the time to sit down with the parents and ask them whether these concerns will pose problems, however, not only initiates problem solving but also allows parents to prepare solutions with a concerned person rather than by themselves at home.

Referral to an appropriate organization can be helpful if a child has a long-term condition. Examples of these are the Arthritis Foundation (www.arthritis.org), the Muscular Dystrophy Association (www.mda.org), the Osteogenesis Imperfecta Foundation (www.oif.org), and the National Scoliosis Foundation (www.scoliosis.org).

Implementation

Many nursing interventions for children with musculoskeletal disorders involve care of a child in a cast or in traction (treatment involving pulling on a body part in one direction against a counterpull exerted in the opposite direction) or teaching about common concerns, such as posture or children's shoes. Parents and children who are kept well-informed in these matters are much more likely to be able to cope with circumstances that occur from growth.

Outcome Evaluation

Children with musculoskeletal disorders invariably need follow-up care after discharge from an ambulatory visit or inpatient care because bone healing is a slow process. Both parents and children may need support at reevaluation visits if they learn that a cast or brace must stay on longer than they thought or if they must continue exercises. Praise for their management so far is an effective intervention for helping parents and the child realize that, because they have coped with the situation so far, they can continue to cope with the situation into the future.

During reevaluation visits, spend time assessing children's body image and self-esteem or the total effect of their condition on growth and development. Do children view themselves as basically well persons who, oh, by the way, have a right leg shorter than their left leg, or as a deformed person who is inferior to others? The success of treatment cannot be achieved if a child's self-concept has been diminished by an injury or disease.

Some examples indicating achievement of outcomes include:

- Child states he feels no pain or numbness in the extremity after the application of a cast.
- Child demonstrates allowable weight-bearing activities with casted lower extremity.
- Parents accurately state the child's care needs both in and out of the hospital.
- Child states positive aspects of self, participates in activities, and establishes friendships with peers.

THE MUSCULOSKELETAL SYSTEM

Bones and Bone Growth

Bones are generally classified by their shape as long (those found in extremities), short (those of the wrist or ankle), flat (those of the skull, ribs, scapula, and clavicle), or irregular (the vertebrae, the pelvis, and the facial bones of the skull).

The mark of a long bone is a lengthy central shaft (the **diaphysis**), a rounded end portion (the **epiphysis**), and a thin area between them (the **metaphysis**) (Fig. 51.1). Increases in the length of long bones occur at the **cartilage** (connective tissue) segment (the **epiphyseal plate**), between the epiphysis and the metaphysis. Injury to this area in a growing child is always potentially serious because it may halt growth, stimulate abnormal growth, or cause irregular or erratic growth.

The central shafts of long bones are covered by an outer sensitive layer of **periosteum**. Bone width increases by growth at the inner surface of this. Injury to the periosteum, such as may occur with osteomyelitis, has the potential to also threaten bone growth (Browne, Guillerman, Orth, et al., 2012).

Although it is easy to think of bones as rigid, solid structures, they are, in fact, active living tissue to which nutrients must be supplied for growth. Calcium, one of the main components of bone, is important for both original bone formation,

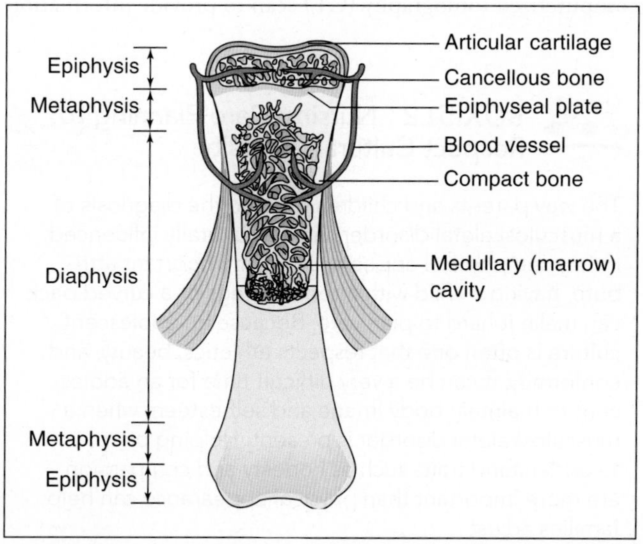

FIGURE 51.1 The structure of a bone.

remodeling (replacement of old by new bone tissue), and **resorption** (bone breakdown). These processes are strongly influenced by vitamin D and the parathyroid hormone calcitonin. "Bone age" in children can be determined by an X-ray of the wrist that shows the ossification level of the bones.

The inner core of long bones is filled with yellow and red marrow and is responsible for the formation of platelets, red blood cells, white blood cells, and adipose (fat) cells. Red marrow is primarily involved in blood component production, whereas yellow marrow is chiefly involved in adipose cell formation. The blood supply to bones is abundant, so that the marrow can actively supply enough blood components for the entire body. As with other tissues, if the blood supply is cut off, bone cells die and blood cell production is hindered.

Muscle

The skeletal muscular system is composed of striated muscle (differentiated from the smooth muscle found in body organs, which is responsible for such activities as intestinal peristalsis). Activation of skeletal muscle occurs with innervation from a motor nerve and is under voluntary control. **Myopathy**, or disease of the muscular system, can be inherited (as in muscular dystrophy) or acquired (as in myasthenia gravis).

ASSESSMENT OF MUSCULOSKELETAL FUNCTION

In addition to a history and physical examination, diagnostic tests are frequently necessary to detect musculoskeletal dysfunction. These may include X-ray and bone scans, bone and muscle biopsies, electromyography, and arthroscopy. Ultrasound and magnetic resonance imaging (MRI) studies are used to reveal soft tissue disorders. Furthermore, obtain information on how parents and children are adjusting to a potential disability because poor acceptance of a condition can limit a child's potential as much as the physical involvement (Box 51.2)

Radiography

Because bones are opaque, they outline well on an X-ray or computerized tomography (CT) scan to provide information about a specific bone or a joint. Other tests, however, are indicated to confirm problems with cartilage, tendons, and ligaments. X-rays in children are limited to the least number necessary for diagnosis or prognosis because excessive radiation is associated with the development of malignancies, such as leukemia (Schmitz-Feuerhake & Pflugbeil, 2011). Radiation of epiphyseal plates can lead to uneven growth.

> **BOX 51.2 Nursing Care Planning to Respect Cultural Diversity**
>
> The way parents and children react to the diagnosis of a musculoskeletal disorder can be culturally influenced. If they see physical appearance as an important attribute, having a child with atrophied legs or a curved back can make it hard to plan care. Because an adolescent culture is often one that respects athletics, beauty, and conformity, it can be a very difficult time for an adolescent to maintain body image and self-esteem when a musculoskeletal disorder is present. Helping people to understand traits such as honesty and compassion are more important than physical appearance can help families adjust.

Bone Scan (Scintigraphy)

A bone scan is a study of the uptake by bone of intravenously injected radioactive substances (Dobrindt, Hoffmeyer, Ruf, et al., 2012). Areas of increased metabolic activity cause the substance to concentrate in that area, often providing information on very early stages of bone disease and healing, possibly before they are visible on an X-ray.

Electromyography

Electromyography studies the electrical activity of skeletal muscle and nerve conduction to determine the location and cause of disorders such as myasthenia gravis, muscular dystrophy, and lower motor neuron and peripheral nerve disorders (Wild, Steele, & Munro, 2012).

For the test, surface electrodes are placed over the muscle, or needle electrodes are inserted into the muscle. The electrical activity of the muscle at rest and in motion is then detected by audioamplification and recorded on an oscilloscope screen. Normally, resting muscle is quiet. If fasciculations are present, abnormal noises or oscilloscope spikes will be observed.

Although the needle electrodes are small, if they are used, the test can be frightening for children because they are pricked by needles. They need support from someone they know during the procedure. Before and after, provide opportunities for therapeutic play so a child can express anxiety and feelings about such an invasive procedure.

Muscle or Bone Biopsy

Both muscle and bone biopsies involve removal of a tissue sample for examination of its microscopic structure. They can provide evidence about infection, malignant bone growth, inflammation, or atrophy of the area. Either type may be done during surgery or as an ambulatory procedure.

Biopsies of these types are usually done using conscious sedation or a local anesthetic. If local anesthesia is used, caution children they will feel the initial prick of an anesthetizing needle; they will then feel additional momentary pressure as the biopsy needle is inserted. You can assure them the amount of tissue that will be taken from them is no larger than the inner bore of the biopsy needle, comparable to the size of the lead in a pencil.

Arthroscopy

Arthroscopy involves direct visualization of a joint with a fiber optic instrument. It is usually done under local anesthesia in an ambulatory care setting. Arthroscopy allows a joint, most commonly the knee, but also the hip, shoulder, elbow, or wrist, to be examined without a large incision. It is most often used to diagnose athletic injuries and to differentiate between acute and chronic joint disorders (Jeong, Lee, & Ko, 2012).

HEALTH PROMOTION AND RISK MANAGEMENT

Health promotion for children with musculoskeletal disorders focuses on thorough assessment at all health maintenance visits. A child's ability to achieve developmental milestones, specifically gross and fine motor abilities, provides important information about musculoskeletal function. Screening for musculoskeletal disorders, such as for scoliosis in the prepubescent child and the adolescent, is an extremely important health promotion nursing role.

Safety precautions and anticipatory guidance for parents is essential to minimize the risk of injury, specifically to extremities. As a child grows and becomes active in sports, parental and child education about the importance of using bike helmets for bike riding, or protective gear for organized sports, takes on an even greater role.

Nutrition education is important to ensure adequate calcium and vitamin D intake for bone growth and healing. However, if a child requires bed rest, calcium intake should be moderated to reduce the risk of renal calculi formation resulting from immobilization. The teenage years are an important time for both males and females to build calcium stores to protect against osteoporosis later in life (Chouinard, Randall, & Buchholz, 2012).

THERAPEUTIC MANAGEMENT OF MUSCULOSKELETAL DISORDERS IN CHILDREN

Various methods are used as therapy for children with musculoskeletal disorders, including casts, traction, distraction, and open reduction. Amputation, a rare necessity, is discussed in Chapter 53.

Casting

Casts are used to treat a wide range of musculoskeletal disorders, from simple fractures in the extremities to correction of congenital structural bone disorders.

Cast Application

Casts are created from either plaster of Paris or fiberglass. Fiberglass is an attractive material to use for children's casts because it is light in weight; comes in attractive colors; and, when a special waterproof liner is used, can be immersed in water. Unfortunately, it is more expensive and may not be practical for casts that need frequent changing, such as those used to correct talipes disorders, a common congenital disorder that requires serial casting.

Children need an explanation of what to expect with casting. To maintain alignment of body parts, a health care provider may gently exert a pull on the body part being casted during the cast application. If a large body cast is being applied, children may be positioned on a special cast table with a traction apparatus at the chin and pelvis to initiate tension. Allow a support person to accompany children to a cast room to hold their hand or talk to them during the application. Most children (and adults) are unaware that casts are formed from strips or rolls of material impregnated with the casting material. The normal curiosity of children as they watch a cast grow and mold to their body part usually makes casting a pleasant procedure. Some children voice that they regard the cast as a badge of courage, or at least, a conversation piece.

Before a cast is applied, a tube of stockinette is stretched over the area and soft cotton padding is placed over bony prominences. At the end of the application, the stockinette will be pulled up and over the raw edges of the cast to create a smooth, padded surface (Fig. 51.2). If a plaster cast is to be applied, caution children that, at first, the wet strips of plaster of Paris feel cool. Almost immediately, however, the strips begin to generate heat as evaporation begins and body parts start to feel warm. If the cast is a full-body cast, children may become uncomfortably warm, with perspiration possibly running from their forehead. Assure them this feeling of warmth is transient and is never enough to cause a burn.

A plaster cast takes 10 to 72 hours to dry depending on its size. Fiberglass casts usually dry within 5 to 30 minutes. A "window" may be placed in a cast if an infection is suspected, so that the area can be observed. If the child has a body or hip spica cast, windowing can prevent uncomfortable abdominal distention and allow bowel sounds to be assessed.

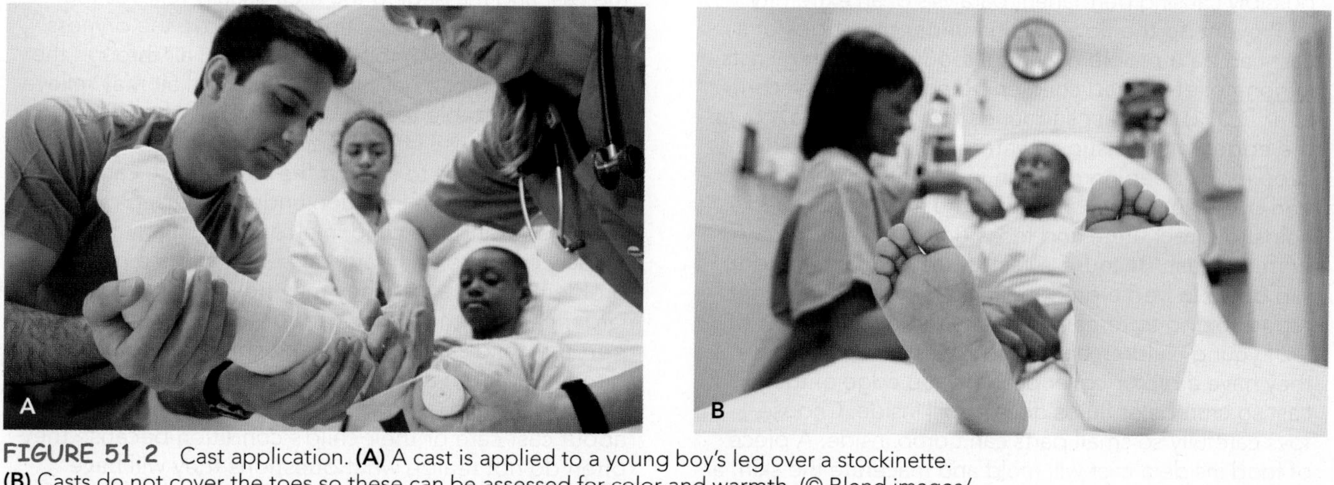

FIGURE 51.2 Cast application. **(A)** A cast is applied to a young boy's leg over a stockinette. **(B)** Casts do not cover the toes so these can be assessed for color and warmth. (© Blend images/ Alamy.)

Compartment syndrome is a phenomenon that can occur when a cast or tight constrictive dressing puts pressure on an enclosed space such as the forearm. This pressure can result in severely decreased blood flow that potentially threatens damage to and necrosis of surrounding soft tissue or nerves (R. M. Rush, Arrington, & Hsu, 2012).

Assess fingers or toes carefully for warmth, pain, and function after application of a cast to be certain a compartment syndrome is not developing. If signs of compartment syndrome are present, the cast will need to be released immediately to prevent permanent nerve and tissue damage. A fasciotomy (surgically opening the compartment) may be necessary to further prevent nerve damage.

Nursing Diagnoses and Related Interventions

Nursing Diagnosis: Risk for ineffective peripheral tissue perfusion related to pressure from cast

Outcome Evaluation: Child states she feels no pain or numbness in extremity; distal nail bed blanches and refills in less than 3 seconds; pedal pulses are palpable.

If an extremity has been casted, keep it elevated by a pillow to prevent edema in the part. Check circulation frequently, such as every 15 minutes during the first hour, hourly for the next 4 hours, and then every 4 hours throughout the first day. Assess for color, warmth, presence of pedal or wrist pulses, and sensations of numbness or tingling. Signs of impaired neurovascular function include pallor (including blueness or coldness of the distal part), pulselessness, pain in the casted part, paresthesia (numbness or tingling in the part, as if it were "asleep"), and paralysis. Children younger than 6 or 7 years of age have difficulty describing paresthesia; however, they may whine or cry with the discomfort of the sensation. Edema that does not improve with elevation is also an important sign. Any of these symptoms requires immediate attention, because neurovascular impairment can lead to nerve ischemia and destruction, possibly causing permanent paralysis of an extremity.

Preventing the flow of urine under the edges of a cast can be a problem with full body or high leg casts in non–toilet-trained children (Reed, Carroll, Baccari, et al., 2011). If a cast surrounds the genital area, cover the edges with plastic or waterproof material to help keep it dry. Keeping children in a semi-Fowler position by using pillows or raising the head of the bed helps to direct urine and feces downward and away from the cast. Because a cast is heavy, infants tend to slip down in bed a great deal, so they need frequent repositioning to remain in this raised position.

If young children have a body cast, make certain they have a bib or cover over the top edge of their cast so crumbs or fluids do not spill inside. Choose toys carefully so small parts can't drop inside. A piece of food inside a cast will mold and macerate the skin; a small part of a toy could cause irritation and a pressure ulcer. If food or fluid is spilled on the outside of the cast, the cast can be cleaned with a damp cloth.

Nursing Diagnosis: Parental health-seeking behaviors related to care of child with cast at home

Outcome Evaluation: Parents state plans for adapting home environment and lifestyle to accommodate child with cast; parents demonstrate measures to check neurovascular status.

If a child has an upper extremity cast, be certain the parents understand how to position the extremity properly, such as with a sling. If the cast is on a lower extremity, be certain parents and the child understand the amount of weight bearing allowed on the affected extremity and how to use crutches safely, if prescribed.

Handling a child in a large cast can seem so overwhelming for parents that they do not see how they will be able to care for their child at home. Assure them the child is quite comfortable in the cast, despite its awkward, constricting appearance. Role model moving the child to show them that it is not an impossible task. Be sure to caution them that, if an abduction bar is used with a cast, it must never be used as a handle for lifting. Such use can break the bar from the cast or weaken its support.

Parents need to use good body mechanics (lift with the thighs, not the back) when turning or positioning the child in a full-body cast. They may appreciate suggestions on ways to move the child from room to room, such as using a toy wagon with a flat board on top or using a skateboard for children to propel themselves forward. Point out that all children thrive on being touched. Children in large body casts need their head and arms stroked (or any areas of the body that are not covered by the cast) so they receive this. Demonstrate how even a child in a large hip spica cast can be held, cuddled, and supported for feeding.

Many children report a sensation of itching inside a cast at about the end of the first week. If the area is immediately under the edge of the cast, the itching is probably the result of dry skin caused by the drying effect of the cast. Reaching a hand under the edge of the cast and massaging the area usually relieves the itching. Applying hand lotion may relieve the dryness. If the area is unreachable, blowing cool air through the cast with a fan or a hair dryer set on cool air may relieve the uncomfortable feeling. Caution both the child and parents not to use implements such as a coat hanger or knitting needle to scratch the area. These can injure the skin, causing an infection under the cast (Box 51.3).

Transporting the child in a car, particularly fitting a bulky cast into an infant car seat, can be a major problem for parents. They may need to purchase a larger car seat than intended for their child to transport the child safely. Before any child with a cast is discharged from a health care facility, give parents a telephone number to call if they have any questions about cast care or their child's condition because they often do not realize what questions they will have until they return home.

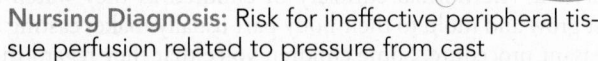

BOX 51.3 Nursing Care Planning to Empower a Family

CAST CARE AT HOME

Q. Jeffrey's sister has a fiberglass cast fitted onto her arm. Her mother ask you, "Is there any special things I have to do?"
A. Some helpful tips to care for your child's cast at home include:

- Keep the casted body part elevated on a pillow for the first day to decrease swelling.
- Observe the hands and fingers (the body part distal to the cast) for swelling or blueness, and ask your child to move her fingers about every 4 hours for the first 24 hours. If she is unable to move her fingers or if she has swelling, blueness, or pain, telephone your health care provider. These signs could mean the cast is pressing on a nerve or constricting a blood vessel.
- Encourage usual activities so your child remains active, but monitor strenuous activities, such as roughhousing, while the cast is in place.
- Ask your child to think through how wearing a cast will change her day, such as making it difficult to eat at preschool or to join in play at the playground, and brainstorm how to solve these problems.
- Be certain your child knows not to put anything inside the cast. If itching occurs, blowing some cool air into it from a hair dryer can be comforting.
- Be certain your child keeps the cast dry (cover it with a plastic bag to shower); no swimming is allowed. Remind her not to use magic markers for autographs because fiberglass is a porous material.
- Keep your return appointment for follow-up care because children can outgrow a cast rapidly. Outgrowing a cast can put pressure on nerves and can lead to permanent disability.

Cast Removal

Most casts remain in place for 4 to 8 weeks and are then removed using an electric cast cutter with a rapidly vibrating, circular disk (Fig. 51.3). Cast cutters are frightening, because the disk makes a very loud noise as it cuts through the cast material and also generates heat. To the child, the disk appears capable of cutting through not only the plaster but also an arm or leg as well. The person removing the cast usually demonstrates that the disk does not cut skin by touching a thumb to the edge of it. Not all children are totally convinced by the demonstration, however, and may require additional support while the disk moves from one end of a cast to the other, such as saying, "It's all right to cry; I know this looks scary" or by holding your hands over the child's ears to lessen the noise.

The skin of the child's extremity looks macerated and dirty after a cast is removed; a good bath usually washes away most of this. If an arm has been casted in flexion, the elbow may feel stiff and even sore when the child is asked to extend it for the first time. Children often continue to use extremities with caution after a cast has been removed. Advise parents to allow children to begin using extremities again at their own pace. As children naturally play and reach for objects, they gradually forget to favor the arm or leg, and full function then returns. Once healing has taken place, the extremity is as strong as it was before the fracture. The child does not need to continue to favor the extremity to protect it from a second fracture.

Medical Boots (Fracture Boots) or Splints

In some instances, a fracture does not require a cast for immobility but can be immobilized by a supportive boot or splint. The child wears the boot or arm splint continuously as if it were a cast; an advantage is that, if a complication should occur, it can be readily removed by its Velcro attachments. Ask at return appointments if children who are prescribed boots or splints are wearing the immobilizer continually. Be certain children who say they take them off "a little" are not actually describing taking them off often and, therefore, are not receiving the support necessary for effective bone healing.

Crutches

Crutches are prescribed for children for one of three reasons: to keep weight off one or both legs, to support weakened legs, or to maintain balance. Usually, a physical therapist measures crutch length and gives beginning instruction in crutch walking. Being familiar with how crutches are measured and having crutch walking supervised not only allows you to offer emotional support to children as they learn to use crutches but also helps you assess progress at follow-up visits.

Fit and Adjustment

If crutches are properly fitted, there should be a space of 1 to 1.5 in. between the axilla crutch pad and the child's axilla. When the child stands upright and places his hands on the hand rests of the crutches, the elbows should flex about 20 degrees. This degree of flexion ensures that, when the child bears weight on the crutch, the body weight will be borne by the arm, not the axilla. Pressure of a crutch against the axilla could lead to compression and damage of the brachial nerve plexus crossing the axilla, resulting in permanent nerve palsy. Teach children not to rest with the crutch pad pressing on the axilla but to always support their weight at the hand grip.

Always assess the tips of crutches to be certain the rubber tip is intact and not worn through because the tip prevents the crutch from slipping. Be certain the child is walking with the crutches placed about 6 in. to the side of the foot. This distance furnishes a wide, balanced base for support.

Before discharge from a health care facility, explore with children any problems crutches may cause with their daily activities. If they carry books to school, for example, they will need to wear a backpack so their hands are free for the hand rests. Caution parents to clear articles such as throw rugs, small footstools, or toys out of paths at home.

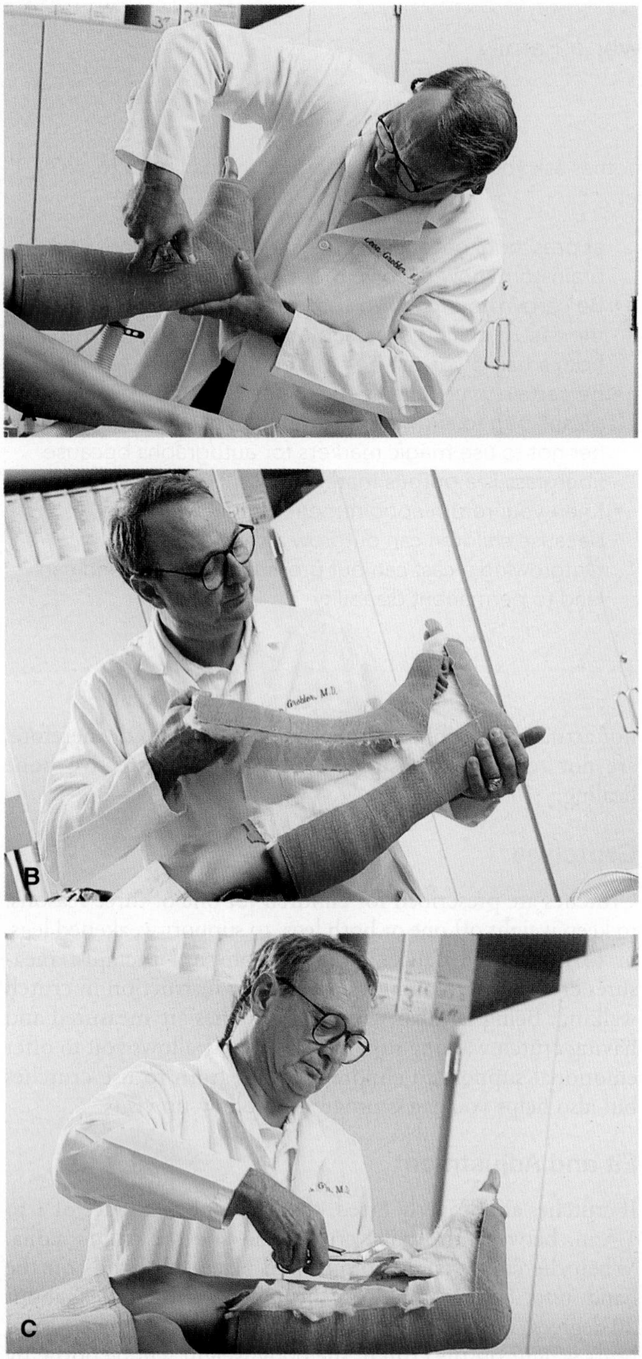

FIGURE 51.3 Cast removal. **(A)** A cast cutter is used to begin the removal of a fiberglass cast on an adolescent's leg. **(B)** The fiberglass cast is lifted off. **(C)** The underlying stockinette and padding are removed. (© Will and Deni McIntyre/Science Source/Photo Researchers.)

Crutch Walking

Two main crutch-walking patterns are used (Fig. 51.4). A two-point gait is used when a child needs support for weakened muscles or balance but may bear weight on both lower extremities. The child places the right crutch and left foot forward, then the left crutch and right foot forward, and so on. Using the crutch opposite a foot provides a wider base of support than using the crutch next to the foot. Caution children to take small steps until they feel confident.

A three-point swing-through gait is used when no weight bearing is allowed on one foot. For this, the crutches are both brought forward. The weight of the body is then shifted forward as both legs are swung through the crutches. The child bears weight on the unaffected (good) leg and moves the crutches forward again. It takes strong arm support to bear full weight on crutches this way. Be certain the child is bearing weight on the hands and not on the axillae. Some children use a swing-through gait rather recklessly and need to be advised to slow their pace to a safer one.

To walk downstairs using a swing-through gait, children place their crutches on the lower step, then swing the unaffected (good) foot forward and down to that step. To go upstairs, they place their unaffected (good) foot on the elevated step, then raise the crutches onto the step and lift themselves up. To help children remember this pattern, the following saying can be taught: "angels" (the good foot) go up; "devils" (the bad foot with the crutches) go down.

QSEN Checkpoint Question 51.1

Informatics

Suppose Jeffrey is prescribed crutches to take weight off his affected leg. What teaching point should you include in his health education?

a. His crutches should be at least 6 in. longer than he is tall.
b. He should lean forward at a 45-degree angle while walking.
c. He should bear weight on his arms to avoid pressure on his axillae.
d. It is unsafe to walk downstairs with crutches; walking upstairs is acceptable.

Look in Appendix A for the best answer and rationale.

Traction

Traction, which is used to reduce dislocations and immobilize fractures, involves pulling on a body part in one direction against a counterpull exerted in the opposite direction. Although still necessary for some conditions, the use of intramedullary rods is making its use unnecessary in many instances. In straight (running) traction, the child's body weight serves as the counterpull. In suspended or balanced traction, the body part is suspended by a sling, and the counterpull and primary pull are accomplished by pulleys and weights. Either skin traction (in which skin provides the counterpull) or skeletal traction (in which bone provides the counterpull) may be used. Skin traction is used if only minimal traction is necessary; the child's skin must be in good condition for this procedure. Skeletal traction is used if a longer period of traction or a greater strength of traction pull is needed. Types of tractions are illustrated in Figure 51.5. Use of traction in the home shortens hospital stays and enables a child to interact with family members, so it should be encouraged when possible.

Skin Traction

Skin traction means a child's extremity is wrapped in a material such as an Ace bandage and then suspended from a nearby pole or frame so the weight of the body part produces traction. Bryant traction, used for fractured femurs in children younger

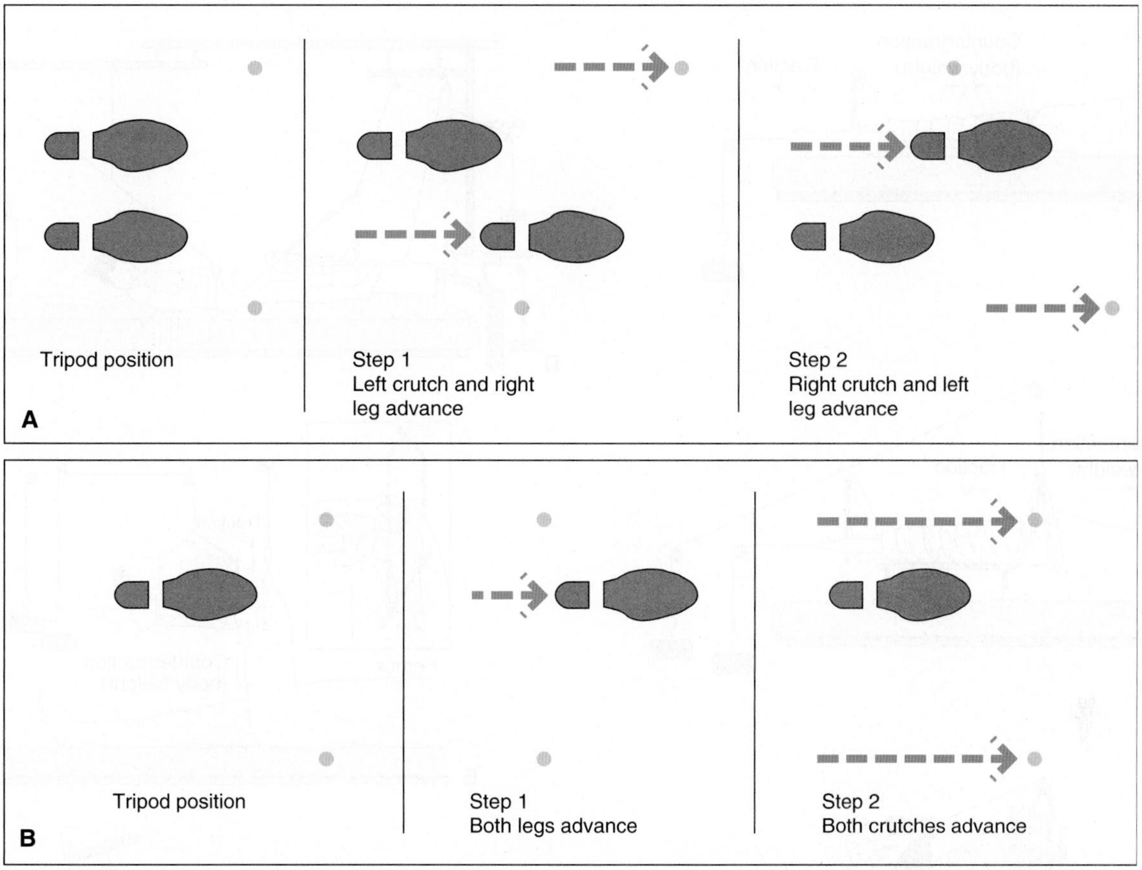

FIGURE 51.4 Crutch-walking patterns. **(A)** The two-point gait. **(B)** The swing-through gait.

than 2 years of age, is an example of skin traction (Fig. 51.6). It also may be used in preparation for surgical repair of congenital developmental disorders, such as developmental hip dysplasia (see Chapter 27). This type of traction is used less frequently now because the elevation of the extremities causes blood to pool at the hips. This and the possible tourniquet effect of the traction strips, bandages, and traction itself increase the risk for vasospasm and avascular hip necrosis.

Buck extension is an example of skin traction used for immobilizing lower extremity fractures in older children. Dunlop traction is used to immobilize an upper extremity. Cervical skin traction may be used to decrease muscle spasms in the back. This type of traction uses a halter-type device attached to weights. The head of the bed is elevated to provide countertraction.

Skeletal Traction

Skeletal traction involves the use of a pin, such as a Steinmann pin, or a wire, such as a Kirschner wire, that is passed through the skin into the end of a bone. The pin or wire can be inserted in an emergency department under local anesthesia if the child can hold absolutely still, but usually it is done under general anesthesia in the operating room. With skeletal traction, ropes strung over pulleys and attached to weights exert a pull on the extremity at the pin site. Cotton gauze squares are usually placed around the ends of the pin on the outside. The sites are cleaned with half strength hydrogen peroxide using sterile technique to keep them free of drainage. Be certain to observe pin sites daily for drainage because odorous or excessive drainage or local erythema may be a sign of infection.

Traction-Related Care

Children in traction need to be assessed carefully for neurovascular impairment, the same as children in casts. Assess the extremity in traction every 15 minutes during the first hour, hourly for 24 hours, and every 4 hours thereafter for signs of pallor (or blueness), lack of warmth, tingling, absent peripheral pulse, edema, or pain. Traction can lead to hypertension because the head typically is positioned lower than the lower extremities. Assess once a day for this possibility by taking blood pressure readings.

Be extremely careful when changing a child's bed linens or carrying out nursing functions that you do not move the weights or interfere with the traction. Provide good skin care on the child's back, elbows, and heels, because they may become irritated from friction against the sheets. A trapeze bar suspended over the bed provides a great deal of mobility and assists children in using a bedpan or positioning themselves in bed.

Being in traction is not as dramatic for children as being placed in a cast. There is an unspoken feeling from other children that "if what you have is really serious, you'd have a cast." Explain to children why this type of treatment is best for them. Keep parents and children informed of X-ray assessments (e.g., "The fracture is being held in just the right position; the bone is beginning to reform"). Although they cannot see progress, this information can help assure them that progress is occurring.

Children in traction usually are not "ill" children. They feel well except for the leg or arm being held in its correct position. Therefore, they have the energy and the need for stimulation of well children. Child life specialists or volunteers can

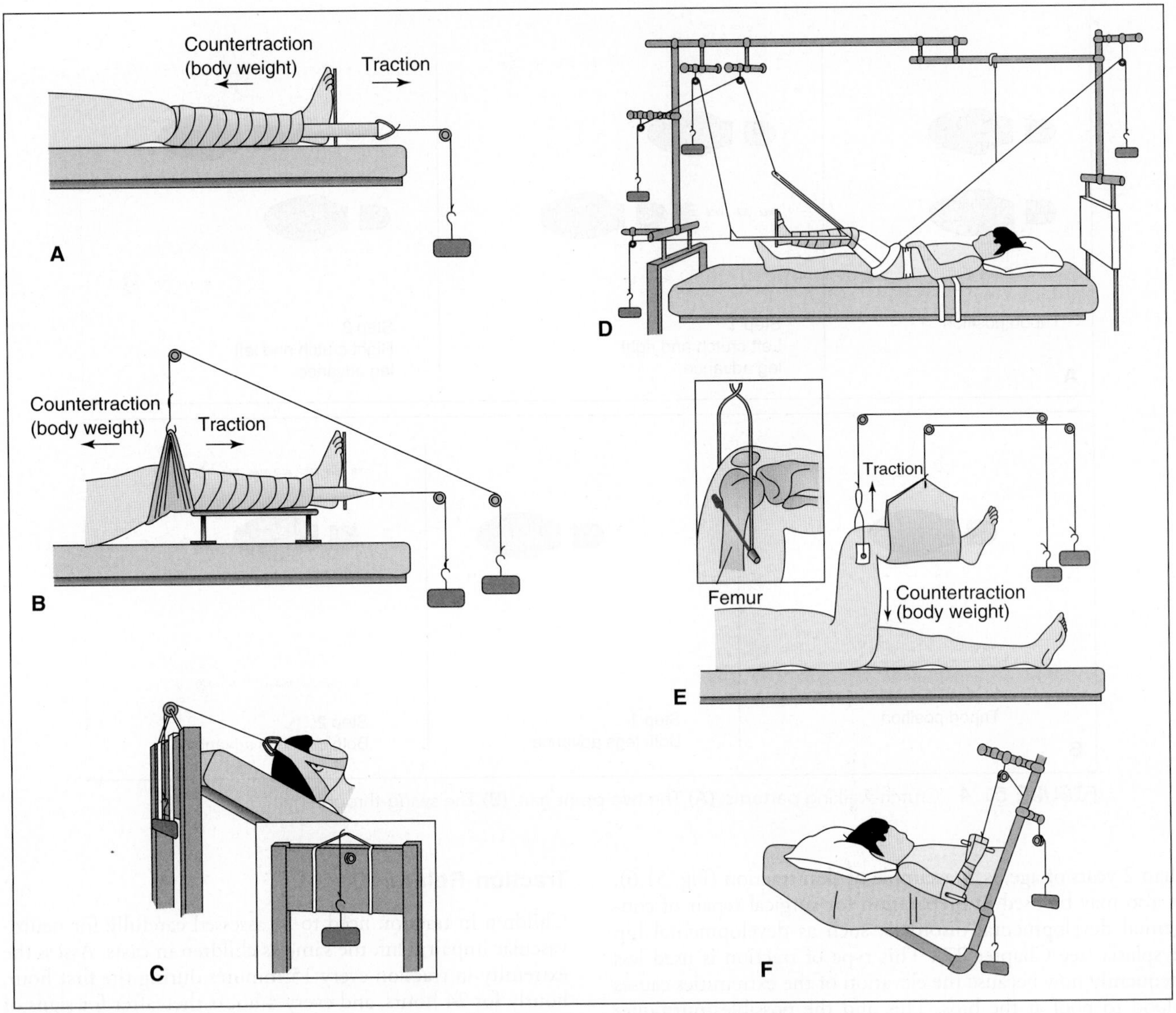

FIGURE 51.5 Types of skin traction: **(A)** Buck extension, **(B)** Russell, and **(C)** cervical skin traction. Types of skeletal traction: **(D)** balanced suspension, **(E)** 90 degrees, and **(F)** Dunlop traction with pin insertion.

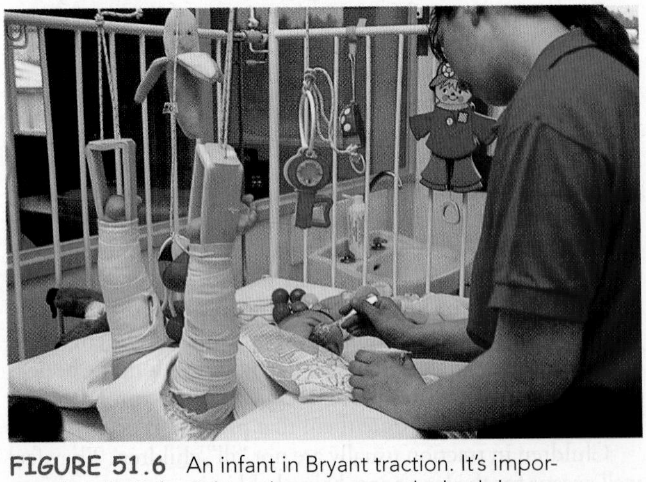

FIGURE 51.6 An infant in Bryant traction. It's important that the infant's hips do not rest on the bed due to bulkiness of a diaper. (© BSIP/Custom Medical Stock Photograph.)

be helpful in keeping them occupied. Being certain they are involved in activities (perhaps using a wireless computer or texting) is an important part of nursing care (Fig. 51.7).

Helping children maintain contact with their school friends through cards, letters, or recorded messages, social media, or texting is also important. If hospitalized, be certain their bed is located so they can see unit activities. Whether at home or in the hospital, encourage frequent visitors of their own age to help maintain peer relationships.

Distraction

Distraction is the use of an external device to separate opposing bones, which then encourages new bone growth. It can be used to lengthen a bone if one limb is shorter than the other. It also can be used to immobilize fractures or to correct defects if the bone is rotated or angled.

A device such as the Ilizarov external fixator is used to achieve distraction (Fig. 51.8). It consists of wires that are inserted through the bone then attached to either full or half rings, which

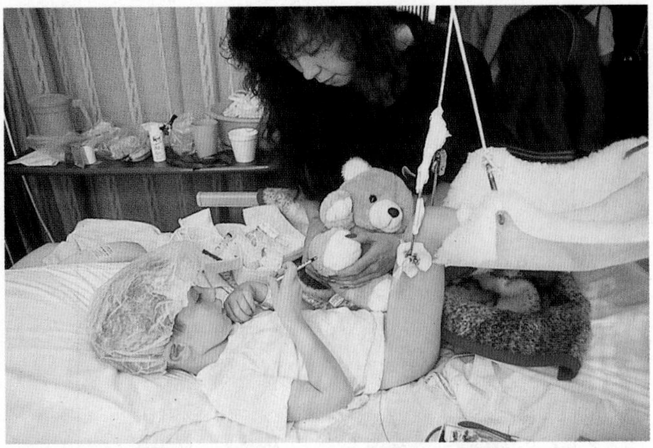

FIGURE 51.7 Children in skeletal traction need engaging activities and therapeutic play so they can remain in this confined position. (© Gary Wagner/Stock Boston.)

are secured to telescoping rods. For bone lengthening, the rods are adjusted approximately 1 mm each day to stimulate bone growth until the desired length is achieved. The device remains in place until consolidation is complete, there is no pain, limp, or edema and the bone is healed and can bear weight.

Both the child and parents need thorough preparation for the surgery, application of the device, how it will appear, and the usual reaction of others to it (surprise). If it seems important to parents, provide suggestions of ways to minimize the device's appearance, such as wide-legged pants with adjustable closures. If parents will be adjusting the telescoping rods, providing care to the wire insertion sites, or restricting activity, be certain they have full and clear instructions on what to do as well as how to assess for signs and symptoms of infection. Be certain also that they have follow-up appointments because continued care is essential to ensure an optimal outcome for their child.

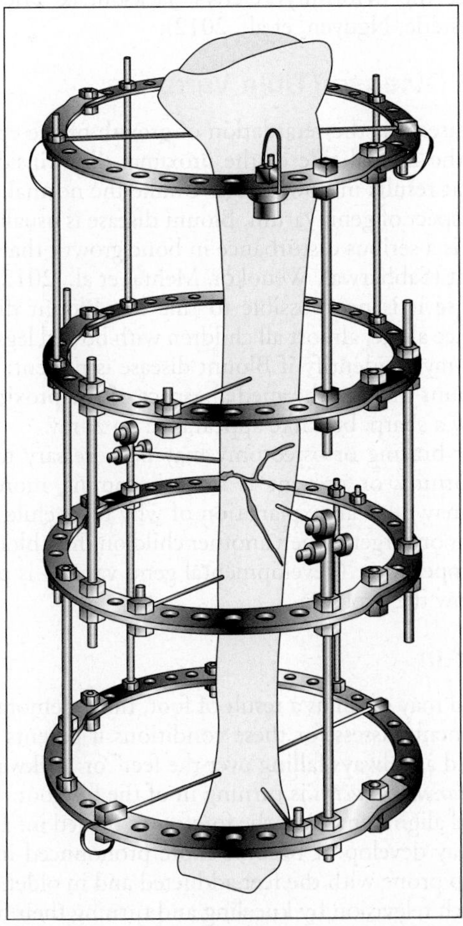

FIGURE 51.8 An Ilizarov device in place to treat a comminuted fracture when bone is splintered or crushed.

Open Reduction

Open reduction is a surgical technique used to align and repair bone. If there is a spinal fracture or both bones of a forearm or lower leg are fractured, open reduction and insertion of a rod or screw (open reduction) stabilizes the bones.

Once an open reduction is completed, the area usually is casted to provide support. Invariably, at least a small amount of serosanguineous fluid oozes from the open reduction site into the cast. Outline with a ballpoint pen any stain that suggests oozing from a surgical incision, so that an increase in the size of the mark can be detected. Do not use a magic marker for this because the fluid tends to penetrate through the cast (use a pen or crayon). Add the time at which you make the mark so you can tell how rapidly the spot is increasing. Because children with an open reduction are prone to infection, the same as any child with a surgical incision, be aware as well of systemic symptoms (e.g., increased pulse, increased temperature, lethargy) as well as local signs (e.g., edema, pain, tingling, blueness or coolness of the distal extremity) of infection.

DISORDERS OF BONE DEVELOPMENT

Many common musculoskeletal disorders in children are first noticed during routine physical exams (Box 51.4).

Flat Feet (Pes Planus)

The term *flat feet* refers to relaxation of the longitudinal arch of the foot (Erickson, Merritt, & Polousky, 2011). Although it is rare, many parents become concerned because their newborn's foot is flatter and proportionately wider than an adult's foot. In actuality, a transverse arch rarely is visible in newborns and a longitudinal arch may not be present until the child has been walking for months.

Evaluate children's feet at health care visits by having them stand on tiptoe. In this position, a longitudinal arch should be visible. Observing whether children are able to stand on their heels with the soles of the feet off the ground is another good assessment. Lastly, examine the ankle joint to be certain a full range of motion is present and the Achilles tendon is not shortened. Tarsal and metatarsal joints should also show a full range of motion.

Some children experience foot pain at the end of the day because of poor arch development. Their arch can be strengthened and the pain diminished if the child walks on tiptoe for 5 to 10 minutes daily or practices picking up marbles with the toes. For an older child, standing pigeon toed (toes pointed in) and throwing the weight forward onto the lateral aspect of the feet also tends to strengthen arches.

BOX 51.4 Nursing Care Planning Using Assessment

Assessing a Child for Signs and Symptoms of a Musculoskeletal Disorder

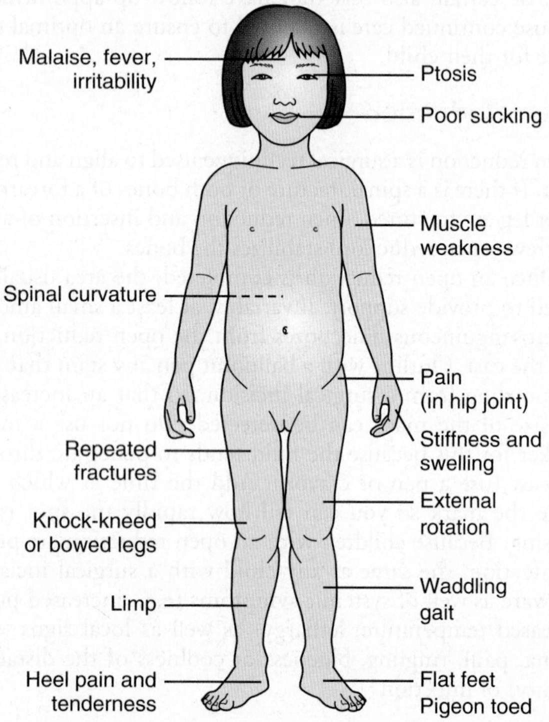

Children do not need a high top or rigid shoe in order for the arch to develop. A sneaker is an example of a shoe that not only offers enough support but that also allows normal arch development.

Bowlegs (Genu Varum)

Genu varum is lateral bowing of the tibia. If this is present, the **malleoli** (rounded prominence on either side of the ankles) will be touching and the medial surfaces of the knees will be more than 2 in. (5 cm) apart (Fig. 51.9A). Children develop this condition as part of normal development; it is seen most commonly in 2-year-olds. It also can occur in athletes who play load-bearing sports such as football (Thijs, Bellemans, Rombaut, et al., 2012).

Record the extent of the bowing at health maintenance visits by approximating the medial malleoli of the ankles and measuring the distance between the patellas (knees) for changes. Genu varum gradually corrects itself in young children by about 3 years of age or, at the latest, by school age. If the problem is unilateral, becomes rapidly worse, or persists beyond this time, the child needs referral to an orthopedist for further evaluation.

Knock Knees (Genu Valgum)

Genu valgum, or knock knee, is the opposite of genu varum. The medial surfaces of the knees touch, and the medial surfaces of the ankle malleoli are separated by more than 3 in. (7.5 cm) (see Fig. 51.9B).

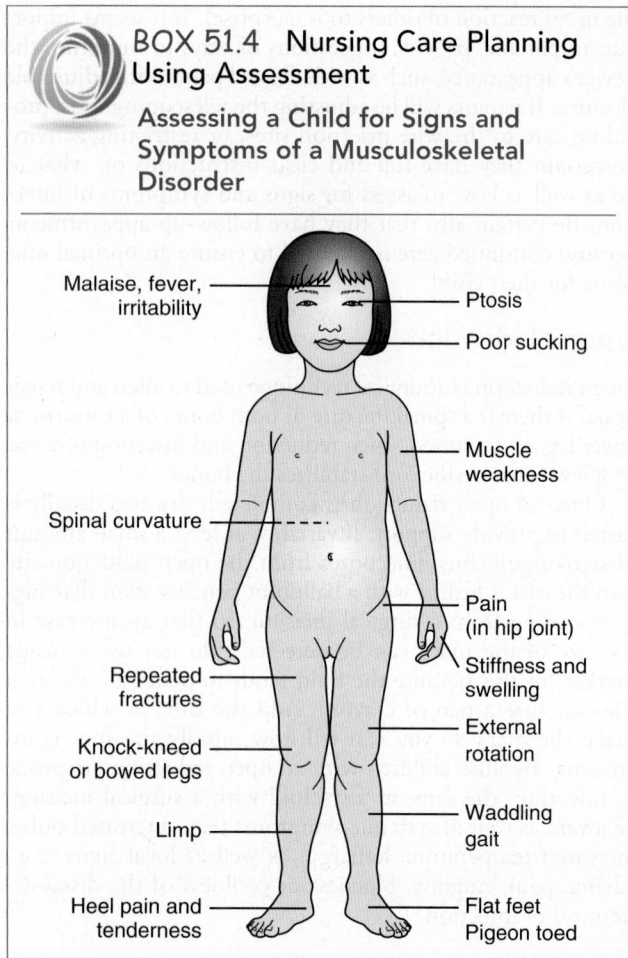

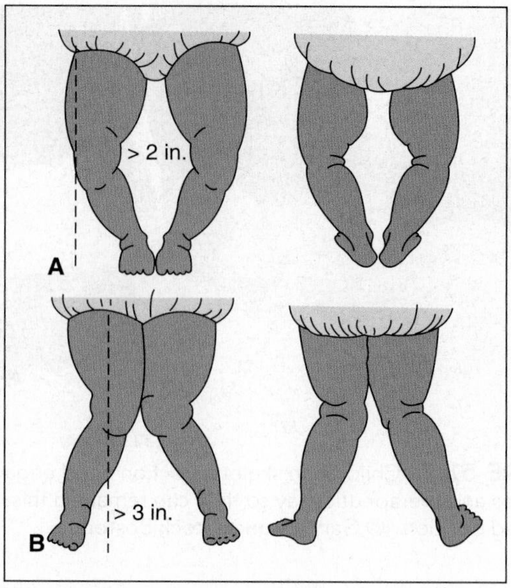

FIGURE 51.9 **(A)** Genu varum. **(B)** Genu valgum.

This is seen most commonly in children 3 to 4 years old and corrects itself by school age as the child grows. Children who continue to have this problem and those in whom the abnormality is unilateral or becomes more pronounced need a referral to an orthopedist for further evaluation because obesity, as well as both vitamin D and calcium deficiencies can cause the deformity (Gettys, Jackson, & Frick, 2011; Voloc, Esterle, Nguyen, et al., 2012).

Blount Disease (Tibia Vara)

Blount disease is the retardation of growth of the epiphyseal line on the medial side of the proximal tibia (inside of the knee) that results in bowed legs. Unlike the normal developmental aspect of genu varum, Blount disease is usually unilateral and is a serious disturbance in bone growth that requires treatment (Sabharwal, Wenokor, Mehta, et al., 2012).

Because it is not possible to rule out Blount disease by appearance alone, almost all children with bowed legs have an initial X-ray to identify if Blount disease is present. In those with Blount disease, the medial aspect of the proximal tibia will show a sharp, beaklike appearance on X-ray.

Either bracing or osteotomy may be necessary to correct this deformity or prevent it from becoming more severe. Parents may need an explanation of why their child requires treatment or surgery when another child on their block with a similar appearance (developmental genu varum) is predicted to outgrow the problem.

Toeing-In

Toeing-in may occur as a result of foot, tibial, femoral, or hip displacement. Assess for these conditions if parents describe their child as "always falling over the feet" or "awkward."

Metatarsus adductus is turning in of the forefoot. The heel is in good alignment; only the forefoot is turned in. This condition may develop or become more pronounced in infants who sleep prone with the feet adducted and in older children who watch television by kneeling and turning their feet in. If you stand the child on a copying machine and make a print, the turning in of the foot can be well demonstrated.

Most instances of metatarsus adductus resolve without therapy. Those that persist beyond 1 year can be corrected by passive stretching exercises; a few infants with extremely rigid, incorrect foot posture may require casts or splints for correction. Early detection of these extreme instances is important because treatment for metatarsus adductus is most effective if it is begun before an infant walks. With early treatment, the prognosis is excellent.

Inward tibial torsion also may be evidenced as toeing-in. This condition is diagnosed when a line drawn from the anterior superior iliac crest through the center of the patella intersects the fourth or fifth toe (or a position even more lateral) (Fig. 51.10) because, ordinarily, such a line should intersect the second toe.

Tibial torsion usually improves as the tibia grows, so this requires no treatment. Parents need a good explanation of why no treatment is necessary, however. Reassure them at periodic health maintenance visits that patience and time will correct tibial torsion (Bazner-Chandler & Brady, 2013).

Inward femoral torsion can be detected if you ask a child to lie supine and attempt to rotate the leg internally and then externally at the hip. Normally, internal rotation is about 30 degrees, and outward rotation is about 90 degrees. With inward femoral torsion, the internal rotation is closer to 90 degrees. In some children, the femur rotates so far that the patellar bones face each other. As with tibial torsion, no treatment is necessary. Inward femoral rotation will not correct itself, but a compensating tibial torsion will develop and make feet appear straight.

A fourth cause of toeing-in may be improper hip placement or developmental hip dysplasia, a problem that is very serious and needs early therapy for correction (see Chapter 27).

Growing Pains

Listen to parents carefully when they state their child has "growing pains" because what they are reporting may be symptoms indicative of rheumatic fever or JRA rather than a simple, transient phenomenon. Growing pains occur most frequently in the muscle of the calf, never in a joint. They are reported most often in preschool and school-age children, who wake at night because of the pain. Such cramping usually follows a day of vigorous activity or wearing new shoes with a heel of a different height than before. Children with genu varum (bowlegs) tend to have more of such pain than do other children. Some children, especially adolescents, who report they have growing pains may actually be reporting restless leg syndrome (Sullivan, 2012). This syndrome (involuntary leg movements that cause insomnia) is thought to be associated with decreased dopamine production. Because iron is an essential component of dopamine, a daily vitamin pill with iron may help relieve the phenomena (Kotagal, 2012).

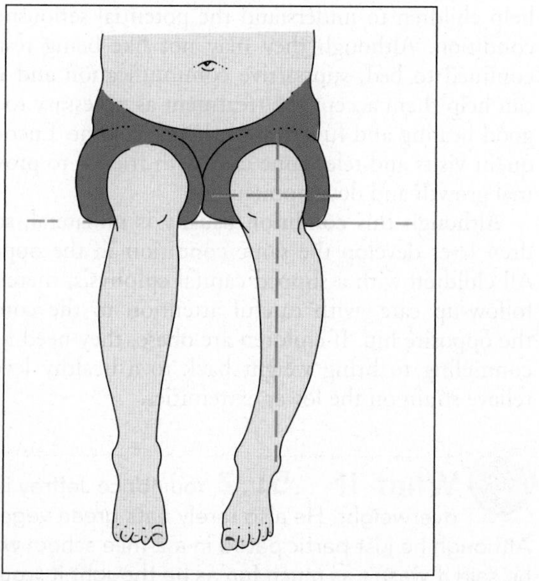

FIGURE 51.10 Toeing-in caused by inward tibial torsion. In good alignment, a line drawn from the anterosuperior iliac crest through the patella should intersect the second toe.

Osteogenesis Imperfecta

Osteogenesis imperfecta is a connective tissue (collagen) disorder in which fragile bone formation leads to recurring (pathologic) fractures (Zhao &Yan, 2011). Although as many as eight types have been identified, the disease occurs most frequently as a severe autosomal dominant form that is recognized at birth (osteogenesis imperfecta type I) or an autosomal recessive form where symptoms, including hearing and cardiovascular anomalies, develop later in life (osteogenesis imperfecta type III).

Children with type I disease may be born with countless fractures already present from the force of birth. They develop many more fractures from the everyday activities of childhood. X-rays reveal a particular ribbonlike or mosaic pattern in their bones, which aids in diagnosis. The sclera of the eye is unusually blue because of poor connective tissue formation.

Children with the type III form may have associated deafness and dental deformities (Santos, McCall, Chien, et al., 2012). In both instances, the major clinical manifestation is a tendency for bones to fracture easily because of the poor collagen formation. In some children, the bones are so fragile that fractures can result not only from trauma, such as a fall, but also from simple walking. Because the child has such frequent injuries, parents may be accused of child maltreatment before the child's condition is firmly diagnosed and documented (Pandya, Baldwin, Kamath, et al., 2011).

As the child grows older, the multiple breaks tend to cause limb and spinal column deformities, interfering with alignment or growth. Lessened rib motility leads to interference with respirations. Bisphosphonates, such as pamidronate, to increase bone mass are helpful in strengthening bones, although it is not curative (E. T. Rush, DeHaai, Kreikemeier, et al., 2012). Lightweight leg braces or intramedullary rod insertion techniques may also be prescribed (Nicolaou, Bowe, Wikinson, et al., 2011).

Parents need to protect children from trauma, fractures need to be aligned and casted, and children need to be educated about a lifestyle that is productive yet minimizes the risk of trauma. Always be careful when caring for a child with this disorder not to cause any trauma to bones. Be certain to raise side rails on cribs or beds. Keep floors dry, and remove objects that could cause falls. Always lift children gently and avoid lifting them by a single arm or leg to avoid placing strain on a bone.

What if...51.1 Jeffrey's parents report that he has been waking up at night because of "growing pains." Is there such a thing?

Legg-Calvé-Perthes Disease (Coxa Plana)

Legg-Calvé-Perthes disease is avascular necrosis (a lack of blood flow resulting in destruction) of the proximal femoral epiphysis (Kim, 2012). The disorder occurs more often in boys than in girls and has a peak incidence between 4 and 12 years of age. It usually occurs unilaterally, but may occur bilaterally.

The child notices pain in the hip joint accompanied by spasm and limited motion. X-ray studies distinguish the condition from simple synovitis (inflammation of the hip joint), which begins with the same symptoms. X-ray changes may not be apparent when a child is first seen, but they appear after about 3 weeks. For this reason, most children seen for synovitis of the hip joint are asked to return in 3 weeks for a repeat film.

Children with Legg-Calvé-Perthes disease pass through four stages. First is the synovitis stage, or a period of painful inflammation. Next is a necrotic stage, during which bone in the femur head shrinks in size and shows increased density on an X-ray. This stage lasts 6 to 12 months. The third stage is a fragmentation stage; resorption of dead bone occurs over a 1- to 2-year period. The fourth stage, a reconstruction stage, marks the final healing, with deposition of new bone.

Treatment for Legg-Calvé-Perthes disease in children under 6 years of age usually focuses on pain reduction with nonsteroidal anti-inflammatory drugs (NSAIDs) plus keeping the head of the femur within the acetabulum by a containment device. The acetabulum then acts as a mold to preserve the shape of the femoral head and maintain range of motion. In children over 6 years of age, reconstructive surgery (an osteotomy to center the femur head in the acetabulum followed by cast application) is most often prescribed. This technique returns the child to normal activity within 3 to 4 months in contrast to many months of restricted activity required by non–weight-bearing devices (Nguyen, Klein, Dogbey, et al., 2012).

Parents and children need thorough education about treatment and care because most of this occurs on an ambulatory basis. It can be difficult for young children to accept the extended treatment period involved with this disorder. Be certain that both parents and children understand there are long-term consequences if rest is not followed conscientiously. Without treatment, the femur head tends to remold into a mushroom shape, making the hip unstable thereafter and leading to degenerative changes later in life, which lead to chronic pain, reduced mobility of the hip joint, and possibly permanent disability. Parents may need assistance with devising appropriate activities for the child during the time that activity is limited and weight bearing is not allowed.

Osgood–Schlatter Disease

Osgood–Schlatter disease is the thickening and enlargement of the tibial tuberosity resulting from microtrauma, probably caused from overuse (Maffulli, Longo, Spiezia, et al., 2011). It occurs more often in boys than girls and at preadolescence or early adolescence, probably because of rapid growth at these times. Children notice pain and swelling just below the knee that is aggravated by running or squatting.

Therapy depends on the extent of the bone changes. Administration of NSAIDs, ice, and limiting strenuous physical exercise may be all that is necessary for effective healing (Kaya, Toprak, Baltaci, et al., 2012). Occasionally, immobilization of the leg in a walking cast or immobilizer for about 6 weeks may be required.

Slipped Capital Femoral Epiphysis

Slipped capital epiphysis is, as the name implies, a slipping of the femur head in relation to the neck of the femur at the epiphyseal line (Novais & Millis, 2012). The proximal femoral head displaces posteriorly and inferiorly, allowing an avascular necrosis—similar to that observed in Legg-Calvé-Perthes disease—to begin. If the cartilage covering the femur head is destroyed, permanent loss of motion of the femoral head in the acetabulum can result. Surgical reconstruction of the hip joint will then be necessary to correct the problem (Loder & Dietz, 2012).

This disorder occurs twice as frequently in young African Americans than in children of other races and twice as frequently in boys as in girls. It occurs most frequently in preadolescence and its highest incidence is in obese children. This suggests that it occurs because of the influence of growth hormone and excessive weight bearing on the hip joint.

The onset of symptoms occurs gradually. Children begin to limp as well as hold the leg on the affected side externally rotated to relieve stress and pain in the hip joint. Although the involvement is actually in the hip, they may report pain first in the knee because favoring the hip joint puts abnormal stress on the knee. On physical examination, internal rotation of the hip is difficult and painful. An X-ray reveals the slipped epiphysis at the femoral head.

Early detection of the condition is important because correction is easiest if it is attempted before the necrosis has progressed to epiphyseal destruction. Surgery with pinning or external fixation, such as with skeletal traction, is used to stabilize the femur head. In some children, a total hip replacement is advised to fully restore hip function (Traina, De Fine, Abati, et al., 2012). With either surgery, the child will have activity restrictions for an extended time afterward.

Because the disease is most common in preadolescence, help children to understand the potential seriousness of the condition. Although they may not like being restricted or confined to bed, supportive communication and education can help them accept the treatment as necessary to maintain good healing and function of their hip joint. Encourage frequent visits and telephone calls with friends to provide optimal growth and development.

Although this condition usually is unilateral, some children later develop the same condition in the opposite hip. All children with a slipped capital epiphysis, therefore, need follow-up care, with careful attention to the condition of the opposite hip. If children are obese, they need nutritional counseling to bring weight back to a healthy level and to relieve strain on the lower extremities.

What if... 51.2 You notice Jeffrey is overweight. He also rarely eats green vegetables. Although he just participated in a 2-mile school walkathon, he said it wasn't as much fun as he thought it would be. Which of his features make him at highest risk for developing slipped capital epiphysis?

INFECTIOUS AND INFLAMMATORY DISORDERS OF THE BONES AND JOINTS

All bone infections are potentially dangerous because bones have such a rich blood supply that infection can easily spread and become systemic (septicemia).

Osteomyelitis

Osteomyelitis is an infection of the bone (Hellmann & Imboden, 2012). It is most often caused by *Staphylococcus aureus* in older children and by *Streptococcus pyogenes* in younger children. Children with sickle-cell anemia have a special susceptibility to *Salmonella* invasion in long bones. The infection may occur after extensive impetigo, burns, or something as simple as a furuncle (skin abscess) when the infectious organism is then carried through the blood supply to the bone. It also may occur directly by outside invasion from a penetrating wound, open fracture, or contamination during surgery.

The infection begins originally as a metaphyseal infection. An abscess forms and spreads along the shaft of the bone under the periosteum, possibly extending to and penetrating into the bone marrow. Sinuses then form between the marrow and the periosteum, or between the infected bone and the skin above. If the epiphyseal plate becomes infected, altered bone growth can result (Dartnell, Ramachandran, & Katchburian, 2012).

Assessment

Osteomyelitis usually begins with acute symptoms. Children show systemic malaise, fever, and irritability. They experience sharp pain at the bone metaphysis site. By the second day, the area of skin over the infected bone feels warm to the touch, and edema is also usually present. Edema formation is serious because it reduces the blood supply to a large expanse of bone, causing the death of bone tissue. This dead bone tissue, which appears dense on an X-ray, is called **sequestrum** and is an important marker for diagnosis. An MRI can be helpful to reveal if the infection has spread to nearby soft tissue (van Schuppen, van Doorn, & van Rijn, 2012).

Blood studies will reveal an increased white blood cell count, C-reactive protein level, and sedimentation rate; blood culture results usually are positive for the offending organism. CT scans are helpful to demonstrate early-stage bone changes. Simple X-rays, in contrast, may not reveal bone changes (the formation of sequestrum) until 5 to 10 days after the beginning of the infection.

Therapeutic Management

Medical therapy includes a limitation on weight bearing on the affected part, bed rest, immobilization, and a short administration of an IV antibiotic such as oxacillin (Bactocill), as indicated by the blood culture. Intravenous therapy is usually initiated in the hospital and then continued at home for as long as 2 weeks, by use of an intermittent infusion device or peripherally inserted central catheter. After this, the child will be prescribed an oral antibiotic for 3 to 4 more weeks.

If pus forms under the periosteum, it may be aspirated using a technique similar to bone marrow aspiration. After the procedure, a catheter may be inserted into the area for instillation of an antibiotic solution. A drainage tube may be inserted and attached to suction to evacuate the subperiosteum area.

Nursing Diagnoses and Related Interventions

Nursing Diagnosis: Parental health-seeking behaviors related to care of the child with osteomyelitis

Outcome Evaluation: Parents accurately identify child's care needs in the hospital and at home; parents demonstrate procedure for IV antibiotic administration.

When planning care for a child with osteomyelitis, because of the long-term immobilization that may be necessary, parents may need to make major changes in their lifestyle such as taking a temporary leave from work or employing a home care nurse.

Parents usually have many questions when osteomyelitis is diagnosed, because the defect may not initially show on a routine X-ray. This can leave them puzzled as they hear their primary health care provider advising them about the need for 6 weeks of antibiotic therapy. They need support to agree to treatment because they may be suspicious, anxious, and afraid that hospitalization and administration of IV antibiotics are excessive. Often, at the point a CT scan or X-ray does reveal the process, they become more supportive and understanding of the care needed for their child.

Keep in mind that young children are active even if they are on bed rest, and so need age-appropriate activities so they maintain rest, not activity. If a child had surgery and drainage tubes are in place, institute infection-control precautions because the drain evacuates infected material. Always handle the extremity gently when giving care because movement can cause pain. Provide instructions to the parents about good food sources of calcium and protein for bone healing.

Most children with osteomyelitis recover without long-term effects (Walter, 2011). When the child is discharged from the hospital, be certain to review with parents measures to care for the antibiotic IV line if this will be continued at home. Also review the signs and symptoms of reinfection, measures for wound care and infection control, and possible adverse effects of the prescribed antibiotic (see Box 51.5, an interprofessional care map for a child with osteomyelitis). Ask if parents would like a referral for home care follow-up to ensure continued support and education.

If osteomyelitis is not entirely eradicated with the initial treatment, it will return and result in a chronic infectious process with open, draining sinuses and bone deformity in years to come. Growth plates can be destroyed, leading to shortening of the affected extremity.

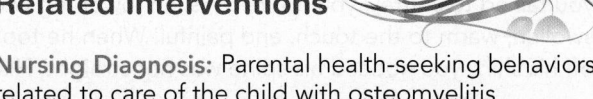

BOX 51.5 Nursing Care Planning

AN INTERPROFESSIONAL CARE MAP FOR A CHILD WITH OSTEOMYELITIS

Jeffrey, a 13-year-old boy, accompanied his mother and 3-year-old sister into the hospital emergency room because his sister had pain in her arm after a fall. As you talked to Jeffrey, you noticed his left lower leg was swollen, warm to the touch, and painful. When he took off his shirt, you noticed his spine was not straight. His mother said she noticed an infected mosquito bite on his leg 2 weeks ago. Jeffrey is diagnosed with osteomyelitis and admitted to the hospital for intravenous antibiotic therapy. His mother asks you, "How could he get a bone infection from such a simple thing as an insect bite? Are you sure he's not just having growing pains?"

Family Assessment Child lives with 10-year-old and 3-year-old sisters and two parents. Father works as a family court judge. Mother works part time as a court reporter. Child rates finances as, "Okay. Although I'd like a better bicycle."

Client Assessment Left lower extremity pale but warm; pedal pulses present. Capillary refill time in toes is 3 seconds. States he had pain on admission, rated at 4 on a numerical scale of 1 to 10. Relieved with prescribed ibuprofen. During morning assessment, child states, "I'm so bored. If I have to stay in bed for a whole week, I'll go stir crazy." Child normally enjoys playing baseball with friends and video games.

Nursing Diagnosis Risk for peripheral neurovascular dysfunction related to the effects of bone infection

Outcome Criteria Child's extremity remains pink and warm with palpable pedal pulses and capillary refill time of 3 seconds or less; pain is no more than 2 on a scale of 1 to 10; states he is complying with bed rest by choosing activities carefully.

Team Member Responsible	Assessment	Intervention	Rationale	Expected Outcome
Activities of Daily Living, Including Safety				
Nurse	Assess whether child understands he should not bear weight on affected leg.	Review with child the importance of not bearing weight on infected leg.	Infected bone is weakened, and so it could fracture more easily than usual.	Child states he understands he should not put pressure on leg.
Teamwork and Collaboration				
Nurse/Primary health care provider	Assess whether orthopedic service will be needed to consult on antibiotic therapy.	Consult with orthopedic service if needed to assure antibiotic regimen is adequate.	Bone infections are deep seated, so antibiotics must be selected for specific organisms and tissue penetration.	Orthopedic service consults as necessary to help decide best therapy.
Procedures/Medications for Quality Improvement				
Nurse	Assess whether child has past experience with intravenous (IV) therapy.	Orient child to IV therapy and importance of small armboard to guard against infiltration.	Infiltration interferes with antibiotic infusion and can cause tissue necrosis.	Child states he understands importance of continuous IV therapy and will work to guard site.
Nutrition				
Nurse/Nutritionist	Meet with child to discuss what are his favorite foods.	Discuss importance of not gaining weight while on bed rest.	Child will be fitted with an orthopedic brace for his back. Gaining weight will interfere with correct fit.	Child states he understands the importance of not gaining weight and will cooperate with nutritionist's recommendations.
Patient-Centered Care				
Nurse	Assess what child understands about the cause of bone infections.	Review association between skin infection and osteomyelitis.	Osteomyelitis is often caused by extension of a skin infection such as impetigo or infected insect bite.	Child and mother state they understand outcome should not result in loss of function.

Psychosocial/Spiritual/Emotional Needs				
Nurse	Assess what activities child would enjoy during bed rest.	Talk to child about importance of keeping busy because he will not feel systemically ill during this time.	Bed rest is difficult for children when they feel well except for one body part.	Child names at least two activities besides schoolwork he could do to keep busy and help relieve boredom.
Informatics for Seamless Health Care Planning				
Nurse	Assess whether child has had experience taking oral medication at home.	Explain necessity to continue antibiotics even though symptoms are lessening.	If child does not understand purpose of long-term therapy, he may neglect to take antibiotic once symptoms fade.	Child and mother state they understand importance of continuing antibiotic and will keep the return appointment.

QSEN Checkpoint Question 51.2

Safety

You are planning care for Jeffrey, who has osteomyelitis. Which of the following interventions should you prioritize in your plan?

a. Maintain Jeffrey's IV antibiotic therapy.
b. Teach his parents about the root causes of his infection.
c. Restrict his fluid intake to increase his hematocrit level.
d. Fully assist Jeffrey with his activities of daily living.

Look in Appendix A for the best answer and rationale.

Synovitis

Synovitis, an acute, nonpurulent inflammation of the synovial membrane of a joint, occurs most commonly in the hip joint in children with a peak age of incidence between 2 and 10 years (Erickson et al., 2011). Children notice pain in the groin, in the lower portion of the thigh or knee, or in the buttocks. Pain is intense and is most noticeable in the morning, when they first awaken. Children may wake at night or in the morning, crying from the pain of turning over. Pain again becomes worse later in the day, when the child becomes tired.

Aside from the localized pain, children feel well except they usually hold the joint flexed in a position of comfort. On physical examination, range-of-motion exercises cause pain. An X-ray or MRI may reveal capsular swelling at the involved joint.

Because this is inflammation, not infection, the treatment of synovitis is the prescription of an NSAID such as ibuprofen (Motrin) and limited activity until muscle spasm from the pain has passed. In most children, 3 days of rest reduces the synovitis. Some children, however, may need as many as 10 to 14 days of rest and a short course of oral corticosteroids to completely reduce the symptoms.

Synovitis must be differentiated from septic arthritis or Legg-Calvé-Perthes disease because septic arthritis will require an antibiotic for therapy and Legg-Calvé-Perthes disease requires a long period of immobilization and perhaps surgery (Kim, 2012). With septic arthritis, a child tends to be systemically ill and blood studies reveal an increased white blood cell count. Legg-Calvé-Perthes disease produces local systems differentiated by an X-ray examination.

Be certain both children and parents understand that synovitis, although painful, is a simple inflammation process that will heal without sequelae. Rest is important for this recovery, however, so they must be prepared to enforce this (which is not easy to do with active children).

Apophysitis and Plantar Fasciitis

Adolescents who are growing rapidly and who are physically active are prone to apophysitis, or inflammation of the epiphysis of a heel bone (Tu & Bytomski, 2011). The heel feels tender, and pain on walking may be acute.

Pain usually can be relieved by adding a lift to the heel of shoe on the affected side, thus reducing the tension on the heel cord and bone. After the pain has subsided, the adolescent needs to practice exercises to stretch the heel cord, such as standing on a slanting board that elevates the foot and toes above the level of the heel, for 20 minutes about three times a day.

Plantar fasciitis is inflammation of the plantar fascia, the ligament that supports the arch of the foot (Klein, Dale, Hayes, et al., 2012). This results in a generalized aching of the foot and a sharp pain in the heel when walking. Although not a serious condition, it can be debilitating for adolescents who want to excel in sports because it may take up to 6 months for healing. Treatment is rest for the foot and insertion of an arch support into the shoe so there is less strain on the affected ligament.

DISORDERS OF SKELETAL STRUCTURE

Spinal disorders in children may include kyphosis (an outward curvature of the spine) or lordosis (an inward curving of the spine), but scoliosis (a sideways curve) is the most commonly seen type of these disorders.

Functional (Postural) Scoliosis

Scoliosis is a lateral (sideways) curvature of the spine. It may involve all or only a portion of the spinal column. It may be functional (a curve caused by a secondary problem) or structural (a primary deformity).

Functional scoliosis occurs as a compensatory mechanism in children who have unequal leg lengths, in children with ocular refractive errors that cause them to constantly tilt their head sideways, or children with accompanying neuromuscular disorders such as cerebral palsy. Spinal deviation results because this is necessary for the child to stand upright. The curve that occurs in functional scoliosis tends to be C-shaped, whereas the curve in structural scoliosis tends to be S-shaped (composed of two separate curves).

Children with noncorrectable neuromuscular conditions that cause a functional scoliosis may need spinal fusion, but to rectify the most simple forms of functional scoliosis, the difficulty causing the spinal curvature can be corrected, eliminating the difficulty (D'Amico, Roncoletta, Di Felice, et al., 2012). A lift inserted in one shoe corrects unequal leg length. Correcting ocular refractive errors improves head tilt problems. In addition, children must be reminded to maintain good posture during everyday activities. Walking with a book on the head for 10 minutes three times a day, hanging by the hands from a door frame (chinning themselves), or doing sit-ups or push-ups are all activities that stretch the back and so are often helpful. Swimming for either enjoyment or as a sport involves stretching the spine and so is a good activity for school-age children and adolescents.

Structural Scoliosis

Structural scoliosis is an idiopathic, permanent curvature of the spine accompanied by damage to the vertebrae. The spine assumes a primary lateral curvature. To allow the child to hold the head level, a compensatory second curve develops, giving the spine an S-shaped appearance (Fig. 51.11). The primary curve is often a right thoracic convexity. As the original curve becomes severe, rotation and angulation of vertebrae also occur. The thoracic rib cage rotates to become very protuberant on the convex curve. Vertebral growth may halt because of extreme pressure changes.

A family history of curvature of the spine is found in up to 30% of children with scoliosis, although no specific inheritance pattern has been documented. It is five times more common in girls than in boys and has a peak incidence at 8 to 15 years of age. As long as the child is growing, the spinal curves will become more severe, which is why the symptoms become most marked at prepuberty (a time of rapid growth). If the child bends forward, the curve becomes even more noticeable.

Assessment

All children older than 10 years of age should be assessed for scoliosis at all health assessment visits (see Chapter 34). Often, the condition develops insidiously and is prominent before it is noticed because of the preadolescent's and adolescent's need for privacy and the lack of pain that accompanies the condition. A parent might notice when doing laundry that a daughter's bra straps are adjusted to unequal lengths. A girl may find it difficult to buy jeans that fit correctly because of uneven iliac crests, or she may notice that a skirt or dress hangs unevenly.

A scoliometer is a commercial device that can be used to document the extent of a spinal curve. With this device (a type of protractor), a reading greater than 7 degrees equals a 20-degree scoliotic curve detected by an X-ray.

MRIs, X-rays and CT scans all play a role in estimating the extent of the deformity and in providing a baseline description. If the child has a vertebral rotation causing rib imbalance, pulmonary function studies and a chest X-ray may be obtained to document the effect on lung capacity. Children's bone age is established by an X-ray of the wrists or iliac bones. If bone

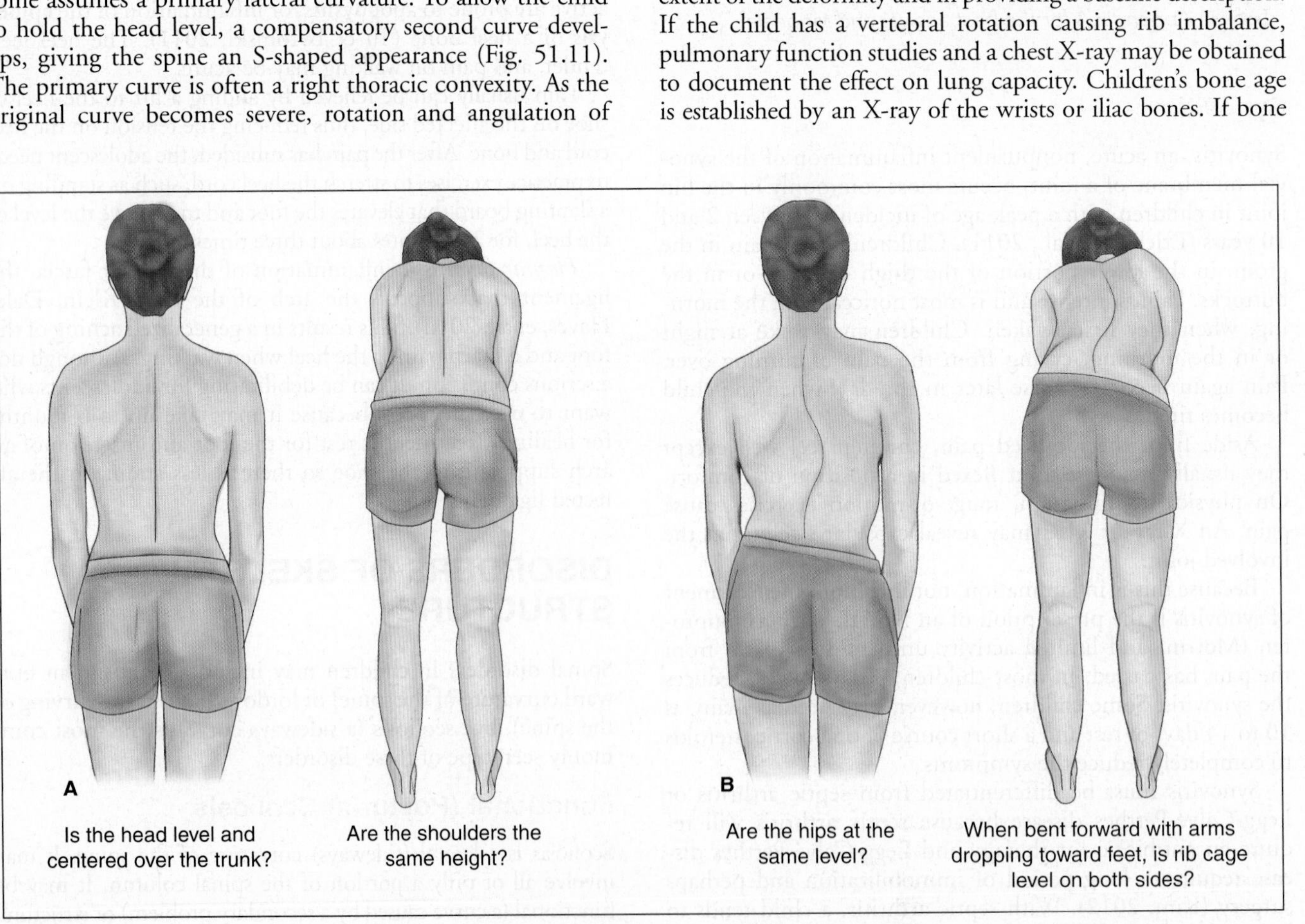

A
B
Is the head level and centered over the trunk?
Are the shoulders the same height?
Are the hips at the same level?
When bent forward with arms dropping toward feet, is rib cage level on both sides?

FIGURE 51.11 Assessing scoliosis. **(A)** Normal position and spinal curves. **(B)** Scoliosis indicators.

growth is complete or almost complete, little more deformity will result, so no correction may be necessary. If the child has 1 to 2 years of bone growth remaining, however, some correction most likely will be recommended.

Therapeutic Management

Usually, if the spinal curve is less than 20 degrees, no therapy is required except for close observation and X-rays about every 6 months until the child reaches 18 years of age. If the curve is greater than 20 degrees, treatment can consist of a conservative, nonsurgical approach using a body brace or traction; it could include surgery or a combination of both surgical and nonsurgical measures. Curves greater than 40 degrees require surgery with spinal fusion. The goal of both surgery and mechanical bracing is to maintain spinal stability and to prevent further progression of the deformity until bone growth is complete. Because of this, regardless of the type of treatment chosen, the child and family must be prepared for long-term treatment.

During prepuberty and adolescence, children tend to be very concerned about body image and so can become very impatient with scoliosis correction. Offering them a great deal of support at health care visits to help them cope can be an important nursing contribution.

Bracing. For slight spinal curves in a child who is still skeletally immature, bracing—one of the oldest forms of correction—is still a prime intervention (Weiss & Werkmann, 2012). The Milwaukee brace was the first type used for this purpose so, although today's braces look much different, they may still be referred to by this name. Originally, these braces extended to the neck and were almost impossible to conceal under clothing; today, they are underarm thoracolumbar supports (e.g., a Boston Brace) that fit under clothing (Fig. 51.12). Newer ones are designed by computer-aided techniques to ensure that the brace will be both comfortable and will accomplish maximum correction (Desbiens-Blais, Clin, Parent, et al., 2012).

The child wears the prescribed brace for 23 hours per day, removed only for showering or participation in a structured athletic program such as soccer. At night, a child may be prescribed a Charleston Bending Brace that confines the spine to an overcorrected position.

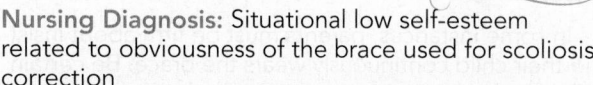

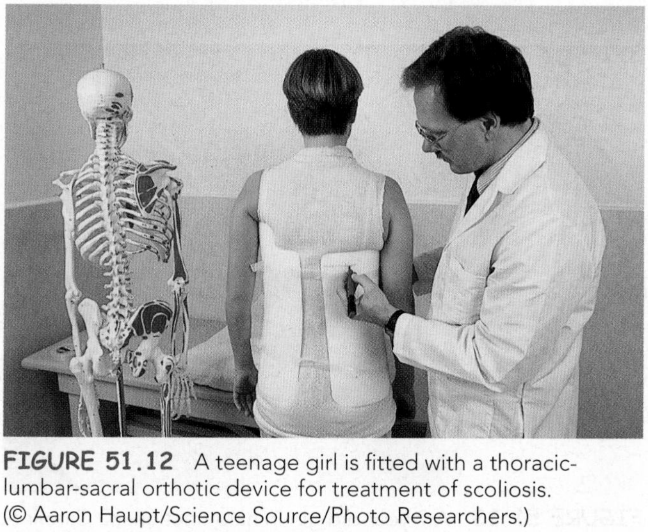

FIGURE 51.12 A teenage girl is fitted with a thoracic-lumbar-sacral orthotic device for treatment of scoliosis. (© Aaron Haupt/Science Source/Photo Researchers.)

Be certain children and parents know how to safely apply these braces. Frequent follow-up health care visits are necessary to check that the device still fits snugly without rubbing on bony prominences, such as the iliac crests. Caution children and parents not to loosen straps if rubbing occurs because this causes the brace to fit loosely, thus not allowing for it to exert adequate compression and traction. Alert parents and children to notify their health care provider instead.

Assess to be certain the child is wearing the brace over a T-shirt to prevent the plastic pads from touching skin surfaces and causing skin excoriation. During the first couple of weeks they wear a brace, children may notice slight muscle aches resulting from the new straighter back alignment. A mild analgesic such as acetaminophen (Tylenol) will decrease this discomfort in most children. Rest also provides considerable relief. Caution children not to remove the brace during this time because taking it off compounds the problem of discomfort by prolonging the period of adjustment.

Nursing Diagnoses and Related Interventions

Nursing Diagnosis: Situational low self-esteem related to obviousness of the brace used for scoliosis correction

Outcome Evaluation: Child states positive aspects of self; participates in activities; establishes friendships with peers.

Adjusting to wearing a brace may be a major problem for some children. Help them to concentrate on things they can do with the brace in place, such as having a friend over or going to the movies, rather than those things they cannot do because of the brace (e.g., playing a contact sport) (Box 51.6).

Encourage children to remain as socially active as possible. They may comment at first that they feel awkward or "so much taller" that they are afraid they will fall. However, the only way to get comfortable with a brace is to walk and get used to the new sensation of actually being a little taller. Braces may be awkward at school if chairs are attached to desks. Advocate for the child with the school nurse for seating arrangements that are comfortable.

Friends typically ask questions about why the child needs the brace. The sooner children expose the brace to friends and family, the sooner these questions cease. A brace may need adjustment about every 3 months to accomplish more alignment, and even more frequent visits may be required so children can express the problems they are having with social and school adjustment. Do not underestimate, however, an adolescent's ability to adjust to new situations. Children can see by looking in a mirror that their spine is curved, and they want this corrected. They will endure necessary discomfort if they have hope they will emerge at the end of the correction period without an obvious physical deformity.

BOX 51.6 Nursing Care Planning Based on Effective Communication

Jeffrey returns to the orthopedic clinic to be fitted with a scoliosis brace.

Less Effective Communication

Jeffrey: I can't wear anything like that!
Nurse: It is awkward, but it's not too bad. You'll see.
Jeffrey: All my friends are going to laugh at me! I'll look like a freak!
Nurse: End of conversation. You need to wear it. Otherwise, your spine will be deformed.

More Effective Communication

Jeffrey: I can't wear anything like that!
Nurse: It is awkward, but it's not too bad. You'll see.
Jeffrey: All my friends are going to laugh at me! I'll look like a freak!
Nurse: Why do you think that?
Jeffrey: How can I wear my clothes? What do I do in gym class?
Nurse: Let's talk about those things. What do you usually wear to school for a start?

In the first scenario, the nurse focuses on stressing the need for wearing the brace but fails to identify and acknowledge the adolescent's concerns about how he will look. This is easy to do because it's easy to be so intent on seeing children follow instructions that you don't ask why they feel they can't follow them. In the second scenario, the nurse recognizes the adolescent's cues about body image and self-esteem and moves to problem solving rather than demanding compliance.

In some instances, parents must be firm about insisting their child continuously wears the brace. Be certain children do not envision spinal surgery (which they will need if bracing is ineffective) as a simple and quick procedure, similar to an appendectomy, because, if they think this, they may deliberately avoid wearing the brace, hoping that surgery will then be prescribed. Do not, however, depict spinal surgery as horrible. In some children, even with conscientious bracing, the scoliosis continues to worsen and surgery will still be necessary.

Scoliosis braces are typically worn until children's spinal growth stops (at about 14.5 years of age in girls, 16.5 years in boys), as demonstrated by a spinal X-ray. The child is usually weaned from the brace gradually, because some demineralization and weakening of vertebrae may have occurred during the long period of bracing. Gradual resumption of activity and wearing the brace for a shorter period of time each day allows both remineralization and continued spinal support.

Halo Traction. Halo traction is the use of opposing forces to straighten and reduce spinal curves that are severe when first diagnosed (over 80 degrees) or that are progressing despite bracing. Halo traction is achieved using a ring of metal (a halo) held in place with about four stainless steel pins inserted into the skull bones (Koller, Zenner, Gajic, et al., 2012). Countertraction is applied by pins inserted into the distal femurs or the iliac crests (Fig. 51.13). A halo traction apparatus is bulky and looks frightening. Children can't help but worry that, when the pins are inserted into their skull (under general anesthesia), they will slip and penetrate their brain. They may worry the apparatus will be so heavy it will strain or break their neck.

Halo traction is typically used for those children who have such severe scoliosis that they experience respiratory involvement, cervical instability, have a high thoracic deformity, or decreased vital capacity from severe spinal curvature and rotation. If at all possible, children need to see photographs of the apparatus or should be able to talk to children who have the apparatus in place before having it applied. This gives them time to express their feelings about being placed in such a cumbersome device. Because it is so cumbersome, some children react to the apparatus physically, with nausea or diarrhea, or emotionally, with chronic sadness, until they realize they can adjust to it. Be certain that orientation is as thorough for the parents as it is for the child. Otherwise, parents may also show symptoms of stress for the first few days after the application of such traction. After application, parents may feel unsure and appreciate practical pointers in how to care for their child. Emphasizing positive aspects, such as what the child can do, and explaining how the traction will help the spinal curvature is helpful to allow both children and parents to accept such extreme traction.

Halo traction is prescribed for about 3 months. For the first 24 hours after application, most children experience a nagging

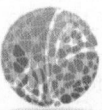

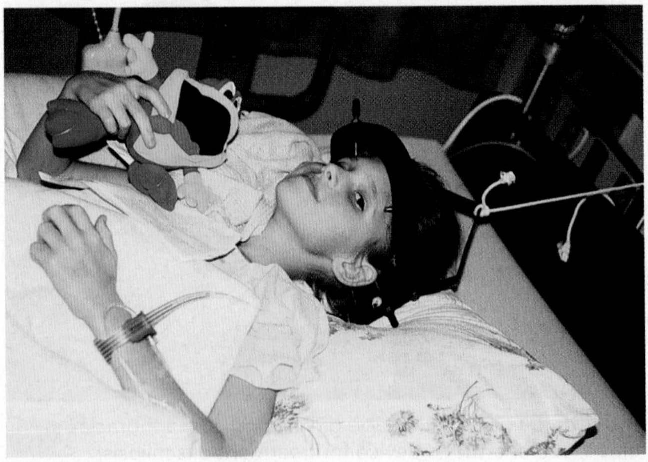

FIGURE 51.13 A 9-year-old girl in halo traction. (© Caroline Brown, RNC, MS, DEd.)

level of pain at the pin insertion sites and perhaps in their back; offer analgesia as prescribed (usually acetaminophen).

Children in halo traction need frequent care at the pin sites by washing with half-strength hydrogen peroxide or another appropriate solution to keep them clear of crusting. Encourage children to be self-sufficient and do as many things as they are able. Be certain parents have a telephone number they can call for advice or if they have questions when caring for their child at home.

After optimal spinal correction has been achieved with the device, the equipment is easily removed. The pin sites in the skull heal within 1 week without obvious scarring.

Surgical Intervention: Spinal Instrumentation. Surgical correction usually is necessary if the spinal curvature is greater than 40 degrees. Instruments such as rods and screws are placed next to the spinal column to provide firm reduction of the curvature; the spine is then fused in the corrected position (Piazzolla, Solarino, De Giorgi, et al., 2011) (Fig. 51.14A). A disadvantage of fusion is that it prevents further spinal growth, a concern that can be solved by the use of fusionless interventions such as intervertebral stapling or expandable rods (Laituri, Schwend, & Holcomb, 2012). Although this is back surgery, the surgical approach may be either from the back of the child or from the front, through the abdomen.

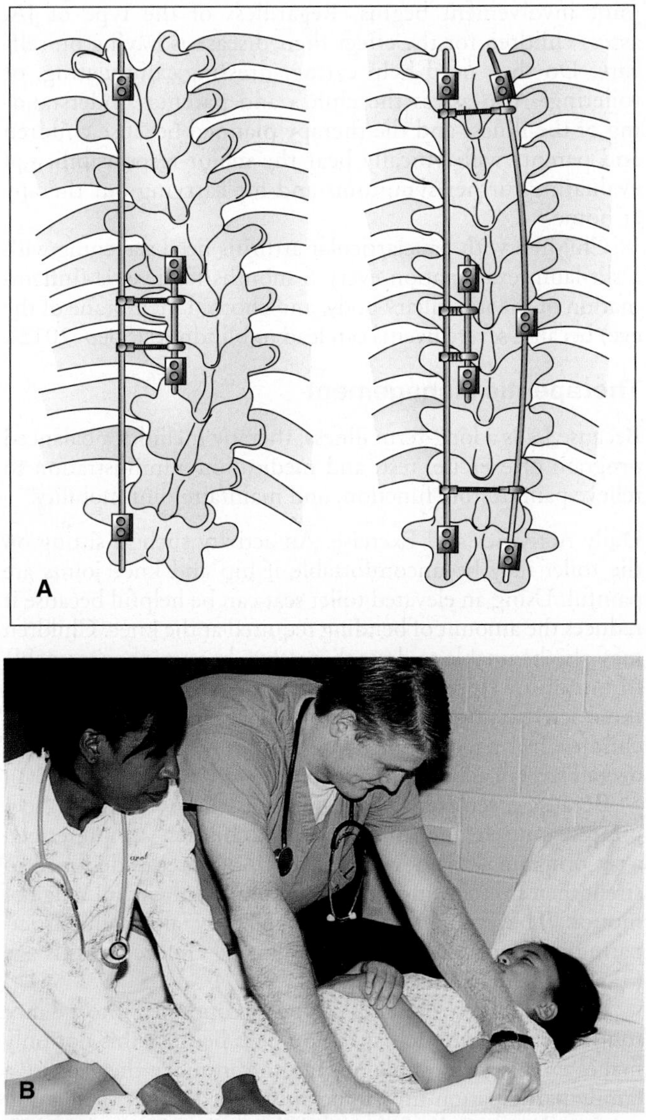

FIGURE 51.14 **(A)** Cotrel-Dubousset rods to correct scoliosis. A short distraction rod is linked to a longer one to correct the major curve. A convex rod is then applied. **(B)** Preparing to log roll. Two nurses use a draw sheet to roll the child in one coordinated movement to the side-lying position.

Preoperative Nursing Care. Before spinal instrumentation, extensive X-rays are taken to plan the exact location of rods or staples. Ensure children have a good explanation of what they can expect after surgery. Deep-breathing exercises will be particularly important for children whose scoliosis has caused chronically reduced lung capacity, so introduce these plus incentive spirometry preoperatively. A nasogastric tube usually is inserted before surgery to prevent abdominal distention because major surgery may cause temporary paralytic ileus and a lack of bowel tone. Because this surgery involves major muscle and tendon shifts, the child will have pain afterward. It is a major operation, so they can also expect to feel tired and "not themselves" for several days. Young adolescents appreciate learning about these feelings before surgery as well as appreciate being treated like adults. Be aware, however, that early adolescents are not adults, and, although they seem eager to breathe deeply and cooperate with routines before surgery, these requests can be overwhelming for them postoperatively; their behavior postoperatively may not be nearly as mature as they anticipated it would be. Epidural anesthesia offers a great deal of pain relief. Allowing children to use an IV or epidural patient-controlled analgesia system offers both pain relief and a feeling of control.

Postoperative Care. After surgery, the head of the child's bed must not be raised because once rods are in place and a spinal fusion has been done, the child's back must not be bent. Tape the latch of the bed in place or unplug electric controls so the head of the bed cannot be raised accidentally by a parent or by uninformed auxiliary personnel.

Depending on the type of rods inserted, when children return from surgery, they may not only need to lie flat but also must be logrolled (always by two people) to a side-lying position every 2 hours to enhance respiratory status (see Fig. 51.14B). Neurologic dysfunction in the legs may result from bleeding or edema compression. Perform neurovascular assessment of lower extremity function every hour for the first 24 hours by assessing the legs for warmth, whether the child can feel you touch a foot, and whether the child can wiggle his or her toes. Circulatory pressure changes resulting from realignment of the chest cage and reduced rotation of the spine may result in circulatory impairment. There is usually extensive blood loss during spinal fusion surgery, so the procedure itself or the blood loss may cause shock and hypotension. To determine these problems, assess and record vital signs frequently. A drainage system, such as a Hemovac, may be inserted next to the incision to evacuate any accumulating blood. The amount collected from this needs to be recorded.

Children are usually prescribed nothing by mouth until bowel sounds return (usually 12 to 24 hours). An indwelling urinary catheter, placed during surgery, is usually left in place for 24 hours, because voiding may be difficult in the horizontal position that must be maintained. This also allows for an assessment of kidney function.

Although a child's parents have been prepared for the fact that spinal rod insertion is major surgery, they may still be shocked by the child's appearance postsurgery. They may be afraid to touch their child at a time when the child would probably enjoy being hugged because of feeling so ill and frightened. Role model touching and talking to the child to help parents overcome their concern as quickly as possible.

As soon as bowel sounds are present, a child can begin to take fluids and then solids. Remember that a lack of exercise can result in rapid release of calcium from bones. Calcium intake should, therefore, be moderate at first rather than extensive to prevent renal calculi from forming.

By 24 to 48 hours after surgery, children are allowed out of bed to sit up, usually with a brace in place. They may feel dizzy at first; therefore, allow them to get used to sitting by attempting it for only short periods at a time at first. Activity is then increased to a normal level with few restrictions.

Because removing rods is as extensive a procedure as inserting them, instrumentation rods are left in place permanently unless they cause irritation later. The average child becomes unaware the rods are in place. Children must always be conscious of good posture, however, such as not slumping in chairs and stooping rather than bending to pick up objects from the floor. Extremely active gymnastics, football, or trampoline work is contraindicated.

Children may be afraid to move freely after rod insertion or stapling because, if they have worn a brace beforehand, they have been in some type of restraining device for a long time. They may need to be reassured frequently that, following surgery, their scoliosis finally is corrected. No further curvature can occur after this point, so it is safe for them to be without support.

Give children opportunities to talk at health care assessments about how they feel to be free of a constrictive brace. If the correction was not as complete as the child wished (children with severe scoliosis cannot expect 100% correction), they need time as well to talk about their disappointment and to adjust to their new appearance. If they believe their disorder has caused them to miss adolescence or "the best time of their lives," assure them that, now with a straightened back, the best years of their life are still to come.

What if...51.3 Jeffrey, who was diagnosed with having scoliosis, was prescribed a brace to wear 23 hours a day. During the last month, he dropped out of the school band and the one after-school club to which he belonged. He tells you he dropped these activities "to have more time to study." Would you be concerned?

DISORDERS OF THE JOINTS AND TENDONS: COLLAGEN VASCULAR DISEASE

Collagen is composed of bundles of protein-rich fibers that form the connective tissue of tendons, ligaments, and bones. Because this tissue is found throughout the body, collagen diseases are systemic. They tend to be painful, involve inflammation, and are long term.

Juvenile Rheumatoid Arthritis

JRA, also called simply juvenile arthritis (JA) or juvenile idiopathic arthritis (JIA), primarily involves the joints of the body, although it also affects blood vessels and other connective tissues (Espinosa & Gottlieb, 2012).

To be classified as JA, symptoms must begin before 16 years of age and last longer than 3 months. Although JA can occur in children as young as 6 months of age, the peak incidence times are 1 to 3 years and 8 to 12 years. It is slightly more common in girls than in boys. The acute changes of the disease rarely continue past 19 years of age.

The cause of JA is unknown, although it is thought to be an autoimmune process in which a child develops circulating antibodies (immunoglobulins) against body cells. This is revealed by the presence of antinuclear antibodies (ANA) in blood serum. A genetic predisposition may also be present and increases the risk in some children (Soep, 2012). Three separate subtypes of JA exist (Table 51.1). The three types differ mainly by the type of joint affected and in the severity of systemic effects.

Assessment

Children with systemic JA are usually brought to a health care facility because of a persistent fever and rash, symptoms that present even before the pain and stiffness of joint involvement begins. Regardless of the type of JA, assess children for the effect their disease is having on self-care. Do they need help eating, dressing, ambulating, or toileting? Also assess the child's and parents' understanding of the illness and the therapy planned because children and parents will typically bear the major responsibility of evaluating further symptoms and for carrying out therapy at home.

Children with pauciarticular arthritis need screening with a slit-lamp examination every 6 months for uveitis (inflammation of the iris, ciliary body, and choroid membrane of the eye) because severe uveitis can lead to blindness (Soep, 2012).

Therapeutic Management

Because JA is a long-term illness, therapy includes a balanced program of exercise, rest, and medication administration to relieve pain, restore function, and maintain joint mobility.

Daily Activities and Exercise. An activity such as sitting on the toilet may be uncomfortable if hip and knee joints are painful. Using an elevated toilet seat can be helpful because it reduces the amount of bending required at the knee. Children may also be unable to dress themselves because they're unable to button or zipper due to painful finger joints. Modifying these activities by using loops or Velcro strips not only helps children feel good about themselves but also increases their overall level of activity despite joint involvement (Fig. 51.12).

Because a set exercise program has the potential to help preserve muscle and joint function, children are prescribed a set program of daily range-of-motion exercises designed to strengthen muscles and put joints through their full range of motion. They can do these independently, although participating in a group is usually appealing to children at this age (Tarakci, Yeldan, Baydogan, et al., 2012).

It is best if these exercises can be incorporated into a dance routine or a game, such as Simon Says because this not only makes exercises enjoyable but it also can make the exercise a family participation time to be anticipated rather than a dull routine that must be followed daily. Swimming and tricycle or bicycle riding are excellent exercises because they provide smooth joint action. Also encourage children to do as much self-care as they can, because the natural motions of activities

TABLE 51.1 Comparing Different Types of Juvenile Arthritis

Characteristic	Polyarticular	Pauciarticular	Systemic Onset
Number of joints involved	Five or more	Four or less	Any number
Joints affected	Small joints of fingers and hands, also possibly weight-bearing joints Often same joint on both sides of body	Usually large joints, such as knees, ankle, or elbow Usually one joint on one side of body	Any joint
Gender affected	More girls than boys	More girls than boys (most common type)	Boys and girls equally
Body temperature	Low-grade fever	Low-grade fever	High spiking fever lasting for weeks or months
Other symptoms	Stiffness and minimal joint swelling, leading to limited motion Rheumatoid nodules or bumps on elbow or other body area receiving pressure from chairs, shoes, or other object (+)Rheumatoid factor (in approximately 20% of children) (+)ANA titer (possible) Elevated white blood cell count, complement, and sedimentation rate	Eye inflammation; painless joint swelling with little redness (+)ANA titer (possible) (+)HLA antigen (possible in boys)	Macular rash on chest, thighs Inflammation of heart and lungs Anemia Enlarged lymph nodes, liver, and spleen Rarely + rheumatoid factor and ANA titer Elevated white blood cell count

ANA, antinuclear antibody; HLA, human leukocyte antigen.

such as dressing and brushing teeth exercise joints. In contrast, to reduce joint destruction, activities that place excessive strain on joints, such as running, jumping, prolonged walking, and kicking, should be avoided. School-age children can cooperate to avoid these activities. Parents of preschool children need to create interesting alternative activities so the child avoids such motions.

Children should continue to attend school if at all possible because this increases activity that hopefully leads to fewer contractures and less decalcification of bones. Children with JA fatigue easily, however, so they may need a shortened school day; moving their starting time to midmorning can be a way to implement this. This late start can allow a

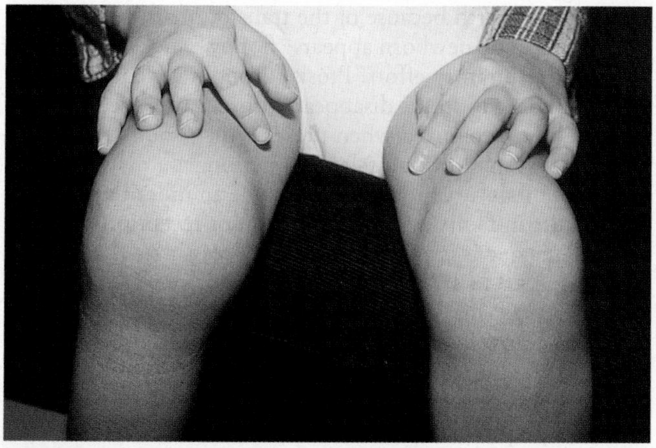

FIGURE 51.15 The knees of a child with juvenile arthritis. Note the degree of joint enlargement and swelling. (Photograph courtesy of A. I. duPont Institute, Children's Hospital, Wilmington, DE.)

child time for a warm bath in the morning, an activity that not only reduces pain but also increases movement in the involved joints.

Heat Application. Heat reduces pain and inflammation in joints and so increases comfort and motion. Heat can be applied by the use of a heating pad or warm water soaks for 20 to 30 minutes. Paraffin soaks can be useful for wrist and finger inflammation. Caution parents that young children frequently play with the controls on a heating pad, so they should tape the control to its medium temperature to help guard against burns.

Medication. NSAIDs such as ibuprofen (Motrin) or naproxen (Naprosyn) are the analgesics of choice for children with JA because they not only control pain and inflammation, thereby reducing joint swelling, joint discomfort, and morning stiffness, but they also may contribute to improvement in malaise and irritability. NSAIDs are taken about four times a day and must be taken for at least 6 to 8 weeks to ensure effectiveness.

Because taking so many NSAIDs can cause gastrointestinal upset and bleeding, be certain parents know to always give the medication with food. Most parents think of NSAIDs as a drug to give children only when they have pain. Teach that they should continue to give the drug even if the child has no noticeable pain at the time of administration because the drug's anti-inflammatory action is just as important as its pain prevention.

Slow-acting antirheumatic drugs (SAARDs), also called disease-modifying antirheumatic drugs (DMARDs), can be used if NSAIDs are ineffective. In contrast to the immediate pain relief or anti-inflammatory effect of NSAIDs, these drugs modify the natural progress of the disease over weeks to months (Beukelman, Ringold, Davis, et al., 2012).

Methotrexate, a cytotoxic drug, is the second drug usually prescribed. Steroids, such as prednisone, are only added to the drug therapy if the disease is extremely severe or is an incapacitating systemic disease that has not responded to other anti-inflammatory agents. Steroids are injected directly into the affected joint.

Newer therapies include the administration of medications called tumor necrosis factor (TNF) inhibitors such as etanercept (Enbrel) or infliximab (Remicade) (Leblanc, Lang, Bencivenga, et al., 2012). These drugs reduce inflammation by blocking the action of TNFs, which cause inflammation. Etanercept is subcutaneously injected every week, so parents need good instructions on the technique to do this as well as the importance of guarding against infections because children are more susceptible to infection than usual while taking these drugs. Infliximab is given IV and so usually requires a short-term health care facility stay for safe administration.

Nutrition. Children with JA, like those with other chronic diseases, may eat poorly because of joint pain and fatigue. Some children experience mild gastric irritation from NSAID therapy. Help parents plan mealtimes at the "best times" of the day to overcome these problems.

Nursing Diagnoses and Related Interventions

Nursing Diagnosis: Deficient knowledge related to care necessary to manage disease symptoms

Outcome Evaluation: Parents and child follow instructions regarding exercise and medication.

Help parents and children to understand the necessity for them to take an active role in therapy by planning exercise and medication programs around school or other activities. Children with JA commonly experience irritability and fatigue, which may interfere with plans. Assist them with devising a schedule that allows for a balance of rest periods with exercise to maximize the possibility of success.

Be certain at health care visits that you evaluate how well children are managing their symptoms in addition to how they view themselves (hopefully feeling well after a long period of pain and illness). The few children who develop joint contractures may require soft-tissue surgery, such as contracture release, tendon reconstruction, and synovectomy, or orthopedic surgery, such as equalization of leg length or orthoplasty, at a later date. Surgery of these types are usually delayed until growth is complete so further growth will not influence the outcome.

About half of children with JA recover at the end of adolescence. The others will continue to have the disease into adulthood. Until the disease does reach remission, children need a great deal of support to perform exercises and take daily medication as prescribed.

QSEN Checkpoint Question 51.3

Patient-Centered Care

Jeffrey's 10-year-old sister has JA and her mother is eager to explore alternative methods of pain control, in addition to standard approaches of analgesia. The standard approach to analgesia with JRA is:

a. Applying ice to painful joints to reduce inflammation
b. Having joints scraped biannually during an arthroscopy
c. Applying topical hydrocortisone to affected joints
d. Taking an NSAID on a daily basis

Look in Appendix A for the best answer and rationale.

DISORDERS OF THE SKELETAL MUSCLES

Myasthenia Gravis

For nerve conduction to cause muscles to contract effectively, a neurotransmitter, acetylcholine (ACh), must be released at synaptic junctions. The release of ACh is governed by the enzyme cholinesterase. With myasthenia gravis, there is interference in ACh processing, which leads to symptoms of progressive muscle weakness or inability to contract. The fault may be impaired synthesis or storage of ACh, insufficient ACh release, inadequate ACh receptors present at motor end plates, opposition of ACh by an anti-ACh factor, or excessive cholinesterase. In adults, the defect is probably most often a motor end plate insufficiency (a decreased number of ACh receptors are present). In children, myasthenia gravis probably occurs most often from an autoimmune process (autoantibodies may block receptor sites for ACh or other still unidentified receptors) (Cavalcante, Bernasconi, & Mantegazza, 2012).

The disease occurs in three forms in childhood: neonatal transient myasthenia, congenital myasthenia, and juvenile myasthenia.

Assessment

With neonatal transient myasthenia, the mother has myasthenia gravis and the infant demonstrates transient disease symptoms at birth because of the transfer of antibodies from the mother. The newborn appears "floppy," sucks poorly, and has weak respiratory effort. Ptosis (drooping eyelids) may be present. The symptoms disappear within 2 to 4 weeks, but if they are not recognized when present, they could prove fatal because of respiratory muscle dysfunction.

Congenital myasthenia appears to be an inherited disorder that results in faulty ACh transmission or reception. Juvenile myasthenia gravis is an autoimmune process that occurs most typically at 10 to 13 years of age and in girls more frequently than in boys. Most children with this form have thymus hypertrophy; this sign helps document the autoimmune process (Bernard, Knupp, & Yang, 2012).

With all forms, children gradually begin to develop double vision (diplopia) and ptosis because of weakness of the extraocular muscles. Symptoms grow intense as facial, neck, jaw, swallowing, and intercostal muscles become affected. Fatigue is extreme, becoming more noticeable as a day progresses.

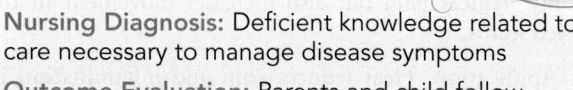

All symptoms increase with emotional stress, fatigue, menstruation, respiratory infections, and alcohol intake. In the most severe form, all muscles, including those of respiration, become unable to contract.

Obtaining an accurate history, especially documenting whether a child can perform repetitive movements, is important. Ask a child to look upward and hold that position. Children with myasthenia gravis, unlike others, will gradually demonstrate ptosis. Other repetitive motions, such as walking up stairs or clapping, may also be tested, although the time spent doing this should not be prolonged because it is tiring and does not reveal much more information. Most children have myography performed to document their poor muscle function. An MRI or a CT scan demonstrates the enlarged thymus gland.

Edrophonium (Tensilon) is a drug that prolongs the action of ACh and therefore increases muscle strength. If the child's muscle strength improves moments after an injection, the child's diagnosis is positive for myasthenia gravis (Karch, 2013).

Therapeutic Management

Myasthenia gravis is treated by the administration of neostigmine (Prostigmin) or pyridostigmine bromide (Mestinon), acetylcholinesterase inhibitors that prolong the action of ACh (Box 51.7). The dosage of these agents must be individually determined. If toxicity occurs, symptoms similar to those of the original disease occur because excessive ACh leads to continued neurotransmitter stimulation and the inability of muscles to repolarize for a new contraction. In some children, prednisone or an immunosuppressant such as azathioprine may be added to their medication regimen to decrease the amount of anticholinesterase medication required. In still others, plasmapheresis to remove immune complexes from the bloodstream or the administration of IV immunoglobulin to provide immune suppression will reduce symptoms (Weeks, 2012).

Excision of the thymus gland may also effectively reduce symptoms, although this is a last resort because it may leave the child open to additional autoimmune disorders in the future.

Teach parents and children that symptoms become worse under stress; therefore, parents need to adequately prepare children for new experiences such as menstruation, high school, a parental divorce, or surgery in order to minimize stress. Help children plan their day to include rest periods, possibly advocating for a special school schedule if necessary. If chewing and swallowing are difficult, ensure a rest period before meals. Even so, children may need to take their medication about an hour before mealtime, eat a soft diet, and learn to eat slowly and cautiously to avoid choking and aspiration. If symptoms of muscle weakness suddenly become very severe, parents should call 911 because the loss of function of intercostal muscles may lead to respiratory arrest. Atropine, an anticholinergic agent and the antidote for an overdose of anticholinesterase drugs, should be available to administer as necessary both for parents at home and on a hospital unit that cares for children with this disease.

Dermatomyositis

Dermatomyositis occurs from the degeneration of skeletal muscle fibers. The cause of the disorder is unknown, although either a viral infection or an autoimmune basis is suspected. It is more common in girls than in boys and occurs between the ages of 5 and 14 years (Soep, 2012).

Symptoms usually begin insidiously, with muscle weakness that presents with difficulty in swallowing or that prevents children from performing tasks they could manage previously, such as competing in gym classes, lifting objects,

BOX 51.7 Nursing Care Planning Based on Responsibility for Pharmacology

NEOSTIGMINE (PROSTIGMIN)

Classification: Neostigmine is a cholinesterase inhibitor that acts as an antimyasthenic agent.

Action: Neostigmine increases the concentration of acetylcholine at nerve endings, prolonging and exaggerating its effects and facilitating neuromuscular transmission (Karch, 2013).

Pregnancy Risk Category: C

Dosage: Orally, 2 mg/kg daily in divided doses every 3 to 4 hours; or 0.01 to 0.04 mg/kg per dose intramuscularly, intravenously, or subcutaneously every 2 to 3 hours, as needed

Possible Adverse Effects: Salivation, dysphagia, increased peristalsis, cardiac arrhythmias, increased respiratory secretions, urinary frequency, pupil constriction, and diaphoresis

Nursing Implications

- Assess the child for increased muscle weakness, indicating possible cholinergic crisis. Keep atropine sulfate readily available as the antidote.
- If giving neostigmine orally, administer the drug with food or milk to minimize gastrointestinal upset. Instruct parents to administer the drug exactly as prescribed.
- Plan to administer larger portions of the divided doses approximately one half hour before anticipated times of greater fatigue.
- Advise parents to watch for signs of excessive salivation, emesis, or frequent urination and to notify their health care provider if these occur.
- Encourage parents to control the child's environmental temperature as much as possible to prevent diaphoresis from too hot or too humid an environment.
- Inform parents an increase in muscle weakness may be related to either drug overdose or exacerbation of the disease. Urge them to report any signs of increased weakness to their health care provider immediately.

or climbing onto a high stool. Skin symptoms such as swollen and discolored upper eyelids, a confluent rash on the cheeks that increases to become telangiectatic, and scaling begin to develop. Subcutaneous calcifications may appear, making the skin feel unusually firm. Muscle breakdown leads to the appearance of creatine phosphokinase and aldolase in the serum. A muscle biopsy or electromyography reveals a lack of electrical activity in muscle fibers.

High-dose corticosteroids, methotrexate, or specific immunosuppressants are the drugs of choice to improve muscle strength. Children who survive beyond the first year after diagnosis have a good prognosis for prolonged remissions, although they are more susceptible to developing cancer later in life.

The Muscular Dystrophies

Muscular dystrophies are a group of inherited disorders that lead to the progressive degeneration of skeletal muscles, apparently caused by a defective gene for dystrophin (a protein in the muscles) that is necessary for muscle contraction (Lewis, 2011).

Types

Muscular dystrophies seen in children are classified into three main types: congenital myotonic dystrophy, facioscapulohumeral muscular dystrophy, and pseudohypertrophic muscular dystrophy (Duchenne disease).

Congenital Myotonic Dystrophy. Congenital myotonic dystrophy is inherited as an autosomal dominant trait. Because the disease process begins in utero, the infant may already have severe myotonia (muscle weakness) at birth. Muscle degeneration continues until adequate respiratory muscle movement becomes difficult. Diagnosis is by serum enzyme analysis and muscle biopsy. Most of these infants die before they are 1 year old because they cannot sustain respiratory function.

Facioscapulohumeral Muscular Dystrophy. Facioscapulohumeral muscular dystrophy is inherited as a dominant trait, carried on chromosome 4. Symptoms begin after the child is 10 years old. The predominant symptom is facial weakness. The child becomes unable to wrinkle the forehead and cannot whistle. Serum enzyme analysis and muscle biopsy are used in diagnosis. The symptoms usually progress so slowly a normal life span is possible.

Pseudohypertrophic Muscular Dystrophy (Duchenne Disease). Duchenne disease, the most common form of muscular dystrophy, is inherited as a sex-linked recessive trait. Therefore, it occurs only in boys although a mother who carries the gene may demonstrate some symptoms. Symptoms are usually apparent by 3 years of age.

Assessment

Children with Duchenne muscular dystrophy usually have a history of meeting motor milestones, such as sitting, walking, and standing, but they reach these milestones later than does the average infant. By about 3 years of age, symptoms become acute and obvious as boys develop a waddling gait and have difficulty climbing stairs. They can rise from the floor only by rolling onto their stomachs and then pushing themselves to their knees. To stand, they press their hands against their ankles, knees, and thighs (they "walk up their front"), called a Gower sign. They may walk on their toes, which leads to the development of a short heel cord. Speech and swallowing become difficult. It may be awkward to lift a young child with this condition by placing your hands under the axillae because the child seems to slip through your hands due to the lax shoulder muscles. In contrast, calf muscles are hypertrophied (measure larger than normal) because the muscles become so degenerated they are replaced by fat and connective tissue.

As the disease progresses, muscle weakness becomes more and more pronounced. Scoliosis of the spine and fractures of long bones may occur from abnormal muscle tension and lack of muscle support. By junior high school age, most boys become wheelchair dependent. Tachycardia can occur as the heart muscle weakens and enlarges. Pneumonia develops easily as the child's cough reflex becomes weak and ineffective. Death from pulmonary dysfunction tends to occur at about 20 years of age (Polat, Sakinci, Ersoy, et al., 2012).

The diagnosis is based on the history and physical findings, a muscle biopsy showing fibrous degeneration and fatty deposits, electromyography showing a decrease in amplitude and duration of motor unit potentials, an increased concentration of serum creatine phosphokinase, and genetic analysis.

Therapeutic Management

Encourage boys with muscular dystrophy to remain ambulatory for as long as possible by a program of active and passive daily range-of-motion exercises. Splinting and bracing may be necessary to maintain lower extremity stability and to avoid contractures. If children become overweight, remaining ambulatory becomes even more difficult for them. Therefore, encourage a low-calorie, high-protein diet to avoid excessive weight gain. In addition, to prevent constipation because of poor abdominal muscle tone, encourage a high intake of fiber and fluids. Advocate for a stool softener if necessary. Drugs or enzymes to help activate dystrophin are being investigated (Abdel-Hamid & Clemens, 2012). In the meantime, corticosteroid therapy is helpful to increase function and strength at least on a short-term basis; be certain parents understand the importance of this and have a set schedule of administration. In the future, stem cell therapy is a strong possibility (Tedesco & Cossu, 2012).

Because the disease is progressive, assist the child and family with achieving the optimal level of activity within the child's limitations. Provide support for parents to assist them with coping because they can become depressed as disease symptoms progress.

QSEN Checkpoint Question 51.4

Quality Improvement

Jeffrey's mother said she was worried her son might be developing muscular dystrophy. A clinical care map for children who have this disease should prioritize which action?

a. Urging them to rest most of the day to avoid systemic fatigue
b. Helping them to avoid weight gain so they can be mobile longer
c. Cautioning them not to eat foods that contain purines
d. Encouraging a diet rich in calcium to prevent osteoporosis

Look in Appendix A for the best answer and rationale.

Fractures

A **fracture** is a break in the continuity or structure of bone. Because children experience falls during their growth years, fractures of long bones are common childhood injuries (Swenson, Henke, Collins, et al., 2012). Various types are described in Table 51.2. Fractures in children tend to be different than in adults because:

- Bone in childhood is fairly porous, allowing bones to bend rather than break.
- The periosteum is thick, so the bone may not break all the way through.
- Epiphyseal lines may cushion a blow so that the bone does not break.
- Healing is rapid as a result of overall increased bone growth.

Because of the high resilience of immature bone, many fractures in early childhood are the greenstick variety (one side of a bone is broken; the other is only bent). These fractures cause minimal pain, swelling, or deformity, the usual hallmarks of a fracture.

Many fractures in children, however, occur at the epiphyseal line. These are always serious because bone growth occurs at this point. Damage to the area can lead to undergrowth, overgrowth, or uneven growth, resulting in angulation. If a fall occurred from a high distance or was caused by a violent force, such as a speeding automobile, breaks may be complex, or the formation may be compounded (the bone pierces the skin) or comminuted (parts of the bone are fragmented). These injuries are always serious because the severed bone may lacerate nerves or blood vessels. The open wound may become infected, and correction will most likely involve surgery with the risks of anesthesia.

The healing of bone is relatively slow compared with other body injuries. Immediately after a fracture, a hematoma forms at the site of the break; over the next several days, granulation tissue is laid down. Over the next several weeks, osteoblasts invade this new tissue, and calcium is deposited (termed *callus*) to form new bone. By the time a callus formation is extensive (enough for movement at the fracture site to be impossible), clinical healing or clinical union has occurred. Complete healing does not occur until all of the temporary callus formation has been replaced by mature bone cells and the bone has once more regained its normal shape and contour.

Several complications may occur during this process. One is fat embolus, which is the release of fat from the marrow of the broken bone into the bloodstream. This embolus then travels to the cerebral vessels and causes symptoms such as confusion or hallucinations as the oxygen supply to brain cells is shut off. It also could become a pulmonary embolus, producing dyspnea, tachycardia, and cyanosis. A second problem that can occur is *compartment syndrome*, which was discussed previously (Najarian, 2013).

If there is a great deal of edema present in the injured part, a cast may not be applied immediately but contained in a splint to avoid compartment syndrome. If the growth plate was involved in the injury, some children may need bone-lengthening or bone-shortening procedures later in life to assure equal and adequate bone growth.

TABLE 51.2 Common Fractures in Children

Type of Fracture	Description
Plastic deformation (bend) 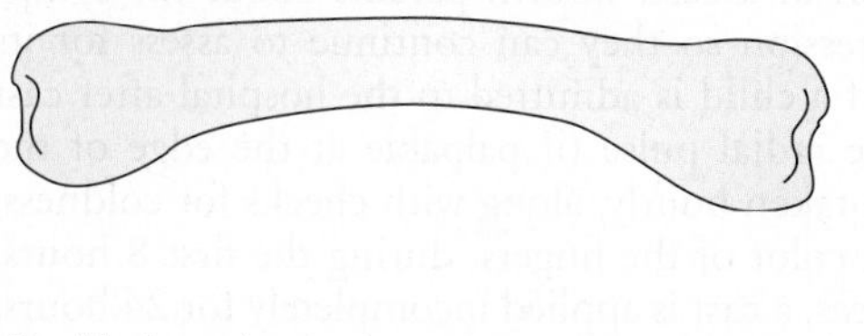	Bone bends, causing a microscopic fracture line that does not cross the bone; most common in the ulna and fibula
Buckle (torus) 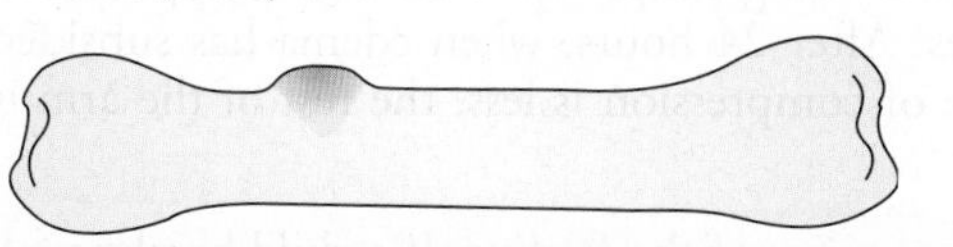	Fracture on the tension side of the bone near softened metaphyseal bone, causing a buckling and raised area on the harder diaphyseal bone (opposite side)
Greenstick 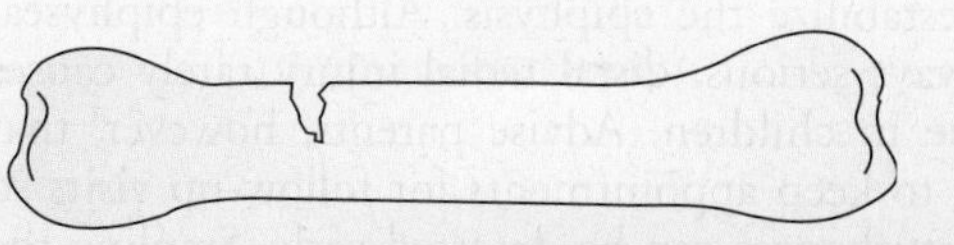	Bone bent with fracture beginning but not crossing through the bone
Complete 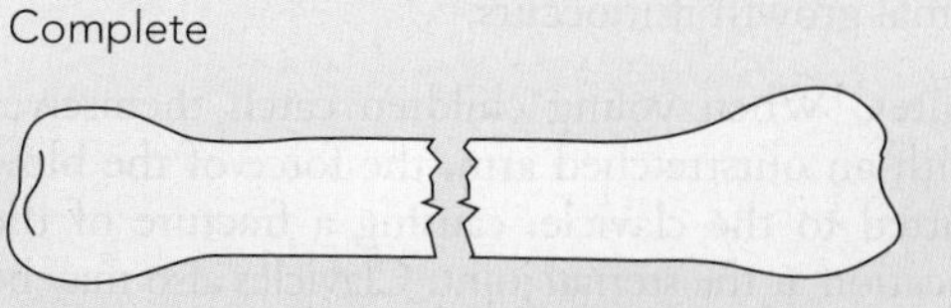	Bone divided (either transversely [crosswise at right angle to long axis of bone], obliquely [slanted but straight], or spirally [slanted and circular]); bone remnants possibly attached by a periosteal hinge

Assessment

When children are seen in an emergency department for multiple trauma, observe the extremities closely for the hallmark signs of fracture (deformity, edema, and pain). If you do suspect a fracture, splint the extremity to avoid further trauma. Splinting also reduces pain because it prevents further movement of the bone. Splints should extend from a joint above to a joint below the suspected fracture site to prevent movement and muscle tension, which could cause further dislocation of the fracture. For example, for a fracture of the forearm, the splint should reach from above the elbow to below the wrist. If an extremity is so seriously deformed by the break that it will not conform to the contour of a splint, do not attempt to move it into a splint position. Immobilize the extremity by placing sandbags on the sides of the arm or leg and leave it in that position.

Be certain you have a thorough history of how the fracture occurred. Some fractures in childhood occur from child maltreatment. This must be ruled out for all unintentional injuries.

Therapeutic Management

All children with a suspected fracture need an X-ray to confirm the diagnosis and to determine the alignment and **apposition** (the amount of end-to-end contact there is of the bone fragments). Apposition is not as important in children as it is in adults, so bayonet or side-to-side apposition may be established for children up to 10 or 12 years old. With this, as the child grows and remodeling occurs, the bone will develop with normal contour and length. Side-to-side apposition has the advantage of allowing for a rapid, strong union and actually is the preferred position for some fractures.

If skin over the fracture site has been broken, the child may need tetanus prophylaxis. A hematocrit determination to estimate blood loss and cross-matching for replacement therapy may be necessary. An IV line may be established to provide a route for fluid or blood replacement or for the administration of an IV antibiotic to reduce the possibility of infection through the open wound.

All children with fractures are in some pain. Usually, they are frightened not only from the pain, the appearance of the fracture, and their inability to use the extremity but also from the frightening situation that led to the fracture such as a fall from a bunk bed or an automobile accident. Spend time comforting and helping children to realize they are now safe and will not be injured further. If they can relax enough to lie still and not move the fractured extremity, the pain will decrease. Reassure both children and parents that, unless the bone has been crushed, bone fragments can be brought back into line, allowing the break to heal with the same strength as before.

Types of Fractures

Forearm Fractures. Because children often fall on an outstretched arm, fractures of the forearm are a common type. Most forearm fractures in children involve the distal third; a smaller number of such accidents occur in the middle or proximal third. Only the radius, both the radius and ulna, or a displacement of the epiphyseal plate of the radius may be involved. In young children, the injury usually is a greenstick or an incomplete fracture.

If a greenstick fracture is slight so that the degree of angulation is not great, it may not be reduced or brought into a straight line; as callus is formed and the bone remodels itself, it will naturally straighten into good alignment. Sometimes greenstick fractures are broken completely before casting to prevent the bone's resuming its "bent" position within the cast. Refer to this as "straightening" the bone, rather than "breaking" the bone so it sounds less frightening.

If the fracture is complete and overriding is excessive, traction to the fingers may be used as a part of the cast. This "banjo" traction is cumbersome and limits the child's use of that hand. You may need to reassure parents that, although the cast is more cumbersome than they anticipated, their child will be able to manage it well with a little practice.

Elbow Fractures. If a child falls and stops the fall with a hand, the elbow may hyperextend, transmitting the force of the blow to the distal humerus and causing a supracondylar fracture of the humerus. Fractures of this kind are reduced and stabilized with an arm cast, a splint, traction, or open surgery depending on the position of the fracture (Yaokreh, Gicquel, Schneider, et al., 2012). Elevating the cast on pillows or suspending the hand by a strip of gauze or traction apparatus reduces edema. Although the fracture may be minor, the child needs to be assessed carefully for signs of blood vessel or nerve compression (Volkmann contracture).

Volkmann Ischemic Contracture. When an arm is flexed and put into a cast, the radial artery and nerve can be compressed at the elbow, causing nerve injury or severe impairment of circulation. If symptoms of compression are present but not detected within 6 hours, Volkmann contracture and possible permanent damage to the arm will result. The arm is left permanently flexed at the elbow. The wrist is hyperextended, and the fingers assume a flexed, clawlike, and useless position. If a child is going to be discharged from a health care facility after application of a cast, inform parents about the symptoms of compression so they can continue to assess for its development. If a child is admitted to the hospital after cast application, the radial pulse (if palpable at the edge of the cast) should be taken hourly, along with checks for coldness, blanching, and color of the fingers, during the first 8 hours. In some instances, a cast is applied incompletely for 24 hours, the elbow portion being simply splinted and wrapped with elastic bandages. After 24 hours, when edema has subsided and the chance of compression is less, the rest of the arm is then casted.

Epiphyseal Separations of the Radius. If a child breaks a fall with an outstretched arm, the separation of the epiphysis of the distal radius may result. When this occurs, the wrist must be casted to restabilize the epiphysis. Although epiphyseal injuries are always serious, distal radial injury rarely causes serious sequelae in children. Advise parents, however, that it is important to keep appointments for follow-up visits so that growth disturbances can be detected early. Stapling the epiphysis or stimulation of the epiphyseal line may be done to arrest abnormal growth if it occurs.

Clavicle Fractures. When young children catch themselves during a fall with an outstretched arm, the force of the blow can be transmitted to the clavicle, causing a fracture of the clavicle or dislocation at the sternal joint. Clavicles also may be

QSEN Checkpoint Question 51.5

Teamwork & Collaboration

You are collaborating with a licensed practical nurse in the care of a child with an elbow cast. What information about an elbow cast would you want all of your care team members to be aware of?

a. The cast must be constructed from fiberglass, not plaster of Paris.
b. Edema at the elbow from a too tight cast can cause severe nerve damage.
c. The child should expect to have low-grade pain following application.
d. These casts often get dirty and so lead to humeral osteomyelitis.

Look in Appendix A for the best answer and rationale.

fractured during birth and are often fractured playing football. These fractures need to be evaluated carefully because they also could be a mark of child maltreatment.

Swelling is often present at the site of the break. In the newborn, a Moro reflex can only be demonstrated on the unaffected side. An older child refuses to use the arm, leaving it hanging at the side. Crepitus (crackling) can be felt over the clavicle. After an X-ray diagnosis, if the bone fragments are not displaced, the child is placed in a commercially manufactured or figure-of-eight splint or stockinette placed over the shoulders and under the axilla, which keeps the arm adducted and flexed across the chest. Caution the parents to keep the splint dry—no swimming or showering during this time—and how to observe it every morning to be certain it is firmly in place or if it needs tightening. Because the splint is left in place for about 3 weeks, the wrap becomes extremely soiled. Parents are usually apologetic about the appearance of the splint when they return for a repeat X-ray. They may be worried the soiled appearance of the splint reflects the quality of their housekeeping or child care. You can assure them that a soiled appearance is expected and proof they followed instructions well to leave the splint in place.

Some parents may need reassurance that a simple splint is adequate therapy. Acknowledge their concern but also assure them that treatment for nondisplaced broken clavicles are the exception to the usual fracture treatment. If the parts of the clavicle are misplaced, especially in adolescents, open surgery can be used to stabilize the bone and assure firm healing (Pandya, Namdari, & Hosalkar, 2012).

Dislocation of the Radial Head. If a small child is lifted by one hand, as happens when a parent pulls on one arm to lift the child over a curb or up a step, the head of the radius may escape the ligament surrounding it and become dislocated (nursemaid's elbow) (Rudloe, Schutzman, Lee, et al., 2012). The child holds the arm flexed at the elbow with the forearm pronated. The child winces with pain when the radial head is palpated.

A simple dislocation of the radial head can be reduced in an emergency room by gentle pressure on the radial head while the arm is flexed and supinated. Relief of pain is immediate, and the child begins to use the arm again.

Parents feel guilty because they caused this dislocation. You can reassure them that this is a common injury in small children, but that they need to avoid lifting their child in this manner again. Be aware, however, that a dislocation of the radial head can occur from extremely rough handling, as is seen in child maltreatment. Investigate the circumstances of the injury closely (Cicero, 2013).

QSEN Checkpoint Question 51.6

Evidence-Based Practice

Young children frequently sustain dislocation of the radial head at the elbow when a parent or caregiver lifts them by an arm. To discover what are the most frequent activities that cause this, researchers studied the records of 2,011 children seen at an urban tertiary care emergency department for this type of traction injury. The median age of children was 2.1 years; 59% of them were female. Activities that most frequently led to the traction and dislocation were lifting the child by the arms (28.3%), "wrestling" (12.3%), swinging the child by the arms (9.2%), and placing the child into and out of a seat (4.3%). Male caregivers were more likely to be involved when a child was swung by the arms, lifted, or "wrestled" with. Injury tended to most often happen with female caregivers when the child pulled away, tripped, or was in the process of getting dressed (Rudloe et al., 2012).

Based on the previous study, which activity would you advise Jeffrey not to do with his preschool sister?

a. Swinging her by the arms to make her laugh
b. Encouraging her to practice hip hop dancing
c. Helping her to fly her kite on a windy afternoon
d. Helping her take off a tight sweater or shirt

Look in Appendix A for the best answer and rationale.

Fracture of the Femur. Children who are involved in automobile accidents or who fall from considerable heights and land on their feet may suffer a fractured femur. Child maltreatment should be considered in an infant who sustains a fractured femur because there are few normal instances when a fracture of this magnitude should occur in an infant. That the break was caused by the presence of a bone malignancy (see Chapter 53) is a third possibility (Norvell, 2012).

Even with closed femoral fractures, blood loss can be extensive because of the size of the bone broken. As the child lies on the examining table in the emergency department, the child tends to hold the leg externally rotated and the thigh may appear abnormally short or deformed. Often, the child is in a great deal of pain, possibly with signs of shock from pain and blood loss. Children are frightened as well by the force of the accident that caused such a severe injury.

In the past, fractured femurs were not casted immediately because strong tendon spasms cause poor alignment and overriding of the femur segments. Only after the muscle spasm had been reduced enough by skeletal or Bryant traction to allow close approximation of the bone edges (7 to 14 days) was the child removed from traction and placed in a hip spica cast. Today, a child may be taken to surgery immediately to have an intramedullary rod placed to align and stabilize the fracture. No cast may be required. Help children and families identify ways for children to continue contact with friends or enjoy usual activities during the time of restricted activity.

What if... 51.4 You are particularly interested in exploring one of the 2020 National Health Goals with respect to musculoskeletal disorders and children (see Box 51.1). What would be a possible research topic to explore pertinent to this goal that would be applicable to Jeffrey's family and that would also advance evidence-based practice?

Key Points for Review

- Bone and muscle disorders tend to be long-term disorders. Help children and their families to think about how the disorder will affect tasks of daily living to help a child better adjust to interventions such as a cast or brace. Help children plan self-diversional activities as necessary so they can continue to grow developmentally while confined to a cast or traction.
- As a rule, children with a broken bone need additional calcium in their diet to aid bone healing. If they are on strict bed rest, however, this should only be a moderate addition to their diet to prevent renal calculi from forming.
- Many children have casts applied to allow broken bones to heal. If broken bones cannot be easily aligned, children are placed in traction.
- Developmental disorders that occur in children include flat feet (pronation), genu varum (bowlegs), and genu valgum (knock knees). The majority of these disorders are corrected naturally by normal growth.
- Slipped capital epiphysis is the slipping of the femur head in relation to the neck of the femur at the epiphyseal line. It occurs most frequently in obese or rapidly growing boys. It may require surgery or possibly a total hip replacement for treatment.
- Osteomyelitis is an infection of the bone. Because it can result in extensive destruction of bone, both IV and oral antibiotic therapy is necessary.
- Scoliosis is a lateral curvature of the spine. It is treated by bracing or surgery.
- JRA occurs in several different forms: polyarticular, pauciarticular, and systemic onset. Therapy includes exercise, heat application, and the administration of medications such as NSAIDs or methotrexate. Stressing the importance of these measures helps in planning nursing care that not only meets QSEN competencies but that also best meets a family's total needs.
- Myasthenia gravis can occur in three types: neonatal transient myasthenia, congenital myasthenia, and juvenile myasthenia. Anticholinesterase drugs such as neostigmine, which prolong ACh action, are used.
- Muscular dystrophies are a group of disorders that lead to progressive degeneration of skeletal muscles. Common types that occur in children include congenital myotonic, facioscapulohumeral, and pseudohypertrophic. Children and parents need support throughout this long-term illness.
- A fracture or bruise of soft tissue can result from any trauma, including child maltreatment. Be certain to secure a detailed history of all injuries to be certain the history is consistent with the degree of injury.
- Volkmann ischemic contracture is a complication that occurs when an arm is casted in a bent position, which causes the radial artery and nerve to become compressed at the elbow. Frequent assessments of finger color and warmth are safeguards to detect if this is occurring when an arm cast is in place.

Critical Thinking Care Study

Bonnie Sue is a 12-year-old who is discovered to have scoliosis during a routine school nurse assessment. She lives with her mother and stepfather on her family's dairy farm. Her chores include helping with milking two times a day and keeping her own room clean. Her mother had "slight scoliosis" as a teenager, which didn't require treatment.

1. Bonnie's mother is concerned that her daughter developed scoliosis because she insists on wearing sneakers, plus she doesn't get enough exercise because she rides a bus to school. Could these factors have contributed to the development of her scoliosis?
2. Bonnie is fitted with a spinal brace. When you see her at a return appointment, her mother tells you Bonnie has to take the brace off at night to be able to sleep and sometimes during the day because it gets too hot. What further health teaching does this family need?
3. When you ask if Bonnie Sue drinks milk daily, her mother answers, "We live on a dairy farm. What do you think?" When you ask if Bonnie Sue is able to do her usual chores, her stepfather answers, "Well, she doesn't help with milking anymore." Could you be certain from these answers that Bonnie Sue is receiving a good source of calcium necessary for strong bone growth and is adjusting well to wearing her brace?

Patient Scenario:
The Cardiff Family

Read about the Cardiff family, a family with a child with a musculoskeletal disorder, then answer the questions to further sharpen your skills and grow more familiar with NCLEX-type questions related to musculoskeletal disorders. Confirm your answers are correct by reading the rationales.

Visit http://thePoint.lww.com

Answers and Rationales

Looking for answers to the What if . . . and Critical Thinking Care Study questions?

Visit http://thePoint.lww.com

References

Abdel-Hamid, H., & Clemens, P. R. (2012). Pharmacological therapies for muscular dystrophies. *Current Opinion in Neurology, 25*(5), 604–608.

Bazner-Chandler, J., & Brady, M. A. (2013). Musculoskeletal disorders. In E. E. Burns & A. M. Dunn (Eds.), *Pediatric primary care* (5th ed., pp. 928–960). Philadelphia, PA: Elsevier/Saunders.

Bernard, T. J., Knupp, K., & Yang, M. L. (2012). Neurologic & muscular disorders. In W. Hay, M. Levin, R. Deterding, et al. (Eds.), *Current diagnosis & treatment pediatrics* (21st ed., pp. 740–829). New York, NY: McGraw-Hill/Lange.

Beukelman, T., Ringold, S., Davis, T. E., et al. (2012). Disease-modifying antirheumatic drug use in the treatment of juvenile idiopathic arthritis: A cross-sectional analysis of the CARRA registry. *Journal of Rheumatology, 39*(9), 1867–1874.

Browne, L. P., Guillerman, R. P., Orth, R. C., et al. (2012). Community-acquired staphylococcal musculoskeletal infection in infants and young children. *AJR: American Journal of Roentgenology, 198*(1), 194–199.

Cavalcante, P., Bernasconi, P., & Mantegazza, R. (2012). Autoimmune mechanisms in myasthenia gravis. *Current Opinion in Neurology, 25*(5), 621–629.

Cicero, M. X. (2013). Musculoskeletal injuries. In D. Cline & O. J. Ma (Eds.), *Tintinalli's emergency medicine* (pp. 287–293). New York, NY: McGraw-Hill.

Chouinard, L. E., Randall Simpson, J., & Buchholz, A. C. (2012). Predictors of bone mineral density in a convenience sample of young Caucasian adults living in southern Ontario. *Applied Physiology, Nutrition, & Metabolism, 37*(4), 706–714.

Copley, L. A., Kinsler, M. A., Gheen, T., et al. (2013). The impact of evidence-based clinical practice guidelines applied by a multidisciplinary team for the care of children with osteomyelitis. *Journal of Bone & Joint Surgery American, 95*(8), 686–693.

D'Amico, M., Roncoletta, P., Di Felice, F., et al. (2012). Leg length discrepancy in scoliotic patients. *Studies in Health Technology & Information, 176*(1), 146–150.

Dartnell, J., Ramachandran, M., & Katchburian, M. (2012). Haematogenous acute and subacute paediatric osteomyelitis: A systematic review of the literature. *Journal of Bone & Joint Surgery, 94*(5), 584–595.

Desbiens-Blais, F., Clin, J., Parent, S., et al. (2012). New brace design combining CAD/CAM and biomechanical simulation for the treatment of adolescent idiopathic scoliosis. *Clinical Biomechanics, 27*(10), 999–1005.

Dobrindt, O., Hoffmeyer, B., Ruf, J., et al. (2012). Estimation of return-to-sports-time for athletes with stress fracture - an approach combining risk level of fracture site with severity based on imaging. *BMC Musculoskeletal Disorders, 13*(1), 139.

Erickson, M. A., Merritt, B. S., & Polousky, J. D. (2011). Orthopedics. In W. Hay, M. Levin, R. Deterding, et al. (Eds.), *Current diagnosis & treatment pediatrics* (21st ed., pp. 830–848). New York, NY: McGraw-Hill/Lange.

Espinosa, M., & Gottlieb, B. S. (2012). Juvenile idiopathic arthritis. *Pediatrics in Review, 33*(7), 303–313.

Gettys, F. K., Jackson, J. B., & Frick, S. L. (2011). Obesity in pediatric orthopaedics. *Orthopedic Clinics of North America, 42*(1), 95–105.

Hellmann, D. B., & Imboden, J. B., Jr. (2012). Musculoskeletal & immunological disorders. In S. J. McPhee & M. Papadakis (Eds.), *Current medical diagnosis & treatment* (51st ed., pp. 787–847). New York, NY: McGraw-Hill Publishing.

Jeong, H. J., Lee, S. H., & Ko, C. S. (2012). Meniscectomy. *Knee Surgery & Related Research, 24*(3), 129–136.

Karch, A. M. (2013). *2013 Lippincott's nursing drug guide.* Philadelphia, PA: Lippincott Williams & Wilkins.

Kaya, D. O., Toprak, U., Baltaci, G., et al. (2012). Long-term functional and sonographic outcomes in Osgood-Schlatter disease. *Knee Surgery, Sports Traumatology, Arthroscopy, 21*(5), 1131–1139.

Kim, H. K. (2012). Pathophysiology and new strategies for the treatment of Legg-Calvé-Perthes disease. *Journal of Bone & Joint Surgery, 94*(7), 659–669.

Klein, S. E., Dale, A. M., Hayes, M. H., et al. (2012). Clinical presentation and self-reported patterns of pain and function in patients with plantar heel pain. *Foot & Ankle International, 33*(9), 693–698.

Koller, H., Zenner, J., Gajic, V., et al. (2012). The impact of halo-gravity traction on curve rigidity and pulmonary function in the treatment of severe and rigid scoliosis and kyphoscoliosis. *European Spine Journal, 21*(3), 514–529.

Kotagal, S. (2012). Treatment of dyssomnias and parasomnias in childhood. *Current Treatment Options in Neurology, 14*(6), 630–649.

Laituri, C. A., Schwend, R. M., & Holcomb, G. W. (2012). Thoracoscopic vertebral body stapling for treatment of scoliosis in young children. *Journal of Laparoendoscopy & Advanced Surgical Techniques, 22*(8), 830–833.

Leblanc, C. M., Lang, B., Bencivenga, A., et al. (2012). Access to biologic therapies in Canada for children with juvenile idiopathic arthritis. *Journal of Rheumatology, 39*(9), 1875–1879.

Lewis, S. W. (2011). Neurology. In K. J. Marcdante, R. M. Kliegman, H. B. Jenson, et al. (Eds.), *Nelson essentials of pediatrics* (6th ed., pp. 671–709). Philadelphia, PA: Saunders/Elsevier.

Loder, R. T., & Dietz, F. R. (2012). What is the best evidence for the treatment of slipped capital femoral epiphysis? *Journal of Pediatric Orthopedics, 32*(Suppl. 2), S158–S165.

Maffulli, N., Longo, U. G., Spiezia, F., et al. (2011). Aetiology and prevention of injuries in elite young athletes. *Medicine & Sport Science, 56*(2), 187–200.

Magee, J. A., Kenney, D. M., & Mullin, E. (2012). Efficacy of and advocacy for postural screening in public schools. *Orthopaedic Nursing, 31*(4), 232–235.

Najarian, S. L. (2013). Compartment syndrome. In D. Cline & O. J. Ma (Eds.), *Tintinalli's emergency medicine* (pp. 615–616). New York, NY: McGraw-Hill.

Nguyen, N. A., Klein, G., Dogbey, G., et al. (2012). Operative versus non-operative treatments for Legg-Calvé-Perthes disease: A meta-analysis. *Journal of Pediatric Orthopedics, 32*(7), 697–705

Nicolaou, N., Bowe, J. D., Wilkinson, J. M., et al. (2011). Use of the Sheffield telescopic intramedullary rod system for the management of osteogenesis imperfecta: Clinical outcomes at an average follow-up of nineteen years. *Journal of Bone & Joint Surgery, 93*(21), 1994–2000.

Norvell, J. G. (2013). Pelvis, hip & femur injuries. In D. Cline & O. J. Ma (Eds.), *Tintinalli's emergency medicine* (pp. 604–608). New York, NY: McGraw-Hill.

Novais, E. N., & Millis, M. B. (2012). Slipped capital femoral epiphysis: Prevalence, pathogenesis, and natural history. *Clinical Orthopedics & Related Research, 470*(12), 3432–3438.

Pandya, N. K., Baldwin, K., Kamath, A. F., et al. (2011). Unexplained fractures: Child abuse or bone disease? *Clinical Orthopaedics & Related Research, 469*(3), 805–812.

Pandya, N. K., Namdari, S., & Hosalkar, H. S. (2012). Displaced clavicle fractures in adolescents: Facts, controversies, and current trends. *Journal of American Academy of Orthopedic Surgeons, 20*(8), 498–505.

Piazzolla, A., Solarino, G., De Giorgi, S., et al. (2011). Cotrel-Dubousset instrumentation in neuromuscular scoliosis. *European Spine Journal, 20*(Suppl. 1), S75–S84.

Polat, M., Sakinci, O., Ersoy, B., et al. (2012). Assessment of sleep-related breathing disorders in patients with Duchenne muscular dystrophy. *Journal of Clinical Medicine Research, 4*(5), 332–337.

Reed, C., Carroll, L., Baccari, S., et al. (2011). Spica cast care: A collaborative staff-led education initiative for improved patient care. *Orthopaedic Nursing, 30*(6), 353–358.

Rudloe, T. F., Schutzman, S., Lee, L. K., et al. (2012). No longer a "nursemaid's" elbow: Mechanisms, caregivers, and prevention. *Pediatric Emergency Care, 28*(8), 771–774.

Rush, E. T., DeHaai, K., Kreikemeier, R. M., et al. (2012). Evaluation and comparison of safety, convenience and cost of administering intravenous pamidronate infusions to children in the home and ambulatory care settings. *Journal of Pediatric Endocrinology & Metabolism, 25*(5–6), 493–497.

Rush, R. M. Jr, Arrington, E. D., & Hsu, J. R. (2012). Management of complex extremity injuries: Tourniquets, compartment syndrome detection, fasciotomy, and amputation care. *Surgical Clinics of North America, 92*(4), 987–1007.

Sabharwal, S., Wenokor, C., Mehta, A., et al. (2012). Intra-articular morphology of the knee joint in children with Blount disease: A case-control study using MRI. *Journal of Bone & Joint Surgery, 94*(10), 883–890.

Santos, F., McCall, A. A., Chien, W., et al. (2012). Otopathology in osteogenesis imperfecta. *Otology & Neurotology, 33*(9), 1562–1566.

Schmitz-Feuerhake, I., & Pflugbeil, S. (2011). 'Lifestyle' and cancer rates in former East and West Germany: The possible contribution of diagnostic radiation exposures. *Radiation Protection Dosimetry, 147*(1–2), 310–313.

Soep, J. B. (2012). Rheumatic diseases. In W. Hay, M. Levin, R. Deterding, et al. (Eds.), *Current diagnosis & treatment pediatrics* (21st ed., pp. 889–896). New York, NY: McGraw-Hill/Lange.

Sullivan, S. S. (2012). Neurotherapeutics. *Current Treatment of Selected Pediatric Sleep Disorders, 9*(4), 791–800.

Swenson, D. M., Henke, N. M., Collins, C. L., et al. (2012). Epidemiology of United States high school sports-related fractures, 2008–09 to 2010–11. *American Journal of Sports Medicine, 40*(9), 2078–2084.

Tarakci, E., Yeldan, I., Baydogan, S. N., et al. (2012). Efficacy of a land-based home exercise programme for patients with juvenile idiopathic arthritis: A randomized, controlled, single-blind study. *Journal of Rehabilitation Medicine, 44*(11), 962–967.

Tedesco, F. S., & Cossu, G. (2012). Stem cell therapies for muscle disorders. *Current Opinion in Neurology, 25*(5), 597–603.

Thijs, Y., Bellemans, J., Rombaut, L., et al. (2012). Is high-impact sports participation associated with bowlegs in adolescent boys? *Medicine & Science in Sports & Exercise, 44*(6), 993–998.

Traina, F., De Fine, M., Abati, C. N., et al. (2012). Outcomes of total hip replacement in patients with slipped capital femoral epiphysis. *Archives of Orthopedic Trauma Surgery, 132*(8), 1133–1139.

Tu, P., & Bytomski, J. R. (2011). Diagnosis of heel pain. *American Family Physician, 84*(8), 909–916.

U.S. Department of Health and Human Services. (2010). *Healthy people 2020.* Washington, DC: Author.

van Schuppen, J., van Doorn, M. M., & van Rijn, R. R. (2012). Childhood osteomyelitis: Imaging characteristics. *Insights Into Imaging, 3*(5), 519–533.

Voloc, A., Esterle, L., Nguyen, T. M., et al. (2012). High prevalence of genu varum/valgum in European children with low vitamin D status and insufficient dairy products/calcium intakes. *European Journal of Endocrinology, 163*(5), 811–817.

Walter, K. D. (2011). Orthopedics. In K. J. Marcdante, R. M. Kliegman, H. B. Jenson, et al. (Eds.), *Nelson essentials of pediatrics* (6th ed., pp. 753–763). Philadelphia, PA: Saunders/Elsevier.

Weeks, B. H. (2012). Myasthenia gravis: Helping patients have better outcomes. *Nurse Practitioner, 37*(9), 30–36.

Weiss, H. R., & Werkmann, M. (2012). Soft braces in the treatment of adolescent idiopathic scoliosis (AIS) - Review of the literature and description of a new approach. *Scoliosis, 7*(1), 11–12.

Wild, C. Y., Steele, J. R., & Munro, B. J. (2012). Insufficient hamstring strength compromises landing technique in adolescent girls. *Medicine & Science in Sports & Exercise, 45*(3), 497–505.

Yaokreh, J. B., Gicquel, P., Schneider, L., et al. (2012). Compared outcomes after percutaneous pinning versus open reduction in paediatric supracondylar elbow fractures. *Orthopedics & Traumatology, Surgery & Research, 98*(6), 645–651.

Zhao, X., & Yan, S. G. (2011). Recent progress in osteogenesis imperfecta. *Orthopaedic Surgery, 3*(2), 127–130.

Chapter 52

Nursing Care of a Family When a Child Has an Unintentional Injury

KEY TERMS

- allografting
- autografting
- contrecoup injury
- debridement
- drowning
- escharotomy
- near drowning
- otorrhea
- plumbism
- rhinorrhea
- sprain
- strain
- stupor

OBJECTIVES

After mastering the contents of this chapter, you should be able to:

1. Describe the causes and consequences of common unintentional injuries in childhood and measures to prevent them.
2. Identify 2020 National Health Goals related to children who have experienced trauma that nurses can help the nation achieve.
3. Assess a child who has been unintentionally injured.
4. Formulate nursing diagnoses related to an unintentionally injured child.
5. Establish expected outcomes for an unintentionally injured child that can help parents manage seamless transitions across differing health care settings.
6. Using the nursing process, plan nursing care that includes the six competencies of Quality & Safety Education for Nurses (QSEN): Patient-Centered Care, Teamwork & Collaboration, Evidence-Based Practice (EBP), Quality Improvement (QI), Safety, and Informatics.
7. Implement nursing care for a child with an unintentional injury, such as providing pain relief.
8. Evaluate expected outcomes for achievement and effectiveness of care.
9. Integrate knowledge of unintentional injury in children with the interplay of nursing process, the six competencies of QSEN, and Family Nursing to achieve quality maternal and child health nursing care.

Jason Varton is 4 years old; his sister Sage is 10 years old. Both are brought into the emergency room because while their parents were playing cards with neighbors next door, they tried to light a fire in their fireplace. Jason jumped out of a window and hit his head on a cement walkway when the carpet caught on fire. Although his only visible sign of trauma is a reddened edematous area on his forehead, his temperature is 99.4°F (37.5°C); respirations are 18 breaths/min; pulse is 62 beats/min; and blood pressure is 110/62 mmHg. His left pupil appears more dilated than his right, and it reacts sluggishly to light. Sage was rescued from the house by her father but not before she suffered third-degree burns on her arms, hands, and neck.

Previous chapters described the growth and development of well children and care of children with disorders of specific body systems. This chapter adds information about the characteristic changes, both physical and psychosocial, that occur when children experience an unintentional injury.

Suppose you are a triage nurse. Would you rate Jason and Sage as children who need to be seen immediately, or could they be given second priority?

TABLE 52.1 Most Common Unintentional Injuries in Children by Age Group

Age (years)	Type of Unintentional Injury
0–1	Falls, inhalation of foreign objects, poisoning, burns, drowning
2–4	Falls, drowning, motor vehicles, poisoning, burns
5–9	Motor vehicles, bicycle injuries, drowning, burns, firearms
10–14	Motor vehicles, drowning, burns, firearms, falls, bicycle injuries
15–18	Motor vehicles, drowning, firearms

National Center for Health Statistics. (2012). *Health data for all ages*. Hyattsville, MD: Author.

Unintentional injuries, such as those that involve motor vehicles, falls, burns, and water immersions, cause more deaths in the 1- to 4-year age group than the next six most prevalent causes combined in that age group. In the 15- to 24-year age group, they cause half of the deaths of the age group (National Vital Statistics Service, 2012). Thus, if unintentional injuries such as these could be prevented, a major cause of childhood morbidity and mortality could be eliminated. Total injury elimination may not be possible, however, because children commonly believe injuries will not happen to them and, as a result, fail to take sensible precautions against them. Some parents may predispose their children to unintentional injuries by overestimating their development and giving them responsibility beyond their capabilities.

The frequency of various types of injuries varies according to age group (Table 52.1). Because the anatomy and physiology of children are different from those of adults, children are not only involved in different types of circumstances than adults, but injuries affect them differently (Latenser, 2013).

Family stress plays a large role in childhood poisoning injuries because these types of injuries tend to occur when parents are stressed or preoccupied. Eliminating unintentional injuries in children, therefore, is not a simple procedure. Box 52.1 shows 2020 National Health Goals related to children and trauma.

BOX 52.1 Nursing Care Planning Based on 2020 National Health Goals

Because prevention of unintentional injuries could have both immediate and long-term effects on the nation's health, several 2020 National Health Goals are concerned with preventing unintentional injuries in children:

- Reduce the number of drowning deaths each year from a baseline of 1.2 per 100,000 to 1.1 per 100,000.
- Reduce sports and recreational injuries from 46.6 per 100,000 to 41.9 per 100,000.
- Reduce the rate of firearm-related deaths from a baseline of 10.2 per 100,000 to 9.2 per 100,000.
- Prevent an increase of poisonings deaths from a baseline of 13.1 per 100,000 (maintain baseline value).
- Reduce the number of deaths caused by suffocation in infants age 0 to 12 months from a baseline of 22.5 per 100,000 to 20.3 per 100,000 infants.
- Reduce unintentional injury deaths from 40.1 per 100,000 to 36.0 per 100,000 (U.S. Department of Health and Human Services [DHHS], 2010; see www.healthypeople.gov).

Nurses can help the nation achieve these goals by providing counseling on safety precautions to parents and children. Always help assess whether injuries were unintentional or possibly a result of child maltreatment or self-injury.

Nursing Process Overview

For Care of a Child With an Unintentional Injury

Assessment

When children are seen at health care facilities because of unintentional injuries, neither they nor their parents may be functioning at their optimal level because of the stress of the situation. Both may be apprehensive and frightened not only about what *has* happened but also about what could have happened. Children often feel guilty and worry they will be scolded or punished. Their parents can feel equally guilty because they realize they could have been watching more closely, causing them to act defensively. Remember people under stress do not process information well, so parents may not perceive the information you give them correctly. All information you supply in an emergency department, therefore, may need to be repeated after the immediate care is completed.

Children are likely to be in pain and may be confused because they count on their parents to keep them safe, but yet they have been hurt. Trust is momentarily broken. How can they be safe in the hospital if their parents are no longer protecting them?

Nursing Diagnosis

Nursing diagnoses need to address not only the physical injury a child sustained but also the psychological or emotional trauma both the child and the parents are experiencing. Examples of possible nursing diagnoses are:

- Pain related to fractured tibia from sports injury
- Ineffective airway clearance related to effect of burned esophageal tissue
- Impaired physical mobility related to severe burn injury
- Disturbed body image related to change in physical appearance from thermal injury
- Parental fear related to outcome after head injury in child
- Interrupted family processes related to child's unintentional injury
- Anxiety related to apprehension and lack of knowledge regarding medical treatment of child

Outcome Identification and Planning

Parents in an emergency department are rarely ready for long-term planning; they often have great difficulty in just answering the most straightforward, immediate questions. As a result, long-term planning may have to be delayed until the shock of the injury has passed.

On discharge from the emergency department, be certain parents have printed as well as oral instructions about the child's care, the name and number of the person to contact if they have questions about care or progress, and an appointment (or the number to call for a return appointment) for follow-up care. If a child is admitted to the hospital from the emergency department, it's helpful if the nurse who cared for the child in the emergency department can accompany the child to the hospital unit because the first person who cares for a child after an injury assumes a very important role to the child and parents, because that person was the first one to recognize their distress. A transition period, or "passing on of care," helps a parent accept the child's new caregivers as being as dependable and trustworthy as the emergency department staff.

A key component of nursing intervention in an emergency department is to help parents understand why an injury happened and plan ways to make their immediate or community environment safe for children. Organizations that might be appropriate for referral are the American Association of Poison Control Centers (www.aapcc.org), the American Burn Association (www.ameriburn.org), the American Academy of Pediatrics (www.aap.org), and, for advice on cardiac resuscitation, the American Heart Association (www.heart.org).

Implementation

The extent of a child's injury depends on the injuring agent, the part of the body that was injured, and often the immediate care, including both physical and psychological management that a child receives.

Be certain to maintain standard infection precautions in emergency situations the same as at any other time. Remember parental consent must be obtained for treatment procedures even in an emergency, except for lifesaving actions, such as cardiopulmonary resuscitation (CPR) (it is assumed parents would consent to lifesaving procedures, and delaying procedures until they can be located could result in permanent disability or death).

Outcome Evaluation

After an injury, children need follow-up care to be certain the immediate interventions were adequate and successful healing is taking place. Evaluation visits are also a time to determine whether the child's environment has been changed so the child is safer now than at the time of the injury (if applicable).

If an injury could not have been anticipated, parents appreciate hearing one more time that such an injury could not have been avoided and that they are good parents because this helps them maintain adequate self-esteem to continue to function well as parents.

Examples of expected outcomes suggesting achievement of goals are:

- The child swallows fluids without distress after esophageal burns.
- The child states pain is at tolerable level within 20 minutes.
- The child demonstrates full range of motion in hand after thermal injury.
- The child states he understands that wearing a seat belt is an important safety measure.
- The child states she will wear a helmet when riding a bicycle in the future.

HEALTH PROMOTION AND RISK MANAGEMENT

In every care setting, nurses have the important opportunity among health care professionals to provide child and family teaching concerning the prevention of unintentional injuries. After an injury has occurred, nurses can provide valuable instruction to families about safeguarding their children against future injuries. In a community setting, nurses have a great opportunity for assessment of the unique threats that are present in particular environments such as lead-based paint or kerosene heaters in older homes, risk of drowning in a home with an unfenced swimming pool, or the danger for children riding in the back of pickup trucks. To teach effective injury prevention, nurses need to be knowledgeable about common measures that prevent injury.

Poisoning is an important cause of serious injuries in children younger than 6 years of age; more than 1 million episodes occur every year, with common household agents often the offending agent (Lee & Marcdante, 2011). Since passage of the Poison Prevention Packaging Act of 1970, which requires potentially hazardous products to be sold in child-resistant containers, a decrease in the incidence of childhood poisonings from common medicines has occurred.

The home environment may still contain products such as plants, cosmetics, and cleaning products that can be hazardous to children if handled improperly. Teaching parents to take such measures as installing child-resistant locks on low cabinets where household products are stored, moving plants to a higher surface, keeping matches in safe places, and teaching street safety so that parents can maintain a safe home environment is an important nursing concern.

QSEN Checkpoint Question 52.1

Evidence-Based Practice

The preadolescent age is a time when children are beginning to do many activities independently, yet it is also an age when their judgment is still not mature. To identify frequent health risk behaviors of this age and what child, family, and environmental factors play into injuries, nurse researchers interviewed 297 Midwestern preadolescents (mean age, 10.5 years) and their parents about health risk behaviors. Results of the study revealed that those children who had a single parent were 2.8 times more likely than children who had two parents (or one parent and a partner) to report intentional risk behaviors; boys were 2 times more likely than girls to engage in common health risk behaviors such as not wearing helmets and not using seat belts (Riesch, Kedrowski, Brown, et al., 2012).

Sage is 10 years old and was burned when she helped set a fire in the fireplace. Based on the previous study, when Sage is well again, which would be the best advice to give Sage's mother to help her family reduce unintentional injuries such as this?

a. Constantly remind Sage that, because of her age, she needs help to make decisions.
b. Stress to Sage that she never did foolish, unsafe things as a child.
c. Don't remind Sage about safety because girls tend to be conscientious about this.
d. When providing safety education, convey that both parents agree it is important.

Look in Appendix A for the best answer and rationale.

THE INJURED CHILD

Because the emergency department nurse is often the first person who sees a child after an injury, nurses need to be prepared to make a preliminary assessment of the extent of a child's injuries. Remember that children may be seriously hurt but not crying because they are in shock. They may be hemorrhaging, but if they are bleeding internally, no blood may be visibly evident. Unintentional injuries become fatal when lung, heart, or brain function becomes inadequate. These three body systems, therefore, must be evaluated first (airway, breathing, circulation, and disability, or an ABCD evaluation). Table 52.2 lists signs and symptoms to assess when determining the respiratory, cardiovascular, and neurologic status of an injured child.

While conducting a preliminary assessment of a child's major body systems, take a brief history of the injury. What happened? How long ago did it happen? Was the child using protective equipment such as a helmet or a secured seat belt? What have the parents done? If the child fell, how far was the fall? On what body part did the child land? What do the parents think is the child's major injury (children may report one body part hurts at first, but then a small cut elsewhere begins to bleed, and they focus on the minor bleeding as their major injury). If parents say, "At first, he acted as if his stomach hurt," this may be the first suggestion that he has a serious abdominal injury such as splenic rupture.

Evaluating children in an emergency department is difficult, because they may be unconscious, too young to communicate, or so frightened that they cannot stop crying to report which body parts are painful or to indicate which parts should be assessed first. Spend a few minutes attempting to calm children and get them past this initial fright, unless symptoms of major body system disturbances require you to direct your immediate efforts elsewhere. Parents need frequent explanations while their care is being evaluated and during care because as long as parents are worried and tense, children cannot be calmed easily.

A proportion of unintentional injuries in children result from child maltreatment. Conflicting histories (a parent and child recounting different stories) are a hallmark of maltreatment. Always ask yourself whether this or intentional self-injury could be a possibility (see Chapter 55).

TABLE 52.2 Important Assessments on Initial Examination of an Injured Child

Body System	Assessment
Respiratory system	Rate and quality of respirations Any sound of obstruction (wheezing, stridor, retractions, coughing?) Color (cyanotic?) Oxygen hunger (restlessness, inability to lie flat?)
Cardiovascular system	Color (pallor from hemorrhage or cardiovascular collapse?) Evident bleeding Pulse rate (increases with hemorrhage) Blood pressure (decreases with hemorrhage) Feeling of apprehension from altered vascular pressure
Nervous system	Level of consciousness (child answers questions coherently, infant attunes to parent's voice?) Pupils (equal and reacting to light?) Bumps or bruises on head or spinal column Loss of motion or sensory function in a body part

HEAD TRAUMA

Children often receive head injuries when they are involved in multiple-trauma injuries, such as automobile crashes, or when they fall from swing sets, porches, or bunk beds. Other children receive head injures by being struck on the head by an object such as a baseball, rock, or hockey puck, or by falling off a bicycle, especially if they're not wearing a protective helmet (Persaud, Coleman, Zwolakowski, et al., 2012).

Head injuries are always potentially serious not only because the immediate injury can be life threatening to the child, but also because the injury can lead to complications that can be equally severe. Following a depressed skull fracture, for example, recurrent seizures and abnormalities on an electroencephalogram (EEG) as a result of scar tissue may occur.

Some children experience minor personality changes, memory deficits, or symptoms such as headache, irritability, and postural vertigo (sensation of feeling faint or unable to maintain normal balance—also known as posttrauma or postconcussion syndrome) (Babcock, Byczkowski, Wade, et al., 2012). Behavioral manifestations may also include aggressiveness or poor school performance, although it may be difficult to determine whether these symptoms are organic or the result of being treated differently than before the injury by anxious parents.

Immediate Assessment

All children with head trauma need to have their neck stabilized with a brace until cervical trauma has been ruled out. They also require a neurologic assessment as soon as they are seen and again at frequent intervals to detect signs and symptoms of increased intracranial pressure (ICP) because increasing pressure puts stress on the respiratory, cardiac, and temperature centers, causing dysfunction in these areas. The mark of increased pressure is a decrease in pulse and respiratory rate and an increase in temperature and pulse pressure (the distance between the diastolic and systolic pressure). The child's pupils also become slow or unable to react immediately. Level of consciousness and motor ability both also decrease.

Important assessments, therefore, are vital signs to detect these changes, observation of children's pupils to be certain they are equal and react to light, level of consciousness, and motor function.

Immediate Management

After a head injury, brain edema is likely to occur because fluid rushes into the inflamed and bruised area so ICP monitoring may be initiated (see Chapter 49). A computed tomography (CT) scan or magnetic resonance imaging (MRI) will be prescribed to determine areas of edema or bleeding. A central venous or central arterial line may be inserted so pressure can be reduced by the administration of a hypertonic intravenous (IV) solution such as mannitol. As this is infused, it increases intravascular pressure and causes the edema fluid to shift back into the blood vessels. Administration of a steroid such as dexamethasone and keeping the child's head elevated are other ways to decrease inflammation and edema and lower ICP.

Nursing Diagnoses and Related Interventions

Nursing diagnoses for children with head injuries address both the physical abnormities that need to be corrected and the psychosocial stress that such a serious injury generates.

Nursing Diagnosis: Risk for excess fluid volume related to administration of hypertonic solution

Outcome Evaluation: Child's respiratory rate remains between 16 and 24 breaths/min; specific gravity of urine is between 1.003 and 1.030; pulse remains between 60 and 100 beats/min; blood pressure remains consistent for age group; lungs are clear to auscultation.

When hypertonic solutions are infused intravenously to reduce cerebral edema, fluid shifts from interstitial spaces into the bloodstream, possibly resulting in blood volume overload. To detect this, assess vital signs frequently. The body evacuates this fluid by the kidneys so it's important to keep an accurate intake and output record to ensure the kidneys are functioning; test the specific gravity of urine to detect whether pituitary compression is leading to over- or underproduction of antidiuretic hormone.

Nursing Diagnosis: Risk for delayed growth and development related to late sequelae of head injury

Outcome Evaluation: Child shows no evidence of any alteration in thought processes, seizure activity, or memory at follow-up visits. Cognitive and physical development proceed appropriately.

Caring for a child after a head injury can be difficult for parents because they are so worried about the child's condition. To help them feel a sense of control, offer information on the child's progress as it becomes available. Urge parents to give as much help as they wish to increase their sense of control.

If parents ask about the possibility that personality changes or seizures will develop later in life from the injury, refer them to their child's primary care provider because that answer is variable and difficult to predict.

Skull Fracture

A skull fracture is a crack in one of the bones of the skull (Mandt & Grubenhoff, 2012). Detecting skull fractures in children is important because associated cerebral injury often occurs under the fracture. Many fractures are simple linear types; most involve the parietal bones. In some children, instead of a bone fracturing, the suture lines separate. This occurs more commonly in the lambdoid suture line; a coronal suture separation is rare and, if present, indicates severe trauma (Fig. 52.1).

Assessment

Skull fractures are confirmed by a skull X-ray. Make sure you have a thorough history of the injury so the strength of the blow to the head can be judged. If the base of the skull is fractured, a child usually exhibits ecchymosis around the eyes or behind an ear. **Rhinorrhea** or **otorrhea** (clear fluid draining from the nose or ear, respectively) may be noticeable. The fluid

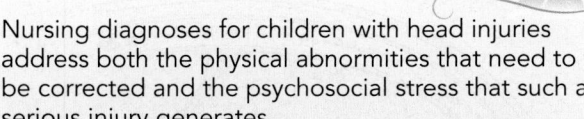

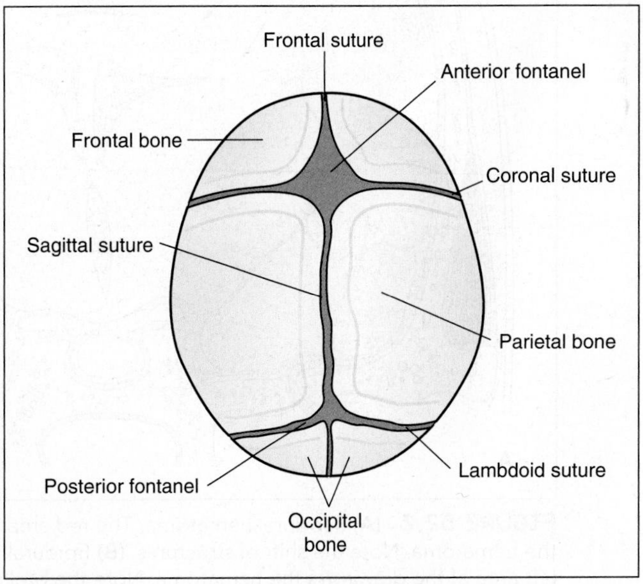

FIGURE 52.1 Location of suture lines of the skull.

is cerebrospinal fluid (CSF) and is a serious finding because it means that the child's central nervous system is open to infection. If it's not clear whether the fluid is CSF or rhinitis from an allergy, test the fluid with a glucose reagent strip. CSF will test positive for glucose, whereas the clear, watery drainage from an upper respiratory tract infection or allergy will not.

If a skull fracture is linear with no underlying pathology, no treatment except observation and prescription of an analgesic is necessary. In about 3 weeks, a repeat X-ray will confirm that healing has taken place. You can assure parents that a second X-ray this soon is not harmful but necessary.

If a fracture is depressed (a bone fragment is pressing inward) or compounded (bone is broken into pieces), surgery will be necessary to remove or repair broken fragments and halt any bleeding that is occurring from a blood vessel being cut by a bone fragment. Cranial surgery of this type is discussed in Chapter 49.

Therapeutic Management

If CSF is draining from the nose or ear, a child will usually be admitted to the hospital for observation because this implies the force of the blow was severe. Keep the child in a semi-Fowler's position so fluid drains out, not inward, to reduce the possibility of introducing infection. Make certain children do not hold their nose or pack their nostrils with something to halt the drainage so the amount escaping can be judged. If the drainage is excoriating to the upper lip, coat the space with an ointment such as petrolatum. Children may be prescribed a prophylactic antibiotic to reduce the risk for meningitis. If the drainage does not stop within a few days, surgery will be necessary to repair the fracture and reduce the danger of meningitis. Air that entered intracranial spaces at the time of the injury usually is absorbed rapidly. If X-rays at 72 hours still show air in the cerebral spaces, this implies a skull defect remains, and surgery may be indicated to close the defect.

Potential Complications

A long-term complication of even a linear fracture may be a *leptomeningeal cyst*. This results from projection of the arachnoid membrane into the fracture site. With the interfering tissue, bone cannot heal and actually erodes, so the fracture site becomes progressively larger, not smaller. That this is happening will be evident on a follow-up X-ray. It may be suspected if a child develops focal seizures or symptoms of increased ICP. The defect may be palpated on the skull as an underlying indentation. Surgical resection is necessary to remove the cyst.

Subdural Hematoma

Subdural hematoma is venous bleeding into the space between the dura and the arachnoid membrane (Fig. 52.2A). This is usually bilateral and occurs when head trauma lacerates minute veins in this area (Nickels, Patel, Merhar, et al., 2013).

Subdural hematomas tend to occur in infants more often than in older children. Symptoms can occur within 3 days or as late as 20 days after trauma. Infants usually have symptoms of increased ICP, such as seizures, vomiting, hyperirritability,

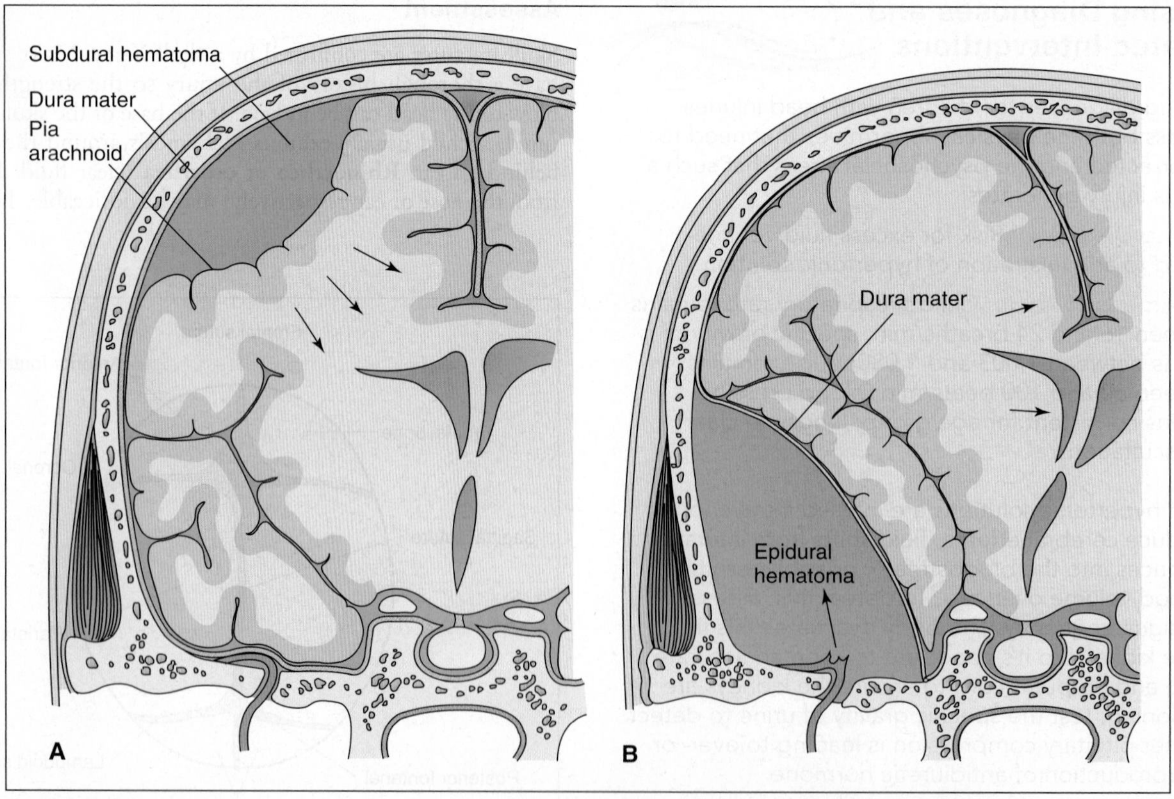

FIGURE 52.2 **(A)** Subdural hematoma. The red area in the upper left area of the drawing is the hematoma. Note the shift of structures. **(B)** Epidural hematoma. The red area in the lower left area of the drawing is the hematoma. Note the broken blood vessel and the shift of midline structures.

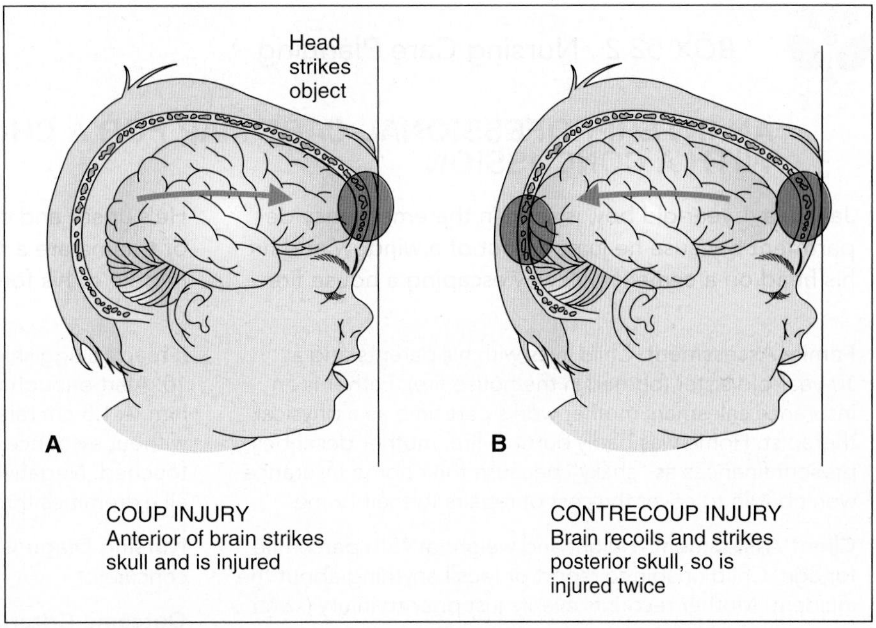

FIGURE 52.3 Etiology of **(A)** coup and **(B)** contrecoup injuries.

and enlargement of the diameter of the head. Anemia caused by the substantial blood loss may occur. Angiography, MRI, or ultrasound will reveal the extent of the hematoma.

In infants, accumulated subdural blood is removed by a subdural puncture through the anterior fontanelle if it is still patent by a procedure similar to a lumbar puncture. Infants receive conscious sedation for the procedure and must be held extremely still so that they do not move and cause the aspiration needle to be inserted incorrectly.

Subdural punctures may need to be repeated daily to empty the subdural space. If bleeding is still present after 2 weeks, surgery usually is necessary to reduce the space and halt bleeding. In older children, surgery usually is necessary from the beginning, because the anterior fontanelle is closed and the space cannot be reached by puncture.

Epidural Hematoma

Epidural hematoma is bleeding into the space between the dura and the skull and happens when head trauma is severe (see Fig. 52.2B). Whereas subdural hemorrhage is usually venous bleeding, epidural hemorrhage is usually a result of rupture of the middle meningeal artery and thus is arterial bleeding. It's usually intense and causes rapid brain compression.

At the time of the injury, children are apt to become momentarily unconscious. They then regain consciousness and, to the untrained eye, appear to be well for minutes or hours. Then signs of cortical compression, such as vomiting, loss of consciousness, headache, seizures, or hemiparesis (paralysis on one side), begin to develop. On physical examination, unequal dilation or constriction of the pupils may be present. Decorticate posturing (see Chapter 49) may be seen, indicating extreme pressure on upper cortical centers. If the pressure is allowed to continue unchecked, it may grow so great that brainstem, respiratory, or cardiovascular function become impaired.

The treatment is surgical removal of the accumulated blood and cauterization or ligation of the torn artery. The earlier the process is recognized and treated, the less the chance of residual damage from extreme pressure or anoxia to the involved portion of the brain.

Concussion

Concussion is the temporary and immediate impairment of neurologic function caused by a hard, jarring shock to the skull (Purcell, 2012). It may occur on the side of the head that was struck (a *coup injury*) or as the brain recoils from the force of the blow and strikes the opposite surface of the skull (a **contrecoup injury**; Fig. 52.3). Children have at least a transient loss of consciousness at the time of the injury and may vomit and show irritability after regaining consciousness. They typically have no memory (amnesia) of the event that led up to the injury or of the injury itself. For some children, this makes being asked questions about the injury extremely upsetting because they do not remember anything that happened and feel a frightening loss of control. A skull X-ray or MRI is needed to rule out skull fracture, and observation for 24 hours is needed to rule out severe brain trauma, edema, or laceration. A child can be observed at home by the parents if they're able to assess the child's level of consciousness every 1 to 2 hours while the child is awake. Parents usually are instructed not to keep waking children during the night, because multiple wakings are disorienting and can make it difficult to tell if the child is confused or not. Parents should wake the child at least once during the night, however, and to be certain they are conscious, ask them to name a familiar object, such as a favorite toy, or to name the color of some object shown to them. Being able to tell parents their name or where they live is equally revealing.

There is an old belief that, if children fall asleep after a head injury, they will die in their sleep; this belief can cause parents to keep shaking their child awake or to make the child walk continually. Be certain they understand that it is okay for children to sleep, but they must wake them at least once to assess their status (see Box 52.2 for an interprofessional care map for a child with a concussion). As a final instruction, be certain parents have a telephone number to call if they have any questions or worries about their child's care.

BOX 52.2 Nursing Care Planning

AN INTERPROFESSIONAL CARE MAP FOR A CHILD WITH A CONCUSSION

Jason, a 4-year-old boy, is seen in the emergency department because he jumped out of a window and hit his head on a cement walkway escaping a house fire. He's upset and crying, although his only visible signs of trauma are a reddened and edematous area on the middle of his forehead.

Family Assessment Child lives with his parents and a 10-year-old sister (burned in the house fire). Father is an insurance salesman; mother works part time as a physical therapist. Home was badly burnt in fire; mother describes present finances as "shaky" because their home insurance won't begin to cover the cost of repairs to their home.

Client Assessment Height and weight at 75th percentile for age. Child unable to report or recall anything about the incident. Mother recounts events just prior to injury (sister reported she and Jason were trying to light a fire in the fireplace).

Vital signs: temperature, 99.4°F (37.5°C); respirations, 18 breaths/min; pulse, 62 beats/min; and blood pressure, 110/62 mmHg. Left pupil is more dilated than his right; it reacts sluggishly to light. Glasgow Coma Scale score is 10. Alert enough to name toy racing car he brought in with him. A 1.5-cm raised area noted on forehead. Skin intact without evidence of bleeding. Child cries when area is touched. Negative otorrhea or rhinorrhea. Able to move all extremities through range of motion.

Nursing Diagnosis Risk for injury related to effects of concussion

Outcome Criteria Child remains alert and oriented; easily arousable. Pupils equal, round, react to light and accommodation; vital signs within age-acceptable parameters; exhibits no signs or symptoms of neurologic dysfunction.

Team Member Responsible	Assessment	Intervention	Rationale	Expected Outcome
Activities of Daily Living, Including Safety				
Nurse	Take history of injury; document distance child fell.	Assess child's vital signs, level of consciousness, and neurologic function initially, and then every 30 minutes until discharge.	Changes in vital signs, level of consciousness, or neurologic function could indicate increasing intracranial pressure.	Parent describes injury and reactions of child since injury.
Teamwork and Collaboration				
Nurse/Primary care provider/Trauma care team	Assess who is available from trauma team for consult; assess if child has ever had magnetic resonance imaging (MRI) before.	Help trauma care team assess child because child has been told not to talk to strangers. Accompany child to MRI service.	Symptoms of concussion can develop slowly over the next few hours after injury. MRI can help detect bleeding and edema.	Trauma care team examines child; prescribes follow-up care. Child cooperates with MRI.
Procedures/Medications for Quality Improvement				
Nurse/Primary care provider	Assess whether child's demeanor (crying) is from fright or pain.	Institute measures to calm the child. Encourage the parents to hold and reassure him.	Crying increases intracranial pressure. Involving the parents provides them with a concrete activity, helping to provide some sense of control over the situation.	Parents are able to calm child to allow for better evaluation of condition.
Nutrition				
Nurse	Assess whether child has vomited since head injury.	If not NPO, offer clear fluid to be certain child does not have vomiting.	Vomiting is a symptom of increased intracranial pressure.	Child drinks some fluid without vomiting.

Patient-Centered Care				
Nurse	Assess what parents understand about concussion in children.	Teach parents how contrecoup injuries occur and symptoms they cause.	A contrecoup injury causes injury or edema to the posterior brain.	Parents state they understand why their child has posterior (eye control) symptoms and the assessment they will need to continue after discharge.
Psychosocial/Spiritual/Emotional Needs				
Nurse	Assess whether child or parents have any questions about care.	Orient the child to his surroundings. Offer explanations about any treatments or procedures that are to come.	Children often have no memory of events with concussion. Orientation and explanation help to minimize a child's fear of the unknown and of his situation.	Parents and child state they understand procedures being carried out. Voice confidence in care.
Nurse	Attempt to identify the meaning and effect of the injury to the child.	Encourage parents to express their feelings about not being in home when injury occurred.	Both child and parents have reasons to feel guilty over injury as child knew not to play with fire and parents were absent from home.	Parents state they understand fire is attractive to children; will make concrete plans for better child care in the future.
Informatics for Seamless Health Care Planning				
Nurse/Primary care provider	Assess whether parents understand why child will be admitted to observation unit overnight.	Child needs continuing care such as being roused every 2 hours during night to ensure he is conscious.	Assessing consciousness is important to assess whether complications are occurring.	Parents state one of them will remain with child in hospital to help reduce child's fear of strangers and better accept needed procedures.

Contusion

A brain *contusion* occurs when there is tearing or laceration of brain tissue (Fig. 52.4). The symptoms are the same type as for a concussion but more severe. In addition, symptoms related to the specific brain area that is lacerated such as a focal seizure, eye deviation, or loss of speech will occur. Surgery may be necessary to halt bleeding. The child's prognosis depends on the extent of the injury and effectiveness of therapy.

What if...52.1 In the emergency department, after Jason's head injury, his parents tell you they both had a gastrointestinal "flu" last week. They assure you the reason Jason is vomiting now is probably because "he's caught their flu." How could you evaluate whether the vomiting is from the head injury or a gastrointestinal infection?

Coma

Coma (unconsciousness from which a child cannot be roused) or **stupor** (grogginess from which a child *can* be roused) may occur in children after severe head trauma. Because these are

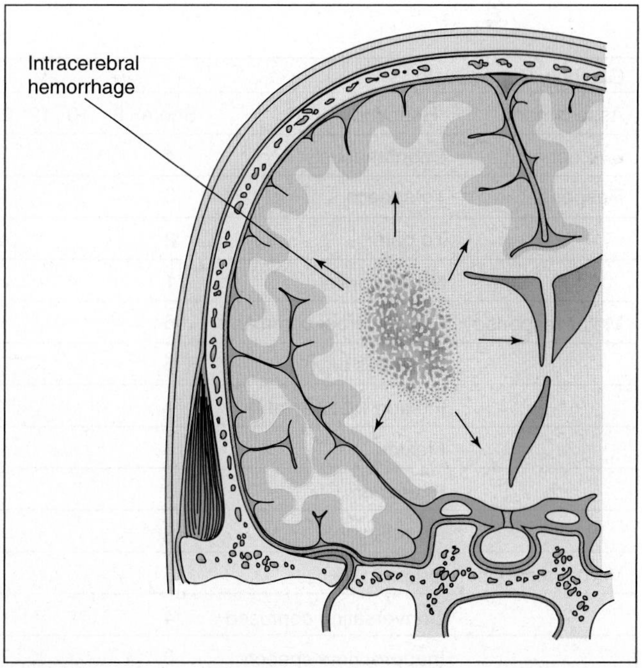

FIGURE 52.4 Intracerebral hemorrhage. The central large dark area represents the hemorrhage. Note the midline shift.

both symptoms of underlying disorders, it's important to obtain a thorough history of the injury so treatment can be directed specifically toward the cause.

Assessment

For assessment, obtain a history from a parent or an observer of the event that caused the injury to determine what happened immediately before the time the child became comatose (e.g., the child fell, was choking, or took a recreational drug).

Undress the child completely so you can inspect all body parts. Although head injury is most likely to be the underlying cause of coma or seizure, metabolic disturbances such as diabetes mellitus, dehydration, severe hemorrhage from another body part, or drug ingestion also must be considered as possible causes. Count respirations and pulse and measure blood pressure to establish baseline values, because changes in these values often provide good clues as to the cause of coma. A child with increased ICP, for example, will show decreased pulse and respiratory rates and increased blood pressure. The child with diabetes, in contrast, will develop increased respirations. Internal hemorrhage will lead to an increased pulse rate and decreased blood pressure. Drug ingestion may lead to either increased or decreased measurements, depending on the drug ingested.

Always turn an unconscious child on the side because, if brainstem compression is present, the child cannot swallow effectively; lying on the side allows saliva to drain from the mouth to prevent aspiration. Observe the child's eyes for signs of dilated pupils from increased ICP. If both pupils are dilated, irreversible brainstem damage is suggested, although such a finding may also be present with poisoning with an atropine-like drug. Pinpoint pupils suggest barbiturate or opiate intoxication. One pupil dilated or the eye deviated downward or laterally more than the other suggests third cranial nerve compression or a tentorial tear (laceration of the membrane between the cerebellum and cerebrum) with herniation of the temporal lobe into the torn membrane. This situation requires immediate surgery to correct temporal compression.

Lack of a doll's eye reflex (see Chapter 49) suggests compression of the oculomotor nerves (third, fourth, or sixth) or of the brainstem is involved. Observe for posturing, such as decerebrate posturing, which suggests cerebral compression and dysfunction. If the retina of the eye reveals papilledema (swelling), it suggests that increased ICP has been longstanding (more than 24 to 48 hours).

Metabolic or renal disorders that cause unconsciousness are revealed by blood analysis, so studies such as blood glucose, electrolytes, blood urea nitrogen (BUN), liver function tests, blood gas studies, and toxicology tests may be prescribed to rule out possible causes. A lumbar puncture and a CT or MRI will be done if a head injury is the most likely cause (Sigurtà, Zanaboni, Canavesi, et al., 2013).

Lumbar puncture may have little value at first in predicting the severity of a head injury, unless there is blood in the CSF because any degree of cerebral contusion causes edema, which leads to increased CSF pressure. The procedure is contraindicated if increased ICP is present because release of fluid with the puncture could cause brainstem compression into the cord, a serious complication.

Coma is graded according to a standard scale so that changes in the level of consciousness can be evaluated and deterioration or improvement can be documented. Figure 52.5 shows the Glasgow Coma Scale, the most commonly used evaluation system for coma (Rhine, Wade, Makoroff, et al., 2012). Because this system was devised as an adult assessment scale, it must be modified for use with children or infants. Such a modification is shown in Box 52.3.

On the scale, a score of 3 to 8 suggests severe trauma (a number less than 5 suggests a very severe prognosis); a score of 9 to 12, moderate trauma; and 13 to 15, slight trauma.

Glasgow Coma Scale			AM		PM					AM				
Assessment	Reaction	Score	8	10	12	2	4	6	8	10	12	2	4	6	8
Eye opening	Spontaneously	4	X						X	X	X	X	X		
Response	To speech	3		X				X							
	To pain	2			X	X	X								
	No response	1													
Motor response	Obeys verbal command	6	X						X	X	X	X	X		
	Localizes pain	5		X	X										
	Flexion withdrawal	4				X		X							
	Flexion	3					X								
	Extension	2													
	No response	1													
Verbal response	Oriented ×3	5	X						X	X	X	X	X		
	Conversation confused	4		X				X							
	Inappropriate speech	3			X										
	Incomprehensible sounds	2				X	X								
	No response	1													

FIGURE 52.5 Glasgow Coma Scale scoring for a child. A score of 3 to 8 denotes severe trauma; 9 to 12, moderate trauma; 13 to 15, slight trauma. Notice the gradual improvement from coma in this example.

BOX 52.3 Scoring for Glasgow Coma Scale

Eye Opening

4. Child opens eyes spontaneously when you approach.
3. Child opens eyes in response to speech (spoken or shouted).
2. Child opens eyes only in response to painful stimuli, such as pressure on a nail bed.
1. Child does not open eyes in response to painful stimuli.

Motor Response

6. Child can obey a simple command such as "hand me a toy" (infant smiles or attunes).
5. Child moves an extremity to locate a painful stimulus applied to the head or trunk and attempts to remove the source.
4. Child attempts to withdraw from the source of pain.
3. Child flexes arms at the elbows and wrists in response to painful stimuli to the nail beds (decorticate rigidity).
2. Child extends arms (straightens the elbows) in response to painful stimuli (cerebrate rigidity).
1. Child has no motor response to pain on any extremity.

Verbal Response

5. Child is oriented to time, place, and person (child >4 years old knows name, date, and where he or she is; infant appears to recognize parent).
4. Child is able to converse, although not oriented to time, place, or person (does not know who or where he or she is; infant says words but does not appear to differentiate parents from others).
3. Child speaks only in words or phrases that make little or no sense ("I want frazzle no"; infant's vocabulary is less than it is normally).
2. Child responds with incomprehensible sounds, such as groans.
1. Child does not respond verbally at all.

Modified from Teasdale, G., & Bennett, B. (1974). Assessment of coma and impaired consciousness: A practical scale. *Lancet, 2*(7872), 81–84.

Therapeutic Management

If children are unconscious for longer than a transient period, they usually are admitted to an observation unit for further assessment. An IV route is established so that, when specific measures such as blood replacement, electrolyte replacement, or fluid replacement are needed, a route for immediate administration is available. Oral suctioning to remove mucus from the mouth and pharynx may be necessary. Measure oxygen saturation by pulse oximetry. If a child has acute signs of respiratory difficulty or oxygen saturation is low, endotracheal intubation may be necessary to ensure respiratory function.

Obtain the child's vital signs and assess neurologic status, such as state of consciousness and the ability of pupils to react to light, every 15 to 20 minutes or as prescribed so a picture of gradual change can be detected.

A child's prognosis after coma depends on the initial cause of the coma and the immediate care the child receives. If the increased ICP can be relieved before any permanent brain damage results, the effects of the coma will be transient. Prognosis is always guarded, however, because coma is a serious, possibly life-threatening response until ruled otherwise.

Nursing Diagnoses and Related Interventions

Care of the child in coma is directed toward maintaining body function in an optimal state until the child reawakens.

Nursing Diagnosis: Risk for ineffective airway clearance related to brainstem pressure

Outcome Evaluation: Child's respiratory rate remains between 16 and 20 breaths/min; no retractions or signs of obstruction are present.

Some children who are comatose require endotracheal intubation or tracheotomy with mechanical ventilation to ensure an open airway and adequate oxygenation. An endotracheal tube may be replaced with a tracheotomy after 3 to 7 days to prevent necrosis of the pharynx from pressure of the endotracheal tube.

Nursing Diagnosis: Risk for impaired skin integrity related to lack of mobility

Outcome Evaluation: Child exhibits no areas of broken or irritated skin.

Bathe children who are comatose daily to stimulate skin circulation; include the hair as part of the bath about every 3 days. Change the child's position at least every 2 hours to prevent pressure ulcer formation or development of hydrostatic pneumonia from pooled secretions in the lungs. Keep the linen on the bed dry and free from wrinkles. Use of a sheepskin, an egg-carton foam, or an alternating-pressure or water mattress also can be important in decreasing pressure to the skin. Perform thorough passive range-of-motion exercises to maintain muscle tone and prevent contractures.

Nursing Diagnosis: Risk for imbalanced nutrition, less than body requirements, related to inability to take in oral food or fluid

Outcome Evaluation: Child has good skin turgor; weight remains within acceptable percentile; hourly urine output remains greater than 1 ml/kg.

Children who are unconscious cannot be fed orally or they might aspirate. Therefore, nutrition is maintained by nasogastric (NG) or gastrostomy tube feedings, IV fluid administration, or total parenteral nutrition (TPN). IV fluid is only a short-term answer, because adequate protein and fat cannot be supplied solely by this route. Always aspirate NG or gastrostomy tubes for stomach contents before giving a feeding to check tube placement and assess gastric residual amounts. As a rule, return any amount of stomach residue aspirated, because if this is discarded each time, a child will lose a large amount of stomach acid, possibly leading to alkalosis. Because children's stomach size is small, check whether the amount of the feeding should be reduced by the amount of fluid remaining in the stomach before feeding the full amount of prescribed formula.

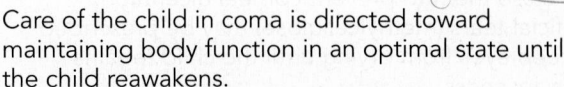

Give mouth care at least twice daily with clear water and a padded tongue blade. Coat lips with petrolatum or a commercial ointment to prevent drying and cracking. If a child's eyes tend to be dry, close them to prevent corneal ulceration. Artificial tears (methylcellulose) may be prescribed to keep eyes from drying until the child regains consciousness.

QSEN Checkpoint Question 52.2

Patient-Centered Care

Jason's parents are in distress because they fear that his ICP is increasing. You want to reassure his parents that you are closely monitoring Jason. Which event would be most indicative that his ICP is increasing?

a. Jason refuses to let you assess his tympanic temperature.
b. Jason asks you to read the same story to him over and over.
c. Jason can't remember a thing about how his injury happened.
d. Jason's temperature and blood pressure are both slowly increasing.

Look in Appendix A for the best answer and rationale.

Choking Games

Adolescents, seeking an inexpensive way to experience a "rush" or euphoria, may induce a partial or complete loss of consciousness in themselves by intentionally depriving their brain of oxygen for a short period of time by extreme hyperventilation, pulling a plastic bag over their head, strangulation, or hanging (Ramowski, Nystrom, Rosenberg, et al., 2012).

The practice may be viewed as a rite of passage or initiation into a gang or club. The practice is also known as erotic asphyxiation because it also induces an orgasm response. Unfortunately, if carried too far, the game results in injuries such as concussion, bone fractures, tongue biting, and even death.

Teach parents, if they are unaware of the game, that it exists and to be aware of signs that their child might be interested or participating in such a game. Common signs are discussion of the game; bloodshot eyes; ligature marks on the neck; severe headaches; disorientation; and the presence of choke collars, ropes, scarves, or belts tied to bedroom furniture. Look for ligature or mark burns and sclera hemorrhages on unconscious children admitted to an emergency room for the possibility that self-injury of this type is the cause of their loss of consciousness.

ABDOMINAL TRAUMA

Abdominal trauma results when an object such as a baseball bat, a seat belt drawn tight in a motor vehicle accident, child maltreatment, or a bicycle handlebar injures the abdomen (Klimek, Lutz, Stranzinger, et al., 2012). Children are more apt to experience injury to their spleen and liver than adults because these organs are more exposed in children than they are in adults. The injury may be difficult to detect, however, because, unlike obvious signs of head or respiratory injuries, abdominal trauma usually presents with much more subtle signs.

Assessment

To detect abdominal trauma, assess vital signs for a baseline and then continue measurements to reveal whether abdominal hemorrhage could be occurring; rapid respirations, hypotension (less than 80 mmHg systolic pressure in an older child; less than 60 mmHg in an infant), and increasing pallor usually suggest that hidden internal bleeding is present. An additional suggestion that internal bleeding is present is that a low blood pressure shows little improvement when IV fluid is administered.

If abdominal trauma is suspected, an NG tube may be passed. Stomach contents are then aspirated to be checked visually for fresh and occult blood and then attached to low intermittent suction to allow for continued stomach observation. An indwelling urinary (Foley) catheter may be inserted into the bladder to evaluate urine for blood and urine output; evidence of blood in the urine suggests bladder damage, and a decreased output suggests accompanying kidney trauma. A paracentesis (introduction of a catheter into the abdomen to aspirate for the presence of blood) is yet another way to detect internal bleeding. Be aware that having NG tubes or catheters passed is extremely frightening for young children (unsure of their anatomy, they have no clear idea where the tubes are going). Offer a great deal of support to help them accept these diagnostic procedures (Box 52.4).

An abdominal X-ray, MRI, or ultrasound may be prescribed to rule out a ruptured liver or spleen or a fractured pelvis, all conditions that could be contributing to blood loss. Air under the diaphragm on an X-ray suggests gastric or intestinal rupture with escape of air from these organs into the peritoneal cavity. Free fluid in the abdomen suggests leakage of bowel fluid, liver or splenic rupture, and pooling of blood.

Parents may not bring their child to an emergency department immediately after abdominal trauma because they are unaware a serious injury has resulted. They may find it difficult to appreciate the seriousness of abdominal trauma so question why so many tests are prescribed, when their child shows no obvious signs of injury. When their child is asked to turn on the X-ray table so that an abdominal fluid level can be revealed, they may perceive this as unnecessary manipulation of an injured child. Without frightening them, explain that an injury need not be obvious at first glance to be serious; because the abdomen holds so many organs, more than one test may need to be prescribed to locate which organ is injured and causing bleeding.

Nursing Diagnoses and Related Interventions

Major features of abdominal injury are pain and a feeling of "fullness," both from edema and possibly internal bleeding. If parents did not recognize their child was injured, guilt and fear on their part may compound the child's care. Goal setting is usually concerned with the immediate diagnostic procedures or anticipated surgery. Interventions differ according to the specific injury present.

BOX 52.4 Nursing Care Planning Based on Effective Communication

Jason, 4 years old, has no memory of how he sustained a head injury and thus needs additional assessments to rule out other trauma.

Less Effective Communication	**More Effective Communication**
Mr. Varton: Why are you looking at his belly? He didn't hurt that. **Nurse:** He needs a thorough assessment to be sure there aren't any other problems. Next I'll be putting in an IV line and urinary catheter, and then taking him for an MRI. **Mr. Varton:** How much will all that cost? **Nurse:** Shame on you. Thinking about money instead of the care your child needs. **Mr. Varton:** Right. Guess it's one more example of what a bad parent I am.	**Mr. Varton:** Why are you looking at his belly? He didn't hurt that. **Nurse:** He needs a thorough assessment to be sure there aren't any other problems. Next I'll be putting in an IV line and urinary catheter, and then taking him for an MRI. **Mr. Varton:** How much will all that cost? **Nurse:** It sounds as if you're worrying about a lot more things than your son. Can I help with any of that? **Mr. Varton:** My daughter is burned. My house is ruined. I shouldn't have been next door . . . **Nurse:** Would you like to speak to a trauma counselor? He probably can't help with finances but he can help you realize that one small decision doesn't make you a bad parent.

In the first scenario, the nurse focuses on getting needed care done but fails to recognize the fear and apprehension and loss of self-esteem the parent is feeling. In the second scenario, the nurse listens and thus recognizes and attends to the parent's fears. By doing so, she helps to establish a sense of support and trust in addition to obtaining consent for procedures.

Nursing Diagnosis: Pain related to abdominal injury

Outcome Evaluation: Child states that level of pain is tolerable or rates it as low on a pain rating scale; does not grimace or guard when abdomen is palpated.

Routinely, analgesics are not administered to children after abdominal trauma, unless their pain is severe, to avoid masking increasing pain and, also, because the location of the pain can help identify which organ may be injured. Offer support until analgesia can be given. Being held by a parent or lying absolutely still on an examining table helps prevent abdominal organs from shifting and thus may help reduce the degree of pain.

Splenic Rupture

In children, the spleen is the most frequently injured organ when there is abdominal trauma, because it is usually palpable under the lower left ribs (McCance & Grey, 2012). Frequent causes of injury are inappropriately applied seat belts in automobiles, handlebar injuries in bicycle accidents, or skateboard or snowboard accidents. The child will have tenderness in the left upper quadrant of the abdomen, especially on deep inspiration, when the diaphragm moves down and touches the spleen. The child may hold the left shoulder elevated so that the diaphragm is raised on the left side to keep this from happening or report radiated left shoulder pain while lying in a supine position (Kehr sign).

An X-ray will show little about the spleen itself but may reveal a broken rib over the spleen, suggesting the extent of the trauma to that area. An MRI will rule out damage not only to the spleen but also to the left kidney just behind the spleen, which may also have suffered trauma. A complete blood count is done to detect blood loss or estimate its extent. An IV line is begun immediately and blood is typed and cross-matched, so blood can be readied for replacement if necessary. Children with suspected splenic injury are usually admitted to an observation unit if the blood loss from rupture appears to be mild. If bleeding is severe, immediate surgery, such as a partial or total splenectomy, may be necessary to halt the bleeding and save the child's life.

After a splenectomy, children are very susceptible to infection, particularly pneumococcal infections. Therefore, a large percentage of children are managed expectantly to see if the bleeding will halt without spleen removal (Lippert, Hartin, Ozgediz, et al., 2013). Children who have their spleen removed are offered *Haemophilus influenzae* type b, pneumococcal, and meningococcal vaccines to protect them against bacterial infections.

Liver Rupture

The liver is also more prone to rupture in children than in adults, because the liver, like the spleen, is not completely sheltered by the rib cage in children (Shao, Zou, Li, et al., 2013).

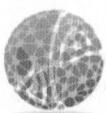

Children with liver rupture or laceration usually have severe abdominal pain that is most marked on inspiration, when the diaphragm descends and touches the liver. They also show symptoms of blood loss, such as tachycardia, hypotension, anxiety, and pallor. Their hematocrit level will be low or falling. Such children need to be prepared for immediate surgery, because the liver is a highly vascular organ, and blood loss from it is acute and possibly life threatening.

Occasionally, a communication between an artery and the bile duct occurs at the time of liver trauma. In this situation, symptoms are not immediate, but gastrointestinal (GI) bleeding, such as hematemesis (vomiting blood) or melena (blood in stool), may occur in a few days. The child may report colicky upper abdominal pain relieved by emesis. An MRI plus a liver study, such as a liver arteriogram, is necessary to reveal the extent of the injured artery.

After either liver or spleen surgery, children need careful observation for return of bowel function, assessment for the possibility of peritonitis, and careful reintroduction of oral nutrition.

DENTAL TRAUMA

Injuries to teeth occur most often from falls in which a child strikes the upper front incisors or from blows to the face by objects such as baseball bats or hockey sticks. Such injuries are always potentially serious, because they can lead to aspiration of the injured teeth or malalignment of future teeth. If a tooth is knocked out of the mouth, parents should rinse the tooth in water, drop it in a salt solution or milk, and bring it to the emergency department with them. Deciduous teeth may not be replaced, but if a permanent tooth can be saved, washed with saline or an antiseptic in the emergency department, and then replaced and wired into place, there is a good chance it will reimplant successfully (McTigue, 2013).

The child will usually be prescribed a course of oral antibiotic, such as penicillin, to prevent infection. Stress to the parents the importance of giving the full course of the antibiotic and allowing only soft food until the tooth has firmly adhered (approximately 2 weeks).

If a blow to a child's teeth was extensive, an X-ray may be taken to rule out an accompanying mandibular or maxillary fracture. If a portion of a tooth cannot be located, the possibility of aspiration must be considered and confirmed or ruled out by a chest X-ray. In young children, often a tooth is not knocked free but is pushed back up into the gum. These teeth gradually regrow, and although they may darken in color, they usually are healthy. If the affected tooth is a deciduous tooth, the permanent tooth is rarely injured even though it is already formed underneath in the gum. At the appropriate time, the permanent tooth will erupt without difficulty.

NEAR DROWNING

Drowning is death caused by suffocation from submersion in liquid when the inhaled water fills the lungs and therefore blocks the exchange of oxygen in the alveoli. More than 3,500 children die from drowning annually, making it one of the most frequent causes of death by unintentional injury among children. The term **near drowning** is used to describe the child with a submersion injury who, because of emergency treatment, survives the first 24 hours after injury (Shields, Pollack-Nelson, & Smith, 2011).

Most infant drownings occur in bathtubs; 1- to 4-year-old children most frequently drown in artificial pools; older children most frequently drown in bodies of fresh water. The majority of drowning injuries that take place outside the home occur in the summer months, when more children are swimming and boating. These may occur in young children because parents overestimate their child's swimming ability (Morrongiello, Sandomierski, Schwebel, et al., 2013). In older children, male adolescents are particularly at risk although both sexes may take dares to swim farther than their ability allows or may swim under the influence of alcohol, which impairs their decision-making ability and their physical coordination.

Pathophysiology of Drowning

When children's heads are submerged so they inhale water, they cough violently from the irritation of the water in their nose and throat. If they cannot get their head out of water at this point, water enters their larynx, causing the larynx to spasm and prevent any further water but also air from entering the trachea, resulting in asphyxia. If a child is ventilated at this point, treatment usually is very effective because there is little water in the lungs.

If treatment is not given at this point, the larynx relaxes from the asphyxia and water enters the lungs. Oxygen can no longer be exchanged as the alveoli fill with water. Hypoxia deepens, and cardiac arrest occurs.

Additional changes that occur when water enters the lungs depend on whether the water is fresh or salt. Salt water is hypertonic, so fluid osmoses from the bloodstream into the alveoli in an attempt to dilute the aspirated water, increasing the amount of fluid in lung tissue and increasing hypoxia. Blood viscosity increases as shown by an increased hematocrit level; both tachycardia and decreased blood pressure from hypovolemia result.

Fresh water is hypotonic, so the aspirated water shifts from the lungs into the bloodstream, again, because of osmotic pressure. This can lead to hemolysis of red blood cells, a dilution of plasma, and possibly hypervolemia with tachycardia and increased blood pressure. If the release of potassium from destroyed red blood cells is great enough with fresh-water drowning, cardiac arrhythmias may occur. In both instances, loss of surfactant from lung alveoli, caused by introduction of the water (adult respiratory distress syndrome), can lead to alveolar collapse on expiration (Varisco, Palmatier, & Alten, 2010).

Urge parents to advocate for neighborhood pools to be fenced; advise against children hyperventilating before swimming. When children hyperventilate before swimming so they "blow off" carbon dioxide and then swim underwater for an extended period of time, carbon dioxide levels will rise, but not adequately enough to cause them to experience distress. Oxygen levels in the meantime decrease because they are breath holding, causing drowsiness and listlessness (children drown without struggling or realizing their danger).

When very young children dive into very cold water, a mammalian diving reflex occurs that helps them survive drowning (immediately after plunging into cold water, a lifesaving bradycardia and shunting of blood away from the periphery of the body to the brain and heart occur). This reflex is triggered when water is 70°F (21°C) or less and the face is submerged first. The phenomenon explains why very young children survive more often than older children after being submerged in icy wintertime water.

Emergency Management

When a child is pulled from the water after near drowning, mouth-to-mouth resuscitation and CPR should be started at once (American Heart Association [AHA], 2011) (discussed in Chapter 41). This is an exception to the advice to use hands-only resuscitation as the child's lungs are filled with water, which must be displaced (AHA, 2011). Assuming CPR is effective, the child then needs follow-up care at a health care facility, because the child is certain to be acidotic from accumulated carbon dioxide and hypoxic from lack of oxygen caused by water retained in the alveoli. There also is a high risk for respiratory infection from contaminants in the water.

Follow-up care aims to increase the child's oxygen and carbon dioxide exchange capacity by using the lung areas that are not filled with water. Attach a pulse oximeter to monitor oxygen saturation. If respiratory efforts remain severely compromised, a child is intubated with a cuffed intratracheal tube; mechanical ventilation with positive end-expiratory pressure may be necessary to force air into the alveoli. A cuffed tube is used because water that has been swallowed will be vomited as the child revives and the cuff will prevent vomitus from being aspirated. The child is usually given 100% oxygen so that as much space as possible in the available lung alveoli can be used. In addition, an NG tube is inserted to decompress the stomach, prevent vomiting, and free up breathing space. A bronchodilator such as albuterol may be administered by aerosol to prevent bronchospasm and, again, to allow the child to make maximum use of the oxygen administered. If the child aspirated salt water, plasma may be administered to replace protein being lost into the lungs and prevent hypovolemia.

If the child's body temperature is very low, it is generally better to allow gradual warming (not using a warming blanket) so the child's metabolic requirement does not rise sharply before alveolar space is ready to accommodate this increased oxygen need. Extracorporeal membrane oxygenation (ECMO) may be necessary if the child has very little lung space free of water able to be used for oxygenation.

Unfortunately, a danger of near drowning is that neurologic damage will occur because of the period when the child was deprived of oxygen. If the child is awake or only lethargic at the scene of the injury and immediately afterward in the hospital, the prognosis is greatly improved over that of the child who is comatose.

Nursing Diagnoses and Related Interventions

Near drowning has both physical (lack of oxygen) and emotional (extreme fright) components, so both areas need to be addressed in planning care.

Nursing Diagnosis: Risk for infection related to foreign substance in respiratory tract

Outcome Evaluation: Child's tympanic temperature remains within normal parameters; rales are absent on lung auscultation; respiratory rate is within age-acceptable parameters.

After near drowning, a child is usually prescribed prophylactic antibiotic therapy to prevent pneumonia or additional airway interference. Assess vital signs and auscultate lung sounds frequently for adventitious sounds, such as rales or fine rhonchi. Turning the child every 2 hours if on bed rest and encouraging deep breathing and incentive spirometry every hour help to aerate the lungs fully and prevent the accumulation of fluid, which promotes infection.

Nursing Diagnosis: Fear related to near-drowning experience

Outcome Evaluation: Child discusses fear; states she understands that, although frightening, the experience is over, and she is now safe.

Children may be admitted to an observation unit for monitoring of oxygenation until water from the alveoli is absorbed and they once again can ventilate effectively on their own. Such children may wake at night or from a nap because of a nightmare they are drowning. Encourage children to verbalize the fright they feel about the experience. Assure them they are now safe and definitely out of the water. Because near drowning is such a frightening experience, a child may need support from parents before they are willing to try swimming again. Stress with parents that keeping the child away from water in the future is not as effective a means of preventing near drowning as being certain the child receives swimming lesions and thus is adept at swimming.

POISONING

Poisoning occurs in all socioeconomic groups and, unlike other unintentional injuries, is entirely preventable. The age group in which it occurs most commonly is children between the ages of 2 and 3 years. Usual agents that are ingested include soaps; cosmetics; detergents or cleaners; plants; over-the-counter drugs, such as vitamins, iron compounds, acetylsalicylic acid (aspirin), or acetaminophen (Tylenol); and prescription drugs, such as antidepressants. Teach the parents of preschool children about the high risk of poisoning in any home and strategies for maintaining a home environment safe for children of all ages. Be aware that poisoning can occur as a form of child maltreatment. When poisoning occurs in a child over about 7 years of age, it may not be poisoning but a self-injury attempt (Dinis-Oliveira & Magalhães, 2013).

Nursing Diagnoses and Related Interventions

Poisoning tends to occur when parents are preoccupied or highly stressed; nursing planning needs to address not only immediate care measures but also education to prevent poisoning from occurring again.

Nursing Diagnosis: Risk for injury related to young maturational age of child and presence of unsecured poisons in the home

Outcome Evaluation: Parents identify poisonous and toxic items in the home and describe how they are stored safely; parents state local poison control center number; parents describe measures to take if poisoning occurs.

Emergency Management of Poisoning at Home

If poisoning occurs, parents should telephone the National Poison Control Center (1-800-222-1222) to ask for advice regarding what to do because not all substances they think are dangerous when swallowed are, in fact, dangerous, and inducing vomiting with caustic substances can compound the poisoning, not help in recovery. Information parents need to provide includes:

- What was swallowed; if the name of a medicine is not known, what it was prescribed for and a description of it (color, size, shape of pills)
- The child's weight and age and how long ago the poisoning occurred
- The route of poisoning (oral, inhaled, sprayed on skin)
- An estimation of how much of the poison the child took (a bottle of cleaner or medicine should say how many pills or how much liquid it originally contained)
- The child's present condition (sleepy, hyperactive, comatose)

If the poison was in pill form, parents should check whether there are pills scattered under a chair before they assume they are all swallowed. If one child in a family has swallowed a poison, parents should investigate whether other children have also poisoned themselves because a preschooler often shares "candy" with a younger sibling. If the poison control center advises parents to make the child vomit, the best way to do this is to place a finger at the back of the child's throat. Old remedies such as giving mustard or salty water are not that effective and waste time that could be spent telephoning an emergency service (911) for help or transporting the child to the hospital.

What if...52.2 You have learned that Jason's older sister, Sage, 10 years old, suffered a mouth burn a year ago when she sprayed her mouth with oven cleaner because she was so sleepy one morning that she thought it was mouthwash. What suggestions could you give her about being more careful when she's sleepy?

Emergency Management of Poisoning at the Health Care Facility

In the emergency department, the best method to deactivate a swallowed poison is the administration of activated charcoal, either orally or by way of an NG tube to halt the action of the poison.

Activated charcoal is supplied as a fine black powder that is mixed with water for administration. Adding a sweet syrup to the mixture can make it more palatable. Caution parents that, as the charcoal is excreted through the bowel over the next 3 days, stools will appear black so they do not mistake the color for blood (Box 52.5).

Always follow immediate emergency measures to neutralize a poison with education for the family on how to prevent poisoning in the future. Specific measures important for each age group are discussed in chapters 29-33, along with problems and concerns of that age group.

Acetaminophen Poisoning

Acetaminophen (Tylenol) is the drug most frequently involved in childhood poisoning today, because parents use acetaminophen to treat childhood fevers and, having been told that acetaminophen is safer than aspirin, parents may not be as careful to put this drug away after use. They may delay bringing the child for emergency care, thinking it is a harmless drug. Acetaminophen in large doses, however, is not innocent; it can cause extreme permanent liver destruction (Ogilvie, Rieder, & Lim, 2012).

Immediately after ingestion, the child develops symptoms of anorexia, nausea, and usually vomiting. Serum aspartate transaminase (AST [SGOT]) and serum alanine transaminase (ALT [SGPT]), liver enzymes, rise. The liver may feel tender on palpation as liver toxicity occurs.

BOX 52.5 Nursing Care Planning Based on Responsibility for Pharmacology

ACTIVATED CHARCOAL

Classification: Activated charcoal is an antidote for poisoning.

Action: Absorbs toxic substances that have been swallowed to prevent them from being absorbed by the stomach (Karch, 2013).

Pregnancy Risk Category: C

Dosage: Provided as a powder that must be mixed with water and administered orally or by way of nasogastric (NG) tube.

Possible Adverse Effects: Vomiting, diarrhea, black stools

Nursing Implications

- Administer orally to conscious victims only.
- Give the drug as soon as possible after poisoning.
- Store the drug in a closed container, because if it absorbs gases from the air, it is inactivated.
- Recognize that the solution feels gritty and tastes disagreeable so young children often have difficulty swallowing it, which is why it may have to be administered by NG tube.
- Caution child and parents that stools will be black for several days after administration.

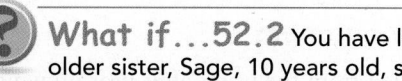

In the emergency department, activated charcoal or acetylcysteine, a mucolytic agent and also the specific antidote for acetaminophen poisoning, will be administered. Acetylcysteine prevents hepatotoxicity by binding with the breakdown product of acetaminophen so that it will not bind to liver cells. Unfortunately, acetylcysteine has an offensive odor and taste. Administering it in a small amount of a carbonated beverage can help the child to swallow it. For small children, it may be administered directly into an NG tube to avoid this difficulty. If the child is admitted to an observation unit, continue to observe for jaundice and tenderness over the liver; assess ALT and AST levels as prescribed.

Nursing Diagnoses and Related Interventions

Parents feel guilty after acetaminophen poisoning because they realize they should have been more careful with storing all medicine out of their child's reach. Be aware that, because it is a drug commonly available in the average home, acetaminophen poisoning may be the cause of unidentified coma or self-injury.

Nursing Diagnosis: Situational low self-esteem of parents related to child's poisoning

Outcome Evaluation: Parents state guidelines for continued assessment of child at home; state ways they can improve "childproofing."

After the child is stabilized following the poisoning, take some time to talk with the parents about the event. Remember poisoning tends to happen in homes where there is stress. If stress was already present, how has this poisoning added to it?

Before the child is discharged from a health care facility, be certain the parents are comfortable with any further assessment measures they will need to continue at home, such as temperature taking and urging a high fluid intake. Be certain they understand the importance of liver function tests for follow-up care to detect any long-term liver injury.

QSEN Checkpoint Question 52.3

Quality Improvement

Suppose you notice Jason was seen in the emergency department last year for acetaminophen poisoning. The hospital's algorithm for dealing with acetaminophen overdose should specify what action?

a. Advise the parents their child must never take acetaminophen again.
b. Be prepared to administer either acetylcysteine or activated charcoal.
c. Palpate the child's abdomen to assess whether the bladder feels tender.
d. Administer potassium chloride elixir immediately.

Look in Appendix A for the best answer and rationale.

Caustic Poisoning

Ingestion of a strong alkali, such as lye, which is contained in certain toilet bowl cleaners or hair care products, causes burns and tissue necrosis in the mouth, esophagus, and stomach. It's very important that parents do not try to make a child vomit after ingestion of these substances, because they can cause additional burning as they are vomited (Rumack & Dart, 2012).

Assessment

After a caustic ingestion, the child has immediate pain in the mouth and throat and drools saliva because of oral edema and an inability to swallow. The mouth turns white immediately from the burn and the child may vomit blood, mucus, and necrotic tissue. The loss of blood from the denuded, burned surface may lead to systemic signs of tachycardia, tachypnea, pallor, and hypotension. Tissue in the mouth turns brown as edema and ulceration develop, although there may be such marked edema of the tongue that it is difficult to examine past the lips. Activated charcoal should not be administered because it is ineffective and obstructs an endoscopic view.

Therapeutic Management

When parents whose child has ingested a caustic substance call a poison control center to ask for advice on how to proceed, they will be advised to immediately take the child to a health care facility for treatment because there is a high possibility that pharyngeal edema will become severe enough to obstruct the child's airway by even 20 minutes after the burn.

In the emergency department, relieving the child's pain is a first step. Advocate for a strong analgesic, such as IV morphine, to achieve pain relief for this level of injury. A chest X-ray may then be prescribed to determine whether the aspirated poison has caused an esophageal perforation that will allow swallowed fluid to seep from the injured esophagus into the mediastinum. A laryngoscopy and esophagoscopy under conscious sedation or general anesthesia may be done to assess the lungs and esophagus, although these must be done cautiously because of the possibility that an examining scope could perforate the burned esophagus or trachea.

Assess vital signs, especially the respiratory rate, and attach a pulse oximeter to establish a baseline and for continued monitoring to help detect if edema of the pharynx is obscuring the child's airway. In infants, increasing restlessness is an important accompanying sign of oxygen deprivation. For some children, intubation or a tracheotomy may be necessary to provide a patent airway, although, again, any intubation must be done cautiously because the throat is edematous and could be injured easily. To protect against stomach reflux against the burned esophageal area, a proton pump inhibitor may be prescribed intravenously. Even though the child has denuded mouth or throat areas, prophylactic antibiotic therapy is not usually necessary. Once a mainstay of therapy to reduce esophageal stricture, the use of a corticosteroid such as dexamethasone (Decadron) is now controversial and may or may not be prescribed.

Nursing Diagnoses and Related Interventions

Poisoning with a caustic substance is a true emergency because care must be initiated to preserve the child's airway. Providing adequate nutrition is a second concern because the child is unable to swallow through an edematous throat or esophagus.

Nursing Diagnosis: Risk for imbalanced nutrition, less than body requirements, related to esophageal stricture from burn scarring

Outcome Evaluation: Child's diet meets recommended daily allowance requirements for age.

Oral intake commonly will be a problem for the first week following a caustic injury because of soreness in the child's mouth; an NG tube is contraindicated so the child may be fed by TPN or gastrostomy feedings during this time. After about a week, liquids are introduced because liquid passing through the burned and scarred esophagus can help maintain esophageal patency or be therapeutic for the burn as well as nutritious for the child. Observe children carefully the first time they attempt to drink something for coughing, choking, or cyanosis, which are signs that suggest the liquid is not able to pass through the esophagus and is being aspirated into the lungs. Be certain parents have clear explanations of how to offer soft food as long as the child's mouth or throat is sore and the need for follow-up care to be certain their child's esophagus has not stenosed. After 2 weeks, a barium swallow or esophagoscopy will be performed to reveal the final extent of the esophageal burns and determine any further therapy needed. Some children require periodic dilation of the esophagus by endoscopy during the first year after the injury. To correct complete obstruction, repeated surgical procedures such as transplantation of intestinal tissue or a synthetic graft will be required to replace the obstructed esophagus. Because there is a correlation with the development of esophageal carcinoma later in life in individuals who swallowed a caustic substance, both the parents and the child need to be alerted to this possibility and to the signs of esophageal cancer (e.g., weight loss, difficulty swallowing) (Mas, Breton, & Lachaux, 2012).

Hydrocarbon Ingestion

Hydrocarbons are substances contained in products such as kerosene and furniture polish. Because these substances are be in volatile, fumes rise from them, causing their major effect to be in the respiratory system, such as the development of pneumonia, not gastric irritation. They are discussed in Chapter 40 with other causes of pneumonia.

Iron Poisoning

Iron is frequently swallowed by small children because it is an ingredient in vitamin preparations, particularly in prenatal vitamins. When ingested, a large amount of iron is corrosive to the gastric mucosa and leads to signs and symptoms of severe gastric irritation in the child (Chang & Rangan, 2011).

The immediate effects include nausea and vomiting, diarrhea, and abdominal pain. After 6 hours, however, these symptoms seem to fade, and the child's condition appears to improve. Internally, however, hemorrhagic necrosis of the lining of the GI tract continues to occur. By 12 hours, melena (blood in stool) and hematemesis (blood in emesis) are revealed. Lethargy and coma, cyanosis, vasomotor collapse, coagulation defects, and hepatic injury may also result. Hypovolemic shock may result from blood loss and decreased cardiac output. Long-term effects include gastric scarring from fibrotic tissue formation.

Assessment

It is difficult to estimate the amount of iron a child has swallowed, because the amount of elemental iron in compounds varies and parents can only guess at the number of pills that were in the bottle before the ingestion. Obtaining blood for a serum iron level analysis should be performed to establish a baseline.

Therapeutic Management

In the emergency department, activated charcoal is not given because it is not effective at neutralizing iron. Stomach lavage is done instead to remove any pills not yet absorbed. A cathartic may be given to help the child pass enteric-coated iron pills before they can be activated. A soothing compound such as Maalox or Mylanta (aluminum hydroxide and magnesium hydroxide) or a proton pump inhibitor can help decrease gastric irritation and pain.

If a child has ingested a potentially toxic dose of iron, an exchange transfusion can be used to remove excess iron from the body. Administration of a chelating agent such as IV or intramuscular (IM) deferoxamine can also be effective because this combines with the iron and allows it to be excreted harmlessly from the body in urine. Caution parents that deferoxamine causes urine to turn orange so they're not concerned about the color change. Parents may be asked to test any stool passed for the next 3 days for occult blood, to assess for stomach irritation and subsequent GI bleeding. Be certain that parents understand how to do this accurately.

For follow-up, an upper GI X-ray series and liver studies may be prescribed 1 week after the ingestion to screen for long-term effects. The hope is that the iron load was removed from the stomach in time so that not all of it was absorbed and long-term effects were prevented.

Nursing Diagnoses and Related Interventions

Many parents are unaware that iron can be toxic because they have been told so often that iron is necessary for good blood cell formation.

Nursing Diagnosis: Deficient parental knowledge related to the danger of iron as a poison

Outcome Evaluation: Parents state they understand the danger of iron ingestion for children; state ways they have safeguarded their child from future iron exposure.

Pregnant women may not realize prenatal vitamins contain more iron than usual (25 to 60 mg compared to 18 mg in usual or children's vitamins) and thus may not be as conscientious about storing these in a safe place, an action that can lead to iron poisoning in a child. Because many children's vitamins are manufactured in the shapes of familiar television or cartoon characters, children can think of these as candy and overdose on them if not supervised.

Whenever you instruct parents on taking an iron supplement for themselves or their children, stress that overdoses can be fatal to small children. Help them think of iron as they would any other medicine and keep it out of the reach of small hands.

Lead Poisoning

When lead enters the body, it interferes with red blood cell function by blocking the incorporation of iron into the protoporphyrin compound that makes up the heme portion of hemoglobin in red blood cells and leads to a hypochromic, microcytic anemia (Lee & Marcdante, 2011). In addition, kidney destruction may occur, causing excess excretion of amino acids, glucose, and phosphates in the urine. The most serious effect, however, is lead encephalitis or inflammation of brain cells because of the toxic lead content. Lead poisoning (**plumbism**), like all forms of poisoning in children, tends to occur most often in the toddler or preschool child. (See Chapter 30 for measures to prevent lead poisoning in the toddler or preschool child.)

Assessment

There is no safe level of lead accumulation in a child's body. Lead poisoning is said to be present when the child has two successive blood serum lead levels greater than 5 μ/dl (Centers for Disease Control and Prevention [CDC], 2012). The usual sources of ingested lead are paint chips or paint dust, home-glazed pottery, or fumes from burning or swallowed batteries (Marom, Goldfarb, Russo, et al., 2010). Paint tastes sweet, so a child will repeatedly pick up paint chips off the floor or off the walls to taste them. If a crib rail or a windowsill is painted with lead paint, a child will ingest it as the child teethes on the rail or sill. In fishing communities, swallowing lead sinkers can be a common source. Restoring an older home saturates the air with lead dust. In such homes, lead plumbing also may contaminate the drinking water.

Many children are asymptomatic until their level of ingested lead rises fairly high. Others show insidious symptoms of anorexia and abdominal pain from the presence of lead in their stomachs. Children with encephalopathy usually have beginning symptoms of lethargy, impulsiveness, and learning difficulties. As the child's blood level of lead increases, severe encephalopathy with seizures and permanent neurologic damage will result.

The most widely used method of screening for lead levels is the blood lead determination (serum ferritin). Unfortunately, this test requires the use of atomic absorption spectrophotometry, which is a costly procedure. The free erythrocyte protoporphyrin test is a simple screening procedure that involves only a finger stick. Because protoporphyrin is blocked from entering heme by the lead, it will be elevated in a child with lead poisoning.

Basophilic stippling (an odd striation of basophils) may be apparent on a blood smear. An X-ray of the abdomen may reveal paint chips in the intestinal tract (Fig. 52.6A). "Lead lines" (areas of increased density) may be present near the epiphyseal line of long bones with the thickness of the line revealing the length of time lead ingestion has been occurring (see Fig. 52.6B). Urine analysis reveals kidney damage. CSF may reveal an increased protein level from the presence of lead.

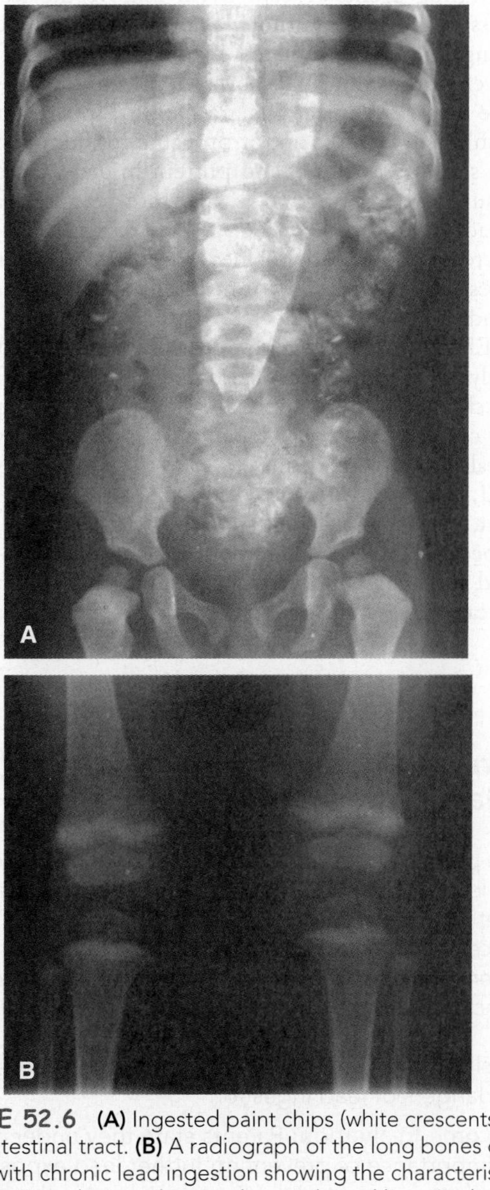

FIGURE 52.6 **(A)** Ingested paint chips (white crescents) in the intestinal tract. **(B)** A radiograph of the long bones of a child with chronic lead ingestion showing the characteristic "lead line" or white marking at the epiphyseal line. (Radiographs courtesy of Dr. Jerald P. Kuhn, Children's Hospital, Buffalo, NY.)

Therapeutic Management

A child with a blood lead level over 5 μg/dl needs to be rescreened to confirm the level, and then active interventions done to prevent further lead exposure such as removal of the child from the environment containing the lead source or removal of the source of lead from the child's environment. Removal of the lead source is not an easy task in homes because simple repainting or wallpapering does not necessarily remove the source of peeling paint adequately. After some months, the new paint will begin to peel because of the defective paint underneath. The walls must therefore be covered by paneling or dry wall or other solid protective material.

All children with lead levels greater than 10 to 20 μg/100 ml will be prescribed an oral chelating agent such as dimercaptosuccinic acid (DMSA) or succimer. Children with blood lead levels of greater than 45 μg/100 ml are treated with stronger chelation therapy such as dimercaprol (BAL) or edetate calcium disodium (CaEDTA) (Karch, 2013).

Chelating agents (except BAL) remove the lead from soft tissue and bone (although not from red blood cells), allowing it to be eliminated in the urine. CaEDTA can be given intravenously or by IM injection into a large muscle mass; IM injections are painful, so the drug may be combined with 0.5 ml of procaine for administration. BUN, serum creatinine, and protein in urine are assessed to ensure kidney function is adequate because CaEDTA can lead to nephrotoxicity or kidney damage if it cannot be excreted. Be certain to measure intake and output as an assessment that kidney function is adequate to excrete the lead.

CaEDTA is so effective as a chelating agent that it unfortunately has the side effect of also removing calcium from the body; children who receive CaEDTA, therefore, must have serum calcium measured periodically to determine whether their calcium level is adequate.

BAL has the advantage over CaEDTA of being able to remove lead from red blood cells, as well as other tissues, but, because of the danger of severe toxicity, it is prescribed only for children who have severe forms of lead intoxication.

Nursing Diagnoses and Related Interventions

Care planning can be difficult when a child is diagnosed with lead poisoning because parents are immediately upset at learning their child has been exposed to a source of lead. They may experience a loss of self-esteem and a sense of powerlessness as they realize their financial circumstances or lifestyle has hurt their child.

Nursing Diagnosis: Deficient knowledge related to the dangers of lead ingestion

Outcome Evaluation: Parents state they understand the importance of preventing further lead exposure; identify measures to take to reduce lead in the environment.

Parental education about the risk of lead poisoning is crucial. Parents may have to move to a new home or locale or extensively renovate their home. As temporary measures, placing the television or an overstuffed chair against a lead-based windowsill or placing the child's crib about 3 ft away from the walls so there is less risk the child will pick at loose wallpaper and expose lead-based plaster can be helpful. Be certain parents understand that all children with elevated lead levels need careful follow-up to determine the seriousness of their condition and to ensure they are being kept from a lead source. Because children who recover from symptomatic lead poisoning have a high incidence of permanent neurologic damage, all children with elevated blood lead levels need appropriate follow-up care to evaluate development and intelligence (CDC, 2012).

Pesticide Poisoning

Pesticide poisoning can occur by unintentional ingestion but usually occurs through skin or respiratory tract contact when children play in an area that has recently been sprayed. Long-term exposure may result from exposure to a parent's clothing if the parent comes home covered with pesticide spray. Although pesticide poisoning was once thought to be only a rural problem, the increase in the use of lawn sprays by commercial lawn care companies now makes this a suburban problem as well (Langley & Mort, 2012).

Many pesticides have an organophosphate base that causes acetylcholine to accumulate at neuromuscular junctions, leading to muscle paralysis. Within a few minutes to 2 hours after exposure, children develop nausea and vomiting, diarrhea, excessive salivation, weakness of respiratory muscles, confusion, depressed reflexes, and possibly seizures.

In the emergency department, activated charcoal is administered if the pesticide was swallowed. If clothing is contaminated, remove it and thoroughly wash the child's skin and hair. To prevent coming in contact with the pesticide, be certain to wear gloves.

IV atropine and the cholinesterase reactivator, pralidoxime chloride (Protopam), are effective antidotes to reverse symptoms. If parents apply a pesticide to children to help avoid mosquito or tick bites, diethyltoluamide (DEET)-based pesticides appear to be safe if they are used once a day, applied by the parent (not the child), not applied to a child's face (so it isn't near their eyes or nose) or on their hands (they may put their hands in their mouth), and washed off when the child returns indoors (Roberts & Karr, 2012).

Plant Poisoning

Plant poisoning (ingestion of a growing plant) occurs because parents commonly do not think of house plants as being poisonous (Matulkova, Gobin, Evans, et al., 2012). Plants served in salads are responsible for bacterial poisoning such as salmonella infection if not washed well before being served (Olaimat & Holley, 2012). Common toxic house plants to which children may be exposed are English ivy, hydrangea, holly berries, mistletoe, and poinsettia.

Poisoning by Drugs of Abuse

Adolescents and even grade-school children are brought to health care facilities by parents or friends because of a drug overdose, an unusual reaction to a drug, or the effect of an unfortunate combination of drugs. Typical drugs seen with overdoses are codeine and antidepressant drugs, often removed from the family medicine cabinet (Viana, Trent, Tull, et al., 2012).

Children are often extremely disoriented and may be hallucinating when seen for this form of ingestion. Obtaining a history may be very difficult because children have no idea what they took except it was a red or a yellow capsule. Others may know the name of what they took but be reluctant to name the drug if it was obtained illegally.

Assessment

Although a child may not appear to understand instructions well or may not seem coherent, avoid shouting or aggravating to obtain a history, because a child having a paranoid reaction to a drug will be unable to cope rationally with this approach. If friends accompany the ill child, point out that your role is not that of a law enforcer. Your role is to help the child, and you cannot do that effectively unless the drug can be identified. If a child is brought in by parents who have no idea what drug could possibly have been taken, assuming the child became ill at home, ask them to have someone at home check the child's bedroom for drugs or what could be missing from the medicine cabinet.

Blood specimens need to be obtained for electrolyte levels and a toxicology screen. If the child vomits, save any vomitus because this can be analyzed for the presence of the drug. Try to determine whether the ingestion was unintentional (perhaps the child was unaware the two drugs would react this way or calculated a wrong dose) or whether the child was actually attempting self-injury. Consider all poisonings or drug ingestions in children older than 7 years of age as potential self-injury until established otherwise.

Therapeutic Management

Children need immediate supportive measures for their specific symptoms, including rapid IV fluid administration in an attempt to dilute the drug, oxygen administration, and electrolyte replacement (particularly if there is accompanying nausea and vomiting). Factors such as reduction of fear and anxiety, increased coping mechanisms, knowledge of the effects of drug use, and availability of referral sources for drug abuse are important follow-up areas to address. (See Chapter 33 for more information related to adolescents and drug use.)

If the ingestion was unintentional, the child will need counseling to avoid drug use for the future. If the incident was attempted self-injury, the child will need observation and counseling toward more effective coping mechanisms in self-care. A potentially lethal ingestion of this type may act as a turning point in the child's life, possibly alerting the child and family for the first time to a drug abuse problem and the need for help.

QSEN Checkpoint Question 52.4

Informatics

Suppose Jason is found to have an elevated serum lead level. What is the most common source of lead poisoning in young children that would contribute to this assessment finding?

a. Smelling lead fumes from cooking utensils
b. Swallowing batteries that fall out of toys
c. Drinking lead-contaminated drinking water
d. Chewing on chips of flaking lead-based paint

Look in Appendix A for the best answer and rationale.

FOREIGN BODY OBSTRUCTION

Foreign bodies can become lodged in children's esophagus, ear canals, noses, or lungs, causing direct obstruction of the airway or long-term stasis of secretions and infection. Whether a foreign substance is inhaled or embedded elsewhere, nursing interventions should focus first on comforting the child and aiding in removal of the substance, and then on teaching the child and parents ways to avoid such occurrences in the future.

Foreign Bodies in the Ear

Any child with a history of draining exudate from the ear canal needs an otoscopic examination to establish the reason this is occurring because, in toddlers and preschoolers, the drainage often is the result of a foreign body such as a small piece of a toy, a piece of paper, a small battery, or food, such as a peanut that was pushed into the ear canal (Sharpe, Rochette, & Smith, 2012).

Removal of a foreign body from the ear can be difficult. Because children are afraid that the instrument used to remove the object will hurt them, they have difficulty lying still for the procedure. Often, it is better to wait for an otolaryngologist to care for the child, because trauma to the ear canal during an attempt to remove a foreign body can cause edema and make removal even more difficult.

In many instances, if the object is in the outer canal, it can be grasped by forceps and easily removed. If there is reason to think the tympanic membrane is intact, irrigating the object from the ear canal with a syringe and normal saline may be possible, although this should not be done if the object is a substance that will swell when wet, such as a peanut. If there is a possibility that the tympanic membrane is ruptured, the ear canal should not be irrigated or fluid will be forced into the middle ear, possibly introducing infection (otitis media).

Foreign Bodies in the Nose

Foreign objects stuffed into the nose eventually cause inflammation and purulent discharge from the nose. The odor accompanying such impaction is often the first sign noticed by a parent. Objects pushed into the nose usually can be removed with forceps. A local antibiotic might be necessary after removal if ulceration resulted from the local irritation.

Foreign Bodies in the Esophagus or Stomach

Children tend not to chew food well or to swallow portions that are too big to pass safely through the esophagus when they are in a hurry. Pieces of candy, such as Lifesavers, are common objects caught in the esophagus in young children; coins may be swallowed by adolescents playing drinking games. Wires of orthodontic appliances that dislodged are also frequently swallowed. The mark of an object lodged in the esophagus is intense pain at the site where the object is located. If the object is one that will dissolve, such as a Lifesaver or a piece of digestible meat, offer the child fluid to drink to help flush the object into the stomach. Even after the object dissolves or passes into the stomach, the child will feel transient pain at the original site of the obstruction.

Magnets, particularly those in watches or hearing aids, are also frequently swallowed by young children. These need to be removed by endoscopy as soon as possible because they can lead to bowel perforation or volvulus from their acid content. Objects, such as a part of a toy, a chicken bone, or a large coin, that will not dissolve and should not be passed are also removed by endoscopy (Avey, Euathrongchit, & Stern, 2012).

Small coins, such as pennies and dimes, usually pass by themselves without difficulty. Parents (or children themselves if adolescents) need to observe stools over the next several days to determine that the coin does pass through the GI tract (about 48 hours after ingestion). Without frightening them, caution parents to observe for signs of bowel perforation or obstruction, such as vomiting or abdominal pain, until the coin has passed. If there is any doubt, an X-ray taken 3 to 7 days after ingestion will establish whether the coin has been evacuated from the body.

Subcutaneous Objects

Children receive many wood splinters in the hands and feet. These usually are removed easily by a probing needle and tweezers after cleaning with an antiseptic solution. If the penetrating object is metal, such as a sewing needle or nail, its presence can be detected by X-ray. If the object is one that would have been in contact with soil, such as a rusty nail, the child will need tetanus prophylaxis after extraction of the object if the child's tetanus immunization is not current.

What if...52.3 Jason's mother tells you she thinks the reason he has an elevated lead level is because he swallowed a penny a month ago and it must still be inside him. Is a penny a likely source of lead poisoning? Is it likely the penny is still in his gastrointestinal tract?

BITES

Children receive bites from snakes and animals such as dogs or raccoons; they occasionally receive bites from other children. In an emergency room, the source of a bite needs to be documented because human bites can also result from child maltreatment.

Mammalian Bites

Dog bites account for approximately 90% of all bites inflicted on humans, and children and adolescents are involved in one third to one half of reported incidents. The dog is usually one owned by the child's family. Cat bites, wild animal bites, and human bites also constitute a threat, although these are less common in children. All of these bites can cause abrasions, puncture wounds, lacerations, and crushing injuries related to the size of the animal and the location of the bite (Dyring-Andersen, Menne, & Skov, 2012).

The biggest concerns associated with animal bites are the possibilities of long-term scarring and disfigurement and the possibility of infection, especially rabies, from the presence of microorganisms in the animal's mouth. Rabies and the vaccine for rabies are discussed in Chapter 43.

Snakebite

Snakebites tend to occur during the warm months of the year, from April to October. A few fatal bites in the United States occur from cottonmouth moccasins or coral snakes (both found in southeastern states), but the majority of fatal snakebites (envenomations) are from copperheads or rattlesnakes. Copperheads are found in eastern and southern states; rattlesnakes are found in almost every state. The effect of the bite of a rattlesnake, copperhead, or cottonmouth moccasin (all pit vipers) is the almost immediate failure of the blood coagulation system (Warrell, 2012).

Coral snakes are known for the small coral, yellow, and black rings encircling their body. Fortunately, they are shy and seldom bite. However, the venom injected through the bite of these snakes leads to neuromuscular paralysis.

Assessment

Immediately after a pit viper bite, a white wheal surrounding the puncture marks begins to appear, accompanied by excruciating pain at the site. Purplish erythema and edema extend rapidly from the site.

By the time a child is seen at a health care facility, sanguineous fluid may be oozing from the bite. Systemic symptoms, such as dizziness, vomiting, perspiration, and weakness, may be present. Because snake venom interferes with blood coagulation, the child may have hematemesis or bleeding from the nose, intestines, or bladder because of subcutaneous or internal hemorrhage. The pupils may be dilated, showing the potent effect on cerebral centers. If the envenomation is not treated, seizures, coma, and death may result.

Emergency Management at the Scene

At the scene of a snakebite, parents should apply a cold compress to the bite, in the hope of slowing the spread of the venom and reducing edema formation. Urging the child to lie quietly, with the bitten extremity dependent also helps to slow circulation. Commercial snakebite kits have rubber suction cups in them that can be used to suction out the venom, so if available, they should be used. Excising the bite with a knife and sucking out the venom orally (often shown in old western movies) is of questionable value and if the person administering the treatment has open mouth lesions, such as carious teeth, the procedure could be dangerous to that person (venom is not dangerous when swallowed, only when absorbed through open lesions). Excising the bite also may lead to secondary infection and, if done too vigorously, may injure tendon or muscle. Parents should waste no time before the child is transported to a health care facility for therapy.

Emergency Management at the Health Facility

In the emergency department, ask the child or a person who was with the child to describe the snake. In areas where snakebites are frequent, keep available photographs of the venomous snakes commonly found because even a preschooler may be able to identify the snake by pointing to a photograph. Specific antivenin depending on the type of snake is then administered. Because rattlesnakes, copperheads, and cottonmouth moccasins are all one type of snake (pit vipers), one form of antivenin acts against all of these bites. Specific antivenin is prepared for coral snake or cobra bites (not typically kept in emergency departments but obtained from most zoos). If a child receives antivenin promptly after a bite, the prognosis for full recovery is good.

Antivenin may contain a horse-serum base. Therefore, before the serum is injected intramuscularly or intravenously, a skin test may need to be performed to prevent a possible anaphylactic reaction to the horse serum. If giving the serum IM, do not inject it into an edematous body part, because medication will be poorly absorbed from edematous tissue; you may need to assure the parents that giving antivenin into the limb opposite the bitten limb is just as effective as administering it into the bitten limb. If the child's immunization status is unknown or it has been more than 10 years since a tetanus immunization was given, ask if tetanus prophylaxis should also be administered.

Nursing Diagnoses and Related Interventions

Snakebites are frightening, so nursing diagnoses need to address both calming the child and parents as well as administering immediate interventions.

Nursing Diagnosis: Fear related to seriousness of child's condition

Outcome Evaluation: Parents and child state they are able to cope with the degree of fear present.

Following a venomous snakebite, children need a great deal of support from health care personnel because their parents may be too frightened to offer adequate support. As a final care measure, teach children the following common safety rules for avoiding snakebites:

- Look for snakes before stepping into underbrush.
- Be aware that snakes sun on warm rocks.
- Do not lift up rocks without looking at what could be under them.
- Listen for the telltale sound of a rattlesnake.
- Know the markings of poisonous snakes to help avoid them.

ATHLETIC INJURIES

Although participating in athletics promotes growth and development and teaches concepts of teamwork and perseverance, this can unfortunately also lead to injury. Playing on backyard trampolines, in particular, is a dangerous sport for children because neck and spine injuries can result (American Academy of Pediatrics Council on Sports Medicine and Fitness, 2012). Strategies to prevent sports injuries include preparticipation health examinations, proper coaching, attention to safety, adequate hydration, proper officiating, availability of first aid and medical coverage at all sporting events, and proper equipment and field or surface playing conditions.

Knee Injuries

Participation in sports such as football, skateboarding or snowboarding, skiing, soccer, and track is a frequent cause of knee injuries in children that usually involve the ligaments surrounding the knee—the medial, lateral, posterior, and cruciate ligaments. Immediately after the injury, the child reports severe pain in the knee, and localized edema becomes evident. An X-ray or MRI will be taken to rule out fracture and the extent of the ligament damage. If the injury is mild (only a few torn fibers), bed rest with an ice pack applied to the knee is often the only therapy needed. After 24 hours, heat is applied to the knee to hasten healing.

If the injury is more severe, the knee joint may fill with fluid. In addition to bed rest and an ice pack applied to the joint, the abnormal synovial fluid may be aspirated and a compression dressing applied to discourage accumulation of further fluid. After 24 hours, heat treatments hasten healing.

If the injury is severe, arthroscopy is necessary to visualize and surgically repair the knee ligaments. Arthroscopic surgery makes repair of ligaments or cartilage a minor procedure and limits the necessity for immobilization and a cast. Children who have one anterior cruciate ligament injury need to be aware that they may suffer another in their other knee and may be more prone to osteoarthritis in the affected knee later in life (Smith, Vacek, Johnson, et al., 2012).

If a child experiences a severe twisting motion to the knee, a dislocation of the patella (kneecap) can result (the kneecap moves to the posterior surface of the knee). The knee appears immediately deformed, and the child feels acute pain. An ultrasound or MRI will reveal if there is accompanying ligament damage. Immediate treatment for a dislocated kneecap is to slide the patella back to the front of the knee. After this realignment, the pain subsides, but the child may have to be fitted with a leg immobilizer for about 1 week to keep the kneecap in good alignment. Quadriceps exercises (straight-leg raising) are important to prevent the dislocation from occurring again because these exercises strengthen the leg muscles and tendons. If the problem becomes chronic or occurs frequently, surgery to strengthen the knee ligaments may be necessary (Felus & Kowalczyk, 2012).

Throwing Injuries

Throwing an object such as a baseball places repeated stress on an upper extremity, particularly the elbow joint. The injury that occurs is caused either by the forward motion of the arm or during the follow-through. After the injury, a child is unable to extend the elbow completely because of minute tears and fibrous contractures in the muscle for about the next 24 to 48 hours. Pain and tenderness are marked. Resting the arm and applying ice packs for 15 to 20 minutes three times a day relieve the pain. An anti-inflammatory agent (nonsteroidal anti-inflammatory drug) will also relieve the pain. A limited number of cortisone injections into the elbow musculature may be necessary for complete healing. Exercises to strengthen flexor muscles help to prevent this type of injury.

"Little leaguer's elbow" is epiphysitis (inflammation) of the medial epicondylar epiphysis caused by too many throwing motions a week. An X-ray of the elbow will reveal increased growth, separation, and fragmentation of the medial epicondylar epiphysis. Children need extra protection against this type of injury by limiting the amount of time spent in practice or games until the epiphyseal growth centers at the elbow have fused at 14 to 17 years of age (Hoang, Coel, Vidal, et al., 2012).

Treatment for little leaguer's elbow is rest and immobilization until pain, tenderness, and limitation of movement have passed. This is important because if the injury is not treated adequately, permanent damage to the epiphyseal line and elbow deformity can occur (Fleisig & Andrews, 2012).

INJURIES OF THE EXTREMITIES

Finger Injuries

It is common for a child to sustain a finger injury from a slammed car door. This injury, which causes a crushing blow to the tip of the finger, is excruciatingly painful. The fingernail may be lacerated and detached. As blood accumulates under the fingernail, pain continues to increase unless an incision under the distal end of the nail or a stab wound through the nail helps to relieve the pain. Fingernails often are lost after these injuries, but they grow back readily with little scarring. You can assure parents that, although the fingernail may be lost, the cosmetic effect will invariably not be a problem.

Parents may feel embarrassed and guilty when they bring a child to a health care facility for this type of injury. The injury usually occurred because they closed a door without looking out for the child's finger. They appreciate how much this hurts and are angry with themselves for being so careless. Reassure parents that this is a common childhood injury and unintentional injuries do happen.

An X-ray of the fingertip may be obtained to be certain the tip of the distal phalanx is not broken. The rule, "If the child can bend it, it's not broken," does not apply to this injury, because the fracture may be distal to the last phalangeal joint. The open wound needs to be cleaned well. If the distal phalanx is fractured, the finger needs a splint applied to stabilize the bone. A follow-up visit will be necessary to ensure healing has occurred.

Bicycle-Spoke Injuries

Children who ride in child bicycle seats or over the back wheel of a bicycle can easily catch a foot or ankle between the spoke and the frame of the bicycle, resulting in a crushing, lacerating injury that quickly becomes edematous (Agarwal & Pruthi, 2010). They can also injure their fingers in bicycle spokes. In both instances, an X-ray may be needed to rule out a fracture.

The wound, which usually is contaminated with spoke grease, needs to be cleaned with an antiseptic. It may be necessary to soak the area first with a solution of lidocaine, a local anesthetic, because of the amount of pain that quickly occurs from edema and ecchymosis. Sutures and a splint may be necessary to stabilize a finger injury. If a foot is injured, the child may need to limit weight bearing by using crutches.

Soft-tissue injuries of this nature continue to be painful until the edema is absorbed (perhaps up to 6 weeks). Elevating the body part on pillows helps to reduce both the pain and edema. Be certain parents understand that healing will be slow or they can worry the child's injury is not healing well. Remind parents about the importance of children wearing helmets when bicycling so they can be instrumental in decreasing the rate of the most serious type of injury from bicycle accidents (head injuries) (Koestner, 2012).

Strains and Sprains

A **strain** is a muscle–tendon injury. A **sprain** is a ligament injury. Strained or sprained ankles are common and slow-to-heal childhood injuries (Tiemstra, 2012). Immediately after an injury, the affected joint feels painful and is swollen. Such injuries typically occur from inline skating or snowboarding or skateboarding. When X-ray reveals no fracture, a child may feel as though someone has said the injury is not serious but "just a sprain." This makes the extent of the swelling and pain baffling. Some children may be accused by parents of "putting on" pain because the injury is "only a sprain."

Help the child and parents to understand that strains and sprains are truly painful. Because a cast is not used and the ankle is not immobilized, but just wrapped in an elastic bandage, strains and sprains can be more painful than fractures.

If the injury is recent, apply an ice pack for approximately 20 minutes to reduce edema at the site; repeat this for 4 to 7 days at home. The child may be fitted for crutches to limit weight bearing for the next 3 or 4 days or fitted with a supportive medical boot. Make certain the parents of the child understand how the elastic bandage is applied so that it can be rewrapped if it loosens, and be certain the child is using the crutches or boot properly before being discharged from the emergency department.

THERMAL INJURIES

Thermal injuries include those caused by either cold (frostbite) or excessive heat (burns).

Frostbite

Frostbite is tissue injury caused by freezing cold; the extreme cold causes peripheral vasoconstriction, cutting off the oxygen supply to surrounding cells (Castellani & Young, 2012). In children, the body parts involved usually are the nose, fingers, or toes.

Assessment

The severity of frostbite is classified by degree:

- First degree: Mild freezing of epidermis; appears erythematous with edema
- Second degree: Partial- or full-thickness injury; appears erythematous; blisters and pain occur after rewarming
- Third degree: Full-thickness injury (epidermis, dermis, and subcutaneous tissue); appears white
- Fourth degree: Complete necrosis with gangrene and possible ultimate loss of body part

Frostbite occurs most frequently in children who have been skiing, snowmobiling, or snowboarding for long periods. Frostbite of the lips or tongue can occur from sucking on a popsicle and from inhalant abuse. Always explore the cause and circumstances of frostbite by careful history taking because it can also result from neglect or child maltreatment.

Therapeutic Management

Always warm frostbitten areas gradually because sudden warming increases the metabolic rate of cells; without adequate blood flow to the area because of still-present vasoconstriction, additional damage could occur. Administration of a vasodilator and use of hyperbaric oxygen may help reduce the effect on body cells.

Nursing Diagnoses and Related Interventions

Frostbite may not be recognized immediately, so children generally have pain and blistering by the time they are seen for emergency care.

Nursing Diagnosis: Pain related to damage of cells because of freezing temperature

Outcome Evaluation: Child states that pain is controlled at a tolerable level.

As soon as warming of the frostbitten body part begins, the part becomes extremely painful because the cells that are injured register their anoxic state. Advocate for a strong analgesic for pain, such as morphine, given IV or epidurally.

During the next few days after severe frostbite, necrosis of destroyed tissue occurs; the affected tissue then sloughs away. Apply or change dressings as necessary to avoid secondary bacterial contamination of the necrotic injury site. Assess body temperature conscientiously to detect early symptoms of infection at the site. Be certain that children understand the cause of the injury so they take more precautions against cold injury in the future.

Burns

Burns are injuries to body tissue caused by excessive heat (heat greater than 104°F [40°C]). Such injuries occur so commonly in children that they are the second greatest cause of unintentional injury in children 1 to 4 years of age and the third greatest cause in children age 5 to 14 years. Toddlers are often burned by biting into electric cords, by pulling pans of scalding water or grease off the stove and onto themselves, or by bath water that is too hot (Laitakari, Pyörälä, & Koljonen, 2012). Older children are more apt to be burned from flames after they move too close to a campfire, heater, or fireplace; touch a hot curling iron; or play with matches or lighted candles. Eye burns occur from splashed chemicals doing home projects or in science classes. Always keep in mind when evaluating burns that some (particularly scalding) can also be caused by child maltreatment (Blackburn, Levitan, MacLennan, et al., 2012).

Burn injuries tend to be more serious in children than in adults, because the same size burn covers a larger surface of a child's body. Many burns can be prevented with improved parent and child education.

Assessment

Because burns are classified as to degree, when children with a burn injury are brought to a health care facility, the first questions asked must be, "Where is the burn?" and "What are its extent and depth?" (Nicole & Huether, 2012). Along with the size and depth, be certain to assess and document the location of the burn. Face and throat burns, for example, are particularly hazardous because there may be accompanying but unseen burns in the respiratory tract that could lead to respiratory tract obstruction. Hand burns are also hazardous because, if the fingers and thumb are not positioned properly during healing, adhesions will inhibit full range of motion in the future. Burns of the feet carry a high risk for secondary infection. Genital burns are also hazardous because edema of the urinary meatus may prevent a child from voiding.

With adults, the "rule of nines" is a quick method of estimating the extent of a burn. For example, each upper extremity represents 9% of the total body surface; each lower extremity represents two 9s, or 18%, and the head and neck represent 9%. Because the body proportions of children are different from those of adults, this rule does not always apply and is misleading in the very young child. Data for determining the extent of burns in children are shown in Figure 52.7. Computer analysis is now available to rapidly assess the extent of burns.

Depth of Burn. When estimating the depth of a burn, use the appearance of the burn and the sensitivity of the area to pain as criteria. Descriptions of tissue at various burn depths are shown in Table 52.3 and illustrated in Figures 52.8 through 52.11.

Many burns are compound, involving first-, second-, and third-degree burns, or there may be a central white area insensitive to pain (third degree), surrounded by an area of erythematous blisters (second degree), surrounded by another area that is erythematous only (first degree).

Be certain to undress children with burns completely so the entire body can be inspected. Because a first-degree burn is painful but a third-degree burn is not, a child may be crying from a superficial burn that is obvious on the arm, although the condition needing the most immediate attention is a third-degree burn on the chest, covered by a jacket.

Be certain to ask also what caused the burn because different materials cause different degrees of burn. Hot water, for example, causes scalding, a generally lesser degree of burn than one caused by flaming clothing. Ask where the fire happened because fires in closed spaces are apt to cause more respiratory involvement than those in open areas.

Lastly, determine whether other family members were burnt as well. Parents, for example, may have burned hands from putting out the fire on the child's clothes and need equal care, but in their anxiety about the child's condition, they do not mention this. If they picked up and brought the burned child to the hospital quickly, they may have left other children unprotected at home. They also may be so concerned

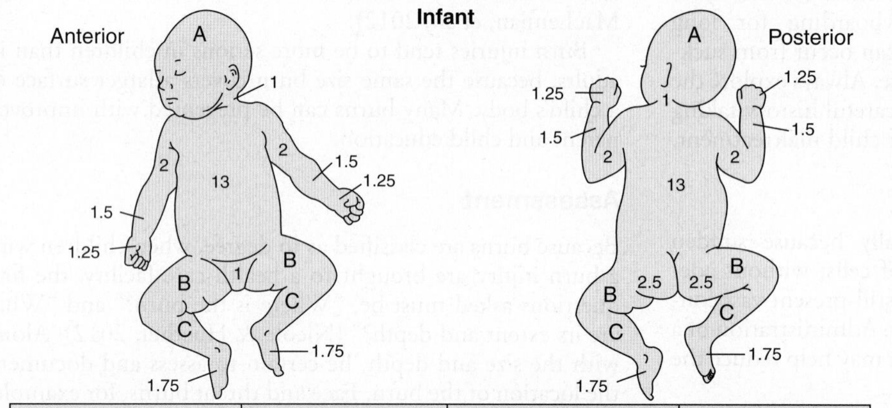

AREA	BIRTH	AGE 1 YEAR	AGE 5 YEARS
A = 1/2 of head	9 1/2	8 1/2	6 1/2
B = 1/2 of one thigh	2 3/4	3 1/4	4
C = 1/2 of one leg	2 1/2	2 1/2	2 3/4

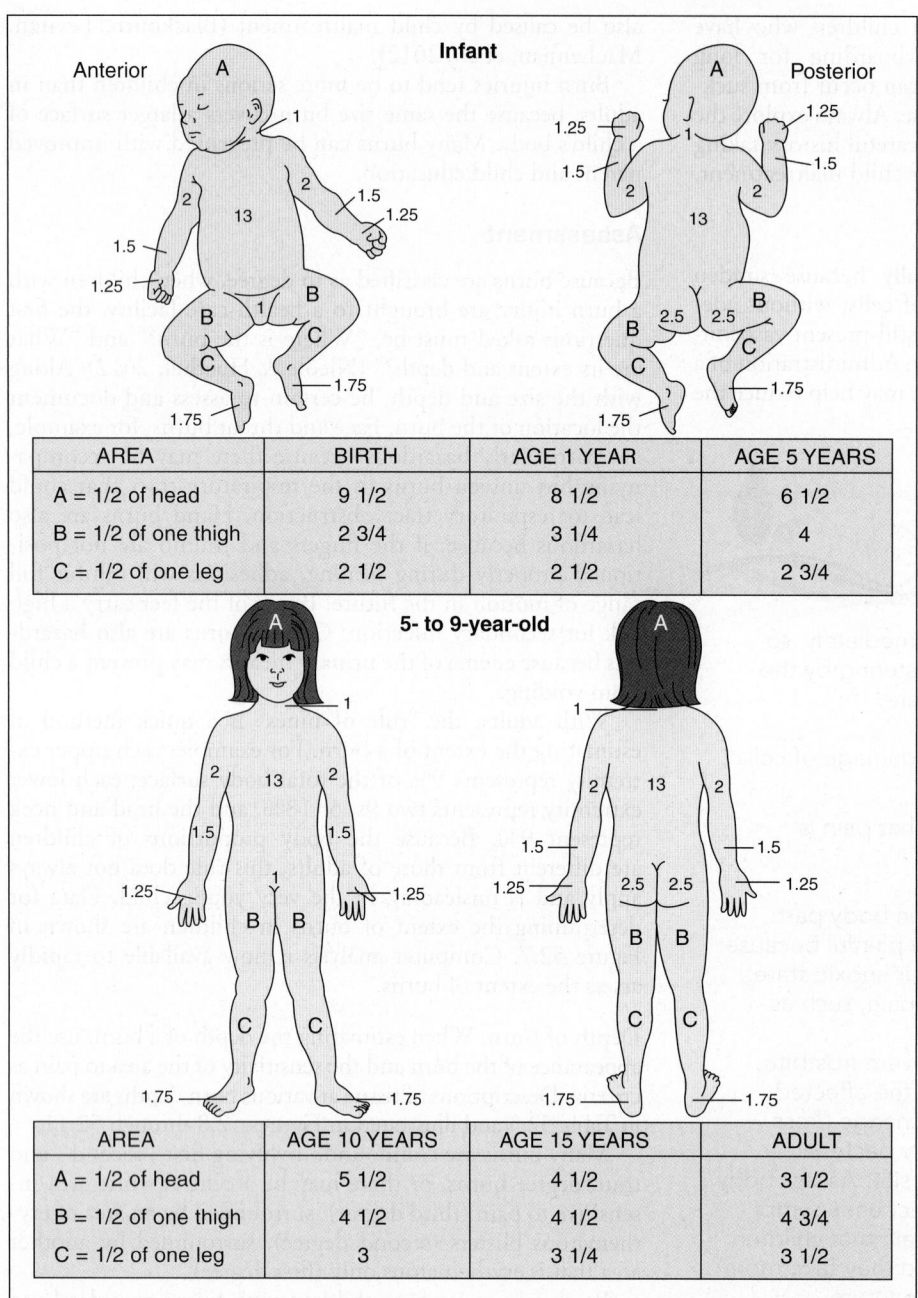

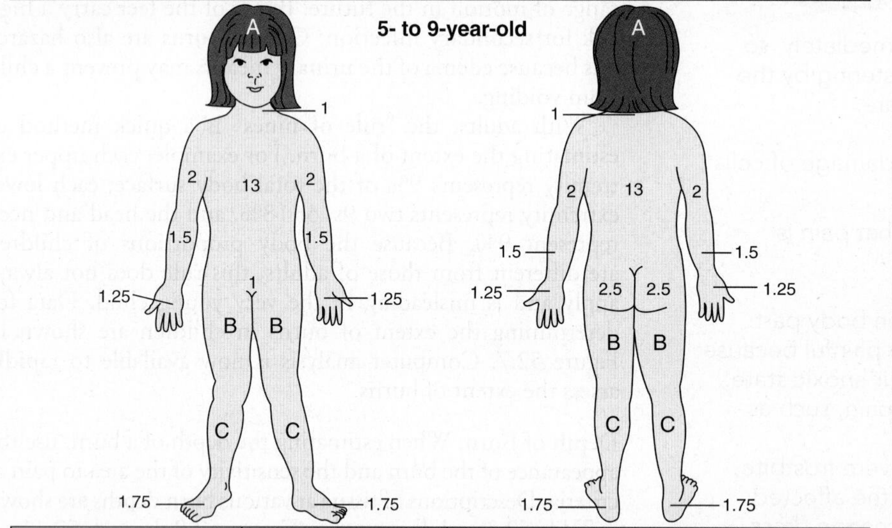

AREA	AGE 10 YEARS	AGE 15 YEARS	ADULT
A = 1/2 of head	5 1/2	4 1/2	3 1/2
B = 1/2 of one thigh	4 1/2	4 1/2	4 3/4
C = 1/2 of one leg	3	3 1/4	3 1/2

FIGURE 52.7 Determination of extent of burns in children.

TABLE 52.3 Common Classifications and Descriptions of Burns

Degree	Description	Common Cause
First degree	Involves the epidermis or outer layer of skin. Appears reddened, dry, and feels mildly painful. Heals by simple regeneration so takes 1–10 days to heal.	Sunburn (Fig. 52.9A)
Second degree	Involves the epidermis and part of the dermis layer of skin. Appears red, blistered, and may be swollen. Very painful. Heals by regeneration of tissue over 2–6 weeks.	Scalding (Fig. 52.9B)
Third degree	Involves the epidermis and full extent of the dermis. Appears white or charred and lacks sensation as the nerve endings are destroyed. Skin grafting is usually necessary, and healing takes months. Scar tissue will cover the final healed site.	Flames (Figs. 52.10 and 52.11)
Fourth degree	Full-thickness burn extending into muscle or bone. Skin grafting is necessary; muscle and bone may be permanently damaged; scarring will cover the healed site.	High-voltage electric or severe fire

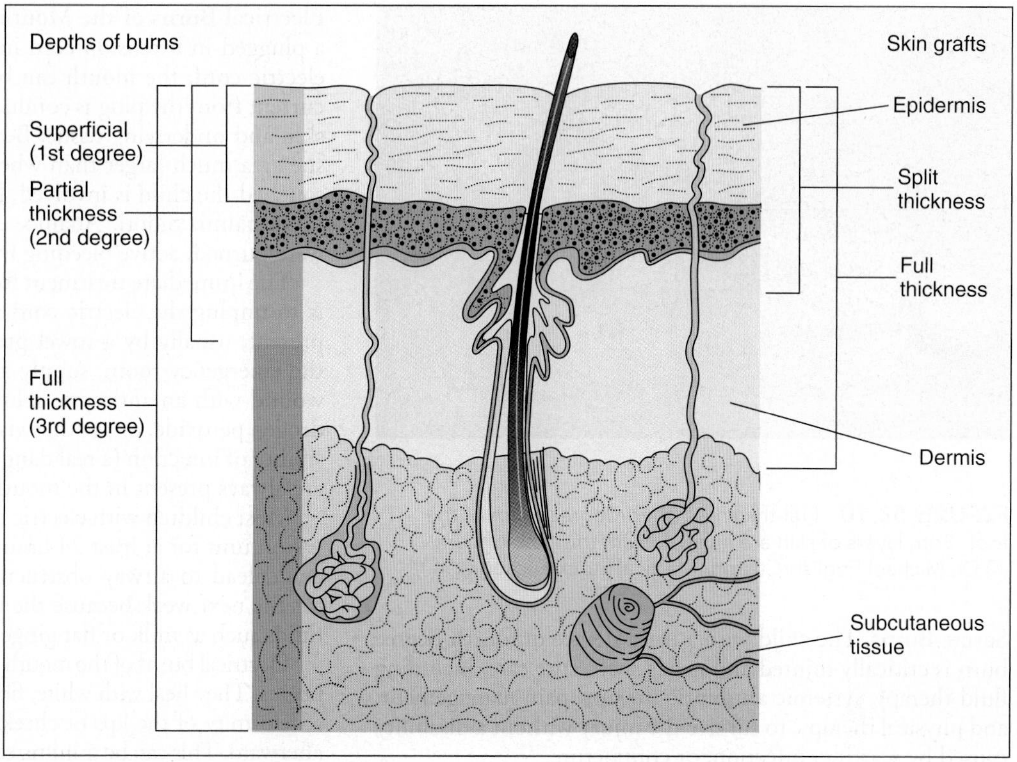

FIGURE 52.8 Depths of burns.

about the burn that they neglect to mention the child has a secondary health concern such as diabetes or allergy to a common drug unless specifically asked.

Emergency Management of Burns

All burns need immediate care because of the potential pain involved (Mandt & Grubenhoff, 2012).

Minor Burns. Although minor burns (typically first-degree partial-thickness burns) are the simplest type of burn, they involve pain and death of skin cells, so they must be treated seriously. Immediately apply cool water to cool the skin and prevent further burning. Application of an analgesic–antibiotic ointment and a gauze bandage to prevent infection is usually the only additional treatment required. Be certain that parents have a follow-up appointment in about 2 days to have the dressing changed and the area inspected for a secondary infection. Caution parents to keep the dressing dry (no swimming or getting the area wet while bathing until the burn is healed—about 1 week).

Moderate Burns. Moderate or second-degree burns typically are blistered. Do not rupture these blisters because doing so denudes the site and invites infection. The burn will be covered with a topical antibiotic such as silver sulfadiazine and a bulky dressing to prevent damage to the burned site and begin healing. The child usually is asked to return in 24 hours to assess that pain control is adequate and there are no signs and symptoms of infection. Broken blisters may be debrided (cut away) to remove possible necrotic tissue as the burn heals.

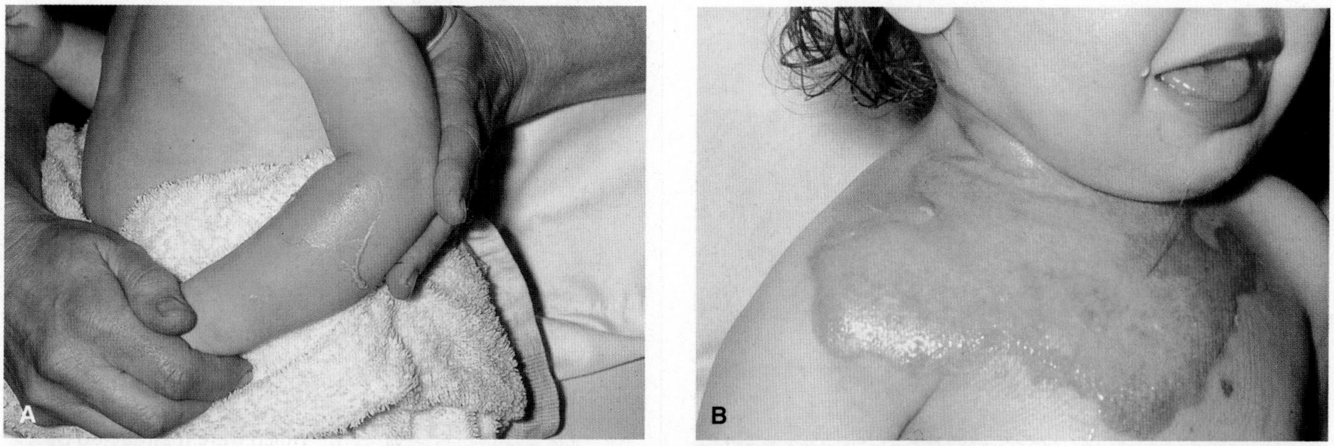

FIGURE 52.9 Partial-thickness burns. **(A)** An infant with a first-degree burn on the arm and chest caused by scalding with hot water. **(B)** A toddler with a second-degree burn caused by scalding. The area appears severely reddened and moist with some blistering. (**A,** © Dr. P. Marazzi/SPL/Science Source/Photo Researchers. **B,** © NMSB/Custom Medical Stock Photograph.)

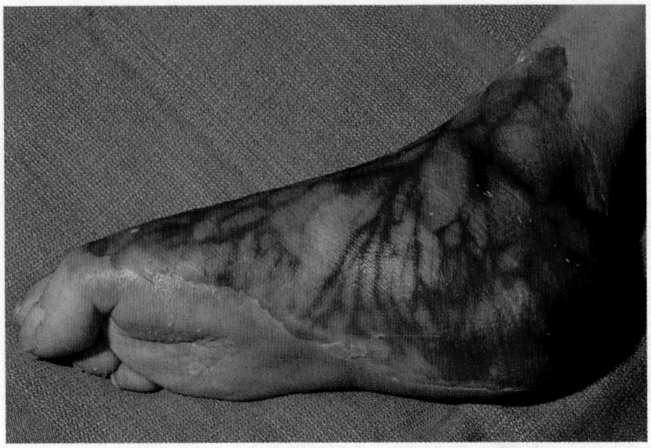

FIGURE 52.10 Full-thickness (third-degree) burn of the foot. Both layers of skin are involved with this type of burn. (© Dr. Michael English/Custom Medical Stock Photograph.)

Severe Burns. The child with a third-degree or fourth-degree burn is critically injured and needs swift, sure care, including fluid therapy, systemic antibiotic therapy, pain management, and physical therapy, to survive the injury without a disability caused by scarring, infection, or contracture.

QSEN Checkpoint Question 52.5

Safety

Suppose you were with Jason when he spilled scalding hot water onto his hand last year. Which of the following would be the best emergency action?

a. Apply a layer of vegetable oil over his hand.
b. Cover his hand with a gauze dressing.
c. Pour cool water from a faucet over his hand.
d. Apply soothing hand lotion to keep the area moist.

Look in Appendix A for the best answer and rationale.

Electrical Burns of the Mouth. If a child puts the prongs of a plugged-in extension cord into the mouth or chews on an electric cord, the mouth can be burned severely as electrical current from the plug is conducted for a distance through the skin and underlying tissue. Because of the conduction, a tissue area much larger than where the prongs or cord actually touched the child is involved, leaving an angry-looking ulcer (Yeroshalmi, Sidoti, Adamo, et al., 2011). If blood vessels were burned, active bleeding from the lesion will be present.

The immediate treatment for electrical burns of the mouth is to unplug the electric cord and control bleeding if this is present, usually by a towel pressed against the burn site. In the emergency room, supply adequate pain relief. Clean the wound with an antiseptic solution, such as half-strength hydrogen peroxide, or as otherwise prescribed to reduce the possibility of infection (a real danger in this area, because bacteria are always present in the mouth).

Most children with electric burns are admitted to an observation unit for at least 24 hours because edema in the mouth could lead to airway obstruction. Eating will be a problem for the next week because the child's mouth is so sore. Bland fluids such as milk or flat ginger ale may be easiest to swallow.

Electrical burns of the mouth turn black as local tissue necrosis begins. They heal with white, fibrous scar tissue, possibly leaving a deformity of the lips or cheeks and difficulty speaking clearly afterward. This can be minimized by the fitting of a mouth appliance, which helps maintain lip contour, but many children need follow-up care by a plastic surgeon to restore their lip contour.

Nursing Diagnoses and Related Interventions

Because pain and anxiety are marks of a burn, relieving them is always an important concern in burn care.

Nursing Diagnosis: Pain and anxiety related to thermal damage to body cells

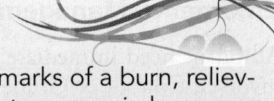

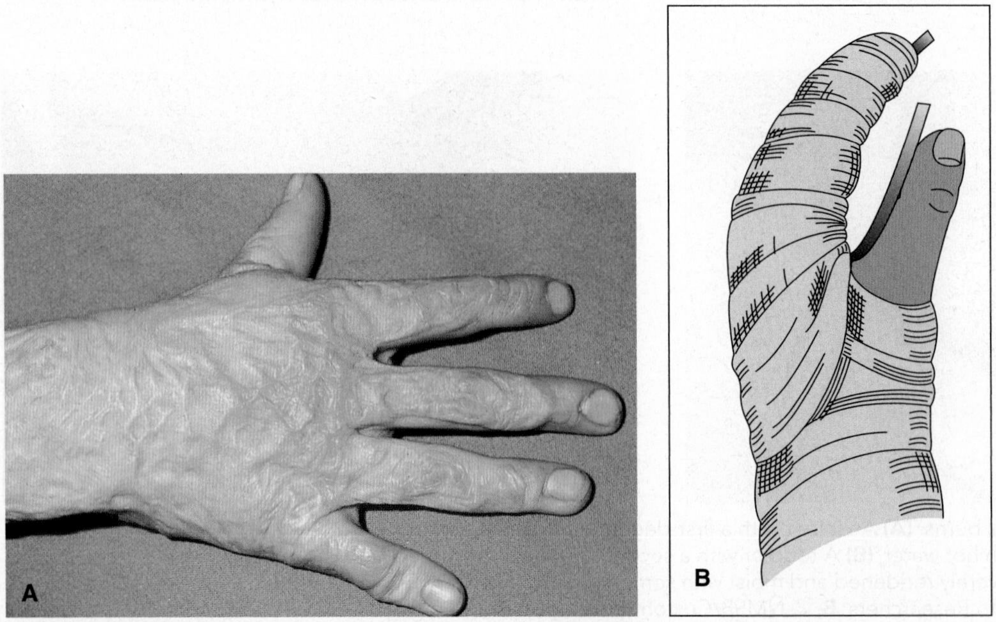

FIGURE 52.11 (A) An adolescent's hand scarred from third-degree burns. Note the proper extension and alignment of the hand and fingers, which were maintained by the use of splints **(B)** during healing. © Dr. P. Marazzi/SPL/Science Source/Photo Researchers.)

Outcome Evaluation: Child states that pain and anxiety are at a tolerable level; rates pain at 2 or below on a pain rating scale.

Morphine sulfate IV or via epidural injection is commonly the agent of choice for pain relief. Performing burn care such as debridement (the removal of necrotic tissue from a burned area) may be done with the use of patient-controlled analgesia or conscious sedation.

In addition to having pain from a burn, children may be required to remain in awkward positions to keep joints overextended so the skin over them does not heal with a contracture. If the anterior throat is burned, for example, the child's head needs to be hyperextended to keep the scar tissue that forms on the anterior neck from pulling the chin down against the chest in a permanent position. If children have burns over extremity joints, they may have splints applied over their burn dressings to maintain the joints in extension. Encourage children to talk about their injury and how it occurred (a form of debriefing) so they can integrate this unexpected event into their life. Be certain parents understand the importance of keeping this type of splint in place so they don't remove them or allow the child to remove them "just once," because "just once" can become many times.

Although most children are awake and very aware of the pain and treatments involved, children who experience smoke inhalation from the fire that caused their injury may become unconscious from brain anoxia. After the first week following a major burn, some children develop symptoms of delirium, seizures, and coma that result from toxic breakdown of damaged cells, sensory deprivation, isolation, and lack of sleep. Nursing care aimed at reducing unnecessary stimuli and providing adequate pain relief helps to prevent these late symptoms from occurring.

Nursing Diagnosis: Deficient fluid volume related to fluid shifts from severe burn

Outcome Evaluation: Skin turgor remains good; hourly urine output is greater than 1 ml/kg, with specific gravity between 1.003 and 1.030; vital signs are within acceptable parameters.

Immediately after a severe burn, there is an increased permeability of capillaries (or direct damage to capillaries). This leads to a loss of plasma, which oozes from blood vessels into the burn site and then sequesters in edematous tissue surrounding the site resulting in hypovolemia. The phenomenon is most marked during the first 6 hours after a burn. It continues to some extent for the first 24 hours.

In addition to hypovolemia, because so much of the child's skin surface may be exposed for examination, a child is prone to hypothermia (keep body parts not burned well covered). Children may also develop a severe anemia following a burn because of injury to red blood cells caused by the heat and loss of blood at the wound site. The large amount of sodium lost from the bloodstream into the edematous burn fluid and the release of potassium from damaged cells can lead to both immediate hyponatremia and hyperkalemia (Table 52.4).

TABLE 52.4 Fluid Shifts After Burn Injury

Fluid Shifts in First 24 Hours	Remobilization of Fluid After 48 Hours
Burn	Edematous tissue surrounding burn area
↓	↓
Increased capillary permeability	Intravascular compartment
↓	↓
Hypoproteinemia	Hypervolemia
Hyponatremia	Hypernatremia
Hyperkalemia	Hypokalemia
Hypovolemia	

To detect whether extreme hypovolemia is occurring, monitor vital signs closely even with relatively minor burns; lactated Ringer's solution is the commercially available solution most compatible with extracellular fluid, so that or normal saline will be administered for fluid replacement. A child may also need plasma replacement and a source of glucose such as 5% dextrose in water. Do not administer a potassium additive immediately after a burn until kidney function is evaluated, to be certain extra potassium can be eliminated. IV fluid is usually administered by the most convenient venous access, so that an analgesic for pain can be administered. A more stable fluid line may then be inserted.

The amount of fluid necessary is calculated carefully, based on predicted insensible fluid loss and loss that can be predicted because of the burn (2,000 ml/M^2 of body surface per 24 hr plus 5,000 ml/M^2 of body surface burned over 24 hr). Fluid is administered rapidly for the first 8 hours (half of the 24-hour load), and then more slowly for the next 16 hours (the second half). It's important that administration is continued beyond the time of increased capillary permeability (at least the first 24 hours), so be certain to protect the administration site to prevent infiltration. A central venous pressure or pulmonary artery catheter may be inserted to determine hemodynamic and fluid volume status and evaluate that the child is receiving adequate fluid. If many red blood cells were destroyed at the burn site, the child may need packed red blood cells to maintain an adequate hemoglobin level.

About 48 hours after the burn, as inflammation decreases, the extracellular fluid at the burn site begins to be reabsorbed into the bloodstream. Edema at the burn site begins to subside; the child begins diuresis and loses weight. The heart rate increases because of temporary hypervolemia. The hematocrit level will be low because red blood cells are diluted. The child needs frequent evaluation of electrolyte levels again at this time to determine the hypervolemia is not overwhelming. Potassium supplements may be necessary to maintain normal heart function, because, although potassium is released into the serum from destroyed cells, it is rapidly excreted by the kidneys.

Nursing Diagnosis: Risk for ineffective tissue perfusion related to cardiovascular adjustments after burn injury

Outcome Evaluation: Child's vital signs stay within normal limits; hourly urine output remains greater than 1 ml/kg of body weight per hour.

A complete blood cell count, blood typing and cross-matching, electrolyte and BUN determinations, and blood gas studies to ascertain blood levels of oxygen and carbon dioxide are important to obtain to monitor the shifts in fluid and electrolytes that occur.

Take height, weight, and vital signs on admission of a child with a burn, and continue to take vital signs every 15 minutes until they are stable. Once these are stabilized, record pulse, blood pressure, and central venous pressure closely until the child passes the immediate danger of shock (at least 24 hours). Another important monitoring period occurs at 48 hours after the injury, when fluid is returning to the bloodstream. Remember that gradual but persistent changes in blood pressure may be as informative as sudden changes.

QSEN Checkpoint Question 52.6

Teamwork & Collaboration

You help a fellow nurse care for Sage, Jason's older sister who has a third-degree burn on her arms and neck. Which statement by your team member on the second day of Sage's care would alert you that your team needs more instruction on burn management?

a. "I'm guarding her IV site so she has an open route for pain management."
b. "I'm measuring her oral and IV fluid intake to help prevent hypervolemia."
c. "I'm monitoring urine output so I can be certain her kidneys are functioning."
d. "I'm urging her not to talk so she doesn't relive the house fire over and over."

Look in Appendix A for the best answer and rationale.

Nursing Diagnosis: Risk for ineffective breathing patterns related to respiratory edema from burn injury

Outcome Evaluation: Child's respiratory rate remains within 16 to 20 breaths/min; lung auscultation reveals no sound of rales.

If a child inhaled smoke from a fire, the injury from the smoke inhalation can be more serious than the skin surface burns received because smoke coming from a fire is at the temperature of the fire or is the same as exposing the upper respiratory tract to open flame. In addition, toxic substances and soot given off by the fire may cause local irritation to the respiratory tract. If carbon monoxide is inhaled with the smoke, it enters red blood cells in place of oxygen, shutting off the oxygen supply to body cells. If this is extensive, it can lead to loss of consciousness because of cerebral anoxia. If the trachea is burned, edema fluid will pass into the injured bronchioles and trachea, causing pulmonary edema or obstruction and limiting air inflow, leading to dyspnea and stridor. About 1 week after the smoke inhalation, the child is at risk for the development of pneumonia because of infection of the denuded tracheal and bronchial tract areas. Because parents are usually relieved that their child has suffered only smoke inhalation from a fire, they may need an explanation of the physiologic consequences that can result from pulmonary injury and why hospitalization is necessary.

To help rule out smoke inhalation, obtain a history to assess whether the fire occurred in a closed space, such as a garage. Assess for burns of the face, neck, or chest, which would indicate the fire was near the nose and respiratory tract. Assess the quality of the child's voice (it will be hoarse if the throat is irritated from smoke). Carefully monitor the respiratory rate of all burned children, because respiratory rate increases with respiratory obstruction. A child also may become restless and thrash about because of lack of oxygen. Measurement of oxygen saturation will demonstrate the degree of hypoxia present from carbon monoxide intoxication. The best therapy for displacing carbon monoxide and providing adequate oxygenation to body cells is the administration of 100% oxygen. The child may need endotracheal intubation or a tracheostomy with assisted ventilation to ensure adequate oxygen is reaching the lungs. Intubation is best, because tracheostomies can lead to infection, and this child is at a much higher risk for pneumonia than the average child.

Bronchodilators and antibiotics may be prescribed as a prophylactic measure because symptoms of smoke inhalation may not occur immediately but only 8 to 24 hours after the burn when the child's temperature increases or a chest X-ray reveals collecting edematous fluid and decreased aeration. High-frequency ventilation may be helpful to keep alveoli functioning. Some children need ECMO support because smoke inhalation has compromised their lung function to such a great extent.

Nursing Diagnosis: Risk for impaired urinary elimination related to burn injury

Outcome Evaluation: Child's urine output is greater than 1 ml/kg of body weight per hour.

Because the child's blood volume can decrease immediately after a burn, renal function can be threatened just when it is needed in order to rid the body of breakdown products from burned cells. Monitor blood volume conscientiously to detect whether hypovolemia is occurring and maintain IV fluid administration so urinary output can be maintained at about 1 ml/kg of body weight per hour. Monitor the specific gravity of urine as well to determine whether the kidneys are able to concentrate urine to conserve body fluid (failing kidneys lose this ability rapidly). In the days after the burn, because products of necrotic tissue and toxic substances must be evacuated by the kidneys and antidiuretic hormone and aldosterone levels may increase in response to low blood pressure, kidney function may fail again. If free hemoglobin from destroyed red blood cells plugs kidney tubules (acute tubular necrosis), urine color will turn red or black because of the hemoglobin present.

Because maintaining kidney function is so important, throughout the child's hospital stay, observing urinary output is a major nursing responsibility. An indwelling urinary (Foley) catheter should be inserted in the emergency department for a child with a large burn to obtain a baseline urine for analysis and allow for continued specimens to be obtained. If hemoglobin in tubules becomes a threat, a diuretic may be administered to flush this from the kidneys (urine will turn to its usual straw color if this is effective).

Nursing Diagnosis: Risk for imbalanced nutrition, less than body requirements, related to burn injury

Outcome Evaluation: Child's weight remains within normal age-appropriate growth percentiles; skin turgor remains good; urine specific gravity remains between 1.003 and 1.030.

After burns, the metabolic rate increases in children as the body begins to pool its resources to adjust to the insult. If children do not receive enough calories in IV fluid to accommodate this increased metabolic need, their body will begin to break down protein for use, a particularly dangerous problem because the child needs protein to be available for burn healing. Additionally, if the breakdown of protein is extreme, it can lead to severe acidosis.

After a severe burn, some children feel nauseated because bowel peristalsis halts (paralytic ileus) from the systemic shock. Symptoms of intestinal obstruction, such as vomiting, abdominal distention, and colicky pain, follow within hours of the burn. To prevent aspiration of vomitus, an NG tube will be inserted and attached to low, intermittent suction. It then remains in place until bowel sounds are detected as assurance the GI tract is again functioning (as long as 24 to 72 hours in severely burned children). Fluid suctioned from an NG tube may appear blood tinged (coffee-ground fluid) because of bleeding caused by stomach vessel congestion. Closely observe this drainage for a change to fresh bleeding, which can be caused by the development of a stress ulcer (Curling ulcer) from the overall trauma of the burn. This type of ulcer can be prevented by administering a histamine-2 receptor antagonist, such as cimetidine (Tagamet) or a proton pump inhibitor such as omeprazole (Prilosec), which reduce gastric acidity (Pilkington, Wagstaff, & Greenwood, 2012). If a bleeding ulcer does occur, gastric lavage with iced saline may be necessary. Blood for transfusion should be readily available, because the blood loss from a GI ulcer can be rapid and severe.

Because of these potential GI concerns, children with severe burns usually are allowed nothing by mouth for 24 hours. After this time, most children are able to eat, so oral feedings are begun as soon as possible. To supply adequate calories for increased metabolic needs and spare protein for repair of cells, the diet is high in calories and protein (Medlin, 2012). Children may also need supplemental vitamins (particularly B and C), iron supplements, and high-protein drinks between meals to ensure an adequate protein intake (Latenser, 2013).

In addition to this oral intake, it may be necessary to supplement the child's diet with IV or parenteral nutrition solutions or gastrostomy tube feedings. As methods of stimulating interest in eating, encourage school-age children to help add intake and output columns, help the dietitian add a calorie-count list, or keep track of their own daily weight (taken at the same time each day in the same clothing). It may be helpful to make contracts with older children to agree to eat at least some of each food offered on their plate.

Nursing Diagnosis: Risk for injury related to effects of burn, denuded skin surfaces, and lowered resistance to infection with burn injury

Outcome Evaluation: Child's temperature remains at 98.6°F (37°C); skin areas surrounding burned areas show no signs of erythema or warmth.

There appears to be some defect in the ability of neutrophils to phagocytize bacteria after burn injury, and the formation of immunoglobulin G antibodies also apparently fails. For these reasons, a child has reduced protection against infection for some time after a severe burn. *Staphylococcus aureus* and group A β-hemolytic streptococci are the gram-positive organisms and *Pseudomonas aeruginosa* is the gram-negative organism most likely to invade burn tissue. In addition to bacteria, fungi such *Candida* also may invade burns (White, Swales, & Butcher, 2012). Children are usually prescribed an antibiotic to prevent these infections and tetanus toxoid to prevent tetanus.

Bacteria and fungi can penetrate the burn eschar readily, so this tissue offers little protection from infection, necessitating nose, throat, and wound cultures to be done immediately and then daily to detect whether offending organisms are present. Fortunately, granulation tissue, which forms under the eschar 3 to 4 weeks after the burn, is resistant to microbial invasion.

Systemic antibiotics are not totally effective in controlling burn-wound infection, probably because the burned and constricted capillaries around the burn site cannot carry the antibiotic to the area. For this reason, any equipment used at the burn site must be sterile, to avoid introducing infection. Children are placed on a sterile sheet on the examining table, and personnel caring for the severely burned child should wear caps, masks, gowns, and gloves, even for emergency care.

Even if their burns are covered by gauze dressings, children usually are cared for in private rooms to help reduce the possibility of infection. Helping children maintain their self-esteem and keeping them from withdrawing from social contacts when such strict infection control precautions are required calls for creative nursing care solutions.

TABLE 52.5 Comparing Open and Closed Burn Therapy

Method	Description	Advantages	Disadvantages
Open	Burn is exposed to air; used for superficial burns or body parts that are prone to infection, such as perineum	Allows frequent inspection of site; allows child to follow healing process	Requires strict isolation to prevent infection; area may scrape and bleed easily and impede healing
Closed	Burn is covered with antibiotic cream and nonadherent gauze; used for moderate and severe burns	Provides better protection from injury; is easier to turn and position child; allows child more freedom to play	Requires dressing changes that can be painful; possibility of infection is still present because of dark, moist environment

Therapy for Burns

Second- and third-degree burns may receive open treatment, leaving the burned area exposed to the air, or closed treatment, in which the burned area is covered with an antibacterial cream and many layers of gauze. These two methods are compared in Table 52.5. As a rule, burn dressings are applied loosely for the first 24 hours to prevent interference with circulation as edema forms. Be certain not to allow two burned body surfaces, such as the sides of fingers or the back of the ears and the scalp, to touch, because, as healing takes place, webbing will form between these surfaces. Do not use adhesive tape to anchor dressings to the skin; it is painful to remove and can leave excoriated areas, which provide additional entry sites for infection. Netting is useful to hold dressings in place, because it expands easily and needs no additional tape.

Topical Therapy. Silver sulfadiazine (Silvadene) is the drug of choice for burn therapy to limit infection at the burn site for children. It is applied as a paste to the burn, and the area is then covered with a few layers of mesh gauze. Because silver sulfadiazine has a sulfa base, it is an effective agent against both gram-negative and gram-positive organisms and even against secondary infectious agents, such as *Candida*. It is soothing when applied and tends to keep the burn eschar soft, making debridement easier. It does not penetrate the eschar (the tough, leathery scab that forms over moderately or severely burned areas) well, however, which is its one drawback.

If *Pseudomonas* is detected in cultures, nitrofurazone (Furacin) cream may be applied. If a topical cream is not effective against invading organisms in the deeper tissue under the eschar, daily injections of specific antibiotics into the deeper layers of the burned area may be necessary.

If a burned area, such as the female genitalia, cannot be readily dressed, the area can be left exposed. The danger of this method is the potential invasion of pathogens.

Escharotomy. As natural protection for a burned area, a rigid scab (an eschar) forms over moderately or severely burned areas. Fluid accumulates rapidly under an eschar, putting pressure on underlying blood vessels and nerves. If an extremity or the trunk has been burned so that both anterior and posterior surfaces both have eschar formation, a tight band may form around the extremity or trunk, cutting off circulation to distal body portions. Distal parts begin to feel cool to the touch and appear pale. The child notices tingling or numbness, pulses are difficult to palpate, and capillary refill is slow (longer than 5 seconds). To alleviate this problem, an **escharotomy** (cut into the eschar) may need to be performed (Kupas & Miller, 2010). Some bleeding will occur after escharotomy. Packing the wound and applying pressure usually relieves this.

Debridement. **Debridement** is the removal of necrotic tissue on which microorganisms could thrive from a burned area to reduce the possibility of infection. This may be done using collagenase (Santyl), an enzyme that dissolves devitalized tissue, or manually. For manual debridement, children may have 20 minutes of hydrotherapy beforehand to soften and loosen eschar, which then can be gently removed with forceps and scissors. Debridement is painful, and some bleeding occurs with it. Premedicate the child with a prescribed analgesic, and help the child use a distraction technique during the procedure to reduce the level of pain. Transcutaneous electrical nerve stimulation (TENS) therapy or patient-controlled analgesia also can be helpful pain management measures. Extensive debridement is done using conscious sedation. Praise any degree of cooperation. Plan an enjoyable activity afterward to aid in pain relief and also to help reestablish some sense of control over the situation (Fig. 52.12).

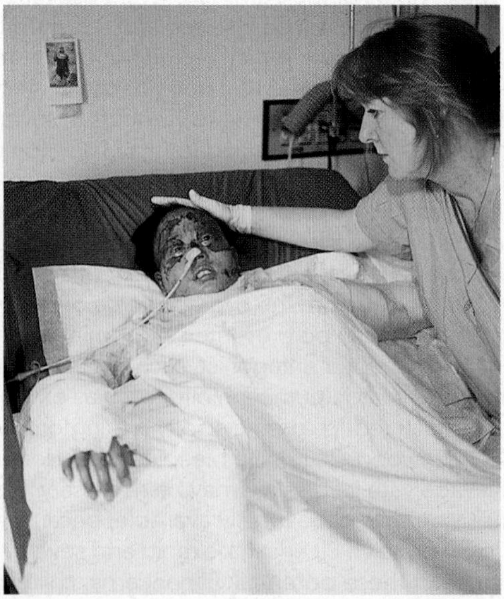

FIGURE 52.12 A nurse provides comfort and support to a child before debridement. (© Kathy Sloane/Science Source/Photo Researchers.)

If burned areas are debrided in this manner day after day, granulation tissue forms underneath. When a full bed of granulation tissue is present (about 2 weeks after the injury), the area is ready for skin grafting. In some burn centers, this waiting period is avoided by immediate surgical excision of eschar and placement of skin grafts.

Grafting. **Allografting** is the placement of skin (sterilized and frozen) from cadavers or a donor on the cleaned burn site. These grafts do not grow but provide a temporary protective covering for the area. In small children, *xenografts*, or skin from other sources, such as porcine (pig) skin, may be used. **Autografting** is a process in which a layer of skin of both epidermis and a part of the dermis (called a *split-thickness graft*) is removed from a distal, unburned portion of the child's body and placed over the prepared burn site, where it will grow and replace the burned skin (Coruh & Yontar, 2012). The advantage of both types of grafting is that they reduce fluid and electrolyte loss, pain, and the chance of infection.

Skin for a split-thickness graft is removed from the buttocks or inner thigh under general anesthesia. Large burn areas may require mesh grafts (a strip of partial-thickness skin is slit at intervals so that it can be stretched to cover a larger area; Fig. 52.13).

After the grafting procedure, the burned area is covered by a bulky dressing. The donor site on the child's body is also covered by a gauze dressing. So that the growth of the newly adhering cells underneath will not be disrupted, don't remove or change the dressings. To detect infection at the sites, observe both the donor and graft dressings for fluid drainage and odor, and assess for pain and body temperature, all of which might indicate infection. Autograft sites heal so quickly that they can be reused every 7 to 10 days, so any one site can provide a great deal of skin for grafting.

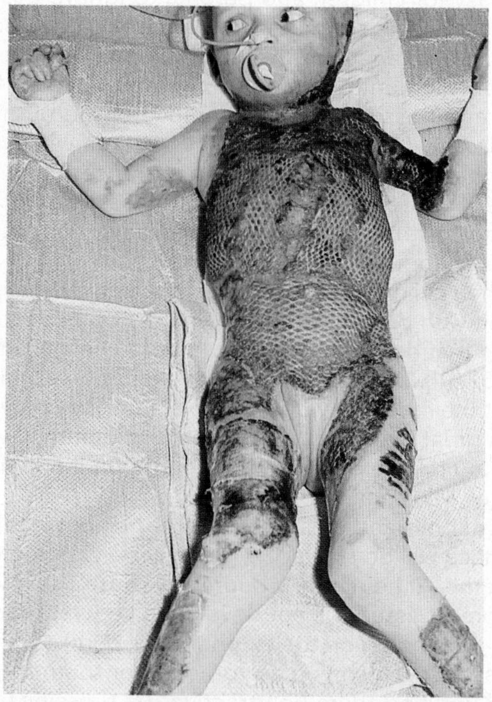

FIGURE 52.13 Mesh grafting is necessary to cover large areas of the body such as in this young child with third-degree burns. (© CC Studio/SPL/Photo Researchers Inc.)

Full-thickness grafts involve both layers of the skin and are used for deep or very severe burned areas. Skin for these is usually removed from the back or abdomen; because the amount of skin removed is so extensive, the donor site may require a split-thickness graft for healing. An alternative to skin grafting in a child who doesn't have enough unburned skin surface for autografting is the technique of using artificial skin to cover the burn. Artificial skin consists of synthetic fibers that, when placed over the denuded burn area, are filled in by fibroblasts and blood vessels and nerve fibers from surrounding healthy tissue to create a new dermal layer. Artificial skin is not rejected as is an allograft or a xenograft, but is dissolved as the new skin replaces it. Another option is removing a small number of the child's skin cells and allowing them to grow in a culture laboratory until a point they can be used as a graft. Because skin cells grow fairly rapidly, this supplies an unlimited supply of available skin for large burn areas.

Nursing Diagnoses and Related Interventions

For children who survive the immediate insult of a large burn, infection becomes their chief threat.

Nursing Diagnosis: Social isolation related to infection control precautions necessary to control spread of microorganisms

Outcome Evaluation: Child states he understands the reason for infection control precautions; accepts it as a necessary part of therapy.

Infection control measures involved in the care of children with major burns consist of more than just placing the child in a private room. Aseptic technique and appropriate barriers are necessary to reduce the risk of exposing the child to infection by the use of gowns, masks, caps, and sterile gloves by health care providers, creating a situation where the child is doubly isolated—by distance and by never being touched directly.

It is easy for children with burns (who were told measures such as not to play with matches or go too close to the fireplace) to interpret confinement in a room as punishment. Make every effort to make the child's environment as warm and comforting as possible, despite infection control procedures. Place children's beds so they can see as much unit activity as possible. Decorate walls in front of them with cards they receive or with a changing gallery of pictures drawn by staff members of things in which the child appears interested.

Provide time for children to discuss their feelings about being kept in a room by themselves. A question such as, "It's hard to understand a lot of things about a hospital; do you understand why your bed is in this special room?" gives children a chance to express their feelings.

Show parents how to put on gowns, gloves, and masks if required so they can feel comfortable participating in the child's care. Parents may not offer to help with care when their child is severely burned because they are still in a state of shock or grief. They may perceive the bulky dressings as making it impossible for them to hold the child. You can assure them the closed bulky dressings on the burned area are what make it *possible* for them to hold the child. If it is not possible for them to do this, help them see how stroking their child's face or touching a hand (even with gloves in place) gives the child a feeling of still being loved and not totally removed from warm contact.

Remember that, even if children's chests, abdomens, and hands are burned, they do not stop thinking and thus need stimulation in their restricted environment. A television set is good for passing time, but for longer than 1 day, it is not adequate as the child's main communication with the outside world. Listening to favorite music with them, reading stories to them, talking about what is going on at home or what they normally do at school, and doing schoolwork are also important.

Make certain to visit a child in isolation to talk or play a game at times other than procedure or treatment times so the child can view the nursing staff as friends and caregivers, not as busy people who can't be interrupted. Frequent visits also convey that the child is not alone and others are aware of important needs.

Nursing Diagnosis: Interrupted family processes related to the effects of severe burns in a family member

Outcome Evaluation: Family members state that they are able to cope effectively with the degree of stress to which they are subjected; family demonstrates positive coping mechanisms.

Children with severe burns always have a difficult hospitalization because of the pain, restrictions, and (at some point) awareness of the disfigurement that accompanies major burns. Some parents have exceptional difficulty adjusting to what has happened because they are grieving so deeply over the child's condition or are so concerned with other upsetting factors in their lives (many burns happen because of situational crises in the family; the family may have lost their home and possessions to the fire that burnt the child) that their interaction with the child seems to falter or be very difficult for them. Because they may not be able to stay with the child constantly because they also have to meet with financial advisors, insurance inspectors, or home construction people to begin to get their home back in repair, assure them their child is in good hands during the time they must be away to help relieve stress at least in this one area.

Nursing Diagnosis: Disturbed body image related to changes in physical appearance with burn injury

Outcome Evaluation: Child expresses fears about physical appearance; demonstrates desire to resume age-appropriate activities.

Children with burns are often forced to become extremely dependent on the nursing staff because of the position in which they must lie and because the bulky dressings that cover their arms or hands prevent them from feeding themselves. They respond to this forced dependence at first with gratitude. They are hurt, and someone is taking care of them. After a period, however, their response may become less healthy; young school-age children or preschoolers may revert to bed-wetting or baby talk. Older children may respond by open aggressiveness such as refusing to eat or to lie in a position that is best for them in order to reestablish independence and counteract their feelings of helplessness. To help avoid these reactions, make certain to allow independent decision making whenever possible. Be careful to avoid questions such as, "Can I change your dressing now?" or "Will you swallow this pill?" because these imply choices when there really are none as these measures are important for healing.

Allow secondary choices instead. Children, for example, must take their 10 o'clock medicine, but they can choose the fluid they want to swallow after it. They must be fed meals because of the bulky dressings over their hands, but they can decide which food they will eat first. They must have their dressings changed, but they can choose the story you will read them afterward.

Immediately after a severe burn, children (if they are old enough to understand) and their parents are most concerned with whether the child will live. After body systems have stabilized and the parents have been assured the child will live, thoughts turn to the child's cosmetic appearance. At first, it is easy for children and parents to ignore this problem, because the burned areas are covered by dressings. Even when the dressings are removed for debridement or whirlpool therapy, it's easy for children to assume the appearance of the burned area is only temporary and that the area will eventually heal and have a good appearance. They have probably never seen anyone with a scar from a second- or third-degree burn and have no reason to worry about it.

When children begin to see others on the hospital unit with burn scars, however, they do begin to realize that healing may result in permanent scarring (Fig. 52.14). Parents and children need time to talk about their feelings about this because they may feel a great deal of guilt about the incident and ways they could have prevented the burn from happening (Bakker, Van Loey, Van Son, et al., 2010).

Both boys and girls are concerned about whether their face will be scarred. A girl may be extremely concerned if her chest is burned because she is worried breast tissue will not develop (a very real concern, depending on the extent of the burn).

Children watch you as you care for them to see if you find them unattractive. As dressings are removed, children may expose parts of their

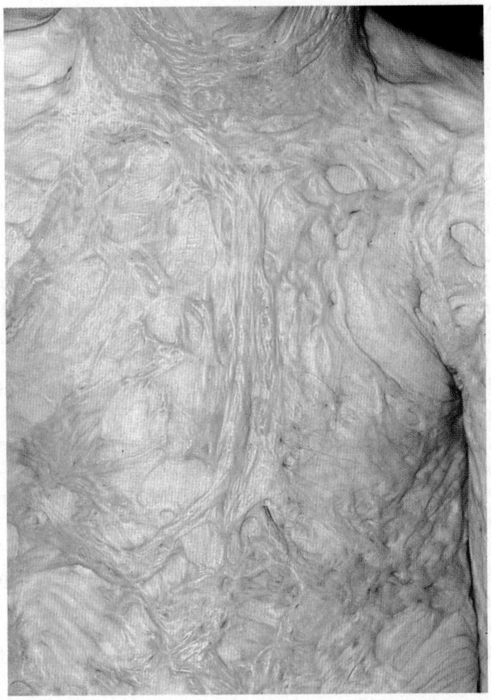

FIGURE 52.14 Extensive scarring on the chest of a 9-year-old boy following a third-degree burn. (© Dr. P. Marazzi/SPL/Science Source/Photo Researchers.)

body seemingly inappropriately, to see if you are shocked or revolted by them. It is easy to think that you will not react this way, but, for everyone, the first sight of a severe burn is a shock and it is difficult not to react accordingly. Imagining how children feel and realizing that this mutilated skin is their skin can help health care providers maintain a professional attitude. As a rule, the appearance of scar formation can be improved by the application of pressure dressings that the child wears 24 hours a day.

Returning to school can be difficult for all children who have been hospitalized or have been receiving home care for a long time. Their old friends have new friends, so they may feel cut out of school activities. It may be particularly difficult if the child is left with burn scars. Ask how the child is adjusting at follow-up visits. Some children need referral for formal counseling to help rebuild their self-image. Some parents need formal counseling also, to help them accept their child's changed appearance and work through lingering guilt.

What if...52.4 You are particularly interested in exploring one of the 2020 National Health Goals related to unintentional injury in children (see Box 52.1). What would be a possible research topic to explore pertinent to this goal that would be applicable to Jason's family and also advance evidence-based practice?

Key Points for Review

- Children need total body assessment after an unintentional injury, because they may be unable to describe other injuries besides the primary one they have suffered.
- Be aware that some trauma in children occurs as a result of child maltreatment. Screen for this by history and physical examination.
- Head injuries are always potentially serious in children. Many different types such as skull fractures, subdural hematomas, epidural hematomas, concussions, and contusions all can occur. Coma (unconsciousness from which a child cannot be roused) may be present after severe head trauma.
- Abdominal trauma can result in rupture of the spleen or liver and may occur in connection with multiple trauma.
- Near drowning can occur in either salt or fresh water. The physiologic basis for complications after drowning differs depending on the type of water in which the child was submerged.
- Common substances children swallow that result in poisoning include acetaminophen (Tylenol), caustic substances, and hydrocarbons. Teach parents to keep the number of the National Poison Control Center next to their telephone or as a contact number in their cell phone (1-800-222-1222) and always call first for advice before administering an antidote for poisoning in order to not only meet QSEN competencies but also best meet the family's total needs.
- Lead poisoning most frequently occurs from the ingestion of paint chips in older housing units. Educating parents so they can prevent this is a major nursing responsibility.
- Burns are classified as first, second, third, and fourth degree—depending on the depth of the burn. Use sterile technique when caring for a child who has been burned so the child does not develop an additional unnecessary infection. Be aware that burns produce systemic body reactions and require long-term nursing care.

Critical Thinking Care Study

Meredith is a 2-year-old girl you see in an emergency room. Meredith lives with her mother, Antoinette, and her mother's boyfriend in a three-bedroom suburban home. Meredith swallowed three of her mother's birth control pills earlier this evening. On the way to the hospital, Antoinette ran her car into a pick-up truck. Meredith was thrown out of the car and trapped against the exhaust pipe of the truck. The dress she was wearing is partially burned away; her chest is reddened and blistered and weeping fluid. She's obviously in pain. "Can anything else go wrong?" Antoinette asks you. "I received my divorce papers today. My college loan wasn't approved. And now my car is ruined."

1. Antoinette doesn't understand why Meredith swallowed the pills. She says, "I've told her over and over medicine is for grown-ups." What factors in this family's background made this a day when poisoning was apt to occur? Did Antoinette take the best first-aid step for an unintentional poisoning?

2. Meredith has a second-degree burn on her chest, so insertion of an IV line with an infusion of normal saline is prescribed. You're concerned that, because the burned area is losing fluid, Meredith needs electrolytes replaced as well as fluid. What do you need to know to safely add a potassium supplement following a severe burn?
3. While hospitalized for her burn, Meredith had her serum lead level assessed, and it was found to be 15 μg/dl. What is the safe level of lead in children? If Meredith is prescribed CaEDTA to be infused IV, what do you need to know before administration? What is the purpose of this drug?

Patient Scenario

The Long Family

Read about the Long family, a family with a child with an unintentional injury, then answer the questions to further sharpen your skills and grow more familiar with NCLEX-type questions related to nursing care of a family with an unintentional injury concern. Confirm your answers are correct by reading the rationales.

Visit http://thePoint.lww.com

Answers and Rationales

Looking for answers to the What if . . . and Critical Thinking Care Study questions?

Visit http://thePoint.lww.com

References

Agarwal, A., & Pruthi, M. (2010). Bicycle-spoke injuries of the foot in children. *Journal of Orthopedic Surgery, 18*(3), 338–341.

American Academy of Pediatrics Council on Sports Medicine and Fitness. (2012). Trampoline safety in childhood and adolescence. *Pediatrics, 130*(4), 774–779.

American Heart Association. (2011). *Two steps to staying alive with Hands-Only™ CPR.* Dallas, TX: Author.

Avey, G., Euathrongchit, J., & Stern, E. J. (2012). Simultaneous cases of traumatic coin aspiration. *Current Problems in Diagnostic Radiology, 41*(4), 118–119.

Babcock, L., Byczkowski, T., Wade, S. L., et al. (2012). Predicting post-concussion syndrome after mild traumatic brain injury in children and adolescents who present to the emergency department. *Archives in Pediatric & Adolescent Medicine,* (12), 1–6.

Bakker, A., Van Loey, N. E., Van Son, M. J., et al. (2010). Mothers' long-term posttraumatic stress symptoms following a burn event of their child. *Journal of Pediatric Psychology, 35*(6), 656–661.

Blackburn, J., Levitan, E. B., MacLennan, P. A., et al. (2012). The epidemiology of chemical eye injuries. *Current Eye Research, 37*(9), 787–793.

Castellani, J. W., & Young, A. J. (2012). Health and performance challenges during sports training and competition in cold weather. *British Journal of Sports Medicine, 46*(11), 788–791.

Centers for Disease Control and Prevention. (2012). *Childhood lead poisoning data, statistics, and surveillance.* Atlanta, GA: Author.

Chang, T. P., & Rangan, C. (2011). Iron poisoning: A literature-based review of epidemiology, diagnosis, and management. *Pediatric Emergency Care, 27*(10), 978–985.

Coruh, A., & Yontar, Y. (2012). Application of split-thickness dermal grafts in deep partial- and full-thickness burns: A new source of auto-skin grafting. *Journal of Burn Care & Research, 33*(3), e94–e100.

Dinis-Oliveira, R. J., & Magalhães, T. (2013). Children intoxications: What is abuse and what is not abuse. *Trauma Violence Abuse, 14*(2), 113–132.

Dyring-Andersen, B., Menne, T., & Skov, L. (2012). Sharply demarcated incisions caused by rat bites. *Archives of Dermatology, 148*(10), 1209–1210.

Felus, J., & Kowalczyk, B. (2012). Age-related differences in medial patellofemoral ligament injury patterns in traumatic patellar dislocation: Case series of 50 surgically treated children and adolescents. *American Journal of Sports Medicine, 40*(10), 2357–2364.

Fleisig, G. S., & Andrews, J. R. (2012). Prevention of elbow injuries in youth baseball pitchers. *Sports Health, 4*(5), 419–424.

Hoang, Q. B., Coel, R. A., Vidal, A., et al. (2012). Sports medicine. In W. Hay, M. Levin, R. Deterding, et al. (Eds.), *Current diagnosis & treatment pediatrics* (21st ed., pp. 849–880). New York, NY: McGraw-Hill/Lange.

Karch, A. (2013). *2013 Lippincott's nursing drug guide.* Philadelphia, PA: Lippincott Williams & Wilkins.

Klimek, P. M., Lutz, T., Stranzinger, E., et al. (2013). Handlebar injuries in children. *Pediatric Surgery International, 29*(3), 269-273.

Koestner, A. L. (2012). ThinkFirst for teens: Finding an injury-prevention approach for teenagers. *Journal of Trauma Nursing, 19*(4), 227–231.

Kupas, D. F., & Miller, D. D. (2010). Out-of-hospital chest escharotomy: A case series and procedure review. *Prehospital Emergency Care, 14*(3), 349–354.

Laitakari, E., Pyörälä, S., & Koljonen, V. (2012). Burn injuries requiring hospitalization for infants younger than 1 year. *Journal of Burn Care & Research, 33*(3), 436–441.

Langley, R. L., & Mort, S. A. (2012). Human exposures to pesticides in the United States. *Journal of Agromedicine, 17*(3), 300–315.

Latenser, B. A. (2013). Burn treatment guidelines. In E. T. Bope & R. D. Kellerman (Eds.), *Conn's current therapy* (pp. 1111–1115). Philadelphia, PA: Elsevier/Saunders.

Lee, K. J., & Marcdante, K. J. (2011). The acutely ill or injured child. In K. J. Marcdante, R. M. Kliegman, H. B. Jenson, et al. (Eds.), *Nelson essentials of pediatrics* (6th ed., pp. 141–166). Philadelphia, PA: Saunders/Elsevier.

Lippert, S. J., Hartin, C. W., Jr., Ozgediz, D. E., et al. (2013). Splenic conservation: Variation between pediatric and adult trauma centers. *Journal of Surgical Research, 182*(2), 17–20.

Mandt, M. J., & Grubenhoff, J. A. (2012). Emergencies & injuries. In W. Hay, M. Levin, R. Deterding, et al. (Eds.), *Current diagnosis & treatment pediatrics* (21st ed., pp. 316–338). New York, NY: McGraw-Hill/Lange.

Marom, T., Goldfarb, A., Russo, E., et al. (2010). Battery ingestion in children. *International Journal of Pediatric Otorhinolaryngology, 74*(8), 849–854.

Mas, E., Breton, A., & Lachaux, A. (2012). Management of caustic esophagitis in children. *Archives of Pediatrics, 19*(12), 1362–1368.

Matulkova, P., Gobin, M., Evans, M., et al. (2012). Gastro-intestinal poisoning due to consumption of daffodils mistaken for vegetables at commercial markets, Bristol, United Kingdom. *Clinical Toxicology, 50*(8), 788–790.

McCance, K. L., & Grey, T. C. (2012). Altered tissue & cellular biology. S. E. Huether & K. L. McCance (Eds.), *Understanding pathophysiology* (5th ed., pp. 59–97). New York, NY: Elsevier Publishing.

McTigue, D. J. (2013). Overview of trauma management for primary and young permanent teeth. *Dental Clinics of North America, 57*(1), 39–57.

Medlin, S. (2012). Nutrition for wound healing. *British Journal of Nursing, 21*(12), S11–S15.

Morrongiello, B. A., Sandomierski, M., Schwebel, D. C., et al. (2013). Are parents just treading water? The impact of participation in swim lessons on parents' judgments of children's drowning risk, swimming ability, and supervision needs. *Accident Analysis & Prevention, 50*(1), 1169–1175.

National Vital Statistics Service. (2012). *Deaths: Preliminary data for 2011.* Washington, DC: Author.

Nickels, D., Patel, T., Merhar, G., et al. (2013). Core curriculum illustration: Subdural hematoma. *Emergency Radiology, 20*(1), 85–86.

Nicole, N. H., & Huether, S. E. (2012). Structure, function & disorders of the integument. In S. E. Huether & K. L. McCance (Eds.), *Understanding pathophysiology* (5th ed., pp. 1038–1069). New York, NY: Elsevier Publishing.

Ogilvie, J. D., Rieder, M. J., & Lim, R. (2012). Acetaminophen overdose in children. *CMAJ: Canadian Medical Association Journal, 184*(13), 1492–1496.

Olaimat, A. N., & Holley, R. A. (2012). Factors influencing the microbial safety of fresh produce: A review. *Food Microbiology, 32*(1), 1–19.

Persaud, N., Coleman, E., Zwolakowski, D., et al. (2012). Nonuse of bicycle helmets and risk of fatal head injury: A proportional mortality, case-control study. *CMAJ: Canadian Medical Association Journal, 184*(17), E921–E923.

Pilkington, K. B., Wagstaff, M. J., & Greenwood, J. E. (2012). Prevention of gastrointestinal bleeding due to stress ulceration: A review of current literature. *Anaesthesia & Intensive Care, 40*(2), 253–259.

Purcell, L. K. (2012). Evaluation and management of children and adolescents with sports-related concussion. *Paediatrics & Child Health, 17*(1), 31–34

Ramowski, S. K., Nystrom, R. J., Rosenberg, K. D., et al. (2012). Health risks of Oregon eighth-grade participants in the "choking game": Results from a population-based survey. *Pediatrics, 129*(5), 846–851.

Rhine, T., Wade, S. L., Makoroff, K. L., et al. (2012). Clinical predictors of outcome following inflicted traumatic brain injury in children. *Journal of Trauma & Acute Care Surgery, 73*(4, Suppl. 3), S248–S253.

Riesch, S. K., Kedrowski, K., Brown, R. L., et al. (2012). Health-risk behaviors among a sample of US pre-adolescents: Types, frequency, and predictive factors. *International Journal of Nursing Studies.* Advance Online Publication.

Roberts, J. R., & Karr, C. K. (2012). Technical report—Pesticide exposure in children. *Pediatrics, 12*(6), 130.

Rumack, B. H., & Dart, R. C. (2012). Poisoning. In W. Hay, M. Levin, R. Deterding, et al. (Eds.), *Current diagnosis & treatment pediatrics* (21st ed., pp. 339–366). New York, NY: McGraw-Hill/Lange.

Shao, Y., Zou, D., Li, Z., et al. (2013). Blunt liver injury with intact ribs under impacts on the abdomen: A biomechanical investigation. *PLoS One, 8*(1), e52366.

Sharpe, S. J., Rochette, L. M., & Smith, G. A. (2012). Pediatric battery-related emergency department visits in the United States, 1990–2009. *Pediatrics, 129*(6), 1111–1117.

Shields, B. J., Pollack-Nelson, C., & Smith, G. A. (2011). Pediatric submersion events in portable above-ground pools in the United States, 2001–2009. *Pediatrics, 128*(1), 45–52.

Sigurtà, A., Zanaboni, C., Canavesi, K., et al. (2013). Intensive care for pediatric traumatic brain injury. *Intensive Care Medicine, 39*(1), 129–136.

Smith, H. C., Vacek, P., Johnson, R. J., et al. (2012). Risk factors for anterior cruciate ligament injury: A review of the literature. *Sports Health, 4*(2), 155–161.

Tiemstra, J. D. (2012). Update on acute ankle sprains. *American Family Physician, 85*(12), 1170–1176.

U.S. Department of Health and Human Services. (2010). *Healthy people 2020.* Washington, DC: Author.

Varisco, B. M., Palmatier, C. M., & Alten, J. A. (2010). Reversal of intractable hypoxemia with exogenous surfactant (calfactant) facilitating complete neurological recovery in a pediatric drowning victim. *Pediatric Emergency Care, 26*(8), 571–573.

Viana, A. G., Trent, L., Tull, M. T., et al. (2012). Non-medical use of prescription drugs among Mississippi youth: Constitutional, psychological, and family factors. *Addictive Behavior, 37*(12), 1382–1388.

Warrell, D. A. (2012). Venomous bites, stings, and poisoning. *Infectious Disease Clinics of North America, 26*(2), 207–223.

White, R., Swales, B., & Butcher, M. (2012). Principles of infection management in community-based burns care. *Nursing Standard, 27*(2), 64–68.

Yeroshalmi, F., Sidoti, E. J., Jr., Adamo, A. K., et al. (2011). Oral electrical burns in children: A model of multidisciplinary care. *Journal of Burn Care & Research, 32*(2), e25–e30.

Chapter 53

Nursing Care of a Family When a Child Has a Malignancy

KEY TERMS

- biopsy
- chemotherapeutic agent
- Ewing sarcoma
- leukemia
- lymphoma
- metastasis
- neoplasm
- nephroblastoma
- neuroblastoma
- oncogenic virus
- osteogenic sarcoma
- rhabdomyosarcoma
- sarcoma
- tumor staging

OBJECTIVES

After mastering the contents of this chapter, you should be able to:

1. Describe usual cellular growth and theories that explain why cells alter to become malignant in children.
2. Identify 2020 National Health Goals related to the care of the child with a malignancy that nurses can help the nation achieve.
3. Assess a child with a common malignant process, such as a rhabdomyosarcoma, neuroblastoma, nephroblastoma, or leukemia.
4. Formulate nursing diagnoses related to a child with a malignancy.
5. Establish expected outcomes for a child with a malignancy to help parents manage seamless transitions across differing health care settings.
6. Using the nursing process, plan nursing care that includes the six competencies of Quality & Safety Education for Nurses (QSEN): Patient-Centered Care, Teamwork & Collaboration, Evidence-Based Practice (EBP), Quality Improvement (QI), Safety, and Informatics.
7. Implement nursing care for a child with a malignancy, such as explaining why chemotherapy is important.
8. Evaluate expected outcomes for achievement and effectiveness of care.
9. Integrate knowledge of malignancy in children with the interplay of nursing process, the six competencies of QSEN, and Family Nursing to achieve quality maternal and child health nursing care.

Gerri is a 6-year-old boy you meet at a health maintenance organization clinic when he arrives for a well-child checkup. His mother tells you that Gerri wakes up every morning with a headache; he usually vomits after breakfast. Immediately after that, though, he seems fine. The problem began just after he started a new school in the fall, so the mother is certain the vomiting is related to this. His teacher has suggested that Gerri needs an eye examination because he cocks his head to see the chalkboard. When you weigh him, you notice he has lost weight. "What do I do for school phobia?" his mother asks you.

Previous chapters described the growth and development of well children and disorders associated with specific body systems. This chapter adds information about the dramatic changes, both physical and psychosocial, that occur when children develop a malignancy, a phenomenon that can happen in any body system. Such information forms a base for care and health teaching.

(Continued on next page)

(Continued from previous page)

Is Gerri's mother describing school phobia, or is this something more serious? What additional questions would you want to ask to help discover whether you need to alert her primary care provider of your concern?

The terms *malignant* and *cancerous* describe cells that are growing and proliferating in a disorderly, chaotic fashion. In adults, cancer usually occurs in the form of a solid tumor. In children, the most frequent type of cancer is that of immature white blood cell (WBC) overgrowth, or leukemia (Brown & Hunger, 2013).

Many parents assume that a diagnosis of cancer means their child's life will be very limited. Because of the tremendous advances in cancer research and treatment over the past 20 years, however, the prognosis for children and the chances for a cure improve daily. Ninety-five percent of children with leukemia, for example, can expect to be cured. To help both parents and children adjust to this serious illness, however, nursing support is necessary from the time of diagnosis throughout the long-term therapy required. Because decreasing the incidence of cancer is important to the nation, 2020 National Health Goals related to malignancies and children address this concern and are shown in Box 53.1.

BOX 53.1 Nursing Care Planning Based on 2020 National Health Goals

Several 2020 National Health Goals concern cancer prevention and children:

- Reduce the overall cancer death rate from a baseline of 178.4 per 100,000 to 160.6 per 100,000 of the population.
- Increase the proportion of adolescents in grades 9 through 12 who follow protective measures that may reduce the risk of skin cancer from 9.3% to 11.2%.
- Reduce the rate of melanoma cancer deaths from a baseline of 2.7 per 100,000 to a target level of 2.4 per 100,000 of the population (U.S. Department of Health and Human Services [DHHS], 2010; see www.healthypeople.gov).

The health goals don't speak to leukemia because there is no screening test available as yet for hematologic types. Nurses can help the nation achieve these goals by careful history taking at health assessments to reveal the symptoms of leukemia, which are often subtle in children, and by active teaching of available self-screening measures, such as testicular examination, and preventive measures, such as avoiding excessive sun exposure.

Nursing Process Overview

For Care of a Child With a Malignancy

Assessment

The symptoms of malignancy in children are often insidious and difficult to identify because headaches or pain at a particular body site can often be explained away by other factors, such as a sports injury or fatigue. Weight loss, however, is a common symptom of cancer and is never normal in healthy children. Therefore, at every health care visit, plot and analyze a child's height and weight carefully to document evidence of this important finding. Refer children with swelling or pain at major joints to their primary health care provider for further assessment so that bone tumors will not go undetected.

Nursing Diagnosis

Nursing diagnoses established for the child with a malignancy address specific symptoms caused by the malignancy itself, side effects of therapy, or coping abilities of the child and family. Examples include:

- Pain related to neoplastic process in bone
- Imbalanced nutrition, less than body requirements, related to mucositis from radiation therapy
- Risk for infection related to immunosuppressive effects of chemotherapy
- Disturbed body image related to loss of hair after radiation treatment
- Compromised family coping, related to long-term chemotherapy program

Outcome Identification and Planning

When a neoplasm (abnormal growth that does not respond to normal growth-control mechanisms) is first diagnosed in their child, parents may be able to deal only with short-term outcomes and plans. They may concentrate on learning about the effect or toxic properties of a particular chemotherapeutic drug prescribed for their child, or they may ask how long the child's surgical incision will be. Dealing with such specifics helps them to control their anxiety because it prevents them from dealing with the overall picture or prognosis—that their child has a potentially fatal illness.

Be certain the family has an overall picture of the treatment protocol. Explain measures they will need to take to make their child more comfortable during therapy such as not forcing food if their child is nauseated and playing games or reading stories while an intravenous (IV) chemotherapy agent is administered.

Parents are usually eager for results of diagnostic tests. They may need support while waiting until all the findings have been assembled for an accurate assessment of staging and prognosis. Establishing a primary relationship with both the child and the parents is important so that, no matter how many hospitalizations are necessary, they know a support person is waiting to help them through this long-term illness. Be certain the child's siblings are included in planning care, because the treatment will be long term, putting stress on the entire family.

Parents can be expected to experience grief if they learn their child's prognosis is poor and move through stages of denial, anger, bargaining, depression, and, hopefully, acceptance. During planning, be certain to take into account their current stage of grief so planning can be successful (see Chapter 56).

Organizations that may be helpful for referral are the American Cancer Society (ACS) (www.cancer.org), the National Cancer Institute (www.cancer.gov), the Children's Oncology Group (www.childrensoncologygroup.org), Candlelighters for Children with Cancer (www.4kidswithcancer.org), and the Leukemia and Lymphoma Society (www.lls.org).

Implementation

Nursing interventions for a child with cancer include supporting the child and parents from the time of diagnosis through procedures such as surgery, radiation therapy, chemotherapy, and continued health supervision. Increasingly, cancer treatment is offered on an ambulatory basis to keep hospitalization to a minimum, so many nursing interventions include teaching the parents how to give care or monitor for recurring signs while at home.

Keep in mind the stress of long-term treatment can put the child and family at risk for developmental or family coping problems. You can be a positive force in encouraging healthy adaptation to the demands of the child's illness and in reassessing the situation periodically during therapy to be certain the child is receiving appropriate stimulation for developmental growth. Providing comfort and alleviating pain are often primary concerns in oncology nursing. Measures for pain relief are discussed in Chapter 39.

Outcome Evaluation

Because cancer therapy includes long-term care, children need to be evaluated periodically to be certain projected outcomes are being met and are still current. Some examples indicating outcome achievement are:

- Child keeps all appointments for chemotherapy treatments.
- Child maintains passing grades in school despite interruptions for therapy.
- Parents state they are able to keep anxiety at an acceptable level between clinic appointments.

Children with cancer need the same well-child maintenance care that all children do, with one exception. While they are undergoing chemotherapy, which causes a decreased immune response, they should not receive live-virus vaccines.

Follow-up visits are usually anxiety filled for both parents and the child. The child seems well, but parents may be apprehensive while a health care provider palpates the child's abdomen or blood specimens are obtained. Some parents may find the strain of returning for follow-up visits too great and miss appointments (not knowing seems better than to be told bad news). Such parents need help in understanding that initial remissions can be maintained and second remissions can be achieved, so maintenance therapy must be continued. Because a child who receives chemotherapy or radiation is more prone than others to develop myocarditis or pericarditis and a second cancer later in life, follow-up becomes an essential detection measure to see if these conditions are occurring (Frew, Lewis, & Lucraft, 2013; Kucharska, Negrusz-Kawecka, & Gromkowska, 2012).

If a child dies, parents may feel a need to return to the health care agency for support to accept the death. This provides an opportunity to evaluate their adjustment and offer support if needed. Being with a child who dies at home appears to make death a more understandable phenomenon for siblings and, in many instances, can be advocated. Care in a separate hospice setting is another option for the child in whom a remission cannot be achieved (see Chapter 56).

HEALTH PROMOTION AND RISK MANAGEMENT

Because childhood cancers do not seem to arise from environmental contaminants as much as adult cancers do, methods to reduce the risk are not as well defined. Urging parents to reduce children's exposure to secondary cigarette smoke and urging adolescents not to begin smoking, including the use of bidis or kreteks (imported and flavored tobacco products that may contain a higher level of nicotine than cigarettes), can help reduce the incidence of lung cancer when they reach adulthood. Although it is not yet known how much sunscreen actually reduces the risk of melanoma, applying sunscreen, reducing the overall time of sun exposure, and avoiding tanning salons are measures to help reduce the development of skin cancer in later life (Quatrano & Dinulos, 2013). Children who receive chemotherapy or radiation for one cancer have a higher incidence of developing another cancer later in life. Therefore, urging these children to continue health appointments so that any additional tumor development can be discovered as soon as it occurs is another important preventive measure. Reminding parents that both boys and girls should receive the vaccine against human papillomavirus (HPV) is an important preventive measure to reduce the incidence of cervical cancer.

Parents of a child with cancer may seek health maintenance care or evaluation for their other children more often than other parents would because they are worried that what seems like just a minor symptom is actually a sign of cancer in that child. They may need greater amounts of reassurance that their other children are well, reflecting the overall stress they feel (Cernvall, Carlbring, Ljungman, et al., 2013).

NEOPLASIA

All body tissue undergoes continuing growth to develop into and maintain that specific type of tissue. Normally, the body is able to balance the proliferation necessary to replace old cells that die plus produce new cells for physical growth needs. Cancerous, or malignant, tissue, however, is unable to maintain this balance and begins to proliferate in disorderly, chaotic ways.

The word **neoplasm** means "new growth," although it is typically used to refer to a new *abnormal* growth that does not respond to normal growth-control mechanisms. Whether this process is one that produces a solid tumor or one that involves blood-forming elements, growth begins insidiously and usually has been happening for some time before the parents or child

BOX 53.2 Nursing Care Planning to Respect Cultural Diversity

People in various cultures have differing beliefs regarding what causes cancer, ranging from evil spirits or evil past lives to totally environmental, genetic, or psychological causes. Talking with the parents and the child, if old enough, about what they think is the cause of cancer can add understanding to their reactions to procedures or medicine; it can make explanations of therapy more meaningful to parents, because explanations can be geared to fit within their beliefs.

realize it is present. Even after they are aware a change exists, some time may pass before they realize the few symptoms they feel are serious enough to require health care (Box 53.2).

Although cancer in children is rare compared to unintentional injury or infection, it is a leading cause of death among children younger than 15 years of age. Fortunately, the overall survival rate for children with cancer today has improved as much as 50% from the 1970s (Smith, Seibel, Altekruse, et al., 2010).

Cell Growth

The normal cell cycle consists of two main divisions: an interphase (resting) phase and a mitosis (dividing) phase. The interphase has four separate stages: G0, G1, S, and G2. Activity during these periods is summarized in Table 53.1. The time span of a cell's life cycle varies based on the type of tissue involved. A bone cell cycle, for instance, is short—about 10 hours; a nerve cell cycle is long—the lifetime of the person. The rate of the cycle is slowed or increased by outside stimuli, such as hypoxia, genetic and immunologic factors, and physical and chemical agents. Normally, an organ has some cells in both resting and active cells.

TABLE 53.1 Phases of the Cell Cycle

Phase	Activity
G	Gap, or the phase between mitosis and synthesis.
G0	Cell at rest. Cells remain in this state until some stimulant, such as death of surrounding cells, triggers the cell to enter an active phase; it is difficult to destroy cells in this resting state.
G1	Period until DNA stabilization is complete; it remains difficult to destroy cells in this phase.
S (synthesis)	Period (6–8 hr) during which DNA and chromosomes are duplicated or a cell readies itself for division into two daughter cells.
G2	Cell doubling in size as preparation for dividing into two daughter cells; if protein synthesis can be stopped at this point so that the cell cannot reach a "critical mass," mitosis (cell division) cannot take place.
M (mitosis)	Period of cell division into two like daughter cells.

Body cells apparently have the ability to recognize their own type, possibly by recognizing surface enzymes or glucose particles on cell membranes. As a result, cells of like type do not migrate away from each other but instead recognize and adhere to each other to form a solid mass. In contrast, neoplastic cells seem to lose this ability to adhere to one another (they are autonomous cells). The reason for this is not well documented but may be related to decreased calcium in the cell membrane or to an increased negative charge that repels other cells rather than bonds them together.

Another feature of healthy cells is that they appear to be able to recognize when they are being crowded for the space they must occupy and, at that point, are able to halt growth to reduce overcrowding. Neoplastic cells do not respond to this communication or cannot receive it, so, despite how crowded they become, they continue to grow. By the time a tumor mass is detected by palpation, it is probably about 30 times the size of its original aberrant cell. In many instances, it may be necessary to kill as many as a billion cells to destroy the entire mass (Kline, 2012).

Neoplastic Growth

Neoplasms are either *benign* (growth is limited) or *malignant* (cancerous or with unlimited growth). Even when a tumor is benign, however, it doesn't mean it is completely harmless because it can cause damage by pressing on adjacent tissue. For example, brain tumors in children are often benign, but they can cause extensive respiratory depression from increased pressure on the respiratory center.

Causes of Neoplastic Growth

The exact origin of neoplastic growth is unknown, and any growth may actually involve more than one cause. As more and more evidence is compiled on the nature of genes, specific markers in tumors that apparently fail to suppress, or stimulate, cancer-causing genes are being identified; almost all childhood cancers have such markers or a genetic trigger or predisposition to cancer (Graham, Maloney, Quinones, et al., 2012; Virshup, 2012).

In adults, tumors may grow because normal cell growth has been altered by environmental irritation, such as chronic exposure to chemical irritants or cigarette smoke. In adults, the skin, bladder, lungs, and intestines involve organs exposed to such outside influences and irritation and thus become common sites for abnormal growths. In children, in contrast, tumors most frequently occur in organs unexposed to the environment such as leukemia of the bloodstream, nephroblastoma of the kidney, tumors of the brain, or neuroblastoma in the abdomen, and because many tumors occur in children younger than 5 years of age who haven't had long-term exposure to environmental carcinogens, this cause of tumors is probably not a great influence in childhood cancer. Another difference in childhood cancer is that it is possible for cancers to begin in utero before direct exposure to harmful substances could have occurred (Sato, Izumi, Minegishi, et al., 2011).

Two substances that are documented as leading to lung cancer later in life and to which children need to be protected from contacting are secondary smoke and asbestos. Asbestos is particularly difficult to avoid if a child's school or home is insulated with this material or a parent works in asbestos removal and brings home particles on clothing (Reid, Franklin, Olsen, et al., 2013). Yet another reason why childhood cancers occur is that a child who has survived one cancer appears to be at a higher than usual risk for the development of a second cancer such as bone cancer.

Another common theory of why neoplasms grow is the cell mutation theory. This suggests that carcinogenic agents and hereditary susceptibility combine to alter the nature of cells. The genetic factor may mark the cells for abnormal growth. The environmental factor actually causes the abnormal growth. Carcinogenic agents capable of doing this can be living (viral), physical (radiation), or chemical. Radiation during intrauterine life, for example, is a documented cause of leukemia (Rajaraman, Simpson, Neta, et al., 2011). Radiation of the thyroid in infancy is associated with thyroid cancer later in life (Sassolas, Hafdi-Nejjari, Casagranda, et al., 2013).

This theory explains why the growth of neoplastic cells is not reversible (the cells cannot return to a normal state because they are intrinsically changed) and why neoplasms occur in some people but not in others (both an intrinsic and an extrinsic factor, or an inherited tendency and an environmental insult, must be present). It is difficult to document this process, however, because if there is a lengthy time span between these steps, the cause-and-effect relationship is difficult to trace.

In other cancers, oncogenic (cancer-causing) viruses such as HPV may be directly responsible for tumor growth (Ciesielska, Nowińska, Podhorska-Okołów, et al., 2012). According to this viral theory, **oncogenic viruses** have the ability to change the structure of DNA or RNA in cells. C-type RNA viruses, for example, have been implicated in leukemia. The Epstein–Barr virus (EBV) is associated with Burkitt lymphoma. This theory is supported by the fact that an immunodeficient state appears to increase the risk for development of a neoplastic growth. In some children, because of their genetics, tumor suppressor cells may not be present, allowing abnormal growth stimulated by viruses to continue.

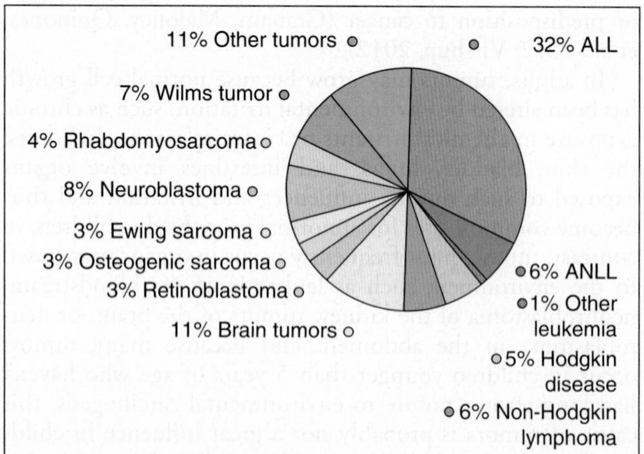

FIGURE 53.1 Approximate incidence of common childhood cancers. ALL, acute lymphocytic leukemia; ANLL, acute nonlymphocytic leukemia.

ASSESSING CHILDREN WITH CANCER

The incidence of various types of childhood cancers is shown in Figure 53.1. Because these cancers involve different body systems, signs and symptoms can vary greatly (Box 53.3).

History

Thorough history taking at health care visits is necessary to reveal the common local symptoms (bruising, nosebleeds, headache, pain in a knee, constipation) of childhood malignancies so that a child can be further evaluated and a cancer discovered early in its growth. Also important is discovering and appreciating systemic effects such as cachexia (loss of weight and anorexia) because these can occur if the tumor is growing so rapidly it is taking nutrients away from normal cells. Other systemic symptoms occur because of excessive hormone production (overproduction of antidiuretic, thyroid, or adrenocorticotropic hormone, for example), which results from tumor growth in a specific body area. Although the signs and symptoms of cancer listed by the ACS (Box 53.4) apply primarily to cancers in adults, they should also be kept in mind as general guidelines when assessing children.

BOX 53.3 Nursing Care Planning Using Assessment

Assessing a Child for Signs of Cancer

History

Chief concern: Weight loss, loss of appetite, easy bruising, swelling in a body part, headache, eye deviations.

Past medical history: Family member with a history of cancer.

Physical examination

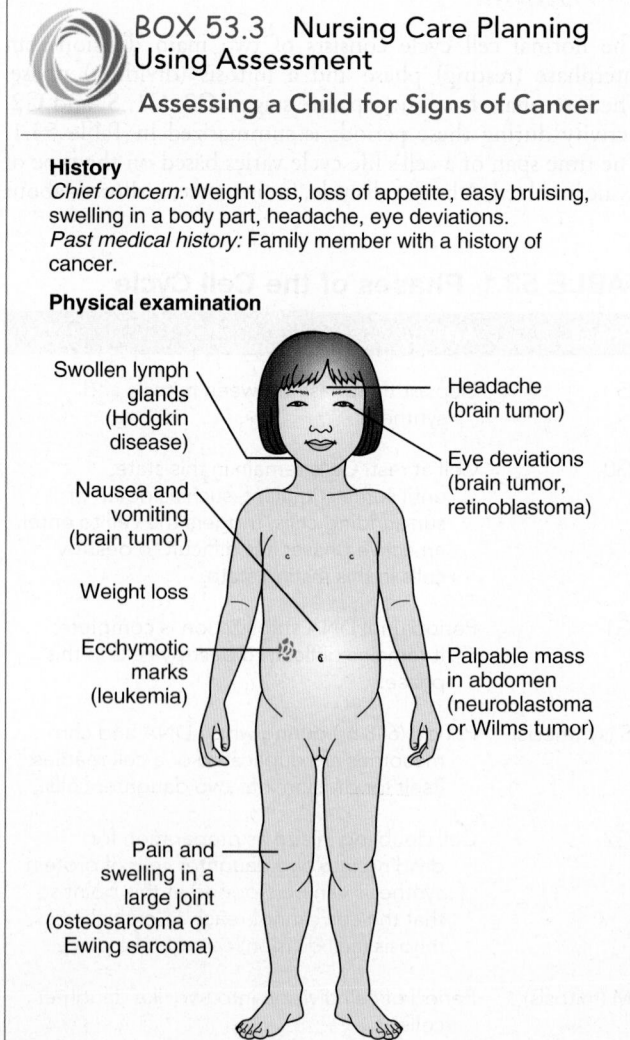

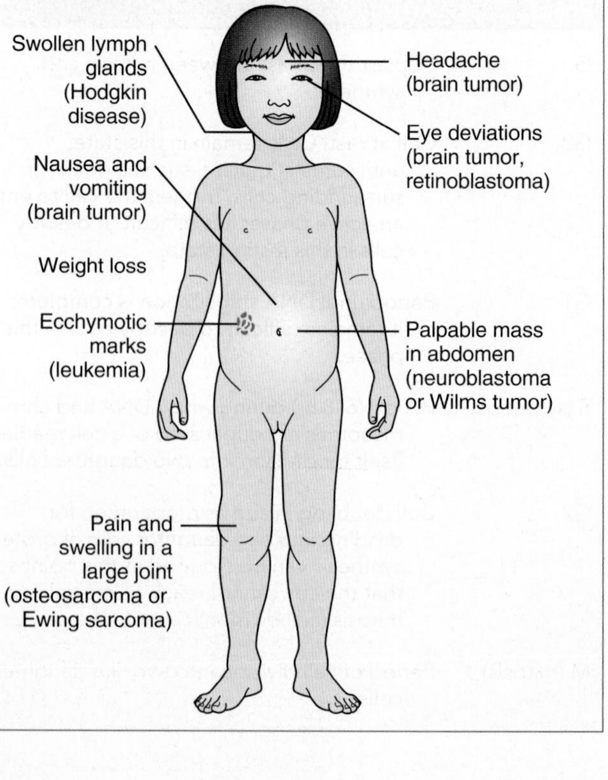

BOX 53.4 Signs and Symptoms of Cancer

General Signs and Symptoms of Cancer
- Unexplained weight loss
- Fever
- Fatigue
- Pain
- Skin changes

Signs and Symptoms of Certain Cancers
Change in bowel habits or bladder function
Sores that do not heal
White patches inside the mouth or white spots on the tongue
Unusual bleeding or discharge
Thickening or lump in the breast or parts of the body
Indigestion or trouble swallowing
Recent change in a wart or mole or any new skin change
Nagging cough or hoarseness

Modified and reprinted by the permission of the American Cancer Society, Inc. from www.cancer.org.

Physical and Laboratory Examination

Assessing height and weight followed by a thorough physical examination of children are instrumental measures in discovering malignancy. To confirm a diagnosis, a number of further diagnostic procedures may be used, including X-ray, ultrasound, magnetic resonance imaging (MRI), blood analysis, and biopsy.

Biopsy

Most children with a possible diagnosis of cancer will have a **biopsy** (the surgical removal of tissue cells for laboratory analysis) performed to confirm the diagnosis (McLean & Wofford, 2011). Although biopsies are classified as minor surgery and usually done on an ambulatory basis, do not treat lightly the meaning of them to a family. In addition to carrying a definite surgical risk if conscious sedation or general anesthesia is used, they are an anxiety-producing procedure because, up to that point, parents can convince themselves their child has something innocent. A biopsy clouds this hope, because the word "biopsy" implies that cancer is at least a possibility. For this reason, be certain parents and children have thorough preparation for the biopsy procedure and any care the child will need afterward. Remember that anxious parents do not "hear" well and thus may need to have postoperative instructions or aftercare repeated. Bone marrow aspiration is an example of a frequent type of biopsy used with children (see Chapter 44).

Staging

Tumor staging is a procedure by which a malignant tumor's extent and progress are documented. Knowing the stage of a tumor helps the health care team design an effective treatment program, establish an accurate prognosis, and evaluate the progress or regression of the disease. In general, stage I refers to a tumor that has not extended into the surrounding tissue and thus can be completely removed surgically; stage II means there is some local spread, but the chance for complete surgical removal is good. Stage III typically means cancer cells have spread to local lymph nodes; stage IV designates tumors that have spread systemically (**metastasis**). There are various staging systems, but one of the most common is known as the TNM system; it describes the tumor's size (T), any presence in the lymph nodes (N), and if the cancer has metastasized or spread to other organs (M). A TNM system is most applicable to carcinomas (tumors of epithelial tissue). Because most childhood tumors tend to be sarcomas (tumors derived from connective tissue), the classification does not apply to all childhood tumors.

OVERVIEW OF CANCER TREATMENT MEASURES USED WITH CHILDREN

Therapy for a child with cancer focuses on devising ways to kill the growth of the abnormal cells while protecting the normal surrounding cells. This is done by a combination of surgery, radiation, chemotherapy, stem cell transplantation, immunotherapy (biologic response modifiers), and general health measures.

Radiation Therapy

Radiation therapy changes the DNA component of a cell nucleus to a point at which the cell cannot replicate DNA material and thereby inhibits further cell division and growth. Radiation is not effective on cells that have a low oxygen content (a proportion of cells in every tumor) nor is it effective at the time of cell division (mitosis). Therefore, radiation schedules are designed so that therapy occurs over a period of 1 to 6 weeks and includes time intervals when cells will be in a susceptible stage.

Immediate Side Effects

Radiation has both systemic and localized effects. Radiation sickness (fatigue, anorexia, nausea, vomiting) is the most frequently encountered systemic effect. This occurs if the gastrointestinal (GI) tract is irradiated. It also occurs to a lesser degree as a result of the release of toxic substances from destroyed tumor cells. To counteract this, a child is prescribed an antiemetic before each procedure. Skin reactions, such as erythema and tenderness, are typical local effects.

Long-Term Side Effects

The long-term side effects of radiation are becoming more apparent as increasing numbers of children who have undergone intense radiation therapy survive years beyond the radiation. Because radiation damages all cells in its path toward the tumor to some extent, any body tissue has the possibility of being affected by radiation.

Effects on Bone. Asymmetric growth of bones, easy fracturing, scoliosis, kyphosis, and spinal shortening are effects that can occur in bones. Bone tissue is most vulnerable during times of rapid growth, such as during the first year of life or during a prepubertal growth spurt. Scoliosis and kyphosis can be avoided if the entire vertebra is irradiated rather than only one side or the other; this means a larger area of bone may be irradiated than was done formerly, so that both sides of the vertebra are in the radiation path.

Effects on Hormones. Radiation to the head and neck can result in long-term thyroid, hypothalamic, and pituitary gland dysfunction, resulting in growth hormone deficiency or hypothalamic–pituitary stimulation to the thyroid gland. For this reason, children's growth and thyroid function need to be evaluated about every 6 months for the next 3 years after cranial radiation to detect these changes. It's possible to treat both hypothyroidism and hypopituitary growth failure with hormone replacement in coming years if these do occur. Radiation to ovaries or testes can also result in complications such as infertility or less estrogen or testosterone production, preventing the development of secondary sexual changes. For children past puberty, pretreatment sperm or oocyte banking may be advocated before they undergo radiation to the testes or ovaries so they have viable sperm or oocytes banked for use later in life (Olatunbosun & Zhu, 2012).

Effects on the Nervous System. Long-term effects of radiation to the nervous system are demyelination and necrosis of the white matter of the brain, which results in symptoms of lethargy, sleepiness, and possibly seizures, and effects on the gray matter, which can result in learning disabilities. In addition, children may show abnormal electroencephalograph (EEG) tracings or experience low-intensity headaches, cataracts, salivary gland damage, and a chronic change in or loss of taste.

Effects on the Organs of the Chest and Abdomen. Extensive radiation to the lungs can result in a chronic pneumonitis and pulmonary fibrosis. Heart effects may include pericardial thickening with reduced heart expandability. Radiation to the GI system can result in chronic malabsorption from changes in intestinal villi; hepatic fibrosis can result in reduced liver function. Radiation to the kidney and bladder can result in nephritis and chronic cystitis.

If the child's head area is involved in therapy, alopecia (hair loss), impaired growth of teeth, or reduced salivary gland function, leading to a constantly dry mouth, may result. Radiation to bone marrow may depress the production of both WBCs and platelets. The possibility of these long-term effects of radiation should be explained to parents when radiation is initially discussed, as a part of obtaining informed consent. At the early stage of diagnosis, however, parents rarely are concerned with these long-term effects. Their thoughts are understandably filled with such short-term outcomes as the achievement of a remission or destruction of the tumor.

Nursing Diagnoses and Related Interventions

Nursing diagnoses related to radiation therapy should include not only the physical preparation or aftercare necessary but also the stress such a procedure places on families.

Nursing Diagnosis: Parental and child anxiety related to radiation therapy

Outcome Evaluation: Parents state they understand the necessity of the therapy and will help support the child during therapy.

Before Treatment. The points where radiation therapy will be directed are usually marked on the child's skin in indelible ink. As a rule, parents shouldn't apply any cream or lotion to the marked areas until the treatment series is complete because if a cream contains a metal base, it could distort or interfere with the entrance of radiation. If the head will be irradiated, a dental consultation may be necessary because radiation therapy can slow healing if a tooth extraction is necessary.

During Treatment. Most children have previously had X-ray films taken by the time that radiation therapy is begun, so they're already familiar with thinking of the radiation machine as a giant nonthreatening camera. Because the procedure requires them to lie still for a period of time, possibly on an uncomfortable table in a room isolated from personnel or their parents, they may experience extreme fear. Reassure the parents and the child that during the treatment, just as there is no sensation from X-ray exposure, the child will experience no sensation from radiation. Infants are usually prescribed a sedative or conscious sedation before therapy to ensure they are able to lie still during the needed time interval. To make this approach effective, if only a sedative will be given, keep the child fairly active early in the day and introduce calming activities after the sedative is administered so the child will be sleepy and fall asleep during irradiation. An older child may want to plan an activity to think about during irradiation, such as selecting 10 people to take on a camping trip (and why), or choosing 10 places to visit next year—mental activities that require no movement but are still stimulating.

After Treatment. Children undergoing radiation therapy need their leukocyte and platelet counts monitored periodically for changes. Teaching points for parents to help their children during therapy are summarized in Box 53.5.

What if...53.1 You find Gerri's mother scrubbing her son's head to remove the purple marks inked there by the radiation department. Would you stop her or let her continue, knowing the radiation department can easily replace them?

Chemotherapy

A **chemotherapeutic agent** is one that is capable of destroying malignant cells. In most instances, several chemotherapeutic agents are used to cause multiple damages to each cell, thereby increasing the chance the cell will no longer be able to reproduce. Like radiation, chemotherapy is scheduled over a period of time so that all malignant cells can eventually be destroyed or cells that are not susceptible on one day because they are undergoing mitosis will be susceptible on the next day.

Types of Chemotherapeutic Agents

Chemotherapeutic agents fall into a number of different categories. Typically, any agent that needs mixing for hospital

BOX 53.5 Nursing Care Planning Based on Family Teaching

CARING FOR THE CHILD RECEIVING RADIATION THERAPY

Q. Gerri's mother asks you, "What sorts of things do we need to do when Gerri begins receiving radiation therapy?"

A. In addition to preventing infection, you need to take some special actions to meet your child's needs. Here are some tips designed to promote radiation's therapeutic benefits and minimize its adverse effects.

Skin Care

- If the area to be radiated is marked on the child's skin, do not erase the marks.
- Expose irradiated area to air but not to direct heat or sunlight.
- Avoid lengthy soaks in bath water or swimming pools.
- If the head is irradiated, use mild shampoo on hair and rinse gently with water. Air dry or pat excess moisture gently. Avoid rough towels and hair dryers.
- Supply a soft toothbrush to protect gums and oral mucous membranes. Keep the mouth moist by offering frequent sips of water—particularly if radiation decreases salivary gland secretions.
- Encourage clothing that fits loosely over irradiated areas.
- Because some skin preparations are drying and some interfere with radiation, do not apply creams or lotions to the irradiated area unless prescribed.

Nutrition

- To promote retention of nutrients, administer antiemetics as prescribed.
- Encourage high-calorie meals when child is least likely to be nauseated. Praise the child's efforts to eat. Strive for peaceful and pleasant meal and snack times.
- Provide foods identified by child as special favorites. Serve easy-to-swallow foods at best liked temperatures.

Hydration

- Reduce amounts of fresh fruit and vegetables rich in cellulose, and eliminate apple juice from the child's diet, because these may contribute to diarrhea and subsequent fluid loss.
- If diarrhea occurs, administer antidiarrheal medication as prescribed.

Activity

- Provide adequate rest periods. Schedule activities to avoid waking the child frequently at night.
- Structure the child's activities to be stimulating but not physically tiring.
- Recommend mild activity that does not stress bones that may be weakened by radiation and, therefore, easily fractured.

Instruction and Distraction

- Prepare the child for the effects of radiation therapy, particularly hair loss, in case they occur. Some comfort measures may include wearing a wig or special cap; introducing play things, such as dolls without hair; and most important, stressing that people like people for themselves, not for their appearance.
- Schedule a tour of the radiation department. If possible, let the child play-act and become familiar with the equipment. Provide ample time to answer questions.
- Encourage active games before the procedure and quiet games afterward.
- Help the child devise "mind games" to play during the procedure such as listing 10 friends to take camping, 10 activities to do, or 10 favorite games to play so the procedure is not boring but a learning experience.

use is prepared under a specialized hood in the pharmacy to prevent airborne drug residue. When administering such agents, wear gloves and wash your hands well afterward to prevent skin exposure and absorption of the drug. Don't pour unused medicine into a sink drain because chemotherapy drugs should be considered hazardous substances. Caution parents, when administering such drugs at home, to use the same precautions.

Alkylating Agents. Alkylating agents work by interfering with DNA synthesis. They are cell-cycle specific or are most effective against cells in the G1 and S phases of growth. An alkylating agent commonly used with children is cyclophosphamide (Cytoxan).

Antimetabolites. Antimetabolites are drugs that so closely resemble natural products that a cell readily incorporates them into its structure. Because they are not the natural product, however, the cell cannot function or replicate with them in its structure and dies. They act only in the S (synthesis) phase of the cell cycle. Methotrexate (Folex PFS), a folic acid antagonist, is an example.

Plant Alkaloids. Plant alkaloids interfere with cell mitosis (M phase). Two commonly used plant alkaloids are vincristine (Oncovin) and vinblastine (Velban).

Antibiotics. Several antibiotics are effective in destroying malignant cells by impairing DNA synthesis. These are not cell-cycle specific, which means they can be effective at any cell phase (resting or dividing). Dactinomycin (Cosmegen) and doxorubicin (Adriamycin) are examples.

Nitrosoureas. Nitrosoureas disrupt protein production, thereby interfering with DNA synthesis. Because these drugs cross the blood–brain barrier, they are effective as chemotherapy agents in brain tumor therapy. A common example is lomustine (CeeNU).

Enzymes. Body cells need a ready supply of L-asparagine (an essential amino acid) in order to grow. L-Asparaginase (Elspar), a chemotherapeutic agent, is an enzyme that converts L-asparagine into L-aspartic acid, thereby making L-asparagine unavailable for cell growth. It is used in the treatment of acute lymphoblastic leukemia.

Steroids. A corticosteroid, most frequently prednisone, binds to DNA to inhibit mitosis and probably RNA synthesis in cells. When it is added to therapy, it helps prevent the formation of new cells.

Immunotherapy. Immunotherapy is the stimulation of the body's immune system to attempt destruction of foreign or malignant cells. The administration of bacille Calmette-Guérin vaccine (the vaccine for tuberculosis) is an example of this type of therapy. The tuberculin antigen stimulates the immune system to identify and destroy an antigen, with the hope that the system will "recognize" foreign tumor cells and act against them as well. Interferon is an antiviral agent that prevents growth of viruses; agents that stimulate the production of interferon may also be used to encourage the immune system to identify and halt malignant cell growth.

Immune therapy of these types is limited if the immune system has been so altered by the malignant process that it cannot respond when stimulated. It is also possible that the immune response to malignant cells is so different from the response to invading microorganisms that specific types of immunotherapy are necessary to stimulate it. Neuroblastoma is an example of a childhood cancer that appears to respond to antibody-based therapy (Parry & Engh, 2013).

Chemotherapy Protocols

Chemotherapy is scheduled for children at set times and days and by various predetermined routes. At first, children may remain in the hospital for a few days of treatment; later, they may report on a specific day for therapy, or parents may administer the designated therapy at home. Parents must learn about the child's treatment protocol so that they know which drug the child will be receiving each day and on which day each drug must be administered. Knowing the protocol and the specific drug therapy not only helps with accurate dosing but also helps parents begin to prepare the child for administration of a particular drug, such as increasing fiber in the child's diet for a few days before the beginning of a constipation-causing drug like vincristine.

Caution parents, while children are receiving chemotherapy, not to give them aspirin for pain because, in addition to increasing the child's susceptibility to Reye syndrome, aspirin may interfere with blood coagulation, a problem that may already be present because of lowered thrombocyte levels. Instead, suggest they use acetaminophen (Tylenol) or ibuprofen (Motrin) to relieve a headache or to reduce fever. A parent who wants to give a child vitamins should check with their child's primary health care provider to be certain the vitamin preparation will not interfere with a chemotherapeutic agent. Administration of a vitamin that contains folic acid, for example, could interfere with the effectiveness of methotrexate, a folic acid antagonist.

A child receiving chemotherapy is particularly susceptible to contracting an infection and thus should be kept away from people with known infections. Zoster immune globulin may be administered if the child has not been immunized against varicella and is exposed to chickenpox during chemotherapy. Caution parents that live-virus vaccines should not be given during chemotherapy because, if the child's immune mechanism is deficient, these vaccines could cause widespread viral disease.

Side Effects and Toxic Reactions to Chemotherapy

All chemotherapeutic agents have both side effects and toxic effects. Table 53.2 lists commonly used chemotherapeutic agents, their specific side effects, and their potential toxic effects. Malnutrition, nausea and vomiting, hair loss, mucositis (mouth irritation), constipation, diarrhea, cushingoid effects, and susceptibility to infection are side effects common to almost all of these agents. A danger of IV infusion of a chemotherapeutic agent is that, if the fluid infiltrates into a child's subcutaneous tissue, there is apt to be extensive tissue sloughing and damage. Therefore, monitor IV infusions of chemotherapeutic vesicants (agents that cause blistering) carefully to prevent tissue infiltration. Discontinue the infusion if it occurs and apply an ice pack to the site, to create vasoconstriction and prevent further spread of the toxic solution. Dexaroxane (Totect) is an example of a U.S. Food and Drug Administration–approved drug that may be injected into the site to speed absorption. After about 20 minutes, application of warm compresses hastens absorption and clearance of the solution from subcutaneous tissue.

QSEN Checkpoint Question 53.1

Evidence-Based Practice

Following hospital discharge, parents assume the responsibility of administering chemotherapy at home. To see whether parents followed adequate protection for themselves while handling chemotherapy drugs, researchers asked 50 parents of children with acute lymphoblastic leukemia to fill in a questionnaire asking about their experience with chemotherapy drugs. Seventy-two percent of parents reported receiving instruction on safe handling of oral chemotherapy. Ninety percent of parents, however, reported they did not use protective gear such as gloves during preparation of oral chemotherapy. Although tablet crushers were designated for use with oral chemotherapy by 61% of parents, 22% used the same device to crush other nonchemotherapy medications. Over 50% of parents disposed of medication waste with regular garbage or poured the remainder down the sink (Held, Ryan, Champion, et al., 2012).

Based on the previous study, which statement by Gerri's mother would cause you to believe she needs additional education about safe administration of Gerri's oral chemotherapy?

a. "I'll call for advice if Gerri vomits a pill or refuses to take one."
b. "I know his pills' side effects and will observe for them carefully."
c. "I know I have to give the medicine according to a schedule."
d. "I know to wash my hands before handling his pills."

Look in Appendix A for the best answer and rationale.

TABLE 53.2 Commonly Used Chemotherapeutic Agents

Drug	Classification	Side Effects and Toxic Effects	Special Considerations
L-Asparaginase (Elspar)	Enzyme; deprives cancer cells of asparagine, leading to cell death	Anorexia, weight loss, nausea, vomiting, hepatotoxicity, central nervous system toxicity, anaphylactic reaction	Staying with child for first hour of infusion is important; take vital signs every 15 min for first hour to detect anaphylactic reaction.
Cisplatin (Platinol)	Alkylating agent; reacts with and injures cell nucleus	Bone marrow depression, nephrotoxicity (renal dysfunction), nausea, vomiting, loss of taste, tinnitus, high-frequency hearing loss	Infusion bag must be covered with aluminum foil or commercial cover to keep out light, or decomposition can result.
Cyclophosphamide (Cytoxan)	Alkylating agent (nitrogen mustard derivative)	Bone marrow depression, anorexia, nausea, vomiting, mucositis, alopecia, cystitis, (hemorrhagic) hepatotoxicity	Encourage high fluid intake; maintain IV line to limit bladder irritation; test urine for blood and specific gravity.
Cytarabine (Ara-C)	Antimetabolite (pyrimidine analog)	Nausea, vomiting, bone marrow depression, mucositis, alopecia, photosensitivity	Child may need to wear sunglasses in bright light.
Dactinomycin (Cosmegen)	Antibiotic; inhibits DNA synthesis	Nausea, vomiting, bone marrow depression, mucositis	Extreme tissue inflammation occurs if it extravasates into tissue.
Daunorubicin (DaunoXome)	Antibiotic; vesicant	Alopecia, bone marrow depression	Extravasation causes severe tissue damage.
Etoposide (Toposar)	Mitotic inhibitor; inhibits DNA synthesis	Fatigue, alopecia, nausea and vomiting	Slow IV administration is necessary to avoid irritation.
Doxorubicin (Adriamycin)	Antibiotic; inhibits DNA synthesis; vesicant	Nausea, vomiting, bone marrow depression, alopecia, mucositis, possible heart toxicity	Urine may turn red; take pulse for full minute to detect arrhythmia; tissue necrosis occurs if extravasated.
Ifosfamide (Ifex)	Alkylating agent; interferes with DNA synthesis	Leukopenia, alopecia, hemorrhagic cystitis	Maintaining hydration is important to prevent cystitis.
Lomustine (CCNU; CeeNu)	Alkylating agent (nitrosourea compound)	Nausea, vomiting, bone marrow depression (after 3–4 weeks)	Administration on an empty stomach enhances absorption.
Mercaptopurine (Purinethol)	Antimetabolite (purine analog)	Bone marrow depression, nausea, vomiting, mucositis, hepatotoxicity	Allopurinol delays the degradation of mercaptopurine and thus increases toxicity; question prescription if both are to be administered.
Methotrexate (MTX)	Antimetabolite	Mucositis, bone marrow depression, nausea, vomiting, alopecia, hepatotoxicity, nephrotoxicity at high dosage	Decreased effect occurs if administered with salicylates; often followed by leucovorin to decrease toxicity to normal cells.
Prednisone	Corticosteroid; suppresses lymphocyte production	Weight gain, cushingoid facies, depressed systemic response to infection	Child may need support to accept changed appearance.
Procarbazine (Matulane)	Antineoplastic; interferes with DNA and RNA synthesis	Nausea, vomiting, bone marrow depression	Drug may cause blurriness of vision; avoid foods with high tyramine content.

(continues on page 1570)

TABLE 53.2 Commonly Used Chemotherapeutic Agents (continued)

Drug	Classification	Side Effects and Toxic Effects	Special Considerations
Thioguanine	Antimetabolite	Bone marrow suppression	Monitoring of hepatic function tests is necessary.
Vincristine (Oncovin)	Plant alkaloid; vesicant	Constipation, alopecia, joint and muscle pain, muscle weakness	Paresthesia of fingers and toes, foot drop may occur; may need stool softener; tissue necrosis occurs if infiltrated.
Additional Agents			
Allopurinol (Lopurin, Zyloprim)	Antigout agent	Nausea, vomiting	Prevents uric acid formation from destroyed cells.
Bacillus Calmette-Guérin (bCG) vaccine	Vaccine	Local inflammation	Stimulates immune system.
Leucovorin (Wellcovorin)	Folic acid derivative		Neutralizes the toxicity of methotrexate.
Interferon	Antiviral agent	Fever	Blocks virus replication.
Filgrastim (Neupogen)	Granulocyte colony-stimulating factor	Nausea, vomiting	Leukocyte count increases.
Epoetin alfa (Procrit)	Recombinant human erythropoietin	Hypertension; headache	Red blood cell count increases.

Nursing Diagnoses and Related Interventions

As with radiation therapy, nursing diagnoses related to chemotherapy need to address both physical and psychosocial aspects of care.

Nursing Diagnosis: Imbalanced nutrition, less than body requirements, related to nausea, vomiting, or anorexia resulting from chemotherapy

Outcome Evaluation: Child is able to eat frequent, small meals; calorie intake is adequate for age and size; child maintains percentile place on growth curve.

It is easy for a child with cancer to become malnourished as the fast-growing malignant cells take more than their share of nutrients from normal cells. Nausea and vomiting resulting from chemotherapy add to the difficulty of maintaining an adequate oral intake. If stomatitis (stomach irritation) or mucositis (mouth irritation) occurs as a result of chemotherapy, eating becomes exceedingly difficult because of stomach or mouth pain (Zur, 2012).

If the effect of the chemotherapy is extreme, stomach and intestinal ulcers can develop and interfere with absorption. Changes in fatty acid metabolism may alter the responsiveness of body cells to insulin metabolism. Unable to use glucose effectively, cells cannot function at an optimum level, and a chronic feeling of fatigue results. Anorexia may occur from a factor produced by the tumor that acts directly on the center for hunger in the hypothalamus or from nausea produced by chemotherapy. Cyclophosphamide, a commonly used chemotherapeutic agent to treat leukemias or lymphomas, is associated with taste changes. Many children taking this drug report that foods taste bitter or do not describe foods as sweet until they are very sweet. Because of these taste changes, foods the child used to enjoy may no longer be enjoyable. Unwilling to try new foods, the child decreases oral intake.

To counteract these taste changes, you may need to suggest different foods or methods of food preparation or include a dietitian as a major health team member. Chicken, for example, may taste less bitter than beef or pork. Sprinkling brown sugar on cereal may offer a sweeter taste than plain sugar. Many children know that excess sugar leads to obesity and therefore are reluctant to use a lot of it to make foods taste better. You can assure them eating is the most important thing to think about now. When they're well there will be time enough to worry about the amount of their sugar intake. Be certain they continue careful cleaning of their teeth after eating to prevent tooth decay even if a great deal of sugar is eaten. However, do not recommend honey as a sweetener. Botulism organisms can grow in honey, placing the immunosuppressed child at risk for infection.

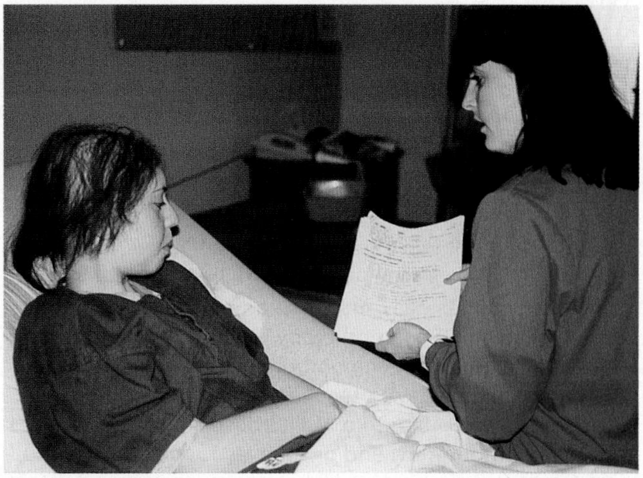

FIGURE 53.2 Children receiving radiation or chemotherapy often have reduced appetites. Here, a nurse discusses nutrition and food choices with a 15-year-old with leukemia. (© Caroline Brown, RNC, MS, DEd.)

Urge parents to be careful that mealtime remains a pleasant time, even if the child isn't eating well. Encourage them to allow the child to make choices whenever possible. Offer small portions because a small meal fully finished is usually more satisfying than a large meal half finished. Being certain snack foods are nutritious (perhaps a malted milkshake rather than a cola beverage) is another way to increase nutrient intake. Suggest eating larger meals early in the day before chemotherapy begins, when the child is less likely to be nauseated (Fig. 53.2).

Nursing Diagnosis: Risk for deficient fluid volume related to nausea and vomiting resulting from chemotherapy

Outcome Evaluation: Skin turgor remains good; mucous membranes are moist; vomiting does not occur more than once a day.

Nausea and vomiting are common side effects of almost all chemotherapy agents because the cells lining the stomach are fast-growing and therefore are among the first cells to incorporate the drug and die. Nausea and vomiting can be prevented by administering an antiemetic, such as hydroxyzine (Atarax) or ondansetron (Zofran), before chemotherapy and at 4- to 8-hour intervals during the course of therapy (Box 53.6). These drugs work best in children to prevent nausea; they do not necessarily relieve it once it is present. Thus, begin these medications prophylactically or before chemotherapy begins for best results.

If children are too nauseated to eat, see if they will accept some clear fluids because this helps prevent uric acid buildup in the kidneys from the number of malignant cells being destroyed. If children are vomiting or cannot take even clear fluid, IV hydration therapy will be necessary. With a drug such as cyclophosphamide (Cytoxan), which is known to cause

BOX 53.6 Nursing Care Planning Based on Responsibility for Pharmacology

ONDANSETRON HYDROCHLORIDE (ZOFRAN)

Classification: Ondansetron is an antiemetic agent.
Action: Blocks central and peripheral serotonin receptor sites to prevent chemotherapy-induced nausea and vomiting in adults and children older than 3 years of age (Karch, 2013).
Dosage: Dependent on weight of child. Typically, 4 mg orally three times daily, first dose administered 30 minutes before beginning chemotherapy, with subsequent doses at 4 and 8 hours after chemotherapy continued every 8 hours for 1 to 2 days after chemotherapy treatment; or three doses of 0.15 mg/kg IV, first dose started 20 minutes before chemotherapy and given over 15 minutes, with subsequent doses at 4 and 8 hours.

Possible Adverse Effects: Dizziness, headache, pruritus, myalgia, pain at injection site

Nursing Implications

- Be aware of timing of chemotherapeutic treatment to ensure that first dose is given 20 to 30 minutes before beginning chemotherapy.
- Instruct parents to continue oral form for 1 to 2 days after completion of chemotherapy to maximize effect.
- Advise parents to administer the oral drug every 8 hours around the clock for maximum results.

cystitis (bladder irritation) if fluid intake is reduced, an IV line for adequate fluid intake is very important.

Nursing Diagnosis: Risk for disturbed body image related to changes in physical appearance caused by chemotherapy

Outcome Evaluation: Child discusses feelings about appearance changes with nurse and parents; child states that, although she does not like them, she understands any changes are temporary.

Because chemotherapy causes changes in body appearance, both children and their parents can benefit from a frank discussion of symptoms and their feelings about these changes both before chemotherapy begins and during the therapy.

Alopecia. Alopecia, or hair loss, is a side effect that occurs with almost all chemotherapeutic drugs, because hair cells, like stomach cells, are fast-growing and easily killed as they incorporate the drug. Even when forewarned that such a consequence is likely, most children and parents are surprised at the suddenness of the hair loss (entire curls may fall out at one time, and a child can become totally bald in 1 to 3 days). For most children, hair loss is a greater problem for the parents than for the child. If a child feels self-conscious, suggest a wig, scarf, or baseball cap. Introducing a doll without hair and reminding the child that those who love the child love the whole person, not just the packaging, are also helpful (Fig. 53.3).

Cushingoid Appearance. Children receiving long-term corticosteroid (prednisone) therapy develop a typical "moon face," red cheeks, and a stocky build. Like the loss of body hair, a cushingoid appearance can be devastating to children or parents, the final insult in light of all the other things happening to them. Provide support and reassurance that this appearance is only temporary and will fade after they are no longer on therapy.

Nursing Diagnosis: Impaired oral mucous membrane related to effects of chemotherapy

Outcome Evaluation: Child states mouth discomfort is at a tolerable level; no signs of ulceration are present.

Mucositis (ulcers of the gum line and mucous membranes of the mouth) is another frequent effect of antimetabolic drugs (Lalla, Brennan, & Schubert, 2011). Because chewing is painful, the child needs a soft or light diet prescribed. Brushing, flossing, and fluoride supplements should continue. Brushing teeth with a soft swab rather than a toothbrush may feel more comfortable for some children. If the child has ulcers present, an antibacterial mouthwash may be prescribed (be certain that the child understand the wash should be spit out afterward, not swallowed; demonstrate this to very young children if necessary so you're certain they understand what "don't swallow" means).

Another caution is to be aware that mucous membrane ulcers can occur throughout the GI tract. For this reason, avoid taking rectal temperatures for children

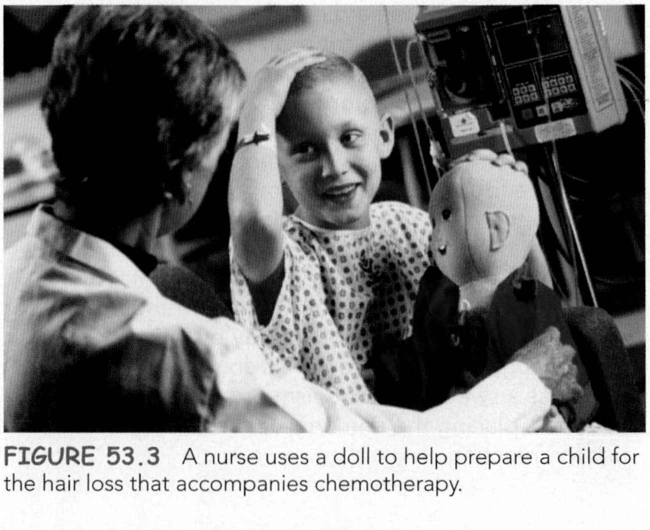

FIGURE 53.3 A nurse uses a doll to help prepare a child for the hair loss that accompanies chemotherapy.

BOX 53.7 Nursing Care Planning to Empower a Family

TIPS FOR RELIEVING THE DISCOMFORT OF MUCOSITIS

Q. Gerri's father tells you, "Our son has developed ulcers in his mouth from the chemotherapy. What can we do to help him feel more comfortable?"

A. Continuing oral care despite discomfort is important to minimize the number of germs in the mouth and ideally prevent infection. Here are some tips for relieving the discomfort:

- Use a soft toothbrush.
- Try to make oral hygiene fun. Make up a game about mouth care such as "Simon Says" (and he says "brush") that the whole family can play.
- Encourage your child to rinse his mouth with lukewarm water about three times a day for comfort and to encourage healing.
- Serve soft foods such as mashed potatoes and pudding, rather than hard ones, such as toast crusts or crunchy cereal, to avoid further abrasions to tender gum lines.
- Provide nonacidic foods, such as gelatin instead of orange juice, which can sting if sores are present.
- Encourage your child to drink as much fluid as possible, because proper hydration helps to keep lips from cracking.
- Keep lips well lubricated with petroleum jelly or a commercial product. This care also prevents cracking.

on antimetabolic therapy to prevent aggravation or perforation of rectal ulcers. General measures to reduce mucositis are summarized in Box 53.7.

Nursing Diagnosis: Risk for constipation or diarrhea related to effects of chemotherapeutic agents

Outcome Evaluation: Child maintains usual pattern of bowel elimination; child reports (and parent confirms) no existence of hard or loose stools.

Some chemotherapeutic agents, particularly vincristine, cause constipation. Record the frequency of bowel movements so that constipation is recognized early in its course. Anticipate the need for increasing the intake of fluids and dietary roughage and prescribing of a stool softener, such as docusate sodium (Colace), to prevent hard stools from exacerbating rectal ulcers. Diarrhea needs to be identified early to prevent dehydration. Care of a child with diarrhea is discussed in Chapter 45.

Nursing Diagnosis: Risk for deficient diversional activity related to neuropathy resulting from chemotherapy

Outcome Evaluation: Child identifies activities in which he can participate that do not require fine motor skills while neuropathy is present.

Almost all children receiving chemotherapy experience fatigue and are unable to participate in their usual activities. If they develop neutropenia (reduced number of WBCs), they may require temporary seclusion from other children to prevent exposure to and subsequent development of infection. Help children who are restricted in these ways to find an activity they enjoy, such as drawing, coloring, or playing handheld electronic games, so they can remain active.

Vincristine, a drug used as therapy for leukemias, results in specific neurologic symptoms of weakness, tingling, and numbing of the extremities and sometimes the inability to walk because of loss of ankle support. While taking the drug, children may be unable to hold a pen or pencil or maneuver small parts of toys because their fingers are so affected. These symptoms subside after the medication is discontinued, but in the meantime, help the child think of games that can be accomplished without fine motor control. Be careful that children on bed rest don't develop foot drop because of nerve involvement of the ankle. In some children, physical therapy may be needed along with special braces or boots to prevent this.

Nursing Diagnosis: Risk for infection related to therapy-induced depression of immune system

Outcome Evaluation: Child's temperature is no higher than 98.6°F (37.0°C); no areas of erythema or other signs or symptoms of infection are present.

Children with cancer are very susceptible to infection, not only because their immune system is depressed by chemotherapy but also because they develop a degree of malnutrition that decreases the effectiveness of macrophage and phagocytosis functions and possibly lowers the production of interferon, which is important for destroying viral invaders. A malignant process in the body also decreases the body's overall ability to recognize foreign invaders and respond with the usual efficient rejection process. When these invade, frequently used IV insertion sites, the development of dry and cracking mucous membranes, and ulcer formation throughout the GI tract provide ready sites for growth of microorganisms.

Although not well studied in children, administration of a colony-stimulating factor such as filgrastim (Neupogen) can help the body quickly begin replacing damaged WBCs (Perkins, Shapiro, Bookout, et al., 2012). Even with the use of this agent, however, gram-negative bacteria such as *Escherichia coli*, *Pseudomonas aeruginosa*, and *Klebsiella pneumoniae*, and gram-positive bacteria such as *Staphylococcus aureus* and streptococci, commonly cause infections. Viral infections such as varicella (chickenpox), varicella zoster (shingles), herpes simplex, viral hepatitis, and cytomegalovirus also are common invaders.

Pneumocystis carinii pneumonia (normally a very rare pneumonia) may occur from protozoal invasion. Treating bacterial infections with antibiotics can cause overgrowth of fungal infections such as candidiasis or aspergillosis.

If infection is discovered in a child with cancer, the causative agent is identified by culture. Specific antibiotics are then prescribed. Box 53.8 identifies interventions to reduce the possibility of infection occurring in a child with a low WBC count (neutropenia).

What if...53.2 Gerri's mother tells you she does not want her child to have an antiemetic drug before chemotherapy, because the nausea and vomiting are proof the chemotherapy is working. Would you hold the drug or administer it?

Stem Cell Transplantation

Transplantation of stem cells from the bone marrow of a well person to a child with cancer has become a frequently used treatment. The procedure allows higher doses of chemotherapy and radiation to be used because, in the event of severe bone marrow depression, the child can have healthy marrow restored. Immune cells in the transplanted marrow may actually help to kill remaining cancer cells in the child's circulation.

If stem cells are donated by someone who is histocompatible (immune compatible) with the child, this is an *allogeneic* transplant. If the child's own cord blood was preserved and frozen since birth or removed prior to chemotherapy, this is an *autologous* transplant. A *syngeneic* transplant is one between twins.

Before transplantation, the child receives a chemotherapy agent, such as cyclophosphamide, or total-body irradiation to kill as many T cells as possible, suppress the child's immune response to the transplanted tissue, and create space in the bone marrow to allow the newly transplanted cells to implant.

Stem cells are removed from the circulating blood of the designated donor or from cord blood. They are then processed and transfused into the child intravenously. The new stem cells enter the bone marrow and begin to function

BOX 53.8 Nursing Care Planning Based on Family Teaching

PREVENTING INFECTION IN THE CHILD WITH NEUTROPENIA

Q. Gerri's mother asks you, "What special things should I do to help prevent my child from developing an infection until his white blood cell count returns to normal?"

A. Here are some suggestions to help prevent infection:

- Arrange for your child to sleep in a single bed and room, if possible, to avoid close contact with other family members who might be developing upper respiratory tract infections.
- Limit the child's exposure to large crowds, such as those at movie theaters.
- Screen and prohibit visitors who have signs of infection such as runny nose, oral herpes, or rashes; who have been exposed to a communicable disease, such as chickenpox; or who have recently been vaccinated.
- Wash your hands frequently before child care and after handling potentially contaminated items such as tissues or diapers.
- Urge the child to wash hands well after using a bathroom and before eating.
- Keep child's immediate surroundings free of plants, flowers, and goldfish, all of which could harbor mold spores.
- Be sure the child has a daily bath or shower. Clean mouth with soft toothbrush to reduce opportunity for bacteria, which are always present in the mouth, to invade.
- Inspect mouth daily for breaks in the tissue, bleeding, or white patches that suggest oral thrush (*Candida*) infection. Apply a moisturizing and protective barrier, such as petroleum jelly, to the lips to help prevent them from cracking.
- Take pulse and respiratory rate and temperature daily. Avoid taking rectal temperatures, to protect against injuring rectal tissue.
- Inspect all skin surfaces daily for scratches that could become entrances for infection. Include intravenous or intramuscular injection sites, venous access device insertion sites, and the diaper area.
- Administer stool softeners, if prescribed, to promote soft stools and bowel movements and avoid rectal tears.
- Provide high-calorie, high-protein foods and food supplements to help rebuild white blood cells. Limit fresh fruits and vegetables, because they have more potential to harbor infectious organisms than cooked foods.
- Assess for respiratory tract infection by listening for cough and throat clearing; inspect throat for redness and nasal passage for discharge. Keep child active and moving through playing a game, such as "Simon Says," that encourages deep breathing.
- Assess for possible genitourinary tract infections. Note the color, clarity, frequency, and concentration of urine. If necessary, obtain a urine specimen using a clean-catch method for testing. Promote increased fluid intake to keep urine flowing. Advise girls to wipe from front to back after voiding or defecating to avoid bringing organisms forward to the urethra. If a girl is menstruating, urge her to change pads or tampons frequently (every 4 hours).
- Question the administration of any vaccine made with a live virus until the child's white blood cell count returns to normal.

after about 3 weeks. Until this time, a child is at extreme risk for infection. Everyone coming in contact with the child must wash their hands well, and specific infection control precautions must be maintained. Transfusion of blood products may be necessary to maintain functional blood components until the transplanted marrow begins to function (Grupp, Asgharzadeh, & Yanik, 2012).

Not all medical centers perform stem cell transplantation, so a family may have to travel a distance for the therapy. Complications of stem cell transplantation are discussed in Chapter 44, because this technique also is used for children with blood dyscrasias.

Pain Assessment

Because growing tumors displace cells, causing anoxia to those cells, pain is a common symptom experienced by children with cancer. Methods to assess pain and interventions to help children deal with pain are discussed in Chapter 39.

THE LEUKEMIAS

Leukemia is the distorted and uncontrolled proliferation of WBCs (leukocytes) and is the most frequently occurring type of cancer in children.

Acute Lymphocytic (Lymphoblastic) Leukemia

Acute lymphocytic leukemia (ALL) accounts for 75% of leukemias (Brown & Hunger, 2013) and involves lymphoblasts (immature lymphocytes). Because of the rapid proliferation of so many immature lymphocytes, the production of red blood cells (RBCs) and platelets falls; invasion of body organs by the rapidly increasing WBC elements begins. The abnormally proliferating cells are so immature that they may be identifiable only at the immature "blast cell" or "stem cell" stage.

The highest incidence of ALL is in children between 2 and 6 years of age. The prognosis in children younger than 1 year or older than 10 years at the time of first occurrence is not as good as in those between 2 and 10 years of age. The prognosis in children who have a WBC count higher than 50,000/mm^3 or who have more than 10% L2 cells (see classification of cells, described later) in bone marrow at the time of diagnosis is not as good as in those with a lower WBC count and fewer L2 cells at first diagnosis. The incidence of ALL is slightly higher in boys than in girls, and the disease is seen more often in Hispanic and white children than in children of other races (McLean & Wofford, 2011).

Although it can be shown that leukemia in mice and cats is of viral origin, the cause of leukemia in children is unknown. Radiation, exposure to chemicals, or genetic factors may have some influence on the occurrence as children with Down syndrome are more likely to develop leukemia than other children. If a twin has leukemia, the other twin (as opposed to a nontwin sibling) is also more likely to develop it as well. Bone irradiation may be implicated, so children should be submitted to as few X-rays as possible, including while in utero. An association between magnetic fields or power lines and leukemia is disputed because different studies show different results (Miller & Green, 2010).

Assessment

With ALL, because the bone marrow overproduces lymphocytes and therefore is unable to continue normal production of other blood components, the first symptoms of ALL in children usually are those associated with decreased RBC production (anemia) such as pallor, low-grade fever, and lethargy. A low thrombocyte (platelet) count will lead to petechiae and bleeding from oral mucous membranes and cause easy bruising on arms and legs. As the spleen and liver begin to enlarge from infiltration of abnormal cells, abdominal pain, vomiting, and anorexia occur. As abnormal lymphocytes invade the bone periosteum, the child experiences bone and joint pain. Central nervous system (CNS) invasion leads to symptoms such as headache or unsteady gait.

On physical assessment, painless, generalized swelling of lymph nodes, especially of the submaxillary or cervical nodes, is revealed. Laboratory studies reveal an elevated leukocyte count with cells almost stopped at the blast cell stage. The platelet count and hematocrit value will be low; RBCs that are present are normocytic and normochromic (of normal size and color) but few in number. X-rays of the long bones may reveal lesions caused by the invasion of abnormal cells. A lumbar puncture may show evidence of blast cells in the cerebrospinal fluid (CSF).

A bone marrow aspiration (performed at the iliac crest rather than the sternum as in adults, both because this is less frightening and because it yields more marrow) will be prescribed to identify the type of WBC involved, which documents the type of leukemia (if there are more than 25% blast cells present, a leukemia diagnosis is established).

✔ QSEN Checkpoint Question 53.2

Informatics

The child in the room next to Gerri's is a boy with ALL. Although his parents knew he wasn't well, they had no idea his diagnosis would be leukemia. A review of this boy's electronic health record would most likely note what early signs commonly seen in a child with ALL?

a. Nodules and an abdominal rash
b. Headaches and sleepiness
c. Fatigue and leg bruises
d. Joint pain and coughing

Look in Appendix A for the best answer and rationale.

Therapeutic Management

Up to 95% of children with ALL will achieve a first remission. If a child experiences a relapse, the chances of long-term survival are reduced to approximately 70%. Although remission can be reinduced, the length of each subsequent remission tends to be shorter and less effective.

Disease Classification and Prognosis. Leukemia is classified to define subgroups of cells and to predict the usual response to treatment. Blasts with B-lymphocyte cell characteristics can be recognized by the presence of immunoglobulin and antigen–antibody receptors on their surfaces. B-lymphocyte cell types account for about 85% of instances of ALL; the other 15% of children have T-lymphocyte cell involvement (Schrappe, Hunger, Pui, et al., 2012).

Cure as Goal. The goal of therapy for leukemia is complete cure, based on the use of chemotherapeutic agents. Parents hear of many questionable cancer cures from the Internet or friends during the course of their child's illness. Help them to voice their hopes and concerns for these cures as they hear them, but urge them to discuss these with their primary health care provider to gain a clear picture. When these questionable cures cannot be discussed with health care personnel, they appear to grow in importance, and parents may turn to them in preference to established therapy (Box 53.9).

A chemotherapy program is aimed at, first, achieving a complete remission or absence of leukemia cells (induction phase); second, preventing leukemia cells from invading or growing in the CNS (sanctuary or consolidation phase); third, administering delayed intensive therapy; and fourth, maintaining the original remission (maintenance phase).

Chemotherapy in children is administered by means of a central venous catheter or port, because administration of drugs into a major vessel helps prevent irritation to the vessel walls. These access devices have the secondary advantage of being able to be clamped or "trapped" so that the child can be ambulatory between treatments.

The drug regimen frequently used to initiate a remission includes vincristine, prednisone or dexamethasone, L-asparaginase, and doxorubicin given over a period of 4 weeks. Because so many cells are destroyed by chemotherapy, a high level of uric acid must be excreted during treatment. Such a high level can lead to plugging of kidney glomeruli and loss of kidney function. To prevent this, keeping a child well hydrated and administering a drug such as allopurinol help to reduce the formation of uric acid and maintain safe uric acid excretion.

Although a chemotherapy protocol will achieve disease remission in 95% of children, because many chemotherapy drugs do not cross the blood–brain barrier in effective concentrations, leukemic cells in the CNS can continue to flourish. Intrathecal administration (injection of methotrexate into the CSF by lumbar puncture) is next instituted to eradicate this source of leukemic cells (termed a *consolidation* or *sanctuary phase*, because no "sanctuary" is given to malignant cells). Cranial radiation, once used extensively for this purpose, is less used today than previously because, over the long term, minimal learning disorders may result from excess brain cell radiation.

The third phase of therapy (instensification phase) strengthens the assault against leukemic cells again using chemotherapeutic agents such as vincristine, prednisone, L-asparaginase, doxorubicin, and methotrexate. A drug such as leucovorin (often called leucovorin rescue) may be administered after systemic methotrexate to neutralize its action and protect normal cells from the effect of the drug.

Maintenance and Monitoring. Maintenance chemotherapy aims to eliminate completely any remaining leukemic cells, so that the child's immune system can complete the eradication. Standard maintenance therapy includes a combination of daily mercaptopurine, weekly methotrexate, sporadic vincristine and prednisone, and intrathecal methotrexate and may be continued for 2 to 3 years. During the maintenance phase, the child's blood values must be monitored at least monthly. If there is serious bone marrow depression, medication levels may be reduced or a transfusion or stem cell transplant may be necessary.

BOX 53.9 Nursing Care Planning Based on Effective Communication

Gerri, 6 years old, was diagnosed with a brain tumor 3 months ago. His mother brings him into the emergency room because of a severe nosebleed. While you are putting pressure on his nose, you notice his eyes seem to have poor alignment.

Less Effective Communication

Nurse: Is Gerri still receiving chemotherapy, Mrs. Miller?
Mrs. Miller: No. He's in remission.
Nurse: Is he taking anything that would lower his platelet count or clotting factors?
Mrs. Miller: He takes asparagus powder we get from Mexico.
Nurse: Asparagus powder?
Mrs. Miller: It's the same as L-asparaginase. And so much cheaper.
Nurse: Sounds good. Let's focus right now on getting this bleeding stopped.

More Effective Communication

Nurse: Is Gerri still receiving chemotherapy, Mrs. Miller?
Mrs. Miller: No. He's in remission.
Nurse: Is he taking anything that would lower his platelet count or clotting factors?
Mrs. Miller: He takes asparagus powder we get from Mexico.
Nurse: Asparagus powder?
Mrs. Miller: It's the same as L-asparaginase. And so much cheaper.
Nurse: Let's get this nosebleed stopped. Then we can take a minute to talk about what chemotherapy means.

Of all known diseases, none has as many false "cures" as cancer. When talking with parents, see whether they are using any of these unproven methods. Some of them do no harm, so parents can continue to give them along with proven therapies. Others actually interfere with the action of a chemotherapy drug so are contraindicated. In the above scenario, the parent has chosen an unproven regimen that closely resembles L-asparaginase. Ignoring the possibility that this choice may be an unhelpful one (L-asparaginase does not come from asparagus) and denying the potential discovery of the recurrence of cancer is not therapeutic and could be detrimental in the long term.

If a bone marrow study during the maintenance phase shows that leukemic cells are again evident, a new induction phase will be initiated, followed by a new sanctuary, intensification, and maintenance phase. Children who are free of disease for 4 years are considered cured, and their maintenance therapy can then be stopped. Newer drugs are constantly being investigated to use for relapse therapy. Stem cell transplantation may significantly shorten the course of therapy

Complications

Throughout therapy, the health care team and family need to be alert for complications of leukemia or of the therapy. Among these problems are CNS, renal, and reproductive system disorders.

Central Nervous System Involvement. If CNS involvement occurs, it can become severe and intense. Blindness, hydrocephalus, and recurrent seizures are possible results, although the meninges and the sixth and seventh cranial nerves are the structures most often affected. With meningeal involvement, the child develops nuchal rigidity, headache, irritability, and perhaps vomiting and papilledema. A lumbar puncture will reveal the presence of blast cells in the CSF. If these are discovered, the child will be treated with intrathecal injections of a drug such as methotrexate. Always check that a child is not prescribed oral and IV methotrexate at the same time, because some of the dose of intrathecal methotrexate will be absorbed systemically and could lead to a toxic reaction. Inserting silicon tubing into a cerebral ventricle and threading it under the scalp (an Ommaya reservoir) provides easy access to the CSF for sampling or injection without the need for repeated lumbar punctures (Fig. 53.4).

Renal Involvement. Kidney involvement, resulting from invasion of leukemia cells or plugging of renal tubules with uric acid crystals, is a second serious complication. The kidneys enlarge, and their function will be impaired. The development of renal involvement this way may limit the further use of chemotherapeutic agents because the metabolites of these can no longer be excreted effectively.

Testicular Invasion. In boys, leukemic cells tend to invade the testes and, unless specifically addressed, these cells will not be destroyed by chemotherapy. As a result, the leukemic cells in the testes may continue to proliferate. In most boys, therefore, the testes will be irradiated to destroy this sanctuary site for cells, therapy that leads to sterilization. If a boy is past puberty and is producing sperm, sperm banking may be suggested before chemotherapy and radiation to preserve sperm for reproduction later in life (Babayev, Arslan, Kogan, et al., 2013).

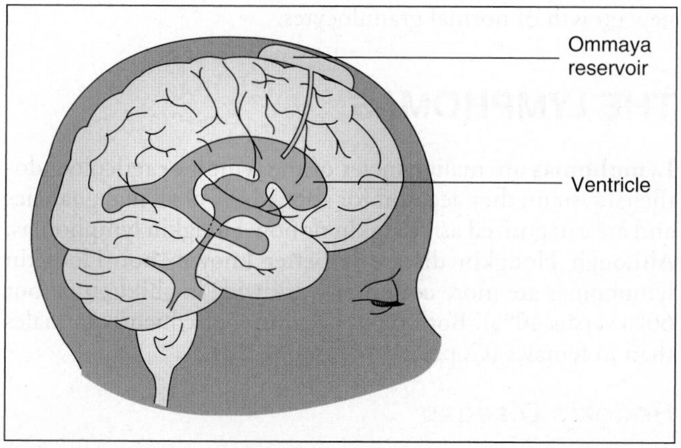

FIGURE 53.4 An Ommaya reservoir. Medication injected into the reservoir flows down to the ventricle and enters the cerebrospinal fluid.

Nursing Diagnoses and Related Interventions

Nursing care for children with leukemia centers both on reducing the number of abnormal cells and helping a young child and parents adjust to the illness.

Nursing Diagnosis: Risk for infection related to nonfunctioning WBCs and immunosuppressive effects of therapy

Outcome Evaluation: Child's temperature remains lower than 98.6°F (37.0°C); no areas of erythema or drainage are present on skin.

Because the number of functioning WBCs is reduced and the drugs used for treatment are immunosuppressive, children with leukemia are at an extremely high risk for infection during chemotherapy. The risk is so high that most deaths in children result from infections, such as septicemia, pneumonia, or meningitis. *Pseudomonas* is also a commonly invading organism.

While children are receiving care at home, teach parents to observe them carefully and to promptly report any indication of infection, such as low-grade fever or behavior that does not seem typical of the child because the sooner the symptoms are reported, the sooner anti-infective therapy can begin.

Some children may be prescribed prophylactic antibiotics to reduce the possibility of infection. Parents may be advised to limit visitors, especially anyone with an infection, until the child's functioning WBC count improves.

If the child has a particularly low functioning leukocyte count, leukocytes may be transfused. Symptoms of fever and chills from leukocyte transfusion tend to be more common than with RBC transfusion and in fact are so common that they are not considered a true transfusion reaction and usually are not a reason to stop the transfusion.

Nursing Diagnosis: Risk for deficient fluid volume related to increased chance of hemorrhage from poor platelet production

Outcome Evaluation: No evidence of hemorrhage is present (no epistaxis, hematuria, or hematemesis); pulse rate and blood pressure remain within parameters for age group.

Because platelet production is limited, children with leukemia are also extremely prone to hemorrhage.

Epistaxis (nosebleed) is the most common kind of bleeding; GI, renal, or CNS bleeding also may occur.

Digital pressure against the nose is usually effective to stop epistaxis, although the application of Gelfoam soaked in topical thrombin may be necessary. In some children, postnasal packing will be necessary, and the child will be transfused with packed RBCs to replace the lost blood volume. Platelet-rich plasma or a concentrated preparation of platelets may be prescribed to improve the platelet count. Because the life span of transfused platelets is short (1 to 3 days), platelets must be infused frequently.

After an intramuscular (IM) injection or the removal of an IV needle, always apply firm pressure to the injection site to prevent bleeding from these sites. Because children with leukemia have blood samples drawn frequently, receive transfusions, and have IV chemotherapeutic drugs administered, provide opportunities for them for therapeutic play with needles and syringes or IV tubing so they can work through some feelings about these intrusive, hurtful procedures (Evans, 2012). Advocate for intermittent infusion devices such as heparin locks or multilumen central venous catheters to minimize the need for repeated venipunctures.

Nursing Diagnosis: Pain related to invasion of leukocytes

Outcome Evaluation: Child rates pain as not above 2 on a pain rating scale (if infant, child is not crying).

Children with acute leukemia experience pain because of the vast number of WBCs that invade the periosteum of the bones. Always assess pain using a standard scale for highest accuracy. Handle legs and arms gently to minimize pain on movement. Use an alternating mattress or sheepskin underneath body joints to help reduce skin irritation caused by resting in a constant position. Administer analgesia as needed (Pound, Clark, Ni, et al., 2012).

Nursing Diagnosis: Ineffective health maintenance related to long-term therapy for leukemia

Outcome Evaluation: Parents and child state importance of regular health maintenance visits; child continues chemotherapy regimen at home and keeps all ambulatory appointments.

During the maintenance phase of therapy, children can participate in usual activities and should attend regular school. Because chickenpox can be fatal to a child who is immunosuppressed, parents should ask the child's school to notify them if any other child in the school develops this disease so appropriate immune protection can be given. If the child has not received immunization against varicella (chickenpox) before this, varicella immune globulin will need to be administered if exposure does occur.

Evaluation of children at follow-up visits includes not only the state of their blood but also whether they are making forward-thinking plans or beginning to think of themselves as well children again. Parents may continue to need a great deal of support during the maintenance phase of therapy as they live from day to day, hoping the remission period will not end (Gibbins, Steinhardt, & Beinart, 2012). If it does end, because they know leukemia is a curable disease today, parents may need a great deal of support to deal with the "bad luck" that their child's therapy was not effective. If death occurs, the reality of what has happened may be extremely difficult for the parents to accept. They may return to the hospital for visits weeks or months after the child's death in an effort to accept reality and work through their grief.

Acute Myeloid Leukemia

Acute myeloid leukemia (AML) involves the overproliferation of granulocytes (neutrophils, basophils, and eosinophils). It is most often seen in adults and accounts for only about 20% of all childhood leukemias. The frequency of the disorder increases in late adolescence as children reach adulthood (Rubnitz & Inaba, 2012).

With AML, granulocytes grow so rapidly that they are forced out into the bloodstream while still in the blast stage. As with ALL, the overproliferation of granulocytes limits the production of RBCs and platelets.

Assessment

Children with AML have the same symptoms as those with ALL. Because they do not have mature granulocytes, they are very susceptible to infection and may have noticed many recent upper respiratory tract infections before the time of diagnosis.

Therapeutic Management

The diagnosis is established by bone marrow aspiration and biopsy. After diagnosis, chemotherapy to effect remission begins. Cytarabine (Ara-C), etoposide (VePesid), and daunorubicin (DaunoXome) make up the drug regimen commonly used for therapy. It may take 1 to 2 months to reach a full remission (Graham et al., 2012). Bone marrow transplantation may be attempted after the initial remission to ensure new growth of normal granulocytes.

THE LYMPHOMAS

Lymphomas are malignancies of the lymph or reticuloendothelial system; they account for about 11% of all malignancies and are categorized as Hodgkin or non-Hodgkin lymphomas. Although Hodgkin disease is better known, non-Hodgkin lymphomas are more common worldwide in children (about 60% versus 40%). Both types occur more frequently in males than in females (Copeland & Younes, 2012).

Hodgkin Disease

With Hodgkin disease, lymphocytes proliferate in the lymph glands, and special *Reed-Sternberg cells* (large, multinucleated cells that are probably nonfunctioning monocyte-macrophage cells) develop. Although these lymphocytes are capable of DNA synthesis and mitotic division, they are abnormal because they lack both B- and T-lymphocyte surface markers and cannot produce immunoglobulins as do usual B-lymphocytes (McLean & Wofford, 2011).

As with all neoplastic diseases, the etiology of Hodgkin disease is unknown, but both genetic and environmental factors probably play a part. It is rarely seen in children younger than 7 years of age, with the incidence increasing greatly during adolescence and young adulthood. Metastasis is through lymphatic channels. Untreated, late in the disease process, it spreads to lung, liver, and bone marrow.

Assessment

Symptoms of Hodgkin disease usually begin with the enlargement of only one painless, enlarged, rubbery-feeling cervical lymph node. Other nodes then become involved, along with the liver, spleen, bone marrow, and, eventually, the CNS. The child usually reports accompanying symptoms of anorexia, malaise, night sweats, and loss of weight. Fever may be present. The sedimentation rate is elevated; anemia is usually present as a result of reduced RBC survival.

Hodgkin disease is confirmed by biopsy of the lymph nodes. Further studies (bone marrow analysis, liver function tests, chest and abdominal computed tomography [CT] or MRI scans, lymphangiography, and abdominal biopsy) are done to classify the clinical stage of the disorder. The chest CT scan may reveal enlarged mediastinal nodes; the abdominal CT may reveal enlarged lymph nodes of the abdomen.

A lymphangiogram, a procedure performed by injecting dye into the hand or foot, allows visualization of the lymphatic system. For this, a catheter is inserted into a lymph vessel, and radiopaque dye is injected into the vessel, as in angiography. The dye then outlines lymphatic channels on X-ray films. The original dye injected into the skin to visualize the lymph vessels stains the skin a bluish green at the point of injection. This dye will remain as a skin stain for about 1 year. Because the lymph system does not eradicate opaque dye readily, in some children, lymph chains can still be outlined on X-ray films for up to 1 year. Nodes opacified by lymphangiogram dye can be used as markers of disease progress on plain, flat-plate X-ray films for 6 to 12 months.

Therapeutic Management

Although the main subcategories of Hodgkin disease that are documented are lymphocyte predominant and nodular sclerosing, mixed cellularity and lymphocyte depletion also occur. The disease is staged according to regional involvement revealed by a CT scan or MRI, followed by multiple lymph node and bone marrow biopsies.

Treatment depends on the clinical stage of the disease at the time of diagnosis. Although Hodgkin disease once was treated mainly with radiation therapy, children today in all stages except stage I receive combination chemotherapy using the agents cyclophosphamide, vincristine, procarbazine, and prednisone. Current therapy results in a 90% 5-year survival rate for children with stage I or stage II disease and 60% to 90% for more advanced disease. If a relapse occurs, additional chemotherapy, radiation, or bone marrow transplantation will be scheduled (Graham et al., 2012).

Children need conscientious follow-up for symptoms of Hodgkin disease relapse during adult life because a relapse is often retreatable, using a chemotherapy course different from that used initially.

Nursing Diagnoses and Related Interventions

The nursing diagnoses most often used with Hodgkin disease address the child's impaired immune defenses and risk for infection, fear and feelings about the diagnosis, or changed body image (particularly in an adolescent). Both the parents and the child need opportunities to express their feelings about the seriousness of this disease and how this has changed their life.

Nursing Diagnosis: Risk for powerlessness related to constant possibility of disease recurrence

Outcome Evaluation: Child states he feels healthy during remission; participates in school and extracurricular activities; voices confidence in health care team to treat symptoms if they recur.

The course of treatment for Hodgkin disease extends over a long time period. For adolescents (in whom the disease is most prevalent), some live from day to day wondering whether symptoms will recur. Encourage adolescents to attend regular school during periods of remission, so that they can lead as normal a life as possible. Some adolescents want to know exactly what stage they are in; others prefer not to be told, so they can continue to believe that a cure will be possible. Both adolescents and their parents need continued support from health care personnel during the long course of therapy because they worry symptoms could be returning (B. L. Jones, 2012).

✔ QSEN Checkpoint Question 53.3

Patient-Centered Care

Gerri's father is a Hodgkin lymphoma survivor, having experienced the active disease as an adolescent. Because of his disturbing memories of having this disease, he is highly anxious that the care team assess Gerri for Hodgkin lymphoma. What is the most likely first sign that Hodgkin lymphoma is beginning to develop in Gerri?

a. A single, enlarged submaxillary lymph node
b. Sharp pain in joints from blocked lymph drainage
c. Easy bruising from a shortage of platelets and RBCs
d. Discolored fingernails from clotting in distal extremities

Look in Appendix A for the best answer and rationale.

Non-Hodgkin Lymphoma

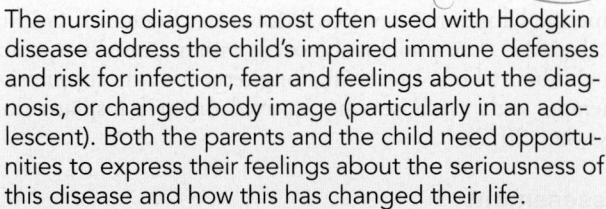

Non-Hodgkin lymphomas are malignant disorders of the lymphocytes (either B or T cells) and occur in a number of forms. Unlike Hodgkin disease, spread from the original site is through the bloodstream rather than directly by lymph flow, making the course of the disease unpredictable. Metastatic spread to CNS tends to occur early in the disease, with the common age of occurrence at 5 to 15 years.

The cause of non-Hodgkin lymphomas is undocumented, but many viruses such as EBV, which causes mononucleosis, *Helicobacter pylori*, which causes stomach ulcers, and HIV, have all been linked to the occurrence of lymphomas. That is not to say that the viruses cause the lymphoma, only that the viruses were recently present or are present at the same time the lymphoma develops (Molyneux, Rochford, Griffin, et al., 2012). Lymphomas also occur with increased frequency in children who are receiving long-term immunosuppressive therapy, such as those who received organ transplantation (Kaplan, 2012).

Assessment

Non-Hodgkin lymphomas tend to involve the lymph glands of the neck and chest most commonly, although axillary, abdominal, or inguinal nodes may be the first involved. If mediastinal lymph glands are swollen, the child may notice a cough or chest "tightness." Because mediastinal nodes press on the veins returning blood from the head, edema of the face may result. Diffuse, undifferentiated types manifest most commonly with an abdominal mass. Children notice abdominal pain; they may have diarrhea or constipation, and a mass may be palpable on examination.

To establish the diagnosis, biopsy of the affected lymph nodes and bone marrow is performed. Both are needed because it is often difficult to distinguish between undifferentiated lymphoma cells and ALL; if a bone marrow biopsy shows more than 25% blasts, the diagnosis is acute leukemia; fewer than this is suggestive of lymphoma. Areas of metastases are identified by X-ray, lymphangiography, gallium (radioactive) scan, or CT scan.

Therapeutic Management

Non-Hodgkin lymphomas are treated with systemic chemotherapy, similar to that used for ALL. The initial phase of therapy is an induction phase (a time during which the child is put into remission, or no tumor can be detected by clinical examination); this is followed by a maintenance phase of up to 2 years. The common drug regimen used is cyclophosphamide, hydroxydaunorubicin (doxorubicin hydrochloride), vincristine (Oncovin), and prednisone (CHOP therapy). Intrathecal chemotherapy may be included because of the tendency for non-Hodgkin lymphoma to metastasize to the CNS. Because the breakdown of cells is so rapid with chemotherapy, assess for hyperkalemia and hyperphosphatemia (because of potassium and phosphorus released from destroyed cells). Anticipate that allopurinol will be added to the therapy to prevent uric acid accumulation and blocking of kidney tubules. A granulocyte colony-stimulating factor may also be prescribed to increase WBC production and prevent neutropenia.

Autologous stem cell transfusion (using bone marrow removed at diagnosis, before the disease has spread to the bone marrow, and then replaced after blood components have been destroyed by chemotherapy) allows more aggressive chemotherapy, a regimen so effective that between 80% and 90% of children with non-Hodgkin lymphoma with minimal symptoms achieve remission.

Burkitt Lymphoma

Burkitt lymphoma (a non-Hodgkin lymphoma involving B-lymphocyte cells) is a specifically named but rare form of lymphoma in the United States; it is seen much more commonly worldwide. Children 2 to 14 years of age have the highest incidence, with a peak at 7 years. The same associations as in non-Hodgkin lymphoma exist regarding infection with *H. pylori*, HIV, or EBV.

The first indication of disease is an enlarged lymph node of the neck or abdomen. It is usually painless unless it blocks some body system. The abnormal cells then grow so rapidly that the cell mass may double in size in as few as 24 hours, so early diagnosis and treatment are important. Surgery is used to remove the primary tumor. This is followed by administration of the same chemotherapy regimen used with other non-Hodgkin lymphomas. To prevent CNS involvement, intrathecal methotrexate may be given (Ngoma, Adde, Durosinmi, et al., 2012).

Because Burkitt lymphoma is such a rapidly growing tumor, the condition responds dramatically to chemotherapy (the cells are almost always in a susceptible state). As with other lymphomas, tissue breakdown may be so voluminous that the uric acid level of the urine may cause renal tubule plugging unless the child is kept well hydrated and a drug such as allopurinol is administered concurrently.

NEOPLASMS OF THE BRAIN

Brain tumor is the second most common form of cancer and the most common solid tumor form in children. Tumors tend to occur between 1 and 10 years of age, with 5 years being the peak age of incidence. In children, brain tumors tend to occur at the midline in the brainstem or cerebellum and be located beneath the tentorial membrane, a contrast to the usual site in adults, which is lateral and above the tentorial membrane. This feature is what makes brain tumors particularly difficult to remove in children without damage to normal brain tissue (Kline, 2012).

Types of Brain Tumors

Common sites for brain tumors in children are shown in Figure 53.5. The most common brain tumors are cerebellar astrocytomas, medulloblastomas, and brainstem gliomas.

Astrocytomas are slow-growing, cystic tumors that arise from the glial or support tissue surrounding neural cells. They account for about one fourth of all brain tumors in children. The peak age of incidence is 5 to 8 years.

Medulloblastomas are fast-growing tumors found most commonly in the cerebellum. The peak age of incidence is 5 to 10 years. Usually found at the midline, they cause fourth-ventricle compression and disturbances in the flow of CSF. Brainstem gliomas often cause paralysis of the fifth, sixth, seventh, ninth, and tenth cranial nerves. They may produce symptoms of ataxia, nystagmus, and changes in respiratory and pulse findings because of pressure on these centers.

Assessment

Children with any form of brain tumor develop symptoms of increased intracranial pressure: headache, vision changes, vomiting, an enlarging head circumference, or papilledema. Lethargy, projectile vomiting, and coma are late signs.

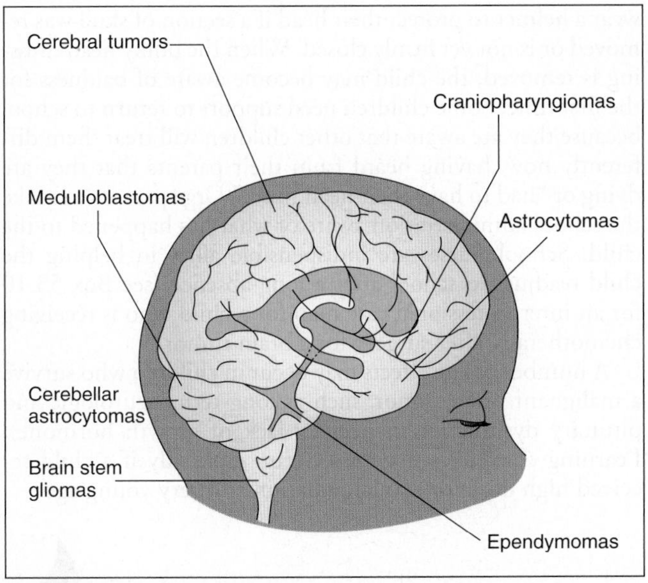

FIGURE 53.5 Common sites for brain tumors in children.

The headache associated with brain tumor usually occurs on arising in the morning. It may be intermittent throughout the day because of pressure changes related to position and the ability of the cranium to expand to some degree and temporarily relieve the associated pressure. It becomes intense on straining, such as occurs with coughing or bowel movements. A parent may report these symptoms as an increasingly irritable young child who is constipated because of reluctance to strain to pass stool. With some tumors, the pain is occipital. This is an important finding, because this is an unusual location for a headache from any other cause.

Vomiting, like headache, most commonly occurs on arising. Unlike the child who vomits because of GI distress, the child with a brain tumor is not usually nauseated and will eat immediately afterward. The vomiting pattern occurs morning after morning. Vomiting eventually will become projectile; projectile vomiting, however, is not an initial symptom. Vomiting early in the morning is easily discounted by parents as school phobia (reluctance to attend school), because the child is able to eat again immediately and seems to recover about half an hour after getting out of bed (at the same time the school bus leaves).

Diplopia or ptosis because of cranial nerve involvement or strabismus because of suppression of vision in one eye may begin to be noticeable as the tumor continues to grow. Children may tilt their head to the side or develop a torticollis (wry neck) to compensate for the suppression and strabismus. Papilledema (swelling of the optic nerve) may be evident on funduscopic examination.

Apart from these generalized symptoms of increased intracranial pressure, a growing tumor produces specific localized signs, such as nystagmus (constant horizontal movement of the eye) or visual field defects. As tumor growth continues, symptoms of ataxia, personality change (e.g., emotional lability, irritability), and seizures may occur.

Four to 6 months may pass, however, from the time of initial symptoms until symptoms become localized enough to arouse suspicion of a brain tumor. When this suspicion arises, a child needs a thorough neurologic examination; skull films, a bone scan, ultrasound or MRI, cerebral angiography, or a CT scan will be performed as needed. Myelography may be done to identify tumors that could have spread into the spinal column. Lumbar puncture must be done cautiously, because the release of CSF can cause the brainstem (under pressure from the tumor) to herniate into the spinal cord, interfering with respiratory and cardiac function.

Therapeutic Management

Therapy for brain tumors includes a combination of surgery, radiation, and chemotherapy, depending on the location and extent of the tumor (Fried, Hawkins, Scheinemann, et al., 2012). Because they are located so deeply, many tumors cannot be completely surgically removed, making radiation and chemotherapy increasingly important. Radiation therapy is carefully staged because, if tumor tissue is not rapidly proliferating, cells are not easily destroyed. Chemotherapy is also limited because many chemotherapeutic agents do not cross the blood–brain barrier. Typical drugs used are carboplatin or a combination of thioguanine, procarbazine, lomustine, and vincristine. Administration of drugs directly into the ventricular system via a reservoir (Ommaya) may increase drug effectiveness.

The diagnosis of brain tumor at any age is always a serious one and a stress for parents (S. Jones, 2012). Closely observe a child who is admitted to the hospital for a possible diagnosis of brain tumor, to detect signs of increased intracranial pressure or new localizing signs as they occur. Record pulse rate, blood pressure, and respiratory rate with extreme accuracy, so that subtle changes are apparent. Note and document episodes of irritability, drowsiness, speech difficulty, and eye involvement. Statements such as, "Child says he sees two forks when I show him one" or "Child is unable to see objects held in her left field of vision" are much more meaningful to a neurosurgeon than "Child has difficulty seeing." Completely describe any seizure activity observed as well, particularly the beginning movements of the seizure, because these can help localize the point of maximum brain pressure. Be certain side rails are in place for protection in case a seizure should occur while the child is in bed.

Preoperative Care

Before brain surgery, a child will usually receive a stool softener to prevent straining with bowel movements. Dexamethasone (Decadron) may be prescribed to reduce cranial edema by shifting fluid from extracellular to intravascular spaces. An anticonvulsant will be prescribed if the child is experiencing seizures or if surgery is apt to induce seizures. Before surgery, a portion of the child's head is shaved. Prepare the child for this in a positive way by emphasizing that this is necessary and hair grows back very rapidly. If the child will be cared for in an intensive care unit (ICU) for the first few days after surgery, include a preoperative visit to meet the ICU staff if at all possible.

Postoperative Care

Following cranial surgery, position the child as prescribed, as the best position for the child depends on the location of the tumor and the extent of surgery. In general, a child is positioned on the side opposite the surgical incision. Keep the bed flat or only slightly elevated, again, as prescribed, because this helps to reduce intracranial pressure from accumulation of increased fluid in the surgical area. Note carefully how much movement of the child's neck is allowed. If surgery was in the low occipital area, the operating surgeon may want the child to be moved as though the head and neck were a single body part. A neck brace or cast may be applied to stabilize the head and neck and prevent movement.

You can expect the child to be comatose or extremely lethargic for several days after surgery because of brain irritation and edema. In addition, a child may require mechanical ventilation because of pressure on the respiratory center. Unless they are being ventilated, are comatose, or have another contraindication, comatose children need to be positioned on their side so that oral secretions drain from the mouth to prevent aspiration. Many children have such extreme facial edema that they cannot close their eyelids completely or their nasal breathing space is impaired. Cool compresses over the eyes may help to reduce edema. Saline eye drops or eye dressings (with the eyes carefully closed under the dressings) may be prescribed to keep the cornea from drying and ulcerating.

Carefully assess the pulse and respiratory rates, pupillary size and ability to react to light, muscle strength (ask children to squeeze your hands), and level of consciousness (ask their name or give a simple instruction to follow) about every 15 minutes, until vital signs are stable and there is no apparent increase in intracranial pressure. A child's temperature may be either elevated or decreased immediately postoperatively because of the effect of the edema on the hypothalamus. Measures to reduce hyperthermia (sponging, antipyretics given by gavage or rectal administration because of lethargy or coma, or a hypothermia blanket) may be necessary to reduce the temperature to less than 101°F (38.4°C).

Be certain to regulate the rate of IV fluid infusions carefully because an increase in the infusion rate has the potential to increase intracranial pressure. Children with increased pressure may have infusions of mannitol or hypertonic dextrose prescribed to aid in evacuating the cerebral hemispheres of edematous fluid. As the child regains consciousness, small amounts of oral fluid can be introduced. Make certain, when introducing fluid, the child is free of nausea from the anesthetic, to help prevent vomiting because this increases intracranial pressure.

Observe head dressings carefully for any drainage. A wet dressing is no longer a sterile dressing because pathologic organisms can filter through its folds to reach the meninges and cause meningitis. Place a sterile towel, therefore, under a wet dressing, or reinforce the dressing with sterile compresses. Report signs of drainage, and estimate the extent of the seepage so that you can tell later whether seepage has increased or stopped.

Children regaining consciousness after brain surgery usually are confused regarding time and place; they may have difficulty performing simple tasks they could do easily before. As the cerebral edema subsides and they begin to regain consciousness, they may need a parent to stay with them or to be restrained to stop them from touching their head dressing or IV line. Use as few restraints as possible, however, because fighting restraints is yet another way to cause intracranial pressure to increase. Help the child gradually regain independence in self-care.

When the child is ready for discharge from the hospital, talk to parents about encouraging their child to begin as near-normal activities as possible. Some children may need to wear a helmet to protect their head if a section of skull was removed or is not yet firmly closed. When the bulky head dressing is removed, the child may become aware of baldness for the first time. Some children need support to return to school because they are aware that other children will treat them differently now, having heard from their parents that they are dying or "had to have their head fixed." Urge parents to make the school administration aware of what has happened to the child. School nurses are indispensible allies in helping the child readjust to school after a long absence (see Box 53.10 for an interprofessional care map for a child who is receiving chemotherapy after surgery for a brain tumor).

A number of late effects may occur in children who survive a malignant brain tumor, such as long-term neurologic and pituitary dysfunction (especially lack of growth hormone). Learning challenges may also occur, especially if a child received high doses of cranial radiation at a very young age.

Nursing Diagnoses and Related Interventions

Because a diagnosis of brain tumor is so frightening to parents and the child, nursing diagnoses need to include both physical and psychosocial aspects.

Nursing Diagnosis: Fear related to diagnosis of brain tumor

Outcome Evaluation: Parents and child continue to maintain function as a family, visit in hospital, and plan appropriately for discharge and continued care.

Because parents bring their child to a health care facility in response to insidious symptoms such as vomiting, headache, or strabismus, they may not be prepared for the severity of their child's diagnosis. This can cause such distress at the time of the initial diagnosis that they cannot think of questions to ask. In the hours or days after the diagnosis, however, they often have a great need to talk to health care professionals who are familiar with the care of children with brain tumors to ask questions about surgery or their child's prognosis.

Most parents want to hear a definite statement about prognosis—for example, "All of the tumor can be removed; your child will be as good as new" or "Your child's chances are 1 in 4 of surviving surgery (or of having permanent effects)." Because the type of tumor, its exact location, and its extent are not fully known until surgery, these predictions are difficult to make with more than an uninformed guess. You can assure parents it is normal in these instances for a surgeon not to give more definitive information; this vagueness does not reflect an unwillingness to offer a definite prognosis or lack of interest. They also may need assurance that if they had realized their child's symptoms were serious earlier, it would not have made a difference in the final outcome. Such assurance is what makes it possible for them to live

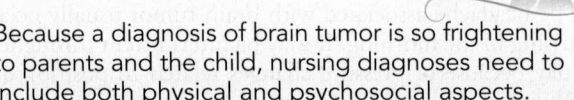

BOX 53.10 Nursing Care Planning

AN INTERPROFESSIONAL CARE MAP FOR A CHILD RECEIVING CHEMOTHERAPY

Gerri, 6 years old, has had surgery to remove a brain tumor. He is now on ambulatory care receiving additional chemotherapy postoperatively. His father states, "He refuses to take his antinausea medicine, so he's vomiting all the time. He says he's never going back to school because he looks so funny. This cure is worse than the disease."

Family Assessment Child lives with parents and two sisters (ages 2 and 12 years) in four-bedroom first-floor home. Father is manager of a local computer store. Mother used to work as a manicurist but is stay-at-home mom since Gerri was diagnosed with cancer. Father rates finances as, "Okay. If nothing unexpected happens."

Client Assessment Sad and pale-appearing school-age child with bald head and recent surgical scar. Weight decreased 5 lb in last 2 weeks. Skin turgor sluggish. Oral mucous membranes red and irritated. Two ulcers noted on inner aspect of left cheek at gum line. Child states, "I look like an old man."

Nursing Diagnosis Disturbed body image related to hair loss and nausea secondary to the effects of chemotherapy

Outcome Criteria Child states effect of hair loss and nausea on appearance and feelings; verbalizes measures to cope with hair loss and nausea; reports continued participation in age-appropriate activities.

Team Member Responsible	Assessment	Intervention	Rationale	Expected Outcome
Activities of Daily Living, Including Safety				
Nurse	Assess whether child is capable of self-care in light of changes that have occurred with chemotherapy.	Encourage child to perform as many self-care activities as he did before becoming ill.	Maintaining self-care activities is a way of maintaining self-esteem and competence.	Child states that although he doesn't feel well, he will try to do self-care.
Teamwork and Collaboration				
Nurse/Oncology nurse specialist	Assess whether oncology nurse specialist is available for consult with parents and child.	Contact oncology nurse, if desired, to review problems with nutrition, self-image, and mouth care during chemotherapy.	An expert can help parents to determine more effective strategies to combat and accept the nausea and appearance caused by chemotherapy.	Oncology nurse specialist arranges a home visit to review child's situation and suggest improvements in quality of life.
Procedures/Medications for Quality Improvement				
Nurse	Assess oral mucous membrane to document oral lesions.	Review importance of oral care with parents. Advise using a soft toothbrush or swabs to cleanse teeth.	Good oral care is essential to prevent further ulceration.	Child is able to maintain nutrition despite oral lesions; cooperates with toothbrushing three times daily.
Nutrition				
Nurse/Primary care provider	Assess whether child is taking prescribed antiemetic and has had any relief at all.	Review with parents importance of giving antiemetic 30 minutes before chemotherapy and every 8 hours.	Antiemetics administered before chemotherapy help to prevent nausea and vomiting.	Child states he will take antiemetic as prescribed to give it a "fair chance" to work.

(continued on page 1584)

BOX 53.10 Nursing Care Planning (continued)

Nurse/Nutritionist	Assess child's intake by a 24-hour recall history.	Encourage parent to offer food early in the day before chemotherapy. Suggest frequent, high-calorie snacks, such as high-energy snack bars.	Eating before chemotherapy enhances nutrition because the child is less likely to be nauseated at this time.	Parent states she will try to have child eat highly nutritious snacks during times he is not nauseated to optimize nutrition intake.
Patient-Centered Care				
Nurse	Assess parents' and child's understanding of the action of chemotherapy.	Teach parents about the type of medications child is receiving and their usual actions and side effects.	Understanding that side effects are expected, not unique, can help parents and child accept the appearance changes that occur.	Parents/child state they understand what changes to expect and they understand these are temporary.
Psychosocial/Spiritual/Emotional Needs				
Nurse	Assess whether child can devise any measures that would make him feel better about his changed appearance.	Brainstorm with child and parents about measures such as wearing a scarf or cap or modeling an action figure.	Fostering a positive outlook can help child accept changed appearance as a mark he is managing a stressful time of life very well.	Child states he will try to view hair loss as a positive feature, not a detrimental one.
Informatics for Seamless Health Care Planning				
Nurse	Assess whether parents or child have any further questions before leaving clinic and have appointment for return visit.	Urge parent to contact clinic if child develops further ulcerations or experiences continued weight loss or an increase in nausea and vomiting.	Continued nausea and vomiting, weight loss, or development of more ulcers requires further evaluation and follow-up to minimize the risk of additional concerns for the child.	Parents and child state they feel confident in managing nutrition adequately during remainder of chemotherapy and will keep return appointment.

with themselves afterward and not be overwhelmed by guilt, thinking they could have prevented a bad outcome. Symptoms of brain tumor *are* insidious, and the average parent cannot be expected to recognize them for what they represent.

Help parents also to understand that, because of the importance of brain tissue, brain surgery is never minor. Be certain they understand their child will have a large, bulky head dressing; may be drowsy or unresponsive; and possibly have extensive facial edema afterward. The child may be intubated and ventilated. Even parents who are well prepared are likely to be shocked at the actual sight of their child. Before you take them to the child's room after surgery, review with them once more how the child will look to be certain they are prepared for the changed appearance of their child.

Some parents may not "hear" the full extent of their child's diagnosis before surgery because they simply cannot believe all of their child's tumor cannot be removed. After surgery, when they are told some of the tumor had to be left to preserve the brain tissue nearby, a very genuine grief reaction can occur. As a result, it may be difficult for them to sit and hold the child's hand or read to the child because their minds have already jumped ahead to the time when the child might die. The child may have difficulty relating to them because they are no longer acting like the parents the child knew before surgery (more like two strangers). Offering parents support from the time a child is first seen, through the days of surgery, chemotherapy, and any remission, is an important nursing responsibility.

Children as young as 5 years old are aware their brain is important for functioning. They become very aware of the tone they detect in the words of parents and health care personnel when they talk about a brain tumor. Because they undergo several diagnostic studies, followed by surgery and prolonged therapy, provide children with opportunities to express their feelings about intrusive procedures through play with puppets or hospital equipment. Remember that, when a person becomes unconscious, hearing is often the last sense lost. Although children do not appear to respond after surgery, they may be able to hear everything that is said in the room.

QSEN Checkpoint Question 53.4

Quality Improvement

Gerri had surgery for a brain tumor 2 weeks ago. Your unit protocol specifies the administration of stool softeners be given before and after surgery when not contraindicated. What is the rationale for this protocol?

a. Constipation stimulates the release of pituitary hormones.
b. Straining with bowel movements increases intracranial pressure.
c. Constipation can lead to anal fissures, which can be a source of infection.
d. Children in Trendelenburg positions cannot effectively move their bowels.

Look in Appendix A for the best answer and rationale.

BONE TUMORS

Tumors derived from connective tissue, such as bone and cartilage, muscle, blood vessels, or lymphoid tissue, are termed **sarcomas**. They are the second most frequently occurring neoplasms in adolescents (only lymphomas occur more frequently). Bone tumors may arise during adolescence because rapid bone growth is occurring at this time. Because girls have a puberty growth spurt a year or two earlier than boys, bone tumors tend to occur slightly earlier in girls than in boys (13 compared with 14 or 15 years of age). The two most frequently occurring types are osteogenic sarcoma and Ewing sarcoma (Fig. 53.6).

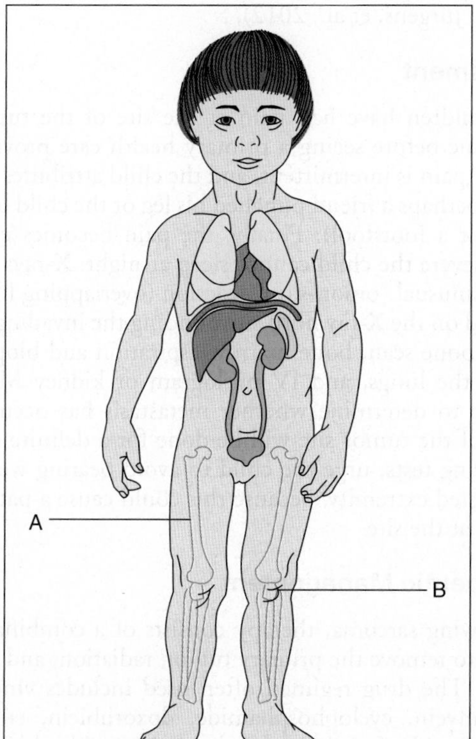

FIGURE 53.6 **(A)** The diaphysis (midshaft) is one of the most frequent sites of Ewing sarcoma. **(B)** The epiphysis of a bone is a common site of osteogenic sarcoma.

Osteogenic Sarcoma

An **osteogenic sarcoma** is a malignant tumor of long bone involving rapidly growing bone tissue (mesenchymal-matrix forming cells). It occurs more commonly in boys than in girls and in children who have had radiation for other malignancies as a later life effect. The most common sites of occurrence are the distal femur (40%–50%), the proximal tibia (20%), and the proximal humerus (10%–15%) (Roth, Mirochna, & Harsha, 2012). Children with retinoblastoma have a higher incidence than usual of developing an osteosarcoma, so a hereditary influence may be present.

Metastasis occurs early with bone tumors because of the extensive vascular system in bones. Metastasis to the lungs is very common; as many as 25% of adolescents will have lung metastasis already by the time of initial diagnosis. When this is present, the adolescent usually has noticed a chronic cough, dyspnea, and chest pain in addition to chronic leg pain. Other common sites of metastasis are brain and other bone tissue.

Assessment

Children with osteogenic sarcoma often are taller than average, suggesting that rapid bone growth helps to create abnormal cells. The area may be painful and swollen; it may be inflamed and feel warm because tumors are highly vascular and therefore call increased blood into the area.

Often, adolescents report a history of recent trauma to the site such as a fall playing basketball or a bump to their knee during soccer practice and attribute pain in the knee to this injury for some time. All adolescents with extremity pain and swelling, particularly near the knee, require evaluation because of the possibility that a malignant process, not the athletic injury, may be the cause. To prevent the adolescent from thinking he caused the tumor, be certain he and his parents understand trauma did not cause the process; it merely called attention to the leg or arm where a malignant process was at work.

For diagnosis, blood serum for alkaline phosphatase will be obtained because rapidly growing bone cells markedly raise the serum level of this enzyme. For final diagnosis, a biopsy will be done of the suspicious site. To determine metastasis, a complete blood cell count, urinalysis, chest X-ray, chest CT scan, and bone scans will be done. Caution children not to bear weight on an affected leg while waiting for tests or surgery because if the bone has become weakened by the growing tumor, weight bearing could result in a fracture at the tumor site.

Therapeutic Management

Chemotherapy may be prescribed to shrink the tumor before surgery. If parents are concerned with this delay, explain that, with bone tumor, this is a helpful intervention because it will make removal of the tumor more successful. A common chemotherapy drug regimen used for treatment includes methotrexate, cisplatin, doxorubicin, and ifosfamide.

If the tumor is small at the time of diagnosis, only the local tumor will be removed. If it is too large for this, and if the child has reached adult height, the single bone involved may be surgically removed and replaced with a bone transplant or metal prosthesis (Puri & Gulia, 2012).

Rarely necessary, if the tumor is extensive at the time of diagnosis, the leg may be amputated at the joint above the tumor (this usually involves a total hip amputation). If the cancer has spread to the lung, metastasis tumors can usually be removed by thoracotomy.

Only a few years ago, a diagnosis of osteogenic sarcoma was ominous; few children survived into adulthood. Today, 70% of adolescents in whom the diagnosis is made early and who are treated rigorously can be cured (Brown & Hunger, 2013).

Nursing Diagnoses and Related Interventions

Diagnosis of malignant bone tumor is a shock to both parents and children because the symptoms began so insidiously the diagnosis doesn't seem real. You can assure parents that any delay in seeking treatment would not have had a marked effect on the chances for a cure. Neither the adolescent nor the parents could have been expected to seek medical attention any earlier than they did. This is important assurance because it can help parents function more effectively to help their child through this extensive illness.

Be certain that outcomes established are realistic. It is not realistic, for example, for an adolescent to accept with understanding leg surgery that could compromise an athletic career. The highest achievable outcome might be that the adolescent realizes surgery is necessary to save her life.

Nursing Diagnosis: Risk for injury related to surgery and bone prosthesis

Outcome Evaluation: Extremity distal to surgical incision remains warm to touch; capillary filling is less than 5 seconds.

The major danger associated with surgery for excising osteosarcoma and placement of a bone prosthesis (limb salvage surgery) is that the swelling that occurs during surgery or immediately afterward can disrupt neurologic or circulatory function to the lower leg. Always position and handle the leg carefully to prevent further disruption. Assess frequently for signs the neurologic and circulatory systems are intact distal to the surgery (toes are warm and pink; capillary filling is less than 5 seconds; adolescent reports no numbness or tingling).

Adolescents who had pain in the leg before surgery may continue to feel this pain even after the involved bone segment has been removed. This is *phantom pain* and occurs because nerve tracts continue to report pain for a time after the pain has been relieved. Although it seems as if phantom limb pain does not need analgesia, the opposite is true. The pain is very real. An adolescent may need an analgesic to control it.

QSEN Checkpoint Question 53.5

Teamwork & Collaboration

Gerri's school nurse informs you that his mother forbids him to play basketball because she heard a friend's son developed osteosarcoma when he was injured playing the sport. You collaborate with your colleague to plan a unified response to her concerns. What would be the best advice to give his mother regarding her understanding of osteosarcoma?

a. Evidence has shown that bone cancer is associated with active, organized sports.
b. Osteosarcoma more often occurs in girls, so the boy's diagnosis is unusual.
c. The sports injury more likely led to diagnosis of the tumor but was not the cause of it.
d. The boy's inadequate calcium intake was a more likely cause of his health problem.

Look in Appendix A for the best answer and rationale.

Ewing Sarcoma

Ewing sarcoma is a malignant tumor associated with a genetic dislocation; it occurs most frequently in the bone marrow of the diaphyseal area (midshaft) of long bones and spreads longitudinally through the bone (Subbiah & Kurzrock, 2012) (see Fig. 53.6). It occurs primarily in young adolescents and older school-age children; it is slightly more common in boys than in girls. Metastasis is usually present at the time of diagnosis, with the lungs, other bones, the CNS, and lymph nodes being the most common sites (Potratz, Dirksen, Jürgens, et al., 2012).

Assessment

Most children have had pain at the site of the tumor for some time before seeing a primary health care provider. At first, the pain is intermittent, and the child attributes it to an injury (perhaps a friend punched his leg or the child bumped it against a footstool). Finally, the pain becomes constant and so severe the child cannot sleep at night. X-rays will reveal an unusual "onion-skin" reaction (overlapping fine lines disclosed on the X-ray film) surrounding the invading tumor cells. A bone scan, bone marrow aspiration and biopsy, CT scan of the lungs, and IV pyelogram or kidney MRI will be done to determine whether metastasis has occurred. A biopsy of the tumor site will be done for a definite diagnosis. During tests, urge the child to avoid bearing weight on the affected extremity, because this could cause a pathologic fracture at the site.

Therapeutic Management

With Ewing sarcoma, therapy consists of a combination of surgery to remove the primary tumor, radiation, and chemotherapy. The drug regimen often used includes vincristine, dactinomycin, cyclophosphamide, doxorubicin, etoposide, and ifosfamide. Irradiation of the entire involved bone may be scheduled.

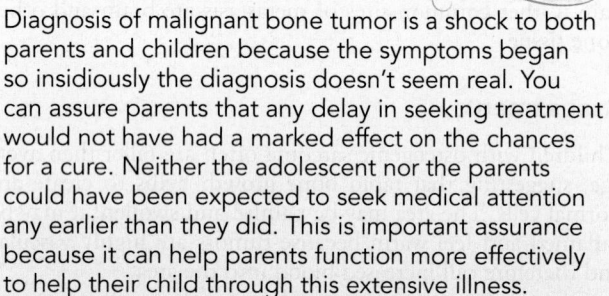

About 50% of children survive for at least 5 years; older children have a better survival rate than younger children. Caution adolescents to continue to be careful about stress on a leg that has received extensive radiation (no football, no weight lifting with pressure on that leg) because it may not be as strong as usual afterward.

OTHER CHILDHOOD NEOPLASMS

Neuroblastoma

Neuroblastomas are tumors that arise from the cells of the sympathetic nervous system; cells are highly undifferentiated and invasive, occur most frequently in the abdomen near the adrenal glands or spinal ganglia, and are the most common abdominal tumor in childhood (Davenport, Blanco, & Sandler, 2012). Neuroblastoma occurs primarily in infants and preschool children; it is slightly more common in boys than in girls. These tumors may occur so early in life, in fact, that they are detected by fetal ultrasound or at birth. Common sites of metastasis include the bone marrow, liver, and subcutaneous tissue.

Assessment

The growing tumor is most often discovered on abdominal palpation as an abdominal mass after general symptoms of weight loss and anorexia are noticed. Pressure on the adrenal glands from the tumor may cause excessive sweating, flushed face, and hypertension. Abdominal pain and constipation may also be present. Compression on the spinal nerves or invasion into the intervertebral foramina may cause loss of motor function in lower extremities.

If the primary lesion is in the upper chest, children will report dyspnea; swallowing may be difficult, and neck and facial edema may occur from compression on the vena cava. If liver metastasis is present, children may have jaundice. If metastasis to the skin has occurred, blue or purplish nodules (prominent raised areas) on arms or legs may be seen.

The extent of the tumor and any metastases present are identified by an IV pyelogram, MRI, or ultrasound (a mass growing on an adrenal gland just above the kidney will demonstrate kidney compression); an arteriogram (neuroblastomas are vascular tumors and incorporate veins and arteries into their structure as they grow); ultrasound, CT, or MRI scan of the chest, abdomen, and pelvis; a gallium bone scan; or bone marrow aspiration and biopsy. If an adrenal tumor is present, it will stimulate production of adrenal gland hormones or catecholamines. To detect these substances, a urine sample will be tested for the presence of catecholamines or vanillylmandelic acid and homovanillic acid (the breakdown products of catecholamines). A biopsy of the tumor site will be planned so the tumor can be definitely identified and staged.

Therapeutic Management

If the tumor is localized (stage I or II), therapy will consist of surgical removal of the primary tumor. If the tumor is stage III (lymph nodes are involved) or stage IV (metastasis has occurred), surgery will be followed by chemotherapy combinations using agents such as doxorubicin, cyclophosphamide, etoposide, and carboplatin.

A "second look" surgical procedure may be scheduled within several months to determine the effectiveness of therapy and to attempt the possible removal of further tumor. If aggressive chemotherapy has decreased bone marrow function, stem cell transplantation to restore functioning bone marrow may be scheduled. Immunotherapy is another possibility to eliminate residual disease after chemotherapy (Park, Bagatell, Hogarty, et al., 2013).

Stage IV disease is a unique form because it has a high rate of spontaneous regression. This occurs because the tumor either spontaneously degenerates or undergoes differentiation to normal tissue (Gains, Mandeville, Cork, et al., 2012).

Overall, children with neuroblastoma have a 5-year survival rate of 70% to 90%. Although most children have a positive initial response to therapy, recurrence is common within the first year. The prognosis is better in children diagnosed before 1 year of age.

Rhabdomyosarcoma

A **rhabdomyosarcoma** is a tumor of striated muscle (Arndt, Rose, Folpe, et al., 2012). It arises from the embryonic mesenchyme tissue that forms muscle, connective, and vascular tissue. The peak age of incidence of these tumors is 2 to 6 years, with a second peak occurring during puberty. Common sites of occurrence include the eye orbit, paranasal sinuses, uterus, prostate, bladder, retroperitoneum, arms, and legs. CNS invasion occurs from direct tumor extension, resulting in cranial nerve palsy, nuchal rigidity, bradycardia, or bradypnea (because of brainstem compromise). Distant metastasis most commonly occurs in lungs, bone, or bone marrow.

Assessment

The symptoms relate to the site of the tumor (Table 53.3). A biopsy specimen of the tumor is taken and examined for tissue identification. Metastasis is ruled out by bone scan, chest X-ray, CT scan, MRI, and bone marrow aspiration.

TABLE 53.3 Common Sites and Associated Symptoms of Rhabdomyosarcoma

Site of Tumor	Symptoms
Orbit	Proptosis (extruding eye); visible and palpable conjunctival or eyelid mass
Neck	Hoarseness, dysphagia; visible and palpable mass in neck
Nasopharynx	Airway obstruction, epistaxis, dysphagia, visible mass in nasal or nasopharyngeal passages
Paranasal sinuses	Swelling, pain, nasal discharge, epistaxis
Middle ear	Pain, chronic otitis media, hearing loss, facial nerve palsy, mass protruding into external ear canal
Bladder and prostate	Dysuria, urinary retention, hematuria, constipation, palpable lower abdominal mass
Vagina	Mass protruding from uterus or cervix into vagina, abnormal vaginal bleeding
Trunk, extremities	Visible and palpable soft-tissue mass
Testicles	Visible and palpable soft-tissue mass

Therapeutic Management

The primary treatment is surgical removal of the tumor, followed by chemotherapy combinations with agents such as vincristine, dactinomycin, cyclophosphamide, doxorubicin, etoposide, topotecan, and ifosfamide. The child receives chemotherapy every 3 or 4 weeks for 18 to 24 months. If CNS extension has occurred, intrathecal chemotherapy may be included in the regimen.

A child's prognosis depends on the size of the tumor and whether metastasis was present at the time of initial diagnosis. If the entire tumor was removed and no lymph node metastasis has occurred, the chances are as high as 80% that the tumor will not recur. If some of the tumor had to be left because of its size or location, the chance of recurrence rises to about 50%. If metastasis to the lungs or bone was present at the time of the initial diagnosis, the prognosis drops still further; about 20% of children in this situation have long-term survival. Among children who do survive, long-term complications such as cardiomyopathy and infertility may occur from the side effects of chemotherapy.

Nephroblastoma (Wilms Tumor)

Nephroblastoma (Wilms tumor) is a malignant tumor that rises from the metanephric mesoderm cells of the upper pole of the kidney (Romão, Pippi Salle, Shuman, et al., 2012). It accounts for 20% of solid tumors in childhood; there is no increased incidence based on sex or race. It occurs in association with congenital anomalies such as aniridia (lack of color in the iris), cryptorchidism, hypospadias, pseudohermaphroditism, cystic kidneys, hemangioma, and talipes disorders. A number of genes have been identified as associated with the disorder, most prominently, a deletion of chromosome 11. Without therapy, metastatic spread by the bloodstream is most often to the lungs, regional lymph nodes, liver, bone, and, eventually, brain.

Assessment

A nephroblastoma is usually discovered early in life (6 months to 5 years; peak at 3 to 4 years), although it apparently arises from an embryonic structure present in the child before birth. Nephroblastomas distort the kidney anteriorly so that the tumor is felt as a firm, nontender abdominal mass. Parents are aware their infant has a mass in the abdomen but bring the infant to their health care provider thinking that it is hard stool from chronic constipation. Fathers may discover the tumor when they toss a baby in the air, catch the infant by the abdomen, and feel the abdominal mass. Parents often report that the mass seemed to appear overnight. This actually can happen, because tumors can hemorrhage into themselves, doubling their size in a matter of hours. If this happens, accompanying signs may be hematuria and a low-grade fever. The child may be anemic from blood loss and lack of erythropoietin formation by the diseased kidney. Although hypertension may also occur because of excessive renin production, blood pressure is not taken routinely in children of this age, so the tumor is rarely discovered by this method.

A CT scan or ultrasound reveals the primary tumor and any points of metastasis. Kidney function studies, such as glomerular filtration rate or blood urea nitrogen, will be done to assess function of the kidneys before surgery. Little time, however, can be allotted for preoperative testing, because these tumors metastasize rapidly as a result of the large blood supply to the kidneys and adrenal glands.

It is important that the child's abdomen not be palpated any more than is necessary for diagnosis, because handling appears to aid metastasis. Place a sign reading "No Abdominal Palpation" over the child's crib to help prevent this.

Therapeutic Management

Nephroblastomas are staged to predict therapy and prognosis. The tumor will be removed by nephrectomy (excision of the affected kidney). This is usually followed immediately by radiation therapy (omitted in stage I tumors) and by chemotherapy with dactinomycin, doxorubicin, or vincristine, cyclophosphamide, and etoposide. Chemotherapy may be given at varying intervals for as long as 15 months. A second surgical procedure may be scheduled after 2 or 3 months to remove any remaining tumor.

If tumor involvement is bilateral, the operative decisions obviously become more complex. If the tumors are small, both tumors may be removed, leaving functioning kidney on both sides intact. In other children, the kidney with the larger tumor is removed and the tumor site in the remaining kidney is then treated with both radiation and chemotherapy.

Overall therapy for nephroblastoma is so effective that about 90% of children who had no metastatic spread at diagnosis survive for at least 5 years. Complications such as nephritis, small bowel obstruction, and hepatic damage caused by fibrotic scarring from radiation can occur. In girls, radiation-related damage to the ovaries may result in sterility. Radiation to the lungs may result in interstitial pneumonia; spine radiation can result in scoliosis.

QSEN Checkpoint Question 53.6

Safety

A child on the same hospital unit as Gerri has nephroblastoma (Wilms tumor). What is an important nursing intervention to ensure the safety of a child with nephroblastoma before surgery?

a. Post a sign over the crib stating, "No Abdominal Palpation."
b. Alert the mother that her child will be infertile after surgery.
c. Be certain the child eats no high-iron vegetables before surgery.
d. Mark the child's head circumference in the electronic record daily.

Look in Appendix A for the best answer and rationale.

Retinoblastoma

Retinoblastoma is a malignant tumor of the retina of the eye (Nagarkatti-Gude, Wang, Ali, et al., 2012). A rare tumor, it accounts for only 1% to 3% of childhood malignancies. In about 10% of children, these tumors develop because of an inherited autosomal dominant pattern that causes an alteration of chromosome 13. Parents who have one child with retinoblastoma have about a 4% chance of having a second child with a similar tumor. If two or more children have the tumor, the parents are probably carriers, and it can be predicted that up to 50% of their children will be affected. Because of the dominant pattern of inheritance, a person who survives retinoblastoma has an elevated chance of having a child with a similar tumor. Parents who may be carriers and children who survive the disease need genetic counseling so that they are aware of the risk to their children. Because the 5-year survival rate for children with retinoblastoma is good (at least 90%), this is an important counseling role (Rowland & Metcalfe, 2013).

Retinoblastoma occurs most often, however, as spontaneous development, not the inherited type. Children with the inherited type tend to develop bilateral disease; those with the spontaneous type may or may not have the tumor in both eyes.

Assessment

Retinoblastoma occurs early in life, from about 6 weeks of age through the preschool period. It occurs equally in boys and girls, and there is no preference for either the right or the left eye. One tumor or many individual tumors may be present. Tumors are located on the retina or in the vitreous fluid or may extend backward into the choroid, the optic nerve, and the subarachnoid space.

On examination, the child's pupil appears white (the red reflex is absent) or is described as a typical "cat's eye." The child develops strabismus as the eye becomes nonfunctional. This tumor metastasizes readily along the course of the optic nerve to the subarachnoid space and brain; it can quickly involve the second eye. Metastasis to distant body sites, such as bone marrow and liver, also occurs because of the rich blood supply to the brain.

Children with a family history should have an ophthalmic exam usually under general anesthesia or conscious sedation at least three times yearly until they reach 5 years of age. CT scanning, MRI, and ultrasound may all be prescribed to detect intraocular calcification or the presence of tumor. The possibility of distant metastasis is evaluated by lumbar puncture, liver and skeletal survey, MRI, or bone marrow biopsy.

Therapeutic Management

Retinoblastomas are serious tumors because they involve the retina of the eye and, if allowed to grow, will cause blindness. If the tumor is very small at the time of diagnosis, it may be treated with cryosurgery (freezing the tumor to destroy local cells), hopefully preserving partial vision in the eye. Photocoagulation using laser surgery to destroy the blood vessels supplying the tumor or localized radioactive applicators or plaques sutured to the sclera over the tumor may also be used. If the tumor has metastasized, the child may also receive radiation treatment and chemotherapy (vincristine, cyclophosphamide, doxorubicin, carboplatin, and etoposide are components of commonly used regimens).

If the tumor is large when first discovered, enucleation of the eye may be necessary. After enucleation, the child has a large pressure dressing applied to the empty socket. Observe for bleeding on the dressing and assess vital signs frequently. To keep young children from tugging at the dressing and removing it, they may need to be restrained if a parent cannot be with them constantly. After about 48 hours, the pressure dressing is removed and a small eye patch is applied. Irrigation of the empty socket with normal saline solution or application of an antibiotic ointment may be prescribed with dressing changes.

An eye prosthesis is fitted about 3 weeks after surgery. Prostheses in children do not need to be removed and cleaned daily, and in children this young, leaving the prosthesis in place prevents the child from removing and playing with it (an interesting, colorful, round ball).

As discussed earlier, the long-term survival rate for children with retinoblastoma is as high as 90%. Evaluation of the child after retinoblastoma must include not only whether metastasis can be detected but whether the child is adjusting to the loss of sight in one or both eyes. Children who do not have binocular vision this early in life usually do not have difficulty adjusting. They notice it most at school age when they may have difficulty participating in sports that require three-dimensional sight, such as baseball. They may be restricted from obtaining a driver's license in some states. If radiation was used for therapy, cataracts may develop several years later. The high incidence of osteogenic and soft-tissue sarcomas that occurs following retinoblastoma therapy may not be related to therapy as much as to a tendency for tumor growth.

Nursing Diagnoses and Related Interventions

A diagnosis of retinoblastoma is a devastating one for parents because, at best, it threatens their child's vision. At worst, it can be fatal.

Nursing Diagnosis: Decisional conflict related to approval of eye removal to save child's life

Outcome Evaluation: Parents and child state they can accept removal of eye to save child's life.

With the diagnosis of retinoblastoma, parents may be asked to make a most difficult decision. To save their child's life, they must agree to the removal of an eye. Even after this procedure, the second eye may become involved or distant metastasis may be detected. Offer parents support in the decision they make because, if there is metastasis at a later date, they may feel guilty they agreed to enucleation, believing they have put the child through surgery for nothing. They may need help managing the degree of guilt they feel because they noticed their child's eye was abnormal but thought the child only needed glasses and so delayed seeking health care. Be certain parents understand fully what the word enucleation means (loss of the eye) before surgery. Provide time for discussion to help them work through this very emotional time in their life.

What if... 53.3 Gerri's mother shows you a photo she took of their family, and you notice that only one of the pupils of Gerri's 2-year-old sister shows a typical red reflex but the other pupil looks white. Would you be concerned, or are you aware that this effect often happens with a phone camera?

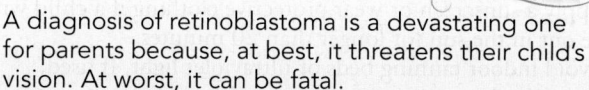

Skin Cancer

One in five people in the United States develop skin cancer in their lifetime (Robinson, Baker, & Hillhouse, 2012). Three common types are involved: basal cell carcinoma (a surface epithelial growth that appears as a small ulcer that does not heal), squamous cell carcinoma (a tumor of the epidermis that appears as a white scaly lesion), and malignant melanoma (a tumor originating in melanocytes or nevi) that appears as a mole changing in appearance. All three types of skin cancer are increasing in incidence, and although the symptoms usually do not appear until late adolescence, the chief cause (excessive sun exposure) begins in childhood (Nicole & Huether, 2012).

Malignant Melanoma

Melanomas can be differentiated from benign moles by an A-B-C-D assessment: **a**symmetry, **b**order irregularity, **c**olor (variable or dark pigmentation), and **d**iameter (over 6 mm). Melanomas are treated with surgery, radiation, and adjuvant interferon-α2b or ipilimumab (immunotherapy) to improve overall survival. Nurses can play a major role in helping to reduce the incidence of skin cancer by teaching parents and adolescents ways to identify these malignancies and better protect against excessive sun exposure using measures such as:

- Apply a sunscreen or wear protective clothing if a child will be out in the sun for longer than 20 minutes.
- Avoid indoor tanning beds or ultraviolet light. If used, maintain the same precautions as with sunlight.
- Avoid sunburn because there is a direct association between two or more episodes of sunburn in adolescence and the development of malignant melanoma in young adulthood (ACS, 2012).

What if . . . 53.4 You are particularly interested in exploring one of the 2020 National Health Goals that address malignancies in children (see Box 53.1). What would be a possible research topic to explore pertinent to this goal that would be applicable to Gerri's family and also advance evidence-based practice?

Key Points for Review

- After a diagnosis of malignancy, parents and children need help to change their thinking from an older concept of cancer as being an always painful, fatal disease to a newer concept of cancer as a condition for which there is therapy and hope.
- Because the therapy for cancer involves so many health care visits and so much parental concern, the entire family needs support, not only to meet QSEN competencies but also to best meet the family's total needs.
- Radiation is an important treatment modality in cancer therapy. Immediate side effects include anorexia, nausea, vomiting, and hair loss if radiation is to the head. Long-term effects may include growth restriction or learning disabilities.
- A chemotherapeutic agent is one that is capable of destroying malignant cells. Common side effects are the same as those for radiation therapy. Help children to use time during chemotherapy treatments in constructive ways, such as playing a game, to keep them mentally stimulated yet quiet.
- Be aware of the need to use gloves when preparing a chemotherapy drug to protect yourself from adverse effects of the medication.
- Leukemia is the distorted and uncontrolled proliferation of WBCs and is the most frequently occurring type of cancer in children. About 90% to 95% of children will achieve remission and have a good prognosis for long-term survival.
- Hodgkin disease and non-Hodgkin lymphomas are malignancies of the lymphatic system. Hodgkin disease occurs most often in adolescents; the initial symptom is often one painless, enlarged lymph node. Therapy is radiation and chemotherapy.
- Brain tumors are the most common solid tumors occurring in childhood. Beginning symptoms are usually those of increased intracranial pressure. Therapy may include a combination of surgery followed by radiation and chemotherapy.
- Bone tumors occur in two main forms: osteogenic sarcoma and Ewing sarcoma. These tumors tend to be fast growing because of the ready blood supply to bone. Therapy consists of surgery followed by radiation and chemotherapy.
- Neuroblastomas are tumors that arise from the cells of the sympathetic nervous system. They are the most common abdominal tumor in childhood. Therapy is surgery and chemotherapy.
- Rhabdomyosarcomas are tumors of striated muscle. The peak age of incidence is 2 to 6 years. Therapy is surgery and chemotherapy.
- Nephroblastoma (Wilms tumor) is a malignancy that arises from the metanephric mesoderm cells of the kidney. It is usually discovered early in life. Therapy is surgery followed by radiation and chemotherapy.
- Retinoblastoma is a malignant tumor of the retina of the eye. It may be inherited as an autosomal dominant pattern. Therapy involves surgery, radiation, chemotherapy, and possibly enucleation if the tumor is large.
- Skin cancer is a type of malignancy that can be prevented beginning in childhood. Cautioning children about sensible sun exposure can be an important health promotion role for nurses.

Critical Thinking Care Study

Damion is a 15-year-old boy recently diagnosed with melanoma occurring on his chest. He lives with his single mom in a beach community and spends long hours in the summer playing beach volleyball. He's had bad sunburn at least two times this past summer because he didn't apply sunscreen. He knew that a small mole under his right nipple had darkened in color and grown bigger but, because he's been doing exercises to strengthen his chest muscles, he thought that was the cause of the change.

1. Damion's mother has always been proud of the way that her son spends so much time at the beach doing "healthy" activities. What precautions should Damion have taken to be sure his beach time was healthy?

2. What are the signs of melanoma Damion should have been aware of?
3. Damion's dream is to earn a sports scholarship, go to college, and hopefully, be an Olympic volleyball player some day. Assuming treatment of his present cancer is successful, would you counsel him to choose another sport or continue with beach volleyball?

Patient Scenario

The Ralston Family

Read about the Ralston family, a family with a child with acute lymphoblastic leukemia, then answer the questions to further sharpen your skills and grow more familiar with NCLEX-type questions related to malignancies in children. Confirm your answers are correct by reading the rationales.

Visit http://thePoint.lww.com

Answers and Rationales

Looking for answers to the What if . . . and Critical Thinking Care Study questions?

Visit http://thePoint.lww.com

References

American Cancer Society. (2012). *Cancer facts and figures*. Atlanta, GA: Author.

Arndt, C. A., Rose, P. S., Folpe, A. L., et al. (2012). Common musculoskeletal tumors of childhood and adolescence. *Mayo Clinical Proceedings, 87*(5), 475–487

Babayev, S. N., Arslan, E., Kogan, S., et al. (2013). Evaluation of ovarian and testicular tissue cryopreservation in children undergoing gonadotoxic therapies. *Journal of Assisted Reproduction & Genetics, 30*(1),3–9.

Brown, P., & Hunger, S. P. (2013). Acute leukemia in children. In E. T. Bope & R. D. Kellerman (Eds.), *Conn's current therapy* (pp. 765–768). Philadelphia, PA: Elsevier/Saunders.

Cernvall, M., Carlbring, P., Ljungman, G., et al. (2013). Guided self-help as intervention for traumatic stress in parents of children with cancer: conceptualization, intervention strategies, and a case study. *Journal of Psychosocial Oncology, 31*(1), 13–29.

Ciesielska, U., Nowińska, K., Podhorska-Okołów, M., et al. (2012). The role of human papillomavirus in the malignant transformation of cervix epithelial cells and the importance of vaccination against this virus. *Advances in Clinical & Experimental Medicine, 21*(2), 235–244.

Copeland, A., & Younes, A. (2012). Current treatment strategies in Hodgkin lymphomas. *Current Opinion in Oncology, 24*(5), 466–474.

Davenport, K. P., Blanco, F. C., & Sandler, A. D. (2012). Pediatric malignancies: neuroblastoma, Wilms' tumor, hepatoblastoma, rhabdomyosarcoma, and sacroccygeal teratoma. *Surgery Clinics of North America, 92*(3), 745–767.

Evans, B. (2012). The power of play. *Journal of Family Health Care, 22*(4), 32–34.

Frew, J. A., Lewis, J., & Lucraft, H. H. (2013). The management of children with lymphomas. *Clinical Oncology, 25*(1), 11–18.

Fried, I., Hawkins, C., Scheinemann, K., et al. (2012). Favorable outcome with conservative treatment for children with low grade brainstem tumors. *Pediatric Blood & Cancer, 58*(4), 556–560.

Gains, J., Mandeville, H., Cork, N., et al. (2012). Ten challenges in the management of neuroblastoma. *Future Oncology, 8*(7), 839–858.

Gibbins, J., Steinhardt, K., & Beinart, H. (2012). A systematic review of qualitative studies exploring the experience of parents whose child is diagnosed and treated for cancer. *Journal of Pediatric Oncology Nursing, 29*(5), 253–271.

Graham, D. K., Maloney, K., Quinones, R. R., et al. (2012). Neoplastic disease. In W. Hay, M. Levin, R. Deterding, et al. (Eds.), *Current diagnosis & treatment pediatrics* (21st ed., pp. 949–979). New York, NY: McGraw-Hill/Lange.

Grupp, S. A., Asgharzadeh, S., & Yanik, G. A. (2012). Neuroblastoma: issues in transplantation. *Biology of Blood & Marrow Transplantation, 18*(1, Suppl.), S92–S100.

Held, K., Ryan, R., Champion, J. M., et al. (2012). Caregiver survey results related to handling of oral chemotherapy for pediatric patients with acute lymphoblastic leukemia. *Journal of Pediatric Hematology & Oncology*. Advance online publication.

Jones, B. L. (2012). The challenge of quality care for family caregivers in pediatric cancer care. *Seminars in Oncology Nursing, 28*(4), 213–220.

Jones, S. (2012). Brain tumours and cancer: Insights as a parent and a nurse. *Nursing of Children & Young People, 24*(7), 14–17.

Kaplan, L. D. (2012). HIV-associated lymphoma. *Best Practice & Research in Clinical Haematology, 25*(1), 101–117.

Karch, A. (2013). *2013 Lippincott's nursing drug guide.* Philadelphia, PA: Lippincott Williams & Wilkins.

Kline, N. E. (2012). Cancers in children. In S. E. Huether & K. L. McCance (Eds.), *Understanding pathophysiology* (5th ed., pp. 288–291). Philadelphia, PA: Elsevier Mosby.

Kucharska, W., Negrusz-Kawecka, M., & Gromkowska, M. (2012). Cardiotoxicity of oncological treatment in children. *Advances in Clinical & Experimental Medicine, 21*(3), 281–288.

Lalla, R. V., Brennan, M. T., & Schubert, M. M. (2011). Oral complications of cancer therapy. In J. A. Yagiela, F. J. Dowd, B. S. Johnson, et al. (Eds.), *Pharmacology and therapeutics for dentistry* (6th ed., pp. 782–798). St. Louis, MO: Mosby/Elsevier.

McLean, T. W., & Wofford, M. M. (2011). Oncology. In K. J. Marcdante, R. M. Kliegman, H. B. Jenson, et al. (Eds.), *Nelson essentials of pediatrics* (6th ed., pp. 585–606). Philadelphia, PA: Saunders/Elsevier.

Miller, A. B., & Green, L. M. (2010). Electric and magnetic fields at power frequencies. *Chronic Diseases in Canada, 29* (Suppl. 1), 69–83.

Molyneux, E. M., Rochford, R., Griffin, B., et al. (2012). Burkitt's lymphoma. *Lancet, 379*(9822), 1234–1244.

Nagarkatti-Gude, N., Wang, Y., Ali, M. J., et al. (2012). Genetics of primary intraocular tumors. *Ocular Immunology & Inflammation, 20*(4), 244–254.

Ngoma, T., Adde, M., Durosinmi, M., et al. (2012). Treatment of Burkitt lymphoma in equatorial Africa using a simple three-drug combination followed by a salvage regimen for patients with persistent or recurrent disease. *British Journal of Haematology, 158*(6), 749–762.

Nicole, N. H., & Huether, S. E. (2012). Structure, function and disorders of the integument. In S. E. Huether, & K. L. McCance (Eds.), *Understanding pathophysiology* (5th ed., pp. 1038–1065). Philadelphia, PA: Elsevier Mosby.

Olatunbosun, O. A., & Zhu, L. (2012). The role of sperm banking in fertility preservation. *Clinical & Experimental Obstetrics & Gynecology, 39*(3), 283–287.

Park, J. R., Bagatell, R., Hogarty, M., et al. (2013). Children's Oncology Group's 2013 blueprint for research: Neuroblastoma. *Pediatric Blood & Cancer, 60*(6), 985–993.

Parry, P. V., & Engh, J. A. (2013). Antibody-based therapeutic targeting of human neuroblastoma. *Neurosurgery, 72*(2), N16–N17.

Perkins, J. B., Shapiro, J. F., Bookout, R. N., et al. (2012). Retrospective comparison of filgrastim plus plerixafor to other regimens for remobilization after primary mobilization failure: Clinical and economic outcomes. *American Journal of Hematology, 87*(7), 673–677.

Potratz, J., Dirksen, U., Jürgens, H., et al. (2012). Ewing sarcoma: Clinical state-of-the-art. *Pediatric Hematology & Oncology, 29*(1), 1–11.

Pound, C. M., Clark, C., Ni, A., et al. (2012). Corticosteroids, behavior, and quality of life in children treated for acute lymphoblastic leukemia: A multicentered trial. *Journal of Pediatric Hematology/Oncology, 34*(7), 517–523.

Puri, A., & Gulia, A. (2012). The results of total humeral replacement following excision for primary bone tumour. *Journal of Bone &Joint Surgery, 94*(9), 1277–1281.

Quatrano, N. A., & Dinulos, J. G. (2013). Current principles of sunscreen use in children. *Current Opinion in Pediatrics, 25*(1), 122–129.

Rajaraman, P., Simpson, J., Neta, G., et al. (2011). Early life exposure to diagnostic radiation and ultrasound scans and risk of childhood cancer: Case-control study. *BMJ: British Medical Journal, 342*(2), d472.

Reid, A., Franklin, P., Olsen, N., et al. (2013). All-cause mortality and cancer incidence among adults exposed to blue asbestos during childhood. *American Journal of Industrial Medicine, 56*(2), 133–145.

Robinson, J. K., Baker, M. K., & Hillhouse, J. J. (2012). New approaches to melanoma prevention. *Dermatology Clinics, 30*(3), 405–412.

Romão, R. L., Pippi Salle, J. L., Shuman, C., et al. (2012). Nephron sparing surgery for unilateral Wilms tumor in children with predisposing syndromes: Single center experience over 10 years. *Journal of Urology, 188*(4, Suppl.), 1493–1498.

Roth, E., Mirochna, M., & Harsha, D. (2012). Adolescent with knee pain. *American Family Physician, 86*(6), 569–570

Rowland, E., & Metcalfe, A. (2013). Communicating inherited genetic risk between parent and child: A meta-thematic synthesis. *International Journal of Nursing Studies, 50*(6), 870–880.

Rubnitz, J. E., & Inaba, H. (2012). Childhood acute myeloid leukaemia. *British Journal of Haematology, 159*(3), 259–276.

Sassolas, G. M., Hafdi-Nejjari, Z., Casagranda, L., et al. (2013). Thyroid cancers in children, adolescents, and young adults with and without a history of childhood exposure to therapeutic radiation for other cancers. *Thyroid.* Advance online publication.

Sato, Y., Izumi, Y., Minegishi, K., et al. (2011). Prenatal findings in congenital leukemia: A case report. *Fetal Diagnosis & Therapy, 29*(4), 325–330.

Schrappe, M., Hunger, S. P., Pui, C. H., et al. (2012). Outcomes after induction failure in childhood acute lymphoblastic leukemia. *New England Journal of Medicine, 366*(15), 1371–1381.

Smith, M. A., Seibel, N. L., Altekruse, S. F., et al. (2010). Outcomes for children and adolescents with cancer: Challenges for the twenty-first century. *Journal of Clinical Oncology, 28*(15), 2625–2634.

Subbiah, V., & Kurzrock, R. (2012). Ewing's sarcoma: Overcoming the therapeutic plateau. *Discovery Medicine, 13*(73), 405–415.

U.S. Department of Health and Human Services. (2010). *Healthy people 2020.* Washington, DC: Author.

Virshup, D. M. (2012). Biology, clinical manifestations & treatment of cancer. In S. E. Huether, & K. L. McCance (Eds.), *Understanding pathophysiology* (5th ed., pp. 222–248). Philadelphia, PA: Elsevier Mosby.

Zur, E. (2012). Oral mucositis: Etiology and clinical and pharmaceutical management. *International Journal of Pharmaceutical Compounding, 16*(1), 22–33.

Unit 8

The Nursing Role in Restoring and Maintaining the Mental Health of Children and Families

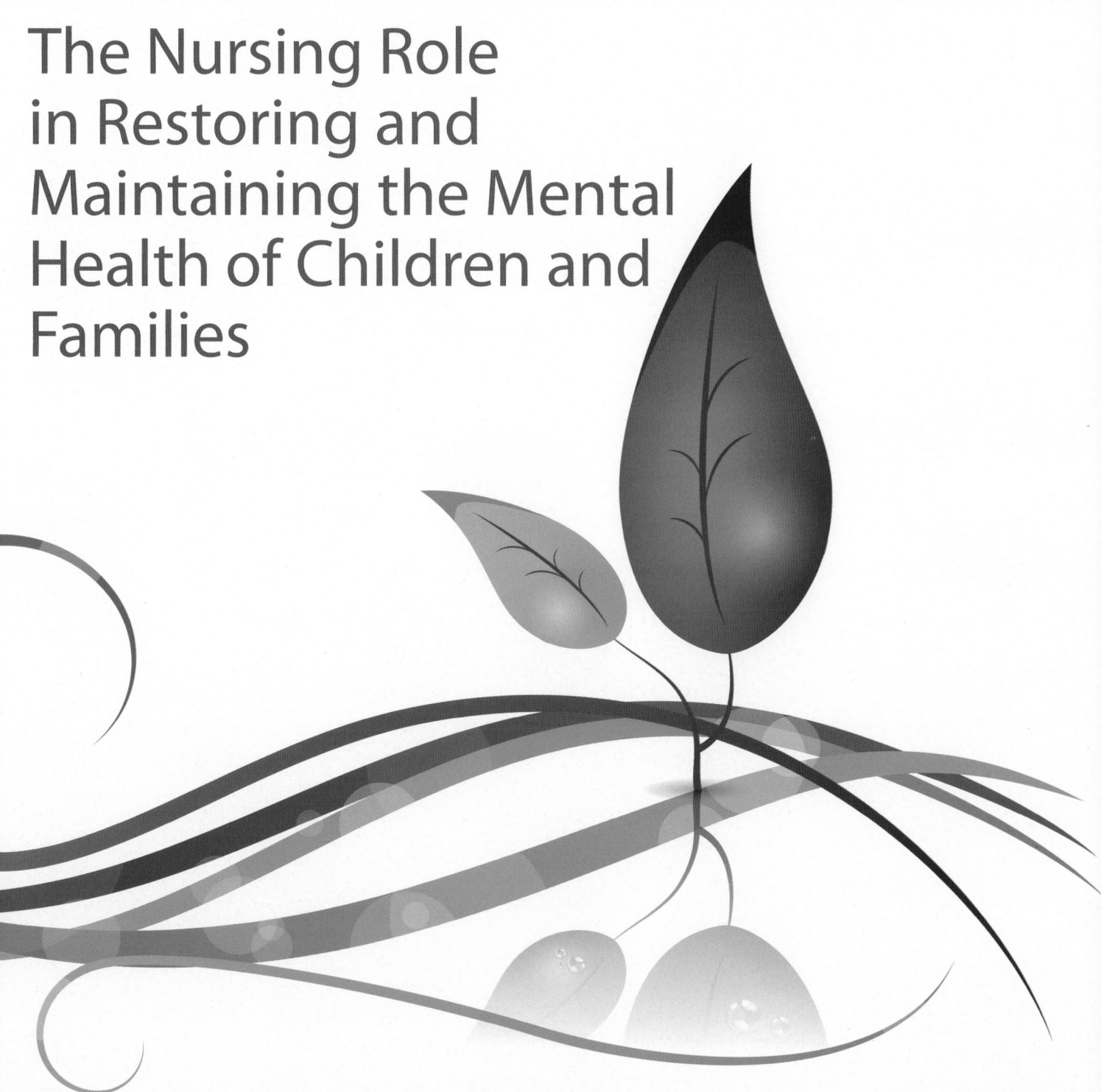

Chapter 54

Nursing Care of a Family When a Child Has a Cognitive or Mental Health Disorder

KEY TERMS

- anhedonia
- binge eating
- catatonia
- choreiform movements
- complex vocal tics
- coprolalia
- dyslexia
- echolalia
- flat affect
- graphesthesia
- hyperactivity
- labile mood
- motor tics
- palilalia
- purging
- stereognosis
- vocal tics

OBJECTIVES

After mastering the contents of this chapter, you should be able to:

1. Describe common cognitive and mental health disorders that occur in children.
2. Identify 2020 National Health Goals related to cognitive or mental health disorders that nurses can be instrumental in helping the nation achieve.
3. Assess a child for a cognitive or mental health disorder.
4. Formulate nursing diagnoses related to the cognitive or mental health disorders of childhood.
5. Establish expected outcomes for a child with a cognitive or mental health disorder that help parents manage seamless transitions across differing health care settings.
6. Using the nursing process, plan nursing care that includes the six competencies of Quality & Safety Education for Nurses (QSEN): Patient-Centered Care, Teamwork & Collaboration, Evidence-Based Practice (EBP), Quality Improvement (QI), Safety, and Informatics.
7. Implement nursing care for a child with a cognitive or mental health disorder, such as explaining ways to remember to take medicine long term.
8. Evaluate expected outcomes for achievement and effectiveness of care.
9. Integrate knowledge of a cognitive challenge or mental illness in children with the interplay of nursing process, the six competencies of QSEN, and Family Nursing to achieve quality maternal and child health nursing care.

You meet Todd, a second grader who was diagnosed last year with autism spectrum disorder, who is admitted to your ambulatory care unit to have plaque removed from his teeth under conscious sedation. You observe Todd coloring, drumming on the table, running to the door, opening and closing the door, and then throwing pamphlets out of an information rack. His sister Cheyenne, 15 years old, who seems very underweight, tells you she is "at her wits' end" trying to babysit Todd in the evenings because his attention span is so short and his behavior is so disruptive. Todd's father tells you he's proud that his son is "all boy."

Previous chapters described the growth and development of well children and the care of children with physiologic disorders. This chapter adds information about the dramatic changes that occur when children demonstrate a cognitive or mental health disorder. Such information builds a base for care and health teaching.

What additional education does Todd's family need to understand him better? Does his older sister need counseling as well?

Children who are mentally healthy successfully master the tasks of each developmental phase of childhood and grow up to possess a positive self-concept and sense of contentment within their own limits. In addition, there is a good emotional relationship between the parents and the child and a sense of safety and security in the home environment. Promoting suggestions for healthy family functioning during health care visits, providing anticipatory guidance about developmental milestones and needs, and listening carefully to both children and parents are important nursing actions to foster both the physical and mental health of children.

Sound mental health implies that a child is able to use adaptive coping mechanisms appropriately to meet the normal stressors of life. When stressors, such as acute illness, hospitalization, natural disasters, or chronic illness, drain a family's resources and go beyond what is considered "the norm," many children and parents are unable to cope adequately, which results in mental illness. It's important for nurses to be able to recognize how situations such as chronic illness or hospitalization affect children and their families and to be prepared to provide interventions to improve coping mechanisms (Brosbe, Faust, & Gold, 2013).

Children can develop the same mental health disorders that affect the adult population, such as depression or schizophrenia. In addition, several disorders such as autism spectrum disorder and separation anxiety begin for the first time in childhood. Current research attributes some of the disorders that occur in children to genetic vulnerability and others to disruption in family life, temperament, or inadequate parent–child bonding and attachment. For best results, children with mental illness, whatever the cause, must be evaluated and treated by specialists in the mental health field as early in their disease process as possible. A child health nurse is often the first health care provider to become aware of such problems and can be instrumental, through appropriate referrals, in helping a child and family adjust to the disorder.

Because mental health is important to the nation, Box 54.1 shows cognitive and mental health disorders addressed by the 2020 National Health Goals.

BOX 54.1 Nursing Care Planning Based on 2020 National Health Goals

Cognitive and mental health disorders in children produce major costs to the nation, as well as to individual families, because these disorders have the potential to reduce the earning power and contributions of the nation's future citizens. Examples of 2020 National Health Goals that speak to this are:

- Decrease the proportion of adolescents 12 to 17 years of age who experience major depressive episodes from a baseline of 8.3% to a target level of 7.4%.
- Increase the proportion of children with mental health problems who receive effective treatment from a baseline of 68.9% to 75.8%.
- Prevent inappropriate weight gain (excessive or inadequate) in adolescents 12 to 18 years of age.
- Increase the incidence of primary care physicians who screen youth age 12 to 18 years for depression during office visits from 2.1% to 2.3% (U.S. Department of Health and Human Services [DHHS], 2010; see www.healthypeople.gov) (APA, 2000).

Nurses can help the nation achieve these goals by educating parents about nutrition and inadequate weight gain; educating families about ways to reduce stress; and helping to identify children in school and health care settings who demonstrate a high level of stress, depression, or other symptoms of mental illness.

Nursing Process Overview

For Care of a Child With a Cognitive Challenge or Mental Illness

Assessment

Both personality and mental growth potential in a child are influenced by several factors, including genetic makeup, cultural background, family environment, and community resources. All of these need to be taken into account when assessing a child's cognitive or mental health. Be certain to assess children for emotional as well as physical problems at regular health maintenance visits. If a mental health or cognitive problem is suspected, obtain a detailed history of the presenting concern, any relevant past history, the child's developmental history including school and social aspects, and the current pattern of family functioning.

Nursing Diagnosis

Nursing diagnoses established for ill children often address mental health or the response of children and their families to their condition or treatment. Examples of these diagnoses are:

- Anxiety related to surgical experience
- Fear related to potential loss of independence secondary to traumatic injury
- Situational low self-esteem related to disfiguring scars after accident
- Powerlessness related to loss of independence and control in hospital environment

Examples of additional nursing diagnoses, which need to be added if a concern of cognitive or mental health is present, include:

- Risk for self-directed violence related to impulsivity
- Impaired social interaction related to short attention span and distractibility
- Interrupted family processes related to inability of child to follow instructions
- Disturbed thought processes related to the effects of schizophrenia
- Impaired verbal communication related to depression and withdrawn behavior
- Ineffective health maintenance related to inattention to food or hygiene needs
- Situational low self-esteem related to lack of successful coping strategies

Outcome Identification and Planning

Although the diagnosis of a mental health disorder or referral to a child guidance or psychiatric clinic does not carry the stigma it once did, many parents still worry such a referral is a mark of inadequacy or a sign of failure for themselves as parents. Help them to see that this type of referral is in their child's best interest and is actually no different from one to a cardiologist or orthopedist for a purely physical reason.

It can help if you remind parents that the world puts many pressures and stresses on children today that parents cannot control or guard against completely. Many parents find it reassuring to be assured their contact with a child guidance clinic, psychologist, or psychiatrist will be kept confidential. They may also feel reassured by knowing health care personnel making the referral will continue to offer episodic or health maintenance care—they are not being "transferred out" but asked to seek additional help only in this one area.

Organizations that can be helpful for referral include Anorexia Nervosa and Related Eating Disorders, Inc. (www.anred.com), the Autism Society (www.autism-society.org), the National Tourette Syndrome Association (www.tsa-usa.org), National Association for Down Syndrome (www.nads.org), and Mental Health America (www.mentalhealthamerica.net).

Implementation

Often, what parents and children need most when a cognitive or mental health disorder is identified is an empathic but uninvolved person to listen to their story objectively and to provide support for them as they try to resolve and manage the situation to a conclusion satisfactory for the family. Serving in this capacity can be a help to families and also personally satisfying.

Outcome Evaluation

Children who have a cognitive or mental health disorder need ongoing evaluation by health care personnel at routine visits, because these disorders tend to be long term and change over time. In addition, it's important to determine whether any circumstance that might have led to a temporary problem has truly been corrected or only superficially changed because, if the circumstance remains the same, the child's problem may return or be manifested later in another way.

Examples suggesting achievement of expected outcomes are:

- Child does not cut himself during the coming month.
- Parents state they are able to cope with child's disruptive behavior since prescription of antipsychotic medication for child.
- Child ingests a minimum of 1,000 calories daily with no binge eating.
- Parents state they accept that their child is cognitively challenged; parents will meet with school psychiatrist to arrange specific schooling.

HEALTH PROMOTION AND RISK MANAGEMENT

Nurses play a key role in assessing and promoting the mental and cognitive health of children and their families at health maintenance visits and during school years and establishing environments for children and families that foster mental health. It's impossible to plan care that keeps children, like adults, completely shielded from stress, but plans can be formulated so that if stress does enter their lives, children can cope with the difficulties that follow. Table 54.1 lists some helpful observational and interview data for assessing these areas.

Various factors have been associated with an increased risk for mental health disorders in children, including trauma, poverty or neglect, difficult temperament or attachment problems, medical illness, or major losses to the family such as divorce or death. A thorough assessment of the child and family can provide clues to the existence of such possible risk factors and suggest strategies to reduce their impact through counseling or early intervention programs, helping to minimize the overall effects of the disorder on the child and family.

CLASSIFICATION OF MENTAL HEALTH DISORDERS

Psychopathology in children is classified according to the American Psychiatric Association (APA) and described in the *Diagnostic and Statistical Manual of Mental Disorders* (4th ed., text rev.; *DSM-IV-TR*) (APA, 2000).

DEVELOPMENTAL DISORDERS

Developmental disorders, although not related by etiology, typically share a common feature in that there is a delay in one or more areas of development such as attention span, cognition, language, affect, and social or moral behavior. Because these behaviors are interrelated, a delay in one area often interferes with development in another area. This category includes cognitive challenge, pervasive developmental disorders, and specific developmental concerns such as learning, developmental coordination, and communication disorders.

Cognitive Challenge (Intellectual Disability)

Cognitive challenge (formerly, mental retardation) is commonly defined based on two criteria: intellectual functioning significantly below average—an intelligence quotient (IQ) of 70 or lower with onset before 18 years of age—and concurrent deficits in adaptive functioning (APA, 2000). The IQ level of 70 was chosen as the upper limit of cognitive challenge because most children who score below this level are so limited in functioning that they require special services, protection, and schooling. For infants, because available intelligence tests do not yield numerical values, a clinical judgment of significant subaverage mental status function is necessary.

Approximately 2% of children in the United States are cognitively challenged. This does not occur as the result of a single cause but from genetic abnormalities such as fragile X syndrome and Down syndrome (trisomy 21) or metabolic disorders such as untreated congenital hypothyroidism. In addition, interplay of several genes with environmental factors (polyfactorial causes) is a possible source in some children (Box 54.2).

Children who are cognitively challenged are seen in health care settings for diagnosis; they continue to come to health settings throughout their lives for the same reasons as other children—for well-child or ambulatory health maintenance visits; for treatment of lacerations or poisoning in emergency departments; or

TABLE 54.1 Guidelines for the Mental Health Interview of a Child

Observational Data	Examples of Possible Findings
General appearance	Height, weight, grooming and hygiene, nutrition, physical health, rhythmic movement or tics
Motor behaviors	Fine and gross balance, unusual motor activity
Speech and language	Receptive, expressive; content, tone, and articulation
Affect	Predominant emotion (depressed, angry, anxious, happy, labile), emotional reactions to content of interview (appropriate, inappropriate)
Thought process	Estimated intellectual level via language and knowledge base (organization and thought content); orientation (to person, place, time); perceptual distortions (hallucinations, illusions, obsessions, delusions); attention span, learning disabilities
Ability to relate to evaluator	Eye contact; attitude toward interviewer (negative, positive, shy, suspicious, withdrawn, friendly, self-centered)
Behaviors displayed during interview	Impulsivity, aggression, inhibition, distractibility, low frustration tolerance, ability to have fun, sense of humor, creativity
Interview Data	
Interpersonal relationships	Attitudes toward and perceptions of family, siblings, peers, transitional objects (inanimate objects used to allay anxiety); social skills and relationships with peers, parents, and siblings; conflicts; behavior problems; adjustment to changes in routine or new situations
Self-concept and image	Self-appraisal (does child like self?), comparison of self with others (siblings, peers). What would the child like to change about self? Sense of pride in accomplishments, sex role, and gender identity
Conscience or moral reasoning	Understands right and wrong; is able to express common judgments or values.

for treatment of illnesses such as pneumonia or appendicitis in in-service units. For these reasons, child health nurses need to be skilled in meeting the needs of these special children.

Classification

It's unfair to categorize children only according to the results of intelligence tests, because children do not always perform well in testing situations and many situations in life require "common sense" reasoning not easily tested. So there is a general understanding of a child's functioning ability, however, cognitive challenge is usually classified as mild, moderate, severe, or profound based on IQ. IQ tests are considered to have an error of measurement of about 5 points. Therefore, many children with an IQ of 75 are included in special schooling or concentrated programs. Assessing for physical illness in children who are cognitively challenged at any level is difficult because they may not appreciate the seriousness of symptoms or be able to report them as well as other children.

BOX 54.2 Common Causes of Cognitive Challenge

- Chromosomal abnormalities such as Down syndrome and fragile X syndrome
- Infection in utero, such as rubella or cytomegalic inclusion disease
- Anoxia at birth from such causes as umbilical cord compression
- Fetal alcohol spectrum disorder
- Inherited metabolic disorders such as phenylketonuria or Tay-Sachs disease
- Head trauma, lead poisoning, or hypothyroidism
- Brain malformations such as anencephaly
- Very low birth weight
- Infections such as measles encephalitis
- Autism spectrum disorder

Mild Cognitive Challenge. About 85% of children who are cognitively challenged have an IQ of 50 to 70 and may be referred to as "educable" by a school system. During early years, these children learn social and communication skills and are often not too distinguishable from average infants or toddlers. They continue to learn academic skills up to about a sixth-grade level. As adults, they can usually achieve social and vocational skills adequate for minimum self-support. They're able to live independently but need guidance and assistance when faced with new situations or unusual stress.

Moderate Cognitive Challenge. Children in this category have an IQ between 35 and 49 and represent about 10% of cognitively challenged children. During preschool years, these children learn to talk and communicate, although they have poor awareness of social conventions. They can learn some vocational skills during adolescence or young adulthood and learn to take care of themselves with moderate supervision. They are unlikely to progress beyond the second-grade level in academic subjects. As adults, they may be able to contribute to their own support by performing unskilled or semiskilled work under close supervision such as in a sheltered workshop setting, although they need close supervision and guidance when in stressful settings.

Severe Cognitive Challenge. Children in this group have an IQ between 20 and 34 and represent only about 4% of cognitively challenged children. During the preschool period, these children develop only minimal communicative speech. They may have accompanying poor motor development. During school years, it may be possible for them to learn to talk as well as basic hygiene and dressing skills. As adults, they may be able to perform simple work tasks under close supervision, but as a group, they do not profit from vocational training. They need constant supervision for safety.

Profound Cognitive Challenge. The IQ of children in this group is less than 20. Fewer than 1% of cognitively challenged children fall into this group. Such children demonstrate only minimal capacity for sensorimotor functioning. Some are able to respond to training in minimal self-care, such as toothbrushing, but only very limited self-care is possible. They need a highly structured environment and a constant level of help and supervision for safety.

Assessment

Assessment regarding whether a child is cognitively challenged is done by history taking and IQ testing. Early assessment is key and should be done as soon as parents become aware their child is evidencing a developmental delay, as this helps prevent parents from developing unrealistic expectations of children or punishing children for doing things they don't understand not to do. Assessment also allows parents to appreciate the things their child can do and to see where they can be of most help.

Intelligence is routinely measured with standardized tests. Adaptive behavioral functioning, which may vary in different environments, is judged according to several methods, including standardized instruments for assessing mental status, social maturity, and adaptive skills. A composite picture of life functioning is drawn from these multiple sources.

Parents may react to the diagnosis of cognitive challenge in the same way as parents who have been told that their child has a chronic or fatal illness—with a grief reaction. This may be manifested as disbelief, anger, or extreme sorrow. The grief may become chronic—always present, always waiting to strike a parent especially hard at times when the child would have reached milestones in life, such as the first day of school or the time the child would have obtained a driver's license. Be certain when working with such families to help them develop plans that are realistic for their individual child that maximize the child's capabilities (Yildirim, Hacihasanoğlu Aşilar, & Karakurt, 2013).

Therapeutic Management

To aid in planning, parents need a realistic prognosis for their child. This may be difficult to offer in early life, because infant intelligence tests are not accurate and more sophisticated tests are difficult to administer until the preschool years. Because prediction based on these early tests involves some subjective input, a child's potential may be overrated or underrated when using these. Once parents have a realistic expectation based on the best judgment possible, however, they are ready, with guidance, to help their child achieve his or her full potential.

Nursing Diagnoses and Related Interventions

Parents of children who are cognitively challenged have several important decisions to make concerning care of their child.

Nursing Diagnosis: Health-seeking behaviors related to increasing knowledge of care needs of a cognitively challenged child

Outcome Evaluation: Parents identify their particular options; identify child's care needs; demonstrate measures to care for child.

Home and Family Environment. Ideally, children with intellectual disabilities are cared for best in a small, caring, family environment because this strengthens a child's ability to relate to other people, receive stimulation, and master a desire to achieve.

Parents shoulder a great deal of responsibility to provide constant watchful care for a child who lacks judgment, a responsibility that increases as both the child and the parents grow older. Parents find that their freedom to go on vacation or to have an adult life apart from the child is restricted. They may need to spend so much time with the child that other children in the family feel left out, unloved, or burdensome.

If parents are unable to care for a child at home, a suitable foster home placement may be possible, offering the child the advantage of a small family setting. Halfway houses or group homes (6 to 12 children living in a home with assigned counselors) offer another option for providing a care setting with a home atmosphere and community experiences.

Health Maintenance Needs. Children who are cognitively challenged need the same health maintenance supervision as all other children. At health care visits, reinforce and review precautions against unintentional injuries. Remind parents to treat their child according to the child's intellectual age, not the chronologic age. All 2-year-old children, for example, would turn on the burners of the stove to see the flame if they could reach them. Most 2-year-olds do not do this, however, because they cannot reach that high. In contrast, a child who is 6 years old but operates at a 2-year-old level can reach the burners, so parents have to maintain constant vigilance to prevent that from happening.

Illness. Children with intellectual disabilities can develop a degree of depression by school age as they attempt to fit into a school system geared for higher functioning children (McGillivray & Kershaw, 2013). It may be more difficult to detect this or other illness in children than usual because they may not appreciate the importance of a symptom or be able to describe the symptom clearly. For example, children experiencing pain may respond to it by generalized crying, the same as infants, because they do not know the terms sharp, nagging, or aching. This puts added responsibility on

Autism spectrum disorder is marked by deficits in language, perceptual, and motor development and the inability to function well in social settings. There often is a lack of responsiveness to people around them, gross impairment in communication skills, and bizarre responses to various aspects of the environment, all developing within the first 30 months of age. It occurs in 1% of U.S. children or occurs as frequently as 1 in 88 children (Autism Society, 2012). As many as 50% of children with the disorder are also cognitively challenged; many have coexistent mental health diagnoses (Stafford, Talmi, & Burstein, 2012). A former concern that immunization may precede or cause the disorder has now been ruled out as a cause (Kirkland, 2012).

Assessment

Common symptoms of autism spectrum disorder are summarized in Box 54.4. Asperger disorder contains aspects of autism spectrum disorder but no language impairment. Rett disorder, which only occurs in girls, also has closely associated symptoms. Although autism spectrum disorders often are not diagnosed until the child is 2 to 3 years of age, parents report they were worried much earlier that the child had the disorder because the infant failed to cuddle, make eye contact, exhibit facial responsiveness, react to pain, or reach to be picked up. As toddlers, their inability to play cooperatively or make friendships becomes apparent. Parents may bring a child to a health care facility for the first time thinking the child is deaf because of this inability to establish usual relationships.

The impairment in communication includes both verbal and nonverbal skills, and communication may be totally absent. If a child does speak, deficiencies in grammatical structure such as the use of "you" when "I" is intended may be noticed as well as an inability to name objects (nominal aphasia) and abnormal speech melody, such as question-like rises at the end of statements. **Echolalia** (repetition of words or phrases spoken by others) and concrete interpretation are also common findings.

Bizarre responses to the environment may include intense reactions to minor changes in the environment (perhaps screaming if a toy box is moved across the room) and attachment to odd objects such as always carrying a string or a shoe. Even as an infant, repetitive hand movements (clapping or flapping) and constant body rocking are often observed. It may be difficult to gain the child's attention as the child becomes intensely preoccupied by music or objects that revolve, such as a fan, the swirling water in the toilet bowl, or a spinning top. Aggressive actions, such as hitting, head banging, and biting, or the inability to feel pain may also be present.

Children are said to have a **labile mood** (crying occurs suddenly and is followed immediately by giggling or laughing or vice versa). They may react with overresponsiveness to sensory stimuli, such as light or sound, but then be unaware of a major event in the room, such as the sound of a fire alarm.

In contrast to these mannerisms, long-term memory and "savant" skills (exceptional skills such as virtuoso piano playing) may be excellent (Bölte, Duketis, Poustka, et al., 2011). For example, autistic children may be able to recall dates and spoken words from conversations that took place years before. This excellent memory previously led to the belief that most of these children have usual intelligence. Actually, the majority of children with autism spectrum disorders have an IQ of less than 70 (APA, 2000). Intelligence testing is difficult, however, because children with the disorder do not respond well to test situations, scoring particularly poorly on the verbal parts of these tests. In contrast, tasks requiring manipulative or visual skills or immediate memory may be performed at above-usual levels.

Therapeutic Management

Autism spectrum disorder is a perplexing condition because of the extreme variability a child may exhibit. As a rule, children need intensive therapy to learn improved communication techniques; they need parental support to learn self-care and proceed with therapy (Carter, Lane, Cooney, et al., 2013). Behavior modification therapy is an example of a social learning technique that may be effective in controlling some of the unusual mannerisms that accompany autism spectrum disorder, but, because children demonstrate such a wide range of behaviors, it will not always succeed (Maglione, Gans, Das, et al., 2012). No specific medication for the disorder is available, but various medications such as selective serotonin reuptake inhibitors (SSRIs) may help reduce aggression, antipsychotic agents such as risperidone may help reduce anxiety, and melatonin may be prescribed to reduce sleep difficulties (Scheffer, 2011). Ask at health care visits if parents are finding time for both care of their child and themselves because there is a danger that excessive parental stress can lead to child maltreatment (Hall & Graff, 2012).

As children mature, they develop greater awareness of and attachment to parents and other familiar adults. A day care program can help promote social awareness. Some children may eventually reach a point where they can become passively involved in loosely structured play groups. Some children may be able to lead independent lives, although social ineptness and awkwardness may remain, especially if accompanied by cognitive challenges. Box 54.5 shows an interprofessional care map for a child with autism spectrum disorder.

BOX 54.4 Common Symptoms in the Child With Autism Spectrum Disorder

- Failure to develop social relations
- Stereotyped behaviors such as hand gestures
- Extreme resistance to change in routine
- Abnormal responses to sensory stimuli
- Decreased sensitivity to pain
- Inappropriate or decreased emotional expressions
- Specific, limited intellectual problem-solving abilities
- Stereotyped or repetitive use of language
- Impaired ability to initiate or sustain a conversation

QSEN Checkpoint Question 54.2

Informatics

Todd has symptoms of autism spectrum disorder. When reviewing Todd's electronic health record, which of these symptoms would you recognize as being most consistent with this disorder?

a. Lack of short-term memory
b. Audio hallucinations
c. Constant whirling around in a circle
d. Severe depression or emotional lability

Look in Appendix A for the best answer and rationale.

BOX 54.5 Nursing Care Planning

AN INTERPROFESSIONAL CARE MAP FOR A SCHOOL-AGE CHILD WITH AUTISM SPECTRUM DISORDER

Todd, a second grader, is admitted to the 1-day surgery unit to have plaque removed from his teeth under conscious sedation. You observe Todd drumming on the table, running to the door, opening and closing the door, and then throwing pamphlets out of an information rack. His sister, who seems very underweight, tells you she is "at her wits' end" trying to babysit Todd in the evenings while their mother works because his behavior is so disruptive. Todd's father tells you he's proud that his son is "all boy."

Family Assessment Child lives with two parents and sister in three-bedroom condominium. Father works as a sail maker; mother works part time in local fish market. Father rates finances as "Not good. My wife wants to work more, but we can't find anyone to watch Todd; he's such a handful."

Client Assessment A 7-year-old, slightly overweight male grasping toy dog tightly in his arms. Mother states, "He talks to the dog when he's upset." Tends not to interact with other children. Often repeats himself, asking "What's your name?" and "How old are you" over and over. Mother feeds him mainly fast-food meals because he throws food if he doesn't like the taste. Toilet trained but sometimes has accidents as he "forgets" to go. Needs supervision dressing because he loses track of task at hand. Refuses to let mother brush teeth. Mother says, "He gets upset and cries easily if his routine changes." Attends special class in public school, as he was too disruptive in regular classroom.

Nursing Diagnosis Impaired social interaction related to easy distractibility

Outcome Criteria Child cooperates to extent possible with IV therapy and bed rest after conscious sedation.

Team Member Responsible	Assessment	Intervention	Rationale	Expected Outcome
Activities of Daily Living, Including Safety				
Nurse	Assess what self-care activities child completes for himself.	Allow child to wear own clothes until under conscious sedation to avoid confrontation.	Self-care can offer a sense of control unless it becomes frustrating.	Child cooperates to help with self-care to the extent he is capable.
Teamwork and Collaboration				
Nurse/Child care specialist	Assess whether child care specialist is available for consultation.	Consult with child care specialist about what activities would be best for child who is easily distracted.	Games can become frustrating if they can't be completed in a short time period.	Child care specialist visits with child and suggests at least two activities for period before surgery.
Procedures/Medications for Quality Improvement				
Nurse	Assess whether child has past experience with IV therapy and whether he took prescribed medication today.	Begin IV line in nondominant hand. Document medication given at home.	Use of nondominant hand allows child to complete small, frequent tasks. Documentation will help avoid medication toxicity.	Mother remains with child to ensure child does not remove IV line.
Nutrition				
Nurse/Nutritionist	Assess what mother means by "fast-food" meals.	Discuss a diet with mother that doesn't involve so many fatty foods because child is overweight.	Child is overweight, a finding that can be caused by eating fat-heavy, fast-food meals.	Mother states she will try to find healthier foods that child will eat.

(continued on page 1604)

BOX 54.5 Nursing Care Planning (continued)

Patient-Centered Care				
Nurse	Assess what parent understands about good tooth care.	Talk to mother about techniques to make toothbrushing a game, not a chore.	Plaque will form again on teeth if they are not brushed after this procedure.	Mother suggests two different ways, such as playing Simon Says, that she could use to interest child in toothbrushing.
Nurse/Primary health care provider	Assess what parents understand about autism spectrum disorder and if they have enough support to care for child with a potentially disruptive disorder.	Educate parents that autism is a disorder, not normal boyish behavior. Explore whether the family is aware of "respite" services in community.	As long as one parent continues to think of the child's behavior as within usual limits, it will be difficult for them to be consistent in care.	Mother and father state they understand their son's condition is one that needs therapy.
Psychosocial/Spiritual/Emotional Needs				
Nurse	Assess whether child can take favorite toy to operating room.	Respect that toy dog is favorite toy and important to child.	Children can find comfort and security in a favorite toy.	Toy is respected by unit and surgery personnel.
Informatics for Seamless Health Care Planning				
Nurse	Assess whether parents have any questions about care at home after dental procedure.	Discuss that child will be sleepy for remainder of day after conscious sedation.	Conscious sedation is necessary because of child's resistance to new procedures.	Mother repeats care needed for next 24 hours to safeguard a still sleepy child.

Specific Developmental Disorders

Specific developmental disorders are characterized by the more narrowed area of development involved with the delay. Typically, these include learning disorders, communication disorders, and motor skills disorders.

Learning disorders occur in approximately 5% of children in the United States. Although the degree may vary, the disorders involve a discrepancy between actual achievement and what is expected based on the child's age and intelligence. Learning disorders may involve **dyslexia** (reading reversal), mathematics, or writing (Batorowicz, Missiuna, & Pollock, 2012). Children need individualized educational plans to help them achieve at the highest level possible and prevent low self-esteem or deficits in social skills (DuPaul, Gormley, & Laracy, 2013).

Communication disorders involve problems of speech (motor aspect) or language (formulation and comprehension of verbal communication) including expressive disorders, phonologic disorders, and stuttering. Like learning disorders, these conditions can lead to a lack of self-esteem unless a child receives support and encouragement from parents, teachers, and health care providers. Speech therapy is usually effective to improve these disorders and allow children to achieve sufficiently to become successful adults.

ATTENTION DEFICIT AND DISRUPTIVE BEHAVIOR DISORDERS

Attention deficit disorder and the disruptive behavior disorders may begin with behavior problems that are not so different from what most families experience. As a result, parents may be initially unaware of the need for interventions. By the time they do seek help, they may be extremely distressed about the seeming unmanageability of their child.

Like autistic behavior, these disorders need to be diagnosed as early as possible, before the child's behavior leads to a deteriorating level of self-esteem, compromised social skills, and complications in family functioning.

Attention Deficit Hyperactivity Disorder

Attention deficit hyperactivity disorder (ADHD) is a persistent pattern of inattention and/or hyperactivity-impulsiveness revealed before the age of 7 years (APA, 2000). It is estimated to occur in 3% to 7% of school-age children, with boys affected more frequently than girls. Although the cause is unknown, it occurs more frequently among some families than in the general population, indicating a combination of possible genetic or environmental etiologic components. Both medication and behavior modification therapy can be used with success, a fact that may support the theory of varying causes.

The disorder is characterized by three major behaviors: inattention, impulsiveness, and hyperactivity. Inattention makes children become easily distracted, and they often may not seem to listen or complete tasks effectively. Impulsiveness causes them to act before they think and therefore to have difficulty with such tasks as awaiting turns. With hyperactivity, children may shift excessively from one activity to another and exhibit excessive or exaggerated muscular activity, such as excessive climbing onto objects, constant fidgeting, or aimless or haphazard running.

Assessment

The disorder is diagnosable by about 36 months of age, although parents may excuse the behavior as "active" or "always on the go" until school age, when it is apparent the child is unable to sit still in school or concentrate on problem solving for long periods. To reveal the extent of the problem, take a thorough initial history. This history of the child's actions is important, because some children have enough control in a one-to-one situation that their extremes of behavior are not apparent at a one-time health care visit.

As part of history taking, review both the pregnancy and birth history, the child's ability to meet developmental milestones, and a typical day for the child. The term **hyperactivity**, or excessive movement, is commonly carelessly used by parents to describe any active child. To reveal true hyperactivity, ask the parent to give an exact description of the child's actions such as being unable to sit still long enough to finish a full meal or running to the window 10 times in 15 minutes.

Ask as well about activity that is not only excessive but also disorganized. For example, during a health care visit, children with ADHD may run from the back of the room to the front of the room, to the window, to the examining table, then back to the door. They perform repetitive activities such as pencil tapping, arm swinging, and finger tapping. At home, they may exhibit driven or compulsive behavior; for example, in the middle of working on a project or listening to a television program, they may run to the refrigerator and repetitively bang the door open and closed.

Variability is another important symptom. Everyone has days when they perform at their peak and days when their performance is less than optimum. Children with ADHD may have behavior so variable that they have good and bad *moments*, causing them to lose track of whole systems and methods, not just answers, leading school performance to falter. When asked to add, for example, a child might add 4 plus 3 correctly, but then lose track of the system and add 2 plus 3 as 23 or 32.

This high level of impulsiveness causes children to make statements without thinking, to touch objects they have just been told not to touch, or to speak or act before they have time to think about what they want to say or do. When angered, they may shout, strike out, or bite. Because they feel they must have things done for them immediately, they may be unable to wait in line for a drink of water or wait to take a turn at a board game.

The usual child is able to filter out stimuli that are not important at that moment. Children with ADHD, however, seem to have an "all-or-none" reaction to stimuli. This leads them to block out all incoming stimuli and, as a result, do not hear parents or a teacher calling them. Their history will reveal they were disciplined at school for something such as not answering a fire drill (unaware the bell was ringing and that children around them were moving toward the exit). At other times, they may be unable to suppress any incoming stimuli. They mean to concentrate on a desk assignment in school, for example, but, outside the window, they hear a bird singing; they smell a girl's perfume; or they feel their watch on their wrist and thus cannot concentrate on the homework problem at hand.

Yet another symptom of children with ADHD is difficulty with concepts such as *right* and *left*, *before* and *after*, *in front of* and *in back of*, and *yesterday* and *tomorrow*, because these concepts call for sequencing, or the process of relating things to one another in time or space. If children cannot tell the difference between left and right, this leads to difficulty forming common letters such as *b* and *d*, which vary only in the direction of the bottom loop. It can cause difficulty with common tasks such as washing their hands, because they never know which way to turn a faucet. Turning door knobs and keys, tying shoelaces, and screwing on bottle caps are other tasks that call for sequencing. Because children have awkward motor movements or cannot work all muscles gracefully in proper sequence, they may reach beyond an object, possibly spilling a glass of milk at the table at every meal.

Long after the average child is speaking in fluent sentences, children with ADHD may still have difficulty using conjunctions or prepositions correctly (sequencing of words). They may have difficulty learning to read because to read words of more than one syllable, they must sound the first syllable and then retain that sound in their mind while they sound the second syllable. If they have difficulty retaining the first syllable long enough to connect it with the second, it's difficult to construct the word. Similarly, they can have difficulty with arithmetic, because they may be unable to retain the sum of two numbers long enough to add a third. Spelling may be equally difficult because not only are they unable to sequence the letters in a word correctly, but they also cannot retain memory rules such as "i before e" to help them.

As a rule, children with ADHD do not have a deficit in intelligence, although they may seem to because of their impulsive behavior and an unawareness that their behavior is upsetting to family, friends, and teachers. On physical assessment, they often show many "soft" neurologic signs, such as difficulty performing tests such as a finger-to-nose test or rapid hand movements (touching one finger after another with the thumb). They also tend to show "mirroring" with these movements (their second hand imitates what the first hand is doing). Cerebellar difficulty may be evidenced by the inability to perform a tandem walk or a heel-to-shin test. They may not show the normal responses of **graphesthesia** (ability to recognize a shape that has been traced on the skin) or **stereognosis** (ability to recognize an object by touch). When asked to stand with arms outstretched, **choreiform movements** (aimless movements), such as rising of the fingers, are often present. More definite neurologic signs, such as a unilateral Babinski reflex, may also be present. Testing children through the use of games may be necessary so that their attention is maintained long enough to complete the assessment.

IQ testing is used to document intelligence. The Wechsler Intelligence Scale for Children (WISC), the test most often chosen, consists of two portions: a verbal scale and a performance scale. A child is given three final scores: verbal IQ, performance IQ, and a combination or full-scale IQ. The child with perceptual and motor deficits tends to do poorly on the performance scale but average or better on the verbal scale. Children with language difficulty typically do poorly on the verbal scale but average or greater on the performance scale. Children with ADHD show a "scatter" pattern on both performance and verbal portions, doing well on some portions and poorly on others.

Because they have difficulty filtering out stimuli, they tend to do poorly on group-administered intelligence tests.

For this reason, test results are more accurate if they take IQ tests individually. Be certain that neurologic examinations are performed in rooms free of distractions such as attractive toys for this same reason.

Children with ADHD are often referred to a health care facility by school personnel because they are having difficulty achieving in school. Parents may have been reassured on previous occasions that, although their child has difficulty settling down to tasks, this is because he's "adventurous" or "every child is different." They may need time to accept the child's diagnosis as one that interferes with learning. Because caring for the child is exhausting for them, they may be unaware themselves of the strain the child's illness has produced in their family until they start to describe it.

Therapeutic Management

A variety of treatment methods are used, often in combination, in the management of ADHD.

Environment. Construction of a stable learning environment is crucial for children with ADHD so instruction can be free from the distractions of an entire class. Some parents may have difficulty accepting special schooling for their child (the intelligence test, after all, said their child was normal or even above average). Health care personnel can be instrumental in helping them understand that their child's condition interferes with intellectual functioning and that a special program will offer their child the best chance to succeed.

Urge parents to construct a home environment that is as free of stimulating distractions as possible. Decorating the child's room with pastel rather than primary colors, for example, can help reduce environmental stimuli. Encourage them to be fair but firm and to set consistent limits to reduce arguments. Teach parents to give instructions slowly and to make certain they have their child's attention before beginning instructions. Breaking down a chore into several steps may help (get the toy box is one step; pick up the toys is a second). If a child has difficulty making decisions because of easy distractibility, a question such as, "Do you want to wear your red or your blue shirt today?" is less effective than a statement such as, "Here is your blue shirt to wear today."

All children like to participate in dinner conversation or discussions about their day. However, children with ADHD often have difficulty telling a story or repeating a joke told to them (a sequencing problem). Suggest that parents help them by asking questions such as "Why?" "Where?" or "Who?" to reach the point of the story. Also encourage parents to be sure, when they correct behavior, that their anger is directed at something the child has deliberately done wrong and not at some incident that happened because of the child's inability to sequence, filter, or integrate concepts. If punishment is necessary, it should follow an offense quickly, before the child forgets what he did wrong. Urge parents to make sure their child understands their anger is at the behavior, not the child. It's easy for children with ADHD to develop poor self-esteem because, although they are intelligent, they cannot succeed. Helping parents build, not hinder, their development of self-esteem at every stage possible is an important nursing action.

Medication. Several medications are helpful in reducing the excessive activity of children with ADHD as well as lengthening the attention span and decreasing distractibility so they can function in school.

Methylphenidate hydrochloride (Ritalin, Concerta [extended-release form]) is the most frequently prescribed medication (Box 54.6). It works by stimulating dopamine receptors so there is more regular nerve transmission. Unfortunately, the drug has side effects of insomnia and anorexia. The insomnia may be relieved by administering the drug early in the day. Be certain at health care visits to measure height and weight to evaluate that long-term anorexia is not causing weight loss. Caution parents that this

BOX 54.6 Nursing Care Planning Based on Responsibility for Pharmacology

METHYLPHENIDATE HYDROCHLORIDE (RITALIN, CONCERTA)

Classification: Methylphenidate is a central nervous system stimulant.

Action: Acts paradoxically in children with attention deficit hyperactivity disorder, possibly by stimulating dopamine receptors to calm rather than stimulate activity (Karch, 2013).

Pregnancy Risk Category: C

Dosage: Initially, 5 mg orally before breakfast and lunch, gradually increased in 5- to 10-mg increments. The extended-release form (Concerta) is administered once daily; dosage is determined by weight and symptoms.

Possible Adverse Effects: Nervousness, insomnia, anorexia, pulse rate changes, hypertension or hypotension, tachycardia, leukopenia, anemia, and growth suppression.

Nursing Implications

- Administer the drug exactly as prescribed, and instruct parents to do the same. Reinforce proper administration of once-daily extended-release form; instruct parents to have child swallow extended-release tablets whole and to refrain from chewing or crushing them.
- Instruct the parents to administer the drug before 6 PM to prevent interference with sleep.
- Advise the parents and child to avoid over-the-counter drugs, such as cold remedies and cough syrups that contain alcohol.
- Obtain baseline vital signs and monitor on follow-up visits for changes.
- Arrange for follow-up laboratory tests, including complete blood count for children on long-term therapy.
- Stress the need for adequate nutrition in light of possible anorexia. Monitor child's weight closely for changes.
- The safety of using methylphenidate for children younger than 6 years of age has not been established.

drug offers a "high" to children who do *not* have ADHD, so their child must be conscientious that the medication is not stolen by other children to use for an euphoria effect (Viana, Trent, Tull, et al., 2012). Other medications that may be useful are atomoxetine (Strattera), a selective norepinephrine reuptake inhibitor, as well as tricyclic antidepressants. Atomoxetine and antidepressants must be used cautiously with children because they have "black box" warnings that the risk of suicide increases with their use by children (Adegbite-Adeniyi, Gron, Rowles, et al., 2012).

Family Support. Parents of a child with ADHD often need frequent health care visits because of small unintentional injuries such as lacerations or simple burns. Ask parents at these visits if they are having difficulty managing the challenge of raising a child who exhibits so much activity. Help them to understand that, because of a very complex and as yet ill-understood syndrome, the behavior is the best their child can achieve. Although hyperactivity fades with late adolescence, some children with ADHD continue to experience problems with impulsivity and inattention into adulthood. They may need counseling to find a career that fits with these behaviors and allows them to succeed as adults.

Oppositional Defiant Disorders

Oppositional defiant disorders consist of long-term hostile, negativistic, or defiant behaviors that result in disturbed functioning in academic and social domains. Children typically have difficulty controlling their temper; such anger is often directed at an authority figure.

The disorder develops most frequently in late preschool or early school age. The cause may be a combination of temperament, inheritance, and adverse social factors. Therapy is individually designed to meet the needs of the child and includes such techniques as family therapy and anger management (Fraire & Ollendick, 2012).

QSEN Checkpoint Question 54.3

Safety

Todd's father had ADHD as a child. Which of his memories from childhood would lead you to believe he was experiencing an adverse effect of methylphenidate hydrochloride (Ritalin)?

a. "I used to play that I was an astronaut for hours on end."
b. "I was the fattest kid in my gym class."
c. "I hardly ever slept; I would just lay awake for what felt like hours."
d. "I found out that I had iron-deficiency anemia in high school."

Look in Appendix A for the best answer and rationale.

Conduct Disorders

Conduct disorders are persistent antisocial acts that involve violations of personal rights or societal rules, such as disobedience, stealing, fighting, destruction of property, fire setting, and early sexual behavior (Buitelaar, Smeets, Herpers, et al., 2013). Symptoms can be clustered as involving aggression toward people and animals, destruction of property, deceitfulness and theft, and serious violations of family and community rules.

Conduct disorders are seen in about 5% to 7% of children and occur more frequently in males than in females, particularly if property or violent crimes are involved; the prevalence of conduct disorders in girls is increasing, however, so the male predominance may reduce over time. Children with the disorder seem to develop an increasing loss of self-regulation or an inability to know when to stop a disruptive action.

A number of etiologic factors are suggested as the cause of the disorder, including genetic predisposition, neurologic deficit correlates, and sociologic factors related to poverty and cultural disadvantage. The home environment may be characterized by rejection, frustration, and harsh and inconsistent discipline. Parents may have marital conflicts or substance abuse problems, or children may have had a series of inconsistent caretaking by stepparents or foster parents.

Therapy for children with conduct disorders focuses on modifying the home environment and educating the child in social skills, anger management, and problem-solving skills so children can appreciate how their behavior affects others. Learning problem-solving skills can also help children learn to generate alternative solutions to situations, sharpen thinking about the consequences of choices, and evaluate responses. In most instances, parental education is also important, but this can be difficult to achieve until the parents realize this is a family concern, not an isolated child concern. If the home environment can't be changed, removing the child from the home to a structured, consistent, and caring day care environment may produce better results.

Numerous medications such as carbamazepine (Tegretol), propranolol (Inderal), and lithium carbonate may be prescribed to reduce the aggressive behavior. Long-term therapy with an agent such as buspirone (BuSpar) may be effective in helping children control temper or explosive outbursts. It's important that conduct disorders be identified in children, or with the weapons available to them today, their aggression can lead to harm to their family, friends or strangers if they try to "make a statement" or "let others know who they are."

ANXIETY DISORDERS OF CHILDHOOD OR ADOLESCENCE

Because childhood anxieties such as stranger anxiety in the 6- to 8-month-old child (discussed in Chapter 29), separation anxiety in the toddler (discussed in Chapter 30), fear of mutilation and fear of the dark in the preschooler (discussed in Chapter 31), and performance anxiety or school avoidance in the school-age child (discussed in Chapter 32) are considered part of usual development, other anxiety disorders in children may be overlooked. If these disorders are left untreated, however, children may cope with their fear by becoming overdependent on others for support or by turning away from the problem and withdrawing into themselves, leaving them socially immature and unable to achieve in school.

Separation Anxiety in the Older Child

Separation anxiety is considered a disorder when an older child shows excessive anxiety about separation or the possibility of separation from parents. This causes them to be so worried they have difficulty falling asleep at night or insist on sleeping with their parents or just outside their parents' bedroom door. They experience acute distress and perhaps frequent nightmares about separation and, when separated, show symptoms of nausea, vomiting, or crying to such a degree that it prevents them from visiting at friends' houses, enjoying a camp experience, or actively participating in school (Santucci & Ehrenreich-May, 2013).

The disorder has a familial history and occurs slightly more frequently in girls than in boys. Temperament may be a contributing factor. Unresolved internal conflicts, insecurity in the home environment, and parent-induced anxious attachment are psychodynamic factors attributed to the disorder.

Treatment for separation anxiety includes individual and family counseling to allow the family to gain greater insight into the dynamics of the problem and aid the child to gain more confidence in the ability to function independently. For some children, antidepressant medication can be helpful. Remind parents that when children take antidepressant medication they need to be observed closely because taking antidepressants can lead to thoughts of suicide (Adegbite-Adeniyi et al., 2012).

Posttraumatic Stress Disorder

Posttraumatic stress disorder occurs in children who have survived an experience that is more traumatic than usual, such as child maltreatment, domestic violence, a natural disaster such as a hurricane, a harrowing accident such as a house fire, a home robbery, or a near-fatal illness. When these events happen, children continue to have recurring recollections or dreams of the event or demonstrate intense psychological symptoms, if a reminder of the initiating event occurs. They may feel guilt they survived the event if a close family member or friend did not.

Absence of effective support people can contribute to symptoms. Therapy consists of cognitive behavior therapy such as family counseling, eye movement desensitization, and psychological debriefing perhaps through play therapy to help a child rework the event and reduce the feeling of threat (Gillies, Taylor, Gray, et al., 2012).

EATING DISORDERS

Eating disorders consist of pica, rumination, and food aversion in young children and anorexia nervosa and bulimia nervosa in older children.

Pica

Pica is the Latin word for magpie (a bird that is an indiscriminate eater). Pica in children is the persistent eating of non-food substances such as dirt, clay, paint chips, crayons, yarn, or paper (Bryant-Waugh, Markham, Kreipe, et al., 2010). It is a potential dangerous disorder because of the possibility of unintentional poisoning. Other complications include constipation, gastrointestinal malabsorption, fecal impaction, and intestinal obstruction. The disorder is seen predominantly between the ages of 2 and 6 years, although it may be present in adolescence, especially with pregnancy. Often, it is not diagnosed until a child presents with a pica-induced complication, such as lead poisoning (see Chapter 52).

The incidence of pica increases in children who are cognitively challenged, possibly because of their inability to distinguish edible from inedible substances. It is highly associated with and may be caused by iron-deficiency anemia (which is why it occurs with a high incidence in pregnant teenage girls, who also may be iron deficient) (Young, 2010). In most instances, correcting the anemia also corrects the pica. In the meantime, devise an individualized therapy plan to keep the child safe from ingesting inedible substances until the phenomenon fades.

Rumination Disorder of Infancy

The term *rumination* comes from the Latin word for "chewing the cud" (as cattle do). It is the act of regurgitation and then reswallowing of previously ingested food. A rare disorder that usually affects infants between the ages of 3 and 12 months, it is seen most often in children who are cognitively challenged and appears to be a pleasurable act (Bredenoord, 2011). Both organic and environmental theories have been investigated to explain the disorder. In some children, an accompanying gastroesophageal reflux disorder may be implicated. It has also been postulated that rumination is a form of self-stimulation by the infant, similar to actions such as head banging and body rocking. It also may be related to an understimulating environment, although attempts to implicate the role of the primary caregiver in contributing to the disorder are not apparent. Attachment between the child and the parents, however, may be at risk because of the anxiety experienced by parents from their infant's constant regurgitation of food and consequent lack of growth.

A parent may report a child is constantly "spitting up" or vomiting or that the child's breath smells sour. Children can lose so much fluid and electrolytes through this process that they show signs of failure to thrive (a distinct problem of undernutrition discussed in Chapter 55). Distracting infants by holding, rocking, and talking to them tends to decrease rumination. Offering cereal thickened with formula or expressed breast milk may be effective in reducing rumination because this is more difficult to regurgitate than simple milk. Parents may need support, reassurance, and education to help them maintain or reestablish a bond with the child.

Food Refusal or Aversion

Food refusal or aversion is, as the name implies, failure to eat adequately because of food dislikes. The persistent failure to eat eventually results in significant failure to gain weight or actual weight loss, although no medical reason or lack of food appears to be present. The disorder begins in infancy and is usually seen in children younger than 6 years of age. It may begin because the child has more sensitive taste buds than usual, making the taste of foods less enjoyable and possibly bitter (Negri, Morini, & Greco, 2011). Because the child doesn't eat, mealtime becomes a battlefield as parents insist on the child's eating and the child persistently refuses food or exhibits extremely faddish or bizarre food preferences.

Therapy is a combination of counseling for the parents, to help them appreciate that food refusal used this way can be a potent controlling measure, and therapy for the child, to learn to recognize hunger as a stimulant to eating rather than using food refusal as a controlling or attention-getting mechanism. By late school age, food aversion seems to fade and, along with it, the parent–child conflict.

Anorexia Nervosa

Anorexia nervosa is characterized by refusal to maintain a minimally usual body weight because of a disturbance in perception of the size or appearance of the body (Clarkin, 2012). It may be genetically based and includes three separate features: self-induced starvation to a significant degree, a relentless drive for thinness, and medical signs and symptoms resulting from starvation. In an era when health care providers concentrate on reducing obesity, it is easy to miss that underweight can be just as unhealthy as too much weight (Bonsergent, Agrinier, Thilly, et al., 2013).

Specific characteristics of a child with anorexia nervosa that are usually present include:

- Severely distorted body image
- Body mass index (BMI) less than 17.5 or less than 85% of expected weight
- Intense fear of gaining weight or becoming fat even though underweight
- Refusal to acknowledge seriousness of weight loss
- Amenorrhea (in girls)

Anorexia nervosa occurs most often in girls (90%), usually at puberty or during adolescence. It is also more common in lesbian, gay, or bisexual youth (Austin, Nelson, Birkett, et al., 2013) and among sisters and daughters of mothers who also had the disorder.

Children with the disorder think of themselves as overweight even though their weight is adequate and thus severely limit their intake, begin excessive exercise, or use emetics, laxatives, enemas, or diuretics (purging) to better reduce their weight to what they envision their weight should be (Sigel, 2012).

Children who develop an eating disorder this way may have a genetic susceptibility to the illness. Stressors in their environment such as parental divorce, social pressure to lose weight, and personal psychological trauma such as attempted rape can then set into motion a chain reaction that, coupled with the genetic tendency, leads to the development of the eating disorder. Adolescents who are "overachievers" or strive to be the best academically or at sports may develop the disorder as a way of helping them improve a poor self-image or feelings of inadequacy (they cannot live up to their own or their parents' expectations) because excessive dieting can offer them a sense of control they otherwise don't feel.

Lack of nutrition can become so extreme in these children that it causes delayed pubertal development. They develop a starved appearance and significant symptoms of dehydration and acidosis. They may develop severe osteoporosis from loss of calcium from bones (Swenne & Stridsberg, 2012).

Assessment

Because of their intense fear of becoming obese, children with anorexia come to perceive food as revolting and nauseating; they refuse to eat or else vomit food immediately after eating. Always ask if, in addition to not eating, the child is using a laxative or diuretic or extensively exercising to further lose weight because it is the lack of food plus these measures that leads eventually not only to the excessive weight loss but also acidosis, dependent edema, hypotension, hypothermia, bradycardia, and the formation of lanugo (fine, neonatal-like hair). If the process is allowed to continue without therapy, it can lead to starvation and death.

By the time most children are seen at health care facilities, they are already extremely underweight, pale, and lethargic, and amenorrhea is present in girls. Often, the child's parents have tried various methods of getting the child to eat, such as threatening, coaxing, and punishing; as a result, parent–child relationships may be strained. Parents may feel guilty for insisting their child lose weight if the girl was once overweight.

Therapeutic Management

Planning and outcome identification for a child with anorexia nervosa needs to be realistic. Remember that, although the condition began as a psychosocial problem, by the time a child is seen for care, physical starvation and its effects have become a second important component. A girl who grows nauseated just looking at food cannot quickly begin to ingest a large amount. For therapy, typically, oral foods are withheld to prevent vomiting, and total parenteral nutrition or enteral feedings (nasogastric or gastronomy) are initiated to supply needed fat, protein, and calories. Children usually accept total parenteral nutrition well because they view it as medicine, not as food.

In addition, identification of emotional triggers, education about normal nutritional needs, antidepressants if warranted, and establishing trust and effective communication are crucial measures to help the child resolve interpersonal issues that are present (Box 54.7).

The goal of therapy is gradual weight gain (1 to 3 lb a week) because a rapid gain of weight can cause a child to begin dieting to reduce this weight gain. Weighing once a week is better than every day, to reduce the focus on weight. An SSRI such as escitalopram (Lexapro) and mood regulators such as risperidone (Risperdal) and quetiapine (Seroquel) may be helpful in some children.

Children who have had anorexia nervosa need continued follow-up after weight is regained to be certain they do not revert to their former dieting pattern (Fig. 54.2). Counseling may need to be continued for 2 to 3 years to be certain self-image is maintained. With adequate counseling, most girls achieve better reactions to stress and achieve full recovery with adulthood.

What if...54.2 Every time you see Todd at the clinic, his teenage sister, Cheyenne, looks more and more underweight to you. Her mother tells you she's lost 20 lb in the past 6 months. "She's the perfect daughter, always getting straight A's in school," the mother adds. Would you be worried about Cheyenne?

Bulimia Nervosa

Bulimia refers to recurrent and episodic **binge eating** and **purging** by vomiting, accompanied by awareness that the eating pattern is abnormal yet the child is not able to stop the pattern (Lock, 2013). A period of depression or guilt usually follows the period of bingeing. Like anorexia nervosa, bulimia typically is seen in adolescence or early adult life and predominantly in girls. The disorder may last for months or years with periods of normal eating interspersed between

BOX 54.7 Nursing Care Planning Based on Effective Communication

Cheyenne, 15 years old, is 5 ft 8 in. tall and weighs 95 lb. She is diagnosed as having anorexia nervosa.

Less Effective Communication

Nurse: Let's talk about your weight, Cheyenne.
Cheyenne: I know I'm fat. Look at this belly of mine.
Nurse: You need to eat at least three good meals a day.
Cheyenne: I do. I eat a lot.
Nurse: You especially should have a healthy breakfast. It's the most important meal of the day.
Cheyenne: I eat huge breakfasts. I'm just so active, I don't gain weight.

More Effective Communication

Nurse: Let's talk about your weight, Cheyenne.
Cheyenne: I know I'm fat. Look at this belly of mine.
Nurse: You feel fat?
Cheyenne: I am fat. I pig out constantly.
Nurse: What did you pig out on for breakfast this morning?
Cheyenne: Well, nothing this morning, but I was in a hurry.

Notice how, in the first scenario, the nurse is intent on persuading the client to eat. In the second scenario, the nurse is attempting to obtain more information about the client, her image of herself, and her diet in the hope that, when she knows more about her, she can help her eat more.

bulimic ones. Food consumed during a binge often has a high caloric content and a texture that facilitates rapid eating. It may be eaten secretly, such as late at night or in the privacy of a bedroom. After ingestion of this food, abdominal pain develops, and the teen will vomit to decrease the physical pain of abdominal distention as well as to improve self-concept that they couldn't possibly lack that much control.

Some teenagers with the disorder rely on laxatives and diuretics and excessive exercise in place of vomiting to maintain their weight (a nonpurging type) (Sigel, 2012). With either type, the combination of frequent vomiting and use of laxative or diuretics can result in such serious physical complications, notably electrolyte abnormalities, that these can ultimately lead to effects as severe as cardiac arrest. Adolescents with purging may develop severe erosion of their teeth because of the constant exposure to acidic gastrointestinal juices from vomiting. Esophageal tears may also result from forceful vomiting.

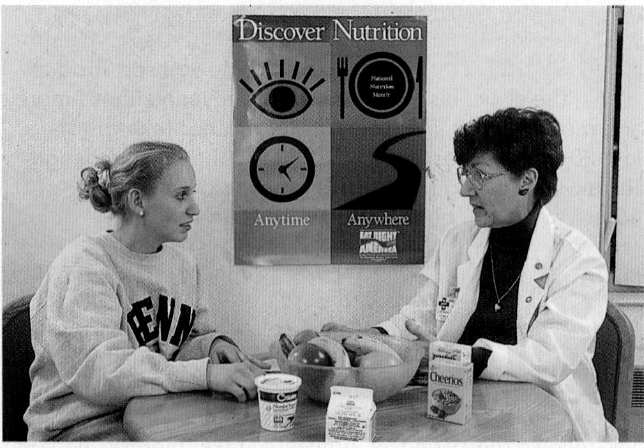

FIGURE 54.2 This anorexic teen, who is in the later stages of treatment, continues to meet with a counselor to discuss her food choices, exercise program, and overall well-being. (© Barbara Proud.)

The cause of the disorder may be related to unusual levels of serotonin but also has psychosocial components as these teens exhibit great concern about their weight and overall body image and appearance. In contrast to children with anorexia, however, most of those with bulimia are only slightly underweight or are of average weight and therefore may be discounted as merely slim unless a thorough history is obtained. As with anorexia nervosa, therapy consists of antidepressants, perhaps the use of ondansetron (Zofran), a serotonin antagonist, and counseling aimed at increasing the child's self-esteem and sense of control.

QSEN Checkpoint Question 54.4

Evidence-Based Practice

Eating disorders have a high incidence in adolescents. To see if this also exists in teenage athletes, researchers asked 966 first-year high school students to complete a questionnaire and then sit for an interview as to whether they have or ever had an eating disorder. Results of the study showed that the prevalence of eating disorders was higher in athletes compared to nonathletes (6.9% versus 2.3%). It was also higher in female than male athletes (13.5% versus 3.2%) (Martinsen & Sundgot-Borgen, 2013).

Based on the previous study, which statement by Cheyenne, Todd's adolescent sister, would make her at highest risk for developing an eating disorder?

a. "I hate sports. Nothing more athletic than poker interests me."
b. "I've played basketball for two years; I like the way I look in uniform."
c. "I don't play a whole lot of sports, but I love watching football games."
d. "I don't know why girls play sports like tennis; they all look so skinny."

Look in Appendix A for the best answer and rationale.

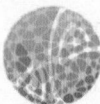

TIC DISORDERS

Tic disorders are abnormalities of semi-involuntary movement that apparently result from dysfunction in the basal ganglia. *Tics* are rapid, repetitive muscle movements, such as rapid eye blinking or facial twitching. They usually become more pronounced during periods of stress and diminish during sleep. **Motor tics** include eye blinking, neck jerking, and facial grimacing. Simple **vocal tics** include coughing, throat clearing, snorting, and barking. Complex motor tics include facial gestures, grooming behaviors, jumping, touching, and smelling objects.

Children are most prone to these disorders between the ages of 9 and 13 years. They occur more frequently in boys than in girls and more frequently in children who demonstrate obsessive–compulsive behavior. Some instances tend to be familial, possibly because of dopamine receptor inhibition. They occur so frequently that as many as 15% of children experience some form of transient tic disorder (Plessen, 2013).

Because transient tics are associated with high stress, treatment usually focuses on reducing areas of stress in the child's life. Pointing out the mannerism to the child is not usually helpful and may intensify the frequency of the manifestation if it increases stress. Behavior modification may be successful in eliminating a particular tic. If the stress is not removed, however, the child may substitute another compulsive mechanism for the original tic.

Tourette Syndrome

Tourette syndrome is an inherited syndrome of motor and phonic vocal tics (Wu & Gilbert, 2013). It occurs three times more frequently in boys than in girls and, because it is inherited, often, there is some other form of tic in another family member. Typically, the age of onset is around 7 years, with motor tics usually occurring before vocal tics. **Complex vocal tics** include the repeated use of words or phrases out of context—specifically, **coprolalia** (use of socially unacceptable words, usually obscenities), **palilalia** (repeating one's own words), and *echolalia* (repeating others' words). Some children with this syndrome have nonspecific electroencephalographic abnormalities and soft neurologic signs that aid in diagnosis. Although most children can suppress their tics for short periods, the syndrome lasts a lifetime. Children with Tourette syndrome can develop low self-esteem because of their uncontrollable actions before the syndrome is fully diagnosed. Fortunately, this syndrome responds to administration of neuroleptic agents such as haloperidol (Haldol) or pimozide (Orap).

QSEN Checkpoint Question 54.5

Quality Improvement

Cheyenne tells you she had a transient tic disorder when she was in grade school. You would rate her subsequent care as most adequate if it included assessment for which of the following?

a. Signs she has developed a convulsive disorder
b. Lack of sensitivity to pain from autistic disorder
c. Gastrointestinal symptoms because she likely has pica
d. Depression because she has a loss of self-esteem

Look in Appendix A for the best answer and rationale.

DEPRESSION AND PSYCHIATRIC DISORDERS AFFECTING CHILDREN

Two mental health illnesses typically thought of as occurring in adults, depression and schizophrenia, have their roots in childhood.

Childhood Depressive Episodes

Children and adolescents can experience depressive episodes similar to those experienced by adults (Hagerty, 2012). The incidence ranges from 1% to 3% before puberty and 3% to 6% among adolescents. A child is considered to be depressed when symptoms such as loss of interest or pleasure, significant weight loss or gain, depressed mood, insomnia, psychomotor agitation, feelings of worthlessness or excessive or inappropriate guilt, diminished concentration, recurrent thoughts of death, and suicidal ideation exist for 2 weeks or longer. Underlying factors that lead to extended depression in children are marital discord or violence, paternal anxiety, and lack of family or social support (Fatori, Bordin, Curto, et al., 2013). Because these symptoms are easily missed, a history should be taken from the child as well as from the parents at well-child health care visits. A major way depression can be differentiated from "usual" sadness is when children report they cannot remember the last time they felt happy or had a good time **(anhedonia)** (Fig. 54.3).

Children who are depressed need therapy to prevent their depression from worsening, such as individual or family counseling time to help children regain self-esteem and the family to understand the level of depression that has occurred. In addition to counseling, some children require antidepressant therapy with an SSRI to relieve the symptoms. Observe carefully any child who is prescribed an antidepressant to detect deepening depression or presuicidal behavior because this is associated with antidepressant use in children. Adolescent self-injury as a result of depression is discussed in Chapter 33 with concerns of the adolescent.

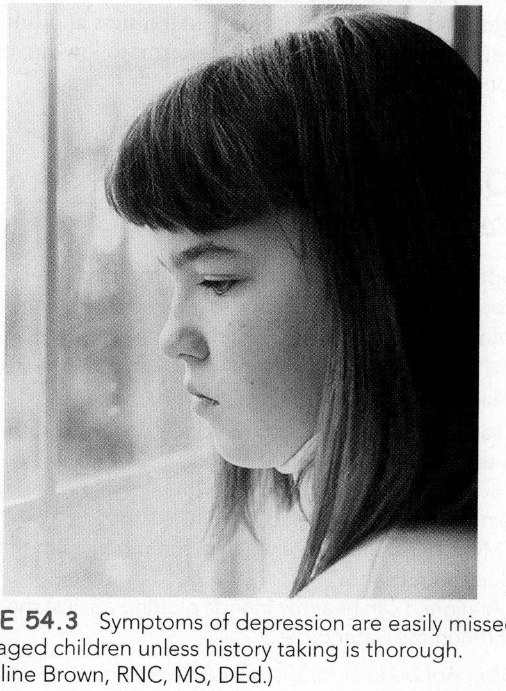

FIGURE 54.3 Symptoms of depression are easily missed in school-aged children unless history taking is thorough. (© Caroline Brown, RNC, MS, DEd.)

What if... 54.3 The parents of Cheyenne, Todd's sister, tell you she seems increasingly tired, so much so that she sleeps almost all day every weekend. Is this usual teenage behavior, or does Cheyenne need a referral to detect whether she is depressed?

Childhood Schizophrenia

Schizophrenia is actually a group of disorders of thought processes characterized by the gradual disintegration of mental functioning; it occurs in about 2 of every 10,000 children (Miller & Buckley, 2013). It is a devastating mental illness that most commonly strikes in adolescence or young adulthood. Symptoms until that time may be undifferentiated or ill defined.

Despite years of investigation, the cause of schizophrenia is unknown. Current evidence suggests there may be both genetic and environmental bases for the disorder. Magnetic resonance imaging has shown that cerebral involvement, such as enlarged ventricles, decreased blood to the frontal lobe, or cortical cell loss, may begin the disorder. Neurochemical mediators may influence or prolong the disorder.

Children with schizophrenia experience hallucinations (hear or see people or objects that other people cannot) and may display rambling or illogical speech patterns. They may not be responsive (have a **flat affect**), may withdraw into themselves so completely they are stuporous **(catatonia),** or be so extremely suspicious that others want to harm them (paranoia) that it is difficult for them to function. Although schizophrenic manifestations may occur suddenly after a major stress in a child's life (such as rejection by a boyfriend or girlfriend), subtle signs of mental illness have usually been present for some time.

The diagnosis of a psychotic disorder of this extent is a shock to parents. Fortunately, therapy with modern antipsychotic drugs such as clozapine is effective in reducing children's hallucinations and bizarre thought processes. Many children who are diagnosed as having schizophrenia in childhood continue to have mental illness as adults, making continuing support and long-term follow-up essential (Malone-Cole, 2012).

QSEN Checkpoint Question 54.6

Teamwork & Collaboration

Symptoms of schizophrenia often begin in adolescence, so you are reviewing Cheyenne's history with a psychiatric–mental health nurse. Which statement by Cheyenne would signal to you and your colleague that she is developing symptoms of schizophrenia?

a. "I absolutely hate babysitting for my younger brother on week nights."
b. "Both my English and math teachers gave me bad marks last quarter. I got so mad."
c. "My father seems more worried about his health than he does about mine."
d. "At night, I can hear my friends plotting against me through the water pipes."

Look in Appendix A for the best answer and rationale.

ELIMINATION DISORDERS

Elimination disorders include functional enuresis (involuntary loss of urine) and encopresis (involuntary loss of feces). Developmental enuresis is discussed in Chapter 31 with the development of the preschooler.

Encopresis

Loss of feces is *encopresis* if there is repeated passage of feces at least once a month in places not culturally appropriate for that purpose. It is more common in boys than in girls and considered primary if the child was never fully toilet trained and secondary if the problem began after effective training (Coehlo, 2011). It is diagnosed only after medical causes such as lactase deficiency, thyroid disease, hypercalcemia, Hirschsprung disease, and infectious diarrhea have been ruled out.

Isolated occurrences of encopresis may happen when a sibling is born (as part of an overall regression reaction) or when a child is visiting at a strange house and is too shy to ask for the bathroom. It can occur in a new school because a child can't locate a bathroom in time or can't use a bathroom because it is "owned" by a school gang.

In a few instances, encopresis occurs because hard bowel movements cause anal fissures. Because it then hurts to move the bowels, children avoid bowel movements, leading to chronically distended rectums. They are then no longer able to sense when they need to defecate, so involuntary or overflow defecation occurs.

Assessment

To document encopresis, take a careful history of usual bowel evacuation habits, the number of bowel accidents, and the times at which they occur. Investigate any recent changes or stress factors in the child's environment. A physical examination that includes a rectal examination should be done to establish whether there is proper anal sphincter control. If anal fissures are present, whether child maltreatment has occurred needs to be investigated.

Therapeutic Management

Reserving time in a busy household for children to evacuate their bowels about two times daily (in the morning and after dinner) may create "habit" periods for them. It's especially advantageous if they're able to evacuate their bowels before they leave for school in the morning, because then they're less likely to experience encopresis and embarrassment in school. The administration of a stool softener such as lactulose, a high-fiber diet, or 1 to 6 tablespoons of mineral oil daily for 2 or 3 months often softens stools so bowel movements are not painful. Remind parents that children receiving long-term mineral oil therapy also need to take water-soluble forms of vitamins A, D, and K, because these vitamins tend to be removed from the gastrointestinal tract with the mineral oil.

Emphasize to parents that children should not be punished for encopresis. Encourage them to pay as little attention as possible to bowel accidents and to give praise for days when encopresis does not occur.

Enuresis

Enuresis is defined as repeated involuntary or intentional urination during the day or at night after an age at which a child has attained or should have attained control over bladder function, when no organic cause for the problem can be found (Deshpande, Caldwell, & Sureshkumar, 2012). Although stress may be a factor in occurrences of enuresis, its primary cause is unknown. Most children outgrow the problem by adolescence. As with encopresis, the most serious result of enuresis is related to the child's feelings of failure with each occurrence and associated rejection by peers. All this contributes to a lowered sense of self-esteem. The problem and associated nursing diagnoses are described in more detail in Chapter 46.

What if...54.4 You are particularly interested in exploring one of the 2020 National Health Goals related to mental illness in children (see Box 54.1). What would be a possible research topic to explore pertinent to this goal that would be applicable to Todd's and Cheyenne's family and also advance evidence-based practice?

Key Points For Review

- Both cognitive and mental health disorders pose long-term care concerns for children and their families.
- For children who are cognitively challenged, a stigma still may be present in many communities, although less so than previously. Help parents to gain the insight that cognitive challenges occur in a proportion of infants in every population and that having a child with this problem merely reflects a chance occurrence not a reflection of their family's capabilities.
- Mental health disorders often begin subtly in children and are often first manifested as behavior problems in school. Assess thoroughly any child who is referred for disruptive behavior in a school class for the possibility the child has a serious mental health problem in order to not only meet QSEN competencies but also best meet the family's total needs.
- Autism spectrum disorder is a pervasive developmental disorder that has a range of behaviors, including fascination with movement, impairment of communication skills, and insensitivity to pain.
- Attention deficit and disruptive behavior disorders, such as oppositional defiant and conduct disorders, may occur in childhood. Children with ADHD may be treated with methylphenidate hydrochloride (Ritalin, Concerta) to reduce the hyperactivity and allow them to achieve better in school and interact successfully at home.
- Eating disorders seen in childhood include pica, rumination, anorexia nervosa, and bulimia. All of these disorders can lead to loss of weight and electrolyte imbalances if left unrecognized and untreated.
- Tic disorders such as Tourette syndrome are abnormalities of semi-involuntary movement that are thought to result from dysfunction of the basal ganglia or distorted dopamine reception.
- Children who are depressed are at high risk for self-injury. They need thorough assessment and close observation to be certain that this does not happen. Monitor children carefully who are prescribed antidepressants to relieve depression because these may actually increase self-injury attempts.
- Schizophrenia often begins in adolescence. It usually presents as disorganized behavior. Long-term therapy with antipsychotic drugs is necessary.
- Encopresis is the repeated passage of feces in places not culturally appropriate for that purpose. Therapy is both physiologic and psychological.

Critical Thinking Care Study

Leonette is an 8-year-old child you see at an ambulatory clinic. She began loud lip smacking and shouting, "Hey! Hey! Hey!" almost constantly when she was 4 years old. That was the time her parents were divorced, so her mother thought for a long time that her behavior was a reaction to the divorce. A childcare teacher suggested that it might be something more significant, and Leonette was diagnosed with Tourette syndrome. Today, she takes haloperidol and still has those mannerisms, but they only occur when she's in a new situation or stressed. Leonette lives with her mother; a new stepfather; two stepbrothers, ages 12 and 14 years; and a new baby sister, age 2 months. Because the house is small, Leonette and her two brothers share a bedroom and bathroom. "Not a good arrangement," Mrs. Firestone tells you, "but workable." Mrs. Firestone works as a teller at a local bank; she has just returned to work after a 10-week maternity leave; her husband sells real estate.

1. "Take Your Daughter to Work Day" is next week, so you ask Leonette's mother if she is going to take Leonette to the bank with her. Mrs. Leonette looks uncomfortable at your question and replies quickly, "No. It's not allowed, because we handle money and everything." Leonette looks disappointed. Would you suggest that Mrs. Firestone take Leonette, or would the visit be too upsetting to suggest?
2. Leonette's mother brought her to the clinic today because she's had two episodes in the past month where the school called her to take Leonette home because of encopresis. When you ask the mother when was the last time Leonette moved her bowels at home, her mother answers, "No idea. I don't have time to keep track of who's going to the bathroom or not." How could you help this family?
3. You notice that Leonette is afraid to leave her mother's side to come into an examining room so you can take her blood pressure. Her mother tells you she has had to stay home from work for the past 3 days because Leonette refused to go to school and even refuses to leave her side, following her from room to room in the house and sleeping on the floor at the foot of her bed. "Her teacher said it's separation anxiety from the new marriage and will pass," the mother tells you. Would you be concerned that this is not as simple a problem as the mother suggests?

Patient Scenario

The Berlinger Family

Read about the Berlinger family, a family with a child with a mental health concern, then answer the questions to further sharpen your skills and grow more familiar with NCLEX-type questions related to nursing care of a family with a cognitive or mental health concern. Confirm your answers are correct by reading the rationales.

Visit http://thePoint.lww.com

Answers and Rationales

Looking for answers to the What if . . . and Critical Thinking Care Study questions?

Visit http://thePoint.lww.com

References

Adegbite-Adeniyi, C., Gron, B., Rowles, B. M., et al. (2012). An update on antidepressant use and suicidality in pediatric depression. *Expert Opinion in Pharmacotherapy, 13*(15), 2119–2130.

American Psychiatric Association. (2000). *Diagnostic and statistical manual of mental disorders* (4th ed., text rev.). Washington, DC: Author.

Austin, S. B., Nelson, L. A., Birkett, M. A., et al. (2013). Eating Disorder symptoms and obesity at the intersections of gender, ethnicity, and sexual orientation in US high school students. *American Journal of Public Health, 103*(2), e16–e22.

Autism Society. (2012). *Facts & statistics*. Bethesda, MD: Author.

Batorowicz, B., Missiuna, C. A., & Pollock, N. A. (2012). Technology supporting written productivity in children with learning disabilities: A critical review. *Canadian Journal of Occupational Therapy, 79*(4), 211–224.

Bölte, S., Duketis, E., Poustka, F., et al. (2011). Sex differences in cognitive domains and their clinical correlates in higher-functioning autism spectrum disorders. *Autism, 15*(4), 497–511.

Bonsergent, E., Agrinier, N., Thilly, N., et al. (2013). Overweight and obesity prevention for adolescents: A cluster randomized controlled trial in a school setting. *American Journal of Preventive Medicine, 44*(1), 30–39.

Bredenoord, A. J. (2011). Belching, aerophagia, and rumination. *Journal of Pediatric Gastroenterology Nutrition, 53*(Suppl. 2), S19–S21.

Brosbe, M. S., Faust, J., & Gold, S. N. (2013). Complex traumatic stress in the pediatric medical setting. *Journal of Trauma Dissociation, 14*(1), 97–112.

Bryant-Waugh, R., Markham, L., Kreipe, R. E., et al. (2010). Feeding and eating disorders in childhood. *International Journal of Eating Disorders, 43*(2), 98–111.

Buitelaar, J. K., Smeets, K. C., Herpers, P., et al. (2013). Conduct disorders. *European Child & Adolescence Psychiatry, 22*(Suppl. 1), 49–54.

Carter, E. W., Lane, K. L., Cooney, M., et al. (2013). Parent assessments of self-determination importance and performance for students with autism or intellectual disability. *American Journal of Intellectual Developmental Disabilities, 118*(1), 16–31.

Casey, A. F., & Rasmussen, R. (2013). Reduction measures and percent body fat in individuals with intellectual disabilities: A scoping review. *Disability & Health Journal, 6*(1), 2–7.

Clarkin, A. (2012). Eating disorders. In K. M. Fortinash & P. A. Holoday Worret (Eds.), *Psychiatric mental health nursing* (5th ed., pp. 416–436). St. Louis, MO: Elsevier/Mosby.

Coehlo, D. P. (2011). Encopresis: A medical and family approach. *Pediatric Nursing, 37*(3), 107–112.

Davies, L., & Oliver, C. (2013). The age related prevalence of aggression and self-injury in persons with an intellectual disability: A review. *Research in Developmental Disabilities, 34*(2), 764–775.

Deshpande, A. V., Caldwell, P. H., & Sureshkumar, P. (2012). Drugs for nocturnal enuresis in children (other than desmopressin and tricyclics). *Cochrane Database of Systematic Reviews,* (12), CD002238.

DuPaul, G. J., Gormley, M. J., & Laracy, S. D. (2013). Comorbidity of LD and ADHD: Implications of DSM-5 for assessment and treatment. *Journal of Learning Disabilities, 46*(1), 43–51.

Fatori, D., Bordin, I. A., Curto, B. M., et al. (2013). Influence of psychosocial risk factors on the trajectory of mental health problems from childhood to adolescence: A longitudinal study. *BMC Psychiatry, 13*(1), 31.

Flanagan, C. M. (2012). Disorders of infancy, childhood & adolescence. In K. M. Fortinash & P. A. Holoday Worret (Eds.), *Psychiatric mental health nursing* (5th ed., pp. 392–415). St. Louis, MO: Elsevier/Mosby.

Fraire, M. G., & Ollendick, T. H. (2012). Anxiety and oppositional defiant disorder: A transdiagnostic conceptualization. *Clinical Psychology Reviews, 33*(2), 229–240.

Gillies, D., Taylor, F., Gray, C., et al. (2012). Psychological therapies for the treatment of post-traumatic stress disorder in children and adolescents. *Cochrane Database of Systematic Reviews,* (12), CD006726.

Hagerty, B. M. (2012). Mood disorders, depression, bipolar & adjustment disorders. In K. M. Fortinash & P. A. Holoday Worret (Eds.), *Psychiatric mental health nursing* (5th ed., pp. 218–258). St. Louis, MO: Elsevier/Mosby.

Hall, H. R., & Graff, J. C. (2012). Maladaptive behaviors of children with autism: Parent support, stress, and coping. *Issues in Comprehensive Pediatric Nursing, 35*(3–4), 194–214.

Kirkland, A. (2012). Credibility battles in the autism litigation. *Social Studies of Science, 42*(2), 237–261.

Lock, J. (2013). Bulimia nervosa. In E. T. Bope & R. D. Kellerman (Eds.), *Conn's current therapy* (pp. 930–932). Philadelphia, PA: Elsevier/Saunders.

Maglione, M. A., Gans, D., Das, L., et al. (2012). Nonmedical interventions for children with ASD: Recommended guidelines and further research needs. *Pediatrics, 130*(Suppl. 2), S169–S178.

Malone-Cole, J. A. (2012). Schizophrenia & other psychiatric disorders. In K. M. Fortinash & P. A. Holoday Worret (Eds.), *Psychiatric mental health nursing* (5th ed., pp. 259–297). St. Louis, MO: Elsevier/Mosby.

Martinsen, M., & Sundgot-Borgen, J. (2013). Higher prevalence of eating disorders among adolescent elite athletes than controls. *Medicine and Science in Sports and Exercise, 45*(6), 1188–1197.

McGillivray, J. A., & Kershaw, M. M. (2013). The impact of staff initiated referral and intervention protocols on symptoms of depression in people with mild intellectual disability. *Research in Developmental Disabilities, 34*(2), 730–738.

Miller, B., & Buckley, P. (2013). Schizophrenia. In E. T. Bope & R. D. Kellerman (Eds.), *Conn's current therapy* (pp. 952–956). Philadelphia, PA: Elsevier/Saunders.

Negri, R., Morini, G., & Greco, L. (2011). From the tongue to the gut. *Journal of Pediatric Gastroenterology & Nutrition, 53*(6), 601–605.

Plessen, K. J. (2013). Tic disorders and Tourette's syndrome. *European Child & Adolescent Psychiatry, 22*(Suppl. 1), 55–60.

Santucci, L. C., & Ehrenreich-May, J. (2013). A randomized controlled trial of the child anxiety multi-day program (cAMP) for separation anxiety disorder. *Child Psychiatry and Human Development, 44*(3), 439–451.

Scheffer, R. (2011). Psychiatric disorders. In K. J. Marcdante, R. M. Kliegman, H. B. Jenson, et al. (Eds.), *Nelson essentials of pediatrics* (6th ed., pp. 63–80). Philadelphia, PA: Saunders/Elsevier.

Sigel, E. J. (2012). Eating disorders. In W. Hay, M. Levin, R. Deterding, et al. (Eds.), *Current diagnosis & treatment pediatrics* (21st ed., pp. 167–178). New York, NY: McGraw-Hill/Lange.

Stafford, B., Talmi, A., & Burstein, A. (2012). Child & adolescent psychiatric disorders & psychosocial aspects of pediatrics. In W. Hay, M. Levin, R. Deterding, et al. (Eds.), *Current diagnosis & treatment pediatrics* (21st ed., pp. 179–222). New York, NY: McGraw-Hill/Lange.

Starke, M. (2011). Young adults with intellectual disability recall their childhood. *Journal of Intellectual Disabilities, 15*(4), 229–240.

Swenne, I., & Stridsberg, M. (2012). Bone metabolism markers in adolescent girls with eating disorders and weight loss: Effects of growth, weight trend, developmental and menstrual status. *Archives of Osteoporosis, 7*(1–2), 125–133.

U.S. Department of Health and Human Services. (2010). *Healthy people 2020*. Washington, DC: Author.

Viana, A. G., Trent, L., Tull, M. T., et al. (2012). Non-medical use of prescription drugs among Mississippi youth: Constitutional, psychological, and family factors. *Addictive Behavior, 37*(12), 1382–1388.

Wu, S. W., & Gilbert, D. L. (2013). Gilles de la Tourette syndrome. In E. T. Bope & R. D. Kellerman (Eds.), *Conn's current therapy* (pp. 605–607). Philadelphia, PA: Elsevier/Saunders.

Yildirim, A., Hacihasanoğlu Aşilar, R., & Karakurt, P. (2013). Effects of a nursing intervention program on the depression and perception of family functioning of mothers with intellectually disabled children. *Journal of Clinical Nursing, 22*(1–2), 251–261.

Young, S. L. (2010). Pica in pregnancy: New ideas about an old condition. *Annual Review of Nutrition, 30*(8), 403–422.

Chapter 55

Nursing Care of a Family in Crisis: Maltreatment and Violence in the Family

KEY TERMS

- failure to thrive
- hebephile
- incest
- intimate partner violence
- learned helplessness
- maltreatment
- mandatory reporters
- molestation
- Munchausen syndrome by proxy
- pedophile
- permissive reporters
- rape trauma syndrome
- shaken baby syndrome
- silent rape syndrome

OBJECTIVES

After mastering the contents of this chapter, you should be able to:

1. Discuss the types of child maltreatment or intimate partner violence seen in families and the theories explaining their occurrence.
2. Identify 2020 National Health Goals related to child maltreatment or intimate partner violence that nurses can help the nation achieve.
3. Assess a family that has experienced physical or emotional child maltreatment or intimate partner violence.
4. Formulate nursing diagnoses related to a family in which child maltreatment or intimate partner violence is present.
5. Develop expected outcomes for a family that has experienced child maltreatment or intimate partner violence to help them manage seamless transitions across differing health care settings.
6. Using the nursing process, plan nursing care that includes the six competencies of Quality & Safety Education for Nurses (QSEN): Patient-Centered Care, Teamwork & Collaboration, Evidence-Based Practice (EBP), Quality Improvement (QI), Safety, and Informatics.
7. Implement nursing care for a family in which child maltreatment or intimate partner violence has occurred, such as ways to role model better parenting.
8. Evaluate expected outcomes for effectiveness and achievement of care.
9. Integrate knowledge of family child maltreatment or intimate partner violence with the interplay of nursing process, the six competencies of QSEN, and Family Nursing to promote quality maternal and child health nursing care.

Hillary Landstrum is a 3-year-old you see in an emergency department. Her mother, who is the city mayor, tells you Hillary fell off a swing in the backyard. Hillary has a broken forearm, a broken rib, and multiple bruises on her chest and back. You notice in her electronic record that Hillary was seen in the same emergency room a month ago for a burn on her hand. When you mention to her mother that Hillary's injuries seem extreme for a simple fall, her mother says, "She isn't very pretty. I guess she's also clumsy."

Previous chapters described the normal growth and development of children and care of children with disorders of specific body systems. This chapter adds information about the effect on children when child maltreatment or intimate partner violence occurs in a family. Such information can build a base for care and for putting into place ways to prevent further maltreatment or violence.

You suspect Hillary is a victim of child maltreatment. What additional questions would you want to ask her mother to help determine whether this is so? What should you do if you feel certain Hillary has been maltreated?

Child protective services in the United States receive 3.3 million reports of children being maltreated or neglected per year, with about 772,000 of those children determined to have been maltreated (Centers for Disease Control and Prevention [CDC], 2012). A nationally representative sample determined that 10.2% of U.S. children are maltreated in some way, and the lifetime cost in medical bills and lost productivity is over $210,000 per child, making the total economic cost of maltreatment as much as $585 billion a year nationally (Fang, Brown, Florence, et al., 2012).

Child maltreatment is associated with stress and has been linked to inability of a family to handle external and internal stressors. Accordingly, maltreatment or violence in a family is rarely an isolated event but rather an indication of how much the family needs overall care (McCloskey, 2013).

Maltreatment, formerly termed *abuse*, is defined as the "willful injury by one person of another" (Helfer & Kempe, 1987) and takes many forms: physical or emotional maltreatment, neglect or sexual maltreatment, intimate partner violence, and maltreatment or violence of the elderly. Maternity, child health, and family care nurses need to be especially observant for signs of possible maltreatment or violence in a family because these increase during pregnancy and possibly during the care of an ill child. In all instances, the victim's safety is paramount, but ensuring this safety must be done with sensitivity to the importance of maintaining and improving overall family functioning.

Child maltreatment has long-term consequences, because as many as 30% of children from families where there is child maltreatment become maltreating parents themselves (A. J. Lang, Garstein, Rodgers, et al., 2010; Valentino, Nuttall, Comas, et al., 2012). It also predisposes victims to numerous psychological problems and induces a persistent sensitization of the stress-response system (Heim, Shugart, Craighead, et al., 2010). Box 55.1 shows 2020 National Health Goals related to child maltreatment and intimate partner violence.

BOX 55.1 Nursing Care Planning Based on 2020 National Health Goals

The mark of a developed nation is the ability to protect the health of its most vulnerable members. This makes both child maltreatment and intimate partner violence both national health concerns. Examples of 2020 National Health Goals that specifically address these issues are:

- Reduce the rate of maltreatment of children younger than 18 years of age from a baseline of 9.4 per 1,000 to a target level of 8.5 per 1,000.
- Reduce the rate of child maltreatment fatalities from a baseline of 2.4 per 100,000 to a target level of 2.2 per 100,000.
- Reduce the rate of physical, sexual, and psychological violence by current or former intimate partners.
- Reduce stalking by former or present intimate partners.
- Reduce abusive sexual conduct and rape (U.S. Department of Health and Human Services [DHHS], 2010; see www.healthypeople.gov).

Nurses can help the nation achieve these goals by educating parents about how to parent more effectively and by identifying children or adults in school or health care agency settings who have been maltreated, neglected, or a victim of violence.

Nursing Process Overview

For Care of a Family That Has Experienced Child Maltreatment or Intimate Partner Violence

Assessment

Nurses are often the first individuals to identify symptoms of possible child maltreatment or intimate partner violence in a family, because they are often the first to take a health history or see a child or woman undressed at a health care visit and recognize significant bruising; they are also often the person to whom a pregnant woman or child confides the problem. If maltreatment or violence in any form is suspected, it is essential to get as full a picture as possible. If child maltreatment is suspected, talk with the parents first, without the child, and then interview the child separately to help to uncover any inconsistencies in the parents' explanations. Remember, however, you are *not* investigating the concern—you are doing an initial screening to assess the need for referral and reporting. Your agency's client protective services department will do the actual investigation.

Nursing Diagnosis

Nursing diagnoses associated with child maltreatment or family violence should address both the physical and the emotional results of the concern. Some examples are:

- Pain related to burn on hand from documented child maltreatment
- Risk for injury related to previous intimate partner violence
- Risk for other-directed violence related to admitted poor self-control
- Impaired parenting related to high level of stress
- Compromised family coping as manifested by child maltreatment related to alcohol use by father
- Disturbed self-esteem related to stalking and sexual maltreatment

Outcome Identification and Planning

Planning must center first on ensuring the safety of the maltreated family member and minimizing the effects of trauma. Second comes reporting the discovery to authorities as nurses are mandated by law to report child maltreatment. Long-term planning includes helping a maltreated family member find safe refuge and reestablishing self-esteem through a self-help or advocacy program. Teaching empowerment, or the ability to take charge of one's life, is particularly important for older children and women in families where there is maltreatment or violence. In addition, the person who maltreated a child or woman needs a program of therapy to help prevent future offenses.

The following organizations can be helpful for referral: Parents Anonymous (www.parentsanonymous.org), the Child Abuse Prevention Network (www.child-abuse.com), the National Coalition Against Domestic Violence (www.ncadv.org), and Women Organized Against Rape (www.WOAR.org).

Implementation

The most important intervention related to family child maltreatment or intimate partner violence is prevention. Nurses can do much in all settings to be particularly observant for families who seem to be at risk for maltreatment or violence and role model optimal ways to handle family stress. Further education is an intervention that can help parents who may not recognize their children's needs or normal child behavior to learn healthy patterns of childrearing.

Outcome Evaluation

Expected outcomes should focus on specific examples of improved family interaction, such as:

- The parent holds baby in a caring manner and maintains good eye contact.
- The parent attends full series of counseling sessions on learning better parenting.
- The parent states she has the Crisis Center telephone number on her cell phone and will call for help if she feels under threat by her partner.
- The adolescent states she can still think of herself with high self-esteem despite rape by stepbrother.
- The parent attends monthly meetings of Parents Anonymous.

HEALTH PROMOTION AND RISK MANAGEMENT

Prevention must be the goal of health care providers to reduce the incidence of child maltreatment (Box 55.2). Because many adults who maltreat children were maltreated themselves, stopping the concern in any one generation helps prevent it in the next.

Identifying parents who may maltreat children if under enough stress is a necessary step in prevention. Listen carefully to the way pregnant women or their partners talk about the child they are expecting. A parent who is overly concerned about the physical appearance or sex of the child ("This had better be a girl" or "He'd better not have his father's nose" or "She better have good hair") may have difficulty accepting a child who does not meet these expectations. Listen for a parent who is concerned about "not letting children get the upper hand" or who says a child "had better be good." Such parents may be conveying worry about how they will act when a child is "bad."

During the postpartum period, be aware of parents who do not touch their infant within 24 hours and those who make disparaging remarks about the child's appearance, as this lack of contact could signal risk. Remember, though, not all parents immediately bond or react warmly to their newborns. Many may only tentatively touch or pick up their infant immediately.

Parents may also be identified as being able to maltreat children during health maintenance visits. By the time a baby is brought to a health care agency for an initial health maintenance visit, you should be able to see that positive parent–child interaction has begun. Listen for parents who say the baby is "nothing but trouble," "cries all the time," or "is bad." Ask new parents how it feels to be a new parent. "I'm exhausted but enjoying it" is a different answer from "it takes too much time" or "it's not much fun." Specific observations to make during postpartum and pediatric health care checkups are summarized in Box 55.3.

Helping parents to seek assistance from support people is another necessary step in prevention. Home visits, family counseling and therapy, and referral to organizations for parents who maltreat children, such as Parents Anonymous, can be highly effective in encouraging parents to reach out for help in times of crisis.

Another nursing responsibility aimed at preventing child maltreatment is helping young parents learn about normal growth and development of children and how to be better parents (Fig. 55.1). Courses in high school or college that describe sound parenting and review normal growth and development and the responsibilities involved in parenting are additional measures in preventing child maltreatment. Classes conducted in high-risk prenatal settings might also have an impact.

BOX 55.2 Measures to Prevent Child Maltreatment or Intimate Partner Violence

1. Advocate for high school or college courses on parenting and growth and development of children so young parents are familiar with usual growth and development of children.
2. Help children learn problem-solving techniques so they are not overwhelmed by mounting problems when they become adults.
3. Foster high self-esteem in children and women so they are not dependent on others but are assertive (to prevent them from becoming passive observers to maltreatment or violence).
4. Help parents with responsible reproductive planning, so children are intended and desired.
5. Help parents locate support people in their community, such as crisis centers or Parents Anonymous or religious or social contacts, so they have ready support people to help them manage stress.
7. Role model caring behaviors with children for parents.
8. Identify children who may be viewed as special in some way by parents, such as those who were separated from the family at birth, were premature, or are physically or cognitively challenged, because these children are at high risk to be victims of maltreatment.
9. Identify parents who were maltreated as children, and offer specific help to them to break the chain of child maltreatment.

BOX 55.3 Questions to Ask to Detect the Potential for Child Maltreatment in New Parents

1. Is the parent enjoying this new role?
2. Does the parent establish eye contact (direct *en face* position) with the baby?
3. How does the parent talk to the baby? Is everything expressed as a demand?
4. Are most of the parent's verbalizations about the child negative?
5. Does the parent remain disappointed about the child's sex or appearance?
6. Are the parent's expectations for the child's development far beyond the child's capabilities?
7. Is the parent very bothered by the baby's crying? Does she or he ignore the baby's demands to be fed? When the baby cries, does the parent or can the parent comfort the child?
8. What is the parent's reaction to the task of changing diapers? Is the parent repulsed by the messiness?
9. Can the parents name a support person they can turn to for advice or assurance?
10. Is sibling rivalry a problem? Is the husband jealous of the baby's claim on the mother's time and affection?
11. When a parent brings the child for health care, does the parent become involved with the baby's needs during the examination and while in the waiting room? Or does the parent relinquish control to the health care provider or nurse such as undressing the child, holding the child, or allowing the child to express fears?
12. Can attention be focused on the child in the parent's presence? Can the parent see something positive in that focus?
13. Does the parent report nonexistent symptoms in the baby? Describe the child in terms that you do not recognize at all? Call with strange stories, such as the child has stopped breathing, changed color, or is doing something "on purpose" to aggravate the parent?

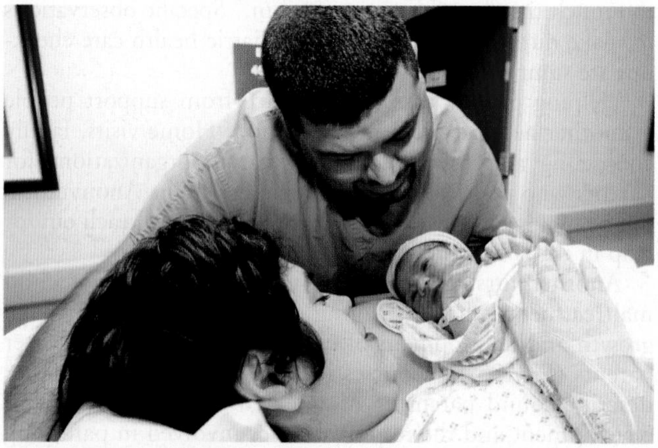

FIGURE 55.1 Teaching that all children have unique characteristics helps to prevent child maltreatment. Here, new parents explore the already noticeable unique aspects of their newborn.

CHILD MALTREATMENT

Because parenting is not an easy task and good parenting is not an automatic or truly instinctive ability, children in every community are injured because of maltreatment. This may be physical (the child is beaten or burned); it may be neglect (the child is not fed, clothed, supervised properly, or offered medical care or educational opportunities); or it also could be psychological or emotional (a child is made to feel unintelligent or inadequate). In some instances, women who threatened the health of their fetus by drug abuse during pregnancy have been viewed by the courts as being guilty of child maltreatment (Goodwin, 2011).

Maltreatment not only places a child at immediate risk for harm but can also lead to long-term effects. For example, physically maltreated children are found to be more angry, noncompliant, and hyperactive than others; they may demonstrate poor self-control and low self-esteem. Children whose parents do not interact with them (emotional maltreatment) are apt to be more withdrawn and to have a flatter affect than others. Because a family where maltreatment occurs is a disrupted one, children often have undiagnosed medical problems, such as anemia, otitis media, or lead poisoning. Children who suffer sexual maltreatment can develop sexually transmitted infections or have long-term effects of depression, guilt, and difficulty enjoying sexual relations (Hornor, 2010).

In addition, when children reach adulthood and begin parenting, they tend to rear their children in basically the same way as they were reared. Parents who themselves received little love or were maltreated as children may never form a basic sense of trust, and so may not be able to form a sense of intimacy or the ability to care for others as young adults.

Theories of Child Maltreatment

The most commonly accepted theory regarding why child maltreatment occurs is that a special triad of circumstances develops (Helfer & Kempe, 1987):

- A parent has the potential to maltreat a child (special parent).
- A child is viewed as "different" in some way by the parent (special child).
- An event or circumstance brings about the maltreatment (special circumstance).

Some health practices or illnesses can be confused with child maltreatment and thus are important to remember in assessment. For example, coin-rolling, a type of massage to draw illness out of the body used by some Asian cultures (a coin is heated and then vigorously rubbed over the body), leaves red welts on the back similar to those that would appear on a child who has been struck repeatedly.

Some infants may bump their head while learning to walk; most toddlers have some ecchymotic spots on their legs from bumping into tables or chairs during normal toddler activities, and preschoolers who actively play may have bruises on multiple bony spots (shin, elbows, knees, etc.). Some childhood diseases, such as leukemia or purpura, begin with easy bruising, which can mimic marks from maltreatment. Children with osteogenesis imperfecta have frequent broken bones as a natural consequence of their disease. Because of inadequate fact-finding in these instances, false reports do occur. When this happens, it can lead to severe stress on the family that has been falsely accused and can interfere with the relationship between the parents of an ill child and the health care personnel who will then give care to the child. Being aware of a practice such as coin-rolling and usual symptoms of illnesses aids understanding of the meaning of illness to parents and helps prevent false reports of child maltreatment.

There are, however, classic "red flags" of nonaccidental trauma that are important to keep in mind, such as spiral fractures of bones (from a twisting force—envision an adult twisting a child's arm, hard) and skull fractures. There are times when these injuries are unintentional injuries, such as a spiral fracture of the leg because the child slipped when climbing down the bunk-bed ladder and the leg was caught while the body twisted and fell, but these injuries always need to be reviewed carefully with an increased index of suspicion. Any fracture in a nonmobile infant is suspicious, especially long bone fractures (Sullivan, 2011). Always assess for injuries that do not match a child's developmental level or abilities or injuries that do not match the explanation of how the injury occurred.

Special Parent: Parents Who Maltreat

Parents who maltreat children seem, on the surface, little different from others. Only a small fraction of them (probably less than 10%) have a history of mental illness, although such parents may have less self-control than others. Many of these parents were maltreated as children. They may be unfamiliar with the normal growth and development of children and so have unrealistic expectations of a child. They also may be socially isolated, with no support people readily available, and so can become overwhelmed by childrearing. The isolation may be by distance (a parent separated from other people in a farmhouse miles from neighbors), or it may be the type that exists in communities or apartment houses where neighbors do not routinely speak to one another. Maltreatment is strongly associated with excessive parental use of drugs such as alcohol, substances that remove inhibitions and self-control. Studies have found that areas with an increased amount of bars per square mile have increased amounts of child neglect, while areas with more off-premises alcohol outlets/liquor stores have increased amounts of child maltreatment, possibly because some parents who drink in bars leave children home alone, whereas some parents who drink at home are more likely to maltreat when the child "misbehaves" (Freisthler, 2011).

Special Child: Children Who Are Maltreated

Maltreated children tend to be viewed by parents as somehow "different." They may be more or less intelligent than other children in the family; they may have been unplanned, or they just may not live up to their parents' expectations in some way. Other reasons are a birth anomaly or an attention span deficit. A category of children who are at high risk are those who were born preterm or who had an illness at birth where they were kept from parents or separated from them by special nurseries or equipment for the first weeks of life, the time during which usual bonding occurs. Because the child is perceived as different, a strong parent–child relationship never develops.

Without an effective relationship, when a child is injured, parents who are unable to deal with stress may not show the usual degree of compassion for their child's pain or offer to comfort. They may appear more concerned with how the injury affects them than how it affects the child, saying: "Don't cry. You'll make me look like a bad parent," rather than, "It's okay to cry. I know that hurts." They may not seek treatment for an injury in an expected amount of time.

To prevent maltreatment, a child may assume a role reversal with the parent or become the comforting, solacing person. They recognize very early in life that when a parent is upset, they will be hurt. They learn to comfort the parent and reduce the parent's stress and anxiety, thereby avoiding the hurt. For this reason, it is important to assess who is comforting whom when a childhood injury occurs.

Special Circumstance: Stress

The third factor in child maltreatment is stress, which may be a response to an event that would not necessarily be stressful for an average parent. It might be something as common as a blocked toilet, an illness in the family, a lost job, a landlord asking for the rent, or a rainstorm that cancels a picnic. Child maltreatment crosses all socioeconomic levels because stress of this nature occurs at all levels. Stress generally has a greater impact on individuals who do not have strong support people around them, so families whose internal support system is faulty or who have not formed outside support systems are apt to have a higher incidence of maltreatment.

Reporting Suspected Child Maltreatment

State laws typically identify two levels of responsibility for reporting child maltreatment: **mandatory reporters** and **permissive reporters**. Nurses are included in the mandatory category in most states; this means they *must* report suspected child maltreatment when they identify it. Failure to do so can result in a fine, jail time, or loss of nursing licensure. The fact that the information was given in a confidential interview does not free a nurse from this responsibility (it is an exception under the confidentiality rules of the Health Insurance Portability and Accountability Act [HIPAA]) (Fraser, Matthews, Walsh, et al., 2010).

All health care institutions and agencies have protocols on how the reporting of child maltreatment should be managed. It is important to learn the protocol required by your particular agency, community, and state. After an official report of child maltreatment has been made to a child protection agency, a health care agency has the right, in most instances, to hold the child for 72 hours for protection, to give an appointed caseworker time to investigate whether maltreatment has occurred. After the 72 hours, a court proceeding will determine whether the child should be returned to the parents' care or kept in a safer location. Because child maltreatment is a crime, the health care record of the child can be subpoenaed and displayed in court. Be certain, therefore, when charting information related to child maltreatment that you make specific and factual notes (observations, not interpretations), such as "Parent spoke loudly and slurred his words," rather than "Parent was intoxicated," or "Mother stated 'This child is nothing but trouble,'" not "I think this mother dislikes this child." Photographs of physical maltreatment enhance the strength of the testimony of maltreatment, so these are usually taken.

A second provision in state laws is protection from having a lawsuit brought against a health care provider for reporting suspected maltreatment "in good faith" that is then proved false. In other words, the laws are written to make it better to err on the side of reporting suspected maltreatment rather than not reporting it, from both a child safety standpoint and from a legal perspective. When maltreatment is officially reported, parents need to be told child maltreatment is suspected, because open lines of communication with parents are important to both protect the child and to arrange counseling for the parent who has maltreated the child. Remember when history taking that maltreatment is not always done by parents, so a parent could really not know how an injury occurred. Alternate caregivers such as day care workers, a babysitter, or a nonbiological parental figure (the new spouse) could be the person at fault.

Physical Maltreatment

Physical maltreatment is the action of a caregiver that causes physical injury to a child. It is commonly revealed by burns or by injuries to the head or hands (Box 55.4).

Assessment

When history taking, always ask caregivers to account for any injury to a child's body. Remember, however, that most childhood injuries are the result of unintentional injuries caused by the child's inability to distinguish safe situations from dangerous ones, or by parents' overestimating their child's ability to do such things as lighting a fire to burn trash or using a saw for a wood project.

An important mark of maltreatment in contrast to an unintentional injury is that the injury is out of proportion to the history given by the parent or caregiver (Fig. 55.2). The parent or caregiver, for example, may report that the child was playing underneath the coffee table when he reared up quickly and hit his head to explain the large hematoma and temporary loss of consciousness the child is experiencing, or that the infant "rolled off the couch" but now has two broken arms. In other instances, the parents may give conflicting stories (the mother says the child fell, but the father says the child broke his arm while throwing a baseball), or they may give no reason for the injury ("He woke up from his nap and couldn't move his arm; I have no idea what could have happened.").

Ask children about the injury as well as the parents because if they did not hear the parent's explanation of the injury, they may say something that is inconsistent with the parent's explanation. They also may cry little in response to a painful procedure, such as an injection, because they are not used to receiving comfort for pain. They may draw back from an examiner more than the average child because they are afraid of adults. These are very subjective observations, however, because children react in different ways to the fear produced by a recent injury or a health examination.

It is often difficult to remain objective when talking to the parents of a child who has been maltreated when you believe the parent is the one who is guilty of the maltreatment. Emotional involvement is not constructive, however; it rarely helps the parents to change, and it may cause them to avoid seeking health care in the future, leaving the child totally unprotected, especially if they were not the one who hurt the child.

To remain objective, always assume the parents have done the best they could under the circumstances in which they found themselves. The fact they have brought the child for care means they are seeking help; it may be their way of saying, "Help me; I don't want this to happen again." In many instances, child maltreatment is not an isolated phenomenon, or a parent is also a victim and needs as much help and protection as the child.

Physical Examination. When children are examined at a well-child visit or because of illness, be certain they are fully undressed (including removing all bandages and Band-Aids) so their entire body can be observed. Plot height and weight on a standard growth chart. Delays in growth may suggest neglect.

Several injuries in children clearly signal probable child maltreatment. Most parents protect their children's hands carefully; in contrast, children who are maltreated have a higher incidence of hand injury. Children who are beaten with electrical cords, belts, or clotheslines have peculiar circular and linear lesions (see Fig. 55.2). Children who are beaten with a belt buckle may have additional curved lacerations from the imprint of the buckle; few other objects produce such contusions. Abrasions or ecchymotic areas on the wrists or ankles may be present if the child was tied to a bed or against a wall.

Burns or scalds are frequent injuries in maltreated children. The peak age at which children unintentionally burn themselves is 2 years; the peak age of burns related to maltreatment is closer to 3 years. When children burn their hand by accident, they usually burn the palm; burns from maltreatment are often on the dorsal surface. Scalding with hot water can occur from a child pulling a hot cup of coffee or a coffee maker off a table. This can, however, be child maltreatment (an adult deliberately scalded the child). Young children do unintentionally step into bathtubs containing water that is hot enough to burn. When this happens, however, the child usually falls forward and so also has burns on the hands and splash marks on the chest or face. If a child is lowered into scalding water as punishment, only the feet and the skin up to the knees

BOX 55.4 Nursing Care Planning Using Assessment

Assessing a Child for Signs of Maltreatment

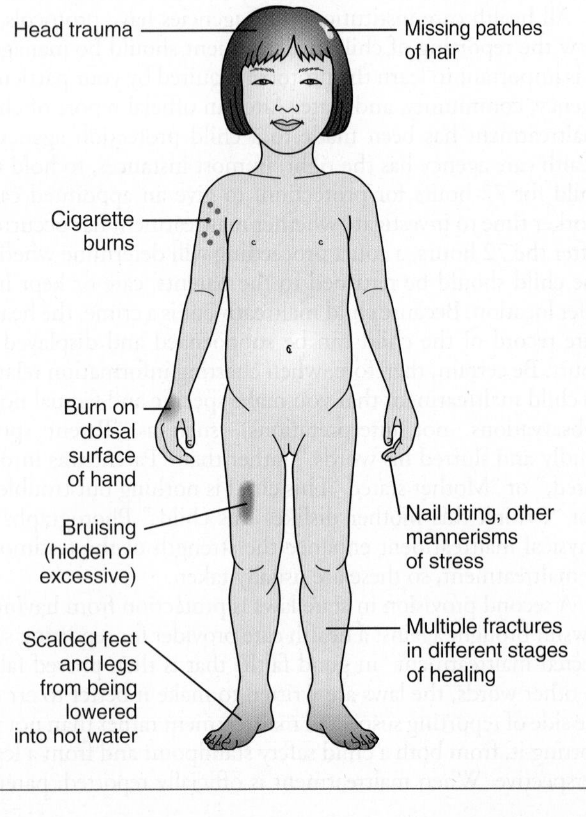

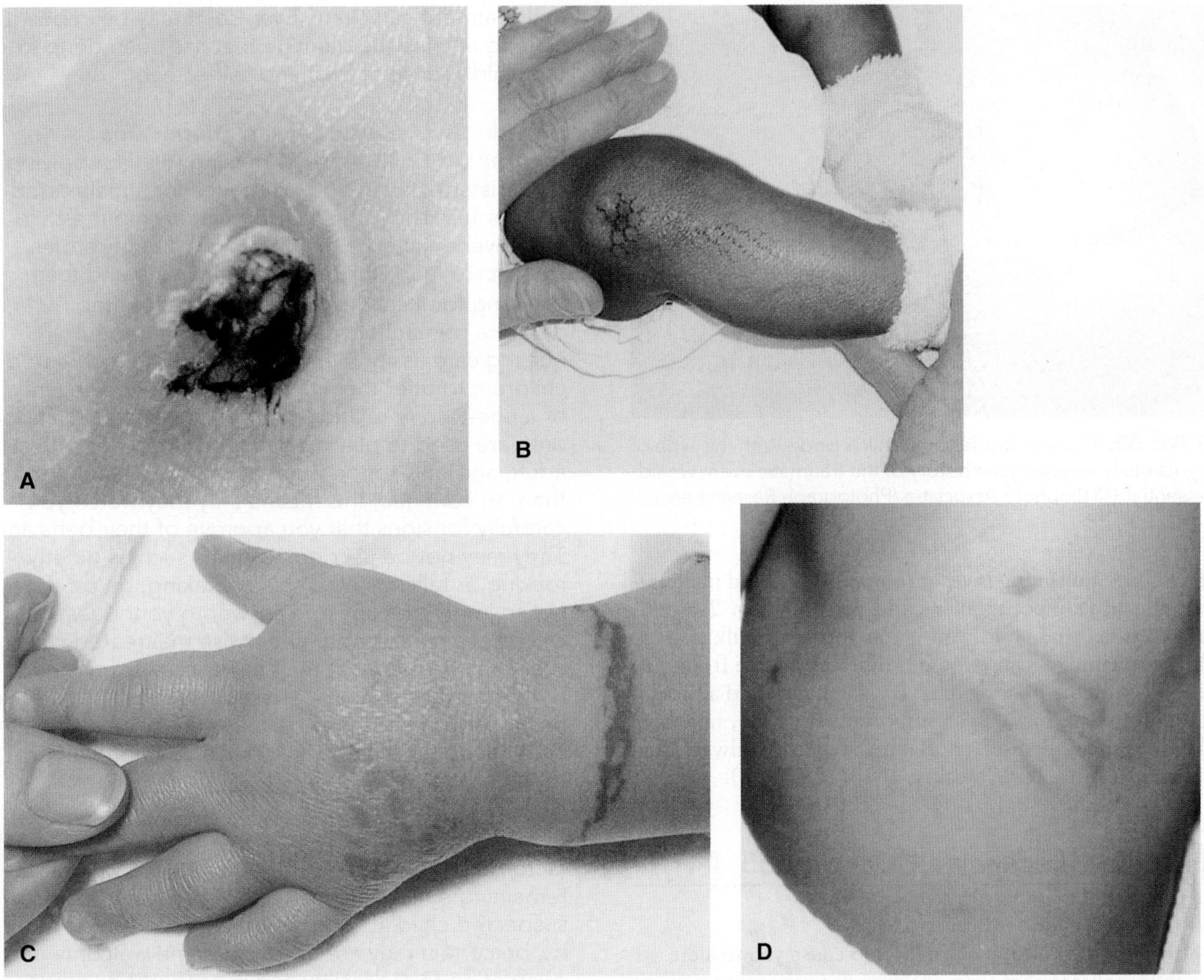

FIGURE 55.2 **(A)** Cigarette burn on child's foot. **(B)** Branding injury showing imprint of radiator cover. **(C)** Rope burn with edema and skin breakdown from being tied to crib rails. **(D)** Imprint marks from beating with a looped electrical cord. (From Zitelli, B. J., & Davis, H. W. [1997]. *Atlas of pediatric physical diagnosis* [3rd ed.]. St. Louis, MO: Mosby–Year Book, Inc.)

are scalded. A child who is placed in a tub of hot water buttocks first by an angry parent usually has no burn in the center of the buttocks because the buttocks touched the bottom of the tub creating a ring of burns or a "doughnut-hole" effect.

Cigarette burns are another common finding on the bodies of physically maltreated children. A fresh cigarette burn causes a blister that resembles the scab of impetigo; differentiation at this stage is often difficult. Impetigo lesions, however, heal without scarring. Cigarette burns heal with a definite circular scar.

Human bites or chunks of hair pulled off the scalp are other signs of maltreatment. Head injuries and broken bones are also frequent findings. Children who are preschool age and younger usually do not fall far enough under normal circumstances to break bones; a broken bone at this age, therefore, suggests the child was thrown or struck so hard the bone broke. Other common findings include multiple fractures in different stages of healing, rib or occipital fractures, and metaphyseal–epiphyseal injuries. Bones are not always broken if a child is shaken roughly, but the periosteum may be torn, so that an X-ray reveals a strange haziness along both sides of the bone shaft. Tibial torsion (twisting) is also often seen (Fig. 55.3).

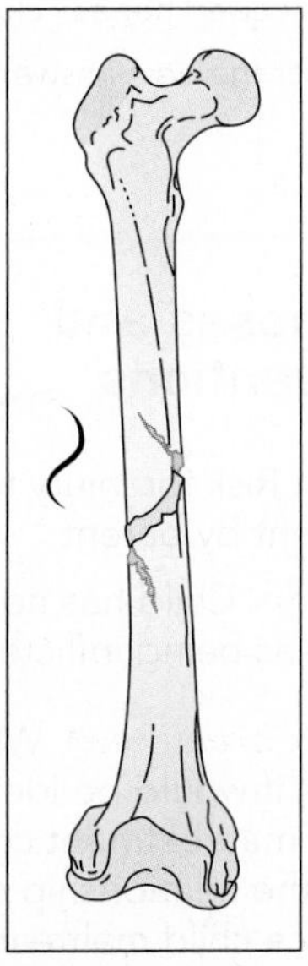

FIGURE 55.3 A spiral fracture around the bone is caused by a wrenching force and is frequently associated with child maltreatment.

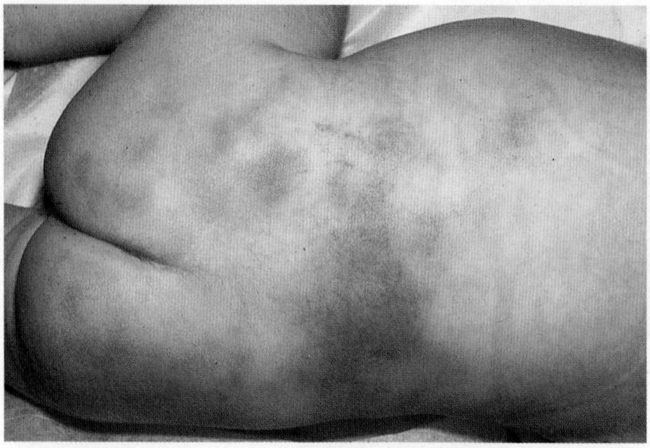

FIGURE 55.4 Large bruises on a child's body. With this type of injury, carefully assessing the history of the traumatic event would be essential. (© Biophoto Associates/Photograph Researchers.)

Deliberate poisoning is yet another form of child maltreatment; this usually occurs in a child younger than 2.5 years of age. Bruises on a child who is too young to walk also are highly suspicious, because those bruises only come from outside sources. Remembering the 3 B's, a light-hearted although meaningful phase for such an important situation, may help with assessment: **B**ruises on **B**abies are nearly always **B**ad (Lazoritz, Rossiter, & Whiteaker, 2010) (Fig. 55.4).

QSEN Checkpoint Question 55.1

Teamwork & Collaboration

Which finding in Hillary's history would cause you to alert the child maltreatment team of your agency because you suspect child maltreatment?

a. Hillary's mother described her as "not pretty."
b. Hillary has a previous health visit for "multiple bruises."
c. Hillary's mother is under severe stress because of her job.
d. Hillary's mother described her as "clumsy."

Look in Appendix A for the best answer and rationale.

Nursing Diagnoses and Related Interventions

Nursing Diagnosis: Risk for injury related to documented maltreatment by parent

Outcome Evaluation: Child has no further physical injuries identifiable as being inflicted by parent.

Prevent Further Maltreatment. When child maltreatment is discovered, it would be ideal if the person responsible for the maltreatment could change behavior and thus the relationship could be kept intact. In reality, once child maltreatment has been discovered, either the child or the abuser usually must be removed from the home so that no more maltreatment can occur. Even so, it may be impossible to reverse the damage that has been done to the child's sense of trust and self-esteem.

Provide Consistent Care and Support for the Maltreated Child. A major nursing role is supplying a consistent, caring adult presence for a maltreated child or furnishing the type of relationship the child has never enjoyed. Box 55.5 shows an interprofessional care map illustrating both nursing and team planning for a child who has been maltreated.

Use a primary or case management type of nursing care assignment, therefore, with maltreated children, to offer them consistency and the security of a one-to-one relationship. Many maltreated children are used to playing by themselves, not with an adult, and only to the point at which a parent wants them to continue; this means they may watch you carefully for signs that you approve of their behavior. They may not be used to activities such as quietly rocking or talking. When history taking, be careful not to imply that any one answer to your question will be the correct one. Otherwise maltreated children may supply what they think you want to hear rather than the truth. (A question such as, "That feels better, doesn't it?" may be followed by an instant "yes" even though the child feels no improvement in symptoms.)

Evaluate and Promote Family Health. An important factor to help evaluate is whether a child will be safe remaining in the parents' care. When parents who are suspected child abusers visit the health care facility, be certain they are given the same welcome and orientation to the facility and procedures as other parents. When caring for a child, point out positive characteristics about the child, as well as growth and development markers and realistic expectations of the child's age, because lack of knowledge of normal growth and development may have contributed to the maltreatment. Take some time as well to talk to the parents away from the child, so that your total attention is focused on them. Praise them for the things they have done well to lay a foundation for them to accept counseling and hopefully change.

For many parents, the response to a charge of child maltreatment is anger. For others, it is relief; now an unwanted child will be taken away from them. In some instances, the diagnosis of maltreatment will force a passive partner to make some important decisions about whether to continue a marriage or relationship with the abusive partner. These are not easy decisions to make; if decision making of any kind were easy for this parent, the circumstances probably would never have reached the point at which child maltreatment occurred.

In most instances, a maltreated child will be removed temporarily from a home and only returned to the home after the person responsible for the maltreatment has been removed or after the stress that led to the maltreatment has been resolved. Such

BOX 55.5 Nursing Care Planning

AN INTERPROFESSIONAL CARE MAP FOR A CHILD WHO HAS BEEN MALTREATED

Hillary is a 3-year-old you see in the emergency department. She has a broken forearm, a broken rib, and multiple bruises on her chest and back. She was seen in the same emergency room a month ago for a burn on the palm of her hand. When you mention to her mother that Hillary's injuries seem extreme for a simple fall, her mother says, "Hillary isn't very pretty. I guess she's also clumsy." You suspect Hillary may be a victim of child maltreatment.

Family Assessment Hillary is an only child. Mother works long hours as city mayor; father (computer consultant) provides child care most evenings. Finances rated as "good." When primary health care provider suggested the child may have been beaten and maltreated, she stated, "Neither of us would ever do that. Not with me running for reelection."

Client Assessment A 3-year-old girl dressed in wool coat and cap even though outside temperature is 80°F. Father protested removal of the child's clothing for examination. Child's right forearm is misaligned and swollen; 3 × 4-in. bruise on right side of anterior ribs, four ½-in. diameter circular lesions on right arm; large 4-cm ecchymotic area on both buttocks and anterior left thigh. Sharp, pointed, triangular blistering and inflamed area noted on back of left hand mother states are "mosquito bites"; mark on hand is a "birthmark." Child remained passive while being examined but drew back when mother approached.

Nursing Diagnosis Fear related to repeated episodes of maltreatment

Outcome Criteria Child expresses fears verbally and through play; interacts with caregivers appropriately; demonstrates positive age-appropriate coping behaviors.

Team Member Responsible	Assessment	Intervention	Rationale	Expected Outcome
Activities of Daily Living, Including Safety				
Nurse	Assess what self-care activities child is able to complete after right arm is casted.	Assist child as necessary with self-care.	Maltreated children may lack self-esteem; allowing them to do as much self-care as able can help improve self-esteem.	Child names tasks she thinks she can do herself; asks for appropriate help for others.
Teamwork and Collaboration				
Nurse/Primary health care provider	Assess physical and history findings to establish suspicion of maltreatment.	Contact hospital child maltreatment team and alert them to suspicious findings.	Child health care providers have an obligation to report maltreatment to proper authorities.	Child maltreatment team meets with parents; documents or rules out maltreatment.
Procedures/Medications for Quality Improvement				
Nurse/Nurse practitioner	Assess whether child has ever had a full physical examination and full body photographs before.	Perform or assist with a complete physical exam and photographs to document child's injuries.	Physical examinations can refresh memories of maltreatment; photographs document extent and type of injuries.	Child cooperates with physical exam and photographer. Photographs are obtained.
Nutrition				
Nurse	Assess whether child is able to manage fork and spoon with cast in place.	Offer help with eating as necessary.	Eating is a self-care activity that can increase self-esteem.	Child demonstrates ability to eat satisfactorily with cast in place.

(continued on page 1624)

BOX 55.5 Nursing Care Planning (continued)

Patient-Centered Care				
Nurse/Primary health care provider	Assess whether parent understands the seriousness of the diagnosis of child maltreatment and need for hospitalization	Explain the reporting procedures and actions that accompany a child maltreatment report.	The parent's cooperation is essential for a successful outcome.	Mother states she will cooperate with procedures. Child understands she will remain in hospital overnight.
Psychosocial/Spiritual/Emotional Needs				
Nurse	Assess which nurse would be the best primary nurse provider for the child.	Arrange for a primary nurse provider; assure child she is now in safe hands.	Removing the child from the threatening environment and providing a consistent caretaker can help reduce fear.	Child states she feels safe in the hospital; participates in therapeutic play.
Informatics for Seamless Health Care Planning				
Nurse/Child maltreatment team	Assess whether parent would like a referral to Parents Anonymous.	Make a referral as appropriate for support people for family. Explain why a restraining order may be issued to prevent one or both parents from visiting child.	Family needs continued follow-up and support because investigation of child maltreatment can be lengthy. Passive parent needs counseling as well as potential maltreating parent.	Parents are cooperative with maltreatment investigation; will attend at least one parents' group meeting.

children need careful follow-up, because an offending parent may return to the home while waiting trial and, if stress occurs again, revert to a maltreatment pattern.

If a child was injured seriously enough to be hospitalized and has had to be removed permanently from the parents' care, urge the foster family to visit before discharge to make the change less frightening for the child. Children who are being removed from their parents in this way can feel an acute sense of loss and may grieve for the nonabusing parent or siblings very much. You may also find maltreated children grieving for an abusing parent, especially if they are convinced that they were the one responsible for the maltreatment or that the parent was not to blame.

Outcome evaluation for maltreated children must include not only whether they are physically safe but also whether they are developing self-esteem, so they can become adults who do not need role reversal with their children.

What if...55.1 You overhear Hillary keep repeating to her mother that she knows the fall was her own fault and she shouldn't be mad because everything will be all right. Is this a typical sign of maltreatment?

Shaken Baby Syndrome

Shaken baby syndrome is the repetitive, violent shaking of a small infant by the arms or shoulders, causing a whiplash injury to the neck, edema to the brainstem, possibly subdural hemorrhage, and distinctive hemorrhages to the retinas (Hitchcock, 2012). A controversial diagnosis, and one difficult to prove, it is a particularly insidious form of child maltreatment, because the damage inflicted on the infant is not readily apparent. Increased use of computed tomography (CT) scans and magnetic resonance imaging is helping to detect children with these internal symptoms. Parents may bring a child for care because they have used a covert camcorder ("a Nanny cam") to reveal that a caregiver shook their baby this way.

Ritual Maltreatment

Ritual maltreatment is cult based or religiously, spiritually, or satanically motivated and typically involves physical, sexual, or psychological maltreatment with bizarre or ceremonial activities. With this type of maltreatment, multiple perpetrators may maltreat multiple victims over an extended period (Schwecke, 2011).

Physical Neglect

Physical neglect is a more subtle form of maltreatment than physical maltreatment, but it can be just as damaging to a child's welfare. A neglected child may appear unwashed, thin, and malnourished or be dressed inappropriately, such as without mittens, a coat, or shoes in cold weather. In some families, no one has a warm coat to wear or receives enough food because there is no money for these things; that is different from the family in which parents do have these things, but the children or one particular child does not.

Failing to bring a child for immunizations or failing to seek early medical care for an infection are other signs of neglect. Not requiring a child to attend school, deliberately keeping a child out of school without setting up a home school program, or allowing a child to go unsupervised after school may also be interpreted as neglect. Such actions may be willful, or they may occur if parents simply do not realize the normal needs of a child. Use of electronic records allowing a child's total health care history to be examined has made identifying neglected children easier (Tonmyr, Jack, Brooks, et al., 2012). Such parents need guidance from health care personnel to better understand their child's needs and how to parent.

Psychological Maltreatment

Psychological maltreatment includes constant belittling or threatening, rejecting, isolating, or exploiting a child or is the absence of positive parenting. Children who are psychologically maltreated this way are likely to have difficulty becoming emotionally confident adults. This type of maltreatment is the most difficult form of maltreatment to detect because it may occur only in the home, and its effects, although severe, may be subtle. It can result, however, in the same type of inability to achieve that occurs in children who are physically maltreated.

Be sure to include enough growth and development questions during a health assessment to reveal this; observe the parent–child interaction to determine whether it is positive and healthy or negative and potentially unhealthy.

Munchausen Syndrome by Proxy

Munchausen syndrome by proxy refers to a parent who repeatedly brings a child to a health care facility and reports symptoms of illness when, in fact, the child is well (Kucuker, Demir, & Oral, 2010). For example, a parent might report symptoms such as seizures, excessive sleepiness, or abdominal pain in a child. Because of these symptoms, the child is submitted to needless diagnostic procedures or therapeutic regimens. Another parent might go so far as to deliberately inflict injury on a child, such as giving a laxative to induce diarrhea or slowly poisoning the child with a prescription drug. Two classic findings of the syndrome are usually present: first, the symptoms are not easily detected by physical examination, only by history; second, the symptoms are present only when the person initiating the symptoms is providing care (they disappear when care is provided by another person). The parent usually has some degree of medical or child care knowledge obtained through formal education, reading, or Internet browsing. In the hospital, the parent tends to stay with the child constantly, offering to give the majority of care. This makes this a difficult to detect form of maltreatment because wanting to stay and give care is also the hallmark of a very conscientious and caring parent.

To diagnose this disorder, covert video surveillance may be necessary. Because this syndrome reveals distorted perceptions on the part of the parent, it is almost always necessary to remove the child from the home to protect the child, even if the parent receives counseling.

QSEN Checkpoint Question 55.2

Safety

If Hillary had been maltreated as an infant, she might have experienced shaken baby syndrome. Which of the following findings is common with this syndrome and would indicate a baby should be evaluated for medical and safety reasons?

a. A baby is fearful of strangers.
b. Retinal hemorrhages develop.
c. A baby develops Crohn disease.
d. A major bone has been broken.

Look in Appendix A for the best answer and rationale.

Failure to Thrive (Reactive Attachment Disorder)

Failure to thrive is a unique syndrome in which an infant falls below the 5th percentile for weight and height on a standard growth chart or is falling in percentiles on a growth chart. The condition is usually divided into two categories: one where severe loss of weight can be explained because of organic causes, such as cardiac disease; and a second that occurs because of a disturbance in the parent–child relationship, resulting in maternal role insufficiency (a nonorganic cause). Sometimes both forms combine to play a role in failure to thrive (Jaffe, 2011).

The nonorganic type is considered a form of child neglect, although this represents a very complex interplay between parent and child. In many instances, the parent feels little emotional attachment to the child and often has a history of frequent moves and little family support. The parent may not be offering enough food because of the lack of attachment, he or she is not aware of the hunger cues the infant is offering, or the parent does not have enough concern for the child to offer food regularly. A child may contribute to the poor parenting interaction by being an irritable, fussy, colicky, or "difficult" child. Some infants are offered sufficient food, but the emotional deprivation they sense makes them so lethargic they do not eat enough. In other instances, the child has a minimal neurologic dysfunction and thus does not respond as a usual child. The mother may interpret this lethargic behavior as lack of response to her and thus does not carry out her half of the interaction adequately.

Failure to thrive begins with subtle signs that need to be identified and taken seriously, because the syndrome can lead to cognitive impairment in the child and even death if allowed to continue.

Assessment

Take a detailed pregnancy history of children at routine health assessments, because in many instances, a breakdown in the development of parenting began in the prenatal period because of such factors as a pregnancy that was unintended or not accepted, a partner who left during the pregnancy, an economic catastrophe such as loss of a job, or a long-distance move that left support people behind.

Always weigh children at routine assessments and plot and compare their weight with standard growth curves so children who are failing to thrive can be identified at the earliest point

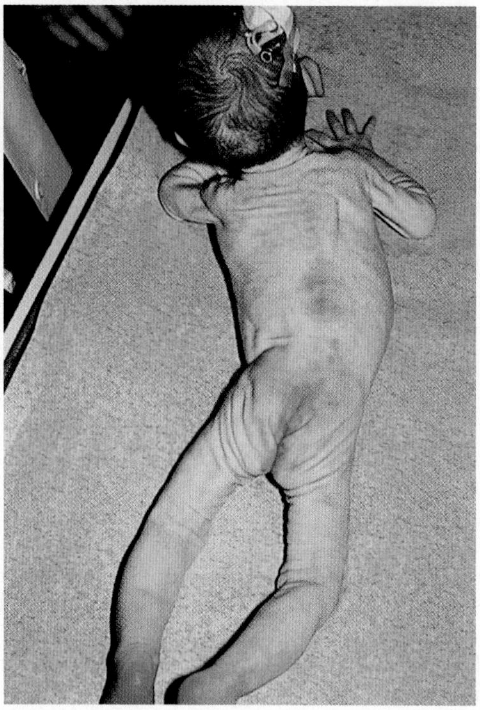

FIGURE 55.5 The child with failure to thrive experiences a loss of subcutaneous fat, muscle wasting, and skin breakdown. (From Zitelli, B. J., & Davis, H. W. [1997]. *Atlas of pediatric physical diagnosis* [3rd ed.]. St. Louis, MO: Mosby–Year Book, Inc.)

possible. On physical examination, these infants usually demonstrate typical characteristics such as:

- Lethargy with poor muscle tone, a loss of subcutaneous fat, or skin breakdown (Fig. 55.5)
- Lack of resistance to the examiner's manipulation, unlike the response of the average infant
- Rocking on all fours excessively, as if seeking stimulation
- Possibly a greater reluctance to reach for toys or initiate human contact than is demonstrated by the average infant; diminished or nonexistent crying
- Staring hungrily at people who approach them as if they are starved for human contact.
- Little cuddling or conforming to being held
- Delays in sitting, pulling to a standing position, crawling, and walking because the child spends so much time alone
- Markedly delayed or absent speech because of the lack of interaction

With advanced failure to thrive, the child's nutritional status may be so extremely poor that the infant is near acidosis from starvation. If an upper respiratory tract infection should develop, the child's resistance to infection may be so low that it could result in death from pneumonia.

Therapeutic Management

With rare exceptions, children with failure to thrive need to be removed from the parents' care for evaluation and therapy. Otherwise, the syndrome may lead to permanent neurologic damage or leave a child cognitively challenged because of protein deficits and interference with brain metabolism. If an infant is admitted to a hospital, studies other than routine admission blood work and urinalysis are usually delayed, to avoid submitting such an understimulated child to pain or unnecessary manipulation.

Infants are immediately placed on a diet appropriate for their ideal weight (the weight they would have been normally for their age). Rapid weight gain on this diet is diagnostic that their presenting illness was nonorganic failure to thrive.

Nursing Diagnoses and Related Interventions

Nursing Diagnosis: Imbalanced nutrition, less than body requirements, related to inadequate intake secondary to emotional deprivation

Outcome Evaluation: Child shows interest in bottle feedings; child is able to establish a regular eating pattern; child begins to gain weight.

Be certain the plan of care designed for the family of a child who is failing to thrive is realistic because parents cannot be made to form a bond with a child instantly, particularly if lack of bonding has gone on for some time. Don't give up hope, however, that this will happen. With the proper support and guidance over time, and when obstacles to bonding are removed, a healthy child–parent relationship could still develop.

Ensure Adequate Nutrition. Keep a careful record of intake and output so the number of calories being consumed every day can be effectively evaluated. Assess stools for pH and reducing substances (glucose) to be certain the infant is absorbing nutrients. If a stool tests positive for glucose or has an acid pH (less than 7.0), it suggests that not even carbohydrates, the easiest food to absorb, are being processed.

Evaluate how well the infant sucks or is able to take food from a spoon and swallow to be certain these reflexes are intact. Record any symptoms, such as pulling up the legs or crying after eating, that suggest gastrointestinal discomfort.

Nurture the Child. Because infants with failure to thrive are suffering from emotional deprivation, they need effective nurturing from the nurses who care for them. This does not mean everyone who passes the crib should stop and play with the child for a few minutes; it means one member of the nursing team should be chosen to care for the child during the hospital stay (a primary nursing or case management pattern of assignment). It's important this nurse reserves time for providing active interactions with the child such as rocking and talking, giving a leisurely bath, offering toys, and "parenting" as passive rocking without talking to the child may be no different than the parents' care.

Support and Encourage the Parents. Encourage the parents of children with failure to thrive to visit as much as possible while the child is hospitalized or in foster care because without encouragement, these parents may visit little or not at all. When they do visit, encourage them to feed and interact with the infant. Parents cannot change their feelings about a child overnight, however, so telling them they ought to pick up the baby more or hold the infant while feeding may only increase the parents' feelings of inadequacy. Giving some suggestions about how the baby tries to communicate with them may be more effective; for example: "Do you know what I think he's trying to say when he stops sucking like that? I think he's saying he's ready to be burped." "Look how he turns his head at the sound of your voice. He recognizes you."

Occasionally, parents are so distraught by such factors as the illness or death of an older child or relative they simply have become unaware of how much energy is being drained from them by these events. These parents quickly can become good parents to a deprived child as soon as they realize what has been happening. More often, however, the disturbance in a parent–child interaction began long before or is so great that a parenting bond cannot be established. If the infant is discharged from the hospital to the parents' care, the parents will need effective follow-up in the months to come to see that they maintain parenting at an acceptable level. There is a very thin line between the child who fails to thrive and one who is maltreated, so some of these children need to be placed in foster homes for their own safety and to ensure that they receive adequate care.

Help Prevent Poor Parenting. Parents who may be at risk for poor parenting need to be identified during pregnancy, so they can receive counseling and close follow-up in the postnatal period. Some parents who are overwhelmed by the task of parenting may need respite care for their children and extended counseling to prevent future parenting breakdown.

What if...55.2 You weigh Hillary's baby cousin at a well-child visit and discover the infant's weight has fallen below the 2nd percentile on a standardized growth chart. What questions would you want to ask the mother? What particular areas would you want to assess on a physical examination?

SEXUAL MALTREATMENT

Sexual maltreatment is broadly defined as any sexual contact between a child and an adult (Neutze et al., 2012). It involves the coercion of dependent, developmentally immature children or adolescents in sexual activities that they do not fully comprehend, to which they are unable to give informed consent, or that violate the social taboos of family roles. Adolescents have a higher rate of rape or sexual maltreatment than any other age group (8% to 10%) (Delacroix, Brown, Kadenhe-Chaweshe, et al., 2011). Remember that boys, as well as girls, can be sexually maltreated. Although their abusers may be seemingly trustworthy coaches or teachers, they also may be people inside the family such as an older sibling, a parent, or a stepparent (Carlson, 2011). Abusers may contact children online through chat rooms, making the monitoring of Web sites an important preventive measure for parents (Briggs, Simon, & Simonsen, 2011). Health professionals who care for children with cognitive disabilities must be especially watchful to protect these vulnerable children from sexual maltreatment (Koetting, Fitzpatrick, Lewin, et al., 2012).

Sexual maltreatment is physically and emotionally destructive because it leaves children unable to trust others and may result in a sense of ambivalence toward intimacy and an overall sense of worthlessness. Remind parents to teach children by preschool age that their bodies are their own and to report anyone who tries to touch them in a way they do not like (Fig. 55.6). Children who have been sexually maltreated may be identified because they have a sexual vocabulary beyond that expected of a child their age. On physical exam, girls will have tears or inflammation of the vagina or perineum; both sexes may have rectal tears or symptoms of a sexually transmitted disease. Both sexes need a great deal of support to consent to an anogenital examination to document the maltreatment.

Megan's Law is a federal law that requires law enforcement authorities to report to neighbors when a sexual abuser moves into a neighborhood. Parents need to be aware of this law and insist that it be enforced so they can take appropriate precautions to protect their children's safety (Neutze, Grundmann, Scherner, et al., 2012). Sexual predators are also listed on Internet Web sites and thus can be tracked by parents. Additional laws parents need to be aware of to keep their children safe are child pornography laws. In some states, for example, "sexting" (texting sexually explicit photos) to friends may violate such laws—even though a minor is doing the texting. Their child could forever be classified as a sexual abuser and listed under Megan's Law (Wastler, 2010).

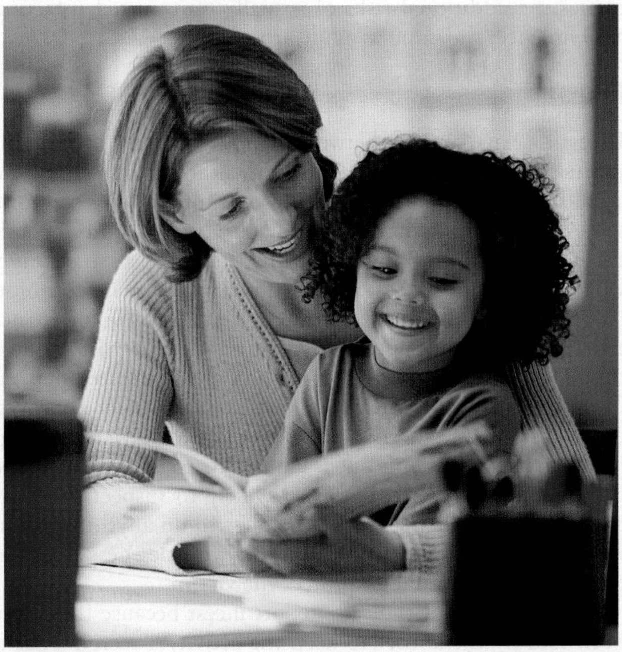

FIGURE 55.6 Teach children their bodies are their own and they have to give permission before anyone can touch them.

Types of Sexual Maltreatment

Sexual maltreatment involves a wide range of diagnoses from molestation to vaginal penetration.

Molestation

Molestation is a vague term that includes "indecent liberties" such as oral–genital contact, genital fondling and viewing, or masturbation. A **pedophile** is an adult who seeks out prepubescent children (Tanner stage 0–1, usually younger than 12 years of age) for sexual gratification, whereas a **hebephile** seeks out pubescent children (Tanner stage 1–4, usually age 11 to 15 years) (Neutze et al., 2012). In contrast to a rapist, whose crime is violent, both pedophiles and hebephiles may be very gentle and limit the involvement to molestation. Such persons are usually male, but sometimes female; they may have suffered sexual maltreatment as a child and thus repeatedly select children or young adolescents who are of the same age at which the maltreatment occurred. The relationship may involve people with either homosexual or heterosexual orientations. Many pedophiles or hebephiles take photos or videos of their activities with children to use for sexual gratification at a later date.

Rehabilitation of pedophiles/hebephiles is difficult because they are fixated emotionally at a childhood level (seeing themselves as children, they do not perceive relationships with children as wrong). Listen carefully to children who report that someone enjoys photographing them; ask children to describe what they mean by someone "touching" or "feeling" them, to detect this type of maltreatment.

Pornography and Prostitution

Child pornography involves photographing or describing sexual acts by any medium involving children, or distributing such material in person or by mail, fax, cell phone, or over the Internet. Child prostitution involves arranging or participating in sexual acts with children. Both of these phenomena are demeaning to children and are illegal. Child prostitution carries the additional risks of sexually transmitted infection and violence, the same as adult prostitution.

Incest

Incest is sexual activity between family members. It often involves an older man and a young girl, although it may involve an older woman and a younger boy, a brother and sister, or a same-sex partner. It may involve foster, adopted, and stepchildren. Incest is a deviation from the norm and is so strongly viewed as such by most people that incest taboos are common to most cultures (Carlson, 2011). Incest results in a destructive relationship because it causes a great deal of guilt and loss of self-esteem in both the abusing and the maltreated person. The abuser is aware that this act is not culturally approved but still is unable to end the relationship; the victim recognizes this act as wrong but is unable to resist the advances. Other members of the family are likely to suspect the maltreatment is occurring but are helpless to do anything about it; this leads to guilt and feelings of worthlessness on their part for not being able to protect the victim.

Children do not typically report incest because they have been told by the abuser to keep the activity a secret. That it has occurred may first be revealed on a routine health examination by the finding of vaginal or rectal lesions.

QSEN Checkpoint Question 55.3

Evidence-Based Practice

It's difficult to know the true incidence of sexual maltreatment in adolescents because it is suspected that many teenagers never report any maltreatment occurred. To investigate whether adolescents who are sexually maltreated confide in their parents, researchers interviewed 26 adolescents (23 girls and 3 boys; age 15 to 18 years) who had been sexually maltreated. Results of the study showed that less than one third of the participants immediately disclosed the maltreatment to another person. More than one third never disclosed the maltreatment to a parent. With most participants, the person whom they did disclose the maltreatment to was a peer. The main motives for nondisclosure to parents were lack of trust or not wanting to burden the parents (Schönbucher, Maier, Mohler-Kuo, et al., 2012).

Mrs. Landstrum's adolescent sister, Andrea, is examined in the emergency room because she has pain and a vaginal discharge. Aside from Andrea herself, based on the previous study, which person would be the most reliable reporter as to whether Andrea has been sexually maltreated?

a. Andrea's mother, because Andrea says she respects her
b. Megan, a soccer teammate and close friend of Andrea
c. Andrea's father, because he is the patriarch of the family
d. Andrea's soccer coach, because she sees Andrea daily

Look in Appendix A for the best answer and rationale.

Assessment

Signs of sexual maltreatment are shown in Box 55.6. In addition to physical signs, a suspicion of sexual maltreatment may first be revealed by a young girl worrying she is pregnant or a child's abnormal anxiety about a parent returning home from a hospital stay or being left with or cared for by a particular individual in the family (Box 55.7). Young children who are the victims of this type of relationship typically have extremely low self-esteem and may believe they are so inadequate they deserve to be treated this way.

Allowing young children to play with anatomically correct dolls is a common method for determining whether sexual maltreatment is occurring (Hlavka, Olinger, & Lashley, 2010). The average reaction of a preschooler or young school-age child who has not been maltreated, for example, is to undress the dolls, giggle for a moment or two about how they look, and then redress or put them aside. The child who is involved in an incestuous relationship may make the dolls perform a sexual act, such as placing the male doll's penis into the female doll's mouth. The use of such dolls is controversial because there is a concern that without a common protocol for their use, the child's actions could be overinterpreted. Asking the child to draw a picture of what happened may also be an effective way of revealing sexual maltreatment.

Therapeutic Management

Sexual maltreatment, like physical maltreatment, must be reported because this is a criminal offense. It's important, as with all child maltreatment, that information about the

BOX 55.6 Nursing Care Planning Based on Family Teaching

IDENTIFYING SIGNS OF SEXUAL MALTREATMENT

Q. Hillary's mother asks you, "What signs should I look for if I suspect my daughter is being sexually maltreated?"

A. Here are some general indications that a child is being sexually maltreated:

- The child reports she has had sexual activity with an adult.
- The child demonstrates an awareness of sex or a sexual vocabulary beyond her age expectations.
- The child participates in sexual expression with dolls.
- A girl younger than 15 years of age is pregnant.
- A perineal, vaginal, or anal exam reveals inflammation or vaginal tears or anal fissures.
- A child younger than 15 years of age has a sexually transmitted infection.
- A child has a history of symptoms of increased anxiety such as a sleep disturbance, development of nervous tics, nail biting, or stuttering.
- There is a change in school performance, school phobia, or truancy.
- The child voices a fear of being left alone with a certain adult.
- A child reports vague abdominal pain or demonstrates acting-out behavior.

maltreatment is collected objectively so the adult's rights are respected and the testimony is therefore admissible in court.

Both the adult and the child involved in a sexual maltreatment relationship need psychological counseling—the child to improve self-esteem and the adult to channel sexual expression to less destructive outlets. To improve the child's self-esteem, the adult in the relationship needs to admit the fault was the adult's, not the child's. Follow-up care is best done by one of the people who sees the child initially, so that the child does not have to recount the incident to strangers again and again. Treatment for sexually transmitted infections or protection against pregnancy should be provided as needed.

BOX 55.7 Nursing Care Planning Based on Effective Communication

You notice during history taking that Hillary uses several four-letter words to describe where she hurts.

Less Effective Communication

Nurse: Mrs. Lindstrum, your daughter seems to know some words that are unusual for a 3-year-old.

Mrs. Lindstrum: She gets that from watching cartoons on TV.

Nurse: Cartoon characters don't usually say the words she uses.

Mrs. Lindstrum: We're proud she's advanced for her age.

Nurse: Okay. I just want you to know I think her vocabulary is advanced. Here is the medicine to apply to her bottom to help the tear there heal.

More Effective Communication

Nurse: Mrs. Lindstrum, your daughter seems to know some words that are unusual for a 3-year-old.

Mrs. Lindstrum: She gets that from watching cartoons on TV.

Nurse: Cartoon characters don't usually say the words she uses.

Mrs. Lindstrum: We're proud she's advanced for her age.

Nurse: Using words with sexual connotations doesn't necessarily mean her vocabulary is advanced. It means she most likely keeps company with an adult who speaks that way.

Mrs. Lindstrum: That's probably her uncle. He babysits once a week.

Nurse: Does she mind staying with him?

Mrs. Lindstrum: Does it matter? A free babysitter doesn't happen every day.

Nurse: Let's talk some more about her vocabulary, especially in light of her infection.

It is often very difficult for families to face the fact a family member could be guilty of child sexual maltreatment. It's necessary to pursue the subject, rather than let yourself be distracted, to help a parent examine what could be happening.

Parents may need as much counseling as the child when their child has been sexually maltreated, so they can help the child work through feelings about the situation. In many instances, because the offender is a family member or a trusted outsider and the relationship has been occurring for some time before it is reported, parents may feel guilty they allowed the family member to have access to the child or did not listen to a child's protestations that being alone with this family member was uncomfortable for them. If incest involves a parent or marriage or relationship partner, it may be extremely difficult for parents or partners to continue to relate to each other effectively enough to help the child. Review with parents and encourage parents to teach children simple rules to help children avoid sexual maltreatment (see Chapter 32, Box 32.4).

QSEN Checkpoint Question 55.4

Quality Improvement

A member of the child maltreatment team offers Hillary anatomically correct male and female dolls for her to play with. When Hillary begins play by placing the male doll's penis in the female doll's mouth, what would your best response be?

a. "Do you think it's wrong that the dolls do that?"
b. "I bet you're playing a game you've seen on TV."
c. "Are the dolls playing a game? Tell me about it."
d. "Okay, can you please put the dolls down now?"

Look in Appendix A for the best answer and rationale.

RAPE

Rape is sexual activity such as intercourse or penetration of a body orifice by a penis or other object under actual or threatened force. *Statutory rape* is sexual activity with a person under the age of consent (in most states, younger than 18 years of age) and is considered to have occurred regardless of the apparent willingness of the underage person. *Sexual assault* is typically used to refer to other forced sexual acts, such as oral–genital or anal–genital acts (Hornor, 2011).

Rape is a crime of violence, not of passion, and includes "date rape," a situation in which an individual forces a date or casual friend into having coitus despite a voiced unwillingness or inability to consent (D. L. Lang, Sales, Salazer, et al., 2011). The increasing misuse of flunitrazepam (Rohypnol), a drug easily dissolved in a drink, has led to an increase in the incidence of date rape because it leaves a victim with little or no memory of the event (see Chapter 33). It may be very difficult for the victim of date rape to find a sympathetic ear if her companion insists he meant no harm; he simply didn't believe her. Urge adolescents to be aware of the danger of the drug and to say "no" convincingly (Makin-Byrd & Bierman, 2013).

Both rape and sexual assault represent deviant behavior. They lack privacy and mutual consent, which are the elements of "normal" or usual sexual behavior, and include violence, causing them to be degrading and dehumanizing and leaving the victim feeling helpless and victimized. Review with teenagers of both sexes ways to prevent rape at routine health visits (Box 55.8).

Determining the actual incidence of rape is difficult; it seems to be more prevalent than formerly, but that may be because more people report it. Many adolescents want to avoid the secondary, but no less severe, trauma associated with reporting rape and therefore do not report it. This leaves them, unfortunately, without the immediate treatment and follow-up care that are so important to a complete recovery.

Although victims can be of any age and either male or female, the average rape victim is an adolescent girl. The rapist may be a relative or family friend, and rapists frequently commit the act in the neighborhood where they live, so up to 75% of girls know their attacker. Based on arrest data, the average rapist is a young adult man with a background of aggressive behavior. His motivation usually relates to expressions of power or anger; sexual satisfaction does not appear to be a dominant motive. An excessive amount of alcohol intake often precedes rape (Thompson, McGee, & Mays, 2012). Rape tends to be a repetitive, planned activity on the part of the attacker, rather than an isolated event.

Assessment

Many rape victims demonstrate immediate physical and emotional symptoms that can last for weeks. These symptoms constitute what has been termed **rape trauma syndrome**, a form of posttraumatic stress syndrome, and they usually occur in two stages: disorganization and reorganization. In the immediate *disorganization phase*, victims feel a combination of humiliation, shame and guilt, embarrassment, anger, and vengefulness. They feel that their lives have been completely disrupted by the crisis because they were unable to protect themselves from the assault. They may tremble from fear or be in great pain from perineal lacerations and are apt to startle visibly at the sound of anyone approaching or touching them. They need gentle, sympathetic support people with them in the days after the event to allow them to feel safe. They may have nightmares of the attack occurring again. This immediate stage of disruption and disorganization usually lasts about 3 days.

The second stage of rape trauma syndrome, termed the *reorganization phase*, may last for months or years. Many rape victims report recurring nightmares, perhaps sexual dysfunction, and continuing inability to relate to the opposite sex or to face new and surprising situations. They may continue to have a great deal of difficulty discussing the rape. Many rape victims, trying to escape from so personal an offense, change their residence at great sacrifice to finances and lifestyle. If not offered constructive counseling, victims may still feel guilt or shame when thinking about the rape as long as 20 to 30 years later.

If victims do not report rape and therefore receive no counseling, symptoms indicative of **silent rape syndrome**, similar to posttraumatic stress disorder (PTSD), can result (Rothbaum, Kearns, Price, et al., 2012). When the subject of rape is mentioned, people with silent rape syndrome may grow increasingly emotionally disturbed; it may be evident in their history that they altered their behavior toward persons who resemble the rapist at a certain point in life and perhaps began to resist actions such as going outside by themselves or being alone in a house after that time. This condition can be devastating to their ability to maintain employment or

BOX 55.8 Nursing Care Planning to Empower a Family

GUIDELINES FOR THE PREVENTION OF RAPE IN ADOLESCENTS

Q. Hillary's mother is concerned about the incidence of rape in her community. She asks you, "What should I teach my adolescent sister to help her avoid rape?"

A. A number of suggestions are:

Home

1. Do not advertise that you stay alone while a parent works or is on vacation.
2. Do not admit anyone to your house when you are home alone, even meter readers or repairmen who produce identification.
3. Insist on adequate lighting for hallways in an apartment building or streetlights around your home.
4. Have your house key in your hand when you approach your door; do not stand fumbling for it by the doorway.
5. Keep your doors and windows locked when you are alone at home.

Car

1. Avoid isolated parking places; park near a building or in a lot with a parking attendant.
2. Lock your car when waiting in it and after parking it.
3. Look in the backseat before unlocking and entering your car to be sure no one is there.
4. Have your car key ready when you approach your car; do not stand fumbling for it.

Work or School

1. Do not enter an elevator with a stranger.
2. Lock the outside door, and do not admit people you do not know when working alone in an office or classroom at night.
3. Ask for security protection to walk out to your car after hours.
4. When going to and from school or work after dark, walk in the street rather than next to shrubs or dark buildings.

Social Settings

1. Be clear with your date that when you say no, you mean no.
2. Limit alcohol use, because it can lead to risk-taking behavior.
3. Make it clear you consider date rape the same as any rape and you will press charges.
4. Rohypnol is a sedative, known as a "date rape" drug. Do not date any individual who brags that he knows how to obtain it or use it.

Personal Actions

1. Do not wear chains around your neck that could be used to strangle you.
2. Learn self-defense; scratch the attacker to obtain skin and blood specimens under fingernails.
3. Be aware that an attacker could take any weapon you hold away and use it on you; use caution carrying a weapon or mace.
4. If an attack occurs, observe the attacker's appearance as carefully as possible. Note identifying characteristics, such as a birthmark, scar, tattoo, words, or manner of speech, to be able to identify the individual later.
5. Press charges in court to make rape a crime of extreme magnitude and as an opportunity to fight back.
6. Work to provide rape prevention information and a united front against rape in your community.

remain independent. They need counseling as much as a person who reported a rape.

Emergency Care

Although most large city police forces have special officers assigned to investigate rape charges, victims can be confused and further traumatized by police officers who imply they provoked the attack because of their manner of dress or could have done more to resist or prevent the event. This increases a victim's feelings of shame and degradation. It may be especially harmful to adolescents, because people they have been taught to respect have no concept of the degree of fright they have experienced or the strength of their attacker. Health care providers usually are the second group of people victims see after an attack, so they need to be extremely cautious that they do not show this same type of callous behavior.

Most health care agencies where many rape victims are seen have a rape trauma team, including specially educated counselors to talk to victims immediately after a rape and to offer long-term counseling as needed. Nurses serve as important members of such teams and may provide primary care after a rape. Any nurse should be able to offer emergency support because it might be a long time before a specifically designated staff member arrives, and such services are not available in every community.

Because rape is a crime, the electronic record of a rape victim is often displayed as part of a court procedure. For the victim to bring charges against the attacker, information concerning the victim's appearance and history needs to be detailed in the record. For that reason, a sexual assault nurse examiner (SANE nurse) should be called if available. Pediatric nurses trained as sexual assault examiners are called P-SANE nurses and are a crucial part of properly examining a child assault victim. Be aware if child advocacy centers (CACs) are available in your area to consult with and examine child maltreatment and child sexual assault victims. If available, *stop* after the initial basic exam and call the CAC team so they can properly interview and examine the victim, observing local laws and evidence requirements.

Table 55.1 summarizes common tests and procedures for emergency care of rape victims. If no CAC team is available,

TABLE 55.1 Common Specimen Procedures After Rape

Procedure	Purpose
Oral washing	Help client rinse mouth with 5 ml sterile water, which is then collected in test tube, analyzed for blood group antigens, or sperm or DNA of attacker.
Fingernail scraping	Scrape under all of client's fingernails so scrapings can be analyzed for blood, skin, DNA, and clothing fibers of attacker.
Blood VDRL, HIV, and HbsAg	Draw blood for antibody titer for syphilis, HIV, and hepatitis B and typing to differentiate it from attacker's type.
Pregnancy test	Obtain blood for analysis; complete vaginal examination before woman voids.
Hair samples	Remove both scalp and pubic hairs of client (about 10) to be compared with attacker's.
Vaginal smear for sperm and DNA	Swab vagina with a dry applicator and smear onto slide so sperm and DNA analysis can be performed.
Gonococcus smear	Culture the client's cervix, vagina, and rectum (also throat if oral coitus was attempted).
Vaginal washing	Place 5 ml of sterile saline into client's vagina and aspirate again to detect sperm, DNA, and acid phosphate.
Skin washings	Touch any dried stains of blood or semen on the client's skin or clothing with a moistened cotton swab to be analyzed for attacker's blood, semen, or DNA.
Clothing	Save any clothing stained or torn as evidence of violent attack.
Label all specimens carefully, indicating where they were obtained, to aid medical therapy and provide legal evidence.	

be certain statements you make in a record are accurate and unbiased. Quote the victim's exact words whenever possible. Describe the victim's physical appearance in unbiased detail, including the presence and location of injuries, such as bruises, lacerations, teeth marks, or abrasions, and the condition of clothing. Be certain to ask whether the victim bathed or washed before coming for care, because this can obscure evidence and obliterate the presence of sperm or DNA material. Ask whether the woman was menstruating or using a tampon as the force of penis penetration with rape can cause a tampon to tear through the posterior vaginal wall into the abdominal cavity, causing an extreme loss of blood internally.

After preliminary observations, a gynecologic or anal examination will be done to evaluate the physical condition of the victim and to document that rape occurred by the presence of any vaginal or perineal lacerations or sperm or DNA left behind by the assailant on the perineum or in the vagina or rectum. Acid phosphate, a component of prostatic fluid, is a substance that is not normally present in vaginal or rectal secretions but is present in semen. Determining the presence of acid phosphate can be extremely important, therefore, if the attacker is infertile or sterile, making DNA analysis difficult. Its presence may be the best evidence that rape occurred. Vaginal and anal cultures are taken for gonorrhea, and a Pap test is also performed. Blood is drawn for a pregnancy test and a VDRL test for syphilis if appropriate. Prophylactic administration of antibiotics against gonorrhea and syphilis may be necessary. If the woman is not menstruating, she may be given "morning after" therapy to avoid pregnancy. The victim may have a baseline blood sample drawn to diagnose HIV and hepatitis B status.

Be certain during emergency care to provide privacy. Many people may want to ask the victim questions, including police officers or detectives, the victim's family, a rape trauma team, and an examining primary health care provider. Describing the experience is good, but lack of privacy during a perineal examination demonstrates little concern for the victim's self-esteem. Many female victims are uncomfortable with a male examiner after rape, because they are temporarily fearful of men. Having a female nurse remain with the victim during this time may be helpful. A male nurse can be equally supportive, however, because it is not the male–female contrast that a victim is seeking so much as a contrast between aggression and caring.

What if... 55.3 Hillary's physical examination reveals she has a purulent vulvovaginitis, and a culture reveals this is caused by a gonorrhea infection. What questions would you want to ask her to determine how she contracted the infection? Would the fact that her mother is influential in the city influence what questions you ask?

Legal Considerations

Nurses working in emergency departments may be asked to testify in court about a rape victim's appearance after the assault, although the documentation in the record is usually all that is necessary. Many victims, especially adolescents, do not press charges against their assailants because they were too frightened or unable at the time to observe the assailant's appearance and therefore cannot identify him later. They may fear that if they name him in court, he will return and kill them. Whether victims follow through with a legal action or not is their choice, but the incidence of rape might be reduced if rapists were aware they are not apt to escape without a penalty for their crime. For that reason, some states have prosecutors press charges even if the victim declines, as with domestic violence charges. Taking the rapist to court may be an opportunity and appropriate time for victims to "fight back" and therefore not be as helpless as they were forced to be during the attack.

QSEN Checkpoint Question 55.5

Informatics

Hillary's mother reveals that she was raped when she was a teenager. Before beginning a physical assessment of an adolescent who has been raped, which would be the most important question to ask?

a. "Have you bathed or showered since the attack?"
b. "Did the rape feel more sexual or more violent?"
c. "Was anything stolen from you during the attack?"
d. "Can you think of a way you could have prevented this?"

Look in Appendix A for the best answer and rationale.

Nursing Diagnoses and Related Interventions

Nursing Diagnosis: Anxiety related to recent rape

Outcome Evaluation: Victim is able to discuss what happened and voice intense feelings about the crime; victim states ability to move forward with life.

One of the major needs of any victim after a violent act is to talk about what happened because a person who can describe an incident can also begin to "put a fence around" the event or bring the event down from "something terrible has happened," a situation that leaves the person with a continuing high anxiety level, to "this specific thing has happened," a situation that allows the traumatic event to be examined and managed (something that is concrete and describable is rarely as frightening as "something out there").

Ask the victim to describe the incident to you with an introduction such as, "Most people find it helps to talk about what happened to them." Be certain victims have a support person to accompany them home. Be sure they know that, if their distress becomes acute, they can return as needed to the health care facility for additional care or counseling. Be certain as well that they have the telephone number of a counseling service.

Because genital bruising may not be apparent until 24 hours after the rape, victims may be asked to return for a re-examination the next day so this can be documented. Syphilis will not be apparent for up to 6 weeks in serum, so they should return for a repeat VDRL at that time. They may be advised to return in 6 weeks and again in 6 months for HIV testing.

Nursing Diagnosis: Disabled family coping related to recent rape of family member

Outcome Evaluation: Partner or other family members express feelings about the rape to health care provider; family members state confidence in ability to support rape victim.

In many instances, the victim's usual sexual partner has difficulty being a support person after a rape because this person has as much difficulty dealing with the rape as the victim. Not infrequently, a relationship that was meaningful before the rape deteriorates because the partner mistakenly believes the victim was somehow responsible for the trauma or actually enjoyed the experience. In other instances, the partner may become so overprotective (not allowing the victim to go out alone; checking on her constantly) that she is not free to maintain her identity. Parents of a young adolescent may feel the same way. Counseling for the victim's partner or family may be necessary to help them to be truly supportive (Box 55.9).

BOX 55.9 Goals of Crisis Intervention for Families of Rape Victims

- Help the family be supportive of and reassuring to the victim to help initiate problem-solving techniques.
- Explain the possibility of future psychological and somatic symptoms that characterize a rape trauma syndrome and what the family can do to minimize these symptoms.
- Eliminate the family's sense of guilt for not protecting the victim by assuring them they could not have anticipated or prevented the rape.
- Educate the family about rape as a *violent crime*, not a sexually motivated act, to eliminate a focus on the victim's guilt or responsibility.
- Discourage violent, destructive, or irrational retribution toward the rapist (under the guise of being on the victim's behalf) by encouraging sharing of feelings of helplessness, sadness, hurt, and anger.
- Encourage discussion of the sexual relationship between partners; suggest that the victim's partner let her know (1) that his or her feelings have not changed (if this is true) and that she is still sexually desirable, (2) that the partner will wait for her to approach, and (3) that sex therapy is available if they have persistent difficulties and want assistance in re-establishing usual sexual relations.
- Explain the possibility of sexually transmitted disease and pregnancy that may result from a rape, the preventive care necessary for the victim and spouse or sexual partner, and the follow-up care indicated.
- Refer the family for direct counseling if members' shared responses to the crisis interfere with their ability to cope adaptively.
- Identify how the family has handled crises in the past, and encourage members to use adaptive coping mechanisms for this crisis. Encourage contact with persons identified as supportive to the family, and offer to contact such persons.

INTIMATE PARTNER VIOLENCE

Intimate partner violence is maltreatment by a family member against another adult living in the household, such as a spouse or significant other. That spouse or partner maltreatment and child maltreatment may both exist in a family strengthens the importance of providing family-centered nursing care so both of these situations can be identified and halted. As many as 20% to 30% of women seen in emergency departments are there because they have been maltreated by their intimate partner. Common injuries suffered include burns, lacerations, bruises, and head injuries. Asking all women at physical examinations to account for any bruise they have helps detect physical maltreatment. Asking them whether they are ever concerned about their safety or well-being helps detect emotional maltreatment.

Like child maltreatment, intimate partner violence affects all ethnic and social groups. If it appears to be more prevalent in lower socioeconomic neighborhoods, it is because these families are more visible to service organizations and law enforcement officials. When it occurs in middle or upper class houses, wives are often too embarrassed to let people know and tend to keep the violence hidden longer.

It occurs at a higher rate during pregnancy than other times, so including questions about this in pregnancy health histories is especially important (Hellmuth, Coop Gordon, Stuart, et al., 2013). The rate of intimate partner violence is so high during pregnancy that homicide from intimate partner violence is the number one cause of death in pregnant women, a finding that probably occurs because stress can be a trigger to violence, and pregnancy, with all that an expected new child entails (another mouth to feed, body to clothe, or dependent to protect), can increase stress.

Maltreated women may have an unintended and unwanted pregnancy because they were unable to fight off sexual advances from their abusive partner. Other women may desire the pregnancy very much even with such a poor beginning because they believe having a child will change the partner and make him a better person or having an infant will offer her someone who loves her.

Why intimate partner violence occurs is perplexing, but violent family situations can be divided into two groups: those in which violence preceded the relationship or children and those in which the violence developed after the relationship was established or children were born.

In the first situation, which is more common, violence is usually brought into the family by a man with a history of violence (although women may also be offenders). His violence-prone characteristics usually erupt early in the courtship and grow progressively worse as he uses violence to handle even small conflicts, which instills a pervasive feeling of powerlessness in the people around him. Such men usually have a history of early and prolonged exposure to family violence as children; alcohol is frequently associated with the expression of violence (Gomez, 2011).

A cycle of violence often follows three phases: tension-building, acute violence, and a "honeymoon" or tranquil, loving phase. During the first phase, the offender displays actions such as anger, arguing, and blaming the victim for external problems or for provoking the violence. The acute violence phase can be triggered by a response from the intimate partner or by an external crisis and can result in extreme physical harm to the victim. The tranquil, loving phase, characterized by kind and contrite behavior, follows the violence, lulling the victim into forgiveness and a wish to continue the relationship. Without intervention, however, this phase ends at some point, and the cycle of violence repeats (Koijpers, van der Knapp, & Winkel, 2012).

TABLE 55.2 Typical Levels of Intimate Partner Violence

Level	Description
I	Maltreatment is occasional; consists of slapping, punching, kicking, verbal maltreatment. Contusions occur.
II	Maltreatment is becoming more frequent; beatings are sustained and cause fractures, such as a broken jaw or rib fracture.
III	Maltreatment is even more frequent, perhaps daily. A weapon, such as a gun, baseball bat, or broom handle, may be used. Permanent disability or death from injuries, such as intracranial hemorrhage or concussion, may occur.

Partners react to the situation in three phases (Table 55.2). During the impact phase (stage I), or the light level of violence, the victim uses denial as a defense mechanism. By not stopping or facing what is happening, however, she is indirectly giving the offender permission to continue. During the second stage, the victim can no longer deny the violence is occurring. At the same time, she cannot stop it because she does not provoke the violence; she is only a convenient recipient of poorly controlled extreme behavior. She is forced to use coping mechanisms such as becoming very obedient and cooperative and doing everything her partner asks in a desperate effort to reduce the violence. The woman is forced to become isolated; she sinks into hopelessness and depression. This phase is often referred to as psychological infantilism or **learned helplessness**. To stop the cycle from repeating after a period of calm, she needs health care personnel to recognize her circumstances and offer her help.

Although it is impossible to predict how any individual woman will respond, pregnant maltreated women may demonstrate typical behaviors that reveal violence. A woman may come for care late in pregnancy or not at all, for example, because her partner controls her transportation or money; she may have been pretending the pregnancy did not exist to reduce stress in her home. She may be noticeable in a prenatal setting because she has purchased no maternity clothing (she has no funds for herself and asking for money may incite violence). For the same reason, she may decline laboratory tests if they involve additional transportation or money.

A maltreated woman may have difficulty following recommended pregnancy nutrition (she must cook what her partner wants or she will be beaten). She may grow anxious if her appointment is running late (she must be home to cook dinner or risk a beating). She may call and cancel appointments frequently (or simply not keep appointments) because she has an obvious black eye or a bleeding facial laceration she does not want to reveal. She may dress inappropriately for warm weather, wearing long-sleeved, tight-necked blouses to cover up bruises on her neck or arms. When undressed for a physical examination, there may be bruises or lacerations on her breasts, abdomen, or back she cannot explain. Her neck may reveal linear bruises from strangulation. Give thoughtful consideration as to whether the explanation the woman gives for a bruise or laceration correlates with the extent and placement of the injury

A woman who has experienced recent violence may be anxious to listen to the baby's heartbeat or have fundal height measured at prenatal visits because she is worried the fetus may have been hurt. If abdominal trauma is present, an ultrasound may be prescribed to further assess fetal health. If an ultrasound reveals minimal placental infarcts from blunt abdominal trauma, this can lead to poor placental perfusion, low birth weight, or pregnancy loss.

QSEN Checkpoint Question 55.6

Patient-Centered Care

Hillary's mother appears to function competently at her high-level job. Suppose you discover, though, by history taking, that she is a victim of intimate partner violence. When addressing this issue, what typical characteristic of an intimate partner who is violent toward a female partner should you be aware of?

a. A man has been raised in a family where the father was violent.
b. A man wants to earn more money but has no education.
c. A man is under severe psychological stress.
d. A man has more than three children younger than 10 years old.

Look in Appendix A for the best answer and rationale.

Nursing Diagnoses and Related Interventions

Nursing diagnoses for a woman who has experienced intimate partner violence may pertain to physical injuries sustained, but they should also address the emotional manifestations of violence. Some examples include:

- Powerlessness related to perception that it is impossible to break away from abusing partner
- Fear related to constant threat of violence
- Social isolation related to client's need to hide evidence of intimate partner violence
- Ineffective denial related to inability to face the fact that partner is sexually violent
- Compromised family coping related to dysfunctional relationship between client and abusive partner

Expected outcomes should address specific tasks a woman could accomplish to keep herself safe from further intimate partner violence, such as:

- Client carries with her telephone numbers of emergency services and a shelter for women who have experienced intimate partner violence.
- Client and abusive partner continue to attend counseling sessions.
- Client states she has filed a restraining order against abusive partner.
- Client states she feels secure living at safe house.

It may be difficult to understand why a woman elects to stay in a violent intimate partner relationship. A common finding is that a woman cannot leave because the guilt and low self-esteem she feels have led her to believe she deserves to be treated this way or because of fear the abusive person will find her and kill her. To free herself from this emotional paralysis, she needs outside help. Unfortunately, she doesn't seek this because her low self-esteem and depression lead her to believe that no one would be interested in helping her.

Until she can develop better self-esteem, a woman may need support to make even simple decisions, so support any ability she has to make constructive decisions. Be familiar with shelters for women who have experienced intimate partner violence in your community; discuss with her how she can call the police at any time and they will take her to the shelter. Help her to file charges or obtain a restraining order to keep the abusive person from coming near her again if this is necessary.

Be careful not to blame the victim or leave a woman who has found the courage to leave her abuser without a support system because without effective support, she may decide that self-injury or returning to the intimate partner is her best recourse. If a woman does return to live with an abusive partner, both she and the infant need frequent health care visits scheduled so their health and welfare can be monitored. A child raised in a home where a member is violent will learn that this is acceptable conduct, and the violence may extend to yet another generation.

Children who have a parent who is violent may be identified because of conduct problems, noncompliance, and aggression in school. They may develop low levels of empathy, or they may display distress behaviors such as clinging, crying, abdominal pain, or sleeping disorders. Effects may be long term if the violence causes teenage girls to shy away from relationships with boys, afraid they will be exposed to the same level of violence as their mother.

What if...55.4 You are interested in exploring one of the 2020 National Health Goals regarding violence or maltreatment of children and families (see Box 55.1). Most government-sponsored money for nursing research is allotted based on these goals. What would be a possible research topic to explore pertinent to these goals that would be applicable to Hillary's family and also advance evidence-based practice?

Key Points for Review

- Child maltreatment can exist in many forms. It may be physical, emotional, or sexual and may encompass neglect.
- A high suspicion for child maltreatment should be present if burns, head injury, or rib fractures are present or if the history of the accident seems out of proportion to the injury.
- Shaken baby syndrome involves repetitive, violent shaking of a small infant by the arms or shoulders, causing a whiplash injury to the neck, edema to the brainstem, and distinct retinal hemorrhages.
- A triad of "special parent, special child, special circumstance" is characteristic of the family in which child maltreatment occurs.
- Failure to thrive is a syndrome in which an infant falls below the 5th percentile for weight and height on a standard growth chart. It is associated with a disturbance in the parent–child relationship.
- Children who comfort parents in emergency settings may just be sensitive children, or they may be demonstrating role reversal, a behavior characteristic of maltreated children.
- In families in which a child is maltreated, a parent may also be a victim of maltreatment. Ask enough questions at health care visits to be certain that this problem does not exist as well as help plan nursing care that not only meets QSEN competencies but also best meets the family's total needs.
- Child maltreatment is reportable by law. Nurses can initiate reporting as an independent action or through their health agency's referral network.
- Methods to prevent maltreatment in which nurses can actively participate include teaching about the expected growth and development of children, educating parents for parenting roles, and teaching empowerment, or a sense that children and adults have control of their own lives.
- Sexual maltreatment of children can be prevented by teaching children to recognize abnormal advances and to know it is right to speak out about wrongs against them.
- Maltreatment is a family problem, not an individual problem. Therapy must include all family members to be effective.
- Rape is a crime of violence, not of sexual intent. Rape victims need both short- and long-term counseling.
- Pregnant women with traumatic injuries need to be carefully assessed to determine whether intimate partner violence was the cause of the trauma.

Critical Thinking Care Study

Nick is 6 years old; his brother Sam is 13 months old. Emergency medical technicians (EMTs) brought them into your emergency room by ambulance after a minor automobile accident involving their family car. They are alert, were in child booster seats with seat belts, and appear uninjured. However, when examined at the accident scene, the EMTs found bruises in various stages of healing on the children. Some were in expected areas, but others indicated potential child maltreatment.

1. Sites of "expected bruising" change with developmental level. How would they differ between Nick, a 6-year-old, and his 13-month-old brother?
2. When the boys' father arrives, you hear him tell the boys, "Don't say a word about the accident." Is this a clue the boys have been maltreated? If these two boys are being maltreated, would they have been so carefully protected by seat belts in the car?
3. Should you alert your agency's child protection team based on the above findings that you suspect child abuse or wait until you talk to the mother to see if there is another side of this story?

Patient Scenario
The Ludlow Family

Read about the Ludlow family, a family with a child who has been maltreated, then answer the questions to further sharpen your skills and grow more familiar with NCLEX-type questions related to child maltreatment and intimate partner violence. Confirm your answers are correct by reading the rationales.

Visit http://thePoint.lww.com

Answers and Rationales

Looking for answers to the What If . . . and Critical Thinking Care Study questions?

Visit http://thePoint.lww.com

References

Briggs, P., Simon, W. T., & Simonsen, S. (2011). An exploratory study of internet-initiated sexual offenses and the chat room sex offender: Has the internet enabled a new typology of sex offender? *Sexual Abuse: A Journal of Research and Treatment, 23*(1), 72–91.

Carlson, B. E. (2011). Sibling incest: Adjustment in adult women survivors. *Families in Society: The Journal of Contemporary Social Services, 92*(1), 77–83.

Centers for Disease Control and Prevention. (2012). *Child maltreatment prevention.* Atlanta, GA: Author.

Delacroix, J., Brown, J., Kadenhe-Chaweshe, A., et al. (2011). Rectal perforation secondary to rape and fisting in a female adolescent. *Pediatric Emergency Care, 27*(2), 116–119.

Fang, X., Brown, D. S., Florence, C. S., et al. (2012). The economic burden of child maltreatment in the United States and implications for prevention. *Child Abuse & Neglect, 36*(2), 156–165.

Fraser, J., Matthews, B., Walsh, K. M., et al. (2010). Factors influencing child abuse and neglect recognition and reporting by nurses: A multivariate analysis. *International Journal of Nursing Studies, 47*(2), 146–153.

Freisthler, B. (2011). Alcohol use, drinking venue utilization, and child physical abuse: Results from a pilot study. *Journal of Family Violence, 26*(3), 185–193.

Gomez, A. M. (2011). Testing the cycle of violence hypothesis: Child abuse and adolescent dating violence as predictors of intimate partner violence in young adulthood. *Youth & Society, 43*(1), 171–192.

Goodwin, M. B. (2011). Precarious moorings: Tying fetal drug law policy to social profiling. *Rutgers Law Journal, 42*(3), 659–694.

Heim, C., Shugart, M., Craighead, W. E., et al. (2010). Neurobiological and psychiatric consequences of child abuse and neglect. *Developmental Psychobiology, 52*(7), 671–690.

Helfer, R. E., & Kempe, R. S. (1987). *The battered child.* Chicago, IL: University of Chicago Press.

Hellmuth, J. C., Coop Gordon, K., Stuart, G. L., et al. (2013). Risk factor for intimate partner violence during pregnancy and postpartum. *Archives of Women's Mental Health, 16*(1), 19–27.

Hitchcock, J. (2012). The debate over shaken baby syndrome. *Journal of Neonatal Nursing, 18*(1), 20–21.

Hlavka, H. R., Olinger, S. D., & Lashley, J. L. (2010). The use of anatomical dolls as a demonstration aid in child sexual abuse interviews: A study of forensic interviewers' perceptions. *Journal of Child Sexual Abuse, 19*(5), 519–553.

Hornor, G. (2010). Child sexual abuse: Consequences and implications. *Journal of Pediatric Health Care: Official Publication of National Association of Pediatric Nurse Associates and Practitioners, 24*(6), 358–364.

Hornor, G. (2011). Medical evaluation for child sexual abuse: What the PNP needs to know. *Journal of Pediatric Health Care: Official Publication of National Association of Pediatric Nurse Associates and Practitioners, 25*(4), 250–260.

Jaffe, A. C. (2011). Failure to thrive: Current clinical concepts. *Pediatrics in Review, 32*(3), 100–108.

Koetting, C., Fitzpatrick, J. J., Lewin, L., et al. (2012). Nurse practitioner knowledge of child sexual abuse in children with cognitive disabilities. *Journal of Forensic Nursing, 8*(2), 72–80.

Koijpers, K. F., van der Knapp, L. M., & Winkel, F. W. (2012). Risk of revictimization of intimate partner violence: The role of attachment, anger and violent behavior of the victim. *Journal of Family Violence, 27*(1), 33–44.

Kucuker, H., Demir, T., & Oral, R. (2010). Pediatric condition falsification (Munchausen syndrome by proxy) as a continuum of maternal factitious disorder (Munchausen syndrome). *Pediatric Diabetes, 11*(8), 572–578.

Lang, A. J., Garstein, M. A., Rodgers, C. S., et al. (2010). The impact of maternal childhood abuse on parenting and infant temperament. *Journal of Child and Adolescent Psychiatric Nursing, 23*(2), 100–110.

Lang, D. L., Sales, J. M., Salazer, L. F., et al. (2011). Rape victimization and high-risk sexual behaviors: Longitudinal study of African-American adolescent females. *Western Journal of Emergency Medicine, 12*(3), 333–342.

Lazoritz, S., Rossiter, K., & Whiteaker, D. (2010). What every nurse needs to know about the clinical aspects of child abuse. *American Nurse Today, 5*(7), 1–3.

Makin-Byrd, K., & Bierman, K. L. (2013). Individual and family predictors of the perpetration of dating violence and victimization in late adolescence. *Journal of Youth & Adolescence, 42*(4), 536–550.

McCloskey, L. A. (2013). The intergenerational transfer of mother-daughter risk for gender-based abuse. *Psychodynamic Psychiatry, 41*(2), 303–328.

Neutze, J., Grundmann, D., Scherner, G., et al. (2012). Undetected and detected child abuse and child pornography offenders. *International Journal of Law and Psychiatry, 35*(3), 168–175.

Rothbaum, B. O., Kearns, M. C., Price, M., et al. (2012). Early intervention may prevent the development of posttraumatic stress disorder: A randomized pilot civilian study with modified prolonged exposure. *Biological Psychiatry, 72*(11), 957–963.

Schönbucher, V., Maier, T., Mohler-Kuo, M., et al. (2012). Disclosure of child sexual abuse by adolescents: A qualitative in-depth study. *Journal of Interpersonal Violence, 27*(17), 3486–3513.

Schwecke, L. H. (2011). Beyond childhood sexual abuse: Ritual abuse—Torture and human trafficking. *Journal of Psychosocial Nursing and Mental Health Services, 49*(1), 8–10.

Sullivan, C. M. (2011). Child abuse and the legal system: The orthopaedic surgeon's role in diagnosis. *Clinical Orthopaedics and Related Research, 469*(3), 768–775.

Thompson, N. J., McGee, R. E., & Mays, D. (2012). Race, ethnicity, substance abuse and unwanted sexual intercourse among adolescent females in the United States. *Western Journal of Emergency Medicine, 13*(3), 283–288.

Tonmyr, L., Jack, S. M., Brooks, S., et al. (2012). Utilization of the Canadian Incidence Study of Reported Child Abuse and Neglect by child welfare agencies in Ontario. *Chronic Disease & Injury in Canada, 33*(1), 29–37.

U.S. Department of Health and Human Services. (2010). *Healthy people 2020.* Washington, DC: Author.

Valentino, K., Nuttall, A. K., Comas, M., et al. (2012). Intergenerational continuity of child abuse among adolescent mothers: Authoritarian parenting, community violence, and race. *Child Maltreatment, 17*(2), 172–181.

Wastler, S. (2010). The harm in "sexting": Analyzing the constitutionality of child pornography statues that prohibit the voluntary production, possession, and dissemination of sexually explicit images by teenagers. *Harvard Journal of Law & Gender, 33*(2), 687–702.

Chapter 56

Nursing Care of a Family When a Child Has a Long-Term or Terminal Illness

KEY TERMS

- anticipatory grief
- death
- complicated grief
- grief process
- vulnerable children

OBJECTIVES

After mastering the contents of this chapter, you should be able to:

1. Describe common concerns of parents of children with a long-term or terminal illness.
2. Identify 2020 National Health Goals related to children with long-term or terminal illnesses that nurses could help the nation achieve.
3. Assess the adjustment of a child or family to a long-term or terminal illness.
4. Formulate nursing diagnoses for a child with a long-term or terminal illness to help him or her manage seamless transitions across differing health care settings.
5. Identify expected outcomes for a child with a long-term or terminal illness.
6. Using the nursing process, plan nursing care that includes the six competencies of Quality & Safety Education for Nurses (QSEN): Patient-Centered Care, Teamwork & Collaboration, Evidence-Based Practice (EBP), Quality Improvement (QI), Safety, and Informatics.
7. Implement nursing care for a child with a long-term or terminal illness, such as helping parents with time management.
8. Evaluate expected outcomes for effectiveness and achievement of care.
9. Integrate knowledge of long-term or terminal illness with the interplay of nursing process, the six competencies of QSEN, and Family Nursing to promote quality maternal and child health nursing care.

Charlie is a 3-year-old who has had a relapse after 18 months of chemotherapy for leukemia. You meet him in the emergency department because he has developed a severe cough and high fever. He is diagnosed as having pneumonia. "We're all so tired," her mother tells you. "And he's been sick for so long. How could he develop something else?"

Previous chapters described the growth and development of well children and the care of children with specific disorders. This chapter adds information about the care of chronically and terminally ill children. This is important information because it builds a base for care and health teaching and support for the parents and child.

How could you best help this parent? What would be important topics to talk to her about?

When children have an acute illness, both they and their parents become frightened by the sudden onset and severity of symptoms. Because human beings have a great capacity for coping with stress, however, as long as they are given adequate support, they can usually adjust to the strain of disrupted daily routines, hospital visits, and home care.

When a child's illness becomes long term or is one that is projected to have a terminal outcome, a family's capacity to cope can become stretched beyond its limits. Support is essential for such a family if it is to survive under this level of pressure and stress (Epelman, 2012; Nikkola, Kaunonen, & Aho, 2013).

People cope with situations depending on their perception of the event, the type and kind of support they receive from people around them, and the ways they have found to be successful in coping with stressful situations in the past. When working with parents of a child with a long-term or terminal illness, discovering how the parents perceive the problem, what resources they have available, and how they plan to use these resources are crucial in planning effective nursing care.

Whether the medical diagnosis involves a permanent disability or impending death, parents' first response may be grief. The parents have either lost the "perfect" child imagined during pregnancy or the well child they had up to the time of diagnosis. Depending on their age and maturity, children may also experience a grief response. Because the quality of life children with long-term or terminal conditions can enjoy is important to the overall health of children, 2020 National Health Goals that speak to this are shown in Box 56.1.

Nursing Process Overview

For Care of a Family With a Child Who Has a Long-Term or Terminal Illness

Assessment

Because a family's coping abilities are best assessed gradually and over a period of many contacts, nurses' assessments of the degree of a family's coping are often the most thorough and meaningful of all health care providers.

Observing children at home, where they are most comfortable, or at school in a familiar atmosphere often reveals a great deal more about a child's present disease status or coping potential than does a formal test situation. Children with a long-term illness, on the whole, have been through many tests and procedures in the diagnosis of their disorder; they may have reason to think of health care providers as people who hurt them, not people from whom they wish to receive care. It may be possible to change their perception by maintaining a reassuring, gentle manner during assessment and subsequent care procedures.

Nursing Diagnosis

A long-term illness can take many forms. A condition that requires daily attention, such as diabetes mellitus (e.g., managing an insulin pump), but that is stabilized may not be as stressful to parents as an illness, such as muscular dystrophy, that, because it slowly progresses in severity, may need many adjustments in care. In the former, although the child and family must adjust their lifestyle to incorporate the child's daily needs into theirs, they feel they have some control over the course of the illness and the child's overall health. In the latter, the child and family feel powerless because they lack any ability to alter the course of the disease; they must simply wait for the next acute crisis to develop. Nursing diagnoses for children with long-term or terminal illnesses need to address both the child and the family and the stage of illness of the child. Some examples of nursing diagnoses when a long-term illness is present include:

- Interrupted family processes related to recent diagnosis of chronic illness in the oldest child
- Compromised family coping related to the child's disability
- Disabling family coping related to the parents' inability to accept the child's long-term illness
- Anticipatory grieving related to chronicity of the child's illness
- Risk for delayed growth and development related to lack of age-appropriate stimulation because of disability

BOX 56.1 Nursing Care Planning Based on 2020 National Health Goals

Long-term illness or early death in children is a major cost to the nation and individual families because it has the potential to reduce the earning power and contribution of future citizens. Examples of 2020 National Health Goals that address this include:

- Increase the proportion of youth with special health care needs whose health care provider has discussed transition planning from pediatric to adult health care from a baseline of 41.2% to a target level of 45.3%.
- Increase the proportion of children with disabilities from birth through age 2 years who receive early intervention services in home or in community-based settings from 91% to 95%.
- Reduce the rate of infant deaths from a baseline of 6.7 per 1,000 live births to a target rate of 6.0 per 1,000.
- Reduce the death rate for children 1 to 4 years of age from a baseline of 28.6 per 100,000 to no more than 25.7 per 100,000 children, and for children aged 5 to 9 years from a baseline of 13.7 per 100,000 to 12.3 per 100,000.
- Reduce the death rate for children 10 to 14 years of age from a baseline of 16.9 per 100,000 to no more than 15.2 per 100,000, and the death rate for adolescents 15 to 19 years of age from a baseline of 61.9 per 100,000 to 55.7 per 100,000 (U.S. Department of Health and Human Services [DHHS], 2010; see www.healthypeople.gov).

Nurses can help the nation achieve these goals by educating women to seek care during pregnancy so that congenital anomalies, a common cause of infant morbidity and mortality, are less frequent and to teach unintentional injury prevention and the importance of immunizations so unintentional injuries and infectious diseases that can lead to long-term illness, such as rubeola and meningitis, can be reduced.

New issues develop when the child's disorder becomes terminal. The family must learn to accept not only the child's illness but also its eventual outcome. Some examples of nursing diagnoses when a terminal illness is present include:

- Hopelessness related to steady progression of the child's disease
- Anticipatory grieving related to the child's terminal illness
- Powerlessness related to inability to prolong the child's life
- Decisional conflict related to treatment options and choice of setting for the child's final care

Outcome Identification and Planning

Be certain when planning care for children with a chronic or fatal illness that the outcomes established are realistic. You probably cannot alter the course of a child's illness, but you can help parents cope with signs and symptoms of the illness or the impending death.

Parents who have not yet accepted the seriousness of their child's illness—who hold on to the hope that their child will eventually be cured or restored to full health—may make plans that the child cannot accomplish. Sometimes this level of denial is necessary so the parents can cope with the child's daily needs and the needs of the rest of the family. If they believe they must shield the child or other family members from the truth, it can be hard for them to plan effective outcomes. Focusing on hopeful but realistic outcomes, such as the desire the child will not experience pain for that day or the child will learn how to move about independently in a wheelchair, can help a family move forward toward a final, realistic acceptance of the seriousness of the child's illness.

Helpful organizations to use for referral are the Candlelighters for Children With Cancer (www.4kidswithcancer.org), The Compassionate Friends (www.compassionatefriends.org), and the National Association of School Psychologists (www.nasponline.org).

Implementation

When children have a long-term or terminal illness, parents may begin to overprotect them so much that they neglect to encourage their development, such as neglecting to provide play materials or other stimulation appropriate for their age. Helping parents to look at their child's capabilities and arranging appropriate activities for the child are ways in which nurses can facilitate parents' acceptance of the diagnosis and the road ahead. Suggestions for helping children achieve developmental milestones are discussed for each age group in Chapters 29 through 33.

Helping parents learn better coping strategies and teaching them ways to remember to give medication for several years, ways to maintain quality care without becoming exhausted, and the importance of maintaining a lifestyle of their own are other important measures.

Outcome Evaluation

Children with a long-term or terminal illness need periodic follow-up care, because plans made for a newborn may no longer be suitable as soon as the child becomes a toddler. Plans made in the early school years may need to be modified by the time the child is 12 years of age, and they must change again with adolescence. You may need to remind parents that, in addition to health care by a specialty clinic, children also need routine health maintenance care. Otherwise, children will be well protected from the complications of their special illness but unprotected from common childhood illnesses that could be even more devastating.

An evaluation of whether expected outcomes for the family of a child who died were met helps to strengthen your planning with the next dying child you care for, to improve your ability make sensitive plans, and to build confidence in your ability to care for dying children. When an evaluation reveals discrepancies between the wish and the reality of care, identifying areas you need to strengthen helps you to grow as a health care provider. Some examples suggesting achievement of outcomes include:

- Parents state realistic plans for their child regarding school placement.
- Parents state they have been able to deal with their grief over their child's diagnosis to maintain near-normal family functioning.
- Parents state they are able to cope with present stressors.
- The child states he is aware his illness is chronic (long term) but thinks of himself as a person who will be able to accomplish many things in life.

THE CHILD WITH A LONG-TERM ILLNESS

Because families have different resources and everyone reacts to situations differently, each child with a long-term illness and the family need to be assessed for their potential to cope with the illness and to provide necessary care. Through such an assessment, appropriate interventions to help the family adapt can be started early in the course of the illness (Longden, 2011).

The Parents' Adjustment

Children have difficulty adjusting to stressful events without good role modeling from their parents. Therefore, an assessment begins with an examination of how well the parents are responding to the diagnosis of a long-term illness.

The Grief Response

Parents can be expected to experience a **grief process**, or the regulated steps in grieving, when they are told their child will be physically or cognitively challenged or is terminally ill. The most commonly accepted steps or stages of grief are those outlined by Kübler-Ross (1969). Table 56.1 summarizes these stages. Many parents with a child who is physically or cognitively challenged never arrive at the final stage of acceptance or they spend years with chronic sorrow (also called **complicated grief**) (Whittingham, Wee, Sanders, et al., 2013). For parents with a terminally ill child, acceptance may come only with the child's death. Reaching a final stage may be particularly difficult when parents grieve in different ways or at different paces (Wender, 2012).

During the first stage of grief (shock or denial), parents are usually unable to plan past immediate or short-term actions

TABLE 56.1 The Stages of Grief

Stage	Parents' Reaction	Description
1	Denial	Parents have difficulty realizing what has occurred. They ask, "How could this have happened?"
2	Anger	Parents react to the injustice of being singled out this way. They say, "It isn't fair this is happening."
3	Bargaining	Parents attempt to work out a "deal" to buy their way out of the situation. They say, "If my child gets well, I'll devote the rest of my life to doing good."
4	Depression	Parents begin to face what is happening. They feel sad and unprotected.
5	Acceptance	Acceptance is being able to say, "Yes, this is happening, and it is all right it is happening." With a child who has a long-term illness, parents may never reach this stage but will always remain in the chronic sorrow of the depression stage.

Based on Kübler-Ross, E. (1969). *On death and dying.* New York: Macmillan.

(e.g., learning to change a dressing, what pills to give each day). Trying to establish long-term outcomes at this point (e.g., what type of school the child will attend, future surgery that will be needed) is rarely productive, because this must all be done again when parents are truly ready to look this far ahead. During the second stage (anger), parents may be unwilling to concentrate on goals (e.g., the whole thing is so unfair; planning is asking too much of them; besides, if you were really helpful, you would cure their child, not talk about ways they have to adjust). Therefore, this may also be a time of waiting. During the bargaining stage of grief, parents are still not ready for planning. They believe that if their bargain is fulfilled (e.g., let their child be able to walk, and they will spend the rest of their life doing good), they do not have to make plans such as purchasing a wheelchair because these will be unnecessary after their wish is granted and the child's condition improves.

During the next stage of grief (depression), parents are ready to make plans but need a great deal of help in planning because they feel so sad and fatigued. Be careful in working with people who are so depressed this way that you do not totally plan *for* them rather than *with* them. Many parents of children who are born physically or cognitively challenged develop low self-esteem as well as depression (they believe that if they were as good as others, they would have had a healthy child). This makes them believe your suggestions must be better than any they could make. After they return home, however, they are the ones who must live with these plans, so they need to participate in making them.

Even after parents reach the final stage of grief (acceptance), some parents need guidance in making plans to avoid becoming so self-sacrificing that the needs and wishes of the spouse and other children are ignored. For example, parents may spend every waking moment with their ill child. Doing this is a way to ease guilt or proving that they are equal to others, or perhaps even the best parents in the entire world. Talking to them about possible reasons why they feel they must push themselves in this manner can be helpful. Help them find a middle-of-the-road approach to their child's care if possible that allows time for all family members as well as some for themselves. Helping them to plan a respite from the care of a sick child, such as an evening out while a babysitter cares for the child, could be part of this approach (Thomas & Price, 2012).

If parents had a chronically ill child late in life, by the time the child is school age, parents need to face one more step in their development as parents of a chronically ill child: to begin to make some concrete plans as to who will care for the child after they die. Like the steps that came before it, this is very difficult for parents; it asks them to contemplate not only their child's vulnerability but also their own (something people rarely want to do). They might consult with family members about guardianship and with a lawyer to help them write a will that will provide future caretaking and economic support for the chronically ill child when they are no longer able to do so.

Factors Influencing Parental Adjustment

Certain circumstances, such as the degree and timing of their child's illness, the experience of the parents, the availability of support people, and the ability to make long-term plans, appear to increase parents' ease or difficulty in adjusting to their child's disabling or long-term illness.

The Degree of Illness. The seriousness of an illness obviously affects the ability of parents to adjust (Whittingham et al., 2013). A child who needs total care, for example, requires a much more radical readjustment of the parents' lives than a child who only needs additional speech therapy for an hour a day. In most instances, the parents' perception of the child's illness is as important as the child's condition itself (Fig. 56.1). For example, a parent who envisioned a son as

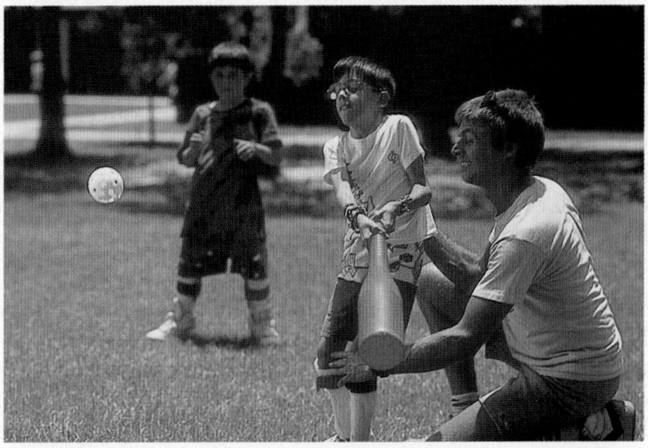

FIGURE 56.1 A parent's perception of a child's disability is important to how well the family adjusts. Often, it is easier to accept a disability that allows for greater functioning in everyday activities. (© Bill Bachman/Science Source/Photo Researchers.)

someday becoming an Olympic runner may perceive a son with developmental hip dysplasia as having a serious physical challenge; a parent whose mental image of the child was that of a lawyer mainly doing desk work may not view the hip problem as a serious illness.

Many parents are not aware of the mental image they carry of their child, an image that began to form the moment the woman realized she was pregnant. Hidden desires are often revealed if you ask parents, "If things could have been different, what kind of person would you have liked your child to be?" A parent who answers, "a kind person" can still have that wish fulfilled, no matter what the degree of illness. A parent who says, "I always assumed my child would take over the family business someday" may have some major mental readjustments to make.

Whether an illness is noticeable (cerebral palsy) or not noticeable (controlled seizures) also can make a difference in how parents adjust to the illness. A mother who takes her child with cerebral palsy shopping, during which the child walks unsteadily and knocks over a display, may hear other shoppers say, "Wouldn't you think a mother would watch her child more carefully?" On days that her child uses a wheelchair, however, shoppers' comments are more apt to be, "Poor little thing. Isn't it wonderful his mother brings him shopping with her?" She is happy to have a signal (the wheelchair) that announces that her child is different and cannot be held to the same standards as other children. Other parents might be more grateful that a child's illness is not a visible one: it makes the illness seem lesser in extent, and therefore easier for them to accept.

The Relationship With Own Parents. When adults are able to relate well to their parents, it suggests they were raised in an atmosphere of love or were able to develop a sense of trust (Erikson, 1993). People with a sense of trust are able to form a firm sense of intimacy as adults and so be better able to give love to children even when the children are handicapped in some way.

The Onset of the Illness. Whether a condition is apparent at birth (such as a myelomeningocele) or occurs at a later time (a child is struck by a car at school age or who develops autism spectrum disorder) is another factor that may make a difference in parents' ability to adjust. For some parents, never having had a well child can make the child's illness easier to accept. In either situation, the long-term care of a child will totally change the parents' lifestyle. They may no longer be able to live in a two-story house because the affected child can not walk upstairs, they have to buy an automobile that is not too high so their child can step up into it, or a parent may have to reduce work hours or give up a career to devote full time to the child's care. They may have to limit such things as vacations to save money for the child's medications or health care visits. They may have to change plans to have a large family so they have the time to devote their lives to the child's care.

The Effect of Parental Experience. First-time parents may have more difficulty caring for a child with a long-term illness than older, more experienced parents because all phases of parenting are new and unique for them. First-time parents, however, have no preconceived opinions and so may be more flexible than other parents or able to adjust more readily to a change in routine. A young parent who has just this one child may have more time to spend in a daily exercise program than does a parent with four other children.

The Availability of Support People. A family that has few close friends and lives some distance from relatives is apt to have more difficulty adjusting to illness in a child than a family that has close support people. People who can locate secondary support systems in their community, such as an organization for parents of children who are physically or cognitively challenged, a local church or synagogue, or who can depend on health care resources usually do better than parents who are without these resources. Whether a family can depend on health care resources is related to:

- The availability of transportation (e.g., it is difficult to take a child in a 50-lb cast on a bus)
- A language barrier (e.g., it is frustrating to go for care and be unable to make your needs known)
- Finances and insurance coverage (e.g., it is disturbing for parents to be told their child needs to see a specialist when they have no money or health coverage to pay for one)
- Past experience with health care providers (e.g., if the best advice that has been given to parents up to that point has been, "Take your baby home and treat him as near normally as possible," the parents may not see health care providers as a source of useful information or help)

Life Events. A child's illness usually appears to be more acute at times when the child would normally reach developmental milestones than at other times such as when the baby should take a first step or when the child would normally begin school, participate in a first communion or bar mitzvah, obtain a driver's license, or vote for the first time. When the child does not reach these traditional milestones, it reminds parents about their child's illness in a particularly painful way. Factors that indicate a family will probably be able to adjust to caring for a child with a long-term illness are summarized in Table 56.2.

QSEN Checkpoint Question 56.1

Informatics

You are reviewing the electronic notes of the social worker who has been involved with the family's care of Charlie, 3 years of age. What noted factor is most apt to help Charlie's parents cope with the stress of his long-term illness?

a. The parents believe in alternative therapies and consequently have many options.
b. Both parents have a good relationship with their own parents.
c. The parents are wealthy, so are not distressed by the cost of his care.
d. The family is private, so they cannot compare Charlie's condition to other ill children.

Look in Appendix A for the best answer and rationale.

The Child's Adjustment

A child's reaction to being physically or cognitively challenged or to having a long-term illness is strongly influenced by the family's reaction to the illness. This may range from overprotectiveness to rejection and from denial to accep-

TABLE 56.2 Factors That Ease Parental Adjustment to a Child's Long-Term Illness

Factor	Rationale
Support people are available.	Caring for a child is a series of crises during which support people become very important.
A strong marital bond exists between the parents.	A marriage partner can serve as the strongest support person.
A good relationship exists between the child's parents and their parents.	The parents (because they had good care) have a firm sense of trust and the ability to give care to another.
The child is other than the first born.	The parents have had practice parenting.
The family lives close to shopping, schools, and transportation.	The family is not isolated.
The family has a strong religious faith or community contacts.	Secondary support systems are important in times of stress.
The parents are told of the child's disability as soon as possible.	A handicap may be easier to accept if the parents never thought of the child as totally well.

tance. The child's adjustment may also be influenced by peers and other support people, such as school personnel or health care providers. Social exclusion, discrimination, and physical barriers at school or in the community make it difficult for a child to adjust to a physical challenge or a long-term illness. Inclusion in school and social activities, acceptance by peers and support people, and the ability to function as normally as possible help the child adjust (Crosland & Dunlap, 2012).

A child's ability to cope is further influenced by personal attitude and temperament, self-concept, age and development, understanding of the condition, and degree of the disorder. As the child grows and life situations change, the ability to cope may improve or worsen. For example, an adolescent who is physically challenged may become more optimistic about her condition because she is successfully working at her first job; another adolescent may become angered by his deteriorating condition because he is suddenly confined to a wheelchair.

The degree of fatigue that a child experiences is also instrumental in how well a child adjusts to a chronic illness because chronic fatigue can play a large role in making even simple tasks seem monumental (Fisher & Crawley, 2012).

Nursing interventions to help a child better adjust to a chronic condition include encouraging optimal growth and development (see Chapters 29 to 33), promoting self-care activities, enhancing self-esteem, preventing social isolation, providing health teaching, preventing fatigue, and aiding the child and family to accept the child's condition.

Siblings' Adjustment

Siblings' reactions to a child with a long-term or terminal illness are influenced by individual circumstances; however, their chief reaction is most profoundly affected by the reactions and perceptions of the parents. Without counseling, siblings may react with jealousy, anger, hostility, resentment, competition, guilt, or withdrawal. They may feel they take second place to the sibling who needs more care. These reactions are common when parents focus most of their attention on the ill child, allow the health problem and its treatment to disrupt family life significantly, or grant the ill child special privileges and minimal discipline.

With counseling and support, however, siblings can develop acceptance, care, concern, and cooperation (Vermaes, van Susante, & van Bakel, 2012). Such reactions are common when parents make it a point to set aside time each day for special activities with the well siblings such as playing a table game, walking in the park, teaching a child to swim, carefully explaining the condition and the necessity for their sibling's special care, including them in the care of the ill child, providing them with respite from care if needed, and establishing realistic rules for all family members.

At any one time, the siblings may experience a mixture of feelings. For example, if a boy's parents must take his sister for chemotherapy during his swim meet, the boy may feel both resentment that his parents missed the meet and sadness that his sister could not compete in that meet or in any others.

The Nurse and the Ill Child

Caring for children with long-term illnesses can be a stressful role for nurses (St. Ledger, Begley, Reid, et al., 2012). To help the parents and child with a long-term illness, review specific aspects of the child's condition and the possible complications that could occur. Over a period of years, parents become experts in the care of a child with a particular condition (Box 56.2). This can make them grow impatient with health care providers who appear to be unaware of things they know well. When young children are seen at an ambulatory care setting or are admitted to a hospital for care, review with the parents their typical way of carrying out a procedure so that you can continue to care for their child in the same way. As the child grows older, do this same review with the child. Be available, however, to show a parent or a child an easier way to do something if it seems appropriate. Frankly admitting to parents, "You're more familiar with Jennifer's care than I am; you'll have to teach me some things" is a refreshing approach; it not only allows parents to feel confidence in you (you are honest) but it also increases their self-esteem (they are knowledgeable people).

Familiarize yourself as well with the community resources that are available for children with long-term illnesses. Advising parents to see a dentist who specializes in caring for children with autism spectrum disorder when there is no one of that description less than 200 miles away, for example, is not only

BOX 56.2 Nursing Care Planning Based on Effective Communication

Charlie is admitted to the hospital and intravenous therapy is begun. You notice his skin where the adhesive tape was removed is unusually reddened. He cries when you touch the irritated site.

Less Effective Communication

Nurse: Look at Charlie's skin. It looks really red and sore.
Mrs. Circuso: That's from the adhesive tape.
Nurse: Oh, I don't think so. I tape this way all the time.
Mrs. Circuso: I never use it, even on myself.
Nurse: Well, it usually works really well. Charlie must have very sensitive skin.

More Effective Communication

Nurse: Look at Charlie's skin. It looks so red and sore.
Mrs. Circuso: That's from the adhesive tape.
Nurse: Has Charlie had this type of reaction before?
Mrs. Circuso: All the time. That's why I never use it, even on myself.
Nurse: I should have asked you how you usually do things for Charlie. You've been caring for him longer than I have.

It is easy to believe that a fellow nurse who has spent a great deal of time caring for a child has become an expert in that child's care. It is often more difficult to remember that a parent can become this type of expert also. Asking parents of children with a long-term illness for their input not only can simplify care but can also add to the parents' feeling of self-esteem, thus improving their parenting.

unhelpful but it also is destructive because it raises expectations in parents that cannot be met, thus accentuating, not solving, a problem.

Most parents of a chronically ill child adhere well to instructions and keep health care appointments consistently. Sometimes, however, you will find parents who do not follow this pattern. This inability to adhere usually is related to their stage of adjustment to the illness. As long as denial, anger, bargaining, or depression is functioning (and there is rarely a parent who has successfully moved completely through these stages of grief to acceptance), coming in for health care or an evaluation is viewed as a major demand. Each visit is more of a reminder of the child's illness than a time of reassuring health assessment.

Developmental Tasks

Children with long-term illnesses often do not meet developmental milestones on schedule because achieving developmental tasks takes practice. When you are helping parents teach a child who is physically or cognitively challenged a new skill, such as toilet training or using a spoon, help them to break the task down into its component parts (e.g., reach for the spoon, grasp it, push it under the chosen food, lift it toward the mouth). Breaking a task down into steps in this way allows parents to appreciate that they are asking their child to learn a task that, although it looks easy, actually encompasses 20 or more coordinated motions. Helping them learn this technique enables them to be patient in teaching additional tasks in future years.

The unique concerns of children who are physically or cognitively challenged and ways to help them achieve developmental tasks are discussed in Chapters 29 to 33. For health care providers, exposing them to usual events during a hospital stay or an ambulatory health care visit can help expand their world (Fig. 56.2).

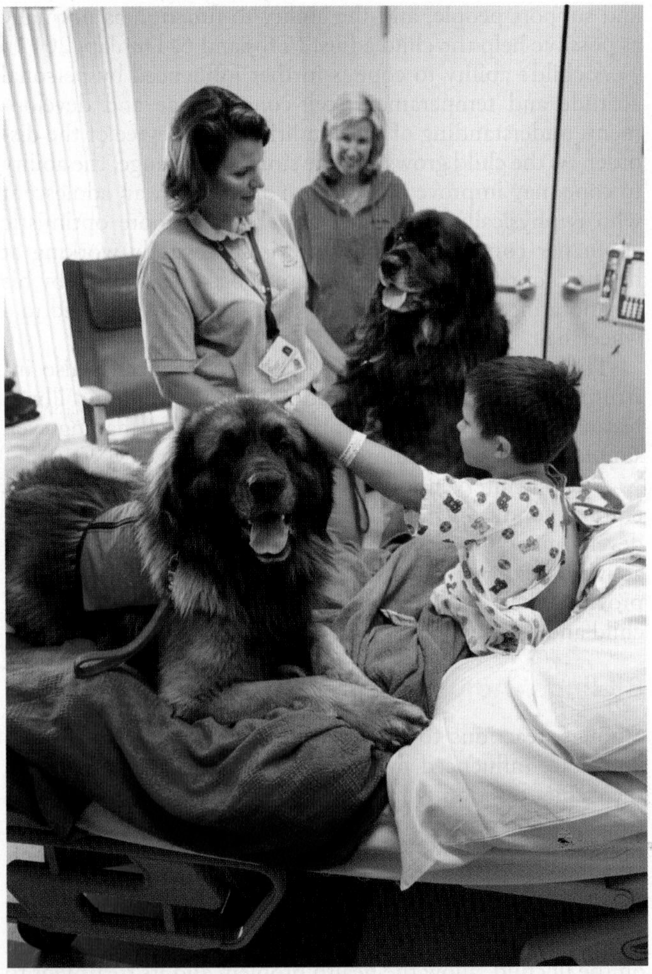

FIGURE 56.2 Therapy dogs can be helpful to keep children with a long-term illness active and in touch with usual events. (© Marmaduke St. John/Alamy)

Education

Children with a long-term illness often need special education programs or at least separate hours of individualized instruction to achieve in school. Most children benefit from preschool programs because these programs offer them a head start on school adjustment and learning. Children with a long-term illness tend to miss school more often than do their healthier classmates because of health care visits and exacerbations of their illness. This can cause them to fall behind in school unless individualized plans to keep them with their school group are made. By federal law (Public Law 99-457, Education of the Handicapped Amendment), a school system must provide educational opportunities in the least structured setting possible for physically and cognitively challenged children, beginning with preschool. You may have to be a strong child advocate to see that the best educational program available is being provided for an individual child (Kirk, Beatty, Callery, et al., 2012).

Home Care

Most children with a long-term illness may be hospitalized for a short term but then receive the bulk of their care at home (Newton & Lamarche, 2012).

Planning for home care is discussed in Chapter 4. Important aspects to consider include the best school setting (home or away?), ways to involve the family in community activities, ways to include the child in a play group if possible (children as young as preschool age may not choose an ill child as a playmate unless urged to do so), how much self-care the child can achieve, and future plans, such as preparing a child for puberty or enrolling in college. Home care or community health nurses can be instrumental in planning this type of care (Peacock & Stanik-Hutt, 2013).

Many parents today seek complementary or alternative therapies for children with long-term illnesses on home care. Always ask what therapies and medications they are using to document the full extent of treatment that a child is receiving (Fowler Braga & Almgren, 2013).

What if...56.1 You arrange for Charlie's mother to spend an afternoon shopping so she can have some respite time away from her ill child, but she spends the time cleaning her kitchen cupboards instead. Would you consider this a good use of respite time?

THE CHILD WHO IS TERMINALLY ILL

Death can come suddenly to some families, such as when an adolescent chooses self-injury as a means to problem solve or when a child is killed in an automobile accident or random shooting, providing no time for parents to prepare for the death (Carr, Nance, Branas, et al., 2012). Most children die after a terminal illness, however, so steps can be taken to help parents prepare for the coming death. This can be one of the hardest tasks in nursing because most people are raised to accept the fact that elderly people die, but such people have also lived a long life. Most people can accept the death of middle-aged people with the same philosophy—they experienced at least a portion of their life. It is often more difficult to accept the death of children because they have had so little opportunity to live. Although difficult, this makes it imperative to work through your own feelings about a child's dying so you can find the strength to care for the child and support the parents.

BOX 56.3 Nursing Care Planning to Respect Cultural Diversity

The way death is viewed and the manner in which people express grief differ greatly across cultures. Some people express grief very loudly and openly, whereas others are very restrained. The way a child's body is handled after death also differs. Some religions, for example, forbid organ donations or transplants. Autopsies are not approved because it is important that a child be buried quickly. Cremation may or may not be permitted. Being aware that people have different expectations for final care and that grief is expressed differently by different cultures enables better understanding of parents' concerns and reactions during a child's terminal illness and when death occurs. Don' t depend on stereotypical descriptions of how parents should react; ask them if they need help resolving a cultural conflict or if there is a care measure based on their cultural beliefs that they would like you to include in care.

Parental Grief Responses

Although the reaction to learning that a child has a terminal illness is strongly culturally influenced, each family reacts in a unique way. Being aware of the usual grief response that occurs in anticipation of a child's death helps in recognizing such a response as grief and supporting a family through this very difficult period (Box 56.3).

Stage 1: Denial

A parent's usual response to the diagnosis of a terminal illness in a child is denial, the same as with long-term illness (see Table 56.1). Although people are aware that children die, most proceed through life thinking, "It won't happen to my child." When they learn it may, they respond with disbelief. The likelihood of this response is enhanced by the fact that many terminal illnesses, such as a brain tumor or leukemia, begin insidiously (e.g., "How can a few black-and-blue marks be the symptoms of a potentially terminal disease?").

How the parents handle this initial disbelief has a great deal to do with their relationship with health care personnel. If they have trusted health care personnel up to this point, they may be able to accept the diagnosis without questioning any further. If they do not have this relationship, they may feel the need to obtain a second opinion. Although this often involves considerable expense, for many parents, it is a necessary step in moving past this first reaction. Parents who feel a need for a third, fourth, or fifth opinion may be having an unusually difficult time resolving a "surely not me" response. Be certain they have received a factual explanation of why it is certain that their child has this disease such as through a copy of the blood or the pathologist's biopsy report. Urge them to talk about how they feel and if they have any questions. Only after people can grasp that their child's illness is definitely present can they begin to accept that the disease will ultimately prove fatal.

During this stage of denial, you may find the parents' actions inappropriate to the child's condition. They may talk of an "upset stomach," for example, when the child is unable to eat anything or "probably just a cold" when the child has been diagnosed as having cystic fibrosis. It is easy to view such denial as a step that should be hurried because parents cannot begin to deal with the problem as long as they deny there is a problem. This is true, but neither can they deal with a problem when it hurts as much as this one. Denial is a temporary pain-relief measure and a necessary step on the way to acceptance.

Stage 2: Anger

Parents can be expected to enter a stage of anger soon—a change from "Surely not me" to "It's not right this is happening to me." When parents are angry about a diagnosis, they may be unable to direct their anger appropriately. They may find themselves angry with the child (e.g., scolding the child for crying during a painful procedure). One parent may be angry with the other parent (e.g., criticizing the other for reckless driving or for eating a fattening food for lunch). They may be angry with you (e.g., for not answering the child's call light immediately). They may be angry with the medical, X-ray, laboratory, and dietary staff or with the entire health care system. It can be difficult to react to this kind of angry attack because it seems unjustified (after all, you came as soon as you could). Be certain your first reaction is not to be angry in return because this could result in your avoidance of the child's room for the rest of the day so as not to undergo that kind of unfair criticism again.

A more therapeutic reaction is to accept this angry response as the stage of grief that it is and respond accordingly: "I'm sorry it seemed to take me so long to answer your call bell, but you seem angry about more than just the light. Would it help to talk about it?"

Some parents may "shop" for another health care provider during the stage of anger, although their reaction will depend to a great extent on their experience with death in the past and the meaning this child has to them. Because grandparents live longer today, for some parents, a fatal illness in a child is their first contact with death. Another influential factor is that different children mean different things to parents. A child born to them at a happy time can represent all that is good and happy in their life, so a loss of that child could also mean a loss of all the joy that the child represents.

When you ask grieving parents to talk, therefore, they may talk not about the child, but about how they felt when a parent died, how hard their job is for them, or how they worry that their marriage is failing. This is part of grief: gathering resources, reworking stress from the past, and arming themselves to face stress in the near future. Parents often receive support from other parents on the hospital unit whose children also are terminally ill. They are helped by seeing parents of other children adjusting to approaching death, or if not adjusting, at least functioning in what passes for a normal manner.

What if...56.2 Charlie's parents, who are both 50 years old and live on a ranch, tell you their two grown children have expressed resentment at the amount of time and money they have spent trying to find a cure for Charlie. Because Charlie's parents have no health insurance, so finances are always tight, would you agree with their children?

Stage 3: Bargaining

Although not everyone progresses through a grief response in a linear fashion, and instead go back and forth between stages, bargaining is often the next stage to occur. This is a time when parents try to correct what is happening by making a bargain to be better people (i.e., a change from "This isn't right" to "I can make it right"). They vow to be better people or to function in a different way in exchange for their child's life. When parents realize that bargaining is ineffective, it brings them to a very low point because they are let down not only by health care providers but also by the superior power with whom they tried to bargain. They may need more support after bargaining fails than at any other point.

Stage 4: Depression

When parents have passed through the stages of denial, anger, and bargaining, developing awareness of the true meaning of what is happening with accompanying depression is the next step to occur. This is a change from "I can keep it from happening" to "It is happening." Frequent crying or projecting an overall sad countenance is the most common sign that this stage has been reached. Parents may ask more questions about care, procedures, or medications than they did before. Be careful you do not interpret this questioning as criticism. Parents are asking why a child must have continuous dialysis not to criticize care, but because this is the first time they are fully aware of its serious implication.

Parents may work through the expected loss of a child at this stage by talking about their plans for the child or how the child was achieving in school. They may suddenly shower the child with expensive gifts or trips. They may have a great deal of difficulty leaving a hospitalized child to go home to care for other children or to report for work. On the surface, this reaction appears to be a step backward (they were accepting the diagnosis so well, and now they seem demanding and overwhelmed by it). Actually, this reflects the first time they have actually begun to appreciate the diagnosis and what it means and, therefore, is a step forward.

At about this stage, parents need to think about preparing other children in the family for the death of the ill child. If the ill child is hospitalized and siblings have not been allowed to visit, siblings may interpret this as meaning that death is such a horrible sight that they are not allowed to be exposed to it, rather than that sibling visitation in the intensive care unit is not allowed. You may need to advocate for sibling visitation to overcome this concern.

Some siblings feel responsible for the death of the ill child. All children wish at one time or another that a sibling were dead (or would simply disappear) so they could have a bedroom all to themselves or so they could have the other child's bicycle. Maybe they were told not to wrestle with the ill sibling, but they did anyway. These children need reassurance that wishing for something does not make it come true, and that the sibling's death is uncontrollable. Assure them that it will happen no matter what they or their parents did or will do to help manage this level of guilt.

Stage 5: Acceptance

The acceptance stage of the grief process is resolution that the child will die (a change from "This is happening" to "It's all right this is happening"). Few parents reach this stage by the time of the child's death; grief work will need to continue for years past the time of the death until this stage can be reached.

QSEN Checkpoint Question 56.2

Patient-Centered Care

Charlie's parents are grieving because they fear he will not survive this recurrence of his illness. You are planning your care with the knowledge that the family is experiencing intense sadness. During which stage of grief do parents usually feel the most intense depression?

a. The first stage, because everything is such a shock
b. The last stage, because they fully accept the death
c. The fourth stage, as they realize death is happening
d. The stage at which the child begins to talk about death

Look in Appendix A for the best answer and rationale.

Parental Coping Responses

Throughout the stages of grieving, parents develop important coping mechanisms to help them through this crisis in their life. Even if they have already learned to cope positively with their child's illness and treatment measures, the determination that the illness is now terminal requires yet another step. Promoting the development of positive coping strategies while being sensitive to the unique needs of each family member is an important nursing responsibility. It may be difficult to determine when a coping strategy is truly helpful and when it has become maladaptive. For instance, seeking information, such as surfing the Internet and asking to have medical library access, is generally a very useful strategy for parents with ill children. Knowing what to expect reduces anxiety. Some parents, however, continue these seeking procedures past the point at which information is helpful to them, believing if they only look hard enough or long enough, they will discover a way to cure their child (prolonged denial), or they may "overintellectualize" their child's illness and impending death to block out their feelings of sadness.

Problem solving is always an effective coping strategy as long as the parents are realistic about which problems they can solve. Seeking the support of others, including health care providers and families with similar needs, is a strategy to encourage. Providing the names of support groups or individual families (with their permission) who have gone through similar experiences can also be a helpful nursing action. You may also need to help parents who are not comfortable accepting the help of others to learn how to do so or to simply learn how to feel comfortable expressing their feelings to others.

Many parents are able to cope by searching for the meaning of their child's life or impending death in philosophical, spiritual, or religious terms. For these parents, body organ donation may be a meaningful way to give themselves some solace that their child will in some way continue to live and contribute to others. Assuring parents that their child will be kept comfortable and will not die in pain can be extremely comforting.

Anticipatory Grief

Parents who have been warned that their child's death should be expected from the time the child's illness is diagnosed may begin a preparatory or **anticipatory grief** phase in which they gradually incorporate the reality of their child's fate into their thoughts. Anticipatory mourning in this way can prepare parents for their child's death and spare them the abrupt, devastating, and intolerable grief reaction that comes to parents whose child dies suddenly from trauma, such as in a car accident or sudden infant death syndrome (see Box 56.4, an interprofessional care map on nursing and team responsibility for care of children when illness has become terminal).

Although anticipatory grief does not shield parents from experiencing renewed grief once their child has died, it can be a useful process for them. A danger of anticipatory grief is that a parent may reach the acceptance stage of the grief process too far in advance of the child's death. If this happens, parents may begin to treat the child as if the child has already died. They stop visiting, or when they do visit, they spend most of their time visiting other children on the unit or sitting in the waiting room talking to other parents. Once they spent time comforting their child; now they may fail to rock or touch the child as much. They may clean out the child's room and throw out or give away toys. They are gradually drawing back from emotional attachment to shield themselves from the abrupt, stabbing pain that death will bring.

Children need a great deal of support if anticipatory grieving blocks out communication this way, just as they did during the initial denial stage. Parents cannot help that the grief process did not time itself to coincide exactly with the child's death. Extend understanding and do not provide criticism for this reaction.

For some parents, because of anticipatory grief, the event seems anticlimactic when the child actually dies. They have anticipated death so long that, when it does occur, they cannot believe it has actually happened. They may be so used to thinking constantly about their child's needs and having their child dependent on them that they feel lost or feel as if there is a hole in their thoughts and life. Some parents are reluctant to leave the hospital this final time because leaving with the child's possessions is the step that will make the death real.

Vulnerable or Fragile Child Syndrome

When anticipatory grief proceeds so effectively that parents begin to think of a youngster as already dead but then the child does not die, parents may find their grief reaction was so complete that they are unable to reverse it and they cannot view the child in the same way as they did before. Instead, they begin to treat the child in a cold and unfeeling way, as if the child were not really there but had actually died. Such children are termed **vulnerable children**, or fragile children (Green & Solnit, 1964). They may develop behavior problems as they grow older (e.g., acting out behavior, such as temper tantrums; stealing in school; shoplifting as adolescents) as if to say, "Notice me! I'm not dead!" They may require skilled counseling so they can feel secure that they are still loved and can learn to react effectively with others.

Children's Reactions to Impending Death

Children's reactions to death are strongly influenced by the previous experiences they have had and the family's attitude toward death. For instance, death can be a new or frightening phenomenon if a child have never had a pet die, was forbidden from visiting a dying relative, or was discouraged from discussing the death of a loved one. Children's reactions to death are also influenced by their stage of development and cognitive ability.

BOX 56.4 Nursing Care Planning

AN INTERPROFESSIONAL CARE MAP FOR THE FAMILY OF A CHILD WITH A POTENTIALLY FATAL ILLNESS

Charlie is a 3-year-old who has had a relapse after 18 months of chemotherapy for leukemia. His parents have arranged for hospice care for him at home. They state, "He's been through so much already. It's very hard on us but we want him to die at home, close to us."

Family Assessment Child lives with parents on their llama ranch. Two older siblings (brother, age 20 years and sister, age 26 years) have left home. Parents report finances as "tight." Family has no health insurance because they are self-employed.

Client Assessment Child is cachexic. Skin cool, damp, and mottled. Pulse rate, 62 beats/min and weak; respirations, 8 breaths/min. Rattling sounds noted from chest. Responsive only to deep pain stimuli. Parents at bedside; older siblings absent.

Nursing Diagnosis Anticipatory grieving related to impending death of child

Outcome Criteria Parents express feelings about anticipated death; demonstrate positive coping mechanisms.

Team Member Responsible	Assessment	Intervention	Rationale	Expected Outcome
Activities of Daily Living, Including Safety				
Nurse	Assess whether the parents have any concerns or special wishes about child's final days of care.	Stay with the family and sit with them quietly if they prefer not to talk, and allow them to cry.	Staying with the family demonstrates caring and concern for their well-being and wishes and offers support.	Parents discuss any concerns or wishes they have with care.
Teamwork and Collaboration				
Nurse/Hospice care staff	Assess whether the parents would like a final visit from their clergy or other support person.	Arrange for visit by the support person if desired.	A visit by the family's support people can provide the family with final needed support.	Parents state whether a support person's visit would be helpful to them. Help plan arrangements.
Procedures/Medications for Quality Improvement				
Nurse	Assess whether the child appears comfortable.	Provide for the child's comfort, including positioning, turning, changing linen, applying lotion, and alleviating pain.	Providing comfort to the child is comforting to the family as well as the child.	Parents state they feel the child is comfortable.
Nurse	Ask whether the parents would like to provide final care.	Allow family members to provide care as desired without forcing them.	Allowing family participation in care provides them with some sense of control over the situation, decreasing their feelings of powerlessness.	Parents state they feel they have had a voice in and are satisfied with child's care.
Nutrition				
Nurse	Assess whether the child could be hungry.	The child is too comatose for oral feeding; intravenous (IV) fluid prescribed only as maintenance.	Hunger is an uncomfortable sensation.	Parents agree they feel the child is comfortable and no food is needed.

Patient-Centered Care				
Nurse	Assess whether parents have any questions about what actions they should take when the child dies.	Inform the family about what to expect, and explore their expectations and clarify any misconceptions.	Providing information helps to ease the family's fears and anxiety about the unknown.	Parents state they feel comfortable caring for child in final minutes and immediately afterward.
Psychosocial/Spiritual/Emotional Needs				
Nurse	Assess whether parents need any type of additional emotional support, and question why older siblings are not present.	Explore as far as parents are willing whether support from their other children would be helpful.	Close family members can supply the most meaningful type of emotional support.	Parents state that although they are disappointed in older siblings' reactions, they understand everyone grieves differently and are managing well.
Nurse	Ask whether parents have begun "grief work" such as reviewing and preserving memories of the child.	Provide the family with opportunities to review special memories or experiences with the child.	Reviewing memories and special experiences provides a positive method for coping with grief.	Parents report they have begun a scrapbook of favorite photos they anticipate will give them solace in years to come.
Informatics for Seamless Health Care Planning				
Nurse	Assess whether parents have made final arrangements for the child's burial, and responsibility for reporting death to hospice group.	Assist the family with making arrangements for what to do when the child dies.	Assistance with planning provides support and aids in grieving, allowing time to be spent with the child rather than on arrangements.	Parents state that they understand obligations for reporting death; and have good relationship with the hospice group to answer questions.
Nurse	Assess whether parents have contacted a community support group other than hospice group.	If parents feel they need this, initiate referral to a community organization for additional support.	Community organizations can supply long-term support after the child dies.	Parents state they have the name of a community support group and will contact group if they feel a need in the future.

Infants and Toddlers

Infants and toddlers are certainly too young to appreciate that their death is about to occur. If the person who cared for them dies, they experience a deep loss and a void in their life. If such a loss interferes with the development of a sense of trust, its implications for the child's ability to achieve warm, close relationships could last a lifetime.

Preschoolers

Preschoolers usually learn about the concept of death when a pet dies or when they discover a dead bird or mouse. They envision death as temporary, however, and appear to have little of adults' fear of it. This casualness toward death is sometimes interpreted as callousness. For example, the first response of a child who is told his brother has just been killed in an automobile accident might be to ask if he can have his brother's cell phone. This happens because he thinks of his brother as being gone for only a short time, making this a chance to take advantage of his property. This concept is strengthened by children's cartoons, in which characters frequently are killed and then immediately revive and go on with the story.

Because preschoolers fear separation greatly, they are stunned by the death of a parent. If children grasp the concept that they themselves are dying, their major worry might be that they will be alone and separated. These children may need someone to stay with them constantly to reassure them that they are loved and that people are caring for them.

School-Age Children

School-age children begin to have additional experiences with death, so their knowledge of it as a final measure increases. They may think of it, however, as something that happens only to adults. Children's books tend to deal only shallowly with the subject, although many books that deal specifically with death are available for children (Box 56.5). As children near

BOX 56.5 Books About Death for Children

Brown, L. K., & Brown, M. (1996). *When dinosaurs die: A guide to understanding death.* Boston, MA: Little, Brown.
Davis, C. (1997). *For every dog an angel.* Portland, OR: Lighthearted Press.
Farrant, N. (2013). *After Iris.* New York, NY: Dial Press.
Isherwood, S., & Isherwood, K. (2000). *Remembering Granddad.* London: Oxford Press.
Koppens, J., & van Lindenhuizen, E. (2013). *Goodbye, fish.* New York, NY: Clavis Publishing.
Millis, J. C. (2003). *Gentle Willow: A story for children about dying.* Warminster, PA: Marco Publishers.
Spergel, H., & Stylou, G. (2013). *Cloud City: A child's journey through bereavement.* Upper Montclair, NJ: Turn the Page Publishing.
Tott-Rizzuti, K. (1992). *Mommy, what does dying mean?* Pittsburgh, PA: Dorrance.
Weitzman, E. (1996). *Let's talk about when a parent dies.* New York, NY: Rosen Group.

8 or 9 years of age, they begin to appreciate that death is permanent. They may experience the same lonesome feeling they experienced when their parents left them at camp or went away for a weekend, but this time, the separation will be permanent.

Most children of school age are aware of what is happening to them when their disorder has a fatal prognosis. Unfortunately, they may learn this from other children on the unit or at school (e.g., "Are you the kid who's dying?"), from their parents' strange responses to questions, or from overhearing snatches of conversation about reports or physical findings. Children, however, are accustomed to meeting new situations (e.g., starting school, visiting a museum for the first time, boarding an airplane for the first time) and they are able to effectively cope with these experiences as long as they know someone they care about will be there to support them. Dying can be viewed in this same light as another new experience for them. They are able to cope with it well if they know there will be someone with them. If the parents become unable to relate to a child of this age because of their grief, a nurse may need to become the person to fill the gap (Fig. 56.3).

FIGURE 56.3 A one-to-one nursing relationship helps children with terminal illnesses to not feel deserted.

Many children associate death with sleep (perhaps that was the explanation they were given for a grandparent's death), so they may be afraid to fall asleep without someone near them. They may need the light left on at night because death is associated with darkness. They may need to have you sit with them while they fall asleep. Often, on a busy care unit, a child who is dying is moved to the end of the hallway, away from the nurses' station so the nearby room can be used for a child who needs frequent procedures (a justifiable move in terms of efficiency). However, this further isolates both a child who needs support and the child's parents, who also need your support and your presence nearby. Advocate as necessary for both the child and the parents so they can have continued interaction not just with each other but also with outside sources.

Adolescents

Although adolescents have an adult concept of death, they also may feel immune to it. Risky activities such as driving at high speeds reflect this judgment. They may deny symptoms that reveal their condition is worsening for longer than you'd expect because they believe it is impossible that anything serious could be happening to them. They appreciate time provided for discussion of how they have contributed to their family or community even though they are dying young. Continuing to participate in typical teenage activities helps them maintain a sense of control.

QSEN Checkpoint Question 56.3

Quality Improvement

Suppose Charlie, 3 years old, asks you what it feels like to die. Assuming you want to improve the way you discuss sensitive topics with children, what would be your best answer?

a. "I think it's like going into a long white tunnel."
b. "It doesn't hurt if you're worrying about that."
c. "Everything probably goes black like it does at night."
d. "Why are you asking a question about dying?"

Look in Appendix A for the best answer and rationale.

Environment for Death

The environment in which children die can influence their acceptance and their family's acceptance of death.

The Hospital

A number of children die each year in emergency departments from unintentional injuries such as automobile accidents or from severe infections (Vaillancourt, Li, Guttman, et al., 2012). A few children who have a terminal illness need such a great deal of physical care (e.g., a new tracheotomy, lung ventilation) they may remain in a hospital for care because their family does not have the skill, energy, or money necessary to care for them at home. In a hospital setting, be certain that visiting hours are adequately extended for parents and other family members so that children are not left alone when they need people around the most. Be certain also that children have opportunities to maintain contact with peers.

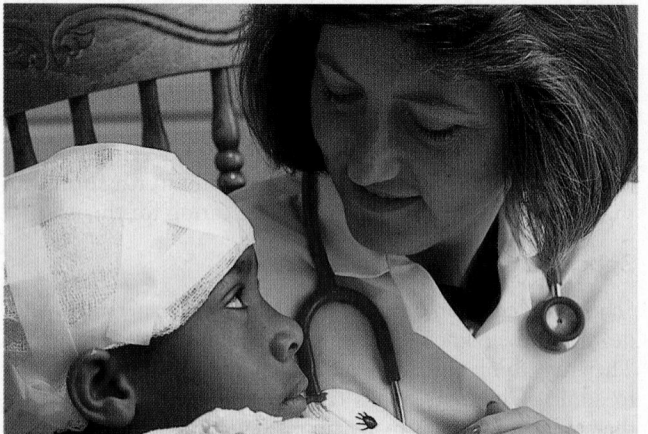

The Home

Today, most children with terminal illnesses are not kept in the hospital past the time when it is determined that therapy is no longer effective. Many families prefer that a child dies at home, surrounded by family and familiar possessions, rather than in a hospital. Time spent talking about arrangements—such as who the parents should contact if the child suddenly becomes more ill than usual, how they will manage periodic checkups, or how they will purchase medicine or supplies—is important preparation for home care. Assess how the family will schedule its time to have some leisure periods free so they can balance the care of the ill child in their lives.

Home care can be an extremely satisfying experience, both for a child who is dying and for the family, as long as safeguards exist for protecting the caregivers' health and for providing good care for the child (discussed further in Chapter 4).

The Hospice

In 1967, St. Christopher's Hospice in London opened as a facility for people who wanted to die in a homelike setting while still receiving skilled professional health care. Most large communities today have hospice settings, although places specifically for children, and especially infants, are still not available in many communities (Price, Dornan, & Quail, 2012).

In a hospice, friends, family, and even younger children and pets are allowed unlimited visiting. Children are invited to bring possessions with them that are important to them. They are urged to choose the degree of pain relief they want. Strong analgesia is often used to make a child pain free (a criticism of hospice care is that this level of analgesia slows the respiratory rate and actually hastens death).

The philosophy of hospice care is that death is an extension or part of life, not a separate entity; therefore, it can be accepted not with separate or awkward rituals, but with the same warm concern as other situations in everyday life. For many children, hospice care is furnished as part of home care, so that they are not separated from their families (Robert, Zhukovsky, Mauricio, et al., 2012).

✔ QSEN Checkpoint Question 56.4

Teamwork & Collaboration

Suppose Charlie's parents were told by his medical care team that he was going to die, but then he didn't die. What is an unexpected consequence of anticipatory grieving you would want your nursing colleagues to know when planning subsequent care for the family?

a. It will have minimal effect, because he did not die.
b. It could disrupt the parents' relationship with Charlie.
c. It teaches the child that heath care providers can be wrong.
d. It breaks the parents' confidence in health care procedures.

Look in Appendix A for the best answer and rationale.

Preparation for a Nursing Role With Dying Children and Their Families

Caring for dying children can be an emotionally draining experience for health care providers as well as family members (Cook, Mott, Lawrence, et al., 2012). Although it is best that nursing assignments be consistent so a child has meaningful support, there is a point at which a health care provider may need a respite from caring for a certain child or help in offering support for the parents.

Self-Awareness

Before you can offer support to children in any circumstance, be aware of your own reactions and feelings. To offer support to a child who is dying, examine how you feel about caring for someone who is dying so young.

Fear. Fear is a natural response to death because the phenomenon is new and strange. To overcome this fear, put it into perspective. In nursing, you care for many people who have illnesses and experiences you will never have, so caring for people with experiences beyond your own is not really strange but almost routine.

People who have never seen someone die are often afraid the moment of death will be terrifying to watch. Death usually occurs gently, however, with body functioning gradually lessening until it stops in a pain-free, quiet manner. People who have been declared dead and were then resuscitated by heroic measures report that death was not at all frightening but actually involved a feeling of exceptional calm and comfort; people have reported afterward they wished they had been allowed to die rather than being called back to their body because death seemed so appealing (Facco & Agrillo, 2012).

Failure. Some health care professionals find themselves drawing back from caring for dying children because death symbolizes failure to them. Unfortunately, this can make children feel as if they have failed—they have not been able to keep their body from dying despite everyone's best efforts.

Remind yourself that death is the ultimate outcome for everyone. At the point that death becomes unpreventable, the only failure that can exist is the failure of health care professionals to help a child achieve death with dignity and consideration, and free of guilt that the child failed caregivers.

Grief

Nursing care is so intense that the relationship formed between a nurse and a child may be closer than you realize until a child is diagnosed as having a terminal illness or dies, and only then do you experience the depth of the relationship. Because nurses develop such close bonds with terminally ill children, they may experience profound grief when a child dies or no longer requires their care. The grief that accompanies caring for dying children can be broken down into the same stages of grief experienced by the children themselves when they learn they are dying.

Denial. There is a danger that a nurse who is in a stage of denial may care for children without mentioning they have more than a simple illness. This includes omitting the use of such common expressions as, "How are you this morning?" to avoid having to hear the answer. Denial may be so extensive that you avoid going into a child's room unless an important procedure must be done. This is unfortunate because it can be confusing and lonely for children because they miss the normal exchange of conversation and contact. Nurses sometimes change professions after the death of a child to whom they felt close because they are unwilling to submit themselves to that level of hurt again.

Anger. Anger may be intense when a young child dies because the death seems so unfair. Nurses who are angry have difficulty offering effective care; they may perceive themselves as giving thorough, comforting care, but actually, they inflict discomfort with sharp, abrupt movements. Anger also clouds nursing judgment, such as to which analgesic would be best to administer or whether a change in vital signs is important. It is disappointing from a child's perspective because dying children cannot approach angry caregivers or ask questions; they are left alone and perhaps left to feel guilty they caused this anger.

Bargaining. Caregivers begin to bargain for life, just as children do. A statement such as, "If Tommy just makes it through the weekend while I'm off, I'll spend all my extra time with him next week" is a bargaining statement. Bargains of this kind are easy to overlook in your coworkers or yourself. Listening for them helps you to evaluate when a fellow worker is having difficulty caring for a particular child and perhaps needs to change assignments. Hearing yourself say them should alert you that you may be more involved with a child than you perhaps have realized. It's a warning that you need to talk to someone about your feelings or ask for help. Remember that, when bargaining fails, people reach their lowest point in grief. Recognizing bargaining statements in yourself, therefore, helps you to be prepared for the depression that will follow.

Depression. Nurses who enter this phase may be ineffective caregivers because depressed people are poor problem solvers (everything seems to be a crisis). It's easy for nurses to make unwise decisions in their personal lives (e.g., drop out of a night school course, file for divorce) because they cannot solve problems effectively.

Depression is doubly destructive because, when you are depressed, your reasoning processes are so distorted that you lose the ability to recognize that depression is the problem. When caring for a child who is expected to die, monitor your behavior to see if you are following your usual pattern. If irregularities occur (e.g., sleeping a great deal, not sleeping, loss of appetite), assess whether depression has overwhelmed you. If you feel you are depressed, try to make no major decisions for at least a week to give your perspective time to change, or you may find later you have made an unwise, irreversible decision.

Acceptance. The average person can reach a stage of acceptance in grief because people are subjected to few true losses in a lifetime. As a nurse on a unit where many terminally ill children come for care, you may find yourself facing loss or death repeatedly. Therefore, a stage of acceptance may never be reached. A caregiver who cannot reach a stage of acceptance is left in a stage of depression and has extreme difficulty functioning.

To achieve a stage of acceptance, you may need to modify what it is you are accepting. You cannot accept the unfairness of death in children, but you can accept your ability to offer care that gives death dignity and compassion, and so maintains quality of life. Be careful you do not compensate for being unable to feel good by not feeling. This is a dangerous attitude because it also blocks your ability to feel happiness, love, and trust. If this happens, you may need to ask for a temporary change of assignment to reestablish your perspective. You may need to concentrate on self-esteem therapy for yourself (doing something special for yourself, such as taking an evening to do nothing but meet your own needs).

What if...56.3 While caring for Charlie for an extended period, you notice yourself going from store to store spontaneously buying items. Could this be an expression of grief?

Caring for the Dying Child

A child may live for days, weeks, or even months in a "dying phase." Attentive physical and emotional care is essential for a child to maintain a sense of security and positive self-esteem during this time. It is also essential to assess if parents are coping well with this long period. Frequent and substantive communication is a major part of providing this care. Children, like their parents, need the opportunity to talk about their fears and feelings about death. Practicing good communication skills when providing any care such as when administering pain medication, starting intravenous lines, or providing basic comfort measures such as a bath help to establish a trusting relationship with the child, hopefully making the child feel more comfortable about sharing feelings with you (Fig. 56.4). Box 56.6 provides some specific guidelines about communicating with a child who is dying.

The Child's Family

For many children, terminal illness involves a series of hospital admissions interspersed with ambulatory care or home visits. Parents need time during these visits to talk about the problems they are having, not only with physical care (e.g., Should the child attend regular school? Could he come on vacation? How many times a day are we supposed to give the immunosuppressant?) but also about how it feels to live with a child who is dying (e.g., How should they answer the child's or siblings' questions about dying?). Although many parents are reluctant to tell a child that he is dying, this is probably the soundest course once the child can see that his or her condition is deteriorating because there is often less anxiety in knowing what is happening than in hearing people whispering or spelling out words.

If a child with a chronic illness experiences an exacerbation of the disease, parents may again begin an anticipatory grief reaction: anger, bargaining, depression, and acceptance. The process will be cut short by improvement, only

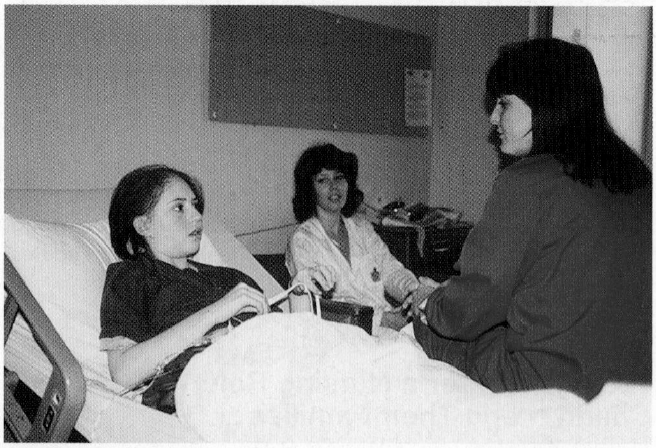

FIGURE 56.4 Good communication skills help build a trusting relationship, allowing a child to share feelings about being terminally ill. (© Caroline Brown, RNC, MS, DEd.)

BOX 56.6 Nursing Care Planning to Empower a Family

MEASURES TO HELP COMMUNICATION WITH CHILDREN WHO ARE TERMINALLY ILL

1. *Continue active conversation.* Children who are dying need to receive stimulation in as near normal a way as possible.
2. *Use moments of silence therapeutically.* Such moments occur normally just as speech occurs normally. Do not feel you have to chatter to fill quiet intervals.
3. *Use the words "death" and "dying" as appropriate in conversation.* Trying to avoid a word makes interchanges awkward. Statements such as, "These flowers are dying," "That's a dead-end job," or "I'm dying to try that" may make it acceptable for the child you are caring for to voice for the first time what is happening—"I'm dying, too; let me tell you about dead-ending."
4. *Preserve dying children's defenses.* If they are using denial or bargaining, do not try to push them to the next step of grieving by confrontation. Children will move on to the next step when they are psychologically ready.
5. *Remember that many children assume that they will die at night.* Therefore, night is "owned" by the dying. A child may talk more freely at night about fears or an unfulfilled life ambition than during the day. Children may also be more frightened at night and enjoy having someone sit beside them until they fall asleep.
6. *Be supportive, not trite.* A statement such as "All of us are dying" is true but not helpful. A supportive statement such as, "This must be hard for you" is better.
7. *Be aware that not all people's beliefs are the same as yours.* It's all right if a statement such as, "God works in mysterious ways," which may explain death for the person saying it, evokes an angry response from you. People grieve and react to grief in many different ways.

to begin again at the next exacerbation. For this reason, the parents of a child who is being admitted to the hospital for the 12th time for a fatal illness may be in the same stage of grief as the parents of a child with a newly diagnosed fatal illness.

During health supervision visits, ask parents how other children in the family are managing. The parents may need to be reminded that, although the dying child does need a lot of their time, other children find this illness in a sibling just as baffling as the parents. When the ill child dies, siblings need the same active support to help them grieve (Siegel, Alpert, & Goldstein, 2011).

QSEN Checkpoint Question 56.5

Evidence-Based Practice

Helping parents survive the death of a child can be a challenging experience in nursing. To investigate what role parents wanted to most play in the care of their terminally ill children, researchers interviewed the parents of 18 children who had recently died in a pediatric intensive care unit. Results of the interviews revealed that parents most wanted to be able to continue to be "good parents" through such means as providing love, comfort, and care; creating security and privacy for the family; and exercising responsibility for procedures or therapy that their child was receiving (McGraw, Truog, Solomon, et al., 2012).

Based on the previous study, which action would probably give Charlie's mother the most satisfaction with his end-of-life care?

a. Participating in keeping him clean and comfortable
b. Being allowed to inspect his health record on a regular basis
c. Interacting with the nursing staff on a personal or friendly level
d. Providing counseling to other parents on the unit

Look in Appendix A for the best answer and rationale.

The Onset of Death

As death nears in children, physiologic changes, such as slowed metabolism, decreased cell oxygenation, and cell dysfunction, begin to occur, thus changing children's appearance.

Stroke volume of the heart decreases, so the power to circulate blood is reduced. The child's skin feels cool and may appear mottled or cyanotic because blood can no longer be pushed to distal sites. Just before death, blood begins to pool in dependent body parts, making them appear purple. As circulation fails, absorption of a drug from a muscle becomes virtually impossible; if emergency drugs need to be administered, they need to be injected intravenously or often don't have an effect.

As peripheral circulation fails, less heat is lost from the body and the internal temperature rises. The child's body compensates for this by increased perspiration to increase heat loss through evaporation. This makes the child's skin feel cool and damp. You may need to change linens frequently because of the increased moisture on the skin. Because perfusion of distal body parts is impaired, turn the child slowly to allow the circulatory system to accommodate to the change in position.

Slowed respirations lead to increased secretions in the lungs and the appearance of rales, the sound of air being pulled through fluid in the alveoli. To compensate for a few minutes of very slow respirations, a child may take several quick or extremely deep inhalations periodically. Be certain the child's chest is not compressed, so that the child has optimal lung expansion to do this.

A decrease in muscular function leads to severe weakness and fatigue. More and more, children maintain the exact position into which they were placed. As the throat muscles become lax, the possibility of aspiration increases. Offer only a small amount of oral fluid until you're certain the child's swallowing reflex is intact before offering a full glass. If the gag or swallowing reflex is impaired, position the child on the side to allow saliva to drain from the mouth to prevent aspiration. An often noticed phenomenon of someone close to death is constant hand movement (e.g., picking at bedclothes), which probably represents the loss of upper centers of voluntary muscular control. Neurologically, deep reflexes, such as the Achilles tendon reflex, begin to fade.

A loss of consciousness occurs as children grow closer and closer to death, although they may remain perfectly alert until seconds before death. Vision apparently blurs because children tend to turn their head toward a light. Touch seems to remain intact because they often quiet to a gentle stroking of the arm or shoulder, and they grasp your hand meaningfully, as if touch is appreciated and felt. Because hearing is one of the last senses lost, you may need to remind family members and, on occasion, other health care personnel, that the child may not be able to respond but may be able to hear. Continue to explain procedures to unconscious children as if they were conscious because they undoubtedly do hear you. Never make any comment in their presence that you would not make if they were alert. Continue to use the same gentle touch and nonverbal communication motions, such as holding a hand or brushing hair from the forehead as if children were fully conscious because they may be fully aware of your actions even though they can give no indication of it.

Another body function that slows is digestion as total body metabolism slows. Constipation because of poor bowel tone and decreased peristaltic action will occur. The abdomen may become distended from intestinal flatus. Dehydration with dry mucous membranes and conjunctivae will occur unless intravenous fluid replacement is initiated. Mouth dryness will lead to cracking, secondary infection, and pain; prevent this by frequently cleaning the mucous membrane with clear water and with the application of an ointment to the lips. If the conjunctivae appear dry, ask for a prescription of moistening eye drops, and keep any crusting at the eyelids washed away so that optimal vision is possible.

Be certain to keep skin surfaces from rubbing against one another by using supportive pillows and good positioning. Keep the skin free of urine or feces from incontinence to prevent painful ulcers. These are normally not a major concern in children, but they are a concern here because of the lessened peripheral blood perfusion. Assess for indications of pain (e.g., thrashing, moaning), and provide relief with appropriate comfort measures.

QSEN Checkpoint Question 56.6

Safety

Children's body functions grow increasingly weaker as death approaches. What would be a safety precaution you would want to remember when caring for Charlie?

a. Children may aspirate easily as their gag reflex begins to fade.
b. Children who are unconscious cannot hear and so like the room quiet.
c. Turning and repositioning children can cause more harm than good.
d. To help them cope, you should avoid asking parents to give any final care.

Look in Appendix A for the best answer and rationale.

Documentation of Death

Defining when death occurs is controversial and involves both legal and ethical issues, but signs of death in a child not receiving ventilatory or mechanical assistance are the same as in adults:

- Absence of respirations
- No audible heart sounds by stethoscope
- No pulse by palpation
- No apparent blood pressure
- Absence of body movement or reflexes
- Dilated, fixed pupils

Death is officially determined by a lack of receptivity and responsivity, no spontaneous muscular movement or breath, no reflex response, and a flat electroencephalogram—again, the same as in adults.

Organ Donation

Parents may be asked by their primary health care provider or by a specifically designated transplantation team before a child's death to grant permission for body organs to be transplanted into other children after death occurs (Brierley & Hasan, 2012). This is particularly important for liver and kidney transplants because it is difficult to transplant adult-size organs into children. If parents decide to allow organ donation, mark this information on the child's electronic record in a conspicuous place and alert the primary care provider about the decision. When death does occur, the child's body will be maintained by a life-support system to ensure that the chosen organ remains perfused until it can be removed. The donation of body organs is not something that all parents can agree too, but it can help parents who choose the option to accept their child's death more easily because it allows them to feel that their child has helped another person live. If, however, parents are reluctant to agree to organ donation, you may need to advocate for them. Donating their child's organs is not a practice for everyone (Siebelink, Albers, Roodbol, et al., 2012).

Aftercare

Before beginning any aftercare for a child who has died in a health care facility or at home, check with family members to see if they want to spend a few minutes with the child or if there are any religious rites they want to complete before the body is transported to the morgue or funeral parlor. Some parents need this time to comprehend that death has really occurred. Some people have special prayers they want to say; others want to say a final, private goodbye. Check that the child's bed and room is orderly before you ask a family whether they would like to spend some time in the room, particularly if a final resuscitation attempt resulted in blood-soaked sponges or scattered equipment.

Remain in the room with the family in case they need your support, but be unobtrusive. Some parents fear touching a child's body after death, but touch is a strong and intimate communication technique that a family member may appreciate being shown how to use. Role model touching by holding the child's hand or brushing hair away from the forehead as if the child were still alive. Some parents may seem unable to leave the room or to let go of the child's hand. It may be necessary for you to gradually separate their hands, saying something such as, "I'll always remember Molly the way she was when I first met her—so full of life and always laughing. I'm sure that's how you'll always remember her, too." This helps parents begin to accept the fact that, in more than a physical sense, it is time to let go.

As a rule, crying is helpful for parents. You may need to tell them that it is all right to cry. Do not, however, interpret a lack of tears as a lack of feeling because crying is not everyone's response to death. It is not unprofessional for nurses to cry when a child dies. A parent's warmest memory of a hospital experience may be that a nurse cried as she said goodbye to their child—the implication being the child made an important impact on people other than the family.

Autopsy Permission

State laws vary, but as a rule, if a child's death is a result of homicide, suicide, death within 24 hours after a hospital admission, suspected harmful death, or death in an institution or home where the child was not under the care of a primary health care provider, an autopsy is required by law and parents have no input regarding whether this is done or not. In other instances, it would be helpful to medical progress or to research if an autopsy could be done. In these instances, parents must give permission for this. Parents may refuse to allow an autopsy for a child, believing that doing so will protect the child from any more hurt or because of religious convictions. Autopsies advance medical science, so they should be done if at all possible; however, parents have every right to refuse permission without being made to feel guilty for their actions, so you may need to advocate for them.

What if...56.4 You are particularly interested in exploring one of the 2020 National Health Goals related to chronic or terminal illness and children (see Box 56.1). What would be a possible research topic to explore pertinent to this goal that would be applicable to Charlie's family and that would also advance evidence-based practice?

Key Points for Review

- Children with long-term illnesses need continual reassessment because, like all children, their needs change as they grow older. Larger doses of medicine will become necessary; care such as additional muscle-strengthening exercises may be necessary.
- Factors that make it easier for parents to accept a long-term illness in a child include having support people present and being told about the child's condition as early as possible.
- Long-term illness in a child is often most difficult for parents to accept at times when the child would have been achieving specific milestones of development such as on what would have been their first day of school. Extra support for both the parents and the child may be necessary at these times because this not only helps in planning nursing care that meets QSEN competencies but also best meets a family's total needs.
- Help children with a long-term disorder to do as much care for themselves as possible within the limits of their illness. Self-care empowers them to be as independent as possible.
- Children are about 9 years old before they are able to understand the meaning of death and that it is permanent. A child and parents can be expected to move through the stages of grief (denial, anger, bargaining, depression, and acceptance) on learning about a potentially fatal diagnosis.
- Children and parents are apt to need help to face a terminal diagnosis in a child. Urge the parents and the child to ask for help to see them through this very difficult time in their lives.

Critical Thinking Care Study

"Skater" is a 16-year-old gang member you meet in the emergency room. He is unconscious from a gunshot wound to his head, which was suffered while he was robbing a convenience store. The police officer who accompanied the ambulance tells you Skater was shot by the store owner. A fellow gang member tells you Skater shot himself to keep from being arrested.

1. Skater was diagnosed with autism spectrum disorder when he was 4 years old. He dropped out of school last year because "he didn't like being told what to do". If you were assigned to accompany him to the X-ray department for a cranial magnetic resonance imaging (MRI), would you need to explain to him what is happening (he doesn't like instructions and he's unconscious)?
2. Skater's mother rushes into the emergency room and describes her son as "a precious child" whom she wants to live. His older brother describes him as "nothing but trouble his whole life" and adds that the family would be better off if Skater died. Would these conflicting opinions affect your care? Would the dispute over whether he was shot or shot himself influence care?
3. Skater's mother and sibling seem to have totally different opinions about the effect Skater has had on his family, probably based on actions related to him being autistic. Why do you suppose these two people have formed such different opinions of Skater?

Patient Scenario

The Bergin Family

Read about the Bergin family, a family with a chronically ill child, then answer the questions to further sharpen your skills and grow more familiar with NCLEX-type questions related to long-term or terminal illnesses. Confirm your answers are correct by reading the rationales.

Visit http://thePoint.lww.com

Answers and Rationales

Looking for answers to the What if . . . and Critical Thinking Care Study questions?

Visit http://thePoint.lww.com

References

Brierley, J., & Hasan, A. (2012). Aspects of deceased organ donation in paediatrics. *British Journal of Anaesthesia, 108*(Suppl. 1), i92–i95.

Carr, B. G., Nance, M. L., Branas, C. C., et al. (2012). Unintentional firearm death across the urban-rural landscape in the United States. *Journal of Trauma & Acute Care Surgery, 73*(4), 1006–1010.

Cook, K. A., Mott, S., Lawrence, P., et al. (2012). Coping while caring for the dying child: Nurses' experiences in an acute care setting. *Journal of Pediatric Nursing, 27*(4), e11–e21.

Crosland, K., & Dunlap, G. (2012). Effective strategies for the inclusion of children with autism in general education classrooms. *Behavior Modification, 36*(3), 251–269.

Epelman, C. L. (2012). End-of-life management in pediatric cancer. *Current Oncology Reports, 14*(2), 191–196.

Erikson, E. (1993). *Childhood and society* (3rd ed.). New York, NY: W.W. Norton.

Facco, E., & Agrillo, C. (2012). Near-death experiences between science and prejudice. *Frontiers in Human Neuroscience, 2012*(6), 209.

Fisher, H., & Crawley, E. (2012). Why do young people with CFS/ME feel anxious? A qualitative study. *Clinical Child Psychology & Psychiatry.* Advance online publication.

Fowler Braga, S. F., & Almgren, M. M. (2013). Complementary therapies in cystic fibrosis: Nutritional supplements and herbal products. *Journal of Pharmacy Practice, 26*(1), 14–17.

Green, M., & Solnit, A. (1964). Reactions to the threatened loss of a child: A vulnerable child syndrome. *Pediatrics, 34*(6), 58.

Kirk, S., Beatty, S., Callery, P., et al. (2012). Perceptions of effective self-care support for children and young people with long-term conditions. *Journal of Clinical Nursing, 21*(13–14), 1974–1987.

Kübler-Ross, E. (1969). *On death and dying.* New York, NY: Macmillan.

Longden, J. V. (2011). Parental perceptions of end-of-life care on paediatric intensive care units: a literature review. *Nursing Critical Care, 16*(3), 131–139.

McGraw, S. A, Truog, R. D., Solomon, M. Z., et al. (2012). "I was able to still be her mom"—Parenting at end of life in the pediatric intensive care unit. *Pediatric Critical Care Medicine, 13*(6), e350–e356.

Newton, K., & Lamarche, K. (2012). Take the challenge: Strategies to improve support for parents of chronically ill children. *Home Healthcare Nurse, 30*(5), E1–E8.

Nikkola, I., Kaunonen, M., & Aho, A. L. (2013). Mother's experience of the support from a bereavement follow-up intervention after the death of a child. *Journal of Clinical Nursing, 22*(7–8), 1151–1162.

Peacock, J., & Stanik-Hutt, J. (2013). Translating best care practices to improve nursing documentation regarding pediatric patients dependent on home mechanical ventilation and tracheostomy tube support: a quality improvement initiative. *Home Healthcare Nurse, 31*(1), 10–17.

Price, J., Dornan, J., & Quail, L. (2012). Seeing is believing—Reducing misconceptions about children's hospice care through effective teaching with undergraduate nursing students. *Nurse Education in Practice.* Advance online publication.

Robert, R., Zhukovsky, D. S., Mauricio, R., et al. (2012). Bereaved parents' perspectives on pediatric palliative care. *Journal of Social Work in End of Life & Palliative Care, 8*(4), 316–338.

Siebelink, M. J., Albers, M. J., Roodbol, P. F., et al. (2012). Children as donors: A national study to assess procurement of organs and tissues in pediatric intensive care units. *Transplant International, 25*(12), 1268–1274.

Siegel, B. S., Alpert, J. J., & Goldstein, R. (2011). Palliative care & end-of-life issues. In K. J. Marcdante, R. M. Kliegman, H. B. Jenson, et al. (Eds.), *Nelson essentials of pediatrics* (6th ed., pp. 8–12). Philadelphia, PA: Saunders/Elsevier.

St. Ledger, U., Begley, A., Reid, J., et al. (2012). Moral distress in end-of-life care in the intensive care unit. *Journal of Advanced Nursing.* Advance online publication.

Thomas, S., & Price, M. (2012). Respite care in seven families with children with complex care needs. *Nursing Children & Young People, 24*(8), 24–27.

U.S. Department of Health and Human Services. (2010). *Healthy people 2020.* Washington, DC: Author.

Vaillancourt, S., Li, Q., Guttman, A., et al. (2012). Children discharged from the emergency department with serious infections: A population-based study in Ontario. *Canadian Journal of Emergency Medicine, 14*(Suppl. 1), 1–3.

Vermaes, I. P., van Susante, A. M., & van Bakel, H. J. (2012). Psychological functioning of siblings in families of children with chronic health conditions: A meta-analysis. *Journal of Pediatric Psychology, 37*(2), 166–184.

Wender, E. (2012). Supporting the family after the death of a child. *Pediatrics, 130*(6), 1164–1169.

Whittingham, K., Wee, D., Sanders, M. R., et al. (2013). Predictors of psychological adjustment, experienced parenting burden and chronic sorrow symptoms in parents of children with cerebral palsy. *Child: Care, Health & Development, 39*(2), 366–373.

Appendix A

Answers to QSEN Checkpoint Questions

CHAPTER 1
A Framework for Maternal and Child Health Nursing

1.1 C. A Magnet hospital is one which stresses exemplary nursing care. It does not necessarily denote care for acute patients. This designation is not conferred by the American Medical Society.

1.2 C. The perinatal period is the time between 20 weeks of pregnancy and 4 to 6 weeks following birth.

1.3 C. Technology can become overwhelming for families if nursing support is not included in care. Premature infants require extensive care, and there are not immunizations for all childhood diseases. Nursing is predicted to maintain an important role in health care.

1.4 A. Skin-to-skin contact is important for newborns and may help fathers bond with their infant. It would be incorrect to withhold this until after discharge.

1.5 B. Acknowledging the patient's concerns while affirming her efforts is a more beneficial response than downplaying her concerns or providing false assurance.

1.6 D. Consent is required for all patients regardless of age. Assuring the mother that this can be done long distance is important.

CHAPTER 2
The Childbearing and Childrearing Family

2.1 B. Because women earn less than men and single-parent families are usually headed by women, finances are a common concern. Communication, emotional engagement, and education are not necessarily lacking as often.

2.2 B. The person who allows information in or out of a family is the gatekeeper.

2.3 D. The oldest child marks a family stage; because the Hanovan's oldest child is 17 years old, they are a family experiencing an adolescent stage.

2.4 D. Automobile accidents are a major cause of death in adolescents.

2.5 B. Teenagers need responsible adult supervision in all custodial settings. It would be inappropriate to suggest shared custody, to suggest quitting work, or to assume that the situation will be independently resolved.

2.6 C. To reduce exposure to violence and to stimulate language development, the American Academy of Pediatrics (AAP) recommends television viewing be restricted until a child is 2 years of age.

CHAPTER 3
Cultural Diversity and Maternal and Child Health Nursing

3.1 C. Women in this study wanted care providers to remember their name. The other listed responses acknowledge the client's presence and priorities, but they do not show that the nurse remembered her identity.

3.2 D. Respecting cultural preferences is important to individualize care. Making an effort to supply a cultural food preference is an example of that.

3.3 A. The care provider should be encouraged to communicate as naturally and clearly as possible; imitating Maria's accent is inappropriate. There is no particular need to avoid movie references if these are contextually appropriate.

3.4 D. It is important to avoid interactions between home remedies and prescribed medicine. The words "you people" is a term of disrespect.

3.5 B. It would be discriminatory to presume that Maria will not "fit in" by virtue of her ethnicity.

3.6 D. Respecting food choices is a way of respecting cultural diversity. Addressing the taste of the food does not focus on Maria's concerns.

CHAPTER 4
The Childbearing and Childrearing Family in the Community

4.1 C. Lisa needs a sedentary activity to interact with friends. Shouting for basketball teams or joining in with cheerleading would contradict bed rest. She is unable to safely go on outings due to her activity restriction. Journaling does not meet her socialization needs.

4.2 A. A first visit will involve gathering a health history, so having a parent present would be helpful. Dictating a time is not an effective way to empower or involve a client in planning care.

4.3 D. Always call for help if you feel you are in danger. Leaving the home would leave your client still in danger. Changing the locks would not solve the immediate problem. It is difficult and often unsafe to reason with angry people.

4.4 A. Privacy rules apply to home care as well as hospital care; health records are not copyrighted.

4.5 C. An adequate fluid intake helps prevent constipation. Walking is contraindicated because Lisa is on bed rest. The size of meals or calcium intake shouldn't make a difference.

4.6 A. Lisa's community is probably safe enough for her to stay alone. "Trying to quit smoking" is not enough to prevent exposure to secondary smoke and toxic tobacco contaminants because these cling to clothing. If the mother "usually" smokes outside, then this implies that she is sometimes smoking in the home.

CHAPTER 5
The Nursing Role in Reproductive and Sexual Health

5.1 C. Thelarche refers to breast development. Adrenarche is the development of other secondary sex characteristics, and menarche is the first menstrual period.

5.2 C. Because the vas deferens is easy to locate, it is the organ blocked/ligated for a vasectomy.

5.3 D. A cystocele is herniation of the bladder into the vagina and can lead to urinary tract infection.

5.4 D. Ovulation usually occurs on the 14th day from the end of the menstrual cycle, or in this instance, 14 days from day 34, or on the 20th day.

5.5 C. Helping an adolescent make independent decisions helps combat peer influence. Smoking cessation and church attendance may be poorly received suggestions and may not lead to meaningful change if they are imposed. Teaching about negative consequences may or may not be effective.

5.6 C. Women who have sex with women have a lower than average risk for sexually transmitted infections (STIs).

CHAPTER 6
Nursing Care for the Family in Need of Reproductive Life Planning

6.1 B. Cervical mucus is thin and watery at ovulation. Subjective sensations of warmth, breast tenderness, and emotional lability are not reliable indicators.

6.2 B. Female condoms should be inserted before any sexual contact, they should not be reused, and they already contain a spermicide.

6.3 D. Severe migraine headaches are a contraindication to combination oral contraceptives (COCs).

6.4 B. Intramuscular injections (depot medroxyprogesterone acetate [DMPA]) are associated with osteoporosis, so recommending a high calcium intake is important.

6.5 C. Fallopian tubes are the organs blocked in tubal ligation.

6.6 C. No ideal method that completely prevents pregnancy, stops menses, and doesn't need a reminder to take is available. DMPA probably comes closest to these specifications.

CHAPTER 7
The Nursing Role in Genetic Assessment and Counseling

7.1 D. Providing health information in a relevant and appropriate manner is an important component of high-quality care. False hope must be avoided. Journals and Web sites are not substitutes for health education provided by nurses and may not meet Amy's learning needs.

7.2 D. So Mrs. Alvarez can make an informed choice about her future, talking to other parents might be helpful. False hope should be avoided, and your own personal views are not relevant.

7.3 B. Amy has an extra chromosome 21 attached to another chromosome, so there is a greater chance than usual her children will inherit an extra chromosome. This is not sex related.

7.4 D. Patients should feel free to ask questions; promoting this implements the principles of patient-centered care. Genetic counseling is confidential and so can't be shared with family members indiscriminately. Health care providers shouldn't inject their own values into counseling.

7.5 C. Children with fragile X syndrome are hyperactive and aggressive, so childproofing will be necessary.

7.6 B. Infants with Down syndrome have one palm crease instead of the usual three; babies tend to be hypotonic, not hypertonic; and sole creases are an indication of any mature fetus.

CHAPTER 8
Nursing Care of the Family Having Difficulty Conceiving a Child

8.1 C. A year is the typical time to wait because, after trying to conceive unsuccessfully for 1 year, a couple is said to be subfertile. Acknowledging the reality of regretting a decision does not directly address her concerns.

8.2 C. Couples with reduced fertility may need to be reminded that just because they are no longer using a contraceptive method, they still need to follow safer sex precautions.

8.3 A. Mild cramping may occur during the procedure, an X-ray is not used, and no bleeding should result.

8.4 D. Endometriosis can block fallopian tubes, interfering with sperm or ovum transport.

8.5 C. Patients who are to undergo intrauterine insemination receive an injection of Clomid or follicle-stimulating hormone (FSH) 1 month prior to the procedure. Estrogen, bed rest, and genetic testing are not indicated.

8.6 C. Women begin breastfeeding well but may need additional support to continue it long term. Telling someone to not worry is not effective counseling. In vitro fertilization (IVF) does not preclude breastfeeding.

CHAPTER 9
Nursing Care of the Growing Fetus

9.1 D. A future baby is an embryo during the period between implantation and 5 to 8 weeks. After that, a baby is termed a fetus.

9.2 B. A normal umbilical cord has one vein and two arteries. Other patterns are associated with cardiac or chromosomal disorders.

9.3 A. Surfactant, produced by the lining of the alveoli, keep lung alveoli from collapsing on expiration, aiding alveoli expansion at birth.

9.4 A. The study reveals that low socioeconomic status and depression contribute to smoking. Stating that she has a constant shortage of money is suggestive of low socioeconomic status.

9.5 C. A full bladder improves the accuracy of the scan. There is no pain involved.

9.6 A. Voiding before an amniocentesis helps to reduce bladder size so it doesn't obstruct a clear view of the uterus.

CHAPTER 10
Nursing Care Related to Psychological and Physiologic Changes of Pregnancy

10.1 A. Women in the study reacted both positively and negatively at the thought of a second pregnancy. Lauren's paradoxical response represents this.

10.2 B. Ensuring safe passage for the fetus consists of accepting the pregnancy (first trimester), accepting the coming baby (second trimester), and preparing for parenthood (third trimester).

10.3 C. Narcissism refers to interest in oneself in contrast to interest in others.

10.4 D. The three positive signs of pregnancy are fetal heartbeat heard by examiner or fetal outline or heartbeat seen on sonogram and fetal movement felt by examiner.

10.5 D. Chadwick's sign is a color change in the vagina from pink to purple because of increased formation of blood vessels and blood flow.

10.6 A. With insulin becoming ineffective, glucose levels rise, serving to safeguard the fetus from hypoglycemia. Maternal insulin does not cross the placenta.

CHAPTER 11
Nursing Care Related to Assessment of a Pregnant Family

11.1 C. The odds of experiencing a medication-free birth are higher when a nurse-midwife leads care. It is inaccurate to characterize nurse-midwives as always being more "patient-friendly" and it is not appropriate to wholly defer teaching or advice when the patient asks for this.

11.2 C. Prenatal care is a prime time for health education; during this time, nurses play an important role in effective prenatal care. Ultimately, this promotes safe pregnancy, labor, and birth. This is more important than collecting statistical data or promoting social interaction. Allergies are not correlated with preterm labor. Despite the patient's wishes, regular prenatal care should be strongly encouraged.

11.3 B. Surgery such as for appendicitis can leave adhesions that then might interfere with uterine growth. Risks of uterine rupture and preterm labor are not higher in women with abdominal surgical history.

11.4 D. Palmar erythema commonly occurs from increasing estrogen levels. It is not a result of Rh incompatibility, edema, or anxiety.

11.5 D. Relaxation is important to reduce pain with a pelvic exam. Holding the breath or pushing down on the diaphragm does not relax abdominal muscles.

11.6 C. A weight gain over 3 lb a week during the second trimester would be a potential sign of gestational hypertension. The other listed changes do not constitute safety risks.

CHAPTER 12
Nursing Care to Promote Fetal and Maternal Health

12.1 C. Julberry can still contact a sexually transmitted infection, so she still needs to use precautions. However, a condom would not tear the membranes. Julberry's other responses reflect a sound understanding of self-care during pregnancy.

12.2 A. Jogging is not recommended during pregnancy because the extra weight of the pregnancy can cause knee injuries. The other health promotion statements are accurate.

12.3 C. All of these things Julberry describes are concerns, but it is the accumulation of symptoms that apparently leads to depression.

12.4 D. Witch hazel feels cool and may shrink hemorrhoids. Mineral oil is contraindicated because it prevents the absorption of vitamin A; eating fiber should not be omitted because it is helpful in preventing constipation; and she can't lie on her stomach because she is pregnant.

12.5 C. Ankle edema is a common occurrence in pregnancy and occurs from increased pressure on lower extremity veins. It can be relieved by resting with the feet elevated.

12.6 C. Pregnant women should check with their health care provider before taking medicine during pregnancy. All over-the-counter medicine is not safe; and the measles vaccine contains a live virus, and so is contraindicated during pregnancy.

CHAPTER 13
The Nursing Role in Promoting Nutritional Health During Pregnancy

13.1 B. Overweight women should gain between 15 and 25 lb with pregnancy.

13.2 D. Iron is absorbed best from an acid medium. Crushing the pills or taking them with milk or carbonated beverages is not advised.

13.3 C. Leafy green vegetables are rich in many of the dietary components that are lacking in women's diets. Protein, fiber, and iron are all important during pregnancy and so should be encouraged; and dieting should normally be discouraged.

13.4 C. A 24-hour recall history usually secures the most accurate nutrition pattern.

13.5 C. Pica is the ingesting of non-food substances, such as chalk or erasers.

13.6 D. Vitamin B_{12} is found only in animal sources.

CHAPTER 14
Preparing a Family for Childbirth and Parenting

14.1 D. The best birth plans are flexible. Rigid expectations can lead to disappointment and anxiety; the partner's wishes are indeed secondary, but they should not be wholly rejected; and interventions such as opioids should not be included solely on the recommendation of a parent.

14.2 B. Squatting or tailor sitting tightens perineal muscles. Tightening and relaxing them (Kegel exercises) would also strengthen them; and vigorous exercise and bearing down forcefully are not recommended, and these actions carry safety risks.

14.3 C. Women who give birth in upright positions have shorter labors. Voicing the fact that she is willing to try different positions should achieve this, and labor in a supine position is normalized in media depictions of birth.

14.4 A. The Lamaze philosophy is based on the gate control theory of pain perception, which states that pain sensations can be interrupted. This philosophy does not deny the reality of pain or the inevitability of pain during labor.

14.5 D. Slow breathing is adequate for early contractions; a cleansing breath is always important. Ice water will not relieve hypoventilation, and rapid breathing is contraindicated.

14.6 C. Emergency care is more readily available in a hospital setting than in other birth settings. Childbirth is not pain free, and the cost of present day hospital stays is typically high; and hospitals, like all birth settings, are not sterile environments.

CHAPTER 15
Nursing Care of a Family During Labor and Birth

15.1 A. An occipitoanterior position means the lie is cephalic—the back of the baby's head is facing the right anterior quadrant of the mother's pelvis; full flexion means the smallest diameter of the fetal head is presenting to the cervix. This position is considered to be ideal and is most conducive to a healthy delivery that requires fewer interventions.

15.2 D. Cervical dilation is a mark of true labor. For the mucus plug to be loosened, cervical dilatation must be occurring.

15.3 A. In the study, a feeling of loss of control severely affected women's impressions of whether labor was traumatic or not.

15.4 D. Pulling on the cord, pushing on the uterine fundus, or hard pushing could all cause additional bleeding. The placenta must normally be delivered spontaneously.

15.5 B. A contraction over 70 seconds long is long enough to compromise fetal oxygenation. In the context of labor, pain is not necessarily indicative of pathophysiology.

15.6 B. A late deceleration means the fetal heart rate decreases as a contraction ends, rather than at the beginning of a contraction, as is usual.

CHAPTER 16
The Nursing Role in Providing Comfort During Labor and Birth

16.1 C. A doula is a second support person in labor. She doesn't replace a woman's partner and does much more than time contractions. The use of a doula is an individual choice.

16.2 D. Music is best used in early labor to help a woman relax.

16.3 C. Slow breathing calls for concentration. Consequently, it can be used as a distraction technique. Women should not lie on their back during labor in order to prevent hypotension, women should not hold their breath as long as possible, and rapid breathing could lead to hyperventilation.

16.4 B. Warm water is comforting during labor, but it may be contraindicated if membranes are ruptured because of the increased risk of infection.

16.5 A. Peripheral relaxation can lead to systemic hypotension with epidural anesthesia. A slowed second stage of labor also may occur.

16.6 C. A drug to increase gastric emptying helps to avoid vomiting. The other listed drugs do not have this therapeutic effect.

CHAPTER 17
Nursing Care of a Postpartal Family

17.1 C. The taking-hold phase means a woman is interested in actively caring for her baby. Encouraging rest or encouraging the naming of the baby do not help to usher in the taking-hold phase.

17.2 A. An "en face" position suggests she is interested in becoming acquainted with the newborn.

17.3 A. Tampons should not be used postpartum in order to help prevent infection.

17.4 B. If the uterine fundus does not grow firm with massage, extreme atony, possibly retained placenta fragments, or an excess amount of blood loss may be occurring; you should notify the woman's primary health care provider. A uterine fundus decreases in size at a rate of one fingerbreadth a day. The fundus should be located midline. Firm massage will result in pain, so this is not acceptable nursing practice.

17.5 D. This statement may suggest that Leana is unprepared for the fact that her infant may spend more time crying than sleeping. Her expectations for her own levels of rest may be unrealistic.

17.6 B. A uterine fundus sinks below the symphysis pubis so is no longer palpable at about 10 days after birth.

CHAPTER 18
Nursing Care of a Family With a Newborn

18.1 D. Conduction is the transfer of body heat to a cold object that touches the infant. Each of the other factors can result in heat loss, but none involves heat loss by conduction.

18.2 C. This action best initiates a Moro reflex. Making a noise or shaking a crib are less effective ways to test the reflex.

18.3 A. Assessment of heart rate, respiratory effort, muscle tone, reflex irritability, and color are used to assess newborn well-being.

18.4 C. Milia are immature sebaceous glands, which will open and drain without therapy. There is no need to alter the infant's bathing routine.

18.5 C. A week is an average time for a dried cord to detach.

18.6 C. Shaking infants is potentially dangerous because it can cause head injury; educating about newborn abilities helps parents better understand why a newborn reacts the way he or she does. This approach is likely more effective than immediately addressing shaken baby syndrome, which may be a premature and "heavy-handed" approach. A sedative is contraindicated with breastfeeding.

CHAPTER 19
Nutritional Needs of a Newborn

19.1 **A.** Assessment of infant nutrition begins during pregnancy with an assessment of the mother's and her partner's attitudes and choices about infant feeding. This is an important aspect of patient-centered care and should normally precede other assessments.

19.2 **A.** Prenatal care is associated with success at exclusive breastfeeding. Smoking, young age, and low income are negatively associated.

19.3 **B.** Breast milk not only provides nutrition but also aspects of immunity. Breastfeeding may reduce the risk of obesity but does not ensure the infant will never become obese, and it does not necessarily prevent cancer.

19.4 **C.** Drinking 12 glasses of fluid a day is extreme; 6 to 8 glasses is a better recommendation.

19.5 **A, B, D.** Formula feeding does not increase calcium density of the spine.

19.6 **D.** Discarding leftover milk discourages the growth of pathogens. The presence of yellowish stools is consistent with breastfeeding. A microwave should not be used to warm breast milk, and propping a bottle increases the risk for aspiration.

CHAPTER 20
Nursing Care of a Family Experiencing a Pregnancy Complication from a Preexisting or Newly Acquired Illness

20.1 **C.** Heparin is administered subcutaneously; it does not cross the placenta and so has no effect on a fetus. Hemoglobin levels do not need to be monitored during therapy.

20.2 **C.** Women with sickle-cell anemia are not usually prescribed iron pills during pregnancy because sickle cells are unable to incorporate as much iron in their structure as normal red cells. The woman's other statements reflect a sound understanding of sickle cell disease.

20.3 **C.** Good perineal care, a generous fluid intake, wearing cotton underwear, and avoiding bath salts are common ways to avoid urinary tract infections and so should be followed during pregnancy.

20.4 **A.** Because the fetus requires calcium to build bones, calcium-surrounded tuberculosis lesions can be activated if a woman doesn't ingest adequate calcium.

20.5 **B.** Women should typically eat a high protein/complex carbohydrate snack such as peanut butter and celery before bedtime to prevent fetal hypoglycemia from ingesting little food during the night.

20.6 **A.** Concerns about gaining weight and having to have a cesarean birth were the two factors most associated with depression following pregnancy with gestational diabetes. Wanting to "shed some pounds" is suggestive of earlier weight gain that is perceived as being excessive.

CHAPTER 21
Nursing Care of a Family Experiencing a Sudden Pregnancy Complication

21.1 **C.** Saving any clots or material passed will help the health care provider assess the amount of bleeding and whether the miscarriage process is incomplete or complete and allows them to be assessed for the possibility of gestational trophoblastic disease. A woman should not use a tampon so the amount of bleeding she is having can be evaluated. Vaginal bleeding always needs to be investigated during pregnancy.

21.2 **B.** Rh immune globulin (RhIG or RhoGAM) is the medication used to minimize the risk of isoimmunization.

21.3 **C.** It is important to assess for vaginal bleeding and clear fluid leakage every shift. Vaginal examinations are contraindicated because this procedure may cause bleeding. If the previa is not total, a cesarean birth may not be necessary.

21.4 **B.** Assessing fetal heart rate and whether she is having contractions are the best first actions. Walking stimulates contractions; and hydration, not dehydration, may reduce contractions.

21.5 **D.** Edema is often a first symptom a woman notes. The edema associated with gestational hypertension can be separated from the typical ankle edema of pregnancy because it begins to accumulate in the upper part of the body as well. Beverly's other statements are not necessarily indicative of gestational hypertension.

21.6 **B.** Activities at work were not associated with the development of gestational hypertension. Not taking time to eat regularly could lead to fetal hypoglycemia and would be a significant concern.

CHAPTER 22
Nursing Care of a Pregnant Family With Special Needs

22.1 **C.** Pregnant adolescents are emancipated minors and so are capable of and appreciate support for making health care decisions. It would be unwise to create a climate that would alienate the mother because, although Mindy is an emancipated minor, she will still need the support and help of her mother.

22.2 **C.** Reticulocytes are immature red blood cells that will start to grow rapidly if sufficient iron is available. Mindy's oral report may or may not be reliable. Urine testing and an assessment of her nail beds are not reliable indicators.

22.3 D. Gestational hypertension is caused by marked vasospasm. Hypertension becomes even more acute if blood vessels have limited elasticity, as in older women.

22.4 C. It is imperative to provide information that is appropriate to the patient's cognitive level. The patient herself must not be excluded from education, and written material is unlikely to be ideal.

22.5 D. Substance dependence is an all-encompassing phenomenon, and such women need support from an interprofessional team because pregnancy is a long time to remain drug free. Toxicology testing will confirm the type of substance being abused but will not give Mindy support to quit. Telling her to quit without providing support could be futile.

22.6 B. Leg veins are under more pressure than usual during pregnancy because of uterine pressure on veins returning to the vena cava, so bleeding can be profuse. Nonsteroidal anti-inflammatory drugs (NSAIDs) are contraindicated during pregnancy, primary health care providers are responsible for obtaining consent for surgery, and hydrogen peroxide is irritating and so is not ideal to use to irrigate an open wound.

CHAPTER 23
Nursing Care of a Family Experiencing a Complication of Labor or Birth

23.1 D. It would be important to document the characteristics of Rosann's contractions to see if they are irregular; even though ineffective, they are still painful, so she needs pain relief.

23.2 C. A large fetus is a reason to question oxytocin administration because cephalopelvic disproportion may be present. Amniocentesis, an elevated blood pressure, and ruptured membranes do not contraindicate the use of oxytocin.

23.3 C. Discontinuing the oxytocin infusion would be the first step in the management of Rosann's change in labor progress. Turning her to the left side and increasing fluid are second and third steps.

23.4 A. Fetal blood sampling can only be done after membranes are ruptured. Fetal position and the mother's blood pressure are important, but secondary, considerations.

23.5 D. Although not evidence based, a hands-and-knees position appears to aid fetal occipital rotation more than the other listed positions.

23.6 B. Check that the arms are warm and an equal length because a dislocated or broken collarbone (from those wide shoulders) could cause them to be an unequal length.

CHAPTER 24
Nursing Care of a Family During a Surgical Intervention for Birth

24.1 C. A danger of amniotomy is that the fetal cord can prolapse, which will interfere with fetal circulation. This makes an immediate assessment of the fetal heart rate important.

24.2 A. The urinary catheter will keep the bladder empty. Oxytocin contracts the uterus, not the bladder; and restricting fluid and administering a diuretic could lead to fluid volume deficit.

24.3 C. Moja will want her dominant hand free to hold her baby after birth so she needs to identify this. Giving Moja this choice exemplifies patient-centered care.

24.4 A. The priority in this situation is to protect confidential health information. Leaving or minimizing the record until the nurse who left it open returns may expose Moja's health information, and reporting this error to the nurse manager is not the immediate priority.

24.5 C. Women rated spontaneous vaginal birth as the most satisfying type. Nurses should be knowledgeable about best evidence and use this knowledge to guide their practice. A coworker's personal experience might not be a reliable opinion. Instrumental vaginal births were rated lower than cesarean births, so it would be inaccurate to describe all vaginal births as being more satisfying than all cesarean births.

24.6 D. Moja needs reassurance that incisional pain only lasts about 4 to 7 days following surgery. Although women need to be comfortable while breastfeeding, many medications are contraindicated. Referral to a lactation consultant may or may not be necessary, and you would not insist on this action.

CHAPTER 25
Nursing Care of a Family Experiencing a Postpartum Complication

25.1 D. Assessing uterine tone and height has the potential to prevent uterine hemorrhage. Collection of this assessment datum is a priority over assessing the patient's perineal care, oxygen saturation, or skin integrity.

25.2 C. Human chorionic gonadotropin (hCG) hormone is produced by the placenta. As a result, it will be present as long as any placenta is present. Estrogen, progesterone, and oxytocin levels are not assessed for this purpose.

25.3 A. An upright position prevents pooling of infected lochia. Supine, prone, and Trendelenburg positions should be avoided.

25.4 D. Early ambulation is a safeguard against the development of blood stasis, which could lead to a blood clot. None of the other listed measures are a prevention against venous thromboembolism.

25.5 B. Being unable to recall the newborn's name suggests loss of short-term memory.

25.6 C. Postpartum psychosis means a woman has separated from reality. Each of the other statements can be linked to Bailey's current reality.

CHAPTER 26
Nursing Care of a Family With a High-Risk Newborn

26.1 A. It is critical to guard against hypothermia in low–birth-weight infants because they are unable to increase their metabolic rate to warm themselves. The study revealed that stockinette caps alone are not adequate to do this.

26.2 C. Developmental care is aimed at instilling a sense of safety and security into the child by reducing stimuli such as loud noises or bright lights. A homemade blanket could give him a feeling of being sheltered. None of the other listed actions would have this beneficial effect.

26.3 B. Surfactant is not a relaxant, and it does not influence respiratory rate. It acts on the surface of the alveoli to help them not collapse upon expiration. Without surfactant, the alveoli collapse, the sides stick together, and they are very difficult to inflate.

26.4 B. Flicking the foot gently stimulates the infant and reminds the baby to breathe. Theophylline would not be an initial intervention; both rectal temperature assessment and vigorous suctioning can produce a vagal stimulation causing bradycardia; in addition, the infant should only be suctioned as needed, not every 2 hours.

26.5 B. Infants should be in a well-lit environment to enhance the binding of bilirubin. Phototherapy is not initiated until the infant's total serum bilirubin level rises to a specific age- and gestational age–dependent level; an older therapy, phenobarbital is rarely used today to combat neonatal jaundice; and early feeding enhances bilirubin clearance.

26.6 A. If a diabetic woman has hyperglycemia during pregnancy, her baby is apt to be born hypoglycemic. Early feeding guards against rebound hypoglycemia from this. The infant will not necessarily have diabetes, impaired respiratory function, or cognitive deficits.

CHAPTER 27
Nursing Care of the Child Born With a Physical or Developmental Challenge

27.1 A. Simple neck stretching should relieve torticollis in infants, giving aspirin with each feeding would result in an overdose and would not alleviate the problem, and application of a warm towel is insufficient.

27.2 C. Pavlik harnesses seem simple, but because they hold the hip in adduction, they are very effective. They should be worn constantly except for bathing. Looking at blog sites for specific care advice could supply misinformation.

27.3 B. Role modeling better interactions would be a subtle but effective way of demonstrating warmer parent–child interactions. Although the mother may not realize she is not reacting warmly to her child, people do not usually change behavior simply by being told to do so.

27.4 D. Keeping the herniated intestines moist helps keep them from drying. Warmth is important but not by a radiant heater because this would dry the bowel, and resting on the abdomen could cause the intestine to twist.

27.5 C. Sitting the infant in an infant chair encourages the herniated bowel to sink against the diaphragm, freeing up lung space. Lying on the left side allows greater respirations in the unaffected lung.

27.6 C. Changes in vital signs with increased cranial pressure are easy to remember because they move in opposite directions: Temperature and blood pressure increase, and pulse and respiratory rate decrease.

CHAPTER 28
Principles of Growth and Development

28.1 B. The lymphatic system reaches such a peak in early school-age children that their throats appear to be "all tonsils."

28.2 B. Young children in the study recognized what overweight was but were unable to apply the concept to themselves. John's inability to link his own appearance with the pictures is consistent with this tendency.

28.3 C. Freud stressed that school age is a latent stage and that it is not a stage of great advancement.

28.4 D. According to Erikson, the developmental task of the school-aged child is to learn industry or to do things well.

28.5 A. Ascribing human properties to inanimate objects is indicative of magical thinking.

28.6 C. Conservation is learning that two different shapes can actually be equal in mass or volume.

CHAPTER 29
Nursing Care of a Family With an Infant

29.1 C. Infants sit steadily at 8 months of age.

29.2 A. Children at 12 months usually say two words besides "ma-ma" and "da-da." They are not incapable of understanding, but they cannot express their needs verbally.

29.3 A. Infants understand permanence when they look for someone or something out of sight.

29.4 D. A mother who "always has a hot cup of coffee in her hand" could easily spill that on the infant while giving care or holding the infant.

29.5 D. Aspiration and falls are the most frequent unintentional injuries in infants.

29.6 D. Focusing on abilities rather than inabilities promotes efficacy and well-being among the family members of a child with unique needs. This practice exemplifies patient-centered care. Lowering the family's expectations is normally inappropriate and unnecessary.

CHAPTER 30
Nursing Care of a Family With a Toddler

30.1 B. Toddlers typically walk with a wide-based gait. Strong arch support would not make a difference.

30.2 B. Two-year-olds should speak with two-word, noun–verb sentences.

30.3 D. Television viewing for toddlers should be carefully limited; they need supervision to prevent pulling a television down onto themselves.

30.4 D. Locking medicine or placing it out of reach are the best safeguards. Young children can occasionally open childproof caps.

30.5 A. This seems like a short time, but for a 2-year-old, sitting still for 2 minutes is a long time.

30.6 C. Reducing the number of questions asked reduces the number of times a toddler can say no. Reasoning with toddlers or mimicking behavior is rarely effective.

CHAPTER 31
Nursing Care of a Family With a Preschool Child

31.1 C. Although this is variable, preschoolers typically ask 300 to 400 questions a day.

31.2 B. Watching chosen DVDs could improve the quality of video material to which Cathy is exposed. Cartoons are often violent, and TV should be carefully limited but does not necessarily need to be withheld until age 5 years.

31.3 C. Allowing a child to use a night-light, inspecting the child's room for objects that look particularly scary after dark, and limiting the child's television viewing to programs not as frightening can help decrease a child's fears.

31.4 D. Children need to know not to leave day care with anyone but a parent. It is not likely necessary to limit Cathy to her own home, and describing kidnapping is likely to elicit fear.

31.5 A. It is important to encourage women to maintain contact with their preschooler during the short time they are hospitalized for the new birth. This fosters family cohesion. Each of the other teaching points may be necessary, but none so clearly promotes family bonding.

31.6 C. Sexual education should be approached in a clear, but age-appropriate, manner. At this age, it is not normally necessary to address sexual intercourse and its consensual nature.

CHAPTER 32
Nursing Care of a Family With a School-Age Child

32.1 D. A sense of industry is best achieved through completing small projects or tasks that offer a reward when completed.

32.2 C. Clubs are frequently single gender, and they do not always have formal rules and regulations. They tend to exclude some children.

32.3 D. Heavy backpacks can put unnecessary strain on the back of school-age children. All ages need to wear seat belts in automobiles. Weight gain is serious. Encouraging self-evaluation is encouraging a sense of industry.

32.4 D. The study documents the fact that injuries occur in cheerleading activities. However, taking part is likely of benefit, provided she is cognizant of some of the risks. No mention is made of weight or calcium intake.

32.5 B. Candy that dissolves rapidly remains in contact with teeth for the shortest time. This may be associated with a reduced risk of dental caries.

32.6 C. Smoking is viewed as an adult activity, so adopting the habit can be considered a giant step on the road to adulthood. Antismoking interventions must acknowledge this reality, and the media are not known to have exaggerated the risks of smoking.

CHAPTER 33
Nursing Care of a Family With an Adolescent

33.1 B. Apocrine glands, found predominantly in the axilla and groin, are responsible for body odor. This problem does not result from sebaceous activity or ethnicity, and hygiene is not the major contributing factor.

33.2 A, B, C, D. All the options represent tasks adolescents must complete to achieve a sense of identity: emancipation, body image, values, and career choice.

33.3 B, C, D. Teenagers may have many misconceptions about the cause of acne. Neither hot water nor chocolate cause it; medicine should not be shared.

33.4 C. Whether stalking is done in person or on the Internet, continuous and unwelcome actions are stalking.

33.5 C. Alcohol is identified as the gateway drug or is the one that is most apt to lead to further substance abuse, especially if parents condone early use. Celebrating a birthday by drinking alcohol is inviting gateway activities.

33.6 D. Sniffing cocaine can cause a loss of nasal hair. The absence of nasal hair would suggest more extensive cocaine use.

CHAPTER 34
Child Health Assessment

34.1 C. Household products were swallowed most commonly by young children. These are often stored below sinks in bathrooms or kitchens.

34.2 B. Parents may be unwilling to discuss a chief concern until they feel comfortable with an interviewer. Providing an open-ended invitation to address any outstanding issues can sometimes reveal important data.

34.3 B. Blood pressure is routinely assessed beginning at 3 years of age.

34.4 B. Gagging a child who has a swollen epiglottis can cause the epiglottis to obstruct breathing.

34.5 D. Although not its anatomical position, mitral valve sounds are heard best at the fourth or fifth left intercostal space at the nipple line.

34.6 D. Human papillomavirus virus (HPV) vaccine is typically administered at 11 to 12 years of age.

CHAPTER 35
Communication and Teaching With Children and Families

35.1 D. Personal space is a distance of about 18 in. to 4 feet, or conversational space. It is most appropriate for face-to-face teaching.

35.2 C. Technology has the potential to enhance learning and communication, but it cannot wholly substitute for the nurse's thoughtful interpersonal communication skills.

35.3 B. Cognitive learning is learning facts or increasing knowledge. A and D are examples of affective learning, and C is an example of skill learning.

35.4 A. Video resources must be vetted by the nurse to ensure that the material presented is evidence based, safe, and age appropriate.

35.5 C. Neither the Web-based program nor the face-to-face instruction was demonstrably superior, so a child could choose which delivery method he or she preferred.

35.6 C. A 3-year-old would probably do best by playing a game. A lecture, group discussion, and reading a pamphlet are all more advanced.

CHAPTER 36
Nursing Care of a Family With an Ill Child

36.1 A. Protest, the first stage of separation anxiety, is marked by loud, intense crying.

36.2 D. The most significant outcome of teaching patients and their families about the perioperative process was a reduction in their anxiety. As an outcome of education, this is more important than being able to adhere to instructions, to describe asepsis, or to explain the rationale for surgery.

36.3 B. School children do best with small tasks and a feeling of reward. This collaborative approach is also more likely to prevent nausea and vomiting, and warning her of negative consequences is less likely to result in positive outcomes.

36.4 D. Of the options suggested, the best way to help make a hospital stay nontraumatic would be to keep the child's bed a safe area by taking her to the playroom.

36.5 C. Any item smaller than the internal roll on toilet paper is a size that is dangerous and could be aspirated. Crayons, especially broken ones, are easily aspirated.

36.6 B. Having Becky handle a bandage addresses specifically what is happening to her. She can apply it to the foot and become more comfortable with the concept of a bandage. Therapeutic play materials are best if they are most relevant to a child's condition or procedures.

CHAPTER 37
Nursing Care of a Family When a Child Needs Diagnostic or Therapeutic Modalities

37.1 C. When using a restraint, restrain only the one body part necessary. Don't ask parents to restrain for painful procedures. Asking a fellow nurse to restrain the child's arm would be the best solution.

37.2 D. Most parents are anxious to have diagnostic tests done so their child's illness can be identified. Asking the mother why she feels the way she does could reveal she needs a better understanding of what computed tomography involves.

37.3 C. The commercial device reduced pain by serving as a distraction. Selecting a distraction technique that would be effective with Felipe would be important, and his mother may know what will work best. A preprocedure and postprocedure assessment will not necessarily reduce his anxiety and pain. Telling him that you will try to distract him may be counterproductive.

37.4 B. Giving a child a choice of fingers can interest them in the procedure. Comparing him to other children his age or threatening the withholding of privileges or treats is inappropriate.

37.5 A. A 24-hour urine collection is timed from the discard of the first urine to ensure it is truly a 24-hour specimen.

37.6 A. Measuring the amount a child vomits (emesis) can be challenging if it spills onto clothing or bed linen. When this happens, estimate the amount in relation to the amount of food or fluid the child recently ate; include the number of episodes and a description of the vomitus. Estimating the quantity should not be delegated to Felipe's mother.

CHAPTER 38
Nursing Care of a Family When a Child Needs Medication Administration or Intravenous Therapy

38.1 C. Many drugs are transported attached to plasma proteins; a deficit of these can interfere with medication distribution. Arterial blood gasses, gallbladder function, and renal function are important assessments, but none directly gauge drug distribution.

38.2 C. In the absence of an ID band, you should ask a parent to identify her. Children may lie about their name or give a false name out of fear or if being playful.

38.3 C. Using something that dissolves easily, like ice, can allow children to practice swallowing in a safe and effective way. Drawing a picture or tipping the child's head forward is not effective, and never refer to medicine as candy.

38.4 D. Keeping the child's head turned to the side will allow the medication to stay in the ear longer and so will increase absorption. Self-administration is unsafe and impractical; and for a child over the age of 2 years, the ear pinna should be pulled up and back.

38.5 D. The point of watching television is to create a distraction. If Terry is absorbed in watching her present program, changing the channel could exacerbate her pain by removing the distraction.

38.6 A. To help guard the stability of the intravenous site while still meeting her psychosocial needs, Terry needs an activity that is quiet and that does not include use of her hands.

CHAPTER 39
Pain Management in Children

39.1 B. Bone pain is somatic pain. Cutaneous pain is skin pain, and visceral pain is from body organs.

39.2 C. Distraction techniques need to be individualized, so asking the mother what technique is apt to be most successful would be helpful. Reassuring the parents before the procedure so they do not radiate extensive fear would be a better action than asking them to leave or not talk.

39.3 C. Imagery requires a child to be able to replace a painful image with a nonpainful one. This requires a working imagination, which is a characteristic of childhood.

39.4 B. Knowing that the doses are correct is a priority; drug doses are based on weight, not age. The mother's opinion is interesting but not a priority in comparison to right dose.

39.5 A. A patient-controlled pump offers the child a sense of control and rapid analgesia. Nursing care is not reduced, and there is still a chance of adverse effects.

39.6 D. This is a comforting and accurate explanation. It is inappropriate to tell a child that he or she will be "knocked out"; and a description of analgesia and anesthetic is too technical for a 3-year-old child.

CHAPTER 40
Nursing Care of a Family When a Child Has a Respiratory Disorder

40.1 B. Because oximeter alarms may not be set accurately, it is important to assess these before beginning care. The other listed actions are all inappropriate and unsafe.

40.2 B. Choanal atresia is blockage of the posterior nares in newborns. This health problem may be assessed by holding the newborn's mouth closed, then gently compressing first one nostril and then the other. If atresia is present, infants will struggle as they experience air hunger when their mouth is closed.

40.3 C. Group A β-hemolytic streptococcus can lead to glomerulonephritis or rheumatic fever.

40.4 D. A cold fluid can be comforting after a tonsillectomy. Don't offer a food that is crunchy and could scratch the denuded surgical surface or any that is red so bleeding can be easily detected.

40.5 D. Because initiating gagging may cause further airway closure, never elicit a gag reflex on children with a high fever, barky cough, and sore throat. Instead, assess his throat with simple inspection.

40.6 C. A child who is undergoing peak flow testing places the meter in his or her mouth and blows out as hard and fast as possible.

CHAPTER 41
Nursing Care of a Family When a Child Has a Cardiovascular Disorder

41.1 C. The QRS spike is a record of ventricular activity. If this is unusually high or wide, it means the electric current took longer than usual to cross enlarged ventricles.

41.2 C. According to the study, the three variables which proved to be most predictive of an infection were age less than 6 months, a PICU stay longer than 48 hours, and open sternum for longer than 48 hours.

41.3 B. A knee–chest position helps relieve extreme cyanosis with tetralogy of Fallot because it traps blood in the lower extremities and allows better oxygenation of the blood left in the upper torso. Chest compressions are not indicated except in the event of cardiac arrest. Sitting the child upright will not adequately relieve symptoms.

41.4 D. Nausea and vomiting are symptoms of toxic effects or may mean the child is receiving too high a dosage of the drug. The other listed statements are accurate.

41.5 A. The nurse should seek to promote Megan's activity, growth, and development while still protecting her health. This will benefit Megan far more than focusing solely on indoor pursuits. Encouraging her to challenge herself could be dangerous.

41.6 D. The first step in cardiopulmonary resuscitation should be chest compressions to quickly supply the brain and heart with blood. Assessment should take no more than 10 seconds.

CHAPTER 42
Nursing Care of a Family When a Child Has an Immune Disorder

42.1 D. Repeated exposures to latex can create allergies in sensitive children. Distraction does not help protect his safety, and the use of a new blood pressure cuff does not prevent allergic reactions.

42.2 B, C. The major blood values that are used in the assessment of HIV are the viral load and CD4 count. Hemoglobin A1C, phosphatase, and C-reactive protein levels are not directly relevant.

42.3 C. Hyposensitization increases the number of immune globulin (Ig)G, which then blocks the action of IgE, which is involved in an allergic response. Immunotherapy does not improve the broader function of the immune system or protect against infection.

42.4 B. Epinephrine is the drug of choice for an anaphylactic reaction because it quickly causes bronchodilation, immediately enlarging a constricted airway. The correct dose is 0.48 mg.

42.5 A. Treatment would be deemed successful if the child is able to maintain age-appropriate activities despite having allergies. "Curing" allergies is not always a possibility.

42.6 B. Many unintentional ingestions occurred because food was offered by another person. A willingness to share may include sharing food and a consequent allergic reaction.

CHAPTER 43
Nursing Care of a Family When a Child Has an Infectious Disorder

43.1 B. Parents' hand-washing practices were noted to influence hand washing in their children. Frequent reminders, teaching children about bacteria, and characterizing hand hygiene as "grown up" were not specifically noted to be effective interventions.

43.2 C. Coughing and sneezing requires droplet precautions (gloves, mask, and gown). If Marty wears a mask, there still may be contaminated surfaces in the room, so you need to guard against these.

43.3 B. Although rating his pain would be informative, to stop the itching, the administration of an antihistamine would be most effective. Children need their hands free to facilitate self-care.

43.4 C. Swelling over the parotid gland (above the jawline and in front of the ear) is the usual symptom of mumps.

43.5 B. The spleen enlarges to destroy the affected cells, so the spleen could rupture easily on pressure. Petechiae should not be massaged, and percussion and the use of a Doppler are unnecessary during assessment.

43.6 D. Scarlet fever is contagious for 24 hours after beginning an antibiotic or, if untreated, 1 to 7 days after the appearance of disease symptoms. A faster return to school may result in the infection of other children.

CHAPTER 44
Nursing Care of a Family When a Child Has a Hematologic Disorder

44.1 C. Bone marrow is infused intravenously, so the child will need to lie still during the infusion. It would be inappropriate to have the child's mother restrain her during a painful procedure; and it would be inaccurate to reassure her that this is a one-time event.

44.2 A. Iron chelation therapy removes excess iron from the body to prevent hemosiderosis. The mother needs to assess voiding, not pulse, before administration.

44.3 B. Swimming would be a healthy and low-risk activity. To protect the father, playing football would be inadvisable. Sedentary activities are not an advantage for either the father or the son.

44.4 B. Pain control is paramount during sickle-cell crises. As a result, evidence of adequate pain control is a priority over positive expressions about his time in the hospital, even though these are certainly desirable. Health education is similarly important, but pain control is the priority.

44.5 D. Autoimmune acquired hemolytic anemia is an autoimmune disorder, or antibodies are reacting against red blood cells.

44.6 A. Idiopathic thrombocytopenia purpura (ITP) is a deficiency of platelets, so Lana will bruise easily. Assessments related to blood glucose levels, headaches, and proteinuria are not priorities.

CHAPTER 45
Nursing Care of a Family When a Child Has a Gastrointestinal Disorder

45.1 C. Metabolic alkalosis occurs because of the loss of gastric acid that occurs with emesis.

45.2 C. Raw chicken is a potential source of *Salmonella*. None of the other listed actions prevent this foodborne illness.

45.3 A. Vomiting associated with pyloric stenosis usually occurs immediately after feeding due to the thickened pylorus muscle that causes a delay in gastric emptying.

45.4 B. Hepatitis A can be transmitted via fecally contaminated shellfish. Parents should be advised to carefully consider the origin of sushi or shellfish served to their family.

45.5 C. The study showed that unaccompanied children received more nursing time than children whose parent was present. The study did not address children's risks of anxiety.

45.6 C. Kwashiorkor results from a deficiency of protein in the diet.

CHAPTER 46
Nursing Care of a Family When a Child Has a Renal or Urinary Tract Disorder

46.1 C. Because preschoolers have recently been taught that voiding is a private activity, voiding while an X-ray is taken may feel uncomfortable. Dye capsules are not used and the test does not occur in a metal tube.

46.2 C. Taking the full antibiotic prescription helps prevent recurrence of infection. Avoidance of dairy and exercise is unnecessary. The use of bath salts is not required.

46.3 B. A first symptom of poststreptococcal glomerulonephritis is often bright red hematuria. Abdominal pain and joint pain are atypical.

46.4 C. Testing for urine protein is important with nephrotic syndrome because a large amount of protein is lost in urine. The other listed actions do not directly address this health problem.

46.5 A, B, C, E. Anemia develops from a lack of erythropoietin in renal failure and vitamin D cannot be synthesized. As well, phosphorus cannot be excreted and fluid overload causes hypertension. Creatinine levels increase, not decrease, with renal failure.

46.6 A. Parents thought support from health care professionals was important; asking the grandmother to keep a journal or ignore family members could make her time management even more stressful.

CHAPTER 47
Nursing Care of a Family When a Child Has a Reproductive Disorder

47.1 C. Although children with precocious puberty appear older, they function at their chronologic age. Both sexes can be fertile even at such a young age, and dietary and activity restrictions are unnecessary.

47.2 C. Yoga may be an effective measure to reduce symptoms of dysmenorrhea. Increased exercise intensity is not a guarantee of a proportionate reduction in pain. The benefits of yoga were not limited to improved coping.

47.3 B. Polycystic ovary syndrome leads to obesity, hirsutism, irregular menstrual cycles, and subfertility. It is not easy to reverse the syndrome.

47.4 C. If having small breasts interferes with self-esteem, a girl can have surgical augmentation, but this needs careful consideration regarding whether it is necessary at this young of an age. There is no increase in disease risk, and breastfeeding is unaffected.

47.5 C. Candidal vaginal infections usually cause a thick, pruritic, white vaginal discharge. All of the listed concerns warrant follow-up, but they are not indicative of candidiasis.

47.6 B. Gonorrhea may be spread by singular sexual contact; the disease has a bacterial etiology; saliva is not bactericidal. It can be spread by penile–anal contact.

CHAPTER 48
Nursing Care of a Family When a Child Has an Endocrine or a Metabolic Disorder

48.1 A, B, C, D. Growth hormone cannot be given orally; it doesn't cause reddened skin, increase urination, or need to be taken after epiphyseal lines of long bones close. Sandy's determination to preserve her quality of life is laudable.

48.2 C. Hyperthyroidism increases metabolism, so it leads to rapid, jittery movements.

48.3 C. A function of aldosterone is to retain sodium in the body.

48.4 D. When children with diabetes first begin injections of insulin, it "reminds" their pancreas to produce insulin, so for a short period, the child may not need exogenous insulin administered or may need minimal amounts.

48.5 B. The total amount of carbohydrates included in this lunch is 75 g. At a ratio of 1 to 10, he would inject 7.5 units of regular insulin.

48.6 A. The study found that loss of friends had a negative effect on quality of life. The other statements do not reflect an influence on quality of life.

CHAPTER 49
Nursing Care of a Family When a Child Has a Neurologic Disorder

49.1 B. Neurologic examinations are lengthy so it's difficult to keep children's attention unless the exam is presented as being interesting. There is no "pass" or "fail." Alluding to the possibility of tumors or an "unhealthy brain" will likely cause undue anxiety.

49.2 A. Before a lumbar puncture is performed, the lumbar region is cleansed with a solution that creates a temporary sensation of cold. The procedure is not necessarily painless and EMLA should be applied approximately 1 hour beforehand. A side-lying position is used to perform a lumbar puncture.

49.3 D. Because the child needs fine motor control to achieve at writing or ambulating, the loss of function may seem more acute. Cognitive and physical effects of the disease do not necessarily exist in the same degree. Vaccinations do not cause cerebral palsy.

49.4 B. Respiratory precautions are necessary for at least 24 hours following the beginning of antibiotic therapy.

49.5 B. Tasha's expression of sadness could be suggestive of symptoms of depression. None of the other listed statements is as clearly suggestive of depression.

49.6 A, C, D. It is not likely a child would require a tracheotomy and using a tongue blade to keep the airway open could break the child's teeth. The call bell, suction, and supplementary oxygen could be important to maintaining safety and the integrity of the child's airway.

CHAPTER 50
Nursing Care of a Family When a Child Has a Vision or Hearing Disorder

50.1 B. Covering the stronger eye will encourage central vision to develop in the weaker eye. Each of the other actions is counterproductive.

50.2 C. Wiping infectious discharge away from the other eye prevents infection from spreading to the second eye. The other listed actions are not indicated.

50.3 C. Increased intraocular pressure from vomiting could disrupt a suture line.

50.4 C. The hallmark of glaucoma is increased intraocular pressure.

50.5 D. The study showed that long exposure to loud noise may be responsible for lowering hearing levels in teenagers. An individual is more likely to listen at high volume when using earphones (as when on a bus or in a subway car). Music from computer speakers may not be as loud.

50.6 B. Otitis media is an infection of the middle ear; otitis externa is infection of the ear canal. Both diagnoses can be painful.

CHAPTER 51
Nursing Care of a Family When a Child Has a Musculoskeletal Disorder

51.1 C. It's important for children to bear weight on their arms, not their axillae, so nerves and blood vessels that cross at the axilla are not injured. If crutches are properly fitted, there should be a space of 1 to 1.5 in. between the axilla crutch pad and the child's axilla; when the child stands upright and places his hands on the hand rests of the crutches, the elbows should flex about 20°; and stairs present a risk of falls.

51.2 A. Osteomyelitis is a severe bone infection that needs intravenous antibiotic therapy to ensure that microorganisms do not cause chronic infection and deformity. Vigilant administration of antibiotics is thus a priority over health education, even though this should be performed; activities of daily living should be encouraged within his current limitations; and fluid restriction is not indicated.

51.3 D. Application of heat and administration of a nonsteroidal anti-inflammatory agent are first-line therapies for children with juvenile arthritis.

51.4 B. Preventing weight gain and encouraging the child to be as mobile as possible are both ways to prolong function in muscular dystrophy as muscles weaken. Purines and calcium are not focuses of dietary modifications.

51.5 B. An elbow cast that is too tight can lead to compartment syndrome and can result in permanent nerve damage. Frequent neurovascular assessment is necessary. Sepsis is not likely, and cleanliness of cast is not a priority over neurovascular assessment.

51.6 A. Holding preschoolers by the arms and swinging them is the most common cause of a traction injury. The other listed activities are not considered to be high risk.

CHAPTER 52
Nursing Care of a Family When a Child Has an Unintentional Injury

52.1 D. The study revealed that fewer injuries occurred when safety precautions were enforced by both parents.

52.2 D. Increasing temperature and blood pressure are marks of increasing intracranial pressure. Amnesia is frequently seen with a head concussion.

52.3 B. Acetylcysteine is the specific antidote for acetaminophen poisoning; activated charcoal may be given if no acetylcysteine is immediately available. Educating the parents is important but is not the immediate priority.

52.4 D. Paint chips taste sweet so children enjoy their taste; they are the most common source of lead poisoning in children.

52.5 C. Applying cool water will reduce the water temperature and stop the burning as well as reduce the pain.

52.6 D. Being burned is such a frightening event, children need "debriefing" afterward so they be assured they are now safe and healing. The other listed actions are inappropriate.

CHAPTER 53
Nursing Care of a Family When a Child Has a Malignancy

53.1 D. Hand hygiene prevents the mother from spreading microorganisms to her son, but it does not protect her from the possible effects of handling toxic drugs. She needs to wear gloves to handle oral chemotherapy agents. The other listed actions are appropriate.

53.2 C. Because so many white blood cells are produced with acute lymphocytic leukemia (ALL), red blood cell and platelet production falls, leading to fatigue and bleeding disorders.

53.3 A. Hodgkin disease usually presents with a single isolated lymph node. The other listed signs and symptoms are not closely associated with this disease.

53.4 B. Straining to pass stool causes increased intracranial pressure. A Trendelenburg position would rarely be used because this would increase intracranial pressure.

53.5 C. Osteosarcoma is often discovered when a sports injury causes an athlete to report pain or a swelling at the injury site for some time. Calcium intake is unrelated.

53.6 A. If Wilms tumors are palpated, they appear to metastasize faster than if not palpated. There is no need to measure head circumference frequently or to avoid iron-rich foods.

CHAPTER 54
Nursing Care of a Family When a Child Has a Cognitive or Mental Health Disorder

54.1 C. Chronic sorrow is apt to be most acute at the time of development milestones such as beginning first grade or high school graduation.

54.2 C. Repetitive movements such as whirling, rocking or watching a spinning top are common symptoms of autism spectrum disorder. The other listed symptoms are not consistent with this health problem.

54.3 C. The most common side effects of Ritalin are insomnia and lack of appetite. Weight gain and iron-deficiency anemia are atypical.

54.4 B. Eating disorders in the study occurred more often in female athletes than in nonathletes.

54.5 D. Because tics are poorly understood, children who have them can be the victim of bullying or teasing and develop low self-esteem.

54.6 D. Hearing voices, or hallucinations, is a prominent symptom of schizophrenia. The other listed statements are not consistent with this disorder.

CHAPTER 55
Nursing Care of a Family in Crisis: Maltreatment and Violence in the Family

55.1 B. A previous emergency department visit for bruising would be an alert for maltreatment in this young of a child.

55.2 B. Shaking a baby causes small hemorrhages in the retina of the eye as well as possibly more serious injuries such as subdural hematoma. Broken bones are associated with maltreatment but not specifically with shaking.

55.3 B. According to this study, most adolescents reveal sexual maltreatment to a trusted peer.

55.4 C. Children who have been physically maltreated may reveal the maltreatment through having dolls simulate a sex act. You want to learn more about their reaction, not stop the play.

55.5 A. It is important to preserve any DNA evidence that could reveal the identity of the rapist so a woman should not bath or shower until after an internal exam. Property loss is comparatively insignificant and it would be highly inappropriate to address prevention at this time.

55.6 A. Intimate partner violent offenders are often men who were raised in a household with violence.

CHAPTER 56
Nursing Care of a Family When a Child Has a Long-Term or Terminal Illness

56.1 B. As with any crisis, support people can offer help and guidance. Privacy and a belief in alternative therapies may not necessarily enhance their coping skills. Wealth can be an asset during treatment but does not necessarily help the family cope with the child's illness.

56.2 C. The fourth stage of grief is depression, or the stage when parents start to realize death will happen.

56.3 **D.** This is a mature question for a 4-year-old child. Before answering, it would be important to know why the child is asking the question. Has he heard he is dying or is he just interested in what happened to a favorite cartoon character he just saw "die" on television?

56.4 **B.** Anticipatory grieving can make it hard for parents to relate to their child because they have already grieved as if the child were dead.

56.5 **A.** The study revealed parents wanted most to just continue to be effective parents. Enhancing Charlie's comfort by keeping him neat and clean is the sort of activity that might meet that need. None of the other listed actions would normally be appropriate.

56.6 **A.** If a gag reflex is not intact, children can aspirate easily. Hearing may not be lost, and parents usually appreciate giving final care.

Index

NOTE: Page numbers followed by *f* indicate figures, page numbers followed by *t* indicate tables, and page numbers followed by *b* indicate boxes.

B

D

E

G

H

I

N

O

Q

R